185

CAFFEY'S
PEDIATRIC
DIAGNOSTIC
IMAGING

CAFFEY'S
PEDIATRIC
DIAGNOSTIC
IMAGING

ELEVENTH EDITION

EDITOR-IN-CHIEF

Thomas L. Slovis, MD
Professor of Radiology and Pediatrics
Wayne State University School of Medicine
Department of Pediatric Imaging
Children's Hospital of Michigan
Detroit, Michigan

Volume 2

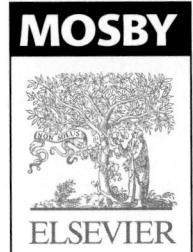

MOSBY

ELSEVIER

ASSOCIATE EDITORS

Brent H. Adler, MD
Clinical Assistant Professor of Radiology
Division of Pediatric Radiology
Ohio State University Medical Center
Chief of Musculoskeletal Radiology
Department of Radiology
Nationwide Children's Hospital, Columbus, Ohio

David A. Bloom, MD
Clinical Associate Professor of Radiology
Wayne State University School of Medicine, Detroit
Staff Pediatric Radiologist
William Beaumont Hospital, Royal Oak, Michigan

Dorothy I. Bulas, MD
Professor of Radiology and Pediatrics
George Washington University School of Medicine and Health Sciences
Department of Diagnostic Imaging and Radiology
Children's National Medical Center
Washington, DC

Brian D. Coley, MD
Clinical Professor of Radiology and Pediatrics
The Ohio State University College of Medicine and Public Health
Assistant Director of Radiology
Nationwide Children's Hospital, Columbus, Ohio

James S. Donaldson, MD
Professor of Radiology
Northwestern University Feinberg School of Medicine
Chairman, Department of Medical Imaging
Children's Memorial Hospital, Chicago, Illinois

Eric N. Faerber, MD
Professor of Radiology and Pediatrics
Drexel University School of Medicine
Director, Department of Radiology
St. Christopher's Hospital for Children, Philadelphia, Pennsylvania

Donald P. Frush, MD
Professor of Radiology and Pediatrics
Faculty, Medical Physics
Duke University
Chief, Pediatric Radiology
Duke University Medical Center
Durham, North Carolina

Marta Hernanz-Schulman, MD
Medical Director, Diagnostic Imaging
Vanderbilt Children's Hospital
Director, Pediatric Radiology
Vanderbilt University Medical Center, Nashville, Tennessee

Peter J. Strouse, MD
Professor of Radiology
Director, Section of Pediatric Radiology
C. S. Mott Children's Hospital
Department of Radiology
University of Michigan Health System, Ann Arbor, Michigan

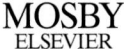

MOSBY
ELSEVIER

1600 John F. Kennedy Blvd.
Ste 1800
Philadelphia, PA 19103-2899

CAFFEY'S PEDIATRIC DIAGNOSTIC IMAGING   ISBN: 978-0-323-04520-9

Notice

Knowledge and best practice in this field are constantly changing. As new research and experience broaden our knowledge, changes in practice, treatment and drug therapy may become necessary or appropriate. Readers are advised to check the most current information provided (i) on procedures featured or (ii) by the manufacturer of each product to be administered, to verify the recommended dose or formula, the method and duration of administration, and contraindications. It is the responsibility of the practitioner, relying on his or her own experience and knowledge of the patient, to make diagnoses, to determine dosages and the best treatment for each individual patient, and to take all appropriate safety precautions. To the fullest extent of the law, neither the Publisher nor the Authors assume any liability for any injury and/or damage to persons or property arising out or related to any use of the material contained in this book.

Library of Congress Cataloging-in-Publication Data

Caffey's pediatric diagnostic imaging. — 11th ed./editor-in-chief, Thomas L. Slovis; associate editors, Donald P. Frush...[et al.].
    p.; cm.
  Includes bibliographical references and index.
  ISBN-13: 978-0-323-04520-9
  ISBN-10: 0-323-04520-0
1. Pediatric diagnostic imaging. I. Slovis, Thomas L. II. Caffey, John. III. Title: Pediatric diagnostic imaging.
  [DNLM: 1. Diagnostic Imaging. 2. Child. 3. Infant. WN 240 C1292 2008]
RJ51.D5C34 2008
618.92'007572—dc22   2007003810

Acquisitions Editor: Rebecca Schmidt Gaertner
Developmental Editor: Kristina Oberle
Publishing Services Manager: Tina Rebane
Senior Project Manager: Linda Lewis Grigg
Design Direction: Ellen B. Zanolle

Printed in the United States of America

Last digit is the print number: 9 8 7 6 5 4 3 2 1

To my wife, Ellie, who, despite the long hours,
weekends, and vacations I spent on this edition,
always supported my efforts. The time
I spent working on "the book" involved sacrifices
by both of us. The 11th edition is "our book."

TRIBUTE to Drs. John P. Caffey and Frederic N. Silverman

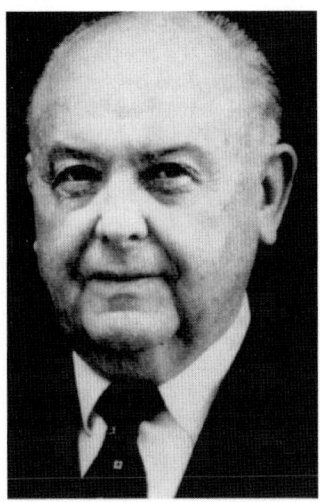

John P. Caffey

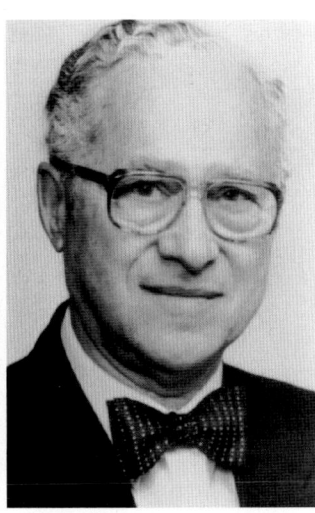

Frederic N. Silverman

Caffey's Pediatric Diagnostic Imaging (titled *Caffey's Pediatric X-ray Diagnosis* for the first nine editions) is the longest continuous comprehensive textbook in this subspecialty (first published in 1945 to the present edition in 2008). It began as a labor of love for John Caffey, the lone author for the first four editions. Let's think about that. In 1945, we didn't have computers, digital images, or Photoshop. Each chapter was meticulously dictated, typed, and corrected and eventually reached the publication stage. Each radiograph was selected from Dr. Caffey's own teaching file at Babies Hospital in New York City. Dr. Caffey had to find perfect images for the books, because they could not be enhanced. The content of the book was focused on the radiographic findings correlated with clinical information. Searching the literature was laborious. There was no PubMed or Google Scholar. For those of us involved in writing textbooks or editing journals, it is hard to imagine the labor that went into that first edition, resulting in the presentation of an incredible amount of clinical and radiologic information. The original text in 1945 had a subtitle: "A textbook for students and practitioners of pediatrics, surgery and radiology." Dr. Caffey devoted over half of his professional life to the book. He was an astute clinician, but, as Dr. Silverman wrote in the preface to the eighth edition, "Dr. Caffey stated that he preferred to title his book 'Radiographic Findings in Infants and Children.' His argument for the change was that a diagnosis is not made from a single type of examination, such as a radiograph, but rather from a 'cluster of findings' that is derived from history, physical examination, and laboratory studies and that may include a radiograph." Dr.

Caffey stressed the normal so that we would recognize the abnormal.

By the 1960s, he realized that there was increasing subspecialization and the use of newer modalities to help diagnose diseases of children. In 1967, with the fifth edition, Dr. Frederic N. Silverman of Children's Hospital of Cincinnati, Ohio, participated in preparation of the text. Dr. Silverman had been a Fellow of Dr. Caffey. Silverman was joined 5 years later by other co-authors for the sixth edition. As Dr. Caffey added authors to the mix, he would say, "We are particularly happy to make available for our readers the special expertise and talents of these younger colleagues, all of whom studied with me or with students of mine." Dr. Silverman devoted an enormous amount of time and effort working with Dr. Caffey over the next several editions. With the passing of Dr. Caffey, Dr. Silverman became editor of the next (eighth) edition in 1985. He carried on the tradition of stressing the need for clinical information and said, "Images without a clinical history are comparable to findings on percussion by a blindfolded examiner—one method of physical examination used to the exclusion of the others." Dr. Silverman also spent over half of his professional life on the book, working well into his emeritus years. He always enjoyed taking care of children and stressed to his fellows and colleagues the importance of the physical examination. He was an advocate for children and thought that if you could make the diagnosis clinically, most likely imaging was not needed. He had a natural sense of inquiry, whether related to medical disease, new discoveries in viruses, or fine wines. He added authors, expanded sections, and selected Dr. Jerald P. Kuhn to join him as co-editor with the ninth edition (1993) and then to succeed him in 2003. The longevity of the Caffey textbook is an important legacy of both John Caffey and Fred Silverman. More important, they taught us the essential need for clinical information when interpreting images. The irony is that most radiologists today have less clinical information, and the physical examination is frequently supplanted by imaging. Drs. Caffey and Silverman imparted to us the value of detail and normal anatomy so as not to make non-diseases into diseases. We need to remember their key messages and work toward improved systems of care. Their impact on thousands of health care providers is immeasurable. This textbook—often called "the bible"—made it possible for today's young pediatric imagers to gain knowledge from "the giants."

Thomas L. Slovis
Editor, 11th edition
2008

CONTRIBUTORS

Denise Adams, MD
Associate Professor, University of Cincinnati; Oncologist and Medical Director of the Hemangioma and Vascular Malformation Center, Cincinnati Children's Hospital and Medical Center, Cincinnati, Ohio

Brent H. Adler, MD
Clinical Assistant Professor of Radiology, Division of Pediatric Radiology, Ohio State University Medical Center; Chief of Musculoskeletal Radiology, Department of Radiology, Nationwide Children's Hospital, Columbus, Ohio

Kimberly E. Applegate, MD, MS
Professor and Director, Pediatric Radiology Research, Department of Pediatric Radiology and Health Services Research, Riley Hospital for Children, Indianapolis, Indiana

Derek Armstrong, MB, BS, FRCPC
Associate Professor, University of Toronto; Pediatric Neuroradiologist, The Hospital for Sick Children, Toronto, Ontario, Canada

E. Michel Azouz, MD, FRCPC
Professor of Radiology, University of Ottawa; Senior Pediatric Radiologist, Diagnostic Imaging, Children's Hospital of Eastern Ontario, Ottawa, Ontario, Canada

Paul S. Babyn, MD, FRCPC
Associate Professor, Department of Medical Imaging, University of Toronto; Radiologist-in-Chief, Diagnostic Imaging, The Hospital for Sick Children, Toronto, Ontario, Canada

James W. Backstrom, MD
Director of Pediatric Radiology, Member of Board of Directors, Lucien Diagnostic Imaging/North Pittsburgh Imaging Specialists, Pittsburgh; Director of Radiology, Head of Armstrong Outpatient Imaging Center, Armstrong Country Memorial Hospital, Kittanning, Pennsylvania

D. Gregory Bates, MD
Clinical Assistant Professor of Radiology, The Ohio State University College of Medicine and Public Health; Section Chief, Fluoroscopy, Department of Radiology, Nationwide Children's Hospital, Columbus, Ohio

Cristie J. Becker, MD
Assistant Professor of Radiology, Pediatric Imaging, Children's Hospital of Michigan, Detroit, Michigan

Mary P. Bedard, MD
Associate Professor of Pediatrics, Wayne State University School of Medicine; Clinical Director, Newborn Intensive Care Unit, Children's Hospital of Michigan, Detroit, Michigan

Tamar E. Ben-Ami, MD
Professor of Radiology, Northwestern University Feinberg School of Medicine; Director of Education, Department of Medical Imaging, Children's Memorial Hospital, Chicago, Illinois

Ellen C. Benya, MD
Assistant Professor of Radiology, Northwestern University Feinberg School of Medicine; Attending, Department of Medical Imaging, Children's Memorial Hospital, Chicago, Illinois

Walter E. Berdon, MD, FACR
Professor of Radiology, Department of Radiology, Morgan-Stanley Children's Hospital of New York; Professor of Radiology, Columbia University College of Physicians and Surgeons, New York, New York

Isaac Binkovitz, BA
Student, McGill University, Montreal, Québec, Canada

Larry A. Binkovitz, MD
Clinical Assistant Professor of Radiology, Ohio State University; Section Chief, Nuclear Medicine, Department of Diagnostic Radiology, Nationwide Children's Hospital, Columbus, Ohio

David A. Bloom, MD
Clinical Associate Professor of Radiology, Wayne State University School of Medicine, Detroit; Staff Pediatric Radiologist, William Beaumont Hospital, Royal Oak, Michigan

Danielle K. B. Boal, MD
Professor of Radiology and Pediatrics, Department of Radiology, Pennsylvania State University College of Medicine; Professor of Radiology and Pediatrics, Department of Radiology, Milton S. Hershey Medical Center, Hershey, Pennsylvania

Timothy N. Booth, MD
Associate Professor, University of Texas Southwestern Medical Center; Director of Head and Neck Imaging, Children's Medical Center of Dallas, Dallas, Texas

Boris Brkljacic, MD, PhD
Professor of Radiology, Department of Radiology,
University of Zagreb Medical School; Professor of
Radiology, Department of Radiology, University
Hospital "Dubrava," Zagreb, Croatia

Dorothy I. Bulas, MD
Professor of Radiology and Pediatrics, George
Washington University School of Medicine and
Health Sciences; Department of Diagnostic Imaging
and Radiology, Children's National Medical Center,
Washington, DC

Marguerite M. Caré, MD
Assistant Professor of Radiology, Division of
Neuroradiology, Cincinnati Children's Hospital
Medical Center, Cincinnati, Ohio

Kim M. Cecil, PhD
Associate Professor of Radiology, Pediatrics and
Neuroscience, Departments of Radiology and
Pediatrics, University of Cincinnati; Associate
Professor and MR Spectroscopist, Department of
Radiology, Cincinnati Children's Hospital Medical
Center, Cincinnati, Ohio

Luisa F. Cervantes, MD
Staff Radiologist, Department of Radiology, Miami
Children's Hospital, Miami, Florida

Frandics P. Chan, MD, PhD
Assistant Professor of Radiology, Department of
Radiology, Stanford University Medical Center;
Pediatric Radiologist, Department of Radiology, Lucile
Packard Children's Hospital, Stanford, California

Harry T. Chugani, MD
Professor of Pediatrics, Neurology, and Radiology;
Chief, Pediatric Neurology; Director of PET Center,
Children's Hospital of Michigan, Detroit, Michigan

Harris L. Cohen, MD
Professor of Radiology, Stony Brook School of
Medicine, Stony Brook, New York; Visiting Professor,
Johns Hopkins Medical Institutions, Baltimore,
Maryland

Ronald A. Cohen, MD
Director, Department of Diagnostic Imaging, Children's
Hospital Oakland, Oakland, California

Brian D. Coley, MD
Clinical Professor of Radiology and Pediatrics, The
Ohio State University College of Medicine and Public
Health; Assistant Director of Radiology, Nationwide
Children's Hospital, Columbus, Ohio

Virgil R. Condon, MD
Emeritus Professor of Radiology, University of Utah;
Chairman, Department of Medical Imaging
(Retired), Primary Children's Medical Center,
Salt Lake City, Utah

Bairbre L. Connolly, MB BCh, FRCP(C)
Associate Professor, Medical Imaging, University of
Toronto; Medical Director of Image Guided Therapy,
Diagnostic Imaging, The Hospital for Sick Children,
Toronto, Ontario, Canada

Moira L. Cooper, MD, FRCP(C)

John J. Crowley, MD
Staff Radiologist, Henry Ford Macomb Hospital,
Clinton, Michigan

J. A. Gordon Culham, MD, FRCP(C)
Professor, Department of Radiology, University of
British Columbia; Radiologist and Co-Director,
Cardiac Catheterization Laboratory, Vancouver,
British Columbia, Canada

Alan Daneman, MB BCh, FRCP(C)
Professor of Radiology and Pediatric, Radiologist,
Department of Diagnostic Imaging, Hospital for
Sick Children, Toronto, Ontario, Canada

Jeffrey W. Delaney, MD
Clinical Associate, Duke University School of Medicine
and Duke University Medical Center, Durham,
North Carolina

Guilherme T. S. Demarchi, MD
Research Assistant in Radiology/Radiologist-in-Training,
Department of Diagnostic Imaging, Federal
University of Sao Paulo, Sao Paulo, Brazil

Michael A. DiPietro, MD
John F. Holt Collegiate Professor of Radiology,
University of Michigan; Pediatric Radiologist, C.S.
Mott Children's Hospital, University of Michigan
Medical Center, Ann Arbor, Michigan

James S. Donaldson, MD
Professor of Radiology, Northwestern University
Feinberg School of Medicine; Chairman, Department
of Medical Imaging, Children's Memorial Hospital,
Chicago, Illinois

Mary T. Donofrio, MD, FAAP, FACC, FASE
Associate Professor of Pediatrics, George Washington
University; Director of the Fetal Heart Program,
Children's National Heart Institute, Children's
National Medical Center, Washington, DC

F. Daniel Donovan, MD
Cardiovascular Imaging Fellow, Stanford University
Medical Center/Lucile Packard Children's Hospital,
Stanford, California

Stephen M. Druhan, MD
Pediatric Radiologist, Department of Radiology,
Columbus Children's Hospital, Columbus, Ohio

Josée Dubois, MD, MsC
Professor of Radiology, Faculty of Medicine, University of Montreal; Radiologist, and Head of the Interventional Radiology Section, Sainte-Justine Hospital, Montreal, Quebec, Canada

Jerry R. Dwek, MD
Adjunct Clinical Assistant Professor of Radiology, University of California at San Diego; Attending Physician, Rady Children's Hospital and Health Center, San Diego, California

Kirsten Ecklund, MD
Assistant Professor of Radiology, Harvard Medical School; Division Director for General Diagnostic Radiology, Director of Body MR Imaging, Department of Radiology, Children's Hospital, Boston, Massachusetts

Eric L. Effmann, MD
Professor of Radiology, and Division Director, Pediatric Radiology, Department of Radiology, University of Washington; Director, Department of Radiology, Children's Hospital and Regional Medical Center, Seattle, Washington

John C. Egelhoff, DO
Professor of Clinical Radiology, University of Cincinnati College of Medicine; Chief, NeuroCT, and Staff Neuroradiologist, Division of Neuroradiology, Cincinnati Children's Hospital, Cincinnati, Ohio

Tamer El-Helw, MD
Cardiovascular Imaging Fellow, Stanford University Medical Center/Lucile Packard Children's Hospital, Stanford, California

Sitaram M. Emani, MD
Instructor in Surgery, Harvard Medical School; Assistant in Cardiac Surgery, Children's Hospital Boston, Boston, Massachusetts

Kathleen H. Emery, MD
Clinical Professor, Departments of Radiology and Pediatrics, University of Cincinnati; Section Chief, Body MRI, Department of Radiology, Cincinnati Children's Hospital Medical Center, Cincinnati, Ohio

Eric N. Faerber, MD
Professor of Radiology and Pediatrics, Drexel University School of Medicine; Director, Department of Radiology, St. Christopher's Hospital for Children, Philadelphia, Pennsylvania

Diana L. Farmer, MD
Professor of Surgery, Pediatrics, Obstetrics and Gynecology, and Reproductive Sciences, University of California at San Francisco; Surgeon-in-Chief, University of California at San Francisco Children's Hospital and Medical Center, San Francisco, California

Kate A. Feinstein, MD, FACR
Associate Professor of Radiology and Surgery, and Chief, Section of Pediatric Radiology, Department of Radiology, Pritzker School of Medicine and University of Chicago Medical Center, Chicago, Illinois

G. Peter Feola, MD
Adjunct Assistant Professor, Department of Radiology, University of Utah; Director of Interventional Radiology, Medical Imaging, Primary Children's Medical Center, Salt Lake City, Utah

Sandra K. Fernbach, MD
Professor of Radiology, Northwestern University Feinberg School of Medicine, Chicago; Staff Radiologist, Evanston Northwestern Healthcare, Evanston, Illinois

Barry D. Fletcher, MD, CM
Former Chairman, Department of Diagnostic Imaging, St. Jude Children's Research Hospital, Memphis, Tennessee

Donald P. Frush, MD
Professor of Radiology and Pediatrics, and Faculty, Medical Physics, Duke University; Chief, Pediatric Radiology, Duke University Medical Center, Durham, North Carolina

Ana Maria Gaca, MD
Associate in Radiology and Pediatrics, Duke University Medical Center, Durham; Attending, Alamance Regional Medical Center, Burlington, North Carolina

Jeffrey G. Gaca, MD
Fellow, Division of Thoracic Surgery, Duke University Medical Center, Durham, North Carolina

Marilyn J. Goske, MD
Staff Radiologist, Department of Radiology, Akron Children's Hospital, Akron, Ohio

P. Ellen Grant, MD
Associate Professor, Harvard Medical School; Chief of Pediatric Radiology, Massachusetts General Hospital, Boston, Massachusetts

S. Bruce Greenberg, MD
Professor of Radiology, University of Arkansas for Medical Sciences and Arkansas Children's Hospital, Little Rock, Arkansas

R. Paul Guillerman, MD
Assistant Professor of Radiology, Department of Radiology, Baylor College of Medicine; Staff Radiologist, Singleton Department of Diagnostic Imaging, Texas Children's Hospital, Houston, Texas

Eric J. Hall, DPhil, DSc, FACR, FRCR
Higgins Professor of Radiation Biophysics, Center for Radiological Research, Columbia University, New York, New York

Jack O. Haller, MD†
Professor Emeritus of Radiology, Albert Einstein
College of Medicine-Beth Israel Campus, and
formerly Director of Pediatric Radiology, Beth Israel
Continuum Hospitals, New York, New York

Edward C. Halperin, MD, FACR
Vice Dean of the School of Medicine, R.J. Reynolds
Professor of Medical Education, Professor of
Radiation Oncology and Pediatrics, Duke University,
Durham, North Carolina

H. Theodore Harcke, MD, FACR, FAIUM
Professor of Radiology and Pediatrics, Department of
Radiology, Jefferson Medical College, Philadelphia,
Pennsylvania; Chief of Imaging Research,
Department of Medical Imaging, Alfred I. DuPont
Hospital for Children, Wilmington, Delaware

Gary L. Hedlund, DO
Adjunct Professor of Radiology, The University of Utah
College of Medicine; Chairman, Department of
Medical Imaging, Primary Children's Medical Center,
Salt Lake City, Utah

Kathleen Jacobson Helton, MD
Neuroradiologist and Associate Professor of Radiology,
University of Tennessee College of Medicine;
Neuroradiologist, Associate Member, Radiological
Sciences, St. Jude Children's Research Hospital,
Memphis, Tennessee

Stephen M. Henesch, DO
Former Pediatric Radiology Fellow, The Children's
Hospital of Philadelphia, Philadelphia, Pennsylvania;
Director, Pediatric Radiology, Good Samaritan
Hospital and Medical Center, West Islip, New York

J. René Herlong, MD
Associate Professor of Pediatric Cardiology, Duke
University School of Medicine; Director of
Noninvasive Imaging for Pediatric Cardiology, Duke
University Medical Center, Durham, North Carolina

Thomas E. Herman, MD, FACR
Associate Professor of Radiology, Washington University
of St. Louis, Mallinckrodt Institute of Radiology;
Associate Radiologist, St. Louis Children's Hospital,
St. Louis, Missouri

Marta Hernanz-Schulman, MD, FAAP
Professor of Radiology and Pediatrics, Vanderbilt
University Medical Center; Medical Director,
Diagnostic Imaging, Monroe Carell, Jr. Children's
Hospital at Vanderbilt, Nashville, Tennessee

Jeanne G. Hill, MD
Associate Professor of Radiology and Pediatrics, Medical
University of South Carolina; Division Director of
Pediatric Radiology, Medical University Children's
Hospital, Charleston, South Carolina

Karin L. Hoeg, MD
Assistant Professor of Radiology, University of
Cincinnati; Staff Radiologist, Cincinnati Children's
Hospital Medical Center, Cincinnati, Ohio

Mark J. Hogan, MD
Clinical Associate Professor, Department of Radiology,
The Ohio State University; Chief, Section of Vascular
and Interventional Radiology, Department of
Radiology, Nationwide Children's Hospital,
Columbus, Ohio

Richard A. Humes, MD
Professor of Pediatrics, Chief, Division of Cardiology,
Wayne State University; The Carman and Ann Adams
Department of Pediatrics, Children's Hospital of
Michigan, Detroit, Michigan

Richard B. Jaffe, MD, FACR
Adjunct Professor of Radiology, Department of Medical
Imaging, Primary Children's Medical Center, Salt
Lake City, Utah

James Jaggers, MD
Associate Professor of Surgery, and Chief, Pediatric
Cardiac Surgery, Duke University Medical Center,
Durham, North Carolina

Charles A. James, MD
Associate Professor of Radiology and Pediatrics,
University of Arkansas for Medical Sciences; Chief of
Pediatric Radiology, Arkansas Children's Hospital,
Little Rock, Arkansas

Diego Jaramillo, MD, MPH
Professor of Radiology, University of Pennsylvania;
Radiologist-in-Chief and Van Alen Chair, Department
of Radiology, Children's Hospital of Philadelphia,
Philadelphia, Pennsylvania

Joseph J. Junewick, MD
Chair, Diagnostic Radiology, Spectrum Health
Hospitals; Helen DeVos Children's Hospital, and
Advanced Radiology Services, Grand Rapids,
Michigan

Ronald J. Kanter, MD
Associate Professor of Pediatrics, Duke University;
Director, Pediatric Electrophysiology, The Heart
Center, Duke University Medical Center, Durham;
Associate Clinical Professor of Pediatrics, University
of North Carolina at Chapel Hill, Chapel Hill, North
Carolina

Sue Creviston Kaste, DO
Professor of Radiology, University of Tennessee, Health
Science Center; Member, Radiological Sciences,
St. Jude Children's Research Hospital, Memphis,
Tennessee

†deceased

Theodore E. Keats, MD
Alumni Professor of Radiology, University of Virginia and University of Virginia Health Systems, Charlottesville, Virginia

Stanley T. Kim, MD
Instructor in Radiology, Northwestern University; Attending Interventional Radiologist, Medical Imaging, Children's Memorial Hospital, and Attending Interventional Radiologist, Radiology, Northwestern Memorial Hospital, Chicago, Illinois

Keith A. Kronemer, MD
Assistant Professor, Washington University School of Medicine, Mallinckrodt Institute of Radiology; Radiologist, Pediatric Radiology, St, Louis Children's Hospital, St. Louis, Missouri

Jerald P. Kuhn, MD
Professor Emeritus of Radiology, State University of New York at Buffalo; Former Radiologist-in-Chief, Children's Hospital Buffalo, Buffalo, New York

Ralph S. Lachman, MD
Professor Emeritus, Radiological Sciences and Pediatrics, University of California at Los Angeles School of Medicine; Co-Investigator, International Skeletal Dysplasia Registry, Cedars-Sinai Medical Center, Los Angeles, California

Tal Laor, MD
Professor of Radiology and Pediatrics, University of Cincinnati College of Medicine; Professor of Radiology and Pediatrics, Cincinnati Children's Hospital Medical Center, Cincinnati, Ohio

Nicole Larrier, MD, MSc
Associate, Department of Radiation Oncology, Duke University Medical Center, Durham, North Carolina

Theodore Lawrence, MD, PhD
Professor and Chair, Department of Radiation Oncology, University of Michigan and University of Michigan Medical Center, Ann Arbor, Michigan

Henrique M. Lederman, MD
Professor of Radiology, Department of Diagnostic Imaging, Federal University of Sao Paulo; Chief, Center of Diagnostic Imaging, Pediatric Oncology Institute, Sao Paulo, Brazil

Andrew J. Lodge, MD
Assistant Professor of Surgery, Division of Cardiovascular and Thoracic Surgery, Duke University School of Medicine and Duke University Medical Center, Durham, North Carolina

Frederick R. Long, MD
Clinical Professor, Department of Radiology, The Ohio State University Medical Center University Hospitals; Section Chief, Body CT and MR Imaging, Department of Radiology, Columbus Children's Hospital; Associate Attending, Radiology, The Arthur G. James Cancer Hospital and Richard J. Solove Research Institute; Adjunct Assistant Professor, Radiology, Medical University of Ohio at Toledo, Columbus, Ohio

Lisa H. Lowe, MD, FAAP
Associate Professor and Academic Chair, Department of Radiology, University of Missouri Kansas City; Pediatric Radiologist and Fellowship Director, Department of Radiology, Children Mercy Hospitals and Clinics, Kansas City, Missouri

Cathy MacDonald, MD, FRCP(C)
Assistant Professor, Department of Medical Imaging, University of Toronto, Staff Radiologist, Department of Diagnostic Imaging, The Hospital for Sick Children, Toronto, Ontario, Canada

Richard I. Markowitz, MD, FACR
Professor of Radiology, University of Pennsylvania; Radiologist, Children's Hospital of Philadelphia, Philadelphia, Pennsylvania

John B. Mawson, MB, ChB, MHB (Hon), FRACR, FRCR(C)
Assistant Professor, Department of Radiology, University of British Columbia; Associate Director, Department of Radiology, British Columbia Children's Hospital, Vancouver, British Columbia, Canada

Charles M. Maxfield, MD
Associate Professor of Radiology and Pediatrics, Duke University Medical Center, Durham, North Carolina

William H. McAlister, MD
Professor of Radiology and Pediatrics, Mallinckrodt Institute of Radiology, Washington University School of Medicine; Radiologist, St Louis Children's Hospital, Barnes Hospital, and Shriners Hospital, St Louis, Missouri

Clare A. McLaren, DCR(R)
Clinical Specialist Radiographer, Department of Radiology, Great Ormond Street Hospital, London, United Kingdom

James S. Meyer, MD
Associate Professor of Radiology, University of Pennsylvania School of Medicine; Associate Radiologist-in-Chief, Department of Radiology, Children's Hospital of Philadelphia, Philadelphia, Pennsylvania

Swati Mody, MD, MBBS
Assistant Professor, Department of Radiology, Wayne State University; Section Head, Neuroradiology, Department of Pediatric Imaging, Children's Hospital of Michigan, Detroit, Michigan

James F. Mooney III, MD
Professor of Orthopaedic Surgery, Medical University of South Carolina, Charleston, South Carolina

Charlotte Waugh Moore, MD
Assistant Professor of Pediatrics, University of Missouri-Kansas City; Pediatric Radiologist, Department of Radiology, Children's Mercy Hospitals and Clinics, Kansas City, Missouri

Kevin R. Moore, MD
Assistant Professor of Radiology, University of Utah School of Medicine; Pediatric Neuroradiologist and Radiologist, Primary Children's Medical Center, Salt Lake City, Utah

Mary Beth Moore, MS, MD
Assistant Professor, Department of Radiology, University of Arkansas for Medical Sciences; Radiologist, Arkansas Children's Hospital, Little Rock, Arkansas

Frank P. Morello, MD
Associate Professor of Radiology, University of Missouri at Kansas City; Radiologist-in-Chief, Department of Radiology, Children's Mercy Hospital, Kansas City, Missouri

Otto Muzik, PhD
Associate Professor of Pediatrics and Radiology, Wayne State University Medical School; Staff Physician, Children's Hospital of Michigan PET Center, Detroit, Michigan

Oscar Navarro, MD
Assistant Professor, Department of Medical Imaging, University of Toronto; Staff Radiologist, Department of Diagnostic Imaging, The Hospital for Sick Children, Toronto, Ontario, Canada

Michael D. Neel, MD
Adjunct Faculty, Department of Orthopaedics, St. Jude Children's Hospital, Memphis, Tennessee

Marvin D. Nelson, MD
Professor of Radiology, University of Southern California Keck School of Medicine; Chairman, Department of Radiology, Children's Hospital Los Angeles, Los Angeles, California

Beverley Newman, BSc, MB BCh, FACR
Associate Professor of Radiology, Department of Radiology, Stanford University; Associate Professor of Radiology and Associate Chief of Pediatric Radiology, Department of Radiology, Lucile Packard Children's Hospital at Stanford, Stanford, California

Julie Currie O'Donovan, MD
Clinical Assistant Professor, Department of Radiology, The Ohio State University College of Medicine and Public Health, Columbus; Pediatric Radiologist, Department of Radiology, Children's Hospital and Children's Radiological Institute, Columbus; Adjunct Assistant Professor, Department of Radiology, Medical College of Ohio, Toledo, Ohio

Joseph H. Piatt, Jr., MD, FAAP
Professor, Department of Pediatrics, Drexel University College of Medicine; Chief, Section of Neurosurgery, St. Christopher's Hospital for Children, Philadelphia, Pennsylvania

Avrum N. Pollock, MD, FRCPC
Assistant Professor of Radiology, University of Pennsylvania School of Medicine; Director of Resident and Fellowship Program and Neuroradiologist, Department of Radiology, Children's Hospital of Philadelphia, Philadelphia, Pennsylvania

Tina Young Poussaint, MD
Associate Professor of Radiology, Harvard Medical School; Attending Neuroradiologist, and Director, PBTC Neuroimaging Center, Department of Radiology, Children's Hospital Boston, Boston, Massachusetts

John M. Racadio, MD
Associate Professor of Radiology and Pediatrics, and Division Chief, Pediatric Interventional Radiology, Cincinnati Children's Hospital Medical Center and University of Cincinnati College of Medicine, Cincinnati, Ohio

Marilyn D. E. Ranson, MD, BSc, FRCP(c)
Assistant Professor, Department of Medical Imaging, University of Toronto; Staff Radiologist, Department of Diagnostic Imaging, The Hospital for Sick Children, Toronto, Ontario, Canada

John F. Rhodes, MD
Assistant Professor of Pediatrics, Duke University School of Medicine; Chief of Clinical Cardiology and Medical Director, Pediatric and Adult Congenital Catheterization Laboratory, Duke University Medical Center, Durham, North Carolina

Michael Riccabona, MD
Professor of Pediatrics and Radiology, and Head of Radiology, Division of Pediatric Radiology, University Hospital Graz, Graz, Austria

Cynthia K. Rigsby, MD
Associate Professor of Radiology, Northwestern University Feinberg School of Medicine; Head, Division of Body Imaging, Medical Imaging, Children's Memorial Hospital, Chicago, Illinois

Derek J. Roebuck, MB BS, FRANZCR
Honorary Senior Lecturer, Institute of Child Health, University College London; Consultant Radiologist, Great Ormond Street Hospital, London, United Kingdom

Lucy B. Rorke-Adams, MD
Clinical Professor of Pathology, Neurology and Pediatrics, Pathology and Laboratory Medicine, University of Pennsylvania School of Medicine; Senior Neuropathologist, Division of Neuropathology, Department of Pathology and Laboratory Medicine, The Children's Hospital of Philadelphia, Philadelphia, Pennsylvania

Arlene A. Rozzelle, MD
Assistant Professor of Surgery, Wayne State University School of Medicine; Chief, Plastic Surgery, and Director, Cleft/Craniofacial Team, Children's Hospital of Michigan, Detroit, Michigan

Craig A. Sable, MD
Associate Professor of Radiology, George Washington University School of Medicine; Director of Echocardiography, Fellowship Training, and Telemedicine, Children's National Medical Center, Washington, DC

Pallavi Sagar, MD
Instructor in Radiology, Harvard Medical School; Assistant Radiologist, Pediatric Radiology, Massachusetts General Hospital, Boston, Massachusetts

Martha C. Saker, MD
Assistant Professor, Pediatric Radiology, Northwestern University; Attending Radiologist, Medical Imaging, Children's Memorial Hospital, Chicago, Illinois

L. Santiago Medina, MD, MPH
Co-Director, Division of Neuroradiology, and Director, Health Outcomes Policy and Economics (HOPE) Center, Miami Children's Hospital, Miami, Florida

Alan E. Schlesinger, MD
Professor, Department of Radiology, Baylor College of Medicine; Staff Radiologist, The Edward B. Singleton Department of Diagnostic Imaging, Texas Children's Hospital, Houston, Texas

Brian E. Schirf, MD
Dept of Radiology, Feinberg School of Medicine Northwestern University, Chicago, Illinois

Erin Simon Schwartz, MD
Associate Professor of Radiology, University of Pennsylvania School of Medicine; Staff Neuroradiologist, Department of Radiology, Division of Neuroradiology, The Children's Hospital of Philadelphia, Philadelphia, Pennsylvania

Richard M. Shore, MD
Associate Professor, Department of Radiology, Northwestern University Feinberg School of Medicine; Head, Division of General Radiology and Nuclear Medicine, Children's Memorial Hospital, Chicago, Illinois

Carlos J. Sivit, MD
Professor of Radiology and Pediatrics, Case Western Reserve School of Medicine; Director of Pediatric Radiology, Rainbow Babies and Children's Hospital, Cleveland, Ohio

Thomas L. Slovis, MD
Professor of Radiology and Pediatrics, Wayne State University School of Medicine; Former Chief, Pediatric Imaging, Children's Hospital of Michigan, Detroit, Michigan

Jennifer D. Smith, MD
Assistant Professor of Radiology, University of Pennsylvania School of Medicine; Radiologist, The Children's Hospital of Philadelphia, Philadelphia, Pennsylvania

Sandeep Sood, MD
Associate Professor, Neurosurgery, Wayne State University School of Medicine; Staff Neurosurgeon, Pediatric Neurosurgery, Children's Hospital of Michigan, Detroit, Michigan

Stephanie E. Spottswood, MD
Associate Professor of Radiology and Pediatrics, Vanderbilt University Medical Center; Medical Director of Nuclear Medicine Section, Diagnostic Imaging, Monroe Carell, Jr. Children's Hospital at Vanderbilt, Nashville, Tennessee

Jan Stauss, MD
Harvard Medical School and Division of Nuclear Medicine, Children's Hospital Boston, Boston, Massachusetts

R. Grant Steen, PhD
Associate Professor, Department of Psychiatry, University of North Carolina at Chapel Hill; President, Medical Communications Consultants, Chapel Hill, North Carolina

Sharon M. Stein, MB ChB
Associate Professor of Radiology and Pediatrics, Radiology and Radiological Sciences, Vanderbilt University Medical Center; Associate Professor of Radiology and Pediatrics, Diagnostic Imaging, Vanderbilt Children's Hospital, Nashville, Tennessee

John Strain, MD, FACR
Chairman, Department of Radiology, The Children's Hospital; Professor of Radiology, University of Colorado at Denver Health Science Center, Denver, Colorado

Peter J. Strouse, MD
Professor of Radiology and Director, Section of
Pediatric Radiology, C.S. Mott Children's Hospital;
Department of Radiology, University of Michigan
Health System, Ann Arbor, Michigan

Joel D. Swartz, MD
President, Germantown Imaging Associates, Gladwyne,
Pennsylvania

Alexander J. Towbin, MD
Fellow in Radiology, University of Cincinnati; Fellow in
Radiology, Cincinnati Children's Hospital Medical
Center, Cincinnati, Ohio

Jeffrey Traubici, MD, FRCP(C)
Assistant Professor, Department of Medical Imaging,
University of Toronto; Staff Radiologist, Department
of Diagnostic Imaging, The Hospital for Sick
Children, Toronto, Ontario, Canada

S. Ted Treves, MD
Professor of Radiology, Harvard Medical School; Chief,
Division of Nuclear Medicine, Children's Hospital
Boston, Boston, Massachusetts

Henry L. Walters III, MD
Professor of Surgery and Chief, Department of
Cardiovascular Surgery, Wayne State University
School of Medicine and Children's Hospital of
Michigan, Detroit, Michigan

Robert G. Wells, MD
Associate Clinical Professor of Radiology and Pediatrics,
Medical College of Wisconsin; Interim Medical
Director, Radiology, Children's Hospital of Wisconsin,
Milwaukee, Wisconsin

Mary R. Wyers, MD
Assistant Professor of Radiology, Northwestern
University, Attending, Children's Memorial Hospital,
Chicago, Illinois

Adam S. Young
Undergraduate Student, Richard T. Farmer School of
Business, Miami University, Oxford; Research Aide,
Department of Radiology, Nationwide Children's
Hospital, Columbus, Ohio

FOREWORD

I am pleased that Dr. Thomas Slovis has asked me to write the foreword for this 11th edition of the most widely used textbook of pediatric imaging. I have served as a link between the real fathers of this text, Dr. John Caffey and Dr. Fred Silverman, and the current editor, Dr. Slovis, who has described in his TRIBUTE their historic contributions both to this book and to our field of pediatric radiology. Because of my interest in pediatric computed tomography, I was asked by Dr. Silverman in 1985 to revise and expand the section on thoracic imaging that previously had been written by Dr. Caffey himself. This was a great and humbling challenge, and I found that while my knowledge of CT allowed me to add to what Dr. Caffey had written, many of his observations based on plain radiography needed no revision or updating. Dr. Silverman then honored me by asking me to serve as co-editor for the ninth edition, published in 1993. It was a major revision and included much new material, particularly in CT and ultrasound. After Dr. Silverman's retirement, the task of organizing the tenth edition fell to me, and I knew that I would need outstanding co-editors to help compensate for the loss of Dr. Silverman's expertise. I asked Dr. Slovis and Dr. Jack Haller to assume the responsibility of composing another major revision that included entirely new sections on radiation risk and neonatal imaging, a complete revision of the GI, GU, and neuroradiology sections, and much new material on magnetic resonance imaging and interventional radiology. This edition was published in 2004; but, tragically, Dr. Haller died prematurely, and it became Dr. Slovis's task to revise the 11th edition to be published only four short years after the tenth. Tom has an unequaled energy level and an uncanny ability to quickly get to the essence of a problem. He recruited eight new section editors and sought contributions from clinicians in diverse fields of pediatrics to strongly re-emphasize the clinical background of this comprehensive text. Tom believes, as do many others, that as imaging has become more technically advanced, our daily interchange with those directly caring for our patients has become more distant and clinical correlation of imaging findings more difficult. To further improve this new edition, he painstakingly reviewed and enhanced all of the older, irreplaceable images and replaced the outdated examples. More than 50% of the images in this edition are new. While some of the text describing classic radiographic findings remains unchanged, updated information and references have been added. A new section discussing perinatal imaging, a completely revised cardiovascular section, and new material on interventional radiology are other highlights of this 11th edition. Another new, important feature is a website that includes an appendix containing many useful tables and measurements and incorporating a self-testing module to aid the learning process. The website includes video and color images that could not be included in a conventional printed text. I am very pleased to see this book continue to evolve and improve, and I am confident that it and its future editions will continue to serve as a cornerstone of learning both for pediatric imagers and our clinical colleagues for many years to come.

Dr. Jerald P. Kuhn
Professor Emeritus of Radiology
State University of New York at Buffalo
Former Radiologist-in-Chief, Children's Hospital
Buffalo, Buffalo, New York

PREFACE

My earliest recollection of *Caffey's Pediatric X-ray Diagnosis* is as a pediatric resident in 1967. I was amazed at the depth of clinical information provided in a radiology book. "The bible" plus the mentoring of Walter Berdon, David Baker, and R. Parker Allen made it easy for me to choose a career in pediatric radiology. Through the years, with huge technical advances (PACS, images circulated throughout the hospital, etc.), imagers have been less involved with their referring physicians, and both groups have lost a valuable learning experience. As noted in the tribute, Drs. Caffey and Silverman both believed that we cannot succeed without a strong clinical background and significant patient history when we read our images.

This 11th edition of *Pediatric Imaging* attempts to bring us back to our clinical roots. The authors are not only pediatric imagers but include a host of referring physicians, such as cardiologists, cardiovascular surgeons, general pediatric surgeons, neonatologists, neurosurgeons, oncologists, orthopedists, perinatologists, pathologists, plastic surgeons, and radiation oncologists. I hope this edition will stimulate more discussion with our referring physicians, leading to mutual gain and, more important, improvement in the care of our patients. With advances in interventional radiology, we anticipate narrowing the gap between surgeons and radiologists—two dynamic disciplines that should and can work together. In selected centers in North America, imagers, interventional cardiologists, and cardiovascular surgeons work together, sharing patients, improving the outcome, and advancing knowledge. More connectivity will follow if we allow it, and all of this will benefit our young patients.

This is the first edition since 1993 in which Dr. Jerald P. Kuhn has not participated as an editor, but I appreciate his advice. The absence of Dr. Jack O. Haller, co-editor of the tenth edition, due to his untimely death is a severe professional and personal loss.

A major innovation in this 11th edition is a new section on interventional radiology and the inclusion of prenatal imaging in the perinatal section. The cardiology section is completely revised, and major advances have been made in all the other sections. Fifty percent of the images are new, and all of the pictures have been enhanced to ensure visual excellence.

For the first time, a website is included with the text. It contains a new section, the appendix, which has crucial charts, measurements, and differentials in one place for easy access. The website also includes selected cases from most chapters so you can test yourself, your resident, or medical student before reading the chapter. There are multiple color images, more than we could include in the book, and a specific section for videos of those examinations in which motion is more instructive than still pictures.

Nine associate editors (eight of whom never worked on this text before) were newly initiated into what it takes to get a textbook of this magnitude put together in a timely manner. It is these individuals who will superbly guide the Caffey-Silverman text into the future.

The editor and associate editors thank Amanda Oberlee, of the medical photography division of Children's Hospital of Michigan, for her enormous help in enhancing the images. We thank Pat Vario for taking on the additional, unexpected job of assisting with the manuscripts and helping us stay organized. We are indebted to Kristina Oberle of Elsevier for taking this on as a personal project and shepherding us through from beginning to end. Rebecca Gaertner and Linda Grigg have worked tirelessly to make sure this publication is as good as it can be.

I hope this book stimulates you to have further discussions with your referring physicians, to answer the many questions posed by our pediatric patients, and to continue to value the opportunity of being a pediatric health care provider.

Thomas L. Slovis

PREFACE TO FIRST EDITION

Shadows are but dark holes in radiant streams, twisted rifts beyond the substance, meaningless in themselves.

He who would comprehend Röntgen's pallid shades need always to know well the solid matrix whence they spring. The physician needs to know intimately each living patient through whom the racing black light darts, and flashing the hidden depths reveals them in a glowing mirage of thin images, each cast delicately in its own halo, but all veiled and blended endlessly.

Man — warm, lively, fleshy man — and his story are both root and key to his shadows; shadows cold, silent and empty. — (JOHN CAFFEY)

Within a few weeks after Röntgen announced his now renowned discovery to the world in December, 1895, the x-ray method of examination was applied to infants and children. The Vienna letter of February 29 (M. Rec. 49:312, 1896) contained a roentgen print of the arm of an infant made of Kreidl in Vienna: this is the second reproduction of a roentgen image in the American literature. Credit for the first recorded roentgen examination of an infant in the United States undoubtedly belongs to Dr. E. P. Davis of New York City, who described the roentgen shadows cast by the trunk of a living infant and the skull of a dead fetus in March, 1896. In his remarkable article (The study of the infant body and the pregnant womb by the roentgen ray, Am. J. M. Sc. 111:263, 1896) Dr. Davis also included three drawings of shadows visualized by means of a skiascope — shadows visualized by means of a skiascope — shadows of the feet, elbows and orbit of a living infant. Feilchenfeld's discussion of spina ventosa in May, 1896, is probably the first roentgen description of morbid anatomy in children (Berlin. Klin. Wchnschr. 33:403, 1896). There were only two roentgen pediatric publications in 1896; the number increased to 14 in 1897.

In 1898, Escherich of Graz had had sufficient experience with pediatric roentgen examinations to write a general exposition on the merits and weaknesses of the method (La valeur diagnostique de la radiographie chez les enfants, Rev. d. mal. de l'enf. 16:233, May 1898). This is a highly interesting and illuminating discussion in which Escherich points out the roentgen examination was already not being used as commonly in young patients as in adults. He states that a roentgen laboratory was established especially for children at Graz in 1897, and it seems probable that this was the first of its kind. A single film is reproduced — a print of an infantile hand and forearm which shows rachitic changes. The uncertainties of the mediastinal shadows, which still bedevil us, were fully appreciated by Escherich, and he was quite unhappy about this baffling structure "in which so many important infantile lesions lie concealed." He was enthusiastic in regard to the possible estimation of the state of hydration of soft tissues in infantile diarrhea from their roentgen densities.

Reyher's German monograph in 1908 is the earliest review of the world literature of pediatric roentgenology which I have found (Reyher, P.: Die roentgenologische Diagnostik in der Kinderheilkunde, Ergebn. d. inn. Med. U. Kinderh. 2:613, 1908). In it there are 276 references to articles published during the first 12 years following Röntgen's discovery, and these furnish a good key for the study of the early writings in this field. The appendix contains 40 small but clear roentgen prints.

Rotch's *The Roentgen Ray in Pediatrics* appeared in 1910 – the first book in any language devoted exclusively to pediatric x-ray diagnosis and still, I believe, the only one in English. Dr. Thomas Morgan Rotch was Professor of Pediatrics, Harvard University, and an outstanding podiatrist of his time.* In this pioneer treatise he stresses the importance of mastering the shadows of normal structure before attempting the recognition and interpretation of the abnormal, and he carefully correlates the clinical findings with the roentgen findings in the cases illustrated; 42 of 264 figures depict the "normal living anatomy of infants and children." This material was taken largely from the files of the Boston Children's Hospital, and the author's statement that more than 2,300 cases were available for study demonstrates that roentgen examination had long been a commonplace in his clinic. Dr. Rotch's early fostering of roentgen examination of infants and children, his appreciation of the special problems in applying this method to the young, his careful anatomicroroentgen studies and his text, monumental for this time, all mark him as the father of pediatric roentgenology in America.

Two years later — 1912 — the first German book, Reyher's *Das Roentgenverfahren in der Kinderheilkunde*, was published. Later and more familiar texts are Gralka's *Roentgendiagnostik im Kindesalter* (1927), Becker's *Roentgendiagnostik und Strahlentherapie in der Kinderheilkunde* (1931) and the *Handbuch der Roentgendiagnostik und Therapie im Kindesalter* by Engel and Schall (1933). As far as I have been able to determine, no book on pediatric roentgen diagnosis has been published in English during the 35 years which have passed since Rotch's unique publication in 1910. The absence of pediatric roentgenology in the flood of medical texts which has streamed from the American and English presses during the last three decades constitutes a dereliction unmatched in other equally important fields of medical diagnosis — a literary developmental hypoplasia which it is hoped *Pediatric X-Ray Diagnosis* will remedy.

---

*Jacobi, A.: In memoriam Thomas Morgan Rotch, Am. J. Dis. Child. 8:245, 1914.

This book stems from the roentgen conferences held semimonthly at the Babies Hospital during the last 20 years. The films reproduced herein were all selected from our own roentgen files save those for which credit to others is indicated in the legends. The purpose of the author is two-fold: description of shadows cast by normal and morbid tissues, and clinical appraisal of roentgen findings in pediatric diagnosis. Roentgen physics, technic and therapy have been omitted intentionally. As references and acknowledgments testify, the writer has borrowed freely from the literature and is indebted to many contributors for subject matter and illustrations. To all of them I am sincerely grateful. In the broad and deep field of pediatric diagnosis, selection of the most appropriate material has posed many dilemmas. In the main, data have been chosen which have proved the most useful and instructive in solving the common and important diagnostic problems which have arisen during two decades in a large and busy pediatric hospital and out-patient clinic.

The limitations of space do not permit adequate recognition here of all those to whom credit is due for the making of this book. The roentgen examinations which are its foundation could not have been made without the cooperation of thousands of patients — many weak and painweary; to all of these I am profoundly thankful. Intimate clinical contacts have been maintained and essential collateral examinations have been made possible through the sustained collaboration of my colleagues — attending physicians and surgeons, resident physicians and nurses. I am under deep and solid obligation to Dr. Rustin McIntosh who read the entire manuscript; his discerning criticism and valuable suggestions are responsible for numerous corrections and improvements in the text. The sympathetic reception given to our early endeavors by Dr. Ross Golden will always be remembered gratefully, as well as his continuing wise and friendly counsel. We have benefited much and often from the discipline of the necropsy table — from the instructive dissections of Dr. Martha Wollstein, Dr. Beryl Paige and Dr. Dorothy Anderson.

To none, however do I owe more than to my loyal coworkers in the roentgen department of the Babies Hospital — Edgar Watts, Cecelia Peck, Moira Shannon, Mary Fennell and Mary Jean Cadman — for their gentle handling of patients, unfailing industry and superlative technical skill. Mrs. Cadman typed the manuscript; I am grateful to her for the speedy completion of a thorny chore. The drawings are the work of Alfred Feinberg, and they reflect his rich experience in medical illustration.

The final phase in the preparation of the manuscript was saddened by the death of Mr. H. A. Simons, President of the Year Book Publishers. His stimulating enthusiasm and generosity were indispensable to the completion of the book during these unsettled war years. His passing was a grievous loss. The task of publication has fallen to the capable and patient hands of Mr. Paul Perles and Mrs. Anabel Ireland Janssen.

John Caffey
Babies Hospital
New York 32
June 10, 1945

CONTENTS

Volume 1

SECTION III
NEURORADIOLOGY
ERIC N. FAERBER

PART 1
OVERVIEW

SECTION IV
THE RESPIRATORY SYSTEM
BRENT H. ADLER

Volume 2

SECTION VI
THE ABDOMEN, PELVIS, AND RETROPERITONEUM
BRIAN D. COLEY and MARTA HERNANZ-SCHULMAN

SECTION VII
MUSCULOSKELETAL SYSTEM
PETER J. STROUSE

APPENDICES
DAVID A. BLOOM, SECTION EDITOR
www.caffeysimaging.com

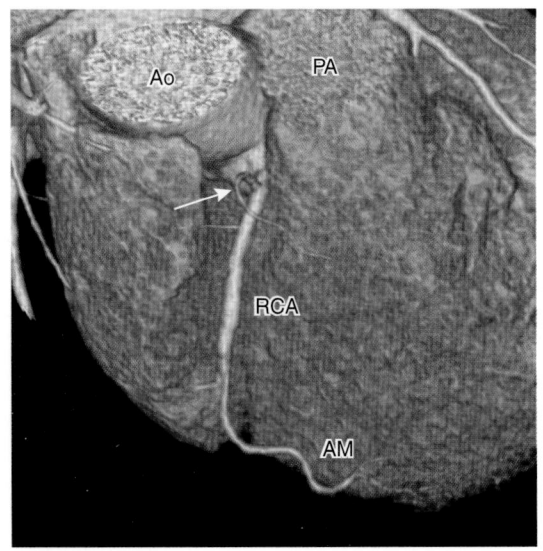

B

FIGURE 98-5B.

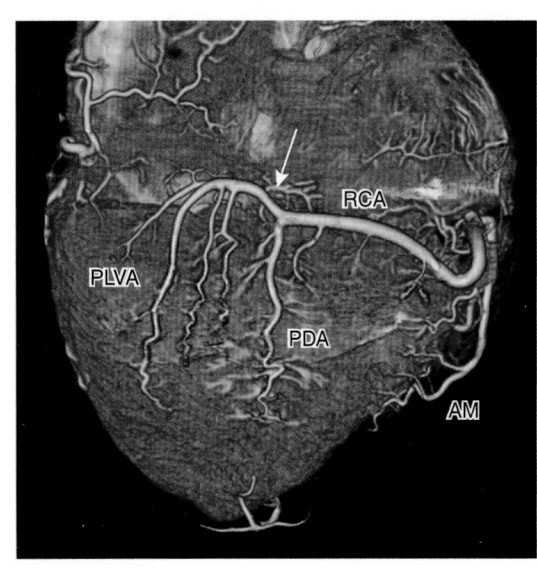

C

FIGURE 98-5C.

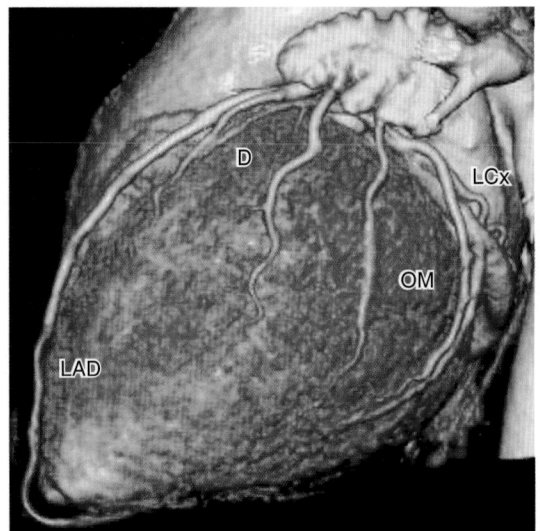

B

FIGURE 98-6B.

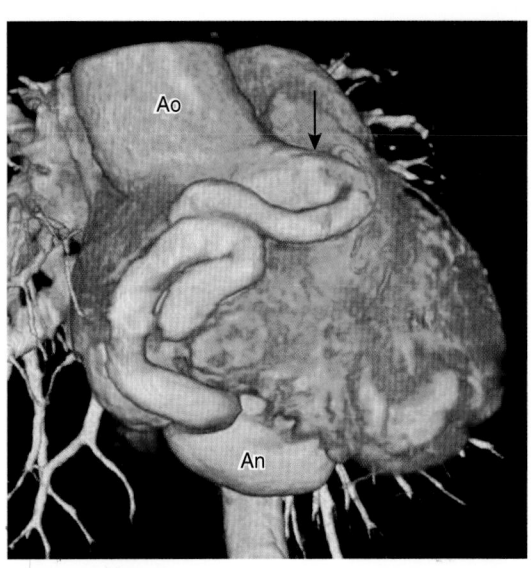

FIGURE 98-10.

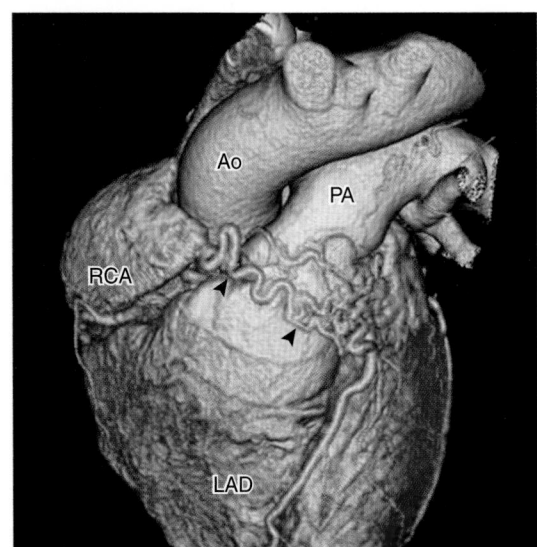

FIGURE 98-11.

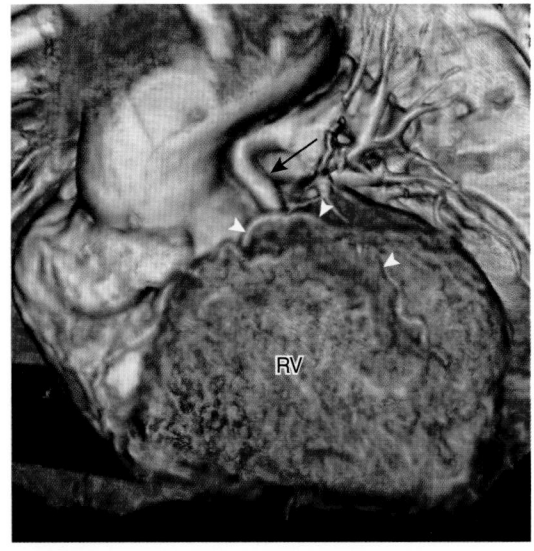

FIGURE 98-12.

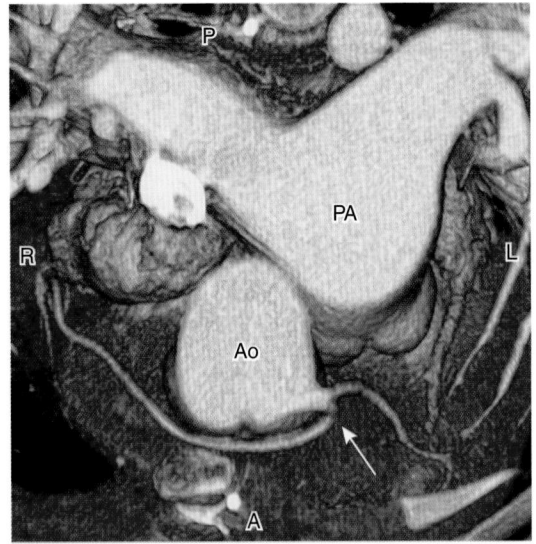

A
FIGURE 98-13A.

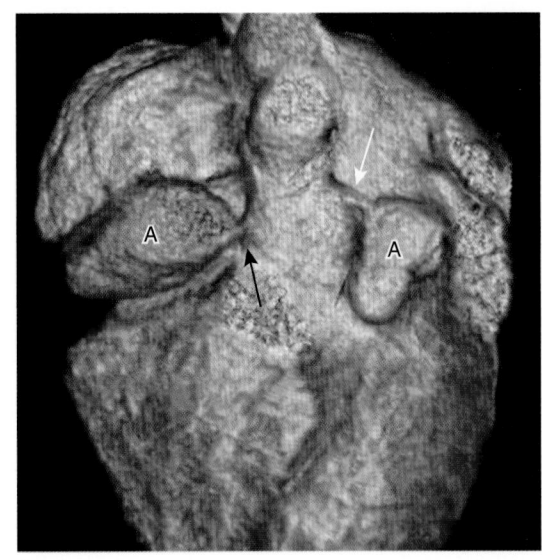

A
FIGURE 98-16A.

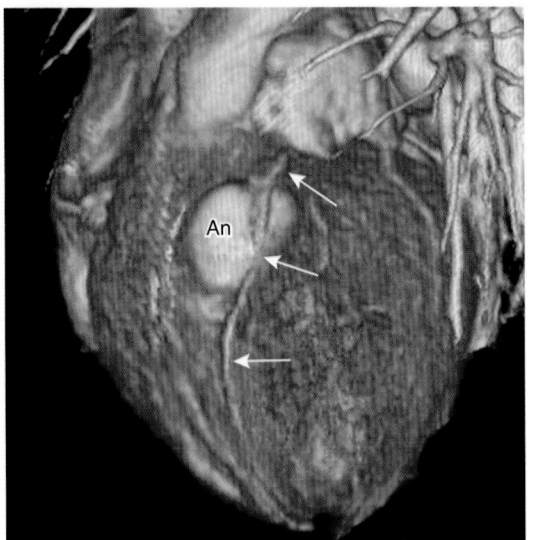

FIGURE 98-18.

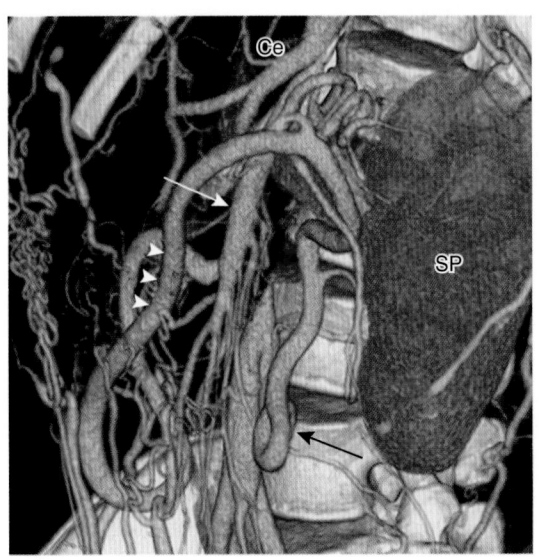

FIGURE 99-9.

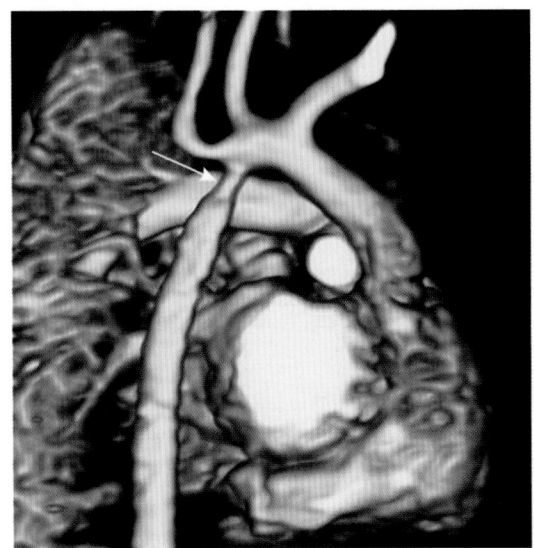

FIGURE 99-10.

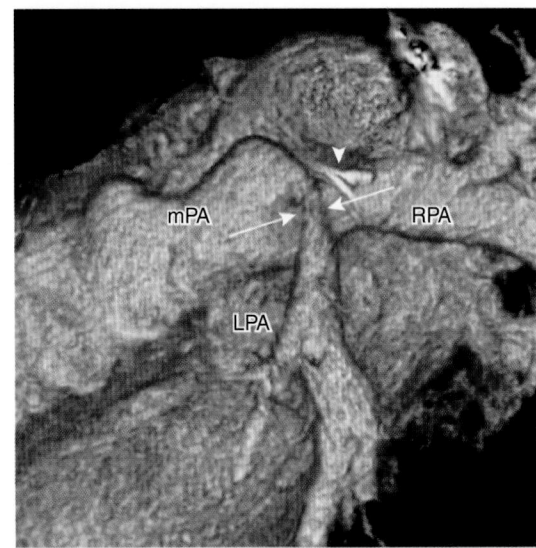

FIGURE 99-13.

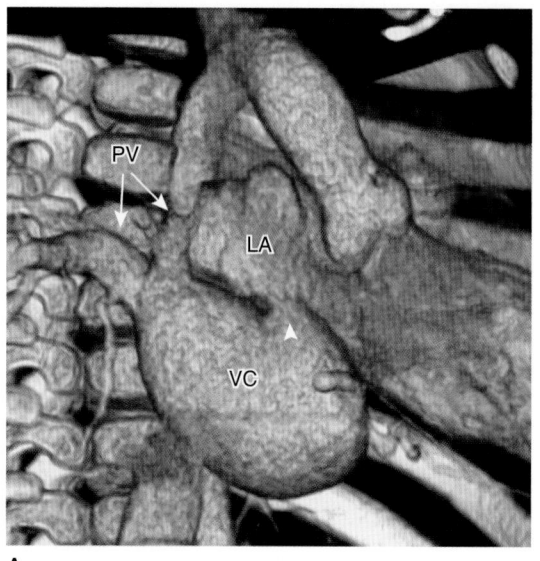

A

FIGURE 99-17A.

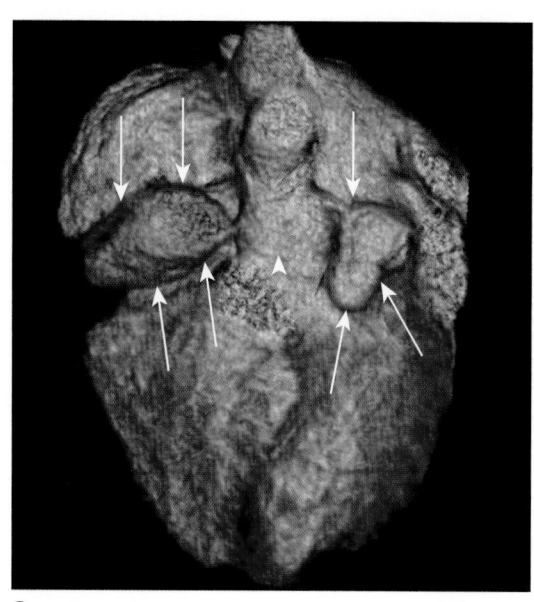

C

FIGURE 100-6C.

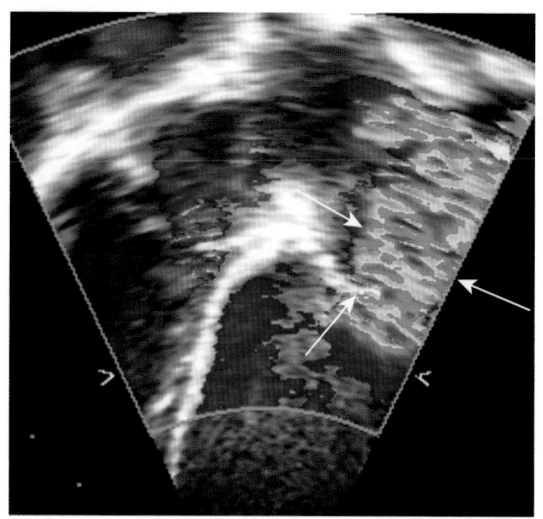

B

FIGURE 100-7B.

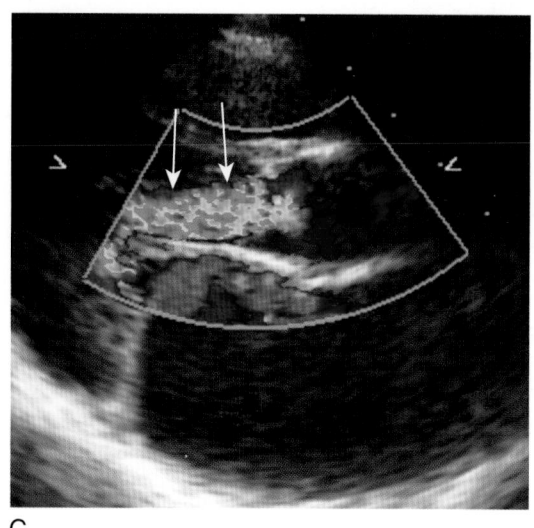

C

FIGURE 100-7C.

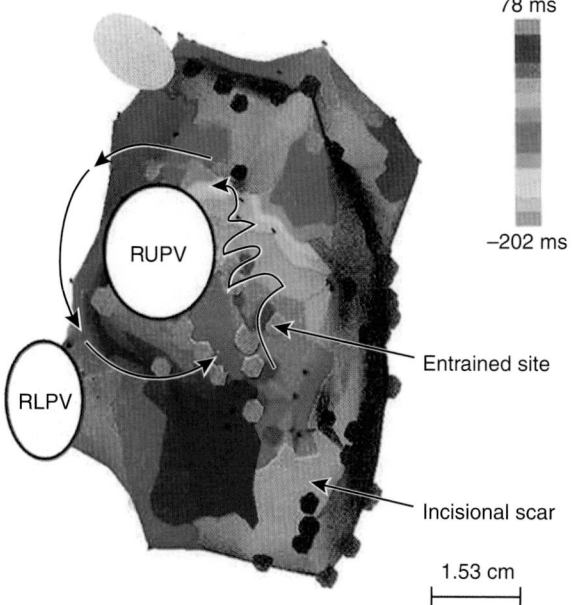

FIGURE 102-3.

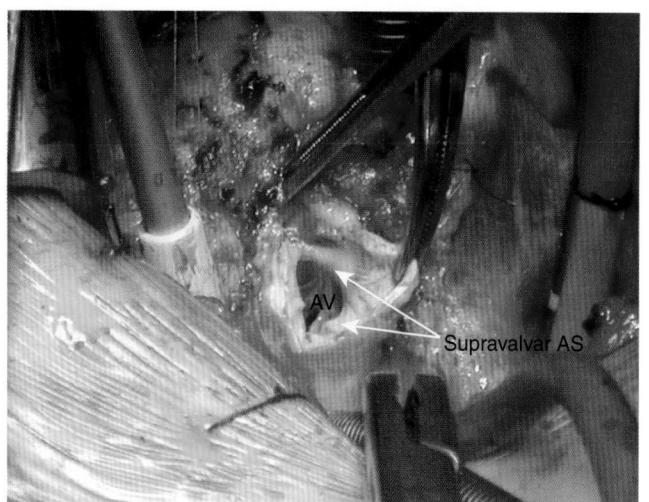

FIGURE 103-4.

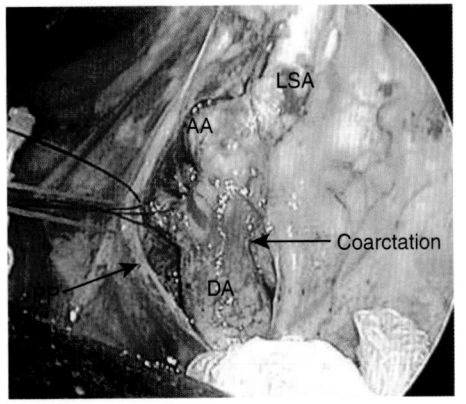

FIGURE 103-5.

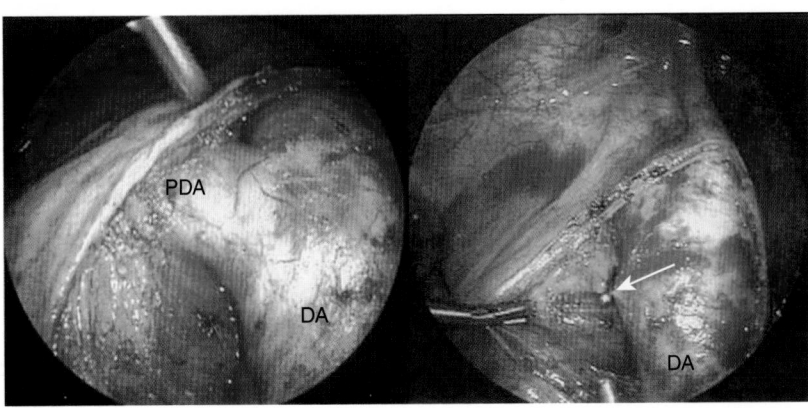

FIGURE 103-6.

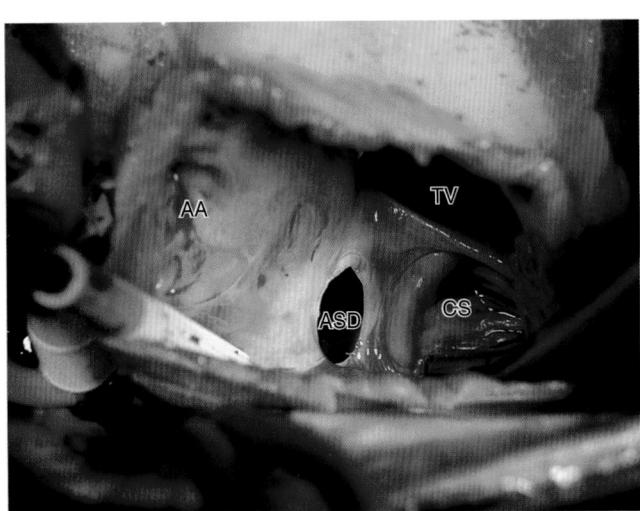

FIGURE 103-7.

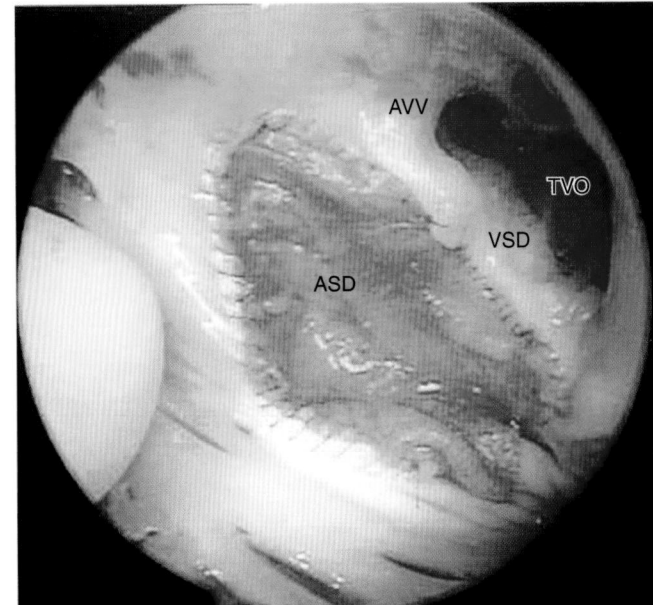

FIGURE 103-8.

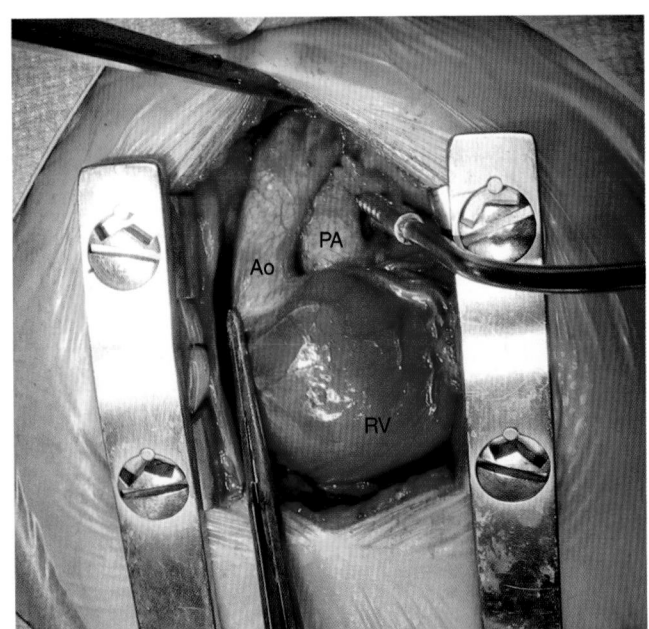

FIGURE 103-9.

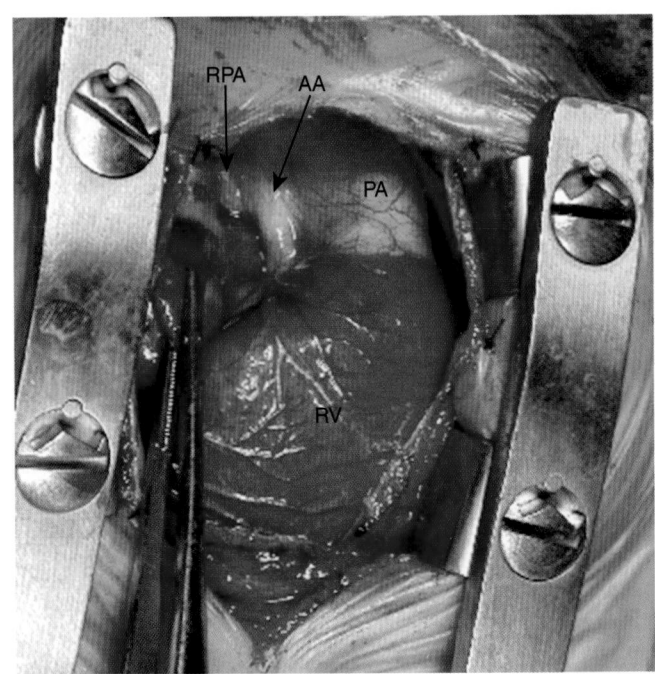

FIGURE 103-10.

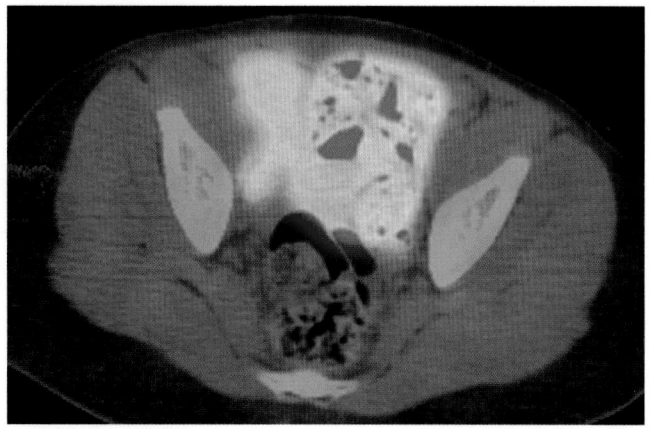

FIGURE 108-17.

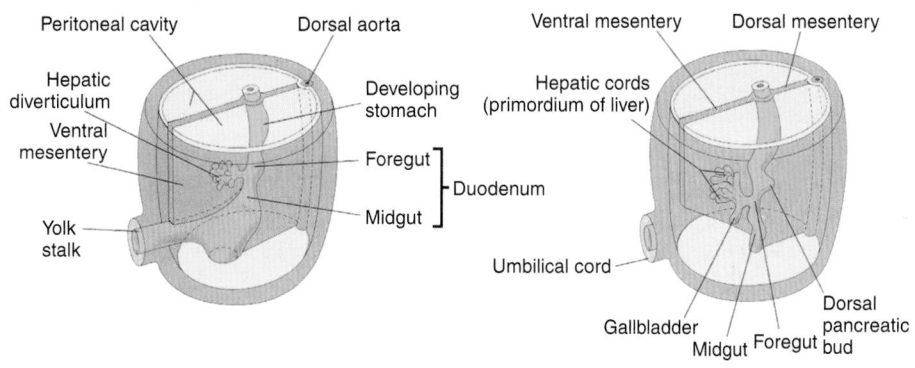

Peritoneal cavity
Dorsal aorta
Hepatic diverticulum
Developing stomach
Ventral mesentery
Foregut
Midgut
Duodenum
Yolk stalk

Ventral mesentery
Dorsal mesentery
Hepatic cords (primordium of liver)
Umbilical cord
Gallbladder
Midgut
Foregut
Dorsal pancreatic bud

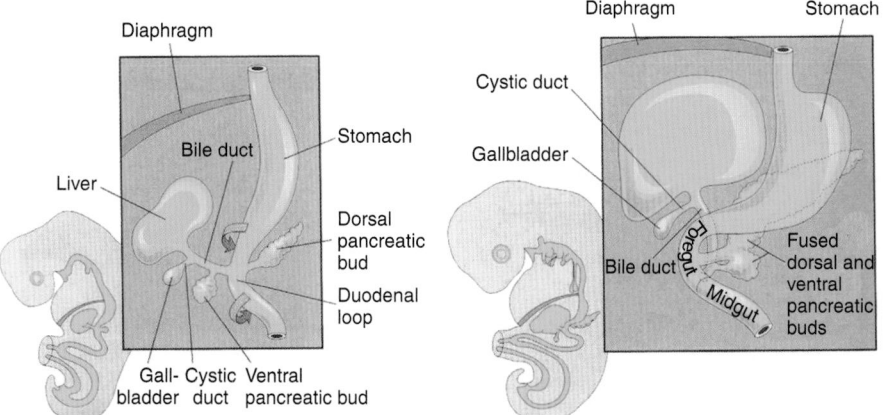

Diaphragm
Bile duct
Stomach
Liver
Dorsal pancreatic bud
Duodenal loop
Gall-bladder
Cystic duct
Ventral pancreatic bud

Diaphragm
Stomach
Cystic duct
Gallbladder
Foregut
Bile duct
Midgut
Fused dorsal and ventral pancreatic buds

FIGURE 111-2.

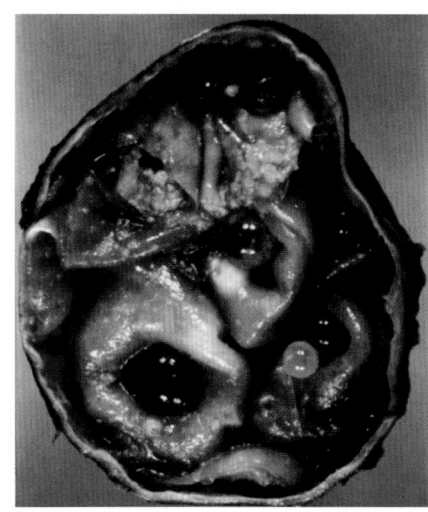

D
FIGURE 113-7D.

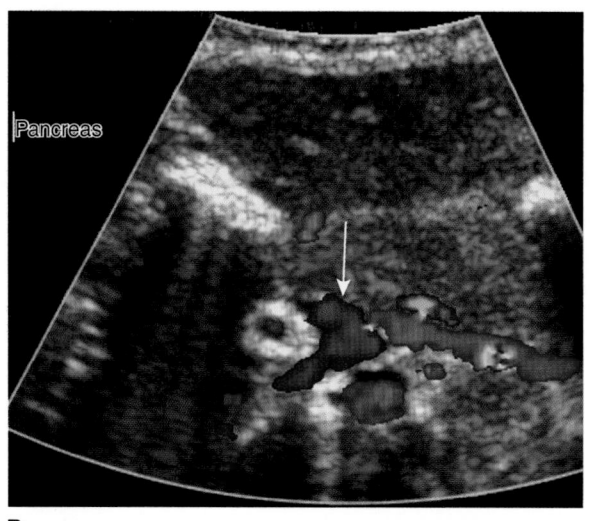

Pancreas

B
FIGURE 115-3B.

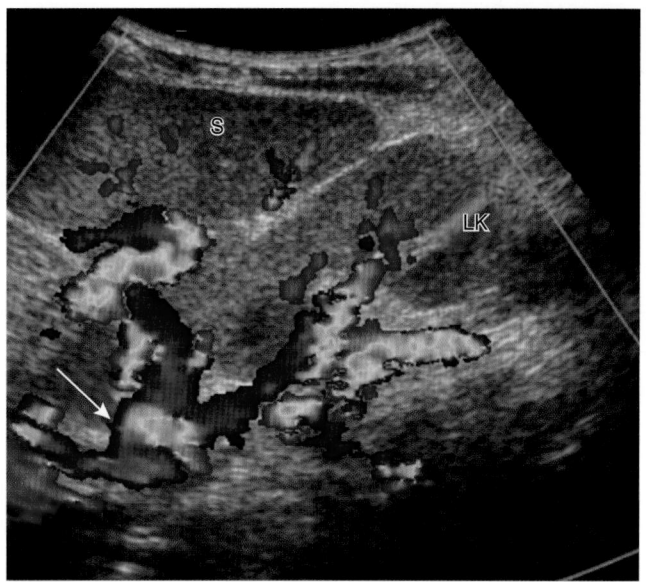

D

FIGURE 115-3D.

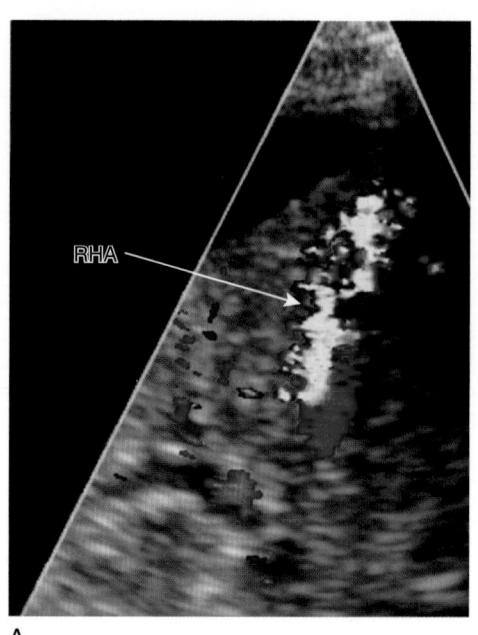

A

FIGURE 115-12A.

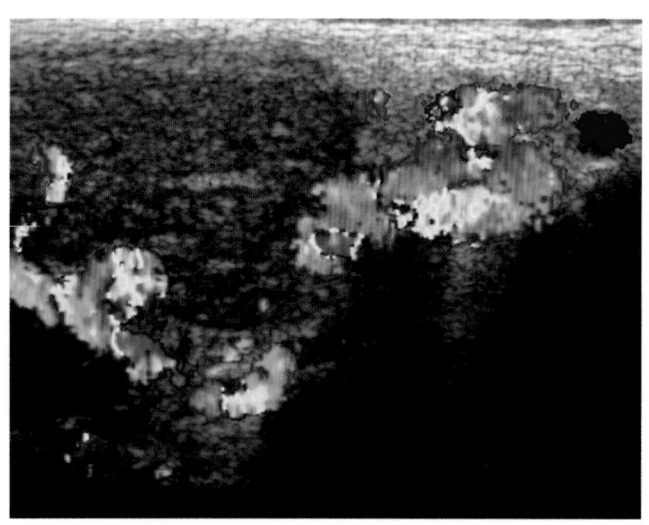

B

FIGURE 115-17B.

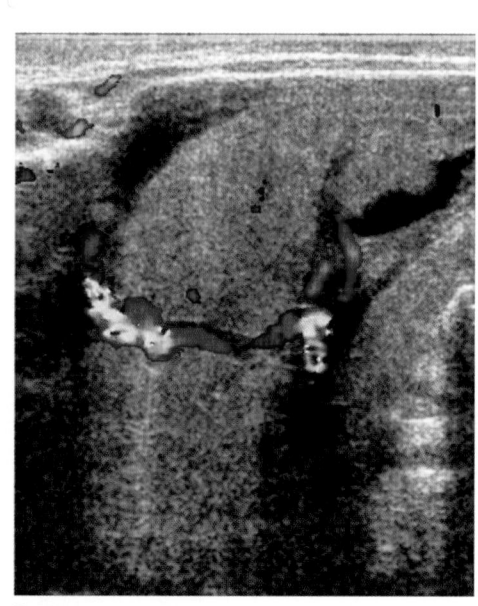

B

FIGURE 115-20B.

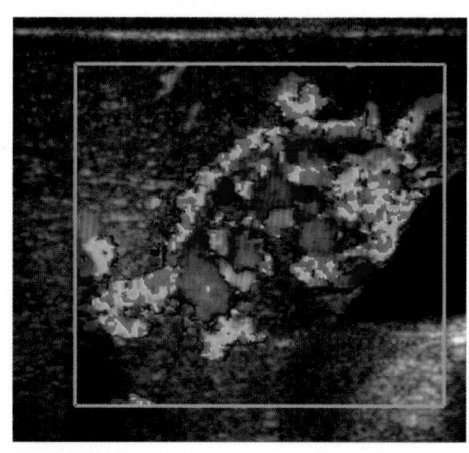

B

FIGURE 117-15B.

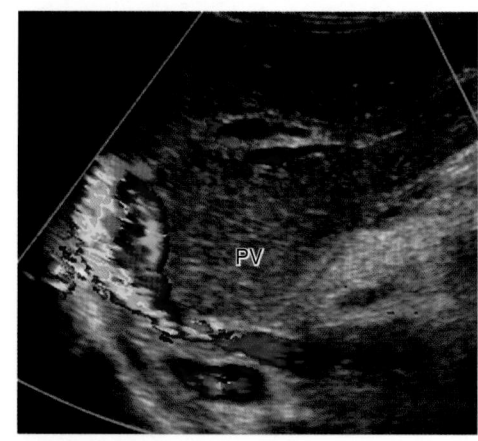

FIGURE 118-12.

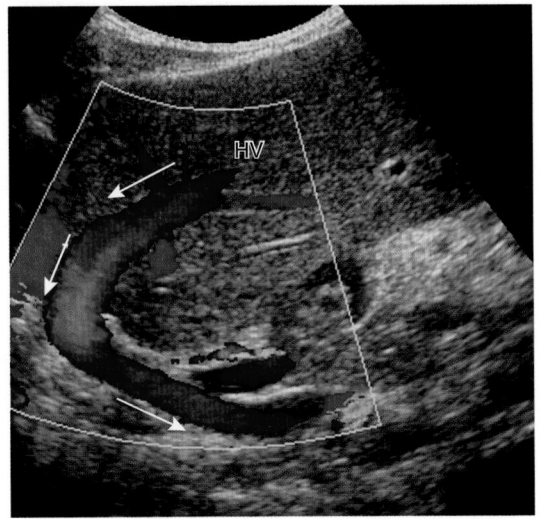

C
FIGURE 118-25C.

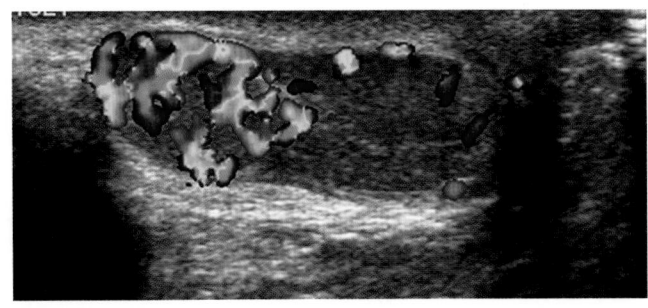

B
FIGURE 119-5B.

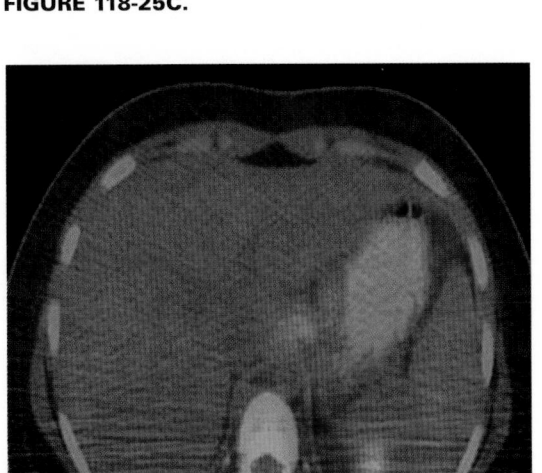

E
FIGURE 119-15E.

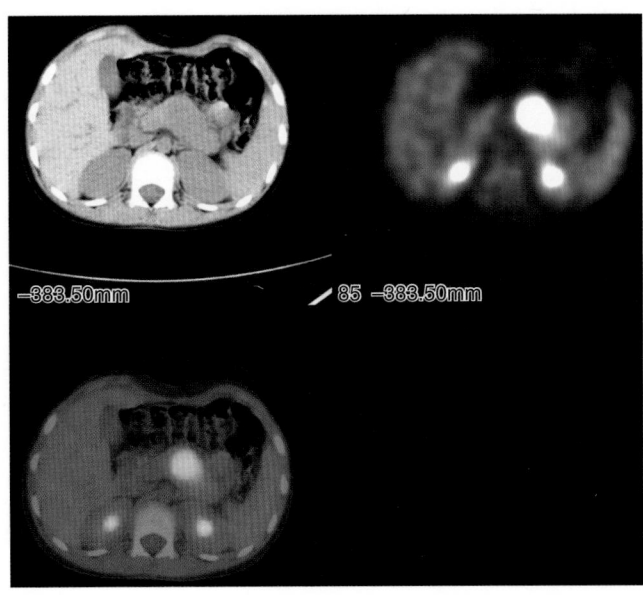

B
FIGURE 120-22B.

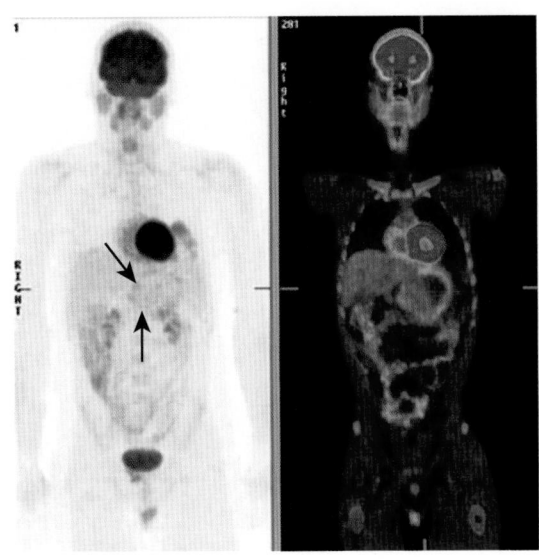

B
FIGURE 120-23B.

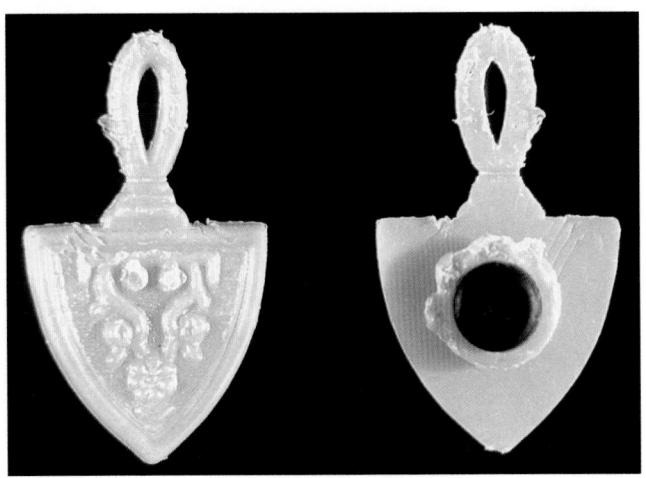

B
FIGURE 124-11B.

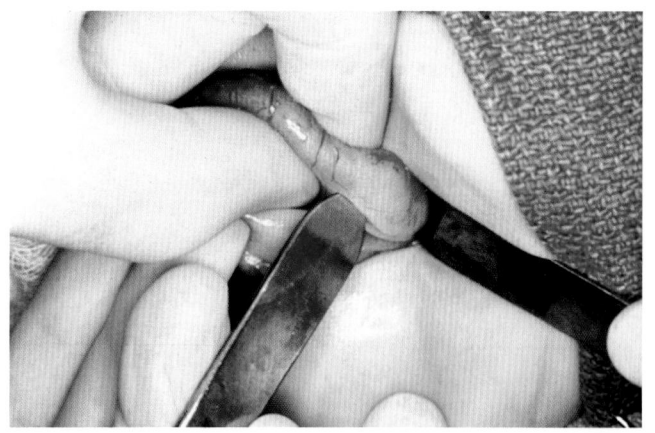

FIGURE 129-3.

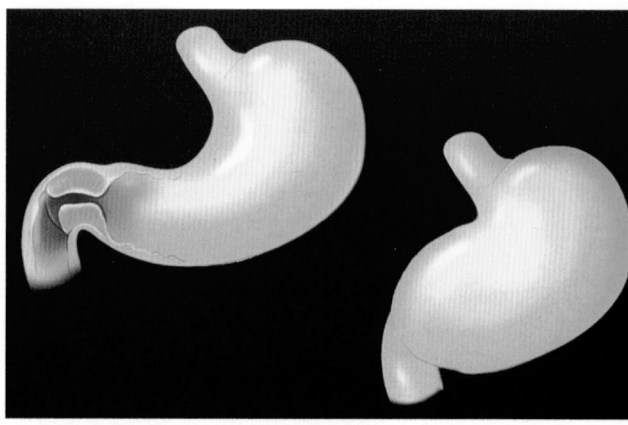

A

FIGURE 129-6A.

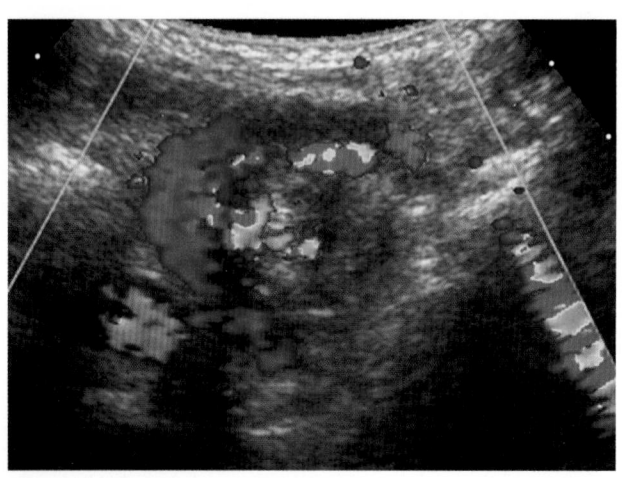

B

FIGURE 133-12B.

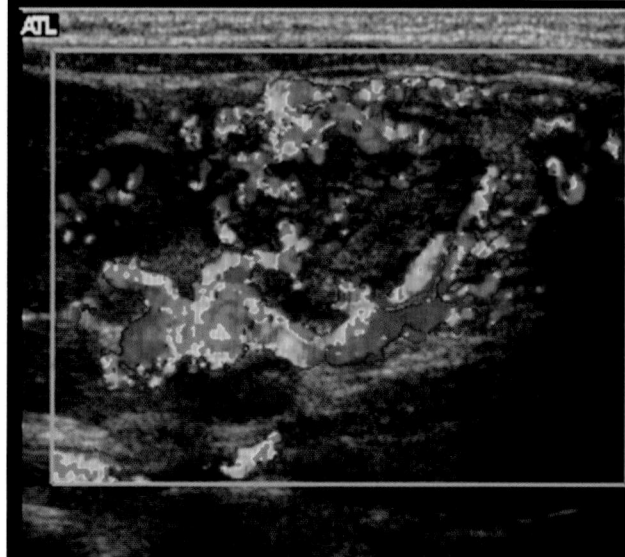

D

FIGURE 137-10D.

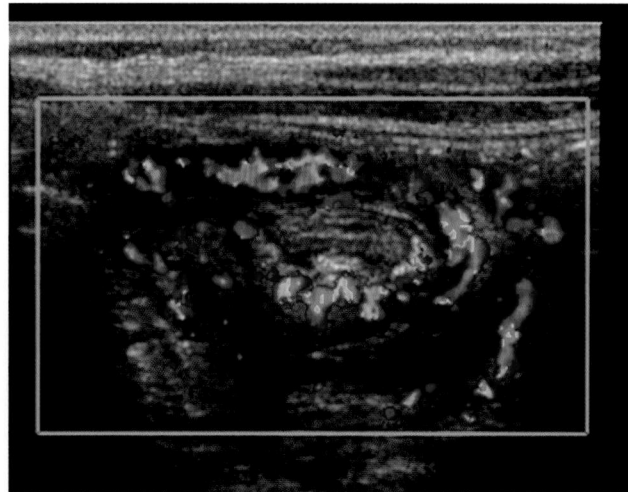

B

FIGURE 141-5B.

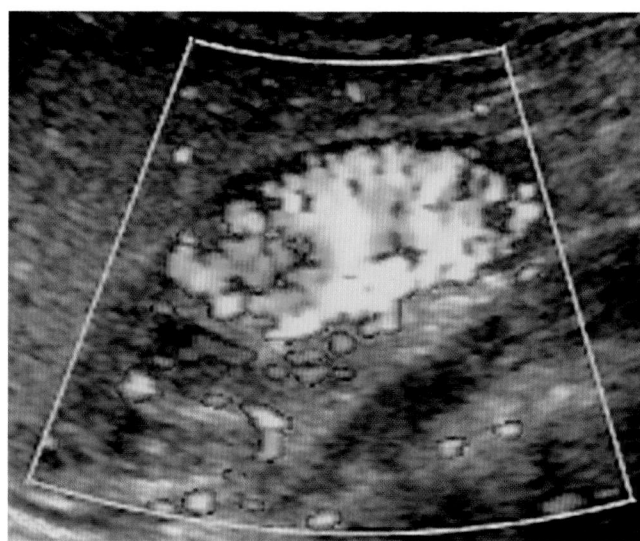

B

FIGURE 151-31B.

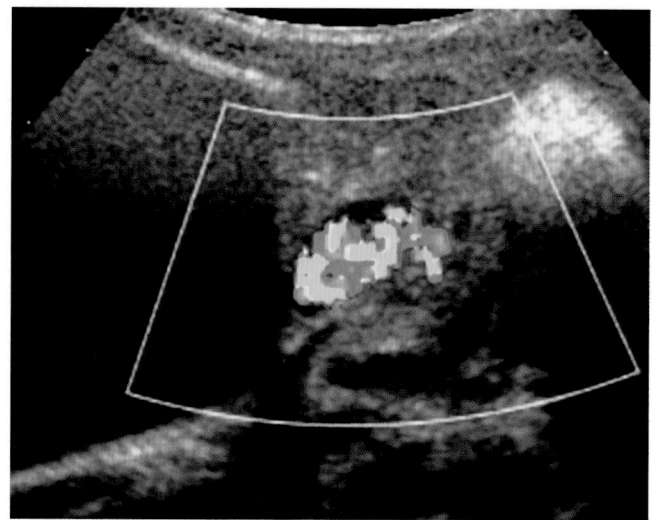

A

FIGURE 151-37A.

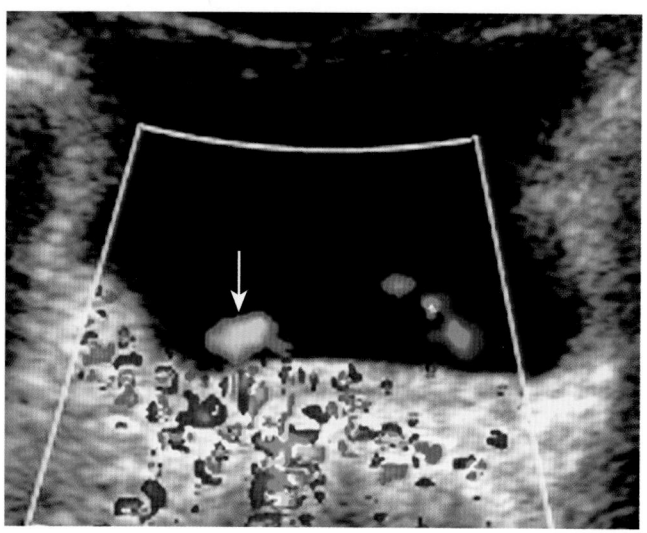

FIGURE 151-44.

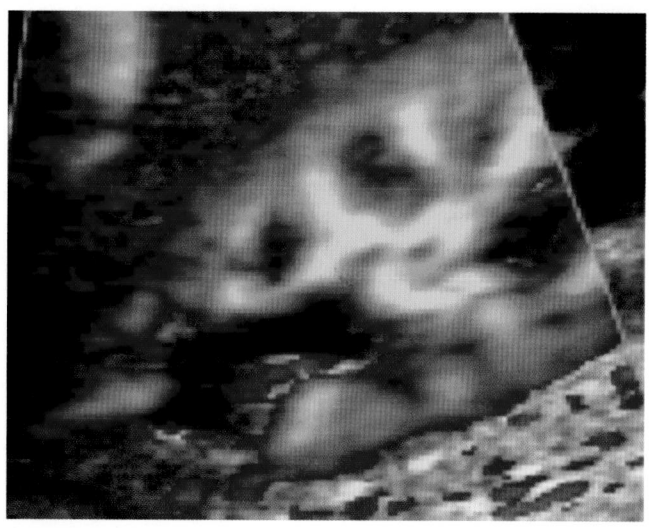

A

FIGURE 151-47A.

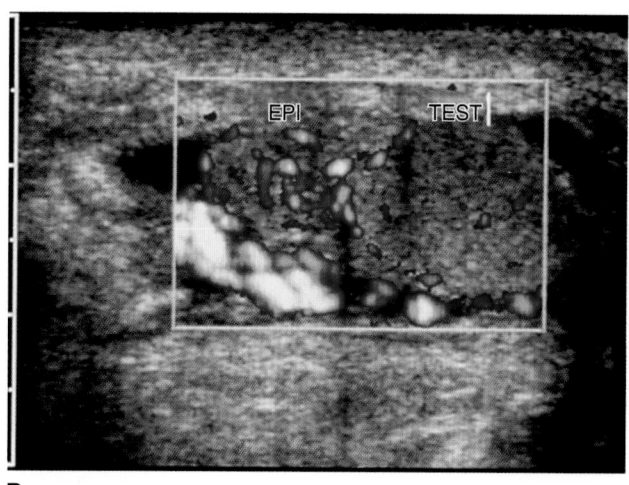

B

FIGURE 154-22B.

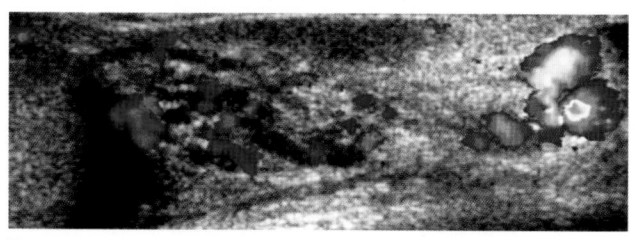

B

FIGURE 154-31B.

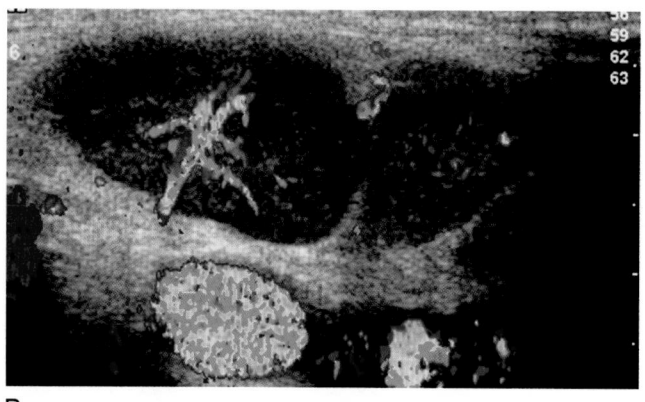

B

FIGURE 160-2B.

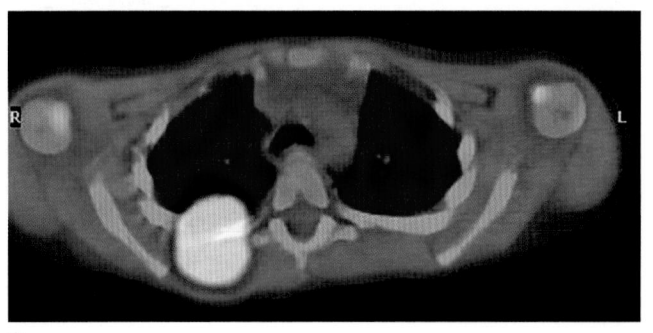

C

FIGURE 160-3C.

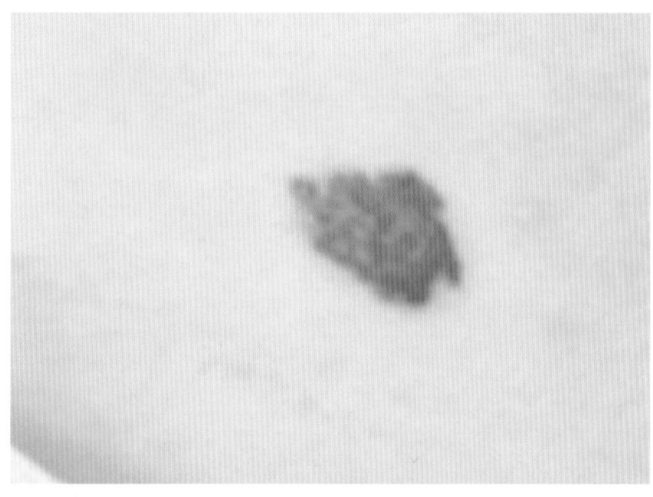

FIGURE 161-2.

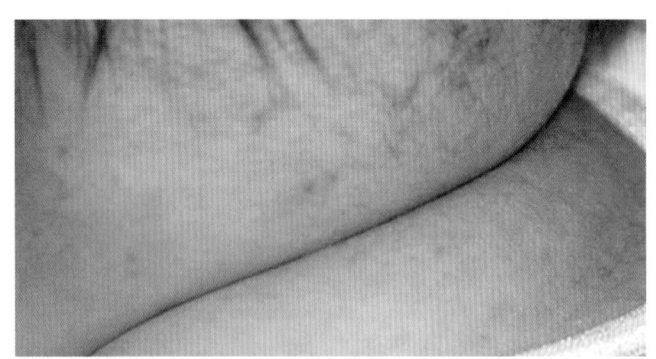

A

FIGURE 161-4A.

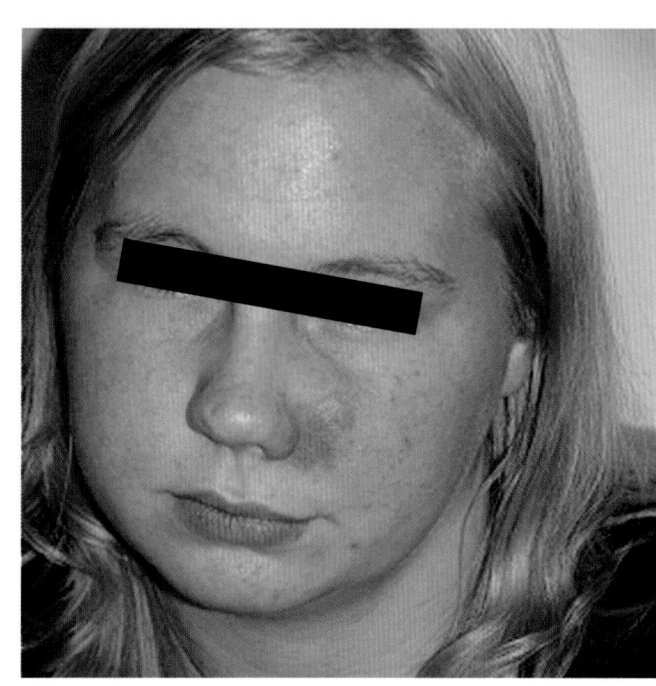

A

FIGURE 161-14A.

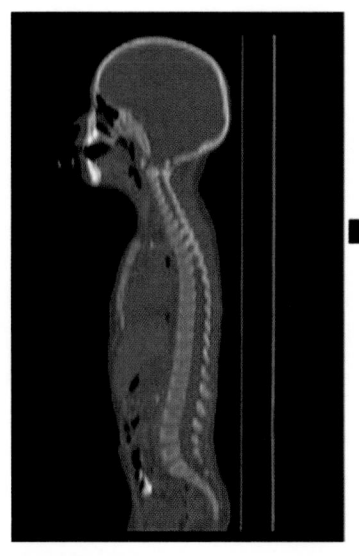

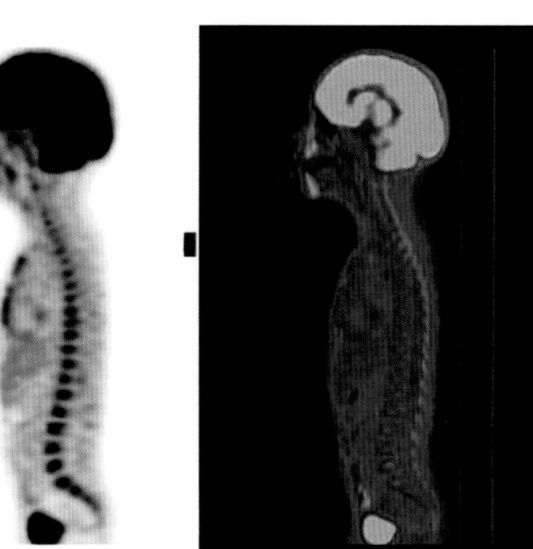

FIGURE 177-17.

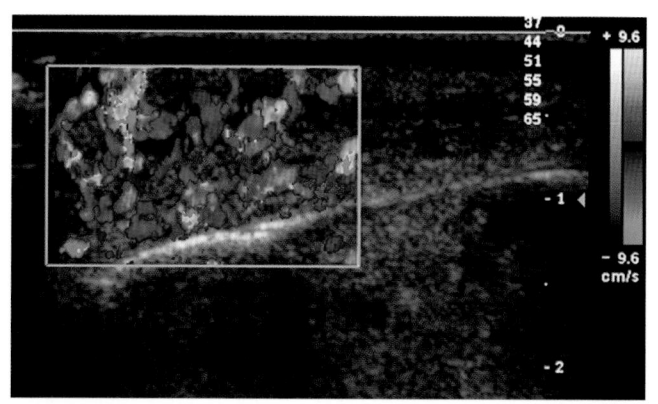

A

FIGURE 186-1A.

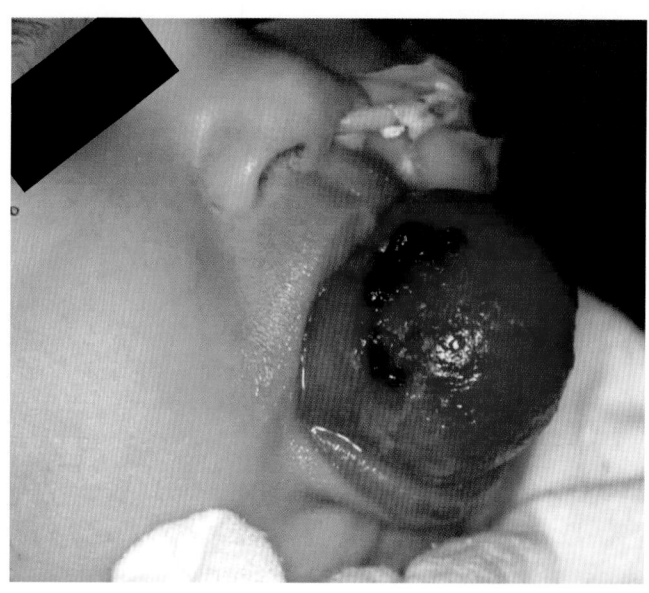

A

FIGURE 186-2A.

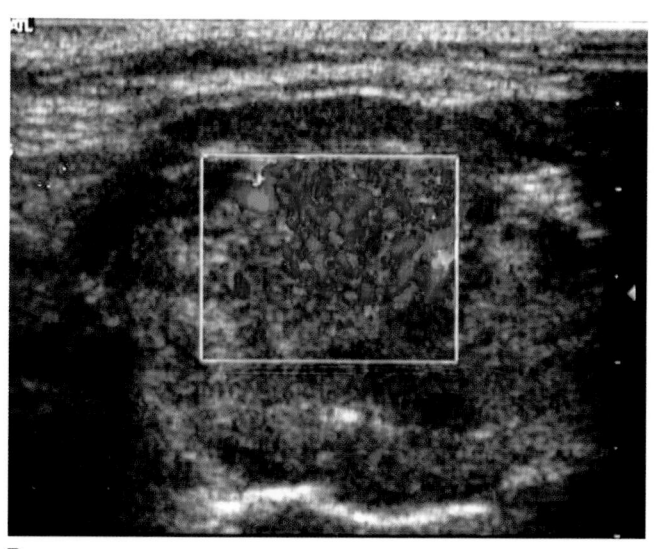

B

FIGURE 186-2B.

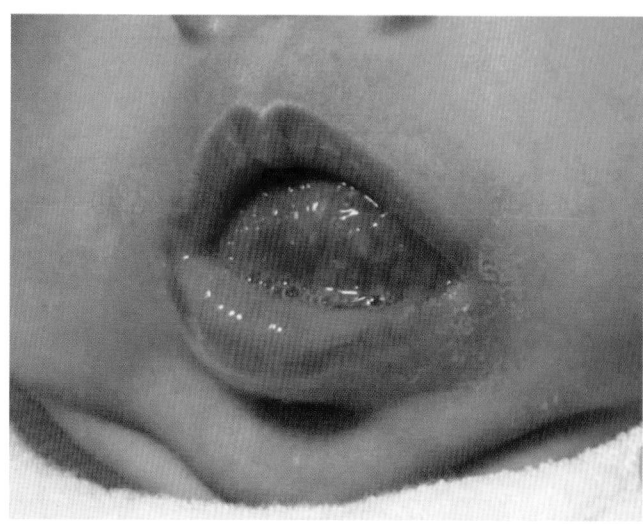

F

FIGURE 186-2F.

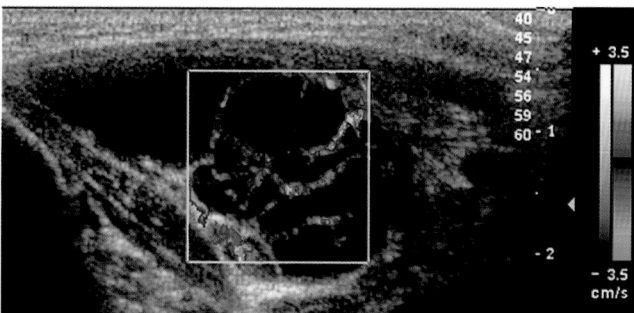

FIGURE 186-6.

PART 3 — ACQUIRED CARDIOVASCULAR DISEASE

CHAPTER 96

Myocardial and Valvular Diseases

ANA MARIA GACA and JEFFREY G. GACA

CARDIOMYOPATHY

Cardiomyopathy is a chronic and often progressive disease of the myocardium, with associated cardiac dysfunction. It is a rare but serious disorder in children, with only 25% of patients surviving more than 5 years after the onset of symptoms. Although our understanding of the causes of pediatric cardiomyopathy has advanced, the prognosis has not changed considerably in the past 30 years and is the same in developing and industrialized nations.

The cardiomyopathies can be classified according to the dominant pathophysiology (Table 96-1). There are four major forms of cardiomyopathy: dilated, hypertrophic, restrictive, and arrhythmogenic. Dilated and hypertrophic cardiomyopathies are the most common forms in children. Patients may be classified as having more than one form of cardiomyopathy, or the classification may change over time. Cardiomyopathies associated with particular cardiac or systemic diseases are referred to as specific cardiomyopathies (see Chapters 95 and 100). Inflammatory and isolated familial cardiomyopathies

---

TABLE 96-1

Types of Cardiomyopathies According to the World Health Organization

MAJOR FORMS
Dilated cardiomyopathy
  Congestive cardiomyopathy
Hypertrophic cardiomyopathy
  Hypertrophic obstructive cardiomyopathy
  Idiopathic hypertrophic subaortic stenosis
  Asymmetric septal hypertrophy
  Nonobstructive hypertrophic cardiomyopathy
Restrictive cardiomyopathy
Arrhythmogenic right ventricular cardiomyopathy
  Arrhythmogenic right ventricular dysplasia
  Right ventricular dysplasia
  Right ventricular cardiomyopathy

SPECIFIC CARDIOMYOPATHIES
Inflammatory
  Idiopathic
  Infectious
  Autoimmune
Metabolic
  Endocrine
    Thyrotoxicosis
    Hypothyroidism
  Adrenal
    Adrenal cortical insufficiency
    Pheochromocytoma

Familial storage or infiltration disorders
  Hemochromatosis
  Glycogen storage disease
  Mucopolysaccharidoses
  Niemann-Pick disease
General systemic diseases
  Connective tissue disorders
    Systemic lupus erythematosus
  Polyarteritis nodosa
  Scleroderma
  Dermatomyositis
  Infiltrative diseases
  Sarcoidosis
  Leukemia
Muscular dystrophies
  Duchenne
  Myotonic dystrophies
Neuromuscular disorders
  Friedreich ataxia
  Noonan syndrome
Sensitivity or toxic reactions
  Alcohol
  Irradiation
  Catecholamines

account for the majority of pediatric cases with a known cause. Other specific cardiomyopathies that are less common in the pediatric population include those associated with metabolic disorders, general systemic diseases, muscular dystrophies, neuromuscular disorders, and sensitivity or toxic reactions (e.g., radiation, chemotherapy). In two thirds of children with cardiomyopathy, no cause is found.

Because of its availability, lack of radiation, and portability, echocardiography is the most common method of classifying cardiomyopathy and evaluating cardiac function. With improvements in technology, however, cardiovascular magnetic resonance imaging (MRI) has become an accepted tool for the assessment of cardiomyopathy. With the multiple techniques available, cardiac MRI can be used to assess myocardial morphology and function (cine sequences), myocardial perfusion reserve (first-pass contrast-enhanced perfusion), and myocardial viability and scar formation (delayed contrast-enhanced sequences).

Dilated Cardiomyopathy

Dilated cardiomyopathy is characterized by dilation and impaired contraction of the left ventricle or both ventricles, and patients typically present with progressive heart failure. The majority of cases in children are idiopathic, but causes include infectious myocarditis, familial disease, and neuromuscular disorders (Duchenne and Becker muscular dystrophies). Coronary artery disease, a common cause of dilated cardiomyopathy in adults, is uncommon in children. The majority of children are diagnosed in the first year of life.

The functional and anatomic changes associated with dilated cardiomyopathy can be well evaluated with cardiac MRI, including acute and chronic changes of myocarditis and changes in left ventricular mass, stroke volume, and ejection fraction.

> **Idiopathic dilated cardiomyopathy is the most common cause of congestive heart failure in children.**

Hypertrophic Cardiomyopathy

Hypertrophic cardiomyopathy is generally characterized by left ventricular hypertrophy without a demonstrable cause. Although any region of the left ventricle can be involved, there is often hypertrophy of the interventricular septum, which may cause obstruction of the left ventricular outflow tract (Fig. 96-1). The right ventricle may also be affected. Hypertrophic cardiomyopathy is commonly familial and is inherited in an autosomal dominant fashion with variable penetrance and expression. Although some children are asymptomatic, hypertrophic cardiomyopathy can present with arrhythmias and sudden cardiac death at any age.

Echocardiography is the standard method of diagnosing hypertrophic cardiomyopathy, but cardiac MRI can be used to assess the location and degree of left ventricular wall thickness, including areas that are difficult to visualize with echocardiography, such as the cardiac apex and portions of the right ventricle. Cine gradient echo sequences can be used to evaluate the flow dynamics of the left ventricular outflow tract both before and after surgery. Contrast-enhanced MRI may also demonstrate delayed enhancement within scarred areas of myocardial hypertrophy—areas thought to play a role in the arrhythmias associated with hypertrophic cardiomyopathy.

Arrhythmogenic Right Ventricular Cardiomyopathy

Arrhythmogenic right ventricular cardiomyopathy (ARVC) is characterized by progressive fibrofatty replacement of right ventricular myocardium. This tissue replacement

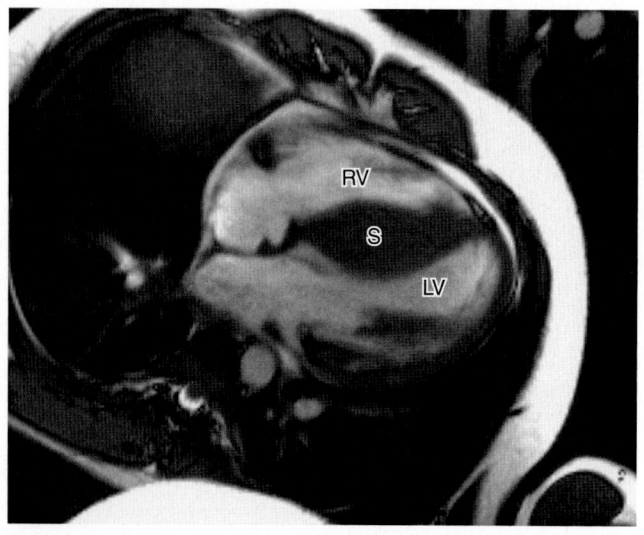

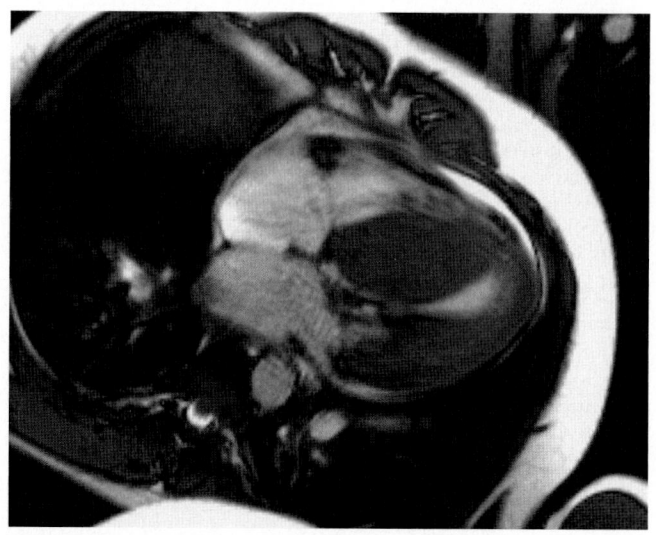

A   B

FIGURE 96-1. Hypertrophic cardiomyopathy. **A,** Four-chamber cine MR view at end-diastole shows marked septal (S) thickening. **B,** During systole, there is near-complete obliteration of the left ventricular chamber. LV, left ventricle; RV, right ventricle. (Courtesy of Laura Heyneman, Duke Medical Center.)

starts focally in the right ventricle but may progress to involve the entire right ventricle; it may involve the left ventricle as well. Areas of spared myocardium may act as foci of instability, resulting in ventricular arrhythmias and sudden death, which become more common in adolescents and young adults. The fibrofatty myocardial replacement and wall thinning of ARVC are well visualized on T1-weighted spin echo MR sequences (Fig. 96-2). Additional findings on MRI include abnormal myocardial wall function and aneurysms.

Restrictive Cardiomyopathy

Restrictive cardiomyopathy, the least common type, is characterized by restricted filling and decreased diastolic volume of one or both ventricles, without ventricular dilation or hypertrophy. Usually idiopathic, restrictive cardiomyopathy may be associated with diseases causing infiltration or fibrosis of the myocardium or endocardium, such as hemochromatosis; glycogen storage diseases; and Gaucher, Hurler, and Fabry disease. Amyloidosis and sarcoidosis may also cause restrictive cardiomyopathy, but these diseases are uncommon in the pediatric population. Because both ventricles may be involved, patients may present with signs and symptoms of right or left ventricular failure or arrhythmias. Restrictive cardiomyopathy should be considered in patients presenting with heart failure but without cardiomegaly or systolic dysfunction. However, it is important to distinguish restrictive cardiomyopathy from constrictive pericarditis, which has a similar clinical appearance but can be cured surgically.

Radiographs of the chest in patients with restrictive cardiomyopathy may demonstrate a normal heart size. Pulmonary congestion, interstitial edema, and pleural effusions may be seen. Cardiac MRI may demonstrate ventricles that are small (Fig. 96-3) to normal in size; there may be signs of poor ventricular filling, including dilation of the atria, superior and inferior venae cavae, and hepatic veins. These findings are similar to those of constrictive pericarditis; however, the pericardial thickening (>4 mm) typical of constrictive pericarditis is absent in restrictive cardiomyopathy.

> Although restrictive cardiomyopathy is rare in the pediatric population, the main diagnostic challenge is to differentiate it from constrictive pericarditis, which can be cured surgically.

Specific Cardiomyopathies

Aside from inflammatory and neuromuscular cardiomyopathies, the other specific cardiomyopathies account for only a small fraction of cases in children. Of these, only cardiomyopathy associated with metabolic abnormalities is addressed here.

INFLAMMATORY CARDIOMYOPATHY

The inflammatory cardiomyopathies include both infectious and familial forms. Among cases with a known cause, nearly 30% are attributed to infection. Although infectious cardiomyopathy, also known as myocarditis, can be caused by bacterial, fungal, or parasitic infection, viral myocarditis is most common. Enteroviruses, particularly coxsackievirus B, are associated with 25% to 40% of cases of pediatric acute myocarditis and dilated cardiomyopathy. The acute clinical presentation of myocarditis is characterized by dyspnea and tachypnea due to congestive heart failure.

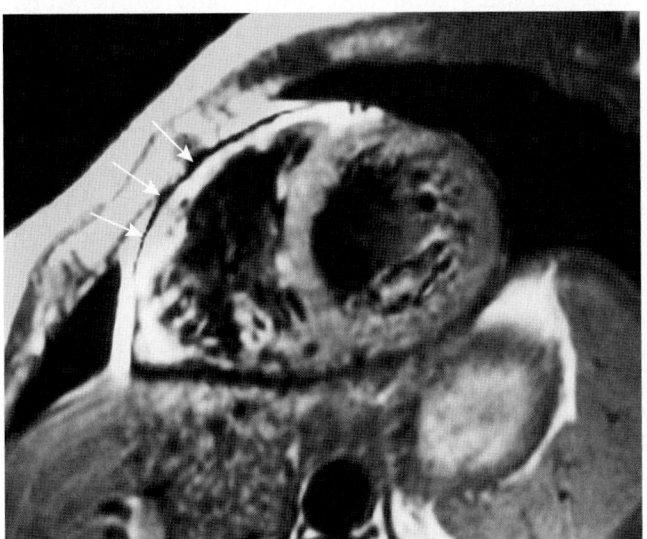

FIGURE 96-2. Arrhythmogenic right ventricular cardiomyopathy in an 18-year-old woman with recurrent supraventricular tachycardia. T1-weighted short-axis image through the heart shows abnormal high signal involving the anterior wall of the right ventricle (arrows) adjacent to the normally high T1 signal of pericardial fat. This appearance is consistent with the fibrofatty myocardial replacement and wall thinning seen with arrhythmogenic right ventricular cardiomyopathy.

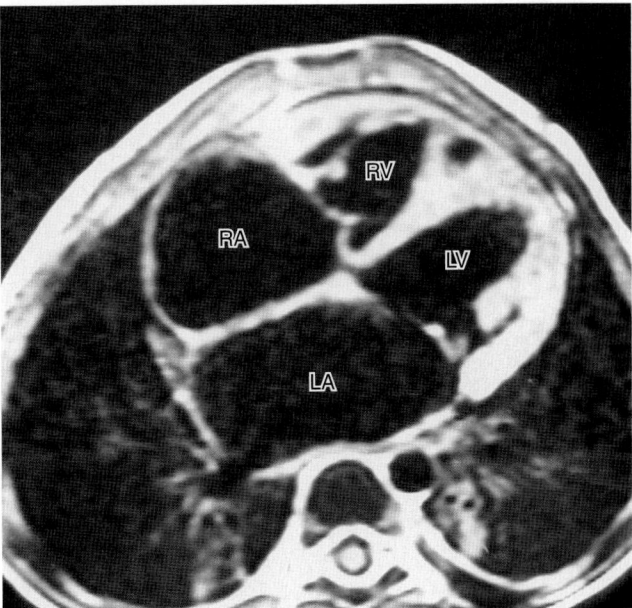

FIGURE 96-3. Restrictive cardiomyopathy. T1-weighted long-axis image in a 3-year-old boy with idiopathic restrictive cardiomyopathy demonstrates the relatively small size of the right (RV) and left (LV) ventricles, with dilation of the right (RA) and left (LA) atria. There is no evidence of pericardial thickening to suggest restrictive pericarditis.

- **Infection accounts for 30% of inflammatory cardiomyopathies with a known cause.**
- **The most common cause of myocarditis is viral infection.**

Isolated familial cardiomyopathy is typically defined as cardiomyopathy with no systemic features occurring in a patient with an identified genetic defect or in multiple family members. Familial cardiomyopathy accounts for approximately 20% to 25% of nonidiopathic cases of cardiomyopathy.

Acute rheumatic fever is an autoimmune response that follows a small percentage of infections with group A beta-hemolytic streptococcus. The sequela, rheumatic heart disease, is significant because of the associated morbidity, including valvular disease (more common) and carditis (pericarditis, myocarditis, endocarditis) in the acute setting (Fig. 96-4).

- **Nearly two thirds of pediatric cases of cardiomyopathy are idiopathic.**
- **Of the cases with an identified cause, 30% are infectious and 20% to 25% are familial.**

NEUROMUSCULAR CARDIOMYOPATHY

This group of cardiomyopathies includes a variety of genetic and acquired disorders. Friedreich ataxia is a rare, autosomal recessive neurologic disorder characterized by progressive ataxia and musculoskeletal abnormalities (scoliosis and foot deformities). The cardiac disease of Friedreich ataxia includes hypertrophic obstructive cardiomyopathy with round cell infiltration and arrhyth-

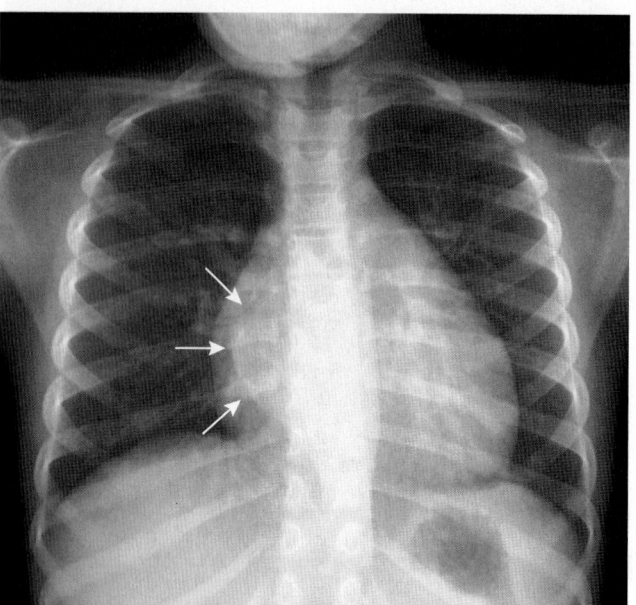

FIGURE 96-4. Rheumatic heart disease. Chest radiograph in an 8-year-old girl with a history of acute rheumatic fever who now has mitral valve insufficiency. Radiographic findings include cardiomegaly with enlargement of the left atrium *(arrows)* and ventricle.

mias. Although patients typically present with neurologic symptoms, a small minority may present with cardiac symptoms.

Duchenne muscular dystrophy, the most common of the muscular dystrophies, is an X-linked recessive neurodegenerative disorder characterized by progressive skeletal muscle weakness. These children develop dilated cardiomyopathy, with alternating areas of hypertrophy, atrophy, and myocardial fibrosis. Interestingly, dilated cardiomyopathy may be the only clinical manifestation of genetic carriers of Duchenne muscular dystrophy.

Noonan syndrome is a relatively common genetic syndrome characterized by typical facies, short stature, and cardiac abnormalities. These include pulmonary valve stenosis and hypertrophic cardiomyopathy, with or without obstruction.

METABOLIC CARDIOMYOPATHY

The glycogen storage diseases (GSDs) constitute a group of rare diseases characterized by abnormal glycogen breakdown, with resultant storage in various tissues. Cardiac involvement is most common in types II (Pompe disease), III, and IV. Pompe disease is discussed in detail in Chapter 100. Nearly all patients with GSD type III have clinically silent heart disease. Patients with GSD type IV typically die of liver disease before their cardiomyopathy becomes clinically obvious. Chest radiographs demonstrate cardiomegaly (Fig. 96-5). Echocardiography demonstrates cardiac hypertrophy, which may result in left ventricular outflow tract obstruction, but no cardiac dilation.

The mucopolysaccharidoses are a group of rare inherited disorders characterized by a deficiency of lysosomal enzymes that results in the abnormal storage of glycosaminoglycans. Of the mucopolysaccharidoses, Hurler, Hunter, Sanfilippo, Scheie, and Hurler-Scheie syndromes may have severe cardiac involvement. The myocardial cells become distended with storage material. These patients may also have valvular thickening and short, thick chordae tendineae, resulting in valvular insufficiency.

Fabry disease is an X-linked recessive storage disorder characterized by the accumulation of glycosphingolipid in different tissues. Patients with classic Fabry disease have diffuse organ involvement, with left ventricular hypertrophy and dilation, conduction abnormalities, valvular dysfunction, and myocardial infarcts. Some patients may have a cardiac variant of the disease that is limited to myocardial hypertrophy. Cardiac Fabry disease may be difficult to differentiate from hypertrophic cardiomyopathy; however, different patterns of enhancement can be seen on enhanced cardiac MRI.

Unspecified Cardiomyopathy

Left ventricular noncompaction, also known as persistence of the spongy myocardium and left ventricular hypertrabeculation, is a rare congenital cardiomyopathy causing heart failure. It is characterized by excessively prominent ventricular trabeculations and deep intertrabecular recesses. These patients demonstrate systolic and diastolic dysfunction, arrhythmias, and embolic

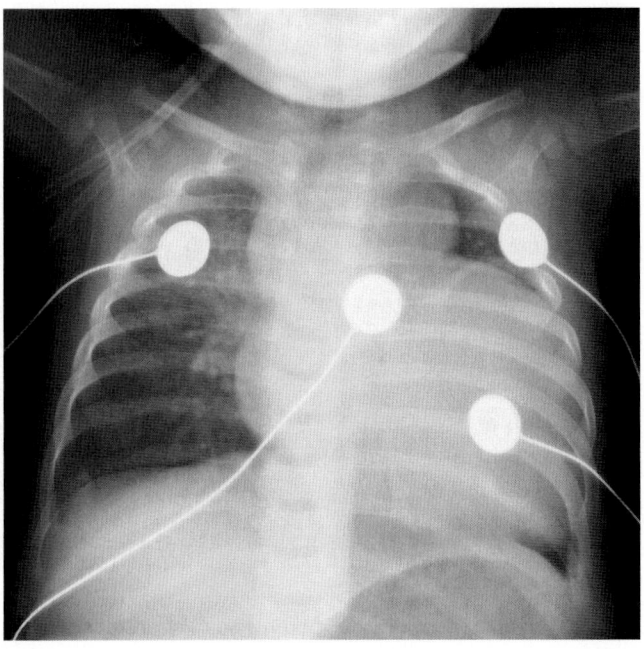

A

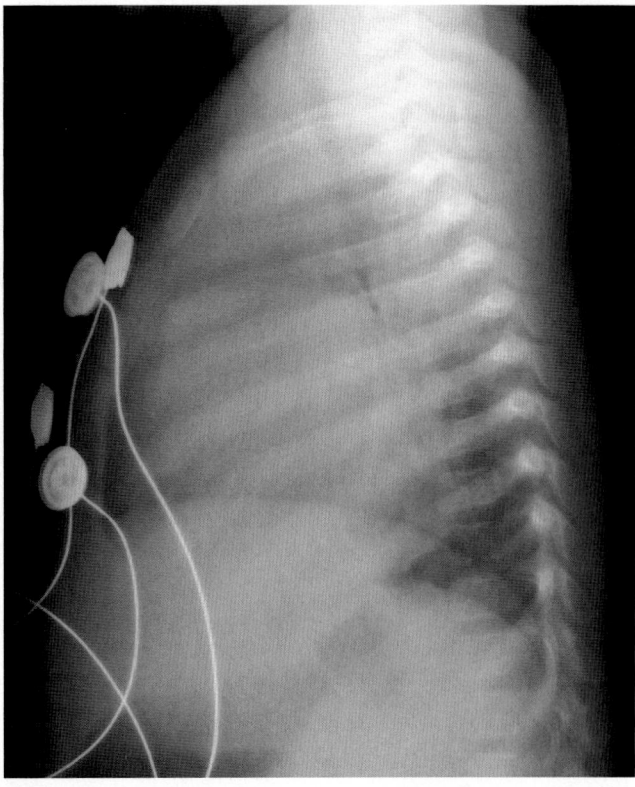

B

FIGURE 96-5. Glycogen storage disease of the heart (Pompe disease) in a 5-month-old girl. There is marked cardiomegaly on frontal **(A)** and lateral **(B)** radiographs. The prominent lobular shape of the superior mediastinum is due to the thymus.

events. MRI can be useful in making the diagnosis, demonstrating thick trabeculae in the left ventricle and deep recesses within the myocardial wall.

ENDOCARDIAL FIBROELASTOSIS

Endocardial fibroelastosis (EFE) is characterized by diffuse thickening of the ventricular endocardium and usually leads to death from congestive heart failure in infancy. EFE is either primary (no associated cardiac disease) or, more commonly, secondary to congenital heart malformations, including hypoplastic left heart, aortic stenosis or atresia, and coarctation of the aorta. As a primary process, there is no underlying cardiac structural abnormality; in these cases, EFE may be familial or associated with an intrauterine process, including infection and autoimmune disorders. Pathologically, there are two forms of EFE: dilated and contracted. With dilated EFE, the heart is markedly enlarged and globular, with endocardial thickening most marked in the outflow tract (Fig. 96-6). Less commonly, the left ventricle is normal or small in size. The right and left atria and the right ventricle, however, are markedly enlarged and hypertrophied. These patients have impaired ventricular filling on hemodynamic studies and mild to moderate reduction in left ventricular contractility.

> **EFE causes diffuse thickening of the endocardium and may result in death from congestive heart failure in infancy.**

HIGH-OUTPUT STATES

Anemia

Chronic severe anemia is an important cause of cardiomegaly and congestive heart failure. Most commonly seen with thalassemia major and sickle cell anemia, chronic anemia leads to high-output failure and generalized enlargement of all cardiac chambers. Clinical findings of anemia include pallor, lethargy, and other specific features, depending on the type of anemia. Heart failure relates not only to volume overload but also to myocardial hypoxia secondary to inadequate coronary oxygen content. Typical features of cardiomegaly and heart failure are common (Fig. 96-7).

> **Heart failure associated with anemia can be due to both volume overload and myocardial hypoxia.**

Arteriovenous Malformation

Arteriovenous malformations are congenital vascular anomalies characterized by abnormal connections between the arterial and venous systems, without normal interposed capillaries. The vascular malformations that present with congestive heart failure in infancy most commonly involve the brain, liver, or lungs. These patients typically demonstrate cardiomegaly (Fig. 96-8). Enlargement of the aorta may be present; with cerebral malformations, the brachiocephalic vessels may also be enlarged. Ultrasonography is helpful not only in evaluating the size of the heart and the vascular structures

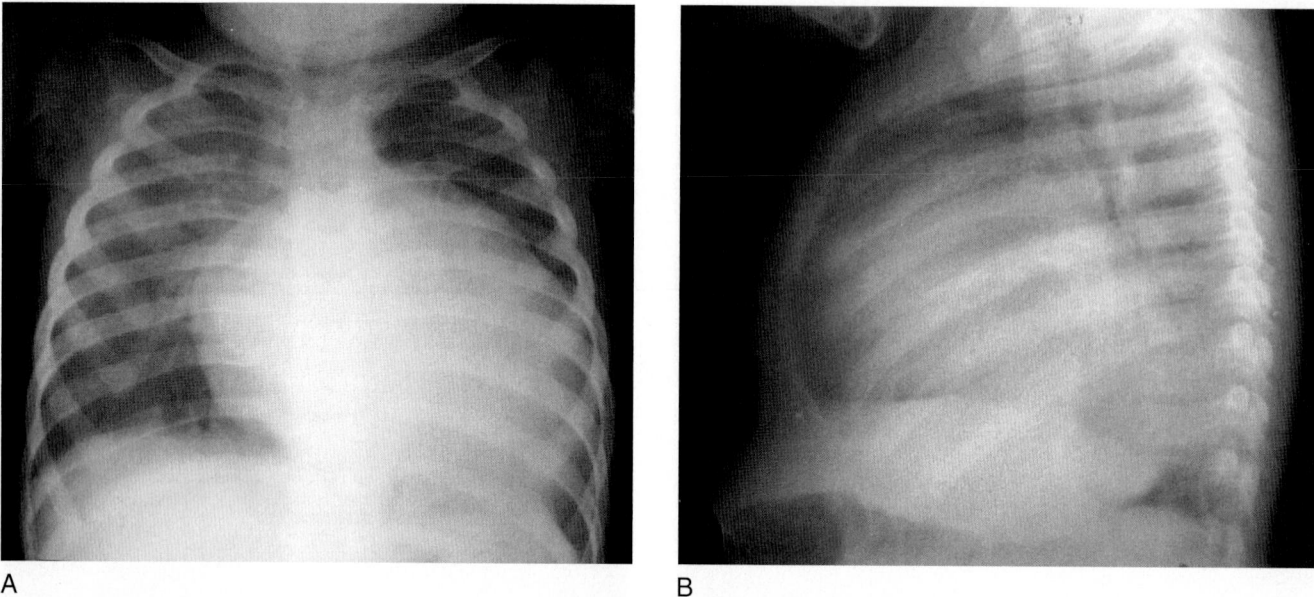

FIGURE 96-6. Frontal (**A**) and lateral (**B**) radiographs in a 13-month-old girl with dilated endocardial fibroelastosis show marked cardiomegaly, with signs of congestive heart failure.

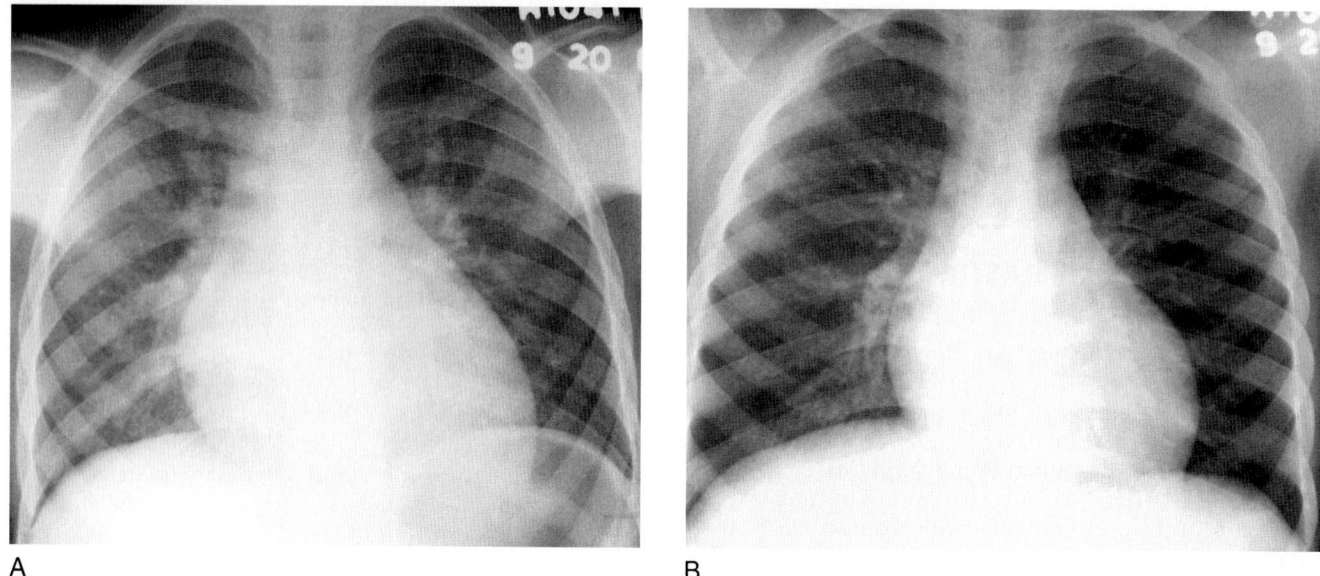

FIGURE 96-7. Anemia. **A,** Frontal chest radiograph in a patient with anemia shows mild enlargement of the cardiac silhouette, with findings of congestive heart failure. **B,** Frontal chest radiograph in the same patient 1 week later, following blood transfusion, shows marked improvement in both the size of the cardiac silhouette and the heart failure.

but also in demonstrating the arteriovenous malformation in the head, liver, or other organs. Angiography, computed tomography (CT), or MRI with angiographic technique may also demonstrate the malformation.

> **Vascular malformations that present in infancy with congestive heart failure most commonly involve the brain, liver, or lungs.**

Chorioangioma of the Placenta

Although chorioangioma is the most common benign tumor of the placenta, it is still a rare lesion. When small, these neoplasms may not cause clinical symptoms; however, when they are large (generally >5 cm), they may result in hydramnios and preterm labor due to arteriovenous shunting between the umbilical artery and vein. This shunting may result in high-output cardiac failure in the neonate, with polyhydramnios, cardiomegaly, and hypoxia. Echocardiography demonstrates

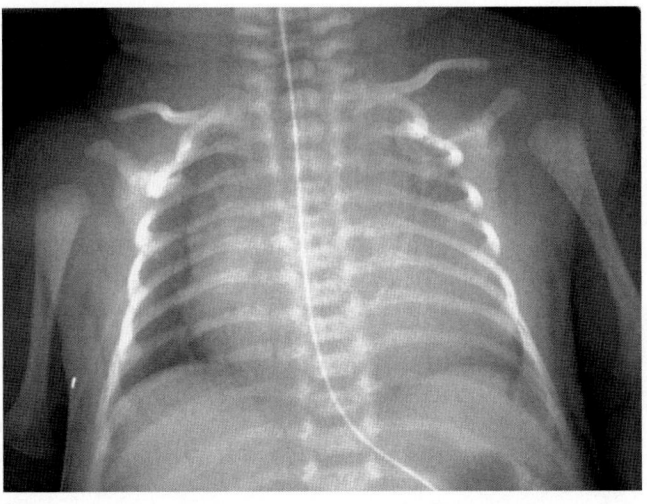
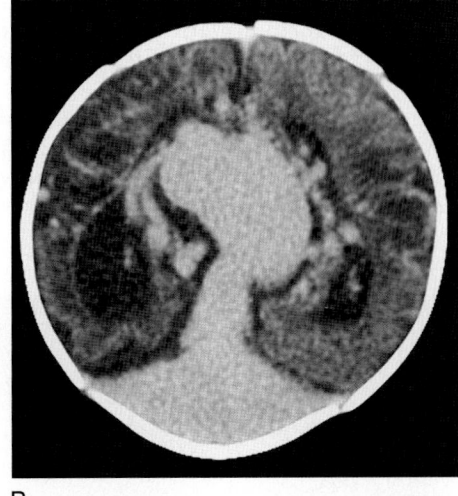

A   B

FIGURE 96-8. Arteriovenous malformation. **A,** Frontal chest radiograph in newborn boy with respiratory distress shows cardiomegaly and pulmonary edema. **B,** Head CT following intravenous contrast administration in the same patient shows the vein of Galen with a large draining vein and numerous feeding vessels.

dilation of the inferior vena cava, cardiac chambers, and thoracic and abdominal aorta secondary to arteriovenous shunting in utero.

Twin-Twin Transfusion Syndrome

Twin-twin transfusion syndrome is caused by unbalanced blood flow that results in significant hemodynamic changes between the twins. With discrepant blood flow, the donor twin pumps blood into the recipient. The donor becomes hypovolemic, hypoxic, and anemic, with oligohydramnios, oliguria, and poor intrauterine growth. The recipient becomes polycythemic with polyhydramnios and may develop hypertension, cardiomegaly, and signs of congestive heart failure. The cardiac disease of the recipient is thought to be the major cause of death for both twins. Chest radiographs may demonstrate cardiomegaly and pleural effusions if hydrops is present. Echocardiography may demonstrate myocardial hypertrophy and dysfunction and valvular insufficiency in either twin.

VALVULAR DISEASE

Pediatric valvular disease includes both congenital and acquired lesions; congenital lesions predominate. For the radiologist, evaluating valvular disease generally involves assessing the consequences of the disorder, such as congestive heart failure with critical aortic stenosis or left ventricular and atrial enlargement with significant mitral regurgitation. The valves themselves are best assessed with echocardiography from both a morphologic and a functional standpoint.

The following discussion provides a general overview of the more common valvular lesions in infants and children, focusing on isolated valve involvement rather than the lesions as part of other structural defects. The individual cardiac valves are addressed (with the exception of the tricuspid valve, which is discussed in Chapter 91), followed by a brief section on valvular involvement

by endocarditis. Further discussion of pediatric valvular disorders can be found in Chapters 91, 92, 94, 95, 99, and 100.

Aortic Valve

Aortic stenosis occurs in up to 1% to 2% of the population, represents about 5% of congenital heart lesions, and is about four times more common in males than females. There are four types of aortic stenosis: valvular, subvalvular, muscular, and supravalvular. Valvular aortic stenosis is the most common form of left ventricular outflow tract obstruction and is the most common type of aortic stenosis; the supravalvular type (occurring as part of Williams syndrome or as familial or idiopathic types) is the least common.

> **Valvular aortic stenosis is the most common form of left ventricular outflow tract obstruction and the most common type of aortic stenosis. The supravalvular type (occurring as part of Williams syndrome or as familial or idiopathic types) is the least common.**

Children with aortic valve stenosis most commonly have a bicuspid valve (fusion of one commissure) or, less commonly, a unicuspid valve (fusion of two or more commissures). Aortic valve stenosis may be associated with other cardiac defects, such as coarctation of the aorta, interrupted aortic arch, and mitral stenosis, and it is often asymptomatic. A minority of patients present with aortic stenosis in the first few weeks of life. These patients usually have a unicuspid aortic valve and severe or critical obstruction. In some neonates, this stenosis is so severe that a patent ductus arteriosus is necessary to ensure adequate systemic perfusion. In these children, either surgical or balloon valvotomy is necessary to allow forward flow from the left ventricle and to allow ductus closure. Children with a bicuspid aortic valve are usually asymptomatic and may remain so well into adulthood. As these patients age, however, the valve leaflets may thicken, and the valve may become stenotic, insufficient, or both.

The aortic valve may also be primarily insufficient. Children with primary insufficiency may have bicuspid or tricuspid valves, and some have connective tissue abnormalities such as Marfan syndrome or Ehlers-Danlos syndrome.

Radiographic findings of aortic stenosis range from normal to poststenotic dilation of the aorta (rare before 5 years of age) and left ventricular hypertrophy (Fig. 96-9). In neonates, critical aortic stenosis can manifest as cardiomegaly and pulmonary edema. Findings of aortic insufficiency may include left ventricular enlargement from volume overload (Fig. 96-10). MRI can be used to assess for aortic stenosis and regurgitation and to determine pressure gradients across the stenotic valve (Fig. 96-11).

Aortic valve repair may be possible in a minority of patients, but valve replacement is usually required. In children, options for valve replacement are limited by their small size and the desire to avoid anticoagulation. Porcine valves and allograft aortic valves are available in annular sizes suitable for small children. However, both these options have limited durability in the aortic position, and frequent reoperation is required. Mechanical valves are unavailable for neonates and infants but are available for older children. The need for lifelong anticoagulation, however, often makes these valves a poor choice in this population. One suitable option in children is the Ross procedure, in which the normal pulmonary valve is translocated to the aortic position, and the pulmonary valve is replaced with a pulmonary allograft. This allows for growth of the newly created aortic valve, places the allograft in the low-pressure pulmonary system, and avoids the need for anticoagulation.

Mitral Valve

Mitral regurgitation is much more common than mitral stenosis and has many causes, including defects (clefts or dysplasia) in the valve leaflets, abnormal chordae or

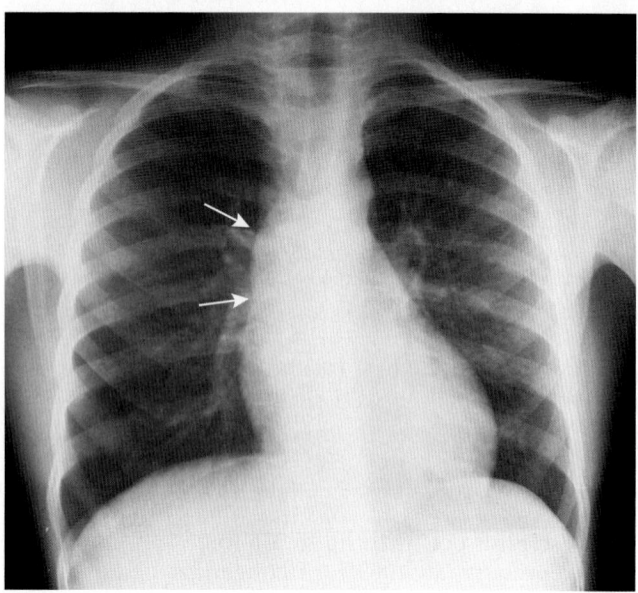

FIGURE 96-9. Aortic valvular stenosis. Chest radiograph in an 8-year-old boy with a history of aortic valvular stenosis shows prominence of the ascending aorta *(arrows)* without significant cardiomegaly.

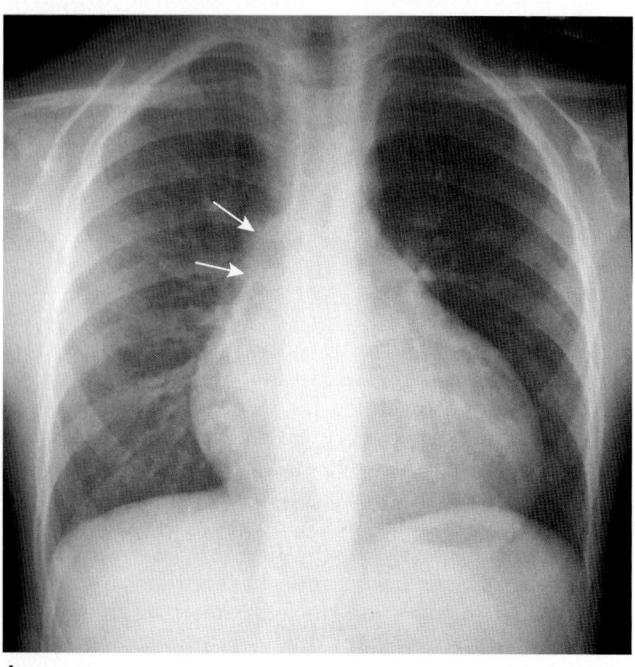

A

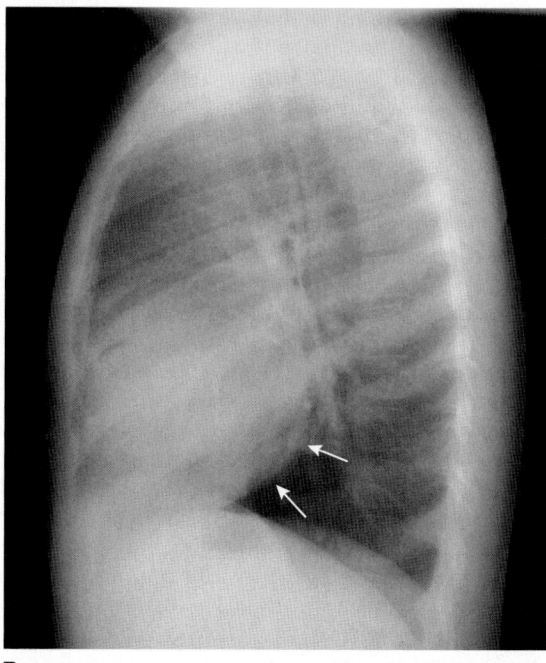

B

FIGURE 96-10. Aortic valvular insufficiency. This 5-year-old boy, diagnosed in infancy with aortic valvular stenosis, developed aortic insufficiency following valvotomy. **A,** Frontal radiograph shows prominence of the ascending aorta *(arrows)*, as well as left ventricular enlargement. **B,** Left ventricular enlargement *(arrows)* is also evident on the lateral view.

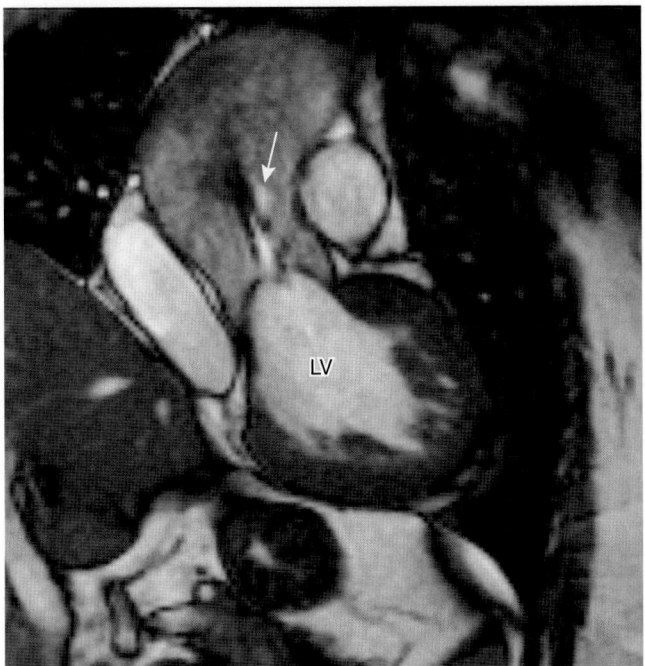

FIGURE 96-11. Cine MR image of aortic stenosis shows a jet *(arrow)* through the stenotic, domed aortic valve. LV, left ventricle. (Courtesy of Laura Heyneman, Duke Medical Center.)

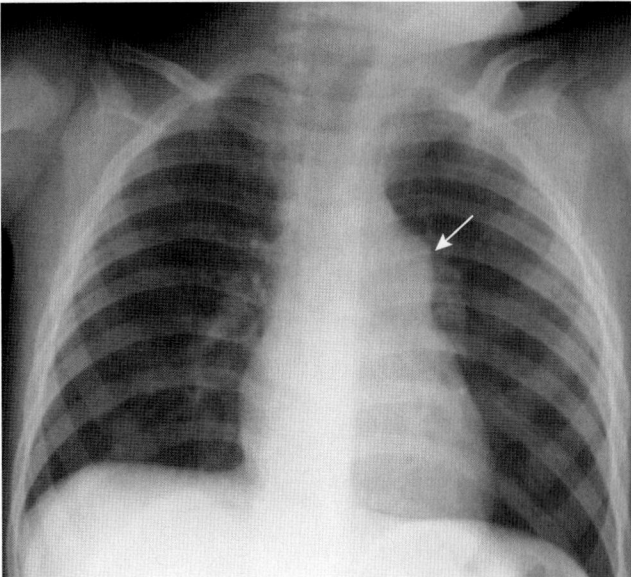

FIGURE 96-12. Pulmonary valvular stenosis. Frontal chest radiograph in a 1-year-old girl with a history of pulmonary stenosis shows prominence of the main pulmonary artery *(arrow)*, with normal pulmonary blood flow and no cardiomegaly.

papillary muscles, or a dilated valve annulus. The first line of therapy typically includes afterload reduction and anticongestive medication. Surgery is reserved for patients who fail medical therapy and is directed at correcting the underlying abnormality. This usually involves closing clefts in the mitral valve, or commissuroplasty. If annuloplasty is needed, prosthetic material is avoided in children who are expected to grow. Valve replacement is reserved for those who fail or are unsuitable for valve repair.

Mitral valve stenosis can occur in isolation, but it is much more commonly associated with other left heart defects. A common association is Shone complex, consisting of left heart obstructive lesions including mitral stenosis, supra–mitral valve ring, hypoplastic left ventricle, aortic valve stenosis, and coarctation of the aorta. Congenital mitral stenosis is often associated with an abnormal sub–mitral valve apparatus, including parachute mitral valve, mitral valve arcade, and single papillary muscle. Surgical repair of congenital mitral stenosis typically involves division or elongation and separation of the chordae and commissurotomy. In the case of a supra–mitral valve ring, simple resection of this abnormal fibrotic tissue may relieve the obstruction. In some situations, the fibrotic ring may involve the mitral leaflets, necessitating repair or replacement of the mitral valve.

Mitral valve prolapse has a prevalence of about 4%, with an approximately 2:1 female-to-male ratio. The disorder can be primary (80% to 90%) or secondary (hereditary or acquired); the latter is associated with other cardiac disease. The chest radiograph is usually normal. In severe cases of mitral valve prolapse, both left atrial and ventricular enlargement can be seen. Congestive heart failure is very rare.

In third-world countries, rheumatic heart disease is the most common cause of mitral valve stenosis and insufficiency.

Pulmonary Valve

As with the aortic valve, pulmonary stenosis consists of several types, including subpulmonary, valvular (pulmonary valve), and supravalvular stenosis. Isolated pulmonary stenosis is responsible for 5% to 10% of congenital heart lesions. Radiographic findings range from a normal examination to enlargement of the main pulmonary artery and proximal left pulmonary artery due to the orientation of the postvalvular jet (Fig. 96-12). Importantly, pulmonary blood flow is not reduced with isolated pulmonary stenosis because, unlike the pulmonary outflow obstruction in tetralogy of Fallot, there is no path for the blood (e.g., ventricular septal defect) to travel other than through the right heart and the lungs. With MRI, the stenotic valve manifests as a signal void with bright blood techniques (Fig. 96-13). Pulmonary insufficiency as an isolated entity is rare; it is generally seen following intervention for pulmonary valve stenosis. Cardiomegaly can be seen with isolated pulmonary regurgitation. MRI also allows the characterization of gradients with stenosis, determination of regurgitant fractions from stroke volumes in the setting of pulmonary valve regurgitation, and assessment of right ventricular wall motion and thickness (superior to echocardiography). Involvement of the stenotic pulmonary valve by endocarditis is infrequent.

Acquired Inflammatory Valvular Disorders

Infectious or rheumatic endocarditis is an inflammatory condition that involves the cardiac valves. In the past, rheumatic heart disease was the chief underlying cause

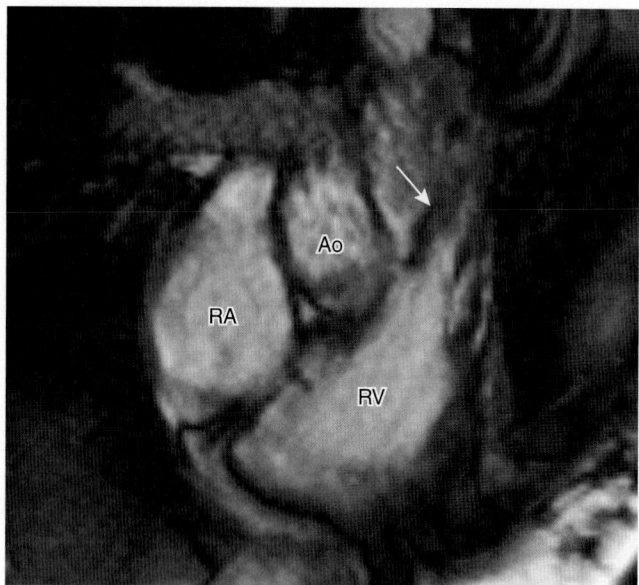

FIGURE 96-13. Pulmonary stenosis. Cine MR image shows signal void *(arrow)* in the main pulmonary artery. The right atrium (RA) and right ventricle (RV) are mildly dilated. Ao, aorta. (Courtesy of Laura Heyneman, Duke Medical Center.)

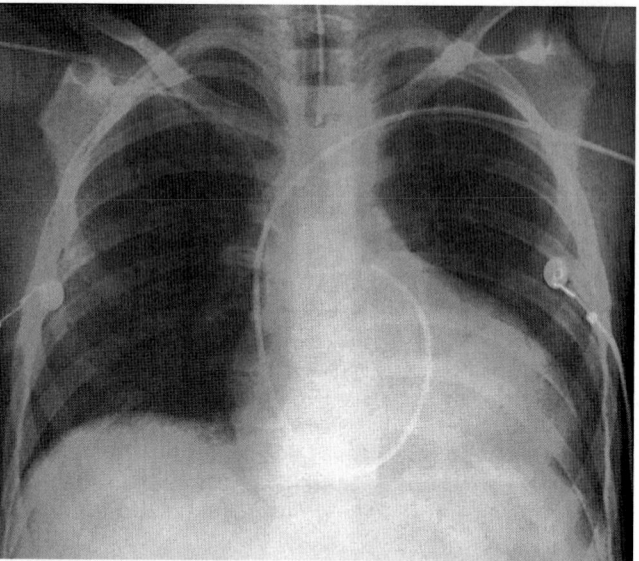

FIGURE 96-14. Bacterial endocarditis. Anteroposterior supine chest radiograph in a patient with bacterial endocarditis superimposed on congenital aortic valve disease. Gross cardiomegaly and left heart dilation with mild congestive heart failure are present. A Swan-Ganz catheter is in the main pulmonary artery, and a central venous line is in the superior vena cava.

of infectious endocarditis with valvular involvement in children. Given the improved survival of children with congenital heart disease and the decrease in rheumatic heart disease in developed countries, congenital heart disease is now a major predisposing factor for infectious endocarditis. Although patients with prosthetic patches, grafts, or valves are at increased risk, all children who have undergone repair or palliation of congenital heart disease are at a higher risk of endocarditis compared with children without congenital heart disease. In the absence of congenital heart disease, infectious endocarditis is often associated with indwelling venous catheters. It is thought that the presence of the catheter traumatizes the endocardium or valve epithelium. Noninfected thrombus develops at the site of injury, which then acts as a site for bacterial growth should the patient become bacteremic. In up to 10% of pediatric cases, infectious endocarditis develops without structural heart disease or other identifiable risk factors and usually involves aortic or mitral valve infection secondary to *Staphylococcus* bacteremia.

> **Major predisposing factors to infectious endocarditis include congenital heart disease and indwelling venous catheters.**

Children with infectious endocarditis may present acutely, with high, spiking fevers. The presentation is typically more indolent, however, with prolonged low-grade fever and nonspecific complaints such as lethargy, weakness, arthralgia, myalgia, and weight loss. In neonates, the symptoms may be even more difficult to recognize, consisting of feeding difficulty and neurologic signs and symptoms, including seizures, hemiparesis, and apnea. Gram-positive cocci are the most common causative agent, usually *Streptococcus*, followed by *Staphylococcus*.

The diagnosis of infectious endocarditis is based on the modified Duke criteria. These involve a combination of major criteria, including positive blood cultures or evidence of endocardial or valve involvement (vegetations, valve function) by transthoracic or transesophageal echocardiography, and minor criteria, including fever, predisposing factors (heart condition or intravenous drug use), and evidence of embolic disease (septic pulmonary emboli, intracranial hemorrhage, conjunctival hemorrhage, Janeway lesions).

Radiographic findings of infectious endocarditis may include cardiomegaly and congestive heart failure (Fig. 96-14). Diagnostic imaging is also beneficial in assessing for sequelae of endocarditis. In the setting of right heart involvement, pulmonary parenchymal opacities may be related to septic emboli. Mycotic aneurysms may develop when infections involve the great arteries or a patent ductus. Prompt diagnosis of these life-threatening aneurysms by echocardiography, CT, angiography, or MRI is critical (Fig. 96-15).

> **Radiographic findings of infectious endocarditis include cardiomegaly and congestive heart failure and pulmonary opacities from septic emboli.**

Surgery is indicated in patients who develop abscesses, mycotic aneurysms, fistulous tracts (into the pericardium, between the cardiac chambers or vascular structures), congestive heart failure, recurrent systemic embolization, acute valvular insufficiency, conduction abnormalities such as complete heart block, or persistent sepsis despite adequate antibiotic therapy. Surgery may also be indicated in patients with indwelling prosthetic material when medical therapy alone is ineffective.

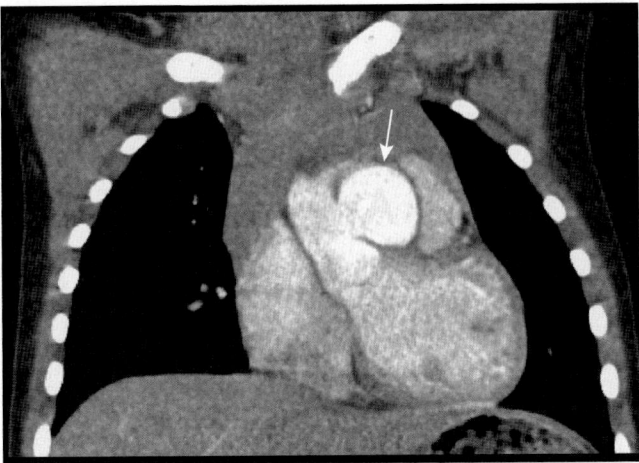

FIGURE 96-15. Mycotic aneurysm. Coronal reformation of CT angiogram shows a wide-necked saccular aneurysm *(arrow)* arising from the ascending aorta.

SUGGESTED READINGS

Cardiomyopathies

Choudhury L, Mahrholdt H, Wagner A, et al: Myocardial scarring in asymptomatic or mildly symptomatic patients with hypertrophic cardiomyopathy. J Am Coll Cardiol 2002;40:2156-2164

Cox GF, Sleeper LA, Lowe AM, et al: Factors associated with establishing a causal diagnosis for children with cardiomyopathy. Pediatrics 2006;118:1519-1531

Hughes SE, McKenna WJ: New insights into the pathology of inherited cardiomyopathy. Heart 2005;91:257-264

Kushwaha SS, Fallon JT, Fuster V: Restrictive cardiomyopathy. N Engl J Med 1997;336:267-276

Lipshultz SE: Ventricular dysfunction clinical research in infants, children and adolescents. Prog Pediatr Cardiol 2000;12:1-28

Lipshultz SE, Sleeper LA, Towbin JA, et al: The incidence of pediatric cardiomyopathy in two regions of the United States. N Engl J Med 2003;348:1647-1655

Macedo R, Schmidt A, Rochitte CE, et al: MRI to assess arrhythmia and cardiomyopathies. J Magn Reson Imaging 2006;24:1197-1206

Masui T, Finck S, Higgins CB: Constrictive pericarditis and restrictive cardiomyopathy: evaluation with MR imaging. Radiology 1992;182:369-373

Nugent AW, Daubeney PE, Chondros P, et al: The epidemiology of childhood cardiomyopathy in Australia. N Engl J Med 2003;348:1639-1646

Richardson P, McKenna W, Bristow M, et al: Report of the 1995 World Health Organization/International Society and Federation of Cardiology Task Force on the Definition and Classification of Cardiomyopathies. Circulation 1996;93:841-842

Rickers C, Wilke NM, Jerosch-Herold M, et al: Utility of cardiac magnetic resonance imaging in the diagnosis of hypertrophic cardiomyopathy. Circulation 2005;112:855-861

Schulz-Menger J, Friedrich MG: Magnetic resonance imaging in patients with cardiomyopathies: when and why. Herz 2000; 25:384-391

Teraoka K, Hirano M, Ookubo H, et al: Delayed contrast enhancement of MRI in hypertrophic cardiomyopathy. Magn Reson Imaging 2004;22:155-161

Towbin JA, Lowe AM, Colan SD, et al: Incidence, causes, and outcomes of dilated cardiomyopathy in children. JAMA 2006;296:1867-1876

Specific and Unspecified Cardiomyopathies

Cardiovascular health supervision for individuals affected by Duchenne or Becker muscular dystrophy. Pediatrics 2005; 116:1569-1573

Freedom RM: Congenital Heart Disease: Textbook of Angiocardiography. Armonk, NY, Futura, 1997

Gilbert-Barness E: Review: metabolic cardiomyopathy and conduction system defects in children. Ann Clin Lab Sci 2004;34:15-34

Leonard EG: Viral myocarditis. Pediatr Infect Dis J 2004;23:665-666

McCrohon JA, Richmond DR, Pennell DJ, Mohiaddin RH: Images in cardiovascular medicine. Isolated noncompaction of the myocardium: a rarity or missed diagnosis? Circulation 2002; 106:e22-e23

Mirabella M, Servidei S, Manfredi G, et al: Cardiomyopathy may be the only clinical manifestation in female carriers of Duchenne muscular dystrophy. Neurology 1993;43:2342-2345

Moon JC, Sachdev B, Elkington AG, et al: Gadolinium enhanced cardiovascular magnetic resonance in Anderson-Fabry disease: evidence for a disease specific abnormality of the myocardial interstitium. Eur Heart J 2003;24:2151-2155

Shaw AC, Kalidas K, Crosby AH, et al: The natural history of Noonan syndrome: a long-term follow-up study. Arch Dis Child 2007; 92:128-132

Endocardial Fibroelastosis

Trastour C, Bafghi A, Delotte J, et al: Early prenatal diagnosis of endocardial fibroelastosis. Ultrasound Obstet Gynecol 2005; 26:303-304

High-Output States

Kawamotoa S, Ogawa F, Tanaka J, et al: Chorioangioma: antenatal diagnosis with fast MR imaging. Magn Reson Imaging 2000; 18:911-914

Kline-Fath BM, Calvo-Garcia MA, O'Hara SM, et al: Twin-twin transfusion syndrome: cerebral ischemia is not the only fetal MR imaging finding. Pediatr Radiol 2007;37:47-56

Aortic Valve Disease

Calhoon JH, Bolton JW: Ross/Konno procedure for critical aortic stenosis in infancy. Ann Thorac Surg 1995;60:S597-S599

Durack DT, Lukes AS, Bright DK: New criteria for diagnosis of infective endocarditis: utilization of specific echocardiographic findings. Duke Endocarditis Service. Am J Med 1994;96:200-209

Ferrieri P, Gewitz MH, Gerber MA, et al: Unique features of infective endocarditis in childhood. Pediatrics 2002;109:931-943

Jonas RA, DiNardo JA: Comprehensive Surgical Management of Congenital Heart Disease. London, Arnold, 2004 (distributed in the United States by Oxford University Press)

Mitral Valve Disease

Wood AE, Healy DG, Nolke L, et al: Mitral valve reconstruction in a pediatric population: late clinical results and predictors of long-term outcome. J Thorac Cardiovasc Surg 2005;130:66-73

Yoshimura N, Yamaguchi M, Oshima Y, et al: Surgery for mitral valve disease in the pediatric age group. J Thorac Cardiovasc Surg 1999;118:99-106

CHAPTER

97

Pericardial Disease

CHARLES M. MAXFIELD

NORMAL PERICARDIUM

The pericardium is a conical structure that contains the heart and juxtacardiac origins of the great vessels. It consists of a tough, outer *fibrous* layer and an inner *serosal* layer; the latter consists of an outer *parietal* layer and an inner *visceral* layer (the *epicardium*), separated by a potential space, the *pericardial cavity*, which normally contains as much as 30 ml of serous fluid in an adult.

A complex three-dimensional arrangement of pericardial reflections extends between the vessels off the principal cavity, forming recesses that contain a small amount of fluid. Familiarity with these normal recesses can avoid misdiagnosis, such as mistaking a pericardial recess for precarinal adenopathy or mistaking the oblique pericardial recess (located dorsal to the left atrium) for a bronchogenic cyst. The thickness of the normal pericardium is less than 2 mm and is best seen radiographically between the epicardial and anterior mediastinal fat, anterior to the right ventricle and just above the diaphragm (Fig. 97-1).

The pericardium and pericardial cavity are most often imaged using echocardiography, but computed tomography (CT) and magnetic resonance imaging (MRI) offer distinct advantages in certain clinical settings. Both modalities provide a larger field of view, superior tissue characterization, and excellent anatomic delineation.

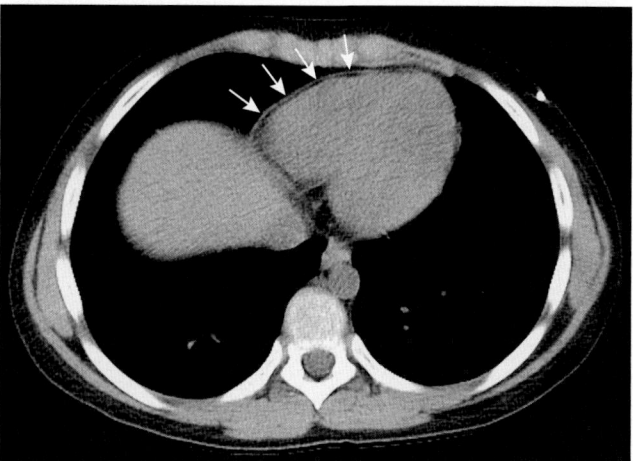

FIGURE 97-1. Axial non–contrast-enhanced CT image shows the normal pericardium (*arrows*) outlined between anterior mediastinal and epicardial fat.

MRI is superior to CT and echocardiography in characterizing pericardial effusions and pericardial masses. CT is most sensitive for pericardial calcifications.

> CT and MRI provide distinct advantages over echocardiography in the characterization of pericardial effusions and masses.

CONGENITAL ABSENCE OF THE PERICARDIUM

Congenital pericardial defects are rare. They are complete (70%) more often than partial, and left-sided more often than right-sided. In approximately 30% of cases, there are associated cardiac and pulmonary anomalies. Clinically, pericardial defects are often discovered incidentally at surgery, at autopsy, or on chest radiography, but they may present with periodic stabbing chest pain. Herniation of the left atrial appendage through a partial defect can be life threatening.

In complete absence of the pericardium, the chest radiograph typically reveals levocardia with varying degrees of prominence of the main pulmonary artery and, characteristically, a thin tongue of lung tissue extending medially between the aorta and the pulmonary trunk and between the inferior border of the heart and the left hemidiaphragm. This is best seen on cross-sectional imaging (Fig. 97-2). Partial defects can be suspected when there is focal prominence of the left atrial appendage along the upper left heart border. MRI can confirm this congenital anomaly by showing a defect in the thin, low signal intensity pericardium, as well as herniation of the left atrial appendage through the defect (Fig. 97-3).

> Partial absence of the pericardium can present with intermittent, stabbing chest pain.

Surgical reconstruction of the pericardium can be performed to reduce the risk of death from strangulation of cardiac structures and to manage symptoms.

PNEUMOPERICARDIUM

Pneumopericardium can be iatrogenic or post-traumatic but is most often seen in premature infants receiving

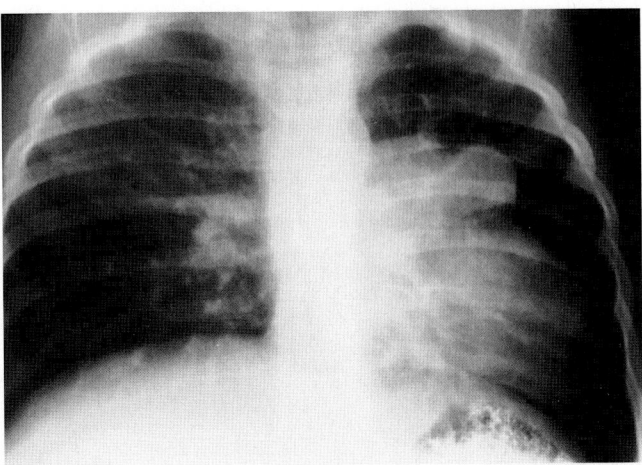

FIGURE 97-2. Complete absence of the left pericardium in a 9-year-old boy. The heart appears to be in the "oblique" position. The caudad surface is separated from the diaphragm (i.e., air between heart and diaphragm). The heart is displaced to the left.

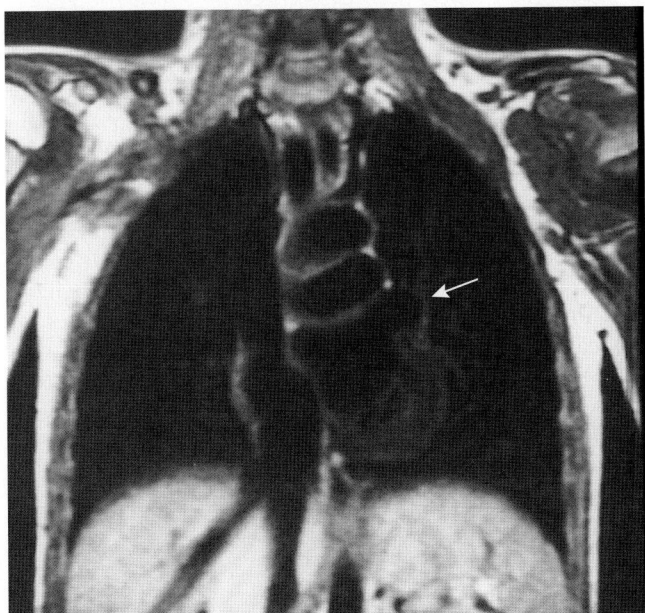

FIGURE 97-3. Nine-year-old girl with partial absence of the pericardium. Coronal T1-weighted image shows herniation of the left atrial appendage *(arrow)* through the partial pericardial defect.

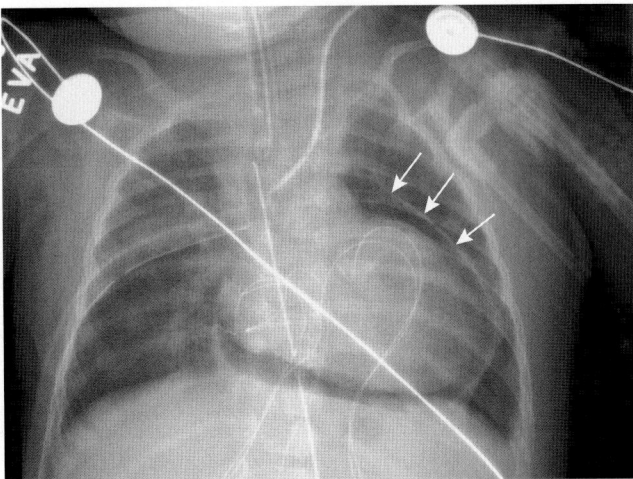

FIGURE 97-4. Sixteen-day-old girl who developed pneumopericardium after surgery for atrioventricular septal defect repair, presumably due to positive pressure ventilation. Note the air encircling the heart but not extending above the origins of the great vessels. The pericardium is visible as a thin white stripe *(arrows)* encircling the heart.

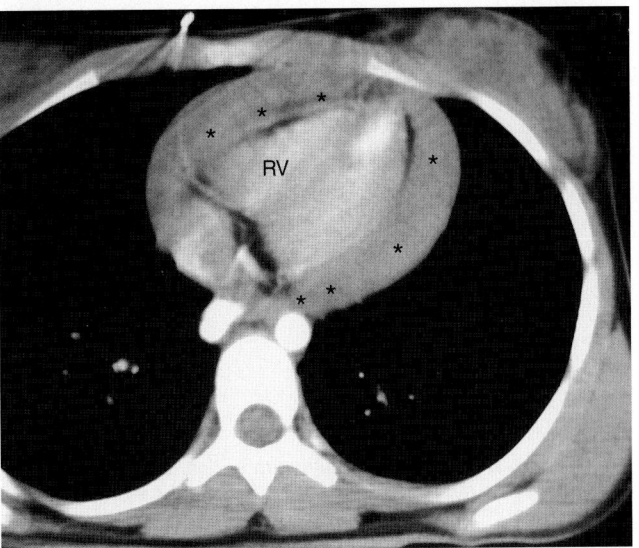

FIGURE 97-5. Traumatic hemopericardium in a juvenile involved in a motor vehicle crash. High-density fluid *(asterisks)* surrounds the heart, distending the pericardial space. Note compression of the right ventricle (RV).

positive pressure ventilation. Radiographs show a lucent halo of air encircling the heart, extending between the heart and diaphragm inferiorly and the origin of the great vessels superiorly (Fig. 97-4). The parietal and fibrous pericardium itself can sometimes be seen as a thin white stripe contrasted between the lung and pericardial air in the pericardial cavity. Pneumopericardium must be distinguished from pneumomediastinum, in which air can also outline the inferior aspect of the heart. In pneumomediastinum, however, air often extends above the origin of the great vessels, surrounding the thymus and occasionally extending into the neck.

The clinical significance of pneumopericardium depends on the amount of air in the pericardium. Large pericardial air collections can cause tamponade and must be evacuated.

PERICARDIAL EFFUSION AND PERICARDITIS

The most common identifiable causes of pericardial effusion in children are infectious and iatrogenic. Neoplastic and connective tissue causes are less common. Infectious pericarditis is most often viral, but those cases associated with significant pericardial fluid are more often of bacterial origin. Tuberculous or fungal pericarditis is unusual. Large pericardial effusions are often due to bacterial pericarditis, malignancy, or immune disorders, but in some cases, the cause is never determined. Hemopericardium is often caused by trauma,

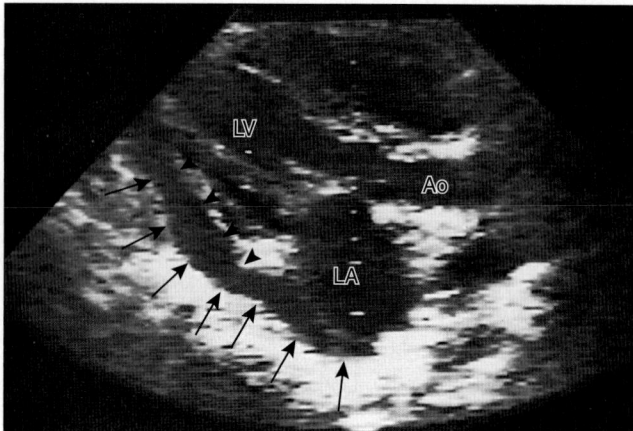

FIGURE 97-6. Echocardiogram shows pericardial effusion between the posterior left ventricular (LV) wall *(arrowheads)* and the pericardium *(arrows).* Ao, aorta; LA, left atrium.

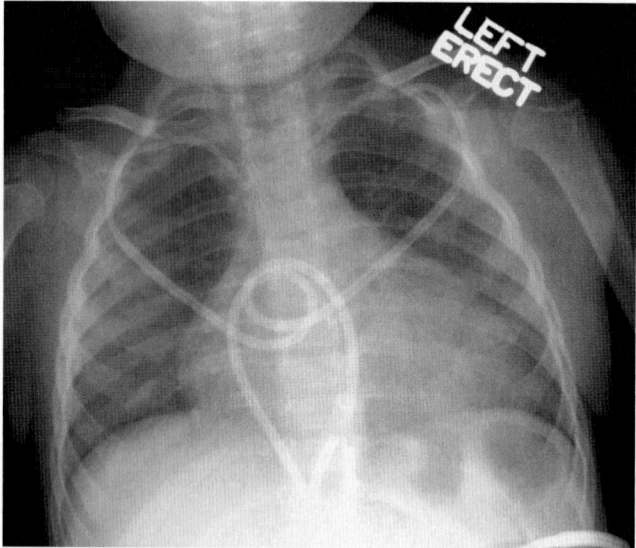

FIGURE 97-7. One-year-old child with pericardial effusion following bone marrow transplantation. Note the symmetric enlargement of the cardiac silhouette. Pericardial fluid was confirmed by echocardiography.

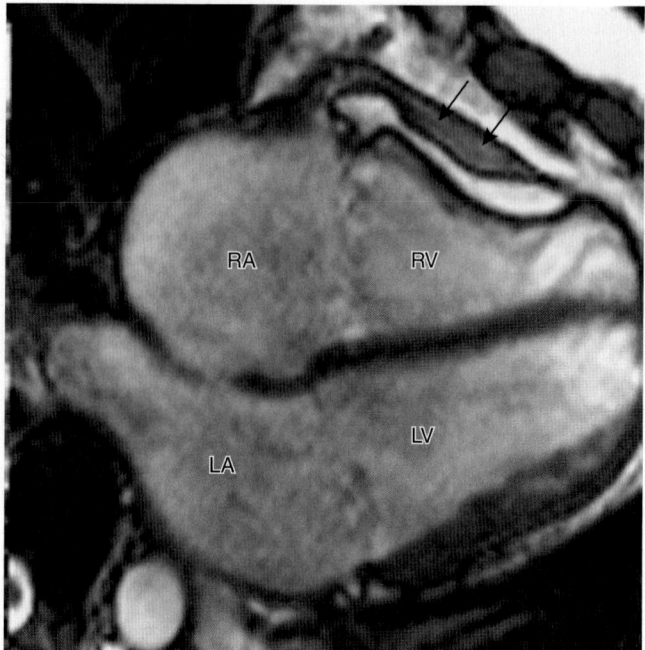

FIGURE 97-8. Four-chamber bright-blood sequence in an 18-year-old with uremic pericarditis. The ventricles are cone shaped, and there is biatrial enlargement. Focal thickening and abnormal signal are noted within the pericardium *(arrows).* LA, left atrium; LV, left ventricle; RA, right atrium; RV, right ventricle.

either accidental (Fig. 97-5) or iatrogenic. Special note should be made of pericardial effusions related to central venous catheter placement in children. Cardiac tamponade can result from vessel perforation, leading to hemopericardium or to intrapericardial infusion of fluids, such as total parenteral nutrition.

Clinically, pericarditis often presents with nonspecific fever, malaise, and chest pain. Echocardiography is the imaging modality of choice to evaluate for pericardial fluid; it is readily available and sensitive and avoids ionizing radiation (Fig. 97-6). Chest radiography is insensitive for pericardial effusion but can document large or rapidly expanding effusions. The typical appearance consists of symmetric enlargement of the cardiac shadow in a characteristic water-bottle configuration (Fig. 97-7). Posterior displacement of the epicardial fat pad on the lateral view can be a specific finding. CT and, especially, MRI offer better soft tissue contrast and anatomic delineation than echocardiography, and these studies

are indicated when pericardial fluid might be loculated or hemorrhagic. Both modalities can also be used to differentiate constrictive pericarditis from restrictive cardiomyopathy. The presence of pericardial thickening or calcification in the setting of restrictive cardiac physiology is suggestive of constrictive pericarditis (Fig. 97-8). This is a rare condition in children but is treatable by pericardial stripping.

> **MRI is indicated when pericardial fluid might be loculated or hemorrhagic.**

PERICARDIAL MASSES

Pericardial cysts are quite rare in children, despite the fact that they are considered congenital. They are typically located in the cardiophrenic angle, especially on the right side. These cysts are most often an incidental finding on chest radiographs and can be further characterized with CT. Pericardial cysts can be followed, aspirated, or resected, depending on their size and the patient's symptoms.

The most common primary pericardial tumor in childhood is the pericardial teratoma, which may be cystic or solid. This tumor is benign but can present dramatically in a newborn with rupture, causing a massive pericardial effusion and resulting in cardiorespiratory distress. Other benign pericardial masses in children include hemangiomas (Fig. 97-9) and mesenchymal tumors. Both primary and secondary malignant pericardial tumors are very rare in children. The most common is lymphoma, which most often produces nodular thickening of the pericardium.

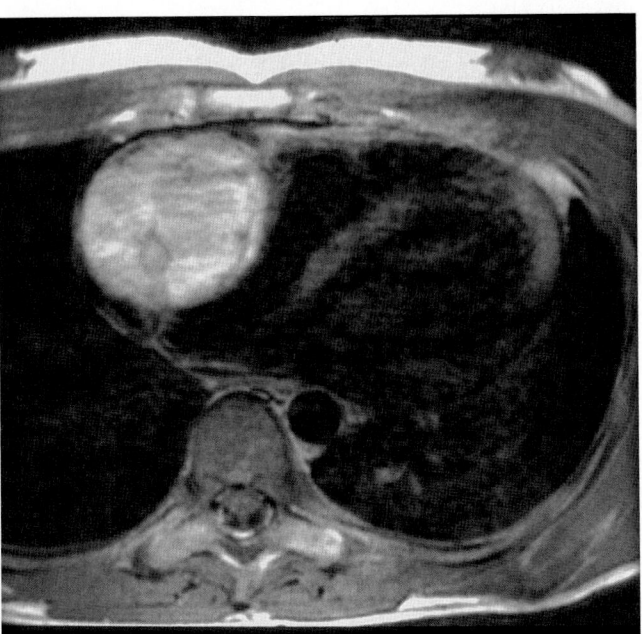

FIGURE 97-9. Postcontrast, cardiac-gated, T1-weighted axial MR image shows a mass (M), identified as a hemangioma, in the pericardium of a 5-year-old boy.

> Pericardial teratomas can present catastrophically in a newborn, with pericardial tamponade secondary to rupture.

SUGGESTED READINGS

Abbas AE, Appleton CA, Liu PT, Sweeney JP: Congenital absence of the pericardium: case presentation and review of literature. Int J Cardiol 2005;19:21-25

Breen JF: Imaging of the pericardium. J Thorac Imaging 2001; 16:47-54

Bull RK, Edwards PD, Dixon AK: CT dimensions of the normal pericardium. Br J Radiol 1998;71:923-925

Chan HS, Sonley MJ, Moes CA, et al: Primary and secondary tumors of childhood involving the heart, pericardium, and great vessels: a report of 75 cases and review of the literature. Cancer 1985; 56:825-836

Demmler GJ: Infectious pericarditis in children. Pediatr Infect Dis J 2006;25:165-166

Ferreira G, Ferreira A, do Nascimento MA, et al: Constrictive chronic pericarditis in children. Cardiol Young 2001;11:210-213

Gatzoulis MA, Munk MD, Merchant N, et al: Isolated congenital absence of the pericardium: clinical presentation, diagnosis, and management. Ann Thorac Surg 2000;69:1209-1215

Grebenc ML, Rosada de Christenson ML, Burke AP, et al: Primary cardiac and pericardial neoplasms: radiologic-pathologic correlation. Radiographics 2000;20:1073-1103

Levy-Ravetch M, Auh RY, Rubenstein WA, et al: CT of the periocardial recesses. AJR Am J Roentgenol 1985;144:707-714

Mok GC, Menahem S: Large pericardial effusions of inflammatory origin in childhood. Cardiol Young 2003;13:131-136

Nowlen TT, Rosenthal GL, Johnson GL, et al: Pericardial effusion and tamponade in infants with central catheters. Pediatrics 2002;110:137-142

Noyes BE, Weber T, Vogler C: Pericardial cysts in children: surgical or conservative approach. J Pediatr Surg 2003;38:1263-1265

Robles P, Rubio A, Olmedilla P: Value of multidetector cardiac CT in calcified constrictive pericarditis for pericardial resection. Heart 2006;92:1112

Trujillo MH, Fragachan CF, Tortoledo F: Cardiac tamponade due to pneumopericardium. Cardiology 2006;105:34-36

Wang ZJ, Reddy GP, Gotway MB, et al: CT and MR imaging of pericardial disease. Radiographics 2003;23:S167-S180

CHAPTER 98

Coronary Artery Disease in Children

FRANDICS P. CHAN and TAMER EL-HELW

Diseases of the coronary arteries are less common in children than in adults. Adult diseases are dominated by atherosclerotic coronary artery disease, whereas most pediatric diseases are congenital. There are a large number of anomalous arrangements of the coronary arteries, but only a few have clinical significance. Among acquired disease of the coronary artery, Kawasaki disease is the most common in children. Others include trauma sequelae, Behçet syndrome, polyarteritis nodosa, radiation injury after oncologic treatment, and rare cases of familial hyperlipidemia and idiopathic infantile arterial calcification. Table 98-1 outlines the two principal manifestations of coronary artery diseases in children, together with the diseases in which they are commonly seen.

In the past, echocardiography and catheter angiography were relied on to study pediatric coronary artery diseases. Both of these techniques are now performed almost exclusively by pediatric cardiologists. As a result,

most radiologists have not been exposed to pediatric coronary artery diseases, nor have they participated in the care of these patients. This situation is changing with the advent of cardiac computed tomography (CT) and cardiac magnetic resonance imaging (MRI). Radiologists who manage these modalities are again being called on to aid in making diagnoses. In practice, patients are usually referred for coronary CT or MRI to diagnose a coronary anomaly in those presenting with syncope, arrhythmia, or sudden death; to confirm and clarify echocardiographic findings of coronary anomalies; to map out the coronary arteries for surgical planning; and to evaluate coronary aneurysm and stenosis. Therefore, radiologists must know how to image the coronary system of children using CT and MRI, how to recognize pathologic abnormalities, and how imaging results affect treatment. Table 98-2 compares the advantages of various coronary imaging modalities.

TABLE 98-1

Principal Manifestations of Coronary Artery Diseases

Manifestation	Disease Examples
Coronary aneurysm or ectasia	High-flow fistula
	Anomalous left coronary artery from the pulmonary artery (ALCAPA) with large collateral flow
	Kawasaki disease
	Behçet disease
	Polyarteritis nodosa
	Trauma (pseudoaneurysm)
Coronary stenosis	Kawasaki disease
	Behçet disease
	Polyarteritis nodosa
	Postsurgical
	Trauma (dissection)
	Radiation
	Williams syndrome
	Congenital coronary hypoplasia
	Homozygous familial hypercholesterolemia
	Idiopathic infantile arterial calcification

TABLE 98-2

Coronary Imaging Modalities: Advantages

Modality	Advantages
Echocardiography	Accessible, noninvasive
	Good visualization in infants
	No ionizing radiation
	Flow imaging with Doppler
Catheter angiography	High spatial and temporal resolutions
	Selective angiography
	Hemodynamic measurements
	Coronary interventions
Computed tomography	Three-dimensional imaging
	Noninvasive
	Good visualization in all ages
	Fast study
Magnetic resonance imaging	Three-dimensional imaging
	Noninvasive
	No ionizing radiation
	Myocardial perfusion and infarct imaging
	Ventricular function quantification
	Flow quantification with phase-contrast imaging

> **Patients are usually referred for CT or MR coronary imaging for:**
> - **Diagnosis of coronary anomaly**
> - **Confirmation and clarification of echocardiographic findings of coronary anomalies**
> - **Mapping out the coronary arteries for surgical planning**
> - **Evaluating coronary aneurysm and stenosis**

IMAGING CONSIDERATIONS

Cardiac-gated multidetector row CT (MDCT) is the latest development in CT technology. It combines the rapid scan rate of an MDCT scanner with methods that synchronize data acquisition with the cardiac cycle. Each image is captured in a brief moment of time at a consistent cardiac phase such that the heart structures can be seen clearly for diagnostic interpretation. The first commercially available cardiac-gated MDCT appeared in 2000, and since then scanner performance has improved dramatically in terms of scan rate, temporal resolution, and spatial resolution. Its principal application is the imaging of atherosclerotic coronary artery disease in adults. However, the same technique has been successfully adapted to image the heart and the coronary arteries in children less than 1 week old.

The currently available 64-slice MDCT scanner with 300-msec gantry rotation time and 0.5-mm detector width can scan through a pediatric heart in 10 to 20 seconds. The through-plane resolution is typically 0.6 mm and the in-plane resolution is 0.3 mm. Using two-sector reconstruction, a temporal resolution of 100 to 130 msec can be routinely achieved. Newer scanner design with multiple x-ray sources promises even better temporal resolution. A typical protocol for coronary CT angiography (CCTA) (Table 98-3) calls for the injection of 2 to 3 ml/kg of intravenous iodinated contrast agent over the period of the scan, followed by a saline chase. Bolus tracking technique can be used to trigger the scan at the arrival of contrast material in the aortic root. Breath holding is generally necessary. If a patient is not old enough to do this voluntarily, an anesthesiologist should be involved to induce transient apnea during the scan. Retrospective electrocardiographic (ECG)-gating and multisector reconstruction should be used to maximize temporal resolution. For a heart rate of greater than 80 beats per minute (bpm), reconstruction at systole (or about 30% RR-interval) usually yields better image quality. For a heart rate of less than 80 bpm, reconstruction at diastole (or about 60% RR-interval) may do better. Coronary arteries have been successfully imaged at a heart rate as high as 160 bpm. Finally, images are analyzed with the aid of three-dimensional-reconstruction workstation.

The greatest concern for CCTA is the ionizing radiation. The exact biologic dose in children depends heavily on the protocol. Based on adult data, the biologic dose presented by CCTA is probably about 10 mSv, comparable to catheter angiography undertaken with ventriculo-

TABLE 98-3

Protocol for Pediatric Coronary CT Angiography

Scan geometry	64-slice MDCT scanner
	0.6 mm or thinnest slice thickness
	Scan range from carina to bottom of the heart
Radiation dose	100 kilovolt peak (kVp)
	Minimum milliampere-second (mAs) per body size
Gating mode	Retrospective ECG gating
	Two-sector reconstruction
	0.3 sec, or shortest gantry rotation time
	Use ECG dose modulation if available
Contrast usage	2-3 ml/kg, >300 mg I/mL (iodinated contrast agent)
	If necessary, dilute contrast to a 15-ml volume minimum
	Calculate injection rate to deliver contrast over the scan period
	10-20 ml saline chase at the same injection rate
Scan trigger	Bolus tracking at the aortic root
Reconstruction	30% RR-interval at heart rate > 80 bpm, adjust for best image
	60% RR-interval at heart rate < 80 bpm, adjust for best image

bpm, beats per minute; CT, computed tomography; ECG, electrocardiography; MDCT, multidetector CT.

grams. There is a small but not negligible risk of oncogenesis over the lifetime of a child. Therefore, every measure must be taken to meticulously reduce the radiation exposure. First, CCTA should be undertaken only if clearly indicated. As much as possible, scanning should be limited to a single pass over the heart only. Tube voltage should be lowered to between 100 and 80 kVp and the tube current should be adjusted to the minimum necessary for each patient's size. If possible, the pitch factor should be increased for higher heart rate. ECG dose-modulation and geometric dose-modulation should be used whenever it is available.

> **Measures to minimize CCTA radiation dose:**
> - **Study must be indicated**
> - **Single pass only, no precontrast scan**
> - **100 to 80 kVp**
> - **Minimize tube current for body size**
> - **Maximize pitch factor**
> - **Geometric dose-modulation**
> - **ECG dose-modulation**

Given this shortcoming of CCTA, coronary MR angiography (CMRA) should have been the better choice for imaging the coronary arteries. Unfortunately, despite intensive research efforts for more than two decades, progress in improving CMRA has been slow. Image quality of CCTA from current technology surpasses that of CMRA in terms of spatial resolution, scan time, and

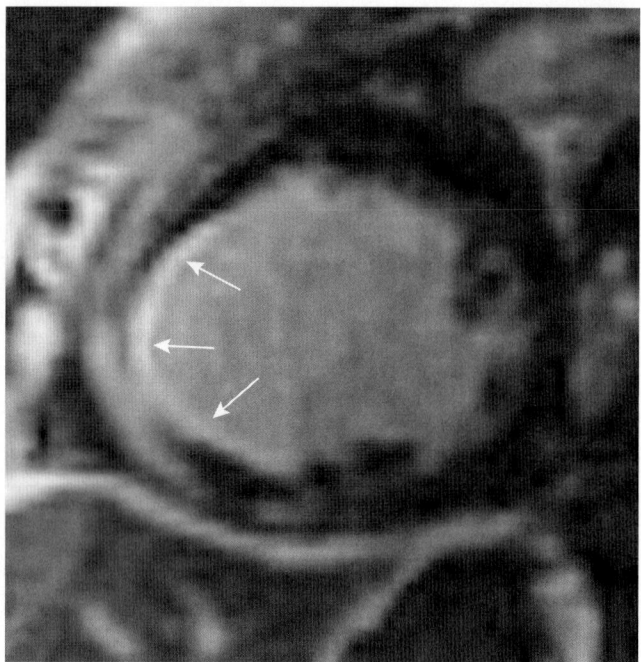
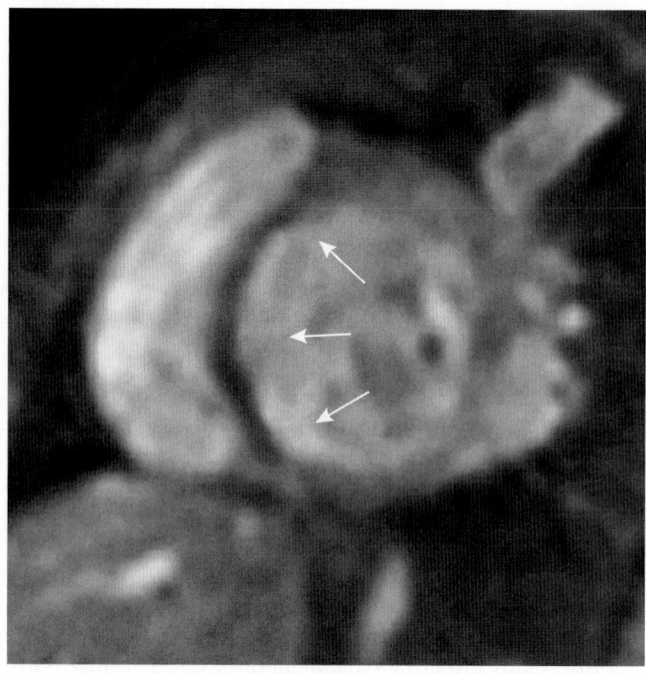

A   B

FIGURE 98-1. Septal myocardial infarction in a 4-year-old boy. **A,** MRI delayed-enhancement imaging in the short-axis plane shows transmural enhancement *(arrows)* of the septum, corresponding to the region of myocardial infarction. The septum is thin and its motion was severely dyskinetic. During systole, when this picture was taken, the septum paradoxically reached the free wall of the right ventricle. **B,** MRI first-pass perfusion scan in the same short-axis plane shows hypoenhancement *(arrows)* of the septum compared with the lateral left ventricular wall, corresponding to hypoperfusion at the region of infarct scar. This image is taken at diastole when the septum returns to its normal position.

consistency across different patient conditions. Available CMRA techniques can be divided into breath-hold methods and free-breathing methods. Breath-hold methods avoid problems with respiratory artifact but are limited by a low signal-to-noise ratio (SNR), low spatial resolution, and small spatial coverage. Free-breathing methods promise better SNR and spatial coverage at the cost of long scan time—up to half an hour to cover the whole heart. A variety of complex algorithms, typically involving navigator echoes to detect the diaphragm position, are used to reduce but not eliminate respiratory artifact. The quality of CMRA implementations varies greatly depending on the manufacturer and the scanner model. For adolescents and young adults who are co-operative and have large coronary arteries, it is reasonable to try CMRA first. If it fails to answer the question, then CCTA or catheter angiography may be used as backup. For infants and small children who must be studied under anesthesia, CCTA is a better choice at this time. The future choice between CCTA and CMRA will depend on technical advancements.

Besides angiography, MRI is helpful evaluating the consequences of ischemia from coronary artery disease. Delayed enhancement imaging is an established technique for imaging myocardial infarction in adults. Similar findings have been demonstrated in children (Fig. 98-1). In addition, delayed enhancement is useful for the diagnosis of endocardial fibroelastosis, myositis, and other infiltrative heart diseases. Less established is the first-pass, contrast-enhanced myocardial perfusion scan in children (see Fig. 98-1). This technique calls for the use of adenosine or dipyridamole to enhance the

coronary perfusion difference between territories supplied by normal coronary artery and those supplied by stenotic coronary artery. Finally, multiplanar cine imaging with or without tagging, helps detect subtle wall-motion abnormalities related to ischemia. From cine images of the ventricles, ventricular volumes and ejection fractions can be measured to assess global ventricular functions.

In infants, transthoracic echocardiography is the first-line imaging tool for the evaluation of coronary anomalies (Fig. 98-2). In this population, the short distance between the aortic root and the ultrasound probe, the lack of intervening lungs, the good sonographic window, and the use of a high-frequency probe all promote good visualization of the proximal coronary arteries. In older children, these advantages lessen and visualization of the coronary arteries becomes unreliable. Transesophageal echocardiography produces better images in older patients. However, neither technique is capable of imaging the entire coronary system.

Catheter angiography is the gold standard for the determination of coronary anomalies, but this technique is not without its problems. It is invasive and carries the risk of infection, hemorrhage, and embolic complications. Engagement of a catheter to anomalous coronary origin can be difficult. For inflammatory diseases, direct contact between the catheter and the inflamed vessel wall can cause vasospasm, thrombosis, and dissection. Finally, complicated anomalies may be difficult to evaluate from a limited number of projections. Although CCTA and CMRA solve some of these problems, catheter angiography remains superior in terms of temporal and

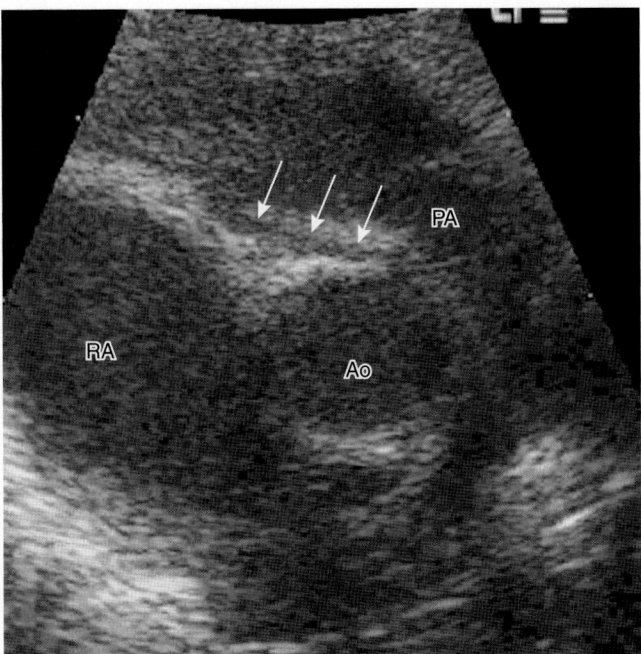

FIGURE 98-2. Gray scale echocardiography of an ectopic right coronary artery (RCA) with interarterial course in a 3-week-old boy. The anomalous RCA (*arrows*) lies between the aorta (Ao) and the pulmonary artery (PA).

spatial resolutions. It can resolve submillimeter vessels reliably. Furthermore, contrast progression imaged by high-speed fluoroscopic cine provides invaluable information about connectivity and hemodynamics of the vascular network. Finally, important hemodynamic parameters, such as pressure and oxygen saturation, can be measured as needed.

EMBRYOLOGY OF CORONARY ARTERIES

A brief overview of the embryologic development of the coronary arteries helps us understand why certain coronary anomalies occur. The coronary arteries develop concurrently with the complex development of the heart, beginning at the third week and completing by the fifth to sixth week of gestation. Development of the coronary arteries can be divided into three consecutive stages. In the first stage, a network of intra-trabecular sinusoids forms within the ventricular cavity and extends into the myocardium. These sinusoids may serve as conduits that deliver blood to the developing myocardium. In the second stage, endothelial precursor cells migrate from the septum transversum to the epicardium to form a mantle of blood islands. These islands coalesce into vascular channels that extend over the surface of the epicardium and penetrate into the myocardium. These myocardial channels communicate with the sinusoidal networks. In the final stage, a capillary plexus forms around the primitive truncus arteriosus. The peripheral portion of this plexus connects with the epicardial vascular channels, and the proximal portion organizes to form large, muscular coronary arteries that penetrate the aortic wall at the sinuses of Valsalva. As the coronary flow from the aorta increases, the intratrabecular sinusoids

regress and are obliterated, thus completing the basic plan of the coronary artery system. Because it is possible to develop a coronary artery that travels between the aorta and the pulmonary artery, truncal separation must be completed before the coronary system is fully developed.

Development of the coronary arteries follows a process that is closely coordinated with the developing heart. For example, in L-loop development of the ventricles, positions of the left and right ventricles are reversed. The coronary artery branching pattern follows the ventricles, and it is similarly reversed. Such coordination is presumed to be mediated by local growth factors, chemotactic factors, extracellular matrix molecules, and myocardial mechanical stress. Alteration of these factors is the basis for anomalous coronary formation. For example, if the intra-trabecular sinusoids fail to regress, then the coronary system communicates directly with the ventricle, forming a coronary-ventricular fistula. If the peritruncal capillary plexus perforates the pulmonary artery instead of the aorta, it develops either a coronary–pulmonary artery fistula or an anomalous origin of the coronary artery from the pulmonary artery. It can be expected that the abnormal development of the truncus arteriosus is associated with an increased incidence in coronary anomalies. Such is indeed the case found in persistent truncus arteriosus, transposition of the great arteries, and tetralogy of Fallot.

NORMAL CORONARY ARTERY ANATOMY

Many anatomic variations of the coronary arteries exist, and the line drawn to separate normal variants from anomalous ones is arbitrary. The coronary artery pattern can be generally divided into a right-dominant system, a left-dominant system, and a codominant system. A right-dominant system, which is found in 85% of the population, has a right coronary artery (RCA) that supplies the inferoseptal and inferior walls of the left ventricle by giving rise to both the posterior descending artery (PDA) and the posterior left ventricular arteries (PLVA) (Fig. 98-3). In this pattern, the myocardial perfusion of the left ventricle is shared between the left and the right coronary arteries. A left-dominant system, which is found in 8% to 10% of the population, has a left circumflex artery (LCx) that supplies the PDA and the PLVA (see Fig. 98-3). In this configuration, the left ventricle is completely supplied by the left main coronary artery (LMCA). In a codominant system, which is found in 5% to 7% of the population, an RCA supplies the PDA and an LCx supplies the PLVA. The left ventricle is perfused predominantly by the LMCA.

> Coronary dominance:
> **Right dominance (85% of population)**
> - **RCA supplies PDA and PLVA**
> **Left dominance (10% of population)**
> - **LCx supplies PDA and PLVA**
> **Codominance (5% of population)**
> - **RCA supplies PDA, LCx supplies PLVA**

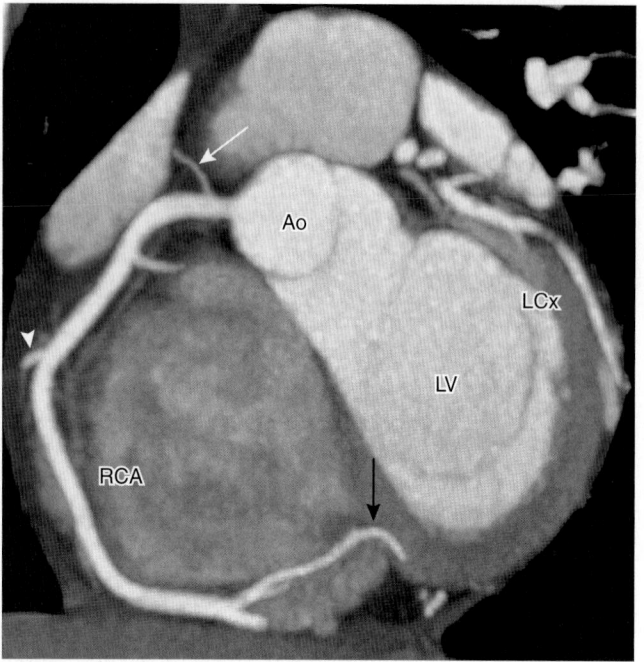
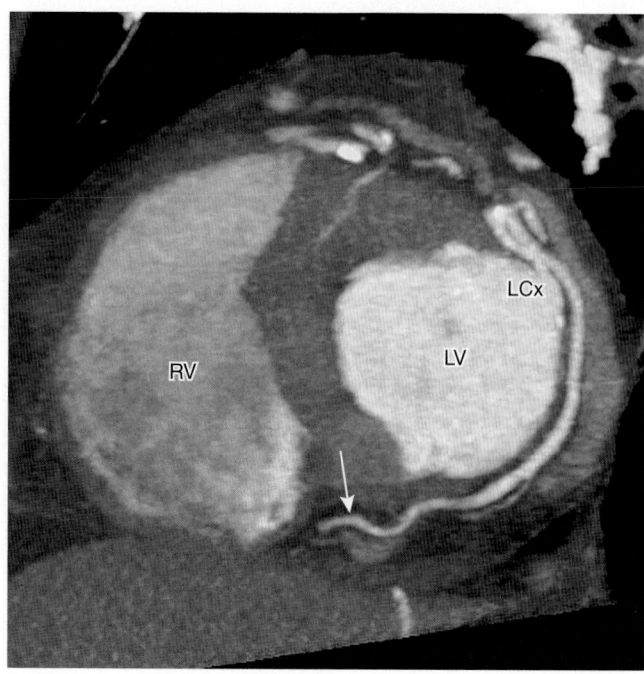

A   B

FIGURE 98-3. Normal coronary CTA in the short-axis plane. **A,** In this right-dominant coronary system, the right coronary artery (RCA) originates from the aorta (Ao), gives off the conal artery (*white arrow*) as its first branch, then gives off an acute marginal branch (*arrowhead)* to the anterior free wall, reaches the crux (*black arrow*), and continues on to the inferior surface of the left ventricle (LV). **B,** In this left-dominant coronary system, the left circumflex artery (LCx) wraps around the left atrioventricular groove to reach the crux (*white arrow*); RV, right ventricle.

The three sinuses of Valsalva line up with the three semi-lunar cusps of the aortic valve. Two of the three sinuses face the pulmonary artery, and from each of the two facing sinuses, a coronary artery normally arises. The three aortic sinuses are anatomically labeled as the right, left, and posterior sinuses, which correspond to the right coronary cusp, the left coronary cusp, and the noncoronary cusp, respectively (Fig. 98-4).

The RCA normally originates from the right sinus of Valsalva and courses anteriorly into the right atrioventricular groove. A conal artery may arise as the first branch of the RCA, although 50% of the time it arises directly from the aorta. This conal artery supplies the myocardium at the right ventricular outflow tract. Although normally small, the conal artery can become large when there is increased coronary flow to a hypertrophic right ventricle, which can be found in tetralogy of Fallot and corrected transposition of the great arteries. A sinoatrial nodal artery may arise from the proximal RCA (Fig. 98-5) or from the LCx, and this occurs at roughly equal frequencies. The middle portion of the RCA gives rise to one or more acute marginal branches. The distal portion of the RCA wraps around the inferior surface of the heart. In a right-dominant system, the RCA gives off a PDA and enters the "crux," the intersection between the interventricular septum and the atrioventricular groove. At the crux, the RCA bends and forms an inverted U before entering the left atrioventricular groove, where it gives off multiple posterior left ventricular arteries and terminates. An atrioventricular nodal (AVN) branch normally arises from the RCA near the apex of the

inverted U. The PDA has many inferior perforator branches that supply the inferior septum.

The LMCA originates from the left sinus of Valsalva and courses to the left for a short distance. In most people, it bifurcates into a left anterior descending (LAD) artery and an LCx. In some, the LMCA trifurcates into an LAD, an LCx, and, in between, a ramus medianus or a ramus intermedius branch (Fig. 98-6). The LAD gives rise to two sets of vessels: an epicardial set called the diagonal branches and an intramuscular set called the anterior perforator branches. The distal LAD typically wraps around the cardiac apex and terminates at the inferior wall of the apex. The LCx may give off a sinoatrial nodal branch before it enters the left atrioventricular groove. The LCx then gives rise to a number of obtuse marginal branches. In a codominant system, the LCx supplies the PLVA. In a left-dominant system, the LCx supplies both the PLVA and the PDA.

Nomenclature of the coronary arteries can be confusing in the presence of severe ventricular malformation. In general, the coronary arteries are named relative to the morphology, not the position, of the underlying ventricles. For example, in L-loop ventricles where the morphologic left ventricle lies to the right, the coronary artery in the right-side atrioventricular groove is named the left circumflex artery. When derangement of the ventricles is so severe that the morphology of the ventricles cannot be clearly identified, then the coronary arteries should be described relative to physical landmarks—for example, left-side atrioventricular branch instead of LCx, right-side atrioventricular branch instead

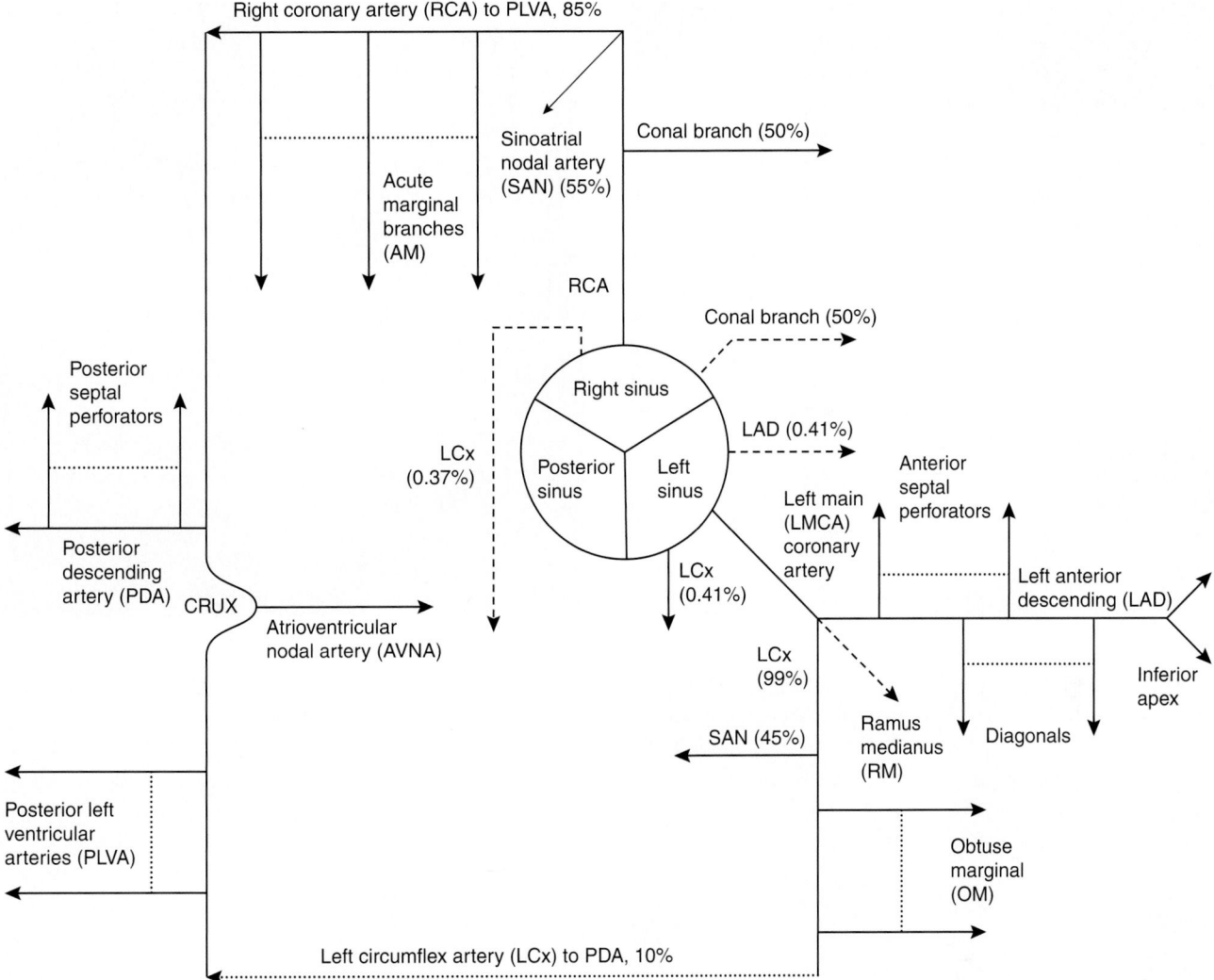

FIGURE 98-4. Coronary artery distribution diagram. *Solid lines* represent the most common coronary artery pattern. *Dashed lines* represent common variants (their prevalence is given).

of RCA, anterior interventricular septal branch instead of LAD, and posterior interventricular septal branch instead of PDA.

CONGENITAL CORONARY ARTERY ANOMALIES

Epidemiology

The true prevalence of congenital coronary artery anomalies is unknown. Using angiographic data from adult patients who underwent catheter coronary angiography, 0.6% to 1.5% of patients were found to have coronary artery anomalies. So far, the largest study of this type reviewed more than 126,000 coronary studies. The prevalence of coronary artery anomalies in this population was 1.3%. Of these anomalous cases, 80% were judged to have no clinical significance. The prevalence for ectopic coronary origin and aberrant course is estimated at 1% and for coronary artery fistulas, at 0.16% in the population. Of the ectopic coronary origin, the most common type is separate origins of the LAD and the LCx arising from the left sinus of Valsalva (0.41%)

(Fig. 98-7). The next most common type is ectopic LCx arising from the right sinus or the RCA and then coursing posterior to the aorta (0.37%). Both configurations are clinically benign. Other examples of benign anomalies are absent LCx with a superdominant RCA that reaches the anterior atrioventricular groove, ectopic right or left coronary artery from the posterior sinus, and ectopic left or right coronary origin from the ascending aorta. Table 98-4 lists the clinically significant coronary artery anomalies.

Coronary Artery with Interarterial Course

The LMCA may originate from the right sinus of Valsalva or from the RCA. Before bifurcating into the LAD and the LCx, the LMCA must travel toward the left by one of three courses: anterior to the right ventricular outflow tract, between the aorta and the pulmonary artery, and posterior to the aorta. Similarly, the RCA may originate from the left sinus of Valsalva or from the LMCA. It must travel toward the right atrioventricular groove by one of these three courses. For both coronary arteries, the anterior and posterior courses are clinically benign,

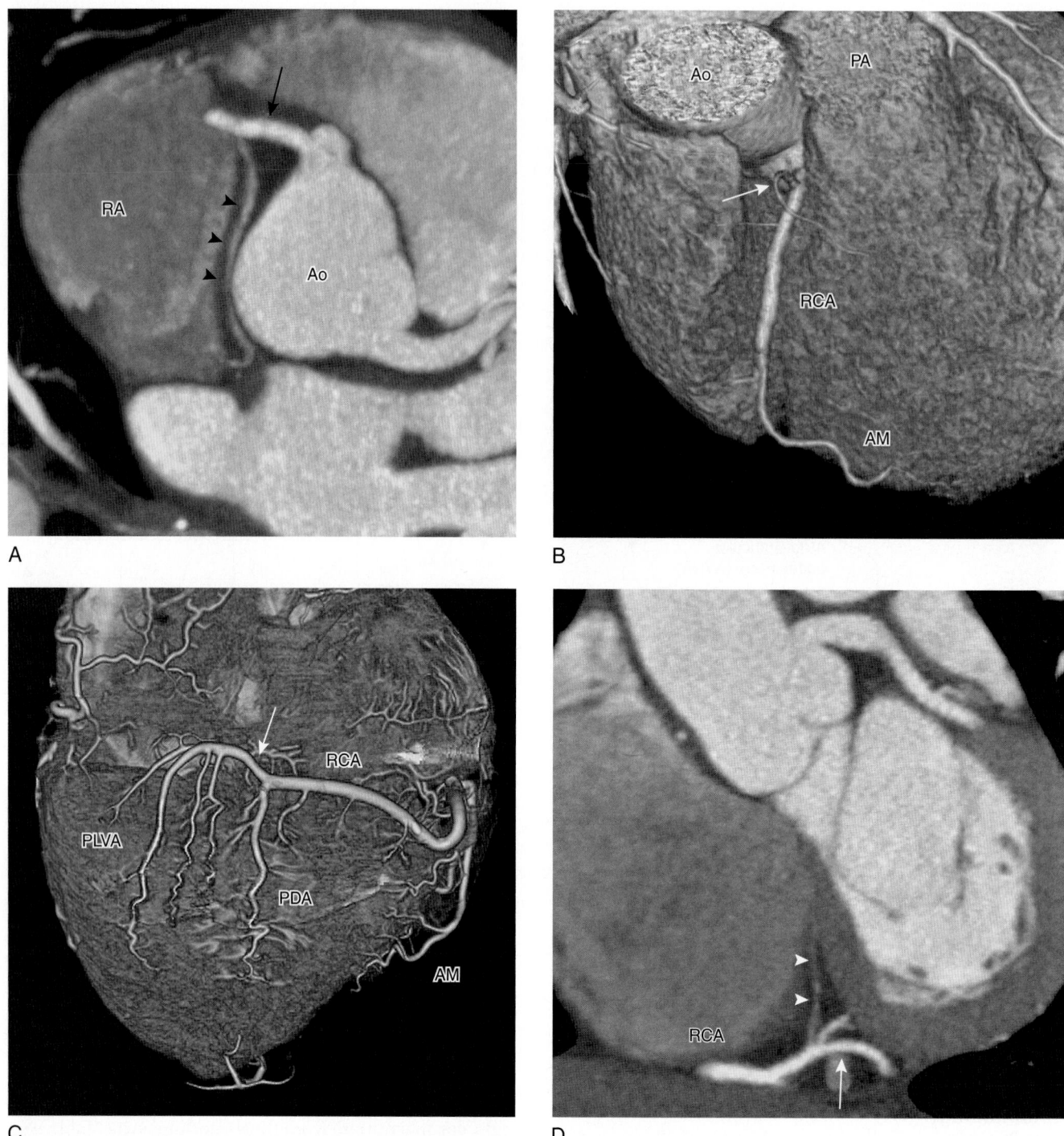

FIGURE 98-5. Major branches of the normal right coronary artery (RCA). **A,** An axial image taken with coronary CTA shows the RCA *(arrow)* originating from the aorta (Ao) and extending toward the right atrioventricular groove. It gives off a sinoatrial nodal branch *(arrowheads)* that terminates at the right atrium (RA) near the atrial septum. **B,** A volume-rendered image shows an acute marginal (AM) branch arising from the RCA at the right ventricular free wall. The conal branch *(arrow)* is the first branch of the RCA. PA, pulmonary artery; Ao, aorta. (*See color plate.*) **C,** A volume-rendered image shows the inferior surface of a heart. The RCA gives off in succession the AM branch, the posterior descending artery (PDA), and the posterior left ventricular arteries (PLVA), which lie on the left side of the crux *(arrow)*. (*See color plate.*) **D,** A short-axis view shows the RCA at the crux *(arrow)* giving off an atrioventricular nodal branch *(arrowheads)*.

whereas the interarterial course—that is, between the aorta and the pulmonary artery (Fig. 98-8)—is associated with sudden death. The prevalence of anomalous LMCA with interarterial course is estimated to be 0.03% to 0.05% of the population. Anomalous RCA with interarterial course is more common, with a prevalence estimated at

0.1%. The interarterial segment of the coronary artery may be intramural within the aortic wall, intramuscular within the myocardium, or free between the aorta and the pulmonary artery.

The association between anomalous coronary artery with interarterial course and sudden death in young

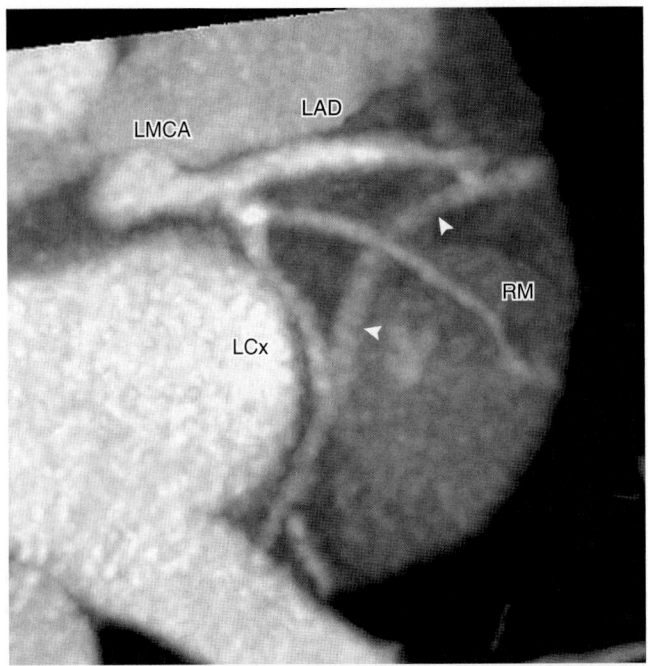

A

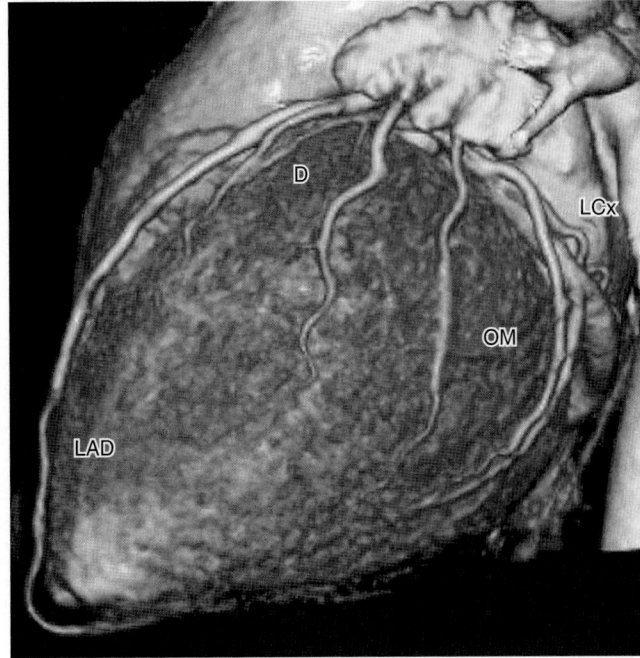

B

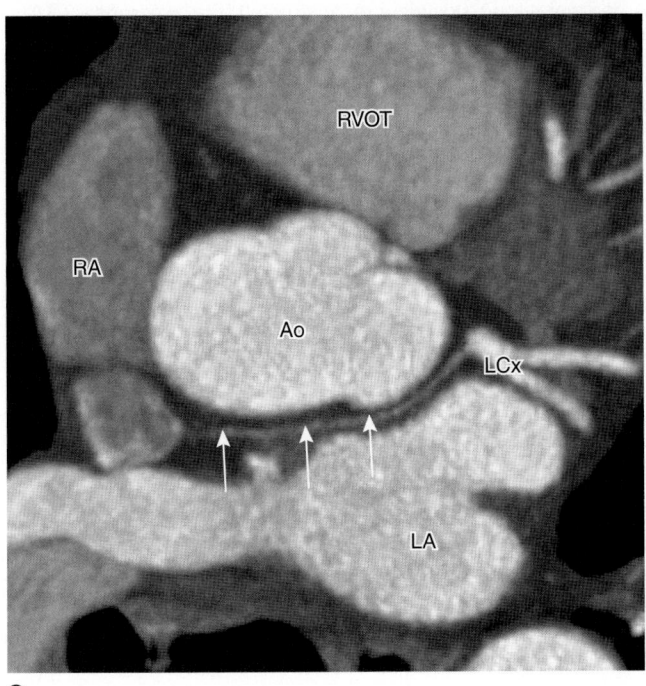

C

FIGURE 98-6. Major branches of the normal left main coronary artery (LMCA). **A,** An oblique axial image taken with coronary CTA shows the trifurcation of the LMCA into a left anterior descending (LAD) artery, a ramus medianus (RM) branch, and a left circumflex (LCx) artery. The crossing vessel *(arrowheads)* is the greater cardiac vein. **B,** A volume-rendered image shows the LAD and several diagonal (D) branches. The LAD wraps around the apex to reach the apical inferior surface. The left circumflex (LCx) artery gives off several obtuse marginal (OM) branches. *(See color plate.)* **C,** An axial image shows the LCx giving off a sinoatrial nodal branch *(arrows)* that travels behind the aorta and terminates at the right atrium (RA) near the atrial septum. Ao, aorta; LA, left atrium; RVOT, right ventricular outflow tract.

athletes was discovered in autopsy series. Sudden death in this otherwise healthy population is rare, with an incidence estimated to be 5 in 1 million people per year. Autopsy series found that the two most common cardiac causes of sudden death are hypertrophic obstructive cardiomyopathy and arrhythmogenic right ventricular dysplasia, followed by anomalous coronary artery in up to 20% of these cases. Most autopsy series report a greater number of anomalous LMCA than anomalous RCA, some by a ratio of 3:1. Given that anomalous RCA is three times more common, the autopsy results suggest that anomalous LMCA is a more lethal lesion. Mortality

rate of these lesions is unknown, because most patients have not been diagnosed and followed prospectively.

In patients with the malignant type of coronary anomalies, sudden death almost always occurs during exertion. The majority of these patients who died had no known premonitory symptoms. In about 30% of the cases, syncope or chest pain occurred within 2 years of death but resting ECG and stress ECG have been reported normal. The pathophysiology of sudden death has not been conclusively determined. A lethal arrhythmia may be triggered by transient ischemia caused by inadequate coronary flow through either the slitlike opening of

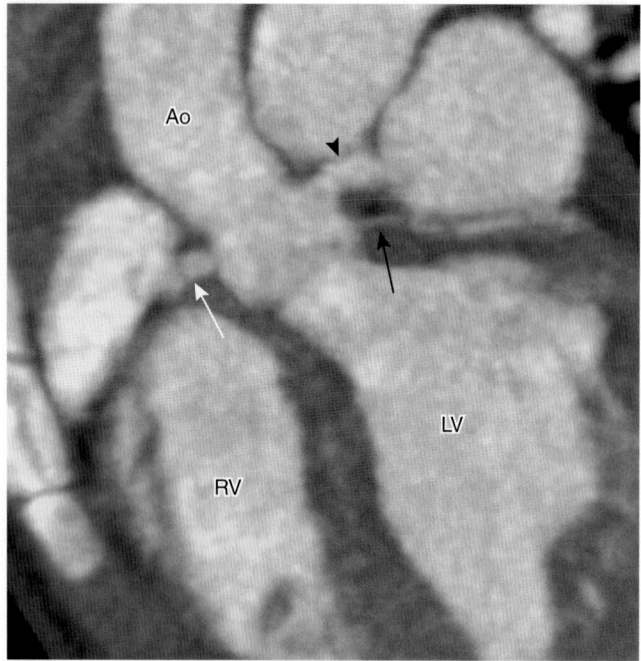

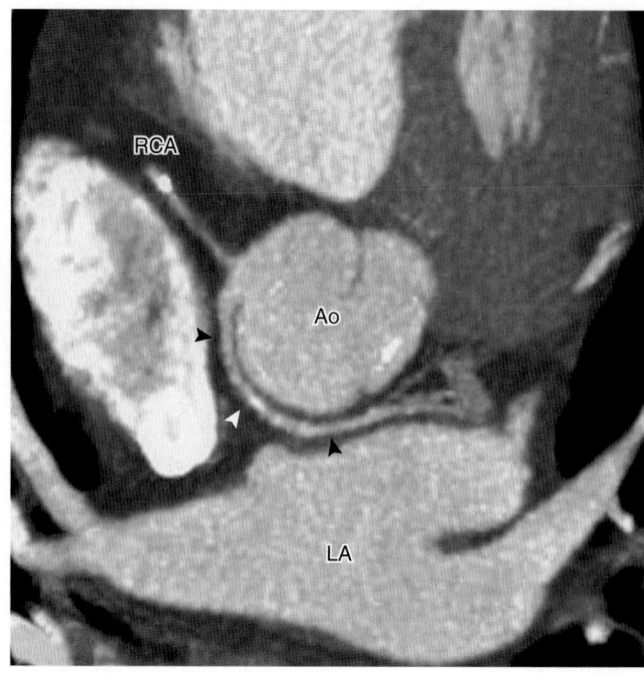

A

B

FIGURE 98-7. Common benign variants of the coronary arteries. **A,** A horizontal long-axis view reconstructed from a coronary CTA of a 1-year-old boy shows separate origins for the LAD *(arrowhead)* and the LCx *(black arrow)* arteries. The RCA *(white arrow)* is in normal position. This variant occurs in 0.41% of the population. Ao, aorta; LV, left ventricle; RV, right ventricle. **B,** A short-axis view from a 40-year-old man shows the LCx and the RCA arising separately from the right sinus. The LCx *(black and white arrowheads)* wraps around posterior to the aorta (Ao) and then enters the left atrioventricular groove. This variant occurs in 0.37% of the population. LA, left atrium.

TABLE 98-4	
Clinically Significant Coronary Artery Anomalies	
Anomaly	**Route**
Coronary artery with interarterial course	LMCA from RCA or right sinus of Valsalva
	RCA from LMCA or left sinus of Valsalva
Coronary artery from pulmonary artery (PA)	LMCA from PA (ALCAPA)
	RCA from PA (ARCAPA)
	LAD from PA
	LCx from PA
Large coronary artery fistula	*From* RCA > LAD > both
	To RV > RA > PA > LV > SVC
Coronary artery–associated cardiac anomalies	Truncus arteriosus
	Tetralogy of Fallot
	Transposition of the great arteries
	Pulmonary atresia with intact ventricular septum
	Coronary artery hypoplasia

ALCAPA, anomalous left coronary artery from the PA; ARCAPA, anomalous right coronary artery from the PA; LAD, left anterior descending; LCx, left circumflex artery; LMCA, left main coronary artery; LV, left ventricle; RA, right atrium; RCA, right coronary artery; RV, right ventricle; SVC, superior vena cava; >, greater in frequency than.

the ectopic coronary artery or the narrowed lumen compressed by the aorta and pulmonary artery.

In adolescents, echocardiography is generally not reliable for detecting anomalous coronary arteries. In the past, catheter angiography was the definitive test.

This role is now taken over by CMRA and CCTA, both having the advantage of being noninvasive. The choice between CMRA and CCTA depends on equipment capability, and size and age of the patient as discussed previously.

Because most deaths occur in patients between 10 and 30 years of age, teenagers and young adults who are diagnosed with anomalous coronary artery with interarterial course should consider surgery with the goal of preventing sudden death. Preventive surgery in patients outside this age group is controversial, as their risk of sudden death is not known. The surgical approach depends on whether the interarterial segment is intramural or free. If it is intramural, then the ostium can be surgically enlarged by unroofing the common wall between the aorta and the coronary segment. Otherwise, the coronary artery must be reimplanted or bypassed.

Coronary Artery from Pulmonary Artery

This condition includes anomalous origin of the LMCA, LAD, LCx, or RCA from the pulmonary trunk or the main branch pulmonary arteries. The most common and clinically most important type is the anomalous left coronary artery from the pulmonary artery (ALCAPA) (Fig. 98-9). The incidence is approximately 1 in 300,000 live births, accounting for 0.24% to 0.5% of congenital cardiac anomalies. Anomalous right coronary artery from the pulmonary artery (ARCAPA) is four times less common than ALCAPA. The embryology of this lesion is thought to be abnormal connection of the peritruncal capillary plexus to the pulmonary artery instead of the

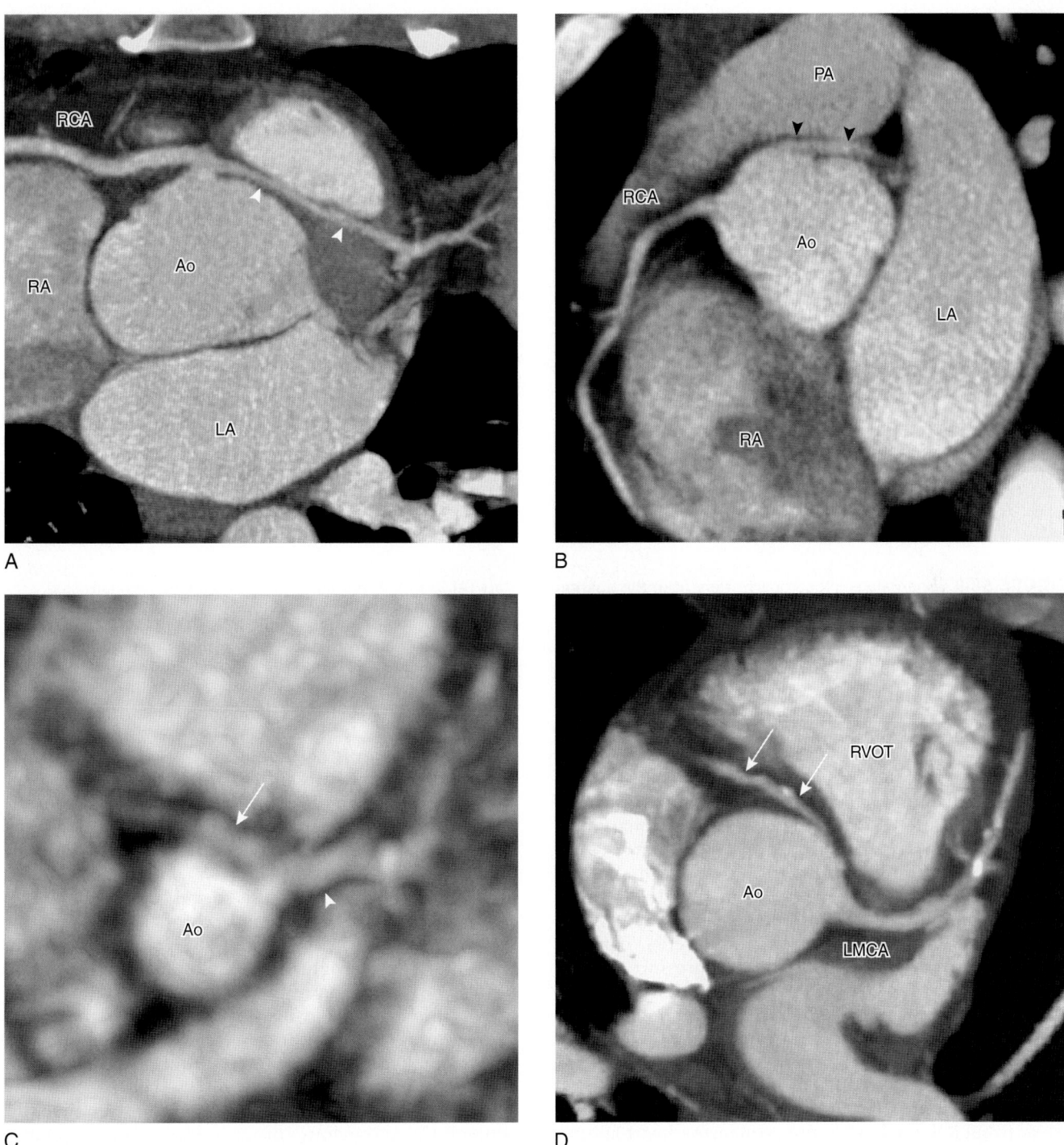

FIGURE 98-8. CT angiogram of ectopic coronary artery with interarterial course. **A,** A short-axis view from a cardiac CTA of an adult patient shows a common origin of the right coronary artery (RCA) and the left main coronary artery (LMCA) *(arrowheads)* arising from the right sinus of the aorta (Ao). The LMCA has a long segment narrowing as it travels between the aorta and the right ventricular outflow tract. LA, left atrium; RA, right atrium. **B,** In this 20-year-old man, an LMCA *(arrowheads)* originates from the right sinus separate from the RCA, then travels between the Ao and the pulmonary artery (PA). **C,** In this 6-week-old infant, the RCA *(arrow)* arises from the LMCA *(arrowhead)*. **D,** In this adult with calcific coronary plaques, an RCA *(arrows)* originates from the left sinus separate from the LMCA. A tapered narrowing is evident at the proximal, interarterial portion of the RCA.

aorta. The clinical presentation depends on how much of the coronary flow to the left ventricle is compromised.

In fetal circulation, the pulmonary artery pressure is higher than the aortic pressure because the pulmonary resistance is high. Furthermore, both the pulmonary artery and the aorta conduct oxygenated blood. Consequently, the coronary flow through the anomalous LMCA is essentially normal, and fetal development is unaffected. Immediately after birth, oxygenation in the pulmonary artery drops. The pulmonary pressure

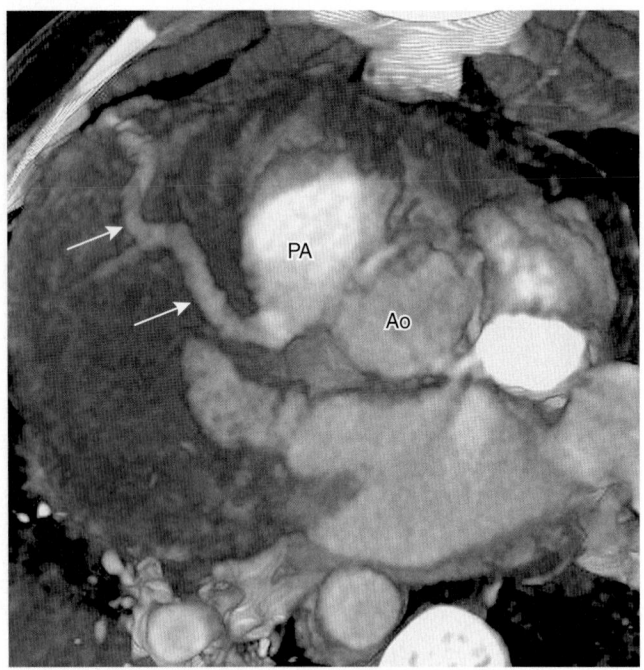

A

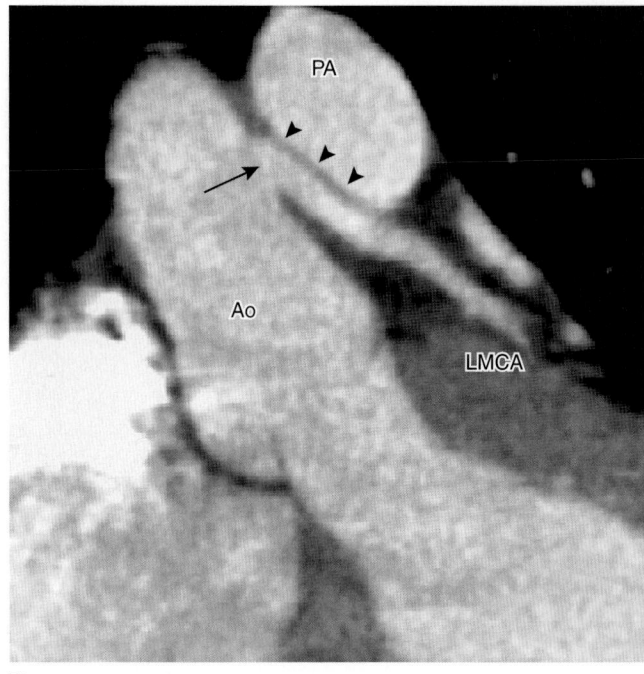

B

FIGURE 98-9. Anomalous left coronary artery from the pulmonary artery (ALCAPA). **A,** A volume-rendered image reconstructed from a routine contrast-enhanced CT shows a left anterior descending artery *(arrows)* arising from the pulmonary artery (PA) in this 17-year-old boy. The coronary artery may not be long enough to reach the aorta (Ao) for reimplantation. **B,** A coronal view from a cardiac CTA shows the result of the Takeuchi operation in a 12-year-old girl. The PA is connected to the Ao through an aortopulmonary window *(arrow)*. A surgically placed baffle *(arrowheads)* creates a channel that connects the Ao to the left main coronary artery (LMCA).

remains high as long as the pulmonary resistance is high and the ductus arteriosus is open, which allows aortic flow into the pulmonary artery. Coronary pressure in the anomalous LMCA stays high, and the coronary flow direction remains antegrade. As the pulmonary resistance drops and the ductus arteriosus closes, the pulmonary pressure and the LMCA pressure gradually drop. Flow through the LMCA slows and myocardial perfusion decreases. Eventually, the pressure difference between the high-pressure RCA and the low-pressure LMCA favors collateral flow from the RCA to the LMCA. Blood in the LMCA flows retrograde into the pulmonary artery. Coronary "steal" deprives myocardium in the LMCA territory of adequate perfusion, ensuring ischemia.

In 90% of these patients, the RCA-to-LMCA collateral flow is not enough to sustain myocardial viability. Myocardial ischemia, infarction, congestive heart failure, ventricular dilation, mitral regurgitation, and pulmonary edema develop early during the sixth to eighth week of life. This is the infantile form of ALCAPA, and the associated clinical syndrome is called the Bland-White-Garland syndrome. Without intervention, mortality can be as high as 90%. In 10% of patients with ALCAPA, collateral flow from RCA to LMCA was large enough to sustain myocardial viability. As a result of the high shunt flow, the coronary arteries can be abnormally large. These patients have few or no symptoms and survive into adulthood. This is the adult form of ALCAPA. ALCAPA is usually an isolated lesion, but it can be associated with ventricular septal defect, atrioventricular canal, tetralogy of Fallot, truncus arteriosus, and aortic stenosis.

ARCAPA, in contrast, is usually asymptomatic in the first 2 years of life and presents with exertional chest pain later in adolescence or adulthood.

For the infantile form of ALCAPA, chest radiographs usually show enlarged cardiac silhouette and signs of pulmonary venous congestion or pulmonary edema. ECG and other laboratory tests suggest myocardial ischemia and infarction. In selective coronary angiography, the catheter fails to engage the LMCA ostium. An aortogram fills a single right coronary artery in early phase, with late opacification of the LMCA and retrograde flow of contrast material into the pulmonary artery. Echocardiography can usually detect the connection between the anomalous coronary artery and the pulmonary artery, and it can visualize the reverse coronary flow by color Doppler imaging. In difficult cases, the connection between the anomalous coronary artery and the pulmonary artery can be readily seen with CCTA.

The definitive treatment is surgery. The most straightforward approach is to reimplant the anomalous coronary artery from the pulmonary artery to the aorta. With ALCAPA, reimplantation of the LMCA can be difficult because the LMCA may be too short to reach the centrally located aorta. This problem is solved by the Takeuchi procedure, in which an aortopulmonary window is created first. Then, a baffled tunnel is created inside the pulmonary trunk to connect the aortopulmonary window to the ostium of the anomalous LMCA (see Fig. 98-9). Blood flows from the aorta, through the aortopulmonary window, into the baffled tunnel, and then into the anomalous LMCA ostium.

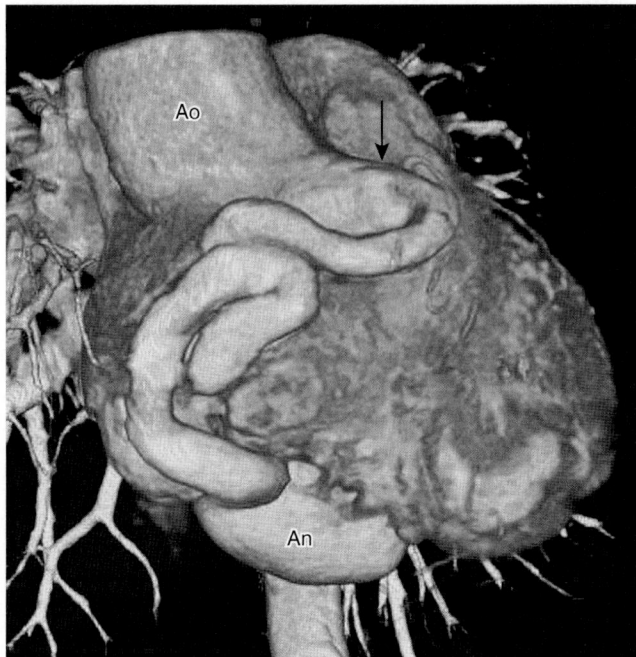

FIGURE 98-10. Coronary fistula to the right ventricle. A volume-rendered image from a coronary CTA of a 22-year-old woman shows a large and extremely tortuous right coronary artery arising *(arrow)* from the aorta (Ao). At the inferior surface of the heart, this coronary fistula connects to a giant aneurysm (An), which empties into the right ventricle (not shown). (*See color plate.*)

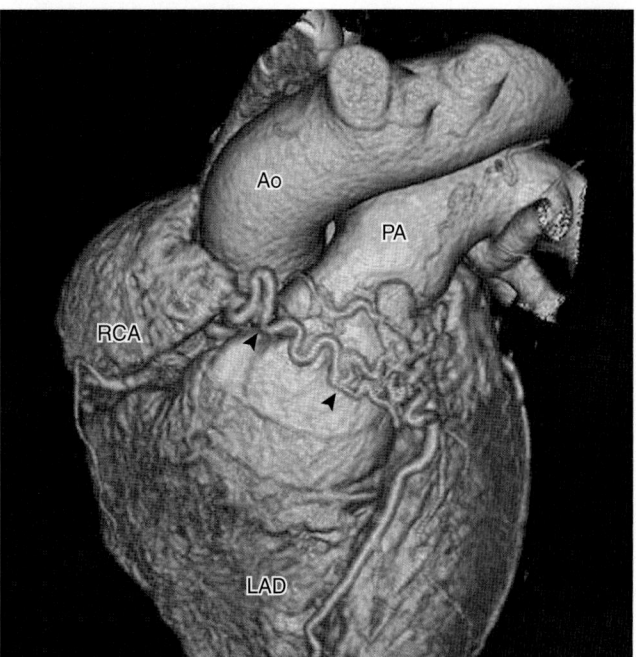

FIGURE 98-11. Coronary fistulas to the pulmonary artery. A volume-rendered image from a coronary CTA of a 30-year-old man shows multiple, small, tortuous coronary fistulas (*arrowheads*) arising from both the right coronary artery (RCA) and the left anterior descending (LAD) artery, feeding into the pulmonary artery (PA). Ao, aorta. (*See color plate.*)

Coronary Artery Fistula

Coronary artery fistula is a common coronary abnormality seen in 0.3% to 0.8% of patients referred for cardiac catheterization. It is an abnormal communication between a normal coronary artery and another cardiovascular structure. Although usually congenital, it can form after trauma or a surgical procedure such as myomectomy. Anatomically, coronary fistula most frequently originates from the RCA (55%), followed in frequency by the LAD (35%), both (5%), and others (5%). Coronary fistula terminates in the right side of the heart far more often than the left. The most common site of termination is the right ventricle (41%) (Fig. 98-10), followed by the right atrium (26%), pulmonary trunk (17%) (Fig. 98-11), left ventricle (3%), and superior vena cava (1%).

Embryologically, fistulous communication with the ventricle is thought to be caused by a failure of regression of the intra-trabecular sinusoids. Fistulous communication with the pulmonary artery may have the same cause as ALCAPA—that is, abnormal connection of the peritruncal plexus to the pulmonary artery. Coronary artery fistula usually occurs as an isolated lesion without associated cardiac anomalies. However, in pulmonary atresia with intact ventricular septum (PAIVS), coronary fistulas to the right ventricle are an integral part of the disease, with important consequences to treatment options. Coronary fistulas in PAIVS are discussed later in the context of complex congenital heart disease.

The clinical significance of a coronary artery fistula depends on the size of the fistulous communication as well as its termination site. Most fistulas are small and conduct too little flow to be clinically significant. These patients are usually asymptomatic and may have a continuous murmur. A large fistula communicating to the right side of the heart is effectively a left-to-right shunt. It behaves clinically like a ventricular septal defect (VSD) and has complications normally associated with VSD, such as endocarditis and pulmonary hypertension. In contrast, a large fistula to the left side of the heart forms a left-to-left shunt. It clinically behaves like aortic regurgitation, with signs and symptoms relating to volume overload of the left ventricle. Chronically, the left ventricle enlarges and fails, leading to symptoms of heart failure: fatigue, dyspnea, and orthopnea. In addition, a large coronary artery fistula can divert flow from myocardial perfusion enough to cause myocardial ischemia and infarction. Finally, a large coronary fistula can expand like an arterial aneurysm, and it can thrombose or rupture.

A small coronary artery fistula may be detected incidentally by screening echocardiography ordered for unexplained murmur or for unrelated symptoms. If the fistula is large, the course and connections of the fistula, as well as aneurysmal or stenotic segments, should be clearly defined with catheter angiography, CCTA, or CMRA. MRI can, in addition, quantify the shunt flow and shunt ratio using phase-contrast techniques.

Patients with fistulas of any size should be given antibiotic prophylaxis against endocarditis. For patients with shunt ratio greater than 1.5, the fistula should be closed to prevent the development of pulmonary hypertension. Some authors advocate elective closure of all fistulas to prevent myocardial ischemia, endocarditis, and aneurysm formation. Fistulas with favorable connections and shapes can be closed with catheter embolization. Otherwise, they can be closed with surgical ligation. Aneurysmal segments should be surgically reduced to prevent rupture.

Cardiac Anomalies Associated with the Coronary Artery

The prevalence of anomalous coronary artery is much greater in the presence of underlying cardiac malformation, especially conotruncal anomalies, such as truncus arteriosus, transposition of the great arteries (TGA), and tetralogy of Fallot (TOF). The origins and courses of the anomalous coronary arteries can affect important surgical decisions, especially in the repair of TOF, TGA, and PAIVS. The role of the imager is to map out the coronary pattern in relationship to other cardiovascular structures as clearly as possible to help a surgeon plan the surgical approach. Instead of describing all the possible coronary variations associated with cardiac malformations, we will attempt to explain the importance of certain coronary anomalies in the surgical repair of TOF, TGA, and PAIVS.

Tetralogy of Fallot

TOF is the most common cyanotic congenital heart disease, accounting for 10% of all congenital heart defects. The standard treatment today is early total correction between 3 and 12 months of age. The surgical repair has two components: a patch closure of the VSD, and a transannular patch augmentation of the right ventricular outflow tract (RVOT) and the pulmonary trunk. In 4% of patients with TOF, an aberrant LAD arises from the RCA and crosses anterior to the RVOT before entering the anterior interventricular septal groove (Fig. 98-12). This LAD lies in the path of the transannular incision and can be accidentally transected. If it cannot be adequately mobilized, it may prevent sufficient augmentation of the RVOT. The alternative operation is the Rastelli procedure, which calls for implantation of an extracardiac pulmonary arterial conduit between the right ventricle and the pulmonary artery, effectively jumping over the aberrant LAD. To accommodate a pulmonary arterial conduit of adequate size, the Rastelli procedure is best done later in life. This anomaly can usually be detected with echocardiography, but some institutions advocate screening catheter angiography. Today, this can be evaluated reliably with CCTA.

TRANSPOSITION OF THE GREAT ARTERIES

TGA accounts for 5% of congenital heart defects and can occur with or without ventricular inversion. The uncorrected TGA is associated with normal ventricular position (D-loop) and dextropositions of the great arteries (D-TGA) (Fig. 98-13). It is uncorrected in the sense that the systemic circulation is uncoupled from the pulmonary circulation. The congenitally corrected TGA is associated with ventricular inversion (L-loop) and levopositions of the great arteries (L-TGA) (see Fig. 98-13). The circulation of oxygenated and unoxygenated blood is correct but the aorta is pumped by the right ventricle

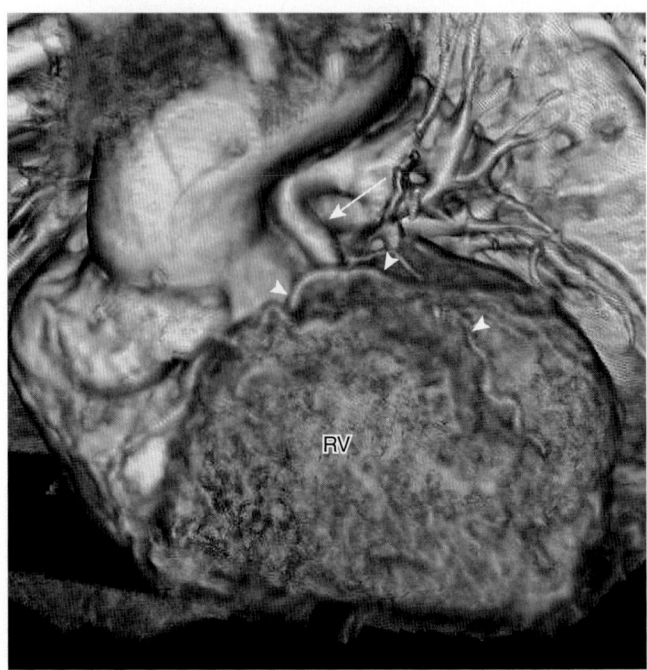

FIGURE 98-12. Aberrant left anterior descending (LAD) artery in tetralogy of Fallot. A volume-rendered image from a 1-year-old boy viewed from the front shows an LAD *(arrowheads)* that travels in front of the stenotic pulmonary trunk *(black arrow).* The position of this LAD may complicate the surgical repair. RV, right ventricle. (*See color plate.*)

and the pulmonary artery is pumped by the left ventricle. Uncorrected TGA is nearly 10 times more common than corrected TGA.

Because the two types of TGA have very different physiologies, they have different clinical presentations and treatment approaches. For uncorrected TGA, patients usually present early with cyanosis. The severity of the cyanosis is dictated by the degree of mixing between oxygenated and deoxygenated blood at the atrial and ventricular levels. The preferred surgical treatment for uncorrected TGA is the arterial switch, or Jatene operation. This is a definitive operation in which the aorta and the pulmonary trunk are surgically transposed, thereby returning the circulatory anatomy to "normal." In this operation, the coronary arteries also have to be reimplanted from the aortic sinuses to the pulmonary sinuses. In normal truncal anatomy, the left and right coronary arteries arise from the aortic sinuses closest to the pulmonary trunk. This relationship is usually preserved even when the aorta and the pulmonary trunk are congenitally transposed. The close proximity of the coronary origins from both great arteries makes surgical translocation of the coronary arteries possible. However, there are variations of coronary origin and course that make this operation difficult or even impossible. Therefore, knowledge of this anatomy before surgery is enormously beneficial.

For congenitally corrected TGA, symptoms are usually mild, depending on coexisting cardiac defects, such as VSD and ventricular outflow obstruction. These patients do have a shortened life span, because they develop right ventricular failure early in their third or fourth decade

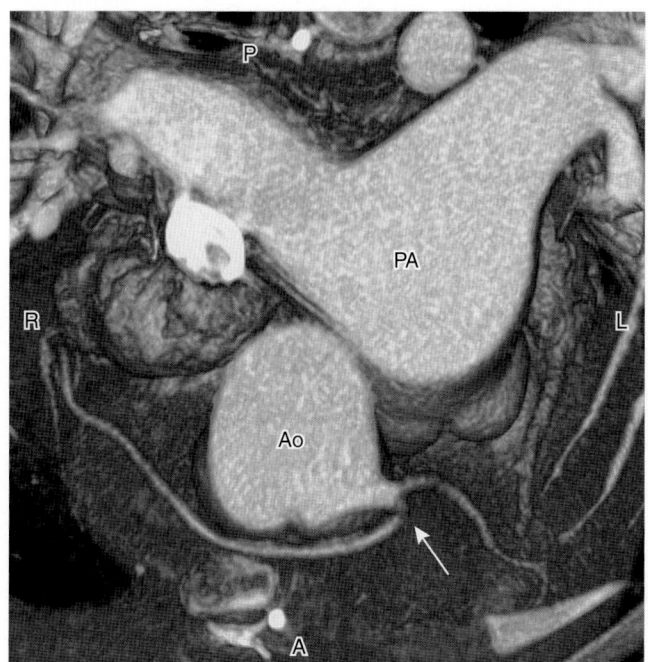

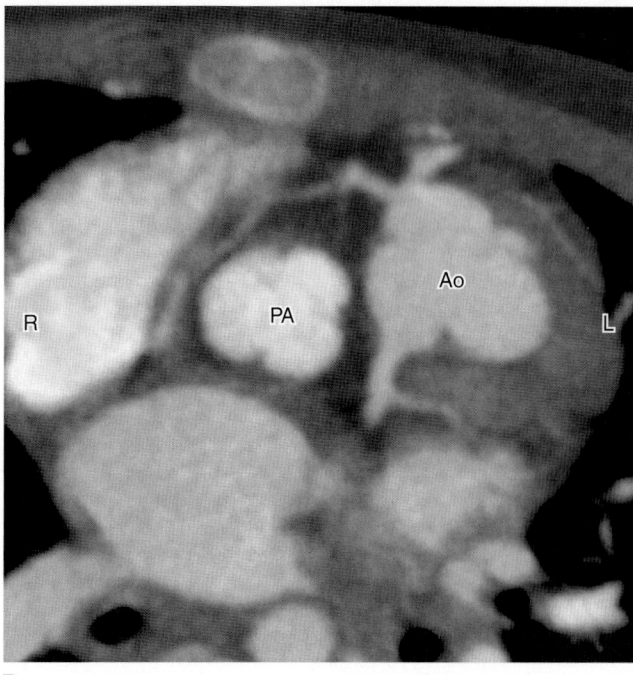

A   B

FIGURE 98-13. Coronary artery arrangements in transposition of the great arteries (TGA). **A,** A volume-rendered image from a coronary CTA of a 12-year-old girl shows an aorta (Ao) that is situated in front and to the right of the pulmonary artery (PA), consistent with a D-TGA. There is a single coronary ostium *(arrow),* and the right coronary artery courses in front of the Ao. This is not a favorable coronary pattern for the arterial switch operation. A, anterior patent; P, posterior patent. (*See color plate.*) **B,** An axial image shows an aorta (Ao) that is situated in front and to the left of the pulmonary artery (PA), consistent with an L-TGA. The coronary arteries arise from the aortic sinuses facing the PA, which is a normal pattern.

of life. Causes of right ventricular failure are many, but in general terms, it seems that the right ventricle is not optimized to handle life-long, systemic pressures. For this reason, some clinicians have advocated for the "double switch" operation, which combines the arterial switch (Jatene) operation with the atrial switch (Mustard-Senning) operation. The double switch operation returns the systemic load to the left ventricle and the pulmonary load to the right ventricle. The feasibility of this operation depends on the feasibility of the arterial switch component, which in turn depends on favorable coronary arterial anatomy. Again, knowledge of the coronary anatomy is very important.

PULMONARY ATRESIA WITH INTACT VENTRICULAR SEPTUM

PAIVS is a rare anomaly accounting for 1% to 1.5% of all congenital heart defects. This lesion is thought to be caused by the in utero obstruction of the pulmonary valve after the formation of the pulmonary infundibulum and the central pulmonary arteries. The reduced right ventricular flow prevents the normal growth of the right ventricle and the tricuspid valve, causing hypoplasia of both structures. Without outlet flow, the right ventricular pressure can rise above the left ventricular pressure and the coronary arterial pressure, impeding normal coronary flow in the myocardium of the right ventricle. This, in turn, disrupts the normal regression of the intratrabecular sinusoids, resulting in coronary fistulas to the right ventricle in 75% of the patients at birth.

After birth, the right ventricular pressure remains high and blood flows from the right ventricle into the coronary system. If the right ventricle is decompressed, for example by surgically relieving the pulmonary obstruction, blood flow in the coronary fistulas abruptly reverses, shunting blood away from the myocardium into the right ventricle, leading to myocardial ischemia and infarction. Normal coronary circulation, then, depends on a pressurized right ventricle. This, in turn, precludes surgery that restores the right ventricle to a functioning pump for the pulmonary circulation. A right-ventricle–dependent coronary circulation is suggested by the presence of coronary fistulas seen on catheter angiography. Classic findings on coronary angiography include systolic retrograde filling of the RCA and the LAD during right ventriculography (Fig. 98-14), and end-diastolic filling of the right ventricle during coronary angiography. This type of coronary fistula can be readily seen in CCTA, although its role in the management of PAIVS has yet to be defined.

Coronary Artery Hypoplasia

Coronary artery hypoplasia (CAH) is a rare condition characterized by diffusely narrowed, underdeveloped major coronary segment or branch. The prevalence of CAH is estimated at 0.03% based on adult coronary angiography, and at 6% of all coronary anomalies. Most reported cases involved the left coronary system (Fig. 98-15). The pathogenesis of this lesion is unknown, but an in utero embolic event to a coronary artery is a possibility. The clinical significance of CAH is also unknown. In a few cases, it was related to sudden death,

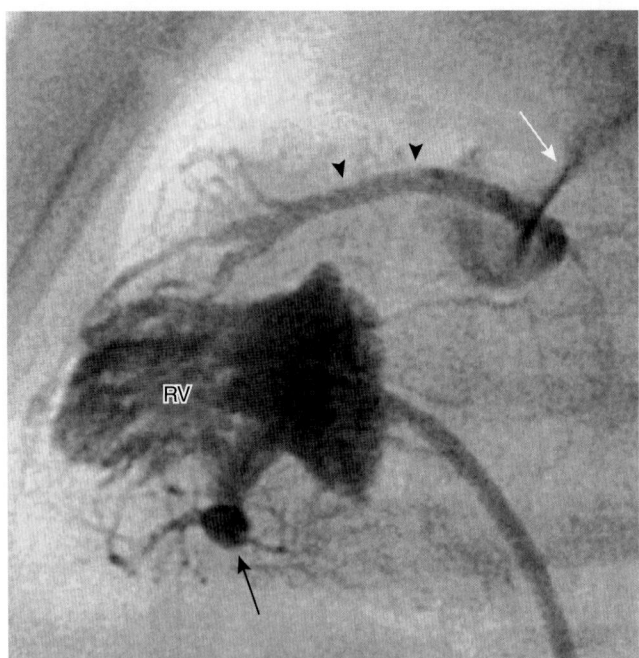

FIGURE 98-14. A catheter angiography of the right ventricle of a 1-year-old boy with pulmonary atresia and an intact ventricular septum. Contrast material injected into the right ventricle *(RV)* flows through the sinusoids *(black arrow)* into the coronary arterial system *(arrowheads)*, and then flows retrograde out the pulmonary artery *(white arrow)*. This coronary circulation is judged right-ventricular dependent.

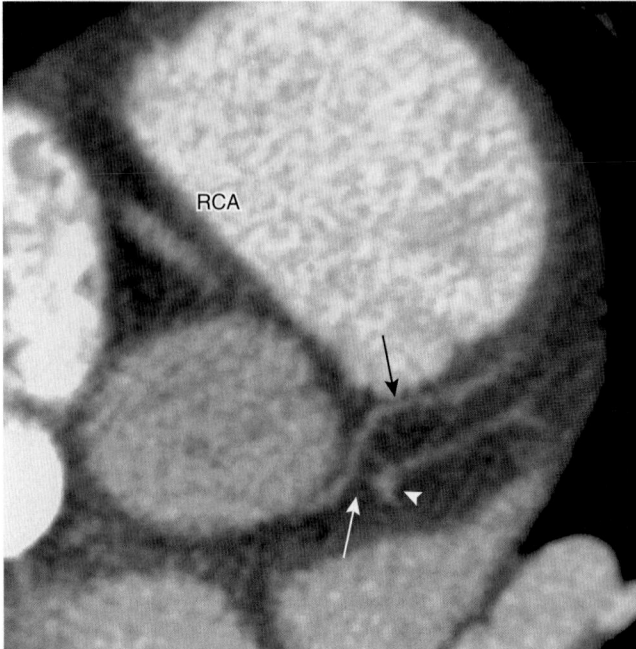

FIGURE 98-15. Coronary artery hypoplasia in a 15-year-old girl with exertional angina. An axial view from a coronary CTA shows diffusely small left coronary arteries compared with the right coronary artery *(RCA)*. The left circumflex artery *(arrowhead)* is occluded *(white arrow)* from the left main coronary artery *(black arrow)*.

but other individuals with this anomaly led normal lives and were diagnosed at autopsy after dying from unrelated causes. CCTA can be used to visualize the threadlike epicardial coronary artery. However, catheter angiography is needed to delineate all collateral vessels. The optimal treatment has not been determined, but in CAH patients with documented arrhythmia or syncope, defibrillator implantation would be a prudent choice.

ACQUIRED CORONARY ARTERY DISEASES

Kawasaki Disease

Kawasaki disease (KD), or mucocutaneous lymph node syndrome, was first described by Tomisaku Kawasaki in 1967. It is an acute, febrile, multisystem vasculitis of unknown etiology that affects primarily children less than 5 years of age, with a slight male predominance. It is most common in Japan, although the number of cases in the United States is increasing. The number of children hospitalized for KD is estimated to be 3000 per year in the United States. KD is the most common acquired coronary artery disease in children. Diagnosis is made by clinical characteristics of prolonged high fever, conjunctivitis, red cracked lips, red oral mucous membrane, strawberry tongue, multiform rash, cervical lymphadenopathy, erythema of the palms and the soles, swollen hands and feet, and desquamation around fingers and toes 1 to 2 weeks after the onset of symptoms. The disease is usually self-limiting, although recurrence has been seen in 3% of the patients.

Diagnostic criteria for Kawasaki disease:

- **Fever persists for 5 days or more, and four of the following findings:**
  - **Changes in the hands and feet: erythema, edema, desquamation**
  - **Bilateral conjunctivitis**
  - **Multiform rash**
  - **Cervical lymphadenopathy**
  - **Oral changes: cracked lips, red mucous membrane, strawberry tongue**

The most important complication of KD is the development of coronary artery aneurysm (Fig. 98-16). Among patients who did not receive gamma globulin therapy, 15% to 30% develop coronary artery aneurysm, usually 1 to 4 weeks after disease onset. In multiple studies, it has been shown that intravenous gamma globulin therapy lowers the risk of aneurysm formation to 5%. High-dose aspirin is used as adjunctive therapy during the acute phase to lower coagulation activation. Thromboembolism of coronary artery aneurysm (see Fig. 98-16) and coronary artery stenosis are the causes of myocardial ischemia, infarction, heart failure, and sudden death. Expanding aneurysm may also rupture. In 1970, the mortality rate of KD was 2%, mostly from cardiac complications, but as a result of treatment improvements, it has dropped to 0.1%.

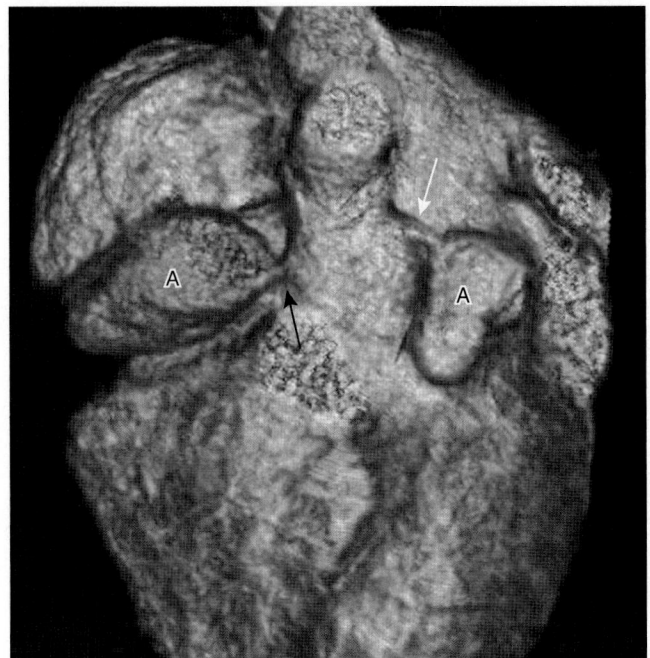
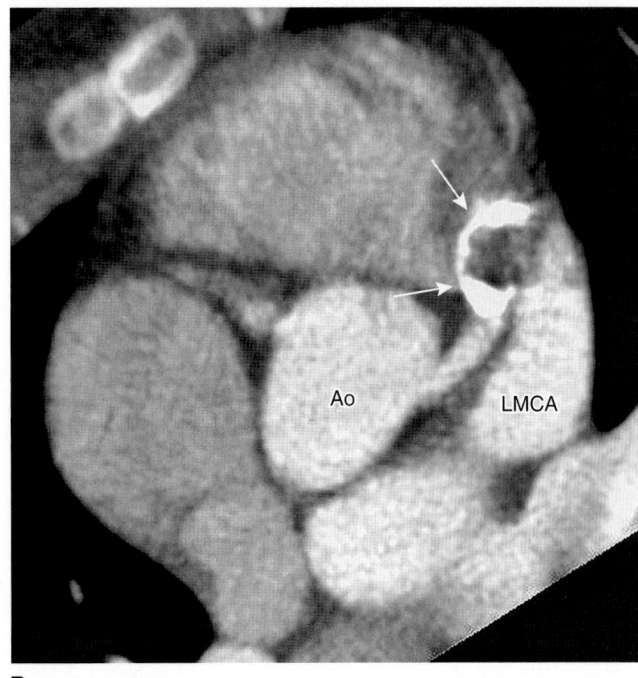

FIGURE 98-16. Kawasaki disease. **A,** A volume-rendered image from a coronary CTA in a 2-year-old girl shows large fusiform aneurysms (A) in both the right coronary artery (*black arrow*) and the left main coronary artery (*white arrow*). (*See color plate.*) **B,** An axial image from another coronary CTA shows chronic changes of Kawasaki disease, which include calcified, thrombosed aneurysm *(arrows)* in the left main coronary artery *(LMCA)*. Ao, aorta.

Echocardiography is the mainstay imaging tool in KD. In young children, it is quite effective in detecting coronary aneurysms. Giant aneurysm (>8 mm in diameter) is associated with increased risk of myocardial infarction and sudden death. Echocardiography is less effective in older children and young adults, and serial angiography is needed to monitor progression of aneurysm and development of stenosis. Cardiac CT may be a useful, noninvasive alternative for this purpose, and its efficacy is being investigated. MRI is useful in the assessment of myocardial infarction and ventricular function.

Behçet Disease

Behçet disease (BD) is a multisystem inflammatory disease of unknown cause. Classically, BD describes a syndrome of recurrent aphthous ulcers, genital ulceration, and uveitis. The vascular system is involved in 10% to 40% of the cases. Its prevalence in the United States is 5 cases per 100,000 people, but BD is 20 times more common in Turkey and Middle Eastern countries. Although BD is typically an adult disease, onset in childhood is well recognized. The mean age of diagnosis is 12 years in one pediatric series.

Vasculitis associated with BD is unusual in that it can affect both the arterial and the venous system, and both the systemic and the pulmonary arteries. Arterial pathology is typically aneurysm and stenosis formation, whereas venous pathology is commonly thrombosis. Vascular manifestation of BD usually affects the abdominal aorta and its branches, but rare cases of coronary artery involvement have been reported. As in Kawasaki disease, BD-related coronary artery aneurysm, thrombosis, and stenosis have led to myocardial ischemia and infarction.

Catheter angiography has been the principal imaging technique for the assessment of the coronary lesions and their follow-up. More recently, BD-related aneurysm has been demonstrated by CCTA (Fig. 98-17). MRI is useful in determining the extent of myocardial infarction and the global ventricular function.

Trauma

Trauma to the chest is relatively common in children, although few reported injuries are specific to the coronary arteries. The most common cause of pediatric trauma is blunt trauma from motor vehicle accident, although in urban areas penetrating injuries from assaults and other violence occur not infrequently. Blunt injury to the coronary artery can cause intimal tear, dissection, and acute thrombosis, leading to myocardial infarction and arrhythmia. Both blunt and penetrating injury can cause rupture of the coronary arteries, resulting in hemorrhage, tamponade, and myocardial infarction. Commotio cordis, or concussion of the heart, has led to dramatic sudden death in otherwise healthy children during play. The pathophysiology is not known, but postulated mechanisms include ventricular fibrillation brought on by mechanical shock to the myocardium during its vulnerable repolarization period, or by myocardial ischemia resulting from coronary vasospasm or dissection. Chronically, the weakened or ruptured coronary vessel wall can form a pseudoaneurysm. Traumatic coronary artery fistulas to the ventricles have been reported. The infarcted or contused myocardium can become aneurysmal (Fig. 98-18), and if the injury to myocardium is extensive, heart failure can result.

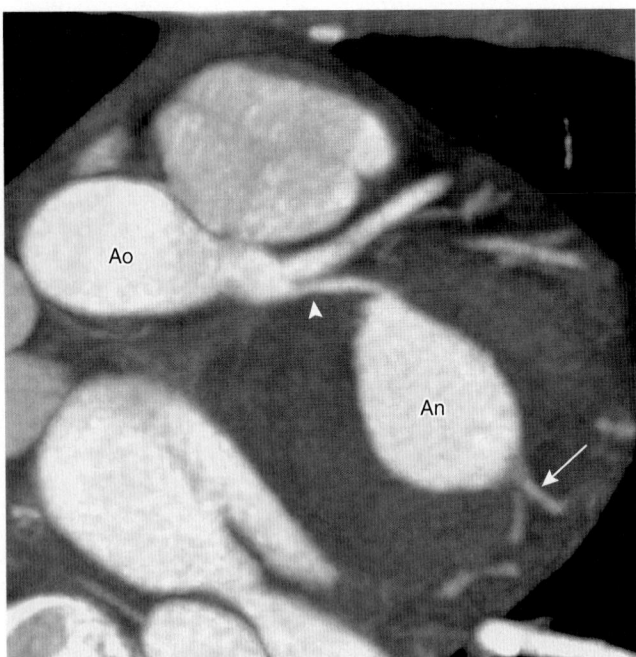

FIGURE 98-17. Coronary aneurysm associated with Behçet disease in a 14-year-old boy. This axial image from a coronary CTA shows a large aneurysm *(An)* supplied by the left circumflex artery *(arrowhead)* with outlet flows *(arrow)* to coronary branches of the lateral wall. The aneurysm has a concentric layer of intraluminal thrombus. Ao, aorta.

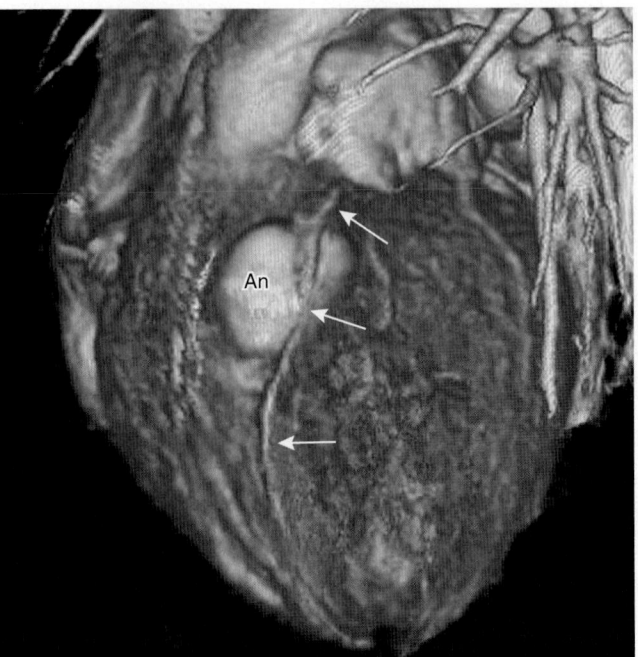

FIGURE 98-18. Ventricular aneurysm *(An)* from blunt trauma to the chest of a 13-year-old boy during a motor vehicle accident. An aneurysm developed at the anterior interventricular septum in close proximity to the left anterior descending artery *(arrows)*. (*See color plate.*)

The initial management of chest trauma focuses on more common lethal injuries such as airway compromise, pneumothorax, aortic rupture, and tamponade. Conventional CTA is now routinely performed to evaluate for these. If signs of cardiac injury, such as abnormal ECG, hemodynamic instability, and elevated myocardial enzymes, are found, echocardiography is performed to evaluate wall motion abnormality, abnormal valvular function, myocardial hematoma, and pericardial effusion or blood. To assess acute injury of the coronary artery, catheter angiography is the imaging modality of choice. Less acutely, CCTA can be used to assess structural damages in the heart, such as traumatic VSD and myocardial aneurysm. MRI is useful for the evaluation of myocardial infarction and ventricular functions.

Management of traumatic coronary artery injuries depends on the type of injury and the degree and extent of myocardial compromise. Initial management should focus on the preservation of viable myocardium. Acutely, dissection, intimal flap, and stenosis of the coronary artery can be stented to maintain coronary patency. Aneurysm of the coronary artery and traumatic coronary fistula, as well as secondary damages in the heart, such as ventricular aneurysm, VSD, and injured valves, require surgical repair.

TREATMENT COMPLICATIONS INVOLVING CORONARY ARTERIES

Surgical manipulation of the coronary arteries always carries the risk of postsurgical stenosis or occlusion of the arteries. Indeed, this was a concern during the early

surgical experience with the arterial switch operation. Other pediatric cardiac operations that affect the coronary arteries are reimplantation of anomalous coronary artery, Takeuchi operation for ALCAPA, surgical augmentation for supravalvular aortic stenosis (Fig. 98-19), composite valve-graft repair (Bentall procedure) for Marfan aortic aneurysm, and aortic valve replacement with autologous pulmonary valve (Ross procedure). Connective tissue disease, such as Marfan syndrome, can develop aneurysm at the coronary ostia after the Bentall procedure. Finally, radiation therapy that includes the aortic root in the radiation mantle causes accelerated atherosclerosis and stenoses of the proximal coronary arteries and the coronary ostia. Symptoms occur typically a decade or more after treatment.

METABOLIC DISEASES AFFECTING THE CORONARY ARTERY

Familial Hypercholesterolemia

Familial hypercholesterolemia (FH) is an autosomal dominant disorder that causes severe elevations in total cholesterol and low-density lipoprotein (LDL). It is caused by mutations in the LDL receptor gene in chromosome 19. The prevalence of the heterozygous form of FH is 1 in 500 people, and the prevalence of homozygous FH is 1 in 1 million people. Children with the heterozygous form usually are asymptomatic. Children with the rare but clinically much more severe homozygous form present with early atherosclerosis of their coronary arteries, leading to acute myocardial

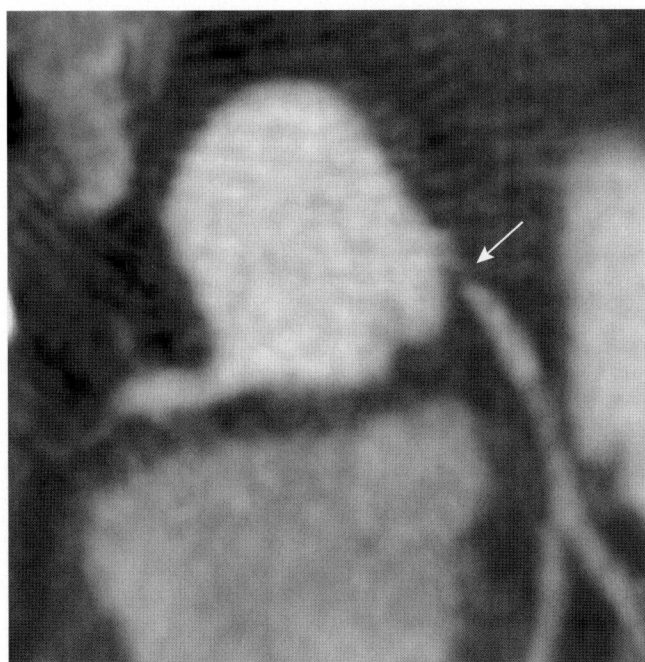

FIGURE 98-19. This 12-year-old girl with Williams syndrome had a supravalvular aortic stenosis surgically repaired. An oblique axial view from a cardiac CTA shows a focal stenosis *(arrow)* at the ostium of the left main coronary artery. The patient has developed sufficient collateral flow to be asymptomatic.

infarction and sudden death at as young as 1 to 2 years of age. They also develop peripheral vascular disease, cerebrovascular disease, aortic stenosis, cutaneous xanthomas, corneal arcus, and an LDL level of greater than 600 mg/dl. The role of imaging, except for echocardiography screening for aortic stenosis, has not been defined for this rare disease. The mainstay of treatment is aggressive cholesterol-lowering medical therapy and treatments of atherosclerosis-related complications. Because FH is a disease of a defective LDL receptor in the liver, liver transplant has been attempted as a curative procedure.

Coronary Calcinosis

Coronary calcification in children is rare, but it can occur in chronic vasculitis, usually Kawasaki disease, radiation, end-stage renal disease, and type I diabetes mellitus. Coronary calcification can be seen as part of idiopathic infantile arterial calcification (IIAC), a very rare disease characterized by extensive depositions of hydroxyapatite in the elastic layer of the large and medium-size muscular arteries, including the coronary arteries. Coronary stenosis is caused by intimal proliferation, and the patients with IIAC suffer myocardial infarction in infancy. Similarly, renal artery stenosis causes hypertension, and carotid stenosis causes cerebral infarction. Patients rarely survive beyond infancy, and many die prenatally. Diagnosis is made by radiologic demonstration of diffuse arterial calcifications, arterial biopsy, or prenatal ultrasound demonstrating dilated cardiac ventricles, hydrops fetalis, and hyperechogenic large vessels. Treatment is etidronate, which inhibits calcific mineralization in

addition to inhibiting bone resorption. Regression of arterial calcification has been shown after treatment, but vascular stenoses may not resolve.

SUGGESTED READINGS

General

De WD, Vercruysse T, Suys B, et al: Major coronary anomalies in childhood. Eur J Pediatr 2002;161:637-642

Frommelt PC, Frommelt MA: Congenital coronary artery anomalies. Pediatr Clin North Am 2004;51:1273-1288

Kruskal JB, Hartnell GG: Nonatherosclerotic coronary artery disease: more than just stenosis. Radiographics 1995;15:383-396

Liberthson RR: Sudden death from cardiac causes in children and young adults. N Engl J Med 1996;334:1039-1044

Ogden JA: Congenital anomalies of the coronary arteries. Am J Cardiol 1970;25:474-479

Werner B, Wroblewska-Kaluzewska M, Pleskot M, et al: Anomalies of the coronary arteries in children. Med Sci Monit 2001;7:1285-1291

Imaging

Dawn B, Talley JD, Prince CR, et al: Two-dimensional and Doppler transesophageal echocardiographic delineation and flow characterization of anomalous coronary arteries in adults. J Am Soc Echocardiogr 2003;16:1274-1286

Fernandes F, Alam M, Smith S, Khaja F: The role of transesophageal echocardiography in identifying anomalous coronary arteries. Circulation 1993;88:2532-2540

Goo HW, Park IS, Ko JK, et al: Computed tomography for the diagnosis of congenital heart disease in pediatric and adult patients. Int J Cardiovasc Imaging 2005;21:347-365

Levin DC, Fellows KE, Abrams HL: Hemodynamically significant primary anomalies of the coronary arteries: angiographic aspects. Circulation 1978;58:25-34

Prakash A, Powell AJ, Krishnamurthy R, Geva T: Magnetic resonance imaging evaluation of myocardial perfusion and viability in congenital and acquired pediatric heart disease. Am J Cardiol 2004;93:657-661

Welker M, Salanitri J, Deshpande VS, et al: Coronary artery anomalies diagnosed by magnetic resonance angiography. Australas Radiol 2006;50:114-121

Epidemiology

Aydinlar A, Cicek D, Senturk T, et al: Primary congenital anomalies of the coronary arteries: a coronary arteriographic study in Western Turkey. Int Heart J 2005;46:97-103

Donaldson RM, Raphael MJ, Yacoub MH, Ross DN: Hemodynamically significant anomalies of the coronary arteries: surgical aspects. Thorac Cardiovasc Surg 1982;30:7-13

Engel HJ, Torres C, Page HL: Major variations in anatomical origin of the coronary arteries: angiographic observations in 4,250 patients without associated congenital heart disease. Cathet Cardiovasc Diagn 1975;1:157

Gol MK, Ozatik MA, Kunt A, et al: Coronary artery anomalies in adult patients. Med Sci Monit 2002;8:CR636-CR641

Harikrishnan S, Jacob SP, Tharakan J, et al: Congenital coronary anomalies of origin and distribution in adults: a coronary arteriographic study. Indian Heart J 2002;54:271-275

Kardos A, Babai L, Rudas L, et al: Epidemiology of congenital coronary artery anomalies: a coronary arteriography study on a central European population. Cathet Cardiovasc Diagn 1997;42:270-275

Rigatelli G, Docali G, Rossi P, et al: Congenital coronary artery anomalies: angiographic classification revisited. Int J Cardiovasc Imaging 2003;19:361-366

Yamanaka O, Hobbs RE: Coronary artery anomalies in 126,595 patients undergoing coronary arteriography. Cathet Cardiovasc Diagn 1990;21:28-40

Coronary Artery with Interarterial Course

Basso C, Maron BJ, Corrado D, Thiene G: Clinical profile of congenital coronary artery anomalies with origin from the wrong aortic sinus leading to sudden death in young competitive athletes. J Am Coll Cardiol 2000;35:1493-1501

Bekedam MA, Vliegen HW, Doornbos J, et al: Diagnosis and

management of anomalous origin of the right coronary artery from the left coronary sinus. Int J Card Imaging 1999;15:253-258

Frescura C, Basso C, Thiene G, et al: Anomalous origin of coronary arteries and risk of sudden death: a study based on an autopsy population of congenital heart disease. Hum Pathol 1998; 29:689-695

Frommelt PC, Frommelt MA, Tweddell JS, Jaquiss RD: Prospective echocardiographic diagnosis and surgical repair of anomalous origin of a coronary artery from the opposite sinus with an interarterial course. J Am Coll Cardiol 2003;42:148-154

Kragel AH, Roberts WC: Anomalous origin of either the right or left main coronary artery from the aorta with subsequent coursing between aorta and pulmonary trunk: analysis of 32 necropsy cases. Am J Cardiol 1988;62:771-777

Roberts WC, Siegel RJ, Zipes DP: Origin of the right coronary artery from the left sinus of Valsalva and its functional consequences: analysis of 10 necropsy patients. Am J Cardiol 1982;49:863-868

Coronary Artery from Pulmonary Artery

Driscoll DJ, Garson A Jr, McNamara DG: Anomalous origin of the left coronary artery from the right pulmonary artery associated with complex congenital heart disease. Cathet Cardiovasc Diagn 1982;8:55-61

Takenaga M, Matsuda J, Miyamoto N, et al: Magnetic resonance imaging of Bland-White-Garland syndrome: a case of anomalous origin of the left coronary artery from the pulmonary trunk in a 22-year-old woman. Jpn Circ J 1998;62:219-221

Wilcox WD, Hagler DJ, Lie JT, et al: Anomalous origin of left coronary artery from pulmonary artery in association with intracardiac lesions: report of two cases. J Thorac Cardiovasc Surg 1979;78:12-20

Coronary Artery Fistula

Carrel T, Tkebuchava T, Jenni R, et al: Congenital coronary fistulas in children and adults: diagnosis, surgical technique and results. Cardiology 1996;87:325-330

Gillebert C, Van Hoof R, Van de Werf F, et al: Coronary artery fistulas in an adult population. Eur Heart J 1986;7:437-443

Gowda RM, Vasavada BC, Khan IA: Coronary artery fistulas: clinical and therapeutic considerations. Int J Cardiol 2006;107:7-10

Said SA, Landman GH: Coronary-pulmonary fistula: long-term follow-up in operated and non-operated patients. Int J Cardiol 1990;27:203-210

Schumacher G, Roithmaier A, Lorenz HP, et al: Congenital coronary artery fistula in infancy and childhood: diagnostic and therapeutic aspects. Thorac Cardiovasc Surg 1997;45:287-294

Sercelik A, Mavi A, Ayalp R, et al: Congenital coronary artery fistulas in Turkish patients undergoing diagnostic cardiac angiography. Int J Clin Pract 2003;57:280-283

Vavuranakis M, Bush CA, Boudoulas H: Coronary artery fistulas in adults: incidence, angiographic characteristics, natural history. Cathet Cardiovasc Diagn 1995;35:116-120

Coronary Artery Associated with Cardiac Anomalies

Berry JM Jr, Einzig S, Krabill KA, Bass JL: Evaluation of coronary artery anatomy in patients with tetralogy of Fallot by two-dimensional echocardiography. Circulation 1988;78:149-156

Chiu IS, Chu SH, Wang JK, et al: Evolution of coronary artery pattern according to short-axis aortopulmonary rotation: a new categorization for complete transposition of the great arteries. J Am Coll Cardiol 1995;26:250-258

Dabizzi RP, Barletta GA, Caprioli G, et al: Coronary artery anatomy in corrected transposition of the great arteries. J Am Coll Cardiol 1988;12:486-491

Dabizzi RP, Caprioli G, Aiazzi L, et al: Distribution and anomalies of coronary arteries in tetralogy of Fallot. Circulation 1980;61:95-102

Giglia TM, Mandell VS, Connor AR, et al: Diagnosis and management of right ventricle-dependent coronary circulation in pulmonary atresia with intact ventricular septum. Circulation 1992; 86:1516-1528

Gremmels DB, Tacy TA, Brook MM, Silverman NH: Accuracy of coronary artery anatomy using two-dimensional echocardiography in d-transposition of great arteries using a two-reviewer method. J Am Soc Echocardiogr 2004;17:454-460

Ismat FA, Baldwin HS, Karl TR, Weinberg PM: Coronary anatomy in congenitally corrected transposition of the great arteries. Int J Cardiol 2002;86:207-216

Jureidini SB, Appleton RS, Nouri S: Detection of coronary artery abnormalities in tetralogy of Fallot by two-dimensional echocardiography. J Am Coll Cardiol 1989;14:960-967

McMahon CJ, el Said HG, Feltes TF, et al: Preoperative identification of coronary arterial anatomy in complete transposition, and outcome after the arterial switch operation. Cardiol Young 2002;12:240-247

Pasquini L, Parness IA, Colan SD, et al: Diagnosis of intramural coronary artery in transposition of the great arteries using two-dimensional echocardiography. Circulation 1993;88:1136-1141

Pasquini L, Sanders SP, Parness IA, et al: Coronary echocardiography in 406 patients with d-loop transposition of the great arteries. J Am Coll Cardiol 1994;24:763-768

Ruzmetov M, Jimenez MA, Pruitt A, et al: Repair of tetralogy of Fallot with anomalous coronary arteries coursing across the obstructed right ventricular outflow tract. Pediatr Cardiol 2005;26:537-542

Shrivastava S, Mohan JC, Mukhopadhyay S, et al: Coronary artery anomalies in tetralogy of Fallot. Cardiovasc Intervent Radiol 1987;10:215-218

Sim EK, van Son JA, Edwards WD, et al: Coronary artery anatomy in complete transposition of the great arteries. Ann Thorac Surg 1994;57:890-894

Coronary Artery Vasculitis

Arishiro K, Nariyama J, Hoshiga M, et al: Vascular Behçet's disease with coronary artery aneurysm. Intern Med 2006;45:903-907

Atzeni F, Sarzi-Puttini P, Doria A, et al: Behcet's disease and cardiovascular involvement. Lupus 2005;14:723-726

Drobinski G, Wechsler B, Pavie A, et al: Emergency percutaneous coronary dilatation for acute myocardial infarction in Behcet's disease. Eur Heart J 1987;8:1133-1136

Freeman AF, Shulman ST: Kawasaki disease: summary of the American Heart Association guidelines. Am Fam Physician 2006;74:1141-1148

Trauma

Anto MJ, Cokinos SG, Jonas E: Acute anterior wall myocardial infarction secondary to blunt chest trauma. Angiology 1984;35:802-804

Cheng TO, Adkins PC: Traumatic aneurysm of left anterior descending coronary artery with fistulous opening into left ventricle and left ventricular aneurysm after stab wound of chest: report of case with successful surgical repair. Am J Cardiol 1973;31:384-390

Cizmarova E, Simkovic I, Zelenay J, Masura J: Post-traumatic coronary occlusion and its consequences in a young child. Pediatr Cardiol 1988;9:117-120

Harada H, Honma Y, Hachiro Y, et al: Traumatic coronary artery dissection. Ann Thorac Surg 2002;74:236-237

Long WA, Willis PW, Henry GW: Childhood traumatic infarction causing left ventricular aneurysm: diagnosis by two-dimensional echocardiography. J Am Coll Cardiol 1985;5:1478-1483

Orliaguet G, Ferjani M, Riou B: The heart in blunt trauma. Anesthesiology 2001;95:544-548

Wang JN, Tsai YC, Chen SL, et al: Dangerous impact: commotio cordis. Cardiology 2000;93:124-126

Miscellaneous

Amabile N, Fraisse A, Quilici J: Hypoplastic coronary artery disease: report of one case. Heart 2005;91:e12

Fuzelier JF, Mauran P, Metz D: Radiation-induced bilateral coronary ostial stenosis in a 17-year-old patient. J Card Surg 2006;21:600-602

Marais AD, Firth JC, Blom DJ: Homozygous familial hypercholesterolemia and its management. Semin Vasc Med 2004;4:43-50

van de Sluis I, Boot AM, Vernooij M, et al: Idiopathic infantile arterial calcification: clinical presentation, therapy and long-term follow-up. Eur J Pediatr 2006;165:590-593

99

Acquired Great Vessel Abnormalities

FRANDICS P. CHAN and F. DANIEL DONOVAN

In this chapter, the epidemiology, pathogenesis, and clinical and imaging findings of acquired pediatric diseases of the thoracic aorta, venae cavae, pulmonary arteries, and pulmonary veins will be reviewed. Acquired pediatric aortic disease is uncommon, but radiologists and imagers play an important role in the care of patients who have sustained traumatic aortic injury, and in the diagnosis and clinical follow-up of the less common infectious, inflammatory, and connective tissue diseases of the aorta.

Acquired diseases of the pulmonary artery can degrade the efficiency of the pulmonary ventilation-perfusion process. Embolic events and vascular stenosis reduce total and regional pulmonary perfusion. Although pulmonary vasculitis is less common than aortic vasculitis, both can lead to vascular stenosis or aneurysm. Other important causes of pulmonary artery enlargement in pediatric patients include pulmonary valve stenosis, severe pulmonary regurgitation, and pulmonary arterial hypertension.

Most pediatric abnormalities of the pulmonary veins and venae cavae are congenital. The most common acquired abnormalities are obstruction or stenosis caused by luminal occlusion or extrinsic compression from mediastinal pathologies. Hemodynamically significant obstruction of the superior vena cava (SVC) leads to SVC syndrome, whereas obstruction of the pulmonary veins leads to pulmonary venous hypertension.

IMAGING CONSIDERATIONS

Historically, evaluation of the thoracic great vessels was performed by catheter-based angiography. Over the past decade, technologic advancements in computed tomography (CT) and magnetic resonance imaging (MRI) produced efficient, three-dimensional angiographic techniques that require only peripheral intravenous access for contrast infusion. These techniques substantially reduce the risks and complications associated with catheterization. Techniques for CT angiography (CTA) in children have been described, and the radiation dose can be comparable to that in catheter angiography. CTA offers a number of benefits, including a very short examination time, avoidance of contact between the catheter and the inflamed vessel wall, and the ability to directly visualize the diseased vessel wall and other extraluminal pathologies. Today, CTA is the first-line imaging modality

for traumatic arterial disease and pulmonary embolism. Important contraindications are allergic reaction to iodinated contrast material and renal insufficiency/failure: these are relatively rare in the pediatric population.

Although spatial resolution of MR angiography (MRA) is generally less than CTA, MRA has unique benefits, which include no ionizing radiation and the ability to quantify flow. Common contraindications for MRA are the presence of pacemakers and other electronic implants, ferromagnetic aneurysm clips, and unstable metallic fragments near vital structures. MRA is especially preferred in situations in which serial imaging studies are necessary for longitudinal follow-ups.

ACQUIRED DISEASES OF THE THORACIC AORTA

The aorta begins at the annulus of the aortic valve. Above the annulus, the aorta expands and forms an onion-shaped structure called the sinus of Valsalva, where the coronary arteries normally originate (Fig. 99-1). The sinus of Valsalva is connected to the tubular portion of the ascending aorta (Fig. 99-2). The transition between these two structures is called the sinotubular junction, and its integrity may be disrupted in connective tissue diseases. Dimensions of the aortic annulus, the sinus of Valsalva, and the sinotubular junction should be carefully evaluated in aneurysmal diseases of the aorta, because they can be affected differently in different disease processes. The ascending aorta turns posteriorly at the aortic arch, where the cervical vessels originate. In the vast majority of the population, the aortic arch travels to the left of the trachea and the esophagus before turning downward and becoming the descending aorta. Pathology of the aorta can be categorized into aortic aneurysm, aortic dissection, and aortic stenosis. Although each aortic disease may cause one or more of these manifestations, it is the clinical consequences of aneurysm, dissection, or stenosis that directly determine mortality and morbidity (Table 99-1).

> Aorta pathology can be categorized as aortic aneurysm, aortic dissection, or aortic stenosis, and the clinical consequences of these three diagnostic entities directly determine mortality and morbidity.

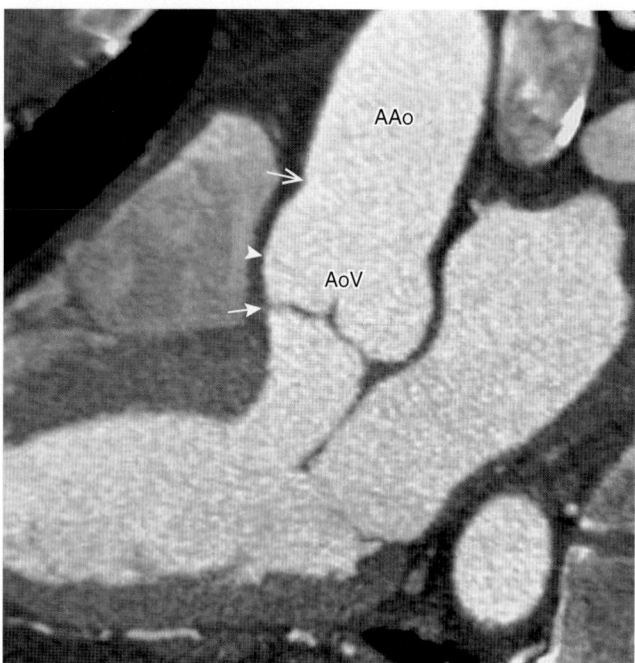

FIGURE 99-1. Normal aortic root as seen in the three-chamber view of a cardiac-gated multidetector CT. The aortic valve (AoV) is circumscribed by the aortic annulus (*lower white arrow*). The sinus of Valsalva (*arrowhead*) is a bulbous extension above the aortic annulus. The ascending aorta (AAo) is connected to the sinus of Valsalva at the sinotubular junction (*upper white arrow*).

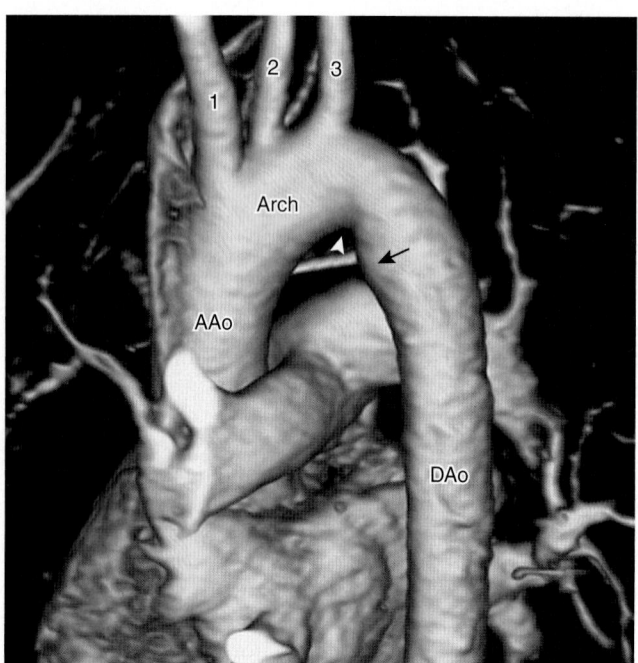

FIGURE 99-2. Normal thoracic aorta as seen in a volume rendering of an aortic CT angiogram. The ascending aorta (AAo) turns posteriorly to become a left aortic arch, from which the right brachiocephalic artery *(1)*, the left carotid artery *(2)*, and the left subclavian artery *(3)* originate. The aortic isthmus *(arrowhead)* is the portion of the distal arch just before the insertion of the ligamentum arteriosum. Beyond the isthmus is a mild aortic dilation of variable prominence called the ductus bump *(arrow)* before the aorta continues as the descending aorta (DAo).

TABLE 99-1
Principal Etiologies of Acquired Aortic Diseases

Manifestation	Causes
Aortic aneurysm	Infectious aortitis
	Inflammatory aortitis
	Takayasu (acute, chronic)
	Systemic lupus erythematosus
	Sarcoid
	Connective tissue disease
	Marfan
	Ehlers-Danlos (vascular type)
	Loeys-Dietz syndrome
	Arterial tortuosity syndrome
	Neurocutaneous disease
	Tuberous sclerosis
	Trauma or postsurgical (pseudoaneurysm)
Aortic dissection	Connective tissue disease
	Marfan
	Ehlers-Danlos (vascular type)
	Trauma
Aortic stenosis	Inflammatory aortitis
	Takayasu (chronic)
	Congenital rubella syndrome
	Radiation
	Neurocutaneous disease
	Neurofibromatosis (type I)
	PHACE complex
	Postsurgical
	Coarctation repair
	Aortopulmonary shunts

Normally, the caliber of the aorta gradually decreases in size from the sinotubular junction to the aortic hiatus. An aortic aneurysm is defined as an abnormal dilation of the aorta, which may undergo progressive expansion. Normal values have been obtained in children by catheter cine angiography, echocardiography, and MRI (Table 99-2). Aortic aneurysm may form if pressure-induced wall stress increases, as in the case of aortic stenosis, or if the aortic wall weakens, as in the case of Marfan syndrome. The expansion rate of an aneurysm is determined by the wall stress, which increases with diameter. Thus, a large aneurysm is more likely to expand than a small aneurysm, and the expansion is an accelerating process until rupture occurs.

Aortic dissection can occur in children as a complication of trauma or connective tissue diseases. A dissection is created when blood forces through a tear in the aortic intima and progressively separates the intimal layer from the media. Dissection thus creates two channels: a true lumen that is completely surrounded by the intima, and a false lumen that is partially surrounded by the intima and the media. The false lumen, lacking adequate outlet for blood flow, may pressurize much like a windsock. The pressurized false lumen may then propagate the dissection. Dissection can cause end-organ ischemia by obstructing branch vessels. It may also rupture the aorta to cause catastrophic hemorrhage.

TABLE 99-2

Normal Dimensions* of the Aorta and Pulmonary Arteries

Structure	Echocardiography[†]	Angiography[‡]
Aortic root	—	$2.49 \times BSA$
Aortic sinus of Valsalva	—	$3.79 \times BSA$
Aortic sinotubular junction	—	$2.90 \times BSA$
Ascending aorta	$0.00427 + 1.454 \times BSA^{0.5}$	—
Aortic arch	$0.0356 + 1.343 \times BSA^{0.5}$	—
Proximal descending aorta	—	$1.58 \times BSA$
Distal descending aorta	—	$1.30 \times BSA$
Pulmonary root	—	$2.53 \times BSA$
Pulmonary sinus of Valsalva	—	$3.52 \times BSA$
Pulmonary sinotubular junction	—	$2.93 \times BSA$
Main pulmonary artery	$0.0946 + 1.544 \times BSA^{0.5}$	—
Right pulmonary artery	$0.00372 + 1.160 \times BSA^{0.5}$	$1.76 \times BSA$
Left pulmonary artery	—	$1.53 \times BSA$

*Vessel diameters are in centimeters, and body surface area (BSA) is in meters squared.
[†]Echocardiographic data adapted from Snider AR, Enderlein MA, Teitel DF, Juster RP: Two-dimensional echocardiographic determination of aortic and pulmonary artery sizes from infancy to adulthood in normal subjects. Am J Cardiol 1984;53:218-224.
[‡]Catheter angiography data adapted from Rammos S, Apostolopoulou SC, Kramer HH, et al: Normative angiographic data relating to the dimensions of the aorta and pulmonary trunk in children and adolescents. Cardiol Young 2005;15:119-124.

Aortic stenosis is defined as a narrowing that limits perfusion to organs supplied by the aorta distal to the stenosis. The body may attempt to compensate by increasing pressure proximal to the stenosis to increase flow, or by developing collateral channels to bypass the obstruction. When severe, the aortic stenosis may cause systemic hypertension, left ventricular pressure overload, and end-organ ischemia. Middle aortic syndrome describes symptoms attributable to stenosis of the descending thoracic and abdominal aorta. In children, Takayasu arteritis is the most common cause of acquired aortic stenosis; other causes include neurofibromatosis, congenital rubella syndrome, and other vasculitides.

> **Common causes of acquired aortic stenosis in children include Takayasu arteritis, neurofibromatosis, congenital rubella syndrome, and other vasculitides.**

Infectious Aortitis

Acute infectious aortitis (Fig. 99-3) in children is often caused by bacterial septicemia originating from infected lines and intravascular devices, and from valvular endocarditis. Predisposing conditions include congenital heart disease and immune compromise. Once in the bloodstream, virulent organisms adhere to and invade the aortic wall. The resulting inflammation leads to suppurative necrosis that weakens the aortic wall and forms an aneurysm. Staphylococci and streptococci are the most frequently responsible organisms. Immune system weakening by varicella has been contributory in 28% of aortitis cases caused by group A streptococci. Besides sepsis, aortitis can be caused by direct spread from an adjacent infection, such as an abscess. When the aortic wall is weakened, infected aortic aneurysm can rupture. Staphylococcal aortitis is particularly prone to this com-

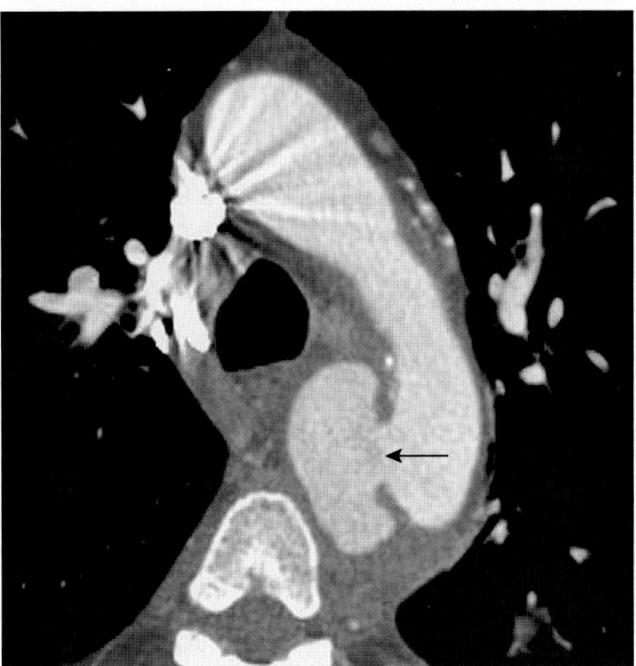

FIGURE 99-3. Infectious aortitis. Axial image from a CT angiogram shows a thick-walled, saccular aneurysm communicating with the aortic arch through a narrow opening *(arrow)*.

plication. In one series infected aneurysms related to an umbilical artery catheter, 86% of cases were caused by *Staphylococcus*. Syphilitic and tuberculous aortic aneurysms are rare complications of chronic infection by syphilis and tuberculosis. Although well known in adults, they are fortunately uncommon in children.

Difficulties arise in diagnosis because many infected aneurysms in children are asymptomatic, or the patients present with nonspecific complaints, such as fever and abdominal or back pain. Commonly used laboratory markers of infection are often normal. Blood cultures were negative in 28% and white blood cell levels were normal in 42% of adult cases. However an elevated erythrocyte sedimentation rate (ESR), a nonspecific finding, was found in 92% of patients.

Few clinical studies have evaluated the imaging appearance and distribution of infected aortic aneurysms in children, but experience from adult patients suggests that these aneurysms are more often saccular (93%) than fusiform (7%). The distribution was found to be as follows: 6% involved the ascending aorta, 23% the descending thoracic, 19% the thoracoabdominal aorta, and 10% the juxtarenal aorta. Periaortic fluid, stranding, or soft tissue mass was present in 48%. Periaortic gas, a specific sign, was present in only 7%. Rapid progression of aneurysm size was found in infected aneurysms in both adults and children.

Antibiotic treatment with the goal of eradicating the offending organism is the first step in the treatment of infectious aortitis. At the same time, imaging to document stability of the aortic lumen is necessary. If an aneurysm has formed, it should be repaired surgically after an adequate period of antibiotic treatment. Deployment of endovascular stent grafts in infected aortic aneurysms has been attempted. Although this is not considered a treatment of choice, it may be useful as a bridge to open surgical repair, especially in the presence of low-virulence organisms or rapidly expanding aneurysms.

Takayasu Aortitis

Takayasu aortitis (TA) (also called Takayasu arteritis), although rare, is the most common large-vessel vasculitis in children (Fig. 99-4). The incidence in the United States is 2.6 cases per 1 million people per year, and it is significantly higher in Asia and in Africa. Patients may present as early as the first year of life, but more commonly they present in teenage years or older. Two thirds of patients are female. Accurate diagnosis is difficult because the symptoms are often subtle and nonspecific. An average delay in diagnosis of 19 months has been reported.

TA affects the large, muscular arteries, including the aorta and its branches. The diseased vessel wall is thickened and shows granulomatous changes from the adventitia to the media. The inflammatory process is thought to be primarily a T cell–mediated mechanism, and the formation of granulomas is stimulated by various cytokines. Giant cell (or temporal arteritis) is identical in appearance pathologically but affects an older population and typically involves the temporal artery.

Classically, TA is divided into an acute (or pre-pulseless) phase and a chronic, pulseless phase. During the acute phase, the arteries are actively inflamed and thickened. The clinical manifestations are nonspecific and the patient may have constitutional symptoms of fever and failure to thrive. Laboratory tests, such as the ESR, show elevated acute-phase reactants. The chronic phase of TA is caused by scarring of the arterial wall and resultant luminal narrowing or occlusion. Occasionally, dilation and aneurysm formation can occur. Clinically, patients in this stage of the disease have diminished and discrepant pulses in the extremities, and symptoms of ischemia in organs supplied by diseased vessels such as renovascular hypertension. Involvement of the carotid arteries can manifest in symptoms of cerebral ischemia, including stroke, dizziness, seizures, and transient blindness. Clinical presentations can be quite variable, and a patient may not experience all the classically described clinical phases.

Diagnosis is based on patient symptoms, physical findings, clinical laboratory values, serologic markers, and vascular findings. The American College of Rheumatology criteria include arm or leg claudication, age less than 40 years, a blood pressure difference between extremities of greater than 10 mm Hg, subclavian or aortic bruit, decreased brachial artery pulse, and aortic or branch narrowing. Three of these criteria provide a diagnosis of Takayasu arteritis with a sensitivity of 90.5% and a specificity of 97.8%. Other clinical manifestations of TA that are not involved in diagnosis include fever, headache, weight loss, postural dizziness, arthralgias, weight loss, myalgias, and hypertension secondary to renal artery stenosis.

Although not part of the diagnostic criteria for TA, vascular stenosis and aneurysm are the primary causes of mortality and morbidity and therefore should be evaluated with angiographic techniques. Noninvasive MRA or CTA has replaced catheter angiography for this purpose. In addition to precisely demonstrating areas of stenosis and aneurysm, CTA and MRA provide information on wall thickening and inflammation activity that can be useful in guiding medical therapy. Imaging findings that indicate active inflammation include increased MRI T2 signal or delayed contrast enhancement in a thickened wall after MRA or CTA.

> **To demonstrate areas of stenosis and aneurysm in patients with TA, MRA and CTA have replaced catheter angiography. The information they provide on wall thickening and inflammation helps guide medical therapy. Active inflammation can be shown by increased MRI T2 signal or delayed contrast enhancement in a thickened wall after MRA or CTA.**

TA in the chronic phase is further subclassified by the location of abnormal findings in the aorta and the aortic branch vessels. Type I involves the cervical vessels: brachiocephalic artery, subclavian arteries, and carotid arteries. Type II involves the thoracic aorta: type IIa affects the ascending aorta and/or the arch vessels, and type IIb affects in addition the descending thoracic aorta. Type III involves the descending thoracic aorta and the abdominal aorta but not the ascending aorta and the aortic arch. Type IV affects only the abdominal aorta and/or the renal arteries, and type V involves the entire aorta and its branches.

Medical therapy of TA initially focuses on the suppression of the immunologic responses with corticosteroids, methotrexate, azathioprine, and cyclophosphamide. In refractory TA, the anti–tumor necrosis factor-alpha (TNF-α) agents etanercept and infliximab have been used to achieve sustained remission. Follow-

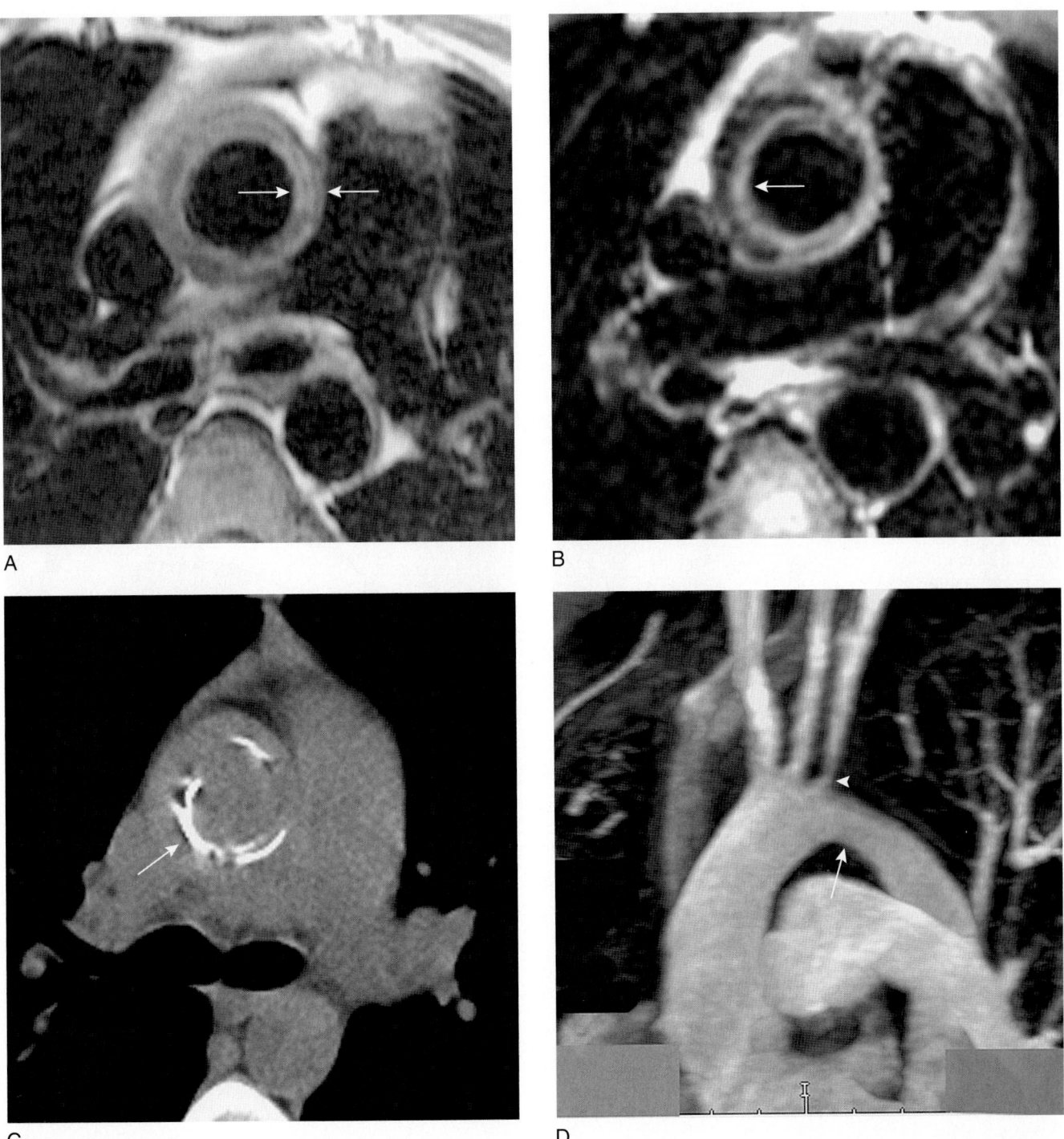

FIGURE 99-4. Takayasu arteritis in a 16-year-old girl. **A,** Axial T1-weighted MR image shows the thickened wall *(arrows)* of the inflamed aorta. **B,** Axial T2-weighted MR image shows hyperintense T2 signal *(arrow)* within the thickened wall, suggesting soft tissue edema and active inflammation. **C,** During the chronic phase, the aortic wall may calcify *(arrow)* as seen in this noncontrast axial CT image. **D,** MR angiography shows a narrowed distal aorta *(arrow)* and tapered narrowing of the left subclavian artery *(arrowhead)*, consistent with a type IIa chronic change.

up with CTA or MRA helps document stability or progression of the vascular abnormalities and their complications. Patients with renovascular hypertension, severe coarctation of the aorta, claudication, progressive aneurysm enlargement, coronary artery disease, or cervicocranial vessel stenosis may benefit from surgical revascularization. Bypass grafts, either synthetic or autologous, can be used, but restenosis occurs in up to one

third of cases in which synthetic grafts were used and in approximately 10% of procedures in which an autologous vessel was used. Other postoperative complications include heart failure, intractable hypertension, and graft deterioration with pseudoaneurysm formation. Postsurgical aneurysm formation at the anastomosis is a known complication and seen in up to 34% of patients. Angioplasty has been used with success in TA patients with vascular stenosis, with an initial success rate of 92% and a restenosis rate of 22%.

Other Vasculitides

Aneurysmal disease of the aorta, which generally afflicts older patients, is a rare complication of systemic lupus erythematosus (SLE). The exact pathophysiology of the aortic aneurysm is unknown. It may be caused directly by the SLE-related inflammation of the vessel wall or secondarily by chronic steroid treatment and the resultant accelerated atherosclerosis of the aorta. Sarcoid has

been reported as a rare cause of large-vessel vascular stenosis and it has been recommended that children with early-onset sarcoid be evaluated for occlusive arterial disease.

Marfan Syndrome

Marfan syndrome is an inherited connective tissue disorder with an autosomal dominant transmission. It is caused by mutations in the *FBN1* gene on chromosome 15, which codes for the fibrillin-1 protein. Prevalence of this disease is 1 per 5000 people, and 25% of cases represent

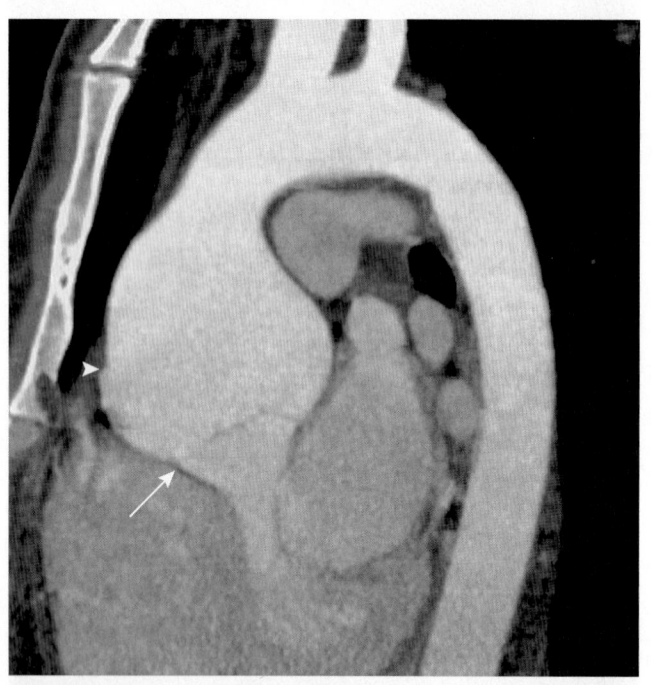

A

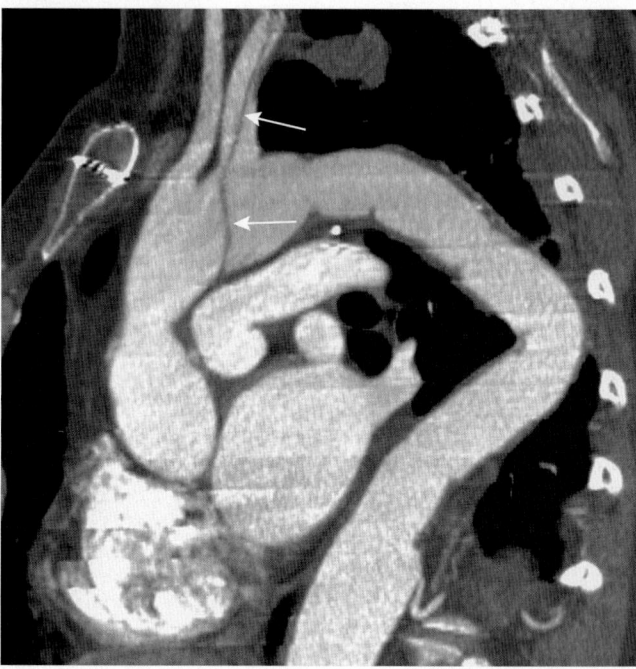

B

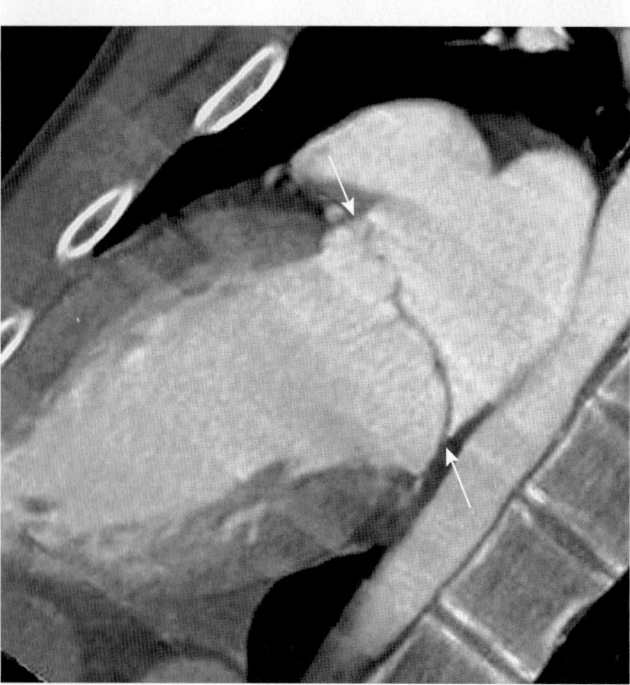

C

FIGURE 99-5. Marfan syndrome. **A,** CT angiogram shows an aneurysmal aortic root in a 15-year-old boy. Dilation begins at the aortic annulus *(arrow)* and expands to the largest at the sinus of Valsalva *(arrowhead).* The sinotubular junction is obliterated. **B,** CTA shows a dissected thoracic aorta that has been partially repaired in a 20-year-old man. The dissection *(arrow)* extends into the left subclavian artery. **C,** Cardiac-gated CT shows the mitral leaflets bulging posterior to the annular line *(arrows),* consistent with mitral valve prolapse, in a 17-year-old boy.

new mutations. A large number of different point mutations can lead to fibrillin protein dysfunction. Diagnosis by gene sequencing is therefore of limited value. As can be expected, the polymorphism of the *FBN1* gene mutation leads to a wide spectrum of clinical presentations and disease severities, from near normal phenotype to severe clinical symptoms.

Fibrillin-1 is a major component of the extracellular microfibrils found in many types of connective tissues and suspensory ligaments, but it is especially prevalent in the elastic fibers of the ascending aorta. Polymerization of fibrillin forms microfibrils that are responsible for the structural strength of the elastic tissue. Dysfunction of the fibrillin molecules, therefore, prevents proper microfibril formation and disrupts elastic tissue integrity. This is the prevailing explanation for many of the clinical manifestations of Marfan syndrome, including vascular aneurysm, dural ectasia, and ligament laxity. Recent evidence suggests that mutation in another gene for the transforming growth factor-beta (TGF-β) may play a role in Marfan syndrome type II.

Clinically, 75% of patients come to attention because of an affected family member and 25% present with characteristic manifestations noticed by a primary care provider. Because of the polymorphism of the mutation and the variable clinical presentation, there is no single diagnostic test for Marfan syndrome. Diagnosis is based on a set of major and minor clinical criteria that have been revised over time. The current criteria are known as the Ghent nosology (Table 99-3), which is a complex algorithm that incorporates findings of cardiovascular abnormalities as well as a family history of Marfan syndrome and skeletal, ocular, pulmonary, skin, and central nervous system abnormalities. Major criteria involving the cardiovascular system are (1) dilation of the ascending aorta and sinuses of Valsalva and (2) ascending aortic dissection. Minor criteria involving the cardiovascular

system are (1) mitral valve prolapse, (2) mitral annular calcification in patients less than 40 years of age, and (3) descending and abdominal aortic dissection in patients less than 50 years of age.

Dilation of the aortic root (Fig. 99-5) is present in at least 60% of patients with Marfan syndrome, and it is an important prognostic factor for aortic dissection and rupture, the major causes of death in Marfan syndrome. Aortic aneurysm in Marfan syndrome typically dilates the ascending aorta on both sides of the sinotubular junction. Dilation of the aortic root may lead to aortic regurgitation. Microscopic findings of the diseased aortic wall show cystic medial necrosis. Aortic dissection in Marfan patients often involves the ascending aorta and the aortic root. The dissection flap can be quite complex, creating multiple false lumina. Other cardiovascular manifestations important in children are mitral valve prolapse and mitral regurgitation. They are caused by malcoaptation of the mitral leaflets, in turn caused by laxity of the leaflets and their supporting chordal structures. The tricuspid valve can be similarly affected.

Because aortic aneurysm is a major determinant of prognosis in Marfan syndrome, vascular imaging is directed toward quantifying the size and the extent of the aneurysm, and detecting aortic rupture or dissection. Routine surveillance can be performed noninvasively with MRA or CTA, and MRA is preferred because it has no ionizing radiation. If an aneurysm is found, diameters of the aortic annulus, the sinus of Valsalva, and the ascending aorta should be recorded and compared with previous studies for any progression in size and for the rate of increase. If dissection is found, involvement of the ascending aorta or cervical arteries, change in the extent of the dissection flap, patency of branch vessels, and evidence for end-organ ischemia should be carefully evaluated. MRA and CTA are also important for evaluating postsurgical complications, such as pseudoaneurysm

TABLE 99-3

Major and Minor Criteria in the Ghent Nosology

Sphere of Abnormalities	Major Criteria	Minor Criteria
Cardiovascular	Dilated aortic root Ascending aortic dissection	Mitral valve prolapse Early mitral annular calcification Early descending or abdominal aortic dissection
Dura	Lumbosacral dural ectasia	
Family history	First-degree relative with Marfan syndrome	
Musculoskeletal	Pectus carinatum or severe pectus excavatum Large ratio of arm span to height Wrist and thumb signs Scoliosis Elbow hyperextension Pes planus Protrusio acetabuli	Typical facies Joint hypermobility High-arched palate
Ocular	Lens dislocation	Myopia Flat cornea Ciliary muscle hypoplasia
Pulmonary		Pneumothorax Apical blebs
Skin		Atrophic striae Recurrent or incisional hernia

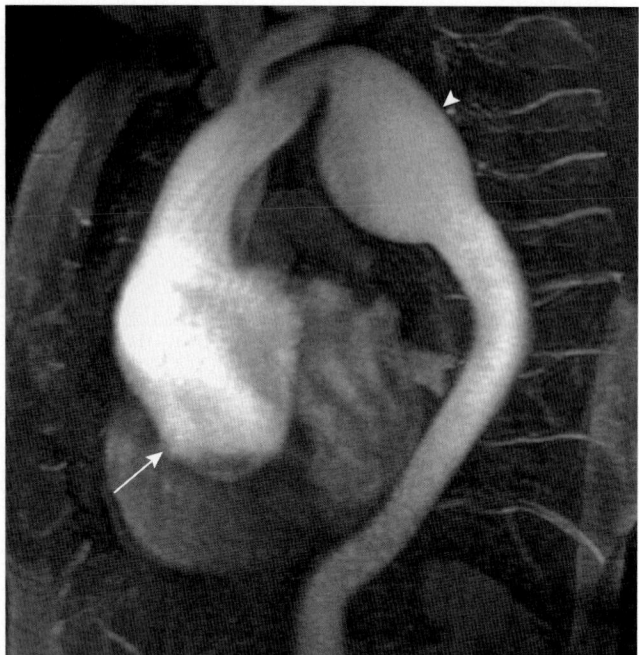

A

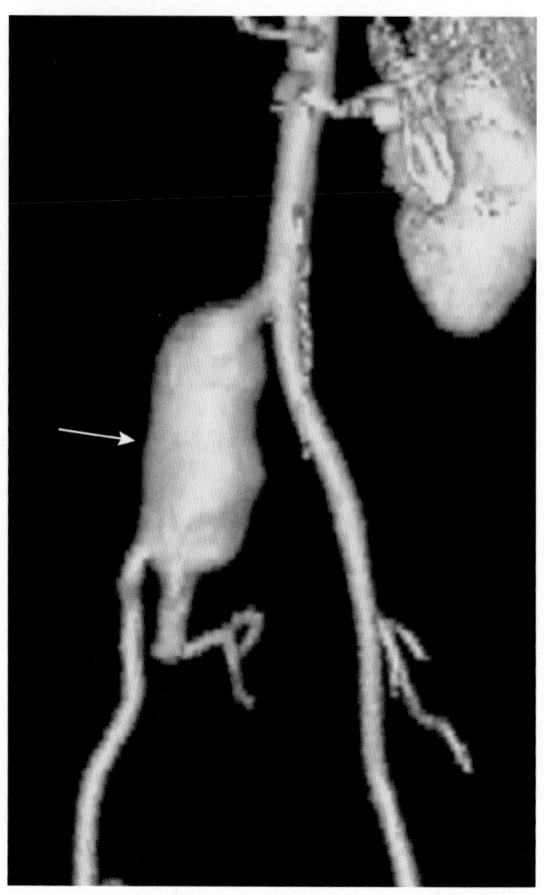

B

FIGURE 99-6. Vascular Ehlers-Danlos syndrome (EDS) in a 14-year-old boy. **A,** MRA shows an aneurysmal aortic root *(arrow)* similar to that found in Marfan syndrome. However, unlike in Marfan syndrome, other fusiform aneurysms may appear anywhere along the aorta *(arrowhead).* **B,** Volume rendering of an MRA shows another EDS aneurysm *(arrow)* in the right common iliac artery.

formation, graft leak, graft thrombosis, and, in the case of combined repair of the aorta and the aortic valve, coronary obstruction and aneurysm.

Treatment of Marfan syndrome consists of beta-blocking agents, exercise restriction, and prophylactic aortic root replacement. Patients of all ages treated with beta-blockade demonstrated slower aortic root growth, fewer cardiovascular complications, and improved survival. The risk of ascending aortic rupture or dissection increases in proportion to the aortic diameter, and therefore surgical prophylactic aortic root replacement is recommended when the ascending aortic diameter reaches 5.0 cm. Indications for earlier surgery include rapid increase in aortic diameter (>1.0 cm/yr), family history of premature aortic dissection (dissection occurring with diameter <5.0 cm), and greater than mild aortic regurgitation. Types of aortic repair include composite valve graft, aortic root remodeling, and aortic root reimplantation.

Ehlers-Danlos Syndrome

Ehlers-Danlos syndrome (EDS) is a group of disorders that affect the synthesis and metabolism of collagen and associated proteins. Patients with EDS typically share clinical features of skin hyperextensibility, joint hypermotility, easy bruising, and poor wound healing. The prevalence of all types of EDS is reported to be in the range of from 1 per 5000 people to 1 per 10,000 people. Historically, over 10 types of EDS with various, over-

lapping clinical findings have been described (Table 99-4). Like Marfan syndrome, EDS is currently diagnosed and classified by major and minor clinical criteria, and a nosology updated by the Ehlers-Danlos National Foundation in 1997 is known as the Villefranche classification.

The vascular type (previously type IV) of EDS is a form that affects primarily the cardiovascular system, producing aneurysms of the large and medium-size arteries (Fig. 99-6). Among all types of EDS, the vascular type has the worst prognosis, with early mortality frequently caused by aneurysm rupture. It is an autosomal dominant disorder of the *COL3A1* gene on chromosome 2, which codes for type III procollagen. The prevalence of the vascular type is estimated to be 1 per 100,000 people, significantly less common than Marfan syndrome. Other types of EDS may have milder presentations of aortic abnormalities.

Diagnosis of the vascular type of EDS is made on the basis of four major clinical criteria: characteristic facial dysmorphism, easy bruising, thin translucent skin, and rupture of arteries, uterus, or intestines. Facial features include thin lips, periorbital pigmentation, prominent cheek bones and eyes, and facial slenderness; however, these features are not always present. Easy bruising is secondary to the fragile nature of the vessels and skin and is frequently seen after trivial trauma. Blood and clotting tests are usually normal. Thin translucent skin with apparent loss of subcutaneous fat and that heals poorly is often present.

TABLE 99-4

Classification in Ehlers-Danlos Syndrome

Classification	Inheritance Pattern	Major Diagnostic Criteria
Classic type	Autosomal dominant	Skin hyperextensibility, wide atrophic scars, joint hypermobility
Hypermobility type	Autosomal dominant	Joint hypermobility
Vascular type	Autosomal dominant	Translucent skin, arterial or intestinal rupture, easy bruising
Kyphoscoliosis type	Autosomal recessive	Joint laxity, hypotonia at birth, scoliosis, globe rupture
Arthrochalasia type	Autosomal dominant	Congenitally dislocated hips, joint hypermobility, recurrent subluxations
Dermatosparaxis	Autosomal recessive	Skin fragility, redundant skin

In the largest study to date of patients with EDS type IV, life expectancy was 48 years, and mortality and morbidity resulted from arterial dissection and rupture (79%), gastrointestinal rupture (8%), and other organ rupture (10%). Although rupture of the gastrointestinal tract occurs earlier than arterial complications, the latter are more commonly lethal. The thoracic and abdominal arteries are involved in half of the cases, with extremity and head-and-neck vessels each contributing 25%. Common neurovascular complications include carotid-cavernous fistula formation, carotid dissection, aneurysm formation, and rupture. Pregnancy is dangerous in patients with vascular EDS: a 6% mortality rate is associated with first pregnancy.

As done in Marfan syndrome, vascular imaging is geared toward defining areas of vascular aneurysm, dissection, and rupture. The size and the rate of growth of each aneurysm should be quantified. Because the neurovascular system may be involved, imaging of the cerebral circulation and the carotid arteries may be necessary. The pattern of aneurysm distribution in EDS differs from that in Marfan syndrome. Whereas Marfan syndrome typically results in dilation of the aortic root and the sinus of Valsalva, EDS produces discrete, fusi-form aneurysms at different locations on the aorta, the iliac arteries, the cervical arteries, and their branches. Dissection in EDS often has complex morphology. Both features are usually well characterized by noninvasive CTA and MRA. Because of the rarity of the vascular form of EDS, there is a lack of data about the proper management of these patients. The substrate of the vascular wall is abnormal, so surgical repair is often complicated by the formation of new aneurysm, rupture, or dissection. As a result, surgery is a last resort.

Other Connective Tissue Diseases

Loeys-Dietz syndrome (LDS) and arterial tortuosity syndrome (ATS) are rare conditions associated with the dysregulation of TGF-β caused by mutations in the TGF-β receptor gene. LDS is an aortic aneurysm syndrome characterized by midline abnormalities such as bifid uvula or cleft palate, widely spaced eyes (hypertelorism), and aortic aneurysm and dissection formation, in addition to brain and skull abnormalities, congenital heart disease, and mental retardation. ATS is an autosomal recessive disorder caused by a mutation in the facilitative glucose transporter GLUT10. Manifestations include

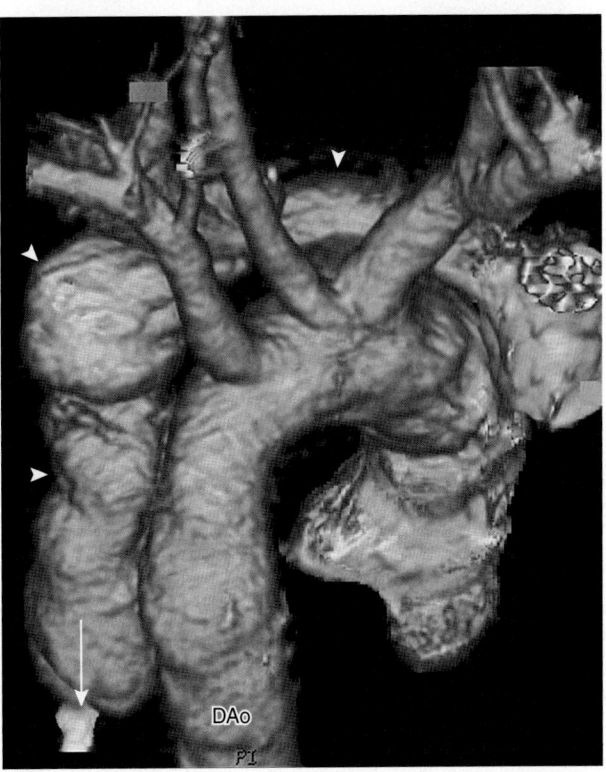

FIGURE 99-7. Gunshot wound in an 18-year-old man. A volume rendering of a CT angiogram shows a false aneurysm *(arrowheads)* that follows the track of a bullet. The bullet first entered the chest horizontally, parallel to the aortic arch, rupturing the aorta. Then it was deflected downward and came to rest *(arrow)* adjacent to the descending aorta (DAo).

elongated and tortuous large arteries, aneurysm formation, and stenosis.

Trauma

Trauma is a major cause of death in the pediatric population and results primarily from motor vehicle accidents, although firearm injury (Fig. 99-7) and child abuse are other important causes. Traumatic aortic injury surviving to the emergency room in the pediatric population, however, is rare accounting for one to two cases per year at large metropolitan level-1 pediatric trauma centers. Operative treatment involves less than 0.14% of all trauma patients, and only 6% of all traumatic ruptures of the aorta occur in patients less than 16 years old. The outcome of traumatic aortic injury in the

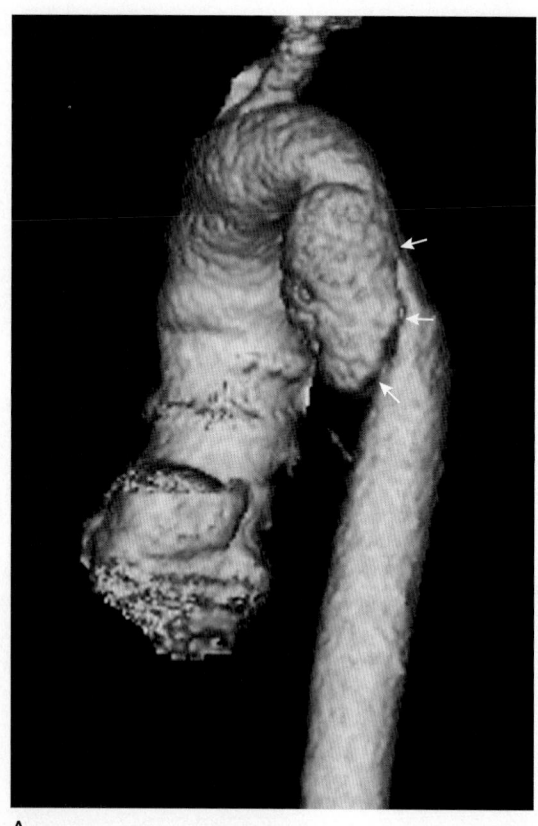
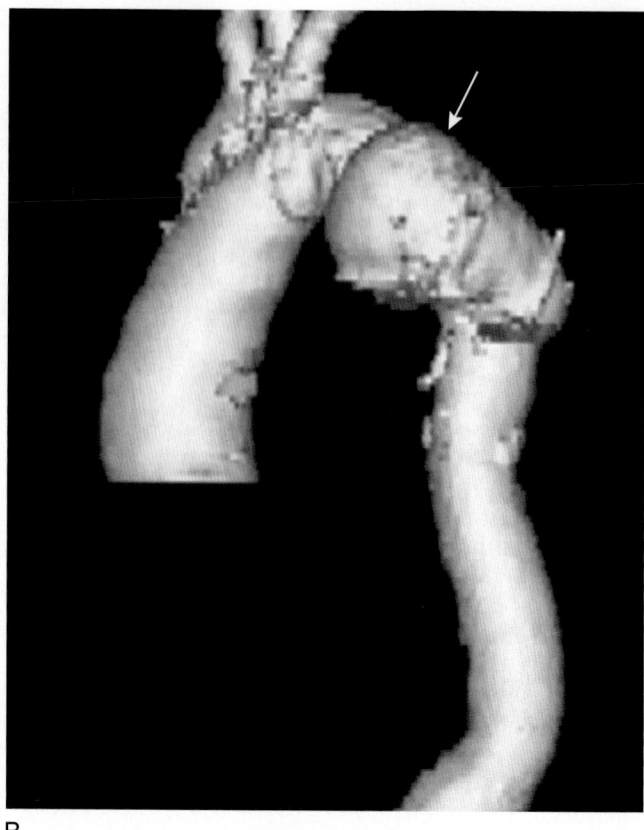

A   B

FIGURE 99-8. Traumatic aortic injury. **A,** Volume rendering of a CT angiogram shows a patch of irregular surface at the proximal descending aorta in a 15-year-old boy. A curvilinear impression *(arrows)* identifies the torn aortic wall intruding into the flow lumen of the aorta. **B,** Volume rendering of a CT angiogram shows a pseudoaneurysm *(arrow)* in another patient, which has a narrow connection (not shown) with the aortic arch.

pediatric population is directly related to timely diagnosis, proper treatment, and hemodynamic status at the time of presentation.

Chest radiographic findings, such as left apical capping, obscuration of the aortic arch, mediastinal widening, pleural effusion, pneumothorax, pulmonary contusion, tracheal and nasogastric tube deviation, and upper rib and clavicle fracture in the setting of blunt trauma, should raise clinical suspicion for aortic injury (Fig. 99-8). Historically, the definitive diagnosis of traumatic injury to the aorta was made by conventional catheter angiography. Today, CTA has supplanted catheter angiography as the diagnostic method of choice. CTA allows speedy and precise visualization of the traumatic aortic injury. Care should be taken to identify the location of aortic rupture, active extravasation of arterial contrast, dissection flap extending to major aortic branches, hemothorax and hemopericardium, and other organ and musculoskeletal injuries.

The goals of treatment of pediatric traumatic aortic rupture are identical to those in adults. The mainstay is operative repair of the aorta. Patients at high risk for surgery have been successfully treated with endovascular stent grafts, with deployment during adenosine arrest. Angiograms should be performed immediately after placement, with follow-up CTA at 48 hours, to document the success of the repair. Rarely, observational management for intimal tear has been utilized in patients with comorbidities too severe for intervention.

Neurocutaneous Diseases

Neurocutaneous diseases affecting the aorta in children include neurofibromatosis type I, tuberous sclerosis complex, and the more recently described PHACE syndrome.

Neurofibromatosis type I (NF-1), or von Recklinghausen disease, is an autosomal dominant disorder with an incidence of 1 per 3000 births. Dysplasia of neuroectodermal and mesodermal tissues leads to a variety of clinical manifestations, including multiple cutaneous tumors and spotty pigmentation. Vascular manifestations of NF-1 are rare, occurring in 1% to 3% of patients, and may manifest as aneurysms, stenosis, occlusions (Fig. 99-9), fistulas, and arteriovenous malformations. Vascular changes affect large, medium, and small vessels, with renal artery stenosis and associated hypertension being among the most common complications. Up to 18.5% of pediatric patients with NF-1 have hypertension resulting from vascular lesions, and these lesions may be treated with drug therapy, angioplasty, or surgery to remove the stenosis. Typically, patients with NF-1 are screened with frequent blood pressure measurements and undergo arterial imaging if hypertension develops. Another

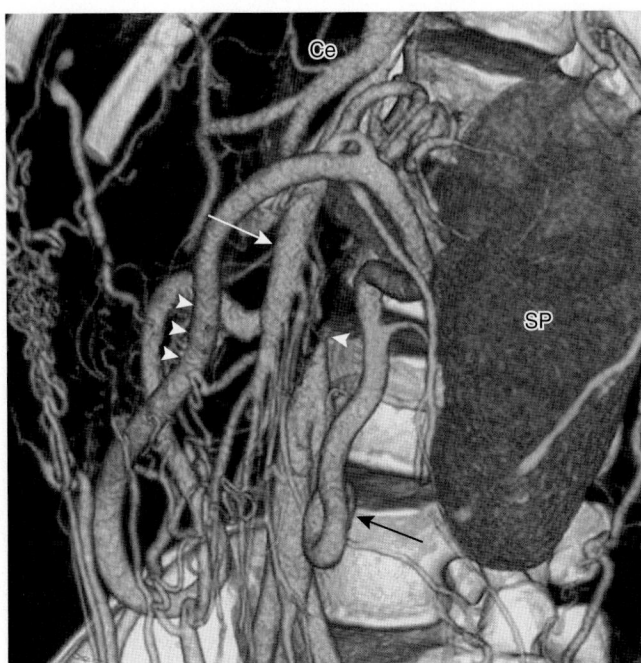

FIGURE 99-9. Aortic obstruction from neurofibromatosis type I in a 14-year-old boy. Volume rendering of an abdominal CT angiogram shows a complete obstruction of the aorta beyond the origins of the celiac trunk (Ce) and the superior mesenteric artery *(white arrow).* The distal aorta *(single arrowhead)* is reconstituted through the superior mesenteric artery, the marginal artery of Drummond *(three arrowheads),* and the inferior mesenteric artery *(black arrow).* SP, spleen. *(See color plate.)*

vascular manifestation, known as middle aortic syndrome, is caused by the narrowing of the distal thoracic or abdominal aorta, leading to renal vascular hypertension and ischemia of the visceral organs and lower extremities. This complication has been treated successfully with aortic bypass with resolution of hypertension and claudication. Development of aneurysm has been reported after stent or stent graft placement, suggesting an underlying disorder of the vascular wall.

Tuberous sclerosis complex, when fully manifest, includes a triad of epilepsy, mental retardation, and facial angiofibromas. The underlying pathologic process is the development of hamartomas of multiple organ systems. Occasionally, however, tuberous sclerosis affects the aorta, and in these cases the pathologic process is medial atrophy and disruption. Patients with tuberous sclerosis develop aortic aneurysms more commonly in the abdomen, but also in the thorax. Aneurysms in the abdomen appear at an earlier age than those in the thorax. Open elective repair is imperative, as one third of patients with tuberous sclerosis complex and aneurysms present with rupture and death. Screening for aortic aneurysms is recommended both at the time of diagnosis and at frequent regular intervals thereafter.

The PHACE association, consisting of posterior fossa malformations, hemangiomas, arterial anomalies, coarctation of the aorta, cardiac defects, and eye abnormalities, is a recently described neurocutaneous complex. There is a striking female predominance. Features overlap with Sturge-Weber syndrome, leading to confusion as to the nature of the disease and associated vascular lesions.

More than 30% of patients have coarctation of the aorta or other congenital aortic abnormalities such as arch atresia, aberrant subclavian origins, hypoplasia of the descending thoracic aorta, and double aortic arch. Other abnormalities, such as progressive stenosis and aneurysm formation of the aorta and the cervical arteries, are thought to be acquired. Patients with PHACE association are at an unusually high risk of stroke secondary to a progressive arterial vasculopathy, and of cerebrovascular abnormalities. Currently, imaging strategy is geared toward identification of vascular lesions, treatment planning, and monitoring of disease progression.

Neoplasms Involving the Aorta

Primary neoplasms involving the aorta have not been described in the pediatric population. However, secondary involvement of the aorta either in the form of invasion or compression from nearby tumor, or of radiation aortitis from radiation treatment, has been described but is uncommon in children. Examples of neoplastic processes that can affect the aorta include mediastinal lymphoma, germ cell tumor, teratoma, rare types of sarcomas, and mediastinal metastasis.

Postoperative Complications

Pseudoaneurysm and stenosis can develop as complications of surgical repair or interventional treatment of pediatric aortic abnormalities, among which coarctation is the best studied. The average restenosis rates are 15% and 2% for balloon angioplasty and surgical repair of coarctation, respectively (Fig. 99-10). Other surgical procedures that can be complicated by aortic aneurysm or stenosis are surgical aortopulmonary shunts, such as Potts shunt, Waterston shunt, and central shunt.

ACQUIRED DISEASES OF THE PULMONARY ARTERY

Pulmonary Embolism

Pulmonary embolism (PE) is an uncommon, but potentially fatal disease in children. In pediatric patients with deep venous thrombosis (DVT) and PE, mortality from all causes has been reported to be as high as 16%, whereas mortality directly attributable to DVT or PE was 2.2%.

> **The most common risk factor for PE is catheter thrombosis, which develops in as many as 50% of patients with central venous catheters.**

The most common risk factor is catheter thrombosis, which develops in as many as 50% of patients with central venous catheters. Other risk factors are peripartum asphyxia, dehydration, septicemia, trauma and burns, surgery, hemolysis, malignancy, and renal disease such as nephrotic syndrome. Rarely, PE can be seen in the setting of intracranial venous sinus thrombosis and Klippel-Trénaunay syndrome. The latter is characterized

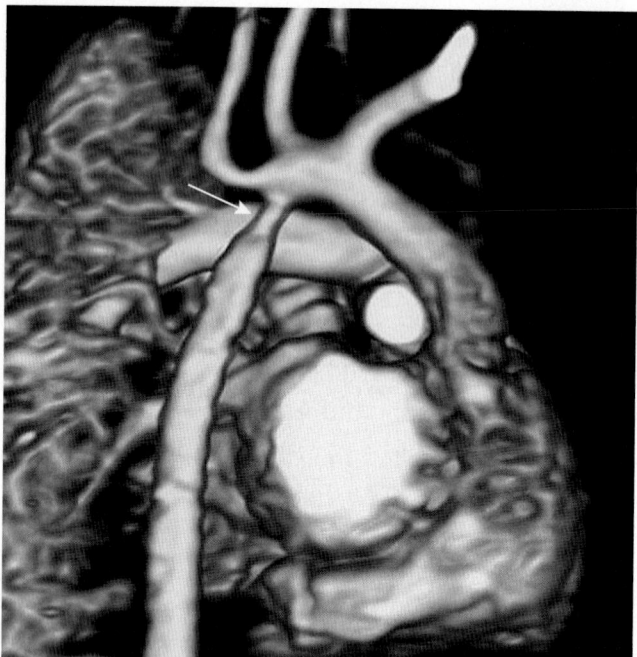

FIGURE 99-10. Restenosis 5 months after a surgical repair for coarctation in a 6-month-old boy. Volume rendering shows a segmental, circumferential narrowing *(arrow)* at the surgical site. *(See color plate.)*

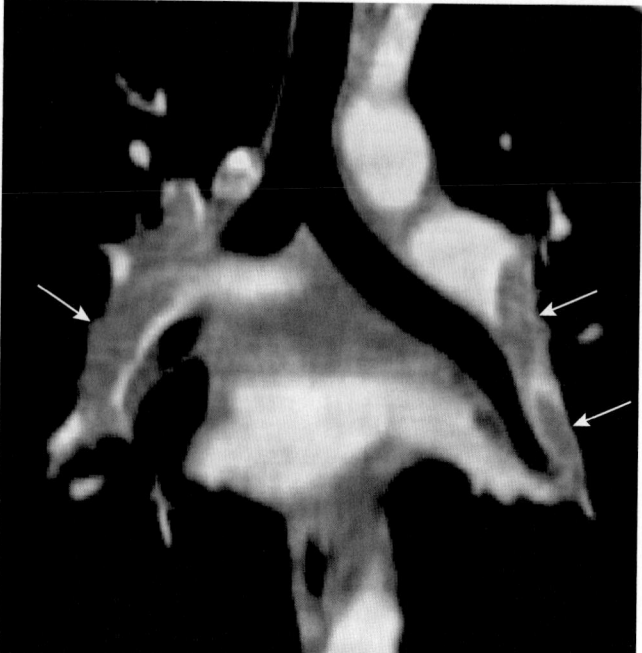

FIGURE 99-11. Pulmonary embolism in a 17-year-old girl. Coronal reformation of a pulmonary CT angiogram shows multiple filling defects *(arrows)* within the central pulmonary arteries.

by systemic capillary malformation, venous varicosities, and unilateral limb overgrowth. Abnormal coagulation factors associated with adult PE that have also been reported in children are antiphospholipid antibodies, factor V Leiden mutation, and deficiencies in protein S, protein C, and antithrombin III.

Clinical diagnosis of PE is often difficult because most cases of venous thrombosis in children are silent. Symptoms of PE may be masked by intrinsic lung disease or other underlying illness. In one series, 40% of proven cases of PE were negative in the D-dimer assay. Therefore, a negative D-dimer assay in pediatric patients cannot exclude PE. A high level of clinical suspicion in the presence of risk factors is imperative.

> **A negative D-dimer assay in pediatric patients cannot exclude PE.**

Catheter pulmonary angiography is considered the diagnostic gold standard. Other imaging methods include nuclear ventilation-perfusion scanning and CT pulmonary angiography (Fig. 99-11). As in adult patients, CT pulmonary angiography is increasingly being used to diagnose PE in children. Although CT pulmonary angiography is noninvasive compared with catheter angiography, its accuracy has not been established. CT pulmonary angiography in children is technically more challenging than in adults. Meticulous attention must be paid to maximize spatial resolution and contrast density in the pulmonary arteries. Wherever possible, breath holding, either voluntary or induced by anesthesia, should be used to minimize respiratory motion artifact.

Anticoagulation is the mainstay of medical therapy for PE. Thrombolytic therapy is reserved for those with hemodynamic instability, and it has a significant risk of hemorrhage. Surgical pulmonary thrombectomy has been successfully performed in those with central or saddle emboli.

Pulmonary embolic events can be caused by materials other than bland thrombus. Septic emboli can be the result of endocarditis and of thrombophlebitis. Lemierre syndrome describes jugular vein thrombosis associated with anaerobic infection of the head and neck, and more than 50% of these cases are complicated by septic emboli to the lungs. Tumor emboli may come from Wilms tumor, neuroblastoma, and hepatocellular carcinoma, because these tumors occasionally invade the inferior vena cava. Rarely, tumor emboli originate from pediatric primary tumor of the heart, such as rhabdomyosarcoma. Foreign bodies that embolize to the lungs include broken catheter tips and guide wires, misplaced embolization coils, and other endovascular devices. Finally, fat emboli may occur after major orthopedic trauma or surgery. In these situations, CT and MRI may help locate the source of emboli.

Vasculitis of the Pulmonary Artery

The most common cause of autoimmune vasculitis in the central pulmonary arteries is Takayasu arteritis. The epidemiology, pathophysiology, and clinical presentation were discussed along with Takayasu aortitis, earlier. TA involvement is more common in the systemic arteries than in the pulmonary arteries. In a series of 44 adult patients diagnosed with TA involvement of the systemic arteries, six (14%) showed abnormalities of their pulmonary arteries. Vascular findings include both aneurysm and stenosis. Severe stenosis or occlusive thrombosis may lead to pulmonary infarction and pulmonary hypertension. Imaging evaluation can be performed with MRA or CTA. Medical treatment is as described previously for Takayasu aortitis. Surgical repair of pulmonary stenosis has been successfully attempted after the inflammatory phase subsided.

Another cause of pulmonary artery vasculitis is Behçet syndrome (BS). BS is a multisystemic inflammatory disease of unknown cause. Classically, BS describes a syndrome of recurrent aphthous ulcers, genital ulceration, and uveitis. It also involves the central nervous system in 10% to 30% of cases, and the vascular system in 10% to 40% of cases. Its prevalence in the United States is probably at less than 5 cases per 100,000 people, but it is much more common in Turkey, with an estimated prevalence of 100 cases per 100,000 people. Although BS is typically an adult disease, onset in childhood is well recognized. In one series, the mean age of diagnosis in Turkish children with BS is 12 years old. When the pulmonary artery is affected by BS, the most common lesion is pulmonary artery aneurysm. Other findings include pulmonary artery stenosis and thrombosis, pulmonary infarct, and hemorrhage. These lesions are readily evaluated with CT pulmonary angiography. Treatment, as for Takayasu arteritis, is focused on immunosuppression. Resolution of aneurysm has been observed after remission of BS.

Other causes of pulmonary artery aneurysm include infectious arteritis secondary to septic emboli or pneumonia, trauma, postsurgical complications (Fig. 99-12), and pulmonary hypertension. Wegener granulomatosis (WG) and granulomatous vasculitis have been reported as rare causes of pulmonary artery stenosis. Both entities, however, are very uncommon in children. Finally, pulmonary artery stenosis or aneurysm can be a complication of surgery that involves manipulation of the pulmonary arteries. The Taussig-Blalock shunt, which classically connects the right subclavian artery to the right pulmonary artery, can lead to stenosis or obstruction of the right pulmonary artery (Fig. 99-13). Potts shunt, which connects the descending aorta to the left pulmonary artery, often results in left pulmonary artery stenosis. Waterston shunt connects the ascending aorta to the pulmonary trunk (Fig. 99-14). Control of shunt flow is difficult, and excessive flow creates massive aneurysm of the pulmonary artery. For these reasons, both Potts and Waterston shunts are rarely performed today.

ACQUIRED DISEASES OF THE SUPERIOR VENA CAVA

Superior Vena Cava Syndrome

Superior vena cava syndrome (SVCS) is a clinical manifestation of gradual obstruction of SVC flow, leading to elevated central venous pressure of the upper extremities and the head, interstitial edema and swelling of the upper body, and development of venous collaterals to the inferior vena cava. In children, although SVCS is rare, it is a medical emergency because swelling of the neck can cause compression and obstruction of the airway more easily than in adults. The most common pediatric

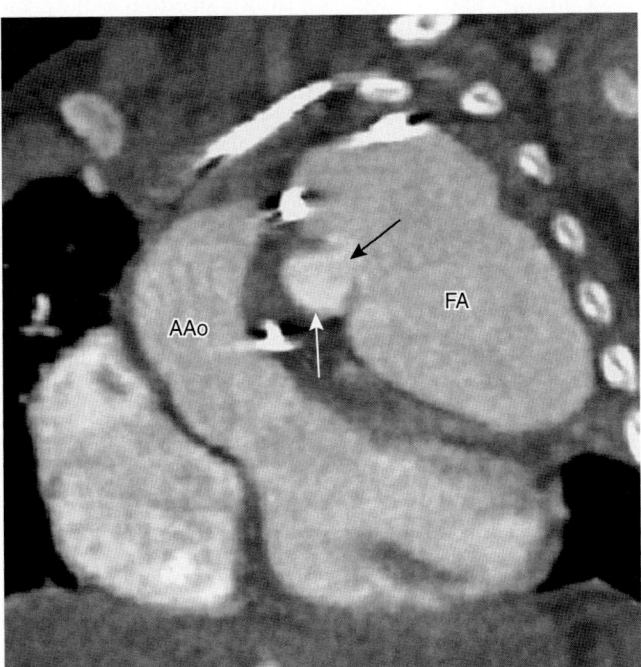

FIGURE 99-12. False aneurysm from pulmonary conduit rupture in a 1-year-old boy. Coronal reconstruction of a CT angiogram shows a large false aneurysm (FA) connected to a pulmonary conduit (*white arrow*) through a narrow opening (*black arrow*). AAo, ascending aorta.

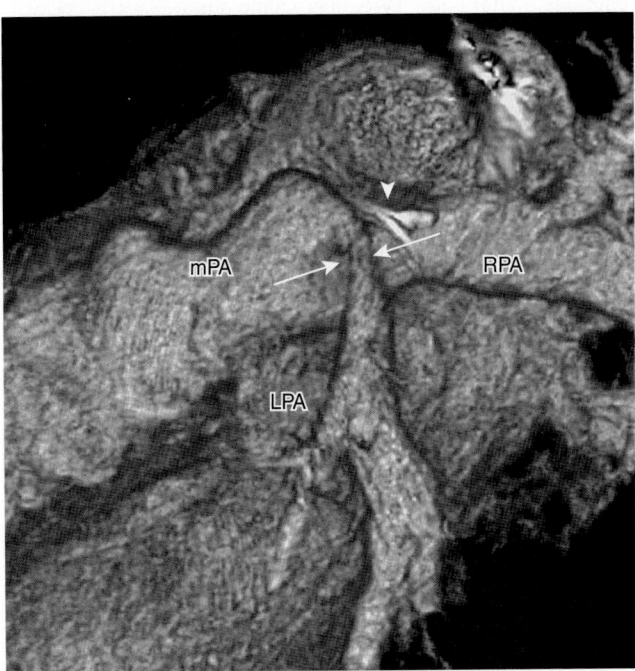

FIGURE 99-13. Postsurgical pulmonary artery stenosis in a 10-year-old boy. Volume rendering of a CT angiogram shows evidence of an arteriopulmonary shunt, now closed, identified by a surgical clip (*arrowhead*). Adjacent to this clip is a kink and a focal narrowing (*arrows*) of the left pulmonary artery (LPA). mPA, main pulmonary artery; RPA, right pulmonary artery. (*See color plate.*)

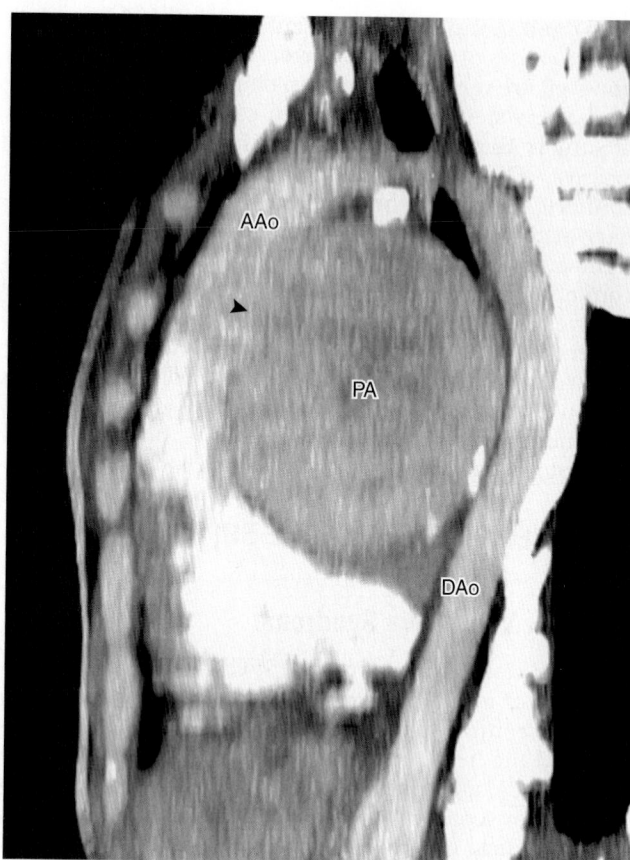

FIGURE 99-14. Pulmonary aneurysm from Waterston shunt in a 20-year-old man. Sagittal reconstruction of a routine contrast-enhanced CT scan shows the anastomosis *(arrowhead)* between the ascending aorta (AAo) and the massively dilated main pulmonary artery (PA). DAo, descending aorta.

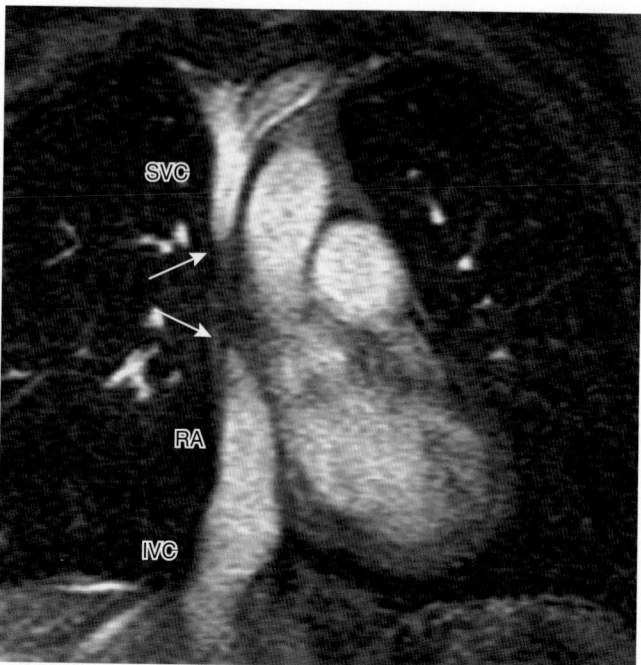

FIGURE 99-15. Superior vena cava (SVC) occlusion in a 14-year-old girl. Coronal reconstruction of an MR angiogram shows a complete obstruction *(arrows)* between the SVC and the right atrium (RA), whereas the inferior vena cava (IVC) drains freely into the right atrium.

cause of SVCS is extrinsic compression of the SVC by non-Hodgkin lymphoma. The SVC can be compressed by other mediastinal masses, including germ cell tumor, infectious lymphadenopathy, aortic aneurysm, and mediastinal fibrosis. Luminal occlusion (Fig. 99-15) can be the result of thrombus forming around a central venous catheter or pacemaker wires, or of venous thrombosis secondary to Behçet syndrome. Intrinsic stenosis of the SVC can be caused by scarring from a chronic indwelling catheter and infusion of caustic agents. Finally, the SVC flow may be obstructed within the atrial baffle after the atrial switch procedure (Mustard-Senning procedure). Obstruction of the SVC above the azygos return precludes decompression by retrograde flow into the azygos vein and leads to more severe symptoms.

> **Superior vena cava syndrome is a medical emergency in children because swelling of the neck can cause compression and obstruction of the airway.**

The gold standard for the diagnosis of SVCS is thoracic venography, in which the level of SVC obstruction, the presence of venous collaterals, and the central venous pressure can be assessed. Noninvasive tomographic techniques such as CT and MR venography can define the SVC stenosis and are helpful in evaluating any extrinsic mass. MRI has the advantage that venography can be done without contrast agent using phase-contrast or time-of-flight inflow enhancement techniques. Treatment of SVCS depends on the underlying cause. Radiation therapy that reduces the tumor size may relieve the SVC obstruction. Thrombosed central venous catheters should be removed. Residual thrombosis may be treated with selective thrombolysis, and residual stenosis may be stented.

Inferior Vena Cava Obstruction

Reasons for acquired obstruction of the inferior vena cava (IVC) are similar to those of the superior vena cava. Thrombosis of the IVC can be the result of catheter access and placement of caval filter, severe illness including sepsis and dehydration, and other hypercoagulopathy. The IVC can be obstructed at its entrance to the right atrium by abdominal tumors, such as Wilms tumor, neuroblastoma, hepatoblastoma, and hepatocellular carcinoma. The Budd-Chiari syndrome is classically attributed to hepatic venous obstruction, but the intrahepatic portion of the IVC can be involved, resulting in symptoms of hepatomegaly, ascites, and abdominal pain (Fig. 99-16). Obstruction is caused by thrombus or web. Imaging evaluation can be performed with abdominal ultrasound, CT, and MRI, with the investigation focused on the location and severity of the obstruction, and on the presence of thrombus or extrinsic mass. Treatment is directed to correct the underlying conditions. In the short term, patency of the IVC can be maintained with an endovascular stent.

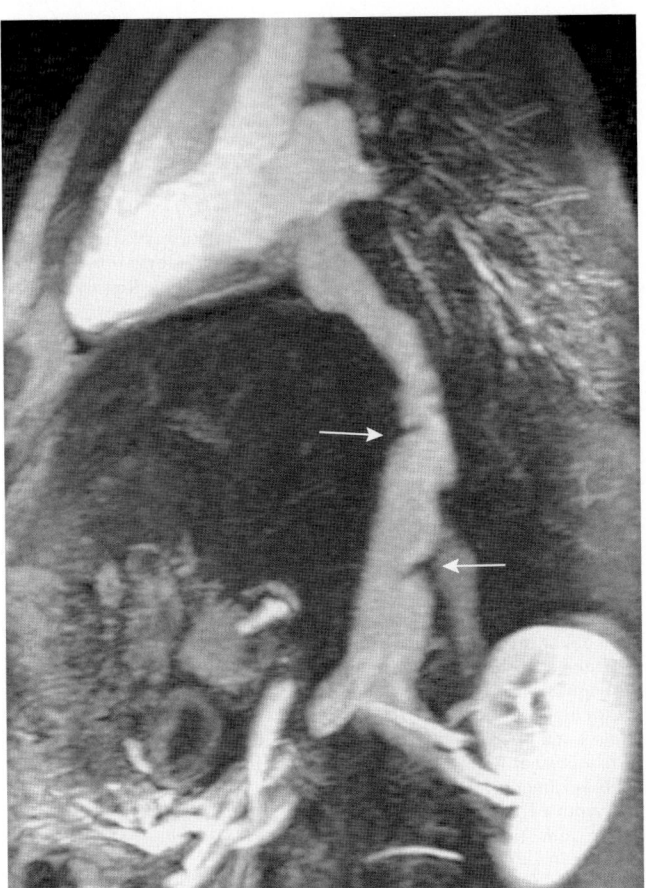

FIGURE 99-16. Inferior vena cava (IVC) stenosis in a 13-year-old boy who developed Budd-Chiari syndrome after trauma. Sagittal reconstruction of an MR angiogram shows a narrowed IVC with multiple webs *(arrows)* protruding into the caval lumen.

Superior Vena Cava Aneurysm

Although true superior vena cava aneurysm is very rare, dilation of the SVC is more commonly seen in elevated central venous pressure secondary to right heart failure or severe tricuspid valve regurgitation. Dilated SVC is also associated with mediastinal cystic hygroma, although the pathophysiology is not known. Patients with saccular SVC aneurysm may be at risk for SVC thrombosis and pulmonary embolism. Surgical resection of SVC aneurysm has been successfully performed. CT and MRI can help surgical planning by defining the extent of the aneurysm and detecting involvement of other draining veins.

ACQUIRED DISEASE OF THE PULMONARY VEINS

Pulmonary Vein Stenosis

Acquired pulmonary vein stenosis in children is uncommon but can be seen in complications of surgical repair of congenital pulmonary vein anomalies. Repairs for total anomalous pulmonary venous return (Fig. 99-17) and scimitar syndrome are at increased risk. Up to 10% of infants who undergo repair of total anomalous pulmonary venous return develop pulmonary stenosis. These patients are often very ill from pulmonary edema and poor oxygen saturation. Mortality is as high as 50%. Prognosis is worse for those who have coexisting complex cardiac anomalies, often as part of the heterotaxy syndrome. Other acquired causes of pulmonary vein stenosis include mediastinal fibrosis and extrinsic compression by mediastinal tumors. Catheter angiography is used to define the location of the pulmonary venous

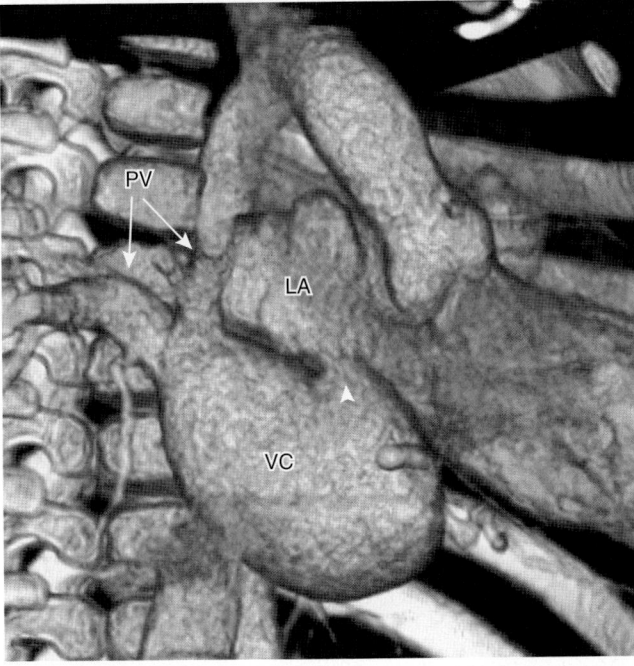

A

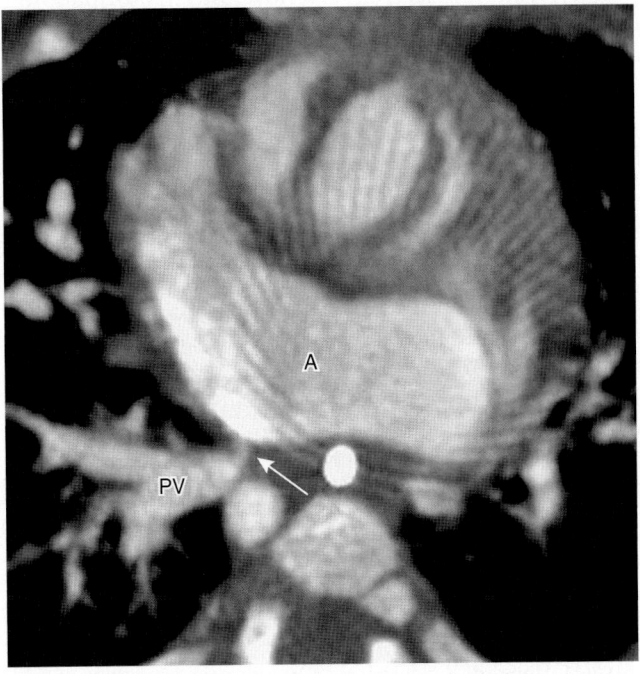

B

FIGURE 99-17. Pulmonary venous stenosis after surgical repair for total anomalous pulmonary venous return. **A,** Volume rendering of a CT angiogram from a 3-year-old boy shows the right pulmonary veins (PV) draining into a dilated venous confluence (VC), which is surgically connected to the left atrium (LA) through a stenosis *(arrowhead)*. (*See color plate.*) **B,** An axial view of a CT angiogram shows a tight stenosis *(arrow)* at the origin of a right PV in a 6-month-old girl.

obstruction, and the severity of the stenosis can be evaluated by measuring the pressure gradient across the stenosis. With their three-dimensional imaging capability, CTA and MRA can often identify the obstruction better than catheter angiography. CTA has the added advantage of evaluating the pulmonary parenchyma and airways for additional complications.

Pulmonary vein stenosis has been treated with angioplasty, endovascular stent placement, and surgical repair. Despite immediate postoperative success, restenosis is frequent and mortality is not substantially improved. The pathophysiology of pulmonary vein restenosis is not well understood. Medial fibrosis of the injured pulmonary veins, endothelial ingrowth into the stent, and abnormal reactivity of the pulmonary vascular bed have been proposed as possible mechanisms of restenosis.

Pulmonary Varix

Pulmonary varices are rare aneurysmal dilations of the pulmonary veins. They may be congenital or acquired. Acquired pulmonary varices are usually the result of pulmonary venous hypertension, caused by central pulmonary vein stenosis, mitral regurgitation, mitral stenosis, and coarctation. Pulmonary varices are generally benign and require no specific treatment. They usually regress with correction of the underlying abnormality. However, it is important to distinguish pulmonary varices from pulmonary arteriovenous malformation, which can have a similar appearance. Pulmonary arteriovenous malformation carries the risk of stroke and other embolic events and requires surgical removal or catheter embolization. Both CTA and MRA can detect pulmonary varices. In difficult cases, catheter angiography may be needed to differentiate varices from arteriovenous malformation.

SUGGESTED READINGS

General

Anderson RH: Clinical anatomy of the aortic root. Heart 2000; 84:670-673

Coady MA, Rizzo JA, Goldstein LJ, Elefteriades JA: Natural history, pathogenesis, and etiology of thoracic aortic aneurysms and dissections. Cardiol Clin 1999;17:615-635

Connolly JE, Wilson SE, Lawrence PL, Fujitani RM: Middle aortic syndrome: distal thoracic and abdominal coarctation, a disorder with multiple etiologies. J Am Coll Surg 2002;194:774-781

Hernandez RJ: Magnetic resonance imaging of mediastinal vessels. Magn Reson Imaging Clin N Am 2002;10:237-251

Lorenz CH: The range of normal values of cardiovascular structures in infants, children, and adolescents measured by magnetic resonance imaging. Pediatr Cardiol 2000;21:37-46

Rammos S, Apostolopoulou SC, Kramer HH, et al: Normative angiographic data relating to the dimensions of the aorta and pulmonary trunk in children and adolescents. Cardiol Young 2005;15:119-124

Snider AR, Enderlein MA, Teitel DF, Juster RP: Two-dimensional echocardiographic determination of aortic and pulmonary artery sizes from infancy to adulthood in normal subjects. Am J Cardiol 1984;53:218-224

Infectious Arteritis

Barth H, Moosdorf R, Bauer J, et al: Mycotic pseudoaneurysm of the aorta in children. Pediatr Cardiol 2000;21:263-266

Gonzalez-Fajardo JA, Gutierrez V, Martin-Pedrosa M, et al: Endovascular repair in the presence of aortic infection. Ann Vasc Surg 2005;19:94-98

Kim HS, Oh YW, Noh HJ, et al: Mycotic pulmonary artery aneurysm as an unusual complication of thoracic actinomycosis. Korean J Radiol 2004;5:68-71

Macedo TA, Stanson AW, Oderich GS, et al: Infected aortic aneurysms: imaging findings. Radiology 2004;231:250-257

Roy N, Azakiea A, Moon-Grady AJ, et al: Mycotic aneurysm of the descending thoracic aorta in a 2-kg neonate. Ann Thorac Surg 2005;80:726-729

Autoimmune Arteritis

Aktogu S, Erer OF, Urpek G, et al: Multiple pulmonary arterial aneurysms in Behcet's disease: clinical and radiologic remission after cyclophosphamide and corticosteroid therapy. Respiration 2002;69:178-181

Arend WP, Michel BA, Bloch DA, et al: The American College of Rheumatology 1990 criteria for the classification of Takayasu arteritis. Arthritis Rheum 1990;33:1129-1134

Clark T, Hoffman GS: Pulmonary artery involvement in Wegener's granulomatosis. Clin Exp Rheumatol 2003;21:S124-126

Dedeoglu F, Sundel RP: Vasculitis in children. Pediatr Clin North Am 2005;52:547-575, vii

Doyle DJ, Fanning NF, Silke CS, et al: Wegener's granulomatosis of the main pulmonary arteries: imaging findings. Clin Radiol 2003;58:329-331

Hiller N, Lieberman S, Chajek-Shaul T, et al: Thoracic manifestations of Behcet disease at CT. Radiographics 2004;24:801-808

Liang P, Hoffman GS: Advances in the medical and surgical treatment of Takayasu arteritis. Curr Opin Rheumatol 2005;17:16-24

Marten K, Schnyder P, Schirg E, et al: Pattern-based differential diagnosis in pulmonary vasculitis using volumetric CT. AJR Am J Roentgenol 2005;184:720-733

Matsunaga N, Hayashi K, Sakamoto I, et al: Takayasu arteritis: MR manifestations and diagnosis of acute and chronic phase. J Magn Reson Imaging 1998;8:406-414

Nakamura T, Hayashi S, Fukuoka M, et al: Pulmonary infarction as the initial manifestation of Takayasu's arteritis. Intern Med 2006;45:725-728

Ohara N, Miyata T, Kurata A, et al: Ten years' experience of aortic aneurysm associated with systemic lupus erythematosus. Eur J Vasc Endovasc Surg 2000;19:288-293

Ozen S, Ruperto N, Dillon MJ, et al: EULAR/PReS endorsed consensus criteria for the classification of childhood vasculitides. Ann Rheum Dis 2006;65:936-941

Rose CD, Eichenfield AH, Goldsmith DP, Athreya BH: Early onset sarcoidosis with aortitis: "juvenile systemic granulomatosis"? J Rheumatol 1990;17:102-106

Schett G, Winkler S, Hollenstein U, et al: Obstruction of the pulmonary artery by granulomatous vasculitis: a clinical, morphological, and immunological analysis. Ann Rheum Dis 2002;61:463-467

Seo JB, Im JG, Chung JW, et al: Pulmonary vasculitis: the spectrum of radiological findings. Br J Radiol 2000;73:1224-1231

Sharma BK, Jain S, Suri S, Numano F: Diagnostic criteria for Takayasu arteritis. Int J Cardiol 1996;54(Suppl):S141-147

Sharma S, Kamalakar T, Rajani M, et al: The incidence and patterns of pulmonary artery involvement in Takayasu's arteritis. Clin Radiol 1990;42:177-181

Shikata H, Sakamoto S, Ueda Y, et al: Reconstruction of bilateral branch pulmonary artery stenosis caused by Takayasu's aortitis. Circ J 2004;68:791-794

Sparks SR, Chock A, Seslar S, et al: Surgical treatment of Takayasu's arteritis: case report and literature review. Ann Vasc Surg 2000;14:125-129

Takagi H, Mori Y, Iwata H, et al: Nondissecting aneurysm of the thoracic aorta with arteritis in systemic lupus erythematosus. J Vasc Surg 2002;35:801-804

Taketani T, Miyata T, Morota T, Takamoto S: Surgical treatment of atypical aortic coarctation complicating Takayasu's arteritis: experience with 33 cases over 44 years. J Vasc Surg 2005;41:597-601

Uzun O, Akpolat T, Erkan L: Pulmonary vasculitis in Behcet disease: a cumulative analysis. Chest 2005;127:2243-2253

Weyand CM, Goronzy JJ: Medium- and large-vessel vasculitis. N Engl J Med 2003;349:160-169

Connective Tissue Disease

Ades LC, Sullivan K, Biggin A, et al: FBN1, TGFBR1, and the Marfan-craniosynostosis/mental retardation disorders revisited. Am J Med Genet A 2006;140:1047-1058

Coucke PJ, Willaert A, Wessels MW, et al: Mutations in the facilitative glucose transporter GLUT10 alter angiogenesis and cause arterial tortuosity syndrome. Nat Genet 2006;38:452-457

De Paepe A, Devereux RB, Dietz HC, et al: Revised diagnostic criteria for the Marfan syndrome. Am J Med Genet 1996;62:417-426

Germain DP: The vascular Ehlers-Danlos syndrome. Curr Treat Options Cardiovasc Med 2006;8:121-127

Judge DP, Dietz HC: Marfan's syndrome. Lancet 2005; 366:1965-1976

Knirsch W, Hillebrand D, Horke A, et al: Aortic aneurysm rupture in infantile Marfan's syndrome. Pediatr Cardiol 2001;22:156-159

Loeys BL, Chen J, Neptune ER, et al: A syndrome of altered cardiovascular, craniofacial, neurocognitive and skeletal development caused by mutations in TGFBR1 or TGFBR2. Nat Genet 2005;37:275-281

Meijboom LJ, Timmermans J, Zwinderman AH, et al: Aortic root growth in men and women with the Marfan's syndrome. Am J Cardiol 2005;96:1441-1444

Milewicz DM, Dietz HC, Miller DC: Treatment of aortic disease in patients with Marfan syndrome. Circulation 2005;111:e150-157

Pepin M, Schwarze U, Superti-Furga A, Byers PH: Clinical and genetic features of Ehlers-Danlos syndrome type IV, the vascular type. N Engl J Med 2000;342:673-680

Trauma

Cox CS Jr, Black CT, Duke JH, et al: Operative treatment of truncal vascular injuries in children and adolescents. J Pediatr Surg 1998;33:462-467

Karmy-Jones R, Hoffer E, Meissner M, Bloch RD: Management of traumatic rupture of the thoracic aorta in pediatric patients. Ann Thorac Surg 2003;75:1513-1517

Lowe LH, Bulas DI, Eichelberger MD, Martin GR: Traumatic aortic injuries in children: radiologic evaluation. AJR Am J Roentgenol 1998;170:39-42

Spouge AR, Burrows PE, Armstrong D, Daneman A: Traumatic aortic rupture in the pediatric population: role of plain film, CT and angiography in the diagnosis. Pediatr Radiol 1991;21:324-328

Takach TJ, Anstadt MP, Moore HV: Pediatric aortic disruption. Tex Heart Inst J 2005;32:16-20

Neurocutaneous Disease

Bronzetti G, Giardini A, Patrizi A, et al: Ipsilateral hemangioma and aortic arch anomalies in posterior fossa malformations, hemangiomas, arterial anomalies, coarctation of the aorta, and cardiac defects and eye abnormalities (PHACE) anomaly: report and review. Pediatrics 2004;113:412-415

Drolet BA, Dohil M, Golomb MR, et al: Early stroke and cerebral vasculopathy in children with facial hemangiomas and PHACE association. Pediatrics 2006;117:959-964

Fossali E, Signorini E, Intermite RC, et al: Renovascular disease and hypertension in children with neurofibromatosis. Pediatr Nephrol 2000;14:806-810

Jost CJ, Gloviczki P, Edwards WD, et al: Aortic aneurysms in children and young adults with tuberous sclerosis: report of two cases and review of the literature. J Vasc Surg 2001;33:639-642

Tatebe S, Asami F, Shinohara H, et al: Ruptured aneurysm of the subclavian artery in a patient with von Recklinghausen's disease. Circ J 2005;69:503-506

Towbin RB, Ball WS, Kaufman RA: Pediatric case of the day: abdominal aortic aneurysm in a patient with tuberous sclerosis. Radiographics 1987;7:818-821

Wendelin G, Kitzmuller E, Salzer-Muhar U: PHACES: a neurocutaneous syndrome with anomalies of the aorta and supraaortic vessels. Cardiol Young 2004;14:206-209

Neoplasm

Bagatell R, Morgan E, Cosentino C, Whitesell L: Two cases of pediatric neuroblastoma with tumor thrombus in the inferior vena cava. J Pediatr Hematol Oncol 2002;24:397-400

Upadhyaya M, Jaffar SM, Tomas-Smigura E: Recurrent immature mediastinal teratoma with life-threatening respiratory distress in a neonate. Eur J Pediatr Surg 2003;13:403-406

Pulmonary Embolism

Babyn PS, Gahunia HK, Massicotte P: Pulmonary thromboembolism in children. Pediatr Radiol 2005;35:258-274

Ceelen W, Kerremans I, Lutz-Dettinger N, et al: Wilms' tumour presenting as a pulmonary embolism. Acta Chir Belg 1997; 97:148-150

Goldenberg NA, Knapp-Clevenger R, Hays T, Manco-Johnson MJ: Lemierre's and Lemierre's-like syndromes in children: survival and thromboembolic outcomes. Pediatrics 2005;116:e543-548

Huang J, Yang J, Ding J: Pulmonary embolism associated with nephrotic syndrome in children: a preliminary report of 8 cases. Chin Med J (Engl) 2000;113:251-253

Huiras EE, Barnes CJ, Eichenfield LF, et al: Pulmonary thromboembolism associated with Klippel-Trenaunay syndrome. Pediatrics 2005;116:e596-600

Journeycake JM, Buchanan GR: Thrombotic complications of central venous catheters in children. Curr Opin Hematol 2003;10:369-374

McBride WJ, Gadowski GR, Keller MS, Vane DW: Pulmonary embolism in pediatric trauma patients. J Trauma 1994;37:913-915

Monagle P, Adams M, Mahoney M, et al: Outcome of pediatric thromboembolic disease: a report from the Canadian Childhood Thrombophilia Registry. Pediatr Res 2000;47:763-766

Nuss R, Hays T, Chudgar U, Manco-Johnson M: Antiphospholipid antibodies and coagulation regulatory protein abnormalities in children with pulmonary emboli. J Pediatr Hematol Oncol 1997;19:202-207

Van Ommen CH, Peters M: Acute pulmonary embolism in childhood. Thromb Res 2006;118:13-25

Caval Diseases

Joseph AE, Donaldson JS, Reynolds M: Neck and thorax venous aneurysm: association with cystic hygroma. Radiology 1989; 170:109-112

Kamath PS: Budd-Chiari syndrome: radiologic findings. Liver Transpl 2006;12:S21-22

Pasic M, Schopke W, Vogt P, et al: Aneurysm of the superior mediastinal veins. J Vasc Surg 1995;21:505-509

Robertson BD, Bautista MA, Russell TS, et al: Fibrosing mediastinitis secondary to zygomycosis in a twenty-two-month-old child. Pediatr Infect Dis J 2002;21:441-442

Santoro G, Ballerini L, Bialkowski J, Bermudez-Canete R: Stent implantation for post-Mustard systemic venous obstruction. Eur J Cardiothorac Surg 1998;14:332-334

Sharoni E, Erez E, Birk E, et al: Superior vena cava syndrome following neonatal cardiac surgery. Pediatr Crit Care Med 2001;2:40-43

Williams BJ, Mulvihill DM, Pettus BJ, et al: Pediatric superior vena cava syndrome: assessment at low radiation dose 64-slice CT angiography. J Thorac Imaging 2006;21:71-72

Yellin A, Mandel M, Rechavi G, et al: Superior vena cava syndrome associated with lymphoma. Am J Dis Child 1992;146:1060-1063

Pulmonary Venous Diseases

Devaney EJ, Chang AC, Ohye RG, Bove EL: Management of congenital and acquired pulmonary vein stenosis. Ann Thorac Surg 2006;81:992-995

Devaney EJ, Ohye RG, Bove EL: Pulmonary vein stenosis following repair of total anomalous pulmonary venous connection. Semin Thorac Cardiovasc Surg Pediatr Card Surg Annu 2006:51-55

Michel-Behnke I, Luedemann M, Hagel KJ, Schranz D: Serial stent implantation to relieve in-stent stenosis in obstructed total anomalous pulmonary venous return. Pediatr Cardiol 2002; 23:221-223

Nishi H, Nishigaki K, Kume Y, Miyamoto K: In situ pericardium repair of pulmonary venous obstruction after repair of total anomalous pulmonary venous connection. Jpn J Thorac Cardiovasc Surg 2002;50:338-340

Platzker J, Goldhammer E, Simon J, Abinader E: Pulmonary varices, benign congenital anomalies simulating perihilar masses of various etiologies. Clin Cardiol 1984;7:295-298

Wax DF, Rocchini AP: Transcatheter management of venous stenosis. Pediatr Cardiol 1998;19:59-65

100 Cardiac Involvement by Systemic Diseases

ALEXANDER J. TOWBIN and BEVERLEY NEWMAN

Numerous systemic diseases can affect the heart and great vessels and are important causes of cardiac dysfunction. These include both prenatal and postnatal toxic and infectious exposures, side effects of therapeutic agents, and various nutritional, metabolic, inflammatory, granulomatous, infectious, and autoimmune entities. Endocrine, circulatory, and blood disorders frequently have secondary cardiac effects. Primary cardiac tumors can occur in association with underlying systemic disorders; although rare, neoplasms elsewhere can metastasize to the heart or locally invade the great vessels or pericardium. Both congenital and secondary lung and chest wall abnormalities are associated with structural and functional cardiac abnormalities.

These entities and the spectrum of their cardiac effects are outlined in Table 100-1. We have included both common diseases that have cardiac features and uncommon lesions in which cardiac manifestations are prominent. Selected entities are discussed in the following paragraphs. Some of the lesions included here overlap with Chapter 95. Some well-known syndromes, such as Marfan syndrome, have both cardiac and other organ manifestations. These entities are omitted here and are covered in Chapter 95.

TOXINS/DRUGS

Doxorubicin

Doxorubicin (Adriamycin) is a drug used to treat a variety of pediatric malignancies, including acute lymphoblastic leukemia, acute myeloblastic leukemia, lymphomas, Wilms tumor, and neuroblastoma. Among its well-known cardiotoxic effects are cardiomyopathy and congestive heart failure (Fig. 100-1). The elapsed time from initial treatment to heart failure is variable and may occur from months to years after termination of therapy. The probability of developing heart failure increases with the cumulative dosage. Female patients and those who have had prior mediastinal radiation that included the left ventricle are at increased risk for developing heart failure.

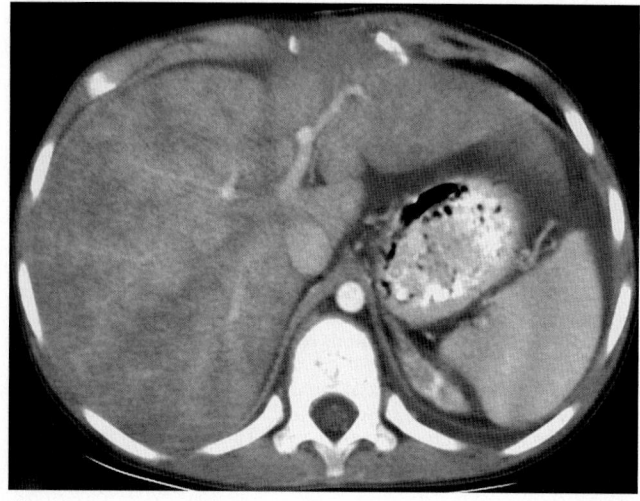
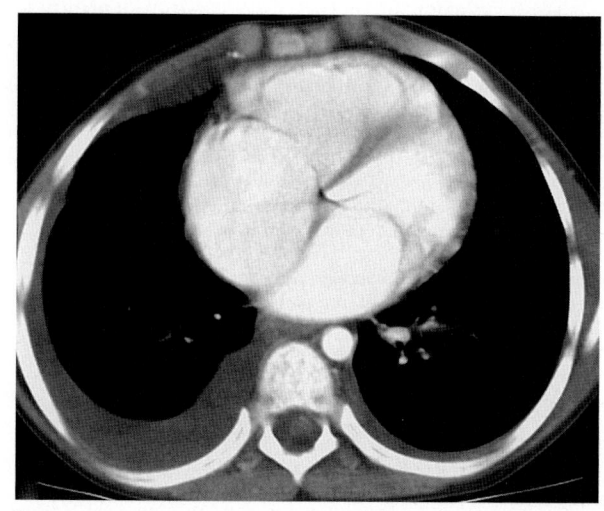

A   B

FIGURE 100-1. Doxorubicin toxicity in a 10-year-old boy with a history of rhabdomyosarcoma of the orbit. His chemotherapy regimen included doxorubicin, and he presented with abdominal pain and hepatomegaly. A CT was obtained to evaluate for metastatic disease. **A,** Contrast-enhanced CT (CECT) of the abdomen shows hepatomegaly and a mottled appearance of the liver caused by passive congestion as well as dilation of the hepatic veins and inferior vena cava. **B,** CECT of the chest shows cardiomegaly, a dilated right atrium and ventricle, and bilateral pleural effusions consistent with right heart failure. These findings were attributed to doxorubicin toxicity.

TABLE 100-1

Cardiovascular Manifestations of Systemic Diseases or Disorders

Disease or Disorder Category	Cardiovascular Manifestations
TOXINS/DRUGS	
Carbon monoxide	Tachycardia, noncardiogenic pulmonary edema
Doxorubicin (Adriamycin) (see Fig. 100-1)	Cardiomyopathy, CHF
Fetal alcohol exposure (see Fig. 100-2)	ASD, VSD, PDA, COA, arch interruption, PA hypoplasia, DORV, DEXTRO, TOF
Fenfluramine and phentermine (Fen-phen)	Valvular regurgitant heart disease, primary pulmonary hypertension
HAART (used to treat HIV)	Cardiomyopathy, CHF
Lead	Myocarditis, atherosclerosis
Radiation	Cardiomyopathy, MI, pericarditis, valvular disease, especially aortic
Steroids (chronic)	Cardiomyopathy, CHF, cardiomegaly
Theophylline	Arrhythmias
METABOLIC	
Alkaptonuria	CAD, aortic and mitral valvulitis
Amyloidosis	Cardiomyopathy, CHF, arrhythmias
Carnitine deficiency	Dilated cardiomyopathy, CHF, endocardial fibroelastosis
Fabry disease	Cardiomyopathy, mitral valve disease, thromboembolism, arrhythmias, coronary aneurysm
Glycogen storage disease	
Type II (Pompe) (see Fig. 100-3)	Cardiomyopathy, CHF, outflow tract obstruction
Type III	Hypertrophic cardiomyopathy
Type IV	Dilated cardiomyopathy
Danon disease (lysosomal glycogen-storage disease)	Hypertrophic cardiomyopathy
Hemochromatosis (see Fig. 100-4)	Cardiomyopathy, arrhythmia, CHF
Gaucher disease (cerebroside lipidosis)	Cardiomyopathy, MR, MS, AS, coagulopathy
GM1 gangliosidosis	Infantile cardiomyopathy
Homocystinuria	Vascular stenoses and occlusions, aneurysms, thromboembolic episodes
Long-chain acyl CoA dehydrogenase deficiency	Cardiomyopathy
Mucolipidosis III	AR, cardiomyopathy
Mucopolysaccharidosis	
IH (Hurler syndrome)	Acute cardiomyopathy associated with endocardial fibroelastosis, AR, MR, coronary narrowing
IS (Scheie)	AS, MS
II (Hunter syndrome)	AR
III (Sanfilippo syndrome)	Functional and morphologic mitral valve deterioration
IV (Morquio syndrome)	AR, MR, CAD
VI (Maroteaux-Lamy syndrome)	AS, MS
Oncocytic (histiocytoid) cardiomyopathy (infantile histiocytic cardiomyopathy, Purkinje cell tumor, focal lipid cardiomyopathy, idiopathic infantile cardiomyopathy)	Cardiomyopathy, ASD, VSD, nodular deposits on the ventricular endocardium or valves
Pseudoxanthoma elasticum	Premature atherosclerosis, MI, restrictive cardiomyopathy, mitral valve disease, AO dilation, vascular, coronary occlusions
Refsum disease (phytanic acid α-oxidase deficiency)	CHF, cardiomyopathy, conduction abnormality
Sitosterolemia (inherited plant sterol storage disease)	CAD, MI, CHF
Uremia	Pericardial effusion, constrictive pericarditis, CHF, cardiomyopathy
GRANULOMATOUS	
Histoplasmosis	Pericardial effusion, tamponade, AR, endocarditis, fibrosing mediastinitis
Sarcoid	Infiltrative cardiomyopathy, pericardial effusion, papillary muscle dysfunction, valvular disease, fibrosing mediastinitis
Tuberculosis (see Fig. 100-5)	Myocarditis, ventricular aneurysms, calcific/constrictive pericarditis, fibrosing mediastinitis
Wegener granulomatosis	Pulmonary vasculitis, pericarditis, coronary arteritis, MI
INFECTIOUS/INFLAMMATORY/AUTOIMMUNE/CONNECTIVE TISSUE DISORDERS	
Behçet syndrome	Aortic, pulmonary and coronary vasculitis and aneurysms, cardiac valvular vegetations
Chagas disease (*Trypanosoma cruzi*) (see Fig. 100-13)	Myocarditis, CHF, apical aneurysm
Dermatomyositis	Cardiomyopathy

Continued

TABLE 100-1, *cont'd*

Cardiovascular Manifestations of Systemic Diseases or Disorders

Disease or Disorder Category	Cardiovascular Manifestations
Diphtheria	Cardiomyopathy, myocarditis
Enterovirus (Coxsackie B)	Myocarditis
Fetal rubella infection	PDA, pulmonary artery stenosis, COA, ASD, VSD, myocarditis, cardiomyopathy
HIV	Cardiomyopathy, CHF
Juvenile rheumatoid arthritis	Pericarditis, myocarditis, CHF
Kawasaki disease (see Fig. 100-6)	Coronary artery aneurysm, coronary thrombosis, MR, papillary muscle dysfunction, MI, myocarditis, CHF, pericarditis, AR, systemic vasculitis
Polyarteritis nodosa	Cardiomyopathy, pericarditis, coronary artery aneurysms, MI, systemic vasculitis
Relapsing polychondritis	CM, AO dilation/aneurysm, AR, TR, MR
Rheumatic fever (see Fig. 100-7)	Pancarditis, valve insufficiency, CHF, valvular stenosis (MS, AS, TS), atrial dilation, left atrial thrombus, constrictive pericarditis
Scleroderma	CM, pericarditis, myocarditis, conduction abnormality, cor pulmonale
Systemic lupus erythematosus	Pericarditis, cardiomyopathy, Libman-Sacks endocarditis, heart block, endocardial fibroelastosis, systemic/coronary vasculitis
Takayasu arteritis (see Figs. 100-8 to 100-10)	Widened mediastinum, AR, CHF, myocarditis, aortitis, pulmonary/coronary vasculitis, aneurysms, stenoses
Toxoplasmosis	Myocarditis
MALNUTRITION	
Anorexia	Decreased ventricular mass, MVP
Bulimia	Arrest, cardiac rupture, pneumomediastinum
Marasmus	Thinning of cardiac muscle, CHF, CHD
Obesity	CM, pulmonary hypertension, early atherosclerotic disease
Selenium deficiency (Keshan disease)	Congestive cardiomyopathy, cardiogenic shock, CHF
Vitamin B$_1$ (thiamine) deficiency (beriberi)	Cardiomyopathy, CHF
CARDIAC TUMORS ASSOCIATED WITH SYSTEMIC DISEASE	
Fibromas (in Beckwith-Wiedemann syndrome, nevoid basal cell carcinoma syndrome or Gorlin syndrome)	Cardiomyopathy, CHF, mass most commonly originates at the intraventricular septum, occasional calcification in the tumor
Myxomas (in Carney complex, LAMB syndrome, and NAME syndrome) (see Fig. 100-14)	Attached to atrial septum and mitral apparatus in LA, can prolapse or embolize, multiple, can occur in any cardiac chamber, can recur at distant intra- and extracardiac sites, intracardiac valvular obstruction leading to CHF
Rhabdomyomas (in tuberous sclerosis) (see Fig. 100-15)	Multiple intramural hamartomas, present in utero, abnormal valve function, outflow obstruction, cardiomyopathy, spontaneously regress
METASTASES	
Lymphoma (see Fig. 100-16)	Great vessel obstruction, SVC syndrome, CHF, pericardial infiltration
Wilms tumor (hepatoblastoma less commonly) (see Fig. 100-17)	IVC extension, CHF, cardiomyopathy
ENDOCRINE	
Cushing disease	Cardiomyopathy, blood vessel fragility
Diabetes (see Fig. 100-11)	*Acquired:* early CAD *Congenital:* cardiovisceral or atrioventricular discordance, outflow tract anomalies, TGA, AVSD, cardiomyopathy, DiGeorge complex
Gigantism/acromegaly	Cardiac hypertrophy, LVH
Hyperthyroidism	CHF, cardiomyopathy
Hypothyroidism	Pericardial effusion, CHF
CIRCULATORY/BLOOD DISORDERS	
Arteriovenous fistula (especially vein of Galen aneurysm, HHT and hepatic hemangioendothelioma) (see Fig. 100-18)	CHF: high output, HHT: skin, visceral, single or multiple pulmonary AVM, angiodysplasia, coronary ectasia, Kasabach-Merritt syndrome (platelet trapping and consumptive coagulopathy)
Fanconi anemia	PDA, VSD, peripheral PS, cardiomyopathy, ASD, TOF, AS, COA, AO atheromas, hypoplastic AO, double AO arch

TABLE 100-1, *cont'd*

Cardiovascular Manifestations of Systemic Diseases or Disorders

Disease or Disorder Category	Cardiovascular Manifestations
Hepatopulmonary syndrome (chronic liver disease, hypoxemia, clubbing)	Pulmonary capillary microshunts, vasodilation, CHF—high output
Abernethy malformation: hepatopulmonary syndrome with no liver disease, portosystemic shunting	*Type I* abnormal portal–systemic (IVC) connection; absent intrahepatic portal vein; associated with VSD, AO arch anomalies *Type II* abnormal portal—systemic (IVC) connection; intrahepatic portal vein present
Leukemia	SVC syndrome, cardiomyopathy, CHF, pericardial effusion
Polycythemia vera	MI, arterial and venous clots, CHF
Sickle cell disease (see Fig. 100-12)	Cardiomyopathy, MI, acute chest syndrome, CHF, vascular thromboses
Thalassemia	CHF, cardiomyopathy
Twin-to-twin transfusion	Shared placental circulation leads to unbalanced flow. Both the anemic and the polycythemic twin may develop CM and CHF.
MUSCULOSKELETAL/NEUROLOGIC	
Abetalipoproteinemia	Arrhythmia, cardiomyopathy, CHF
Duchenne muscular dystrophy	Cardiomegaly, progressive cardiomyopathy, conduction abnormalities, CHF, MVP
Friedreich ataxia (spinocerebellar degeneration)	CM, cardiomyopathy, CHF, cardiac thrombus
Kyphoscoliosis	Cardiac, vascular, and airway displacement and compression
Osteogenesis imperfecta	MVP, AR, enlarged AO root
Pectus excavatum (see Fig. 100-19)	Cardiac displacement, MVP, anterior compression of right ventricle
CONGENITAL THORACIC LESIONS	
Congenital pulmonary airway malformation (CPAM), a.k.a. congenital cystic adenomatoid malformation (CCAM)	MR, TR, cardiomyopathy, pericardial effusion, ASD, VSD, PDA, sequestration
Congenital diaphragmatic hernia	HPLH, cardiac shift and compression, sequestration
Congenital lobar hyperinflation (congenital lobar emphysema)	Cardiomegaly, ASD, VSD, PDA
Pulmonary agenesis or hypoplasia	Cardiomediastinal shift, primary pulmonary vascular abnormalities, scimitar, TOF, PAT, hypoplastic right heart
Pulmonary sling	ASD, PDA, VSD, left SVC, hypoplastic or absent right lung, scimitar
Scimitar syndrome (see Fig. 100-20)	Small or absent RPA, PAPVR, hypoplastic right lung, CHF, ASD, PDA, TOF, COA, PFO, pulmonary sling
Sequestration	TRU, TAPVR, scimitar, CHF, ASD, PDA, DEXTRO, pericardial defect

Abbreviations: AO, aorta/aortic; AR, aortic regurgitation; AS, aortic stenosis; ASD, atrial septal defect; AVM, arteriovenous malformations; AVSD, atrioventricular septal defect; CAD, coronary artery disease; CHD, congenital heart disease; CHF, congestive heart failure; CM, cardiomegaly; COA, aorta coarctation; DEXTRO, dextrocardia; DORV, double outlet right ventricle; HHT, hereditary hepatic telangiectasia; HPLH, hypoplastic left heart; IVC, inferior vena cava; LA, left atrium; LVH, left ventricular hypertrophy; MI, myocardial infarction; MR, mitral regurgitation; MS, mitral stenosis; MVP, mitral valve prolapse; PA, pulmonary artery; PAT, pulmonary atresia; PAPVR, partial anomalous pulmonary venous return; PDA, patent ductus arteriosus; PFO, patent foramen ovale; PS, pulmonary stenosis; RPA, right pulmonary artery; SVC, superior vena cava; TAPVR, total anomalous pulmonary venous return; TGA, transposition of great arteries; TOF, tetralogy of Fallot; TR, tricuspid regurgitation; TRU, truncus arteriosus; TS, tricuspid stenosis; VSD, ventricular septal defect.
Acronyms: HAART, highly active anti-retroviral therapy; HIV, human immunodeficiency virus; LAMB, lentigines, atrial myxoma, mucocutaneous myxomas, blue nevi; NAME, nevi, atrial myxoma, myxoid neurofibromas, ephelides.

> *Doxorubicin*
> - **Well-known cardiotoxicity, cardiomyopathy**
> - **Related to cumulative dosage, female sex, and cardiac radiation**
> - **Time to manifest: variable**

Fetal Alcohol Exposure

Fetal alcohol syndrome is a common disorder affecting 0.5 to 2.0 children per 1000 live births. Affected infants have moderate to severe growth retardation both in the prenatal and postnatal period and a characteristic facies. In most children, there are associated neurologic problems including mental retardation and learning deficiencies, as well as altered behavior.

Cardiac malformations are common with fetal alcohol exposure, the most frequent being ventricular septal defect (VSD). Other cardiac anomalies include pulmonary artery hypoplasia, coarctation or interruption of the aortic arch, atrial septal defect (ASD), patent ductus arteriosus (PDA), and tetralogy of Fallot (TOF) (Fig. 100-2).

METABOLIC DISORDERS

Pompe Disease

Pompe disease, or glycogen storage disease type II, is an autosomal recessive, lysosomal storage disease associated

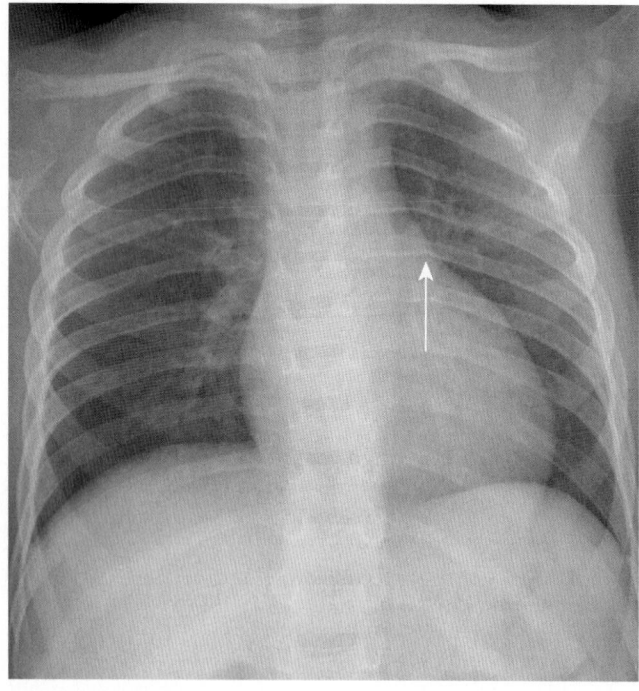
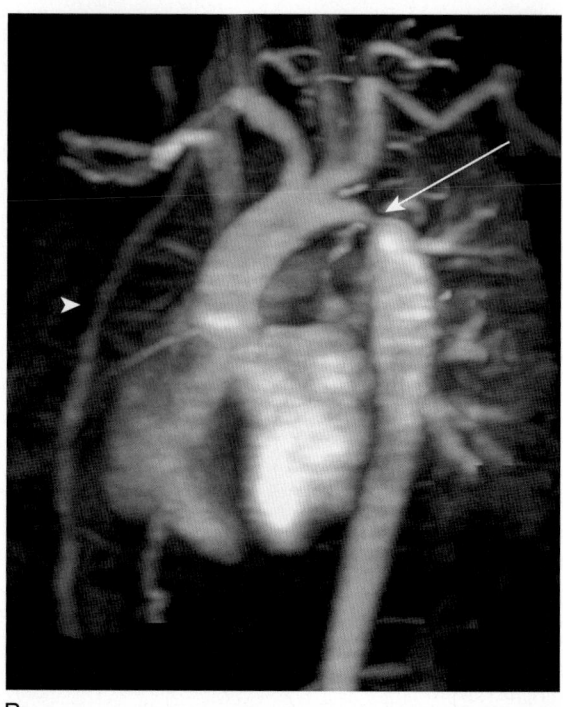

A   B

FIGURE 100-2. Fetal alcohol syndrome and aortic coarctation in a 4-year-old boy. **A,** Chest radiograph shows a prominent aortic arch and descending aorta. There is notching of the posterior left sixth rib *(arrow)* from an aortic collateral vessel. **B,** Oblique sagittal three-dimensional MR angiography image demonstrates marked coarctation of the aorta *(arrow)* distal to the left subclavian artery. Multiple large intercostal collateral vessels are present, as well as enlarged internal mammary collaterals *(arrowhead)*.

with a deficiency of acid α-glucosidase. Its incidence is 1 in 40,000 live births.

There are three major forms of the disease: infantile, juvenile, and adult. A complete deficiency of α-glucosidase leads to the most severe form of the disease, the infantile form. Its symptoms include failure to thrive, feeding difficulties, hypotonia, weakness, motor retardation, respiratory difficulties, and cardiac problems. The cardiac features include congestive heart failure, arrhythmias, cardiomegaly, biventricular hypertrophy, and outflow tract obstruction. Marked cardiomegaly, with or without congestion, in an infant beyond the immediate newborn period should raise this entity as a differential diagnostic possibility (Fig. 100-3).

Hemochromatosis

Hemochromatosis is a disorder of abnormal absorption and organ deposition of iron. Two types of primary hemochromatosis affect the young: juvenile hemochromatosis and neonatal hemochromatosis. Juvenile hemochromatosis is a severe form of hereditary hemochromatosis. Two subtypes have been described, both with an autosomal recessive inheritance pattern. Common features of the disease include liver involvement, diabetes, hypogonadotropic hypogonadism, cardiomyopathy, arrhythmias, and heart failure. Systemic manifestations of the disease are present by the second or third decade. Death, resulting from intractable heart failure, often occurs before the age of 30. A restrictive cardiomyopathy can be present because of myocardial iron deposition.

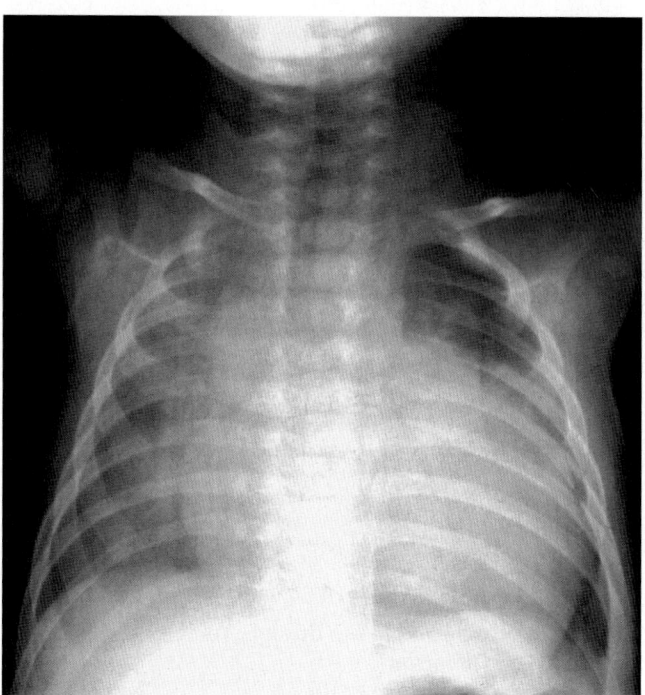

FIGURE 100-3. Pompe disease. This 3-month-old infant boy presented with shortness of breath. The chest radiograph demonstrates congestive heart failure including cardiomegaly with frank alveolar edema.

Neonatal hemochromatosis is a disease of uncertain and complex etiology. Patients present with neonatal onset of liver failure, and this is one of the more common reasons for neonatal liver transplantation. Affected infants are small for gestational age. The fetal period is complicated by oligohydramnios, placental edema, and intrauterine growth restriction. By the first several weeks of life, neonates have usually been diagnosed with the disorder. At this time, liver failure, hypoalbuminemia, hypoglycemia, coagulopathy, low fibrinogen, thrombocytopenia, anemia, ascites, and hyperbilirubinemia are present. Although the liver is the most common organ for iron deposition, other affected organs include the heart, pancreas, exocrine and endocrine organs, intestines, stomach, and salivary glands (Fig. 100-4).

Both juvenile and neonatal hemochromatosis have similar findings with magnetic resonance imaging (MRI) due to the paramagnetic effects of iron. Any iron-containing tissue will have low signal intensity on T1-weighted and especially T2-weighted and T2*-weighted sequences. Fetal MRI can be used in the third trimester of high-risk pregnancies as well as postnatally to evaluate the infant and help plan treatment options. In primary hemochromatosis, iron deposition is present in the liver, myocardium, and pancreas, but not the spleen (see Fig. 100-4). In the secondary form, which is often the result of repeated blood transfusions, excess iron intake, or cirrhosis, splenic iron deposition is present.

INFECTIOUS, INFLAMMATORY, AND AUTOIMMUNE DISORDERS

Tuberculosis

Tuberculosis is a significant cause of morbidity and mortality in children worldwide; however, the majority of cases occur in developing countries. In general, children have less specific symptomatology and fewer positive cultures, and they are at increased risk for both disease progression and dissemination. In 2002, the World Health Organization reported that rates of smear-positive cases among children ranged from 0 per 100,000 in Europe, to 43 and 45 per 100,000 in South Africa and Zambia, respectively. In the United States, the incidence of childhood tuberculosis was 1.5 per 100,000. Tuberculosis most commonly affects the lungs, but extrapulmo-

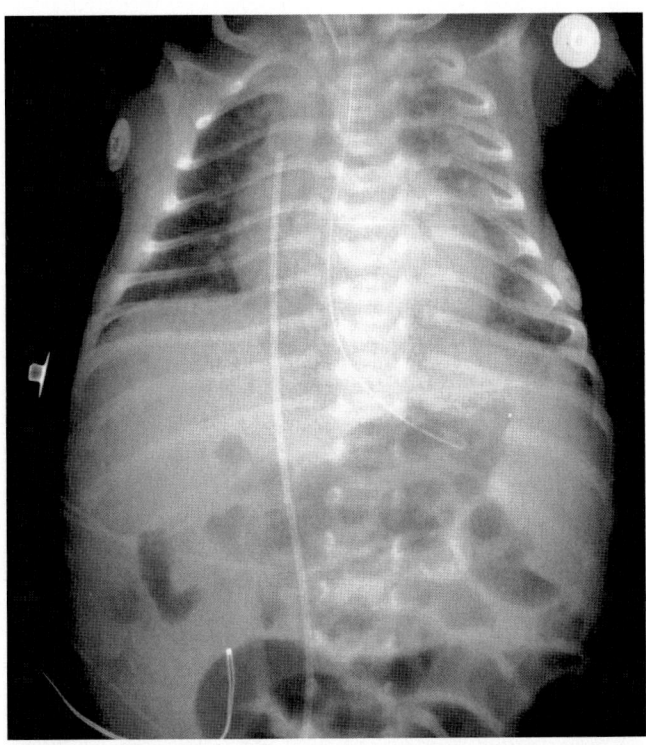

A

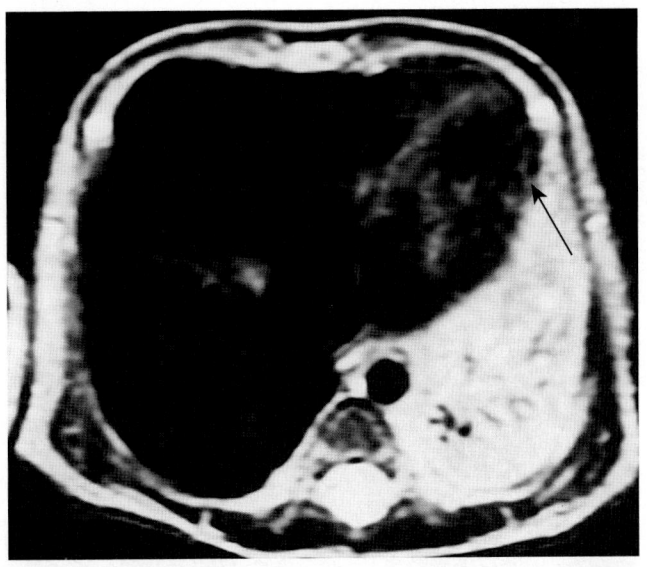

B

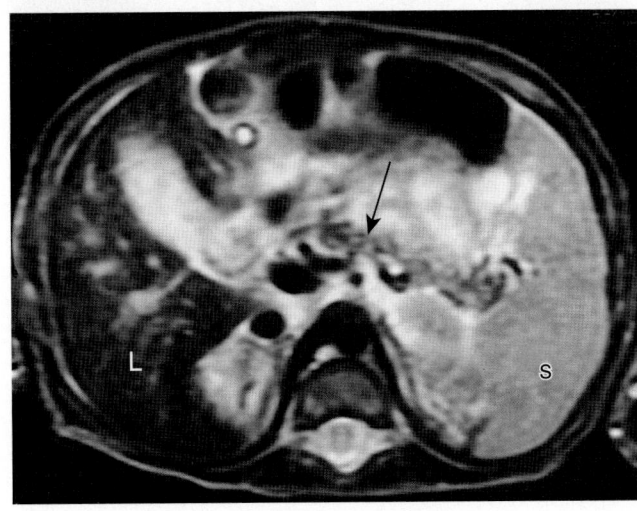

C

FIGURE 100-4. This 2-week-old infant boy presented with liver failure and a distended abdomen and was later diagnosed with neonatal hemochromatosis. **A,** Radiograph of the chest and abdomen shows mild cardiomegaly and mild splenomegaly. The liver is small and the flanks are bulging with ascites. Multiple dilated loops of small bowel are present and represent an ileus. **B,** T2-weighted axial MR image of the chest shows the "disappearing heart" sign, a feature of hemochromatosis. The near-complete signal dropout of the myocardium *(arrow)* is caused by iron deposition. High signal intensity in the left hemithorax is the result of atelectasis of the left lower lobe. **C,** T2-weighted axial MR image of the upper abdomen shows marked low signal intensity of the liver (L) and pancreas *(arrow)* compared with the relatively normal signal in the spleen (S). These findings are typical of primary hemochromatosis.

nary disease does occur in 9% to 23% of pediatric cases. Superficial lymphadenopathy is the most common form of extrapulmonary tuberculosis, followed by pleural, meningeal, osteoarticular, and miliary tuberculosis.

Cardiac involvement is rare. Disseminated tuberculosis can cause myocarditis and lead to heart failure. Although pericardial involvement with tuberculosis is unusual, it is a predominant cause of constrictive calcific pericarditis, which can present with fever, weight loss, dyspnea, cough, chest pain, palpitations, congestive heart failure, and atrial fibrillation.

Chest radiography shows an enlarged heart with pericardial calcification, pleural and pericardial effusion, and signs of congestive failure. The size and nature of the pericardial effusion is usually well demonstrated by ultrasound; however, ultrasound is limited in diagnosing constrictive findings or calcification. Computed tomography (CT) and MRI are used in select cases to evaluate pericardial thickening, calcifications (CT), and signs of cardiac tamponade (Fig. 100-5). Symptomatic constrictive pericarditis is treated with pericardiectomy.

> *Tuberculosis*
> - **Cardiac involvement in TB is uncommon.**
> - **TB is an important cause of pericardial calcification and constrictive pericarditis.**
> - **CT and MRI are used for diagnosis.**

Sarcoid

Sarcoidosis is a multiorgan disease typified by non-caseating granulomas. It is uncommon in childhood, occurring most often in adolescents, but it has been reported in children as young as 2 years old. Clinical manifestations vary according to age. In children younger than 5 years, the disease involves mainly the skin, eyes, and joints, whereas in older children, involvement of the lymph nodes, lungs, or eyes is more common.

Cardiac disease is uncommon but has a wide spectrum of manifestations, including cardiomegaly, heart block,

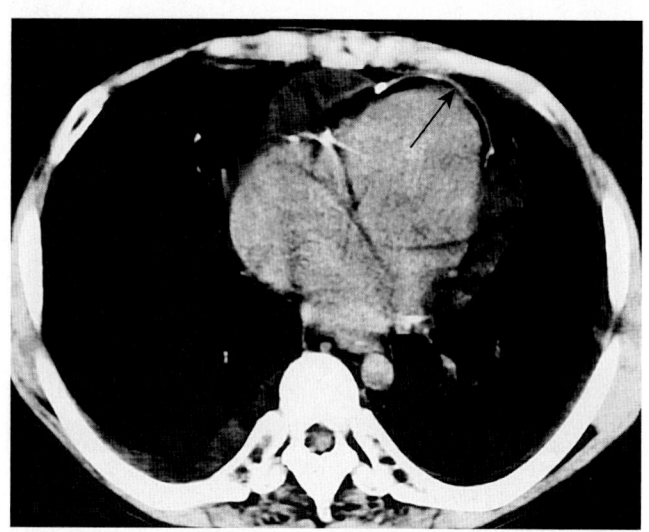

A

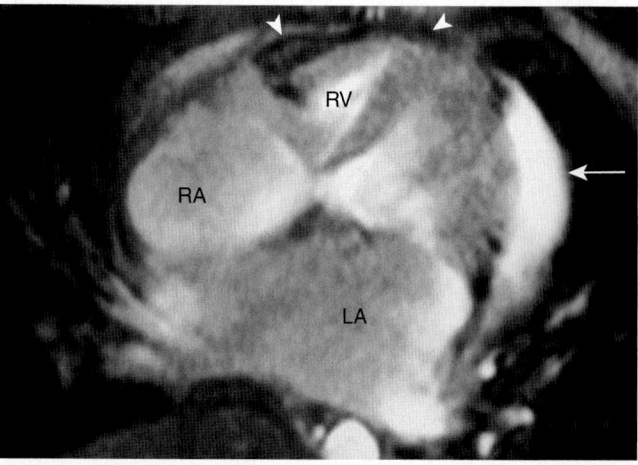

B

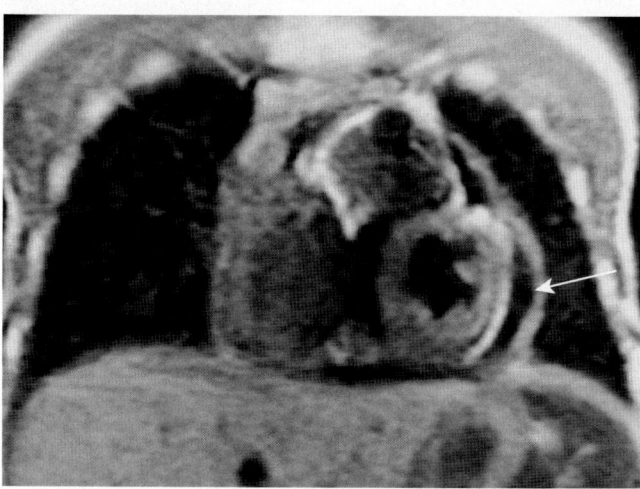

C

FIGURE 100-5. This 18-year-old man presented with liver failure due to constrictive pericarditis. **A,** An unenhanced CT of the chest shows the partially calcified and thickened pericardium *(arrow)* typical of constrictive pericarditis. **B,** Gradient echo cardiac MR image in the axial plane shows a thickened, low signal intensity pericardium, most prominent in the atrioventricular groove and at the apex *(arrowheads).* The right and left atria (RA, LA) are dilated, and the right ventricle (RV) is small. A small, high signal pericardial effusion is also present *(arrow).* These findings are consistent with constrictive pericarditis. **C,** Coronal T1-weighted MR image shows thickened, low signal intensity pericardium *(arrow).*

dilated cardiomyopathy, and ventricular arrhythmias. Other cardiovascular manifestations include pericardial effusion, papillary muscle dysfunction, valvular disease, and fibrosing mediastinitis. MRI has been used to make the diagnosis of cardiac involvement with infiltration of the myocardium.

Kawasaki Disease

Kawasaki disease is an acute vasculitis of childhood that presents with persistent fever, polymorphous rash, conjunctival injection, cervical lymphadenitis, inflammation of the lips and oral cavity, and erythema, edema, and desquamation of the hands and feet. The diagnostic criteria include fever for more than 5 days plus four of the other features in the preceding list. Fewer signs are needed when a coronary abnormality is present. It is currently the most common cause of acquired heart disease in children. It is more common in boys, and 76% of children are younger than 5 years of age. The incidence is variable depending on the child's ethnicity and ranges from 112 per 100,000 Japanese children less than 5 years old, to 9.1 per 100,000 white children in the same age range.

> *Kawasaki disease*
> - **Of affected children, 76% are less than 5 years old.**
> - **More common in boys.**
> - **Fever plus four additional signs for diagnosis.**
> - **Coronary dilation and aneurysms are most important factors for morbidity and mortality.**

Mortality from Kawasaki disease almost always occurs as a result of myocardial ischemia. The most serious complication is coronary artery aneurysm or ectasia (Fig. 100-6), which occurs in up to 25% of children not treated with intravenous immunoglobulin (IVIg), and which is more common in very young children with acute Kawasaki disease. Even in patients treated promptly with IVIg, coronary artery abnormalities develop in 5%, with giant aneurysms in 1%. Because of this complication, baseline echocardiography should be performed at the time of diagnosis and then followed up 2 to 6 weeks later. Children with coronary artery aneurysms should be assessed with periodic stress testing to evaluate for reversible ischemia. MRI and CT have also proved useful for imaging complex cases, both to directly image the coronary arteries and to assess cardiac function.

Approximately half to two thirds of coronary aneurysms regress over time. This is more likely if the initial aneurysm is small, the age at the onset of illness is less than 1 year, and the aneurysm is saccular and located distally.

Other cardiac complications of Kawasaki disease include myocarditis and valvular disease. Myocarditis is present in the early phase of the disease and can be diagnosed by abnormal gallium-67 citrate scans or using white blood cells labeled with technetium-99m. The myocarditis resolves rapidly after IVIg infusion. Both mitral and aortic regurgitation can be present.

Systemic vasculitis including aortitis and involvement of renal and mesenteric vessels can also occur. Ultrasound imaging is typically used to evaluate abdominal pain, often caused by hydrops of the gallbladder, which occurs in association with a systemic small-vessel vasculitis.

Rheumatic Fever

Rheumatic heart disease was once the leading cause of childhood-acquired heart disease in the United States and remains preeminent in many parts of the world. Rheumatic heart disease is the most serious manifestation of rheumatic fever, an autoimmune disease seen following pharyngitis with group A beta-hemolytic *Streptococcus*. The incidence of rheumatic fever and rheumatic heart disease has dramatically decreased with improved living conditions and the prompt use of antibiotics.

Diagnosis of rheumatic fever is based on the Jones criteria. Major criteria include migratory arthritis of the large joints, carditis, Sydenham chorea, erythema marginatum, and subcutaneous nodules. Minor criteria for diagnosis include arthralgia, fever, elevated erythrocyte sedimentation rate (ESR), presence of C-reactive protein, prolonged PR interval on the electrocardiogram, and leukocytosis. Rheumatic fever is diagnosed if the child has two major criteria or one major and two minor criteria.

Rheumatic heart disease has been described in the past as a pancarditis. More recent studies have described the primary abnormality as occurring at the valvular level. Specifically, dilation of the mitral valve annulus may be the initial cardiac manifestation.

The mitral valve is most commonly affected (65% to 70%), followed by the aortic valve (25%) and the tricuspid valve (10%) (Fig. 100-7). Severe valvular insufficiency in the acute phase can result in congestive heart failure and death. Noninfectious vegetations can be present on the valve leaflets. Other abnormalities that can be seen in rheumatic heart disease include pericardial effusion and left atrial enlargement, characteristically involving the atrial appendage. In chronic disease, valve deformity can occur, with fusion, stenosis, or insufficiency (see Fig. 100-7).

> *Rheumatic heart disease*
> - **Valvular disease is the most common manifestation of rheumatic heart disease.**
> - **The mitral valve is the most frequently affected valve, followed by the aortic and tricuspid valves.**

Takayasu Arteritis

Takayasu arteritis is also known as pulseless arteritis. It is a chronic inflammatory arteritis of large vessels. The aorta is the most commonly involved artery. The abdominal aorta is involved in 59% to 75% of cases, and the thoracic aorta is involved in 40% to 56%.

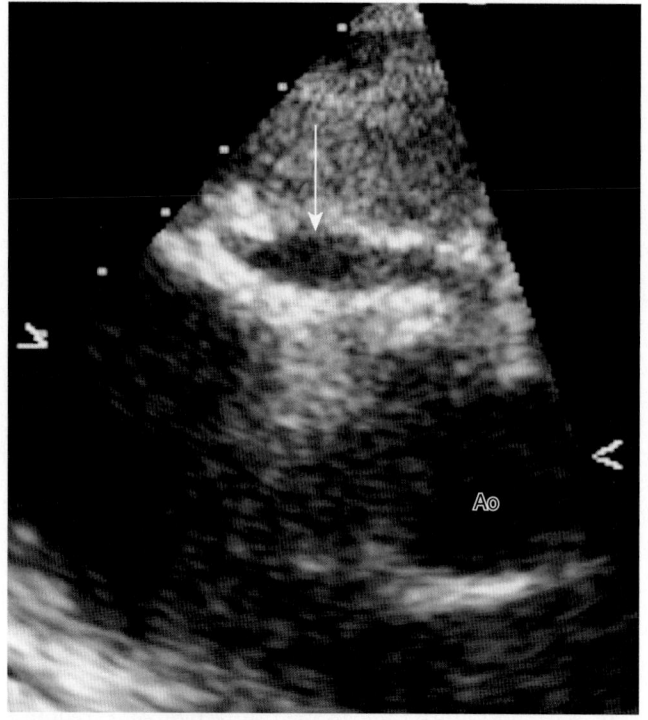

A

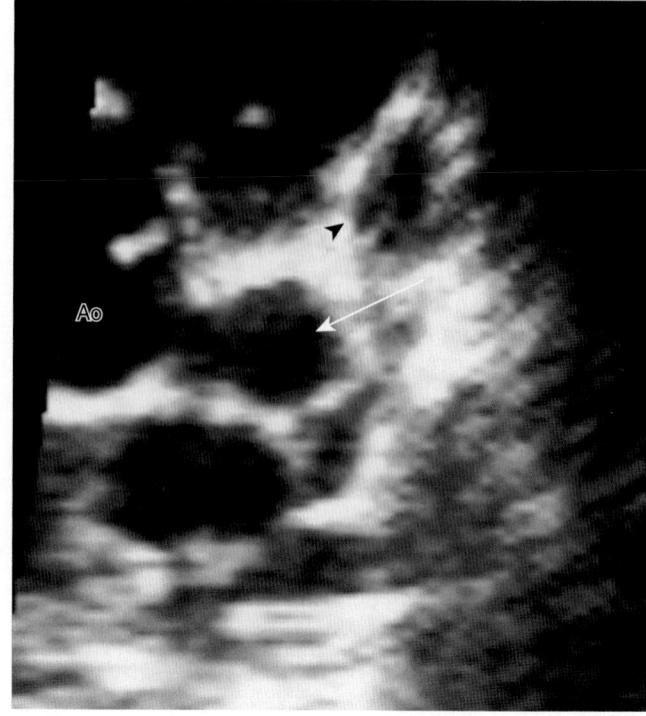

B

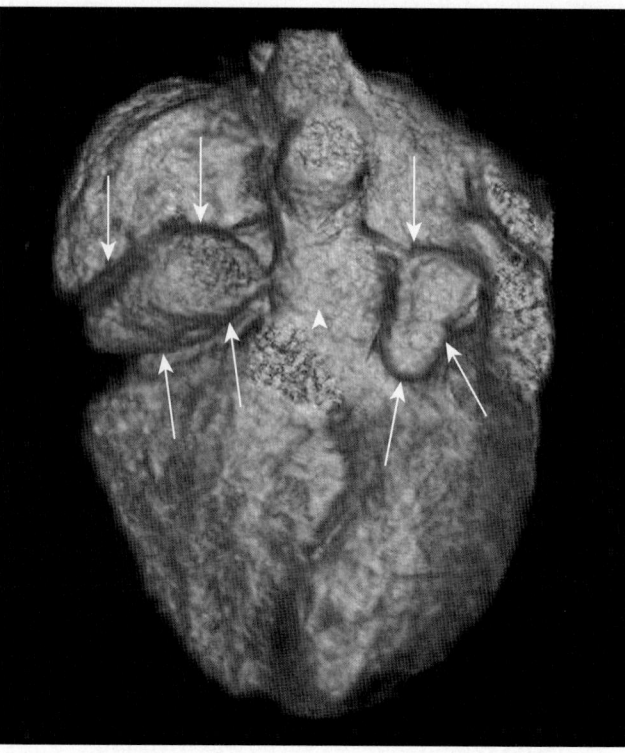

C

FIGURE 100-6. A 17-year-old boy with a remote history of Kawasaki disease. **A,** Echocardiogram shows a fusiform aneurysm of the right coronary artery *(arrow)* in its long axis near the origin of the aorta (Ao). **B,** Transverse echocardiogram shows an aneurysm of the left main coronary artery *(arrow)* near its origin from the aorta (Ao). In addition, a second aneurysm *(arrowhead)* is present in the proximal portion of the left anterior descending coronary artery. **C,** Three-dimensional volume rendering of an electrocardiography-gated CT angiogram in a 3-year-old child with prior Kawasaki disease. The right ventricular outflow tract and pulmonary arteries have been removed to expose the aortic root *(arrowhead).* The proximal-most portions of the right and left coronary arteries are normal. Giant aneurysms *(arrows)* of both coronary arteries are present just distal to the origins. *(See color plate.)* (**A** and **B** courtesy of Lizabeth Lanford, MD, Children's Hospital of Pittsburgh. **C** courtesy of Frandics Chan, MD, Stanford University.)

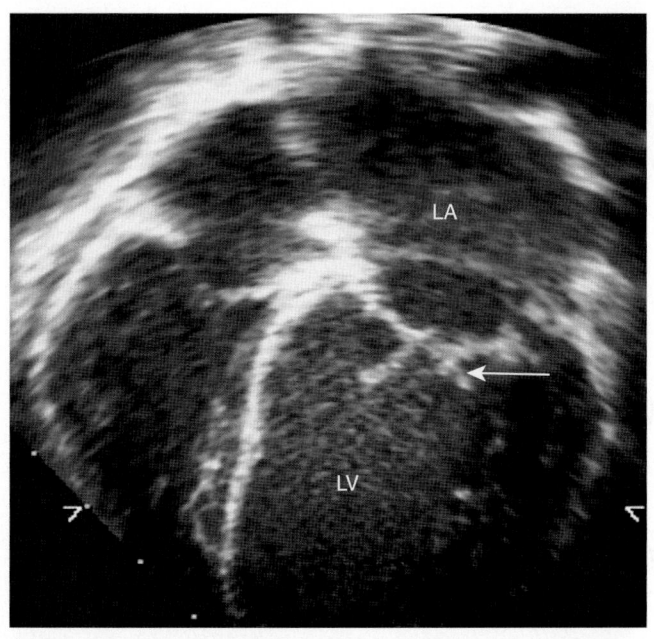

A

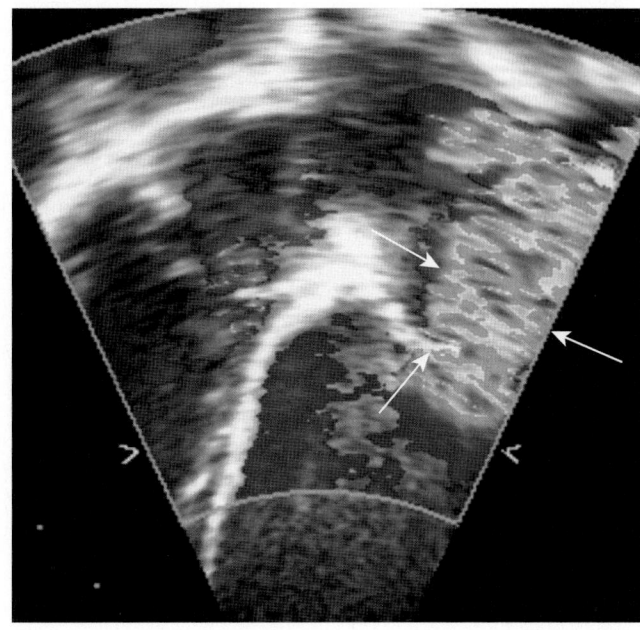

B

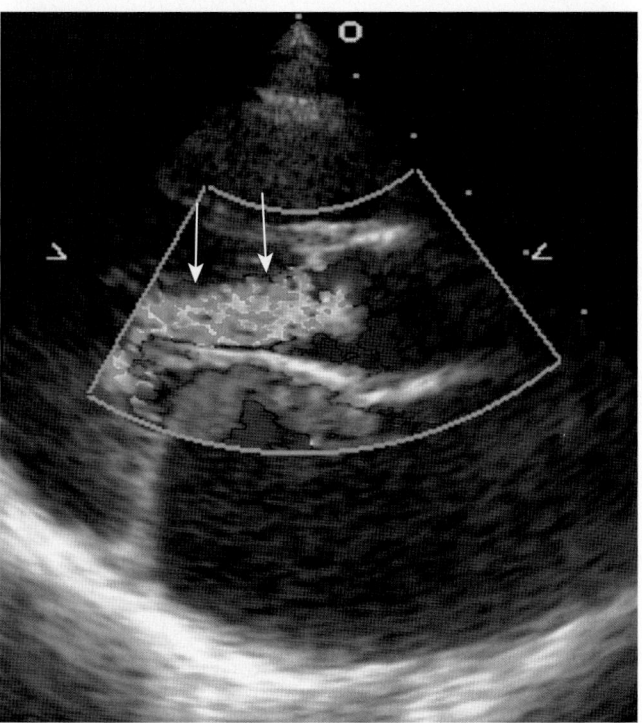

C

FIGURE 100-7. A 6-year-old boy with rheumatic heart disease. **A,** A four-chamber view from an echocardiogram shows a dilated left atrium (LA) and ventricle (LV), as well as a thickened mitral valve *(arrow).* **B,** Moderate mitral regurgitation *(arrows)* is also seen. **C,** A long-axis view shows aortic regurgitation *(arrows).* (**B** and **C,** *See color plate.*) (Courtesy of Lizabeth Lanford, MD, Children's Hospital of Pittsburgh.)

Takayasu arteritis is a rare disease, occurring in 2.6 per 1,000,000 people. It is more common in patients of Asian descent, and females make up 80% to 90% of patients. The specific cause of this condition is unknown, but it is probably an autoimmune process. Infection, particularly tuberculosis, has been linked to the development of Takayasu arteritis, especially in children.

The disease is currently divided into six types. Coronary (C+) or pulmonary (P+) involvement may occur in all types (Fig. 100-8).

Type I	Aortic arch branches only
Type II a	Ascending aorta, aortic arch, and its branches
Type II b	Descending thoracic aorta, with or without involvement of the ascending aortic arch and its branches
Type III	Descending thoracic aorta, abdominal aorta, and the renal arteries
Type IV	Abdominal vessels only
Type V	Generalized

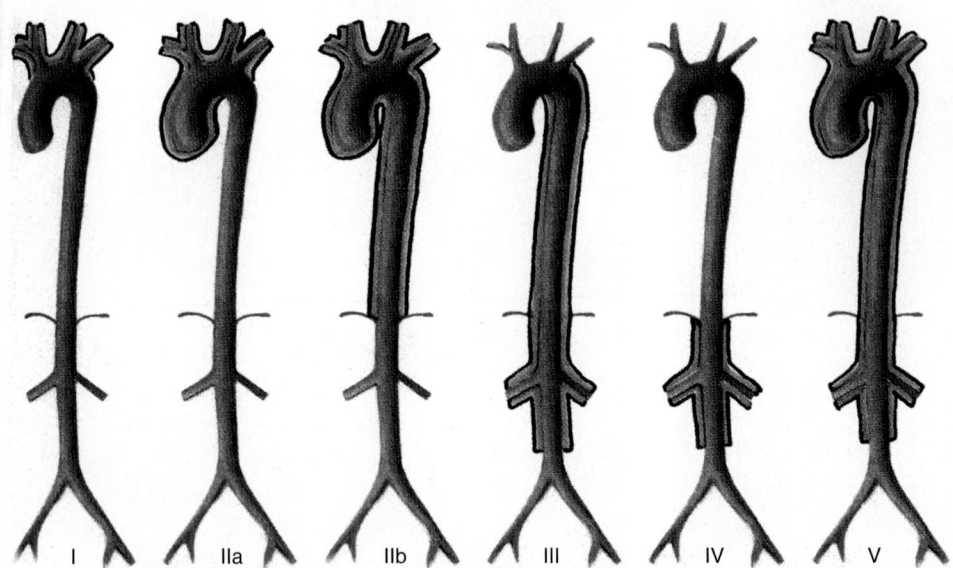

FIGURE 100-8. Diagram illustrating the classification schema of Takayasu arteritis as described in the text. Coronary (C+) and/or pulmonary (P+) involvement can occur in all types. (From Nastri MV, Baptista LPS, Baroni RH, et al: Gadolinium-enhanced three-dimensional MR angiography of Takayasu arteritis. Radiographics 2004;24:773-786.)

> ***Takayasu arteritis***
> - **Predominantly in females and Asians**
> - **Diagnosis often difficult and hence delayed, especially in children**
> - **Aorta most common, particularly in children**
> - **Systemic, vascular inflammatory, and fibrotic phases**
> - **Vascular stenosis, occlusion, and aneurysms**
> - **MRI/CT: T2-weighted images and enhancement to gauge activity; angiographic imaging for anatomy**

Takayasu arteritis has a triphasic pattern: a systemic nonvascular phase, a vascular inflammatory phase, and a quiescent "burnt out" phase, although the inflammatory and fibrotic changes often overlap. In children, there is often a long delay in diagnosing Takayasu arteritis, especially when systemic symptoms predominate.

The lesions of Takayasu arteritis are segmental with a patchy distribution. The vasculitis can lead to stenosis, occlusion, and aneurysm formation. Characteristic findings in the late phase include decreased or absent pulses, limb claudication, blood pressure discrepancies, vascular bruits, hypertension, and neurologic symptoms secondary to stroke.

Cardiac symptoms include aortic regurgitation, dilated cardiomyopathy, myocarditis, pericarditis, congestive heart failure, and myocardial ischemia. Conventional angiography has been the gold standard for diagnosis; however, this is being supplanted by MR angiography (MRA) (Figs. 100-9 and 100-10). MRA has several advantages, including its lack of ionizing radiation, its noninvasive nature, and its ability to show abnormal vascular wall signal and thickening before luminal narrowing becomes apparent. It also does not require iodinated contrast agents. Active inflammation produces a high T2 signal within the vessel wall (see Fig. 100-10). Vessel wall enhancement can be seen with the administration of gadolinium and is also used to gauge the activity of the inflammatory process (see Fig. 100-9).

Other imaging studies can be used to show the abnormalities of Takayasu arteritis. Gallium-67 scanning may show increased uptake within the aorta and its branches during active disease, and ultrasound can show vessel wall thickening. Contrast-enhanced CT may demonstrate mural thickening and wall enhancement as well as luminal dilation, narrowing, or occlusion (see Fig. 100-10).

High-dose steroids remain the mainstay of therapy to control and curtail the inflammatory process. Cytotoxic agents are occasionally needed. Angioplasty or vascular surgery may be necessary and is preferably performed during disease remission.

MALNUTRITION

Anorexia

Anorexia is a common eating disorder. It is characterized by an intense fear of gaining weight, undue influence of body shape or weight on self-image, the refusal to maintain a body weight of greater than 85% of predicted weight, and the absence of at least three consecutive menstrual periods. It is 10 times more common in girls, occurring mostly during adolescence.

Cardiovascular complications are frequent and occur in up to 80% of patients. Approximately one third of deaths are the result of cardiac complications. The most common cardiac abnormality is decreased ventricular wall thickness caused by a loss of cardiac muscle. Other cardiac manifestations include sinus bradycardia, hypotension, arrhythmias, QT-interval prolongation, and even sudden death. These abnormalities are reversible in the early stages of disease.

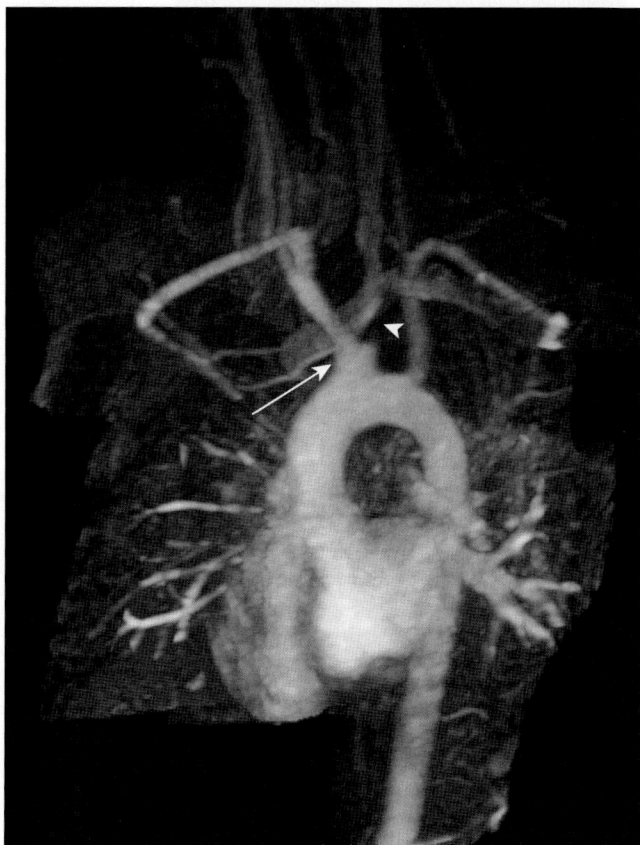

A

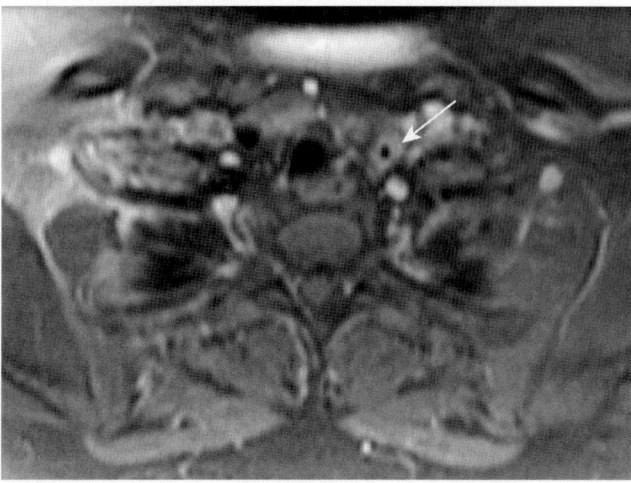

B

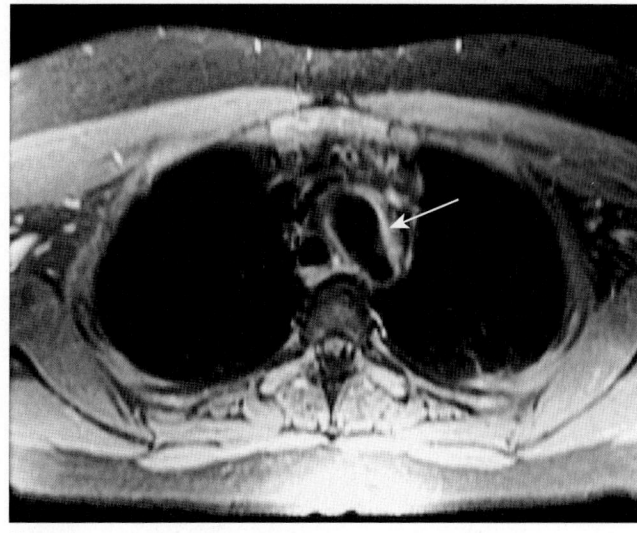

C

FIGURE 100-9. A 14-year-old girl with active, type IIa Takayasu arteritis. **A,** An oblique sagittal, thin, maximum-intensity projection from an MR angiogram shows a common origin of the left common carotid artery and the brachiocephalic artery *(arrow)*. There is severe stenosis of the left common carotid artery at its origin *(arrowhead)*, with only a small amount of flow extending superiorly. **B,** T1-weighted axial MR image with contrast shows thickening and enhancement of the wall of the left common carotid artery *(arrow)*. **C,** T1-weighted axial MR image with contrast shows thickening and enhancement of the wall of the aortic arch *(arrow)*, suggestive of active inflammation.

Anorexia

- **Most often affects adolescent girls.**
- **Cardiovascular disease is an important cause of morbidity.**
- **Cardiac complications are responsible for a third of deaths.**

Obesity

There has been a worldwide epidemic of obesity among people of all ages. The Obesity Consensus Working Group reported that the prevalence of overweight status has doubled among children 6 to 11 years of age and tripled in those 12 to 17 years of age from 1980 to 2000. Approximately 15% of all 15-year-olds can be classified as obese in the United States. Children are thought to be obese if their body mass index (BMI) is greater than the 95th percentile.

Obesity in children has led to an increase in type 2 diabetes mellitus, hypertension, and possibly asthma. Heart disease is a significant cause of morbidity in the obese. Excessive adipose accumulation induces increased blood volume and cardiac output, leading to cardiomegaly. Decreased alveolar ventilation and sleep apnea may contribute to both cardiomegaly and pulmonary hypertension (Pickwickian syndrome). Obesity (as well as type 2 diabetes) leads to the development of early atherosclerotic disease. It is uncertain whether childhood obesity increases the risk of myocardial infarction or stroke in adulthood.

The high incidence of obesity has led to a corresponding increase in the number of bariatric procedures used to treat patients, including children. Large, rapid weight loss and decreased absorption of nutrients postoperatively puts individuals at risk for nutritional deficiencies. Beriberi, a disorder of thiamine deficiency, has been reported after gastric bypass surgery. The wet form of beriberi is associated with cardiac failure and edema.

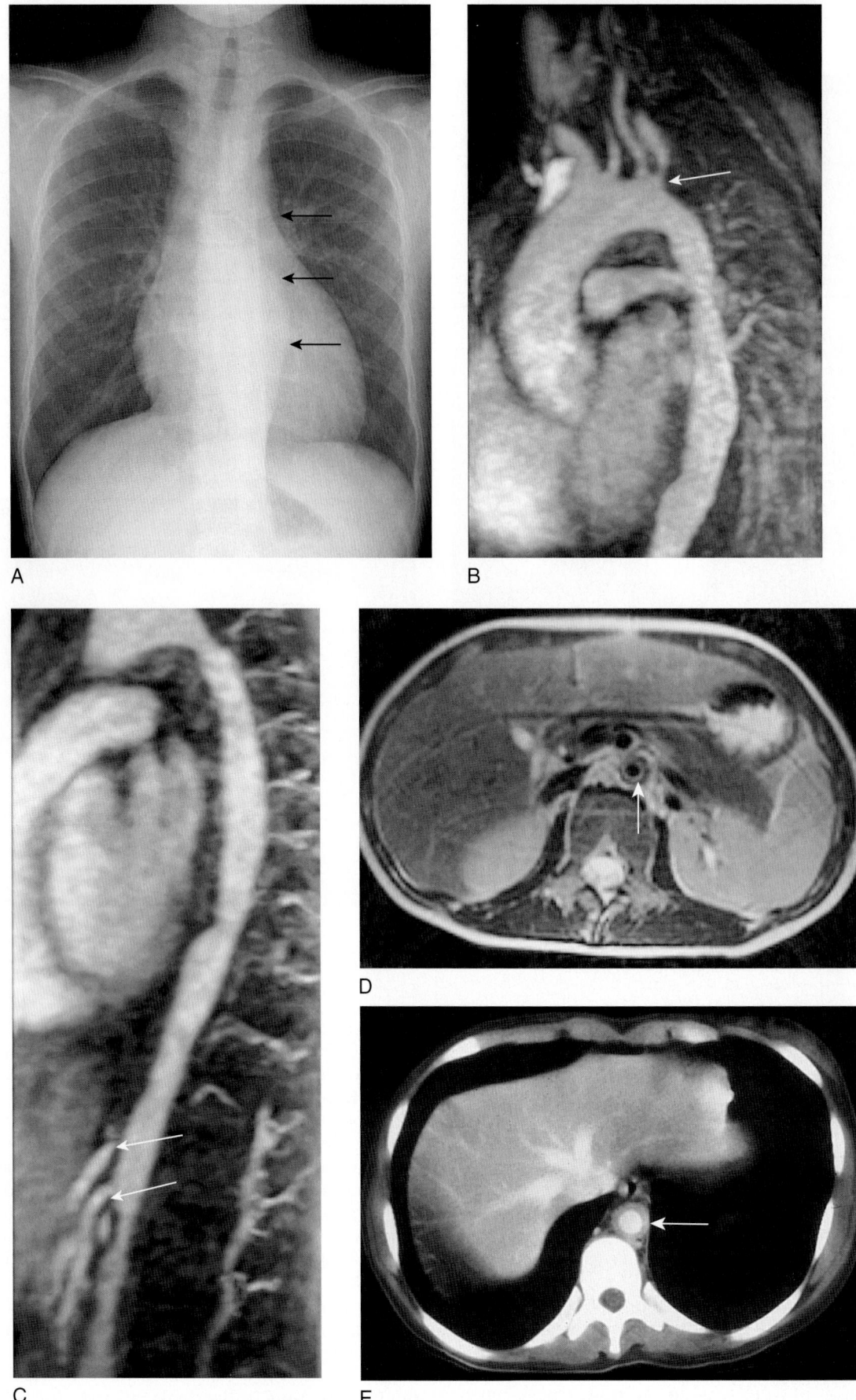

FIGURE 100-10. An 11-year-old girl with type V Takayasu arteritis. **A,** Chest radiograph shows a heart that is top-normal in size and an abnormal wavy contour to the descending thoracic aorta *(arrows)*. **B,** Oblique sagittal thin maximum-intensity projection (MIP) from an MRA image shows four vessels arising from the aortic arch: the brachiocephalic artery, left common carotid artery, left vertebral artery, and left subclavian artery. There is stenosis at the origin of the left subclavian artery *(arrow)* as well as areas of stenosis and aneurysmal dilation of the visible portions of the descending aorta. **C,** Thin sagittal MIP from an MRA image shows an irregular contour and narrowing of the descending aorta as well as at the origins of the celiac and the superior mesenteric arteries *(arrows)*. **D,** T2-weighted axial MR image shows increased signal and thickening of the wall with a narrowed lumen *(arrow)* of the inframesenteric abdominal aorta. **E,** Contrast-enhanced CT of a different patient shows wall thickening and enhancement *(arrow)* of the abdominal aorta.

ENDOCRINE DISORDERS

Type 1 Diabetes Mellitus

Type 1 insulin-dependent diabetes mellitus (IDDM) occurs relatively frequently in the United States, with an estimated 3 out of 1000 children developing IDDM by age 20. The precise etiology of diabetes is unknown, but it is thought to be an autoimmune disorder of islet cells, possibly related to prior viral infection. Most children present with polyuria, polydipsia, polyphagia, and weight loss with hyperglycemia, glycosuria, ketonemia, and ketonuria.

Cardiovascular complications are the most common causes of morbidity and mortality in diabetes in childhood and are mainly the result of atherosclerotic disease. There is an increased prevalence of symptomatic cardiovascular disease in patients with type 1 diabetes. Diabetics are more likely than nondiabetic individuals to have severe narrowing of the coronary arteries, stenosis in all three major coronary vessels, and disease in more distal segments.

> **Type I diabetes**
> - **May have a viral or autoimmune etiology.**
> - **Cardiovascular complications resulting from atherosclerotic disease are the most common causes of morbidity and mortality in children.**

In addition to its acquired effects, diabetes is also associated with congenital abnormalities in infants born to affected mothers. As part of the Baltimore-Washington Infant Study, Loffredo and colleagues calculated the odds ratio of cardiovascular malformations in children born to women with preconceptional diabetes. They found that maternal diabetes was strongly associated with early cardiovascular malformations (Fig. 100-11) and with cardiomyopathy. Early cardiovascular malformations refer to defects in early cardiac development such as laterality and cardiac looping defects, outflow tract anomalies with or without transposed great vessels, and atrioventricular septal defects. The data from this study also showed that maternal diabetes was not associated with obstructive and simple shunting defects.

Visceromegaly, hypoglycemia, and cardiomegaly occur commonly in neonates born to diabetic mothers (see Fig. 100-11). The severity of findings may be related to how well the maternal blood sugar was controlled during pregnancy. Left ventricular septal wall thickening and hypertrophic subaortic stenosis are characteristic and often transient features in affected neonates (see Fig. 100-11).

> **Infant of a diabetic mother**
> - **Increased incidence of congenital heart disease.**
> - **Cardiomyopathy at birth is usually transient.**

BLOOD DISORDERS

Sickle Cell Anemia

Sickle cell anemia is the most common single gene disorder of African Americans and affects 1 in 375. Almost 1 in 12 African Americans are heterozygous for the trait. Children with sickle cell anemia constitute the largest subgroup of patients with chronic anemia in the United States. Cardiac enlargement is the most common cardiac feature related to the chronic anemia. These children may also develop cardiomyopathy from coronary sickling and ischemia.

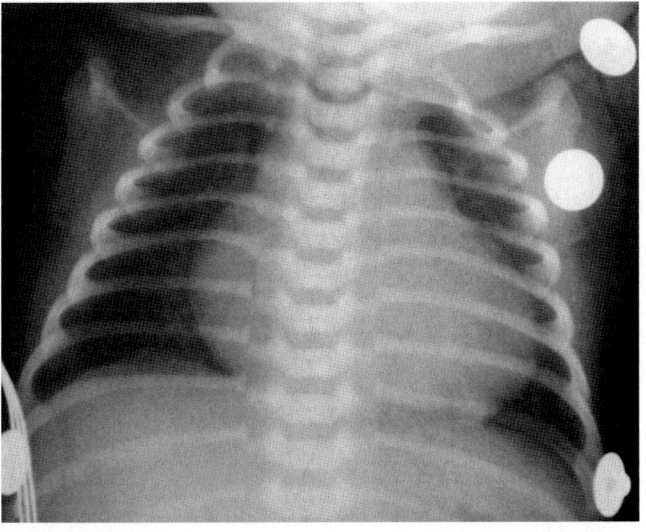

A

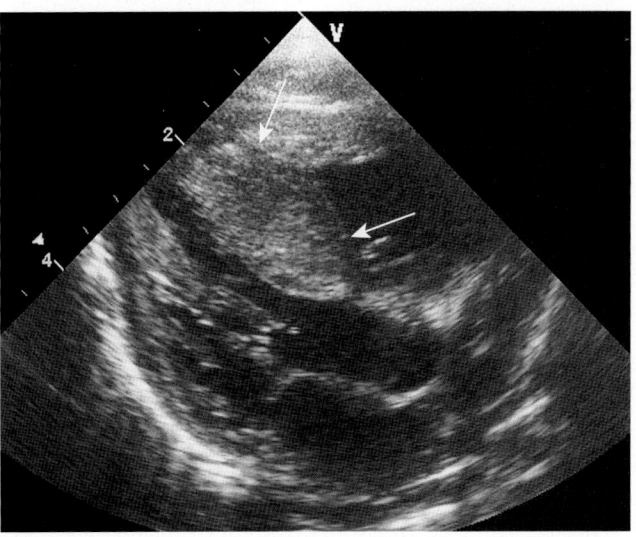

B

FIGURE 100-11. Newborn boy born to a diabetic mother. **A,** Chest radiograph shows an enlarged heart and mild congestive heart failure. A hypoplastic left heart malformation was diagnosed on echocardiography. **B,** Long-axis echocardiogram from another patient with neonatal diabetic cardiomyopathy shows septal hypertrophy *(arrows),* which partially impinges on the left ventricular outflow tract. (**B** courtesy of Fred Sherman, MD, Children's Hospital of Pittsburgh.)

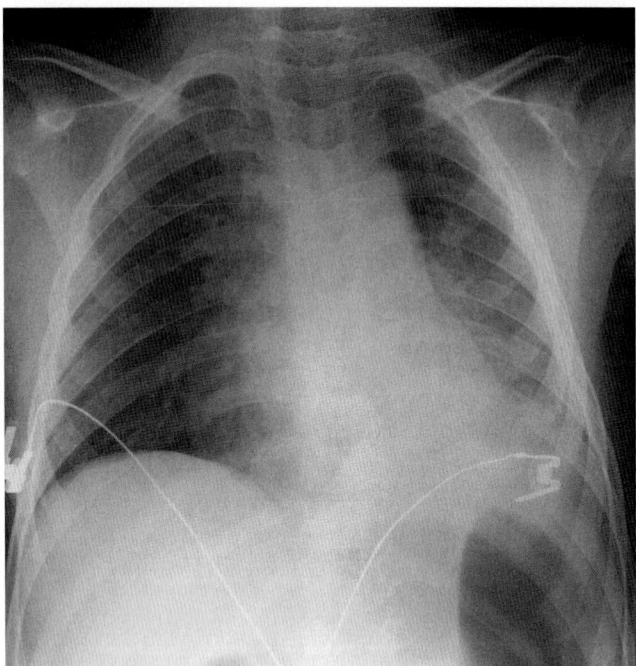

FIGURE 100-12. This 5-year-old boy with a history of sickle cell anemia presented with acute onset of chest pain. The chest radiograph shows mild cardiomegaly, bibasilar opacity that is worse on the left, and a small left pleural effusion. These findings are consistent with acute chest syndrome.

TABLE 100-2	
Causes of Endocarditis, Myocarditis, and Pericarditis in Children	
Infection	**Cause**
Endocarditis	Bacterial
	Fungal
	Rheumatic fever
	Systemic lupus erythematosus
Myocarditis	Bacterial
	Chagas disease
	Diphtheria
	Juvenile rheumatoid arthritis
	Kawasaki disease
	Lead
	Rubella
	Takayasu arteritis
	Toxoplasmosis
	Tuberculosis
	Viral (esp. Coxsackie B)
Pericarditis	Amebic
	Bacterial (esp. staphylococci, pneumococci)
	Congestive failure
	Fungal
	Histoplasmosis
	Hypothyroidism
	Juvenile rheumatoid arthritis
	Kawasaki disease
	Lymphangiomatosis
	Lymphoma/leukemia
	Polyarteritis nodosa
	Postsurgical
	Protozoan
	Radiation therapy
	Rheumatic fever
	Systemic lupus erythematosus
	Takayasu arteritis
	Trauma
	Tuberculosis
	Uremic
	Viral
	Wegener granulomatosis

Children with sickle cell disease and specific risk factors have been shown by de Montalembert and coworkers to be at risk for myocardial ischemia. The risk factors include chest pain, heart failure, or a ventricular arrhythmia. Thallium-201 single-photon emission CT (SPECT) scans showed that almost one third of the symptomatic children had a fixed perfusion defect. These perfusion defects were not in a specific vascular pattern and suggested involvement of the cardiac microcirculation.

Sickle cell chest syndrome is a common cause of hospitalization, morbidity, and mortality in children with sickle cell disease (Fig. 100-12). Clinical presentation includes chest pain, leukocytosis, and fever. Typical radiographic manifestations are a combination of features including cardiomegaly, venous congestion, new radiographic opacity (atelectasis or consolidation), and pleural effusion. The inciting etiology is not always apparent, but possibilities include infection, pulmonary sickling and infarction, and fat emboli from marrow infarction. Infection appears to be a more common underlying factor in younger children, whereas infarction is more common in older individuals.

OTHER SYSTEMIC DISORDERS

Many other systemic disorders affect the cardiovascular system. These are listed in Table 100-1. Causes of endocarditis, myocarditis, and pericarditis are listed in Table 100-2 (see also Figs. 100-13 to 100-20).

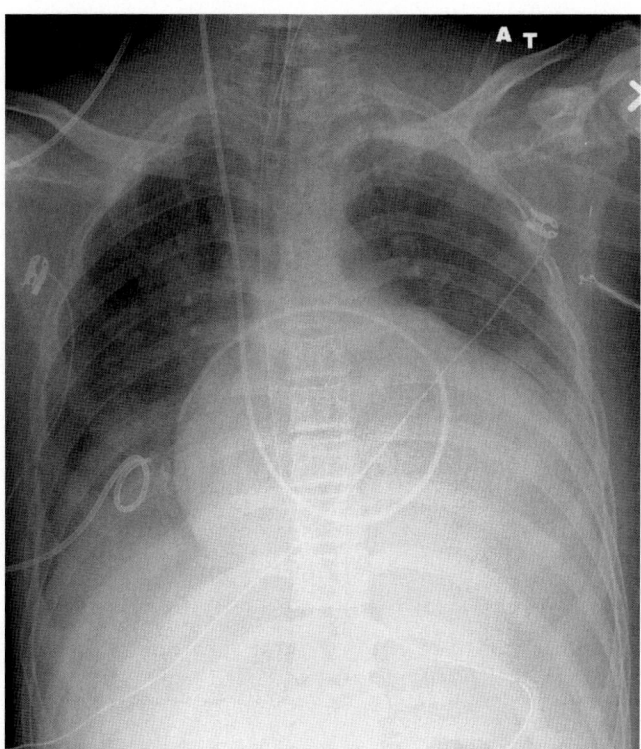

FIGURE 100-13. This 18-year-old man from Honduras presented with end-stage heart failure requiring cardiac transplant. The etiology is thought to be Chagas disease. The chest radiograph shows marked cardiomegaly and congestive heart failure. Cardiac involvement with Chagas disease occurs in the chronic phase and can occur anywhere from 10 to 40 years after infection. Cardiac involvement is an important element of the disease and includes cardiomegaly, arrhythmias, heart failure, and cardiac arrest.

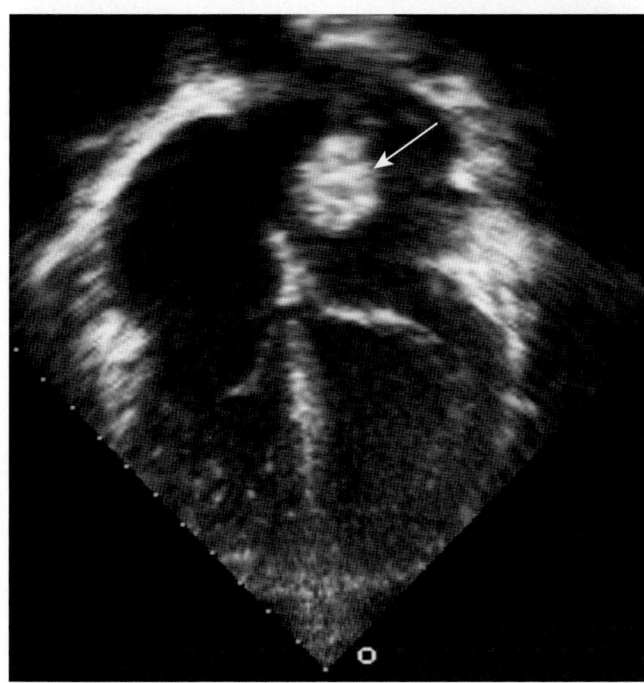

A

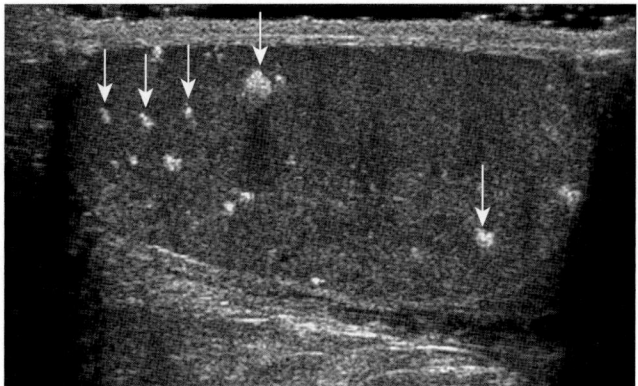

B

FIGURE 100-14. A 12-year-old boy with a family history of cardiac myxomas and a diagnosis of Carney complex. **A,** Four-chamber view from an echocardiogram shows an echogenic mass in the left atrium *(arrow)* that on resection was a cardiac myxoma. **B,** Ultrasound of the right testis shows multiple echogenic foci with posterior acoustic shadowing *(arrows).* Similar findings were present on the left (not shown). Carney complex is a rare autosomal dominant disorder that has a constellation of findings, including spotty skin pigmentation, endocrine hyperactivity, and cardiac myxomas. Common endocrine gland manifestations are acromegaly, thyroid and testicular tumors, and adrenocorticotropic hormone–independent Cushing syndrome. The large-cell calcifying Sertoli cell tumor is the most common testicular tumor and can have macrocalcifications. (**A** courtesy of Lizabeth Lanford, MD, Children's Hospital of Pittsburgh.)

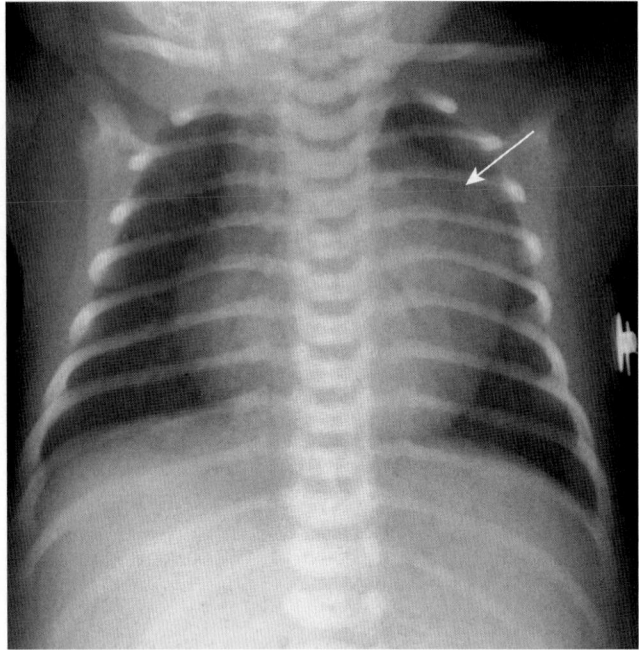

A

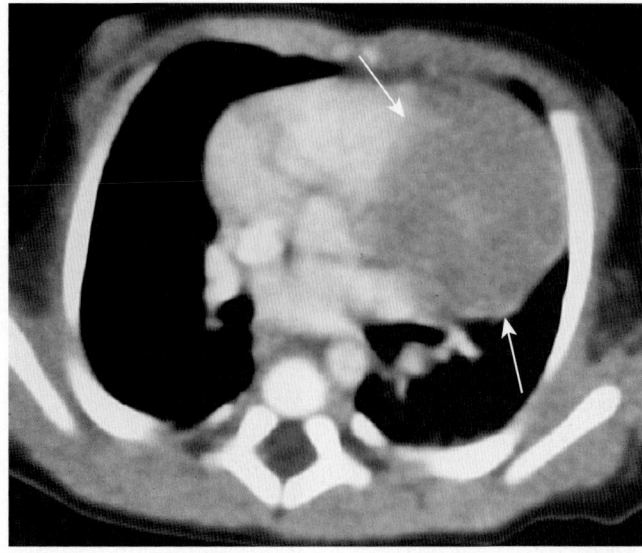

B

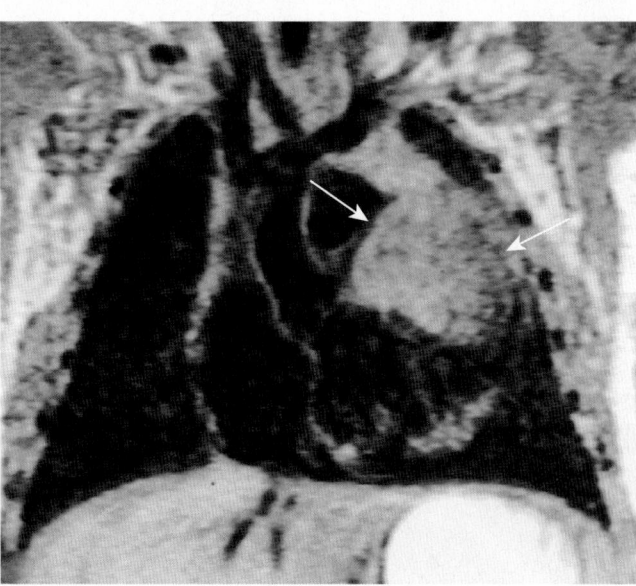

C

FIGURE 100-15. This 3-day-old boy with an abnormal fetal ultrasound (not shown) was later diagnosed with tuberous sclerosis and cardiac rhabdomyoma. **A,** Chest radiograph shows a prominent left superior heart border *(arrow)*. **B,** Contrast-enhanced CT of the same patient shows a large, soft-tissue density mass of the left ventricular wall *(arrows)*. **C,** Coronal T1-weighted MR image demonstrates the large, isointense-to-muscle rhabdomyoma in the left ventricular free wall *(arrows)*.

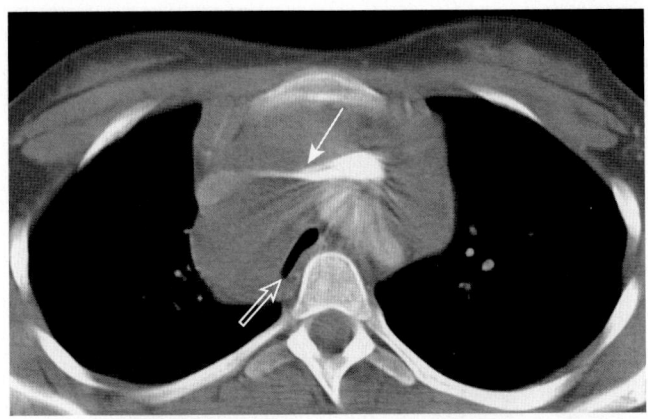

A

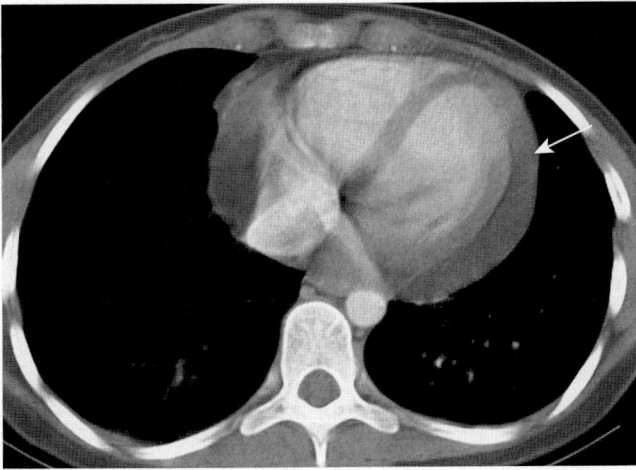

B

FIGURE 100-16. A 15-year-old girl with Hodgkin lymphoma.
A, Contrast-enhanced CT shows hypodense mediastinal
lymphadenopathy of the upper mediastinum that compresses
the vasculature *(arrow)* and trachea *(open arrow)*. **B,** There is
also extension of tumor inferiorly, producing diffuse pericardial
thickening *(arrow)*.

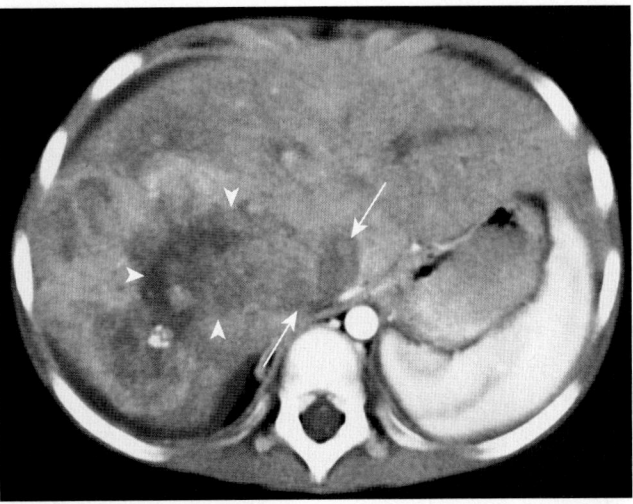

A

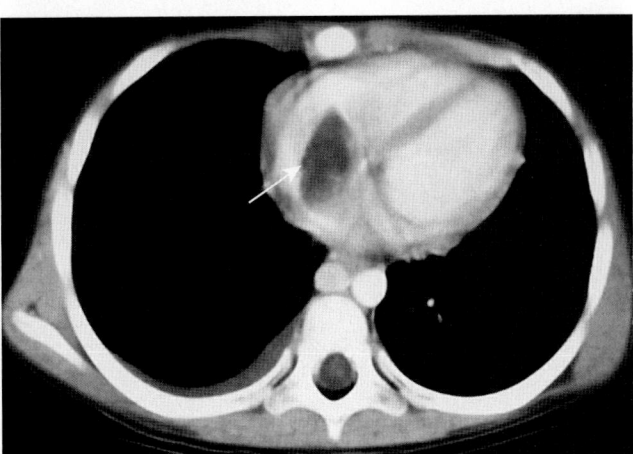

B

FIGURE 100-17. A 4-year-old girl with a hepatoblastoma.
A, Contrast-enhanced CT of the abdomen shows a
heterogeneously enhancing, infiltrative mass of the right lobe of
the liver. The right hepatic vein *(arrowheads)* as well as the
intrahepatic portion of the inferior vena cava *(arrows)* is dilated
and occluded with tumor thrombus. **B,** Contrast-enhanced CT of
the chest in the same child shows extension of the tumor
thrombus from the inferior vena cava into the right atrium
(arrow). The azygos vein is enlarged, allowing systemic blood
return.

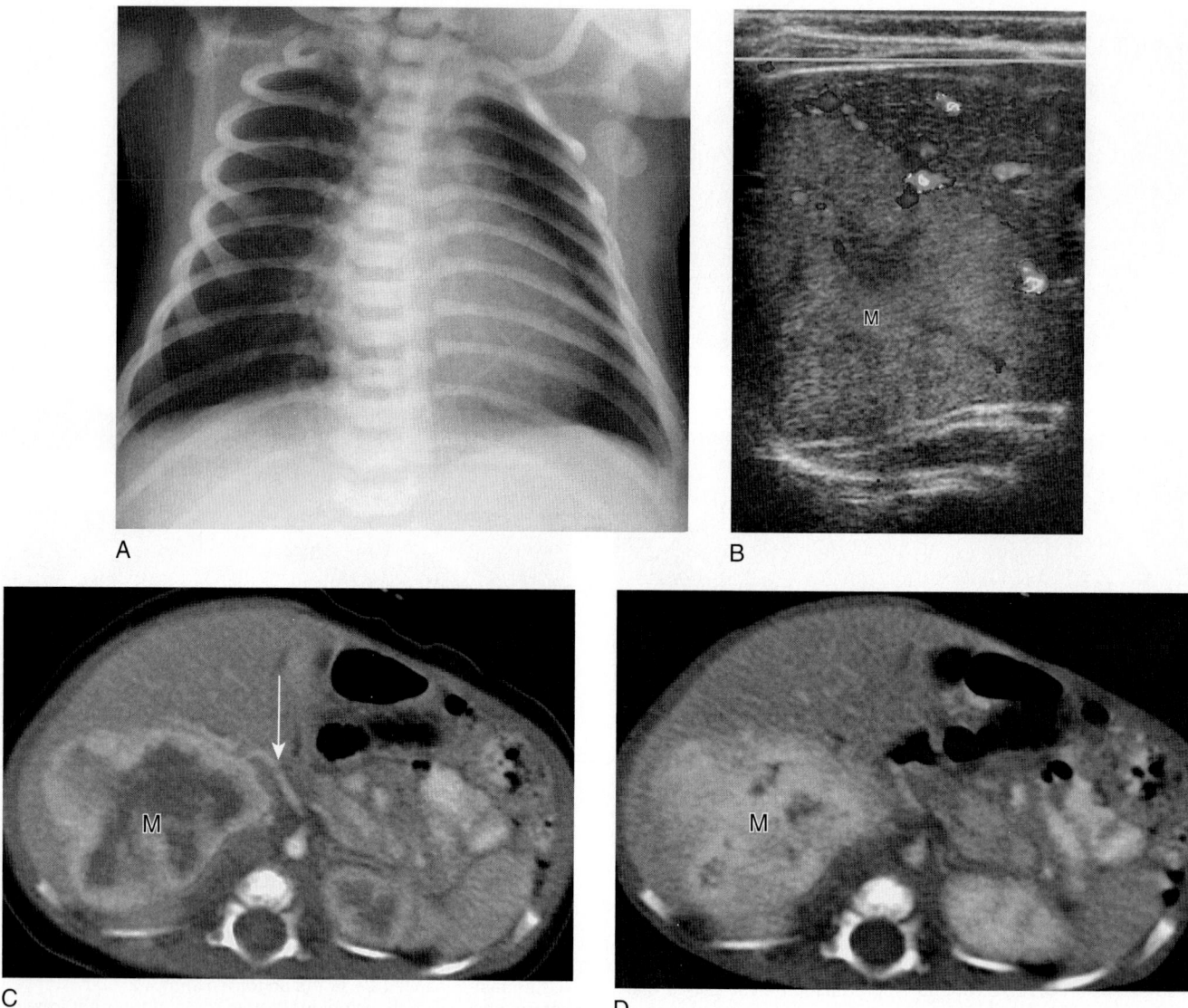

FIGURE 100-18. This 4-day-old infant girl presented with signs of heart failure and was later diagnosed with a hepatic hemangioendothelioma. **A,** Chest radiograph shows mild cardiomegaly and indistinctness of the pulmonary vasculature, suggesting mild congestion. **B,** An ultrasound of the liver in the same patient shows a large, hyperechoic, moderately vascular mass (M) occupying most of the right lobe of the liver. Contrast-enhanced CT images of the abdomen in the arterial **(C)** and portal venous **(D)** phases show a large mass (M) in the right lobe of the liver. This mass has early, peripheral arterial enhancement that fills in on the delayed, portal venous images. In the arterial phase, a mildly enlarged hepatic artery is present (*arrow* in **C**). These findings are characteristic of hepatic hemangioendothelioma.

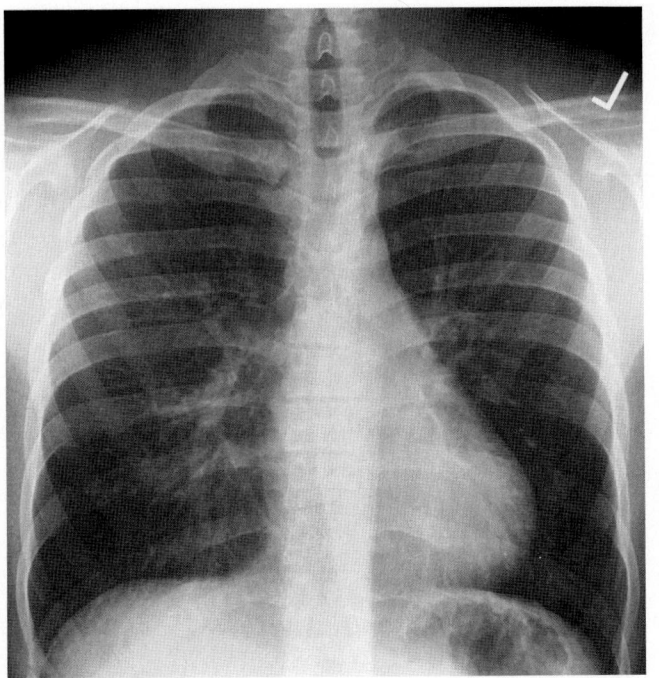

A

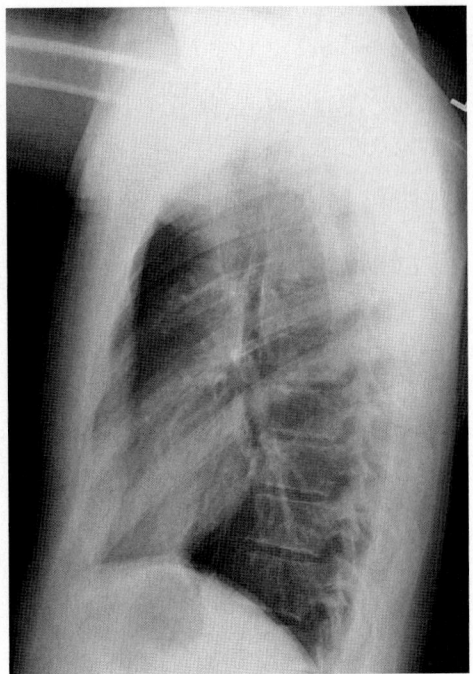

B

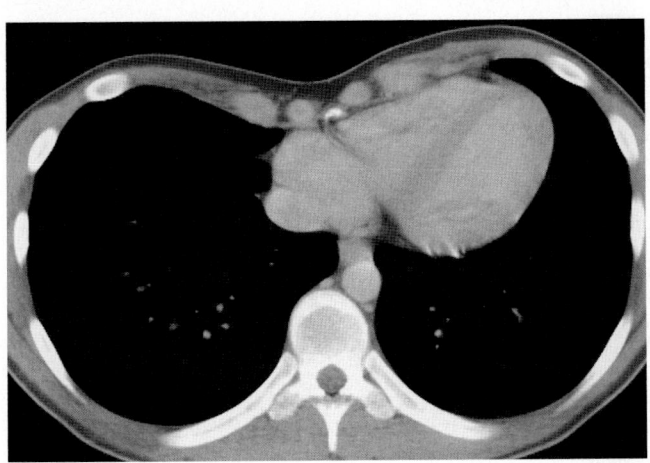

C

FIGURE 100-19. A 20-year-old man with a pectus excavatum deformity. **A,** Posteroanterior view of the chest shows indistinctness of the right heart border and prominence of the left heart border. The anterior ribs are oriented vertically. **B,** The lateral view of the chest shows narrowing of the anteroposterior diameter of the chest and compression of the heart by the inwardly bowing lower sternum. **C,** Contrast-enhanced CT of the same patient shows compression of the right atrium and ventricle by the sternum, and cardiac displacement to the left.

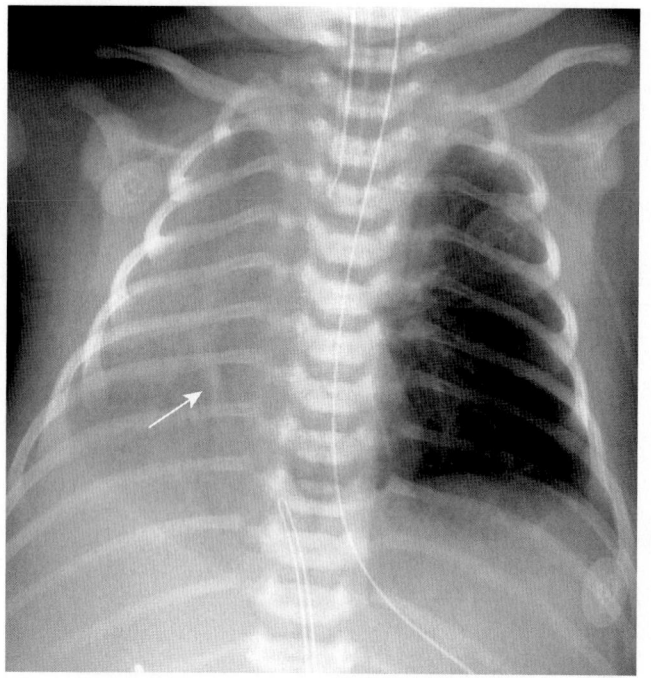

A

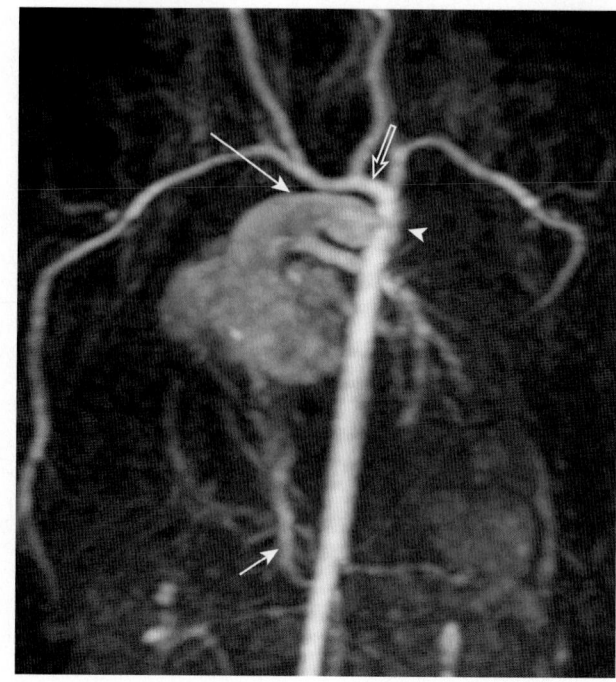

B

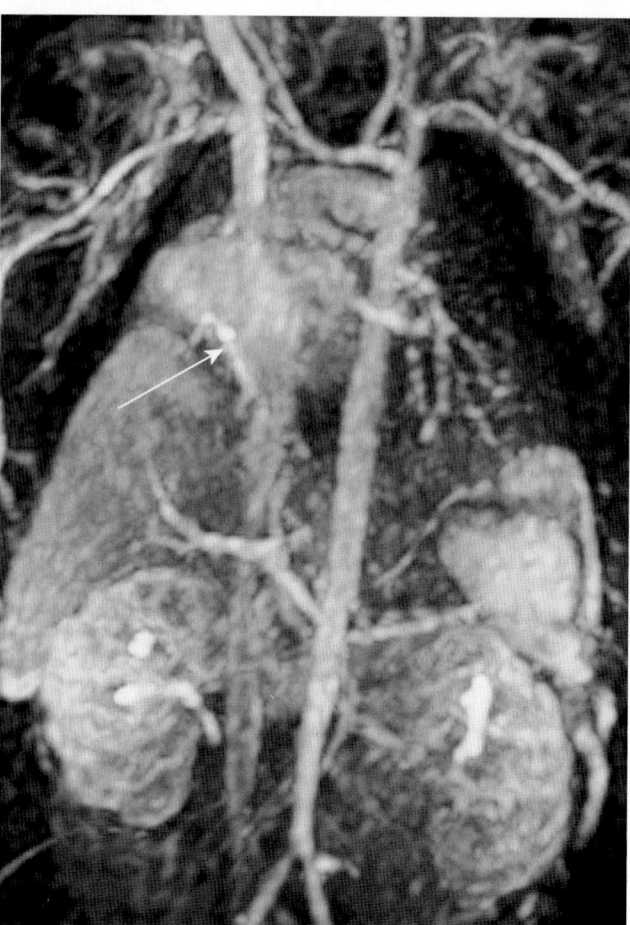

C

FIGURE 100-20. A 4-day-old infant with respiratory distress and complex anomalies including scimitar syndrome. **A,** Chest radiograph shows a small, opacified right lung with rightward mediastinal shift, and a subtle linear, tubular density that suggests a scimitar vein *(arrow)*. **B,** Coronal three-dimensional volumetric maximum-intensity projection (MIP) MR angiography image shows multiple abnormalities. The right lung is hypoplastic, and its arterial supply is systemic, arising entirely from multiple branches of the celiac artery *(short arrow)*; no right pulmonary artery is present. The heart is shifted to the right and there is a large patent ductus arteriosus *(long arrow)*. The aortic arch is hypoplastic *(open arrow)*, and an aortic coarctation is present *(arrowhead)*. The right pulmonary opacification seen on the chest radiograph is probably caused by the high-volume flow to the right lung, perhaps with venous obstruction. **C,** Venous-phase thin coronal MIP MRA image shows the small right scimitar vein *(arrow)* draining to the inferior vena cava.

SUGGESTED READINGS

Toxins/Drugs

Bertrand J, Floyd LL, Weber MK: Guidelines for identifying and referring persons with fetal alcohol syndrome. MMWR Recomm Rep 2005;54:1-14

Chaudhuri JD: Alcohol and the developing fetus: a review. Med Sci Monit 2000;6:1031-1041

Davidson DM: Cardiovascular effects of alcohol. West J Med 1989;151:430-439

Green, DM: Late effects of treatment for cancer during childhood and adolescence. Curr Probl Cancer 2003;27:127-142

Simbre VC, Duffy SA, Dadlani GH, et al: Cardiotoxicity of cancer chemotherapy: implications for children. Paediatr Drugs 2005;7:187-202

Zareba KM, Lavigne JE, Lipshultz SE: Cardiovascular effects of HAART in infants and children of HIV-infected mothers. Cardiovasc Toxicol 2004;4:271-279

Metabolic Disorders

Dangel JH: Cardiovascular changes in children with mucopolysaccharide storage diseases and related disorders: clinical and echocardiographic findings in 64 patients. Eur J Pediatr 1998;157:534-538

Desai MY, Lima JA, Bluemke DA: Cardiovascular magnetic resonance imaging: current applications and future directions. Methods Enzymol 2004;386:122-148

Moses SW, Wanderman KL, Myroz A, Frydman M: Cardiac involvement in glycogen storage disease type III. Eur J Pediatr 1989;148:764-766

Murray KF, Kowdley KV: Neonatal hemochromatosis. Pediatrics 2001;108:960-964

Phornphutkul C, Introne WJ, Perry MB, et al: Natural history of alkaptonuria. N Engl J Med 2002;347:2111-2121

Pietrangelo A: Hereditary hemochromatosis—a new look at an old disease. N Engl J Med 2004;350:2383-2397

van den Hout HM, Hop W, van Diggelen OP, et al: The natural course of infantile Pompe's disease: 20 original cases compared with 133 cases from the literature. Pediatrics 2003;112:332-340

Wippermann CF, Beck M, Schranz D, et al: Mitral and aortic regurgitation in 84 patients with mucopolysaccharidoses. Eur J Pediatr 1995;154:98-101

Infectious, Inflammatory, and Autoimmune Disorders

Aluquin VPR, Albano SA, Chan F, et al: Magnetic resonance imaging in the diagnosis and follow up of Takayasu's arteritis in children. Ann Rheum Dis 2002;61:526-529

Bozbuga N, Erentug V, Eren E, et al: Pericardiectomy for chronic constrictive tuberculous pericarditis: risks and predictors of survival. Tex Heart Inst J 2003;30:180-185

Brogan PA, Dillon MJ: Vasculitis from the pediatric perspective. Curr Rheumatol Rep 2000;2:411-416

Fauroux B, Clement A: Paediatric sarcoidosis. Paediatr Respir Rev 2005;6:128-133

Feja K, Saiman L: Tuberculosis in children. Clin Chest Med 2005;26:295-312

Ferrieri P, for the Jones Criteria Working Group: Proceedings of the Jones Criteria workshop. Circulation 2002;106:2521-2523

Fulton DR, Newburger JN: Long-term cardiac sequelae of Kawasaki disease. Curr Rheumatol Rep 2000;2:324-329

Harisinghani MG, McLoud TC, Shepard JO, et al: Tuberculosis from head to toe 2000;20:449-470

Jain S, Sharma N, Singh S, et al: Takayasu arteritis in children and young Indians. Int J Cardiol 2000;75:S153-157

Nastri MV, Baptista LPS, Baroni RH, et al: Gadolinium-enhanced three-dimensional MR angiography of Takayasu arteritis. Radiographics 2004;24:773-786

Newburger JW, Fulton DR: Kawasaki disease. Curr Opin Pediatr 2004;16:508-514

Pemberton J, Sahn DJ: Imaging of the aorta. Int J Cardiol 2004; 97:53-60

Prager RL, Burney DP, Waterhouse G, Bender HW Jr: Pulmonary, mediastinal, and cardiac presentations of histoplasmosis. Ann Thorac Surg 1980;30:385-390

Rose AG: Cardiac tuberculosis: a study of 19 patients. Arch Pathol Lab Med 1987;111:422-426

Special Writing Group of the Committee on Rheumatic Fever, Endocarditis, and Kawasaki Disease, Council on Cardiovascular Disease in the Young, American Heart Association: Guidelines for the diagnosis of rheumatic fever: Jones criteria, 1992 update. JAMA 1992;268:2069-2073

Tani LY, Veasy LG, Minich LL, Shaddy RE: Rheumatic fever in children younger than 5 years: is the presentation different? Pediatrics 2003;112:1065-1068

Veasy LG, Tani LY: A new look at acute mitral regurgitation. Cardiol Young 2005;15:568-577

Malnutrition

American Psychiatric Association: Diagnostic and Statistical Manual of Mental Disorders, 4th ed, text revision. Washington, DC, American Psychiatric Association, 2000:589

Bergqvist AG, Chee CM, Lutchka L, et al: Selenium deficiency associated with cardiomyopathy: a complication of the ketogenic diet. Epilepsia 2003;44:618-620

Mont L, Castro J, Herreros B, et al: Reversibility of cardiac abnormalities in adolescents with anorexia nervosa after weight recovery. J Am Acad Child Adolesc Psychiatry 2003;42:808-813

Olivares JL, Vázquez M, Fleta J, et al: Cardiac findings in adolescents with anorexia nervosa at diagnosis and after weight restoration. Eur J Pediatr 2005;164:383-386

Speiser PW, Rudolf MCJ, Anhalt H, et al: Consensus statement: childhood obesity. J Clin Endocrinol Metab 2005;90:1871-1887

Towbin A, Inge TH, Garcia VF, et al: Beriberi after gastric bypass surgery in adolescence. J Pediatr 2004;145:263-267

US Preventive Services Task Force: Screening and interventions for overweight in children and adolescents: recommendation statement. Pediatrics 2005;116:205-209

Endocrine Disorders

Berger E, Sochett EB, Peirone A, et al: Cardiac and vascular function in adolescents and young adults with type 1 diabetes. Diabetes Technol Ther 2004;6:129-135

Dahl-Jørgensen K, Larsen JR, Hanssen KF: Atherosclerosis in childhood and adolescent type 1 diabetes: early disease, early treatment? Diabetologia 2005;48:1445-1453

Loffredo CA, Wilson PD, Ferencz C: Maternal diabetes: an independent risk factor for major cardiovascular malformations with increased mortality of affected infants. Teratology 2001; 64:98-106

Raggi P, Bellasi A, Ratti C: Ischemia imaging and plaque imaging in diabetes. Diabetes Care 2005;28:2787-2794

Segni M, Gorman CA: The aftermath of childhood hyperthyroidism. J Pediatr Endocrinol Metab 2001;14(Suppl 5):1277-1282

Silverstein J, Klingensmith G, Copeland K, et al: Care of children and adolescents with type 1 diabetes: a statement of the American Diabetes Association. Diabetes Care 2005;28:186-212

Zimmerman D: Fetal and neonatal hyperthyroidism. Thyroid 1999;9:727-733

Blood Disorders

Batra AS, Acherman RJ, Wong W, et al: Cardiac abnormalities in children with sickle cell anemia. Am J Hematol 2002;70:306-312

de Montalembert M, Maunoury C, Acar P, et al: Myocardial ischaemia in children with sickle cell disease. Arch Dis Child 2004;89:359-362

Ferrara M, Matarese SM, Borrelli B, et al: Cardiac involvement in beta-thalassemia major and beta-thalassemia intermedia. Hemoglobin 2004;28:123-129

Lonergan GJ, Cline DBZ, Abbondanzo SL: From the archives of the AFIP: sickle cell anemia. Radiographics 2001;21:971-994

General and Other Systemic Disorders

Araoz PA, Eklund HE, Welch TJ, Breen JF: CT and MR imaging of primary cardiac malignancies. Radiographics 1999;19:1421-1434

Bertherat J: Carney complex (CNC). Orphanet J Rare Dis 2006;1:21

Chandramohan NK, Hussain MB, Nayak N, et al: Multiple cardiac metastases from Ewing's sarcoma. Can J Cardiol 2005;21:525-527

Corbet HJ, Humphrey GME: Pulmonary sequestration. Paediatr Respir Rev 2004;5:59-68

Harding CO, Pagon RA: Incidence of tuberous sclerosis in patients with cardiac rhabdomyoma. Am J Med Genet 1990;37:754-755

Isaacs H Jr: Fetal and neonatal cardiac tumors. Pediatr Cardiol 2004;25:252-273

Mahle WT, Rychik J, Tian ZY, et al: Echocardiographic evaluation of the fetus with congenital cystic adenomatoid malformation. Ultrasound Obstet Gynecol 2000;16:620-624

Newman B: Congenital bronchopulmonary foregut malformations: concepts and controversies. Pediatr Radiol 2006;36:773-791

Platonov MA, Turner AR, Mullen JC, et al: Tumour on the tricuspid valve: metastatic osteosarcoma and the heart. Can J Cardiol 2005;21:63-67

Reeder MM: Gamuts in Radiology: Comprehensive Lists of Roentgen Differential Diagnosis, 3rd ed. New York, Springer-Verlag, 1993

Sparrow PJ, Kurian JB, Jones TR, Sivananthan MU: MR imaging of cardiac tumors. Radiographics 2005;25:1255-1276

Taybi H, Lachman RS: Radiology of syndromes, metabolic disorders, and skeletal dysplasias, 4th ed. St. Louis, Mosby-Year Book, 1996

Tworetzky W, McElhinney DB, Margossian R, et al: Association between cardiac tumors and tuberous sclerosis in the fetus and neonate. Am J Cardiol 2003;92:487-489

101 Cardiac Tumors

S. BRUCE GREENBERG and CATHY MacDONALD

Primary cardiac tumors are rare in infants and children, with a reported prevalence of up to 0.32%. Use of echocardiography has resulted in more frequent detection of cardiac tumors in the fetus and neonate. Greater than 90% of cardiac tumors in infants and children are benign. Symptoms are variable and usually depend on tumor location and size. Intracavitary cardiac tumors can cause cardiac valve obstruction or result in spread of tumor emboli into either the pulmonary or systemic vascular beds. These children present with heart failure, dyspnea, or neurologic symptoms. Myocardial tumors compress the cardiac lumen, leading to obstruction or heart failure, and can be associated with arrhythmias. Pericardial tumors are associated with pericardial effusions. Conventional radiographs may show cardiomegaly, an abnormal cardiac shape, or pulmonary edema from congestive heart failure (Fig. 101-1). Cardiac tumors in children can be associated with several syndromes, as shown in Table 101-1. Computed tomography (CT) and magnetic resonance (MR) findings can help differentiate tumor types (Table 101-2).

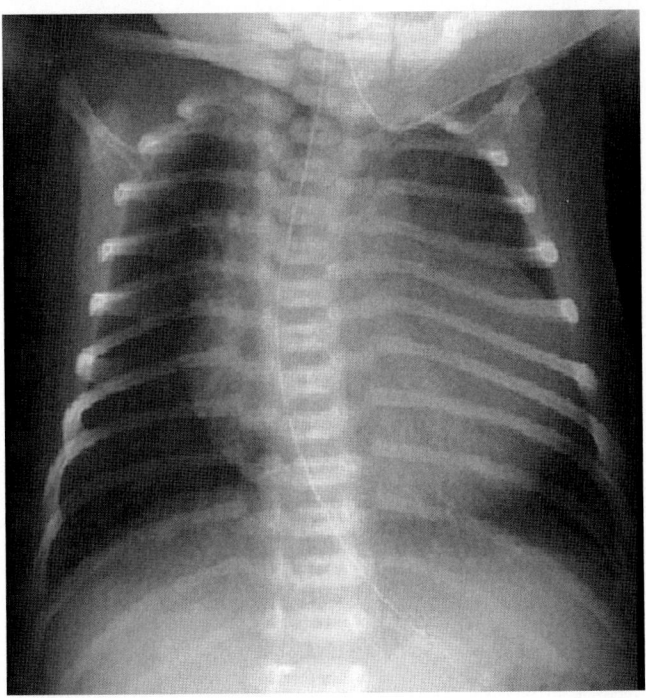

FIGURE 101-1. Cardiomegaly in a child with a cardiac fibroma.

INTRINSIC TUMORS

Rhabdomyoma is the most common primary cardiac tumor of childhood and accounts for up to 90% of all cardiac tumors during the first year of life. Rhabdomyomas are hamartomas that regress and have no malignant potential. More than half of fetuses with rhabdomyomas are asymptomatic. Patients with rhabdomyomas can present with nonimmune fetal hydrops, outflow tract obstruction, or arrhythmia. At least 50% of patients with rhabdomyomas have tuberous sclerosis, and rhabdomyomas can be the first detectable manifestation of tuberous sclerosis.

> At least 50% of patients with rhabdomyomas have tuberous sclerosis, and rhabdomyomas can be the first detectable manifestation of tuberous sclerosis.

Rhabdomyomas are round, hyperechoic, solid masses on echocardiography (Fig. 101-2). They are frequently multiple and occur most commonly in the ventricular tissue but can arise from atrial walls. The rhabdomyoma signal characteristics on MR T1-weighted and T2-weighted imaging are similar to those of myocardium. Signal is increased on contrast-enhanced T1-weighted and proton-weighted imaging. Rhabdomyomas are easier to detect when they extend into the cardiac lumen (Fig. 101-3). They have increased attenuation compared with myocardium on noncontrast-enhanced CT scans, and they enhance slightly with contrast. Small fat globules may be detected in rhabdomyomas.

Cardiac fibroma is the second most common primary cardiac tumor of childhood. The tumors are frequently detected in the first year of life but can present throughout childhood. Fibromas are solitary tumors located in

TABLE 101-1	
Cardiac Tumors Associated with Syndromes	
Cardiac Tumor	**Association**
Rhabdomyoma	Tuberous sclerosis
Fibroma	Gorlin (basal cell nevus) syndrome
Myxoma	Carney syndrome

TABLE 101-2

Cardiac Tumors: Computed Tomography (CT) and Magnetic Resonance Imaging (MRI) Findings

Tumor	Location	Number	CT	MRI Signal Intensity
Rhabdomyoma	Myocardium	Multiple	– Calcification Increased* attenuation ↑ Enhancement	Isointense T1- and T2-weighted ↑ Signal proton density ↑ Enhancement
Fibroma	Myocardium	Solitary	+ Calcification Heterogeneous enhancement	↓ T2-weighted ↓ Early enhancement ↑ Delayed enhancement
Myxoma	Intracavitary	Solitary†	+ Calcification Decreased attenuation, outlined by intracavitary contrast	↑ T2-weighted; irregular enhancement
Teratoma	Pericardium	Solitary	+ Calcification + Fat, heterogeneous attenuation	Heterogeneous T1- and enhancement

*Relative to myocardium.
†Multiple and recurrent tumors associated with familial forms.

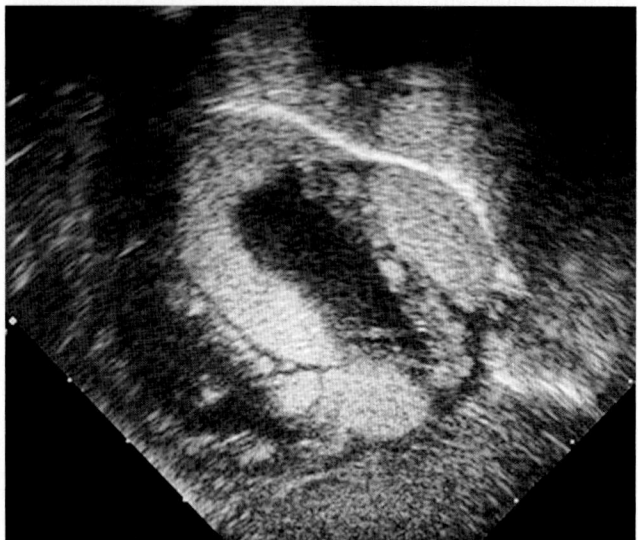

FIGURE 101-2. Cardiac ultrasound of multiple rhabdomyomas shows hyperechogenic foci in the left ventricle. (Courtesy of Renee Bornemeier, MD, Little Rock, AR).

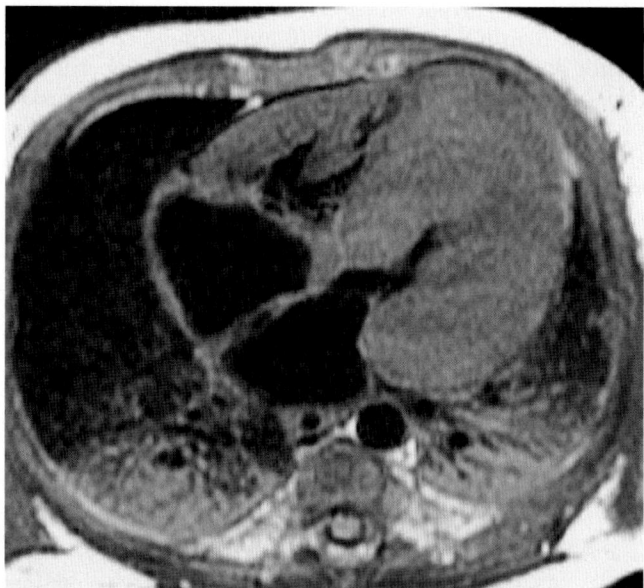

FIGURE 101-3. Rhabdomyomatosis in an infant shows multiple bulging tumors with isosignal to the left ventricular myocardium on T1-weighted imaging.

the myocardium, and they are composed of fibroblasts and collagen. Calcifications are present in half. The tumor can be associated with Gorlin (basal cell nevus) syndrome. Children can present with heart failure and arrhythmia. Echocardiography reveals a heterogeneous, echogenic, solitary mass. Cardiac fibroma signal intensity is lower on T2-weighted imaging than other cardiac tumors. Classically, contrast-enhanced MR imaging of fibromas initially shows less enhancement than myocardium, but enhancement is increased on delayed imaging. The contrast enhancement pattern can be variable, with increased initial contrast enhancement or heterogeneous contrast enhancement (Fig. 101-4). Calcifications may be detected by CT (Fig. 101-5).

> **Signal is lower on T2-weighted imaging for fibroma than for other cardiac tumors.**

Myxomas are the most common cardiac tumor in adults, but they are rare in children. Myxoma is an exophytic mass extending into a cardiac chamber. Most are pedunculated, irregular masses attached to the atrial septum, but myxomas can originate from other locations on the endocardium. Calcifications are common. Myxomas occurring in children are frequently associated with Carney syndrome. Myxomas in children are more likely to be multiple and to recur than in adults. Clinical symptoms include obstructive cardiac symptoms, embolic phenomena, and constitutional symptoms.

Echocardiography identifies a heterogeneous, spherical mass attached to the endocardial surface. The pedunculated mass can be seen to prolapse across the mitral or tricuspid valve during the cardiac cycle. Myxomas have high signal on T2-weighted imaging and enhance with gadolinium (Fig. 101-6). Prolapse of the pedunculated mass can be identified with cine imaging. Tumor attenua-

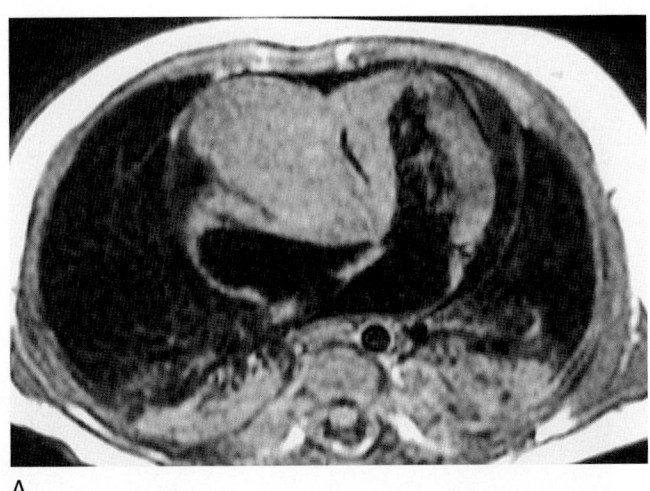
A

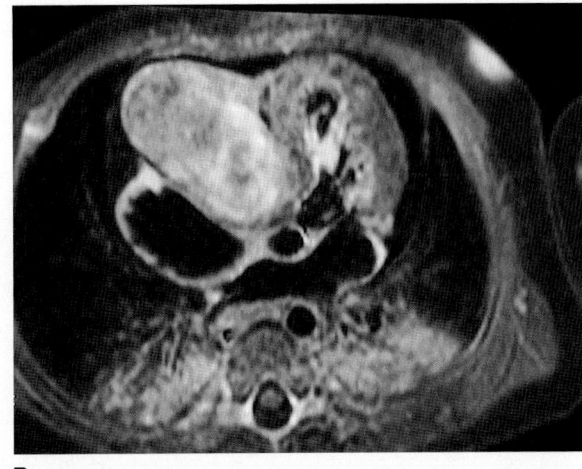
B

FIGURE 101-4. A solitary cardiac fibroma in a child obliterates the right ventricle on T1-weighted MR imaging **(A)** and demonstrates heterogeneous enhancement on the contrast-enhanced T1-weighted sequence **(B)**.

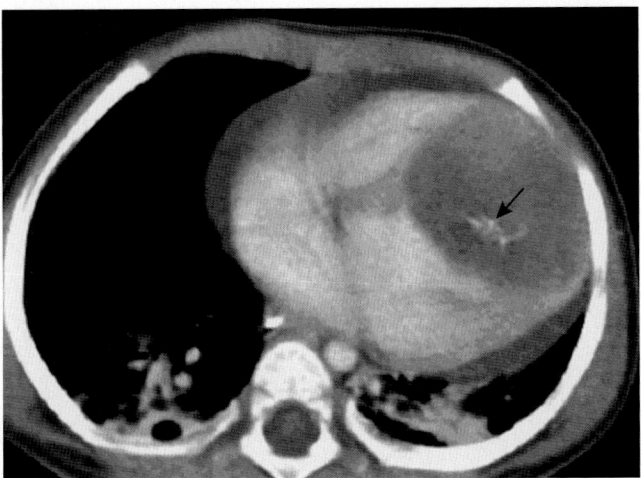

FIGURE 101-5. Cardiac fibroma. CT shows calcification *(arrow)* in the low-attenuation mass in the left ventricular apex.

tion is lower than nonopacified blood on CT sections. The mass is well outlined on contrast-enhanced CT scans.

Other benign tumors, such as fibroelastosis, teratomas, hemangioma, and lipoma, are extremely rare in children. Fibroelastoma is another intracavitary tumor rarely found in children. Unlike myxomas, fibroelastomas are usually attached to cardiac valves. Cardiac teratomas overall are rare, but they are the most common pericardial tumors in infants and most are identified during infancy. Teratomas are typically attached to the pulmonary artery and aorta root and extend into the pericardium. Pericardial effusions are usually present. Fetal hydrops

from caval obstruction can lead to spontaneous abortion. Echocardiography, CT, and MR images show a mixed, solid, and multicystic tumor in the pericardium with a pericardial effusion (Fig. 101-7). Calcification may be present. Hemangiomas can occur in the pericardium and are also associated with pleural effusion (Fig. 101-8).

Lipomas can occur at any age but are rare in children. CT and MR demonstration of fat allows the specific diagnosis (Fig. 101-9).

MALIGNANT TUMORS

Primary malignant tumors are so rare that they are frequently absent from series of cardiac tumors in children, appearing only in case reports. Only four malignant, primary cardiac tumors were confirmed in Great Britain during a 21-year period. Rhabdomyosarcoma, leiomyosarcoma, fibrosarcoma, angiosarcoma, and primary lymphoma of the heart have been reported in children. Primary cardiac lymphoma is defined as lymphoma restricted to the heart and pericardium (Fig. 101-10). Metastatic tumors are more common than primary cardiac malignancies. Metastatic tumors are secondary to leukemia, lymphoma, Wilms tumor, hepatoblastoma, neuroblastoma, Ewing sarcoma, and osteosarcoma. Spread may be from direct extension, by tumor extension through the inferior vena cava (Fig. 101-11), or via hematogenous metastases.

> Metastatic tumors are more common than primary cardiac malignancies.

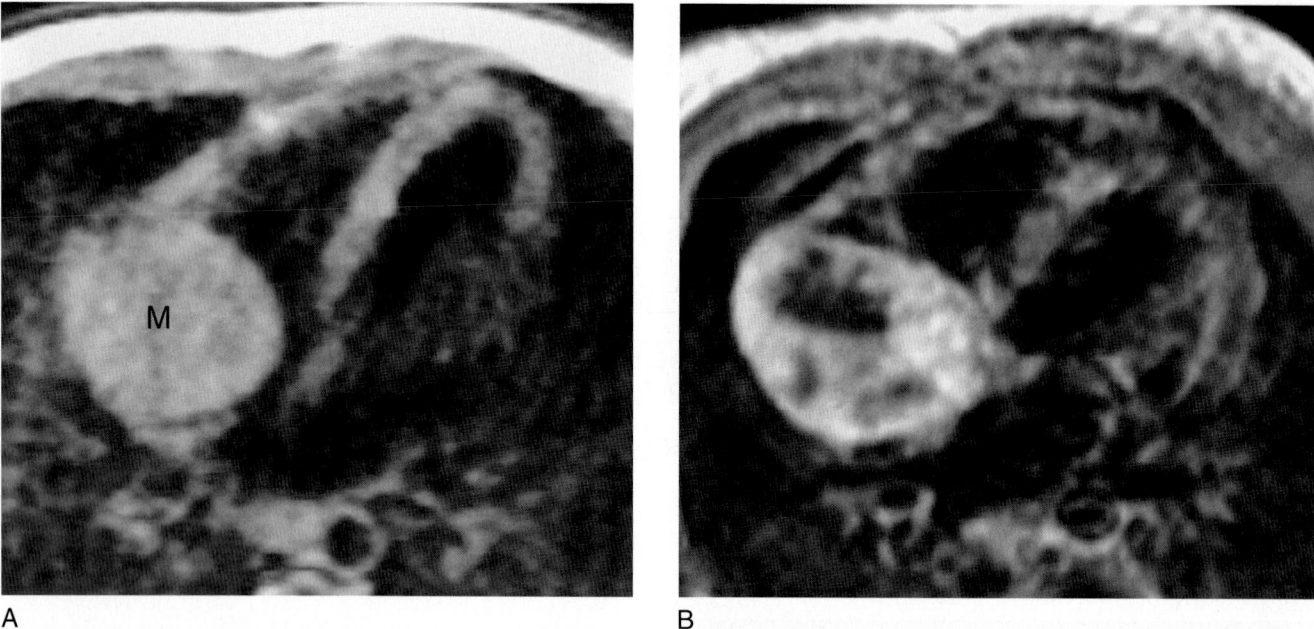

A   B

FIGURE 101-6. Right atrial myxoma in a child. **A,** MRI shows an intraluminal right atrial mass (M). **B,** The mass enhances heterogeneously with gadolinium.

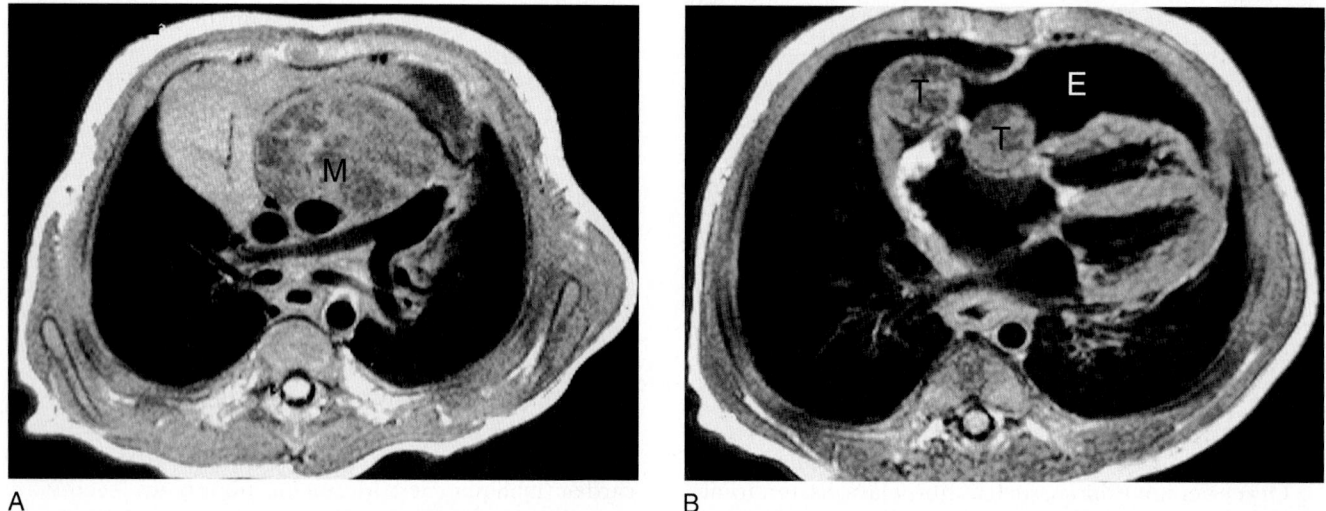

A   B

FIGURE 101-7. Pericardial teratoma in a child. **A,** MRI shows a pericardial mass (M) with low-signal cystic components in a child with a pericardial teratoma. **B,** Daughter tumors (T) are present in the pericardial space. Note large pericardial effusion (E).

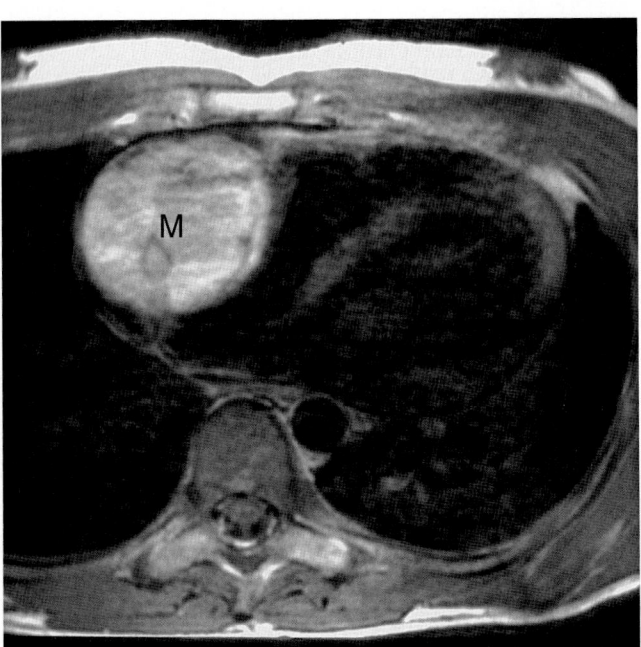

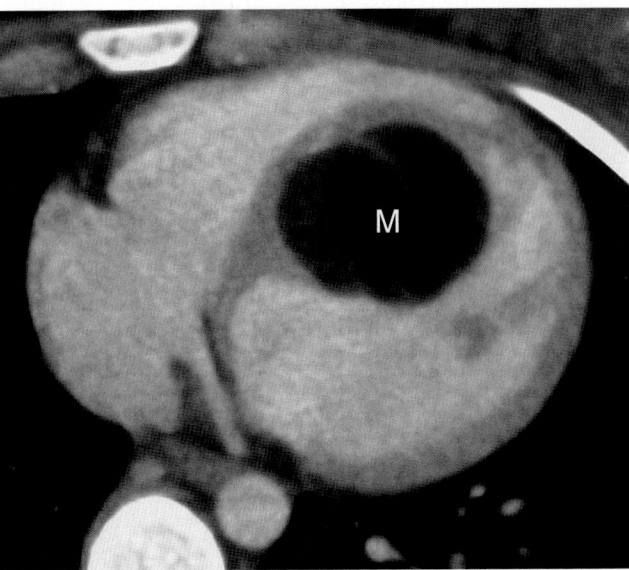

FIGURE 101-9. Intracardiac lipoma in a teenager. CT shows a fatty low-attenuation mass (M) extending into the left ventricular lumen from the ventricular septum in a teenager with a lipoma.

FIGURE 101-8. Pericardial hemangioma in an 8-year-old child. MR shows a high-signal mass on T1-weighted imaging. The mass (M) impinges on the right ventricle.

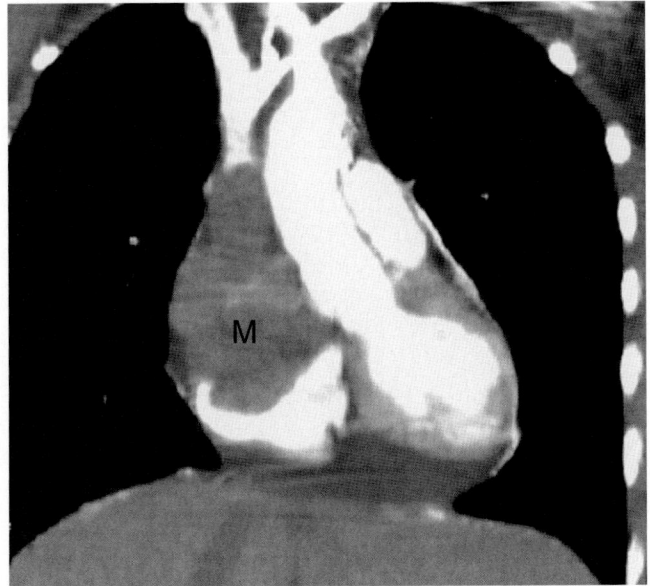

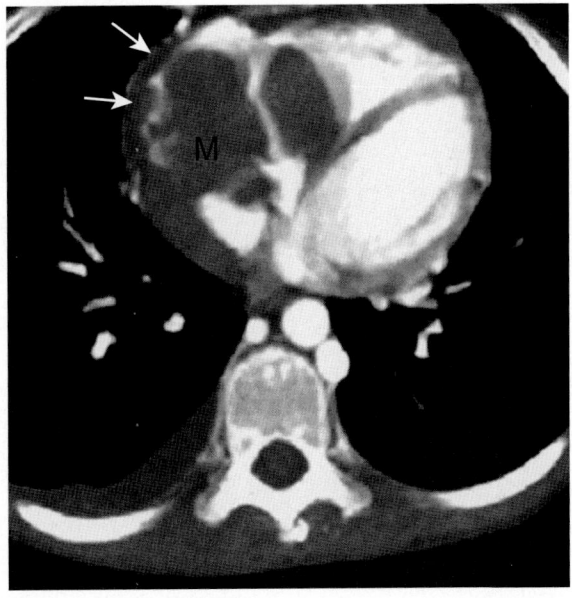

A   B

FIGURE 101-10. Primary cardiac lymphoma in a child. Axial **(A)** and coronal **(B)** CT images show a low-attenuation mass (M) involving the pericardium (*arrows* in **B**) and right heart.

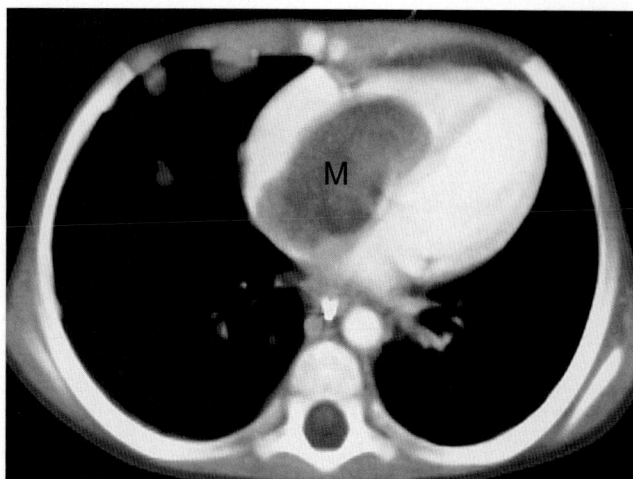

FIGURE 101-11. Wilms tumor thrombus extending into the heart in a child. CT image shows a right atrial mass (M) that prolapses across the tricuspid valve in a child with Wilms tumor. Lung metastases are also evident in the right lung.

SUGGESTED READINGS

De Cobelli F, Esposito A, Mellone R, et al: Images in cardiovascular medicine: late enhancement of a left ventricular fibroma assessed with gadolinium-enhanced cardiovascular magnetic resonance. Circulation 2005;112:e243-e252

Elderkin RA, Radford DJ: Primary cardiac tumours in a paediatric population. J Paediatr Child Health 2002;38:173-177

Freedom RM, Lee K, MacDonald C, Taylor G: Selected aspects of cardiac tumors in infancy and childhood. Pedatr Cardiol 2000;21:299-316

Gilkeson RC, Chiles C: MR evaluation of cardiac and pericardial malignancy. Magn Reson Imaging Clin N Am 2003;11:173-186

Grebenc ML, Rosado de Christenson ML, Burke AP, et al: Primary cardiac and pericardial neoplasms: radiologic-pathologic correlation. Radiographics 2000;20:1073-1103

Hoffmann U, Globits S, Schima W, et al: Usefulness of magnetic resonance imaging of cardiac and paracardiac masses. Am J Cardiol 2003;92:890-895

Isaacs H: Fetal and neonatal cardiac tumors. Pediatr Cardiol 2004;25:252-273

Kaminaga T, Takeshita T, Kimura I: Role of magnetic resonance imaging for evaluation of tumors in cardiac region. Eur Radiol 2003;13:L1-10

Kiaffas MG, Powell AJ, Geva T: Magnetic resonance imaging evaluation of cardiac tumor characteristics in infants and children. Am J Cardiol 2002;89:1229-1233

Mahilmaran A, Seshadri M, Nayar PG, et al: Familial cardiac myxoma: Carney's complex. Tex Heart Inst J 2003;30:80-82

Pipitone S, Mongiovi M, Grillo R, et al: Cardiac rhabdomyoma in intrauterine life: clinical features and natural history: a case series and review of published reports. Ital Heart J 2002;1:48-52

Schvartzman P, White R: Imaging of cardiac and paracardiac masses. J Thorac Imaging 2000;15:265-273

Sridhar AV, Bulock F, Hickey MS, et al: Papillary fibroelastoma of the tricuspid valve presenting as neonatal pulmonary haemorrhage. Acta Paediatr 2004;93:1254-1256

Sugiyama H, Naito H, Tsukano S, et al: Evaluation of cardiac tumors in children by electron-beam computed tomography: rhabdomyoma and fibroma. Circ J 2005;69:1352-1356

PART 4 INTERVENTIONAL PROCEDURES

CHAPTER

102 Pediatric Electrophysiology

RONALD J. KANTER

The clinical practices of the pediatric radiologist and the pediatric electrophysiologist intersect in several regards. Both subspecialists are interested in detailed internal anatomy; and both subspecialties have evolved toward performing therapeutic procedures. In addition, both disciplines require knowledge of the application and effects of ionizing radiation. The radiologist should also have a fundamental understanding of arrhythmias and a basic working knowledge of emergency arrhythmia management, in case such should occur during a radiologic procedure. Moreover, advanced interventional skills, such as transhepatic vascular access for ablation, have been in the armamentarium of the radiologist for some time and may benefit the electrophysiologist. The radiologist must also be able to recognize the types and appropriate positions of various devices used for management of arrhythmias and to understand the effects of electromagnetic fields on implanted cardiac devices in order to prevent harm to patients.

This chapter is divided into three sections: (1) a brief description of tachyarrhythmias that may be encountered in the radiology department, and emergency management strategies for treating them; (2) indications for catheter ablation of cardiac arrhythmias, newer imaging technologies to guide catheter ablation, and radiation exposure risks during catheter ablation; and (3) cardiac device therapy and special concerns in the radiology department.

TACHYARRHYTHMIAS IN CHILDREN

Here we highlight only those clinically relevant tachyarrhythmias that may occur during radiologic procedures and their recommended treatment: atrial flutter (AFl), supraventricular tachycardias (SVTs) using the atrioventricular (AV) node as a part of the reentry circuit, and ventricular tachycardia (VT). Figure 102-1 illustrates the mechanisms and surface electrocardiographic (ECG) manifestations of these arrhythmias, as well as initial medical management. Atrial flutter is very rare in children, except following certain types of congenital heart surgery, especially Fontan, Mustard, and Senning operations; other complex atrial surgeries; or tetralogy

of Fallot repair. Atrioventricular node–dependent SVTs are the most common pathologic tachycardia in children who do not have other heart disease, and they are hemodynamically well tolerated in the absence of comorbid conditions. When sustained VT occurs after congenital heart surgery, it must be regarded as life-threatening. Ventricular tachycardia in an otherwise normal heart is not uncommon, is hemodynamically well tolerated, is the only one of the aforementioned tachycardias that may not use reentry as its mechanism, and, hence, may not respond to direct current cardioversion.

Tachyarrhythmias that most often occur during radiologic procedures:

- **Atrial flutter**
- **Supraventricular tachycardias using the AV node as part of the reentry circuit**
- **Ventricular tachycardia**

Reentry tachycardias of any type may be induced by premature beats (atrial for AFl, atrial or ventricular for SVT, and ventricular for VT). This should be kept in mind when an at-risk patient is undergoing central vascular catheter manipulation in the radiology department. Sudden alterations in autonomic tone, as may occur during oropharyngeal stimulation from orogastric/duodenal or nasogastric/duodenal tube placement, may have either provocative or suppressive effects on arrhythmogenesis. For children known to be at risk for any of these arrhythmias, secure venous access and appropriate monitoring equipment should be present before entering the radiology suite for these types of procedures.

Sudden alterations in autonomic tone (e.g., during oropharyngeal stimulation from tube placement) may have provocative or suppressive effects on arrhythmogenesis. When children are at risk for these arrhythmias, secure venous access and appropriate monitoring equipment should be available in the radiology suite.

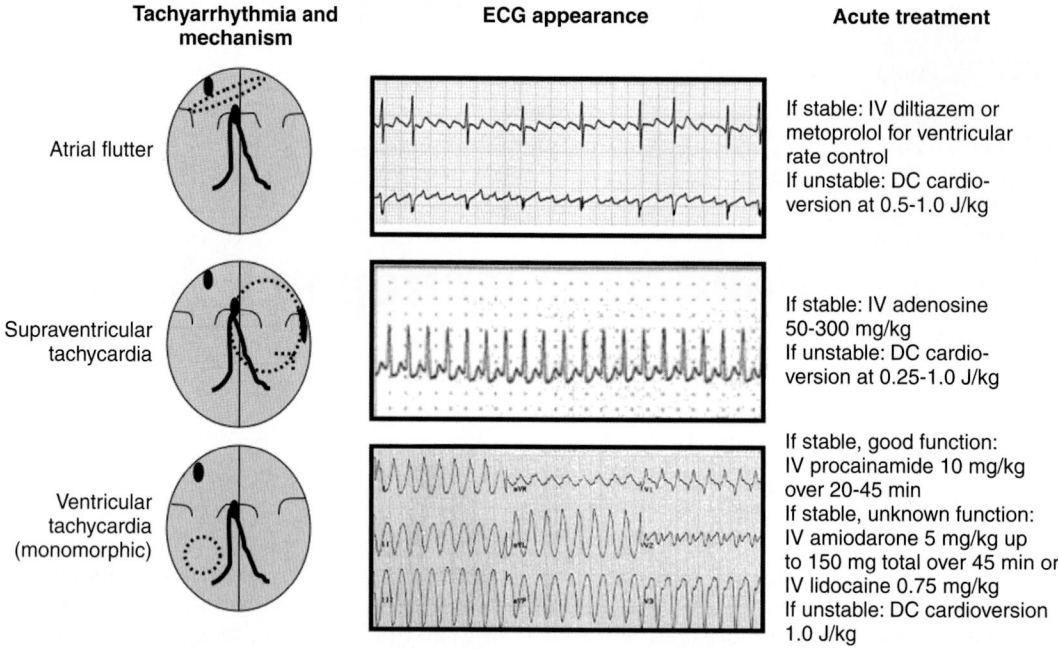

FIGURE 102-1. The most commonly encountered clinically important paroxysmal tachycardias in children who appear in the radiology department are atrial flutter, supraventricular tachycardia, and ventricular tachycardia. They are depicted mechanistically in the left column; electrocardiographic (ECG) rhythm strips of these tachycardias are shown in the center column; and initial medical management is provided in the right column.

CATHETER ABLATION IN CHILDREN

History and Indications

Ablative therapy for tachycardia substrates was first performed surgically for Wolff-Parkinson-White syndrome in 1968. The use of transvascular catheter delivery of direct current (DC) to create AV block in adults with troublesome atrial fibrillation was first reported in 1983. However, the lesions created by this technique proved to be dangerously proarrhythmic. The modern era of catheter ablation truly began with back-to-back reports from the University of Oklahoma and the University of Michigan in 1991. The original arrhythmia substrates were accessory AV connections, and the energy used was alternating current in the radiofrequency range (RF) of about 550 kHz. As this current passes from the low impedance catheter tip through the higher impedance tissue, electrical energy is dissipated in the form of heat by the mechanism of resistance heating. Energy at much lower frequencies (e.g., 60 Hz, used as household electricity) can cause arrhythmias and is painful, whereas frequencies above 1 MHz are less efficient. The lesion volume is created by a combination of resistance heating and deeper convective heating. Because current density diminishes inversely with the square of the distance from the source, this technique creates a fairly well circumscribed lesion and minimizes collateral damage. Since those original reports, this technology has expanded to include children and patients of all ages with congenital heart disease. Almost no tachyarrhythmia substrate is now considered exempt from catheter ablation therapy thanks to newer catheter designs, new electroanatomic mapping technologies, and additional energy sources, including microwave, cryotherapy, and ultrasound. Indi-cations to perform catheter ablation in children remain somewhat limited by the benign natural history of some tachyarrhythmia substrates, continued concern about damage to nearby structures, and concern about scar expansion with somatic growth. The arrhythmia substrates commonly ablated in children appear in Table 102-1, and published indications to perform ablation appear in Table 102-2.

Technical Considerations

The guiding principle of electrophysiologic testing and catheter ablation involves coupling of anatomic structures to electrical phenomena. The majority of cases can be accomplished with standard fluoroscopy and three to five multielectrode catheters positioned in the right ventricle, right atrium, coronary sinus, and His bundle region of the tricuspid valve annulus, and one for mapping and ablation (Fig. 102-2). Quadripolar catheters down to 2F and creative catheter designs now enable electrophysiologic testing in neonates. These anatomic sites can be easily accessed from a combination of femoral, internal jugular, and subclavian venous approaches. However, in some patients having complex congenital cardiovascular anomalies (e.g., interrupted inferior vena cava in some heterotaxy patients) and in others having undergone certain congenital heart operations (e.g., cavopulmonary connection or extracardiac conduit in patients having single-ventricle physiology), some or all of these venous sites do not allow access to the heart. Moreover, patients who have undergone multiple prior procedures may have permanent venous occlusion of some of these sites. In these instances, alternate approaches may include transhepatic venous access,

---

TABLE 102-1

Tachyarrhythmia Substrates Targeted by Catheter Ablation

Tachyarrhythmia Type	Substrate Target
Atrial flutter (postoperative)	Zone of slow conduction between conduction barriers
Atrial ectopic tachycardia	Focus of earliest activation
Focal atrial tachycardia	Focus of earliest activation
Atrioventricular (AV) reciprocating tachycardia	Accessory pathway
AV node reentry tachycardia	"Slow inputs" to AV node
Ventricular tachycardia in normal heart	Focus of earliest activation
Ventricular tachycardia (postoperative)	Zone of slow conduction between conduction barriers

---

TABLE 102-2

Indications for Radiofrequency Catheter Ablation in Pediatric Patients

Class I: There is consistent agreement and/or supportive data that catheter ablation is likely to be medically beneficial or helpful for the patient.
  1. WPW syndrome after an episode of aborted sudden cardiac death.
  2. The presence of WPW syndrome associated with syncope when there is a short pre-excited RR interval during atrial fibrillation (pre-excited R-R interval, 250 msec), or when the antegrade effective refractory period of the AP measured during programmed electrical stimulation is <250 msec.
  3. Chronic or recurrent SVT associated with ventricular dysfunction.
  4. Recurrent VT that is associated with hemodynamic compromise and is amenable to catheter ablation.

Class IIA: There is a divergence of opinion regarding the benefit or medical necessity of catheter ablation, but the majority of opinions/data are in favor of the procedure.
  1. Recurrent and/or symptomatic SVT refractory to conventional medical therapy and age > 4 years.
  2. Impending congenital heart surgery when vascular or chamber access may be restricted after surgery.
  3. Chronic (occurring for >6-12 months after an initial event) or incessant SVT in the presence of normal ventricular function.
  4. Chronic or frequent recurrences of intra-atrial reentrant tachycardia.
  5. Palpitations with inducible sustained SVT during electrophysiologic testing.

Class IIB: There is clear divergence of opinion regarding the need for the procedure.
  1. Asymptomatic pre-excitation (WPW pattern on an electrocardiograph), age > 5 years, with no recognized tachycardia, when the risks and benefits of the procedure and arrhythmia have been clearly explained.
  2. SVT, age > 5 years, as an alternative to chronic antiarrhythmic therapy that has been effective in control of the arrhythmia.
  3. SVT, age < 5 years (including infants), when antiarrhythmic medications, including sotalol and amiodarone, are not effective or are associated with intolerable side effects.
  4. IART, one to three episodes per year, requiring medical intervention.
  5. AVN ablation and pacemaker insertion as an alternative therapy for recurrent or intractable IART.
  6. One episode of VT associated with hemodynamic compromise and that is amenable to catheter ablation.

Class III: There is agreement that catheter ablation is not medically indicated and/or the risk of the procedure may be greater than benefit for the patient.
  1. Asymptomatic WPW syndrome, age < 5 years.
  2. SVT controlled with conventional antiarrhythmic medications, age < 5 years.
  3. Nonsustained, paroxysmal VT that is not considered incessant (i.e., present on monitoring for hours at a time or on nearly all strips recorded during any 1-hour period), and where no concomitant ventricular dysfunction exists.
  4. Episodes of nonsustained SVT that do not require other therapy and/or are minimally symptomatic.

AP, accessory pathway; AVN, atrioventricular node; IART, intra-atrial reentrant tachycardia; SVT, supraventricular tachycardias; VT, ventricular tachycardia; WPW, Wolff-Parkinson-White.

---

arterial and retroaortic access, and even transthoracic access.

Even high-resolution fluoroscopy in multiple projections is insufficient to display the internal cardiac topography after complex congenital heart surgery. Therefore, new technologies using mathematically derived reconstructions have been developed for real-time creation of three-dimensional cardiac chambers and associated structures. These technologies have also been shown to reduce duration of fluoroscopic exposure in routine cases.

The CARTO system (Biosense Webster, Inc.) allows development of an endocardial map using a low-energy, triple-source transmitter located on a position pad mounted beneath the patient, a receiver in the tip of the specialized mapping/ablation catheter, and global positioning system technology. A second electrode catheter in a fixed intracardiac position serves as a temporal reference, thus permitting electroanatomic coupling by the mapping catheter, as it is manipulated to create a point-by-point rendition of the chamber of interest. Iso-

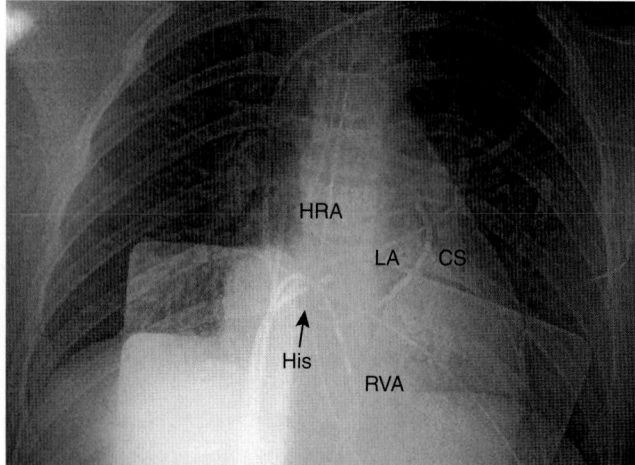

FIGURE 102-2. Anteroposterior projection of a chest fluorograph during a radiofrequency catheter ablation procedure in a teenager with Wolff-Parkinson-White syndrome and a left lateral accessory pathway. Standard multipole electrode catheters are positioned in the high right atrium (HRA), across the tricuspid valve in the His bundle region (His), in the right ventricular apex (RVA), in the coronary sinus (CS), and at the mapped location of the accessory pathway along the mitral valve annulus (accessed from the left atrium [LA] via transseptal puncture).

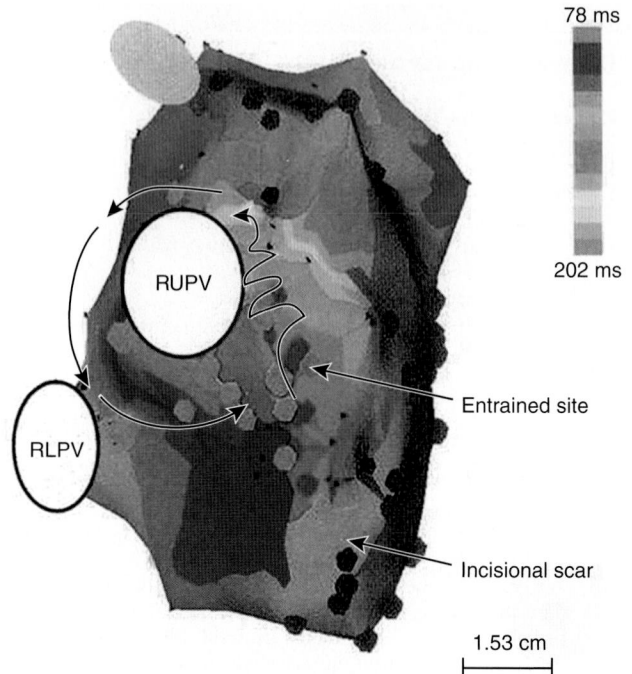

Isochronal step: 20 ms

FIGURE 102-3. Electroanatomic reconstruction of the pulmonary venous atrium from a right posterior oblique projection, using the CARTO system (Biosense-Webster, Inc.), from a patient with atrial flutter who underwent the Mustard operation for D-transposition of the great arteries. The color-coded isochrones indicate a reentry circuit around the ostium of the right upper pulmonary vein (RUPV). Areas colored *gray* are regions whose voltage is low enough to suggest scar. RLPV, right lower pulmonary vein ostium. (*See color plate.*) (From Zrenner B, Dong J, Schreieck J, et al: Delineation of intra-atrial reentrant tachycardia circuits after mustard operation for transposition of the great arteries using biatrial electroanatomic mapping and entrainment mapping. J Cardiovasc Electrophysiol 2003;14:1302-1310.)

chronal activation, isopotential, and animated activation maps may be produced (Fig. 102-3).

The Ensite system (Endocardial Solutions, Inc.) uses a noncontact multielectrode array, which is mounted on a balloon catheter and centrally positioned in the chamber of interest (intracavitary). Ring electrodes on this catheter, proximal and distal to the array, serve as receivers from a low-current locator signal delivered from any second standard electrode catheter. As this second catheter is rapidly swept along all endocardial surfaces of the chamber of interest, a three-dimensional computer model of the endocardium is generated. Far-field electrical activity recorded from each electrode on the array is enhanced and resolved based on an inverse solution to the Laplace equation. The inverse solution considers how a signal detected at a remote point (the array) will appear at its source (endocardial surface), thus superimposing a real-time isopotential map on the geometry matrix, even from a single heartbeat (Fig. 102-4).

Less robust electroanatomic mapping systems include LocaLisa (Medtronic, Inc.) and the Realtime Position Management system (RPM), and they will not be discussed. All of these systems permit only an anatomic approximation. However, both Biosense Webster, Inc., and Endocardial Solutions, Inc., are developing systems that will allow DICOM-formatted computed tomography (CT) or magnetic resonance (MR) images from a patient to be merged into the previously described virtual image of the chamber.

This technology has been of greatest value in the mapping and ablation of atrial or ventricular muscle tachycardias whose substrates are within the wall of a chamber, defined by areas of slow or absent conduction and not only by structural conduction boundaries, such as venous ostia or valve annuli. Each system has its own

idiosyncrasies and limitations, and all of them require extra equipment with attendant cost.

Radiation Exposure

Despite the introduction of newer imaging techniques as just described, and even MRI-guided ablation procedures, fluoroscopy remains the workhorse for cardiac catheter ablation procedures in most institutions. Under the direction of Dr. John Kugler, the Pediatric Electrophysiology Society began a pediatric radiofrequency registry in 1990, which has demonstrated a progressive reduction in procedural fluoroscopy duration, from 61.5 minutes in 1994 to 38.3 minutes in 2004, at least among patients having SVT. Most operators limit x-ray exposure by reducing frame rates to 15 and even 7.5 frames per second and by minimizing the use of magnification.

Data on x-ray exposure during catheter ablation procedures come largely from adult series, in which thermoluminescent dosimeters and/or anthropomorphic radiologic phantoms were used. Considering fluoroscopy times ranging from 41 to 60 minutes, a single procedure has been estimated to carry risk of a fatal malignancy in 0.03% to 0.13% of individuals, and to result in birth defects in 0.00012%. This is approximately

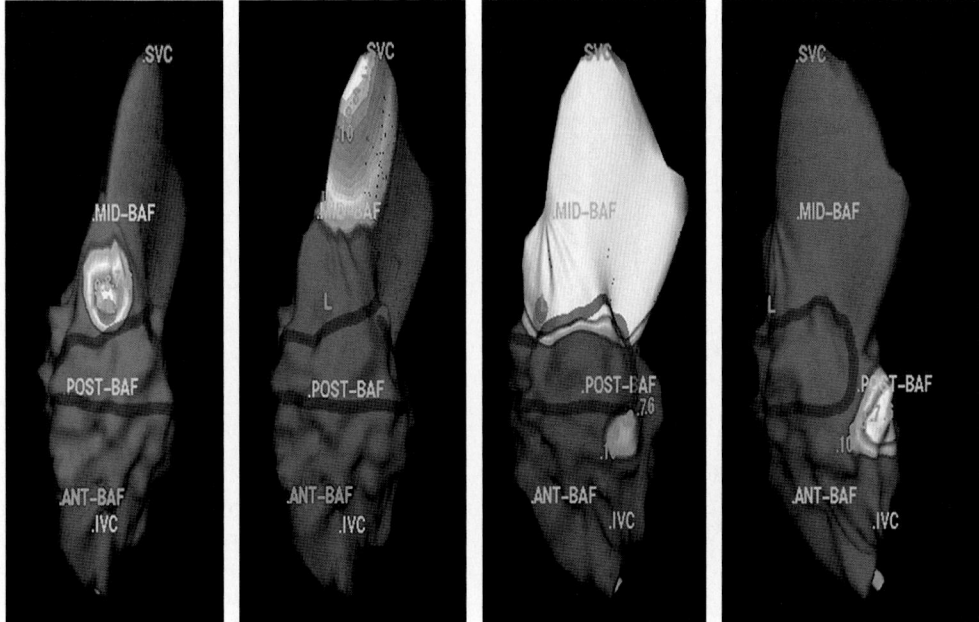

FIGURE 102-4. Electroanatomic reconstruction of the systemic venous atrium (intercaval region) from a left posterior oblique projection, using the Ensite system (Endocardial Solutions, Inc.) from a patient who underwent the Mustard operation for D-transposition of the great arteries and who has atrial flutter. This is an isopotential map, with brighter colors (white = brightest) representing higher voltages, and illustrating regions of depolarization over time (reading from left to right). The *purple* regions are presumably electrically refractory or inexcitable. Ant.-Baf., anterior portion of baffle; IVC, inferior vena cava; Mid.-Baf., midportion of baffle; Post.-Baf., posterior portion of baffle; SVC, superior vena cava. (Courtesy of Dr. Maully Shah; adapted.)

equivalent to 1% of the spontaneous incidence of fatal malignancy and 0.1% of the spontaneous incidence of birth defects. Giese and colleagues reported radiation doses to exposed skin to be 6.2 to 49 mGy/min in nine children. This calculated to total doses of 0.09 to 2.35 Gy. In our laboratory, our median fluoroscopy time is 32 minutes/case, and we limit fluoroscopy times to 120 minutes, even for complicated cases.

DEVICE THERAPY IN CHILDREN

Fundamentals of Pacing Hardware

Bradycardia devices (pacemakers) and antitachycardia devices (implantable cardioverter-defibrillators [ICDs]) require two basic hardware components, the pulse generator and conductors (primarily, "leads"). The pulse generator consists of an energy source (usually, lithium iodide battery), microcircuitry, a titanium alloy housing, and a plastic connector block for conductor attachment. In addition, the ICD contains capacitors to store deliverable energy. The lead consists of one (unipolar) or two (bipolar) wires, silicon or polyurethane insulation, a connector pin or pins that insert into the pulse generator connector block, and a fixation end that attaches to myocardium (via a tiny screw, "fish-hook," plaque, or other). Transvenous bipolar leads generally have a radiodense distal electrode and a slightly more proximal ring electrode, whereas the unipolar lead has only a distal electrode. Epicardial leads are mostly unipolar, but bifurcated plaque electrodes and in-line bipolar leads have just become available. In addition, the ventricular lead for an ICD may have one or two additional insulated conductors that are exposed on the outer surface of the

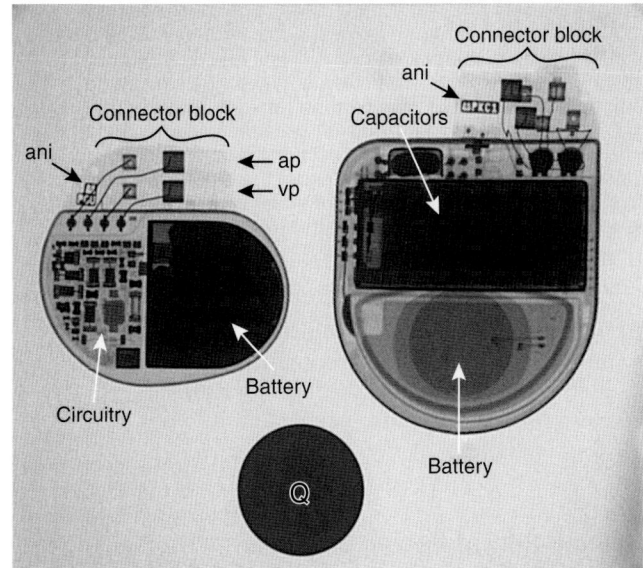

FIGURE 102-5. Radiograph of a modern dual-chamber pacemaker *(left)* and implantable cardioverter-defibrillator *(right)*. ani, alphanumeric identifier; ap, atrial port (portion of connector block that accepts connector pin of atrial lead); vp, ventricular port (portion of connector block that accepts connector pin of ventricular lead; Q, quarter (for size comparison).

lead ("coils") and that are vital components of cardioversion or defibrillation. When other conductors, including arrays and patches, are necessary to optimize cardioversion or defibrillation, they are inserted in subcutaneous or intrapericardial sites. Figures 102-5 and 102-6 illustrate the radiographic appearance of this hardware.

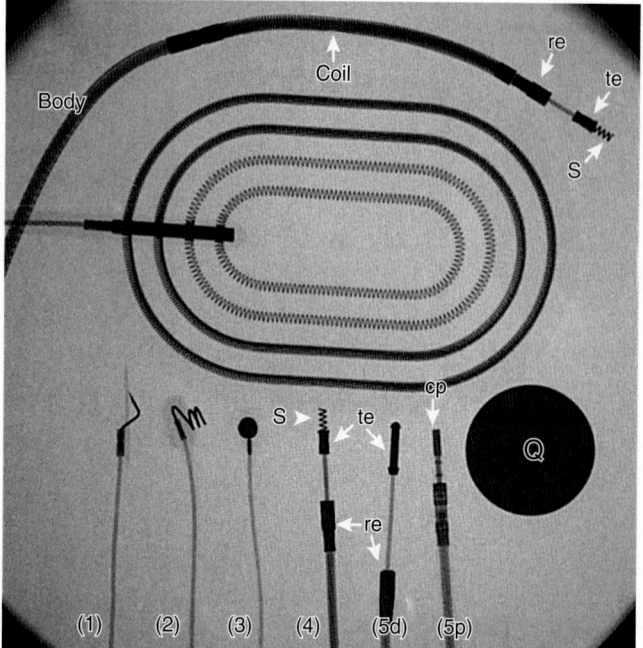

FIGURE 102-6. Radiograph of several types of conductors used for cardiac device therapy in children and teenagers, including: **Top,** Transvenous, active fixation, bipolar, ventricular lead used with implantable cardioverter-defibrillators (ICDs) and containing a coil for participation in shock delivery. **Middle,** Patch that is placed in either pericardial or subcutaneous locations and used with ICDs for participation in shock delivery. **Bottom,** Variety of leads used with either pacemakers or ICDs. *1,* Distal (cardiac) end of a unipolar, epicardial active fixation ("stab-on" or "fish-hook") lead. *2,* Distal end of a unipolar, epicardial active fixation ("screw-in") lead. *3,* Distal end of a unipolar, epicardial passive fixation (plaque, "suture-on") lead. *4,* Distal end of a bipolar, transvenous active fixation lead (with retractable screw). *5d* and *5p,* Distal (cardiac) and proximal (connector block of pacemaker) ends of a bipolar, passive fixation lead, respectively. cp, connector pin; re, ring electrode; s, screw; te, tip electrode, Q, quarter (for size comparison).

> Bradycardia devices (pacemakers) and antitachycardia devices (implantable cardioverter-defibrillators) require two basic hardware components, the pulse generator and conductors (i.e., leads).

Radiography of Pacing Systems

There are three main circumstances in which radiologists are called on to interpret radiographs from children with implanted devices: immediately after device implantation, during routine outpatient follow-up, and when component failure is suspected.

> Radiologists interpret radiographs from children with implanted devices:
> - **Immediately after device implantation**
> - **During routine outpatient follow-up**
> - **When component failure is suspected**

Although most immediate postoperative chest radiographs are ordered simply to rule out a pneumothorax, a systematic approach will enable the radiologist to interpret the appearance of the new hardware also. Three critical responsibilities for the radiologist are to identify the location of the pulse generator, describe each conductor, and correlate the congenital and surgical anatomy with lead locations and courses.

> Three critical responsibilities of the radiologist:
> - **Identify the location of the pulse generator**
> - **Describe each conductor**
> - **Correlate the congenital and surgical anatomy with lead locations and courses**

IDENTIFY THE LOCATION OF THE PULSE GENERATOR. When the device is infraclavicular, the conductors are usually transvenous. Epicardial leads are generally tunneled to a subcutaneous abdominal device, but subcostal and flank locations may also be used (especially for premature infants). Hybrid systems imply that there is a combination of transvenous, epicardial, and subcutaneous conductors, configured to accommodate restricted venous access, with or without a pre-existing lead that is considered valuable, and with or without an optimized shock vector in the case of ICDs. The pulse generator is positioned in the best location for the complex configuration of the conductors.

DESCRIBE EACH CONDUCTOR. The description includes the type (lead, lead with coils, array, patch), its course from the pulse generator to the heart or other thoracic site, its form of attachment to the heart in the case of leads, and whether the lead is unipolar or bipolar. Magnification of the lead tip may be required to identify a distal screw or other attachment device. In young children, redundant lead body is often coiled anterior to the heart in the case of epicardial leads and partially looped within the right atrium in the case of transvenous leads (the so-called growth loop).

CORRELATE THE CONGENITAL AND SURGICAL ANATOMY WITH LEAD LOCATIONS AND COURSES. Understanding the appropriateness of the course of each lead often requires some knowledge of the surgical anatomy. For example, in a person who has undergone the Mustard operation for D-transposition of the great arteries and who has sinus node dysfunction, a transvenous atrial lead is usually attached to the anatomic left atrium, leftward of the spine, and yet in the systemic venous circulation. As a second example, a patient with a single ventricle who has undergone a Fontan-type operation and who has heart block may have a transvenous atrial lead and an epicardial ventricular lead (a hybrid system). Finally, having leads attached to both right and left ventricles suggests an attempt at ventricular resynchronization for clinical ventricular dysfunction. The left ventricular lead may be transvenous to the coronary sinus or epicardial. Figures 102-7 through 102-9 illustrate the radiographic appearance of patients having complex cardiac device therapy.

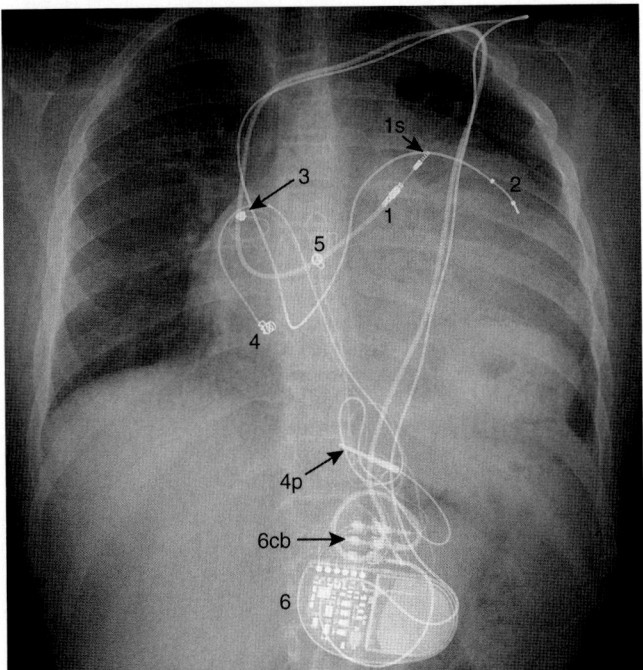

FIGURE 102-7. Posteroanterior chest radiograph from an 11-year-old girl after repair of atrioventricular septal defect. She has postoperative heart block and severe mitral regurgitation and left ventricular dysfunction. *1,* Transvenous, bipolar, active fixation (*1s,* screw) lead, positioned in the right ventricular outflow tract. *2,* Transvenous, bipolar, passive fixation lead, positioned in the posterolateral cardiac vein via the coronary sinus for the purpose of synchronizing ventricular activation. *3,* Epicardial, unipolar, passive fixation (plaque electrode) lead, positioned on the right atrium. *4,* Epicardial, unipolar, active fixation (screw-in) lead, positioned on the right atrium abandoned, with proximal end (*4p,* connector pin) in abdominal pacemaker pocket. *5,* Epicardial, unipolar screw fragment positioned on the right ventricle. *6,* Pacemaker (*6cb,* pacemaker connector block).

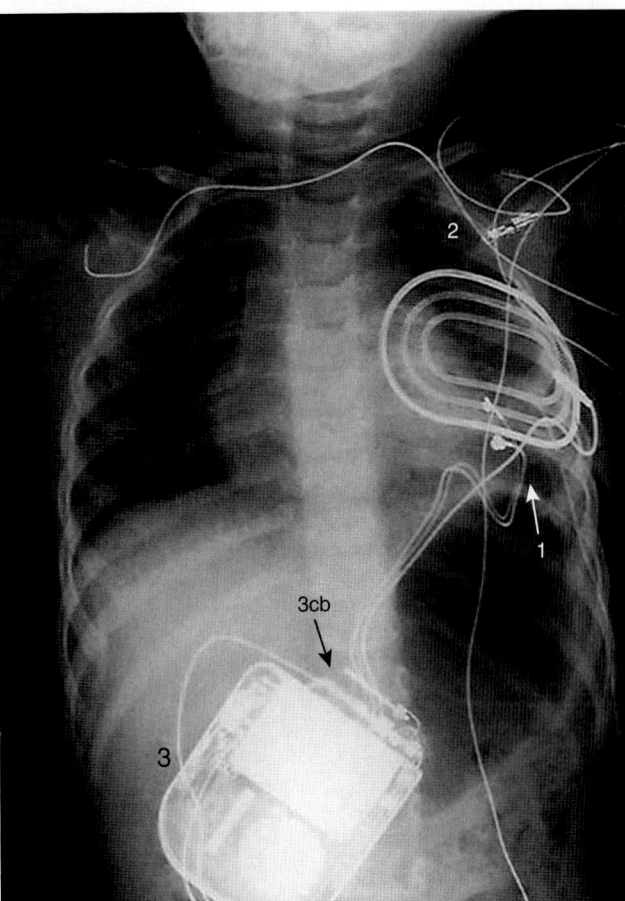

FIGURE 102-8. Posteroanterior chest radiograph from a 3-month-old male infant who has ventricular tachycardia associated with Brugada syndrome, a genetically determined sodium channel defect that can result in fatal ventricular tachycardia. *1,* Epicardial, bifurcated (thus bipolar), passive fixation (plaque electrodes) lead, positioned on the left ventricle for purposes of ventricular pacing and sensing. *2,* Patch placed posteriorly and in a subcutaneous location for participation in possible shock delivery. *3,* Implantable cardioverter-defibrillator in a subcutaneous pocket over the left abdomen. *3cb,* Implantable cardioverter-defibrillator connector block.

Children with chronic device therapy may develop symptoms suggestive of device malfunction: syncope, skeletal muscle twitching, hiccoughs, new onset of fatigue, palpitations, and, in the case of ICDs, inappropriate shocks. Radiographic abnormalities that suggest the etiology of device malfunction include lead conduction fracture, lead dislodgement (especially if soon after implantation), lead stretch caused by somatic growth, and connector pin separation from pulse generator. Transvenous leads most often fracture beneath the clavicle, but the appearance may be very subtle. Epicardial leads tend to fracture at the level of the diaphragm or within the active fixation component (especially when it is a screw). There is one caveat. The Medtronic model 4968 bifurcated, epicardial, double-plaque lead always has the appearance of near-fracture at the union of the two conductors. This is its normal appearance (Fig. 102-10). Finally, the radiologist may be called on to identify the type of implanted device (manufacturer and model number), particularly in a patient who appears in an emergency department and is new to the institution. Each pulse generator has a radiodense alphanumeric identifier (often its model number), which can be referenced in any of the major companies' device encyclopedias (see

Fig. 102-5). Unfortunately, if the face of the device is facing posteriorly or if there is sufficient obliquity, it may not be readable.

> **Radiographic abnormalities that suggest device malfunction:**
> - **Lead conduction fracture**
> - **Lead dislodgement (especially if soon after implantation)**
> - **Lead stretch caused by somatic growth**
> - **Connector pin separation from pulse generator**

Caring for Children with Devices While in the Radiology Department

Cardiac devices became interactive with the first inclusion of demand circuitry, developed in 1965 to allow sensing of intrinsic electrical activity. We now communicate with these devices for purposes of reprogramming, functional testing, and telemetry using a computerized programmer and radiofrequency waves. Hence, despite various forms of protective shielding and electronic filters, all devices may be affected by certain sources of electromagnetic interference (EMI) that may be present in the radiology department. Radiation used for diagnostic procedures is *not a source* of EMI. However, repeated high-dose *radiation therapy* may damage the silicone and silicone oxide insulation necessary for the complementary metal oxide semiconductor chip technology of cardiac devices. Device manufacturers have provided guidelines to minimize the risk of damage to ICDs from radiotherapy. Interactions between EMI and the device may result from MRI, defibrillation, electrocautery, neurostimulation and peripheral nerve stimulation, transcutaneous electrical nerve stimulation (TENS), diathermy, radiofrequency ablation, and lithotripsy. Untoward responses by the device may include oversensing, noise reversion, power on reset, permanent circuit failure, and damage to the lead–tissue interface that causes a permanent rise in the stimulation threshold. A glossary of these terms is in Table 102-3. Table 102-4 shows some potentially harmful medical procedures that are performed in the radiology department, specific responses to EMI, and ways to prevent the responses.

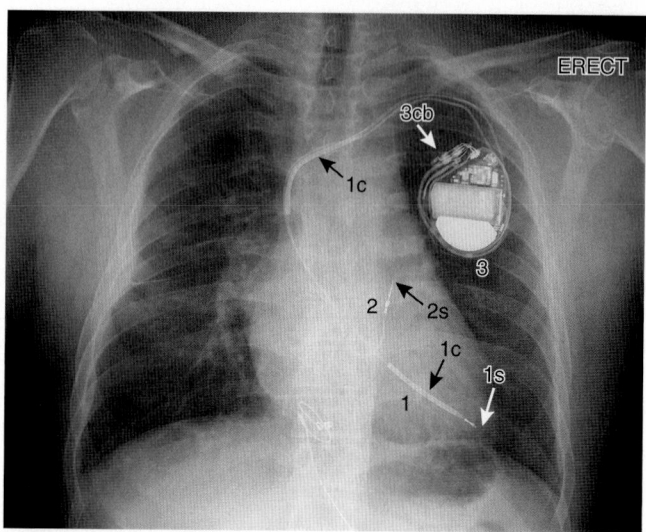

FIGURE 102-9. Posteroanterior chest radiograph from a 19-year-old man after a Senning operation for D-transposition of the great arteries, sinus node dysfunction, and a history of ventricular tachycardia. *1,* Transvenous, active fixation lead, which is attached to the left ventricular apex (systemic venous ventricle) by a retractable screw *(1s).* The lead contains two coils *(1c),* which will participate in possible shock delivery. *2,* Transvenous, bipolar, active fixation lead, which is attached to the roof of the left atrium (systemic venous atrium) by a retractable screw *(2s). 3,* Implantable cardioverter-defibrillator. *3cb,* Implantable cardioverter-defibrillator connector block.

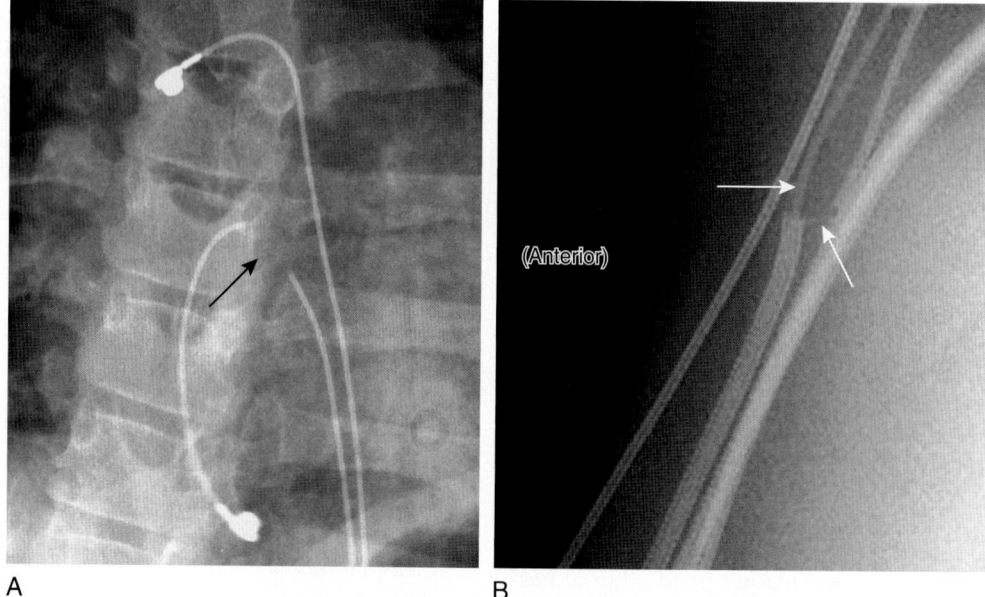

FIGURE 102-10. A, Posteroanterior projection of the chest, showing an epicardial lead fracture *(black arrow).* **B,** Lateral projection of the upper abdomen in a different child, showing pseudofracture in the Medtronic 4968 epicardial lead. The proximal conductors are identified by *white arrows* just superior to their union at the bifurcation. The *lower arrow* identifies the smallest-caliber component of the conductor. This is the normal appearance of this lead.

TABLE 102-3

Glossary of Terms Applicable to Interactions between Electromagnetic Interference and Cardiac Devices*

Activity sensor: A pacing device component that responds to a physiologic or nonphysiologic patient parameter (e.g., motion, minute ventilation) to provide a faster pacing rate.

Asynchronous mode: A mode of operation in which the pacemaker is insensitive to incoming signals from the chamber being paced.

Back-up mode: Pacing mode typically similar to that observed when the device battery has reached critical depletion; usually VVI (see below).

DDD mode: Dual-chamber mode of operation, in which pacing and sensing occur in both the atrium and the ventricle. AV synchrony is thus maintained from the lower programmed rate to the upper p-wave tracking (sensing) rate.

Inhibition: A pacemaker response in which a stimulus is withheld in response to a sensed event.

Noise reversion mode: Pacing mode activated when electrical noise is sensed. Mode usually consists of "fixed-rate pacing" for one pacing cycle, but in some devices this mode may continue as long as the electrical noise is sensed, and normal pacemaker function resumes when the noise is no longer sensed.

OOO mode: A programmable mode in some devices, in which no chambers are sensed and no chambers can be paced. In essence, the device is "off."

Oversensing: When the sensing circuitry of a pacemaker senses noncardiac electrical activity (such as electromagnetic interference [EMI]) and interprets it as cardiac activity. This may result in inappropriate inhibition (see above) or inappropriate pacing, depending on the underlying programmed pacing mode.

Pacing mode: A programmable feature of all cardiac devices that defines the cardiac chamber or chambers that can be paced and sensed from, and how the device will respond to a sensed intrinsic electrical event. The mode is abbreviated using an internationally recognized three- to five-letter code.

Pacing threshold: The minimum programmable energy output required to obtain a propagated response by the cardiac chamber of interest. This value depends on complex lead, tissue, and metabolic interactions.

Reed switch: A magnetically activated component of most pacemakers that "closes" when exposed to certain magnetic fields. Typically, this results in asynchronous pacing (see above), thus ensuring pacemaker output in the presence of possible EMI-induced oversensing (see above) and inappropriate inhibition.

Sensing threshold: The minimum cardiac chamber electrogram amplitude that can still be identified by the pacemaker circuitry as an intrinsic electrical event. This value depends on complex lead orientation, tissue, and metabolic interactions.

VDD mode: Dual-chamber mode of operation in which pacing can occur only in the ventricle but sensing can occur in both chambers.

VOO mode: Single-chamber mode of operation that is asynchronous, and pacing occurs only in the ventricle at the programmed rate, irrespective of the intrinsic ventricular rate.

VVI mode: Single-chamber mode of operation in which both pacing and sensing occur in the ventricle. Intrinsic ventricular beats are sensed by the pacemaker, resetting the lower rate timing circuitry and thus avoiding competitive pacing.

*See Table 102-4.

TABLE 102-4

Electromagnetic Interference: Potential Procedure Source, Effects on Cardiac Devices, and Prevention of Those Effects

Procedure	Possible Effects	Prevention of Untoward Effects
Cardioversion/ defibrillation	Reprogramming to back-up mode Local tissue or lead damage (increasing pacing and sensing thresholds)	Paddles should be >4-6 inches from device. Patches should be placed in anteroposterior orientation. Cardiologist should reevaluate device afterward.
Diathermy	Oversensing and inhibition Heating and destruction of device components (if placed directly over device)	Avoid application directly over device.
Electrocautery	Oversensing and inhibition (if brief) Noise reversion mode (if prolonged) Reprogramming to back-up mode Inappropriate tachycardia recognition (ICD)	Place ground patch distant from device. Use bipolar cautery. Never apply cautery within 4-6 inches of device. Program to asynchronous mode during duration of procedure (or tape magnet over device). Program tachycardia recognition "off" (ICDs).
Extracorporeal shock wave lithotripsy	Oversensing and inhibition Noise reversion mode Malfunction of reed switch Activity sensor-driven pacing Inappropriate tachycardia recognition (ICDs)	Synchronize lithotripter to patient's R wave. Maintain focal point of lithotripter >6 inches from device. Program pacemaker to VVI or VOO mode for duration of procedure. Program tachycardia recognition "off" (ICDs). Cardiologist should reevaluate device afterward.

Magnetic resonance imaging	Reed switch closure and reversion to asynchronous mode
	Theoretical (from RF scanning):
	  Rapid pacing (>300)
	  Heating of conductors with local lead or tissue damage
	  Oversensing and inhibition (pacers)
	  Inappropriate tachycardia recognition (ICDs)
	  Back-up mode
		If not pacemaker dependent:
		  Program output to < pacing threshold.
		  Program to OOO mode.
		Avoid procedure, if possible.
		Explant device first.

Transcutaneous electrical nerve stimulators	Oversensing and inhibition Reprogramming Rapid ventricular pacing if VDD or DDD modes Inappropriate tachycardia recognition (ICDs) [All rare]	Probably safe, if bipolar cardiac device. Avoid stimulation using vector parallel to leads. Program tachycardia recognition "off" (ICDs).

ICD, implantable cardioverter-defibrillators; RF, radiofrequency.

SUGGESTED READINGS

Calkins H, Sousa J, el-Atassi R, et al: Diagnosis and cure of the Wolff-Parkinson-White syndrome or paroxysmal supraventricular tachycardias during a single electrophysiologic test. N Engl J Med 1991;324:1612-1618

Cobb FR, Blumenschein SD, Sealy WC, et al: Successful surgical interruption of the bundle of Kent in a patient with Wolff-Parkinson-White syndrome. Circulation 1968;38:1018-1029

Dickfield T, Calkins H, Zviman M, et al: Anatomic stereotactic catheter ablation on three-dimensional magnetic resonance images in real time. Circulation 2003;108:2407-2413

Fischbach P, Campbell RM, Hulse E, et al: Transhepatic access to the atrioventricular ring for delivery of radiofrequency energy. J Cardiovasc Electrophysiol 1997;8:512-516

Friedman RA, Walsh EP, Silka MJ, et al: NASPE Expert Consensus Conference: radiofrequency catheter ablation with and without congenital heart disease: report of the writing committee. North American Society of Pacing and Electrophysiology. Pacing Clin Electrophysiol 2002;25:1000-1017

Giese RA, Peters NE, Dunnigan A, Milstein S: Radiation doses during pediatric radiofrequency catheter ablation procedures. Pacing Clin Electrophysiol 1996;19:1605-1611

Jackman WM, Wang XZ, Friday KJ, et al: Catheter ablation of

accessory pathways (Wolff-Parkinson-White syndrome) by radiofrequency current. N Engl J Med 1991;324:1605-1611

Kovoor P, Ricciardello M, Collins L, et al: Radiation exposure to patient and operator during radiofrequency ablation for supraventricular tachycardia. Aust N Z J Med 1995;25:490-495

Kovoor P, Ricciardello M, Collins L, et al: Risk to patients from radiation associated with radiofrequency ablation for supraventricular tachycardia. Circulation 1998;98:1534-1540

Kugler JD, Danford DA, Deal BJ, et al: Radiofrequency catheter ablation for tachyarrhythmias in children and adolescents. The Pediatric Electrophysiology Society. N Engl J Med 1994; 330:1481-1487

Lickfett L, Mahesh M, Vasamreddy C, et al: Radiation exposure during catheter ablation of atrial fibrillation. Circulation 2004;110:3003-3010

Lindsay BD, Eichling JO, Ambos HD, Cain ME: Radiation exposure to patients and medical personnel during radiofrequency catheter ablation for supraventricular tachycardia. Am J Cardiol 1992; 70:218-223

Naheed ZJ, Strasburger JF, Benson DW Jr, et al: Natural history and management strategies of automatic atrial tachycardia in children. Am J Cardiol 1995;75:405-407

Nehgme RA, Carboni MP, Care J, Murphy JD: Transthoracic percutaneous access for electroanatomic mapping and catheter ablation of atrial tachycardia in patients with a lateral tunnel Fontan. Heart Rhythm 2006;3:37-43

Perisinakis K, Damilakis J, Theocharopoulos N, et al: Accurate assessment of patient effective radiation dose and associated detriment risk from radiofrequency catheter ablation procedures. Circulation 2001;104:58-62

Saul JP, Hulse JE, Papagiannis J, et al: Late enlargement of radiofrequency lesions in infant lambs: implications for ablation procedures in small children. Circulation 1994;90:492-499

Schilling RJ, Peters NS, Davies DW: Simultaneous endocardial mapping in the human left ventricle using a non-contact catheter. Circulation 1998;98:887-898

Solan AN, Solan MJ, Bednarz G, Goodkin MB: Treatment of patients with cardiac pacemakers and implantable cardioverter-defibrillators during radiotherapy. Int J Radiat Oncol Biol Phys 2004;59:897-904

Sporton SC, Earley MJ, Nathan AW, Schilling RJ: Electroanatomic versus fluoroscopic mapping for catheter ablation procedures: a prospective randomized study. J Cardiovasc Electrophysiol 2004;15:310-315

Sweesy MW, Holland JL, Smith KW: Electromagnetic interference in cardiac rhythm management devices. AACN Clin Issues 2004;15:391-403

Van Hare GF, Javitz H, Carmelli D, et al: Prospective assessment after pediatric cardiac ablation: demographics, medical profiles, and initial outcomes. J Cardiovasc Electrophysiol 2004;15:759-770

Van Hare GF, Lesh MD, Stanger P: Radiofrequency catheter ablation in patients with congenital heart disease: results and technical considerations. J Am Coll Cardiol 1993;22:883-890

Wood DL, Hammill SC, Holmes DR Jr, et al: Catheter ablation of the atrioventricular conduction system in patients with supraventricular tachycardia. Mayo Clin Proc 1983;58:791-796

103 Surgical Considerations for Congenital Heart Defects

SITARAM EMANI, JAMES JAGGERS, and ANDREW J. LODGE

Congenital cardiac defects may be categorized in a variety of ways. One is to separate them on the basis of the presence or absence of cyanosis in the patient presenting to the pediatric cardiologist or cardiac surgeon. Cyanotic lesions are associated with shunting of deoxygenated blood into the systemic arterial circulation or with severely reduced pulmonary blood flow. Acyanotic lesions include obstructions to left ventricular outflow and defects involving shunting of blood from the systemic circulation to the pulmonary circulation. Often, a combination of lesions exists, and preoperative imaging studies must thoroughly identify associated anomalies. This chapter reviews a variety of common congenital heart defects and includes summary discussions on the nature of the lesion, including the pathophysiology, and clinical and imaging evaluation, as these are important aspects of surgical planning. We emphasize treatment, especially operative intervention of lesions, including intraoperative and postoperative considerations pertinent for radiologists.

GENERAL CONSIDERATIONS

Many congenital heart defects are fatal if not corrected surgically. Others can lead to long-term complications or a shortened life expectancy if timely surgical treatment is not undertaken. Surgery for congenital heart disease has advanced quite rapidly in the past several decades. This process has involved progress with surgical techniques and instrumentation, but it has also included substantial improvements in anesthesia and critical care. As a result, many congenital heart defects can be effectively treated, and results are consistently improving.

Surgical Approaches

Surgery for congenital heart disease is most commonly performed via a median sternotomy incision. Exceptions to this include some relatively simple extracardiac defects such as patent ductus arteriosus or vascular rings. These are typically approached through a thoracotomy incision, usually on the left side. In recent years, as techniques have been refined, there has been increasing interest in repairing more simple defects through minimally invasive incisions. Examples include the partial median sternotomy, where the skin incision is kept small and only the upper or lower sternum is

divided, and small anterior thoracotomy incisions. Defects that can be addressed through such incisions include atrial and simple ventricular septal defects (VSDs), and certain cardiac valve abnormalities. There is frequently radiographic evidence of the surgical approach. Patients who have had median sternotomy incisions often have steel wires reapproximating the sternum, although in children sutures that are not radiopaque are sometimes used. Thoracotomy incisions can produce distortion of the ribs on the operated side, and can lead to scoliosis in children. In the current era, ribs are not usually cut or sectioned during thoracotomy procedures, but sometimes inadvertent rib fractures occur.

CARDIOPULMONARY BYPASS AND ECMO

The majority of operations for congenital heart defects are performed using cardiopulmonary bypass (CPB) to support the circulation (Fig. 103-1). This apparatus has become progressively sophisticated and includes many built-in safety features, such as continuous online blood gas monitoring, bubble detectors, biocompatible surfaces, and filters, all of which have contributed to a decrease in CPB-related complications. The principal components of the system are a blood pump and an artificial lung. The pump is most commonly a roller pump, which compresses flexible tubing within the pump housing, or a centrifugal pump, which uses a spinning impeller within the pump housing to propel the blood. The artificial lung in modern CPB contains a network of microporous membranes through which oxygen and carbon dioxide can be added to or removed from the blood. These are more efficient and safe than the original bubble and screen oxygenators. CPB is accomplished by the placement of arterial and venous cannulas to deliver blood to the heart-lung machine and return it to the patient. Arterial access is generally obtained via cannulation of the ascending aorta, but large peripheral arteries such the femoral or axillary arteries are sometimes used. Venous return is most commonly obtained by a single cannula in the right atrium. Procedures in which the right side of the heart is opened require separate cannulation of the superior and inferior venae cavae. CPB completely replaces the function of the heart and lungs during surgery, so that ventilation is stopped and the heart is emptied of blood and can be arrested completely when necessary, facilitating accurate repair.

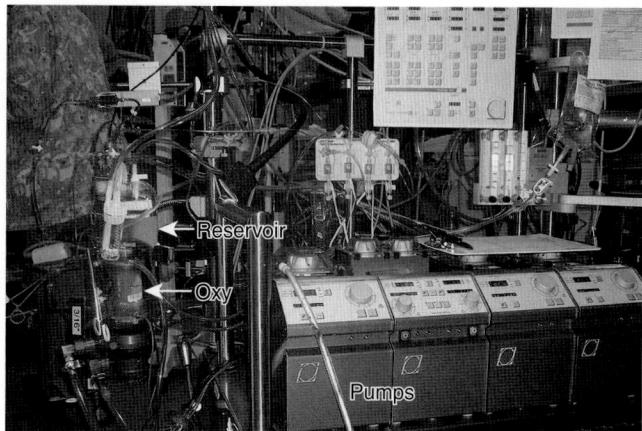

FIGURE 103-1. Pediatric cardiopulmonary bypass (heart-lung) machine. The blood reservoir, oxygenator (oxy), and pumps are labeled. The blood tubing connecting the components can be seen. Below the oxygenator is a temperature coil, to which water lines are attached allowing control of the patient's body temperature. Some of the monitoring equipment for the apparatus can be seen in the upper right of the picture.

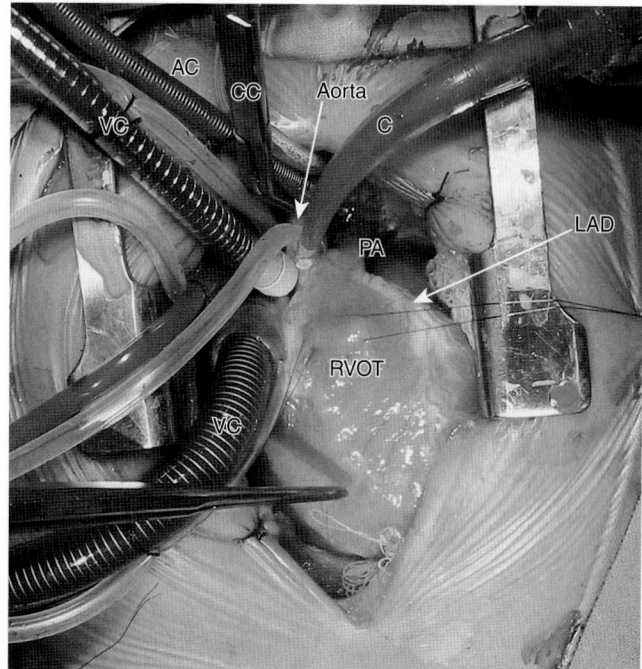

FIGURE 103-2. Intraoperative photograph of an infant with tetralogy of Fallot (TOF) demonstrates a typical setup for cardiopulmonary bypass. The patient's head is toward the top of the picture. A cross-clamp (CC) has been applied to the aorta between the arterial cannula (AC) and the cardioplegia catheter (C). Venous cannulas (VC) are positioned in the superior vena cava and right atrium. The surface of the right ventricle is visible and sutures are present in the right ventricular infundibulum (RVOT). The diminutive main pulmonary artery (PA), which is typical of TOF, is seen. The left anterior descending coronary artery (LAD) is seen at the left lateral margin of the field. The left ventricle is typically not visible without retraction through a median sternotomy, as this is a posterior structure.

Surgery for congenital heart defects can occasionally be performed without CPB when the procedure exclusively involves extracardiac structures, and when it does not require complete occlusion of either the aorta or the main pulmonary artery. Examples of such procedures include modified Blalock-Taussig shunts and pulmonary artery banding. More complex extracardiac operations or those in which the patient becomes unstable require the use of CPB. In addition, any procedure involving an intracardiac structure such as a heart valve or septal defect requires CPB. Sometimes, extracorporeal circulatory support is necessary after surgery to allow recovery of the heart over an extended period, or as a bridge to transplant in the case of an unsuccessful repair. In these cases, a modified CPB circuit is used for extracorporeal membrane oxygenation (ECMO). ECMO can be continued for days to weeks if necessary. Survival in patients who require ECMO after surgery is approximately 50%.

CARDIOPLEGIA AND CIRCULATORY ARREST

In general, most intracardiac procedures are facilitated by cardioplegia, which is accomplished by administering a potassium-rich solution that induces a diastolic cardiac arrest and thus produces a motionless and relatively bloodless field inside the heart. This cardioplegic solution is administered after clamping the aorta between the arterial inflow cannula and the coronary arteries (Fig. 103-2). Because the heart is ischemic during this time, it is usually cooled to approximately 4° C by making the solution cold and bathing the heart in cold saline or slush. These measures allow the heart to tolerate even relatively prolonged periods of ischemia. In very complex cases, such as those involving small neonates or complex aortic arch reconstruction, it is occasionally desirable to temporarily stop the entire circulation. This technique, termed deep hypothermic circulatory arrest, employs total-body cooling to approximately 18° C, allowing the circulation to be safely suspended for 30 to 45 minutes.

Chest Radiography

Chest radiographs are critical after cardiac surgery and are by far the most common radiographic study obtained in the postoperative period. The initial postoperative chest radiograph is obtained immediately on arrival to the recovery room or intensive care unit. Important considerations on this film include verifying the proper position of support equipment such as central venous lines, chest tubes, and the endotracheal tube, assessing the degree of lung expansion, and ruling out unsuspected pleural effusions or pneumothoraces (Fig. 103-3). In small children with limited percutaneous vascular access, pressure-monitoring lines are sometimes inserted directly into the cardiac chamber (and later removed at the bedside). The most common points of insertion, in decreasing order of frequency, are the right atrium, left atrium (usually via the right superior pulmonary vein), and pulmonary artery. The immediate postoperative film must be obtained and interpreted in a timely fashion, as delays can be life-threatening.

Other surgically relevant features of the postoperative chest film include the integrity or stability of items such as sternal wires and prostheses. Many patients have mild pulmonary edema or small pleural effusions related to the inflammatory response to CPB. These findings

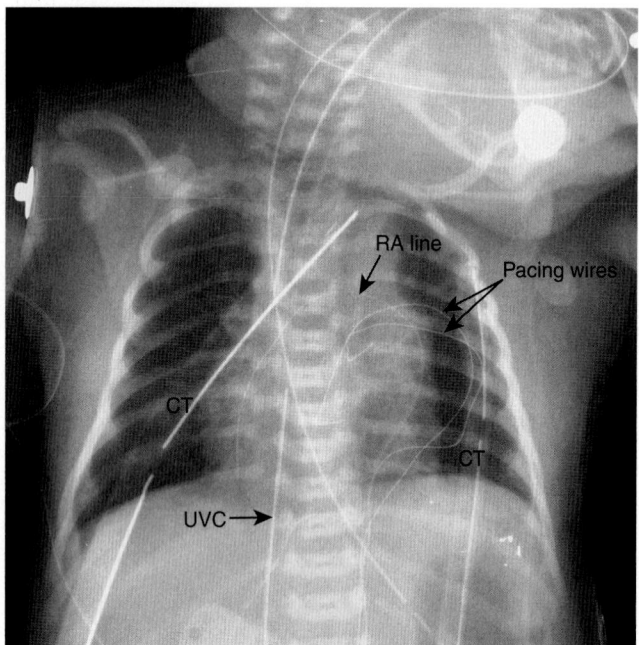

FIGURE 103-3. A typical postoperative infant's chest radiograph. The tip of the endotracheal tube can be seen above the carina. Other support equipment is labeled. The pacing wires can appear similar to the transthoracic pressure lines. The wires can be identified by their typical termination in a J configuration, whereas the pressure lines are straight. There is typically some redundant length of each in the pericardial space. The right chest tube (CT) traverses the right pleural space and terminates in the pericardium/mediastinum. The right atrial (RA) line tip is near the RA-to-inferior vena cava junction. UVC, umbilical vein catheter.

generally resolve with diuretic treatment. Most current valve prostheses (Table 103-1) are visible on chest radiographs because of the presence of metal in the sewing ring, the stent, or the valve itself. Homografts or autografts are the exception. Daily chest radiographs are frequently obtained after cardiac surgery. Posteroanterior and lateral films are generally preferred for patients stable enough to travel, including those with indwelling appliances such as chest tubes. Follow-up films are usually obtained immediately after the removal of pleural chest tubes (which are generally placed only if the pleural space is entered during the procedure), but they are not routinely necessary after the removal of intracardiac lines, pacing wires, and pericardial (mediastinal) drains.

Many procedures used to correct congenital heart defects are designed to be anatomically corrective. Despite this, it is not uncommon for children who have had surgery for congenital heart disease to need subsequent intervention for residual or recurrent lesions. Reasons for this include scarring and the use of conduits or valves that do not grow with the child. Most children with repaired congenital heart defects need life-long follow-up with a cardiologist.

ACYANOTIC LESIONS

Aortic Stenosis

Congenital aortic stenosis (AS) accounts for about 5% to 10% of cardiac malformations recognized in childhood, and it occurs with an incidence of 6.1 per 10,000 births. This entity is to be distinguished from bicuspid aortic valve, which is identified in autopsy series in up to 2% of adults and is often clinically silent. Aortic stenosis is more common in males than in females (3:1).

ANATOMY AND PATHOPHYSIOLOGY

Congenital aortic stenosis is classified according to the location of the stenosis. Valvar stenosis (70%) is associated with commissural fusion and valvular deformity. Subvalvar stenosis (10% to 20%) is usually seen in older children and is most commonly the result of a fibromuscular shelf. Supravalvar stenosis is caused by a thickening of the aortic media at the sinotubular junction (Fig. 103-4).

Valvar aortic stenosis in the neonate has a high mortality, partly because of the association with hypoplastic left ventricle and other left heart obstructive lesions. From a surgical standpoint, small ventricular size is a predictor of mortality and may contraindicate isolated aortic valvotomy. The natural history in older children presenting with valvar aortic stenosis depends on the degree of stenosis. Patients with mild stenosis (peak gradient <50 mm Hg) exhibit an actuarial survival close to

TABLE 103-1			
Cardiac Valve Prostheses			
Prosthesis Type	**Synonym**	**Definition**	**Characteristics**
Bioprosthetic	Xenograft, heterograft	Manufactured valve; uses tissue from other species such as pig or cow	Does not require long-term anticoagulation; subject to structural deterioration
Mechanical	—	Manufactured valve, generally composed of metal and pyrolytic carbon	Requires long-term anticoagulation; the most durable prosthesis; MRI compatible
Homograft	Allograft	Cryopreserved human valve or valved conduit	Included segment of aorta or pulmonary artery offers greater reconstructive potential; subject to structural deterioration; aortic valve particularly prone to calcification
Autograft	—	Patient's own tissue	Pulmonary autograft used to replace aortic valve in Ross procedure
Stentless	—	Bioprosthetic valve that does not have a rigid plastic or metal stent built in	Technically more difficult to implant; may have greater effective orifice area

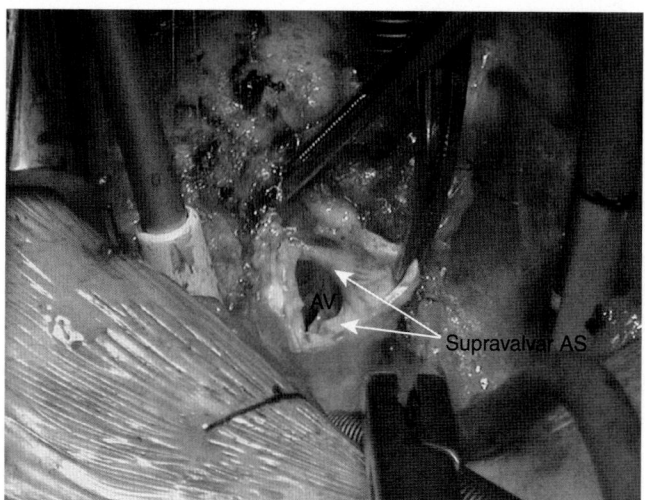

FIGURE 103-4. Intraoperative photograph of a patient with supravalvar aortic stenosis. The aortic cannula and cross-clamp can be seen toward the bottom of the photo (cephalad). The aorta has been opened. The aortic valve (AV) can be seen below the fibrous ridge of supravalvar aortic stenosis (AS; *arrows*). (*See color plate.*)

that of a matched population, with only 15% coming to surgical intervention. Patients presenting with moderate stenosis (peak gradient between 50 and 75 mm Hg), however, demonstrate a diminished actuarial survival and require aortic valvotomy or valve replacement in at least two thirds of cases.

> Valvar aortic stenosis in the neonate has a high mortality. Small ventricular size is a predictor of mortality and may contraindicate isolated aortic valvotomy.

Subvalvar stenosis, if left untreated, can progress from a simple obstructive membrane to a fibromuscular tunnel. Tunnel-like obstruction may also occur after previous surgery for subvalvar AS. The incidence of aortic regurgitation at the time of presentation is higher in patients with subvalvar AS than in those with other forms of aortic stenosis, and it may be caused by valvular trauma secondary to turbulent flow. Subvalvar AS is rarely diagnosed during early infancy. It often arises after previous documentation of an unobstructed left ventricular outflow tract, and it may develop after surgery for other congenital heart defects, particularly atrioventricular septal defects.

In the setting of supravalvar AS, pathologic changes in the coronary arteries located proximal to the area of obstruction may be present. These include intimal hyperplasia, medial hypertrophy, and luminal obstruction. Coronary dysplasia with concomitant left ventricular (LV) hypertrophy increases the risk of developing myocardial ischemia. Supravalvar AS is commonly associated with Williams syndrome.

All forms of AS increase the afterload on the left ventricle and lead to left ventricular hypertrophy (LVH). This can lead to diastolic dysfunction and heart failure symptoms. If untreated, LVH can be progressive and lead

to subendocardial ischemia, systolic LV dysfunction, and eventually death.

CLINICAL PRESENTATION

Approximately 10% of patients with valvar AS present within the first weeks of life with signs of congestive heart failure (CHF) such as irritability, difficulty feeding, and tachypnea. Poor peripheral perfusion and metabolic acidosis indicate a low cardiac output. Cyanosis, particularly in the lower extremities, may be noted in patients with a patent ductus arteriosus and right-to-left shunting. The electrocardiogram may occasionally be normal even with more severe obstruction, but evidence of left ventricular hypertrophy and strain (inverted T waves in the left precordial leads) is usually present if severe stenosis is long-standing.

Diagnosis

Chest radiography may demonstrate cardiomegaly and pulmonary edema. A prominent ascending aorta due to poststenotic dilation may be present if severe aortic stenosis is long-standing. The chest radiograph may be normal in the neonate. Echocardiography identifies both the location and the severity of the obstruction. Left ventricle size, morphology of the aortic valve, and the presence of a subaortic membrane or supravalvar stenosis must be assessed. The endocardium may be echo-bright, indicating the development of endocardial fibroelastosis. Doppler studies determine the peak and mean systolic LV outflow tract gradients. Echocardiography is also useful for assessing the size of other left-sided structures (mitral valve, LV cavity), which can sometimes represent limitations to surgical repair. Most infants with critical AS do not require cardiac catheterization for diagnostic purposes but may undergo the procedure for a balloon valvuloplasty.

Treatment

Intervention is indicated for children having moderate (50 to 80 mm Hg) to severe (>80 mm Hg) valvar AS. For critical aortic stenosis in the neonate, administration of prostaglandin E_1 is begun immediately to maintain ductal patency and systemic cardiac output. The echocardiographic findings determine feasibility of surgical (two-ventricle) repair, using criteria such as those developed by Rhodes and colleagues: (1) the ratio of the left ventricular long axis to the heart long axis is greater than 0.8, (2) the aortic root diameter is greater than $3.5 \, cm/m^2$, (3) the mitral valve area is greater than $4.75 \, cm^2/m^2$, and (4) the left ventricular mass is greater than $35 \, g/m^2$. Valvotomy in patients failing to meet two or more of these criteria resulted in 100% mortality, compared with only 8% in patients with only one risk factor or none. If two-ventricle repair is not feasible, patients may undergo single-ventricle palliation, similar to that for hypoplastic left heart syndrome (see later).

Percutaneous transluminal balloon valvotomy has been successfully applied to selected patients with valvar AS and is becoming the first-line therapy in centers experienced with interventional catheter techniques. Complications include the development of aortic insufficiency, which may require surgical intervention. Although balloon dilation provides excellent short-term palliation, 50% require reintervention within 5 years. Surgical treatment for valvar AS involves CPB with open valvotomy or valve replacement.

When aortic valve replacement is necessary, the choices include cryopreserved aortic homograft (allograft), bioprosthetic, mechanical, and pulmonary autograft valve replacement. Bioprosthetic and mechanical valves are limited to use in larger patients, and mechanical valves require anticoagulation. Autograft replacement (Ross procedure) and homografts are better-suited for neonates and infants. Root enlargement can be added to valve replacement if the annular size or subaortic area is small (Konno-Rastan procedure).

Indications for intervention for either subvalvar and supravalvar stenosis include the presence of symptoms and a gradient of greater than 40 mm Hg. Aortic insufficiency in the presence of subvalvar obstruction may constitute an indication for surgery to relieve the source of the turbulent flow damaging the aortic valve. These lesions are not amenable to percutaneous intervention, and treatment is transaortic surgical resection of obstruction (subaortic stenosis) or patch augmentation of the ascending aorta (supravalvar stenosis). For severe concentric subaortic stenosis, augmentation of the LV outflow tract with a Dacron patch can be performed through the right ventricle (modified Konno procedure).

> Indications for intervention for either subvalvar and supravalvar stenosis include symptoms and a gradient of greater than 40 mm Hg. Aortic insufficiency in the presence of subvalvar obstruction may be an indication for surgery to relieve the source of turbulent flow damaging the aortic valve.

Mortality as low as 0% has been reported for neonates with isolated critical aortic stenosis, but patients requiring concomitant repair of other cardiac lesions may experience an operative mortality approaching 50%. Whether surgical or catheter treatment has been carried out, aortic insufficiency or calcification with restenosis is likely to occur years or even decades later, eventually requiring reoperation and often aortic valve replacement.

Coarctation of the Aorta

Coarctation of the aorta comprises 5% to 8% of cases of congenital heart disease, with an incidence in the general population estimated at 1 per 1200 live births. The anomaly occurs twice as often in males as in females. It can occur in association with a variety of other heart defects.

ANATOMY AND PATHOPHYSIOLOGY

The location of aortic coarctation in 98% of patients is just below the origin of the left subclavian artery at the insertion of the ductus arteriosus (juxtaductal coarctation) (Fig. 103-5). Nearly half of patients with coarctation develop symptoms within the first month of life and often have the preductal subtype of coarctation with

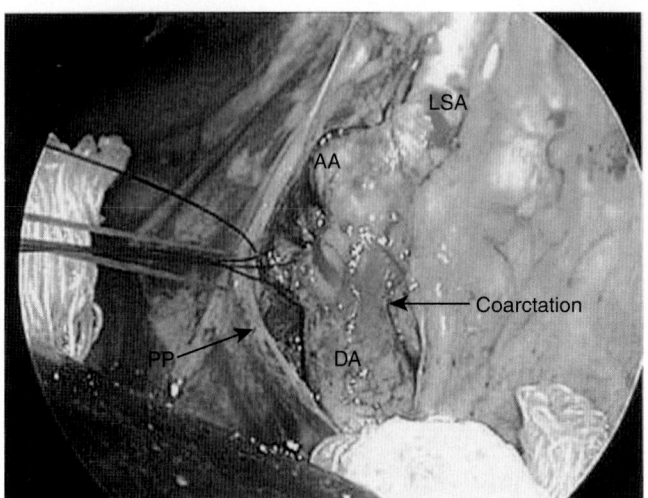

FIGURE 103-5. Intraoperative photograph during repair of aortic coarctation. The parietal pleura (PP) has been opened to expose the aorta. This flap of tissue contains the vagus and recurrent laryngeal nerves. The sutures are around the ductus arteriosus. The coarctation is visible as a subtle indentation externally. The internal diameter will be substantially smaller. AA, aortic arch; DA, descending aorta; LSA, left subclavian artery. (See color plate.)

hypoplasia of the arch. This form is associated with high early mortality if left untreated.

Collateral vessels may develop in patients who do not develop CHF within 3 to 6 months of age. Most of these patients become asymptomatic into adolescence or early adulthood. The most common symptom is hypertension. Untreated coarctation is associated with a substantially diminished long-term survival. Death in these patients usually results from systemic effects of hypertension, including heart failure, coronary artery disease, or aortic rupture or dissection.

CLINICAL PRESENTATION

Age of presentation follows a bimodal distribution. Infants present with symptoms of CHF such as tachypnea or difficulty feeding. Young adults may present with hypertension refractory to pharmacotherapy, headaches, or angina. The classic physical findings are the presence of brachiofemoral pulse delay, diminished or absent femoral pulses, and a blood pressure gradient between the upper and lower extremities. The electrocardiogram may reveal evidence of left ventricular hypertrophy in older patients.

DIAGNOSIS

Infants with severe coarctation may demonstrate radiographic signs of cardiac enlargement and pulmonary congestion. During adolescence or adulthood, the findings may include a figure-3 configuration resulting from proximal and poststenotic dilation of the aorta. Notching of the inferior border of the ribs from the development of intercostal collateral vessels is common by late childhood.

The segment of coarctation can usually be visualized in children by two-dimensional echocardiography. As mentioned earlier, associated defects must be ruled out. VSD is a common associated lesion. Anomalies of the mitral and aortic valves can also be demonstrated. Bicuspid aortic valve is the most common associated valvular lesion. Pulsed and continuous-wave Doppler determine the pressure gradient directly at the area of coarctation. However, in the presence of a patent ductus arteriosus, proximal obstruction such as aortic stenosis, or low cardiac output, the severity of the narrowing may be underestimated. A peak gradient greater than 20 mm Hg, especially if accompanied by continuous forward flow during diastole in the descending or abdominal aorta, suggests significant aortic coarctation. Pressure gradients as measured by Doppler imaging correlate with those measured by angiography.

In older children and adults, the anatomy may be difficult to define by echocardiography because of poor sonographic windows. Computed tomography angiography (CTA) as well as magnetic resonance imaging angiography (MRA) have become valuable diagnostic tools in these patients. The use of catheterization with aortography is currently limited to determining the diagnosis and severity of coarctation in patients with disparate clinical and echocardiographic findings. It is also used to determine the degree of coronary artery stenosis in adult patients requiring surgical repair, although evolution in CTA coronary artery evaluation with electrocardiographic gating may change this algorithm.

TREATMENT

In neonates with severe coarctation of the aorta, prostaglandin E_1 is given to establish and maintain ductal patency to ensure adequate visceral and lower extremity blood flow. All patients with significant coarctation or recoarctation warrant intervention to reduce or eliminate the obstruction. This includes patients with an arm-to-leg systolic blood pressure difference of 10 mm Hg or greater, brachiofemoral pulse delay, peak transcoarctation gradient greater than 20 mm Hg at angiography, and long-standing hypertension (regardless of age), whether symptomatic or asymptomatic. Several techniques have been used to repair coarctation of the aorta: balloon angioplasty with or without stent placement, end-to-end anastomosis, prosthetic patch angioplasty, subclavian artery flap angioplasty, interposition grafts, and bypass procedures.

Primary treatment is extended end-to-end anastomosis for neonates, patch angioplasty or interposition graft for adults, and balloon dilation for recoarctation. Although balloon dilation and stenting has been used in adolescents and children for primary coarctation, the long-term results of this approach are not yet known. Complications following coarctation repair include rebound hypertension, mesenteric arteritis, spinal cord ischemia, aneurysm formation, and late restenosis.

> **Primary treatment for coarctation is extended end-to-end anastomosis for neonates, patch angioplasty or interposition graft for adults, and balloon dilation for recoarctation. Although balloon dilation and stenting has been used in adolescents and children for primary coarctation, its long-term results are not yet known.**

Management of coarctation in the presence of a VSD is controversial and is therefore tailored to the individual patient. In many cases, coarctation is the more symptomatic anomaly, and resection of the coarctation segment results in marked improvement. Repair of the VSD is performed when symptoms of CHF develop. Other options include repair of the coarctation and placement of a pulmonary artery band through a left lateral thoracotomy, or simultaneous repair of both the VSD and the coarctation through a midline sternotomy using CPB.

Patent Ductus Arteriosus

Patent ductus arteriosus (PDA) is a common lesion. It is frequently noted in combination with other heart defects, but it can occur in isolation. It is most commonly seen in premature infants. The incidence in this population is several times higher than that in full-term infants.

PATHOPHYSIOLOGY

The detailed pathophysiology of PDA is covered in Chapters 9, 28, and 90. When the ductus remains patent after birth, increasing left-to-right shunting of blood occurs as the pulmonary vascular resistance falls. This leads to pulmonary overcirculation. If the condition persists, CHF can develop, and eventually pulmonary vascular obstructive disease can occur. Patients with a PDA also have a higher risk of endocarditis.

DIAGNOSIS

On physical examination, a continuous murmur may be heard. Patients who have CHF may have pulmonary rales and an extra heart sound (gallop). Bounding pulses can occasionally be felt. Premature infants are especially susceptible to the hemodynamic effects of PDA. They may have hypotension, particularly diastolic hypotension, and are at increased risk of developing visceral malperfusion, which can lead to renal insufficiency and necrotizing enterocolitis.

Chest radiography may show cardiomegaly, signs of pulmonary congestion, and pulmonary edema. In older patients, calcification in the wall of the ductus or enlarged pulmonary arteries characteristic of pulmonary hypertension may be noted. Transthoracic echocardiography is used to make the diagnosis. This is very sensitive in children. In adults, echo windows may be suboptimal, and CT or MRA may be helpful. Cardiac catheterization is necessary only if pulmonary hypertension is suspected.

TREATMENT

PDA is one of the few congenital heart lesions that can be definitively managed medically. Prostaglandin inhibitors such as indomethacin or ibuprofen can be successfully used to produce ductal closure. Situations in which such treatment is contraindicated include the presence of renal insufficiency, intestinal compromise, and significant intracranial hemorrhage.

If medical treatment fails or is contraindicated, surgical therapy is appropriate. Preoperative evaluation is critical, particularly in the premature infant who is likely to have multiple comorbidities. Emphasis should be on medical stabilization, exclusion of active infections, and appropriate treatment of pre-existing infections.

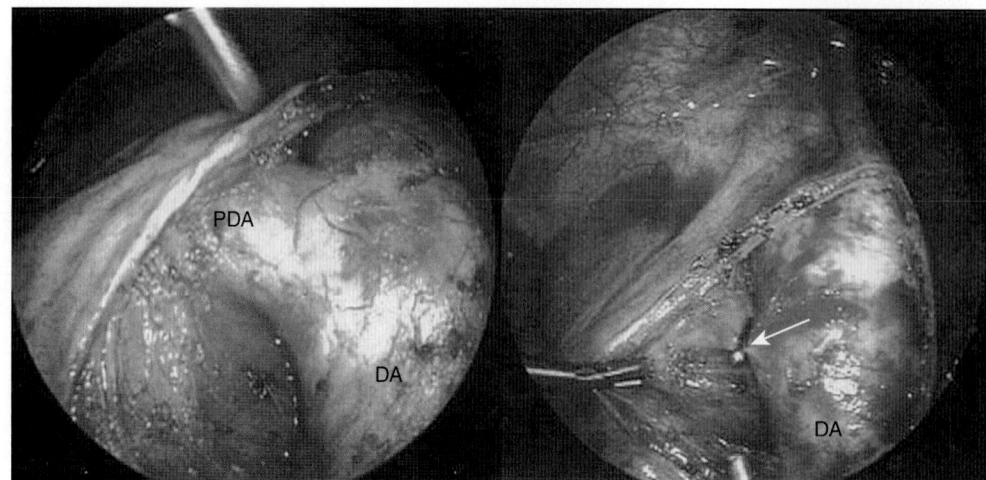

FIGURE 103-6.
Thoracoscopic ligation of a patent ductus arteriosus (PDA). The parietal pleura has been opened to expose the PDA and descending aorta (DA). In the photo on the right, the PDA has been ligated with a single titanium hemoclip (*arrow*). These clips are generally MRI compatible. (*See color plate.*)

Because these infants may be unstable with stimulation or transport, surgery is frequently performed at the bedside in the intensive care nursery.

In the case of isolated PDA, the preferred surgical approach is a posterolateral left thoracotomy. A preoperative echocardiogram should be obtained to confirm the presence of a left aortic arch and normal ductal anatomy. Variations may necessitate an alternative approach. In patients undergoing the repair of associated cardiac defects, the PDA can be accessed via the median sternotomy incision. Some have advocated the use of video-assisted thoracoscopy to allow a minimally invasive approach to the PDA. In older patients in whom the ductus is calcified, CPB may be necessary.

The ductus may be simply ligated with suture or clips (Fig. 103-6). This approach is favored in the premature infant because of the fragility of the vessels. Alternatively, ligation and division of the PDA may be performed. This approach minimizes the chances of a persistent communication. In the case of a calcified PDA, closure with a patch from within the pulmonary artery (using CPB) may be necessary. Newer techniques involve transcatheter device closure in adequately sized patients.

PROGNOSIS

Operative mortality related to PDA ligation is very low. Premature infants with multiple comorbidities may have a higher mortality, but the cause of death is rarely related to the procedure. Complications include left recurrent laryngeal nerve injury, bleeding (which is rare), and postoperative chylothorax.

Atrial Septal Defect

Atrial septal defect (ASD) is one of the most common congenital cardiac abnormalities, occurring in 10% to 15% of all patients with congenital heart disease. It may occur as an isolated lesion or be associated with other congenital heart defects. It was the first intracardiac defect to be successfully repaired using CPB.

ANATOMY AND PATHOPHYSIOLOGY

Three types of ASDs are commonly recognized: ostium primum, ostium secundum, and sinus venosus. The most

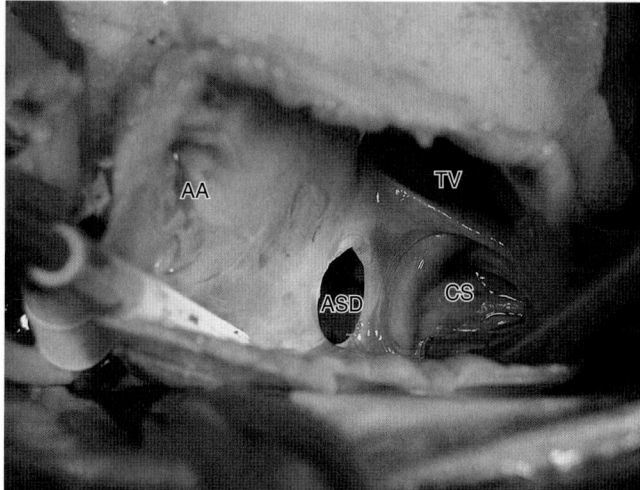

FIGURE 103-7. Intraoperative view of a secundum atrial septal defect (ASD) is shown via a right atriotomy. The patient's head is to the left, and the feet toward the right. Also visible are the entrance to the right atrial appendage (AA), the tricuspid valve orifice (TV), and the ostium of the coronary sinus (CS). (*See color plate.*)

common type of defect is the secundum ASD, a defect in the region of the fossa ovalis, which comprises over 80% of cases (Fig. 103-7). This is usually distinguished from a patent foramen ovale, which is a relatively common finding in the general population, by a true deficiency of atrial septum primum tissue.

Primum ASDs result from a lack of closure of the ostium primum near the endocardial cushions during cardiac development. This defect is in the spectrum of endocardial cushion (atrioventricular septal) defects, and it is essentially always associated with abnormalities of the atrioventricular valves, notably a cleft in the anterior leaflet of the mitral valve. This is a substantially more complex lesion than a secundum ASD and is discussed later.

Sinus venosus ASDs usually occur in the postero-superior aspect of the atrial septum. Embryologically, sinus venosus ASD results from a deficiency of the right portion of the common pulmonary vein, which contributes to the formation of the atrial septum. For this reason, this defect is associated with partial anomalous drainage of the right superior pulmonary vein to the right atrium or superior vena cava. Much less commonly, the sinus venosus ASD occurs in the posteroinferior portion of the atrial septum near the inferior vena cava orifice and may involve anomalous drainage of the right lower pulmonary vein.

ASDs do not generally spontaneously close. For example, an estimated 15% or less of secundum ASDs close by 4 years of age. Uncomplicated ASDs rarely cause severe symptoms at an early age, and there is little likelihood that pulmonary arterial obstructive disease will develop in the first few years of life. However, longer-standing unrepaired ASDs can lead to chronic pulmonary overcirculation or enlargement of the right atrium and ventricle, and eventually they can lead to irreversible pulmonary vascular disease.

CLINICAL PRESENTATION

Younger patients are asymptomatic, and the defect is found on routine physical examination. Most commonly, a systolic murmur is present secondary to increased flow across the pulmonary valve. The second heart sound may exhibit fixed splitting. Rarely, young children with ASDs present with failure to thrive attributed to heart failure. Older patients may be symptomatic, with either subtle signs of heart failure, exercise intolerance, or palpitations. Complications such as paradoxical embolus or atrial arrhythmias may be the presenting feature.

DIAGNOSIS

Chest radiography usually reveals enlargement of the right atrium and ventricle, enlargement of the pulmonary artery and its branches, and increased pulmonary vascular markings. Prominence of the proximal portion of the superior vena cava is occasionally noted in patients with a sinus venosus defect. Left atrial enlargement is extremely rare but may be observed when significant mitral regurgitation exists.

Transthoracic echocardiography (TTE) provides excellent visualization of defects of the atrial septum in children and has been used for diagnosis in adults with suspected ASD. A bubble study can be performed by intravenously injecting agitated saline as a contrast medium and observing for microbubbles crossing the septum into the left atrium. Transesophageal echocardiography is superior to TTE for the diagnosis of sinus venosus defects, and it may also be useful in adults with poor transthoracic echo windows.

Experience is being accumulated with the use of cardiac MR imaging for the diagnosis of ASD. Cardiac catheterization is recommended for adults if there is a question of elevated pulmonary vascular resistance or concomitant coronary artery disease.

TREATMENT

Traditionally, indications for closure of atrial septal defects included diameter larger than 1 cm in children, and in adults, symptoms or the presence of a left-to-right shunt (Qp:Qs of 1.5:1 or greater). The lesion is repaired in children before they begin school (at age 3 to 5 years), and in adults at the time of diagnosis if there are symptoms or a significant left-to-right shunt is identified.

Repair involves the use of CPB and exposure of the defect by an incision in the right atrium (right atriotomy). In most cases of secundum ASD, the repair is sufficiently straightforward that a minimally invasive surgical approach can be used. More recently, closure of ASDs using a percutaneous transcatheter device method has gained popularity. This technique has essentially become the standard of care in most heart centers for simple ASDs. Contraindications to device closure include prohibitively large defect size and lack of a sufficient tissue rim to anchor the device. Severe, irreversible pulmonary vascular obstructive disease (resistance greater than 8.0 Wood units · m^2) is a contraindication to closure.

> Traditionally, indications for ASD closure included diameter larger than 1 cm in children, and symptoms or the presence of a left-to-right shunt in adults. The lesion is repaired in children before school age, and in adults at the time of diagnosis if symptoms or a significant left-to-right shunt is identified.

Ventricular Septal Defect

Isolated VSD is one of the most common congenital heart defects, occurring at a rate of approximately 2 per 1000 live births. VSD, either in isolation or associated with other congenital abnormalities, is present in approximately 50% of patients with congenital heart disease.

Anatomy and Pathophysiology

Abnormal development of the ventricular septum during the first 8 weeks of gestation results in a VSD. The ventricular septum is formed by a muscular partition that extends from the primitive ventricle of the cardiac tube to the endocardial cushions, as well as a conal septum component (the tissue that separates the great vessels). A defect in the membranous area of the ventricular septum results in a perimembranous VSD, the most common type. A defect in endocardial cushion formation results in an inlet (atrioventricular septal or canal) VSD. A defect in the conal septum results in a subarterial (supracristal) VSD. These are rare and seen more often in those of Asian descent. Finally, a defect in the muscular portion of the interventricular septum is termed a muscular VSD.

The natural history of a VSD depends on the size and location. Some VSDs close spontaneously. Those most likely to do so are in the perimembranous region or muscular septum. Muscular VSDs are more likely to close if they are smaller, but VSDs located in the subarterial position are unlikely to close no matter how small they are. Perimembranous or subarterial VSDs may be associated with aortic insufficiency when flow beneath the aortic valve disturbs valve function, or with prolapse of an aortic valve leaflet into the defect itself. Whereas all isolated VSDs are associated with a left-to-right shunt, the magnitude of this shunt depends on the size of the defect and on the downstream pulmonary vascular resistance. As pulmonary vascular resistance falls in infancy, the degree of left-to-right shunting increases. Thus, symptoms of CHF may not become apparent until then.

If the VSD is left unrepaired, there is a relatively high risk of developing pulmonary hypertension. When the pulmonary vascular resistance becomes sufficiently elevated, shunting through the defect may become right-to-left shunting, leading to cyanosis (Eisenmenger syndrome).

DIAGNOSTIC STUDIES

Chest radiography may demonstrate signs of CHF if the degree of left-to-right shunting is significant. This is manifested by pulmonary vascular congestion and cardiomegaly. Left atrial and ventricular enlargement may be prominent. With long-standing VSD, the pulmonary arteries may be enlarged, suggesting pulmonary hypertension.

Echocardiography is used to make the diagnosis. Information that must be obtained from this study includes the size and location of the VSD, the presence of aortic valve regurgitation, and an estimation of pulmonary artery pressure if possible. Associated anomalies, including additional VSDs, must also be ruled out. Cardiac catheterization is not routinely necessary, but it is indicated in older patients or if there is clinical suspicion of elevated pulmonary vascular resistance.

TREATMENT

Medical therapy and observation are indicated for patients who have a restrictive VSD or one that has features suggestive of a high probability of closure. This includes small defects in the muscular and perimembranous ventricular septum that are not associated with aortic valve pathology. These patients should be followed closely. Their likelihood of developing bacterial endocarditis is greater than that of the general population.

Surgical repair for large VSDs is generally recommended between 3 and 6 months of age. Most of these are the perimembranous type. Surgical therapy may be necessary earlier if there are findings suggestive of a large left-to-right shunt or in the presence of symptoms that are refractory to medical therapy.

> **Surgical repair for large VSDs (mostly the perimembranous type) is generally recommended at 3 to 6 months of age. Surgery may be necessary earlier if there is a large left-to-right shunt or if symptoms are refractory to medical therapy.**

CHF very often comes in the form of failure to thrive even if symptoms of pulmonary congestion are adequately managed medically. Another indication for intervention is the presence of aortic insufficiency caused by leaflet prolapse into the septal defect. This is unusual in infants. A VSD in the teenager or young adult may be closed provided that the patient has not developed prohibitive pulmonary hypertension and right-to-left shunting. Surgical closure in these patients may reduce the risk of bacterial endocarditis.

Surgical treatment can be divided into complete repair and palliative procedures. Most VSDs closed today are approached through a right atriotomy with CPB. Deep hypothermic circulatory arrest is occasionally used in very small infants. Some defects must be approached through a right ventricular or pulmonary artery incision

to allow better visualization. A patch of polyethylene terephthalate (Dacron) or polytetrafluoroethylene (PTFE; Gore-Tex) is typically used to close the defect. Rarely, the presence of multiple muscular defects and significant CHF mandates palliative treatment. This can be performed by placement of a restrictive band around the pulmonary artery to reduce the amount of left-to-right shunting, and to allow for subsequent complete repair after the child has grown sufficiently.

Transcatheter device closure of VSDs is a developing field. VSDs are more complicated, and the technology is not yet as advanced as for ASDs. At present, device closure is most appropriate for some muscular VSDs. Devices for perimembranous defects are under development and are the subject of ongoing clinical trials.

Prognosis

Early mortality for repair of isolated VSD in infants is less than 2%. Complications of surgery are related to the proximity of the defect to several important cardiac structures, including the aortic and tricuspid valve, and the conduction system. The incidence of complete heart block requiring a permanent pacemaker should be 1% or less of cases of uncomplicated VSD. Small residual VSDs are not uncommon, but the majority close spontaneously. The incidence of postoperative aortic or tricuspid valve insufficiency is very low.

Long-term outcomes after VSD repair are good, with an approximately 87% overall probability of 25-year survival. Good results can be obtained with definitive repair even in neonates. Low-birth-weight infants who undergo repair often return to normalized growth parameters within 6 to 12 months after surgery.

Atrioventricular Septal Defects

Atrioventricular septal defects (AVSDs), also known as atrioventricular (AV) canal defects, are relatively common lesions and are the most common heart defect in children with trisomy 21. They represent approximately 4% of all congenital heart defects and over 50% of those in children with trisomy 21.

ANATOMY AND PATHOPHYSIOLOGY

The three commonly recognized types of AVSD represent a spectrum of severity. They occur when the embryologic endocardial cushions fail to properly fuse to form the AV canal portion of the heart. This results in abnormalities of atrial and ventricular septation and atrioventricular (mitral and tricuspid) valve formation. The most commonly recognized form is the complete AVSD, which is characterized by a primum atrial septal defect, a common AV valve, and a large inlet VSD. The second most commonly recognized type is the partial or incomplete AVSD in which there is a primum ASD and a cleft in the anterior leaflet of the left AV (mitral) valve. The least commonly recognized type is the transitional AVSD. This is similar to a partial AVSD, except there is also a small VSD.

In all of these lesions, left-to-right shunting is the predominant pathophysiology. As in other lesions with left-to-right shunting, pulmonary overcirculation and

CHF result. In the case of the complete AVSD, some bidirectional shunting may occur, resulting in slight arterial desaturation. In addition, there may be varying degrees of AV valve insufficiency. Symptoms develop earliest in patients with complete AVSDs. This typically occurs in early infancy as the pulmonary vascular resistance falls after birth and more left-to-right shunting occurs. It is unusual for patients with incomplete or transitional defects to develop early heart failure. However, symptoms in any of the three types are accelerated by significant AV valve insufficiency. In patients with complete AVSD who do not develop CHF symptoms in the first few months of life, concern is raised for persistently elevated pulmonary vascular resistance.

Chronic pulmonary overcirculation can lead to irreversible pulmonary hypertension. These changes occur most rapidly in patients with complete AVSD and are accelerated in patients with trisomy 21. Long-standing left AV valve insufficiency can contribute to this process. If these changes are sufficiently advanced, operative repair may be precluded.

DIAGNOSIS

Typically, the diagnosis of AVSD is made in infancy. Patients usually present with signs of CHF such as failure to thrive, tachypnea, and hepatomegaly. A systolic ejection murmur secondary to increased flow across the pulmonary valve may be present. A holosystolic murmur from AV valve regurgitation may also be heard.

Chest radiography shows cardiomegaly and signs of increased pulmonary blood flow. As in many other congenital heart defects, echocardiography is the mainstay of diagnosis. All of the important features of AVSDs can be well visualized by this technique in children. It is important to characterize the septal defects, identify additional atrial or ventricular septal defects, and fully assess the AV valves for morphology and regurgitation. As aortic coarctation and PDA may be associated, these lesions also must be sought. Cardiac catheterization is reserved for those patients with suspected pulmonary hypertension or other hemodynamic concerns.

TREATMENT

Initially, the therapy of AVSD is medical. Agents such as loop diuretics and digoxin are used to control the symptoms of CHF. If there is significant AV valve regurgitation, angiotensin-converting enzyme inhibitors may be of benefit. Careful attention must be paid to the nutritional status of the child, and supplemental feedings are sometimes necessary.

Surgical repair is the definitive treatment. For complete AVSD, repair is most commonly performed between 3 and 6 months of age. Earlier repair may be indicated for patients who fail to respond to medical therapy. Patients with trisomy 21 are prone to the early development of pulmonary vascular disease. Repair for these patients should generally not be delayed beyond 6 months. The defect is exposed through a right atriotomy. Complete repair includes closure of the VSD with a prosthetic patch, partitioning of the common AV valve into right (tricuspid) and left (mitral) components, closure of the cleft in the left-sided AV valve, and repair of the primum

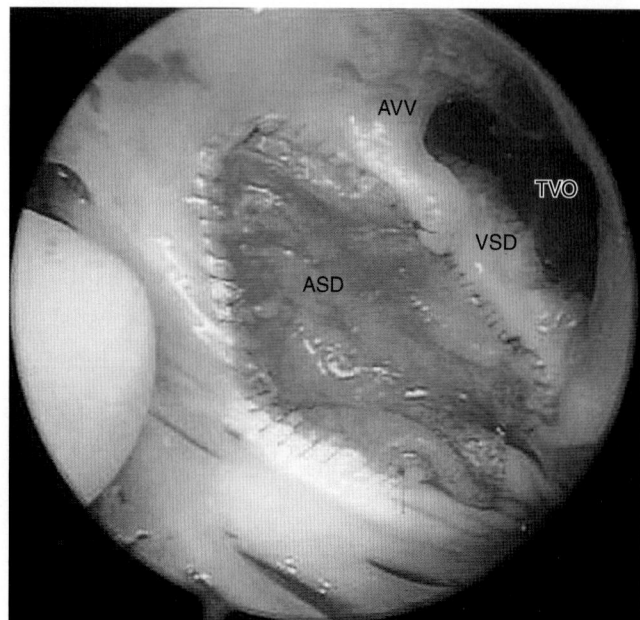

FIGURE 103-8. Repaired complete atrioventricular septal defect seen through a right atriotomy. The pericardial atrial septal defect patch (ASD) and prosthetic inlet ventricular septal defect patch (VSD) can be seen. The patches are connected at the level of the atrioventricular valves (AVV). The right-sided (tricuspid) component of the AVV is labeled, as is the tricuspid valve orifice (TVO). (*See color plate.*)

ASD with an autologous pericardial patch (Fig. 103-8). In very young or premature infants, pulmonary artery band placement is occasionally performed to limit pulmonary blood flow and allow the child to reach a larger size when definitive repair will be performed.

> **For complete AVSD, surgical repair is the definitive treatment and is most commonly performed at age 3 to 6 months, or earlier for patients who fail to respond to medical therapy. For patients with trisomy 21, who are prone to early development of pulmonary vascular disease, repair should generally not be delayed beyond 6 months.**

The physiology of partial AV septal defects is more like that of an ASD, and repair can usually be delayed until the child is older. Repair should not be delayed, however, if significant symptoms of heart failure or significant AV valve regurgitation develops. Repair of these defects involves closure of the cleft in the left AV valve and closure of the primum ASD. In the case of transitional defects, the VSD component is sufficiently small that it can be repaired primarily with sutures.

PROGNOSIS

Contemporary series report operative mortalities in the range of 1% to 6%. Five-year survival is approximately 90%. Survival is not appreciably different for children with and those without trisomy 21. Residual septal defects requiring reoperation are rare. There is a small but appreciable incidence of complete heart block requiring a permanent pacemaker. By far the most common significant clinical issue after repair of AVSD is residual or recurrent AV valve regurgitation, particularly of the left-sided AV valve. This is the most common reason for reoperation. Children who do not have trisomy 21 seem to be at higher risk of needing eventual reoperative mitral valve repair or replacement.

CYANOTIC LESIONS

Transposition of the Great Arteries

Transposition of the great arteries (TGA) is a relatively common heart defect, representing almost 10% of all cases of congenital heart disease in selected series. It is the most common cyanotic heart defect recognized in the neonate.

ANATOMY AND PATHOPHYSIOLOGY

In typical TGA, the aorta arises from the right ventricle, and the pulmonary artery from the left ventricle (Fig. 103-9). The etiology of this abnormality is thought to relate to failure of the common arterial trunk to spiral and septate in the usual fashion. This results in ventriculoarterial discordance. The spatial relationship between the great arteries is variable, but the aorta is usually rightward and anterior of the pulmonary artery. Associated anomalies include VSD in 25% of patients, and VSD with left ventricular outflow tract obstruction in up to 25%. The presence of two separate parallel circulations results in cyanosis. For the infant to survive, there must be mixing between the circulations. This occurs

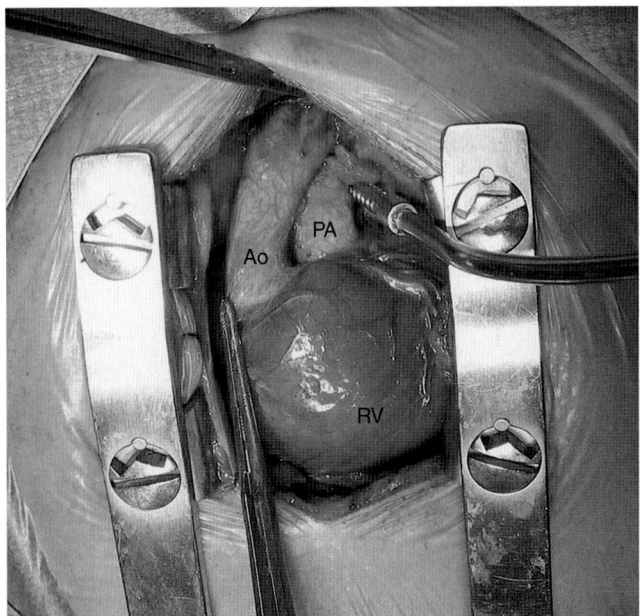

FIGURE 103-9. Intraoperative photograph before repair of transposition of the great arteries is shown. The patient's head is toward the top of the photograph. The aorta (Ao) can be seen to be arising from the right ventricle (RV) and giving off the brachiocephalic branches distally. The pulmonary artery (PA) is leftward and posterior, arising from the left ventricle (not visible in this illustration). The coronary arteries, some of which can be seen on the surface of the heart, arise from the anterior aorta. (*See color plate.*)

through either the ASD, the VSD (if present), or PDA, or via a combination of these. Patients with inadequate mixing have more profound hypoxia.

CLINICAL PRESENTATION

Patients with transposition and an intact ventricular septum show symptoms of cyanosis in the neonatal period or early in infancy (see Chapter 28). Patients with transposition and VSD may show symptoms later because of the presence of adequate pulmonary blood flow and improved mixing. If pulmonary overcirculation occurs, these patients may present with CHF.

DIAGNOSIS

The usual relationship of the great vessels in transposition —the aorta lying anterior to the pulmonary artery—leads to the appearance of a narrow mediastinum on chest radiography, which represents the classic "egg on a string." The chest radiograph may be normal at birth in patients with an intact ventricular septum, but those with a large VSD may display cardiomegaly and other signs of CHF.

The diagnosis of transposition is generally made with echocardiography. The presence of a posterior great artery that divides into right and left pulmonary arteries but arises from the left ventricle is generally seen. The aorta is anterior and arises from the right ventricle. Doppler techniques are used to evaluate the integrity of the ventricular septum and the status of the atrial septal defect or patent foramen ovale, and to confirm the patency of the ductus arteriosus. It is important to identify the coronary arteries, because several variations of right and left coronary artery anatomy are possible with this lesion, and these may affect surgical management.

TREATMENT

Initial medical management of the neonate with TGA and intact ventricular septum involves prostaglandin infusion to increase pulmonary blood flow as well as correction of acid-base deficits in preparation for surgery. Atrial balloon septostomy (Rashkind procedure) can be performed to allow improved mixing before surgical intervention. This can be done percutaneously via the femoral or umbilical vein. Successful balloon atrial septostomy sometimes obviates prostaglandin stabilization before surgery.

Timing of surgery depends on the presence or absence of a VSD. If a VSD is absent, the left ventricle can become deconditioned as a consequence of pumping into the lower-resistance pulmonary circulation. Left ventricular muscle mass can be lost, resulting in failure of the left ventricle once corrective surgery is performed and the LV is exposed to the increased work of pumping against systemic vascular resistance. Surgery should therefore be performed within the first 2 weeks of life to avoid this situation. If a nonrestrictive VSD is present, systemic pressure is maintained in the left ventricle, LV mass is preserved, and it is sometimes possible to delay surgery somewhat.

Historically, an atrial switch operation (Mustard or Senning procedure) was performed for this anomaly. These procedures reroute the venous return at the atrial level into the opposite ventricle, and thereby into the appropriate great artery. This was an effective operation, but it leaves the right ventricle and tricuspid valve in the systemic circulation. Eventually, a substantial percentage of these patients develop heart failure secondary to systemic (right) ventricular dysfunction or tricuspid valve insufficiency, or both.

The arterial switch procedure is a more anatomically correct option and is now considered the standard operative approach. This operation involves CPB, division of the aorta distal to the coronary arteries, translocation of the distal aorta and pulmonary artery to the appropriate proximal great vessel, and reimplantation of the coronary arteries onto the neoaorta. The neopulmonary artery is reconstructed, generally using autologous pericardium, anterior to the aorta. The ASD is closed at the same operation.

> **The more anatomically correct arterial switch procedure, now the standard operative approach, involves CPB, division of the aorta distal to the coronary arteries, translocation of the distal aorta and pulmonary artery to the appropriate proximal great vessel, and reimplantation of the coronary arteries onto the neoaorta. The neopulmonary artery is reconstructed anterior to the aorta. The ASD is closed at the same time.**

Patients with transposition and VSD should undergo simultaneous arterial switch and VSD closure during infancy. Occasionally, they are treated with a temporary pulmonary artery band to reduce excessive pulmonary blood flow until the patient grows to an adequate size, but this approach is unusual in the current era. Patients with left ventricular outflow tract obstruction require more sophisticated reconstructive techniques.

PROGNOSIS

In general, procedural mortality for the arterial switch operation is less than 5%. Operative mortality is generally higher if there is a VSD present. The 5-year survival rate is approximately 80%. The most common late complication of the arterial switch is supravalvar pulmonary stenosis. This is related to reconstruction of the pulmonary artery anterior to the aorta, which results in some tension on the branch pulmonary arteries. If evaluation of this condition is insufficiently addressed by echocardiography, CTA or MRA can be performed. Late stenosis or occlusion of a coronary artery has also been seen, albeit less frequently.

> **Supravalvar pulmonary stenosis, the most common late complication of the arterial switch, is related to reconstruction of the pulmonary artery anterior to the aorta and results in some tension on the branch pulmonary arteries. If evaluation of this condition is insufficiently addressed by echocardiography, CTA or MRA can be performed. Late stenosis or occlusion of a coronary artery is seen less frequently.**

Tetralogy of Fallot

Tetralogy of Fallot is the most common congenital cardiac anomaly producing cyanosis. It was the first complex congenital heart defect to be successfully repaired.

ANATOMY AND PATHOPHYSIOLOGY

The classic description of tetralogy of Fallot includes four anatomic features: ventricular septal defect, right ventricular outflow tract obstruction (RVOTO), overriding aorta, and right ventricular hypertrophy. Essentially all of this results from anterior displacement of the infundibular septum into the right ventricular outflow tract.

Obstruction of the right ventricular outflow tract results in right-to-left shunting at the ventricular level. There is a spectrum of severity of tetralogy of Fallot primarily related to the degree of RVOTO. Patients on the mild end of the spectrum may have very little RVOTO, and the pulmonary valve and pulmonary arteries are relatively normal in size. The more typical patient has a small pulmonary annulus and pulmonary arteries as well as some degree of subpulmonary (infundibular) stenosis. In its most severe form, there is atresia of the pulmonary valve, and there may be discontinuity or absence of the pulmonary arteries. This is also referred to as pulmonary atresia with VSD. Cyanosis results from RVOTO and ventricular-level right-to-left shunting. Its severity is related to the degree of obstruction.

CLINICAL PRESENTATION

Cyanosis is the main physical finding in patients with tetralogy of Fallot. Children are typically well nourished (as opposed to other children with large VSDs), as the RVOTO prevents pulmonary overcirculation and CHF. The systolic ejection murmur seen on physical examination is related to the degree of RVOTO. In addition, patients may present with hypercyanotic "tet spells." These episodes represent acute arterial desaturation and result primarily from conditions that decrease systemic vascular resistance and enhance right-to-left shunting. If severe, they can lead to profound hypoxemia, metabolic acidosis, hemodynamic collapse, and death.

DIAGNOSIS

With chest radiography, the heart size is usually normal, but it may have a characteristic boot-shaped appearance from elevation of the cardiac apex and from right ventricular hypertrophy. This is particularly prominent in older infants and children.

Echocardiography is used to establish the diagnosis of tetralogy of Fallot. The key features are the presence of an anterior malalignment VSD, aortic override, and RVOTO. The presence of an anomalous coronary artery such as the left anterior descending arising from the right coronary artery should be identified, as this may alter surgical management. The size of the pulmonary annulus and the anatomy of the pulmonary arteries dictate intraoperative management. Left pulmonary artery narrowing at the site of ductal insertion is relatively common. Occasionally, in more severe forms of the disease, the pulmonary arteries can be discontinuous.

Most patients do not need cardiac catheterization. Indications for this procedure include lack of visualization of the pulmonary arteries on echocardiography or inability to delineate the coronary artery anatomy.

TREATMENT

Initial medical management consists of observation until the patient reaches an appropriate age and size for surgical repair. Conditions that may trigger tet spells, including acidosis or dehydration, are avoided. If such spells do occur, treatment includes supplemental oxygen, sedation, hydration, and maneuvers to increase the systemic vascular resistance, such as the knee-to-chest position or the administration of intravenous vasoconstrictor agents.

Surgery is generally indicated when the patient begins to experience oxygen desaturation to less than 75%, or when hypoxemia spells begin to occur. Asymptomatic patients generally undergo repair between 3 and 6 months of life. Surgical management of tetralogy of Fallot can be divided into palliative procedures and complete repair. Palliative procedures are generally reserved for patients with severe hypoplasia of the pulmonary arteries or pulmonary valve, and occasionally for those with coronary anomalies. In general, palliation takes the form of a modified Blalock-Taussig shunt. In this procedure, a PTFE tube graft is placed between the subclavian or innominate artery and the pulmonary artery to increase pulmonary blood flow. Definitive repair is performed at a later date when the child is larger.

> **Surgery is indicated when the patient begins to experience oxygen desaturation to less than 75%, or when hypoxemia spells begin to occur. Asymptomatic patients undergo repair between 3 and 6 months of life.**

Complete repair is recommended for most patients and entails closure of the VSD and relief of RVOTO. Many patients can be repaired using a combined approach through the right atrium and pulmonary artery. This avoids a right ventriculotomy, a procedure that may lead to late complications. In patients with a very small pulmonary annulus or significant infundibular stenosis, an incision that extends from the main pulmonary artery to the right ventricular cavity must be made and is closed with a transannular patch. In the case of pulmonary atresia, reconstruction of the pulmonary arteries and placement of a valved conduit between the right ventricle and the pulmonary artery may be required. The latter group of patients may require early and frequent reinterventions for conduit replacement or pulmonary artery stenoses.

PROGNOSIS

Hospital mortality after repair is less than 5%. The 5-year survival is greater than 90% in most series. Late complications include the occurrence of pulmonary insufficiency, which requires reoperation for pulmonary valve replacement. This is particularly common after repairs involving a transannular patch, because pulmonary valve function is eliminated with this procedure. Other late complications include atrial and ventricular arrhythmias and sudden death. Atrial arrhythmias are probably related to right atrial dilation, which occurs as a result of pulmonary and tricuspid insufficiency. Ventricular arrhythmias are more likely to be related to scar in the ventricle related to the VSD repair and transannular patch. Early morbidity and mortality are higher for patients with pulmonary atresia and those requiring operation in the neonatal period. Surgery should not be excessively delayed, however, as repair later in childhood has been shown to be a risk factor for later poor outcome.

Truncus Arteriosus

Truncus arteriosus is a relatively uncommon congenital heart defect, representing 0.21% to 0.34% of cases.

ANATOMY AND PATHOPHYSIOLOGY

Persistent truncus arteriosus results from defective separation and spiral septation of the primordial truncus arteriosus into the pulmonary artery and aorta. As a result, a common arterial trunk arises from the heart and is associated with a common truncal valve that connects to both the right and left ventricles, with a VSD that is usually anterosuperior in position. The resultant physiology involves a large left-to-right shunt with pulmonary overcirculation as the pulmonary vascular resistance decreases postnatally. Cyanosis occurs because of the mixing of oxygenated and deoxygenated blood at the ventricular level. In the setting of chronic pulmonary overcirculation, eventual pulmonary vascular obstructive disease can develop. Classification schemes for truncus arteriosus depend on the site of origin of the pulmonary arteries from the common trunk. In the simplest form, there is a main pulmonary artery segment that arises from the common trunk and gives rise to the right and left pulmonary arteries. In more complex forms, the right and left pulmonary arteries arise separately from the common trunk.

CLINICAL PRESENTATION

Most patients present in early infancy. Initial symptoms typically include the development of tachypnea, diaphoresis with feeding, failure to thrive, and cyanosis. On physical examination, signs of CHF such as an active precordium and hepatomegaly are present. A holosystolic murmur can be heard. Subcostal retractions may be present, and rales may be present on lung examination. The presence of a diastolic murmur suggests the presence of truncal valve regurgitation.

DIAGNOSIS

Chest radiography typically shows evidence for CHF with increased pulmonary vascular markings, and cardiomegaly. The presence of a right aortic arch may be seen in approximately 30% of patients. The diagnosis is confirmed by echocardiography. Attention must be paid to the site of origin of the pulmonary arteries, coronary arteries, and the competence of the truncal valve. As with most congenital heart defects, initial diagnostic cardiac catheterization is not usually necessary.

TREATMENT

Medical therapy is indicated initially. Anticongestive medications such as those used in patients with AVSD are employed. Operative repair is the definitive treatment, usually performed at 2 weeks to 1 month of age. Waiting longer than this is not constructive, as most children have failure to thrive due to CHF. An excessively long wait risks the development of pulmonary vascular obstructive disease.

Repair involves the use of CPB. The pulmonary arteries are separated from the common trunk, and the resulting defect in the neoaorta is repaired primarily (with sutures) or with a patch. The VSD is closed with a Dacron or PTFE patch. A valved conduit is then placed between the right ventricle and the pulmonary arteries to reconstruct the right ventricular outflow tract. The conduit may be a cryopreserved pulmonary homograft, or a xenograft such as bovine jugular vein.

> **Repair involves CPB. The pulmonary arteries are separated from the common trunk and the resulting defect in the neoaorta is repaired primarily (with sutures) or with a patch. The VSD is closed with a Dacron or PTFE patch. A valved conduit is then placed between the right ventricle and the pulmonary arteries to reconstruct the right ventricular outflow tract. The conduit may be a cryopreserved pulmonary homograft, or a xenograft such as bovine jugular vein.**

PROGNOSIS

The natural history of unrepaired truncus arteriosus is poor, with a 1-year mortality rate of 75%. Results of complete repair in infancy are now good, with a greater than 90% early survival. All long-term surviving patients will require reoperation for right-ventricle-to-pulmonary-artery conduit replacement as they outgrow the conduit placed at the initial procedure. This is necessary, on average, approximately three times during the patient's life. Conduits may be replaced with another homograft, a bioprosthetic valved conduit, or a xenograft. If the patient is large enough, a bioprosthetic valve and outflow tract patch may be used. Reoperation for late truncal valve insufficiency is also occasionally necessary. Usually, mechanical valve replacement is performed in this circumstance.

Total Anomalous Pulmonary Venous Connection

Total anomalous pulmonary venous connection (TAPVC) is another unusual cyanotic congenital heart defect in which the pulmonary veins do not connect directly to the heart. It represents 1% to 5% of congenital cardiac anomalies.

ANATOMY AND PATHOPHYSIOLOGY

Development of normal pulmonary venous drainage into the left atrium requires a series of events during fetal development, including connection between the splanchnic plexus and common pulmonary vein, incorporation of the common pulmonary vein into the left atrial body, and degeneration of the pulmonary venous connection to the cardinal and umbilicovitelline veins. If this process fails, TAPVC can occur. In this defect, the pulmonary venous confluence does not connect to the left atrium directly, and the pulmonary venous blood must return to the heart via an alternative route. Classification is according to location of drainage of the pulmonary veins.

Supracardiac TAPVC (type 1) usually involves connection of the common pulmonary vein confluence to the innominate vein and then the superior vena cava via an ascending vertical vein. The vertical vein is usually located to the left of midline, approximately in the location of a persistent left superior vena cava. This type of TAPVC is the most common type observed. In cardiac TAPVC (type 2), the pulmonary vein confluence connects directly to the right atrium or coronary sinus. Infracardiac TAPVC (type 3) involves pulmonary venous drainage into the portal vein via a descending connecting vein. Type 4 (mixed) TAPVC includes multiple sites of anomalous pulmonary venous drainage. All patients with anomalous pulmonary venous connection have an associated ASD, which is required to sustain the systemic cardiac output. If this were not present, no blood would return to the left heart, a situation incompatible with life.

Various degrees of obstruction to pulmonary venous drainage may occur and influence the clinical presentation. Obstructed TAPVC most commonly occurs in the infracardiac type, followed by the supracardiac and cardiac types. Obstruction of the anomalous connection leads to more severe hypoxia.

CLINICAL PRESENTATION

Cyanosis is always present in TAPVC. The presentation ranges from mild tachypnea to hemodynamic collapse, depending on the degree of obstruction present either at the level of the atrial septal defect or the pulmonary vein confluence connection to the systemic venous circulation. In the absence of obstruction at either level, tachypnea results from increased pulmonary blood flow. Patients with obstruction at either level may present with hemodynamic compromise from decreased systemic blood flow. This leads to metabolic acidosis, shock, and death if not corrected. This sequence of events can evolve fairly rapidly if the diagnosis is not made and steps are not taken to correct it.

DIAGNOSIS

The chest radiograph may show evidence of pulmonary edema in the setting of venous obstruction, or pulmonary arterial engorgement from increased pulmonary blood flow. In cases of severe obstruction, the diffuse reticular pattern seen in pulmonary lymphangiectasia can be observed. Later in infancy, when the thymus involutes, patients with the supracardiac connection appear on radiographs to have a rounded shadow in the superior mediastinum, producing a "snowman" appearance.

Echocardiography is used to establish the diagnosis and the type of anomalous pulmonary venous connection. Information that must be provided by the echocardiographer includes the pressure gradient across the atrial septum and the presence of obstruction of the anomalous pulmonary venous connection. Cardiac catheterization is rarely indicated. If information is incomplete regarding the anomalous venous connections (including the postoperative status), CTA or MRA can be performed.

TREATMENT

There is no effective medical treatment for obstructed TAPVC, making it one of the few surgical emergencies in congenital heart surgery. Medical therapy should focus on proper resuscitation and support to optimize the patient's condition before surgical correction. This may include initiation of prostaglandins, intubation and ventilation with 100% oxygen, and correction of electrolyte and acid-base abnormalities. In some cases, severe hemodynamic compromise in the setting of venous obstruction mandates emergent surgical treatment despite the medical condition. Extracorporeal membrane oxygenation (ECMO) can be used for hemodynamic support and recovery of compromised end-organ function in extreme circumstances.

Definitive surgical treatment involves reconnection of the pulmonary veins to the left atrium, and closure of the ASD. For patients with the supracardiac or infracardiac type, this involves a direct anastomosis between the common pulmonary vein confluence and the left atrium/atrial appendage, with ligation of the connecting vein. If the common pulmonary vein drains into the coronary sinus (cardiac TAPVC), the coronary sinus can be unroofed into the left atrium by removing the common wall between them. The atrial septum is then closed so that the pulmonary veins and the coronary sinus both empty into the left atrium. This results in a small amount of deoxygenated blood returning to the left side of the heart, but this seems to be clinically insignificant.

> If the common pulmonary vein in TAPVC drains into the coronary sinus, the coronary sinus can be unroofed into the left atrium by removing the common wall between them. The atrial septum is then closed so that the pulmonary veins and the coronary sinus both empty into the left atrium. The small amount of deoxygenated blood that then returns to the left side of the heart seems to be clinically insignificant.

PROGNOSIS

Operative mortality after repair of TAPVC ranges from 5% to 10%, and it is worse for patients presenting with pulmonary venous obstruction and shock. Long-term complications include pulmonary venous stenosis in at least 10% of patients. This can take the form of anastomotic stenosis, but it can also be caused by more peripheral pulmonary vein obstruction. Late sinus node dysfunction or atrial arrhythmias can also occur.

Hypoplastic Left Heart Syndrome and Other Single-Ventricle Lesions

A variety of heart defects are characterized by the presence of a single functional ventricle, including tricuspid atresia, pulmonary atresia with intact ventricular

septum, hypoplastic left heart syndrome (HLHS), and other more complex anatomic defects (see Chapter 28). Among these, HLHS is relatively common. It is seen in approximately 7% to 9% of infants who are diagnosed with congenital heart disease in the first year of life. As the treatment strategies for the vast majority of single-ventricle lesions are similar, and as a discussion of the complex physiology of different single-ventricle lesions is beyond the scope of this text, this section will focus on HLHS.

ANATOMY AND PATHOPHYSIOLOGY

In HLHS, a combination of aortic and mitral valve hypoplasia or atresia is seen and is associated with hypoplasia of the left ventricle, most likely from decreased forward flow to the left ventricle in utero. The ascending aorta and transverse arch are also variably hypoplastic, and there is coarctation of the aorta (Fig. 103-10). The ventricular septum is intact. The right ventricle is the dominant ventricle and is responsible for supplying both the pulmonary and systemic circulations. Other lesions (HLHS variants) may have features of HLHS, but to meet the criteria for the actual syndrome, all of the stated criteria must be met. In HLHS and essentially all single-ventricle lesions, a balanced circulation is maintained by intracardiac mixing at the atrial level through a patent foramen ovale or an atrial septal defect, and a PDA.

CLINICAL PRESENTATION

Fetal echocardiography has allowed early-stage diagnosis of this lesion before delivery, and it has allowed improved

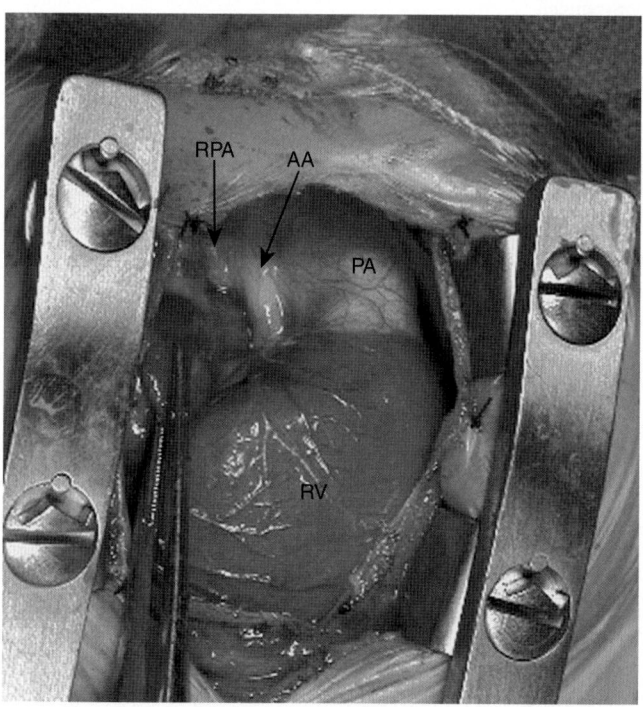

FIGURE 103-10. Intraoperative photograph of hypoplastic left heart syndrome before first-stage palliation (Norwood procedure). The enlarged main pulmonary artery (PA) arises normally from the right ventricle (RV). The very hypoplastic ascending aorta (AA) can be seen. The forceps are retracting the right atrial appendage. The large right pulmonary artery (RPA) is seen in its normal location posterior to the aorta. (See color plate.)

prenatal counseling, as well as planning for immediate postnatal care. If such a diagnosis is made, delivery at a tertiary care center is recommended. Cyanosis is present shortly after birth. If ductal patency is maintained, tachypnea and other signs of CHF typically occur within 24 to 48 hours of birth as the pulmonary vascular resistance falls and more left-to-right shunting occurs. If the ductus arteriosus closes, the infant will develop progressive cyanosis and shock as a result of poor systemic circulation. This presentation may be observed if the diagnosis is unrecognized before hospital discharge of the newborn infant.

DIAGNOSIS

Chest radiography shows cardiomegaly and increased pulmonary vascular markings. A reticular pattern of obstructed pulmonary venous return may be seen in the presence of a restrictive atrial septal defect. This is an ominous sign.

The diagnosis is made by echocardiography, which may show a diminutive left ventricular cavity, mitral and aortic stenosis or atresia, a small ascending aorta, and aortic coarctation. It is important to assess the status of the atrial communication and the ductus arteriosus. Often, retrograde flow is seen in the ascending aorta as the coronary arteries are supplied by ductal-dependent flow. Abnormalities of systemic or pulmonary venous return must be identified, as they can have a significant impact on the surgical reconstruction and prognosis.

TREATMENT

Initial medical management includes a prostaglandin infusion to maintain ductal patency. To avoid pulmonary overcirculation, oxygen supplementation is avoided and hypoventilation may be maintained, which promotes an elevated pulmonary vascular resistance. Some infants need to be intubated or maintained on inotropes before surgery to achieve stability, but some have suggested that outcomes are better if these interventions are avoided or when they are not required.

Surgical management of HLHS includes either staged reconstruction toward a Fontan procedure or cardiac transplantation. Staged single-ventricle palliation is considered when right ventricular function is thought to be adequate, whereas cardiac transplantation may be pursued if right ventricular dysfunction is seen, or if there is severe tricuspid valve regurgitation. The first stage of reconstruction, known as the Norwood procedure, involves augmentation of the ascending aorta and aortic arch with amalgamation of the proximal aortic and pulmonary artery trunks, atrial septectomy, and construction of either a systemic-to-pulmonary artery shunt or right-ventricle-to-pulmonary artery shunt. At approximately 4 to 6 months of age, after pulmonary vascular resistance has decreased, the second stage involves division of the systemic-to-pulmonary artery shunt and creation of an anastomosis between the superior vena cava and the pulmonary artery (the bidirectional Glenn procedure or hemi-Fontan). This allows passive flow from the superior systemic venous circulation to the pulmonary arteries. Subsequently, at approximately 2 years of age or older, the final stage of reconstruction, or

Fontan procedure, involves completion of a total cavo-pulmonary connection by routing the inferior vena cava to the pulmonary artery, with either an extracardiac conduit or an intracardiac tunnel. Some institutions have implemented a strategy of neonatal heart transplantation for patients with HLHS. Limitations of this strategy include a small donor pool, which often results in a 25% mortality of patients awaiting transplantation.

> **Surgical management of HLHS includes either staged reconstruction toward a Fontan procedure or cardiac transplantation. Staged single-ventricle palliation is considered when right ventricular function is adequate, whereas cardiac transplantation may be pursued if right ventricular dysfunction is seen, or if there is severe tricuspid valve regurgitation.**

PROGNOSIS

Without surgical intervention, mortality is nearly 100% within the first year of life. Hospital mortality after the Norwood procedure has improved substantially in recent years but is still quite variable. A generally accepted average survival estimate is 80%. At subsequent stages of the reconstruction, hospital survival is reported to be up to or exceeding 90%. There is significant interstage mortality, particularly between the first and second stages. This cumulative mortality leads to an estimated 5-year survival in the range of 50% to 60%. Complications associated with surgical palliation of hypoplastic left heart syndrome include recurrent aortic arch obstruction, neurodevelopmental delay, and eventual CHF due to single ventricle dysfunction. Cardiac transplantation is considered if CHF develops. Primary cardiac transplantation is felt to have a survival similar to that of staged palliation.

OTHER DEFECTS

Ebstein Anomaly

Ebstein anomaly is an exceedingly rare condition, and the exact incidence in the general population is unknown, primarily because of a large variation in the spectrum of clinical presentations.

ANATOMY AND PATHOPHYSIOLOGY

Ebstein anomaly is characterized by downward displacement of the tricuspid valve leaflets, as well as by failure of delamination of these leaflets (separation of leaflets from the endocardium). The effect is greatest on the septal leaflet, followed by the posterior, then the anterior leaflet. This results in an "atrialized" portion of the right ventricle, or the portion of the right ventricle that is above the downwardly displaced tricuspid annulus. Also seen are tricuspid valve insufficiency and, occasionally, RVOTO resulting from underdevelopment secondary to a low flow state. Enlargement of the right ventricle causes left ventricular dysfunction due to compression, and this results in diminished cardiac output. These latter effects are seen in patients at the more severe end of the spectrum. Ebstein anomaly is commonly associated with an ASD and supraventricular arrhythmias. Cyanosis results from decreased pulmonary blood flow and right-to-left shunting at the atrial level.

CLINICAL PRESENTATION

Neonates and infants presenting with Ebstein anomaly are frequently morbidly ill and display symptoms of heart failure, hypoxia, and cardiac arrhythmias (see Chapter 28). Patients with less severe forms of the anomaly have mild valvular dysfunction and may remain asymptomatic for a long period of time. Eventually, symptoms of cyanosis or dyspnea on exertion may develop.

DIAGNOSIS

Neonates presenting with Ebstein anomaly have a characteristic appearance on chest radiography. The cardiac silhouette is massively enlarged, and opacification of both lung fields is often seen. The enlarged cardiac silhouette is primarily the result of enlargement of the right atrium and atrialized portion of the right ventricle.

Echocardiography is performed to confirm the clinical diagnosis. Right ventricular size, right ventricular outflow tract dimensions, degree of tricuspid regurgitation, pulmonary artery size, and left ventricular function can be assessed. The tricuspid valve anatomy is important in planning therapy and can usually be fairly accurately assessed. In older patients with arrhythmias, electrophysiologic evaluation may be necessary.

TREATMENT

Infants presenting with Ebstein anomaly are often severely symptomatic and must undergo repair. Neonates presenting in extremis have a poor prognosis and limited options. Medical management rarely provides stabilization because of the dangerous combination of cyanosis and impaired left ventricular function. Often, prostaglandin infusion is initiated to ensure adequate pulmonary blood flow. Maneuvers to reduce the pulmonary vascular resistance may improve pulmonary blood flow; however, in patients with RVOTO, this is often futile. Surgical management ranges from palliative options, such as placement of a systemic-to-pulmonary shunt with right ventricular exclusion, to complete repair with plication of the atrialized right ventricle, tricuspid valve annuloplasty, and closure of the ASD. Consideration is sometimes given to primary heart transplantation.

Indications for surgery in older patients include the onset of symptoms such as dyspnea on exertion, cyanosis, or arrhythmias. In these patients, complete repair is more commonly performed. Tricuspid valve replacement is necessary in many cases when tricuspid valve repair fails to produce a functional valve. The need for valve replacement is related primarily to the severity of tricuspid valve dysplasia.

PROGNOSIS

Reported mortality early after repair of Ebstein anomaly ranges from 6% to 20%, with the large variability caused by the inclusion of both neonates and adults in the same study group. Older patients undergoing repair tend to have a durable result, although approximately 20% having tricuspid valve repair may require late reoperation for tricuspid valve insufficiency.

Vascular Rings

Vascular rings are unusual abnormalities of the aorta and arch vessels. Although variability in arch sidedness and of branching of the aorta may be commonly observed, true vascular rings are not. Their true incidence is difficult to determine, as symptoms are variable and many may go undiagnosed. They have been estimated to constitute approximately 1% of all cardiovascular abnormalities.

ANATOMY AND PATHOPHYSIOLOGY

During normal embryologic development of the thoracic great vessels, regression of specific segments of the embryologic aortic arch results in normal development of a left-sided aorta with a typical branching pattern and a normal pulmonary artery. Abnormal regression of these segments leads to abnormalities of the aortic arch and may lead to compression of the trachea and esophagus. There are four types of vascular rings. Persistence of the right and left fourth arch leads to development of a double aortic arch. In this abnormality, two separate arches from the distal ascending aorta travel on opposite sides of the trachea and esophagus, and join the descending aorta. The trachea and esophagus are compressed by the two arches, which are connected proximally and distally, thus forming a ring. In many cases, one of the arches, typically the left, is either hypoplastic or atretic. The right-sided arch is dominant in most patients (70% to 75% of the time), whereas the left arch is dominant in approximately 20% of patients. Regression of the left fourth arch and persistence of the right fourth arch results in the development of a right aortic arch. In the case of a right aortic arch, a complete vascular ring is formed if there is a left ligamentum arteriosum. This commonly occurs if there is an anomalous left subclavian artery arising from the descending aorta. The ligamentum arteriosum arises from the base of this vessel, which may look like a diverticulum (of Kommerell), and connects to the pulmonary artery, forming a ring. The former two lesions are complete vascular rings. Incomplete vascular rings are formed in the cases of a right aortic arch with mirror-image branching and a right ligamentum arteriosum, and with a left aortic arch and anomalous (retroesophageal) right subclavian artery. The latter is the most common aortic arch vessel anomaly and rarely causes symptoms requiring intervention.

Two other lesions are commonly grouped with vascular rings. The first is a pulmonary artery sling, which is formed when the left pulmonary artery arises from the right pulmonary artery and courses between the trachea and the esophagus. This results in compression of the trachea. It is commonly associated with tracheal stenosis due to complete tracheal rings. The second is innominate artery compression syndrome. This is thought to be caused by an unusual (leftward and posterior) takeoff of the innominate artery from the aorta, causing compression of the airway.

CLINICAL PRESENTATION

A child with a vascular ring may present with respiratory distress, stridor, or dysphagia, or a combination of these symptoms. The symptoms are variable in severity, and some patients may be asymptomatic. The symptoms of dysphagia become most pronounced when the child begins to eat solid food, whereas symptoms may be less prominent when the child is on formula or breast milk only. Occasionally, a history of recurrent respiratory infections can be elicited.

DIAGNOSIS

With chest radiography, the findings include tracheal narrowing at the level of the aortic arch, and unclear delineation of the aortic knob. Unilateral hyperinflation of the right lung may suggest the presence of a pulmonary artery sling.

Before the diagnostic capability of CTA or MRA in the evaluation of patients with vascular rings, the barium esophagogram was the most reliable initial study for establishing the diagnosis. With a barium swallow, the typical appearances consisted of posterior extrinsic esophageal compression in the presence of a right aortic arch, anterior esophageal compression in the presence of a pulmonary artery sling, and anterior and posterior extrinsic compression of the esophagus in the setting of double aortic arch.

Echocardiography is helpful for delineating the arch anatomy, but it cannot definitely make the diagnosis of a vascular ring unless there is a double aortic arch and both arches are patent. CT scanning is used by many surgeons to help confirm the diagnosis and to plan an operative procedure. Specific information that must be obtained includes the course and origin of arterial branches and the location of the ligamentum arteriosum in the case of right aortic arch. CT also provides necessary information on the degree of airway compression.

Other studies that are used to aid in the diagnosis of vascular rings include bronchoscopy and MRA. Bronchoscopy is particularly useful in the diagnosis of innominate artery compression, which is diagnosed by observation of anterior tracheal compression at the level of the innominate artery. The information provided by MRA is similar to that from CT, but MRA may be more difficult to perform in infants and small children because of the study time required and the increased need for sedation.

TREATMENT

Vascular rings should be repaired if there are symptoms. Virtually all vascular rings can be approached through a left thoracotomy incision. In the case of double aortic arch, this requires division of the smaller of the two arches at the insertion with the descending aorta to preserve flow to the branch vessels. If one of the aortic arches has an atretic segment (with no flow), it is divided at that point. Repair of right aortic arch with left ligamentum arteriosum simply involves division of the ligamentum arteriosum. Occasionally, the left subclavian artery arises from abnormal aortic tissue (Kommerell diverticulum). If present, the diverticulum may be resected or plicated to prevent esophageal compression or aneurysmal dilation in the future. Treatment of innominate artery compression syndrome involves an anterior right thoracotomy with suspension of the innominate artery to the posterior aspect of the sternum. Pulmonary artery sling is typically approached via median sternotomy and involves the use of CPB. Repair consists of division of the left pulmonary artery from the right pulmonary artery, and reimplantation into the main pulmonary artery anterior to the trachea. Alternatively, the trachea can be divided and brought posterior to the pulmonary artery. This approach is particularly useful if tracheal resection or reconstruction is necessary because of the presence of complete tracheal rings and tracheal stenosis.

> Virtually all vascular rings can be approached through a left thoracotomy incision.

PROGNOSIS

In general, the results of repair for vascular ring defects have been very good, with relief of symptoms noted in over 95% of patients. Recurrence of symptoms of esophageal compression has been noted after repair of right aortic arch with left ligamentum arteriosum because of the presence of an enlarging Kommerell diverticulum. Occasionally, reoperation in such patients has been required.

SUMMARY

Congenital heart disease can appear with a variety of clinical features in patients at any age. Table 103-2 lists some common eponyms and definitions used in congenital heart disease. Diagnosis is established by echocardiography in most circumstances, although MRA and CTA may be useful in a number of preoperative and postoperative circumstances. Management decisions are based on the overall clinical picture, which takes into consideration patient symptoms, physical findings, and results of imaging studies. Surgical and catheter-based techniques, as well as pediatric cardiac anesthesiology, have evolved over the past 30 years, and interventions are being performed at an earlier age and through smaller incisions, with improving short- and long-term survival.

TABLE 103-2

Congenital Heart Defects: Select Eponyms and Definitions

Eponym	Definition
Williams syndrome	Rare genetic condition characterized by elfin facial features, variable developmental delay, an overfriendly personality, and a tendency to have supravalvar aortic stenosis, pulmonary artery stenoses, and pulmonary hypertension
Ross procedure	Pulmonary autograft replacement of the aortic valve or root with homograft replacement of the pulmonary root; named for Donald Ross
Konno-Rastan procedure	Replacement of the aortic valve with enlargement of the subaortic area by incision into the ventricular septum. Procedure is performed through a right ventriculotomy.
Modified Konno procedure	Enlargement of the left ventricular outflow tract by incision and patching of the ventricular septum, sparing the aortic valve. Procedure is performed through a right ventriculotomy.
Wood units	Measure of vascular resistance usually used to quantify pulmonary vascular resistance according to the formula (PAP–PCWP)/CO
Eisenmenger syndrome	Pulmonary hypertension and cyanosis resulting from right-to-left shunting through an unrepaired septal defect
Rashkind procedure	Balloon atrial septostomy performed by advancing balloon catheter via a systemic vein across an ASD and withdrawing the catheter with balloon inflated to enlarge the atrial defect and improve mixing of systemic and pulmonary venous blood; most commonly used in infants with TGA for stabilization before arterial switch operation
Mustard procedure	Atrial switch operation for TGA; uses *prosthetic* material to create intra-atrial baffle to route systemic venous blood to mitral valve/left ventricle to lungs, and pulmonary venous blood to tricuspid valve/right ventricle to body; RV is systemic ventricle
Senning procedure	Atrial switch operation for TGA; uses *autologous* material to create intra-atrial baffle to route systemic venous blood to mitral valve/left ventricle to lungs, and pulmonary venous blood to tricuspid valve/right ventricle to body; RV is systemic ventricle
Tetralogy of Fallot	Cyanotic congenital heart defect characterized by anterior malalignment of the infundibular septum resulting in VSD, over-riding aorta, RV outflow tract obstruction, and RV hypertrophy
Blalock-Taussig (BT) shunt	Classically, a shunt created by anastomosis of the subclavian artery to the PA; modified form used most commonly today employs a PTFE tube graft between the subclavian or innominate artery to the PA (usually right)
Norwood procedure	First-stage palliative operation for HLHS or related single-ventricle lesions, involves creating common outflow from heart by amalgamation of aorta and main PA, creation of systemic-to-PA shunt (BT or Sano), and atrial septectomy
Sano	Name frequently used to refer to RV-to-pulmonary artery shunt in modification of Norwood procedure
Bidirectional Glenn shunt	End-to-side SVC to right PA anastomosis; intermediate stage to Fontan procedure; classic Glenn was end-to-end SVC to right PA (unidirectional); usually followed by extracardiac conduit Fontan
Hemi-Fontan	Alternative to bidirectional Glenn, wherein RA is connected to underside of PA but excluded from pulmonary circulation in addition to the superior cavopulmonary connection; usually followed by lateral tunnel Fontan
Fontan procedure	Operation that creates total cavopulmonary connection wherein all of the systemic venous return flows directly into the pulmonary arteries; exists in the classic atriopulmonary connection, lateral tunnel, and extracardiac conduit types
Ebstein anomaly	Congenital abnormality of tricuspid valve characterized by apical displacement of the septal and posterior leaflets and an atrialized portion of the right ventricle; wide spectrum of severity
Kommerell diverticulum	Remnant of the left fourth embryonic aortic arch from which the left subclavian artery may arise in patients with a right aortic arch

ASD, atrial septal defect; CO, cardiac output; HLHS, hypoplastic left heart syndrome; PA, pulmonary artery; PAP, mean pulmonary artery pressure; PCWP, pulmonary capillary wedge pressure; PTFE, polytetrafluoroethylene (Gore-Tex); RA, right atrium; RV, right ventricle; SVC, superior vena cava; TGA, transposition of the great arteries; VSD, ventricular septal defect.

SUGGESTED READINGS

Bichell DP, Geva T, Bacha EA, et al: Minimal access approach for the repair of atrial septal defect: the initial 135 patients. Ann Thorac Surg 2000;70:115

Daebritz SH, Nollert GDA, Zurakowski D, et al: Results of Norwood stage I operation: comparison of hypoplastic left heart syndrome with other malformations. J Thorac Cardiovasc Surg 2000; 119:358

Danton MHD, Barron DJ, Stumper O, et al: Repair of truncus arteriosus: a considered approach to right ventricular outflow tract reconstruction. Eur J Cardiothorac Surg 2001;20:95

Derby CD, Pizarro C: Routine primary repair of tetralogy of Fallot in the neonate. Expert Rev Cardiovasc Ther 2005;3:857-863

Dodge-Khatami A, Tulevski II, Hitchcock JF, et al: Vascular rings and pulmonary arterial sling: from respiratory collapse to surgical cure, with emphasis on judicious imaging in the hi-tech era. Cardiol Young 2002;12:96-104

Formigari R, Di Donato RM, Mazzera E, et al: Minimally invasive or interventional repair of atrial septal defects in children: experience in 171 cases and comparison with conventional strategies. J Am Coll Cardiol 2001;37:1707

Frid C, Bjorkhem G, Jonzon A, et al: Long-term survival in children with atrioventricular septal defect and common atrioventricular valvar orifice in Sweden [see comment]. Cardiol Young 2004; 14:24-31

Hernanz-Schulman M: Vascular rings: a practical approach to imaging diagnosis. Pediatr Radiol 2005;35:961-979

Hokanson JS, Moller JH: Adults with tetralogy of Fallot: long-term follow-up. Cardiol Rev 1999;7:149-155

Hopkins RA, Bert AA, Buchholz B, et al: Surgical patch closure of atrial septal defects. Ann Thorac Surg 2004;77:2144

Kanter KR: Surgical repair of total anomalous pulmonary venous connection. Semin Thorac Cardiovasc Surg Pediatr Card Surg Ann 2006:40-44

Losay J, Hougen TJ: Treatment of transposition of the great arteries [see comment]. Curr Opin Cardiol 1997;12:84-90

Mahle WT, Spray TL, Wernovsky G, et al: Survival after reconstructive surgery for hypoplastic left heart syndrome: a 15-year experience from a single institution. Circulation 2000;102:III136-141

Meisner H, Guenther T: Atrioventricular septal defect. Pediatr Cardiol 1998;19:276-281

Quaegebeur JM, Cooper RS: Surgery for atrioventricular septal defects. Adv Cardiol 2004;41:127-132

Rao PS: Coarctation of the aorta. Curr Cardiol Rep 2005;7:425-434

Rhodes LA, Colan SD, Perry SB, et al: Predictors of survival in neonates with critical aortic stenosis [erratum in Circulation 1995;92:2005]. Circulation 1991;84:2325-2335

Sarris GE, Chatzis AC, Giannopoulos NM, et al: The arterial switch operation in Europe for transposition of the great arteries: a multi-institutional study from the European Congenital Heart Surgeons Association. J Thorac Cardiovasc Surg 2006;132:633

Shih MC, Tholpady A, Kramer CM, et al: Surgical and endovascular repair of aortic coarctation: normal findings and appearance of complications on CT angiography and MR angiography. AJR Am J Roentgenol 2006;187:W302-312

Spitaels SE: Ebstein's anomaly of the tricuspid valve complexities and strategies. Cardiol Clin 2002;20:431-439

Tweddell JS, Hoffman GM, Mussatto KA, et al: Improved survival of patients undergoing palliation of hypoplastic left heart syndrome: lessons learned from 115 consecutive patients. Circulation 2002;106:I82-89

104 Introduction to Cardiovascular Catheterization for Congenital Abnormalities

JOHN F. RHODES and JEFFREY W. DELANEY

Cardiovascular catheterization is used predominantly either for diagnostic procedures to assess the patient with complex congenital abnormalities, or for interventional procedures that offer therapeutic options to patients, thus allowing them to avoid surgery. The procedures are not without risk, and risks are discussed with families before signing consent forms for the procedure. Risks of interventional cardiac catheterization procedures include bleeding, infection, damage to the blood vessels or cardiac structures, thromboembolic events, arrhythmias, and embolized devices. Overall, the risk for any complication from an interventional catheterization procedure is less than 5%, and the risk for a major complication is 1% to 2%. Each patient's risk may be higher or lower, depending on patient-specific circumstances and on the planned procedure.

Over the past few decades, with the evolution of noninvasive imaging techniques including echocardiography and magnetic resonance (MR) and computed tomography (CT) angiography, the catheterization laboratory has come to be used mainly for interventional procedures. These include ballooning of stenotic valves or blood vessels and occlusion of abnormal shunting lesions. Because many transcatheter techniques for congenital heart disease were adapted from adult practice, most of the procedures are similar for children and adults. The types of interventional devices and their expected radiographic appearances are found in Table 104-1.

> Over the past few decades, with the evolution of noninvasive imaging techniques including echocardiography and MR and CT angiography, the catheterization laboratory has come to be used mainly for interventional procedures.

GENERAL PROCEDURAL TECHNIQUES AND CONSIDERATIONS

The catheterization procedures for diagnostic or interventional radiologic procedures are similar. Catheterizations are performed with either general anesthesia or moderate sedation with a combination of opiates (fentanyl or morphine) and benzodiazepines (midazolam or lorazepam). The procedures start by obtaining percutaneous access using standard Seldinger technique in the femoral artery or vein. Alternative venous accesses include the internal jugular, subclavian, and transhepatic approaches. Arterial access may also be obtained from the arteries of the upper extremities or the carotid, but this is typically restricted to larger patients or emergency conditions. Hemodynamic measurements and angiograms may further delineate the anatomy or lesion severity. For therapeutic procedures, a catheter is passed across the target area, such as a stenosis or an abnormal shunt. A guide wire is then passed through the catheter to provide a track over which therapeutic devices are delivered. Balloon catheters are threaded directly, whereas stents and occlusion devices are protected or constrained within long delivery sheaths. Anticoagulation is managed with heparin (80 to 100 units/kg) for a goal activated clotting time (ACT) of 200 to 250 seconds, depending on the procedure to be performed. In addition, antibiotics are given to patients who receive an implanted device.

BALLOON ATRIAL SEPTOSTOMY AND SEPTAL DEFECT CREATION FOR INTACT ATRIAL SEPTUM

Infants born with any combination of complex congenital heart disease that requires mixing or pooling of the blood for adequate delivery of oxygenated blood to the tissues must have an intracardiac communication for this to occur. Although balloon and catheter technology has evolved since this procedure was first introduced by Dr. Rashkind nearly four decades ago, the overall procedural technique has changed little. The Rashkind balloon septostomy procedure is still standard palliation practice for any neonate with a restrictive atrial septum and a need for unrestrictive mixing. Balloon septostomy is now used for infants with all variants of single-ventricle physiology, right heart lesions, such as tricuspid atresia and pulmonary atresia with intact ventricular septum, and all variants of hypoplastic left heart syndrome.

> The Rashkind balloon septostomy procedure is standard palliation practice for neonates with a restrictive atrial septum and a need for unrestrictive mixing. Balloon septostomy is used

TABLE 104-1	
Interventional Devices	
Devices	Location on Chest Radiographs
CLOSURE DEVICES	
PDA closure devices	Left hilar region on anteroposterior view, centered over the anterior aspect of the trachea on lateral view
ASD closure devices	To the right of the spine, just anterior to the spine; in a more superior location on lateral view
VSD closure devices	To the left of the spine, closer to the chest wall, in a more inferior location on lateral view
VASCULAR OCCLUSION DEVICES	
Internal mammary artery to pulmonary artery collaterals	Anterior location; parallel to the spine
Aortopulmonary collaterals	Variable
Venous collaterals	Indistinguishable from arterial vessels on plain radiographs; clinical history necessary for detailed assessment
STENTS	
PDA	Left hilum, seen en face on anteroposterior views
ASD	To the right of the spine, more superior
Pulmonary artery	Midline, horizontal, hilar region
Pulmonary vein	Either side of the midline, mid-heart, posterior
Descending aorta	To the left of the spine (in left arch) along the axis of the descending aorta

ASD, atrial septal defect; PDA, patent ductus arteriosus; VSD, ventricular septal defect.
From Williams RJ, Levi DS, Moore JW, Boechat MI: Radiographic appearance of pediatric cardiovascular transcatheter devices. Pediatr Radiol 2006;36:1231-1241.

for infants with single-ventricle physiology, right heart lesions (e.g., tricuspid atresia and pulmonary atresia with intact ventricular septum), and hypoplastic left heart syndrome.

The Neonate with Transposition of the Great Vessels

The goal is to improve mixing of oxygenated and deoxygenated blood in neonates with transposition physiology. Balloon atrial septostomy is typically performed at the bedside or in the catheterization laboratory and may involve either fluoroscopic or echocardiographic guidance, or both. Venous access is required and the procedure is quite successful from either the femoral or umbilical vein. The balloon septostomy catheter (Fig. 104-1) is passed across the existing atrial communication, and its position in the left atrium is verified by fluoroscopy and echocardiography. The balloon is inflated with saline or a mixture of saline and contrast, placed against the atrial septal communication, and pulled firmly across, tearing a larger hole and allowing free mixing of the venous return from both atrial chambers. A large atrial communication should be palliative, stabilizing the neonate with transposition physiology until definitive surgical repair can be done. Outside the neonatal period, when the atrial septum is much tougher, enlargement of the atrial communication is accomplished by first cutting the atrial septum with a blade septostomy catheter or cutting balloon (Boston Scientific, Inc.) (see Fig. 104-1), or by using a modified stent technique such as the butterfly-shaped stent, accomplished by suturing the center of the stent to a fixed diameter.

The Neonate with Hypoplastic Left Heart Syndrome or Single-Ventricle Physiology

All infants with single-ventricle physiology require two sources of mixing before surgical repair: both an atrial communication to allow the venous return access to the functional ventricle for ejection, and a patent ductus arteriosus for delivery of the blood to the lungs or to the body, depending on which ventricle is deficient. Hypoplastic left heart syndrome with mitral, or mitral and aortic, atresia is one of the most severe forms of single-ventricle physiology and will be used as the model for this discussion.

Standard balloon septostomy, using the technique just described, may be performed when an atrial communication exists but is believed to be inadequate. As with the neonate with transposition of the great vessels, if the atrial septum is completely intact, the infant will be dramatically ill and a more complex transseptal puncture and septoplasty procedure must be emergently performed (Fig. 104-2). The initial puncture of the atrial septum is performed by placing a curved (Mullins) transseptal sheath firmly against the atrial septum, in the area of the fossa ovalis, with biplane fluoroscopic guidance. A hollow needle and stylet (Brockenbrough needle, Medtronic, Inc.) with the same contour as the sheath is then advanced a few millimeters out of the sheath to puncture and cross the atrial septum and into the left atrium. Hand injections of contrast through the needle confirm the appropriate location. The sheath is

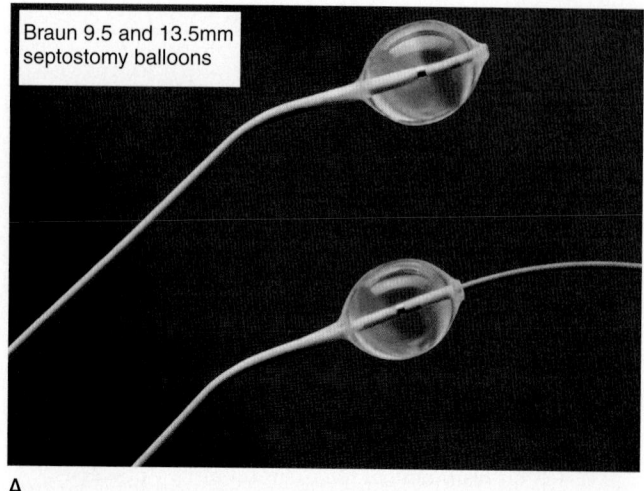

A

Braun 9.5 and 13.5mm
septostomy balloons

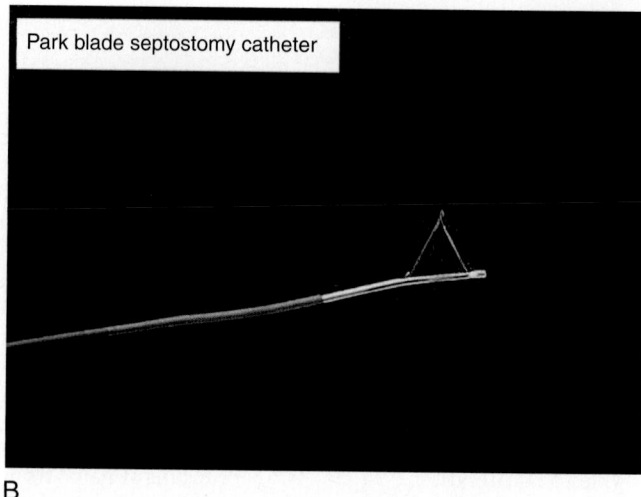

B

Park blade septostomy catheter

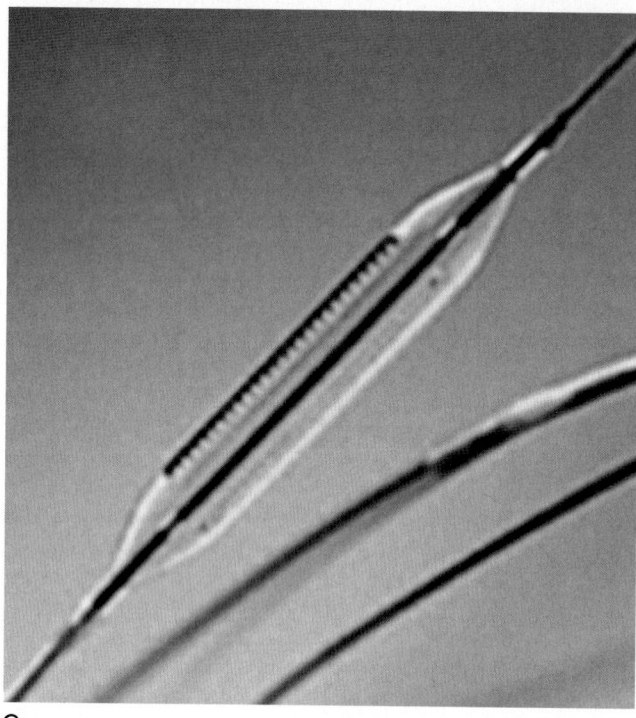

C

FIGURE 104-1. Types of septostomy catheters **A,** Braun septostomy balloon catheter. **B.** Blade septostomy catheter. **C.** Cutting balloon catheter. (**A** from B. Braun; **B** from Cook Medical; **C** from Boston Scientific.)

then advanced across the septum, allowing delivery of the tools for creating a large stable communication. Stent septoplasty with or without a butterfly modification is commonly used to maintain an open atrial communication in the patient with an intact atrial septum. Defects created with standard angioplasty balloons have had less reliable results and a tendency to become restrictive during follow-up. Another technique is to create a larger defect using a cutting balloon (Boston Scientific, Inc.), which is an angioplasty balloon with 2 to 4 thin blades oriented at 90-degree angles along the length of the balloon. This results in small circumferential tears in the atrial septum, which prevents the septum from simply stretching and subsequently recoiling. The cutting balloon septoplasty is then followed by a static inflation using an 8- to 14-mm Tyshak II angioplasty balloon (3 to 5 atmospheres of pressure), or a standard 13.5-mm

septostomy balloon is pulled through the smaller hole (with the technique described earlier) to further extend the tear and enlarge the hole. Either stent or nonstent septoplasty is effective, with a very high immediate success rate and a sustainable defect diameter. For the neonate who will not require a subsequent surgical procedure, the nonstent technique is our preference, with plans to use a septal occluder to close the defect later.

The Child, Teenager, or Young Adult with Dilated Cardiomyopathy or Myocarditis

Patients who present acutely with a severe myopathy or myocarditis may need to be placed on an extracorporeal membrane oxygenation (ECMO) circuit to sustain them while they await recovery or as a bridge to cardiac transplantation. ECMO provides an adequate cardiac output

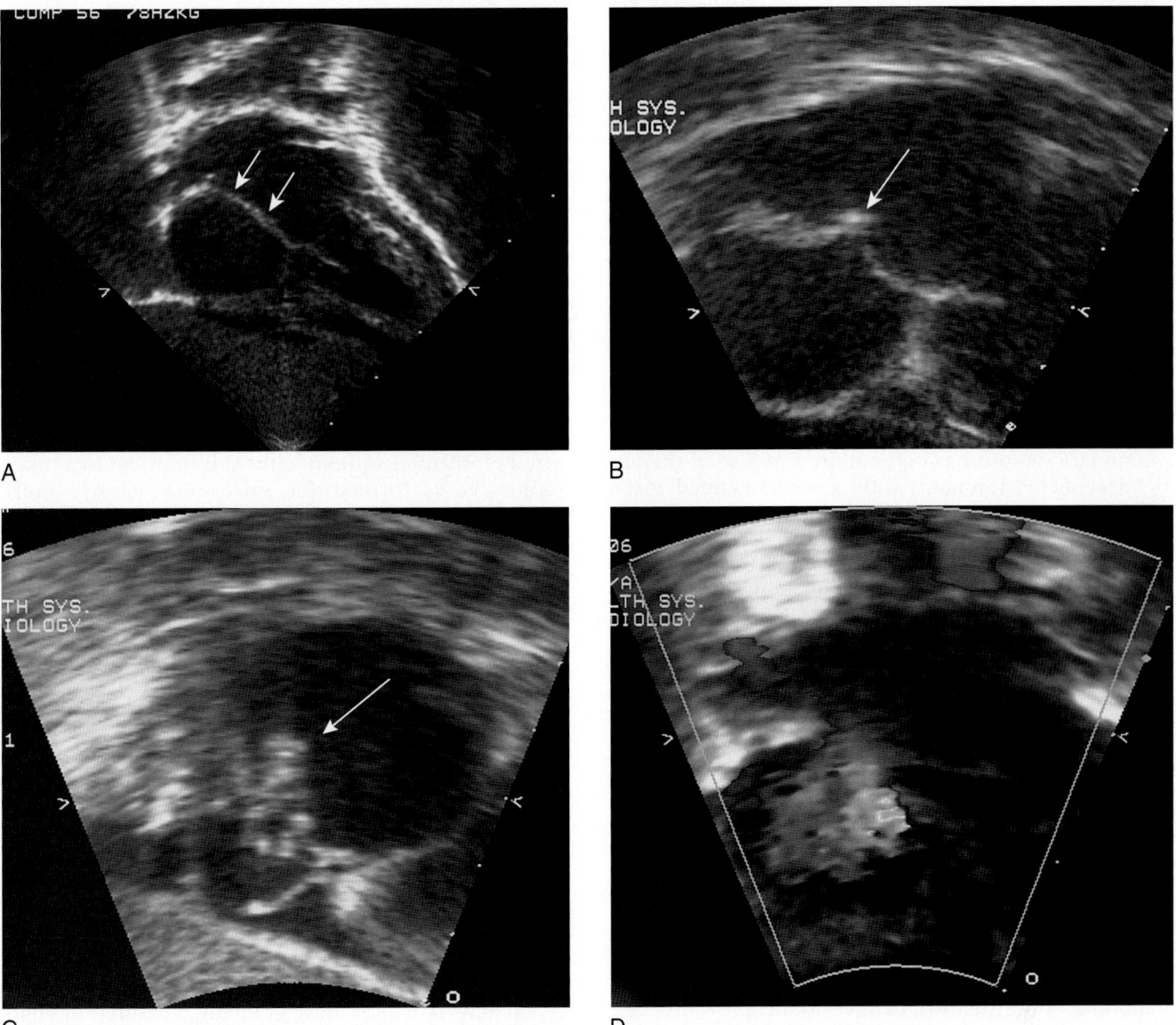

FIGURE 104-2. Echocardiographic views of transseptal or cutting balloon septostomy procedure. **A,** Preprocedure intact atrial septum *(arrows)*. **B,** Transseptal puncture with Brokinbrough transseptal puncture needle *(arrow)*. **C,** Cutting balloon inflation through transseptal puncture site *(arrow)*. **D,** Color Doppler image, final result, with low-velocity left-to-right shunt.

and oxygenates the blood, but pressures in the left ventricle and left atrium may still be unacceptably high. Left ventricular recovery may be compromised if the workload and wall stress are not further reduced by providing an atrial communication. Left atrial hypertension can also cause other significant complications, such as worsening pulmonary edema and pulmonary hemorrhage. The bleeding can be quite severe because the patient must be anticoagulated to be maintained on the ECMO circuit. Patients with a small or no communication in the atrial septum are approached in a manner similar to that described for infants with intact atrial septum (as described previously). Additional care must be taken when performing the transseptal puncture and septal cutting procedure, as the hypertensive left atrium will cause the septum to bow into the right atrium, significantly altering the anatomy and the surface for puncture. Also, any bleeding complication with the transseptal

needle is likely to be more severe and more difficult to control with the anticoagulated patient. The operator needs to be especially vigilant to treat bleeding into the pericardial space, and the cardiothoracic surgical team should be readily available.

BALLOON VALVULOPLASTY OR VALVOTOMY

Pulmonary Valve Stenosis

Valvar pulmonary stenosis is found in 8% to 10% of patients with congenital heart disease. The refinement of two-dimensional and Doppler echocardiography over the past two decades has had a dramatic impact on the role of cardiac catheterization in the management of valvar pulmonary stenosis. In the past, catheterization was required to make a definitive diagnosis, exclude other associated lesions, and measure the pressure gradient across the pulmonary valve. Because all of this can now be accomplished noninvasively, the role of catheterization has become largely therapeutic, and balloon pulmonary valvuloplasty has supplanted surgical valvotomy as the treatment of choice for this lesion.

> The role of catheterization has become largely therapeutic, as balloon pulmonary valvuloplasty has supplanted surgical valvotomy as the treatment of choice for pulmonic stenosis.

Transcatheter balloon pulmonary valvuloplasty for valvar pulmonary stenosis in infants was first reported in the early 1980s. Since this initial report, balloon pulmonary valvuloplasty for infants with isolated valvar pulmonary stenosis has become the first line of therapy in most medical centers, with a recommended mean balloon annulus ratio of 120%. The reported success rate is greater than 90%, with complications occurring in less than 1% of the procedures.

Balloon pulmonary valvuloplasty is performed and hemodynamic data are obtained with the patient sedated and breathing room air. A sheath is placed in the femoral vein and a monitoring catheter in the femoral artery of each patient. Hemodynamic measurements include the right ventricular pressure in comparison to systemic arterial pressure and the pressure gradient across the pulmonary valve. An end-hole catheter is used to carefully obtain withdrawal pressure recordings from the pulmonary artery to the body of the right ventricle, to assess the severity and location of any stenoses. In infants with relatively high pulmonary artery pressures, classification of severity of pulmonary stenosis is based on measurements of right ventricular pressure compared with systemic arterial pressure rather than valve gradient. Indications for balloon pulmonary valvuloplasty are at least moderate pulmonary valve stenosis, defined as a right ventricular pressure greater than one half of the systemic pressure, or a peak-to-peak gradient of 50 mm Hg or greater.

Right ventricular angiography in the anteroposterior view angled cephalad and in the lateral view is performed to provide information about location and severity of pulmonary stenosis for diagnostic and therapeutic purposes. The diameter of the pulmonary valve annulus is measured digitally. The angiographic diagnosis of dysplastic pulmonary valve stenosis is confirmed when the valve leaflets are markedly thickened and relatively immobile, with little excursion during the cardiac cycle and hypoplasia of the annulus.

For infants who meet the hemodynamic criteria, balloon pulmonary valvuloplasty is performed using a standard technique. The balloon pulmonary valvuloplasty is deemed successful if the estimated peak right ventricular pressure is less than 50 mm Hg or less than 0.5 of the peak systemic pressure, and the peak-to-peak gradient across the pulmonary valve is less than 30 mm Hg. Also, procedures are deemed successful only if the infant had a stable saturation with a closed ductus arteriosus and no immediate operative intervention is necessary before discharge from the hospital.

Aortic Valve Stenosis

Fusion of two of the three aortic valve leaflets, creating a "bicuspid" or functionally two-leaflet aortic valve, is the most common congenital heart lesion, occurring in 1% to 2% of the population. However, only 0.5% of these children will have a significant valve function abnormality (stenosis or regurgitation) by adolescence. Patients with aortic valve stenosis can be classified into two groups: those with disease severe enough that they present at birth or within 1 year of age (10% to 15%), and those who are not diagnosed until after age 2 and will progress much more slowly if at all. The mortality and need for intervention is significantly skewed toward the infantile group. As with pulmonary stenosis, noninvasive imaging techniques have advanced to the point that nearly all anatomic and functional information about the valve may be obtained without catheterization, and catheterization is performed for valves that clearly merit intervention, or when symptoms and imaging findings are incomplete or confounding.

> Because of improvements in noninvasive imaging techniques, nearly all anatomic and functional information about the stenotic aortic valve can be obtained without catheterization, which is performed for valves that clearly merit intervention, or when symptoms and imaging findings are incomplete or confounding.

Aortic valve stenosis is classified into the following categories: trivial, mild, moderate, severe, and critical. Critical aortic stenosis is not defined by a specific pressure gradient or valve orifice size, but on the basis of physiologic manifestations. If the stenosis is such that the patient cannot produce and maintain an adequate cardiac output, the stenosis is critical. Patients in this group may have a low valve gradient, measured by echo, because of decreased cardiac function and low cardiac output. Although some controversy still exists as to the most beneficial treatment method for this population (surgical valvotomy versus percutaneous balloon valvuloplasty), most centers have adopted balloon valvuloplasty as the initial treatment of choice. Patients in this category do not tolerate the stress of any procedure well, but catheterization has immediate results (reduction in gradient and resultant valve regurgitation) that are comparable to surgery, and a shorter postprocedure intensive care unit course and overall hospital stay. Balloon valvuloplasty has been associated with an increased rate of reintervention over surgical valvotomy, secondary to recurrent stenosis or worsening regurgitation. Because residual aortic valve disease, especially regurgitation, may progress over time, recommendations for valvuloplasty technique are more conservative, with a smaller maximal balloon diameter (80% to 100% of the annulus) than that recommended for the pulmonary valve (100% to 120%).

The valve may be approached retrograde from the aorta, using a soft-tipped J-wire to cross the narrowed valve orifice, with arterial access in the femoral (more common) or carotid artery. The valve may also be approached prograde by crossing an existing atrial communication or by performing a transseptal puncture to access the left heart. Once in the left ventricle, angiography is performed to measure the annulus of the valve and obtain landmarks for valvuloplasty. The typical camera angles are right anterior oblique (about 20 degrees rightward on the frontal camera) and long axial oblique (70 degrees leftward, 25 degrees cranial angulation with the lateral camera). A low-pressure balloon should be chosen that is at least 2 cm in length. The diameter of the balloon should not exceed 80% to 100% of the valve annulus. The smaller balloon diameter, compared with a similar-sized pulmonary valve annulus, is recommended to decrease the amount of valve tearing and resultant regurgitation. Many centers have adopted rapid right ventricular pacing at the time of balloon inflation. This rapid pacing transiently reduces cardiac output and the shearing force transmitted to the balloon as it is inflated across the valve annulus. The goal is to reduce the motion on the fragile valve leaflets and prevent excessive damage and regurgitation. Repeat angiography and echocardiography after the inflation are essential to evaluate the success of the valvuloplasty and monitor for regurgitation or other complications.

The differentiation between noncritical stenosis categories is made by noninvasive echocardiographic measurements of valve area and Doppler gradient. Normal valve area is $2 \text{ cm}^2/\text{m}^2$. Mild obstruction is consistent with valve areas of less than $2 \text{ cm}^2/\text{m}^2$, but greater than $0.7 \text{ cm}^2/\text{m}^2$, and severe obstruction at valve areas of less than $0.5 \text{ cm}^2/\text{m}^2$. Mean echocardiographic Doppler gradients are good predictors of the peak-to-peak pressure gradient measured at catheterization. Gradients of less than 25 mm Hg are considered trivial, 25 to 50 mm Hg are mild, 50 to 75 mm Hg are moderate, and severe is greater than 75 mm Hg. These measurements are made with the understanding that the cardiac function and cardiac output are normal. Catheterization is not recommended for trivial or mild stenosis. Moderate and severe stenoses are approached with primary balloon valvuloplasty using the techniques described previously.

ANGIOPLASTY

General Techniques for Standard Balloon, Cutting Balloon, and Stent Angioplasty

Beginning in the late 1980s, balloon angioplasty was used at low pressure, or less than 5 atmospheres, but balloons capable of dilations at higher pressure were later introduced. Since the introduction of high-pressure balloons, standard balloon angioplasty has resulted in a greater than 70% successful result for pulmonary artery angioplasty. For coarctation or recoarctation, balloon angioplasty has also been used with some success.

Patients with severely hypoplastic, multiply stenotic pulmonary arteries that are refractory to high-pressure angioplasty may not be treatable using currently available medical, surgical, or catheter-based tools. In such cases, a "waist" persists during angioplasty at the maximal recommended inflation pressure, or even at pressures

exceeding the recommended maximum, because of inadequate stretching or tearing of the vessel wall. For this patient population, cutting balloon angioplasty has become a therapeutic option, using balloons up to 8 mm in diameter. Often, cutting balloon angioplasty is followed by standard angioplasty for the best final result.

Balloon expandable stents have improved results in proximal vessels, eliminating the need for surgery in most patients, but they are of limited value in distal pulmonary vessels. Furthermore, stents are contraindicated in noncompliant vessels that cannot be expanded using high-pressure balloons. Stent angioplasty has also been used for coarctation of the aorta in postoperative and native lesions. Stents rarely migrate after appropriate deployment.

Pulmonary Artery Angioplasty

Pulmonary artery stenosis is a form of congenital heart disease that can occur in isolation or as part of more complex malformations such as tetralogy of Fallot. Although obstructions confined to the main or proximal branches can be repaired surgically, many patients can receive adequate palliation with transcatheter balloon angioplasty techniques. In addition, more distal obstructions that cannot be repaired operatively require angioplasty with balloons delivered to the distal stenotic segments, as described earlier. The inflation of a balloon that is two to three times the lesion diameter will tear the vessel wall within the stenotic segment, resulting in an increase in lumen diameter. Although balloon catheters have not been approved by the U.S. Food and Drug Administration (FDA) as a treatment for pulmonary artery stenoses, transcatheter techniques have become the mainstay of treatment for distal vessel obstruction.

Aortic Angioplasty: Ascending Aorta, Transverse Arch, and Isthmus

Few data exist regarding stent angioplasty for ascending aortic obstruction. The majority of reports involve either single-ventricle patients with arch obstruction resulting from the Norwood repair or a previously placed bypass cannula, or the patient with Williams syndrome and supravalvar aortic stenosis. Although a few case reports have described the use of stent angioplasty for supravalvar aortic stenosis, the risk for aortic valve leaflet entrapment has also been reported, so this has yet to become an accepted therapy.

Often, the aortic obstruction after an end-to-end surgical repair at the isthmus is caused by aortic narrowing within the transverse arch. These obstructive lesions are further defined as being either in the proximal transverse arch (between the innominate artery and left carotid artery) or in the distal transverse arch (defined as the region between the left carotid artery and the left subclavian artery). Although few data exist regarding stent angioplasty within the distal transverse aortic arch, general experience has been that this is a safe and effective procedure. An arterial monitoring catheter is placed in the right upper extremity, and a 4F sheath is used to advance a 4F pigtail to the aorta from the right radial artery. This catheter is used to monitor pressures during stent angioplasty of the distal transverse arch and to monitor cine angiograms to determine appropriate stent placement distal to the takeoff of the left carotid artery.

Transcatheter stent angioplasty for postoperative recoarctation of the aorta at the isthmus has been demonstrated to be safe and effective. The technique usually involves a femoral arterial approach. The exchange-length wire is placed in the ascending aorta or right subclavian artery. An angioplasty balloon is used whose diameter is equal to or less than that of the normal aortic segments around the stenosis or the diameter of the descending thoracic aorta at the diaphragm. The stent is mounted on the angioplasty balloon and a sheath at least 1F to 2F larger than that required by the balloon is used. The stent length depends on the lesion length but is usually at least 36 mm in adults. The stent is fully dilated in most cases, but at times it is deemed safer to dilate the lesion over two procedures.

OCCLUSION DEVICES

Atrial Septal Communications

Although diagnosing the presence of an atrial septal defect (ASD) rarely requires cardiac catheterization, today many patients undergo cardiac catheterization for device closure. These patients require an investigation to assess associated anomalies such as those of pulmonary venous connection. In addition, for older patients or patients with trisomy 21, catheterization may be indicated to measure pulmonary artery pressures and pulmonary vasculature resistance to ensure that closure can be performed safely. A step-up in oxygen saturations in the right atrium and the pulmonary arteries is characteristic for an ASD, and the degree of left-to-right shunting or the pulmonary-to-systemic blood flow ratio ($Q_p:Q_s$) can be determined. In cases of elevated pulmonary vascular resistance (PVR), 100% oxygen or nitric oxide can be administered during catheterization to confirm reversibility. If the PVR falls below 5 Wood units, ASD closure is usually safe. The ideal age or timing for elective ASD closure is 2 to 5 years of age, or within 6 to 12 months of diagnosis. Although it is uncommon, occasionally a child with an ASD and severe CHF requires intervention in the first year of life.

> The ideal age or timing for elective ASD closure is 2 to 5 years of age or within 6 to 12 months of diagnosis. Occasionally, a child with an ASD and severe CHF requires intervention in the first year of life.

Percutaneous ASD closure is a safe and effective alternative to operative repair. The technique involves transcatheter delivery of a device in its retracted state via the femoral vein under fluoroscopic and echocardiographic guidance. Echocardiographic guidance can be transthoracic in young children, or transesophageal, intracardiac, and even three-dimensional in older children. The most commonly available devices consist of a double-disk design made of nickel and titanium (Nitinol). The first disk is deployed on the left atrial aspect of the septum, and then a second opposing disk is deployed on the right atrial wall. The expanded disks are tightly approximated, thus closing the defect. The device becomes endothelialized over the next 3 to 12 months while the patient is treated with antiplatelet medications. Limitations include the size of the defect, the absence of adequate margins, proximity to vital cardiac structures, and overall size of the child. ASD devices require an adequate tissue margin (minimum, 7 to 8 mm) for deployment. The ASD must be small enough that the device can be deployed and held in the atrial septum (adequate margin must be present on all sides other than the anterior superior rim by the aorta, where some splay of the device around the aorta compensates for a deficient rim) without impingement on adjacent structures or significant pressure on the walls of the atrium. Venous inflow to both the right and left atrium must not be impeded, and the tricuspid and mitral valve should not come in contact with the device.

The world experience of transcatheter ASD closure using the FDA-approved Amplatzer septal occluder has been reported, with a greater than 97% immediate success. The occlusion rate reached 100% by 3 years. There is an overall 2.8% adverse event rate, with no procedural mortalities. Several studies providing comparisons of device occlusion versus surgical closure have been performed prospectively. These reports include the Amplatzer and Helex devices for ASD closure. Findings include a shorter hospital stay and much less discomfort, and the time required for convalescence is reduced for patients undergoing successful device closure. Hospital costs are similar. Regression of right ventricular dilation was similar for both groups of patients but depended on what age the patient underwent closure: greater success was reported with earlier intervention.

Procedural adverse events are uncommon but include embolization into either the right or left atrium, pulmonary artery, left ventricle; and aorta; stroke caused by clot or air embolization; and bleeding complications. Both acute and late embolizations have been reported. It is therefore critical that the radiologist be familiar with the location of the intra-atrial septum on radiography to ascertain the correct device position in the anteroposterior and lateral chest radiographs (Fig. 104-3). The atrial septal occluder, like the ventricular septal occluder, has an oblique orientation on the frontal and lateral radiographs but is positioned higher and more medial than the appropriately located ventricular septal defect (VSD) occluder.

Patent Ductus Arteriosus

Closure of a persistently patent ductus arteriosus (PDA) was the first transcatheter interventional procedure, performed by Portsmann in 1967. Since that time, a number of different PDA closure devices have been studied, and some of these are no longer available. The goal of the procedure has always been to achieve 100% closure of the PDA without obstruction of either adjoining blood vessel (the aorta or the left pulmonary artery) with min-

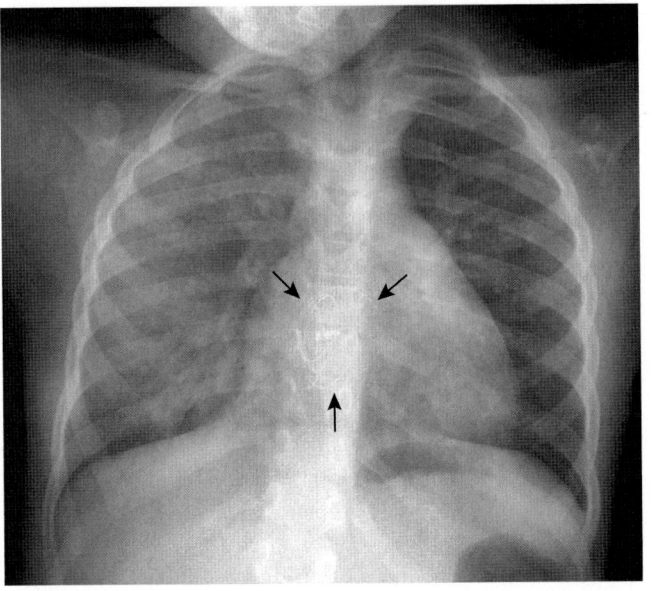

A

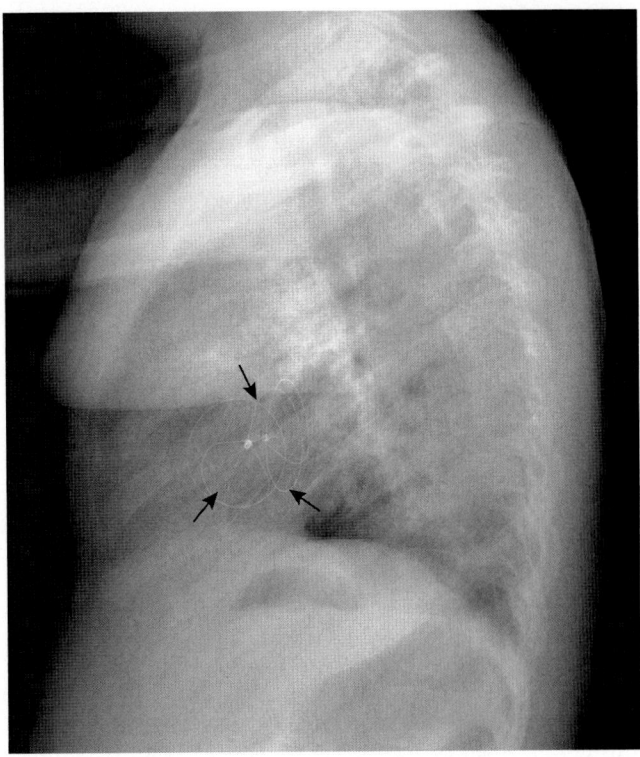

B

FIGURE 104-3. Atrial septal occluder device (Helex) for a secundum defect is evident on the frontal **(A)** and lateral **(B)** radiographs *(arrows)* in a 5-year-old girl with trisomy 21.

imal risk for complications. The difficulty is that PDAs exhibit extreme variability in size and shape. Krichenko and colleagues classified PDAs into five different atatomic types based on the lateral aortic angiogram. The most common (type A) ductus is conical with a narrowed pulmonary arterial end and large aortic ampulla. Other types include a narrowed aortic end, narrowing at both ends, and a tubular configuration. Early device closure procedures were complicated by a lack of choices for different size and shape vessels. The early devices had unsatisfactory rates of complications and residual leak and were abandoned. In 1992, the first report was published using the Gianturco embolization coil (Cook, Bloomington, IN) for closure of small PDAs. The Gianturco coil, which is available in multiple lengths and diameters, has now been in use for more than 30 years for blood vessel occlusion of collateral vessels, fistulas, and arteriovenous malformations. The successful use of the coil in PDA closure, combined with individual operators sharing ingenious techniques to deploy multiple coils and secure the coils before deployment, provided the needed variety of approaches to close PDAs successfully. Tens of thousands of PDAs have now been closed with embolization coils around the world.

As expected, the recommended technique for coil embolization is variable and depends on the size and shape of the ductus. In general, PDA coil embolization techniques share features with coil procedures discussed elsewhere in this text. The vessel can be approached from the venous or arterial side, and the coils may be deployed "free-hand" or secured with a bioptome or modified catheter. Smaller coils, such as the Flipper coil (Cook, Bloomington, IN), are also available that are attached

to the delivery system and released once their position is verified.

The only recent additions to the interventional cardiologist's armamentarium for PDA closure are the Gianturco-Grifka vascular occlusion device (GGVOD; Cook, Bloomington, IN) and the Amplatzer duct occluder (AGA Medical Corp., Golden Valley, MN). The GGVOD addressed one of the main problem areas with coil embolization. Moderate to large PDAs, especially if the ductus was tubular, were very difficult to close with coils; the high pressure flow would not allow for stable coil placement until multiple coils were in place, and coils embolized easily. Closure of these types of PDAs with coils was largely abandoned. The GGVOD uses a nylon sack that is secured to a delivery sheath and a 0.025-inch wire is pushed forward, filling the sack. This sack is then pulled securely into the PDA and released. It requires an 8F Mullins transseptal sheath for deployment, so the size of the delivery system is somewhat limiting.

The duct occluder is a fundamentally different device and procedure from coil embolization. The PDA occluder is a self-expanding wire-mesh device that is attached to a delivery cable and deployed through a long sheath from the venous system (Fig. 104-4). The device has a retention skirt to occupy the aortic ampulla, and it tapers slightly to the pulmonary artery end. The device is filled with a polyester mesh that stimulates thrombus formation within the lumen of the PDA. The shape of the device and its self-expanding properties exert radial force on the walls of the PDA, holding the device in place until endothelialization occurs. The device has excellent closure rates, approaching 100% at 1 month after the

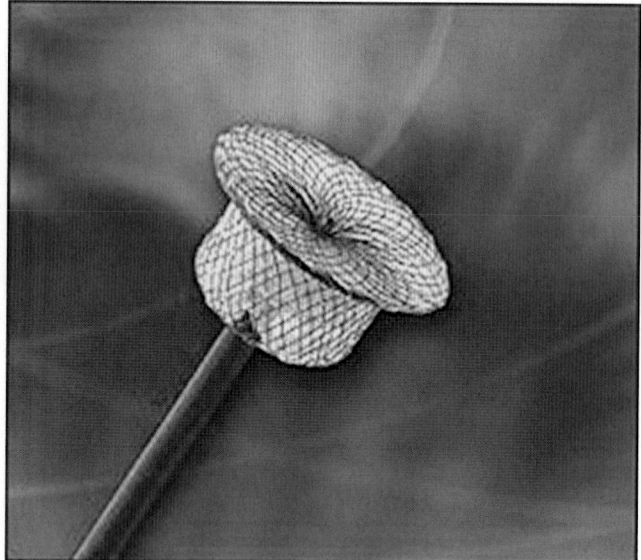

FIGURE 104-4. Amplatzer duct occluder, connected to delivery cable deployed through delivery sheath. (From AGA Medical Corporation, Golden Valley, MN.)

procedure. The limitation of the duct occluder is also the size and bulky nature of the device. The PDA must have an aortic ampulla adequate to accommodate the retention skirt without creating aortic obstruction, and the device can create left pulmonary artery stenosis by compressing adjoining structures once released.

Most PDAs (other than large PDAs in newborn or premature infants) can be closed safely and effectively in the cardiac catheterization laboratory using the devices detailed here, as long as the operator is familiar with the use and limitations of each device and has a good understanding of the anatomy of the patent ductus.

> Most PDAs (other than large PDAs in newborn or premature infants) can be closed safely and effectively in the cardiac catheterization laboratory using devices.

Ventricular Septal Defects

For children with moderate defects and no clinically significant CHF, pulmonary overcirculation, or pulmonary hypertension, echocardiography suffices as the definitive preoperative study. Cardiac catheterization may be indicated when echocardiographic data are unsatisfactory and in patients with large defects and significant pulmonary hypertension, or when there is doubt about the anatomy of associated lesions.

Cardiac catheterization can demonstrate the location, size, and number of defects, along with associated cardiac anomalies. It facilitates direct measurement of left and right heart pressures and oxygen saturations (Fig. 104-5), from which quantification of the intracardiac shunt and PVR can de derived.

The shunt fraction is the ratio of pulmonary blood flow (Q_p) to systemic blood flow (Q_s). It is calculated according to the following formula:

$$Q_p/Q_s = (Ao_2 - MVo_2) \div (PVo_2 - Pao_2)$$

where Ao_2 is the aortic oxygen saturation, MVo_2 is the mixed venous oxygen saturation, Pao_2 is the pulmonary arterial saturation, and PVo_2 is the pulmonary venous saturation.

Patients with elevated PVR (5 to 10 U/m^2) are administered 100% oxygen or nitric oxide to test for reversibility. If recalculated PVR falls below 7 U/m^2, VSD repair can be safely performed. Persistent elevation of PVR suggests irreversible pulmonary hypertension and that VSD closure will very likely result in acute right heart failure and death. Heart-lung transplantation and single lung transplantation with VSD closure are the only surgical options for this group of patients.

Transcatheter device closure has recently been considered in investigational trials for muscular and membranous defects. Although the frequency of heart block has precluded general use of devices in the membranous septum, the muscular defect closure technique with the Amplatzer device may be FDA approved early in 2007.

Collateral Vessels and Arteriovenous Malformations

Accessory blood vessels are a common area of concern for the interventional radiologist and interventional cardiologist. These may include aortopulmonary or venovenous collaterals (Fig. 104-6), arteriovenous fistula (Fig. 104-7), and malformations, surgically placed shunts, and transhepatic access tracts. Techniques for closure are similar to that described for the PDA, predominantly involving Gianturco coils, the Amplatzer duct occluder, or the Amplatzer vascular plug (Fig. 104-8). The vascular plug is similar to the duct occluder in that it has a self-expanding wire mesh design. It differs in that it is cylindrical in shape with no retention skirt, no tapering through its length, and no polyester mesh interior fabric. The device has excellent occlusion results, but it has been unsuccessful in short arterial vessels such as aortopulmonary collaterals and PDAs. It is thought that the lack of occlusive material through the center of the device does not provide enough restriction to arterial blood flow to stimulate thrombosis and occlude the vessel.

CONCLUSIONS

Cardiac catheterization for congenital heart disease has evolved from its early days as an exclusively diagnostic tool to a dynamic and continuously growing field of therapeutic interventional procedures for children and adults with cardiac abnormalities. The physicians and industry have a history of working together to push the field forward, finding novel solutions to difficult problems, while making the products to accomplish these goals smaller and safer. The interventional cardiologist and cardiothoracic surgeon have truly become an organized team in the treatment of once uniformly fatal conditions to offer longer life and a better quality of life to a diverse group of complex and rewarding patients.

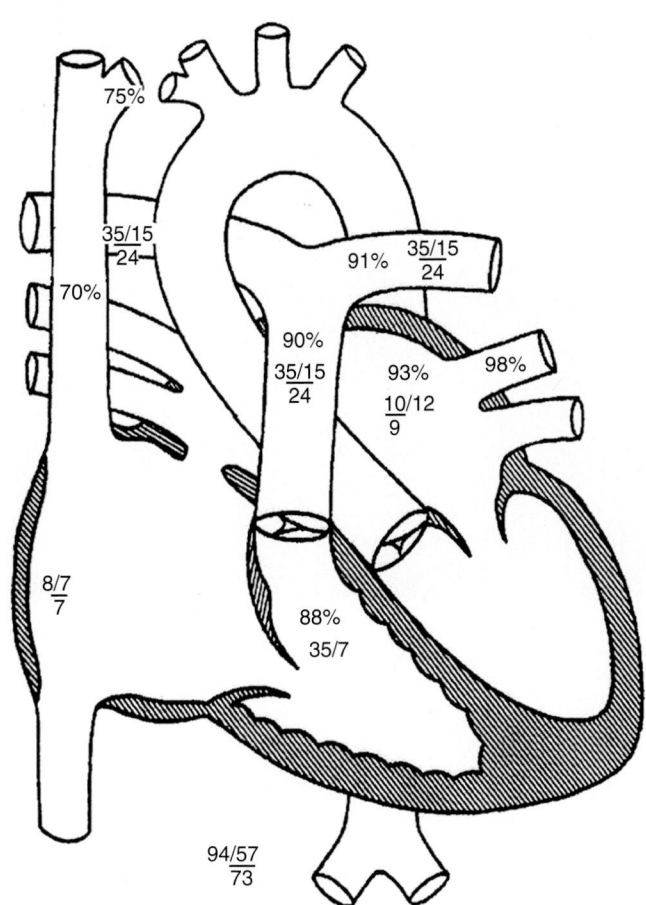

Height: 140.0 cm Weight: 28.0 kg
BSA = 1.07 m^2

Fluoro: 13.80 min Contrast: 36.00 mL
Vein: 9Fr-RFV/11Fr-LFV
Artery: None

Conscious sedation
Qp = 9.30 L/min (8.69 L/min/m^2)
Qs = 3.24 L/min (3.02 L/min/m^2)
Rp = 1.61 units (1.73 units x m^2)
Rs = 20.40 units (21.82 units x m^2)
Qp/Qs = 2.87 : 1 | Rp/Rs=0.08

Heart rate: 84 bpm
VO2: 140 ml/min/m^2
Hemoglobin: 14.8 gm/dL

Inspired O2: 21%
pH: 7.31
pCO2: 50.0
pO2: 82.0
HCO3: 24.0

Thermo CO:

%O2	Site	Sys/A	Dias/V	Mean
70	SVC			
	RA	8	7	7
88	RV	35	7	
90	PA	35	15	24
	RPA	35	15	24
91	LPA	35	15	24

Right		Left	
	Wedge mean		

%O2	Site	Sys/A	Dias/V	Mean
93	LA	10	12	9
	LV			
	aAO			
	dAO			

INN: O2%: 75

LUPV: O2%: 98

NIBP
 Sys/A: 94 Dias/V: 57 Mean: 73

FIGURE 104-5. Mullin's diagram depicting the results of a cardiac catheterization for a child with an atrial septal defect. Pressure measurements and oxygen saturation measurements are recorded. Calculation results of the cardiac index and shunt fraction are shown on the right.

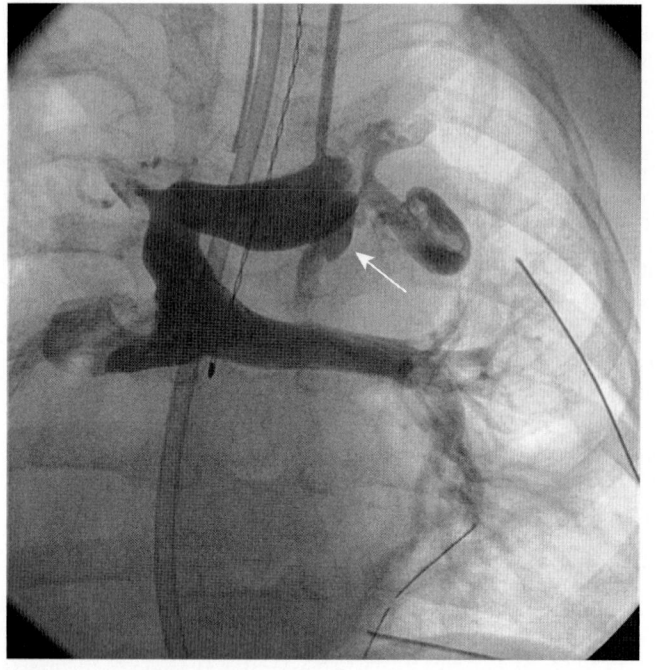

A

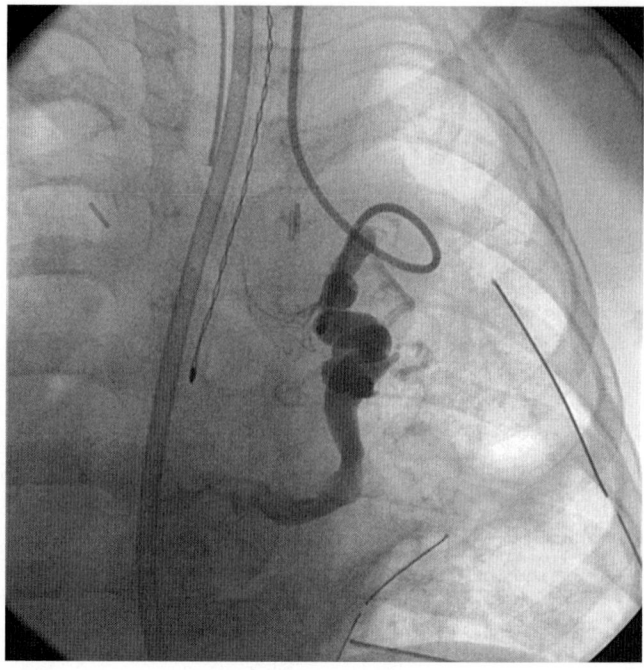

B

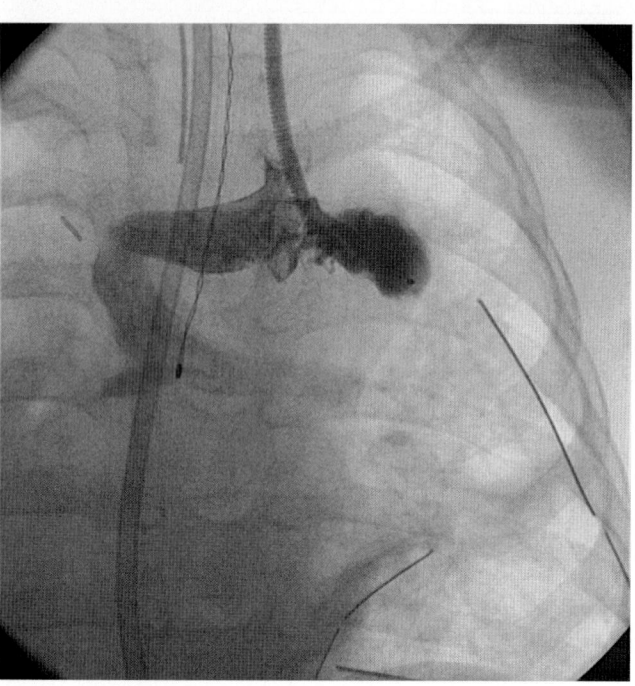

C

FIGURE 104-6. Angiograms of venovenous collateral in a single-ventricle patient who has undergone the Fontan procedure, before intervention **(A)** and **(B)**. **C,** The venovenous collateral (*arrow* in **A**) occluded with a vascular plug.

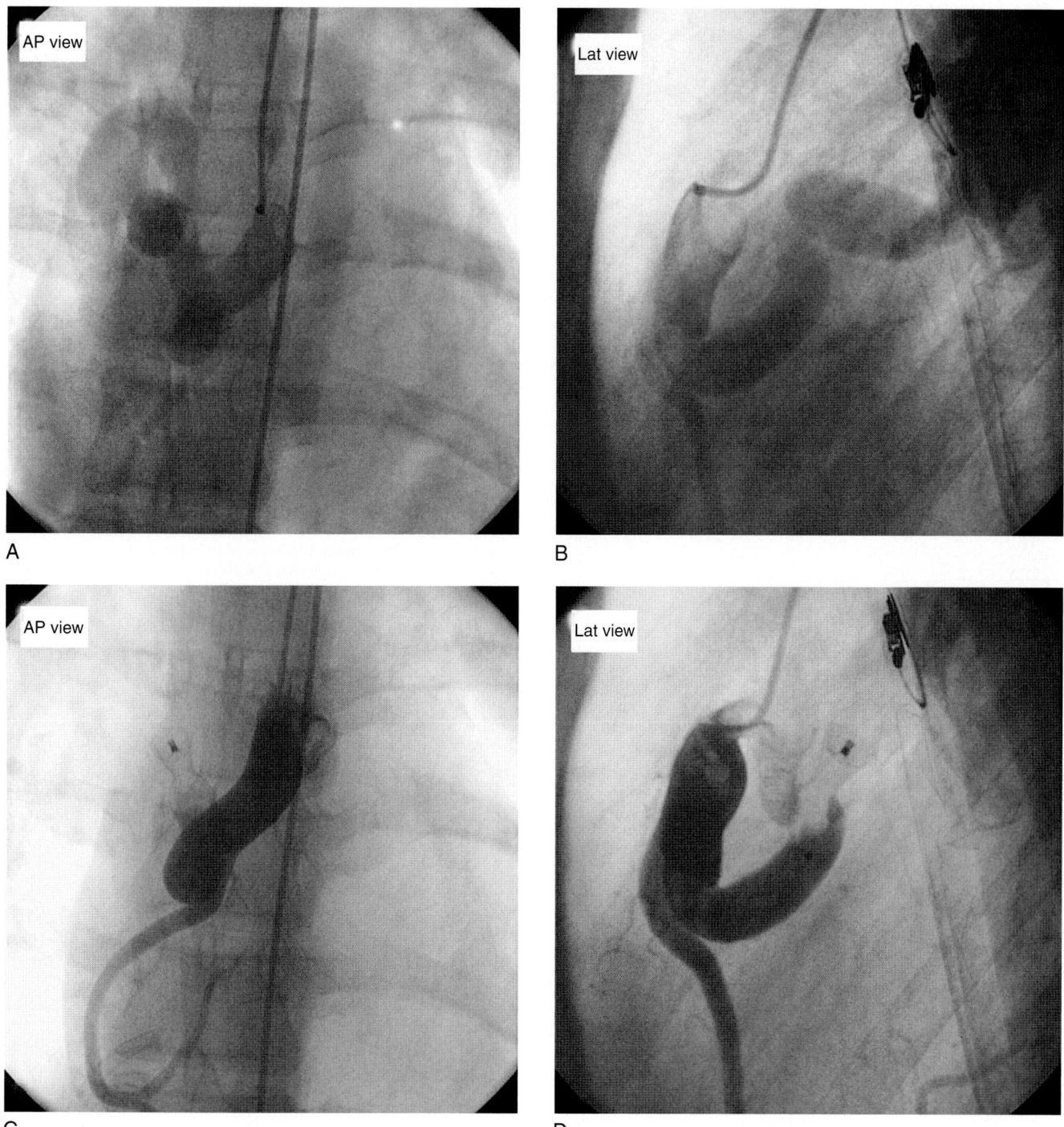

FIGURE 104-7. Angiograms of a coronary fistula, AP and lateral views, before intervention **(A, B)** and after successful occlusion **(C, D)**.

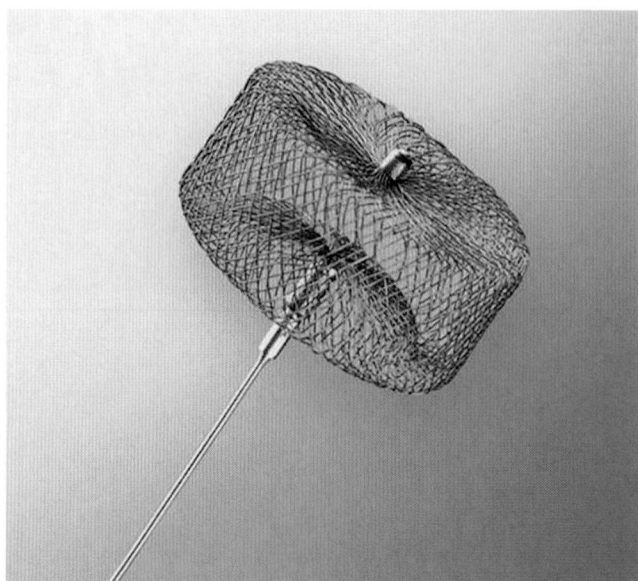

FIGURE 104-8. Figure of the vascular plug, connected to delivery cable, deployed through a standard long sheath or guide catheter. (From AGA Medical Corporation, Golden Valley, MN.)

SUGGESTED READINGS

ACC/AHA 2006 guidelines for the management of patients with valvular heart disease: a report of the American College of Cardiology/American Heart Association Task Force on Practice Guidelines (writing committee to revise the 1998 Guidelines for the Management of Patients With Valvular Heart Disease): developed in collaboration with the Society of Cardiovascular Anesthesiologists: endorsed by the Society for Cardiovascular Angiography and Interventions and the Society of Thoracic Surgeons. Circulation 2006;114:e84-231

Cambier PA, Kirby WC, Moore JW: Percutaneous closure of the small (less than 2.5 mm) patent ductus arteriosus using coil embolization. Am J Cardiol 1992;69:815-816

Fiser WP, Yetman AT, Gunselman RJ, et al: Pediatric arteriovenous extracorporeal membrane oxygenation (ECMO) as a bridge to cardiac transplantation. J Heart Lung Transplant 2003;22:770-776

Grifka RG: Transcatheter closure of the patent ductus arteriosus. Catheter Cardiovasc Interv 2004;61:554-570

Hill SL, Mizelle KM, Vellucii SM, et al: Radiofrequency perforation and cutting balloon septoplasty of intact atrial septum in a newborn with hypoplastic left heart syndrome using transesophageal ICE probe guidance. Catheter Cardiovasc Interv 2005;64:214-217

Krichenko A, Benson LN, Burrows, et al: Angiographic classification of the isolated, persistently patent ductus arteriosus and implications for percutaneous catheter occlusion. Am J Cardiol 1989;63:877-880

Lababidi Z, Wu JR: Percutaneous balloon pulmonary valvuloplasty. Am J Cardiol 1983;52:560-562

Matsura J, Walsh KP, Thanpoulous B, et al: Catheter closure of moderate to large sized patent ductus arteriosus using the new Amplatzer duct occluder: immediate and short-term results. J Am Coll Cardiol 1998;31:878-882

Rashkind WJ, Miller WW: Creation of an atrial septal defect without thoracotomy. JAMA 1966;196:991-992

Roccini AP, Kveselis DA, Crowley D, et al: Percutaneous balloon valvuloplasty for treatment of congenital pulmonary valvular stenosis in children. J Am Coll Cardiol 1984;3:1005-1012

Seib PM, Faulkner SC, Erickson CC, et al: Blade and balloon atrial septostomy for left heart decompression in patients with severe ventricular dysfunction on extracorporeal membrane oxygenation. Catheter Cardiovasc Interv 1999;46:179-186

Vida VL, Bottio T, Milanesi O, et al: Critical aortic stenosis in early infancy: surgical treatment for residual lesions after balloon dilation. Ann Thorac Surg 2005;79:47-52

Williams RJ, Levi DS, Moore JW, Boechat MI: Radiographic appearance of pediatric cardiovascular transcatheter devices. Pediatr Radiol 2006;36:1231-1241

Zain Z, Zadinello M, Menahem S, Brizard C: Neonatal isolated critical aortic valve stenosis: balloon valvuloplasty or surgical valvotomy. Heart Lung Circ 2006;15:18-23

Zellers TM, Hijazi ZM, Sandhu S, et al: Catheter closure of patent ductus arteriosus using the Amplatzer device: interim report on US phase I and II clinical trial. Circulation 2000;102:II587

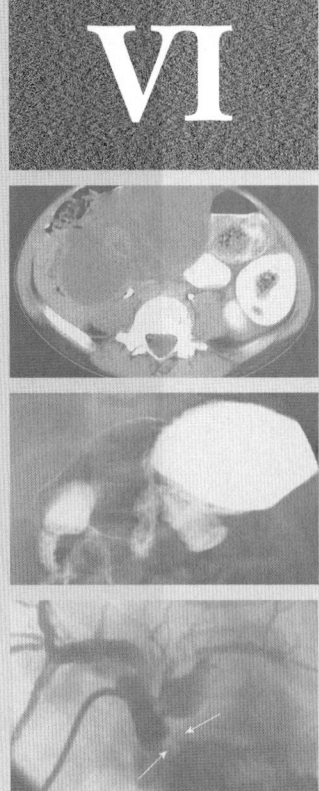

THE ABDOMEN, PELVIS, AND RETROPERITONEUM

BRIAN D. COLEY AND MARTA HERNANZ-SCHULMAN

PART 1 OVERVIEW

CHAPTER

105 Overview

MARTA HERNANZ-SCHULMAN and BRIAN D. COLEY

The gastrointestinal system is extensive and complex, encompassing an area from the mouth to the anal sphincter. It includes both hollow and solid viscera and is affected by a wide spectrum of pathology. The genitourinary system, though less extensive, has its own complexities and disease features. In children, congenital anomalies present a specific set of findings and diagnostic possibilities not typically encountered in adults, and the pediatric manifestations of acquired disease are often unique. The application of new imaging techniques has had a significant impact on the diagnostic approach to sick children, underscoring the key role of the radiologist in the management of pediatric patients. This chapter presents an overview of the relevant general principles; the diagnosis of specific conditions is covered in other chapters.

Although a wide array of imaging techniques is currently available, radiographs are still a mainstay in the imaging armamentarium; they can be used as definitive diagnostic tools or to guide further investigations. Chest radiographs can identify the findings of esophageal atresia or of chronic aspiration, suggesting the presence of an H-type fistula. Abdominal radiographs, often supplemented by a decubitus or prone view, can provide valuable information. For instance, the well-known double-bubble sign is diagnostic of duodenal atresia. Abdominal radiographs can suggest the presence of pyloric stenosis, intussusception, ileus, obstruction, and masses, as well as identify intramural air, portal venous air, and free intraperitoneal air. Calcifications may be seen in meconium peritonitis, as manifestations of genitourinary tract stone disease, or with tumors such as neuroblastoma.

Fluoroscopic examinations retain an important role in the evaluation of the gastrointestinal tract, although newer contrast agents are often used. Other modalities, notably ultrasonography and computed tomography (CT), complement or supersede fluoroscopic procedures in specific cases, such as pyloric stenosis, intussusception, appendicitis, and inflammatory bowel disease. Barium is the mainstay among gastrointestinal contrast agents, with nonionic water-soluble media used when there is concern about contrast extravasation. Hyperosmolar agents should be used cautiously, and never in the setting of potential aspiration. These agents are useful in therapeutic enemas for uncomplicated meconium ileus, with close monitoring of electrolytes and fluid status. Therapeutic enemas for the reduction of intussusception are performed with air insufflation or with isotonic water-soluble media. Fluoroscopy is also important in the evaluation of the genitourinary tract, particularly in cases of vesicoureteral reflux and urethral pathology.

Sonography, CT, and magnetic resonance imaging (MRI) are extremely useful for the evaluation of gastrointestinal and genitourinary pathology in pediatric patients. Sonography offers exquisite detail of bowel anatomy and blood flow and can be used effectively in many situations, including in the assessment of inflammatory bowel disease, appendicitis, intussusception with or without lead points, pyloric stenosis, masses, and the solid viscera. Sonography is the initial modality of choice for investigating the genitourinary tract, reliably depicting renal anomalies, hydronephrosis, masses, and bladder pathology. Coupled with contrast agents, ultrasonography provides a method of assessing vesicoureteral reflux without radiation exposure. The main limitations of sonography are the interposition of air and bone, the small tomographic field of view, and operator dependence. CT is not limited by air or bone; it offers angiographic data, multiplanar and three-dimensional reconstructions, rapid scanning time, and tomographic capability with no limitation of field of view; and it is much less operator dependent. Disadvantages of CT include the need for sedation in some cases and radiation exposure. The role of CT in pediatric gastrointestinal, abdominal, and genitourinary imaging; in the evaluation of abdominal masses; and in the evaluation of patients with abdominal pain, continues to expand. It is important that the choice of CT be optimized and that appropriate pediatric imaging parameters be used. MRI requires the patient to be perfectly still for prolonged periods, which usually translates to a need for sedation in infants and young children. However, MRI can outline inflammatory processes and delineate and map abdominal masses without radiation exposure. MR cholangiopancreatography has become widely used in imaging both the dilated and the nondilated biliary tree. Dynamic MR urography couples anatomic detail with the functional information traditionally obtainable only with nuclear medicine studies.

Nuclear medicine is employed in the evaluation of gastric emptying and reflux; the assessment of gastrointestinal bleeding, particularly that associated with gastric mucosa in Meckel diverticulum; and in the evaluation of the liver and biliary tree in jaundiced infants. In the evaluation of hydronephrosis, nuclear medicine assists in assessing obstruction and renal function. Cortical scintigraphy allows the evaluation of pyelonephritis and renal scarring. Although nuclear medicine cystography does not have the spatial resolution of other modalities, it reliably evaluates vesicoureteral reflux with less radiation exposure than fluoroscopy.

As technology pushes the envelope of diagnostic modalities, choosing the "correct" imaging evaluation can be complex and confusing. It is incumbent on the pediatric radiologist to remain focused and to analyze the clinical history. For example, in a patient presenting with an abdominopelvic mass, age may be the most important determinant of the differential diagnosis (Table 105-1). The primary site of a lesion changes with age, as does the kind of lesion (e.g., hydronephrosis versus Wilms tumor). Knowledge of the mechanism of metastatic spread may also influence the choice of imaging; for example, in neuroblastoma, we want to see the extent of neuroforaminal and intraspinal disease, rendering MRI or multidetector CT with multiplanar reconstructions the primary imaging tools.

The imaging workup of a child with acute abdominal pain further emphasizes the importance of the imager as a diagnostician. There are multiple causes of abdominal pain in childhood, but several predominate in each age group (Table 105-2). Our knowledge of the differential diagnosis allows us to discuss with referring physicians the need for imaging based on the child's age, presentation, and laboratory evaluation. Together, we can choose the correct test (if indicated) and expedite the diagnosis.

TABLE 105-1

Most Common Abdominal and Pelvic Masses by Age

Age and Type of Mass	Incidence (%)
NEONATE	
Renal	55
Hydronephrosis	
Ureteropelvic junction obstruction	
Ureterovesical junction obstruction	
Reflux (includes valves)	
Multicystic kidney	
Genital	15
Hydrometrocolpos	
Ovarian lesions	
Gastrointestinal	15
Duplications	
Nonrenal retroperitoneal	10
Adrenal hemorrhage	
Neuroblastoma	
Teratoma	
Hepatosplenobiliary	5
1 MONTH TO 2 YEARS	
Renal	55
Wilms tumor	
Hydronephrosis	
Nonrenal retroperitoneal	23
Neuroblastoma	
Teratoma	
Gastrointestinal (including biliary masses, appendiceal abscess, and intussusception)	18
Genital, miscellaneous	4
OLDER THAN 2 YEARS*	
Visceromegaly secondary to infection, leukemia, lymphoma; splenomegaly secondary to portal hypertension	Frequent
Wilms tumor and neuroblastoma	Frequent up to age 5; decreases thereafter
Pregnancy	Common pelvic mass in adolescent girls

*It is difficult to obtain precise numbers for this age group.
Modified from Griscom NT: The roentgenology of neonatal abdominal masses. AJR Am J Roentgenol 1965;93:447; and Kasper TE, et al: Urological abdominal masses in infants and children. J Urol 1967;116:629; reprinted from Haller JO, Slovis TL, Joshi A (eds): Pediatric Radiology, 3rd ed. Berlin, Springer, 2005.

Once a decision is made to image, the imager uses all the data to formulate the relevant questions and identify the correct modality to provide the pertinent answers, bearing in mind that no one way is always best. As members of the clinical care team, pediatric radiologists can navigate the complex choice of imaging techniques, translating into the delivery of optimal care for our children.

TABLE 105-2

Principal Causes of Acute Abdominal Pain Based on Age

INFANT (<2 YEARS)
Colic (<3 mo)
Acute gastroenteritis or "viral syndrome"
Traumatic perforation of viscus (nonaccidental trauma)
Intussusception
Incarcerated hernia
Volvulus (malrotation)
Sickling syndromes

INFANT AND CHILD (2-13 YEARS)
Acute gastroenteritis or "viral syndrome"
Urinary tract infection
Appendicitis
Trauma
Constipation
Pneumonia
Sickling syndromes

ADOLESCENT
Acute gastroenteritis or "viral syndrome"
Urinary tract infection
Appendicitis
Trauma
Constipation
Pelvic inflammatory disease
Pneumonia
Mittelschmerz

Adapted from Boyle JT: Abdominal pain. *In* Walker WA, Goulet O, Kleinman RE, et al (eds): Pediatric Gastrointestinal Disease, 4th ed. Hamilton, Ontario, Decker, 2004:225-231.

CHAPTER

106

Gastrointestinal Tract

MARTA HERNANZ-SCHULMAN and STEPHANIE SPOTTSWOOD

When the first edition of this textbook was published in 1945, the title was *Caffey's Pediatric X-ray Diagnosis*, denoting the single modality in existence at the time. Since then, there have been nine additional editions of the book, and the title was changed to *Caffey's Pediatric Diagnostic Imaging* to reflect the diversity of tools now available to the pediatric radiologist. Indeed, technological advances have been achieved at an accelerating rate, and the capabilities and applications of existing modalities have increased as well. This expansion has been coupled with an increasing awareness of the importance of safety in the application of both older and newer techniques, adding to the complexity of choosing and implementing optimal pediatric imaging. This chapter is an overview of the applicability of the various modalities to the gastrointestinal (GI) tract; their application to specific entities is outlined in the chapters that follow.

PLAIN RADIOGRAPHY

The GI system includes the hollow viscera from esophagus to rectum; the solid viscera—liver, spleen, and pancreas; and the peritoneal cavity and retroperitoneal spaces in which all these organs are contained. Although there is considerable overlap among the various imaging modalities, and new applications continue to be defined, plain films are usually an excellent starting point in the assessment of the GI system. The chest radiograph can show some abnormalities of the esophagus, such as achalasia and, notably, esophageal atresia, which requires no further imaging for diagnosis. The abdominal radiograph can assess calcifications, which would be expected in cases of meconium peritonitis and can be present in abdominal masses such as hepatoblastoma or in appendicitis. Intramural air, free intraperitoneal air, portal venous air, and the double-bubble sign of duodenal atresia are identified on plain films, pointing to the correct diagnosis in the appropriate clinical setting. Inflammatory conditions, such as Crohn disease, may be suspected by assessing the gas pattern. Dilated bowel loops typically direct the radiologist toward a consideration of an ileus pattern or obstruction. In such cases, decubitus views and prone cross-table lateral views of the rectum can differentiate between these possibilities and direct further diagnostic imaging.

Air is the inherent contrast medium in plain film diagnosis, and the abdominal series is based on the distribution and movement of gas. The basic plain film evaluation typically consists of supine and horizontal-beam images. The prone film is helpful in directing gas to the rectum for the assessment of its caliber when bowel obstruction is a concern; a prone horizontal-beam (cross-table lateral) film of the rectum is particularly helpful in these cases. Left-side-down decubitus and upright views evaluate for free intraperitoneal air and air-fluid levels. The left-side-down decubitus view further directs air toward the right colon, for evaluation of the right lower quadrant, and into the rectum, for evaluation of obstruction.

FLUOROSCOPY

For further assessment of suspected pathology of the hollow viscera, fluoroscopy is the mainstay, although sonography, scintigraphy, computed tomography (CT), and, in some cases, magnetic resonance imaging (MRI) are increasingly applicable. Fluoroscopy should be intermittent, to limit the radiation dose; pulsed fluoroscopic techniques can decrease the radiation dose substantially without the loss of clinical information. Fluoro grab images can be used liberally to document such findings as viscus distention, course of contrast, and peristaltic activity; spot films are reserved for areas where mucosal detail is of diagnostic importance.

Contrast Media

Fluoroscopic studies are occasionally performed without contrast media, such as fluoroscopy of the diaphragm. However, enteric contrast is typically required for diagnosis, and there are a number of choices. Barium, an inert substance that is not absorbed and has physical properties well suited to the roentgen ray, is the contrast medium used most often in fluoroscopic procedures, whether administered orally to evaluate the esophagus and upper GI tract or rectally as a contrast enema. Several barium preparations are available: barium sulfate powder (96% weight/weight) can be diluted with sterile water for infant upper gastrointestinal (UGI) examinations to the desired concentration of 40% to 60% weight/volume. Premixed suspensions (60% weight/volume) can be used in older children and adolescents as well as in adults. Enema kits containing 97% barium weight/weight can be mixed with water to a final concentration of 15% to 33% barium weight/volume for infants, older children, and adolescents.

Barium is contraindicated when viscus perforation is suspected. In such cases, low-osmolality, nonionic, water-soluble iodinated media, such as iohexol, are indicated (Table 106-1). It is important that hypertonic media, such as ionic or high-osmolality media (diatrizoate, iothalamate), not be used orally, owing to the risk of aspiration and consequent danger of pulmonary edema. Further, such hypertonic media are diluted by increased luminal fluid; they have also been associated with mucosal injury and large fluid shifts, which are potentially dangerous in young infants and in patients with obstruction. Therefore, they are unsuitable for small bowel evaluation, particularly in patients with suspected obstruction.

Meglumine diatrizoate (Gastrografin) is an ionic, markedly hypertonic iodine solution with an osmolality of approximately 1600 mOsm/kg. A 1:5 dilution would be needed to approximate serum osmolality (285), which would render the iodine concentration quite low. Ionic hyperosmolar media can be absorbed from the GI tract, which poses a risk in patients with a history of hypersensitivity, particularly to iodine, and potentially in those with thyroid disease. Hyperosmolar media cause severe pulmonary complications (edema, pneumonitis) if aspirated, as well as major fluid shifts into the bowel lumen, leading to a decrease in intravascular volume, increase in serum osmolarity, and decrease in cardiac output. In patients with underlying bowel disease, additional injury is possible.

Iohexol (Omnipaque) is a nonionic, water-soluble, iodinated contrast medium that is available in concentrations of 140, 180, 240, 300, and 350 mg of iodine. It is poorly absorbed from the intact GI tract, with renal excretion of 0.1% to 0.5% of the administered dose. Iopamidol (Isovue) has also been used to evaluate the pediatric GI tract, but currently only Omnipaque is officially approved for this purpose. It must be emphasized that the osmolality of both these media is greater than that of blood, and no agent is safe in the tracheobronchial tree. Therefore, great care and close fluoroscopic monitoring are necessary in all patients in whom aspiration is a potential complication.

Barium is the standard agent for the evaluation of the colon. However, in cases of potential perforation, water-soluble agents are used. Iothalamate meglumine 30% (with an osmolality of 600) can be diluted 1:1 with water to achieve a nearly iso-osmolal solution with a diagnostic iodine concentration. Higher osmolality contrast media are used rectally for therapeutic purposes in cases of uncomplicated meconium ileus, after the diagnosis has been made with a low-osmolarity agent. Gastrografin was the original agent described for this purpose; however, its use can be associated with large fluid shifts and systemic complications in severely ill infants. Full-strength iothalamate meglumine 30% can also be used successfully for this purpose. Close attention to water and electrolyte balance and standby for surgical intervention are mandatory.

Air, the contrast medium in abdominal radiographs, can also be used during fluoroscopic procedures. It is an excellent way to distend a viscus during fluoroscopic transpyloric tube placement without obscuring the tube or adjacent bowel loops, and it is the preferred agent for the reduction of intussusception.

Esophagogram and Upper Gastrointestinal Series

The esophagogram and UGI series are usually performed in conjunction; they include an evaluation of the

TABLE 106-1				
Commonly Used Contrast Media in the Gastrointestinal Tract				
Contrast Medium	**Organically Bound Iodine (mg/ml)**	**Osmolality (mOsm/kg)**	**Viscosity (37°C)**	**Comments**
HIGH OSMOLAR, IONIC				
Gastrografin (meglumine diatrizoate; diatrizoate sodium)	367	1600		Potential for aspiration, dehydration, precarious electrolyte balance May cause problems if underlying bowel injury
Conray 30 (iothalamate meglumine)	141	600	1.5	Lower gastrointestinal tract
LOW OSMOLAR, NONIONIC				
Omnipaque (iohexol)				Upper gastrointestinal tract
140	140	322	1.5	Young infants
180	180	408	2	Infants and young children
240	240	520	3.4	Young children or ostomy evaluations
300	300	672	6.3	Not used
350	350	844	10.4	Not used

Source: package inserts.

swallowing mechanism, esophagus, stomach, and duodenum to the duodenojejunal junction. The examination is begun in the lateral projection, with the child lying on his or her left side to maintain the barium within the fundus of the stomach. Images of the esophagus are obtained from the nasopharynx to the esophagogastric junction, with special attention to nasopharyngeal aspiration, tracheal aspiration, masses, fistulas, and esophageal peristalsis and distensibility. The child is then laid supine, and the esophagus is examined in the anteroposterior projection. When the evaluation of the esophagus is completed, the barium in the fundus is directed into the duodenum by laying the child in the prone, right anterior oblique position. Gastric emptying is assessed, as well as distensibility of the antrum, pylorus, duodenal bulb, and descending duodenum. Once the contrast material has reached the junction of the second and third portions of the duodenum, the infant is rapidly placed in the supine position for assessment of the duodenojejunal junction, which is visible through the air-filled antrum. This should lie to the left of the spine, at approximately the same level as the duodenal bulb. Once this is accomplished, the child is quickly turned again, this time into the lateral position, for documentation of the posterior course of the ascending and descending limbs of the normally rotated retroperitoneal duodenum. If no small bowel follow-through procedure is scheduled, the infant may be allowed to eat his or her usual formula ad libitum, and evaluation for reflux is carried out after feeding with intermittent fluoroscopy over a 5-minute period, with the child calm and lying in the supine position. A final image documents gastric emptying (Fig. 106-1).

Small bowel follow-through usually requires the ingestion of a larger amount of contrast agent, typically barium; in premature infants, however, we use a nonionic, water-soluble contrast medium. Radiographs are obtained at regular intervals based on the course of the contrast agent through the bowel loops, with fluoroscopic evaluation as indicated. Images of the terminal ileum with and without compression are obtained once the contrast material has reached the cecum.

Contrast Enema

The contrast medium and the technique used vary with the indications for contrast enema (described in detail in the appropriate chapters). Barium is the usual contrast medium used unless perforation is suspected, in which case a water-soluble medium, usually diluted to near iso-osmolal concentration, is employed. In newborns suspected of having distal bowel obstruction, we usually use a water-soluble medium diluted to a near iso-osmolal concentration and change to a hyperosmolal medium if meconium ileus is encountered. Air is the contrast material of choice in patients with intussusception.

A small-tipped catheter is placed in the rectum and secured with tape to both buttocks, which are then taped together using manual pressure. Use of a balloon-tipped catheter is usually unnecessary, and it is inadvisable in young infants owing to the potential for rectal injury. Fluoro grab images can be recorded liberally to docu-

ment the progression of the barium and to document any findings dependent on temporal change; spot filming is needed in areas where mucosal detail is important.

SONOGRAPHY

Despite its inability to circumvent air and calcium, sonography is extraordinarily useful in the evaluation of patients with GI symptoms. In addition to spectral Doppler, color Doppler, and so-called power Doppler, advances in equipment now allow the recording of motion cine images on an electronic picture-archiving system; harmonic imaging, which can be helpful in delineating echo-free structures; extended field of view imaging, which can outline large structures and masses on a single image; and three-dimensional capability.

The primary role of sonography in the diagnosis of pyloric stenosis has been firmly established. Sonography is also extremely useful in the assessment of patients with clinically equivocal symptoms of appendicitis (Fig. 106-2), although this setting underscores sonography's well-known operator dependence, with published sensitivity ranging between 40% and 100%. The major advantage of sonography over CT is the lack of ionizing radiation. Sonography is also extremely useful in the evaluation of mesenteric adenopathy (Fig. 106-3), the bowel wall (Fig. 106-4), small and large bowel intussusception (Fig. 106-5), and, coupled with Doppler, disease activity in patients with Crohn disease.

The role of sonography in the diagnosis of solid organ pathology is extensive, and it can be the final diagnostic tool in many abnormalities affecting the solid abdominal viscera. Sonographic detail is particularly good in young children, in whom high-frequency and linear transducers can be used to access even the deeper abdominal structures. Biliary tract abnormalities—either congenital, such as choledochal cyst, or acquired, such as gallstones—are ideally evaluated with sonography. The examination is accurate, rapid, and accomplished with relative ease. Liver masses can be evaluated with sonography, although in the case of malignant disease, CT is typically performed. Nevertheless, sonography may be the initial modality used to investigate the patient's symptoms, and the CT protocol can be tailored based on the sonographic findings. The sonographic characteristics and location of a mass can be evaluated by localization of adjacent hepatic vasculature, and real-time evaluation of movement with respiration can help determine the origin of a large mass.

Although vascular structures are easily seen with contrasted CT, the direction and velocity of flow can be evaluated with Doppler sonography, and the findings in these two modalities are often complementary. Analysis of waveform patterns can identify hepatofugal flow in collateral vessels in patients with portal hypertension, as well as vascular stenosis or thrombus. In patients with heterotaxy, abdominal sonography is helpful in assessing the splenic mass located along the greater curvature of the stomach (see Fig. 119-7 in Chapter 119) and associated vascular anomalies, such as interruption of the inferior vena cava, preduodenal portal vein, and infra-

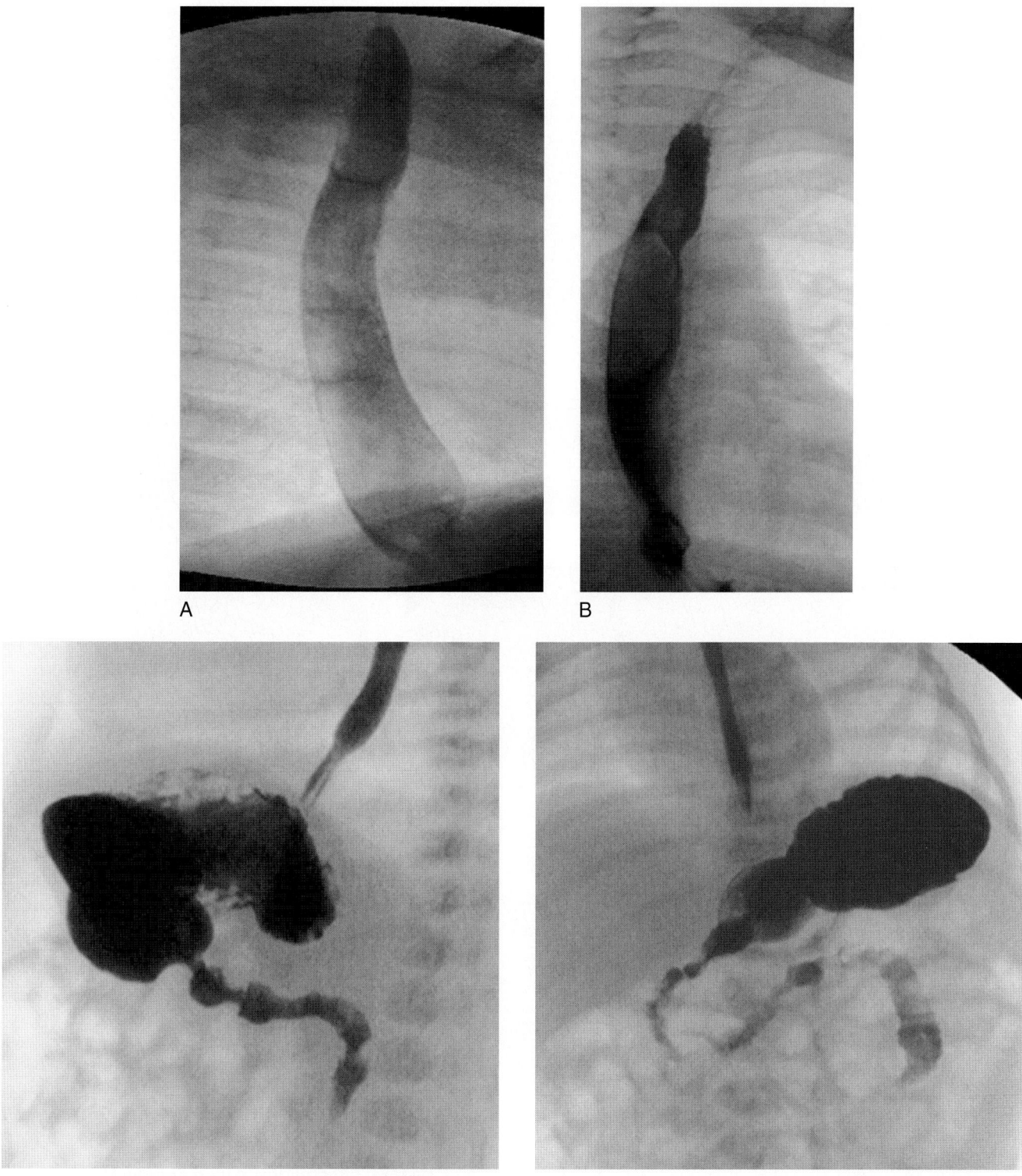

FIGURE 106-1. Typical upper gastrointestinal examination shows reflux in an otherwise normal infant. **A** and **B,** Lateral **(A)** and anteroposterior **(B)** views of the esophagus during drinking show full distensibility without intrinsinc or extrinsic mass lesions. **C,** Right anterior oblique imaging directs barium to the gastric outlet and shows prompt emptying and a normal pylorus and first and second portions of the duodenum. **D,** Anteroposterior image immediately following **C** shows the progress of contrast material to the normally located gastroduodenal junction at the ligament of Treitz. *Continued*

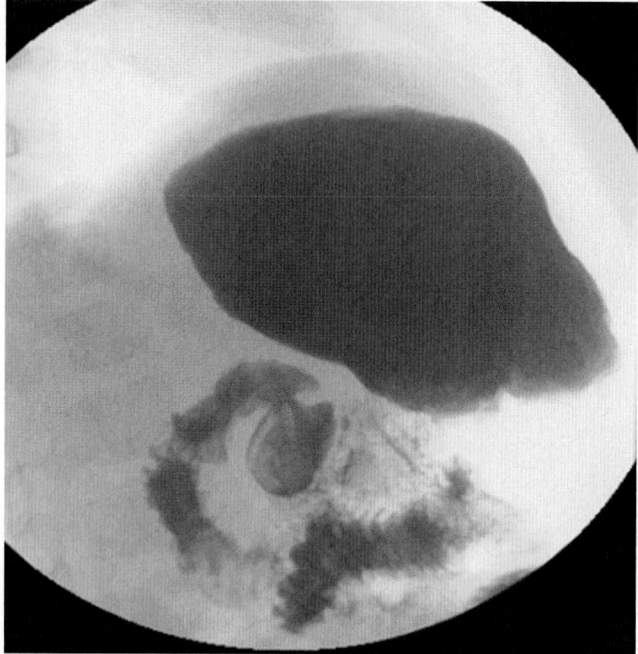

E

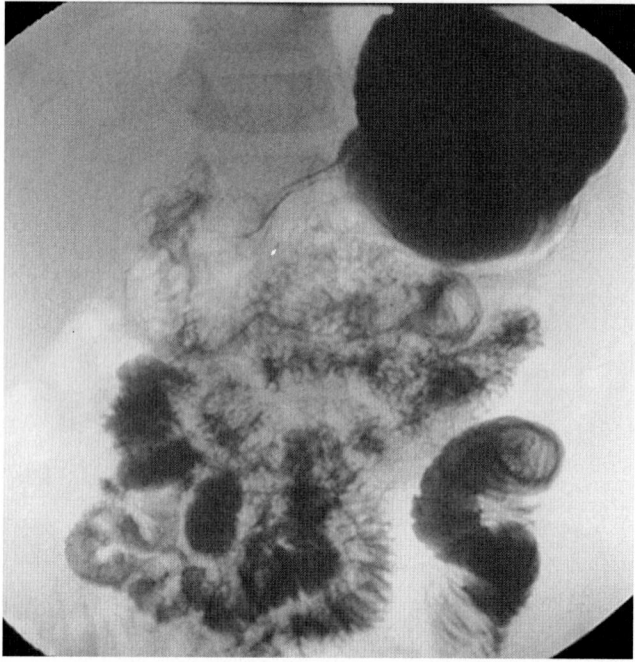

G

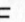

F

FIGURE 106-1, *cont'd.*
Typical upper gastrointestinal examination shows reflux in an otherwise normal infant. **E,** Subsequent lateral view of duodenum shows its posterior location anterior to the spine. **F,** After further drinking and gastric filling, an episode of reflux to the cervical esophagus is documented. Note the wide-open gastroesophageal junction, which is typical during reflux. **G,** Image recorded at the completion of the study shows good progress of contrast material through the small bowel.

diaphragmatic total anomalous pulmonary venous connection (Fig. 106-6).

Common indications for sonography of the GI tract:
- Bowel: pyloric stenosis, appendicitis, inflammatory bowel disease, intussusception
- Liver: masses, infection, biliary disease, congenital anomalies
- Spleen: heterotaxy, masses, wandering spleen

- Pancreas: pancreatitis, pancreatic ductal dilation, masses
- Doppler: portal hypertension, portosystemic shunt, congenital malformations

COMPUTED TOMOGRAPHY

CT is a particularly useful modality in pediatric abdominal imaging. The introduction of scanners with multichannel technology (16, 32, and 64 detectors)

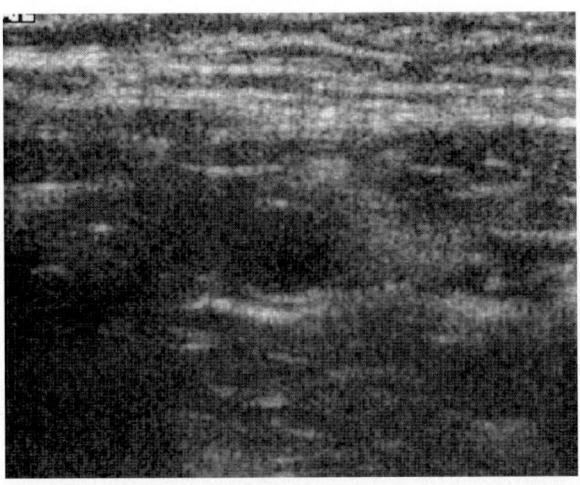 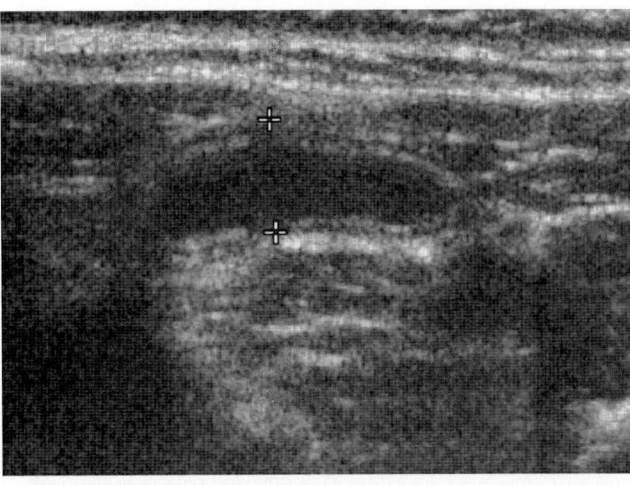

FIGURE 106-2. Appendicitis. Transverse **(A)** and longitudinal **(B)** images of unruptured appendicitis. The appendix measures 8 mm in diameter and is fluid filled, with an intact hyperechoic mucosal layer.

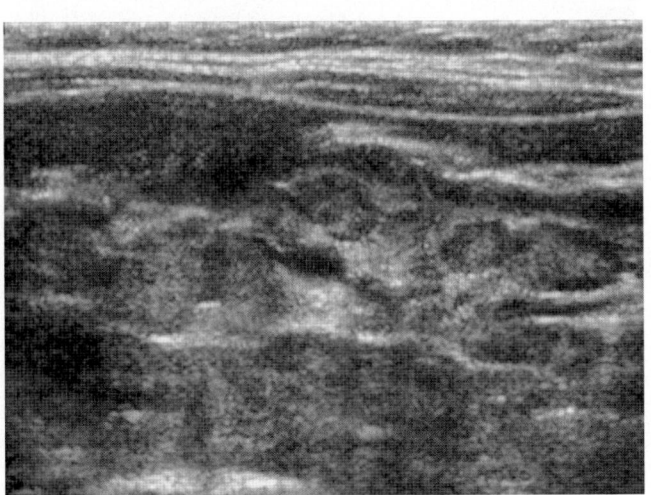 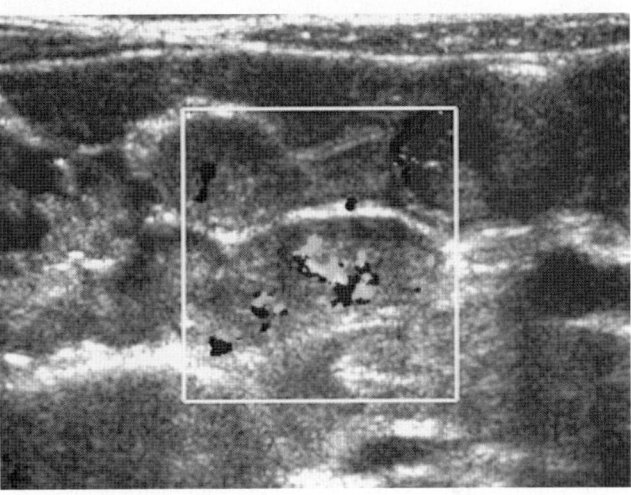

FIGURE 106-3. Mesenteric adenopathy. **A,** Transverse image through the right lower quadrant with a linear transducer shows multiple enlarged mesenteric nodes in an 8-month-old child with gastroenteritis. **B,** Doppler interrogation reveals flow into the nodal hila.

permits rapid examinations with isotropic reconstructions in multiple orthogonal and curved planes, in many cases without the need for sedation. These new capabilities, however, require new protocols to accommodate the more complex and sophisticated diagnostic methods. For instance, the timing and rate of contrast administration, with the ability to scan during a specific phase of intravascular contrast distribution, demand attention to technical details and new approaches to image interpretation. The pediatric radiologist is further challenged by the need to balance image detail with radiation dose and implementation of the ALARA (as low as reasonably achievable) concept.

The administration of intravenous contrast agents is extremely important to obtain diagnostic images, particularly in pediatric patients, in whom the paucity of intra-abdominal fat decreases the intrinsic contrast. The type of contrast agents used and their dosages are similar to those outlined in Chapter 107. Precontrast images are seldom necessary; they generally increase the radiation

dose without providing additional diagnostic information. If precontrast images are necessary (e.g., to identify calcifications in an abdominal mass), the radiation dose delivered can be decreased significantly, to one third or less of the diagnostic contrasted scan. The use of oral contrast material is important when outlining intraperitoneal pathology, such as an abscess or mass. In the evaluation of the bowel, the use of oral contrast agents is more controversial; it is important to bear in mind that positive oral contrast material masks mucosal enhancement, and water-density contrast may be more appropriate in such cases. We review images at 3-mm collimation in most patients, and at 2-mm collimation in infants. When reformats are needed, 50% overlap of the data set is essential to obtain good image quality.

Unlike sonography, CT images are sequential, standardized, and much less operator dependent. Therefore, CT is particularly useful in patients with complex disease affecting multiple organ systems, such as malignancies, and it provides reliable monitoring of changes in the

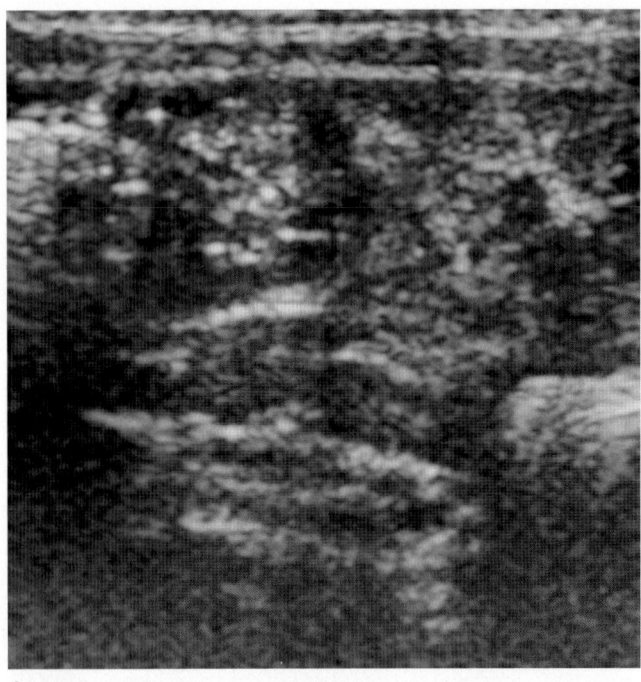

A

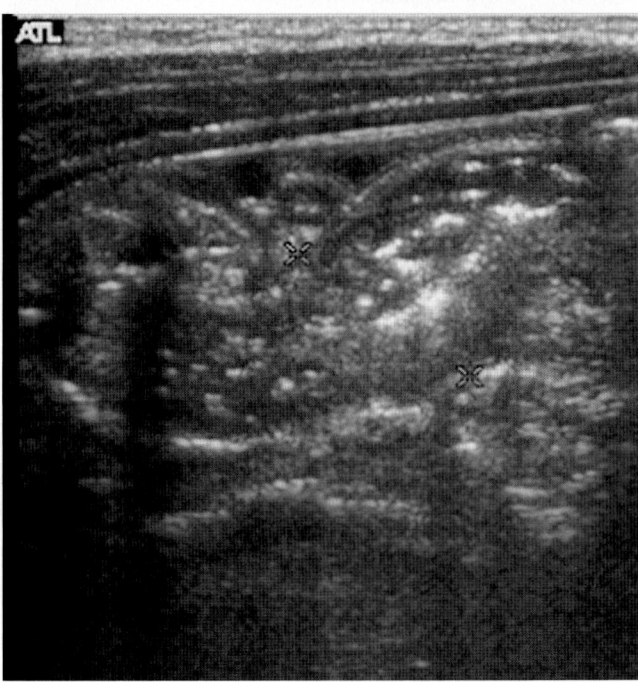

B

C

FIGURE 106-4. Normal right lower quadrant. **A,** Transverse image through right lower quadrant shows normal, collapsed loops of small bowel. **B,** Transverse image through the right lower quadrant in an infant with gastroenteritis shows several fluid-filled, moderately distended loops of bowel (*cross hairs*). **C,** Transverse image through the right lower quadrant in the same infant as in **B** shows a fluid-filled, distended terminal ileum at the ileocecal valve. The normal appendix is seen in cross section anterior to the terminal ileum.

extent of disease during therapy and follow-up. CT is also a good problem-solving technique in patients with unusual multiorgan abnormalities (Figs. 106-7 and 106-8). The evaluation of solid organ pathology, such as hepatic portal hypertension, trauma, pancreatitis, and tumors, is rapidly accomplished and results in extensive anatomic detail and physiologic information. CT is also widely and successfully applied to pathology of the hollow viscera and peritoneal cavity. The lack of operator dependence and high sensitivity and specificity in the diagnosis of appendicitis has led to the increasing use of CT in cases that are clinically equivocal. CT is also helpful in the evaluation of patients with inflammatory bowel disease, such as Crohn disease; it identifies areas of bowel wall thickening, enhancement, and abscess, although it does not provide the mucosal detail of fluoroscopy and spot films.

> **Common indications for CT of the GI tract:**
> - **Trauma**
> - **Masses, particularly malignant disease**
> - **Peritoneal disease: abscess, tumor, loculated collections**
> - **Complications of inflammatory bowel disease**

NUCLEAR MEDICINE

Nuclear medicine plays a significant role in the evaluation of hepatobiliary dysfunction and disorders of the GI tract in infants and children. It has clinical applications for both the pediatrician and the pediatric surgeon in daily, routine practice. Although some of the

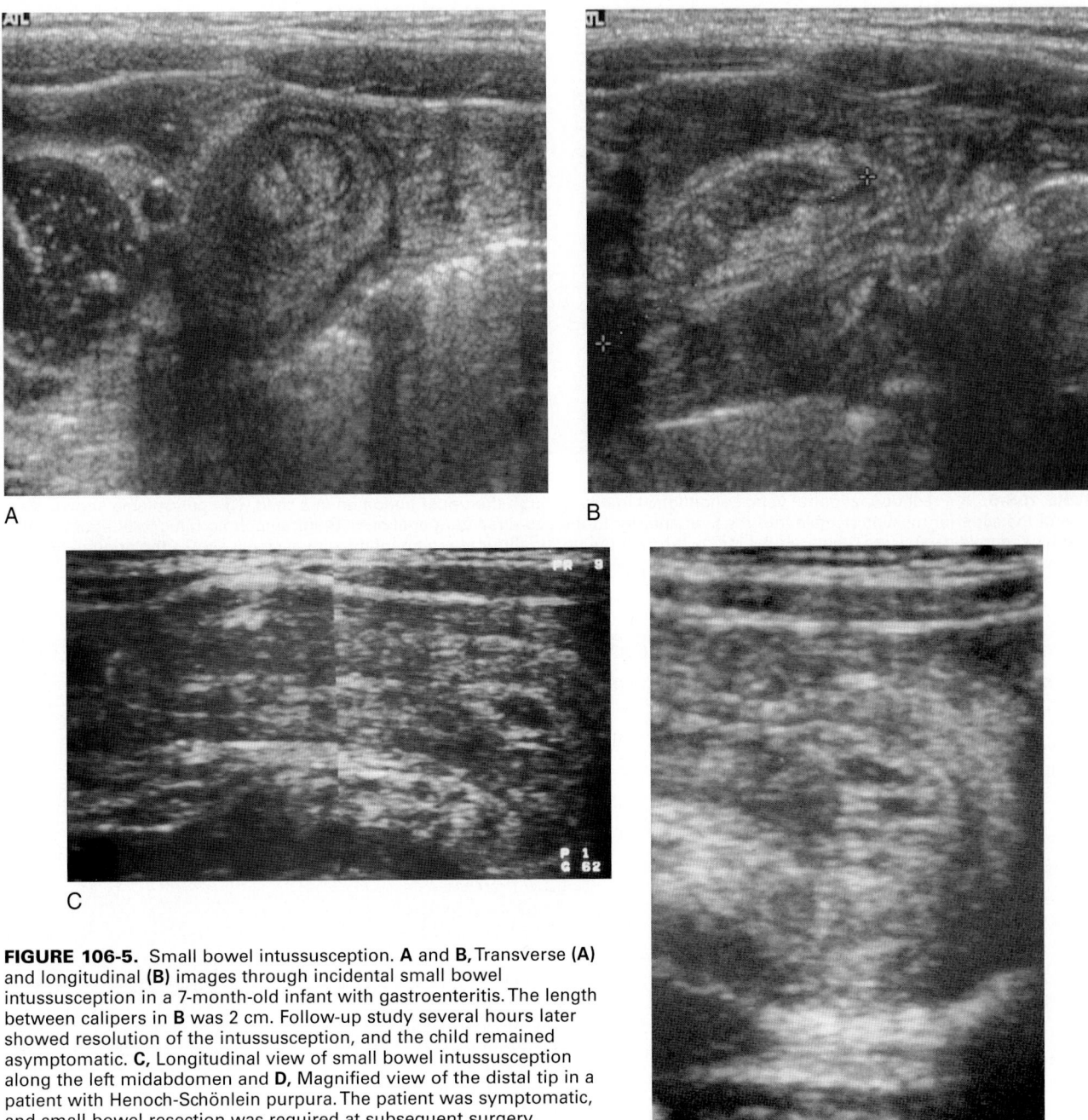

FIGURE 106-5. Small bowel intussusception. **A** and **B,** Transverse **(A)** and longitudinal **(B)** images through incidental small bowel intussusception in a 7-month-old infant with gastroenteritis. The length between calipers in **B** was 2 cm. Follow-up study several hours later showed resolution of the intussusception, and the child remained asymptomatic. **C,** Longitudinal view of small bowel intussusception along the left midabdomen and **D,** Magnified view of the distal tip in a patient with Henoch-Schönlein purpura. The patient was symptomatic, and small bowel resection was required at subsequent surgery.

studies offer unique diagnostic information, others provide functional information complementary to that obtained with sonography, CT, MRI, and routine contrast-enhanced fluoroscopy.

Radionuclide imaging of the GI system can be divided into two categories: imaging of the hepatobiliary system and spleen (Table 106-2), and imaging of the GI tract (Table 106-3). Hepatobiliary scintigraphy provides an anatomic and dynamic physiologic evaluation of biliary function. GI scintigraphy allows the dynamic assessment of swallowing, gastric emptying, gastroesophageal reflux, and aspiration. In addition, the in vivo or in vitro radiolabeling of the child's red blood cells allows the anatomic localization of intestinal bleeding, and the

labeling of white blood cells can be used for the localization of sites of abdominal infection.

The radionuclide used in all studies is technetium-99m (Tc-99m), which is administered either intravenously or orally, usually combined with a nonradioactive compound (pharmaceutical). The resulting radiopharmaceutical (e.g., Tc-99m sulfur colloid) is directed to the target tissue (e.g., reticuloendothelial system of the liver, spleen, and bone marrow), which can be visualized with the use of a gamma camera. Pediatric radiopharmaceutical dosage is carefully calculated on the basis of either body surface area or weight. Standard imaging parameters vary, but children are usually imaged in the supine position with either a single-head

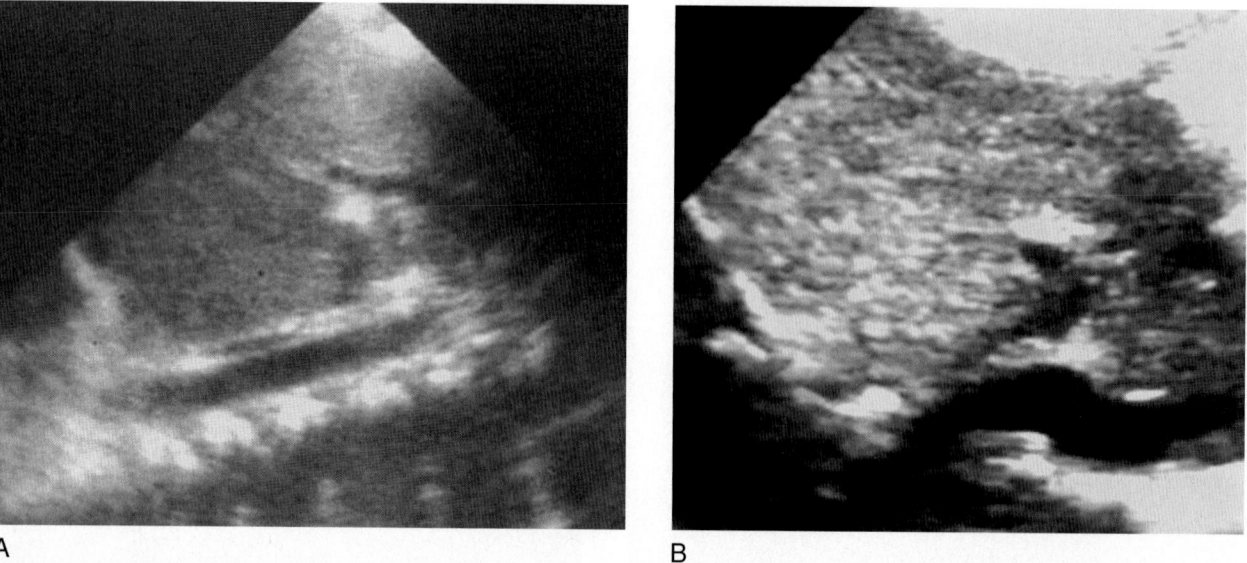

A

B

FIGURE 106-6. A, Preduodenal portal vein. Longitudinal image through the upper abdomen in a child with polysplenia shows the course of the superior mesenteric vein into the liver anterior to the gas-filled duodenal bulb. **B,** Infradiaphragmatic total anomalous pulmonary venous connection. Longitudinal image through the upper abdomen in an infant with asplenia shows the anomalous vessel entering the abdomen from the chest at the esophageal hiatus.

TABLE 106-2

Radionuclide Imaging of the Liver, Biliary System, and Spleen

Study	Radiopharmaceutical	Indication
Hepatobiliary scan	Tc-99m IDA	Hepatitis
		Biliary atresia
		Choledochal cyst
		Acute cholecystitis
		Bile plug syndrome
		Caroli disease
		Trauma—bile leak
		Liver transplantation
		Assess vascularity, parenchymal function
		Evaluate bile drainage, possible bile leak, possible obstruction
Liver-spleen scan	Tc-99m sulfur colloid	Hepatitis
		Hepatic mass (e.g., FNH)
		Diffuse hepatic disease
		Abnormal LFTs
		Congenital abnormalities
		Diaphragmatic hernia
		Splenogonadal fusion
		Wandering spleen
		Ectopic or accessory spleen
		Functional asplenia
Hemangioma scan	Tc-99m–labeled RBCs	Liver hemangioma
Splenic sequestration scan	Tc-99m–labeled, heat-damaged RBCs	Hypersplenism

FNH, focal nodular hyperplasia; LFT, liver function test; RBC, red blood cell; Tc, technetium.

or dual-head gamma camera, using a low-energy all-purpose collimator or a low-energy high-resolution collimator. Correct anatomic positioning is essential, and some type of restraint is usually required, even with co-operative children. Rarely, patient sedation is necessary for lengthy examinations. Some of the studies discussed in this section require a period of fasting before imaging.

Hepatobiliary Scintigraphy

Hepatobiliary scintigraphy is a useful adjunct to sonography in the evaluation of infants with jaundice and older children with hyperbilirubinemia. This study is also useful in assessing the patency of the cystic duct in children with suspected acute cholecystitis. Other

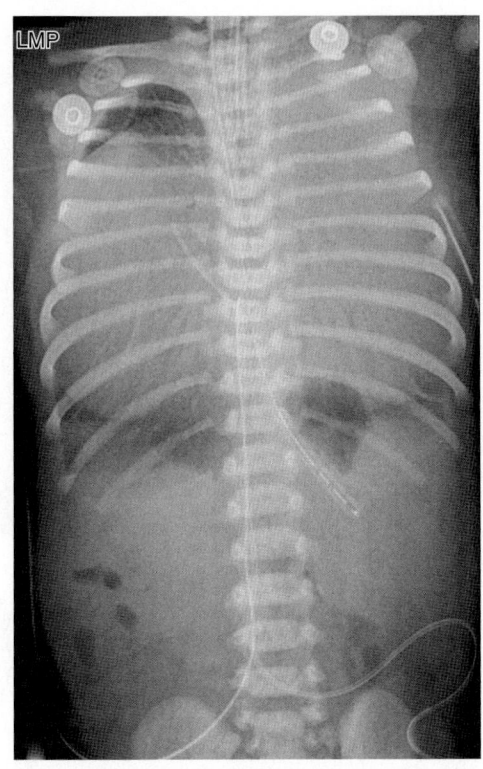

A

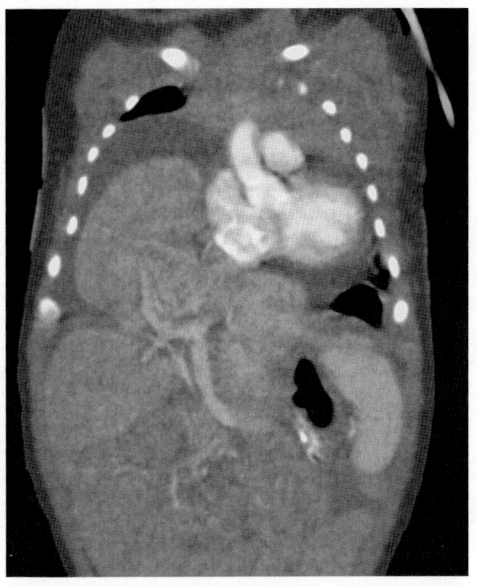

B

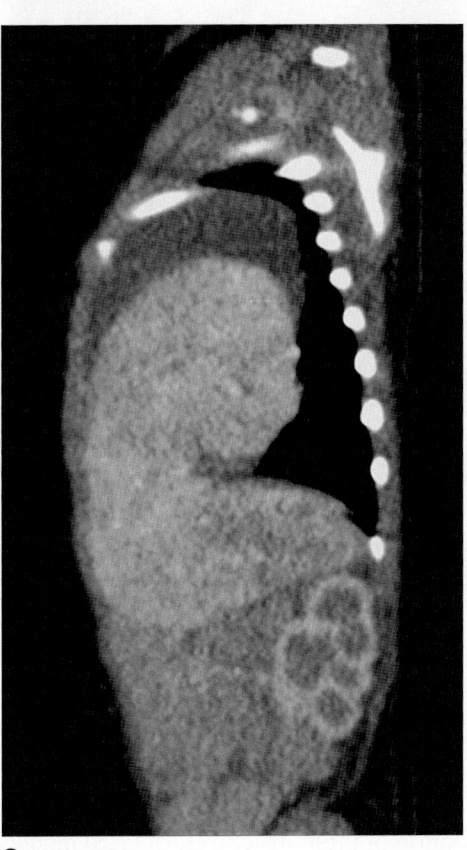

C

FIGURE 106-7. Unusual presentation of Morgagni hernia. **A,** Abdominopelvic radiograph of a newborn infant with the prenatal diagnosis of hydrothorax. The radiograph suggests the absence of most of the liver shadow from the right upper quadrant. The posterior costophrenic sulci are well outlined, indicating that chest density is not related to bilateral hydrothorax. **B** and **C,** Coronal (**B**) and sagittal (**C**) reformats of contrasted CT outline an intrapericardial foramen of Morgagni hernia and hepatic herniation.

clinical indications are listed in Table 106-2. Its value in jaundiced neonates is the timely differentiation of neonatal hepatitis and biliary atresia, because surgical intervention with the Kasai procedure in patients with biliary atresia is most successful when performed early in life.

Premedication with phenobarbital (5 mg/kg per day for 5 days) was reported by Majd and coworkers to improve hepatic extraction of tracer. The child should fast for 2 to 4 hours; prolonged fasting is not recommended.

Radiopharmaceuticals used for hepatobiliary imaging are Tc-99m–labeled iminodiacetic acid derivatives. Those with the highest hepatic extraction, such as disofenin or mebrofenin, are preferred. Currently, Tc-99m mebrofenin is widely used for hepatobiliary imaging because it has a higher hepatic extraction (98%) than disofenin (88%). The radiopharmaceutical is administered intravenously, and static images of the abdomen are acquired in the supine position every 5 minutes for 30 minutes. The radiopharmaceutical is transported into the hepato-

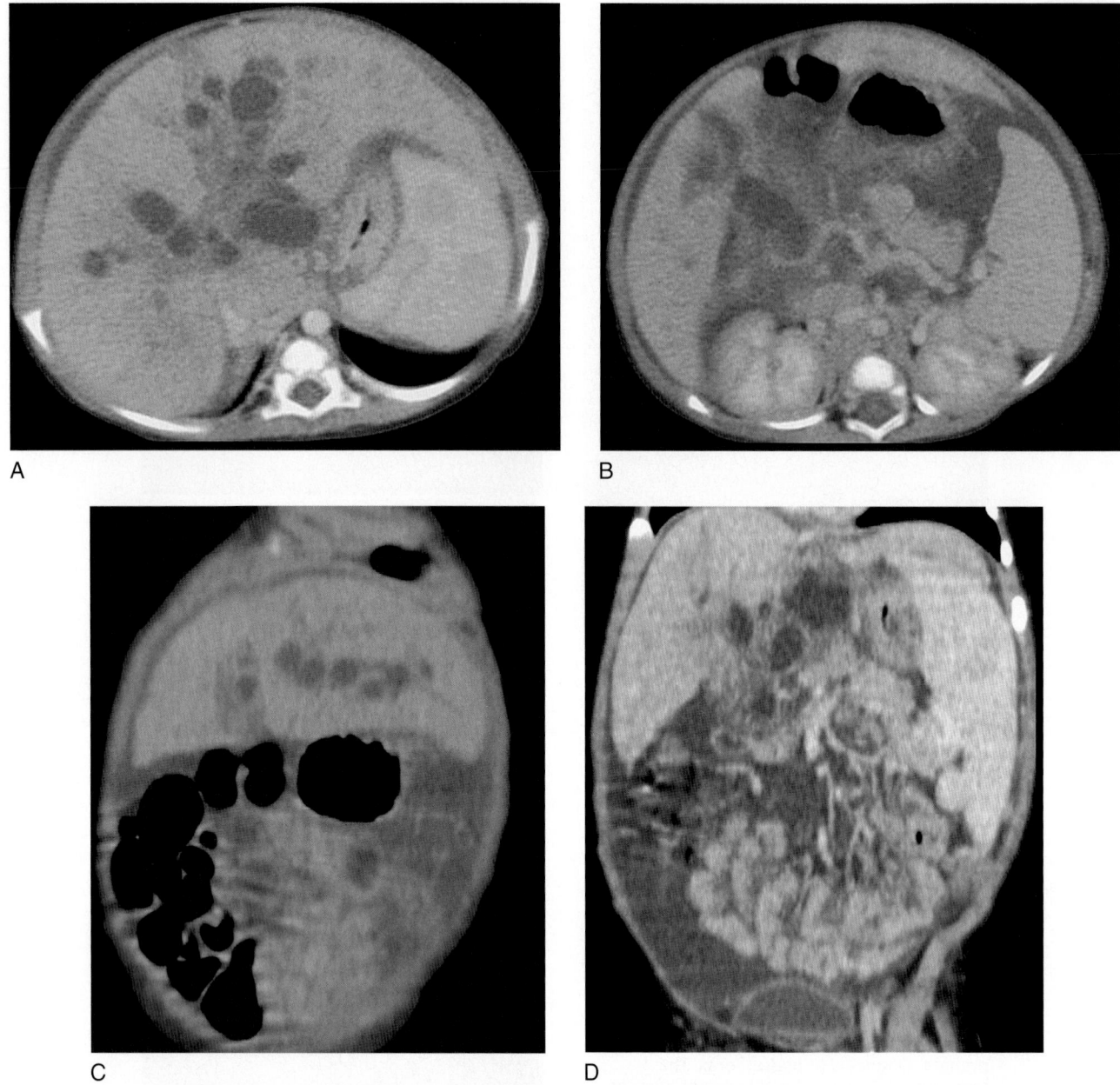

FIGURE 106-8. Choledochal cyst with intrahepatic ductal dilation and absence of the portal vein. **A** and **B,** Axial contrasted CT images through the liver and porta hepatis outline intrahepatic cystic dilation of the biliary tree (Caroli disease) and cystic dilation of the common bile duct at the porta hepatis in **B. C** and **D,** Coronal reconstructions better define the cystic intrahepatic ductal dilation, absence of the portal vein, and splenomegaly.

cytes and then excreted with bile into the bile ducts, allowing visualization of these structures. Delayed images may be obtained at 45 minutes, 60 minutes, and up to 24 hours, as necessary, to visualize the gallbladder and biliary tree and excretion into the duodenum.

A normal scan typically demonstrates radiopharmaceutical uptake in the liver by 5 minutes, the biliary tree by 15 minutes, and the small bowel by 15 to 45 minutes (Fig. 106-9). Renal and urinary bladder activity is normal as well. In *neonatal hepatitis,* there is delayed and diminished uptake by the liver, but the radiopharmaceutical eventually reaches the small bowel. Liver uptake can also be diminished with prolonged cholestasis from long-term total parenteral nutrition administration and bile

plug syndrome, other forms of hepatocellular dysfunction, and biliary atresia. In *biliary atresia,* radiopharmaceutical uptake by the liver is usually adequate, but the radiotracer never reaches the bowel, even on delayed 24-hour images (Fig. 106-10).

Choledochal cysts present with a classic triad of jaundice, pain, and abdominal mass, although this triad is present in a minority of patients; older children may present with pancreatitis. Imaging with sonography, CT, and MRI is frequently diagnostic, but hepatobiliary imaging is a useful adjunct. Initial images reveal a rounded focus of photopenia near the medial aspect of the liver, with delayed accumulation of the radiopharmaceutical within the initial photopenic area. *Acute cholecystitis* is charac-

TABLE 106-3

Radionuclide Imaging of the Gastrointestinal Tract

Study	Radiopharmaceutical	Indication
GE reflux	Tc-99m sulfur colloid	Gastric regurgitation Early satiety Recurrent pneumonia Pulmonary aspiration Preoperative: Nissen fundoplication, gastrostomy tube
Salivagram	Tc-99m sulfur colloid	Pulmonary aspiration
Meckel scan	Tc-99m pertechnetate	GI bleeding
GI bleeding (labeled RBCs)	Tc-99m pertechnetate	GI bleeding Asplenia
Infection (labeled WBCs)	Tc-99m HMPAO	Inflammatory bowel disease Appendicitis Abscess

GE, gastroesophageal; GI, gastrointestinal; RBC, red blood cell; Tc, technetium; WBC, white blood cell.

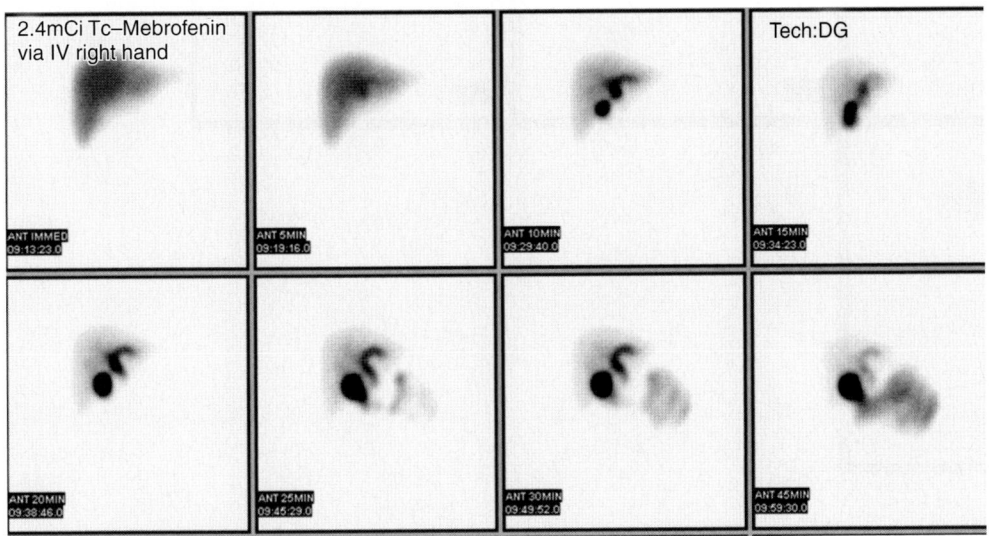

FIGURE 106-9. Normal hepatobiliary study in a 5-year-old with right upper abdominal pain. Anterior static images of the abdomen were obtained every 5 minutes for 60 minutes following the intravenous administration of technetium-99m mebrofenin. There is homogeneous radiotracer accumulation throughout the liver, with prompt visualization of the intrahepatic ducts by 5 minutes, common bile duct and gallbladder by 10 minutes, and small bowel by 25 minutes.

terized scintigraphically by prompt hepatic extraction and excretion into the biliary system and bowel, but lack of gallbladder visualization.

Liver-Spleen Scintigraphy

With the advent of sonography, CT, and MRI and the improved technical quality of cross-sectional abdominal imaging studies, the liver-spleen scan is seldom used. These other modalities exhibit far greater spatial and contrast resolution and provide more precise anatomic details of the liver and spleen. However, there are still several important indications for the liver-spleen scan, including the evaluation of congenital anomalies, such as the location of accessory or ectopic spleens; the evaluation of functional asplenia; the functional evaluation of hepatitis and cirrhosis; and the diagnostic differentiation of certain hepatic masses, such as focal nodular hyperplasia (see Table 106-2). Some authors have reported its utility in the assessment of children with heterotaxy syndrome; however, differentiating a normal abdominal situs from asplenia with a midline, transverse

liver extending into both upper quadrants or a prominent left hepatic lobe can be difficult when the splenic fossa is occupied by liver tissue. This distinction is better made by CT or MRI. Scintigraphically, evaluation of a transverse liver or functional asplenia is better documented with Tc-99m–labeled, heat-damaged red blood cell imaging.

No patient preparation is necessary for the liver-spleen scan. The child receives an intravenous injection of Tc-99m sulfur colloid, and static images are obtained from multiple projections approximately 15 minutes after injection, with the child lying supine. Dynamic images may also be acquired, depending on the clinical indication.

The physiologic basis of this study is the phagocytosis of radioactive colloid particles by the reticuloendothelial cells of the liver, spleen, and bone marrow. Normal images reveal homogeneous distribution of the radiopharmaceutical in the liver and spleen, which can be evaluated for size, position, configuration, and any focal areas of radiotracer deficit. (See Fig. 119-5 in Chapter 119, which shows the splenogonadal fusion anomaly imaged with Tc-99m sulfur colloid.)

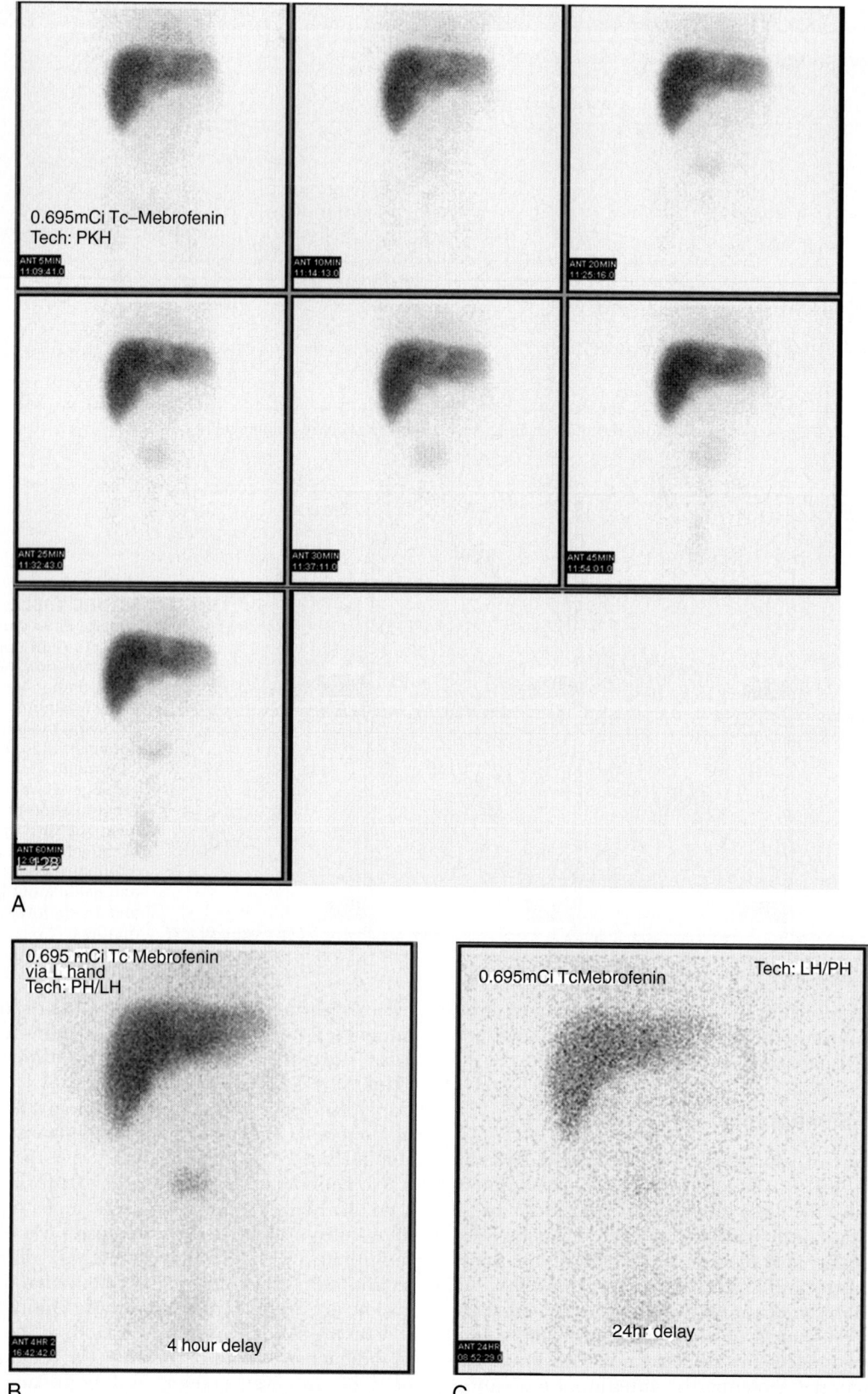

FIGURE 106-10. Biliary atresia in an 8-week-old infant with jaundice and conjugated hyperbilirubinemia. Technetium-99m mebrofenin biliary scintigraphy shows good hepatic extraction of the radiotracer, nonvisualization of the biliary system, and no evidence of radiotracer passage into the bowel. Anterior projection images are shown at 0 to 60 minutes **(A)**, 4 hours **(B)**, and 24 hours **(C)**. All images reveal normal, faint radiopharmaceutical accumulation in the urinary bladder.

In children with hepatitis, the liver-spleen scan may be normal. However, when abnormal, the images may demonstrate hepatomegaly, heterogeneous radiotracer accumulation, or hepatosplenomegaly. When hepatic disease is severe, there is a redistribution of the colloidal radiotracer, with diminished uptake by the liver, greater than normal uptake by the spleen, and visualization of the bone marrow ("colloid shift").

Splenic Sequestration Scintigraphy

Splenic sequestration scintigraphy is used in children with hypersplenism, which results in acceleration of the normal sequestration and phagocytosis of abnormal erythrocytes, neutrophils, and platelets. The child receives an intravenous injection of Tc-99m–labeled, heat-damaged red blood cells. Diagnostic images reveal rapid clearance of the radiolabeled red blood cells from the blood pool and greater than normal splenic uptake.

Gastrointestinal Tract Scintigraphy

Radionuclide imaging of the GI tract is a sophisticated, systematic technique that allows anatomic and functional imaging of the esophagus and stomach, with evaluation of gastroesophageal reflux, secondary pulmonary aspiration, and gastric emptying. Anatomic location of GI bleeding or GI infection can be accomplished with dynamic imaging of the entire GI tract. These studies are usually more sensitive than conventional radiographic and fluoroscopic studies because dynamic, uninterrupted imaging can be performed for longer periods and with less radiation exposure.

> GI scintigraphy involves less radiation exposure to the child than conventional radiography and fluoroscopy, and the physiologic information obtained complements the anatomic information provided by radiography.

GASTROESOPHAGEAL REFLUX SCINTIGRAPHY

Gastroesophageal reflux in infants and young children manifests clinically with vomiting and failure to thrive; it is associated with recurrent bronchitis and pneumonia, peripheral airway disease, esophagitis, and GI bleeding. Radionuclide imaging can detect and quantify gastroesophageal reflux, as well as pulmonary aspiration. The sensitivity is greater than with conventional barium fluoroscopy because the chest and abdomen are monitored continuously without additional radiation exposure. The only disadvantage is the lack of resolution compared with that provided by conventional radiography.

Patient preparation requires fasting for 2 to 4 hours. A radiolabeled liquid or solid meal is administered using Tc-99m sulfur colloid. Infants can be fed infant formula or saved breast milk. The child is then placed supine, and a computer acquisition is immediately obtained dynamically at 60 seconds/image for 30 minutes. At our institution, we image 15 minutes in the supine position, followed by 15 minutes in the prone position. A 3- to 4-hour delayed image over the lungs is then obtained to evaluate for pulmonary aspiration.

A normal study shows the radiopharmaceutical in the stomach, but no activity in the esophagus or lungs. If reflux is detected, the number of episodes is counted over the entire imaging period. Additional imaging of the chest with a transmission scan is useful to detect pulmonary aspiration (Fig. 106-11).

Gastric Emptying Scintigraphy

Gastric emptying imaging is useful in the evaluation of early satiety, bloating, or abdominal pain and for the preoperative assessment of children with reflux undergoing Nissen fundoplication and gastrostomy tube placement. The gastric emptying study can be performed with a liquid or solid meal. Liquid gastric emptying studies can be performed in combination with a gastroesophageal reflux study. When performed separately, images are obtained in the left anterior oblique position for 90 to 120 minutes. When performed in combination with the gastroesophageal reflux study, images are obtained with a dual-head camera in the anterior and posterior projections in the supine position only. In the case illustrated in Figure 106-11, we imaged every 2 minutes for 16 minutes, then every 10 minutes for 60 minutes, then every 10 minutes for another 30 to 60 minutes, until much of the gastric activity had ceased. The child can move between images, but walking about is discouraged.

A normal study reveals radiotracer in the stomach on the initial images, followed by progressive emptying of the stomach. Computer processing is performed by drawing a region of interest around the stomach at selected time points, to calculate fractional emptying. A time-activity curve is then generated and plotted on a linear scale using the geometric mean of the anterior and posterior counts (see Fig. 106-11). A half-time for emptying ($T_{1/2}$) is calculated: the length of time required for the initial number of counts to decrease by 50%. Normal values for gastric emptying cannot be readily established because of the ethical issues involved in studying normal subjects and because of the difficulty in standardizing imaging technique as well as the size and composition of the ingested meal. However, the time-activity curve should exhibit a continuous decline in activity over time. A study performed by Seibert and colleagues on patients with underlying diseases who were fed a radiolabeled milk formula revealed normal 60-minute gastric emptying values of 48% ± 16% in infants and 51% ± 7% in children (roughly, a gastric emptying $T_{1/2}$ of 60 minutes in each age group). A different study performed on normal infants who were fed radiolabeled milk demonstrated a $T_{1/2}$ of 87 ± 29 minutes. Normal values are typically established by each individual nuclear medicine laboratory or imaging department.

SALIVAGRAM

The salivagram allows the dynamic assessment of swallowing in patients suspected of having primary aspiration with feeding. It is often used in children who are unable to handle their secretions.

Fasting is not required. The child is positioned supine, and a small dose of Tc-99m sulfur colloid mixed

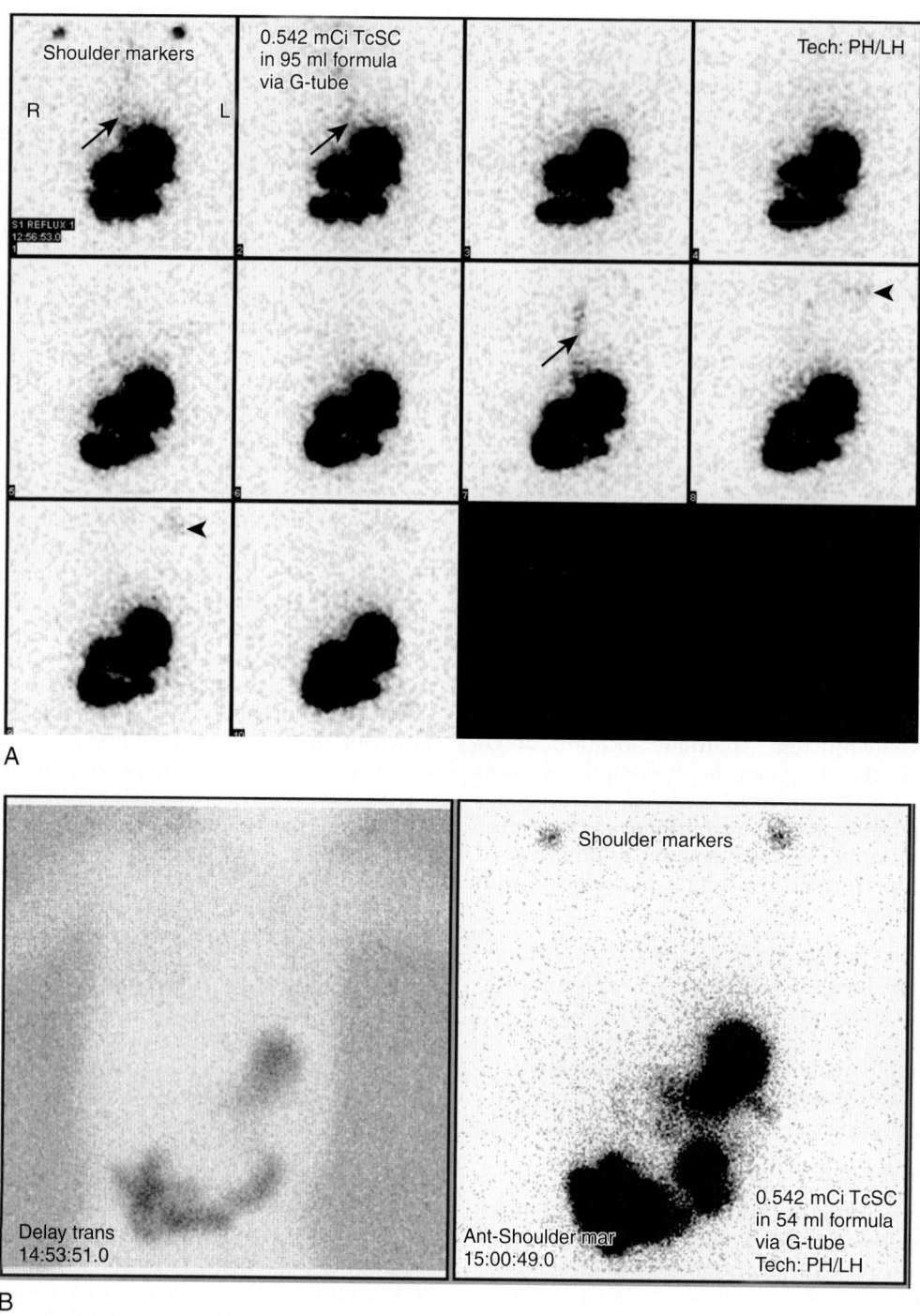

FIGURE 106-11. Combined gastroesophageal reflux and gastric emptying studies in a 1-year-old child with persistent emesis. **A,** Initial images of the chest and abdomen reveal three episodes of reflux (*arrows* in first, second, and seventh images), with subsequent visualization of radiopharmaceutical in the child's mouth (*arrowheads* in eighth and ninth images). **B,** Three-hour delayed transmission and routine images of the chest and upper abdomen reveal no pulmonary aspiration. *Continued*

in 0.1 to 0.5 ml of water or saline is placed on the anterior tongue and allowed to mix with oral secretions. Rapid dynamic images of the neck, chest, and upper abdomen are acquired from the posterior projection every 60 seconds for 1 hour. Static images are then obtained at 1 hour and 3 hours. Detection of any radiopharmaceutical in the tracheobronchial tree is abnormal (Fig. 106-12).

GASTROINTESTINAL BLEEDING SCINTIGRAPHY

Lower GI bleeding has many causes in infants and children, and the causes are largely age specific. Conventional fluoroscopy is indicated for the evaluation of suspected malrotation with midgut volvulus or bowel polyp or for the reduction of an intussusception. When these entities are excluded, radionuclide imaging is useful for the localization of a bleeding source. Tc-99m–

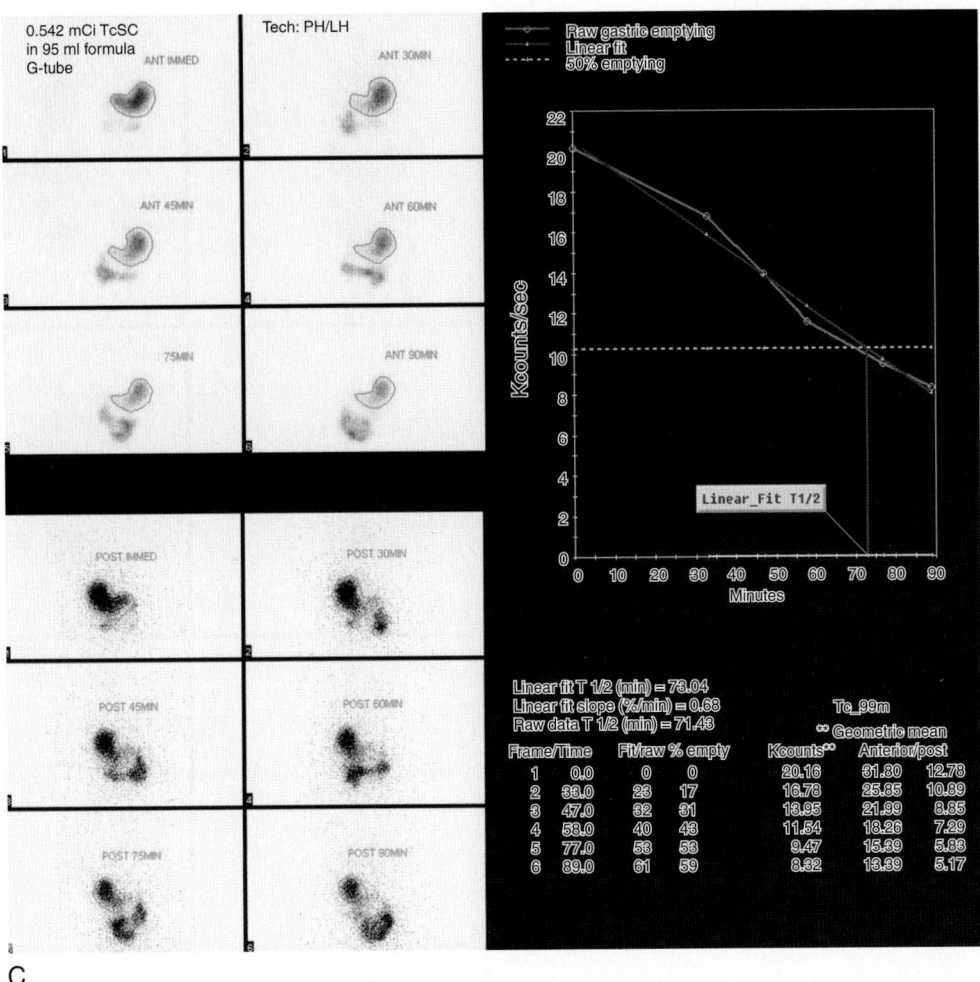

C

FIGURE 106-11, *cont'd.* Combined gastroesophageal reflux and gastric emptying studies in a 1-year-old child with persistent emesis. **C,** There is progressive gastric emptying. A time-activity curve constructed from regions of interest drawn around the stomach reveals a half-time for emptying of 73 minutes, which is within normal limits.

labeled red blood cells are useful in patients who are bleeding slowly or intermittently. In vitro labeling of the patient's red blood cells is usually performed with a technique that involves subsequent reinjection of the tagged autologous cells. The child is placed supine on the table, with the imaging camera positioned over the abdomen. Following a bolus intravenous injection of Tc-99m–labeled red blood cells, a dynamic flow study is performed for 1 minute, followed by a static image obtained every 5 minutes for 30 minutes. If the images do not immediately reveal bleeding, delayed images are obtained at 45 minutes and 60 minutes; they can be obtained up to 24 hours after injection. A cinematic display is also processed when bleeding is detected. A positive study reveals activity in a location and configuration consistent with bowel, displays progressively increased intensity over time, and exhibits movement through the GI tract over time.

An additional, infrequent use of Tc-99m–labeled red blood cells is the differentiation of hepatic tumor from hemangioma. After the intravenous administration of tagged red blood cells, the typical scintigraphic appearance of a hemangioma is the initial rapid appearance of radiotracer at the periphery of the lesion, with gradual internal accumulation over time. The same imaging concept applies to CT imaging of hemangiomas, with better anatomic resolution.

MECKEL SCINTIGRAPHY

Meckel diverticulum is a congenital anomaly resulting from incomplete closure of the omphalomesenteric duct; it is present in approximately 2% of the population. It is usually located approximately 2 feet from the ileocecal valve, on the antimesenteric border of the ileum. Most of these diverticula are asymptomatic and are lined by ileal mucosa. However, those that contain ectopic gastric mucosa are capable of producing hydrochloric acid and pepsin, thereby inducing ulceration of the gastric and adjacent ileal mucosa. Peptic ulceration causes acute GI hemorrhage in children, usually in the first 2 years of life. A Meckel diverticulum can be quite small, making evaluation by barium small bowel series difficult. The ectopic mucosa can be detected with scintigraphy because the radiopharmaceutical accumulates within the ectopic gastric mucosa and is therefore "hot" in contrast to the low-activity background of the normal small bowel. The Meckel scan is the study of choice for unexplained GI bleeding in children.

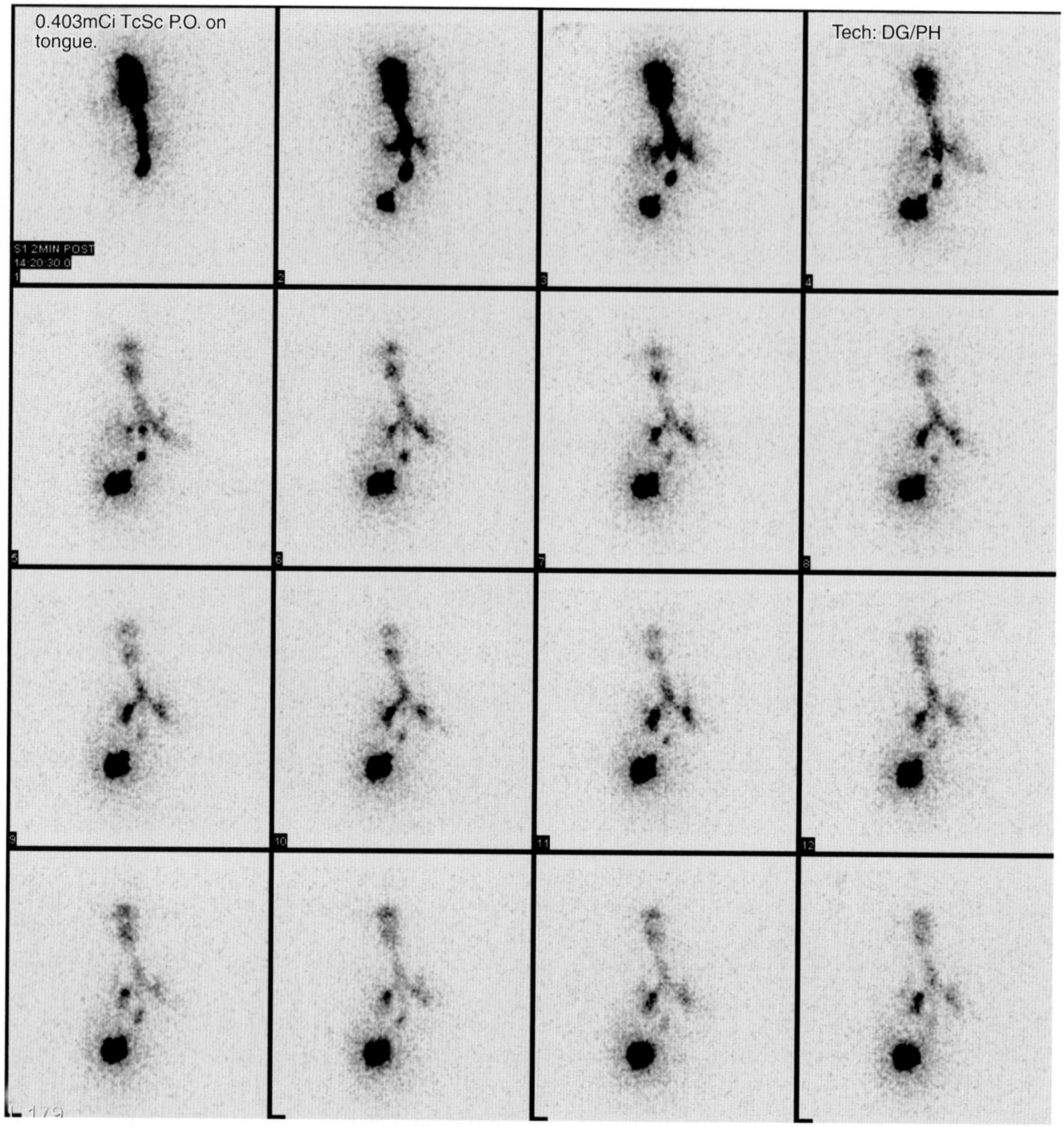

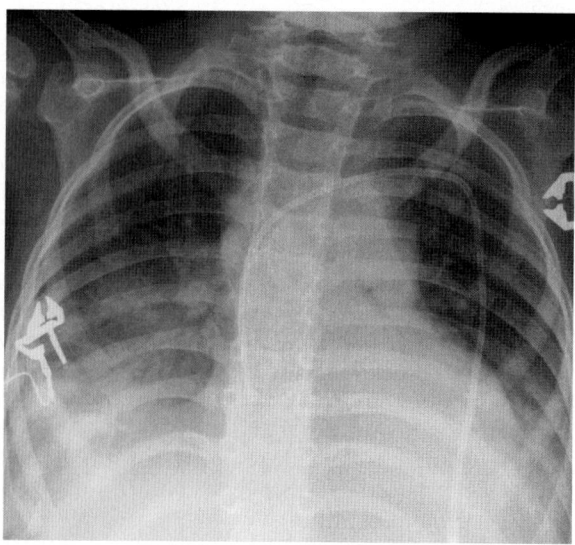

0.403mCi TcSc P.O. on tongue.
Tech: DG/PH
S1 2MIN POST
14:20:30.0
1
2
3
4
5
6
7
8
9
10
11
12

A

B

FIGURE 106-12. A, Radionuclide salivagram (posterior images) obtained in a child with recurrent pneumonia and neuromuscular incoordination demonstrates technetium-99m sulfur colloid outlining the tracheobronchial tree. Some swallowed radiopharmaceutical is seen in the stomach. **B,** Chest radiograph obtained the same day reveals bibasilar lung opacity.

The child is placed supine under the camera and receives an intravenous injection of Tc-99m pertechnetate. Multiple static anterior images of the abdomen are obtained for 30 minutes. A normal study reveals radiotracer accumulation in the stomach as well as the urinary bladder, sometimes with faint uptake by the kidneys. An abnormal study demonstrates accumulation of radiotracer in ectopic tissue simultaneously with the appearance of gastric mucosa, usually between 6 and 10 minutes after injection. The abnormality is usually a small, rounded focus of radiopharmaceutical uptake in the right lower abdomen (Fig. 106-13). An important differential diagnostic consideration is ectopic mucosa in a duplication cyst.

GASTROINTESTINAL INFLAMMATION AND INFECTION SCINTIGRAPHY

The radiopharmaceutical used is Tc-99m hexamethyl-propyleneamine oxime (HMPAO). In children, the minimal amount of blood needed for labeling is 10 to 15 ml, depending on the child's size and circulating leukocyte count. A normal study reveals uptake of the radio-labeled leukocytes by the liver, spleen, bone marrow, kidneys, and urinary bladder. Normal bowel activity due to hepatobiliary excretion is seen in 20% to 30% of children by 1 hour. Abnormal bowel activity may be seen in 15 to 30 minutes and usually increases in intensity over the next 2 to 3 hours. Focal abdominal activity identified outside of the liver, spleen, and bowel may indicate focal infection or an abscess; however, this finding should be correlated with cross-sectional imaging.

According to guidelines published by the Society of Nuclear Medicine, the indications for Tc-99m HMPAO–labeled leukocyte scintigraphy include the detection and determination of extent of inflammatory bowel disease. Charron and associates have published data suggesting that Tc-99m HMPAO–labeled leukocyte imaging is superior to contrast radiology for assessing the extent and activity of inflammatory bowel disease. The utility of this study as an initial screening modality in children suspected of having inflammatory bowel disease is controversial, however. Charron and associates reported a sensitivity of 94% compared with colonoscopy; however, Grahnquist and colleagues found a lower sensitivity of 75%, with a low negative predictive value of 50%.

MAGNETIC RESONANCE IMAGING

MRI is the most recent modality to be added to the radiologist's diagnostic tools, with additional applications paralleling the development of new imaging sequences and more efficient and specialized coils. The lack of ionizing radiation is a major advantage in pediatric patients; however, this is often counterbalanced by the length of the examination and the need for sedation in young children. Unlike multidetector CT, in which multiplanar imaging can be performed retrospectively after a single pass, each plane in MRI often necessitates an additional sequence. Motion artifacts, which can be considerable in children, particularly with respiratory motion along the anterior abdominal wall, can be ameliorated with appropriately placed saturation bands and changes in the direction of the phase-encoding gradient.

MRI is helpful in the evaluation of liver disease, particularly hepatic steatosis and hemochromatosis, as well as in patients with portal hypertension. Hepatic steatosis can result in impaired hepatocyte function and is commonly associated with obesity. Gradient echo sequences with in-phase and out-of-phase images demonstrate diminished hepatic signal on the out-of-phase images, by cancellation of the fat signal. MRI is extremely sensitive to iron because of its paramagnetic properties, with shortening of the T2 relaxation time; it is far

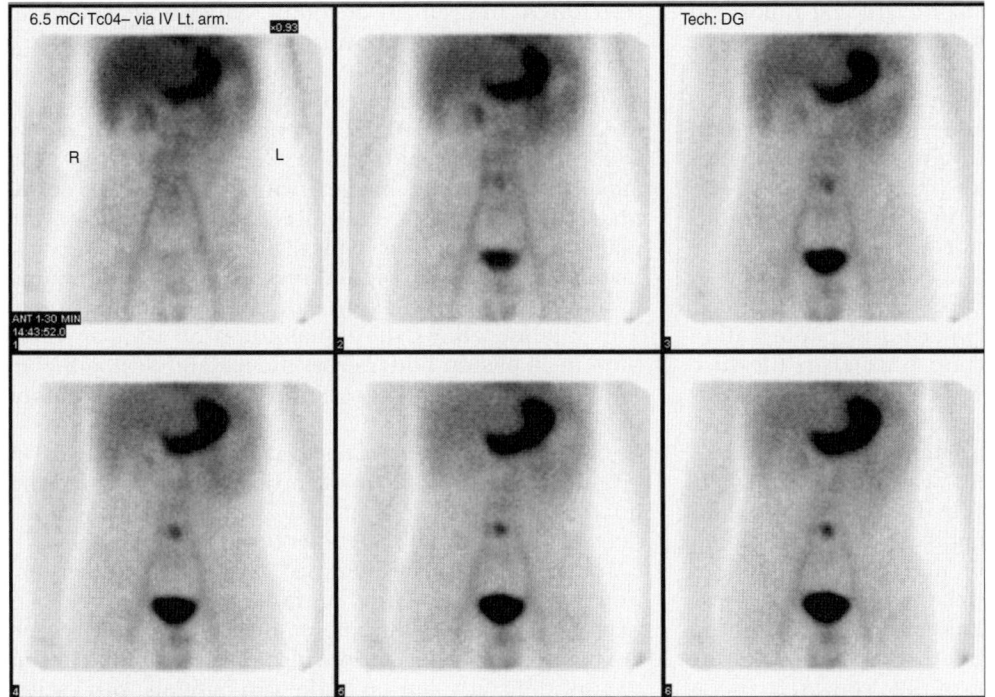

FIGURE 106-13. Meckel scan in an 11-year-old with lower gastrointestinal bleeding shows ectopic gastric mucosa in the midline of the lower abdomen. The timing coincides with the appearance of the stomach, with increasing conspicuity over time. Lateral views (not shown) revealed abnormal uptake anteriorly in the lower abdomen.

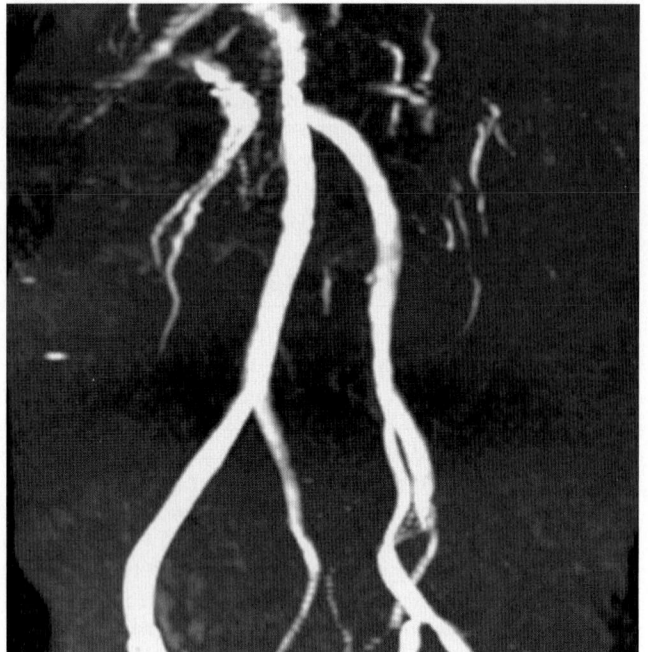
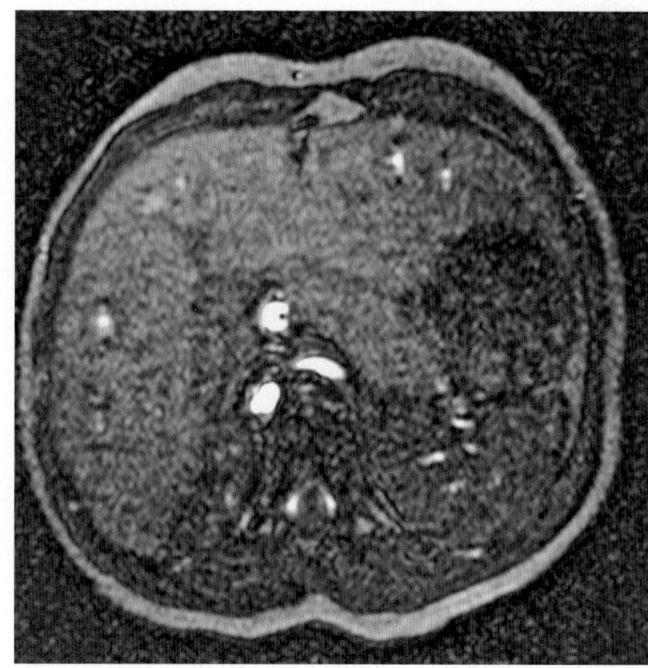

A   B

FIGURE 106-14. Venous anomaly. **A,** Coronal time of flight venogram shows duplication of the infrahepatic inferior vena cava in a 5-year-old child with multiple congenital anomalies, including a single midline kidney in the lower abdomen. **B,** Axial, two-dimensional, 1-mm source image shows the communicating vein coursing from left to right behind the pancreas.

superior to CT, which can detect only very high concentrations of iron and may be unsuitable in cases of coincident fatty deposition. MRI can be used to diagnose neonatal hemochromatosis, hereditary hemochromatosis, and secondary iron deposition disease with excellent correlation with biopsy and spectrophotometry. T2 decay in spin echo sequences can detect high levels of iron concentration, whereas T2 decay in gradient echo sequences without refocusing pulses is more sensitive and potentially quantitative. Liver-to-muscle ratios are believed to be more accurate than liver-to-fat ratios and should be determined on the same slice.

Magnetic resonance angiography (MRA) can be performed with or without contrast, and multiplanar reconstructions of angiograms with variable temporal resolution can be postprocessed in a relatively short time. Time of flight (TOF) techniques involve repeated pulses to the tissues within the slice volume, so that flowing protons entering the image that are not saturated are able to emit a bright signal. The signal is brightest when the flow plane is perpendicular to the plane of the slice; therefore, this technique is limited in acquiring information from vessels with a flow direction parallel to the slice plane. In two-dimensional TOF techniques, very thin (1 to 1.5 mm) images are obtained, which can then be used to create angiographic reconstructions in various planes (Fig. 106-14). Arteries and veins can be separated by applying a saturation pulse in the direction of the flowing blood that needs to be eliminated. The reformatted images provide an overview of the anatomy, but it is important to review the source images carefully. Whereas in TOF angiography the signal intensity is related to the amplitude of the signal, in phase contrast angiography the signal is related to the phase of the protons. In phase

contrast imaging, two equal but separate gradients are applied to a specific site. This has the effect of canceling the signal from stationary protons, but the phase shift and signal from moving protons are proportional to their velocity, because their net residual phase varies with their position in the field during the application of the two gradients. Phase contrast is widely applied in cardiac imaging; it is less widely used in the abdomen but can be helpful in analyzing flow direction and velocity in specific vessels, such as the portal vein. Appropriate selection of the velocity encoding values is important, to avoid artifacts. Phase contrast images can also assess for the presence of stationary thrombus, which can show high signal on TOF images despite saturation pulses.

Contrast-enhanced MRA derives the vascular signal from intravascular gadolinium. Rapid image acquisition allows time-resolved images, with arterial and venous phases. The images are acquired as thin sections in the plane of major interest, typically the coronal plane, and maximal intensity projection images can be reformatted in any plane, as well as in a three-dimensional format. This method allows the visualization of vascular structures in all planes, both perpendicular and orthogonal to the field of view, and separation of arterial and venous structures.

Magnetic resonance cholangiopancreatography (MRCP) is becoming more widely used to visualize the dilated and nondilated biliary tree; it can also outline congenital ductal anomalies such as choledochal cysts (Fig. 106-15), Caroli disease, ductal stenosis, and pancreas divisum. The examination is based on fat-suppressed, heavily T2-weighted sequences that highlight the static fluid within the biliary tree while suppressing adjacent signal. For this reason, the study can be limited in patients with ascites

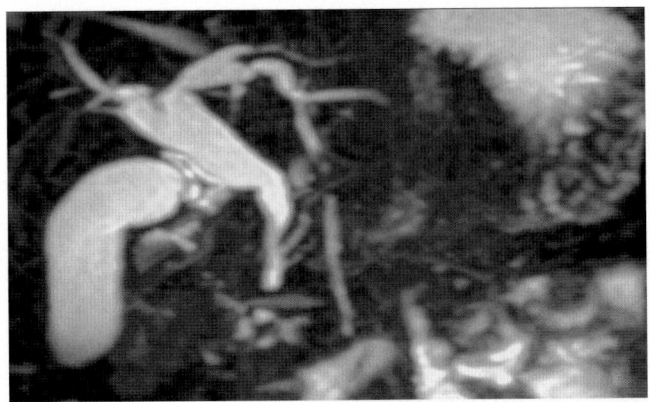

FIGURE 106-15. Choledochal cyst with long common channel. Maximal intensity projection oblique reconstruction from MRCP in a 5-year-old girl with jaundice shows dilation of the common duct, hepatic duct, and right and left intrahepatic branches. The pancreatic ducts of Santorini and Wirsung empty separately into the common bile duct, with a long common channel.

or bowel dilation. Patients must fast before the study to eliminate interference from fluid within the stomach and adjacent bowel loops. Breath-holding techniques can be used in older cooperative patients; in younger patients, single-shot fast spin echo (SSFSE) and respiratory gating may be used. Based on the initial image sets, angled images can be prescribed to demonstrate the specific areas of concern in individual patients. For increased signal-to-noise ratio and excellent MRCP and angiographic studies, 3T field strength magnets hold promise.

FETAL IMAGING

Ultrasonography is the primary modality for prenatal imaging. MRI is increasingly used after the 18th week of gestation to evaluate complex anomalies that are difficult to define on a sonogram and in specific cases in which oligohydramnios, fetal lie, or maternal body habitus obstruct an optimal ultrasonographic evaluation. The examination may be difficult and prolonged in patients with polyhydramnios, owing to excessive fetal motion.

Routine fetal MRI is performed on a 1.5T magnet, with pillows supporting the mother's knees; in cases of late gestation, polyhydramnios, or multiple pregnancies, the mother should lie on her left side to relieve pressure on the inferior vena cava. Fast imaging techniques allow for rapid image acquisition without the need for sedation. T2-weighted images are most commonly employed, consisting of SSFSE or half-Fourier acquisition single-shot turbo spin echo (HASTE) sequences performed in the axial, coronal, and sagittal planes of the fetus, with a 3- to 5-mm slice thickness. T1-weighting may be achieved with fast low-angle shot (FLASH) sequences, typically performed during maternal breath-holding. Steady-state free precession images can be performed with T2-weighted contrast; these are helpful in the assessment of vascular structures.

Patients with esophageal atresia may demonstrate a distended esophageal pouch and an empty or small stomach bubble. In patients with diaphragmatic hernia, lung volume and position of the liver within the chest can be evaluated (Fig. 106-16). Similarly, patients with omphalocele can be evaluated (see Fig. 106-16). Dilation of bowel loops and caliber of the rectum can also be evaluated in patients with bowel obstruction. Meconium shows high signal intensity on T1-weighted images and low signal intensity on T2-weighted images, rendering the colon dark in most routine SSFSE sequences. T1-weighted sequences are helpful in evaluating the colon and liver owing to the increased signal of these structures with this pulse sequence.

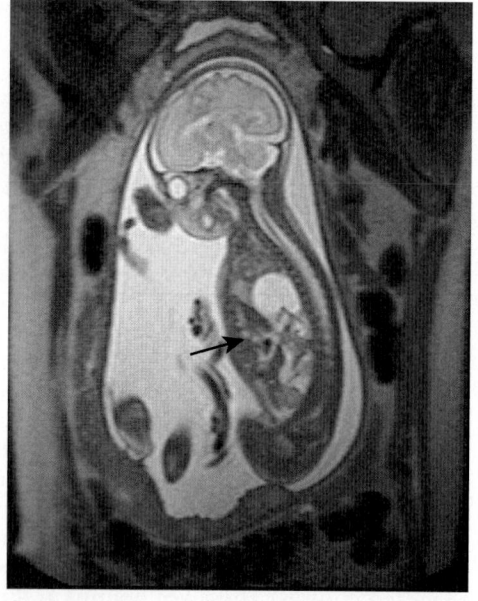

A

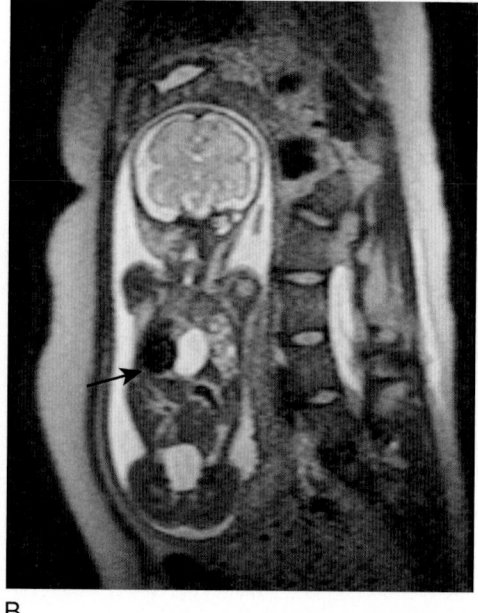

B

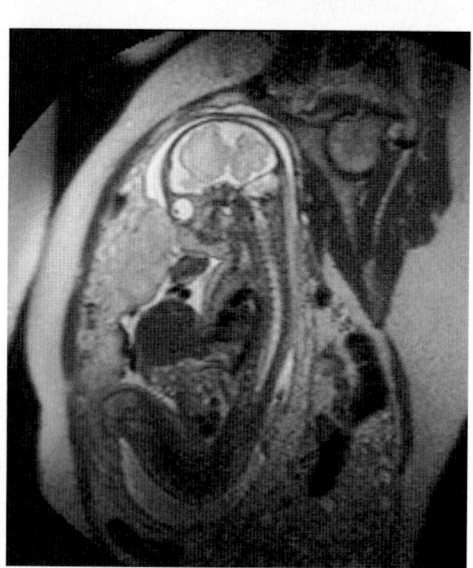

C

FIGURE 106-16. Fetal imaging. **A** and **B**, Sagittal **(A)** and coronal **(B)** SSFSE sequences of a fetus with diaphragmatic hernia. Intrathoracic portion of the left lobe of the liver *(arrow)* is noted as a dark triangular structure anterior to the intrathoracic, fluid-filled stomach in **A**, showing high signal intensity on this T2-weighted sequence. Intrathoracic stomach and nondilated, fluid-filled small bowel loops are seen filling the left chest cavity in **B**. Note the marked contralateral deviation of the heart *(arrow* in **B)**. **C,** Sagittal SSFSE image of a fetus with omphalocele shows the liver and small bowel within the sac. A normal aortic arch is noted incidentally.

SUGGESTED READINGS

Fluoroscopy

Cohen MD: Choosing contrast media for the evaluation of the gastrointestinal tract of neonates and infants. Radiology 1987;162:447-456

Cohen MD: Choosing contrast media for pediatric gastrointestinal examinations. Crit Rev Diagn Imaging 1990;30:317-340

Hollingsworth C, Frush DP, Cross M, Lucaya J: Helical CT of the body: a survey of techniques used for pediatric patients. AJR Am J Roentgenol 2003;180:401-406

Leonidas JC, Burry VF, Fellows RA, Beatty EC: Possible adverse effect of methylglucamine diatrizoate compounds on the bowel of newborn infants with meconium ileus. Radiology 1976;121:693-696

Moore DE, Carroll FE, Dutt PL, et al: Comparison of nonionic and ionic contrast agents in the rabbit lung. Invest Radiol 1991; 26:134-142

Rowe MI, Furst AJ, Altman DH, Poole CA: The neonatal response to Gastrografin enema. Pediatrics 1971;48:29-35

Tuladhar R, Daftary A, Patole SK, Whitehall JS: Oral Gastrografin in neonates: a note of caution. Int J Clin Pract 1999;53:565

Sonography

Coley BD: Pediatric applications of abdominal vascular Doppler imaging: part I. Pediatr Radiol 2004;34:757-771

Coley BD: Pediatric applications of abdominal vascular Doppler: part II. Pediatr Radiol 2004;34:772-786

Hernanz-Schulman M: Infantile hypertrophic pyloric stenosis. Radiology 2003;227:319-331

Khong PL, Peh WCG, Lam CHL, et al: Ultrasound-guided hydrostatic reduction of childhood intussusception: technique and demonstration. Radiographics 2000;20:1e

Riccabona MG: Paediatric ultrasound. I. Abdominal. Eur Radiol 2001;11:2354-2368

Spalinger J, Patriquin H, Miron MC, et al: Doppler US in patients with Crohn disease: vessel density in the diseased bowel reflects disease activity. Radiology 2000;217:787-791

Computed Tomography

Donnelly LF, Emery KH, Brody AS, et al: Minimizing radiation dose for pediatric body applications of single-detector helical CT: strategies at a large children's hospital. AJR Am J Roentgenol 2001;176:303-306

Donnelly LF, Frush DP: Pediatric multidetector body CT. Radiol Clin North Am 2003;41:637-655

Frush DP: Pediatric CT: practical approach to diminish the radiation dose. Pediatr Radiol 2002;32:714-717; discussion 751-754

Frush DP, Yoshizumi T: Conventional and CT angiography in children: dosimetry and dose comparisons. Pediatr Radiol 2006;36:154-158

Hollingsworth C, Frush DP, Cross M, Lucaya J: Helical CT of the body: a survey of techniques used for pediatric patients. AJR Am J Roentgenol 2003;180:401-406

Lowe LH, Penney MW, Stein SM, et al: Unenhanced limited CT of the abdomen in the diagnosis of appendicitis in children: comparison with sonography. AJR Am J Roentgenol 2001;176:31-35

Pappas JN, Donnelly LF, Frush DP: Reduced frequency of sedation of young children with multisection helical CT. Radiology 2000;215:897-899

Thomton FJ, Paulson EK, Yoshizumi TT, et al: Single versus multi-detector row CT: comparison of radiation doses and dose profiles. Acad Radiol 2003;10:379-385

Nuclear Medicine

Balon HR, Fink-Bennett DM, Brill DR, et al: Procedure guideline for hepatobiliary scintigraphy. Society of Nuclear Medicine. J Nucl Med 1997;38:1654-1657

Ben-Haim S, Seabold JE, Kao SC, et al: Utility of Tc-99m mebrofenin scintigraphy in the assessment of infantile jaundice. Clin Nucl Med 1995;20:153-163

Brayton D: Gastrointestinal bleeding of unknown origin. Am J Dis Child 1964;107:288-292

Charearnrad P, Chongsrisawat V, Tepmongkol S, et al: The effect of phenobarbital on the accuracy of technetium-99m diisopropyl iminodiacetic acid hepatobiliary scintigraphy in differentiating biliary atresia from neonatal hepatitis syndrome. J Med Assoc Thai 2003;86(Suppl 2):S189-S194

Charron M: Pediatric inflammatory bowel disease imaged with Tc-99m white blood cells. Clin Nucl Med 2000;25:708-715

Charron M, DiLorenzo C, Kocoshis S: Gastric and small bowel Crohn's disease assessed with leukocytes-Tc(99m) scintigraphy. Pediatr Surg Int 1999;15:500-504

Charron M, DiLorenzo C, Kocoshis S: Are ^{99m}Tc leukocyte scintigraphy and SBFT studies useful in children suspected of having inflammatory bowel disease? Am J Gastroenterol 2000;95:1208-1212

Datz FL, Seabold JE, Brown ML, et al: Procedure guideline for technetium-99m-HMPAO-labeled leukocyte scintigraphy for suspected infection/inflammation. J Nucl Med 1997;38:987-990

Dolgin SE: Answered and unanswered controversies in the surgical management of extra hepatic biliary atresia. Pediatr Transplant 2004;8:628-631

Emamian SA, Shalaby-Rana E, Majd M: The spectrum of heterotopic gastric mucosa in children detected by Tc-99m pertechnetate scintigraphy. Clin Nucl Med 2001;26:529-535

Esmaili J, Izadyar S, Karegar I, et al: Biliary atresia in infants with prolonged cholestatic jaundice: diagnostic accuracy of hepatobiliary scintigraphy. Abdom Imaging (in press)

Ford PV, Bartold SP, Fink-Bennett DM, et al: Procedure guideline for gastrointestinal bleeding and Meckel's diverticulum scintigraphy. Society of Nuclear Medicine. J Nucl Med 1999;40:1226-1232

Gilmour SM, Hershkop M, Reifen R, et al: Outcome of hepatobiliary scanning in neonatal hepatitis syndrome. J Nucl Med 1997; 38:1279-1282

Grahnquist L, Chapman SC, Hvidsten S, et al: Evaluation of 99mTc-HMPAO leukocyte scintigraphy in the investigation of pediatric inflammatory bowel disease. J Pediatr 2003;143:48-53

Heyman S: Hepatobiliary scintigraphy as a liver function test. J Nucl Med 1994;35:436-437

Heyman S: Pediatric gastrointestinal motility studies. Semin Nucl Med 1995;25:339-347

Heyman S, Eicher PS, Alavi A: Radionuclide studies of the upper gastrointestinal tract in children with feeding disorders. J Nucl Med 1995;36:351-354

Heyman S, Respondek M: Detection of pulmonary aspiration in children by radionuclide "salivagram." J Nucl Med 1989; 30:697-699

Kim OH, Chung HJ, Choi BG: Imaging of the choledochal cyst. Radiographics 1995;15:69-88

Leonidas JC, Germann DR: Technetium-99m pertechnetate imaging in diagnosis of Meckel's diverticulum. Arch Dis Child 1974;49:21-26

Levin K, Colon A, DiPalma J, Fitzpatrick S: Using the radionuclide salivagram to detect pulmonary aspiration and esophageal dysmotility. Clin Nucl Med 1993;18:110-114

Love C, Palestro CJ: Radionuclide imaging of infection. J Nucl Med Technol 2004;32:47-57

Lugo-Vicente HL: Trends in management of gallbladder disorders in children. Pediatr Surg Int 1997;12:348-352

Majd M: Radionuclide imaging in clinical pediatrics. Pediatr Ann 1986;15:396-402, 407-408

Majd M, Reba RC, Altman RP: Effect of phenobarbital on the 99m Tc scintigraphy in the evaluation of neonatal jaundice. Semin Nucl Med 1981;11:194-204

Markisz JA, Treves ST, Davis RT: Normal hepatic and splenic size in children: scintigraphic determination. Pediatric Radiol 1987; 17:273-276

Marsh GW, Lewis SM, Szur L: The use of ^{51}Cr-labeled heat-damaged red cells to study splenic function. II. Splenic atrophy in thrombocytopenia. Br J Haematol 1966;12:167-171

Nadel HR: Hepatobiliary scintigraphy in children. Semin Nucl Med 1996;26:25-42

O'Hara S: Pediatric gastrointestinal nuclear imaging. Radiol Clin North Am 1996;34:845-862

Omar AM, Al-Saee'd TA, Elgazzar A: Scintigraphic pattern of intestinal duplication on a Meckel's diverticulum scan. Clin Nucl Med 1998;23:708-709

Palestro CJ, Torres MA: Radionuclide imaging of nonosseous infection. J Nucl Med 1999;43:45-60

Reyhan M, Yapar AF, Aydin M, Sukan A: Gastroesophageal scintigraphy in children: a comparison of posterior and anterior imaging. Ann Nucl Med 2005;19:17-21

Roddie ME, Peters AM, Danpure HJ, et al: Inflammation: imaging with Tc99m HMPAO-labeled leukocytes. Radiology 1988; 166:767-772

Seabold JE, Forstrom LA, Schauwecker DS, et al: Procedure guideline for indium-111-leukocyte scintigraphy for suspected infection/inflammation. J Nucl Med 1997;38:997-1001

Seibert JJ, Byrne WJ, Euler AR: Gastric emptying in children: unusual patterns detected by scintigraphy. AJR Am J Roentgenol 1983;141:49-51

Sfakianakis CH, Conway JJ: Detection of ectopic gastric mucosa in Meckel's diverticulum and in other aberrations of scintigraphy. 1. Pathophysiology and 10-year clinical experience. J Nucl Med 1981;22:647-654

Signer E, Fredrich R: Gastric emptying in newborns and young infants. Acta Pediatr Scand 1975;64:525-530

Smart RC: The use of technetium-99m labeled heat-damaged red cells for the quantitative measurement of splenic function. Eur J Nucl Med 1976;1:211-214

Swaniker F, Soldes O, Hirschl RB: The utility of technetium 99m pertechnetate scintigraphy in the evaluation of patients with Meckel's diverticulum. J Pediatr Surg 1999;34:760-764

Taylor GA: Acute hepatic disease. Radiol Clin North Am 1997; 35:799-814

Thomas EJ, Kumar R, Dasan JB, et al: Prevalence of silent gastroesophageal reflux in association with recurrent lower respiratory tract infections. Clin Nucl Med 2003;28:476-479

Magnetic Resonance Imaging

Anupindi S, Jaramillo D: Pediatric magnetic resonance imaging techniques. Magn Reson Imaging Clin N Am 2002;10:189

Danrad R, Martin DR: MR imaging of diffuse liver diseases. Magn Reson Imaging Clin N Am 2005;13:277-293

Elsayes KM, Narra VR, Mukundan G, et al: MR imaging of the spleen: spectrum of abnormalities. Radiographics 2005;25:967-982

Elsayes KM, Staveteig PT, Narra VR, et al; MRI of the peritoneum: spectrum of abnormalities. AJR Am J Roentgenol 2006; 186:1368-1379

Gandon Y, Olivie D, Guyader D, et al: Non-invasive assessment of hepatic iron stores by MRI. Lancet 2004;363:357-362

Laissy JP, Trillaud H, Douek P: MR angiography: noninvasive vascular imaging of the abdomen. Abdom Imaging 2002;27:488-506

Martin DR, Danrad R, Herrmann K, et al: Magnetic resonance imaging of the gastrointestinal tract. Top Magn Reson Imaging 2005;16:77-98

Martin DR, Danrad R, Hussain SM: MR imaging of the liver. Radiol Clin North Am 2005;43:861-886

Metreweli C, So NM, Chu WC, Lam WW: Magnetic resonance cholangiography in children. Br J Radiol 2004;77:1059-1064

Pereles FS, Baskaran V: Abdominal magnetic resonance angiography: principles and practical applications. Top Magn Reson Imaging 2001;12:317

Strouse PJ: Magnetic resonance angiography of the pediatric abdomen and pelvis. Magn Reson Imaging Clin N Am 2002;10:34

Fetal Imaging

Brugger PC, Prayer D: Fetal abdominal magnetic resonance imaging. Eur J Radiol 2006;57:278

Brugger PC, Stuhr F, Lindner C, Prayer D: Methods of fetal MR: beyond T2-weighted imaging. Eur J Radiol 2006;57:172

CHAPTER 107

Genitourinary Diagnostic Procedures

ADAM S. YOUNG, LARRY A. BINKOVITZ, and BRIAN D. COLEY

Imaging investigations of the genitourinary tract are common in pediatric practice. In past years, the choices were rather limited, but advances in all modalities have increased the number of techniques available. The ability to delineate anatomy with current imaging methods is impressive, and the functional information obtainable is becoming more sophisticated through nuclear medicine and magnetic resonance imaging (MRI) techniques. Acquiring the necessary information for proper patient treatment must be tempered with patient safety and minimization of radiation exposure. Advances in ultrasonography (US), nuclear medicine, and MRI have helped in this regard. Although there are generally accepted approaches to many genitourinary diseases, the tests performed vary among institutions, countries, and individual radiologists. Our practices change as we learn and understand more about the conditions we investigate, but the goal of obtaining clinically relevant, high-quality diagnostic data in the safest manner possible remains constant.

FETAL UROLOGIC IMAGING

Prenatal US examination of the fetus is performed with increasing frequency in cases of suspected fetal abnormalities (see Chapter 12). More than one third of the anomalies detected in the fetus are urogenital. Fetal kidneys and bladder can be visualized by US as early as 13 weeks of gestation. The pelvicalyceal systems and ureters are not seen unless dilated. Urinary anomalies are discovered incidentally during routine screening or in cases of oligohydramnios, abnormal serum α-fetoprotein, abnormal fetal growth pattern, or family history of renal disease. Suspicion of urinary tract abnormalities identifies those infants who require a more complete investigation and possible treatment soon after birth. On occasion, early delivery or prenatal therapeutic intervention is warranted.

In the second half of gestation, fetal urine plays a major role in the formation of amniotic fluid. Oligohydramnios in the second trimester commonly reflects bilateral severe renal malformations or severe urinary tract obstruction. These infants present with Potter facies, hypoplastic lungs and thorax, abnormalities of the limbs, and severe bilateral renal dysplasia. The kidneys may be difficult to visualize, although a large fluid-filled bladder and ureters are seen. Bilateral multicystic kidneys or severe cystic renal dysplasia is identified in utero, appearing much as it does postnatally. Posterior urethral valves or prune-belly syndrome is suggested by dilated ureters. Unfortunately, by the time in utero diagnosis is possible, significant damage has occurred to the parenchymal development of the kidneys, and intervention does not significantly improve the outcome. It is noteworthy that moderate dilation of the calyces and pelvis is often identified early in the third trimester, representing normal fetal diuresis and not a pathologic process.

After delivery, significant dilation of the pelvicalyceal system may not be apparent in the first 24 to 48 hours of life because of low glomerular filtration and relative dehydration of the neonate. Studies before this time may appear falsely normal, whereas studies after this time identify collecting system dilation that was previously obscure.

US is the primary modality for prenatal imaging, but in complex or difficult cases, fetal MRI provides additional capabilities. Large maternal size or oligohydramnios makes US more difficult but does not severely limit MRI. Multiplanar imaging allows a thorough evaluation of the kidneys and bladder and provides some information about the renal parenchyma. Associated anomalies can be sought and evaluated, providing much-needed information regarding these complicated pregnancies.

CONTRAST MEDIA

Radiographic and Computed Tomographic Contrast Media

Contrast media are pharmaceuticals that alter tissue characteristics to enhance information obtained on diagnostic images. The contrast media used in radiography are based on the interruption of x-ray beam transmission by iodine; they are categorized as high-osmolality contrast media (HOCM) and low-osmolality contrast media (LOCM). When choosing a contrast agent, considerations include the concentration of iodine needed, economic factors, and safety issues. HOCM are rarely used as intravascular agents in current pediatric practice, but low-iodine-concentration formulations are frequently used for nonvascular fluoroscopic studies. LOCM have an iodine content ranging from 128 to 320 mg/ml and an osmolality ranging from 290 to 702 mOsm/kg. Normal serum osmolality is 285 mOsm/kg. Those with an iodine content of 240 to 300 mg/ml are used intravascularly for computed tomography (CT) and excretory urography. LOCM with a high iodine content (320 to 370 mg/ml) are used for CT and angiography.

The intravenous (IV) dosage of contrast material is based on grams of iodine in relation to body mass. It is appropriate to use a dosage of approximately 300 mg iodine per kilogram body weight. This represents approximately 1 ml/kg in the most commonly used forms of LOCM. However, with newer CT scanners and rapid scanning techniques, adequate contrast enhancement can often be achieved with smaller doses. Intravenous urography (IVU), though rarely required in current practice, may require higher doses of contrast agent (especially in infants) for adequate opacification of the collecting system.

After the IV injection of contrast material, a peak plasma level occurs within the first minute. This peak is followed by a rapid decline resulting from renal excretion, dilution of the material from mixing within the vascular space, and rapid diffusion into the extravascular and extracellular compartments. Contrast material is filtered by the glomerulus and concentrated in the proximal tubules. Contrast excretion begins immediately on initial circulation through the kidney and peaks at 10 to 20 minutes. At least 50% of injected contrast material is excreted within 2 to 3 hours of injection, and 100% is cleared within 24 hours. In patients with renal failure, contrast material remains in the circulation for much longer and may eventually be excreted vicariously from mucosal surfaces, including the small bowel and gallbladder.

The quality of radiographic renal visualization is related to the initial plasma level of contrast material. This is affected by the iodine concentration of the agent used and by the speed of contrast injection. Collecting system visibility on IVU is related to the concentration of contrast material in the urine, the volume of pre-existing urine, and the diuretic effect of the contrast medium used.

Evidence suggests that there are definite advantages to the use of LOCM. Current indications for the use of LOCM as advised by the American College of Radiology are as follows:

1. Patients with a history of a previous allergic reaction to contrast material
2. Patients with a history of asthma or allergy
3. Patients with known cardiac dysfunction, including recent or potentially imminent cardiac decompensation, severe arrhythmias, unstable angina pectoris, recent myocardial infarction, and pulmonary hypertension
4. Patients with generalized severe debilitation
5. Any other circumstances in which, after due consideration, the radiologist believes that there is a specific indication for the use of LOCM

In infants and children, considerations include very small size, prematurity, significant cardiac disease, congestive failure, dehydration, severe asthma or allergies, previous reaction to contrast material, renal insufficiency, and sickle cell anemia. In general, only LOCM should be used for intravascular administration in pediatric practice.

> **Only low-osmolality contrast media should be used for intravascular administration in children.**

ADVERSE REACTIONS

Factors affecting the chemotoxicity of contrast material include concentration, site of injection, injection rate, specific chemical action, and osmolality. The physiologic effects related to osmolality include hypervolemia, cellular diuresis, urinary diuresis, altered vascular and glomerular endothelial permeability, vessel dilation with decreased resistance and blood pressure, increased blood flow, pain, and sinus bradycardia and cardiac conduction delays.

Compared with HOCM, LOCM have little or no effect on serum osmolality, serum sodium, vasodilation, hemodilation, red blood cell morphology, or vascular permeability. There is little or no effect on the blood-brain barrier; there are fewer electrocardiographic changes and fewer alterations in myocardial contractility, cardiac output, and left ventricular, pulmonary artery, and aortic pressures. LOCM cause less endothelial damage, less release or activation of vasoactive substances, and diminished effects on coagulation pathways. Of importance is the reduction in the nephrotoxic effects, including proteinuria, altered renal blood flow, and urinary enzyme excretion. There is a notable improvement in the patient's experience, with less or no pain, heat, nausea, vomiting, or anxiety. Improved patient comfort results in diminished motion and improved image quality.

Contrast reactions represent the most common complications of intravascular contrast administration. Katayama and colleagues' study of 337,647 cases found that use of LOCM significantly reduces the incidence of all adverse reactions and specifically the incidence of severe and potentially life-threatening reactions. The incidence of adverse reactions was 3.13% among patients given LOCM, compared with 12.66% among those given HOCM. Severe reactions occurred in 0.04% of LOCM patients, compared with 0.22% of HOCM patients. In children younger than 1 year, the incidence of all adverse reactions was 0.7% with HOCM and 0.4% with LOCM. The risk of death is very low with either HOCM or LOCM.

Most contrast reactions are minor and do not require treatment. Life-threatening reactions such as laryngeal and facial edema, cardiac arrhythmias, severe bronchospasm, pulmonary edema, and cardiovascular collapse are detected in 1 in 3000 to 1 in 14,000 patients undergoing contrast studies. Most patients with potentially fatal reactions are successfully resuscitated. Contrast reactions are classified as idiosyncratic and nonidiosyncratic. Idiosyncratic reactions are allergic-type reactions and include hives, itching, facial and laryngeal edema, bronchospasm, and circulatory collapse. Although there is significantly greater contrast binding by serum globulin in patients who experience contrast reactions, it has been suggested that most reactions are not the result of immunoglobulin

E–antigen interactions. Contrast reactions are considered to be anaphylactoid, or allergy-like, rather than anaphylactic. Contrast material may induce histamine release from basophils and mast cells and may affect both the complement and coagulation systems. Nonidiosyncratic reactions result from direct toxic effects of contrast material and contrast hyperosmolality and include nausea, vomiting, cardiac arrhythmias, pulmonary edema, and cardiovascular collapse. The existence of a known allergy doubles the frequency of contrast reactions and quadruples the rate of severe reactions. Recurrent reactions have been reported in 15% to 60% of patients with a history of previous contrast reaction, and nearly 20% of such patients developed identical severe reactions. There is a higher frequency of reactions when the total iodine dose exceeds 20 g.

Several disease processes may be aggravated by the administration of intravascular contrast material. Hypertensive crisis, related to catecholamine release, may occur in patients with pheochromocytoma. Contrast-induced crisis can occur in patients with sickle cell anemia, and patients with hyperthyroidism may develop thyroid storm. Contrast nephropathy may occur following intravascular contrast administration; patients at risk for this complication are those with azotemia, diabetes mellitus, severe congestive failure, multiple contrast studies, or renal tubules filled with uric acid precipitates (e.g., those undergoing rapid tumor lysis). It is inadvisable to administer contrast media for CT in patients at risk for azotemia. Patients taking oral hypoglycemic agents containing metformin who continue the medication after IV contrast media administration may develop fatal metabolic lactic acidosis; these drugs are not commonly prescribed to children, however.

It is important to be aware that both mild and severe adverse reactions may occur with any IV contrast material. Immediate treatment of contrast reactions includes the use of antihistamines, epinephrine, intravascular volume expansion, and oxygen. Patients with a history of iodinated contrast allergy should undergo alternative imaging procedures. However, if the use of iodinated contrast media cannot be avoided, pretreatment with corticosteroids should be considered. Pretreatment with a two-dose corticosteroid regimen given 12 and 2 hours before HOCM administration lowered the reaction rate in high-risk patients to that observed in a large group of patients receiving LOCM without pretreatment. H_1 blockers may provide some benefit. This regimen does not protect completely against reactions to contrast material, and high-risk patients should receive LOCM with resuscitation personnel, medication, and equipment immediately available.

CONTRAST EXTRAVASATION

If, during IV contrast administration, there is any indication of extravasation, such as swelling or pain, the injection must be halted. Extravasated contrast material produces an inflammatory response causing pain, edema, and necrosis of subcutaneous tissues and skin. Such reactions are less severe with LOCM than with HOCM. Unfortunately, a definitive treatment strategy is lacking. Treatment regimens include elevation and warm or cold compresses, and some have advocated the subcutaneous injection of saline or hyaluronidase for larger extravasations. If the local reaction is severe, or if there are any questions, surgical consultation should be sought.

Magnetic Resonance Imaging Contrast Media

In uroradiology, MRI contrast media are used to improve the inherent contrast differences between magnetically similar tissues, to directly evaluate organ function, and to estimate perfusion of an organ. MRI contrast agents in the proximity of tissue protons stimulate relaxation of nuclei, decreasing T1 and T2 relaxation times. These paramagnetic substances are ions, atoms, or molecules that align with an external magnetic field, then return to their random orientation when the field is removed. Strongly paramagnetic substances, such as the Gd^{3+} in gadopentetate dimeglumine (with seven unpaired electrons), produce proton relaxation enhancement, resulting in a significant reduction in T1 and T2 times for neighboring protons and a resultant increase in MR signal intensity. Binding of metal ions to multidentate chelates by electrostatic forces effectively reduces their toxicity, prevents intracellular deposition, facilitates rapid and complete renal excretion, and controls biodistribution. The paramagnetic substances considered for use as contrast agents include transition series metals (Fe^{3+} or Mn^{2+}, with up to five unpaired electrons), lanthanide metals (Gd^{3+}, with up to seven unpaired electrons), or nitroxide spin labels (pyrroxiamide, one or more unpaired electrons).

The most commonly used IV contrast agent for MRI, gadolinium-diethylenetriaminepenta-acetic acid (Gd-DTPA) dimeglumine, was approved in 1988 for clinical use. Gd-DTPA dimeglumine has a high T1 relaxivity of 4.5 to 5.1 mmol/sec and a half-life of 90 minutes. It is highly water soluble and, although hyperosmolar (1900 mOsm/kg), requires only small volumes (0.1 mmol/kg) to be effective. Gd-DTPA is excreted by glomerular filtration, with 90% excreted within 24 hours. Rapid renal clearance and low toxicity are important features of this contrast material.

Gadolinium-based MRI contrast media are generally quite safe. Adverse reactions occur in less than 0.5% of patients; severe reactions occur in around 0.01%. Risk factors for reactions are similar to those for iodinated contrast agents and respond to similar treatments. Traditionally, gadolinium agents were considered safe in case of renal insufficiency where iodinated contrast agents were contraindicated. Recently, however, an association between gadolinium contrast agents and a rare disease, nephrogenic systemic fibrosis (NSF), has been described. NSF affects the skin, muscle, and viscera, causing debilitation and sometimes death. Although the pathogenesis is still not entirely clear, all patients developing NSF after gadolinium administration had severe acute or chronic renal insufficiency. Most reported cases are in adults, although cases in children have also occurred. Patients scheduled for contrast MRI studies should thus be carefully questioned about renal disease and, if necessary, undergo serum testing prior to having gadolinium administered. If renal insufficiency is discovered or suspected, noncontrast MRI, alternative imaging modalities, and/or nephrology consultation should be considered, depending on clinical conditions.

Ultrasonography Contrast Media

US contrast media promise to be an exciting addition to the diagnostic capabilities of this modality. Although they have existed for many years, these agents have only recently become widely available and approved for use. The specific compositions of these agents vary by manufacturer, but all are microbubbles of air or perfluorocarbon gas contained within a lipid or proteinaceous shell. When insonated, these bubbles resonate, increasing both gray scale and color Doppler signal. Specific US pulse strategies have been developed to optimize signal from these contrast agents, further improving their utility.

Used intravenously, US contrast media can help evaluate tissue perfusion and assess normal structures as well as masses. Used intravesically, these agents provide a method to evaluate vesicoureteral reflux (VUR) without the use of ionizing radiation.

RADIOGRAPHIC PROCEDURES

Intravenous Urography

IVU uses the physiologic excretion of injected iodinated contrast media for visualization of the renal cortex, medulla, and collecting system. Anatomic details of the renal parenchyma and collecting system and general information concerning renal function are obtained. The study requires good excretion of iodinated contrast material and appropriate filming to document the nephrographic phase and excretion of contrast material into the pelvicalyceal collecting system. IVU was previously the imaging method of choice for the kidneys and collecting system, but it has been supplanted by US, radionuclide studies, MRI, and CT and is rarely the preferred imaging method in current practice.

Bowel preparation is unnecessary in infants and children, except for extremely constipated patients. Dehydration should be avoided. A light meal or clear fluids several hours before the study, followed by the withholding of feeding for 2 to 4 hours, is helpful in decreasing the stomach contents and reducing the risk of aspiration if vomiting occurs. Imaging begins with a frontal radiograph of the abdomen to identify any calcifications or masses. Following this preliminary radiograph, high-iodine-content LOCM are given intravenously at a dose of 2 to 3 ml/kg (maximum, 150 ml) to obtain adequate iodine concentration in the renal tubules and collecting system.

The filming sequence is tailored to the individual examination. An initial frontal radiograph within 1 to 2 minutes of injection, collimated over the region of the kidneys, is used for visualization of the nephrographic phase. Assessment of this radiograph determines subsequent filming. On routine examination, a radiograph at

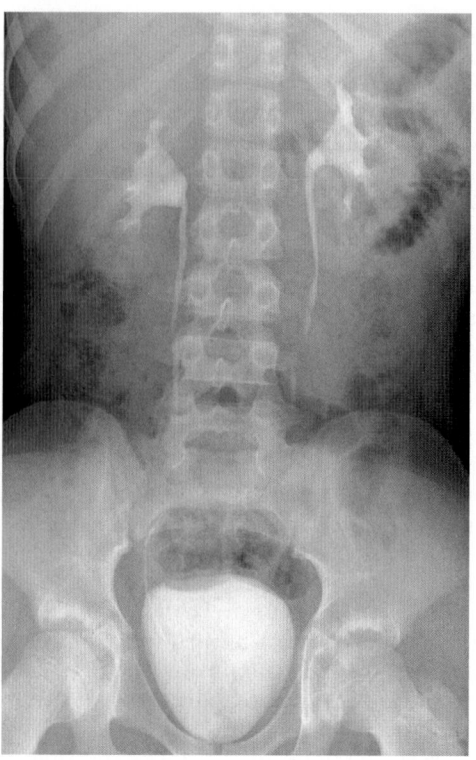

FIGURE 107-1. Normal intravenous urography. Five-minute image shows opacification of the upper collecting system with normal thin, delicate calyces; normal nondilated ureters; and filling of the bladder.

approximately 5 to 10 minutes allows visualization of the kidneys and their collecting systems, including the bladder (Fig. 107-1). This is collimated over the entire abdomen with the patient prone or supine. In many circumstances, an abbreviated examination with only two or three images is adequate to answer the clinical question. In the prone position, the higher specific gravity of the contrast material allows better visualization of the anteriorly positioned renal pelves and proximal ureters. Oblique views may provide visualization of the more anterior and posterior aspects of the kidneys and the lower ureters and trigonal region of the bladder. Upright and postvoid images may facilitate the visualization of the lower ureters. The ingestion of carbonated beverages can lead to better visualization of the kidneys through the window of the distended stomach.

The nephrographic phase provides a gross estimate of renal function, as well as information on renal size and parenchymal contour. A poorly visible nephrogram may indicate a technical problem in achieving optimal plasma concentration of contrast material or some degree of renal failure or diminished renal function. A dense and prolonged nephrogram indicates obstruction of the renal collecting system or renal tubules, hypotension, hypovolemia, or acute tubular necrosis. In these conditions there is diminished tubular flow and increased water resorption, with resultant higher tubular concentration of iodine. The dense nephrogram may remain for a prolonged period, often 24 hours or longer, with little or no opacification of the collecting system.

> **Causes of a dense and prolonged nephrogram: hypotension, obstruction, hypovolemia, tubular dysfunction.**

Opacification of urine in the pelvicalyceal collecting system reflects the plasma concentration of contrast material and is enhanced by dehydration and diminished by dilution during diuresis and high tubular flow. Diminished glomerular filtration also results in reduced opacification. The normal reduced glomerular filtration in neonates limits the utility of IVU in these patients.

Voiding Cystourethrography

Antegrade voiding cystourethrography (VCUG) is the examination of choice for detailed anatomic evaluation of the bladder, for study of the anatomy of the male urethra, and for identification of VUR. After sterile preparation, a well-lubricated small catheter is advanced through the urethra into the bladder. Prefilling the urethra with an anesthetic gel reduces discomfort. The bladder is filled by gravity pressure (fluid at a height of approximately 1 m) using dilute sterile contrast media with an iodine concentration of 80 to 100 mg/ml. Sufficient contrast is introduced into the bladder to produce the urge to void in older children, often visible fluoroscopically by relaxation of the internal sphincter. The predicted bladder capacity (in milliliters) for children younger than 1 year is the child's weight in kilograms multiplied by 7. In children older than 1 year, the predicted capacity is the child's age in years plus 2, multiplied by 30.

> **Predicted bladder capacity (in milliliters):**
> - **Age younger than 1 year: Patient weight (kg) × 7**
> - **Age older than 1 year: [Patient age (years) + 2] × 30**

Imaging begins with a scout view to search for abnormal masses, calcifications, or bony abnormalities and may consist of an overhead or fluoroscopic image. An early bladder filling image is obtained to evaluate for ureteroceles or masses. Images with a full urinary bladder are obtained in anteroposterior and both lateral oblique projections to look for reflux. Voiding images that include the bladder trigone and urethra are obtained in an anteroposterior projection in girls and in a steep oblique position in boys. Initial voiding images are obtained with the catheter in place, followed by images with the catheter removed. Voiding films are useful to evaluate the bladder and urethra (particularly the male urethra) and for the diagnosis of VUR, which may occur only during voiding. Following voiding, an image of the bladder documents any postvoid residual, and an image of the kidneys documents any reflux that occurred during the examination. If there has been VUR, a delayed image documenting the clearing of contrast material from the upper collecting system should be obtained. Neonates should undergo at least two filling and voiding cycles to increase the chance of detecting VUR.

Fluoroscopic time should be kept to the minimum required for diagnostic purposes. The fluoroscope tower should be kept as close to the patient as possible, because reducing the distance from the radiation source to the image intensifier decreases exposure. Pulsed fluoroscopy, last image hold recording, and videotaping can also reduce exposures (see Chapter 1).

In patients with neurogenic bladder and myelomeningocele, voiding is usually impossible, and detecting reflux is the most important part of the study. In these cases, the bladder is filled to a volume appropriate for age or corresponding to typical volumes obtained during catheterization, with images obtained over the kidneys and ureters to evaluate for reflux. The bladder is then emptied through the catheter.

Vesicostomy Study

In patients with a simple vesicostomy, a small Foley catheter is inserted into the bladder through the stoma, and the balloon is inflated and used to occlude the vesicostomy site. A cystogram is then performed, filling the bladder by gravity introduction of contrast material. Bladder size and morphology, VUR, and bladder outlet can be evaluated.

Retrograde Urethrography

Retrograde urethrograms are obtained infrequently in children but are performed in boys to evaluate possible urethral injury or rupture following straddle injury or pelvic trauma. A small catheter is introduced into the anterior urethra to or slightly past the fossa navicularis, and the meatus is occluded. With the patient in a steep oblique position, a small amount of contrast material is injected through a syringe to allow evaluation of the urethra to the level of the external sphincter. Spasm of the external sphincter sometimes prevents filling of the most proximal portion of the posterior urethra. Though urethrograms are rarely performed for girls, the tip of a small Foley catheter with the balloon distended can be placed into the urethra and then taped to the perineum to allow retrograde evaluation of the urethra.

Vaginography

A vaginogram is used to evaluate vaginal size, a common urogenital orifice, the presence of a cervix, or a vaginal mass. The technique is used in cases of ambiguous genitalia or common urogenital sinus. A small catheter is introduced into the vagina and taped. If possible, another catheter is introduced anteriorly into the urethra and bladder, particularly when evaluating a common urogenital sinus. Contrast material is injected under fluoroscopic control with the patient in a steep oblique or lateral position to establish the interrelationships of the urogenital structures.

Genitography

Genitography is most useful in children with suspected intersex or whose sexual differentiation is indeterminate by external genitalia. Most of these children are masculinized females. US or MRI can establish the presence of a uterus and gonads, but genitography is used to detail the anatomy of the urethra, vagina, and bladder. Genitography is carried out by catheterization of the urethra and urinary bladder; a second catheter may then be placed just dorsally and enter a vagina that communicates with the proximal urethra. Some examiners also prefer to place a catheter within the rectum, possibly with a small amount of contrast material. A standard cystourethrogram is performed to evaluate the bladder and urethra. During this procedure, there may be reflux of contrast material into the vagina that enters a masculinized urethra. If this does not occur, use of a second posterior catheter is helpful. Injection by hand into the urethra, with the tip of the catheter placed in the posterior urethra, often delineates a vagina and its associated cervix. These studies are best performed with the patient in the true lateral position and are discussed in Chapter 153.

Retrograde Pyelography

This procedure is usually done as an adjunct to cystoscopy, with the urologist placing retrograde catheters within the ureter. The examination is performed most frequently in children with a blind-ending ureter (either duplex or single) and before ureteropelvic junction repair to ensure that no ureteral anomalies exist. Following placement of the ureteral catheters by the urologist, sterile contrast medium is injected, and images are obtained to identify the anatomic relationships.

Nephrostomy and Ureterostomy Studies

These examinations are performed by gravity introduction or low-pressure manual injection of iodinated contrast material into an indwelling catheter, or through a small catheter inserted into the stoma with the tip advanced to the desired location. Both procedures are performed with fluoroscopic guidance.

ULTRASONOGRAPHY

Real-Time Gray Scale Ultrasonography

US is the most widely used general examination of the urinary system in infants and children. The widespread use of obstetric US has resulted in the early detection of many urinary tract abnormalities, allowing early treatment and the prevention of adverse sequelae.

US is an inexpensive and easily accessible technique for screening, identifying, and characterizing urinary tract abnormalities and for postoperative and post-treatment follow-up. Common indications for US of the urinary tract include the following:

- Possible fetal anomalies (in utero screening)
- Palpable abdominal mass
- Renal enlargement
- Unexplained infection, fever, pyuria, failure to thrive
- Urinary tract infection
- Hematuria
- Abnormal pattern of urination
- Presence of anomalies that may be associated with urinary anomalies: limb, vertebral, cardiac, anal
- Physical characteristics associated with renal neoplasia: hemihypertrophy, visceromegaly, sporadic aniridia
- Hypertension
- Serologic findings of diminished renal function or impending renal failure
- Positive family history of urinary abnormalities

Owing to the small physical habitus of infants and children and their lack of abdominal fat, along with the lack of ionizing radiation, US is an ideal method for examining the kidneys and bladder. There is no specific preparation for an ultrasound examination, although patients are encouraged to drink fluids so as to have a full bladder at the start of the study. Variable transducer frequencies and transducer design (sector, phased, curvilinear, and linear array) allow for individualized approaches. Children are scanned in the supine, decubitus, or prone position. The liver provides an excellent acoustic window for the upper pole of the right kidney, and the spleen may be useful as an acoustic window for the left kidney. On occasion, bowel gas may obscure part of the kidney on supine views, but a posterolateral approach can be used to improve visualization.

In young children, it is advisable to initiate the urogenital ultrasound examination with an examination of the bladder. The full bladder of an infant usually empties when the transducer is placed in the suprapubic region. Kidneys are imaged in the longitudinal and transverse planes. The highest frequency transducer that allows adequate penetration should be used to provide the best spatial resolution possible. Examination with high-frequency linear transducers can provide information about the renal cortex and medulla (e.g., dysplasia, cysts, scars) that may be missed during a more cursory examination. The use of harmonic imaging may improve visualization in larger patients and may help discriminate cysts from hypoechoic masses.

The kidneys are ovoid solid organs with fine, medium-level echoes arising from the cortex; a well-delineated corticomedullary junction with brightly echoic arcuate arteries; and pyramid-shaped, relatively large medullary rays that are hypoechoic. Cortical echogenicity in neonates and young infants is higher and the medullary pyramids are more hypoechoic than in older children (Fig. 107-2). The cortical echogenicity is increased compared with the liver and spleen in preterm infants, isoechoic in neonates and young infants, and diminishes progressively in older children. The transition from the infant renal echo pattern to that of the child typically occurs between 6 and 9 months (Fig. 107-3). The central, highly echoic sinus results from vascular structures interfacing with fat around the renal pelvis. In infants and young children, the kidneys typically have minimal central sinus echoes. With maturity, the highly echoic hilar structures develop and are similar to those of adults by the time children reach adolescence. Separation of the hyperechoic renal sinus echo can be seen with collecting system obstruction, but it can also be seen with diuresis and prone positioning.

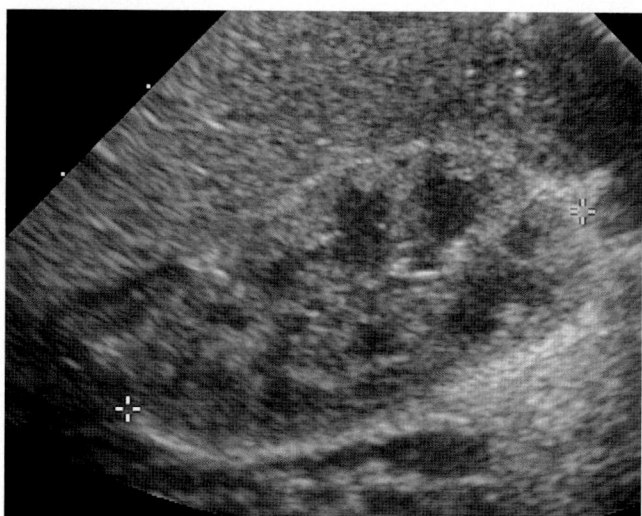

FIGURE 107-2. Normal newborn kidney. Longitudinal sonogram shows the right renal cortex to be slightly more echogenic than the adjacent liver. The hypoechoic medullary pyramids are quite distinct.

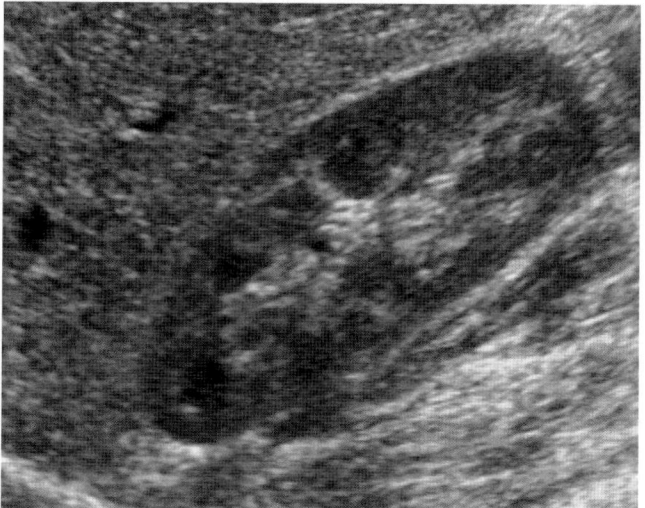

FIGURE 107-3. Normal pediatric kidney. Longitudinal sonogram in a 5-year-old child shows that the renal cortex is hypoechoic relative to the adjacent liver. The medullary pyramids are still distinct. Note the minimal echogenicity of the renal sinus owing to a paucity of renal sinus fat.

The adrenal glands of full-term neonates are one third the size of the kidneys at birth, but they decrease in size by 50% in the first 3 weeks of life. On a longitudinal ultrasound examination, the adrenal gland appears as an inverted Y- or V-shaped structure; on a transverse scan, it appears as an oval structure superior and slightly medial to the upper pole of each kidney. The adrenal cortex is hyperechoic, and the central medulla is hypoechoic. Adrenal imaging is discussed in Chapters 24 and 144.

The uterus and ovaries are visualized using the fluid-filled bladder as an acoustic window. Structures are easily identified in newborns because of residual maternal hormonal stimulation, which may continue if the child is breastfed. During childhood, the ovaries become smaller and more difficult to visualize until puberty. With puberty,

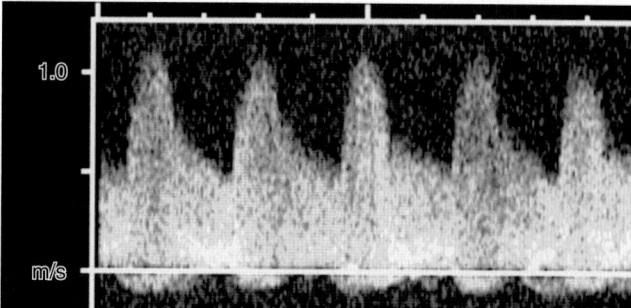

FIGURE 107-4. Normal renal Doppler waveform. There is a prompt systolic upstroke and normal forward flow through diastole.

the uterine fundus begins to develop, and the endometrium becomes more visible. These appearances are discussed in Chapter 155. Although it is often avoided in pediatric imaging, endovaginal sonography is a valuable technique in adolescents. Patients who have had gynecologic examinations, who use tampons, or who are sexually active should be considered for an endovaginal examination if transabdominal scanning is unrewarding.

The testis can be visualized within the scrotum or in the inguinal canal up to the internal inguinal ring. High-frequency linear transducers provide excellent resolution. The testis is ovoid, with the comma-shaped epididymis and appendix identified superiorly. A homogeneous medium-echo pattern is present throughout the testis, and a slightly hyperechoic central hilum is identified. Fine septations are occasionally seen. Chapter 154 discusses testicular evaluation in detail.

Doppler Ultrasonography

Although gray scale US provides excellent anatomic detail, it does not provide functional data. The use of color and pulsed-wave Doppler, however, can provide important information about renal perfusion and indirect information about the renal parenchyma. Doppler US is valuable for the detection of blood flow, to confirm arterial perfusion, or to exclude venous thrombosis. Measurable blood flow parameters from spectral Doppler analysis include peak systolic velocity, end-diastolic velocity, and acceleration times. Calculated values such as mean velocity, volume flow rate, flow impedance, and pulsatility can also be obtained.

The normal renal artery has a prompt systolic upstroke with an acceleration time of 70 msec or less and a visible early systolic peak (Fig. 107-4). The normal resistive index depends on patient age; it may be as high as 0.9 in a preterm infant and falls to around the adult value of 0.7 in the first few months of life. Elevated renal artery velocities relative to the aorta, or a delayed systolic upstroke, may indicate renal artery stenosis (see Chapter 150). Diminished diastolic or reversed diastolic arterial flow indicates increased renovascular impedance, which can be seen in medical renal diseases, venous obstruction, and renal transplant dysfunction (see Chapter 149). Abnormally increased diastolic flow may indicate renal artery stenosis or abnormal arteriovenous communication.

Color Doppler is also useful for evaluating potential ureteric obstruction. The impedance in an acutely obstructed kidney may be increased, leading to decreased renal arterial diastolic flow and an increase in the resistive index. Additionally, ureteric inflow to the bladder can be assessed by looking for ureteral "jets" with color Doppler. A unilateral diminished frequency or absence of ureteric flow may indicate ipsilateral ureteral obstruction.

In evaluating scrotal pain, testicular torsion and ischemia can be differentiated from epididymitis, tumor, orchitis, or appendix torsion using color Doppler sonography. This technique is accurate in older children and adolescents and can also be used successfully in infants and young children.

Contrast-Enhanced Ultrasonography

Ultrasound contrast agents are widely available worldwide, except in North America. Most of these agents are variations of gas-filled microbubbles that are injected intravenously. These agents increase signal on both gray scale and Doppler imaging, enhancing the depiction of parenchymal and vascular structures. Contrast-enhanced US provides better anatomic information in difficult patients and permits the evaluation of renal perfusion.

Contrast-Enhanced Cystosonography

The intravesical instillation of ultrasound contrast agents in the urinary bladder allows the sonographic evaluation of VUR. The ultrasound transducer is positioned intermittently over the bladder, ureters, and kidneys while the bladder is filled, as with VCUG. Refluxed fluid appears brightly echogenic and is thus detectable by US, especially with the use of harmonic imaging and contrast-specific sonographic pulse techniques. Although this technique does not avoid catheterization, it does eliminate radiation exposure. Results indicate that the sensitivity for VUR detection is comparable to that of standard techniques, although urethral visualization is more difficult.

COMPUTED TOMOGRAPHY

CT is one of our most powerful imaging tools. High-quality CT can be performed in patients of all ages and sizes and is not limited by bone or bowel gas. Relative immobility is required, and reassurance, explanation of the procedure, the presence of a parent, sedation, and immobilization all contribute to a successful diagnostic study. Faster multidetector scanners obviate the need for sedation in most patients. Mutliplanar reformatting, especially in the coronal plane, can depict the entire course of the collecting system.

Noncontrast imaging is performed for calcifications or nephrolithiasis (see Chapter 147), but most CT imaging is performed with IV contrast. Contrast enhancement is required for the evaluation of renal lesions and the vessels of the abdomen. Delayed imaging is useful for assessing the integrity of the collecting system (such as after trauma), for assessing the course of the ureter, and

for evaluating renal masses and cysts. As with all ionizing radiation, CT doses should be reduced and optimized based on patient size and purpose of the study.

In small children, contrast material is administered by hand injection, although a power injector should be considered in older patients to provide more controlled contrast administration. Careful visual monitoring of the IV line is important during injection to ensure that extravasation is not occurring. Scanning begins based on the speed of the particular CT scanner and the information being sought. By showing the progression of contrast enhancement of the cortex, medulla, and collecting system of the kidney, CT provides some assessment of renal function as well as anatomy.

MAGNETIC RESONANCE IMAGING

MRI is a sectional diagnostic technique that depends on proton density, T1 and T2 relaxation, flow phenomena, magnetic susceptibility, and diffusion to produce images. Advantages include good spatial resolution, excellent contrast resolution, multiplanar imaging, and lack of ionizing radiation. Lipid suppression techniques are helpful in the abdomen, particularly after contrast enhancement, by removing the contribution of high signal from fat. Degradation resulting from metallic foreign material and patient motion can have a significant effect on the image. Use of surface coils, the ability to reduce motion artifact, and the development of appropriate contrast materials and faster scanning times have resulted in improved imaging. Patient sedation is required in very young or agitated patients to obtain sufficient immobility during the scan.

MRI is not always readily available, and because of its cost and requirement for sedation in younger patients, it may not be considered a primary imaging modality. However, its superior tissue characterization, multiplanar capabilities, and ability to gather functional as well as anatomic information without ionizing radiation make it an increasingly important tool in pediatric imaging. Rapid scan techniques—such as rapid acquisition relaxation enhancement (RARE), half-Fourier acquisition single-shot turbo spin echo (HASTE), and single-shot fast spin echo (SSFSE)—gradient echo and fast spin echo techniques, and three-dimensional acquisitions all improve the speed of data acquisition and image quality. The use of surface coils results in improved resolution, with an improved signal-to-noise ratio but limitations in the field of view. However, the pediatric urogenital tract can often be evaluated effectively.

The standard planes in which MRI is performed are the axial, coronal, and sagittal; in addition, oblique imaging or off-axis reconstructed images are often useful for the optimal display of anatomy. Blood within vessels may be bright or dark, depending on the sequence or contrast technique used. Urine in the collecting system and ureter and other water-density structures have low signal intensity on T1-weighted images and higher signal intensity on T2-weighted scans. The kidney is easily visualized with intermediate signal on T1-weighted sequences. The renal cortex has an intermediate signal close to that of the spleen, and the medullary pyramids show a lower

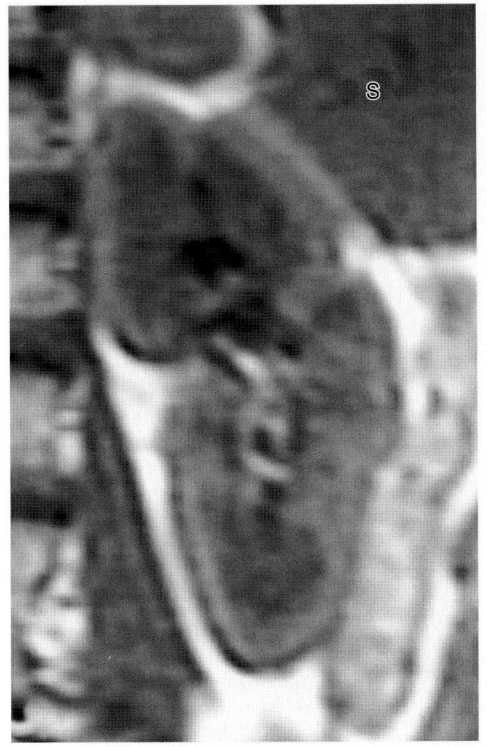

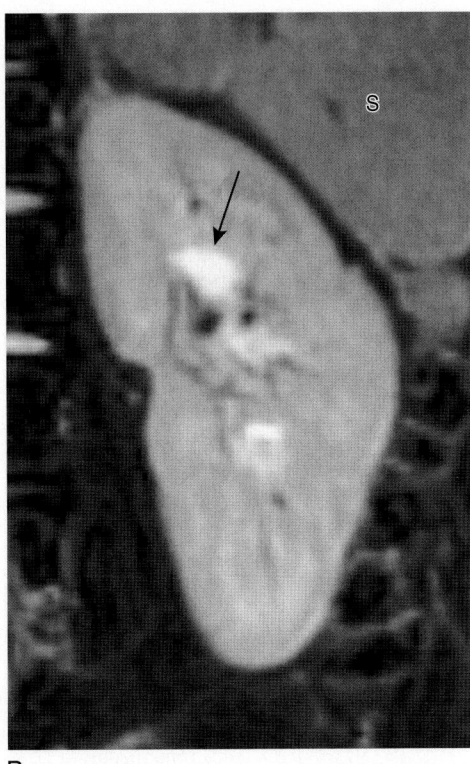

A

B

FIGURE 107-5. Normal renal MRI. **A,** Coronal T1-weighted image shows the renal cortex to be isointense to the adjacent spleen (S) and the medulla to be hypointense relative to the cortex. **B,** Coronal T2-weighted fat-saturated image shows diffuse hyperintensity of the renal parenchyma relative to the spleen (S), with the urine in the central pelvis appearing quite hyperintense (arrow).

TABLE 107-1

Radiopharmaceutical Dosage Guidelines and Dosimetry for a Five-Year-Old Child

Radiopharmaceutical	Administered Activity, MBq/kg (mCi/kg)	Minimum and Maximum Doses	Organ Receiving the Largest Radiation Dose, mGy (rad)	Effective Dose, mSv (rem)	Other Affected Critical Organs (rad/mCi)
Tc-99m MAG3	3.2-4.2 (0.08-0.12)	min: 1 mCi max: 10 mCi	Bladder wall, 0.17 (0.63)	0.015 (0.056)	Ovaries (0.0327) Testes (0.0306)
Tc-99m DTPA	3.2-4.2 (0.08-0.12)	min: 1 mCi max: 2 mCi	Bladder wall, 0.086 (0.32)	0.012 (0.044)	Kidneys (0.055) Ovaries (0.0325)
Tc-99m sulfur colloid	18.5-37 (0.5-1.0)	600 μCi	Bladder, 0.028 (0.10)	0.0024 (0.0089)	Ovaries (0.025) Testes (0.0048)
Tc-99m DMSA	1.5-1.9 (0.04-0.05)	min: 1 mCi max: 6 mCi	Kidneys, 0.45 (1.67)	0.039 (0.14)	Renal cortex (2.00) Kidneys (1.60) Ovaries (0.069)

---

intensity signal on T1-weighted images. On T2-weighted scans, renal signal is uniformly high (Fig. 107-5).

Although MRI is usually performed to obtain anatomic information, it is proving to be a powerful dynamic imaging modality capable of providing functional information as well. Magnetic resonance urography (MRU) provides exquisite anatomic information, and by using rapid scanning techniques to track the progress of contrast material from the vascular space to the collecting system, renal functional information can be obtained. With the administration of diuretics, washout information analogous to that achieved with nuclear medicine studies can be obtained. Though still undergoing refinement, these MRU techniques hold great promise in terms of providing a complete and detailed renal evaluation.

After US, MRI is the modality of choice for imaging pelvic structures, including the uterus and ovaries in girls and the testes in boys. The bladder wall is imaged against the low water signal of urine. The uterus shows an intermediate signal on both T1- and T2-weighted images; this is variable, however, depending on degree of maturation and phase of the menstrual cycle. MRI is particularly well suited for the evaluation of pelvic structures because of its excellent soft tissue discrimination, anatomic detail, multiplanar capabilities, and absence of respiratory degradation.

NUCLEAR MEDICINE

Nuclear medicine imaging of the pediatric urinary system serves a vital role, providing both anatomic and physiologic information for the evaluation of pediatric urologic disorders. These studies are most commonly performed during the evaluation or follow-up of urinary

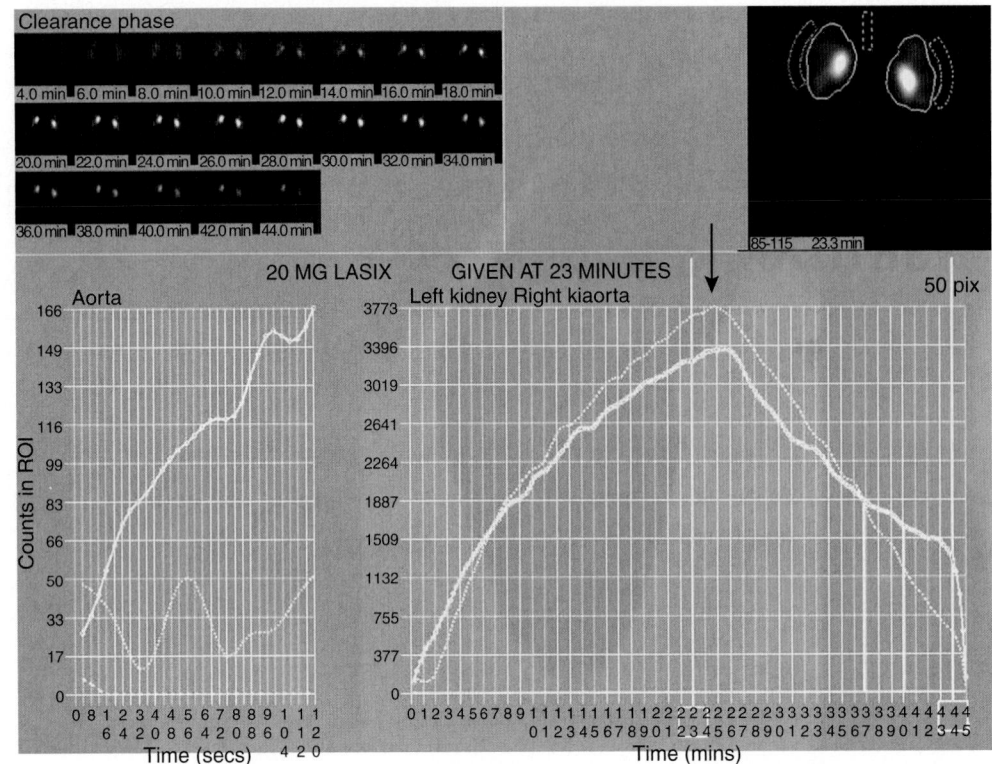

FIGURE 107-6. Time versus activity graph shows a steady accumulation of tracer in the renal region of interest until washout occurs, starting 3 minutes after diuretic injection *(arrow)*. Note the superolateral background region of interest adjacent to both kidneys. Also note mild urinary stasis and hydronephrosis, with no spontaneous excretion until after diuretic administration. The diuretic $T^{1/2}$ is approximately 10 minutes, which is considered normal in the presence of mild hydronephrosis.

dilatation or obstruction (hydronephrosis or hydro-ureter), urinary tract infection (acute pyelonephritis or pyelonephritic scarring), VUR, or congenital urinary anomalies (duplex, ectopic, or dysplastic kidneys). This section covers the basic technical and interpretive aspects of the nuclear renogram, cystogram, and cortical scan as they apply to pediatric patients.

The pediatric patient requires special considerations when performing nuclear medicine studies. Specifically, radiopharmaceutical dosage adjustments—based on body weight (Table 107-1) (From Society of Nuclear Medicine Guidelines Manual, March 2003) or body surface area—must be made to achieve satisfactory images while keeping radiation doses as low as possible. In particular, efforts should be made to minimize the time tracer-laden urine remains in the bladder. This is especially important in girls, to minimize the ovarian absorbed dose. This can be achieved with bladder catheterization or hydration and frequent voiding.

For most children, nuclear studies of the urinary tract can be performed without sedation. Very young infants can be swaddled gently for immobilization. Older children can be distracted during imaging by the parents or with cartoons or movies. Sedation may be necessary for some studies, such as renal cortical single-photon emission computed tomography (SPECT) imaging, and a standard protocol should be followed, including continuous cardiorespiratory monitoring.

For all nuclear studies discussed in this chapter, the agent used is technetium-99m. This agent is ideal for nuclear imaging because it is readily available, has an appropriate half-life (6 hours) with a low-energy photopeak (140 keV), and has excellent chemical binding to the agents used to image the kidney parenchyma (dimer-captosuccinic acid [DMSA] or glucoheptonate), urinary system (mertiatide [MAG3] or DTPA), or VUR (sulfur colloid). The radiation doses associated with this agent are well within the diagnostic ranges for other uroradiologic studies (see Table 107-1).

Standard imaging parameters include a single-head gamma camera for planar acquisitions using either a low-energy all-purpose or low-energy high-resolution collimator with 128×128 matrix. Optimal evaluation of the renal parenchyma in young children with cortical scintigraphy requires pinhole collimation; SPECT acquisitions may be preferred by some radiologists in older children.

Diuretic Renography

Diuretic renography was first described in the late 1970s and is used to distinguish obstructive from nonobstructive hydronephrosis. It attempts to quantify urinary obstruction based on the relative function of the hydronephrotic kidney compared with the normal kidney and the rate of urinary excretion of radiotracer from the renal pelvis (and, in the presence of hydroureter, from the ureter) after a diuretic challenge. The graphic presentation of renal excretion using a time versus intensity curve is termed a *renogram* (Fig. 107-6); normal, equivocal, and obstructed patterns of excretion following a diuretic challenge, termed *washout*, have been described (Fig. 107-7). Additionally, the time required for half the tracer in the collecting system to pass across the ureteropelvic junction, termed *diuretic* $T^{1/2}$, is stratified to indicate a normal (0 to 10 minutes), equivocal (10 to 20 minutes), or obstructed (>20 minutes) pattern. These values are useful in distinguishing obstructive from nonobstructive

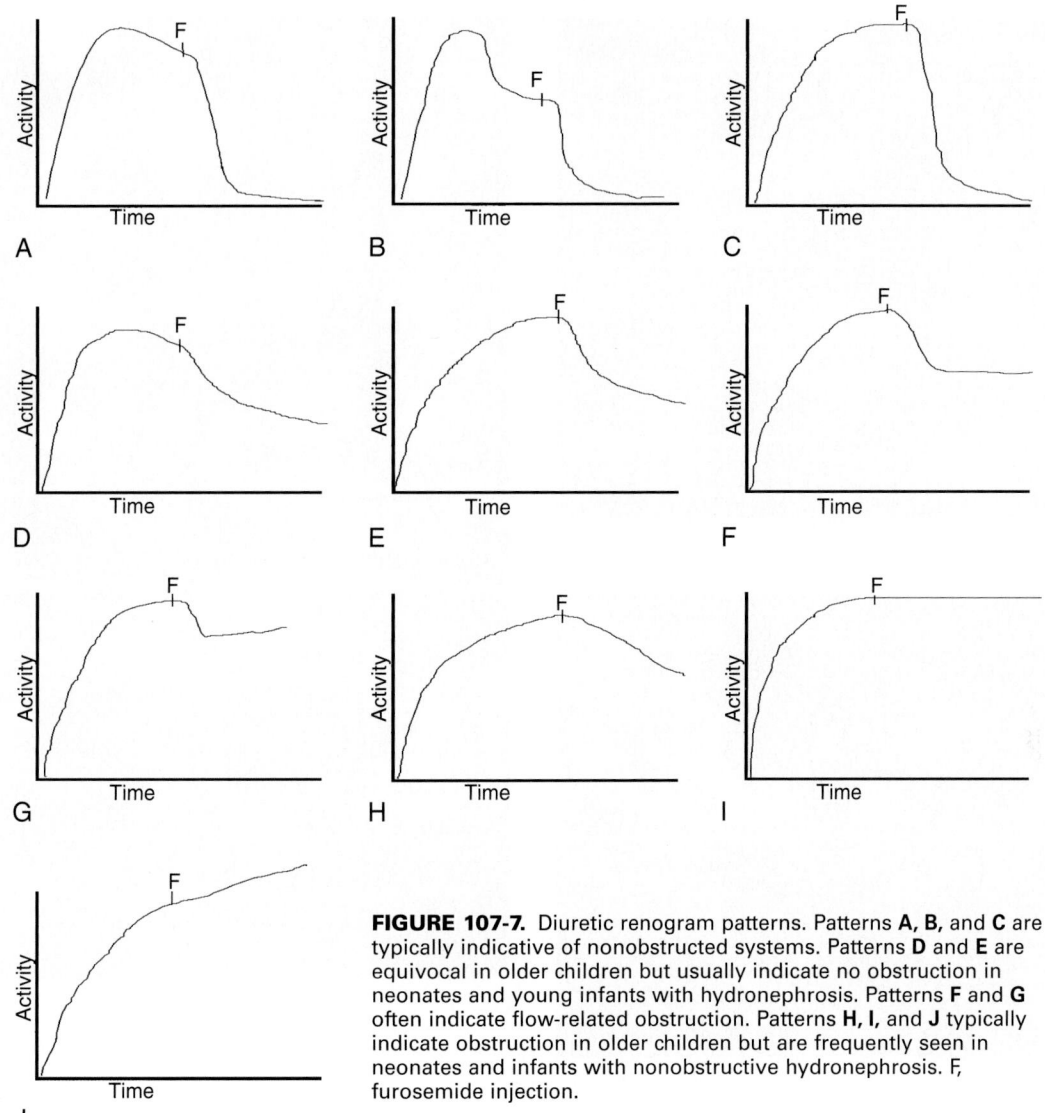

FIGURE 107-7. Diuretic renogram patterns. Patterns **A, B,** and **C** are typically indicative of nonobstructed systems. Patterns **D** and **E** are equivocal in older children but usually indicate no obstruction in neonates and young infants with hydronephrosis. Patterns **F** and **G** often indicate flow-related obstruction. Patterns **H, I,** and **J** typically indicate obstruction in older children but are frequently seen in neonates and infants with nonobstructive hydronephrosis. F, furosemide injection.

hydronephrosis in older children and adults. However, application of these guidelines can lead to the misdiagnosis of obstruction in a large number of young infants with hydronephrosis demonstrated on routine prenatal sonography (Fig. 107-8). Some clinicians challenged the need for surgical intervention in the majority of these patients and showed that conservative management was appropriate in more than 80% of them. In the hope of increasing the utility of the diuretic renogram in neonates and infants, specialists in multiple fields have attempted to standardize its performance and refine the diagnostic criteria for obstruction so as to better predict which patients with prenatally diagnosed hydronephrosis require surgical correction and which can be managed conservatively. Despite numerous modifications, there continues to be considerable controversy regarding the performance and interpretation of the diuretic renogram in these patients. The high capacitance of the dilated renal pelvis and relatively low renal urine output in young infants limit the accuracy of this test in the setting of hydronephrosis in children younger than 2 years.

Optimization of the renogram technique includes the following key points:
- Adequate patient hydration is required before and during the examination (10 ml/kg IV 5% dextrose solution with 0.45% normal saline in children older than one year, or oral hydration and dextrose solution with 0.22% normal saline in children less than one year of age).
- Adequate bladder drainage is achieved with frequent voiding in older children who are able to cooperate and with bladder catheterization in infants. An alternative to bladder catheterization is the addition of a supine postvoid planar image after upright positioning.
- Adequate diuretic challenge is achieved using 1 mg/kg IV furosemide. The timing of the diuretic injection is controversial. Recommendations include 15 minutes before the tracer injection so as to image renal perfusion and extraction during maximal diuresis (termed F–15), at the time of tracer injection to minimize

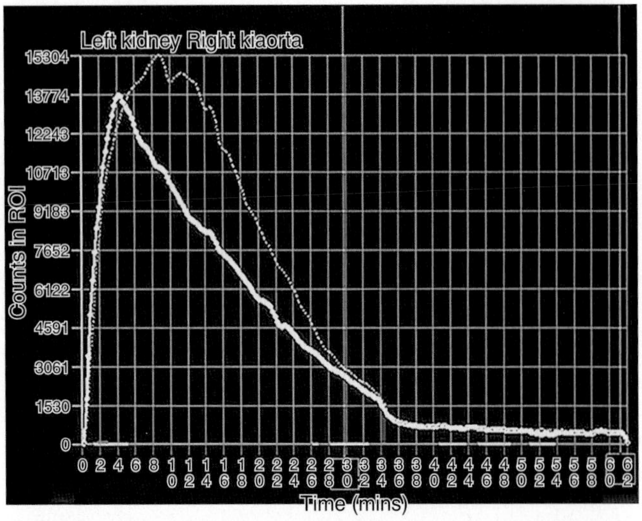

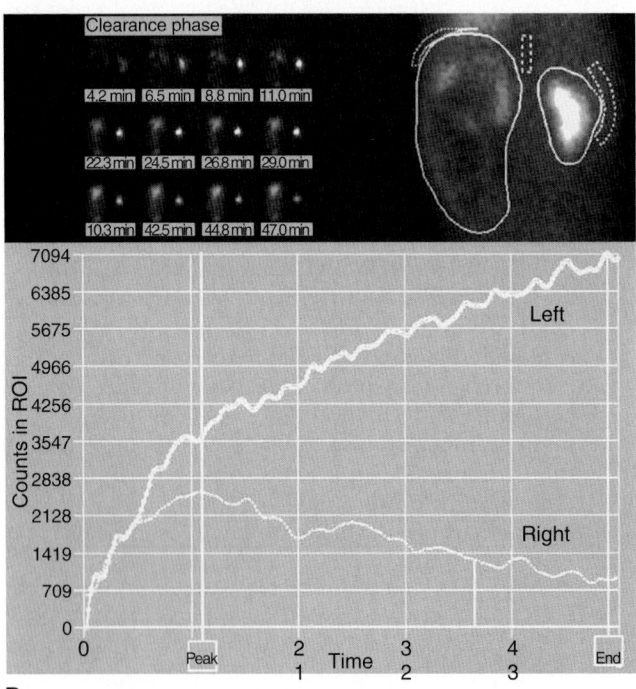

FIGURE 107-8. Diuretic renogram patterns. **A,** Washout curve shows prompt diminution of counts in both kidneys, with $T_{1/2}$ values less than 10 minutes bilaterally. Split function is equal, and the renogram is normal. **B,** Marked right and moderate left hydronephrosis with prompt washout on the left and reduced washout on the right. Split function is equal, and the findings are equivocal for obstruction. Follow-up studies showed improvement, and surgery was not necessary. **C,** Moderate left hydronephrosis with prompt but limited washout that levels off. This pattern is worrisome for impending deterioration of renal function. Follow-up studies showed deterioration, and pyeloplasty was performed. **D,** Severe left hydronephrosis with progressive accumulation of tracer throughout the study and no washout. This is often diagnostic of ureteropelvic obstruction.

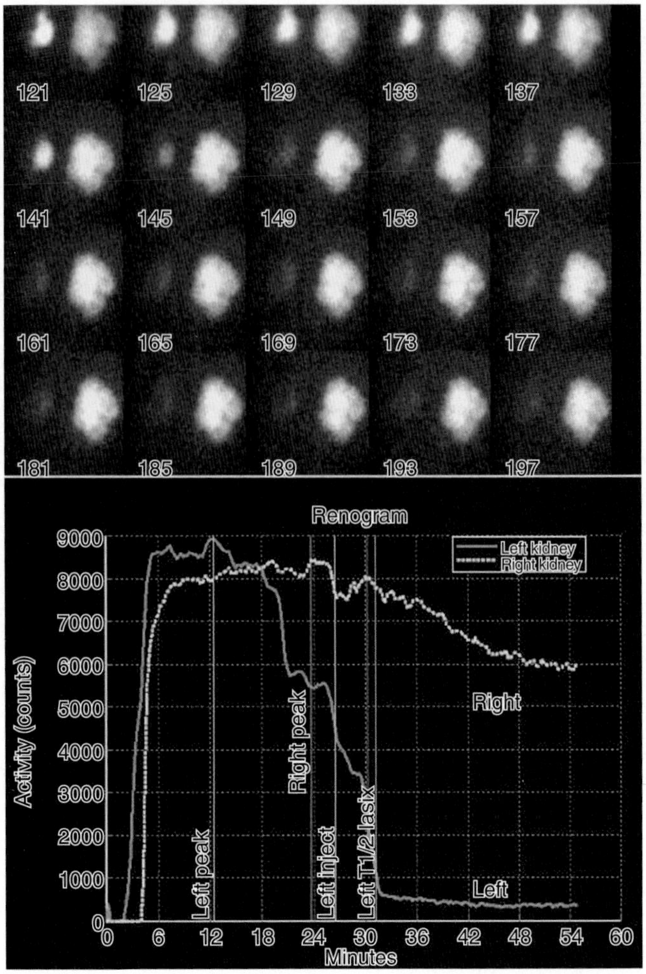

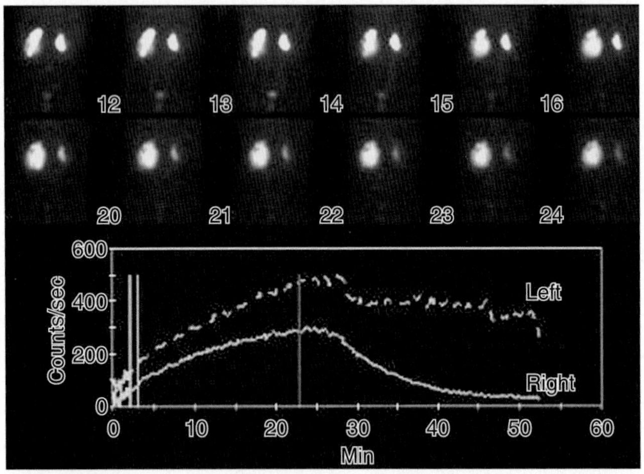

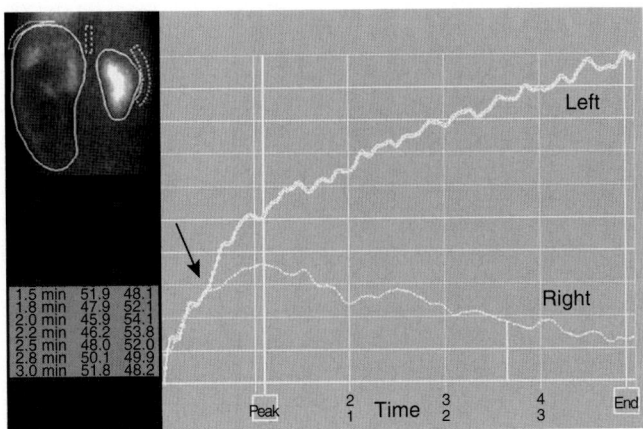

1.5 min	51.9	48.1
1.8 min	47.9	52.1
2.0 min	45.9	54.1
2.3 min	46.2	53.8
2.5 min	48.0	52.0
2.8 min	50.1	49.9
3.0 min	51.8	48.2

FIGURE 107-9. Markedly enlarged left kidney with central photopenic regions consistent with marked hydronephrosis. The renogram shows tracer accumulation and retention throughout, with no discernible washout after diuretic administration. Note that the renogram tracings of the two kidneys are superimposed during the first few minutes after injection of the tracer *(arrow)*. This indicates nearly equal split renal function, as shown on the function table between 1.5 and 3 minutes.

acquisition time (termed F–0), and after maximal urinary distention (termed F+20).

- Adequate renal-to-background visualization is achieved with technetium-99m MAG3. This agent has better renal extraction than DTPA, substantially reducing background activity (especially important with respect to the liver and spleen) and optimizing renal parenchymal visualization, even in the presence of reduced renal function. MAG3 can be used to determine effective renal plasma flow. For children older than 2 years, technetium-99m DTPA is an adequate and less expensive alternative; it can be used to determine glomerular filtration rate (GFR).

Additional technical factors that have been optimized for diuretic renography include appropriate renal parenchymal and pelvic regions of interest, as well as background subtraction regions of interest.

In general, the diuretic renogram is useful in the evaluation of hydronephrosis in adults and older children. In infants, the examination is less accurate but can be optimized with consistent application of a standard technique, correlation of the renogram washout curve with the split renal function, and correlation with serial ultrasound examinations. Increasing hydronephrosis, decreasing split renal function of the hydronephrotic kidney, and worsening washout curve all suggest the possibility of significant obstruction (Fig. 107-9).

> Renography requires strict attention to technical details, including patient hydration, bladder drainage, adequate diuretic challenge, and appropriate choice of radiopharmaceutical.

Nuclear Cystography

Nuclear cystography is performed for the assessment of VUR and is an alternative to fluoroscopic VCUG. The examination can be performed *directly* with instillation of tracer and sterile saline into the bladder (following sterile catheterization or suprapubic puncture) or *indirectly* following nuclear renography with planar images obtained during voiding. Catheterization should be performed by an experienced individual, and care should be taken to maintain sterile technique throughout. Anesthetic gel should be applied to the female urethral orifice or injected into the male urethral meatus to decrease the discomfort of catheterization. The risk of catheterization-induced infection is very small when the procedure is performed by experienced personnel and can be further minimized by delaying the study in a child with fever or a newly diagnosed urinary tract infection for at least 24 hours after the initiation of antibiotics. Bladder puncture for cystography is rarely performed in North America.

Technical features of the direct nuclear cystogram include the use of a technetium-99m–labeled agent, typically sulfur colloid, instilled into the bladder during the earliest phase of bladder filling, gravity-assisted infusion of saline into the bladder to the expected bladder capacity, and dynamic imaging of the bladder and kidney regions using a posterior gamma camera throughout the filling and voiding cycle. The data can be grouped (in 10- or 60-second intervals) as well as viewed dynamically. VUR is documented when tracer is shown to ascend into a tubular structure corresponding to the ureter or when there is visualization of the renal collecting system. The catheter is left in the bladder to minimize the amount of tracer remaining in the patient after voiding. In older children without VUR, discomfort caused by catheter manipulation can be decreased by allowing it to be expelled during voiding. The voiding phase can be performed supine or upright, depending on the child's ability to cooperate and the physician's preference. As with VCUG, mean bladder capacity for children 1 year of age or older is predicted by this formula: [Patient age (years) + 2] × 30 ml. For infants younger than 1 year, the formula is as follows: 7 ml × Patient weight (kg). The dose of tracer is dependent on bladder volume: 300 μCi for bladder volumes up to 300 ml, and 600 μCi for larger bladder volumes. A cyclic cystogram is recommended for children younger than 2 years, for those with previously documented or high suspicion for VUR, and for children who void well before the expected bladder capacity is reached. The procedure is identical to the standard cystogram; however, the catheter is left in the bladder after the first voiding cycle and is used to refill the bladder for a repeat void. As with VCUG, cyclic studies increase the diagnostic yield (Fig. 107-10), identifying an additional 10% to 15% of children with VUR compared with noncyclic voiding studies.

> Cyclic voiding studies increase the detection of VUR in infants.

The major technical pitfalls of nuclear cystography include tracer-laden urine contamination within the field of the gamma camera and motion artifact. Tracer may contaminate clothing or linens and can obscure or be

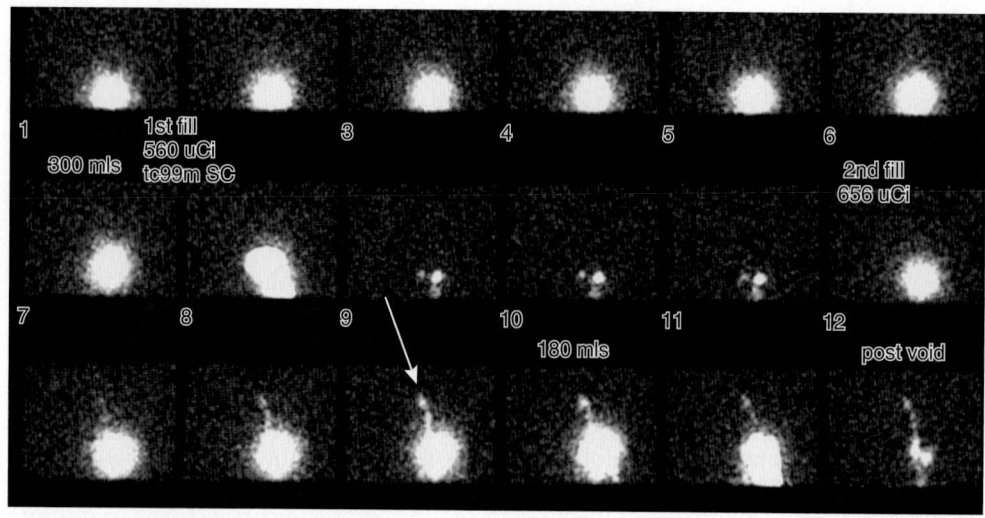

FIGURE 107-10. Cyclic nuclear cystogram demonstrates a normal first cycle, with intermediate-grade reflux present on the second cycle only *(arrow).*

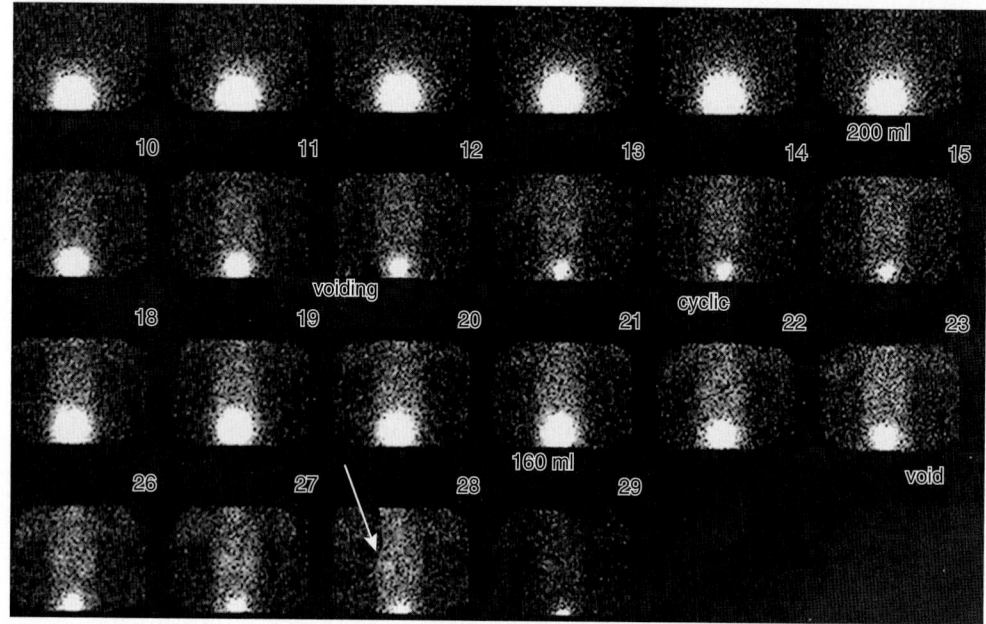

FIGURE 107-11. Nuclear cystogram performed with technetium-99m pertechnetate shows progressive soft tissue accumulation of tracer during the study owing to absorption of the tracer across the bladder wall. Late in the study, renal excretion may be mistaken for vesicoureteral reflux *(arrow).*

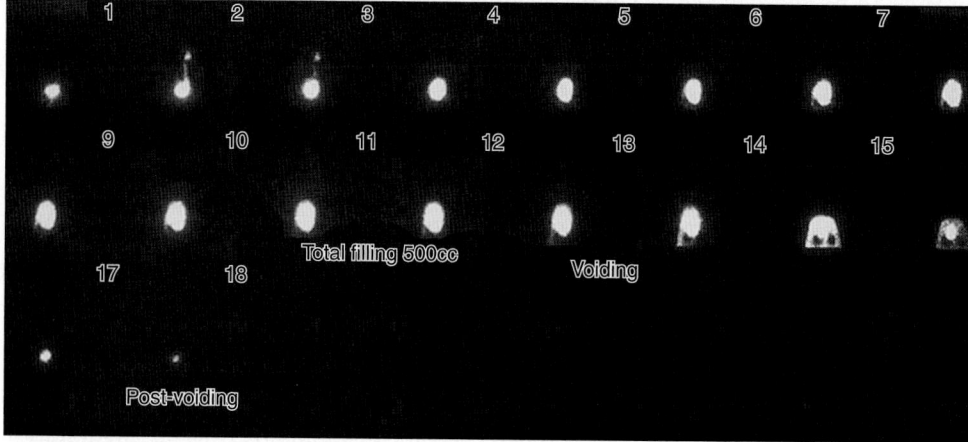

FIGURE 107-12. Early in the study, this nuclear cystogram shows intermediate-grade vesicoureteral reflux that later fully drains and does not recur through voiding. Continuous acquisition of the nuclear cystogram allowed the demonstration of this transient reflux, which likely would have been missed with fluoroscopic voiding cystourethrography.

confused with VUR. Rarely, the use of nonlabeled tracer, in the form of technetium-99m pertechnetate, can result in the systemic absorption of tracer and mimic reflux (Fig. 107-11).

Nuclear cystography offers two main advantages over fluoroscopic VCUG. First, with continuous imaging throughout the filling and voiding cycles, there is increased detection of VUR (Fig. 107-12). Second, with standard techniques, nuclear cystography has a substantially reduced radiation dose compared with VCUG. With modern fluoroscopic equipment, VCUG has approximately a 10-fold greater radiation dose than nuclear cystography.

Disadvantages of nuclear cystography include a lack of detailed anatomic visualization of the urethra and collecting systems; if these structures need to be evaluated more thoroughly, VCUG is the procedure of choice. For this reason, boys whose urethra must be examined for posterior urethral valves or strictures or patients with dysfunctional voiding should have a standard fluoroscopic VCUG as part of the initial workup. If VUR is confirmed, follow-up with nuclear cystography is sufficient. Nuclear cystography does not show bladder abnormalities, such as periureteric diverticula, that may result in VUR. Additionally, the classification of VUR with nuclear cystography is less refined than that with VCUG; the nuclear grades of low, intermediate, and high roughly correspond to the fluoroscopic grades of 1, 2 or 3, and 4 or 5, respectively.

Cortical Scintigraphy

The renal cortical scan is performed for the assessment of acute pyelonephritis or its sequela, atrophic pyelonephritic scarring. In the United States, the clinical utility of this study is limited by the fact that urinary tract infections, whether cystitis or pyelonephritis, are treated with the same course of antibiotics. However, in some practices in Europe and Australia, localization of the infection is clinically relevant because pyelonephritis is treated more aggressively; this is thought to decrease the incidence of subsequent scarring. A common indication for this examination is to assess for renal parenchymal involvement in the setting of recurrent urinary tract infections, such as a patient with neurogenic bladder or one in whom VUR is being managed medically, in which case a positive study would lead to an alteration in clinical management. The cortical scan can also be used to identify renal anomalies of fusion or location, although sonography is the examination of choice because of its lack of ionizing radiation, increased availability, better anatomic detail, and lower cost.

The cortical scan is typically performed with technetium-99m–labeled DMSA. This agent is extracted by and then binds to cells of the proximal convoluted tubule. It does not accumulate in the medulla or collecting system, thus accounting for the scan appearance of cortical uptake with relative central photopenia (Fig. 107-13). Imaging typically occurs 2 to 3 hours after injection and should be performed with pinhole collimation or SPECT acquisition with a dual-headed camera. The accuracy in demonstrating acute pyelonephritis is

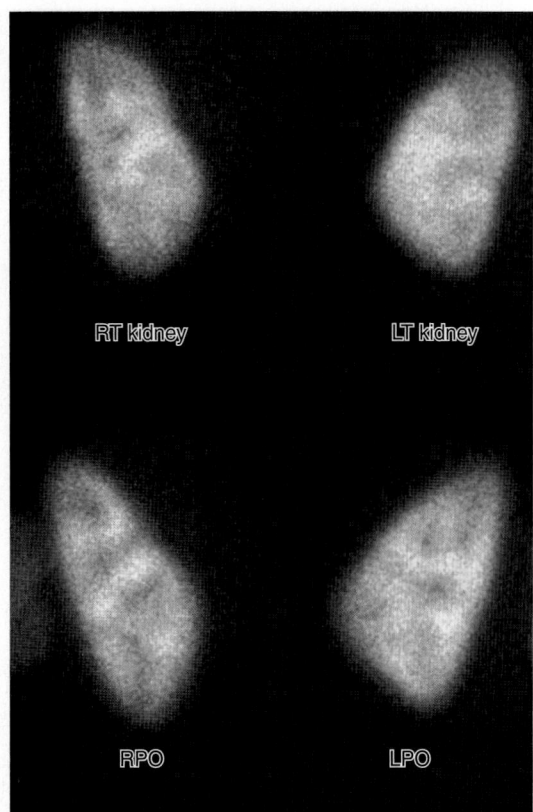

FIGURE 107-13. Normal DMSA pinhole images. Note the relative photopenia of the medulla due to a lack of uptake by the deeper portions of the loop of Henle. Also note the decreased intensity of the polar regions due to the relatively thinner polar cortex when compared with the midpolar region. LPO, left posterior oblique; RPO, right posterior oblique.

excellent, reported to exceed 95%. The pinhole images, obtained in both posterior and posterior oblique positions, have a higher specificity but lower sensitivity than SPECT images. A defect that appears as a vague area of photopenia not associated with volume loss is more consistent with acute pyelonephritis, whereas a triangular, well-demarcated photopenic focus with volume loss is typically considered an atrophic scar (Fig. 107-14), although it may also be related to focal renal dysplasia. Most areas of infection resolve without residual scarring, especially in older children, but this may take 6 months or longer after the acute infection. Therefore, a definitive diagnosis of scar requires a follow-up study at least 6 months after the acute infection. Scarring can also result from trauma, and recovery of function in a fractured kidney can be documented with cortical scinitigraphy (Fig. 107-15). Rounded defects identified with cortical scintigraphy should be further characterized with US to assess for cyst or mass (Fig. 107-16).

Miscellaneous Renal Nuclear Studies

Quantitation of renal function is possible with nuclear imaging techniques. The relative function of each kidney can be assessed during the renogram before tracer exits the renal pelvis, or with cortical scintigraphy. Regions of interest for each kidney are drawn from a posterior

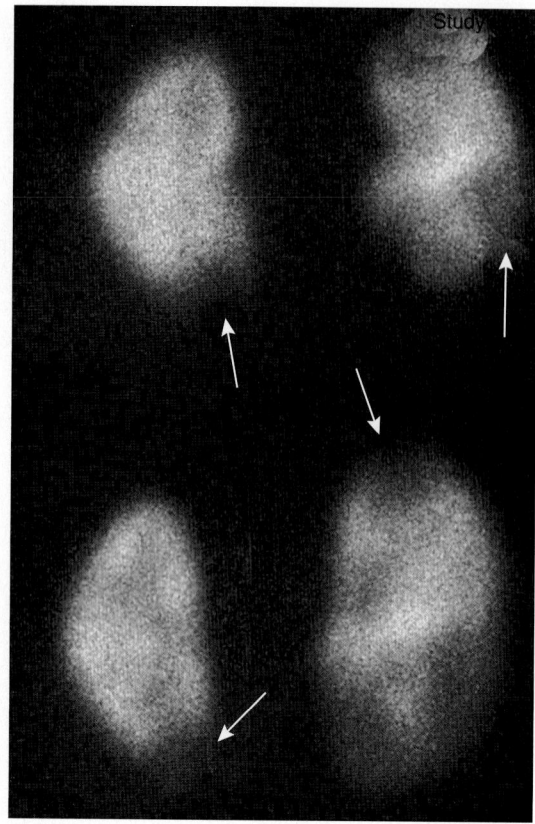

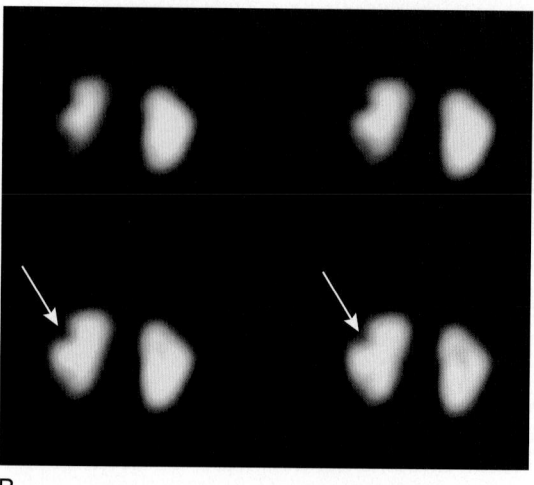

A

B

A

FIGURE 107-14. Pyelonephritis versus scarring. **A,** Pinhole DMSA images obtained for split uptake assessment show bilateral photopenic defects that are rather poorly defined and not associated with renal parenchymal volume loss *(arrows)* indicating pyelonephritis. **B,** Coronal SPECT glucoheptonate images show sharply defined wedge-shaped defects *(arrows)* indicative of renal scars. Glucoheptonate has been largely replaced by DMSA for cortical scintigraphy because of better binding characteristics.

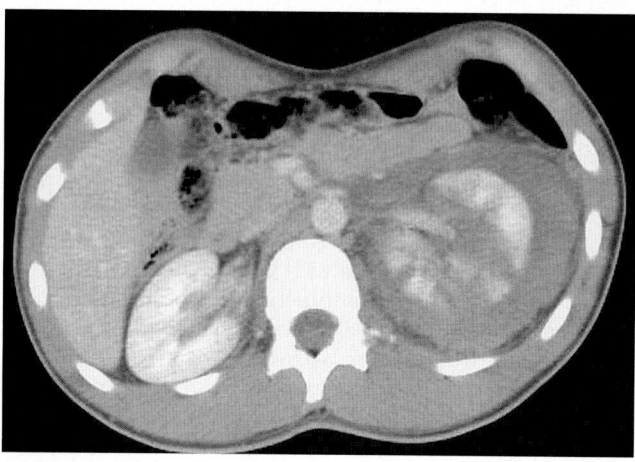

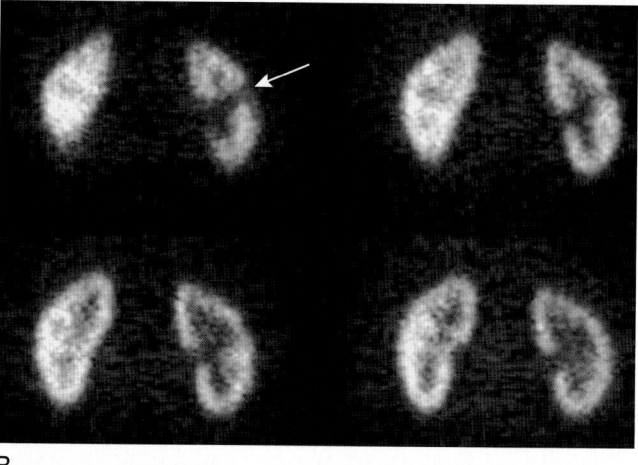

A

B

FIGURE 107-15. Renal scarring after trauma. **A,** Axial CT images show left renal fractures with multiple perfused renal fragments and a large perirenal hematoma. **B,** Three-month follow-up coronal SPECT DMSA images show a small persistent transverse scar *(arrow)* in the midpolar region.

image, and relative function is given in terms of a percentage of total renal counts. The normal value is $50\% \pm 5\%$. Camera-based techniques for absolute renal function are inaccurate in children owing to factors related to patient size and renal depth correction. Absolute renal function quantitation in terms of GFR or effective renal plasma flow can be performed with technetium-labeled MAG3 and DTPA, respectively, but these techniques require one to four blood samples. These measurements can assist in the evaluation of patients with chronic renal disease, the assessment of those

requiring potentially nephrotoxic medications (chemotherapy), or to follow patients with hydronephrosis of a solitary kidney or with bilateral hydronephrosis. In the latter case, individual renal GFR can be obtained with a combination of camera-based techniques to determine relative renal function and laboratory-based techniques for assessment of total GFR. Renal function increases rapidly in the first 2 years of life and reaches adult values, when normalized to body surface area (normal values range from 80 to 140 ml/min/1.73m^2), by age 2 years.

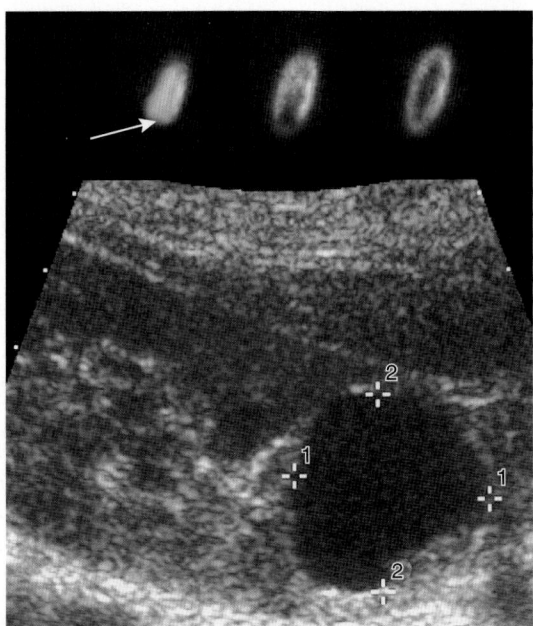

FIGURE 107-16. Sagittal SPECT DMSA images show a rounded, photopenic defect in the lower pole *(arrow)*, shown to be a cyst on follow-up US.

Immediately after renal transplantation, nuclear renography can be used to evaluate graft perfusion, urinary leak, and obstruction, although Doppler US has largely replaced nuclear techniques for these indications. Subacute rejection and acute tubular necrosis may have identical renograms and are differentiated by their time course and differences from baseline renograms. Nephrotoxic drug reaction and chronic rejection may be difficult to differentiate based on alterations in the renogram perfusion, extraction, and excretion phases and may coexist. Biopsy is often required in these cases.

Systolic hypertension affects 1% to 3% of children, and a specific cause is more frequently found in children than in adults, especially in neonates and infants; up to 48% of these young patients have secondary hypertension. The most frequently identified causes of secondary hypertension in children are abnormalities of renal vascular supply or drainage. These abnormalities are termed *renal vascular hypertension* and account for approximately 5% to 25% of pediatric hypertension. Identifying which children should undergo imaging evaluation and determining the specific imaging studies that should be performed are discussed in Chapter 150.

An underperfused kidney maintains filtration across the glomerulus by increasing the pressure in the postglomerular arteriole. This process is mediated by angiotensin. The renogram of such a kidney may be abnormal at baseline or become abnormal (tracer retention or decreased split function) following the administration of an angiotensin-converting enzyme (ACE) inhibitor. Nuclear renography using an ACE inhibitor is performed in some pediatric centers, either before or after angiography. Angiography reportedly finds a renal vascular lesion in approximately 85% of kidneys with ACE inhibitor–induced abnormal renograms. Additionally, approximately 15% of stenoses demonstrated angiographically are not confirmed to be the source of the patient's hypertension, and an abnormal ACE inhibitor renogram can be used to determine whether a stenosis is functionally significant.

ACE inhibitor renography requires strict attention to the patient's hydration status, as well as a consideration of antihypertensive medications that may affect the results. The use of a baseline renogram to compare with the ACE inhibitor study has been recommended. Specific interpretive criteria have been suggested, and they vary depending on the specific agent used. A more thorough discussion of ACE inhibitor renography is beyond the scope of this text and can be found in nuclear medicine references.

VASCULAR STUDIES

Diagnostic vascular procedures performed in children include inferior vena cava cavography, abdominal aortography, selective renal arteriography, digital subtraction angiography, renal venography, and selective venous renin studies. These studies have largely been supplanted by CT and MRI, which allow diagnostic information to be obtained noninvasively and provide superior depiction of adjacent anatomy. The remaining indications for angiographic evaluation and intervention are discussed in Chapter 185.

ACKNOWLEDGMENTS

The authors wish to recognize the work of Dr. Jack O. Haller, Dr. Beverly P. Wood, Dr. Guido Currarino, and Dr. Douglas F. Eggli from prior editions of this book.

SUGGESTED READINGS

Fetal Urologic Imaging

Cassart M, Massez A, Metens T, et al: Complementary role of MRI after sonography in assessing bilateral urinary tract anomalies in the fetus. AJR Am J Roentgenol 2004;182:689-695

Ismaili K, Avni FE, Wissing KM, et al: Long-term clinical outcome of infants with mild and moderate fetal pyelectasis: validation of neonatal ultrasound as a screening tool to detect significant nephrouropathies. J Pediatr 2004;144:759-765

Witzani L, Brugger PC, Hormann M, et al: Normal renal development investigated with fetal MRI. Eur J Radiol 2006;57:294-302

Contrast Media

American College of Radiology: Manual on Contrast Media. www.acr.org/s_acr/sec.asp?CID=2131&DID=16687

Aspelin P, Stacul F, Thomsen HS, et al: Effects of iodinated contrast media on blood and endothelium. Eur Radiol 2006;16:1041-1049

Bagg MNJ, Horwitz TA, Bester L: Comparison of patient responses to high- and low-osmolality contrast agents injected intravenously. AJR Am J Roentgenol 1986;147:185-187

Barrett BJ, Parfrey PS: Clinical practice: preventing nephropathy induced by contrast medium. N Engl J Med 2006;354:379-386

Bettmann MA: Frequently asked questions: iodinated contrast agents. Radiographics 2004;24(Suppl 1):S3-S10

Bettmann MA, Holzer JF, Trombly ST: Risk management issues related to the use of contrast agents. Radiology 1990;175:629-631

Brasch RC: Allergic reactions to contrast media: accumulated evidence. AJR Am J Roentgenol 1980;134:797-801

Caro JJ, Trindade E, McGregor M: The risks of death and of severe nonfatal reactions with high- vs low-osmolality contrast media: a meta-analysis. AJR Am J Roentgenol 1991;156:825-832

Choyke PL, Kobayashi H: Functional magnetic resonance imaging of the kidneys using macromolecular contrast agents. Abdom Imaging 2006;31:224-231

Cochran ST: Anaphylactoid reactions to radiocontrast media. Curr Allergy Asthma Rep 2005;5:28-31

Cohan RH, Dunnick NR, Bashore TM: Treatment of reactions to radiographic contrast material. AJR Am J Roentgenol 1988; 151:253-270

Delaney A, Carter A, Fisher M: The prevention of anaphylactoid reactions to iodinated radiological contrast media: a systematic review of randomized controlled trials. BMC Med Imaging 2006;27:2

DeRidder F, DeMaeseneer M, Stadnik T: Severe adverse reactions with contrast agents for magnetic resonance: clinical experience in 30,000 MR examinations. JBR-BTR 2001;84:150-152

Elam EA, Door RT, Lagel KE, et al: Cutaneous ulceration due to contrast extravasation: experimental assessment of injury and potential antidotes. Invest Radiol 1991;26:13-16

FDA/Center for Drug Evaluation and Research: Information on Gadolinium-Containing Contrast Agents. Available at: http://www.fda.gov/cder/drug/infopage/gcca/default.htm. Last accessed on 8/14/2007

Federle MP, Chang PJ, Confer S, et al: Frequency and effects of extravasation of ionic and nonionic CT contrast media during rapid bolus injection. Radiology 1998;206:637-640

Grobner T, Prischl FC: Gadolinium and nephrogenic systemic fibrosis. Kidney Int 2007;72:260-264

Harvey L, Caldicott WJH, Kuruc A: The effect of contrast media on immature renal function. Radiology 1983;148:429-432

Katayama H, Yamaguchi K, Kozuka T, et al: Adverse reactions to ionic and nonionic contrast media: a report from the Japanese Committee on the Safety of Contrast Media. Radiology 1990;175:621-628

Kaufmann HJ (ed): Contrast Media in Pediatric Radiology. Berlin, Schering AG, 1987

Lasser EC: Pretreatment with corticosteroids to prevent reactions to IV contrast material: overview and implications. AJR Am J Roentgenol 1988;150:257-259

Lasser EC, Berry CC, Talner LB: Pretreatment with corticosteroids to alleviate reactions to IV contrast material. N Engl J Med 1987;317:845-849

Li A, Wong CS, Wong MK: Acute adverse reactions to magnetic resonance contrast media—gadolinium chelates. Br J Radiol 2006;79:368-371

Miller DL, Chang R, Wells WT, et al: Intravascular contrast media: effect of dose on renal function. Radiology 1988;167:607-611

Moore RD, Steinberg EP, Powe NR, et al: Frequency and determinants of adverse reactions induced by high osmolality contrast media. Radiology 1989;170:727-732

Morcos SK: Acute serious and fatal reactions to contrast media: our current understanding. Br J Radiol 2005;78:686-693

Mortele KJ, Oliva MR, Ondategui S: Universal use of nonionic iodinated contrast medium for CT: evaluation of safety in a large urban teaching hospital. AJR Am J Roentgenol 2005;184:31-34

Newman B, Caldicott WJH, Michelow P: Contrast media and renal function in the immature kidney. Invest Radiol 1987;22:608-612

Reuter SR: The use of conventional vs lower-osmolar contrast agents: a legal analysis. AJR Am J Roentgenol 1988;151:529-531

Runge VM, Dickey KM, Williams NM: Local tissue toxicity in response to extravascular extravasation of magnetic resonance contrast media. Invest Radiol 2002;37:393-398

Sadowski EA, Bennett LK, Chan MR, et al: Nephrogenic systemic fibrosis: risk factors and incidence estimation. Radiology 2007;243:148-157

Saini S, Modic MT, Hamm B, et al: Advances in contrast-enhanced MR imaging. AJR Am J Roentgenol 1991;156:235-254

Thomsen HS, Morcos SK: ESUR guidelines on contrast media. Abdom Imaging 2006;31:131-140

Urography

Diament M, Kangarloo H: Dosage schedule for pediatric urography based on body surface area. AJR Am J Roentgenol 1983; 140:815-816

Leppert A, Nadalin S, Schirg E: Impact of magnetic resonance urography on preoperative diagnostic workup in children affected by hydronephrosis: should IVU be replaced? J Pediatr Surg 2002;37:1441-1445

Persliden J, Helmrot E, Hjort P: Dose and image quality in the comparison of analogue and digital techniques in pediatric urology examinations. Eur Radiol 2004;14:638-644

Riccabona M, Lindbichler F, Sinzig M: Conventional imaging in pediatric uroradiology. Eur J Radiol 2002;43:100-109

Voiding Cystourethrography and Other Procedures

Al Jurayyan NA, Patel PJ, al Herbish AS: Ambiguous genitalia: comparative role of pelvic ultrasonography and genitography. Ann Trop Paediatr 1995;15:203-207

Darge K, Riedmiller H: Current status of vesicoureteral reflux diagnosis. World J Urol 2004;22:88-95

Lederman HM, Khademian ZP, Felice M: Dose reduction fluoroscopy in pediatrics. Pediatr Radiol 2002;32:844-848

McEwing RL, Anderson NG, Hellewell S: Comparison of echo-enhanced ultrasound with fluoroscopic MCU for the detection of vesicoureteral relfux in neonates. Pediatr Radiol 2002;32:853-858

Medina LS, Aguirre E, Altman NR: Vesicoureteral reflux imaging in children: comparative cost analysis. Acad Radiol 2003;10:139-144

Papdopoulou F, Efremidis SC, Oiconomou A, et al: Cyclic voiding cystourethrography: is vesicoureteral reflux missed with standard voiding cystourethrography. Eur Radiol 2002;12:666-670

Persinakis K, Raissaki M, Damilakis J, et al: Fluoroscopy-controlled voiding cystourethrography in infants and children: are the radiation risks trivial? Eur Radiol 2006;16:846-851

Persliden J, Helmrot E, Hjort P, et al: Dose and image quality in the comparison of analogue and digital techniques in paediatric urology examinations. Eur Radiol 2004;14:638-644

Piaggio G, Degl' Innocenti ML, Toma P: Cystosonography and voiding cystourethrography in the diagnosis of vesicoureteral reflux. Pediatr Nephrol 2003;18:18-22

Riccabona M, Lindbichler F, Sinzig M: Conventional imaging in pediatric uroradiology. Eur J Radiol 2002;43:100-109

Riccabona M, Mache CJ, Lindbichler F: Echo-enhanced color Doppler cystosonography of vesicoureteral reflux in children: improvement by stimulated acoustic emission. Acta Radiol 2003;44:18-23

Sukan A, Bayazit AK, Kibar M, et al: Comparison of direct radionuclide cystography and voiding direct cystography in the detection of vesicoureteral reflux. Ann Nucl Med 2003;17:549-553

Ward VL, Barnewolt CE, Strauss KY, et al: Radiation exposure reduction during voiding cystourethrography in a pediatric porcine model of vesicoureteral reflux. Radiology 2006;238:96-106

Ultrasonography

Aso C, Enriquez G, Fite M: Gray-scale and color Doppler sonography of scrotal disorders in children: an update. Radiographics 2005;25:1197-1214

Avni EF, Brion LE: Ultrasound of the neonate urinary tract. Urol Radiol 1983;5:177-183

Coley BD: Pediatric applications of abdominal vascular Doppler: part II. Pediatr Radiol 2004;34:772-786

Correas JM, Claudon M, Tranquart F: The kidney: imaging with microbubble contrast agents. Ultrasound Q 2006;22:53-66

Haller JO, Berdon WE, Friedman AP: Increased renal cortical echogenicity: a normal finding in neonates and infants. Radiology 1982;142:173-174

Hricak H, Slovis TL, Callen CW, et al: Neonatal kidneys: sonographic-anatomic correlation. Radiology 1983;147:699-702

Jequier S, Paltiel H, Lafortune M: Ureterovesical jets in infants and children: duplex and color Doppler US studies. Radiology 1990;175:349-353

Karmazyn B, Steinberg R, Kornreich L: Clinical and sonographic criteria of acute scrotum in children: a retrospective study of 172 boys. Pediatr Radiol 2005;35:302-310

Keller MS: Renal Doppler sonography in infants and children. Radiology 1989;172:603-604

Kraus RA, Gaisie G, Young LW: Increased renal parenchymal echogenicity: causes in pediatric patients. Radiographics 1990;10:1009-1018

Nelson TR, Pretorius DH: The Doppler signal: where does it come from and what does it mean? AJR Am J Roentgenol 1988; 151:439-447

Oppenheimer DA, Carroll BA, Yousem S: Sonography of the normal neonatal adrenal gland. Radiology 1983;146:157-160

Riccabona M: Modern pediatric ultrasound: potential applications and clinical significance: a review. Clin Imaging 2006;30:77-86

Scoutt LM, Zawin ML, Taylor KWJ: Doppler US. Part II. Clinical applications. Radiology 1990;174:309-319

Wiener JS, O'Hara SM: Optimal timing of initial postnatal ultrasonography in newborns with prenatal hydronephrosis. J Urol 2002;168:1826-1829

Computed Tomography

Bjorkman H, Eklof H, Wadstrom J, et al: Split renal function in patients with suspected renal artery stenosis: a comparison between gamma camera scintigraphy and two methods of measurement with computed tomography. Acta Radiol 2006;47:107-113

Dachner JN, Boillot B, Eurin D, et al: Rational use of CT in acute pyelonephritis: findings and relationships with reflux. Pediatr Radiol 1993;23:281-285

Donnelly LF, Frush DP: Pediatric multidetector body CT. Radiol Clin North Am 2003;41:637-655

Frush DP: Pediatric CT: practical approach to diminish the radiation dose. Pediatr Radiol 2002;32:714-717

Frush DP: Review of radiation issues for computed tomography. Semin Ultrasound CT MR 2004;25:17-24

Huang J, Kim YH, Shankar S, et al: Multidetector CT urography: comparison of two different scanning protocols for improved visualization of the urinary tract. J Comput Assist Tomogr 2006;30:33-36

Kaste SC, Young CW: Safe use of power injectors with central and peripheral venous access devices for pediatric CT. Pediatr Radiol 1996;26:499-501

Kawamoto S, Horton KM, Fishman EK: Opacification of the collecting system and ureters on excretory-phase CT using oral water as contrast medium. AJR Am J Roentgenol 2006;186:136-140

Kirks DR: Computed tomography of pediatric urinary tract disease. Urol Radiol 1983;5:199-210

Kocakoc E, Bhatt S, Dogra VS: Renal multidetector row CT. Radiol Clin North Am 2005;43:1021-1047

Larsen AS, Pedersen R, Sandbaek G: Computed tomography of the urinary tract: optimalization of low-dose stone protocol in a clinical setting. Acta Radiol 2005;46:764-768

Nakayama Y, Awai K, Funama Y, et al: Abdominal CT with low tube voltage: preliminary observations about radiation dose, contrast enhancement, image quality, and noise. Radiology 2005;237:945-951

Quillin SP, Brink JA, Heiken JP, et al: Helical (spiral) CT angiography for identification of crossing vessels at the ureteropelvic junction. AJR Am J Roentgenol 1996;166:1125-1130

Siegel MJ: Protocols for helical CT in pediatrics. In Silverman PM (ed): Helical (Spiral) Computed Tomography: A Practical Approach to Clinical Protocols. New York, Lippincott-Raven, 1998:179-224

Smith RC, Rosenfield AT, Choe KA, et al: Acute flank pain: comparison of non-contrast-enhanced CT and intravenous urography. Radiology 1995;194:789-794

Strouse PJ, Bates DG, Bloom DA, Goodsitt MM: Non-contrast thin-section helical CT of urinary tract calculi in children. Pediatr Radiol 2002;32:326-332

Magnetic Resonance Imaging

Bennett HF, Debiao L: MR imaging of renal function. Magn Reson Imaging Clin N Am 1997;5:107-126

Boechat MI: MR imaging of the pediatric pelvis. Magn Reson Imaging Clin N Am 1996;4:679-696

Borthne A, Pierre-Jerome C, Gjesdal KI: Pediatric excretory MR urography: comparative study of enhanced and non-enhanced techniques. Eur Radiol 2003;13:1423-1427

Fukuda Y, Watanabe H, Tomita T, et al: Evaluation of glomerular function in individual kidneys using dynamic magnetic resonance imaging. Pediatr Radiol 1996;26:324-328

Grant PE, Matsuda KM: Applications of new MR techniques in pediatric patients. Magn Reson Imaging Clin N Am 2003;11:493-522

Jones RA, Easley K, Little SB, et al: Dynamic contrast-enhanced MR urography in the evaluation of pediatric hydronephrosis. Part 1. Functional assessment. AJR Am J Roentgenol 2005;185:1598-1607

Jones RA, Perez-Brayfield MR, Kirsch AJ, Grattan-Smith JD: Renal transit time with MR urography in children. Radiology 2004;233:41-50

Kocaoglu M, Ilica AT, Bulakbasi N, et al: MR urography in pediatric uropathies with dilated urinary tracts. Diagn Interv Radiol 2005;11:225-232

Lang IM, Babyn P, Oliver GD: MR imaging of paediatric uterovaginal anomalies. Pediatr Radiol 1999;29:163-170

McDaniel BB, Jones RA, Scherz H, et al: Dynamic contrast-enhanced MR urography in the evaluation of pediatric hydronephrosis. Part 2. Anatomic and functional assessment of ureteropelvic junction obstruction. AJR Am J Roentgenol 2005;185:1608-1614

Nolte-Ernsting CC, Bucker A, Adam GB, et al: Gadolinium-enhanced excretory MR urography after low-dose diuretic injection: comparison with conventional excretory urography. Radiology 1998;209:147-157

Regan F, Bohlman ME, Khazan R, et al: MR-urography using HASTE imaging in the assessment of ureteric obstruction. AJR Am J Roentgenol 1996;167:1115-1120

Reuther G, Kiefer B, Wandl E: Visualization of urinary tract dilatation: value of single-shot MR urography. Eur Radiol 1997;7:1276-1281

Riccabona M: Pediatric MRU—its potential and its role in the diagnostic work-up of upper urinary tract dilatation in infants and children. World J Urol 2004;22:79-87

Riccabona M, Ruppert-Kohlmayr A, Ring E, et al: Potential impact of pediatric MR urography on the imaging algorithm in patients with a functional single kidney. AJR Am J Roentgenol 2004;183:795-800

Rohrschneider WK, Becker K, Hoffend J, et al: Combined static-dynamic MR urography for the simultaneous evaluation of morphology and function in urinary tract obstruction. II. Findings in experimentally induced ureteric stenosis. Pediatr Radiol 2000;30:523-532

Rohrschneider WK, Haufe S, Clorius JH: MR to assess renal function in children. Eur Radiol 2003;13:1033-1045

Rohrschneider WK, Hoffend J, Becker K, et al: Combined static-dynamic MR urography for the simultaneous evaluation of morphology and function in urinary tract obstruction. I. Evaluation of the normal status in an animal model. Pediatr Radiol 2000;30:511-522

Sigmund G, Stoever B, Zimmerhackl LB, et al: RARE-MR-urography in the diagnosis of upper urinary tract abnormalities in children. Pediatr Radiol 1991;1991:416-420

Staatz G, Nolte-Ernsting CC, Adam GB, et al: Feasibility and utility of respiratory-gated, gadolinium-enhanced T1-weighted magnetic resonance urography in children. Invest Radiol 2000;35:504-512

Verswijvel GA, Oyen RH, Van Poppel HP, et al: Magnetic resonance imaging in the assessment of urologic disease: an all-in-one approach. Eur Radiol 2000;10:1614-1619

Nuclear Medicine

Conway JJ, Maizels M: The "well tempered" diuretic renogram: a standard method to examine the asymptomatic neonate with hydronephrosis or hydroureteronephrosis. A report from combined meetings of the Society for Fetal Urology and members of the Pediatric Nuclear Medicine Council–Society of Nuclear Medicine. J Nucl Med 1992;33:2047-2051

Dubovsky EV, Russell CD, Bischof-Delaloye A, et al: Report of the Radionuclides in Nephrourology Committee for evaluation of transplanted kidney (review of techniques). Semin Nucl Med 1999;9:175-188

Gelfand MJ, Koch BL, Elgazzar AH, et al: Cyclic cystography: diagnostic yield in selected pediatric populations. Radiology 1999;213:118-120

Gordon I: Diuretic rengography in infants with prenatal unilateral hydronephrosis: an explanation for the controversy about poor drainage. BJU Int 2001;87:551-555

Koff SA, Binkovitz L, Coley B, Jayanthi VR: Renal pelvis volume during diuresis in children with hydronephrosis: implications for diagnosing obstruction with diuretic renography. J Urol 2005;174:303-307

Lagomarsino E, Orellana P, Munoz J, et al: Captopril scintigraphy in the study of arterial hypertension in pediatrics. Pediatr Nephrol 2004;19:66-70

Mandell GA, Cooper JA, Leonard JC, et al: Society of Nuclear Medicine procedure guideline for diuretic renography in children. Society of Nuclear Medicine, 1999. http://interactive.snm.org/index.cfm?PageID=1110&RPID=808&FileID=1330

Mandell GA, Eggli DF, Gilday DL, et al: Society of Nuclear Medicine procedure guideline for radionuclide cystography in children. Society of Nuclear Medicine, 2003. http://interactive.snm.org/index.cfm?PageID=1110&RPID=810&FileID=1342

Mandell GA, Eggli DF, Gilday DL, et al: Society of Nuclear Medicine procedure guideline for renal cortical scintigraphy in children. Society of Nuclear Medicine, 2003. http://interactive.snm.org/index.cfm?PageID=1110&RPID=811&FileID=1333

Mandell GA, Majd M, Shalaby-Rana EI, et al: Society of Nuclear Medicine procedure guideline for pediatric sedation in nuclear medicine. Society of Nuclear Medicine, 2003. http://interactive.snm.org/index.cfm?PageID=1110&RPID=809&FileID=1341

Piepsz A, Colarinha P, Gordon I, et al: Guidelines for glomerular filtration rate determination in children. European Association of Nuclear Medicine. http://www.eanm.org/scientific_info/guidelines/gl_paed_gfrd.php?navId=54

Piepsz A, Colarinha P, Gordon I, et al: Guidelines on ^{99m}Tc-DMSA scintigraphy in children. European Association of Nuclear Medicine. http://www.eanm.org/scientific_info/guidelines/guidelines_intro.php?navId=54

Taylor AT, Blaufox D, Dubovsky EC, et al: Society of Nuclear Medicine procedure guideline for diagnosis of renovascular hypertension. Society of Nuclear Medicine, 2003. http://interactive.snm.org/index.cfm?PageID=772&RPID=10

Taylor A, Thakore K, Folks R, et al: Background subtraction in technetium-99m-MAG3 renography. J Nucl Med 1997;38:74-79

Turkolmez S, Atasever T, Turkolmez K, Gogus O: Comparison of three different diuretic renal scintigraphy protocols in patients with dilated upper urinary tracts. Clin Nucl Med 2004;29:154-160

Ulman I, Jayanthi VR, Koff SA: The long-term followup of newborns with severe unilateral hydronephrosis initially treated nonoperatively. J Urol 2001;164:1101-1105

Wong DC, Rossleigh MA, Farnsworth RH: Diuretic renography with the addition of quantitative gravity-assisted drainage in infants and children. J Nucl Med 2000;41:1030-1036

Vascular Studies

Chan FP, Rubin GD: MDCT angiography of pediatric vascular diseases of the abdomen, pelvis, and extremities. Pediatr Radiol 2005;35:40-53

Siegel MJ: Pediatric CT angiography. Eur Radiol 2005;15(Suppl 4):D32-D36

Strouse PJ: Magnetic resonance angiography of the pediatric abdomen and pelvis. Magn Reson Imaging Clin N Am 2002;10:345-361

108 Oncology: Imaging Gastrointestinal and Genitourinary Tumors

SUE C. KASTE

Recent technological advances in diagnostic imaging have improved the precision in diagnosing abdominal masses, assessing tumor size and spread, and guiding interventions. These advances in imaging have occurred in parallel with a rapid rise in the survival rates of children treated for malignant diseases. Currently, the overall expected survival rate for pediatric patients with any type of cancer is 80%. Incorporating these technological advances in imaging into the evaluation and treatment of children with masses, whether benign or malignant, requires increased knowledge and expertise on the part of the imager. These technologies are also associated with more costly equipment and increased complexity in terms of selecting the most appropriate modality for a given patient. Factors to be considered in such decisions include access to new technologies, accuracy, expediency, cost, radiation exposure, and patient condition.

Along with an understanding of contemporary technology, radiologists must be knowledgeable about the clinical presentations and natural courses of benign and malignant abdominal and pelvic masses. For example, ovarian masses may present with abdominal complaints that mimic appendicitis. Gastrointestinal masses may present as nonspecific abdominal complaints. Renal masses may present with pain after trauma. Even if an abdominal or pelvic mass is not palpable, it may be discovered by the radiologist when searching for unrelated pathology.

Diagnostic imaging plays a major role in the diagnosis and management of pediatric masses, the staging of disease, the identification and monitoring of complications of therapy, the monitoring of response to therapy, and the guiding of therapy. However, imaging techniques are not always accurate in distinguishing benign from malignant masses. Further, imaging characteristics of malignant tumors can vary, based on technique, and they may be discrepant from histologic staging, as noted by Gow and colleagues in a study of Wilms tumor using 10-mm contiguous sections.

This chapter addresses many of the technological innovations and new modalities that have been refined or developed over the past several years, as well as their relative merits and limitations. Specific characteristics of individual tumors are addressed in organ-specific chapters.

IMAGING GOALS IN PEDIATRIC ONCOLOGY

The goals of imaging in pediatric oncology can be considered in four stages: initial diagnosis, assessment of therapeutic response, end-of-therapy evaluation, and monitoring after completion of therapy. Each phase of imaging has a purpose, and the imaging techniques chosen reflect the phase of therapy. Further, imaging choices should reflect the patient population, the risks and benefits of the modality, and the information desired from the study (Tables 108-1 and 108-2).

Imaging goals in pediatric oncology:
- **Initial diagnosis and staging**
- **Assessment of therapeutic response**
- **End-of-therapy evaluation**
- **Post-therapy monitoring**

Several issues must be considered when diagnosing pediatric malignancies. Most important, children should not be treated like small adults. The child's knowledge base should always be considered, particularly when the child is very ill and the parents are severely stressed by the concept of their child having cancer. Each patient and his or her family are unique, and imaging personnel should be specially qualified to work with this patient cohort. We must also be cognizant of the fact that the effects of radiation exposure are cumulative and make an effort to adjust techniques to optimize information while minimizing patient doses (see Chapters 1 and 2). In addition, malignancies may present differently in children versus adults. Masses of similar size may present more acutely in a child than in an adult, owing to greater compromise of smaller structures. Although many tumors have a predisposition for certain age groups, we must remember that adult tumors may occasionally be seen in children and adolescents; typical examples include hepatocellular carcinoma (Fig. 108-1), renal cell carcinoma (Fig. 108-2), malignant melanoma, and colon cancer.

At initial diagnosis, imaging is used to identify and characterize the mass, provide a differential diagnosis, and determine the extent of disease, both locally and distantly (Table 108-3). As a member of the interdisci-

TABLE 108-1

Comparison of Diagnostic Imaging Modalities

Modality	Anatomic Information	Physiologic Information	Cost	Cautions
Radiography	X	X (with contrast)	Low	Pregnancy
Ultrasonography	X		Moderate	Contrast*
Computed tomography	X	X (with contrast)	Moderate to high	Pregnancy IV contrast
Magnetic resonance imaging	X	X (with contrast)	High	Pregnancy for >3T IV contrast Ferromagnetic metal
Nuclear imaging		X	Moderate	Pregnancy
Fused imaging	X	X	High	Pregnancy IV contrast

*Ultrasound contrast is not yet widely used.

TABLE 108-2

Characteristics of Different Imaging Techniques

Type of Study	Type of Contrast	Time to Complete (min)	Sedation Needed	Patient Preparation	Sensitivity to Motion	Risk to Patient
Radiography (x-ray)	Oral; intravenous	5-20	No	Sometimes	Yes	Ionizing radiation
Computed tomography	Oral; intravenous	0.5-15	Sometimes	Yes	Yes	Ionizing radiation Contrast
Magnetic resonance imaging	Intravenous	30-120	Frequently	Yes	Yes	Ferromagnetic metal Contrast
Ultrasonography	None	10-40	No	Yes	Yes	None
Nuclear medicine	Intravenous tracer	60-90	Sometimes	Sometimes	Yes	Ionizing radiation
Positron emission tomography–computed tomography	Intravenous; oral	60-90 (includes equilibrium phase)	Frequently	Yes	Yes	Ionizing radiation Contrast if used

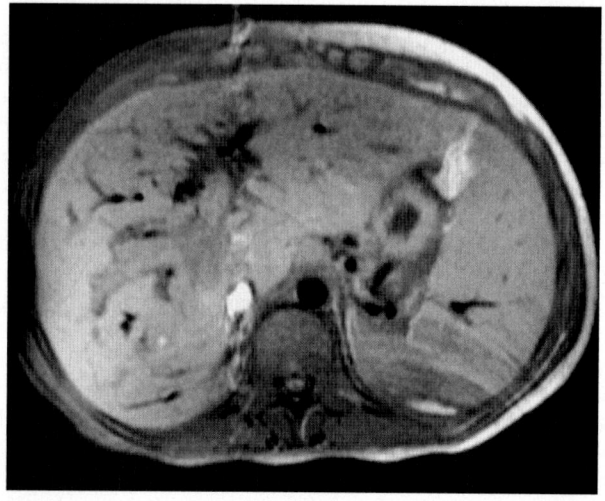 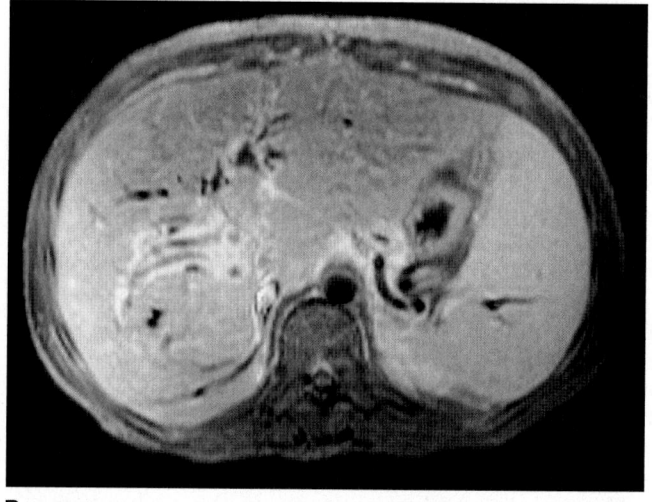

A   B

FIGURE 108-1. Fibrolamellar hepatocellular carcinoma of the liver in a 13-year-old boy. **A** and **B,** Axial images through the liver. Noncontrast T1-weighted image **(A)** and contrast-enhanced image **(B)** show poorly defined low signal infiltrating along the portal architecture, which enhances with intravenous contrast administration.

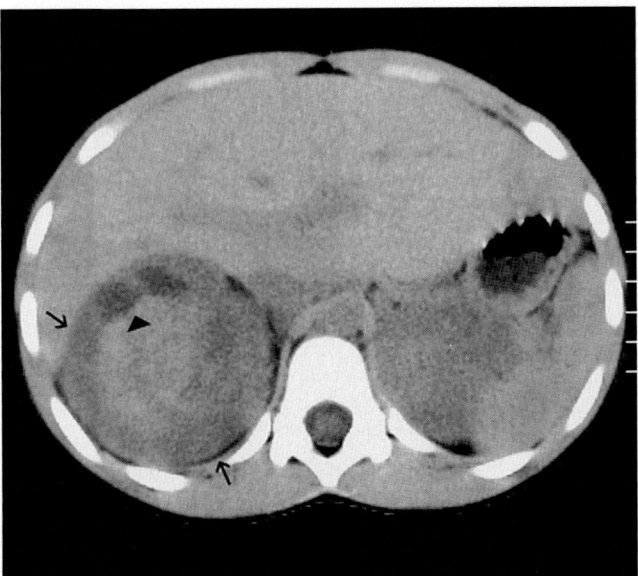

FIGURE 108-2. Renal cell carcinoma in a 7-year-old girl who developed hematuria after being kicked in the right side. Axial, noncontrast abdominal CT image obtained after trauma shows a large solid mass *(arrows)* involving the upper pole of the right kidney. The low-density areas *(arrowhead)* may represent blood or distended calyces.

TABLE 108-3

Imaging Goals for Tumor Staging at Diagnosis

Define the lesion or process
  Benign or aggressive
  Aggressive or quiescent
Determine extent of disease
  Primary
  Metastatic
Identify and characterize mass
Identify organ of origin
Identify other involved structures
Delineate metastatic sites of disease

---

plinary care team, the radiologist should prioritize the differential diagnosis, orchestrate additional imaging as needed, and assist with surgical and radiation planning. Important information for surgical planning includes whether the tumor invades or abuts vessels or other critical structures and whether the mass invades or merely displaces adjacent solid organs. The radiologist is in the unique position of understanding the advantages and limitations of the wide variety of imaging modalities available, allowing him or her to determine the best protocol for obtaining the key information needed by the oncology and surgical teams.

> **At initial diagnosis and staging, imaging is integral for:**
> - **Defining the nature and extent of disease**
> - **Detecting distant metastases**
> - **Planning therapy and surgery**

TABLE 108-4

Imaging Goals during Tumor Therapy

Assess tumor response in "upfront window" studies
Determine nonresponse in a timely manner, allowing
  management changes
Determine therapeutic value of treatment protocols
  New front-line therapy
  Relapse therapy
Differentiate residual active disease from fibrosis
Assess complications of therapy
  Hemorrhage
  Toxicity
  Acute abdominal or pelvic events
  Infection
Assess tumor: use same modalities as for initial staging

Imaging during therapy is the primary method of assessing tumor response in "upfront window" studies (Table 108-4). Timely determination of a lack of response allows management changes to be made, with the purpose of better controlling and eradicating the disease. Imaging during therapy also helps determine the therapeutic value of treatment protocols, which is particularly important in trials of new front-line and relapse therapy. In assessing tumor response to treatment, however, standard imaging methods have a limited ability to differentiate residual active disease from fibrosis.

Many complications can occur while a patient is on therapy. Although these complications are often symptomatic, some may be occult. Imaging is used to identify, quantify, and characterize these complications. Examples of on-therapy complications include hemorrhage, mucositis, cystitis (Fig. 108-3), acute abdominal events such as typhlitis or perforation, pneumoperitoneum (Fig. 108-4), infection, pneumatosis intestinalis (Figs. 108-5 and 108-6), and other less common conditions, such as acquired vaginal obstruction. (Fig. 108-7).

> **Complications of therapy include:**
> - **Hemorrhage**
> - **Mucositis**
> - **Cystitis**
> - **Typhlitis**
> - **Perforation**
> - **Infection**

End-of-therapy imaging is dictated by the primary diagnosis and stage of disease, treatment protocol, and initial imaging findings (Table 108-5). The intended purpose is to assess the therapeutic response, including identifying the presence of residual disease, early relapse, or progressive disease.

Imaging for long-term follow-up after completion of therapy is also dictated by the primary disease and its treatment (Table 108-6). Certain tumors can recur after completion of therapy; others increase the patient's risk of additional malignancies, such as familial adenomatous

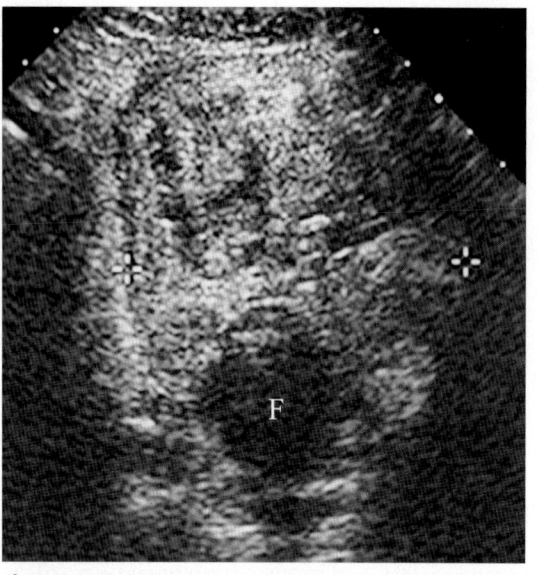
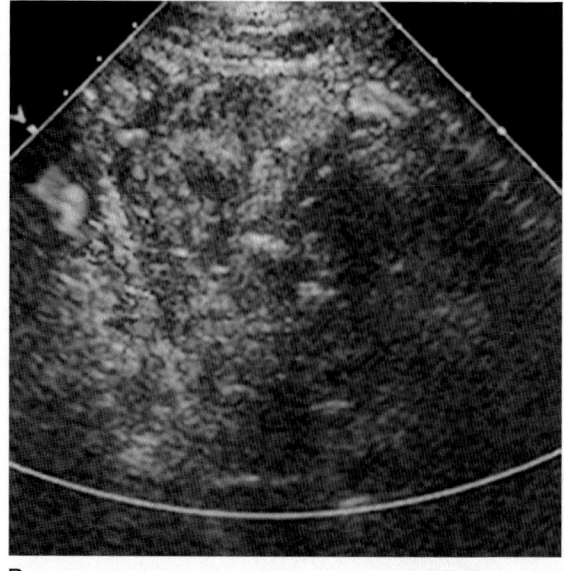

A   B

FIGURE 108-3. Hemorrhagic cystitis after bone marrow transplantation for relapsed Ewing sarcoma. **A** and **B,** Transverse **(A)** and color Doppler **(B)** ultrasound images through the pelvis show that the bladder is filled with heterogeneous echogenic material, indicative of extensive clot. The transverse diameter of the bladder in **A** is demarcated by the cursors (+). Note the hypervascularity of the bladder wall in **B**. F, Foley catheter balloon.

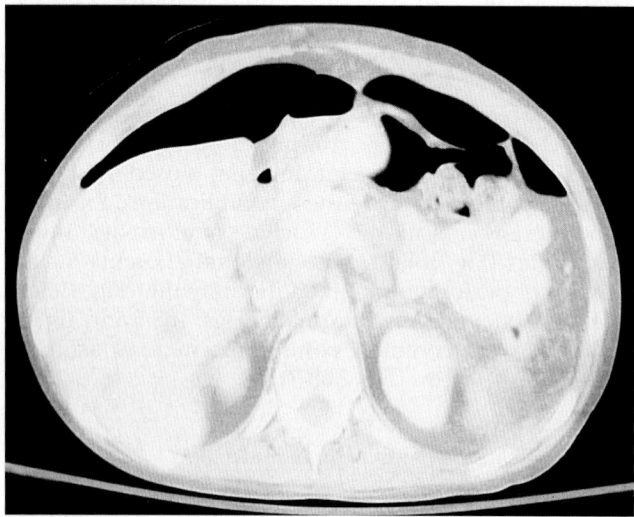

FIGURE 108-4. This teenage boy with multiply relapsed Hodgkin disease and known involvement of the liver and spleen underwent contrast-enhanced CT of the abdomen for evaluation of abdominal pain. Review of abdominal image with lung windows indicates the presence of unexpected pneumoperitoneum.

TABLE 108-5
Imaging Goals at Completion of Therapy
Choose imaging modalities based on the primary disease, treatment protocol, and initial imaging
Assess therapeutic response
Determine presence of residual disease
Identify early relapse or progressive disease

TABLE 108-6
Follow-up Imaging
Choose imaging modalities based on the primary disease and its treatment
Perform surveillance for recurrence
Identify and monitor expected treatment sequelae (e.g., scoliosis), cardiac and pulmonary function
Perform surveillance for second malignant neoplasms

polyposis (Gardner syndrome). Similarly, exposure to chemotherapy and radiation places the childhood cancer survivor at risk for late treatment-related toxicities (see Chapter 2). Thus, long-term follow-up imaging provides surveillance for recurrence of primary tumor, second malignant neoplasms, and expected sequelae of treatment.

RADIOGRAPHY

Despite the upsurge in technological complexity, abdominal radiographs continue to play a prominent role in the initial assessment of abdominal masses. Radiography is readily available and can be performed without sedation, making it ideal for the initial investigation of the patient's symptoms and the initial characterization of the mass. Radiographs can differentiate an abdominal mass from such entities as constipation (Fig. 108-8). Plain radiography provides information about a wide variety of structures that can aid in the clinical management of gastrointestinal and genitourinary masses and tumors. For instance, the bowel gas pattern, if displaced, can suggest the location of a mass (see Fig. 108-8). A bowel obstruction can indicate gastrointestinal involvement by disease, the approximate level of obstruction (Fig. 108-9), and the presence of calcifications. The integrity of the bony skeleton (including bony mineralization) and the

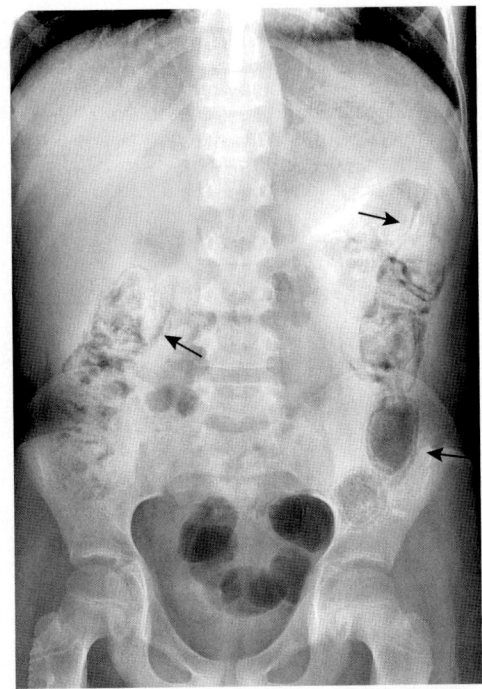
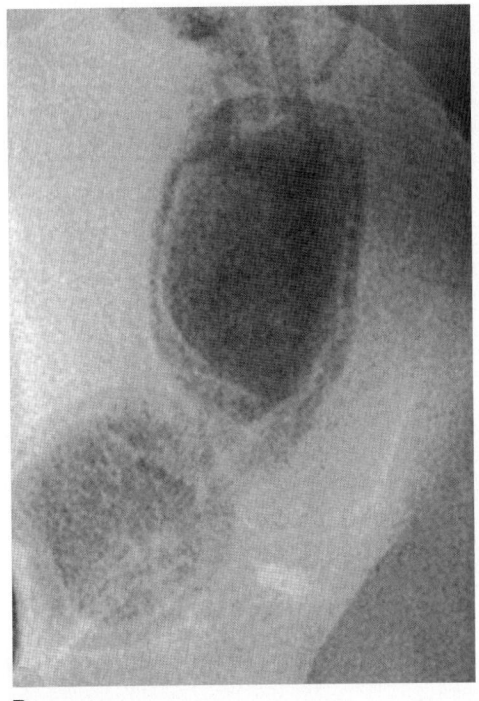

A   B

FIGURE 108-5. This 9-year-old boy with recurrent neuroblastoma underwent follow-up imaging to assess his response to therapy. **A,** CT scout view of the abdomen and pelvis shows pneumatosis intestinalis involving the colon (*arrows*). The patient's only complaint was diarrhea. **B,** Close-up view shows air lucencies in the wall of the descending colon.

presence of congenital or developmental abnormalities may suggest an associated mass. For example, the suggestion of nephromegaly or hepatomegaly in a patient with skeletal asymmetry associated with Beckwith-Wiedemann syndrome may indicate Wilms tumor or hepatoblastoma, respectively. Hepatoblastoma may also be associated with periostitis; thus, periosteal reaction seen on included ribs in the presence of right upper quadrant pain may lead to the inclusion of hepatoblastoma in the differential diagnosis. Diffuse or focal bony demineralization or vertebral compression fractures may suggest widespread metastases, such as those that occur in neuroblastoma, rhabdomyosarcoma, or leukemia. Radiographic information can direct subsequent studies using more sophisticated technology (Fig. 108-10). This allows more complete staging of primary and metastatic sites, delineation of associated congenital abnormalities, and better assessment of tumor response to therapy.

> **Plain films can be used to:**
> - **Identify other conditions (e.g., constipation)**
> - **Evaluate the skeleton**
> - **Assess bowel gas pattern and displacement**
> - **Assess calcifications**

ULTRASONOGRAPHY

Ultrasonography (US) is a particularly attractive imaging modality in pediatrics because of the lack of ionizing radiation. As such, US plays a significant role in the preliminary evaluation of abdominal and pelvic masses.

Ultimate tumor staging and preoperative planning usually involve additional cross-sectional imaging such as computed tomography (CT) or magnetic resonance imaging (MRI); however, US provides information about tumor characteristics, organ of origin, involvement of adjacent structures, and characteristics of ascites (Fig. 108-11), allowing subsequent imaging studies to be planned in an expeditious manner. US is an excellent method for assessing not only the abdomen and pelvis but also tumor vascularity and supply (Fig. 108-12) and scrotal contents.

Mass Characterization

The evaluation of a gastrointestinal or genitourinary mass is often initiated by clinical symptoms such as abdominal pain, nausea, vomiting, or weight loss or by the clinical discovery of an abdominal mass by palpation. Normal structures, such as bowel distended by excessive stool, can be assessed by radiography. However, further characterization is often necessary to identify and characterize a lesion. For example, an upper quadrant mass may be identified as a ureteropelvic junction obstruction, necessitating a functional imaging study and surgical management. Alternatively, US might identify a solid mass, such as a Wilms tumor, and show tumoral invasion of the renal vein and the inferior vena cava with Doppler capability.

US readily differentiates cystic from solid masses and is particularly valuable for imaging the solid organs of the abdomen, gallbladder, bladder, and abdominal vessels. US is also an exquisite modality for the assessment of ascites (see Fig. 108-11), which is associated with several

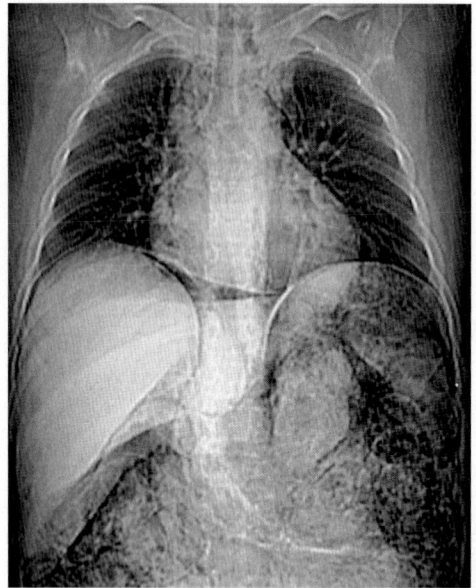

A

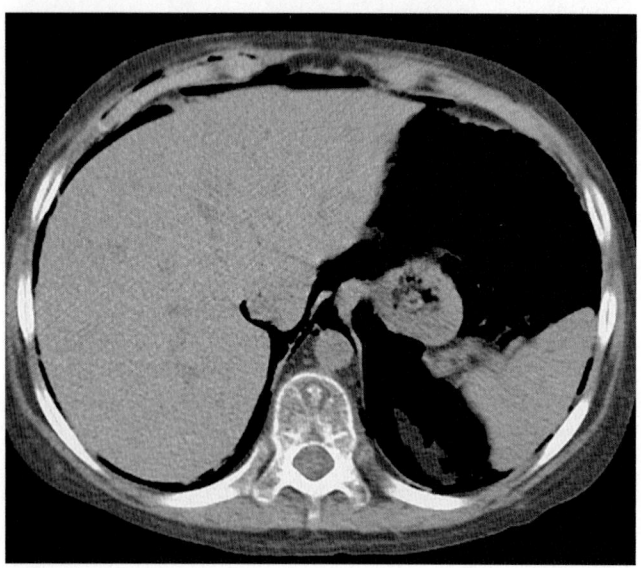

B

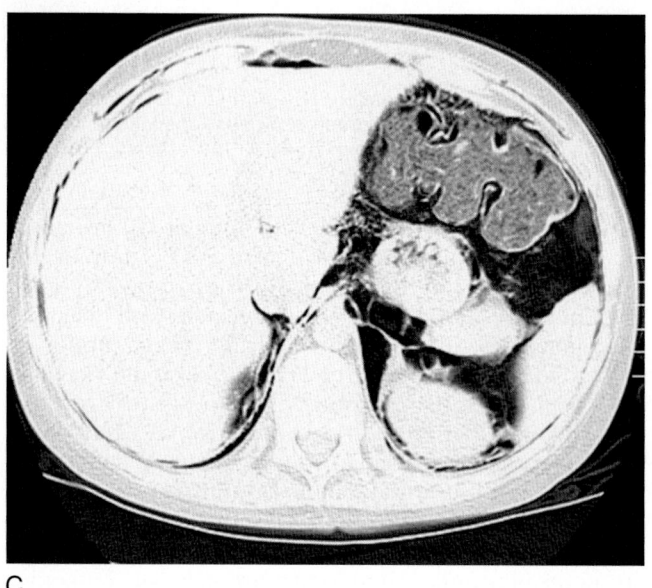

C

FIGURE 108-6. This 13-year-old boy, who underwent allogeneic bone marrow transplantation for acute lymphoblastic leukemia almost 1 year earlier, had follow-up CT for the evaluation of pulmonary fungal disease. **A-C,** Extensive pneumatosis intestinalis is accompanied by pneumoperitoneum, pneumomediastinum, and pneumoretroperitoneum. Note the limited ability to detect the abnormal distribution of air when images are recorded with narrow soft tissue windows **(B)** compared with lung windows **(C).**

pediatric tumors that involve the gastrointestinal and genitourinary tracts. Optimal imaging of the uterus and adnexa is achieved with US, possibly coupled with MRI. US is also an ideal technique for directing image-guided biopsies. Prenatally, US can identify and characterize lesions in the fetus, allowing appropriate parental counseling, delivery planning, and, if warranted, prenatal surgery. In a multicenter study of 53 suprarenal masses, Sauvat and coworkers detected 30 prenatally and 23 postnatally; of these masses, 58% were histologically proven neuroblastoma.

Limitations of US include the inability to image through interposed bone or bowel gas (which is particularly difficult to circumvent in a crying child) and profound operator dependence. Reproducibility of ultrasound findings is difficult because of both operator dependence and the multiplicity of planes at which the

pathology can be scanned. Very large masses may be difficult to include in a single field of view for measurement. Retroperitoneal adenopathy can be assessed with US but, because of overlying structures, is more reliably demonstrated with CT or MRI. Intraperitoneal lesions, especially when very small, may be obscured. Ultrasound contrast agents, though not universally available, may permit further tissue characterization.

Monitoring Primary Tumor Treatment Response

US can be used to monitor tumor response to therapy; however, its utility may be limited by a lack of standardization and reproducibility of images. In other words, measuring the same tumor in the same plane after it has decreased in size or after resolution of ascites may be impossible.

Post-Treatment Monitoring

After therapy, few tumors are monitored by US because of its limited field of view, difficulty in reliably identifying small but important sites of intraperitoneal disease, and limited visualization of intra-abdominal structures by overlying bowel gas. Wilms tumor is routinely monitored by US for recurrence of disease in the surgical bed, metachronous contralateral disease, and potential hepatic metastases. Nephroblastomatosis can also be monitored with US or with MRI (Fig. 108-13).

> US can be used to:
> - **Confirm the presence of a lesion**
> - **Identify the organ of origin**
> - **Assess tumor vascularity**
> - **Assess vascular invasion**
>
> **Disadvantages of US include:**
> - **Inability to image through air or calcium**
> - **Operator dependence, poor reproducibility**

COMPUTED TOMOGRAPHY

Cross-sectional imaging using CT provides sensitive, detailed anatomic evaluation of the organ of interest, tumor involvement of the adjacent structures, and detection of metastases; it also routinely contributes to disease staging and preoperative planning. Perhaps the greatest drawback of CT is the use of ionizing radiation to generate the images. With the advent of multichannel scanning techniques, allowing rapid image acquisition, sedation or general anesthesia is required much less frequently than in the past.

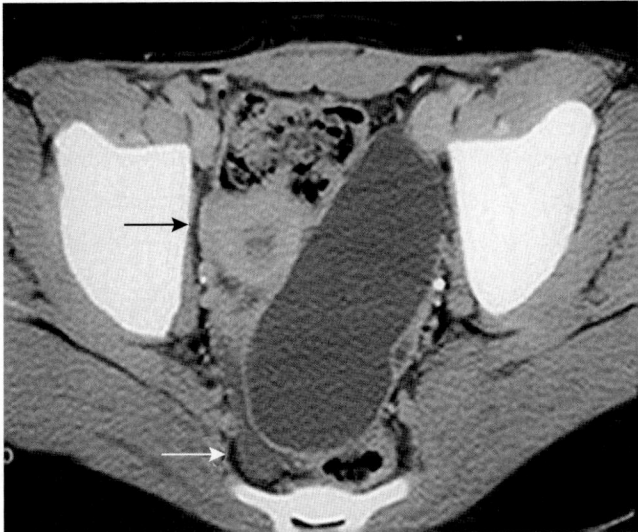

FIGURE 108-7. Acquired vaginal occlusion in a young woman who survived pelvic rhabdomyosarcoma and presented with pelvic pain. Axial contrast-enhanced CT image through the pelvis shows a large, low-density tubular structure displacing the uterus *(black arrow)* to the right. There is a tiny amount of deep pelvic fluid *(white arrow)*.

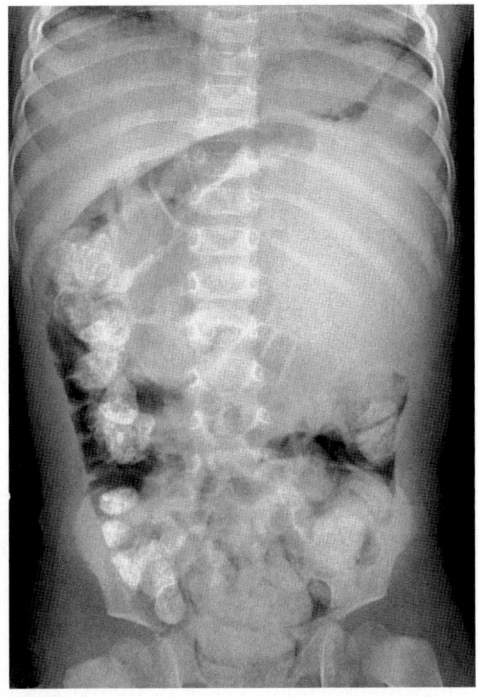
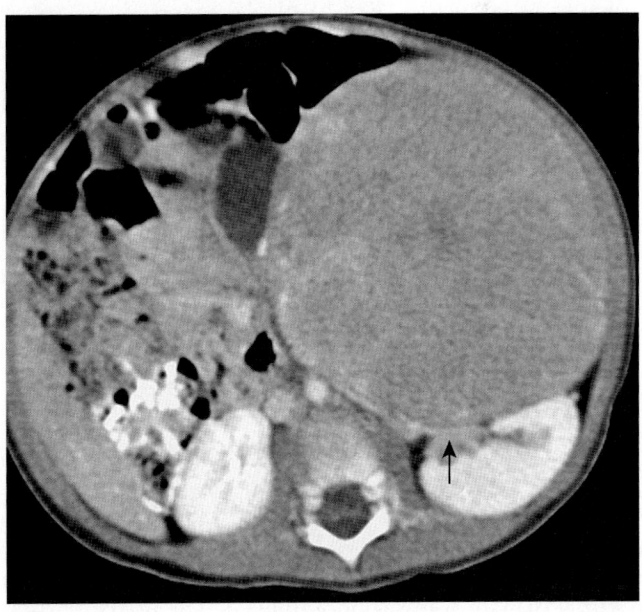

A   B

FIGURE 108-8. Favorable-histology neuroblastoma. Fifteen-month-old girl with an abdominal mass. **A,** Frontal radiograph shows marked displacement of the splenic flexure by a large, noncalcified soft tissue mass. Note the line of demarcation between the mass and the spleen, the absence of rib destruction, and inferior displacement of the colon. **B,** Contrast-enhanced CT confirms the location of the mass in the left anterior pararenal space and its solid character. Note stretching of the left renal artery posteriorly around the mass *(arrow).* This tumor was histologically proved to be favorable-histology neuroblastoma.

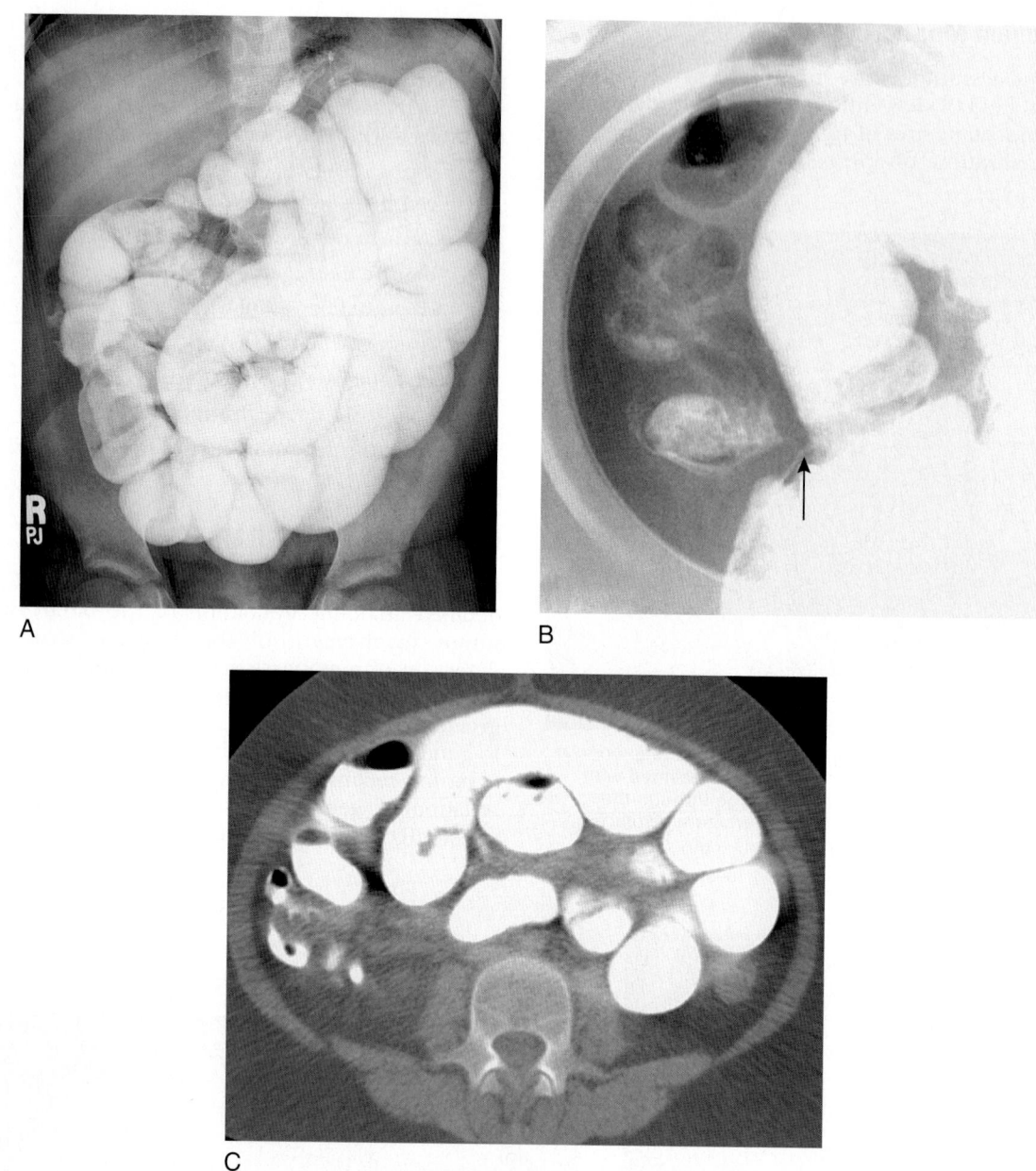

FIGURE 108-9. This teenage boy with treated non-Hodgkin lymphoma of the ileocecal valve developed small bowel obstruction resulting from persistent narrowing and scarring of the involved site. **A,** Upper gastrointestinal series with small bowel follow-through shows lack of progression of barium through the small bowel. **B,** Spot image from the same study confirms narrowing of the distal ileum *(arrow).* **C,** Although the ingested contrast from the upper gastrointestinal series is far more dense than typically used for CT, cross-sectional imaging confirmed the location of the partial obstruction and contributed to surgical planning for resection of the involved segment.

Mass Characterization

CT, particularly if precontrast images are obtained, identifies the presence of calcifications and background density of the lesion, such as fat content. The use of intravenous contrast material is essential to better define adjacent anatomic structures, particularly in young children with a paucity of intra-abdominal fat. The use of intravenous contrast also contributes functional information about organs and adjacent tissues (Fig. 108-14) and may suggest the distribution of necrosis in tumors. Its use is tailored to the information needed. Modifications using intravenous contrast include dynamic enhance-ment coupled with three- or four-phase imaging as an aid in distinguishing tumor from vascular malformations. Postprocessing images with state-of-the-art technology can also create three-dimensional angiographic studies that contribute to preoperative planning, tumor staging, assessment of adjacent tissue involvement, and radiation treatment planning, obviating the use of inva-sive standard angiography. Newer nonionic, low-osmolar intravenous contrast agents are safer, with less risk of renal compromise.

Oral contrast material is often critical in differentiat-ing lymph nodes from loops of bowel in defining tumor margins. This is particularly important in young children

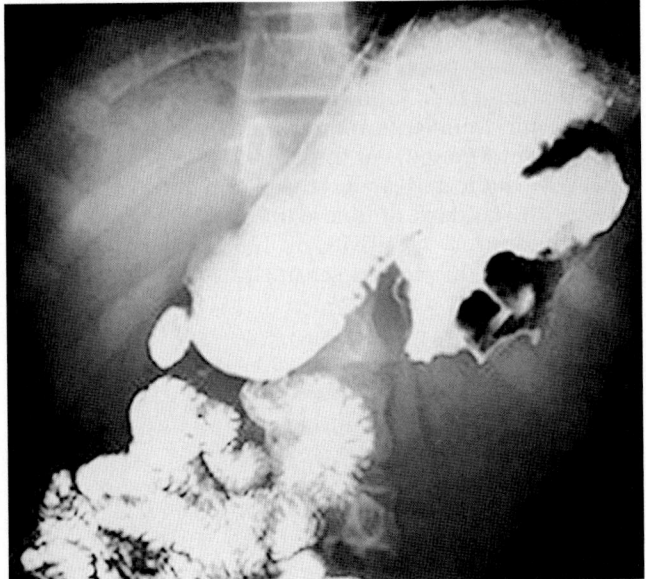

FIGURE 108-10. Non-Hodgkin lymphoma. Teenage boy with progressive abdominal pain and anemia. Upper gastrointestinal series shows a large exophytic ulcerating gastric mass, suggesting CT as subsequent examination. Histologically diagnosis was non-Hodgkin lymphoma.

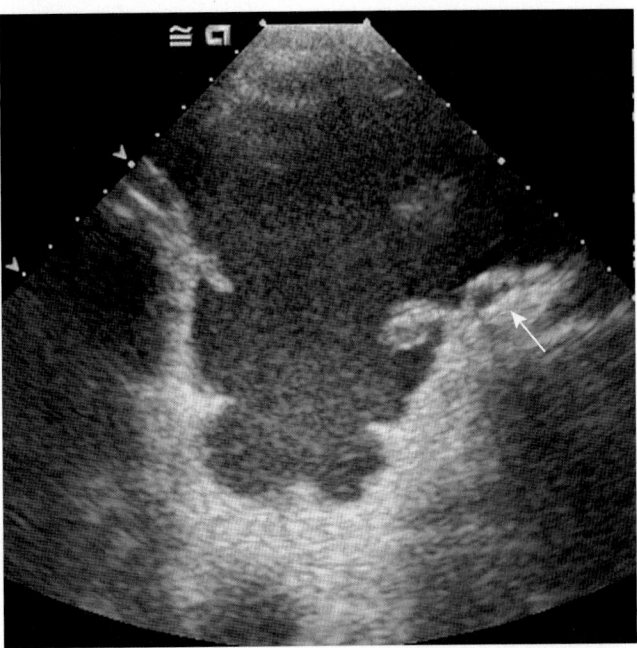

FIGURE 108-11. Peritoneal implants. This 6-year-old girl presented with constipation of 1 week's duration and a 15-pound weight loss over 4 months. Transverse ultrasound image through the pelvis shows a large collection of complex ascites associated with multiple peritoneal implants *(arrow)*.

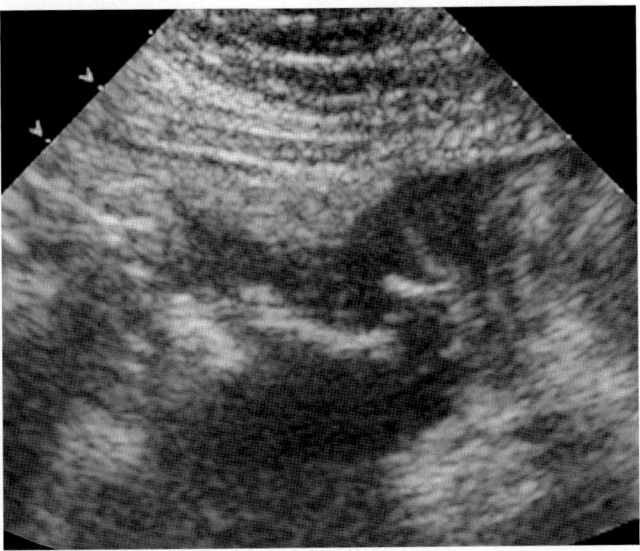

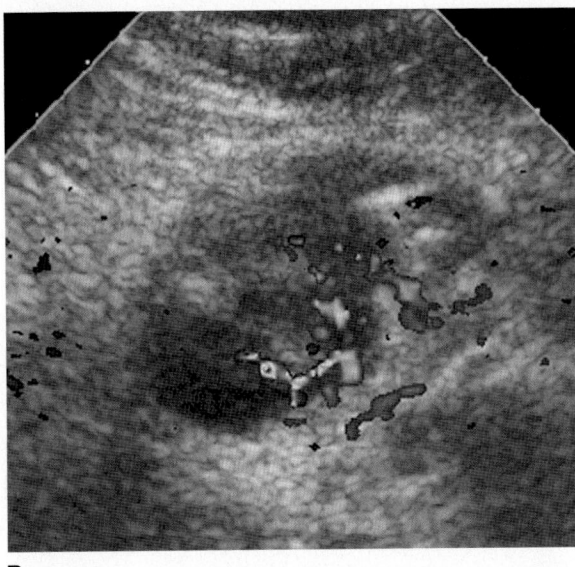

A   B

FIGURE 108-12. Relapsed non-Hodgkin lymphoma in a teenage boy with subacute right lower quadrant pain. Real-time **(A)** and color Doppler **(B)** ultrasound images demonstrate abnormal thickening of the distal ileum *(cursors)* associated with hypervascularity.

and small, lean patients who lack the inherent contrast of adequate retroperitoneal and mesenteric fat. Although CT is able to identify lymph nodes as small as 1 to 2 mm in diameter, it cannot always differentiate benign reactive nodes from those with malignant involvement. The specificity of assessing malignancy in lymph nodes is low owing to the presence of reactive hyperplasia in 12% of children younger than 12 years and 19% of children younger than 11 years. As with any other modality, the origin of very large abdominal or pelvic masses may be particularly difficult to discern, as

in some cases of Burkitt lymphoma or ovarian neoplasm (Fig. 108-15). Demonstration of ingested oral contrast as it courses through a thinned bowel lumen supports the bowel as the organ of origin of the mass. Allowing oral contrast to course to the level of the rectum can aid in differentiating low-lying deep pelvic structures. Occasionally, rectal contrast may be helpful; however, rectal contrast should not be administered to patients with neutropenia because of the possibility of inducing septicemia from dissemination of gastrointestinal flora.

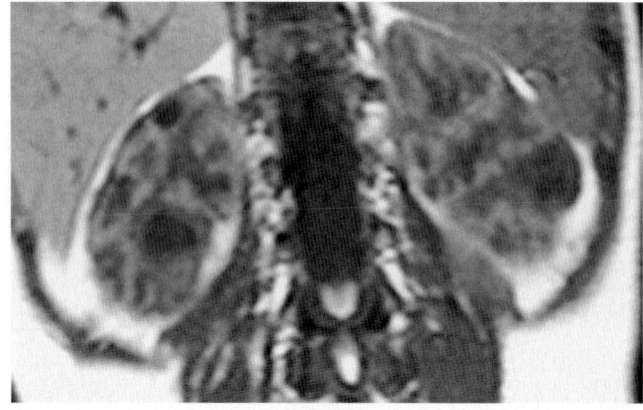

A

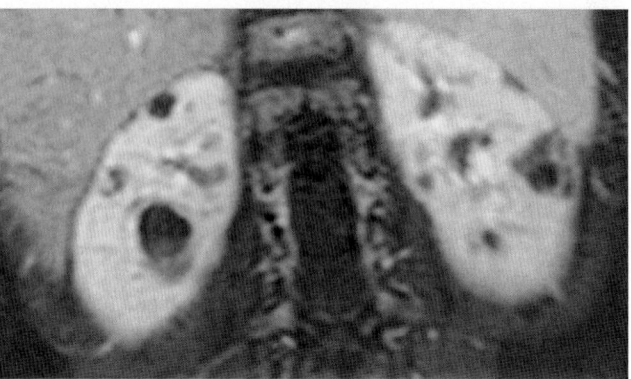

B

FIGURE 108-13. Nephroblastomatosis imaged with MRI. **A** and **B,** Coronal, noncontrast T1-weighted **(A)** and short tau inversion recovery **(B)** images through the kidneys show dark signal in the majority of the many round lesions of nephroblastomatosis. These lesions had decreased in size and become more sclerotic with chemotherapy.

Contemporary CT fluoroscopic capabilities allow for "real-time" imaging; "virtual" endoscopic techniques are being explored, but little experience has been published in pediatric cases, and their impact on diagnostic imaging and interventional techniques in pediatrics has yet to be determined. An initial report by Anupindi and colleagues indicated a decreased radiation dose compared with standard double contrast barium enemas in small children, a sensitivity of 100% for 5- to 10-mm polyps, and a moderate sensitivity of about 67% for larger lesions.

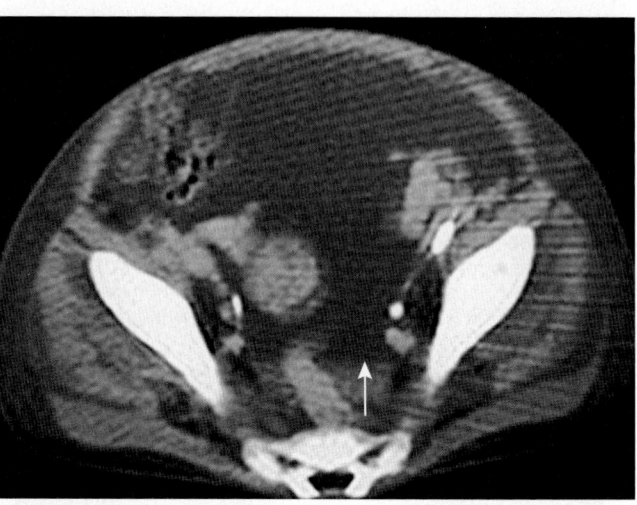

FIGURE 108-14. This 2-year-old girl with a newly diagnosed large retroperitoneal neuroblastoma surrounding and displacing the celiac axis presented with acute abdominal distention and decrease in hemoglobin to 2 mg. Axial CT image through the pelvis shows abundant pelvic ascites, with a blood-fluid level in pelvis *(arrow)*, indicative of tumor hemorrhage.

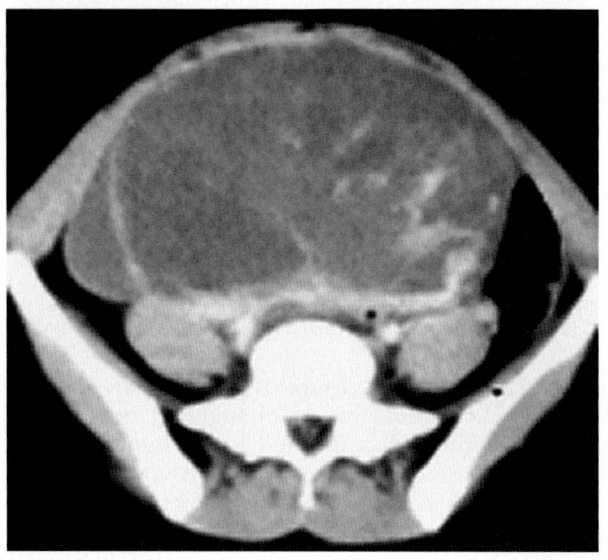

A

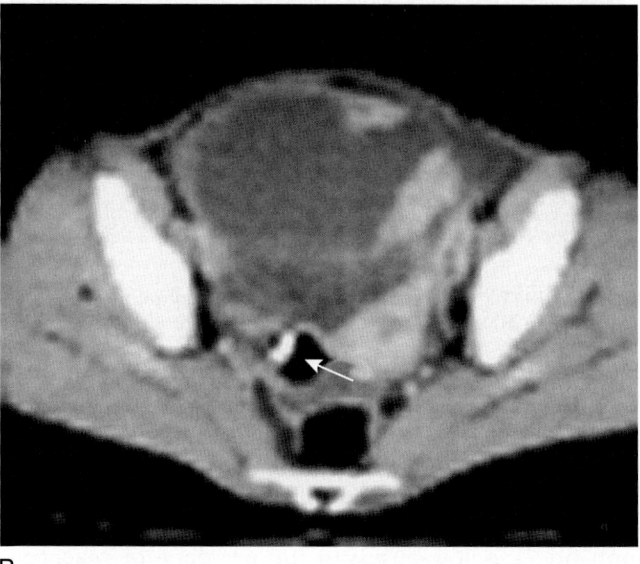

B

FIGURE 108-15. Yolk sac tumor. Abdominopelvic mass in 18-year-old girl. **A,** Axial contrast-enhanced CT image through the upper pelvis shows a massive, heterogeneous, predominantly low-density mass. Because of the tumor's size, the organ of origin cannot be determined. **B,** Imaged more inferiorly, the low-density appearance, the associated tooth surrounded by fat density *(arrow)*, and the displacement of the uterus suggest an adnexal origin.

Monitoring Primary Tumor Treatment Response

Most abdominal and pelvic tumors that respond favorably to therapy decrease in size, demonstrate increasing necrosis, and are associated with decreasing ascites and adenopathy. In the case of very large tumors, the site of origin may be masked until tumor shrinkage allows it to be defined.

> **Advantages of CT include:**
> - **Rapid evaluation and potential avoidance of sedation**
> - **Postprocessing multiplanar capabilities**
>
> **Disadvantages of CT include:**
> - **Radiation exposure**
> - **Need for administration of contrast material**

NUCLEAR MEDICINE

Nuclear scintigraphy provides functional information about the targeted tissues but is limited in its anatomic delineation of tumors. The information sought in the evaluation of a suspected mass involving the gastrointestinal and genitourinary tracts dictates the radiopharmaceutical used.

Technetium methylenediphosphonate is used primarily to identify skeletal metastatic disease in the presence of a primary abdominal or pelvic tumor. Gallium-67 can identify a potential site of infection (subacute and chronic) that may mimic a tumor and is a mainstay for assessing abdominal and pelvic lymphomas; it is also routinely used to monitor response to therapy for lymphoma. Coupling single-photon emission computed tomography (SPECT) with planar imaging optimizes image acquisition, particularly in the abdomen, where overlying bowel excretion can obscure sites of avidity.

Liver-spleen scans are seldom used for tumor staging but may be useful in the differential diagnosis of an infiltrative process such as lymphoma or leukemia. This imaging modality is less sensitive than CT, US, or MRI for the detection of small lesions and metastatic foci and is inferior at characterizing a primary lesion of the liver or spleen.

Indium-111 (or technetium-99m) white blood cell infection imaging (acute) is not used for tumor diagnosis. However, it may be beneficial in differentiating an infectious focus from a malignancy. Iobenguane sulfate (MIBG) iodine-131 and MIBG iodine-123 are useful in assessing primary, metastatic, and residual neuroblastoma (Fig. 108-16) and pheochromocytoma. Radiation exposure is less with MIBG iodine-123, making it the preferred agent for diagnostic imaging. MIBG iodine-131 may also be used for tumor-specific radiotherapy.

Positron emission tomography (PET) is increasingly used in the evaluation of pediatric patients with lymphoma. This modality identifies sites of increased metabolic activity. The most commonly used radiopharmaceutical, fluorodeoxyglucose (FDG), a glucose surrogate, identifies sites where glucose metabolism exceeds baseline levels. Although nonspecific for types of metabolically active

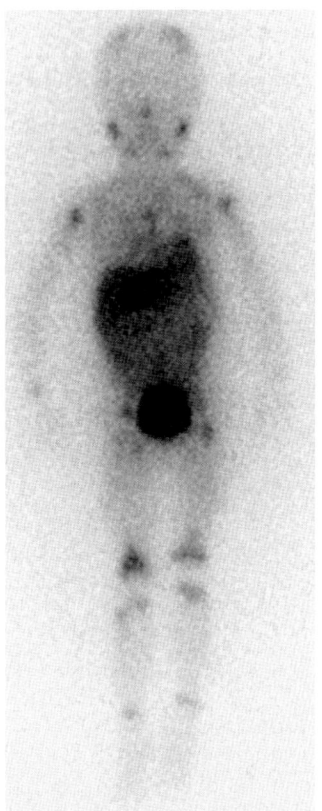

FIGURE 108-16. Anterior whole-body planar image from a 24-hour MIBG scan obtained for staging of metastatic neuroblastoma in a young child. Multiple sites of abnormal uptake of tracer are shown. (Courtesy of Dr. M. Elizabeth McCarville, Memphis, TN.)

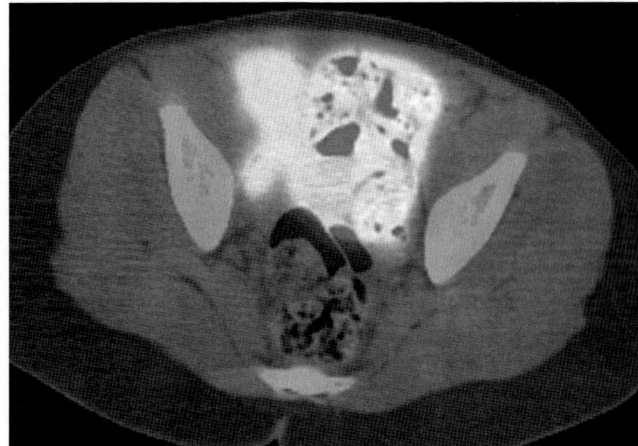

FIGURE 108-17. PET-CT defines tumor extent. Axial fused image from a staging PET scan shows abundant tracer-avid adenopathy in the right pelvis, metastatic from the patient's rhabdomyosarcoma of the right thigh. (*See color plate.*) (Courtesy of Dr. M. Elizabeth McCarville, Memphis, TN.)

tissue, FDG is very sensitive and useful for assessing primary, metastatic, and residual disease, including soft tissue and skeletal lesions. This technique can identify an unknown primary site in patients who present with abdominal or pelvic adenopathy or solid organ metastases (Fig. 108-17).

Contemporary technology now readily merges anatomic and functional imaging in the form of PET-CT. Although not yet routine in all centers, this modality is increasingly being used to evaluate pediatric tumors. Its identification of metabolically active sites of disease can also serve as a guide for surgical or percutaneous biopsy.

Currently, FDG is the most commonly used radiopharmaceutical for PET and PET-CT imaging. However, there is a growing armamentarium of tumor-specific agents with yet-to-be-defined roles in pediatric imaging.

> **Uses of nuclear medicine include:**
> - **Technetium methylenediphosphonate to identify skeletal disease**
> - **MIBG iodine-123 to evaluate primary, metastatic, and residual neuroblastoma and pheochromocytoma**
> - **SPECT, particularly in the abdomen**
> - **PET and PET-CT, particularly in children with lymphoma**

MAGNETIC RESONANCE IMAGING

Over the past 30 years, the role of MRI has rapidly expanded, and it has become integral to the initial evaluation and staging of many pediatric tumors. Like US, MRI does not require ionizing radiation; like CT, it can encompass a large field of view and produce standardized, reproducible multiplanar images.

Disadvantages of MRI include the frequent requirement for sedation in young children and older claustrophobic patients; longer study times than CT or US; more limited availability compared with CT and US; and potential patient safety hazards in the presence of ferromagnetic devices. The latter may become more problematic with the clinical use of higher strength equipment such as 3T and 7T. The discrimination between intra-abdominal pathology and bowel may be compromised without oral contrast material in some cases.

Mass Characterization

The inherent tissue contrast provided by MRI can be particularly helpful in characterizing abdominal and pelvic masses, even without the use of intravenous contrast enhancement. MRI exceeds the capability of CT in discriminating between normal and abnormal tissue.

Multiplanar image acquisition and reformatting using MRI provides information about the anatomic location of masses and the involvement of adjacent tissues—information that is key to strategic preoperative planning. Imaging guidance for biopsies and drainage procedures is becoming more frequent with the refinement and development of MRI-compatible biopsy equipment and advances in open magnet technology.

MRI sequences are continually being developed and revised and their applications evaluated. For example, diffusion-perfusion sequences and magnetic resonance spectroscopy are standard in neuroimaging, but their potential use in body imaging has not yet been fully explored. Similarly, dynamic-enhanced MRI, used with musculoskeletal tumors, has not been investigated in abdominal and pelvic tumors. In addition, the creation of tissue-specific sequences could aid in differential diagnosis and therapeutic planning, and as the technology improves and sequences are developed, tumor-specific protocols are likely to evolve.

An additional advantage of MRI is its exquisite ability to detect distant metastases, particularly those in the skeleton. This sensitivity has prompted interest in using whole-body MRI protocols as an initial staging method for specific tumor types. Peritoneal involvement, complicating such tumors as colon cancer, lymphoma, or desmoplastic small round cell tumors, is readily demonstrated by MRI without or with intravenous contrast enhancement.

Angiographic information may be important for tumor staging and preoperative planning; vascular MRI frequently provides the necessary information, obviating the need for more invasive standard angiography (Fig. 108-18). Modification of sequences to include breath-hold and "time-resolved" contrast-enhanced magnetic resonance angiography can optimize imaging results in selected patients.

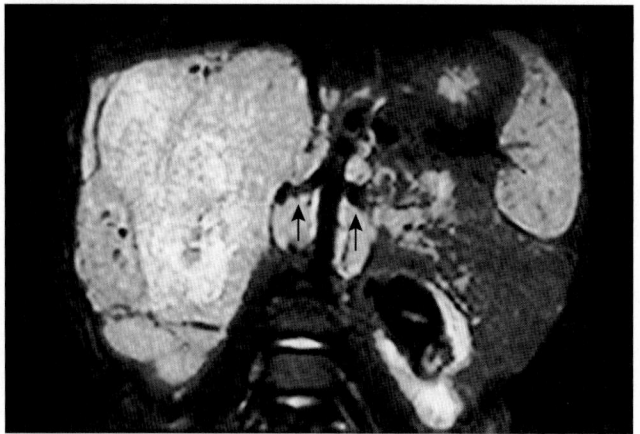
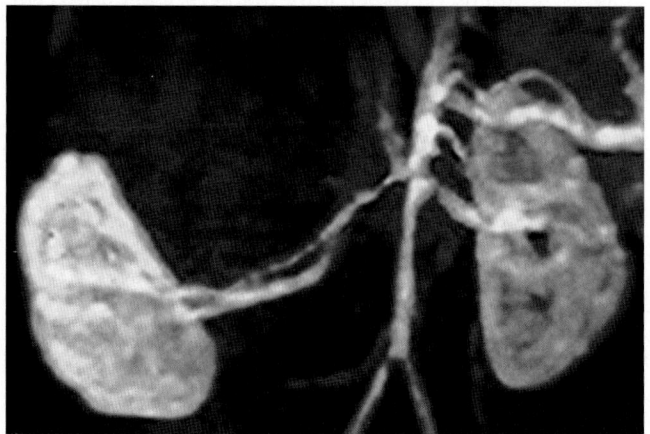

A   B

FIGURE 108-18. Magnetic resonance angiography for preoperative planning in a 1-year-old boy with right adrenal neuroblastoma. **A,** Coronal, turbo short tau inversion recovery MRI of the midabdomen shows encasement and stretching of the abdominal aorta and the renal arteries *(arrows).* **B,** Oblique maximal intensity projection of the arterial phase of a non-breath-hold magnetic resonance angiogram shows a stretched appearance of the right renal artery and marked displacement of the right kidney. (Courtesy of Dr. Fred Hoffer, Memphis, TN.)

Finally, MRI is increasingly being used to further characterize abnormalities identified on prenatal screening US, to optimize parental counseling and strategic perinatal planning. Although currently limited to several referral centers for complex obstetrics, the role of MRI in prenatal diagnosis is likely to continue to expand.

Monitoring Primary Tumor Treatment Response

In addition to detecting a change in size of the primary mass, the soft tissue contrast inherent in MRI readily demonstrates areas of tumor necrosis in response to therapy. Knowledge of imaging patterns of response based on specific tumor type is imperative for the accurate interpretation of any examination. However, the understanding of MRI findings may be complicated by postoperative and post–radiation therapy changes adjacent to primary sites of disease. Merging MRI findings with functional imaging information such as FDG PET can refine radiation therapy portals and direct surgical planning.

Advantages of MRI include:
- **Absence of radiation**
- **Exquisite tissue contrast**
- **Ability to identify distant metastases (e.g., skeleton, peritoneum)**
- **Provision of time-resolved angiographic data**

Disadvantages of MRI include:
- **Long imaging time**
- **Need for sedation**
- **Limited in the presence of ferromagnetic devices**

In summary, imaging plays a key role in the diagnosis, treatment, and follow-up of children and adolescents with cancer. The role of the radiologist as a member of the multidisciplinary team is increasingly complex and requires familiarity with the technology and knowledge of the pathophysiology of disease and its multimodality manifestations.

ACKNOWLEDGMENTS

The author thanks Sandra Gaither for manuscript preparation.

SUGGESTED READINGS

Anupindi S, Perumpillichira J, Israel EJ, et al: Low-dose CT colonography in children: initial experience, technical feasibility, and utility. Pediatr Radiol 2005;35:518-524

Bartsch EMP, Paek BW, Yoshizawa JK, et al: Giant fetal hepatic hemangioma: case report and literature review. Fetal Diagn Ther 2003;18:59-64

Braverman RM, Parker BR: Imaging studies in the diagnosis and management of pediatric malignancies: relative merits of imaging procedures. In Pizzo PA, Poplack DG (eds): Principles and Practice of Pediatric Oncology, 4th ed. Philadelphia, Lippincott Williams & Wilkins, 2002:206-220

Chan FP, Rubin GD: MDCT angiography of pediatric vascular diseases of the abdomen, pelvis, and extremities. Pediatr Radiol 2005; 35:40-53

Chung T: Magnetic resonance angiography of the body in pediatric patients: experience with a contrast-enhanced time-resolved technique. Pediatr Radiol 2005;35:3-10

Ciftci AO, Senocak ME, Tanyel FC, Buyukpamukcu N: Adrenocortical tumors in children. J Pediatr Surg 2001;36:549-554

Constantine S, Kaye J: Metastatic renal abscess mimicking Wilms' tumour. Pediatr Radiol 2004;34:924-926

Czauderna P, Schaarschmidt K, Komasara L, et al: Abdominal inflammatory masses mimicking neoplasia in children—experience of two centers. Pediatr Surg Int 2005;21:346-350

Foglia RP, Fonkalsrud EW, Feig SA, Moss TJ: Accuracy of diagnostic imaging as determined by delayed operative intervention for advanced neuroblastoma. J Pediatr Surg 1989;24:708-711

Golden CB, Feusner JH: Malignant abdominal masses in children: quick guide to evaluation and diagnosis. Pediatr Clin North Am 2002;49:1369-1392

Gow KW, Roberts IF, Jamieson DH, et al: Local staging of Wilms' tumor—computerized tomography correlation with histological findings. J Pediatr Surg 2000;35:677-679

Haliloglu M, Hoffer FA, Gronemeyer SA, Rao BN: Applications of 3D contrast-enhanced MR angiograpy in pediatric oncology. Pediatr Radiol 1999;29:863-868

Hamada Y, Sato M, Sanada T, et al: Spiral computed tomography for biliary dilatation. J Pediatr Surg 1995;30:694-696

Irsutti M, Puget C, Baunin C, et al: Mesoblastic nephroma: prenatal ultrasonographic and MRI features. Pediatr Radiol 2000;30:147-150

Karmazyn B, Ash S, Goshen Y, et al: Significance of residual abdominal masses in children with abdominal Burkitt's lymphoma. Pediatr Radiol 2001;31:801-805

Ko SF, Ng SH, Lee TY, et al: Hepatic focal nodular hyperplasia: the "star sign" on gadolinium-enhanced magnetic resonance angiography. Hepatogastroenterology 2002;49:1377-1381

Konen O, Rathaus V, Dlugy E, et al: Childhood abdominal cystic lymphangioma. Pediatr Radiol 2002;32:88-94

Kurosawa H, Matsunaga T, Shimaoka H, et al: Burkitt lymphoma associated with large gastric folds, pancreatic involvement, and biliary tract obstruction. J Pediatr Hematol Oncol 2002;24:310-312

Meyers RL, Scaife ER: Benign liver and biliary tract masses in infants and toddlers. Semin Pediatr Surg 2000;9:146-155

Nicolau C, Vilana R, Catala V, et al: Importance of evaluating all vascular phases on contrast-enhanced sonography in the differentiation of benign from malignant focal liver lesions. AJR Am J Roentgenol 2006;186:158-167

Nikou GC, Toubanakis C, Nikolaou P, et al: VIPomas: an update in diagnosis and management in a series of 11 patients. Hepatogastroenterology 2005;52:1259-1265

Pomeranz AJ, Sabnis S: Misdiagnoses of ovarian masses in children and adolescents. Pediatr Emerg Care 2004;20:172-174

Qayyum A, Coakley FV, Westphalen AC, et al: Role of CT and MR imaging in predicting optimal cytoreduction of newly diagnosed primary epithelial ovarian cancer. Gynecol Oncol 2005;96:301-306

Reddy SC, Reddy SC: Hemangiosarcoma of the spleen: helical computed tomography features. South Med J 2000;93:825-827

Sauvat F, Sarnacki S, Brisse H, et al: Outcome of suprarenal localized masses diagnosed during the perinatal period: a retrospective multicenter study. Cancer 2002;94:2474-2480

Savci G, Yazici Z, Sahin N, et al: Value of chemical shift subtraction MRI in characterization of adrenal masses. AJR Am J Roentgenol 2006;186:130-135

Shek TWH, Chan GCF, Khong PL, et al: Ewing sarcoma of the small intestine. J Pediatr Hematol Oncol 2001;23:530-532

Skiadas VT, Koutoulidis V, Eleytheriades M, et al: Ovarian masses in young adolescents: imaging findings with surgical confirmation. Eur J Gynaecol Oncol 2004;25:201-206

Stringer MD: Liver tumors. Semin Pediatr Surg 2000;9:196-208

Traubici J, Daneman A, Hayes-Jordan A, Fecteau A: Primary germ cell tumor of the diaphragm. J Pediatr Surg 2004;39:1578-1580

Xu H, Jiang D, Yang L, et al: The value of in-phase and opposed-phase T1-weighted breath-hold FLASH sequences for hepatic imaging. J Tongji Med Univ 2000;20:290-293

Yang Y-S, Huang Q-Y, Wang W-F, et al: Primary jejunoileal neoplasms: a review of 60 cases. World J Gastroenterol 2003;9:862-864

PART 3

ABDOMINAL WALL AND PERITONEAL CAVITY

CHAPTER

109 Abdominal Wall and Its Abnormalities

SUE C. KASTE

NORMAL ANATOMY

The anterior abdominal wall is composed of several layers: skin, superficial fascia (Camper and Scarpa fascia), subcutaneous fat, muscles, transversalis fascia (Gallaudet or innominate fascia), properitoneal fat, and peritoneal membrane. The muscular layer consists of the paired rectus muscles in the midline and the paired anterolateral muscles, which consist of the external and internal oblique muscles and the transversus abdominis. The aponeurosis of the external oblique muscles splits at the anterior border of the muscle to form the spigelian fascia, which in turn forms the anterior and posterior rectus sheaths (Fig. 109-1). These sheaths join in the midline to form the linea alba, which separates the rectus muscles for a variable distance, as long as 6 mm. The lowest portion of the aponeurosis of the external oblique muscles ends in a thickened free border, the inguinal ligament, which extends from the anterior superior iliac spine to the pubic tubercle. The subcutaneous or external inguinal ring is an opening in the aponeurosis of the external oblique muscle, between the inguinal ligament inferiorly and the tendinous portion superiorly. The spermatic cord in males, and the round ligament in females, passes through the inguinal canal. The diaphragms form the roof of the abdomen. The posterior abdominal wall is composed of the spine, psoas muscles, quadratus lumborum, iliacus, and paraspinal musculature.

HERNIAS

Herniation of abdominal contents can occur superiorly into the thorax via diaphragmatic defects, inferiorly through the femoral and inguinal canals, anteriorly through abdominal wall defects or the umbilical ring, and, rarely, posteriorly through defects in the posterior abdominal wall musculature. Internal hernia occurs when bowel herniates through the peritoneum or mesentery. Herniation of the stomach through the esophageal hiatus is the most common type of hernia. A

sliding hiatus hernia in which the esophagogastric junction is located above the hiatus occurs most frequently. A paraesophageal hernia occurs when the gastric fundus and proximal body herniate into the chest, leaving the esophagogastric junction in a near-normal position (see Chapters 122 and 124).

Hernias may occur through:

- **Diaphragmatic defects**
- **Gastroesophageal hiatus**
- **Anterior abdominal wall (groin, ventral, incisional)**
- **Posterior wall defects**

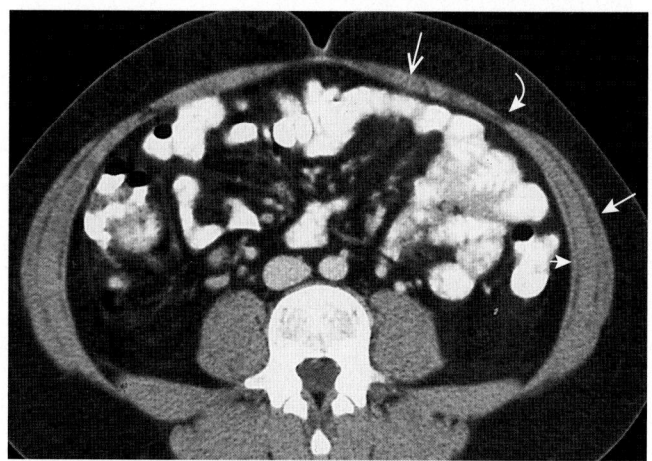

FIGURE 109-1. Normal anatomy. CT scan at the level of the umbilicus in an obese 11-year-old boy shows the abdominal musculature to good advantage. The external oblique muscle *(straight arrows)* and the transversus abdominis muscle *(small arrow)* are seen on either side of the internal oblique muscle. The aponeurosis of the external oblique muscle becomes the spigelian fascia *(curved arrow)*, which splits to form the anterior and posterior sheaths of the rectus abdominis muscle.

Diaphragmatic Hernias

Diaphragmatic hernias may occur posteriorly and laterally through patent pleuroperitoneal canals, also known as the *foramina of Bochdalek*. Bochdalek hernias usually occur during fetal development and present in the newborn; however, delayed Bochdalek hernias in older children are being reported with increasing frequency (Fig. 109-2). In newborns, the hernias are more commonly left-sided, but the opposite has been suggested in patients with a delayed presentation, although this is not confirmed in all series. Berman and coworkers reported 26 patients with Bochdalek hernias diagnosed more than 8 weeks after birth. Twenty-two were left-sided, three were right-sided, and one was bilateral. Misdiagnosis had occurred in 16 patients. Only one third of the patients had pulmonary hypoplasia, consistent with a later onset of herniation. Delayed right-sided Bochdalek hernias have also been reported in neonates with group B streptococcal infection.

The diagnosis of congenital Bochdalek hernia is usually made by clinical means and plain radiographs, which show loops of bowel and portions of abdominal organs in a hemithorax, with corresponding contralateral displacement of the mediastinum and paucity of intra-abdominal bowel loops. If the diagnosis is in doubt, ultrasound or contrast studies can document the intrathoracic location of the herniated structures. Computed tomography (CT) is useful in the diagnosis of delayed congenital Bochdalek hernia, particularly with the use of coronal and sagittal reformats. In traumatic diaphragmatic hernias, CT, magnetic resonance imaging (MRI), and oral contrast studies play a role, but a high index of suspicion of traumatic hernia is crucial. MRI can aid in the prenatal diagnosis of Bochdalek hernia and can differentiate herniated bowel loops from other chest lesions (see Fig. 109-16).

The *foramen of Morgagni* is an anterior and medial diaphragmatic defect through which hernias can occur,

typically with a delayed presentation beyond the neonatal period. Small hernias are difficult to diagnose definitively on plain radiographs because the most common structure to herniate through the foramen is the transverse mesocolon, which appears as a solid mass in the cardiophrenic angle. The liver commonly herniates through the foramen in young children (Fig. 109-3). If bowel (usually the transverse colon) herniates through the foramen, an air-filled structure may be seen in the same location. Morgagni hernias are more common on the right side than the left, but they may extend to both sides of the midline. Ultrasonography (US), CT, and MRI have all been used to confirm the diagnosis and identify the contents of the hernia (see Fig. 109-3).

A rare type of diaphragmatic hernia involves a defect of the central tendon of the diaphragm, with herniation of abdominal contents into the pericardial sac via an incompletely closed pericardioperitoneal canal (see Fig. 106-7; Chapter 9).

Groin and Pelvic Hernias

Indirect inguinal hernias are the most common form of inferior abdominal wall herniation. If the processus vaginalis remains open, bowel can herniate through the inguinal ring into the scrotum in boys (Fig. 109-4) or through the canal of Nuck into the labia majora in girls, the latter being relatively infrequent. Ovarian tissue can also herniate through the canal of Nuck (see Fig. 109-4). Most inguinal hernias in children are asymptomatic, but incarceration or strangulation can cause intestinal obstruction. A sliding hernia may cause sufficient bowel irritation to lead to ileus or even intermittent functional obstruction.

Inguinal hernias may be seen coincidentally on plain radiographs, usually presenting as a loop of bowel in the scrotum, although this is often obscured by gonadal shielding in boys. In cases in which the loop is persistently fluid filled, US can identify the intestinal wall surround-

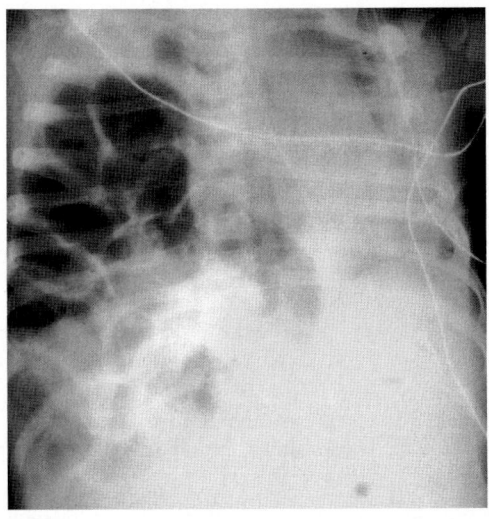 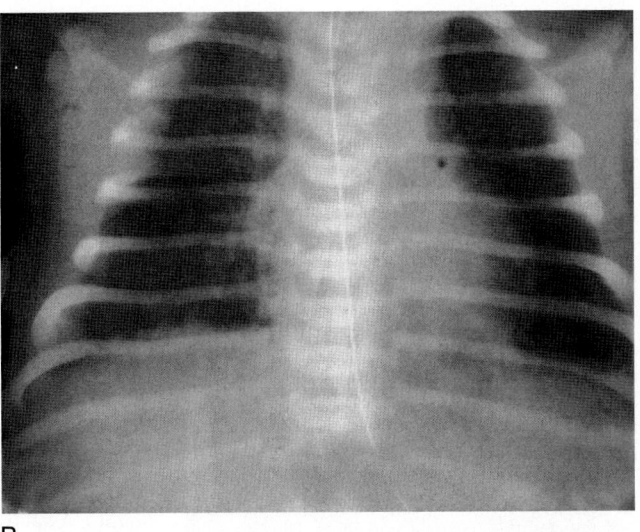

A   B

FIGURE 109-2. Delayed presentation of Bochdalek hernia in an 18-month-old infant with respiratory distress. **A,** Chest radiograph at presentation reveals a large right diaphragmatic hernia. **B,** Prior chest radiograph at 1 day of age (obtained because of transient tachypnea of the newborn) shows no hernia.

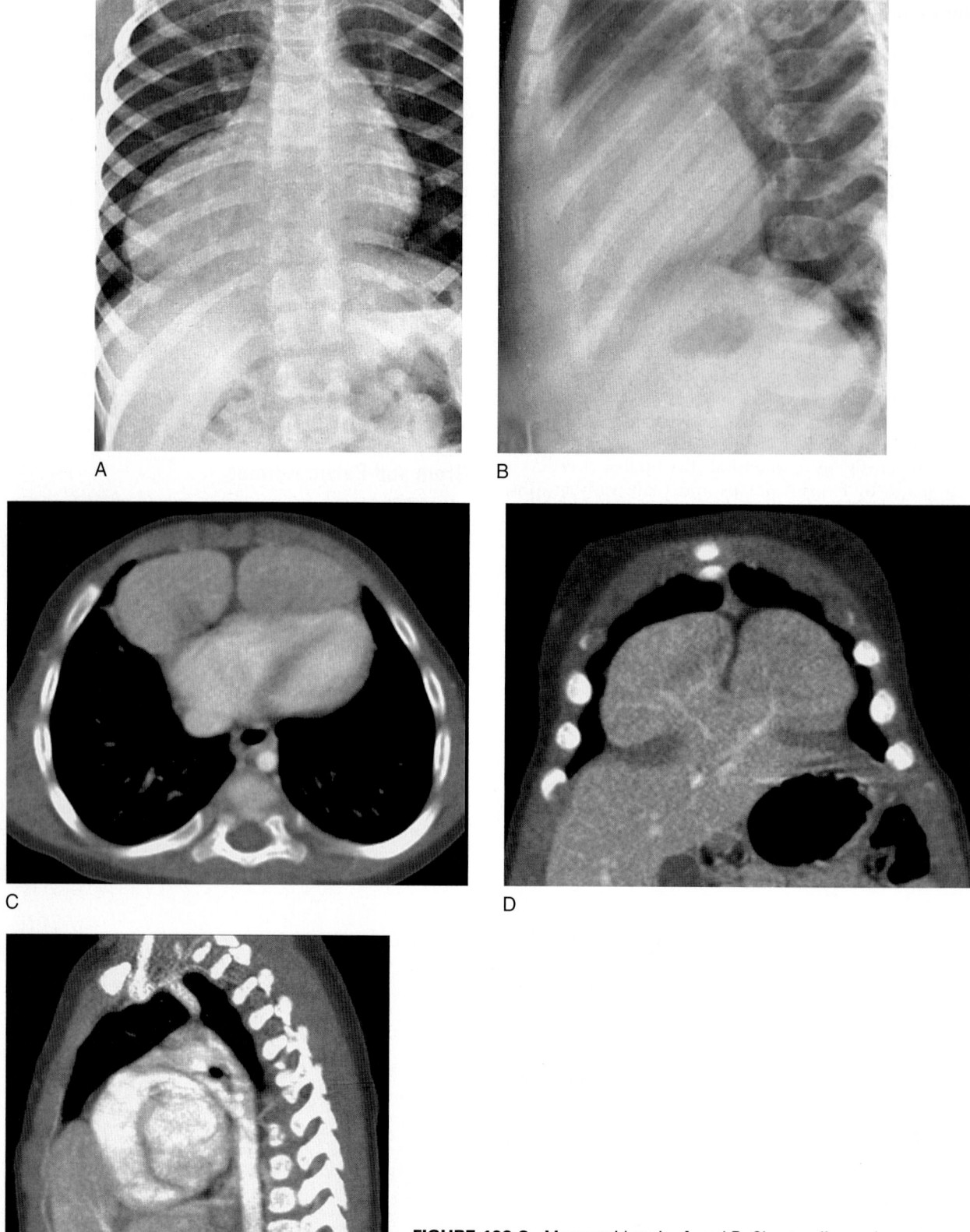

FIGURE 109-3. Morgagni hernia. **A** and **B,** Chest radiographs were obtained in this 4-year-old girl because of symptoms of upper respiratory infection. Frontal **(A)** and lateral **(B)** chest radiographs reveal a right-sided anterior soft tissue mass representing the herniated portion of the liver. **C-E,** Morgagni hernia in a 3-year-old with a similar history. Axial **(C),** coronal reformat **(D),** and sagittal reformat **(E)** show herniation of a portion of the liver through a foramen of Morgagni defect. (**C-E** courtesy of Marta Hernanz-Schulman, Nashville, TN.)

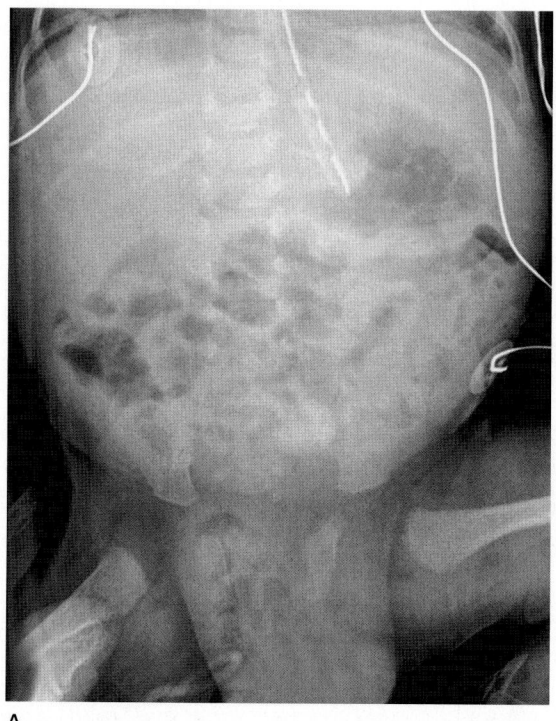
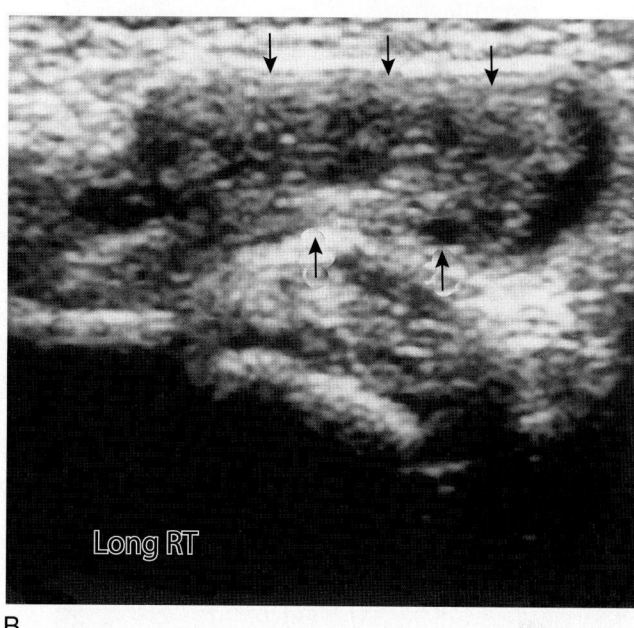

FIGURE 109-4. Inguinal hernia. **A,** Anteroposterior view of the abdomen and pelvis in a newborn boy shows an enlarged scrotum with multiple air-filled loops of intestine within it, secondary to indirect right inguinal hernia. **B,** US in the inguinal region of an infant girl with a labial mass confirms a herniated ovary *(arrows)* in the canal of Nuck. (**A** courtesy of Marta Hernanz-Schulman, Nashville, TN.)

ing the intraluminal fluid and may show small bubbles of air or peristalsis. Color Doppler US may show blood flow in the wall of the herniated bowel loop. These findings help differentiate a hernia from a hydrocele, which results from incomplete closure of the processus vaginalis. Contrast studies are rarely needed, but a small bowel series may demonstrate the herniated loop. Contrast enema with reflux into the small intestine in infants with intestinal obstruction may show a pinched-off loop at the entrance to the inguinal canal. Contrast peritoneography (herniography) is no longer used. Wechsler and colleagues demonstrated the CT and MRI appearance of inguinal hernias, but these studies are rarely needed for diagnostic purposes in children. Hernias may be incidental findings when these examinations are performed for other reasons.

Direct inguinal hernias, those in which the hernia sac is medial to the epigastric vessels, are acquired rather than congenital and are uncommon in children. *Femoral hernias* are also uncommon in the pediatric age group. The intestine herniates through the femoral ring and presents at the saphenous opening. Wechsler and colleagues demonstrated the value of CT in differentiating femoral hernias from other abdominal wall masses that may have similar clinical presentations. *Hernias through the obturator foramen* typically occur in elderly women and are rarely, if ever, found in children. *Sciatic hernias* pass through the sciatic foramen into the buttock. Though unusual in childhood, they should be included in the differential diagnosis of pelvic masses that extend through the sciatic foramen into the buttock, such as rhabdomyosarcoma and endodermal sinus tumor.

Anterior Abdominal Wall Defects with Herniation

The majority of patients with anterior wall defects and herniation present in the newborn period and are discussed more thoroughly in Chapter 8. *Omphaloceles* occur when the midgut does not return to the intraembryonic coelomic cavity by the 10th week of gestation. This leads to failure of infolding of the lateral abdominal walls. In infants, the gut appears outside the anterior abdominal wall in the base of the umbilical cord and is surrounded by a translucent sac of peritoneum and amnion (Fig. 109-5). With larger defects, the liver may also partially herniate into the sac. When the cephalic fold as well as the lateral fold fails to develop, the result is *ectopia cordis,* which is associated with congenital heart disease and defects in the pericardium, diaphragm, abdominal wall, and sternum—termed pentalogy of Cantrell. *Cloacal exstrophy* results from failure of development of the caudal fold.

Gastroschisis, unlike omphalocele, is a paraumbilical herniation through the abdominal wall. The cause is unknown, and approximately half of the affected patients are premature. Clinical differentiation from omphalocele can be made by noting the presence of a normal umbilical cord and the lack of a covering sac.

Umbilical hernias are common protrusions through the umbilical ring (Fig. 109-6). The majority regress as the child grows, and in most cases, no diagnostic or therapeutic procedures are required. The hernia may rarely become incarcerated or strangulated, but the clinical diagnosis is obvious, and imaging studies are not needed.

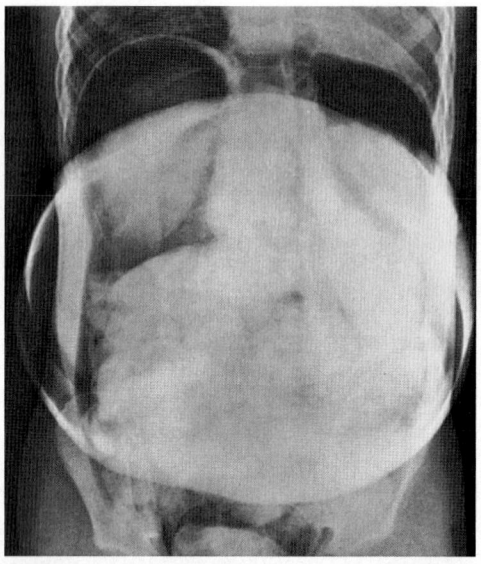
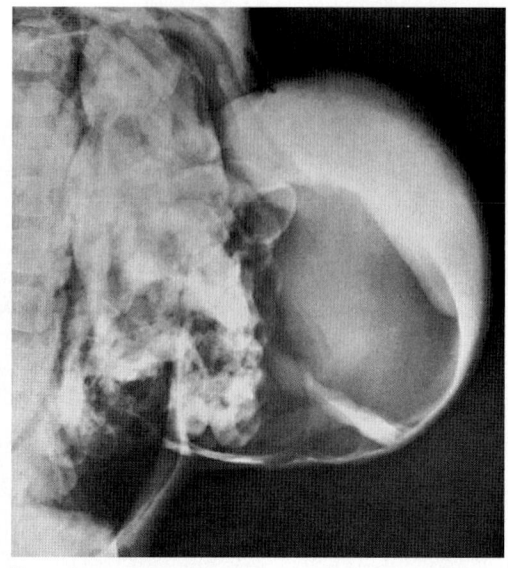

A   B

FIGURE 109-5. Omphalocele. Frontal **(A)** and lateral **(B)** views of the abdomen in a patient with omphalocele and pneumoperitoneum. Note that both loops of bowel and the liver are within the enclosed sac.

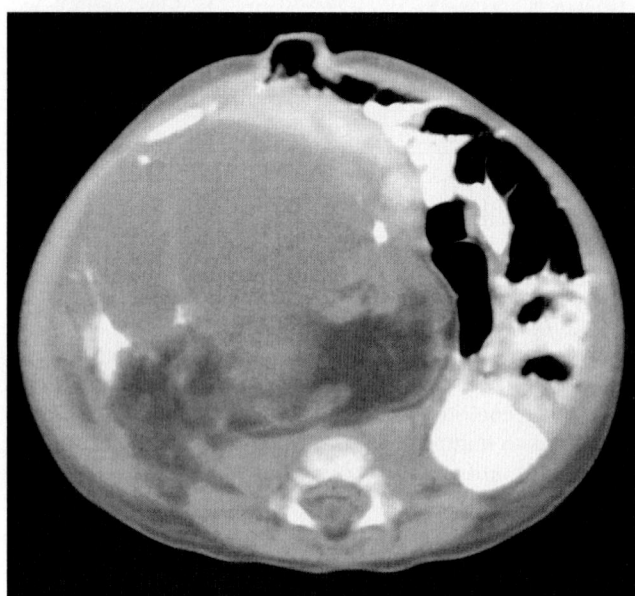

FIGURE 109-6. Umbilical hernia in a 3-month-old girl with teratoma. Although spontaneous umbilical hernias are common, there is an increased incidence in patients with abdominal masses.

Other abdominal wall hernias are rare in childhood. *Paraumbilical hernias* after infancy are unusual until adulthood. *Epigastric hernias* are defects in the linea alba between the xiphoid and umbilicus. *Spigelian hernias* are herniations through defects in the aponeurosis of the external oblique muscle lateral to the ipsilateral rectus muscle; they frequently become incarcerated and strangulated. CT is diagnostic in most cases. *Prune-belly syndrome* is the result of failure of development of the anterior wall musculature (Fig. 109-7) and is discussed in Chapter 19.

An *internal hernia* occurs when a portion of viscera protrudes through the peritoneum of mesentery. Most of these children present with small bowel obstruction. These are unusual hernias but may be suggested when an older child presents with small bowel obstruction without obvious etiology (no adhesions, etc.).

UMBILICAL REMNANT ABNORMALITIES

Omphalomesenteric Duct Remnant

The omphalomesenteric (or vitelline) duct can remain open throughout its length, at either end, or only in the midportion (Fig. 109-8). DiSantis and associates defined the completely open duct as type 1, the open-ended variant (open at either the ileum or the umbilicus) as type 2, and the open midportion as type 3. In type 1, enteric luminal contents can pass through the open duct from the terminal ileum to the umbilicus (Fig. 109-9). The opening at the umbilicus can often be probed and contrast material injected that passes directly into the ileum. In type 2, open at the umbilical end, there is a sinus tract from the umbilicus to the closed portion of the omphalomesenteric duct. A discharge may be present, consisting of secretions from the lining of the tract. Contrast injection reveals a blind-ending sinus tract. Type 2, open at the ileal end, is a Meckel diverticulum. Type 3, a vitelline duct cyst open only in the midportion, is usually asymptomatic. Type 3 vitelline duct cysts and some Meckel diverticula (type 2) may be large enough to be identified on US and CT as subumbilical cystic masses.

Meckel diverticulum is not only the most commonly identified omphalomesenteric duct remnant but also the most common congenital anomaly of the gastrointestinal tract, occurring in up to 4% of the population, according to autopsy studies. As an omphalomesenteric duct remnant, it projects from the antimesenteric side of the ileum, anywhere from 16 to 80 cm proximal to the ileocecal valve, depending somewhat on the age of the

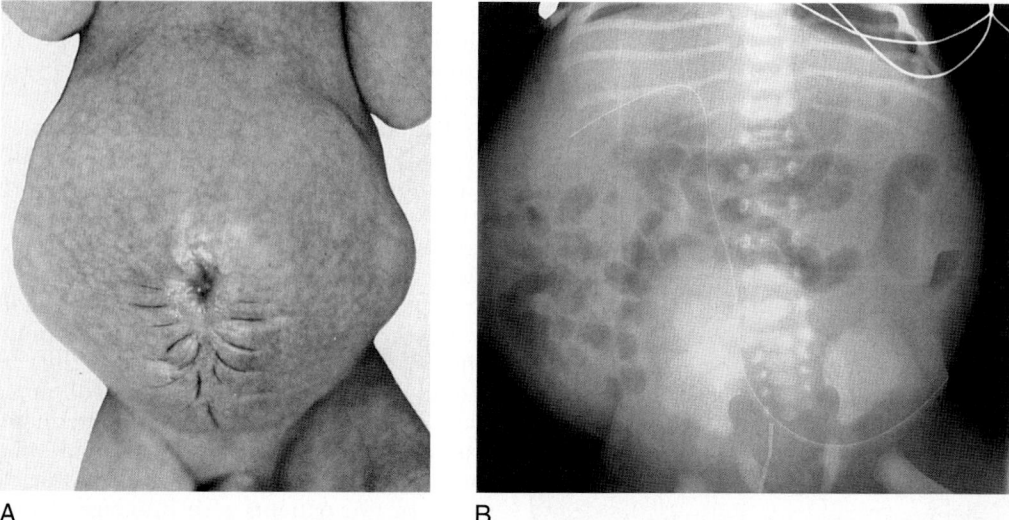

FIGURE 109-7. Prune-belly syndrome. **A,** Photograph of a 5-week-old boy with prune-belly syndrome shows congenital absence of the abdominal musculature. **B,** Abdominal radiograph of a different patient with prune-belly syndrome shows flaccidity of the abdominal wall, with marked dilation of the bladder. An umbilical venous catheter has been misplaced in the right portal vein.

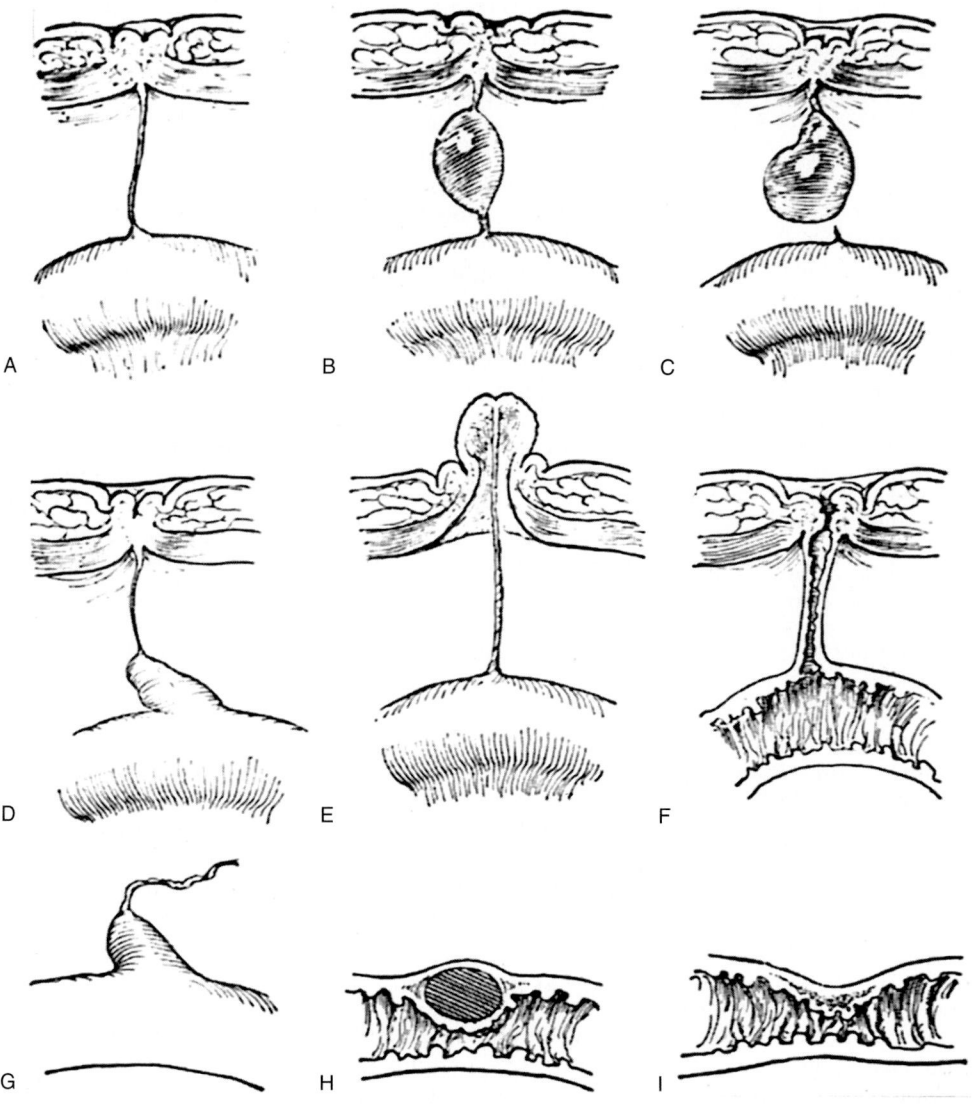

FIGURE 109-8. Variants of omphalomesenteric duct remnants. **A,** Persistent cord between the ileal wall and the closed umbilicus. **B,** Cyst in the same cord. **C,** Cyst anchored at the umbilical end of the cord but free at the ileal end. **D,** Meckel diverticulum attached to the closed umbilicus by a closed cord. **E,** Everted mucocele of the umbilicus with the cord attached to the ileal wall. **F,** Fecal fistula open at both the umbilical and ileal ends. **G,** Meckel diverticulum open at the ileal end but blind at the umbilical end, which is unattached. **H,** Intramural cystic diverticulum. **I,** Local stenosis of the ileum at the site of the mouth of the omphalomesenteric duct. (From Cullen TS: Embryology, Anatomy and Diseases of the Umbilicus. Philadelphia, Saunders, 1916.)

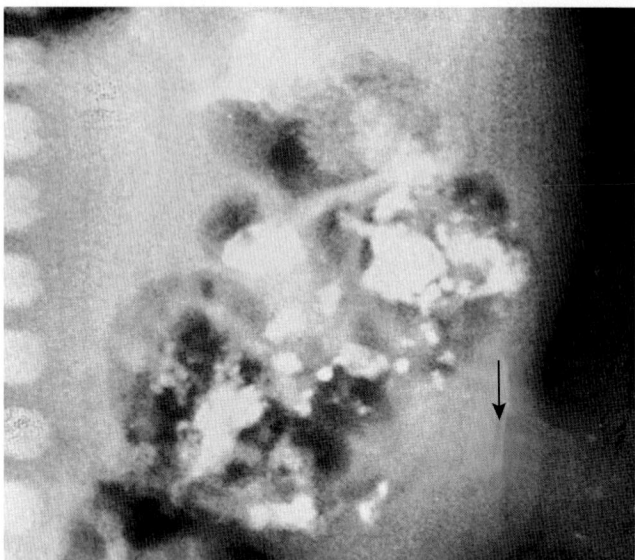

FIGURE 109-9. Patent omphalomesenteric duct remnant. Lateral film of the abdomen from an upper gastrointestinal series demonstrates barium flowing from the ileum through a patent omphalomesenteric duct *(arrow)* to the umbilicus and the anterior abdominal wall.

TABLE 109-1

Findings in Meckel Diverticulum

PLAIN RADIOGRAPHS AND CONTRAST STUDIES
Common
   Obstruction
   Contrast studies may show point of obstruction
   Filling defect on contrast studies if diverticulum is
     inverted
Less common
   Enteroliths in giant diverticulum

ULTRASOUND (US) AND COMPUTED TOMOGRAPHY (CT) STUDIES
Common
   Target-like mass with central echogenic fat on US if
     diverticulum is inverted
   Double target sign of inverted diverticulum and
     associated intussusceptum on US (diverticulum may
     also be fluid filled)
   Mass with fat attenuation and surrounding collar of soft
     tissue attenuation on CT if diverticulum is inverted
Less common
   Enteroliths in giant diverticulum on CT or US

---

patient. Because the diverticulum represents an opening into the embryonic duct, it contains all four intestinal wall layers, making it a true diverticulum (Table 109-1).

Most Meckel diverticula are asymptomatic and are found incidentally on imaging studies or at surgery or autopsy. Giant Meckel diverticula containing enteroliths may be seen on plain radiographs, CT, or US. Meckel diverticulum can result in intestinal obstruction by acting as a lead point for intussusception (inverting into the ileal lumen) or causing segmental small bowel volvulus around a persistent vitelline duct remnant leading from the diverticulum to the umbilicus. Because 15% of Meckel diverticula contain heterotopic gastric mucosa,

patients may present with abdominal pain or gastrointestinal hemorrhage secondary to peptic ulceration. Less commonly, the diverticula may include duodenal or jejunal mucosa or pancreatic tissue.

Patients with intestinal obstruction present with typical plain radiographic findings of obstruction. Contrast studies or CT scans may demonstrate the point of obstruction, but the diverticulum or vitelline duct remnant is usually not seen. An inverted Meckel diverticulum may occasionally be visualized as a filling defect on upper gastrointestinal series and small bowel follow-through. Inverted Meckel diverticula contain invaginated mesenteric fat centrally. Therefore, they can present as a target-like mass with a central area of increased echogenicity on US and a mass of fatty attenuation with a surrounding collar of soft tissue attenuation on CT. Itagaki and coworkers reported an ultrasonic "double target sign" in two patients with intussusception secondary to inverted Meckel diverticula. The two targets were adjacent to each other but of differing sizes. The larger target represented the intussusceptum and the smaller target the inverted Meckel diverticulum, which acted as a lead point. Daneman and colleagues described five patients with intussusception secondary to inverted Meckel diverticula imaged with US. In four of the five children, US demonstrated the fluid-containing or fat-containing diverticulum at the apex of the intussusceptum.

Patients with symptoms suspicious of peptic disease of the diverticulum are best examined initially with technetium-99m pertechnetate scintigraphy. Because the pertechnetate ion is secreted by gastric mucosa, the scan may show abnormal accumulation of radiopharmaceutical in the right midabdomen or right lower quadrant, coincident with the appearance of the stomach (see Fig. 106-13; Chapters 106 and 137). False-positive scans may result from the presence of ectopic gastric mucosa in other parts of the intestinal tract. False-negative results can be caused by a variety of factors. The false-negative rate can be reduced by pretreating the patient with cimetidine and glucagon. CT scans may show inflammatory changes around the diverticulum (Fig. 109-10). Small bowel series or contrast enema may demonstrate a Meckel diverticulum (Figs. 109-11 and 109-12), but the sensitivity is very low, and routine barium studies are of limited value. Angiography has been used to evaluate active gastrointestinal bleeding from Meckel diverticulum and can be enhanced by the use of digital subtraction techniques; however, scintigraphic nuclear medicine studies may also be of value. Routh and colleagues reported abnormal, irregular vessels supplied by an elongated, nonbranching ileal artery in two patients with Meckel diverticulum who had a history of gastrointestinal bleeding but were not actively bleeding at the time of angiography. Arterial embolization in patients bleeding from Meckel diverticulum has been reported.

Urachal Remnant

The residuum of the embryonic allantois is known as the urachus. In a manner analogous to omphalomesenteric duct remnants, the urachus can be open throughout

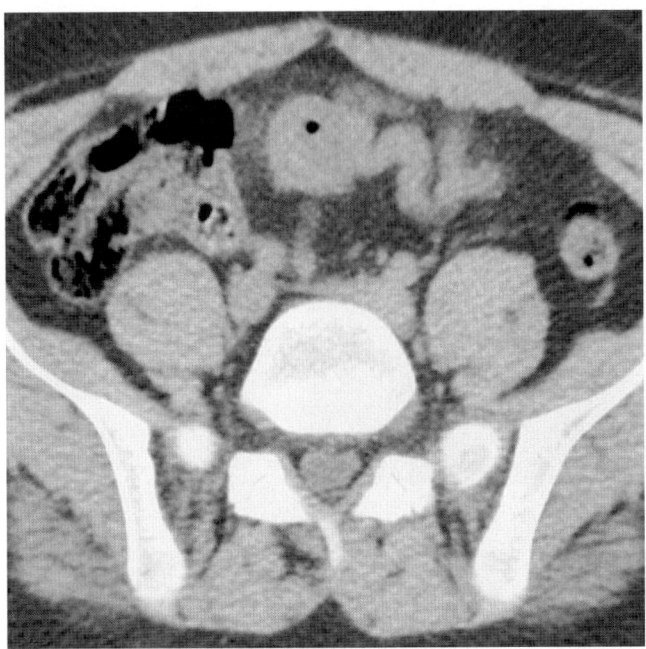 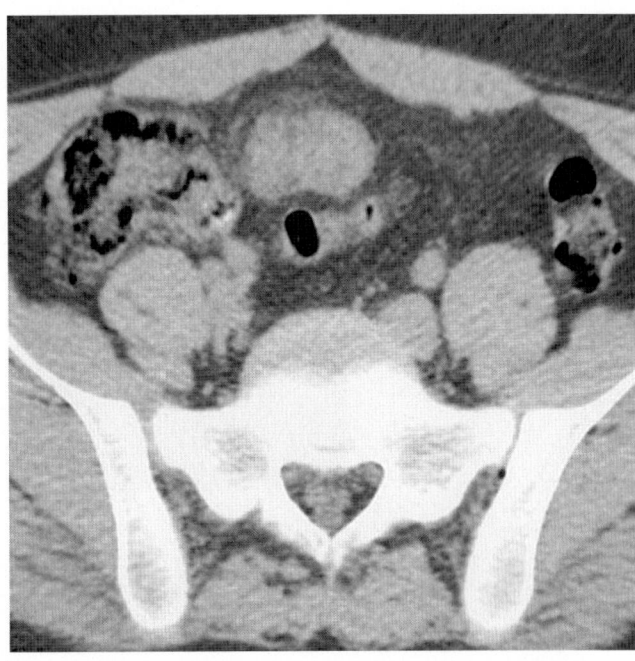

A   B

FIGURE 109-10. Meckel diverticulum. **A** and **B,** Infraumbilical images from uncontrasted CT in an adolescent boy with abdominal pain reveal a Meckel diverticulum with a small amount of intraluminal air and surrounding inflammatory changes in the adjacent fat. (Courtesy of Marta Hernanz-Schulman, Nashville, TN.)

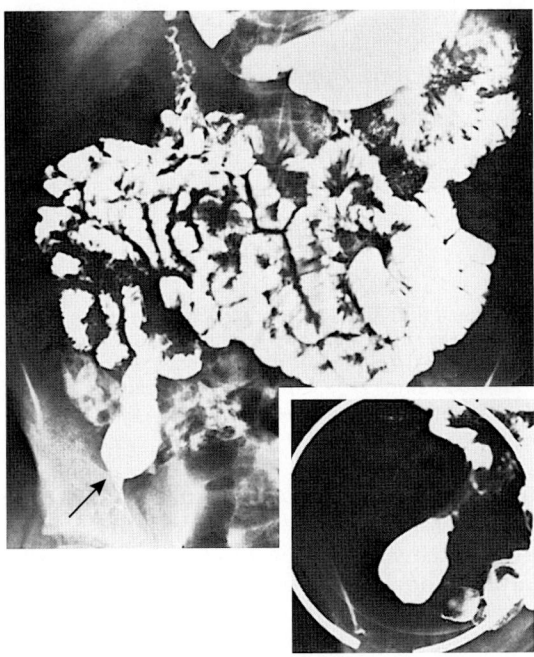

FIGURE 109-11. Meckel diverticulum. Delayed abdominal radiograph following upper gastrointestinal series in a 9-year-old child with abdominal pain shows filling of a Meckel diverticulum *(arrow). Inset,* Pressure spot film of the involved area.

its course from the bladder to the skin surface at the umbilicus; a portion of the urachus can be open as a blind-ending sinus from either the dome of the bladder or the umbilical skin surface; or only the midportion may remain patent as a urachal cyst that does not communicate with the bladder or the skin surface. A fully patent urachus connects the bladder to the umbilicus,

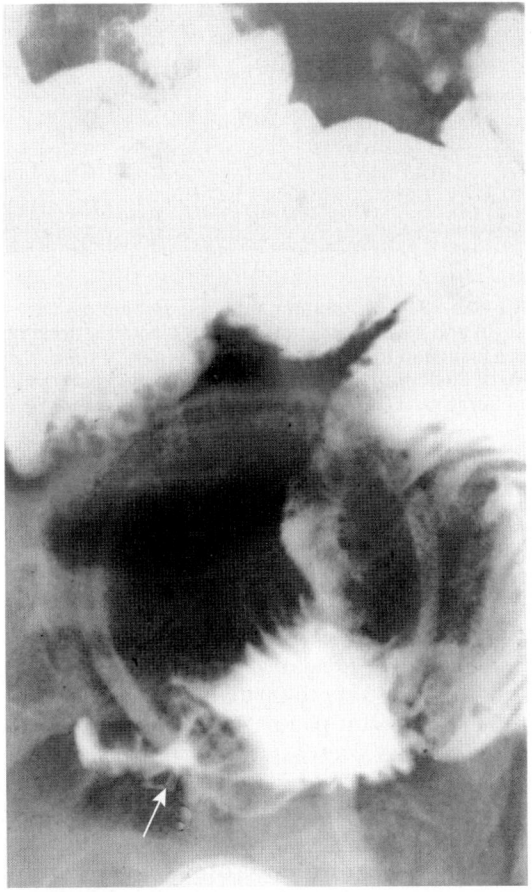

FIGURE 109-12. Pressure spot image of a Meckel diverticulum from an upper gastrointestinal series in a patient with a history of gastrointestinal bleeding shows a characteristic peptic ulcer with a barium-filled niche and radiating folds *(arrow).*

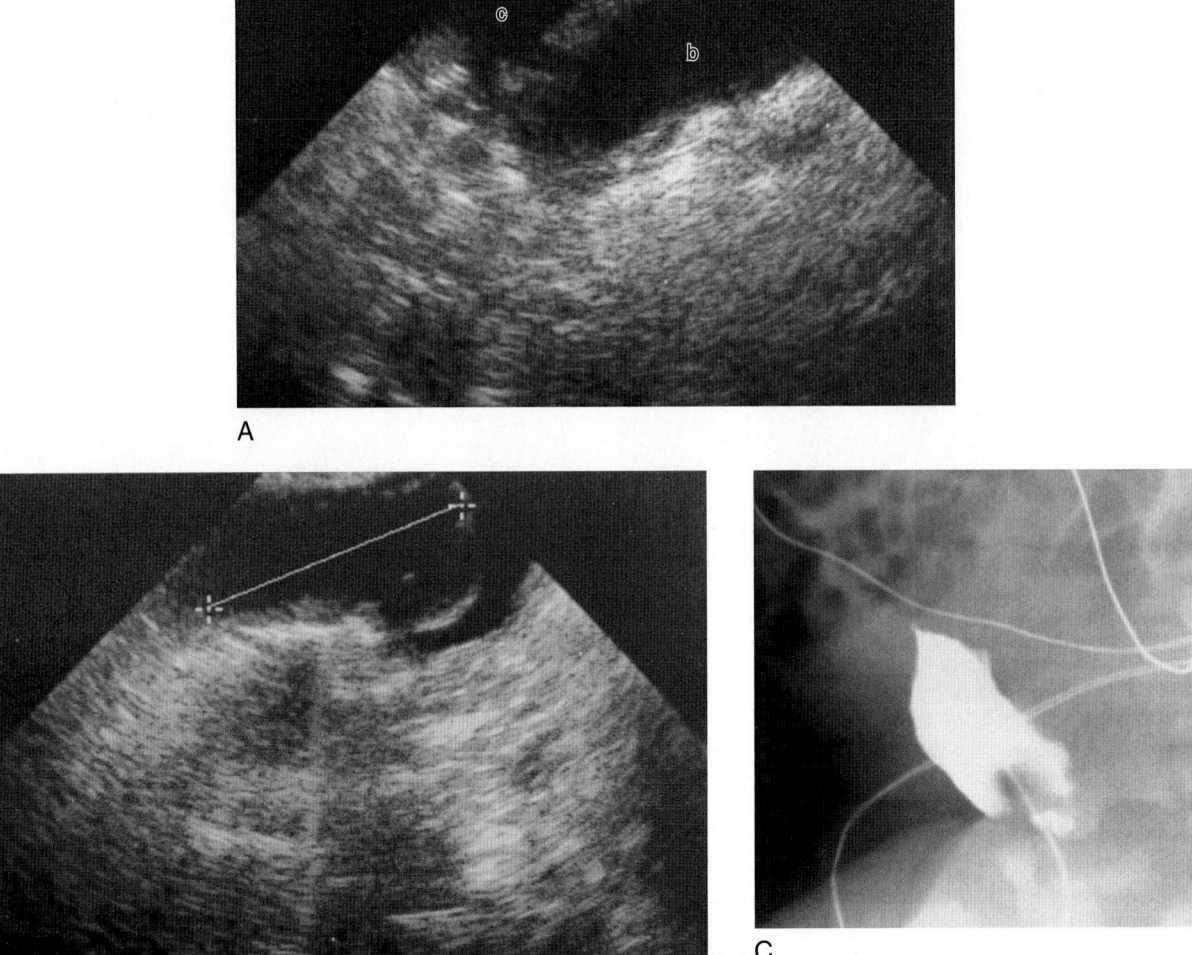

FIGURE 109-13. Urachal remnants. **A,** Longitudinal ultrasound scan demonstrates a fluid-filled tubular structure between the bladder (b) and a cystic structure (c) in the anterior abdominal wall. **B,** Transverse scan at the level of the umbilicus shows a cystic structure just deep to the umbilicus. At surgery, a urachal cyst directly connecting the skin surface at the umbilicus to the bladder was excised. **C,** Cystogram in another patient shows characteristic beaking of the anterosuperior aspect of the bladder caused by a patent proximal urachus. The remainder of the urachus from this point to the umbilicus was completely closed.

permitting urine to pass between them (Fig. 109-13). Leaking of urine is typically first noticed in the neonatal period. Other urologic abnormalities, such as hypospadias or renal ectopia, may be present in a few cases. The umbilical opening may be difficult to catheterize because of its small size, but often the bladder can be filled in this way. Alternatively, a voiding cystourethrogram may demonstrate the patent connection.

A urachal remnant patent only to the skin surface at the umbilicus may present with an umbilical discharge, especially when infected (Fig. 109-14). This is often identified by US. When open at the proximal end only, the urachal remnant appears as an extension of the bladder, most commonly at its anterosuperior portion (see Fig. 109-13). Cacciarelli and associates described a normal remnant of the closed urachus seen sonographically as a small, elliptical, hypoechoic structure at the anterosuperior aspect of the urinary bladder in 62 of 100 children.

A vesicourachal diverticulum results when the vesical end of the urachus fails to close, forming a lesion in which the urachus communicates only with the dome of the bladder. These lesions are usually asymptomatic and discovered incidentally on a voiding cystourethrogram or other imaging study; they are often associated with prune-belly syndrome. Urachal lesions are discussed more fully in Chapter 23.

> **Incomplete involution of the umbilical structures (omphalomesenteric duct or urachus) can lead to a spectrum of congenital anomalies, persistent communication between the umbilicus and either the ileum or the bladder, cysts, or blind-ending sinuses.**

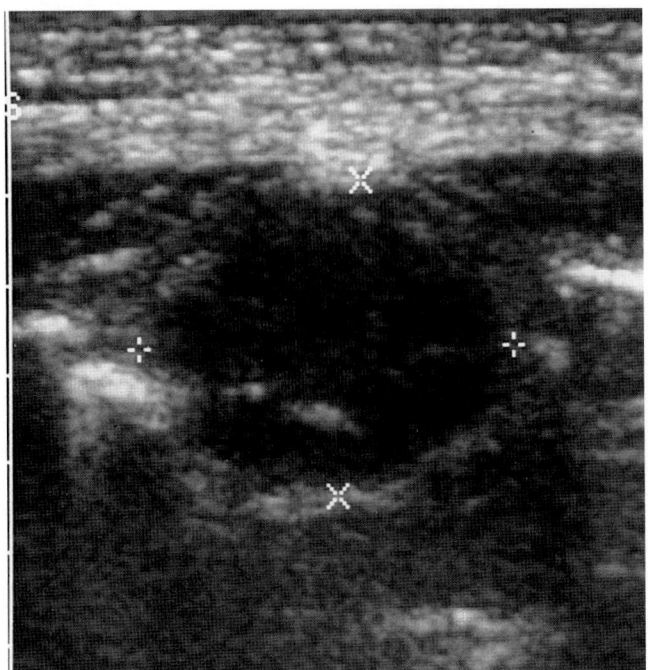

FIGURE 109-14. Infected urachal cyst. Transverse sonogram at the level of the umbilicus shows a hypoechoic structure just deep to the abdominal wall. When the transducer was placed on the abdomen, purulent material was expressed from the umbilicus. An infected urachal cyst was removed at surgery.

ABDOMINAL WALL MASSES

Masses of the abdominal wall, whether primary or metastatic, are rare and of diverse histology at all ages. Their rarity is even more striking in pediatric patients. Little information is available regarding tumors originating in the abdominal wall as independent entities. When tumors in this location are reported, they are typically presented based on histology, and the site of origin is grouped with other sites. Those originating in or involving the urachus are discussed in association with the genitourinary system. The extensive overlap of imaging findings between benign and malignant processes precludes a definitive imaging diagnosis; the vast majority of cases require biopsy for definite diagnosis.

Benign Masses

Included as benign masses are neoplasms such as angiomyolipoma, lymphangioma, hemangioma, and entities that may masquerade as masses, such as hematomas. Several of these lesions are discussed here.

Angiomyolipoma is a typically benign soft tissue tumor comprising mature adipose tissue (Fig. 109-15); tortuous, thick-walled blood vessels lacking elastic lamina; bundles of smooth muscle that seem to emanate from the vessel walls; and perivascular epithelioid cells. Tumors composed solely of perivascular epithelioid cells belong to a family of tumors known as perivascular epithelioid cell

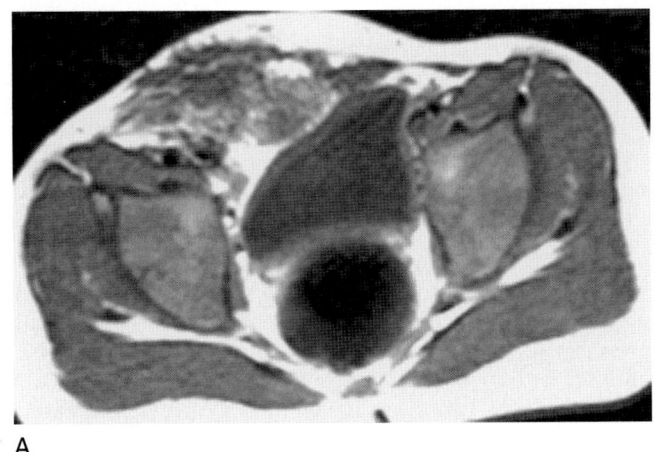

A

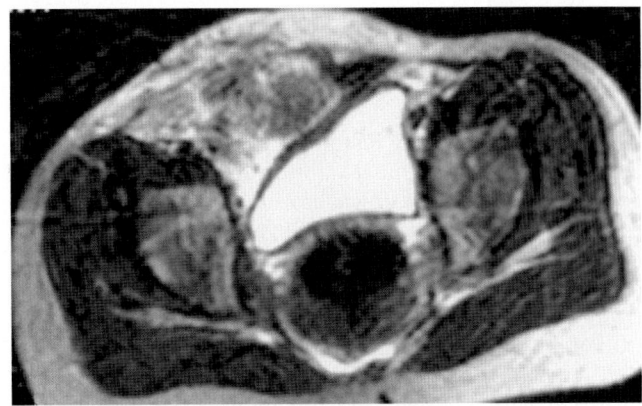

B

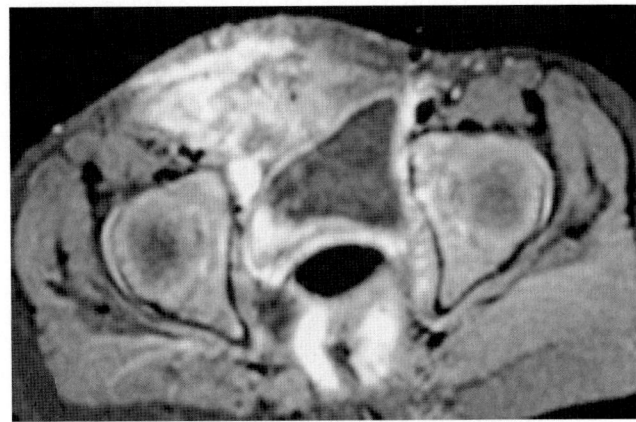

C

FIGURE 109-15. Angiomyolipoma in a 5-year-old girl. **A,** Axial, noncontrast T1-weighted MR image shows a poorly defined, heterogeneous, infiltrative process involving both subcutaneous soft tissues and muscles in the right anterior abdominopelvic wall. Note the mass effect on the right anterolateral margin of the bladder. **B,** Angiomyolipoma demonstrates heterogeneously increased signal on a T2-weighted sequence. **C,** Heterogeneous enhancement with intravenous contrast administration is shown on this postcontrast T1-weighted MR image with fat saturation.

neoplasms (PEComas). Occasionally, PEComas may be associated with tuberous sclerosis. A defining feature of angiomyolipoma and its variants is expression of the melanocytic marker HMB-45 by the perivascular epithelioid cells. Strict criteria for malignancy have not been established; however, tumors with highly pleomorphic, mitotic activity with foci of necrosis suggest malignancy. Controversy exists about the development of metastasis versus multifocality, although there are some cases that have clearly become metastatic. Folpe and colleagues found a heavy female predominance and a wide variety of primary sites of disease. Of the 26 PEComas they presented, only 2 arose in the abdominal wall. The median age at time of presentation was 46 years (range, 15 to 97 years).

Hematoma of the abdominal wall is a rare cause of abdominal pain, particularly in healthy pediatric patients. It may be more common in the elderly. Titone and coworkers reported that up to 90% of abdominal wall hematomas are misdiagnosed as tumors. On US, a hematoma is seen as a solid or cystic mass with septations. Characteristic findings on CT are those of a soft tissue mass, possibly with areas of increased density; hematomas may appear to be homogeneous or heterogeneous. The MRI appearance of an abdominal wall hematoma varies with the age of the lesion. Unger and associates found that subacute and chronic hematomas present for up to 10 months had areas of increased signal on both T1- and T2-weighted images.

Lymphangioma is a malformation of the lymphatics and can arise almost anywhere in the body. These tumors typically occur in the head and neck and are frequently associated with chromosomal abnormalities. Rarely, lymphangiomas occur in the anterior abdominal wall (Fig. 109-16).

Desmoid tumors are histologically benign but locally aggressive, nonmetastasizing tumors that belong to a group of disorders known as the fibromatoses. These tumors account for 3.5% of fibrous tissue tumors and can occur at any age but are more common in the third decade. In the abdominal wall, desmoid tumors arise from the aponeuroses of fascia, such as those associated with the rectus abdominis and internal oblique muscles; they may be single or multiple. Such tumors typically occur in young gravid females and have a recurrence rate after resection of about 20% to 30%.

Mesenteric desmoids are the most common mesenteric tumor. Although most often sporadic, these masses are seen with increased frequency in patients receiving estrogen therapy, those with Gardner syndrome (occurring in 9% to 18% of cases), and patients with a history of surgical trauma.

Histologically, desmoid tumors are poorly defined and infiltrative; they are composed of fibroblastic proliferation without evidence of malignancy or inflammation. Imaging characteristics of desmoid tumors vary, depending on the amount of collagen, proliferating fibroblasts, fibrosis, and vascularity. The fibrous and cellular composition of desmoid tumors varies with their stage at evaluation. On US, the margins may be ill-defined or irregular, and the echogenicity is variable. CT density, enhancement pattern, and margins likewise vary. On

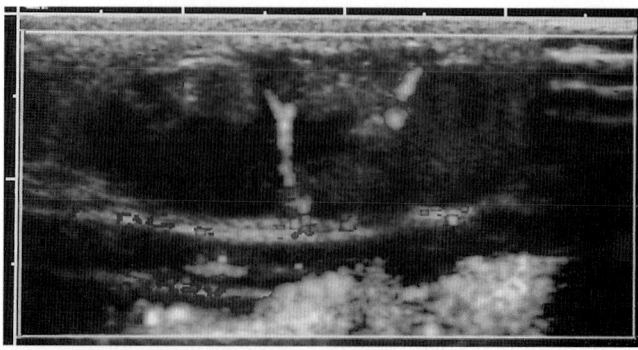

A

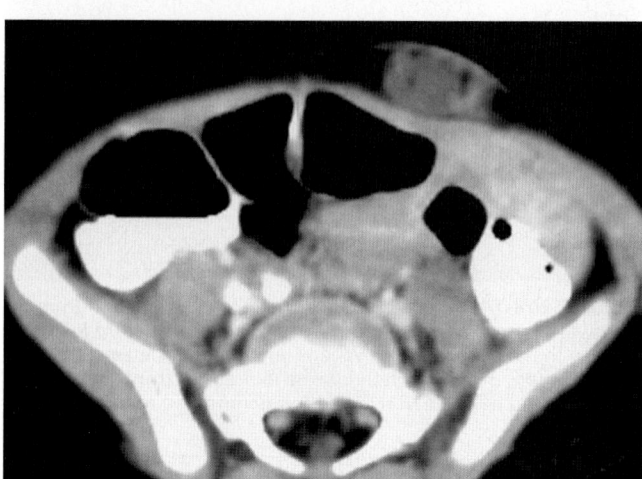

B

FIGURE 109-16. Lymphangioma in a 20-month-old boy with a new abdominal mass. **A,** Longitudinal ultrasound image of the abdominal mass shows that a large central area of the mass is anechoic, surrounded by solid tissue. Small arteries course into the center of the mass. **B,** Axial contrast-enhanced CT image through the lower abdomen shows a heterogeneous superficial left anterior abdominal wall mass located in the subcutaneous fat and extending to the skin.

MRI, desmoid tumors typically demonstrate decreased signal intensity on T1-weighted images and variable signal intensity on T2-weighted sequences compared with muscle. Enhancement patterns are also variable. Healy and coworkers found an association between increased tumor cellularity as shown on T2-weighted images and a tendency for rapid tumor growth. MRI is a useful method for staging desmoid tumors, assessing their stage of activity, and detecting recurrence. The role of positron emission tomography (PET) and PET-CT in determining tumor activity has yet to be determined.

Desmoid tumors have the following characteristics:

- **Histologically benign but locally aggressive**
- **Most common mesenteric tumor**
- **Occur with increased frequency in patients receiving estrogen therapy and in those with Gardner syndrome**

Infantile myofibromatosis is a benign entity distinct from desmoid-type fibromatosis and is the most common fibromatosis of infancy. This entity is now considered to be synonymous with *hemangiopericytoma.* Stanford and Rogers found that 80% of these lesions are solitary, and 60% were present at or soon after birth. The prognosis is favorable in patients with solitary lesions and no visceral involvement. The lack of a specific clinical appearance leads to frequent misdiagnosis. Lesions are usually dermal or subcutaneous in location and have prominent vascularity that may mimic hemangioma. Tumors may also be intramuscular or intraosseous in location.

Bronchogenic cyst of the anterior abdominal wall was reported by Kim and colleagues in an interesting single case report. The authors suggest that this unusual location of a bronchogenic cyst resulted from downward migration of a sequestered tracheobronchial tree bud during embryologic development.

Malignant Masses

Primary or metastatic subcutaneous tumors are extremely rare, as reported by De la Luz Orozco-Covarrubias and coworkers. In a 20-year review of 36,207 pediatric dermatology patients, these authors found that the most common such tumors were leukemia and lymphoma

(32%), rhabdomyosarcoma (25%), basal and squamous cell carcinoma (19%), and neuroblastoma (10%). However, other primary tumors do occur in the pediatric population.

Malignant mesenchymomas are rare soft tissue tumors seen predominantly in adults, but they can occur in patients of any age. These tumors contain at least two distinct histologic sarcoma subtypes and are typically considered to be high-grade tumors with an overall poor prognosis. Variability in prognosis is dependent on the histologic components, and because of the rarity of this tumor, information on morbidity and mortality is incomplete. Death is often due to local recurrence and pulmonary metastases. The most common sites of primary malignant mesenchymoma are the retroperitoneum or the thigh, but these tumors can occur anywhere. Treatment of malignant mesenchymoma is dependent on the tumor's histologic cell type but typically includes a combination of surgical incision, radiation therapy, and chemotherapy.

There are limited reports addressing the imaging features of malignant mesenchymoma. CT findings include a soft tissue mass with mixed attenuation and often containing areas of necrosis and calcification (Fig. 109-17). Lesions are typically greater than 10 cm in size, well circumscribed, and heterogeneous; however, lesions as

FIGURE 109-17. Recurrent mesenchymoma in a 5-year-old girl originally diagnosed at age 3 years. **A,** Abdominal radiograph from a barium enema demonstrates a normal colon, with displacement of the right colon *(arrow)* from the adjacent abdominal wall mesenchymoma. **B** and **C,** Axial CT images after intravenous and oral contrast administration show expansion of the anterolateral abdominal wall by heterogeneous infiltrative soft tissue *(asterisk).* There is extension from the subcutaneous location **(B** and **C)** into the abdomen, with mass effect on adjacent structures, most notably the right colon, as depicted in **A.**

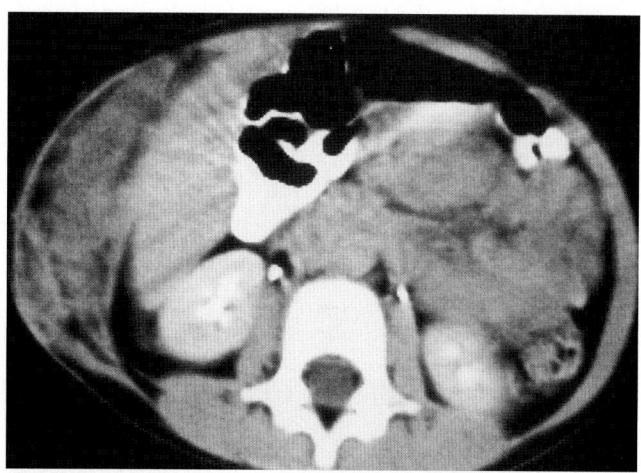

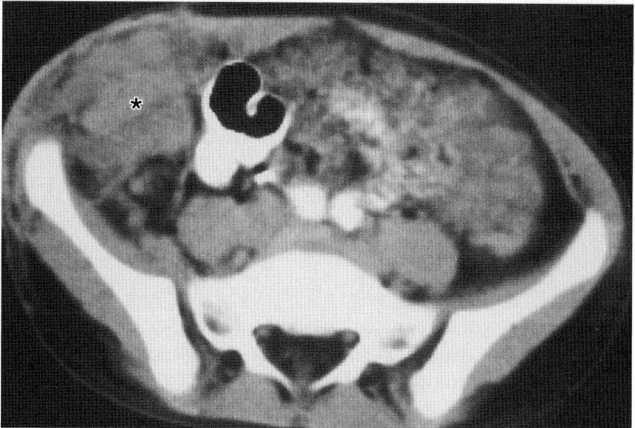

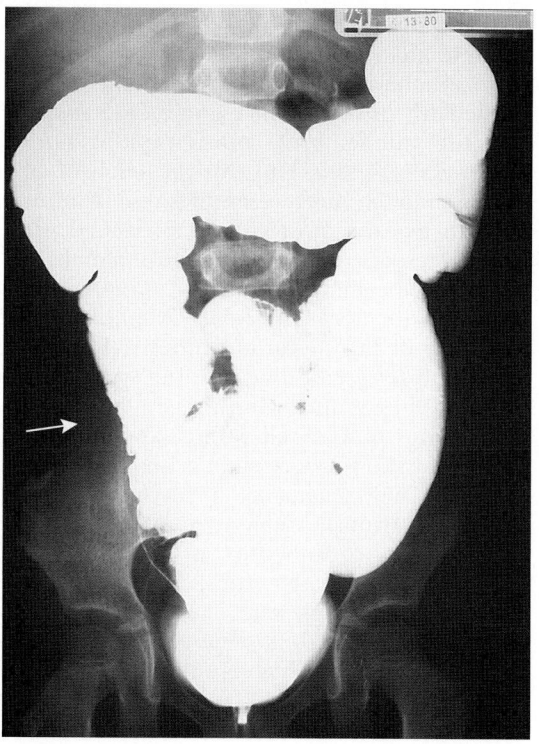

A

B

C

small as 3 cm have been reported. By CT, malignant mesenchymoma demonstrates heterogeneous enhancement and moderate vascularity. On MRI, these lesions are typically heterogeneous in appearance, particularly on T2-weighted images.

Primitive neuroectodermal tumors (PNETs) are members of the Ewing sarcoma family of tumors. This tumor group represents the second most common pediatric sarcoma of bone and soft tissue in most series. PNETs are reported to occur in the age range of 14 to 22 years, with peak presentation during adolescence. There is no gender bias. Most of the extraskeletal soft tissue tumors present as a painless mass. Histologically, a PNET is a small round cell tumor; translocation of the *EWS* gene at 22q12 and either the *FLI1* gene at 11q24 or the *ERG* gene at 21q22 is characteristic of the Ewing sarcoma family of tumors and PNETs.

Imaging characteristics of PNETs are heterogeneous and nonspecific. On US, lesions typically show multiple septations with cystic spaces. These masses are heterogeneous when imaged with CT and are iso- to slightly hypodense compared with muscle. Calcifications may be present (Fig. 109-18). Hyperdense areas of hemorrhage may be seen. The tumors enhance heterogeneously with intravenous contrast administration. Khong and colleagues found that MRI readily demonstrates hyperintense loculi on T2-weighted sequences, separated by hypodense septa. On T1-weighted sequences, the masses are heterogeneously hypointense to muscle and enhance heterogeneously. The tumor masses may be surrounded by a hypodense rim of hemosiderin deposition.

- **PNETs are members of the Ewing sarcoma family of tumors**
- **This tumor family represents the second most common pediatric sarcoma of soft tissue and bone**

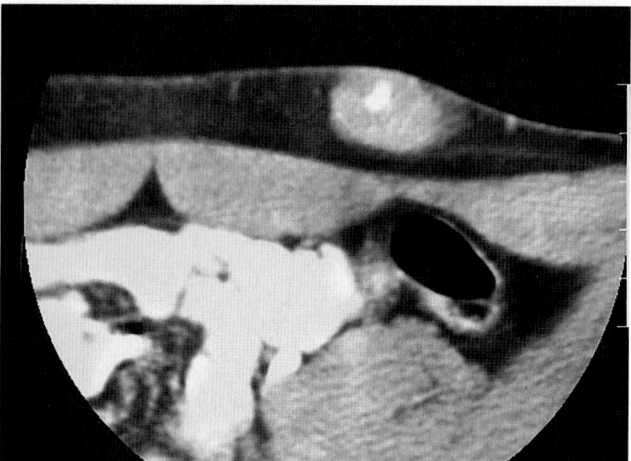

FIGURE 109-18. Primitive neuroectodermal tumor in a 15-year-old boy with a 1-year history of a small left anterior abdominal wall "lump." Axial contrast-enhanced CT image shows a soft tissue mass with central calcifications in the subcutaneous fat of the left anterior abdominal wall. The lateral margin suggests some local infiltration into the adjacent fat.

- **PNETs are heterogeneous by US, CT, and MRI and enhance heterogeneously**

Desmoid-type fibromatosis (aggressive fibromatosis) is a rare, histologically benign, but locally infiltrative and aggressive soft tissue tumor for which surgery is the mainstay of treatment. There is a high risk of local recurrence, reported by Phillips and associates to approach 21% at a median of 39 months. Although they carry no malignant potential, because of their likelihood of recurrence, these tumors are classified with malignant soft tissue tumors, of which they constitute approximately 4%. Desmoid-type fibromatosis has a slight female predominance and typically occurs in the fourth decade of life, but scattered pediatric cases have been reported. Desmoid-type fibromatosis is more likely to recur and develop at an older age than are desmoid tumors.

On MRI studies, Lee and colleagues found that 52% of desmoid-type fibromatosis masses were ovoid, 34.5% were infiltrative, 76% had an irregular or lobulated contour, 54% had well-defined margins, and the tumor crossed the fascial plane in 31%. These investigators found that the majority of cases (83%) had a signal intensity iso- or hyperintense to skeletal muscle on T1-weighted sequences, with homogeneous or mostly homogeneous signal in 79%. In 77% of cases, increased signal relative to skeletal muscle was shown on T2-weighted sequences; this was heterogeneous in 65% of cases. Moderate or intense enhancement was demonstrated with intravenous contrast administration.

Fibrosarcoma is a mesenchymal tumor of fibroblast derivatives that varies in terms of histologic subtype and clinical behavior. It represents approximately 10% of pediatric soft tissue sarcomas, not including rhabdomyosarcoma, and has a bimodal distribution in patients younger than 2 years and in the second decade. The clinical behavior of adult tumors and pediatric tumors, particularly those presenting in infants, is quite different; infantile tumors grow more rapidly, but the overall prognosis is better. The clinical behavior of fibrosarcomas in older children resembles that in adults. Prognosis in both types is most closely associated with complete primary resection. Low-grade fibrosarcomas may resemble desmoid fibromatosis tumors. Hansen and coworkers proposed the term *low-grade fibrosarcoma fibroblastic type* for some of the low-grade tumors that are difficult to classify under established grading systems; these include fibromyxoid sarcoma, sclerosing epithelioid fibrosarcoma, hyalinizing spindle cell tumor, and myxofibrosarcoma, which may show progression to high-grade tumors. Fibrosarcomas may occur as a secondary malignancy in patients previously treated for other tumors. Dermatofibrosarcoma protuberans is a skin malignancy that presents largely in the trunks and extremities of young adults; it has a high rate of recurrence and metastatic potential. On imaging, tumors have been described as similar to muscle in echogenicity on US, slightly hypodense on uncontrasted CT, isointense on T1-weighting, and hyperintense on T2-weighting, with heterogeneous enhancement (Fig. 109-19).

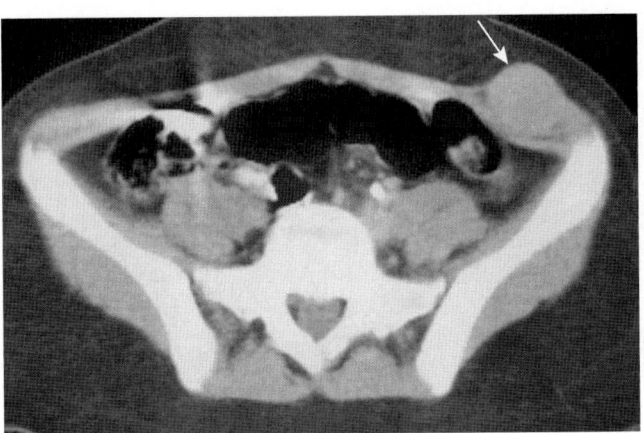

FIGURE 109-19. Fibrosarcoma of the anterior abdominal wall in a 14-year-old girl. Axial contrast-enhanced CT image through the upper pelvis shows a well-defined, round, 3-cm mass in the left anterior abdominal wall. The mass expands and is isointense with the left lateral oblique muscles (arrow).

- **Fibrosarcomas have a bimodal distribution, occurring in patients younger than 2 years and in those in the second decade of life**
- **Infantile tumors are larger but tend to have a better prognosis**
- **Long-term prognosis is dependent on complete resection**

Rhabdomyosarcoma is the most common soft tissue sarcoma in children, accounting for about half of all such tumors. As with rhabdomyosarcoma arising elsewhere in the body, Chui and associates reported that event-free and overall survival in patients with primary abdominal wall rhabdomyosarcoma is predicted by tumor size at diagnosis, nodal disease, and gross total tumor resection (those up to 5 cm could be totally resected). These tumors may develop in association with syndromes such as Beckwith-Wiedemann syndrome, phakomatosis pigmentokeratotica, and others.

Imaging demonstrates a solid soft tissue mass with variable enhancement (Fig. 109-20). Tumor margins also vary. There may be associated soft tissue edema. The involved muscle of origin is expanded at the site of the mass.

- **Rhabdomyosarcoma is the most common pediatric soft tissue sarcoma**
- **Event-free and overall survival is predicted by tumor size at diagnosis, complete tumor resection, and nodal disease**
- **These tumors are associated with Beckwith-Wiedemann syndrome and phakomatosis pigmentokeratotica**

Synovial sarcoma of the abdominal wall is a rare malignancy constituting 5% to 6% of pediatric soft tissue sarcomas. It is the fourth most common soft tissue malignancy; the vast majority originate in the extremities. Fetsch and Meis reported a series of 27 synovial sarcomas

arising in the abdominal wall identified in the Soft Tissue Registry of the Armed Forces Institute of Pathology, with patients ranging in age from 8 to 58 years. As with synovial sarcoma in other locations, in patients with primary disease in the abdominal wall, a poor prognosis is associated with high mitotic rate and poorly differentiated subtype. Lesions 5 cm or larger also have a less favorable prognosis. Imaging characteristics vary widely and cannot differentiate between benign tumors and malignant synovial sarcoma; these are discussed in greater detail in Chapter 16.

Metastatic tumors of the abdominal wall result from hematogenous spread and are quite rare; these metastatic deposits may involve the muscles of the abdominal wall or the subcutaneous tissues. Little information is available regarding abdominal wall metastases of non-hematologic pediatric malignancies. When the metastases involve the subcutaneous tissues, they are often nodular. Those involving the abdominal wall muscles typically cause muscular expansion and enlargement and may cause heterogeneous density, signal intensity, or enhancement in the involved distribution.

Wesche and coworkers reported 40 cases from 34 patients identified in a 30-year series of nearly 2000 pathology specimens that were coded as cutaneous metastases of nonhematologic malignancies. Among these patients, only eight had involvement of the abdominal skin. The primary diagnosis was neuroblastoma in two cases, rhabdomyosarcoma in five cases, and sarcoma not otherwise specified in one case. Imaging by US may aid in characterizing such lesions and, when necessary, provide localization for biopsy. CT or MRI may be required for disease staging.

In addition to solid tumors delineated earlier, malignant melanoma and, extremely rarely, medulloblastoma can metastasize to the abdominal wall.

- **Metastases to the abdominal wall are rare and result from hematogenous dissemination**
- **Metastases are often nodular when subcutaneous tissues are involved**
- **Neuroblastoma, rhabdomyosarcoma, malignant melanoma, medulloblastoma, and sarcoma (not otherwise specified) have been reported as the primary tumors**

INFLAMMATORY CONDITIONS

Myositis of the abdominal wall is a rare occurrence. Cheon and colleagues reported two cases in which children undergoing intra-arterial chemotherapy for proximal femoral osteosarcoma developed signs of an acute abdomen evidenced by localized rebound tenderness; laboratory values were normal. US examination revealed unilateral thickening of the rectus abdominis muscle. The authors hypothesized that this inflammatory response occurred as a result of repositioning of the intra-arterial catheter into an artery supplying the rectus abdominis or as a result of incomplete admixture of agents.

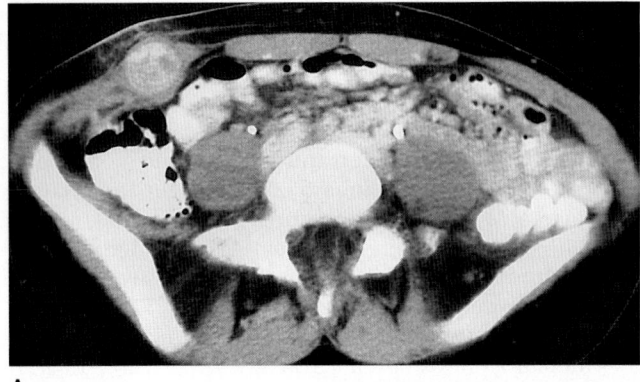

A

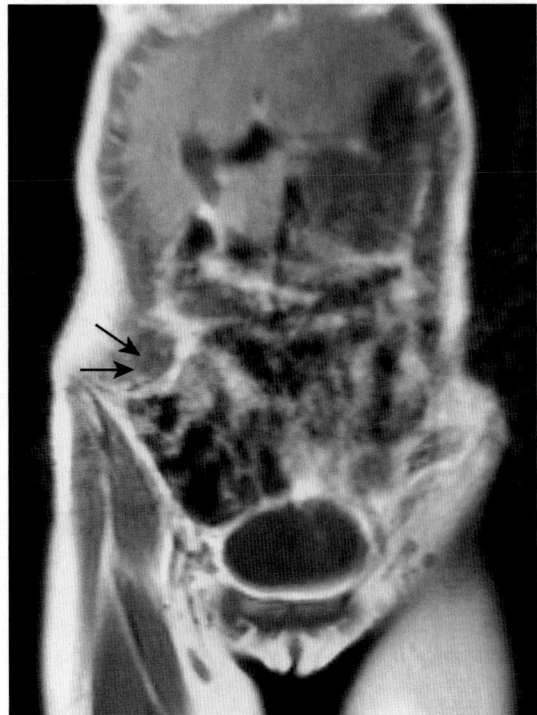

B

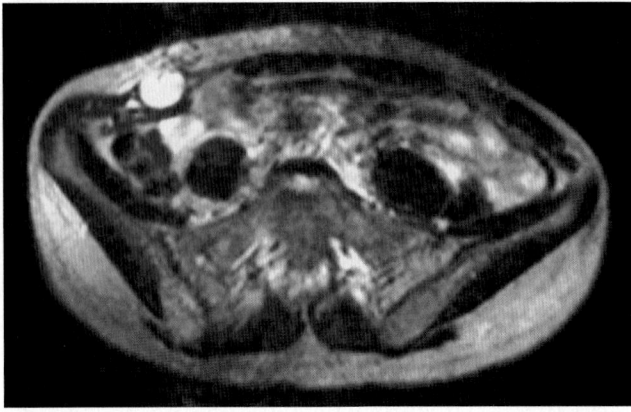

C

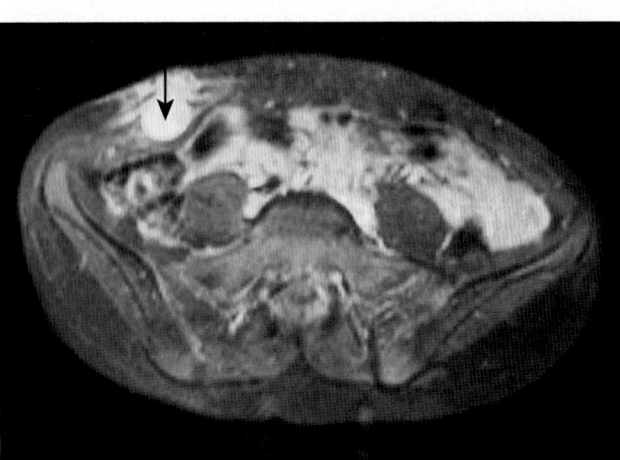

D

FIGURE 109-20. Rhabdomyosarcoma (embryonal) in a 13-year-old girl with a firm subcutaneous mass in the right lower abdominal wall. **A,** Axial contrast-enhanced CT image of the lower abdomen shows a heterogeneously enhancing mass that causes focal enlargement of the right lateral oblique muscles. There is evidence of edema within the subcutaneous fat overlying the mass. Local infiltration by tumor cannot be excluded on this image. **B,** Oblique, coronal, noncontrast T1-weighted MR image shows the 3-cm round soft tissue mass within the right lateral oblique muscles *(arrows).* **C,** On an axial T2-weighted MR image, the mass exhibits intense signal (as it did on short tau inversion recovery, not shown). **D,** There is intense enhancement with intravenous contrast administration in the soft tissue mass, as well as in the overlying subcutaneous fat *(arrow).* This finding leads to concern about tumor infiltration.

Other causes of inflammatory processes of the abdominal wall are infection, surgery, and accidental trauma. Cellulitis and myositis can be exquisitely demonstrated by MRI. Areas of involvement demonstrate markedly increased signal on T2-weighted and short tau inversion recovery sequences and enhance with intravenous contrast administration.

ACKNOWLEDGMENTS

I thank Drs. Bruce Parker and Al Schlesinger for their work on the previous version of this chapter and Sandra Gaither for assistance in manuscript preparation.

SUGGESTED READINGS

Hernias

Aguirre DA, Santosa AC, Casola G, Sirlin CB: Abdominal wall hernias: imaging features, complications, and diagnostic pitfalls at multi-detector row CT. Radiographics 2005;25:1501-1520

Bair JH, Russ PD, Pretorius DM, et al: Fetal omphalocele and gastroschisis: a review of 24 cases. AJR Am J Roentgenol 1986;147:1047-1051

Balthazar EJ, Dubramanyam BR, Megibow A: Spigelian hernia: CT and ultrasonography diagnosis. Gastrointest Radiol 1984;9:81-84

Berman L, Stringer D, Ein SH, et al: The late-presenting pediatric Bochdalek hernia: a 20-year review. J Pediatr Surg 1988;23:735-739

Chou TY, Chu CC, Diau GY, et al: Inguinal hernia in children: US versus exploratory surgery and intraoperative contralateral laparoscopy. Radiology 1996;201:385-388

Currarino G: Incarcerated inguinal hernia in infants: plain films and barium enema. Pediatr Radiol 1974;2:247-250

Fogata ML, Collins HB 2nd, Wagner CW, Angtuaco TL: Prenatal diagnosis of complicated abdominal wall defects. Curr Probl Diagn Radiol 1999;28:101-128

Franken EA Jr: Anomalies of the anterior abdominal wall: classification and roentgenology. Am J Roentgenol Radium Ther Nucl Med 1971;112:58-67

Gayer G, Bilik R, Vardi A: CT diagnosis of delayed presentation of congenital diaphragmatic hernia simulating massive pleuropneumonia. Eur Radiol 1999;9:1672-1674

Hubbard AM, Adzick NS, Crombleholme TM, et al: Congenital chest lesions: diagnosis and characterization with prenatal MR imaging. Radiology 1999;212:43-48

McCarten KM, Rosenberg HK, Borden S 4th, et al: Delayed appearance of right diaphragmatic hernia associated with group B streptococcal infections in newborns. Radiology 1981; 139:385-388

Miller PA, Mezwa DG, Feczko PJ, et al: Imaging of abdominal hernias. Radiographics 1995;15:333-347

Munden M, McEniff N, Mulvihill D: Sonographic investigation of female infants with inguinal masses. Clin Radiol 1995;50:696-698

Newman B, Davis PL: Sonographic and magnetic resonance imaging of an anterior diaphragmatic hernia. Pediatr Radiol 1989;20:110-112

Oh KS, Condon VR, Norst RP, et al: Peritoneographic demonstration of femoral hernia. Radiology 1978;127:209-211

Ramos CT, Koplewitz BZ, Babyn PS, et al: What have we learned about traumatic diaphragmatic hernias in children? J Pediatr Surg 2000;35:601-604

Siegel MJ, Shackelford GD, McAlister WH: Left-sided diaphragmatic hernia: delayed presentation. AJR Am J Roentgenol 1981;137:43-46

Toyama WM: Combined congenital defects of the anterior abdominal wall, sternum, diaphragm, pericardium, and heart: a case report and review of the syndrome. Pediatrics 1972;50:778-792

Wechsler RJ, Kurtz AB, Needleman L, et al: Cross-sectional imaging of abdominal wall hernias. AJR Am J Roentgenol 1989;153:517-521

Umbilical Remnant Abnormalities

Aggarwal S, Kumar A, Nijhawan S, et al: Bleeding Meckel's diverticulum demonstrated by digital subtraction angiography. Pediatr Radiol 1989;19:438

Cacciarelli AA, Kass EJ, Yang SS: Urachal remnants: sonographic demonstration in children. Radiology 1990;174:473-475

Cullen TS: Embryology, Anatomy, and Diseases of the Umbilicus. Philadelphia, Saunders, 1916

Daneman A, Lobo E, Alton DJ, et al: The value of sonography, CT, and air enema for the detection of complicated Meckel diverticulum in children with nonspecific clinical presentation. Pediatr Radiol 1998;28:928-932

Daneman A, Myers M, Shuckett B, et al: Sonographic appearances of inverted Meckel diverticulum with intussusception. Pediatr Radiol 1997;27:295-298

Diamond RH, Rothstein RD, Aloni A: Role of cimetidine-enhanced technetium-99m pertechnetate imaging for visualizing Meckel's diverticulum. J Nucl Med 1991;32:1422-1424

DiSantis DJ, Siegel MJ, Katz ME: Simplified approach to umbilical remnant abnormalities. Radiographics 1991;11:59-66

Grosfield JL, Franken EA: Intestinal obstruction in the neonate due to vitelline duct cysts. Surg Gynecol Obstet 1974;138:527-532

Itagaki A, Uchida M, Ueki K, et al: Double targets sign in ultrasonic diagnosis of intussuscepted Meckel diverticulum. Pediatr Radiol 1991;21:148-149

Little DC, Shah SR, St Peter SD, et al: Urachal anomalies in children: the vanishing relevance of the preoperative voiding cystourethrogram. J Pediatr Surg 2005;40:1874

Okazaki M, Higashihara H, Yamasaki S, et al: Arterial embolization to control life-threatening hemorrhage from a Meckel's diverticulum. AJR Am J Roentgenol 1990;154:1257-1258

Pantongrag-Brown L, Levine MS, Elsayed AM, et al: Inverted Meckel's diverticulum: clinical, radiologic, and pathologic findings. Radiology 1996;199:693

Rossi P, Gourtsoyiannis N, Bezzi M, et al: Meckel's diverticulum: imaging diagnosis. AJR Am J Roentgenol 1996;166:567

Routh WD, Lawdahl RB, Lund E, et al: Meckel's diverticula: angiographic diagnosis in patients with non-acute hemorrhage and negative scintigraphy. Pediatr Radiol 1990;20:152-156

Salomonowitz E, Wittich G, Hajek P, et al: Detection of intestinal diverticula by double-contrast small bowel enema: differentiation from other intestinal diverticula. Gastrointest Radiol 1983;8:271-278

Sfakianakis GN, Haase GM: Abdominal scintigraphy for ectopic gastric mucosa: a retrospective analysis of 143 studies. AJR Am J Roentgenol 1982;138:7-12

Torii Y, Hisatsune I, Imamura K, et al: Giant Meckel diverticulum containing enteroliths diagnosed by computed tomography and sonography. Gastrointest Radiol 1989;14:167-169

Abdominal Wall Masses

Adachi T, Oda Y, Sakamoto A, et al: Prognostic factors in the so-called malignant mesenchymoma: a clinicopathological and immunohistochemical analysis. Oncol Rep 2003;10:803-811

Alaminos-Mingorance M, Sanchez-Lopez-Tello C, Castejon-Casado J, et al: Scrotal lymphangioma in children. Urol Int 1998;61:181-182

Al-Salem AH: Lymphangiomas in infancy and childhood. Saudi Med J 2004;25:466-469

Beech TR, Moss RL, Anderson JA, et al: What comprises appropriate therapy for children/adolescents with rhabdomyosarcoma arising in the abdominal wall? A report from the Intergroup Rhabdomyosarcoma Study Group. J Pediatr Surg 1999;34:668-671

Brady MS, Perino G, Tallini G, et al: Malignant mesenchymoma. Cancer 1996;77:467-473

Carpentieri DF, Qualman SJ, Bowen J, et al: Protocol for the examination of specimens from pediatric and adult patients with osseous and extraosseus Ewing sarcoma family of tumors, including peripheral primitive neuroectodermal tumor and Ewing sarcoma. Arch Pathol Lab Med 2005;129:866-873

Casillas J, Sais GJ, Greve JL, et al: Imaging of intra- and extraabdominal desmoid tumors. Radiographics 1991;11:959-968

Cecchetto C, Carli M, Alaggio R, et al: Fibrosarcoma in pediatric patients: results of the Italian Cooperative Group Studies (1979-1995). J Surg Oncol 2001;78:225

Chui CH, Billups CA, Pappo AS, et al: Predictors of outcome in children and adolescents with rhabdomyosarcoma of the trunk—the St Jude Children's Research Hospital experience. J Pediatr Surg 2005;40:1691-1695

De la Luz Orozco-Covarrubias M, Tamayo-Sanchez L, Duran-McKinster C, et al: Malignant cutaneous tumors in children: twenty years of experience at a large pediatric hospital. J Am Acad Dermatol 1994;30:243

Donaldson SS, Anderson J: Factors that influence treatment decisions in childhood rhabdomyosarcoma. Intergroup Rhabdomyosarcoma Study Group of the Children's Cancer Group, the Pediatric Oncology Group, and the Intergroup Rhabdomyosarcoma Study Group Statistical Center. Radiology 1997;203:17-22

Eich GF, Hoeffel JC, Tschappeler H, et al: Fibrous tumours in children: imaging features of a heterogeneous group of disorders. Pediatr Radiol 1998;28:500-509

Fetsch JF, Meis JM: Synovial sarcoma of the abdominal wall. Cancer 1993;72:469-477

Folpe AL, Mentzel T, Lehr H-A, et al: Perivascualr epithelioid cell neoplasms of soft tissue and gynecologic origin. Am J Surg Pathol 2005;29:1558-1575

Galarza M, Sosa FP: Pure subcutaneous seeding from medulloblastoma. Pediatr Neurol 2003;29:245-249

Godambe SV, Rawal J: Blueberry muffin rash as a presentation of alveolar cell rhabdomyosarcoma in a neonate. Acta Paediatr 2000;89:115-117

Goldblum J, Fletcher JA: Desmoid-type fibromatosis. In Fletcher CDM, Unni KK, Mertens F (eds): World Health Organization Classification of Tumours: Pathology and Genetics of Tumours of Soft Tissue and Bone. Lyon, IARC Press, 2002:83-84

Gruson LM, Orlow SJ, Schaffer JV: Phacomatosis pigmentokeratotica associated with hemihypertrophy and a rhabdomyosarcoma of the abdominal wall. J Am Acad Dermatol 2006;55:S16-S20

Hansen T, Katenkamp K, Brodhum M, Katenkamp D: Low-grade fibrosarcoma: report on 39 not otherwise specified cases and comparison with defined low-grade fibrosarcoma types. Histopathology 2006;49:152

Healy JC, Reznek RH, Clark SK, et al: MR appearances of desmoid tumors in familial adenomatous polyposis. AJR Am J Roentgenol 1997;169:465-472

Israels SJ, Chan HSL, Daneman A, Weitzman SS: Synovial sarcoma in childhood. AJR Am J Roentgenol 1984;142:803-806

Johnson GL, McCarthy EF, Fishman EK: Clinical image: malignant mesenchymoma of the buttock. J Comput Assist Tomogr 1996;20:999-1001

Karadag O, Altundag K, Elkiran ET, et al: Anterior abdominal wall synovial sarcoma: a rare presentation. Am J Clin Oncol 2005; 28:323-324

Kaste SC, Hill A, Conley L, et al: Magnetic resonance imaging after incomplete resection of soft tissue sarcoma. Clin Orthop Relat Res 2002;397:204-211

Kew CCY, Putti TC, Razvi K: Malignant mesenchymoma arising from a uterine leiomyoma in the menopause. Gynecol Oncol 2004; 95:712-715

Khong PL, Chan GCF, Shek TWH, et al: Imaging of peripheral PNET: common and uncommon locations. Clin Radiol 2002;57:272-277

Kim NR, Kim HH, Suh Y-L: Cutaneous bronchogenic cyst of the abdominal wall. Pathol Int 2001;51:970-973

Klijanienko J, Caillaud JM, Lagace R: Fine-needle aspiration of primary and recurrent dermatofibrosarcoma protuberans. Diagn Cytopathol 2004;30:261

Knudsen AL, Bulow S: Desmoid tumour in familial adenomatous polyposis: a review of literature. Fam Cancer 2001;1:111-119

Kransdorf MJ: Malignant soft-tissue tumors in a large referral population: distribution of diagnoses by age, sex, and location. AJR Am J Roentgenol 1995;164:129-134

Kransdorf MJ, Jelinek JS, Moser RP Jr, et al: Soft-tissue masses: diagnosis using MR imaging. AJR Am J Roentgenol 1989; 153:541-547

Kudawara I, Araki N, Nakanishi H, et al: Malignant mesenchymoma of the lower leg. J Clin Pathol 2001;54:877-879

Kulaylat MN, Karakousis CP, Keaney CM, et al: Desmoid tumour: a pleomorphic lesion. Eur J Surg Oncol 1999;25:487-497

Lee JC, Thomas JM, Phillips S, et al: Aggressive fibromatosis: MRI features with pathologic correlation. AJR Am J Roentgenol 2006;186:247-254

Oguzkurt P, Kayaselcuk F, Arda IS, et al: Anterior abdominal wall malignant peripheral nerve sheath tumor in an infant. J Pediatr Surg 2001;36:1866-1868

Phillips SR, Hern RA, Thomas JM: Aggressive fibromatosis of the abdominal wall, limbs and limb girdles. Br J Surg 2004; 91:1624-1629

Reitamo JJ, Scheinin TM, Hayry P: The desmoid syndrome: new aspects in the cause, pathogenesis and treatment of the desmoid tumor. Am J Surg 1986;151:230-237

Robbin MR, Murphey MD, Temple HT, et al: Imaging of musculoskeletal fibromatosis. Radiographics 2001;21:585-600

Sato N, Sato N, Matoba N, Inoue T: Malignant mesenchymoma arising in an incisional scar of the abdominal wall. Eur J Surg Oncol 1998;24:449-450

Sheth S, Horton KM, Garland MR, Fishman EK: Mesenteric neoplasms: CT appearances of primary and secondary tumors and differential diagnosis. Radiographics 2003;23:457-473

Somers GR, Shago M, Zielenska M, et al: Primary subcutaneous primitive neuroectodermal tumor with aggressive behavior and an unusual karyotype: case report. Pediatr Dev Pathol 2004; 7:538-548

Stanford D, Rogers M: Dermatological presentations of infantile myofibromatosis: a review of 27 cases. Australas J Dermatol 2000;41:156-161

Sutton RJ, Thomas JM: Desmoid tumours of the anterior abdominal wall. Eur J Surg Oncol 1999;25:398-400

Suzuki N, Tsuchida Y, Takahashi A, et al: Prenatally diagnosed cystic lymphangioma in infants. J Pediatr Surg 1998;33:1599-1604

Taylor LJ: Musculoaponeurotic fibromatosis: a report of 28 cases and review of the literature. Clin Orthop Relat Res 1987;224:294-302

Teo HEL, Peh WCG, Shek TWH: Case 84: desmoid tumor of the abdominal wall. Radiology 2005;236:81-84

Titone C, Lipsius M, Krakauer JS: "Spontaneous" hematoma of the rectus abdominis muscle: critical review of 50 cases with emphasis on early diagnosis and treatment. Surgery 1972;72:568-572

Unger EC, Glazer HS, Lee JK, Ling D: MRI of extracranial hematomas: preliminary observations. AJR Am J Roentgenol 1986;146:403-407

Van Rijswijk CSP, Geirnaerdt MJA, Hogendoorn PCW, et al: Soft-tissue tumors: value of static and dynamic gadopentetate dimeglumine-enhanced MR imaging in prediction of malignancy. Radiology 2004;233:493-502

Votta TJ, Fantuzzo JJ, Boyd BC: Peripheral primitive neuroectodermal tumor associated with the anterior mandible: a case report and review of the literature. Oral Surg Oral Med Oral Pathol Oral Radiol Endod 2005;100:592-597

Wesche WA, Khare VK, Chesney TM, Jenkins JJ: Non-hematopoietic cutaneous metastases in children and adolescents: thirty years experience at St Jude Children's Research Hospital. J Cutan Pathol 2000;27:485-492

Windfuhr JP: Primitive neuroectodermal tumor of the head and neck: incidence, diagnosis, and management. Ann Otol Rhinol Laryngol 2004;113:533-543

Yu JS, Kim KW, Lee HJ, et al: Urachal remnant diseases: spectrum of CT and US findings. Radiographics 2001;21:451-461

Inflammatory Conditions

Bennett HF, Balfe DM: MR imaging of the peritoneum and abdominal wall. Magn Reson Imaging Clin N Am 1995;3:99-120

Cheon JE, Kim IO, Kim WS, et al: Abdominal-wall myositis secondary to intra-arterial chemotherapy for femoral osteosarcoma. Pediatr Radiol 1999;29:546-548

Crim JR, Seeger LL, Yao L, et al: Diagnosis of soft-tissue masses with MR imaging: can benign masses be differentiated from malignant ones? Radiology 1992;185:581-586

Irifune H, Kawaguchi S, Wada T, et al: Abdominal wall haematoma in an adolescent javelin thrower. Injury 2001;32:339-340

Shih WJ, Han JK, Brandenburge S, et al: Localization of a bone imaging agent in a calcified hematoma. J Nucl Med Technol 1999;27:45-47

CHAPTER 110

The Peritoneal Cavity

SUE C. KASTE

The peritoneal cavity is a potential space bounded by the largest serous membrane in the body and covered by a layer of epithelium. The surface area of the peritoneum is similar to that of the skin, estimated at about 2 m² in adults. *Parietal peritoneum* refers to the portion of the membrane that covers the abdominal wall, and *visceral peritoneum* refers to the portions covering the abdominal solid and hollow viscera. The peritoneal cavity contains the gastrointestinal viscera, the hepatobiliary structures, the spleen and pancreas, with the associated blood vessels, nerves, and supporting mesenteries. Specific disease entities of these structures are discussed in other chapters.

Situs solitus refers to the normal asymmetric position of the intra-abdominal organs, such that the liver lies in the right upper quadrant, and the spleen and stomach in the left upper quadrant. Abnormalities of abdominal situs, often defined in terms of asplenia and polysplenia, are discussed in Chapter 119.

IMAGING TECHNIQUES

Plain film evaluation of the peritoneum is limited in its resolution and sensitivity. Cross-sectional imaging has replaced complex plain film evaluation of the peritoneal cavity as performed by instillation of intraperitoneal air. However, plain films offer a clue to pathologic intraperitoneal processes. Displacement of intraperitoneal fat stripes may suggest a localized mass, inflammatory process, or hemorrhage. The identification of intraperitoneal and retroperitoneal air may indicate a perforated viscus or may be the result of dissection of intrathoracic air (Figs. 110-1 and 110-2), and these entities can be differentiated by the presence of air-fluid levels. Several of these conditions are discussed later in greater detail.

Ultrasound (US) evaluation is the most sensitive method of detecting even very small amounts of intraperitoneal free fluid. Abnormal peritoneal lining may be seen in cases of peritonitis or peritoneal metastases as focal areas of surface irregularity or larger, peritoneum-based masses, or they may be suggested by complex ascites containing debris or septations (Fig. 110-3).

Computed tomographic (CT) evaluation of the abdomen and pelvis provides detailed assessment of the peritoneum but is less sensitive than US for the detection of small physiologic amounts of ascites. Intravenous contrast administration enhances visualization of the peritoneal surface and associated masses (Figs. 110-4 and 110-5). Scans with multidetector capability allow reformats in multiple planes. A significant advantage of CT over US is the ability of CT to identify abdominal and pelvic disease located between bowel loops and within the retroperitoneum.

Magnetic resonance (MR) imaging is probably the most sensitive method for assessing the peritoneal surface itself because of its inherent soft tissue contrast and multiplanar capabilities. The peritoneal surface is normally isointense with muscles of the abdominal wall. Abnormally increased peritoneal permeability associated with carcinomatosis or peritonitis allows differentiation of the peritoneal surface from the abdominal wall. Thus, contrast enhancement and subtraction techniques, particularly when coupled with fat suppression, can further enhance assessment of the peritoneal surfaces (see Fig. 110-5). Sagittal imaging can be particularly helpful for examining the serosal surfaces of deep pelvic organs and can improve detection of small peritoneal metastases. Although the lack of ionizing radiation and the soft tissue contrast are significant advantages of MR compared with CT, differentiating between fluid collections and fluid within bowel may be difficult. Respiratory motion and bowel peristalsis may further compromise the MR, a problem that can be circumvented in many cases with fast scanning techniques, breath hold, and saturation bands.

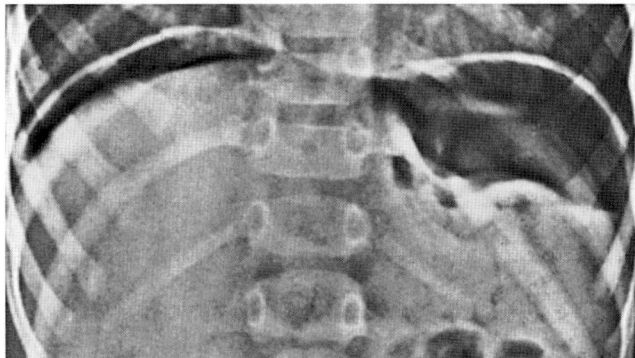

FIGURE 110-1. Free intraperitoneal air on an upright examination of the abdomen in a 2-year-old boy with perforated gastric ulcer. Air is easily shown between the diaphragm and the liver on the right side, and between the diaphragm and the spleen and stomach on the left.

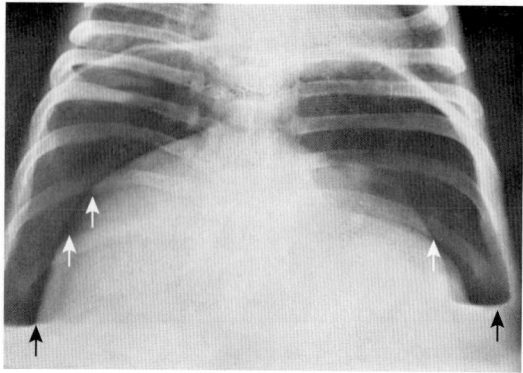

A

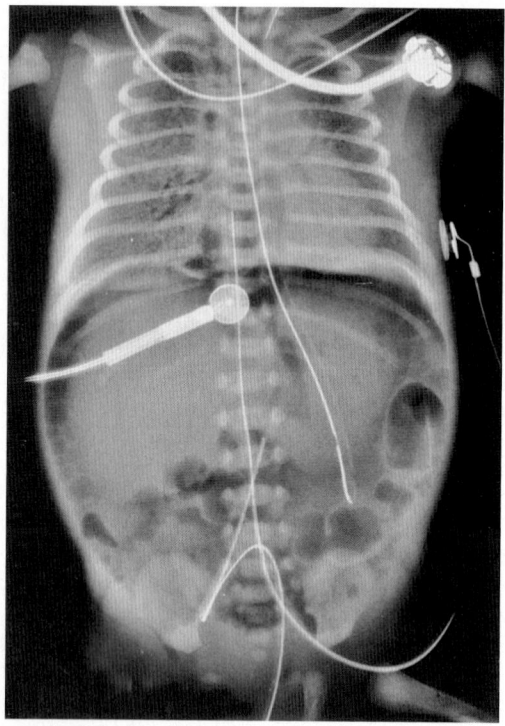

B

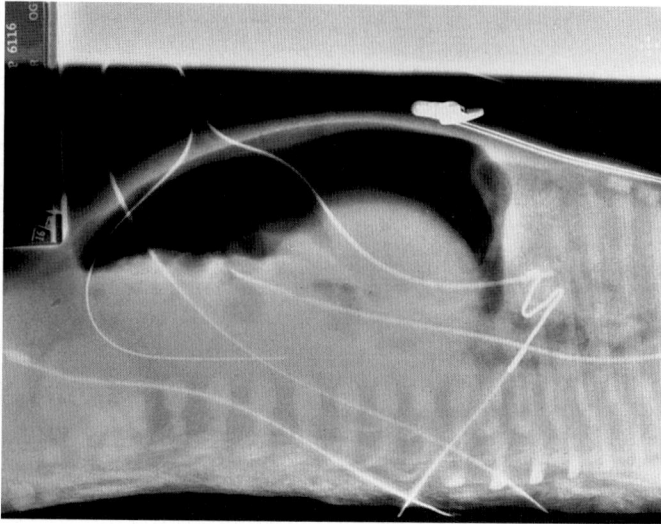

C

FIGURE 110-2. **A,** Massive amount of free air in the abdomen below the diaphragm *(white arrows)* with air-fluid levels *(black arrows)* on an upright radiograph in a patient with pyopneumoperitoneum. **B,** Digitally enhanced anteroposterior view of the chest and abdomen in a newborn with pulmonary interstitial emphysema, pneumomediastinum, and pneumoperitoneum. There is a large amount of gas in the peritoneal cavity with a positive Rigler sign (see text), as well as decreased density of the liver compared with the extraperitoneal soft tissues. The falciform ligament per se is not visualized because of the obscuring umbilical venous catheter. **C,** Digitally enhanced cross-table lateral view of the same patient shows large pneumoperitoneum without air-fluid levels, suggesting that the air could have dissected into the peritoneum from the chest.

PNEUMOPERITONEUM

Free intraperitoneal air is most commonly a consequence of the perforation of a hollow viscus. In the neonate, this occurs most frequently when there is intestinal obstruction, necrotizing enterocolitis, or gastric perforation. In children beyond the neonatal period, perforated peptic ulcers and inflammatory bowel disease may produce pneumoperitoneum. It is rarely found with appendiceal perforation. Trauma, both accidental and nonaccidental, may cause pneumoperitoneum (see Chapter 157). Free air in the chest can pass into the abdomen in various ways and cause pneumoperitoneum. Tension pneumomediastinum can dissect along the retroperitoneum and the subadventitial layer of the mesenteric vessels, rupturing freely into the peritoneal cavity. Its differentiation from perforated viscus can be difficult and will be discussed further.

Pneumoperitoneum may be suspected clinically because of a history of an underlying disease that predisposes to bowel perforation, by detection of acute abdominal distention with increased tympany on physical examination, or fortuitously on imaging examinations of the chest or abdomen. Benign postoperative pneumoperitoneum may be detected after abdominal surgery, although the free peritoneal air clears more rapidly in children than in adults. Several studies have demonstrated clearing of free air in 68% to 90% of postoperative children by 24 hours, but free air was seen as long as 6 to 7 days postoperatively in 2% to 3% of the cases reported by Wiot and coworkers.

The diagnosis of pneumoperitoneum is most easily made on horizontal-beam plain radiographs. Upright radiographs show air collecting between the diaphragm and the liver on the right and between the diaphragm and the liver, spleen, stomach, or colon on the left. The intra-abdominal viscera fall away from the diaphragm in the upright position, making visualization of the free peritoneal air relatively easy (see Figs. 110-1 and 110-2).

Young children and children too ill to sit or stand can be examined in the decubitus or supine position using

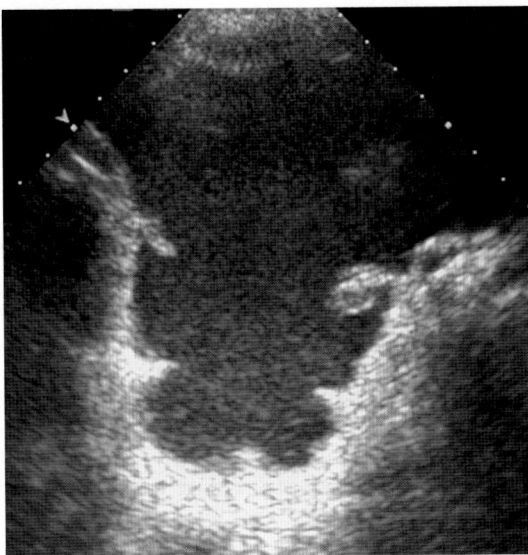

FIGURE 110-3. Complex ascites in 6-year-old patient with epithelioid sarcoma. Transverse ultrasound image through the deep pelvis shows abundant complex ascites. The thickening of the lateral peritoneal surface indicates peritoneal disease.

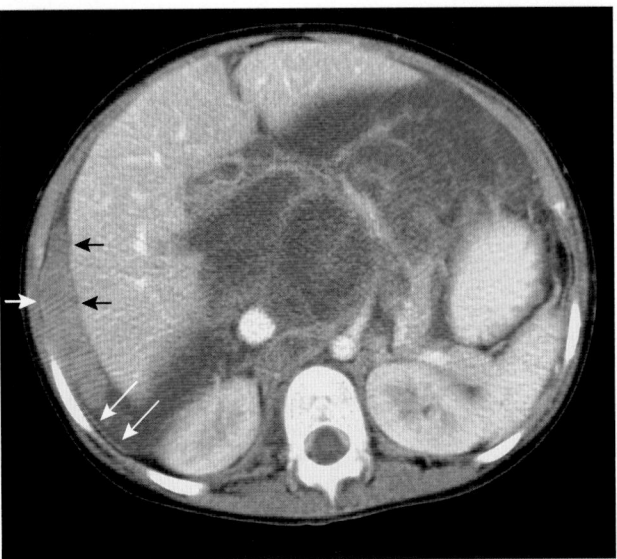

FIGURE 110-4. Transverse contrast-enhanced CT image through the midabdomen of the patient described in Figure 110-3 shows exaggerated enhancement of the peritoneal surface *(long arrows)* adjacent to the larger solid peritoneal metastasis *(short arrows)* of epithelioid sarcoma.

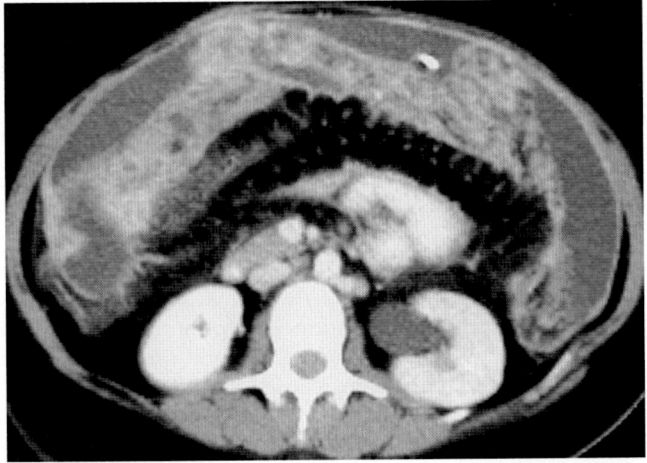

A

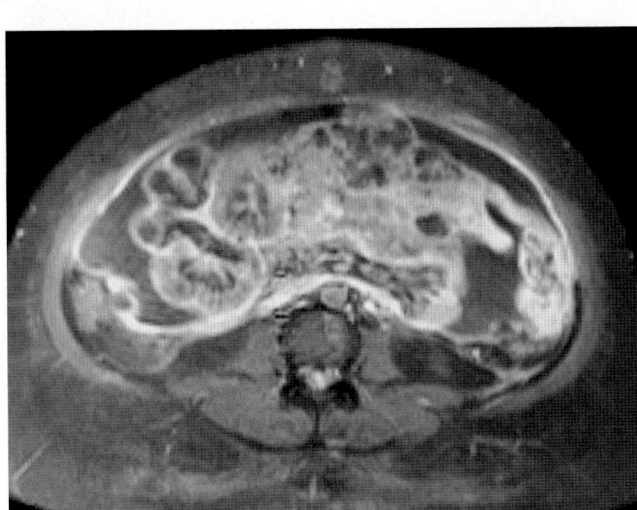

C

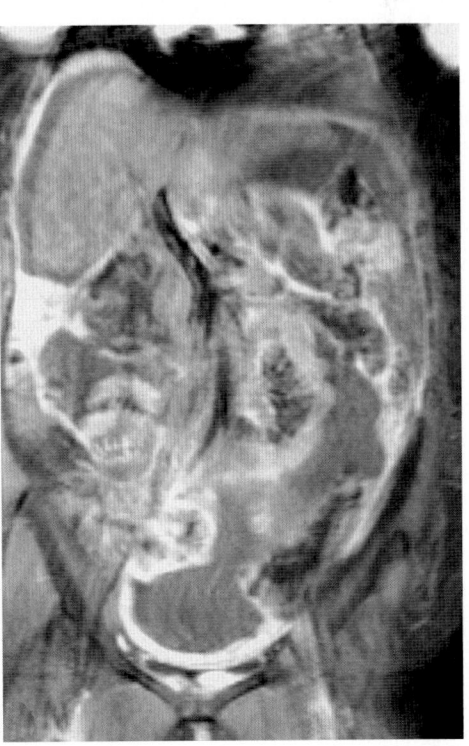

B

FIGURE 110-5. Peritoneal mesothelioma in an 18-year-old patient with a past history of posterior fossa medulloblastoma, presenting with new onset of hemorrhagic ascites. **A,** Contrast-enhanced CT image through the midabdomen shows abundant ascites and abnormal enhancement of the peritoneal surfaces. Note diffuse enhancing omental caking. Coronal **(B)** and axial **(C)** contrast-enhanced T1-weighted MR images of the abdomen and pelvis exquisitely show the thickened, intensely enhancing peritoneal surfaces and abundant ascites.

the horizontal-beam technique. The decubitus view should be obtained with the right side up, to allow the liver to fall away from the wall of the peritoneal cavity, permitting free peritoneal air to be seen between the liver and the abdominal wall. Identification of small amounts of free air is easier and more specific when viewed against the solid surface of the liver than against gas-filled bowel loops; such small amounts therefore may be difficult to distinguish from intraluminal air if the left-side-up decubitus view is obtained. On the horizontal-beam supine radiograph, free peritoneal air often collects between the anterior surface of the liver and the anterior abdominal wall (see Fig. 110-2). Small amounts of free air may be more difficult to define than by the right-side-up decubitus or upright views, particularly if located over loops of bowel. Seibert and Parvey described a "telltale triangle" sign of free peritoneal air; the three sides of the triangle of extraluminal air are created by the external surface walls of adjacent bowel loops and the anterior abdominal wall, as the air collects at the highest point in the peritoneal space.

Horizontal-beam images are also useful to differentiate pneumoperitoneum caused by a perforated viscus from that caused by downward dissecting air. The latter is usually suspected because of the history of assisted ventilation and the presence of pneumomediastinum, pulmonary interstitial emphysema, or pneumothorax. A ruptured viscus permits both air and fluid to escape into the peritoneal cavity, causing extraluminal air-fluid levels (see Fig. 110-2). Dissecting air causes only air in the peritoneal space, and thus a significant air-fluid level is not typically identified in the peritoneal space on horizontal-beam examination (see Fig. 110-2). However, the differentiation may remain difficult in patients with pre-existent ascites.

Pneumoperitoneum should be diagnosed on a supine radiograph because a single supine abdominal image may be the only study requested when free peritoneal air is not clinically suspected. A sufficiently large amount of free air can be seen as a large ovoid lucency overlying the abdominal contents (Fig. 110-6, and see Fig. 110-2). As the liver falls away from the anterior peritoneal surface in the supine position, free peritoneal air dissects along both sides of the falciform ligament. The ligament, which attaches the liver to the anterior abdominal wall, appears as a very thin opaque line running vertically just to the right of the spine when outlined by free peritoneal air (see Fig. 110-6). The distension of the flanks caused by the free intraperitoneal air, together with the outline of the falciform ligament centrally, has been termed the football sign because of its similarity to a rugby ball, with the falciform ligament representing the central thread in the ball.

Pneumoperitoneum leads to visualization of the outer edge of the bowel wall. This makes the bowel wall look like an arciform line rather than having its usual appearance of an arciform edge. The line is caused by the presence of air on both sides of the bowel wall and is known as the Rigler sign (see Fig. 110-2). A pseudo-Rigler sign is a potential pitfall in the supine film diagnosis of free peritoneal air, and it occurs when two loops of dilated air-filled bowel lie adjacent to one another. The line seen in the pseudo-Rigler sign is thicker than with free peritoneal air because it represents a double thickness of bowel wall (from the two adjacent bowel loops), whereas the line in patients with free peritoneal air (a true Rigler sign) represents a single bowel wall. However, this is not always a reliable differentiation, because the underlying disease causing perforation may lead to a thickened bowel wall. In equivocal cases, a horizontal-film radiograph should be obtained for clarification. The tell-tale triangle sign may also be seen on supine radiographs, wherever free air collects between adjacent loops of bowel.

The lucency caused by the free air rising to an anterior position in the abdomen is most easily appreciated where it projects over the liver. The normal liver is the same radiographic density as the abdominal wall musculature. The overlying air on a supine radiograph renders the liver (or a portion of the liver, depending on the amount of free air) more lucent than the adjacent muscles. When there is a smaller amount of free air, the portion of the liver beneath the free air will be more lucent than the remainder of the liver. Smaller amounts of free air may look like a rounded lucent bubble projecting over the midabdomen.

Small amounts of free air may appear only as localized collections in the right upper quadrant on supine radiographs. According to Levine and colleagues, linear collections represent air in the right subhepatic space, whereas triangular collections are seen with air in a Morison pouch (the hepatorenal fossa). The linear collection of air may represent air in the fissure of the ligamentum teres, as described by Cho and Baker. The collections are invariably medial within the right upper quadrant, and they are more likely to be seen in older children and adults than in infants, although Brill and coworkers described six newborns with necrotizing enterocolitis in whom air in a Morison pouch was the only compelling evidence of pneumoperitoneum. A less commonly encountered sign of pneumoperitoneum is the inverted-V sign, caused by air outlining the medial umbilical folds in the pelvis.

Although not typically performed for assessment of pneumoperitoneum, CT is an exquisite method to identify small amounts of intraperitoneal or extraperitoneal air, and intraperitoneal air-fluid levels. Detection of small amounts can be optimized by reviewing abdominal images using lung window parameters (Figs. 110-7 and 110-8).

Radiographic signs of pneumoperitoneum:
- "Football" sign on supine radiograph
- Rigler sign (visualization of external surface of bowel wall)
- "Telltale triangle" sign (air collecting between adjacent bowel loops)
- Linear collection in subhepatic space
- Triangular collection in Morison pouch
- Extraluminal air-fluid levels with ruptured viscus on horizontal-beam image

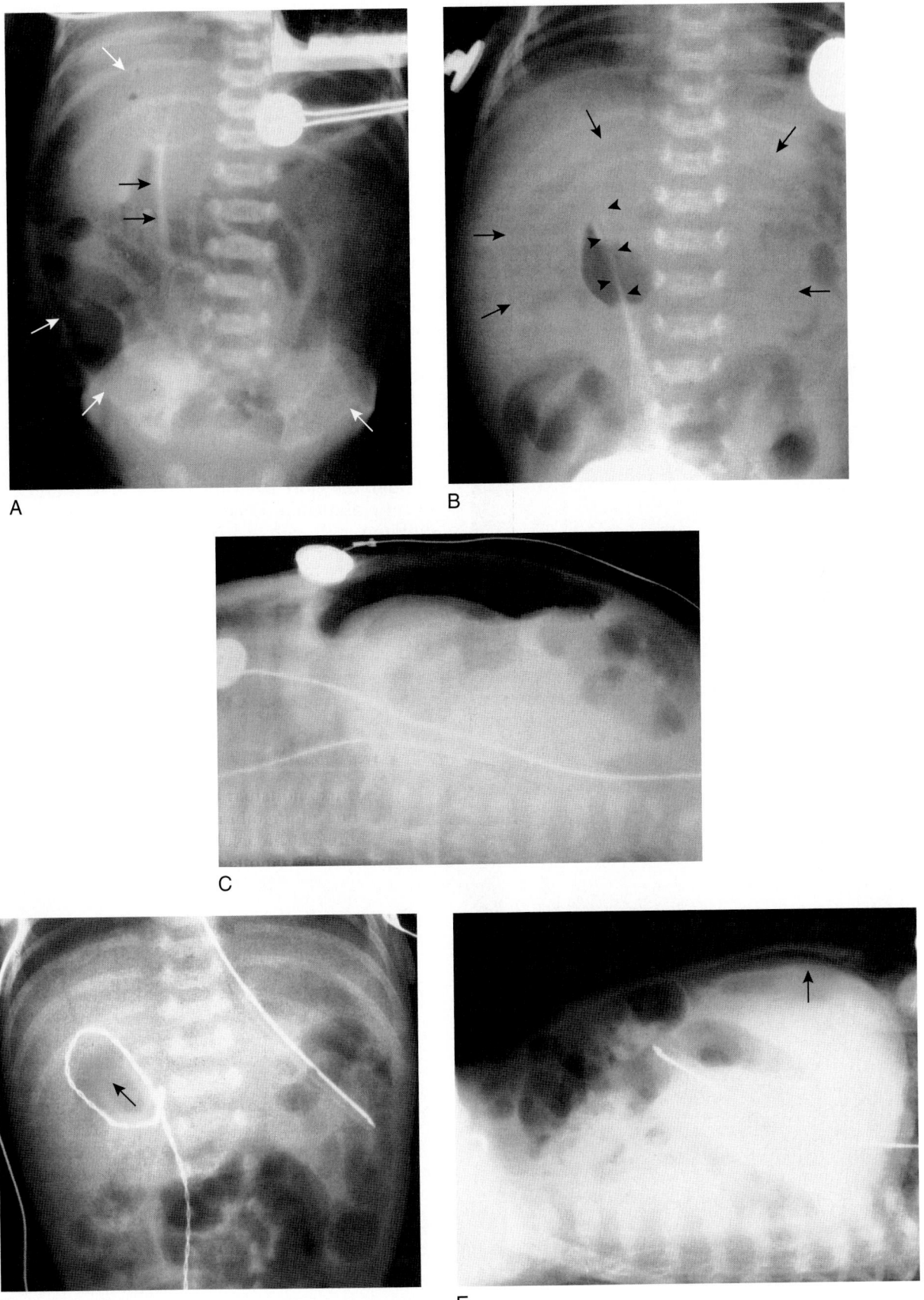

FIGURE 110-6. **A,** Supine view of the abdomen of an infant with a perforated viscus. The large oval lucency *(white arrows)* overlying the entire abdomen coupled with the dense line of the falciform ligament *(black arrows)* outlined by air on both sides represent the "football" sign. **B,** Supine view of the abdomen in another infant with free peritoneal air reveals a smaller oval lucency *(arrows)* and the falciform ligament surrounded by air *(arrowheads).* **C,** Cross-table lateral view in the infant seen in **B** confirms free peritoneal air below the anterior abdominal wall. **D,** Supine view of the abdomen in a third infant with free air resulting from necrotizing enterocolitis. A small collection of gas is noted in the Morison pouch (the hepatorenal recess) *(arrow).* **E,** Same patient as in **D** in the supine position using horizontal-beam technique. Air is demonstrated between the liver and anterior abdominal wall *(arrow).*

ASCITES

A small amount of fluid can normally be present in the peritoneal cavity and may be seen incidentally on cross-sectional imaging. Pathologic intraperitoneal fluid collections stem from a variety of causes and include blood, usually from trauma; urine, secondary to rupture of an obstructed collecting system or the bladder; pus in cases of peritonitis; bile from biliary tract rupture; and cerebrospinal fluid (CSF) in patients with ventriculo-peritoneal shunts for treatment of hydrocephalus. Transudative ascites is most commonly found in patients with hepatobiliary disease (especially cirrhosis), heart failure, hyponatremia, renal failure, peritonitis, and

Budd-Chiari syndrome. Peritoneal metastases are less common in children than adults but, when present, usually cause an exudative ascites. Exudative ascites may also be seen with certain intraperitoneal infections. Rupture of the gastrointestinal tract results in air as well as fluid escaping into the peritoneal cavity.

Fluid can be found in a variety of intraperitoneal locations and may change rapidly with changes in patient position. The greater peritoneal cavity, the lesser sac, a Morison pouch, the paracolic gutters, the pelvis, and recesses formed by many of the peritoneal ligaments are all sites where fluid can collect (see Fig. 110-3). Typically, small amounts of ascites collect in the pelvis when the patient is supine. As the amount of fluid increases, it moves cephalad along the paracolic gutters into the subhepatic spaces and the Morison pouch. It can sometimes be identified in the fossa of the ligamentum teres (Fig. 110-9). A sufficient volume of ascites eventually spreads through the peritoneal cavity, surrounding the outer wall of bowel loops, and extending into the mesenteric recesses (Fig. 110-10). The larger the amount of fluid, the more likely the fluid is to be found throughout the abdomen. Loculated ascites is less common in children, although encysted collections of CSF may be seen adjacent to the tip of a ventriculoperitoneal shunt tube ("CSF pseudocyst"), usually as a result of an inflammatory response around the shunt tube tip (Fig. 110-11).

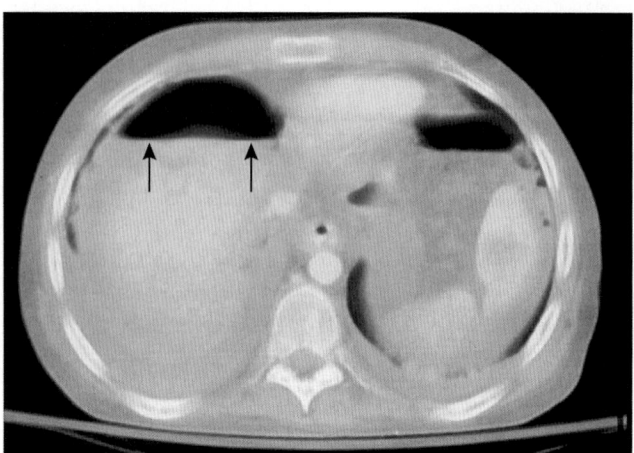

FIGURE 110-7. Axial abdominal CT images at lung window settings, showing hydropneumoperitoneum in a 19-year-old man with relapsed Hodgkin disease and severe abdominal pain. Note air-fluid levels *(arrows).*

Abdominal ascites:
- **Fluid can be found in a variety of intraperitoneal locations.**
- **Location may change rapidly with changes in patient position.**

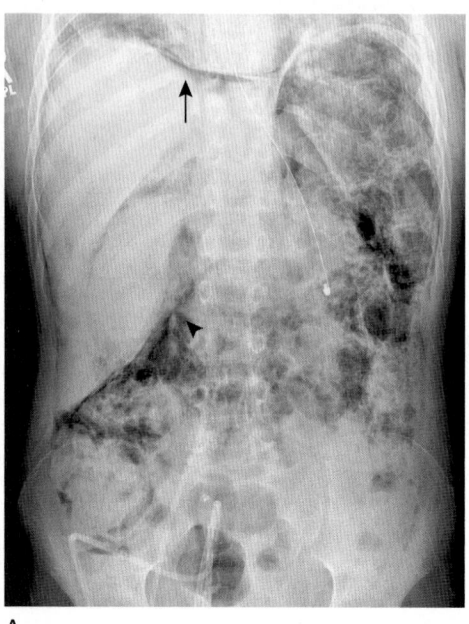

A

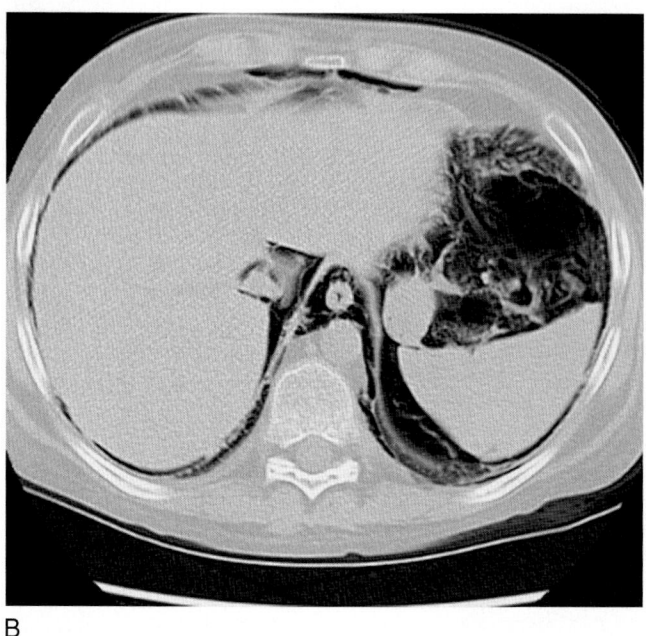

B

FIGURE 110-8. Pneumatosis intestinalis in a patient who underwent bone marrow transplantation for refractory recurrent neuroblastoma. **A,** CT scout image of the abdomen and pelvis shows abundant pneumatosis intestinalis that has resulted in pneumoperitoneum *(arrow)* and pneumoretroperitoneum *(arrowhead).* **B,** Axial CT image through the upper abdomen recorded with lung windows confirms the pneumoperitoneum, pneumoretroperitoneum and pneumomediastinum. Note absence of air-fluid levels.

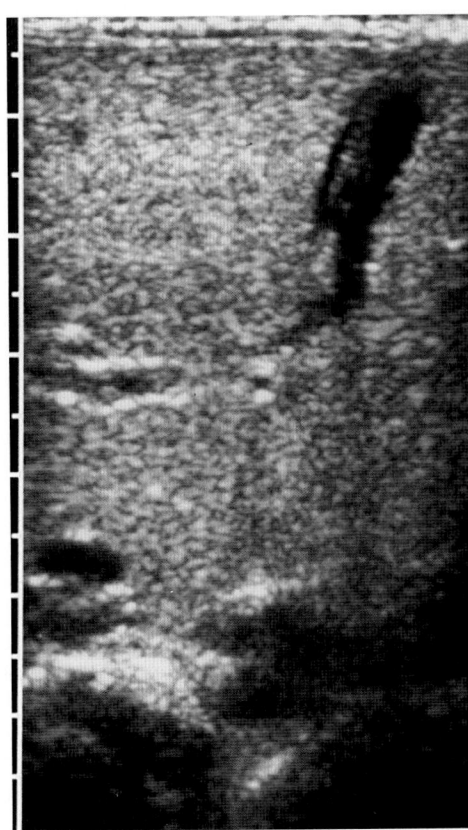

FIGURE 110-9. Oblique sonogram through the liver shows ascitic fluid in the fissure of the ligamentum teres. The ligament and the obliterated umbilical vein can be seen within the fluid collection.

- Larger amounts of fluid are more likely to be found throughout the abdomen.
- Exudative ascites is typically seen with infection and neoplastic disease.

Plain radiographs are sensitive only to large amounts of intraperitoneal fluid. In such cases, the gas-filled bowel loops appear to be centrally located, with widened paracolic gutters. Although fluid-filled distended colon

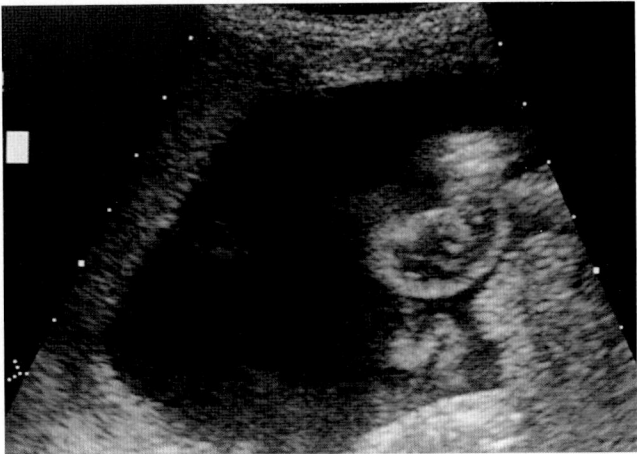

FIGURE 110-10. Transverse sonogram through the left lower quadrant shows a massive ascitic fluid collection outlining thick-walled loops of intestine in a patient with graft-versus-host disease after bone marrow transplantation.

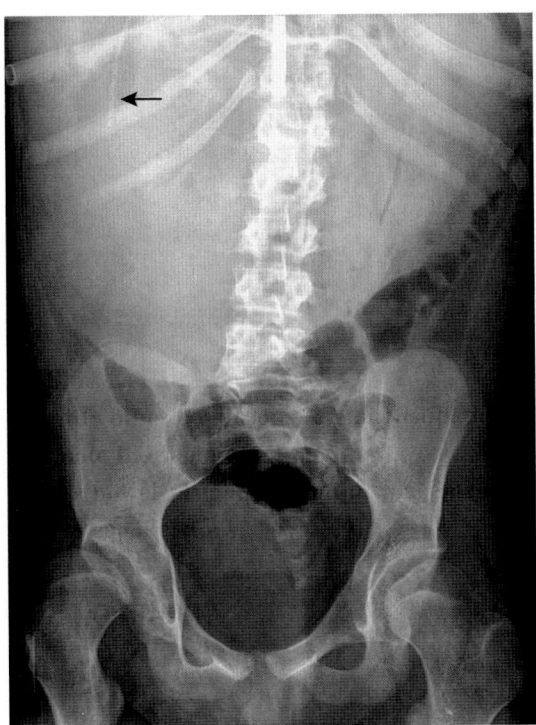

A

FIGURE 110-11. Cerebrospinal fluid pseudocyst. **A,** Abdominal radiograph shows a large soft tissue mass occupying the entire upper abdomen, especially the right abdomen. The tip of a ventriculoperitoneal shunt is seen in the right upper quadrant *(arrow)*. **B,** Transverse ultrasound image through the entire upper abdomen confirms a large cystic mass surrounding the tip of the shunt *(arrow)*.

could simulate this finding, a large amount of ascites shows a characteristic appearance on plain radiographs (Fig. 110-12). Separation of bowel loops may also occur as a result of ascites, but this can be simulated by large amounts of intraluminal fluid combined with relatively small amounts of intraluminal gas, or by thick-walled

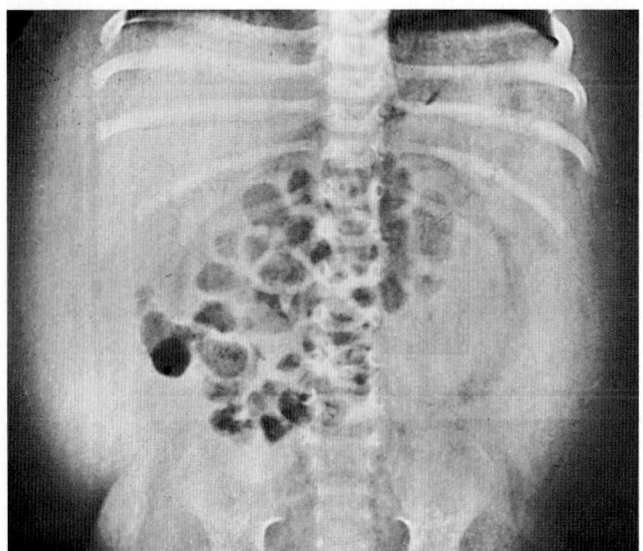

FIGURE 110-12. Anteroposterior views of the abdomen in a 16-month-old infant with severe nephrotic syndrome. Abdominal distention is noted, with numerous loops of gas-containing intestine floating in the center of the abdomen.

bowel loops (Fig. 110-13). In such equivocal cases, ultrasound can be done for confirmation.

Ultrasound is the most sensitive imaging modality for ascites, often allowing visualization of even physiologic amounts of intraperitoneal fluid. Abnormal free fluid can be seen in the various peritoneal recesses and in the pelvis and may cause apparent thickening of the gallbladder wall. Most transudates are anechoic collections. Complex fluid collections suggest blood, chyle, inflammatory cells, or peritoneal metastases (Fig. 110-14; see Fig. 110-3). Ascites occasionally pass through the esophageal hiatus or through patent pleuroperitoneal canals to present as intrathoracic fluid. CT is particularly useful in identifying the individual fluid-filled spaces, and it gives useful diagnostic information if the ascites is secondary to an intra-abdominal process. However, CT is not as sensitive as US to small volumes of fluid.

Abdominal compartment syndrome is an uncommon sequela of excessive ascites but may arise secondary to a collection of any material, such as blood, which leads to intra-abdominal hypertension. It is most commonly described after trauma but has also been noted in medical and surgical cases. More recently, it has been reported in a patient who presented with abdominal Burkitt lymphoma. The criteria for diagnosis of abdominal compartment syndrome vary but generally include elevation of intra-abdominal pressure to 20 mm Hg or greater, coupled with impaired respiratory or renal function. Radiographically, this syndrome can be diagnosed by a ratio of anteroposterior-to-transverse diameters of the abdomen exceeding 0.81 (Fig. 110-15).

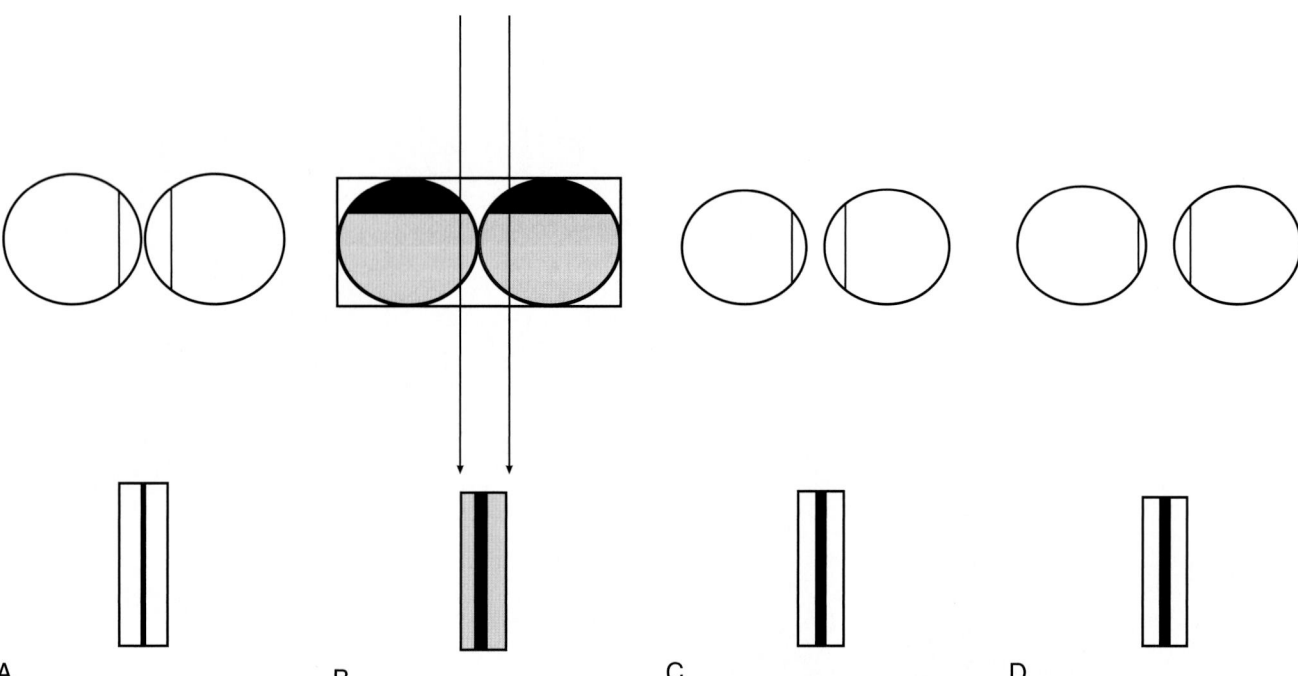

A   B   C   D

FIGURE 110-13. Pseudoseparation and true separation of bowel loops. The x-ray beam detects gas with intervening fluid density. *Dark gray,* air; *light gray,* fluid; thickness of the shadow cast on the film is represented by the thickness of the black line in the box below. **A,** Adjacent bowel loops filled with air cast a shadow of a normal, thin bowel wall. **B,** Adjacent loops filled largely with dependent fluid and a small amount of air cast a shadow equivalent to fluid-wall-wall-fluid, which appears as a thick line simulating separation of bowel loops, falsely suggesting the presence of ascites. **C,** Thick-walled bowel loops filled with gas cast a shadow of two thick adjacent walls, again falsely simulating ascites. **D,** If the gas-filled loops are separated by ascites, gas-filled bowel also casts a thick shadow, equivalent to two bowel walls and intervening ascitic fluid between the intraluminal air columns. Note that the thickness of the shadow cast is the same in **B, C,** and **D.**

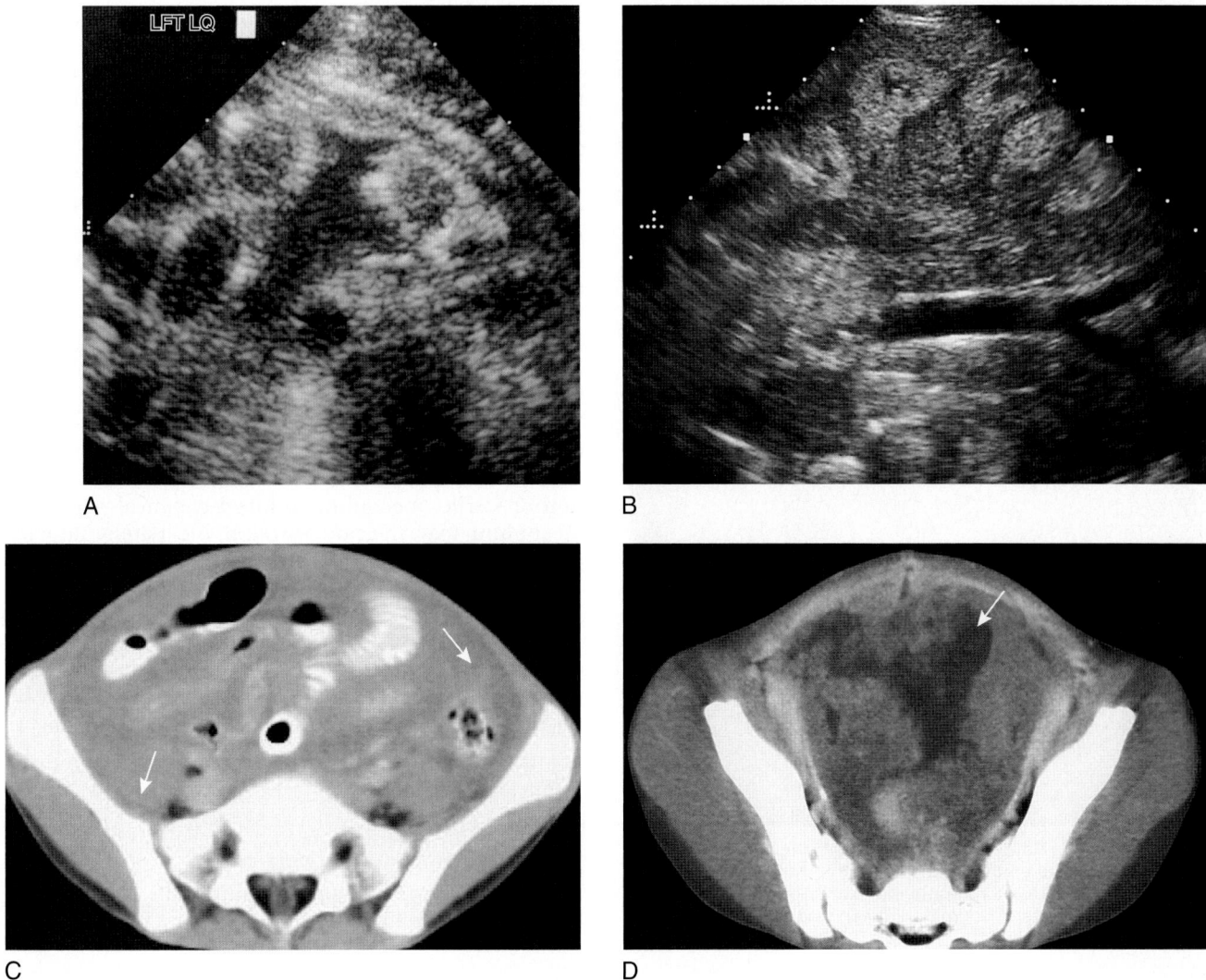

FIGURE 110-14. Peritoneal fluid. **A,** Transverse sonogram through the left lower quadrant of a 1-year-old boy with disseminated intravascular coagulation and thrombocytopenia after surgery for congenital heart disease. A fluid collection separates multiple loops of bowel. However, the fluid is not anechoic as in simple ascites but contains some internal echoes. Paracentesis revealed a hematocrit level within the ascitic fluid. **B,** Peritoneal mesothelioma in a 7-year-old boy who had been treated at age 3 years for non-Hodgkin lymphoma; treatment included whole abdominal radiation therapy. Coronal US image through the midabdomen shows echogenic material surrounding, separating, and displacing small bowel loops, which are also hyperechoic. **C,** Axial CT image through the same area shows ascites and peritoneal soft tissue densities and masses *(arrows)*. **D,** Axial CT through the pelvis shows intense peritoneal enhancement and numerous soft tissue masses *(arrow)*.

> *Abdominal compartment syndrome:*
> - **More commonly post-traumatic**
> - **Intra-abdominal pressure of ≥20 mm Hg**
> - **Impairment of respiratory or renal function**
> - **Abdominal anteroposterior-to-transverse diameter ratio of >0.81**

ACUTE GENERALIZED PERITONITIS

Peritonitis is a diffuse inflammatory process, usually of infectious etiology. The most common cause in children is ruptured appendix. Patients with inflammatory bowel disease also may develop peritonitis after rupture of the bowel. Chemical peritonitis can occur with bile leak and in patients with pancreatitis. Plain radiographs in patients with peritonitis often show a nonspecific adynamic ileus pattern with dilated bowel and multiple intraluminal air-fluid levels (Fig. 110-16). The signs of associated ascites may be seen, and the properitoneal fat plane may be obliterated.

Because of the ease of flow of fluid within the peritoneal cavity, abscesses may develop at sites distant from the perforation as well as in the immediate area. The subhepatic and subphrenic spaces are the most common distant sites for abscess formation. US identifies a focal collection of mixed echogenicity. CT shows a focal lesion, often with attenuation greater than that of clear fluid. The thickened walls of the abscess enhance after the intravenous injection of contrast material. CT and US are particularly useful as a guide for percutaneous drainage of abscesses (see Chapter 190). Peritoneal abscesses can be detected with MR imaging, but this modality is not typically employed for this purpose. Both gallium citrate–labeled and indium-labeled white blood cells have been used as scintigraphic agents in the diagnosis of abscesses.

ABDOMINAL WALL AND PERITONEAL CALCIFICATION

Abdominal wall calcification is uncommon in infants and children. Although some cases of fat necrosis are idio-

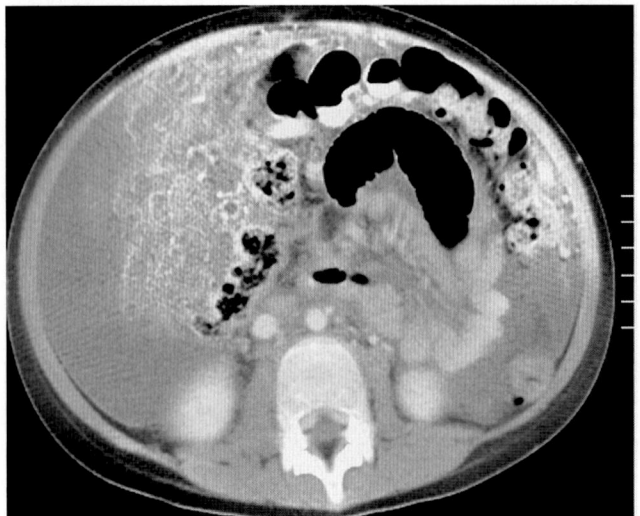

FIGURE 110-15. Abdominal compartment syndrome in 6-year-old with abdominal epithelioid sarcoma (the child described in Figures 110-3 and 110-4). The ratio of the anteroposterior to transverse diameters of the midabdomen was abnormally increased, at 0.84.

pathic, the majority are associated with neonatal sepsis. Older children with hypothermia, hepatic failure, and renal failure may also present with findings of subcutaneous fat necrosis. Abdominal wall calcification in infants has been described after subcutaneous emphysema and in prune-belly syndrome.

In children, abdominal wall calcification may be seen in fibrodysplasia ossificans progressiva and myositis ossificans, but these lesions are more common in the thoracic wall than in the abdominal wall, where they are usually located posteriorly in the paraspinal region. Calcifications secondary to dermatomyositis are more likely to be in the extremities than in the trunk, but they can be found in the abdominal wall. Subcutaneous hemangiomas may contain phleboliths.

The most common cause of *peritoneal calcification* in the neonate is meconium peritonitis (see Chapter 14). This occurs secondary to intrauterine intestinal perforation or sterile, meconium-induced chemical peritonitis. Meconium may migrate through the patent neonatal processus vaginalis and cause scrotal calcification.

Peritoneal calcification in older children is quite rare. Intestinal perforation with subsequent peritonitis may cause calcification. Tuberculous peritonitis may result in minimal to extensive calcification. Most causes of *intraabdominal calcification* are related to specific organs and are discussed in the appropriate chapters.

Etiology of calcification:
- **Abdominal wall**
  - **Subcutaneous fat necrosis**
  - **Fibrodysplasia and myositis ossificans (more common in thoracic wall)**

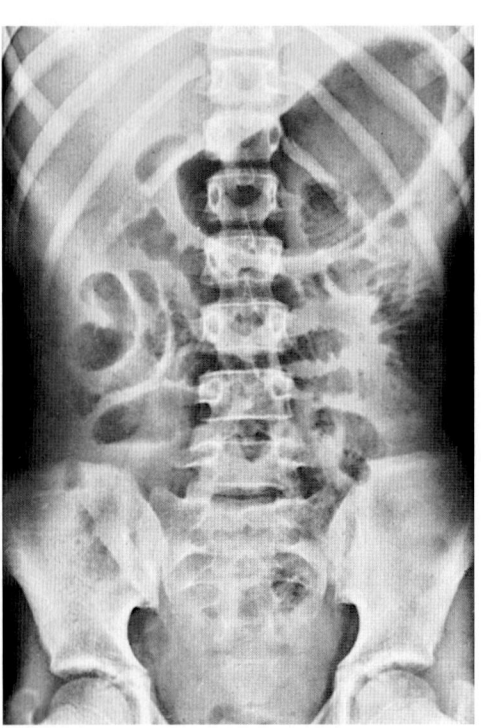

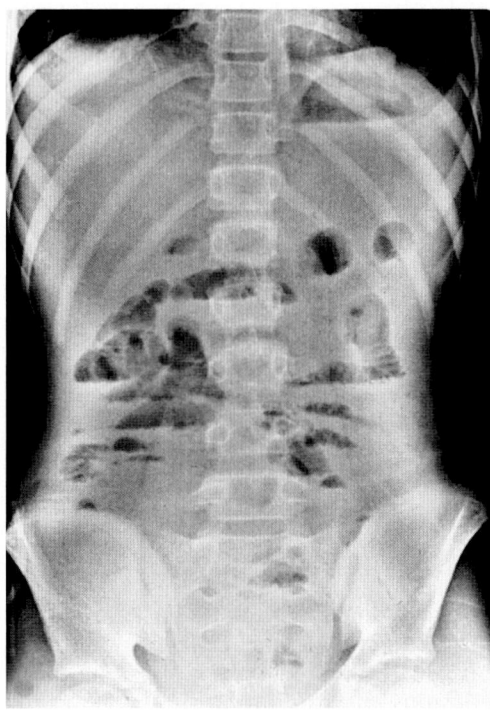

FIGURE 110-16. Purulent peritonitis. Supine **(A)** and upright **(B)** views of the abdomen in a teenage patient with purulent peritonitis. The gas-filled loops of small intestine are mildly dilated and separated from one another, and multiple scattered air-fluid levels can be seen throughout the intestine.

A   B

- Dermatomyositis (more common in extremities)
- Subcutaneous hemangiomas (phleboliths)
- Peritoneum
  - Meconium peritonitis
  - Intestinal perforation
  - Tuberculosis

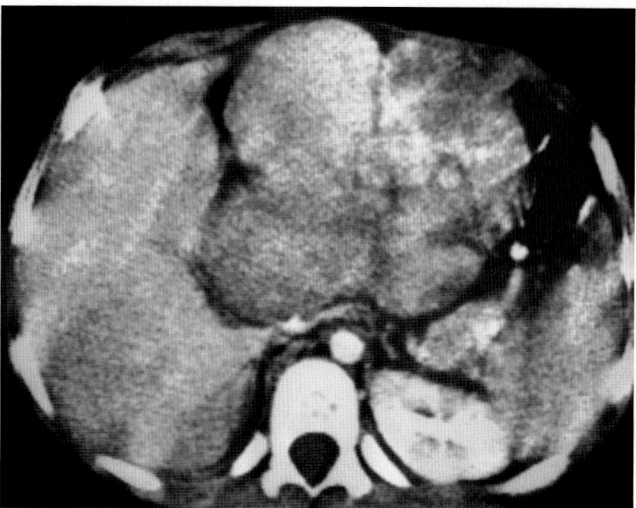

FIGURE 110-17. Benign fibrous mesothelioma in a 10-year-old boy with a large midepigastric mass found on routine physical examination. Axial contrast-enhanced CT image shows a large, multilobulated midepigastric soft tissue mass that shows very little enhancement. Image is somewhat degraded by patient motion. The mass was found at surgery to arise from the rectus sheath.

PERITONEAL TUMORS AND TUMOR-LIKE CONDITIONS

Benign Lesions

Cystic mesothelioma of the peritoneum (CMP) is a rare, benign, cystic peritoneal tumor that should not be confused with *malignant peritoneal mesothelioma* (discussed later). A single case in which the histologic features were interpreted as a low-grade malignancy has been reported by Moriwaki and colleagues. CMP arises from the mesothelium of the serosal surfaces of the peritoneal space, pericardium, and pleura. In contrast to malignant peritoneal mesothelioma, there has been no reported association between CMP and radiation or asbestos exposure. CMP occurs more often in girls and most commonly arises in the pelvis; it does not metastasize but recurs locally.

On imaging, CMP is seen as a well-defined, thin-walled, unilocular or multilocular cystic mass. A solid projection extends into the central portion of the cyst. The cystic components have increased intensity on T2-weighted and proton density–weighted MR sequences, and low intensity on T1-weighted sequences. The solid projection is of decreased signal on T2-weighted and proton density–weighted sequences, has mildly decreased signal on T1-weighted images, and enhances well with contrast administration. However, radiographically, this lesion can be indistinguishable from lymphangiomas or other cysts.

Benign fibrous mesothelioma is typically a tumor arising from the pleura, although it can rarely arise within the peritoneum (Fig. 110-17).

Benign mesenchymal tumors of the abdomen and pelvis arise from the subperitoneal space along its intraperitoneal interface. They include tumors of the lymphatics (Fig. 110-18), vascular system, adipose tissues (Fig. 110-19), and neuromuscular system. The mesenchymal subperitoneal space allows widespread tumor extension along multiple peritoneal compartments. Those tumors likely to be seen in children are described below.

Lymphangiomas are benign developmental abnormalities or benign tumors of the lymphatic system; mesenteric and omental lymphangiomas are termed mesenteric and omental cysts, respectively. Most lymphangiomas (95%) occur in the head and neck. Lymphangiomas from the mesentery and abdominal wall are relatively rare, and omental origin is less common than mesenteric. When evaluated with US, lymphangiomas are typically seen as single or multiple cysts; septations may or may not be present. In the presence of hemorrhage or infection, these lesions may mimic a solid mass by US, although Doppler interrogation reveals no internal flow within the echogenic but cystic component. By CT, lymphangiomas appear as cysts, with the cyst walls often being imperceptible. Attenuation coefficients of the cyst contents may be less than water because of their chylous nature. In the abdomen, such lesions appear to be poorly marginated. By MR, lymphangiomas are typically of decreased signal on T1-weighted and increased signal on T2-weighted sequences. The presence of complexity, such as hemorrhage, within the cyst may be manifested as increased signal intensity on both T1-weighted and T2-weighted sequences. Fibrous septa are seen as focal linear inhomogeneities that may enhance. MR may aid in distinguishing large lymphangiomatous masses that have hemorrhaged from complex intraperitoneal fluid.

Hemangiomas may involve the mesentery and are often identified incidentally. Mesenteric cavernous hemangiomas consist of large, blood-filled spaces lined by endothelium, with interspersed vascular structures. Internal calcifications consisting of phleboliths may be seen on ultrasound or precontrast CT imaging. Doppler interrogation and postcontrast images often demonstrate vascular structures coursing through the lesions. Stover and colleagues suggest that hemangiomas can be differentiated from lymphangiomas by MR using RARE (rapid acquisition with relaxation enhancement) MR sequences; like lymphangiomas, hemangiomas are hyperintense on T2-weighted sequences, but hemangiomas lack signal on RARE sequences.

Lipoblastoma (see Fig. 110-19) is a rare benign mesenchymal tumor seen exclusively in infants and young children. It arises from embryonal white fat and was recently reported to contain the 8q11-13 clonal chromosomal rearrangement affecting *PLAG1*. Lipoblastoma occurs with a 3:1 male-to-female predominance. Approx-

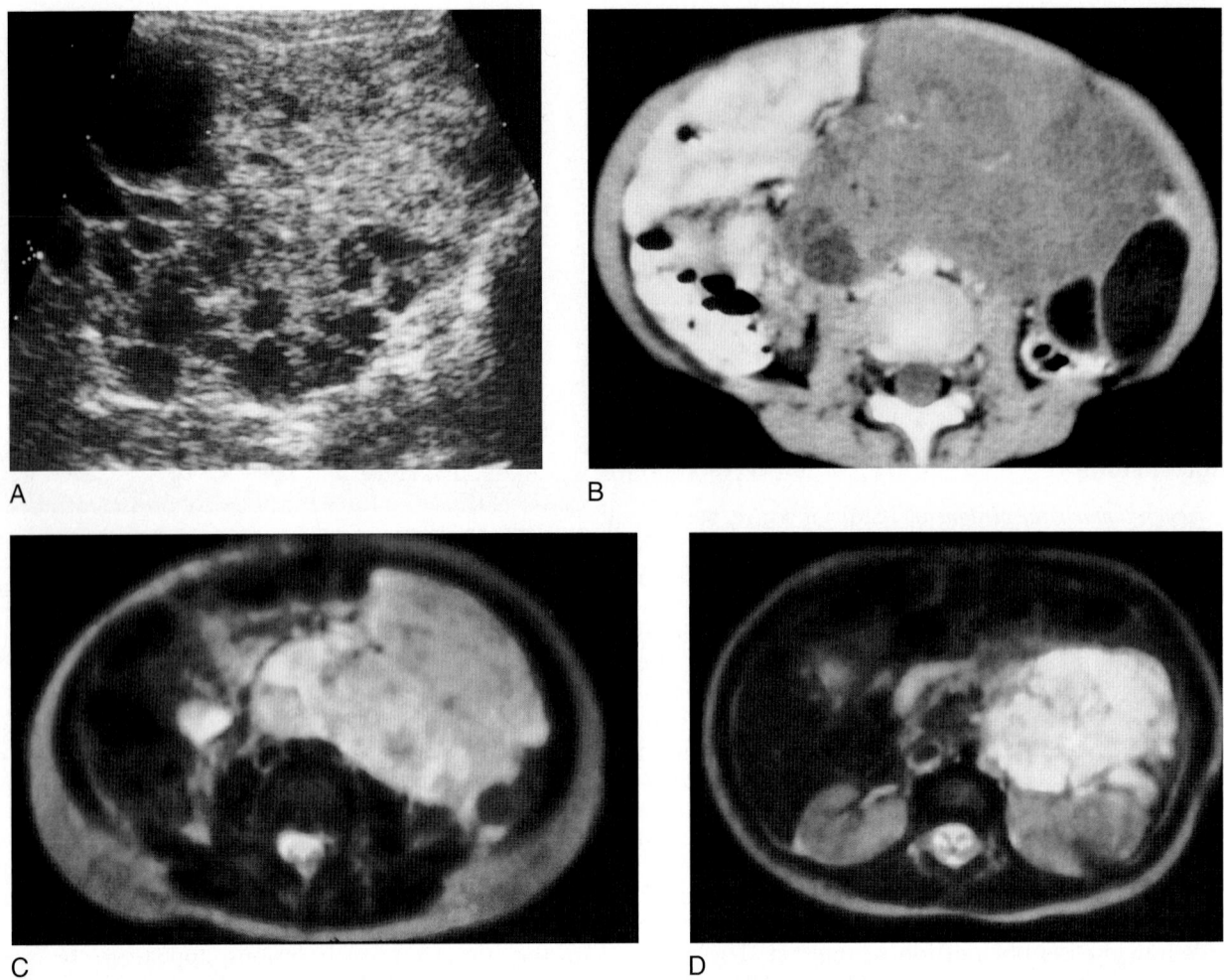

FIGURE 110-18. Lymphangioma arising from the mesentery in an asymptomatic 2-year-old girl. Ultrasound **(A)** and contrast-enhanced CT **(B)** images show a very large heterogeneous solid and cystic mass of indeterminate origin. **C** and **D**, Axial T2-weighted MR images with fat saturation confirm the extent and heterogeneity of the mass.

imately 50% are diagnosed at less than 1 year of age and almost 90% are diagnosed before the age of 3 years. Clinical manifestations depend on the size and location of the mass and its effect on adjacent structures. Lipoblastomas frequently manifest as rapidly growing, painless masses.

Lipoblastoma is different from lipoblastomatosis, but both entities are benign with no malignant potential. Lipoblastoma is a discrete mass and lipoblastomatosis is a diffuse infiltrating process without a defined capsule. Treatment of both lesions has historically been complete surgical resection, but both tumors may locally recur—which occurs in up to 20% of cases. Contemporary management suggests that mutilating surgery is not justified to achieve complete resection. Spontaneous regression and maturation into lipoma have both been described.

Imaging features of lipoblastoma reflect the underlying pathology: they are composed primarily but often not completely of fat. Radiographically, the mass is radiolucent, reflecting internal fat content. On US, these masses are echogenic. On CT, a lipoblastoma appears as a large, hypodense, well-circumscribed mass, often with internal septations. MR images show the mass signal

tracking that of subcutaneous fat on both fat-saturated and non–fat-saturated pulse sequences (see Fig. 110-19).

Nerve sheath tumors are typically seen in the setting of neurofibromatosis type 1, and are discussed in greater detail in Chapters 160 and 166.

Pseudomyxoma peritonei is a rare entity in which the omental and peritoneal surfaces are caked with a benign gelatinous material; this entity should be considered separate from peritoneal metastases from a primary malignancy that does not itself arise from the peritoneum. Confusion may arise between this discrete entity and the same term used to describe peritoneal metastases associated with mucinous ovarian or appendiceal tumors. Pseudomyxoma peritonei is typically low in density by CT and most frequently occurs in the right lower quadrant of the abdomen.

Malignant Lesions

Desmoplastic small round cell tumor (DSRCT) is a very rare, highly malignant tumor characterized by nests of small round cells that are surrounded by fibrous tissue. It occurs in the serosal surfaces of body cavities, much more commonly in the abdomen and retroperitoneum.

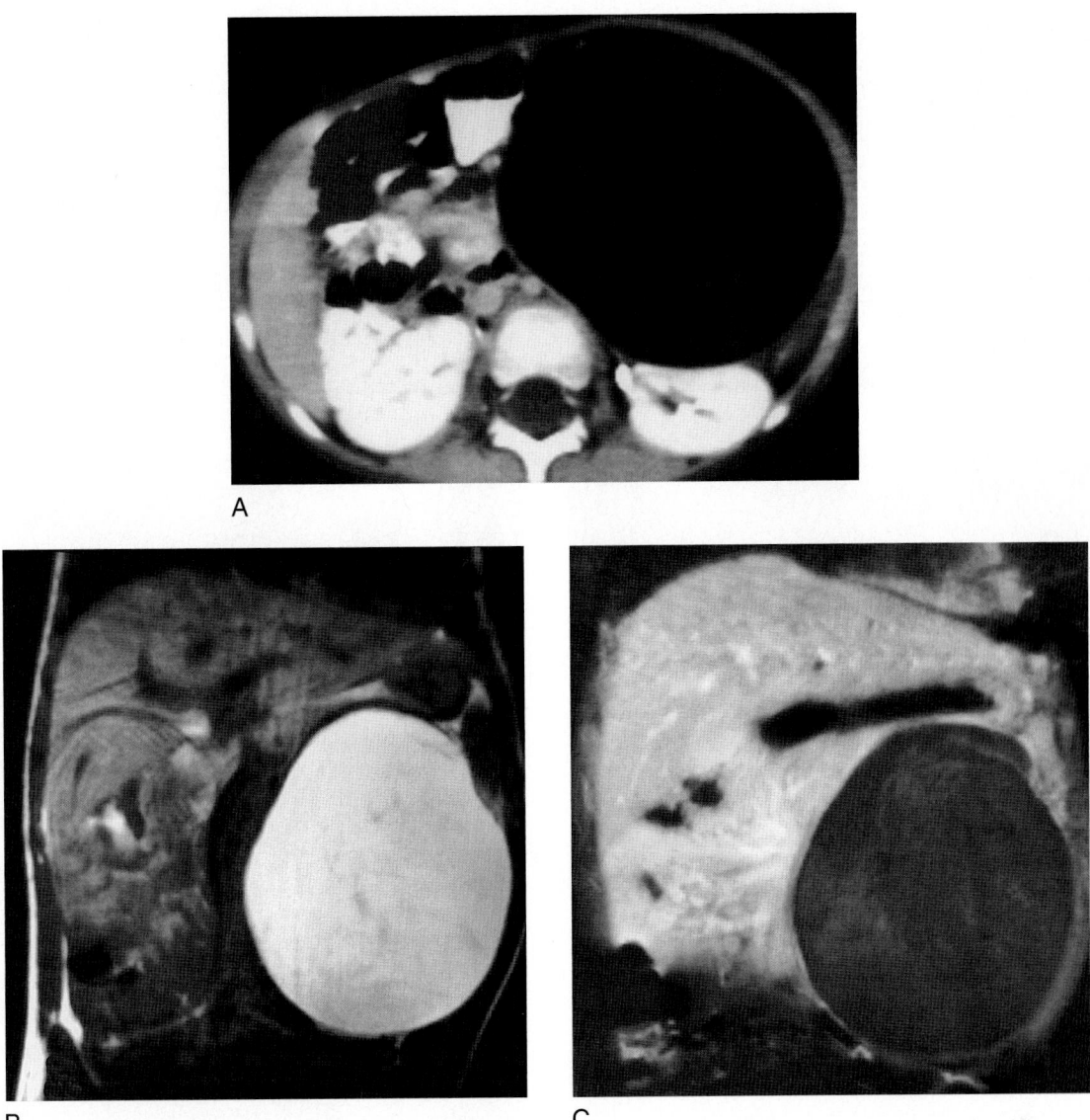

FIGURE 110-19. Encapsulated left upper quadrant lipoblastoma attached to the pancreatic tail of a 2-year-old girl. **A,** Axial contrast-enhanced CT image through the midabdomen shows a large fatty mass. Coronal noncontrast T1-weighted sequence without **(B)** and with **(C)** fat saturation depicts the fatty nature of the entire mass, as well as some internal septations seen in **B.**

Survival is poor, with approximately 30% 3-year and 18% 5-year survival rates. About 96% of cases are in males, typically seen in adolescent and young adults. Gerald and associates reported fusion between the *WT1* Wilms tumor gene and *EWS* Ewing sarcoma gene t(11;22)(p13;q12), which they consider a consistent "genetic event of primary importance in development of DSRCT."

If examined early in the course of disease, a dominant mass, usually located deep in the pelvis, may be identified. With disease progression, imaging often shows multiple solid masses studding surfaces of intra-abdominal organs (Figs. 110-20 and 110-21), a process that may be diffuse and not readily localized to a primary site. Chouli and colleagues describe 73% of masses to be bulky and heterogeneous in appearance. Local regional adenopathy has been reported by the same group in about 50% of cases.

Pickardt and coworkers found these tumors to be well-defined but hypoechoic by US. Some masses were heterogeneous as a result of hemorrhage and necrosis. About one third of cases were associated with ascites and less commonly with lymphadenopathy, hepatic metastases, hydronephrosis, punctate calcifications, bowel obstruction, or nodular peritoneal thickening. Ascites has been reported in about half of patients in other series.

By MR (see Figs. 110-20 and 110-21), DSRCTs show heterogeneous intermediate signal on T1-weighted sequences, increased signal on T2-weighted sequences, and enhancement with contrast administration. In some cases, diffuse peritoneal carcinomatosis without discrete masses is demonstrated. Distant metastases in the lungs, liver, bone, and brain may also be identified.

Malignant peritoneal mesothelioma has an overall poor prognosis, and it is very rare in children and adolescents. Peritoneal mesothelioma is more common in girls, and pleural mesothelioma in boys. Pediatric cases and abdominal tumors are not necessarily associated with asbestos or radiation exposure. As examined with MR,

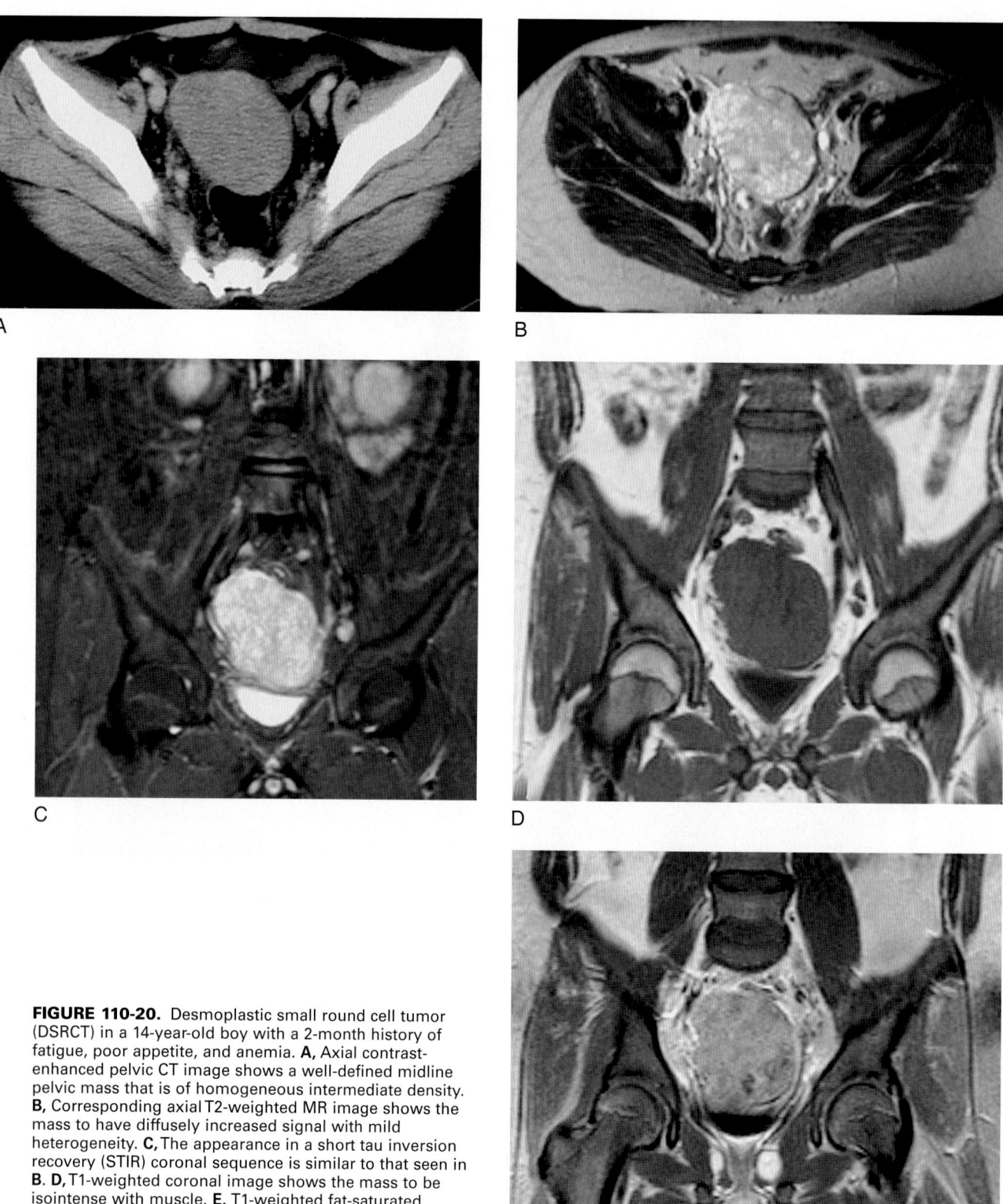

FIGURE 110-20. Desmoplastic small round cell tumor (DSRCT) in a 14-year-old boy with a 2-month history of fatigue, poor appetite, and anemia. **A,** Axial contrast-enhanced pelvic CT image shows a well-defined midline pelvic mass that is of homogeneous intermediate density. **B,** Corresponding axial T2-weighted MR image shows the mass to have diffusely increased signal with mild heterogeneity. **C,** The appearance in a short tau inversion recovery (STIR) coronal sequence is similar to that seen in **B. D,** T1-weighted coronal image shows the mass to be isointense with muscle. **E,** T1-weighted fat-saturated coronal image with contrast shows mild heterogeneous enhancement of the lesion.

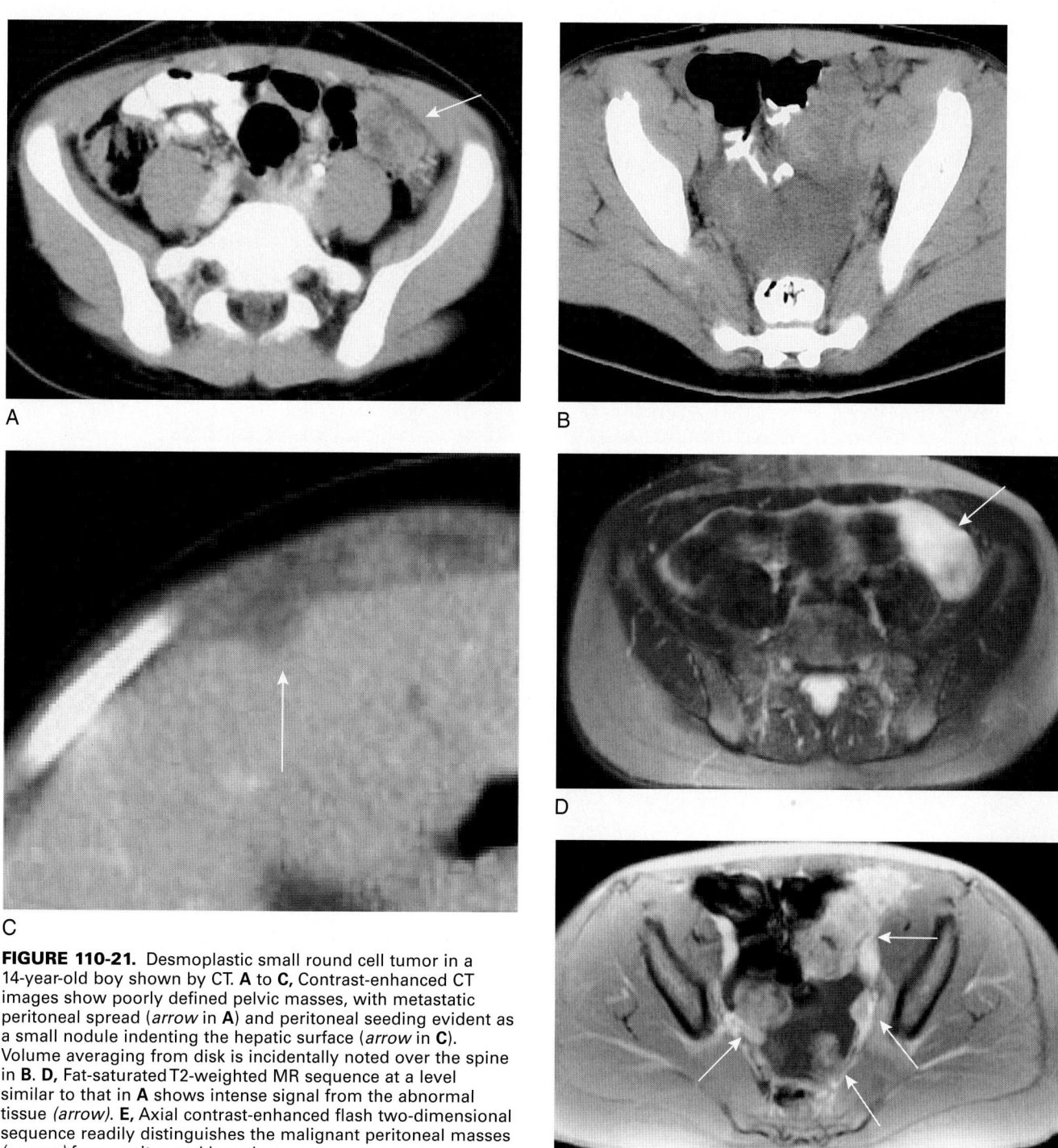

FIGURE 110-21. Desmoplastic small round cell tumor in a 14-year-old boy shown by CT. **A** to **C,** Contrast-enhanced CT images show poorly defined pelvic masses, with metastatic peritoneal spread (*arrow* in **A**) and peritoneal seeding evident as a small nodule indenting the hepatic surface (*arrow* in **C**). Volume averaging from disk is incidentally noted over the spine in **B. D,** Fat-saturated T2-weighted MR sequence at a level similar to that in **A** shows intense signal from the abnormal tissue *(arrow).* **E,** Axial contrast-enhanced flash two-dimensional sequence readily distinguishes the malignant peritoneal masses *(arrows)* from ascites and bowel.

CT, or US, malignant peritoneal mesothelioma has been described as peritoneal thickening, ascites, omental masses, peritoneal nodules, and mesenteric involvement (see Figs. 110-5 and 110-14). In two reported cases, teenage girls presented with malignant mesothelioma as ovarian masses. One additional case has been described involving an intermittent history of abdominal pain for several weeks, with acute exacerbation mimicking an acute abdomen. Calcifications in peritoneal mesothelioma are uncommon, in contrast to the calcified plaques seen in pleural mesothelioma. By MR with contrast enhance-

ment and spin echo fat-saturated T1-weighted sequences, diffuse peritoneal enhancement associated with ascites, peritoneal nodules, and omental masses has been described in patients with this disease.

Malignant abdominal mesothelioma is not typically associated with asbestos exposure as is seen in intrathoracic mesothelioma.

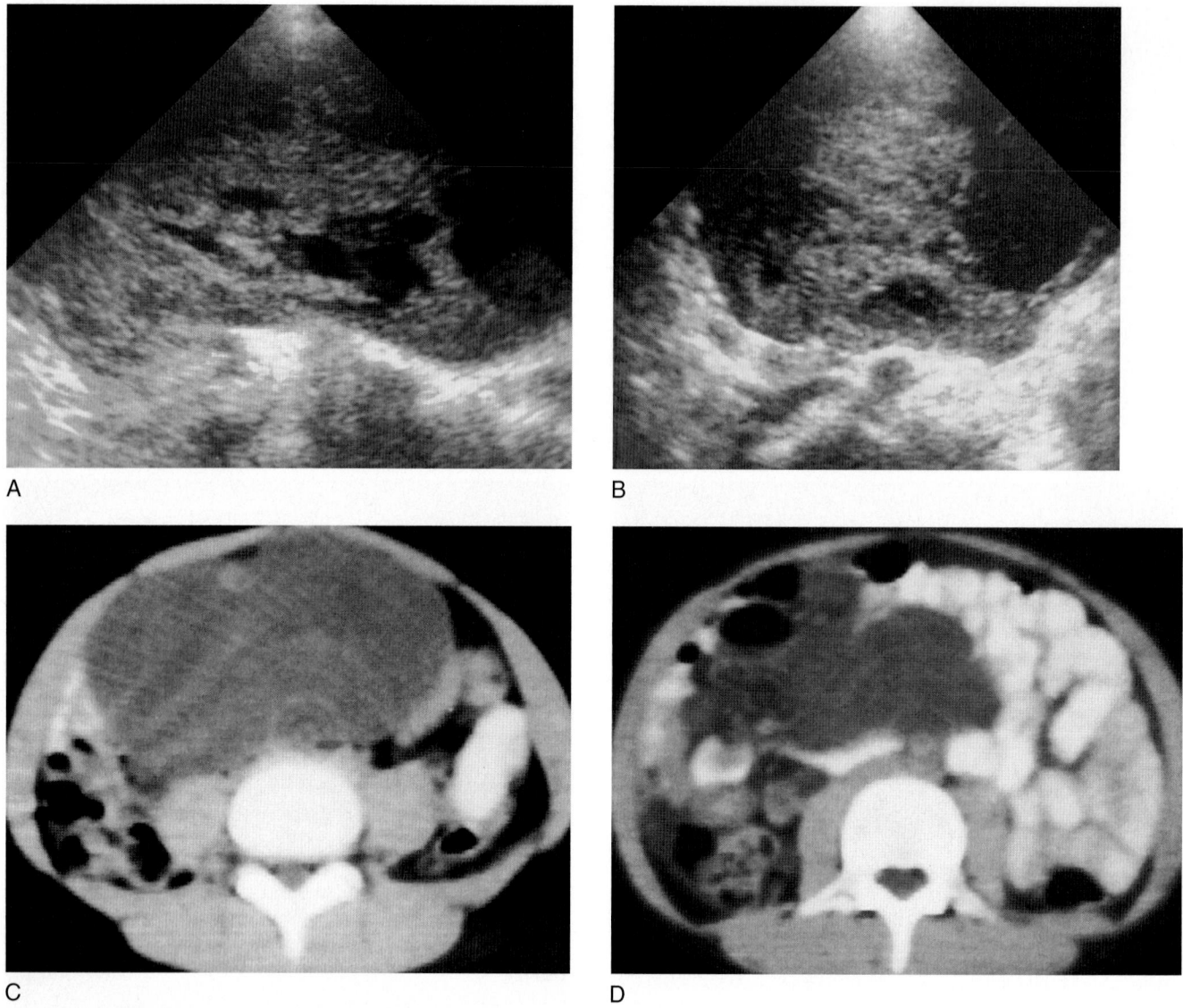

FIGURE 110-22. Leiomyosarcoma in a 10-year-old boy. Longitudinal **(A)** and transverse **(B)** ultrasound images through the midabdomen show a large heterogeneous solid and cystic mass, very similar in ultrasound appearance to the complex lymphangioma seen in Figure 110-18A. **C** and **D,** Axial CT images without intravenous contrast show a large homogeneous low-density midline soft tissue mass displacing bowel.

Malignant mesenchymal tumors of the peritoneum and subperitoneal space are extremely rare, particularly in children. These tumors include primary sarcomas such as leiomyosarcoma (Figs. 110-22 and 110-23), liposarcoma, and malignant fibrous histiocytoma. With the exception of liposarcoma, these tumors generally have few features that allow them to be distinguished from one another by imaging, and they typically appear as large single solid masses.

Leiomyosarcoma of the peritoneum (see Figs. 110-22 and 110-23) may be considered an adult disease, as it very rarely occurs in pediatric patients. These tumors occur in smooth muscle, often originating in the retroperitoneum, genitourinary tract, or gastrointestinal tract. In a large series of soft tissue tumors archived at the Armed Forces Institute of Pathology, Kransdorf found the retroperitoneum to be the most common primary site of leiomyosarcoma, followed by the lower extremity.

Rarely, such a lesion may arise in the omentum. The age range of Kransdorf's reported cases was 35 to 79 years. Lane and colleagues reported a mild female (6:4) predominance of this tumor. Leiomyosarcomas metastasize hematogenously to liver, lung, and peritoneum. Lymphatic metastases are less common. Metastases to soft tissues and spleen may occur; bone metastases are osteolytic. Intraperitoneal spread of disease may occur by direct spread along mesenteric reflections, by ascitic seeding of the peritoneum, or hematogenously. Peritoneal leiomyosarcomatosis may result and appears as multiple discrete nodules or masses, as massive lesions and as infiltration of the omentum.

The degree of vascularity varies with the primary site of abdominal disease. Leiomyosarcomas originating in small bowel are typically well-circumscribed hypervascular masses associated with large feeding arteries and draining veins. Those originating in the colon and

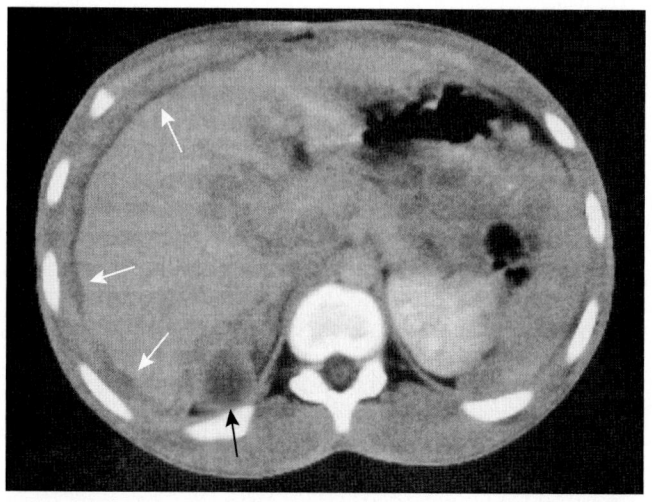

A

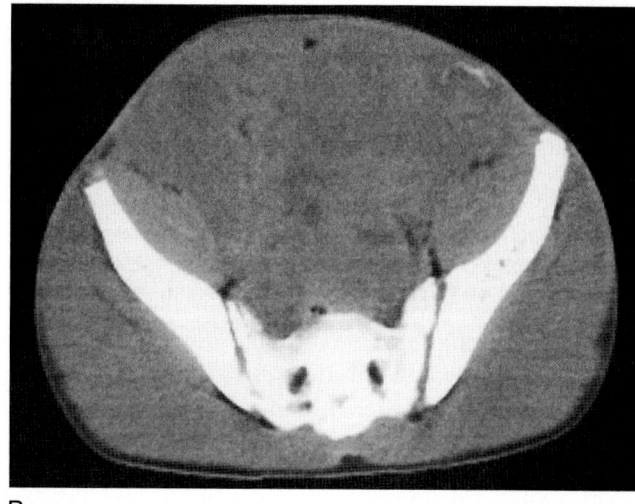

B

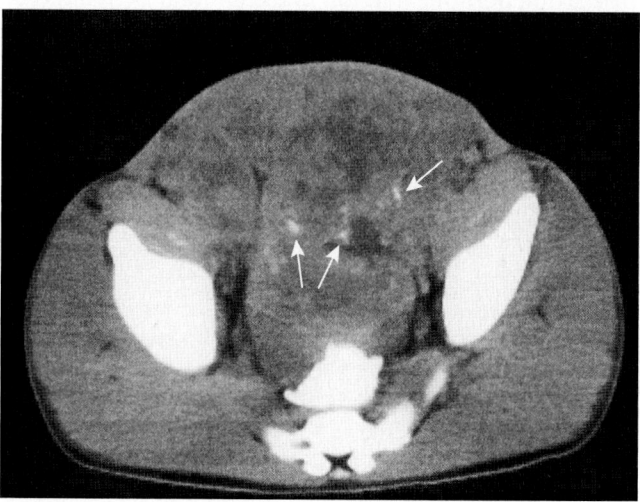

C

FIGURE 110-23. Abdominal leiomyosarcoma in a 16-year-old boy. **A,** Axial contrast-enhanced CT image shows extensive peritoneal metastases around the liver *(arrows)* and surrounding the pancreas, and a cystic peritoneal metastasis *(black arrow).* **B,** Lower image in the upper pelvis shows that the mass occupies most of the lower abdomen and pelvis. **C,** Image in the lower pelvis shows scattered calcifications *(arrows).* Bowel contrast is present in the rectum.

stomach have moderate vascularity, whereas those originating in the retroperitoneum may be hypovascular or moderately vascular and displace major vessels, particularly the inferior vena cava. Metastatic sites usually have vascularity similar to the primary tumor.

The CT appearance is not specific. The lesions may be homogeneously isointense with muscle, but more often they have necrotic areas of decreased density with variable degree of heterogeneity. Tumor necrosis may lead to communication with gastrointestinal tract and to perforation into the peritoneal cavity. Calcification within the mass occurs but is uncommon. Contrast enhancement varies with the vascularity of the tumor. Some large primary or metastatic lesions may show moderate peripheral enhancement.

Liposarcoma occurs more commonly in the retroperitoneum than in the peritoneal cavity. In some cases of liposarcoma, CT attenuation may suggest areas of fat. However, areas of fat attenuation are likely to be seen in high-grade liposarcomas.

Malignant fibrous histiocytoma is a mesenchymal soft tissue sarcoma that may occur at multiple sites, most commonly in the extremities and retroperitoneum, and more rarely within the abdomen. It is most often seen in

adults, but it has been reported in children and infants. The tumor is aggressive and metastasizes widely, particularly to the liver. Imaging has been described as showing lobulated echogenic masses and cystic areas, with heterogeneous enhancement on CT.

Peritoneal tumors:
- **Mesenchymal tumors: subperitoneal space**
  - **Benign**
    - **Lymphatic: lymphangioma**
    - **Adipose: lipoblastoma, lipoma; fat density**
    - **Vascular: hemangioma, calcifications, phleboliths**
    - **Nerve sheath tumors: neurofibromatosis type 1**
  - **Malignant**
    - **Smooth muscle: leiomyosarcoma**
    - **Fat: liposarcoma: fat density decreases with malignancy**
    - **Malignant fibrous histiocytoma**

TABLE 110-1

Routes of Peritoneal Metastatic Spread

Spread along peritoneal ligaments, omenta, mesenteries
Seeding through ascites
Lymphatic dissemination
Hematogenous spread

TABLE 110-2

Pediatric Malignancies Associated with Peritoneal Metastases

Colon carcinoma
Rhabdomyosarcoma
Teratoma
Germ cell tumor
Ovarian germ cell tumor
Wilms tumor
Small blue round cell tumor
Non-Hodgkin lymphoma
Melanoma
Endodermal sinus tumor
Desmoplastic small round cell tumor
Juvenile granulosa cell tumor
Peripheral neuroepithelioma
Pineoblastoma
Leiomyosarcoma
Neuroblastoma
Epithelioid carcinoma

Peritoneal tumors:

- **Benign**
  - **Cystic mesothelioma**
  - **Pseudomyxoma peritonei (distinct from mucinous metastases)**
- **Malignant**
  - **Desmoplastic small round cell tumor (DSRCT)**
  - **Malignant mesothelioma**
  - **Metastases**

Peritoneal metastases are the most common malignancy involving the peritoneum. They occur with a wide variety of primary pediatric malignancies and may be detected at the time of initial staging or during follow-up imaging. Malignancy disseminates throughout the peritoneum via four routes: through the lymphatics; direct spread along peritoneal ligaments, omentum, and mesenteries; by seeding through ascites; and via hematogenous routes

(Table 110-1). Peritoneal metastases frequently occur in the presence of other sites of metastatic disease. Intra-abdominal spread of intracranial disease may be prompted by the presence of a ventriculoperitoneal shunt catheter. Although the tumors most commonly associated with peritoneal metastases are those with mucinous histology, a wide variety of tumors are associated with peritoneal disease (Table 110-2).

The most common CT appearance of peritoneal metastases is that of solid masses adherent to the peritoneal surfaces. Alternative appearances include diffuse or patchy peritoneal enhancement, peritoneal studding by small implants, diffuse peritoneal caking, or a combination of these (Fig. 110-24 and 110-21).

Identification of peritoneal implants has improved with contemporary CT imaging. Even so, CT has been reported to detect only about half the lesions that were as small as 5 mm and determined surgically. In pediatrics, peritoneal lesion detection may be hampered by lesion size, presence or absence of ascites, contiguity with a site of primary disease, paucity of intra-abdominal fat, location of peritoneal implant, and adequacy of bowel opacification.

MR detection of peritoneal implants may be improved over CT because of the inherent tissue contrast and multiplanar capabilities (see Fig. 110-21). However, respiratory and bowel motion may degrade identification of peritoneal and serosal lesions. Contrast enhancement and subtraction techniques may improve detection (Fig. 110-25).

Peritoneal metastatic disease:

- **Solid masses adherent to peritoneal surfaces**
- **Patchy peritoneal enhancement**
- **Irregular peritoneal surface secondary to studding by small implants**
- **Diffuse peritoneal caking**

Detection may be hampered by the following:

- **Lesion size and location**
- **Ascites**
- **Contiguity with primary disease**
- **Paucity of intra-abdominal fat**
- **Suboptimal contrast enhancement**

ACKNOWLEDGEMENTS

The author gratefully thanks Sandra Gaither for manuscript preparation and the Department of Biomedical Communications for the preparation of the images. I particularly thank Bruce Parker and Al Schlesinger for their chapter contribution in the prior edition.

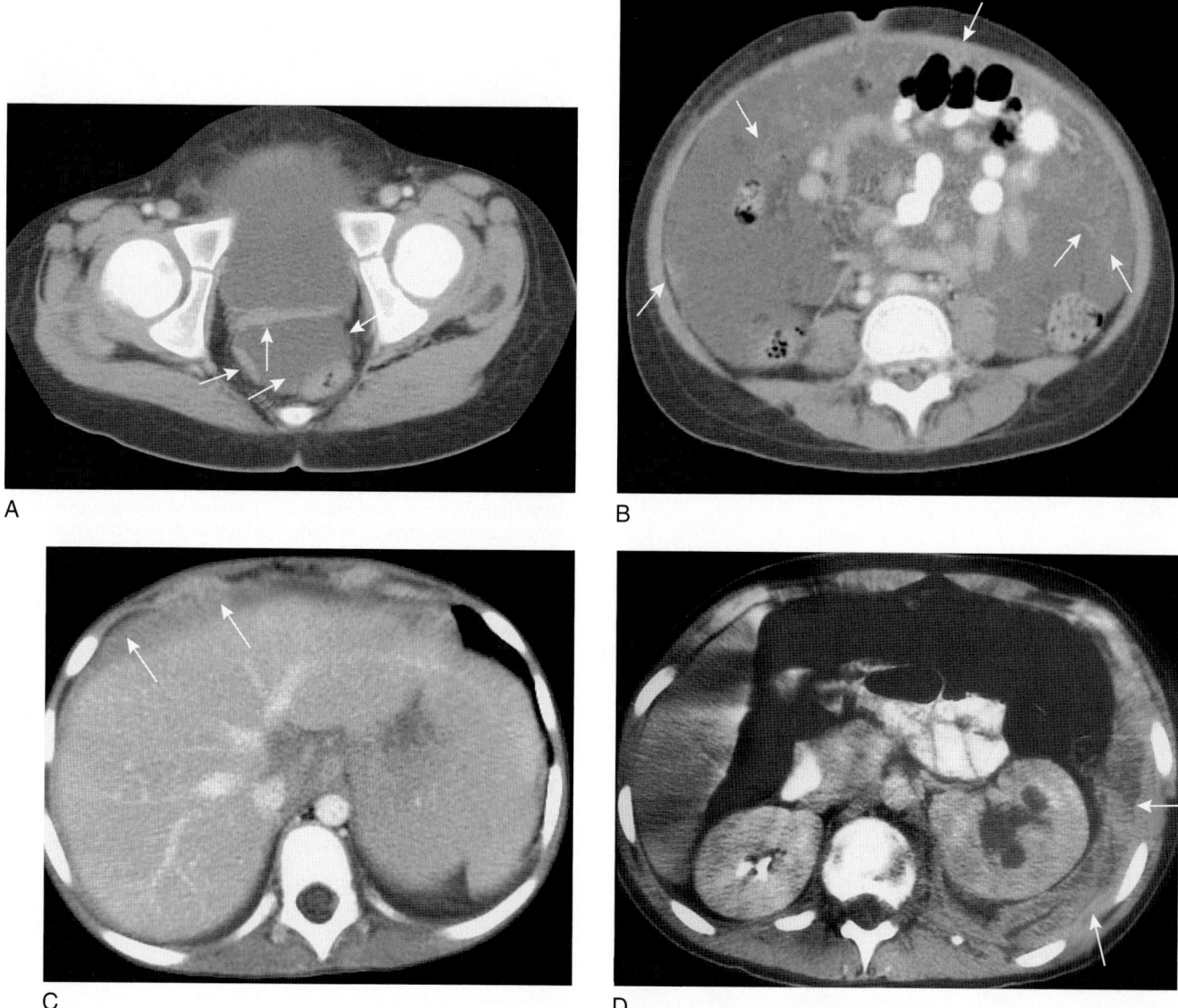

FIGURE 110-24. Peritoneal metastases may have varied appearance. **A,** Axial contrast-enhanced CT image of the deep pelvis shows a moderate amount of pelvic ascites *(arrows)* resulting from the peritoneal metastases evidenced by abnormal thickening and enhancement of the peritoneal surface *(arrows)* in a patient with a history of desmoplastic small round cell tumor and recurrent ascites. **B,** Contrast-enhanced CT through the midabdomen in a patient with epithelioid sarcoma shows more extensive peritoneal disease and complex ascites. Note tiny masses studding the peritoneum *(arrows)* and numerous strands of solid disease throughout the ascites *(arrows)*. Contrast-enhanced CT images in patient with Burkitt lymphoma **(C)** and patient with metastatic melanoma **(D)** show diffuse thickening of the peritoneal surface (*arrows* in **C** and **D**).

Continued

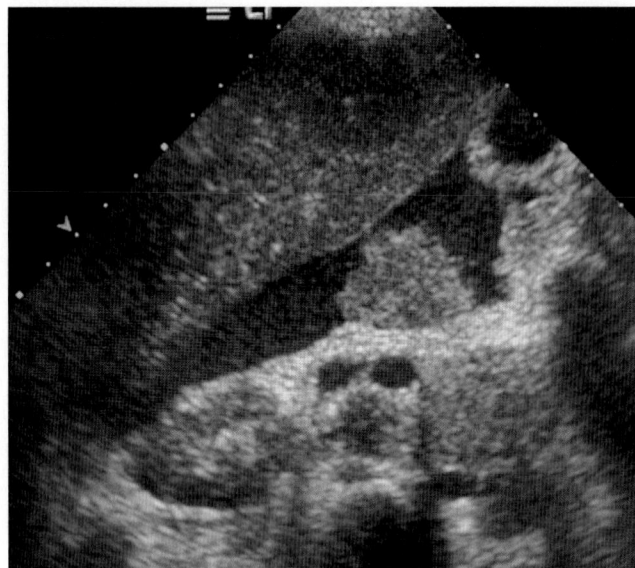

E

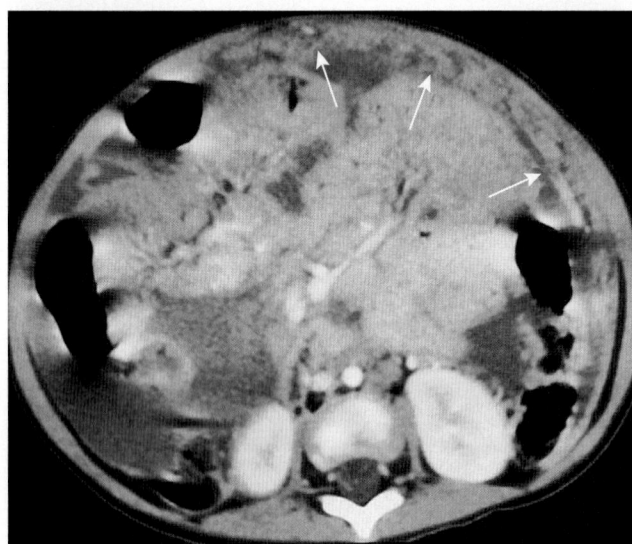

F

FIGURE 110-24, *cont'd*. Peritoneal metastases may have varied appearance. **E,** Transverse ultrasound image shows metastatic disease manifested as a discrete mass surrounded by ascitic fluid. **F,** Contrast-enhanced CT image shows a cystic peritoneal metastasis *(arrow)* in a patient with neuroblastoma.

FIGURE 110-25. Tuberculous peritonitis mimics malignant disease in this 14-month-old girl. Axial contrast-enhanced CT image shows a large amount of ascites displacing bowel loops centrally, with studding of the peritoneal surface *(arrows)*.

SUGGESTED READINGS

Pneumoperitoneum

Bray JF: The "inverted V" sign of pneumoperitoneum. Radiology 1984;151:45

Brill PW, Olson SR, Winchester P: Neonatal necrotizing enterocolitis: air in Morison pouch. Radiology 1990;174:469

Cho KC, Baker SR: Air in the fissure for the ligamentum teres: new sign of intraperitoneal air on plain radiographs. Radiology 1991;178:489

Levine MS, Scheiner JD, Rubesin SE, et al: Diagnosis of pneumoperitoneum on supine abdominal radiographs. AJR Am J Roentgenol 1991;156:731

Menuck L, Siemans PT: Pneumoperitoneum: importance of right upper quadrant features. AJR Am J Roentgenol 1980;127:753

Miller RE: Perforated viscus in infants: a new roentgen sign. Radiology 1960;74:65

Rigler LG: Spontaneous pneumoperitoneum: a roentgenologic sign found in the supine position. Radiology 1941;37:604

Seibert JJ, Parvey LS: The telltale triangle: use of the supine cross table lateral radiograph of the abdomen in early detection of pneumoperitoneum. Pediatr Radiol 1977;5:209

Wind ES, Pillari GP: Lucent liver in the newborn: a roentgenographic sign of pneumoperitoneum. JAMA 1977;237:2218

Wiot JF, Benton C, McAlister WH, et al: Postoperative pneumoperitoneum in children. Radiology 1967;89:285

Ascites and Acute Generalized Peritonitis

Churchill RJ: CT of intra-abdominal fluid collections. Radiol Clin North Am 1989;27:653

Colli A, Cocciolo M, Buccino G, et al: Thickening of the gallbladder wall in ascites. J Clin Ultrasound 1990;19:357

Dinkel E, Lehnart R, Troger J, et al: Sonographic evidence of intraperitoneal fluid: an experimental study and its clinical implications. Pediatr Radiol 1984;14:299

Gruenebaum M, Ziv N, Kornreich L, et al: The sonographic signs of the peritoneal pseudocyst obstructing the ventriculo-peritoneal shunt in children. Neuroradiology 1988;30:433

Hoffman RB, Wankmuller R, Rigler LG: Pseudoseparation of bowel loops: a fallacious sign of intraperitoneal fluid. Radiology 1966;87:845

Meyers MA, Oliphant M, Berne AS, et al: The peritoneal ligaments and mesenteries: pathways of intraabdominal spread of disease. Radiology 1987;163:593

Meyers MA: Dynamic Radiology of the Abdomen: Normal and Pathologic Anatomy, 5th ed. New York, Springer Verlag, 2000

Newman B, Teele RL: Ascites in the fetus, neonate and young child: emphasis on ultrasonographic evaluation. Semin Ultrasound CT MR 1984;5:85

Pandolfo I, Gaetta M, Scribano E, et al: Mediastinal pseudotumor due to passage of ascites through the esophageal hiatus. Gastrointest Radiol 1989;14:209

Ruess L, Frazier AA, Sivit CJ: CT of the mesentery, omentum, and peritoneum in children. Radiographics 1995;15:1995

Abdominal Compartment Syndrome

Epelman M, Soudack M, Engel A, et al: Abdominal compartment syndrome in children: CT findings. Pediatr Radiol 2002;32:319

Hendrick JM, Kaste SC, Tamburro RF, et al: Abdominal compartment syndrome in a newly diagnosed patient with Burkitt lymphoma. Pediatr Radiol 2006;36:254

Hsu HH, Lin JY, Hsu SC, et al: Neglected cause of renal failure in cancer patients: spontaneous tumor lysis syndrome inducing acute uric acid nephropathy. Dialysis Transplant 2004;33:316

Malbrain ML: Different techniques to measure intra-abdominal pressure (IAP): time for a critical re-appraisal. Intensive Care Med 2004;30:357

Malbrain ML, Chiumello D, Pelosi P, et al: Prevalence of intra-abdominal hypertension in critically ill patients: a multicentre epidemiological study. Intensive Care Med 2004;30:822

Malbrain ML, Chiumello D, Pelosi P, et al: Incidence and prognosis of intraabdominal hypertension in a mixed population of critically ill patients: a multiple-center epidemiological study. Crit Care Med 2005;33:315

Pickhardt PJ, Shimony JS, Heiken JP, et al: The abdominal compartment syndrome: CT findings. AJR 1999;173:575

Schein M, Wittman DH, Aprahamian CC, Condon RE: The abdominal compartment syndrome: the physiological and clinical consequences of elevated intra-abdominal pressure. J Am Coll Surg 1995;180:745

Sieh KM, Chu KM, Wong J: Intra-abdominal hypertension and abdominal compartment syndrome. Langenbecks Arch Surg 2001;386:53

Abdominal Wall and Peritoneal Calcification

Blane CE, White SJ, Braunstein EM, et al: Pattern of calcification in childhood dermatomyositis. AJR Am J Roentgenol 1984; 142:397

Kirks DR, Taybi H: Prune-belly syndrome: an unusual cause of neonatal abdominal calcification. Am J Roentgenol Radium Ther Nucl Med 1975;123:778-782

Naidech HJ, Chawla HS: Soft-tissue calcification after subcutaneous emphysema in a neonate. AJR Am J Roentgenol 1982;139:374

Taybi H: Thoracic and abdominal calcification in children: a review. Perspect Radiol 1989;2:135

Peritoneal Tumors and Tumor-Like Conditions

Al-Salem A: Lymphangiomas in infancy and childhood. Saudi Med J 2004;25:466

Bani-Hani KE, Gharaibeh KA: Malignant peritoneal mesothelioma. J Surg Oncol 2005;91:17

Brandal P, Bjerkehagen B, Heim S: Rearrangement of chromosomal region 8q11-13 in lipomatous tumours: correlation with lipoblastoma morphology. J Pathol 2006;208:388

Chouli M, Viala J, Dromain C, et al: Intra-abdominal desmoplastic small round cell tumors: CT findings and clinicopathological correlations in 13 cases. Eur J Radiol 2005;54:438

Clement PB, Young RH, Scully RE: Malignant mesotheliomas presenting as ovarian masses: a report of nine cases, including two primary ovarian mesotheliomas. Am J Surg Pathol 1996;20:1067

De Perrot M, Rostan O, Morel P, Coultre LE: Abdominal lymphangioma in adults and children. Br J Surg 1998;85:395

Fetsch JF, Miettinen M, Laskin WB, et al: A clinicopathologic study of 45 pediatric soft tissue tumors with an admixture of adipose tissue and fibroblastic elements, and a proposal for classification as lipofibromatosis. Am J Surg Pathol 2000;24:1491

Fultz PJ, Hampton WR, Skucas J, Sickel JZ: Differential diagnosis of fat-containing lesions with abdominal and pelvic CT. Radiographics 1993;13:1265

Gerald WL, Ladanyi M, de Alava E, et al: Clinical, pathologic and molecular spectrum of tumor associated with t(11;22)(p13;q12): desmoplastic small round-cell tumor and its variants. J Clin Oncol 1998;16:3028-3036

Granmayeh M, Jonsson K, McFarland W, Wallace S: Angiography of abdominal leiomyosarcoma. AJR Am J Roentgenol 1978;130:724

Haliloglu M, Hoffer FA, Fletcher BD: Malignant peritoneal mesotheliomas in two pediatric patients: MR imaging findings. Pediatr Radiol 2000;30:251

Hibbard MK, Kozakewich HP, Cin PD, et al: PLAG1 fusion oncogenes in lipoblastoma. Cancer Res 2000;60:4869

Kaste SC, Marina N, Fryrear R, et al: Peritoneal metastases in children with cancer. Cancer 1998;83:385

Kataoka ML, Togashi K, Yamaoka T, et al: Posterior cul-de-sac obliteration associated with endometriosis: MRI imaging evaluation. Radiology 2005;234:815

Kim OH, Lee KY: Malignant fibrous histiocytoma of primary omental origin in an infant. Pediatr Radiol 1994;24:285

Kransdorf MJ: Malignant soft-tissue tumors in a large referral population: distribution of diagnoses by age, sex, and location. AJR Am J Roentgenol 1995;164:129

Kransdorf MJ: Benign soft-tissue tumors in a large referral population: distribution of specific diagnoses by age, sex, and location. AJR Am J Roentgenol 1995;164:395

Kretschmar C, Colbach C, Bhan I, Crombleholme TM: Desmoplastic small cell tumor: a report of three cases and a review of the literature. J Pediatr Hematol Oncol 1996;18:293

Kurugoglu S, Ogut G, Mihmanli I, et al: Abdominal leiomyosarcomas: radiologic appearances at various locations. Eur Radiol 2002;12:2933

Lane RH, Stephens DH, Reiman HM: Primary retroperitoneal neoplasms: CT findings in 90 cases with clinical and pathologic correlation. AJR Am J Roentgenol 1989;152:83

McLeod AJ, Zornoza J, Shirkhoda A: Leiomyosarcoma: computed tomographic findings. Radiology 1984:152:133

Mingo L, Seguel F, Rollan V: Intraabdominal desmoplastic small round cell tumour. Pediatr Surg Int 2005;21:279

Moholkar S, Sebire NJ, Roebuck DJ: Radiological-pathological correlation in lipoblastoma and lipoblastomatosis. Pediatr Radiol 2006;36:851

Mohta A, Anand RK: Lipoblastoma in infancy. Indian Pediatr 2006;43:78

Morerio C, Panarello C, Russo I, et al: A further cases of chromosome 8q rearrangement in lipoblastoma. J Pediatr Hematol Oncol 2000;22:484

Moriwaki Y, Kobayashi S, Harada H, et al: Cystic mesothelioma of the peritoneum. J Gastroenterol 1996;31:868-874

Murphey MD, Carroll JF, Flemming DJ, et al: Benign musculoskeletal lipomatous lesions. Radiographics 2004;24:1433

Nishimura H, Zhang Y, Ohkuma K, et al: MR imaging of soft-tissue masses of the extraperitoneal spaces. Radiographics 2001;21:1141

Nishino M, Hayakawa K, Minami M, et al: Primary retroperitoneal neoplasms: CT and MR imaging findings with anatomic and pathologic diagnostic clues. Radiographics 2003;23:45

Niwa K, Hashimoto M, Hirano S, et al: Primary leiomyosarcoma arising from the greater omentum in a 15-year-old girl. Gynecol Oncol 1999;74:308

Oliphant M, Berne AS, Meyers MA: The subperitoneal space of the abdomen and pelvis: planes of continuity. AJR Am J Roentgenol 1996;167:1433

Outwater E, Schiebler ML, Brooks JJ: Intraabdominal desmoplastic small cell tumor: CT and MR findings. J Comput Assist Tomogr 1992;16:429

Pickhardt PJ, Bhalla S: Primary neoplasms of peritoneal and sub-peritoneal origin: CT findings. Radiographics 2005;25:983

Pickhardt PJ, Fisher AJ, Balfe DM, et al: Desmoplastic small round cell tumor of the abdomen: radiologic-histopathologic correlation. Radiology 1999;210:633

Qureshi N, Hallisey M, Fielding J, Gourevitch D: Primary intra-abdominal malignant fibrous histiocytoma presenting as pyrexia of unknown origin: report of a case with review of the literature. Int Semin Surg Oncol 2006;3:15

Rha SE, Ha HK, Kim AY, et al: Peritoneal leiomyosarcomatosis originating from gastrointestinal leiomyosarcomas: CT features. Radiology 2003;227:385

Seidel FG, Magill HL, Burton EM, et al: Cases of the day: pediatric: lipoblastoma. Radiographics 1990;10:728

Signorelli M, Cerri V, Groli C, et al: Cystic lymphangioma of the greater omentum and ascites: an unusual combination. Prenat Diagn 2004;24:745

Soin S, Andronikou S, Lisle R, et al: Omental lipoblastoma in a child: diagnosis based on CT density measurements. J Pediatr Hematol Oncol 2006;28:57

Stover B, Laubenberger J, Hennig J, et al: Value of RARE-MRI sequences in the diagnosis of lymphangiomatosis in children. Magn Reson Imaging 1995;13:481

Surendrababu NRS, Rao A, Samuel R: Primary hepatic leiomyosarcoma in an infant. Pediatr Radiol 2006;36:366

Ukihide T, Hasegawa T, Kusumoto M, et al: Desmoplastic small round cell tumor: imaging findings associated with clinicopathologic features. J Comput Assist Tomogr 2002;26:579

CHAPTER 111

Introduction to the Hepatobiliary System

LISA H. LOWE and ALAN E. SCHLESINGER

NORMAL ANATOMY

The liver is the largest of the abdominal organs, occupying most of the right upper quadrant and extending across the midline. It is larger in neonates and infants than it is in older children and adults. The right lobe is larger than the left, and the caudate and quadrate lobes are substantially smaller. The superior portion of the liver is in direct contact with the diaphragm at the bare area without intervening peritoneum. The posterior margin is in contact with the inferior vena cava, the right adrenal gland, and the distal esophagus. Inferiorly, the liver is in contact with the colon, the gallbladder, and the right kidney. The left lobe is in contact with the stomach. The visceral surface of the liver contains the porta hepatis with its vessels and biliary ducts. The two major intrahepatic biliary ducts join to form the common hepatic duct, which is joined by the cystic duct from the gallbladder to form the common bile duct. The common bile duct drains into the descending limb of the duodenum.

Cross-sectional imaging studies can identify the landmarks that divide the hepatic lobes and their respective segments. Traditional nomenclature used in the United States divides the liver into five segments: the right anterior and posterior, left lateral and medial, and caudate lobes. The right and left lobes are divided by the middle hepatic vein, and by a line between the inferior cava and the gallbladder fossa (Cantlie line); the anterior and posterior segments of the right lobe are separated by the right hepatic vein; and the medial (quadrate lobe) and lateral segments of the left lobe are segmented by the falciform ligament. However, hepatic segmental anatomy, as described by Couinaud, is currently more useful in defining surgically resectable segments (Fig. 111-1). In Couinaud's system, the right and left lobes of the liver are again divided by the middle hepatic vein and the Cantlie line. The caudate lobe is segment I. Segments II to IV are in the left lobe; segments V to VIII in the right lobe. On the right, the right hepatic vein divides the right lobe into posterior segments VI and VII, and anterior segments V and VIII. The superior segments (VII and VIII) are separated from the inferior segments (V and

VI) by the horizontal course of the right portal vein. On the left, the left hepatic vein divides the left lobe into posterior segment II and anterior segments III and IV; III and IV are in turn separated by the umbilical fissure and falciform ligament, which contains the left portal pedicle. Ultrasound (US), computed tomography (CT), CT arterial portography, and magnetic resonance imaging (MRI) have been used to identify the hepatic segments as defined by Couinaud's nomenclature for segmental anatomy of the liver.

> *Segmental hepatic anatomy:*
> - **The caudate lobe is segment I.**
> - **The middle hepatic vein and Cantlie line separate the right and left hepatic lobes.**

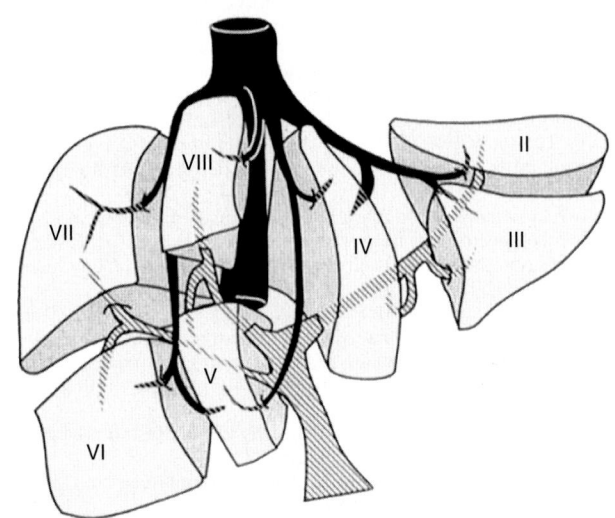

FIGURE 111-1. Schematic of hepatic segmental anatomy according to Couinaud. *Diagonally shaded* vessels indicate the portal venous supply to each segment. Hepatic veins are *solid black*. Not shown are the bile ducts, which drain within the portal triads parallel with the portal venous system and hepatic arteries. (From Gazelle GS, Lee MJ, Mueller PR: Cholangiographic segmental anatomy of the liver. Radiographics 1994;14:1005.)

- **The right hepatic vein separates the right lobe into anterior and posterior segments.**
- **The right portal vein separates the right lobe into superior and inferior segments.**
- **The left hepatic vein divides the left lobe into anterior and posterior segments.**
- **The fissure for the round ligament (plane of the left portal vein) divides the anterior left lobe into medial and lateral segments.**

EMBRYOLOGY OF THE LIVER

According to Moore and Persaud, the liver and biliary duct system, including the gallbladder, arise from the most caudal part of the foregut as a ventral bud early in the fourth week of embryonic life (Fig. 111-2). This bud, known as the hepatic diverticulum, extends into the ventral mesentery of the septum transversum, which is the future diaphragm. It divides into two parts as it grows between the layers of the ventral mesentery. The larger cranial part of the hepatic diverticulum develops into the hepatic primordium. The proliferating endodermal cells develop into hepatocytes and into the epithelial cells lining the biliary system. The reticuloendothelial portions of the liver develop from the splanchnic mesenchyme of the septum transversum. The smaller caudal part of the hepatic diverticulum expands to form the gallbladder, and its stalk becomes the cystic duct. The stalk that connects the cystic and hepatic ducts becomes the common bile duct (CBD) connecting to the duodenum, which also arises from the caudal foregut.

The liver grows very rapidly, with the right lobe becoming the larger of the two lobes. The caudate and quadrate lobes are thought to develop as subdivisions of the right lobe, although this has been questioned by Dodds and colleagues, who have suggested an alternative embryologic scheme for development of the caudate lobe. By the ninth week, the liver represents 10% of the embryo's weight, primarily because of the hematopoietic function of the embryonic liver. The liver accounts for 5% of the newborn infant's weight. Bile formation by hepatocytes begins during the 12th embryonic week, and bile pigments begin to develop between the 13th and

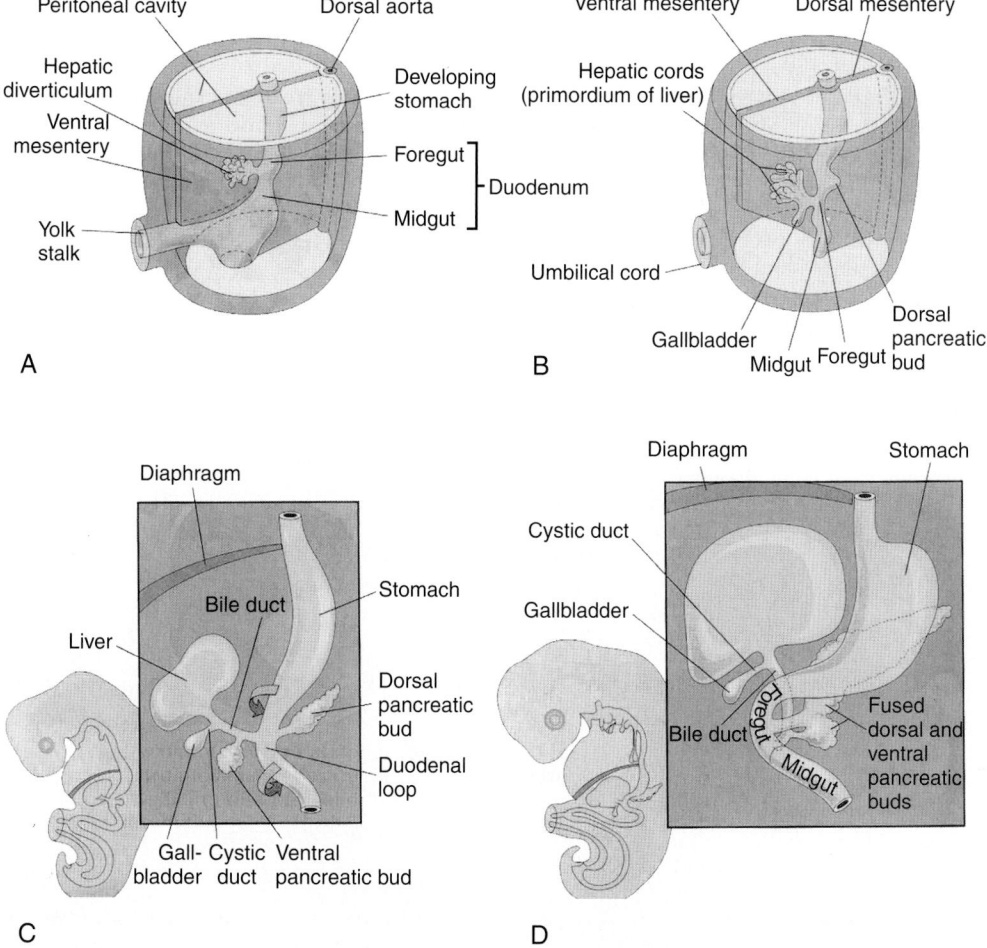

FIGURE 111-2. Schematic illustrations of hepatic embryology. **A,** At 4 weeks. **B** and **C,** At 5 weeks. **D,** At 6 weeks. Note hepatic diverticulum extending into the ventral mesentery and dividing into cranial (liver primordium) and caudal (gallbladder and common bile duct) buds. Also note that the entrance of the bile duct into the duodenum shifts gradually to a posterior position, which explains why the bile duct passes posterior to the duodenum. (From Moore KL, Persaud TVN: The digestive system. *In* Moore KL, Persaud TVN [eds]: The Developing Human: Clinically Oriented Embryology, 7th ed. Philadelphia, WB Saunders, 2003:262.) *(See color plate.)*

16th weeks. These pigments enter the duodenum, giving the intraintestinal meconium its characteristic green color. The ventral mesentery is a double-layer membrane that becomes the gastrohepatic, hepatoduodenal, and falciform ligaments. The falciform ligament extends from the liver to the anterior abdominal wall. Its inferior free border contains the umbilical vein. The ventral mesentery also gives rise to the hepatic visceral peritoneum that fully covers the liver except for the bare area in contact with the diaphragm.

HEPATOBILIARY IMAGING

Plain Radiography

Plain radiographs play a relatively small role in the evaluation of hepatobiliary diseases. Although hepatomegaly can be identified on plain radiographs, liver size is usually sufficiently evaluated on physical examination. Because there is insufficient perihepatic fat in neonates and infants to identify the hepatic outline on plain radiographs, the radiologist must rely on being able to identify displacement of adjacent bowel, but this can be impossible to do when it is filled with fluid. Plain radiographs are useful, however, for identifying calcifications in the liver parenchyma (Fig. 111-3) or in the biliary system, and air in the portal venous system or biliary tree (Fig. 111-4). Profound fatty replacement of the liver may reduce its radiographic density, but cross-sectional imaging is much more sensitive to the presence of fatty replacement.

Ultrasound

US has been an extraordinarily useful tool in the evaluation of the liver and biliary system in children because it requires no sedation or anesthesia, and it provides excellent anatomic definition without ionizing radiation. Because the liver lies superficially in infants, curved or linear transducers are superior to sector transducers; usually, 5 to 7 MHz is optimal in neonates and infants. A 3.5- or even a 2.0-MHz transducer may be necessary in older, larger children and adolescents, and sector footprints become useful in older patients. When the possibility of superficial subcapsular disease, such as metastases or hematoma, is being considered, a high-resolution linear transducer is typically necessary.

The echogenicity of the liver should be homogeneous and uniform throughout. A complete examination requires evaluation of the hepatic parenchyma, the portal venous system, the hepatic veins, intrahepatic bile ducts, the common bile duct, and the gallbladder. Hernanz-Schulman and colleagues studied the CBD diameter by US in 173 children ranging in age from 1 day to 13 years. They found that it was less than or equal to 3.3 mm in all patients, less than or equal to 1.6 mm in all patients 1 year or younger, and less than or equal to 1.2 mm in all infants 3 months of age or younger.

> *Common bile duct diameter:*
> - **1.2 mm in children younger than 3 months**
> - **1.6 mm in children 3 months to 1 year**
> - **3.3 mm in children 1 to 13 years**

Doppler US is especially valuable in patients with portal hypertension and other vascular diseases. Color Doppler sonography is useful to rapidly differentiate the hepatic artery from the biliary ducts, to assess for portal vein thrombosis, and to identify the hepatic arterial system. It is essential in the evaluation of transplanted livers. Although the examination may be requested for suspected liver disease, a full evaluation of the upper abdomen, including spleen, pancreas, and other upper abdominal organs and vascular structures, should always be performed.

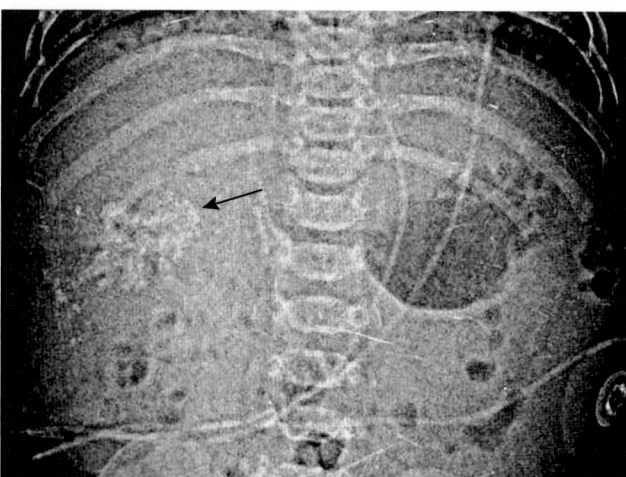

FIGURE 111-3. Hepatic calcification in a 5-month-old boy, a former 23-week premature infant, after placement of an umbilical venous catheter that was complicated by a hepatic hematoma. A large, ill-defined focus of calcification is noted over the liver *(arrow)*.

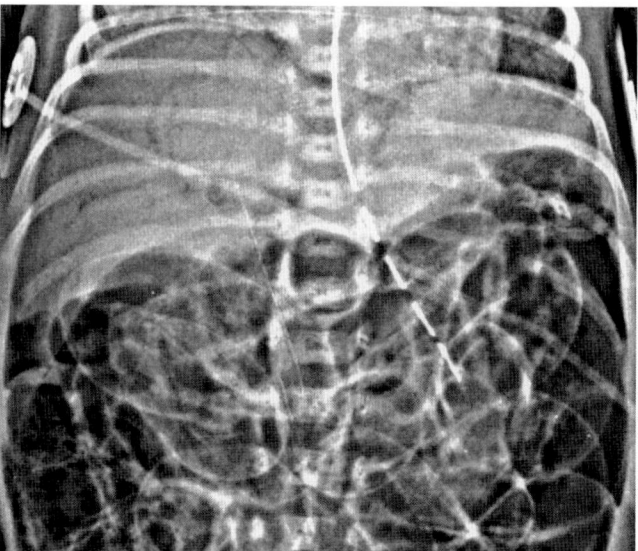

FIGURE 111-4. Portal venous gas and free air secondary to necrotizing enterocolitis in a 3-week-old premature infant girl. Radiolucent branching air is seen within the portal radicles of the right hepatic lobe. Dilated bowel is seen in addition to free air with radiolucency over the liver and a Rigler sign (air on both sides of the bowel wall).

Nuclear Medicine Studies

Nuclear medicine studies offer physiologic as well as some anatomic information. The Kupffer cells of the reticuloendothelial system of the liver and spleen take up technetium-99m sulfur colloid, providing information about the hepatic parenchyma. Single-photon emission CT increases the sensitivity of the procedure and the ability to evaluate hepatic function. Nevertheless, US, CT, and MRI have replaced the sulfur colloid scan in the evaluation of hepatic masses.

Hepatobiliary patency studies are useful for differentiating neonatal hepatitis from congenital biliary atresia. The most commonly used agents are derivatives of iminodiacetic acid. These compounds are taken up by hepatocytes and secreted into the biliary ductules (Fig. 111-5). Hepatobiliary scanning in these infants is optimally performed after pretreatment with phenobarbital to optimize hepatic excretion. Biliary scanning may play a role in any disorder in which it is important to determine the patency of the biliary tree, such as choledochal cysts and acute and acalculous cholecystitis (see Chapter 107).

Computed Tomography

Helical CT has become widely used in the evaluation of hepatobiliary disease. With the advent of multidetector technology, the need for sedation or anesthesia in young children has markedly decreased. However, the dramatic increase in CT use has meant that more patients are exposed to ionizing radiation, which is an important concern. CT of the liver is most often used in patients in

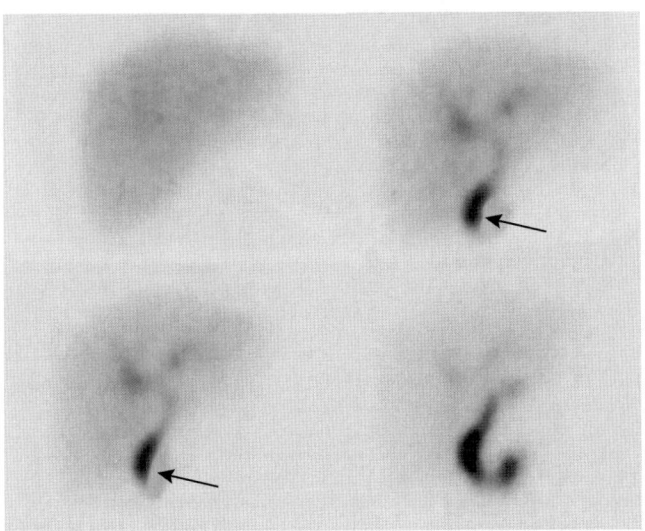

A   B

C   D

FIGURE 111-5. Normal biliary scintigram in a 2-month-old male infant with jaundice. **A,** Hepatobiliary scintigrams using technetium-99m dimethylisopropyliminodiacetic acid show immediate radionuclide uptake in the liver. **B** and **C,** Scans at 20 and 30 minutes demonstrate radionuclide in the small intestine (*arrow* in **B** and in **C**). **D,** One hour after injection, radionuclide is largely cleared from the liver.

whom a mass has been identified clinically or on US. Although performing sonography before CT is not required, it is very useful to have an initial impression of the most likely differential diagnoses before performing the CT. This allows the CT scan to be tailored to the type of mass suspected. Imaging choices include precontrast, an arterial phase, a portal venous phase, equilibrium (delayed) phase images, or a combination of phases. By tailoring the examination with US, the routine performance of multiple-phase CT examinations on children who do not need them can be avoided.

Better characterization of various liver lesions is possible with CT, and if appropriate, CT-guided biopsy or abscess drainage may be contemplated. CT is less useful for diffuse parenchymal liver disease, although fatty liver, hemachromatosis, hemosiderosis, and changes in parenchymal attenuation secondary to cirrhosis and fibrosis can be identified. Dynamic CT scanning may be particularly useful in the evaluation of highly vascular neoplasms.

Magnetic Resonance Imaging

With the advent of multidetector CT and CT angiography, the advantages that MR imaging (MRI) previously had over CT are becoming less significant. Often, the choice between CT and MRI is more a personal or institutional preference, based on type and availability of resources and expertise. The advantage of MRI over CT is that it does not use ionizing radiation, which is important to consider. MRI is certainly more costly, the examination is significantly longer, motion artifact is a greater problem with young children, and sedation is more often required. In older, more cooperative children, newer breath-hold pulse sequences, especially useful for biliary ductal disease and for MR cholangiopancreatography, can significantly shorten the scan time and eliminate motion artifact caused by respiration. MRI of the liver is especially useful for evaluation of diffuse infiltrative diseases such as hemochromatosis and Gaucher disease.

Generally, the closest-fitting coil should be used to improve signal-to-noise ratio and resolution. Standard spin-echo pulse sequences are most commonly used. Both T1-weighted and T2-weighted sequences are useful for full evaluation. Fat-suppression techniques and chemical shift imaging can be used to evaluate masses that may contain fat. Gradient recalled echo sequences are especially useful for evaluation of the vascular structures. Magnetic resonance angiography (MRA), both with and without intravenous contrast, can be used to better evaluate the vascular structures. Heavily T2-weighted images are widely used for MR cholangiopancreatography (MRCP) to evaluate the biliary tree and pancreatic ducts (Fig. 111-6).

Endoscopic Retrograde Cholangiopancreatography

Endoscopic retrograde cholangiopancreatography (ERCP) is used less frequently in children than in adults. The examination has the advantage of allowing diagnosis and therapeutic interventions simultaneously. Although it

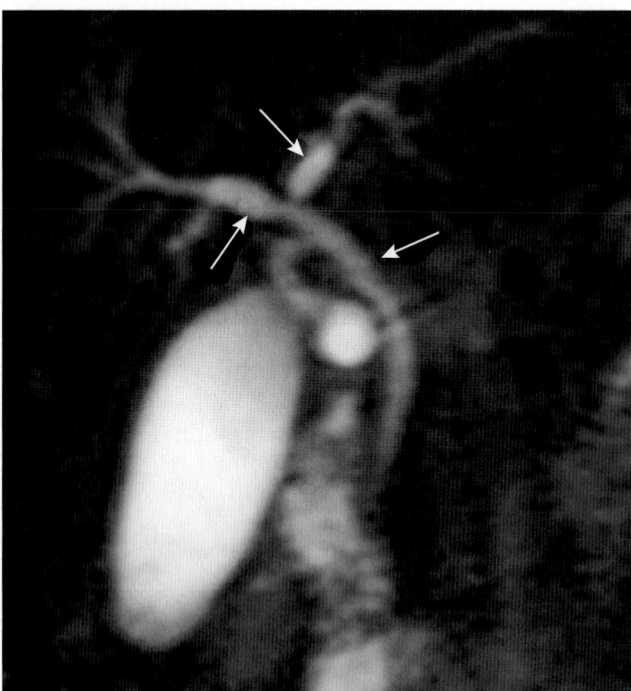

FIGURE 111-6. Normal MR cholangiopancreatography in a 12-year-old-girl with mild dilation of the biliary tree. Two-dimensional, thick-slab, heavily T2-weighted, fast spin echo pulse sequence shows the common bile duct and proximal intrahepatic ducts *(arrows).*

can demonstrate anatomic detail in various congenital and acquired diseases of the biliary tree and pancreas, its major role is interventional: sphincterotomy to relieve obstruction and allow passage of a stone, and biopsy of the biliary tree. The disadvantages of ERCP are that it is difficult to perform in children and usually requires general anesthesia. *Percutaneous transhepatic cholangiography* (PTC) is often better than ERCP for demonstrating the intrahepatic ducts, and it can often accomplish similar goals, such as stent placement and biopsy.

Arteriography

Diagnostic arteriography is rarely performed since the advent of MRA and CT angiography. Arteriography of the pediatric hepatobiliary system is now performed when intervention is required, such as embolization of vasoproliferative lesions, vascular tumors before surgery, post-traumatic or postoperative hemorrhage, arteriovenous fistulas, or angioplasty of vascular stenoses, such as hepatic arterial stenosis in patients with transplanted livers.

SUGGESTED READINGS

Normal Anatomy and Embryology of the Liver

Dodd GD 3rd: An American's guide to Couinaud's numbering system. AJR Am J Roentgenol 1993;161:574

Gazelle GS, Lee MJ, Mueller PR: Cholangiographic segmental anatomy of the liver. Radiographics 1994;14:1005

Moore KL, Persaud TVN: The digestive system. *In* Moore KL, Persaud TVN (eds): The Developing Human: Clinically Oriented Embryology, 7th ed. Philadelphia, WB Saunders, 2003:259-265

Hepatobiliary Imaging

Akisik MF, Sandrasegaran K, Aisen AA, et al: Dynamic secretin-enhanced MR cholangiopancreatography. Radiographics 2006;26:665

Ashida K, Nagita A, Sakagichi M, et al: Endoscopic retrograde cholangiopancreatography in paediatric patients with biliary disorders. J Gastroenterol Hepatol 1998;13:598

Bonetti MG, Castriota-Scanderberg A, Criconia GM, et al: Hepatic iron overload in thalassemic patients: proposal and validation of an MRI method of assessment. Pediatr Radiol 1996;26:650

Carneiro RC, Fordham LA, Semelka RC: MR imaging of the pediatric liver. MRI Clin N Am 2002;10:137

Elsayes KM, Narra VR, Yin Y: Focal hepatic lesions: diagnostic value of enhancement pattern approach with contrast enhanced 3D gradient-echo MR imaging. Radiographics 2005;25:1299

Graham KS, Ingram JD, Steinberg SE, et al: ERCP in the management of pediatric pancreatitis. Gastrointest Endosc 1998;47:492

Hainaux B, Christophe C, Hanquinet S, et al: Gaucher's disease: plain radiography, US, CT and MR diagnosis of lungs, bone and liver lesions. Pediatr Radiol 1992;22:78

Hernanz-Schulman M, Ambrosino MM, Freeman PC, et al: Common bile duct in children: sonographic dimensions. Radiology 1995;195:193

Hill SC, Damaska BM, Ling A, et al: Gaucher disease: abdominal MR imaging findings in 46 patients. Radiology 1992;184:561

Irie H, Honda H, Jimi M, et al: Value of MR cholangiopancreatography in evaluating choledochal cysts. AJR Am J Roentgenol 1998;171:1381

Lafortune M, Madore F, Patriquin H, et al: Segmental anatomy of the liver: a sonographic approach to the Couinaud nomenclature. Radiology 1991;181:443

Matos C, Nicaise N, Deviere J, et al: Choledochal cyst: a comparison of findings at MR cholangiopancreatography and endoscopic retrograde cholangiopancreatography in eight patients. Radiology 1998;209:443

Miyazaki T, Yamashita Y, Tang Y, et al: Single-shot MR cholangiopancreatography of neonates, infants, and young children. AJR Am J Roentgenol 1998;170:33

Mukai JK, Stack CM, Turner DA, et al: Imaging of surgically relevant hepatic vascular and segmental anatomy. Part 1: Normal anatomy. AJR Am J Roentgenol 1987;149:287

Norton KI, Glass RB, Kogan D, et al: MR cholangiography in children and young adults with biliary disease. AJR Am J Roentgenol 1999;172:1239

Parulekar SG: Ligaments and fissures of the liver: sonographic anatomy. Radiology 1979;130:409

Ramm GA, Ruddell RG. Hepatotoxicity of iron overload: mechanisms of iron-induced hepatic fibrogenesis. Semin Liver Dis 2005;25:433

Rosenthal DI, Barton NW, McKusick KA, et al: Quantitative imaging of Gaucher disease. Radiology 1992;185:841

Siegel MJ: MR imaging of the pediatric abdomen. Magn Reson Imaging Clin N Am 1995;3:161-182

Smith D, Downey D, Spouge A, et al: Sonographic demonstration of Couinaud's liver segments. J Ultrasound Med 1998;17:375

Soyer P, Bluemke DA, Bliss DF, et al: Surgical segmental anatomy of the liver: demonstration with spiral CT during arterial portography and multiplanar reconstruction. AJR Am J Roentgenol 1994;163:99

Tagge EP, Tarnasky PR, Chandler J, et al: Multidisciplinary approach to the treatment of pediatric pancreatobiliary disorders. J Pediatr Surg 1997;32:158

Teele RL, Share JC: Ultrasonography of the biliary tree in infants and children. Appl Radiol 1992;21:15

Teo EL, Strouse PJ, Prince MR: Applications of magnetic resonance imaging and magnetic resonance angiography to evaluate the hepatic vasculature in the pediatric patient. Pediatr Radiol 1999; 29:238

Terk MR, Esplin J, Lee K, et al: MR imaging of patients with type 1 Gaucher's disease: relationship between bone and visceral changes. AJR Am J Roentgenol 1995;165:599

Waggenspack GA, Tabb DR, Tiruchelvam V, et al: Three-dimensional localization of hepatic neoplasms with computer-generated scissurae recreated from axial CT and MR images. AJR Am J Roentgenol 1993;160:307

Yamataka A, Kuwatsuru R, Shima H, et al: Initial experience with non-breath-hold magnetic resonance cholangiopancreatography: a new noninvasive technique for the diagnosis of choledochal cyst in children. J Pediatr Surg 1997;32:1560

LISA H. LOWE and ALAN E. SCHLESINGER

PARTIAL HEPATIC AGENESIS AND GALLBLADDER ANOMALIES

Agenesis or hypoplasia of a hepatic lobe is an uncommon abnormality, although it is being identified with higher frequency as a result of the increased use of cross-sectional imaging. Most commonly, the right lobe is absent, with compensatory hypertrophy of the left lobe of the liver and the caudate lobe. This anomaly can be associated with gallbladder agenesis or abnormal retrohepatic or suprahepatic position of the gallbladder. Associated congenital anomalies, especially those of the biliary tract, have been reported, as well as portal hypertension. Most reported cases have been in adults, in whom the differential diagnosis should include atrophy of the right lobe secondary to cirrhosis or tumor. In children, these latter conditions are less likely, and agenesis is the probable diagnosis when the right lobe cannot be identified. Agenesis of the left lobe is less frequent. The gallbladder may be congenitally absent (without associated biliary atresia), ectopically positioned, duplicated, or septated.

ALAGILLE SYNDROME (ARTERIOHEPATIC DYSPLASIA)

Paucity and hypoplasia of interlobular bile ducts in association with other congenital abnormalities is known as Alagille syndrome or arteriohepatic dysplasia. Alagille and colleagues described five major components of this autosomal dominant disorder: (1) abnormal facies (large forehead, small pointed chin, hypertelorism, poorly developed nasal bridge), (2) chronic cholestasis, (3) ocular abnormalities, (4) butterfly vertebrae, and (5) pulmonary artery hypoplasia or stenosis (Fig. 112-1). The last may be either isolated or associated with complex cardiac anomalies. Less commonly seen vascular abnormalities occur frequently, suggesting a broader spectrum of potential vascular anomalies in patients with Alagille syndrome. Half of the cases have four of these abnormalities, 30% will have all five features, and 15% will have three of the abnormalities. A number of other congenital abnormalities are seen less frequently, including caudal dysplasia. The bones may show osteopenia and undertubulation.

> *Major components of Alagille syndrome:*
> - **Abnormal facies**
> - **Chronic cholestasis**
> - **Ocular abnormalities**
> - **Butterfly vertebrae**
> - **Pulmonary artery hypoplasia or stenosis**

Affected patients usually present with jaundice in early infancy that is distinguished from biliary atresia by the presence of other components of this syndrome. Patients presenting beyond the newborn period may have ultrasound findings of cirrhosis, with heterogeneous echogenicity in the liver and evidence of regenerating nodules. Typically, scintigraphic biliary imaging fails to show normal excretion of radioisotope into the gastrointestinal tract. Definitive diagnosis is usually made on liver biopsy. Intraoperative cholangiogram usually shows patency of the extrahepatic biliary tree. Most patients with Alagille syndrome die before the end of the third decade as a result of complex congenital heart disease, intracranial hemorrhage, or hepatic disease. Hepatocellular carcinoma as a complication of Alagille syndrome has been reported in both children and adults. Liver transplantation can be performed in patients with Alagille syndrome, but the results are better if surgery occurs before the development of hepatic tumors.

Hypoplasia of the interlobular bile ducts without other associated congenital anomalies has been described as well. The differentiation from biliary atresia can be made by the later age at presentation, hepatic wedge biopsy, and demonstration of a patent extrahepatic biliary tree.

FIBROCYSTIC DISEASES

Fibrocystic liver diseases (see Chapter 15) are a group of entities characterized by a spectrum of hepatic cysts and hepatic fibrosis, believed to be a result of abnormal development and resorption of the ductal plates. Depending on the timing of the event, the abnormality may involve the extrahepatic ducts, or the small, medium-sized, or large intrahepatic ducts, and result in chole-

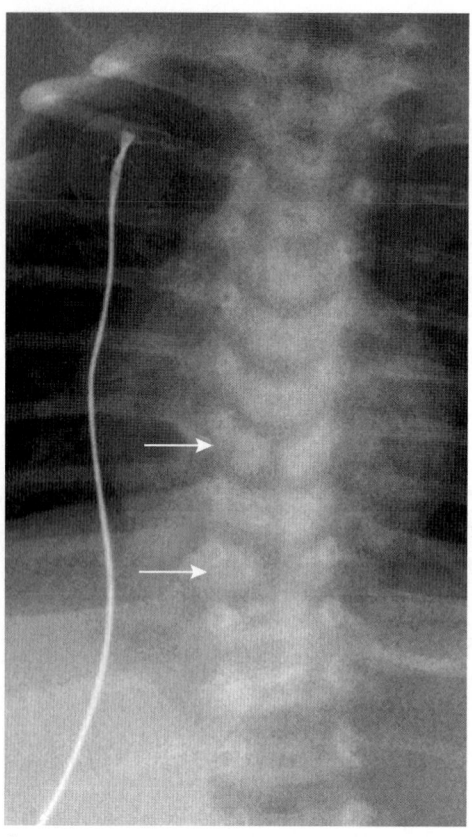

A

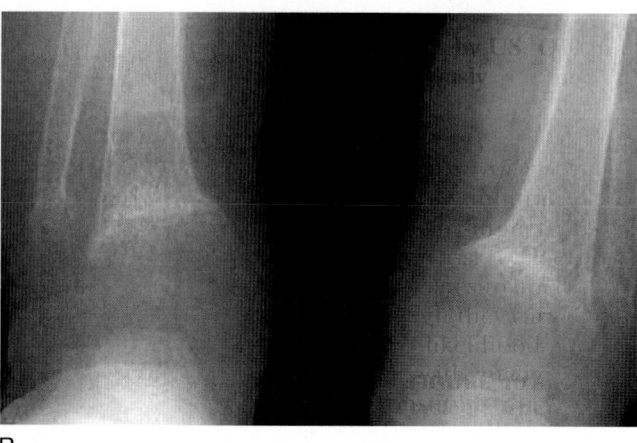

B

FIGURE 112-1. Alagille syndrome in a male infant with abnormal liver function tests. **A,** Frontal view of the spine shows butterfly vertebrae at T7 and T9 *(arrows).* **B,** Rachitic changes are seen as flared, cupped, irregular, poorly ossified distal tibial metaphyses. Bile duct hypoplasia was found on liver biopsy, compatible with Alagille syndrome.

dochal cysts, Caroli disease, hepatic fibrosis, hepatic cysts, or microhamartomas.

Choledochal Cyst

Choledochal cyst refers to dilation of the common bile duct, which can be saccular or fusiform. A frequently used classification is that of Todani and colleagues describing five general types (with several subtypes) of choledochal cysts, which differ in etiology, pathogenesis, appearance, and presentation (Fig. 112-2). Various theories for the pathogenesis of the type I choledochal cysts exist, with the leading theories invoking obstruction of the distal biliary duct and/or reflux of pancreatic enzymes into the biliary tree as a result of anomalous proximal insertion of the pancreatic duct into the common bile duct (ductal malunion). Ductal malunion permits reflux of pancreatic enzymes into the common bile duct, with subsequent inflammation and weakening of the wall, a pathogenetic mechanism that occurs in about 60% of patients. This anomalous ductal connection has been demonstrated on endoscopic retrograde cholangiopancreatography (ERCP), rendering it the most plausible theory to explain the pathogenesis of type I choledochal cysts (Fig. 112-3). Furthermore, the development of an acquired choledochal cyst has described in a 6-year-old boy with previously documented ductal malunion, who initially had normal biliary ducts. Type I choledochal cyst is more common in girls than boys in Western countries, but the sex ratio is equal in Asia. About 65% of all reported cases are from Japan.

> Todani type I choledochal cyst is likely caused by either distal ductal obstruction or ductal malunion, with abnormally proximal insertion of the pancreatic duct into the common duct, and reflux of pancreatic enzymes.

The most common form, found in 80% to 90% of cases, is Todani type I, consisting of dilation of the common bile duct over a variable length and in varying degrees (Figs. 112-4 and 112-5). Todani type IA involves dilation of the common bile duct extending above the insertion of the cystic duct. Conversely, in Todani type IB, common bile duct dilation, occurs below the level of the cystic duct. Todani type II choledochal cyst consists of one or more diverticula of the common bile duct and is found in 2% of cases. Some theorize that this form of choledochal cyst may be caused by prenatal rupture of the common bile duct with subsequent healing. Todani type III is a choledochocele—a dilation of the intraduodenal portion of the duct with both the common bile duct and pancreatic duct emptying into it—and is found in 1.5% to 5.0% of cases (Fig. 112-6). This form of choledochal cyst may be the sequela of ampullary obstruction, or may be the result of a congenital duplication of the duodenum in the region of the ampulla. Todani type IVA consists of multiple intrahepatic and extrahepatic cysts, and it occurs in approximately 10% of patients (Fig. 112-7). Type IVA of Todani may represent a form of Caroli disease, but it has also been called type I with intrahepatic involvement. Type IVB involves multiple

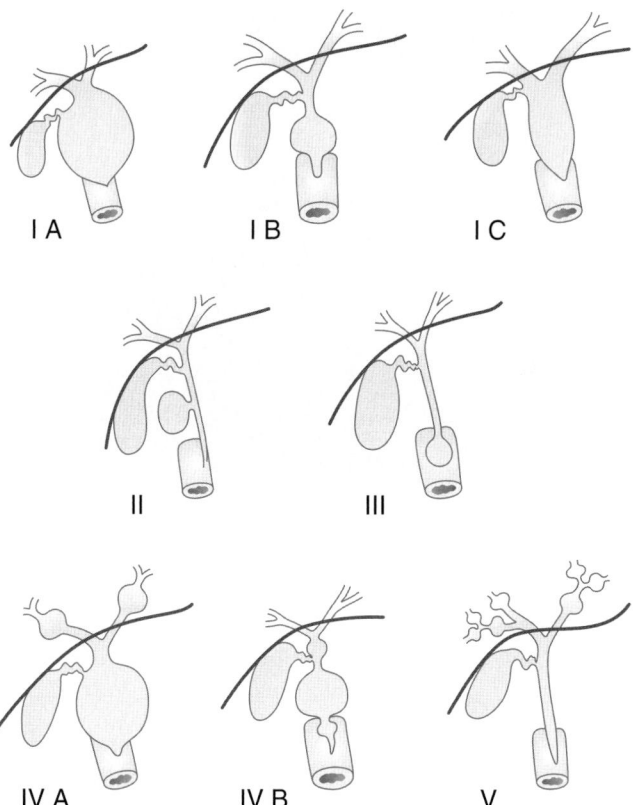

FIGURE 112-2. Schematic of Todani classification of choledochal cysts based on cholangiographic morphology. Type IA and IB involve dilation of the common bile duct, type II is a saccular diverticulum from the common bile duct, type III is a cyst at the ampulla of Vater, type IVA and IVB are multiple fusiform cysts of the intrahepatic and extrahepatic biliary tree, and type V is equivalent to Caroli disease with numerous intrahepatic bile lakes throughout the biliary tree and liver. (From Kim OH, Chung HJ, Choi BG: Imaging of the choledochal cyst. Radiographics 1995;15:69-88.)

ductal extrahepatic cysts, and it is rare. Todani type V is synonymous with Caroli disease, which is discussed later. The intrahepatic cysts seen in types IV and V may be the result of primary ductal ectasia.

Choledochal cysts may present in infancy with cholestatic jaundice and may be clinically inseparable from neonatal hepatitis or biliary atresia. However, sonographic and radionuclide studies, demonstrating the cysts and continuity with the biliary tree, usually suggest the correct diagnosis, which can be confirmed, if necessary, by magnetic resonance cholangiopancreatography (MRCP). In older children and young adults, the clinical presentation is quite variable. A characteristic triad of

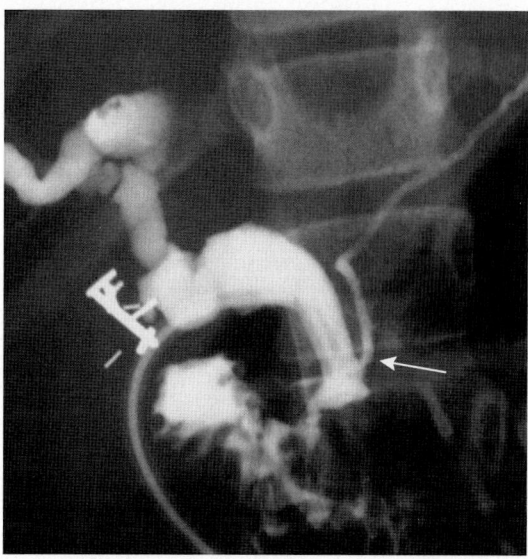

FIGURE 112-3. Endoscopic retrograde cholangio-pancreatography in a child with a choledochal cyst reveals dilation of the common bile duct and a relatively proximal insertion of the pancreatic duct *(arrow)*.

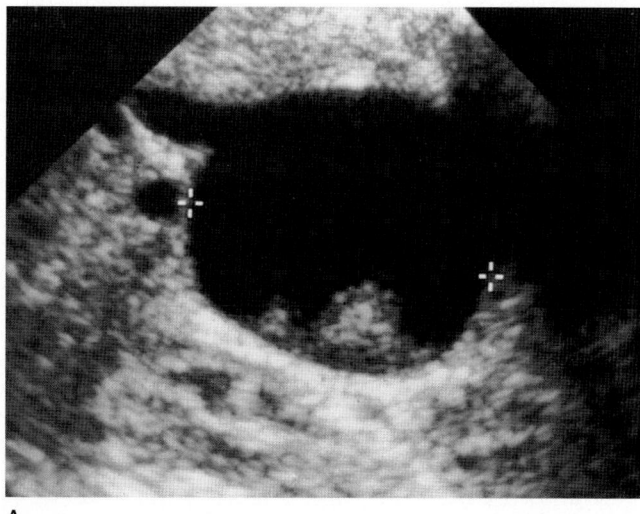

A

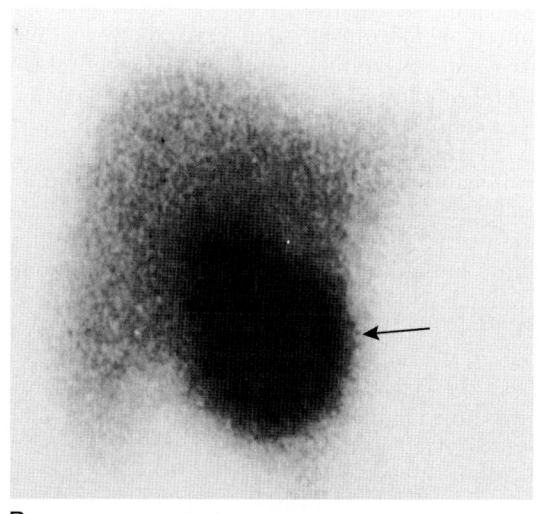

B

FIGURE 112-4. Choledochal cyst (Todani type I). **A,** Ultrasound shows a large cyst in the porta hepatis, communicating with the biliary tree. There is dependently layering sludge within the cyst. **B,** Delayed image from a technetium-99m–labeled hepatoiminodiacetic acid confirms communication with the biliary tree, as radiotracer accumulates in the cyst *(arrow).* This area was photopenic on early scans (not shown).

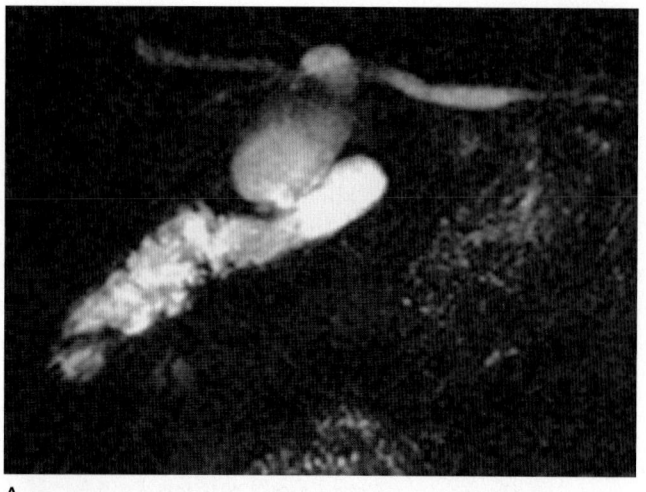
A

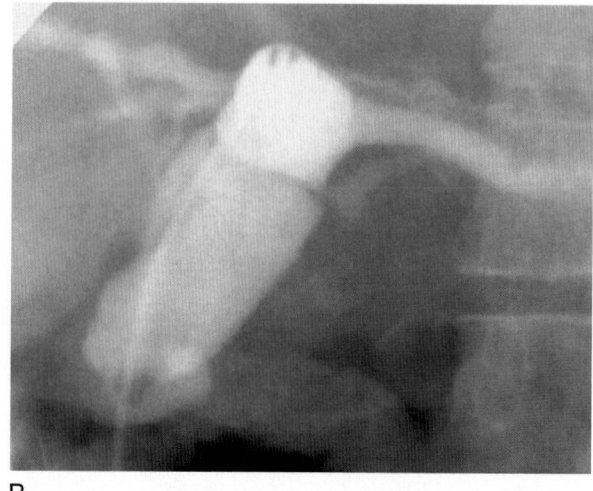
B

FIGURE 112-5. Choledochal cyst (Todani type I) in a 6-year-old boy with abdominal pain. **A,** Magnetic resonance cholangiopancreatography (MRCP) and **B,** endoscopic retrograde cholangiopancreatography (ERCP) reveal fusiform dilation of the common bile duct, consistent with a choledochal cyst.

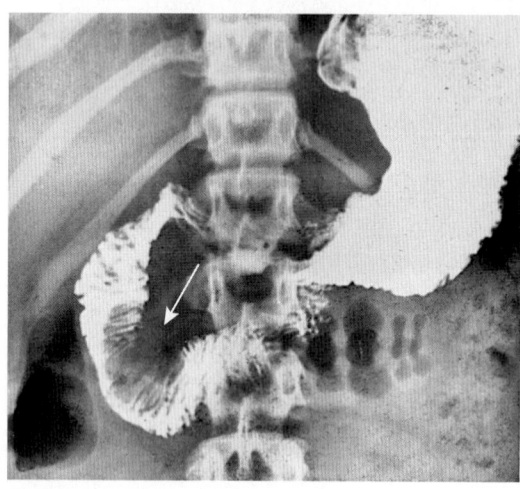
A

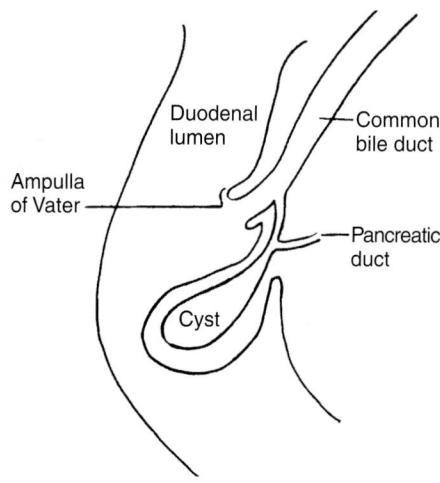
B

FIGURE 112-6. Choledochocele (Todani type III). **A,** Spot film of upper gastrointestinal tract in 12-year-old girl with abdominal pain, shows a large filling defect *(arrow)* coincident with the site of the ampulla of Vater. **B,** Drawing of findings of choledochocele identified at surgery.

abdominal pain, obstructive jaundice, and fever has been reported, but only a minority of patients present with all three components of the triad. Abdominal pain is the most characteristic presentation, and obstructive jaundice, fever, pale stools, hepatomegaly, palpable mass, and splenomegaly are other common presenting symptoms.

Sonography is usually the first imaging study requested, because nearly all of the possible modes of presentation point to a hepatobiliary problem. The markedly dilated common bile duct in type I choledochal cyst is readily discernible. The gallbladder can usually be identified adjacent to the dilated common duct, and the cystic duct may also be seen. Most frequently, the intrahepatic ducts are normal, but varying degrees of dilation may be present. Sludge or stones may be identified within the dilated duct. Biliary scintigraphy shows that the dilated cystic structure communicates with the biliary tree.

Computed tomography (CT) does not demonstrate the ductal anatomy as well as cholangiography, but it may be quite useful in evaluating intrahepatic cysts and identifying abscesses. More recently, CT cholangiography has been performed after intravenous administration of meglumine iodoxamic acid (Endobil; Bracco, Milan, Italy), which is excreted by the liver into the biliary system. Magnetic resonance imaging (MRI) and MRCP have been advocated with increasing frequency for the evaluation of children with choledochal cysts, because these modalities can noninvasively provide imaging information comparable to that of ERCP, including demonstration of ductal malunion. Sedation is required in younger patients.

Percutaneous transhepatic cholangiography (PTC) and ERCP have been reported useful, but are rarely necessary. Some authors prefer PTC, which may better delineate the intrahepatic ducts and has less chance of leading to cholangitis than ERCP.

> **Sonography, hepatobiliary scintigraphy, and MRCP are usually sufficient for the imaging workup of patients with choledochal cysts.**

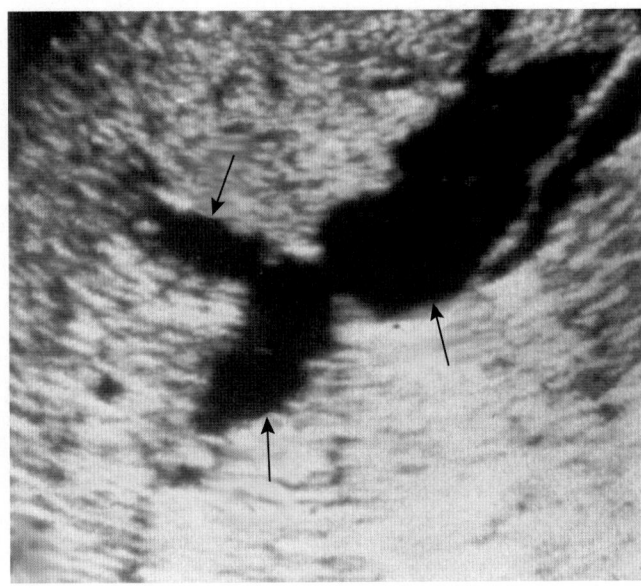 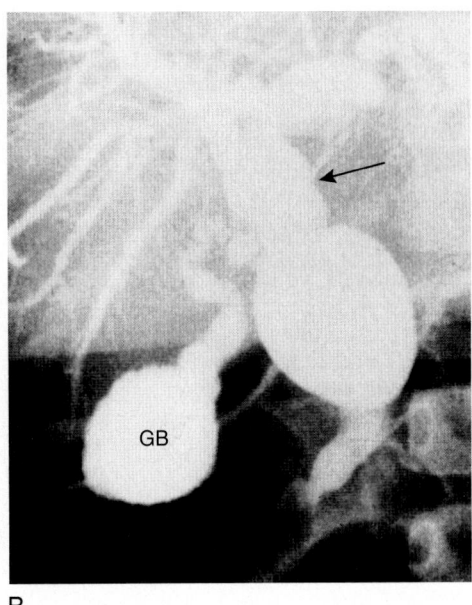

A   B

FIGURE 112-7. Choledochal cyst (Todani type IV) in a 1-year-old boy. **A,** Longitudinal sonogram shows marked saccular dilation of the intrahepatic and extrahepatic bile ducts *(arrows)*. **B,** Operative cholangiogram confirms dilation of intrahepatic biliary tree and common bile duct *(arrow)*. Gallbladder *(GB)* is noted.

The most common complication of type I choledochal cyst is ascending cholangitis. Eventually, hepatic cirrhosis can occur, with subsequent portal hypertension. Spontaneous cyst rupture has been reported. There is a 20-fold increased incidence of carcinoma of the biliary tree in patients with choledochal cyst. The risk is low in the first decade of life but increases with advancing age.

> *Complications of type I choledochal cyst:*
> - **Ascending cholangitis**
> - **Cirrhosis**
> - **Spontaneous cyst rupture**
> - **Carcinoma of the biliary tree**

Caroli Disease

Caroli disease, also classified as Todani type V choledochal cyst, involves segmental nonobstructive dilation of the intrahepatic bile ducts. The cause of Caroli disease is unknown. Leading theories state that it represents a maldevelopment of the ductal plates, involving the large intrahepatic bile ducts. It is characterized by multiple hepatic cysts in continuity with the biliary system, representing ectatic intrahepatic ducts. Other postulated mechanisms include occlusion of the hepatic artery in the neonatal period with associated ischemia of the bile ducts, abnormal growth rate of the biliary epithelium and supporting connective tissues, with lack of the normal involution of ductal plates, leading to biliary cysts surrounding the portal triads. In the "pure" form of Caroli disease, there is only ectasia of the intrahepatic biliary tree. This form is often associated with stone formation, cholangitis, and hepatic abscesses. More commonly, in a condition termed Caroli syndrome,

which involves ductal plate abnormalities in both large and small ducts, there is associated hepatic fibrosis. Caroli hepatic ductal ectasia may also be associated with extrahepatic ductal plate abnormalities and choledochal cysts (Todani IVA choledochal cyst) as discussed previously. There is also an association with renal disease in autosomal recessive polycystic kidney disease, medullary sponge kidney, and nephronophthisis with cysts in the renal medulla and corticomedullary junction.

> *Abnormalities commonly associated with Caroli disease:*
> - **Stone formation, cholangitis, abscess**
> - **Hepatic fibrosis**
> - **Choledochal cyst**
> - **Medullary sponge kidney**
> - **Infantile polycystic kidney disease**
> - **Nephronophthisis**

Although the disease is present from birth, most patients do not present until later in life when abdominal pain secondary to cholangitis leads them to seek medical attention. The abdominal pain may also be related to hepatic abscesses secondary to cholangitis or to biliary stones secondary to stasis. Patients with associated hepatic fibrosis may present with symptoms and signs of secondary portal hypertension. Although typically a diffuse process, monolobar Caroli disease has been reported, and 88% of the cases involve the left lobe.

In most patients, sonography reveals very large, irregularly ectatic ducts (Fig. 112-8). Recognition of the connection of the ectatic ducts with one another and with the rest of the ductal system is useful to distinguish Caroli disease from hepatic cysts, or from autosomal

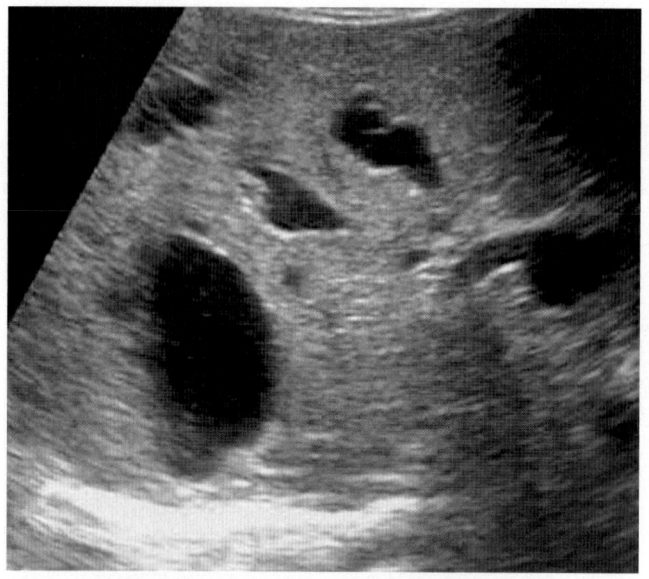

A

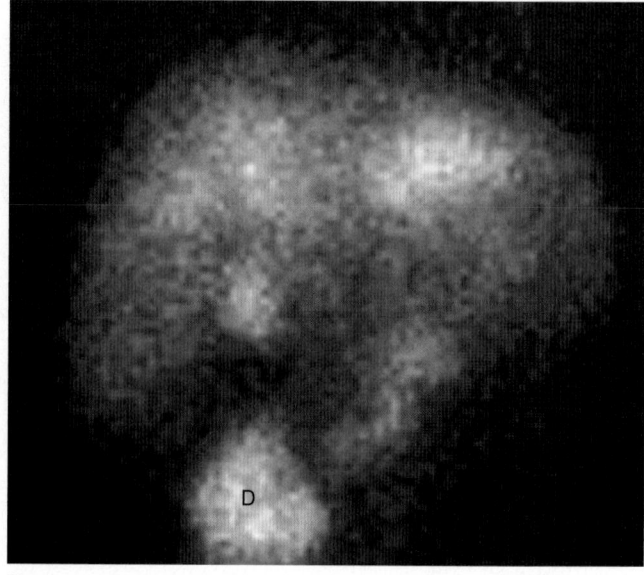

B

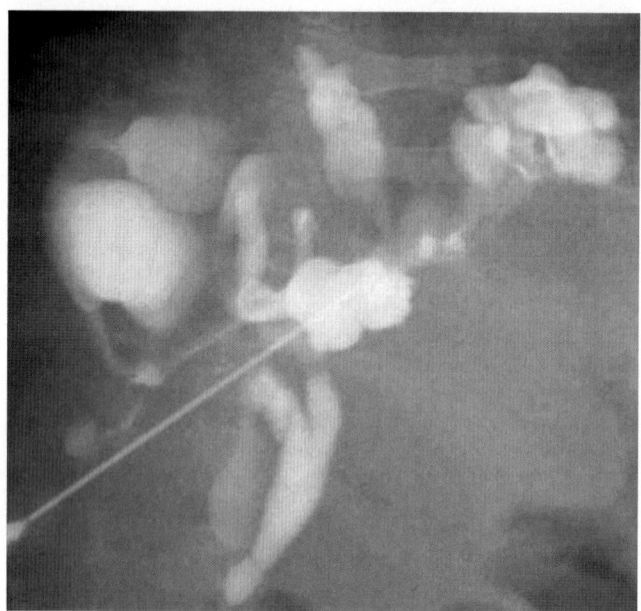

C

FIGURE 112-8. Caroli disease in a 6-month-old girl with associated autosomal recessive polycystic kidney disease, presenting with failure to thrive. **A,** Transverse hepatic sonogram shows multiple scatted large hypoechoic spaces throughout the liver. **B,** Nuclear scintigraphy (technetium-99m–labeled hepatoiminodiacetic acid) confirms focal areas of bile stasis seen as pooled increased activity on a background of good hepatic uptake. Note the normal excretion into the duodenum *(D)*. **C,** Percutaneous cholangiogram also confirms large bile lakes throughout the liver.

dominant polycystic disease. The dilated ducts may give the appearance of surrounding the portal vein radicles, producing the intraluminal portal vein, or central dot sign, believed to be pathognomonic for Caroli disease. Blood flow can be confirmed within these portal venous branches on Doppler interrogation. Biliary sludge and calculi are common findings within the anechoic dilated ducts. Both the gallbladder and the common bile duct may be enlarged. If an abscess is present, one or more cysts will show mixed echogenicity rather than the anechoic appearance of the uncomplicated cysts. In all patients in whom Caroli disease is identified, the kidneys should be examined as well. Such examination may reveal them to be normal, frankly polycystic, or they may show increased medullary echogenicity with loss of corticomedullary differentiation.

Ultrasound findings in Caroli disease:
- **Common**
  - **Dilated, ectatic bile ducts (bile lakes)**
  - **"Intraluminal portal vein," or central dot sign with flow on Doppler (pathognomonic)**
  - **Biliary sludge and calculi**
  - **Enlarged gallbladder and common bile duct**
- **Less common**
  - **Abscesses**
  - **Associated renal anomalies (cysts or abnormal echogenicity)**

Routine hepatic scintigraphy may show multiple filling defects if the ducts are sufficiently dilated. Biliary imaging with technetium-99m iminodiacetic acid compounds shows focal defects during the hepatic phase that gradually increase in activity as the radiopharmaceutical collects in the dilated ducts, whereas the remainder of the liver shows decreased activity with time. Radiotracer activity in the gastrointestinal tract is seen, but this is frequently delayed because of bile stasis. Patients with supervening hepatic fibrosis have hepatomegaly and, frequently, splenomegaly.

CT is an excellent modality to show the extent of disease, especially the intrahepatic ductal ectasia. An enhancing "central dot" may be seen that corresponds to the portal vein seen sonographically. If an abscess is present, the affected cyst may show higher attenuation than the remaining cysts and peripheral enhancement. The common duct is typically dilated, and the gallbladder distended. Cystic disease of the kidneys may be identified, as is splenomegaly in patients with supervening hepatic fibrosis.

Cholangiography, MRCP, PTC, and ERCP show the abnormalities, with communicating cystic and tubular ductal ectasia. Stones and biliary sludge may also be identified. The incidence of biliary duct and pancreatic cancer in patients with Caroli disease and choledochal cyst is increased.

Congenital Hepatic Fibrosis

Congenital hepatic fibrosis is a ductal plate malformation involving the small interlobular ducts. Histologically, periportal fibrosis and scarring bridge adjacent tracts, with ductal plate remnants resembling bile ducts. It is a progressive condition resulting in portal hypertension, and it is associated with renal abnormalities in approximately 50% of patients, most typically autosomal recessive polycystic kidney disease (ARPKD). It is less often identified in patients with other renal entities, such as autosomal dominant polycystic kidney disease (ADPKD) and medullary cystic disease or nephronophthisis. Patients with ARPKD with severe renal involvement present as newborns or infants, with very large kidneys, hypertension, and impairment of renal function (see Chapter 145). Those patients who present later in childhood or in adulthood have mild renal involvement and frequently come to attention because of splenomegaly and portal hypertension related to liver disease. In

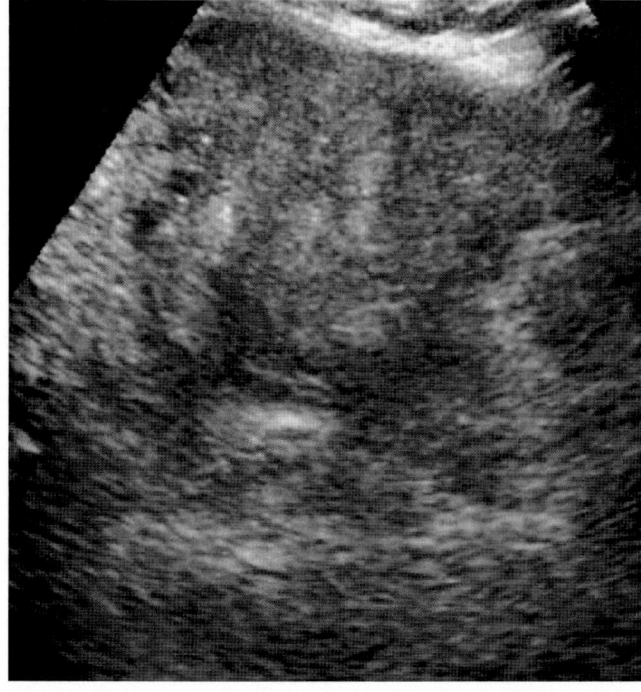

A

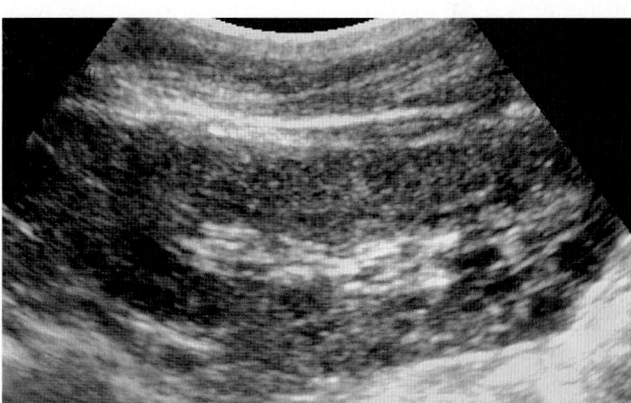

B

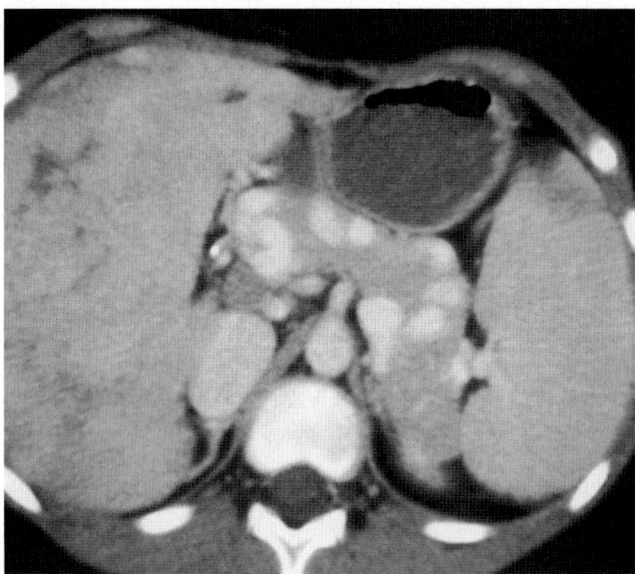

C

FIGURE 112-9. Congenital hepatic fibrosis complicated by portal hypertension with extensive collateral flow in a 14-year-old girl. **A,** Transverse sonogram shows heterogeneous echogenicity of the liver resulting from chronic hepatic fibrosis. **B,** Longitudinal renal sonogram reveals loss of corticomedullary differentiation, and multiple tiny cysts, with some larger macrocysts, diffusely throughout the kidney. **C,** CT image shows heterogeneous enhancement of liver, splenomegaly, and extensive peripancreatic collateral vessels caused by portal hypertension. Hypodense area in anterior spleen resulted from partial volume artifact.

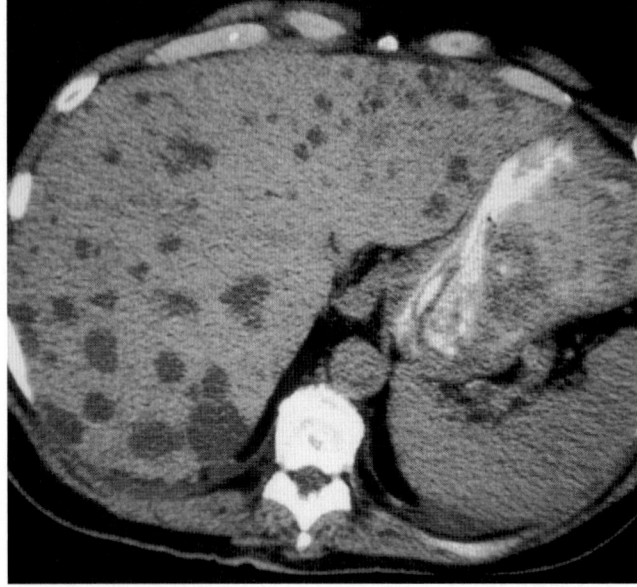

A

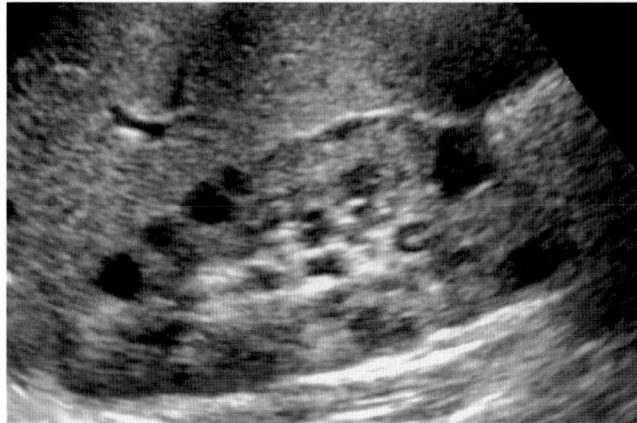

B

FIGURE 112-10. Cystic liver disease in a 16-year-old boy with a family history of autosomal dominant polycystic kidney disease (ADPKD). **A,** CT image reveals numerous, well-defined cysts throughout the liver. **B,** Longitudinal sonogram of the right kidney shows numerous cysts consistent with associated ADPKD.

patients with ADPKD, hepatic fibrosis typically predates the appearance of the renal cysts. There is a low incidence of hepatocellular carcinoma in patients with congenital hepatic fibrosis.

The sonographic characteristics of congenital hepatic fibrosis include hepatomegaly, with or without splenomegaly, depending on the presence or absence of portal hypertension. Hepatic echogenicity is heterogeneous, with increased echogenicity in the portal triads and poorly defined portal vessels on gray scale (Fig. 112-9). If associated with Caroli disease in Caroli syndrome, the typical findings of large cysts representing ectatic biliary ductal segments can be identified. Characteristic imaging findings of portal hypertension may be seen, and associated renal lesions should always be investigated. CT sections show areas of heterogeneously increased and decreased attenuation in the liver, and they outline collateral circulation in portal hypertension very well. MRI of the liver shows low signal intensity on T1-weighted and T2-weighted spin echo pulse sequences, and stigmata of portal hypertension including splenomegaly when present. MR angiography can demonstrate vascular sequelae of portal hypertension, and MRCP can be used to detail the status of the biliary tree when associated with Caroli disease.

Polycystic Liver Disease

Multiple hepatic cysts can be present in both autosomal recessive and autosomal dominant polycystic renal disease. In patients with ARPKD, cysts found in the liver consist of ectatic ductal segments, or Caroli disease. In patients with ADPKD liver disease, the hepatic cysts consist of biliary segments that have become isolated from, and do not communicate with, the biliary tree. When patients present with liver disease, symptoms may result from cyst complications (infection, hemorrhage, torsion, or rupture), mass effect related to cysts (increased intra-abdominal pressure, distention, pain,

biliary duct dilation), or associated hepatobiliary abnormalities, such as hepatic fibrosis, as discussed in the preceding section.

Hepatic biliary cysts are typically round but may be polygonal, and they may be scattered throughout the liver, or they may appear as a string of cysts along portal triads. On ultrasound, one may see echogenic debris due to bile stasis, infection, or hemorrhage complicating the normally anechoic cysts. On CT, the intrahepatic cysts are of lower attenuation than the surrounding parenchyma, usually of uniform attenuation, although of differing size and sharply demarcated from the surrounding parenchyma (Fig. 112-10). On MRI, the cysts have characteristically decreased signal on T1-weighted and increased signal on T2-weighted spin echo sequences, although heterogeneous signal intensity within the cysts, presumably because of hemorrhages of varying age, has been reported.

Microhamartomas

Microhamartomas are small ductlike structures that are lined by biliary epithelium and are considered part of the ductal plate maldevelopment complex. Because of their small size, they are more commonly identified at pathologic examination than on imaging studies. When visible on imaging examinations, they are typically small, although they may be as large as 15 mm in diameter, and typically uniform in size. These characteristics differentiate these structures from hepatic cysts.

Congenital Solitary Cysts

Solitary cysts are uncommon in children. They are benign and usually found incidentally on imaging studies or at surgery. Symptoms may occur when the cysts are large; patients present with a palpable abdominal mass or with obstructive jaundice caused by mass effect on adjacent structures.

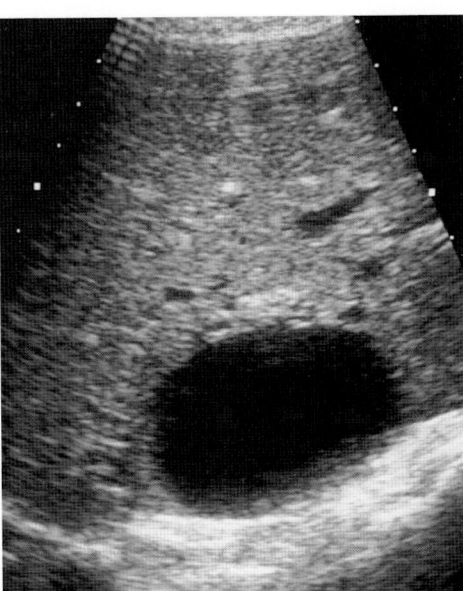

FIGURE 112-11. Hepatic cyst. Longitudinal ultrasound image reveals an asymptomatic simple cyst in the posterior portion of the right hepatic lobe, which was an incidental finding.

Sonography is usually diagnostic, showing an intrahepatic anechoic lesion sharply demarcated from the surrounding liver parenchyma, often incidentally (Fig. 112-11). Rarely, a cyst may be exophytic and extend into the porta hepatis, in which case biliary scintigraphy can be useful in differentiating it from cystic dilation of the biliary tree. The cyst appears as a photopenic area on the hepatic phase and, unlike a choledochal cyst, it does not show increase in activity on delayed scans during the biliary excretion phase on hepatobiliary scintigraphy. Both CT and MRI show the characteristics of a cyst. Neither study is indicated in the workup of a sonographically solitary cyst.

SUGGESTED READINGS

Agenesis of a Hepatic Lobe and Anomalies of the Gallbladder

Coughlin JP, Rector FE, Klein MD: Agenesis of the gallbladder in duodenal atresia: two case reports. J Pediatr Surg 1992;27:1304

Inoue T, Ito Y, Okauchi Y, et al: Hypogenesis of the right hepatic lobe accompanied by portal hypertension: case report and review of 31 Japanese cases. J Gastroenterol 1997;32:836

Ishibashi T, Sato A, Hama H, et al: Liver scarring associated with congenital absence of the right hepatic lobe: CT and MR findings. J Comput Assist Tomogr 1995;19:997

Mortele KJ, Rocha TC, Streeter JL, et al: Multimodality imaging of the pancreatic and biliary congenital anomalies. Radiographics 2006;26:715

Pradeep VM, Ramachandran K, Sasidharan K: Anomalous position of the gallbladder: ultrasonographic and scintigraphic demonstration in four cases. J Clin Ultrasound 1992;20:593

Wu TC, Lee RC, Chiang JH, et al: Reappraisal of left-sided gallbladder and its accompanying anomalies: a report of two cases and literature review. Acta Radiol 2005;46:233

Alagille Syndrome (Arteriohepatic Dysplasia)

Alagille D, Estrada A, Hadchouel M, et al: Syndromic paucity of interlobular bile ducts (Alagille syndrome or arteriohepatic dysplasia): review of 80 cases. J Pediatr 1987;110:195

Emerick KM, Rand EB, Gordmuntz E, et al: Features of Alagille syndrome in 92 patients: frequency and relation to prognosis. Hepatology 1999;29:822

Rachmel A, Zeharia A, Neuman-Levin M, et al: Alagille syndrome associated with moyamoya disease. Am J Med Genet 1989;33:89

Rosenfield NS, Kelley MJ, Jensen PS, et al: Arteriohepatic dysplasia: radiologic features of a new syndrome. AJR Am J Roentgenol 1980;135:1217

Suchy FJ: Neonatal cholestasis. Pediatr Rev 2004;25:388

Fibrocystic Disease, Choledochal Cyst, Caroli Disease

Brancatelli G, Federle MP, Vilgrain V, et al: Fibropolycystic liver disease: CT and MR imaging findings. Radiographics 2005;25:659

Chan YL, Yeung CK, Lam WW, et al: Magnetic resonance cholangiography: feasibility and application in the pediatric population. Pediatr Radiol 1998;28:307

Gupta S, Seith A, Dhiman RK, et al: CT of liver cysts in patients with autosomal dominant polycystic kidney disease. Acta Radiol 1999;40:444

Guy F, Cognet F, Dranssart M, et al: Caroli's disease: Magnetic resonance imaging features. Eur Radiol 2002;12:2730

Horton KM, Bluemke DA, Hruban RH, et al: CT and MR imaging of benign hepatic and biliary tumors. Radiographics 1999;19:431

Johnson K, Alton HM, Chapman S: Evaluation of mebrofenin hepatoscintigraphy in neonatal-onset jaundice. Pediatr Radiol 1998;28:937

Jung G, Benz-Bohm G, Kugel H, et al: MR cholangiography with autosomal recessive polycystic kidney disease. Pediatr Radiol 1999;29:463

Kim OH, Chung HJ, Choi BG: Imaging of the choledochal cyst. Radiographics 1999;15:69

Lam WW, Lam TP, Saing H, et al: MR cholangiography and CT cholangiography of pediatric patients with choledochal cysts. AJR Am J Roentgenol 1999;173:401

Levy AD, Rohrmann CA Jr, Murakata LA, et al: Caroli's disease: radiologic spectrum with pathologic correlation. AJR Am J Roentgenol 2002;179:1053

Lipschitz B, Berdon WE, Defelice AR, Levy J: Association of congenital hepatic fibrosis with autosomal dominant polycystic kidney disease. Pediatr Radiol 1993;23:131

Mas A, Almirall J, Rodriguez A, et al: Microhamartomatosis of the liver associated with autosomal dominant polycystic kidney disease: CT and US appearance. J Comput Assist Tomogr 1994;18:972

O'Neill JA Jr: Choledochal cyst. In O'Neill JA Jr, Rowe MI, Grosfeld JL, et al (eds): Pediatric Surgery, 5th ed. St. Louis, Mosby, 1998:1483-1493

Pirson Y, Lannoy N, Peters D, et al: Isolated polycystic liver disease as a distinct genetic disease, unlinked to polycystic kidney disease 1 and polycystic kidney disease 2. Hepatology 1996;23:249

Sugiyama M, Baba M, Atomi Y, et al: Diagnosis of anomalous pancreatobiliary junction: value of magnetic resonance cholangiopancreatography. Surgery 1998;123:391

Voyles CR, Smadja C, Shands WC, et al: Carcinoma in choledochal cysts: age-related incidence. Arch Surg 1983;118:986

Congenital Solitary Cysts

Athey PA, Lauderman JA, King DE: Case report: massive congenital solitary nonparasitic cyst of the liver in infancy. J Ultrasound Med 1986;5:585

Pliskin A, Cualing H, Stenger RJ: Primary squamous cell carcinoma originating in congenital cysts of the liver: report of a case and review of the literature. Arch Pathol Lab Med 1992;116:105

113

Infections of the Liver

LISA H. LOWE and ALAN E. SCHLESINGER

Viral hepatitis is the most common diffuse infection of the liver in otherwise healthy children. Parasites are more common worldwide, but they typically involve the biliary tree, as in ascariasis, or produce focal infections of the liver, as in echinococcosis or amebiasis. Immuno-compromised patients are most susceptible to various infections, especially fungal.

VIRAL HEPATITIS

Beyond the neonatal period, viral hepatitis is most commonly caused by the hepatitis A, hepatitis B, and hepatitis C viruses. A number of other viruses have been implicated in childhood hepatitis, including mumps, measles, varicella-zoster, herpes simplex, cytomegalo-virus, adenovirus, Coxsackie virus, and Epstein-Barr virus. Most affected patients have a short-lived acute disease with complete recovery. Complications include subacute and chronic active hepatitis, evolution into cirrhosis, and development of hepatocellular carcinoma.

Diagnosis is made clinically and on the basis of lab-oratory data. If imaging is performed during the acute phase of the illness, the liver is often found to be enlarged. Sonography most commonly demonstrates heterogeneity of hepatic parenchymal echogenicity and increased thickness of the portal triads related to peri-portal edema. The wall of the gallbladder may appear thickened, and lymphadenopathy may be present at the porta hepatis (Fig. 113-1). Computed tomography (CT) scans may show heterogeneous changes in attenuation, but they more commonly show hepatomegaly and peri-portal low attenuation. Similarly, magnetic resonance (MR) imaging may show nonspecific increased signal intensity in the periportal region on T2-weighted images, in addition to hepatomegaly. In patients with fulminant hepatitis and subsequent hepatic regeneration, imaging differences have been described between necrotic areas and regenerating nodules. Regions of necrosis have central low attenuation on precontrast CT relative to regions of regeneration. After intravenous (IV) contrast administration, areas of necrosis and regeneration may enhance similarly so that they become indistinguishable, or the regenerating nodules may show diminished enhancement, which can simulate a neoplastic lesion. On MR, areas of nodular regeneration show high signal on T1-weighted and low signal on T2-weighted images relative to adjacent necrotic parenchyma.

Sonography findings in acute viral hepatitis:
- **Heterogeneous increased echogenicity**
- **Periportal edema with increased periportal echogenicity**
- **Thickening of gallbladder wall**
- **Periportal lymphadenopathy**

PYOGENIC ABSCESS

Pyogenic infection with hepatic abscess formation is most commonly found in immunocompromised patients. Patients with chronic granulomatous disease of child-hood, a syndrome of leukocyte dysfunction, or those who have had bone marrow transplantation are at high risk for pyogenic abscesses. Other susceptible patients are those on immunosuppressive chemotherapy, those with congenital or acquired immunodeficiency states, and those with intra-abdominal infection, such as appendici-tis and inflammatory bowel disease. *Staphylococcus aureus* is the most common pathogen secondary to hemato-genous spread to the liver. In more than 50% of cases, multiple microorganisms are found in hepatic abscesses. Blood cultures may be normal or may contain pathogens that differ from those aspirated from the abscess.

Risk factors for pyogenic liver infection:
- **Chronic granulomatous disease**
- **Bone marrow transplant**
- **Immunosuppressive chemotherapy**
- **Congenital or acquired immunodeficiency**
- **Appendicitis or other intra-abdominal infection**

Hepatic abscesses are most common in the right lobe of the liver, and approximately 50% are solitary. The imaging appearance of hepatic abscesses is variable, but they are readily detected on imaging studies. Hepatic abscesses range from single, well-defined, homogeneous, circular masses, to heterogeneous, poorly defined, multi-loculated, septated, debris- or gas-filled masses. Air-fluid levels are found in less than 20% of cases and should raise concern for gastrointestinal connection. Enhanced

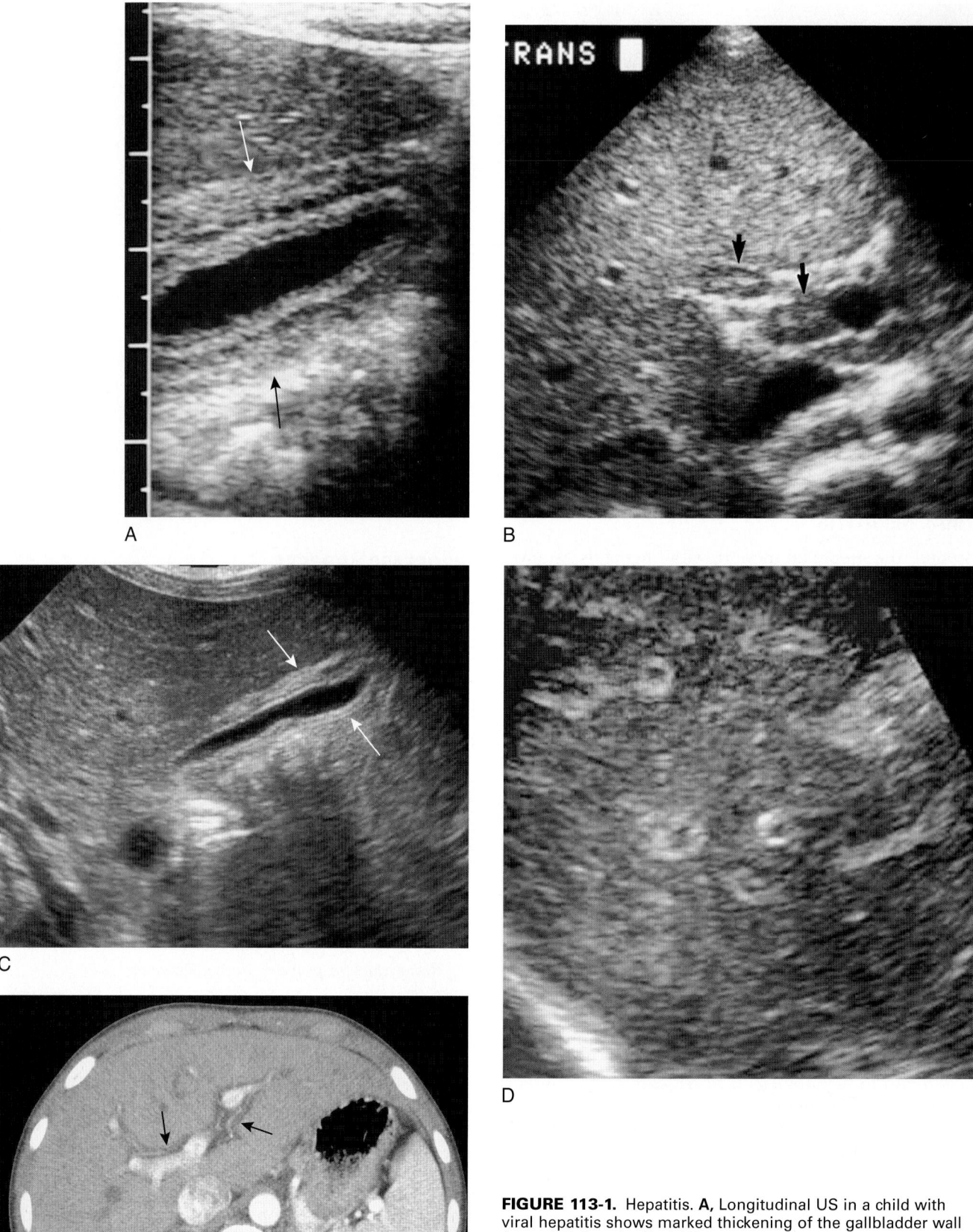

FIGURE 113-1. Hepatitis. **A,** Longitudinal US in a child with viral hepatitis shows marked thickening of the gallbladder wall *(arrow).* **B,** Longitudinal US image through the porta hepatis in another child with hepatitis reveals periportal lymphadenopathy *(arrows).* **C** to **E,** Hepatitis caused by cytomegalovirus. Sonograms show gallbladder wall thickening *(arrows* in **C)** and periportal edema **(D),** seen as increased echogenicity at the portal triads. **E,** CT with intravenous contrast confirms periportal edema *(arrows)* and shows diffusely diminished hepatic attenuation.

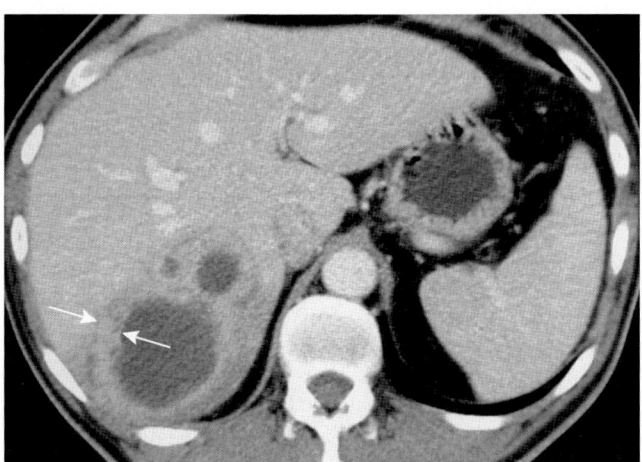

FIGURE 113-2. Liver abscess in a 12-year-old girl receiving steroids for treatment of inflammatory bowel disease. CT scan shows a multiloculated hypoattenuating abscess in the right lobe of the liver, with a thick enhancing capsule (*arrows*) and surrounding low-attenuation edema.

through-transmission on gray scale sonography, lack of central flow with Doppler sonography, and lack of central enhancement on CT are useful findings for confirming a cystic rather than solid lesion. Contrast-enhanced CT shows peripheral enhancement of the wall, at times surrounded by a low-attenuation ring of edema (Fig. 113-2). Abscesses in patients with chronic granulomatous disease may heal with formation of granulomas, which frequently calcify. MR images of hepatic abscesses typically show decreased or nearly isointense signal on T1-weighted images, increased signal on T2-weighted images, and a peripheral ring of contrast enhancement.

Sonography findings in pyogenic liver abscess:
- **Common**
  - **Hypoechoic cystic mass with increased through-transmission**
  - **Surrounding hypoechoic ring of edema**
  - **Internal debris**
- **Less common**
  - **Hyperechoic mass with increased through-transmission**
  - **Anechoic mass**
  - **Fluid-debris levels**
  - **Septations**
- **Common CT findings in pyogenic liver abscess**
  - **Low attenuation relative to hepatic parenchyma after contrast enhancement**
  - **Enhancing abscess wall**
  - **Low-attenuation hepatic edema surrounding abscess**

Multiple abscesses are most commonly the result of biliary disease, biliary obstruction, or hepatic trauma. Hematogenous spread of pyogenic organisms may result in multiple abscesses (Fig. 113-3). Tuberculous abscess cannot be differentiated on imaging studies from other pyogenic infections. Resolved tuberculosis may result in hepatic calcifications.

Treatment of pyogenic abscesses ranges from antibiotics alone for small lesions (usually <5 cm) to percutaneous aspiration and catheter drainage for larger lesions. Percutaneous abscess drainage, often performed under sonographic or CT guidance, is successful in 85% to 90% of patients. The techniques used for children are the same as those used for adults, although IV sedation or general anesthesia may be necessary for children. Hepatic abscesses often have an insidious presentation, leading to a delay in diagnosis. With the introduction of cross-sectional imaging and earlier diagnosis, mortality rates have dropped from 32% to 2%. Amebic abscess should be excluded before percutaneous intervention, as only IV antibiotics are required for their treatment. The rare complications that occur after percutaneous drainage include bleeding, peritonitis, and, less often, septicemia, pneumothorax, and empyema. Surgical drainage is used only if catheter drainage fails or treatment of an underlying cause of abscess is required, such as biliary tree stenosis with stent placement.

FUNGAL INFECTIONS

Fungal infection also occurs most frequently in immunocompromised patients, particularly those with acquired immunodeficiency syndrome (AIDS), leukemia, lymphoma, and lymphoproliferative disorders. The most common causative organism is *Candida albicans*, but other ubiquitous fungi, such as *Aspergillus*, *Histoplasma*, *Coccidioides immitis* (in endemic areas), and *Nocardia* have been identified in fungal hepatitis.

Candida may affect any organ system. The imaging appearance depends on the host's immune response. In neutropenic patients, disease is microscopic and lesions are occult on imaging. Formation of microabscesses is possible when the patient recovers from neutropenia and mounts an immune response.

On sonography, four imaging patterns of candidiasis within the liver are reported. All four have multiple, small (<3- to 4-mm) lesions scattered diffusely throughout the liver parenchyma. Early in the disease process, the wheel-within-a-wheel appearance is seen, representing a hyperechoic nidus of necrotic fungus, surrounded by echogenic inflammatory cells, in turn surrounded by a peripheral zone of fibrosis. The bull's-eye or target appearance, consisting of an echogenic center with a hypoechoic rim, is seen when the host mounts an immune response. The most common appearance is seen later and consists of diffuse uniform hypoechoic foci throughout the liver resulting from formation of tiny microabscesses (<4 mm) and fibrosis (Fig. 113-4). Last is the pattern of calcified, hyperechoic tiny foci in healed or healing candidiasis (1 to 4 mm) (Fig. 113-5).

CT findings are nonspecific and include multiple foci of low attenuation and of variable size (2 to 20 mm), with or without peripheral enhancement and calcification. MR imaging may reveal tiny lesions missed with CT, but the appearance is nonspecific compared with the more distinct patterns found on sonography.

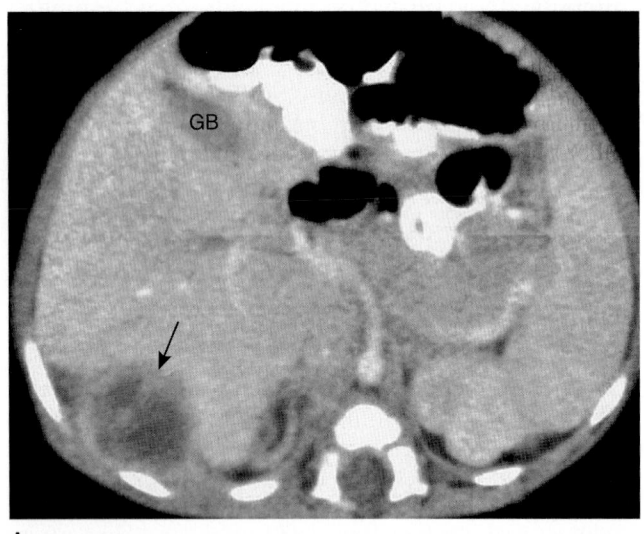

A

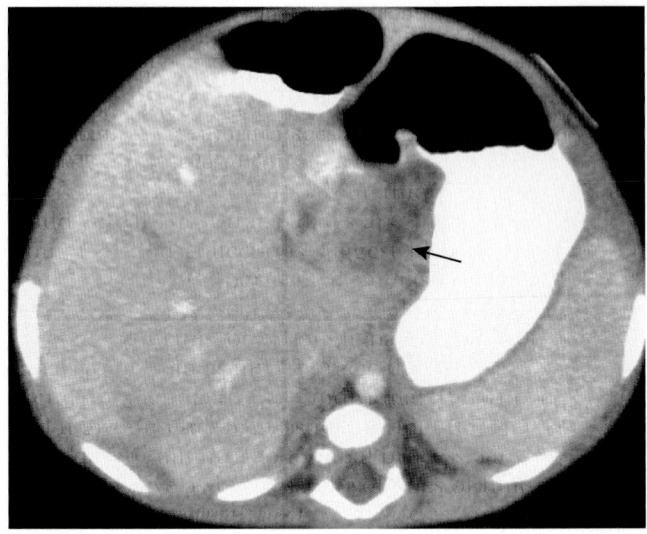

B

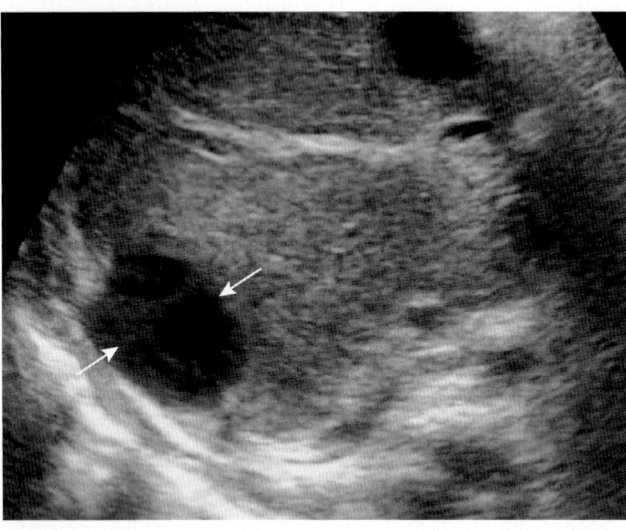

C

FIGURE 113-3. Multiple hepatic abscesses. **A** and **B,** CT images with intravenous contrast material show a multiseptated abscess in the right lobe of the liver (*arrow* in **A**), and a second lesion in the left lobe (*arrow* in **B**). GB, gallbladder. **C,** Transverse sonogram of lesion shown in **A** reveals a hypoechoic, multiseptated lesion in the right lobe of the liver (*arrows*).

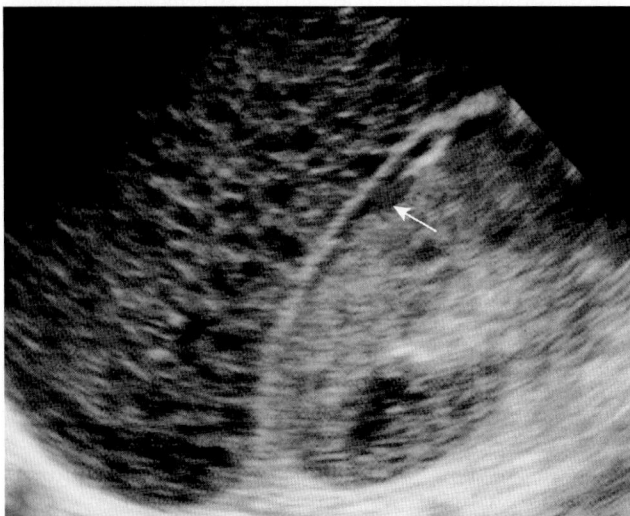

FIGURE 113-4. Hepatic candidiasis. Longitudinal sonogram shows diffuse, homogeneous, hypoechoic foci consistent with microabscesses throughout the liver. Tiny amount of fluid in Morrison pouch is noted *(arrow)* adjacent to the right kidney.

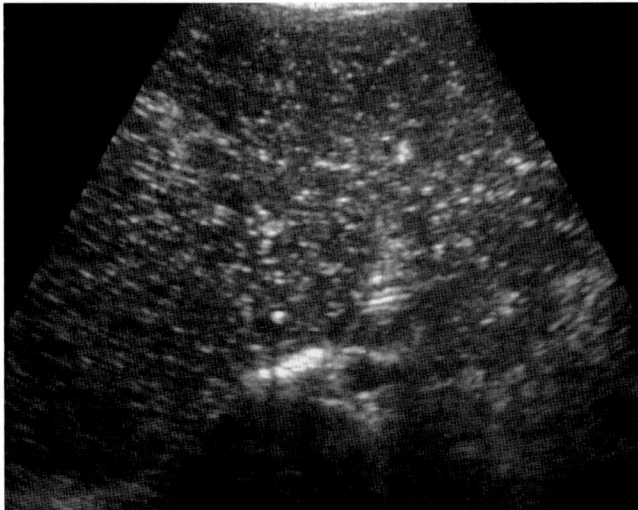

FIGURE 113-5. Hepatic candidiasis. Transverse sonogram of the liver shows tiny discrete foci of punctate hyperechogenicity resulting from extensive diffuse calcified microabscesses in a child with severe combined immune deficiency syndrome.

CAT-SCRATCH DISEASE

Cat-scratch disease, caused by *Bartonella henselae* (a gram-negative bacillus), is a self-limited infection transmitted to the patient's lymphatic system by a cat scratch. It most often involves the lymph nodes, and in 5% to 10% of cases it spreads systemically to involve the liver, spleen, bone, and, less often, the brain.

Children usually present with painful lymphadenopathy; however, systemic spread may cause low-grade fever and various complaints related to the involvement of virtually any organ system. It is important to elicit a history of recent contact or exposure to a cat or kitten. The typical course of cat-scratch disease involves formation of granulomas, which heal spontaneously and may calcify. Diagnosis of cat-scratch disease with an indirect serum fluorescent antibody assay of blood and tissue is 85% to 100% sensitive and specific. Definitive diagnosis requires biopsy to detect organism DNA, but it is rarely performed.

Sonography of a patient with cat-scratch disease reveals numerous small hypoechoic, well-marginated, circular, homogeneous foci within the liver or spleen, in many cases associated with lymphadenopathy (Fig. 113-6). On CT, small lesions (<3 cm) of low attenuation are found before contrast administration. Variable attenuation is seen after contrast, and there is often marginal enhancement. Skeletal lesions may demonstrate increased activity on bone scintigraphy. On plain radiographs, skeletal lesions are lytic when visible. Brain parenchymal involvement is rare but most often shows multifocal nonspecific areas of bright signal intensity on T2-weighted sequences.

> **Cat-scratch disease:**
> - **Self-limited infection**
> - **Caused by *Bartonella henselae***
> - **Multifocal lesions in liver and spleen**
> - **Adenopathy**

PARASITIC INFESTATIONS

Ascariasis

Ascariasis, an intestinal infection caused by *Ascaris lumbricoides,* is the most common human worm infestation in the world. Rare in the United States, ascariasis is most prevalent in regions of the world with poor sanitation. It occurs when eggs are ingested, growing into larvae and

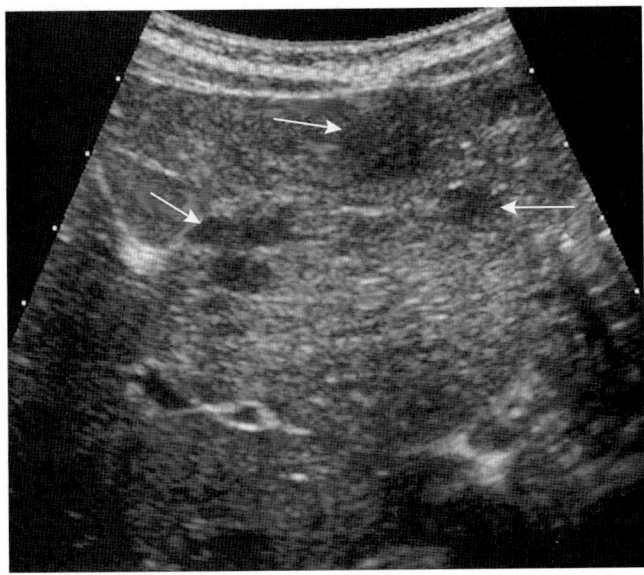

A

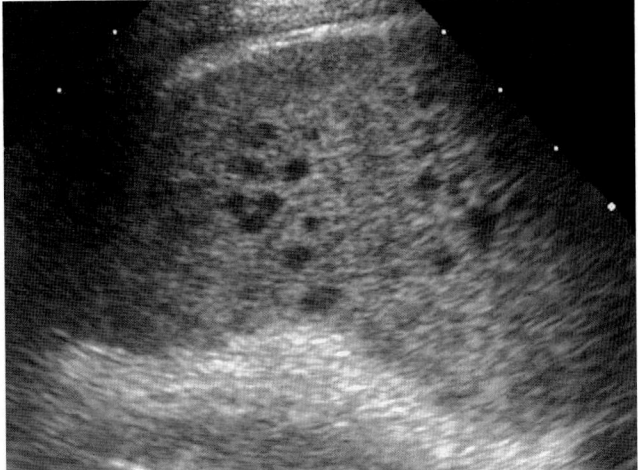

B

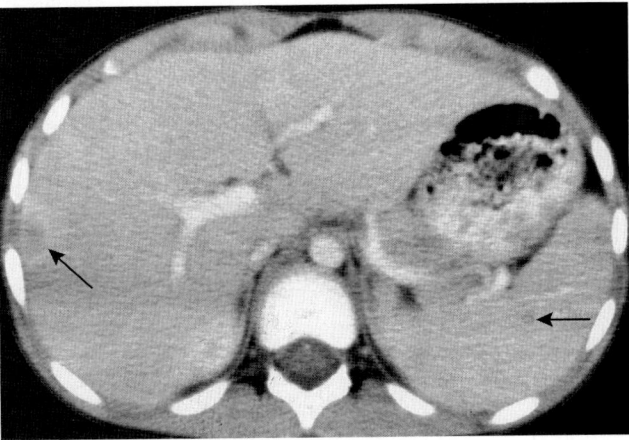

C

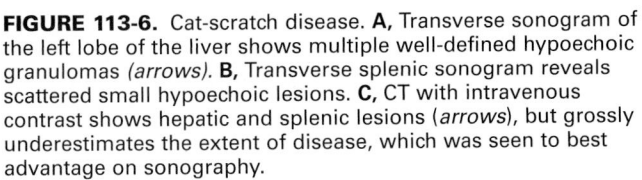

FIGURE 113-6. Cat-scratch disease. **A,** Transverse sonogram of the left lobe of the liver shows multiple well-defined hypoechoic granulomas *(arrows).* **B,** Transverse splenic sonogram reveals scattered small hypoechoic lesions. **C,** CT with intravenous contrast shows hepatic and splenic lesions *(arrows),* but grossly underestimates the extent of disease, which was seen to best advantage on sonography.

then pencil-shaped round worms within the intestine. Larvae that penetrate through the intestinal wall enter the bloodstream and travel to the liver and may continue on to the lungs. Symptoms depend on the organ involved and are caused by mass effect of the larvae and adult worms. Worms may obstruct the biliary system, causing dilation and pain as well as risk for bacterial superinfection. On imaging studies, the characteristic vermiform (worm-shaped) defects are seen inside the small intestine and dilated biliary ducts. The worms are echogenic on sonography. Treatment with antiparasitic medications is usually effective, with rapid improvement of symptoms.

Echinococcosis

Echinococcosis (hydatid disease) is an infestation by the larval form of two main varieties of *Echinococcus* tapeworms. The disease is worldwide in distribution, with the major endemic regions being the Middle East, Mediterranean nations, and all sheep-grazing countries. *Echinococcus granulosus* is more common than *Echinococcus multilocularis*.

The definitive host is the dog and other carnivores; ruminants, particularly sheep, are intermediate hosts. Humans become infected when they ingest the eggs of the parasite from food or water contaminated with fecal material from the definitive host. The larvae are released after ingestion of the eggs, and they pass through the duodenal mucosa into portal venous radicles, to become lodged in the liver. In the liver, the embryos may die or slowly, over a period of years, grow to produce hydatid cystic disease. The embryos that can cross the hepatic capillary bed proceed to, and enter, the lungs. The liver is the most common organ of involvement. In less than 5% of cases, hematogenous dissemination may lead to pulmonary disease, and less often to splenic, renal, adrenal, musculoskeletal, or cerebral disease.

The imaging appearances of *E. granulosus* and *E. multilocularis* are different. *E. granulosus* forms a cyst with three histopathologic layers. The outer pericyst is a tough, collagenous outer membrane formed by the host response to the parasite; the ectocyst is an acellular, thin, lucent and easily ruptured membrane; the endocyst, or germinal layer, is the layer from which brood capsules and scolices are secreted into cyst fluid, forming hydatid sand. Daughter cysts may arise from brood capsules along the periphery of the endocyst. Hydatid cysts may be single or multiple, and an individual cyst may appear multilocular because of internal daughter cysts (Fig. 113-7). The right lobe is most commonly involved. Superinfection occurs only after cyst rupture, because the intact ectocyst is resistant to bacterial invasion. Cyst rupture may be clinically silent or may result in eosinophilia or anaphylaxis.

Echinococcal cysts have been classified into three types, reflecting cyst contents and findings during various stages of development. Type I cysts are simple fluid-filled cysts without matrix or daughter cysts. Type I cysts may, however, contain a central undulating membrane resulting from the disproportionate growth of endocyst and ectocyst within the rigid pericyst. Type II cysts contain daughter cysts or internal matrix. Type III cysts have peripheral pericyst calcification or internal calcification as a result of parasite death (Fig. 113-8).

CT can be used to characterize the cyst type, and it may show peripheral enhancement or adjacent bile duct enlargement resulting from mass effect or rupture into the biliary tree. Cyst rupture can occur at any stage of development. When the rupture is contained, the delaminated endocyst membrane may be seen as a wavy floating central band, known as the "water lily" sign. Rupture into adjacent liver allows formation of new juxtaposed hydatid cysts. Rupture of both the endocyst and the pericyst allows spillage of cyst contents into the peritoneal cavity, which often leads to life-threatening anaphylaxis.

On MR images, hydatid cyst fluid is hypointense to isointense on T1-weighted and hyperintense on T2-weighted sequences. If the lesion is multilocular, the mother cyst tends to have higher signal than the daughter cysts on T2-weighted images. A low-signal-intensity rim of fibrotic pericyst tissue is suggestive of *Echinococcus*. The fibrous pericyst is of low signal intensity on T1-weighted and T2-weighted MR imaging sequences. High signal within the cyst on T1-weighted images (a result of lipid or protein macromolecules) suggests the possibility of a cyst rupture into the biliary tree, or infection.

In general, treatment of echinococcal cysts requires removal of the entire cyst and its contents. Previously thought to be inadvisable, percutaneous aspiration and drainage with a large-bore catheter (14 French) is now the treatment of choice. Exophytic cysts or those associated with bile duct dilation may not be amenable to percutaneous drainage, in which case surgical resection is needed. However, the diagnosis of echinococcal cysts must be made serologically before percutaneous drainage, because the differential diagnosis includes uncomplicated amebic and small pyogenic abscesses, which are treated with medical therapy alone.

E. multilocularis, which is less common than *E. granulosus*, shows different imaging features. Common features of *E. multilocularis* include irregular hepatomegaly, multiple lesions with increased echogenicity on sonography, decreased attenuation on CT, microcalcifications, and dilation of intrahepatic bile ducts. Involvement of parahepatic structures, portal hypertension, and involvement of the spleen, hepatic veins, and inferior vena cava are also described.

Amebic Abscess

The protozoan *Entamoeba histolytica* colonizes 10% of the world population and causes death in 100,000 people per year, especially in developing countries. In the United States, about 1200 cases occur per year. Less than 10% of affected persons become symptomatic, but 3% to 8.5% of clinically symptomatic patients develop liver abscess. Amebic abscesses are most often solitary (85%) and are often found within the right lobe of the liver (75%). The infection is primarily intestinal, with diarrhea and dysentery at presentation. The liver may be involved secondary to spread via the portal vein. Extension across the diaphragm to involve the lungs is not uncommon.

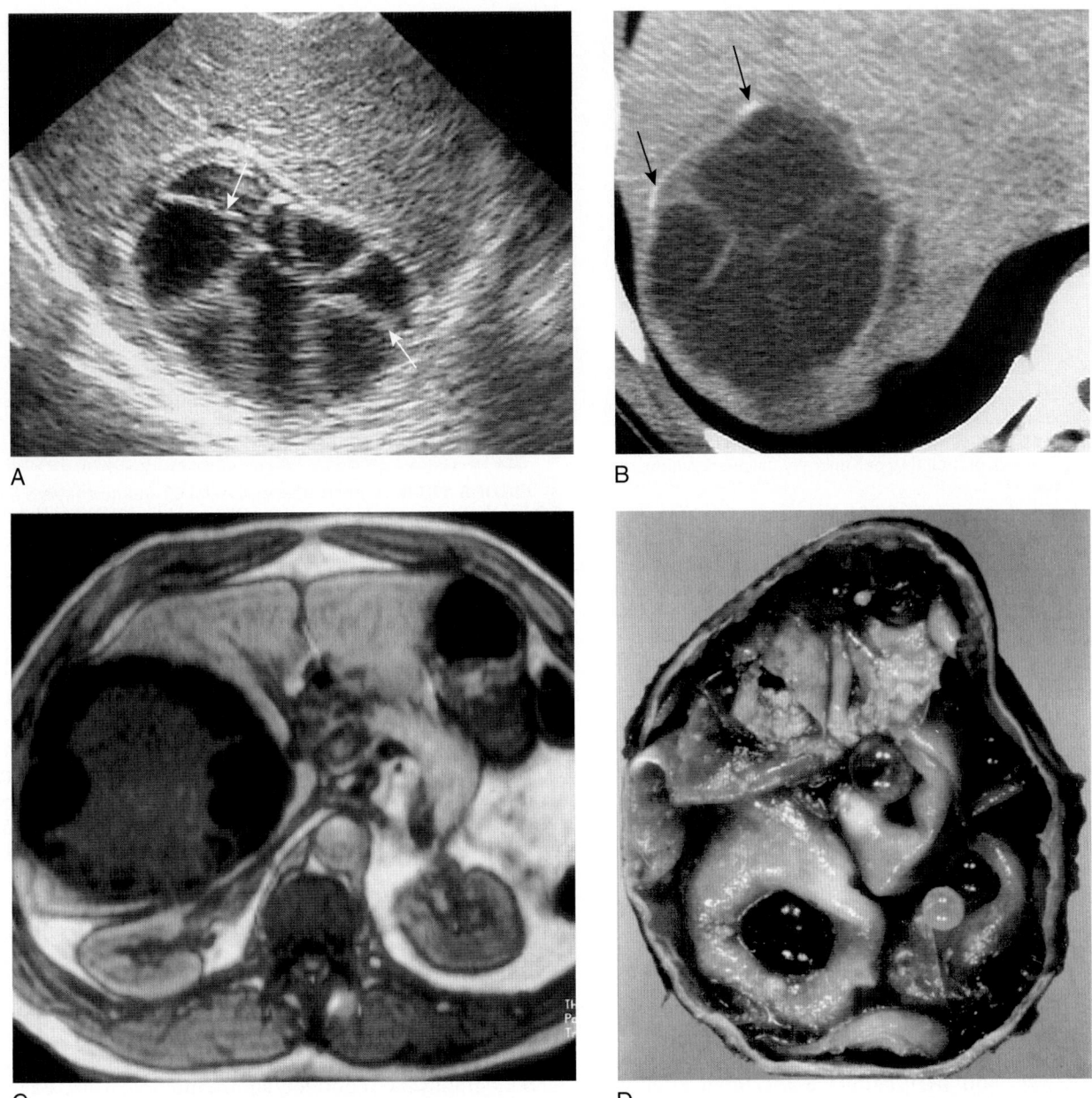

FIGURE 113-7. Echinococcal (hydatid) cyst. **A,** Longitudinal hepatic sonogram shows a well-defined multiseptated (*arrows*), multilocular lesion. **B,** Axial unenhanced CT image of the liver confirms the cystic mass with multiple septations and peripheral calcification *(arrows)*. **C,** Axial T1-weighted gradient echo MR image shows a hepatic hydatid cyst with a hypointense fibrous pericyst, and extensive peripheral low-signal-intensity daughter cysts surrounding central intermediate-signal-intensity material that was bright on T2-weighted images (not shown). **D,** Gross specimen of resected hydatid cyst reveals numerous daughter cysts intermingled with wavy endocyst. (From Mortele KJ, Segatto E, Ros PR: The infected liver: radiologic-pathologic correlation. Radiographics 2004;24:937-955.) (*See color plate.*)

Other extraintestinal sites of amebic disease are rare but include the brain, skin, and genital disease.

Amebic abscesses can occur at any age, but in children they are most common at less than age 3 years. The presentation of hepatic amebic abscesses is usually acute in children, with right upper quadrant pain resulting from cyst rupture or mass effect. Treatment of amebic abscesses is medical only, in contradistinction to pyogenic abscesses, which may require percutaneous or surgical drainage. Amebic abscesses are diagnosed in 90% of patients with a positive hemagglutination test or amebic titers. Stool examination is unreliable. If the diagnosis of amebic abscess is likely but difficult to confirm, empiric antibiotic treatment is useful because the patient usually defervesces and clinically improves quickly.

The cross-sectional imaging appearance of amebic abscesses is variable and depends on the stage of disease. Sonography, the initial imaging modality of choice, reveals a homogeneous round or oval mass with internal debris. Lesions are usually peripheral in location near the

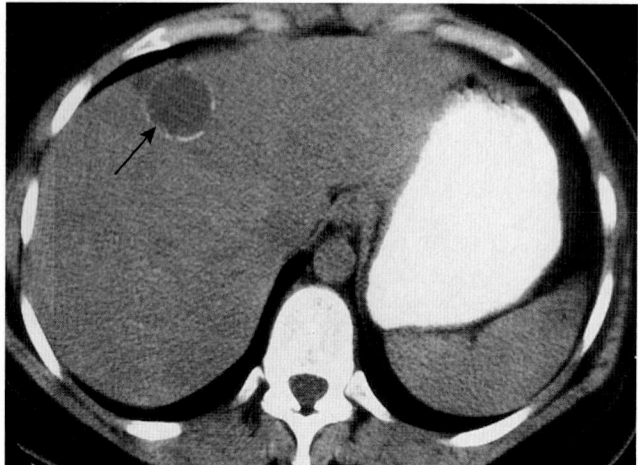

FIGURE 113-8. Echinococcal (hydatid) cyst. Axial unenhanced CT image shows an inactive peripherally calcified echinococcal cyst *(arrow)*.

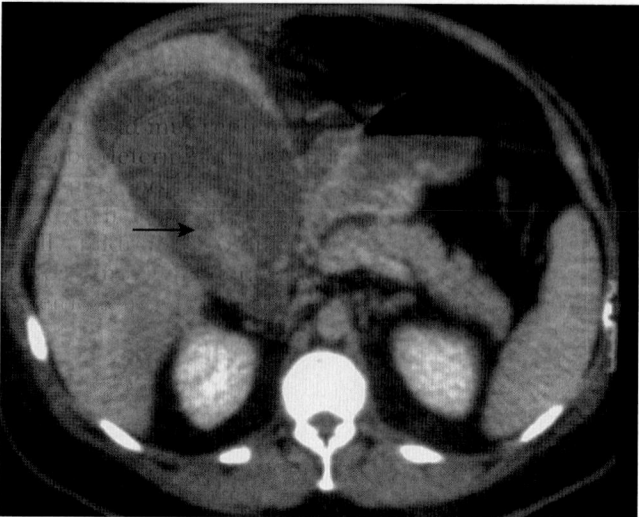

FIGURE 113-9. Amebic abscess. Axial CT image shows a large, exophytic low-attenuation cyst with hyperdense central debris *(arrow)*.

hepatic capsule and have enhanced through-transmission. Early in the course of the lesion, the amebic abscess may be hyperechoic and could be mistaken for a solid mass. However, no internal flow is identified on Doppler interrogation. CT shows a low-attenuation area with peripheral enhancement and a rim of surrounding edema, and it may show internal septations (Fig. 113-9).

> **Ultrasound findings in amebic abscess:**
> - **Peripheral location in contact with liver capsule**
> - **Round or oval hypoechoic lesions with increased through-transmission**
> - **Subtle low-level echoes within lesion**
> - **Peripheral hypoechoic "halo"**

MR imaging of amebic abscesses shows heterogeneous low signal intensity on T1-weighted and high signal intensity on T2-weighted sequences with a double-layered wall, and peripheral enhancement after gadolinium administration. Perforation of amebic abscesses and intraperitoneal spread may occur in up to 35% of cases. Percutaneous aspiration may be useful if impending rupture is an immediate clinical concern. Surgery is reserved for complicated cases, including those that fail medical therapy. More than 90% of patients do well with prolonged antibiotic therapy (most often metronidazole). The initial response to antibiotics is generally rapid, and failure to respond in 24 to 72 hours may indicate superimposed bacterial infection, which occurs in 15% of patients.

Schistosomiasis

Schistosomiasis, a rare disease in North America, affects 200 million people worldwide. Three forms affect humans, *Schistosoma japonicum, Schistosoma mansoni,* and *Schistosoma hematobium.* Infection results from bathing in contaminated waters; humans are the definitive hosts. Mature female worms swim against blood flow to the venules of the urinary bladder (*S. hematobium*) or gastrointestinal tract (*S. mansoni* and *S. japonicum*) to deposit eggs. Eggs deposited in the gastrointestinal tract spread via the mesenteric venules to the portal vein, where they incite an inflammatory granulomatous response, resulting in fibrosis and presinusoidal portal hypertension. Schistosomiasis may remain in the portal system for up to 10 years and may live in the definitive host for up to 30 years.

Little information is known about the imaging findings of acute-phase hepatic schistosomiasis infection. Sonography has reportedly shown multiple scattered hypoechoic foci within the liver and spleen and associated adenopathy. Changes of chronic hepatic involvement resulting from septal fibrosis and calcification are seen on ultrasound, CT (Fig. 113-10), and MR imaging. On CT, dense fibrous and calcific septa distributed at right angles to the hepatic surface produce the classic CT appearance of "turtle back calcification" in *S. japonicum* infection. MR imaging may show isointense periportal bands on T1-weighted images, which are bright on T2-weighted images and enhance after gadolinium contrast administration.

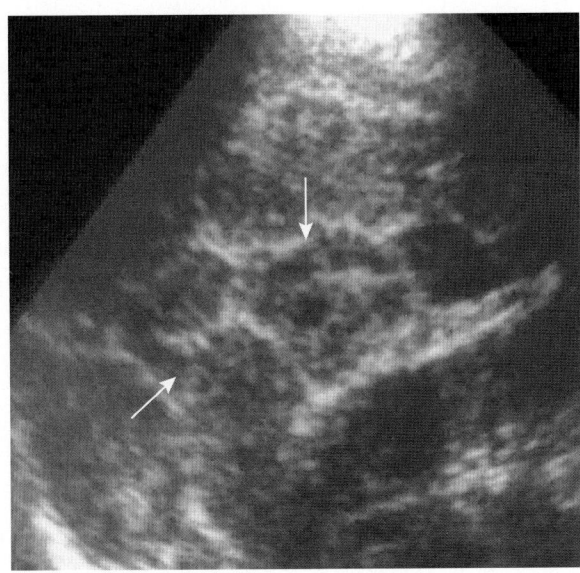
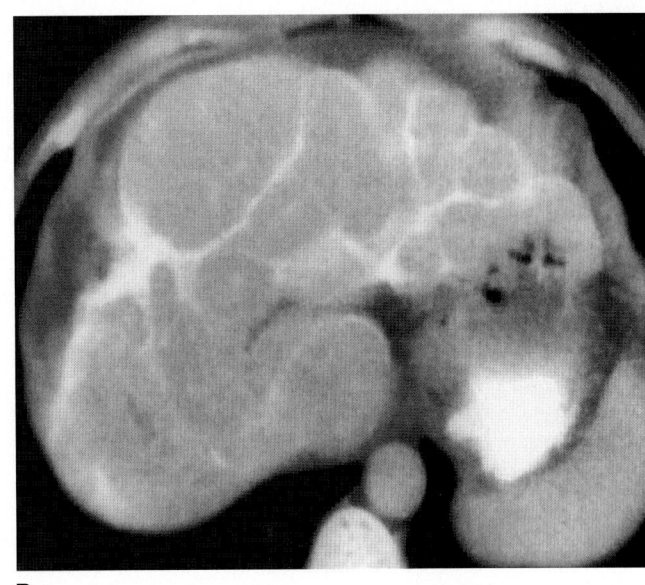

A   B

FIGURE 113-10. Schistosomiasis. **A,** Longitudinal sonogram of the right lobe of liver reveals hyperechoic septations *(arrows)* between polygonal areas of hepatic parenchyma. **B,** Axial CT image of the liver confirms characteristic "turtle back" or "tortoise shell" appearance of the liver resulting from septal fibrosis with calcification. (From Mortele KJ, Segatto E, Ros PR: The infected liver: radiologic-pathologic correlation. Radiographics 2004;24:937-955.)

SUGGESTED READINGS

Viral Hepatitis

Itoh H, Sakai T, Takahashi N, et al: Periportal high intensity on T2-weighted MR images in acute viral hepatitis. J Comput Assist Tomogr 1992;16:564

Murakami T, Baron RL, Peterson MS: Liver necrosis and regeneration after fulminant hepatitis: pathologic correlation with CT and MR findings. Radiology 1996;198:239

Murat A, Akarsu S, Cihangiroglu M, et al: Assessment of Doppler wave form patterns and flow velocities of hepatic veins in children with acute viral hepatitis. Diagn Interv Radiol 2006;12:85

Siegel MJ, Herman TE: Periportal low attenuation at CT in childhood. Radiology 1992;183:685

Pyogenic Abscess

Barnes PF, De Cock KM, Reynolds TN: A comparison of amebic and pyogenic abscess of the liver. Medicine 1987;66:472

Cerwinka H, Bacher H, Werkgartner G, et al: Treatment of patients with pyogenic liver abscess. Chemotherapy 2005;51:366

Francis IR, Glazer GM, Amendola MA, et al: Hepatic abscesses in the immunocompromised patient: role of CT in detection, diagnosis, management, and follow-up. Gastrointest Radiol 1986;11:257

Garel LA, Pariente DM, Nezelof C, et al: Liver involvement in chronic granulomatous disease: the role of ultrasound in diagnosis and treatment. Radiology 1984;153:117

Mortele KJ, Segatto E, Ros PR: The infected liver: radiologic-pathologic correlation. Radiographics 2004;24:937-955

Fungal Infections

Grünebaum M, Ziv N, Kaplinsky C, et al: Liver candidiasis: the various sonographic patterns in the immunocompromised child. Pediatr Radiol 1991;21:497

Lin PC, Chang TT, Jang RC, et al: Hepatosplenic microabscesses in pediatric leukemia: a report of five cases: Kaohsiung J Med Sci 2003;19:368

Miller JH, Greenfield LD, Wald BR: Candidiasis of the liver and spleen in childhood. Radiology 1982;142:375

Cat-Scratch Disease

Hopkins KL, Simoneaux SF, Patrick LE, et al: Imaging manifestations of cat-scratch disease. AJR Am J Roentgenol 1996;166:435

Mortele KJ, Segatto E, Ros PR: The infected liver: radiologic-pathologic correlation. Radiographics 2004;24:937-955

Ascariasis

Akata D, Ozmen MN, Kaya A, et al: Radiological findings of intraparenchymal liver Ascaris (hepatobiliary ascariasis). Eur Radiol 1999;9:93

Bahu Mda G, Baldisseroto M, Custodio CM, et al: Hepatobiliary and pancreatic complications of ascariasis in children: a study of seven cases. J Pediatr Gastroenterol Nutr 2001;33:271

Koumanidou C, Manoli E, Anagnostara A, et al: Sonographic features of intestinal and biliary ascariasis in childhood: case report and review of the literature. Ann Trop Paediatr 2004;24:329

Ng KK, Wong HF, Kong MS, et al: Biliary ascariasis: CT, MR cholangiopancreatography, and navigator endoscopic appearance: report of a case of acute biliary obstruction. Abdom Imaging 1999;24:470

Echinococcus (Hydatid Disease)

Coskun A, Ozturk M, Korahan OI, et al: Alveolar echinococcus of the liver: correlative color Doppler US, CT, and MRI study. Acta Radiol 2004;45:492

Etlik O, Bay A, Arslan H, et al: Contrast enhanced CT and MRI findings of atypical hepatic echinococcus alveolaris infestation. Pediatr Radiol 2005;35:546

Goktay AY, Secil M, Gulcu A, et al: Percutaneous treatment of hydatid liver cysts in children as a primary treatment: long-term results. J Vasc Interv Radiol 2005;16:831

Mortele KJ, Segatto E, Ros PR: The infected liver: radiologic-pathologic correlation. Radiographics 2004;24:937-955

Polat P, Kantarci M, Alper F, et al: Hydatid disease from head to toe. Radiographics 2003;23:475

Amebic Abscess

Balci NC, Sirvanci M: MR imaging of infective liver lesions. Magn Reson Imaging Clin N Am 2002;10:121-135

Kimura K, Stoopen M, Reeder MM, et al: Amebiasis: modern diagnostic imaging with pathological and clinical correlation. Semin Roentgenol 1997;32:250

Kurland JE, Brann OS: Pyogenic and amebic liver abscesses. Curr Gastroenterol Rep 2004;6:273

Mortele KJ, Segatto E, Ros PR: The infected liver: radiologic-pathologic correlation. Radiographics 2004;24:937-955

Oleszczuk-Raszke K, Cremin FJ, Fisher RM, et al: Ultrasonic features of pyogenic and amoebic hepatic abscesses. Pediatr Radiol 1989;19:230

Schistosomiasis

Balci NC, Sirvanci M: MR imaging of infective liver lesions. Magn Reson Imaging Clin N Am 2002;10:121-135

Cesmeli E, Vogelaers D, Voet D, et al: Ultrasound and CT changes of liver parenchyma in acute schistosomiasis. Br J Radiol 1997;70:758

Mortele KJ, Segatto E, Ros PR: The infected liver: radiologic-pathologic correlation. Radiographics 2004;24:937-955

Palmer PE: Schistosomiasis. Semin Roentgenol 1998;33:6

CHAPTER 114

Diffuse Parenchymal Disease

LISA H. LOWE

Many conditions cause diffuse imaging abnormalities in the liver. Although some of these entities are congenital, the hepatic manifestations are acquired as complications of the disease process or its treatment.

FATTY LIVER

Fatty replacement of the liver (steatosis) may be due to a variety of metabolic disorders and hepatic toxins (Table 114-1). Metabolic derangements include obesity and extreme malnutrition, cystic fibrosis, exogenous or endogenous steroids (e.g., Cushing syndrome), familial hyperlipoproteinemia, glycogen storage disease, total parenteral nutrition, Wilson disease, Reye syndrome, poorly controlled diabetes mellitus, severe hepatitis, chronic tuberculosis, chronic congestive heart failure, and, rarely, trauma. Hepatic toxins are more often encountered in adults and include alcohol, carbon toxins, phosphorus, chemotherapy, and amiodarone. Fatty infiltration may be diffuse or localized; further,

islands of uninvolved parenchyma, or focal fatty sparing, may be present within livers with generalized steatosis.

Depending on the cause of the condition, liver function test results may be normal. Hepatomegaly is common (75% of cases). Changes associated with fatty liver may be insidious or may evolve rapidly in a few days to months. Histologically, hepatocytes contain large cytoplasmic fat vacuoles filled with triglycerides. Pathologic diagnosis of hepatic steatosis is made when more than 5% of the total liver weight is replaced by fat.

As noted, focal fatty sparing is seen occasionally and should not be mistaken for a mass. On sonography, focal sparing is hypoechoic relative to surrounding fatty liver and demonstrates no mass effect. On computed tomography (CT) and magnetic resonance imaging (MRI), it maintains normal attenuation and signal intensity, respectively, relative to adjacent changes of fatty liver, and shows no mass effect.

Imaging findings in hepatic steatosis include hepatomegaly; on plain radiographs, the liver may appear lucent in severe cases, but radiographs are otherwise nonspecific. On sonography, fatty infiltration leads to increased hepatic echogenicity, poor parenchymal penetration requiring lower frequency transducers, and poor definition of hepatic vascular borders (Fig. 114-1). On CT, liver attenuation is diminished 10 Hounsfield units or greater compared with the spleen on unenhanced scans, and 25 Hounsfield units or greater after intravenous contrast administration (see Fig. 114-1). In severe cases, hepatic parenchymal attenuation is less than that of the vascular structures, leading to an angiographic effect on unenhanced scans. If fatty infiltration is focal rather than generalized, differences in echogenicity are seen on sonography; on CT, the difference in attenuation is more pronounced after intravenous contrast enhancement (Fig. 114-2). Sonography and CT are 85% to 97% accurate in diagnosing fatty liver. Conventional spin echo MRI of hepatic steatosis is less sensitive; fatty replacement of 10% of the liver weight is required to alter the parenchymal signal intensity by only 5% to 10%. Characteristic MRI findings include increased signal intensity on T1-weighted images and decreased signal intensity on fat-saturated or short tau inversion recovery images. However, chemical shift imaging, with in-phase and out-of-phase images, is highly specific in terms of diagnosing fatty infiltration and differentiating this condition from neoplastic disease in confusing or equivocal cases, parti-

TABLE 114-1

Causes of Hepatic Steatosis

Metabolic and genetic disorders
  Obesity
  Extreme malnutrition
  Total parenteral nutrition
  Cystic fibrosis
  Steroids (exogenous and endogenous; e.g., Cushing syndrome)
  Familial hyperlipoproteinemia
  Glycogen storage disease
  Wilson disease
  Galactosemia
  Reye syndrome
  Severe hepatitis
  Poorly controlled diabetes mellitus
  Chronic tuberculosis
  Chronic congestive heart failure
Hepatotoxins (mostly adults)
  Alcohol
  Chemotherapy
  Carbon toxins
  Phosphorus
  Amiodarone

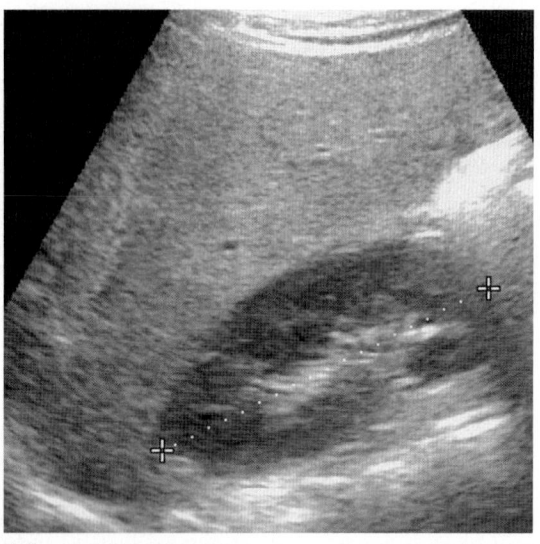
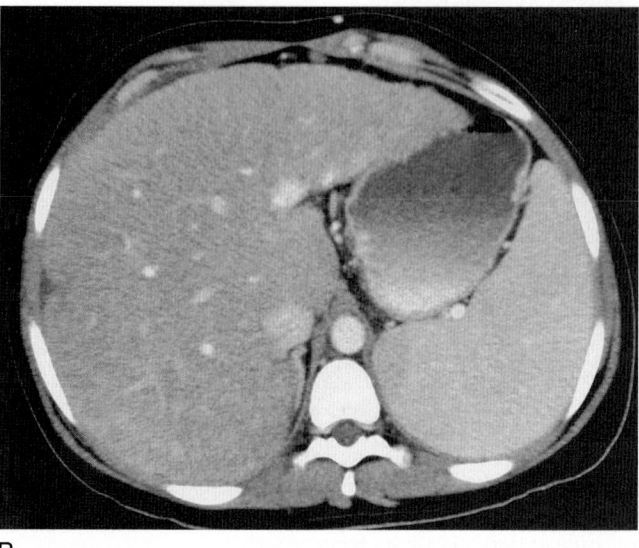

A
B

FIGURE 114-1. Diffuse fatty liver. **A,** Five-year-old boy with cystic fibrosis and hepatomegaly. Longitudinal sonogram reveals increased echogenicity throughout the liver. Note the marked difference in echogenicity between the abnormally bright liver and the normal right kidney. **B,** Sixteen-year-old girl with glycogen storage disease. CT after intravenous contrast administration shows diffuse low attenuation of the enlarged liver. Splenomegaly is also noted, in addition to nodular liver margins, consistent with cirrhotic change.

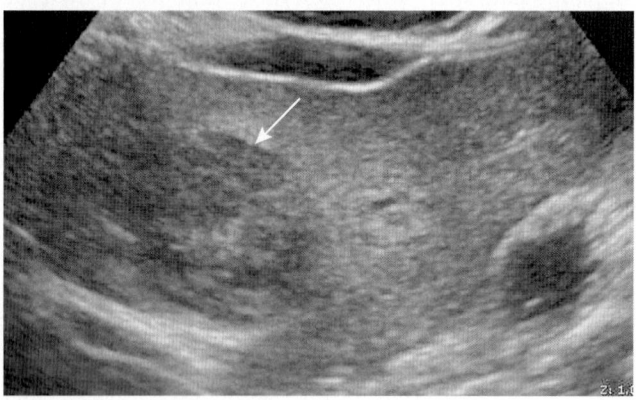

A

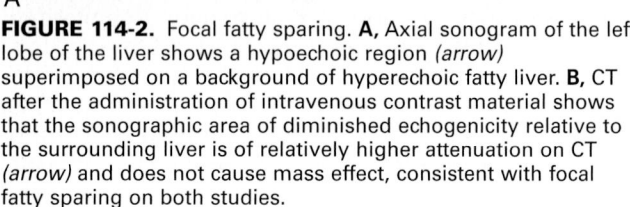

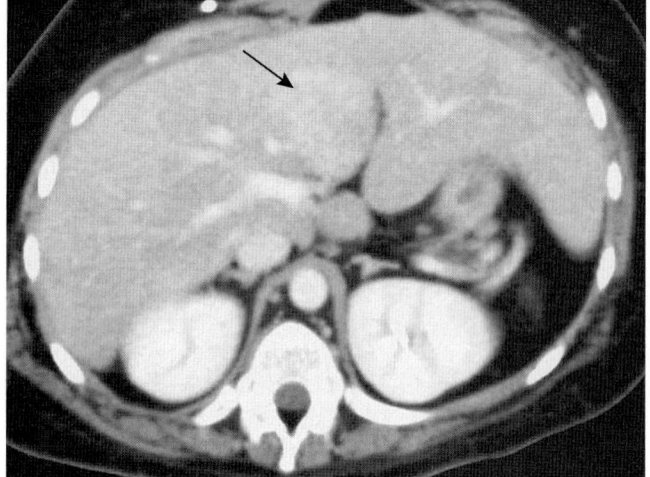

B

FIGURE 114-2. Focal fatty sparing. **A,** Axial sonogram of the left lobe of the liver shows a hypoechoic region *(arrow)* superimposed on a background of hyperechoic fatty liver. **B,** CT after the administration of intravenous contrast material shows that the sonographic area of diminished echogenicity relative to the surrounding liver is of relatively higher attenuation on CT *(arrow)* and does not cause mass effect, consistent with focal fatty sparing on both studies.

cularly in those with focal fatty infiltration or focal fatty sparing.

The cause of focal fatty replacement is unknown. Theories include a variant blood supply or focal hypoxia. The right lobe, caudate lobe, and perihilar locations are most frequently involved. Imaging studies may show one or more areas of focal fat that typically extend to the periphery of the liver and are without mass effect. Focal fat is hyperechoic on sonography, low attenuation (–40 to +10 Hounsfield units) without enhancement on CT, hyperintense on T1-weighted MR images, and isointense to hypointense on T2-weighted MR images. Chemical shift imaging can be used in cases of focal fat to increase diagnostic confidence, as mentioned earlier. Nuclear scintigraphy is generally not performed, but it may be normal or show a focal defect.

IRON DEPOSITION IN THE LIVER

Approximately 80% of the normal iron stores of 2 to 6 g are in the form of hemoglobin, myoglobin, and iron-containing enzymes; the remaining 20% are in the form of ferritin and hemosiderin. Normally, trace levels of iron are found in the liver, spleen, and bone marrow. With excess body iron, deposition may occur in the liver, spleen, lymph nodes, pancreas, kidneys, pituitary, and gastrointestinal tract. The body can compensate for some excess iron (10 to 20 g) without the occurrence of tissue damage, in which case the term *hemosiderosis* is applied. However, if functional and structural impairment of organs occurs as a result of excess iron (50 to 60 g), the term *hemochromatosis* is applied.

> Hemosiderosis refers to compensatory storage of moderate amounts (10 to 20 g) of excess iron without associated tissue damage.
>
>   Hemochromatosis is present when excess iron stores exceed the body's capacity to compensate (50 to 60 g), leading to functional and structural organ impairment.

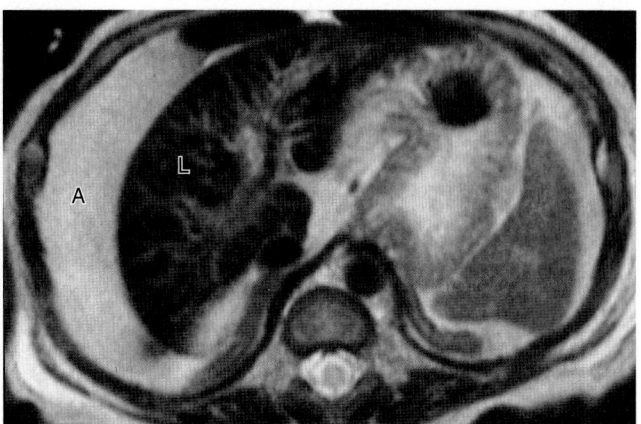

FIGURE 114-3. Primary hemochromatosis in an infant with multiorgan system failure. Axial T2-weighted MR image reveals extensive ascites (A) surrounding a liver of low signal intensity (L). (Courtesy of Lynn Fordham, MD, University of North Carolina–Chapel Hill.)

Primary and secondary types of hemochromatosis are described, based on the cause. Primary hemochromatosis is a rare, autosomal recessive disorder in which a mucosal defect of the duodenum and jejunum leads to excess iron absorption. This iron becomes bound to transferrin and is eventually stored as crystalline iron oxide within the cytoplasm of periportal hepatocytes. With progressive disease, the pancreas, heart, and pituitary may be involved, but the Kupffer cells and reticuloendothelial cells of the bone marrow and spleen are spared.

Patients with primary hemochromatosis usually become symptomatic in the second decade. Symptoms are related to organ injury and replacement with excess iron and may include hyperpigmentation (90% of cases), hepatomegaly (90%), arthralgia (50%), diabetes due to pancreatic beta cell damage (30%), and congestive heart failure and arrhythmia (15%). Other complications of chronic hemochromatosis include periportal fibrosis, cirrhosis, and hepatocellular carcinoma. However, with early diagnosis and treatment, patients may have a normal life expectancy.

A neonatal form of primary hemochromatosis exists in which newborns (often less than 12 hours old) present with fulminant hepatic failure and pancreatic and heart involvement (Fig. 114-3). Hepatic biopsy is diagnostic but is often impossible to perform owing to coexistent coagulopathy.

Secondary hemochromatosis is more common than primary disease and has three general causes related to increased iron ingestion or infusion: erythrogenic, transfusion related, and Bantu siderosis. Erythrogenic hemochromatosis is caused by increased iron absorption in the small bowel in response to defective erythropoiesis and erythroid hyperplasia. Thalassemia (but not sickle cell anemia) is a classic example of this type of hemochromatosis, which resembles hereditary hemochromatosis in that iron is first deposited in the hepatocytes rather than the Kupffer cells. Transfusional iron overload may occur in patients who receive more than 40 units of blood, exceeding the iron storage capacity of the reticuloendothelial system (10 g). Bantu siderosis is also caused by increased absorption of iron and is secondary to cooking food in iron cookware. Secondary hemochromatosis is much more common in adults than in children and occurs in men more often than women, in a ratio of 10:1.

With secondary hemochromatosis, phagocytosis of intact red blood cells causes initial iron deposition within the reticuloendothelial system (liver, spleen, and bone marrow). Once the storage capacity of the reticuloendothelial system is exceeded, iron may accumulate in paren-chymal cells of the organs, including the liver hepatocytes, pancreas, and myocardium, in a pattern similar to primary hemochromatosis.

Sonography is generally unrevealing in hemochromatosis. Unenhanced CT (60% sensitive for iron detection) shows prominent-appearing hepatic vasculature against a background of hyperattenuated liver of up to 135 Hounsfield units (normal range, 45 to 65 Hounsfield units at 120 kVp). Although hemochromatosis is the most common cause of this appearance in children, it is not specific, and the differential diagnosis includes thorotrast, gold therapy, and Wilson disease.

Dual-energy CT has been used to quantitate the amount of liver iron, using the spleen as an internal reference. In the normal situation, a decrease in the kilovolt peak (kVp) on CT leads to a proportionate increase in the attenuation of the liver and spleen, in a linear relationship. However, if there is increased iron within the liver, this proportionate linear increase is replaced by a much larger and markedly disproportionate increase in liver attenuation compared with the normal, linear change in the spleen. This disproportionate increase in hepatic attenuation with a decrease in the kVp is due to the high atomic number of iron, because attenuation is proportionate to the cube of the atomic number. One caveat is that dual-energy CT is not reliable in advanced hemochromatosis because the spleen may also contain excess iron. CT has the additional disadvantage of requiring ionizing radiation.

MRI is becoming the imaging modality of choice to evaluate iron overload because it is highly accurate in detecting clinically significant hepatic, splenic, and pancreatic iron deposition. Skeletal muscle is unaffected by iron overload and is normally isointense with the liver on conventional spin echo MR sequences, so it can be used as an internal reference. Normally, the spleen is slightly more hypointense than the liver on T1-weighted images and hyperintense on T2-weighted images. Owing to the paramagnetic susceptibility of ferritin and ferric ions, which leads to loss of phase coherence of adjacent protons, there is a resultant signal loss of involved tissues

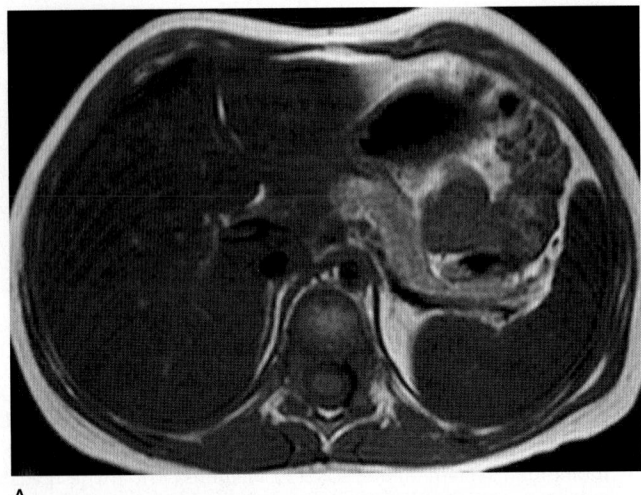
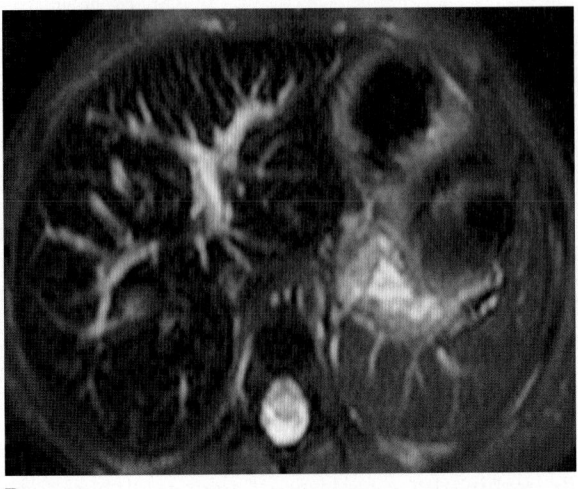

A   B

FIGURE 114-4. Hemosiderosis secondary to multiple transfusions in a 3-year-old boy. T1-weighted **(A)** and T2-weighted **(B)** axial MR images show low signal intensity within the liver and spleen due to iron deposition. Also note the low signal intensity of bone marrow in **B** and a normal pancreatic signal in **A**. (Courtesy of Paul Guillerman, MD, Texas Children's Hospital, Houston, TX.)

on MRI; this is best appreciated on T2-weighted and gradient echo images. The key finding in primary hemochromatosis is low signal intensity within the liver (90%) and pancreas (20%) on T2-weighted images. When changes are mild, signal loss may be seen only on T2-weighted sequences; however, more severe changes result in signal loss on T1-weighted sequences as well.

Imaging features of secondary hemochromatosis include abnormalities in the spleen as well as the liver, because of the early involvement of the reticuloendothelial system in both organs. In many cases, MRI can discriminate between parenchymal iron deposition resulting from primary hemochromatosis and secondary iron deposition in the reticuloendothelial (Kupffer) cells of the liver. There is sparing of the pancreas in most cases of secondary hemochromatosis (Fig. 114-4).

> In primary hemochromatosis, excess iron is stored in the periportal hepatocytes of the liver, pancreas, heart, and pituitary. The spleen is spared except in severe cases complicated by cirrhosis.
>
> In secondary hemochromatosis, excess iron is usually stored in the Kupffer cells of the liver, spleen, and bone marrow (reticuloendothelial system). The pancreas and heart are spared, except in severe disease.

GLYCOGEN STORAGE DISEASES

Glycogen storage diseases are autosomal recessive disorders that involve the abnormal storage and synthesis of glycogen and the catabolism of glucose. Six major types have been described: Von Gierke (type I), Pompe (type II), Cori (type III), Anderson (type IV), McArdle (type V), and Hers (type VI).

Von Gierke disease (VGD), due to glucose-6-phosphatase deficiency, is the most common glycogen storage disease that involves the liver. In VGD, histopathology shows excess intracytoplasmic accumulations of glycogen and small amounts of lipid within the hepatocytes and proximal renal tubules. The clinical presentation of VGD includes failure to thrive, hepatomegaly, hypoglycemia, nephromegaly, jaundice, hyperlipidemia, and hyperuricemia. Complications of VGD include hepatic adenomas (up to 40%), which may be multiple and generally increase in number and size with age, and hepatocellular carcinoma. Hepatic adenomas are believed to result from the chronic hormonal imbalance between glucagon and insulin secondary to prolonged hypoglycemia, with low insulin levels and elevated glucagon. Serial screening is required to monitor for neoplasia.

Plain radiographs and cross-sectional imaging reveal hepatomegaly (Fig. 114-5). Sonography shows diffuse hepatic hyperechogenicity owing to the combination of fatty replacement and glycogen deposition. Superimposed hepatic adenomas are common. They are seen as well-defined masses with variable echogenicity (depending on the relative change in liver echotexture), often demonstrating increased sound transmission and refractory shadowing at the margins (Fig. 114-6); this appearance is a useful diagnostic sign. Because hepatic attenuation is increased by glycogen but decreased by fat, the CT findings are variable and conflicting. When fatty infiltration predominates, the result is diffuse low attenuation of the liver. Hepatic adenomas are hypodense when found in a liver of normal attenuation but are variably hyperdense in the setting of a fatty liver. Hepatic adenomas should be followed with serial imaging to monitor their typical pattern of slow growth. Malignant neoplasia should be suspected in hyperattenuating or rapidly growing liver masses. Enlarged, dense kidneys, with decreased corticomedullary differentiation, are also identified due to cortical glycogen deposition. Nuclear scintigraphy is not usually performed in patients with glycogen storage diseases, but it shows hepatomegaly, heterogeneous hepatic uptake, and colloid shift to the spleen in older children. Focal defects are seen with hepatic adenomas and hepatocellular carcinoma.

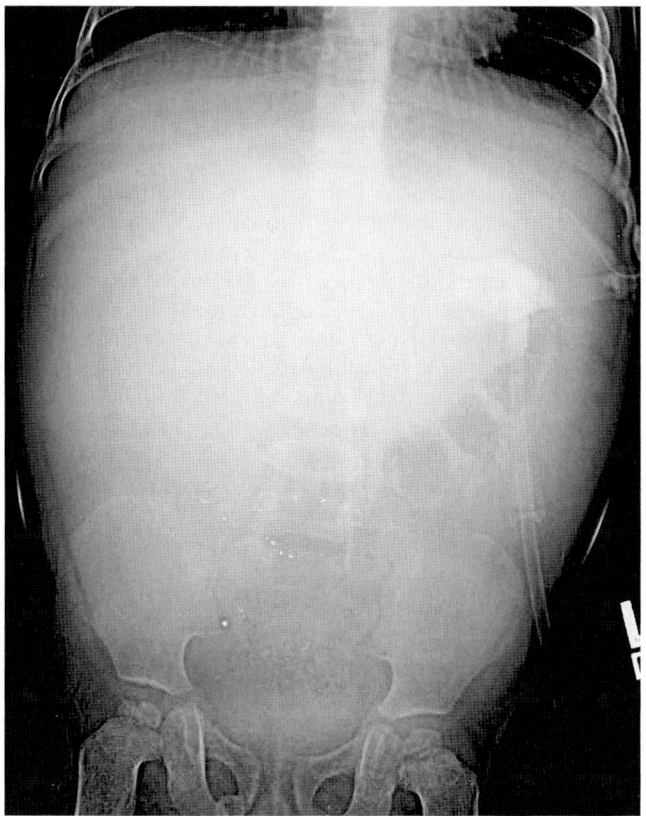

A

FIGURE 114-5. Glycogen storage disease in a 3-year-old boy presenting with abdominal distention and elevated liver function test results. **A,** Abdominal radiograph after insertion of gastrostomy tube shows marked hepatomegaly, with depression of the right side of the transverse colon. **B,** Longitudinal sonogram of the liver shows diffusely increased hepatic echogenicity and hepatomegaly. Renal cortex is also hyperechoic. **C,** Axial contrast-enhanced CT reveals hepatomegaly and nephromegaly. Short-segment small bowel intussusception is noted incidentally in this child without acute gastrointestinal symptoms.

B

C

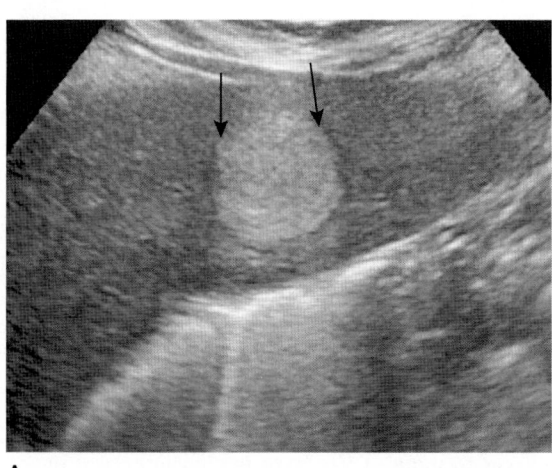

A

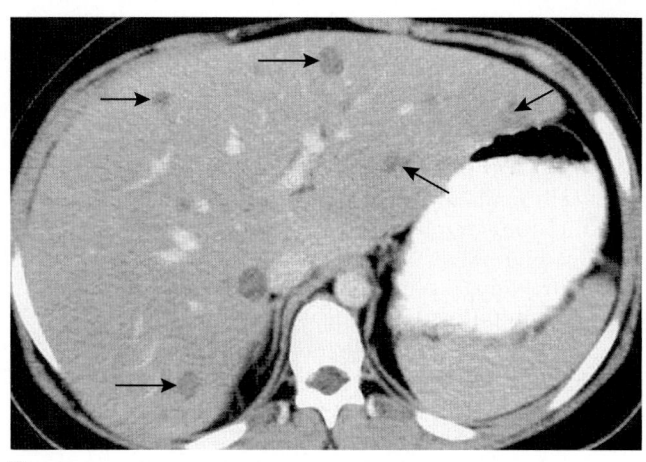

B

FIGURE 114-6. Glycogen storage disease in a 9-year-old boy with hepatic adenomas. **A,** Longitudinal sonogram reveals a hyperechoic mass with enhanced through-transmission and refractory shadowing at the margins *(arrows)*, typical of hepatic adenoma. **B,** Enhanced axial CT demonstrates numerous scattered, low-attenuation, well-defined hepatic adenomas *(arrows)*.

> **Cross-sectional imaging findings in type I (von Gierke) glycogen storage disease vary owing to the combination of fatty replacement and glycogen deposition within the liver, which often have conflicting imaging findings.**
>
> **Hepatic adenomas are common and increase in frequency and number with patient age.**

Glycogen storage disease type III results from a deficiency of amylo-1,6-glucosidase debranching enzyme. Type IIIa is more common and involves both the liver and muscle, whereas type IIIb involves only the liver. Its clinical course parallels that of type I disease, but it is milder; hepatomegaly results from increased glycogen stores, without fat deposition. Hepatic involvement may progress to cirrhosis, but adenomas are less frequent than in type I disease.

Glycogen storage disease type IV is rare and results in the accumulation of both glycogen and amylopectin in hepatocytes. Presentation typically occurs between 3 and 15 months of age, but patients can present with fetal hydrops. Approximately half of patients have abnormal neuromuscular development. Hepatomegaly may progress to cirrhosis and liver failure; adenomas are rare.

GAUCHER DISEASE

Gaucher disease is a rare autosomal recessive lysosomal storage disorder resulting from a deficiency of the enzyme β-glucocerebrosidase. There are three forms of Gaucher disease. Type 1 is the chronic non-neuropathic form; it may present in childhood but is more commonly recognized in the third to fourth decade. Type 2, the acute neuropathic or infantile form, is rapidly fatal and presents with severe hepatosplenomegaly, progressive seizures, mental retardation, spasticity, strabismus, and, rarely, skeletal manifestations. Type 3, the subacute neuropathic or juvenile form, is the rarest and presents between 2 and 6 years of age with hepatosplenomegaly, mild neurologic symptoms, and late-onset skeletal disease. The abnormalities are the result of the accumulation of glucocerebroside in cells of the reticuloendothelial system and in the brain. The disease occurs world wide, most commonly in Ashkenazi Jews. Histopathology of bone marrow aspirates reveals Gaucher cells (kerasin-laden histiocytes).

Significant replacement of liver parenchyma by Gaucher cells leads to hepatomegaly. The course of the disease includes regenerating nodules and hepatic fibrosis, leading to cirrhosis and portal hypertension. Hepatic ultrasonography, CT, and MRI demonstrate findings of hepatosplenomegaly and cirrhosis. In addition, MRI may show focal areas of decreased signal on T1-weighted sequences that are isointense to hyperintense on T2-weighted sequences, presumably due to foci of Gaucher cells or fibrosis.

Splenic manifestations include infarcts and focal clusters of glucosylceramide-laden cells. On sonography, splenic lesions have variable echogenicity. They are usually hypodense on CT before contrast and are most often isointense on T1-weighted and hyperintense on T2-weighted MR images (Fig. 114-7).

Bone complications due to marrow replacement are common, including pathologic fractures, avascular necrosis, and osteomyelitis. Plain radiographs of the extremities reflect marrow packing and replacement. Findings include osteopenia, cortical thinning, and marrow space expansion, with the Erlenmeyer flask deformity of the distal femur being characteristic. MRI has been used to quantify the degree of fatty marrow replacement. Instead of the normal hyperintense fat within the marrow seen on T1-weighted images, the marrow signal decreases to become isointense with muscle. T2-weighted images can confirm marrow packing (bright signal) and show areas of avascular necrosis (bright signal lesions with low signal margins). Lung changes manifest as diffuse, predominantly basilar, reticulonodular infiltrates by Gaucher cells.

Treatment of Gaucher disease with enzyme replacement therapy is possible but costly. In general, the degree of liver and spleen enlargement correlates with the severity of fatty marrow replacement and avascular necrosis. Thus, quantification of hepatosplenomegaly (measurement of liver and spleen volume) has been used to determine the therapeutic enzyme dosage. Liver volume can be measured with sonography, CT, and MRI (Fig. 114-8). The prognosis varies with the type, extent, and severity of disease.

> **Liver and spleen volume is quantified to determine enzyme replacement therapy, because the degree of hepatosplenomegaly correlates with the severity of bone marrow replacement.**

PELIOSIS HEPATIS

Peliosis hepatis, a rare disorder that can occur at any age, is characterized by multiple blood-filled cavities within reticuloendothelial system organs. The cause is unknown, but theories include acquired chronic infection, hepatotoxic drugs, steroids, diabetes mellitus, chronic renal failure, and bacillary peliosis hepatis in acquired immunodeficiency syndrome (*Rochalimaea* species), a form that responds to antibiotic therapy. Liver involvement is more common than spleen involvement, which in turn is more common than bone marrow, lymph node, and lung involvement. Peliosis hepatis is associated with hormonally induced benign and malignant liver tumors.

Imaging features include hepatosplenomegaly, focal liver lesions of variable echogenicity on sonography, and focal enhancing round hepatic lesions on CT (Fig. 114-9). Signal intensity on MRI is mixed owing to repeated hemorrhage within focal hepatic parenchymal lesions.

> **Peliosis hepatis of the liver is characterized by hepatosplenomegaly and multiple blood-filled cavities of variable echogenicity, attenuation, and**

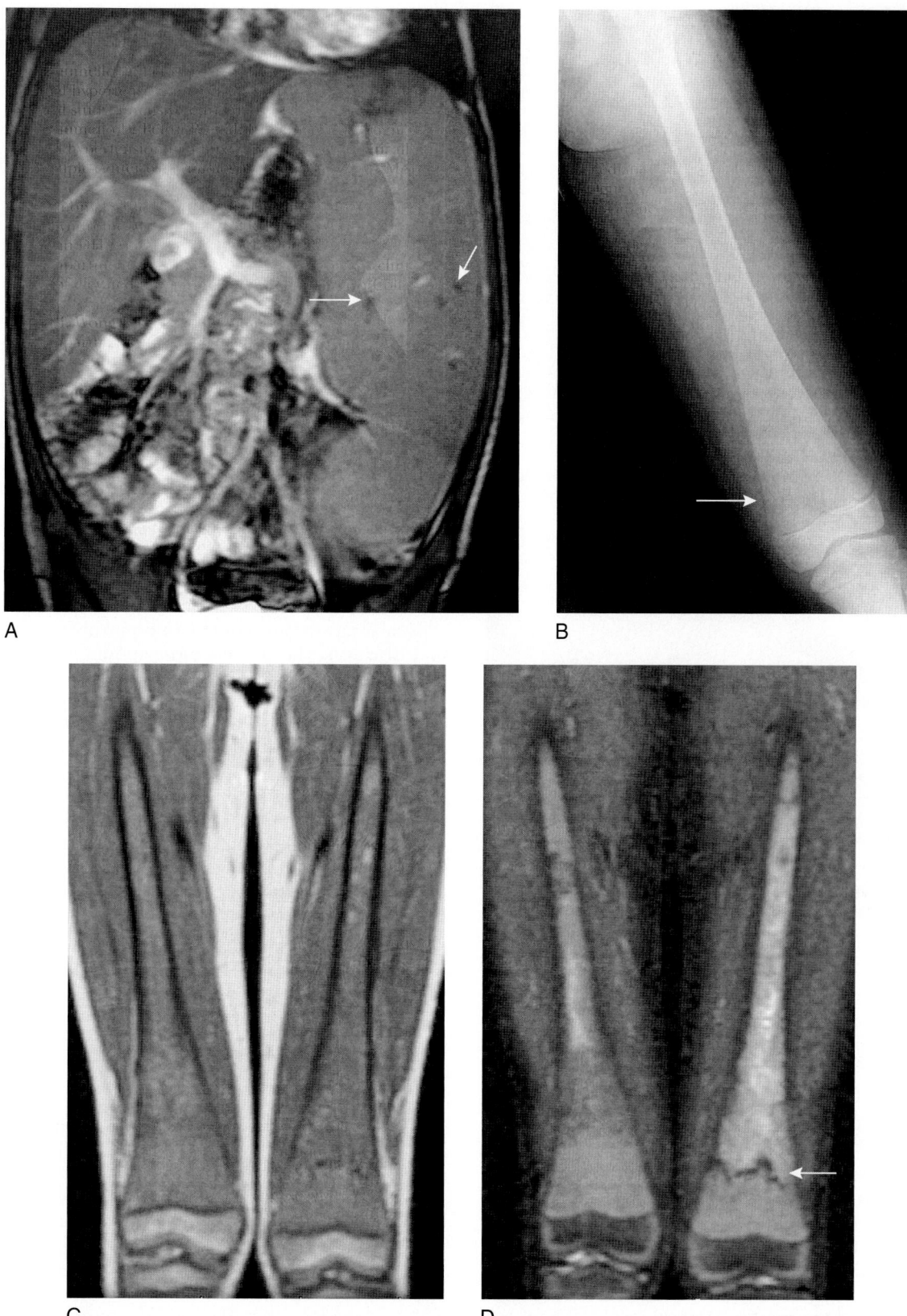

FIGURE 114-7. Gaucher disease in a 9-year-old girl with hepatosplenomegaly and left leg pain. **A,** Coronal T2-weighted MR image shows massive splenomegaly, in addition to several tiny foci of infarct or Gaucher cells *(arrows)*. **B,** Plain radiograph of the femur shows a classic Erlenmeyer flask deformity *(arrow)*, seen as distal femoral metaphyseal widening. **C,** T1-weighted MR image reveals bilateral loss of bright fat signal throughout the femoral diaphyses and metaphyses and, to a lesser degree, the epiphyses. **D,** T2-weighted MR image confirms bright diaphyseal signal, consistent with marrow packing, in addition to a rim of low signal intensity that suggests avascular necrosis *(arrow)*.

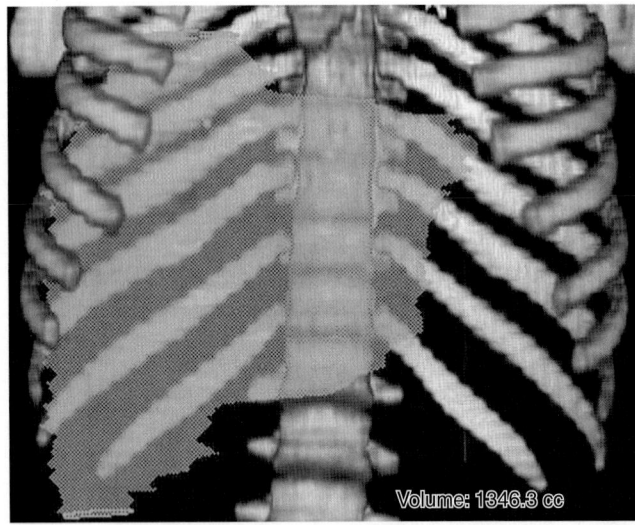

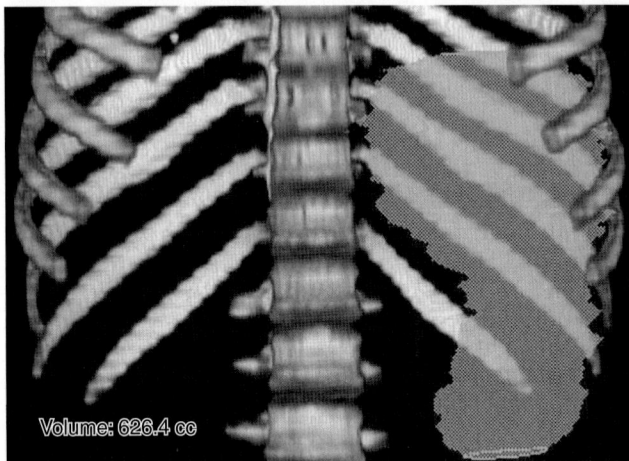

FIGURE 114-8. Gaucher disease in an 11-year-old girl. **A** and **B,** CT shows volumetric measurements of the liver **(A)** and spleen **(B),** which are used to guide therapy.

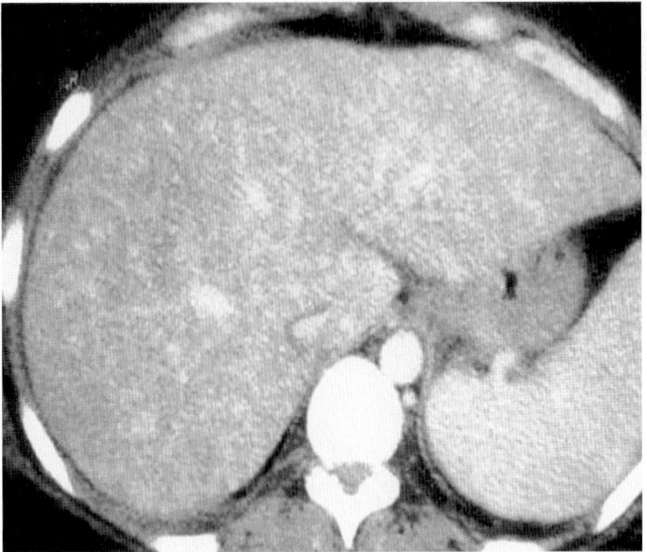

FIGURE 114-9. Peliosis hepatis due to human immunodeficiency virus infection (bacilliary angiomatosis). Contrast-enhanced axial CT shows innumerable tiny, hypervascular nodules through the liver. (From Kawamoto S, Soyer PA, Fishman EK: Nonneoplastic liver disease: evaluation with CT and MR imaging. Radiographics 1998;18:827-848.)

Nearly any organ system can be involved, but abdominal disease is the second most common manifestation after thoracic disease. Abdominal sarcoidosis is associated with marked angiotensin-converting enzyme elevation in 91% of patients. Hepatosplenomegaly occurs in 18% to 29% of sarcoidosis patients, with tiny (<5 mm) hepatosplenic nodules in 5% to 15% of cases within 5 years of diagnosis (Fig. 114-10). Lymphadenopathy is found in 10% to 31% of cases (average node size is 2.6 cm). Fatty changes in the liver may occur as a result of therapy. Other locations of abdominal disease are less common, including the pancreas, gastrointestinal tract, scrotum, or genitourinary tract.

> The imaging appearance of hepatic sarcoidosis includes hepatosplenomegaly, tiny hepatosplenic granulomas, and lymphadenopathy.

> signal intensity. The spleen and, less often, other reticuloendothelial system organs may also be involved.

SARCOIDOSIS

Sarcoidosis is an immunologically mediated multisystem granulomatous disease of unknown cause that occasionally involves the pediatric liver. It is most common in black girls of West African descent and presents most commonly in the second to third decades. The presentation, disease progression, and prognosis are highly variable, depending on the organs involved and the severity of disease. Histology shows noncaseating epithelioid granulomas with occasional central necrosis. Diagnostic studies include angiotensin-converting enzyme levels (elevated in 70% of cases), Kveim-Siltzbach test (positive in 70% of cases), elevated calcium in the blood and urine, and biopsy, which is rarely required.

α_1-ANTITRYPSIN DEFICIENCY

α_1-Antitrypsin deficiency, the second most common cause of chronic severe liver disease in children, is a rare autosomal recessive disorder caused by deficient serum levels of α_1-antitrypsin enzyme, 90% of which is produced in the hepatocytes. The cause of the liver injury is believed to be the inability of the synthesized protein to migrate from the endoplasmic reticulum of the hepatocytes, with secondary accumulation of α_1-antitrypsin, which generates an inflammatory response within the liver. Damage to lung tissue is thought to be due to unhindered neutrophil elastase digestion of collagen, secondary to a lack of protease inhibitors. Although presentation is most commonly in the second decade due to lung disease (panacinar emphysema, bullae, bronchiectasis), α_1-antitrypsin deficiency can also present in

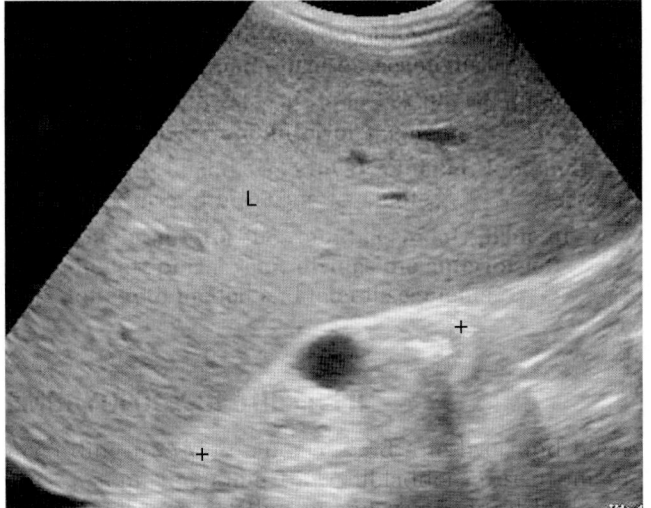

A

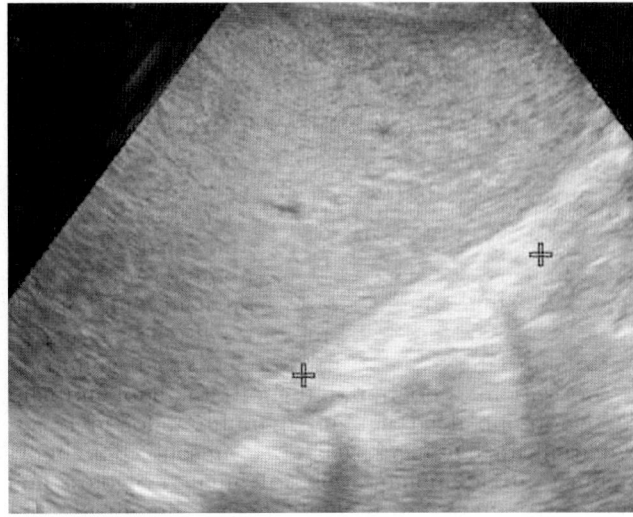

B

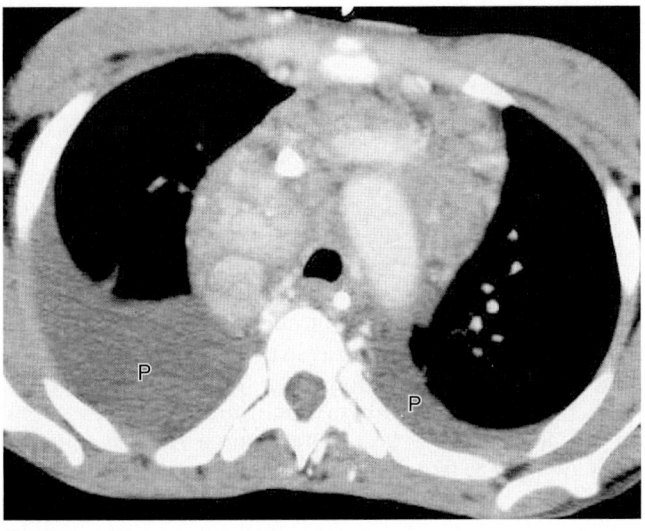

C

FIGURE 114-10. Sarcoidosis in a 16-year-old girl with a history of chronic renal failure. **A** and **B,** Longitudinal sonograms reveal an enlarged, hyperechoic liver (L) in **A** and spleen in **B.** Hyperechoic, tiny kidneys *(calipers)* are also noted. **C,** Contrast-enhanced axial chest CT shows extensive mediastinal lymphadenopathy, bilateral pleural effusions (P), and extensive collateral vascular flow due to portal hypertension.

the neonatal period with jaundice mimicking biliary atresia. Other symptoms related to the liver include feeding difficulties, failure to thrive, ascites, and elevated liver enzymes. Rarely, children may present with symptoms of cirrhosis or a rare skin disorder, panniculitis (inflammation of the subcutaneous fat). The diagnosis can be made by measuring the serum α_1-antitrypsin level and confirmed with biopsy.

Infants presenting in the first months of life with elevated direct bilirubin may undergo scintigraphy with the intention of excluding biliary atresia. In these cases, scintigraphy cannot distinguish biliary atresia from α_1-antitrypsin deficiency because both conditions may show good hepatocyte uptake without biliary excretion. The lack of biliary excretion seen in some cases of α_1-antitrypsin deficiency is due to an associated congenital paucity of intralobular bile ducts (Fig. 114-11). Sonographic correlation may be helpful, because infants with α_1-antitrypsin deficiency generally have normal sonography of the liver and gallbladder. Abdominal cross-sectional imaging in older children generally reveals nonspecific findings of cirrhosis.

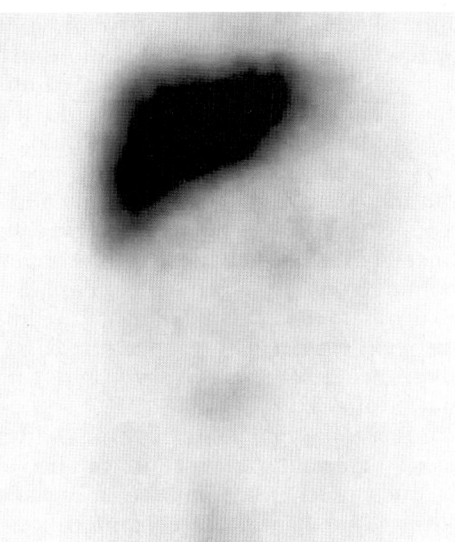

FIGURE 114-11. α_1-Antitrypsin deficiency in a 6-week-old girl with poor weight gain and hyperbilirubinemia. Biliary scintigraphy shows uptake of radiopharmaceutical in the liver without excretion into the biliary tree.

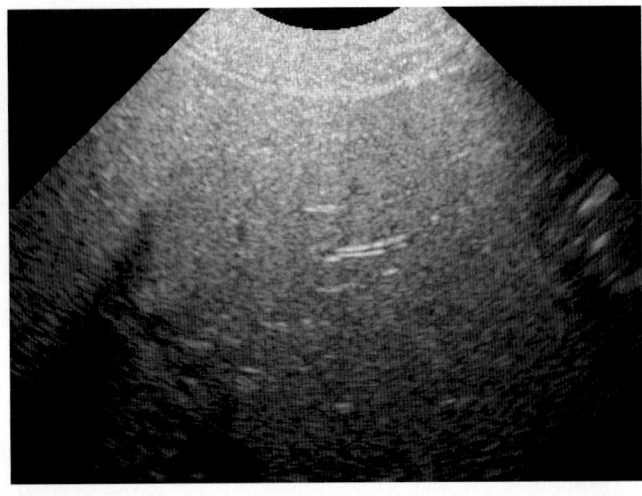
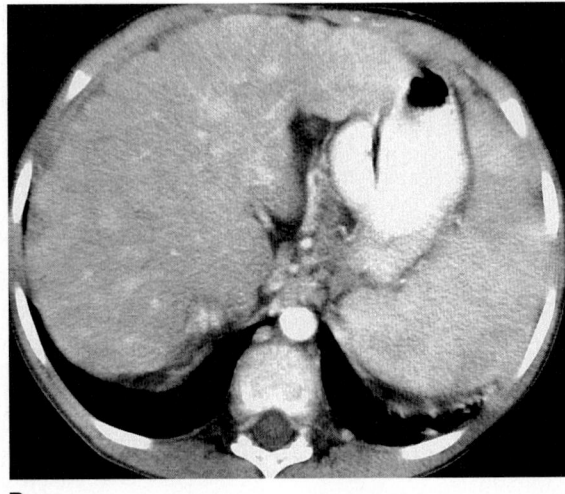

A   B

FIGURE 114-12. Wilson disease in an 8-year-old girl. **A,** Transverse hepatic sonogram shows diffuse hyperechogenicity with poor sound transmission due to steatosis or copper storage. **B,** Contrast-enhanced CT reveals hepatopleuromegaly with diffuse architectural changes of the liver.

There is no cure for α_1-antitrypsin deficiency, and the prognosis is extremely variable, depending on disease severity, age at diagnosis, and therapeutic interventions. It is crucial that patients not smoke, owing to the accelerated lung disease. α_1-Antitrypsin deficiency is the most common genetic disorder for which liver transplantation is performed.

> When deficiency of α_1-antitrypsin presents in infants, it may mimic the clinical and scintigraphic findings of biliary atresia: neonatal jaundice and hepatic radionuclide uptake without biliary excretion.

WILSON DISEASE

Wilson disease (hepatolenticular degeneration) is a rare autosomal recessive disorder of copper metabolism caused by several possible genetic alterations in chromosome 13. In all the genetic variations of Wilson disease, the normal liver excretion of copper into the biliary system is prevented. Specific genetic alterations include a hepatocyte lysosomal defect, deficient copper binding proteins in the biliary tree, hepatic production of high-affinity copper binding proteins, and persistent fetal copper metabolism. Normally, 95% of copper in the body is bound to the serum protein ceruloplasmin. With copper toxicosis, accumulation begins in the liver; when its copper binding capacity is reached, the basal ganglia, renal tubules, corneas, bones, joints, and parathyroid glands may be affected.

Wilson disease presents most often in children older than 7 years and in young adolescents with hepatic manifestations, such as jaundice and hepatomegaly. Older adolescents and adults with unrecognized liver involvement present with Parkinson-like movement disorder (tremor, rigidity, dysarthria, dysphagia) or psychosis if the liver disease remains subclinical. Kayser-Fleischer rings—greenish brown copper deposits in the corneal limbus—

are diagnostic when present. Elevated urine copper levels and low ceruloplasmin are the best screening tests for Wilson disease. Serum ceruloplasmin levels are low in 95% of cases (normally <20 mg/100 ml). Biopsy can be performed as well, in which case hepatic copper content is elevated (>200 pg/g dry weight).

Hepatic changes are poorly seen with cross-sectional imaging owing to the multiple processes occurring in the liver concurrently: copper accumulation, fatty infiltration, hepatitis, cirrhosis, and liver necrosis. The liver is hyperechoic on ultrasonography (Fig. 114-12). Copper has a high atomic number, which increases attenuation on CT. However, hepatic attenuation usually remains normal owing to fatty infiltration, which lowers attenuation and thus cancels out the hyperattenuation of copper. Hepatic MRI early in the course of the disease demonstrates hyperintensity on T1 weighting and hypointensity on T2 weighting, but these changes may be overshadowed once cirrhosis supervenes. Radioactive copper studies have been helpful in demonstrating prolonged turnover of body copper and a decreased rate of hepatic uptake owing to reduced incorporation of copper into ceruloplasmin.

> Hepatic cross-sectional imaging in Wilson disease produces relatively nonspecific and variable findings owing to concurrent copper accumulation, fatty infiltration, hepatitis, cirrhosis, and liver necrosis.

Other imaging findings of Wilson disease involve bone (osteopenia in 85%, pathologic fractures, subarticular cysts), joints (knee, hip, wrist, second through fourth metacarpals), and brain. In the brain, findings reflect the type of presentation: either hepatic failure, typically in younger patients, or neuropsychiatric symptoms in adolescents. In children with hepatic failure, cerebral findings on MRI include bilateral, symmetric, T1 high signal in the globus pallidus and dorsal midbrain. In

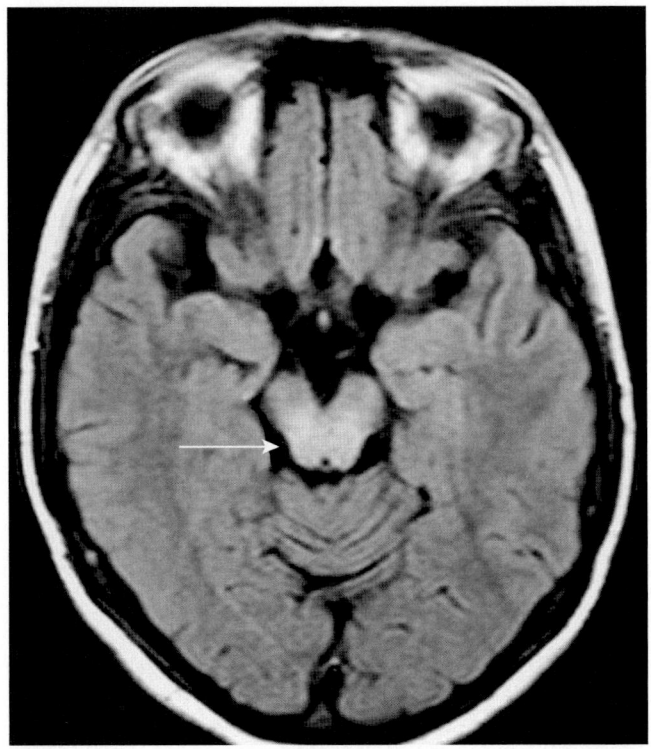

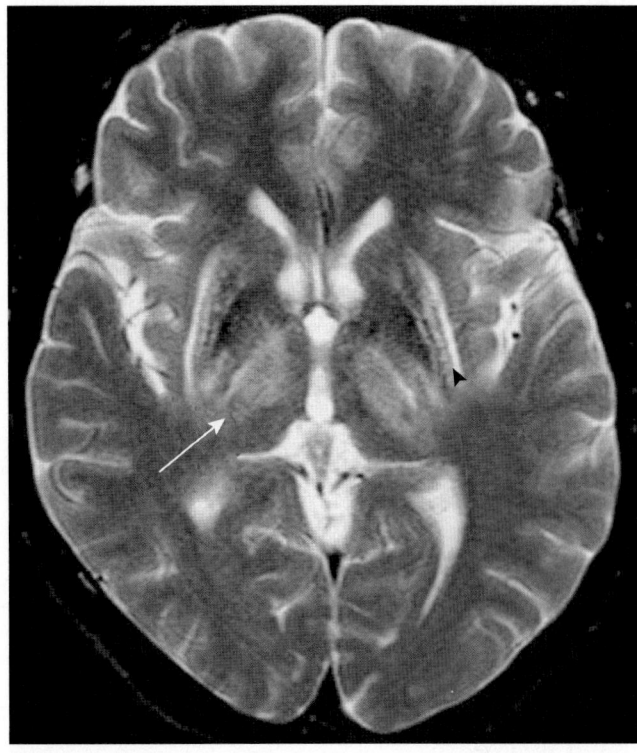

A   B

FIGURE 114-13. Cerebral MR images in Wilson disease. **A,** Fluid attenuated inversion recovery image in a child who presented with hepatic failure shows bright signal in the dorsal midbrain *(arrow)*. **B,** T2-weighted image in a young adult with Kayser-Fleischer rings and mental status changes shows hyperintensity of the claustrum *(arrowhead),* lateral thalamus *(arrow),* globus pallidus, and putamen. (**B** courtesy of Mauricio Castillo, MD.)

teenagers and young adults, cerebral MRI changes are related to copper accumulation and include bilateral, symmetric low density on CT, prolongation of T1 and T2 relaxation times in the putamen, globus pallidus, thalamus, dorsal midbrain, claustrum, and cerebral and superior cerebellar peduncles (Fig. 114-13). White matter changes, such as atrophy, are especially common in the frontal and temporal lobes.

Early treatment, optimally before the patient is symptomatic, is important, because chelation with penicillamine and zinc is effective in preventing toxic copper deposition in the liver and brain. Treatment of symptomatic patients should result in rapid improvement. Lifelong chelation therapy is required, and severe cases may require liver transplantation.

TYROSINEMIA TYPE 1

Tyrosinemia type 1 (hepatorenal tyrosinemia) is a rare autosomal recessive metabolic disorder that is more common in Caucasians, especially those from the Canadian province of Quebec and from Scandinavia. It is most often due to a deficiency of the enzyme fumarylacetoacetate hydroxylase, which is required for the catabolic pathway of tyrosine (a precursor of dopamine, norepinephrine, epinephrine, melanin, and thyroxine) and is largely present in the liver and kidneys. Two main forms of tyrosinemia—acute and chronic— were previously described, based mostly on age at presentation and severity of disease. This classification had limited utility owing to the variation in disease

severity among individuals. However, the age at onset predicts prognosis. Infants who present at younger than 2 months have a 1-year survival rate of 38%, whereas those who present at older than 6 months have a 1-year survival rate of 96%. In the chronic form of tyrosinemia, Fanconi syndrome with renal tubular dysfunction is present, in addition to vitamin D–resistant rickets and intermittent porphyria–like symptoms.

Children with hepatorenal tyrosinemia usually present with progressive liver failure in early childhood with symptoms of anemia, elevated α-fetoprotein, hepatosplenomegaly, altered clotting mechanisms, infantile micronodular progressing to macronodular cirrhosis, hepatic fibrosis, steatosis, nephromegaly with uniform thickening of the renal cortex, and nephrocalcinosis (Fig. 114-14). Hepatic imaging findings are relatively nonspecific and are similar to those of many hepatic disorders that can lead to cirrhosis. Regenerating nodules are common and may be difficult to distinguish from neoplasm without biopsy. Hepatocellular carcinoma complicates tyrosinemia in 37% of children younger than 2 years and is the cause of death in the majority of patients.

Variable renal disease is associated with hepatorenal tyrosinemia, ranging from mild tubular dysfunction to renal failure. Toxic effects on the proximal renal tubules can lead to Fanconi syndrome due to poor resorption of many substances, including phosphate, glucose, amino acids, urate, potassium, and bicarbonate. Phosphate wasting often leads to vitamin D–resistant rickets, which may be identified on the plain radiographs. The presence

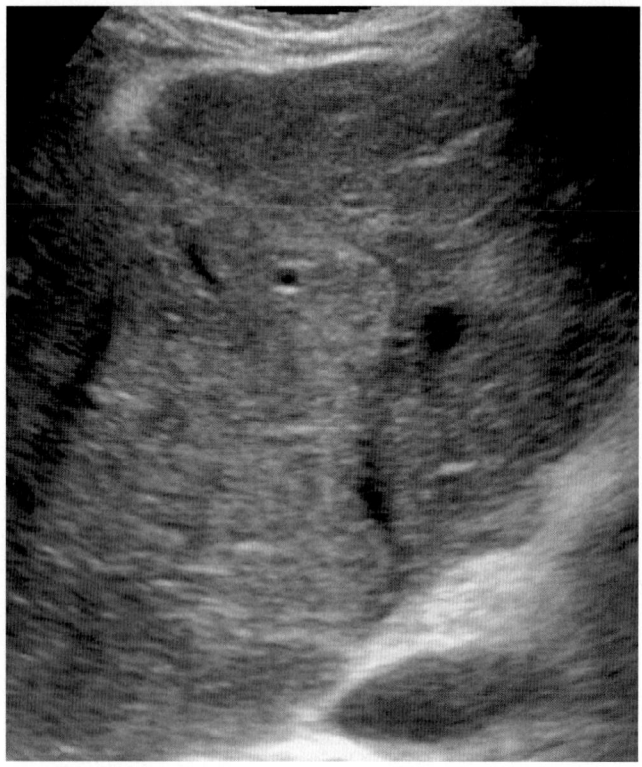

A

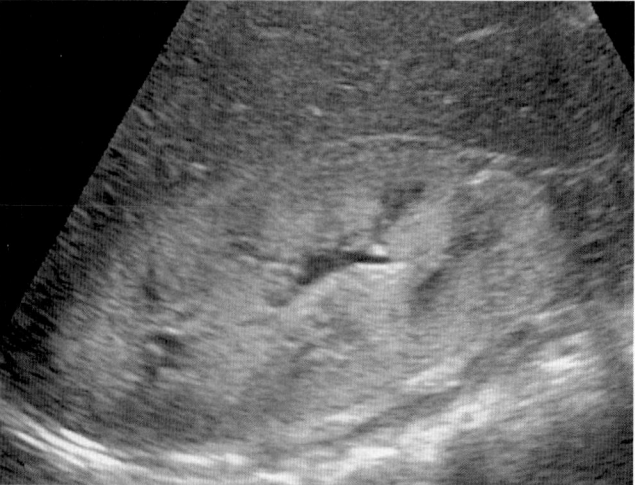

B

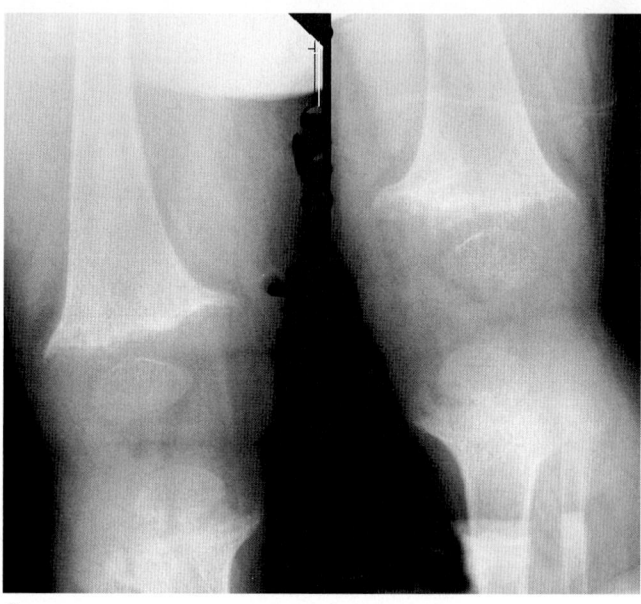

C

FIGURE 114-14. Tyrosinemia in an 8-month-old boy with hepatomegaly. **A,** Transverse sonogram of the liver shows diffusely increased echogenicity and architectural distortion. **B,** Longitudinal sonogram of the right kidney shows diffuse cortical hyperechogenicity and nephromegaly (the left kidney, not shown, was similar). **C,** Plain radiograph of the knees show changes related to rickets (osteopenia, frayed and cupped metaphyses). (**A-C** courtesy of Cindy Taylor, MD.)

of nephromegaly may suggest a diagnosis of hepatorenal tyrosinemia, but it can also be seen in type I glycogen storage disease (VGD). Other organs occasionally affected by tyrosinemia include the pancreas, peripheral nerves, and heart.

Treatment consists of restricted dietary phenylalanine and tyrosine, which helps alleviate but does not cure the liver disease. Promising new medical therapy with 2-2-nitro-4-trifluoromethylbenzoyl-1,3-cyclohexanedione has been effective in many patients. The only hope of cure is liver and renal transplantation before the development of hepatocellular carcinoma. However, even transplantation is not 100% effective due to the fact that succinylacetone is made in small amounts in nonliver tissues.

> **The combination of hepatomegaly, enlarged echogenic kidneys, and rickets should raise concern for hepatorenal tyrosinemia.**

GALACTOSEMIA

Galactosemia is an autosomal recessive disorder occurring in 1 in 60,000 Caucasian births; it results in the inability to metabolize galactose. Three types of galactosemia are described: classic galactosemia, the most common and severe form (galactose-1-phosphate uridyltransferase deficiency); galactokinase deficiency; and galactose-6-phosphate epimerase deficiency. Galactose is found in human and animal milk. In classic galactosemia secondary to transferase deficiency, galactose-1-phosphate accumulates and causes tissue damage in the liver, central nervous system, kidneys, and eyes.

Newborns with galactosemia present with jaundice, hypotonia, vomiting, failure to thrive, diarrhea, lethargy, irritability, seizure, hypoglycemia, hepatomegaly, and aminoaciduria. Chronic galactose exposure may lead to cirrhosis, ascites, metal retardation, cerebral edema, and cataracts as early as 1 month of age. Diagnosis is possible by testing the urine for galactose metabolites, galactose, and ketones. Enzyme assays can give a definitive diagnosis (red cells, leukocytes, urine).

Imaging manifestations in the liver include hepatomegaly and cirrhosis. Diffuse cerebral edema occurs in newborns, in addition to multiple small, hyperintense white matter lesions on T2-weighted images; loss of or decrease in peripheral white matter signal intensity on T2-weighted images in children older than 1 year; cerebral and cerebellar atrophy; and skeletal osteopenia.

Treatment includes lifelong avoidance of milk-containing products and dietary calcium supplementation. The prognosis for a normal life may be favorable when the diagnosis is made early and the child is compliant. However, mild intellectual impairments may occur even under the best of circumstances. Without treatment, death is likely.

> **Children with galactosemia present at birth with jaundice, hypotonia, hypoglycemia, seizures, aminoaciduria, and cataracts.**

CIRRHOSIS

Cirrhosis is a generic term used to describe the end-stage appearance of any chronic liver disease in which there is parenchymal necrosis, nodular regeneration, and active parenchymal fibrosis that distorts normal lobular and vascular architecture. In children, cirrhosis is a secondary phenomenon due to a variety of congenital and acquired diseases, including chronic hepatitis, congenital hepatic fibrosis, biliary atresia, cystic fibrosis, Budd-Chiari syndrome, chronic biliary obstruction, and metabolic disorders such as hemochromatosis, glycogen storage disease, α_1-antitrypsin deficiency, Wilson disease, tyrosinemia, and galactosemia (Table 114-2).

Cirrhosis has traditionally been classified into three main categories: micronodular (Laënnec), with equal-sized nodules up to 3 mm; macronodular (postnecrotic), with variable-sized nodules ranging from 3 mm to 3 cm; and mixed cirrhosis. Disorders that cause micronodular cirrhosis in children include biliary obstruction, hemochromatosis, and venous outflow obstruction. Viral hepatitis, Wilson disease, and α_1-antitrypsin deficiency are pediatric causes of macronodular cirrhosis.

The sonographic features of cirrhosis include diffusely increased echogenicity and decreased hepatic parenchymal beam penetration, leading to poor visualization of the hepatic vasculature and distortion of normal architecture in the cirrhotic liver (Fig. 114-15). Regenerative nodules may have relatively decreased echogenicity. The echogenicity of the liver is heterogeneous, and the surface is irregular. The right lobe of the liver may be relatively small, with compensatory enlargement of the caudate lobe and left lateral segment. The gallbladder may be small, not seen, or contain stones, depending on the primary disease leading to the cirrhosis. Findings of portal hypertension are often seen, with collateral vessels and hepatofugal flow identified on Doppler interrogation.

TABLE 114-2
Causes of Cirrhosis in Children
Viral hepatitis
Hepatic fibrosis
Biliary atresia
Primary biliary cirrhosis
Cystic fibrosis
Budd-Chiari syndrome
Iron overload
Chronic biliary obstruction
α_1-Antitrypsin deficiency
Glycogen storage disease
Tyrosinemia
Wilson disease
Galactosemia
Juvenile polycystic kidney disease
Osler-Weber-Rendu syndrome

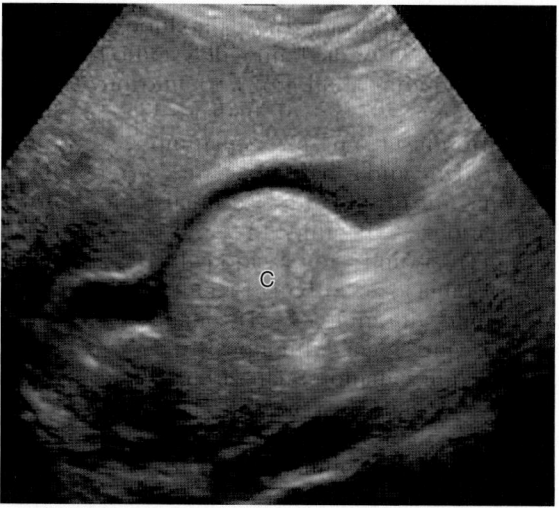
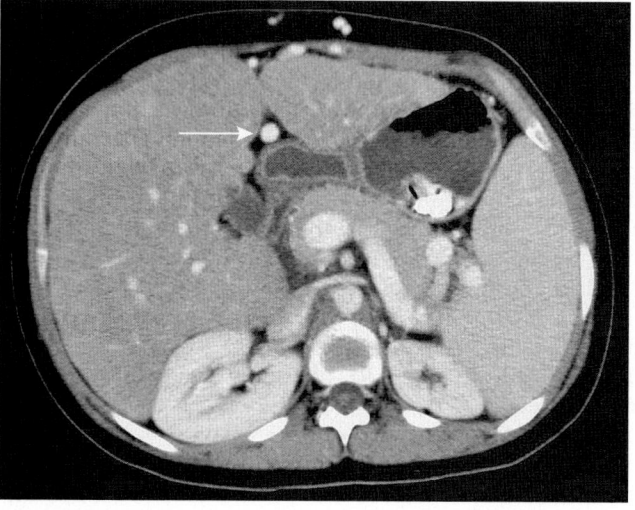

A   B

FIGURE 114-15. Cirrhosis in a 16-year-old girl with type I glycogen storage disease. **A,** Longitudinal sonogram of the liver shows diffuse increased echogenicity and an enlarged caudate lobe (C). **B,** Axial CT after contrast administration shows hepatic steatosis with collaterals due to portal hypertension.

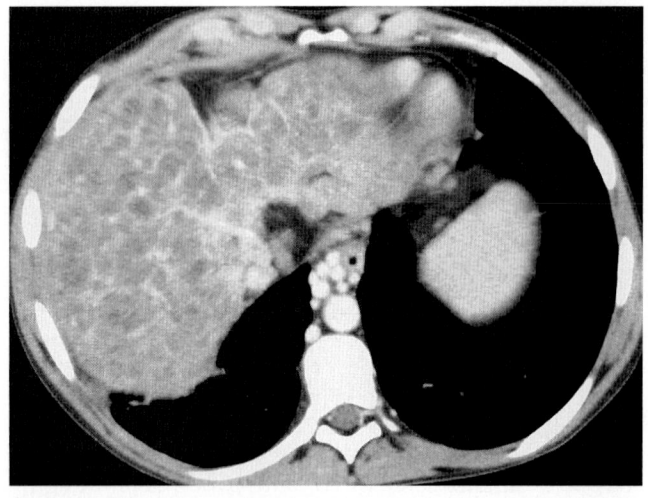

A

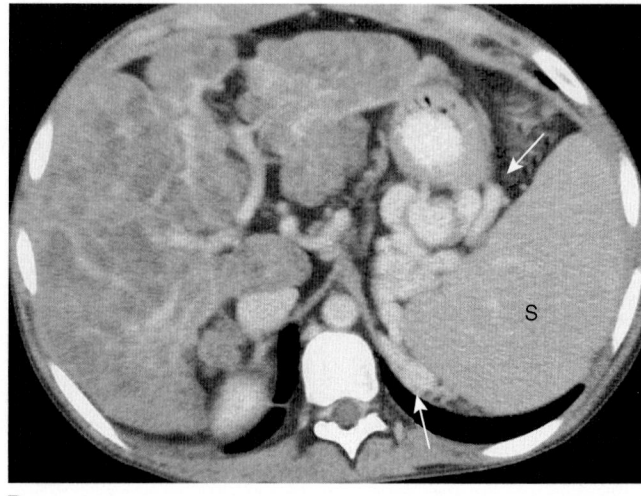

B

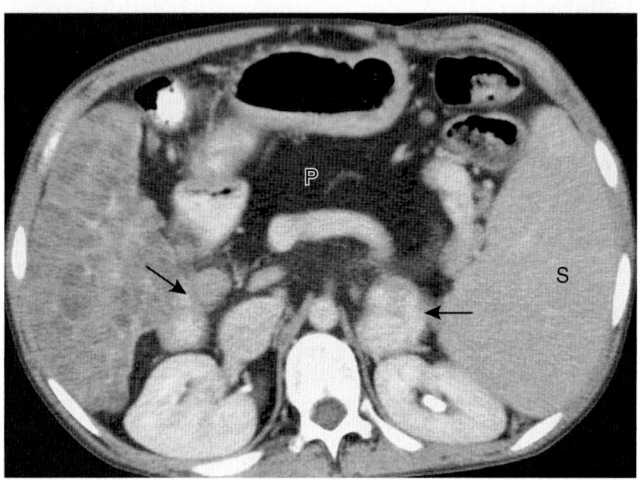

C

FIGURE 114-16. Cirrhosis in an 18-year-old woman with cystic fibrosis. **A,** CT image of the liver after contrast administration shows marked fatty replacement and hepatic surface nodularity. Gastroesophageal varices are also seen. **B,** More caudal CT image shows the abnormal liver, in addition to splenomegaly (S) and extensive gastrosplenic and retroperitoneal collaterals vessels *(arrows)* due to portal venous hypertension. **C,** Section through the pancreas (P) shows that it is entirely replaced by fat. Again noted are changes of cirrhosis, including splenomegaly (S) and extensive collateral flow through the renal and gonadal vessels *(arrows)*.

CT shows a small or normal-sized liver with surface nodularity and heterogeneous attenuation that is exaggerated by the administration of contrast material. Decreased attenuation in areas of fatty infiltration and normal attenuation in areas of fibrosis and regenerating nodules are common (Fig. 114-16). CT may also demonstrate vascular changes, including an enlarged, tortuous hepatic artery due to compensatory increased arterial flow; arterioportal shunting through trans-sinusoidal shunts at the liver periphery in the arterial phase; and findings of portal hypertension. The most common collateral pathways are coronary to gastroesophageal and paraumbilical, followed by splenorenal, gastrorenal, and hemorrhoidal varices.

Typical findings on MRI include the morphologic changes already described on sonography and CT. The hepatic parenchymal signal may be normal or altered, depending on the degree of steatosis, fibrosis, or iron deposition. Regenerating nodules are typically isointense with liver or show reduced signal intensity on T2-weighted and gradient recalled echo sequences secondary to iron deposition, and they enhance less than the surrounding parenchyma. Dysplastic nodules are iso- to hyperintense on T1-weighted images and iso- to hypointense on T2-weighted images, with delayed enhancement after 2 to 3 minutes. Hepatocellular carcinoma complicating cirrhosis is more common in adults than in children and is characterized by variable signal on T1-weighted images and hyperintense signal on T2-weighted images, in addition to enhancement after contrast material administration.

Hepatic scintigraphy has little role in cirrhosis, but it shows a normal-sized or small liver with heterogeneously decreased uptake of the isotope-labeled colloid. Regenerating nodules show increased activity between areas of photopenic fibrosis. Increased activity (colloid shift) within an enlarged spleen, bone marrow, and lungs may be seen.

Complications of cirrhosis include ascites, portal hypertension, hepatocellular carcinoma in up to 12% of cases, and cholangiocarcinoma. Mortality is most often related to bleeding esophageal varices (up to 25%), hepatorenal syndrome (10%), spontaneous bacterial peritonitis (5% to 10%), and treatment related to ascites (10%).

SUGGESTED READINGS

General

Galli G, Valenza V: Is there still a role for functional radionuclide study of the liver? Rays 1997;22:228-248

Genovese E, Maghnie M, Maggiore G, et al: MR imaging of CNS involvement in children affected by chronic liver disease. AJNR Am J Neuroradiol 2000;21:845-851

Gore RM, Levine MS, Laufer I: Hemachromatosis. In Gore RM, Levine MS, Laufer I (eds): Textbook of Gastrointestinal Radiology. Philadelphia, Saunders, 1994:1788

Henschke CI, Goldman H, Teele RL: The hyperechogenic liver in children: cause and sonographic appearance. AJR Am J Roentgenol 1982;138:841

Katz AJ: Diagnostic procedures in the evaluation of hepatic diseases: metabolic errors. Lab Res Methods Biol Med 1983;7:145-152

Kawamoto S, Soyer PA, Fishman EK: Nonneoplastic liver disease: evaluation with CT and MR imaging. Radiographics 1998; 18:827-848

Kawamura E, Shiomi S, Ishizu H, et al: Natural course of changes in hepatic functional reserve in patients with chronic liver diseases evaluated by scintigraphy with GSA. Hepatol Res 2003;27:129-135

Martin DR, Semelka RC: Magnetic resonance imaging of the liver: review of techniques and approach to common diseases. Semin Ultrasound CT MR 2005;26:116

Mergo PJ, Ros PR, Burtow PC, et al: Diffuse disease of the liver: radiologic-pathologic correlation. Radiographics 1994;14:1291

Mitchell DG: Focal manifestations of diffuse liver disease at MR imaging. Radiology 1992;185:1

Mortele KJ, Segatto E, Ros PR: The infected liver: radiologic-pathologic correlation. Radiographics 2004;24:937

Weinreb JC, Cohen JM, Armstrong E, et al: Imaging the pediatric liver: MRI and CT. AJR Am J Roentgenol 1986;147:785

Westra SJ, Zaninovic AC, Hall TR, et al: Imaging in pediatric liver transplantation. Radiographics 1993;13:1081-1099

Fatty Liver

Baker MK, Schauwecker DS, Wenker JC, et al: Nuclear medicine evaluation of focal fatty infiltration of the liver. Clin Nucl Med 1986;11:503

Baldridge AD, Perez-Atayde AR, Graeme-Cook F, et al: Idiopathic steatohepatitis in childhood: a multicenter retrospective study. J Pediatr 1995;127:700-704

Brunt EM: Nonalcoholic steatohepatitis. Semin Liver Dis 2004; 24:3-20

Carneiro RC, Fordham LA, Semelka RC: MR imaging of the pediatric liver. Magn Reson Imaging Clin N Am 2002;10:116

Chaudry G, Navarro OM, Levine DS, Oudjhane K: Abdominal manifestations of cystic fibrosis in children. Pediatr Radiol 2006;36:233-240

Fishbein MH, Miner M, Mogren C, Chalekson J: The spectrum of fatty liver in obese children and the relationship of serum aminotransferases to severity of steatosis. J Pediatr Gastroenterol Nutr 2003;36:54-61

Fishbein MH, Stevens WR: Rapid MRI using a modified Dixon technique: a non-invasive and effective method for detection and monitoring of fatty metamorphosis of the liver. Pediatr Radiol 2001;31:806-809

Kane AG, Redwine MD, Cossi AF: Characterization of focal fatty change in the liver with a fat-enhanced inversion-recovery sequence. J Magn Reson Imaging 1993;3:581-586

Okka WH, Aguirre DA, Casola G, et al: Fatty liver: imaging patterns and pitfalls. Radiographics 2006;26:1637-1653

Pilleul F, Chave G, Dumortier J, et al: Fatty infiltration of the liver: detection and grading using dual T1 gradient echo sequences on clinical MR system. Gastroenterol Clin Biol 2005;29:1143

Quinn SF, Gosink BB: Characteristic sonographic signs of hepatic fatty infiltration. AJR Am J Roentgenol 1985;145:753

Radetti G, Kleon W, Stuefer J, Pittschieler K: Non-alcoholic fatty liver disease in obese children evaluated by magnetic resonance imaging. Acta Paediatr 2006;95:833

Roberts EA: Non-alcoholic fatty liver disease (NAFLD) in children. Front Biosci 2005;10:2306-2318

Tchelepi H, Ralls PW, Radin R, Grant E: Sonography of diffuse liver disease. J Ultrasound Med 2002;21:1023

Iron Deposition in the Liver

Angelucci E, Giovagnoni A, Valeri G, et al: Limitations of magnetic resonance imaging in measurement of hepatic iron. Blood 1997;90:4736-4742

Bonetti MG, Castriota-Scanderberg A, Criconia GM, et al: Hepatic iron overload in thalassemic patients: proposal and validation of an MR method of assessment. Pediatr Radiol 1996;26:650

Carneiro AA, Fernandes JP, de Araujo DB, et al: Liver iron concentration evaluated by two magnetic methods: magnetic resonance imaging and magnetic susceptometry. Magn Reson Med 2005;54:122-128

Carneiro AA, Vilela GR, Fernandes JB, et al: In vivo tissue characterization using magnetic techniques. Neurol Clin Neurophysiol 2004;2004:85

Carneiro RC, Fordham LA, Semelka RC: MR imaging of the pediatric liver. Magn Reson Imaging Clin N Am 2002;10;137-164

Emy PY, Levin TL, Sheth SS, et al: Iron overload in reticuloendothelial systems of pediatric oncology patients who have undergone transfusions: MR observations. AJR Am J Roentgenol 1997;168:1011-1015

Flyer MA, Haller JO, Sundaram R: Transfusional hemosiderosis in sickle cell anemia: another cause of an echogenic pancreas. Pediatr Radiol 1993;23:140-142

Freeny PC, Grossholz M, Kaakaji K, Schmiedl UP: Significance of hyperattenuating and contrast-enhancing hepatic nodules detected in the cirrhotic liver during arterial phase helical CT in pre-liver transplant patients: radiologic-histopathologic correlation of explanted livers. Abdom Imaging 2003;28:333-346

Gomori JM, Horev G, Tamary H, et al: Hepatic iron overload: quantitative MR imaging. Radiology 1991;179:367-369

Gore RM, Levine MS, Laufer I: Hemachromatosis. In Gore RM, Levine MS, Laufer I (eds): Textbook of Gastrointestinal Radiology. Philadelphia, Saunders, 1994:1978

Graghorm E, Richter A, Burdelski M, et al: Neonatal hemochromatosis: long-term experience with favorable outcome. Pediatrics 2006;118:2060

Kornreich L, Horev G, Yaniv I, et al: Iron overload following bone marrow transplantation in children: MR findings. Pediatr Radiol 1997;27:869

Levin TL, Sheth SS, Hurlet A, et al: MR marrow signs of iron overload in transfusion-dependent patients with sickle cell disease. Pediatr Radiol 1995;25:614-619

Mazza P, Giua R, De Marco S, et al: Iron overload in thalassemia: comparative analysis of magnetic resonance imaging, serum ferritin and iron content of the liver. Haematologica 1995;80:398-404

Olynyk JK, St Pierre TG, Britton RS, et al: Duration of hepatic iron exposure increases the risk of significant fibrosis in hereditary hemochromatosis: a new role for magnetic resonance imaging. Am J Gastroenterol 2005;100:837

Papakonstantinou O, Kostaridou S, Maris T, et al: Quantification of liver iron overload by T2 quantitative magnetic resonance imaging in thalassemia: impact of chronic hepatitis C on measurements. J Pediatr Hematol Oncol 1999;21:142

Pomerantz S, Siegelman ES: MR imaging of iron depositional disease. Magn Reson Imaging Clin N Am 2002;10:105

Siegelman ES, Mitchell DG, Rubin R, et al: Parenchymal versus reticuloendothelial iron overload in the liver: distinction with MR imaging. Radiology 1991;179:361

Stark DD, Moseley ME, Bacon BR, et al: Magnetic resonance imaging and spectroscopy of hepatic iron overload. Radiology 1985;154:137

St Pierre TG, Clark PR, Chua-anusom W, et al: Noninvasive measurement and imaging of liver iron concentrations using proton magnetic resonance. Blood 2005;105:855

Wang ZJ, Haselgrove JC, Martin MB, et al: Evaluation of iron overload by single voxel MRS measurement of liver T2. J Magn Reson Imaging 2002;15:395-400

Glycogen Storage Diseases

Bowerman RA, Samuels BI, Silver TM: Ultrasonographic features of hepatic adenomas in type I glycogen storage disease. J Ultrasound Med 1983;2:51

Brunelle F, Tammam S, Odievre M, et al: Liver adenomas in glycogen storage disease in children: ultrasound and angiographic study. Pediatr Radiol 1984;14:1091

Debaere C, Op de Beeck B, De Maeseneer M, Osteaux M: Magnetic resonance imaging findings of hepatic adenomas in von Gierke (type I) glycogen storage disease: case report. Can Assoc Radiol J 1999;50:161-164

Doppman JL, Cornblath M, Dwyer AJ, et al: Computed tomography of the liver and kidneys in glycogen storage disease. J Comput Assist Tomogr 1982;6:67

Grazioli L, Federle MP, Brancatelli G, et al: Hepatic adenomas: imaging and pathologic findings. Radiographics 2001;21:877

Heyman S: Liver-spleen scintigraphy in glycogen storage disease (glycogenoses). Clin Nucl Med 1985;10:839-843

Lee PJ: Glycogen storage disease type I: pathophysiology of liver adenomas. Eur J Pediatr 2002;161(Suppl 1):S46-S49

Miller JH, Gates GF, Landing BH, et al: Scintigraphic abnormalities in glycogen storage disease. J Nucl Med 1978;19:354-358

Parker P, Burr I, Slonim A, et al: Regression of hepatic adenomas in type Ia glycogen storage disease with dietary therapy. Gastroenterology 1981;81:534-536

Tchelepi H, Ralls PW, Radin R, Grant E: Sonography of diffuse liver disease. J Ultrasound Med 2002;21:1023

Gaucher Disease

Altarescu G, Hill S, Wiggs E, et al: The efficacy of enzyme replacement therapy in patients with chronic neuronopathic Gaucher's disease. J Pediatr 2001;138:539-547

Beutler E, Demina A, Laubscher K, et al: The clinical course of treated and untreated Gaucher disease: a study of 45 patients. Blood Cells Mol Dis 1995;21:86-108

Elstein D, Hadas-Halpern I, Azuri Y, et al: Accuracy of ultrasonography in assessing spleen and liver size in patients with Gaucher disease: comparison to computed tomographic measurements. J Ultrasound Med 1997;16:209

Figueroa ML, Rosenbloom BE, Kay AC, et al: A less costly regimen of alglucerase to treat Gaucher's disease. N Engl J Med 1992; 327:1632-1636

Glenn D, Thurston D, Garver P, et al: Comparison of magnetic resonance imaging and ultrasound in evaluating liver size in Gaucher patients. Acta Haematol 1994;92:187

Hainaux B, Christophe C, Hanquinet S, Perlmutter N: Gaucher's disease: plain radiography, US, CT and MR diagnosis of lungs, bone and liver lesions. Pediatr Radiol 1992;22:78-79

Hill SC, Damaska BM, Ling A, et al: Gaucher disease: abdominal MR imaging findings in 46 patients. Radiology 1992;184:561

Lanir A, Hadar H, Cohen I, et al: Gaucher disease: assessment with MR imaging. Radiology 1986;161:239-244

Mariani G, Filocamo M, Giona F, et al: Severity of bone marrow involvement in patients with Gaucher's disease evaluated by scintigraphy with 99mTc-sestamibi. J Nucl Med 2003;44:1253-1262

McHugh K, Olsen OE, Vellodi A: Gaucher disease in children: radiology of non-central nervous system manifestations. Clin Radiol 2004;59:117-123

Rosenthal DI, Barton NW, McKusick KA, et al: Quantitative imaging of Gaucher disease. Radiology 1992;185:841-845

Terk MR, Esplin J, Lee K, et al: MR imaging of patients with type 1 Gaucher's disease: relationship between bone and visceral changes. AJR Am J Roentgenol 1995;165:599

Peliosis Hepatis

Gouya H, Vignaux O, Legmann P, et al: Peliosis hepatis: triphasic helical CT and dynamic MRI findings. Abdom Imaging 2001;26:507

Hiorns MP, Rossi UG, Roebuck DJ: Peliosis hepatis causing inferior vena cava compression in a 3-year-old child. Pediatr Radiol 2005;35:209-211

Iannaccone R, Federle MP, Brancatelli G, et al: Peliosis hepatis: spectrum of imaging findings. AJR Am J Roentgenol 2006; 187:W43

Kawamoto S, Soyer PA, Fishman DA, Blumke DA: Nonneoplastic liver disease: evaluation with CT and MR imaging. Radiographics 1998;18:827-848

Mortele KJ, Segatto E, Ros PR: The infected liver: radiologic-pathologic correlation. Radiographics 2004;24:937

Saatci I, Coskun M, Boyvat F, et al: MR findings in peliosis hepatis. Pediatr Radiol 1995;25:31

Schmidt H, Ullrich K, von Lenglerke HJ, et al: Peliosis hepatis with type I glycogen storage disease. J Inherit Metab Dis 1991;14:831

Tsukamoto Y, Nakata H, Kimoto T, et al: CT and angiography of peliosis hepatis. AJR Am J Roentgenol 1984;142:539

Sarcoidosis

Bean MJ, Horton KM, Fishman EK: Concurrent focal hepatic and splenic lesions: a pictorial guide to differential diagnosis. J Comput Assist Tomogr 2004;28:605-612

Collins MH, Jiang B, Croffie JM, et al: Hepatic granulomas in children: a clinicopathologic analysis of 23 cases including polymerase chain reaction for Histoplasma. Am J Surg Pathol 1996;20:332

Koyama T, Ueda H, Togashi K, et al: Radiologic manifestations of sarcoidosis in various organs. Radiographics 2004;24:87-104

Mortele KJ, Ros PR: Imaging of diffuse liver disease. Semin Liver Dis 2001;21:195

Sarigol SS, Hay MH, Wyllie R: Sarcoidosis in preschool children with hepatic involvement mimicking juvenile rheumatoid arthritis. J Pediatr Gastroenterol Nutr 1999;28:510

α_1-Antitrypsin Deficiency

Alfire ME, Treem WR: Nonalcoholic fatty liver disease. Pediatr Ann 2006;35:290-297

Ishak KG: Inherited metabolic diseases of the liver. Clin Liver Dis 2002;6:455

Kelly DA, McKiernan PJ: Metabolic liver disease in the pediatric patient. Clin Liver Dis 1998;2:1

Odievre M, Martin JP, Hadchouel M, Alagille D: Alpha 1-antitrypsin deficiency and liver disease in children: phenotypes, manifestations, and prognosis. Pediatrics 1976;57:226-231

Shaker SB, Stavngaard T, Stolk J, et al: Alpha1-antitrypsin deficiency. 7. Computed tomographic imaging in alpha1-antitrypsin deficiency. Thorax 2004;59:986

Teckman JH, Lindblad D: Alpha-1-antitrypsin deficiency: diagnosis, pathophysiology, and management. Curr Gastroenterol Rep 2006;8:14

Wilson Disease

Alfire ME, Treem WR: Nonalcoholic fatty liver disease. Pediatr Ann 2006;35:290-297

Chu WC, Leung TF, Chan KF, et al: Wilson's disease with chronic active hepatitis: monitoring by in vivo 31-phosphorus MR spectroscopy before and after medical treatment. AJR Am J Roentgenol 2004;183:1339-1342

Dhawan A, Ferenci P, Geubel A, et al: Genes and metals: a deadly combination. Acta Gastroenterol Belg 2005;68:26-32

Genovese E, Maghnie M, Maggiore G, et al: MR imaging of CNS involvement in children affected by chronic liver disease. AJNR Am J Neuroradiol 2000;21:845-851

Gill HH, Shankaran K, Desai HG: Wilson's disease: varied hepatic presentations. Indian J Gastroenterol 1994;13:95-98

Johnson RC, DeFord JW, Gebhart RJ: Chronic active hepatitis and cirrhosis in Wilson's disease. South Med J 1977;70:753-754

Kawamoto S, Soyer PA, Fishman EK: Nonneoplastic liver disease: evaluation with CT and MR imaging. Radiographics 1998; 18:827-848

Ko S, Lee T, Ng S, et al: Unusual liver MR findings of Wilson's disease in an asymptomatic 2-year-old girl. Abdom Imaging 1998;23:56

Lawler GA, Pennock JM, Steiner RE, et al: Nuclear magnetic resonance (NMR) imaging in Wilson disease. J Comput Assist Tomogr 1983;7:1-8

Lo Curto AG, Marchi A, Grasso M, et al: Early diagnosis of Wilson disease in a six-year-old child. J Pediatr 2006;148:141

Sternlieb I, Scheinberg IH: The role of radiocopper in the diagnosis of Wilson's disease. Gastroenterology 1979;77:138-142

Walshe JM, Potter G: The pattern of the whole body distribution of radioactive copper (67Cu, 64Cu) in Wilson's disease and various control groups. QJM 1977;46:445-462

Walshe JM, Waldenstrom E, Sams V, et al: Abdominal malignancies in patients with Wilson's disease. QJM 2003;96:657-662

Zietz BP, Dieter HH, Lakomek M, et al: Epidemiological investigation on chronic copper toxicity to children exposed via the public drinking water supply. Sci Total Environ 2003;302:127-144

Tyrosinemia

Dubois J, Garel L, Patriquin H, et al: Imaging features of type 1 hereditary tyrosinemia: a review of 30 patients. Pediatr Radiol 1996;26:845-851

Forget S, Patriquin HB, Dubois J, et al: The kidney in children with tyrosinemia: sonographic, CT and biochemical findings. Pediatr Radiol 1999;29:104

Gallant JM, Barnewolt CE, Buonomo C: Pediatric case of the day. Hepatorenal tyrosinemia (tyrosinemia type I). Radiographics 1996;16:1221

Kelly DA, McKiernan PJ: Metabolic liver disease in the pediatric patient. Clin Liver Dis 1998;2:1

Lam R, Armenta A, Kilic M, et al: Tyrosinemia. Liver Transpl 2002;8:500

Macvicar D, Dicks-Mireaux C, Leonard JV, Wight DG: Hepatic imaging with computed tomography of chronic tyrosinaemia type 1. Br J Radiol 1990;63:605-608

Russo PA, Mitchell GA, Tanguay RM: Tyrosinemia: a review. Pediatr Dev Pathol 2001;4:212

Galactosemia

Cox PJ: Galactosaemia. BMJ 1954;2:613-618

Fournier A, Cathala J, Polonovski C, Demassieux R: [On an infectious syndrome with hepatomegaly and glycosuria simulating a congenital galactosemia and terminated by a thrombosis of the cerebral veins with nervous diabetes.] Nourrisson 1959;47:103-112

Gitzelmann R, Steinmann B: Galactosemia: how does long-term treatment change the outcome? Enzyme 1984;32:37-46

Kahler SG, Fahey MC: Metabolic disorders and mental retardation. Am J Med Genet C Semin Med Genet 2003;117:31

Nelson MD, Wolff JA, Cross CA: Galactosemia: evaluation with MR imaging. Radiology 1992;184:255

Pozzato C, Curti A, Radaelli G, et al: Abdominal ultrasonography in inherited diseases of carbohydrate metabolism. Radiol Med (Torino) 2005;109:139-147

Cirrhosis

Akata D, Akhan O, Ozcelik U, et al: Hepatobiliary manifestations of cystic fibrosis in children: correlation of CT and US findings. Eur J Radiol 2002;41:26-33

Chaudry G, Navarro OM, Levine DS, et al: Abdominal manifestations of cystic fibrosis in children. Pediatr Radiol 2006;36:233

Efrati O, Barak A, Modan-Moses D, et al: Liver cirrhosis and portal hypertension in cystic fibrosis. Eur J Gastroenterol Hepatol 2003;15:1073-1078

Gorka W, Kagalwalla A, McParland BJ, et al: Diagnostic value of Doppler ultrasound in the assessment of liver cirrhosis in children: histopathological correlation. J Clin Ultrasound 1996;24:287-295

Gubernick JA, Rosenberg HK, Hakan I, Kessler A: US approach to jaundice in infants and children. Radiographics 2000;20:173-195

MacSween RN, Fell GS: Familial cirrhosis. Scott Med J 1974;19:25-30

Ohtomo K, Itai Y, Ohtomo Y, et al: Regenerating nodules of liver cirrhosis: MR imaging with pathologic correlation. AJR Am J Roentgenol 1990;154:505

Semelka RC, Chung JJ, Hussain SM, et al: Chronic hepatitis: correlation of early patchy and late linear enhancement patterns on gadolinium-enhanced MR images with histopathology initial experience. J Magn Reson Imaging 2001;13:385-391

Simonovsky V: The diagnosis of cirrhosis by high resolution ultrasound of the liver surface. Br J Radiol 1999;72:29-34

Vitellas KM, Tzalonikou MT, Bennett WF, et al: Cirrhosis: spectrum of findings on unenhanced and dynamic gadolinium-enhanced MR imaging. Abdom Imaging 2001;26:601

Zhu JA, Hu B: Ultrasonography in predicting and screening liver cirrhosis in children: a preliminary study. World J Gastroenterol 2003;9:2348-2349

115 Vascular Abnormalities of the Liver

TAMAR BEN-AMI

HEPATIC VASCULAR BED

The paired vitelline veins from the yolk sac form a vascular plexus within the developing liver by the fifth week of gestation. Normally, the left vitelline vein involutes. The right vitelline vein eventually participates in the formation of the hepatic veins, the terminal portion of the inferior vena cava (IVC), and the portal vein. The umbilical veins participate in the formation of the left portal vein and the ductus venosus. Errors in the complex evolution of this intricate network may result in anomalous connections between these structures and in an absent intrahepatic segment of the IVC.

The liver has a dual blood supply, receiving both hepatic arterial and portal venous blood. Both systems are drained by the hepatic veins. A single hepatic artery is present in 57% of patients. It arises from the celiac axis in 90% of cases, from the superior mesenteric artery in 5%, and from other visceral aortic branches in 5%. A separate origin of the hepatic artery from the aorta is less common. After giving rise to the gastroduodenal artery, the hepatic artery enters the liver and branches into right and left lobar and segmental branches. The right and left hepatic arteries originate separately in 43% of patients, arising from the celiac axis, superior mesenteric artery (right), or left gastric artery.

The normal portal vein forms from the splenic, superior mesenteric, and left gastric (coronary) veins. It branches into the right and left portal veins and then into their segmental branches. Prenatally, the left portal vein receives blood from the umbilical vein. Flow in the umbilical vein ceases once the cord is ligated. However, the lumen of the umbilical vein may be recognized within the falciform ligament of the liver for a few days after birth. Following this, the umbilical vein obliterates to form the ligamentum teres. Twenty percent to 30% of portal venous flow enters the ductus venosus, which drains into the infra-atrial IVC adjacent to the hepatic veins. The ductus venosus plays an important regulatory role in the fetus; flow within it increases during hypoxia. Postnatally, the ductus venosus responds to increased oxygen tension by closing within 6 days; it may take longer in infants of younger gestational age, remaining open as long as 37 days in small premature infants. Agenesis of the ductus venosus has been reviewed by Sau and coworkers. This entity is associated with direct insertion of the umbilical vein into the heart and a high incidence of cardiac anomalies.

Normal anatomic variants include absence of the horizontal portion of the left portal vein, with left lobe portal supply from the right portal vein, and absence of the right portal vein, with variable origins of the right anterior and posterior portal veins arising as a trifurcation from the main or left portal vein. Vascular variations are important when planning segmental hepatic resections or ligation of intrahepatic portosystemic shunts, and these variations should be differentiated from portal branch occlusion and thrombosis.

Normal flow velocity in the main portal vein in non-fasting children is 0.1 to 0.3 m/sec. Flow increases in the postprandial state. Portal venous flow may demonstrate some modulation by cardiac systole in some patients.

Because of its dual blood supply, the vascular bed of the liver is unusually complex. Both arterial and portal vascular beds are interconnected through sinusoids and potential communications via the peribiliary plexus and portal vasa vasorum. A decrease in the contribution of one allows an increased contribution from the other. Normally, 75% of the liver's blood supply is received from the portal vein. However, if intrahepatic resistance increases, the portal vein's contribution may decrease, and the hepatic arterial contribution correspondingly increases. With severe cirrhosis, the portal vein may become a draining vein for the hepatic arterial vascular bed.

Variations in hepatic blood flow are well demonstrated by Doppler ultrasonography (US), computed tomography angiography (CTA), and magnetic resonance angiography (MRA). The vessel size and the flow volume and direction best reflect hemodynamic changes. When portal venous flow decreases and hepatic arterial flow increases, areas of increased enhancement appear in the hepatic arterial phase of CTA; these equalize in the portal phase, owing to arterioportal shunting. Variable focal attenuation in the hepatic arterial phase may be caused by other factors as well, such as obstruction of the draining hepatic vein, trauma, tumor, vascular malformation, and aberrant blood supply.

Each cross-sectional modality offers unique advantages when evaluating the hepatic portal and arterial systems. However, computed tomography (CT) and magnetic resonance imaging (MRI) are better suited than US for demonstrating collateral vessels and spontaneous porto-systemic shunts because of the wide field of view and multiplanar capabilities. In general, MRI is better than both CT and US for visualizing the IVC and hepatic veins, and CT and MRI are better than US for demonstrating intrahepatic portal vein branches.

CONGENITAL ANOMALIES OF LIVER VASCULATURE

Anomalies of the Portal Vein

Congenital anomalies of the portal vein include pre-duodenal portal vein, double portal vein, and agenesis of the portal vein. Intrahepatic portal vein anatomy is deficient in the case of congenital absence of the right or left hepatic lobes. True agenesis of a lobe should be differentiated from lobe atrophy, in which case diminutive residual portal branches would be expected. Some portal vein aneurysms are considered congenital, and at least one has been described in utero. Portal vein aneurysms occur most frequently at bifurcation sites—splenomesenteric junction, main portal vein, and intrahepatic branches.

Preduodenal portal vein is a rare anomaly in which the portal vein courses ventral to the duodenum and pancreatic head. The preduodenal portal vein is well identified by US, CT, and MRI. The proposed embryology is nonregression of the caudal anastomotic vein that connects the two vitelline veins ventral to the duodenum, where it then participates in the formation of the portal vein.

The anomaly is closely associated with the heterotaxy syndrome, particularly polysplenia; malrotation; and splenic, pancreatic, cardiac, and duodenal anomalies. In approximately 50% of patients, there is associated duodenal obstruction: atresia, Ladd bands with malrotation, duodenal stenosis, annular pancreas, and duodenal membrane; in a minority of these cases, duodenal obstruction may be caused by the anomalous course of the portal vein. In the other 50% of patients, there is no duodenal obstruction and the lesion is discovered incidentally. Approximately 10% of patients with biliary atresia have an associated situs abnormality; in these patients, the preduodenal portal vein has potential surgical hazards during portoenterostomy for biliary atresia and during liver transplantation and other hepatobiliary procedures and should be recognized preoperatively.

> **Preduodenal portal vein is associated with heterotaxy syndrome; malrotation; and splenic, cardiac, and pancreatic anomalies. Fifty percent of patients have associated duodenal obstruction.**

Congenital Portosystemic Shunts

EXTRAHEPATIC SHUNTS

Abernethy first described an extrahepatic portosystemic connection in 1793, and this is now known as the Abernethy malformation. These extrahepatic portosyste-

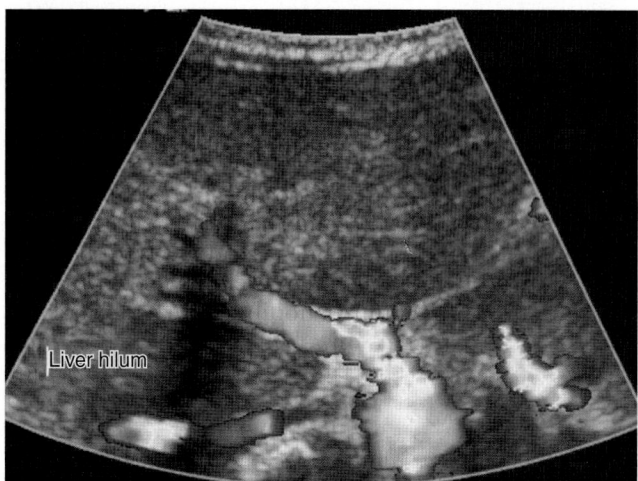

FIGURE 115-1. Congenital extrahepatic portosystemic fistula. Gray scale depiction of color Doppler US shows only a hepatic artery in the liver hilum.

mic shunts were classified by Morgan and Superina into two types:

Type 1: complete shunt—no portal blood reaches the liver, as in congenital absence of the portal vein

Type 2: partial shunt—shunt to the portal vein, hepatic vein, or IVC

The splenic and superior mesenteric veins may become confluent before joining the IVC, right atrium, renal vein, or iliac vein or may drain separately into systemic veins.

Most patients with extrahepatic portosystemic shunt and hypoplastic or absent portal vein demonstrate hyperammonemia and some disturbance of liver function. However, hyperammonemic encephalopathy is less common in children than in adults. Reportedly, most patients with encephalopathy have a greater than 60% shunt. There are reports if hyperinsulinism and hyperandrogenism in teenage girls with portosystemic shunts.

On imaging studies in patients with extrahepatic shunts, the liver is smaller than normal. When the portal vein is absent, a single vascular channel is seen in the hilum by all modalities; this represents the hepatic artery, which is larger than expected relative to the size of the liver and the patient's age (Fig. 115-1). When the portal vein is present, it is small (Fig. 115-2). The shunt's vascular connection may be demonstrated by US, but CTA and MRA are more likely to demonstrate its complete course and anatomy (Figs. 115-3 and 115-4). Associated hepatic parenchymal nodules may be demonstrated by all cross-sectional imaging modalities (Fig. 115-5).

Extrahepatic portosystemic shunts have a high association with absence (rare) or hypoplasia of the portal vein. Absence of the portal vein may be noted prenatally, with congenital agenesis of the ductus venosus and umbilical vein drainage into the IVC or directly into the heart. Postnatally, the anomaly was once considered to be more common in girls, who also have a greater incidence of associated anomalies (predominantly cardiac and genitourinary), heterotaxy, or biliary atresia; alternatively, the anomaly may present as a component of Goldenhar syndrome. Associated liver masses are also

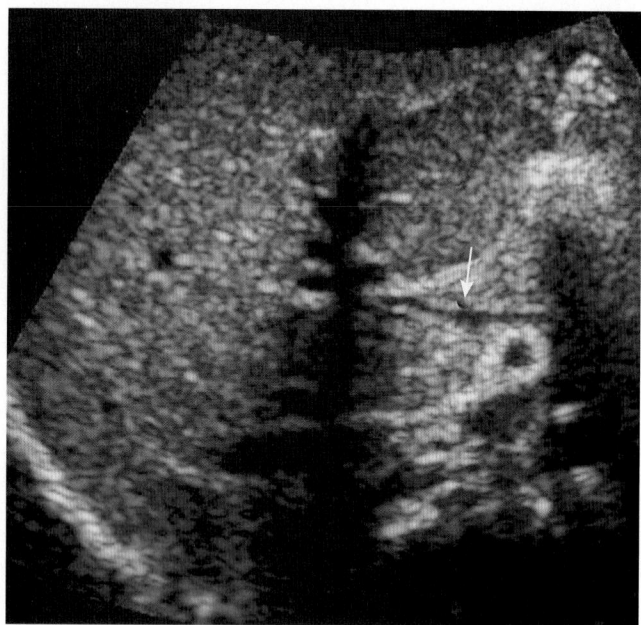

FIGURE 115-2. Congenital extrahepatic portosystemic shunt. A diminutive main portal vein is present *(arrow)*.

more frequent in girls. However, since the widespread use of US and Doppler, there have been numerous reports of asymptomatic children with this anomaly, many of whom are boys. The associated portosystemic shunt may involve the confluence of the left renal vein, splenic vein, and superior mesenteric vein to join the IVC (see Fig. 115-3) or separate drainage of an isolated superior mesenteric vein into the suprarenal IVC (see Fig. 115-4).

INTRAHEPATIC SHUNTS

One or more intrahepatic shunts may be present, representing persistent communications between the portal and hepatic venous derivatives of the embryologic vitelline veins, or between the vitelline and subcardinal veins. A patent ductus venosus represents a form of portosystemic shunt from the left portal vein into the IVC. When diagnosed in neonates, some of these shunts may resolve spontaneously; there are multiple reports of intrahepatic portal vein–to–hepatic vein communications that resolved within a few months.

Intrahepatic portosystemic shunts have been classified by Park and associates into four types:
Type I: single large vein connecting the right portal and hepatic veins
Type II: peripheral single or multiple communications in one segment
Type III: aneurysm connecting a peripheral portal vein and hepatic vein branch
Type IV: diffuse communications in multiple lobes
Type I is the most common. The first three types may be asymptomatic and resolve spontaneously. Type IV may be associated with massive shunt and heart failure.

Although children appear to be relatively resistant to hyperammonemic encephalopathy, a shunt ratio greater than 60% can cause encephalopathy and liver dysfunction and should be corrected. The shunt ratio can be calculated by dividing shunt flow volume by portal vein

flow volume. Asymptomatic children with mild metabolic abnormalities can be treated conservatively by dietary means and Doppler follow-up.

This anomaly is often demonstrated by US, sometimes during the screening of infants with cutaneous hemangiomas. Nonuniform size of the portal vein and hepatic vein branches may locate additional communications. The flow pattern in the portal and even splenic veins may demonstrate a bi- or triphasic pattern. Intrahepatic shunts are well demonstrated by CTA and MRA (Fig. 115-6).

> A larger than normal portal vein or hepatic vein branch should prompt a search for an intrahepatic portosystemic shunt.

Anomalous Connections to the Portal Vein

Pulmonary veins develop in the fourth week of gestation as a plexus that initially drains into both the cardinal veins and the umbilicovitelline venous system. The connection to the umbilicovitelline system is gradually lost, and the pulmonary plexus and pulmonary veins drain into the common pulmonary vein, which becomes incorporated into the left atrium. Any of these embryonal connections may persist as congenital anomalies. Total anomalous venous return into the portal vein and the rare extralobar pulmonary sequestration with venous drainage into the portal system represent the anomalous persistence of the pulmonary-vitelline connection. Total anomalous pulmonary venous return below the diaphragm drains most frequently into the portal vein or ductus venosus.

Imaging of the liver in children with total anomalous pulmonary venous return may demonstrate a larger than normal portal vein. The anomalous common pulmonary vein is seen as a large vascular channel that enters the diaphragmatic hiatus anterior to the esophagus and inserts into the left portal vein or ductus venosus (Fig. 115-7). Doppler evaluation of the anomalous vein shows hepatopetal flow.

This anomaly can be a surgical hazard during portoenterostomy for biliary atresia. It may be associated with portal hypertension and esophageal varices.

VASCULAR MASSES AND MALFORMATIONS

Mulliken and Glowacki divided vascular anomalies of the liver into two categories: vasoproliferative tumors and vascular malformations. This distinction is based on clinical findings, histology, and behavior of the lesions.

Vasoproliferative Tumors

Tumors included in this category are infantile hemangioma, hemangioendothelioma, angiosarcoma, and epithelioid hemangioendothelioma. These lesions are also discussed in Chapter 117.

Hemangioendothelioma and infantile hemangioma of the liver are distinguishable pathologically but have similar clinical and imaging characteristics. They are true

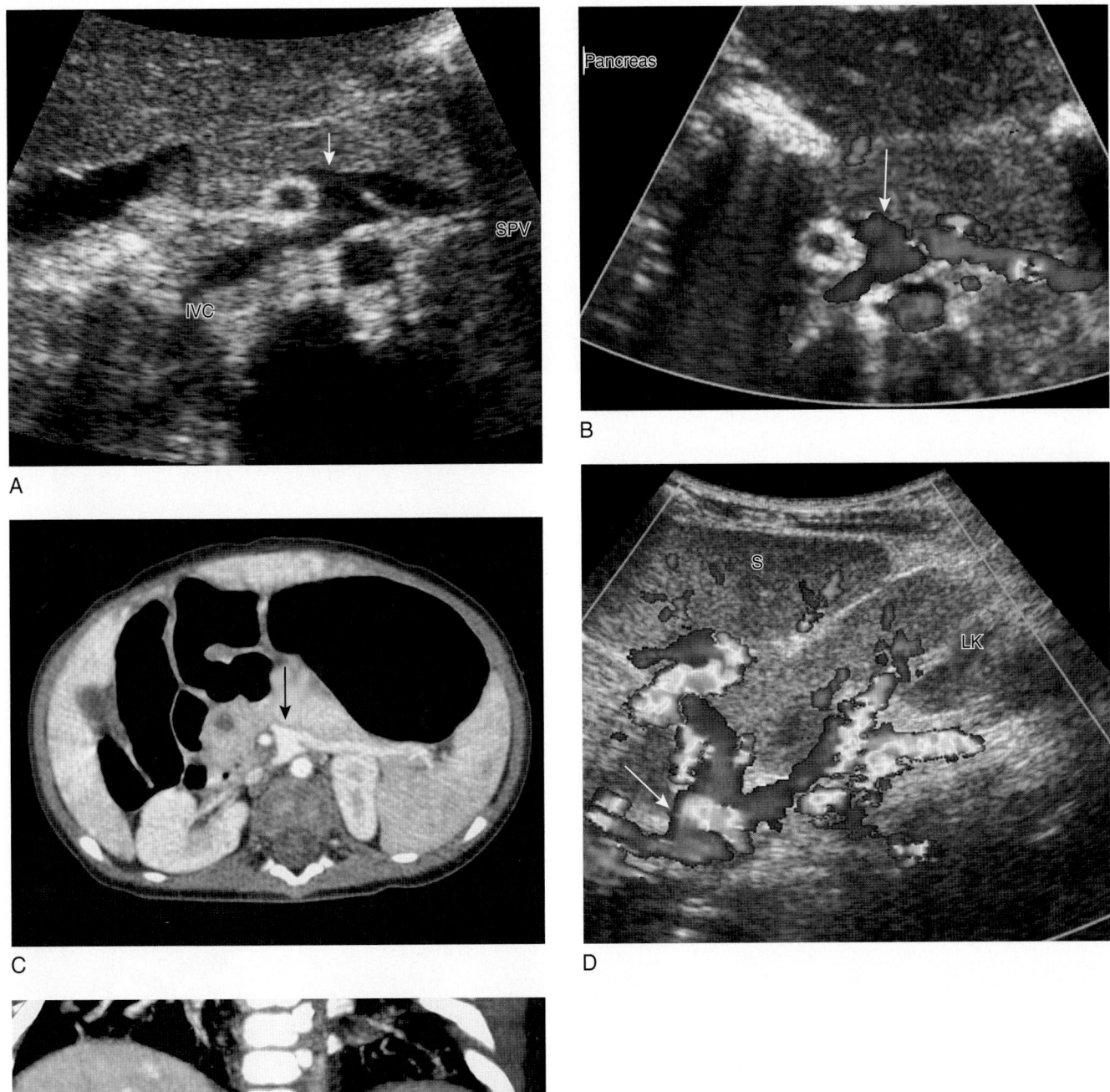

FIGURE 115-3. This 6-month-old anorchic, XY, phenotypically female patient with an interrupted aortic arch had US to evaluate abnormal liver function. An extrahepatic portosystemic shunt is present. **A,** Transverse US image shows the splenic vein (SPV) joining a left-sided superior mesenteric vein *(arrow)*, both draining into the left renal vein and inferior vena cava (IVC). **B,** Color Doppler image shows flow in the appropriate direction in the splenic vein (red), which then turns dorsally to join the left renal vein toward the IVC (*See color plate.*) **C,** Axial CT shows the portosystemic shunt *(arrow)* and the diminutive main portal vein. **D,** Coronal color Doppler image shows the splenic and left renal veins joining to form the shunt *(arrow)*. LK, left kidney; S, spleen. (*See color plate.*) **E,** CTA coronal reconstruction shows that the small splenic vein and left renal vein *(arrowhead)* join the superior mesenteric vein to form a large joint channel that enters the IVC. The arrows mark converging flow in the splenic vein *(upper arrow)* and superior mesenteric vein *(vertical arrow)* to the IVC.

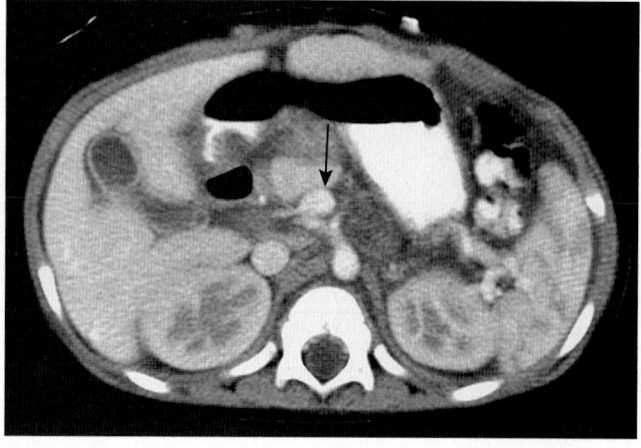

A

FIGURE 115-4. Extrahepatic portosystemic shunt and absence of the portal vein. The superior mesenteric and splenic veins drain into the upper inferior vena cava. **A,** The large shunt vessel *(arrow)* courses in a cranial direction anterior to the celiac axis bifurcation. **B,** CTA coronal reconstruction shows that the portosystemic shunt connects the superior mesenteric vein to the inferior vena cava above the diaphragm.

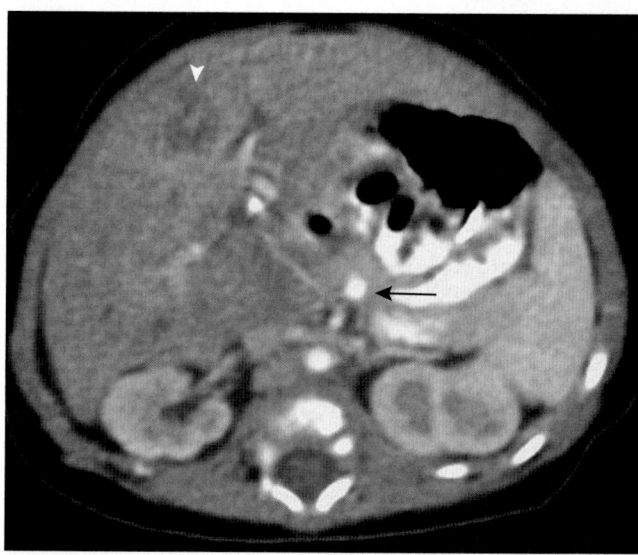

B

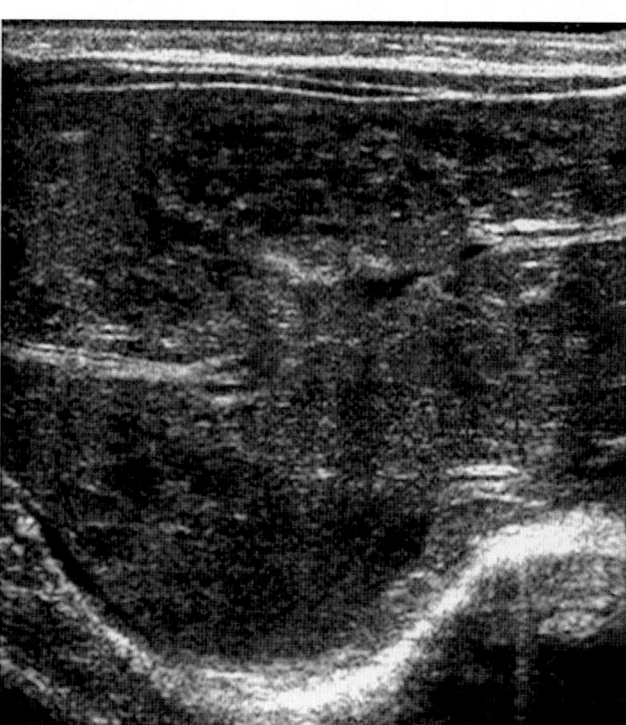

A

B

FIGURE 115-5. Infant with extrahepatic portosystemic shunt and absent portal vein. The liver parenchyma is inhomogeneous and nodular. **A,** Transverse ultrasound image. **B,** Axial CT image. The portosystemic shunt *(arrow)* courses cephalad toward the inferior vena cava. A liver nodule is present *(arrowhead)*. A single vessel in the liver hilum represents the hepatic artery.

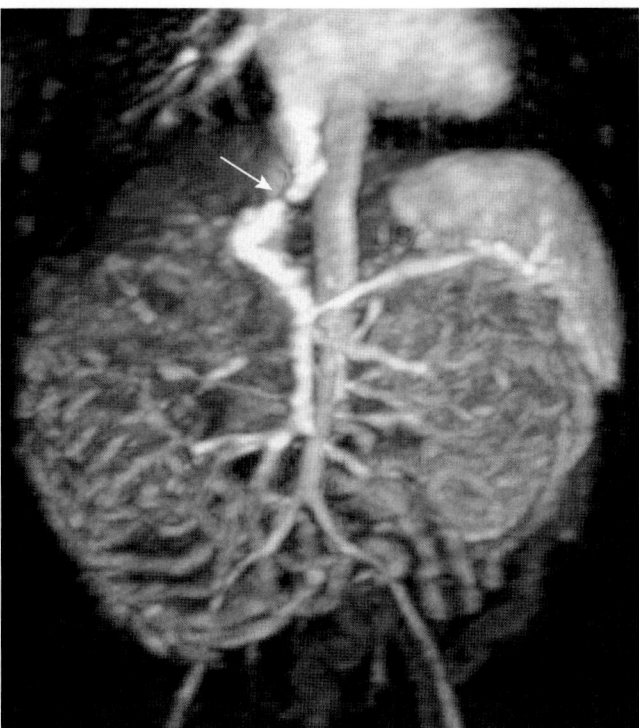

FIGURE 115-6. Intrahepatic portosystemic shunt in an infant with hyperammonemia. Magnetic resonance venography shows the anomalous connection *(arrow)* between the intrahepatic portal vein and the inferior vena cava. The portal vein was larger than normal on US.

benign neoplasms that may occupy variable portions of the liver; hepatic infantile hemangiomas may be single or multiple. The natural history is similar to that of other infantile hemangiomas elsewhere in the body. There is an early proliferative phase in the first few months of life, followed by gradual involution after the first year. Histologically, these lesions have extensive vascular spaces lined with plump endothelial cells of variable appearance, with intervening fibromyxomatous stroma; infantile hemangiomas have been shown to express glucose transporter protein isoform 1. Hemangioendotheliomas are distinguished by slightly more aggressive features.

The presentation of infantile hemangioma or hemangioendothelioma is predominantly a consequence of vascular hemodynamics. When diffuse, multifocal, or single and large, hemangioendotheliomas usually demonstrate extensive hepatovenous shunting—arteriovenous, arterioportal, or portovenous—resulting in hepatomegaly and high-output congestive heart failure. When not hemodynamically significant, such lesions may be asymptomatic or present as an incidental abdominal mass. Burrows and colleagues classified hepatic hemangiomas according to their angiographic findings and the presence and degree of shunting.

Clinically, most patients present before 6 months of age. Some are asymptomatic and have cutaneous hemangiomas. The larger and more hemodynamically active the lesion, the earlier the presentation. Single, large lesions with high-output heart failure tend to present at birth. Multifocal lesions may present between 1 and 16 weeks of age. The infant may exhibit abdominal distention, palpable mass, respiratory distress, congestive heart failure, hepatomegaly, jaundice, anemia, or consumptive manifestations with thrombocytopenia and hemorrhagic diathesis.

Clinical presentation of infantile hemangioma or hemangioendothelioma:

- **Shunt related—high-output congestive heart failure**

- **Bulk related—respiratory distress, abdominal distention, palpable mass**

- **Hematologic—jaundice, anemia, thrombocytopenia**

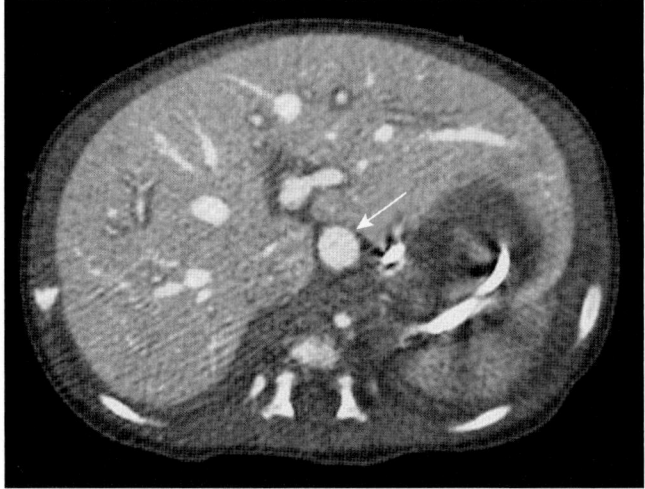

A

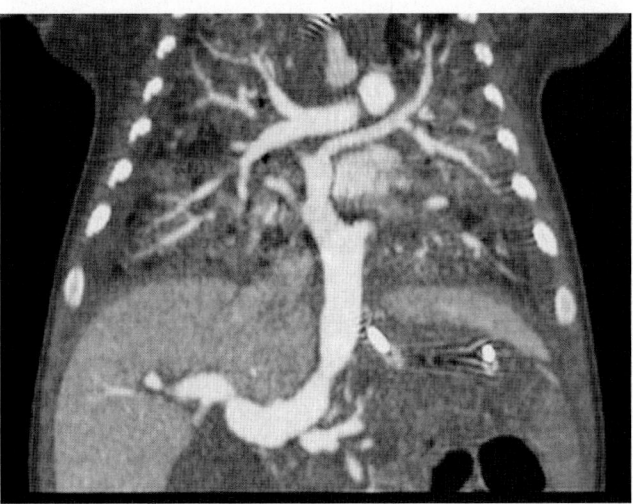

B

FIGURE 115-7. Total anomalous pulmonary venous return into the portal vein. **A,** Axial image from CTA shows the large common pulmonary vein *(arrow)* coursing caudad toward the portal vein. The portal vein branches are much larger than normal. Note the small caliber of the aorta relative to the common pulmonary vein and portal system. **B,** Coronal reconstruction in the same patient shows the pulmonary veins converging to form the common pulmonary vein, which takes a vertical course to join the portal vein.

Plain films of patients with hemodynamically significant hepatic hemangioendothelioma may demonstrate cardiomegaly, hepatomegaly, and sometimes congestive heart failure. US demonstrates multiple parenchymal liver lesions or a single lesion. The lesions are typically hypoechoic, but occasionally they may demonstrate mixed echogenicity or calcifications, particularly hemangioendotheliomas. Doppler characteristics are variable, depending on the lesion's size, flow, and degree and type of shunting. There may be broadening of the hepatic arterial systolic peaks (Fig. 115-8), with increased peak systolic velocity and diastolic flow velocity, and a low resistive index. Draining hepatic venous flow is increased; portal venous flow is variable and may be reversed. As the lesions involute spontaneously or in response to therapy, these flow parameters improve. In patients with multiple lesions, differences in vascularity and stages of involution produce variable Doppler flow patterns.

In hemodynamically significant lesions, the aorta is enlarged proximally and tapers after the takeoff of the celiac. The hepatic artery is larger than normal, frequently larger than the portal vein. The draining hepatic

veins are dilated. These features can be seen on all cross-sectional modalities.

CT demonstrates single or multiple low-attenuation lesions with occasional calcifications on pre-enhanced scans. The enhancement pattern in children may be variable, but dramatic peripheral early enhancement that progresses centripetally is common, particularly in large lesions (Fig. 115-9). There may be variable degrees of central necrosis, preventing central enhancement of the lesion. On delayed scanning, enhancement of the lesion may be greater than or similar to that of the surrounding liver parenchyma (Fig. 115-10).

MRI provides the most complete anatomic and hemodynamic information (Fig. 115-11). Infantile hemangiomas show hyperintense signal on T2 sequences, sharp demarcation from the surrounding parenchyma, and low signal on T1 images. Multiple flow voids in and around the lesions represent the vascular channels. Gadolinium-enhanced MR images parallel CT enhancement patterns. Low central signal in larger lesions represents necrosis, fibrosis, or hemorrhage.

Vascular malformations may be similar hemodynamically and should be considered in the differential diagnosis. However, whereas infantile hemangiomas demonstrate abnormal signal and contrast enhancement in the mass surrounding the lesion, arteriovenous malformations do not. Hemangiomas tend to involute; vascular malformations do not. Pediatric liver masses that must be differentiated are hepatoblastoma, mesenchymal hamartoma, and metastatic disease from neuroblastoma and Wilms tumor. Hepatoblastoma, occasionally mesenchymal hamartoma, and rarely angiosarcoma may be hypervascular and manifest arteriovenous shunting. Hepatocellular carcinoma, focal nodular hyperplasia, adenoma, and lymphoma tend to present in older children.

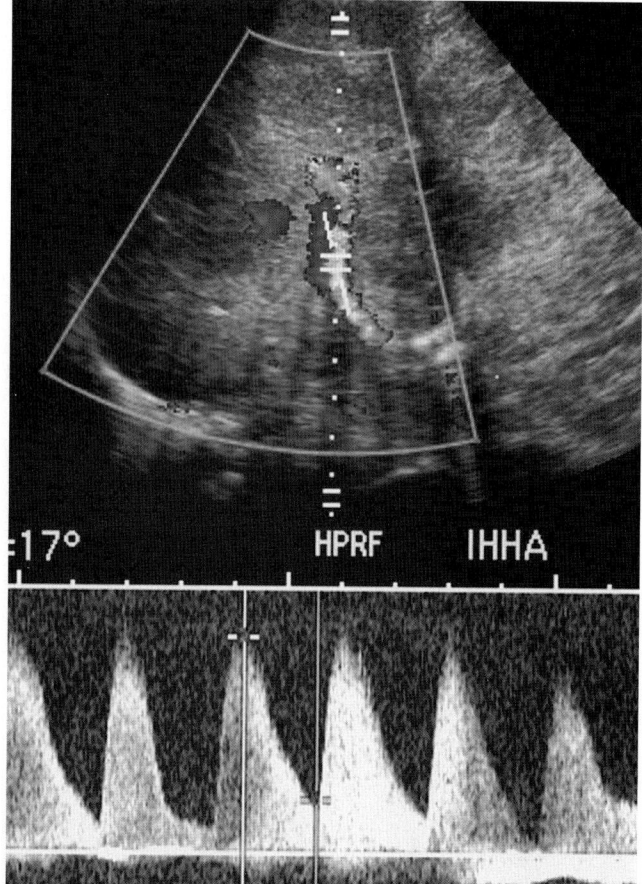

FIGURE 115-8. Infantile hepatic hemangioendothelioma. Color and spectral Doppler show a large, dominant hepatic artery. There is broadening of the hepatic artery systolic peak and increased peak velocity. The diastolic flow is not increased, suggesting relatively little hepatovenous shunting. However, the portal venous flow is reversed, suggesting microscopic arterioportal shunting.

> **Differentiation between infantile hemangioma and arteriovenous malformation:**
> - **Infantile hemangioma demonstrates abnormal signal and contrast enhancement in the mass surrounding the lesion; arteriovenous malformations have no associated mass**
> - **Hemangiomas tend to involute; vascular malformations do not**

Hemodynamically insignificant infantile hemangiomas can be followed expectantly until involution. Mildly symptomatic patients can be treated with corticosteroids or α-interferon. More aggressive intervention with embolization therapy may be performed in patients with refractory congestive heart failure. In patients with therapy-resistant congestive heart failure, liver transplantation may be considered.

Vascular Malformations

Hepatic vascular malformations can be divided into arteriovenous malformations and arterioportal fistulas. Arteriovenous malformations are much less common

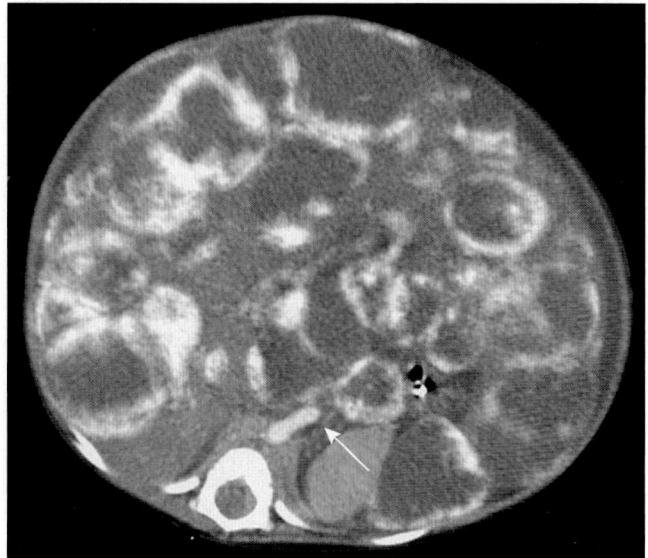 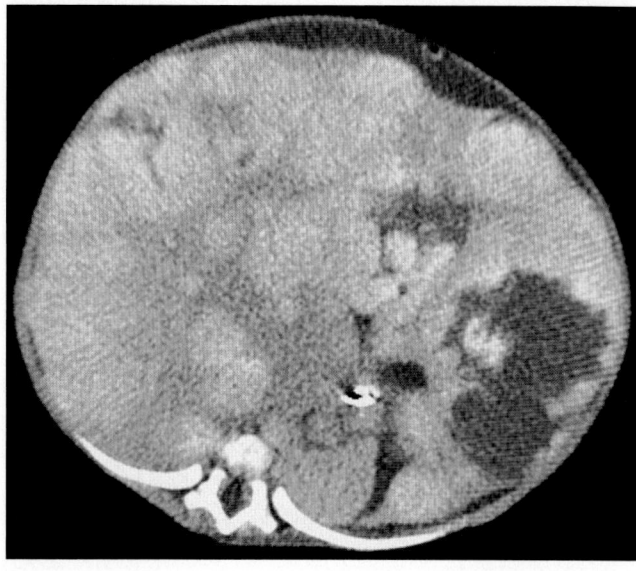

A

B

FIGURE 115-9. Multifocal hepatic hemangioendothelioma in an infant with congestive heart failure. **A,** Axial CT shows innumerable liver lesions with centripetal enhancement, creating nodular, intense peripheral enhancement. Note that the celiac axis diameter *(arrow)* is nearly equal to that of the abdominal aorta. **B,** On delayed images, the nodules became diffusely and homogeneously enhancing.

than infantile hemangiomas. They are non-neoplastic collections of vessels with feeding hepatic artery branches and hepatic venous drainage. Unlike hemangioma or hemangioendothelioma, arteriovenous malformations do not regress; they grow proportionately with the child. They do not respond to medical therapy. Clinical manifestations include congestive heart failure, anemia, hepatomegaly, and portal hypertension.

US demonstrates a tangle of vessels of variable sizes. The size of the hepatic artery is proportional to the size of the shunt; the draining hepatic veins are distended, and the aorta may taper after the takeoff of the hepatic artery. The hepatic artery demonstrates very high systolic Doppler shifts and high diastolic flow, whereas the hepatic veins demonstrate pulsatile or arterialized high-velocity flow. Prenatal sonographic diagnosis of hepatic arteriovenous fistula has been reported.

CT and CTA demonstrate a hypodense precontrast appearance, intense enhancement, and rapid washout. The enlarged arterial supply and venous drainage are well demonstrated by CTA, with early appearance of the draining veins. The excellent temporal resolution of fast sequence MRA allows differentiation between the longer parenchymal uptake in infantile hemangioendothelioma and the absence of tissue stain and fast clearance in arteriovenous malformation.

Arterioportal fistulas are usually acquired lesions, but congenital fistulas have been described. They can be intrahepatic or extrahepatic. Acquired fistulas may be post-traumatic or iatrogenic (postoperative after liver transplantation, liver biopsy, or percutaneous cholangiography), or they may be associated with liver neoplasms such as hepatoblastoma or hepatocellular carcinoma.

Congenital arteriovenous fistulas and malformations may be isolated lesions, or they may be part of the spectrum of Rendu-Osler-Weber syndrome (hereditary hemorrhagic telangiectasia), Ehlers-Danlos syndrome,

biliary atresia, and cirrhosis. Hereditary hemorrhagic telangiectasia affects the liver in the majority of patients and is most often asymptomatic. Lesions include arterioportal shunts in the majority of patients, followed by arteriosystemic and combined lesions.

Clinically, congenital arteriovenous fistulas frequently manifest within the first year of life with rapidly progressive portal hypertension—splenomegaly, hypersplenism, bleeding varices, ascites, and intestinal manifestations of malabsorption. High-output heart failure may be seen in infants, mainly when the ductus venosus is patent. If left untreated, further liver damage with hepatoportal sclerosis may aggravate the portal hypertension.

Clinical symptoms of acquired arteriovenous fistulas depend on their size and location. Postbiopsy fistulas that are generally small and peripheral produce no symptoms and are usually self-limited. Infants with biliary atresia and arterioportal shunt may pose a challenge, owing to the liver's dependence on the hepatic arterial supply and the risk of fatal hepatic necrosis following hepatic artery embolization. For such infants, early liver transplantation may be the treatment of choice.

On imaging, Doppler usually demonstrates a single feeding artery. Portal venous flow is reversed in the draining vein of an arterioportal fistula and may be reversed in the main portal vein, depending on shunt size. The reversed portal venous flow is usually arterialized, with a high flow velocity. Flow may also be reversed in the superior mesenteric and splenic veins. The hepatic artery, or the branch that leads into the fistula, demonstrates high velocity and a decreased resistive index (Fig. 115-12). There may be ascites and bowel wall thickening. The fistula is intensely visible by color and power Doppler, with vibration artifact in the hepatic vein.

CTA and MRA demonstrate arteriovenous fistulas and malformations well. Angiography is reserved for therapeutic embolization.

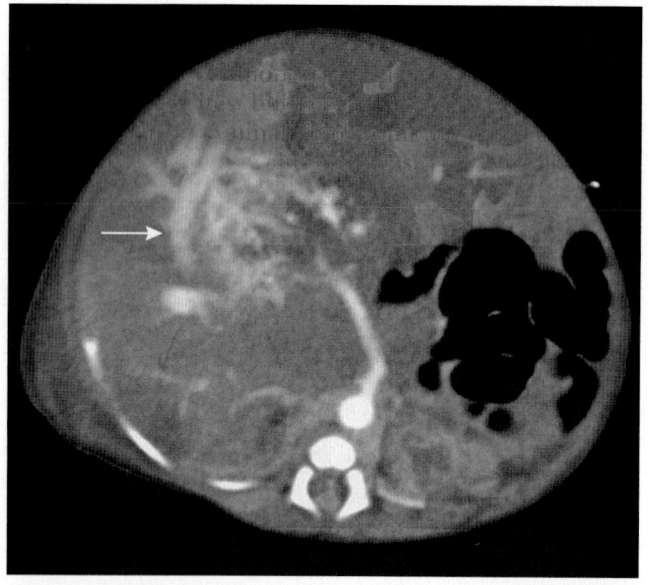

A

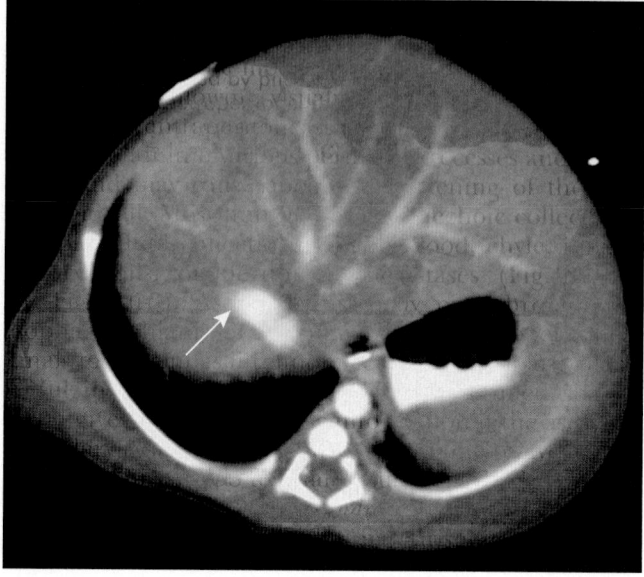

B

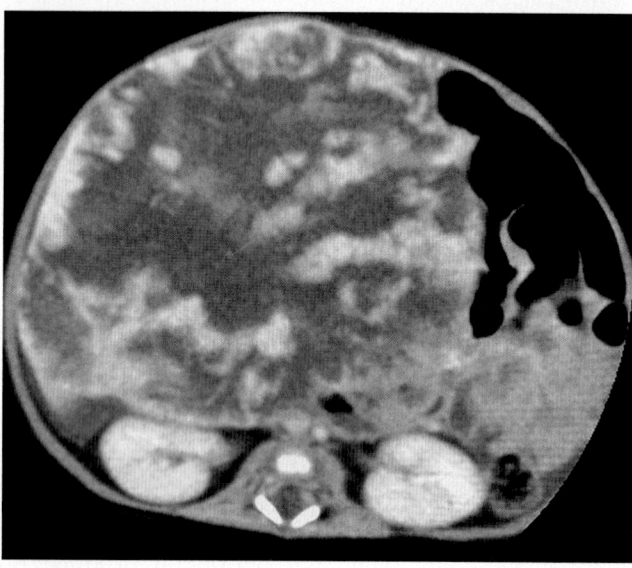

C

FIGURE 115-10. Single large hemangioendothelioma in an infant with congestive heart failure. **A,** On early arterial phase CTA, the hepatic artery is enlarged, and there is a tangle of vessels, with the early appearance of a draining right hepatic vein *(arrow)*. At this phase, it is impossible to differentiate hemangioendothelioma from hepatic arteriovenous malformation. **B,** The right hepatic vein *(arrow)* is disproportionately larger than the middle and left hepatic veins, providing the principal drainage of the hemangioma. **C,** A later phase image demonstrates inhomogeneous enhancement of the large liver mass, with multiple unenhanced areas that did not fill in subsequently, possibly representing hemorrhage or necrosis.

Treatment consists of embolization, surgical ligation, and hepatic lobectomy. As noted earlier, infants with biliary atresia and arterioportal shunt present a special problem; they are unlikely to tolerate interruption in hepatic arterial flow, and early liver transplantation may be the treatment of choice.

Pure venous malformations are usually associated with the blue rubber bleb nevus syndrome, with multisystem focal venous malformations, including focal lesions in the liver.

PORTAL HYPERTENSION

Portal hypertension is defined as a rise in pressure within the splanchnic venous system above 10 mm Hg. This increase in pressure may result from either increased resistance to hepatic venous drainage (postsinusoidal) or

an increase in inflow pressure. Table 115-1 lists causes of portal hypertension in children.

Cirrhosis

Cirrhosis is the scarring that results from the hepatic response to chronic injury. It is associated with deterioration of liver function as well as the development of portal hypertension. The Child-Turcotte-Pugh classification provides a severity score that plays a part in treatment decisions. Patients are stratified into grades A through C based on bilirubin elevation, albumin level, prothrombin time, ascites, and severity of encephalopathy. In pediatric patients, cirrhosis can result from a variety of conditions, including biliary atresia, cystic fibrosis, hemochromatosis, and Wilson disease (see Chapters 15 and 114).

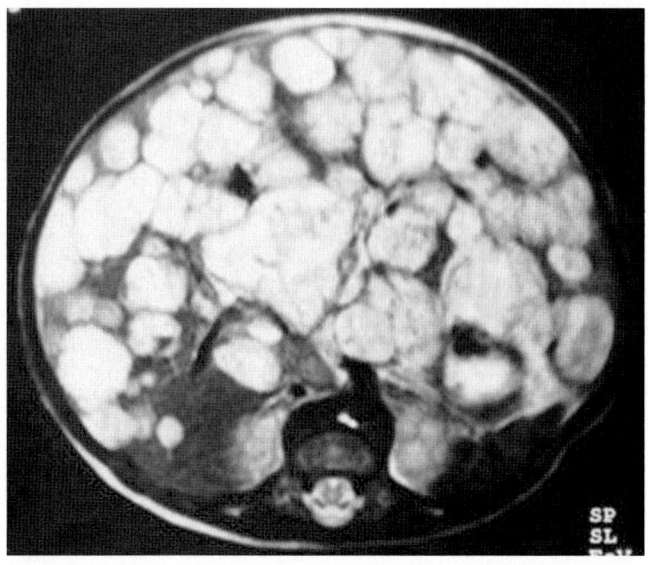

A

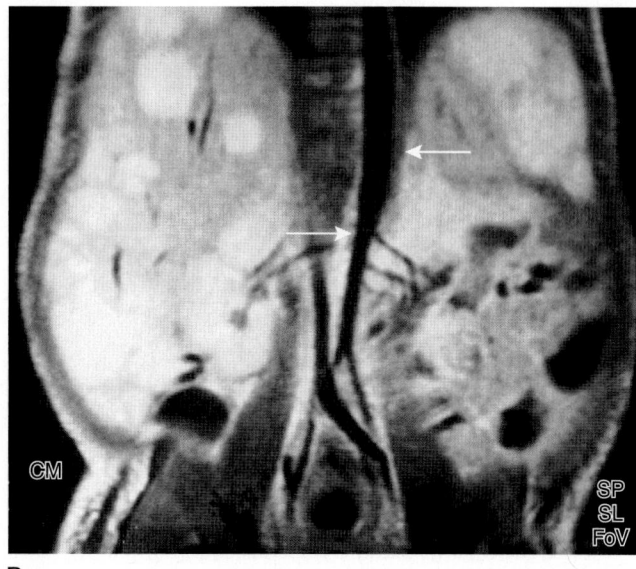

B

FIGURE 115-11. Multifocal hemangioendothelioma. This infant with intractable congestive heart failure did not respond to medical therapy and eventually underwent successful liver transplantation. **A,** T2-weighted axial MRI sequence shows diffuse, extensive involvement of the liver, with multifocal hyperintense lesions as well as massive hepatomegaly. **B,** Coronal T2-weighted sequence shows an enlarged upper abdominal aorta *(upper arrow),* which tapers *(lower arrow)* distal to the origin of the celiac axis.

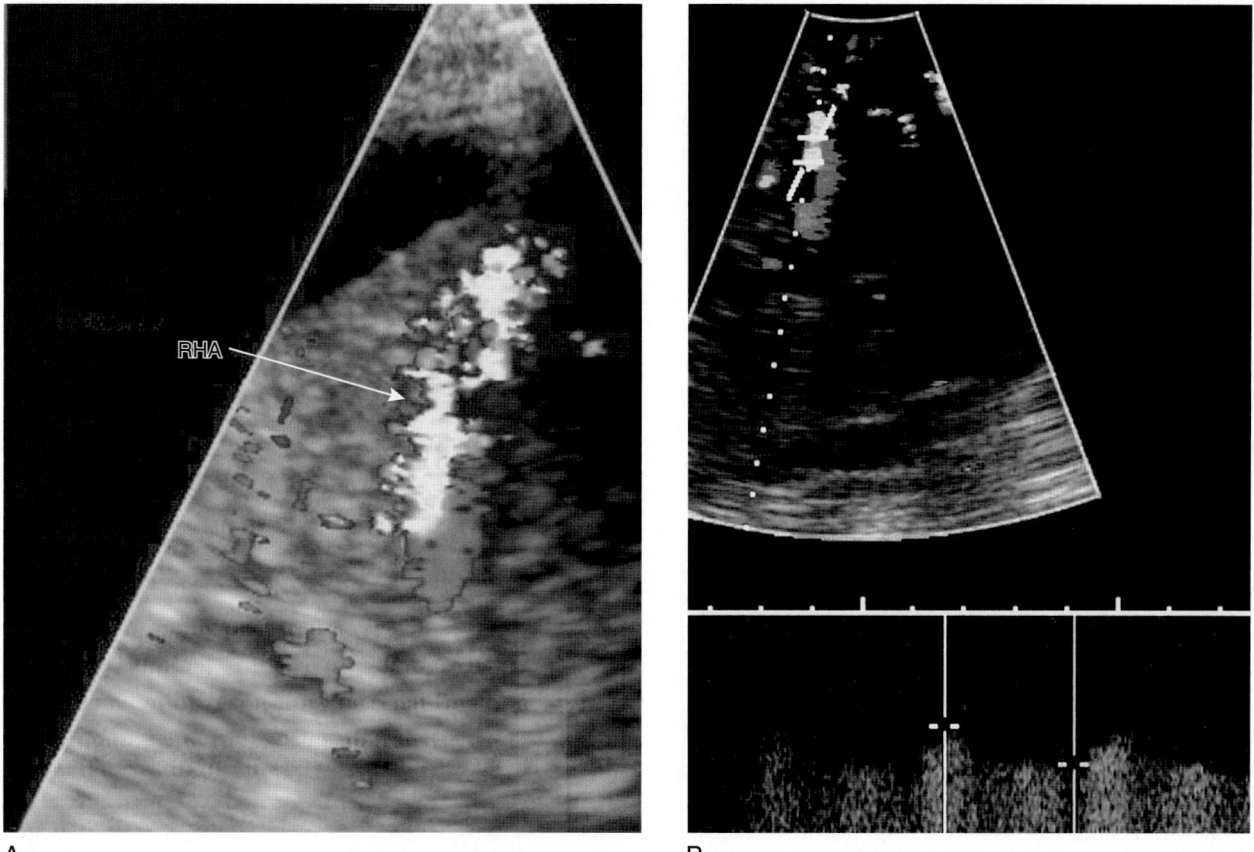

A

B

FIGURE 115-12. Postbiopsy arterioportal fistula in an 8-year-old boy with a liver transplant. **A,** Color Doppler image shows intense Doppler shift in a peripheral, small arteriovenous fistula arising from a right hepatic artery (RHA) branch *(arrow),* at the site of a previous liver biopsy. Ascites is also seen, outlining the liver *(See color plate.)* **B,** Color and spectral Doppler show a very high diastolic flow and a low resistive index in the hepatic artery branch leading into the fistula.

TABLE 115-1

Pediatric Causes of Portal Hypertension

Increased inflow pressure or volume
    Hepatic artery–to–portal vein fistula
    Total anomalous pulmonary venous return below the
      diaphragm
    Pulmonary sequestration with portal venous drainage
Presinusoidal venous obstruction
    Splenic vein occlusion (sinistral portal hypertension)
    Extrahepatic portal vein thrombosis—cavernous
      transformation of portal vein
    Post-transplantation portal vein stenosis, thrombosis, and
      occlusion
    Congenital hepatic fibrosis
    Schistosomiasis
Increased sinusoidal resistance
    Biliary atresia
    Cirrhosis
    Hepatitis C; non-A, non-B hepatitis; autoimmune
      hepatitis; neonatal hepatitis
    Sclerosing cholangitis
Postsinusoidal obstruction
    Budd-Chiari syndrome
    Glenn or Fontan systemic-to-pulmonary venous shunt
    Medications: 6-thioguanine
Idiopathic portal hypertension

Extrahepatic Portal Vein Occlusion—Cavernous Transformation of the Portal Vein

Cavernous transformation of the portal vein (CTPV) represents occlusion and replacement of the portal vein with portoportal venous collaterals along the course of the thrombosed portal vein, directing blood from the high-pressure prethrombotic splanchnic veins to the lower pressure intrahepatic branches. In many patients, the underlying cause cannot be identified. The incidence of portal vein thrombosis is increased in complicated umbilical vein catheterization, sepsis, dehydration, shock, and coagulopathy. CTPV can also be seen in patients with long-standing liver disease, such as congenital hepatic fibrosis with portal hypertension, particularly if complicated by intra-abdominal infection or inflammation such as omphalitis, appendicitis, pancreatitis, Crohn disease, or ulcerative colitis.

Portal vein thrombosis has been reported on prenatal US. Most thrombosed portal veins recanalize; however, thrombosed portal veins in children with severe liver disease tend to remain occluded. The evolution of cavernous transformation has been observed in a few patients with portal vein thrombosis, more often in those with an underlying healthy liver, and most recently in patients with liver transplantation. De Gaetano and colleagues observed the formation of cavernous transformation within 6 to 20 days of acute portal vein thrombosis in 9 of 65 patients. In most young children, the liver distal to the obstruction remains functionally normal; however, many older children with long-standing CTPV demonstrate parenchymal abnormalities. Changes in the hepatocytes can be detected with electron microscopy, and deranged liver function and cholestasis with biliary strictures, biliary sludge, and stones have been described

in children with CTPV. Gallbladder wall thickening, decreased contractility, and increased incidence of cholelithiasis have also been described.

> **In most patients with extrahepatic portal vein thrombosis and cavernous transformation, there is no underlying liver disease.**

Many children present clinically with the consequences of portal hypertension: gastrointestinal bleeding, unexplained splenomegaly and hypersplenism without jaundice, or disturbed liver function. Other children present as a consequence of underlying liver disease, ascites, or cholestasis.

US, contrasted CT, CTA, MRI, and MRA demonstrate a tangle of venous channels in the liver hilum, with no demonstrable hilar portal vein (Fig. 115-13). The tangle also contains some arterial components. Such collaterals may extend only into the liver hilum, but in the majority of patients (76%), they extend for a variable distance along the course of the intrahepatic portal branches. In extreme cases, no portal vein branches can be demonstrated (Fig. 115-14). Preserved intrahepatic portal vein branches may be present, some of which may demonstrate hepatofugal flow toward the cavernous vessels. These intrahepatic branches may represent sinusoidal supply from the hepatic artery or transcapsular collaterals directing flow from the liver periphery toward the lower pressure center, sometimes across segments or lobes. Transcapsular collaterals are frequently seen in patients with portal vein occlusion following liver transplantation. Collateral veins may traverse the liver parenchyma to enter hepatic and capsular veins (Fig. 115-15). Dynamic, contrast-enhanced CT and MRI may demonstrate uneven attenuation of the hepatic parenchyma.

Flow within the cavernous transformation is slow, 0.02 to 0.08 m/sec, compared with 0.2 to 0.4 m/sec in the normal portal vein. Portosystemic collaterals are also seen, with the exception of paraumbilical collaterals, which depend on the patency of the main and left portal veins. Hepatic arterial peak systolic velocity is increased, and the resistive index decreases.

> **Although there is hepatopetal portal flow in CTPV, all patients have portal hypertension.**

Collateral Pathways

When portal venous pressure increases, splanchnic venous return finds alternative drainage pathways connecting the portal circulation to the systemic circulation. Left gastric (coronary) and splenic vein branches drain into the azygos system through esophageal and gastric varices and to the IVC through the left renal vein (Fig. 115-16). Paraumbilical veins (Fig. 115-17) communicate with inferior epigastric and internal mammary abdominal wall venous networks to drain into the inferior and superior vena cavae, respectively. A visible umbilical varix or caput medusae (Courvalhier-Baumgartner syndrome) may be seen clinically.

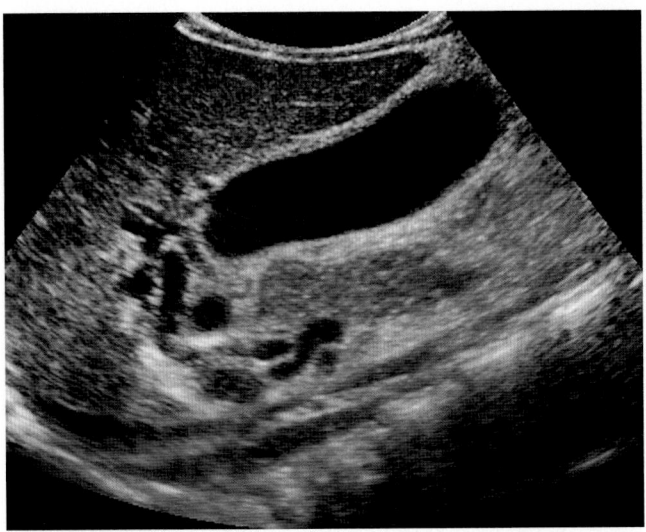

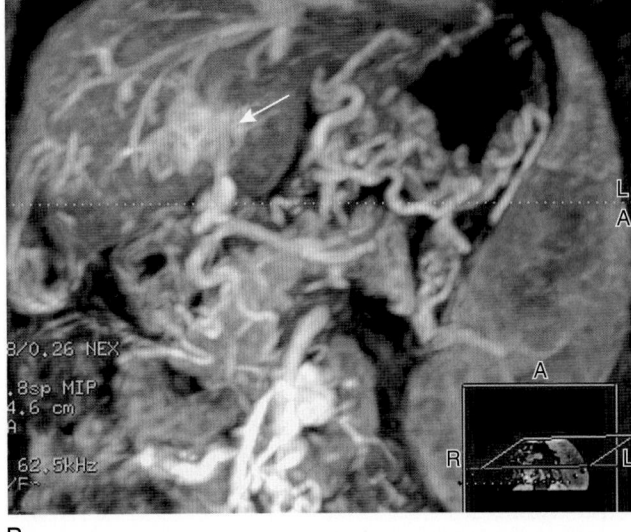

A   B

FIGURE 115-13. Cavernous transformation of the portal vein. **A,** Oblique intercostal image of the liver hilum shows a tangle of collateral veins along the course of the expected portal vein. **B,** MRA performed in preparation for a Rex shunt. There is a tangle of collaterals at the liver hilum *(arrow)*, representing the cavernous transformation; extensive venous collaterals in the liver hilum and gastric walls; and transcapsular collaterals in the liver.

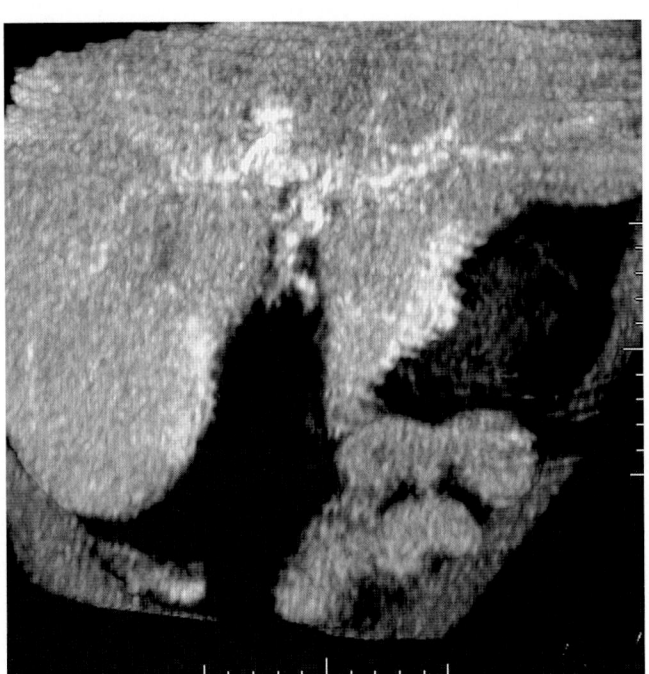

FIGURE 115-14. In this patient with cavernous transformation of the portal vein, no intrahepatic portal vein branches are seen anywhere in the liver. Tangles of collaterals follow the expected course of the entire intrahepatic portal system. It is possible that the system is patent but receives too little flow to be visualized.

Retroperitoneal and peripancreatic collaterals drain through renal and gonadal veins into the IVC and into paraspinal veins, leading into the azygos system (Fig. 115-18). Inferior mesenteric branches drain into superior to middle and inferior hemorrhoidal veins that lead to the iliac veins. Portosystemic collaterals may also form at enterocutaneous junctions in fistulas and enterostomies. Surgical anastomoses, such as a Roux-en-Y

biliary-enteric anastomosis, may serve as sites of portoportal collaterals (Fig. 115-19). Intercostal and phrenic veins may also serve as a means of portosystemic communication across the diaphragm. Collateral veins may traverse the liver, bypassing the intrahepatic portal vein branches to drain into capsular, phrenic, and hepatic veins (Fig. 115-20).

When the severity of hepatic disease is uneven (often with the right lobe affected more severely than the left), portal flow may create lobe-to lobe or segment-to-segment shunting from regions of higher resistance to those of lower resistance.

On imaging, the earliest sign of portal hypertension is splenic enlargement. In portal hypertension originating beyond the main portal vein, the next stage is enlargement of the main portal vein, with an increase in portal volume flow. As resistance to portal flow increases, portal venous flow slows down, portal vein diameter decreases, and, with high resistance, portal venous flow may become reversed or even arterialized. The normal portal vein has a larger cross-sectional area than the splenic vein. If the reverse is seen, the presence of collaterals diverting portal flow away from the liver must be assumed (Fig. 115-21). Reversal of venous flow in the superior mesenteric and splenic veins is also suggestive of collaterals and spontaneous portosystemic shunts. Multiple segmental portal veins should be examined within the liver. Quantitative flow parameters measured by dynamic, contrast-enhanced MRI have been reported to correlate better with the severity of cirrhosis and the severity of portal hypertension as determined by the Child-Turcotte-Pugh classification than do portal venous velocity and hepatic artery resistive index. Hepatofugal flow is a late finding in portal hypertension, and hepatopetal flow in the main portal vein does not exclude severe portal hypertension when collaterals are present or when there is lobe-to-lobe shunting.

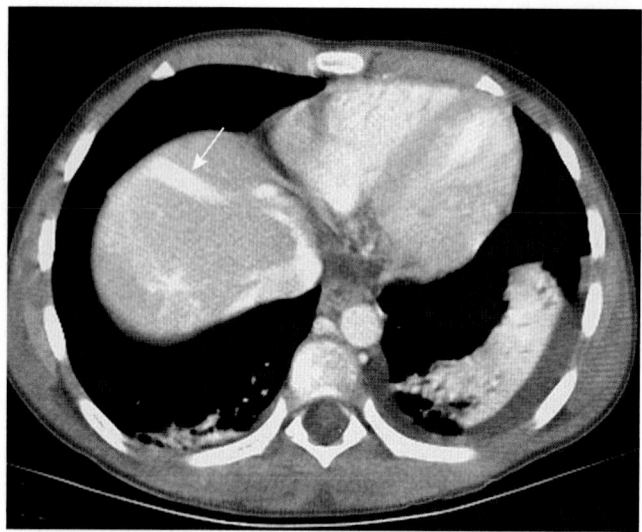

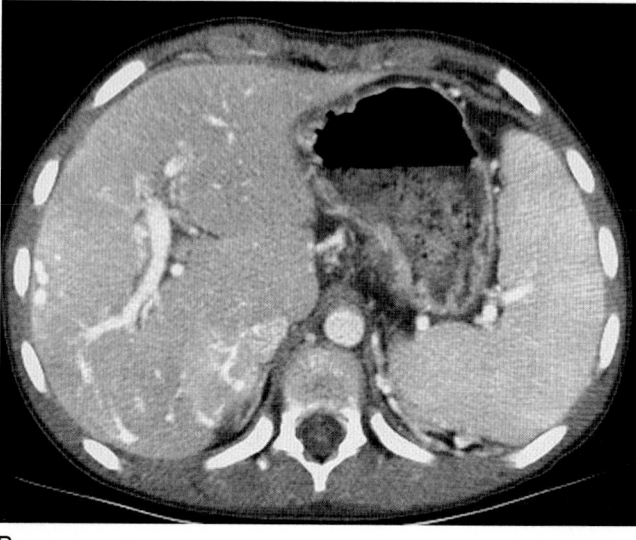

A   B

FIGURE 115-15. Extrahepatic portal vein obstruction with cavernous transformation of the portal vein. There are portovenous and transcapsular connections across the liver parenchyma. **A,** High axial slice at the liver dome shows a peripheral large collateral vein *(arrow)* communicating with the left hepatic vein. **B,** Lower axial CT slice shows numerous transcapsular venous collaterals that communicate with the intrahepatic portal vein branches.

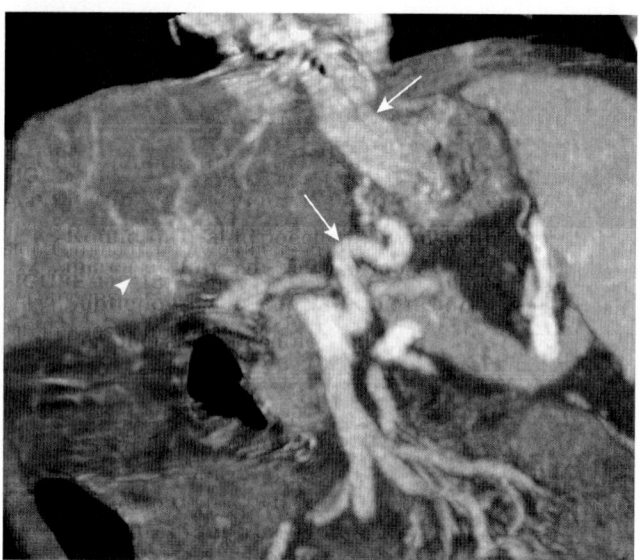

FIGURE 115-16. Patient with extrahepatic portal vein occlusion and cavernous transformation of the portal vein. MRA performed in preparation for a Rex shunt shows a cluster of hilar collaterals *(arrowhead)*. A large left gastric vein *(lower arrow)* leads to gastric and esophageal varices *(upper arrow)*.

The lesser omentum can become thickened due to prominence of the left gastric and short gastric veins, which lead to gastric and esophageal varices. Brunelle and coworkers and Patriquin and colleagues (1985) reported that in portal hypertension, the lesser omental thickness between the aorta and the left lobe of the liver on sagittal ultrasound images exceeds 1.7 times the diameter of the aorta, in the absence of excessive fat or lymphadenopathy.

The presence of a patent paraumbilical vein allows hepatopetal flow in the main portal vein even in the presence of extreme portal hypertension, potentially creating a misleadingly normal portal venous flow. However, because the paraumbilical veins are supplied by the left portal vein, intrahepatic portal flow may be directed toward them, causing reversal of flow in the right portal vein. The paraumbilical veins are well seen in the falciform fossa by color and power Doppler, as well as by CTA and MRA. Hepatic decompression by those veins may serve as relative protection against large esophageal varices and variceal hemorrhage.

The portal system is evaluated equally well by cross-sectional imaging and by conventional angiography. Kreft and associates found no significant differences between digital subtraction angiography and MRA in terms of sensitivity, specificity, and accuracy of assessing vessel patency. Collateral veins in the gastric and esophageal walls, lesser omentum, retroperitoneum, paravertebral regions, pancreas, liver hilum, mesentery, abdominal wall, and pelvis are much better delineated in toto by CT or MRI than by US. It is reported that CTA demonstrates collaterals earlier than endoscopic evaluation of visible varices.

> **Portal vein flow is diminished, reversed, or arterialized in severe portal hypertension. When paraumbilical veins are patent, main portal venous flow may be hepatopetal and normal in spite of severe portal hypertension.**

Surgical and Percutaneous Shunt Procedures

Therapeutic options for children with portal hypertension include percutaneous transjugular intrahepatic portosystemic shunts, sclerotherapy and variceal ligation, and surgical portosystemic shunts.

Surgical portosystemic shunts include splenorenal shunts, mesocaval shunts, and the recently introduced

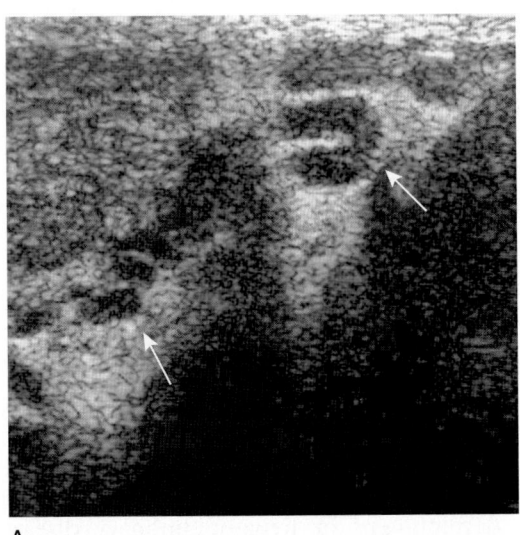

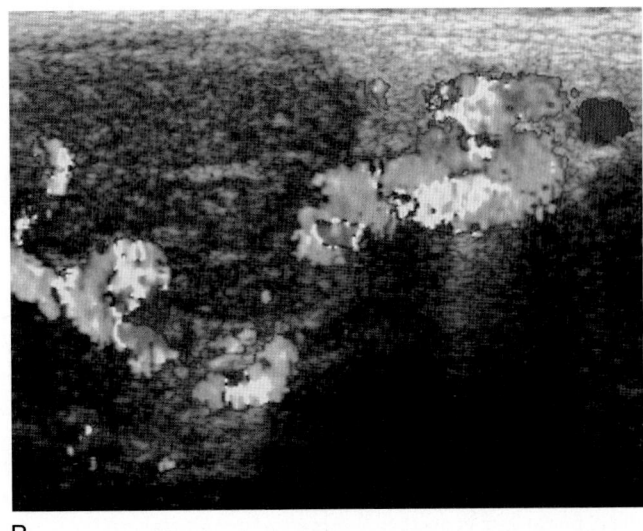

A   B

FIGURE 115-17. Two-year-old girl with biliary atresia, cirrhosis, and portal hypertension. **A,** Longitudinal US of the liver shows tortuous venous collaterals *(arrows)* along the falciform ligament. The veins could be followed to the umbilical region. **B,** Color Doppler shows prominent hepatofugal flow within the paraumbilical venous collaterals. (*See color plate.*)

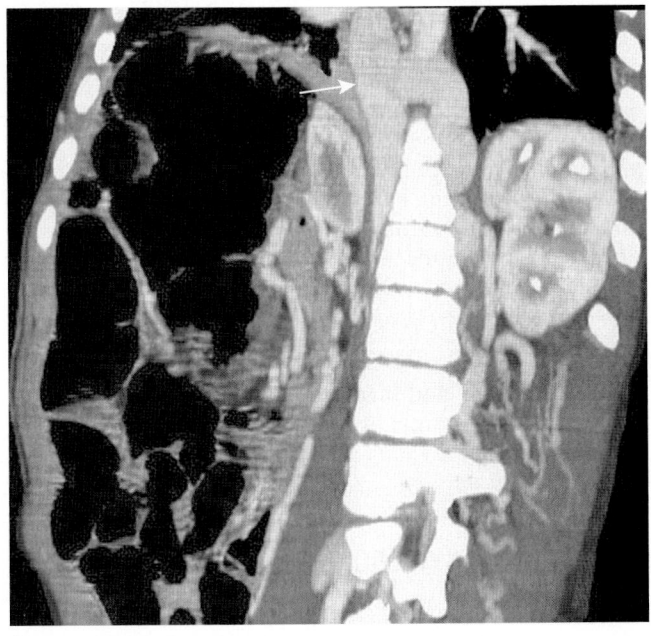

A

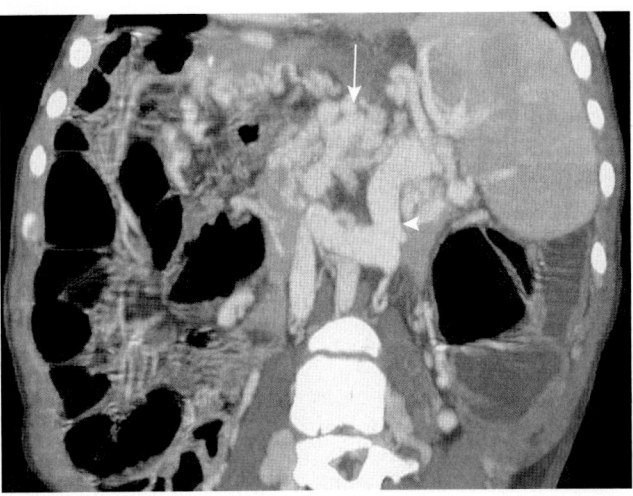

B

FIGURE 115-18. Liver transplant with an occluded portal vein and inferior vena cava. **A,** Retroperitoneal, paraspinal, and intraspinal venous collaterals are present. The azygos and hemiazygos veins are massively enlarged *(arrow)*. **B,** There are extensive pancreatic *(arrow)* and perisplenic collaterals and a splenorenal shunt *(arrowhead)*.

mesoportal (Rex) shunt. The distal splenic vein is connected end-to-side to the left renal vein in distal splenorenal shunts (Fig. 115-22), leaving the superior mesenteric vein to drain into the liver. Portal vein flow is hepatofugal in patent mesocaval and proximal spleno-renal shunts; it may be hepatopetal in distal splenorenal shunts. These shunts may provide long-term palliation in children with portal hypertension and prevent further gastrointestinal hemorrhages, as well as improve hypersplenism. In children with severe underlying liver disease, these shunts are temporizing procedures before liver transplantation.

> In a distal splenorenal shunt, portal vein flow is derived from the superior mesenteric vein, and the entire splenic flow enters the shunt.

The mesoportal (Rex) shunt was first described in 1992 by de Ville de Goyet and coworkers for children with portal vein obstruction following segmental liver transplantation. It was extended to patients with extrahepatic portal vein obstruction over the next few years. In this shunt, a venous graft from the patient's left jugular vein courses from the superior mesenteric vein

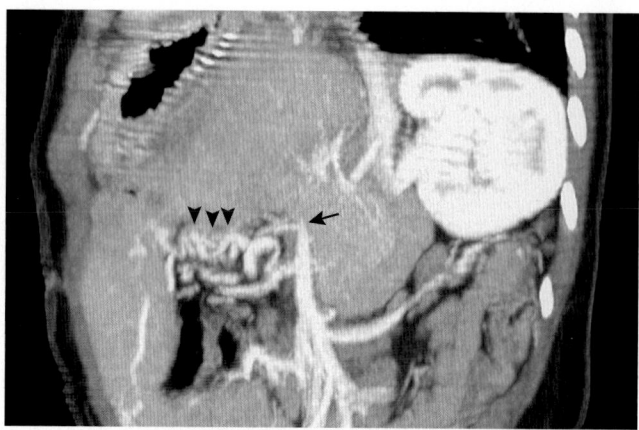

FIGURE 115-19. Oblique semisagittal reformat of contrast-enhanced CT in an 11-year-old boy with a left lateral segment liver transplant and nonacute portal vein thrombosis. The extrahepatic portal vein is occluded *(arrow)*, and multiple corkscrew collaterals from jejunal branches of the superior mesenteric vein are seen at the Roux-en-Y loop *(arrowheads)* used for the biliary anastomosis. The reconstituted central portal vein was identified on other images. Capsular collaterals are seen at the inferior edge of the liver.

inferior to the pancreas to the left portal vein (Fig. 115-23). The Rex shunt may be definitive therapy for children with extrahepatic portal vein obstruction. It cures portal hypertension and restores portal venous flow into the liver, preventing encephalopathy and pulmonary vascular changes. The collapsed intrahepatic portal system, which may be difficult to image before surgery because of exuberant intrahepatic collaterals that dominate portal flow, was shown to distend rapidly and accommodate the large volume of flow from the shunt. The shunt can be seen by all vascular imaging modalities and should demonstrate hepatopetal flow.

> With the mesoportal (Rex) shunt for extrahepatic portal vein occlusion, the entire splanchnic circulation bypasses the main portal vein obstruction to enter the intrahepatic portal system.

HEPATOPULMONARY SYNDROME AND PULMONARY HYPERTENSION

Portal hypertension and cirrhosis, as well as other vascular abnormalities that alter normal portosystemic circulation and normal delivery of hepatic venous blood to the lungs, are associated with pulmonary vascular abnormalities, predominantly right-to-left intrapulmonary shunting and pulmonary hypertension. Hepatopulmonary syndrome is defined as an elevated age-adjusted alveolar-arterial oxygen gradient, often leading to hypoxemia and pulmonary vascular dilation in patients with chronic liver disease. Pulmonary vascular changes have been described in children with cirrhosis, biliary atresia, and portal hypertension; in extrahepatic occlusion of the portal vein; and in children with congenital portosystemic shunts, mainly those with an absent portal vein. Pulmonary hypertension is less common than intra-

pulmonary shunting but may be devastating in patients with liver disease and portal hypertension; it is associated with a poor prognosis and decreased life expectancy.

Although the pathophysiology of human hepatopulmonary syndrome has not been fully described, hypotheses agree on the role of hepatic metabolites in the regulation of normal pulmonary vascularity. In the setting of liver failure and abnormal hepatopulmonary circulation, there is increased pulmonary expression of endothelin B receptor, leading to nitric oxide overproduction mediated by endothelin-1 and nitric oxide synthetase. Endothelial and arterial wall changes produce either ventilation-perfusion mismatch through vasodilation and arteriovenous shunting or pulmonary hypertension.

Clinically, patients may be relatively asymptomatic or develop cyanosis and clubbing. Occasionally, pulmonary manifestations precede the diagnosis of liver disease. Rapid development of hepatopulmonary disease has been documented within months of initial presentation. The pulmonary vascular changes may regress following correction of the portal vascular abnormality. Chiu and colleagues observed regression of pulmonary arteriovenous connections following embolization of a congenital superior mesenteric–to–left renal vein fistula.

Contrast echocardiography demonstrates echogenic bubbles in the pulmonary veins and left atrium after antecubital injection. The bubbles, normally trapped in pulmonary capillaries, reach the left circulation when right-to-left shunting occurs. Perfusion lung scans using microaggregate albumin also demonstrate uptake in the systemic circulation, such as brain, kidney, and bone, in the presence of a right-to-left shunt.

Plain radiographs may demonstrate increased basal vascular markings and cardiomegaly (Fig. 115-24). CT may outline enlarged vessels, predominantly in the bases.

> Cardiomegaly and increased vascular markings in a child with chronic liver disease or a portal vascular anomaly may represent intrapulmonary right-to-left shunts.

BUDD-CHIARI SYNDROME

Obstruction of hepatic veins and the IVC above the hepatic veins results in severe liver congestion, ascites, and portal hypertension. As sinusoidal pressure increases, it reverses the pressure gradient between the portal venous system and the sinusoidal system, causing the portal vein to become a draining system for the hepatic artery. In complete Budd-Chiari syndrome, the liver is supplied solely by the hepatic artery. Because the caudate lobe has separate venous drainage, it is spared in most patients with Budd-Chiari syndrome.

The cause of Budd-Chiari syndrome is often unknown. IVC obstruction at or above the hepatic veins may be caused by a congenital caval web; thrombosis secondary to hypercoagulability states, such as in nephrotic syndrome; tumor extension into the IVC in hepatoblastoma or Wilms tumor; or external compression. Yonekuran and associates reported caval compression by liver herniation through a hernia of Morgagni. Hepatic vein

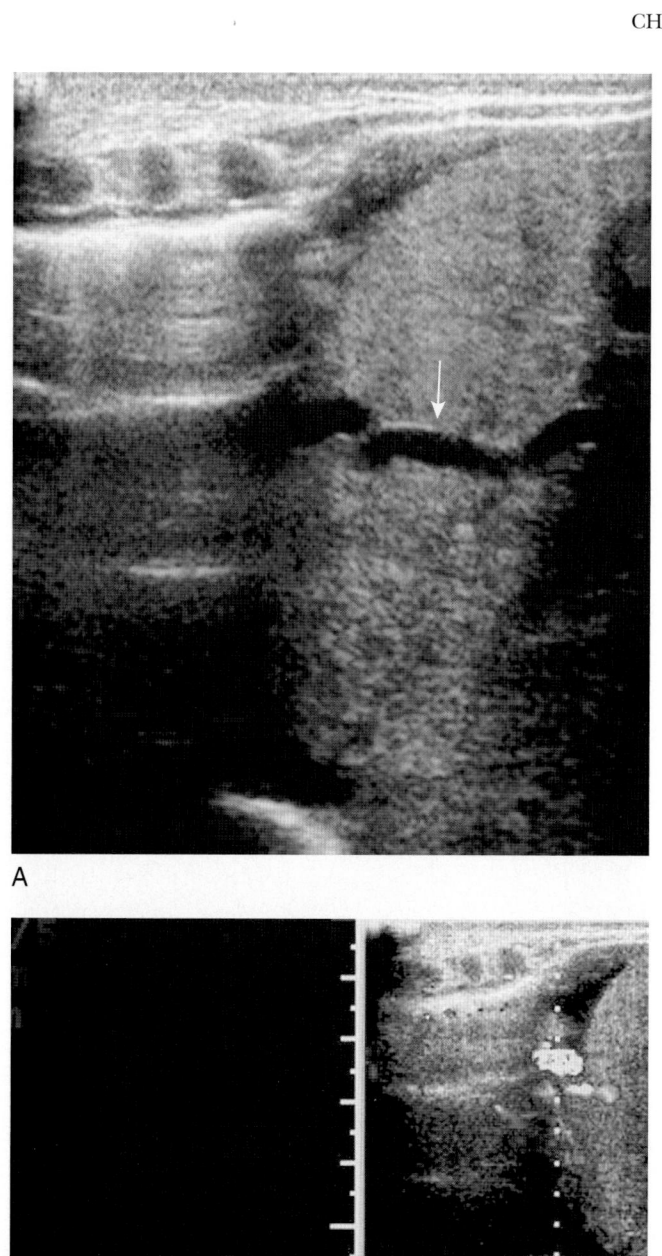

A

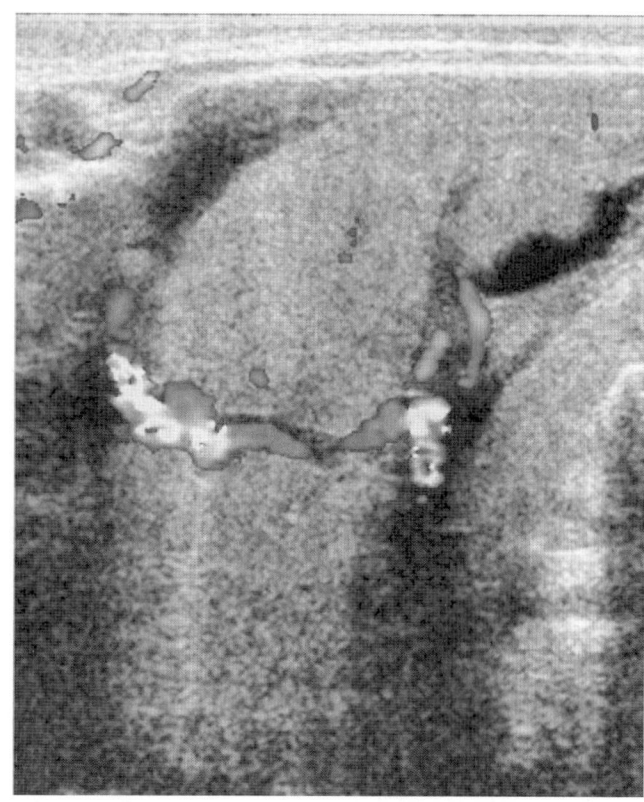

B

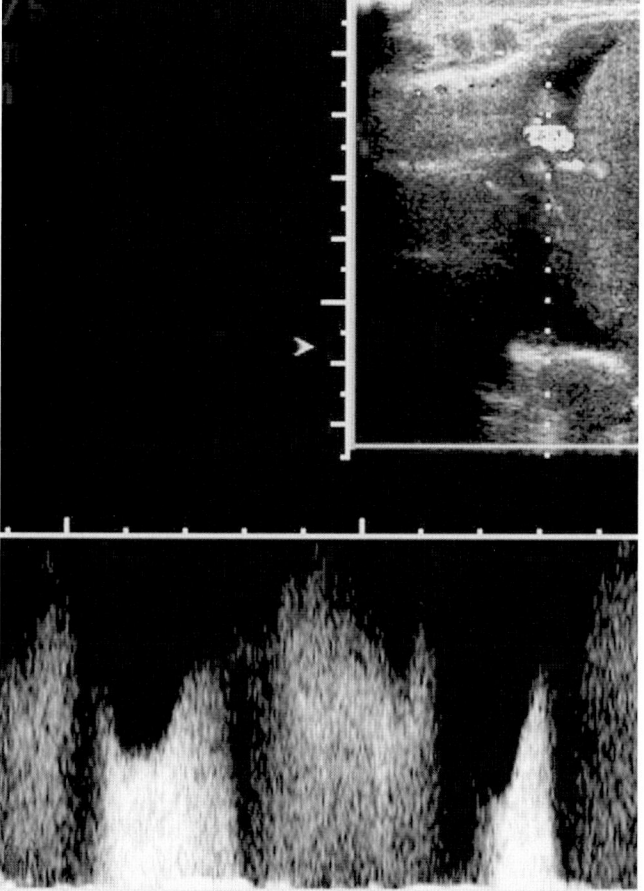

C

FIGURE 115-20. One-month-old boy with liver failure and portal hypertension. **A,** Longitudinal ultrasound image of the liver shows a portovenous collateral *(arrow)* through the liver coursing toward the superior liver surface. **B,** Color Doppler shows hepatofugal flow in the venous collateral *(See color plate.)* **C,** Higher color Doppler image with spectral Doppler tracing shows the vein directed toward the diaphragm and the high-velocity systemic venous flow pattern in a hepatofugal direction.

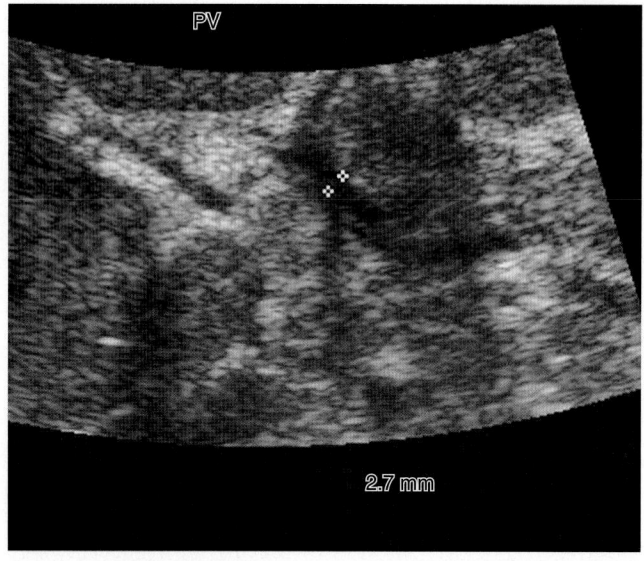

A

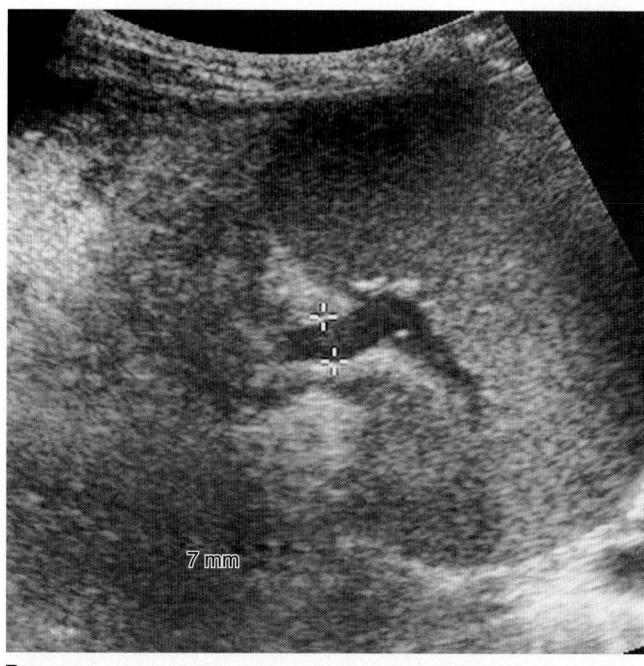

B

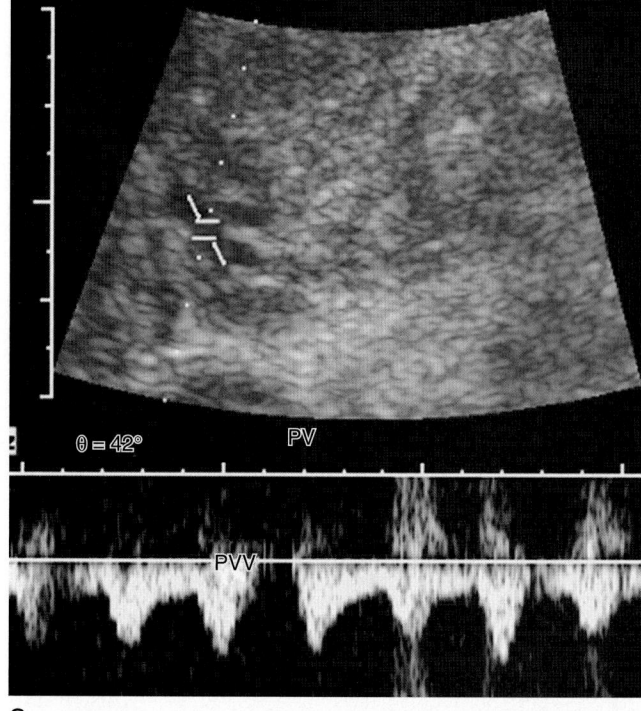

C

FIGURE 115-21. Severe portal hypertension in a 2-year-old girl with biliary atresia following a Kasai portoenterostomy. US was performed in preparation for liver transplantation. **A,** The main portal vein is very small, measuring 2.7 mm in diameter *(calipers)*. Note the lobulated outline of the liver. **B,** The splenic vein is much larger, measuring 7 mm in diameter *(calipers)*. This combination alerts one to the presence of collateral veins and varices. **C,** Spectral Doppler of the main portal vein (PV) reflects severe liver disease with high resistance to flow, causing the portal vein to become a draining vein to the hepatic artery through arterioportal communications. The portal vein flow is reversed and arterialized.

occlusion may result from thrombosis, ostial stenosis, or tumor extension from Wilms tumor or hepatoblastoma. Both hepatic vein and caval obstruction are known complications of liver transplantation.

Clinically, some patients develop collateral venous drainage and may be relatively asymptomatic. Others present with intractable ascites, liver failure, or gastrointestinal hemorrhage. Children who develop hepatic vein or IVC obstruction following liver transplantation may experience a recurrence of portal hypertension.

On imaging, the liver may be enlarged, with ascites and poorly or nonvisualized hepatic veins. Portal venous flow is usually reversed in complete cases; however, in partial hepatic vein occlusion, the flow may shunt from higher resistance segments into lower resistance segments, such as the caudate lobe. Intrahepatic portal-to-systemic collaterals may occur via transcapsular and paraumbilical veins, and extrahepatic collaterals occur via esophageal and gastric varices. These hemodynamic changes can be well demonstrated by Doppler US and MRI.

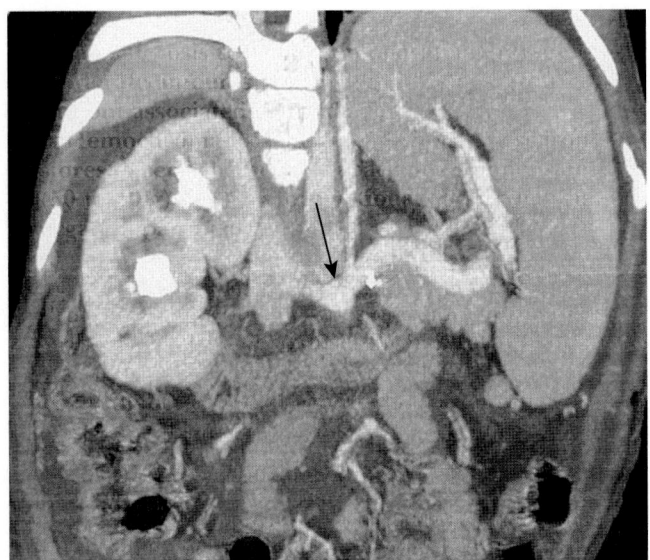

FIGURE 115-22. Surgical distal splenorenal shunt. Oblique reconstruction from CTA shows the splenic vein severed from the superior mesenteric vein, which continues to drain into the portal vein. The splenic vein is connected end-to-side *(arrow)* to the left renal vein.

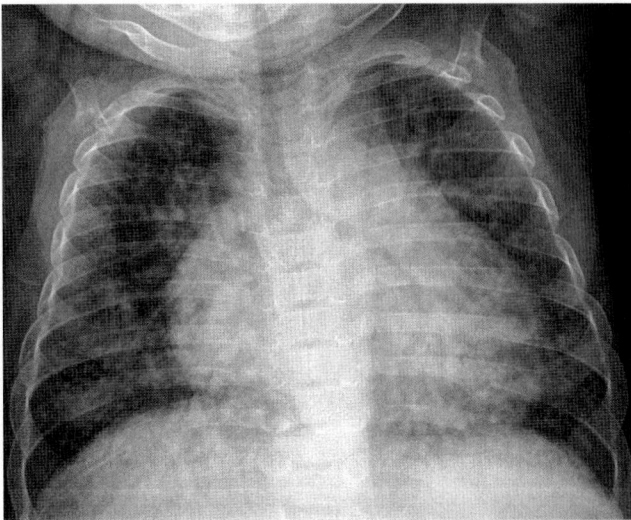

FIGURE 115-24. Hepatopulmonary syndrome in an 8-month-old boy with extrahepatic portal vein occlusion and cyanosis. Chest radiograph shows cardiomegaly and extensively increased pulmonary vascularity, representing diffuse pulmonary arteriovenous shunts.

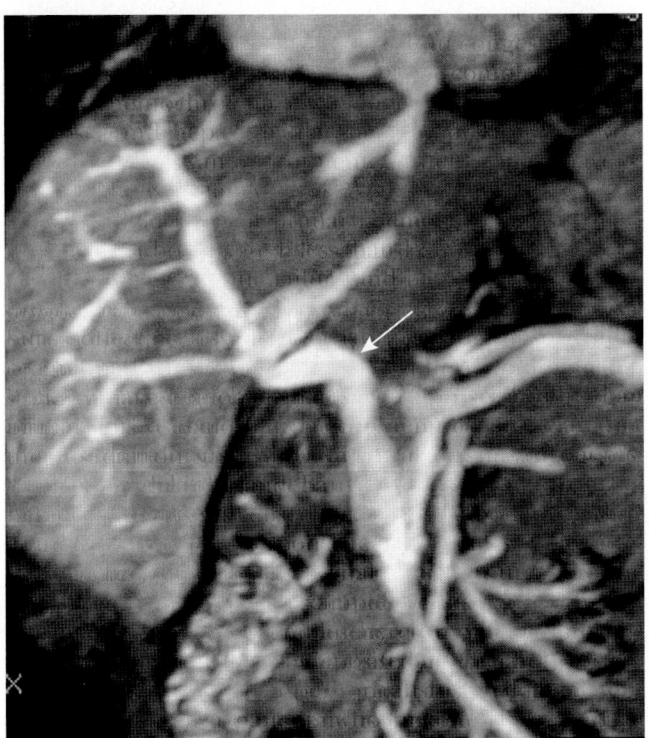

FIGURE 115-23. Rex (superior mesenteric–to–left portal vein) shunt. Angled coronal MRA shows the jugular vein shunt *(arrow)* connecting the superior mesenteric vein below the pancreas to the left portal vein.

On CT and CTA (Fig. 115-25), the liver parenchyma may demonstrate patchy, abnormal wedge-shaped areas of attenuation whose apex points to the IVC, or a heterogeneous, reticular, or mosaic pattern in the hepatic arterial phase that persists during the portal phase. The caudate lobe retains a normal appearance, and the

hepatic veins are not visualized. The portal vein may fill before its tributaries owing to intrahepatic flow reversal. As in other vascular abnormalities of the liver, hepatic nodules may be present.

> **Patients with Budd-Chiari syndrome demonstrate hepatomegaly, nonvisualized hepatic veins, venous collaterals, ascites, and reversal of portal vein flow.**

Treatment consists of medical control of ascites, percutaneous angioplasty when feasible, mesoatrial shunt, and liver transplantation.

HEPATIC VENO-OCCLUSIVE DISEASE

Patients undergoing myeloablative therapy for bone marrow or stem cell transplantation may develop severe endothelial and perivascular hepatocyte damage, followed by fibrosis and obliteration of the terminal hepatic venules—termed hepatic veno-occlusive disease (VOD). McDonald and colleagues established the clinical criteria for VOD: jaundice, ascites or fluid retention, and painful hepatomegaly within the first 20 days after bone marrow transplantation. The clinical diagnosis requires the presence of two of these criteria. The reported frequency of VOD in bone marrow transplant patients varies from 1% to 54% and is greater in patients undergoing bone marrow transplantation for malignant than for nonmalignant indications.

On US, a constellation of findings may be identified, including hepatomegaly, ascites, and thickening of the gallbladder wall. On Doppler, decreased or reversed flow in the portal vein, increased resistive index of the hepatic artery, and appearance of hepatofugal flow in paraumbilical veins have been described in patients with VOD (Fig. 115-26). In some early cases, there may

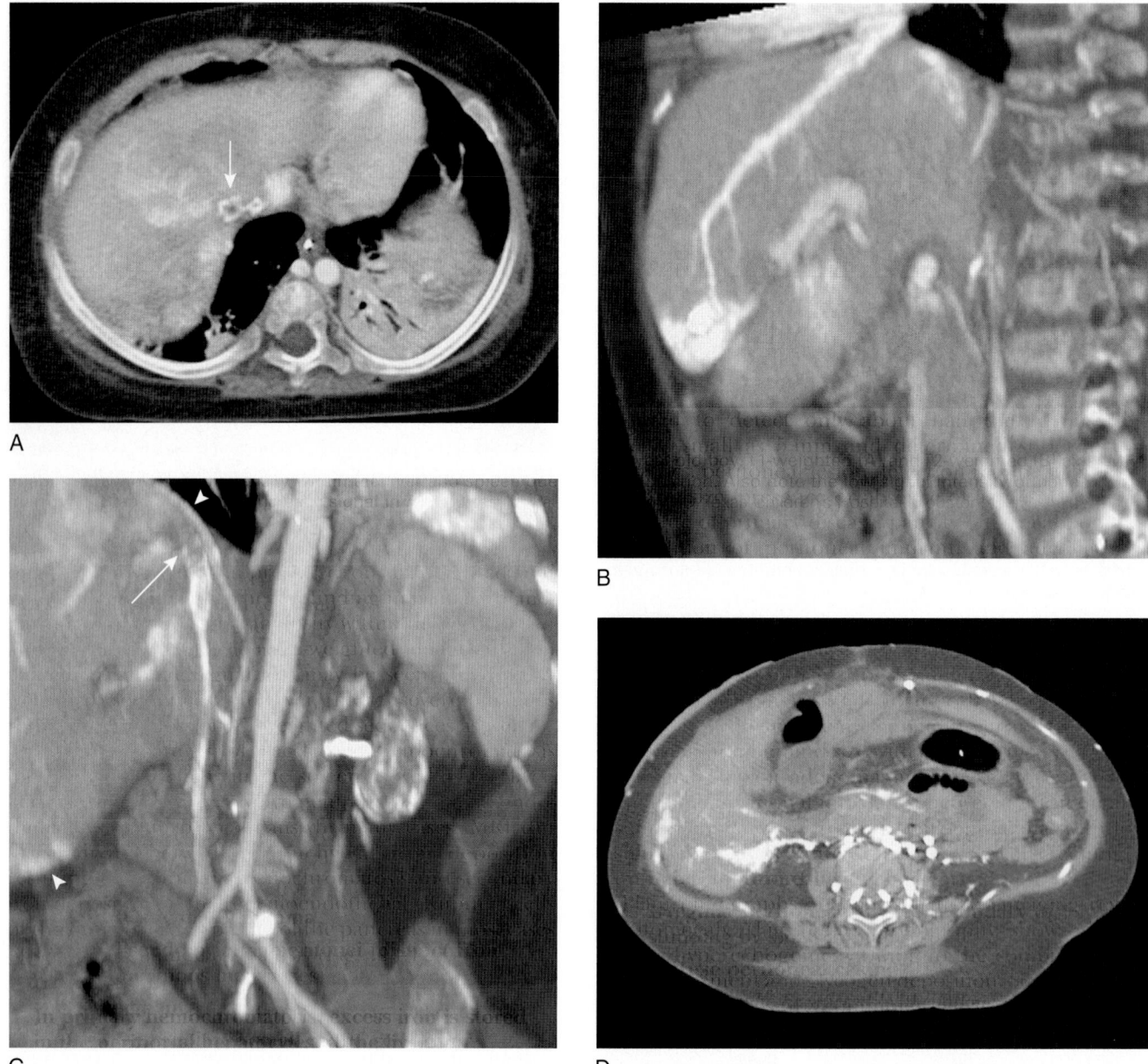

FIGURE 115-25. Budd-Chiari syndrome due to inferior vena cava (IVC) thrombosis. **A,** Axial image from CTA shows a filling defect within the intrahepatic IVC *(arrow)*. Note the patchy, inhomogeneous enhancement of the liver. **B,** Sagittal reconstruction from CTA shows intense contrast retention peripherally, in the territory of the obstructed hepatic vein and transcapsular collateral. **C,** Thrombus is seen in the IVC *(arrow)* in this coronal reconstruction. Transcapsular collaterals are seen at the liver dome and lower lateral edge *(arrowheads)*. **D,** On an axial lower CT slice, extensive retroperitoneal, paraspinal, and transcapsular collaterals enhance brightly.

be partial hemodynamic involvement resulting in flow reversal in only one segmental or lobar portal vein branch. The entire constellation of findings is seldom present, and in many patients, there are no specific ultrasound findings. Lassau and coworkers found that a composite score that includes seven gray scale and seven Doppler criteria may be useful prognostically and diagnostically to differentiate VOD from other potential causes of liver dysfunction and abdominal pain in bone marrow recipients, such as hepatic graft-versus-host disease and infectious hepatitis. In contrast, McCarville and associates concluded that none of the described ultrasound findings was as useful as the clinical McDonald criteria for diagnosing VOD. Similarly, Teefey and coworkers

found no substantial difference in Doppler criteria between patients with VOD and a cohort of patients without VOD.

MRI findings include hepatomegaly, narrowing of hepatic veins, periportal cuffing, gallbladder wall thickening with intense wall signal on T2-weighted sequences, ascites, and pleural effusion.

> **Ultrasound findings of hepatic veno-occlusive disease—hepatomegaly, thickened gallbladder wall, reversed or decreased portal venous Doppler flow signal—are infrequent.**

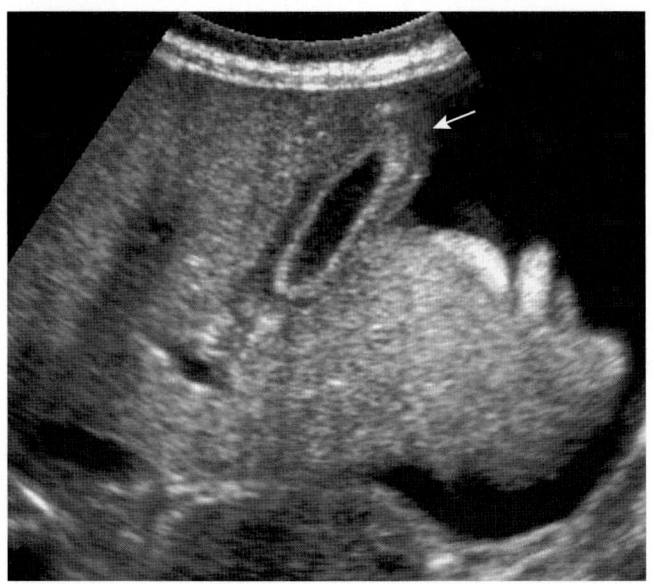

A

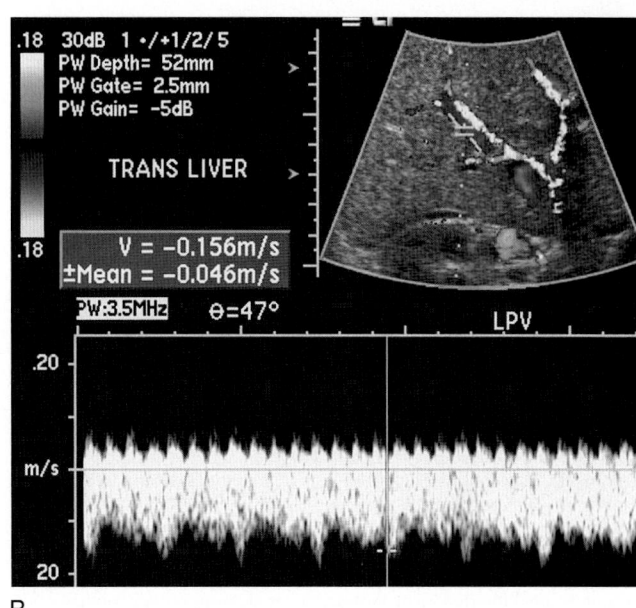

B

FIGURE 115-26. Hepatic veno-occlusive disease. **A,** Longitudinal ultrasound image shows thickening of the gallbladder wall *(arrow)* and ascites. **B,** Color and spectral Doppler with the color velocity threshold adjusted to show the slow flow within the portal vein. The much faster hepatic artery flow velocity causes aliasing. Note the reversal of portal venous flow.

SUGGESTED READINGS

Hepatic Vascular Bed

Atri M, Bret PM, Frazier-Hill MA: Intrahepatic portal venous variations: prevalence with US. Radiology 1992;184:157-158

Frazier-Hill MA, Atri M, Bret PM, et al: Intrahepatic portal venous system: variations demonstrated with duplex and color Doppler US. Radiology 1990;177:523-526

Fugelseth D, Lindemann R, Liestol K, et al: Postnatal closure of the ductus venosus in preterm infants < or +32 week: an ultrasonographic study. Early Hum Dev 1998;53:163-169

Gallego C, Velasco M, Marcuello P, et al: Congenital and acquired anomalies of the portal venous system. Radiographics 2002; 22:141-159

Kiserud T: Physiology of the fetal circulation. Semin Fetal Neonatal Med 2005;10:493-505

Kondo M, Itoh S, Kunikata T, et al: Time of closure of ductus venosus in term and preterm neonates. Arch Dis Child Fetal Neonatal Ed 2001;85:F57-F59

Kraus BB, Ros PR, Abbitt PL, et al: Comparison of ultrasound, CT and MR imaging in the evaluation of candidates for TIPS. J Magn Reson Imaging 1995;5:571-578

Loberant N, Herskovitz M, Barak M, et al: Closure of the ductus venosus in premature infants: findings on real-time grey scale, color-flow Doppler, and duplex Doppler sonography. AJR Am J Roentgenol 1999;172:227-229

Quiroga S, Sebastia C, Pallisa E, et al: Improved diagnosis of hepatic perfusion disorders: value of hepatic arterial phase imaging during helical CT. Radiographics 2001;21:65-81

Sau A, Sharlan G, Simpson J: Agenesis of the ductus venosus associated with direct umbilical vein return into the heart—case report and review of the literature. Prenat Diagn 2004;24:418-423

Tchirikov M, Schroder HJ, Hecher K: Ductus venosus shunting in the fetal venous circulation: regulatory mechanisms, diagnostic methods and medical importance. Ultrasound Obstet Gynecol 2006;27:452-461

Teo EL, Strouse PJ, Prince MR: Applications of magnetic resonance imaging and magnetic resonance angiography to evaluate the hepatic vasculature in the pediatric patient. Pediatr Radiol 1999;29:238-243

Congenital Anomalies of the Portal Vein

Gallager DM, Leiman S, Hux CH: In utero diagnosis of a portal vein aneurysm. J. Clin Ultrasound 1993;21:147-151

Gallego C, Velasco M, Marcuello P, et al: Congenital and acquired anomalies of the portal venous system. Radiographics 2002; 22:141-152

Gray SW, Skandalakis JH: Embryology for Surgeons: The Embryological Basis for Treatment of Congenital Defects. Philadelphia, Saunders, 1972:177-178

Hernanz-Schulman M, Genieser NB, Ambrosino MM, et al: Evaluation of the patient with abnormal visceroatrial situs—an update. AJR Am J Roentgenol 1990;154:747-802

Ito K, Matsunaga N, Mitchell DG, et al: Imaging of congenital abnormalities of the portal vein AJR Am J Roentgenol 1997;168:233-237

Kamata S, Sawai T, Nose K, et al: Extralobar pulmonary sequestration with venous drainage to the portal vein: a case report. Pediatr Radiol 2000;30:492-494

Lallier M, St-Vill D, Vobecky SJ, et al: Total anomalous pulmonary venous return complicating portoenterostomy for biliary atresia. J Pediatr Surg 1994;29:1242-1244

Shuford WH, Sybers RG: Bronchopulmonary sequestration with venous drainage to the portal vein AJR Am J Roentgenol 1969;106:118-120

Congenital Portosystemic Shunts

Abernethy J: Account of two instances of uncommon formation in the viscera of the human body. Philos Trans R Soc Lond Biol 1793;83:59-66

Gallego C, Miralles M, Marin C, et al: Congenital hepatic shunts. Radiographics 2004;24:755-772

Gray SW, Skandalakis JH: Embryology for Surgeons: The Embryological Basis for Treatment of Congenital Defects. Philadelphia, Saunders, 1972:177-178

Howard ER, Davenport M: Congenital extrahepatic portocaval shunts—the Abernethy malformation. J Pediatr Surg 1997; 32:494-497

Jabra AA, Taylor GA: Ultrasound diagnosis of congenital intrahepatic portosystemic venous shunt. Pediatr Radiol 1991;21:529-530

Kohda E, Saeki M, Nakano M, et al: Congenital absence of the portal vein in a boy. Pediatr Radiol 1999;29:235-237

Morgan G, Superina R: Congenital absence of the portal vein: two cases and a proposed classification system for portosystemic vascular anomalies. J Pediatr Surg 1994;29:1239-1241

Paley MR, Farrant P, Kane P, et al: Developmental intrahepatic shunts of childhood: radiological features and management. Eur Radiol 1997;7:1377-1382

Park JH, Cha SH, Han JK, Han MC: Intrahepatic portosystemic venous shunt. AJR Am J Roentgenol 1990;155:527-528

Satoh M, Yokoya S, Hachiya M, et al: Two hyperandrogenic girls with congenital portosystemic shunts. Eur J Pediatr 2001;160:307-311

Scheer I, Kivelitz D, Taupitz M, et al: Patent ductus venosus: diagnosis by MR angiography. Pediatr Radiol 2001;31:279-282

Valls E, Ceres L, Urbaneja A, et al: Color Doppler sonography in the diagnosis of neonatal intrahepatic portosystemic shunts. J Clin Ultrasound 1999;28:42-46

Vascular Masses and Malformations

Burrows PE, Dubois J, Kassarjian A: Pediatric hepatic vascular anomalies. Pediatr Radiol 2001;31:533-545

Hughes JA, Hill V, Patel K, et al: Cutaneous haemangioma: prevalence and sonographic characteristics of associated hepatic haemangioma. Clin Radiol 2004;59:273-280

Ianora AAS, Memeo M, Sabba C, et al: Hereditary hemorrhagic telangiectasia: multi-detector row helical CT assessment of hepatic involvement. Radiology 2004;230:250-259

Ingram JD, Yerushalmi B, Connel J, et al: Hepatoblastoma in a neonate: a hypervascular presentation mimicking hemangioendothelioma. Pediatr Radiol 2000;30:794-797

Kassarjian A, Dubois J, Burrows PE: Angiographic classification of hepatic hemangiomas in infants. Radiology 2002;222:693-698

Kumar N, de Ville de Goyer J, Sharif K, et al: Congenital, solitary, large, intrahepatic arterioportal fistula in a child: management and review of the literature. Pediatr Radiol 2003;33:20-23

Lima M, Lalla M, Aquino A, et al: Congenital symptomatic intrahepatic arteriovenous fistulas in newborns: management of 2 cases with prenatal diagnosis. J Pediatr Surg 2005;40:e1-e5

Morele KJ, Vanzieleghem B, Mortele B, et al: Solitary hepatic infantile hemangioendothelioma: dynamic gadolinium-enhanced MR imaging findings. Eur Radiol 2002;12:862-865

Mulliken JB, Glowacki J: Hemangiomas and vascular malformation in infants and children: a classification based on endothelial characteristics. Plast Reconstr Surg 1982;69:412-422

Nazir Z, Pervez S: Malignant vascular tumors in neonates J Pediatr Surg 2006;41:e49-e51

Quiroga S, Sebastia C, Pallisa E, et al: Improved diagnosis of hepatic perfusion disorders: value of hepatic arterial phase imaging during helical CT. Radiographics 2001;21:65-81

Regiers TS, Ramji FG: Pediatric hepatic hemangioma. Radiographics 2004;24:1719-1724

Roos JE, Pfiffner R, Stallmach T, et al: Infantile hemangioendothelioma. Radiographics 2003;23:1649-1655

Vauthey JN, Tomczak RJ, Helmberger T, et al: The arterioportal fistula syndrome: clinicopathologic features, diagnosis and therapy. Gastroenterology 1997;113:1390-1401

Portal Hypertension

Annet L, Materne R, Danse E, et al: Hepatic flow parameters measured with MR imaging and Doppler US: correlation with degree of cirrhosis and portal hypertension. Radiology 2003;229:409-414

Bambini DA, Superina R, Almond PS, et al: Experience with the Rex shunt (mesenteric-left portal vein bypass) in children with extrahepatic portal hypertension. J Pediatr Surg 2000;35:13-18

Bayraktar Y, Balkan F, Kayhan B, et al: Congenital hepatic fibrosis associated with cavernous transformation of the portal vein. Hepatogastroenterology 1997;44:1588-1594

Botha JF, Campos BD, Grant WJ, et al: Portosystemic shunts in children: a 15 year experience. J Am Coll Surg 2004;199:179-185

Broxson EH, Dole M, Wong R, et al: Portal hypertension develops in a subset of children with standard risk acute lymphoblastic leukemia treated with oral 6-thioguanine during maintenance therapy. Pediatr Blood Cancer 2005;44:226-231

Brunelle F, Alagille D, Pariente D, Chaumont P: Etude echographique de l'hypertension portale chez l'enfant. Ann. Radiol (Paris) 1981;24:121-130

Chen HY, Chen YW, Li MH, et al: Esophageal varices in congenital heart disease with total anomalous pulmonary venous connection. Int J Card Imaging 2000;16:405-409

Dauherty CC, Yazigi N, Bove K, Balistreri W: Mitochondrial enlargement and crystalloid matrix arrays: distinctive findings in childhood portal hypertension due to cavernous transformation of the portal vein. Pediatr Pathol Lab Med 1996;16:263-274

De Gaetano AM, LAfortune M, Patriquin H, et al: Cavernous transformation of the portal vein: patterns of intrahepatic and splanchnic collateral circulation detected with Doppler sonography. AJR Am J Roentgenol 1995;165:1151-1155

De Ville de Goyet J, Alberti D, Clapuyt P, et al: Direct bypass of extrahepatic portal venous obstruction in children: a new technique for combined hepatic portal revascularization and treatment of extrahepatic portal hypertension. J Pediatr Surg 1998;33:597-601

De Ville de Goyet J, Claypuyt P, Otte JD, et al: Extrahilar mesenterico–left portal vein shunt to relieve extrahepatic portal hypertension after partial liver transplant. Transplantation 1992;53:231-232

Dhiman R, Puri P, Chawla Y, et al: Biliary changes in extrahepatic portal venous obstruction: compression by collaterals or ischemic? Gastrointest Endosc 1999;50:646-652

Gauthier-Villars M, Franchi S, Gauthier F, et al: Cholestasis in children with portal vein obstruction. J Pediatr 2005;146:568-573

Gehrke I, John P, Blundell J, et al: Meso-portal bypass in children with portal vein thrombosis: rapid increase of the intrahepatic portal venous flow after direct portal hepatic reperfusion. J Pediatr Surg 2003;38:1137-1140

Gulati MS, Paul SB, Arora NK, et al: Esophageal and gastric vasculature in children with extrahepatic portal hypertension: evaluation by intravenous CT portography. Clin Imaging 2000;24:351-356

Gupta D, Chawala YK, Dhiman RK, et al: Clinical significance of patent paraumbilical vein in patients with liver cirrhosis. Dig Dis Sci 2000;45:1861-1864

Haugen G, Kiserud T, Godfrey K, Hanson M: Portal and umbilical venous blood supply to the liver in the human fetus near term. Ultrasound Obstet Gynecol 2004;24:599-605

Henseler KP, Pozniak MA, Lee FT Jr, Winter TC III: Three-dimensional CT angiography of spontaneous portosystemic shunts. Radiographics 2001;21:691-704

Kader HA, Baldassano RN, Harty MP, et al: Ruptured retrocecal appendicitis in an adolescent presenting as portal-mesenteric thrombosis and pylephlebitis. J Pediatr Gastroenterol Nutr 1998;27:584-588

Kang HK, Jeong YY, Choi JH, et al: Three dimensional multi-detector row CT portal venography in the evaluation of portosystemic collateral vessels in liver cirrhosis Radiographics 2002;22:1053-1061

Khare R, Sikora SS, Srikanth G, et al: Extrahepatic portal venous obstruction and obstructive jaundice: approach to management. J Gastroenterol Hepatol 2005;20:56-61

Kreft B, Strunk H, Flacke S, et al: Detection of thrombosis in the portal venous system: comparison of contrast-enhanced MR angiography with intra-arterial digital subtraction angiography. Radiology 2000;216:86-92

Kuroiwa M, Suzuki N, Hatakeyama S, et al: Magnetic resonance angiography of portal collateral pathways after hepatic portoenterostomy in biliary atresia: comparison with endoscopic findings. J Pediatr Surg 2001;36:1012-1016

Mitchell AWM, Jackson JE: Trans-anastomotic porto-portal varices in patients with gastrointestinal hemorrhage. Clin Radiol 2000; 55:207-211

Nakao N, Miura K, Takahashi H, et al: Hepatic perfusion in cavernous transformation of the portal vein: evaluation by using CT angiography. AJR Am J Roentgenol 1989;152:985-986

Nishimori H, Ezoe E, Ura H, et al: Septic thrombophlebitis of the portal and superior mesenteric veins as a complication of appendicitis: report of a case. Surg Today 2004;34:173-176

Pacifico L, Panero A, Colarizi P, et al: Neonatal *Candida albicans* septic thrombosis of the portal vein followed by cavernous transformation of the vessel. J Clin Bacteriol 2004;42:4379-4382

Patriquin H, Lafortune M, Burns PN, Dauzat M: Duplex Doppler examination in portal hypertension. AJR Am J Roentgenol 1987;149:71-76

Patriquin H, Tessier G, Grignon A, Boisvert J: Lesser omental thickness in normal children: baseline for detection of portal hypertension. AJR Am J Roentgenol 1985;145:693-696

Perlmutter G, Benjamin H, Fritsch J, et al: Biliary obstruction caused by portal cavernoma: a study of 8 cases. J Hepatol 1996;25:58-63

Primignani M, Martinelli T, Bucciarelli P, et al: Risk factors for thrombophilia in extrahepatic portal vein obstruction. Hepatology 2005;41:603-608

Rangari M, Gupta R, Jain M, et al: Hepatic dysfunction in patients with portal venous obstruction. Liver Int 2003;23:434-439

Reyes J, Mazariegos GV, Bueno J, et al: The role of portosystemic shunting in children in the transplant era. J Pediatr Surg 1999;34:117-122

Ryckman FC, Alonso MH: Causes and management of portal hypertension in the pediatric population. Clin Liver Dis 2001; 5:789-818

Stiller RJ, Neale D, Schwartz D, et al: Prenatal diagnosis of portal vein thrombosis by ultrasound. Ultrasound Obstet Gynecol 2003; 22:295-298

Tung JY, Johnson JL, Liacouras CA: Portal-mesenteric thrombosis with hepatic abscesses in a patient with Crohn's disease treated successfully with anticoagulants and antibiotics. J Pediatr Gastroenterol Nutr 1996;23:474-478

Vanamo K, Kiekara O: Pyelophlebitis after appendicitis in a child. J Pediatr Surg 2001;36:1574-1576

Westra SJ, Zaninovic AC, Vargas J, et al: The value of portal vein pulsatility on duplex sonogram as a sign of portal hypertension in children with liver disease. AJR Am J Roentgenol 1995;165:167-172

Yamada RM, Hessel G: Ultrasonographic assessment of the gallbladder in 21 children with portal vein thrombosis. Pediatr Radiol 2005;35:290-294

Hepatopulmonary Syndrome and Pulmonary Hypertension

Chiu SN, Ni YH, Wang JK, et al: Resolution of secondary pulmonary arteriovenous malformations after embolization of a congenital superior-mesenteric-to-left-renal-vein shunt. J Vasc Interv Radiol 2002;13:333-336

Fallon MB: Mechanisms of pulmonary vascular complications of liver disease: hepatopulmonary syndrome. J Clin Gastroenterol 2005;34(Suppl 2):S138-S142

Kimura T, Hasegawa T, Sasaki T, et al: Rapid progression of intrapulmonary arteriovenous shunting in polysplenia syndrome associated with biliary atresia. Pediatr Pulmonol 2003;35:494-498

Schraufnagel DE, Kay JM: Structural and pathologic changes in the lung vasculature in chronic liver disease. Clin Chest Med 1996; 17:1-15

Budd-Chiari Syndrome

Barakat M: Unusual hepato-portal-systemic shunting demonstrated by Doppler sonography in children with congenital hepatic vein ostial stenosis. J Clin Ultrasound 2004;32:172-178

Brancatelli G, Federle MP, Grazioli L, et al: Large regenerative nodules in Budd Chiari syndrome and other vascular disorders of the liver: CT and MR findings with clinicopathologic correlation. AJR Am J Roentgenol 2002;178:877-883

Quiroga S, Sebastia C, Pallisa E, et al: Improved diagnosis of hepatic perfusion disorders: value of hepatic arterial phase imaging during helical CT. Radiographics 2001;21:65-81

Valla DC: Hepatic vein thrombosis (Budd Chiari syndrome). Semin Liver Dis 2002;22:5-14

Yonekuran T, Kubota A, Hoki M, et al: Intermittent obstruction of the IVC by congenital anteromedial diaphragmatic hernia: an extremely rare cause of Budd-Chiari syndrome in an infant. Surgery 1997;124:109-111

Hepatic Veno-occlusive Disease

Ghersin E, Brook OR, Gaitini D, Engel A: Color Doppler demonstration of segmental portal vein flow reversal: an early sign of hepatic veno-occlusive disease in an infant. J Ultrasound Med 2003;22:1103-1106

Lassau N, Auperin A, Leclere J, et al: Prognostic value of Doppler ultrasonography in hepatic veno-occlusive disease. Transplantation 2002;74:60-66

Lassau N, Leclere J, Auperin A, et al: Hepatic veno-occlusive disease after myeloablative treatment and bone marrow transplantation: value of grey-scale and Doppler US in 100 patients. Radiology 1997;204:545-552

McCarville MB, Hoffer FA, Howard SC, et al: Hepatic veno-occlusive disease in children undergoing bone-marrow transplantation: usefulness of ultrasound findings. Pediatr Radiol 2001; 31:102-105

McDonald GB, Sharma P, Matthews DB, et al: Venooclusive disease of the liver after bone marrow transplantation. Hepatology 1984;4:116-122

Teefey SA, Brink JA, Borson RA, Middleton WD: Diagnosis of venoocclusive disease of the liver after bone marrow transplantation: value of duplex sonography. AJR Am J Roengenol 1995;164:1397-1401

Van den Bosch MAAJ, van Hoe L: MR imaging findings in two patients with hepatic veno-occlusive disease following bone marrow transplantation. Eur Radiol 2000;10:1290-1293

Acquired Biliary Tract Disease

LISA H. LOWE and ALAN E. SCHLESINGER

CHOLELITHIASIS AND CHOLEDOCHOLITHIASIS

Cholelithiasis, previously thought rare in children without hemolytic anemia, is diagnosed with increasing frequency since the advent of real-time sonography. In fact, gallstones may be seen sonographically in the fetus, although most resolve spontaneously.

Development of gallstones in infants has been attributed to immature physiologic regulation of bile salt secretion, because infants form bile salts at 50% the rate of adults. Chronic cholestasis probably plays a role in the pathophysiology of the disorder as well. Bilirubinate stones are most common. Although many infantile gallstones (Fig. 116-1) are discovered incidentally, many predisposing conditions have been described (Table 116-1). Infantile gallstones resolve spontaneously less often than in the fetus. Occasionally, infantile stones may be complicated by biliary tract perforation and peritonitis. Treatment is generally conservative and includes addressing the underlying cause of disease.

Although most of the stones seen in older children are idiopathic, a number of underlying states have been associated with gallstones (Table 116-2). Prominent among these are sickle cell disease and intestinal problems that interfere with normal enterohepatic circulation, such as inflammatory bowel disease, cystic fibrosis (bile stasis due to cystic duct obstruction with inspissated secretions), and the short-gut syndrome. Gallstones have also been reported after surgery and antibiotic therapy. Patients with sickle cell disease have an increasing incidence of gallstones with increasing age. Stones occur in 12% of 2- to 4-year-olds with sickle cell compared with 42% of 15- to 18-year-olds.

The clinical presentation of gallstones ranges from asymptomatic in most infants and young children to an increased incidence of symptoms in older children. When symptoms occur, they are similar to those seen in adults and include bloating, nausea, vomiting, and postprandial right upper quadrant colicky pain that radiates to the shoulder.

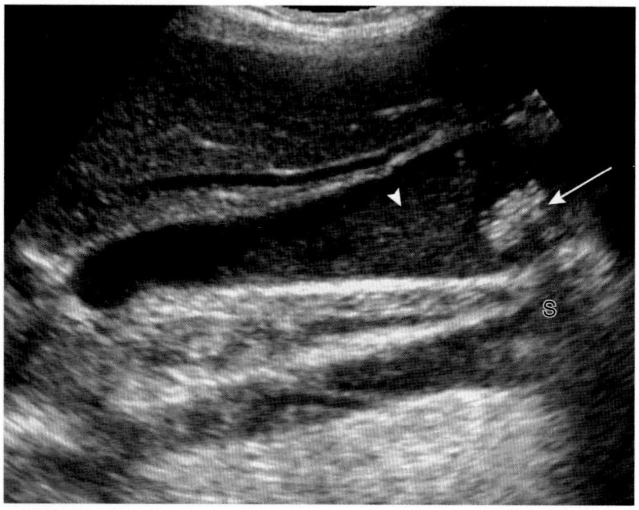

FIGURE 116-1. Cholelithiasis in an infant. Longitudinal sonogram of the gallbladder shows sludge *(arrowhead)* and cholelithiasis *(arrow)* with an associated acoustic shadow (S).

TABLE 116-1

Causes of Infantile Gallstones

Obstructive congenital biliary tree anomalies
Total parenteral nutrition
Diuretics (furosemide)
Gastrointestinal dysfunction (short-gut syndrome or
    terminal ileal disease)
Prolonged fasting
Phototherapy
Dehydration
Infection
Hemolytic anemia
Umbilical venous catheterization
Antibiotic therapy

TABLE 116-2

Causes of Gallstones in Children

Sickle cell disease
Cystic fibrosis or other pancreatic disease
Malabsorption
Total parenteral nutrition
Inflammatory bowel disease (Crohn disease)
Short-gut syndrome (intestinal resection)
Hemolytic anemia
Choledochal cyst
Antibiotics

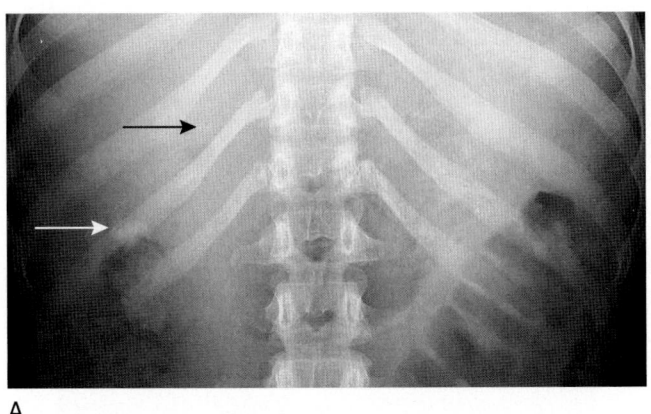

A

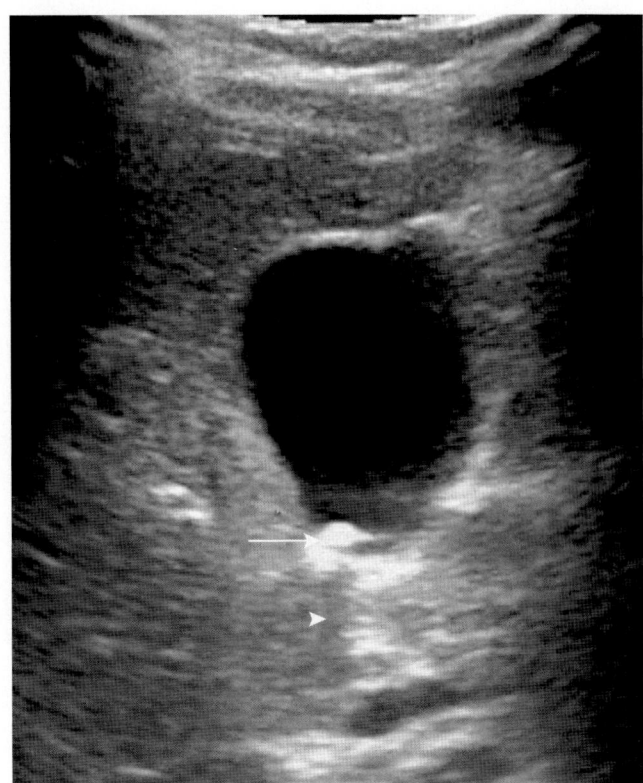

B

FIGURE 116-2. Cholelithiasis in a 13-year-old girl with elevated liver function tests. **A,** Abdominal radiograph shows two gallstones *(arrows)*. The most cranial is found at the gallbladder neck, and the caudalmost gallstone is seen at the gallbladder fundus. **B,** Transverse sonogram shows the echogenic stone *(arrow)* with posterior acoustic shadowing *(arrowhead)* in the dependent portion of the gallbladder.

> **Gallstones in infants and young children are usually asymptomatic; older children are more likely to have symptoms similar to those seen in adults.**

Sonography is the primary imaging modality for the evaluation of cholelithiasis; accuracy is reportedly 90%. However, 50% of gallstones are visible on plain radiography in children (compared with 20% in adults). The higher incidence of stone visibility in children is thought to be due to the fact that radiolucent cholesterol stones, the most common type overall, are rare in children. Three main sonographic criteria are used to diagnose gallstones: (1) echogenic focus, (2) prominent acoustic shadowing, and (3) gravitational dependence (Fig. 116-2). Most stones move with change in patient position, which should be a routine maneuver during sonography. Three general sonographic patterns of cholelithiasis are described. The first pattern includes the simple echogenic, shadowing, mobile stone, which may be single or multiple. When multiple, the number of gallstones identified at sonography is usually less than the number actually found at surgery. The second pattern of cholelithiasis describes collections of very tiny, sandlike stones, termed *milk of calcium*, which may mimic gallbladder sludge; acoustic shadowing may be seen only in the aggregate (Fig. 116-3) and at times may be subtle. Occasionally, if bile within the gallbladder is of high density, the stones may seem to float on the surface, giving an apparent fluid-fluid level. The last pattern of cholelithiasis described with sonography relates to stones within a contracted gallbladder, in which case the stones produce an echogenic double arc known as the *wall echo shadow complex*. This pattern is often seen in patients who have not fasted sufficiently (Fig. 116-4). Careful scrutiny must be employed so as not to confuse the wall echo shadow complex with emphysematous cholecystitis (air in the gallbladder wall), which is far more common in adults than in children.

Choledocholithiasis is usually the result of migration of stones from the gallbladder into the common duct. Stones are more likely to be symptomatic when they pass into the cystic duct or the common bile duct. Sonography is less successful at revealing choledocholithiasis than it is at detecting cholelithiasis, typically because of interference by gas in the duodenum (Fig. 116-5). Dilated extrahepatic bile ducts may be the only sign of a more distal obstructing stone. Hepatobiliary scintigraphy has been used to confirm the diagnosis of gallstones by revealing delayed excretion of radiopharmaceutical into the gastrointestinal tract, although its use is diminishing. Computed tomography (CT) scans are often obtained in children with biliary stones when there is initial clinical suspicion of other abdominal processes. CT is poor at revealing the actual stone, but it easily shows biliary dilation. If biliary ductal dilation is suspected, but no stone is seen on sonography, magnetic resonance (MR) cholangiopancreatography is often used. In these cases, stones are seen as filling defects within the gallbladder and the biliary tree (Fig. 116-6). If direct visualization and intervention (i.e., drainage, stent placement, sphincterotomy, or biopsy) are planned to address an underlying

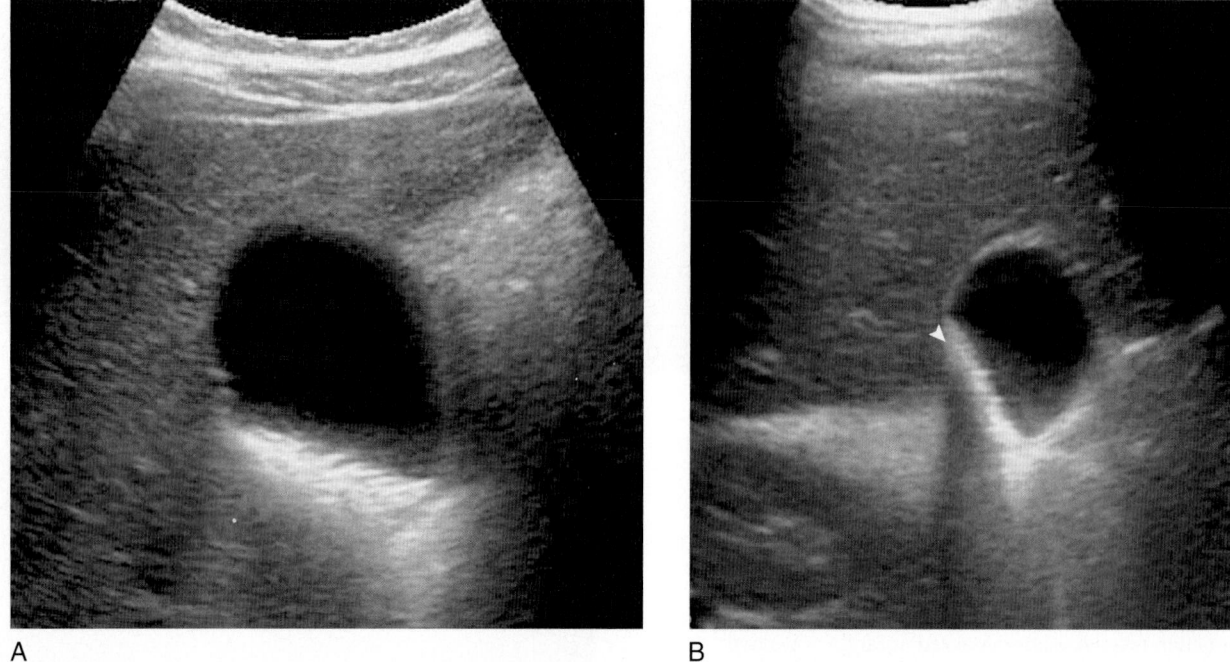

FIGURE 116-3. Cholelithiasis in a 16-year-old girl with right upper quadrant pain. Transverse sonograms in the **(A)** supine and **(B)** decubitus positions reveal echogenic layering of tiny stones with posterior acoustic shadowing *(arrowhead in B)*. Note the change in stones with change in patient position, as well as diffuse shadowing of the stone aggregate, in **B**.

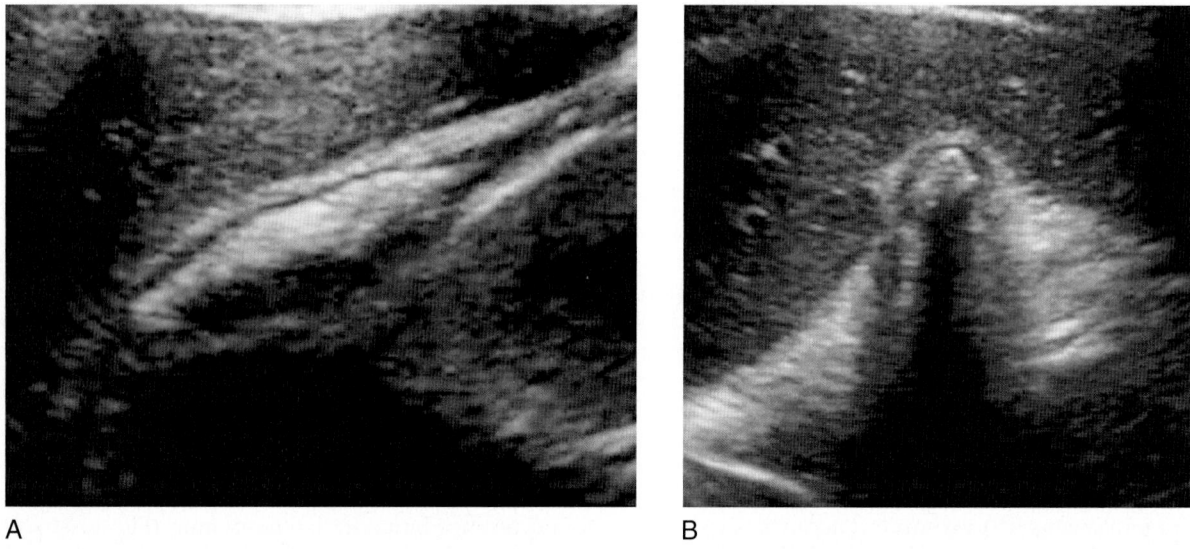

FIGURE 116-4. Cholelithiasis in a 16-year-old girl with abdominal pain. **A,** Longitudinal and **B,** transverse sonograms performed without fasting show the anterior gallbladder wall and multiple echogenic stones with posterior acoustic shadowing (wall-echo-shadow triad).

condition, percutaneous transhepatic cholangiography (PTC) or endoscopic retrograde cholangiopancreatography (ERCP) may be considered. Generally, however, nonoperative interventional treatment of children with choledocholithiasis is rarely performed.

BILIARY SLUDGE

Biliary sludge, particulate matter within the bile produced by cholestasis, is of debated clinical significance. Although the vast majority of biliary sludge is a transient finding, evolution of sludge into gallstones has been documented. Sludge is formed predominantly of calcium bilirubinate particles and, depending on the underlying process, cholesterol crystals. Predisposing conditions, which share the common pathway of biliary stasis, include biliary outflow obstruction, intravenous hyperalimentation, hemolysis, and prolonged fasting.

On sonography, sludge is echogenic without acoustic shadowing; it typically layers in the dependent portion of the biliary tree or gallbladder and may exhibit a fluid-sludge level (Fig. 116-7). Occasionally, sludge coalesces within the gallbladder lumen, forming a tumefactive "sludge ball" that, when fixed, may mimic a polyp or

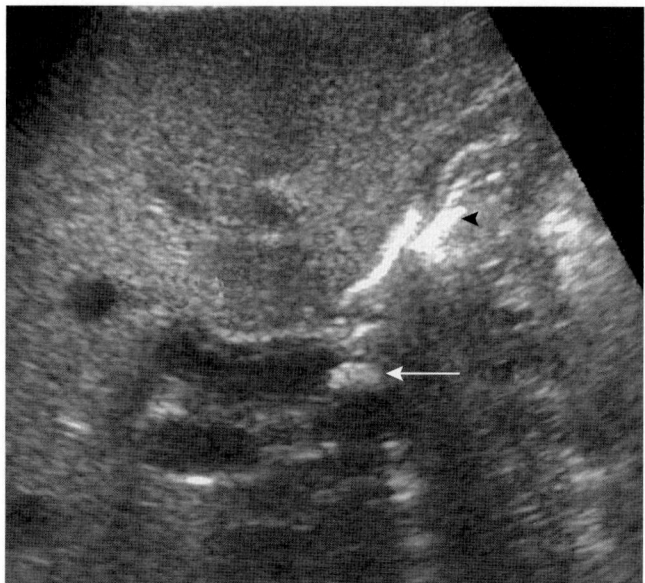

FIGURE 116-5. Choledocholithiasis and emphysematous cholecystitis in a 15-year-old obese female with abdominal pain. Transverse sonogram shows a stone *(arrow)* in the distended common bile duct, in addition to extensive air in the gallbladder lumen and wall *(arrowhead)*, worrisome for emphysematous cholecystitis. Note poorly defined "dirty" shadowing with air compared with stone. The wall of the common bile duct is slightly thickened, consistent with edema.

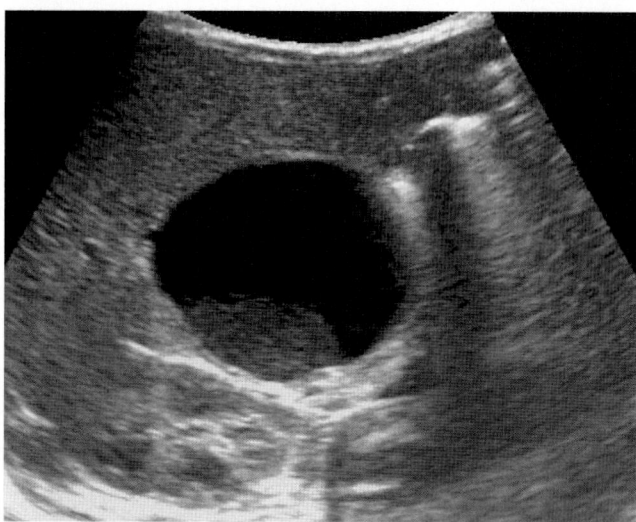

FIGURE 116-7. Biliary sludge in a 1-year-old boy with a choledochal cyst. Transverse sonogram shows layering echogenic material within the cyst; its echogenicity, which is less than that of stone, and lack of shadowing distinguish it from a calculus.

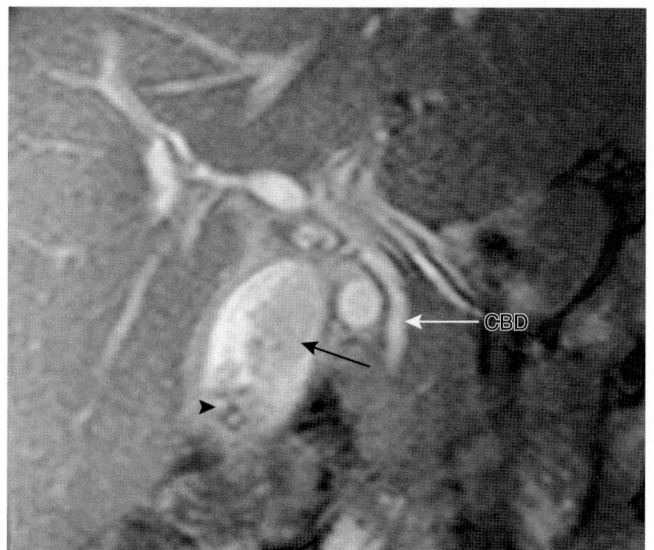

A

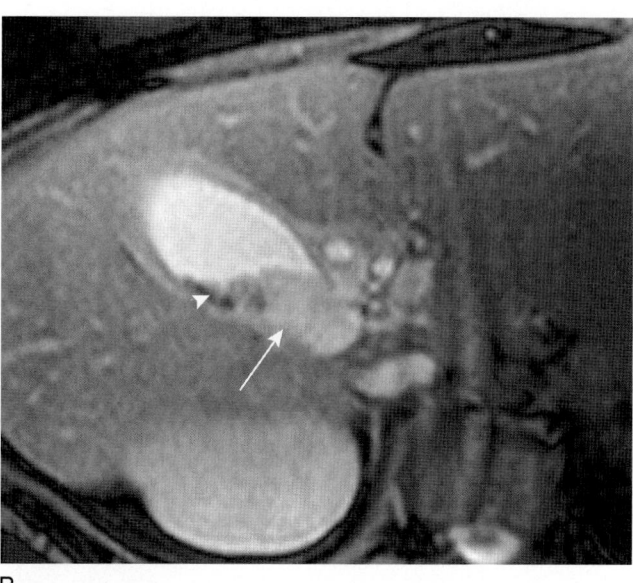

B

FIGURE 116-6. Cholelithiasis in a 12-year-old girl with abdominal pain. **A,** Coronal, and **B,** axial T2-weighted magnetic resonance images reveal low signal intensity gallstones *(arrowheads)* and isointense sludge *(arrows)* within the gallbladder lumen. Note the normal common bile duct (CBD).

mass (Fig. 116-8). Because biliary sludge is asymptomatic and resolves spontaneously with treatment of the underlying condition, it does not require treatment. Differential diagnostic possibilities are uncommon conditions that include hemobilia, biliary mucus, and parasitic infection.

ACUTE CHOLECYSTITIS

Acute cholecystitis is uncommon in infants and children compared with adults. A small percentage of children with cholelithiasis develop cholecystitis, and 30% of cases are acalculous. In most cases, the pathophysiology of

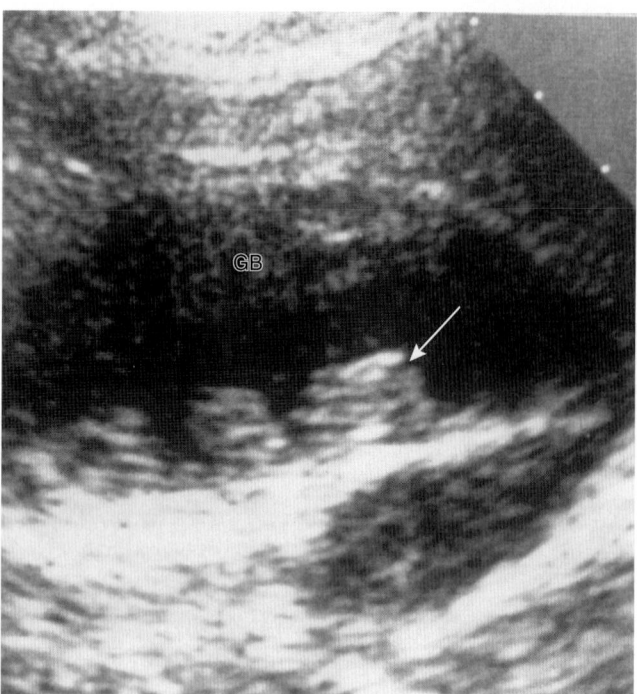

FIGURE 116-8. Sludge balls (tumefactive sludge) in a 6-year-old girl receiving parenteral nutrition. Longitudinal sonogram shows multiple echogenic, nonshadowing balls of sludge *(arrow)* within the gallbladder (GB).

acute cholecystitis involves obstruction of the cystic duct, which leads to gallbladder distention, followed successively by edema, ischemia, mural necrosis, and, in severe cases, perforation. The pathophysiology of acalculous cholecystitis is uncertain, but gallbladder ischemia, alterations in bile flow, and elevated ampullary pressures have been hypothesized as causes or contributing factors.

Episodes of colic without significant inflammation remit in a matter of hours with steroids and antispasmodics. However, biliary colic that lasts longer than 24 hours is not likely to resolve spontaneously. In neonates with acute cholecystitis, the diagnosis may not be suspected, leading to a high mortality rate of 20%.

Urgent imaging of possible acute cholecystitis is useful for rendering a diagnosis, determining the severity of disease, or discovering other potential causes of abdominal pain. Which study to perform depends on the specific clinical concern. If one is seeking to diagnose gallstones, sonography is the imaging modality of choice. However, if one wishes to assess for acute cholecystitis, biliary scintigraphy is preferred (Fig. 116-9). The sonographic findings of calculous and acalculous cholecystitis are identical except for the lack of gallstones in the latter condition (Fig. 116-10). Sonographic findings of cholecystitis when viewed individually are nonspecific, but when combined, they may indicate a specific diagnosis. The best indicators of acute cholecystitis include chole-

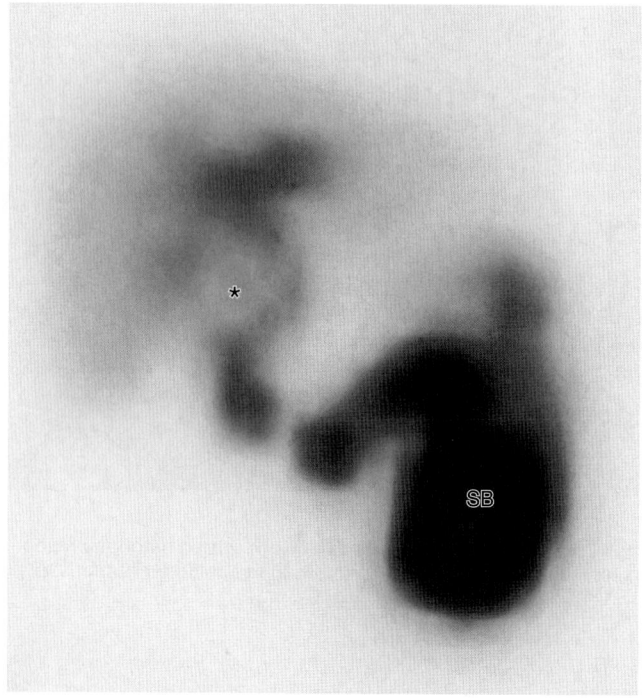
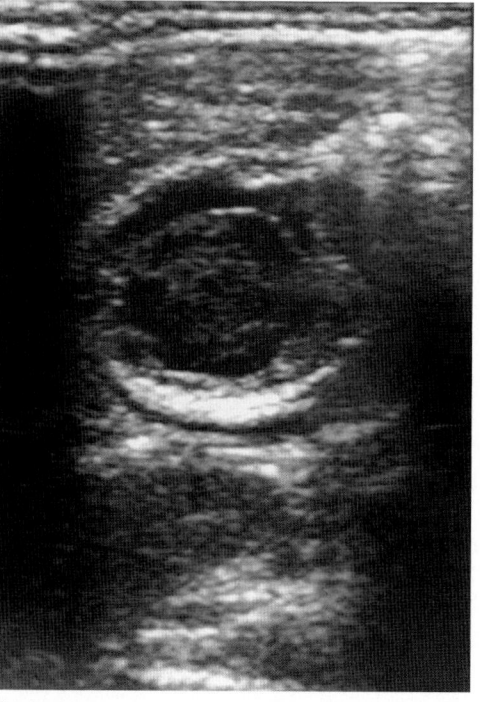

A   B

FIGURE 116-9. Cholecystitis. **A,** Acute cholecystitis in a 15-year-old girl with a history of cholelithiasis. Four-hour image from a biliary patency scan shows hepatic uptake and excretion of technetium-99m–labeled iminodiacetic acid into the biliary tree and small bowel (SB) without gallbladder *(asterisk)* opacification. A halo of increased activity surrounds the gallbladder fossa—known as the rim sign—and is consistent with hyperemia. **B,** Chronic cholecystitis. Transverse sonogram through the gallbladder reveals a markedly thickened, edematous gallbladder wall with echogenic material in the lumen. The patient had a history of chronic, recurrent abdominal pain.

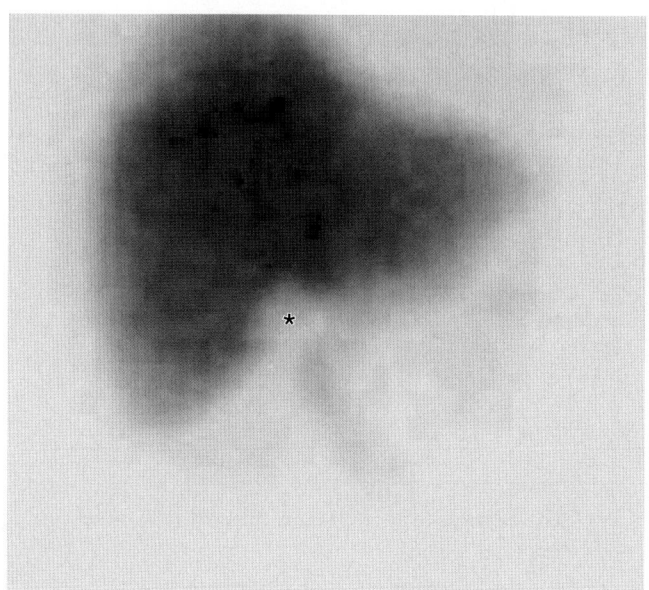

A

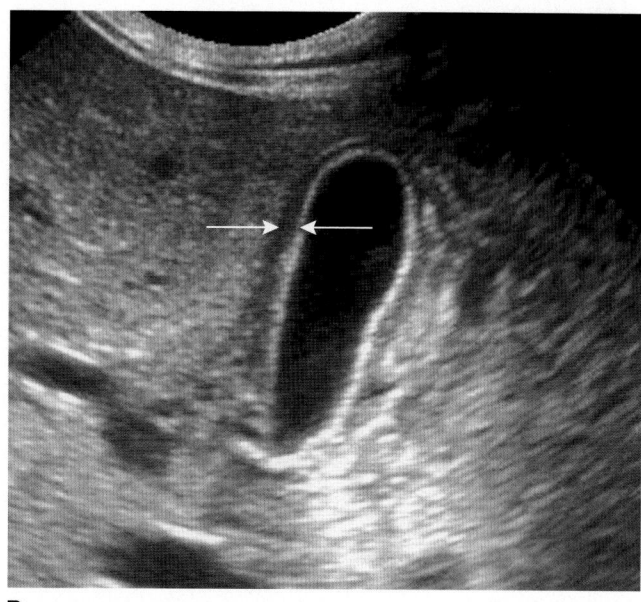

B

FIGURE 116-10. Acalculous cholecystitis in a 17-year-old girl with right upper quadrant pain and a history of lupus. **A,** One-houre image from a biliary patency scan shows hepatic uptake and excretion of technetium-99m–labeled iminodiacetic acid into the biliary tree without gallbladder *(asterisk)* opacification. **B,** Longitudinal sonogram shows gallbladder wall thickening *(arrows)* without gallstones.

lithiasis, a sonographic Murphy sign (tenderness when the gallbladder is compressed), and gallbladder wall edema. Intramural edema related to acute cholecystitis is usually striated, with multiple interrupted bands of hypoechogenicity. This appearance has been associated with gangrenous cholecystitis, but it does not necessarily indicate *Clostridium* infection.

The interrupted layers of intramural edema seen with acute cholecystitis should not be confused with homogeneous gallbladder wall thickening, a common nonspecific finding seen in a variety of disorders such as ascites, hypoalbuminemia, congestive heart failure, hepatitis, portal hypertension, and gallbladder wall varices. Other sonographic findings of acute cholecystitis include gallbladder distention, pericholecystic fluid (especially with perforation), adjacent rim of hypoechogenicity or hypervascularity in the liver, biliary sludge, and, rarely, dirty shadowing due to air-producing infection (found most often in adults with diabetes).

Hepatobiliary scintigraphy with technetium-99m–labeled iminodiacetic acid derivative is highly sensitive for the diagnosis of acute cholecystitis in adults and children. Normally, the gallbladder is opacified with radiopharmaceutical in the first 30 minutes of the study, or in the first hour with slow injection of intravenous (IV) morphine. However, with acute cholecystitis, gallbladder opacification does not occur in the first 30 minutes or within 1 hour after IV morphine. Occasionally, a rim of increased activity is seen in the liver surrounding the gallbladder (the rim sign), and peritoneal activity may be seen with perforation. Gallbladder perforation is a surgical emergency that occurs in 3% to 15% of patients with acute cholecystitis.

Ultrasonographic findings in cholecystitis include the following:

- **Thickened, striated edematous gallbladder wall**
- **Distention of the gallbladder**
- **Pericholecystic fluid**
- **Biliary sludge**
- **Gallbladder wall edema**
- **Irregularity of the gallbladder wall**
- **Air in the gallbladder lumen or wall (emphysematous cholecystitis)**

CHOLANGITIS

Cholangitis, or *ascending cholangitis,* is a nonspecific term that refers to biliary duct obstruction with associated biliary infection. Causes of ascending cholangitis are numerous and range from neoplasms (benign and malignant) to infection (suppurative, nonsuppurative, human immunodeficiency virus [HIV]) to autoimmune, or chemotherapy-induced, disorders. Appropriate therapy is directed toward relief of the underlying cause of obstruction, whether congenital or acquired.

Primary sclerosing cholangitis, an idiopathic insidious obliterative inflammatory fibrosis of the intrahepatic and extrahepatic biliary ducts, is a rare cause of chronic liver disease in children. Its features suggest an autoimmune mechanism, but the pathophysiology of tissue damage has not been definitively determined. Associated disorders in children with sclerosing cholangitis include inflammatory bowel disease, especially ulcerative colitis, and, less often, Crohn disease (up to 57%), idiopathic causes (25%), Langerhans cell histiocytosis (15%), and other immune system disorders (10%). The association between sclerosing cholangitis and ulcerative colitis is not as strong in children as it is in adults. Sclerosing cholangitis has also been associated with cystic fibrosis. The common bile duct is always involved.

Disorders associated with pediatric sclerosing cholangitis include the following:

- **Inflammatory bowel disease (ulcerative colitis)**
- **Langerhans cell histiocytosis**
- **Immune disorders**
- **Cystic fibrosis**

On sonography, nonspecific dilation of the biliary system, hyperechoic portal triads, portal casts, thickened gallbladder wall, and cholelithiasis may be identified in sclerosing cholangitis. CT findings include focal dilation of the biliary tree and contrast enhancement of the bile duct walls caused by inflammatory changes. Magnetic resonance imaging (MRI) may reveal peripheral wedge-shaped areas of high signal in association with dilated bile ducts. T1 and T2 shortening along the periportal triads due to inflammation may also be detected. A definitive diagnosis is possible with cholangiopancreatography, including percutaneous, endoscopic, or, more recently, MR cholangiopancreatography. Key findings on cholangiopancreatography include multifocal stricture of the biliary tree with alternating areas of dilation, forming a classic "string of beads" appearance (Fig. 116-11). Other described appearances include the "pruned tree" appearance (opacification of central ducts without visualization of peripheral ducts), "cobblestone" appearances (coarse nodular mural irregularities), and pathognomonic pseudodiverticula (small saccular outpouchings of the biliary tree). New strictures or elongation of old strictures occurs in less than 20% of cases, and marked ductal dilation is seen in 24% of cases. Although cholangitis is occasionally segmental, the entire biliary tract is usually involved. The gallbladder is rarely involved.

Sonographic findings in sclerosing cholangitis include the following:

- **Dilation of the biliary tree**
- **Thickened gallbladder wall**
- **Stones**

Findings on cholangiopancreatography include those listed here:

- **String of beads (multifocal strictures with intervening dilation)**

TABLE 116-3

Causes of Hydrops of the Gallbladder

Obstruction
Mucocutaneous lymph node syndrome (Kawasaki disease)
Familial Mediterranean fever
Scarlet fever
Leptospirosis
Ascariasis
Typhoid fever
Sepsis
Total parenteral nutrition

- **Pruned tree (opacification limited to central ducts)**
- **Cobblestone appearance (coarse mural irregularities)**
- **Pseudodiverticula (small saccular outpouchings of ducts)**

The differential diagnosis of sclerosing cholangitis includes sclerosing biliary cholangiocarcinoma, which is rare in children. Primary biliary cirrhosis may be considered as well, but it involves only the intrahepatic ducts. Complications of sclerosing cholangitis include portal hypertension, biliary cirrhosis, secondary cholangitis, and cholangiocarcinoma. Treatment is aimed at palliation and may include medical therapy (ursodeoxycholic acid), interventional dilation of dominant strictures, and drainage of infected obstructed ducts. Liver transplantation provides the only possible cure for sclerosing cholangitis.

HYDROPS OF THE GALLBLADDER

Gallbladder hydrops, a rare right upper quadrant mass in children, is thought to be related to transient cholestasis and obstruction of the biliary tree. It is associated with preceding infectious disorders elsewhere in the body (Table 116-3), most notably the mucocutaneous lymph node syndrome, Kawasaki disease, and parenteral hyperalimentation. It is more frequent in boys, with a mean age of 5 years, and can lead to acute abdominal pain. Sonography is striking for marked gallbladder dilation without gallbladder wall thickening. The gallbladder may resemble a balloon in which normal contours are lost (Fig. 116-12). Sludge is seen in some cases, and the biliary tree is otherwise normal. Hydrops generally responds to conservative therapy, although gallbladder perforation has been reported in Kawasaki disease. In infants, gallbladder hydrops is usually due to transient bile plugging, which resolves spontaneously.

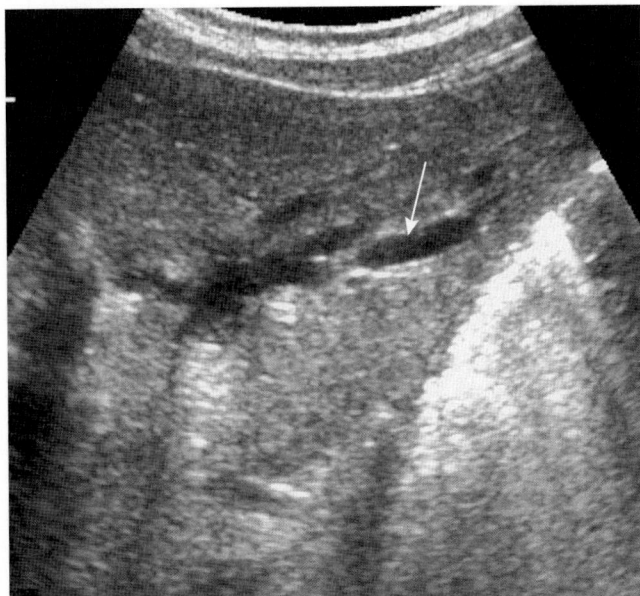

A

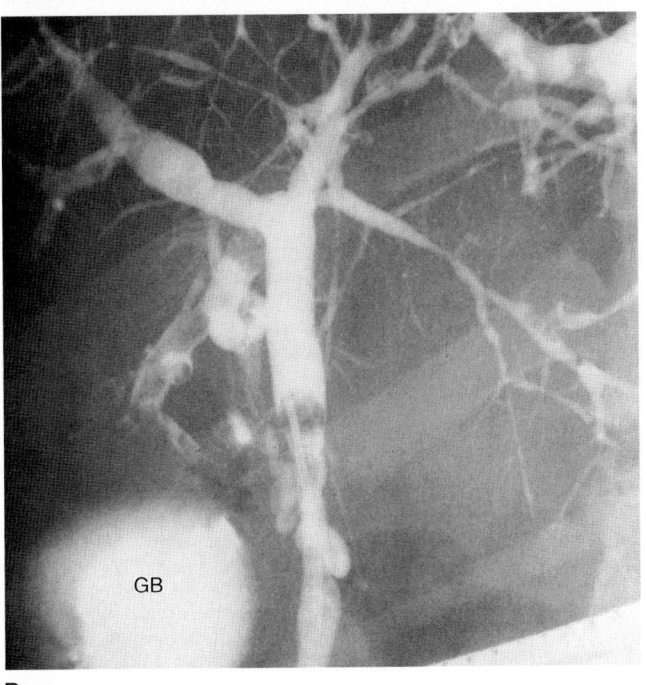

B

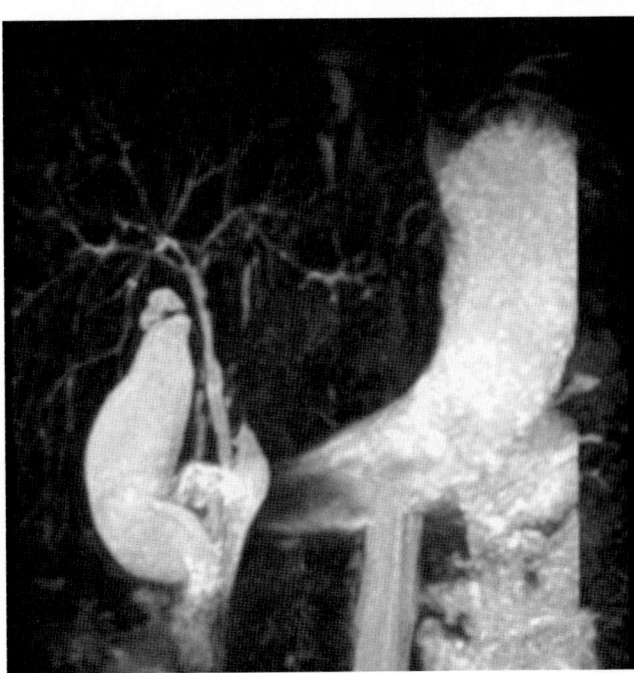

C

FIGURE 116-11. Sclerosing cholangitis in a 13-year-old girl with ulcerative colitis. **A,** Transverse sonogram of left lobe of liver reveals irregular bile duct dilation *(arrow).* **B,** Endoscopic retrograde cholangiopancreatography shows scattered areas of narrowing alternating with areas of dilation. GB, gallbladder. **C,** MR cholangiopancreatography. Single shot fast spin-echo coronal image of a 16-year-old boy with ulcerative colitis and jaundice demonstrates extensive beading of the biliary tree with little dilation. The common bile duct measured 6 mm. (**C,** Courtesy of Marta Hernanz-Schulman, MD, Nashville, TN.)

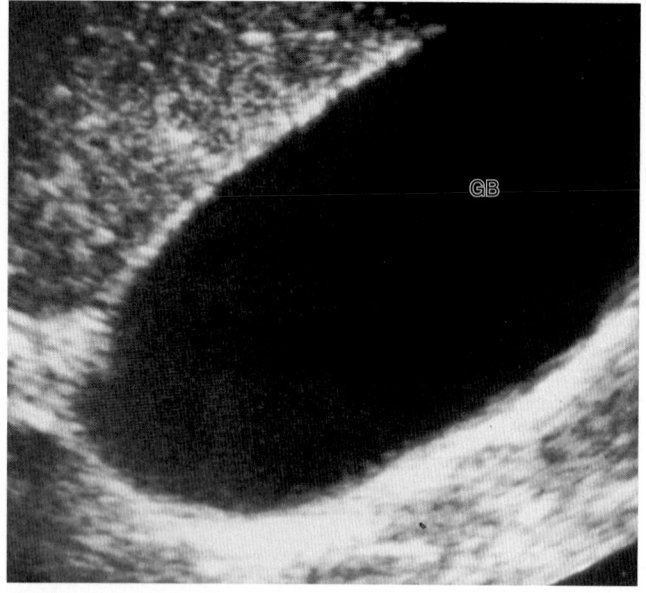

A

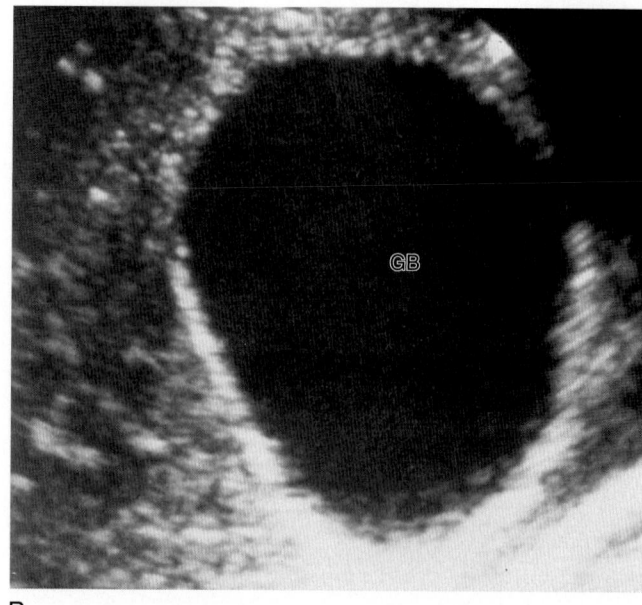

B

FIGURE 116-12. Hydrops of the gallbladder in a child with Kawasaki disease. Longitudinal **(A)** and transverse **(B)** sonograms show a markedly enlarged, balloon-shaped gallbladder (GB). Hydrops resolved spontaneously as the patient's condition improved.

SUGGESTED READINGS

General

Gubernick JA, Rosenberg HK, Ilaslan H, et al: US approach to jaundice in children. Radiographics 2000;20:173

Metreweli C, So NM, Chu WC, Lam WW: Magnetic resonance cholangiography in children. Br J Radiol 2004;77:1059-1064

Rosenthal SJ, Cox GG, Wetzel LH, Batnitzky S: Pitfalls and differential diagnosis in biliary sonography. RadioGraphics 1990;10:285-311

Cholelithiasis

Boraschi P, Neri E, Braccini G, et al: Choledocholithiasis: diagnostic accuracy of MR cholangiopancreatography. Three year experience. Magn Reson Imaging 1999;17:1245

Descos B, Bernard O, Brunelle F, et al: Pigment gallstones of the common bile duct in infancy. Hepatology 1984;4:678

Reif S, Sloven DG, Lebenthal E: Gallstones in children: characterization by age, etiology, and outcome. Am J Dis Child 1991;145:105

Stringer DA, Lim P, Cave M, et al: Fetal gallstones. J Pediatr Surg 1996;31:1589

Suma V, Marini A, Bucci N, et al: Fetal gallstones: sonographic and clinical observations. Ultrasound Obstet Gynecol 1998;12:439

Wu SS, Casas AT, Abraham SK, Billmire DF, Smergel EM, de Chadarevian JP. Milk of calcium cholelithiasis in children. J Pediatr Surg 2001;36:644-647

Biliary Sludge

Barton P, Maier A, Steininger R, et al: Biliary sludge after liver transplantation: 1. Imaging findings and efficacy of various imaging procedures. AJR Am J Roentgenol 1995;164:859-864

Brown DL, Teele RL, Doubilet PM, et al: Echogenic material in the fetal gallbladder: sonographic and clinical observations. Radiology 1992;182:73

Kumar R, Nguyen K, Shun A: Gallstones and common bile duct calculi in infancy and childhood. Aust N Z J Surg 2000; 70:188-191

Sty JR, Wells RG, Schroeder BA: Comparative imaging: bile-plug syndrome. Clin Nucl Med 1987;12:489-490

Cholecystitis

Alobaidi M, Gupta R, Jafri SZ, et al: Current trends in imaging evaluation of acute cholecystitis. Emerg Radiol 2004;10:256-258. Epub 2004 Mar 17

Lemonick DM, Garvin R, Semins H: Torsion of the gallbladder: a rare cause of acute cholecystitis. J Emerg Med 2006;30:397-401

Mirvis SE, Vainright JR, Nelson AW, et al: The diagnosis of acute acalculous cholecystitis: a comparison of sonography, scintigraphy, and CT. AJR Am J Roentgenol 1986;147:1171

Patriquin H, DiPietro M, Barber FE, et al: Sonography of thickened gallbladder wall: causes in children. AJR Am J Roentgenol 1983;141:57

Acalculous Cholecystitis

Barie PS, Eachempati SR: Acute acalculous cholecystitis. Curr Gastroenterol Rep 2003;5:302-309

Imamoglu M, Sarihan H, Sari A, et al: Acute acalculous cholecystitis in children: diagnosis and treatment. J Pediatr Surg 2002;37:36-39

Mariat G, Mahul P, Prev TN, et al: Contribution of ultrasonography and cholescintigraphy to the diagnosis of acute acalculous cholecystitis in intensive care unit patients. Intensive Care Med 2000;26:1658-1663

Cholangitis

Dienes HP, Erberich H, Dries V, et al: Autoimmune hepatitis and overlap syndromes. Clin Liver Dis 2002;6:349-362, vi

Haider MA, Bret PM: The role of magnetic resonance cholangiography in primary sclerosing cholangitis. J Hepatol 2000;33:659-660

Sisto A, Feldman P, Garel L, et al: Primary sclerosing cholangitis in children: study of five cases and review of the literature. Pediatrics 1987;80:918

Hydrops of the Gallbladder

Neu J, Arvin A, Ariagno L: Hydrops of the gallbladder. Am J Dis Child 1980;134:891

Zins M, Boulay-Coletta I, Molinie V, et al: [Imaging of a thickened-wall gallbladder.] J Radiol 2006;87(4 Pt 2):479-493

Zissin R, Osadchy A, Shapiro-Feinberg M, et al: CT of a thickened-wall gallbladder. Br J Radiol. 2003;76:137-143

117

Hepatic Tumors and Tumor-like Conditions

CHARLOTTE WAUGH MOORE and LISA H. LOWE

Hepatic neoplasms constitute about 2% of all childhood tumors and approximately 6% of pediatric abdominal neoplasms. Many imaging modalities are used to evaluate liver masses, including plain films, ultrasonography (US), computed tomography (CT), magnetic resonance imaging (MRI), radionuclide scintigraphy, and catheter angiography. Plain radiographs have a limited role but may reveal calcifications, mass effect, and the source of the mass. Sonography is the study of choice in the initial investigation of pediatric abdominal masses and hepatomegaly to confirm the organ of origin and characterize the lesion. This information can be used to form a preliminary differential diagnosis, which is helpful in deciding on the appropriate subsequent imaging approach. Additional cross-sectional imaging with CT, MRI, nuclear scintigraphy, and, rarely, angiography, may be required to fully characterize a hepatic lesion in anticipation of biopsy and treatment.

MALIGNANT HEPATOBILIARY TUMORS

Hepatoblastoma

Hepatoblastoma is the third most common abdominal tumor in children after Wilms tumor and neuroblastoma; it is the most common primary malignant liver tumor in children younger than 3 years. The peak incidence of hepatoblastoma is between 18 and 24 months. It disproportionately affects former premature infants and is the most common malignancy in these infants. It rarely presents in newborns, and there is a 2:1 male predominance.

There are two histologic types of hepatoblastoma: epithelial, which contains small cells that resemble the embryonic or fetal liver, and mixed, which contains epithelial and mesenchymal cells.

Hepatoblastoma usually presents as a palpable mass in the right upper quadrant and may be confused with hepatomegaly. Other findings at presentation include jaundice, pain, weight loss, irritability, vomiting, diarrhea, and congestive heart failure with large masses. Serum α-fetoprotein is markedly elevated in approximately 90% of patients with hepatoblastoma, and monitoring these levels is helpful in tracking residual disease. Presentation with acute abdomen secondary to tumor rupture is rare. An increased incidence of hepatoblastoma is associated with hemihypertrophy, Beckwith-

Wiedemann syndrome, familial adenomatous polyposis, glycogen storage disease, Gardner syndrome, and trisomy 18. Hepatoblastoma has also been reported in infants born of mothers taking oral contraceptives and gonadotropins and in the setting of fetal alcohol syndrome. Hepatoblastomas are usually solitary, but they may be multifocal or diffusely infiltrative. Multifocal disease may consist of a dominant mass with satellite nodules or multiple small masses. When solitary, hepatoblastoma is most common in the right hepatic lobe (60%). Distant metastases are present in less than 10% of cases at diagnosis, with the lungs being the most common site, followed by local lymph nodes, ovaries, bone, and brain.

> **Conditions in which hepatoblastoma occurs with increased frequency include:**
> - **Beckwith-Wiedemann syndrome**
> - **Familial adenomatous polyposis**
> - **Glycogen storage disease**
> - **Gardner syndrome**

Plain radiographs in patients with hepatoblastoma may show hepatomegaly or calcifications. On sonography, the tumor demonstrates variable echogenicity; is usually well defined; may contain echogenic foci with acoustic shadowing, indicating calcifications; and may have hypoechoic or anechoic areas of necrosis or hemorrhage (Fig. 117-1). Intravascular tumor thrombus may be seen within the hepatic veins or portal vessels and may exhibit flow on color flow Doppler imaging, differentiating it from non-neoplastic thrombus. Infiltrative hepatoblastomas show diffuse heterogeneous echogenicity, with loss of normal parenchymal architecture.

On unenhanced CT, the tumor is of decreased attenuation relative to the surrounding liver parenchyma. Rarely, hepatoblastomas are of equal attenuation to the liver and are not well visualized. Occasionally, the tumor's attenuation is equal to or greater than that of the adjacent normal liver parenchyma. Depending on the cell type, the tumor tends to be more homogeneous (epithelial) or heterogeneous (mixed mesenchymal-epithelial). Calcifications of various size and number may be present. After intravenous (IV) contrast administration, the tumor typically enhances in a heterogeneous

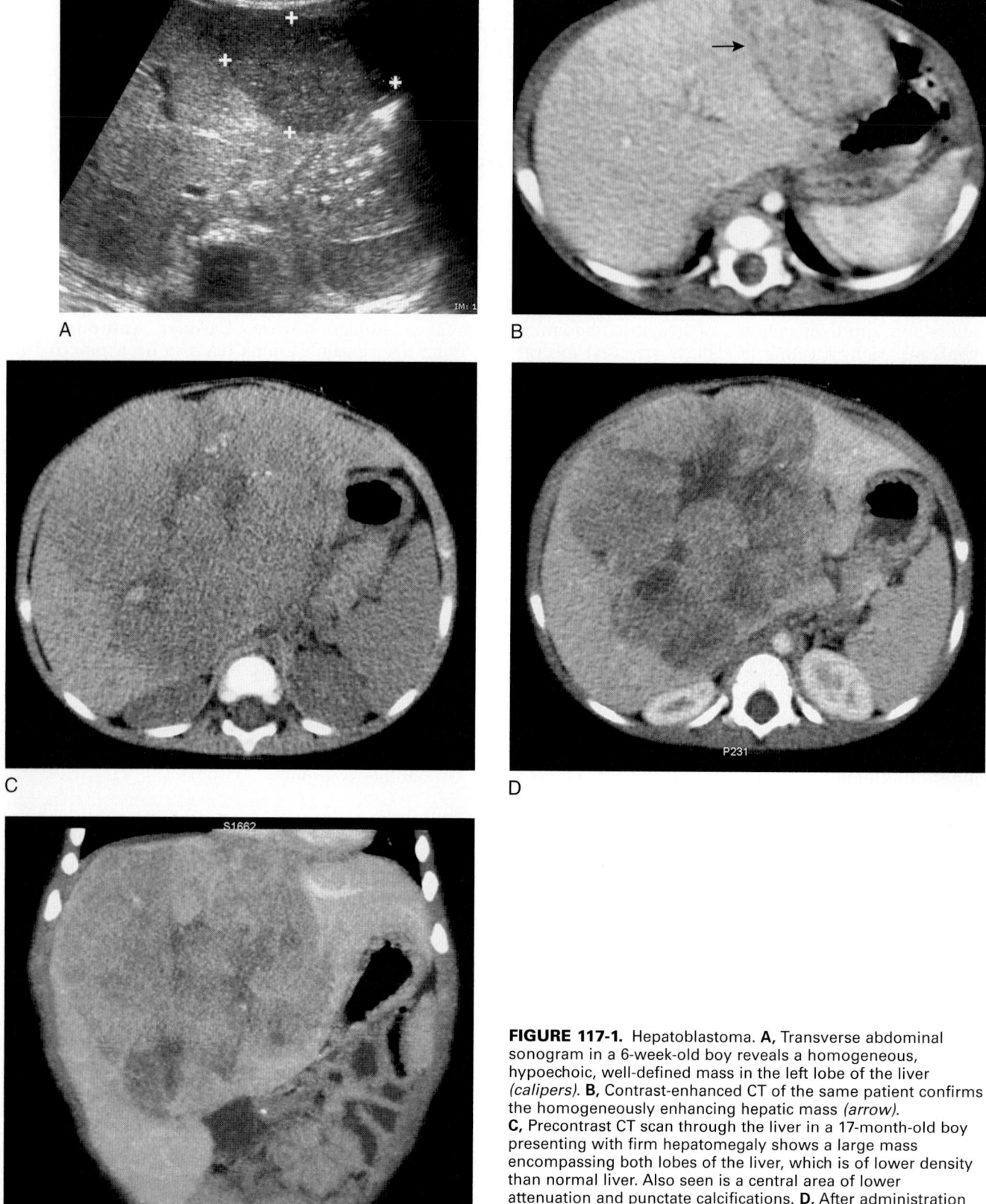

FIGURE 117-1. Hepatoblastoma. **A,** Transverse abdominal sonogram in a 6-week-old boy reveals a homogeneous, hypoechoic, well-defined mass in the left lobe of the liver *(calipers).* **B,** Contrast-enhanced CT of the same patient confirms the homogeneously enhancing hepatic mass *(arrow).* **C,** Precontrast CT scan through the liver in a 17-month-old boy presenting with firm hepatomegaly shows a large mass encompassing both lobes of the liver, which is of lower density than normal liver. Also seen is a central area of lower attenuation and punctate calcifications. **D,** After administration of intravenous contrast material, the mass appears to be multinodular, with heterogeneous enhancement less than that of the surrounding liver. **E,** Reformat shows the extent of the large hepatoblastoma in the coronal plane. (**C-E** courtesy of Dr. Marta Hernanz-Schulman, Nashville, TN.)

fashion, sometimes with peripheral rim enhancement. Computed tomography angiography (CTA) can help further define vascular invasion when present.

On MRI, the appearance of hepatoblastoma varies, depending on the histological tissue type and the character of the mass. The tumor mass is hypointense on T1- and hyperintense on T2-weighted images. Epithelial-type hepatoblastomas tend to enhance more homogenously, whereas mixed-type tumors tend to be more heterogeneous. However, areas of calcification, necrosis, hemorrhage, and septation may influence the signal intensity. Hemorrhage is most often hyperintense on T1-weighted images, and bands of fibrosis or septation are hypointense on T1- and T2-weighted images. Magnetic resonance angiography (MRA) may be useful to evaluate vascular invasion and the tumor's relationship to the hepatic vasculature.

Hepatic scintigraphy is rarely performed, but it may demonstrate increased activity on the initial angiographic phase, due to tumor vascularity, and photopenia on the delayed images. Rarely, increased uptake of the radiopharmaceutical may be seen on delayed images, a finding more typical of focal nodular hyperplasia. Catheter angiography is rarely performed but usually shows tumor hypervascularity except in areas of necrosis, which are hypovascular.

The treatment for hepatoblastoma includes surgical resection of local disease and chemotherapy for inoperable or metastatic disease. Liver transplantation can be considered if there is residual unresectable disease and no metastases after chemotherapy. The survival rate is 60% with complete resection, and overall mortality is 75%. Prognostic considerations include absence of vascular invasion, resectability at diagnosis, favorable epithelial histology, and rapid postsurgical decline of α-fetoprotein levels.

Hepatocellular Carcinoma

Hepatocellular carcinoma, the second most common liver tumor in children after hepatoblastoma, accounts for 35% of primary pediatric hepatic malignancies and occurs much more commonly in children older than 5 years. It has two age peaks in childhood: 4 to 5 years, and (more commonly) 12 to14 years. Is the most common hepatic malignancy in adolescents. The clinical symptoms and presentation are similar to those of hepatoblastoma. Levels of α-fetoprotein are elevated in 50% of patients. On histology, hepatocellular carcinomas range from well-differentiated to anaplastic tumors. The well-differentiated tumors may resemble hepatic architectural patterns, whereas anaplastic tumors show a pleomorphic appearance. Hepatocellular carcinomas may be solitary, multifocal, diffuse, or infiltrative, and the right lobe is involved more commonly than the left. These tumors have a high propensity for vascular invasion and intrahepatic spread of disease.

The majority of hepatocellular carcinomas occur in patients with underlying liver disease—usually in those with a background of cirrhosis, although the association in children is weaker than in adults. Hepatocellular carcinoma has been reported in children with cirrhotic liver disease following parenteral nutrition early in life. The incidence of hepatocellular carcinoma is greater in countries with a high rate of hepatitis B infection, with vertical transmission of the virus from mother to infant conferring as much as a 200-fold risk of developing hepatocellular carcinoma later in life. Specific chronic liver diseases associated with the development of hepatocellular carcinoma include hereditary tyrosinemia, glycogen storage disease, α_1-antitrypsin deficiency, biliary atresia, Alagille syndrome, hemachromatosis, Wilson disease, galactosemia, and viral hepatitis (hepatitis B and C).

Hepatocellular carcinoma is associated with the following chronic liver diseases in children:

- **Tyrosinemia**
- **Glycogen storage disease**
- **α_1-Antitrypsin deficiency**
- **Biliary atresia**
- **Alagille syndrome**
- **Hemachromatosis**
- **Wilson disease**
- **Galactosemia**
- **Viral hepatitis (hepatitis B and C)**

The ultrasound findings of hepatocellular carcinoma are similar to those of hepatoblastoma, but calcifications are less common (Fig. 117-2). As with hepatoblastoma, vascular invasion can be identified in the portal vein, hepatic veins, inferior vena cava, or hepatic arteries. Again, color Doppler US is useful to distinguish bland thrombus from tumor thrombus by identifying blood flow within the substance of tumor thrombus.

On unenhanced CT, hepatocellular carcinoma is hypo- to isodense with adjacent liver and is typically well defined. The tumor shows variable enhancement after IV contrast administration and may contain hypoattenuated regions of necrosis. Tumor thrombus may be seen as intraluminal filling defects with a surrounding meniscus of contrast and can be better evaluated with angiographic sequences. When the tumor arises in a cirrhotic liver, differentiation from regenerating nodules may be difficult.

The MRI appearance of hepatocellular carcinoma is variable. The tumor is hypointense on T1- and hyperintense on T2-weighted images. Hyperintense areas of fat or hemorrhage may be seen on T1-weighted images. When a fibrous pseudocapsule is present, it is of low signal intensity on T1- and T2-weighted pulse sequences. Vascular invasion can be evaluated with MRA. Hepatocellular carcinomas exhibit variable enhancement after gadolinium, depending on the presence and degree of internal necrosis, hemorrhage, or calcifications.

Nuclear scintigraphy is rarely performed in patients with hepatocellular carcinoma but typically shows decreased uptake. Gallium scans, however, are characteristic and may help distinguish hepatocellular carcinoma (gallium avid) from regenerating nodules (not gallium

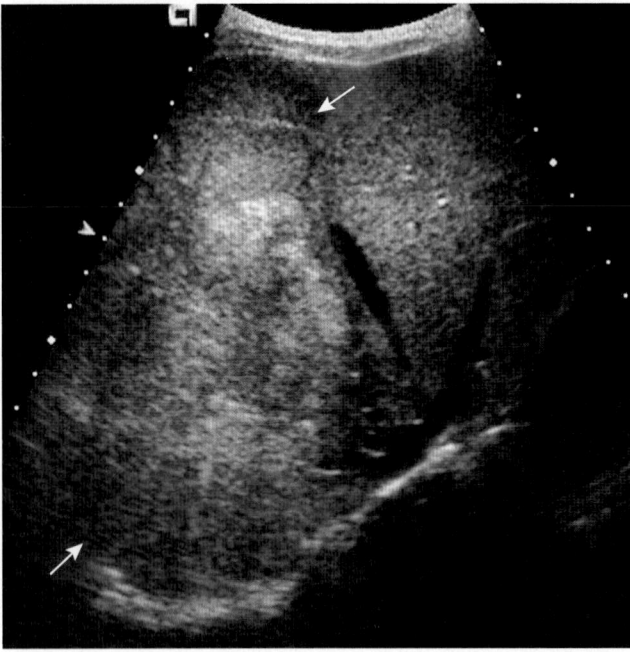

A

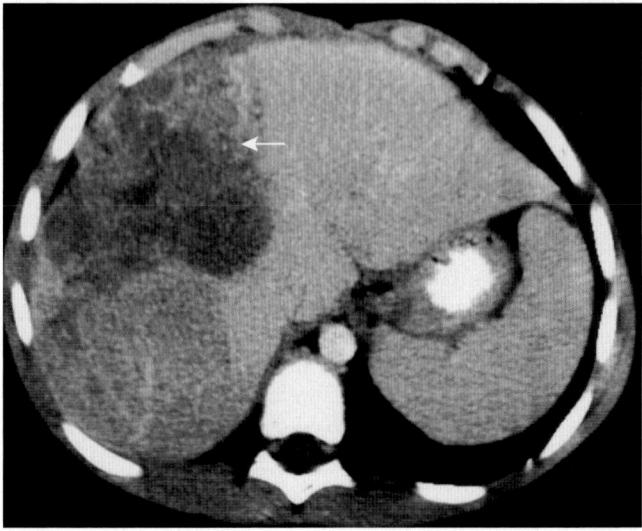

B

FIGURE 117-2. Hepatocellular carcinoma in an 8-year-old boy with abdominal pain. **A,** Abdominal sonogram reveals a heterogeneous mass in the liver *(arrows)*, demarcated by the middle hepatic vein medially. **B,** Contrast-enhanced CT shows the extensive, heterogeneously enhancing liver mass *(arrow)*.

avid). Fluorodeoxyglucose (FDG) positron emission tomography (PET) is useful in evaluating the degree of tumor differentiation. Although the uptake of FDG is variable in hepatocellular carcinomas, markedly elevated uptake is usually seen in poorly differentiated tumors. FDG PET may be used to evaluate for metastatic disease when staging hepatocellular carcinoma or to distinguish regenerating nodules in cirrhotic livers from hepatocellular carcinoma. One caveat is that FDG PET may show normal uptake in well-differentiated tumors. Combining FDG PET and gallium scintigraphy can be useful when grading tumors. For example, low-grade tumors typically show normal uptake on PET and increased uptake on gallium scans. However, gallium uptake is also seen in other processes, such as metastatic disease (lymphoma) and hepatic adenoma.

The treatment for hepatocellular carcinoma is complete surgical resection when possible, with chemotherapy for residual or metastatic disease. The prognosis is variable and is directly related to the resectability and histology of the lesion. In tumors with favorable histology and complete resection, the 2-year survival rate may exceed 97%. However, without complete resection and with unfavorable histology, the 2-year survival rate may be less than 20%.

Fibrolamellar Carcinoma

Fibrolamellar carcinoma is a distinct form of hepatocellular carcinoma. Histologically, it contains large sheets of hepatocyte-like cells with eosinophilic cytoplasm that are separated by lamellae of fibrous stroma. Fibrolamellar carcinoma is typically found in young adults, but the age range is between 5 and 35 years. The tumor is not associated with chronic liver disease or risk factors such as hepatitis B or C, and it is usually not associated with elevated α-fetoprotein levels (11%). A central scar

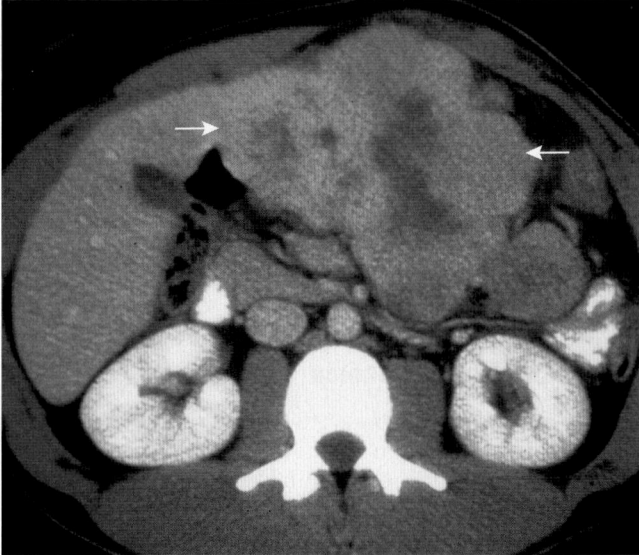

FIGURE 117-3. Fibrolamellar carcinoma in an 18-year-old girl. Axial contrast-enhanced CT shows a lobulated mass *(arrows)* with a central scar in the left lobe of the liver.

that typically does not enhance after contrast administration is common (30% of cases), and calcifications are seen in 40% of the lesions.

> **Fibrolamellar carcinoma is pathologically distinct from hepatocellular carcinoma.**

On US, a lobulated mass with well-defined borders and a heterogeneous echotexture is typical. If a central scar is present, it tends to be hyperechoic. CT shows a well-defined, lobulated mass with calcifications in 30% to 55% of cases and a central scar in 45% to 60% of cases (Fig. 117-3). Adjacent lymphadenopathy is often present at diagnosis. The mass enhances heterogeneously during the arterial phase of contrast administration and is more homogeneous or isodense during the portal venous phase of enhancement. The central scar is of low attenuation, with little or no enhancement on CT.

On T1-weighted MRI, the tumor tends to be homogeneous and iso- to mildly hypointense; on T2-weighted images, the tumor is usually heterogeneous and iso- to hyperintense. The fibrous scar is hypointense on T1- and T2-weighted images, a feature which can be used to distinguish fibrolamellar carcinoma from focal nodular hyperplasia; in focal nodular hyperplasia, the central scar has increased signal on T2-weighted sequences. The central scar enhances with intravenous contrast in focal nodular hyperplasia, but not typically in fibrolamellar carcinoma.

> **Fibrolamellar carcinoma and focal nodular hyperplasia both have central scars. In fibrolamellar carcinoma, the scar lacks contrast enhancement and has low signal intensity on T1- and T2-weighted MRI. In focal nodular hyperplasia, the scar typically enhances after IV contrast and is hyperintense on T2-weighted images.**

The treatment for fibrolamellar carcinoma is surgical resection, which is possible in 48% of cases. The prognosis is better for fibrolamellar carcinoma than for hepatocellular carcinoma, likely because of the higher resectability rate at presentation in some published series. However, when the tumor is not resectable, the overall prognosis does not appear to be affected. The 5-year survival rate ranges from 30% to 67%.

Undifferentiated Embryonal Sarcoma

Undifferentiated embryonal sarcoma, previously called malignant mesenchymoma, embryonal sarcoma, or fibromyxosarcoma, is a rare, extremely malignant tumor of mesenchymal origin affecting children between the ages of 5 and 10 years (90% of cases occur in those younger than 15 years). On histology, undifferentiated embryonal sarcoma shows primitive spindle-shaped, sarcomatous satellite cells, closely packed in sheets or whorls and scattered throughout a background of loose myxoid tissue, which contains foci of hematopoiesis in 50% of cases. The tumor has no gender predilection. The presenting symptoms include abdominal pain, distention, right upper quadrant mass, vomiting, anemia, weight loss, fever, and jaundice. Undifferentiated embryonal sarcoma is usually large at presentation, is solitary, involves the right lobe of the liver (75%) more commonly than the left, and is predominantly solid with occasional cystic, necrotic, or hemorrhagic areas.

On sonography, the tumor is a solid and isoechoic to hyperechoic, with internal anechoic regions of cystic necrosis. On CT, the tumor is often of low attenuation, appearing to be cystlike and mimicking fluid. This misleading appearance may be due to water being attracted by the hydrophilic acid mucopolysaccharides in the

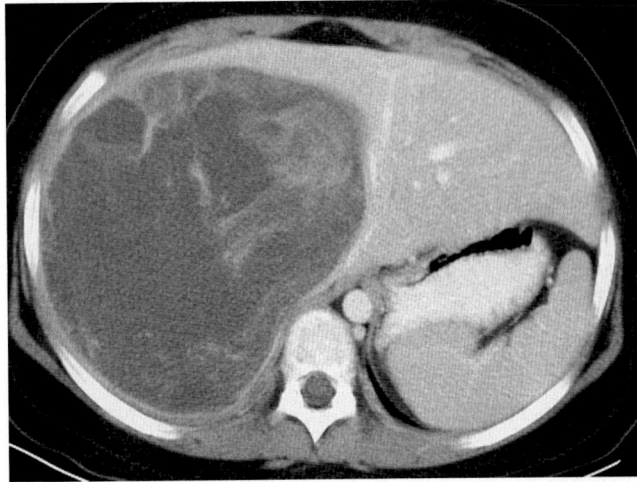

FIGURE 117-4. Undifferentiated embryonal sarcoma in a 9-year-old girl. Postcontrast CT image shows a large, well-defined, heterogeneously enhancing, low-attenuation mass in the right hepatic lobe. (Courtesy of Robert P Guillerman, MD.)

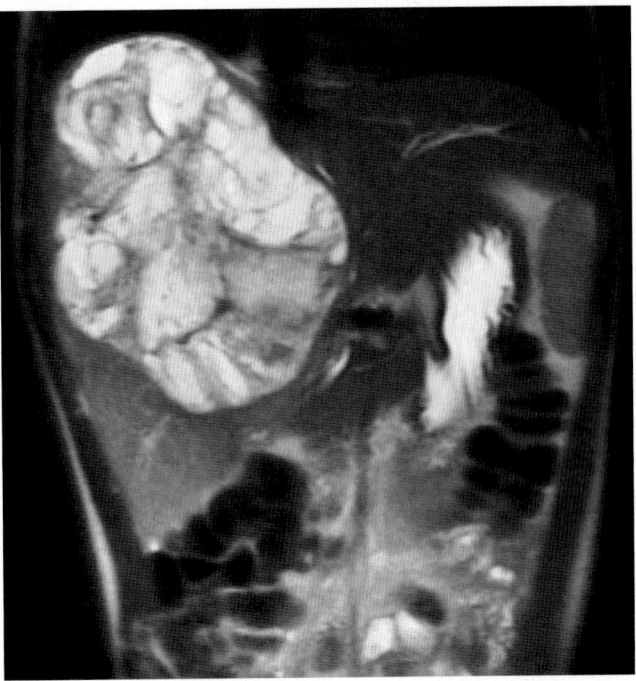

FIGURE 117-5. Undifferentiated embryonal sarcoma in a 13-year-old girl. Coronal T2-weighted MR image shows a multiloculated mass of heterogeneous signal intensity in the right lobe of the liver. (Courtesy of Lynn Fordham, MD.)

myxoid components of the tumor. Hyperattenuated regions may indicate hemorrhage, and enhancement after IV contrast administration is variable (Fig. 117-4). The features of the tumor on MRI are low intensity on T1- and increased intensity on T2-weighted sequences (Fig. 117-5). Bright areas on T1-weighted images can occur in regions of hemorrhage. Peripheral enhancement, corresponding to a pseudocapsule; enhancement of solid tumor components; and enhancement of septa may be seen. Vascular invasion may occur, and metastases are usually to the lung and bone.

> Undifferentiated embryonal sarcoma is a rare, extremely malignant tumor of mesenchymal origin that is solid on sonography but may mimic fluid on CT.

The treatment is similar to that for hepatoblastoma and hepatocellular carcinoma; however, the prognosis is very poor, with death occurring within 12 months in many cases.

Rhabdomyosarcoma of the Biliary Tree

Although rhabdomyosarcoma can be found throughout the body, involvement of the biliary ducts is one of rarest forms of this mesenchymal tumor. In children, however, it is the most common neoplasm of the biliary tree. Histologically, biliary rhabdomyosarcoma demonstrates undifferentiated blue cells with scant cytoplasm and primitive nuclei that form a firm, lobulated mass with infiltrative margins and a well-defined pseudocapsule. Rhabdomyosarcoma tends to occur in children younger than 5 years, with a median age at presentation of 3 years. Patients typically present with jaundice and abdominal distention or, less likely, pain, nausea, vomiting, or fever. The tumor can arise in the intrahepatic bile ducts, gallbladder, cystic duct, extrahepatic biliary tree, or ampulla of Vater or within a choledochal cyst.

US typically reveals biliary duct dilation and an intraductal mass. Larger masses may have areas of cystic necrosis. CT shows an intraductal mass with variable contrast enhancement and associated biliary ductal dilation (Fig. 117-6). MRI usually shows low signal intensity on T1- and high signal intensity on T2-weighted sequences, with intense, heterogeneous enhancement after IV contrast administration. Magnetic resonance cholangio-pancreatography is useful in demonstrating dilated bile ducts.

The treatment of rhabdomyosarcoma may involve complete surgical resection before or after chemotherapy. In some anatomic locations, radiotherapy may be useful as well. The overall survival rate is approximately 65%, but it depends on the stage of disease, the anatomic location of the primary lesion, and its resectability.

Cholangiocarcinoma

Cholangiocarcinoma is a rare hepatic neoplasm accounting for less than 1% of all carcinomas. It may complicate disorders that affect children, such as choledochal cysts and sclerosing cholangitis, but it usually occurs late in the disease process and thus presents mainly in adults.

Hepatic Metastases

Hepatic metastases in children are most often due to Wilms tumor, neuroblastoma, lymphoma, and leukemia. The appearance of hepatic metastatic disease is highly variable, ranging from one or more focal lesions to a diffuse infiltrative pattern, with loss of normal hepatic architecture. Most hepatic metastases are multiple; hypo-

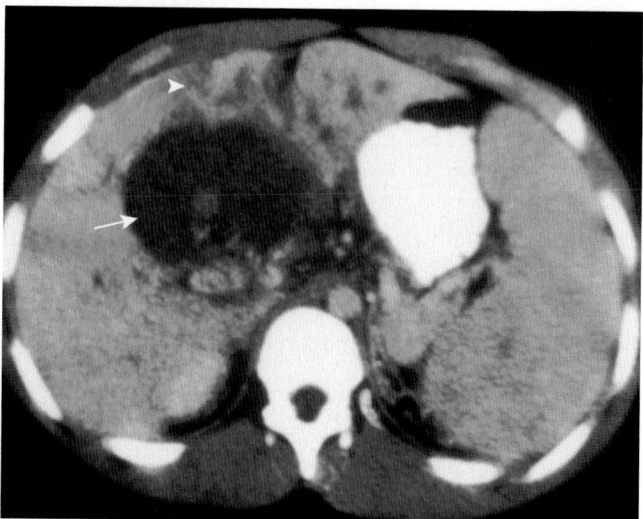

FIGURE 117-6. Rhabdomyosarcoma in a 14-year-old boy. Axial postcontrast CT image reveals a focal hepatic mass *(arrow)* near the porta hepatis, with associated peripheral bile duct enlargement *(arrowhead)*.

echoic on sonography; of low attenuation on CT, with a tendency toward peripheral enhancement; and hypointense on T1- and hyperintense on T2-weighted MRI.

> Hepatic metastases in children are most often due to Wilms tumor, neuroblastoma, lymphoma, and leukemia.

Wilms tumor metastases are most commonly found in the lungs and adjacent lymph nodes. Hematogenous spread of Wilms tumor to the liver occurs in 15% of cases; however, primary renal lesions are often very large at presentation, abutting the liver and making direct hepatic invasion by the primary renal mass impossible to exclude. Most hepatic metastatic lesions due to Wilms tumor are hematogenous and tend to be multifocal and heterogeneously enhancing; they may have central necrosis, calcifications, or vascular invasion (Fig. 117-7).

Neuroblastoma may present with metastatic spread to bone, regional lymph nodes, liver, brain, and lung. Metastatic neuroblastoma to the liver has two typical patterns: (1) numerous discrete lesions of variable echogenicity, attenuation, and enhancement; and (2) diffuse infiltration with distortion of the normal hepatic architecture, leading to hepatomegaly (Fig. 117-8). The latter pattern is especially common with stage IV-S disease (primary lesion limited to the organ of origin or primary lesion with regional spread but without extension across the midline, and involvement of the liver, skin, or bone marrow).

Leukemia often involves the liver at autopsy but is not typically visible with imaging. Lymphoma may present with multiple discrete lesions or an infiltrative pattern similar to that of neuroblastoma. In addition, lymphoma is often associated with lymphadenopathy and splenic lesions (Fig. 117-9).

BENIGN HEPATIC NEOPLASMS

Mesenchymal Hamartoma

Mesenchymal hamartoma, a rare benign hepatic tumor, is considered by many to be a developmental anomaly rather than a true neoplasm. Histologically, it is composed of disordered, primitive, fluid-filled mesenchyma, hepatic parenchyma, and bile ducts, in addition to stromal cysts of variable size without capsules. The tumor presents most often in children younger than 2 years,

with an age range from newborn to 5 years. Mesenchymal hamartomas affect boys slightly more often than girls and have been diagnosed on prenatal US. Most children present with an otherwise asymptomatic palpable abdominal mass; liver function studies are usually within normal limits. The mass may be pedunculated and attached to the inferior surface of the liver.

On US and CT, mesenchymal hamartomas are typically multicystic, heterogeneous masses with septa. The cysts vary in size and may contain internal echogenic or hyperdense material due to hemorrhage. Less often, the tumor may be solid and vascular, similar to hemangioma. On CT, the septations and solid components

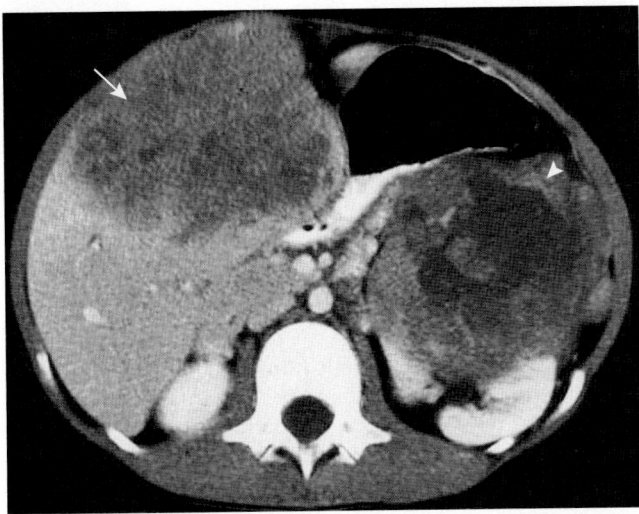

FIGURE 117-7. Metastatic Wilms tumor in a 4-year-old boy with suspected hepatomegaly. Postcontrast CT image demonstrates heterogeneous enhancement within a hepatic metastasis *(arrow)* from a Wilms tumor arising in the left kidney *(arrowhead)*.

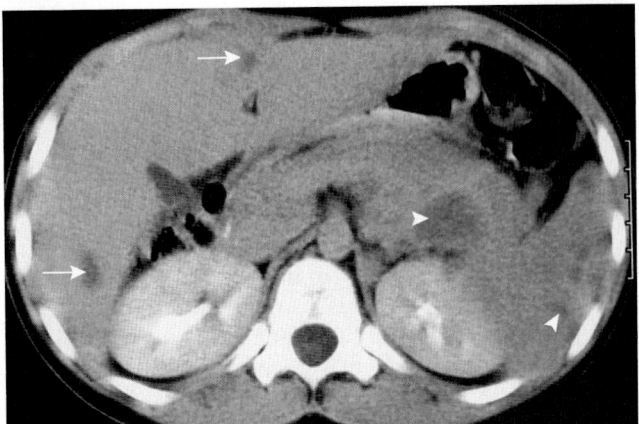

FIGURE 117-9. Lymphoma in a 9-year-old boy. CT image during the equilibrium (delayed) phase of intravenous contrast administration reveals multiple foci of low attenuation within the liver *(arrows)*, in the tail of the pancreas, and in the spleen *(arrowheads)*.

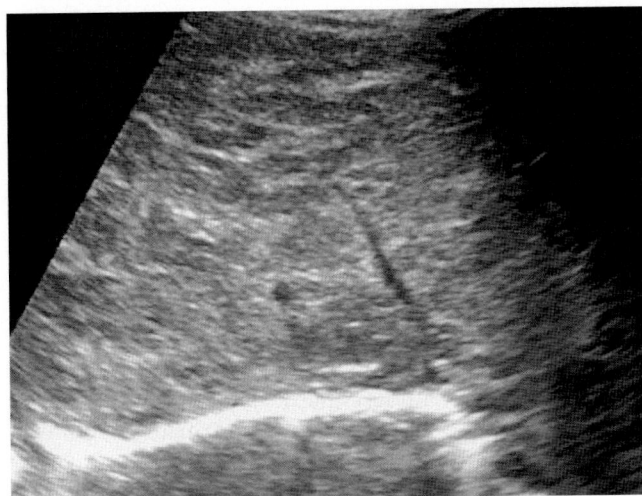

A

FIGURE 117-8. Metastatic infiltrative neuroblastoma in a 10-month-old girl with hepatomegaly. **A,** Axial hepatic sonogram shows diffusely increased echogenicity and loss of normal architecture throughout the enlarged liver. **B,** Coronal CT reconstruction after contrast administration confirms hepatomegaly, loss of normal hepatic architecture, diffusely heterogeneous hepatic enhancement, and a primary, partially calcified thoracic lesion *(arrow)*.

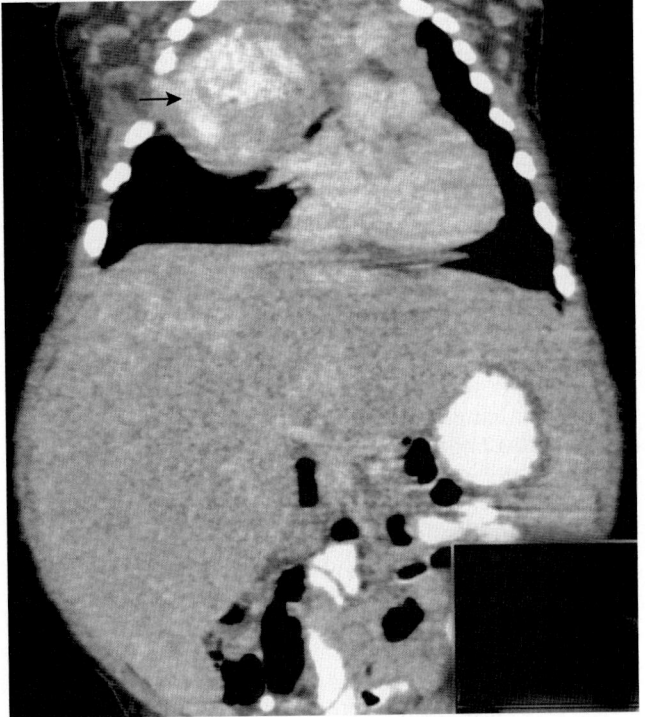

B

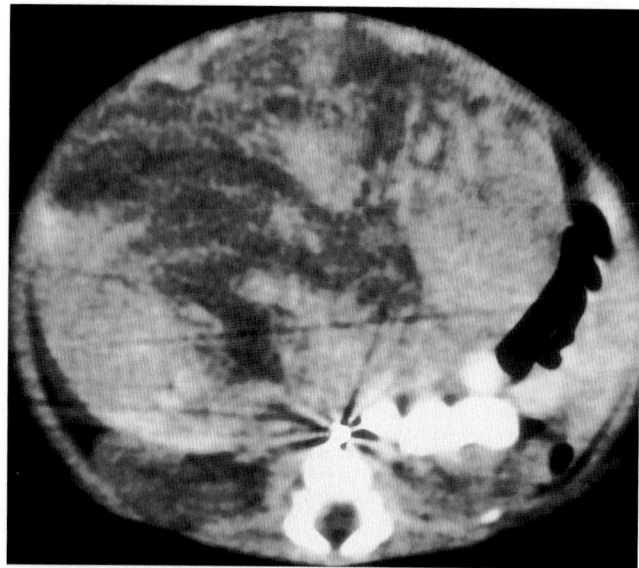

FIGURE 117-10. Mesenchymal hamartoma. Axial postcontrast CT image reveals a large, heterogeneously enhancing mass replacing the right lobe of the liver, representing a mesenchymal hamartoma.

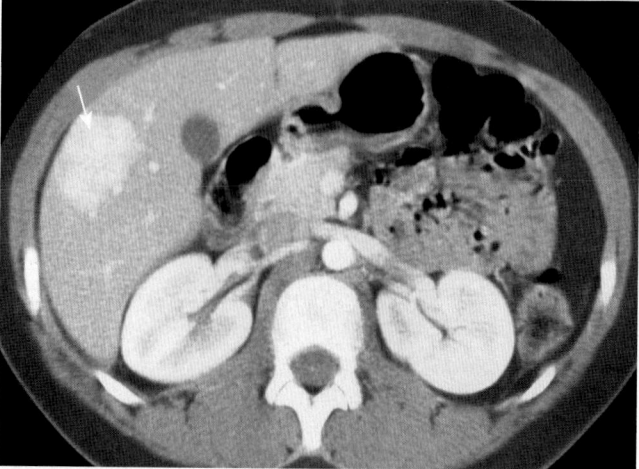

FIGURE 117-11. Focal nodular hyperplasia in an 11-year-old girl. Axial, postcontrast, arterial phase CT shows a well-defined hypervascular mass in the right hepatic lobe *(arrow)*.

enhance after IV contrast administration (Fig. 117-10). On MRI, the cystic regions are hypointense on T1- and hyperintense on T2-weighted images. The signal intensity varies, depending on the stromal content, amount of protein within the cyst fluid, and presence or absence of hemorrhage within the cyst. The septa are usually of decreased signal on T2-weighted images.

> **Mesenchymal hamartomas are typically multicystic, heterogeneous masses with septa, presenting in children younger than 5 years.**

The treatment for mesenchymal hamartoma is surgical resection. The lesion does not have malignant potential, and resection is curative.

Focal Nodular Hyperplasia

Focal nodular hyperplasia (FNH), a rare hamartomatous malformation in children, is the second most common benign pediatric hepatic tumor after hemangioma. It accounts for 4% of all primary pediatric hepatic masses. Histologically, FNH is composed of hepatocytes (filled with fat, triglyceride, and glycogen), Kupffer cells, radial fibrous septa with bile ducts unconnected to the biliary tree, and a central scar that contains an arteriovenous-type malformation, which is important in the enhancement pattern of this lesion after IV contrast administration. FNH is more common in girls and has been reported following the Kasai operation for biliary atresia. Although this tumor is associated with oral contraceptive use, it has been shown that the oral contraceptives promote lesion growth but do not induce its formation. The lesion is usually asymptomatic, is usually located in the right hepatic lobe, is multiple in 20% of cases, and is often identified incidentally on studies done for other reasons. The lesion has

malignant potential and a low tendency for hemorrhagic complications.

> **Focal nodular hyperplasia is composed of hepatocytes, Kupffer cells, and biliary elements unconnected to the biliary tree. The central scar demonstrates delayed enhancement after contrast administration.**

On imaging, FNH is composed of a single, well-defined, often subcapsular mass with a characteristic enhancing central scar. On US, the echogenicity of FNH varies. The central scar, seen in approximately 33% of cases on US, is usually hypoechoic and hypervascular with Doppler interrogation. On CT, the central scar is found in up to 60% of cases. Before contrast administration, the mass and the central scar are hypo- to isodense with liver. After the administration of contrast material, the mass enhances brightly (Fig. 117-11), with delayed enhancement and washout of the central scar. On MRI, FNH is iso- to hypointense on T1-weighted images, mildly hyperintense on T2-weighted images, and enhances after the administration of gadolinium contrast material. The central scar also enhances after contrast, a feature that distinguishes it from fibro-lamellar carcinoma, as discussed previously. Only FNH contains sufficient Kupffer cells to cause normal to increased uptake on sulfur colloid scintigraphy, a finding that is nearly pathognomonic. Because of this fact, sulfur colloid scans may be used to verify the diagnosis of FNH, helping to avoid other unnecessary interventions.

The treatment for focal nodular hyperplasia includes discontinuation of offending drugs, such as oral contraceptives, resection of pedunculated hepatic masses, and, occasionally, excisional biopsy.

Angiomyolipoma

Hepatic angiomyolipoma (AML) is a rare, benign hamartomatous tumor found in the liver or kidney in 5% to 10% of pediatric patients with tuberous sclerosis.

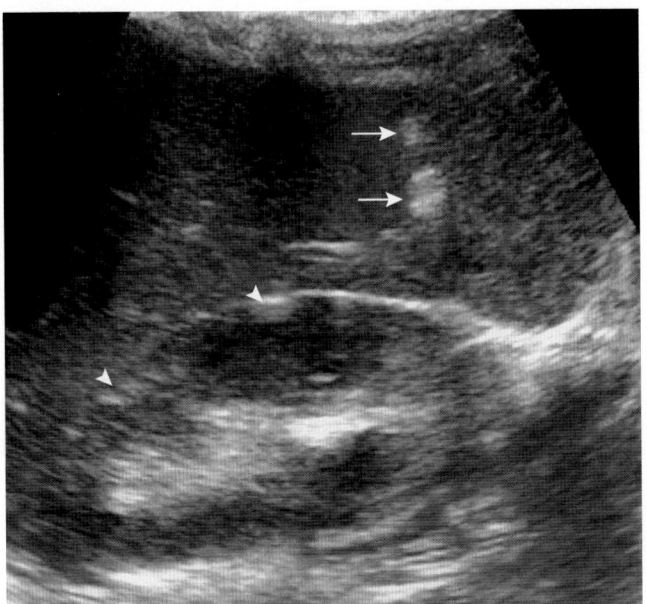

FIGURE 117-12. Angiomyolipomas of the liver and kidney in a 2-year-old girl with tuberous sclerosis. Longitudinal sonogram of the liver and right kidney shows multiple hyperechoic foci in the liver *(arrows)* and kidney *(arrowheads)*, consistent with angiomyolipomas.

Histologically, it contains a combination of smooth muscle, fat, and blood vessels. It affects girls four times as often as boys. In children, it is nearly always associated with tuberous sclerosis and rarely occurs spontaneously. By age 10 years, more than 80% of children with tuberous sclerosis have either renal or hepatic angiomyolipomas.

On imaging, the masses, which are often multiple, contain fat and vigorously enhancing soft tissue. On US, the lesions are hyperechoic and well defined, and the vascular portions enhance on color Doppler interrogation (Fig. 117-12). On CT, the mass is well defined and enhancing and contains mixed areas of fat and soft tissue attenuation. MRI signal characteristics follow those of fat or soft tissue in various portions of the lesion.

> **Hepatic angiomyolipomas in children are nearly always associated with tuberous sclerosis.**

The treatment is conservative, because the lesions are often multiple and involve more than one lobe of the liver. Large lesions may hemorrhage, in which case embolization may be useful. Surgical resection may be possible in the case of single lesions but may not be practical due to multifocal disease.

Hepatic Adenoma

Hepatic adenoma, a rare tumor of the liver in young children, occurs more often in adult women than in children. Hepatic adenomas (called *adenomatosis* when there are four or more adenomas) are associated with anabolic steroids in men and are directly related to the long-term use of oral contraceptives in women. On histology, hepatic adenoma consists of a solitary, spherical growth of hepatocytes within a pseudocapsule. The hepatocytes contain increased amounts of fat and glycogen and are organized in sheets, along with thin-walled vessels, bile ducts, and dysfunctional Kupffer cells. The tumor can be found in patients with type I and, less commonly, type IV glycogen storage disease, as well as diabetes mellitus. Patients with hepatic adenomas usually have normal liver function and may present with a right upper quadrant mass or pain; occasionally, symptoms are due to rupture and bleeding.

> **Hepatic adenoma is associated with:**
> - **Glycogen storage disease**
> - **Diabetes mellitus**
> - **Anabolic steroids**
> - **Long-term oral contraceptive use**

On imaging, hepatic adenomas are solitary in approximately 80% of cases and multiple in 20%. They may be found incidentally on cross-sectional imaging performed for unrelated reasons.

The ultrasound appearance of hepatic adenoma is variable (Fig. 117-13). The hyperechoic masses may have a surrounding hypoechoic rim, and some may lack a well-defined wall. On unenhanced CT, hepatic adenomas are usually hypodense with a low-attenuation capsule (25%) and a well-defined border; the presence of hemorrhage or fat can result in heterogeneous attenuation (7%). Homogeneous early enhancement is seen during the arterial phase of contrast injection, and the mass becomes isodense on delayed CT images. On MRI, hepatic adenomas are mildly hypointense to moderately hyperintense with surrounding liver on T1-weighted images and may have a more hypointense rim. On T2-weighted images, the mass is usually mildly hyperintense. As on CT, heterogeneity may be due to hemorrhage, necrosis, or fat. On fat-suppressed images, the mass may be hyperintense to liver on T1- and T2-weighted sequences. Similar to CT, after the administration of gadolinium contrast, the hepatic adenoma enhances during the arterial phase and becomes nearly isointense to liver on delayed MR images. Gallium uptake in hepatic adenomas is decreased, and they do not usually take up sulfur colloid, appearing as photopenic defects on both studies. Rarely, a hepatic adenoma contains enough Kupffer cells to show uptake of sulfur colloid on scintigraphy, a finding typically associated with FNH. With hepatobiliary agents, hepatic adenomas usually have early uptake, which persists on delayed images.

HEPATIC VASOPROLIFERATIVE ANOMALIES

Vasoproliferative anomalies of the liver include infantile hemangioma, infantile hemangioendothelioma, angiosarcoma, and hepatic epithelioid hemangioendothelioma, all of which are ultimately distinguished on a pathologic basis.

When discussing hemangiomas in children, it important to be aware that they are different in terms of presentation and imaging characteristics from what have

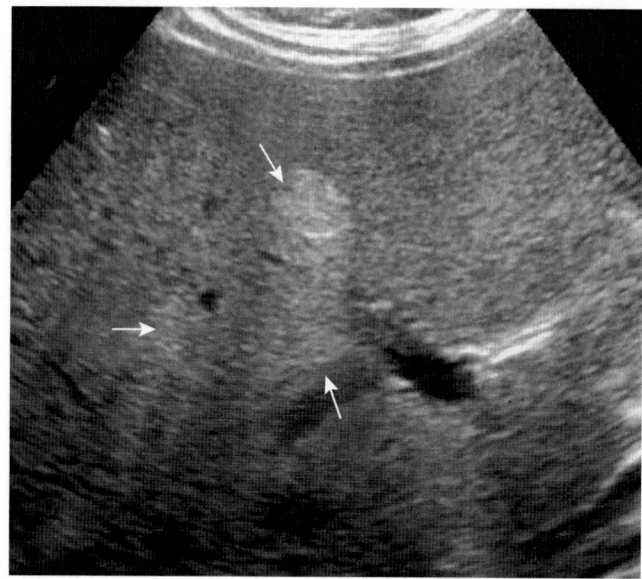

A

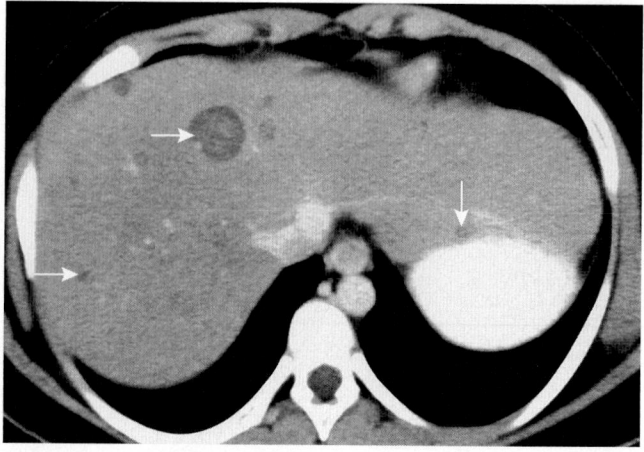

B

FIGURE 117-13. Hepatic adenoma in a 9-year-old girl with glycogen storage disease. **A,** Axial sonogram reveals hyperechoic foci within the liver *(arrows)*. **B,** Axial contrast-enhanced CT confirms multiple well-defined, hypoattenuating masses of varied size throughout the liver *(arrows)*.

traditionally been described as hemangiomas in adults. Indeed, the pathology of adult hemangiomas is currently being reconsidered and debated. In any case, application of adult criteria to hemangiomas in children is likely to cause confusion, result in an erroneous imaging approach, and may lead to incorrect diagnosis and treatment.

> **Hemangiomas in children differ from those in adults in terms of presentation and imaging characteristics.**

Classification

It is important to be familiar with changes that have taken place over the past two decades in the classification of vascular anomalies in children. In this discussion, we use nomenclature from the binary (or biologic) classification system of vascular anomalies according to the International Society for the Study of Vascular Anomalies. This classification system, described by Mulliken and Glowacki, is gradually gaining acceptance among radiologists, dermatologists, pathologists, surgeons, and other clinicians. Although a detailed description of this classification system is beyond the scope of this text, a brief comment should suffice to alleviate confusion about the classification of hemangiomas and other vascular anomalies in children. Vascular anomalies can be divided into two broad types: vasoproliferative anomalies, characterized by an increased endothelial cell cycle, and vascular malformations, which have normal endothelial turnover (Table 117-1). This system does not include descriptive terms used in the past, such as *cavernous* or *strawberry*. Other terms used in the literature that may cause confusion include *kaposiform*, which is typically applied to distinct pathologic lesions found

TABLE 117-1
Classification of Vascular Lesions

VASOPROLIFERATIVE TUMORS
Infantile hemangioma
Hemangioendothelioma
Angiosarcoma

VASCULAR MALFORMATIONS
Slow flow
  Capillary
  Lymphatic
  Venous
Fast flow
  Arterial: aneurysm, coarctation, ectasia
  Arteriovenous fistula
  Arteriovenous malformation
Complex combined (associated with skeletal overgrowth)
Regional syndrome
  Sturge-Weber: facial capillary malformations; intracranial capillary, venous, or arteriovenous malformations
  Klippel-Trénaunay: limb or truncal capillary, lymphatic, or venous malformations
  Parkes Weber: complex combined capillary arteriovenous malformations or fistulas with asymmetric extremity overgrowth and cutaneous port-wine stain
Diffuse syndrome
  Maffucci: lymphatic or venous malformations and enchondromas
  Solomon: capillary or venous malformations, intracranial arteriovenous malformations, epidermal nevi
  Proteus: capillary or venous malformations, macrodactyly, hemihypertrophy, lipomas, pigmented nevi, scoliosis
  Blue rubber bleb nevus (rare, familial): multiple cutaneous, musculoskeletal, and gastrointestinal tract venous malformations

Modified from Mulliken JB: Cutaneous vascular anomalies. Semin Vasc Surg 1993;6:204-218.

on the extremities and trunk and does not refer to vasoproliferative anomalies of the liver. In addition, *epithelioid hemangioendothelioma* is a pathologic term used to describe a rare lesion that occurs in various organs (including the liver) in older children and adults; it should not be confused with the term *infantile hemangioendothelioma*, which is discussed in the following paragraphs. Unfortunately, the nomenclature used in various textbooks and articles by various authors, including pathologists, is still evolving and not always consistent.

> **Based on the biologic classification system, vascular anomalies are divided into two broad types:**
> - **Vasoproliferative anomalies, which are characterized by an increased endothelial cell cycle**
> - **Vascular malformations, which have normal endothelial turnover**

Although this classification system makes it easier to understand vasoproliferative anomalies in children, the system is not perfect. Indeed, the descriptions will likely evolve as these lesions are better understood and the literature on the subject grows.

Currently, vasoproliferative hepatic lesions are thought to represent varying manifestations of etiologically similar entities, with overlapping imaging characteristics. For the purposes of this discussion, hepatic vasoproliferative lesions can be thought of as a heterogeneous spectrum of disorders ranging from *infantile hemangioma* to the intermediate lesion *infantile hemangioendothelioma* to *angiosarcoma* and *epithelioid hemangioendothelioma*, aggressive lesions with poor prognoses.

> **Hepatic vasoproliferative lesions can be thought of as a heterogeneous spectrum of disorders ranging from *infantile hemangioma* to the intermediate *infantile hemangioendothelioma* to the aggressive *angiosarcoma* and *epithelioid hemangioendothelioma*, which have poor prognoses.**

Familiarity with hepatic vasoproliferative anomalies in children is important to distinguish them from vascular anomalies and other hepatic lesions, such as neuroblastoma and hepatoblastoma, so that the appropriate treatment can be pursued. By correlating the age of presentation with the imaging appearance, the radiologist can suggest a specific diagnosis in many cases. This aids greatly in guiding the imaging evaluation and planning appropriate treatment, and in some cases, it may avoid the premature performance of aggressive, unnecessary interventions.

Infantile Hemangioma and Hemangioendothelioma

The terms *infantile hemangioma* (also termed congenital hemangioma, or simply hemangioma) and *infantile hemangioendothelioma* have been used interchangeably in the literature to describe the same vascular lesion. Because differentiation between the two entities requires pathologic analysis and cannot be reliably accomplished based on clinical presentation or imaging features, they are discussed together (see also Chapter 115).

Infantile hemangiomas are most common in premature Caucasian girls. They occur in up to 12% of infants, present before 6 months of age (usually before 2 months of age), and are rarely present at birth. Histologically, hemangiomas are composed of rapidly proliferating endothelial cells and pericytes that form vascular lumina of various sizes during the proliferative phase. In addition, North and coworkers (2000) have shown that infantile hemangioma cells strongly express the immunohistochemical marker glucose transporter protein isoform 1 (GLUT-1). On histology, infantile hemangioendotheliomas are distinguished from hemangiomas by the presence of slightly more aggressive features.

Infantile hemangiomas occur most often on the skin and are associated with liver lesions in approximately 13% of cases. When hemangiomas involve three or more organs, the term *disseminated hemangiomatosis* is applied. Hepatic infantile hemangioendotheliomas may be focal or multiple. Multiple hepatic hemangiomas, also termed *hemangiomatosis*, occur in up to 45% of cases (Fig. 117-14). Recently, it has been discovered that what were previously described as focal hemangiomas are actually GLUT-1 negative; thus, based on histology, they may not be true infantile hemangiomas at all. This terminology remains in transition.

The clinical presentation varies, depending on the size and number of hepatic lesions, and ranges from no symptoms in most cases to various combinations of hepatomegaly, coagulopathy, high-output congestive heart failure (due to high-flow arteriovenous shunting within the lesions), respiratory distress (due to heart failure and bulky hepatomegaly with mass effect), hypothyroidism (thought to be related to increased expression of type 3 iodothyronine deiodinase), and jaundice (see Chapters 15 and 16). Infants presenting with congestive heart failure tend to have large focal lesions present at birth. These focal lesions are now known to be GLUT-1 negative and have recently been termed *rapidly involuting congenital hemangiomas (RICHs)*. They often have direct arteriovenous connections, resulting in misdiagnosis as arteriovenous malformations. They frequently undergo rapid involution and resolution of large vascular channels and often contain calcifications. Rapidly involuting congenital hemangiomas complicated by congestive heart failure respond extremely well to embolization.

Infants with multiple hepatic lesions tend to present between 1 and 3 months of age. In some infants with large focal or numerous multifocal lesions, a microvascular consumptive coagulopathy may develop secondary to intralesional thrombosis, hemorrhage, and hemolysis. Many authors have somewhat inappropriately termed this coagulopathy the *Kasabach-Merritt phenomenon*. However, according to Zukerberg and colleagues, this microvascular coagulopathy is distinct from Kasabach-

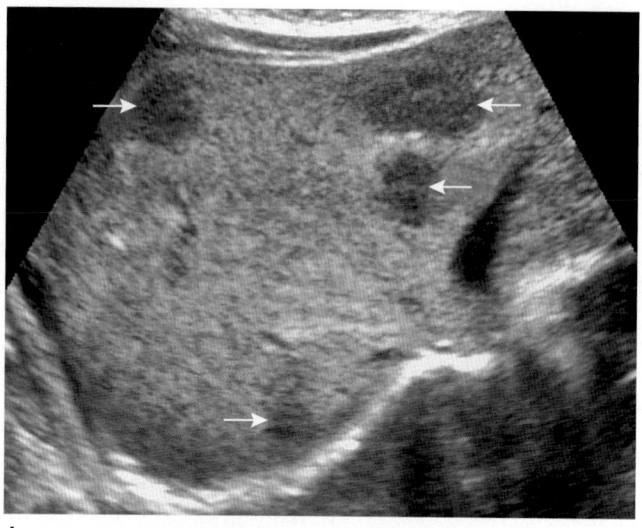

A

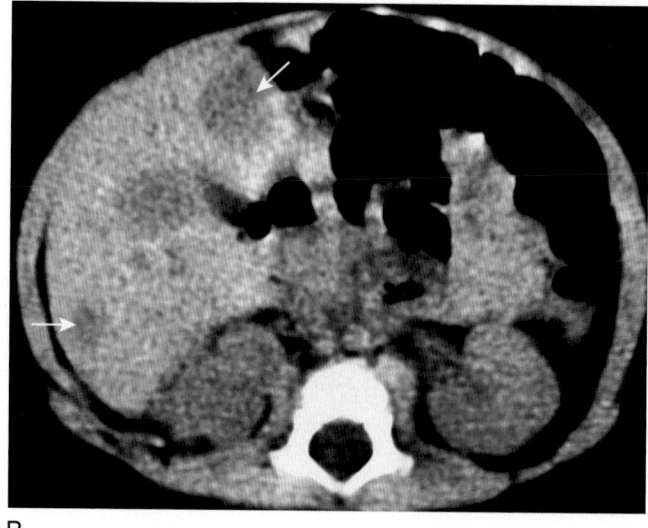

B

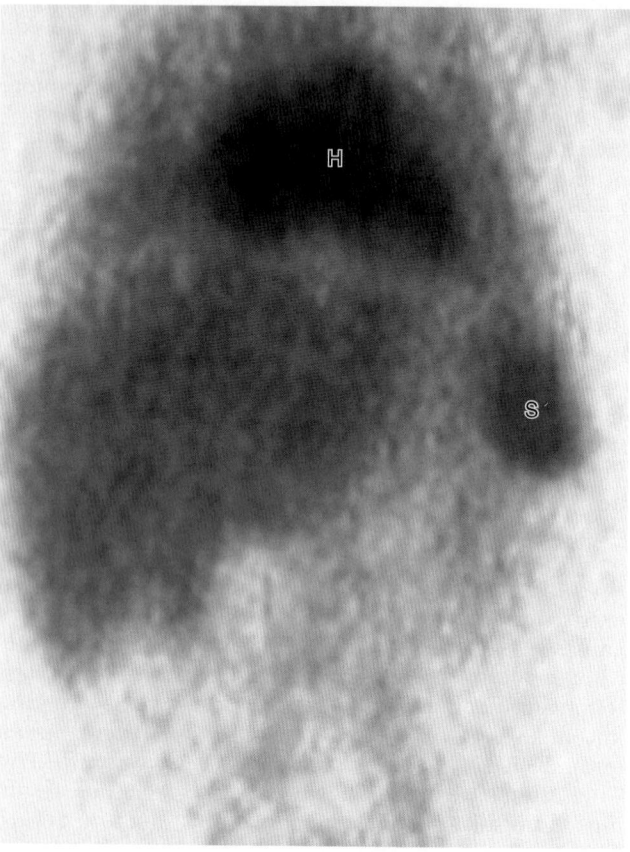

C

FIGURE 117-14. Hemangiomas (hemangiomatosis) in a 4-week-old girl with numerous cutaneous skin hemangiomas. **A,** Axial hepatic sonogram shows multiple well-defined hypoechoic lesions of varied size scattered throughout the liver *(arrows)*. Color Doppler (not shown) demonstrated variable hypervascularity. **B,** Uncontrasted CT confirms multiple lesions of low attenuation *(arrows)*. **C,** Planar image from a technetium-99m–labeled red blood cell study shows heterogeneous uptake in the liver due to scattered areas of increased uptake within hemangiomas on a background of normal parenchymal uptake. Normal physiologic uptake is noted throughout the body, heart (H), and spleen (S).

Merritt syndrome, which is caused by platelet sequestration and occurs in kaposiform hemangioendotheliomas of the trunk and extremities. Rarely, spontaneous rupture of surface hepatic hemangiomas may lead to presentation with potentially life-threatening hemoperitoneum. In contradistinction to some hepatic neoplasms, the α-fetoprotein level is usually normal in vasoproliferative liver anomalies. However, because infants have elevated α-fetoprotein levels normally, and because the normal levels vary widely in infants, this clinical marker is not always reliable.

Initially, infants with multiple hemangiomas or hemangioendotheliomas may be suspected of having neuroblastoma because both present with multiple skin and liver lesions. In this situation, rather than embarking on an extensive radiologic workup to distinguish between the two entities, the urine should be screened for catecholamines to exclude neuroblastoma. Because the imaging appearance of focal hemangiomas and hemangioendotheliomas is highly variable, a number of other lesions may be suspected initially, including mesenchymal hamartoma, hepatoblastoma, or metastatic disease.

The treatment of these masses varies considerably; therefore, in some problematic cases, biopsy may be required. In general, however, biopsy should be avoided in infants younger than 6 months with a clinical presentation and imaging appearance typical for hemangioma.

> **In infants presenting with multiple skin and liver lesions suggesting hemangiomas, the major differential diagnosis is neuroblastoma. The two entities can be distinguished by screening the urine for catecholamines.**

The clinical course of infantile hemangiomas and hemangioendotheliomas is predictable. Lesions appear between 1 and 3 months of age, undergo a rapid proliferative growth phase during the first year of life, and gradually involute over a period of months to years. Because they regress spontaneously, observation is the only treatment required for most hemangiomas. However, steroids (intralesional or systemic), chemotherapy (vincristine), embolization, and, less often, chemotherapy, radiotherapy, or surgical resection may be applied, depending on the specific clinical circumstances. Indications for treatment of complicated hemangiomas and hemangioendotheliomas include hemorrhage, mass effect on vital structures, congestive heart failure, consumptive coagulopathy, and severe respiratory distress.

Plain radiographs of hepatic vasoproliferative lesions may show congestive heart failure, hepatomegaly, or scattered right upper quadrant calcifications (present in up to 40% of hemangioendotheliomas). Imaging should begin with US because it is a noninvasive and cost-effective method of screening, diagnosing, and monitoring hepatic lesions. Multifocal hemangiomas have a characteristic hypoechoic and well-defined appearance on sonography. Solitary hemangiomas and hemangioendotheliomas are much more varied in size and echogenicity (Fig. 117-15). Secondary signs of high flow may be seen in large focal or multifocal lesions, such as craniocaudal tapering of the aorta after the origin of feeding arteries and dilation of the feeding arteries. Spectral Doppler shows highly variable arteriovenous waveforms.

MRI and, less often, CT may be used to better characterize large or complicated lesions. On both modalities, hemangiomas are well-defined and lobulated, enhance intensely, and may contain internal vascular flow voids or calcifications. Multiple hemangiomas tend to be low in attenuation on precontrast CT; after contrast administration, they enhance homogeneously or centripetally (peripheral to central) and may show enlarged feeding arteries and draining veins. The larger the lesion, the more likely it is to have centripetal enhancement or an avascular center owing to prior hemorrhage or necrosis. On MRI, multifocal hemangiomas and hemangioendotheliomas tend to be lower in signal intensity than the adjacent liver on T1-weighted images and have increased signal intensity on T2-weighted images. Focal lesions tend to be more heterogeneous on T1-weighted images but are still hyperintense on T2 sequences. With focal lesions, the pattern of enhancement on MRI is similar to that described on CT (diffuse or centripetal). The technetium-99m–labeled red blood cell scan with single-

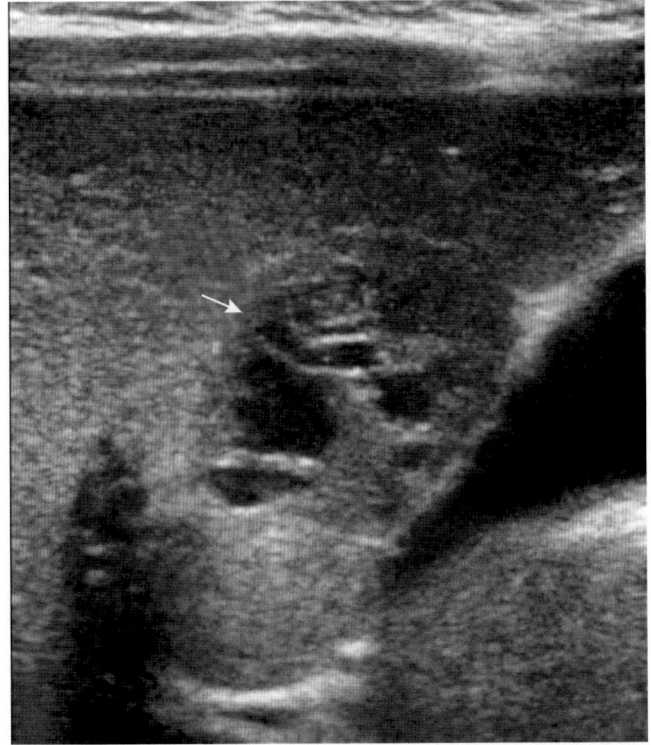

A

B

FIGURE 117-15. Single large hemangioma in a 7-month-old girl with several cutaneous hemangiomas. Longitudinal gray scale **(A)** and color Doppler **(B)** sonograms reveal a well-circumscribed mass in the left hepatic lobe *(arrow)*, with focal hypoechoic areas that demonstrate flow on color Doppler interrogation. **(B,** *see color plate.*)

photon emission computed tomography (SPECT) has been described by some authors as having close to 100% specificity for the diagnosis of hemangiomas in adults. The scan is diagnostic when it demonstrates normal to decreased flow on initial dynamic images, followed by gradual increased activity on delayed images. A delay of several hours may be required in some cases for a diagnostic study. However, a significant number of lesions lack convincing central enhancement due to

regions of necrosis and hemorrhage, in which case scintigraphy is not diagnostic (Fig. 117-16).

Although most vasoproliferative anomalies are asymptomatic and do not require angiography, an angiographic classification system has been described by Kassarjian and coworkers (2002) and is typically applied to complicated anomalies requiring intervention. Focal hemangiomas, similar to other congenital hemangiomas, often have direct arteriovenous, arterioportal, or

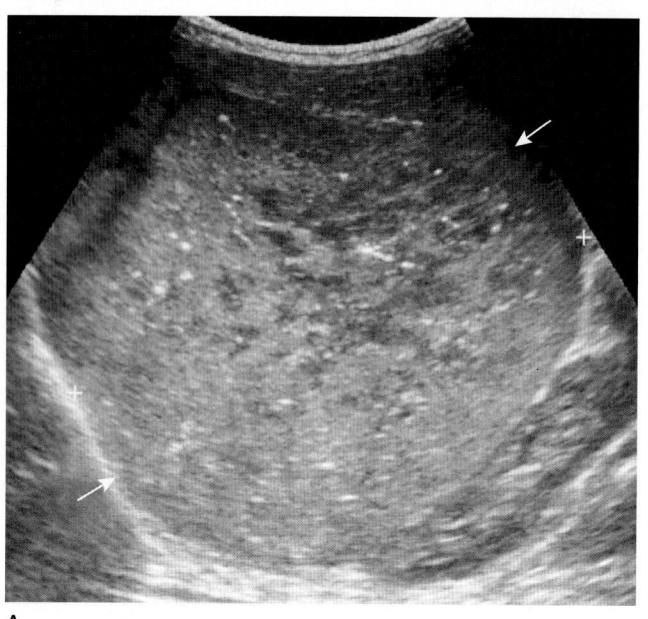

A

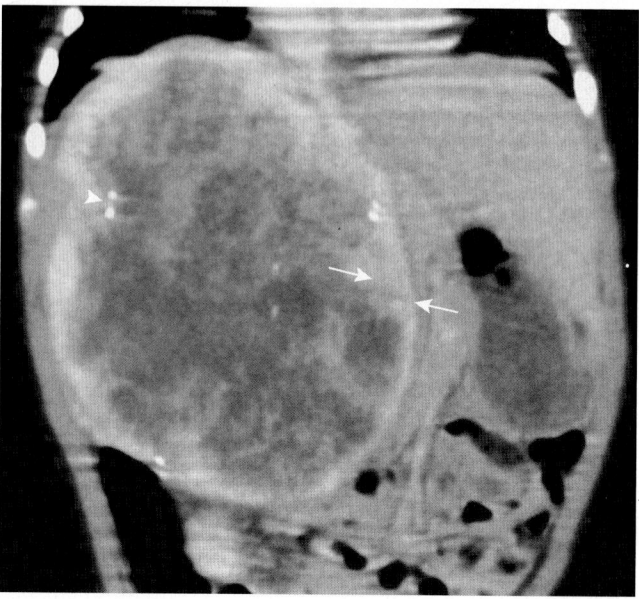

B

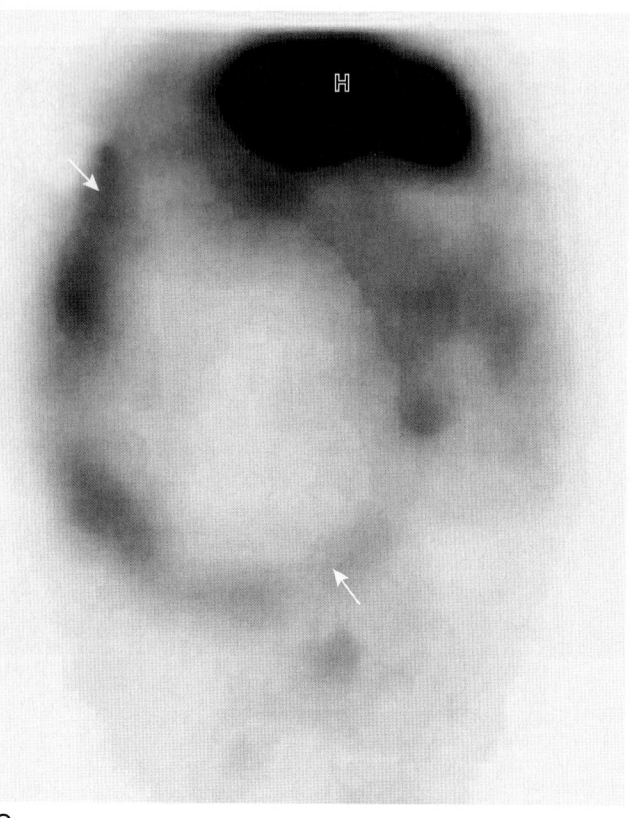

C

FIGURE 117-16. Hemangioendothelioma in a 2-week-old boy with hepatomegaly. **A,** Axial sonogram shows a large hyperechoic mass in the right lobe of the liver *(arrows)* containing numerous punctate hyperechoic foci, suggesting tiny calcifications. **B,** Axial contrast-enhanced CT confirms a large hepatic mass with scattered calcifications *(arrowhead)* and a peripheral rind of nodular enhancement *(arrows)*. **C,** Coronal technetium-99m–labeled red blood cell scan shows peripheral activity within the mass *(arrows)* that failed to fill in on delayed images. H, heart.

portovenous fistulas and may contain a central venous varix or circumferential draining veins. Multifocal hemangiomas have variable patterns of increased flow on hepatic arteriography and often contain portovenous fistulas on portal venography. These portovenous fistulas may be detected on US and MRI, where they may appear as large flow voids, usually within the tumor nodules. The significance of portovenous fistulas is related to hepatic perfusion; in patients with portovenous fistulas, the liver is perfused solely by the hepatic arteries, and hepatic artery embolization carries a significant risk of hepatic necrosis.

> **Multiple hemangiomas tend to be low in attenuation on precontrast CT. After contrast, hemangiomas and hemangioendotheliomas enhance either homogeneously or centripetally (peripheral to central) and may show enlarged feeding arteries and draining veins.**

The prognosis of infantile hemangiomas and hemangioendotheliomas is generally very good. Embolization is reserved for patients with intractable cardiac failure who do not respond to pharmacologic therapy. Unfortunately, deaths related to complications such as congestive heart failure, consumptive coagulopathy, and hemorrhage are possible.

Angiosarcoma

Angiosarcoma is a rare, aggressive vasoproliferative lesion that has been described in a small number of patients who were initially thought to have hemangiomas. The presentation is similar to that of multiple or large hemangiomas or hemangioendotheliomas. Although the imaging features of angiosarcomas are variable, these lesions tend to be large, multifocal hepatic masses with variable central hemorrhage and necrosis (Fig. 117-17). The mass typically demonstrates contrast enhancement, but the pattern varies. Centripetal enhancement may be seen in some cases. The prognosis of angiosarcoma is poor, with a median survival ranging from 6 to 13 months.

Epithelioid Hemangioendothelioma

Epithelioid hemangioendothelioma is a rare vasoproliferative lesion that may involve multiple visceral organs (brain, bone, lung, lymph nodes) and soft tissues, including the liver. It is most common in the second to fourth decades (median age, 41 years; range, 3 to

80 years) and rarely affects children. The presentation is similar to that of other vasoproliferative lesions, and the prognosis lies between that of infantile hemangioendothelioma and angiosarcoma. The hepatic lesions often have a characteristic appearance on MRI, with the main intrahepatic vessels (hepatic artery and portal vein) appearing to pass directly into the nodules ("lollipop" sign).

INFLAMMATORY PSEUDOTUMOR OF THE LIVER

Inflammatory pseudotumor of the liver occurs in adults and children. Patients have a typical clinical presentation of low-grade fever, abdominal pain, and weight loss. Single or multiple well-defined hepatic masses occur. The lesion is hypoechoic on sonography and of low attenuation on CT (Fig. 117-18). It is not possible to reliably distinguish inflammatory pseudotumor from hepatic malignancy with imaging. In some cases, the lesion may be resected based on a high preoperative probability of neoplasm, although a percutaneous biopsy may be diagnostic. Inflammatory pseudotumor is a self-limited condition with an excellent prognosis. Therefore, it is important for clinicians, surgeons, and radiologists to be familiar with its diagnosis and consider it in the appropriate clinical setting.

> **It is important to be familiar with the diagnosis of inflammatory pseudotumor and consider it in the appropriate clinical setting; it is a self-limited condition with an excellent prognosis.**

NODULAR REGENERATIVE HYPERPLASIA OF THE LIVER

Nodular regenerative hyperplasia of the liver is a lesion of unknown cause that develops in noncirrhotic livers. On imaging, it may be confused with FNH, adenomas, or metastases. This entity has been associated with vasculitis, collagen vascular diseases, hematologic disorders, cardiovascular diseases, neoplasms, metabolic disorders, and some drugs. Histologically, regenerative nodules are composed of focal proliferations of cells resembling hepatocytes within a supporting stroma. The nodules may bleed or lead to portal hypertension from pressure on portal radicles, and the liver may or may not be enlarged. On US, the nodules are of variable echogenicity. On CT, the lesions are of lower attenuation than normal liver and do not enhance significantly after IV contrast (Fig. 117-19). The MRI appearance is nonspecific and variable.

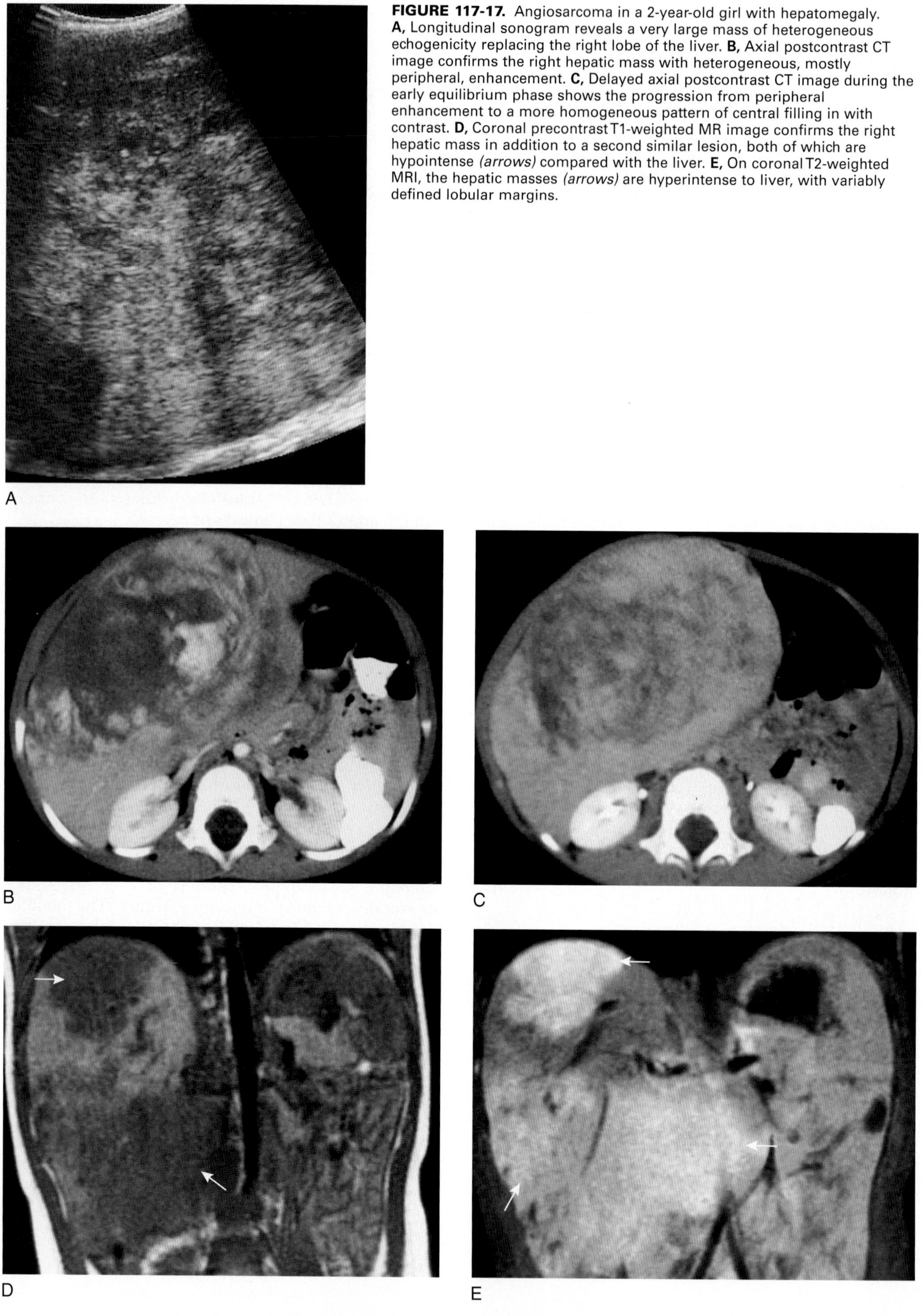

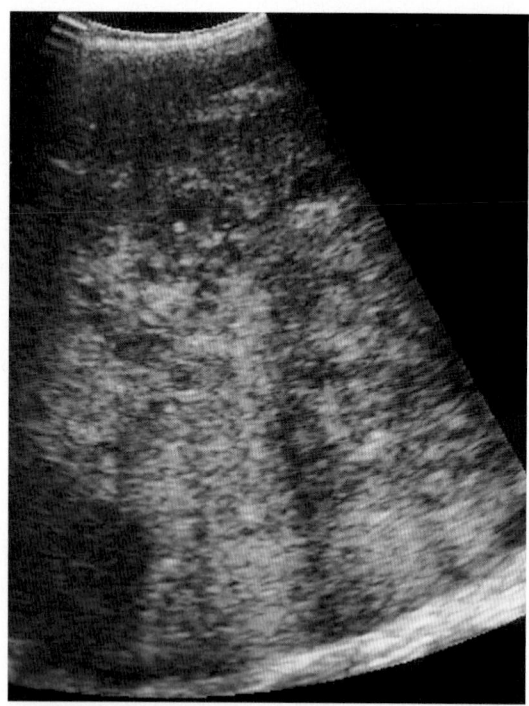

A

FIGURE 117-17. Angiosarcoma in a 2-year-old girl with hepatomegaly. **A,** Longitudinal sonogram reveals a very large mass of heterogeneous echogenicity replacing the right lobe of the liver. **B,** Axial postcontrast CT image confirms the right hepatic mass with heterogeneous, mostly peripheral, enhancement. **C,** Delayed axial postcontrast CT image during the early equilibrium phase shows the progression from peripheral enhancement to a more homogeneous pattern of central filling in with contrast. **D,** Coronal precontrast T1-weighted MR image confirms the right hepatic mass in addition to a second similar lesion, both of which are hypointense *(arrows)* compared with the liver. **E,** On coronal T2-weighted MRI, the hepatic masses *(arrows)* are hyperintense to liver, with variably defined lobular margins.

B

C

D

E

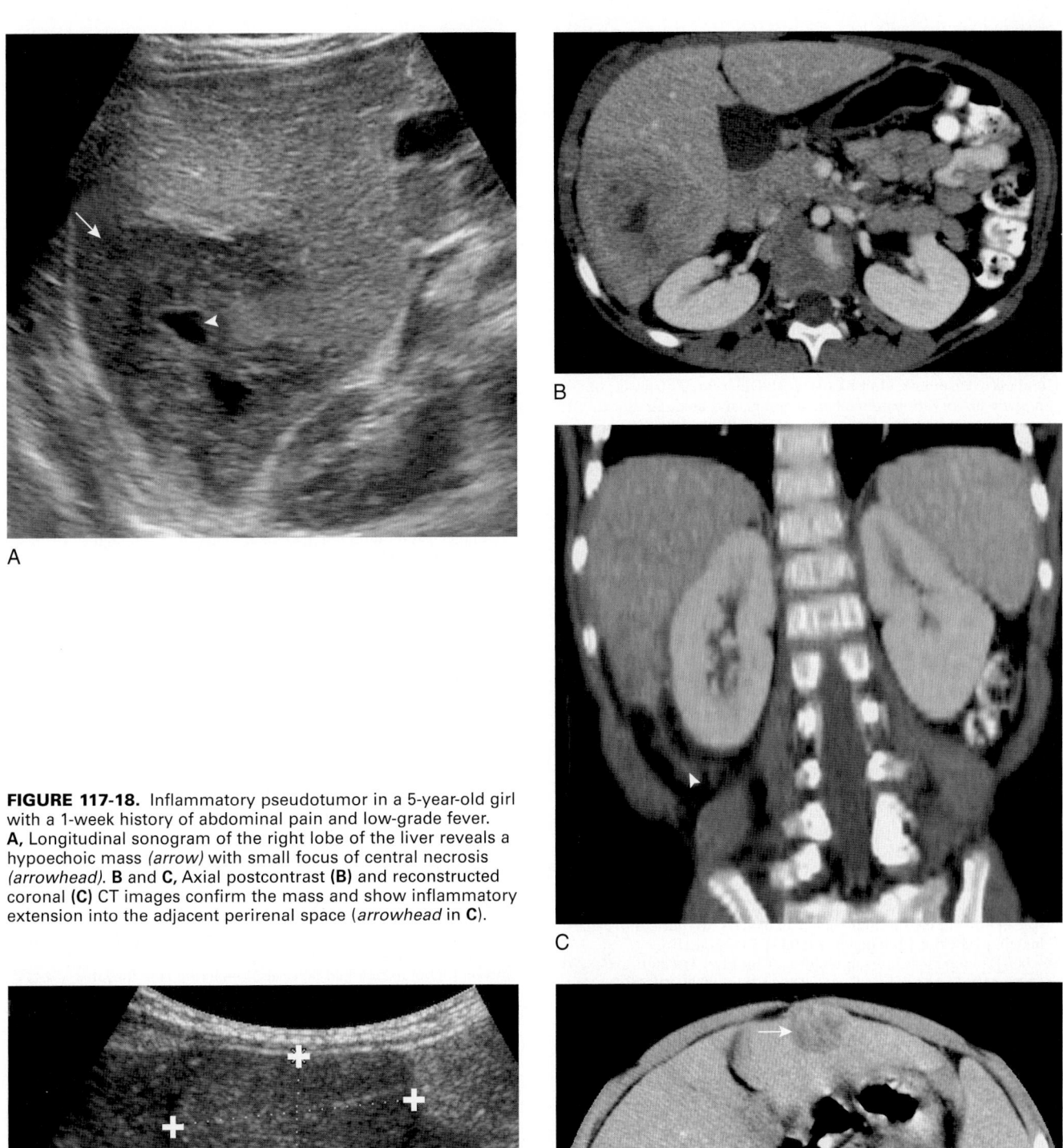

FIGURE 117-18. Inflammatory pseudotumor in a 5-year-old girl with a 1-week history of abdominal pain and low-grade fever. **A,** Longitudinal sonogram of the right lobe of the liver reveals a hypoechoic mass *(arrow)* with small focus of central necrosis *(arrowhead)*. **B** and **C,** Axial postcontrast **(B)** and reconstructed coronal **(C)** CT images confirm the mass and show inflammatory extension into the adjacent perirenal space *(arrowhead in* **C***)*.

FIGURE 117-19. Regenerative nodule in a 16-year-old girl. **A,** Longitudinal sonogram shows a near-isoechoic lesion in the left lobe of the liver *(calipers)*. **B,** Axial postcontrast CT image confirms a low-attenuation mass in the left lobe of the liver *(arrow)*. Pathology was diagnostic of a regenerative nodule.

SUGGESTED READINGS

General

Arcement CM, Towbin RB, Meza MP, et al: Intrahepatic chemoembolization in unresectable pediatric liver malignancies. Pediatr Radiol 2000;30:779-785

DeMatteo RP, Fong Y: Imaging of hepatobiliary neoplasms. Surg Oncol Clin N Am 1999;8:59-89

Freeny PC, Grossholz M, Kaakaji K, Schmiedl UP: Significance of hyperattenuating and contrast-enhancing hepatic nodules detected in the cirrhotic liver during arterial phase helical CT in pre-liver transplant patients: radiologic-histopathologic correlation of explanted livers. Abdom Imaging 2003;28:333-346

Galli G, Valenza V: Is there still a role for functional radionuclide study of the liver? Rays 1997;22:228-248

Genovese E, Maghnie M, Maggiore G, et al: MR imaging of CNS involvement in children affected by chronic liver disease. AJNR Am J Neuroradiol 2000;21:845-851

Honda H, Matsuura Y, Onitsuka H, et al: Differential diagnosis of hepatic tumors (hepatoma, hemangioma, and metastasis) with CT: value of two-phase incremental imaging. AJR Am J Roentgenol 1992;159:735-740

Hussein A, Wyatt J, Guthrie A, Stringer MD: Kasai portoenterostomy: new insights from hepatic morphology. J Pediatr Surg 2005; 40:322-326

Katz AJ: Diagnostic procedures in the evaluation of hepatic diseases: metabolic errors. Lab Res Methods Biol Med 1983;7:145-152

Kawamura E, Shiomi S, Ishizu H, et al: Natural course of changes in hepatic functional reserve in patients with chronic liver diseases evaluated by scintigraphy with GSA. Hepatol Res 2003;27:129-135

Lam CY, Chan KF, Fan TW, et al: Intrahepatic hematoma: hepatic lesion in a newborn with high alpha-fetoprotein level. Pediatr Radiol 2005;35:1139-1141

Mody RJ, Pohlen JA, Malde S, et al: FDG PET for the study of primary hepatic malignancies in children. Pediatr Blood Cancer 2006; 47:51-55

Plumley DA, Grosfeld JL, Kopecky KK, et al: The role of spiral (helical) computerized tomography with three-dimensional reconstruction in pediatric solid tumors. J Pediatr Surg 1995;30:317-321

Soyer P, Bluemke DA, Hruban RH, et al: Primary malignant neoplasms of the liver: detection with helical CT during arterial portography. Radiology 1994;192:389-392

Soyer P, de Givry SC, Gueye C, et al: Detection of focal hepatic lesions with MR imaging: prospective comparison of T2-weighted fast spin-echo with and without fat suppression, T2-weighted breath-hold fast spin-echo, and gadolinium chelate-enhanced 3D gradient-recalled imaging. AJR Am J Roentgenol 1996;166:1115-1121

Stocker JT: Hepatic tumors in children. Clin Liver Dis 2001;5:259-281

Stringer MD: Liver tumors. Semin Pediatr Surg 2000;9:196-208

Westra SJ, Zaninovic AC, Hall TR, et al: Imaging in pediatric liver transplantation. Radiographics 1993;13:1081-1099

Hepatoblastoma

Czauderna P, Otte J-B, Roebuck DJ, et al: Surgical treatment of hepatoblastoma in children. Pediatr Radiol 2006;187-191

Figarola MS, McQuiston SA, Wilson F, Powell R: Recurrent hepatoblastoma with localization by PET-CT. Pediatr Radiol 2005;35:1254-1258

King SJ, Babyn PS, Greenberg ML, et al: Value of CT in determining the resectability of hepatoblastoma before and after chemotherapy. AJR Am J Roentgenol 1993;160:793-798

Morland B: Commentary on hepatoblastoma minisymposium. Pediatr Radiol 2006;36:175

Philip I, Shun A, McCowage G, Howman-Giles R: Positron emission tomography in recurrent hepatoblastoma. Pediatr Surg Int 2005;21:341-345

Roebuck DJ, Olsen O, Pariente D: Radiological staging in children with hepatoblastoma. Pediatr Radiol 2006;36:176-182

Roebuck DJ, Perilongo G: Hepatoblastoma: an oncological review. Pediatr Radiol 2006;36:183-186

Slovis TL, Roebuck DJ: Hepatoblastoma: why so many low-birth-weight infants? Pediatr Radiol 2006;36:173-174

Xianliang H, Jianhong L, Xuewu J, Zhongxian C: Cure of hepatoblastoma with transcatheter arterial chemoembolization. J Pediatr Hematol Oncol 2004;26:60-63

Hepatocellular Carcinoma

Chen JC, Chen CC, Chen WJ, et al: Hepatocellular carcinoma in children: clinical review and comparison with adult cases. J Pediatr Surg 1998;33:1350-1354

Esquivel CO, Gutierrez C, Cox KL, et al: Hepatocellular carcinoma and liver cell dysplasia in children with chronic liver disease. J Pediatr Surg 1994;29:1465-1469

Fibrolamellar Carcinoma

Bedi DG, Kumar R, Morettin LB, Gourley K: Fibrolamellar carcinoma of the liver: CT, ultrasound and angiography: case report. Eur J Radiol 1988;8:109-112

Friedman AC, Lichtenstein JE, Goodman Z, et al: Fibrolamellar hepatocellular carcinoma. Radiology 1985;157:583-587

Khoo JJ, Clouston A: Fibrolamellar hepatocellular carcinoma: a case report. Malays J Pathol 2001;23:115-118

Yamaguchi R, Tajika T, Kanda H, et al: Fibrolamellar carcinoma of the liver. Hepatogastroenterology 1999;46:1706-1709

Undifferentiated Embryonal Sarcoma

Buetow PC, Buck JL, Pantongrag-Brown L, et al: Undifferentiated (embryonal) sarcoma of the liver: pathologic basis of imaging findings in 28 cases. Radiology 1997;203:779-783

Psatha EA, Semelka RC, Fordham L, et al: Undifferentiated (embryonal) sarcoma of the liver (USL): MRI findings including dynamic gadolinium enhancement. Magn Reson Imaging 2004;22:897-900

Rhabdomyosarcoma

Balkan E, Kiristioglu I, Gurpinar A, et al: Rhabdomyosarcoma of the biliary tree. Turk J Pediatr 1999;41:245-248

Cholangiocarcinoma

Tanaka S, Kubota M, Yagi M, et al: An 11-year-old male patient demonstrating cholangiocarcinoma associated with congenital biliary dilatation. J Pediatr Surg 2006;41:e15-e19

Tsuchida A, Kasuya K, Endo M, et al: High risk of bile duct carcinogenesis after primary resection of a congenital biliary dilatation. Oncol Rep 2003;10:1183-1187

Walshe JM, Waldenstrom E, Sams V, et al: Abdominal malignancies in patients with Wilson's disease. QJM 2003;96:657-662

Lymphoma

Huang CB, Eng HL, Chuang JH, et al: Primary Burkitt's lymphoma of the liver: report of a case with long-term survival after surgical resection and combination chemotherapy. J Pediatr Hematol Oncol 1997;19:135-138

Kuroda J, Omoto A, Fujiki H, et al: Primary hepatic Burkitt's lymphoma with chronic hepatitis C. Acta Haematol 2001; 105:237-240

Salmon JS, Thompson MA, Arildsen RC, Greer JP: Non-Hodgkin's lymphoma involving the liver: clinical and therapeutic considerations. Clin Lymphoma Myeloma 2006;6:273-280

Neuroblastoma

Inagaki J, Yasui M, Sakata N, et al: Successful treatment of chemoresistant stage 3 neuroblastoma using irinotecan as a single agent. J Pediatr Hematol Oncol 2005;27:604-606

Wilms Tumor

Sripathi V, Muralidharan KV, Ramesh S, Muralinath S: Wilms' tumor with vena caval, atrial, and middle hepatic vein tumor thrombus. Pediatr Surg Int 2000;16:447-448

Szavay P, Luithle T, Graf N, et al: Primary hepatic metastases in nephroblastoma: a report of the SIOP/GPOH study. J Pediatr Surg 2006;41:168-172

Mesenchymal Hamartoma

Ros PR, Goodman ZD, Ishak KG, et al: Mesenchymal hamartoma of the liver: radiologic-pathologic correlation. Radiology 1986; 158:619-624

Ye BB, Hu B, Wang LJ, et al: Mesenchymal hamartoma of liver: magnetic resonance imaging and histopathologic correlation. World J Gastroenterol 2005;11:5807-5810

Focal Nodular Hyperplasia

Shortell CK, Schwartz SI: Hepatic adenoma and focal nodular hyperplasia. Surg Gynecol Obstet 1991;173:426-431

Tajada M, Nerin J, Ruiz MM, et al: Liver adenoma and focal nodular hyperplasia associated with oral contraceptives. Eur J Contracept Reprod Health Care 2001;6:227-230

Angiomyolipoma

Chung CJ, Fordham L, Little S, et. al: Intraperitoneal rhabdomyosarcoma in children: incidence and imaging characteristics on CT. AJR Am J Roentgenol 1998;170:1385

Lowe LH, Taboada EM: Pediatric kidney cancer. In Guermazi A (ed): Imaging of Kidney Cancer. Berlin, Springer, 2006:351-369

Adenoma

Brummett D, Burton EM, Sabio H: Hepatic adenomatosis: rapid sequence MR imaging following gadolinium enhancement: a case report. Pediatr Radiol 1999;29:231-234

Debaere C, Op de Beeck B, De Maeseneer M, Osteaux M: Magnetic resonance imaging findings of hepatic adenomas in von Gierke (type I) glycogen storage disease: case report. Can Assoc Radiol J 1999;50:161-164

Grazioli L, Federle MP, Brancatelli G, et al: Hepatic adenomas: imaging and pathologic findings. Radiographics 2001;21:877-892

Grazioli L, Federle MP, Ichikawa T, et al: Liver adenomatosis: clinical, histopathologic, and imaging findings in 15 patients. Radiology 2000;216:395-402

Howell RR, Stevenson RE, Ben-Menachem Y, et al: Hepatic adenomata with type 1 glycogen storage disease. JAMA 1976;236:1481-1484

Ishak KG: Hepatic neoplasms associated with contraceptive and anabolic steroids. Recent Results Cancer Res 1979;66:73-128

Mathieu D, Bruneton JN, Drouillard J, et al: Hepatic adenomas and focal nodular hyperplasia: dynamic CT study. Radiology 1986;160:53-58

Parker P, Burr I, Slonim A, et al: Regression of hepatic adenomas in type Ia glycogen storage disease with dietary therapy. Gastroenterology 1981;81:534-536

Paulson EK, McClellan JS, Washington K, et al: Hepatic adenoma: MR characteristics and correlation with pathologic findings. AJR Am J Roentgenol 1994;163:113-116

Shortell CK, Schwartz SI: Hepatic adenoma and focal nodular hyperplasia. Surg Gynecol Obstet 1991;173:426-431

Small WC, Chezmar JL, Bernardino ME: CT angiography and CT arterial portography in evaluation of hepatic adenomas. J Comput Assist Tomogr 1994;18:266-268

Tajada M, Nerin J, Ruiz MM, et al: Liver adenoma and focal nodular hyperplasia associated with oral contraceptives. Eur J Contracept Reprod Health Care 2001;6:227-230

Infantile Hemangioma

Burrows PE, Dubois J, Kassarjian A: Pediatric hepatic vascular anomalies. Pediatr Radiol 2001;31:533-545

Burrows PE, Laor T, Palteil H, Robertson RL: Diagnostic imaging in the evaluation of vascular birthmarks. Pediatr Dermatol 1998;16:455-488

Danet IM, Semelka RC, Braga L, et al: Giant hemangioma of the liver: MR imaging characteristics in 24 patients. Magn Reson Imaging 2003;21:95-101

Dubois J, Garel L: Imaging and therapeutic approach of hemangiomas and vascular malformations in the pediatric age group. Pediatr Radiol 1999;29:879-893

Fishman SJ, Mulliken JB: Hemangiomas and vascular malformations of infancy and childhood. Pediatr Clin North Am 1993; 40:1177-1200

Frischer JS, Huang J, Serur A, et al: Biomolecular markers and involution of hemangiomas. J Pediatr Surg 2004;39:400-404

Huang SA, Tu HM, Harney JW, et al: Severe hypothyroidism caused by type 3 iodothyronine deiodinase in infantile hemangiomas. N Engl J Med 2000;343:185-189

Kassarjian A, Dubois J, Burrows PE: Angiographic classification of hepatic hemangiomas in infants. Radiology 2002;222:693-698

Kassarjian A, Zurakowski D, Dubois J, et al: Infantile hepatic hemangiomas: clinical and imaging findings and their correlation with therapy. AJR Am J Roentgenol 2004;182:785-795

Kim TK, Choi BI, Han JK, et al: Optimal MR protocol for hepatic hemangiomas: comparison of conventional spin-echo sequences with T2-weighted turbo spin-echo and serial gradient-echo (FLASH) sequences with gadolinium enhancement. Acta Radiol 1997;38:565-571

Mulliken JB: A biologic approach to cutaneous vascular anomalies. Pediatr Dermatol 1992;9:356-357

Mulliken JB: Cutaneous vascular anomalies. Semin Vasc Surg 1993;6:204-218

Mulliken JB, Anupindi S, Ezekowitz RA, Mihm MC Jr: Case 13-2004: a newborn girl with a large cutaneous lesion, thrombocytopenia and anemia. N Engl J Med 2004;350:1764-1775

Mulliken JB, Glowacki J: Classification of pediatric vascular lesions. Plast Reconstr Surg 1982;70:120-121

Mulliken JB, Glowacki J: Hemangiomas and vascular malformations in infants and children: a classification based on endothelial characteristics. Plast Reconstr Surg 1982;69:412-422

North PE, Waner M, Mizeracki A, Mihm MC Jr: GLUT1: a newly discovered immunohistochemical marker for juvenile hemangiomas. Hum Pathol 2000;31:11

North PE, Waner M, Mizeracki A, et al: A unique microvascular phenotype shared by juvenile hemangiomas and human placenta. Arch Dermatol 2001;137:559

Prokurat A, Kluge P, Chrupek M, et al: Hemangioma of the liver in children: proliferating vascular tumor or congenital vascular malformation? Med Pediatr Oncol 2002;39:524-529

Soyer P, Gueye C, Somveille E, et al: MR diagnosis of hepatic metastases from neuroendocrine tumors versus hemangiomas: relative merits of dynamic gadolinium chelate-enhanced gradient-recalled echo and unenhanced spin-echo images. AJR Am J Roentgenol 1995;165:1407-1413

Zukerberg LR, Nickoloff BJ, Weiss SW: Kaposiform hemangioendothelioma of infancy and childhood: an aggressive neoplasm associated with Kasabach-Merritt syndrome and lymphangiomatosis. Am J Surg Pathol 1993;17:321

Infantile Hemangioendothelioma

Han SJ, Tsai CC, Tsai HM, Chen YJ: Infantile hemangioendothelioma with a highly elevated serum alpha-fetoprotein level. Hepatogastroenterology 1998;45:459-461

Lu M, Greer MLC: Hypervascular multifocal hepatoblastoma: dynamic gadolinium-enhanced MRI findings indistinguishable from infantile hemangioendothelioma. Pediatr Radiol 2007;37:587-591

Mulliken JB, Anupindi S, Ezekowitz RA, Mihm MC Jr: Case 13-2004: a newborn girl with a large cutaneous lesion, thrombocytopenia, and anemia. N Engl J Med 2004;350:1764-1775

Roos JE, Pfiffner R, Stallmach T, et al: Infantile hemangioendothelioma. Radiographics 2003;23:1649-1655

Sarkar M, Mulliken JB, Kozakewich HP, et al: Thrombocytopenic coagulopathy (Kasabach-Merritt phenomenon) is associated with kaposiform hemangioendothelioma and not with common infantile hemangioma. Plast Reconstr Surg 1997;100:1377-1386

Angiosarcoma

Awan S, Davenport M, Portmann B, Howard ER: Angiosarcoma of the liver in children. J Pediatr Surg 1996;31:1729-1732

Dimashkieh HH, Mo JQ, Wyatt-Ashmead J, Collins MH: Pediatric hepatic angiosarcoma: case report and review of the literature. Pediatr Dev Pathol 2004;7:527-532

Nord KM, Kandel J, Lefkowitch JH, et al: Multiple cutaneous infantile hemangiomas associated with hepatic angiosarcoma: case report and review of the literature. Pediatrics 2006;118:e907-e913

Peterson MS, Baron RE, Rankin SC: Hepatic angiosarcoma: findings on multiphasic contrast-enhanced helical CT do not mimic hepatic hemangioma. AJR Am J Roentgenol 2000;175:165-170

Selby DM, Stocker JT, Ishak KG: Angiosarcoma of the liver in childhood: a clinicopathologic and follow-up study of 10 cases. Pediatr Pathol 1992;12:485-498

Epithelioid Hemangioendothelioma

Burrows PE, Dubois J, Kassarjian A: Pediatric hepatic vascular anomalies. Pediatr Radiol 2001;31:533-545

Mehrabi A, Kashfi A, Fonouni H, et al: Primary malignant hepatic epithelioid hemangioendothelioma: a comprehensive review of the literature with emphasis on the surgical therapy. Cancer 2006;107:2108-2121

Mehrabi A, Kashfi A, Schemmer P, et al: Surgical treatment of primary hepatic epithelioid hemangioendothelioma. Transplantation 2005;80:S109-S112

Weiss SW, Enzinger FM: Epithelioid hemangioendothelioma: a vascular tumor often mistaken for carcinoma. Cancer 1982; 50:970-981

Inflammatory Pseudotumor

Gosavi A, Agashe S, Phansopkar M, et al: Inflammatory pseudotumour of liver: a case report. Indian J Pathol Microbiol 1997;40:81-83

Hata Y, Sasaki F, Matuoka S, et al: Inflammatory pseudotumor of the liver in children: report of cases and review of the literature. J Pediatr Surg 1992;27:1549-1552

Lee SL, DuBois JJ: Hepatic inflammatory pseudotumor: case report, review of the literature, and a proposal for morphologic classification. Pediatr Surg Int 2001;17:555-559

Passalides A, Keramidas D, Mavrides G: Inflammatory pseudotumor of the liver in children: a case report and review of the literature. Eur J Pediatr Surg 1996;6:35-37

Nodular Regenerative Hyperplasia

Brisse H, Servois V, Bouche B, et al: Hepatic regenerating nodules: a mimic of recurrent cancer in children. Pediatr Radiol 2000; 30:386-393

Dachman AH, Ros PR, Goodman ZD, et al: Nodular regenerative hyperplasia of the liver: clinical and radiologic observations. AJR Am J Roentgenol 1987;148:717-722

Day DL, Letourneau JG, Allan BT, et al: Hepatic regenerating nodules in hereditary tyrosinemia. AJR Am J Roentgenol 1987;149:391-393

Ozgenc F, Aydogdu S, Aksoylar S, et al: Regenerative nodule mimicking hepatocellular carcinoma in a cirrhotic child due to hepatitis B: an imaging dilemma. Pediatr Transplant 2004; 8:198-200

CHAPTER 118

Liver Transplantation in Children

TAMAR BEN-AMI

The first liver transplantation was attempted in a 3-year-old boy with biliary atresia, end-stage cirrhosis, and portal hypertension in Denver, Colorado, by Thomas E. Starzl in 1963. The same group reported the first liver transplantation with longer than 1-year survival in 1968.

Liver transplantation increased worldwide with the introduction of the immune suppressant cyclosporine in 1979. Better surgical and organ procurement techniques, along with the introduction of tacrolimus (FK-506), improved transplantation outcomes further. Currently, survival rates of recipients and transplanted organs exceed 90% in elective transplants. Although rejection has become a rare cause of transplant loss, this has been counterbalanced by the introduction of post-transplantation lymphoproliferative disease (PTLD) and susceptibility to opportunistic infections. The incidence of PTLD was reduced when OKT-3 treatment for rejection was abandoned.

Appropriate size-matched donors for pediatric recipients are scarce, and organs are allocated using a severity score to prioritize patients on a national waiting list. The organ pool has been increased, however, by reduced-size liver transplants, the sharing of organs between two recipients, and living related-donor transplantation. Organ handling has been improved by in situ procurement of liver segments from heart-beating cadaveric donors. Decreased use of vascular conduits and the introduction of microsurgery for hepatic artery anastomosis have decreased the rate of complications. However, transplantation in newborns is still less successful than in children older than 6 months.

INDICATIONS

Liver transplantation is indicated in children with irreversible liver disease with liver failure, nonresectable liver tumors, and some metabolic diseases and vascular abnormalities (Table 118-1). Emergency transplantation may be performed for fulminant hepatic failure.

Biliary atresia with cirrhosis and portal hypertension following Kasai portoenterostomy accounts for more than 60% of liver transplants in children younger than 5 years. More than two thirds of patients with biliary atresia eventually require liver transplantation—about one third in the first year of life; approximately 10% of these patients have associated polysplenia.

Other cholestatic causes of cirrhosis include bile duct hypoplasia syndromes (e.g., Alagille, Byler), cystic fibrosis without severe lung involvement, and primary sclerosing cholangitis. Children with cholestasis related to total parenteral nutrition may have underlying short-bowel syndrome and may require combined liver and small bowel transplantation.

TABLE 118-1

Indications for Pediatric Liver Transplantation

CHOLESTATIC LIVER DISEASES
Biliary atresia
α_1-Antitrypsin deficiency
Bile duct hypoplasia syndromes (e.g., Alagille syndrome, Byler syndrome)
Cirrhosis secondary to chronic total parenteral nutrition
Cirrhosis secondary to cystic fibrosis
Sclerosing cholangitis associated with Langerhans cell histiocytosis
Cystic fibrosis

METABOLIC DISEASES
Tyrosinemia
Urea cycle disorders
Glycogen storage diseases
Wilson disease
Maple syrup urine disease
Primary hyperoxaluria
Crigler-Najjar syndrome
Mitochondrial disease
Hyperammonemia

DIFFUSE, NONBILIARY LIVER DISEASES
Viral hepatitis
Congenital hepatic fibrosis
Neonatal hepatitis
Neonatal hemochromatosis
Autoimmune hepatitis
Medication-induced liver failure
Graft-versus-host disease
Acute liver failure
Idiopathic portal hypertension

NEOPLASTIC DISEASES AND LIVER MASSES
Hepatoblastoma
Hepatocellular carcinoma
Extensive hepatic hemangioendothelioma
Hilar inflammatory pseudotumor
Metastatic neuroendocrine tumor

Diffuse nonbiliary liver diseases necessitating transplantation include infectious and autoimmune hepatitis, neonatal hemochromatosis, graft-versus-host disease, and fulminant liver failure. Congenital hepatic fibrosis is associated with autosomal recessive polycystic kidney disease; these patients may require combined liver and kidney transplantation.

Liver transplantation in metabolic diseases remains controversial. In some diseases, it is a well-established therapeutic option. These include glycogen storage disease, which involves a risk of liver adenomas and hepatocellular carcinoma, and tyrosinemia and Wilson disease, which have a risk of neurologic damage and cirrhosis. In some inborn errors of metabolism, such as maple syrup urine disease, the advantage of transplantation over nutritional restrictions may not be sufficient. In others, such as primary hyperoxaluria, liver transplantation has not proved to make a significant difference. In urea cycle disorders, transplantation is the main mode of therapy, but there is hope that it can be avoided when gene therapy becomes available. Liver transplantation may provide relief in children with hyperammonemia due to congenital portosystemic shunts and congenital absence of the portal vein.

PRETRANSPLANT IMAGING

Preoperative imaging is tailored to the patient's underlying disease and coexistent conditions. The goals are to document vascular patency (Fig. 118-1), define visceral and vascular anatomy, exclude contraindications, and evaluate the extent of liver disease, portal hypertension, and venous collaterals.

Advances in surgical technique have eliminated many previous contraindications to transplantation. However,

the following conditions require modifications of surgical technique: small, absent, or occluded portal vein; inferior vena cava (IVC) thrombosis; biliary atresia associated with polysplenia syndrome and absent intrahepatic IVC, with hepatic veins draining into the right atrium (Fig. 118-2); systemic drainage of the splenic veins; congenital portosystemic shunts; and malrotation. Transplantation may be impossible when both the portal and superior mesenteric veins are occluded or in cases of nonresponsive metastatic hepatoblastoma. If hepatocellualr carcinoma is detected in patients with cirrhosis, this changes the transplant urgency and requires staging and decisions about pretransplant therapy and the timing and feasibility of transplantation.

Ultrasonography (US) is the method used most often in the preoperative evaluation of pediatric transplant candidates. Doppler US assesses vessel patency and hemodynamics. Computed tomography (CT) is excellent for showing vascular and visceral anatomy. Magnetic resonance imaging (MRI) may supply hemodynamic information and is superior to US in depicting varices, collaterals, and spontaneous splenorenal shunts. Bone radiographs may detect rickets, osteopenia, and fractures; chest radiographs may show cardiomegaly and vascular prominence in patients with hepatopulmonary disease. Angiography is seldom performed and is reserved for patients in whom noninvasive imaging provides insufficient information.

Imaging before liver transplantation should provide accurate information on the following:

- **Patency and size of the portal vein and IVC**
- **Abdominal anatomic anomalies**
- **Coexisting conditions**
- **Absence of hepatic neoplasm**

SURGICAL ANATOMY

The majority of liver transplants performed in older children involve the use of a whole cadaveric liver (Fig. 118-3). Most young children receive reduced transplants. Liver segments are defined according to the segmental and vascular anatomy described by Couinaud. The majority of living donor transplants use the donor's left lateral segment or left lobe, although use of the right lobe has recently been reported. A cadaveric liver may be split between two recipients. Both situations result in challenging vascular and biliary connections owing to limited pedicle lengths.

Left lobe and left lateral segment hila and their cut surfaces face to the right. They can be differentiated by the presence of the falciform ligament separating lateral segments 2 and 3 from medial segment 4 in the left lobe transplant, which is absent in left lateral segment grafts (Fig. 118-4). Small bowel and duodenum migrate into the vacated liver bed; cecum and right colon ascend, imitating malrotation. The right kidney usually migrates superiorly (Fig. 118-5).

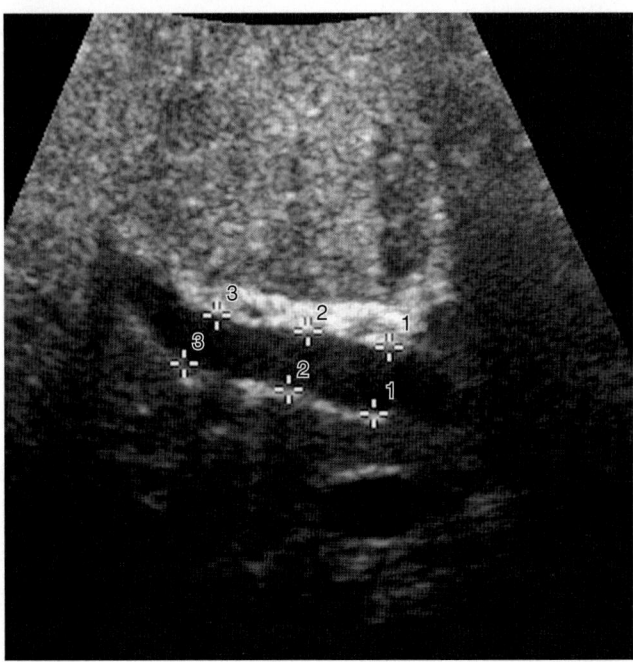

FIGURE 118-1. Preoperative ultrasound evaluation for liver transplantation. Oblique right image shows the measurements of the portal vein. *Calipers* outline portal vein measurements at three separate points.

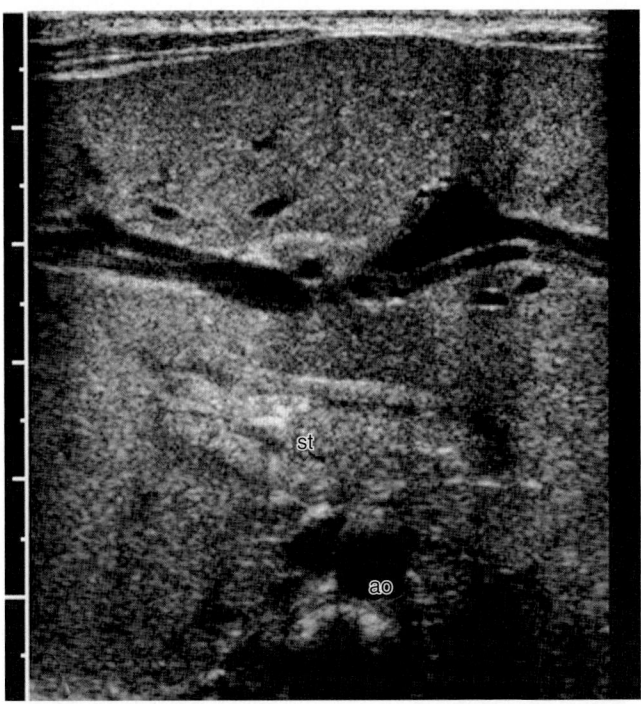

A

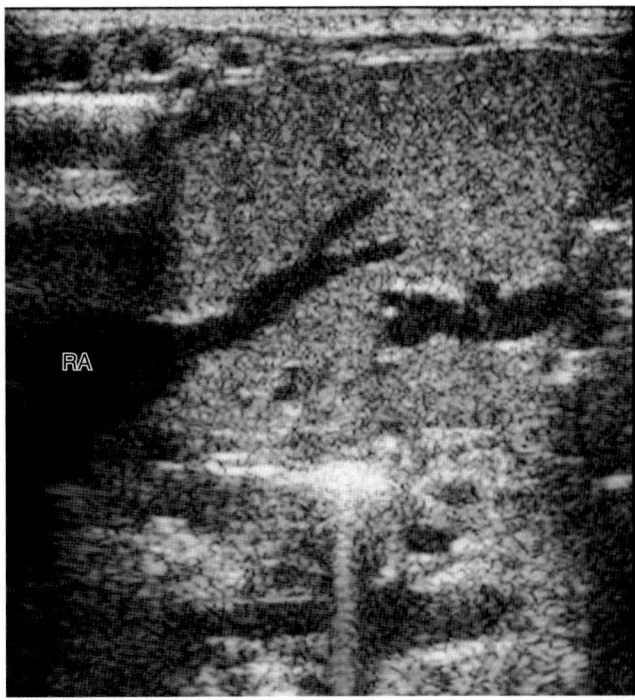

B

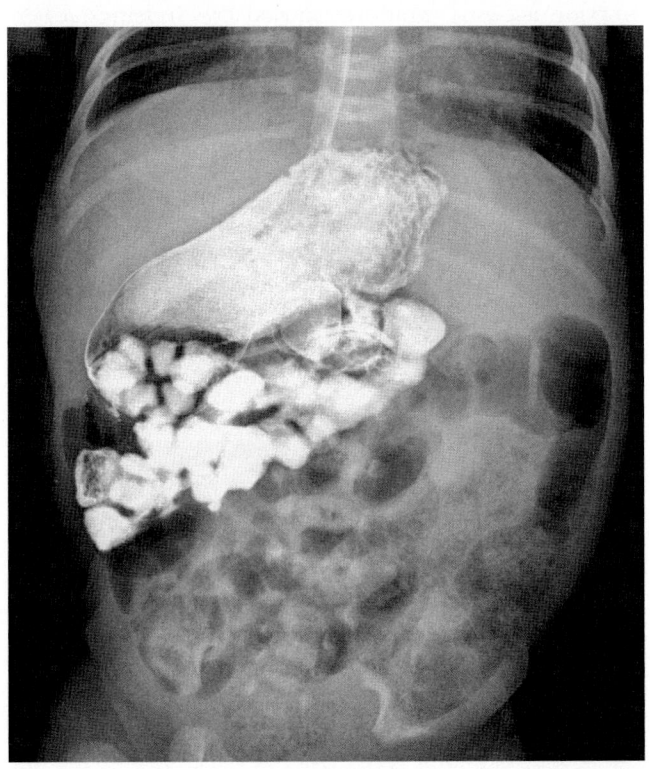

C

FIGURE 118-2. This infant presented initially with congenital heart disease and was found to have situs ambiguous with polysplenia and biliary atresia. **A,** Transverse ultrasound image of the upper abdomen shows a dome-shaped liver and symmetric right and left portal veins. Their anterior confluence represents a preduodenal portal vein. **B,** Longitudinal ultrasound image. The hepatic veins drain directly into the right atrium (RA). **C,** Upper gastrointestinal barium study shows a left-sided cardiac apex, a central stomach, and malrotation.

> **Differentiation of segmental transplants: in a left lobe transplant, the falciform ligament is preserved, and two hepatic vein are usually present. In a left lateral segment transplant, the falciform ligament is absent, and one hepatic vein is present. The hilum faces to the right in both cases.**

The portal vein is usually connected end-to-end to the recipient portal vein (Fig. 118-6). To avoid the need for extension grafts, much of the native portal vein is preserved during hepatectomy. Children with older grafts may have had extension grafts, and these may still be used in patients with unsuitable native portal veins. Today, the donor hepatic artery is usually anastomosed to the recipient's hepatic artery or celiac axis. Previously, or when technically dictated, the hepatic artery may be connected to the infrarenal aorta, sometimes using a cadaveric donor aorta. In such cases, the native hepatic artery is ligated and should not be confused with arterial occlusion on imaging (Fig. 118-7). In most young children, the bile duct is attached to a Roux-en-Y jejunal loop (Fig. 118-8). In reduced-size transplants, the donor hepatic vein is connected to the recipient's modified hepatic vein orifice.

In full-size liver grafts, the donor liver is removed with the intrahepatic IVC, which is then interposed between the infra-atrial and distal native IVC. The donor IVC may be sutured distally and connected proximally, piggyback fashion, to the preserved native IVC. In patients with polysplenia and biliary atresia, these vascular techniques must be modified owing to the frequent absence of the

hepatic segment of the IVC and azygos continuation, malrotation, preduodenal portal vein, and other anomalies (Fig. 118-9).

POSTOPERATIVE IMAGING

Portable sonography may be used during surgery, mainly when vascular anastomoses are difficult or revised and their patency is uncertain. In addition, most transplant centers evaluate vascular patency daily with US and Doppler for the first few days; the fate of the transplant is much improved if vascular occlusions are diagnosed and managed early. The frequency of US then decreases, based on local preference. Periodic screening of liver recipients is mandatory, however, because vascular complications may be clinically silent. US is the main screening tool during follow-up. CT, computed tomography angiography (CTA), magnetic resonance cholangio-pancreatography (MRCP), and magnetic resonance angiography (MRA) are used to determine the need for biliary and vascular interventions in selected patients. MRI also has a role in evaluating neurologic complications. CT is the main modality for evaluating suspected fluid collections, intra-abdominal infection, and PTLD.

Early postoperative US may be challenging owing to poor acoustic windows caused by dressings, open incisions, free intra-abdominal air, and body wall edema. The flow pattern in all vessels varies in the early postoperative period owing to edema of the anastomosis and surrounding tissues, as well as hemodynamic changes in the graft's vascular bed.

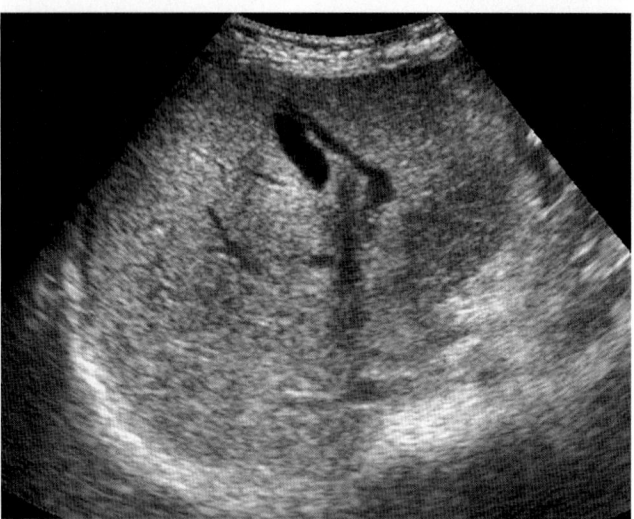

FIGURE 118-3. Transverse ultrasound image of a whole liver transplant. Fluid along the falciform ligaments demarcates the left lateral and medial segments. A right lobe is present.

> **Early post-transplantation flow patterns may suggest vascular stenosis due to edema of the anastomosis and surrounding tissues. These changes are usually reversible but should be followed.**

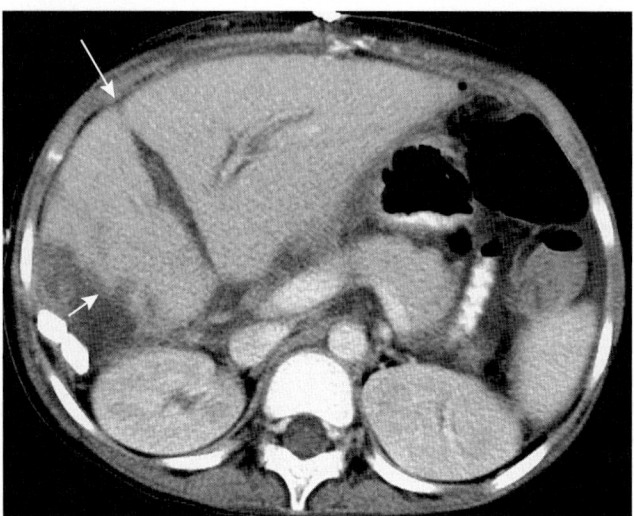

A

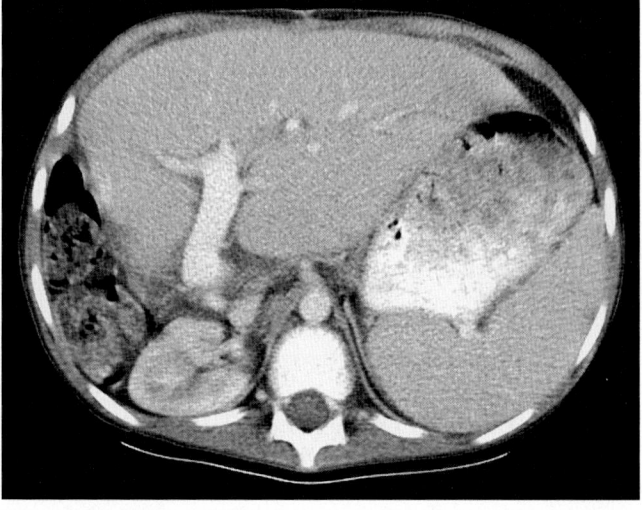

B

FIGURE 118-4. Segmental liver grafts. **A,** CT of a left lobe liver graft. Note the ill-defined, irregular cut edge with adjacent fluid. Fluid along the falciform ligament *(arrow)* separates the left lateral segment (segments 2 and 3) from the medial segment (segment 4). **B,** CT of a left lateral segment graft. Note the course of the portal vein entering from the right and the absence of the falciform ligament.

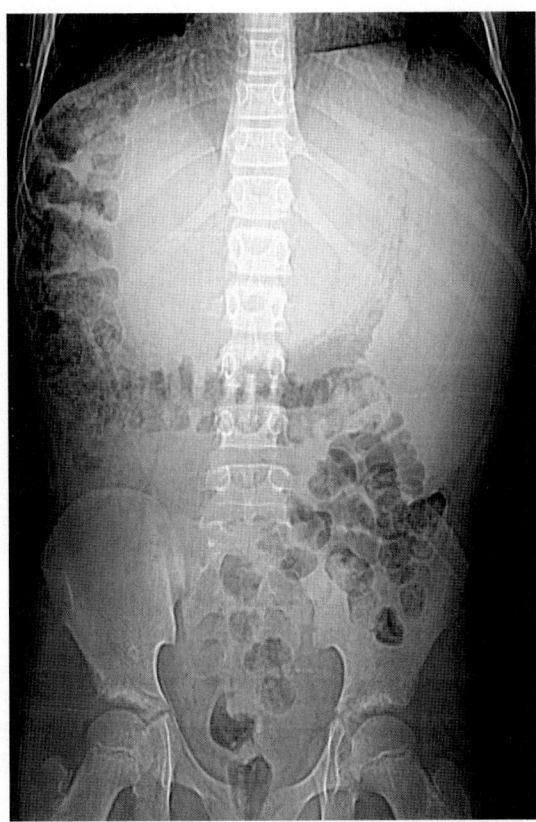

A

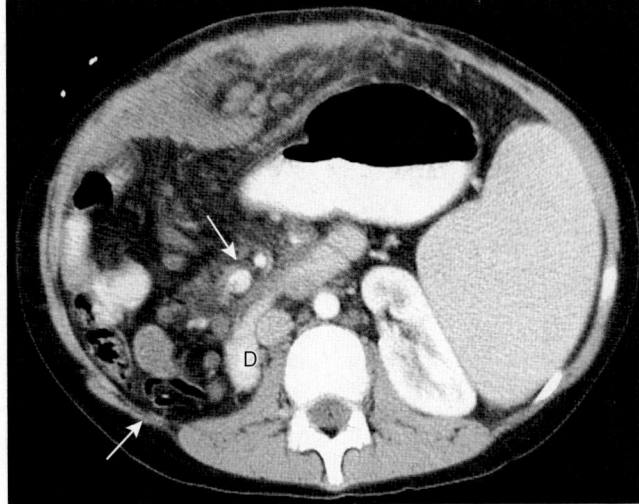

B

FIGURE 118-5. Organs migrate into the vacated space in the right abdomen following left lobe liver transplantation. **A,** Kidney, ureter, bladder scan shows the colon and right flexure in the right upper abdomen. Splenomegaly is also present. **B,** CT scan of the same patient. The duodenum (D) and the superior mesenteric vessels *(upper arrow)* are displaced into the right abdomen. The appendix *(lower arrow)* and cecum are at the level of the duodenum, imitating malrotation. **C,** Coronal CT reconstruction shows the right colonic flexure and the right kidney have migrated cephalad and are located under the right diaphragm.

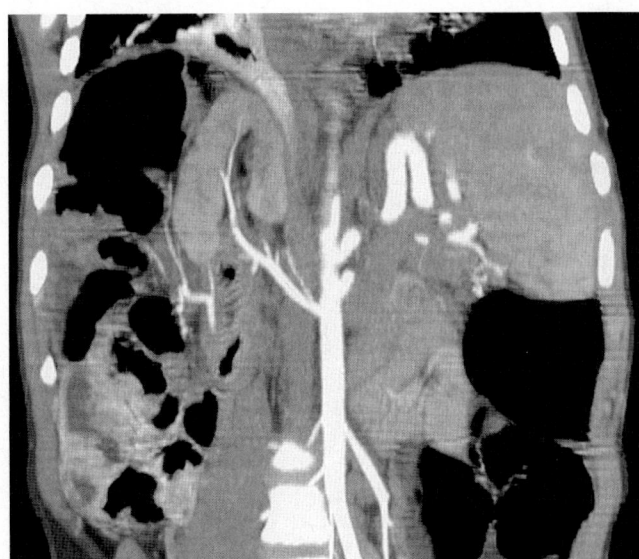

C

Vascular patency and flow direction, pattern, and velocity must be evaluated using both spectral and color Doppler. The color Doppler velocity scale must be adjusted for each vessel separately to avoid aliasing in the faster flowing vessels and ambiguity of flow direction. Efforts must be made to interrogate at the anastomoses, where stenosis, thrombosis, and occlusion are most likely.

Early findings in normal liver grafts include transient lymphatic engorgement, seen as increased periportal echogenicity on US, low attenuation on CT (Fig. 118-10), or high signal on T2-weighted MRI; right pleural effusion; small subhepatic fluid collections; and biliary air in recipients with choledochojejunostomies.

COMPLICATIONS

Vascular, biliary, infectious, and immunosuppression-related complications may befall liver recipients both early and late in the postoperative course. The most common complication of liver transplantation is infection, but vascular thrombosis and primary graft nonfunction account for most cases of graft loss leading to retransplantation. Death in most pediatric liver recipients is caused by infection, neurologic complications, or multisystem organ failure. Enteric complications include bowel perforation and obstruction, gastrointestinal hemorrhage, and infectious enteritis. Neurologic complications include cerebral hemorrhage and infarction, infection, drug toxicity, and PTLD. Immunosuppressive drug-induced nephrotoxicity is common but has no specific imaging features.

More minor complications include hepatic parenchymal defects, pleural effusions, and splenic infarcts, which may occur after splenic artery ligation. Right adrenal hemorrhage and right phrenic nerve injury are complications seen after the standard transplant operation but rarely occur after a cava-sparing operation.

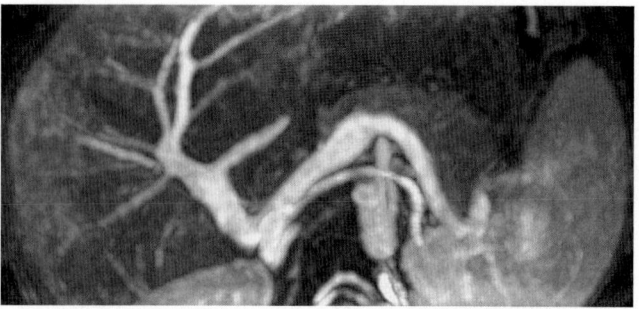

A

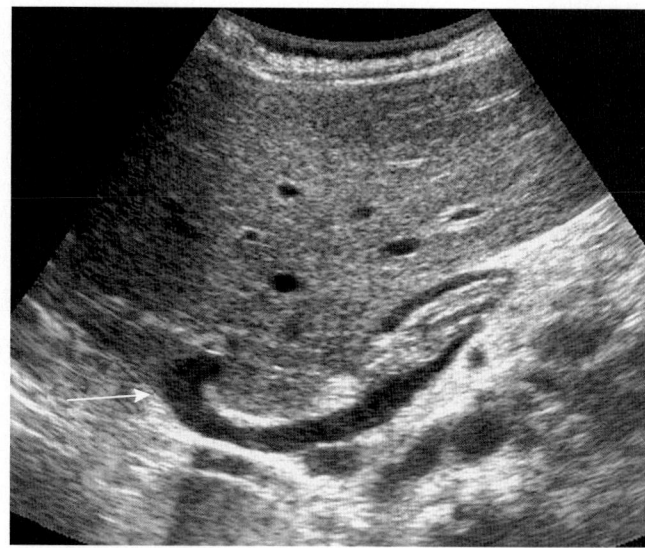

B

FIGURE 118-6. Portal vein anatomy following left lobe liver transplantation. **A,** In the same patient as in Figure 118-4A, magnetic resonance venography shows the course and branching of the portal vein in a left lobe transplant. Note the absence of the right portal vein and its branches. **B,** Transverse ultrasound image of a left lateral segment transplant. Note the curved course of the extrahepatic portal vein. This frequently makes it technically difficult to visualize its entire length.

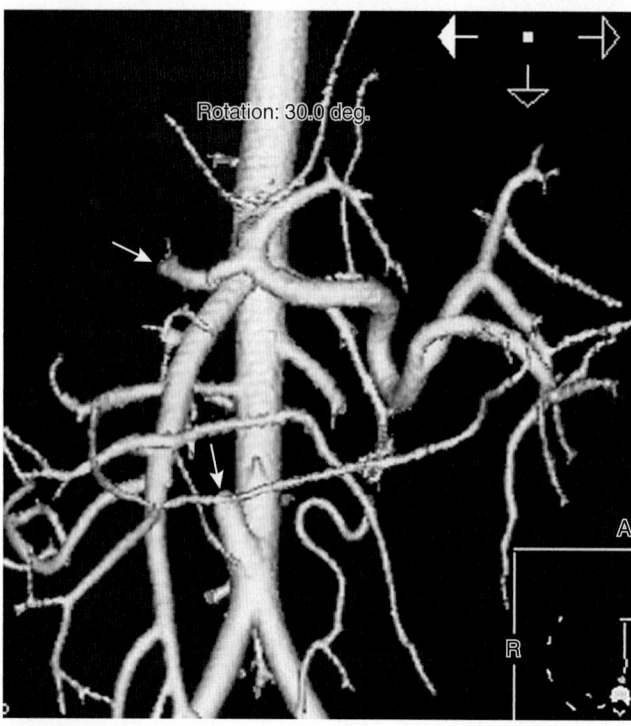

FIGURE 118-7. Hepatic artery anatomy after transplantation on a three-dimensional reconstruction from MRA. The native hepatic artery was ligated at the time of native hepatectomy *(upper arrow)*. The transplant hepatic artery was anastomosed to the infrarenal aorta. It is now occluded *(lower arrow)*.

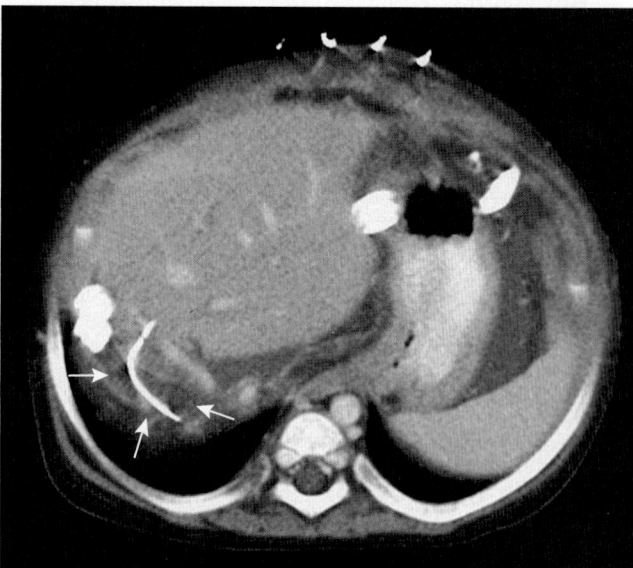

FIGURE 118-8. The Roux-en-Y biliary anastomosis and loop are marked early after transplantation by a small biliary stent *(arrows)*. Being an efferent loop from the liver, it frequently does not fill with intestinal contrast, making it difficult to differentiate from a pathologic fluid collection.

Obstructive lesions of the portal vein, hepatic vein, or IVC may manifest with progressive ascites, deterioration of liver function, gastrointestinal bleeding, decreased platelet count, and increased spleen size. Some patients may develop pulmonary hypertension and intrapulmonary shunting. Doppler signal in the intrahepatic portions of the hepatic artery and portal vein may be present, in spite of stenosis or obstruction in the extrahepatic segment, owing to collateral formation. Portal vein, hepatic vein, or IVC stenosis results in flow acceleration and a jet at the post-stenotic segment. The jet of increased flow velocity appears as a contrasting color owing to aliasing when the color scale is adjusted to the velocity below the stenosis. The jet velocity is proportional to the pressure gradient across the stenosis. The spectral Doppler sampling box must be placed at the site of maximal velocity.

> **Doppler signal in the intrahepatic portions of the hepatic artery and portal vein may be present in spite of stenosis or obstruction in the extrahepatic segment, owing to collateral formation.**

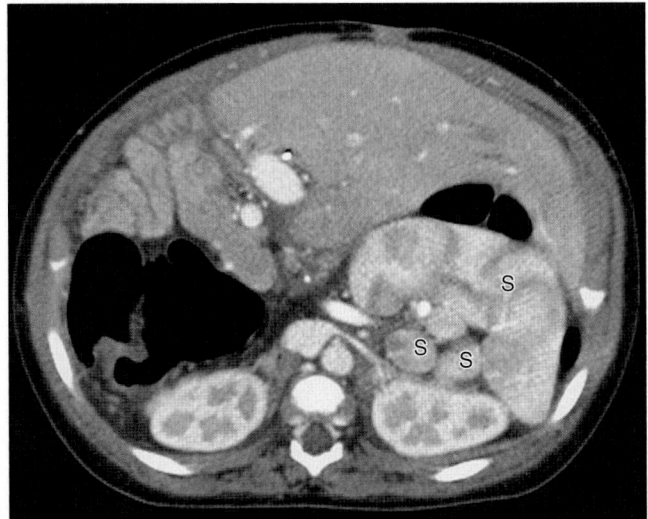

A

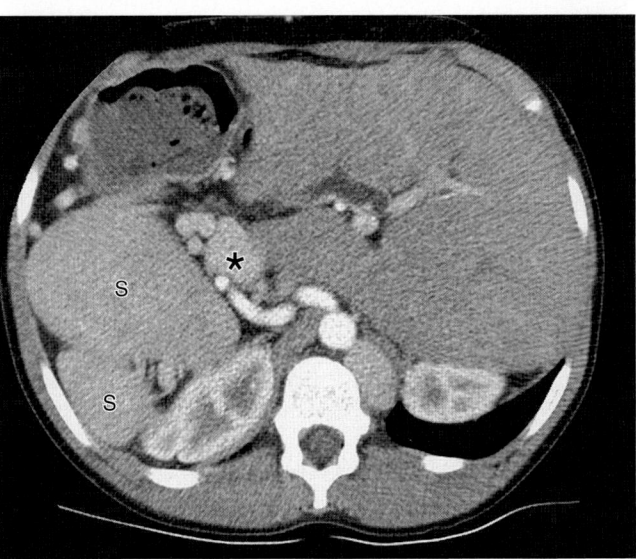

B

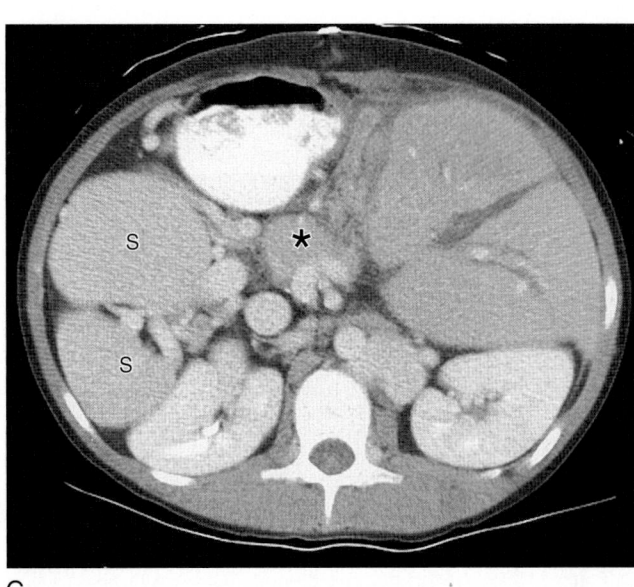

C

FIGURE 118-9. Technical variations in transplantation technique in patients with major visceral anomalies. **A,** In a patient with biliary atresia and polysplenia, a left lateral segment graft was placed anterior to the spleens (S). **B,** Pretransplant CT in a girl with right-sided polysplenia and a left-sided, abnormally lobed liver with biliary atresia. **C,** Post-transplant CT shows that a left lobe liver graft was placed in the vacated liver fossa. Note the right-sided polysplenia and an anomalous short, rounded pancreas (*).

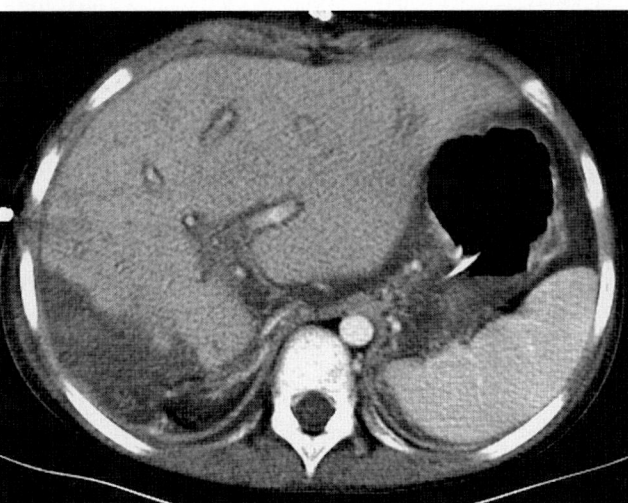

FIGURE 118-10. Early CT findings in liver transplantation. There is diffuse periportal lucency, irregularity of the cut surface edge, and adjacent fluid.

> When evaluating transplant veins, spectral Doppler must be performed at the anastomosis, the narrowest portion, and at the site of maximal jet seen by color Doppler.

Vascular Complications

Portal Vein

US of the transplant portal vein should visualize its entire course, measure the diameter at any site of narrowing, and interrogate the portal vein by spectral and color Doppler along its extrahepatic and hilar course, as well as its major intrahepatic branches. The curved course of the portal vein in left lobe and left lateral segment transplants and the size discrepancy between donor and recipient veins frequently cause dilation at the neohilum due to altered flow dynamics (Fig. 118-11), with a "yin-

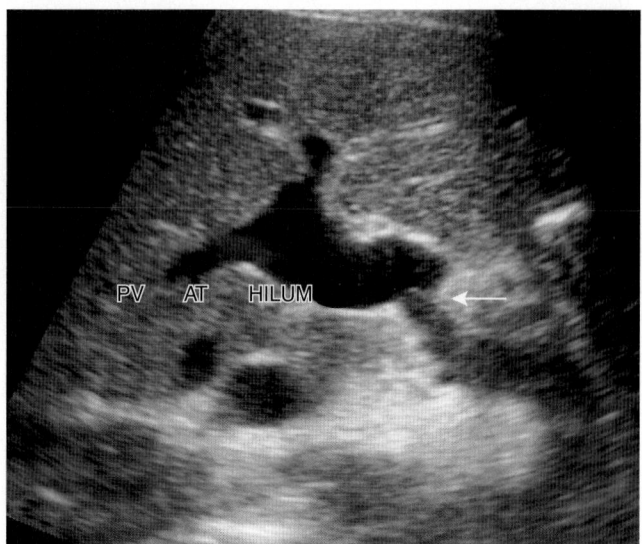
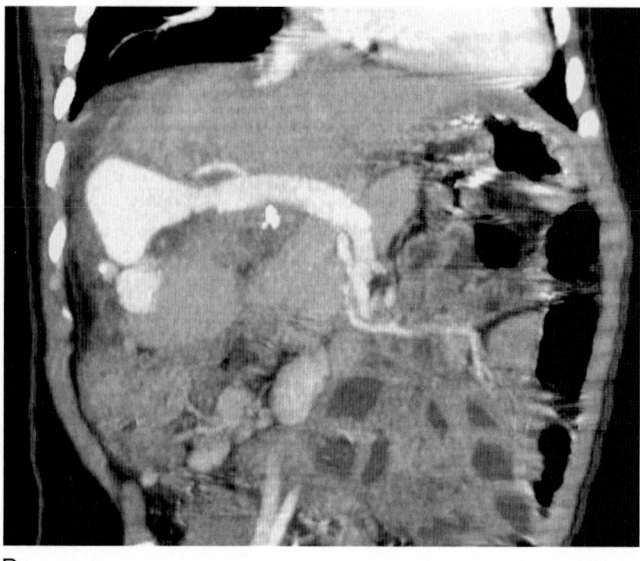

A   B

FIGURE 118-11. Portal vein in segmental transplantation. **A,** Ultrasound image shows a size discrepancy (*arrow*) between the native and donor portal veins and dilation of the donor portal vein (*PV at Hilum*). **B,** Coronal reconstruction from CTA shows the extrahepatic portal vein coursing from the left to the right edge of the transplant, near the right abdominal wall. The portal vein is dilated at the neohilum. Note the slight narrowing at the anastomosis in this early transplant.

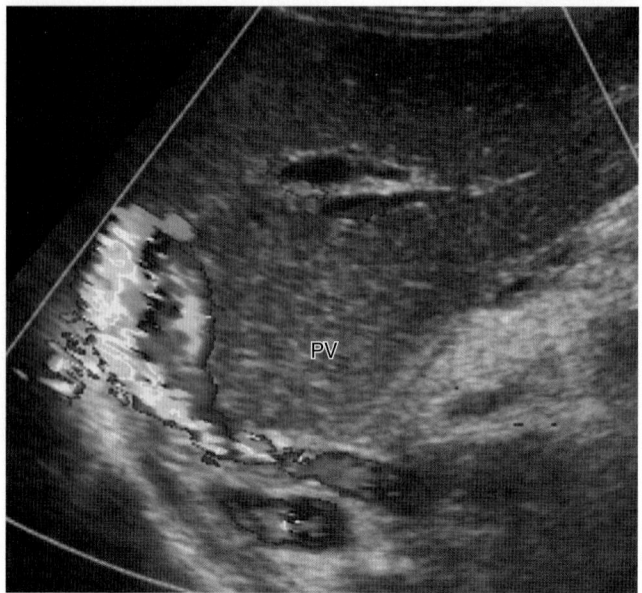

FIGURE 118-12. Color Doppler at the liver hilum in a patient with a left lateral segment liver transplant. The portal vein (PV) is dilated at the hilum, and portal flow swirls in the dilated segment, creating a "yin-and-yang" flow configuration. (*See color plate.*)

and-yang" swirling pattern on color Doppler (Fig. 118-12). This pattern has not been proved to be clinically important. Anastomotic and periportal edema causing relative narrowing with jet formation are very common in the early postoperative period; these are most often transient but may progress or persist and should be followed. Complications include early thrombosis, stenosis, and late occlusion (Fig. 118-13).

An early hypoechoic thrombus may not be recognized by gray scale US. Color Doppler shows absence of color signal and reversal of superior mesenteric or splenic vein

flow. Early thrombosis is usually treated by surgical thrombectomy and revision. Reversal of flow within the entire portal vein in the early post-transplant period may reflect extensive hepatic necrosis and arterioportal shunting—an ominous sign associated with frequent organ loss.

Later, the onset of portal vein thrombosis or occlusion may be clinically silent, manifesting with increasing plasma levels of hepatic enzymes, an enlarging spleen, and gastrointestinal bleeding. Intrahepatic portal venous flow is frequently reconstructed from collaterals recruited from superior mesenteric vein branches via varices in the Roux-en-Y loop and from transcapsular collaterals. In the latter event, flow in the receiving portal vein branches may be reversed with segment-to-segment shunt (Fig. 118-14).

> **Reversal of portal venous flow in a lobar or segmental branch is a strong indication of main portal vein occlusion.**

Stenosis usually occurs at anastomoses and extension grafts (Fig. 118-15). The incidence of stenosis decreased when the use of cryopreserved cadaveric venous extension grafts was abandoned. Because of the curved extrahepatic course of the portal vein, it may be difficult to demonstrate stenosis by US. The jet created at the stenotic site dissipates, such that flow velocity measured at the hilum is frequently normal despite a hemodynamically significant portal vein stenosis more proximally. The jet may also exaggerate the dilation of the portal vein at the hilum. Following successful angioplasty, the jet velocity decreases, and the diameter at the stenotic site increases (Fig. 118-16).

Although more invasive than US, CT and MRI are exceedingly useful in these patients. Intravenous contrast

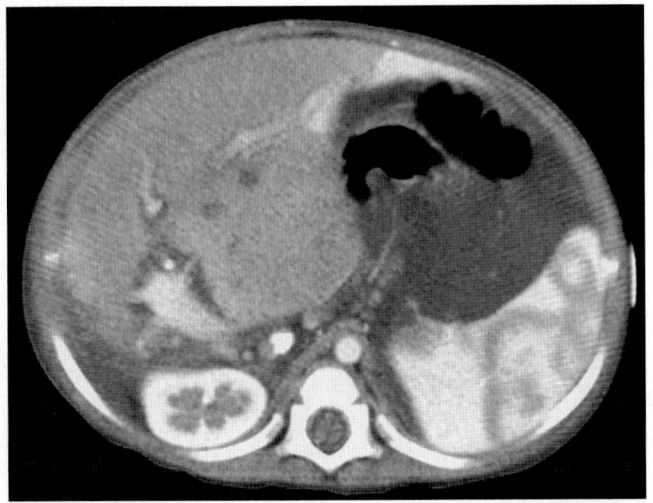

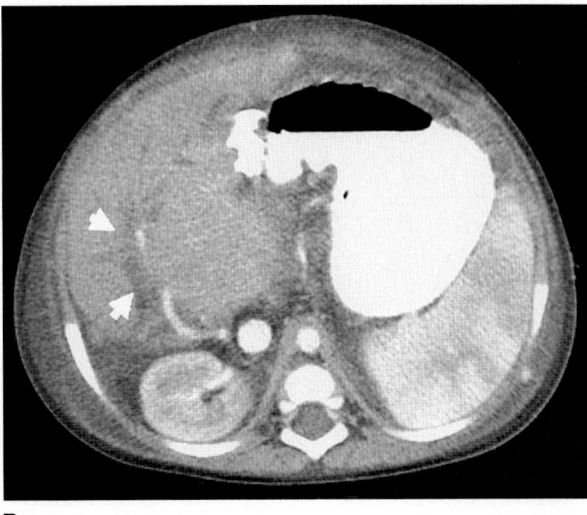

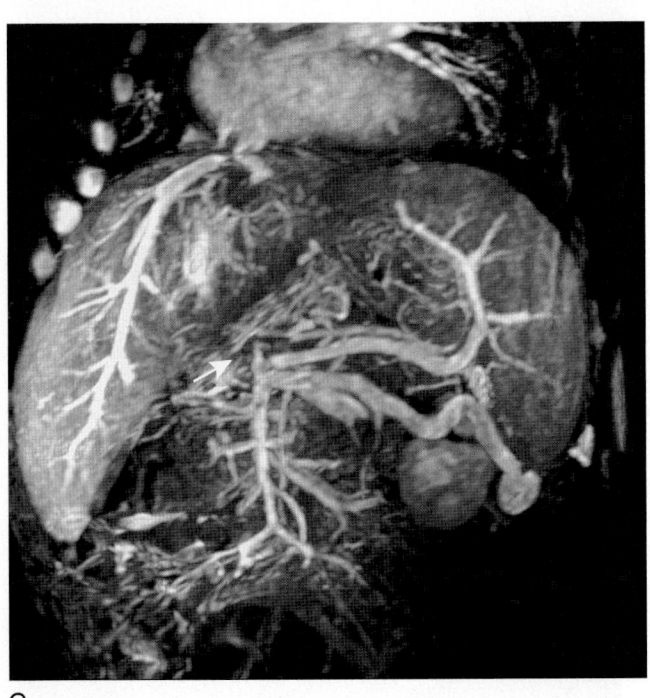

FIGURE 118-13. Portal vein occlusion. **A,** Contrast-enhanced CT in an infant with a left lateral segment graft. Both the portal vein and the hepatic artery are well seen in the neohilum. **B,** Acute portal vein thrombosis 4 months later. Contrast-enhanced CT shows a lucent band where the portal vein was previously seen *(arrows)*. The patient had thrombosis superimposed on portal vein stenosis. He underwent successful angioplasty and thrombolysis. **C,** Long-standing portal vein occlusion. Magnetic resonance venography shows occlusion of the entire portal vein from the splenomesenteric confluence *(arrow)*. A large venous collateral is seen from the confluence to the left flank.

and their multiplanar capabilities render CT and MRI more consistent than US in the evaluation of portal vein occlusion and stenosis.

> Portal vein Doppler signal may appear normal in the intrahepatic portion in the presence of a high-grade stenosis or occlusion of the extrahepatic portion.

HEPATIC ARTERY

Complications in the hepatic artery include thrombosis, occlusion, stenosis, peripheral arteriovenous fistula, and aneurysm. The incidence of hepatic artery complications has decreased with improved surgical techniques, the use of microvascular surgery, and the decreased use of interposition grafts. The hepatic artery is much more difficult to visualize by gray scale US than the portal vein owing to its small caliber. It is best evaluated by color and power Doppler. It is easier to follow the artery to its anastomosis when it is attached to the native hepatic artery or celiac axis rather than to the infrarenal aorta, where much of its course is obscured by bowel gas. Both CTA and MRA are effective in demonstrating hepatic artery anatomy, course, and complications (Fig. 118-17; see Fig. 118-7).

The hepatic artery flow pattern may vary considerably in the early postoperative days, demonstrating both high and low resistive indices, without consistent prognostic implications. High-grade narrowing is usually manifested by turbulence; severely attenuated velocity, with narrow systolic peaks and absent diastolic flow beyond the anastomosis; or a parvus-tardus pattern in intrahepatic branches.

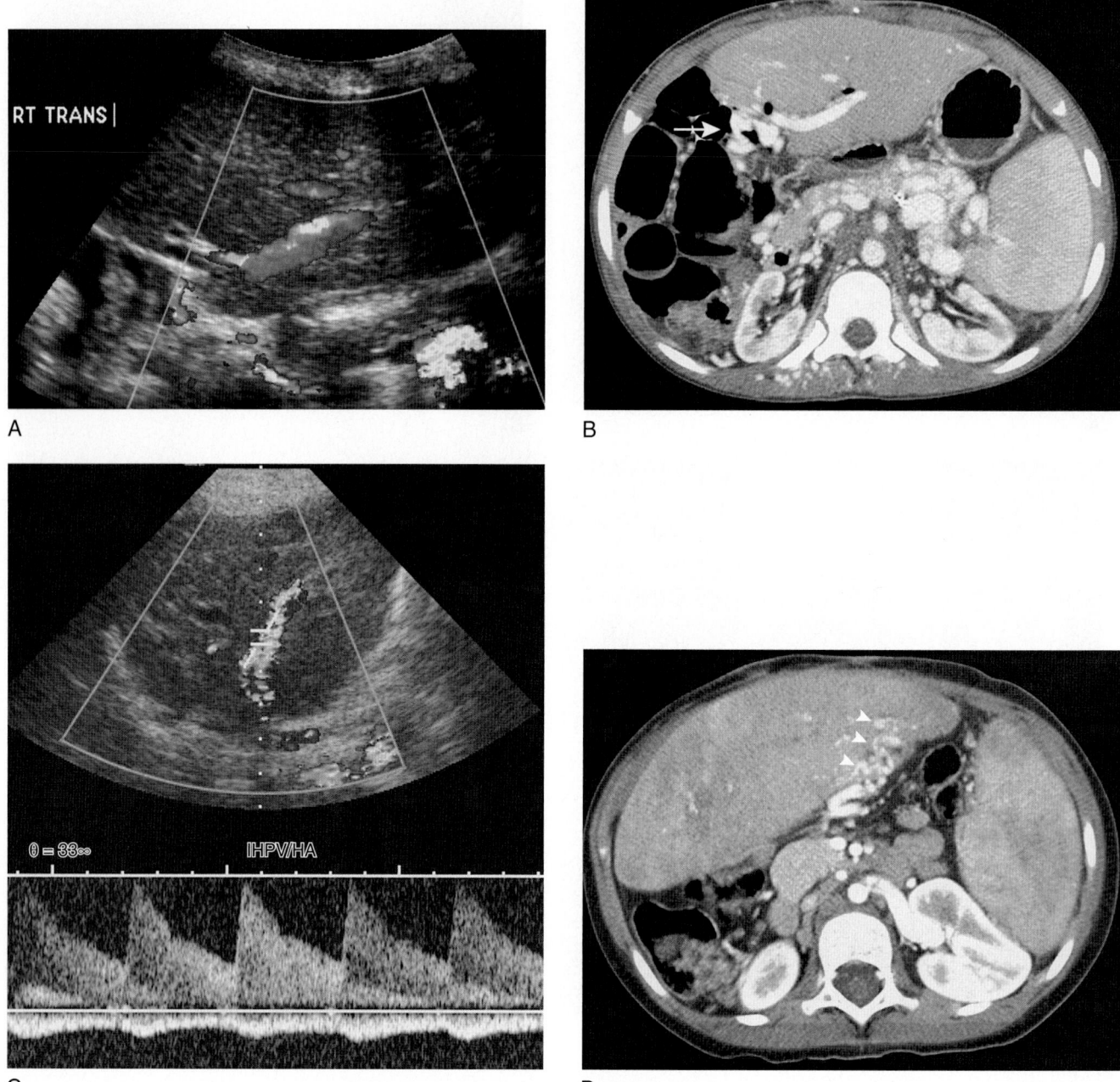

FIGURE 118-14. Flow within the intrahepatic portal venous branches in portal vein occlusion. Both patients had recurrence of pretransplant portal hypertension and gastrointestinal bleeding. **A,** Color Doppler in patient 1 shows that the transplant portal vein is occluded, yet there is hepatopetal flow in the intrahepatic segment. **B,** CTA in the same patient shows venous collaterals (varices) within the Roux-en-Y loop, providing flow into the liver *(arrow)*. **C,** Color and spectral Doppler in patient 2 shows hepatofugal flow (in the opposite direction to the adjacent hepatic artery branch) in the segment 2 portal branch. Note the dominant hepatic artery flow, typical of portal vein occlusion. **D,** Coronal reconstruction from CTA in the same patient shows transcapsular portal vein collaterals penetrating into the same segment.

Acute arterial thrombosis may be catastrophic and result in acidosis, sepsis, and organ necrosis. Early hepatic artery thrombosis is associated with a high incidence of transplant loss. If the problem is diagnosed within the first 2 to 3 days and the patient is still asymptomatic, the majority (78%) of transplanted livers with hepatic artery thrombosis may be salvaged. However, if elevated liver function tests, bile leak, liver abscess, or sepsis have supervened, graft loss may reach 75%. The diagnosis is made by the inability to detect hepatic artery signal on color and spectral Doppler. Acute arterial thrombosis is treated by thrombectomy, revision, and sometimes retransplantation.

Later onset hepatic artery occlusion is less dramatic. Because the biliary tree depends on hepatic arterial supply, arterial compromise may manifest with biliary leaks, strictures, and infection, including peribiliary abscess, liver abscess, and sepsis (Fig. 118-18). Hilar or transcapsular collaterals are frequently present, resulting in detectable arterial Doppler signal (Fig. 118-19).

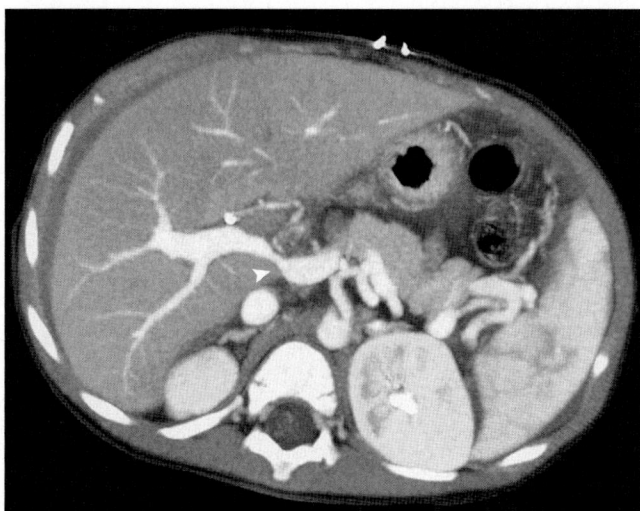

FIGURE 118-15. Portal vein stenosis. Contrast-enhanced CT shows anastomotic stenosis *(arrowhead)* in a patient with a whole liver transplant.

In long-standing hepatic artery occlusion, there is frequently a detectable Doppler arterial signal at the liver hilum and intrahepatic branches, owing to collateral formation. The flow pattern is abnormal, with a low-amplitude, parvus-tardus phenomenon representing a systolic acceleration time longer than 0.08 second and a resistive index lower than 0.5.

Although transplant survival may be extended, almost all transplanted livers with arterial obstruction are eventually lost.

Stenosis of the hepatic artery may be silent or manifest with biliary complications and infection. High velocity and turbulence may be seen at the stenotic site. The flow pattern distal to the stenosis demonstrates a parvus-tardus phenomenon and increased diastolic flow. Very high-grade stenosis manifests with narrow and low-amplitude systolic peaks and absence of diastolic flow. The stenosis is usually extrahepatic and hard to demonstrate directly by Doppler US (Fig. 118-20). The hemodynamic changes of hepatic artery stenosis may be more dramatic than its appearance on CTA or MRA (Fig. 118-21).

Hepatic artery pseudoaneurysm may occur at the anastomosis or within the liver, at a biopsy site. Liver biopsy has also been incriminated in the production of intrahepatic arteriovenous fistulas.

HEPATIC VEIN

Hepatic vein stenosis occurs mainly in reduced-size transplants at the anastomosis to the recipient IVC. In a post-transplant patient with the onset of portal hypertension, special efforts must be made to evaluate the hepatic veins and IVC if a portal vein complication is not seen. Stenosis is invariably near the diaphragm, making it difficult to demonstrate by US (Fig. 118-22). Doppler US demonstrates increased flow velocity and jet, with loss of previous triphasic flow. It should be remembered that triphasic flow may be absent without obstruction. CTA and MRA with multiplanar reconstructions are excellent modalities for diagnosis.

INFERIOR VENA CAVA

IVC stenosis and obstruction may be anastomotic or long segment or may result from compression or torsion (Fig. 118-23). The clinical manifestations of IVC stenosis or obstruction depend on location. If the problem is at or above the hepatic veins, it manifests with ascites and portal hypertension; if the problem is at a lower level, it may be clinically silent.

IVC obstruction can be diagnosed by all cross-sectional modalities; however, several pitfalls may be encountered with Doppler US. Flow in the hepatic veins may be normal and triphasic if the IVC obstruction is distal to their insertion (Fig. 118-24). When the obstruction is proximal to the hepatic vein insertion, hepatic venous blood may enter the IVC and flow retrogradely to decompress into systemic collaterals (Fig. 118-25). In patients with a surgical portosystemic shunt, IVC obstruction prevents adequate decompression, sometimes reversing flow in the shunt and increasing pre-existent varices (Fig. 118-26).

> Hepatic vein flow may be detected in patients with complete IVC obstruction. The entire length of the hepatic segment of the IVC and the flow pattern and direction in the hepatic vein and IVC should be assessed.

Biliary Complications

Bile leaks and strictures occurring early after transplantation are related to technical surgical problems, such as anastomotic leak and narrowing or kinking. Biliary complications with a later onset are commonly associated with ischemia and infection secondary to arterial occlusion or stenosis. Biliary strictures are more common in reduced-size liver transplants than full-sized ones. Inspissated bile may further complicate biliary stasis. Biliary compression by mucocele or cystic duct remnant has also been described. Chronic rejection may be associated with loss of bile ducts and mild chronic dilation.

US and CT demonstrate biliary dilation (Fig. 118-27). MRCP and percutaneous transhepatic cholangiography demonstrate strictures directly. US is the primary screening imaging modality. When bile duct dilation is found, further imaging is indicated. MRCP is increasingly used to assess biliary obstruction and the need for intervention. Direct cholangiogram is usually performed as part of a therapeutic approach (Fig. 118-28).

Fluid Collections

Early postoperative bleeding from leaking anastomoses or inadequate hemostasis leading to visible fluid collections occurs in as many as 15% of recipients. Up to half of these patients undergo operative exploration.

Mycotic arterial pseudoaneurysms at anastomoses may rupture, producing abrupt exsanguination. Any collection of fluid near an artery should be interrogated with Doppler US.

Most fluid collections following pediatric liver transplantation occur at the cut edge; contain serous fluid,

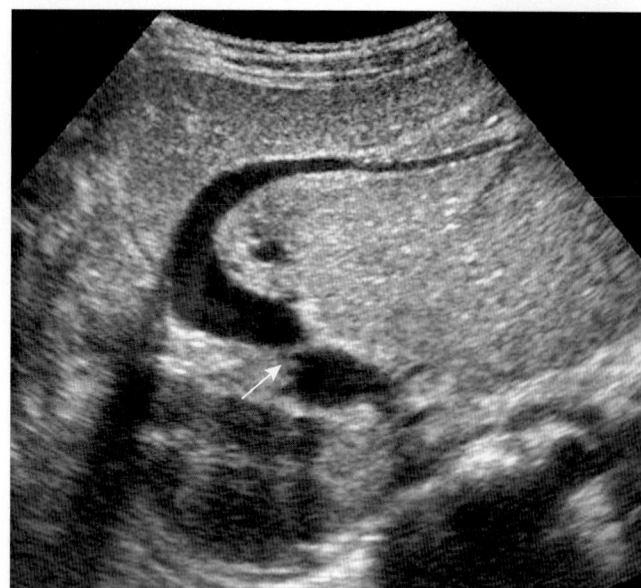

A

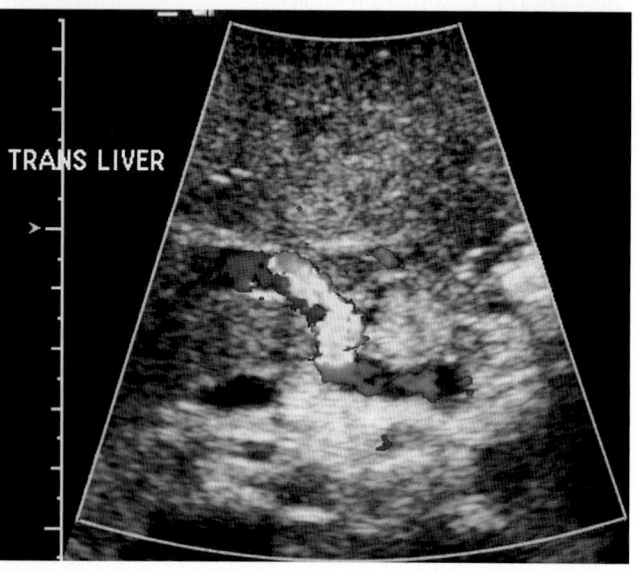

B

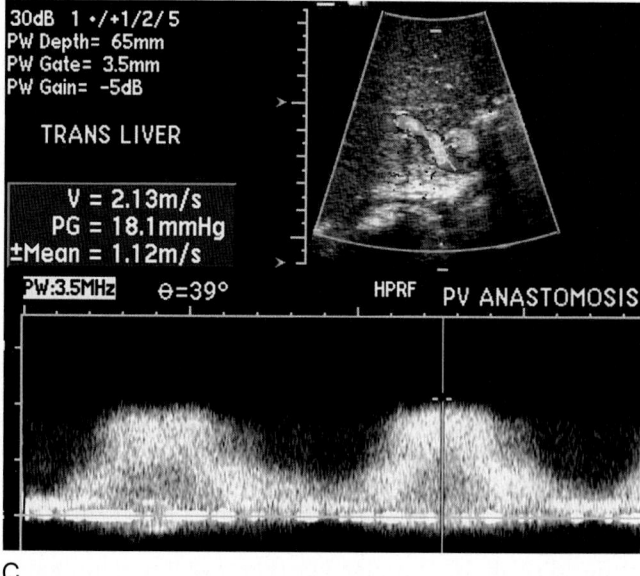

C

FIGURE 118-16. Ultrasound and Doppler characteristics of portal vein stenosis. **A,** US of a child with a left lateral segment graft. The stenosis *(arrow)* is outside the liver hilum, beyond the portal vein curvature. **B,** On color Doppler, the velocity scale is adjusted to demonstrate the jet by aliasing. The jet is seen exiting the stenotic site. **C,** On spectral and color Doppler with sampling at the jet, maximal flow velocity is obtained to assess the hemodynamic impact of the stenosis. The jet velocity exceeds 2 m/sec.

blood, or bile; and are transient and clinically insignificant. Other collections may represent anastomotic bile leak, abscess, or bowel perforation. The imaging appearance of perihepatic fluid collections is nonspecific; most contain some debris. Specific diagnosis may require fluid aspiration or surgery (Fig. 118-29).

Although the blind end of the Roux-en-Y loop may dilate, it is important to be aware that the normal loop at the hilum of the transplanted liver may mimic a fluid collection on US and may not fill with oral contrast during CT scanning.

Ascites is very common in the early days after transplantation and is usually self-limited. If large in amount or prolonged in duration, an evaluation for the cause may be required.

Infection

The majority of liver recipients develop postoperative infection at some time, although the consequent mortality is less than 10%. Bacterial and fungal infections are most common during the first postoperative month. Risk factors include hepatic artery occlusion, immunosuppression, central venous catheters, and nosocomial exposure. Viral and opportunistic infections most often occur between 30 and 180 days after transplantation. Standard imaging techniques are used to evaluate suspected infections. CT is the mainstay for assessing intra-abdominal infections, particularly abscesses. Cholangitis may prompt evaluation with MRCP or percutaneous transhepatic cholangiography.

Rejection

Rejection was a major concern in the early days of transplantation. The introduction of cyclosporine and more recently tacrolimus has resulted in a decrease in the incidence and severity of hepatic transplant rejection. Imaging plays a relatively minor role in the diagnosis of

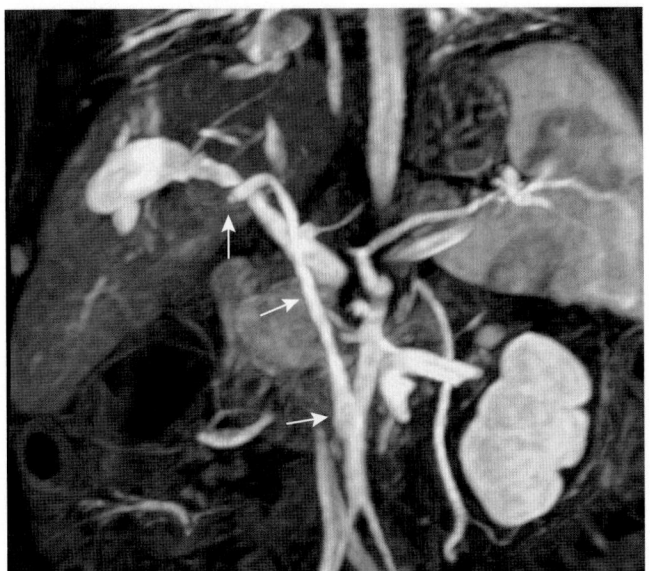

FIGURE 118-17. Hepatic artery occlusion (same patient as in Fig. 118-11B). MRA shows the origin of the transplant hepatic artery from the infrarenal aorta *(arrows)*. It is occluded near the liver.

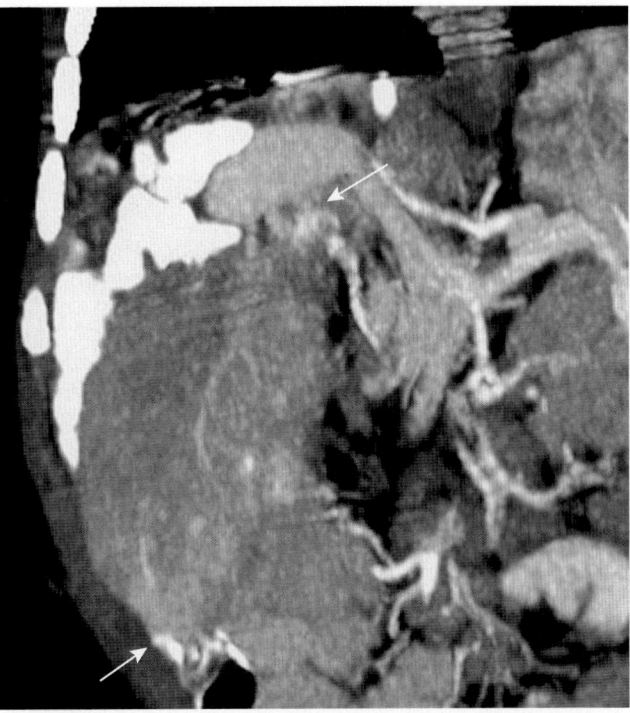

FIGURE 118-19. Hepatic artery occlusion. Doppler US (not shown) detected hepatic arterial signal in the hilum and intrahepatic branches. Coronal reconstructions from CTA show transcapsular arterial collaterals *(arrows)*.

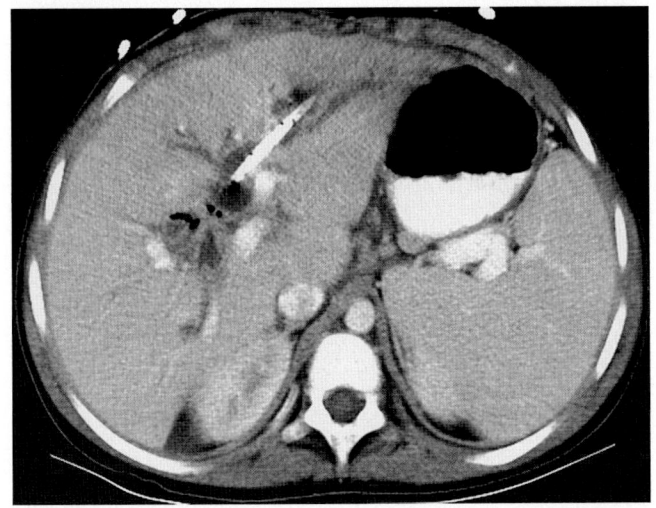

A

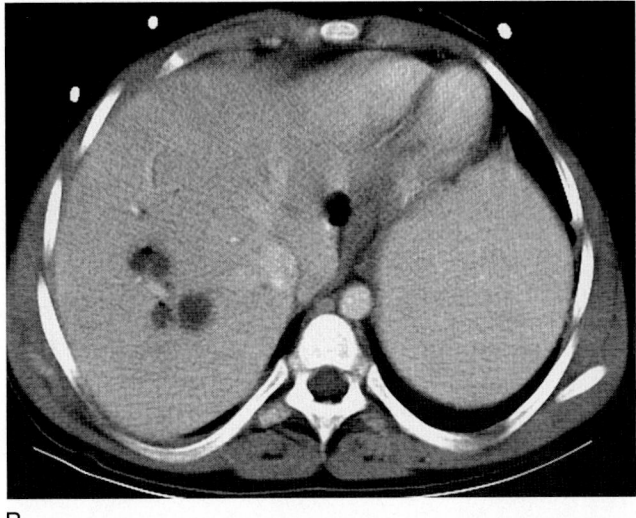

B

FIGURE 118-18. Hepatic artery occlusion with suppurative biliary infection and liver abscesses. **A,** CT at the level of the biliary drain shows the peribiliary nature of the abscesses. **B,** Higher CT slices show additional liver abscesses containing fluid and gas.

rejection, which is established mainly by liver biopsy. Neither hepatic arterial waveforms nor flow pattern in the hepatic veins proved to be significantly predictive of rejection. Rejection may be associated with mild degrees of nonobstructive bile duct dilation and an increase in hepatic arterial resistive indices.

Post-transplantation Lymphoproliferative Disease

PTLD represents a spectrum of abnormalities of lymphoid proliferation linked with Epstein-Barr virus (in 98% of pediatric patients) and immune cell proliferation that ranges from polyclonal reversible B cell proliferation to aggressive monoclonal B cell lymphoma. T cell and Burkitt lymphoma and Hodgkin disease are much less common.

Risk factor for the development of PTLD are seronegativity for Epstein-Barr virus at transplantation; young age; intensity and type of immunosuppression, especially antilymphocyte antibody; and type of transplant. Children develop PTLD about three times as often than adults. In the Pittsburgh experience, 9.7% of children

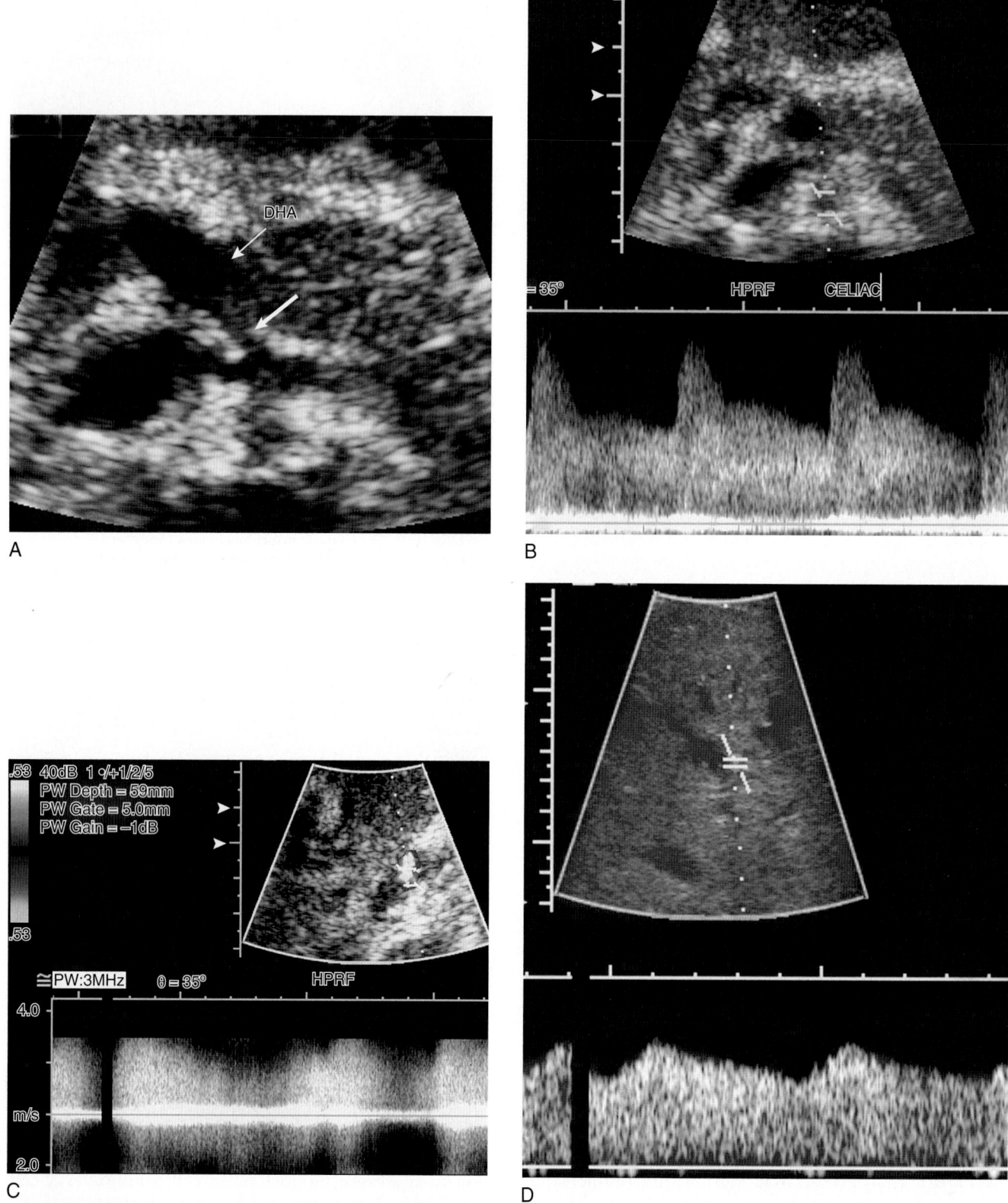

FIGURE 118-20. US and Doppler characteristics of hepatic artery stenosis. **A,** Transverse US shows stenosis immediately distal to the celiac axis *(thick arrow)*. The donor hepatic artery (DHA) distal to the anastomotic stenosis is marked by a *thin arrow*. **B,** Spectral and color Doppler in the celiac axis proximal to the stenosis shows a normal arterial flow pattern. **C,** Spectral and color Doppler at the stenosis shows extreme turbulence and high velocity. A typical arterial signal is hard to recognize due to aliasing. **D,** Spectral and color Doppler in an intrahepatic hepatic artery branch shows a slow systolic upstroke (parvus-tardus phenomenon), low resistive index, and relatively high diastolic flow.

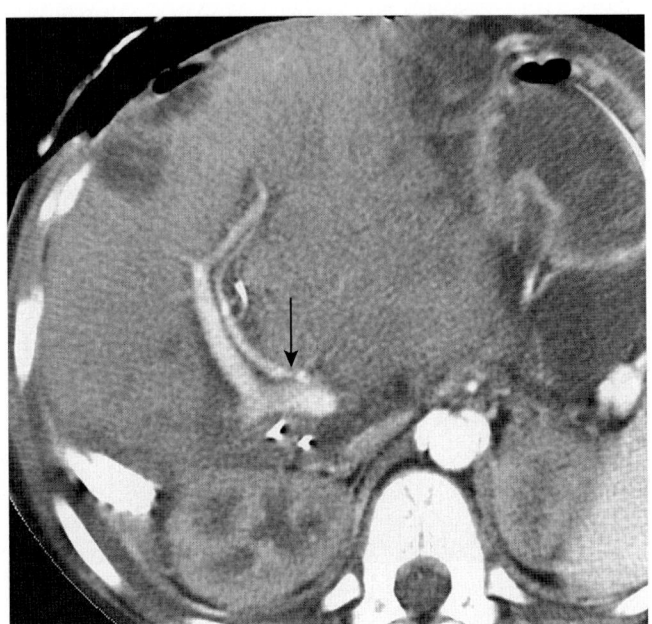

FIGURE 118-21. Hepatic artery stenosis. The CTA appearance of hepatic artery stenosis *(arrow)* may be subtle relative to its hemodynamic significance.

developed this condition, compared with 2.9% of adults. The time from transplantation to the development of PTLD averages about 8 months in children; the time may be shorter in patients treated with tacrolimus, and in our experience, it may be as short as a few weeks. Survival is better in patients with polyclonal PTLD and in those with limited disease. In patients with polyclonal disease, PTLD may reverse completely with a modification of immune suppression. Monoclonal lymphoma usually requires specific therapy.

Sites of involvement in children include any lymphoid tissue (particularly Waldeyer ring and pericardial and mesenteric nodes), the gastrointestinal tract, and the transplanted liver and spleen (Fig. 118-30). Finding newly enlarged tonsils and adenoids in a child with a transplanted liver should raise suspicion of PTLD. Unusually large mesenteric nodes are common in children with PTLD, although lack of normal standards makes it hard to set a threshold size for diagnosis. Central nervous system involvement is uncommon. The appearance of PTLD in the transplanted liver consists of multiple focal lesions and is thus nonspecific if viewed in isolation.

> **Lymphadenopathy in PTLD may be nonspecific, but it has a predilection for Waldeyer ring and mesenteric and pericardial nodes.**

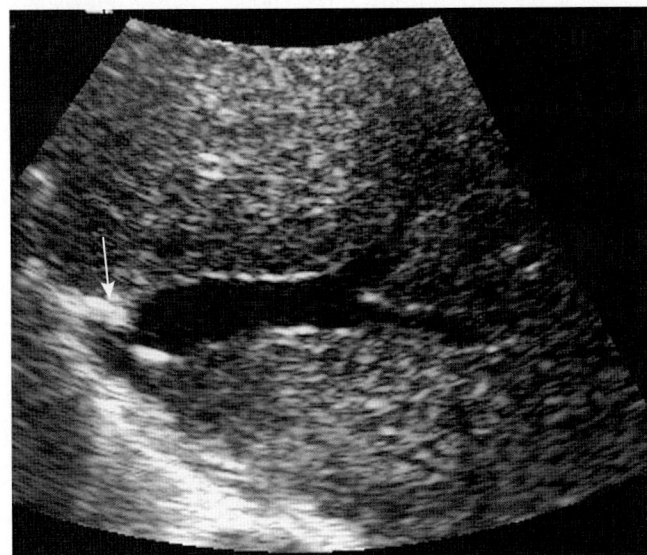

A

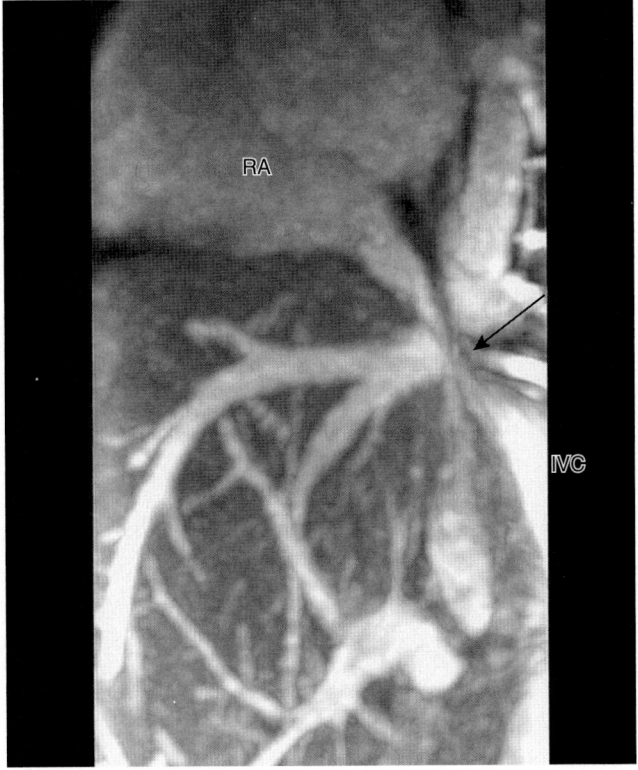

B

FIGURE 118-22. Hepatic vein stenosis. **A,** US demonstrates stenosis *(arrow)* at the typical high location near the diaphragm, where it may be exceedingly difficult to identify. **B,** Sagittal plane magnetic resonance venography shows tight stenosis *(arrow)* and retraction of both the hepatic veins and the inferior vena cava (IVC). RA, right atrium.

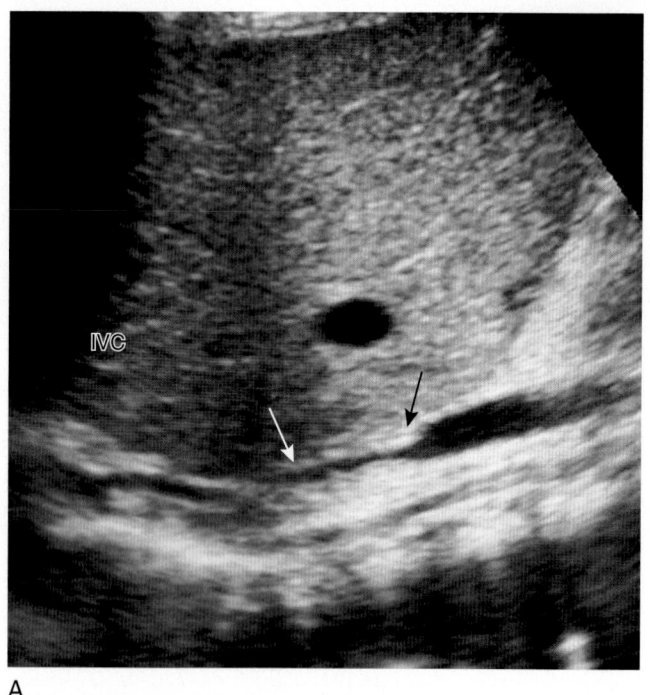

A

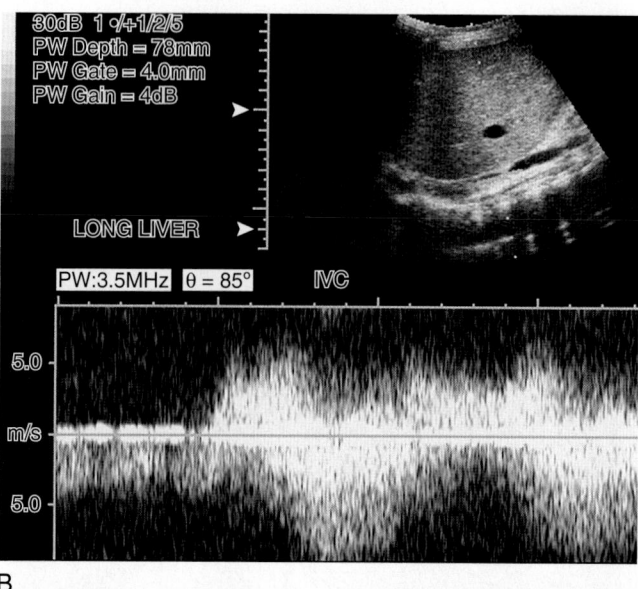

B

FIGURE 118-23. Long-segment inferior vena cava (IVC) stenosis. **A,** Longitudinal ultrasound image shows a long-segment IVC narrowing *(arrows)* along the posterior aspect of the transplanted liver graft. **B,** Spectral Doppler shows an extremely high-velocity turbulence at the stenotic site. **C,** Sagittal reconstruction of CTA shows the long-segment IVC narrowing *(arrows)*.

C

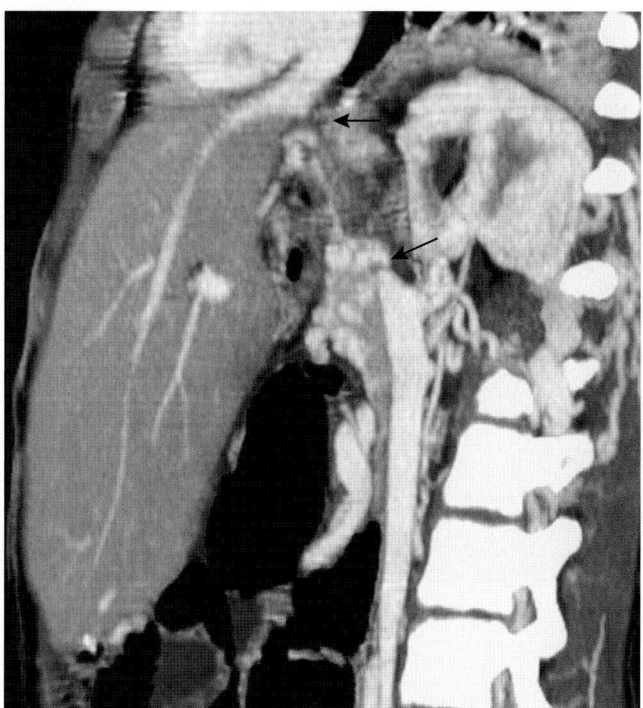

FIGURE 118-24. Complete occlusion of the inferior vena cava along the posterior aspect of the liver segment *(arrows)*. Note that the obstruction is distal to the hepatic veins, which drain into the proximal inferior vena cava and right atrium undisturbed.

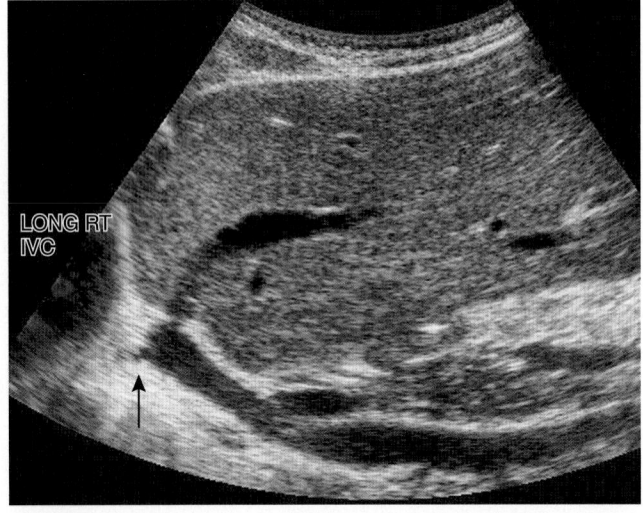

A

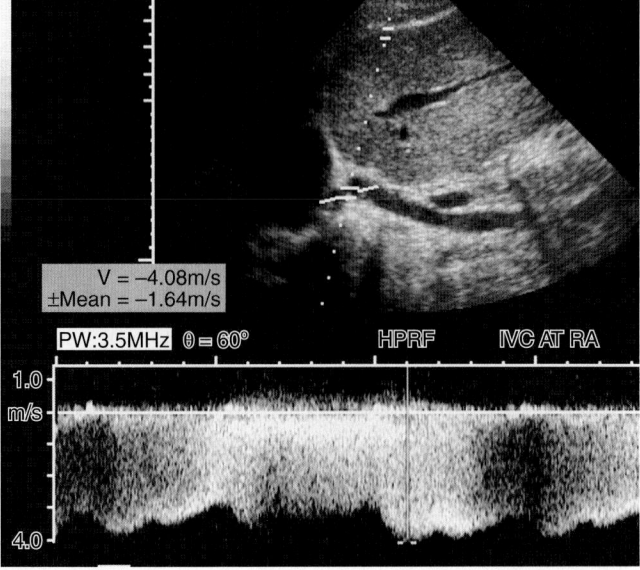

B

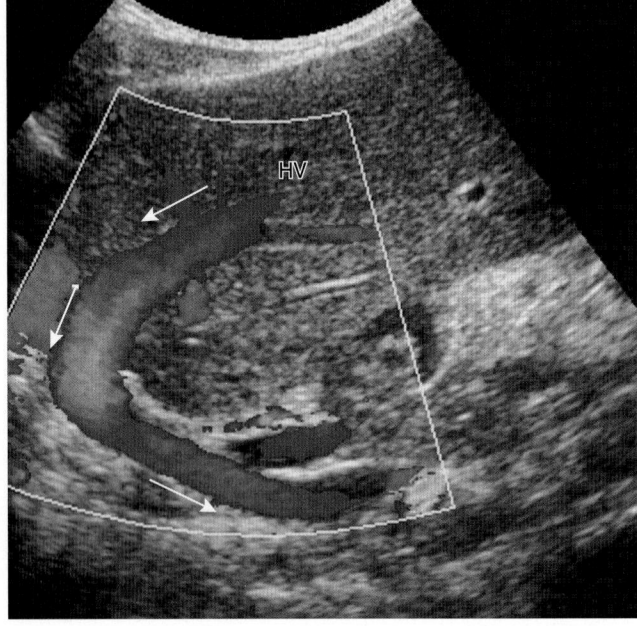

C

FIGURE 118-25. Stenosis of the inferior vena cava (IVC) proximal to the hepatic vein anastomosis. **A,** Longitudinal ultrasound image shows a tight, discrete IVC stenosis *(arrow)* between the hepatic vein anastomosis and the right atrium. **B,** Spectral and color Doppler interrogation shows a high-velocity jet of greater than 4 m/sec. **C,** Color Doppler shows easily identified flow in the hepatic vein (HV), which continues retrogradely *(arrows)* down the IVC distal to the stenosis. (*See color plate.*)

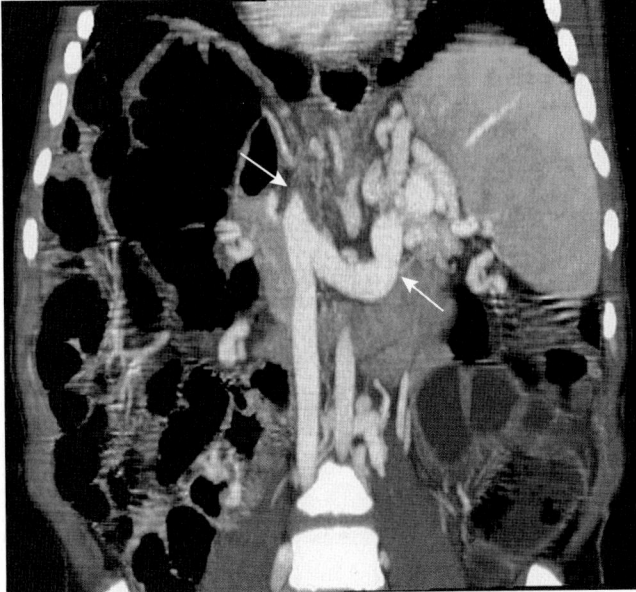

FIGURE 118-26. Inferior vena cava occlusion in a patient with a distal splenorenal shunt. Coronal reconstruction from CTA shows that both systemic venous return and splenic venous blood drain through the splenorenal shunt in a retrograde fashion, into an extensive collateral venous bed. The inferior vena cava obstruction is marked by *arrows*.

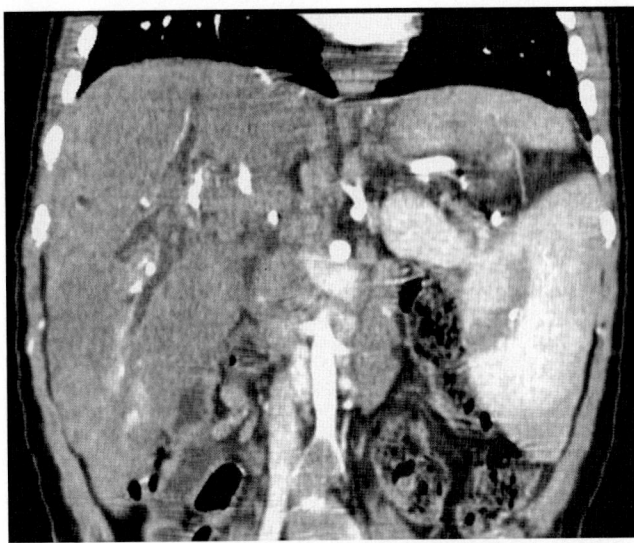

FIGURE 118-27. Bile duct stricture. Coronal reconstruction from CTA shows bile duct dilation.

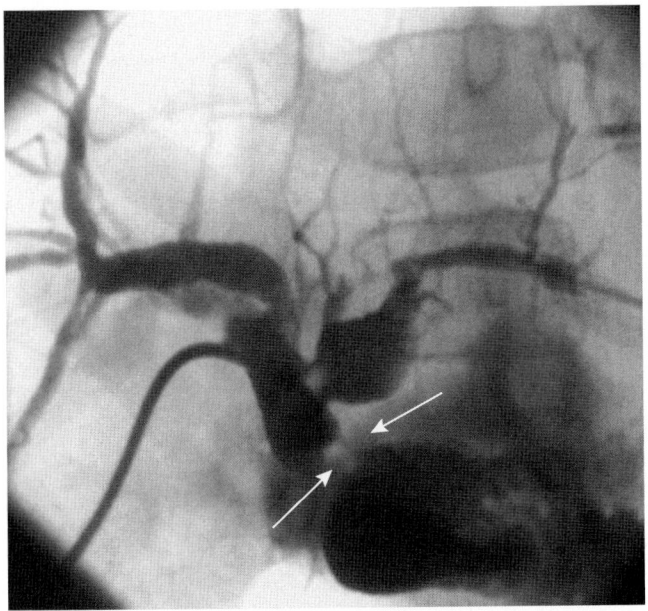

FIGURE 118-28. Percutaneous cholangiogram shows a tight stricture at the anastomosis between the donor left bile duct and the recipient Roux-en-Y loop *(arrows)*. A second branch stricture is also present. The image was obtained during percutaneous dilation of the stenosis.

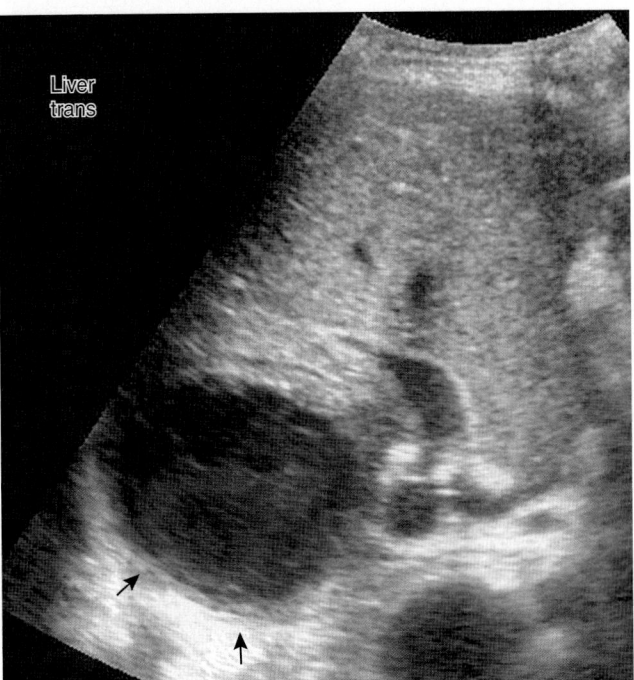

A

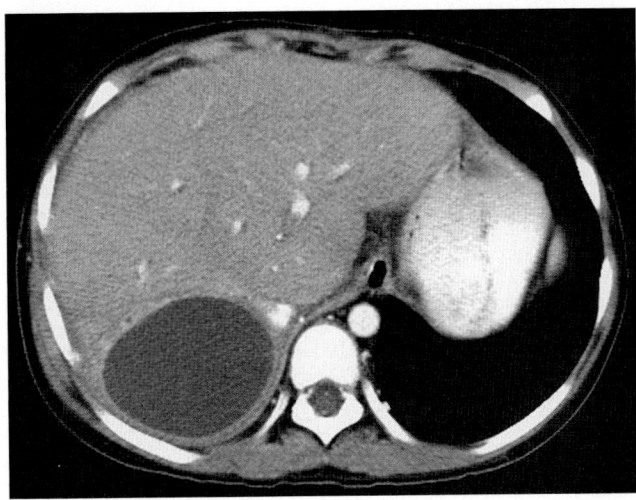

B

FIGURE 118-29. Infected bile collection at the cut edge of the transplanted left lobe graft. **A,** US shows a nonspecific fluid collection *(arrows)* containing ample debris. **B,** CT of the same patient shows the fluid collection, but the fluid characteristics are less apparent.

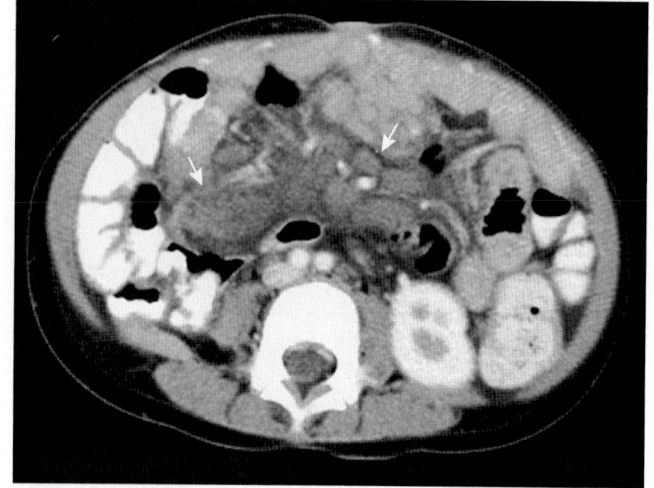

A

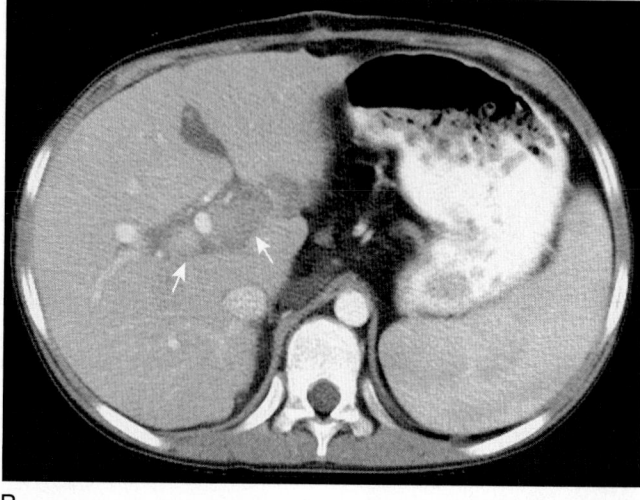

B

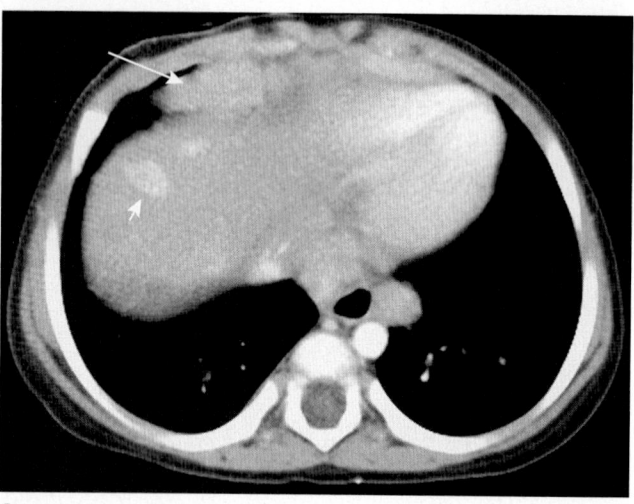

C

FIGURE 118-30. Post-transplantation lymphoproliferative disease. **A,** CT scan of the abdomen shows multiple enlarged mesenteric lymph nodes *(arrows).* **B,** High CT slice shows lymphadenopathy in the transplanted liver hilum *(arrows).* **C,** CT slice at the level of the diaphragm shows an enhancing liver nodule *(short arrow)* and pericardial *(long arrow)* and posterior mediastinal lymphadenopathy.

SUGGESTED READINGS

General

Freeman RB Jr, Weisner RH, Roberts JP, et al: Improving liver allocation: MELD and PELD. Am J Transplant 2004; 4(Suppl 9):114-131

Keefe EB: Liver transplantation at the millennium: past, present and future. Clin Liver Dis 2000;4:241-255

McDiarmid SV, Merion RM, Dykstra DM, Harper AM: Selection of pediatric candidates under the PELD system. Liver Transplant 2004;10(Suppl 2):S23-S30

Millis MJ, Cronin DC, Brady LM, et al: Primary living-donor liver transplantation at the University of Chicago: technical aspects of the first 104 recipients. Ann Surg 2000;232:104-111

Otte JB: History of pediatric liver transplantation. Where are we coming from? Where do we stand? Pediatr Transplant 2002; 6:378-387

Renz JF, Yersiz H, Reichert PR, et al: Split-liver transplantation: a review. Am J Transplant 2003;3:1323-1335

Rogiers X, Malago M, Gawad K, et al: In-situ splitting of the cadaveric livers: the ultimate expansion of a limited donor pool. Ann Surg 1996;224:331-339

Starzl TE, Groth C, Brettschneider L, et al: Orthotopic transplantation of the human liver. Ann Surg 1968;168:392-415

Starzl TE, Marchiaro TL, Von Kaulla K, et al: Homotransplantation of the liver in humans. Surg Gynecol Obstet 1963;117:659-676

Indications

Baerg J, Zuppan C, Klooster M: Biliary atresia—a fifteen year review of clinical and pathologic factors associated with liver transplantation. J Pediatr Surg 2004;39:800-803

Barshes NR, Myers GD, Lee D, et al: Liver transplantation for severe graft-versus-host disease: an analysis of aggregate survival data. Liver Transplant 2005;11:525-531

Dasgupta D, Guthrie A, McClean P, et al: Liver transplantation for hilar inflammatory myofibroblastic tumor. Pediatr Transplant 2004;8:517-521

Fridell JA, Bond GJ, Mazariegos GV, et al: Liver transplantation in children with cystic fibrosis: a long-term longitudinal review of a single center's experience. J Pediatr Surg 2003;38:1152-1156

Lang H, Oldhafer KJ, Weinman A, et al: Liver transplantation for metastatic neuroendocrine tumors. Ann Surg 1997;225:347-354

Lee B, Goss J: Long term treatment of urea cycle disorders. J Pediatr 2001;138(Suppl 1):S62-S71

McDiarmid SV, Millis MJ, Otloff KM, So KM: Indications for pediatric liver transplantation. Pediatr Transplant 1998;2:106-116

Mieli-Vergani G, Vergani D: Immunological liver disease in children. Semin Liver Dis 1998;18:271-279

Noble-Jamieson G, Barnes N, Jamieson N, et al: Liver transplantation for hepatic cirrhosis in cystic fibrosis. J R Soc Med 1996; 89(Suppl 27):31-37

Otte JB, Pritchard J, Aronson DC, et al: Liver transplantation for hepatoblastoma: results from the International Society of Pediatric

Oncology (SIOP) study SIOPEL—and review of the world experience. Pediatr Blood Cancer 2004;42:74-83

Podgaetz E, Chan C: Liver transplantation for Wilson disease. Ann Hepatol 2003;2:131-134

Shinkai M, Ohhama Y, Nishi T, et al: Living related liver transplantation for hyperammonemia due to congenital absence of portal vein. Transplant Proc 2000;32:2184

Tiao GM, Bobey N, Allen S, et al: The current management of hepatoblastoma: a combination of chemotherapy, conventional resection and liver transplantation. J Pediatr 2005;146:204-211

Wendell U, Saudubray JM, Bodner A, Schadewaldt P: Liver transplantation in maple syrup urine disease. Eur J Pediatr 1999;158(Suppl 2):S60-S64

Pretransplant Imaging

Bisset GS, Strife JL, Balisteri WF: Evaluation of children for liver transplantation: value of MR imaging and sonography. AJR Am J Roentgenol 1990;155:351-356

Cheng YF, Chen CL, Jawan B, et al: Multislice computed tomography angiography in pediatric liver transplantation. Transplantation 2003;76:353-357

Cheng YF, Huang TL, Lui CC, et al: Magnetic resonance venography in potential pediatric liver transplant recipients. Clin Transplant 1997;11:121-126

Esquivel CO, Gutierrez C, Cox KL, et al: Hepatocellular carcinoma and liver cell dysplasia in children with chronic liver disease. J Pediatr Surg 1994;29:1465-1469

Ledesma-Medina J, Dominguez R, Bowen A, et al: Pediatric liver transplantation. Part I. Standardization of preoperative diagnostic imaging. Radiology 1985;157:335-338

Naik KS, Ward J, Irving HC, Robinson PJ: Comparison of dynamic contrast enhanced MRI and Doppler ultrasound in the pre-operative assessment of the portal venous system. Br J Radiol 1997;70:43-49

Surgical Anatomy

Caron KH, Strife JL, Babcock DS, Ryckman FC: Left-lobe hepatic transplants: spectrum of normal imaging findings. AJR Am J Roentgenol 1992;158:497-501

Couinaud C: Definition of hepatic anatomical regions and their value during hepatectomy [author's trans; in French.] Chirurgie 1980;106:103-108

Martich V, Ben-Ami TE, Yousefzadeh DK, et al: Anatomic features of reduced-size liver transplant: postsurgical imaging characteristics. Radiology 1993;187:165-170

Postoperative Imaging and Complications

Buell JF, Funaki B, Cronin DC, et al: Long-term venous complications after full-size and segmental pediatric liver transplantation. Ann Surg 2002;236:658-666

Cao S, Cox KL: Epstein Barr virus lymphoproliferative disorders after liver transplantation. Clin Liver Dis 1997;1:453-469

Cheng YF, Chen CL, Huang TL, et al: 3DCT angiography for detection of vascular complications in pediatric liver transplantation. Liver Transplant 2004;10:248-252

De Gaetano AM, Controneo AR, Maresca G, et al: Color Doppler sonography in the diagnosis of arterial complications after liver transplantation. J Clin Ultrasound 2000;28:373-380

Friedewald SM, Molmenti EP, DeLong MR, Hamper UM: Vascular and nonvascular complication of liver transplants: sonographic evaluation and correlation with other imaging modalities and findings at surgery and pathology. Ultrasound Q 2003;19:71-85

George TI, Berquist W, Cherry AM, et al: Epstein-Barr virus-associated peripheral T-cell lymphoma and hemophagocytic syndrome arising after liver transplantation. Pediatr Blood Cancer 2005;44:270-276

Hall TR, McDiarmid SV, Grant EG, et al: False-negative duplex Doppler studies in children with hepatic artery thrombosis after liver transplantation. AJR Am J Roentgenol 1990;154:573-575

Holmes RD, Sokol RJ: Epstein-Barr virus and post-transplantation lymphoproliferative disease. Pediatr Transplant 2002;6:456-464

Kim BS, Kim TK, Jung DJ, et al: Vascular complications after living related liver transplantation: evaluation with gadolinium-enhanced three dimensional MR angiography. AJR Am J Roentgenol 2003;181:467-474

Kuang AA, Renz JF, Ferrell LD, et al: Failure patterns of cryopreserved vein grafts in liver transplantation. Transplantation 1996;62:742-747

Laor T, Hoffer FA, Vacanti JP, Jonas MM: MR cholangiography in children after liver transplantation from living related donors. AJR Am J Roentgenol 1998;170:683-687

Lee J, Ben-Ami TE, Yousefzadeh DK, et al: Extrahepatic portal vein stenosis in recipients of living donor allografts: Doppler sonography. AJR Am J Roentgenol 1996;167:85-90

Norton KI, Lee JS, Kogan D, et al: The role of magnetic resonance cholangiography in the management of children and young adults after liver transplantation. Pediatr Transplant 2001;5:410-418

Pariente D, Bihet MH, Tammam S, et al: Biliary complications after transplantation in children: role of imaging modalities. Pediatr Radiol 1991;21:175-178

Pasquale MA, Weppler D, Smith J, et al: Burkitt's lymphoma variant of post-transplantation lymphoproliferative disease(PTLD). Pathol Oncol Res 2002;8:105-108

Sheiner PA, Varma CV, Guarrera JV, et al: Selective revascularization of hepatic artery thromboses after liver transplantation improves patient and graft survival. Transplantation 1997;64:1295-1299

Someda H, Moiyasu F, Fujimoto M, et al: Vascular complications of living related liver transplantation detected with intraoperative and postoperative Doppler US. J Hepatol 1995;22:623-632

Ueda M, Egawa K, Ogawa K, et al: Portal vein complications in the long term course after living donor liver transplantation. Transplant Proc 2005;37:1138-1140

PART 5   THE SPLEEN

CHAPTER 119

The Spleen

STEPHANIE E. SPOTTSWOOD, SHARON M. STEIN, and JEANNE G. HILL

ANATOMY AND EMBRYOLOGY

The spleen is the largest of the body's lymphatic structures and the second largest organ of the reticuloendothelial system. Situated in the left upper quadrant, the spleen normally lies between the stomach and the diaphragm. In adults, the spleen is comparable in length to the kidney. The superolateral surface of the spleen approximates the diaphragm, which separates it from the 9th through 11th ribs and from the inferior left lung and pleura. The inferior pole of the spleen abuts the splenic flexure of the colon. The visceral surface has a renal portion in relation to the superior pole of the left kidney and to the left adrenal gland. The gastric portion is in contact with the posterior wall of the stomach and the tail of the pancreas. The splenic hilum is a depression along the medial surface through which the splenic artery and vein and the splenic nerves pass. The spleen is maintained in its normal position by ligaments formed by peritoneal folds. The two major ligaments are the gastrosplenic ligament, which runs between the spleen and the stomach and contains the short gastric and gastroepiploic arteries, and the splenorenal ligament, which reflects onto the splenic hilum and envelops the pancreatic tail and the proximal splenic vein. The phrenicosplenic ligament contains the major splenic vessels. Other ligaments that help support the spleen are the splenocolic, pancreaticosplenic, phrenocolic, and pancreaticocolic.

The spleen consists of a larger red pulp and a white pulp composed of lymphocytes and macrophages. The spleen is responsible for filtering red blood cells that lack contractility, as well as antigen-coated cells, bacteria, and foreign particles. The spleen also acts as a platelet reservoir, releasing platelets in response to epinephrine release or consuming platelets in case of splenomegaly.

The spleen appears in the fifth week of embryonic life as a localized thickening of the mesoderm in the dorsal mesogastrium above the pancreatic tail. Normally, the spleen forms from the coalescence of multiple small splenic masses. Accessory spleens are therefore not uncommon, particularly in children. As the stomach rotates its greater curvature to the left, the spleen is carried with it into the left upper quadrant. The gastrosplenic ligament is derived from the residuum of the dorsal mesogastrium. The primary function of the embryonic spleen is erythropoiesis, which is maximal in the middle of the second trimester and subsequently diminishes.

IMAGING THE SPLEEN

On plain films of the abdomen, the spleen may be seen in the left upper quadrant, displacing the stomach medially and the colon inferiorly. The spleen may be obscured when large amounts of gas are present in the gastrointestinal tract.

The spleen is easily identified on abdominal ultrasonography (US). It has a homogeneous sonographic texture. The splenic hilar vessels are usually well seen, but intrasplenic vessels typically require Doppler for identification. Using coronal scans, Rosenberg and coworkers measured the normal spleen length in children during quiet respiration and correlated the results with age, height, and weight. The upper limit of normal was 6.0 cm at 3 months, 6.5 cm at 6 months, 7.0 cm at 12 months, 8.0 cm at 2 years, 9.0 cm at 4 years, 9.5 cm at 6 years, 10.0 cm at 8 years, 11.0 cm at 10 years, and 11.5 cm at 12 years. The upper limit of normal at age 15 years and older was 12.0 cm for girls and 13.0 cm for boys. As a general rule, the tip of the spleen should not extend below the inferior pole of the left kidney (Fig. 119-1).

On computed tomography (CT), the normal spleen has a higher attenuation than the liver. A uniform increase in attenuation occurs after the administration of intravenous contrast agents. Transient heterogeneous splenic enhancement patterns are commonly encountered during the first minute of contrast-enhanced CT, particularly with the rapid bolus technique (Fig. 119-2). This splenic enhancement pattern is a normal phenomenon thought to be secondary to variations in blood flow through the red and white pulp of the spleen; it is more pronounced with contrast injection rates of 1 ml/sec or greater and in children older than 1 year. Common patterns of heterogeneity include (1) arciform, consisting of ringlike or zebra-stripe bands of alternating density; (2) focal areas of low density; and (3) diffuse, mottled

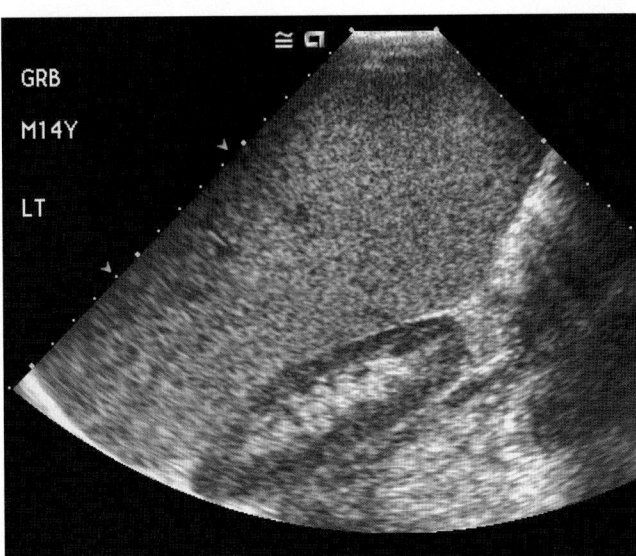

FIGURE 119-1. Splenomegaly in a 14-year-old boy with anemia. Coronal ultrasound image shows that the spleen extends below (caudad to) the lower pole of the left kidney.

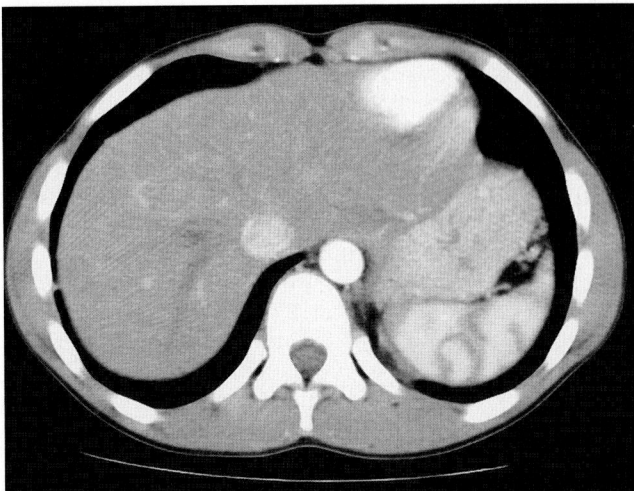

FIGURE 119-2. Contrast bolus artifact on CT. An arciform contrast enhancement pattern is seen in the spleen, with ringlike or zebra-stripe bands of alternating density.

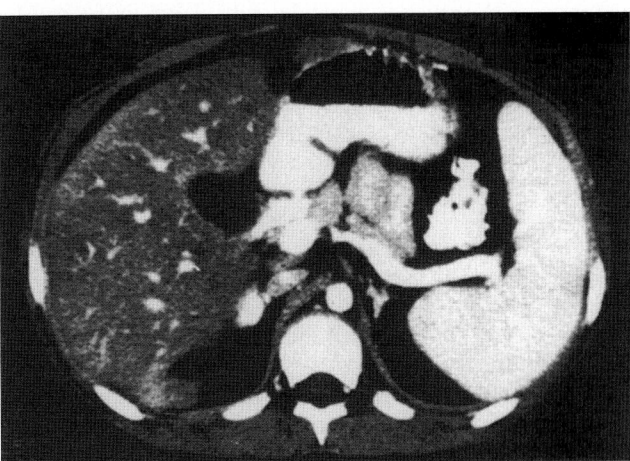

FIGURE 119-3. Normal spleen in an obese 11-year-old boy on CT photographed at narrow window settings after intravenous contrast enhancement. There is uniform enhancement of the spleen and excellent visualization of the splenic vein. There is low attenuation of the liver, consistent with fatty replacement.

areas of inhomogeneity. Paterson and colleagues described a pattern-oriented approach to imaging of the spleen, assessing abnormalities in shape, location, and size and the presence of solitary versus multiple lesions through various techniques.

> **Transient heterogeneous splenic enhancement patterns are commonly encountered during rapid bolus techniques on contrast-enhanced CT.**

Computed tomography angiography (CTA) demonstrates the splenic vessels remarkably well. On dynamic contrast-enhanced CT scans, the splenic vein is well identified and can usually be followed across the abdomen to its juncture with the superior mesenteric vein, forming the portal vein (Fig. 119-3). The splenic artery can also be seen on dynamic scans. Because the artery is less tortuous in children than in adults, it can often be identified throughout much of its course.

On T1-weighted spin echo magnetic resonance imaging (MRI) sections, the spleen has lower signal intensity than the liver and slightly greater signal intensity than muscle. On T2-weighted images, the spleen has higher signal intensity than the liver. The major splenic vessels are well demonstrated because of the characteristic signal void of flowing blood. Magnetic resonance angiography (MRA) also demonstrates the splenic vessels to excellent advantage.

Technetium-99m–labeled sulfur colloid is removed from the blood by the spleen's reticuloendothelial system, permitting its visualization. Isotopic splenic scanning is useful for the identification of splenic ectopia, as well as numerous disease states (described later). It is not as useful in cases of heterotaxy, because splenic and hepatic tissue can be confused, particularly when neither location nor shape is a distinguishing criterion.

Angiography is rarely used for intrasplenic disease, but arterial portography to evaluate the portal venous system offers excellent visualization of the spleen and its vessels. This technique has been largely superseded by CTA and MRA.

CONGENITAL ANOMALIES

Accessory Spleen

The most common congenital anomaly of the spleen is the presence of one or more *accessory spleens,* or splenuli. These occur in 10% to 15% of the normal population and are usually found incidentally at autopsy or on imaging studies. They number six or fewer and are most commonly located in the splenic hilum, in association with the splenic vessels, or in the gastrosplenic ligament. They can be found, however, virtually anywhere in the abdomen. They rarely exceed 2 cm in diameter and are often confused with splenic hilar or parapancreatic lymph nodes. They can be identified on US or CT, but the definitive imaging study is technetium-99m sulfur colloid liver-spleen scans.

Wandering Spleen

Normally, the residuum of the dorsal mesogastrium fuses with the posterior peritoneum, helping to support the spleen in its normal position. When this fusion does not take place, the dorsal mesogastrium may persist as a long mesentery, allowing the spleen to migrate, the so-called *wandering spleen*. The most common location for these ectopic spleens is the left lower quadrant. This congenital anomaly consists of maldevelopment of the splenic suspensory ligaments, including the gastrosplenic, splenorenal, and phrenicocolic ligaments. Acquired cases have also been described and can result from splenomegaly, traumatic injury, or ligamentous laxity.

The abnormal position and orientation of the spleen can be identified by US, CT, or radionuclide imaging with technetium-99m sulfur colloid scan. It is important to pay close attention to the abnormal orientation and location of the spleen. Typically, no splenic tissue can be identified in the left upper quadrant, although a small accessory spleen may remain in the normal anatomic location. The wandering spleen may undergo torsion, causing severe pain secondary to ischemia. A "whorled" appearance of the splenic artery in the splenic pedicle has been described as a characteristic CT sign of torsion. The twisted spleen has little uptake on radionuclide scans and no contrast enhancement on CT (Fig. 119-4). Color Doppler sonography shows lack of flow in the splenic hilar vessels and may also demonstrate the whorled appearance at the splenic hilum.

Treatment is operative, consisting of splenopexy if the spleen is viable or splenectomy if it is nonviable. Because of the defective ligamentous support, gastric volvulus has been associated with wandering spleen (see Fig. 119-4).

> **A "whorled" appearance of the splenic artery and vein in the splenic pedicle is a characteristic CT sign of splenic torsion.**

Splenogonadal Syndrome

The splenogonadal syndrome is a rare anomaly in which a portion of the splenic anlage fuses with primitive left gonadal tissue between the fifth and eighth weeks of gestation. Despite the fused splenic tissue, a normal spleen is present in the left upper quadrant. The splenogonadal fusion is continuous in approximately 56% of cases, with the splenic cord continuous with the ectopic, fused splenic tissue; it is discontinuous in approximately 44% of cases. Splenogonadal fusion is much more common in males, with a male-female ratio of 16:1. The condition may be asymptomatic and discovered incidentally or at autopsy. It may be associated with left cryptorchidism, inguinal hernia, or testicular torsion, particularly when continuous. Multiple other anomalies may be present, particularly in the continuous type. In females, there is fusion of splenic tissue with the left

ovary or mesovarium; this connection does not result in ovarian ectopia.

Although this is an uncommon congenital anomaly, its identification is important because 30% to 50% of cases result in unnecessary orchiectomy for suspicion of extratesticular neoplasm. When the diagnosis is confirmed by means of imaging and the child is asymptomatic, no treatment is necessary. However, if surgical exploration is performed, the splenic tissue can be dissected safely off the tunica albuginea, and the testis can be preserved.

Sonography can reliably demonstrate the extratesticular location of a palpable scrotal mass in these cases. The mass is typically oval or round and of similar echotexture to the adjacent normal testis (Fig. 119-5). It usually has a slightly different size or configuration from the testis. Color Doppler sonography shows abundant vascularity in the splenic tissue (see Fig. 119-5). Radionuclide imaging with technetium-99m sulfur colloid adds specificity to the diagnosis by revealing radiopharmaceutical uptake in the ectopic splenic tissue either in the left hemiscrotum or in the left inguinal canal when associated with cryptorchidism. A linear pattern extending from the left upper quadrant of the abdomen to the pelvis or scrotum may also be detected in the continuous type (see Fig. 119-5).

> **Splenogonadal fusion can be readily detected with technetium-99m sulfur colloid scintigraphy by revealing radiopharmaceutical uptake in the ectopic splenic tissue in the left hemiscrotum.**

Although it is not the imaging modality of choice, contrast-enhanced CT may reveal a rounded, enhancing, well-circumscribed soft tissue mass in the left hemiscrotum or left hemipelvis that may or may not continue cephalad toward the spleen. MRI may be useful to distinguish testicular from extratesticular lesions and solid from cystic lesions.

Abnormal Visceroatrial Situs

Abnormal visceroatrial situs is an intriguing set of entities in which the spleen plays a prominent role. The normal visceroatrial anatomy is known as situs solitus, or usual position. Situs inversus refers to mirror-image visceroatrial anatomy. Patients with situs inversus are frequently asymptomatic, although there is a slightly higher incidence of congenital heart disease. Situs ambiguus, or visceroatrial heterotaxia, refers to deranged visceroatrial symmetry. Patients with this abnormality are divided into two major groups: those with a tendency toward right-sided symmetry and asplenia, and those with a tendency toward left-sided symmetry and polysplenia. Each patient has a unique constellation of anatomic findings, and each must be evaluated and described individually. However, broad categorizations can be made.

Patients with *asplenia* have right-sided isomerism. The spleen is absent, and the liver may appear to have two mirror-image right lobes with a midline gallbladder. The ambiguous atrium resembles the right atrium, and

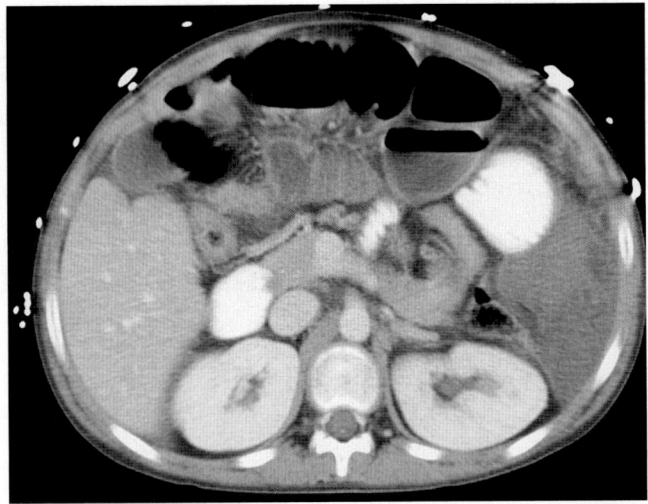

FIGURE 119-4. Wandering spleen in a 14-year-old girl with Niemann-Pick disease and the acute onset of abdominal pain. **A,** Contrast-enhanced CT images of the abdomen show a "whorled" appearance of the splenic vessels and pancreatic tail. There is low attenuation of the spleen, consistent with diminished or absent perfusion, and surrounding edema. **B,** Coronal reconstruction shows displacement of the spleen and lack of contrast enhancement. **C,** One year after splenectomy, the child presented with hypotension and abdominal distention. Coronal reconstruction of abdominal CT performed with oral contrast reveals reversal of the usual relationship of the gastric fundus and gastric outlet, consistent with gastric volvulus. Note the gastric pneumatosis.

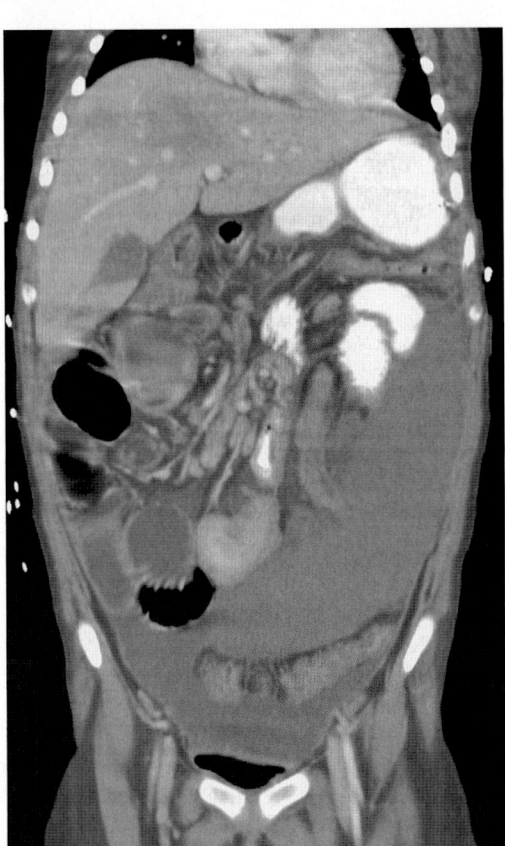

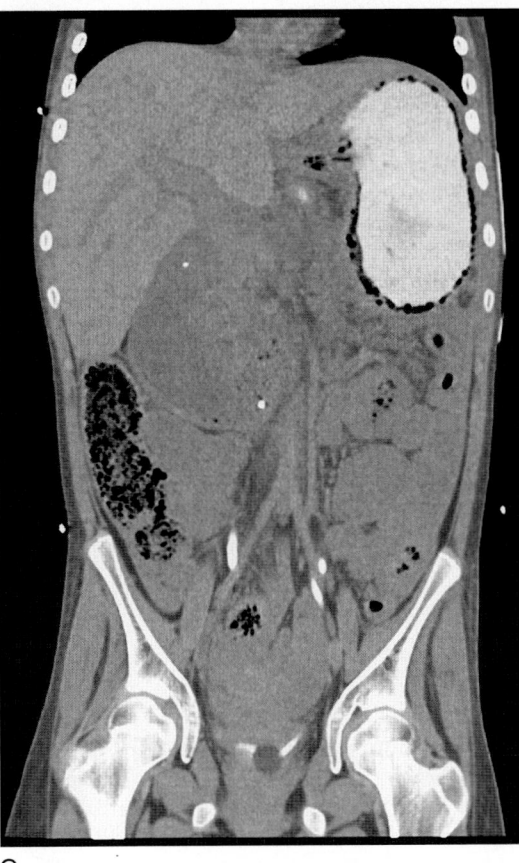

severe congenital cardiac lesions are typically present, usually with diminished pulmonary blood flow. Total anomalous venous connections may be seen. Two trilobed lungs with bilateral eparterial bronchi resembling two right lungs and two right hila are typically present. Midgut malrotation is typical, with the stomach on the right, left, or midline. The inferior vena cava (IVC) is nearly always present and may lie to the right or left of the aorta, crossing the midline anterior to the aorta to enter the atrium, if necessary.

Patients with *polysplenia* have left-sided isomerism. Multiple splenules are typically present (Figs. 119-6 and

119-7); however, there is a spectrum of anomalies, and there may be merely septations of the splenic mass. Because splenic tissue develops in the dorsal mesogastrium, the splenules are found dorsal to the stomach, along the greater curvature, whether the stomach lies on the left or the right. Interruption of the intrahepatic IVC is seen in approximately half of patients, with either right-sided or left-sided azygos continuation. When the IVC is present, it may lie to the right or left of the aorta. A preduodenal portal vein may be seen. Approximately 10% of infants with biliary atresia have polysplenia. In these patients, it is important to evaluate the continuity

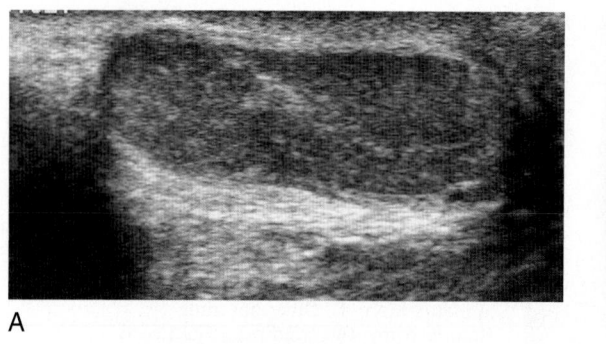

A

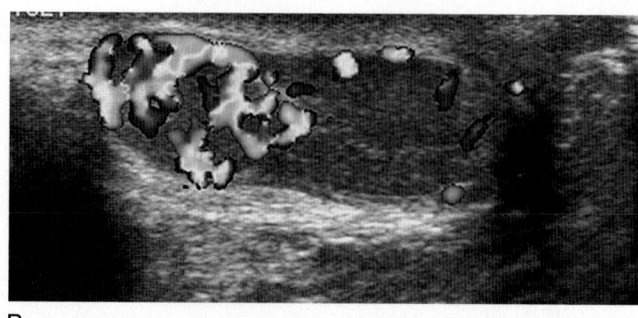

B

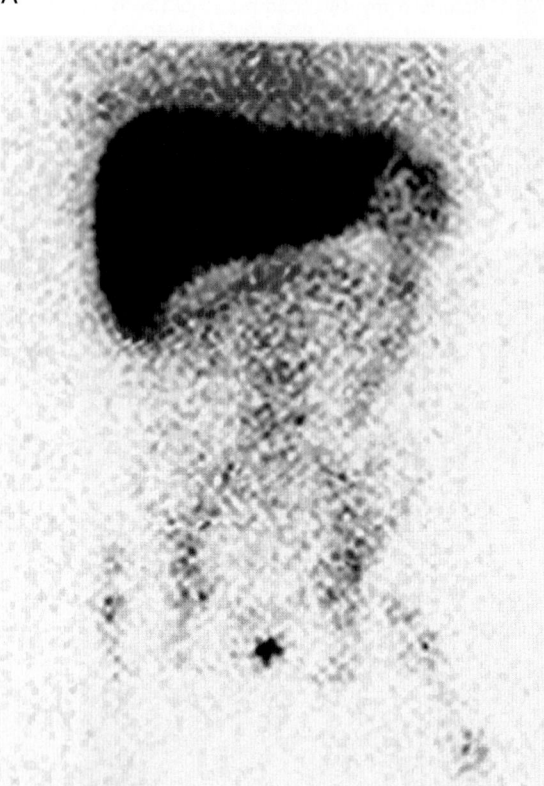

C

FIGURE 119-5. Splenogonadal fusion in a boy with a painless left scrotal mass. **A,** Longitudinal ultrasound image in the left hemiscrotum reveals round-shaped splenic tissue cephalad to the testicle, isoechoic and fused to the more oval-shaped testis. **B,** Color Doppler image shows marked vascularity of the splenic tissue compared with the testicle. (*See color plate.*) **C,** Technetium-99m sulfur colloid liver-spleen scan shows radiopharmaceutical uptake in the expected location of the spleen, as well as within a persistent cord of tissue connecting the spleen with the left testis. Note continuous radiopharmaceutical uptake in the left hemiscrotum, representing splenic tissue next to the testis. (Courtesy of A. Schlesinger, Houston, TX.)

of the IVC and the course of the portal vein, because these vascular derangements are important in patients later referred for liver transplantation. Bilateral bilobed lungs with hyparterial bronchi resembling two left lungs are usually present. Congenital heart disease is often present, although some patients with polysplenia are asymptomatic, and the diagnosis may be made incidentally. Midgut malrotation is typical. Other anomalies, including duodenal atresia or stenosis and renal anomalies, are occasionally present. A short pancreas has been described secondary to failure of development of the dorsal pancreatic bud. Rare anomalies include central nervous system malformations, palatal abnormalities, and a congenitally absent left adrenal gland.

Noninvasive imaging can correctly identify the major anomalies of asplenia and polysplenia syndromes. Combinations of US, CT, and MRI can delineate the extent of the viscerovascular anomalies.

- Situs ambiguous or heterotaxy may present as a right-sided tendency and asplenia or a left-sided tendency and polysplenia.

- Splenules in polysplenia may be multiple or show septations within a larger splenic mass. They are typically located along the greater curvature of the stomach.

- Polysplenia may be associated with biliary atresia, azygos continuation of the intrahepatic IVC, and preduodenal portal vein.

SPLENOMEGALY

Splenomegaly refers to enlargement of the spleen, usually as a result of excessive destruction of abnormal blood cells, excessive antigenic stimulation, storage or infiltrative disorders, or portal venous congestion. *Hypersplen-*

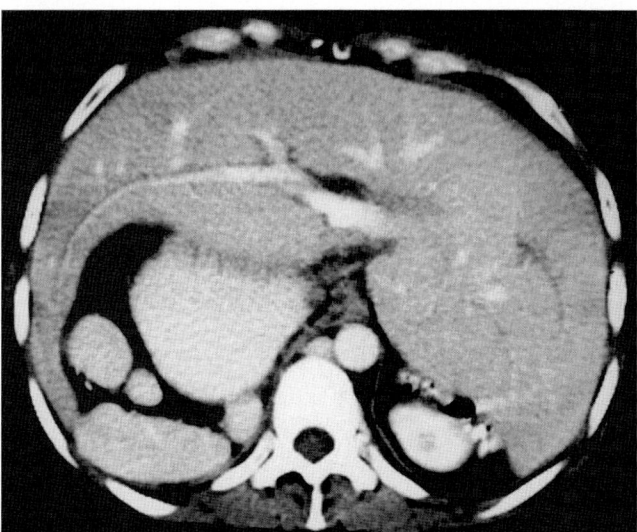

FIGURE 119-6. Multiple splenules in the right upper quadrant of the abdomen. in a child with situs ambiguous and polysplenia. Contrast-enhanced CT also shows the abnormally positioned liver and stomach and azygos continuation of the IVC. (Courtesy of Henrique Lederman, Sao Paulo, Brazil.)

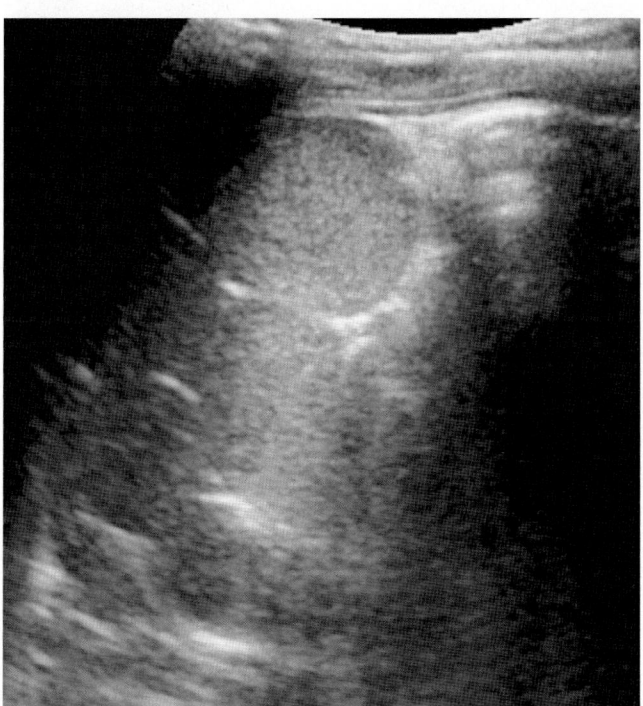

FIGURE 119-7. Multiple splenules in the right upper quadrant of a 2-year-old with polysplenia syndrome are identified on a transverse sonogram of the abdomen. (Courtesy of Marta Hernanz-Schulman, Nashville, TN.)

ism, in contrast, refers to the syndrome of sequestration of blood cell lines by an enlarged spleen, particularly platelets.

The spleen may become enlarged in several inherited conditions (Table 119-1). The hemolytic anemias frequently cause splenomegaly, with hereditary spherocytosis, hereditary elliptocytosis, and thalassemia being the most common. Sickle cell anemia initially leads to

TABLE 119-1
Differential Diagnosis of Splenomegaly

Portal hypertension
Extramedullary hematopoiesis
Hemolytic anemia
Infection
Cyst
  Congenital
  Acquired (usually infectious)
Benign neoplasms
  Hemangioma
  Lymphangioma
  Hamartoma
Malignant neoplasms
  Leukemia
  Lymphoma
  Metastases

splenomegaly, followed by splenic atrophy secondary to multiple infarcts. In some cases, iron deposition secondary to transfusion therapy results in increased attenuation of the spleen on CT and decreased signal intensity on MRI. Patients with portal hypertension from a number of causes, including biliary atresia or absence of the portal vein, have congestive splenomegaly. The imaging findings are nonspecific as to cause, unless there is evidence of extramedullary hematopoiesis or infarcts. Extramedullary hematopoiesis may demonstrate focal areas of increased echogenicity on sonography, whereas infarcts may appear as hypoechoic areas. The storage diseases generally cause nonspecific splenomegaly, but Gaucher disease may lead to focal hypoechoic foci, reflecting collections of Gaucher cells, as described by Hill and associates. The focal collections may occasionally be hyperechoic secondary to fibrosis.

Splenomegaly can also occur in a variety of acquired disorders, including infection and neoplasm (discussed later). Acquired causes of portal hypertension, such as cavernous transformation of the portal vein or secondary cirrhosis of the liver in patients with cystic fibrosis, may present with splenomegaly. Imaging studies can sometimes determine the cause of splenic enlargement through the identification of ancillary findings, such as varices in patients with congestive splenomegaly (Fig. 119-8).

Sequestration in sickle cell disease normally occurs in children younger than 5 years but can occur up to adolescence. The pathophysiology is sequestration of impaired red blood cells by the spleen, leading to splenomegaly, anemia, and thrombocytopenia. It can present as an acute emergency and necessitate transfusion to counteract hypotension and severe anemia. Splenectomy is used sparingly. Once a child has a sequestration crisis, there is a higher risk of recurrence. The long-term management consists of increased awareness of symptoms (primarily worsening anemia) and signs (enlarging spleen) and, in some cases, short-term chronic transfusion. In most sickle cell patients, splenic function is diminished because of splenic infarcts, and autosplenectomy is frequent by age 5 to 6 years. Recent evidence suggests

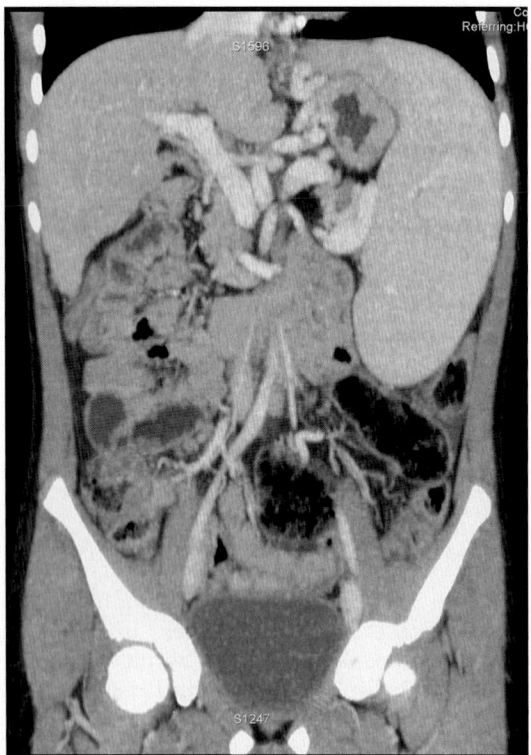

FIGURE 119-8. Portal hypertension in an 11-year-old girl with liver disease. Coronal reconstruction of contrast-enhanced CT of the abdomen shows splenic extension to the left lower quadrant. Multiple variceal collaterals are clearly depicted.

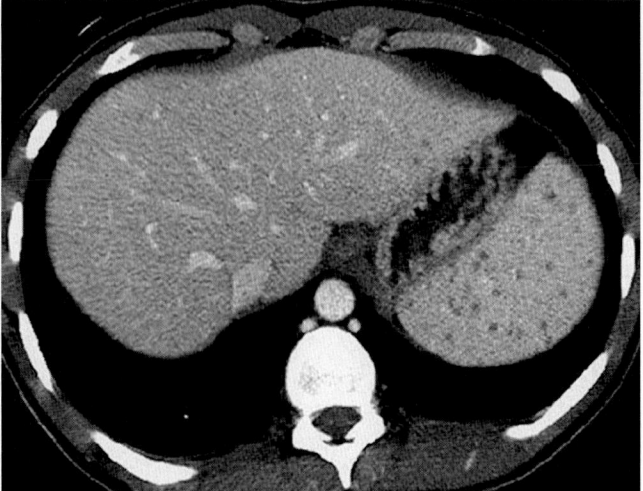

FIGURE 119-9. Candidiasis in an immune-suppressed child. Contrast-enhanced CT of the abdomen shows multiple tiny, low-attenuation lesions diffusely distributed in the spleen.

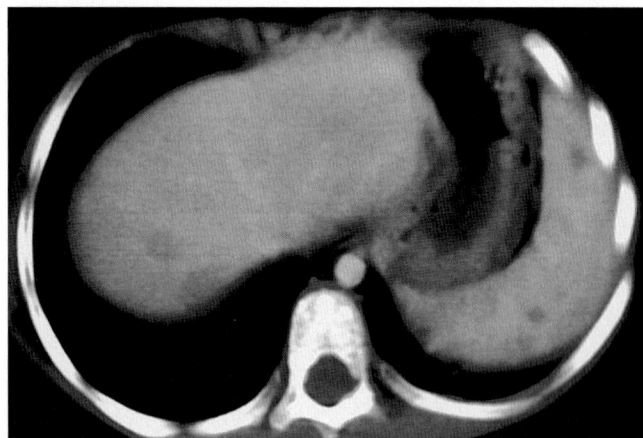

FIGURE 119-10. Cat-scratch fever in a child with fever and abdominal pain. Contrast-enhanced CT reveals several well-circumscribed, round and oval, low-attenuation lesions in the spleen. Similar larger foci were seen in the liver. The pathologic diagnosis was *Bartonella henselae.*

that a transfusion program and bone marrow transplantation can reverse splenic hypofunction.

> - **Splenomegaly is usually a manifestation of an underlying systemic condition**
> - **Hypersplenism refers to the syndrome of sequestration of blood elements within an enlarged spleen**

Infectious Diseases

Involvement of the spleen in systemic infectious disease is most common in immunocompromised patients. Bacterial, fungal, and granulomatous agents are frequently involved. Microabscesses are most commonly seen, especially with a fungal infection such as candidiasis. If large enough, the microabscesses may be seen on sonograms, but CT may be necessary in some cases (Fig. 119-9). Larger, solitary abscesses may also occur with candidiasis. They may be seen as hypoechoic areas on US and as low-attenuation areas on CT. In rare instances, calcification may be seen on CT. Serial CT scans are of value in patients undergoing anticancer chemotherapy.

Splenic involvement can also occur in immune-competent hosts with cat-scratch fever, granulomatous diseases such as histoplasmosis, parasitic diseases such as hydatid cysts, and viral infections. In cat-scratch fever, US may show hypoechoic lesions ranging from well-defined

and homogeneous to indistinct and heterogeneous. Contrast-enhanced CT may show hypoattenuating lesions, isoattenuating lesions, or lesions with marginal enhancement (Fig. 119-10). On MRI, lesions demonstrate low signal intensity on T1-weighted sequences and high signal intensity on T2-weighted sequences. Viral infections, including infectious mononucleosis, are more likely to cause nonspecific splenomegaly due to reactive hyperplasia of the spleen's reticuloendothelial tissue. Hydatid cysts, caused by echinococcal infection, may rarely involve the spleen. Plain films may show calcification of the cyst wall. The cysts are generally anechoic, although the presence of daughter cysts and membranes may induce septations and internal echoes. CT shows a focal lesion of lower attenuation than the surrounding splenic tissue, and it is the best modality to show rim calcification, when present. Tuberculosis, histoplasmosis, and coccidioidomycosis may produce multiple splenic granulomas, almost always associated with diffuse organ involvement

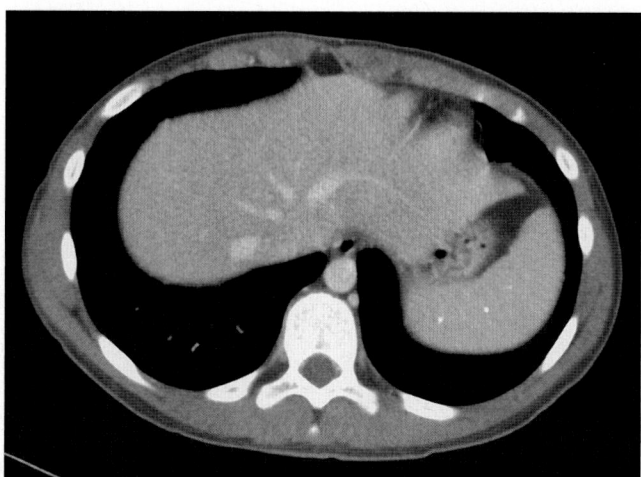

FIGURE 119-11. Splenic granulomas in a 13-year-old girl with histoplasmosis. Two small foci of calcification representing calcified granulomas are seen within the spleen.

secondary to hematogenous spread (Fig. 119-11). Splenic granulomas may be also be found in patients with chronic granulomatous disease of childhood.

Bacterial splenic abscesses can be acquired by several routes. These include hematogenous spread, such as in subacute bacterial endocarditis; spread from a contiguous infection, such as pancreatitis or perinephric abscess; and seeding in a spleen compromised by infarction or trauma.

Neoplasms

BENIGN NEOPLASMS

Benign neoplasms of the spleen are most commonly cystic in nature. Primary splenic cysts may be of epithelial lines, such as epidermoid, dermoid, or transitional cell cysts, or of endothelial lines, such as lymphangiomas and hemangiomas. Acquired cysts may be post-traumatic or infectious, such as hydatid disease.

Epidermoid cysts are the most common noninfectious focal space-occupying lesions of the spleen, accounting for approximately 10% of all nonparasitic splenic cysts worldwide. They are frequently large enough to visibly enlarge the spleen on plain films as a left upper quadrant mass displacing the stomach and colon (Fig. 119-12). A rim of calcification may be seen. On US, the cysts are characteristically anechoic and sharply demarcated from the surrounding normal splenic tissue. However, hemorrhage, inflammatory debris, or internal fat droplets may cause the cyst to contain internal echoes, at times resembling a hypoechoic solid mass (see Fig. 119-12); real-time scanning may show movement of the internal material, and Doppler interrogation reveals no internal flow, disclosing the cystic nature of the lesion. Liver-spleen scintigraphy demonstrates a focal photopenic defect. CT may be best at identifying calcifications (see Fig. 119-12). On CT and MRI, an uncomplicated epidermoid cyst appears as a rounded, sharply demarcated, nonenhancing mass with cystic imaging characteristics. If it is complicated by hemorrhage, the internal signal intensity of the lesion on MRI reflects the chemical state

of the hemoglobin within it. Familial occurrence of epidermoid cysts has been reported.

Some cystic lesions of the spleen lack an epithelial lining and are therefore *pseudocysts*. Acquired nonneoplastic splenic pseudocysts occur after trauma, infarct, or intrasplenic hemorrhage (Fig. 119-13).

Lymphangiomas may be single or multiple and may cause splenic enlargement. Splenic lymphangiomatosis is usually associated with lymphangiomas found elsewhere. On US, CT, and MRI, they are most commonly septated, nonenhancing cystic lesions. Though typically anechoic on US, they may occasionally be hypoechoic because of floating debris. The cysts generally have low signal intensity on T1-weighted images and high signal intensity on T2-weighted images (Fig. 119-14); however, they may have high signal intensity on T1-weighted images secondary to internal hemorrhage or proteinaceous fluid.

Hamartomas, also known as splenomas or nodular hyperplasia of the spleen, are non-neoplastic lesions composed of an anomalous mixture of normal splenic red pulp. Most patients are asymptomatic, and the lesion is found incidentally; if it is large, there is the potential for rupture and hemoperitoneum. They may occur in association with tuberous sclerosis and hamartomas elsewhere. Because they are composed of normal splenic tissue, they may not be detected with US or CT unless they alter the contour of the spleen, producing a focal bulge. Those that are identified by US are most commonly echogenic, although cystic and heterogeneous hamartomas have been reported. On Doppler interrogation, they typically show increased flow. Ramani and coworkers reported that hamartomas are isointense to normal splenic parenchyma on T1-weighted MR images, are heterogeneously hyperintense on T2-weighted images, and demonstrate diffuse heterogeneous enhancement on postcontrast imaging. On scintigraphy, they may have radiopharmaceutical uptake greater than that in the surrounding normal spleen.

Splenic *hemangiomas*, the most common primary neoplasm of the spleen, are usually small and may be associated with a generalized angiomatosis, such as in Klippel-Trénaunay-Weber syndrome. They are sometimes large and associated with hypersplenism, thrombocytopenia, and consumption coagulopathy, and they occasionally rupture. The lesions are predominantly solid but may be cystic or complex. The solid lesions are typically echogenic and well-marginated on US and demonstrate internal vascular flow. Enhancement of splenic hemangiomas may show a centripetal or a mottled attenuation on delayed contrast enhancement. On MRI, splenic hemangiomas are hypo- to isointense on T1-weighted images and hyperintense on T2-weighted images.

Peliosis is an uncommon entity, typically associated with peliosis hepatis. The condition consists of multiple blood-filled spaces and is associated with hematologic disorders and cachexia. If it occurs along the periphery of the spleen, there is a potential for rupture and hemoperitoneum. On US, splenic peliosis may demonstrate multiple foci of abnormal echogenicity and occasionally fluid-fluid levels within the nodules. On CT, it appears as multiple lesions of low attenuation without calcification.

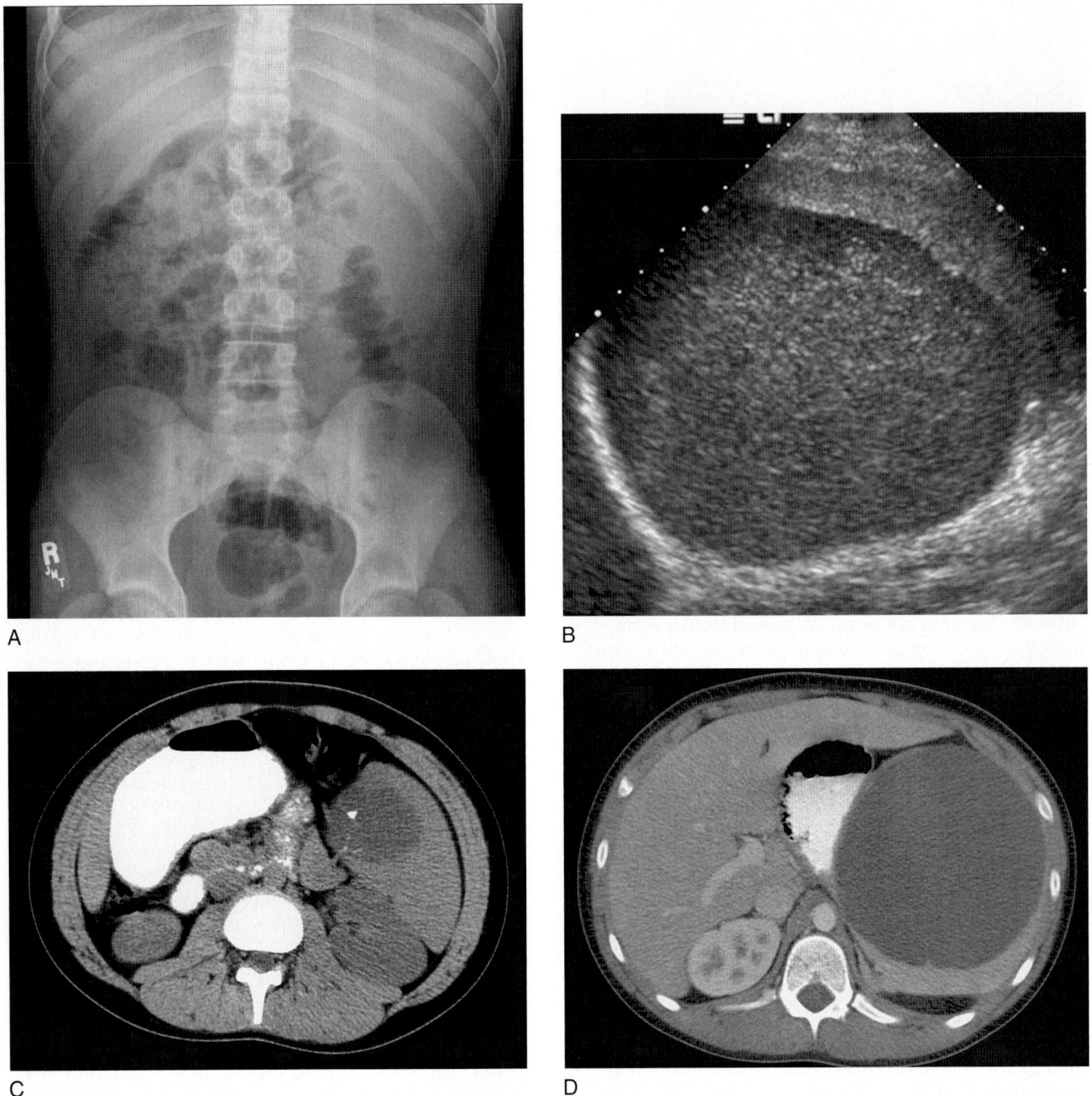

FIGURE 119-12. Twelve-year-old boy with an epidermoid cyst. **A,** A left upper quadrant mass was discovered incidentally on a plain film obtained during the workup of hematuria. **B,** Sagittal ultrasound image of the spleen shows a large, well-circumscribed lesion with internal echoes. **C,** Noncontrasted CT shows the intrasplenic cyst with focal, punctate calcification. **D,** Postcontrast CT shows a well-circumscribed, nonenhancing mass of water attenuation enlarging and distorting the spleen and displacing the stomach medially.

MALIGNANT NEOPLASMS

Malignant neoplasms of the spleen are usually metastatic or related to multifocal neoplastic disorders such as leukemia and lymphoma. Angiomatous tumors include littoral cell angioma, hemangiopericytoma, and angiosarcoma. *Acute lymphocytic leukemia* and other childhood leukemias are usually accompanied by splenomegaly secondary to diffuse infiltration of the spleen. *Chronic myelogenous leukemia* is rare in children but is frequently

accompanied by massive splenomegaly. Imaging studies of the spleen are rarely performed in children with leukemia because the diagnosis is made by other means, and the results of splenic imaging have no impact on staging or prognosis. US demonstrates an enlarged spleen with homogeneous or heterogeneous echogenicity.

Non-Hodgkin lymphoma often has a similar appearance to leukemic infiltration but may also have focal lesions large enough to be seen on US as ill-defined hypoechoic areas, especially in patients with high-grade malignancy

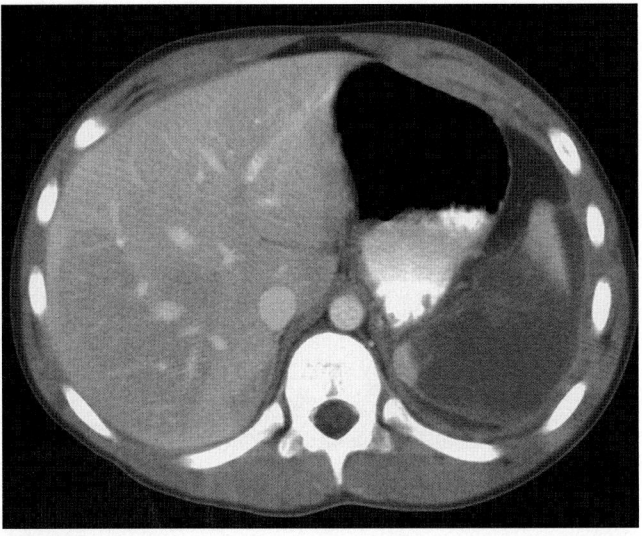
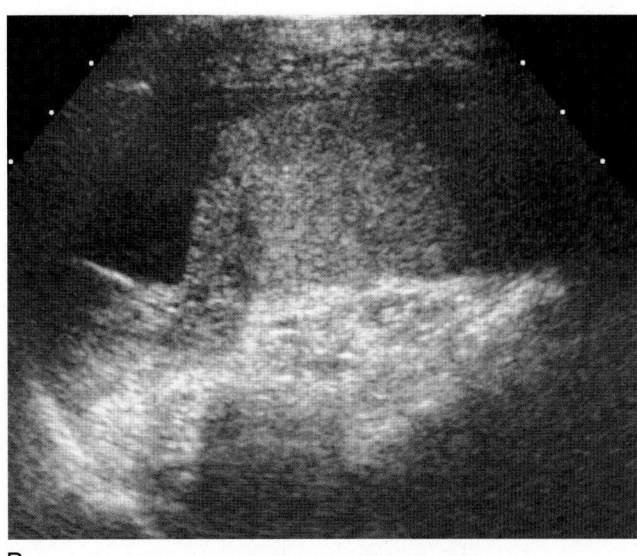

A   B

FIGURE 119-13. Twelve-year-old baseball player with traumatic splenic pseudocyst. **A** and **B,** Axial CT **(A)** and coronal US **(B)** several weeks after trauma show a wedge-shaped hypodense (CT) anechoic (US) lesion at the site of previous injury, consistent with a post-traumatic pseudocyst.

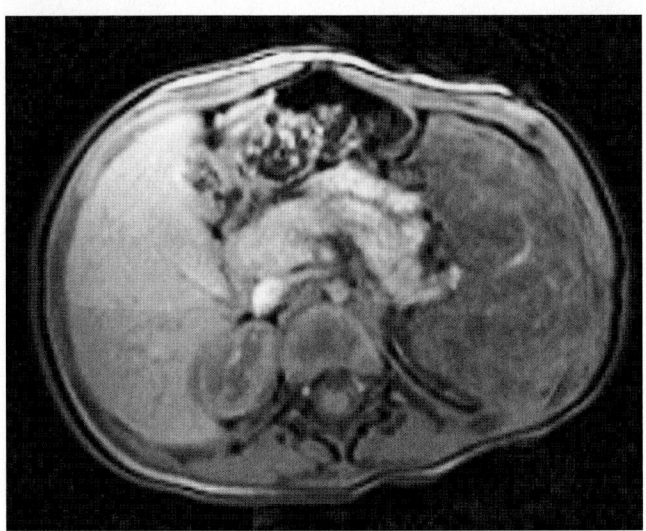
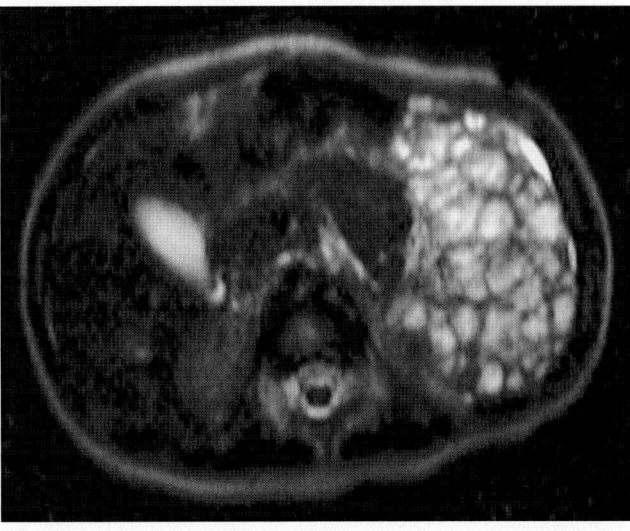

A   B

FIGURE 119-14. Eighteen-month-old girl with massive splenomegaly and multiple lymphangiomas. **A,** T1-weighted MR image shows numerous lesions of low signal intensity diffusely involving the splenic parenchyma. **B,** On a T2-weighted MR image, the lesions have high signal intensity.

at histologic examination. On CT, the low-attenuation lesions do not show appreciable enhancement compared with adjacent parenchyma after intravenous contrast administration. *Hodgkin disease* can also cause diffuse splenic infiltration that may not be detectable on imaging studies, but it is more likely than non-Hodgkin lymphoma to result in focal splenic masses (Fig. 119-15). If splenic involvement is the only subdiaphragmatic site, its detection is important for purposes of staging and prognosis. However, false-negative US, CT, and MRI examinations are common because these modalities depend on morphologic changes of enlargement or discrete nodules to diagnose lymphomatous involvement. Unfortunately, the imaging tissue characteristics of Hodgkin disease lesions are similar to those of normal spleen when the organ is diffusely infiltrated with disease

that is only microscopically detectable. Metabolic imaging with ^{18}F fluorodeoxyglucose (FDG) positron emission tomography (PET) may prove to be superior to US, CT, and MRI in identifying splenic involvement with lymphoma. FDG PET detects lymphomatous involvement of the spleen by identifying elevated glucose metabolism in tumor cells, regardless of whether there are gross morphologic changes. In a recent small series of seven patients, Rini and colleagues reported that FDG PET correctly identified all patients with and without splenic disease with an accuracy of 100%; the accuracy of CT alone was only 57%.

Littoral cell angiosarcoma is an uncommon tumor arising from red pulp cells that can occur at any age and may have some malignant potential. Patients may present with splenomegaly, thrombocytopenia, and systemic

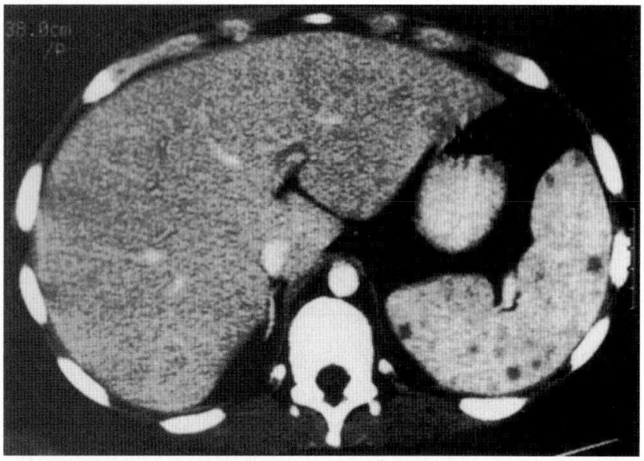

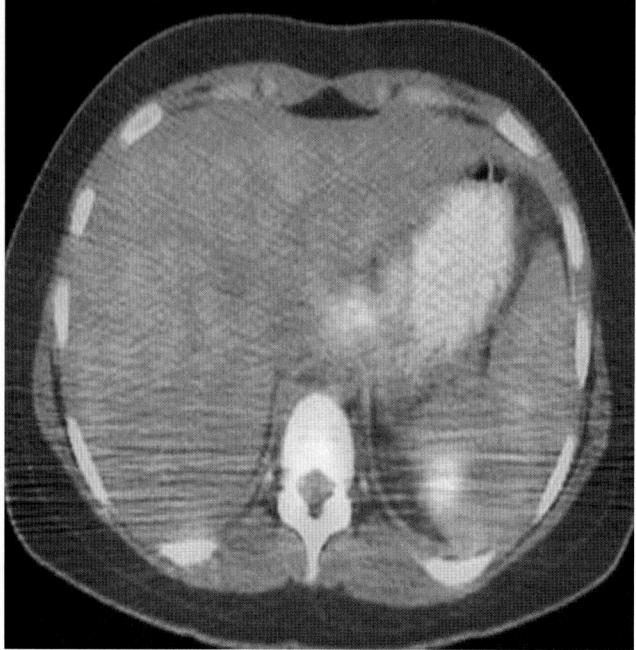

FIGURE 119-15. Hodgkin disease involving the spleen. **A,** Contrast-enhanced CT performed as part of a staging evaluation in a 14-year-old boy with Hodgkin disease shows numerous low-attenuation lesions throughout the spleen. **B,** Contrast-enhanced abdominal CT in a 19-year-old with multiple episodes of relapsing disease and new left upper quadrant pain reveals multiple large, round, hypodense, nonenhancing masses in the spleen. Note additional foci of disease in the right and left hepatic lobes. **C-E,** Nonsclerosing splenic Hodgkin disease in a 19-year-old at presentation. Axial PET image of the upper abdomen (**C**) reveals a focus of intense splenic uptake of fluorodeoxyglucose (FDG). Multiple FDG-avid foci are also evident between the liver and the stomach. Transmission CT with oral contrast (**D**) suggests multiple lymph nodes in the gastrohepatic ligament, which correlates with the multiple FDG-avid foci on the PET image. The spleen shows no focal lesion. Coregistered FDG PET and CT axial image of the upper abdomen (**E**) exhibits marked FDG avidity in the spleen and in the region of the gastrohepatic ligament. (**E,** *see color plate.*) (**B-E** courtesy of Sue Kaste, Memphis, TN.)

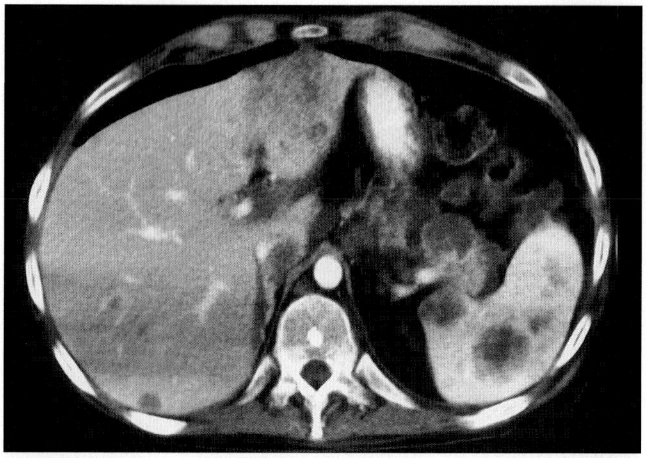

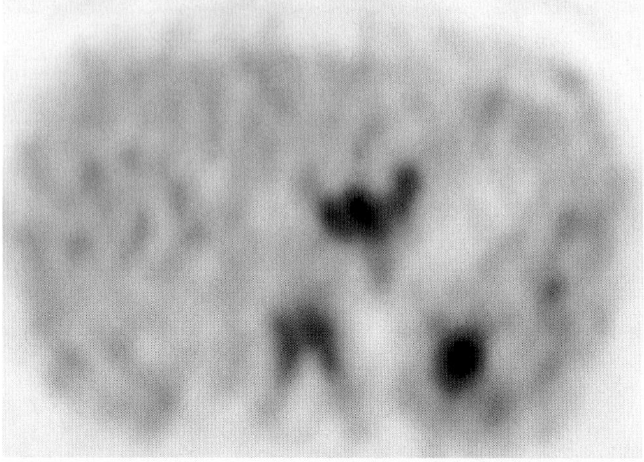

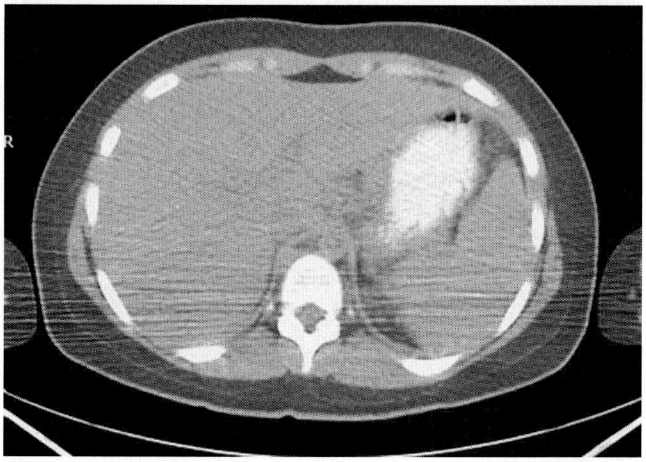

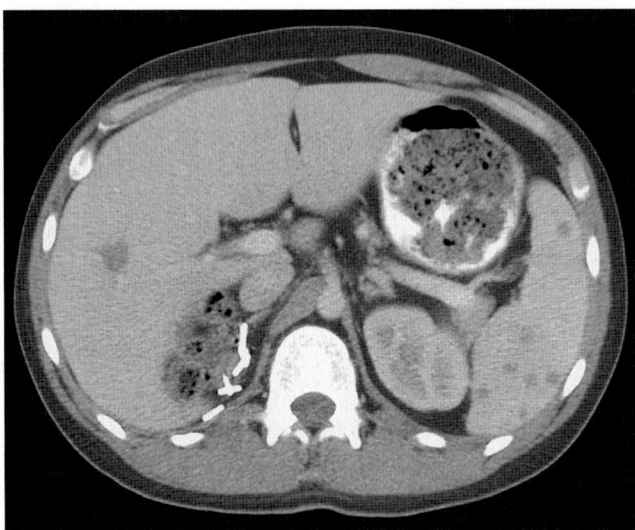

FIGURE 119-16. Splenic metastases in a 24-year-old man with Wilms tumor. CT shows multiple hypodense lesions in the spleen that were pathologically proved to be metastases. An additional lesion is seen in the liver.

symptoms. This entity presents as multiple lesions within an enlarged spleen that are initially of low attenuation on CT but typically become isodense on delayed images after contrast enhancement.

Hemangiopericytoma most commonly occurs in the soft tissues of the extremities. In the spleen, it may appear as a single large mass with smaller lesions within the parenchyma. Contrast enhancement of the solid portions may be seen on CT.

Angiosarcoma is a rare, highly malignant neoplasm that can occur at any age but is less common in children than in adults. The presentation may include left upper quadrant pain, anemia, and thrombocytopenia. Metastases are most common in the liver, lungs, bone, and lymph nodes. Most reports suggest that splenic lesions tend to be multifocal, with lower attenuation than the surrounding spleen on CT.

Splenic metastases from solid primary tumors are less common with childhood tumors than with adult tumors. The most common primary tumors are lung, melanoma, breast, and testicular germ cell tumors, particularly choriocarcinoma. Metastases may be single or multiple and frequently do not cause splenomegaly (Fig. 119-16). Splenic metastases portend a poor prognosis.

SUGGESTED READINGS

Imaging the Spleen

Adler DD, Glazer GM, Aisen AM: MRI of the spleen: normal appearance and finding in sickle-cell anemia. AJR Am J Roentgenol 1986;147:843

Dittrich M, Milde S, Dinkel E, et al: Sonographic biometry of liver and spleen size in childhood. Pediatr Radiol 1983;13:206

Donnelly LF, Foss JN, Frush DP, Bissett GS: Heterogeneous splenic enhancement patterns on spiral CT images in children: minimizing misinterpretation. Radiology 1999;210:493

Hilmes MA, Strouse PJ: The pediatric spleen. Semin Ultrasound CT MRI 2007;28:3-11

Koga T, Morikawa Y: Ultrasonographic determination of the splenic size and its clinical usefulness in various liver diseases. Radiology 1975;115:157

Markisz JA, Treves ST, Davis RT: Normal hepatic and splenic size in children: scintigraphic determination. Pediatr Radiol 1987;17:273

Megremis S, Alegakis A, Koropouli M: Ultrasonographic spleen dimension in preterm infants during the first 3 months of life. J Ultrasound Med 2007;26:329-335

Mirowitz SA, Brown JJ, Lee JKT, et al: Dynamic gadolinium-enhanced MR imaging of the spleen: normal enhancement patterns and evaluation of splenic lesions. Radiology 1991;179:681

Paterson A, Frush DP, Donnelly LF, et al: A pattern-oriented approach to splenic imaging in infants and children. Radiographics 1999;19:1465

Rosenberg HK, Markowitz RI, Kolbert H, et al: Normal splenic size in infants and children: sonographic measurement. AJR Am J Roentgenol 1994;157:119

Vick CS, Hartenberg MA, Allen HA, et al: Abdominal pseudotumor caused by gastric displacement of the spleen: sonographic demonstration. Pediatr Radiol 1985;15:253

Congenital Anomalies

Abramson SJ, Berdon WE, Altman RP, et al: Biliary atresia and noncardiac polysplenic syndrome: US and surgical considerations. Radiology 1987;163:377

Akbar SA, Sayyed TA, Zafar S, et al: Multimodality imaging of paratesticular neoplasms and their rare mimics. Radiographics 2003;23:1461

Applegate KE, Goske MJ, Pierce G, Murphy D: Situs revisited: imaging of the heterotaxy syndrome. Radiographics 1999;19:837

Bakir B, Poyanli A, Yekeler E, et al: Acute wandering spleen: imaging findings. Abdom Imaging 2004;9:707

Bollinger B, Lorentzen T: Torsion of a wandering spleen: ultrasonographic findings. J Clin Ultrasound 1990;18:510

Cirillo RL Jr, Coley BD, Binkovitz LA, et al: Sonographic findings in splenogonadal fusion. Pediatr Radiol 1999;29:73

Dodds WJ, Taylor AJ, Erickson SJ, et al: Radiologic imaging of splenic anomalies. AJR Am J Roentgenol 1990;155:805

Fujiwara T, Takehara Y, Isoda H, et al: Torsion of the wandering spleen: CT and angiographic appearance. J Comput Assist Tomogr 1995;19:84

Groshar D, Israel A, Barzilai A, et al: The value of scintigraphy in evaluation of a wandering spleen. Clin Nucl Med 1986;11:42

Herman TE, Siegel MJ: CT of acute spleen torsion in children with wandering spleen. AJR Am J Roentgenol 1991;156:151

Herman TE, Siegel MJ: Polysplenia syndrome with congenital short pancreas. AJR Am J Roentgenol 1991;156:799

Hernanz-Schulman M, Ambrosino MM, Genieser NG, et al: Current evaluation of the patient with abnormal visceroatrial situs. AJR Am J Roentgenol 1990;154:797

Hill SC, Reinig JW, Barranger JA, et al: Gaucher disease: sonographic appearance of the spleen. Radiology 1986;160:631

Hsu J, Chen H, Lin C, et al: Primary angiosarcoma of the spleen. J Surg Oncol 2005;92:312

Jequier S, Hanquinet S, Lironi A: Splenogonadal fusion. Pediatr Radiol 1998;28:526

Karaman MI, Gonzales ET Jr: Splenogonadal fusion: report of 2 cases and review of the literature. J Urol 1996;155:309

Mandell GA, Heyman S, Alavi A, et al: A case of microgastria in association with splenic-gonadal fusion. Pediatr Radiol 1983;13:95

McLean GK, Alavi A, Ziegler MM, et al: Splenic-gonadal fusion: identification by radionuclide scanning. J Pediatr Surg 1981;16(4 Suppl 1):649

Nemcek AA, Miller FH, Fitzgerald SW: Acute torsion of a wandering spleen: diagnosis by CT and duplex Doppler and color flow sonography. AJR Am J Roentgenol 1991;157:307

Phillips GWL, Hemingway AP: Wandering spleen. Br J Radiol 1987;60:188

Pomara G: Splenogonadal fusion: a rare extra-testicular scrotal mass. Radiographics 2004;24:417

Rodkey ML, Macknin ML: Pediatric wandering spleen: case report and review of the literature. Clin Pediatr 1992;31:289

Schon CA, Gorg C, Ramaswamy A, Barth PJ: Splenic metastases in a large unselected autopsy series. Pathol Res Pract 2006;202:351

Setiawan H, Harrell RS, Perret RS: Ectopic spleen: a sonographic diagnosis. Pediatr Radiol 1982;12:152

Shiels WE II, Johnson JF, Stephenson SR, et al: Chronic torsion of the wandering spleen. Pediatr Radiol 1989;19:465

Spector JM, Chappell J: Gastric volvulus associated with wandering spleen in a child. J Pediatr Surg 2000;35:641

Subraanyam BR, Balthazar EJ, Horii SC: Sonography of the accessory spleen. AJR Am J Roentgenol 1984;143:47

Swischuk LE, Williams JB, John SD: Torsion of wandering spleen: the whorled appearance of the splenic pedicle on CT. Pediatr Radiol 1993;23:476

Tonkin ILD, Tonkin AK: Visceroatrial situs abnormalities: sonographic and computed tomographic appearance. AJR Am J Roentgenol 1984;138:509

Walther MM, Trulock TC, Finnerty DP, et al: Splenic gonadal fusion. Urology 1988;32:521

Winer-Muram HT, Tonkin IL: The spectrum of heterotaxic syndromes. Radiol Clin North Am 1989;27:1147

Acquired Abnormalities

Abbott RM, Levy AD, Aguilera NS, et al: From the archives of the AFIP: primary vascular neoplasms of the spleen: radiologic-pathologic correlation. Radiographics 2004;24:1137

Abramowsky C, Alvarado C, Wyly JB, Ricketts R. "Hamartoma" of the spleen (splenoma) in children. Pediatr Dev Pathol 2004;7:231

Andronikou S, Welman CJ, Kader E: Classic and unusual appearances of hydatid disease in children. Pediatr Radiol 2002;32:817

Balthazar EJ, Hilton S, Naidich D, et al: CT of splenic and perisplenic abnormalities in septic patients. AJR Am J Roentgenol 1985;144:53

Bartley DL, Hughes WT, Parvey LS, et al: Computed tomography of hepatic and splenic fungal abscesses in leukemic children. Pediatr Infect Dis 1982;1:317

Bradley MJ, Metreweli C: Ultrasound appearances of extramedullary hematopoiesis in the liver and spleen. Br J Radiol 1990;63:816

Cornaglia-Ferraris P, Perlino GF, Barabino A, et al: Cystic lymphangioma of the spleen: report of CT scan findings. Pediatr Radiol 1982;12:94

Cox F, Perlman S, Sathyanarayana: Splenic abscesses in cat scratch disease: sonographic diagnosis and follow-up. J Clin Ultrasound 1989;17:511

Dachman AH, Ros PR, Murari JP, et al: Nonparasitic splenic cysts: a report of 52 cases with radiologic-pathologic correlation. AJR Am J Roentgenol 1986;147:37

Daneman A, Martin DJ: Congenital epithelial splenic cysts in children: emphasis on sonographic appearances and some unusual features. Pediatr Radiol 1986;12:119

Danon O, Duval-Arnould M, Osman Z, et al: Hepatic and splenic involvement in cat-scratch disease: imaging features. Abdom Imaging 2000;25:182

Duddy MJ, Calder CJ: Cystic hemangioma of the spleen: findings on ultrasound and computed tomography. Br J Radiol 1989;62:180

Ferrozzi F, Bova D, Campodonico F, et al: Cystic fibrosis: MR assessment of pancreatic damage. Radiology 1996;198:875

Flynn PM, Shenep JL, Crawford R, et al: Use of abdominal computed tomography for identifying disseminated fungal infection in pediatric cancer patients. Clin Infect Dis 1995;4:964

Franquet T, Montes M, Lecumberri FJ: Hydatid disease of the spleen: imaging findings in nine patients. AJR Am J Roentgenol 1990;154:525

Goerg C, Schwerk WB, Goerg K: Sonography of focal lesions of the spleen. AJR Am J Roentgenol 1991;156:949

Goerg C, Schwerk WB, Goerg K, et al: Sonographic patterns of the affected spleen in malignant lymphoma. J Clin Ultrasound 1990;18:569

Gore RM, Skolnik A: Abdominal manifestations of pediatric leukemias: sonographic assessment. Radiology 1982;143:207

Hahn PF, Weissleder R, Stark DD, et al: MR imaging of focal splenic tumors. AJR Am J Roentgenol 1988;150:823

Harris RD, Simpson W: MRI of splenic hemangioma associated with thrombocytopenia. Gastrointest Radiol 1989;14:308

Johnson MA, Cooperberg PL, Boisvert J, et al: Spontaneous splenic rupture in infectious mononucleosis: sonographic diagnosis and follow-up. AJR Am J Roentgenol 1981;136:111

Keidl CM, Chusid MJ: Splenic abscesses in childhood. Pediatr Infect Dis J 1989;8:368

King DJ, Dawson AA, Bayliss AP: The value of ultrasonic scanning of the spleen in lymphoma. Clin Radiol 1985;36:473

Kuykendall JD, Shanser JD, Sumner TE, et al: Multimodal approach to diagnosis of hamartoma of the spleen. Pediatr Radiol 1977;5:239

Magid D, Fishman EK, Siegelman SS: Computed tomography of the spleen and liver in sickle cell disease. AJR Am J Roentgenol 1984;143:245

Miller JH, Greenfield LD, Wald BR: Candidiasis of the liver and spleen in childhood. Radiology 1982;142:375

Okada J, Yoshikawa K, Uno K, et al: Increased activity on radiocolloid scintigraphy in splenic hamartoma. Clin Nucl Med 1990;15:112

Orduna M, Gonzalez de Orbe G, Gordillo MI, et al: Chronic granulomatous disease of childhood: report of two cases with unusual involvement of the gastric antrum and spleen. Eur J Radiol 1989;9:67

Pastakia B, Shawker TH, Thaler M, et al: Hepatosplenic candidiasis: wheels within wheels. Radiology 1988;166:417

Paterson A, Frush DP, Donnelly LF, et al: A pattern-oriented approach to splenic imaging in infants and children. Radiographics 1999;19:1465

Pawar S, Kay CJ, Gonzalez R, et al: Sonography of splenic abscess. AJR Am J Roentgenol 1982;138:259

Polat P, Kantarci M, Alper F, et al: Hydatid disease from head to toe. Radiographics 2003;23:475

Rabushka LS, Kawashima A, Fishman E: Imaging of the spleen: CT with supplemental MR examination. Radiographics 1994;14:307

Ramani M, Reinhold C, Semelka RC, et al: Splenic hemangiomas and hamartomas: MR imaging characteristics of 28 lesions. Radiology 1997;202:166

Rao BK, AuBuchon J, Lieberman LM, et al: Cystic lymphangioma of the spleen: a radiologic-pathologic correlation. Radiology 1981;141:781

Rini JN, Leonidas JC, Tomas MB, Palestro CJ. ^{18}F-FDG PET versus CT for evaluation the spleen during initial staging of lymphoma. J Nucl Med 2003;44:1072

Rose SC, Kumpe DA, Manco-Johnson ML: Radiographic appearance of diffuse splenic hemangiomatosis. Gastrointest Radiol 1986;11:342

Siniluto T, Paivansalo M, Lahde S: Ultrasonography of splenic metastases. Acta Radiol 1989;30:463

Strijk SP, Wagener DJ, Bogman MJ, et al: The spleen in Hodgkin disease: diagnostic value of CT. Radiology 1985;154:753

Von Sinner WN, Stridbeck H: Hydatid disease of the spleen: ultrasonography, CT and MR imaging. Acta Radiol 1992;33:459

Wadsworth DT, Newman B, Abramson SJ, et al: Splenic lymphangiomatosis in children. Radiology 1997;202:173

Younger KA, Hall CM: Epidermoid cyst of the spleen: a case report and review of the literature. Br J Radiol 1990;63:652

CHAPTER

120

The Pancreas

SUE C. KASTE

ANATOMY AND EMBRYOLOGY

The pancreas lies transversely in the retroperitoneum. It is divided into the head, body, and tail (Fig. 120-1). The head is to the right of midline, situated in the curve of the duodenum. At the junction of the inferior and left margins of the pancreatic head is an extension of the gland substance—the uncinate process. The anterior surface of the pancreatic head is in contact with the transverse colon, gastroduodenal artery, and several loops of small intestine. The anterior surface of the uncinate process is in contact with the superior mesenteric artery and vein. The posterior surface of the head is adjacent to the inferior vena cava, common bile duct, renal veins, and abdominal aorta.

The pancreatic body is in contact with the stomach anterosuperiorly. Its posterior portion abuts the abdominal aorta, splenic vein, left kidney, adrenal gland, and origin of the superior mesenteric artery. The small intestine lies inferior to the pancreatic body. The tail may be more bulbous in children than the head or body and is narrower in adults. The pancreatic tail lies in the phrenicolienal ligament in contact with the gastric surface of the spleen and the splenic flexure of the colon.

The pancreas arises from two anlagen. The dorsal part develops from a diverticulum to the dorsal aspect of the duodenum caudal to the hepatic diverticulum. It grows upward and backward into the dorsal mesogastrium, forming part of the head and the entire body and tail. The ventral pancreatic bud is a diverticulum from the primitive bile duct and forms part of the head and the uncinate process. The ventral pancreas rotates counterclockwise posterior to the duodenum at day 37. The two portions fuse at about the sixth week of embryonic life. The ductal systems fuse; the duct from the dorsal bud becomes the accessory pancreatic duct, and that from the ventral bud enlarges to become the main duct after it fuses with the distal two thirds of the dorsal duct. The opening of the accessory duct is often obliterated. Developmental deviation from this embryologic pattern can give rise to duodenal obstruction, pancreaticobiliary maljunction pancreatitis, and biliary cysts.

Pancreatic function is both exocrine and endocrine. The exocrine functions are directed toward digestion, with secretions exiting through the pancreatic duct into the duodenum. The islets of Langerhans are endocrine tissue containing several types of hormone-producing cells.

IMAGING THE PANCREAS

The pancreas itself is not seen on plain radiographs, although calcifications present in patients with chronic pancreatitis or cystic fibrosis may be identified on abdominal radiographs (Fig. 120-2). A pancreatic mass may be sufficiently large to displace adjacent gas-filled portions of the gastrointestinal tract.

Ultrasonography (US) usually provides good visualization of the pancreas in children because the relatively large left lobe of the liver can be used as an acoustic window. The pancreas is most easily seen if the stomach and duodenum are not distended with gas. Ingestion of water devoid of gas bubbles may also aid in visualization by serving as an acoustic window. The body of the pancreas can be located anterior to the splenic vein. The tail is relatively larger in children than in adults and is usually larger than the body. Siegel and colleagues have developed normal dimensions of the pancreas according to age (Table 120-1). Pancreatic size correlates best with its body height, but there is sufficient individual variation that caution must be used when determining pancreatic enlargement. Teele and Share concluded that enlargement of the pancreas should be diagnosed when the anteroposterior dimension of the body is greater than 1.5 cm. The normal duct may be seen as a single- or double-track echogenic line anterior to the junction of the splenic and mesenteric veins (see Fig. 120-1). There is a spectrum of pancreatic echogenicity relative to that of the liver, but in most children, the pancreas is hypoechoic or nearly isoechoic with the liver. However, in neonates, particularly premature infants, the pancreatic gland is more echogenic. US can evaluate the biliary tree prenatally and has led to the prenatal diagnosis of congenital dilation of the bile duct in at least two cases. US is also helpful for image-guided biopsy, and its successful

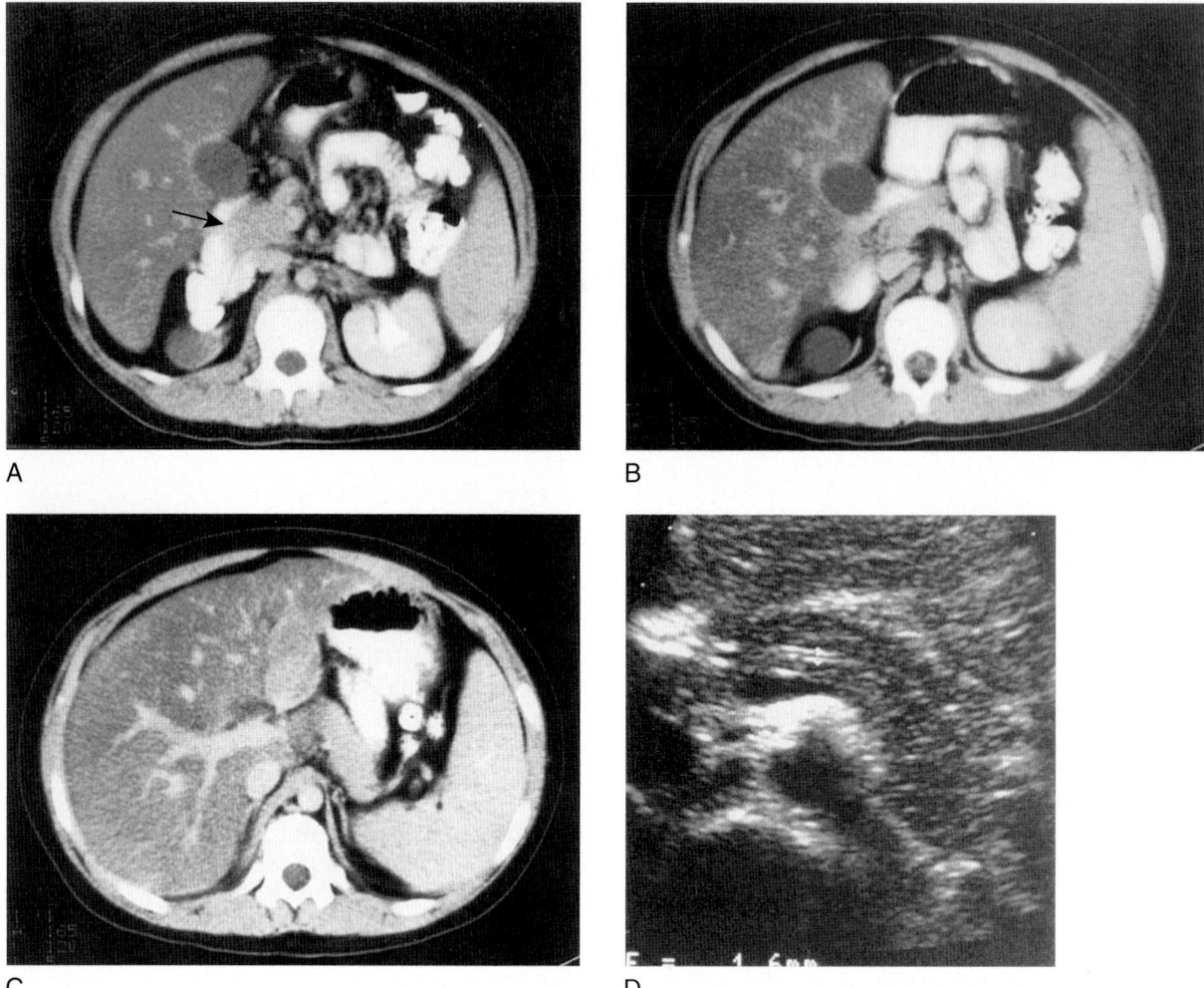

FIGURE 120-1. Normal pancreas in an 11-year-old boy. **A-C,** CT scan sections of the pancreas. The head of the pancreas (*arrow* in **A**) is slightly bulbous and distinct from the contrast-filled duodenal sweep. The body of the pancreas (**B**) is narrower than the head or tail and is seen anterior to the aorta, from which the superior mesenteric artery arises. The tail of the pancreas (**C**) is thicker in children than in adults and extends to the spleen. **D,** Transverse US shows the double track of a normal pancreatic duct.

use in aligning intensity-modulated radiotherapy in upper abdominal malignancies has been reported in children and adults.

Computed tomography (CT) of the pancreas is indicated less frequently than US, but it is valuable in certain conditions, particularly tumors and pseudocysts with uncommon features. The pancreas is best visualized on CT during bolus injection of intravenous contrast material, which readily identifies the adjacent vessels, and with meticulous administration of gastrointestinal contrast to opacify the adjacent stomach and duodenum. The pancreas has lower attenuation than the liver both with and without intravenous contrast. Because the pancreas in children is oblique to the axial plane, multiple thin sections may be necessary for optimal visualization on CT; reconstructions, particularly from axial data obtained with multichannel equipment, can image the pancreas in its own oblique plane. Imaging of the pancreatic head may be optimized by scanning the patient in the right lateral decubitus position soon after the oral ingestion of gastrointestinal contrast material. With this technique, the opacified duodenal C-loop outlines the

pancreatic head. CT is the best modality for assessing neoplasms, pancreatic trauma, and pancreatitis and its complications. Multichannel spiral CT with thin collimation coupled with curved planar reformations produces high-quality imaging of pancreatic and peripancreatic tissues.

Magnetic resonance imaging (MRI) of the pancreas is more difficult in children than in adults because of adjacent gas-filled loops of intestine and motion artifact from peristalsis and respiration. Nevertheless, MRI is a powerful tool for imaging pediatric developmental abnormalities. The pancreas normally has signal intensity equal to that of liver on T1- and T2-weighted spin echo images with midfield strength magnets. Pancreatic images produced with high field strength magnets may have greater signal intensity than liver. To some degree, the signal varies with age. Although normal children do not have as much intrapancreatic fat as adults, adolescents have more fat in the pancreatic septa than do preadolescent children. The amount of intrapancreatic fat may be increased in children with cystic fibrosis. The value of MRI of the pancreas is enhanced by the use

TABLE 120-1

Normal Sonographic Dimensions of the Pancreas in Childhood

Age	Head*	Body*	Tail*
<1 mo	1.0 ± 0.4	0.6 ± 0.2	1.0 ± 0.4
1 mo-1 yr	1.5 ± 0.5	0.8 ± 0.3	1.2 ± 0.4
1-5 yr	1.7 ± 0.3	1.0 ± 0.2	1.8 ± 0.4
5-10 yr	1.6 ± 0.4	1.0 ± 0.3	1.8 ± 0.4
10-19 yr	2.0 ± 0.5	1.1 ± 0.3	2.0 ± 0.4

*Maximal anteroposterior dimension (cm) ± standard deviation.
Modified from Siegel MJ, Martin KW, Worthington JL: Normal and abnormal pancreas in children: US studies. Radiology 1987;165:15.

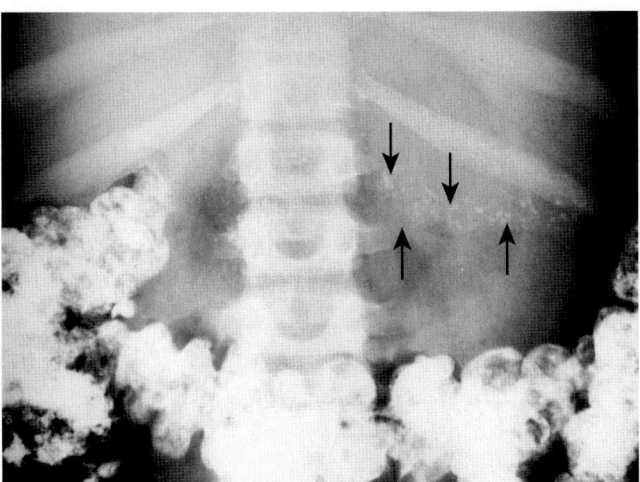

FIGURE 120-2. Cystic fibrosis in a 9-year-old girl with multiple pancreatic calcifications *(arrows)*, seen on an upper gastrointestinal examination.

of breath-holding techniques (generally not possible in younger children), fat-suppression sequences, contrast enhancement, and respiratory gating.

Endoscopic retrograde cholangiopancreatography (ERCP) is useful for identifying the pancreatic duct and associated abnormalities. It is performed much less commonly in children than in adults. When ERCP is performed to evaluate the common bile duct—a more common indication in children than pancreatic disease—the pancreatic duct is also visualized, and related or incidental abnormalities may be identified.

Magnetic resonance cholangiopancreatography (MRCP) may be more useful than ERCP in children because of its noninvasive nature (Fig. 120-3). MRCP has been described in the evaluation of ductal disease. Bolog and associates reported its sensitivity, specificity, and accuracy as 87%, 90%, and 89%, respectively, for stones; 100%, 98%, and 98% for cholangitis; 92%, 97%, and 96% for bile duct tumors; and 89%, 96%, and 95% for periampullary stenosis. The procedure is also useful in certain congenital abnormalities, such as pancreas divisum, and after pancreatic trauma. More recently, MRCP has been compared with intravenous cholangiography spiral CT in children with choledochal cysts who underwent postoperative evaluation. Although intravenous cholangiography spiral CT was superior to MRCP in delineating postoperative anatomy, MRCP was highly accurate (84%) in depicting the anastomotic site, intrahepatic biliary tree, and reconstructed bowel, and it clearly demonstrated pancreaticobiliary maljunction, residual distal common bile duct, common channel, and pancreatic duct. Secretin stimulation with MRCP further enhances the information obtained. Similarly, MRCP accurately depicts the postoperative anatomy and complications after orthotopic liver transplantation with excellent sensitivity, specificity, accuracy, and positive and negative predictive values.

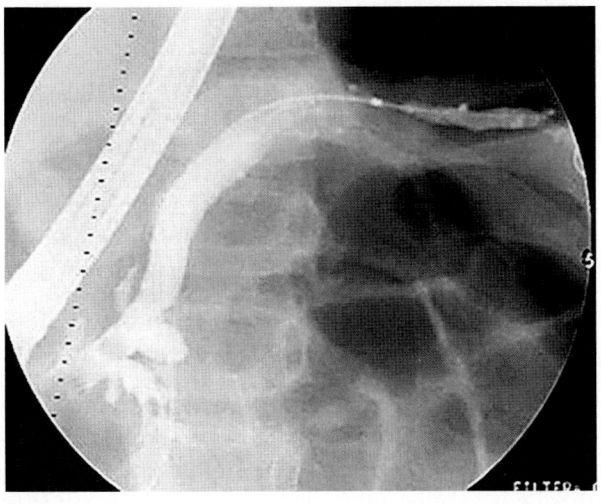
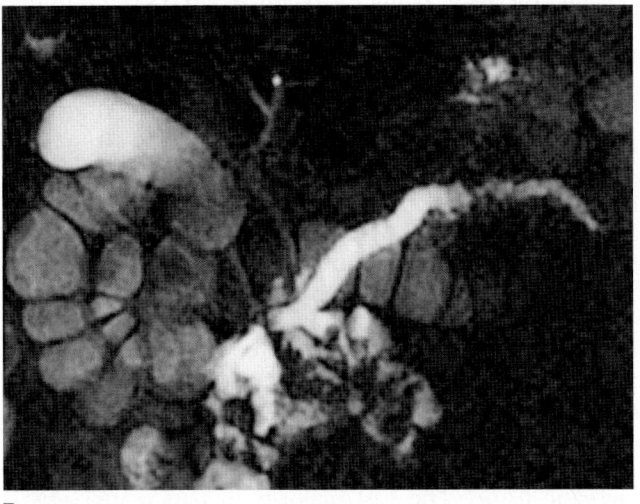

A B

FIGURE 120-3. ERCP and MRCP in a 9-year-old with recurrent pancreatitis and stones. **A,** Anteroposterior image from ERCP shows abnormal dilation of the proximal pancreatic duct and narrowing, irregularity, beading, and an undulating caliber of the distal pancreatic duct. **B,** Anterior MRCP image of the same patient exquisitely defines the abnormal caliber and irregularity of the pancreatic duct, consistent with recurrent pancreatitis. The common bile duct is normal. (Courtesy of Dr. Kimberly Applegate, Indianapolis, IN.)

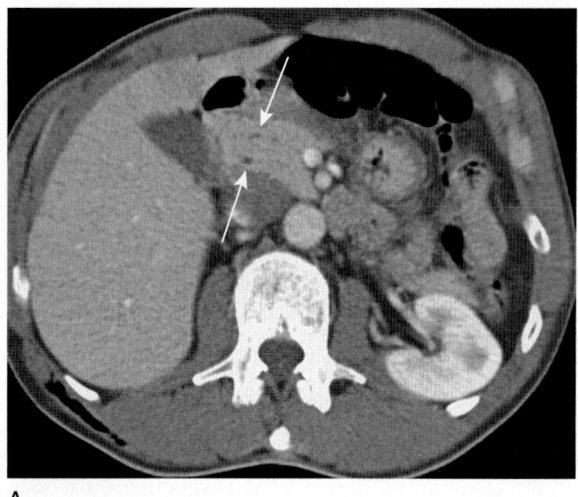
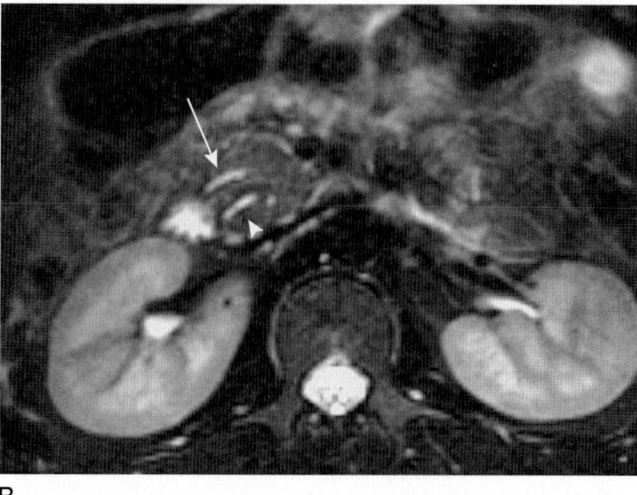

A   B

FIGURE 120-4. Pancreas divisum. **A,** Axial contrast-enhanced CT image through the pancreas shows two pancreatic ducts *(arrows)*. **B,** Axial fast spin echo T2-weighted MR image from a teenager with recurrent pancreatitis shows separate ducts of Santorini *(arrow)* and Wirsung *(arrowhead)* in the pancreatic head. (Courtesy of Dr. Marilyn Siegel, St. Louis, MO.)

CONGENITAL AND HEREDITARY ABNORMALITIES

Pancreas divisum occurs when the dorsal and ventral ducts fail to fuse, although the pancreas is otherwise anatomically normal. This anomaly has been described in 4% to 14% of the population, depending on the method of evaluation. In such cases, the accessory ampulla drains the major portion of the gland, and when this is stenotic, it may predispose to pancreatitis; however, the most recent literature refutes the claim of a higher incidence of pancreatitis in patients with pancreas divisum. CT examinations in children with pancreas divisum and pancreatitis demonstrate enlargement of both ducts, in addition to the characteristic findings of pancreatitis. Further enlargement of the duct can be provoked with secretin stimulation, a technique used in association with CT and MRCP. Increased thickness of the pancreatic head has been described. Zeman and colleagues reported that thin-section CT demonstrated the unfused ducts in 5 of 12 patients (Fig. 120-4); two distinct pancreatic moieties separated by a fat cleft could be seen in 4 patients.

Congenital short pancreas, also known as agenesis of the dorsal pancreatic anlage, occurs when the portion of the pancreas derived from the dorsal embryonic bud is absent, and only the smaller portion derived from the ventral anlage is present. Thus, the pancreatic neck, body, and tail are absent. This anomaly has been described in patients with polysplenia syndrome, or it may be a solitary finding. Only a globular pancreatic head can be identified on CT (Fig. 120-5). Patients with this abnormality have an increased risk of developing diabetes mellitus because of the paucity of islet cells, most of which are located in the distal pancreas.

Ectopic pancreatic tissue is an aberrant rest of normal pancreatic tissue. The vast majority of pancreatic rests (about 70%) are located in the stomach, duodenum, and jejunum, but they can occur anywhere, including the appendix and Meckel diverticulum. This tissue does not communicate with the pancreatic body. The abnormality occurs in 1% to 13% of the population, depending

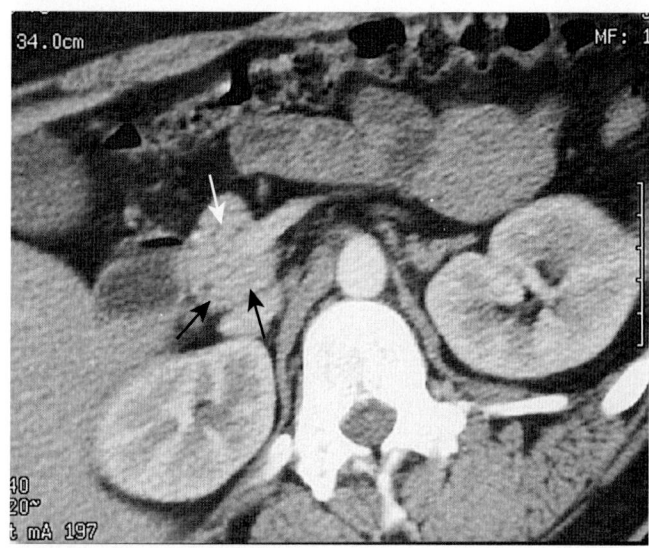

FIGURE 120-5. Congenitally short pancreas. Axial contrast-enhanced abdominal CT image through the pancreatic bed shows a congenitally short pancreas, with only a bulbous pancreatic head present *(arrows).* (Courtesy of Dr. George Taylor, Boston, MA.)

on the study. A noncommunicating gastric duplication cyst has been described that contained ectopic pancreatic ducts and islets without acini. Most pancreatic rests are incidental findings and are asymptomatic.

Annular pancreas in children is frequently diagnosed in infancy because of associated duodenal obstruction. However, in approximately half the cases, the diagnosis is made beyond infancy (Fig. 120-6). Several theories of embryonic dysgenesis have been proposed, but most suggest some form of rotational anomaly of the ventral bud, which may be bifid. The pancreatic annulus, the portion surrounding the duodenum, frequently has a separate duct entering the duodenum opposite the ampulla of Vater. Duodenal contents may reflux through this duct into the annulus. Affected patients may have associated duodenal stenosis or atresia and may present

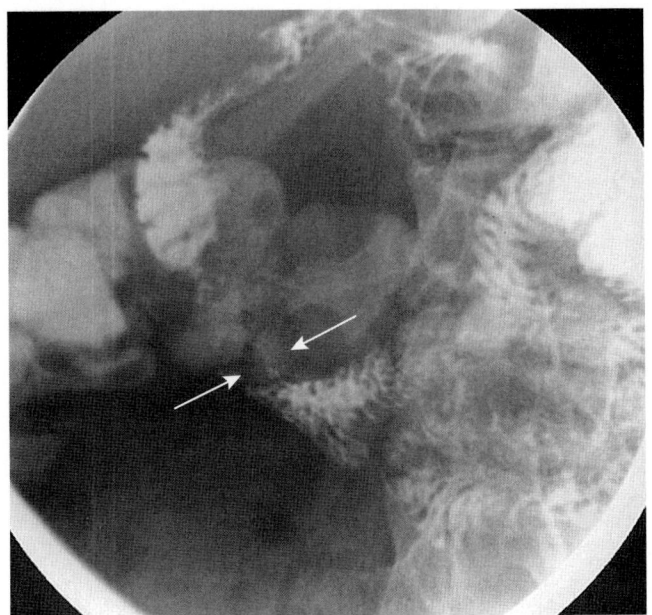 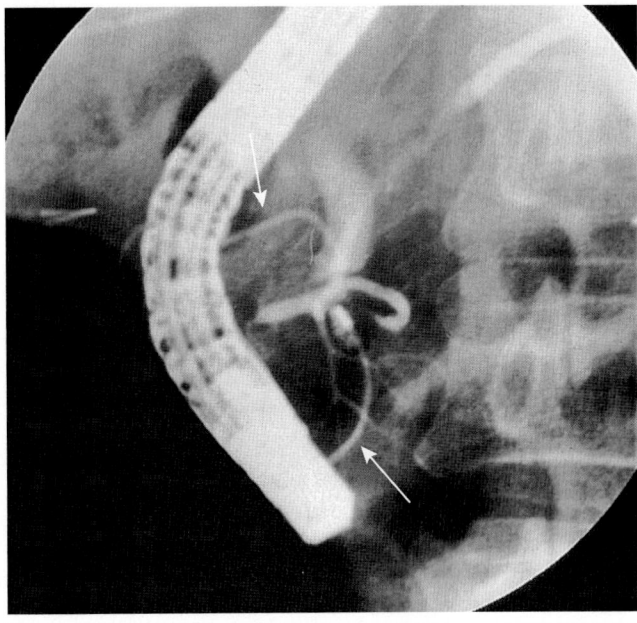

A
B

FIGURE 120-6. Annular pancreas. **A,** Oblique view during an upper gastrointestinal series shows extrinsic narrowing of the duodenal C-loop *(arrows)*. **B,** MRCP confirms the presence of small ducts *(arrows)* encircling the duodenum, consistent with an annular pancreas. (Courtesy of Dr. George Taylor, Boston, MA.)

with duodenal obstruction in infancy. Many other associated abnormalities have been described, the most common being intestinal malrotation, tracheoesophageal fistulas, cardiac abnormalities, and anal atresia. These associated lesions are most common in patients who also have trisomy 21. Annular pancreas has also been described in de Lange syndrome, with heterotaxy, and as a cause of extrahepatic biliary obstruction. Pancreatitis affecting solely the annulus has been reported in adults. ERCP and MRCP are the imaging modalities of choice to investigate the ductal anatomy associated with annular pancreas.

Congenital pancreatic abnormalities include the following:

- **Pancreas divisum**
- **Congenitally short pancreas**
- **Annular pancreas**
- **Congenital cysts**
- **Ectopic pancreatic tissue (anywhere in the gastrointestinal tract)**

Cystic fibrosis (CF) leads to exocrine pancreatic insufficiency in 80% of affected patients. As is the case in the biliary tree, the pancreatic ductules contain goblet cells that produce thickened mucus, leading to obstructive changes in patients with CF. In young patients with CF, US shows pancreatic enlargement, but chronic obstruction ultimately results in shrinkage of the gland with fatty infiltration and fibrosis. On US, these histopathologic changes lead to increased echogenicity of the gland. CT shows a shrunken pancreas with reduced attenuation

secondary to fatty infiltration. Fibrosis without fatty infiltration is found infrequently. Unenhanced scans may show pancreatic calcifications, ductal dilation, and pancreatic cysts (Fig. 120-7). In the MRI study by Tham and coworkers, 9 of 17 patients with CF had an enlarged, lobulated pancreas with fatty infiltration, 5 had an atrophic pancreas with fatty infiltration, 1 had atrophy without fatty replacement, and 2 were normal. In a series of 18 patients who underwent MRI, Murayama and colleagues identified 12 with high signal intensity on T1-weighted spin echo images, indicative of fatty replacement; 3 with low signal intensity; and 3 with normal findings. Their results corresponded well with the clinical stage of disease. Ferrozzi and associates described several MRI patterns of pancreatic changes in patients with CF.

Shwachman–Diamond syndrome is an autosomal recessive disorder resulting in short stature, exocrine pancreatic insufficiency, metaphyseal chondrodysplasia, and bone marrow dysfunction. Sonographic and CT evaluations of the pancreas demonstrate fatty replacement (pancreatic lipomatosis) as described earlier in patients with CF (Fig. 120-8).

Von Hippel–Lindau disease is an autosomal dominant disorder characterized by hemangioblastomas of multiple organs, especially the retina and central nervous system; skin lesions; and cysts of numerous organs, including the pancreas. Mustafa and coworkers reported pancreatic involvement in approximately 21% of patients with von Hippel–Lindau disease. The pancreatic lesions are usually multiple (Fig. 120-9). The cysts are typically anechoic on US and have reduced attenuation on CT compared with the surrounding pancreatic tissue. Multiple cysts as well as serous and mucinous cystadenomas of the pancreas, carcinoma, adenocarcinoma, and islet cell tumors are associated with this disease. Adenocarcinoma occurs in

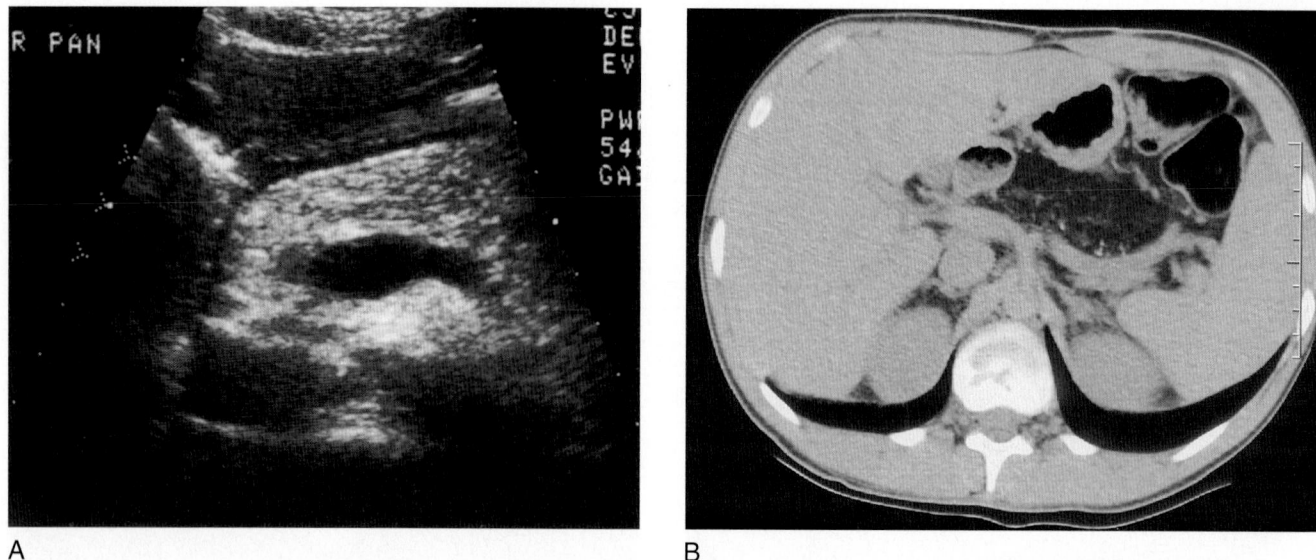

FIGURE 120-7. Cystic fibrosis with diffuse fatty replacement of the pancreas. **A,** Markedly hyperechoic pancreas on US in an 18-year-old woman with cystic fibrosis and fatty infiltration of the pancreas. **B,** Axial noncontrast abdominal CT shows diffuse fatty replacement of the pancreas, with multiple tiny calcifications. (Courtesy of Dr. Robert Kaufman, Memphis, TN.)

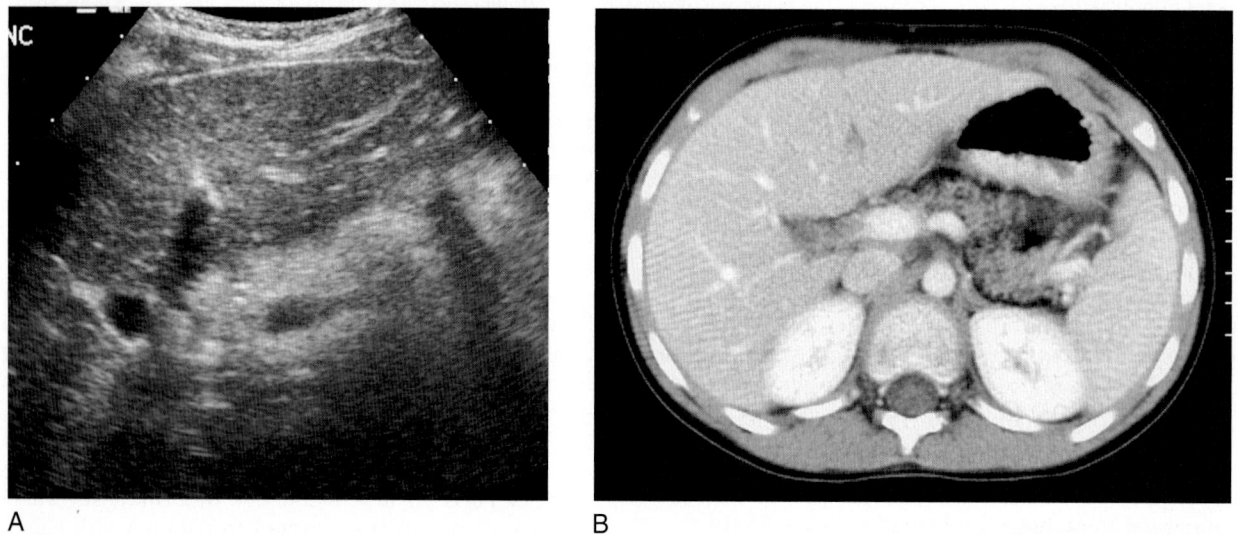

FIGURE 120-8. Shwachman-Diamond syndrome in an 8-year-old boy with anemia. **A,** Transverse US through the pancreas shows increased echogenicity of the pancreas, consistent with fatty infiltration. **B,** Corresponding axial contrast-enhanced CT confirms partial fatty replacement of the pancreas. The patient also had coxa valga (not shown).

affected adults. Pancreatic calcifications can be seen on unenhanced CT scans.

Hereditary pancreatitis is an autosomal dominant disease in which patients have recurrent episodes of pancreatitis. The findings are described later in this chapter, under the discussion of pancreatitis.

Beckwith-Wiedemann syndrome is a relatively frequent overgrowth syndrome with an incidence estimated at 1 in 14,000 births. It is probably an autosomal dominant disorder with variable transmission. The *BWS* gene has been identified on the short arm of chromosome 11 (11p15.5). The syndrome is characterized by visceromegaly, hemihypertrophy, and the development of malignant tumors in 10% to 15% of affected patients; benign tumors are also found. Cross-sectional imaging studies may show nonspecific pancreatic enlargement.

Patients may develop pancreatoblastoma or nesidioblastoma, as discussed later under pancreatic neoplasms. Because of this risk, routine US is initiated at an early age.

Congenital cysts of the pancreas are rare and are often confused with choledochal, omental, or mesenteric cysts when large (Fig. 120-10). Single congenital pancreatic cysts are very rare and occur predominantly in females. They are usually asymptomatic, but when symptoms do occur, they are related to compression of adjacent structures. Such cysts are anechoic by US; they are usually unilocular, are located in the pancreatic tail, and range in size from microscopic to 5 cm. They may rarely be associated with ductal communication. In contrast to single congenital pancreatic cysts, multiple congenital cysts may be associated with a polycystic disorder such as von Hippel–Lindau disease, as discussed earlier.

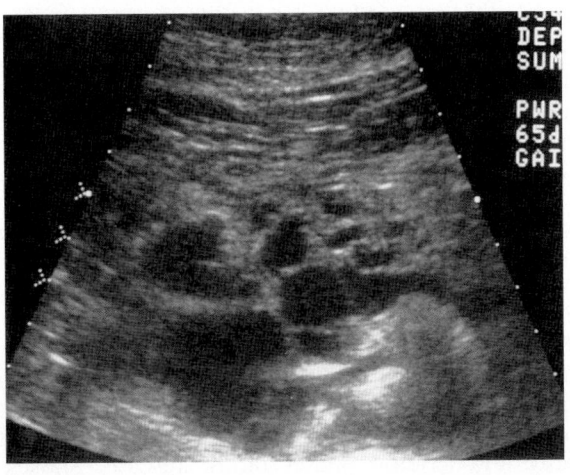
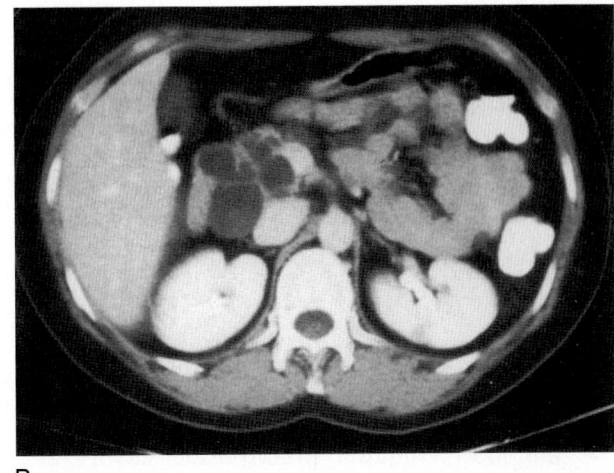

A

B

FIGURE 120-9. Von Hippel–Lindau disease in a young woman. Multiple pancreatic cysts are well demonstrated on US (**A**) and CT (**B**).

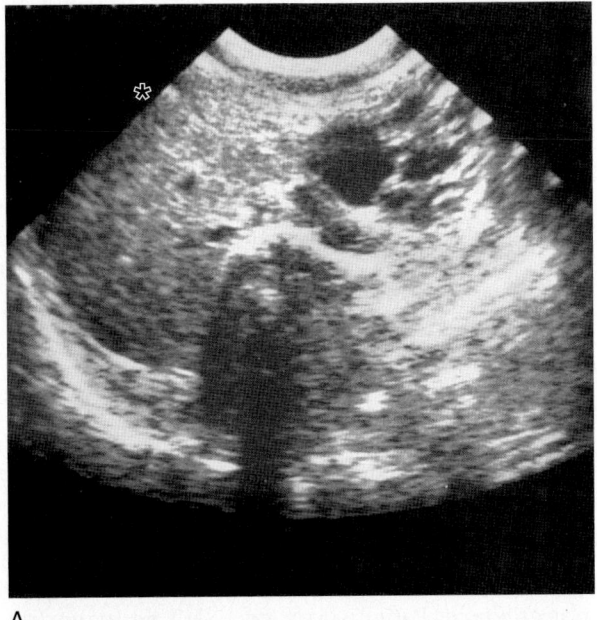

A

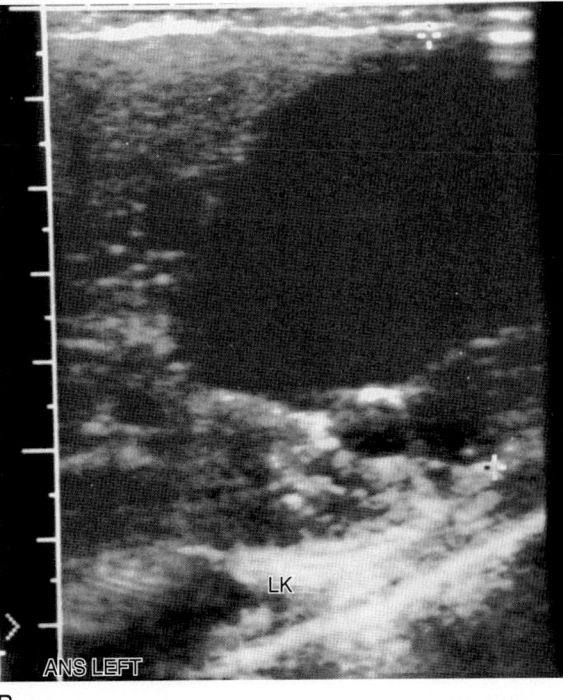

B

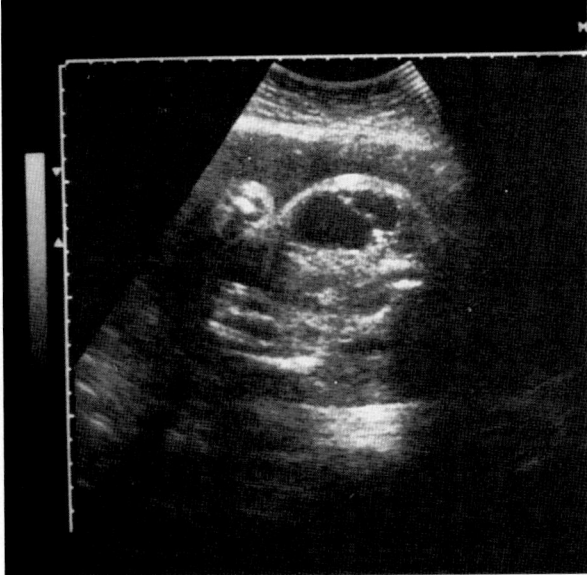

C

FIGURE 120-10. Congenital pancreatic cyst. **A** and **B,** Transverse sonograms of the midabdomen in a newborn girl reveal a large anechoic mass. **C,** Antenatal US shows the cyst in the fetus. At surgery, a large congenital pancreatic cyst was found. LK, left kidney. (**C** courtesy of Dr. D. McCallum, Palo Alto, CA; from Baker LL, Hartman GE, Northway WH Jr: Sonographic detection of congenital pancreatic cysts in the newborn: report of a case and review of the literature. Pediatr Radiol 1990;20:488.)

> **Hereditary systemic conditions with pancreatic involvement include the following:**
> - **Hereditary pancreatitis**
> - **Cystic fibrosis**
> - **Shwachman-Diamond syndrome**
> - **Von Hippel–Lindau disease**
> - **Beckwith-Wiedemann syndrome**

ACUTE PANCREATITIS

Acute pancreatitis is uncommon in childhood, possibly because the most common predisposing factors in adults—alcoholism and cholelithiasis—are seldom encountered in children. In Weizman and Durie's series of 61 children with acute pancreatitis, the most common cause was multisystem disease, including Reye syndrome, sepsis, shock, hemolytic uremic syndrome, and viral infection (specifically, mumps has been implicated). Other causes included blunt trauma in 15% of patients, congenital anatomic abnormalities in 10%, metabolic diseases in 10%, and drug toxicity in 3%. No cause was identified in 25% of patients. As mentioned earlier, MRCP is useful in identifying unsuspected abnormal ductal anatomy in patients with idiopathic pancreatitis.

Anatomic abnormalities associated with pancreatitis include pancreas divisum (discussed earlier), congenital choledochal dilation with pancreaticobiliary malunion, duodenal web, congenital pancreatic cyst, and choledochal cyst. The last may cause pancreatitis because of the abnormal insertion of the common bile duct into the pancreatic duct, which may permit reflux of bile into the pancreas. Associated metabolic disorders include hypercalcemia, hyperlipidemia, and CF; the drugs implicated most frequently are L-asparaginase (Fig. 120-11), steroids, and acetaminophen. Lee and colleagues reported an increased incidence of biliary sludge in their adult patients with pancreatitis and concluded that sludge was the probable cause of idiopathic acute pancreatitis in as many as 70% of patients.

Patients with nontraumatic acute pancreatitis typically present with abdominal pain, most frequently in the epigastrium. Nausea and vomiting are common companion symptoms. Elevation of serum concentrations of pancreatic enzymes (amylase, lipase, trypsinogen) is common. Although abnormal laboratory values are typically considerably more sensitive than imaging in identifying pancreatitis, imaging studies may be useful to confirm the diagnosis and to determine the extent of associated inflammatory changes and complications. Very rarely, pancreatitis may be the presenting symptom of a pancreatic malignancy in children and adolescents.

Abdominal radiographic findings are nonspecific, but certain findings are suggestive. Reactive ileus of nearby gastrointestinal structures may lead to air-fluid levels in the stomach and duodenum, focal dilation of the duodenal sweep, and dilation of the transverse colon ending abruptly at the splenic flexure. Left pleural effusion may occur. Although ascites is common, the amount is rarely sufficient to be appreciated on abdominal radiographs.

US may be the initial imaging procedure for the evaluation of possible pancreatitis. Jeffrey has emphasized the value of semierect and coronal scans, as well as the standard scanning planes, for the optimal evaluation of an abnormal pancreas. The edema that accompanies acute pancreatitis often results in a hypoechoic gland that is diffusely enlarged. A minority of affected patients have increased pancreatic echogenicity (see Fig. 120-11), and some have a normal-appearing pancreas. The pancreatic duct may be dilated; however, this is an inconstant finding, especially when the gland is markedly swollen, causing compression of the duct. When the duct is dilated, there is a correlation with serum lipase in the acute and healing phases of the disease. Masses may be identified in the pancreas, representing focal areas of fluid, hemorrhage, or phlegmon formation, seen as a focal inflammatory hypoechoic mass. Ascites is usually identified on US.

The presence of acute fluid collections in the peripancreatic areas is evidence of acute pancreatitis. The most commonly involved areas are the lesser sac, anterior pararenal space, transverse mesocolon, and perirenal space. US is excellent in demonstrating these fluid collections. Fluid collections may be found as far from the pancreas as the mediastinum and the inguinal regions. Fluid and inflammation may involve the adjacent splenic vein. Doppler examination is useful to rule out splenic vein thrombosis.

CT may show pancreatic abnormalities to better advantage than US. The findings mirror those seen with US and include pancreatic swelling, ductal dilation, mass effect from phlegmon or hemorrhage, peripancreatic fluid collections, thickening of adjacent fascial planes, and ascites. Abscesses are particularly well delineated on CT. Balthazar and associates used dynamic CT scanning to evaluate necrosis in adults with acute pancreatitis. Necrosis was diagnosed when all or part of the gland did not enhance. Patients with necrosis had higher rates of morbidity, mortality, and complications than those without necrosis.

ERCP is excellent for examining the pancreatic duct but is seldom needed in children. It is useful to evaluate complicated or recurrent pancreatitis or in cases of unusual pseudocyst formation. The findings range from mild irregularity of the duct to ductal narrowing with acinar enlargement, which has been likened to a string of beads. Marked ductal ectasia is usually not seen in acute pancreatitis. MRCP may replace ERCP in the evaluation of childhood pancreatitis because of its noninvasive nature (see Fig. 120-3). Enhanced image acquisition has been reported in children as well as adults with the administration of secretin during MRCP. This technique seems to optimize visualization of the pancreatic duct and its radicles and increases the sensitivity for identifying structural abnormalities. An alternative procedure is intravenous contrast-enhanced spiral CT of the biliary tree in patients with a dilated system.

Pseudocyst formation is a potential complication of pancreatitis regardless of cause. Although most pseudocysts are in the region of the pancreas itself (Fig. 120-12;

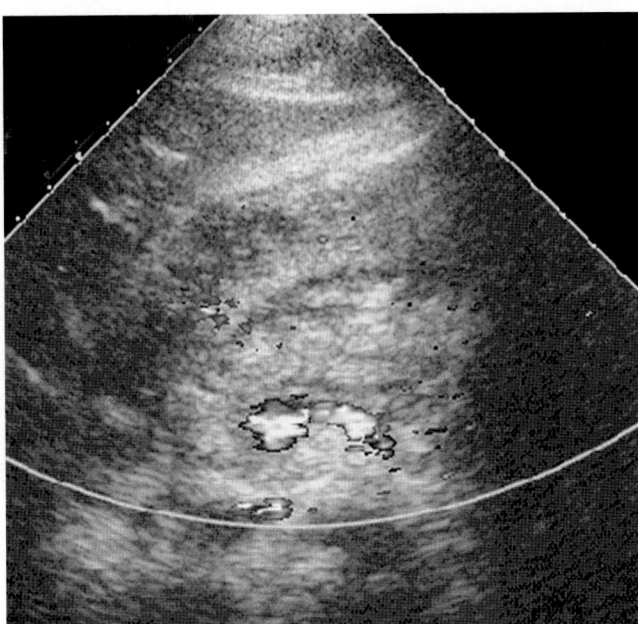

A

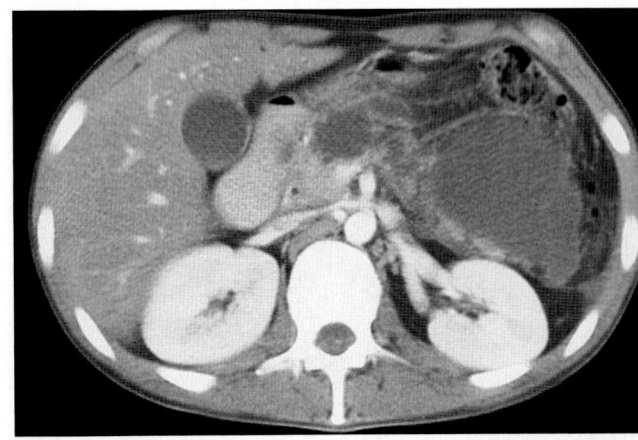

B

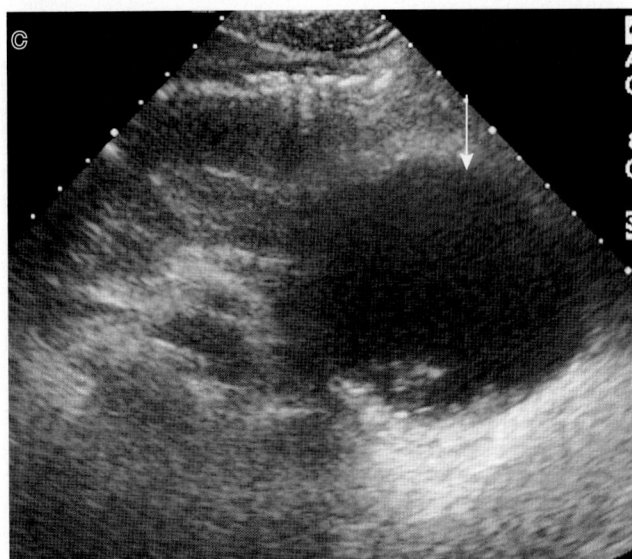

C

FIGURE 120-11. Asparaginase-induced pancreatitis and pseudocyst formation. **A,** Transverse US in a 17-year-old boy undergoing treatment for acute lymphoblastic leukemia who developed acute pancreatitis. The body of the pancreas is enlarged and mildly hyperechoic, with indistinct margins. Doppler signal indicates the splenic vein dorsal to the pancreas. **B,** Axial CT scan 2 days later shows peripancreatic edema and two pseudocysts in the body and tail. **C,** Additional follow-up with US shows a large pseudocyst *(arrow)* involving the pancreatic tail and containing complex debris.

see Fig. 120-11), they can appear nearly anywhere in the abdomen and in the mediastinum (Figs. 120-13 and 120-14). In adults, approximately 5% of patients with acute pancreatitis develop pseudocysts. Although most pseudocysts resolve spontaneously within an average of 5 months, some persist and require surgical intervention. Features associated with spontaneous resolution include a pseudocyst diameter less than 7.5 cm, absence of internal debris, and total pseudocyst volume less than 250 ml. Pseudocysts may be large enough to identify on radiographs. They frequently cause mass effect on adjacent structures, especially the stomach and duodenum, and this may be seen on upper gastrointestinal studies performed for unexplained abdominal pain. Imaging is indicated when a pseudocyst is suspected. Pseudocysts are typically anechoic, although some may contain debris. Their effect on adjacent organs may be identified on US but is seen to better advantage with CT. ERCP usually shows the irregular ductal dilation of chronic inflammation (see Figs. 120-3A and 120-14G). Percutaneous drainage of pseudocysts may provide a nonsurgical alternative.

Skeletal changes, particularly bone marrow infarcts, have long been recognized as a complication of pancreatitis, possibly related to increased levels of circulating lipase and to generalized enzymatic dysfunction of the pancreas. Radiographs generally show late changes with characteristic medullary calcification. Haller and colleagues described MRI findings that preceded radiographic findings in an adult.

CHRONIC PANCREATITIS

Chronic pancreatitis in children is less common than acute pancreatitis. Although it occurs as a sequela of the acute disease, chronic pancreatitis can also be found in association with other entities, such as CF (discussed earlier). Familial hereditary pancreatitis is an autosomal dominant disease that usually presents in childhood or during the teenage years. Ductal dilation, pseudocysts, and calcifications are the most common imaging abnormalities in chronic hereditary pancreatitis. Spencer and coworkers described a 2-year-old boy with abdominal pain and a large hemorrhagic pancreatic mass who was found to have chronic pancreatitis at surgery. Subsequent

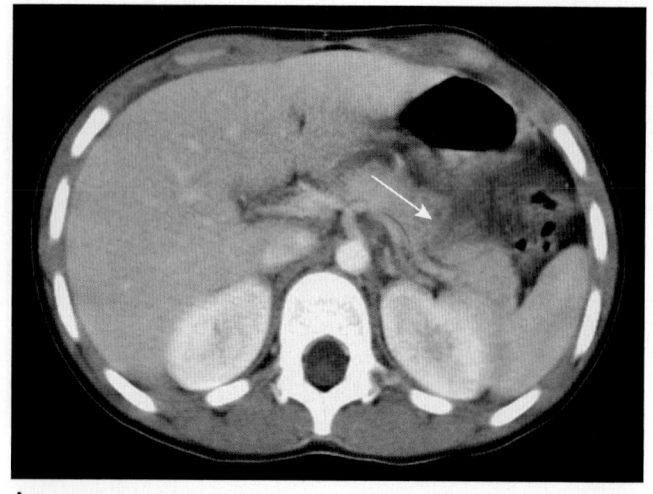

A

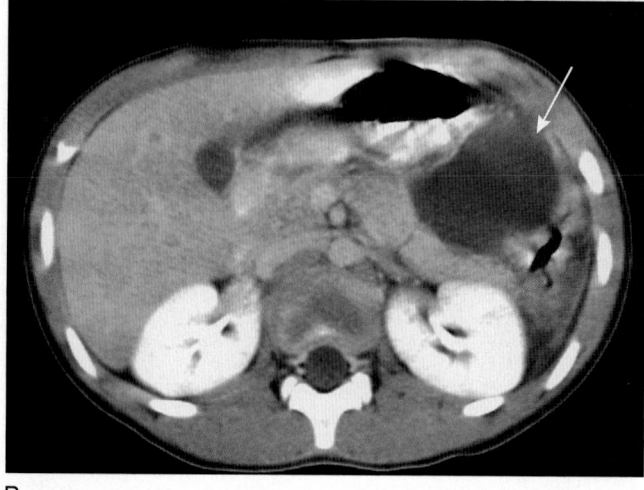

B

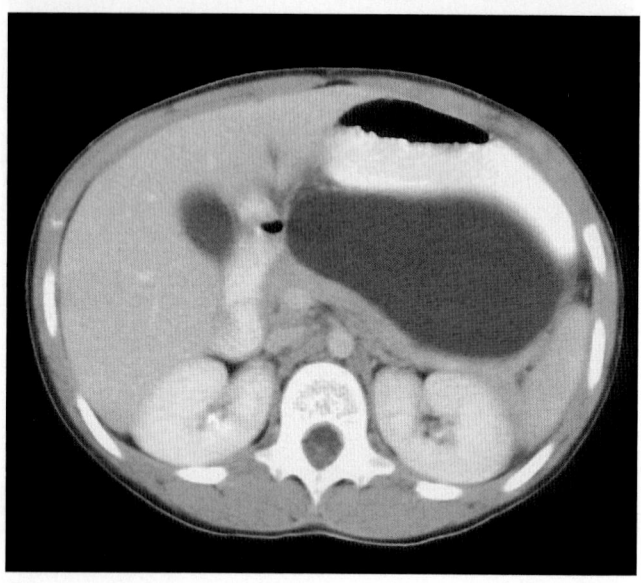

C

FIGURE 120-12. Post-traumatic pseudocyst in a 7-year-old. Ten days after blunt epigastric trauma, the patient continued to have vomiting and rising amylase levels. **A,** Axial contrast-enhanced abdominal CT shows a pancreatic laceration *(arrow)* in the midbody. **B** and **C,** Pseudocyst formation *(arrow)* is shown on follow-up imaging 10 days **(B)** and 20 days **(C)** after the initial imaging study **(A).** (Courtesy of Dr. Robert Kaufman, Memphis, TN.)

abdominal US of the patient's mother revealed pancreatic ductal dilation and calcifications. Chronic fibrosing pancreatitis is characterized by bands of collagen enclosing normal acini. The result is a mass effect that simulates a tumor. Chronic pancreatitis may result in jaundice secondary to biliary duct stricture.

PANCREATIC NEOPLASMS

Primary pancreatic tumors, both benign and malignant, are very rare in childhood and adolescence. Pancreatic tumors that occur in pediatric patients include solid-cystic pseudopapillary tumor (Frantz tumor), pancreaticoblastoma, and islet cell tumors; carcinomas are rare and include acinar cell carcinoma and ductal adenocarcinoma. Other tumors that typically occur elsewhere but can arise within the pancreas include lymphoma and rhabdomyosarcoma.

Solid-Cystic Papillary Tumor

Solid-cystic papillary tumor is also known by many other terms, including Frantz tumor, solid pseudopapillary tumor, papillary epithelial neoplasm, solid and papillary epithelial neoplasm, solid and cystic acinar cell tumor, papillary and solid neoplasm, papillary-cystic epithelial neoplasm, papillary-cystic carcinoma, solid and cystic tumor, solid and papillary neoplasm, papillary cystic tumor, and low-grade papillary neoplasm. This tumor seems to have a predilection for women and for persons of Asian extraction; it is probably the most common pancreatic tumor in Asian children. Solid-cystic papillary tumor is histologically low grade, with a reported 5-year survival of 97%. It accounts for about 0.2% to 2.7% of all nonendocrine pancreatic tumors. Although the median age at diagnosis is 26 years, approximately 20% of cases have been reported in children. Children usually have

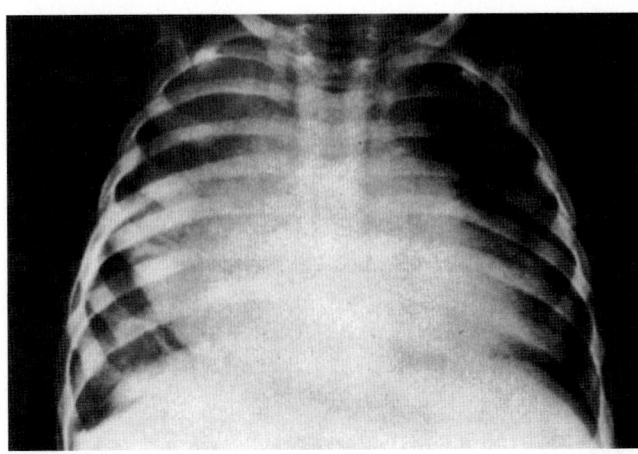

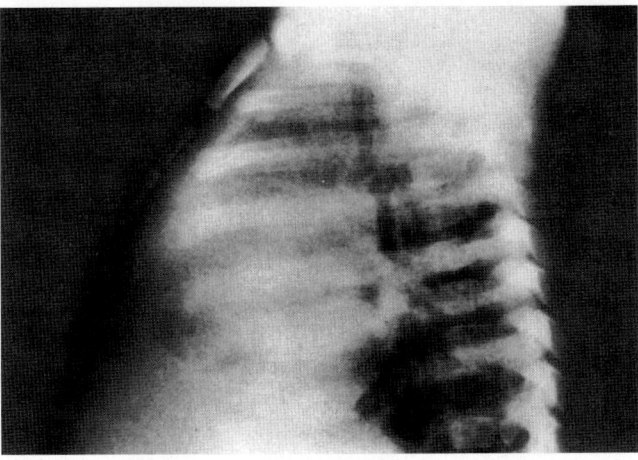

FIGURE 120-13. Mediastinal pancreatic pseudocyst on frontal (**A**) and lateral (**B**) radiographs in a 10-month-old girl who presented with wheezing and tachypnea. (Courtesy of Dr. S. Kirchner, Nashville, TN.)

a better prognosis than adults, owing to less frequent metastatic disease in children. Abdominal pain is the presenting symptom in about one third of cases, and there is typically a palpable abdominal mass; jaundice is extremely rare.

Imaging findings include a large, well-defined solid mass with varying degrees of cystic components that usually represent necrosis but are unrelated to tumor size (Fig. 120-15). Slight peripheral rim enhancement was reported by D'Onofrio and coworkers with the use of microbubble US contrast enhancement. Calcifications may be present. On T1-weighted MR sequences, a low signal rim may represent either a fibrous capsule or compressed pancreatic parenchyma; central high signal areas that may represent debris or hemorrhagic necrosis have also been reported. Almost half of all lesions occur in the pancreatic head. Invasion of adjacent structures occurs and is often associated with liver and lymph node metastases.

Pancreaticoblastoma

Pancreaticoblastoma arises from the pancreatic acinar cells, usually in the head or tail of the gland. The cells of these tumors represent persistence of the fetal anlage of the pancreatic acinar cells. It is one of the most common exocrine tumors in pediatric patients and represents about 0.5% of pancreatic epithelial tumors. These tumors are found in boys twice as often as in girls. There is a relatively high incidence of pancreaticoblastoma in East Asia. Serum α-fetoprotein is elevated in 25% to 55% of cases.

Dhebri and associates reviewed 153 patients with pancreaticoblastoma and found that the median age at presentation was 5 years, although this tumor has been diagnosed in patients as old as 68 years. The liver is the most common site of metastatic disease (88% of metastatic sites), which was found in 17% of the patients in their series. Factors associated with a worse prognosis included metastatic disease, nonresectable disease, and age older than 16 years at diagnosis. Pancreaticoblastomas are often large at presentation (up to 12 cm), with areas of central necrosis in some cases. US and CT findings are often indistinguishable from those of pancreatic adenocarcinoma. Dhebri and associates described the mass as typically hypoechoic and heterogeneous on US. On CT, pancreaticoblastoma is hypodense and appears to be multiloculated, with enhancing septa (Fig. 120-16). Calcifications are not uncommon. When vascular encasement is present, it usually involves the inferior vena cava or mesenteric vessels. Although variable, MRI characteristics of pancreaticoblastoma include typically low signal intensity compared with the liver on T1-weighted spin echo images and iso- to hyperintensity on T2-weighted images; enhancement varies. Although findings are nonspecific as to tumor type, imaging suggests the malignant nature of the tumor and can clearly exclude the kidney and adrenal glands as organs of origin.

Islet Cell Tumors

Hormonally active tumors arise from the islet cells and may be benign or malignant. The B cells produce insulin; A cells produce glucagon; G cells, gastrin; D cells, somatostatin; and D_1 cells, vasoactive intestinal peptide (VIP) and secretin. Those tumors secreting VIP (VIPomas) are associated with the syndrome of secretory diarrhea, hypokalemia, and achlorhydria. VIPomas are rare functioning tumors with an estimated annual incidence of 0.2 to 0.5 per million population. A recent publication by Nikou and colleagues indicated that the most common tumor site is the pancreatic head. These authors also demonstrated the utility of indium-111-pentetreotide (Octreoscan) scintigraphy in the diagnosis of these primary or metastatic tumors.

Islet cell tumors are named after the hormone produced. Insulinoma is the most common islet cell tumor in children (Figs. 120-17 and 120-18). Patients with insulinoma present with hypoglycemia, which typically manifests in children as erratic behavior and seizures. The symptoms are relieved by intravenous glucose administration and reproduced by fasting under controlled circumstances. Nesidioblastosis refers to diffuse islet cell hyperplasia and can also present with hypoglycemia. In a series published by Synn and coworkers, only 3 of 12

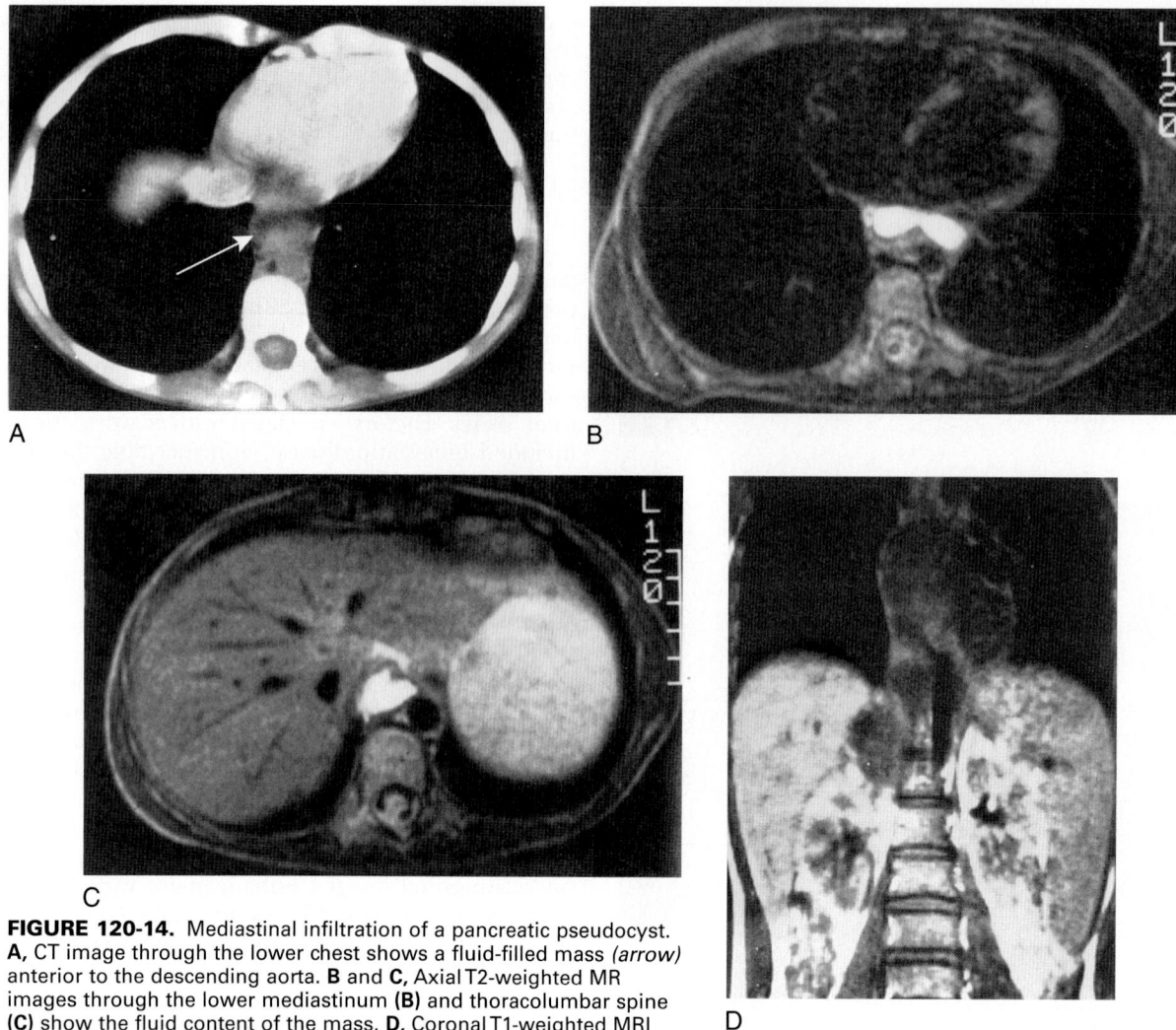

FIGURE 120-14. Mediastinal infiltration of a pancreatic pseudocyst. **A,** CT image through the lower chest shows a fluid-filled mass *(arrow)* anterior to the descending aorta. **B** and **C,** Axial T2-weighted MR images through the lower mediastinum **(B)** and thoracolumbar spine **(C)** show the fluid content of the mass. **D,** Coronal T1-weighted MRI shows the low signal intensity mass extending from a position superior to the right kidney into the posterior mediastinum.

pediatric patients with profound hypoglycemia had identifiable islet cell tumors; the others had islet cell hyperplasia or nesidioblastosis on histologic examination of specimens obtained after partial pancreatectomy.

Islet cell tumors are round or oval and well circumscribed on US. They are hypoechoic but may have a hyperechoic rim. Isoechoic and hyperechoic lesions have also been described in children and young adults. The tumors may be located superficially or deep within the pancreas. On CT, contrast enhancement may cause markedly increased attenuation in the tumors, particularly in the arterial phase (see Fig. 120-17). Because these tumors are hypervascular, arteriography may be necessary in high-risk patients in whom US and CT are nondiagnostic, although magnetic resonance angiography may replace this invasive technique. Intraoperative US has been used successfully to locate functioning islet cell tumors in children. Brunelle and colleagues have performed transhepatic venous sampling in children with hyperinsulinism. They found that 15 of 19 patients had elevated insulin levels when sampling the portal, splenic,

superior mesenteric, inferior mesenteric, and pancreatic collateral veins.

Other islet cell tumors are rare in children. They may be found in association with tumors in other organs as part of the multiple endocrine neoplasia syndromes. Gastrinomas may be found in children with Zollinger-Ellison syndrome. According to Grosfeld and associates, 2 of 56 reported cases of VIP-producing tumors in children were islet cell tumors; neurogenic tumors generated the hormone in the other patients. Glucagonomas and somatostatinomas have not been reported in children. McClain and colleagues reported a case of inflammatory pseudotumor of the pancreas in an 11-year-old child.

Other Pancreatic Tumors

The exocrine tissues of the pancreas give rise to benign and malignant tumors that are hormonally inactive, such as cystadenoma, adenocarcinoma, and adenosarcoma. The most common presenting symptoms include

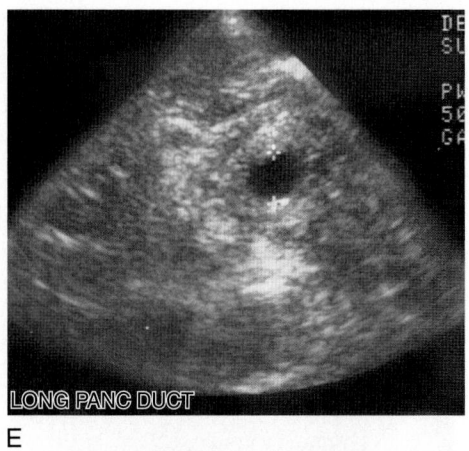

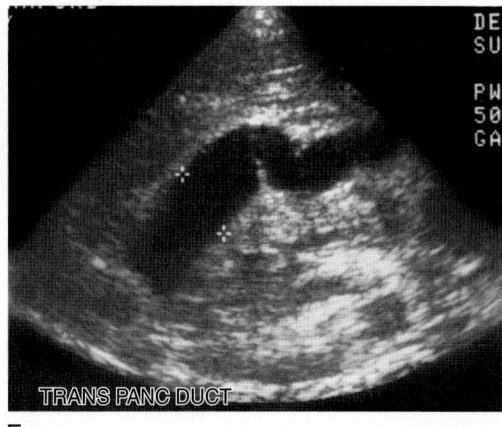

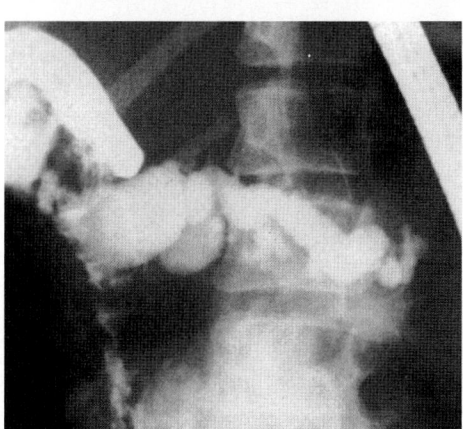

FIGURE 120-14, cont'd. Mediastinal infiltration of a pancreatic pseudocyst. **E** and **F,** Longitudinal (**E**) and transverse (**F**) sonograms of the midabdomen show marked dilation of the pancreatic duct. **G,** ERCP shows a dilated pancreatic duct, characteristic of chronic pancreatitis.

abdominal pain in 55.8%, nausea or vomiting in 32.6%, fatigue in 25.6%, and an abdominal mass in 23.3%, as reported by Liang and coworkers. Cystadenomas and adenocarcinomas of the pancreas occur in children and have been described in infants as well. Pancreatic adenosarcoma has been described in an adolescent boy with Peutz-Jeghers syndrome; Giardiello and colleagues noted a 100-fold increased risk of pancreatic adeno-carcinoma in patients with this syndrome. On US, solid tumors are typically hyperechoic, and cystic lesions are anechoic or hypoechoic. Adenocarcinomas may have cystic or hemorrhagic areas, resulting in mixed echogen-icity. CT usually identifies a pancreatic mass of variable size, often causing obstruction of the bile duct. In a recent study by Luttges and associates, pancreatic ductal adenocarcinomas were identified in only 3 patients younger than 20 years among a total cohort of 439 cases, corresponding to an incidence of 0.1% in this age group. Two of these patients had a mucinous component. Such tumors are often associated with a genetic predisposition. Because the diagnosis of pancreatic carcinoma is so rare in children (only about 50 cases have been reported), imaging evaluation is often delayed, and vascular invasion and metastases to lymph nodes and liver may be noted on imaging.

Rhabdomyosarcoma may arise primarily in the pancreas (Fig. 120-19), as may lymphoma (Fig. 120-20). Neuro-blastoma has been reported in the pancreas secondary to direct extension. A single case of abdominal desmoid tumor presenting in the pancreas has been reported in a 17-year-old boy with familial adenomatous polyposis syndrome.

Lymphangiomas of the pancreas are extremely rare, accounting for less than 1% of all lymphangiomas. They may occur in any portion of the pancreas at any age and are more frequent in females than in males. On imaging, lymphangiomas appear as septated, fluid-filled masses. Clinical presentation is nonspecific and includes nausea, vomiting, vague abdominal pain, and a palpable mass.

Exceptionally rare tumors of the pancreas include anaplastic large cell lymphoma (one case reported by Fraser and colleagues), infantile myofibromatosis (a single case reported by Rohrer and coworkers), and mature cystic teratoma. Anaplastic large cell lymphoma pre-sented in a 13-year-old boy with epigastric pain, nausea, vomiting, and weight loss. Abdominal US and CT demonstrated a large, solid soft tissue mass involving the pancreatic head. Cystic teratoma of the pancreas has been reported in at least seven pediatric cases, ranging in age from 2 to 16 years. These tumors arise from pluripotential cells of ectodermal cell lines and, like other extragonadal teratomas, likely originate from aberrant germ cells. Such cases may be indistinguishable from other cystic abdominal masses.

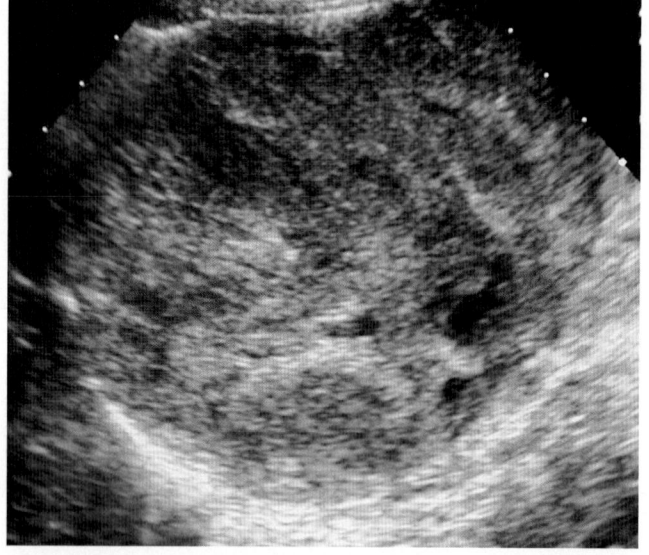

A

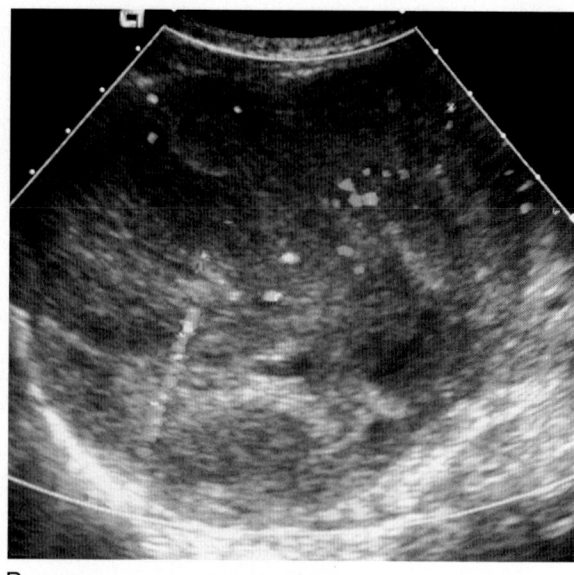

B

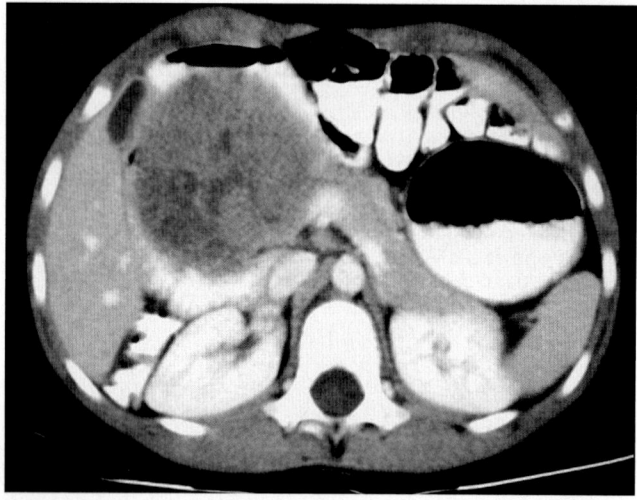

C

FIGURE 120-15. Solid-cystic papillary tumor (Frantz tumor). **A,** Axial US through the midabdomen shows a large, heterogeneous, solid mass that arises from the pancreatic head. **B,** The mass is mildly vascular, as shown with gray scale depiction of the color Doppler image. **C,** Axial contrast-enhanced CT through the midabdomen shows the mildly heterogeneous enhancement pattern of the mass and its origin from the head of the pancreas, widening and displacing the duodenal loop.

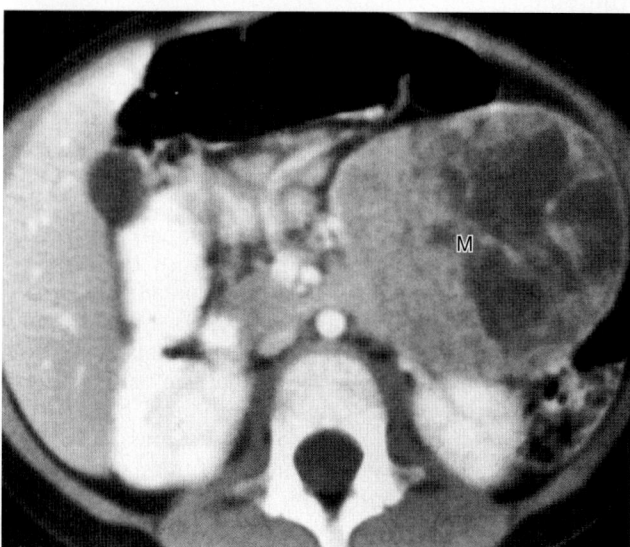

FIGURE 120-16. Pancreaticoblastoma. Axial contrast-enhanced CT in a child shows a large, heterogeneously enhancing mass (M) arising from the pancreatic tail. (Courtesy of Dr. Marilyn Siegel, St. Louis, MO.)

Pancreatic involvement with metastatic disease is also rare but includes malignant melanoma, lymphoma (Fig. 120-21), rhabdomyosarcoma (Fig. 120-22), acute lymphoblastic leukemia, and osteosarcoma (Fig. 120-23).

Tumors found in the pancreas include:

• **Solid-cystic papillary tumor (Frantz tumor)**
• **Pancreaticoblastoma**
• **Islet cell tumors—insulinoma most common**
• **Cystadenoma, adenocarcinoma, adenosarcoma**
• **Lymphoma**
• **Rhabdomyosarcoma**

HYDATID DISEASE

Hydatid cysts of the pancreas are neither congenital nor true neoplasms, and they are extremely rare. However,

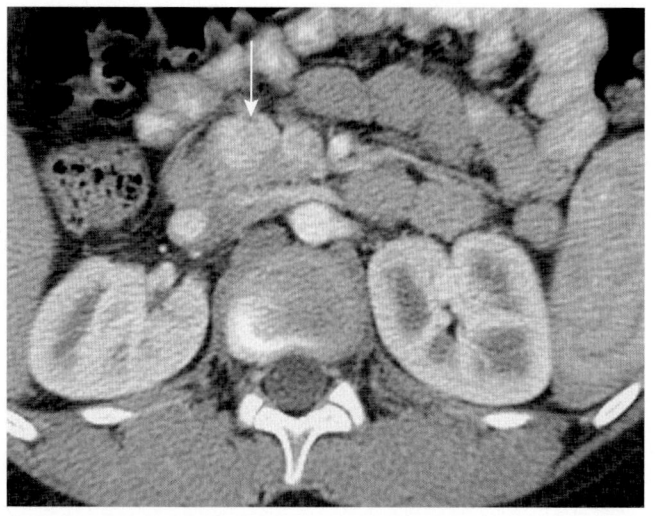

A

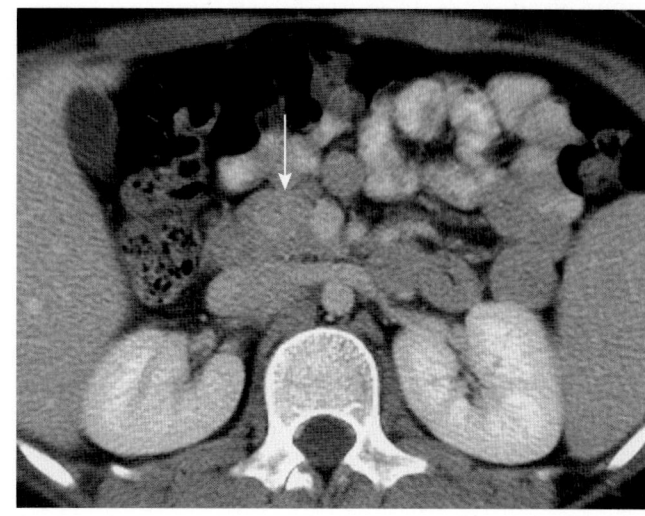

B

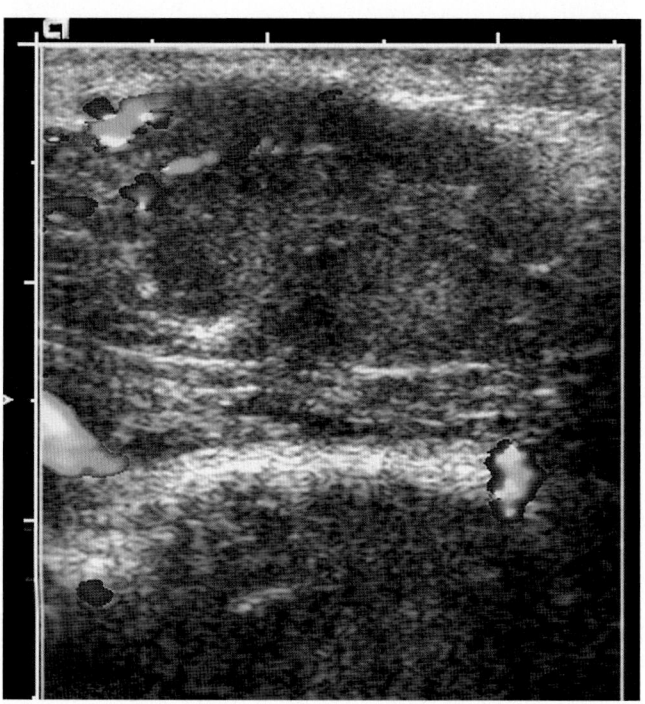

C

FIGURE 120-17. Insulinoma. **A** and **B,** Axial contrast-enhanced CT images through the pancreas during the arterial **(A)** and venous **(B)** phases show a well-defined, ovoid, enhancing mass at the junction of the head and body of the pancreas (to the left of the superior mesenteric vein; *arrows*), which is particularly conspicuous on the arterial phase. **C,** Intraoperative US confirms the mass as a well-defined lesion of intermediate echogenicity within the pancreas. (Courtesy of Dr. George Taylor, Boston, MA.)

they have been reported in 0.1% to 0.2% of patients with hydatid disease. Krige and colleagues reported pancreatic hydatid disease without other associated hydatid disease in two teenagers and two adults. In each of these cases, jaundice and abdominal pain were the presenting symptoms. Abdominal CT demonstrated a complex cystic pancreatic head mass in all four cases; there was a second similar lesion in the pancreatic tail in one

patient. Hydatid disease of the pancreas may also be a rare cause of recurrent pancreatitis.

ACKNOWLEDGMENTS

I thank Sandra Gaither for manuscript preparation and the Department of Biomedical Communications for the preparation of figure images.

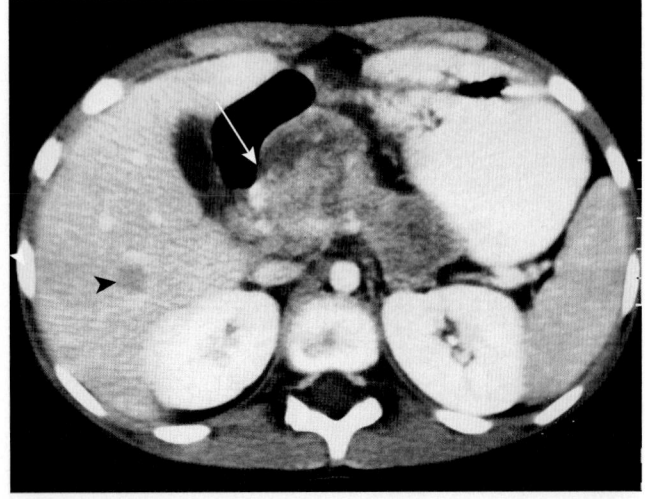

A

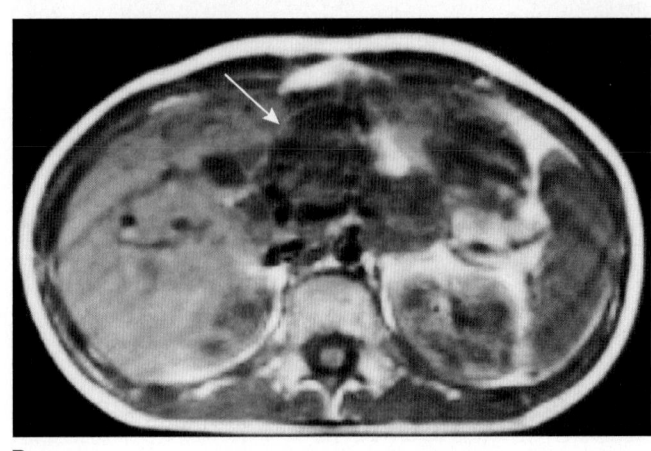

B

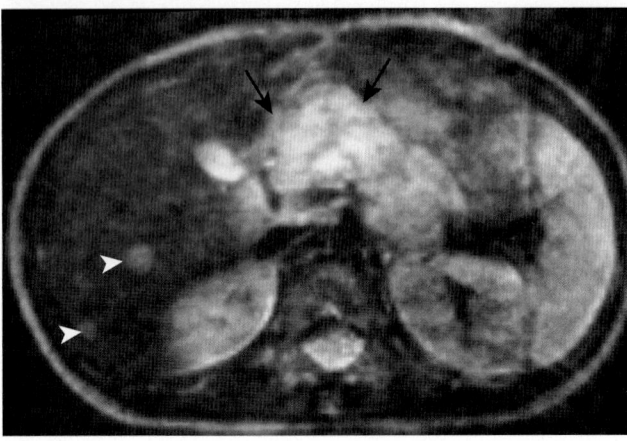

C

FIGURE 120-18. Insulinoma. **A,** Axial contrast-enhanced CT through the pancreas in a 10-year-old girl with hypoglycemia. There is a large, heterogeneously enhancing mass involving the pancreatic head *(arrow)*. The remainder of the pancreas is also somewhat enlarged. Note the low-density hepatic metastasis *(arrowhead)*. **B,** Axial T1-weighted MR image at the same level shows the intermediate-density pancreatic mass *(arrow)*. **C,** T2-weighted sequence shows intensely increased signal *(arrows)*. Note also the conspicuity of the liver metastases on T2 weighting and a second, smaller metastatic focus more peripherally *(arrowheads)*.

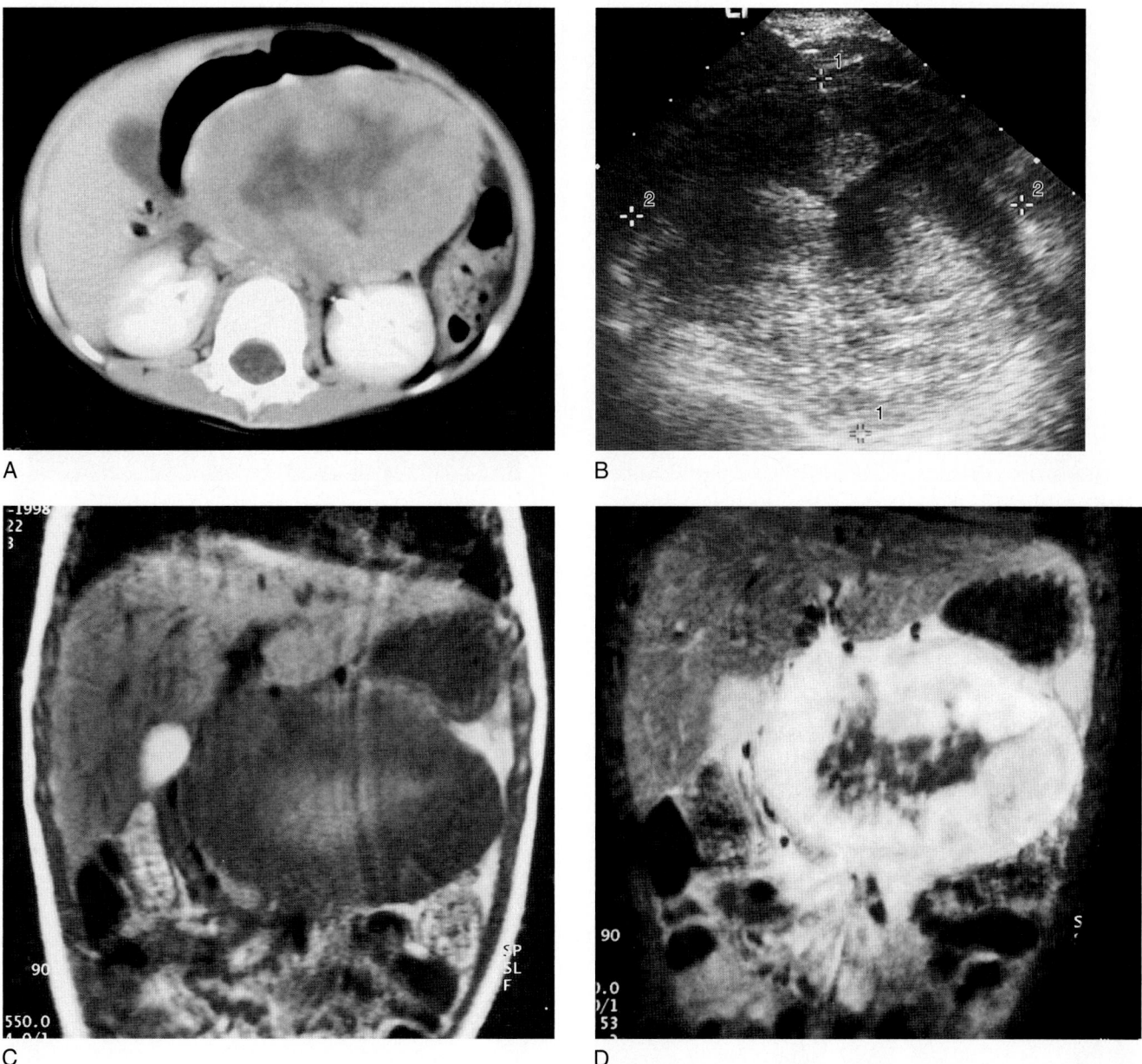

A

B

C

D

FIGURE 120-19. Primary alveolar rhabdomyosacroma of the pancreas in a 3-year-old boy. **A,** Axial, contrasted abdominal CT shows a large midabdominal mass that arises from the pancreatic body, with a central hypodense area. **B,** Axial US through the upper abdomen shows the mass to be of heterogeneous echogenicity. **C,** Coronal, noncontrast, T1-weighted MR image shows irregular high signal centrally, surrounded by decreased signal in the bulk of the mass. **D,** Coronal, contrast-enhanced, T1-weighted image with fat saturation shows diffuse, intense peripheral enhancement of the bulk of the mass around the central area, as well as surrounding edema.

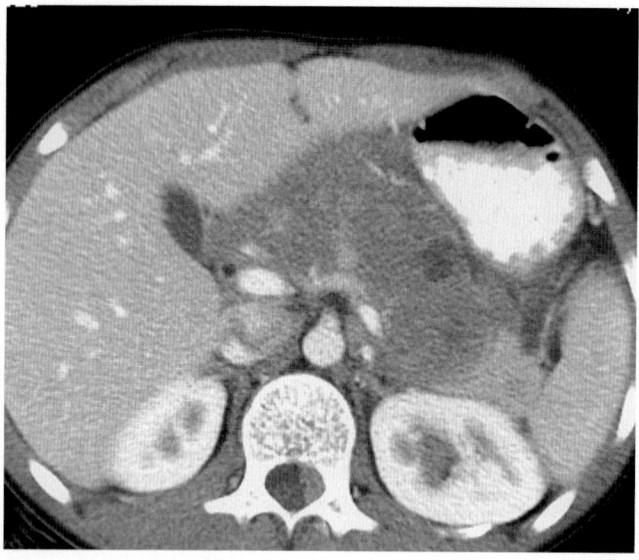
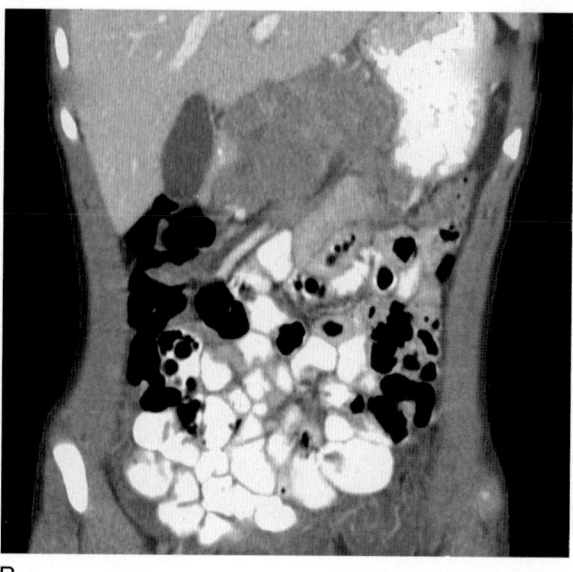

A   B

FIGURE 120-20. Primary pancreatic non-Hodgkin lymphoma. **A** and **B**, Axial **(A)** and reconstructed coronal **(B)** contrasted-enhanced CT images through the abdomen show diffuse enlargement of the pancreas with focal low-density regions, suggesting necrosis. Mass effect on the stomach from this primary pancreatic Burkitt lymphoma is best seen on the coronal reconstruction. (Courtesy of Dr. George Taylor, Boston, MA.)

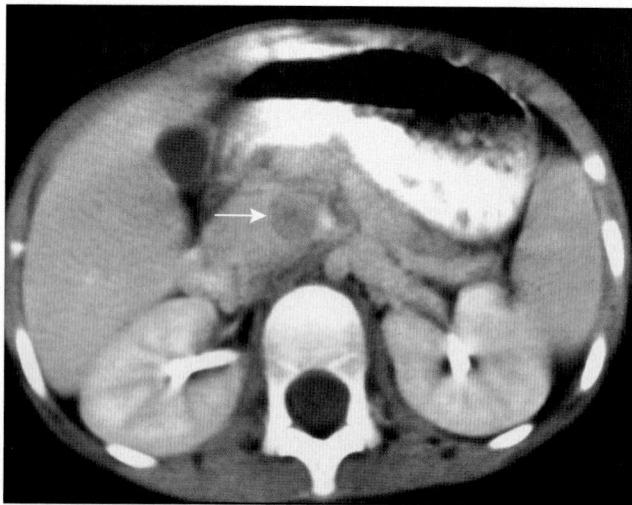

FIGURE 120-21. Primary lymphoma of bone, metastatic to the pancreas. Axial CT of the abdomen in an 8-year-old boy with known lymphoma of bone shows a focal, well-defined, low-density mass within the body of the pancreas *(arrow)*. This lesion showed mild gallium uptake on a staging gallium scan (not shown).

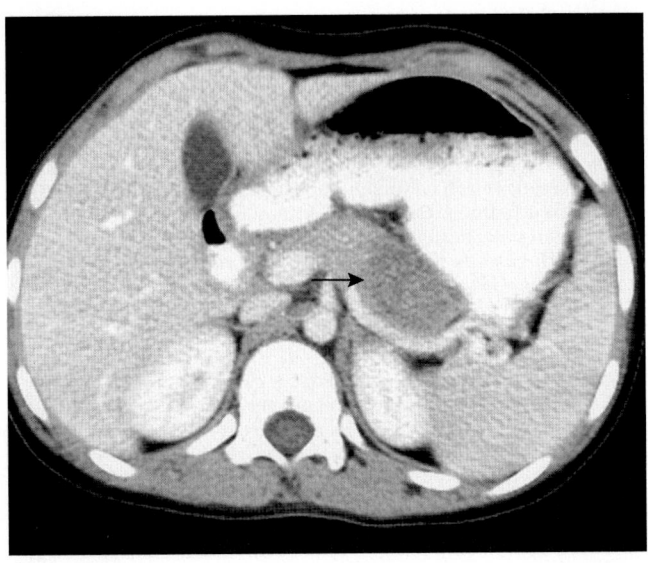
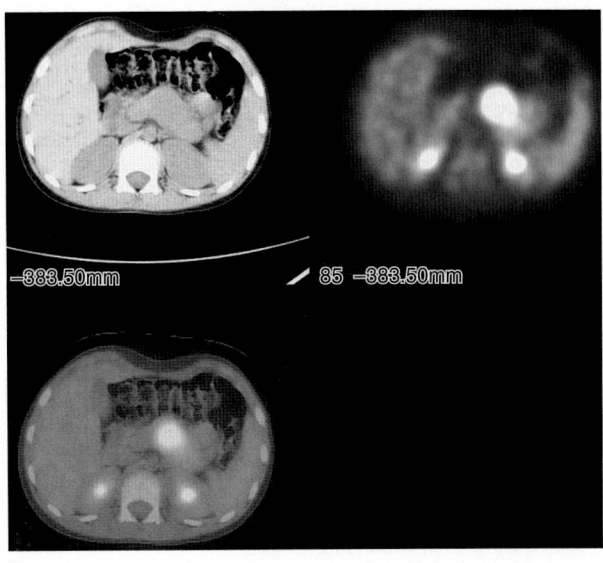

A   B

FIGURE 120-22. Recurrent rhabdomyosarcoma, metastatic to the pancreas. Three years earlier, this 10-year-old girl had been treated for alveolar rhabdomyosarcoma of the calf. **A,** Axial, contrast-enhanced abdominal CT shows a well-defined low-density mass in the pancreas *(arrow)*. **B,** Axial fluorodeoxyglucose positron emission tomography-CT image shows the lesion as a focal mass with intense uptake of radiopharmaceutical in the midbody of the pancreas. (*See color plate.*)

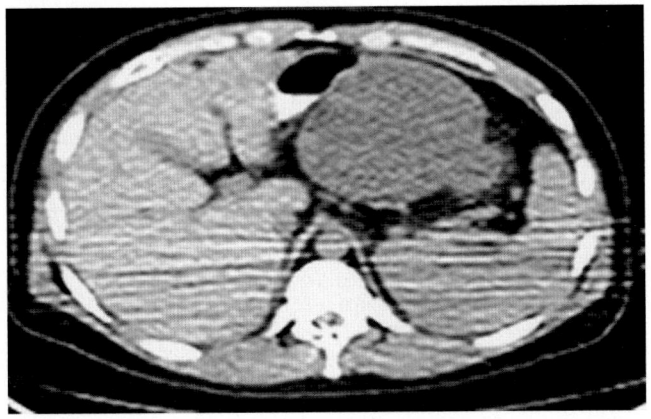

A

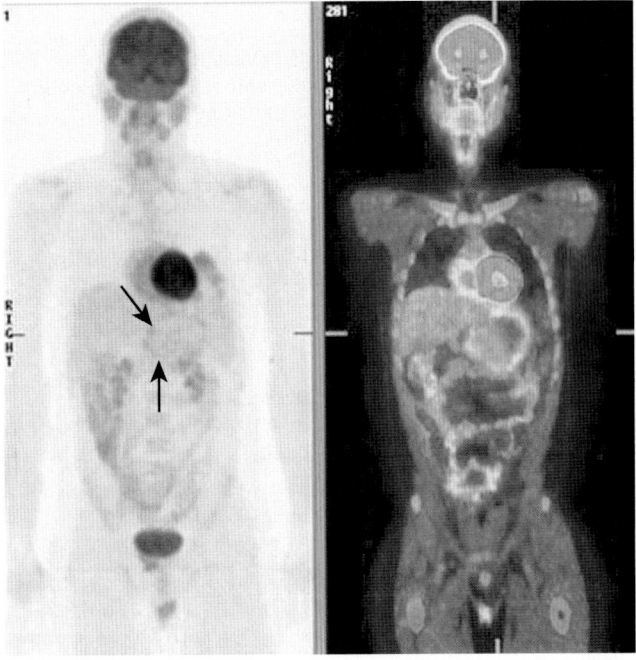

FIGURE 120-23. Recurrent osteosarcoma in 19-year-old man, metastatic to the pancreas. Five years earlier, the patient had been treated for nonmetastatic primary femoral osteosarcoma with multiagent chemotherapy and limb-sparing surgery. He had been well until presenting with abdominal pain and fatigue. **A,** Noncontrast axial CT through the upper abdomen as part of a fluorodeoxyglucose (FDG) positron emission tomography (PET) examination shows a large, low-density midabdominal mass arising from the midbody of the pancreas. **B,** Anterior planar technetium-99m bone scan *(left)* shows a subtle blush of uptake in the distribution of the mass *(arrows)*. Fused FDG PET-CT image *(right)* shows minimal peripheral uptake in the mass and central photopenia, consistent with central necrosis; this was confirmed by aspiration and biopsy. (*See color plate.*)

B

SUGGESTED READINGS

Imaging the Pancreas

Allendorph M, Werlin SL, Geenen JE, et al: Endoscopic retrograde cholangiopancreatography in children. J Pediatr 1987;110:206

Arcement CM, Meza MP, Arumania S, et al: MRCP in the evaluation of pancreaticobiliary disease in children. Pediatr Radiol 2001;31:92

Bolog N, Constantinescu G, Oancea I, et al: Magnetic resonance imaging of bile and pancreatic ducts: a retrospective study. Rom J Gastroenterol 2004;13:91

Fukukura Y, Fujiyoshi F, Sasaki M, Nakajo M: Pancreatic duct: morphologic evaluation with MR cholangiopancreatography after secretin stimulation. Radiology 2002;222:674

Fulcher AS, Turner MA: Orthotopic liver transplantation: evaluation with MR cholangiography. Radiology 1999;211:715

Fuss M, Salter BJ, Cavanaugh SX, et al: Daily ultrasound-based image-guided targeting for radiotherapy of upper abdominal malignancies. Int J Radiat Oncol Biol Phys 2004;59:1245

Gong J-S, Xu J-M: Role of curved planar reformations using multidetector spiral CT in diagnosis of pancreatic and peripancreatic diseases. World J Gastroenterol 2004;10:1943

Hamada Y, Sato M, Sanada T, et al: Spiral computed tomography for biliary dilatation. J Pediatr Surg 1995;30:694

Hamada Y, Tanano A, Takada K, et al: Magnetic resonance cholangiopancreatography on postoperative work-up in children with choledochal cysts. Pediatr Surg Int 2004;20:43

Hanninen EL, Amthauer H, Hosten N, et al: Prospective evaluation of pancreatic tumors: accuracy of MR imaging with MR cholangiopancreatography and MR angiography. Radiology 2002;224:34

Herman TE, Siegel MJ: CT of the pancreas in children. AJR Am J Roentgenol 1991;1547:375

Laor T, Hoffer FA, Vacanti JP, et al: MR cholangiography in children after liver transplantation from living related donors. AJR Am J Roentgenol 1998;170:683

Lawson TL, Berland LL, Foley WD, et al: Ultrasonic visualization of the pancreatic duct. Radiology 1982;144:865

Manfredi R, Lucidi V, Gui B, et al: Idiopathic chronic pancreatitis in children: MR cholangiopancreatography after secretin administration. Radiology 2002;224:675

Matos C, Cappeliez O, Winant C, et al: MR imaging of the pancreas: a pictorial tour. Radiographics 2002;22:e2

Nijs E, Callahan MJ, Taylor GA: Disorders of the pediatric pancreas: imaging features. Pediatr Radiol 2005;35:358

Siegel MJ, Martin KW, Worthington JL: Normal and abnormal pancreas in children: US studies. Radiology 1987;165:15

Teele RL, Share JC: Ultrasonography of Infants and Children. Philadelphia, Saunders, 1990:389

Ueda D: Sonographic measurement of the pancreas in children. J Clin Ultrasound 1989;17:417

Walsh E, Cramer B, Pushpanthan C: Pancreatic echogenicity in premature and newborn infants. Pediatr Radiol 1990;20:323

Congenital and Hereditary Abnormalities

Baggott BB, Long WB: Annular pancreas as a cause of extrahepatic biliary obstruction. Am J Gastroenterol 1991;86:224

Baker LL, Hartman GE, Northway WH Jr: Sonographic detection of congenital pancreatic cysts in the newborn: report of a case and review of the literature. Pediatr Radiol 1990;20:488

Camoglio FS, Forestler C, Zanatta C, et al: Complete pancreatic ectopia in a gastric duplication cyst: a case report and review of the literature. Eur J Pediatr Surg 2004;14:60

Choyke PL, Filling-Katz MR, Shawker TH, et al: Von Hippel–Lindau disease: radiologic screening for visceral manifestations. Radiology 1990;174:815

Clavon M, Verain AL, Bigard MA: Cyst formation in gastroheterotopic pancreas: report of two cases. Radiology 1988;169:659

Daneman A, Gaskin K, Martin DJ, et al: Pancreatic changes in cystic fibrosis: CT and sonographic appearances. AJR Am J Roentgenol 1983;141:653

Eras M, Yenigun M, Acar C, et al: Pancreatic involvement in von Hippel–Lindau disease. Indian J Cancer 2004;41:159

Ferrozzi F, Bova D, Campodonico F, et al: Cystic fibrosis: MR assessment of pancreatic damage. Radiology 1996;198:875

Hernanz-Schulman M, Teele RL, Perez-Atayde A, et al: Pancreatic cystosis in cystic fibrosis. Radiology 1986;158:629

Itoh Y, Hada T, Terano A, et al: Pancreatitis in the annulus of annular pancreas demonstrated by the combined use of computed tomography and endoscopic retrograde cholangiopancreatography. Am J Gastroenterol 1989;84:961

Kamisawa T, Yoshiike M, Egawa N, et al: Classification of choledochocele. Hepatogastroenterology 2005;52:29

Kilman WJ, Berk RN: The spectrum of radiographic features of aberrant pancreatic rests involving the stomach. Radiology 1977;123:291

Lindstrom E, Ihse I: Dynamic CT scanning of pancreatic duct after secretin provocation in pancreas divisum. Dig Dis Sci 1990;35:1371

Liu P, Daneman A, Stringer DA, et al: Pancreatic cysts and calcification in cystic fibrosis. J Can Assoc Radiol 1986;37:279

Manfredi R, Costamagna G, Brizi MG, et al: Pancreas divisum and "satorincele": diagnosis with dynamic MR cholangiopancreatography with secretin stimulation. Radiology 2000;217:403

Marsh TD, Farach L, Wood BP: Radiological case of the month: obstructing annular pancreas. Am J Dis Child 1990;144:505

Matos C, Metens T, Deviere J, et al: Pancreas divisum: evaluation with secretin-enhanced magnetic resonance cholangiopancreatography. Gastrointest Endosc 2001;53:728

McHugo JM, McKeown C, Brown MT, et al: Ultrasound findings in children with cystic fibrosis. Pediatr Radiol 1990;20:536

Murayama S, Robinson AE, Mulvihill DM, et al: MR imaging of pancreas in cystic fibrosis. Pediatr Radiol 1990;20:536

Mustafa E, Mustafa Y, Cengiz A, et al: Pancreatic involvement in von Hippel–Lindau disease. Indian J Cancer 2004;41:159

Nguyen KT, Pace R, Groll A: CT appearance of annular pancreas: a case report. J Can Assoc Radiol 1989;40:322

Rahmah R, Yong JF, Sharifa NA, et al: Bilateral adrenal cysts and ectopic pancreatic tissue in Beckwith-Wiedemann syndrome: is a conservative approach acceptable? J Pediatr Endocrinol Metab 2004;17:909

Sodhi KS, Thapa BR, Khadelwal S, Suri S: Pancreatic lipomatosis in an infant with cystic fibrosis. Pediatr Radiol 2005;35:1157

Soulen MC, Zerhouni EA, Fishman EK, et al: Enlargement of the pancreatic head in patients with pancreas divisum. Clin Imaging 1989;13:51

Tham RTOT, Heyerman HGM, Falke THM, et al: Cystic fibrosis: MR imaging of the pancreas. Radiology 1991;179:183

Tillig B, Gerein V, Coerdt W, et al: Large supraumbilical pseudocystic tumour due to ectopic pancreatic tissue located in a rest of the omphaloenteric duct. Eur J Pediatr Surg 2004;14:126

Ueda D, Taketazu M, Itoh S, et al: A case of gastric duplication cyst with aberrant pancreas. Pediatr Radiol 1991;21:379

Werlin SL: Pancreatitis. In McMillan JA, DeAngelis CD, Feigin RD, Warshaw JB (eds): Oski's Pediatrics: Principles and Practice, 3rd ed. Philadelphia, Lippincott Williams & Wilkins, 1999:1712-1713

Willi UV, Reddish JM, Teele RL: Cystic fibrosis: its characteristic appearance on abdominal sonography. AJR Am J Roentgenol 1980;134:1005

Zeman RK, McVay LV, Silverman PM, et al: Pancreas divisum: thin-section CT. Radiology 1988;169:395

Acute and Chronic Pancreatitis

Albu E, Buiumsohn A, Lopez R, et al: Gallstone pancreatitis in adolescents. J Pediatr Surg 1987;22:960

Amundson GM, Towbin RB, Mueller DL, et al: Percutaneous transgastric drainage of the lesser sac in children. Pediatr Radiol 1990;20:590

Atkinson GO Jr, Wyly JB, Gay BB Jr, et al: Idiopathic fibrosing pancreatitis: a cause of obstructive jaundice in childhood. Pediatr Radiol 1988;18:28

Balthazar EJ, Robinson DL, Megabow AJ, et al: Acute pancreatitis: value of CT in establishing prognosis. Radiology 1990;174:331

Chao HC, Lin SJ, Kong MS, et al: Sonographic evaluation of the pancreatic duct in normal children and children with pancreatitis. J Ultrasound Med 2000;19:757

Crombleholme TM, deLorimier AA, Adzick NS, et al: Mediastinal pancreatic pseudocysts in children. J Pediatr Surg 1990;25:843

Crombleholme TM, deLorimier AA, Way LW, et al: The modified Puestow procedure for chronic relapsing pancreatitis in children. J Pediatr Surg 1990;25:749

Fleischer AC, Parker P, Kirchner SG: Sonographic findings of pancreatitis in children. Radiology 1986;146:151

Ford EG, Hardin WD Jr, Mahour GH, et al: Pseudocysts of the pancreas in children. Am Surg 1990;56:384

Garel L, Burnelle F, Lallemand D, et al: Pseudocysts of the pancreas in children: which cases require surgery? Pediatr Radiol 1983;13:120

Haller J, Greenway G, Resnick D, et al: Intraosseous fat necrosis associated with acute pancreatitis: MR imaging. Radiology 1989;173:193

Handrich SJ, Hough DM, Fletcher JG, Sarr MG: The natural history of the incidentally discovered small simple pancreatic cyst: long-term follow-up and clinical implications. AJR Am J Roentgenol 2005;184:20

Huntington DK, Hill MC, Steinberg W: Biliary tract dilatation in chronic pancreatitis: CT and sonographic findings. Radiology 1989;172:47

Jeffrey RB Jr: Sonography in acute pancreatitis. Radiol Clin North Am 1989;27:5

Jeffrey RB Jr, Laing FC, Wing VW: Extrapancreatic spread of acute pancreatitis: new observations with real-time US. Radiology 1986;159:707

Jeong JB, Whang JH, Ryu JK: Risk factors for pancreatitis in patients with anomalous union of pancreatobiliary duct. Hepatogastroenterolgy 2004;51:1187

Lee SP, Nicholls JF, Park HZ: Biliary sludge as a cause of acute pancreatitis. N Engl J Med 1992;326:589

Mehta R, Survarna D, Sadasivan S, et al: Natural course of asymptomatic pancreatic pseudocyst: a prospective study. Indian J Gastroenterol 2004;23:140

Millward SF, Breatnach E, Simpkins KC, et al: Do plain films of the chest and abdomen have a role in the diagnosis of acute pancreatitis? Clin Radiol 1983;34:133

Mortele KJ, Wiesner W, Intriere L, et al: A modified CT severity index for evaluating acute pancreatitits: Improved correlation with patient outcome. AJR Am J Roentgenol 2004;183:1261

Ozmen MM, Moran M, Karakahya M, Coskun F: Recurrent acute pancreatitis due to a hydatid cyst of the pancreatic head: a case report and review of the literature. JOP 2005;6:354

Rollins MD, Meyers RL: Frey procedure for surgical management of chronic pancreatitis in children. J Pediatr Surg 2004;39:817

Sadry F, Hausen H: Fatal pancreatitis secondary to iatrogenic intramural hematoma: a case report and review of the literature. Gastrointest Radiol 1990;15:296

Shimizu T, Suzuki R, Yamashiro Y, et al: Magnetic resonance cholangiopancreatography in assessing the cause of acute pancreatitis in children. Pancreas 2001;2:196

Slovis TL, von Berg VJ, Mikelic V: Sonography in the diagnosis and management of pancreatic pseudocysts and effusions in childhood. Radiology 1980;135:153

Sonnenberg E, Wittich GR, Casola G, et al: Percutaneous drainage of infected and noninfected pancreatic pseudocysts: experience in 101 cases. Radiology 1980;170:757

Spencer JA, Lindsell DRM, Isaacs D: Hereditary pancreatitis: early ultrasound appearances. Pediatr Radiol 1990;20:293

Stoler J, Biller JA, Grand RJ: Pancreatitis in Kawasaki disease. Am J Dis Child 1987;141:306

Stringer MD: Pancreatic trauma in children. Br J Surg 2005;92:467

Stringer MD, Davison SM, McClean P, et al: Multidisciplinary management of surgical disorders of the pancreas in childhood. J Pediatr Gastroenterol Nutr 2005;40:363

Suarez F, Bernard O, Gauthier F, et al: Bilio-pancreatic common channel in children: clinical, biological and radiological findings in 12 children. Pediatr Radiol 1987;17:206

Swischuk LE, Hayden CK Jr: Pararenal space hyperechogenicity in childhood pancreatitis. AJR Am J Roentgenol 1985;145:1085

Weizman Z, Durie PR: Acute pancreatitis in childhood. J Pediatr 1988;113:24

Wheatley MJ, Coran AG: Obstructive jaundice secondary to chronic pancreatitis in children: report of two cases and review of the literature. Surgery 1988;104:863

Yin WY: The role of surgery in pancreatic pseudocyst. Hepatogastroenterology 2005;52:1266

Ziegler DW, Long JA, Philippart AI, et al: Pancreatitis in childhood. Ann Surg 1988;207:257

Pancreatic Neoplasms

Bowlby LS: Pancreatic adenocarcinoma in an adolescent male with Peutz-Jeghers syndrome. Hum Pathol 1986;17:97

Brenner RW, Sank LI, Kerner MB, et al: Resection of a VIPoma of the pancreas in a 15-year-old girl. J Pediatr Surg 1986;21:983

Brunelle F, Negre V, Barth MO, et al: Pancreatic venous samplings in infants and children with primary hyperinsulinism. Pediatr Radiol 1989;19:100

Carricaburu E, Enezian G, Bonnard A, et al: Laparoscopic distal pancreatectomy for Frantz's tumor in a child. Surg Endosc 2003;17:2028

Cheng D-F, Peng C-G, Zhou G-W, et al: Clinical misdiagnosis of solid pseudopapillary tumour of pancreas. Chin Med J 2005;118:922

Choi BI, Kim KW, Han MC, et al: Solid and papillary epithelial neoplasms of the pancreas: CT findings. Radiology 1988;166:413

Dhebri AR, Connor S, Campbell F, et al: Diagnosis, treatment and outcome of pancreatoblastoma. Pancreatology 2004;4:441; discussion 452

D'Onofrio M, Malago R, Vecchiato F, et al: Contrast-enhanced ultrasonography of small solid pseudopapillary tumors of the pancreas: enhancement pattern and pathologic correlation of 2 cases. J Ultrasound Med 2005;24:849

Fraser CJ, Chan YF, Heath JA: Anaplastic large cell lymphoma of the pancreas: a pediatric case and literature review. J Pediatr Hematol Oncol 2004;26:840

Friedman AC, Lichtenstein JE, Fishman EK, et al: Solid and papillary epithelial neoplasm of the pancreas. Radiology 1985;154:333

Galiber AK, Reading CC, Charboneau JW: Localization of pancreatic insulinoma: comparison of pre- and intraoperative ultrasound with CT and angiography. Radiology 1988;166:405

Giardiello FM, Welsh SB, Hamilton SR, et al: Increased risk of cancer in the Peutz-Jeghers syndrome. N Engl J Med 1987;316:1151

Grant CS, Heerden J, Charboneau W: Insulinoma: the value of intraoperative ultrasonography. Arch Surg 1988;123:843

Grosfeld JL, Vane DW, Rescorla FJ, et al: Pancreatic tumors in childhood: analysis of 13 cases. J Pediatr Surg 1990;25:1057

Hassan I, Celik I, Nies C, et al: Successful treatment of solid-pseudopapillary tumor of the pancreas with multiple liver metastases. Pancreatology 2005;5:289

Hecht ST, Barsch RC, Styne DM: CT localization of occult secretory tumors in children. Pediatr Radiol 1982;12:67

Huang H-L, Shih S-C, Chang W-H, et al: Solid-pseudopapillary tumor of the pancreas: clinical experience and literature review. World J Gastroenterol 2005;11:1403

Kim SJ, Choi J-A, Lee SH, et al: Imaging findings of extrapulmonary metastases of osteosarcoma. J Clin Imaging 2004;28:291

Kosmahl M, Pauser U, Peters K, et al: Cystic neoplasms of the pancreas and tumor-like lesions with cystic features: a review of 418 cases and a classification proposal. Virchows Arch 2004; 445:168

Krige JE, Mirza K, Bornman PC, Beningfield SJ: Primary hydatid cysts of the pancreas. S Afr J Surg 2005;43:37

Lau ST, Kim SS, Lee SL, Schaller RT: Mucinous cystadenoma of the pancreas in a one-year-old child. J Pediatr Surg 2004;39:1574

Liang H, Wang P, Wang X-N, et al: Management of nonfunctioning islet cell tumors. World J Gastroenterol 2004;10:1806

Luttges J, Stigge C, Pacena M, Kloppel G: Rare ductal adenocarcinoma of the pancreas in patients younger than age 40 years: an analysis of its features and a literature review. Cancer 2004;100:173

McClain MB, Burton EM, Day DS: Pancreatic pseudotumor in an 11-year-old child: imaging findings. Pediatr Radiol 2000;30:610

Miller DV, Coffin CM, Zhou H: Rhabdomyosarcoma arising in the hand or foot: a clinicopathologic analysis. Pediatr Dev Pathol 2004;7:361

Moholkar S, Sebire NJ, Roebuck DJ: Solid-pseudopapillary neoplasm of the pancreas: radiological-pathological correlation. Pediatr Radiol 2005;35:819

Montemarano H, Lonergan GJ, Bulas DI, et al: Pancreatoblastoma: imaging findings in 10 patients and review of the literature. Radiology 2000;214:476

Moynan RW, Neehout RC, Johnson TS: Pancreatic carcinoma in childhood: case report and review. J Pediatr 1964;65:711

Nikou GC, Toubanakis C, Nikolaou P, et al: VIPomas: an updated diagnosis and management in a series of 11 patients. Hepatogastroenterology 2005;52:1259

Paal E, Thompson LD, Heffess CS: A clinicopathologic and immunohistochemical study of ten pancreatic lymphangiomas and a review of the literature. Cancer 1998;82:2150

Pho LN, Coffin CM, Burt RW: Abdominal desmoid in familial adenomatous polyposis presenting as a pancreatic cystic lesion. Fam Cancer 2005;4:135

Raffel A, Cupisti K, Krausch M, et al: Therapeutic strategy of papillary cystic and solid neoplasm (PCSN): a rare non-endocrine tumor of the pancreas in children. Surg Oncol 2004;13:1

Robey G, Daneman A, Martin DJ: Pancreatic carcinoma in a neonate. Pediatr Radiol 1983;13:284

Roebuck DJ, Yuen MK, Wong YC, et al: Imaging features of pancreatoblastoma. Pediatr Radiol 2001;31:501

Rohrer K, Murphy R, Thresher C, et al: Infantile myofibromatosis: a most unusual cause of gastric outlet obstruction. Pediatr Radiol 2005;35:808

Rossi P, Allison DJ, Bezzi M: Endocrine tumors of the pancreas. Radiol Clin North Am 1989;27:129

Salimi J, Karbakhsh M, Dolatshahi S, Ahmadi SA: Cystic teratoma of the pancreas: a case report. Ann Saudi Med 2004;24:206

Sato A, Imaizumi M, Chikaoka S, et al: Acute renal failure due to leukemic cell infiltration followed by relapse at multiple extramedullary sites in a child with acute lymphoblastic leukemia. Leuk Lymphoma 2004;45:825

Stephenson CA, Kletzel M, Seibert JJ, et al: Pancreatoblastoma: MR appearance. J Comput Assist Tomogr 1990;14:492

Sty JR, Wells RG: Other abdominal and pelvic masses in children. Semin Roentgenol 1988;23:216

Synn AY, Mulvihill SJ, Fonkalsrud EW: Surgical disorders of the pancreas in infancy and childhood. Am J Surg 1988;156:201

Tang LH, Aydin H, Brennan MF, Kimstra DS: Clinically aggressive solid pseudopapillary tumors of the pancreas: a report of two cases with components of undifferentiated carcinoma and a comparative clinicopathologic analysis of 34 conventional cases. Am J Surg Pathol 2005;29:512

Telander RL, Charboneau JW, Haymond MW: Intraoperative ultrasonography of the pancreas in children. J Pediatr Surg 1986;21:262

Tien Y-W, Ser K-H, Hu R-H, et al: Solid pseudopapillary neoplasms of the pancreas: is there a pathologic basis for the observed gender differences in incidence? Surgery 2005;137:591

To'o KF, Raman SS, Yu NC, et al: Pancreatic and peripancreatic diseases mimicking primary pancreatic neoplasia. Radiographics 2005;25:949

Turkish A, Levy J, Kato M, et al: Pancreatitis and probable paraneoplastic cholestasis as presenting manifestations of pancreatic lymphoma in a child. J Pediatr Gastroenterol Nutr 2004;39:552

Yakovac WC, Baker L, Hummeler K: Beta cell nesidioblastosis in idiopathic hypoglycemia of infancy. J Pediatr 1971;79:226

PART 7 THE ESOPHAGUS

CHAPTER 121

The Normal Esophagus

HENRIQUE M. LEDERMAN and GUILHERME T. S. DEMARCHI

NORMAL ANATOMY

The esophagus is a musculomembranous tubular structure that extends from the distal hypopharynx, at the level of the cricopharyngeus muscle and 7th cervical vertebra, to the esophagogastric junction, normally at the level of the 10th thoracic vertebra (Fig. 121-1). The caliber of the esophagus varies with peristaltic activity but is usually slightly narrower at both ends than along most of its intrathoracic course. Normal extrinsic impressions on the esophagus are caused by the aorta and the left main stem bronchus (Fig. 121-2). The esophagus frequently deviates slightly to the right at the level of the left atrium, just before entering the esophageal hiatus of the diaphragm. In rare cases, a hemiazygous venous impression can be seen in barium swallow studies on the left esophageal wall below the aortic arch. As the esophagus traverses the diaphragmatic hiatus, a sharply defined impression may also be evident, usually on the left, representing compression of the distal esophagus by the diaphragm.

> **Normal esophageal contour landmarks:**
> - **Cricopharyngeus muscle**
> - **Postcricoid impressions**
> - **Aortic impression**
> - **Left main stem bronchus impression**
> - **Left atrium**
> - **Diaphragm**

At its upper end, the esophagus is bounded by an anatomic sphincter, which creates a high-pressure zone and consists partly of fibers of the cricopharyngeus muscle. A second high-pressure region, with no anatomically distinct muscle sphincter, bounds the lower esophagus as it passes from the thoracic to the abdominal cavity.

The esophageal mucosa is composed of squamous epithelium except at a variable and short region at its distal end, where columnar epithelium is present. Underlying the submucosa are two relatively distinct muscle

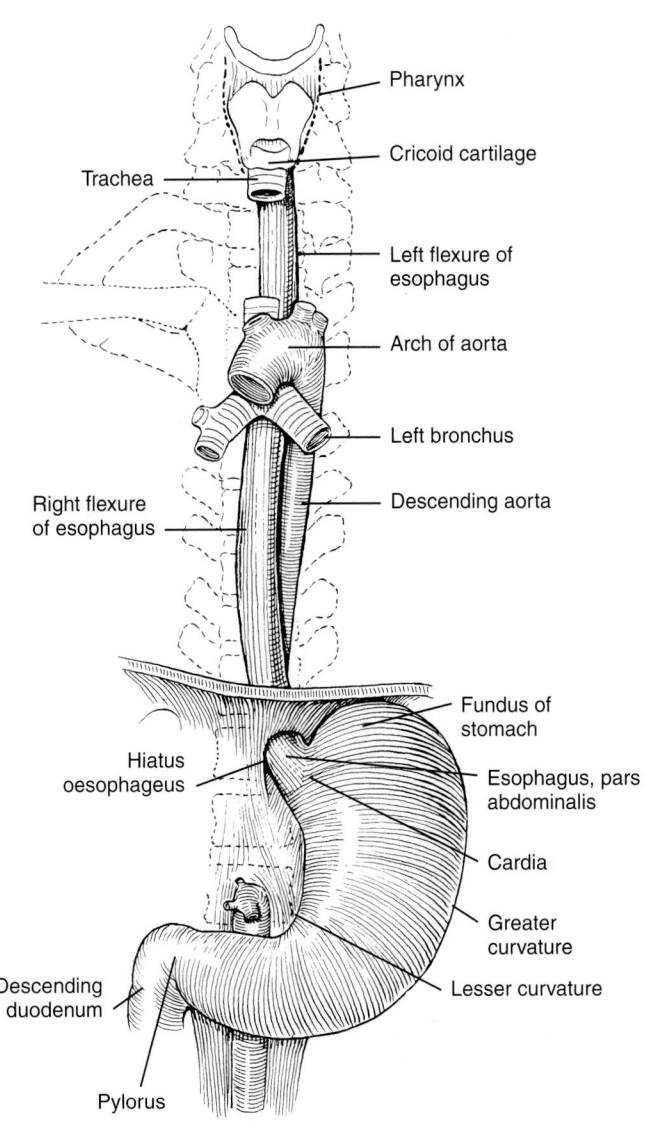

FIGURE 121-1. Semischematic drawing of the normal esophagus depicts its relation to the trachea, aorta, diaphragm, and stomach. (Modified from Schaeffer JP: Morris's Human Anatomy, 10th ed. New York, McGraw-Hill, 1943.)

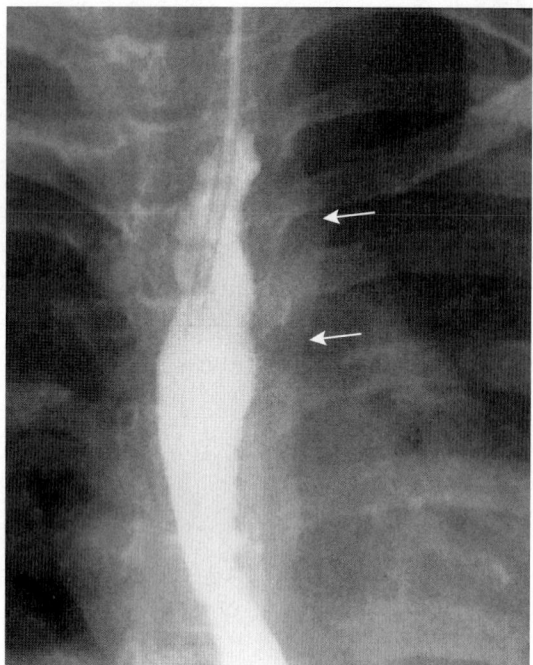

FIGURE 121-2. Barium swallow study demonstrates the impression of the aortic knob *(upper arrow)* and the left main stem bronchus *(lower arrow)* on the barium-filled esophagus. These are normal impressions and are not to be confused with mediastinal abnormalities.

groups enveloping the esophagus like coiled springs. These external muscle bundles usually consist of striated muscle in the upper fourth to third of the esophagus and of smooth muscle more distally. With the exception of its most distal region, the esophagus is not surrounded by serosa, and the absence of such a barrier contributes to the rapid spread of primary esophageal neoplasms and other disorders to the mediastinum and adjacent tissues.

When collapsed, the mucosa has thin, smooth longitudinal folds that, when coated with barium, should measure no more than 3 mm. As the esophagus distends, these folds flatten, and so a smooth outline is normally present. When fully distended by gas or barium, the very distal esophageal end enlarges to a greater diameter than the more proximal tube-shaped esophagus. This distal fusiform shape is commonly termed the *esophageal vestibule* or *phrenic ampulla*. The upper margin of the vestibule is radiographically delineated by a transient contractile area that forms a bilateral semilunar indentation termed the *A ring, inferior esophageal sphincter*, or *Wolf ring*. The lower margin of the vestibule is delineated by yet another transient short contractile region termed the *B ring, transverse mucosal fold, lower esophageal ring, Schatzki ring*, or *lower esophageal diaphragm*. The B ring is formed by a fold of mucosa overlying the upper margin of the gastric sling fibers and is usually best seen with the esophagus maximally distended. Thus, the A and B rings delineate the upper and lower limits of the radiographically defined vestibule, a region approximating the manometrically determined high-pressure zone found in the lower esophagus. The B ring is not usually identifiable when it lies below the diaphragmatic hiatus.

In young infants and children, the vestibule spans the diaphragmatic hiatus so that its upper part lies within the thorax and its distal part within the abdomen.

The mucosal esophagogastric junction (Z line) is occasionally visible as a thin, minimally radiolucent line on double contrast esophagograms. A sharp transition is occasionally seen between the normally featureless squamous portion of the esophagus and the more nodular pattern representing gastric columnar epithelium on the distal side of the esophagogastric junction.

METHODS OF EXAMINATION

General Principles

Standard fluoroscopy and radiographic examination with opaque contrast media continue to be the primary imaging modalities used in evaluation of the esophagus. The radiation dose has been reduced by the use of video fluoroscopy instead of cinefluoroscopy and by the use of 100-mm and 105-mm spot-film cameras in place of standard spot-film devices and conventional film-screen combinations. Further dose reduction during acquisition of fluoroscopic spot images is achieved with relatively insignificant image degradation by the use of digital fluoroscopy. Pulsed fluoroscopy at variable low frame rates can also decrease doses even further. "Last image hold" features on fluoroscopic monitors can lower doses by decreasing total fluoroscopic time, and multiple "grab images" can be saved and later reviewed without the need for continuous patient irradiation.

> **Techniques for fluoroscopy dose reduction:**
> - **Videofluoroscopy**
> - **Spot film cameras or digital spot images**
> - **Low-rate pulsed fluoroscopy**
> - **"Last image hold" on fluoroscopy monitor**

Infants and small children generally must be immobilized for optimal results. Various commercial devices are available, but they may make patient rotation under the fluoroscope difficult. Gonadal shielding is important. A large lead shield on the fluoroscopic table also helps shield parents or personnel who may help in restraining the patient's lower extremities.

Barium suspensions remain the contrast medium of choice unless esophageal perforation or tracheoesophageal fistula is suspected or if there is a high probability of aspiration. The typically small amounts of contrast medium aspirated as a result of unexpected swallowing dysfunction, reflux, and tracheoesophageal fistulas are usually cleared naturally from the normal airway with coughing. Nevertheless, careful fluoroscopic monitoring and small doses of oral contrast should be used at the initiation of the examination to preclude aspiration of significant amounts of contrast material. When barium is contraindicated, low-osmolar nonionic contrast media, although more expensive, are used.

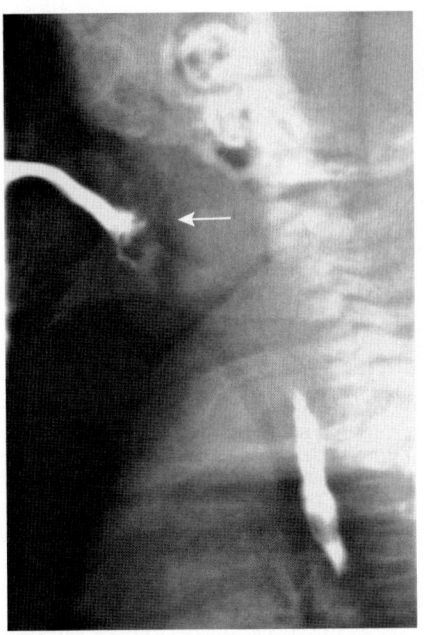 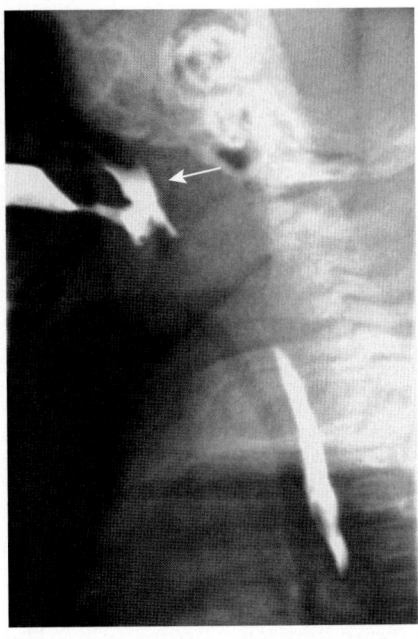 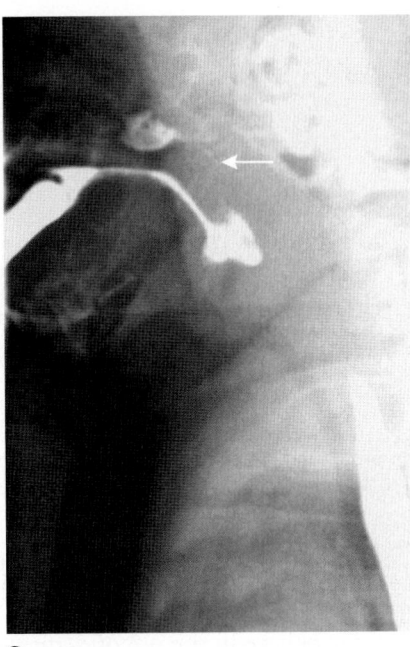

A   B   C

FIGURE 121-3. Swallowing. **A,** As the nipple is inserted into the infant's mouth, the tongue and soft palate are relaxed and the nasopharynx opens *(arrow).* **B,** Normally, the tongue elevates, pushing the nipple to the roof of the mouth and the soft palate elevates. In this example, the soft palate did not elevate and close off the nasal pharynx. Therefore, there was nasopharyngeal reflux *(arrow).* **C,** The infant finally did close the nasal pharynx by elevation of the soft palate against the adenoid tissue *(arrow).* There remains contrast material in the nose and in the hypopharynx.

Techniques for Evaluating Swallowing

General evaluation of swallowing should always be part of an esophageal imaging study. Swallowing is a complex process that requires integrity of many structures and functions. In the dynamic imaging study of swallowing (DISS) for swallowing dysfunction, the function of the structures of the digestive and respiratory tracts during swallowing is radiologically evaluated and the evaluation is documented on videocassette or digitally (compact disk). Our protocol consists of detailed history of feeding habits and clinical condition of the child, which is then followed by the videofluoroscopic evaluation; this evaluation includes swallowing of foods of different consistencies and volumes mixed with contrast material, documented on lateral and posteroanterior views. This is followed by the study of esophageal motility and characterization of gastroesophageal reflux. The DISS is considered the "gold standard" examination for the evaluation of swallowing because it allows the examiner to fully and continuously evaluate swallowing in its three phases (oral, pharyngeal, and esophageal), without interruption.

The history related to feeding aspects and clinical conditions of the child must be very detailed and must include data about the acute clinical complaint, the child's feeding history, ability to suck, use of utensils, positioning and irritability during and after feeding, usual appetite, and signs of fatigue during feeding. Information regarding weight loss and changes in diet, presence of a tracheotomy, changes in voice (e.g., during crying), gastroesophageal reflux, respiratory aspects, medication, and sleep patterns is also needed. All this information should help tailor the DISS, helping deter-

mine the consistency of feeding to be given, volume, utensils used, or specific foods that should be offered first, in order to decrease risks related to tracheal aspiration. The protocol can be modified or shortened according to the child's clinical condition and degree of compromise.

Respiratory aspects must be addressed especially carefully because children with respiratory problems have a higher risk of pulmonary aspiration and more difficulty in clearance of pharyngeal recesses during the DISS. All fluoroscopic rooms should have equipment for suction, oxygen, and a nearby resuscitation cart.

The mean time for the complete DISS protocol in our institution is 6 minutes, and the speech pathologist must participate. However, the examination can be terminated at any moment, according to the clinical conditions of the patient. We first place a metal mark at the mastoid of the patient, to serve as reference for later objective computerized measurements. The infant is fed by a bottle and nipple for this part of the study, while swallowing is evaluated with video fluoroscopy. If the child presents specific difficulties in swallowing, the DISS examination must be initiated with paste consistency, which presents a smaller risk of laryngeal penetration and/or pulmonary aspiration. The examination starts in the lateral projection (Fig. 121-3) and continues with frontal views during swallowing. If the infant will not take barium from the nipple, contrast material can be carefully injected into the baby's mouth (between the cheek and the lateral aspect of the teeth or gums), or a feeding tube can be inserted through the nipple into the baby's mouth and controlled injections under fluoroscopic guidance and control can be made on the back of the tongue to initiate swallowing (Fig. 121-4).

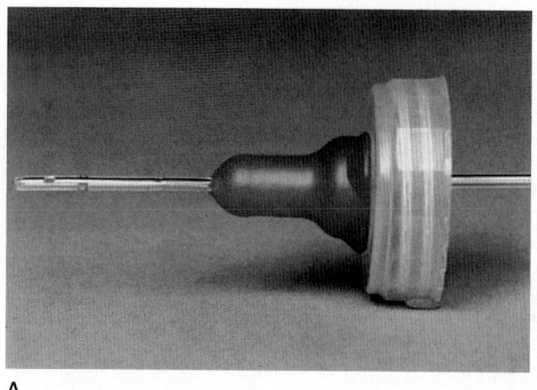
A

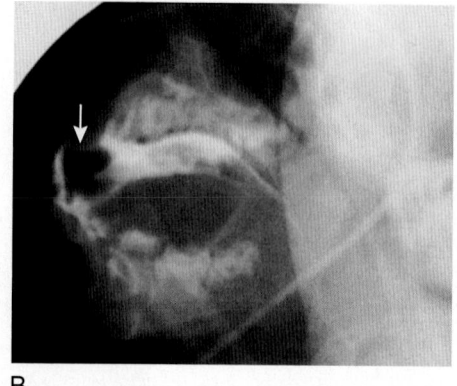
B

FIGURE 121-4. Modified technique. **A,** A No. 8 Silastic feeding tube is placed through a nipple so that a controlled introduction of contrast material can be made into the mouth and the swallowing mechanism observed. **B,** Barium outlines the nipple (*arrow*) and the tube. (Modified from Poznanski A: A simple device for administering barium to infants. Radiology 1969;93:1106.)

Registration of images on videotape makes it possible to review them later frame by frame, allowing a more detailed analysis and a better study of aspiration. The authors believe in the use of dedicated software to reach objective measurements through examination-acquired data, such as degree of laryngeal elevation, cricopharyngeal opening, and hyoid displacement.

To sum up, the main aspects that should be observed during the DISS examination are (1) the oral phase: food capture and apprehension, oral control of the bolus, tongue mobility, and presence of residue in oral cavity; (b) the pharyngeal phase: velopharyngeal motility and closure, presence of laryngeal penetration and/or pulmonary aspiration, laryngeal vertical movement, residue in vallecula or pyriform sinus, cricopharyngeal incoordination, fatigue during or after feeding, pharyngeal constriction, and ability to protect the airway; and (c) the esophageal phase, described in the next section.

Technique for Evaluating the Pharynx and Entire Esophagus

Although radiologists have historically paid primary attention to anatomy, physiology, and pathologic conditions of the esophagus itself, the importance of pharyngeal and esophageal motility disorders requires an understanding of the anatomy and physiology of the pharynx as well. The three components of the pharynx are the nasopharynx, the oropharynx, and the hypopharynx. The nasopharynx and oropharynx communicate through the velopharyngeal portal. Through a highly complex, coordinated neuromuscular mechanism, the portal closes during both speech and swallowing, although the specific neurologic pathways are different during these two physiologic functions. The hypopharynx extends to the level of the larynx, including the epiglottis.

The oral phase of swallowing occurs when the patient chews and mixes food with saliva. This phase is very rapid during the injection of liquid contrast material, but the thrust of the tongue forward and superiorly can be seen. The bolus is transported quickly to the pharyngeal inlet along the dorsum of the tongue by extremely complicated peristalsis-like activity of the tongue muscles (see Fig. 121-3).

During the pharyngeal phase of swallowing, numerous muscles contract in rapid progression to propel the bolus and elevate the soft palate, protecting the nasopharynx from reflux. The larynx and hyoid bone can be seen elevating secondary to the action of muscles that contract to seal off the oropharynx as the bolus is propelled into the cervical esophagus. The epiglottis concurrently seals off the trachea.

Evaluation of the esophagus beyond the pharynx can be accomplished in a similar manner. It is important that the esophagus be distended for optimal evaluation; in the occasional patient who does not ingest sufficient contrast material for adequate distension of the esophagus beyond the pharynx, the remainder of the examination may be performed through a nasoesophageal tube placed within the esophagus under fluoroscopic control. In general, an 8F feeding tube is satisfactory; smaller caliber tubes do not allow rapid injection of sufficient volume. If a tube is used, it is important that the tube have only one opening, at the tip; tubes with side holes may introduce contrast rapidly into the oropharynx with the potential risk of aspiration.

During fluoroscopy, saving of the last image holds, as fluoro grabs, is very helpful. This allows documentation of multiple fluoroscopic observations and of changes such as effectiveness of peristalsis. Images of the esophagus in anteroposterior and lateral projections should be obtained. Pediatric studies are typically performed with single contrast material; double-contrast esophagography is difficult to accomplish in patients younger than 8 years and is seldom performed. Younger patients, even those who are otherwise cooperative, usually let the gas escape by eructation before satisfactory images can be obtained. However, as demonstrated by Levine and colleagues, the double-contrast examination is most useful in patients with mucosal lesions, such as infectious esophagitis, which occur more commonly in older children (Fig. 121-5). Unplanned double-contrast esophagus studies are frequently obtained in infants who cry, swallow air, and eructate during the examination.

More than 50 muscle groups contract during the oral and pharyngeal phases, but the esophageal phase of swallowing is relatively simpler. Distention of the cervical esophagus elicits peristalsis. The upper third of the

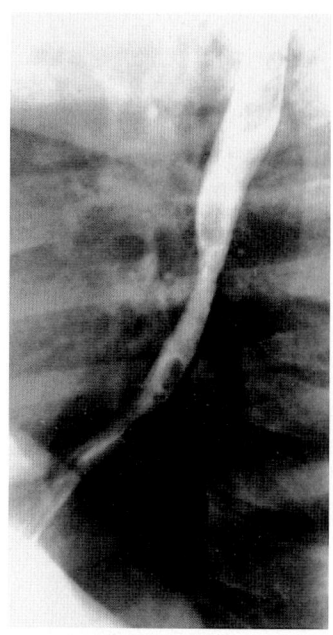

A

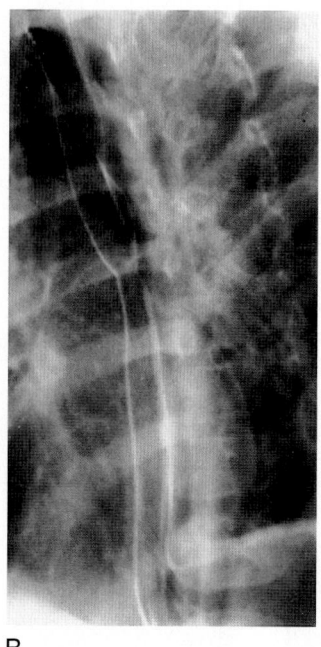

B

FIGURE 121-5. Single- (**A**) and double-contrast (**B**) esophagograms in a 5-year-old boy, performed 6 months after lye ingestion, demonstrate narrowing of the midesophagus. On fluoroscopic study, distal aperistalsis was observed. The mucosa is intact.

esophagus has a striated muscle layer, and the effectiveness of peristalsis here is most dependent on medullary neural reflexes and the vagus nerve. Peristalsis in the lower esophagus, with its smooth muscle layer, relies predominantly on an intrinsic peristaltic mechanism that is modulated by vagus activity. Although this description is oversimplified, it does clarify the variability of peristaltic activity in the upper and lower esophagus that can be observed in a variety of pathologic states.

Swallowing a barium bolus normally initiates primary peristalsis, which is a distally progressive, lumen-obliterating contraction wave. In young adults, the primary peristaltic wave traverses the esophagus from the cricopharyngeus through the vestibule and clears the entire esophagus of barium.

Secondary peristalsis is initiated when residues are left behind in the esophagus or when there is reflux from the stomach. The secondary peristaltic wave usually cleans the esophagus of barium entirely or leaves only residual barium in the cervical and upper thoracic regions.

Tertiary waves are nonpropulsive, uncoordinated esophageal contractions. Their incidence increases with age, and they are usually seen in elderly persons. Tertiary waves are rarely of clinical significance in the absence of symptoms of dysphagia.

The normal thoracic portion of the esophagus shows smooth primary stripping by peristaltic waves during the passage of a single large bolus. Because each swallow elicits a new peristaltic wave, the normal peristaltic mechanism appears to be interrupted during repetitive swallowing. Tertiary contractions are not seen in normal infants and children. When older children are studied in the erect position, gravity plays an important role in the passage of contrast material.

On the lateral view, the impression of the contracted cricopharyngeus muscle may be observed indenting the cervical esophagus posteriorly (Fig. 121-6). This is a normal variant in a patient without swallowing; however,

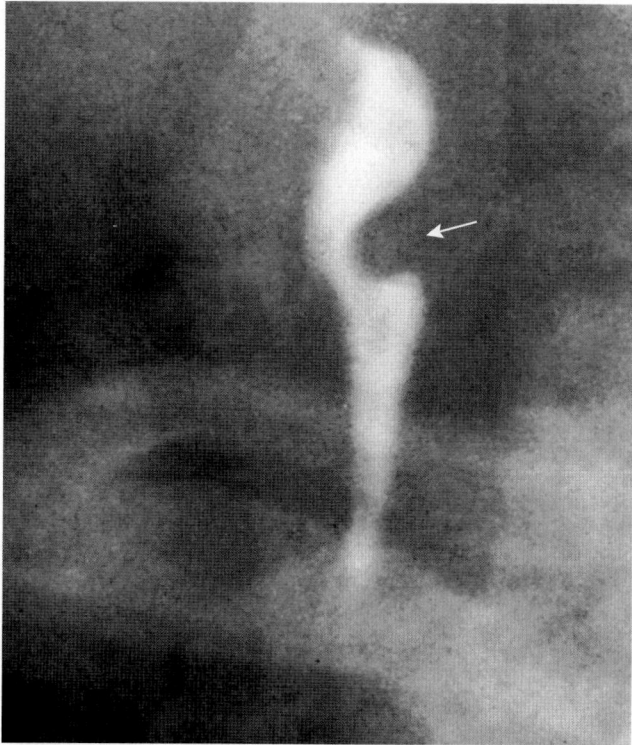

FIGURE 121-6. Lateral view of a barium swallow study demonstrates a normal posterior impression (arrow) by the contracted cricopharyngeus muscle. This is a normal variant in a patient without swallowing difficulties.

in symptomatic infants it can be abnormal (see Chapter 123). Deviation by the aorta and the left atrium, as well as the impression by the left main stem bronchus, is usually seen (see Fig. 121-2).

The course of the esophagus may be affected by spinal and aortic abnormalities such as severe kyphoscoliosis and aortic ectasia. Aortic arch anomalies (Fig. 121-7) such

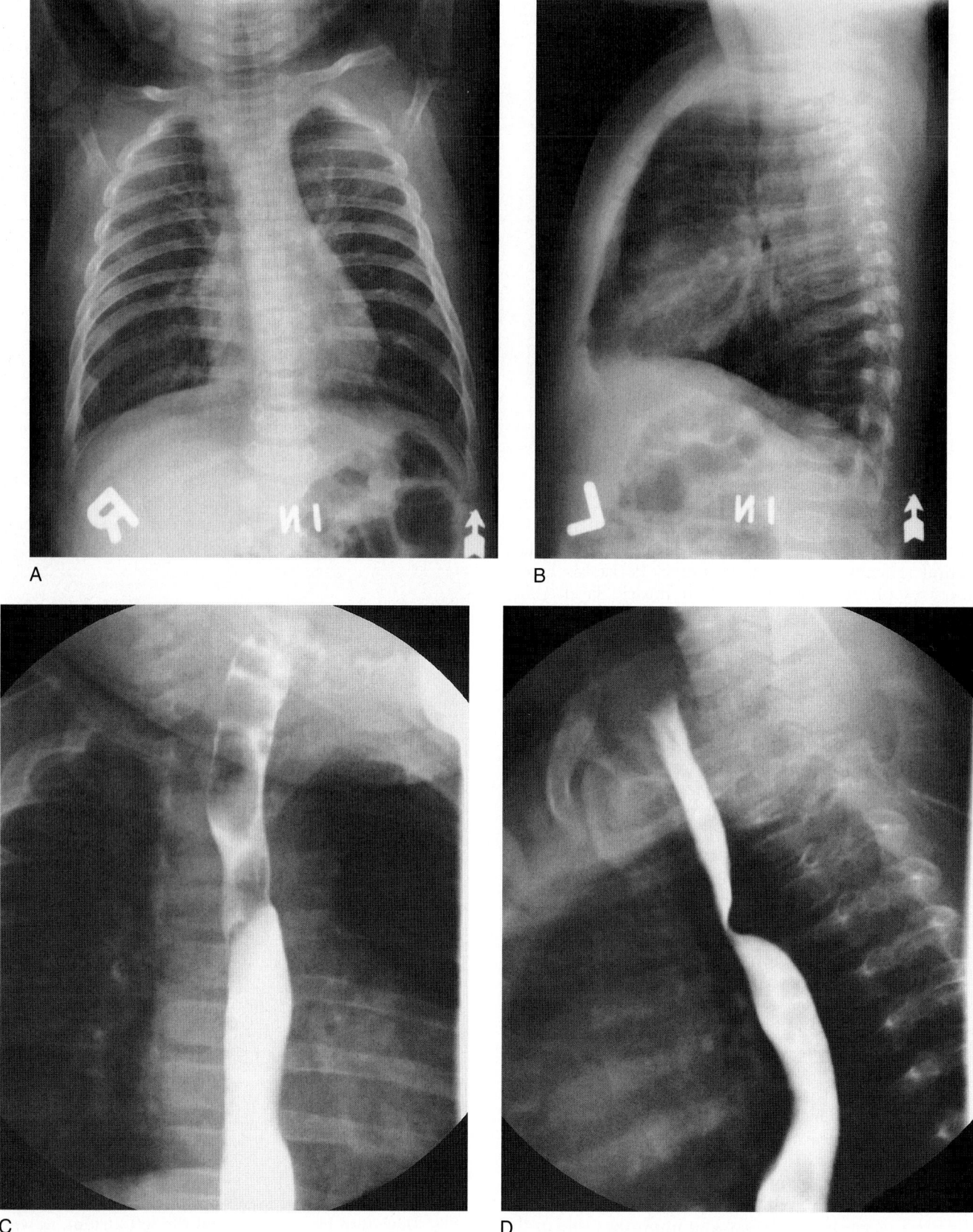

A

B

C

D

FIGURE 121-7. Extrinsic lesions causing deviations in esophageal contour. **A,** Chest film in an infant reveals that the airway is not well seen from the level of T2 to the carina and that the carina is central, not over the right pedicles. **B,** Lateral view shows bowing of the airway anteriorly. Barium swallow study in the frontal (**C**) and lateral (**D**) projections depict a mass impression on the right and left sides of the frontal projection of the contrast material–filled esophagus and, in the lateral view, an enlarged mass behind the esophagus that causes the esophagus and the airway to deviate forward. These findings are diagnostic of a vascular ring.

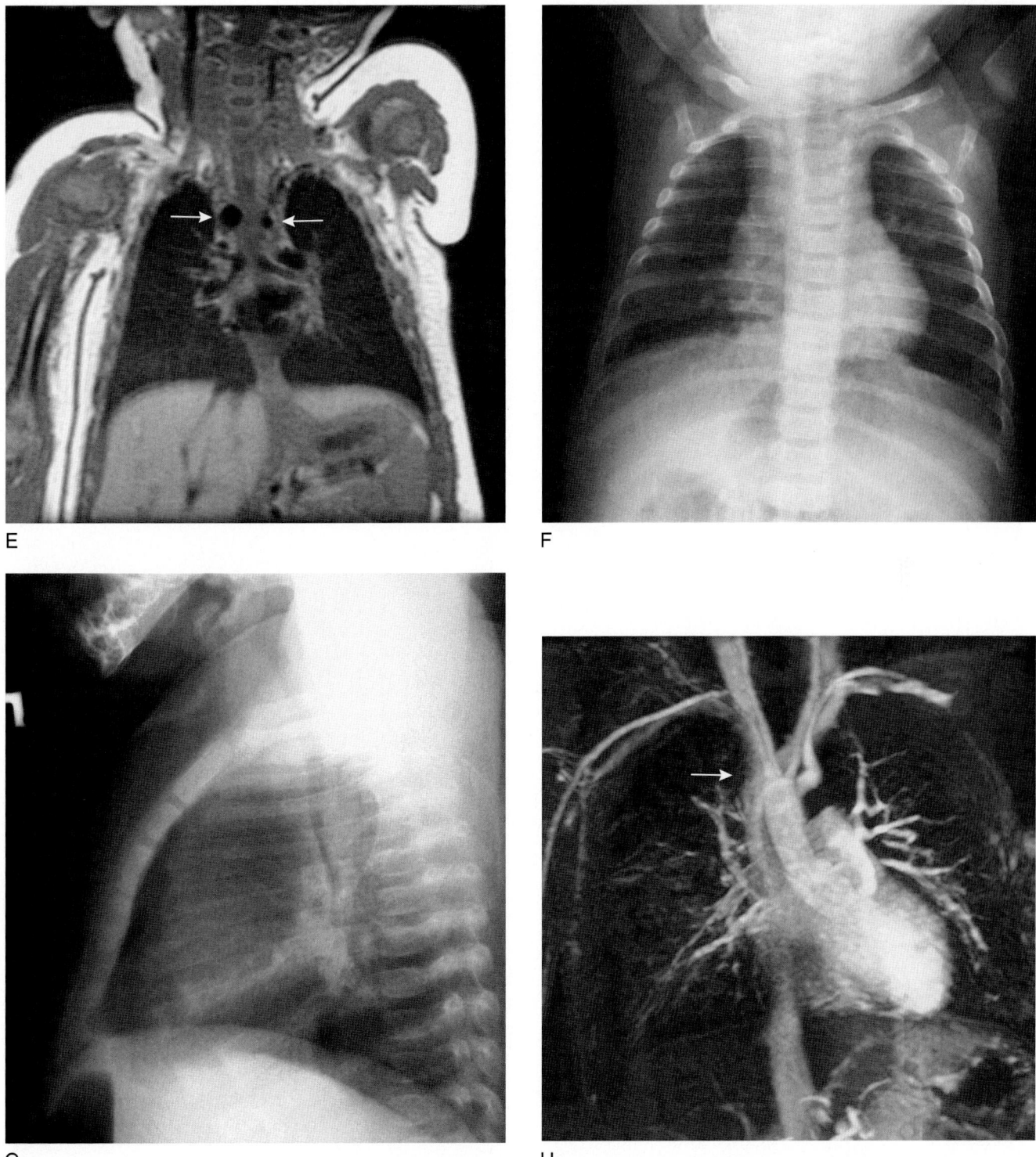

E

F

G

H

FIGURE 121-7, *cont'd*. E, Coronal T1-weighted magnetic resonance image demonstrates the right and left arches (*arrows*). **F,** In a plain film in another child, the carina is not well seen. **G,** Lateral film reveals that the airway is bowed forward. **H,** Cardiac magnetic resonance image depicts the right arch and right descent (*arrow*).

as aberrant vessels, right aortic arch, and double aortic arch cause extrinsic effects on the lateral and posterior aspects of the esophagus. Aberrant left pulmonary artery typically causes an anterior extrinsic compression defect.

SUGGESTED READINGS

Cohen MD: Choosing contrast media for the evaluation of the gastrointestinal tract of neonates and infants. Radiology 1987;162:447-456

Deane MGM, Burton EM, Harlow SA, et al: Swallowing dysfunction in infants less than 1 year of age. Pediatric Radiol 2001;31:423-428

Dodds WJ: The physiology of swallowing. Dysphagia 1989;3:171-178

Donner MW, Bosma JF, Robertson DL: Anatomy and physiology of the pharynx. Gastrointest Radiol 1985;10:196-212

Ginai AZ, Tenkate FJW, Ten Berg RGM, et al: Experimental evaluation of various available contrast agents for use in the upper gastrointestinal tract in case of suspected leakage: effects on lungs. Br J Radiol 1984;57:895-901

Ginai AZ, Tenkate FJW, Ten Berg RGM, et al: Experimental evaluation of various available contrast agents for use in the upper gastrointestinal tract in case of suspected leakage: effects on mediastinum. Br J Radiol 1985;58:585-592

Girdany BR: The esophagus in infancy: congenital and acquired diseases. Radiol Clin North Am 1963;1:557-569

Girdany BR, Lee FA: X-ray examination of the gastrointestinal tract. Pediatr Clin North Am 1967;14:3-19

Hernandez RJ, Goodsitt MM: Reduction of radiation dose in pediatric patients using pulsed fluoroscopy. AJR Am J Roentgenol 1996;167:1247-1253

Hur J, Yoom C-S, Kim M-J, Kim O-H: Imaging features of gastrointestinal tract duplications in infants and children: from oesophagus to rectum. Pediatr Radiol 2007;37:691-699

Jones B, Gayler BW, Donner MW: Pharynx and cervical esophagus. In Levine MS (ed): Radiology of the Esophagus. Philadelphia, Saunders, 1989:311-336

Kendall KA, McKenzie S, Leonard RJ, et al: Timing of events in normal swallowing: a videofluoroscopic study. Dysphagia 2000;15:74-83

Kramer SS: Swallowing in children. In Jones B, Donner MW (eds): Normal and Abnormal Swallowing: Imaging in Diagnosis and Therapy. New York, Springer-Verlag, 1991:173-188

Leonard RJ, Kendall KA, McKenzie S, et al: Structural displacements in normal swallowing: a videofluoroscopic study. Dysphagia 2000;15:146-152

Levine MS, Rubesin SE, Ott DJ: Update on esophageal radiology. AJR Am J Roentgenol 1990;155:933-941

McAlister WH, Askin FB: The effect of some contrast agents in the lung: an experimental study in the rat and dog. AJR Am J Roentgenol 1983;140:245-251

McAlister WH, Siegel MJ: Fatal aspirations in infancy during gastrointestinal series. Pediatr Radiol 1984;14:81-83

Congenital Esophageal Malformations

HENRIQUE M. LEDERMAN and GUILHERME T. S. DEMARCHI

Certain congenital esophageal malformations, such as esophageal atresia, are identified in neonates and discussed in Chapter 14. However, other congenital lesions, such as isolated tracheoesophageal fistulas and duplications cysts, most often manifest in older patients.

ISOLATED TRACHEOESOPHAGEAL FISTULAS: THE N- OR H-TYPE FISTULA

Congenital tracheoesophageal fistula without atresia is difficult to identify, both clinically and radiographically. Affected patients typically present with recurrent pneumonias either in infancy or later in childhood. Patients with unexplained chronic respiratory distress and recurrent pneumonia should always be considered at risk for the presence of a tracheoesophageal fistula, and radiographic examination is warranted.

Esophageal Abnormalities May Manifest with Respiratory Symptoms

Congenital tracheoesophageal fistula without atresia is often termed an *H-type fistula* because of its appearance on an esophagogram, connecting the trachea and esophagus. However, the fistula typically runs cephalad from the esophagus to the trachea and looks more like an *N* (Fig. 122-1). Large fistulas usually manifest very early in life and are relatively easy to diagnose on an esophagogram (Fig. 122-2). More commonly, the fistulas are small and inconstantly patent, and repeated examinations may be necessary to identify them.

Horizontal-beam fluoroscopy, with the patient lying prone on the footboard with the fluoroscopic table in the upright position, is probably not necessary in most cases. Such positioning is possible only in infants. In our institution, the examination is performed after passage of a nasoesophageal catheter, particularly in patients with normal prior examination findings in whom a fistula remains suspect. A major reason for inconstant patency of the fistula is that the normal esophageal mucosa is quite redundant and usually occludes the esophageal side of the fistula. Normal active swallowing may not distend the esophagus sufficiently to allow passage of contrast material into the fistula. The patient should be kept in the lateral recumbent position (with the right side down). The examiner withdraws the catheter from the distal esophagus cephalad, forcefully injecting contrast material to distend the esophagus maximally under constant fluoroscopic monitoring. The catheter should have an end hole, without more proximal side holes, for adequate control of the contrast infusion. If a fistula is present, it is seen in the lateral projection extending anteriorly and cephalad from the esophagus to the trachea. Slightly oblique views may be necessary to see its full course. Unless a fistula is seen, the injection should continue until the catheter is withdrawn into the hypopharynx, but contrast material must not be allowed to spill over into the trachea. The examination should be terminated as soon as a fistula is identified, in order to minimize the amount of contrast material leaking into the airway.

Although there is a danger of spilling contrast material into the airway with injection high in the cervical esophagus, it is important to examine this area because many of these fistulas occur at the level of the lower cervical or upper thoracic spine (see Fig. 122-2). Slow retraction of the catheter and careful fluoroscopic monitoring help prevent overflow into the trachea. Multiple fistulas without atresia have been reported but are extraordinarily rare. Filston and associates catheterized tracheoesophageal fistulas per ora, but this method is little used by other investigators. In rare cases, bronchoscopy can complement esophagography. Fistulas can be extremely difficult to identify, and repetitive examinations should be considered if the presence of a fistula is strongly suspected. Another approach to identify this fistula is through a routine contrast swallow study with the patient in the prone or prone oblique position. Laffan and colleagues were extremely successful with this method. As stated previously, if this does not demonstrate the fistula and if one is strongly suspected, a tube study is performed.

In rare cases, the airway originates from the esophagus, resulting in an anomaly called *esophagotrachea* or *esophageal bronchus* (Fig. 122-3). This anomaly leads to severe respiratory distress with feeding and may be associated with esophageal atresia, tracheoesophageal fistula, or both. A bronchoesophageal fistula between the esophagus and a normal bronchial tree has also been described.

LARYNGOTRACHEOESOPHAGEAL CLEFTS

Laryngotracheoesophageal clefts are high fistulous communications between the hypopharynx and larynx

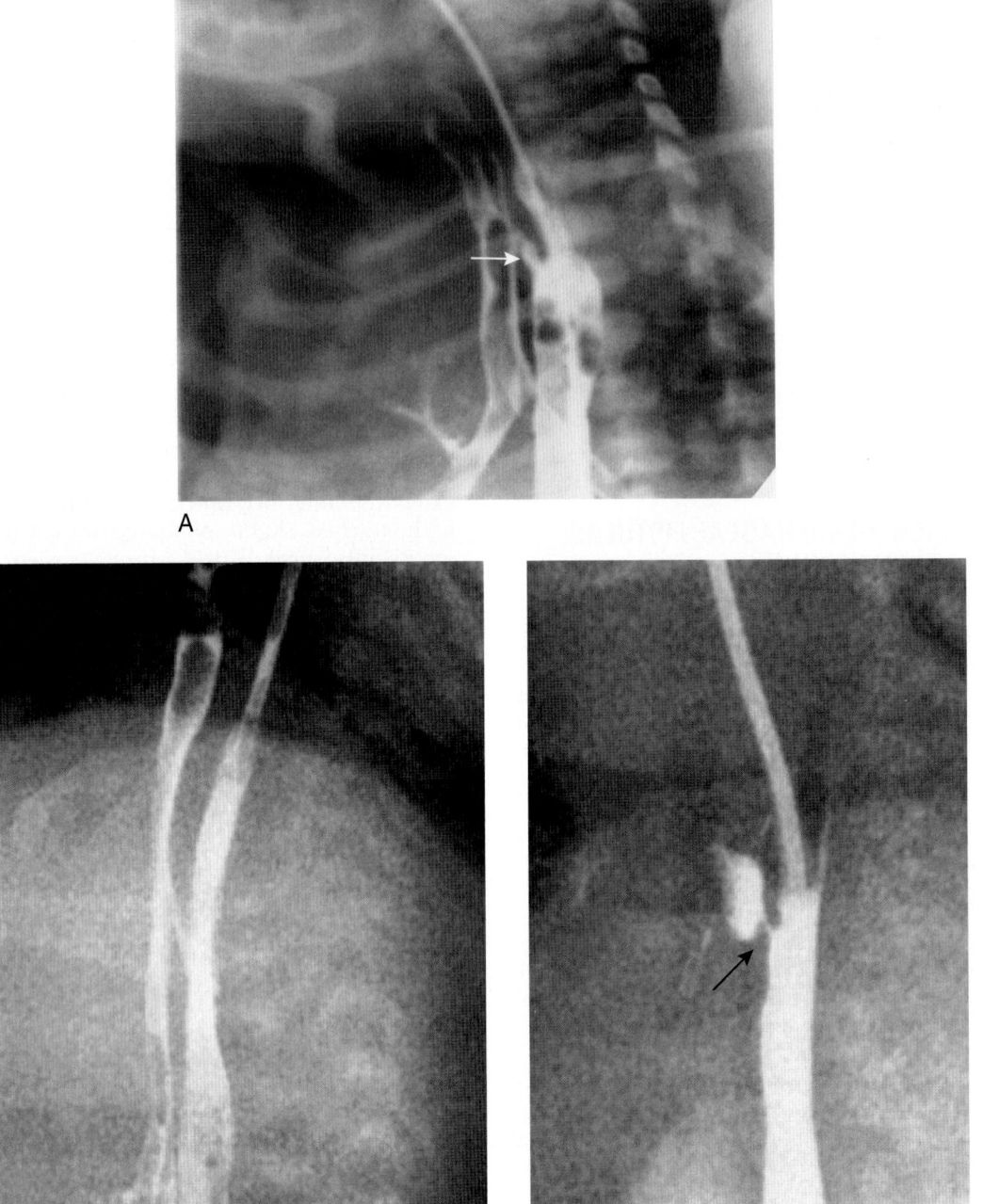

FIGURE 122-1. N- or H-type tracheoesophageal fistula. **A,** Contrast injection reveals the tracheal esophageal fistula (*arrow*). Unfortunately, too much contrast material was injected, and the airway has significant filling. **B,** A second H- or N-type tracheoesophageal fistula is demonstrated. The tube is higher and difficult to see in the cervical esophagus. The fistula is high, well above the carina. Again, there is too much filling of the airway. **C,** A third H- or N-type fistula. There is limited contrast material in the airway, and the fistula is quite small (*arrow*). The examiner must be exceedingly careful when watching fluoroscopically to make sure that only a small amount of contrast material gets into the airway.

(Fig. 122-4). The clefts vary from a small communication between the larynx and esophagus to complete absence of the wall between esophagus and trachea ("persistent esophagotrachea"). Patients with such clefts typically present in infancy with choking during feeding, respiratory distress, aspiration pneumonia, and cyanosis. Stridor has been reported. Diagnosis is usually made by laryngoscopy. Wilkinson and coworkers reported a case of complete laryngotracheoesophageal cleft in an infant boy in whom bronchoscopy could not be performed because of a narrow tracheal orifice. Computed tomography (CT) of the thorax demonstrated a common tracheal and esophageal lumen extending inferiorly to the carina, with hypoplasia of the right lung and cardiac dextroposition. Contrast studies also demonstrated a hypoplastic intrathoracic stomach.

Anomalies such as esophageal atresia and tracheo-esophageal fistulas may occur in association with laryngotracheoesophageal clefts.

ESOPHAGEAL STENOSIS

Congenital esophageal stenosis is a rare lesion, most commonly subdivided into three subtypes: fibromuscular thickening, membranous web, or tracheobronchial remnants or choristoma, often associated with esophageal atresia and fistula. A choristoma in this location is a distinct osseous/cartilaginous tissue proliferation that partially or completely encircles the lower esophagus. Congenital esophageal stenosis caused by a choristoma is a rare lesion, usually resulting from faulty embryologic separation of the respiratory (tracheobronchial) and

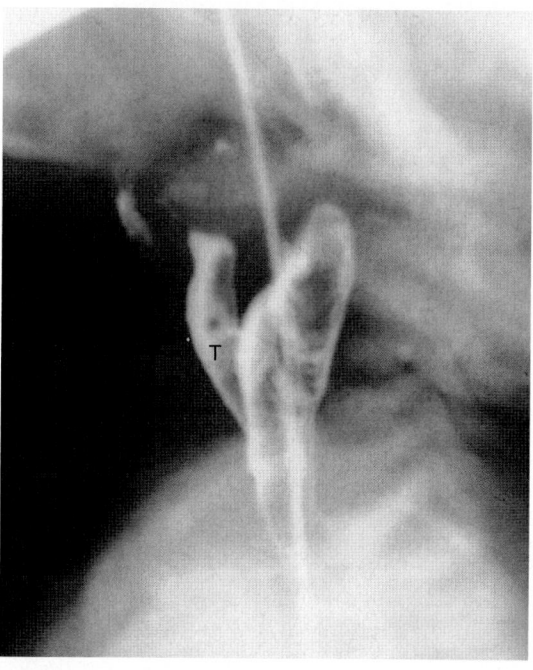

FIGURE 122-2. Large H-type fistula from the upper cervical esophagus to the trachea (T).

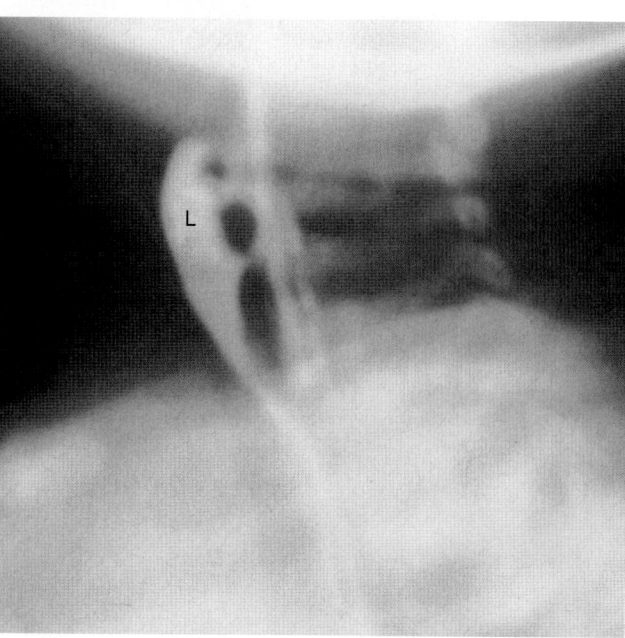

FIGURE 122-4. Laryngotracheoesophageal cleft. Barium swallow study reveals several defects on the posterior wall of the larynx (L) with large volume aspiration.

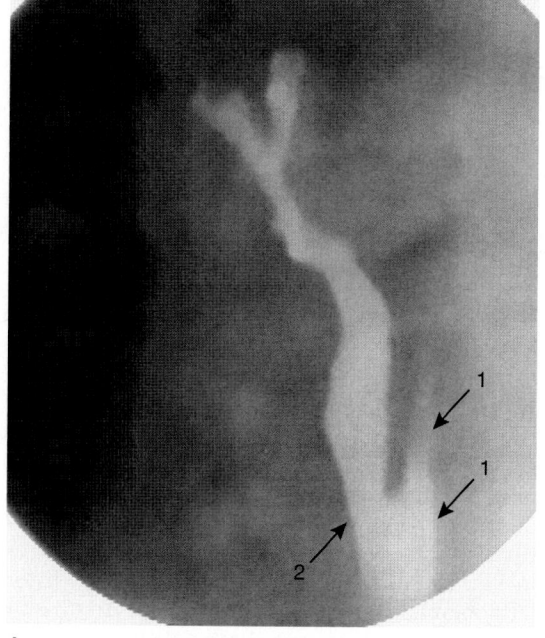

A

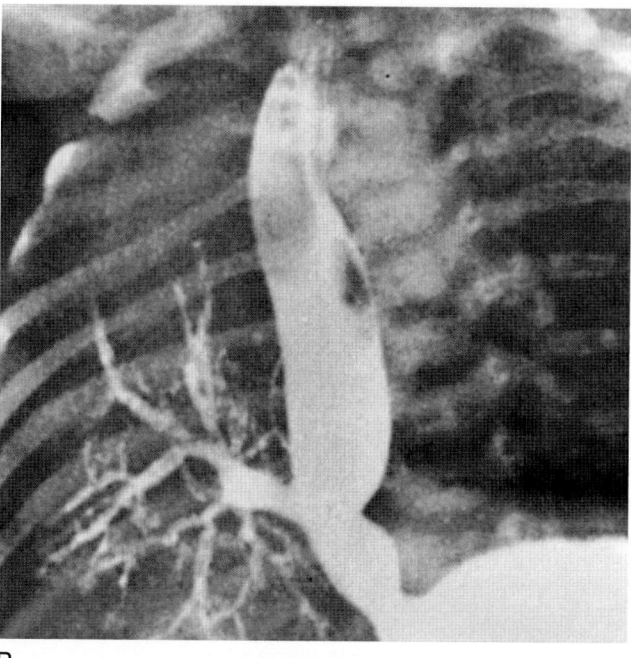

B

FIGURE 122-3. Congenital esophageal bronchial fistula. **A,** Oblique view shows the esophagus (1) and the bronchus to right upper lobe (2). **B,** Esophageal bronchus. An oblique film from an esophagogram in an infant demonstrates the origin of the right main bronchus from the distal esophagus.

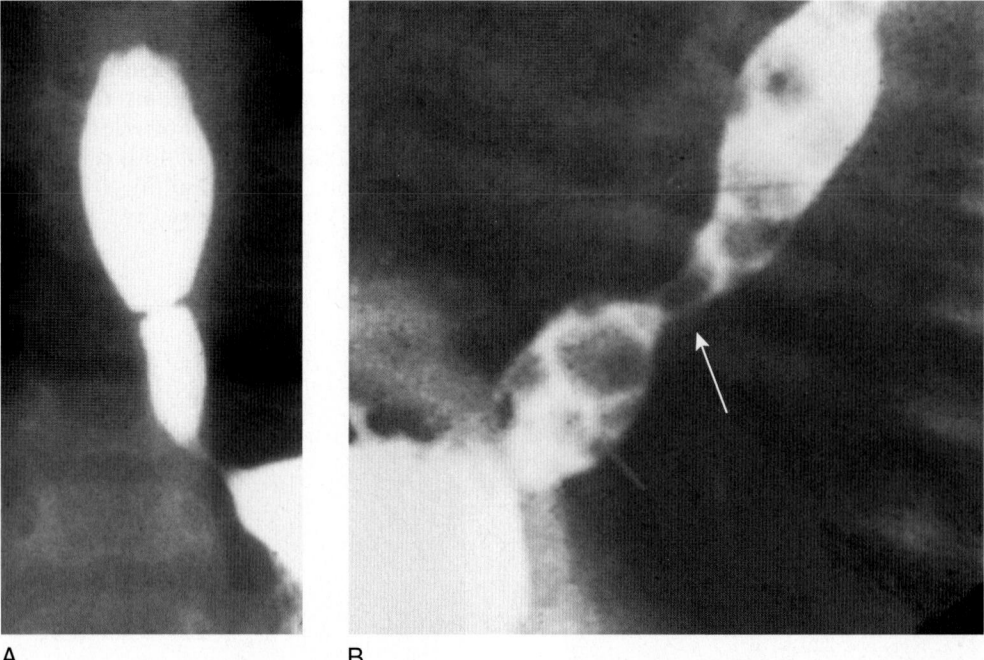

FIGURE 122-5. Esophageal obstructive lesions. **A,** Esophagogram revealing a weblike narrowing of the distal esophagus with large proximal dilation secondary to esophageal cartilaginous rests (choristoma). The diagnosis is suggested by the location of the narrowed segment. **B,** Another esophagogram demonstrating stenosis, this time in the distal portion of the esophagus (*arrow*) secondary to cartilaginous remnants. (Courtesy of Dr. E. Afshani, Buffalo, New York.)

gastrointestinal (esophageal) systems. According to Ibrahim and Sandry, the first case was described by Frey and Duschl who reported a case of congenital esophageal stenosis resulting from a heterotopic tracheobronchial remnant in a 19-year-old girl who died with a diagnosis of achalasia. Worldwide, approximately 150 cases have been reported so far.

The typical manifestation of tracheobronchial remnants is that of dysphagia after ingestion of solids, regurgitation/choking, vomiting of esophageal contents, gradual dysphasia, and weight loss. The diagnosis can be implied by an esophagogram showing a stenotic ring-shaped area on the distal third of the esophagus with proximal dilatation (Fig. 122-5) or by endoscopy and confirmed by histopathologic study. There may be impaction of food proximal to the stenotic site. Treatment is surgical: resection of the stenotic segment and reanastomosis combined with antireflux surgery. Dilation by balloon through endoscopy has been described as alternative therapeutic procedure.

Choristoma versus hamartoma:

- *Choristoma:* histologically normal tissue proliferation not normally found in the particular anatomic site in question
- *Hamartoma:* disorganized overgrowth of mature cells and tissues normally found in the affected site, often with one predominating element

---

ESOPHAGEAL DUPLICATION CYSTS

Duplication cysts usually do not cause symptoms and are often identified incidentally on chest radiographs. Occa-

TABLE 122-1
Differential Diagnosis of Esophageal Duplication Cyst
Bronchogenic cyst Neurogenic tumors Neuroblastoma Ganglioneuroblastoma Ganglioglioma Hiatal hernia Aortic arch congenital anomaly Aortic aneurysm

sional patients present with symptoms of dysphagia as a result of esophageal compression. A differential diagnosis of esophageal duplication is listed in Table 122-1.

Duplication cysts associated with the esophagus can occur by three distinct embryologic processes leading to three types of duplications and/or cysts: esophageal duplication cysts with respiratory epithelium, neurenteric cysts, and true tubular duplications of the esophagus.

Esophageal duplication cysts with respiratory epithelium represent bronchopulmonary foregut malformations that occur earlier in embryonic life than paratracheal, hilar, or carinal "bronchogenic" cysts. These cysts arise from the posterior portion of the foregut and contain intestinal mucosa that, according to histologic examination, is usually gastric or, occasionally, intestinal (Figs. 122-6 and 122-7).

Neurenteric cysts, in contrast, have a distinct embryologic origin that is part of the "split notochord syndrome." The notochord forms during the third embryonic week and separates the ectoderm from the endoderm. If this

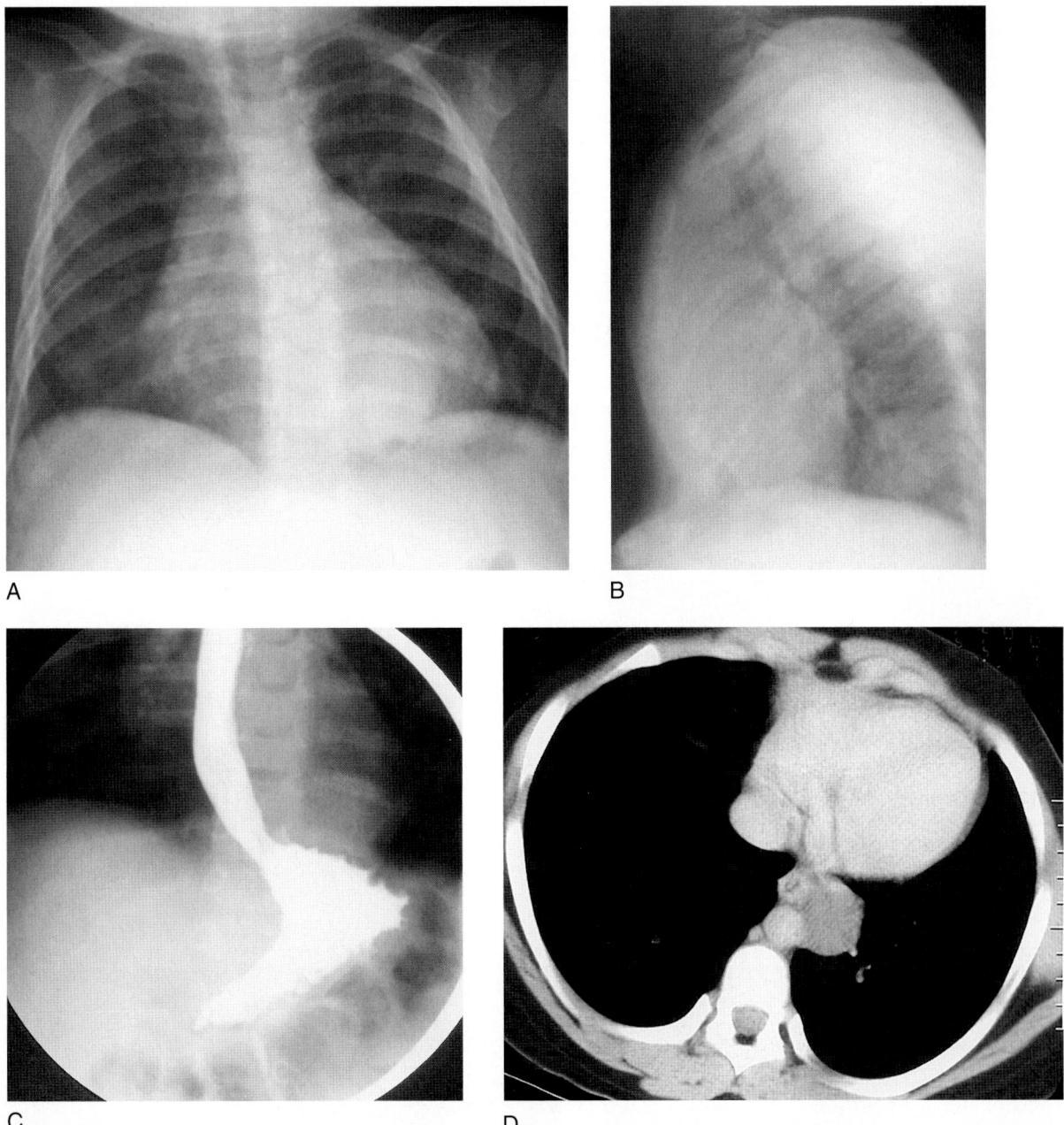

FIGURE 122-6. Esophageal duplication cyst. **A,** Front chest film reveals a mass to the left of the spine behind the heart. It is quite round. **B,** Lateral film reveals the mass posteriorly. The vertebral bodies should become darker the closer they are to the diaphragm. However, there is a large opacity, making the vertebral bodies whiter. **C,** An esophagogram shows the impression on the wall of the distal esophagus. **D,** The computed tomographic examination shows the low attenuation esophageal duplication cyst. Note there is some mild thickening of the esophageal wall adjacent to it.

separation is incomplete and leaves an adhesion between the endoderm and ectoderm, the notochord either splits to encircle the adhesion or deviates to the left or right of the adhesion. The archetype of this spectrum of anomalies is the dorsal enteric fistula, a patent communication between the gut and the dorsal midline skin surface that traverses the vertebral body (or interspace), the spinal canal and its contents, and the posterior vertebral elements (Fig. 122-8). As in the analogous urachal or vitelline duct remnants, some or all of the patent communication in the dorsal enteric fistula can become obliterated, which leads to residual diverticula, cysts, and fibrous cords that give rise to a spectrum of anomalies (Fig. 122-9). These anomalies include

A dorsal enteric sinus (a blind-ending, enteric-lined tract from the dorsal skin surface).

An isolated dorsal enteric cyst (enteric-lined cyst derived from the intermediate portion of the tract with obliteration of the communication with the gut and skin surface), which can be prevertebral, intraspinal, or postvertebral (Fig. 122-10).

A dorsal enteric diverticulum (a blind-ending diverticulum from the gut), which may be intrathoracic or intra-abdominal or may cross the diaphragm.

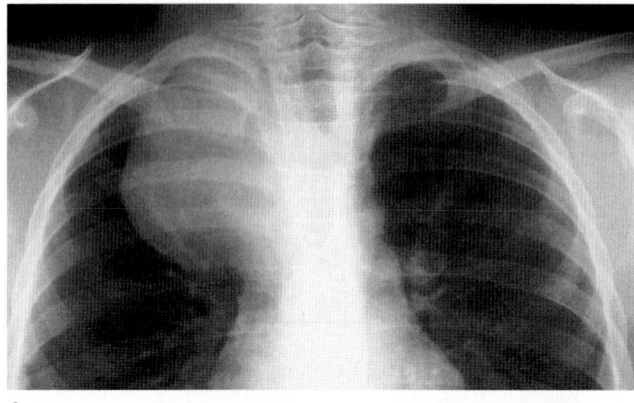

A

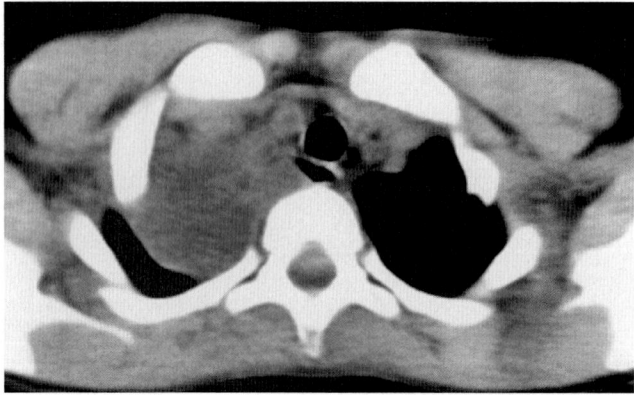

B

FIGURE 122-7. Esophageal duplication cyst. An incidental finding during a chest examination revealed a large posterior mass (**A**), which on computed tomographic scan (**B**) was seen to be cystic. At surgery, the diagnosis of esophageal duplication was confirmed.

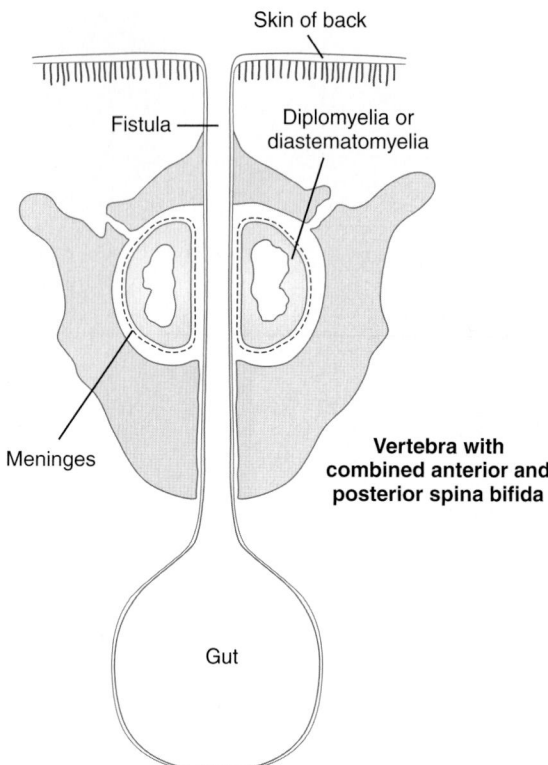

FIGURE 122-8. Diagrammatic representation of the archetypical dorsal enteric fistula. (From Naidich TP, McLone DG, Harwood-Nash DC: Spinal dysraphism. *In* Newton TH, Potts DG [eds]: Computed Tomography of the Spine and Spinal Cord. San Anselmo, CA, Clavadel Press, 1983:299-353.)

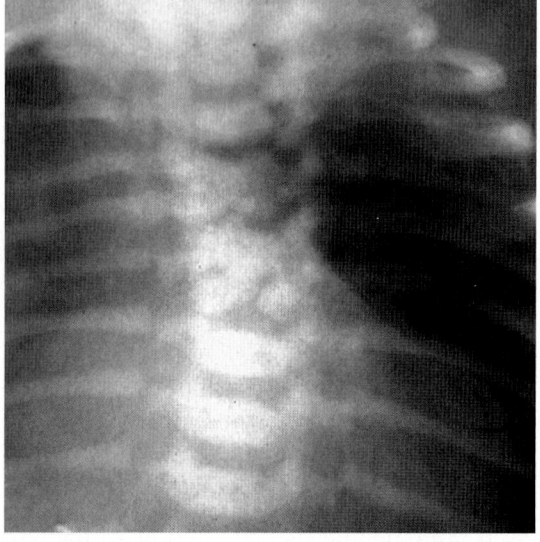

A

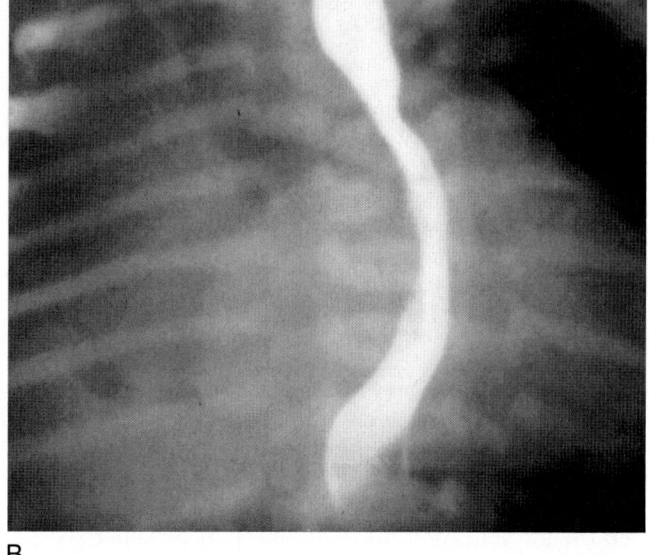

B

FIGURE 122-9. Neurenteric cyst. Frontal cone down view of spine on chest radiograph (**A**) and esophagogram (**B**) demonstrates vertebral body malformations, paravertebral soft tissue masses, and displacement of the esophagus, which are consistent with neurenteric cyst.

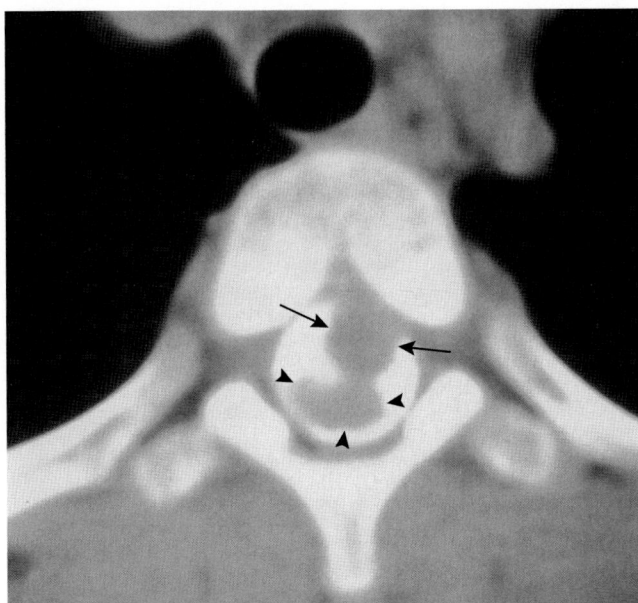

FIGURE 122-10. Intraspinal neurenteric cyst. Axial computed tomography section with intrathecal contrast material demonstrates an intraspinal mass (*arrows*) anterior to the compressed spinal cord (*arrowheads*), surgically proven to represent an intraspinal neurenteric cyst. Note the associated congenital cleft in the vertebral body.

TABLE 122-2
Esophageal Duplication Cyst

FINDINGS ON CHEST RADIOGRAPH/ESOPHAGOGRAM

Common
   Posterior mediastinal mass
   Sharp margins
   Displacement of esophagus on esophagogram
   Intramural esophageal mass
Less common
   Congenital vertebral anomalies (neurenteric cyst)
   Communication with esophagus on esophagogram

FINDINGS ON COMPUTED TOMOGRAPHY/MAGNETIC RESONANCE IMAGING

Common
   Cystic posterior mediastinal mass
   Sharp margins
   Avascular after intravenous contrast
Less common
   Higher attenuation (CT), elevated signal (T1-weighted MRI) associated with hemorrhage, infection, or elevated protein
   Tubular duplications extending below diaphragm to include stomach
   Associated vertebral anomalies in neurenteric cysts
   Intraspinal neurenteric cysts
   Dorsal enteric diverticula (thoracic and/or abdominal diverticula communicating with gastrointestinal tract)

Neurenteric cysts almost always are accompanied by congenital vertebral anomalies (which can help differentiate these congenital anomalies from other posterior mediastinal masses such as neuroblastoma), as well as spinal cord and meningeal anomalies. These cysts are more common in the right hemithorax.

True tubular duplications (see Fig. 122-6) of the esophagus are even rarer than enteric cysts. Nakao and associates reported a rare case of rapidly enlarging esophageal duplication cyst in a 12-year-old girl who presented with fever and cough, probably caused by infection of the cystic structure, which was resected along with adjacent lung parenchyma. These cysts may extend below the diaphragm to involve the stomach as well. They may communicate with the stomach or esophagus and be directly demonstrable on an esophagogram. These duplications probably develop from faulty recanalization of the esophageal lumen.

The choice of imaging modalities for the evaluation of esophageal duplication cysts and neurenteric cysts is influenced by the patient's presentation. Plain radiographs may demonstrate a sharply demarcated posterior mediastinal mass or congenital vertebral anomalies associated with neurenteric cysts (Table 122-2). An esophagogram reveals an intramural mass or displacement of the esophagus by the mass but typically no connection between the two structures. CT and magnetic resonance imaging (MRI) are the modalities of choice for confirming the cystic nature of the mass and for best delineating the abnormality (see Table 122-2). The cyst fluid typically has attenuation of water on CT (0 to 20 Hounsfield units) and signal characteristics of water on MRI (low signal on T1-weighted images and high signal on T2-weighted images). However, attenuation on CT and signal intensity on T1-weighted MRI may be increased as a result of hemorrhage, infection, or increased protein. CT and MRI may be helpful in evaluating vertebral or intraspinal abnormalities associated with neurenteric cysts. Enteric cysts that contain gastric mucosa with acid and pepsin secretion can be identified by nuclear imaging. They may ulcerate or hemorrhage, leading to draining sinuses in the thoracic wall, esophageal necrosis and perforation, and communication with other intrathoracic structures. Massive hemorrhage from ulceration has been reported.

SUGGESTED READINGS

Isolated Tracheoesophageal Fistulas

Crabbe DC: Isolated tracheo-oesophageal fistula [review]. Paediatr Respir Rev 2003;4:74-78

Filston HC, Rankin JS, Kirks DR: The diagnosis of primary and recurrent tracheoesophageal fistulas: value of selective catheterization. J Pediatr Surg 1982;17:144-148

Harmon CM, Coran AG: Congenital anomalies of the esophagus. *In* O'Neill JA, Rowe MI, Grosfeld JL, et al (eds): Pediatric Surgery, 5th ed. St. Louis, Mosby, 1998:941-967

Johnson JF, Sueoka BL, Mulligan ME, et al: Tracheo-esophageal fistula: diagnosis with CT. Pediatr Radiol 1985;15:134-135

Karnack I, Senocak ME, Hicsonmez A, et al: The diagnosis and treatment of H-type tracheoesophageal fistula. J Pediatr Surg 1997;32:1670-1674

Kemp JL, Sullivan LM: Bronchoesophageal fistula in an 11-month-old boy. Pediatr Radiol 1997;27:811-812

Lacasse JE, Reilly BJ, Mancer K: Segmental esophageal trachea: a potentially fatal type of tracheal stenosis. AJR Am J Roentgenol 1980;134:829-831

Laffan EE, Daneman A, Ein SH, et al: Tracheoesophageal fistula without esophageal atresia: are pull-back tube esophagograms needed for diagnosis? Pediatr Radiol 2006;36:1141

Lallemand D, Quignodon JF, Courtel JV: The anomalous origin of bronchus from the esophagus: report of three cases. Pediatr Radiol 1996;26:179-182

McMullen KP, Karnes PS, Moir CR, et al: Familial recurrence of tracheoesophageal fistula and associated malformations. Am J Med Genet 1996;63:525-528

Sieber WK, Girdany BR: Tracheo-esophageal fistula without esophageal atresia, congenital and recurrent. Pediatrics 1956;18:935-942

Laryngotracheal Cleft

Alabdulgader A, Patten D, Harder J, et al: Laryngotracheoesophageal cleft type 3 and double outlet right ventricle: unique combination. Ann Diagn Pathol 2005;9:323-326

Burroughs N, Leape LL: Laryngotracheoesophageal cleft: report of a case successfully treated and review of the literature. Pediatrics 1974;53:516-522

Chitkara AE, Tadros M, Kim HJ, et al: Complete laryngotracheoesophageal cleft: complicated management issues. Laryngoscope 2003;113:1314-1320

Griscom NT: Persistent esophagotrachea: the most severe degree of laryngotracheo-esophageal cleft. Am J Roentgenol Radium Ther Nucl Med 1966;97:211-215

Kawaguchi AL, Donahoe PK, Ryan DP: Management and long-term follow-up of patients with types III and IV laryngotracheoesophageal clefts. J Pediatr Surg 2005;40:158-164; discussion, pp 164-165

Morgan CL, Grossman H, Leonidas J: Roentgenographic findings in a spectrum of uncommon tracheoesophageal anomalies. Clin Radiol 1979;30:353-358

Sandu K, Monnier P: Endoscopic laryngotracheal cleft repair without tracheotomy or intubation. Laryngoscope 2006;116:630-634

Wilkinson AG, Mackenzie S, Hendry GMA: Complete laryngotracheoesophageal cleft: CT diagnosis and associated abnormalities. Clin Radiol 1990;41:437-438

Esophageal Stenosis

Deiraniya AK: Congenital oesophageal stenosis due to tracheobronchial remnants. Thorax 1974;29:720-725

Ibrahim NB, Sandry RJ: Congenital oesophageal stenosis caused by tracheobronchial structures in the oesophageal wall. Thorax 1981;36:465-468

Pumberger W, Geissler W, Horcher E: Congenital oesophageal stenosis due to tracheobronchial remnants. Chirurg 1999;70:1031-5

Takamizawa S, Tsugawa C, Mouri N, et al: Congenital esophageal stenosis: therapeutic strategy based on etiology. J Pediatr Surg 2002;37:197-201

Yeung CK, Spitz L, Brereton RJ, et al: Congenital esophageal stenosis due to tracheobronchial remnants: a rare but important association with esophageal atresia. J Pediatr Surg 1992;27:852-855

Zhao LL, Hsieh WS, Hsu WM: Congenital esophageal stenosis owing to ectopic tracheobronchial remnants. J Pediatr Surg 2004; 39:1183-1187

Esophageal Duplication Cysts

Aoki S, Machida T, Sasaki Y, et al: Enterogenous cyst of cervical spine: clinical and radiological aspects (including CT and MR). Neuroradiology 1987;29:291-293

Chang SH, Morrison L, Shaffner L, et al: Intrathoracic gastrogenic cysts and hemoptysis. J Pediatr 1976;88:594-596

Chitale AR: Gastric cysts of the mediastinum. J Pediatr 1969; 75:104-110

Fitch SJ, Tonkin ILD, Tonkin AK: Imaging of foregut duplication cysts. Radiographics 1986;6:189-201

Hemalatha V, Batcup G, Brereton RJ, et al: Intrathoracic foregut cyst (foregut duplication) associated with esophageal atresia. J Pediatr Surg 1980;15:178-180

Hernandez RJ: Role of CT in the evaluation of children with foregut cysts. Pediatr Radiol 1987;17:265-268

Kamoi I, Nishitani H, Oshiumi Y, et al: Intrathoracic gastric cyst demonstrated by ^{99m}Tc pertechnetate scintigraphy. AJR Am J Roentgenol 1980;134:1080-1081

Kantrowitz LR, Pais MJ, Burnett K, et al: Intraspinal neurenteric cyst containing gastric mucosa: CT and MR findings. Pediatr Radiol 1986;16:324-327

Kitano Y, Iwanaka T, Tsuchida Y, Oka T: Esophageal duplication cyst associated with pulmonary cystic malformations. J Pediatr Surg 1995;30:1724-1727

Michel JL, Revillon Y, Montupet P, et al: Thoracoscopic treatment of mediastinal cysts in children. J Pediatr Surg 1998;33:1745-1748

Naidich TP, McLone DG, Harwood-Nash DC: Spinal dysraphism. In Newton TH, Potts DG (eds): Computed Tomography of the Spine and Spinal Cord. San Anselmo, CA, Clavadel Press, 1983:299-353

Nakao A, Urushihara N, Yagi T, et al: Rapidly enlarging esophageal duplication cyst. J Gastroenterol 1999;34:246-249

Rafal RB, Markisz JA: Magnetic resonance imaging of an esophageal duplication cyst. Am J Gastroenterol 1991;86:1809-1811

Rhee RS, Ray CG, Kravetz MH, et al: Cervical esophageal duplication cyst: MR imaging. J Comput Assist Tomogr 1988;12:693-695

Skandalakis JE, Gray SW, Ricketts RR: Esophagus. In Skandalakis JE, Gray SW (eds): Embryology for Surgeons, 2nd ed. Baltimore, Williams & Wilkins, 1994:64-112

Snyder ME, Luck SR, Hernandez R, et al: Diagnostic dilemmas of mediastinal cysts. J Pediatr Surg 1985;20:810-815

Sumner TE, Auringer ST, Cox TD: A complex communicating bronchopulmonary foregut malformation: diagnostic imaging and pathogenesis. Pediatr Radiol 1997;27:799-801

Superina RA, Ein SH, Humphreys RP: Cystic duplications of the esophagus and neurenteric cysts. J Pediatr Surg 1984;19:527-530

Wootton-Gorges SL, Thomas KB, Harned RK, et al: Giant cystic abdominal masses in children. Pediatr Radiol. 2005;35:1277-1288

CHAPTER 123

Disorders of Deglutition, Peristalsis, and the Velopharyngeal Portal

HENRIQUE M. LEDERMAN and GUILHERME T. S. DEMARCHI

DISORDERS OF DEGLUTITION AND PERISTALSIS

Most swallowing disorders in children are secondary to neurologic abnormalities, of which cerebral palsy is the most common. Other neuromuscular disorders to be considered are brainstem dysfunction, cranial nerve abnormalities, intracranial neoplasms, meningomyelocele, muscular dystrophy, and myasthenia gravis. Familial dysautonomia (Riley-Day syndrome) leads to autonomic dysfunction with esophageal dysmotility and frequent aspiration pneumonia. Disorders of the mouth and jaw such as micrognathia and macroglossia may also cause abnormal swallowing. Bulbar polio may occur in patients who have not been properly immunized.

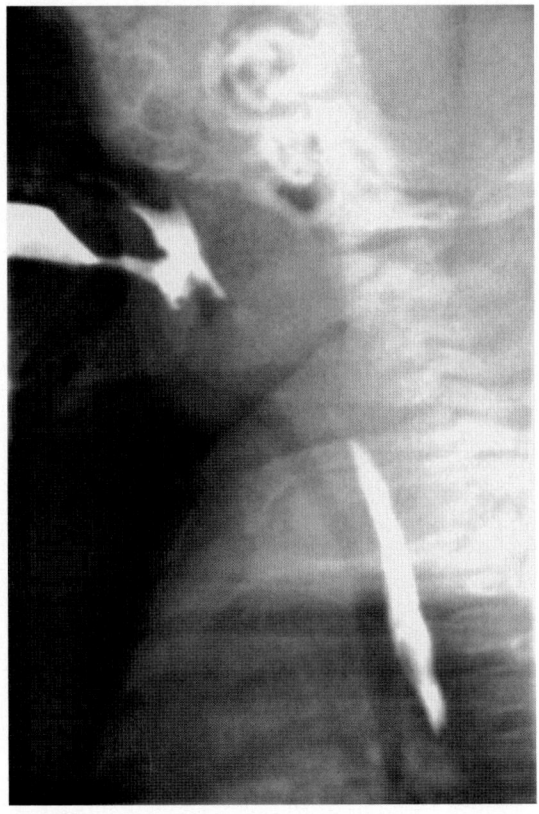

FIGURE 123-1. Abnormal swallowing with nasopharynx incoordination. Contrast material is seen in the nasal cavity.

Depending on the specific neurologic defect, any or all components of the swallowing mechanism may be affected. Some infants with severe damage cannot even suck, and most of the barium used in contrast examinations drools out of their mouths. Moreover, their tongues may not elevate to help initiate the swallowing mechanism. Abnormality of the neuromuscular mechanism elevating the soft palate may lead to reflux of contrast material into the nasopharynx (Fig. 123-1), with subsequent drooling and potential aspiration into the airway. Abnormalities of other muscle groups lead to defective function of the epiglottis and upper esophageal sphincter; aspiration into the airway is common (Fig. 123-2).

Defective peristalsis may be found in patients with the aforementioned neurologic disorders, as well as in patients with connective tissue disorders and esophagitis. Patients with a history of repaired esophageal atresia frequently show abnormal peristalsis in the portion of the esophagus distal to the repair. Patients with disordered esophageal motility may show aperistalsis or hypoperistalsis with or without tertiary contractions (Fig. 123-3). Hypoperistalsis is more common in cases of esophagitis, including those secondary to gastroesophageal reflux.

Specialized radiographic studies of deglutition performed with the help of speech therapist, have been popularized by the Johns Hopkins Swallowing Center. The patient is placed in the position in which he or she is usually fed. Contrast medium is mixed with increasingly thicker food mixtures, ranging from liquid barium to solid food mixed with barium (if age appropriate). Videotaping in the lateral projections allows evaluation of the patient's ability to handle differently textured foods and is of enormous value in planning appropriate diet and therapy (Chapter 122).

Failure of relaxation of the cricopharyngeus muscle can occasionally be seen in asymptomatic infants, as discussed in Chapter 122. However, cricopharyngeal achalasia has been thought to be a primary cause of dysphagia in symptomatic infants. Most experts now agree that primary cricopharyngeal achalasia is probably uncommon. Secondary cricopharyngeal achalasia has been reported after trauma and in patients with autoimmune collagen disorders such as scleroderma and dermatomyositis. The results of studies from the Johns Hopkins Swallowing Center suggest that most cases of cricopharyngeal achalasia are secondary to gastroesophageal reflux (Fig. 123-4).

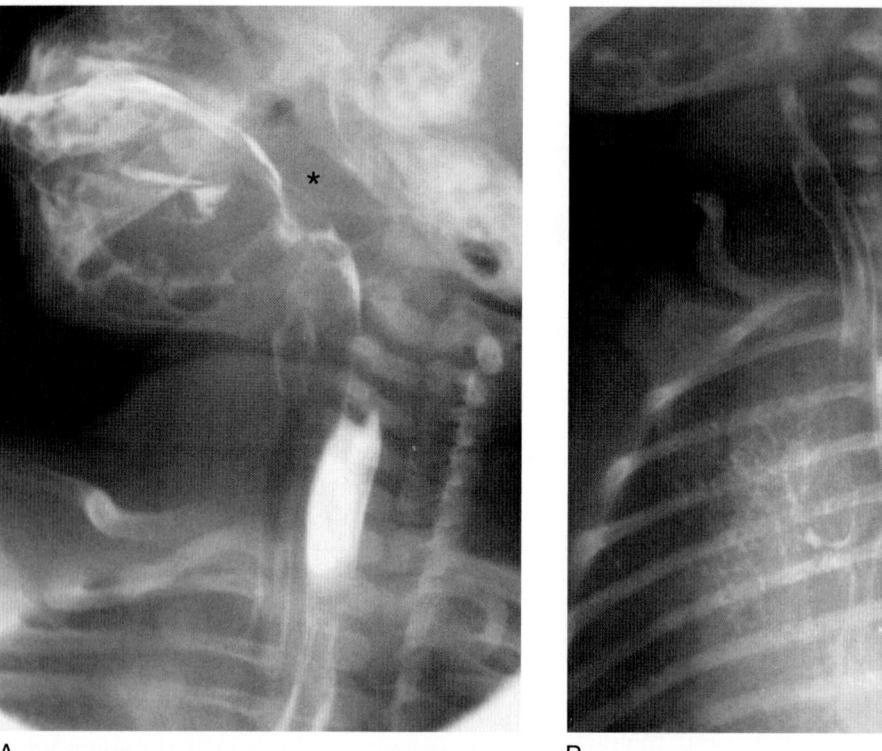

A

B

FIGURE 123-2. Swallowing incoordination and aspiration. **A,** There is complete closure of the nasopharynx and no nasopharyngeal reflux, but there is aspiration of contrast into the larynx and trachea during this barium swallow study. **B,** Oblique view reveals the extensive airway aspiration during a routine barium swallow study. This occurs because of swallowing incoordination. There is barium coating of the lung parenchyma.

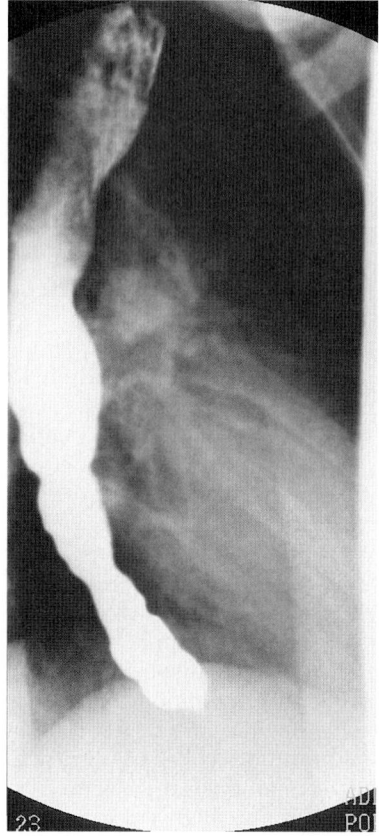

FIGURE 123-3. Lateral esophagogram in which irregular tertiary peristaltic waves are seen in the distal esophagus.

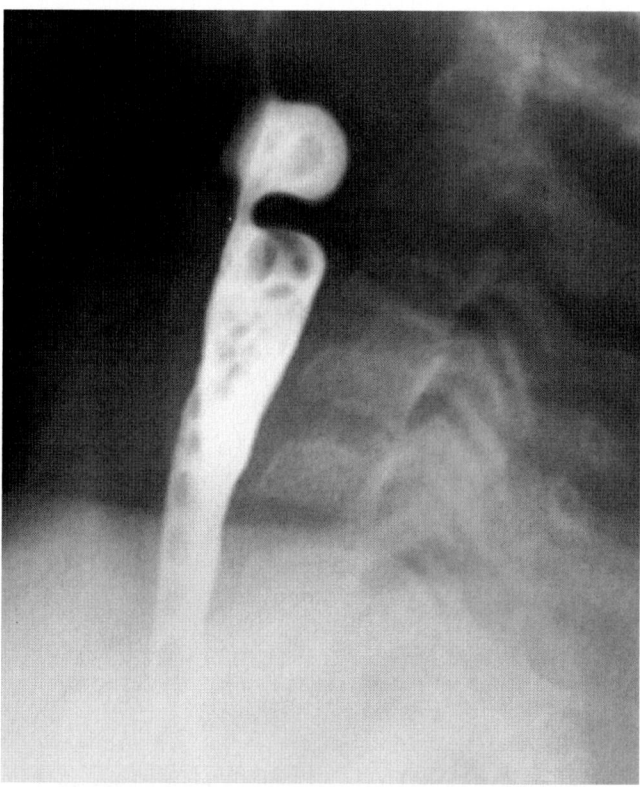

FIGURE 123-4. Posterior impression on the esophagus secondary to contraction of the cricopharyngeal muscle. The patient has cricopharyngeal achalasia and signs of dysphagia and had had associated gastroesophageal reflux.

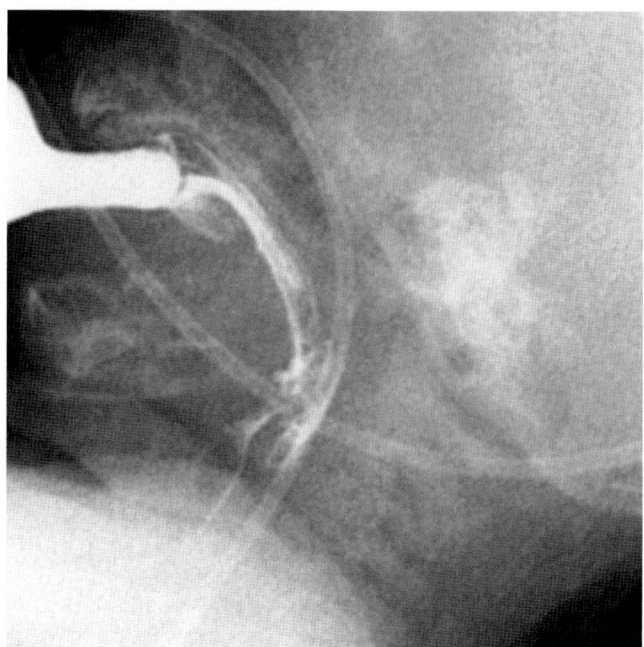

FIGURE 123-5. Laryngotracheal aspiration occurring during swallowing in a patient with a nasogastric feeding tube.

Causes of cricopharyngeal achalasia:
- **Primary (rare)**
- **Secondary**
  - **Gastroesophageal reflux**
  - **Trauma**
  - **Autoimmune disorders**

Direct pharyngeal trauma is an uncommon cause of disordered swallowing but may be seen after instrumentation, especially the passage of endotracheal, nasogastric, or orogastric tubes (Fig. 123-5). Disordered peristalsis may be seen in patients with obstructive lesions such as strictures and achalasia. Dysphagia with disordered esophageal motility may be seen in psychogenic disorders (*globus hystericus*), but in many of these patients, an organic lesion is eventually found. The diagnosis of psychogenic dysphagia should be made only after an exhaustive investigation, especially of the central nervous system, fails to yield a diagnosis of an underlying organic disorder.

Retropharyngeal masses are rare causes of dysphagia. Hemangiomas, teratomas, lymphangiomas (cystic hygromas), and lymphomas may occur at different ages. Retropharyngeal abscesses (Fig. 123-6) cause stridor and

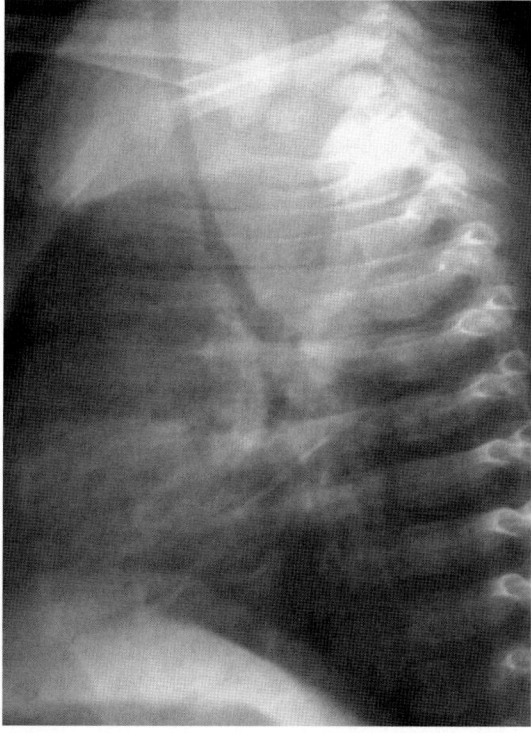
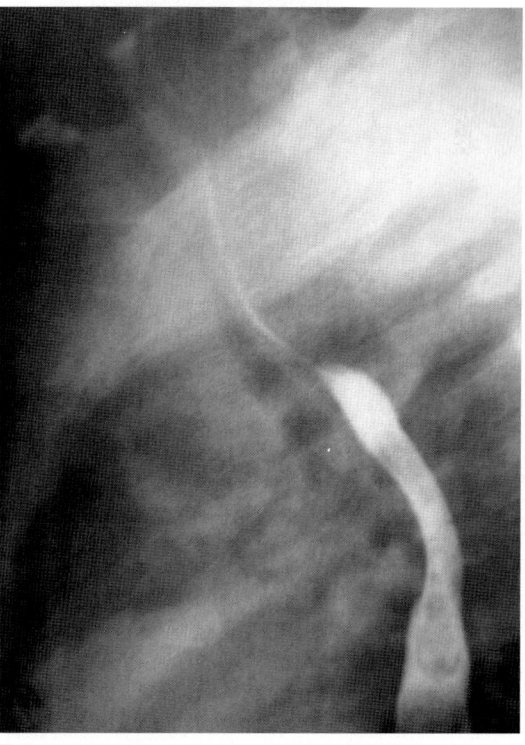

A   B

FIGURE 123-6. Retropharyngeal abscess. **A,** Lateral chest radiograph shows a soft tissue density in the posterior mediastinum that displaces the trachea anteriorly. The trachea is compressed. **B,** Barium swallow study demonstrates the anterior displacement of the esophagus and trachea. The patient had a retropharyngeal abscess that dissected down into the posterior mediastinum.

that usually leads to the correct diagnosis. Congenital pharyngeal diverticula are quite rare. Spinal anomalies may rarely cause dysphagia in children.

> **Retropharyngeal masses include:**
> - **Hemangioma**
> - **Teratoma**
> - **Lymphangioma**
> - **Lymphoma**
> - **Abscess**

Scleroderma and mixed collagen disorders are rare in childhood; they occur most frequently in young adults. Pharyngeal and cervical esophageal function is usually normal. Esophageal dysmotility typically begins at the level of the aortic arch, where the esophageal muscle layer begins to change from striated to smooth muscle. Primary peristalsis is poor to absent in the distal two thirds of the esophagus (Fig. 123-7). Secondary esophageal reflux, with or without esophagitis, may occur. Levine and Ilowite described abnormal motility, diagnosed by esophageal manometry and esophageal endoscopy with biopsy, with a pattern similar to that seen in scleroderma, in breastfed children of mothers with silicone breast implants.

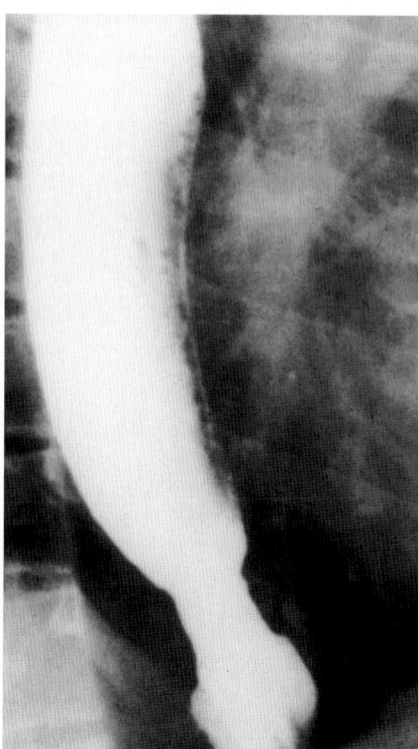

FIGURE 123-7. Dilatation of the distal esophagus in a patient with scleroderma. In addition, emptying was slowed and delayed, and peristaltic activity was decreased.

Dermatomyositis, in contrast, affects primarily the striated muscle of the pharynx and upper esophagus. Dilatation of these structures frequently occurs, as does reflux into the nasopharynx. The associated vasculitis may result in esophageal ulceration and perforation.

VELOPHARYNGEAL INCOMPETENCE

Disorders of the velopharyngeal portal are observed most commonly during evaluation of speech disorders. Although technically simple to perform, these studies are not part of the repertoire of most radiologists. They are most useful in patients being considered for cleft palate surgery and in those with speech disorders secondary to neurologic abnormalities. Because the muscles used in speech and swallowing are largely similar, useful information can be obtained from speech studies. The studies are feasible in most patients aged 5 years or older and can be performed in cooperative children as young as 3 years. The patient is placed in an upright lateral or seated position. A small amount of barium is injected into the nose to coat the soft palate for easier visualization. Combined audio-video recording is obtained while the patient repeats a series of words and phrases designed to maximize function of the pharyngeal muscles. During speech, the soft palate should elevate, becoming nearly horizontal in its proximal two thirds (Fig. 123-8). The distal third remains approximately vertical and should make contact with the posterior pharyngeal wall throughout its course. The motion of the tongue can also be evaluated.

The procedure is then repeated with the patient's head in a modified Towne projection, allowing direct visualization of the oropharynx and nasopharynx (Fig. 123-9). Skolnick and Cohn recommended performing this portion of the study with the patient prone, but we have found that younger patients tolerate the procedure better if kept in a sitting or standing position. The nasopharyngeal walls are seen to function during speech like the iris of a camera. In patients with velopharyngeal incompetence, failure of normal excursion of the soft palate and the muscular pharyngeal side walls is identified. A barium swallow study, which completes the examination, is conducted to evaluate for nasopharyngeal reflux and fistulous communication between the oropharynx and nasopharynx. Speech studies have also proved quite valuable in the evaluation of patients after surgical repair of cleft palate. These studies are quite useful in differentiating primary neuromuscular lesions, such as those seen in central nervous system disorders, from structural lesions, such as those in patients with craniofacial anomalies.

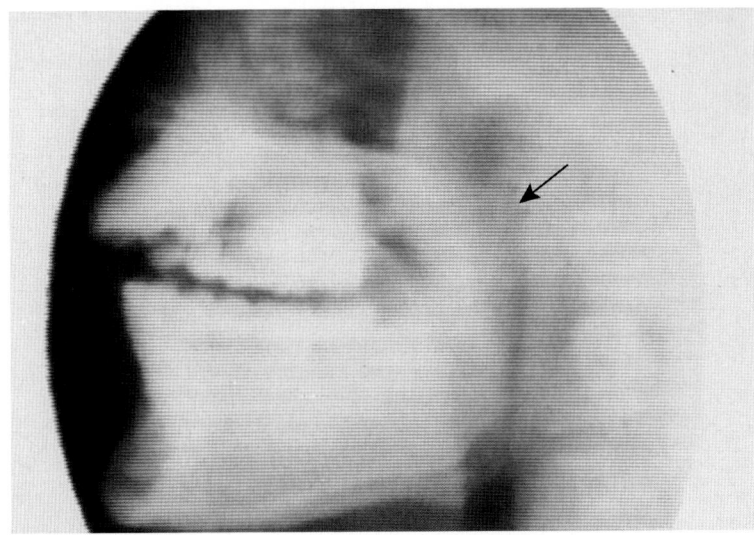

A

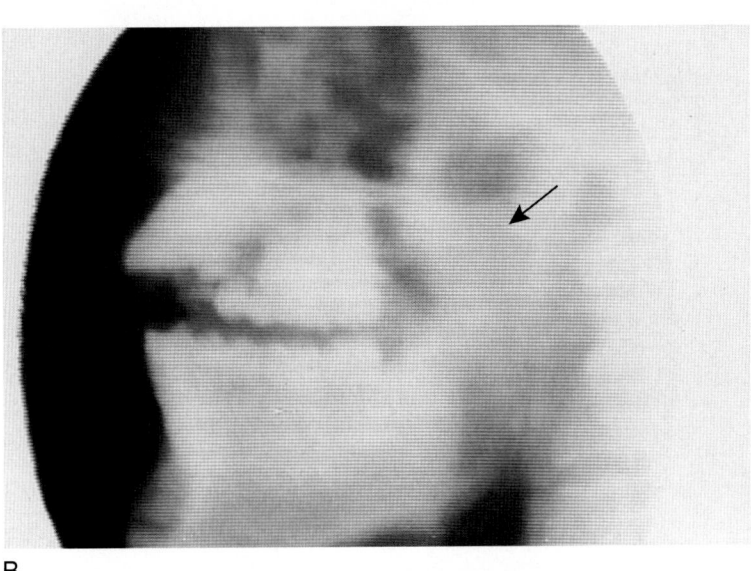

B

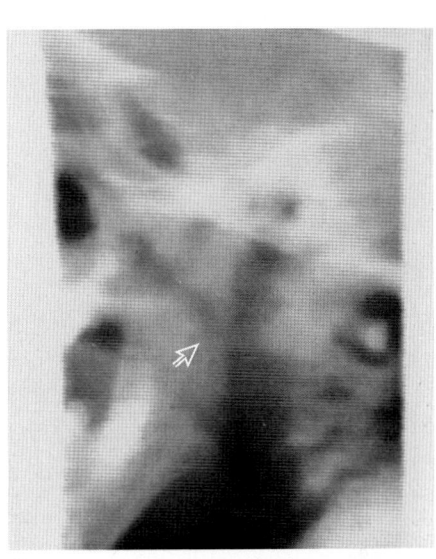

C

FIGURE 123-8. Videofluorography during speech. **A,** During quiet breathing, the soft palate is relaxed and the nasopharyngeal air column is open (*arrow*). **B,** During phonation, the soft palate is elevated and extends posteriorly, completely closing off the nasopharyngeal air column. **C,** In a younger patient with severely nasal speech, the soft palate forms a normal right angle (*arrow*) but does not close off the patent nasopharyngeal air column; this leads to resonant speech.

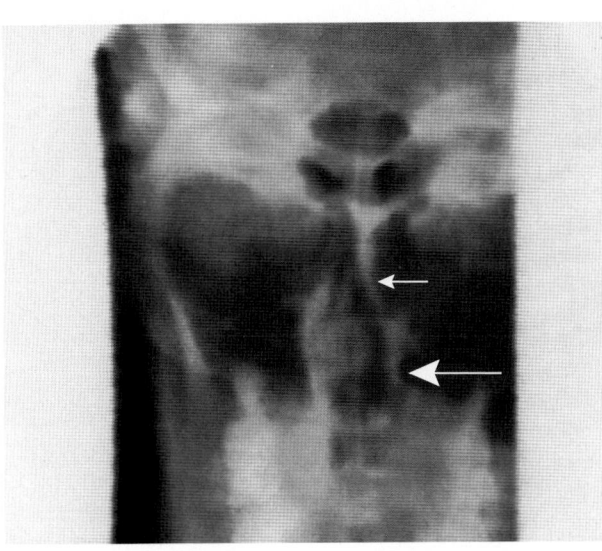

A

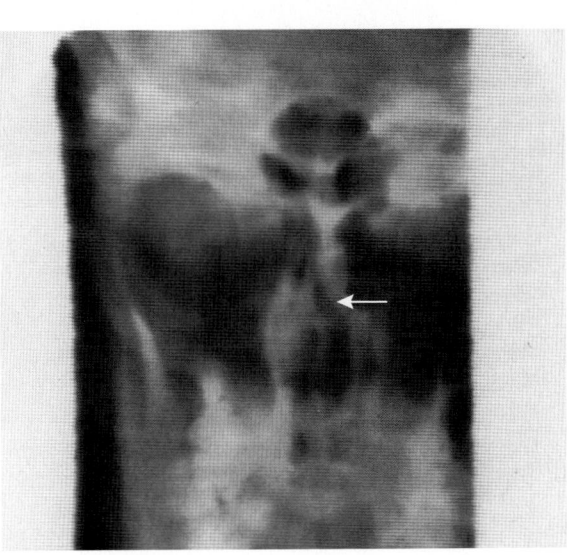

B

FIGURE 123-9. Videofluorography in the modified Towne projection. **A,** During quiet breathing, the nasopharyngeal air column (*small arrow*) and the oropharyngeal air column (*large arrow*) are well demonstrated. **B,** During speech, the nasopharyngeal air column (*arrow*) is reduced in diameter but does not close completely in a patient with nasal speech.

SUGGESTED READINGS

Fisher SE, Painter M, Milmoe G: Swallowing disorders in infancy. Pediatr Clin North Am 1981;28:845-853

Gyepes MT, Linde LM: Familial dysautonomia: the mechanism of aspiration. Radiology 1968;91:471-475

Kramer SS: Special swallowing problems in children. Gastrointest Radiol 1985;10:241-250

Kramer SS: Radiologic examination of the swallowing impaired child. Dysphagia 1989;3:117-125

La Rossa D, Brown A, Cohen M, et al: Video-radiography of the velopharyngeal portal using the Towne's view. J Maxillofac Surg 1980;8:203-205

Levine JJ, Ilowite NT: Sclerodermalike esophageal disease in children breast-fed by mothers with silicone breast implants. JAMA 1994; 271:213-216

Mihailovic T, Perisic VN: Balloon dilatation of cricopharyngeal achalasia. Pediatr Radiol 1992;22:522-524

Nohara K, Tachimura T, Wada T: Prediction of deterioration of velopharyngeal function associated with maxillary advancement using electromyography of levator veli palatini muscle. Cleft Palate Craniofac J 2006;43:174-178

Pryor LS, Lehman J, Parker MG, et al: Outcomes in pharyngoplasty: a 10-year experience. Cleft Palate Craniofac J 2006;43:222-225

Skinner MA, Shorter NA: Primary neonatal achalasia: a case report and review of the literature. J Pediatr Surg 1992;27:1509-1511

Skolnick ML: Video velopharyngography in patients with nasal speech, with emphasis on lateral pharyngeal motion in velopharyngeal closure. Radiology 1969;93:747-755

Skolnick ML, Cohn ER: Videofluoroscopic Studies of Speech in Patients with Cleft Palate. New York, Springer-Verlag, 1989.

Sonmez A, Ersoy B, Numanoglu A: Acute onset of velopharyngeal insufficiency and dysphagia after sternocleidomastoid myotomy for congenital muscular torticollis. Ann Plast Surg 2006;56:348-349

Stringer DA, Witzer MA: Velopharyngeal insufficiency on multiview videofluoroscopy: a comparison of projections. AJR Am J Roentgenol 1986;146:15-19

Tuchman DN: Cough, choke, sputter: the evaluation of the child with dysfunctional swallowing. Dysphagia 1989;3:111-116

Acquired Esophageal Lesions

HENRIQUE M. LEDERMAN and GUILHERME T. S. DEMARCHI

NONINFECTIVE ESOPHAGITIS

The most common cause of noninfective esophagitis in children is gastroesophageal reflux. This entity is discussed separately in Chapter 125. Less common causes include traumatic lesions, such as caustic ingestion, and inflammatory lesions of various origins.

Caustic Ingestion

Ingestion of caustic agents is becoming less common as parents and other caregivers have become more aware of the dangers of careless storage of household agents. Nevertheless, the effects of caustic ingestion are still seen and can be devastating. Acidic compounds typically affect the stomach, whereas caustic esophagitis is usually secondary to ingestion of alkalis, most commonly household lye compounds, which are a mixture of sodium and potassium hydroxide. Burns of the mouth may not be seen or may be superficial because of the short time of contact. The upper portion of the esophagus is less likely to be affected than the middle or lower portions for the same reason, whereas transient cardiospasm may increase the time of contact between liquid alkalis and the esophageal mucosa in the distal third, the most affected segment (Fig. 124-1). Granulated materials, in contrast, may adhere to the more proximal esophageal mucosa and are more likely to affect that portion of the esophagus. Ulcerations are more likely to be seen in acute stages (Fig. 124-2).

> Caustic ingestion with acidic compounds typically affects the stomach, whereas alkali ingestion usually causes caustic esophagitis.

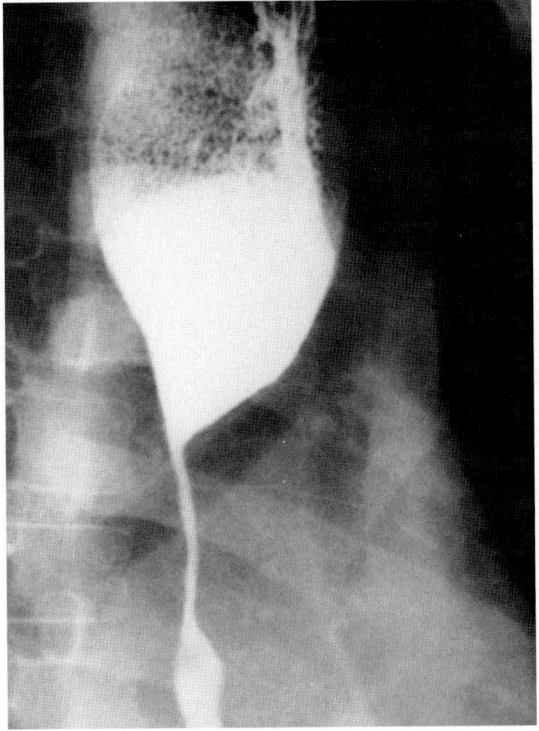 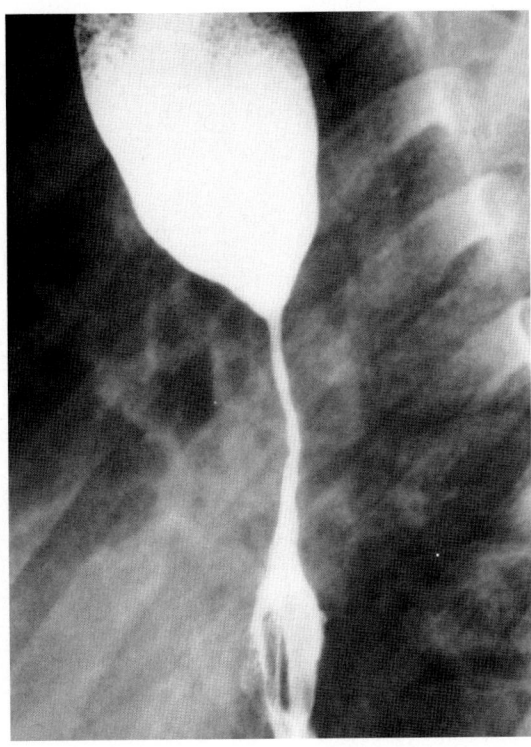

A

B

FIGURE 124-1. Midesophageal stricture. Barium swallow study in the frontal (**A**) and lateral (**B**) projections demonstrates severe stricture at the middle to lower portions of the esophagus, with proximal dilatation and food residues secondary to caustic ingestion.

SECTION VI — THE ABDOMEN, PELVIS, AND RETROPERITONEUM

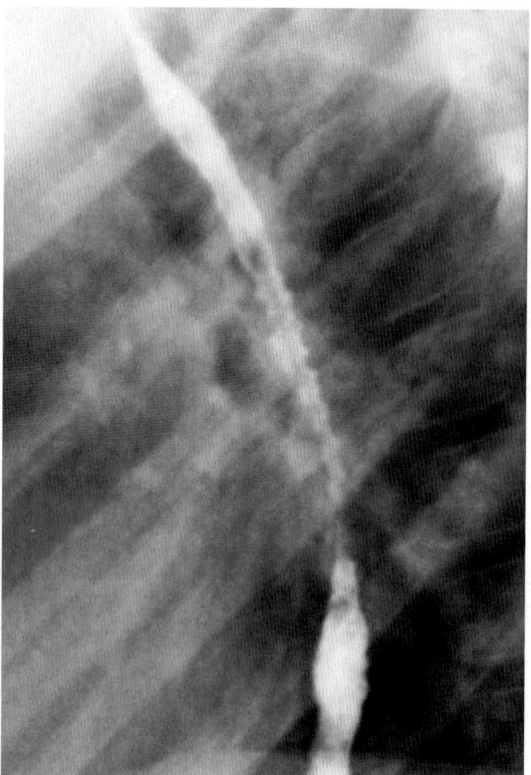

FIGURE 124-2. Caustic ingestion causing lengthy esophageal irregularity. This image was obtained in the more acute stage and shows the multiple ulcerations.

Swelling of the epiglottis indicates that the caustic agent has reached the hypopharynx and probably has been swallowed into the esophagus (Fig. 124-3). In fact, with decreasing incidence of bacterial epiglottitis as a result of the development of the *Haemophilus influenzae* type B vaccine, more "unusual" causes of epiglottic enlargement, such as caustic ingestion and nonaccidental trauma when a child is forced to drink scalding water, should be considered in a young child with epiglottic enlargement. Initial chest radiographs may reveal evidence of mediastinitis with mediastinal widening and a dilated, gas-filled esophagus. Inflammation of the pharynx may cause disordered swallowing with subsequent aspiration. Contrast esophagography is preferable to endoscopy because traumatic perforation may occur with the latter. Spontaneous perforation may occur, as may deep ulceration and tracheoesophageal fistulas. Therefore, the initial examination is performed with low-osmolar, nonionic contrast material, because inert barium can be retained for long periods of time. If no perforation or fistula is seen, barium provides better coating for thorough evaluation of the mucosa.

Caustic ingestions:

- **Swelling of the epiglottis indicates that the ingested agent has reached the hypopharynx and probably the esophagus.**

- **In cases in which fistulas or perforations are suspected, low-osmolar, nonionic contrast material should be used initially.**

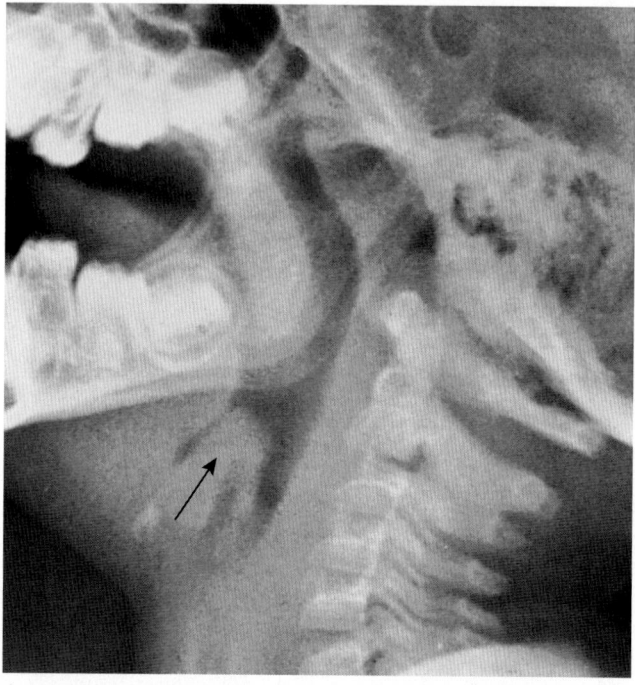

A

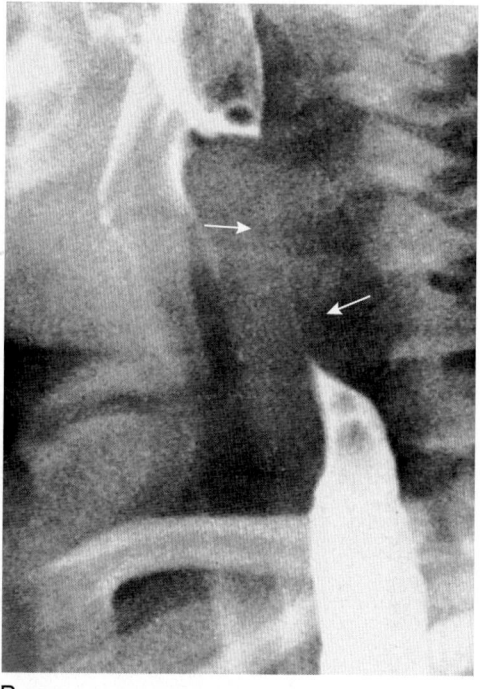

B

FIGURE 124-3. Caustic ingestion with epiglottic involvement. **A,** Lateral neck film shows the swollen epiglottis *(arrow).* This image was obtained 20 hours after the ingestion of caustic material. **B,** Esophagogram 2 weeks later demonstrates the proximal segment of the cervical esophagus to be narrow *(arrows),* with aspiration of contrast material into the trachea. This was a fixed narrowing.

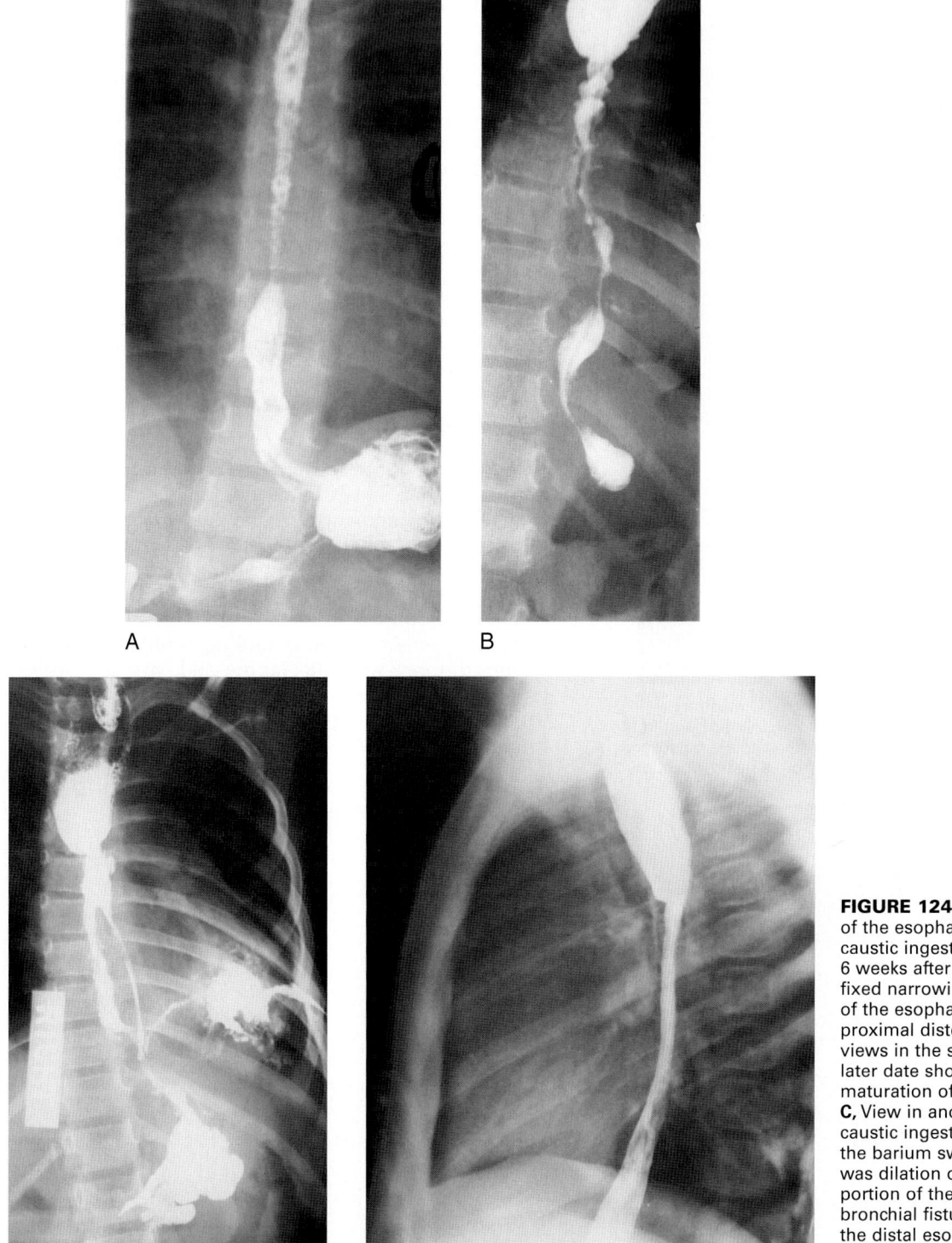

A

B

C

D

FIGURE 124-4. Fixed narrowing of the esophagus secondary to caustic ingestion. **A,** Frontal view 6 weeks after ingestion shows a fixed narrowing of the midportion of the esophagus. There is some proximal distention. **B,** Oblique views in the same patient at a later date shows a continuing maturation of this process. **C,** View in another child after caustic ingestion. At the time of the barium swallow study, there was dilation of the proximal portion of the esophagus with a bronchial fistula and stricture of the distal esophagus. **D,** Lateral view of another patient with a long esophageal stricture several months after caustic ingestion.

Mucosal irregularity, esophageal dysmotility, and ulceration may all be seen in the acute or subacute phase (see Fig. 124-2). Reactive fibrosis of the esophageal wall may cause the appearance of a stenotic, rigid tube on fluoroscopy (Fig. 124-4D). Ultimately, esophageal stricture develops, necessitating dilatation and, in worst cases, esophagectomy and esophageal replacement (typically with ileum or colon tissue or both) (Fig. 124-5). Epithelial metaplasia (Barrett esophagus) may occur, as may development of esophageal carcinoma later in adulthood.

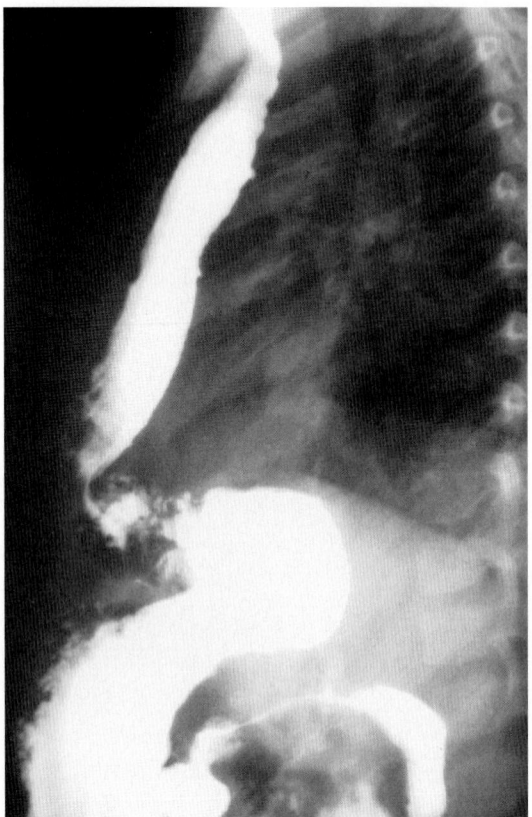

FIGURE 124-5. Lateral view of upper gastrointestinal series, showing a bowel loop: esophageal colonic interposition in the anterior mediastinum. Surgery was performed after a severe narrowing of the esophagus resulted from caustic ingestion.

Epidermolysis Bullosa Dystrophica

Epidermolysis bullosa dystrophica is a congenital disease affecting squamous epithelium and causing esophagitis. In this disease, the skin has numerous bullous lesions that are friable and easily abraded, with sloughing of the skin even after the most minimal contact. Affected patients should not be restrained unless supervised by a dermatologist. Every effort must be made to have the child drink spontaneously during esophagography, because even the minimal trauma caused by a Silastic feeding tube may damage the esophageal epithelium. Loss of motility, mucosal irregularity, ulceration, and stenosis may occur in these children (Fig. 124-6). Esophageal replacement may be necessary in children with severe strictures.

Miscellaneous Causes

Crohn disease of the esophagus is rarely observed on imaging studies but is being described with increasing frequency by endoscopists. Comparisons of endoscopy with esophagography confirm increased sensitivity of endoscopic evaluation. When abnormalities are identified on esophagograms, ulceration and stricture are the most common findings.

Behçet syndrome produces findings similar to those of Crohn disease, with ulceration and stricture in the esophagus, and ileocolitis resembling Crohn disease, with similar findings. The additional multisystem findings of Behçet syndrome affecting skin, mucous

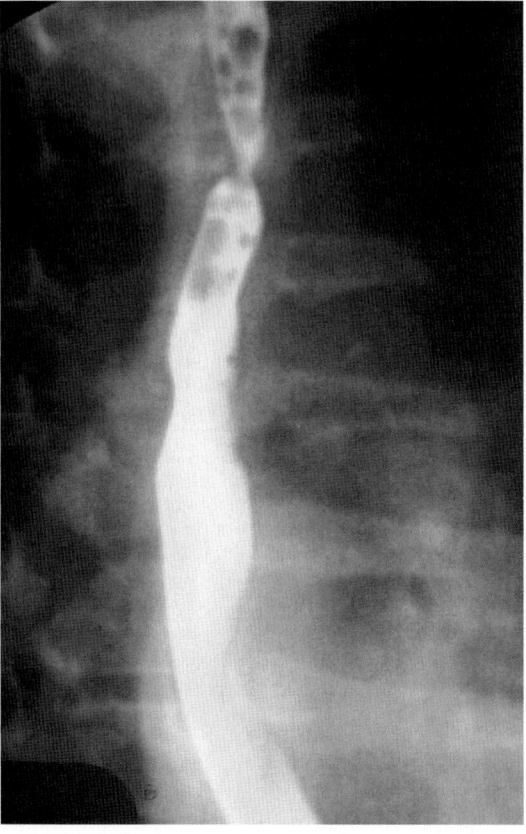

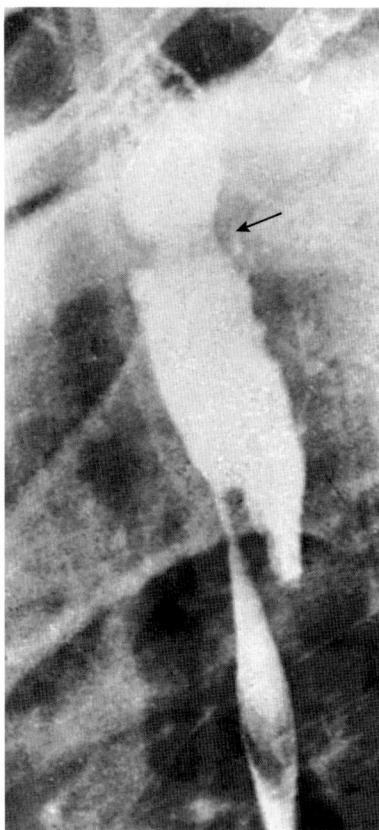

FIGURE 124-6. Epidermolysis bullosa dystrophica. **A,** Anteroposterior view of esophagogram demonstrates focal stricture formation in a 3-year-old girl. **B,** Esophagogram in a different patient demonstrates an annular stenosis just below the thoracic inlet (*arrow*). Below this and posteriorly, a barium-filled pocket suggests an ulcer and submucosal abscess. (**B** courtesy of Dr. Melvin Becker, New York, NY.)

A

B

membranes, uvea, and central nervous system, although not always present in children, can help differentiate these two entities.

Chronic granulomatous disease of childhood can in rare cases produce focal areas of esophageal narrowing, with esophageal stricture caused by the primary disease rather than by opportunistic infection.

Graft-versus-host disease in patients who have undergone bone marrow transplantation at times can produce esophageal lesions, as described by McDonald and colleagues. Webs, ringlike narrowing, and smoothly tapering strictures may be observed on barium studies.

Radiation esophagitis caused by low-dose radiation therapy may be manifested by esophageal inflammation with resultant dysmotility, but it rarely produces long-term effects. High-dose (>25 Gy) radiation therapy, uncommonly used in young children, may lead to dysmotility, mucosal edema, superficial and deep ulceration, and stricture at any age. Similar findings have been described in patients exposed to a variety of chemotherapeutic agents, including antibiotics, quinidine, and anticancer agents. The combined effects of radiation therapy and doxorubicin (Adriamycin) are especially likely to lead to esophagitis, as well as cardiac and other complications, because of their synergistic actions.

Eosinophilic esophagitis was first described in 1977 by Dobbins and associates in a patient with eosinophilic gastroenteritis and esophageal involvement. This pathologic process affects boys more commonly than girls, often with prolonged duration of symptoms before clinical recognition. Symptoms of dysphagia occur almost exclusively with solids, and simultaneous atopic conditions are the rule. Eosinophilic esophagitis is characterized by an inflammatory reaction confined to the esophagus. The expression of eosinophils, T cells, and mast cells in the mucosa of eosinophilic esophagitis is characteristic of the disorder and very similar to that seen within the lungs of patients with asthma. Straumann and coworkers demonstrated that the T-helper type 2 cytokine and interleukin-5 allergic response to inhaled allergens occur consistently in patients suffering from this disease. This suggests a link between allergic asthma and eosinophilic esophagitis.

Carefully conducted skin testing for food allergies among large reported series of children with eosinophilic esophagitis has identified food allergies in about 80%. With meticulous dietary elimination, the investigators demonstrated marked and durable improvement in dysphagia symptoms, with normalization of the esophageal mucosa and decrease in mucosal eosinophil count in many children with positive pinprick or patch testing. This further supports the theory that extrinsic allergens may be responsible for some cases of eosinophilic esophagitis. Long-standing eosinophilic esophagitis appears to be associated with a wide range of radiographic and endoscopic findings. Findings on barium esophagograms may range from short- and high-grade stenosis to very subtle narrowing, often extending the entire length of the esophagus. Of importance is that the finding of a long "small-caliber" esophagus reported by Vasilopoulos and colleagues appears to be correlated with the probability of long, painful mucosal tears with esophageal dilation. Many endoscopists now recommend cautious dilatation in patients with eosinophilic esophagitis only with dilators smaller than those usually used with peptic or acid reflux–related esophageal strictures. However, transient chest pain and odynophagia after esophageal dilatation are common, even with gentle and conservative esophageal dilatation. The resemblance of the inflammatory reaction of eosinophilic esophagitis to allergic asthma has led many investigators to attempt treatment with systemic or topical corticosteroid and leukotriene antagonists. Langdon and others reported a decrease in the number of mucosal eosinophils with such therapy, but dysphagia symptoms did not improve without dilatation. The diagnosis of eosinophilic esophagitis should be considered in children with coincident atopic conditions and symptoms of solid dysphagia. Similarly, the absence of reflux in the child with solid dysphagia is suggestive of eosinophilic esophagitis, and the examiner should carefully inquire about atopic conditions. Esophagogram findings of subtle diffuse esophageal narrowing in the absence of neoplasia or reflux should suggest the diagnosis. Endoscopic findings are described as coiled-spring ("feline") esophagus, segmental stricture, and vertical lined esophagus. For biopsy specimens, the pathologist should be alerted to the possible diagnosis of eosinophilic esophagitis, so that the number of eosinophils per high-power field is carefully counted, because acid reflux esophagitis has been associated with increased numbers of eosinophils, but usually fewer than five per high-power field.

Eosinophilic esophagitis:

- **More common in boys**
- **Dysphagia with solids**
- **Associated atopic conditions are typical**
- **Eosinophils >5 per high-power field**
- **Stricture dilatation with small-diameter dilators**

INFECTIVE ESOPHAGITIS

Although occasionally reported in immunocompetent children, these lesions are usually caused by opportunistic organisms and are seen in children who are immunocompromised as a result of congenital or acquired immunodeficiency syndromes or immunosuppressive drugs. The most common infective agent is *Candida albicans* (*Monilia*), but viral agents such as cytomegalovirus and herpes simplex virus may also cause esophagitis. In older children and adult patients with acquired immunodeficiency syndrome, esophageal infection with human immunodeficiency virus and with mycobacteria has been reported. Although some authorities have advocated routine use of endoscopy in immunocompromised children with symptoms of esophagitis, this position is controversial, and esophagography is still performed in some centers.

Double-contrast examinations of the esophagus are more likely to be diagnostic than are single-contrast studies, but these may be difficult to perform in young or

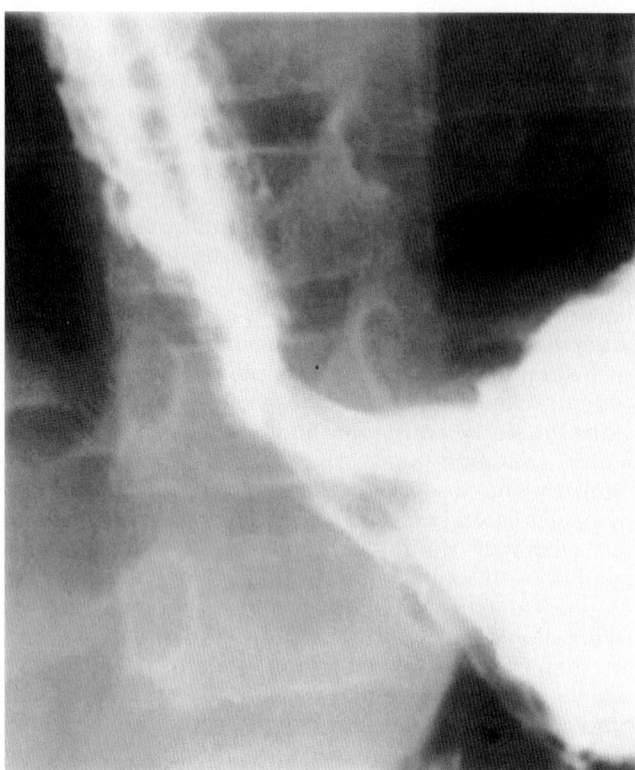

FIGURE 124-7. Candidiasis. Frontal view of the distal esophagus shows multiple small ulcerations and mucosal edema.

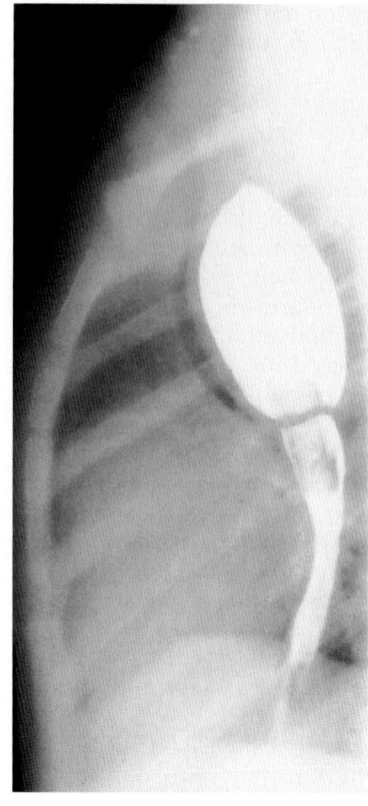

FIGURE 124-8. Cytomegalovirus infection. A midesophageal weblike narrowing, a foreign body impacted proximal to the narrowing, proximal dilation of the esophagus, and anterior displacement of the trachea are present. The patient had had previous cytomegalovirus infection, which caused the weblike narrowing.

uncooperative children. In children with candidal esophagitis, dysmotility, elevated focal lesions (nodules or plaques), and mucosal edema are the common findings (Fig. 124-7). A "shaggy mucosa" or "cobblestone" appearance may result from barium filling the interstices between plaques or necrotic debris. However, the characteristic "shaggy mucosa" of candidiasis is actually nonspecific and may be seen in the viral esophagitides as well. Eventually, deep ulcerations may develop, but frank ulcers are more common with herpes and cytomegalovirus esophagitis. Even if cultures are positive for *Monilia* species, concomitant viral infection should be suspected if ulcers are seen. Pseudodiverticula may form as well.

Cytomegalovirus causes vasculitis by invading the capillary endothelial cells and eventually leads to ischemic necrosis and ulceration. In addition to the classical large ulcers, linear ulcers, nodular thickening, "cobblestone" appearance, pseudodiverticula, and strictures may occur (Fig. 124-8). *Herpes simplex virus* typically causes shallow ulcers that are stellate or diamond-shaped and rarely causes linear or longitudinal ulcers (Fig. 124-9). *Mycobacterium tuberculosis* can invade the esophagus by direct spread from adjacent mediastinal lymph nodes and may cause fistulas or sinus tracts.

Candida albicans (*Monilia*) **is the most common cause of infective esophagitis.**

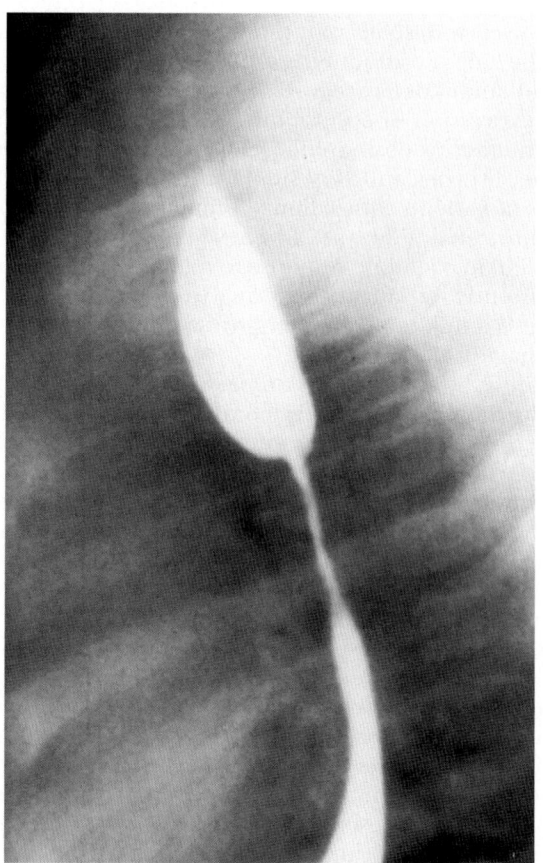

FIGURE 124-9. Herpetic esophagitis. Midesophageal stricture with proximal dilation secondary to herpetic esophagitis.

DIVERTICULA

Diverticula of the esophagus are rare in children. Pulsion or pressure diverticula are herniations of the mucosa and submucosa through congenitally weak sites of the esophageal wall; little or none of the muscular layer is incorporated into the walls of such diverticula. Simple pressure diverticula are usually located above the clavicles and extend from a lateral wall of the esophagus posteriorly, where, when enlarged, they may displace and compress the esophageal channel anteriorly. They are best seen in the lateral and oblique projections, in which they appear as rounded pouches filled with barium; they fill quickly and empty relatively slowly. Traction diverticula are anterior or, less commonly, lateral projections of the esophageal lumen. Their walls may be made up of mucosa alone. More typical, however, is that all of the esophageal mural layers are present. They usually occur just below the tracheal bifurcation. The traction is caused by the fibrous contraction of fibrotic lymph nodes and paraesophageal areolar tissue. Roentgenographically, they appear as triangular pouches that empty quickly. They are usually of little clinical importance except that they may be the sites of impaction and perforation of foreign bodies.

FOREIGN BODIES AND TRAUMA

Foreign bodies may be swallowed at any age. Even the youngest infants may be fed unusual articles by an obliging older sibling. Although the older child or parent may give a history of foreign body ingestion, young children often present with unexplained drooling, inability to swallow solids, or, less commonly, with chest pain. Young patients with an esophageal foreign body commonly present with respiratory problems such as wheezing or stridor. Radiopaque foreign bodies are easily identified on plain radiographs. Smooth objects, such as coins, the most commonly ingested foreign bodies, are usually seen at the thoracic inlet. Less commonly, they become lodged at the level of the left main stem bronchus or just above the esophagogastric junction. If coins are seen at other levels, underlying esophageal abnormalities should be considered. Sharp objects, pins being the most common, may become lodged anywhere along the course of the esophagus and can penetrate the mucosa (Fig. 124-10). Food, plastic, and aluminum articles and buttons are the most common nonopaque esophageal foreign bodies. The examiner must always bear in mind that an opaque image may correspond to only a part of the swallowed object, which may, for instance, be composed of a tiny metal part and a much larger plastic, nonopaque portion (Fig. 124-11).

> An esophageal foreign body can manifest with airway symptoms: stridor, wheezing, and cough.

Plain radiographs of the chest and neck (including a lateral view of the upper airway that includes the nasopharynx, because foreign bodies can be placed in the nose or can be carried by reflux into the nasopharynx once placed in the mouth) should be the first imaging examination. Coins in the esophagus generally lie in the coronal plane (Fig. 124-12), whereas those in the trachea lie in the sagittal plane, presumably because of the anatomy of the tracheal rings, although this is not invariably the case (Fig. 124-13). Increased distance between the trachea and the esophagus, particularly if accompanied by tracheal narrowing, indicates a long-standing foreign body and precludes attempts by balloon removal (see Fig. 124-12). Long-standing foreign bodies may have caused thickening or perforation of the esophageal walls, leading to pneumomediastinum or mediastinal mass. A foreign body such as incompletely chewed food may cause high-grade obstruction with air-fluid levels in the esophagus or a frothy appearance from mixed air and fluid. Impacted food most often occurs in patients who have underlying esophageal abnormalities.

Infants with nonopaque foreign bodies or unexplained respiratory symptoms may require esophagograms for diagnosis. Because the degree of potential obstruction is unknown before the examination, only a small amount of opaque material should be given initially. Contrast studies generally are not performed when an opaque foreign body is identified; however, they may be useful if there is concern about edema, stricture, or perforation. Low-osmolarity contrast material should be used in such cases. Currarino and Nikaidoh reported four cases of foreign bodies in patients with vascular rings and suggested that esophagograms be performed if there is clinical suspicion of such an anomaly. Herman and McAlister reported two cases of traumatic diverticula in patients with unsuspected foreign bodies.

The removal of radiopaque esophageal foreign bodies by radiologists with Foley catheters is a contentious subject. The procedure was initially popularized by Campbell and colleagues, who reported high success rates with no significant complications. Using their patient selection criteria and methods, many pediatric radiologists enjoyed great success with the procedure, which reduced hospitalization and cost. More recent reports, especially in the surgical literature, have raised doubts in the minds of many radiologists as to the wisdom of continuing to remove foreign bodies by this method because of the risk of complications. Furthermore, the higher success rate of esophagoscopy in comparison to this technique has led some radiologists to recommend esophagoscopy as the primary method for esophageal foreign body extraction. Other authors have continued to report a high degree of success and few complications with the Foley catheter technique (Fig. 124-14). This procedure typically is contraindicated if an underlying esophageal abnormality is present or if edema is identified on a lateral chest or airway radiograph (as evidenced by increased soft tissue between the esophageal foreign body and the air-filled adjacent trachea) (see Fig. 124-12). In general, balloon-catheter removal is not recommended if the foreign body has been present for 24 hours or longer, because of the greater likelihood of associated edema. Nonopaque foreign bodies, identified on esophagogram, can also be removed by this method, but only if rounded or oval in shape.

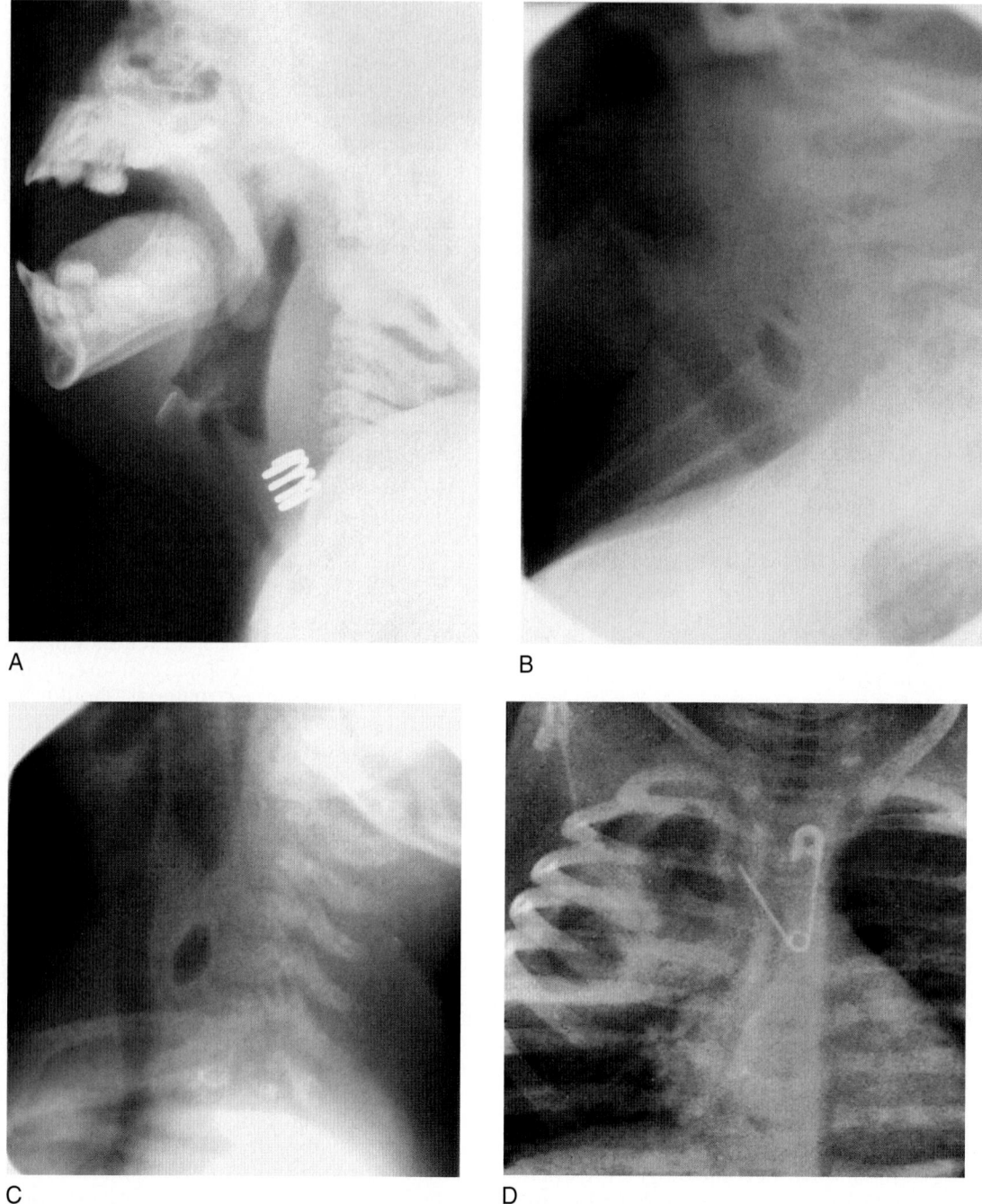

FIGURE 124-10. Opaque, partially opaque, and lucent esophageal foreign bodies. **A,** Lateral neck film in a 1-year-old with a coiled spring in the proximal esophagus. **B** and **C,** Swallowed peach pit in two views in an older child. Note the central lucency surrounded by soft tissue opacity and then a partial lucency around a peach pit in the proximal esophagus. The oblique view (**C**) clearly displays the foreign body. **D,** An open safety pin is visible in the midesophagus of a young child. The esophagus was perforated, which caused mediastinitis and fluid in the pleural cavity surrounding the upper lobe.

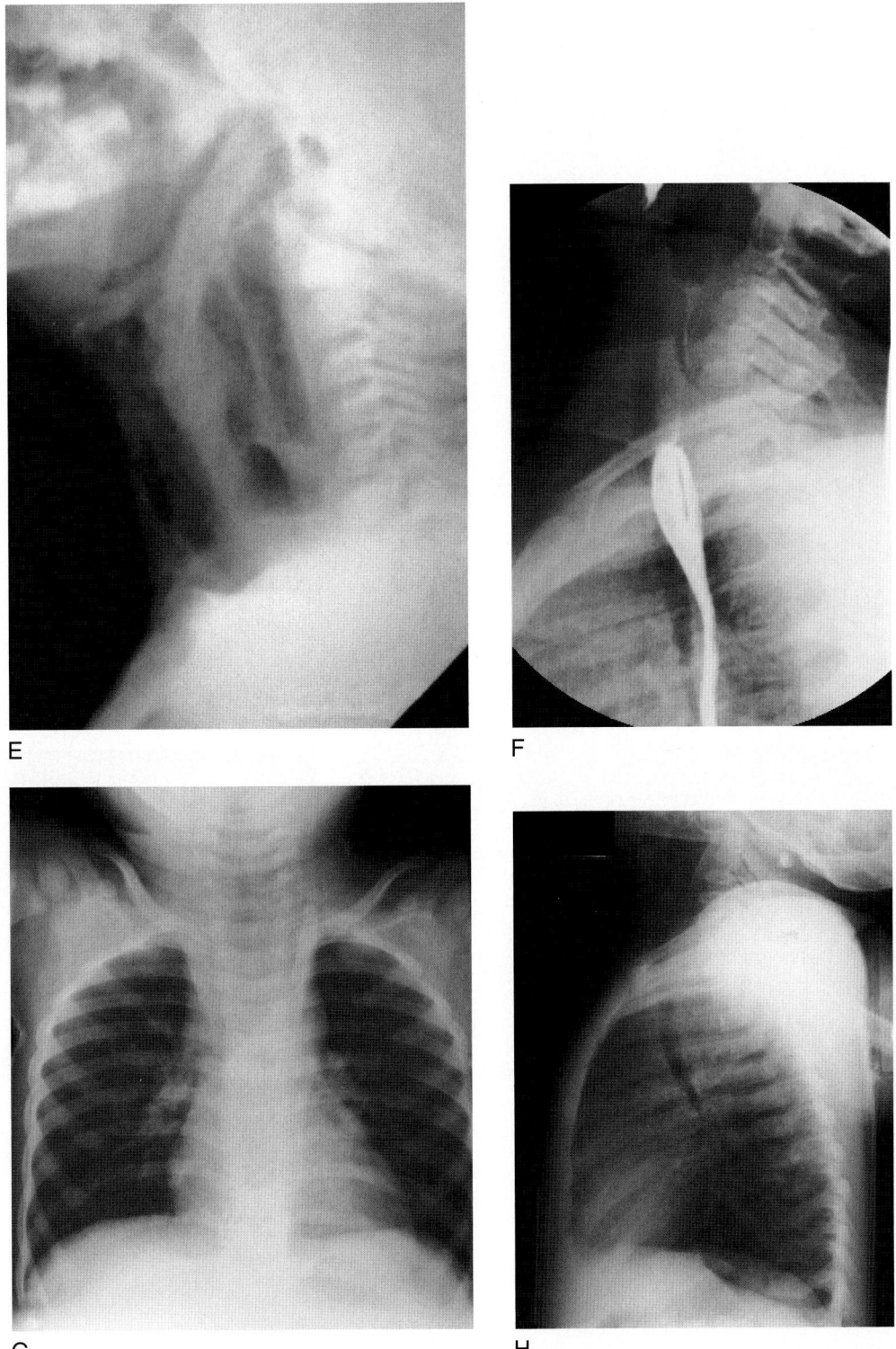

E

F

G

H

FIGURE 124-10, *cont'd.* Opaque, partially opaque, and lucent esophageal foreign bodies. **E,** In the same patient as in **D,** a pneumomediastinum with dissection of air into the neck is visible. **F,** Barium swallow study in a child who was gagging. There is a radiolucent Tiddlywink in the proximal intrathoracic esophagus. This object would be invisible on the plain film. **G** to **J,** A young infant has a widened mediastinum on frontal film but, more impressive, an anteriorly bowed trachea on lateral film. The esophagogram (**I** and **J**) shows extravasation of contrast material into the mediastinum secondary to erosion by a foreign body in the esophagus. Note the narrowing and anterior position of the airway on the lateral film.

Continued

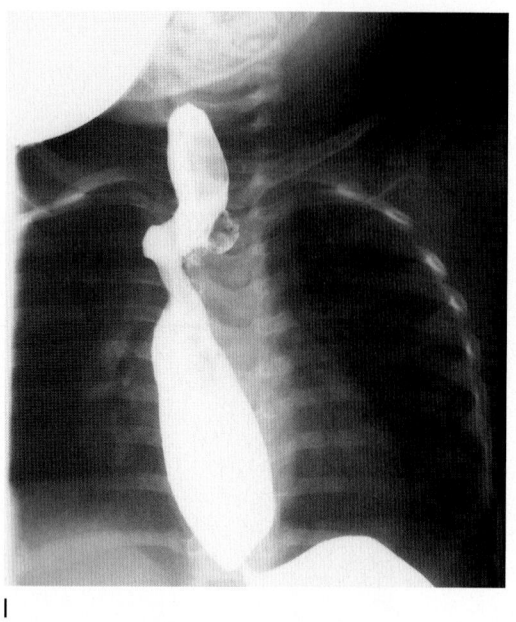
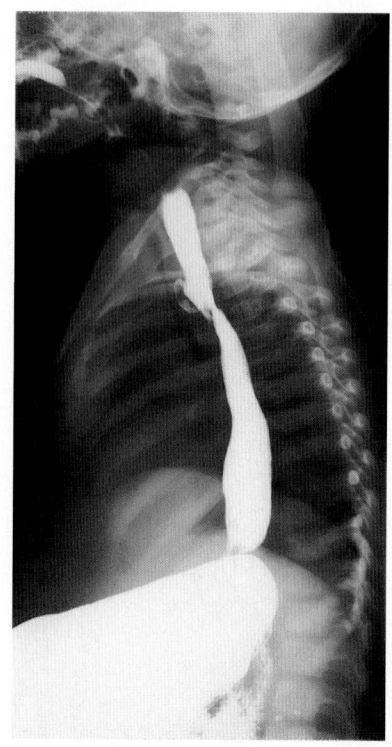

FIGURE 124-10, *cont'd.*

I

J

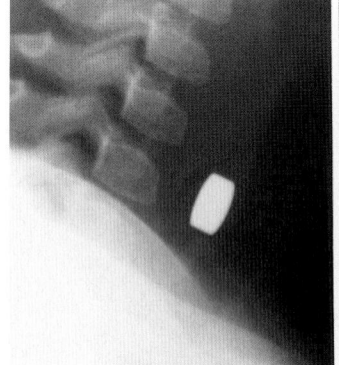
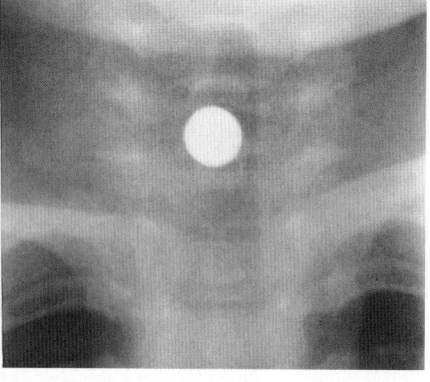
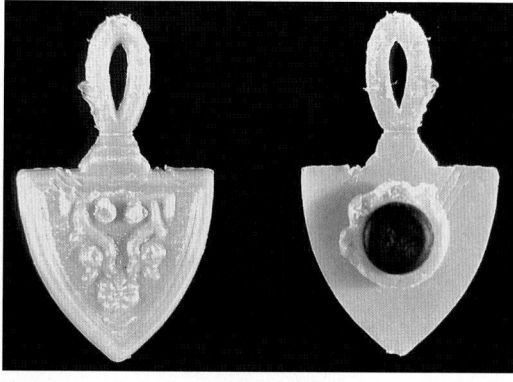

A

B

FIGURE 124-11. Esophageal foreign body. **A,** Small, metallic, round foreign body. This appearance can fool the examiner: When the object was removed (**B**), it was found to be a much larger, radiolucent plastic component of what turned out to be a refrigerator ornament, the opaque portion being the magnet. (**B,** *see color plate.*)

> **Edema of the esophageal wall on lateral chest radiograph suggests that foreign body extraction with Foley catheter will probably be unsuccessful, and complications more likely.**

The other common cause of esophageal trauma is placement of tubes and catheters, which may perforate the pharynx or esophagus. Abrupt onset of new respiratory symptoms; unusual catheter position; air in the soft tissues of the neck, chest, or mediastinum; and unexplained malfunction of the tube or catheter should lead the examiner to suspect possible perforation (Fig. 124-15). Uncomplicated perforations usually resolve, but strictures may occur. A traumatic pseudodiverticulum may result. If a contrast study is necessary after inconclusive plain film radiograph examination, low-osmolar, non-ionic water-soluble contrast material should be used. In patients with prior esophageal strictures, perforation may also occur as a result of dilatation therapy.

Severe vomiting may lead to esophageal mucosal tears and hematemesis (the Mallory-Weiss syndrome). Spontaneous esophageal rupture (Boerhaave syndrome) may occur in infants, presumably secondary to increased esophageal pressure from any one of several causes, and

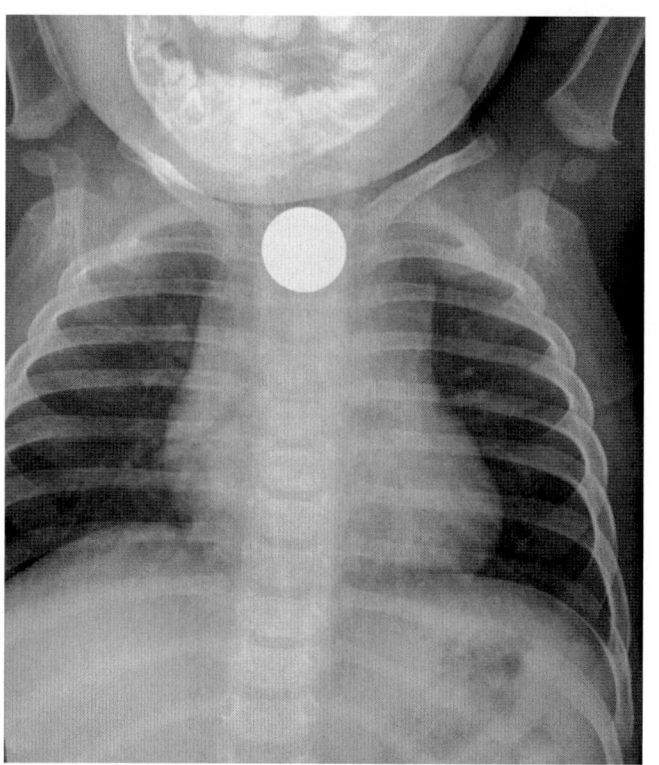
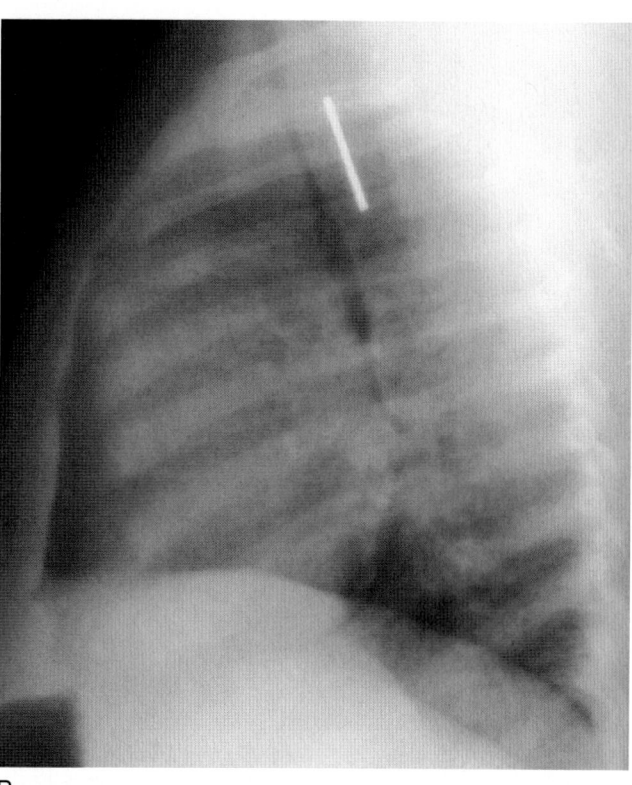

A

B

FIGURE 124-12. Ingested coin. **A,** Typical coronal position on a frontal chest film of a coin lodged in the esophagus. **B,** Lateral chest view showing the coin in the esophagus with associated esophageal wall edema and narrowing of the trachea, a sign that precludes removal by balloon.

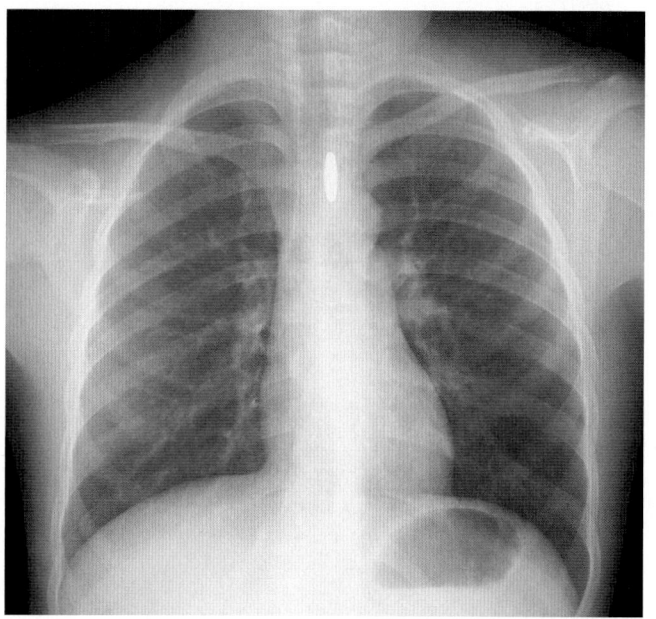
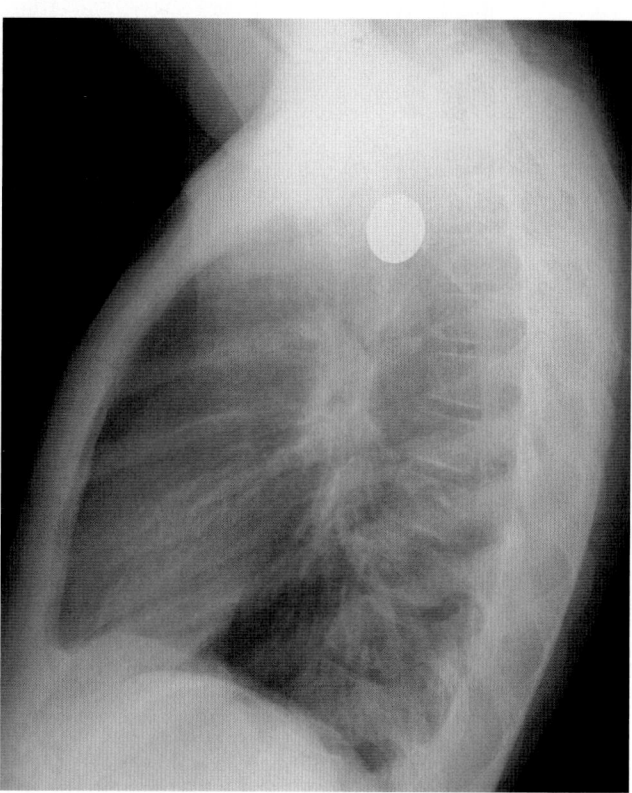

A

B

FIGURE 124-13. Unusual coin position. Frontal (**A**) and lateral (**B**) chest films in a 12-year-old girl who accidentally swallowed a coin. Although the coin is in the esophagus, the orientation is perpendicular to what is typically seen. (Courtesy of Dr. Marta Hernanz-Schulman, Vanderbilt University, Nashville, TN.)

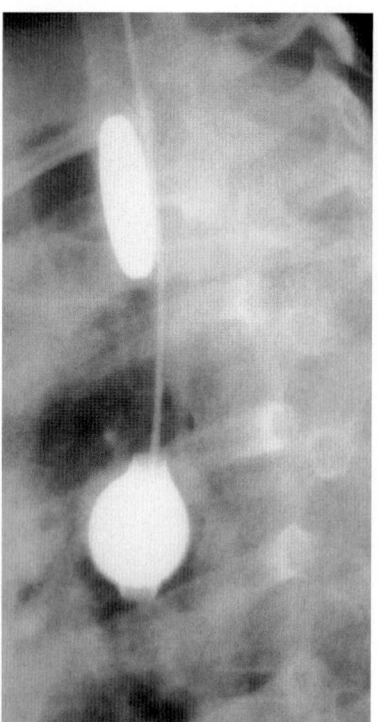

typically manifests with hydropneumothorax. Both syndromes are extraordinarily rare in childhood. When postoperative esophageal ruptures occur, they usually manifest in a similar manner (Fig. 124-16).

EXTRINSIC LESIONS ON THE ESOPHAGUS

Many diseases can cause lymphadenopathy and mass impression on the esophagus (Fig. 124-17). These include congenital, infectious, and neoplastic lesions and are covered in Sections II (Part 4) and IV.

FIGURE 124-14. Balloon removal technique for an esophageal foreign body (coin). A Foley catheter with water-soluble contrast is seen distal to the foreign body, before removal.

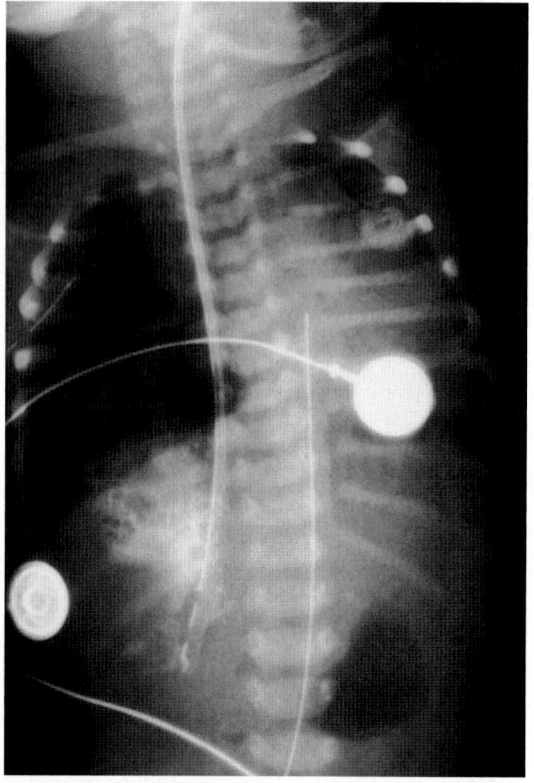

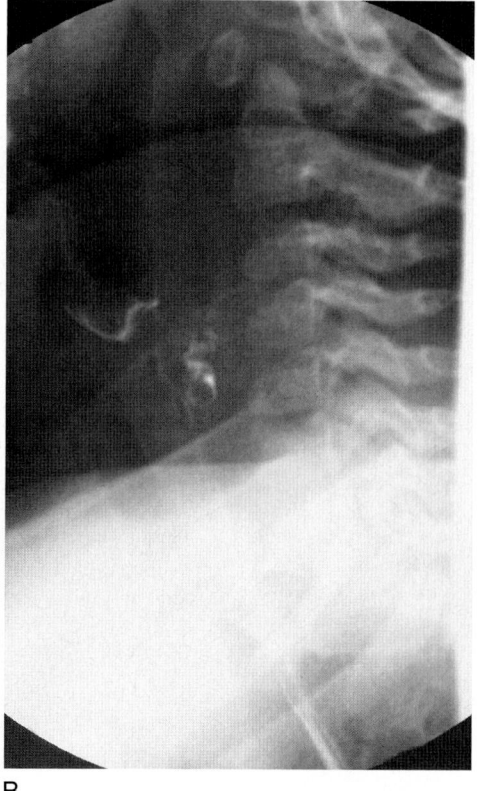

A   B

FIGURE 124-15. Perforation of the esophagus. **A,** Frontal chest film after accidental perforation of the esophagus at the cricoesophageal region. There is a pneumothorax, and the tube enters into the chest cavity to rest in the posterior costophrenic sulcus. **B,** Lateral neck film in a 15-year-old who swallowed an earring. The earring perforated the retropharyngeal region, and there is contrast material behind the esophagus in the retropharyngeal space.

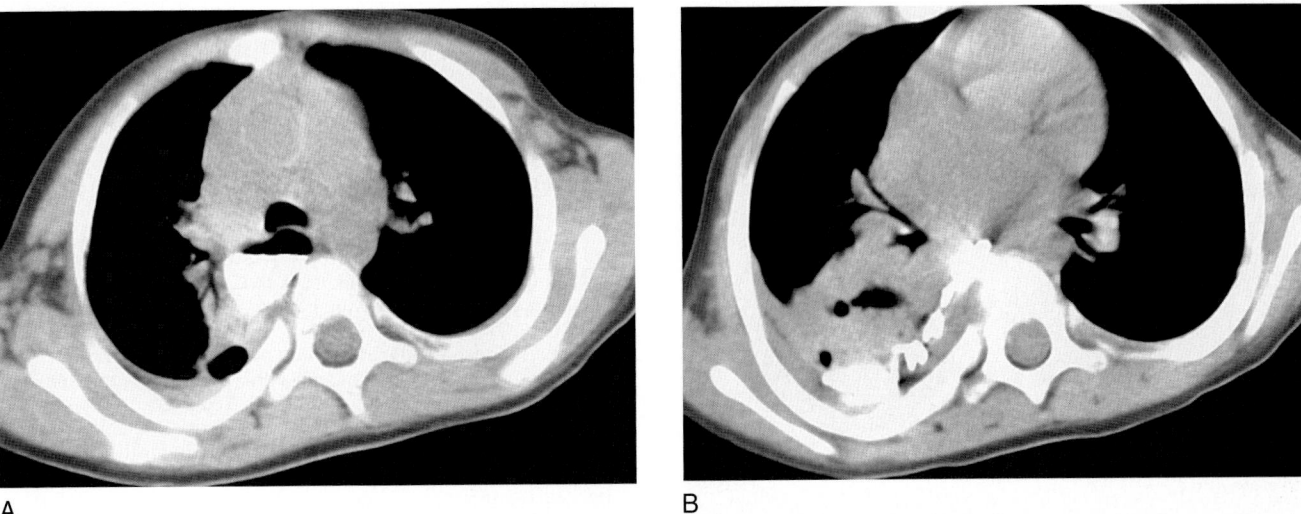

FIGURE 124-16. Esophageal perforation. **A** and **B,** Chest computed tomogram with introduction of nonionic water-soluble contrast into the distal esophagus demonstrates an esophageal rupture, with mediastinal and pulmonary abscess, secondary to previous chest trauma.

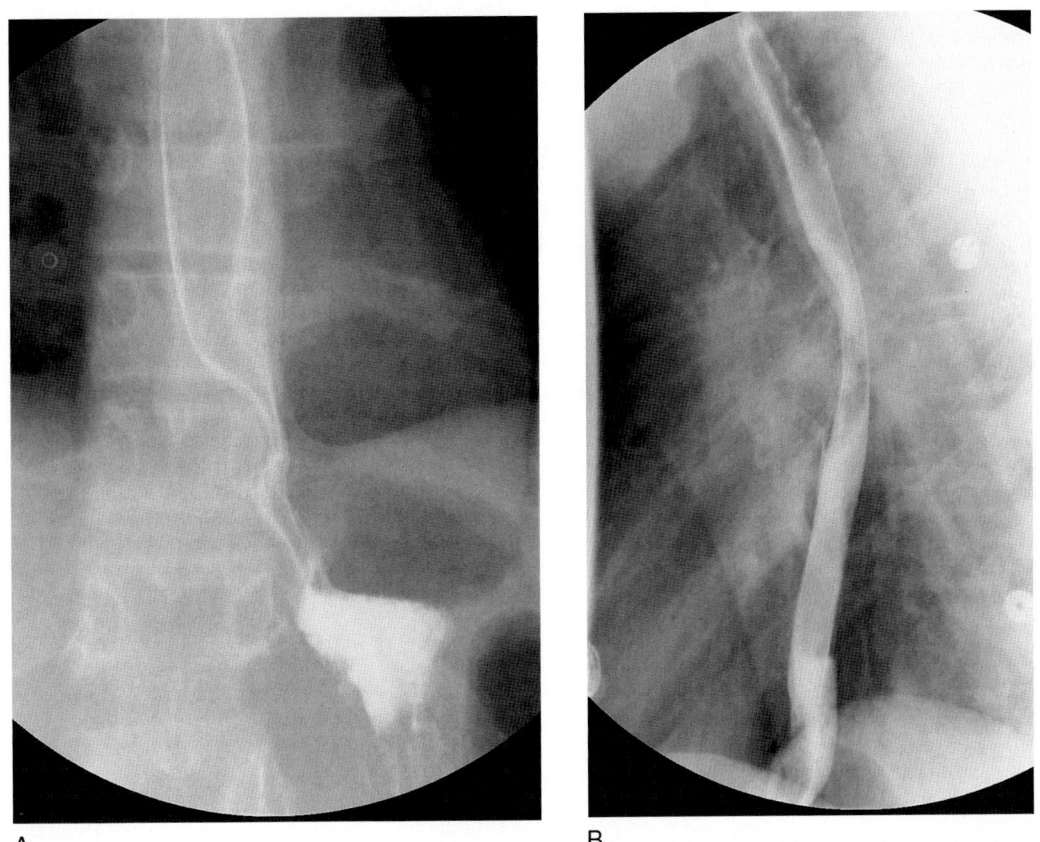

FIGURE 124-17. A child with histoplasmosis. **A,** Esophagogram demonstrates a mass impression on the medial wall of the esophagus distally at the gastroesophageal junction. **B,** There is a second impression at the level of the hilum anteriorly on the esophagus. This is below the level of the carina.

Continued

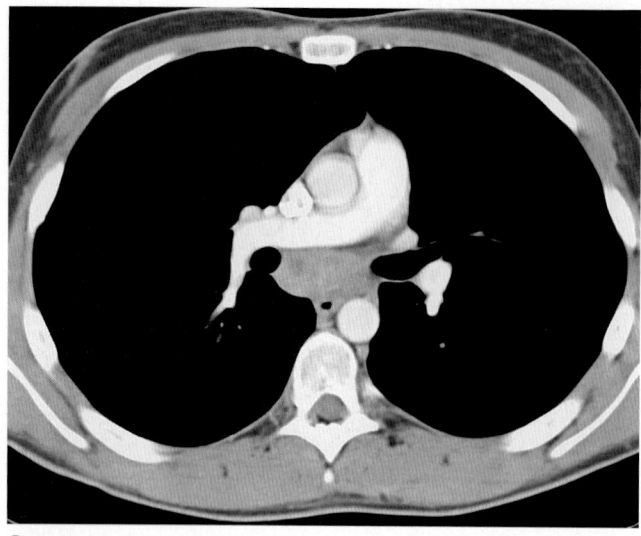

C

FIGURE 124-17, cont'd. A child with histoplasmosis.
C, Enhanced computed tomogram at this level displays the
massive adenopathy.

SUGGESTED READINGS

Noninfective Esophagitis

Abdullah BA, Gupta SK, Croffie JM, et al: The role of
esophagogastroduodenoscopy in the initial evaluation of childhood
inflammatory bowel disease: a 7-year study. J Pediatr Gastroenterol
Nutr 2002;35:636-640

Amoury RA, Hrabovsky EE, Leonidas JC, et al: Tracheo-esophageal
fistula after lye ingestion. J Pediatr Surg 1975;10:273-276

Appelvist P, Salmo M: Lye corrosion carcinoma of the esophagus.
Cancer 1980;45:2655-2658

Becker MH, Swinyard CA: Epidermolysis bullosa dystrophica in
children: radiologic manifestations. Radiology 1968;90:124-128

Canty TG, LoSasso BE: One-stage esophagectomy and in situ colon
interposition for esophageal replacement in children. J Pediatr
Surg 1997;32:334-336; discussion, 337

Creteur V, Laufer I, Kressel HY, et al: Drug-induced esophagitis
detected by double-contrast radiography. Radiology 1983;
147:365-368

Daunt N, Brodribb TR, Dickey JD: Oesophageal ulceration due to
doxycycline. Br J Radiol 1985;58:1209-1211

Franken EA Jr: Caustic damage of the gastrointestinal tract: roentgen
features. Am J Roentgenol Radium Ther Nucl Med 1973;118:77-85

Hillemeier C, Touloukian R, McCallum R, et al: Esophageal web: a
previously unrecognized complication of epidermolysis bullosa
dystrophica. Pediatrics 1981;67:678-682

Hiller N, Fisher D, Abrahamov A: Esophageal involvement in chronic
granulomatous disease: a case report and review. Pediatr Radiol
1995;25:308-309

Janousek P, Kabelka Z, Rygl M, et al: Corrosive injury of the
oesophagus in children. Int J Pediatr Otorhinolaryngol
2006;70:1103-1107

Lenaerts C, Roy CC, Vaillancourt M, et al: High incidence of upper
gastrointestinal tract involvement in children with Crohn disease.
Pediatrics 1989;83:777-781

Lepke RA, Libshitz HI: Radiation-induced injury of the esophagus.
Radiology 1983;148:375-378

Mattos GM, Lopes DD, Mamede RC, et al: Effects of time of contact
and concentration of caustic agent on generation of injuries.
Laryngoscope. 2006;116:456-460

Matziner MA, Daneman A: Esophageal involvement in eosinophilic
gastroenteritis. Pediatr Radiol 1983;13:35-38

Mauro MA, Paker LA, Hartley WS, et al: Epidermolysis bullosa:
radiographic findings in 16 cases. AJR Am J Roentgenol 1987;
149:925-927

McDonald GB, Sullivan KM, Plumley TF: Radiographic features of
esophageal involvement in chronic graft-vs-host disease. AJR Am J
Roentgenol 1984;142:501-506

O'Connor AE, Cooper J: Case of the month: Complete transection of
the trachea and oesophagus in a 10 year old child: a difficult airway
problem. Emerg Med J 2006;23:156-57

Parsons DS, Smith RB, Mair EA, et al: Unique case presentations of
acute epiglottic swelling and a protocol for acute airway
compromise. Laryngoscope 1996;106:1287-1291

Raffensperger JC, Luck SR, Reynolds M, et al: Intestinal bypass of the
esophagus. J Pediatr Surg 1996;31:38-46; discussion, pp 46-47

Ramaswamy K, Jacobson K, Jevon G, et al: Esophageal Crohn disease
in children: a clinical spectrum. J Pediatr Gastroenterol Nutr
2003;36:454-458

Renner WR, Johnson JF, Lichtenstein JE, et al: Esophageal
inflammation and stricture: complication of chronic granulomatous
disease of childhood. Radiology 1991;178:189-191

Ruuska T, Vaajalahti P, Arajarvi P, et al: Prospective evaluation of
upper gastrointestinal mucosal lesions in children with ulcerative
colitis and Crohn's disease. J Pediatr Gastroenterol Nutr
1994;19:181-186

Ryan F, Witherow H, Mirza J, Ayliffe P: The oral implications of
caustic soda ingestion in children. Oral Surg Oral Med Oral Pathol
Oral Radiol Endod 2006;101:29-34

Schmidt-Sommerfield E, Kirschner BS, Stephens JK: Endoscopic
and histologic findings in the upper gastrointestinal tract of children
with Crohn's disease. J Pediatr Gastroenterol Nutr 1990;11:448-454

Tischler JM, Helman CA: Crohn's disease of the esophagus. J Can
Assoc Radiol 1984;35:28-30

Toulokian RJ, Schonholz SM, Gryboski JD, et al: Perioperative
considerations in esophageal replacement for epidermolysis
bullosa: report of two cases successfully treated by colon
interposition. Am J Gastroenterol 1988;83:857-861

Vlymen WJ, Moskowitz PS: Roentgenographic manifestations of
esophageal and intestinal involvement in Behçet's disease in
children. Pediatr Radiol 1981;10:193-196

Eosinophilic Esophagitis

Cherry K: Eosinophilic esophagitis in children. Nat Clin Pract
Gastroenterol Hepatol 2006;3:184.

Dobbins JW, Sheehan DG, Behar J: Eosinophilic gastroenteritis with
esophageal involvement. Gastroenterol 1977;72:1312-1316

Gupta S, Fitzgerald JF, Chong SK, et al: Vertical lines in esophageal
mucosa: a true endoscopic manifestation of esophagitis in children.
Gastrointest Endosc 1997;45:485-489

Kaplan M, Mutlu EA, Kakate S, et al: Endoscopy in eosinophilic
esophagitis: "feline" esophagus and perforation risk. Clin
Gastroenterol Hepatol 2003;1:433-437

Langdon DE: "Congenital" esophageal stenosis, corrugated ringed
esophagus, and eosinophilic esophagitis. Am J Gastroenterol 2000;
95:2123-2124

Noel RJ, Tipnis NA: Eosinophilic esophagitis—a mimic of GERD.
Int J Pediatr Otorhinolaryngol 2006;70:1147-1153

Straumann A, Bauer M, Fischer B, et al: Idiopathic eosinophilic
esophagitis is associated with a T(H)2-type allergic inflammatory
response. J Allergy Clin Immunol 2001;108:954-961.

Thompson DM, Arora AS, Romero Y, et al: Eosinophilic esophagitis:
its role in aerodigestive tract disorders. Otolaryngol Clin North Am
2006;39:205-221

Vasilopoulos S, Murphy P, Averbach A, et al: The small-caliber
esophagus: an unappreciated cause of dysphagia for solids in
patients with esinophilic esophagitis. Gastrointest Endosc 2002;
55:99-106

Infective Esophagitis

Ashenburg C, Rothstein FC, Dahms BB: Herpes esophagitis in the
immunocompetent child. J Pediatr 1986;108:584-587

Bathazar EJ, Megibow AJ, Hulnick D, et al: Cytomegalovirus
esophagitis in AIDS: radiographic features in 16 patients. AJR Am J
Roentgenol 1987;149:919-923

Chusid MJ, Oechler HW, Werlin SL: Herpetic esophagitis in an
immunocompetent boy. Wisc Med J 1992;91:71-72

Goodman P, Pinero SS, Rance RM, et al: Mycobacterial esophagitis in
AIDS. Gastrointest Radiol 1989;14:103-105

Grattan-Smith D, Harrison LF, Singleton EB: Radiology of AIDS in the
pediatric patient. Curr Prob Diagn Radiol 1992;21:79-109

Haller JO, Cohen HL: Gastrointestinal manifestations of AIDS in children. AJR Am J Roentgenol 1994;162:387-393

Isaac DW, Parham DM, Patrick CC: The role of esophagoscopy in diagnosis and management of esophagitis in children with cancer. Med Pediatr Oncol 1997;28:229-303

Lallemand D, Huault G, Laboureau JP, et al: Laryngeal and oesophageal lesions in patients with herpetic disease. Ann Radiol 1974; 17:317-325

Levine MS: Radiology of esophagitis: a pattern approach. Radiology 1991;179:1-7

Levine MS, Laufer I, Kressel HY, et al: Herpes esophagitis. AJR Am J Roentgenol 1981;136:863-866

Levine MS, Macones AJ Jr, Laufer I: *Candida* esophagitis: accuracy of radiographic diagnosis. Radiology 1985;154:581-587

Lewicki AM, Moore JP: Esophageal moniliasis. Am J Roentgenol Radium Ther Nucl Med 1975;125:218-225

Diverticula

Meadows JA Jr: Esophageal diverticula in infants and children. South Med J 1970;63:691-694

Foreign Bodies and Trauma

Beer S, Avidan G, Viure E, et al: A foreign body in the oesophagus as a cause of respiratory distress. Pediatr Radiol 1982;12:41-2

Berdon WE: Editorial commentary on the manuscript entitled: Potential hazards of esophageal foreign body extraction, by CM Myer. Pediatr Radiol 1991;21:99

Campbell JB, Condon VR: Catheter removal of blunt esophageal foreign bodies in children: survey of the Society for Pediatric Radiology. Pediatr Radiol 1989;19:361-5

Campbell JB, Davis WS: Catheter technique for extraction of blunt esophageal foreign bodies. Radiology 1973;108:438-40

Campbell JB, Quattromani FL, Foley LC: Foley catheter removal of blunt esophageal foreign bodies: experience with 100 consecutive children. Pediatr Radiol 1983;13:116-8

Cetinkursun S, Sayan A, Demirbag S, et al: Safe removal of upper esophageal coins by using Magill forceps: two centers' experience. Clin Pediatr (Phila) 2006;45:71-3

Currarino G, Nikaidoh H: Esophageal foreign bodies in children with vascular ring or aberrant right subclavian artery: coincidence or causation? Pediatr Radiol 1991;21:406-8

Dubos JP, Bouchez MC, Kacet N, et al: Spontaneous rupture of the esophagus in the newborn. Pediatr Radiol 1986;16:317-319

Fernbach SK, Tucker GF: Coin ingestion: unusual appearance of the penny in a child. Radiology 1986;158:512

Harell GS, Friedland GW, Daily WJ, et al: Neonatal Boerhaave's syndrome. Radiology 1970;95:665-668

Harned RK, Strain JD, Hay TC, et al: Esophageal foreign bodies: safety and efficacy of Foley catheter extraction of coins. AJR Am J Roentgenol 1997;168:443-446

Herman TE, McAlister WH: Esophageal diverticula in childhood associated with strictures from unsuspected foreign bodies of the esophagus. Pediatr Radiol 1991;21:410-414

MacPherson RI, Hill JC, Othersen HB, et al: Esophageal foreign bodies in children: diagnosis, treatment, and complications. AJR Am J Roentgenol 1996;199:919-924

Myer CM: Potential hazards of esophageal foreign body extraction. Pediatr Radiol 1991;21:97-98

Schulz M, Wild L, Konig C, et al: An esophagobronchial fistula caused by an unusual foreign body in the esophagus leading to mediastinitis with fatal outcome. Klin Padiatr 2006;218:85-87

Smith MT, Wong RK: Esophageal foreign bodies: types and techniques for removal. Curr Treat Options Gastroenterol 2006;9:75-84

Touloukian RJ, Beardsley GP, Ablow RC, et al: Traumatic perforation of the pharynx in the newborn. Pediatrics 1977;59:1019-1022

Towbin R, Lederman HM, Dunbar JS, et al: Esophageal edema as a predictor of unsuccessful balloon extraction of esophageal foreign body. Pediatr Radiol 1989;19:359-360

Disorders of the Esophagogastric Junction

HENRIQUE M. LEDERMAN and GUILHERME T. S. DEMARCHI

ANATOMY AND PHYSIOLOGY

Although the anatomy and physiology of the esophagogastric junction have been studied for decades, the mechanisms of normal and abnormal function, especially with regard to gastroesophageal reflux (GER), are still incompletely understood. There is general agreement that the lower esophageal sphincter represents the true distal end of the esophagus, and its most distal point is the true esophagogastric junction. This point may be radiographically identifiable on mucosal relief studies of the stomach (Fig. 125-1) but may be difficult to identify during active swallowing studies. The lower esophageal sphincter is 3 to 4 cm long in adults and shorter in infants and progresses toward its adult length throughout childhood.

There are several antireflux mechanisms operating at the gastroesophageal junction. The resting lower esophageal sphincter pressure is about 15 to 30 mm Hg higher than the resting pressure in the gastric fundus. During the initiation of swallowing, the intrasphincteric pressure drops rapidly, apparently mediated by the vagus nerve, to a level equal to fundal pressure. Thus, the pressure gradient between lower esophagus and stomach disappears during "dry swallowing," as occurs with a pacifier or thumb sucking, as well as during true feedings. Antireflux activity is also provided by the muscle of the esophageal hiatus of the diaphragm and by the membranous attachments of the lower esophagus to the diaphragm.

The angle between the esophagus and stomach is less acute in infants than in adults. This may be an additional factor in the occurrence of GER even in normal infants. The intra-abdominal portion of the esophagus is probably shorter in infants than in adults, but this varies with phases of respiration and swallowing and is probably not related to the pathophysiology of GER.

GASTROESOPHAGEAL REFLUX

Anyone who has ever fed and burped an infant recognizes that GER occurs in virtually all normal infants. As with any physiologic mechanism, a wide range of normal occurrences can be observed, varying from eructation with no vomiting of gastric contents to persistent "spitting up" during and after feedings. Although sometimes alarming to parents, even persistent GER in otherwise healthy infants with normal weight gain and without chronic respiratory disease is usually physiologic. If extreme, physiologic GER often responds to thickened feedings and maintenance of the semi-upright posture, as in an infant seat. Excessive spitting up usually resolves spontaneously by 9 months of age.

Pathologic GER may be difficult to differentiate from physiologic GER in the first weeks to months of life. However, progressively severe GER after 6 weeks of age may be the first sign of a truly abnormal state. Lack of response to simple dietary and postural therapy, especially if accompanied by weight loss or deceleration of weight gain, may necessitate evaluation for abnormal GER. Pathologic GER has been associated with failure to thrive, hematemesis, a variety of postural and neurologic disorders, torticollis, rumination, acute life-threatening events (apnea), and sudden infant death syndrome.

In patients with severe reflux, chronic respiratory symptoms caused by aspiration into the upper airway and even into the lungs may occur. GER, with or without aspiration, often triggers bronchospasm (laryngeal "asthma").

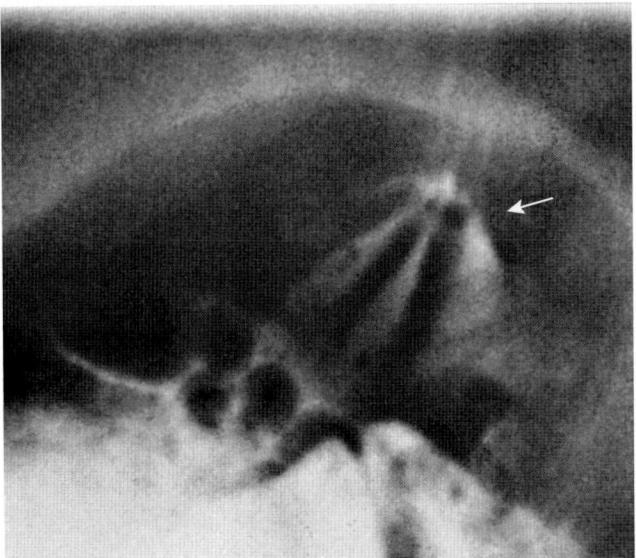

FIGURE 125-1. Fluoroscopic spot film demonstrates the normal esophagogastric junction. The *arrow* points to the convex margin of the "umbrella." The gastric folds diverge below. The parallel longitudinal esophagus folds are seen through the fundus above the margin of the umbrella.

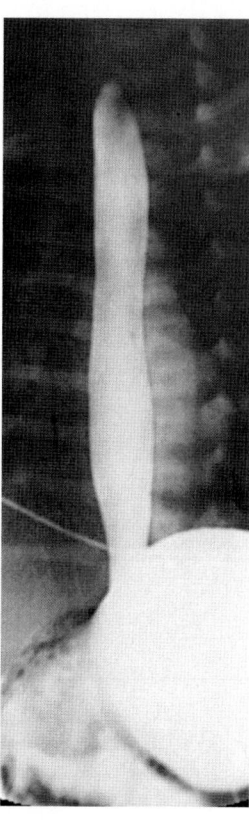

FIGURE 125-2. Gastroesophageal reflux demonstrated during an upper gastrointestinal series. Note the patulous esophagogastric junction, an appearance not seen on views of the esophagus obtained during antegrade flow of contrast while the patient is drinking.

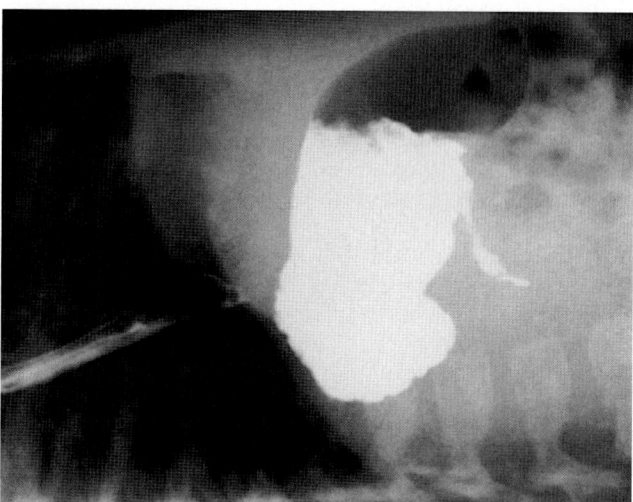

FIGURE 125-3. Lateral cross-table view of the stomach demonstrates barium in the dependent fundus, in the body, and in the distal esophagus, and air in the antrum. Note that if the stomach were sufficiently distended with barium, insufficient barium would pool in the fundus below the esophagogastric junction and might lead to a false-negative conclusion in a reflux study.

Therefore, evaluation for GER in children with unexplained reactive airway disease is indicated because many of the pulmonary symptoms improve when the reflux is treated. Recurrent pneumonia can occur in patients with reflux and aspiration. The incidence of pathologic GER is higher in patients with trisomy 21, cystic fibrosis, and organic brain disease, especially cerebral palsy.

Indicators of pathologic GER include

- **Progressively severe reflux after 6 weeks of age**
- **Lack of response to dietary and postural therapy**
- **Weight loss or deceleration of weight gain**
- **Failure to thrive**
- **Hematemesis**
- **Postural or neurologic disorders**
- **Torticollis**
- **Rumination**
- **Acute life-threatening event**
- **Sudden infant death syndrome**
- **Chronic respiratory symptoms**
- **Bronchospasm**

Imaging Studies

The barium esophagogram is the traditional imaging study for identification of GER (Fig. 125-2). The exami-

nation yields important anatomic information and is used primarily to search for and document organic causes of GER. The examination should include evaluation of swallowing, particularly aspiration; esophageal peristalsis; and other causes of vomiting, such as gastric outlet or duodenal obstruction. The total amount of barium given should be equivalent to a normal feeding volume. Because reflux is best identified with the patient in the supine position, sufficient barium must be given to reach the esophagogastric junction, which is anterior to most of the fundus. Insufficient barium may fill the dependent fundus and lead to reflux of air rather than contrast material (Fig. 125-3).

If a nasogastric tube is present, the tip should be repositioned well above the esophagogastric junction during this evaluation period, to avoid reflux possibly related to the tube crossing the junction. Some pediatric radiologists have suggested that the presence of three episodes of reflux to the level of the aortic arch within 5 minutes is pathologic. However, this much reflux can occur in infants who are growing normally and are asymptomatic. The suggestion has been made that the only significant findings on barium swallow study are continuous reflux, so-called chalasia, or signs of esophagitis.

Some radiologists advocate rolling the infant from side to side or increasing intra-abdominal pressure by external means. These maneuvers are nonphysiologic, however, and reflux elicited by them is of questionable significance. A pacifier may elicit reflux by simulating contrast swallowing. Although not strictly physiologic, the use of a pacifier simulates real-life conditions in a majority of infants; furthermore, because crying has been shown to decrease GER, the pacifier has an additional advantage. In the experience at our institution, reflux should be investigated only after normal burping has occurred, particularly in children younger than 1 year. Our experience is that reflux documented immediately after the ingestion of barium is irrelevant because it translates only to regurgitation/burping, which may occur physiologically in all normal individuals.

Many staging systems for GER have been developed. Typically, they differentiate between reflux to the level of the aortic arch, considered insignificant, and significant reflux above that level. However, few radiologists find staging useful, because there is virtually no correlation between staging and clinical prognosis. Normal infants may, in fact, fill the entire esophagus and pharynx without ever showing clinical evidence of abnormalities. If GER is seen, careful evaluation for aspiration into the airway is important. Hiatal hernias are uncommonly identified.

The major purpose of the barium esophagogram is to yield as much anatomic and physiologic information as possible, document aspiration, and enable the radiologist to rule out organic or anatomic causes of reflux such as obstruction.

The 24-hour intraesophageal pH probe monitoring is a more invasive but sensitive examination; comparison with the barium esophagogram reveals disappointingly high rates of false-negative contrast examinations. A chest radiograph is frequently obtained at the beginning of a pH probe study to document the level of the probe, which should be at the plane of the midleft atrium. When two electrodes are used, one is located at the distal portion of the esophagus and the other in the proximal to middle third. One advantage of all imaging studies over pH probe studies is that the pH examination may not record immediate postprandial GER, because the milk or formula may partially neutralize the refluxing gastric acid. One advantage of esophagography (in comparison with the pH probe and many other imaging modalities used to evaluate for GER) is the demonstration of anatomic information that may identify complications of GER (such as esophagitis or strictures) or an alternative explanation for reflux-like symptoms such as esophageal obstruction, gastric outlet obstruction, or malrotation. We believe pH probe studies should be performed only with precise clinical indications (i.e., in a child with respiratory findings of wheezing, no known allergies, and negative results from other examinations).

Radionuclide studies for the evaluation of GER are more sensitive than barium esophagograms in documenting reflux and more precise in documenting gastric emptying. On the other hand, lack of anatomic information is a limitation of scintigraphy in comparison with upper gastrointestinal series. Food, milk, or formula containing the radionuclide is given orally, after which images are taken immediately and, usually for a period of 2 hours, after a delay (Fig. 125-4). The radionuclide is added to the formula midway through the feeding session, and plain formula is given at the end, in order to wash the radionuclide from the esophagus. Concomitant gastric emptying studies can also be performed, and significant aspiration into the lungs can be identified. Although nuclear scintigraphy is highly sensitive for GER, the reflux episodes detected by this method do not tend to be correlated with falls in measured pH on pH probe studies.

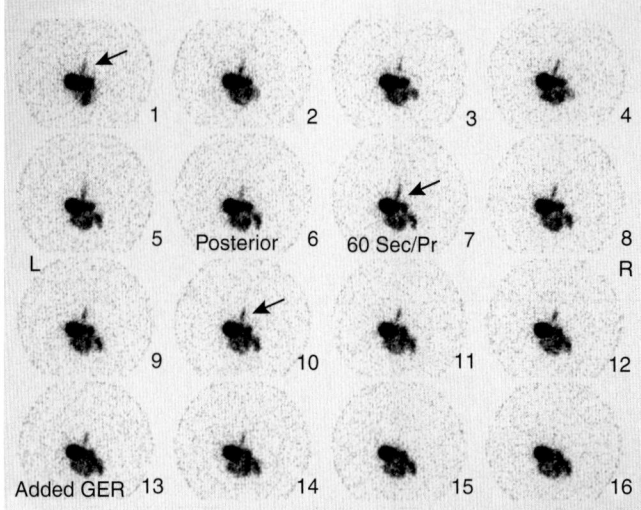

A

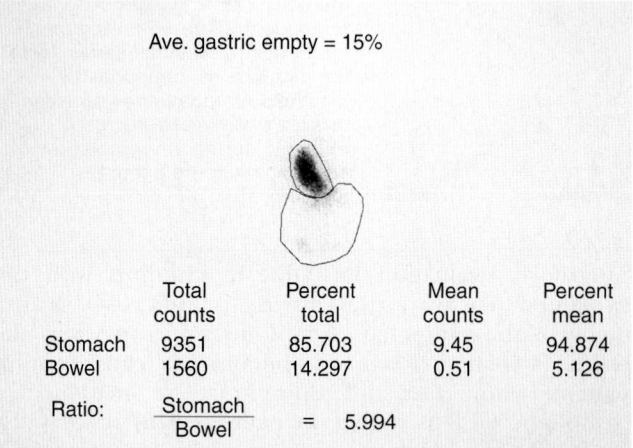

B

FIGURE 125-4. Gastroesophageal reflux. **A,** Multiple views in a technetium-99m milk scan, showing gastroesophageal reflux. *Arrows* point to gastroesophageal reflux. **B,** Failure of gastric emptying with 15% emptying after 1 hour (normal is approximately 50% emptying).

> **Radionuclide studies for evaluation of GER are more sensitive than the esophagogram.**

Ultrasonography can be used to assess for reflux by imaging the gastroesophageal junction at the diaphragmatic hiatus and can also yield anatomic information regarding gastric outlet obstruction, such as hypertrophic pyloric stenosis. Results of these examinations show a high correlation with pH probe studies. Westra and associates reported 81% to 84% agreement between the two studies. Riccabona and coworkers found that sonography identified GER with sensitivity of 100% and specificity of 87.5% in comparison with pH monitoring and manometry. Gomes and Menanteau described an ultrasound scoring system for GER that was well correlated with results of pH probe studies and endoscopy. For ultrasound evaluation, the infant is supine, and the area of the gastroesophageal junction is identified

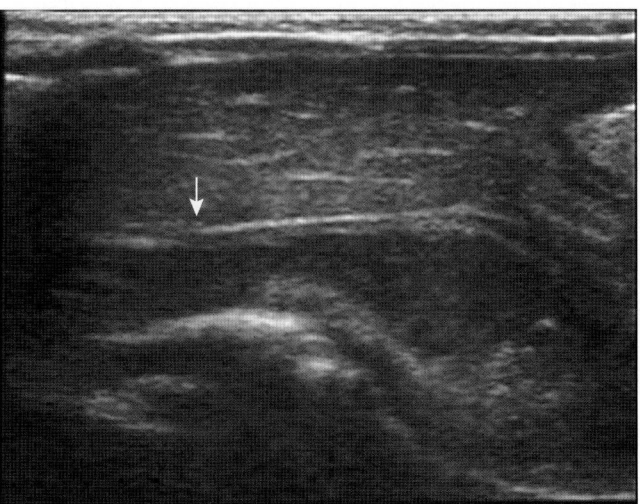

FIGURE 125-5. Ultrasound study of the esophagogastric junction in supine infant demonstrates distention of the esophagus (*arrow*) during active gastroesophageal reflux. (Courtesy of Dr. Marta Hernanz-Schulman, Vanderbilt University, Nashville, Tenn.)

anterior to the aorta. Formula or dextrose/electrolyte solution, such as Pedialyte, is given in an amount equal to a normal feeding. Longitudinal imaging can identify reflux, consisting of fluid mixed with air bubbles, into the distal esophagus (Fig. 125-5). Ultrasonography can be more sensitive than barium esophagography by virtue of the ability to observe for a longer period; the lack of ionizing radiation permits longer continuous monitoring than is possible with fluoroscopy. The disadvantages are that it is time consuming and highly observer dependent, and the level of the reflux and aspiration may not be documented.

The most common complications of significant GER are failure to thrive, chronic and recurrent respiratory symptoms, and esophagitis. The imaging characteristics of reflux esophagitis are nonspecific, dysmotility being the most common finding. This may vary from mild loss of normal primary stripping waves to tertiary contractions or aperistalsis. Frank ulceration can occur but is more common in adults with peptic esophagitis than in children. If ulcers are present, they are typically in the lower third of the esophagus, near the esophagogastric junction. Reflux esophagitis may lead to strictures, most commonly in the midesophagus or lower third (Fig. 125-6). Barrett esophagus, with metaplasia of the esophageal epithelium, which is premalignant in some cases, is less common than in adults.

Pseudodiverticula are seen as small intramural collections of barium. Less commonly seen in children than in adults, they represent excretory ducts of intramural mucous glands in patients suffering from reflux or peptic esophagitis.

Treatment

Although medical therapy may be satisfactory for most cases of significant infantile GER, surgery may be necessary for some infants with severe respiratory symptoms or profound failure to thrive. The most commonly performed procedure is the Nissen fundoplication, in

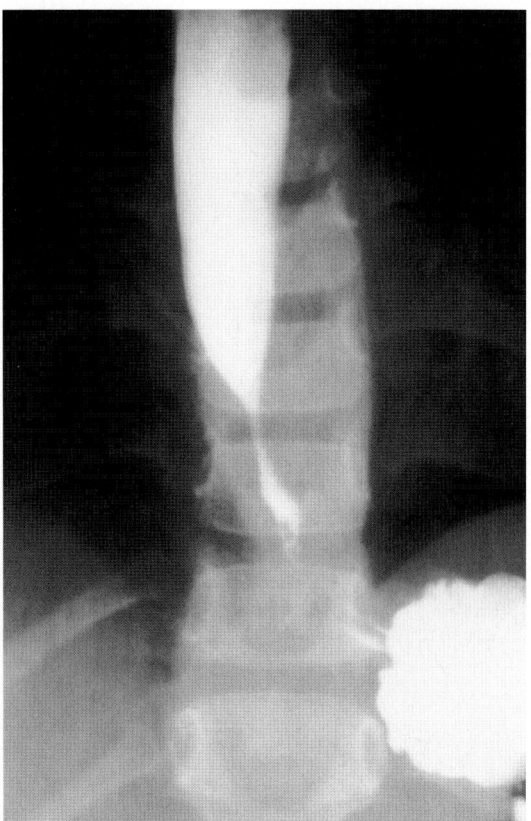

FIGURE 125-6. Narrowing of the distal esophagus with irregular peristalsis secondary to gastroesophageal reflux.

which the upper fundus is wrapped around the distal esophagus (Fig. 125-7). Partial wraps (such as the Thal and Toupet) may also be performed. Fundoplication (with or without gastrostomy) can now be achieved laparoscopically. The results of fundoplication are variable, but long-term cessation of GER can be accomplished in 60% to 70% of patients. In one large multi-institutional study of 7467 patients from seven children's hospitals, Fonkalsrud and colleagues reported good to excellent results in 95% of neurologically normal children and in 85% of neurologically impaired children.

Complications of fundoplication may be encountered. If the wrap is too tight, distal esophageal obstruction occurs (Fig. 125-8); if it is too loose, reflux may persist. On follow-up upper gastrointestinal series, if the wrap loosens, contrast material may enter the potential space between the walls of the stomach used to form the wrap (see Fig. 125-8). This may or may not result in recurrent reflux. In a small percentage of patients, a hiatal hernia (see Fig. 125-8) or paraesophageal hernia may develop. If distal bowel obstruction develops in a patient with a fundoplication, a closed-loop obstruction may be created by the loss of ability to decompress the obstruction by eructation. A relatively high rate of postoperative small bowel intussusception has been described after Nissen fundoplication in one study. The cause of small bowel intussusception in these patients is unclear but may be related to abnormal bowel peristalsis in a patient population already at risk for altered gut motility.

Although surgical antireflux procedures traditionally were commonly performed routinely in all neurologi-

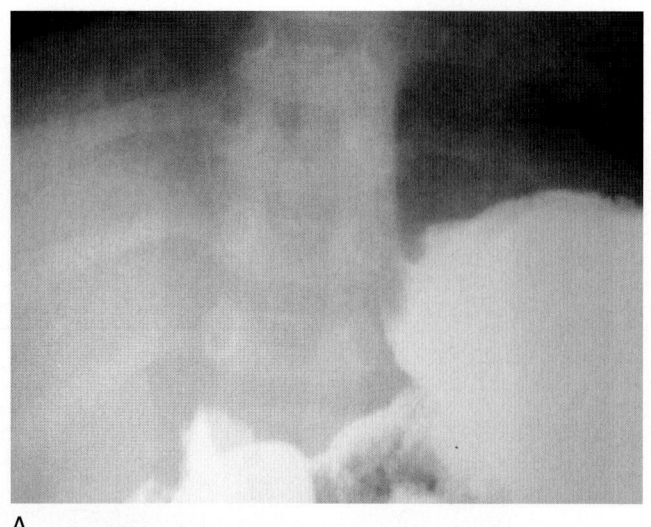

A

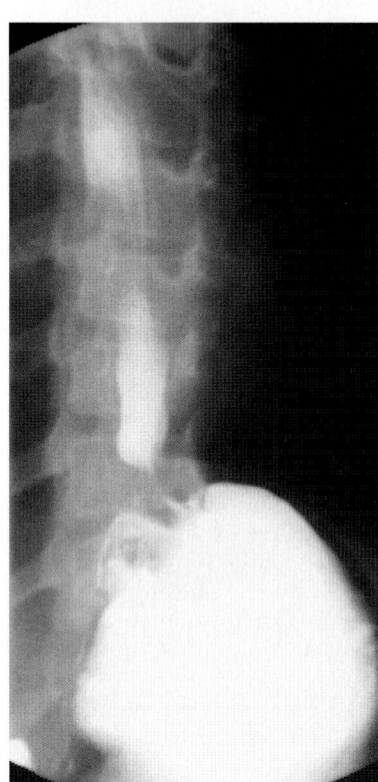

B

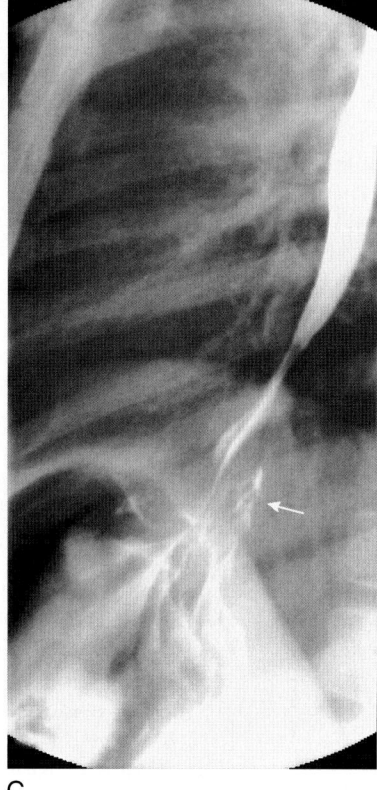

C

FIGURE 125-7. Normal appearance of a Nissen fundoplication with the "shoulder appearance" and irregular outline of the cardia. **A** and **B,** Two frontal films showing the normal appearance of a Nissen fundoplication. **C,** Lateral film in which there is a small amount of barium within the wrap. There is no evidence of leaking or loosening.

cally impaired children referred for feeding gastrostomy, more recent evidence suggests that the potential complications may not justify this approach. Therefore, antireflux surgery in these children at the time of gastrostomy is reserved for those with documented reflux.

In extreme cases of esophagitis and stricture, esophagectomy with colonic interposition may be required. Marked GER may be seen in patients with complicated large congenital diaphragmatic hernias. These infants may require more aggressive treatment with fundoplication and pyloroplasty.

HIATAL HERNIA

Small hiatal hernias may be seen with or without GER, may be transient, and may be of no clinical significance in the absence of GER (Fig. 125-9). Larger hernias may be associated with symptoms but are uncommon. Paraesophageal hernias are very uncommon in children who have not undergone prior gastroesophageal surgery. Partial or complete intrathoracic stomach displacement is rare, but the findings on upper gastrointestinal series are dramatic (Fig. 125-10).

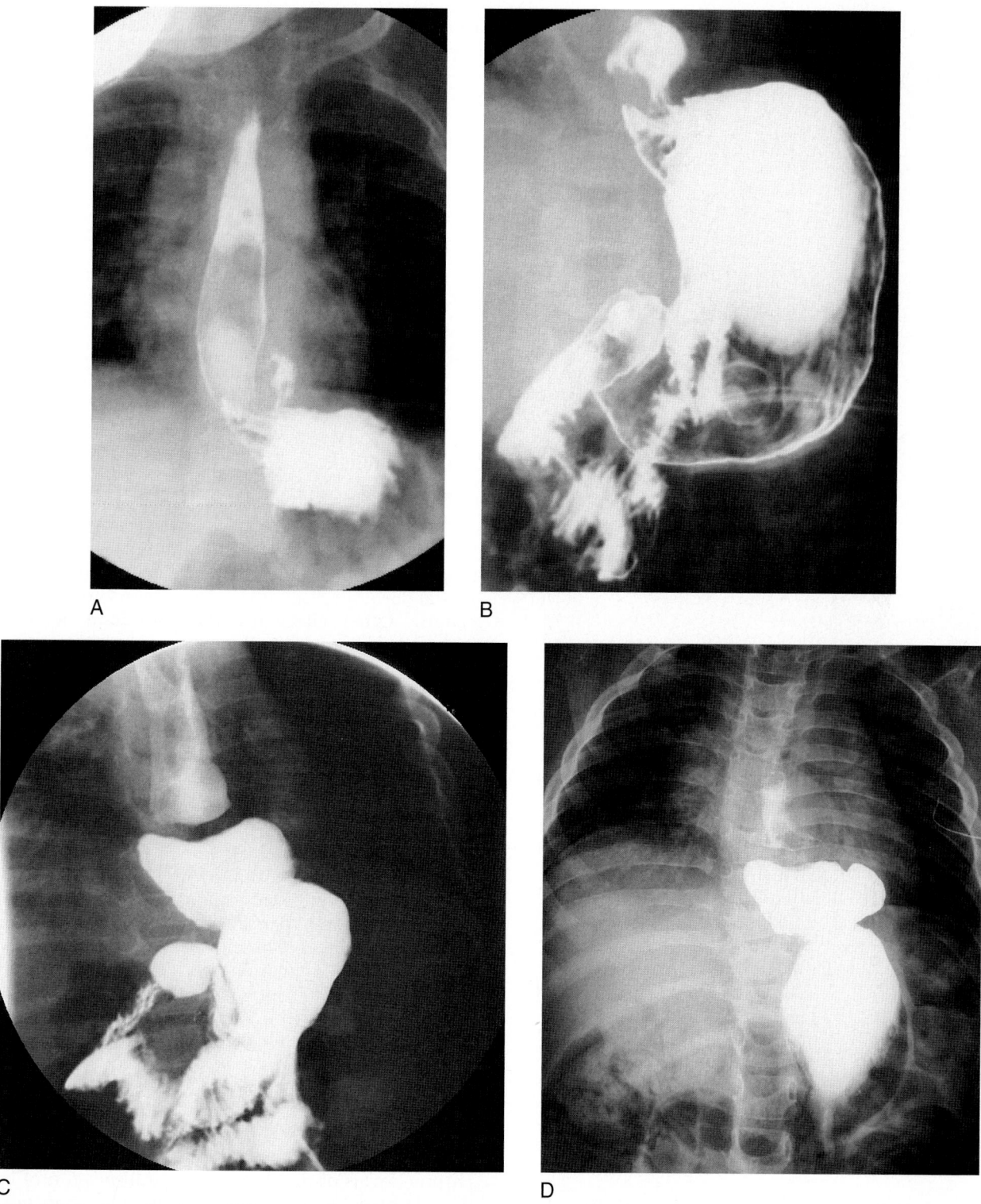

FIGURE 125-8. Complications of Nissen fundoplication. **A,** Tight Nissen fundoplication with partial obstruction and secondary megaesophagus: After fundoplication, signs of dilation of the distal and midesophagus started to appear, along with abnormal peristaltic waves and narrowing of the distal end at the surgical site. **B,** Slipped fundoplication. Loss of the shoulder appearance, and development of a paraesophageal hernia. **C** and **D,** Failed Nissen with stomach in the chest.

ACHALASIA

Failure of relaxation of the lower esophageal sphincter (achalasia or cardiospasm) is rare in children, although it has been described even during infancy. There is often a deficiency of cells in the Auerbach plexus. Defective vagus nerve function or innervation is the most common pathophysiologic mechanism. Patients usually complain of dysphagia, chest pain, and symptoms related to lower esophageal obstruction; in severe cases, regurgitation of undigested food is virtually diagnostic. The differential diagnosis is listed in Table 125-1.

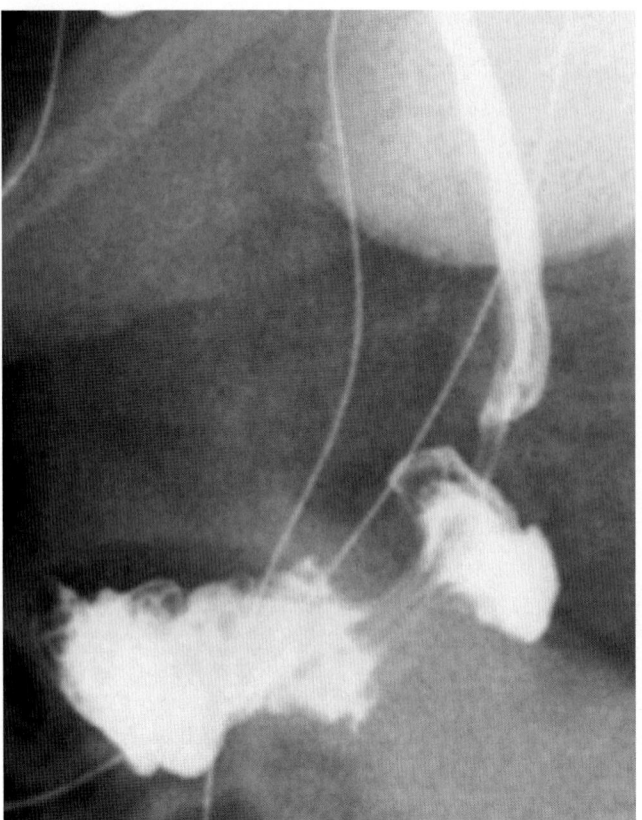

FIGURE 125-9. Lateral view during an upper gastrointestinal series demonstrates a sliding stomach hiatal hernia, with the gastric fundus above the diaphragm.

Although the definitive diagnosis is made by esophageal manometry, characteristic radiographic findings are typically seen. Upright chest radiographs may show an air-filled esophagus, often containing an air-fluid level (Fig. 125-11). Esophagograms demonstrate normal swallowing and, frequently, normal peristalsis to the level of the aortic arch and abnormal peristalsis below. Early cases may show vigorous but uncoordinated peristaltic activity in the esophagus. A characteristic "beaking" of the distal esophagus (Fig. 125-12; see Fig. 125-11C) has been described. Ultimately, the esophagus may become completely atonic and remain markedly dilated, almost continuously filled with ingested material.

> **Chest radiograph findings in achalasia commonly include:**
> - **Esophageal dilation resembling a mediastinal mass**
> - **Air-fluid level in dilated esophagus**
>
> **Esophagogram findings in achalasia include the following:**
> - **Common**
>   1. **Dilated esophagus**
>   2. **"Beaking" of distal esophagus**
>   3. **Normal peristalsis above aortic arch with abnormal peristalsis below aortic arch**

TABLE 125-1

Differential Diagnosis of Achalasia

When esophageal dilation resembles a mediastinal mass
  Neurogenic tumors
  Neuroblastoma
  Ganglioneuroblastoma
  Ganglioglioma
  Tubular esophageal duplication cyst
  Hiatal hernia
When dysphagia is present
  Esophageal stricture
  Gastroesophageal reflux
  Caustic ingestion
  Crohn disease
  Chronic granulomatous disease
  Epidermolysis bullosa

> - **Uncommon**
> - **Completely atonic esophagus in severe cases**

Treatment strategies include thoracoscopic or laparoscopic repair, which can be performed as an alternative to standard surgical repair (with or without fundoplication). Other alternative therapies have been used, including balloon dilatation and endoscopically guided injection of botulinum toxin into the lower esophageal sphincter.

CHAGASIC ESOPHAGOPATHY

South American trypanosomiasis, also known as Chagas disease, is a protozoosis caused by the flagellate protozoa *Trypanosoma cruzi*. The infection is usually transmitted via the feces of blood-sucking insects called *barbeiros* (reduviid bugs). The Brazilian physician Carlos R. J. Chagas discovered American trypanosomiasis in 1909. He identified the parasite in the vector insect and described all the epidemiological and clinical aspects of the infection, a singular feat in the history of medicine.

Vectorial transmission of Chagas disease is responsible for 80% of human infections. Transfusion of infected blood is responsible for 5% to 20% of the human cases of Chagas disease, mainly in urban centers in endemic areas. The maternal vertical transmission occurs in 2% to 10% of infected pregnant women. In contrast to toxoplasmosis, the vertical transmission of *T. cruzi* may occur during each pregnancy, in both the acute and chronic forms of the disease. The transmission of infection via breast milk is extremely rare. Oral transmission can occur and is related to the ingestion of food contaminated by feces of infected insects, or by infected insects themselves such as in sugarcane juice, which caused a recent outbreak of the disease in southern Brazil. Human disease in children born in the United States is rare, despite the occurrence of a sylvatic cycle in some areas. However, infection is found frequently in immigrants from Mexico, other Central American countries, and South America. According to estimates, 100,000 to 675,000 immigrants from Latin America are

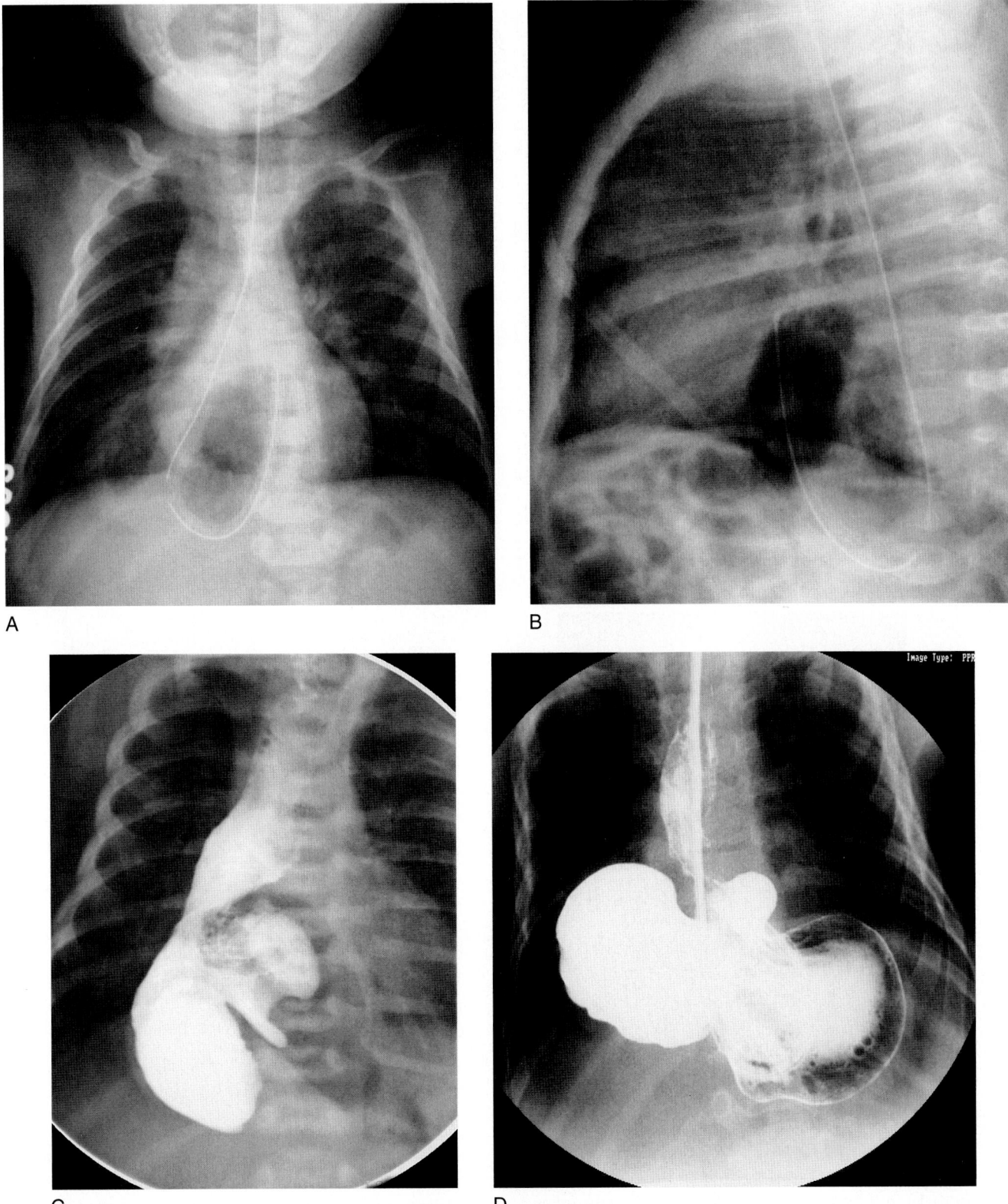

FIGURE 125-10. Hiatal hernia. Frontal chest radiographs before (**A**) and after (**B**) barium ingestion display a very large hiatal hernia; the stomach and duodenum are within the chest, and there is associated malrotation of the stomach. Note the enlarged, partially obstructed esophagus. **C,** Esophagogram depicts the stomach in the chest and a dilated obstructed esophagus. **D,** Barium swallow study performed through a nasogastric tube reveals the stomach with contrast media above and below the diaphragm. Note the volvulated stomach with the fundus to the patient's left and the antral portion higher and to the right.

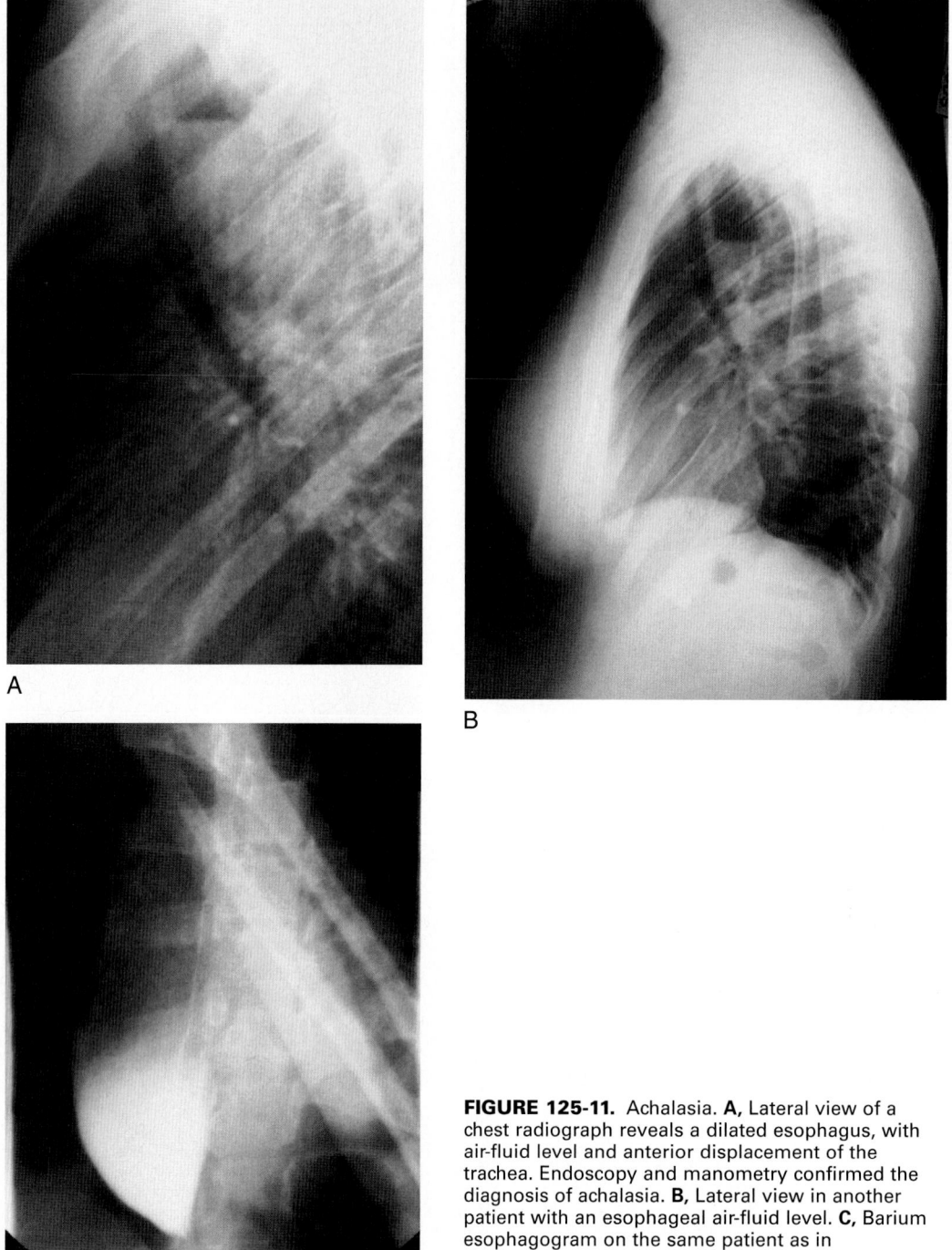

FIGURE 125-11. Achalasia. **A,** Lateral view of a chest radiograph reveals a dilated esophagus, with air-fluid level and anterior displacement of the trachea. Endoscopy and manometry confirmed the diagnosis of achalasia. **B,** Lateral view in another patient with an esophageal air-fluid level. **C,** Barium esophagogram on the same patient as in **B,** demonstrating the classic "beaking" of the distal esophagus with proximal dilation.

infected with *T. cruzi.* Internationally, an estimated 16 million to 18 million people are infected in 18 countries of Latin America. Chagas disease results in 45,000 to 50,000 deaths per year.

The parasite plays a fundamental role in the genesis and development of organ lesions by sequentially inducing an inflammatory response, cellular lesions, and fibrosis. Such pathological processes may occur in many organs but appear more frequently and more intensively in the heart, esophagus, and colon, where it affects mainly nerve cells from the cardiac conductive system and autonomic nervous system (myenteric plexus).

In the gastrointestinal tract the lesions (parasympathetic intramural denervation) are dispersed irregularly and affect mainly the esophagus and the sigmoid colon. The involved segment may appear normal with only functional peristaltic changes, or it may appear markedly narrowed and aperistaltic. Over time, the proximal normal portions dilate, which results in a megaesophagus (Fig. 125-13) or megacolon, or they may appear

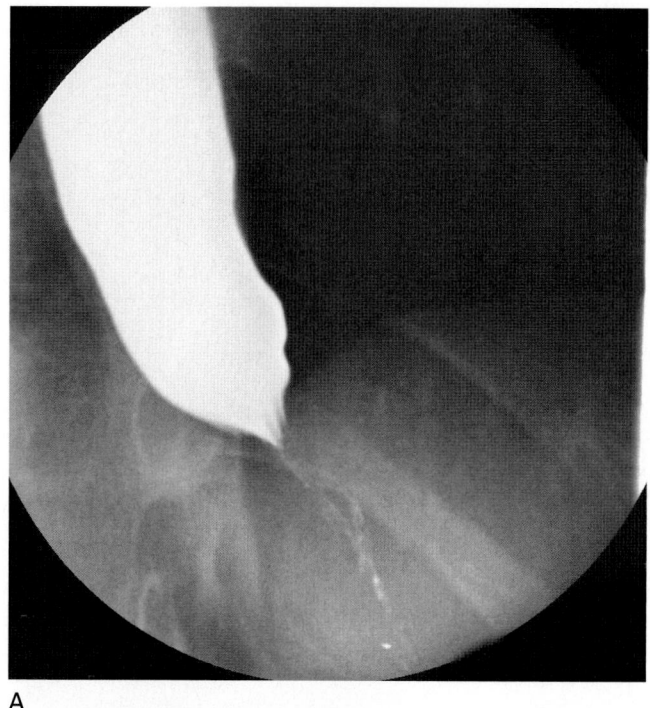

A

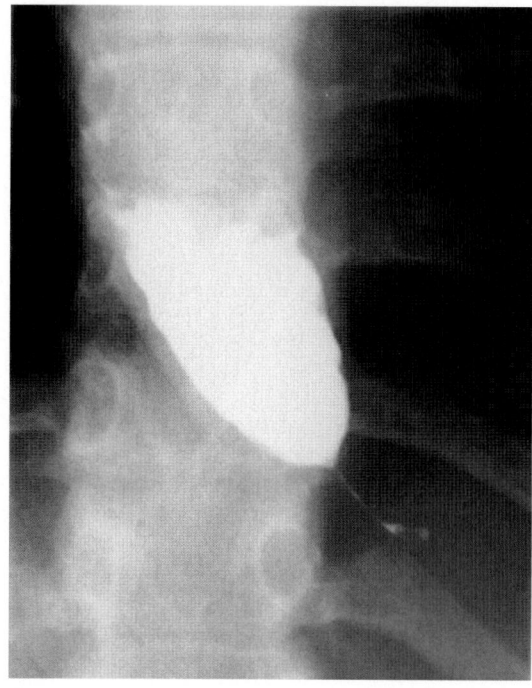

B

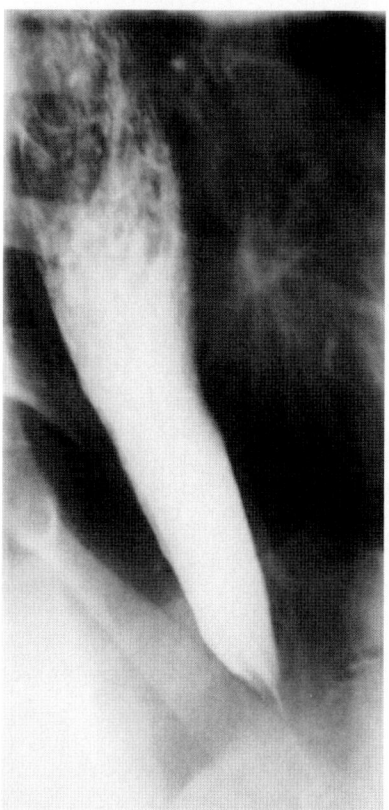

C

FIGURE 125-12. Achalasia. **A** and **B,** Marked "beaking" of the distal esophagus with large proximal dilation. **C,** Another view in a patient with achalasia and food debris in the esophagus. Chagas disease with esophagopathy could have the same appearance.

both dilated and elongated (dolichomegaesophagus). A hypertonia of the cardia is present at the onset of esophageal dysfunction, although an organic stenosis at the level of the cardia cannot be found.

Symptomatic acute phases occur mainly in newborns (congenital infection) or young children. The acute phase is characterized by intense peripheral neuronal destruction. It is reported that the destruction of cells causes the release of self-antigens, which leads to an auto-immune response of the host with even greater tissue damage. Extraesophageal complications of the acute phase include myocarditis and meningoencephalitis.

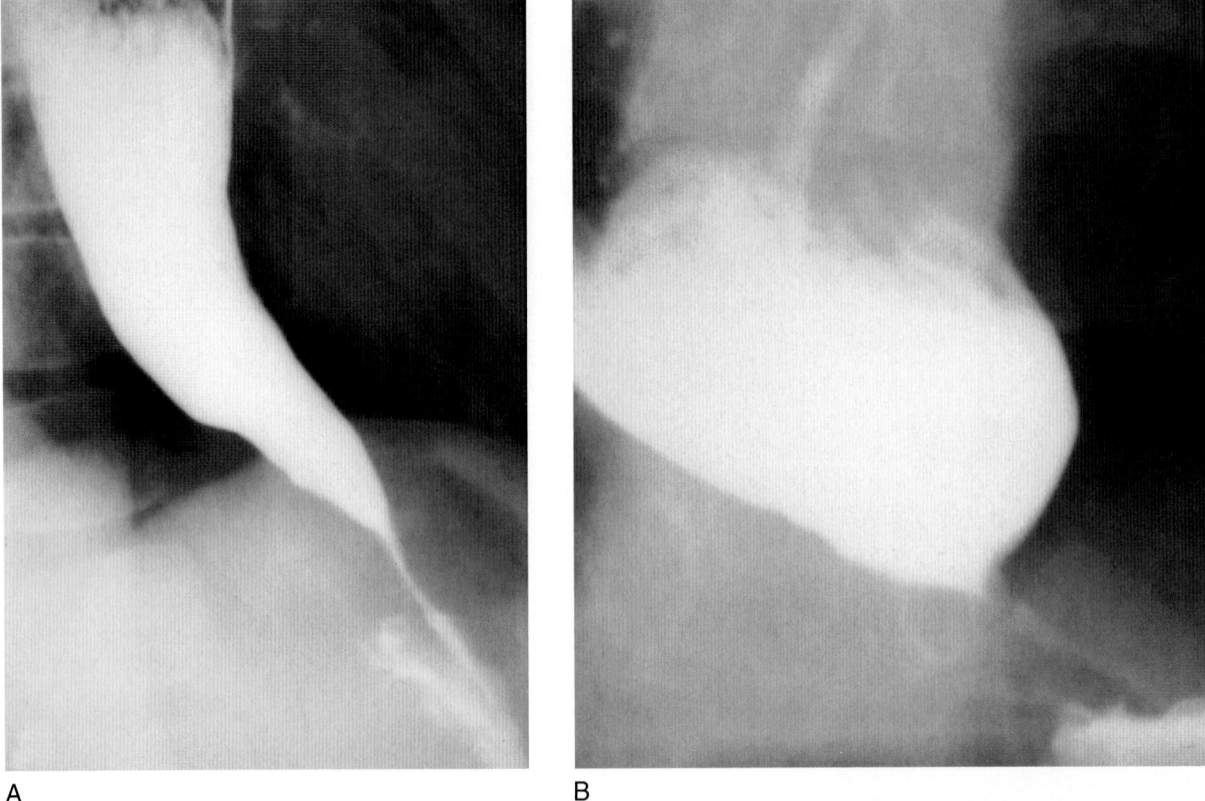

FIGURE 125-13. Chagasic esophagopathy. **A** and **B,** Typical narrowing of the distal esophagus (rat-tail appearance) with proximal dilation and air fluid level.

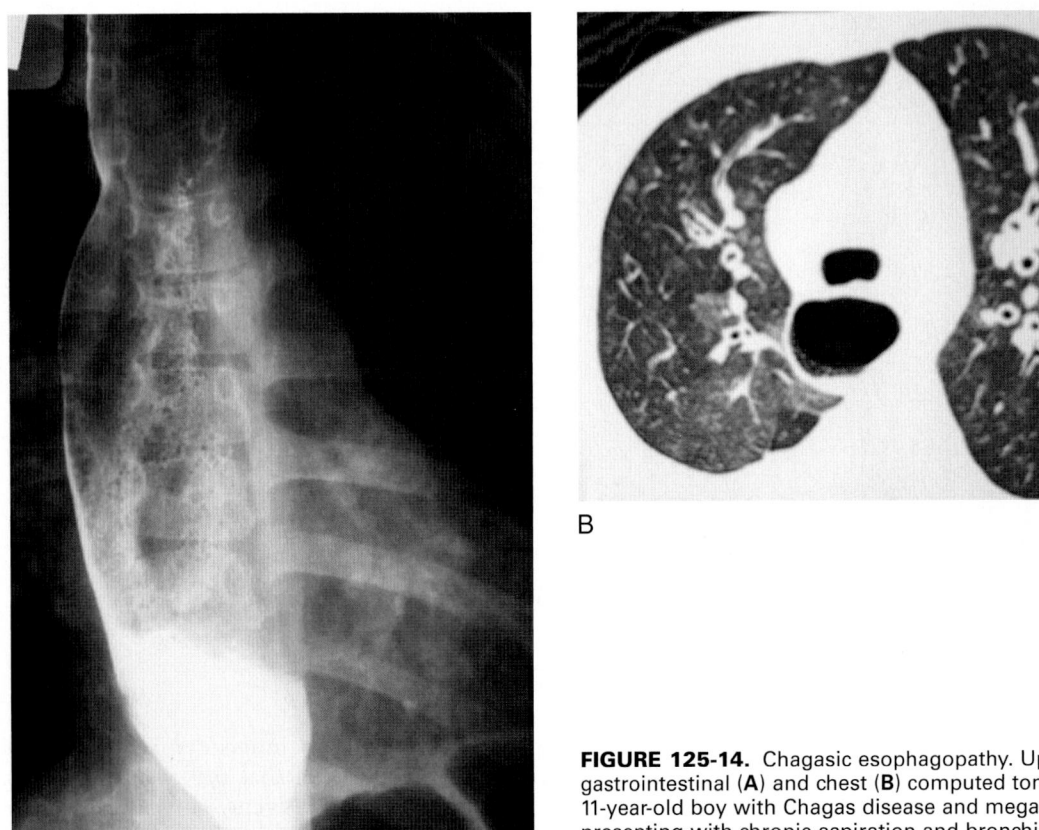

FIGURE 125-14. Chagasic esophagopathy. Upper gastrointestinal (**A**) and chest (**B**) computed tomograms of an 11-year-old boy with Chagas disease and megaesophagus presenting with chronic aspiration and bronchiectasis.

Chagasic esophagopathy clinically manifests as chronic dysphagia after uncoordinated esophageal motility. Over time, dilation and elongation of the esophagus ensues, and the child may present with regurgitation or large volumes, odynophagia, and failure to thrive. Barium studies may reveal a spectrum of esophageal changes ranging from an apparently normal appearance to great enlargement and elongation, with the distal esophagus tapering in a rat-tail appearance and food rests accumulated in its end (Fig. 125-14). Chagasic esophagopathy is observed more frequently in the second decade of life but can occur in children as young as 9 years of age, according to our experience, and chronic chagasic cardiomyopathy and colonopathy are generally detected later, in the third, fourth, or fifth decades of life.

The diagnosis can be suggested by clinical presentation, barium esophagograms, endoscopy with biopsy, and electromanometry. Chagas disease is a chronic, irreversible disorder, and treatment and esophagopathy includes surgical dilation of the cardia with an antireflux procedure. Complications of chronic chagasic esophagopathy include esophagitis and esophageal cancer.

SUGGESTED READINGS

Gastroesophageal Reflux

Argon M, Duygun U, Daglioz G, et al: Relationship between gastric emptying and gastroesophageal reflux in infants and children. Clin Nucl Med 2006;31:262-265

Balson BM, Kravitz EK, McGeady SJ: Diagnosis and treatment of gastroesophageal reflux in children and adolescents with severe asthma. Ann Allergy Asthma Immunol 1998;81:159-164

Blane CE, Turnage RH, Oldham KT, et al: Long-term radiographic follow-up of the Nissen fundoplication in children. Pediatr Radiol 1989;19:523-526

Boix-Ochoa J, Lafuente JM, Gilvernet JM: Twenty-four hour esophageal pH monitoring in gastroesophageal reflux. J Pediatr Surg 1980;15:74-78

Bowen AD: The vomiting infant: recent advances and unsettled issues in imaging. Radiol Clin North Am 1988;26:377-392

Braun P, Nussie D, Roy CC, et al: Intramural diverticulosis of the esophagus in an eight-year-old boy. Pediatr Radiol 1978;6:235-237

Chelimsky G, Shanske S, Hirano M, et al: Achalasia as the harbinger of a novel mitochondrial disorder in childhood. J Pediatr Gastroenterol Nutr 2005;40:512-517

Chung DH, Georgeson KE: Fundoplication and gastrostomy. Semin Pediatr Surg 1998;7:213-219

Cleveland RH, Kushner DC, Schwartz AN: Gastroesophageal reflux in children: results of a standard fluoroscopic approach. AJR Am J Roentgenol 1983;141:53-56

Darling DB, McCauley RGK, Leape LL, et al: The child with peptic esophagitis: a correlation of radiographic signs with esophageal pathology. Radiology 1982;145:673-676

Davies RP, Morris LL, Savage JP, et al: Gastroesophageal reflux: the role of imaging in diagnosis and management. Australas Radiol 1987;31:157-163

Di Ciaula A, Portincasa P, Di Terlizzi L, et al: Ultrasonographic study of postcibal gastro-esophageal reflux and gastric emptying in infants with recurrent respiratory disease. World J Gastroenterol 2005;11:7296-7301

Eid NS, Shepherd RW, Thomson MA: Persistent wheezing and gastroesophageal reflux in infants. Pediatr Pulmonol 1994;18:39-44

Euler AR, Ament ME: Detection of gastroesophageal reflux in the pediatric-age patient by esophageal intraluminal pH probe measurement (Tuttle test). Pediatrics 1977;60:65-68

Festen C: Paraesophageal hernia: a major complication of Nissen's fundoplication. J Pediatr Surg 1981;16:496-499

Fonkalsrud EW, Ashcraft KW, Coran AG: Surgical treatment of gastroesophageal reflux in children: a combined hospital study of 7467 patients. Pediatrics 1998;101:419-422

Frantzides CT, Richards C: A study of 362 consecutive laparoscopic Nissen fundoplications. Surgery 1998;124:651-654; discussion, Surgery 1998;124:654-655

Gold BD: Is gastroesophageal reflux disease really a life-long disease: do babies who regurgitate grow up to be adults with GERD complications? Am J Gastroenterol 2006;101:641-644

Gomes H, Menanteau B: Gastro-esophageal reflux: comparative study between sonography and pH monitoring. Pediatr Radiol 1991;21:168-174

Guill MF: Respiratory manifestations of gastroesophageal reflux in children. J Asthma 1995;32:173-189

Harnsberger JK, Corey JJ, Johnson DG: Long-term follow-up of surgery for gastroesophageal reflux in infants and children. J Pediatr 1983;102:505-508

Hayden CK: Ultrasonography of the gastrointestinal tract in infants and children. Abdom Imaging 1996;21:9-20

Heyman S: Esophageal scintigraphy (milk scans) in infants and children with esophageal reflux. Radiology 1982;144:891-893

Koot VC, Bergmeijer JH, Bos AP, et al: Incidence and management of gastroesophageal reflux after repair of congenital diaphragmatic hernia. J Pediatr Surg 1993;28:48-52

Leape LL, Holder TM, Franklin JD, et al: Respiratory arrest in infants secondary to gastroesophageal reflux. Pediatrics 1977;60:924-928

Levine ML: Pneumatic dilation for the treatment of achalasia in untreated patients and patients with failed Heller myotomy. J Clin Gastroenterol 2005;39:549

Maclean AD, Houghton-Allen BW: Upper esophageal web in childhood. Pediatr Radiol 1975;3:240-241

Marshall JB, Kretschmar JM, Diaz-Arias AA: Gastroesophageal reflux as a pathogenic factor in the development of symptomatic lower esophageal rings. Arch Intern Med 1990;150:1669-1672

McCauley RGK, Darling DB, Leonidas JC, et al: Gastroesophageal reflux in infants and children: a useful classification and reliable physiological technique for its demonstration. AJR Am J Roentgenol 1978;130:47-50

McVeagh P, Howman-Giles R, Kemp A: Pulmonary aspiration studies by radionuclide milk scanning and barium swallow roentgenology. Am J Dis Child 1987;141:917-921

Noel RJ, Tipnis NA: Eosinophilic esophagitis—a mimic of GERD. Int J Pediatr Otorhinolaryngol 2006;70:1147-1153

O'Hara SM: Pediatric gastrointestinal nuclear imaging. Radiol Clin North Am 1996;34:845-862

Peters ME, Crummy AB, Wojtowycz MM, et al: Intramural esophageal pseudodiverticulosis: a report in a child with a sixteen-year-old follow-up. Pediatr Radiol 1982;12:262-263

Piepsz A, Georges B, Perlmutter N, et al: Gastroesophageal scintiscanning in children. Pediatr Radiol 1981;11:71-74

Riccabona M, Maurer U, Lackner H: The role of sonography in the evaluation of gastro-oesophageal reflux-correlation to to pH-metry. Eur J Pediatr 1992;151:655-657

Scott RB, O'Laughlin EV, Gall DG: Gastroesophageal reflux in patients with cystic fibrosis. J Pediatr 1985;106:223-227

Seibert JJ, Byrne WJ, Euler AR, et al: Gastroesophageal reflux-the acid test: scintigraphy or the pH probe? AJR Am J Roentgenol 1983;140:1087-1090

Sigalet DL, Nguyen LT, Adolph V: Gastrointestinal reflux associated with large diaphragmatic hernias. J Pediatr Surg 1994;29:1262-1265

Smith CD, Othersen B, Gogan NJ, et al: Nissen fundoplication in children with profound neurologic diability: high risk and unmet goals. Ann Surg 1992;215:654-658; discussion 658-659

Stolar CJ, Berdon WE, Dillon PW, et al: Esophageal dilation and reflux in neonates supported by ECMO after diaphragmatic hernia repair. AJR Am J Roentgenol 1988;151:135-137

Stolar CJ, Levy JP, Dillon PW, et al: Anatomic and functional abnormalities of the esophagus in infants surviving congenital diaphragmatic hernia. Am J Surg 1990;159:204-207

Thoeni RF, Moss AA: The radiographic appearance of complications following Nissen fundoplication. Radiology 1979;131:17-21

Tolia V, Calhoun JA, Kuns LR, et al: Lack of correlation between extended pH monitoring and scintigraphy in the evaluation of infants with gastroesophageal reflux. J Lab Clin Med 1990;115:559-563

Trinh TD, Benson JE: Fluoroscopic diagnosis of complications after Nissen antireflux fundoplication in children. AJR Am J Roentgenol 1997;169:1023-1028

Vandenplas Y, Derde MP, Peipsz A: Evaluation of reflux episodes during simultaneous esophageal pH monitoring and gastroesophageal reflux scintigraphy in children. J Pediatr Gastroenterol Nutr 1992;14:256-260

Weaver JW, Kaude JV, Hamlin DJ: Webs of the lower esophagus: a complication of gastroesophageal reflux? AJR Am J Roentgenol 1984;142:289-292

Wesley JR, Coran AG, Sarahan TM, et al: The need for evaluation of gastroesophageal reflux in brain-damaged children referred for feeding gastrostomy. J Pediatr Surg 1981;16:866-871

West KW, Stephens B, Rescorla FJ, et al: Postoperative intussusception: experience with 36 cases in children. Surgery 1988;104:781-787

Westra KW, Derkx HH, Taminiau JA: Symptomatic gastroesophageal reflux: diagnosis with ultrasound. J Pediatr Gastroenterol Nutr 1994;19:58-64

Winters C Jr, Spurling TJ, Chobanian SJ, et al: Barrett's esophagus: a prevalent, occult complication of gastroesophageal reflux disease. Gastroenterology 1987;92:118-124

Wolfson BJ, Allen JL, Panitch HB, et al: Lipid aspiration pneumonia due to gastroesophageal reflux: a complication of nasogastric lipid feedings. Pediatr Radiol 1989;19:545-547

Yulish BS, Rothstein FC, Halpin TC Jr: Radiographic findings in children and young adults with Barrett's esophagus. AJR Am J Roentgenol 1987;148:353-357

Hiatal Hernia

Astley R, Carre IJ, Langmead-Smith R: A 20-year prospective follow-up of childhood hiatal hernia. Br J Radiol 1977;50:400-403

Achalasia

Ambrosino MM, Genieser NB, Banguru BS, et al: The syndrome of achalasia of the esophagus, ACTH insensitivity and alacrima. Pediatr Radiol 1986;16:328-329

Berquist WE, Byrne WJ, Ament ME, et al: Achalasia: diagnosis, management, and clinical courses in 16 children. Pediatrics 1983;71:798-805

Hammond PD, Moore DJ, Davidson GP, et al: Tandem balloon dilation for childhood achalasia. Pediatr Radiol 1997;27:609-613

Holzman MD, Sharp KW, Lapido JK, et al: Laparoscopic surgical treatment for achalasia. Am J Surg 1997;173:308-311

Lelli JL, Drongowski RA, Coran AG: Efficacy of transthoracic modified Heller myotomy in children with achalasia—a 21 year experience. J Pediatr Surg 1997;32:338-341

Starinsky R, Berlovitz J, Mores AJ, et al: Infantile achalasia. Pediatr Radiol 1984;14:113-115

Walton JM, Tougas G: Botulinum toxin use in pediatric esophageal achalasia: a case report. J Pediatr Surg 1997;32:916-917

Chagasic Esophagopathy

Benchimol Barbosa PR: The oral transmission of Chagas' disease: An acute form of infection responsible for regional outbreaks. Int J Cardiol 2006;112:132-133

Carlier Y, Luquetti AO, Nettleman M: Chagas disease (American trypanosomiasis). Emedicine 2003, available at http://www.emedicine.com/MED/topic327.htm

Cruz RE, Macedo AM, Barnabe C, et al: Further genetic characterization of the two Trypanosoma cruzi Berenice strains (Be-62 and Be-78) isolated from the first human case of Chagas disease (Chagas, 1909). Acta Trop 2006;97:239-246

Dantas RO, Aprile LR: Esophageal contractions in Chagas' disease and in idiopathic achalasia. J Clin Gastroenterol 2005;39:863-868

Martínez S, Restrepo CS, Carrillo JA: Thoracic manifestations of tropical parasitic infections: a pictorial review. Radiographics 2005;25:135-155

CHAPTER 126

Miscellaneous Esophageal Abnormalities

HENRIQUE M. LEDERMAN and GUILHERME T. S. DEMARCHI

ESOPHAGEAL VARICES

Esophageal varices occur secondary to portal hypertension and are discussed in Chapters 115 and 131. At present, the primary modality for identifying esophageal varices is endoscopy, rather than imaging studies. However, varices may be found in the evaluation of hematemesis or coincidentally when imaging studies are performed for other reasons. In rare cases, paraesophageal varices cause sufficient irregularity of the esophagus that they can be seen as paraspinous widening on chest radiographs (Fig. 126-1). On barium swallow studies, they appear as serpentine filling defects in the distal esophagus (see Fig. 126-1). Computed tomography and magnetic resonance imaging will identify varices when performed in patients with portal hypertension or for other indications (see Fig. 126-1). Angiography (see Fig. 126-1) is typically reserved for patients undergoing embolization procedures. Ultrasonography, especially color Doppler ultrasonography, performed for the evaluation of hepatic disease, may demonstrate esophageal varices at the esophageal hiatus, anterior to the aorta. Endoluminal ultrasonography with 20-MHz transducers have been shown to be more sensitive than endoscopy in the detection of esophageal varices. Complete filling of the esophagus on barium esophagogram may demonstrate varices extending high into the esophagus, again with the appearance of serpentine filling defects in the barium column (Fig. 126-2). Barium paste provides better mucosal relief than does liquid barium, but children do not always find it palatable.

The primary treatment modality for esophageal varices, other than treatment of the underlying portal hypertension, is endoscopic sclerotherapy. Agha described acute complications after sclerotherapy, including mucosal ulceration, luminal narrowing, sinuses, fistulas, dissec-tion, and perforation. Chronic complications that may be found include strictures, mural defects, dysmotility, and obstruction.

NEOPLASMS

Esophageal tumors are extraordinarily rare in children and are usually benign. Hamartomas, leiomyomas, and hemangiomas have all been reported. Leiomyomatosis, a rare neoplastic disorder causing leiomyomatous thickening of all or a portion of the esophagus, has been reported in children as well, manifesting as large filling defects on barium studies or marked esophageal thickening on computed tomography. One of the most common pseudoneoplasms to be found is an inflammatory polyp secondary to chronic gastroesophageal reflux (Fig. 126-3). Carcinomas are even rarer and have been reported after caustic esophagitis, achalasia, and chagasic esophagopathy. Mediastinal tumors, such as lymphoma, teratoma, or neuroblastoma, may displace the esophagus but usually do not primarily involve it.

> **Esophageal neoplasms:**
> - **Benign**
>   - **Hamartomas**
>   - **Leiomyomas**
>   - **Hemangiomas**
>   - **Leiomyomatosis**
> - **Malignant**
> - **Carcinoma (rare, but can be seen after caustic esophagitis, achalasia, or chagasic esophagopathy)**

2055

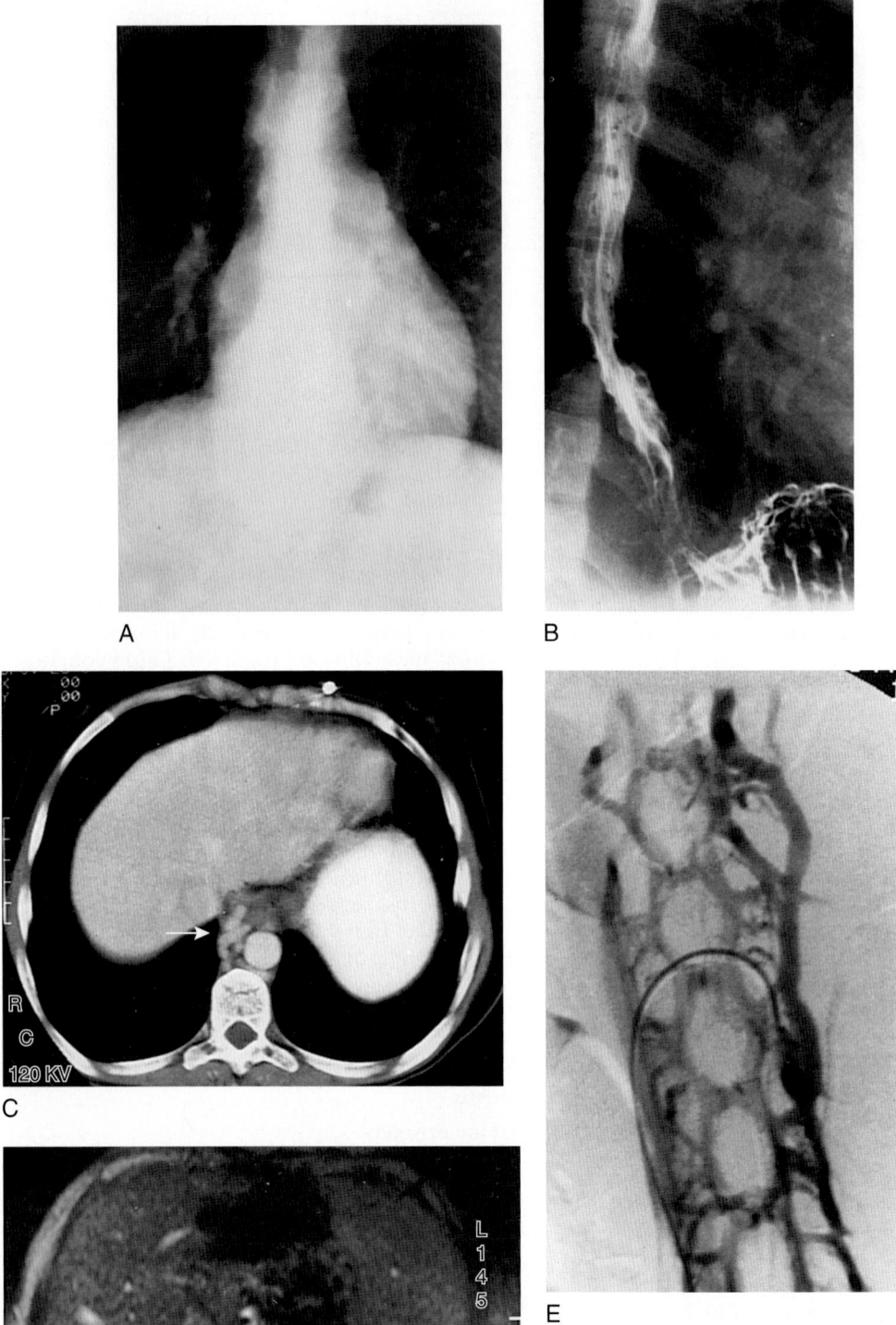

FIGURE 126-1. Marked esophageal and paraesophageal collateral circulation in a 15-year-old girl with cavernous transformation of the portal vein. **A,** Coned-down anteroposterior view of the chest reveals paravertebral widening at the level of the diaphragm. **B,** Esophagogram demonstrates serpentine filling defects in the distal esophagus and the gastric fundus that are consistent with varices. **C,** Computed tomographic scan at the thoracoabdominal junction demonstrates multiple varices in the paraesophageal region (*arrow*). **D,** Magnetic resonance imaging using gradient-recalled echo sequence clearly demonstrates right paraesophageal varices. **E,** Angiography with digital subtraction technique demonstrates massive bilateral paravertebral collateral venous flow.

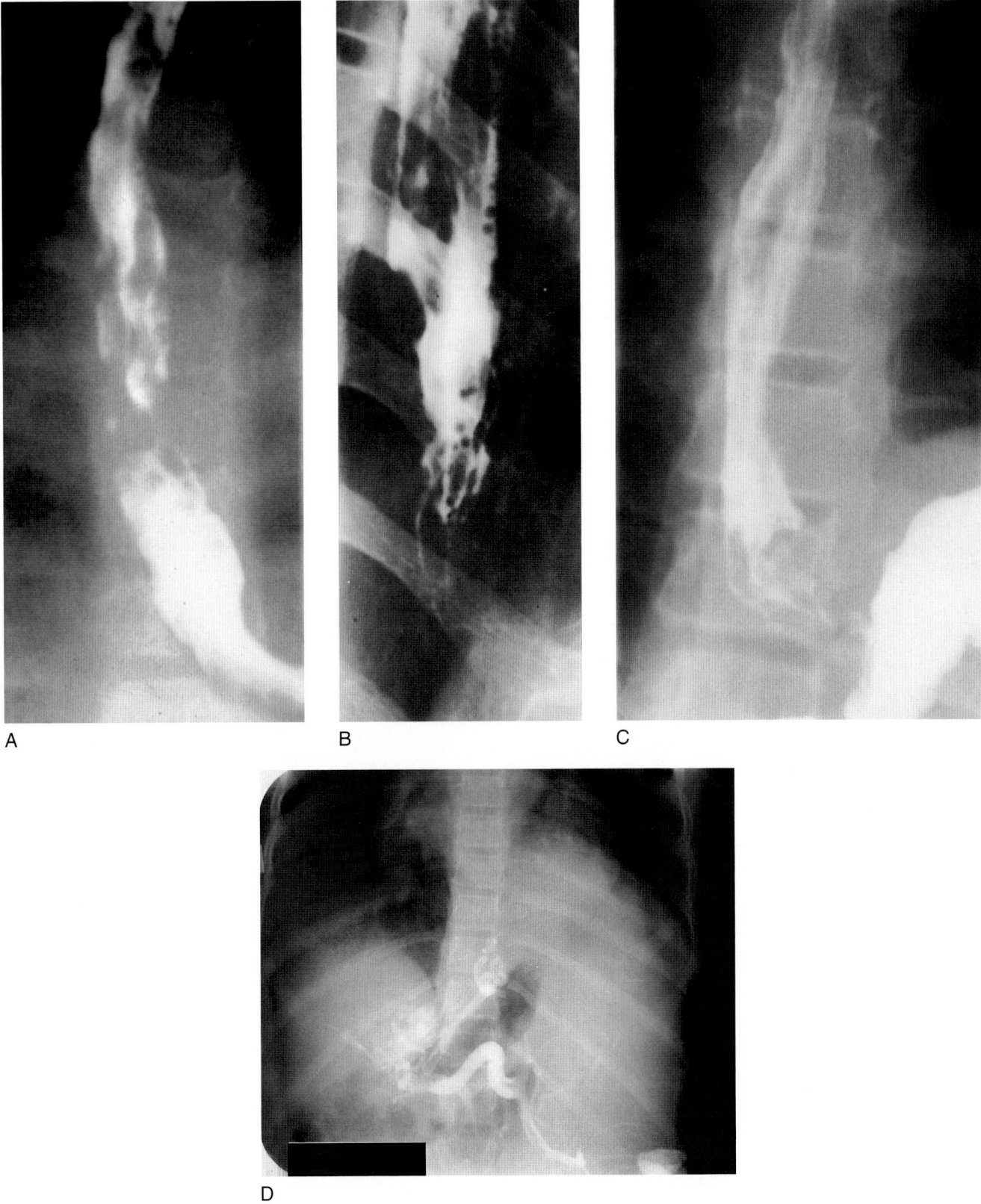

A   B   C

D

FIGURE 126-2. Esophageal varices. **A** and **B,** Esophagogram demonstrates multiple serpentine filling defects in the esophagus resulting from varices secondary to portal hypertension. Another patient shows varices on esophagogram **(C)** and angioscopic evidence **(D)** of the varices.

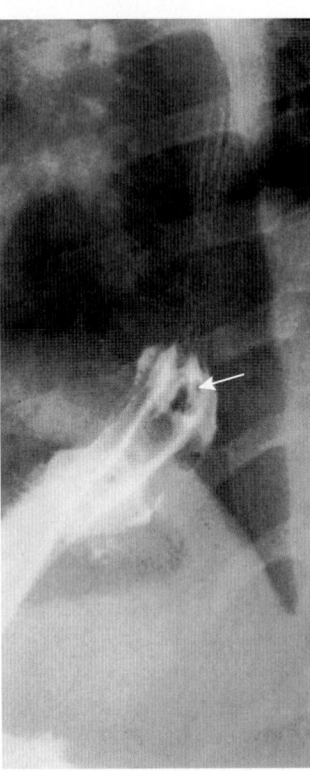

FIGURE 126-3.
Inflammatory gastroesophageal polyp (*arrow*) depicted as a filling defect on upper gastrointestinal series in a 10-year-old boy with hiatal hernia. (Courtesy of Dr. S. Kirschner, Nashville, TN.)

SUGGESTED READINGS

Esophageal Varices

Agha FP: The esophagus after endoscopic injection sclerotherapy: acute and chronic changes. Radiology 1984;153:37-42

Chaudry G, Navarro OM, Levine DS, et al: Abdominal manifestations of cystic fibrosis in children. Pediatr Radiol 2006;36:233-240

Isikawa T, Saeki M, Tsukune Y, et al: Detection of paraesophageal varices by plain film. AJR Am J Roentgenol 1985;144:701-704

Itha S, Yachha SK: Endoscopic outcome beyond esophageal variceal eradication in children with extrahepatic portal venous obstruction. J Pediatr Gastroenterol Nutr 2006;42:196-200

Rose JD, Robert GM, Smith PM: The radiological appearance of the esophagus after sclerotherapy for varices. Clin Radiol 1985; 36:355-358

Neoplasms

Buratti S, Savides TJ, Newbury RO, et al: Granular cell tumor of the esophagus: report of a pediatric case and literature review. J Pediatr Gastroenterol Nutr 2004;38:97-101

Federici S, Ceccarelli PL, Bernardi F, et al: Esophageal leiomyomatosis in children: report of a case and review of the literature. Eur J Pediatr Surg 1998;8:358-363

Guest AR, Strouse PJ, Hiew CC, et al: Progressive esophageal leiomyomatosis with respiratory compromise. Pediatr Radiol 2000;30:247-250

Killian AK, Ringle T, Waag K, et al: Pre- and postoperative MRI of esophageal and gastric leiomyomatosis in a pediatric patient. AJR Am J Roentgenol 2005;184(3 Suppl):S129-S131

Koyluoglu G, Yildiz E, Koyuncu A, et al: Management of an esophagogastric fibromatosis in a child: a case report. J Pediatr Surg 2004;39:640-642

CHAPTER

127

The Stomach: Normal Anatomy and Imaging Techniques

MARTA HERNANZ-SCHULMAN and ALAN E. SCHLESINGER

NORMAL ANATOMY

The stomach normally lies below the left hemidiaphragm and extends obliquely caudally and medially to the duodenal junction. The stomach begins embryologically as a straight tube that rotates clockwise 90 degrees around its long axis; therefore, the dorsal portion of the stomach becomes the left margin. The growth of the left margin is greater than that of the opposite side, which results in a longer, greater curvature to the left and a shorter, lesser curvature to the right. The stomach is relatively fixed at its proximal end by the esophagogastric junction and at its distal end by the fixed retroperitoneal position of the first portion of the duodenum. In addition, the stomach is attached to neighboring structures and organs by four major peritoneal folds, or ligaments: the gastrophrenic, the gastrohepatic, the gastrosplenic, and the gastrocolic ligaments. These attachments are important in maintaining the normal position and orientation of the stomach.

The stomach thus has two openings, one at the esophagogastric junction and the second at the pyloric orifice, and is divided into three major portions: fundus, body, and antrum. The fundus is the most bulbous portion and is the part superior to the esophagogastric junction, normally the most cephalad and posterior portion of the stomach. The body of the stomach is the segment bounded on either side by the greater and lesser curvatures, typically becoming slightly narrower in caliber as it reaches the distal portion. The gastric antrum begins at the incisura angularis, and typically has a more horizontal course. The sulcus intermedius divides the antrum into the prepyloric portion, immediately proximal to the pyloric orifice. The normal shape, size, and position of the stomach are variable, depending on the volume of gastric content and the position, age, and body habitus of the individual. In infancy, the stomach appears high and transverse on contrast studies in most patients (Fig. 127-1). The more longitudinal, J-shaped stomach is uncommon in infants but is characteristic in older children and adults (Fig. 127-2). Although the appearance of the fundus and body may vary, the posi-

tion and appearance of the pylorus are relatively similar from patient to patient.

The fundus and the greater curvature of the body normally exhibit marginal indentations caused by the normal folds in the mucosa, the gastric rugae. The pattern is inconstant, but rugal folds can usually be seen in most normal stomachs unless they are overdistended during barium examination, or obscured by pre-existent gastric contents. The rugae are least prominent in early infancy and become progressively more obvious in older patients (see Figs. 127-1 and 127-2). The mucosal

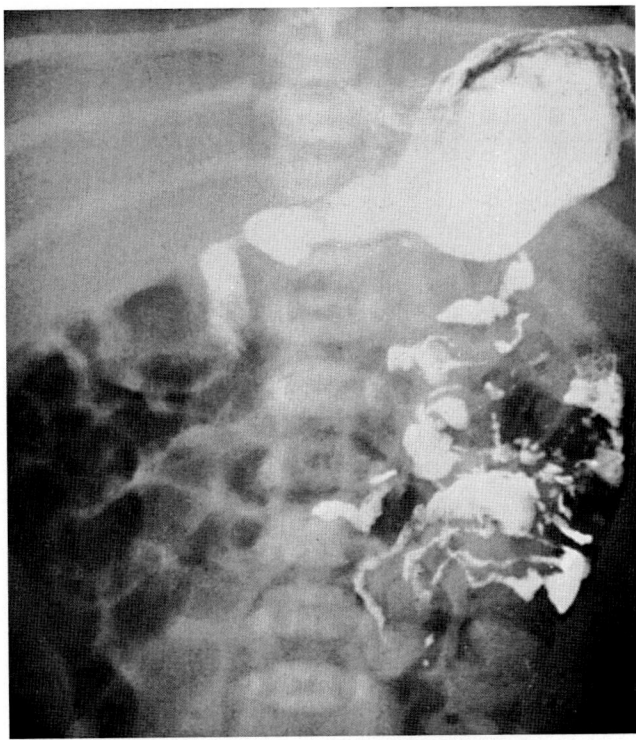

FIGURE 127-1. Changes in the radiographic appearance of the stomach during childhood. Radiographic appearance of the normal stomach in early life. This stomach, in a 6-day-old infant, is high and conical in shape, and transverse rugal markings are not prominent.

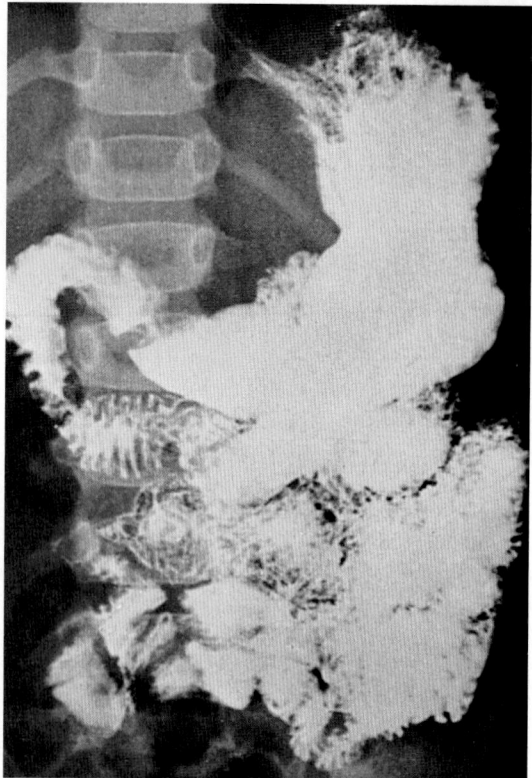

FIGURE 127-2. The stomach in a 4-year-old boy is J-shaped with prominent rugal folds in the fundus.

contour is best evaluated with a small amount of contrast material spread over the surface. Double-contrast studies of the stomach bring the mucosa into sharp relief but cannot always be performed in young children and are seldom necessary.

Normal peristaltic waves can typically be seen even in neonates, although gastric motor activity increases with age. Normally, peristalsis is coordinated from the proximal to the distal stomach and is propulsive. The gastric antrum and pyloric region frequently exhibit muscular spasm, which interrupts the normal peristaltic propulsive waves (Fig. 127-3). Gastric emptying time is far more variable in children than in adults, especially in infants. Although maintenance of the supine position and gaseous distention of the stomach, which typically occur in infants, may have a role in delayed gastric emptying, the effect of the delayed opening of the antrum and pylorus is probably most significant. On occasion, a normal infant may have sufficient antropyloric spasm for contrast material to remain in the stomach for as long as 20 or 25 minutes before finally passing into the small intestine. It is important to be patient, and pulsed and intermittent fluoroscopic techniques are particularly important in these cases to control radiation exposure.

Imaging Techniques

Plain radiographs, fluoroscopic studies, scintigraphy, and cross-sectional imaging, particularly sonography, are valuable in evaluation of abnormalities of the stomach.

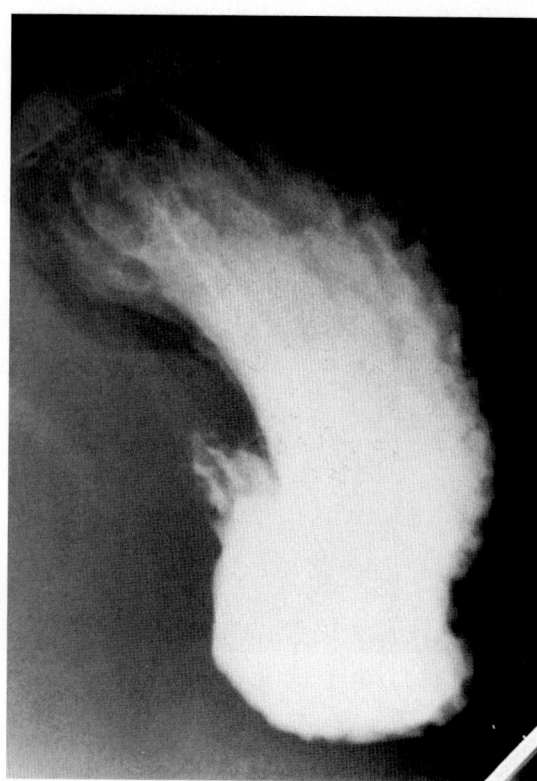

A

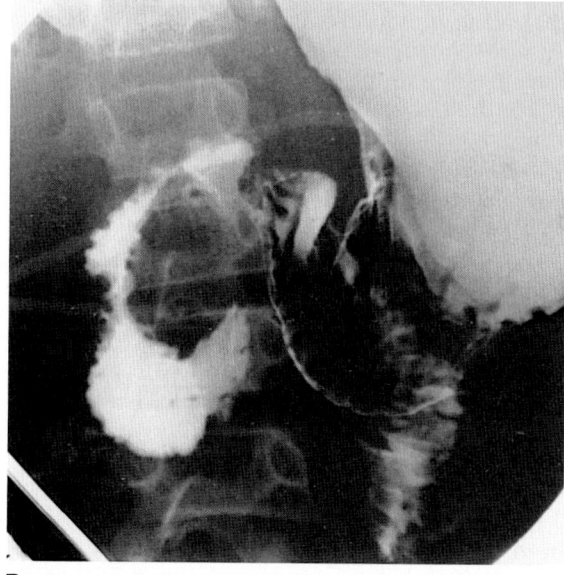

B

FIGURE 127-3. Pyloric spasm. **A,** Upper gastrointestinal tract series in a 7-year-old girl with crampy abdominal pain shows antropyloric spasm 30 minutes after barium ingestion. **B,** After parenteral administration of an anticholinergic agent, there was easy passage of barium through an anatomically normal pylorus and duodenum.

PLAIN RADIOGRAPHS

The appearance of the stomach on plain radiographs varies, depending on the position of the child (i.e., supine versus upright) and the degree of gastric distention. On upright images, air gravitates to the fundus, which is below the diaphragm, medial to the splenic shadow. On supine images, the stomach is outlined by air within the more anterior antrum. On plain radiographs, the stomach should be evaluated for both size and orientation. Distention of the stomach is normal after a full meal but is abnormal if the patient presents with a history of vomiting.

FLUOROSCOPIC EXAMINATION

Contrast studies of the upper gastrointestinal tract under fluoroscopic control (upper gastrointestinal [UGI] series) continue to be the standard examination for most abnormalities of the stomach. Barium is the most commonly used contrast material. In cases in which perforation is a concern, iso-osmolal nonionic contrast media should be used. Hyperosmolal contrast agents should never be used, because of the risk of aspiration and severe pulmonary edema. The advantages of isotonic solutions of low-osmolality nonionic contrast include lack of large fluid shifts, absence of contrast dilution, lack of injury to the bowel mucosa, low absorption from the bowel, and relatively lower risk of pulmonary edema if the isotonic contrast is aspirated. In patients with subtle bowel perforation not identified by contrast extravasation at the time of the examination, perforation can be detected on delayed radiographs from renal excretion of the contrast that is absorbed by the peritoneum.

The UGI examination in children should be tailored to the specific clinical question to be answered in order to limit the radiation exposure. Intermittent fluoroscopy should always be used instead of constant fluoroscopy; careful collimation should be used; and, when available, fluoro grabs should be used liberally, with spot films reserved for areas in which documentation of mucosal detail is needed. If available, pulsed fluoroscopy should be used instead of continuous fluoroscopy. In young infants, the grid should be removed, and the beam should be filtered appropriately for the size of the patient being examined. These maneuvers result in very significant reduction in radiation dose with improvement in diagnostic quality of the study. Infants and young children, of necessity, are studied in the recumbent position. Upright images can be performed in older patients if needed.

Preparation for the examination varies with the age of the patient. In infants, we withhold food so that the child fasts for 3 hours or longer. In older children, breakfast is withheld if the study is to be performed in the morning, and a light breakfast is permitted for patients to be examined in the afternoon. However, when the major concern is documentation of reflux, a strict fasting status is not of paramount importance if the patient can be induced to drink contrast material; an empty stomach is most important for evaluation of mucosal detail and of gastric masses.

Most infants who have fasted through the schedule for feeding, or for at least 3 hours, are hungry and readily take barium from a bottle. We begin the study with the patient lying on his or her left side, for optimal evaluation of the esophagus while maintaining the contrast material within the gastric fundus. This is very important because evaluation of the location of the duodenojejunal junction (ligament of Treitz) (described in Chapter 133) is most reliable and successful if assessed during the first pass of contrast through the pylorus. The child is then turned into the right-side-down decubitus position, in order to assess the antrum. Fluoro grabs and a spot film to document the mucosa or any abnormalities that necessitate detailed evaluation are recorded. Fluoro grabs can document a normal lumen without filling defects, and multiple fluoro grabs recorded in rapid succession can document peristaltic activity.

Evaluation of reflux is one of the major concerns originating the request for the UGI examination. Evaluation for reflux is discussed in detail in Chapter 125.

ULTRASONOGRAPHY

Ultrasonography has become a very useful adjunct in evaluation of the stomach, and its use is discussed under the specific disease category (see Chapters 128 to 131). Ultrasound studies can be helpful in evaluating masses, such as gastric duplication cysts, and luminal abnormalities, such as antral webs, particularly if the stomach is distended with fluid after an initial 3- to 4-hour fast. Ultrasonography is also helpful in evaluation of reflux and is used particularly in Europe. The technique entails the use of an appropriately focused transducer, preferably linear configuration, to visualize the distal esophagus at the gastroesophageal junction. This allows the angle of insertion to be visualized, as well as documentation of episodes of reflux without radiation exposure. This study can be coupled to the evaluation for pyloric stenosis; if the pylorus is found to be normal, reflux can be documented. Unlike the UGI series, the ultrasound study does not allow visualization of the level of the reflux or of aspiration if it occurs. In addition, full evaluation of the esophagus for other causes of feeding difficulties, such as vascular rings or duplication cysts, also cannot be accomplished with sonography. However, it is a useful technique in documentation of reflux. Details on reflux are discussed in Chapter 125.

SCINTIGRAPHY

Radionuclide gastric emptying studies are usually performed at the time of evaluation for gastroesophageal reflux. The infant is fed a liquid meal of approximately the same volume as a normal feeding. Technetium-99m sulfur colloid is typically added to the midportion of the feeding, to prevent emptying of the radionuclide early in the examination while allowing its washout from the esophagus during the later portion of the feeding. The dose of radionuclide is based on the child's age and weight. The examination time varies by institution. Gelfand and Wagner favored the increased accuracy of a 2-hour examination, whereas Miller evaluated the infants for 90 minutes. According to Miller, the lower limits of normal gastric emptying are 45% at 60 minutes and 60% at 90 minutes (Fig. 127-4). See also Fig. 106-11, Chapter 106.

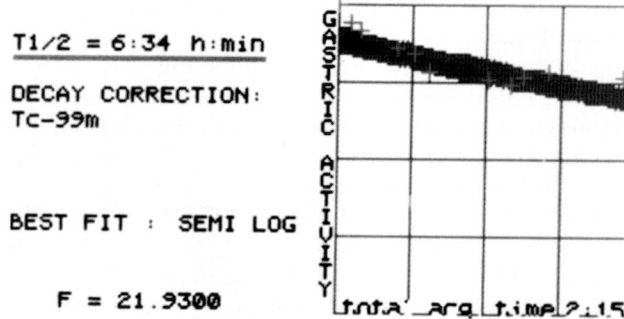

T1/2 = 6:34 h:min

DECAY CORRECTION:
Tc-99m

BEST FIT : SEMI LOG

F = 21.9300

FIGURE 127-4. Delayed gastric emptying after administration of technetium-99m sulfur colloid in formula. Half-gastric emptying time was 6½ hours; normal is 60 to 90 minutes. See also Fig. 106-11, Chapter 106) (Courtesy of Michael L. Goris, MD, Stanford, CA.)

COMPUTED TOMOGRAPHY AND MAGNETIC RESONANCE IMAGING

There are reports of computed tomography and magnetic resonance imaging findings in benign diseases of the stomach in the pediatric population. These are often incidental to an examination being performed for other reasons. Most authors agree that these studies for gastric lesions in children are most useful when gastric or juxtagastric masses are being evaluated or when a proven malignancy is being staged. On the other hand, certain conditions, such as gastric volvulus, could be more rapidly diagnosed with multidetector computed tomography and reconstructions, without need for drinking contrast material. These techniques, when applicable, are discussed with the specific conditions described (see Chapters 128 to 131).

SUGGESTED READINGS

Brown PH, Silberberg PJ, Thomas RD, et al: A multihospital survey of radiation exposure and image quality in pediatric fluoroscopy. Pediatr Radiol 2000;30:236-242

Gelfand MJ, Wagner GC : Gastric emptying in infants and children: limited utility of 1-hour measurement. Radiology 1991;178:379

Koumanidou C, Vakaki M, Pitsoulakis G, et al: Sonographic measurement of the abdominal esophagus length in infancy: a diagnostic tool for gastroesophageal reflux. AJR Am J Roentgenol 2004;183:801-807

Miller J: Upper gastrointestinal tract evaluation with radionuclides in infants. Radiology 1991;178:326

Miller JH, Kemberling CR: Ultrasound of the pediatric gastrointestinal tract. Semin Ultrasound CT MR 1987;8:349-365

Stringer DA, Daneman A, Brunelle F, et al: Sonography of the normal and abnormal stomach (excluding hypertrophic pyloric stenosis) in children. J Ultrasound Med 1986;5:183-188

Tiao MM, Ko SF, Hsieh CS, et al: Antral web associated with distal antral hypertrophy and prepyloric stenosis mimicking hypertrophic pyloric stenosis. World J Gastroenterol 2005;11:609-611.

128 Congenital Gastric Abnormalities

MARILYN J. GOSKE

Congenital anomalies of the stomach encompass a variety of conditions, including duplication cysts; diverticula; anomalies of size and position, such as microgastria; anomalies of the antropyloric area, such as webs; anomalies of fixation leading to volvulus; and ectopic tissue rests.

GASTRIC DUPLICATION CYSTS

Duplications of the gastrointestinal tracts are uncommon (1 per 10,000 births) and duplications of the stomach are even rarer. Less than 4% of intestinal duplications arise from the stomach. The embryologic origin of gastric duplications is speculative. Various theories include the "diverticular theory" (diverticular outpouching of the stomach) and the "split notochord theory" (anomalous separation of the endoderm from the notochord); according to the latter, the duplication originates partially in the occasional association of vertebral anomalies with gastric duplications. Embryologically, smaller submucosal cysts may be secondary to "abnormal vacuolization" of the stomach. Typical gastric duplications are thin walled and cystic, occur along the greater curvature, and do not communicate with the gastric lumen. They are occasionally tubular and can occur anywhere along the stomach from the esophagogastric junction to the pylorus. Because duplication cysts may contain gastric or pancreatic tissue, they may become inflamed, bleed, and eventually perforate (Fig. 128-1). On occasion, pneumoperitoneum may be seen at presentation.

Clinically, newborns may present with vomiting caused by the mass's indenting and partially or completely obstructing the gastric lumen. A palpable mass may be noted on physical examination. Patients typically present before 1 year of age with hematemesis, melena, or anemia. Gastric duplication cysts have been recognized prenatally, with both fetal ultrasonography and magnetic resonance imaging, as fluid-filled structures adjacent to the stomach. Postnatally, the first imaging study is ultrasonography with a high-frequency linear transducer. Careful scanning along the greater curvature reveals the cystic mass that demonstrates "gut signature" on ultrasonography, consisting of a hyperechoic inner mucosal layer and a thinner outer hypoechoic muscular layer. A connection to the stomach may or may not be seen, but the mass abuts its greater curvature. The duplication cyst is often small, approximately 2 cm in diameter, and may contain a variable amount of fluid or debris, representing hemorrhage or proteinaceous material. Cysts containing ectopic gastric tissue may be inflamed and thick walled.

Most notably, Kumar and colleagues discussed the use of technetium-99m pertechnetate in the demonstration of gastric mucosa within gastric duplication cysts and emphasized the spectrum of scintigraphic findings. Gastric duplication cysts are expected to visualize simultaneously with the normal stomach. The sensitivity of technetium-99m pertechnetate imaging varies from 85% to 91% but is reported to yield a high number of false-negative results.

In rare cases, the mass from the gastric duplication cyst may be seen on abdominal radiograph as outlined by gas in the adjacent stomach and colon (Fig. 128-2). Upper gastrointestinal series (UGI) series may demonstrate the mass effect on the stomach or the even rarer communication between the stomach and cyst. If incidentally found on computed tomographic scan, the cystic mass is seen in the left upper quadrant and is usually thin walled and filled with fluid (computed tomographic density <10 Hounsfield units) unless hemorrhage has occurred.

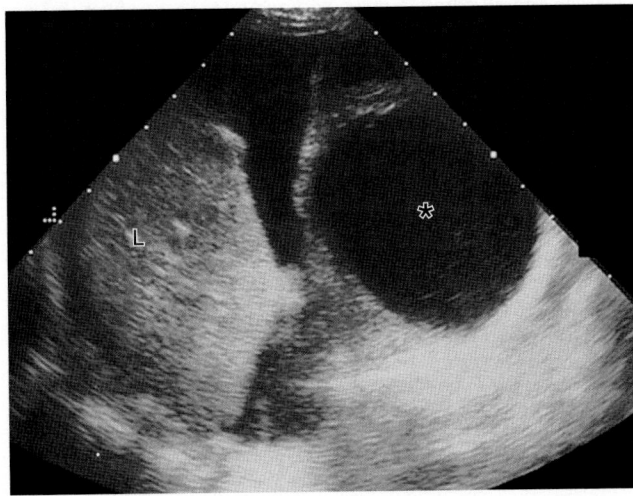

FIGURE 128-1. Ruptured gastric duplication cyst. Sagittal ultrasound image through the medial portion of the right lobe of the liver (L) demonstrates a thin-walled, approximately 4-cm simple cyst (*asterisk*). Free fluid, complex in its dependent portion, was found at surgery to represent hemorrhage secondary to rupture. (Courtesy of Dr. C. Mitchell, Peoria, IL.)

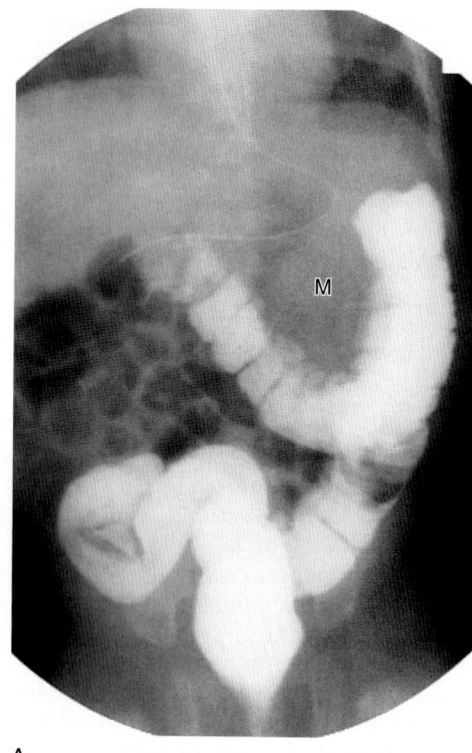

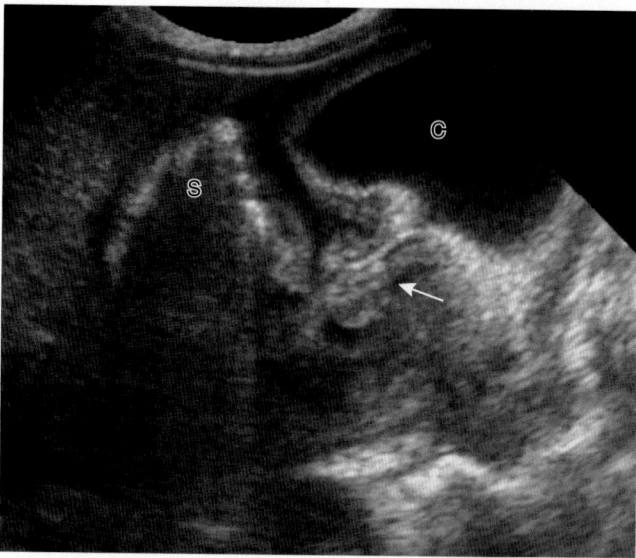

A

B

FIGURE 128-2. Gastric duplication in a 6-week-old with hematemesis. **A,** Barium enema study demonstrates a mass (M) between the greater curvature of the stomach and the contrast-filled transverse colon. **B,** Ultrasound study demonstrates typical findings of fluid-filled cyst (C) with "gut signature" consisting of thick outer hypoechoic muscular layer and echogenic inner layer of mucosa. The stomach (S) contains shadowing gas. The connection of the cyst with the gas-filled stomach is seen *(arrow)* **C,** Upper gastrointestinal study performed after barium enema adminstration demonstrates mass effect (M) on the greater curvature of the stomach. (Courtesy of Dr. D. Barlev, New York, NY.)

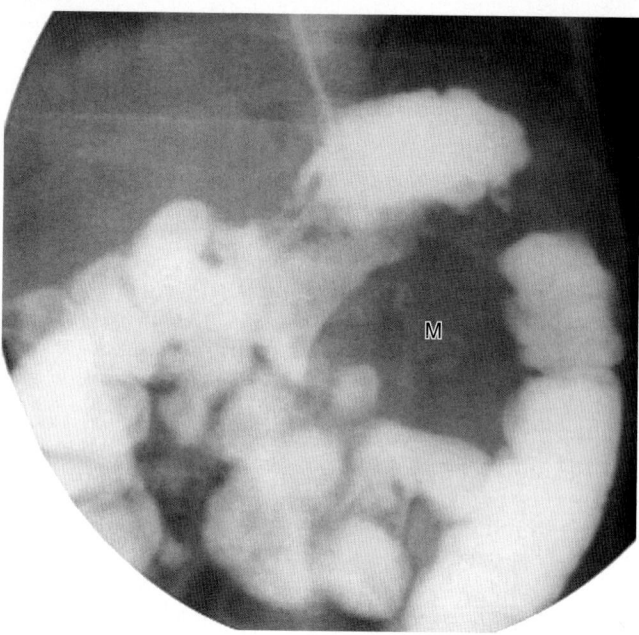

C

T1-weighted magnetic resonance imaging depicts low signal, and T2-weighted imaging depicts high signal, in the cyst in classic cases without hemorrhage.

Gastric duplication cysts
- **Are rare**
- **May bleed and perforate**

Imaging findings:
- **Cystic mass along greater curvature**
- **Gut signature on ultrasonograms**
- **May contain internal echoes or altered attenuation and signal characteristics from hemorrhage, infection, or proteinaceous fluid**

GASTRIC DIVERTICULA

Gastric diverticula are rare and incidental findings that occur more frequently in adults. True gastric diverticula contain all layers of the gastric wall, typically occur within a few centimeters of the esophagogastric junction, are 2 to 4 cm in size, and communicate with the gastric lumen. The partial gastric diverticulum (intramural diverticulum) is a projection of mucosa into, but not through, the muscular wall of the stomach. These two entities change shape during the UGI series when filled with barium and should be differentiated from gastric ulcers. Gastric diverticula are quite rare in children and are usually asymptomatic. In rare cases, food impaction or hemorrhage has been described in adults. Large antral partial diverticula can cause partial gastric outlet obstruction

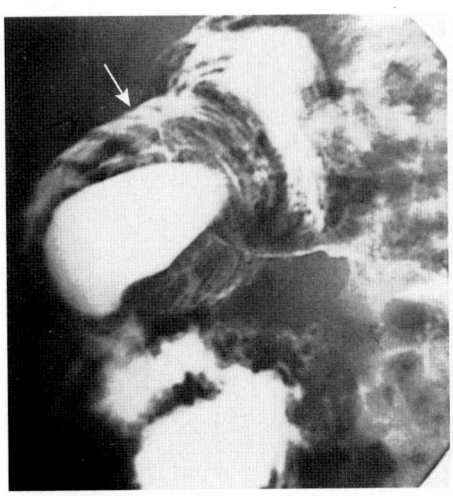 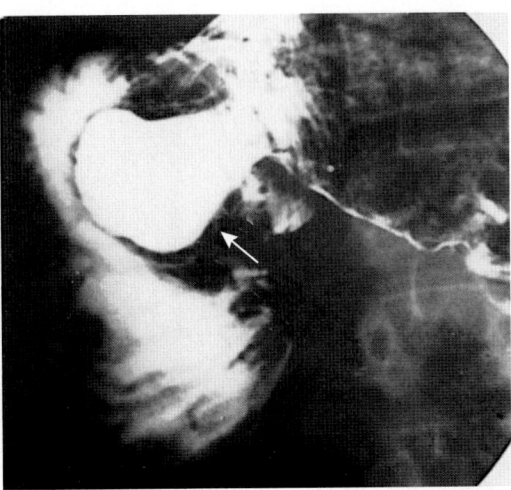

A   B

FIGURE 128-3. Gastric diverticulum. **A,** On upper gastrointestinal series, the coiled-spring appearance of intussusception is identified *(arrow).* **B,** The barium-filled diverticulum is seen to be featureless, with air-filled antrum *(arrow)* proximal to it and barium-filled duodenal sweep distal to it. The diverticulum originated at the gastroduodenal junction and was lined with gastric mucosa.

by compression or intussusception on the antropyloric region (Fig. 128-3).

MICROGASTRIA

Congenital microgastria is a rare abnormality of the pediatric gastrointestinal tract; only approximately 41 patients have been reported to date. The hallmark of the malformation is a small, tubular or saccular, midline stomach with gross gastroesophageal reflux into a megaesophagus, and failure of rotation. The lower esophageal sphincter is incompetent in most affected patients, which leads to free reflux, often complicated by tracheal aspiration and pneumonia. Agastria, or complete lack of gastric development, is the most extreme form of microgastria. Associated anomalies include malrotation and vertebral, tracheoesophageal, renal, limb, and cardiac anomalies. The association of asplenia is not surprising, in view of the development of the spleen from the dorsal mesogastrium during the fifth week of fetal life, when microgastria is thought to occur.

Clinical presentation is variable, depending on the size of the stomach and associated anomalies. The most common presentation is that of a severely ill newborn with a tiny stomach, congenital heart disease, asplenia, renal disease, and limb anomalies, such as can be seen within the VACTERL (vertebral, anal atresia, cardiac, tracheal, esophageal, renal, limb) association (see Chapter 14). Other associations include malrotation and diaphragmatic hernia. Isolated microgastria is exceedingly rare.

The milder side of the spectrum of microgastria is documented in a report of an otherwise normal 6-week-old infant presenting with stridor and presumed respiratory syncytial virus–related pneumonia, who was incidentally found to have microgastria on UGI series in the routine evaluation for gastroesophageal reflux. Only 2 of the approximately 41 patients reported to date have had isolated microgastria. Affected infants usually exhibit vomiting, feeding intolerance, respiratory infection, and malnutrition.

Chest and abdominal radiographs may demonstrate a dilated air-filled esophagus. UGI series reveals an abnormally small stomach oriented in the midsagittal plane. Gross gastroesophageal reflux into a megaesophagus is seen (Fig. 128-4).

Treatment of patients is individualized and initially conservative. In less severe cases, frequent small feedings may be tolerated. In most cases, the infant is treated with a Hunt-Lawrence pouch (double-lumen roux-en-Y jejunal pouch) to increase the size of the "gastric reservoir." After surgery, a marked decrease in the size of the esophagus may be seen, inasmuch as the megaesophagus has been shown to be the result of gastric "overflow," although gastroesophageal reflux is still present.

PYLORIC WEB, DIAPHRAGM, AND ATRESIA

The pyloric web, membrane, or diaphragm is part of a continuum of thin circumferential mucosal septa composed of two layers of gastric mucosa and a central core of submucosa and muscularis mucosa that protrudes into the lumen of the stomach, perpendicular to its long axis. The membrane is usually between 2 and 4 mm thick and is located within 2 cm of the pylorus in children. The size of the aperture within the web is variable, ranging from 2 to 30 mm. The variable size of the aperture may relate to the timing and onset of clinical manifestations. Apertures smaller than 1 cm are typically symptomatic earlier in life and manifest with symptoms of gastric outlet obstruction (Fig. 128-5). The pyloric web or membrane is thought to be congenital in origin, although proven cases of webs in adults secondary to peptic ulcer disease have been documented. When fluid (or barium) is trapped just distal to the membrane, the appearance on fetal ultrasonography or postnatal UGI examination may simulate a gastric "double bubble." A classic appearance on UGI series is a radiolucent band that persists throughout the study (Fig. 128-6). Tiao and associates described a patient with a web and antral muscular hypertrophy, which on UGI mimicked pyloric stenosis, but the child was 3 years old. Ultrasound study of a pyloric web after administration of water reveals four characteristics described by Chew: an echogenic, diaphragm-like structure in the antropyloric region; gastric dilatation; delay in gastric emptying; and

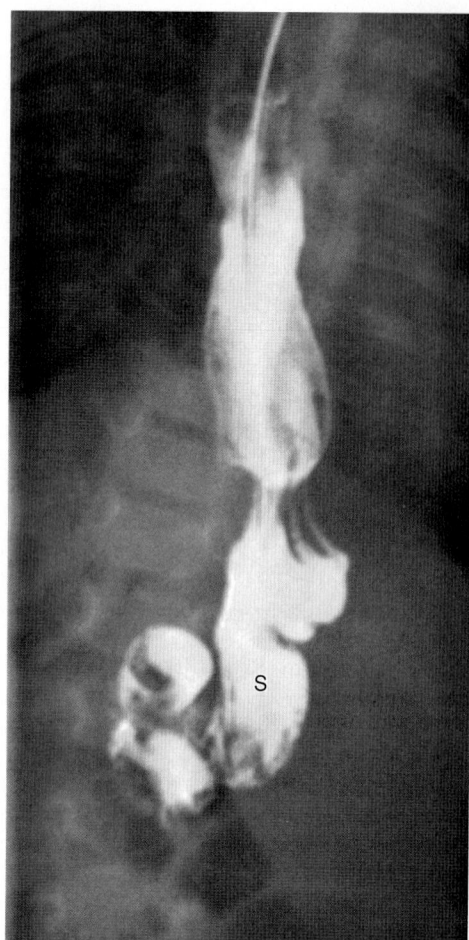

FIGURE 128-4. Microgastria. Frontal chest view, which includes the upper abdomen from an upper gastrointestinal series performed with a nasogastric tube, demonstrates a small midline stomach (S) with grossly patent gastroesophageal junction and megaesophagus. The patient also has malrotation of the bowel.

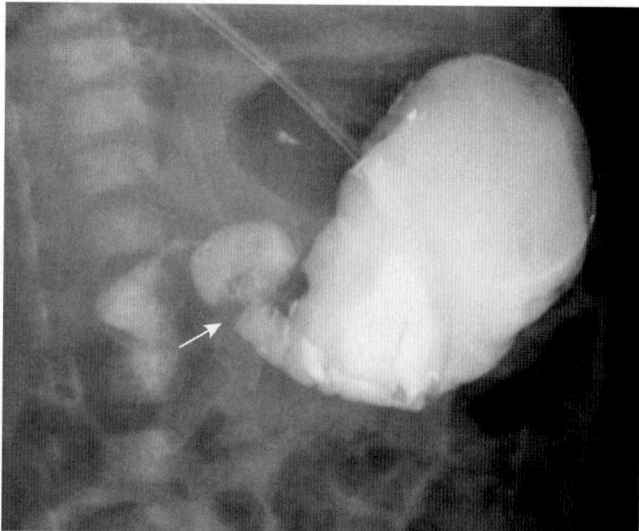

FIGURE 128-5. Pyloric web in an infant who presented with vomiting since birth. Introduction of barium via nasogastric tube demonstrates circular band or indentations in the distal antrum (*arrow*). Endoscopy demonstrated a pyloric web. (Courtesy of Dr. Stuart C. Morrison, Cleveland, Ohio.)

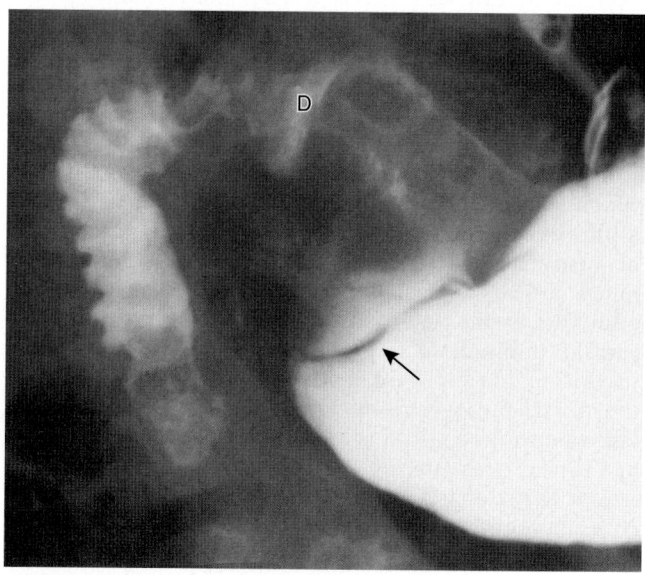

FIGURE 128-6. Antropyloric web. Spot image from upper gastrointestinal series demonstrated barium in the antrum with a thin radiolucent band (*arrow*) representing a web in an older child who presented with long history of intermittent vomiting. D, duodenal bulb.

a normal pylorus. Endoscopy confirms the diagnosis, and, depending on the size of the membrane, the patient may be treated with endoscopic transection or laser lysis of the diaphragm or web; surgical intervention may be necessary.

Pyloric atresia, or complete obliteration of the pylorus, is extremely rare. It is most often associated with epidermolysis bullosa, an autosomal recessive disease with heterogeneous presentation of blistering skin lesions occurring at birth or within the first several years of life. Indirect immunofluorescence study of the affected skin provides prognostic information. Lethal forms of the disease are associated with complete negative staining for integrin β4. Prenatally, this disease has been suggested in affected families when polyhydramnios in association with gastric distention is present. The amniotic fluid during second trimester has characteristic "snowflake" particles, suggestive of this entity.

GASTRIC VOLVULUS

Gastric volvulus is an uncommon condition of which two types have been described (Fig. 128-7). As mentioned previously, the stomach is fixed by four ligaments that represent peritoneal folds. If the stomach is not fixed properly, it can rotate along an axis perpendicular to its long axis, so that the pylorus comes to lie superiorly. This is known as *mesenteroaxial* volvulus and is associated with eventration of the left hemidiaphragm (Fig. 128-8). There may be obstruction of both the gastric inlet and gastric outlet. Plain radiographs of the chest and abdomen reveal a large distended stomach below an elevated left hemidiaphragm.

The stomach may also rotate around its long axis, a condition known as *organoaxial* volvulus. This is most

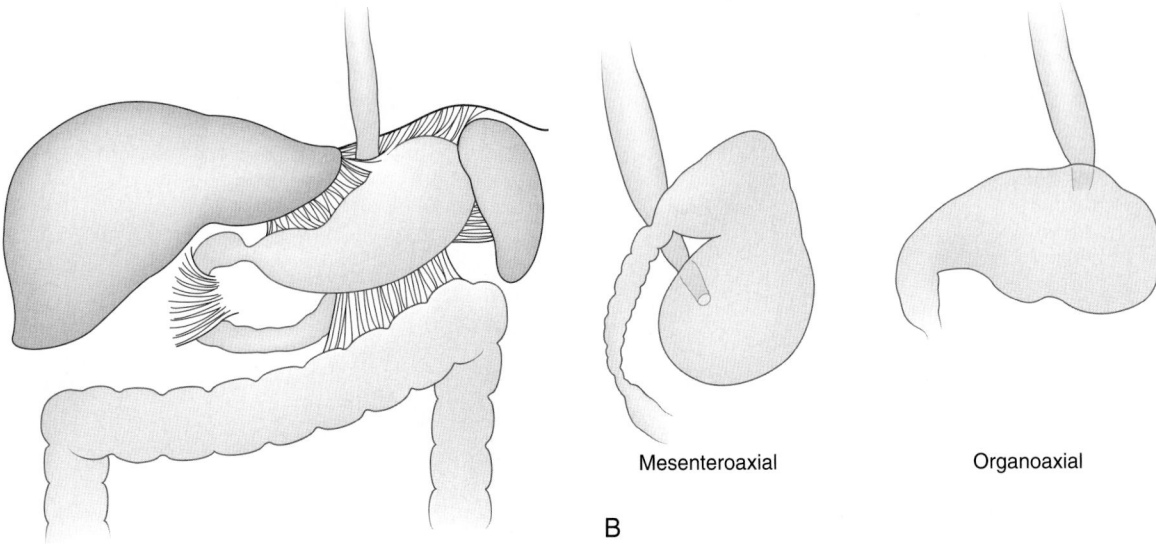

FIGURE 128-7. Gastric fixation. **A,** This drawing demonstrates the anatomic attachments of the stomach at the esophagogastric junction through the diaphragmatic hiatus and the retroperitoneal portion of the duodenum, as well as ligamentous fixation at the gastrohepatic, gastrophrenic, gastrocolic, and gastrosplenic ligaments. **B,** Rotation of the stomach about the short axis results in mesenteroaxial volvulus, and rotation of the stomach about the long axis results in organoaxial volvulus.

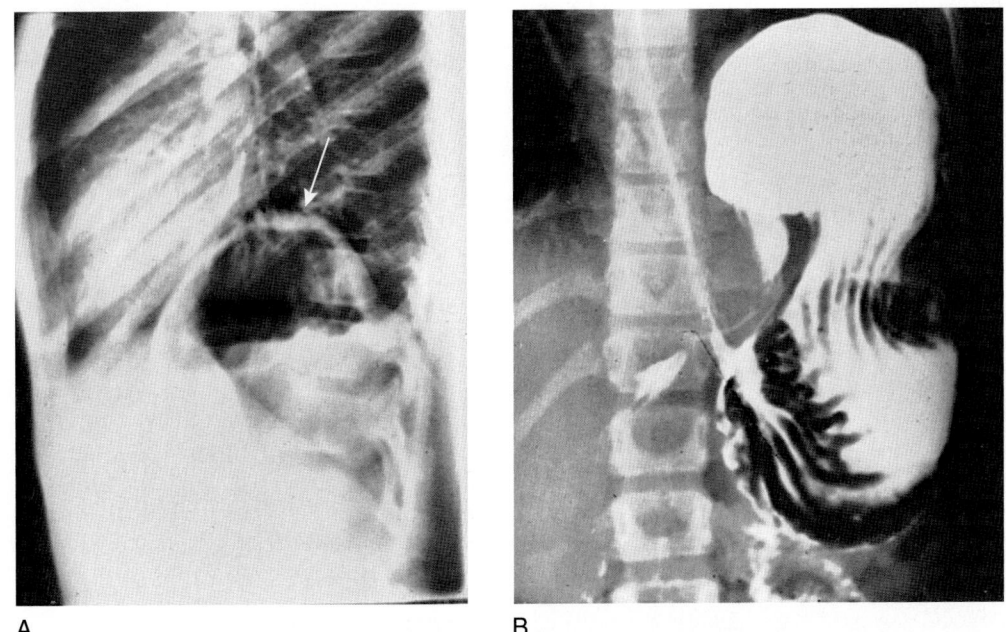

FIGURE 128-8. Mesenteroaxial volvulus in a 7-year-old girl with abdominal pain and distention. **A,** Lateral chest radiograph demonstrates eventration of the left diaphragm (*arrow*). **B,** Frontal radiograph from the upper gastrointestinal series demonstrates the gastroesophageal junction to be normal to slightly low in position. The pylorus has flipped superiorly and is now higher than the gastroesophageal junction. At surgery, the volvulus was easily reduced, and the diaphragmatic eventration was repaired. (Courtesy of Dr. V. Condon, Salt Lake City, UT.)

commonly seen in association with large hiatal hernias, particularly of the paraesophageal type. Of the two types of gastric volvulus, the mesenteroaxial type represents a true emergency because the twist can compromise the blood supply to the stomach. Organoaxial volvulus is much less common and may, in fact, be chronic in nature. UGI examination is usually necessary to make the diagnosis of organoaxial volvulus. Uc and colleagues described a patient with both gastric volvulus and wandering spleen, both of which are caused by anomalous intraperitoneal visceral attachments. Horst and associates reported a 3-month-old with a large congenital diaphragmatic hernia and tension gastrothorax without volvulus (Fig. 128-9). This entity is included in this section as it may be a life-threatening emergency and associated with volvulus.

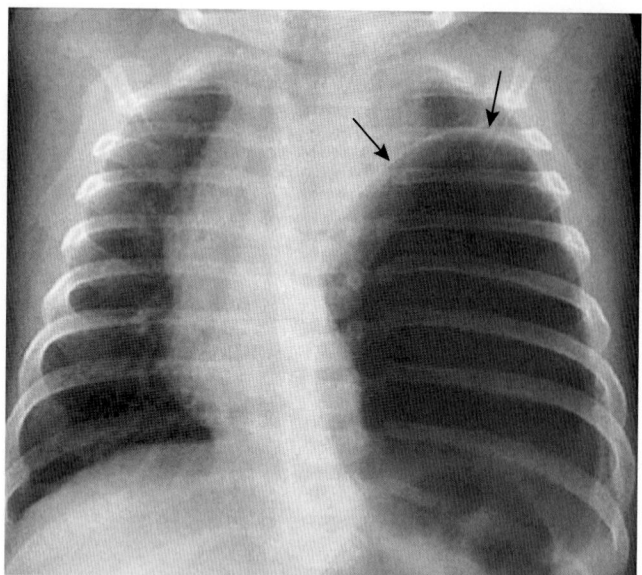

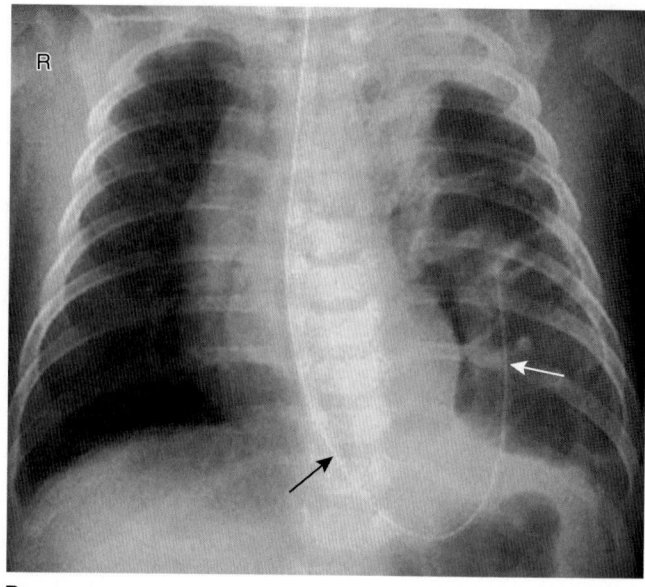

A

B

FIGURE 128-9. Tension gastrothorax. **A,** Massively distended stomach (*arrows*) in the left hemithorax is displacing the mediastinum to the right, causing moderate respiratory distress in a 3-month-old boy. The left diaphragm is not identified. **B,** Insertion of a nasogastric tube (*arrows*) caused prompt decompression of the intrathoracic stomach and prompt resolution of respiratory symptoms. (From Horst M, Sacher P, Molz G, et al: Tension gastrothorax. Pediatr Surg 2005;40:1501.)

FIGURE 128-10. Ectopic pancreas in a teenage girl with chronic vomiting. Air contrast upper gastrointestinal series demonstrates a small mass in the pylorus with central umbilication, proven at surgery to represent ectopic pancreas (*arrowhead*). Annular pancreas/duodenal stenosis was also diagnosed, as demonstrated by narrowing along the second portion of the duodenum, also confirmed at surgery (*arrow*).

- **Mesenteroaxial volvulus represents a true emergency because ischemia of the stomach may occur.**
- **Organoaxial volvulus is much less common and may be chronic.**

ECTOPIC PANCREAS

Ectopic pancreas (Fig. 128-10) is an uncommon anomaly in which pancreatic tissue is found in the antropyloric region or, less commonly, in the duodenum or proximal jejunum and more distally in the bowel. Typically, ectopic pancreas is an incidental finding, but symptoms such as pain, gastrointestinal bleeding, or obstruction occasionally occur. Gastroduodenal prolapse has also been reported. Typically, on UGI series, an intramural mound of tissue is seen projecting into the barium-filled lumen. The mass is umbilicated, and a central niche representing an attempt at duct formation may be seen. This entity can also be identified sonographically, although it is most often described at endoscopy. On computed tomography, it can be identified as a localized thickening of the gastric wall, at times with increased enhancement and thickening of the overlying mucosa, best seen with "negative" oral contrast, such as water.

SUGGESTED READINGS

Gastric Duplication Cysts

Barlev DM, Weinberg G: Acute gastrointestinal hemorrhage in infancy from gastric duplication: imaging findings. Emerg Radiol 2004;10:204-206

Camoglio FS, Forestieri C, Zanatta C: Complete pancreatic ectopia in a gastric duplication cyst: a case report and review of the literature. Eur J Pediatr Surg 2004;14:60-62

Fitzgerald JF, Riccardo, Harnsberger JK: Clinical quiz: Gastric duplication on CT scan. J Pediatr Gastroenterol 2000;31:553-571

Ford WDA, Guelfand M, Lopez PJ: Laparoscopic excision of a gastric duplication cyst detected on antenatal ultrasound scan. J Pediatr Surg 2004;39:e8-e10

Kumar R, Tripathi M, Chandrashekar N: Diagnosis of ectopic gastric mucosa using [99]Tcm-pertechnetate: spectrum of scintigraphic findings. Br J Radiol 2005;78:714-720

Master V, Woods RH, Morris LL, Freeman: Gastric duplication cyst causing gastric outlet obstruction. Pediatric Radiol 2004;34:574-576

Ratan SK, Ratan J, Lohan A: Unusual presentation of gastric duplication cyst in a neonate with pneumoperitoneum and vertebral anomalies. Am J Perinatol 2002;19:361-365

Gastric Diverticula

Bhattacharya K: Gastric diverticulum—"Double pylorus" appearance. J Min Access Surg 2005;1:39.

Flacks K, Stelman HH, Matsumoto PJH: Partial gastric diverticula. Am J Roentgenol Radium Ther Nucl Med 1965;94:339-342

Keet AD: Partial or intramural gastric diverticulum. *In* Keet AD: The Pyloric Sphincteric Cylinder in Health and Disease. PLiG 1998;100; available at http://med.plig.org/22/100/about.html

Microgastria

Chandra Sharma S, Menon P: Congenital microgastria with esophageal stenosis and diaphragmatic hernia. Pediatr Surg Int 2005;21:292-294

Herman TE, Siegel MJ: Asplenia syndrome with congenital microgastria and malrotation. J Perinatol 2004;24:50-52

Kroes EJ, Festen C: Congenital microgastria: a case report and review of literature. Pediatr Surg Int 1998;13:416-418

Waasdorp CE, Rooks V, Sullivan C: Congenital microgastria presenting as stridor. Pediatr Radiol 2003;33:662-663

Pyloric Web, Diaphragm, and Atresia

Bronsther B, Nadeau MR, Abrams MW: Congenital pyloric atresia: a report of three cases and review of the literature. Surgery 1971;69:130-136

Chew AL, Friedwald JP, Donovan C: Diagnosis of congenital antral web by ultrasound. Pediatr Radiol 1992;22:342-343

De Jenlis Sicot B, Deruelle P, Kacet N: Prenatal findings in epidermolysis bullosa with pyloric atresia in a family not known to be at risk. Ultrasound Obstet Gynecol 2005;25:607-609

Felson B, Berkman YM, Hoyumpa AM: Gastric mucosal diaphragm. Radiology 1969;92:513-517

Keet AD: Congenital anomalies. *In* Keet AD: The Pyloric Sphincteric Cylinder in Health and Disease. PLiG 1998;98; available at http://med.plig.org/21/98/about.html

Orense M, Garcia Hernandez JB, Celorio C, et al: Pyloric atresia associated with epidermolysis bullosa. Pediatr Radiol 1987;17:435

Tiao M, Ko S, Hsieh C: Antral web associated with distal antral hypertrophy and prepyloric stenosis mimicking hypertrophic pyloric stenosis. World J Gastroenterol 2005;11:609-611

Gastric Volvulus

Campbell JB, Rappaport LN, Skerket LB: Acute mesentero-axial volvulus of the stomach. Radiology 1972;103:153-156

Horst M, Sacher P, Molz G, et al: Tension gastrothorax. J Pediatr Surg 2005;40:1500-1504

Uc A, Kao SC, Sanders KD: Gastric volvulus and wandering spleen. Am J Gastroenterol 1998;93:1146

Ziprkowski MN, Teele RL: Gastric volvulus in childhood. Am J Gastroenterol 1979;132:921-925

Ectopic Pancreas

Allison JW, Johnson JF, Barr LL, et al: Induction of gastroduodenal prolapse by antral heterotopic pancreas. Pediatr Radiol 1995;25:50-51

Eklof O, Lassrich A, Stanley P, et al: Ectopic pancreas. Pediatr Radiol 1973;1:24-27

Hayes-Jordan A, Idowu O, Cohen R: Ectopic pancreas as the cause of gastric outlet obstruction in a newborn. Pediatr Radiol 1998;28:868

Kilman WJ, Berk RN: The spectrum of radiographic features of aberrant pancreatic rests involving the stomach. Radiology 1977;123:291-296

Matsushita M, Hajiro K, Okazaki K, et al: Gastric aberrant pancreas: EUS analysis in comparison with the histology. Gastrointest Endosc 1999;49:493-497

Cho J-S, Shin K-S, Kwon S-T, et al. Heterotopic pancreas in the stomach: CT findings. Radiology 2000;217:139-144

129

Hypertrophic Pyloric Stenosis

MARILYN J. GOSKE and ALAN E. SCHLESINGER

Hypertrophic pyloric stenosis (HPS) is a common entity in young infants, characterized by hypertrophy of the circular muscle and narrowing of the antropyloric canal (channel), caused in part by crowded and edematous mucosa within the lumen (Fig. 129-1). Hypervascularity of the hypertrophied muscle and mucosa is also seen. The resultant gastric outlet obstruction leads to intractable vomiting, typically described as projectile.

HPS is the most common cause of gastric outlet obstruction and the most common condition necessitating surgery in the first few months of life. HPS affects 2.5% to 3% of liveborn infants in the United States and 2 to 5 per 1000 liveborn infants per year worldwide, depending on geographic area. HPS is less common in children of African-American and Asian descent, with a frequency of one third to one fifth that in white infants of European extraction. Although the age of the child at the onset of symptoms is usually 3 weeks to 3 months, HPS has been described in the first week of life and occasionally in older children. The disease is unusual in premature infants. The incidence of HPS in boys is approximately four times that in girls. In the United States, 80% to 85% of affected patients are boys. There is a positive family history in 5% to 7% of cases, with increased incidence of HPS in infants whose mothers had a diagnosis of the condition. There is also an increased incidence of pyloric stenosis in twin siblings of affected patients. Firstborns seem to be more affected than their younger siblings.

ETIOLOGY

The cause of this intriguing disease is unknown. A genetic component in the etiology of this disease is well established, but the precise genetic locus has not been determined. The pathophysiology seems to be one of work hypertrophy of the circular muscle of the pylorus, as if under constant stimulation. The mucosa also becomes markedly hypertrophied, sometimes simulating a polypoid mass (Fig. 129-2). Although various theories about the cause of this work hypertrophy have been put forward, none has been proven. Hernanz-Schulman

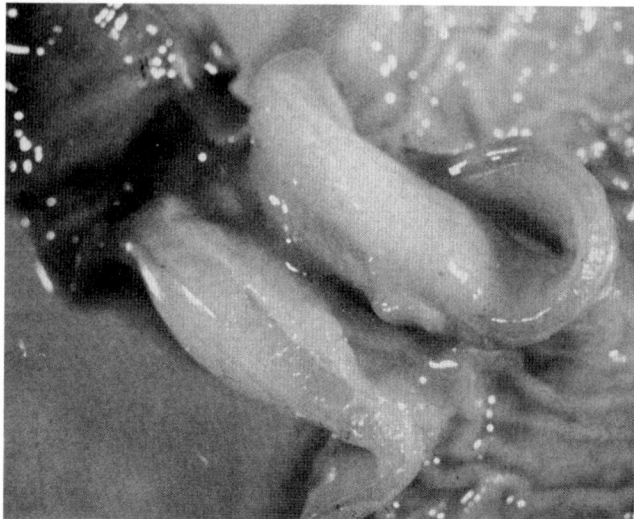

FIGURE 129-1. The morbid anatomic changes in hypertrophic pyloric stenosis. Pathologic section of antropyloric junction from an infant who died as a result of pyloric stenosis. The specimen shows thickening of the pyloric muscle between the base of the duodenal cap and the more proximal antrum and thickening of the mucosa, which fills and obstructs the canal. (Courtesy of Marta Hernanz-Schulman, MD, Nashville, TN. Adapted from Kissane J: Stomach and duodenum. In Pathology of Infancy and Childhood. St. Louis, CV Mosby, 1975:175-178.)

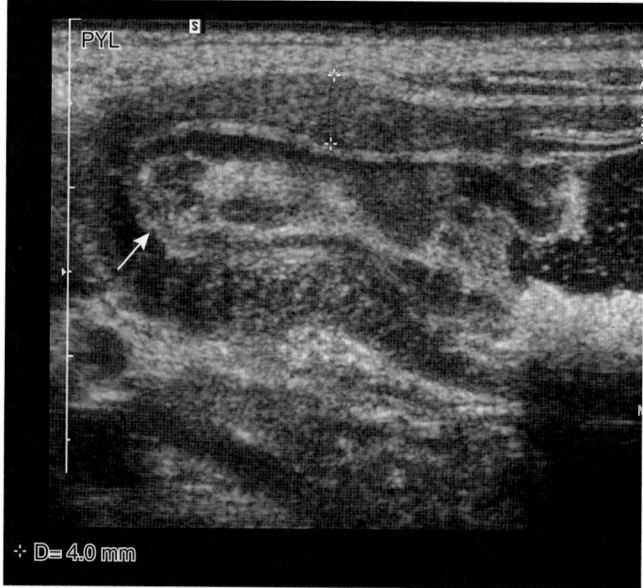

FIGURE 129-2. Hypertrophic pyloric stenosis in a 4-month-old. Scan through the length of the canal shows marked muscle hypertrophy (calipers), as well as mucosal redundancy (arrow).

and colleagues in reporting increased vascularity to the pylorus summarized some of the current thinking on the pathogenesis of HPS: "The thickened muscle is depleted of inhibitory peptides such as vasoactive polypeptide; of synaptic vesicles, presynaptic terminals and neural cell adhesion molecules; of markers for enteric glia; of interstitial cell of Cajal and of nitric oxide synthase activity at the messenger RNA level, with increases in insulin-like and platelet-derived growth factors." They discussed the possible role of increased vascular flow seen in the hypertrophied muscle and mucosa and proposed that the increased vascularity may "conceivably represent an integral component of the changes that occur with HPS."

Harald Hirschsprung, when originally describing the entity, assumed that this disease was congenital in nature. However, HPS is now believed to represent an acquired disease, developing over the first few weeks of life, possibly in response to feeding. Weiskittel and associates reported two cases of evolving HPS in which normal upper gastrointestinal (UGI) series was followed 1 to 2 weeks later by ultrasound findings diagnostic of HPS. Rollins and coworkers examined 1400 neonates with normal ultrasound findings at birth; in 9, pyloric stenosis later developed. These findings lend credence to the belief that the disease evolves over a course of days to weeks. There are case reports of the diagnosis of HPS suggested on prenatal ultrasound studies, secondary to observation of a dilated, fluid-filled stomach and polyhydramnios. Singh and colleagues suggested that HPS could start antenatally with a congenital disturbance of gastropyloric muscular physiology. However, in their patient, despite the subjective prenatal diagnosis of gastric hyperperistalsis and polyhydramnios, HPS did not develop until the time of a second ultrasound study, on day 19 of life.

In addition to classic HPS, there may a "secondary" form of pyloric stenosis, as proposed by Callahan and associates. Latchaw and coworkers described three older infants in whom classical pyloric stenosis developed after prolonged transpyloric jejunal feeding tube placement, which suggests that the late manifestation of HPS may have been related directly to the presence of the partially obstructing feeding tubes. Other reports of HPS in association with congenital webs, prostaglandin-induced foveolar hyperplasia, eosinophilic gastroenteritis, and antral polyps lend credence to the "work hypertrophy" theory of HPS in predisposed patients.

CLINICAL FINDINGS

Infants with HPS typically present with a history of nonbilious vomiting that is initially mild and is often interpreted as gastroesophageal reflux with excessive "spitting up." Careful history often reveals that the vomiting started relatively soon after birth, although the child may not have received medical attention until 3 weeks of age or older. In the classic case, as the relative degree of obstruction increases, the vomiting ultimately becomes projectile. This forceful vomiting may relate to the hypertrophied pyloric muscle or to the progressive gastric outlet obstruction over time. In patients with undiagnosed disease, protracted vomiting eventually leads to a hypo-

chloremic metabolic alkalosis, dehydration, malnutrition, and death, which is seldom seen today. In 1999, Papadakis and colleagues emphasized the changing pattern of presentation of HPS, with no evidence of metabolic abnormality in 90% of infants, and suggested that the increased availability of ultrasonography may be a factor in earlier diagnosis. Approximately 5% of the patients have mild jaundice, secondary to diminished hepatic glucuronyl transferase activity in the presence of starvation.

DIAGNOSIS

Physical examination is often diagnostic. Classically, in thin infants, peristaltic waves may be seen on the abdominal wall, progressing from the left upper quadrant across the epigastrium. The hypertrophied pyloric muscle mass is described as an "olive" or pyloric pseudotumor (Fig. 129-3). An experienced examiner, typically a pediatric surgeon or pediatrician, may palpate it in the midepigastrium. If the olive is palpated by the experienced surgeon, the patient may proceed to surgery without imaging. However, with the ease and accuracy of ultrasound evaluation of pyloric stenosis, there has been a definite trend toward reliance on imaging rather than clinical history and physical examination. In one large children's hospital, the introduction of a clinical guideline to proceed directly for surgical evaluation did not result in a decrease in imaging volume, as might have been anticipated. Although some authorities have lamented the documented loss of clinical skills in the evaluation of this entity and have argued that imaging increases the financial cost of the workup of HPS, ultrasound diagnosis is rapid, noninvasive, and highly accurate.

Some experts have advocated the UGI series as the first examination in patients with symptoms of HPS, for two reasons: although ultrasonography may be quite accurate in the diagnosis of HPS, it is not always diagnostic in infants with vomiting from other causes, and

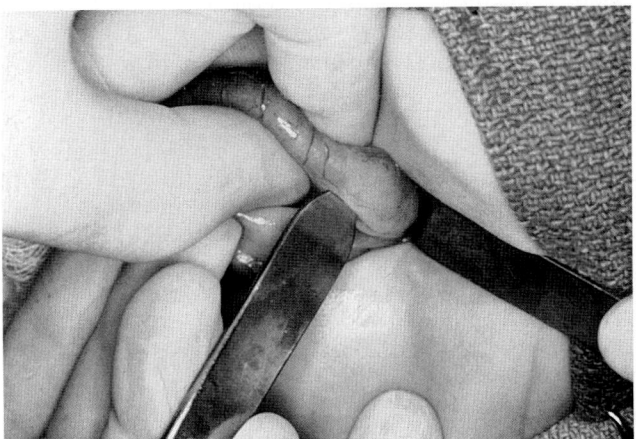

FIGURE 129-3. Intraoperative photograph of infant with hypertrophic pyloric stenosis. The surgeon is demonstrating the "olive" caused by the muscular hypertrophy of the pylorus. This is what the clinician would palpate on physical examination through the abdominal wall. (*See color plate.*) (Courtesy of Frederick Alexander, MD, Cleveland, Ohio.)

UGI examination is deemed by some experts to be more cost effective as the first imaging examination than ultrasonography, inasmuch as a follow-up UGI series may be requested for up to 50% of patients after negative ultrasound findings. An "ultrasonography first" approach has other benefits, such as no radiation, better patient and parental acceptance, and lack of oral contrast material. We recommend ultrasonography as the first imaging study in patients with nonpalpable olives if the clinician wishes to distinguish between HPS and gastroesophageal reflux *and* will treat reflux empirically if the ultrasound findings are negative. If the referring clinician wishes to document or quantitate reflux and the ultrasound findings are negative, such documentation can be performed with UGI examination or scintigraphy, as clinically indicated in the individual patient.

Ultrasonography

Ultrasonography is performed typically with linear transducers with a frequency of 7.5 MHz or higher. We start our examination with a 10-MHz transducer and frequently increase the transducer frequency once the pylorus is found and if depth of penetration is adequate. We start the examination by talking with the parents and inquiring about the history of vomiting, weight loss or lack of weight gain, and positive family history of HPS. We inquire as to when the last meal was given, type of meal (breast milk versus formula), and when the child last vomited. The time of the last feeding may be annotated on the image. The examination is started with the patient in the supine position. The transducer is placed transversely near the left lobe of the liver and the esophagogastric junction. The normal thickness of the wall of the lesser curvature is then noted (2 mm or less) and the volume of retained material in the stomach is documented (Fig. 129-4). Although a large volume of retained fluid is consistent with gastric outlet obstruction, frequent vomiting may empty the stomach in a minority of patients. The typical gray scale appearance of the hypertrophied pylorus is one of retained material within the stomach, with a rather abrupt change to increased muscle thickness at the antropyloric junction, just proximal to the duodenal cap, and variable thickening of the mucosa filling the antropyloric lumen (see Fig. 129-4). If the stomach is empty, or if there is difficulty in identifying the pylorus, the child may be given fluid such as Pedialyte (Fig. 129-5). With the patient in the supine or right posterior oblique position, the examiner follows the stomach to the duodenal cap, thus identifying the pylorus; typically, the pylorus is found just medial to the gallbladder, anterior to the right kidney. Even if air- or barium-filled bowel obscures the pylorus, the pylorus can often be visualized by using the liver as an acoustic window. Sargent and associates described a posterior approach in which the patient is placed prone and scanned from a right posterior direction although we have not found this necessary. Care should be taken not to mistake the gastric antrum for the pylorus; we identify the duodenum on the ultrasonogram to ensure that the correct region (pylorus) is evaluated. When the stomach is markedly distended as a result of retained secretions, the pylorus may "fold" posteriorly (Fig. 129-6). In this instance, placing the child in the left posterior oblique position may improve visualization of the pylorus. Images of the pylorus should be obtained in both transverse and longitudinal projections.

Much emphasis has been placed on the measurements used to diagnose pyloric stenosis. These are certainly helpful and necessary, but they can be confusing because they vary among patients, and even in the same patient. Although an experienced examiner can frequently make the diagnosis by qualitative assessment of the thickness of the pyloric wall and length of the abnormal pyloric channel, great interest has been focused on trying to determine accurate measurements of the pyloric muscle thickness, pyloric muscle length, and length of the pyloric channel. Like Cohen and coworkers, we emphasize that pylorospasm may appear to mimic HPS in both appearance and measurement if the examination is performed quickly. Evaluation of the patient in real time to obtain a "fluoroscopic" look at the stomach is very important. In pylorospasm, the pylorus may initially demonstrate thickened pyloric musculature, retained secretions, and even abnormal measurements as a result of transient muscular contraction. Patients with pylorospasm, however, demonstrate a change in shape of the pylorus with observation (Fig. 129-7). In contrast, intermittent observation over 10 to 15 minutes in patients with HPS fails to demonstrate relaxation of the pylorus. The shape of the pyloric mass remains elongated and thickened, the lumen remains filled with mucosa, and the muscle mass remains parallel, without relaxation to allow significant gastric contents to pass. In patients with HPS, mucosal hypertrophy and increased vascularity of the pyloric musculature typically are identified (Fig. 129-8).

In order to perform pyloric measurements accurately, the pylorus must be imaged carefully and properly. A linear transducer appropriately focused is very important. On the transverse scans, the hypertrophied pylorus appears as a doughnut, with the relatively sonolucent hypertrophied muscle surrounding the more echogenic luminal mucosa (Fig. 129-9). Although asymmetry in the "doughnut" is sometimes seen, careful positioning usually reveals a high degree of symmetry. The sonolucent ring of hypertrophied muscle may sometimes appear nonuniform on the transverse scan. Typically, the near and far fields appear more echogenic than the sides. Spevak and colleagues demonstrated this to be secondary to the anisotropic effect of the sound waves encountering the circular muscle fibers in a perpendicular orientation in the near and far fields and in a more tangential orientation laterally. On longitudinal scans, the hypertrophied muscle should be of equal thickness on both sides of the thickened, echogenic, and typically hyperemic central mucosa.

The pyloric muscle thickness should be measured on both transverse and longitudinal scans, and these measurements should be in close agreement. The boundary between the antrum and pyloric muscle can usually be identified, with an appearance similar to that seen on barium studies (described later). The length of the pyloric muscle can then be measured (Fig. 129-10). Because the

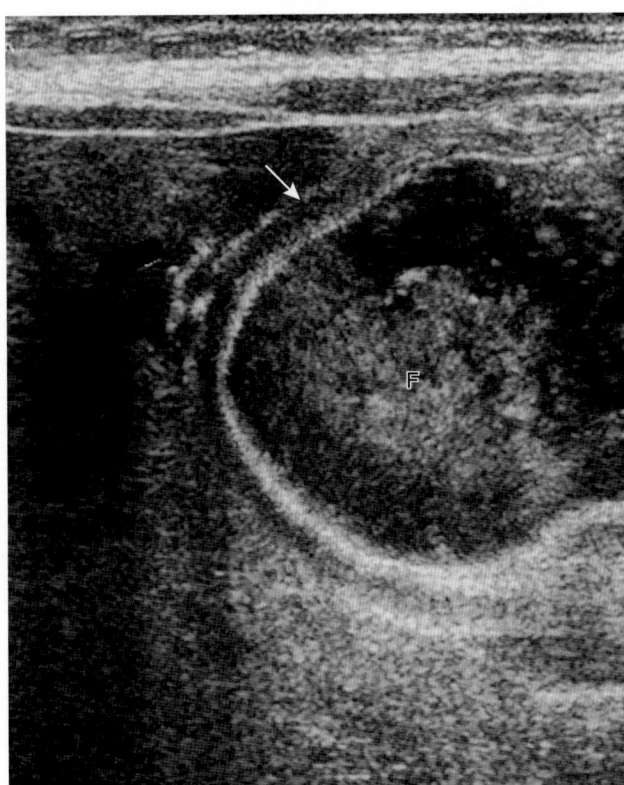

A

B

FIGURE 129-4. Hypertrophic pyloric stenosis (HPS). **A,** Sagittal ultrasound image through the body of the stomach in a child with HPS. Note the sonolucent muscle in the wall of the stomach (*arrow*). There is retained formula (F) in the stomach as a result of partial gastric outlet obstruction from HPS. **B.** Ultrasonogram (**left**) and labeled ultrasound image (**right**) in a patient with HPS. The stomach was filled with retained fluid. The normal gastric wall (G) thickness was 2 mm or less. The pyloric muscle (P) thickening is well seen adjacent to the thickened mucosa. Note the difference in mucosal thickness from normal stomach in the antrum in comparison with the pylorus. D, duodenal cap. (Courtesy of Omar Lababede, MD, Cleveland, Ohio.)

pylorus may be curved, the pylorus may be measured through a "trace" method, which may be more accurate. Keller and coworkers compared ultrasound measurements of the thickened pylorus with measurements at surgery, finding excellent correlation in each of 17 cases. The sonographic measurement was slightly smaller than the anatomic measurement in all cases.

In the original descriptions of the technique by Teele and Smith and by Blumhagen and colleagues, a measurement of pyloric wall thickness of 4 mm was judged to be the upper limit of normal. Since the initial reports, results of a number of studies have suggested that the difference between the pyloric measurements of normal and abnormal patients was somewhat smaller than originally anticipated. Stunden and associates studied 200 consecutive infants with persistent vomiting and determined measurements for overall diameter of the pylorus, thickness of the pyloric muscle, and length of the pyloric canal. Although there was a statistically significant difference in all measurements between the

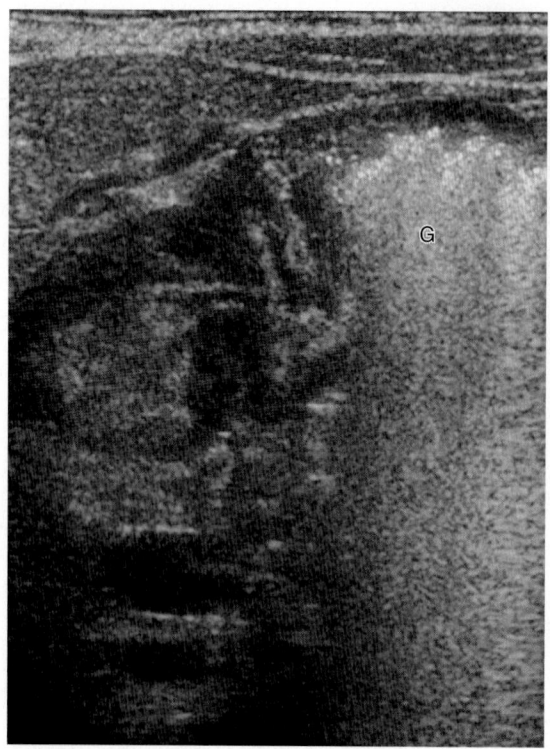

A

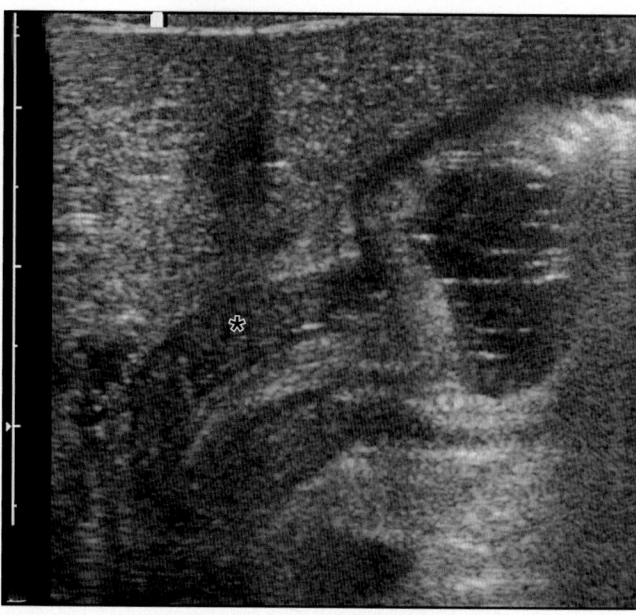

B

FIGURE 129-5. Hypertrophic pyloric stenosis. **A,** Initial transverse scan was suboptimal as a result of shadowing gas (G) and lack of fluid in the stomach. **B,** Ten minutes after dextrose solution was given, the pyloric muscle (*asterisk*) was better seen, and the canal length was easier to evaluate.

normal infants and those with pyloric stenosis, there was a very small overlap between normal and abnormal in diameter and muscle wall thickness. It is possible that some of the patients without HPS may have had pylorospasm. However, there was complete distinction between the two groups in channel length. Blumhagen and colleagues performed a similar study on 319 infants, in whom they measured the thickness of the pyloric muscle, the length of the pyloric muscle, and the length of the pyloric channel. In their study, there was significant overlap between normal and abnormal in measurement of channel length, less overlap in measurement of muscle length, and no overlap in measurement of muscle thickness. The actual values from both studies are given in Table 129-1.

O'Keefe and colleagues studied antropyloric muscle wall thickness in 145 infants with vomiting or regurgitation. All infants with measurements of 3 mm or more had pyloric stenosis, whereas none of the infants with measurements less than 2 mm had HPS. Of the six infants with measurements between 2.0 and 2.9 mm, two developed HPS, two had pylorospasm, and one each had milk allergy and gastritis.

Although the value of measurements of the pylorus varies from one study to another, most experienced sonographers have become very comfortable with the technique, particularly when attention is paid to the real-time aspects of the examination as emphasized earlier in this discussion. In our experience, ultrasound diagnosis of HPS has proved extremely accurate. However, the age of the patient and the duration of the patient's symptoms should be considered in the interpretation of a case of possible HPS with borderline measurements on ultrasonography, because HPS is a progressive process that

evolves with time. Therefore, a borderline measurement in a very young infant (1 to 2 weeks of age) with a very short duration of symptoms may represent very early HPS, even though the pyloric muscle thickness or pyloric canal length measurements do not meet the strict criteria for HPS. In such cases, the study can be repeated in 5 to 7 days if the patient's symptoms persist or progress. Ultrasonography has definitely been shown to improve the ability to correctly diagnose HPS in patients with nonpalpable olives. A large study in 1994 by Hernanz-Schulman and colleagues of 152 infants with suspected HPS and nonpalpable olives demonstrated 100% accuracy of sonography in categorizing the patients as normal, having HPS, or having pylorospasm. Van der Schouw and coworkers demonstrated the utility of ultrasonography when used in conjunction with clinical and laboratory data in children with suspected HPS. In a study of 105 infants with possible HPS, they analyzed the utility of history, clinical signs and symptoms, and laboratory data with and without ultrasound data. Their study demonstrated that addition of ultrasound data greatly increased the ability to predict HPS in the study group.

Swischuk and associates also pointed out the need for careful examination technique, because inaccurate placement of the transducer in a plane tangential to the wall of the normal pylorus or antrum can produce an image simulating a thickened pylorus, and an overfilled stomach with a posteriorly directed antrum may lead to a false-negative diagnosis, as discussed earlier. Other diseases that can mimic pyloric stenosis on sonographic examination are antropyloric gastritis, with or without ulcer disease, and chronic granulomatous disease of childhood.

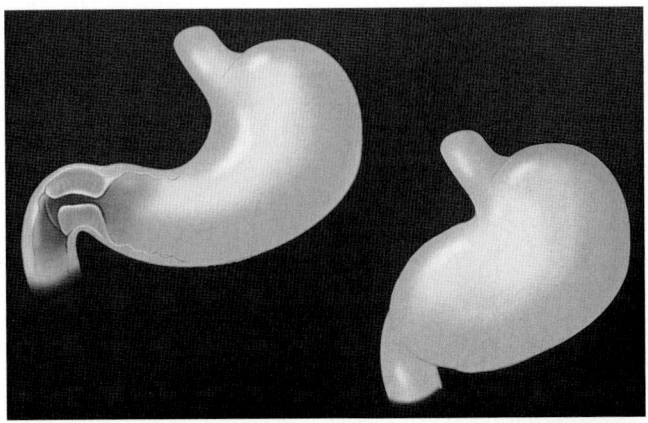

A

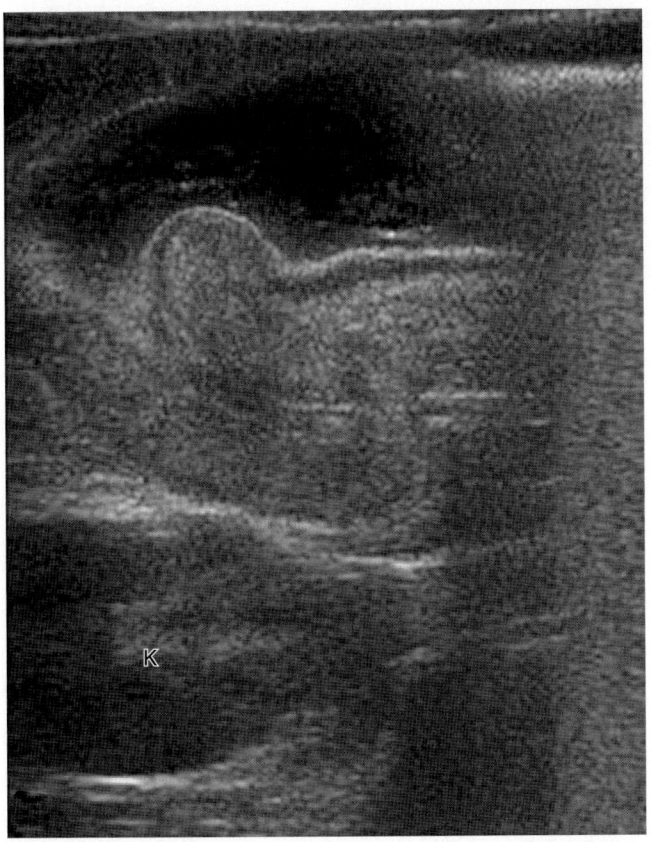

B

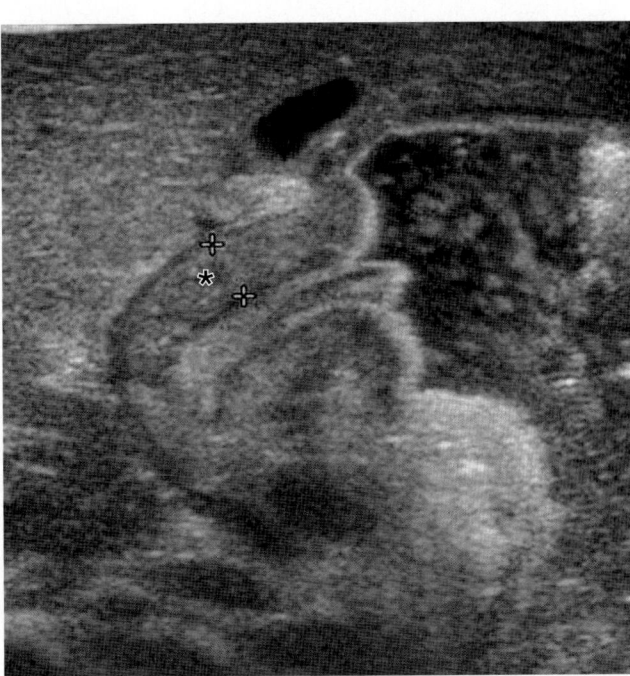

C

FIGURE 129-6. Pitfall of scanning an overdistended stomach with HPS. **A,** In the schematic illustration of the undistended stomach of an infant with HPS (**left**), the pylorus is easy to find. The schematic illustration on the **right** demonstrates the pylorus folding posteriorly as a result of a large volume of retained material, which leads to a potentially false-negative result. (*See color plate.*) **B,** Transverse image of the distal stomach in an infant with HPS demonstrates a distended, fluid-filled stomach; the hypertrophied pylorus is folded behind the distended stomach, anterior to the right kidney (K), and easy to overlook. **C.** After the patient is turned to the left posterior oblique position, the hypertrophied pylorus rises anteriorly and is much more easily detailed. *Calipers* mark the anterior width of the pyloric muscle. Note the pyloric mucosa protruding into the fluid-filled antrum (antral nipple sign). (**A,** courtesy of The Cleveland Clinic, Cleveland, Ohio. **B** and **C,** courtesy of Marta Hernanz-Schulman, MD, Nashville, TN.)

Ultrasound findings in HPS may include the following:

- **Retained gastric secretions**
- **Thickened pyloric muscle measuring ≥3 mm**
- **Fixed narrow, elongated, or curved antropyloric channel**
- **Redundant mucosa measuring ≥3 mm**
- **Hyperemia of mucosa, muscular layer, or both**

Contrast Upper Gastrointestinal Series

Before the advent of real-time ultrasound imaging, the contrast UGI series was used for diagnosis and may still be more widely used than ultrasonography by radiologists with limited pediatric sonographic experience. The UGI series is also sometimes used when ultrasonography findings are normal or equivocal. Riggs and Long described eight plain radiographic findings that are suggestive of the diagnosis when present, but we have never found an instance when an abnormal scout radiograph has precluded the need for ultrasonography or

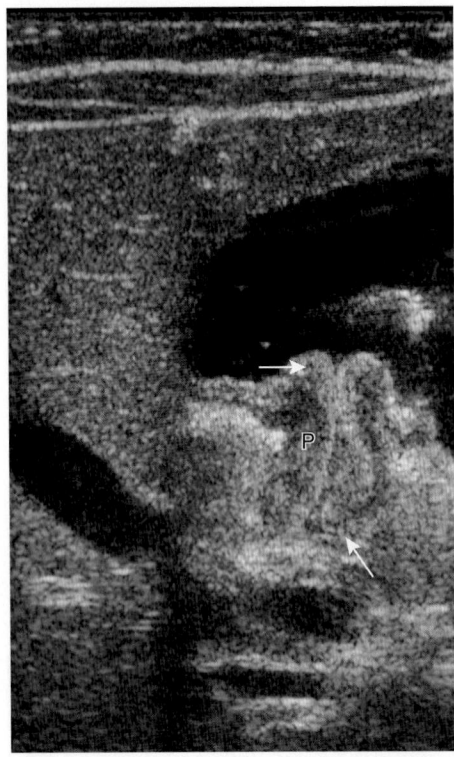

A

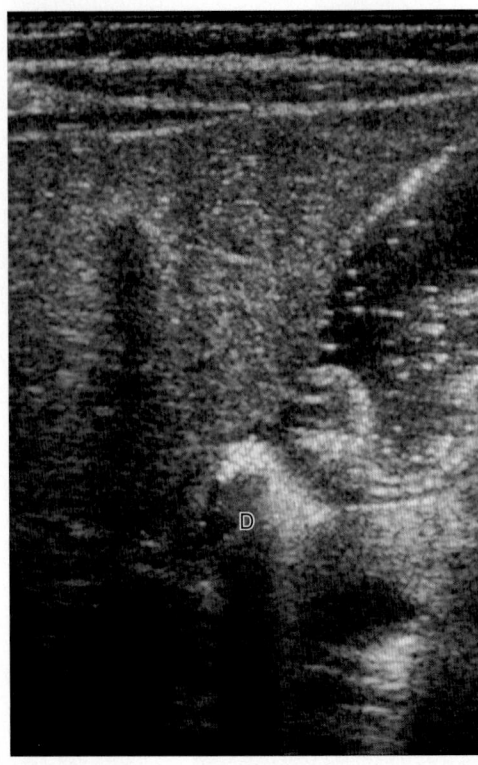

B

FIGURE 129-7. Pylorospasm simulating pyloric stenosis. **A,** Initial scan demonstrates pyloric muscle wall thickening (P) and a suggestion of an elongated canal (*arrows*). **B,** Five minutes after dextrose water was given, the pylorus changed shape, and bubbles within the water are seen freely passing through the pyloric lumen into the duodenum. Gas is also seen in the air-filled duodenal bulb (D).

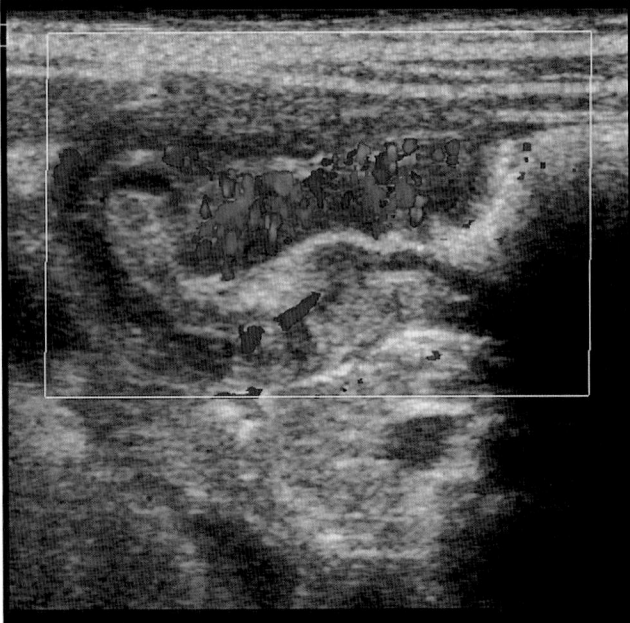

FIGURE 129-8. Color Doppler evaluation in the patient depicted in Figure 129-2 demonstrates marked hyperemia of the mucosa, as seen on this image converted to black-and-white format.

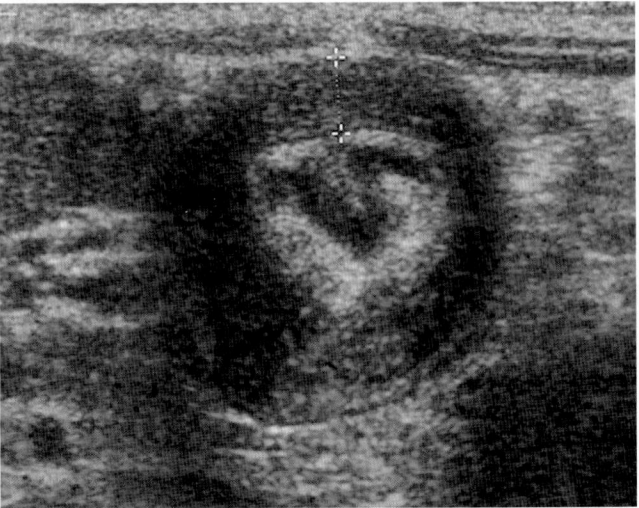

FIGURE 129-9. "Doughnut" sign of hypertrophic pyloric stenosis, in the infant imaged in Figure 129-8. The fixed circumferential thickening of the pylorus may resemble a doughnut in an image taken perpendicular to the long axis of the stomach. *Calipers* mark the anterior muscle, which measures greater than 3 mm. Thickened mucosa is seen centrally. Note that the echogenicity of the muscle perpendicular to the ultrasound beam in the near field and far field is greater than that seen in the lateral aspects of the thickened pyloric muscle.

UGI study. Indeed, the plain radiographs may appear quite normal even when HPS is present (Fig. 129-11). In rare instances, pyloric stenosis is associated with isolated gastric pneumatosis that disappears after the stomach is decompressed (Fig. 129-12).

In order to obtain a technically satisfactory UGI study, many authorities suggest that a nasogastric tube should be passed and the stomach emptied. When we use a tube, we try to place the tube in the antrum with the patient in the prone oblique position so as not to require large amounts of contrast material. Water-soluble contrast or barium is introduced via the tube under fluoroscopic control, and spot images are obtained as needed.

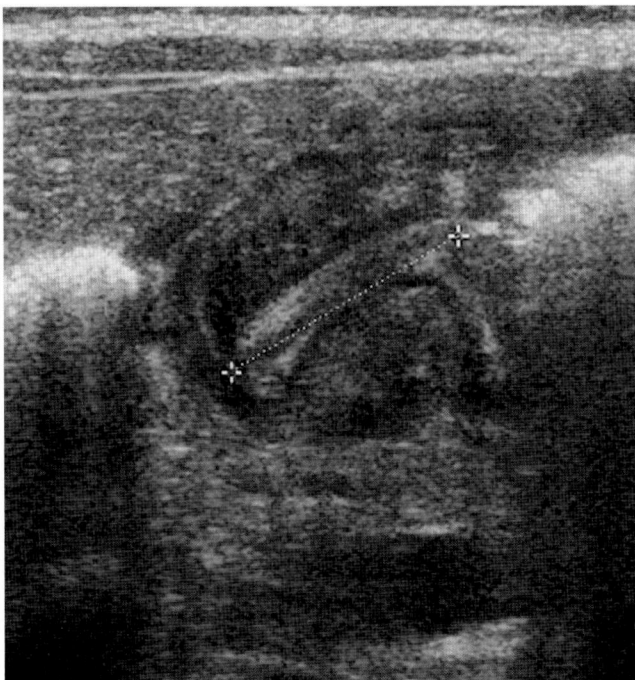

FIGURE 129-10. Difficulty in measuring channel length. This ultrasound image demonstrates the difficulty in measuring the channel length with a straight line. The pyloric channel is often curved. The trace method may aid in more accurate measurements of canal length.

TABLE 129-1

Pyloric Measurements in the Diagnosis of Hypertrophic Pyloric Stenosis (HPS)*

	Stunden et al.	Blumhagen et al.
Pyloric muscle thickness (mm)		
With HPS	3-5	3.5-6.0
Without HPS	1-3	1.0-3.1
Pyloric canal length (mm)		
With HPS	18-28	11-25
Without HPS	5-14	5-22
Pyloric muscle length (mm)		
With HPS	NA	14-29
Without HPS	NA	5.0-26.5
Pyloric diameter (mm)		
With HPS	9-19	NA
Without HPS	7-12	NA

*Data from Stunden RJ, LeQuesne GW, Little KET: The improved ultrasound diagnosis of hypertrophic pyloric stenosis. Pediatr Radiol 1986;16:200; and from Blumhagen JD, Maclin L, Krauter D, et al: Sonographic diagnosis of hypertrophic pyloric stenosis. AJR Am J Roentgenol 1988;150:1367.
NA, not assessed.

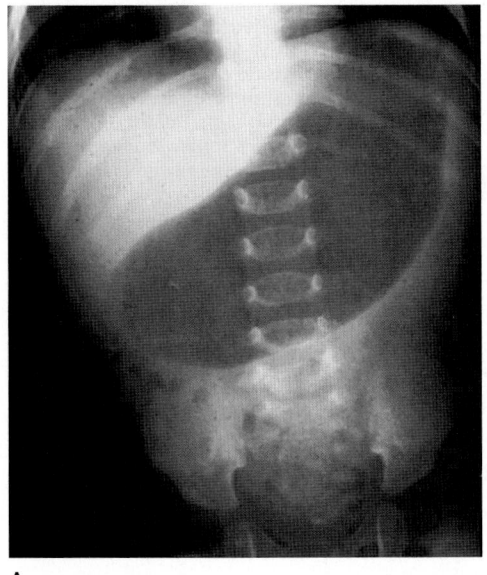

A

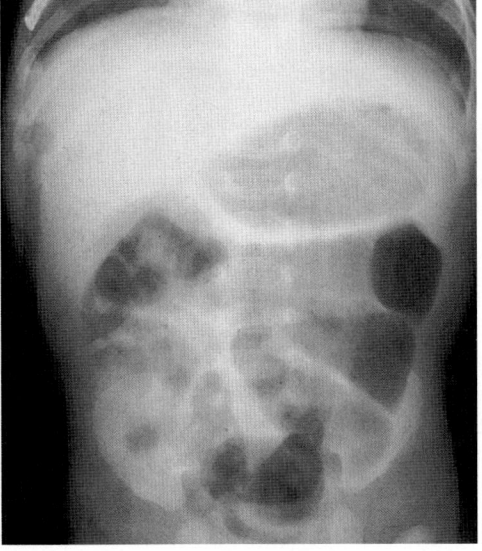

B

FIGURE 129-11. Plain radiographs in pyloric stenosis. **A,** Abdominal radiograph demonstrating marked dilatation of the stomach with little gas in the distal bowel in a patient with documented pyloric stenosis. **B,** Abdominal radiograph in a child with surgically documented pyloric stenosis, demonstrating a relatively normal-sized gastric air bubble for a crying infant and gas throughout the rest of the gastrointestinal tract, including the colon.

Most of the infants with a clinical history suggestive of HPS, both actually with and without HPS, exhibit some degree of pylorospasm. In general, contrast material finally passes the antropyloric region within 1 to 10 minutes in the normal infant, but its passage may be delayed as long as 25 minutes because of pylorospasm; spasm may mimic HPS on the contrast study. With HPS, the pyloric muscle mass pushes into the contrast material– and air-filled antrum of the stomach, enabling diagnosis. If the barium does not pass out of the stomach because of severe HPS,

an ultrasound study may be confirmatory and appears markedly abnormal even to the less experienced sonographer.

The radiographic signs of HPS on UGI series are remarkably constant from one patient to another. The pyloric channel is narrowed (the string sign) and almost always curved upward posteriorly (Fig. 129-13). Barium may be caught between folds of mucosa within the hypertrophied muscle, and parallel lines (the double string sign) may be seen (see Fig. 129-13). The enlarged

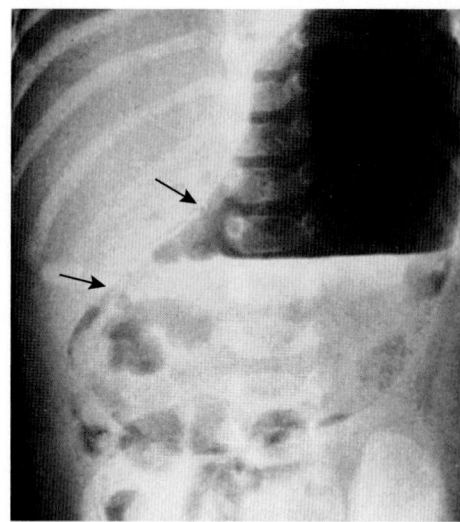
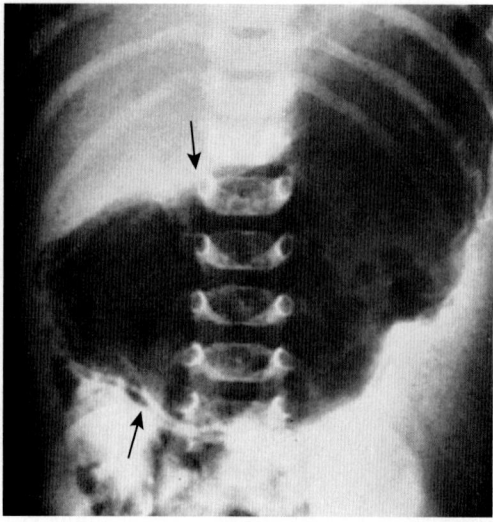

FIGURE 129-12. Gastric pneumatosis. Upright (**left**) and supine (**right**) views of the stomach in a 6-week-old girl with pyloric stenosis. The stomach is distended with gas and liquid. Intramural gas can be identified (*arrows*). The pneumatosis disappeared within 24 hours after decompression with gastric intubation. (Courtesy of Dr. J. Leonidas, New Hyde Park, NY.)

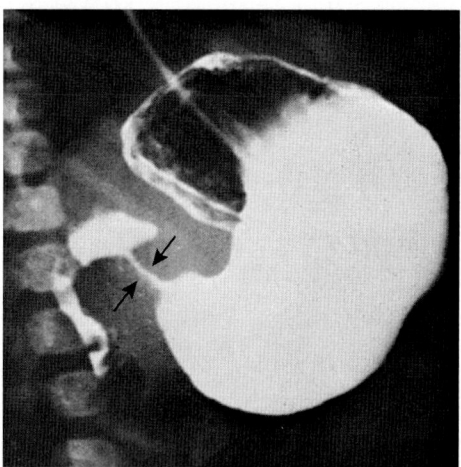
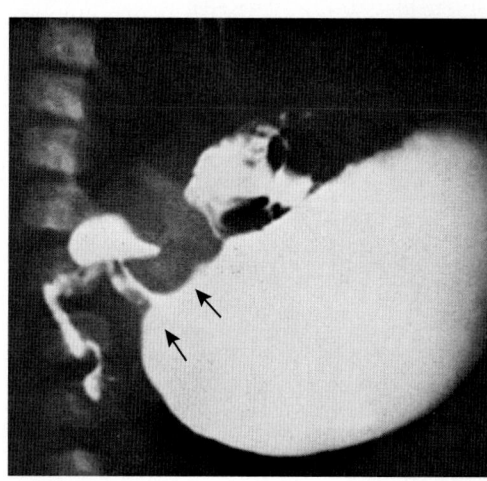

A   B

FIGURE 129-13. Characteristic findings of hypertrophic pyloric stenosis in a 7-week-old boy with a 4-week history of vomiting. **A,** The pyloric canal is narrowed and elongated (*arrows*), and the base of the duodenal bulb is stretched by the pyloric mass. **B,** The pyloric canal is narrow, demonstrating a double string sign. Indentation of the hypertrophied muscle on the lesser curvature is identified by the *double arrows*.

muscle mass looks much like an apple core lesion, with undercutting of the distal antrum and proximal duodenal bulb, although the latter may be seen in normal patients. The shoulder sign is caused by impression of the hypertrophied muscle on the air- or barium-filled antrum at the juncture of the stomach wall and hypertrophied pyloric muscle. The "pyloric tit" can be seen along the lesser curve just proximal to the impression of the pyloric mass and may be the result of a persistent peristaltic wave blocked by the mass of the hypertrophied pyloric muscle (Fig. 129-14). The beak sign is noted where the thick muscle narrows the barium column as it enters the pyloric channel. Virtually all of the signs just mentioned can be seen transiently in infants, especially those with some degree of pylorospasm. The study should be continued long enough to document the persistence of the findings in order to ensure the diagnosis of pyloric stenosis. On occasion, an associated antral web or diaphragm may be identified (see Fig. 129-14).

> **UGI series findings in HPS may include the following:**
> - Gastric distention on scout view
> - Narrowed, elongated, curved pyloric channel
> - Single or double string sign
> - Undercutting of distal antrum and proximal duodenal bulb
> - Shoulder sign
> - "Pyloric tit" on lesser curve
> - Beak sign

Differential Diagnosis

The most common antropyloric abnormality mimicking HPS on UGI series is pylorospasm. Although spasm may also cause the pyloric muscle to appear thicker on ultrasonography, this is a transient phenomenon usually

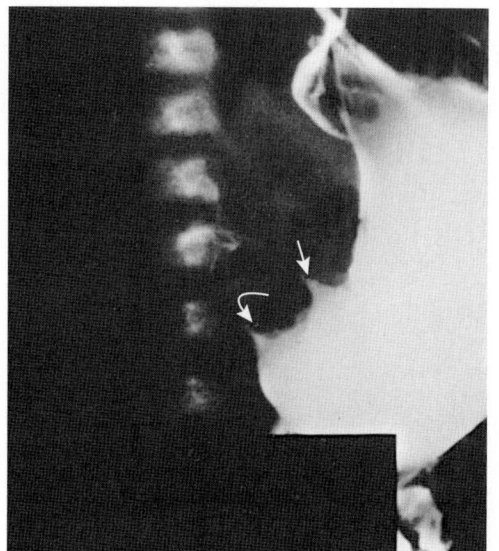

A

FIGURE 129-14. **A,** Typical upper gastrointestinal (UGI) series in a patient with pyloric stenosis. The markedly narrowed pylorus curves upward and posteriorly to the duodenal bulb, which shows an impression of the hypertrophied muscle in the base. The hypertrophied muscle can also be seen impressing itself on the lesser curvature of the stomach, causing the "pyloric tit" (*straight arrow*) to appear slightly above it. The barium column narrows sharply as it enters the pylorus, causing the beak sign (*curved arrow*). **B.** A portion of a UGI examination in a patient with pyloric stenosis demonstrates a linear filling defect in the barium column, suggestive of an antral web. **C.** A little later in the study, the characteristic string sign (*arrow*) of pyloric stenosis is seen. Both the pyloric stenosis and antral web were corrected at surgery.

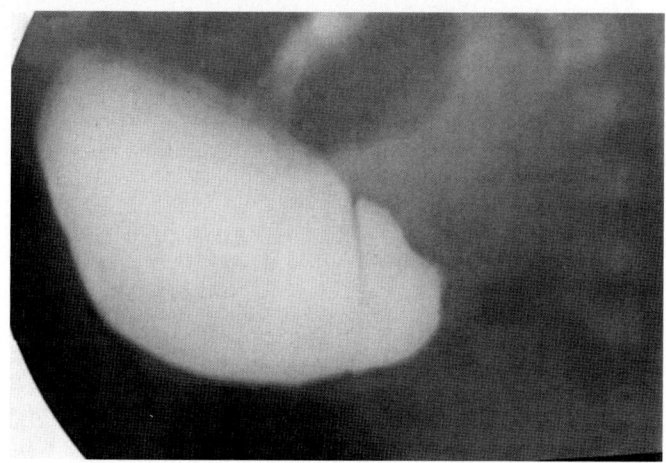

B

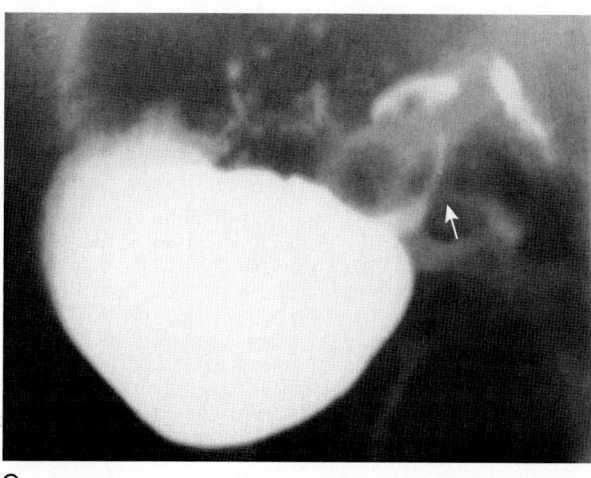

C

distinguishable from HPS. Gastric and duodenal ulcers and gastritis (see Chapter 130) can mimic the findings of HPS, especially on ultrasonography. Rarer entities, such as eosinophilic gastroenteritis, have also been shown to mimic or coexist with HPS (Fig. 129-15). Focal foveolar hyperplasia, a polypoid antral mass that can extend into the pylorus, is a rare entity in children and is usually associated with a history of congenital heart disease and prostaglandin therapy. Although the UGI appearance may mimic that of HPS, sonography can differentiate this entity from HPS because the lobulated lesion causing the increased diameter of the pylorus is located within the lumen and the muscle layer is normal (Fig. 129-16). However, as previously mentioned, co-existence of HPS and focal foveolar hyperplasia has been reported.

> **It is important to confirm the persistence of findings of HPS on UGI series or ultrasonography to avoid false-positive diagnosis of HPS as a result of pylorospasm. Patience is key.**

TREATMENT

Introduced by Conrad Ramstedt in 1912, surgical pyloromyotomy is the traditional therapy for infants with HPS. In this procedure, the muscle is incised, and the mucosa is allowed to protrude through the incision, without resuturing. However, laparoscopic pyloromyotomy has been advocated more recently by some pediatric surgeons. Several attempts have been made to treat HPS by per os balloon dilatation. Hayashi and coworkers performed this procedure on six patients. In five patients, the muscular ring was incompletely disrupted, and pyloromyotomy was still necessary. In the sixth patient, the ring was disrupted but the mucosa was torn, necessitating surgical repair.

After surgical pyloromyotomy, both the ultrasonographic and the UGI examination findings may remain abnormal for several months, even in asymptomatic patients. Thus, the diagnosis of incomplete surgical repair requires a history of persistent vomiting, as well as a positive imaging study (Fig. 129-17). Jamroz and associates suggested that the UGI series may be more sensitive than ultrasonography in detecting incomplete

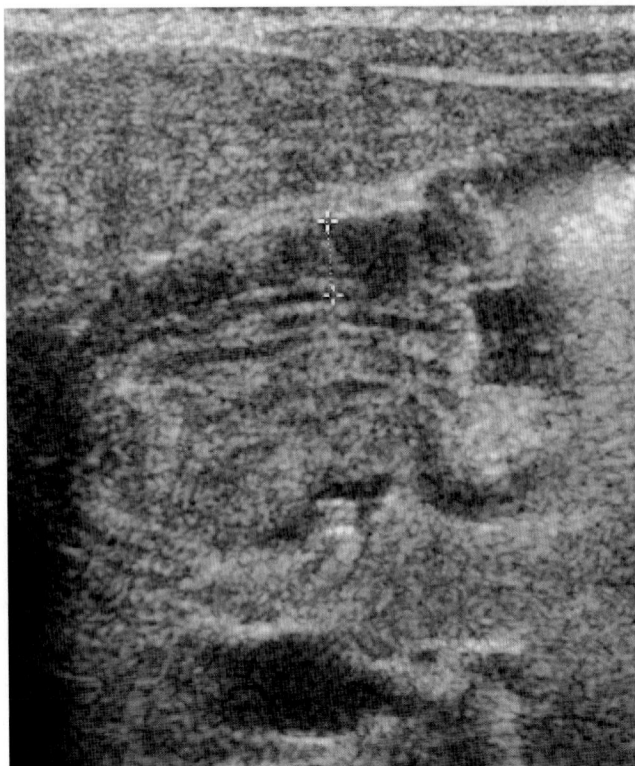

FIGURE 129-15. Hypertrophic pyloric stenosis and eosinophilic gastroenteritis in the same patient. The infant had biopsy-proven eosinophilic gastroenteritis, visible on endoscopy, as well as subsequent development of pyloric stenosis. *Calipers* mark the thickened muscle anteriorly.

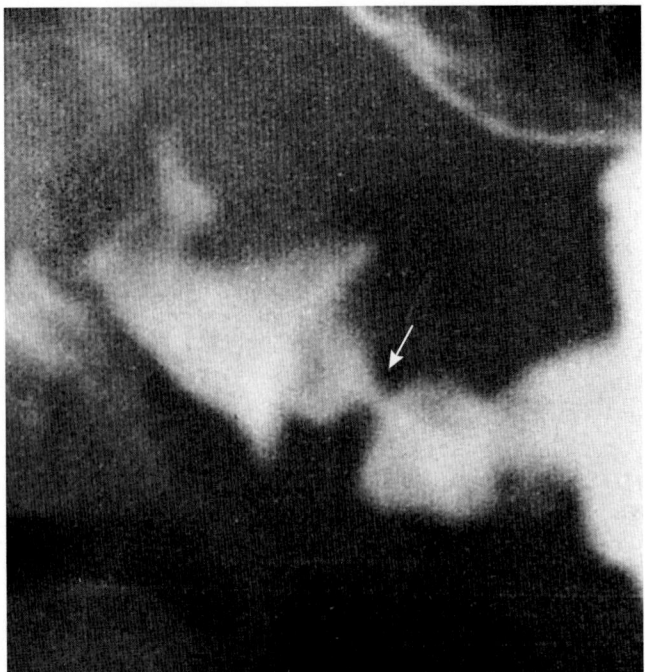

FIGURE 129-17. Incomplete pyloromyotomy. The patient, a 9-month-old infant, had been treated surgically for pyloric stenosis 7½ months earlier. He continued to vomit and did not gain weight adequately. The distal portion of the pyloric channel *(arrow)* at the base of the duodenal bulb did not widen under lengthy fluoroscopic observation. The site of incomplete pyloromyotomy was identified and corrected with surgery.

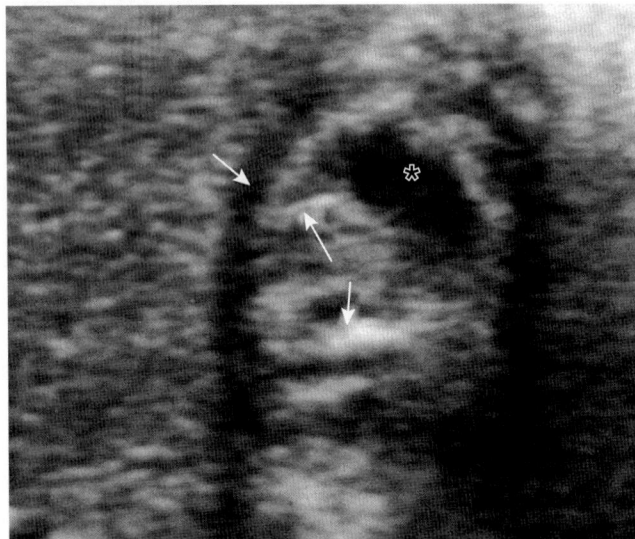

FIGURE 129-16. Foveolar alveolar hyperplasia. Transverse ultrasound image in an infant with congenital heart disease who received prostaglandins and subsequently developed vomiting. Note the fluid *(asterisk)* in the lumen, redundant hyperechoic mucosa *(lower arrows)*, and normal thin pyloric muscle *(upper arrow)*.

pyloromyotomy. Yoshizawa and colleagues described an early transient increase in muscle thickness on ultrasound study in the first few days after surgery. All measurements approached normal at 5 months. Tander and coworkers monitored 22 children with HPS up to 6 months after surgery and believed that muscle thickness measurement on ultrasound study, which returned to normal by 3 months in their study, was the optimal parameter to monitor postoperatively.

In most countries, patients are treated with pyloromyotomy, although in Austria there has been some success with successful nonsurgical therapy of younger infants with oral atropine. In Japan, Kawahara and associates treated 19 infants with intravenous atropine, which was successful in 17. In their study, there was significant decrease in pyloric muscle thickness (not in channel length) after completion of atropine treatment.

SUGGESTED READINGS

Atwell JD, Levick P: Congenital hypertrophic pyloric stenosis and associated anomalies in the genitourinary tract. J Pediatr Surg 1981;16:1029

Bidair M, Kalota SJ, Kaplan GW: Infantile hypertrophic pyloric stenosis and hydronephrosis: is there an association? J Urol 1993;150:153

Blumer RME, Hessel NS, Kuyper CF, et al: Comparison between umbilical and transverse right upper abdominal incision for pyloromyotomy. J Pediatr Surg 2004;39;1091-1093

Blumer SL, Zucconi WB, Cohen HL, et al: The vomiting neonate: a review of the ACR appropriateness criteria and ultrasound's role in the workup of such patients. Ultrasound Q 2004;20:79-89

Blumhagen JD: The role of ultrasonography in the evaluation of vomiting in infants. Pediatr Radiol 1986;16:267-270

Blumhagen JD, Maclin L, Krauter D, et al: Sonographic diagnosis of hypertrophic pyloric stenosis. AJR Am J Roentgenol 1988;150:1367

Breaux CS Jr, Georgeson KE, Royal SA, et al: Changing patterns in the diagnosis of hypertrophic pyloric stenosis. Pediatrics 1988;81:213

Bufo AJ, Merry C, Shah R, et al: Laparoscopic pyloromyotomy: a safer technique. Pediatr Surg Int 1998;13:240

Callahan MJ, McCauley RGK, Patel H, et al: The development of hypertrophic pyloric stenosis in a patient with prostaglandin induced foveolar hyperplasia. Pediatr Radiol 1999;29:748-751

Chen EA, Luks FI, Gilchrist BF, et al: Pyloric stenosis in the age of ultrasonography: fading skills, better patients? J Pediatr Surg 1996;31:829

Cohen HL, Blumer SL, Zucconi WB: The sonographic double track sign: Not pathognomonic for hypertrophic pyloric stenosis; can be seen in pylorospasm. J Ultrasound Med 2004; 23:641-646

Cohen HL, Zinn HL, Haller JO et al. Ultrasonography of pylorospasm: findings may simulate hypertrophic pyloric stenosis. J Ultrasound Med 1998 ;17:705-711

Fernbach SK, Morello FP: Renal abnormalities in children with hypertrophic pyloric stenosis—fact or fallacy? Pediatr Radiol 1993;23:286

Foley LC, Slovis TL, Campbell JB, et al: Evaluation of the vomiting infant. Am J Dis Child 1989;143:660

Geer LL, Gaisie G, Mandell VS, et al: Evolution of pyloric stenosis in the first week of life. Pediatr Radiol 1985;15:205-206

Greason KL, Thompson WR, Downey EC, et al: Laparoscopic pyloromyotomy for hypertrophic pyloric stenosis: report of 11 cases. J Pediatr Surg 1995;30:1571

Haller JO, Cohen HL: Hypertrophic pyloric stenosis: diagnosis using US. Radiology 1986;161:335

Hayashi AH, Giocomantonio JM, Lau HYC, et al: Balloon catheter dilatation for hypertrophic pyloric stenosis. J Pediatr Surg 1990;25:1119

Helton KJ, Strife JL, Warner BW, et al: The impact of imaging guidelines on imaging children with hypertrophic pyloric stenosis. Pediatr Radiol 2004;34:733-736

Hernanz-Schulman M. Infantile hypertrophic pyloric stenosis. Radiology 2003;227:319-331

Hernanz-Schulman M, Neblett WW, Polk DB, et al: Hypertrophied pyloric mucosa in patients with hypertrophic pyloric stenosis [letter]. Pediatr Radiol 1998;28:901

Hernanz-Schulman M, Sells LL, Ambrosino MM, et al: Hypertrophic pyloric stenosis in the infant without a palpable olive: accuracy of sonographic diagnosis. Radiology 1994;193:771

Hernanz-Schulman M, Zhu Y, Stein SM, et al: Hypertrophic pyloric stenosis in infants: US evaluation of vascularity of the pyloric canal. Radiology 2003;229:389-393

Holland AJ, Freeman JK, LeQuesne GW, et al: Idiopathic focal foveolar hyperplasia in infants. Pediatr Surg Int 1997;12:497

Hummer-Ehret BH, Rohrschneider WK, Oleszczuk-Raschke K, et al: Eosinophilic gastroenteritis mimicking hypertrophic pyloric stenosis. Pediatr Radiol 1998;28:711

Jamroz GA, Blocker SH, McAlister WH: Radiographic findings after incomplete pyloromyotomy. Gastrointest Radiol 1986;11:139-141

Katz ME, Blocker SH, McAlister WH: Focal foveolar hyperplasia presenting as an antral-pyloric mass in a young infant. Pediatr Radiol 1985;15:136

Kawahara H, Imura K, Nishikawa M, et al: Intravenous atropine treatment in infantile hypertrophic pyloric stenosis. Arch Dis Child 2002;8:71-74

Keller H, Waldmann D, Greiner P: Comparison of preoperative sonography with intraoperative findings in congenital hypertrophic pyloric stenosis. J Pediatr Surg 1987;22:950

Konvolinka CW, Wernuth CR: Hypertrophic pyloric stenosis in older infants. Am J Dis Child 1971;122:76-79

Latchaw LA, Jacir NN, Harris BH: The development of pyloric stenosis during transpyloric feedings. J Pediatr Surg 1989;24:823

Mandell GA: Association of antral diaphragms and hypertrophic pyloric stenosis. Am J Roentgenol Radium Ther Nucl Med 1978;131:203-206

McAlister WH, Katz ME, Perlman JM, et al: Sonography of focal foveolar hyperplasia causing gastric outlet obstruction in an infant. Pediatr Radiol 1988;18:79

Mercado-Deane MG, Burton EM, Brawley AV, et al: Prostaglandin-induced focal foveolar hyperplasia simulating pyloric stenosis in an infant with cyanotic heart disease. Pediatr Radiol 1994;24:45

O'Keefe FN, Stansberry SD, Swischuk LE, et al: Antropyloric muscle thickness at US in infants: what is normal? Radiology 1991;178:827

Okorie NM, Dickson JA, Carver RA, et al: What happens to the pylorus after pyloromyotomy? Arch Dis Child 1988;63:1339

Olson AD, Hernandez R, Hirschi RB: The role of ultrasonography in the diagnosis of pyloric stenosis: a decision analysis. J Pediatr Surg 1998;33:676-681

Ozsvath RR, Poustchi-Amin M, Leonidas JC, et al: Pyloric volume: an important factor in the surgeon's ability to palpate the pyloric "olive" in hypertrophic pyloric stenosis. Pediatr Radiol 1997;27:175

Papadakis K, Chen EA, Luks FI, et al: The changing presentation of pyloric stenosis. Am J Emerg Med 1999;17:67-69

Riccabona M, Weitzer C, Lindbichler F, et al: Sonography and color Doppler sonography for monitoring conservatively treated hypertrophic pyloric stenosis. J Ultrasound Med 2001;20:997-1002

Riggs W Jr, Long L: The value of the plain film roentgenogram in pyloric stenosis. Am J Roentgenol Radium Ther Nucl Med 1971;112:77-82

Rohrschneider WK, Mittnacht H, Darge K, et al: Pyloric muscle in asymptomatic infants: sonographic evaluation and discrimination from idiopathic hypertrophic pyloric stenosis. Pediatr Radiol 1998;28:429-434

Rollins MD, Shields MD, Quinn RJM, et al: Pyloric stenosis: congenital or acquired. Arch Dis Child 1989;64:138-147

Sargent SK, Foote SL, Shorter NA: The posterior approach to pyloric sonography. Pediatr Radiol 2000;30:256-257

Singh SJ, Trudinger B, Lam A, et al: Antenatal prediction of hypertrophic pyloric stenosis. Pediatr Surg Int 2001;17:560-562

Spevak MR, Ahmadjian JM, Kleinman PD, et al: Sonography of hypertrophic pyloric stenosis: frequency and cause of nonuniform echogenicity of the thickened pyloric muscle. AJR Am J Roentgenol 1992;158:129

Steinicke O, Roelsgaard M: Radiographic follow-up in hypertrophic pyloric stenosis. Acta Paediatr Scand 1960;49:4-16

Stunden RJ, LeQuesne GW, Little KET: The improved ultrasound diagnosis of hypertrophic pyloric stenosis. Pediatr Radiol 1986;16:200

Swischuk LE, Hayden CK Jr, Stansberry SD: Sonographic pitfalls in imaging of the antropyloric region in infants. Radiographics 1989;9:437

Tander B, Akalin A, Abbasoglu L, et al: Ultrasonographic follow-up of infantile hypertrophic pyloric stenosis after pyloromyotomy: a controlled prospective study. Eur J Pediatr Surg 2002;12:379-382

Tashjian DB, Konefal SH: Hypertrophic pyloric stenosis in utero. Pediatr Surg Int 2002;18:539-540

Teele RL, Smith EH: Ultrasound in the diagnosis of idiopathic hypertrophic pyloric stenosis. N Engl J Med 1977;296:1149-1150

van der Schouw YT, van der Velden MT, Hitge-Boetes C, et al: Diagnosis of hypertrophic pyloric stenosis: value of sonography when used in conjunction with clinical findings and laboratory data. AJR Am J Roentgenol 1994;163:905

Vasavada PV: Ultrasound evaluation of acute abdominal emergencies in infants and children. Radiol Clin North Am 2004;42:445-456

Weiskittel DA, Leary DL, Blane CE: Ultrasound diagnosis of evolving pyloric stenosis. Gastrointest Radiol 1989;14:22

White MC, Langer JC, Don S, et al: Sensitivity and cost minimization analysis of radiology versus olive palpation for the diagnosis of hypertrophic pyloric stenosis. J Pediatr Surg 1998;33:913

Yamamoto A, Kino M, Sasaki T, et al: Ultrasonic follow-up of the healing process of medically treated hypertrophic pyloric stenosis. Pediatr Radiol 1998;28:177

Yoshizawa J, Takao E, Yasuyuki H, et al: Ultrasonographic features of normalization of the pylorus after pyloromyotomy for hypertrophic pyloric stenosis. J Pediatr Surg 2001;36:582-586

CHAPTER

130

Gastritis, Gastropathy, and Ulcer Disease

MARILYN J. GOSKE

The term *gastritis* indicates the presence of inflammatory cells and represents a histologic diagnosis made only by biopsy; interestingly, the mucosa may appear normal at endoscopy. *Ulcers* are deep lesions that penetrate into the muscularis mucosa. *Gastropathies* show evidence of epithelial damage and regeneration, have little in the way of inflammatory infiltrate, and are often associated with specific conditions, such as portal hypertensive gastropathy. *Peptic diseases* are acid-related disorders in which gastric acid and pepsin are involved in the pathogenesis. According to Dohill and Hassall, "gastritis and gastropathy are not diagnosed clinically or on radiologic studies. Symptoms that do occur are seldom specific. Upper gastrointestinal studies (upper gastro-intestinal series, UGI) can only define gross mucosal changes." The role of imaging is most helpful in the setting of peptic ulcer disease, in patients with known conditions such as Crohn disease, or in patients with severe vomiting suggestive of gastric outlet obstruction.

ULCER DISEASE AND *HELICOBACTER PYLORI*

The terminology of peptic ulcer disease, gastritis, and gastropathy and our understanding of these disorders have changed dramatically with the elucidation of the involvement of *Helicobacter pylori*, along with the availability of pediatric endoscopy and medical treatments for these illnesses.

New information regarding the role of the gel layer, a protective bicarbonate-mucous barrier that lines the stomach, has furthered our understanding of the continuum of ulcer disease. The gel layer is a 0.2- to 0.5-mm-thick barrier composed of 95% water and 5% mucin glycoprotein, which forms a protective layer against harmful H^+ and pepsin. Any breach in the gel layer caused by *H. pylori*, anti-inflammatory drugs, or ischemia, for example, causes damage to the underlying mucosa. More extensive and severe inflammation extending to the muscular layer results in ulceration. The result is a continuum of disease that makes classification challenging. These complex pathophysiologic and histologic changes, simplified for this discussion, can be further investigated in the suggested readings listed at the end of this chapter.

Peptic ulcers can be classified based on region of involvement (gastric or duodenal) and presence or absence of a known cause (primary or secondary). According to

Sylvester, children who present with gastritis or ulcers with no known underlying condition have primary gastritis, a form of infectious gastritis caused by *H. pylori*. *H. pylori* is a gram-negative spiral organism that lives in the mucous layer covering the gastric epithelial cells. It was first described by Warren and Marshall in 1983, for which they received the Nobel Price in Medicine in 2005. Humans are the only known reservoir for this pathogen. There is evidence that although gastritis and peptic ulcer disease are more prevalent in adults, colonization with *H. pylori* likely occurs during childhood in most cases. This organism is present in the stomachs of 10% of children in developed countries (but in 30% to 40% of those from lower socioeconomic groups) and in 80% to 100% of children in developing countries. There is mounting evidence linking *H. pylori*–associated chronic antral gastritis to gastric adenocarcinoma and mucosa-associated lymphoid tissue (MALT) lymphoma. Secondary gastritis is most often seen in a setting of an underlying systemic condition. See Table 130-1 for a list of conditions that may cause active gastritis or ulcers. These are discussed in greater detail later.

Clinically, patients with *H. pylori* infection may be asymptomatic, unless a peptic ulcer has occurred. Other presentations of the disease include poorly localized abdominal pain, hematemesis, melena, or vomiting, which can also be seen with gastric outlet obstruction. The classic ulcer symptoms of epigastric pain alleviated by food are not commonly seen. Interestingly, the prevalence of *H. pylori* in adult patients with acquired immunodeficiency syndrome (AIDS) is lower than in age-matched human immunodeficiency virus (HIV)–negative controls. Postulated explanations include antimicrobial therapy or HIV-related host factors, such as hypochlorhydria or inadequate inflammatory response, causing impaired colonization of the organism.

> Although antral gastritis and peptic ulcer disease associated with *H. pylori* are more common in adults, colonization with *H. pylori* likely occurs in childhood in most cases. It is the primary cause of gastritis in children.

Endoscopy is the gold standard in the diagnosis of *H. pylori* infection. Antral micronodules and ulceration are seen. Antral gastritis is present in virtually every

Differential Diagnosis of Gastritis

Infection
  Helicobacter pylori
  Opportunistic infection
  Cytomegalovirus
  Toxoplasmosis
  Cryptosporidium
Crohn disease
Chemical gastritis
Ménétrier disease
Eosinophilic gastritis
Chronic granulomatous disease
Graft-versus-host disease
Gastropathy (stress, NSAID-induced, other)

NSAID, nonsteroidal anti-inflammatory drug.

patient—adult or child—from whom the organism is cultured, and gastric or duodenal ulcers have been described in many. Biopsy with tissue staining can detect the organism and rate the intensity and chronicity of the gastritis. UGI studies have demonstrated gastric fold thickening, narrowing, enlarged areae gastricae, and gastric and duodenal ulcers. Morrison and coworkers described a pattern of enlarged gastric folds in the body and antropyloric regions of the stomach in half of their patients with biopsy-proven *H. pylori* infection. Although fold thickening is generally mild, there have been reports of marked gastric fold thickening mimicking malignancy on both UGI series and computed tomography (CT). These findings often reverse after medical therapy

for *H. pylori*. Lee and colleagues reported a 7-year-old with lymphoid hyperplasia of the gastric antrum and fundus that corresponded to endoscopic findings. Nuclear medicine gastric emptying tests do not demonstrate delayed gastric emptying of solids in adult patients with *H. pylori* infection who have clinical dyspepsia without ulcer disease.

Ulcers may or may not be present in patients with *H. pylori*, and there are no explicit characteristics that suggest a specific cause on UGI studies. When present, the radiographic appearance of ulcers in children is much like that in adults (Fig. 130-1). Gastric ulcers are more likely to be in the antrum than in the body or fundus of the stomach. Marked deformity of the pylorus or duodenum is typically seen, with thickening of folds and distortion of normal anatomy. Contrast material pools in the ulcers and, with close observation, does not change shape over time. Ulcer size varies from a few millimeters to centimeters. Ulcers in both the stomach and the duodenum demonstrate a barium-filled niche with radiating folds, representing surrounding mucosal inflammation. In the gastric antrum, "button" ulcers may be seen. Narrowing and fibrosis may occur later, as the disease progresses (Fig. 130-2). Barium is the contrast material of choice unless perforation is suspected, in which case a low-osmolar nonionic contrast agent should be used.

Single-contrast barium studies are insensitive in the detection of ulcer disease compared with endoscopy. Drumm and associates (1988) confirmed that the high false-negative rate of single-contrast barium studies in adults also applies to children. Double-contrast studies of

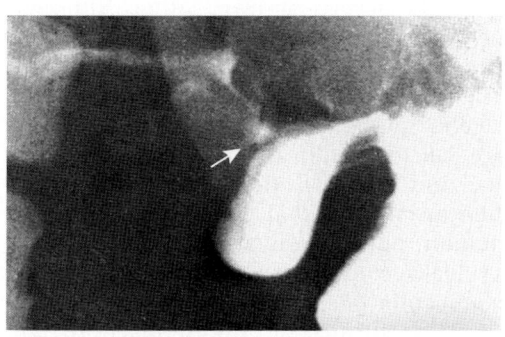

A

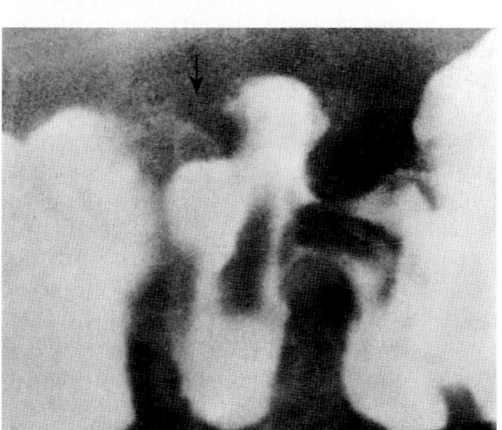

C

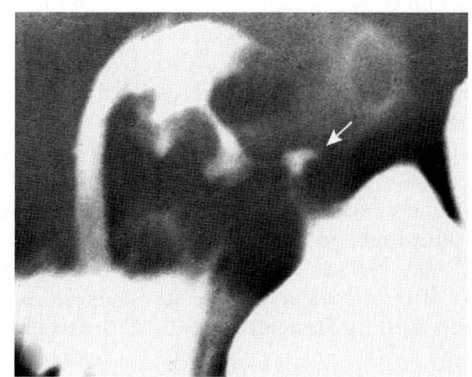

B

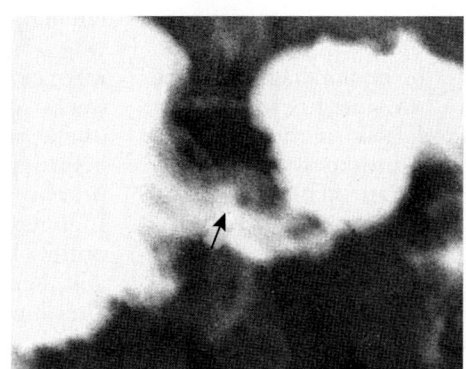

D

FIGURE 130-1. Peptic ulcers. **A,** Postbulbar ulcer *(arrow)* in a 9-year-old girl with a long history of vomiting and weight loss. **B,** Pyloric channel ulcer *(arrow)* in a 6-year-old boy. **C,** Large duodenal ulcer *(arrow)* in the bulb of a 9-year-old boy. Note the marked deformity of the duodenal bulb and the edematous folds. **D,** Small channel ulcer *(arrow)* in an 11-year-old boy with abdominal pain and melena.

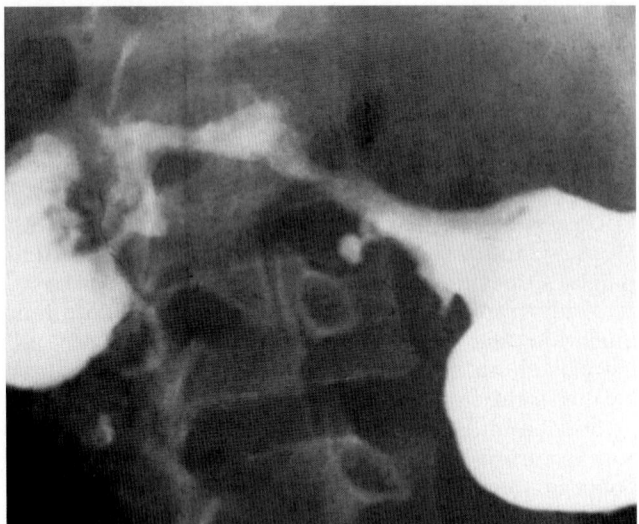

FIGURE 130-2. Polypoid "button" gastric ulcer in the pyloric channel, with marked narrowing and fibrosis of the chronically inflamed pylorus.

the stomach and duodenum may have a higher sensitivity but are difficult to perform in young children.

Although ultrasonography (US) is not used routinely in the evaluation of ulcer disease, Hayden and colleagues found ultrasound abnormalities in 7 of 600 children with vomiting in whom gastric ulcers had been demonstrated by other means. These abnormalities included thickening of the antropyloric mucosa, elongation of the antropyloric canal, persistent spasm, and delayed gastric emptying. Although other authors have reported ultrasound findings in gastritis and peptic ulcer disease in children, US has not been widely accepted for imaging these entities.

Treatment of patients with *H. pylori* is limited to those who have gastric or duodenal ulcers, atrophic gastritis with intestinal metaplasia, or MALT lymphoma. Therapy for the eradication of *H. pylori* disease in children includes at least two antibiotics and a potent antacid given for 2 weeks. This results in complete eradication of the pathogen in most instances, although gross pathologic changes such as nodularity may persist for months. Fortunately, earlier treatment of peptic ulcer disease in children has resulted in a decreased incidence of ulcers identified on UGI series.

STRESS GASTROPATHY

Stress gastropathy may be present in asymptomatic patients who have mild erosive or hemorrhagic gastritis on endoscopy. More severe physiologic stress may result in a reduction of blood flow to the stomach, with resultant mucosal ischemia, breakdown of the gel barrier, and stress erosions. Stress gastropathy in infants, termed *neonatal gastropathy*, is usually associated with respiratory distress or cardiac insufficiency, sepsis, or dehydration. Newborn infants appear to be more prone to gastric perforation. In older children, stress ulcers are seen in the setting of a serious illness such as shock, burns, major surgery, head injury, multiple organ failure, acidosis, and sepsis.

TRAUMATIC GASTROPATHY

Forceful vomiting may result in subepithelial hemorrhage due to prolapse of the gastric cardia into the distal esophagus. Mallory-Weiss tears near the gastroesophageal junction may accompany this entity. Long-term use of a nasogatric tube or prolonged suction may cause subepithelial hemorrhage that results in bleeding. "Buried bumper syndrome," due to migrating indwelling gastric feeding devices, may cause gastric ulceration and hemorrhage.

NONSTEROIDAL ANTI-INFLAMMATORY DRUG GASTROPATHY

Nonsteroidal anti-inflammatory drugs (NSAIDs) are the most common class of drugs prescribed worldwide and are used in a wide variety of pediatric illnesses. Although there are no specific radiographic findings in patients who have ingested aspirin or other NSAIDs, the mucosal damage they can cause ranges from mild histologic changes to frank hemorrhage and perforation secondary to ulcers. The length of treatment and the dosage do not necessarily correlate with the histologic findings. According to Dohill and Hassall, "although all regions of the stomach may be involved, ulceration of the incisura presenting with ulceration is a typical NSAID lesion."

CHEMICAL GASTRITIS

Ingestion of corrosive agents may be associated with suicidal intent in teenagers, is most often accidental in children, and is uncommon in adults. Ingestion of a variety of caustic substances can precipitate a chemical gastritis that may be severe or even lethal. Although alkali ingestion commonly causes esophagitis, about 20% of patients who ingest these substances also develop mild-to-moderate degrees of antral gastritis.

Common agents implicated in the direct production of gastritis are calcium chloride, zinc chloride, iron sulfate tablets, and acids. Button batteries typically contain alkaline electrolytes that can cause esophageal or gastric irritation, but there is also a theoretical risk from mercury leakage. The most common corrosive agent is calcium chloride. It is likely that some free hydrochloric acid is formed in the stomach by the hydrolysis of calcium chloride, and this acid is the direct cause of severe gastritis. Usually, by the time contrast studies are performed, there has already been severe edema, spasm, and narrowing of the distal stomach (Fig. 130-3). Secondary calcification in the gastric wall, with cicatricial constrictions, has been found several weeks after the original ingestion. Extensive necrosis of the stomach, with almost complete obstruction, has been reported from the ingestion of zinc chloride, with primary involvement of the distal body and the antrum. Ingested iron sulfate tablets can lead to complete gastric outlet obstruction with scarring of the antrum. Vomiting and hematemesis generally occur almost immediately after ingestion, and death has been reported. Intramural air in the stomach has been reported in cases of gastritis of various causes, although it is more common in adults than in children.

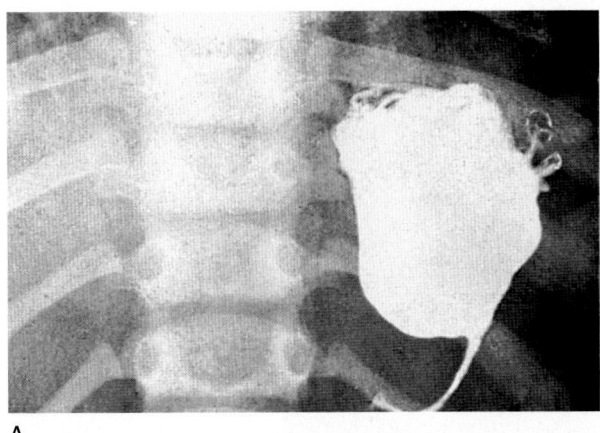
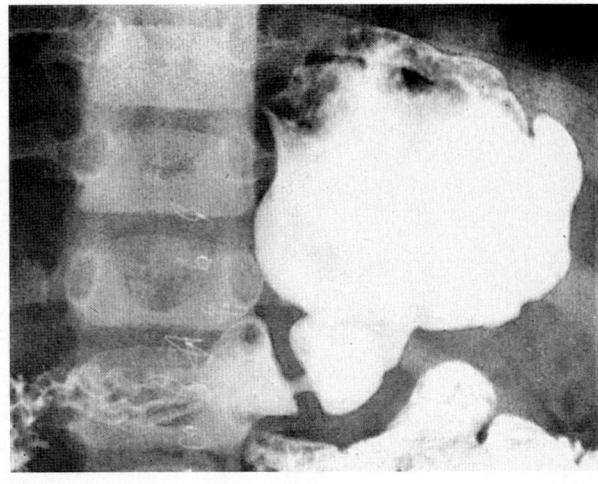

FIGURE 130-3. Severe necrotizing gastritis caused by zinc chloride. **A,** Eight weeks after the ingestion of soldering solution, the distal third of the stomach is constricted to a lumen a few millimeters in diameter, with almost complete obstruction of the pylorus. **B,** Thirteen months after surgery, function of the deformed, remaining portion of the stomach is normal.

Following the ingestion of corrosive agents, plain radiographs, including horizontal-beam views, should be obtained to exclude free air before performing contrast studies. If perforation is suspected, water-soluble contrast material can be administered initially. If there is no evidence of perforation, double-contrast studies of the stomach are most useful. There is limited experience with US of the stomach in patients with corrosive gastritis. A single case report by Aviram and coworkers discusses "localization of gastric injury, and assessment of gastric wall by assessment of its thickness and loss of layering."

MÉNÉTRIER DISEASE

Ménétrier disease, or protein-losing gastropathy with hypertrophic gastric folds, is a rare condition that behaves differently in adults than in children. In adults, the disease is chronic and premalignant, whereas it is usually a self-limited condition in children. The disease is characterized by markedly enlarged gastric folds, excess mucus secretion, decreased acid secretion, and hypoproteinemia. In children, the disease is most frequently associated with cytomegalovirus (CMV); other infectious agents implicated in this illness include *Giardia*, herpes simplex virus, and *H. pylori*. Mean age at presentation is 5 years, and the illness usually lasts 2 weeks. Children usually present with abdominal pain or with nausea and vomiting. Because of the associated protein-losing enteropathy, peripheral edema, ascites, and pleural effusions are frequently found. Immunoglobulin E levels may be elevated. Gastric hemorrhage is rare.

> Ménétrier disease in children is usually self-limited and has an infectious cause; in adults, it is chronic and premalignant.

On UGI series, there is marked enlargement of the fundal rugae, especially along the greater curvature, with sparing of the antropyloric region (Fig. 130-4). US demonstrates thickened mucosa and rugal hypertrophy, according to Gassner and colleagues. High-resolution sonography suggests that gastric wall thickening may occur maximally in the deep mucosal or submucosal layer of the stomach, and serial sonography may be useful in following the course of the disease. Okanobu and associates used high-resolution transabdominal US to depict gastric wall stratification and thus diagnose giant gastric folds. In their series, five adult patients with Ménétrier disease demonstrated thickening in the second layer of the stomach, corresponding to the deep mucosa; wall stratification was preserved. Smet and coworkers reported hyperemia of the mucosal gastric layer on color Doppler US in a 1½-year-old girl with protein-losing gastropathy with hypertrophic gastric folds.

Gastrointestinal lymphangiectasia involving the stomach demonstrates markedly enlarged gastric rugae (Fig. 130-5). The differential diagnosis on imaging includes gastric lymphoma or scirrhous carcinoma, anisakiasis if there is a history of raw fish ingestion, acute gastric mucosal lesion, eosinophilic gastroenteritis, Crohn disease, and inflammatory pseudotumor. Of these disorders, only eosinophilic gastroenteritis, lymphangiectasia, and protein-losing gastropathy with hypertrophic gastric folds cause hypoproteinemia in children, and this laboratory finding helps narrow the differential diagnosis.

> **The differential diagnosis of markedly enlarged gastric rugae includes:**
> - **Gastrointestinal lymphangiectasia**
> - **Gastric malignancy, such as lymphoma**
> - **Anisakiasis**
> - **Eosinophilic gastroenteritis**
> - **Crohn disease**
> - **Inflammatory pseudotumor**

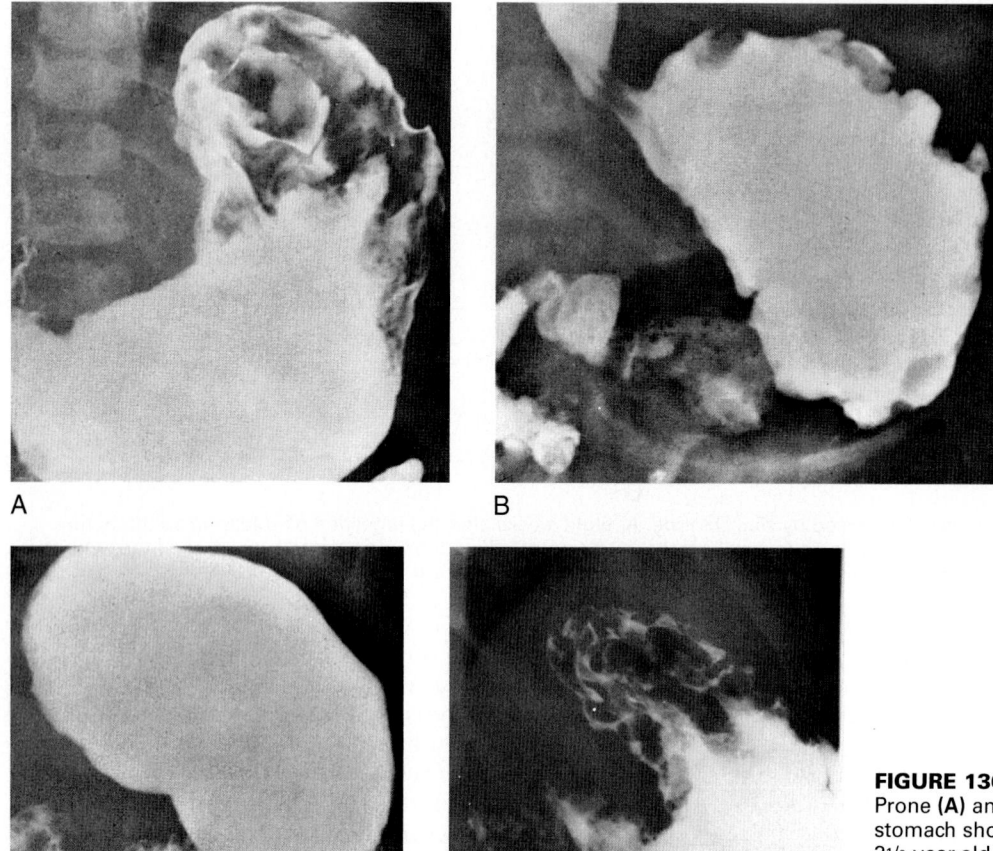

FIGURE 130-4. Ménétrier disease. **A** and **B,** Prone **(A)** and supine **(B)** projections of the stomach show rugal hypertrophy in a 3½-year-old girl with periorbital edema. Hypoproteinemia was found on laboratory studies. **C,** Three months later, serum protein values were normal, as were the gastric rugae. **D,** Giant rugal hypertrophy in a 2-year-old boy with hypoproteinemia, diffuse edema, and pleural effusions. Note that the body and antrum of the stomach are normal.

INFECTIOUS GASTRITIS

Helicobacter pylori is a major cause of gastritis and was discussed in detail earlier in this chapter. Other causes of infectious gastritis have been described in immunocompromised patients with AIDS, particularly in adults. Falcone and coworkers described 11 patients with AIDS who had gastric abnormalities. Five of these patients had infection with CMV, *Toxoplasma gondii,* or *Cryptosporidium;* the other six had Kaposi sarcoma or lymphoma. These authors found that in their patient population, inflammatory processes typically demonstrated thickened gastric folds, whereas neoplastic entities tended to consist of nodular lesions.

CMV is one of the most common causes of gastritis in patients with AIDS, and in the stomach, it typically involves the esophagogastric junction and the antropyloric segment. CMV involvement of the antropyloric portion of the stomach reportedly caused pyloric obstruction in a child with HIV infection. CMV gastritis often causes deep ulcerations, submucosal masses resulting from edema, or focal abscesses. Perforation can occasionally occur.

Cryptosporidium, a protozoan, can also cause antral narrowing and thickened gastric folds in children with AIDS. The differential diagnosis includes *H. pylori* and gut-associated lymphoid tissue, a lymphoproliferative disorder.

EOSINOPHILIC GASTRITIS

Eosinophilic gastroenteritis is a cluster of rare and poorly understood illnesses; their hallmark is gastric and intestinal eosinophilic infiltration and peripheral eosinophilia in more than 50% of patients. Serum immunoglobulin E is elevated. The disease is chronic and may be debilitating. It may be caused by an allergy or hypersensitivity; there is some overlap with the dietary protein hypersensitivity disorders. Eosinophilic gastritis has been reported either alone or, more commonly, as part of a diffuse gastroenteritis involving the esophagus and colon—the small intestine in particular. Eosinophilic gastroenteritis involves all layers of the bowel wall but may be difficult to diagnose; because of the patchy infiltrate, endoscopic biopsy may miss the pathology. In some patients, the disease responds to elimination diets, steroids, or cromolyn.

Eosinophilic gastritis usually causes a strikingly nodular pattern in the gastric antrum, with relative sparing of the body and fundus; this is well seen on UGI series

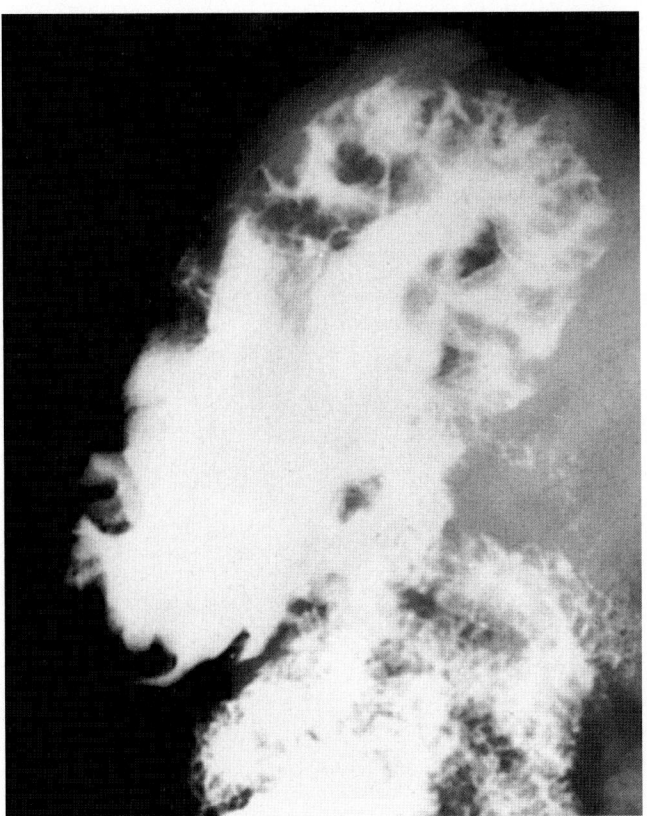

FIGURE 130-5. Lymphangiectasia of the stomach demonstrates giant rugal hypertrophy involving all parts.

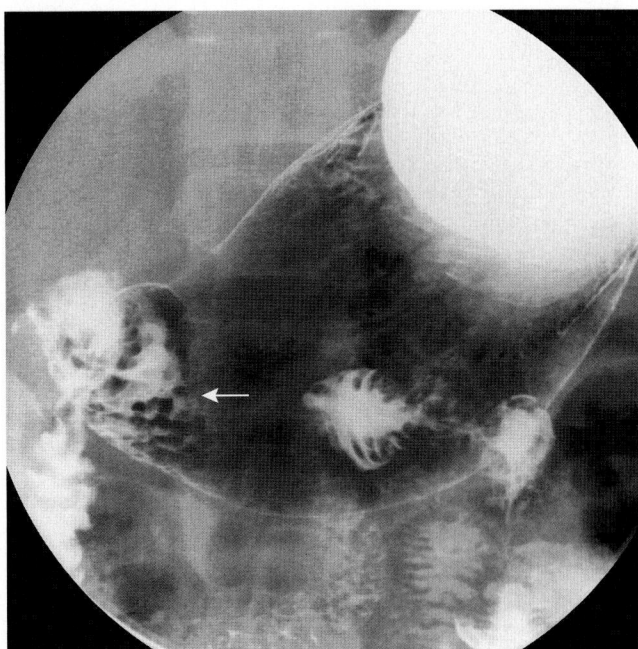

FIGURE 130-6. Eosinophilic gastritis. The gastric antrum is narrowed, with polypoid filling defects *(arrow)*, on this air-contrast upper gastrointestinal series in an adolescent girl with peripheral eosinophilia. Diagnosis was documented by biopsy. Note that the proximal portion of the stomach is entirely normal.

(Fig. 130-6). Several cases have been reported in older children in which the ultrasound findings mimicked those of hypertrophic pyloric stenosis.

CHRONIC GRANULOMATOUS DISEASE OF CHILDHOOD

Chronic granulomatous disease of childhood is a rare group of X-linked or autosomal genetic disorders characterized by the inability of phagocytes to generate oxygen radicals. This cellular failure results in recurrent infection by catalase-positive bacteria and fungi. According to Ruiz-Contreras and associates, "the lack of digestion causes prolonged intracellular survival of microbes, which in turn, results in chronic inflammation and formation of granulomata throughout the body." Patients present with pneumonia, hepatomegaly, dermatitis, osteomyelitis, lymphadenitis, or abscess, usually by age 2 years. Formation of chronic granulomas leads to thickening of the gastrointestinal wall and may lead to gastric outlet obstruction. Pathology demonstrates noncaseating granulomas of the gastric epithelium, with pigmented lipid histiocytes and submucosal edema and fibrosis. The most common gastrointestinal manifestation is chronic antral gastritis (Fig. 130-7). A review by Barton and colleagues emphasized that the entire gastrointestinal tract may be involved. Patients present with vomiting, weight loss, and epigastric pain. US demonstrates an abnormally thickened antropyloric wall greater than 3 mm. This finding simulates hypertrophic pyloric stenosis but occurs in patients beyond infancy. UGI series reveal

a dilated stomach, narrowing of the antropyloric lumen, wall thickening, thickened mucosal folds, distention with a triangular antrum, and gastroesophageal reflux. A thickened gastric wall has been described on CT. Rarely, surgical intervention is required.

CROHN DISEASE

Crohn disease is a chronic, often debilitating illness of unknown cause that is diagnosed in the appropriate clinical setting by the histologic identification of non-caseating granulomas in the stomach or elsewhere in the gastrointestinal tract. According to Dohill and Hassall, Crohn disease is the second most common cause of gastritis in children after *H. pylori* infection. Approximately 25% of new cases of Crohn disease occur in individuals younger than 20 years, with most presenting between the ages of 10 and 16 years. Five percent of children with Crohn disease are younger than 5 years. They often present with atypical and variable symptoms, leading to a delay in diagnosis.

Although isolated gastric involvement in pediatric patients is rare compared with gastroduodenal involvement, Crohn disease is more common in the upper gastrointestinal tract in children than was previously thought. A review of several studies of pediatric patients with Crohn disease demonstrates histologic evidence of gastric involvement in approximately 30%. Two thirds of those patients had visually normal endoscopic examinations. Therefore, radiologists would not expect to identify gross macroscopic changes in many patients on UGI series. The relatively high prevalence of Crohn disease in the stomach and duodenum (with a relatively low radiographic detection rate) has been confirmed

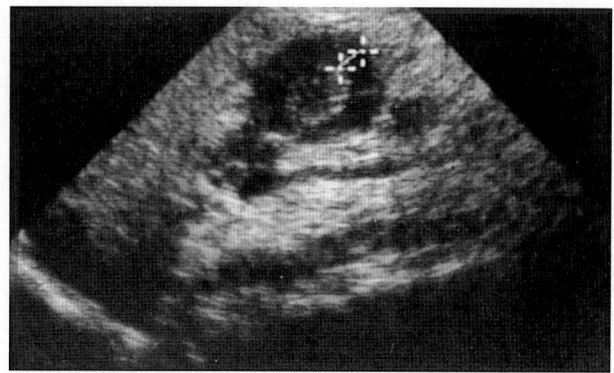

A

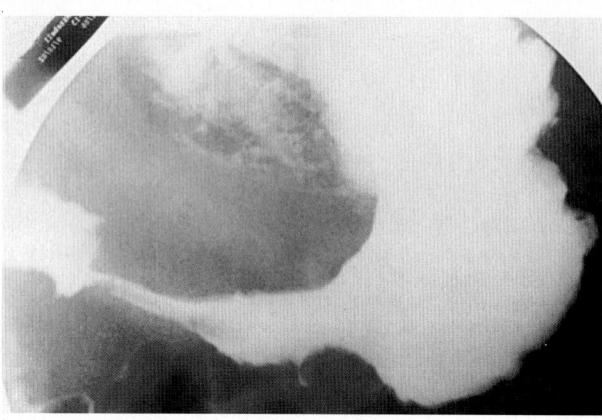

B

FIGURE 130-7. Chronic granulomatous disease of childhood in a 2-year-old boy. **A,** US shows persistently marked thickening of the antropyloric wall. **B,** Upper gastrointestinal series shows a long, narrowed antrum and pylorus, which were noted to be fixed on fluoroscopic observation.

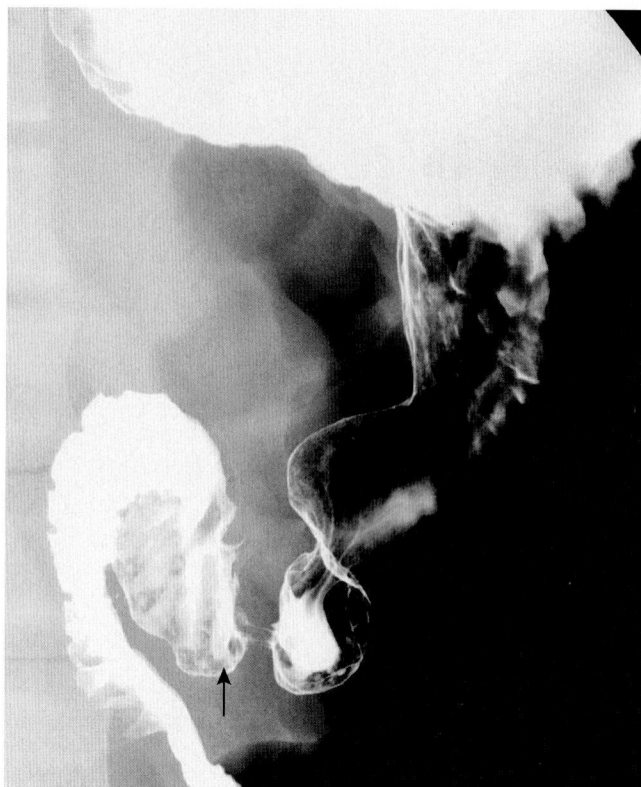

FIGURE 130-8. Crohn disease. Aphthous ulcers *(arrows)* are seen in the antrum and duodenal bulb in this adolescent with newly diagnosed Crohn disease. Air-contrast studies can demonstrate these subtle ulcers to the best advantage.

in more recent studies. In Cameron's prospective endoscopic study in children and adolescents with Crohn disease, biopsies demonstrated evidence of disease in the esophagus in 16%, the gastric body in 46%, the gastric antrum in 36%, and the duodenum in 21%. In a prospective study of 31 children with presumed Crohn disease by Mashako and colleagues, clinical symptoms of upper gastrointestinal tract involvement were present in 5 (16%), radiographic findings in only 1 (3%), and endoscopic abnormalities in 13 (42%); specific histologic evidence of granulomas was found on endoscopic biopsies in 12 children (39%).

Lenaerts and coworkers reported endoscopic involvement of the esophagus, stomach, and duodenum in 69 of 230 children (30%) with Crohn disease; radiographic studies were negative in 13. However, these studies were not performed using a double-contrast technique, which is imperative to find the aphthous ulcers that characterize the early stages of the disease. Radiographically, these are typically found in the antrum, pylorus, and duodenum (Fig. 130-8), but they can be seen in the more proximal stomach as well as the distal esophagus. Crohn disease of the stomach may present with partial or complete gastric outlet obstruction. The stomach may be grossly enlarged on abdominal radiographs at the time of presentation. After adequate gastric emptying with

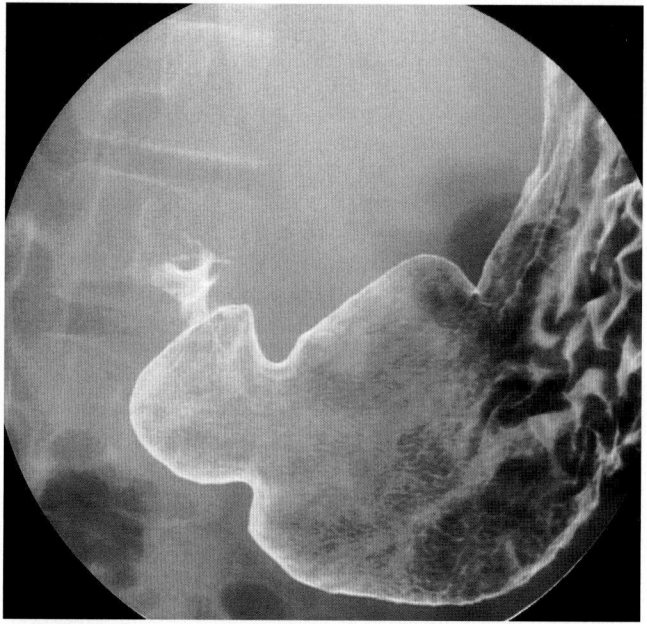

FIGURE 130-9. Crohn disease. This adolescent girl presented to the emergency room with new-onset vomiting. Air-contrast upper gastrointestinal study after adequate gastric emptying shows complete obstruction of the gastric antrum, with narrowing and fold distortion. Endoscopy and biopsy confirmed that this was secondary to previously undetected Crohn disease.

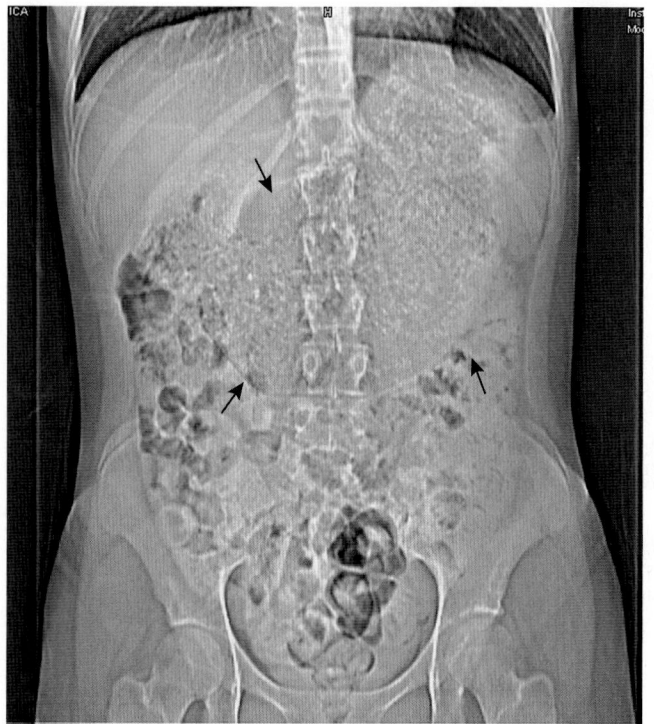

A

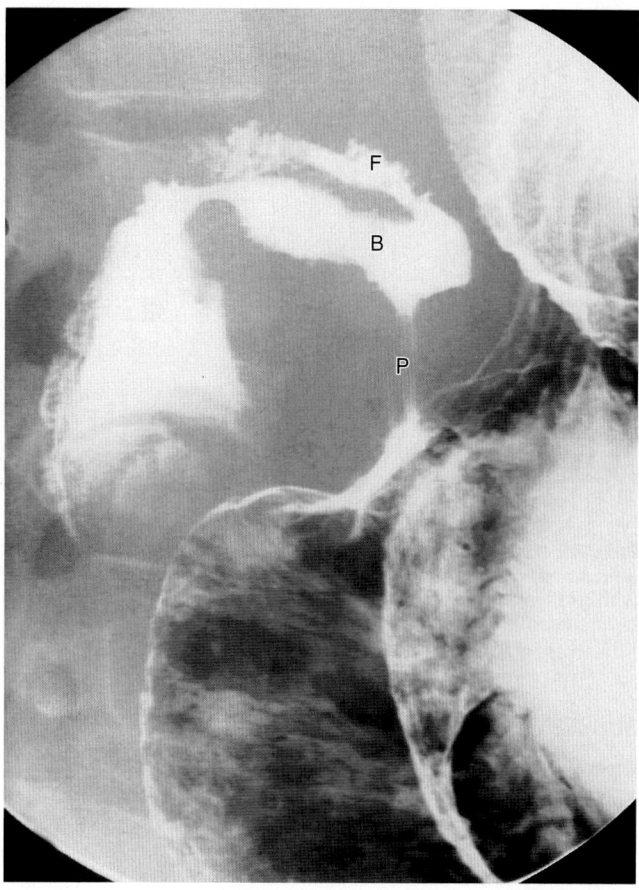

B

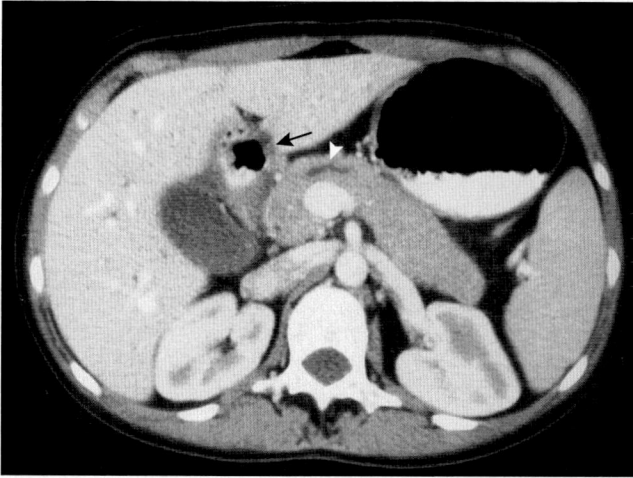

C

FIGURE 130-10. Crohn disease. This adolescent girl with known Crohn disease developed severe vomiting. **A,** Scout film from the initial CT scan shows a massively distended stomach *(arrows)*. **B,** Air-contrast upper gastrointestinal study after several days of nasogastric tube suction and steroids reveals severe pyloric channel (P) narrowing, with a "double channel" at the level of the duodenal bulb (B) secondary to Crohn disease and a fistulous tract (F). **C,** One year later, the patient developed elevated liver and pancreatic enzymes. CT scan reveals thickening of the wall of the duodenum *(arrow)* and mild intrahepatic bile duct and pancreatic duct dilation *(arrowhead)* secondary to partial obstruction at the ampulla, caused by Crohn disease involvement at this site.

nasogastric suction, a double-contrast UGI series shows the gastric antrum to be distorted and narrowed, with thickened folds or even completely obstructed (Fig. 130-9). If the disease also involves the duodenum, wall thickening may cause partial obstruction of the common bile duct or the pancreatic duct (Fig. 130-10).

Technetium-99m hexamethylpropyleneamine oxime (HMPAO) leukocyte scintigraphy is not reliable for detecting Crohn disease in the proximal gastrointestinal tract in comparison to other sites of bowel involvement.

GRAFT-VERSUS-HOST DISEASE

Graft-versus-host disease (GVHD) is a common complication of allogeneic bone marrow transplantation and frequently affects the skin, liver, and gastrointestinal tract due to damage to the lining cells by donor T lymphocytes. The disease typically affects the small intestine and the colon, but it can affect the stomach as well. The findings are nonspecific but are suggestive when other clinical signs of GVHD are present. Mucosal irregularity may be identified on UGI series; CT, US, and UGI series may demonstrate thickening of the gastric wall (Fig. 130-11). Involvement of the stomach is more common in the acute or subacute phase of GVHD than in the chronic phase. In the acute phase, this is related to edema; in the chronic phase, fibrosis is a more likely cause. Patients with GVHD may also acquire CMV gastroenteritis, with the imaging findings being indistinguishable from those of GVHD itself.

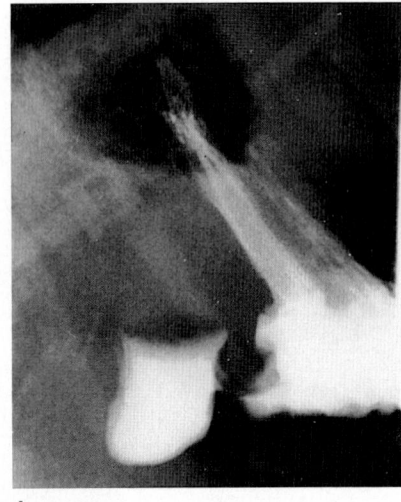
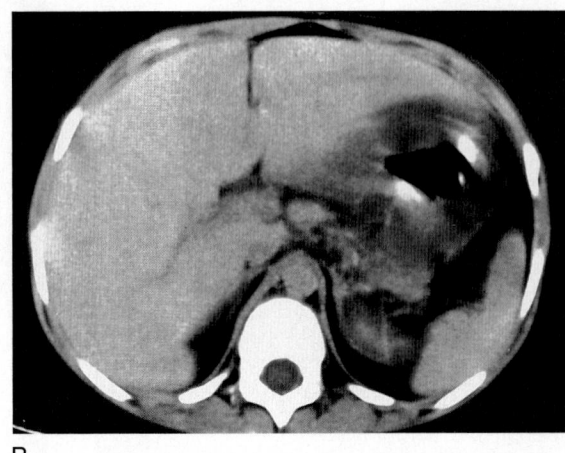

A   B

FIGURE 130-11. Graft-versus-host disease. **A,** Upper gastrointestinal series shows that the body of the stomach is rigid, with effacement of the mucosa secondary to submucosal infiltration. **B,** CT scan shows edema of the gastric wall in this 14-year-old girl with graft-versus-host disease who underwent bone marrow transplantation for acute lymphocytic leukemia. Similar findings have been described elsewhere in the gastrointestinal tract.

SUGGESTED READINGS

Ulcer Disease and *Helicobacter pylori*

Azarow K, Kim P, Shandling B, et al: A 45-year experience with surgical treatment for peptic ulcer disease. J Pediatr Surg 1996;31:750

Blecker U: *Helicobacter pylori* disease in childhood. Clin Pediatr (Phila) 1996;35:175

Blecker U: *Helicobacter pylori*-associated gastroduodenal disease in childhood. South Med J 1997;90:570

Block WM: Chronic gastric ulcer in childhood: a critical analysis of the literature with report of a case in an eleven-year-old boy. Am J Dis Child 1963;85:566-574

Bujanover Y, Reif S, Yahav J: *Helicobacter pylori* and peptic ulcer disease in the pediatric patient. Pediatr Clin North Am 1996;43:213

Chan KL, Tam PK, Saing H: Long-term follow-up of childhood duodenal ulcers. J Pediatr Surg 1997;32:1609

Chang C, Chen G, Kao C, et al: The effect of *Helicobacter pylori* infection on gastric emptying of digestible and indigestible solids in patients with nonulcer dyspepsia. Am J Gastroenterol 1996; 91:474-479

Dohill R, Hassall E: Gastritis, gastropathy and ulcer disease. *In* Wyllie R, Hyams JS (eds): Pediatric Gastrointestinal and Liver Disease: Pathophysiology, Diagnosis and Management, 3rd ed. Philadelphia, Saunders, 2006:367-401

Drumm B, Rhoads JM, Stringer DA, et al: Peptic ulcer disease in children: etiology, clinical findings and clinical course. Pediatrics 1988;82:410-414

Dunn S, Weber TR, Grosfeld JL, et al: Acute peptic ulcer in childhood. Arch Surg 1983;118:656-660

Farthing MJ: *Helicobacter pylori* infection: an overview. Br Med Bull 1998;54:1

Girdany BR: Peptic ulcer in childhood. Pediatrics 1953;12:56

Goggin N, Rowland M, Imrie C, et al: Effect of *Helicobacter pylori* eradication on the natural history of duodenal ulcer disease. Arch Dis Child 1998;79:502

Gormally SM, Kierce BM, Daly LE, et al: Gastric metaplasia and duodenal ulcer disease in children infected by *Helicobacter pylori*. Gut 1996;38:513

Hayden CK Jr, Swischuk LE, Rytting JE: Gastric ulcer disease in infants: US findings. Radiology 1987;164:131-134

Huang FC, Chang MH, Hsu HY, et al: Long-term follow-up of duodenal ulcer disease in children before and after eradication of *Helicobacter pylori*. J Pediatr Gastroenterol Nutr 1999;28:76

Jones NL, Sherman PM: *Helicobacter pylori* infection in children. Curr Opin Pediatr 1998;10:19

Kato S, Abukawa D, Furuyama N, et al: *Helicobacter pylori* reinfection rates in children after eradication therapy. J Pediatr Gastroenterol Nutr 1998;27:543

Kuipers EJ, Uyterlinde AM, Pena AS, et al: Long-term sequelae of *Helicobacter pylori* gastritis. Lancet 1995;345:1525

Kumar D, Spitz L: Peptic ulceration in children. Surg Gynecol Obstet 1987;159:63-66

Lee EY, Brady L, Yousefzadeh DK, Benya EC: Lymphoid hyperplasia of the stomach caused by *Helicobacter pylori:* upper gastrointestinal findings. AJR Am J Roentgenol 1999;173:362-363

Marshall BJ, Warren JR: Unidentified curved bacilli in the stomach of patients with gastritis and peptic ulceration. Lancet 1984; 2390:1311-1315

Meining A, Behrens R, Lehn N, et al: Different expression of *Helicobacter pylori* gastritis in children: evidence for a specific pediatric disease? Helicobacter 1996;1:92

Purelekar SG, Lubert J: Ultrasound demonstration of giant duodenal ulcer. Gastrointest Radiol 1983;8:29-31

Rosenquist CJ: Clinical and radiographic features of giant duodenal ulcer. Clin Radiol 1969;20:324

Rowland M, Drumm B: *Helicobacter pylori* infection and peptic ulcer disease in children. Curr Opin Pediatr 1995;7:553

Rowland M, Drumm B: Clinical significance of *Helicobacter pylori* infection in children. Br Med Bull 1998;54:95

Sherman PM: Peptic ulcer disease in children: diagnosis, treatment, and the implication of *Helicobacter pylori*. Gastroenterol Clin North Am 1994;23:707

Stringer DA, Daneman A, Brunelle F, et al: Sonography of the normal and abnormal stomach (excluding hypertrophic pyloric stenosis) in children. J Ultrasound Med 1986;5:183

Sylvester FA: Peptic ulcer disease. *In* Berhman RE, Kliegman RM, Jenson HB (ed): Nelson Textbook of Pediatrics, 17th ed. Philadelphia, Saunders, 2004:1244-1247

Warren JR, Marshall BJ: Unidentified curved bacilli on gastric epithelium in active chronic gastritis. Lancet 1983;8336:1273-1275 (Letters-to-the-Editor)

Other Causes of Gastritis and Gastropathy

Ali SI, McCarty HML: Paediatric Crohn's disease: a radiologic review. Eur Radiol 2000;10:1085-1094

Aviram G, Kessler A, Reif S, et al: Corrosive gastritis: sonographic findings in the acute phase and follow-up. Pediatr Radiol 1997;27:805-806

Baker A, Volberg F, Summer T, et al: Childhood Menetrier's disease: four new cases and discussion of the literature. Gastrointest Radiol 1986;11:131

Barton LL, Moussa SL, Villar RG, Hulett RL: Gastrointestinal complications of chronic granulomatous disease: case report and literature review. Clin Pediatr 1998;37:231-236

Bar-Ziv J, Barki Y, Weizman Z, Urkin J: Transient protein-losing gastropathy (Menetrier's disease) in childhood. Pediatr Radiol 1988;18:82-84

Bass DH, Millar AJ: Mercury absorption following button battery ingestion. J Pediatr Surg 1992;27:1541

Berhman RE, Kliegman RM, Jenson HB (eds): Nelson Textbook of Pediatrics, 17th ed. Philadelphia, Saunders, 2004:1257

Bowen A III, Gibson MD: Chronic granulomatous disease with gastric antral narrowing. Pediatr Radiol 1980;10:119-120

Burns B, Gay BB: Menetrier's disease of the stomach in children. Am J Roentgenol Radium Ther Nucl Med 1968;103:300-306

Cameron DJ: Upper and lower gastrointestinal endoscopy in children and adolescents with Crohn's disease: a prospective study. J Gastroenterol Hepatol 1991;6:355

Chalouplea JC, Gay BB, Caplan D: *Campylobacter* gastritis simulating Menetrier's disease by upper gastrointestinal radiography. Pediatr Radiol 1990;20:200-201

Coad NAG, Shah KJ: Menetrier's disease in childhood associated with cytomegalovirus infection: a case report and review of the literature. Br J Radiol 1986;59:515-620

Davison SM, Chapman S, Murphy MS: 99m Tc-HMPAO leucocyte scintigraphy fails to detect Crohn's disease in the proximal gastrointestinal tract. Arch Dis Child 2001;85:43-46

Derchi LE, Biggi GARE, Cicio GR, et al: Sonographic findings of Menetrier's disease: a case report. Gastrointest Radiol 1982;7:323-325

Dohill R, Hassall E: Gastritis, gastropathy and ulcer disease. *In* Wyllie R, Hyams JS (eds): Pediatric Gastrointestinal and Liver Disease: Pathophysiology, Diagnosis and Management, 3rd ed. Philadelphia, Saunders, 2006:367-401

Dohmen K, Harada M, Ishibashi M, et al: Ultrasonographic studies on abdominal complications in patients receiving marrow-ablative chemotherapy and bone marrow or blood stem cell transplantation. J Clin Ultrasound 1991;19:321

Donnelly LF: CT Imaging of immuno-compromised children with acute abdominal symptoms. AJR Am J Roentgenol 1996;167:909-913

Drumm B, O'Brien A, Cutz E, Sherman P: *Campylobacter pylori*-associated primary gastritis in children. Pediatrics 1987;80:192-195

Edwards PD, Carrick J, Turner J, et al: *Helicobacter pylori*-associated gastritis is rare in AIDS: antibiotic effect or a consequence of immunodeficiency? Am J Gastroenterol 1991;86:1761

Falcone S, Murphy BJ, Weinfeld A: Gastric manifestations of AIDS: radiographic findings on upper gastrointestinal examination. Gastrointest Radiol 1991;16:95

Franken EA Jr: Caustic damage of the gastrointestinal tract: roentgen features. Am J Roentgenol Radium Ther Nucl Med 1973;118:77-85

Gassner I, Strasser K, Bart G, et al: Sonographic appearance of Menetrier's disease in a child. J Ultrasound Med 1990;9:537

Gelfand DW, Dale WJ, Ott DJ, et al: Duodenitis: endoscopic-radiologic correlation in 272 patients. Radiology 1985;157:577-581

Granot E, Matoth I, Korman SH, et al: Functional gastrointestinal obstruction in a child with chronic granulomatous disease. J Pediatr Gastroenterol Nutr 1986;5:321

Gratten-Smith D, Harrison LF, Singleton EB: Radiology of AIDS in the pediatric patient. Curr Probl Diagn Radiol 1992;21:79

Griscom NT, Kirkpatrick, JA, Girdany BR, et al: Gastric antral narrowing in chronic granulomatous disease of childhood. Pediatrics 1974;54:456-460

Haller JO, Cohen HL: Gastrointestinal manifestations of AIDS in children. AJR Am J Roentgenol 1994;162:387

Hummer-Ehret BH, Rohrschneider WK, Oleszczuk-Raschke K, et al: Eosinophilic gastroenteritis mimicking hypertrophic pyloric stenosis. Pediatr Radiol 1998;28:711

Kopen PA, McAliser WH: Upper gastrointestinal and ultrasound examinations of gastric antral involvement in chronic granulomatous disease. Pediatr Radiol 1984;14:91-93

Kost KM, Shapiro RS: Button battery ingestion: a case report and review of the literature. J Otolaryngol 1987;16:252

Lenaerts C, Roy CC, Vaillancourt M, et al: High incidence of upper gastrointestinal tract involvement in children with Crohn disease. Pediatrics 1989;83:777

Leonidas JC, Beatty EC, Wenner HA: Menetrier disease and cytomegalovirus infection in childhood. Am J Dis Child 1973;126:806-808

Manson DE, Sikka S, Reid B, et al: Primary immunodeficiencies: a pictorial immunology primer for radiologists. Pediatr Radiol 2000;30:501-510

Manson DE, Stringer DA, Durie PR, et al: The radiologic and endoscopic investigation and etiologic classification of gastritis in children. J Can Assoc Radiol 1990;41:201

Marks MP, Lanza MV, Kahlstrom EJ, et al: Pediatric hypertrophic gastropathy. AJR Am J Roentgenol 1986;147:1031-1034

Mashako MN, Cezard JP, Navarro J, et al: Crohn's disease lesions in the upper gastrointestinal tract: correlation between clinical, radiological, endoscopic, and histologic features in adolescents and children. J Pediatr Gastroenterol 1989;8:442

McDonald GB, Shulman HM, Sullivan KM, et al: Intestinal and hepatic complications of human bone marrow transplantation. Part I. Gastroenterology 1986;90:460

Morrison S, Dahms BB, Hoffenbert E, et al: Enlarged gastric folds in association with *Campylobacter pylori* gastritis. Radiology 1989;171:819-821

Narla LD, Hingsbergen EA, Jones JE: Adult diseases in children. Pediatr Radiol 1999;29:244

Okanobu H, Hata J, Haruma K, et al: Giant gastric folds: differential diagnosis at US. Radiology 2003;226:686-690

Ott DG, Gelfand DW, Wu WC, et al: Sensitivity of single- vs double-contrast radiology in erosive gastritis. AJR Am J Roentgenol 1982;138:263-266

Paciorek M, D'Altorio R, Gleeson G: Resolution of giant gastric folds after eradication of *Heliocobacter pylori*. J Clin Gastroenterol 1997;25:696

Pugh TF, Fitch SJ: Invasive gastric candidiasis. Pediatr Radiol 1986;16:67-68

Ruiz-Contreras J, Bastero R, Serrano C, et al: Oesophageal narrowing in chronic granulomatous disease. Eur J Radiol 1998;27:149-152

Ruuska T, Vaajalahti P, Arajarvi P, et al: Prospective evaluation of upper gastrointestinal mucosal lesions in children with ulcerative colitis and Crohn's disease. J Pediatr Gastroenterol Nutr 1994;19:181

Scharschidt BF: The natural history of hypertrophic gastropathy (Menetrier's disease): report of a case with 16-year follow-up and review of 120 cases from the literature. Am J Med 1977;63:644-652

Smet MH, Mussen E, Ectors N, Breysem L: High-resolution real-time compound ultrasound imaging of transient protein-losing gastropathy of childhood. Eur Radiol 2003;13:L142-L146

Smith FJ, Taves DH: Gastroduodenal involvement in chronic granulomatous disease of childhood. Can Assoc Radiol J 1992;43:215

Stringer DA, Daneman A, Brunelle F, et al: Sonography of the normal and abnormal stomach (excluding hypertrophic pyloric stenosis) in children. J Ultrasound Med 1986;5:183-188

Takaya J, Kawamura Y, Kino M, et al: Menetrier's disease evaluated serially by abdominal ultrasonography. Pediatr Radiol 1997;27:178

Teele RL, Katz AJ, Goldman H, et al: Radiographic features of eosinophilic gastroenteritis (allergic gastroenteropathy) of childhood. AJR Am J Roentgenol 1979;132:575-580

Tekant G, Eroglu E, Erdogan E, et al: Corrosive induced gastric outlet obstruction: a changing spectrum of agents and treatments. J Pediatr Surg 2001;36:1004-1007

Theoni RF, Goldberg HI, Ominsky S, et al: Detection of gastritis by single and double contrast radiography. Radiology 1983;148:621-626

Tio TL: Large gastric folds evaluated by endoscopic ultrasonography. Gastrointest Endosc Clin N Am 1995;5:683

Tootla F, Lucas RJ, Bernacki EG, et al: Gastroduodenal Crohn's disease. Arch Surg 1976;3:855-857

Turner CJ, Lipitz LR, Pastore RA: Antral gastritis. Radiology 1974;113:305-312

Urban BA, Fishman EK, Hruban RH: *Heliocobacter pylori* gastritis mimicking gastric carcinoma at CT evaluation. Radiology 1991;179:689

Victoria MS, Nangia BS, Jindrak K: Cytomegalovirus pyloric obstruction in a child with acquired immune deficiency syndrome. Pediatric Infect Dis 1985;4:550

Tumors and Tumor-Like Conditions, Bezoars, and Varices

MARILYN J. GOSKE and ALAN E. SCHLESINGER

BEZOARS

Bezoars are foreign bodies in the stomach or other parts of the gastrointestinal (GI) tract that form from the accretion of nondigestible material such as hair (trichobezoars), plant matter (phytobezoars), or inspissated milk (lactobezoars) and increase in size over long periods. The word *bezoar* originates from the Arabic word *badzehr*, which originally meant "antidote for poisons"; bezoars from animals were thought to have healing or magical powers and were used as homeopathic treatment for a wide variety of maladies, such as seizure disorders and leprosy. Patients with bezoars present with vomiting, early satiety, a palpable upper abdominal mass, anemia, or bloody stools.

Trichobezoars usually result from the swallowing of multiple small amounts of hair plucked from the head or fibers from fur, rugs, or garments. The single hairs or fibers become lodged in the gastric mucosal folds, and over time, an intraluminal mass develops. The bezoar assumes the shape of the stomach and proximal duodenum, where it becomes lodged (Fig. 131-1). Trichobezoars are seen in patients with mental retardation and in young children and adolescents with pica.

Phytobezoars are the most common type of bezoar, composed of plant matter such as cellulose and fruit tannins. They develop most frequently after the ingestion of high-fiber vegetables and fruits, and in adults, they are seen most frequently in patients who have had prior surgery. Phytobezoars tend to pass into the small bowel and, rarely, as far as the colon and may fragment. Therefore, it is important to look for more than one bezoar on imaging.

Lactobezoars are formed from undigested milk curds. Most are seen in preterm infants who received formulas with high casein-whey ratios, but they have also been described (rarely) in infants receiving breast milk. Delayed gastric emptying and decreased acid production may play a role in their development. On upper GI series, they may appear similar to a trichobezoar but tend to have less air trapped within (Fig. 131-2).

> Look for more than one bezoar on imaging, because they may fragment and pass into the distal bowel.

On plain radiographs, the appearance of a bezoar may be similar to that of the stomach shortly after the ingestion of a normal meal. On occasion, normal food contents may mimic a bezoar (Fig. 131-3). Bezoars are difficult to see in the stomach with ultrasonography (US) but have been described as an "arc" of bright echoes with shadowing, owing to the trapped air or calcium in the mass (Fig. 131-4). Computed tomography (CT) is most helpful. If oral contrast is given, a free-floating mass is seen in the stomach that contains an unusual gas pattern within the interstices. Calcification may be present. Ripolles and colleagues cautioned that a gastric bezoar may be missed if no oral contrast is used. They suggested that altering the window level to −100 Hounsfield units allows the air-filled bezoar to be identified. Small bezoars may float within the oral contrast material and appear similar to retained food on CT and be missed. A case report of a trichobezoar in a child described a low signal mass on both T1- and T2-weighted magnetic resonance imaging (MRI).

Treatment of any bezoar includes removal and prevention of recurrence through education or behavioral therapy. A number of treatments have been used, including nasogastric lavage and suction for smaller bezoars and therapy with digestive enzymes, but these methods may not be fully successful. Novel treatments such as lithotripsy or endoscopic removal may be used in some cases. There is the potential for distal migration of a fragment, which might produce small bowel obstruction. Gastrotomy may be required in severe cases.

TUMORS AND TUMOR-LIKE CONDITIONS

True neoplasms of the stomach are relatively uncommon in childhood (Table 131-1). These include various types of polyps, inflammatory pseudotumor, teratoma, lymphoma, and stromal tumors. Carcinoma is extremely rare.

Isolated gastric polyps (without an underlying polyposis syndrome) are typically benign hyperplastic polyps or are related to pancreatic heterotopias. Hyperplastic polyps may overlap with the variable mucosal thickening found in the majority of patients with hypertrophic pyloric stenosis. Intussuscepted hyperplastic gastric polyps may also masquerade as duodenal duplication cysts. There have been rare reports of gastric hamartomatous polyps, including associated gastroduodenal intussusception. Double-contrast studies of the stomach are most useful for evaluating the various types of polyps (Fig. 131-5).

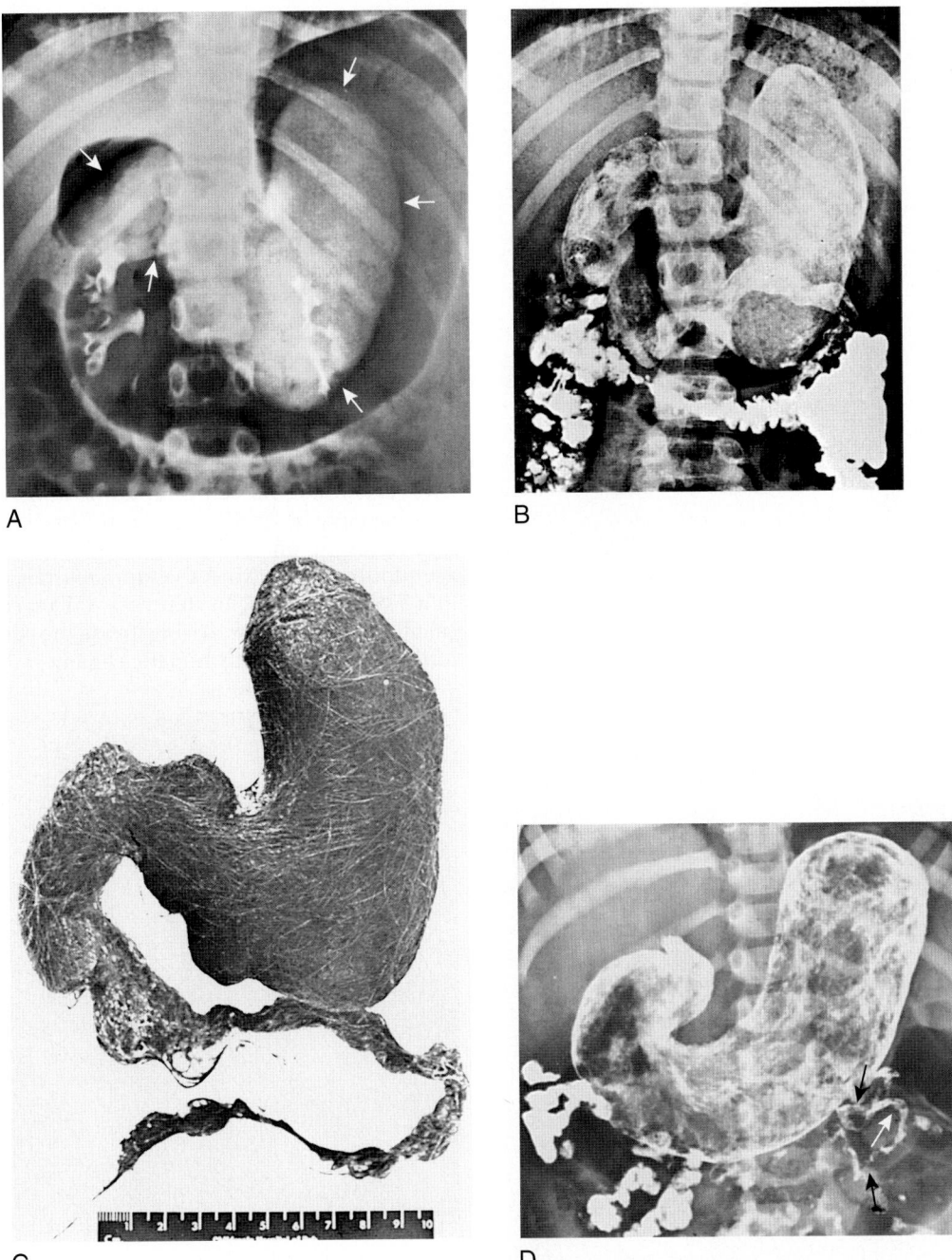

FIGURE 131-1. Trichobezoar in a 10-year-old girl with anemia and a left upper quadrant mass. **A,** A large soft tissue mass *(arrows)* is seen in the dilated, air-filled stomach. **B,** Barium is trapped in the trichobezoar, demonstrating the mass extending through the duodenum and into the proximal jejunum. **C,** Surgical specimen. **D,** Trichobezoar in a 20-month-old girl. The mass of hair fills the gastric lumen. The *arrows* demonstrate pieces of the trichobezoar in the duodenum and jejunum.

Polyps have been described in several of the polyposis syndromes, including Peutz-Jeghers syndrome (hamartomatous polyps), Gardner syndrome (adenomatous polyps), familial polyposis (adenomatous polyps), and juvenile polyposis (juvenile polyps). Recent studies have shown that gastroduodenal polyps may be seen in up to 83% of patients with familial polyposis syndrome, a finding that suggests that lifelong endoscopic surveillance of the upper GI tract is warranted because of the well-known potential for malignant transformation of adenomatous polyps. An increased risk of malignancy (both GI and extraintestinal) has been reported in patients with Peutz-Jeghers syndrome as well, including a case report of gastric adenocarcinoma in a child. Gastroduodenal intussusception has been described in patients with Peutz-Jeghers syndrome and hamartomatous gastric polyps.

Gastric hemangiomas are rare, with only a few case reports in the literature. Patients present with GI bleeding and anemia; they often have an associated cutaneous hemangioma. Large phleboliths may be associated with the gastric mass.

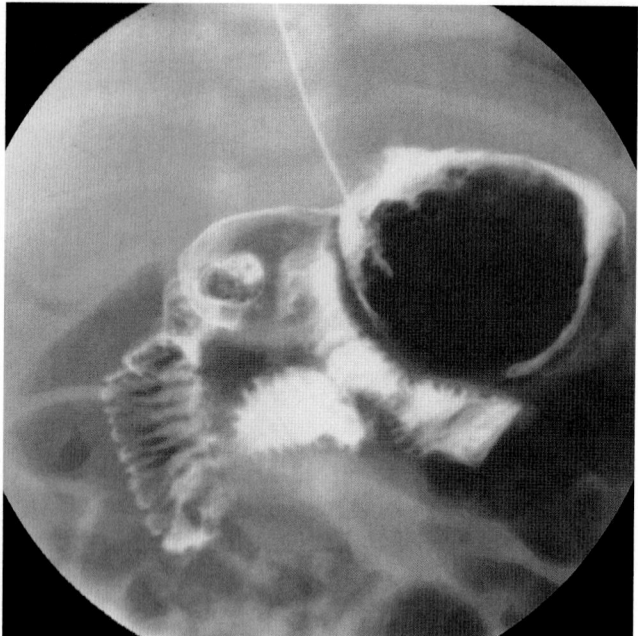

FIGURE 131-2. Lactobezoar in an infant with vomiting. The bezoar is identified as a large, circular filling defect within the barium; the filling defect moved with patient positioning.

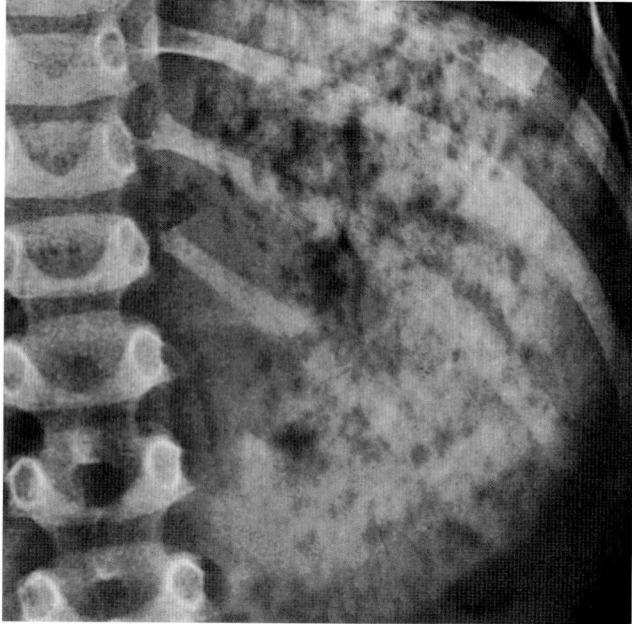

A

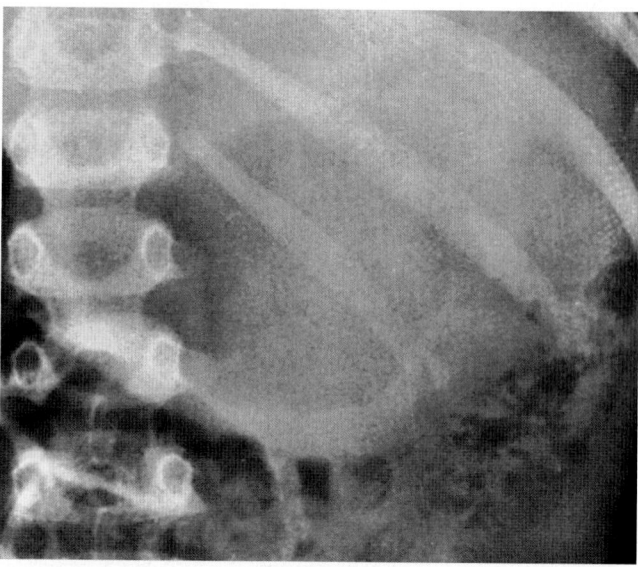

B

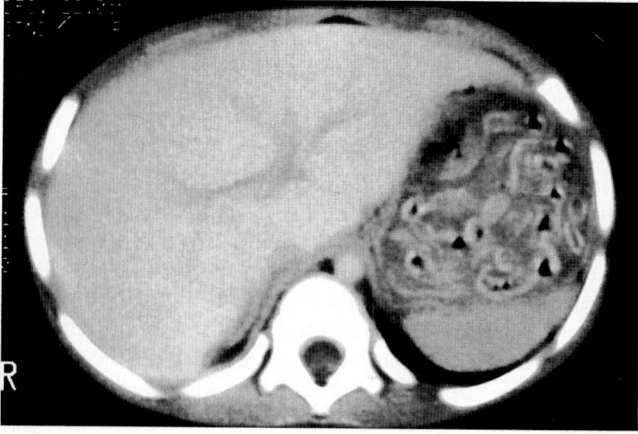

C

FIGURE 131-3. Food simulating a gastric bezoar in a 3-year-old girl. **A,** Radiograph of the left upper quadrant shortly after four bowls of dry cereal were consumed. **B,** Twenty-four hours later, the stomach appears normal. **C,** CT section without contrast in another patient shows a heterogeneous "mass" containing air and curvilinear regions of higher attenuation. This patient had recently eaten macaroni and cheese, and delayed scans confirmed resolution of this pseudomass.

Inflammatory fibroid polyps are typically seen in the small intestine but can appear anywhere in the upper GI tract, including the stomach and duodenum. In fact, reports of these lesions in the stomach and duodenum have been appearing with increasing frequency. Their cause is unclear, and they have been known by a variety of names in the past. The histologic appearance varies slightly, depending on the part of the GI tract involved; gastric lesions frequently contain elements that are histologically characterized as neurilemmomas. These lesions are always benign, can be either polypoid or sessile, originate in the submucosa, and are best seen on double-contrast studies of the stomach or duodenum. They are also easily identified on CT.

Inflammatory pseudotumor is a benign mass of unclear cause (either reactive or neoplastic) that has been reported in most organ systems (Fig. 131-6). It has also been called plasma cell granuloma and is characterized histologically by proliferative myofibroblasts, fibroblasts, histiocytes, plasma cells, and lymphocytes. Inflammatory pseudotumor involving the stomach has been reported in a 5-year-old child. In that case, CT revealed a partially calcified gastric mass arising from the lesser curve and infiltrating the gastrohepatic ligament. MRI demon-

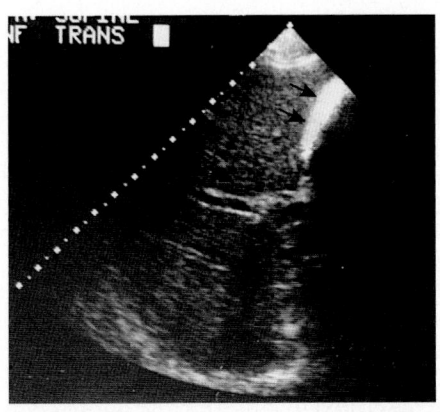

FIGURE 131-4. Gastric bezoar. **A,** Transverse US in the epigastrium demonstrates a broad band of increased echogenicity in the region of the stomach *(arrows),* with clear shadowing posteriorly. This appearance persists regardless of the angle or plane of imaging. **B** and **C,** Axial CT sections through the fundus and antrum of the stomach show an intragastric mass consisting of compressed concentric rings with entrapped air, debris, and barium (from an upper gastrointestinal series 10 days previously). (From Newman B, Girdany BR: Gastric bezoars—sonographic and computed tomographic appearance. Pediatr Radiol 1990;20:526.)

A

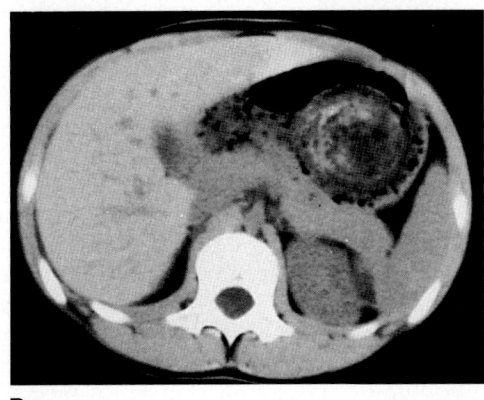

B

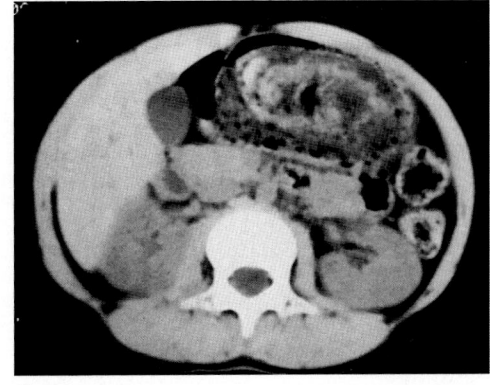

C

TABLE 131-1

Differential Diagnosis of Gastric Mass

Polyp
   Hamartomatous
   Adenomatous
   Juvenile
   Hyperplastic
Inflammatory fibroid
Inflammatory pseudotumor (plasma cell granuloma)
Teratoma
Leiomyoma
Leiomyoblastoma
Leiomyosarcoma
Gastrointestinal stromal tumor, including gastrointestinal
   autonomic nerve tumor
Carcinoma
Lymphoma

strated a mass that was lower in signal intensity than the adjacent stomach on both T1- and T2-weighted images; the mass enhanced after intravenous gadolinium administration.

Gastric teratomas have been described in neonates and young infants, predominantly boys. They most commonly present with evidence of proximal GI obstruction or GI hemorrhage (Fig. 131-7). Cross-sectional imaging has been described of a malignant gastric teratoma in a 4-month-old child; CT and US demonstrated a multilobulated mass.

Rarely, a gastric lipoma may present as a submucosal tumor and is usually indistinguishable from a GI stromal tumor or lymphoma on plain radiography. CT demonstrates fat attenuation within the lesion, which is diagnostic. Lipomas larger than 3 cm may be symptomatic because of proplase, ulceration, and bleeding.

- **Neoplasms of the stomach are uncommon in childhood**
- **Malignant tumors of the stomach are extremely rare**

Malignant lesions of the stomach are extremely rare. Bethel and coworkers' comprehensive review of GI malignancies in children found that only 5.5% (3 of 54) were gastric in origin. Lymphoma and sarcoma are the most common malignant tumors of the stomach in childhood, with mucosa-associated lymphoid tissue (MALT) being the most common. According to Kurugoglu and associates, "MALT lymphoma arises in response to a stimulus. Recently, it has been emphasized that infection with *Helicobacter pylori* triggers the development of gastric MALT and provides the background for MALT-type lymphoma." Non-MALT primary gastric lymphomas are even rarer. This type of lymphoma, usually of the non-Hodgkin variety, is a high-grade, nodal, B cell lymphoma, usually of the Burkitt type. Burkitt lymphoma is generally found in the ileocecal region but has rarely been

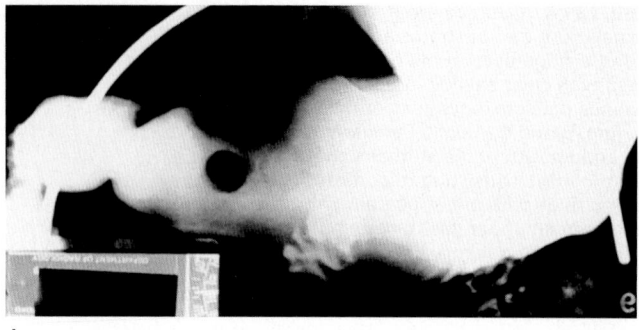

A

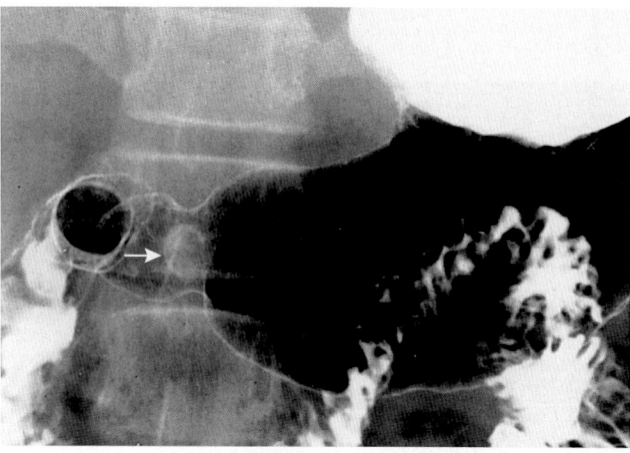

B

FIGURE 131-5. Solitary benign gastric polyp in a 14-year-old boy. Single-contrast (A) and double-contrast (B) upper gastrointestinal series show the intragastric polyp (*arrow in B*). No evidence of polyposis syndromes was found after an extensive evaluation.

reported as a primary malignancy arising in the stomach. These lesions present with marked mucosal nodularity, rugal thickening, shallow or deep ulcers, a mass, or enlarged gastric folds, usually in the body or pyloric region. CT typically shows marked thickening of the gastric wall as a result of diffusely infiltrative tumor (Fig. 131-8). Rarely, they may present as "bull's-eye" lesions, simulating melanomatous lesions in adults (Fig. 131-9).

Both benign and malignant stromal tumors can occur in the stomach in children, but they are rare. *Gastrointestinal stromal tumors* (GISTs) are mesenchymal tumors that typically occur in adults older than 40 years but have been described in children and adolescents (Fig. 131-10). Histologically, GISTs have phenotypic similarities to the interstitial cells of Cajal, and a histogenetic origin from these cells or a pluripotential stem cell is possible. A recent study by Prakash and coworkers revealed an increased incidence of this tumor in girls. Multifocal tumors with a wild-type KIT/PDGFRA genotype are seen. These tumors are less well-differentiated stromal tumors of the GI tract; the term *gastrointestinal stromal sarcoma* is used to describe their malignant counterpart. More recently, a broader spectrum of the phenotypic expression of GISTs has been appreciated, including smooth muscle, peripheral nerve sheath, or neuronal differentiation. A specific subset of GIST that has received attention recently in both adults and children is the gastrointestinal autonomic nerve tumor (GANT), which shows immunohistochemical reaction for markers of neurons of the autonomic enteric plexus. A report of four pediatric patients with GANT involving the stomach described imaging with plain radiographs, upper GI series, and CT. These studies revealed intramural gastric masses; one was multilobular, and one had a large exophytic component.

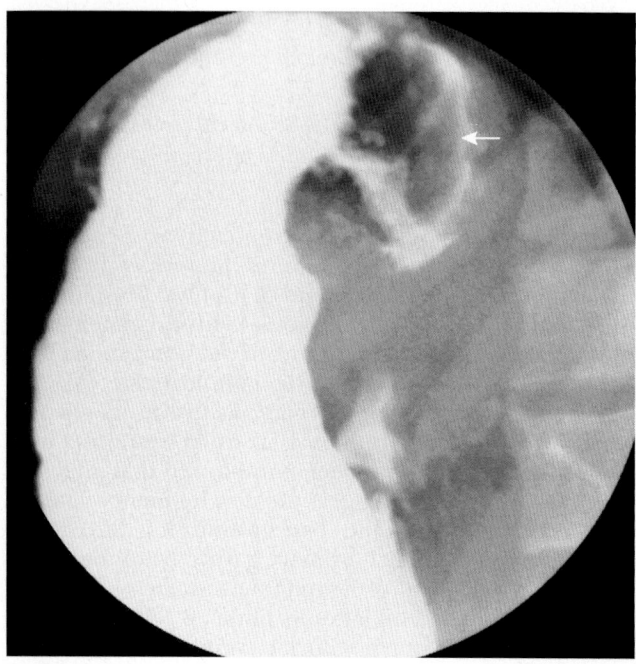

A

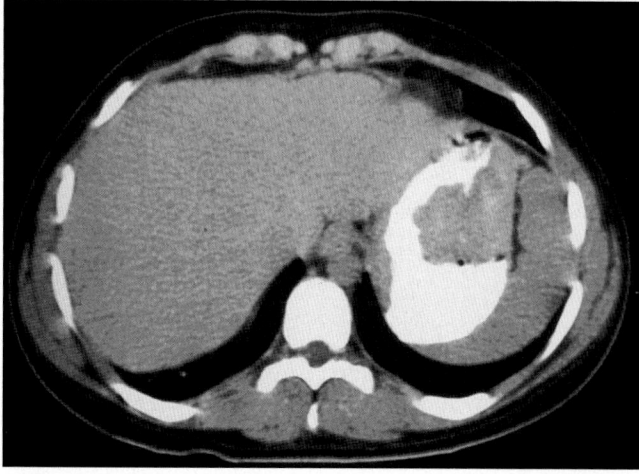

B

FIGURE 131-6. Inflammatory pseudotumor in an 18-year-old girl who presented with abdominal pain. **A,** Upper gastrointestinal series shows a filling defect in the stomach (*arrow*) that did not move with patient positioning. **B,** CT scan after oral contrast shows a large lobular mass in the lateral wall of the stomach.

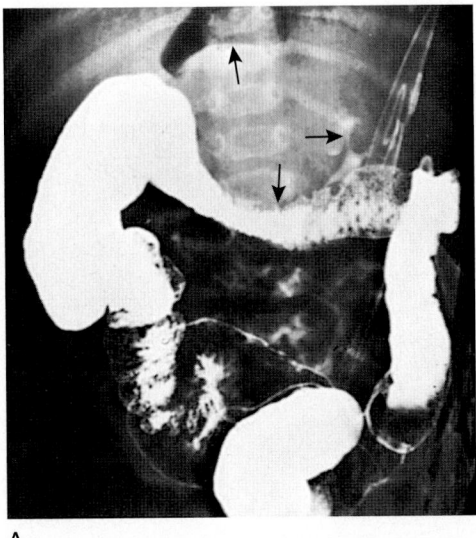
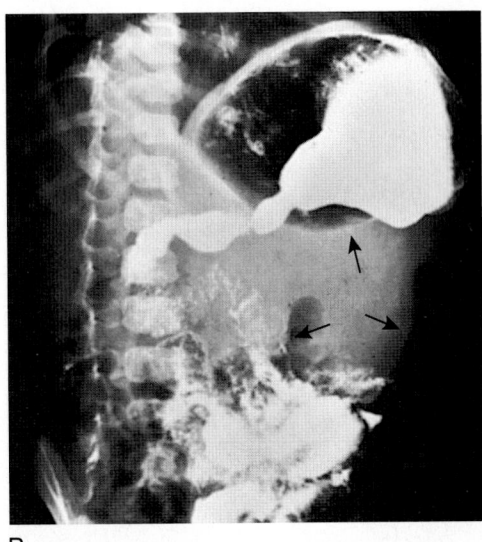

A   B

FIGURE 131-7. Gastric teratoma. Frontal **(A)** and oblique **(B)** views from a barium enema and upper gastrointestinal series show a large mass impinging on the stomach and transverse colon *(arrows)*. At surgery, the mass was found to arise directly from the stomach, and teratoma was documented histologically.

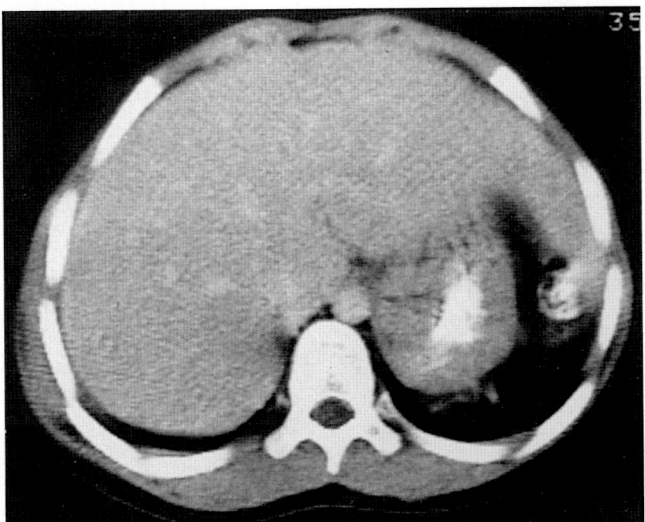

FIGURE 131-8. Non-Hodgkin lymphoma of the stomach in a 14-year-old boy. The wall of the entire stomach is uniformly thickened on CT. Findings were confirmed at laparotomy.

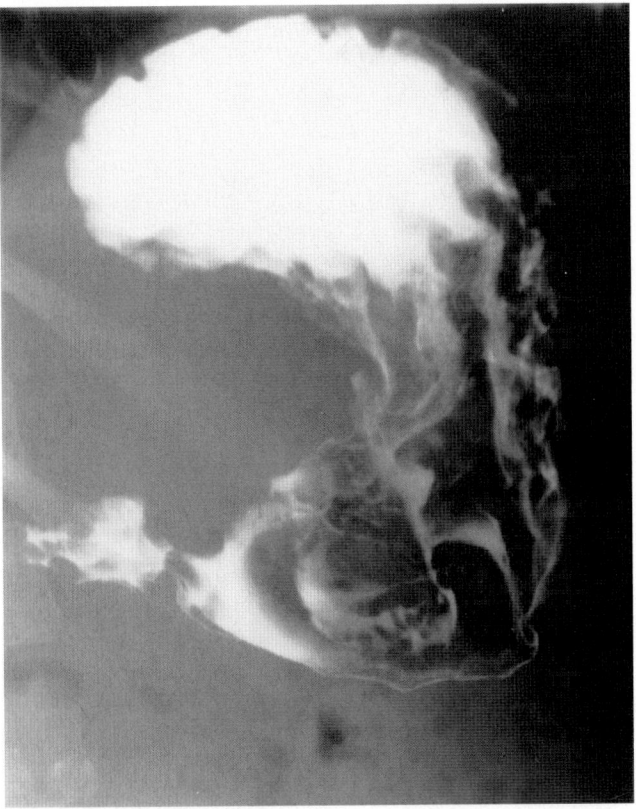

FIGURE 131-9. Upper gastrointestinal series in a 10-year-old boy with non-Hodgkin lymphoma shows a "bull's-eye" lesion and thickened folds in the stomach. The lesion was confirmed as lymphoma at endoscopic biopsy.

With advances in immunohistochemical and molecular genetic techniques, well-differentiated smooth muscle tumors such as leiomyosarcoma are now believed to be rare in the stomach. Because they are typically submucosal, they may be detected on upper GI series. Thickening of the submucosal region on US or CT is suggestive of the diagnosis. CT is particularly useful to demonstrate the extragastric component of the tumor, particularly in those that are malignant. Leiomyomas and leiomyosarcomas have been reported with increasing frequency in the GI tract (including the stomach and duodenum), as well as in various extragastrointestinal sites in immunocompromised patients (both those with acquired immunodeficiency syndrome and those who are human immunonodeficiency virus negative).

Carcinomas have been described in teenagers. There is evidence that gastric carcinoma in children may have more aggressive clinical and pathologic features compared with those in older patients.

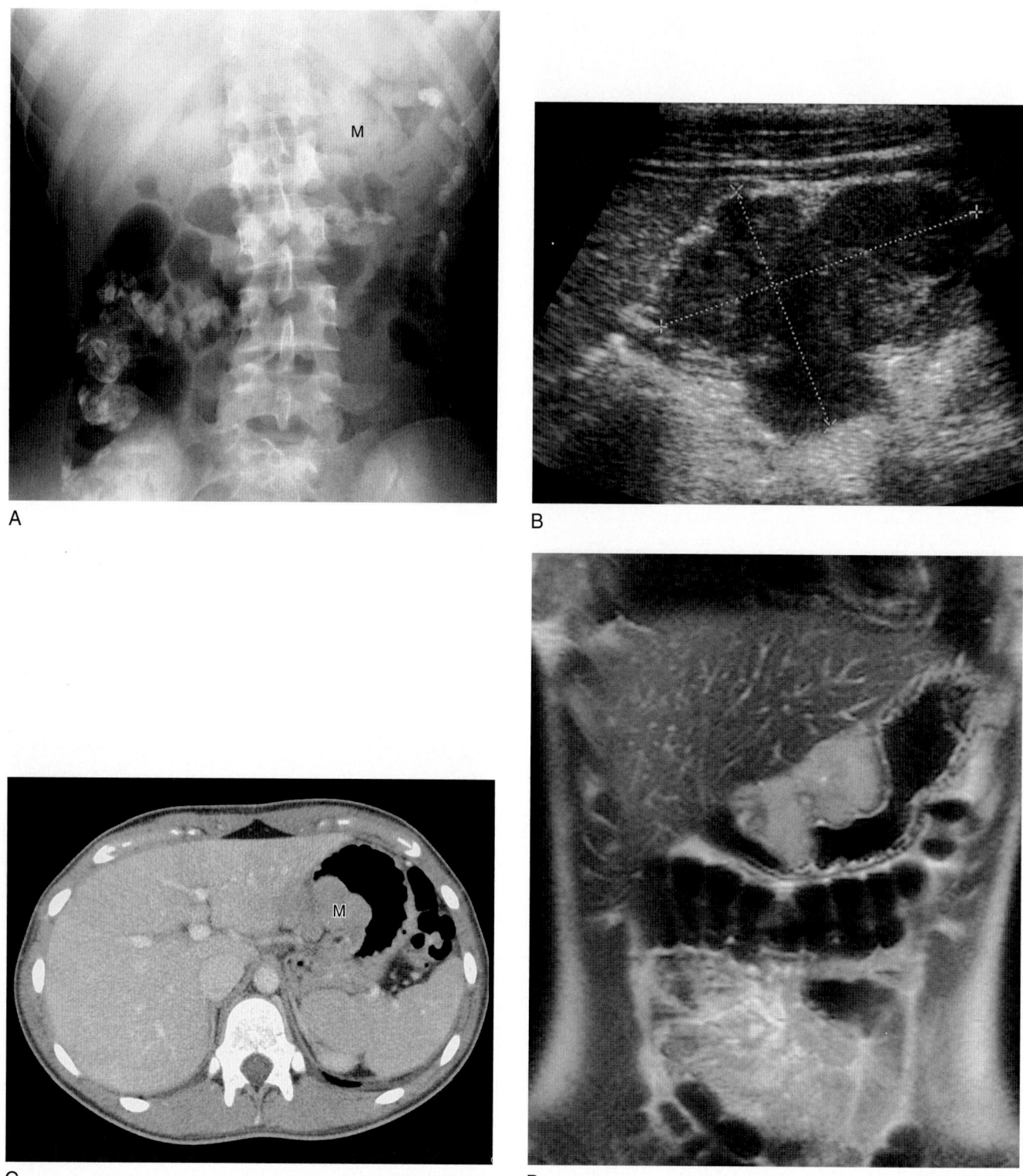

FIGURE 131-10. Sixteen-year-old girl with gastrointestinal stromal tumor. **A,** Abdominal radiograph shows a subtle soft tissue mass (M) impinging on the gas-filled stomach. Residual contrast is seen in the colon. **B,** Transverse US in the midline, at the level of the left lobe of the liver, shows the lobular mass, which was highly vascular on color Doppler. **C,** Axial CT after oral and intravenous contrast administration reveals a soft tissue mass (M) with heterogeneous enhancement originating from the wall of the lesser curvature of the stomach. **D,** Coronal T1-weighted MR image shows the lobular mass arising from the lesser curvature.

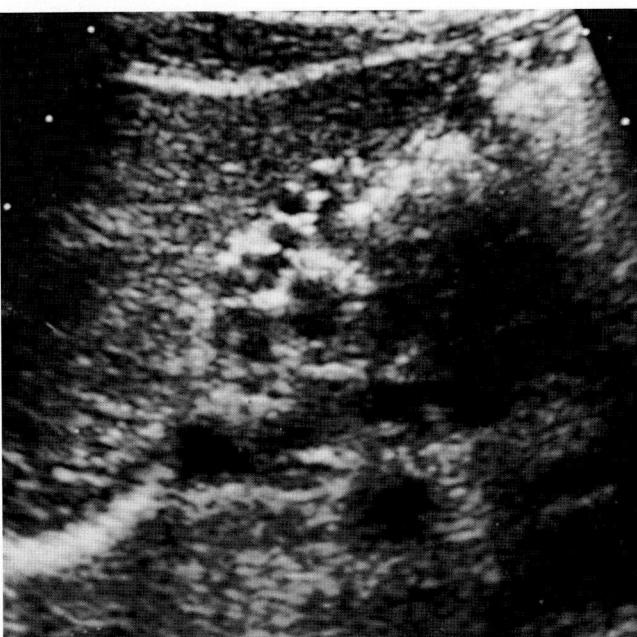

FIGURE 131-11. US of the gastrohepatic ligament shows multiple dilated vessels within the ligament—an appearance virtually diagnostic of varices.

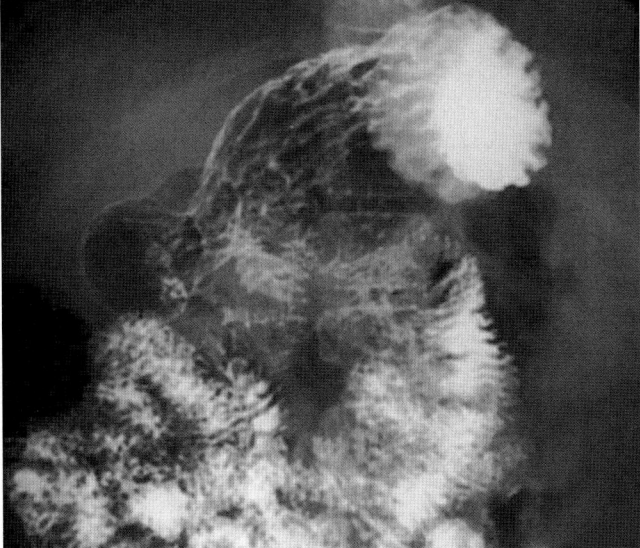

FIGURE 131-12. Gastric varices in an 8-year-old boy with cavernous transformation of the portal vein and massive splenomegaly. Note the serpentine filling defects throughout the fundus and lesser curvature of the stomach. Varices were confirmed by endoscopy.

VARICES

Patients with portal hypertension may develop gastric and duodenal varices in addition to those in the esophagus. On US or CT, varices may be found in the gastrohepatic ligament (Fig. 131-11) and along the gastric wall. On upper GI series, gastric varices are most commonly found in the fundus and along the lesser curvature, appearing as serpentine filling defects (Fig. 131-12). Less commonly, a similar appearance may be seen in the antrum of the stomach or the proximal duodenum. On color Doppler sonography, multiple slow-flowing vessels are seen in the thickened stomach wall. In a series of patients described by Komatsuda and colleagues, which included children, the flow direction of the left gastric vein can help identify patients at high risk for variceal hemorrhage. Patients with hemorrhagic gastric varicosities showed hepatofugal flow on Doppler interrogation.

SUGGESTED READINGS

Bezoars

Chen MK, Beierle EA: Gastrointestinal foreign bodies. Pediatr Ann 2001;30:736

Ciampa A, Moore BE, Listerud RG, et al: Giant trichophytobezoar in a pediatric patient with trichotillomania. Pediatr Radiol 2003;33:219

Krol CM: Small bowel obstruction due to migratory trichobezoar in a child: CT diagnosis. AJR Am J Roentgenol 2001;177:255

Mandel D, Lubetzky R, Mimouni FB, Dollberg S: Lactobezoar and necrotizing enterocolitis in a preterm infant. Isr Med Assoc J 2003;5:895

Phillips MR, Zaheer S, Drugas GT: Gastric trichobezoar: case report and literature review. Mayo Clin Proc 1998;73:653

Ripolles T, Garcia-Aguayo JG, Martinez MJ, et al: Gastrointestinal bezoars: sonographic and CT characteristics. AJR Am J Roentgenol 2001;177:65

Sinzig M, Umschaden HW, Haselbach H, et al: Gastric trichobezoar with gastric ulcer: MR findings. Pediatr Radiol 1998;28:296

Steinberg R, Schwatz M, Gelber E, et al: A rare case of colonic obstruction by cherry tomato phytobezoar: a simple technique to avoid enterotomy. J Pediatr Surg 2002;37:794

Tumors and Tumor-Like Conditions

Aideyan UO, Kao SC: Gastric adenocarcinoma metastatic to the testes in Peutz-Jeghers syndrome. Pediatr Radiol 1994;24:496

Bahk YW, Ahn JC, Choi HJ: Lymphoid hyperplasia of the stomach presenting as umbilicated polypoid lesions. Radiology 1971;100:277

Balsam D, Segal S: Two smooth muscle tumors in the airway of an HIV-infected child. Pediatr Radiol 1992;22:552

Bethel CA, Bhattacharyya N, Hutchinson C, et al: Alimentary tract malignancies in children. J Pediatr Surg 1997;32:1008

Bourke CJ, Mackay AJ, Payton D: Malignant gastric teratoma: case report. Pediatr Surg Int 1997;12:192

Bowen B, Ros PR, McCarthy MJ, et al: Gastrointestinal teratomas: CT and US appearance with pathologic correlation. Radiology 1987;162:431

Brooks GS, Frost ES, Wesselhoeft C: Prolapsed hyperplastic gastric polyp causing gastric outlet obstruction, hypergastrinemia, and hematemesis in an infant. J Pediatr Surg 1992;27:1537

Buck JL, Harned RK, Lichtenstein JE, et al: Peutz Jeghers syndrome. Radiographics 1992;12:365

Cacciaguerra S, Miano AE, Di Benedetto A, et al: Gastric carcinoma with ovarian metastases in an adolescent. Pediatr Surg Int 1998;14:98

da Santos G, Zucoloto S: Inflammatory fibroid polyp: review of the literature. Arq Gastroenterol 1993;30:107

Defago MR, Higa AL, Campra JL, et al: Carcinoma in situ arising in a gastric hamartomatous polyp in a patient with Peutz-Jeghers syndrome. Endoscopy 1996;28:267

Denzler TC, Harned RK, Pergam CJ: Gastric polyps in familial polyposis coli. Radiology 1979;130:63

Desai DC, Neale KF, Talbot IC, et al: Juvenile polyposis. Br J Surg 1995;82:14

Dixon WL, Fazzari PJ: Carcinoma of the stomach in a child. JAMA 1976;235:2414

Domizio P, Talbot IC, Spigelman AD, et al: Upper gastrointestinal pathology in familial adenomatous polyposis: result from a prospective study of 102 patients. J Clin Pathol 1990;43:738

Dunnick NR, Harell GS, Parker BR: Multiple "bull's-eye" lesions in gastric lyphoma. AJR Am J Roentgenol 1976;126:965

Gengler JS, Ashcraft KW, Slattery P: Gastric teratoma: the sixth reported case in a female patient. J Pediatr Surg 1995;30:889

Goedde TA, Rodriguez-Bigas MA, Herrera L, et al: Gastroduodenal polyps in familial adenomatous polyposis. Surg Oncol 1992;1:357

Ha C, Haller JO, Rollins NK: Smooth muscle tumors in immunocompromised (HIV negative) children. Pediatr Radiol 1993;23:413

Hernanz-Schulman M, Dinauer P, Ambrosino MM, et al: The antral nipple sign of pyloric mucosal prolapse: endoscopic correlation of a new sonographic observation in patients with pyloric stenosis. J Ultrasound Med 1995;14:283

Hernanz-Schulman M, Lowe LH, Johnson J, et al: In vivo visualization of pyloric mucosal hypertrophy in infants with hypertrophic pyloric stenosis: is there an etiologic role? AJR Am J Roentgenol 2001;177:843

Hizawa K, Iida M, Matsumoto T, et al: Cancer in Peutz-Jeghers syndrome. Cancer 1993;72:2777

Kerr JZ, Hicks MJ, Nuchtern JG, et al: Gastrointestinal autonomic nerve tumors in the pediatric population: a report of four cases and a review of the literature. Cancer 1999;85:220

Kim S, Chung CJ, Fordham LA, et al: Coexisting hyperplastic antral polyp and hypertrophic pyloric stenosis. Pediatr Radiol 1997;27:912

Kodet R, Snajdauf J, Smelhaus V: Gastrointestinal autonomic nerve tumor: a case report with electronic microscopic and immunohistochemical analysis and review of the literature. Pediatr Pathol 1994;14:1005

Komatsuda T, Ishida H, Konno K, et al: Color Doppler findings of gastrointestinal varices. Abdom Imaging 1998;23:45

Kurugoglu S, Mihmanli I, Celkan T, et al: Radiological features in paediatric primary gastric MALT lymphoma and association with Helicobacter pylori. Pediatr Radiol 2002;32:82

Lauwers GY, Erlandson RA, Casper ES, et al: Gastrointestinal autonomic nerve tumors: a clinicopathological, immunohistochemical, and ultrastructural study of 12 cases. Am J Surg Pathol 1993;17:887

Lee ES, Locker J, Nalesnik M, et al: The association of Epstein-Barr virus and smooth-muscle tumors occurring after organ transplantation. N Engl J Med 1995;332:19

Levy AD, Abbott RM, Rohrmann CA, et al: Gastrointestinal hemangiomas: imaging findings and pathologic correlation in pediatric and adult patients. AJR Am J Roentgenol 2001;177:1073

Lichtman S, Hayes G, Stringer DA, et al: Chronic intussusception due to antral myoepithelioma. J Pediatr Surg 1986;21:955

Marcello PW, Asbun HJ, Veidenheimer MC, et al: Gastroduodenal polyps in familial adenomatous polyposis. Surg Endosc 1996;10:418

McClain KL, Leach CL, Jenson HB, et al: Association of Epstein-Barr virus with leiomyosarcomas in young people with AIDS. N Engl J Med 1995;332:12

McGill TW, Downey EC, Westbrook J, et al: Gastric carcinoma in children. J Pediatr Surg 1993;28:1620

McLoughlin LC, Nord KS, Joshi VV, et al: Disseminated leiomyosarcoma in a child with acquired immune deficiency syndrome. Cancer 1991;67:2618

Megibow AJ, Balthazar EJ, Hulnick DH, et al: CT evaluation of gastrointestinal leiomyomas and leiomyosarcomas. AJR Am J Roentgenol 1985;144:727

Miettinen M, Lasota J: Gastrointestinal stromal tumors—definition, clinical, histological, immunohistochemical, and molecular genetic features and differential diagnosis. Virchows Arch 2001;438:1

Nakamura S, Yao T, Aoyagi K, et al: Helicobacter pylori and primary gastric lymphoma: a histopathologic and immunohistochemical analysis of 237 patients. Cancer 1997;79:3

Odes HS, Krawiec J, Yanai-Inbar I, et al: Benign lymphoid hyperplasia of the stomach. Pediatr Radiol 1981;10:244

Orlow SJ, Kamino H, Lawrence RL: Multiple subcutaneous leiomyosarcomas in an adolescent with AIDS. Am J Pediatr Hematol Oncol 1992;14:265

Prakash S, Sarran L, Socci N, et al: Gastrointestinal stromal tumors in children and young adults: a clinicopathologic, molecular, and genomic study of 15 cases and review of the literature. J Pediatr Hematol Oncol 2005;27:179

Rugge M, Busatto G, Cassaro M, et al: Patients younger than 40 years with gastric carcinoma: Helicobacter pylori genotype and associated gastritis phenotype. Cancer 1999;85:2506

Sanna CM, Loriga P, Dessi E, et al: Hyperplastic polyp of the stomach simulating hypertrophic pyloric stenosis. J Pediatr Gastroenterol Nutr 1991;13:204

Scafidi DE, McLeary MS, Young LW: Diffuse neonatal gastrointestinal hemangiomatosis: CT findings, Pediatr Radiol 1998;28:512

Schneider K, Kickerhoff R, Bertele RM: Malignant gastric sarcoma—diagnosis by ultrasound. Pediatr Radiol 1986;16:69

Schroeder BA, Wells RG, Sty JR: Inflammatory fibroid polyp of the stomach in a child. Pediatr Radiol 1987;17:71

Sharon N, Kenet G, Toren A, et al: Helicobacter pylori-associated gastric lymphoma in a girl. Pediatr Hematol Oncol 1997;14:177

Shimer GR, Helwig EB: Inflammatory fibroid polyps of the intestine. Am J Clin Pathol 1984;81:708

Siegel MJ, Shackelford GD: Gastric teratomas in infants: report of 2 cases. Pediatr Radiol 1978;7:197

Spigelman AD, Williams CB, Talbot IC, et al: Upper gastrointestinal cancer in patients with familial adenomatous polyposis. Lancet 1989;2:783

Suster S: Gastrointestinal stromal tumors. Semin Diagn Pathol 1996;13:297

Taratuta E, Krinsky G, Genega E, et al: Pediatric inflammatory pseudotumor of the stomach: contrast-enhanced CT and MR imaging findings. AJR Am J Roentgenol 1996;167:919

Theuer CP, Kurosaki T, Taylor TH, et al: Unique features of gastric carcinoma in the young: a population-based analysis. Cancer 1998;83:25

Thomas JR, Mrak RE, Linuit N: Gastrointestinal autonomic nerve tumor presenting as a high-grade sarcoma: case report and review of the literature. Dig Dis Sci 1994;39:2051

Thompson WM, Kende AI, Levy AD: Imaging characteristics of gastric lipomas in 16 adult and pediatric patients. AJR Am J Roentgenol 2003;181:981

Uddin N, Abernethy LJ: Gastroduodenal intussusception with a gastric antral polyp. Pediatr Radiol 1998;28:460

Wu YK, Tsai CH, Yang JC, et al: Gastroduodenal intussusception due to Peutz-Jeghers syndrome: a case report. Hepatogastroenterology 1994;41:134

Wurlitzer FP, Mares AJ, Isaacs H Jr, et al: Smooth muscle tumors of the stomach in childhood and adolescence. J Pediatr Surg 1973;8:421

CHAPTER

132 | The Duodenum and Small Intestine: Normal Anatomy and Imaging Techniques

ALAN E. SCHLESINGER and KIMBERLY APPLEGATE

NORMAL ANATOMY

The small intestine is a long, convoluted, musculomembranous tube that begins at the pylorus and ends at the ileocecal valve. Its length and pattern are variable; its three major divisions are the duodenum, jejunum, and ileum.

The duodenum, the most proximal portion of the small intestine, begins at the pyloroduodenal junction. The first portion of the duodenum begins at the pylorus and ends approximately at the neck of the gallbladder. It is almost completely covered by peritoneum but is the only portion of the normal duodenum that is relatively mobile. The second, third, and fourth portions of the duodenum are retroperitoneal. The second or descending portion extends from the neck of the gallbladder and is in intimate contact with the head of the pancreas. The common bile duct enters its midportion. The third portion is horizontal and courses back to the left across the spine. Anteriorly, it is covered by peritoneum and is crossed by the superior mesenteric artery and vein. The fourth portion ascends along the left side of the aorta, where it turns ventrally to become the jejunum at the level of the duodenojejunal flexure. The flexure is retroperitoneal, where it is normally fixed, and is further secured in place by the ligament of Treitz. The duodenojejunal flexure is typically to the left of the left vertebral pedicle at this level, at or near the craniocaudal level of the duodenal bulb. It is important to recall that the proximal portion of the duodenum receives its blood supply from the celiac axis, while the superior mesenteric artery supplies blood to the distal duodenum. Thus, whereas the stomach and the first and second portions of the duodenum are derived from the embryonic foregut, most of the third and all of the fourth portions of the duodenum are of midgut origin and are often involved in midgut volvulus, which is discussed in detail in Chapters 14 and 133.

The jejunum accounts for approximately three fifths of the remaining small bowel; the other two fifths is

ileum. The length of the small bowel is approximately 6 m in adults and 220 cm in term infants. The proximal third of the small intestine commonly fills the left upper abdominal quadrant, the middle third occupies the midportion of the abdomen and the right upper quadrant, and the terminal third lies on the right side of the abdomen and pelvis. The caliber of the lumen gradually diminishes from proximal to distal, with the diameter of the terminal ileum being about one third smaller than that of the first portion of the jejunum. The external surface of the tube is smooth and devoid of permanent folds or creases. The internal surface has transverse and spiral folds, the plicae circulares of the submucosa, which are covered by the villous folds of mucous membrane. These folds greatly increase the secreting and absorbing surface and facilitate digestion by retarding the passage of intestinal contents. The jejunum has more visible folds than the relatively featureless ileum (Fig. 132-1).

IMAGING TECHNIQUES

Plain Radiographs

Plain radiographs are often nonspecific in patients with duodenal and small intestinal disease, but they are extremely useful in identifying intestinal obstruction, intramural air, free peritoneal air secondary to intestinal perforation, pathologic calcification, and masses large enough to displace normal structures.

Fluoroscopic Contrast Studies

Single-contrast studies of the upper gastrointestinal tract under fluoroscopic control—the upper gastrointestinal (GI) series—are the standard examinations for most abnormalities of the stomach and duodenum. A small bowel follow-through is included if the small intestine distal to the duodenojejunal flexure is to be evaluated.

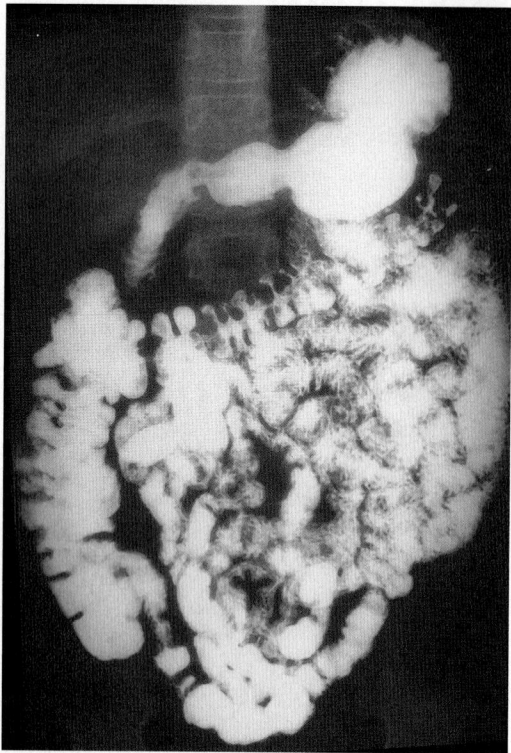

FIGURE 132-1. Normal small intestine. Overhead radiograph from an upper gastrointestinal series with small bowel follow-through shows contrast in the stomach, duodenum, jejunum, ileum, and ascending portion of the colon. The jejunal loops in the left upper quadrant have normal visible folds, and the ileum is relatively featureless.

Barium is the most commonly used contrast material. Water-soluble contrast is typically used when intestinal perforation is suspected. Although more expensive, low-osmolar nonionic contrast agents have largely replaced the older forms of water-soluble contrast media used in the GI tract, especially in neonates and young infants, in whom smaller volumes are needed. These contrast materials are sometimes used for upper GI examinations in patients with intestinal obstruction as well. Low-osmolar contrast is used predominantly in newborns, especially those who are suspected of having necrotizing enterocolitis or who have feeding intolerance that may be secondary to strictures from previous necrotizing enterocolitis. The advantages of isotonic solutions of low-osmolar nonionic contrast media include lack of large fluid shifts, absence of contrast dilution, lack of injury to the bowel mucosa, low absorption from the bowel, and relatively lower risk of pulmonary edema if aspirated. Premature infants may benefit from the use of iso-osmolar contrast agents when evaluating the small bowel, although they are more expensive than low-osmolar agents. Higher osmolar contrast agents are still cautiously used for therapeutic purposes in some neonates with meconium plug syndrome or meconium ileus (see Chapter 14) and in older patients with cystic fibrosis who have distal intestinal obstruction syndrome.

In patients with subtle bowel perforation that is not identified by contrast extravasation at the time of the examination, perforation can be detected on delayed radiographs by renal excretion of the contrast absorbed by the peritoneum.

> **Advantages of isotonic solutions of low-osmolar nonionic contrast media include:**
> - **Lack of large fluid shifts**
> - **Absence of contrast dilution**
> - **Lack of injury to bowel mucosa**
> - **Low absorption from bowel**
> - **Relatively low risk of pulmonary edema if aspirated**

In patients who are old enough to cooperate, double-contrast examinations may be useful. In these cases, a higher density barium is used, and effervescent agents are ingested to produce the double contrast. Double-contrast studies are generally accepted as the upper GI imaging method of choice in adults; however, they require longer fluoroscopy times and a greater number of films than the standard single-contrast examinations. We do not routinely use double-contrast examinations in children; in pediatric patients, the examination should be tailored to the specific clinical question to be answered to limit the radiation exposure. Intermittent, pulsed fluoroscopy (rather than constant fluoroscopy), careful collimation, and photo spot-film cameras or digital fluoroscopy and fluoro grab image recording (in place of the standard film-screen combination spot films) should be used in children, if possible. Pulsed fluoroscopy has become the standard in most children's hospitals because it decreases radiation exposure. Infants and young children, of necessity, are studied in the recumbent position. In older children, especially when double-contrast studies are performed, the examination can be performed with a combination of recumbent and upright spot images.

Older children can be asked to fast overnight if the study will be performed early in the morning. In children younger than 1 year, dehydration is possible with this length of restriction, and we have found that a 3-hour fast is sufficient to empty the normal stomach of food material. In infants with retained material in the stomach, a nasogastric tube should be placed to withdraw most of the retained material, or the examination can be postponed. If the gastric contents are aspirated through a tube, the aspirate should be examined for the presence of bile or blood as a possible diagnostic clue.

Most infants who have fasted for 3 hours will readily take barium from a bottle. They are generally more accepting of the bottle in the supine position, even though this may introduce more air than if they were fed in the prone position.

The routine upper GI examination includes an evaluation of the esophagus, stomach, and duodenum to the duodenojejunal junction. We routinely obtain spot images of the duodenal bulb in the right anterior oblique position (Fig. 132-2) and the anteroposterior supine view of the duodenal sweep demonstrating the duodeno-jejunal junction, the anatomic marker for the location of

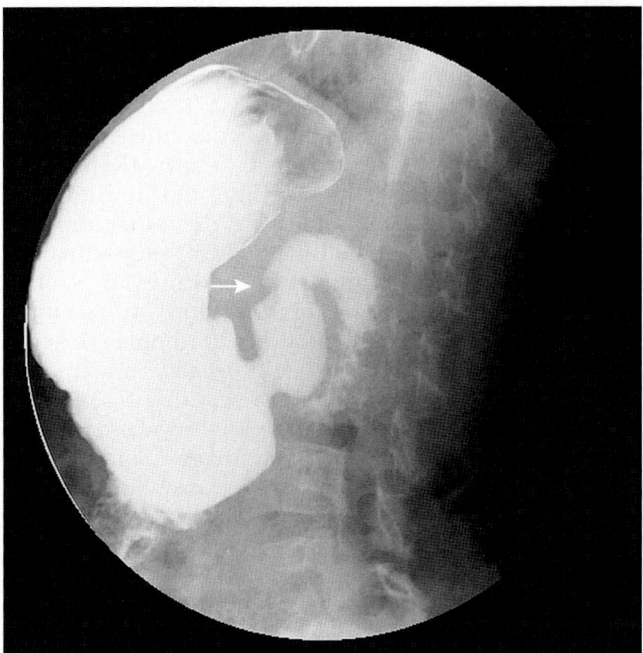

FIGURE 132-2. Normal duodenal bulb. Right anterior oblique view of the duodenal bulb from an upper gastrointestinal series shows a well-distended duodenal bulb just distal to the contracted pylorus *(arrow)*. More proximal constriction in the antrum represents a normal peristaltic wave.

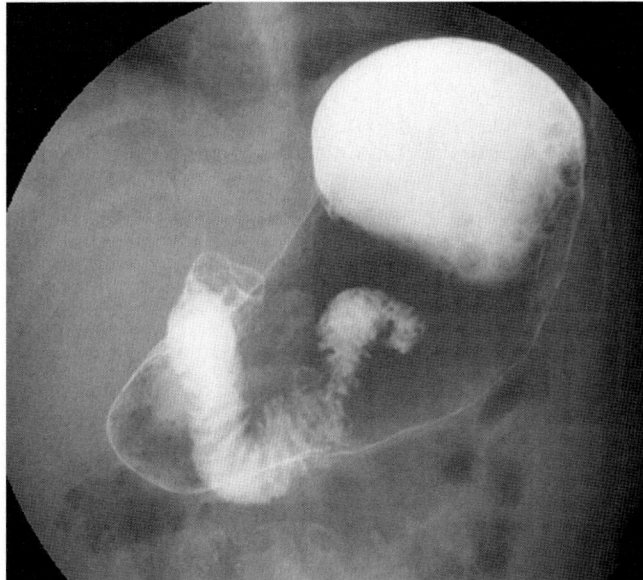

FIGURE 132-3. Anteroposterior supine view of the duodenal sweep. The duodenojejunal flexure is seen through the gas-filled antrum, located to the left of the left pedicle of the vertebra, at or near the level of the duodenal bulb.

the ligament of Treitz (Fig. 132-3). In addition, we obtain a true lateral view of the duodenal sweep to confirm the posterior, retroperitoneal position of the ascending and descending portions of the normally rotated duodenum (Fig. 132-4). We typically obtain a supine spot image of the abdomen at the completion of the study to include the opacified, proximal jejunal loops, in place of an

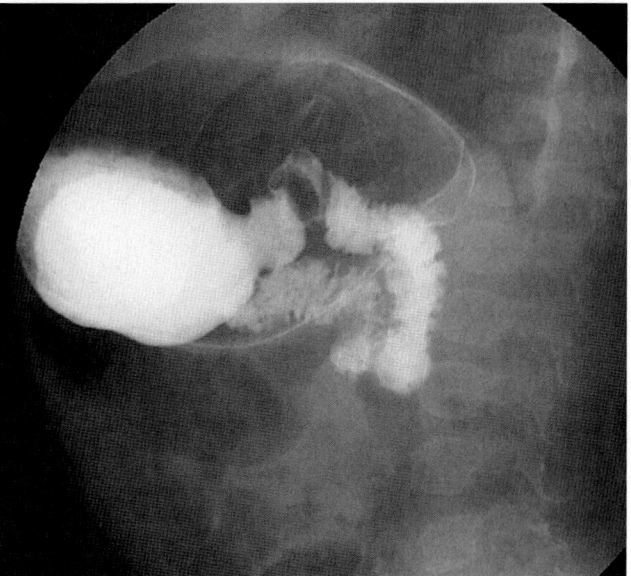

FIGURE 132-4. Lateral view of the duodenal sweep. The posterior (and, therefore, retroperitoneal) position of the duodenal sweep is confirmed.

overhead radiograph. Other specific views are obtained, depending on the results of the fluoroscopic examination. Because it is not necessary to include the pelvis in the radiographic field during upper GI examination, it is imperative that gonadal shielding be used in all children.

When a small bowel follow-through is performed in addition to the upper GI series, sequential overhead images of the abdomen are obtained, typically every 30 to 45 minutes until contrast medium is seen in the cecum, but modified as needed in individual cases (see Fig. 132-1). Some pediatric radiologists alternate these small bowel radiographs between the supine and prone positions. When the contrast agent has reached the cecum, the entire small bowel is viewed fluoroscopically while compressed with a compression paddle, and spot images (with and without compression) are obtained of the terminal ileum. Additional spot images of the remainder of the small bowel are obtained as needed in individual cases. We occasionally perform a small bowel series without the upper GI portion if the esophagus, stomach, and duodenum have been evaluated previously or if only an evaluation of the jejunum or ileum is required. In these cases, the child is given oral contrast material to drink (the amount determined by the child's size and clinical condition), and sequential overhead radiographs are obtained. Spot images of the terminal ileum are performed if needed. Small bowel enteroclysis examinations are rarely performed in young pediatric patients but may be accomplished in cooperative children (Fig. 132-5).

> **A true lateral view of the duodenal sweep (to confirm the posterior, retroperitoneal position of the duodenal C-loop) should be obtained, in addition to the frontal view of the duodenum.**

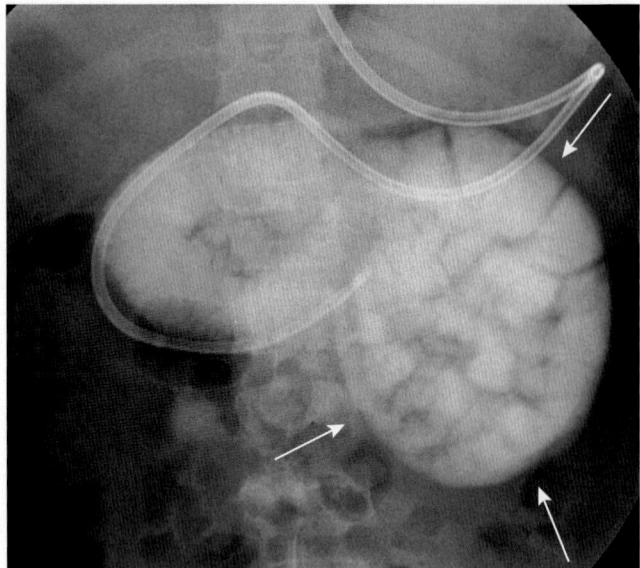

FIGURE 132-5. Enteroclysis image in a 10-year-old girl with recurrent abdominal pain and nonbilious vomiting with surgically confirmed paraduodenal hernia. Prior imaging tests had been negative. The image shows proximal small bowel loops contained within a round sac in the left upper quadrant *(arrows)*, diagnostic of internal hernia. There was no malrotation.

Ultrasonography

Ultrasonography (US) is useful in the evaluation of duodenal and small bowel duplication cysts and duodenal hematomas. US can demonstrate the twist of duodenum and superior mesenteric vein about the superior mesenteric artery in some patients with volvulus, and it can be used to evaluate the orientation of the superior mesenteric artery and vein in patients with presumed malrotation; however, reversal of the normal orientation of these vessels is not entirely sensitive or specific for that condition. In patients with bilious vomiting and suspected malrotation, the upper GI examination is the most expedient method of diagnosis. In the evaluation of suspected appendicitis in children (see Chapter 142), US may identify alternative diagnoses, such as ovarian lesion, inflammatory bowel disease, infectious enteritis, or abnormalities related to the mesentery or omentum, such as mesenteric adenitis, mesenteric or omental cysts, mesenteric masses, or omental infarction. US has become a common screening tool for ileocolic intussusception (see Chapter 141). Doppler US is increasingly being used to assess disease activity in children with Crohn disease involving the small intestine.

> An abnormal relationship of the superior mesenteric artery and vein on US is neither entirely sensitive nor specific for malrotation.

Computed Tomography and Magnetic Resonance Imaging

Computed tomography (CT) and magnetic resonance imaging (MRI) have limited utility in imaging the duo-denum. Although MRI avoids ionizing radiation, it may be more technically challenging to ensure diagnostic quality. Many traumatic duodenal hematomas are diagnosed initially with CT or MRI, and duodenal duplication cysts are occasionally encountered on CT or MRI scans of the abdomen. CT and MRI are the preferred imaging modalities in children with duodenal masses potentially extending beyond the duodenum.

CT and MRI have increasing roles in the evaluation of the small intestine. When CT is performed to evaluate the bowel, adequate bowel opacification with contrast agent is usually necessary. Although the upper GI series with small bowel follow-through usually remains important in the evaluation of children with inflammatory bowel disease, CT is often used to identify abscesses and provide image guidance for drainage. Small bowel injuries may be encountered on CT scans obtained after trauma. CT or MRI is also indicated for the diagnosis and staging of malignancies.

Enterography, Enteroclysis, and Capsule Endoscopy

The use of these newer imaging techniques in children is beginning to grow, following studies demonstrating their utility in adults. CT and MR enterography uses the oral ingestion of high-volume, high-osmolar, and negative contrast agents to distend the bowel for the evaluation of partial small bowel obstruction, intraluminal masses, and inflammatory bowel disease. CT enteroclysis is a more invasive technique that requires the passage of a nasoduodenal tube to administer the contrast agent in a controlled, rapid infusion. Available since 2001, capsule endoscopy has proved to be safe and effective in diagnosing inflammatory and neoplastic disorders in adults and in identifying the cause of obscure bowel hemorrhage. Many pediatric GI specialists are beginning to use capsule endoscopy in children.

Scintigraphy

Scintigraphy plays a limited role in duodenal and small bowel disease but may be useful in cases of abdominal pain or intestinal bleeding, especially when ectopic gastric mucosa is suspected. The value of scintigraphy in inflammatory disease of the intestinal tract is discussed in Chapter 106.

SUGGESTED READINGS

Albert JG, Martiny F, Krummenerl A, et al: Diagnosis of small bowel Crohn's disease: a prospective comparison of capsule endoscopy with magnetic resonance imaging and fluoroscopic enteroclysis. Gut 2005;54:1721-1727

Bodily KD, Fletcher JG, Solem CA, et al: Crohn disease: mural attenuation and thickness at contrast-enhanced CT enterography—correlation with endoscopic and histologic findings of inflammation. Radiology 2006;238:505-516

Brown DM, Schlesinger AE, Komppa GH: Ileal duplication cyst: repeated spontaneous decompression delays diagnosis. Mil Med 1989;154:553-555

Carty HML: Pediatric emergencies: non-traumatic abdominal emergencies. Eur Radiol 2002;12:2835-2848

Cohen MD: Choosing contrast media for the evaluation of the

gastrointestinal tract of neonates and infants. Radiology 1987;162:447-456

Cohen MD, Weber TR, Grosfeld JL: Bowel perforation in the newborn: diagnosis with metrizamide. Radiology 1984; 150:65-69

Guibaud L, Fouque P, Genin G, et al: CT and ultrasound of gastric and duodenal duplications. J Comput Assist Tomogr 1996; 20:382-385

Guilhon de Araujo Sant'Anna AM, Dubois J, Miron MC, Seidman EG: Wireless capsule endoscopy for obscure small-bowel disorders: final results of the first pediatric controlled trial. Clin Gastroenterol Hepatol 2005;3:264-270

Hernanz-Schulman M, Genieser NB, Ambrosino MM: Sonographic diagnosis of intramural duodenal hematoma. J Ultrasound Med 1989;8:273-276

Megramis S, Segkos N, Andrianaki A, et al: Sonographic diagnosis and monitoring of an obstructing duodenal hematoma after blunt trauma. J Ultrasound Med 2004;23:1679-1683

Narlawar RS, Rao JR, Karmarkar SJ, et al: Sonographic findings in a duodenal duplication cyst. J Clin Ultrasound 2002;30:566-568

Puylaert JB: Mesenteric adenitis and acute terminal ileitis: US evaluation using graded compression. Radiology 1986; 161:691-695

Rajesh A, Maglinte DD: Multislice CT enteroclysis: technique and clinical applications. Clin Radiol 2006;61:31-39

Rotondo A, Scialpi M, Pellegrino G, et al: Duodenal duplication cyst: MR imaging appearance. Eur Radiol 1999;9:890-893

Schlesinger AE, Dorfman SR, Braverman RM: Sonographic appearance of omental infarction in children. Pediatr Radiol 1999;29:598-601

Siegel MJ, Carel C, Surratt S: Ultrasonography of acute abdominal pain in children. JAMA 1991;266:1987-1989

Spalinger J, Patriquin H, Miron MC, et al: Doppler US in patients with Crohn disease: vessel density in the diseased bowel reflects disease activity. Radiology 2000;217:787-791

Tiao M-M, Wan Y-L, Ng S-H, et al: Sonographic features of small-bowel intussusception in pediatric patients. Acad Emerg Med 2001;8:368-373

Touloukian RJ, Smith GJ: Normal intestinal growth in preterm infants. J Pediatr Surg 1983;18:720

Vayner N, Coret A, Polliack G, et al: Mesenteric lymphadenopathy in children examined by US for chronic and/or recurrent abdominal pain. Pediatr Radiol 2003;33:864-867

Zerin JM, DiPietro MA: Superior mesenteric vascular anatomy at US in patients with surgically proved malrotation of the midgut. Radiology 1992;183:693-694

ALAN E. SCHLESINGER

Congenital anomalies of the duodenum consist of intrinsically obstructing lesions, such as duodenal atresia and stenosis, malrotation, and duplication cysts.

DUODENAL ATRESIA, STENOSIS, AND WEB

Duodenal atresia typically presents in the newborn period and is discussed in detail in Chapter 14. Duodenal obstructive lesions, including complete atresia and partial obstruction from stenosis or web, are associated with trisomy 21. Whereas duodenal atresia always presents in the immediate newborn period with bilious vomiting, stenosis or partial obstruction from a duodenal web may present later in life. Older patients may present with chronic intermittent vomiting, retention of foreign bodies at the level of the web, or pancreatitis secondary to reflux into the pancreatic duct proximal to the site of duodenal obstruction.

Plain radiographs typically demonstrate a "double-bubble" appearance in duodenal atresia, with a dilated, air-filled stomach and proximal duodenum and a gasless appearance of the remainder of the gastrointestinal (GI) tract (Fig. 133-1). In these cases, the plain radiograph is diagnostic; occasionally, however, contrast material is introduced into the stomach to confirm the diagnosis (see Fig. 133-1). Rarely, air can be seen distally even in a complete atresia; the atresia may occur in conjunction with a congenitally anomalous bifid termination of the common bile duct, with separate insertions into the duodenum above and below the point of atresia. This allows gas to bypass the atresia via the biliary ductal system. Air may then be seen in the pancreatic or biliary tree as well. In patients with duodenal stenosis, dilation of the stomach and proximal duodenum with a paucity of distal gas is typically seen, depending on the degree of stenosis and obstruction (Fig. 133-2). If the stenosis is mild, the distal duodenum, jejunum, and ileum may be of normal caliber.

> In rare cases, air can be seen in the distal GI tract in patients with complete duodenal atresia and bifid biliary duct insertion above and below the site of duodenal atresia.

Contrast studies are usually not necessary in cases of suspected duodenal atresia. However, malrotation, espe-cially if associated with an obstructing band, can simulate duodenal stenosis or atresia. Further, malrotation can coexist with duodenal stenosis or atresia. Therefore, if surgery will be delayed for any reason, it is reasonable to perform a careful upper GI series in patients with duodenal obstruction to assess for the possibility of malrotation. A contrast enema can also be considered to document a normal cecal position, rendering malrota-tion a less likely possibility; however, a normal position of the cecum does not exclude malrotation (see the later section on barium enemas).

Just as air can bypass a complete atresia if there is an associated biliary duct anomaly (see earlier), in such cases contrast material may be seen distal to a complete duodenal atresia. Contrast material can also be seen in the pancreatic duct or the biliary tree (because the biliary tree is in communication with the pancreatic duct; Fig. 133-3).

In duodenal stenosis or duodenal web, an upper GI series confirms the partial obstruction. If contrast is seen on both sides of a web, the thin membrane may be visualized as a linear filling defect (Fig. 133-4). In older patients with duodenal stenosis secondary to a web, the web may become stretched over time, presenting as a "windsock" or intraluminal duodenal diverticulum. Occasionally, older patients with duodenal webs present with retained foreign bodies in the "windsock" created by the web—a sign of the underlying obstruction (Fig. 133-5).

ANNULAR PANCREAS

Annular pancreas may cause extrinsic duodenal obstruc-tion. The head of the pancreas encircles the duodenum because of incomplete migration of the dorsal and ventral pancreatic anlage. Intrinsic duodenal obstruction typically coexists with annular pancreas.

MALROTATION

Malrotation, another potential cause of congenital duo-denal obstruction, often presents in the newborn period and is also discussed in Chapter 14.

Embryology

The midgut is the portion of the bowel that herniates into the extraembryonic coelomic cavity early in the first

CHAPTER 133 — DUODENUM: CONGENITAL ANOMALIES

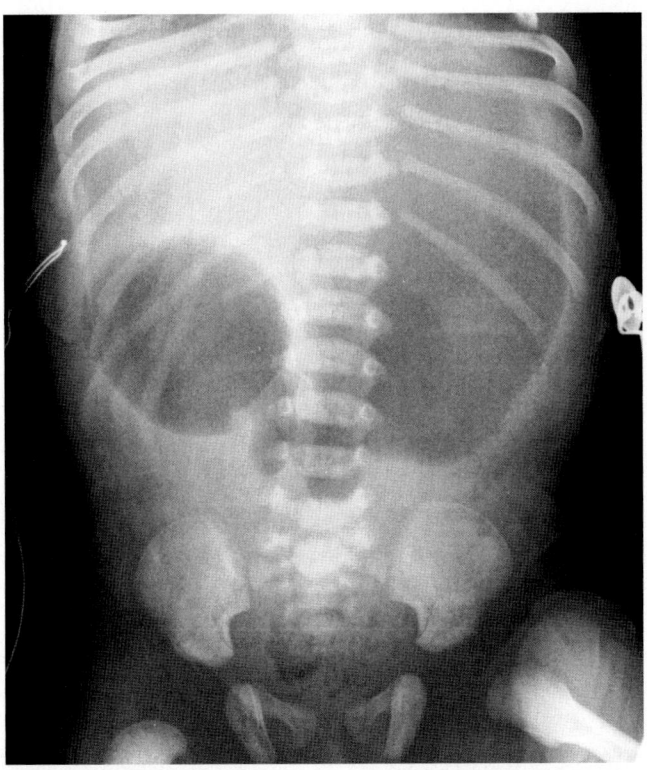 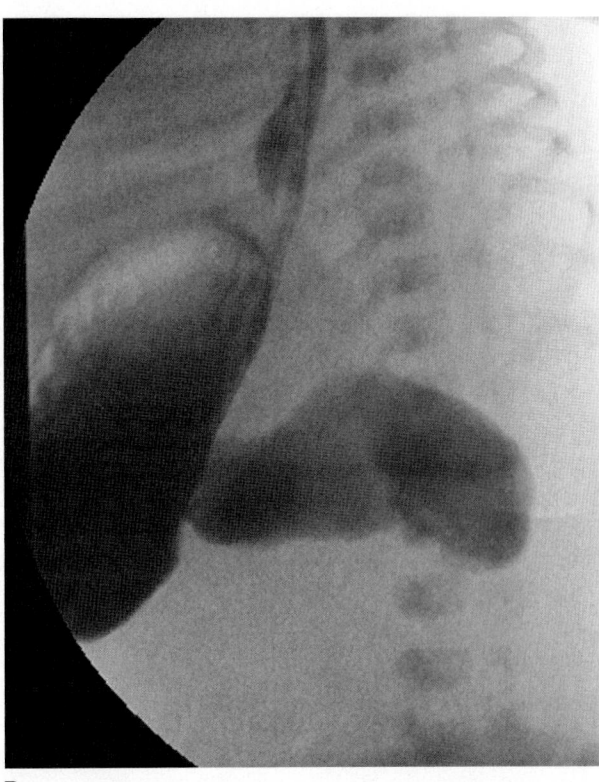

A   B

FIGURE 133-1. Newborn with duodenal atresia. **A,** Portable abdominal radiograph shows a dilated stomach and proximal duodenum ("double-bubble" sign), with absent distal gas. **B,** Right anterior oblique view from an upper gastrointestinal series in the same patient confirms complete obstruction at the site of atresia.

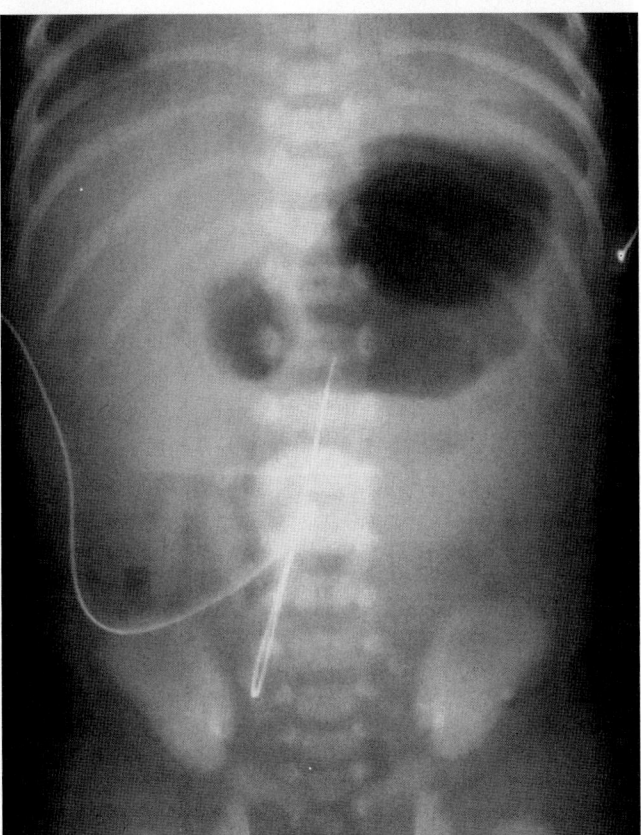

FIGURE 133-2. Infant with duodenal stenosis. Abdominal radiograph shows a dilated stomach and proximal duodenum, with a paucity of gas in the small intestine distal to the partial obstruction.

trimester. The bowel rotates 90 degrees counterclockwise as it herniates into the yolk sac and rotates another 180 degrees as it re-enters the embryonic coelomic cavity, for a total counterclockwise rotation of 270 degrees. This process can be arrested at any point. If the bowel fails to return to the embryonic abdominal cavity, the infant is born with an omphalocele. The bowel may return but fail to undergo some or all of the normal rotation. This can result in an appearance ranging from complete midgut malrotation to normal anatomy except for a high-riding cecum in the right upper quadrant.

The term *malrotation* traditionally refers to the entire spectrum of congenital anomalies. (For an excellent review of the embryology of malrotation, see Strouse.) Briefly, if the rotation of the bowel is arrested after the initial 90 degrees, the result is *nonrotation.* The small intestine lies within the right abdomen, and the colon lies within the left abdomen (Fig. 133-6). *Incomplete rotation* is an arrest during the final 180-degree rotation of the small bowel or colon and represents a spectrum from near nonrotation to near normal. In *reversed rotation,* the caudal midgut returns to the abdomen first (instead of the cephalad midgut in normal rotation), and the duodenum rotates in a clockwise rather than counterclockwise direction; therefore, the duodenum courses anterior and the colon courses posterior to the superior mesenteric artery (opposite of normal anatomy). An *undescended cecum* results from failure of the cecum to elongate, and an incompletely fixed ascending colon may result in a *mobile cecum.*

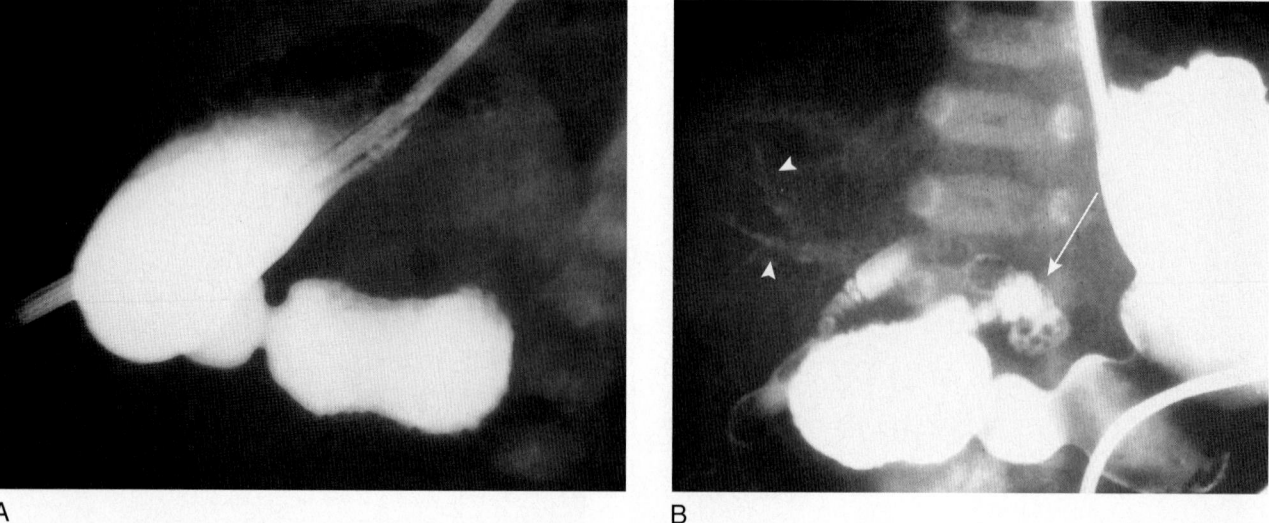

FIGURE 133-3. Duodenal atresia with separate insertions of the biliary tree through the main and accessory pancreatic ducts on either side of the atresia. The plain radiographs (not shown) in this newborn were interpreted as consistent with duodenal stenosis, with a "double-bubble" appearance and a paucity of distal small bowel gas. **A,** Initial right anterior oblique image from an upper gastrointestinal series is consistent with complete obstruction. **B,** Later anteroposterior spot image shows contrast in the normal-caliber, more distal duodenum *(arrow)*, as well as the biliary ducts *(arrowheads)*.

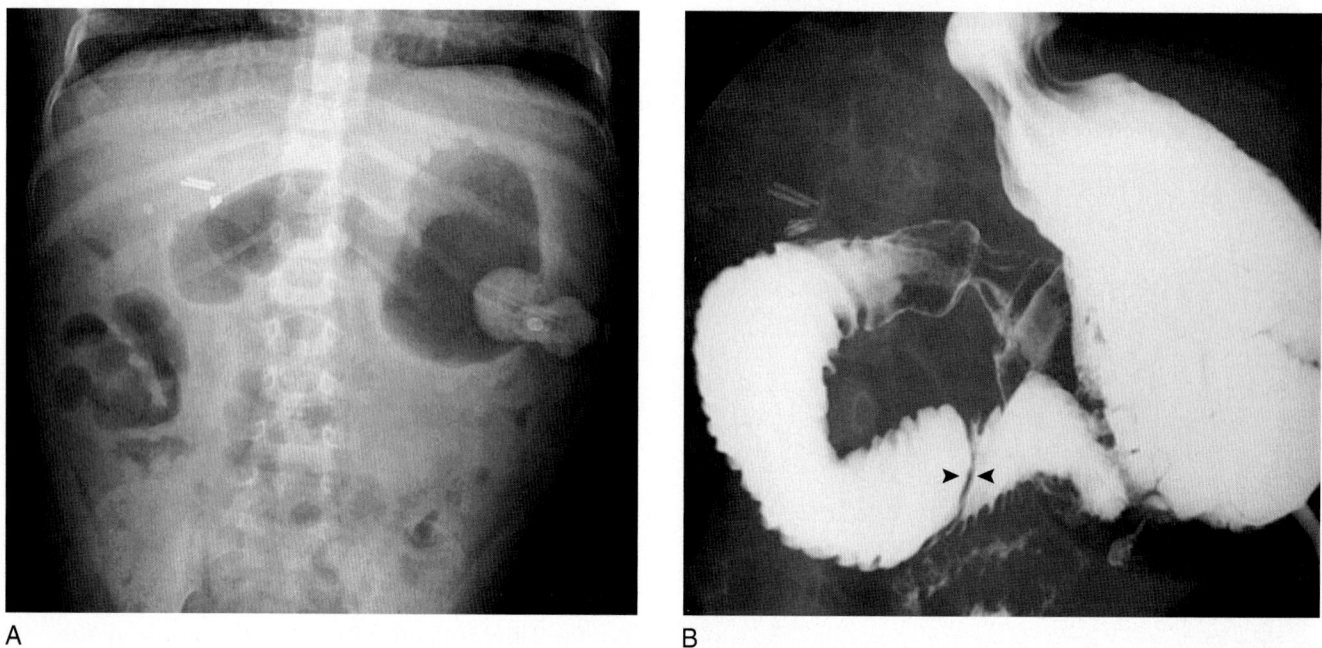

FIGURE 133-4. Nine-month-old girl with duodenal stenosis secondary to a web. **A,** Upright radiograph of the upper abdomen shows an air-filled, dilated duodenum. **B,** Spot image from an upper gastrointestinal series shows the thin web *(arrowheads)* and confirms the proximal duodenal dilation.

In the normally rotated bowel, the mesenteric attachment runs obliquely from a fixed point behind the superior mesenteric artery to a fixed point behind the cecum. The bowel is thus suspended from a long mesentery, with attachments at both ends. The importance of abnormal rotation is that because the cecum and duodenojejunal junction are not properly located, the mesentery is short and improperly attached; thus it may twist on itself, resulting in midgut volvulus. Because the mesentery contains the vessels supplying and draining the small

intestine, this twisting of the mesentery can result in bowel ischemia within a very short time. Malrotation is a surgical emergency when it is accompanied by volvulus.

Abnormal peritoneal bands (Ladd bands) are a result of disordered attempts during embryologic development to fix the anomalously positioned bowel. These bands, as they course from the region of the cecum to the right upper quadrant, may cause a variable degree of obstruction at the level of the descending or transverse duodenum (Fig. 133-7).

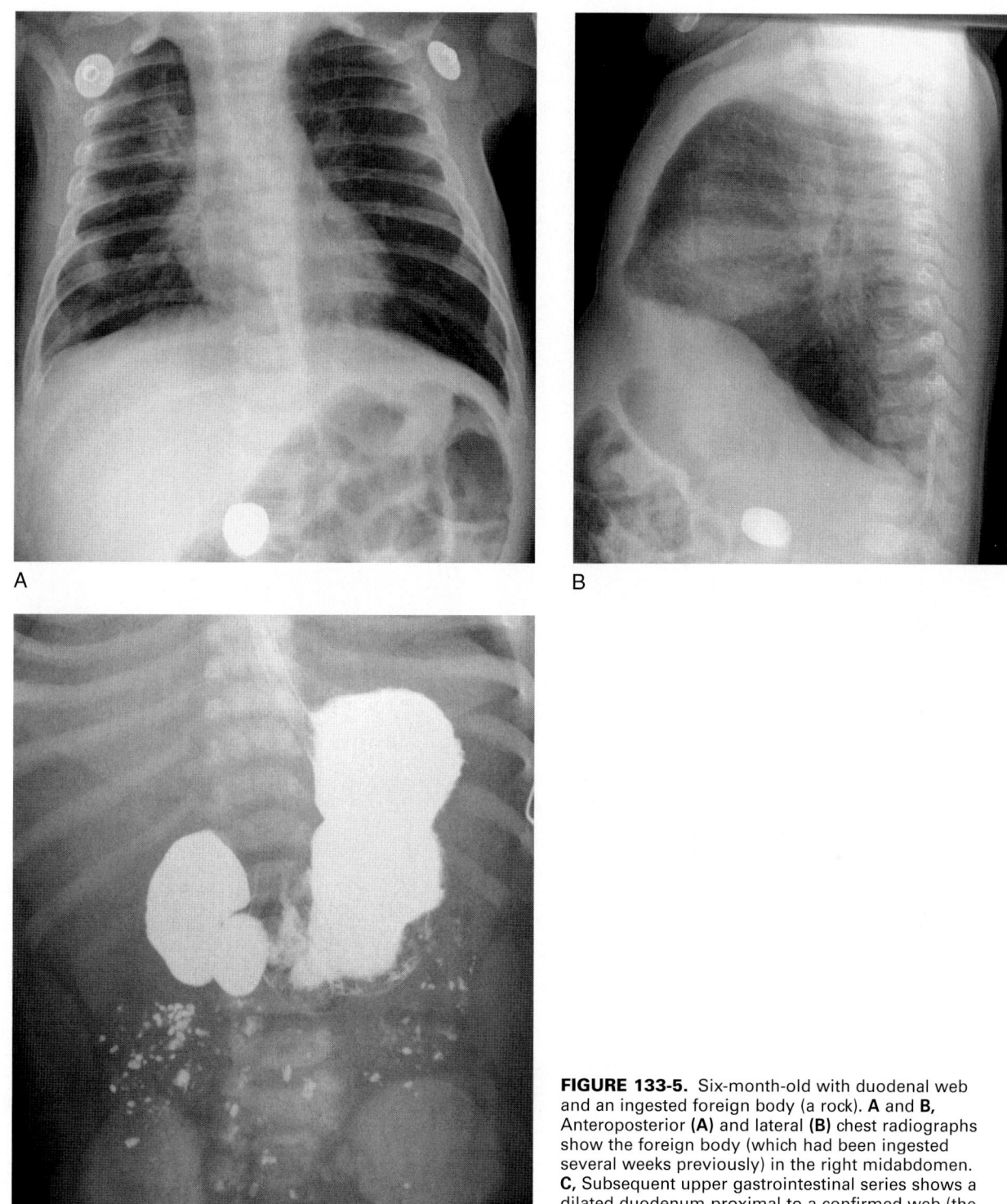

FIGURE 133-5. Six-month-old with duodenal web and an ingested foreign body (a rock). **A** and **B,** Anteroposterior **(A)** and lateral **(B)** chest radiographs show the foreign body (which had been ingested several weeks previously) in the right midabdomen. **C,** Subsequent upper gastrointestinal series shows a dilated duodenum proximal to a confirmed web (the rock is obscured by the barium).

Clinical Associations

Although most cases of malrotation are isolated events, there are many potentially associated congenital anomalies. Malrotation occurs in all patients with omphalocele, gastroschisis, or diaphragmatic hernia and in most patients with heterotaxy. Malrotation has been reported in 28% of patients with duodenal atresia and in 19% of those with jejunal or ileal atresia. Other disorders associated with malrotation include megacystis-microcolon-intestinal hypoperistalsis syndrome, cloacal exstrophy, prune-belly syndrome, Hirschsprung disease, and trisomy 21.

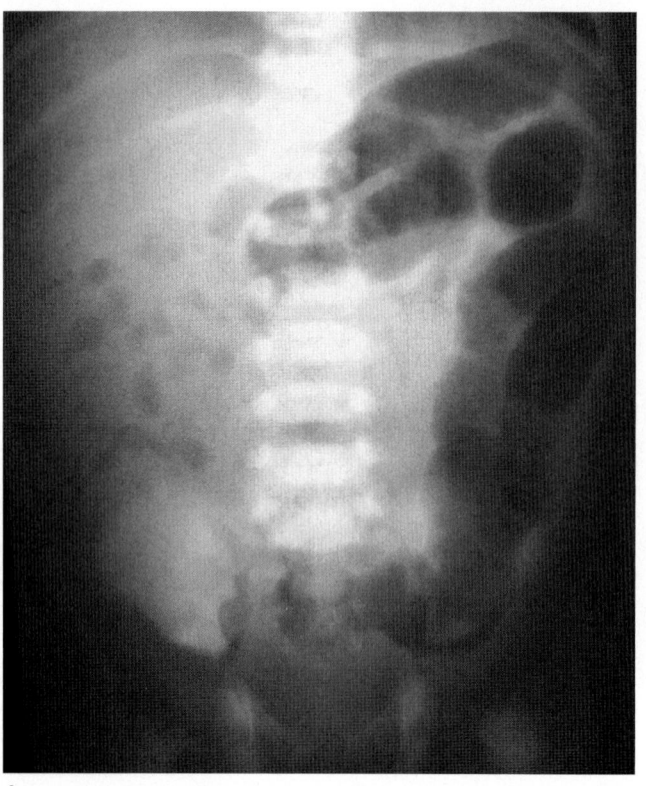
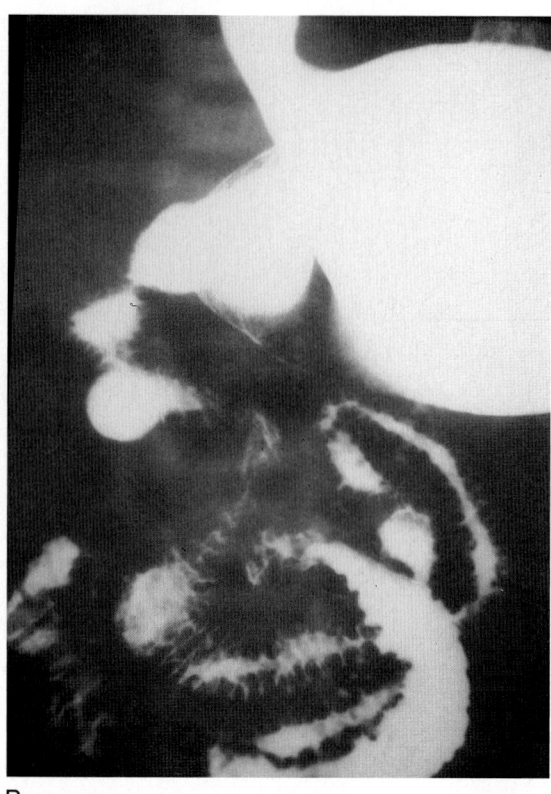

A   B

FIGURE 133-6. Four-month-old boy with nonrotation of the bowel. **A,** Plain radiograph of the abdomen shows an air-filled colon in the left abdomen and small bowel loops in the right abdomen. **B,** Spot image from an upper gastrointestinal series shows an abnormal location of duodenojejunal flexure, confirming malrotation.

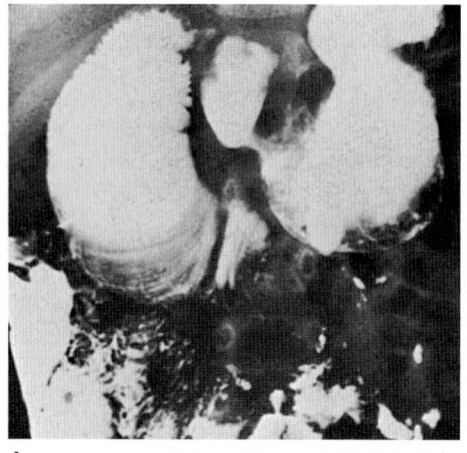
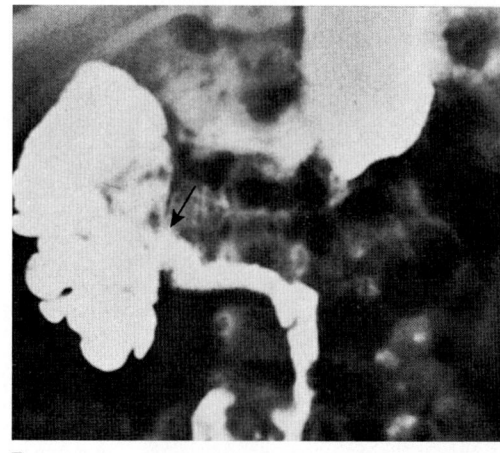

FIGURE 133-7. Incomplete obstruction of the third portion of the duodenum secondary to duodenal bands in a 5-year-old boy. **A,** The first and second portions of the duodenum are markedly dilated. The small intestine distal to the usual site of the ligament of Treitz lies below the duodenum and to the right. **B,** Delayed image shows the terminal ileum and cecum to be on the right, although the cecum is higher than usual *(arrow).*

A   B

Conditions associated with malrotation include:

- Duodenal atresia or stenosis
- Jejunal atresia
- Omphalocele
- Gastroschisis
- Congenital diaphragmatic hernia

- Cloacal exstrophy
- Hirschsprung disease
- Trisomy 21
- Megacystis-microcolon-intestinal hypoperistalsis syndrome

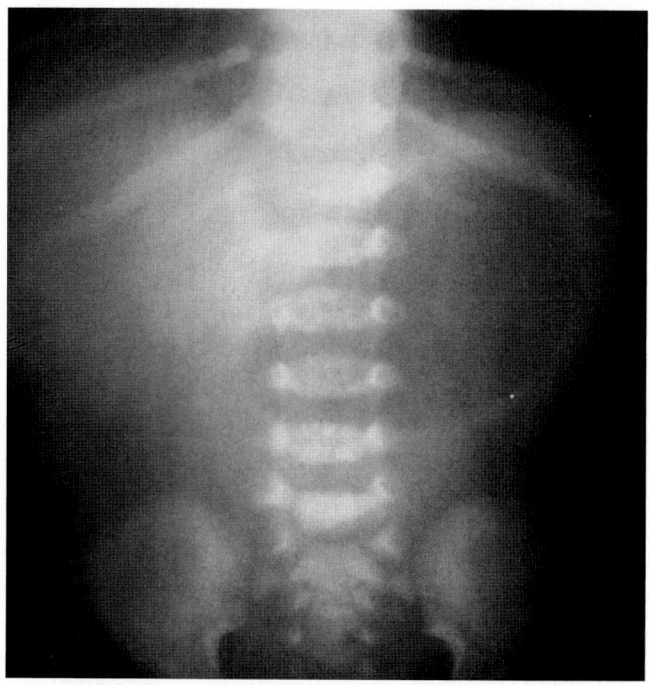

A

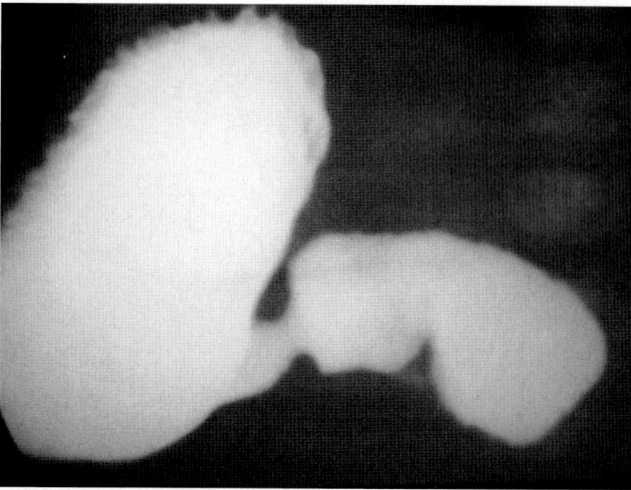

B

FIGURE 133-8. Malrotation with complete duodenal obstruction in a newborn with bilious vomiting. **A,** Abdominal radiograph shows a dilated, air-filled stomach; the dilated proximal duodenum is fluid filled and is therefore not visualized. **B,** Spot image from an upper gastrointestinal series shows complete duodenal obstruction, indistinguishable from duodenal atresia in this case.

Imaging

PLAIN RADIOGRAPHS

Malrotation without volvulus tends to present either as an incidental finding or in children with intermittent symptoms related to repeated episodes of transient, intermittent volvulus (but who are currently asymptomatic). Malrotation without volvulus is rarely diagnosed on plain radiographs but may be suspected when the distribution of the air-filled small bowel and colon appears unusual (see Fig. 133-6).

Most patients with malrotation and midgut volvulus present in the neonatal period (80% in the first month of life), but increasing numbers of cases are being reported in older children. The presentation is usually one of bilious emesis with or without abdominal distention. Plain radiographs typically demonstrate high-grade proximal obstruction, but they may be normal. An appearance mimicking duodenal atresia or stenosis ("double-bubble" sign) can occur, especially with obstructing bands. However, if the dilated proximal duodenum is fluid filled, only a dilated stomach may be seen (Fig. 133-8). A gasless abdomen may occur in cases of volvulus with strangulation of the midgut. Rarely, there is a whirled appearance. More ominous plain radiographic findings of ischemia in patients with volvulus include abdominal distention, separation of bowel loops, tubular appearance of bowel loops, fold thickening, and thumb-printing. Diffuse fluid and gaseous distention of the bowel suggests gangrenous bowel and a poor prognosis.

UPPER GASTROINTESTINAL SERIES

The upper GI series is the standard examination to evaluate for malrotation. In addition to its ability to confirm or exclude malrotation, this examination may demon-

strate other potential causes of duodenal obstruction, such as duodenal atresia, duodenal stenosis, duodenal web, or annular pancreas. Barium can be used if there is no concern about perforation. If bowel ischemia or perforation is suspected, a water-soluble contrast agent should be used. The water-soluble contrast agent should be isotonic to prevent pulmonary edema in case of aspiration.

The normal duodenum has four portions, and the duodenal sweep normally has a C-shaped course (see Chapter 132). The first portion consists of the bulb and the immediate postbulbar duodenum, which are not fixed in the retroperitoneum. The remaining portions are fixed and retroperitoneal: the descending (second) portion, the transverse (third) portion, and the ascending (fourth) portion. The duodenojejunal flexure (or junction) normally is near the craniocaudal level of the pylorus and to the left of the left pedicle of the vertebral body at this level. In malrotation, the sweep does not have the typical C-shaped appearance and the duodeno-jejunal flexure is to the right of the left pedicle (Fig. 133-9). A lateral view is important, because the fixed and retro-peritoneal second through fourth portions of the duodenum should maintain a posterior course anterior to the spine. The proximal jejunal loops usually reside in the left upper quadrant, but in patients with malrotation, the jejunal loops are typically in the right upper quadrant. However, this finding in isolation is not diagnostic of malrotation.

In malrotation with volvulus, a "corkscrew" appearance of the duodenum and proximal jejunum is typical because of the twisted mesentery (Fig. 133-10). However, if complete obstruction at the level of the duodenum occurs in severe volvulus, the corkscrew appearance is not seen (see Fig. 133-8). At times, it may be replaced by

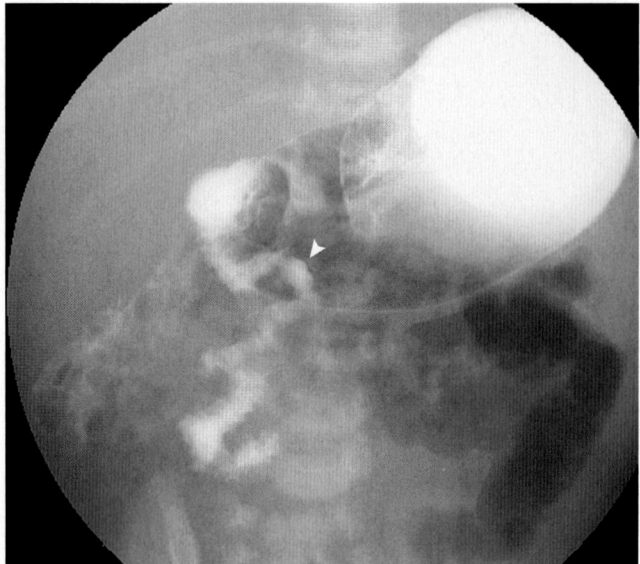

FIGURE 133-9. Abnormal position of the duodenojejunal flexure in a 7-month-old girl with malrotation without volvulus. Spot anteroposterior image from an upper gastrointestinal series shows that the duodenojejunal flexure *(arrowhead)* is low and to the right of midline.

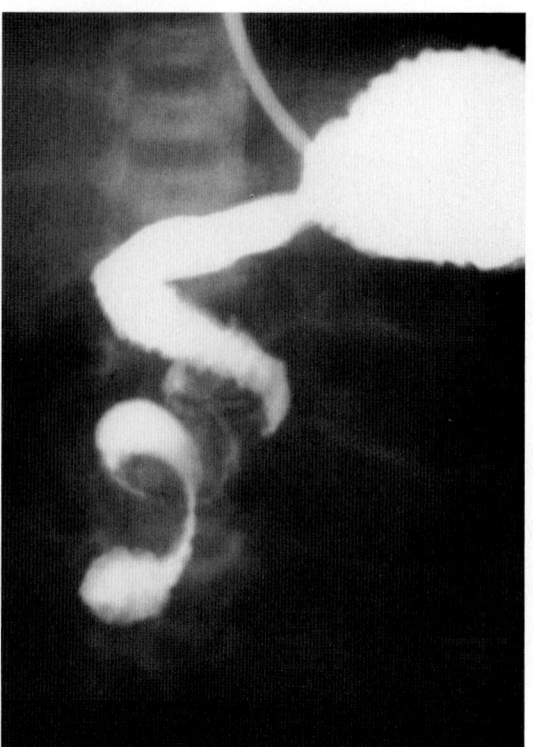

FIGURE 133-10. Midgut volvulus. Spot image from an upper gastrointestinal series shows a "corkscrew" appearance of the distal duodenum and proximal jejunum in an infant with midgut volvulus.

a beak configuration as the contrast column attempts to enter the twisted, obstructed segment. Ladd bands may also contribute to complete or partial obstruction of the duodenum in patients with malrotation with or without volvulus. Ladd bands are bands of peritoneum that, because of cecal malposition, cross anterior to the bowel rather than posterior to it. The third portion of the duodenum is most frequently affected (Fig. 133-11), but other areas of obstruction, even in the colon, have been described. These obstructing bands may cause a Z-shaped configuration of the duodenal sweep, sometimes resembling the corkscrew appearance of volvulus.

Classic findings in malrotation on upper GI series include:

- **Anomalous location of the duodenojejunal flexure**
- **Corkscrew appearance (in the presence of volvulus)**
- **Proximal jejunal loops in the right upper quadrant**

BARIUM ENEMA

In the past, contrast enema was the initial imaging modality used to diagnose malrotation by documenting an anomalous cecal position. Barium enema was favored over an upper GI series because of concerns about vomiting and aspiration during the performance of the latter and about adding a barium burden to an obstructed patient. However, these concerns appear to be unwarranted, and upper GI series is now the preferred initial imaging study. Up to 20% of patients with malrotation may have a normal cecal position, thereby

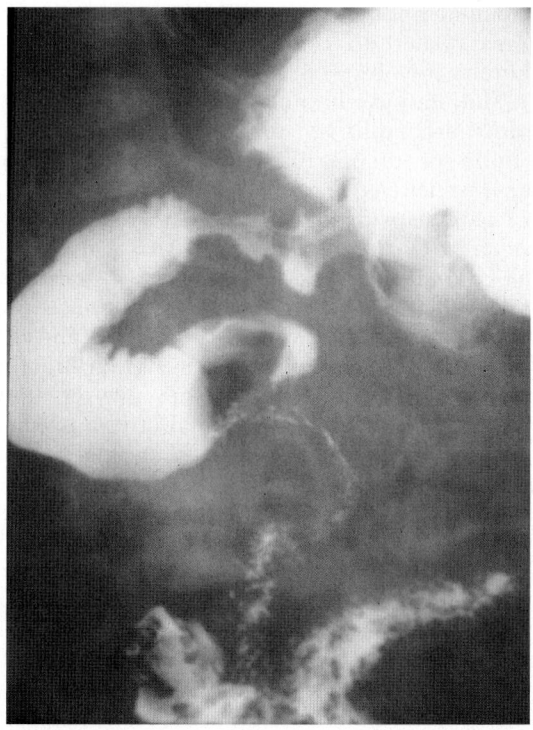

FIGURE 133-11. Ladd bands in a 2-month-old girl with malrotation. Left posterior oblique spot image from an upper gastrointestinal series shows a dilated proximal duodenum due to crossing bands at the level of the third portion of the duodenum. The duodenojejunal flexure is low. Because of the left posterior oblique positioning, the flexure is artifactually projected to the left of midline.

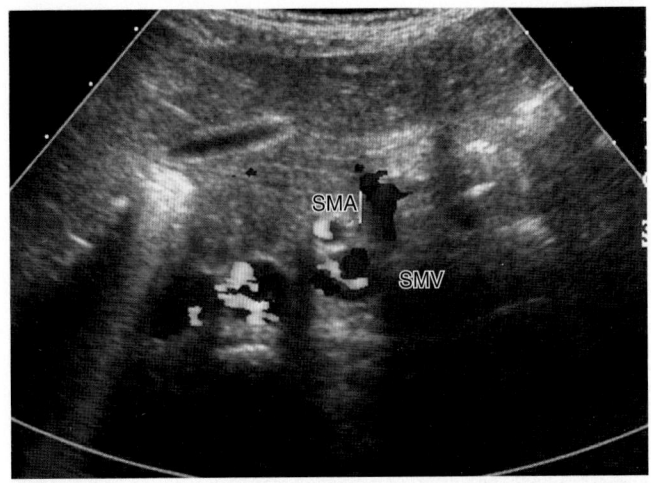

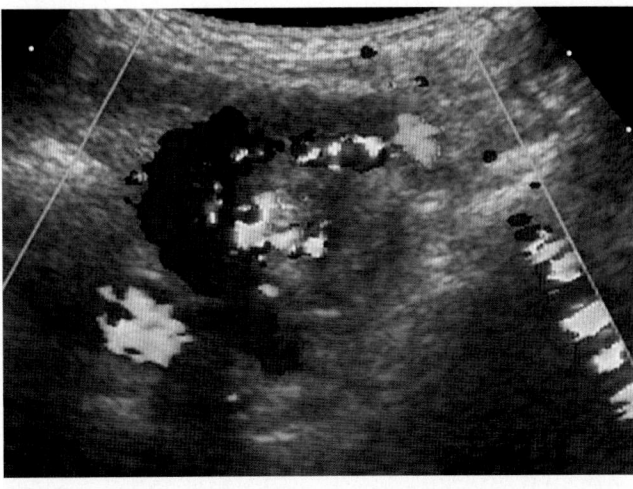

A

B

FIGURE 133-12. Color Doppler US findings in malrotation. **A,** Color Doppler US shows the superior mesenteric artery (SMA) anterior to and to the right of the superior mesenteric vein (SMV). **B,** Single static image from a dynamic clip shows the swirling motions of the mesenteric vessels around the volvulated loop of bowel ("whirlpool" sign). (*B, see color plate.*)

lowering the sensitivity of barium enema; also, in young children, the cecum may be mobile normally, which can lead to the misdiagnosis of malrotation. However, a clearly abnormal cecal position, especially in children with an equivocal location of the duodenojejunal flexure, is diagnostic of malrotation.

CROSS-SECTIONAL IMAGING

Although rarely the first imaging modality used, computed tomography (CT), ultrasonography (US), or magnetic resonance imaging (MRI) is occasionally used in patients with malrotation. This usually occurs when US is performed for presumed hypertrophic pyloric stenosis or when CT is performed in patients with unexplained abdominal complaints or symptoms of obstruction. Inversion of the normal relationship of the superior mesenteric artery and vein can be seen on all cross-sectional imaging and has been described in patients with malrotation; however, it is neither entirely sensitive nor specific for malrotation. Complete inversion of the vessels can occur secondary to adjacent masses, and partial inversion of the vessels can be found in normal persons. In cases of volvulus, US may demonstrate the abnormality with the "whirlpool" sign, a swirling pattern as the duodenum and the superior mesenteric vein twist about the superior mesenteric artery (Fig. 133-12).

> *Cross-sectional imaging findings in malrotation:*
> - Inversion of the superior mesenteric artery and vein
> - "Whirlpool" sign

Atypical and Challenging Cases

It is important to remember that although malrotation most often presents in infancy, it can present later, with more cryptic signs and symptoms. Malrotation with volvulus in neonates or young infants typically presents with

bilious vomiting; although this classic presentation may occur in older children or adults with malrotation, less typical symptoms may be encountered, including intermittent abdominal pain, intermittent vomiting, diarrhea, constipation, and melena. Repeated bouts of vomiting can result in aspiration pneumonia (Fig. 133-13). Chronic intermittent volvulus may impede lymphatic and venous drainage, with resultant failure to thrive or malabsorption. Occasionally, malrotation without volvulus is found incidentally in an asymptomatic patient.

> **Atypical presenting signs and symptoms in older children and adults with malrotation include:**
> - **Intermittent abdominal pain**
> - **Intermittent vomiting**
> - **Diarrhea**
> - **Constipation**
> - **Melena**
> - **Aspiration pneumonia**
> - **Failure to thrive**
> - **Malabsorption**

When malrotation is accompanied by volvulus, emergency surgery is indicated in older children and adults. When malrotation in the absence of volvulus is found in an older child or adult, surgery is indicated if the patient is symptomatic. The role of surgery versus conservative management in asymptomatic older patients with malrotation without volvulus is controversial.

Whereas a clearly abnormal course of the duodenum renders the diagnosis of malrotation straightforward, there are subtle cases that predispose to false-negative interpretations, as well as normal variants that may lead to false-positive results. False-positive interpretations usually result from failure to recognize normal variants, including positioning of the proximal jejunum in the right upper quadrant as an isolated finding, positioning

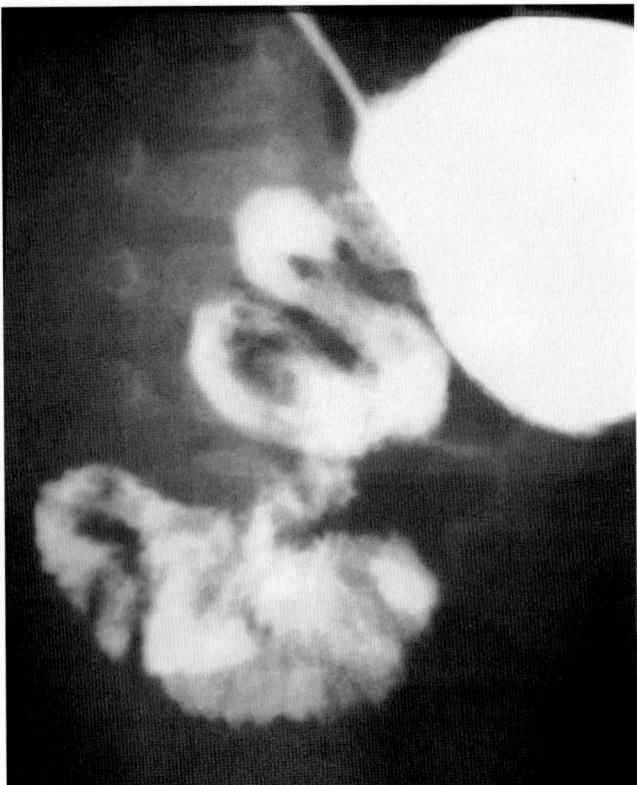

FIGURE 133-13. Malrotation in a 2-month-old boy presenting with recurrent aspiration pneumonia. Spot image from an upper gastrointestinal series shows a low duodenojejunal flexure with spiraling of the duodenum, consistent with malrotation and volvulus (because the patient is rotated to the left, the duodenal sweep is projected to the left of midline).

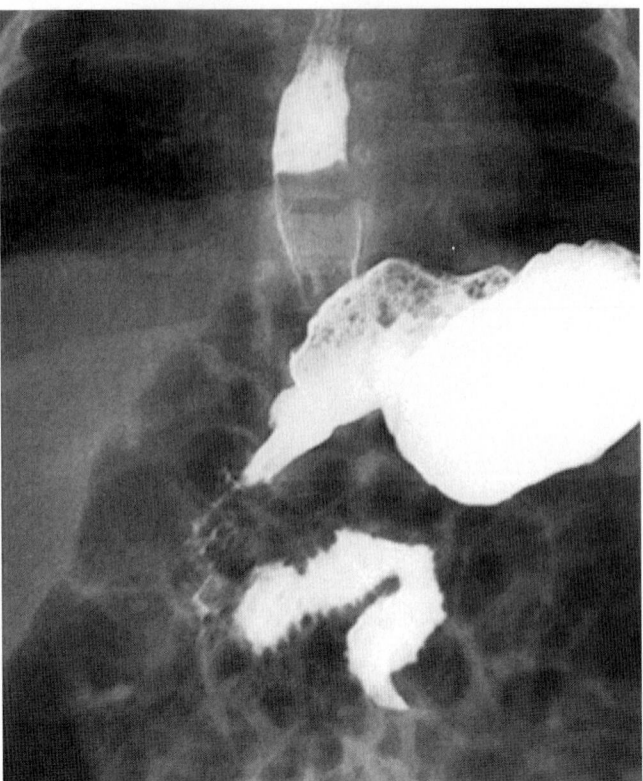

FIGURE 133-14. Normal variant that may be misinterpreted as malrotation. Spot image from an upper gastrointestinal series in a 6-week-old girl without symptoms of malrotation reveals that the duodenojejunal flexure is to the left of midline but slightly depressed. This appearance is often seen in infants with a transverse orientation of the stomach, typically a normal variant. Small bowel follow-through demonstrated a normal cecal position.

of the duodenojejunal junction over the left pedicle rather than to its left, slight depression of the duodeno-jejunal junction (Fig. 133-14), duodenum inversum (the distal duodenum ascends to the right of midline before crossing to the left, with the duodenojejunal flexure in its normal position; Fig. 133-15), redundant postbulbar duodenum (with a normal position of the duodeno-jejunal flexure; Fig. 133-16), and a mobile cecum on barium enema or delayed images of an upper GI series. Potential false-negative outcomes usually result from the misinterpretation of subtle findings of malrotation, such as redundancy of the duodenum with the duodeno-jejunal flexure medial to the left pedicle of the spine. Other clues that the redundancy is not a normal variant include an angular or kinked appearance of the redundant loop or the formation of more than one loop. If the appearance of the duodenal sweep or the duodeno-jejunal flexure is at all suspicious, the contrast material can be followed through the small bowel to identify the position of the cecum (a clearly abnormal cecal position confirms malrotation), or a barium enema can be performed.

DUPLICATION CYSTS

Duodenal duplication cysts account for only 2% to 12% of enteric duplication cysts. They are usually spherical and occur on the mesenteric side of the first or second

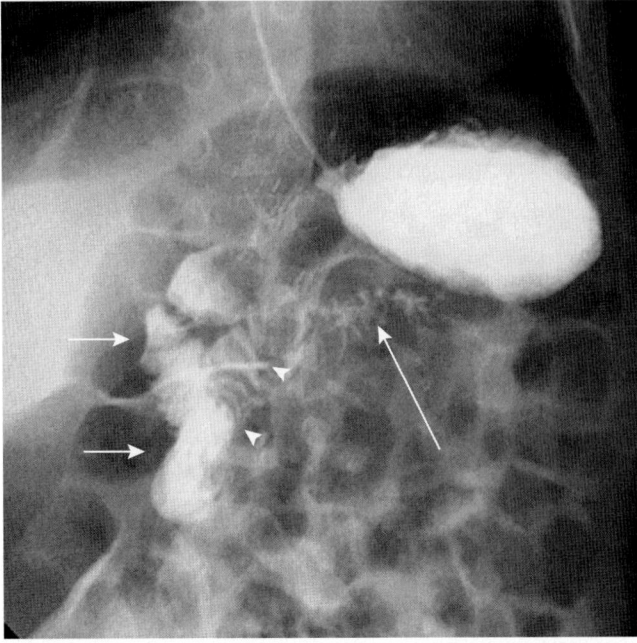

FIGURE 133-15. Duodenum inversum. Anteroposterior spot image from an upper gastrointestinal series shows that the proximal duodenum descends normally *(short arrows),* but the distal duodenum ascends to the right of midline *(arrowheads)* before crossing to the left, where the duodenojejunal flexure is in a normal position *(long arrow).*

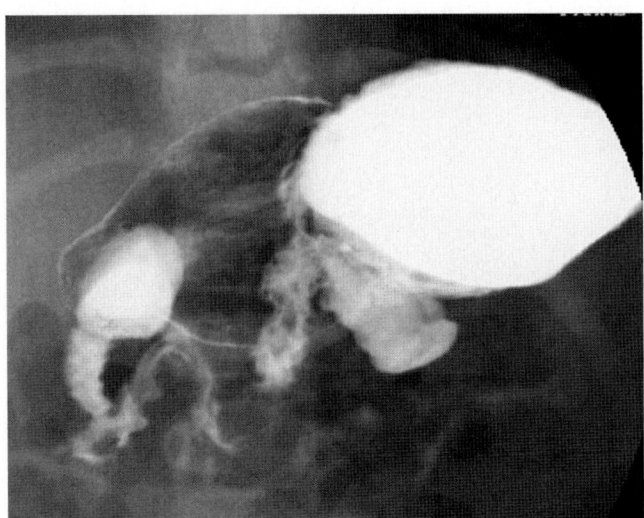

FIGURE 133-16. Normal variant that may be misinterpreted as malrotation. Spot image from an upper gastrointestinal series in a 4-month-old boy shows a normal position of the duodenojejunal junction, but some redundancy in the duodenal sweep.

portion of the duodenum. Duodenal duplication cysts contain gastric or duodenal epithelium and may occasionally contain pancreatic or respiratory epithelium. Typical presentations include obstruction, GI bleeding, or pancreatitis. Bleeding is usually caused by ulceration related to acid secretion from ectopic gastric mucosa. Pancreatitis is likely a result of cyst enlargement with subsequent compression and obstruction of the pancreatic duct. The cysts rarely communicate with the GI tract.

Plain radiographs are usually noncontributory but may demonstrate a soft tissue mass or evidence of duodenal obstruction. Upper GI series reveals a filling defect along the mesenteric wall of the duodenum or extrinsic compression (Fig. 133-17). Rarely, the duplication communicates with the lumen of the duodenum, and contrast material enters the cyst. Cross-sectional imaging can confirm the diagnosis of a duplication cyst suspected from an upper GI series, or it may be the initial imaging modality. US typically reveals an anechoic cyst, but the fluid may contain debris if there has been infection or hemorrhage from associated ectopic gastric mucosa and ulceration. The typical "bowel wall signature" of an enteric duplication cyst is usually present, which helps differentiate a duodenal duplication cyst from a pancreatic pseudocyst if the cyst is located within the pancreatic head. CT demonstrates a discrete fluid-filled cyst on the mesenteric (medial) duodenal margin (see Fig. 133-17). MRI has also been used to evaluate patients with duplication cysts. The signal characteristics are those of fluid (low signal on T1-weighted images and high signal on T2-weighted spin echo pulse sequences), unless there has been hemorrhage or infection. Magnetic resonance cholangiopancreatography can be useful to demonstrate that the cyst is not related to the biliary tree (excluding choledochal cyst from the differential diagnosis) or the pancreatic duct. Antenatal diagnosis of duodenal duplication cysts with fetal US has been reported.

Sonographic findings in duodenal duplication cyst include:

- **Anechoic cyst**
- **Debris in the cyst, if there has been hemorrhage or infection**
- **"Bowel wall signature"**

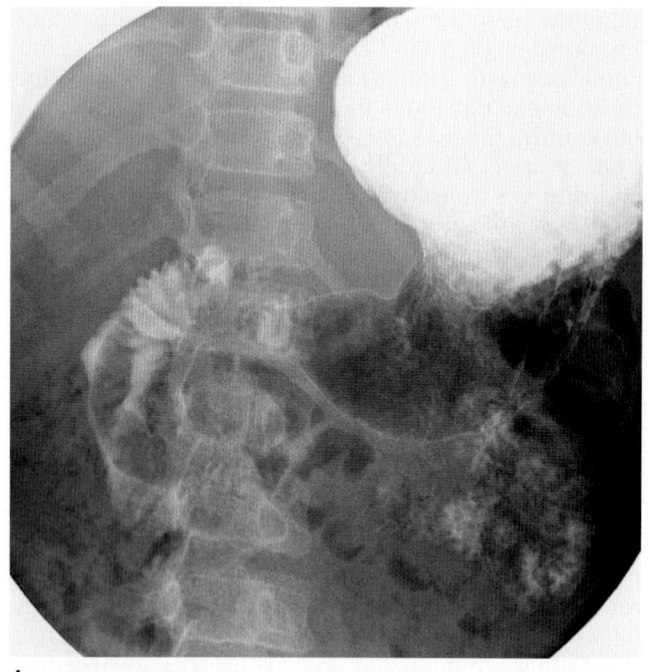

A

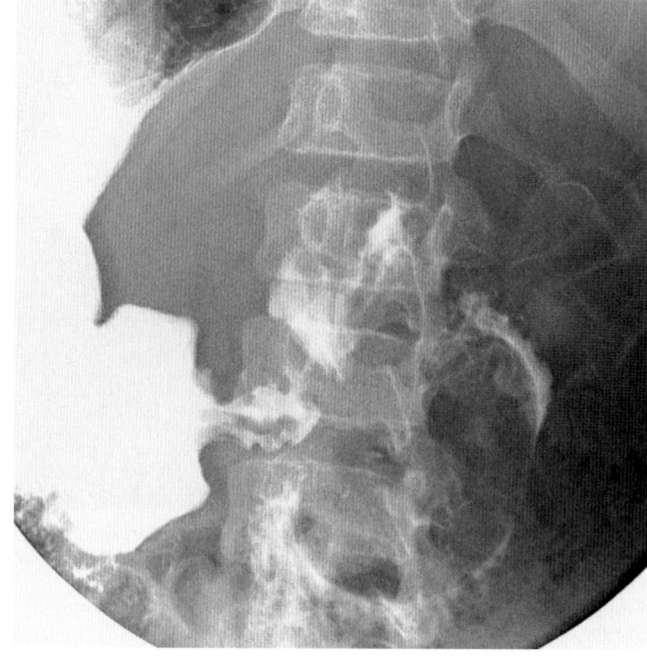

B

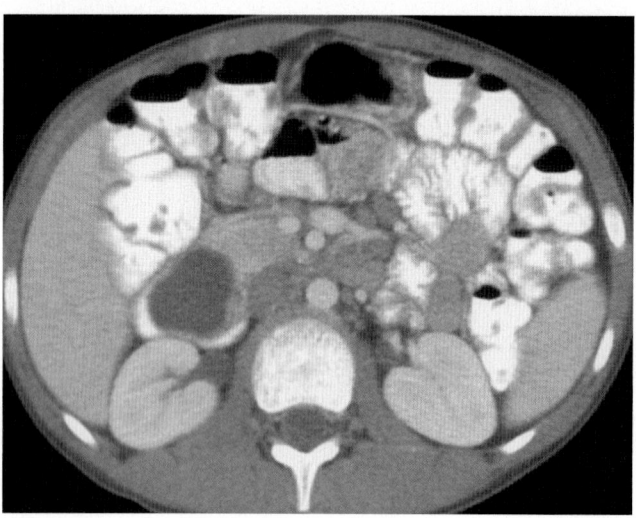

C

FIGURE 133-17. Duodenal duplication cyst in an 11-year-old boy. **A** and **B,** Anteroposterior **(A)** and right anterior oblique **(B)** views from an upper gastrointestinal series show an intramural filling defect. **C,** Axial CT image confirms the cystic nature and location of the mass.

SUGGESTED READINGS

Duodenal Atresia, Stenosis, and Web

Knechtle SJ, Filston HC: Anomalous biliary ducts associated with biliary atresia. J Pediatr Surg 1990;25:1266-1269

Tashjian DB, Moriarty KP: Duodenal atresia with an anomalous common bile duct masquerading as midgut volvulus. J Pediatr Surg 2001;36:956-957

Tasu JP, Rocher L, Amouyal P, et al: Intraluminal duodenal diverticulum: radiological and endoscopic ultrasonography findings of an unusual cause of acute pancreatitis. Eur Radiol 1999; 9:1898-1900

Vecchia LKD, Grosfeld JL, West KW, et al: Intestinal atresia and stenosis. Arch Surg 1998;133:490-497

Malrotation

Beasley SW, DeCampo JF: Pitfalls in the radiological diagnosis of malrotation. Australas Radiol 1987;33:376-383

Dilley AV, Pereira J, Shi ECP, et al: The radiologist says malrotation: does the surgeon operate? Pediatr Surg Int 2000;16:45-49

Frye TR, Mah CL, Schiller M: Roentgenographic evidence of gangrenous bowel in midgut volvulus with observations in experimental volvulus. Am J Roentgenol Radium Ther Nucl Med 1972;114:394-401

Houston CS, Wittenborg MH: Roentgen evaluation of anomalies of rotation and fixation of the bowel in children. Radiology 1965; 84:1-16

Katz ME, Siegel MJ, Shackelford GD, et al: The position and mobility of the duodenum in children. AJR Am J Roentgenol 1987;148:947-951

Koplewitz BZ, Daneman A: The lateral view: a useful adjunct in the diagnosis of malrotation. Pediatr Radiol 1999;29:144-145

Long FR, Kramer SS, Markowitz RI, et al: Radiographic patterns of intestinal malrotation in children. Radiographics 1996;16:547-556

Pasil P, Flageole H, Shaw KS, et al: Should malrotation in children be treated differently according to age? J Pediatr Surg 2000;35:756-758

Pracros JP, Sann L, Genin G, et al: Ultrasound diagnosis of midgut volvulus: the "whirlpool" sign. Pediatr Radiol 1992;22:18-20

Schey WL, Donaldson JS, Sty JR: Malrotation of the bowel: variable patterns with different surgical considerations. J Pediatr Surg 1993;28:96-101

Simpson AJ, Leonida JC, Krasna IH, et al: Roentgen diagnosis of midgut malrotation: value of the upper gastrointestinal radiographic study. J Pediatr Surg 1972;7:243-252

Slovis TL, Klein MD, Watts FB: Incomplete rotation of the intestine with a normal cecal position. Surgery 1987;87:325-330

Strouse PJ: Disorders of intestinal rotation and fixation ("malrotation"). Pediatr Radiol 2004;34:837-851

Vecchia LKD, Grosfeld JL, West KW, et al: Intestinal atresia and stenosis. Arch Surg 1998;133:490-497

Weinberger E, Winters WD, Lidell RM, et al: Sonographic diagnosis of intestinal malrotation in infants: importance of the relative positions of the superior mesenteric vein and artery. AJR Am J Roentgenol 1992;159:825-828

Zerin JM, DiPietro MA: Superior mesenteric vascular anatomy at US in patients with surgically proved malrotation of the midgut. Radiology 1992;183:693-394

Duplication Cysts

Foley PT, Sithasanan N, McEwing R, et al:L Enteric duplications presenting as antenatally detected abdominal cysts: is delayed resection appropriate? J Pediatr Surg 2003;38:1810-1813

Keller MS, Weber TR, Sotelo-Avila C, et al: Duodenal duplication cysts: a rare cause of acute pancreatitis in children. Surgery 2001;130:112-115

Narlawar RS, Rao JR, Karmarkar SJ, et al: Sonographic findings in a duodenal duplication cyst. J Clin Ultrasound 2002;30:566-568

Rotondo A, Scialpi M, Pellegrino G, et al: Duodenal duplication cyst: MR imaging appearance. Eur Radiol 1999;9:890-893

Tang S-J, Raman S, Reber HA, et al: Duodenal duplication cyst. Endoscopy 2002;34:1028-1029

Wong AM-C, Wong H-F, Cheung Y-C, et al: Duodenal duplication cyst: MRI features and the role of MR cholangiopancreatography in diagnosis. Pediatr Radiol 2002;31:124-125

Duodenum: Acquired Obstruction

ALAN E. SCHLESINGER

Acquired duodenal obstruction can be caused by relatively common conditions, such as superior mesenteric artery syndrome; by rare entities, such as duodenal intussusception; and by trauma.

SUPERIOR MESENTERIC ARTERY SYNDROME

The superior mesenteric artery (SMA) syndrome is a condition in which the third portion of the duodenum is compressed between the SMA and the aorta. The mechanism of the obstruction is believed to be secondary to either loss of fat around the SMA, which allows the artery to apply itself more closely to the duodenum at its crossing, or external pressure on the SMA itself, which is transmitted to the underlying duodenum. In either situation, there is a resultant decrease in the angle between the aorta and the SMA, with consequent duodenal obstruction. SMA syndrome was originally described in young adult women, usually occurring in asthenic individuals who developed vomiting following sudden weight loss secondary to either illness or voluntary dieting. The syndrome was subsequently described in children and even prenatally. Marchant and coworkers reviewed their experience with 13 patients ranging in age from 4 to 18 years; SMA syndrome was treated surgically in 9 children, with resolution of symptoms. Ortiz and colleagues described SMA syndrome in five members of a family of eight, raising the question of genetic predisposition.

An acute form of SMA syndrome has been called the *cast syndrome* because it was initially identified in children receiving full-body casts for scoliosis. Presumably, the abrupt straightening of the spine changes the angle at which the SMA branches from the aorta, causing duodenal compression. SMA syndrome that develops in these patients may also be related, in part, to postoperative weight loss. Massive gastric dilation is the rule, and gastric perforation has been described in patients with SMA syndrome related to body casts.

Plain radiographs may show gastric dilation, but the stomach may be decompressed by vomiting. Barium study shows a high-grade partial obstruction of the third portion of the duodenum (Fig. 134-1). Fluoroscopy demonstrates a to-and-fro motion of the barium in the dilated proximal portions of the duodenum. These findings are not specific and may be seen with Ladd bands, focal ileus, or functional obstruction of the proximal jejunum (which may be seen with inflammatory bowel disease), although the straight line at the point of obstruction at the level of the SMA is very suggestive. A useful maneuver to confirm that the obstruction is a consequence of SMA syndrome is to place the patient in the prone position. In true SMA syndrome, prone positioning relieves the compression of the duodenum between the SMA and the aorta, and contrast more readily passes into the more distal duodenum and the proximal jejunum (see Fig. 134-1). Both computed tomography (CT) and ultrasonography have been used to diagnose SMA syndrome. In addition to subjectively identifying a diminished distance between the aorta and the SMA and apparent duodenal compression with these modalities, some have advocated measuring the distance or angle between the two vessels.

> A useful maneuver to confirm that duodenal obstruction is due to SMA syndrome is to place the patient in the prone position, which relieves the obstruction.

DUODENAL INTUSSUSCEPTION

Antegrade Duodenal Intussusception

Antegrade intussusception has been reported in the duodenum in association with gastrojejunostomy tubes in children. Although the intussusception usually occurs at the tip of the tube in the jejunum, it can occasionally be seen along the course of the catheter in either the duodenum or the jejunum. This complication is more common with gastrojejunostomy tubes than with gastrostomy tubes. In one large study by Friedman and associates, 20 of 41 patients with percutaneously placed gastrojejunostomy tubes had jejunal or duodenal intussusception, whereas none of the 208 children with percutaneously placed gastrostomy tubes had intussusception. Patients typically present with bilious emesis. The sonographic appearance is identical to that seen in idiopathic small bowel: small bowel intussusception with a target appearance. Contrast studies reveal the typical "coiled-spring" appearance of intussusception. The intussusception may be reduced by the insufflation of air and contrast through the tube or by removing the tube; in some cases, surgery may be required.

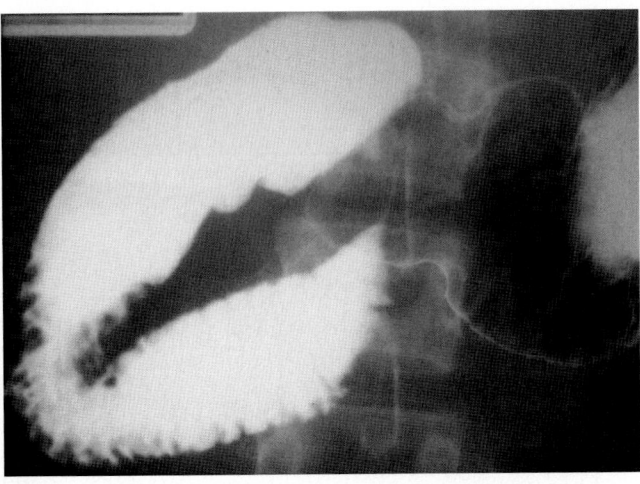

A

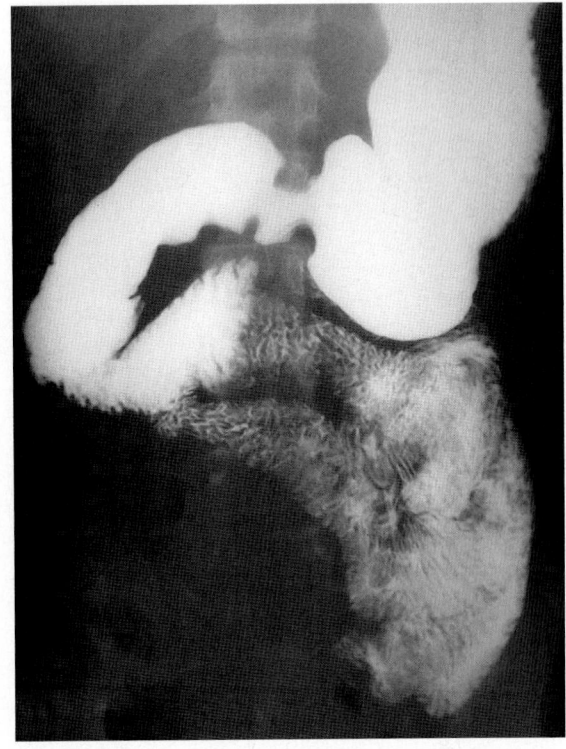

B

FIGURE 134-1. Superior mesenteric artery syndrome in a 15-year-old girl with rapid weight loss. **A,** Anteroposterior spot image from an upper gastrointestinal series shows complete obstruction at the third portion of the duodenum. **B,** Overhead radiograph after placing the patient in the prone position reveals that the complete obstruction has been converted into a partial obstruction.

Retrograde Duodenogastric Intussusception

Retrograde duodenogastric intussusception is a rare complication in children with gastrostomy tubes. The presumed mechanism is antegrade migration of the tube into the pylorus, followed by retrograde intussusception of the duodenum into the stomach when repositioning of the tube is attempted. Jejunogastric intussusception has also been reported. Plain radiographs and upper gastrointestinal series reveal gastric outlet obstruction. Sonography demonstrates the typical target sign of intussusception, and the distal portion of the gastrostomy may be identified within the intussusception (Fig. 134-2). If the gastrostomy tube has migrated distally into the duodenum or jejunum without intussusception, and repositioning of the tube into the stomach is contemplated, the balloon should first be deflated to prevent retrograde intussusception. If intussusception has already occurred when the patient presents, deflating the balloon may aid in reduction; however, surgery may be required.

DUODENAL HEMATOMA

Duodenal hematoma in children is usually associated with bleeding diathesis or, more commonly, with trauma, both accidental and nonaccidental, and is covered in detail in Chapter 157. As opposed to adults, in whom most duodenal injury is related to penetrating trauma, most children suffer from blunt duodenal trauma. Motor vehicle accidents, accidents involving nonmotorized vehicles (especially bicycle handlebars), and direct blows (often nonaccidental) are common causes of duodenal trauma. Compression of the duodenum against the spine is the mechanism of injury, and the result is typically duodenal hematoma or duodenal rupture (due to the rapid rise in intraluminal pressure). CT is typically the initial imaging method in children with trauma; however, duodenal hematoma may be diagnosed by other modalities, especially if the trauma is occult. Plain radiographs and upper gastrointestinal series typically reveal obstruction at the level of the transverse portion of the duodenum, where the duodenum crosses the spine. The presence of an obstructing intramural mass with a "coiled-spring" appearance (due to fold thickening, likely related to extravasation of blood into the valvulae conniventes) is characteristic on upper gastrointestinal series (Fig. 134-3). Ultrasonography may reveal a hypoechoic mural mass. Findings of duodenal hematoma on CT include thickening of the duodenal wall with a mural hematoma; there is often free peritoneal fluid or retroperitoneal fluid.

In a study by Kleinman and colleagues, resolving duodenal hematomas in abused children were imaged on upper gastrointestinal examinations. Although the "coiled-spring" appearance was found to be an acute phenomenon, localized mural masses along the lateral aspect of the duodenum and fold thickening were seen on later studies, after the resolution of symptoms. The authors suggested that this appearance, when seen in a child with nonspecific abdominal symptoms, should raise the suspicion of child abuse. Similarly, in children with suspected occult abdominal trauma who have not been previously imaged, an upper gastrointestinal series should be considered, even if abdominal symptoms have resolved.

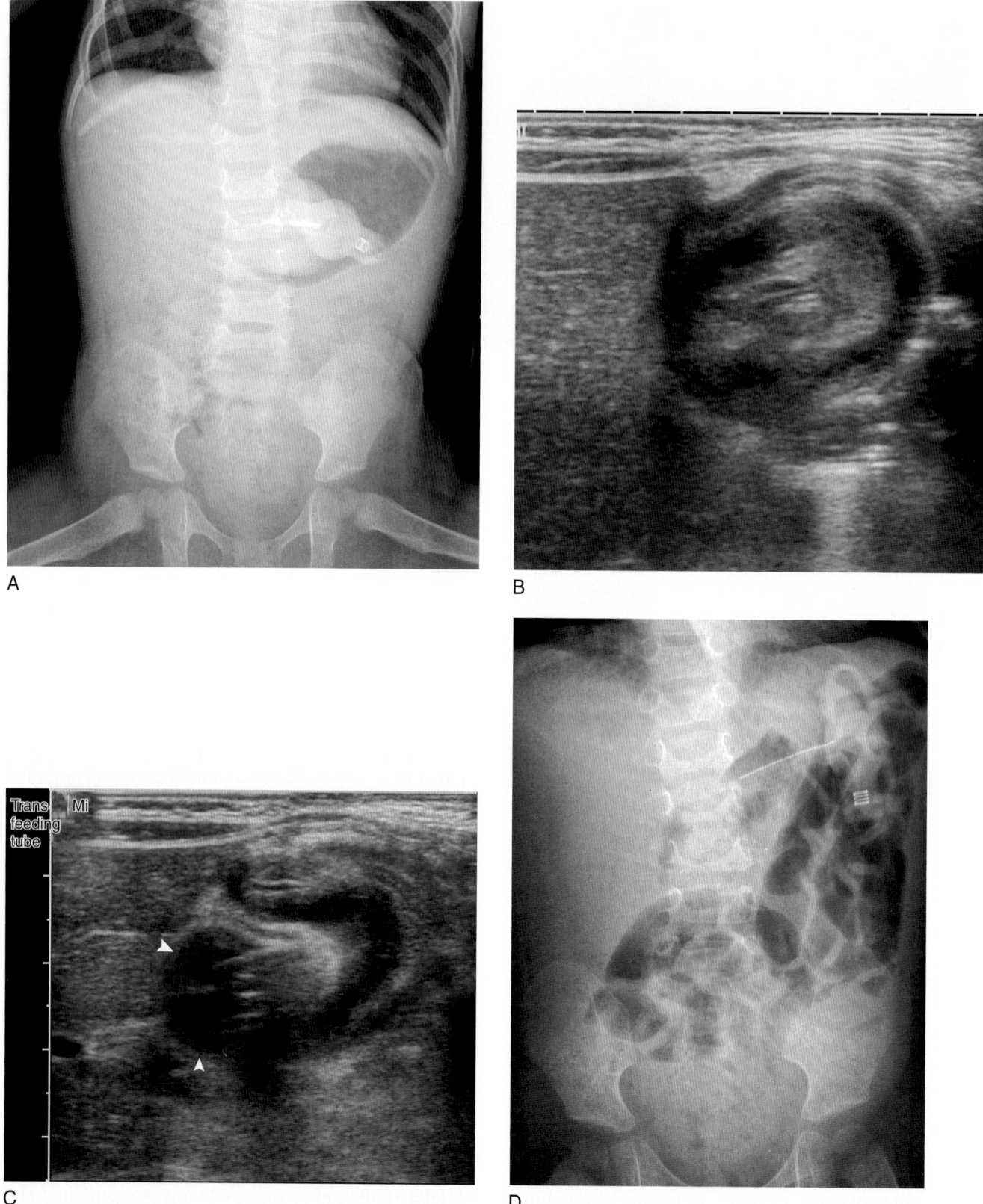

FIGURE 134-2. Retrograde duodenogastric intussusception in a 3-year-old boy with a gastrostomy tube who presented with vomiting. **A,** Anteroposterior view of the abdomen shows the gastrostomy tube; a dilated, air-filled stomach with a masslike lesion at the antrum; and a paucity of distal bowel gas, consistent with gastric outlet obstruction. **B,** Image from right upper quadrant ultrasonography shows intussusception. **C,** Ultrasound image immediately adjacent to **B** confirms that the gastrostomy tube balloon *(arrowheads)* is intimately related to the intussusception. **D,** Follow-up abdominal radiograph after deflating the gastrostomy balloon shows complete resolution of the gastric outlet obstruction.

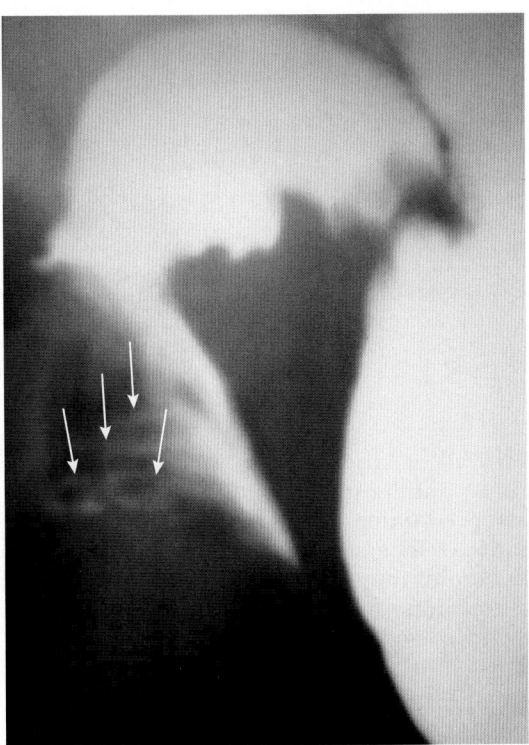

FIGURE 134-3. Duodenal hematoma. Left anterior oblique view from an upper gastrointestinal series shows near-complete obstruction of the duodenum from an intramural hematoma. There are linear collections of barium trapped between thickened folds *(arrows)*, creating a "coiled-spring" appearance.

As opposed to adults, most duodenal injury in children is the result of blunt trauma rather than penetrating trauma.

SUGGESTED READINGS

Superior Mesenteric Artery Syndrome

Ahmed AR, Taylor I: Superior mesenteric artery syndrome. Postgrad Med J 1997;73:776-778

Caspi B, Deutsch H, Grunshpan M, et al: Prenatal manifestation of superior mesenteric artery syndrome. Prenat Diagn 2003;23:932-934

Marchant EA, Alvear DT, Fagelman KM: True clinical entity of vascular compression of the duodenum in adolescence. Surg Gynecol Obstet 1989;168:381-386

Ortiz C, Cleveland RH, Blickman JG, et al: Familial superior mesenteric artery syndrome. Pediatr Radiol 1990;20:588-590

Unal B, Aktas A, Kemal G, et al: Superior mesenteric artery syndrome: CT and ultrasonography findings. Diagn Interv Radiol 2005; 11:90-95

Duodenal Intussusception

Connolly BL, Chait PG, Siva-Nandan R, et al: Recognition of intussusception around gastrojejunostomy tubes in children. AJR Am J Roentgenol 1998;170:467-470

Friedman JN, Ahmed S, Connolly B, et al: Complications associated with image-guided gastrostomy and gastrojejunostomy tubes in children. Pediatrics 2004;114:458-461

Gasparri MG, Pipinos II, Kralovich KA, et al: Retrograde jejunogastric intussusception. South Med J 2000;93:499-500

Osuntokun B, Falcone R, Alonso M, Cohen MB: Duodenogastric intussusception: a rare cause of gastric outlet obstruction. J Pediatr Gastroenterol Nutr 2004;39:299-301

Duodenal Hematoma

Hernanz-Schulman M, Yeneser N, Ambrosino M: Sonographic diagnosis of duodenal hematoma. J Ultrasound Med 1989; 8:273-276

Kleinman PK, Brill PW, Winchester P: Resolving duodenal-jejunal hematoma in abused children. Radiology 1986;160:747-750

Megremis S, Segkos N, Andrianaki A, et al: Sonographic diagnosis and monitoring of an obstructing duodenal hematoma after blunt trauma: correlation with computed tomographic and surgical findings. J Ultrasound Med 2004;23:1679-1683

Shilyanski J, Pearl RH, Kreller M, et al: Diagnosis and management of duodenal injuries in children. J Pediatr Surg 1997;32:880-886

135 Duodenum: Inflammatory Conditions

ALAN E. SCHLESINGER

Infectious and noninfectious causes of inflammation in the duodenum are relatively rare in children compared with adults, but these conditions are being diagnosed more frequently with the increased use of upper endoscopy. In many cases, endoscopy (usually with biopsy) can determine a specific diagnosis. However, in some cases, no infectious agent or other cause of the inflammatory process is found on biopsy, and the diagnosis of *duodenitis* is made; the term *nonspecific duodenitis* or *idiopathic duodenitis* would be preferable in these cases (Fig. 135-1).

INFECTION

The causes of infection (viral, bacterial, and parasitic) in the duodenum are typically the same as those in the stomach and the remainder of the small intestine and are discussed in detail in Chapters 130 and 137. Viral and fungal infections are seen with increased frequency in immunosuppressed patients, especially those with acquired immunodeficiency syndrome (AIDS). As in the stomach, *Helicobacter pylori* infection is associated with

duodenal ulcer disease. The imaging appearance in infectious duodenitis is extremely nonspecific and consists predominantly of mucosal fold thickening, nodularity, or ulceration. Because the collapsed, normal duodenal folds may appear thickened on nondistended views, it is important to evaluate both distended and collapsed views of the duodenum (see Fig. 135-1).

DUODENAL ULCER DISEASE

Peptic ulcer disease can involve the stomach, the duodenum, or both. Gastritis and gastric ulcers are discussed in detail in Chapter 130. Although the incidence is low compared with that in adults, duodenal ulcers do occur in children. Duodenal ulcers are more common than gastric ulcers in the pediatric age group.

The understanding of peptic ulcer disease in children and adults has changed dramatically during the last two decades with elucidation of the involvement of *H. pylori* in chronic antral gastritis and peptic ulcer disease. Although gastritis and peptic ulcer disease are more prevalent in adults, there is evidence that colonization

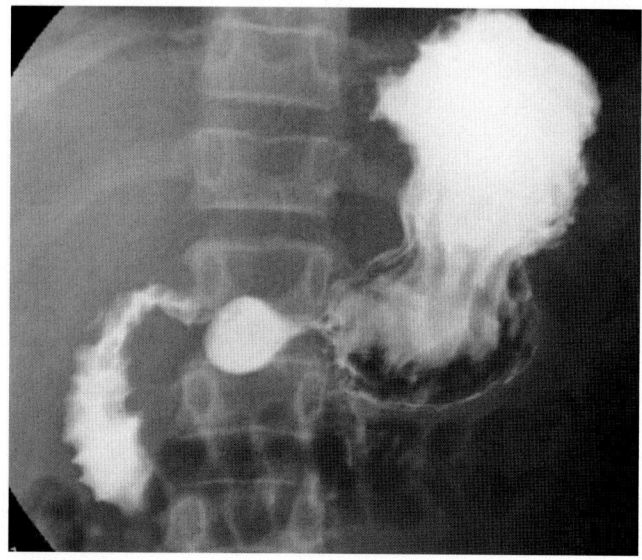

A

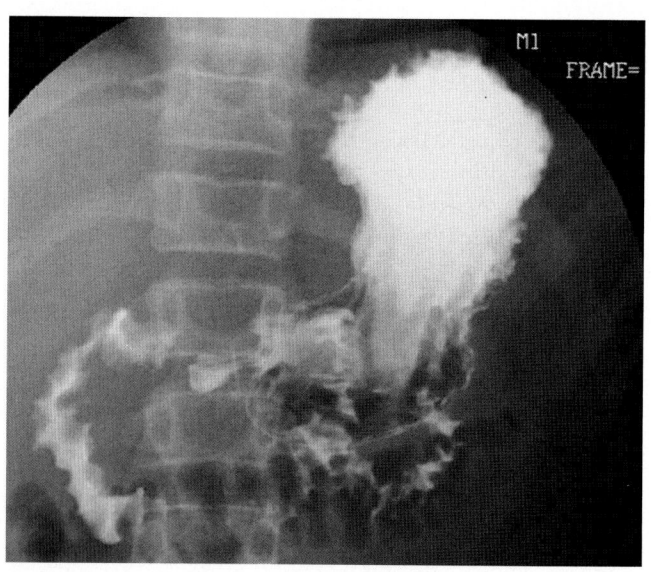

B

FIGURE 135-1. Nonspecific duodenitis in a 14-year-old boy with abdominal pain. Filled **(A)** and collapsed **(B)** views of the duodenal sweep from an upper gastrointestinal series show fold thickening. Biopsy revealed nonspecific inflammation. Cultures were negative, and no specific diagnosis was made.

with *H. pylori* is more likely during childhood and is correlated with socioeconomic status. Eradication of the organism with antibiotic therapy is associated with the resolution of antral gastritis and ulcers and a low recurrence rate of symptoms. Despite the high rate of *H. pylori*–associated gastritis and gastric and duodenal ulcer disease, recent evidence in adults and children suggests a relatively high incidence of idiopathic duodenal ulcer disease as well (unrelated to *H. pylori* or to nonsteroidal anti-inflammatory medications). With further eradication of *H. pylori*, there may be an increasing proportion of cases of idiopathic duodenal ulcer disease.

> **Colonization of the stomach with *H. pylori* likely occurs during childhood in most cases, although gastritis and peptic ulcer disease are more prevalent in adults than in children.**

Ulcer disease in the past has been described as either primary or secondary to chronic diseases or medications. However, the terms *primary* and *secondary* are somewhat archaic in light of the new understanding of the involvement of *H. pylori* in ulcer disease; a majority of what were considered primary ulcers in the past were likely the result of *H. pylori* infection.

Most children with duodenal ulcer disease present with abdominal pain or gastrointestinal (GI) bleeding. In those younger than 10 years, bleeding may occur without pain; abdominal pain is the main complaint in those older than 10 years. Younger children with ulcer disease have a higher mortality rate and are more likely to require emergency surgery than are older children.

Imaging of duodenal ulcer disease is performed predominantly by upper GI series. Although ultrasonography (US) and computed tomography (CT) occasionally detect ulcers incidentally, they are not the preferred methods for investigating duodenal ulcer disease. There continues to be debate regarding the ability of upper GI examinations to detect duodenal ulcers compared with endoscopy. Single-contrast examinations may miss up to 33% of duodenal ulcers, whereas endoscopy misses peptic ulcer disease in only 8% of children undergoing both examinations. Double-contrast upper GI examinations are more sensitive than single-contrast examinations in adults with ulcers; there have been conflicting reports regarding double-contrast upper GI series versus endoscopy for detecting ulcers in adults. To our knowledge, no large series comparing double-contrast upper GI series and endoscopy have been reported in children.

The imaging appearance of duodenal ulcers in children is similar to that in adults. Barium is the contrast agent of choice unless there is concern about perforation, in which case water-soluble contrast media should be used (typically low-osmolar nonionic agents due to risk of aspiration). The most common finding on upper GI series is contrast within an ulcer crater (Fig. 135-2). Radiating folds representing surrounding mucosal edema may also be seen. When the ulcer is on the nondependent wall of the duodenum, air fills the ulcer outlined by barium. Chronic duodenal ulcers may lead to a scarred and deformed duodenum, but this appearance is less common in children than in adults. Free peritoneal air may be seen if there is associated perforation (see Fig. 135-2). Giant duodenal ulcers are even rarer in children than in adults (Fig. 135-3).

INFLAMMATORY BOWEL DISEASE

Crohn disease more commonly involves the distal small bowel than the duodenum and is discussed in detail in Chapters 137 and 142. When Crohn disease involves the duodenum, the imaging findings on upper GI series are the same as those in the distal small bowel, including ulceration, duodenal fold thickening, luminal narrowing, wall thickening, and fistula and sinus tract formation (Fig. 135-4). CT is useful in unusual cases when complications are suspected. CT findings in Crohn disease include bowel wall thickening, obstruction, lymphadenopathy, abscess, and extraluminal contrast in fistulas or sinus tracts (or contrast that has entered the genitourinary tract through a fistula). CT may also demonstrate the complications of Crohn disease or its therapy, including sacroiliitis, gallstones, sclerosing cholangitis, and avascular necrosis of the femoral heads. US demonstrates bowel wall thickening and hyperemia, with surrounding inflammatory changes. Magnetic resonance imaging (MRI) has a more limited role in the evaluation of Crohn disease to date.

> **Complications of Crohn disease include:**
> - **Fistula and sinus tract formation**
> - **Abscess**
> - **Sacroiliitis**
> - **Gallstones**
> - **Sclerosing cholangitis**
> - **Avascular necrosis**

Crohn disease is more common in the upper GI tract than was previously thought, and proximal disease is more common in children than in adults. Lenaerts and colleagues reported endoscopic involvement of the esophagus, stomach, and duodenum in 69 of 230 children with Crohn disease. In 13 of these patients, radiographic studies were negative. However, the double-contrast technique was not used, which is more likely than single-contrast techniques to identify the aphthous lesions that characterize the early stages of the disease. These lesions are typically found in the antrum, pylorus, and duodenum, but they can also be seen in the more proximal stomach as well as the distal esophagus.

This relatively high prevalence of Crohn disease in the stomach and duodenum (with a low radiographic detection rate) has been confirmed in other more recent studies. In Cameron's prospective endoscopic study in children and adolescents with Crohn disease, biopsies demonstrated evidence of disease in the esophagus in 16% of patients, the gastric body in 46%, the gastric antrum in 36%, and the duodenum in 21%. In a prospective study of 31 children with presumed Crohn disease by Mashako and coworkers, clinical symptoms of

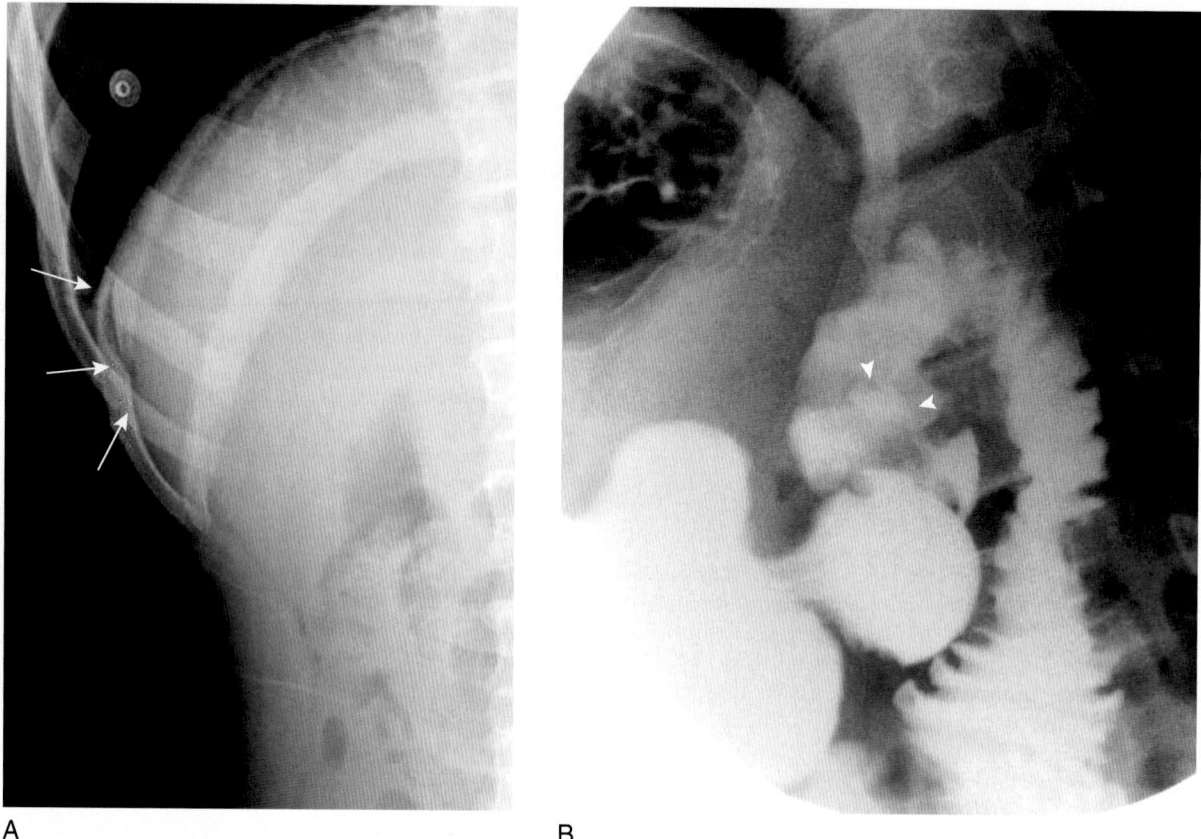

FIGURE 135-2. Duodenal ulcer in a boy with a 1-week history of abdominal pain. **A,** Left lateral decubitus radiograph shows a pneumoperitoneum lateral to the liver *(arrows)*. **B,** Spot image of the duodenal bulb from an upper gastrointestinal series with a water-soluble contrast agent reveals a collection of contrast in the ulcer crater *(arrowheads)*. (Courtesy of Dr. Tamar Ben-Ami, Chicago, IL.)

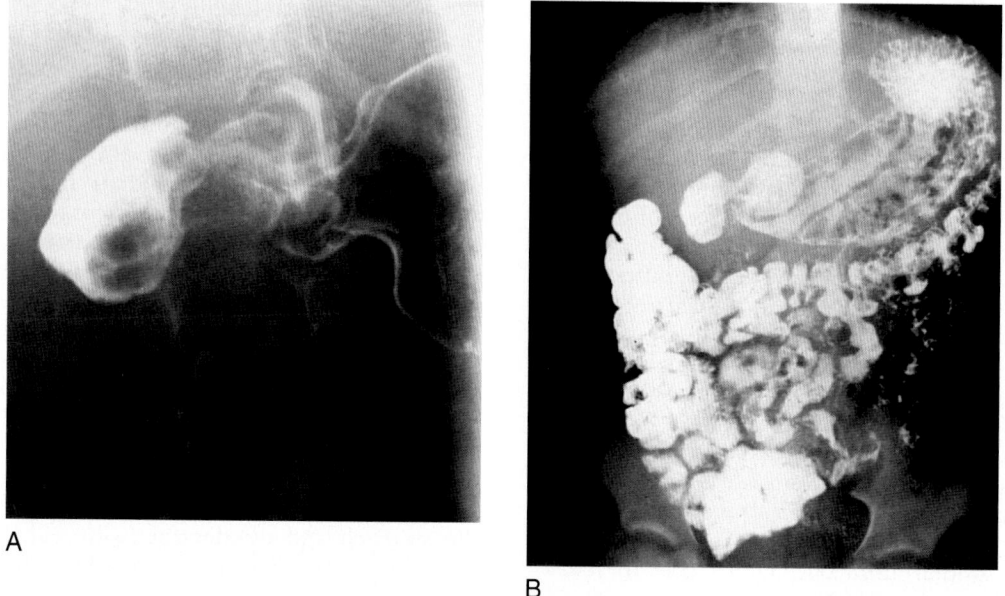

FIGURE 135-3. Giant duodenal ulcer confirmed at endoscopy in a 7-year-old boy with vomiting and hematemesis. **A,** Upper gastrointestinal series shows a large collection of contrast agent in the ulcer. **B,** Persistent barium in the ulcer 2 hours after the ingestion of contrast agent is a useful diagnostic sign.

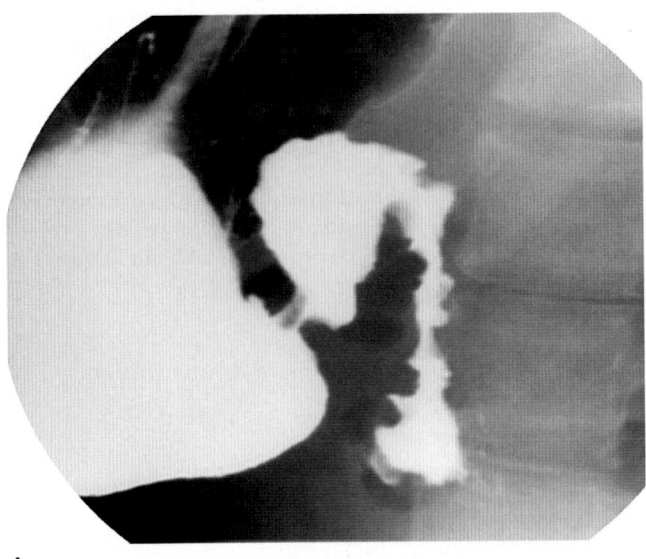

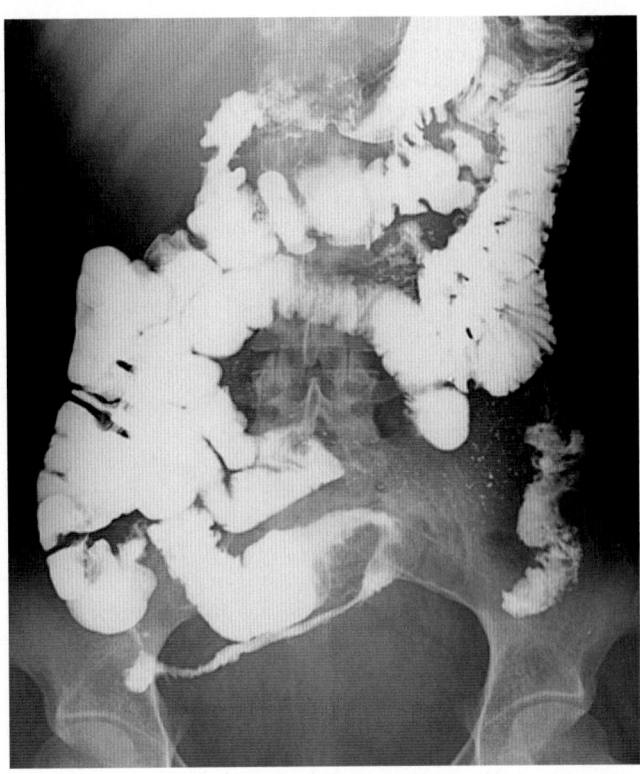

FIGURE 135-4. Crohn disease. **A,** Right anterior oblique spot image from an upper gastrointestinal series shows mucosal fold thickening in the duodenum. **B,** Small bowel follow-through image confirms duodenal changes and also reveals typical involvement of the terminal ileum, with luminal narrowing and spiculation. (Courtesy of Lakshmana Das Narla, Richmond, VA.)

upper GI tract involvement were present in 5 patients (16%) and radiographic findings in only 1 (3%); however, endoscopic abnormalities were found in 13 patients (42%), and specific histologic evidence of granulomas was found on endoscopic biopsies in 12 children (39%). In a study of 41 children with Crohn disease by Ruuska and associates, upper GI endoscopy revealed espohagitis in 16, esophageal ulcer in 2, gastritis in 22, duodenal inflammation or ulcers in 18, and granulomas on biopsy in 10 children. These studies suggest that endoscopy with biopsy may be helpful to evaluate the extent of involvement or to confirm the diagnosis in children with Crohn disease. This approach was recently confirmed in a study by Castellaneta and coworkers, who reported a series of 54 patients with inflammatory bowel disease, all of whom initially had lower endoscopy. Lower endoscopy diagnosed ulcerative colitis in 18 patients and Crohn disease in 23. In the 13 patients with indeterminate findings on lower endoscopy, 11 were shown to have unequivocal evidence of Crohn disease on upper endoscopy.

CELIAC DISEASE

Celiac disease is the most common cause of intestinal malabsorption in childhood. The disease is also known as nontropical sprue or gluten enteropathy because the cause is gluten intolerance. Gluten is a protein present in the food grains most commonly consumed by humans. Most affected children present with failure to thrive, abdominal distention, and diarrhea. Symptoms usually begin before 2 years of age. Diarrhea is considered one of the hallmarks of the disease but is not present in 10% of patients with celiac disease. Affected adolescents have delayed puberty, anorexia, and clinical findings related to hypocalcemia and malabsorption with hypoproteinemia. Although celiac disease classically involves the more distal small intestine (see Chapter 137), duodenal involvement does occur.

Imaging studies are only adjunctive at best, and diagnosis relies on a combination of clinical findings and small bowel biopsy. Plain films in patients with celiac disease may show nonspecific small bowel dilation. The classic findings on barium small bowel series are dilation, thickened mucosal folds, delay of barium transit through the GI tract, flocculation, and segmentation; the last two findings are rarely seen with modern-day barium preparations. There may be reversal of the normal jejunoileal fold pattern, with prominent transverse folds in the ileum and a featureless jejunum. Small bowel intussusception is a common complication in celiac disease.

CT is not indicated for evaluation, but if it is performed, it may demonstrate small bowel dilation; featureless, atonic small bowel loops; and dilution of contrast. Mesenteric lymphadenopathy (which resolves with a gluten-free diet) may also be documented by CT. There are rare reports of the use of US and MRI to evaluate celiac disease.

Involvement of the duodenum in celiac disease is characterized by mucosal erosions, diffusely thickened folds, or nodular folds. Duodenal involvement may be more common than is typically described. In fact, in one series reported by Marn and colleagues, of 16 adult patients with celiac disease evaluated with upper GI series and small bowel follow-through, 81% of the patients had duodenal abnormalities; nonspecific small bowel dilation was seen in only 69% of cases, and the classically described signs of flocculation and segmentation occurred in less than 20%. The findings on plain radiographs and upper GI series in duodenal celiac disease are nonspecific; therefore, biopsy confirmation is crucial.

- **Duodenal involvement in celiac disease may be more common than was previously thought.**
- **Upper GI findings include mucosal erosions and thickened, nodular folds.**
- **Biopsy confirmation is necessary.**

EOSINOPHILIC ENTERITIS

Eosinophilic gastroenteritis is an uncommon inflammatory disease that affects children and young adults and is believed to be caused by allergy or hypersensitivity reactions. Eosinophilic infiltration of the wall of the esophagus, stomach, duodenum, or more distal small bowel occurs, accompanied by peripheral eosinophilia. The disease has alternating periods of exacerbation and remission and generally responds to steroids. Eosinophilic gastroenteritis usually causes a strikingly nodular pattern in the gastric antrum, with relative sparing of the body and fundus when it involves the stomach. Thickening and nodularity of the folds of the duodenum and more distal small bowel can be seen on upper GI series or CT. Pseudomass lesions in the periampullary region of the duodenum presenting with biliary duct dilation have been reported in adults.

ZOLLINGER-ELLISON SYNDROME

Zollinger-Ellison syndrome is usually caused by a gastrin-secreting tumor in the pancreas, but the gastrinoma may be located in the duodenal wall, lymph nodes in the region of the head of the pancreas, or, rarely, other more remote locations. The resulting increased acid production by the stomach leads to peptic ulcers. Although a majority of ulcers occur in the proximal duodenum (the usual site of duodenal peptic ulcers), ulcers in atypical locations, such as the distal duodenum and the jejunum, are very suggestive of Zollinger-Ellison syndrome. Other characteristics that should raise concern for Zollinger-Ellison syndrome are ulcers larger than 2 cm, at multiple locations, and refractory to conventional medical treatment. Zollinger-Ellison syndrome is more common in adults, but isolated cases and small series have been reported in children. Patients typically present with abdominal pain or GI bleeding from ulceration or with diarrhea related to increased acid secretion. Zollinger-Ellison syndrome is caused by isolated gastrinomas in 75% of cases; 25% of patients have multiple endocrine neoplasia type I (MEN I). Most gastrinomas grow slowly, but 60% to 90% are malignant, and 25% demonstrate rapid growth.

Imaging of the duodenum plays a twofold role in patients with Zollinger-Ellison syndrome: evaluation of complications of increased acid production, and evaluation of gastrin-secreting tumors located within the duodenum. The classic imaging finding in the duodenum related to hypersecretion of acid is the presence of duodenal ulcers. As mentioned previously, the presence of multiple ulcers, large ulcers, and ulcers distal to the bulb are suggestive of the diagnosis. Fold thickening can also be seen due to edema.

Findings in Zollinger-Ellison syndrome related to increased acid production:
- **Ulcers larger than 2 cm**
- **Multiple ulcers**
- **Ulcers distal to the duodenal bulb**
- **Fold thickening due to edema**

Findings related to gastrinomas themselves:
- **Gastrinomas typically in the pancreas, duodenal wall, or adjacent lymph nodes (the "gastrinoma triangle")**
- **Rare gastrinomas in remote sites**

Gastrinomas arising within the duodenal wall were once considered rare compared with those in the pancreas, but new data suggest that duodenal gastrinomas are more common than previously thought. This new information is likely related to the increased rate of surgical exploration in patients with Zollinger-Ellison syndrome. Approximately 30% of gastrinomas are found in the pancreas and 60% in the duodenal wall. Approximately 70% to 80% are found in the "gastrinoma triangle"—the region bounded by the confluence of the cystic and common bile ducts, the second and third portions of the duodenum, and the neck and body of the pancreas. Tumors in the duodenum tend to be smaller (many are <1 cm) than those arising in the pancreas. Duodenal gastrinomas metastasize to regional lymph nodes, while pancreatic tumors tend to metastasize to the liver.

Imaging with CT, MRI, and US is less sensitive than somatostatin-receptor scintigraphy. The total-body imaging capability of somatostatin-receptor scintigraphy is an added benefit in the identification of tumors outside the gastrinoma triangle. A recent report of 151 patients with gastrinomas (123 sporadic, 28 associated with MEN I), all of whom underwent laparotomy, reported on the sensitivity of various imaging techniques. In this study, gastrinomas were found at surgery in 93% of patients. The investigators found that in patients with sporadic gastrinomas, US had a sensitivity of 24% for tumor detection; CT, 39%; MRI, 46%; and somatostatin-receptor scintigraphy, 79%. All the imaging studies were negative in one third of the patients with sporadic gastrinomas. The sensitivity of each imaging modality was higher in patients with gastrinomas associated with MEN I because the study design required that these patients have imaged tumors larger than 3 cm. Patients with sporadic gastrinomas without hepatic metastases or with limited hepatic metastases had better disease-free survival rates than those with gastrinomas associated with MEN I or with sporadic gastrinomas with diffuse metastases. The authors concluded that in the absence of MEN I or diffuse hepatic metastases, surgery should be performed in patients with presumed gastrinomas, even if imaging is negative. However, with the improved ability to medically prevent the hyperacidity caused by gastrinomas, surgical therapy remains controversial.

> Gastrinomas arising in the duodenal wall were once considered rare (compared with those in the pancreas), but new data suggest that they may be more common than previously thought.

GRAFT-VERSUS-HOST DISEASE

Graft-versus-host disease (GVHD) is a reaction of donor T lymphocytes against host cells, most commonly in the skin, liver, and GI tract. Involvement in the GI tract can occur anywhere from the esophagus to the rectum, and involvement in the duodenum is similar to that in the remainder of the small intestine. In Donnelly and Morris's series of 16 children with GVHD studied by abdominal CT, all 16 patients had diffuse involvement from the duodenum to the rectum.

Although GVHD can be seen in patients who have undergone solid organ transplantation, it is more common in those who have received bone marrow transplants. Further, bone marrow transplantation is more commonly performed in children than solid organ transplantation; it is useful in hematologic and immunodeficiency states as well as in leukemia, lymphoma, and widespread pediatric malignancies such as metastatic neuroblastoma.

Acute GVHD occurs within the first 3 months after transplantation. Patients typically present with watery diarrhea and crampy abdominal pain. Skin rash, liver dysfunction, and hematologic complications are frequently associated. Plain radiographs may demonstrate bowel wall and mucosal thickening, bowel dilation, gasless abdomen, or air-fluid levels; pneumatosis intestinalis and ascites are less commonly encountered. Contrast studies are usually not necessary, but in the acute phase they show thickened or flattened folds, bowel wall thickening, poor coating of the mucosa due to increased intraluminal fluid, luminal narrowing, and rapid transit time. US reveals thickening of the bowel wall, sometimes with a sonolucent ring in the submucosal layer. The bowel lumen is filled with fluid, and ascites can be identified. CT reveals mucosal enhancement, bowel dilation, fold enlargement, bowel wall thickening, stranding of the mesenteric fat, gallbladder and urinary bladder wall enhancement, periportal low attenuation, and ascites (Fig. 135-5). If there is submucosal edema or hemorrhage, a low-attenuation zone may be seen within the bowel wall, leading to a "target" sign. Chronic changes with fibrosis, not unlike those seen in chronic radiation enteritis, may occur.

> CT findings in graft-versus-host disease include:
> - **Mucosal enhancement**
> - **Bowel dilation**
> - **Fold enlargement**
> - **Bowel wall thickening**
> - **Stranding of the mesenteric fat**
> - **Gallbladder and urinary bladder wall enhancement**
> - **Periportal low attenuation**
> - **Ascites**

CHRONIC GRANULOMATOUS DISEASE

Chronic granulomatous disease of childhood is a syndrome of recurrent infection, usually bacterial or fungal, whose underlying pathophysiology is one of disordered phagocytosis secondary to phagocytes' inability to generate oxygen radicals. The most common GI manifestation is chronic antral gastritis (see Chapter 130); however, involvement of the proximal duodenum may also occur. US typically demonstrates an abnormally thickened antropyloric wall. This finding simulates hypertrophic pyloric stenosis but occurs in patients beyond infancy. Upper GI series reveals narrowing of the antropyloric lumen secondary to chronic inflammation and fibrosis.

CYSTIC FIBROSIS

The genetic mutations responsible for cystic fibrosis have been identified. The gene is located on the long arm of chromosome 7 and encodes for a 1480–amino acid protein that regulates transmembrane ion transport (cystic fibrosis transmembrane conductance regulator). Defects in this protein lead to abnormal permeability of the epithelium to chloride ions, which is the underlying physiologic abnormality in cystic fibrosis.

Duodenal inflammation is seen in children and adults with cystic fibrosis, but the cause is unclear and likely multifactorial. Hypersecretion of acid by the stomach occurs in some of these patients. Decreased bicarbonate levels in the duodenum in patients with cystic fibrosis lead to increased levels of unbuffered gastric acid. The decrease in bicarbonate is caused by both impaired exocrine pancreatic function and decreased bicarbonate secretion by the duodenal mucosa (where bicarbonate production is dependent on transmembrane ion transport). Medications may play a role, and new evidence suggests that the immune system may also be involved. In the lungs, alteration of the normal immune response to infectious agents in patients with cystic fibrosis leads to a chronic inflammatory process. In the duodenum (and other portions of the small intestine), the chronic inflammation is believed to be the result of alimentary antigenic challenge. This was originally thought to be merely a consequence of decreased pancreatic exocrine function, with an associated lack of breakdown of antigens in ingested food. However, there is new evidence

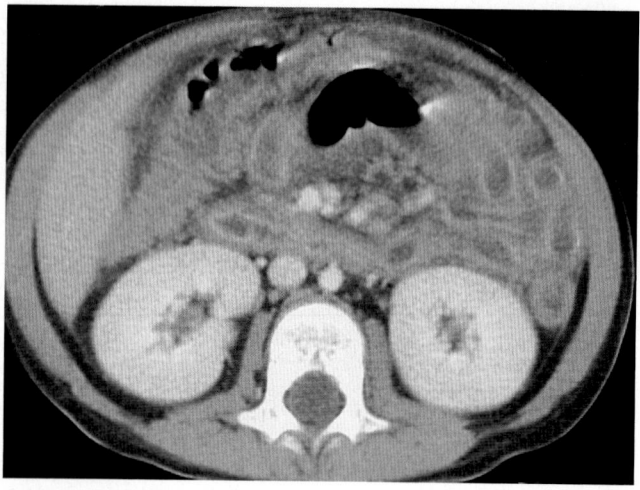
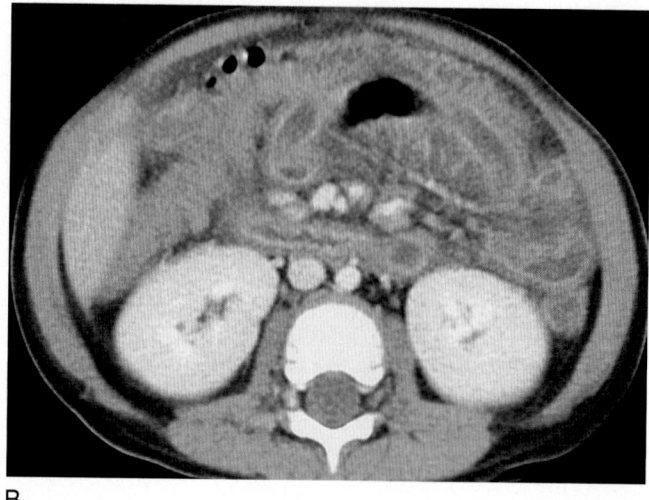

A   B

FIGURE 135-5. Eleven-year-old boy with graft-versus-host disease after bone marrow transplantation. **A** and **B,** Sequential axial CT images show mucosal enhancement, bowel wall thickening, and mesenteric edema involving the duodenum and the more distal small intestine.

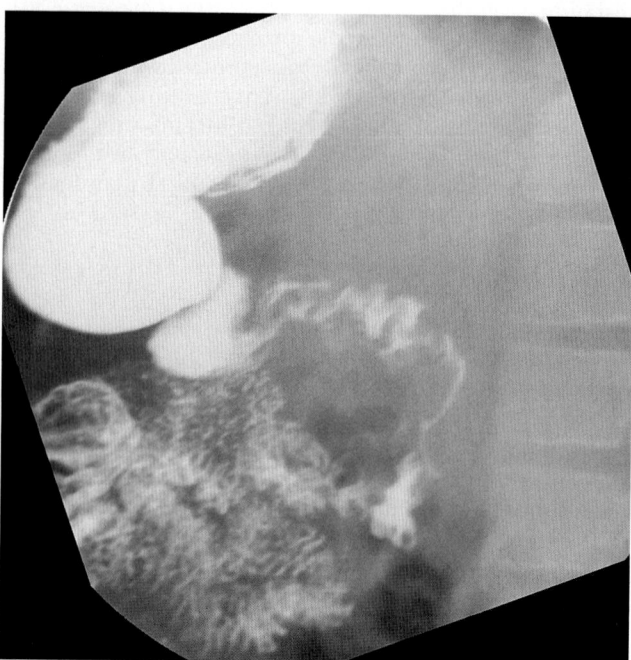

FIGURE 135-6. Duodenal inflammation related to cystic fibrosis. Lateral spot image from an upper gastrointestinal series shows duodenal fold thickening. (Courtesy of Steven Kraus, Cincinnati, OH, and R. Paul Guillerman, Houston, TX.)

that these patients have diminished luminal digestion of proteins that is unrelated to pancreatic exocrine insufficiency, and they also have an underlying impaired immune response.

Imaging manifestations are nonspecific and include fold thickening (Fig. 135-6), nodularity, and ulcers. Ulcers may be underdiagnosed, with 10% of cystic fibrosis patients having duodenal ulcers at autopsy.

DERMATOMYOSITIS

Vasculitis in children with dermatomyositis can involve the GI tract, and GI perforation is a recognized complication. Although perforation can occur throughout the GI tract, there are several reports of a predilection for the duodenum, in particular, the posterior portion of the distal descending duodenum. Spread of the inflammatory process related to perforation from the paraduodenal retroperitoneum may suggest primary right lower quadrant pathology, which can lead to clinical confusion and a delay in diagnosis (Fig. 135-7).

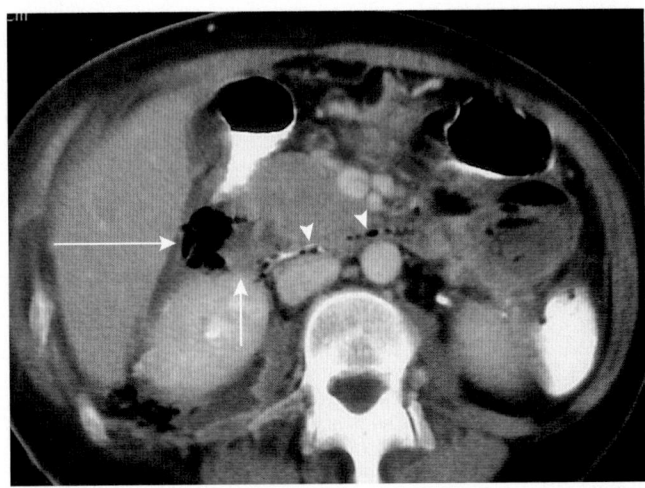
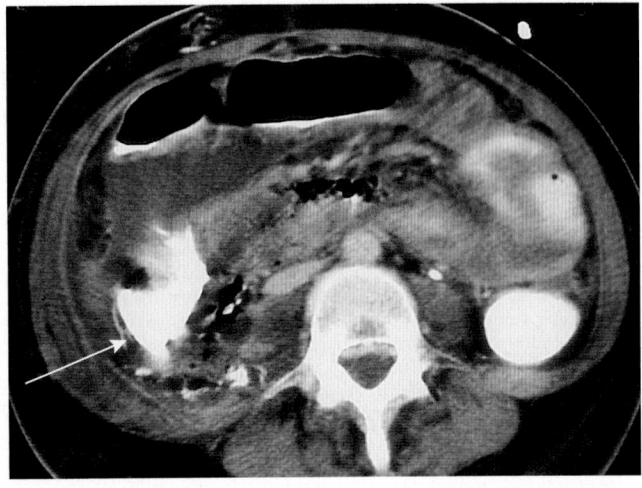

A   B

FIGURE 135-7. Eighteen-year-old girl with juvenile dermatomyositis presenting with right lower quadrant pain and fever. **A,** Axial CT image after oral and intravenous contrast administration reveals pneumatosis involving the distal duodenum *(arrowheads)* and air *(long arrow)* and fluid *(short arrow)* in the right pararenal retroperitoneum. **B,** More inferior axial CT image reveals contrast in the retroperitoneum *(arrow)* as well as fluid and air. Pathology revealed ischemic enteropathy secondary to multifocal occlusive arteriopathy. (Courtesy of R. Paul Guillerman, Houston, TX.)

SUGGESTED READINGS

Infection

Lichtenstein JE: Inflammatory conditions of the stomach and duodenum. Radiol Clin North Am 1993;31:1315-1333

Stringer DA, Babyn PS: Pediatric Gastrointestinal Imaging and Intervention, 2nd ed. Hamilton, Ontario, Decker, 2000

Duodenal Ulcer Disease

Dooley CP, Larson AW, Stace NH, et al: Double contrast barium meal and upper gastrointestinal endoscopy. Ann Intern Med 1984;101:538-545

Drumm B, Rhoads JM, Stringer DA, et al: Etiology, presentation, and clinical course of endoscopically diagnosed peptic ulcer disease in children. Pediatrics 1988;82:410-414

Drumm B, Sherman P, Cutz E, Karmali M: *Campylobacter pylori* associated with primary antral gastritis and duodenal ulcers in children: a prospective study. Paper presented at the annual meeting of the American Society of Microbiology, Atlanta, 1987

Elitsur Y, Lawrence Z: Non-*Helicobacter pylori* related duodenal ulcer disease in children. Helicobacter 2001;6:239-243

Gelfand DW, Dale WJ, Ott DJ, et al: Duodenitis: endoscopic-radiologic correlation in 272 patients. Radiology 1985;157:577-581

Herlinger H, Glanville JN, Kreel L: An evaluation of the double contrast barium meal (DCBM) against endoscopy. Clin Radiol 1977;28:307-314

Laufer I: Assessment of the accuracy of double contrast gastroduodenal radiology. Gastroenterology 1976;71:874-878

Long FR, Kramer SS, Markowitz RI, et al: Duodenitis in children: correlation of radiologic findings with endoscopic and pathologic findings. Radiology 1998;206:103-108

Pun E, Firkin A: Computed tomography and complicated peptic ulcer disease. Australas Radiol 2004;48:516-519

Stringer DA, Babyn PS: Pediatric Gastrointestinal Imaging and Intervention, 2nd ed. Hamilton, Ontario, Decker, 2000

Stringer DA, Daneman A, Brunelle F, et al: Sonography of the normal and abnormal stomach (excluding hypertrophic pyloric stenosis) in children. J Ultrasound Med 1986;5:183-188

Inflammatory Bowel Disease

Cameron DJ: Upper and lower gastrointestinal endoscopy in children and adolescents with Crohn's disease: a prospective study. J Gastroenterol Hepatol 1991;6:355-358

Castellaneta SP, Afzal NA, Greenberg M, et al: Diagnostic role of upper gastrointestinal endoscopy in pediatric inflammatory bowel disease. J Pediatr Gastroenterol 2004;39:257-261

Kirks DR, Currarino G: Regional enteritis in children: small bowel disease with normal terminal ileum. Pediatr Radiol 1978;7:10-14

Lenaerts C, Roy CC, Vaillancourt M, et al: High incidence of upper gastrointestinal tract involvement in children with Crohn disease. Pediatrics 1989;83:777-781

Mashako MN, Cezard JP, Navarro J, et al: Crohn's disease lesions in the upper gastrointestinal tract: correlation between clinical, radiological, endoscopic, and histologic features in adolescents and children. J Pediatr Gastroenterol 1989;8:442-446

Ruuska T, Vaajalahti P, Arajarvi P, et al: Prospective evaluation of upper gastrointestinal mucosal lesions in children with ulcerative colitis and Crohn's disease. J Pediatr Gastroenterol Nutr 1994;19:181-186

Stringer DA, Babyn PS: Pediatric Gastrointestinal Imaging and Intervention, 2nd ed. Hamilton, Ontario, Decker, 2000

Tootla F, Lucas RJ, Bernacki EG, et al: Gastroduodenal Crohn's disease. Arch Surg 1976;3:855-857

Celiac Disease

Horton KM, Fishman EK: Uncommon inflammatory diseases of the small bowel: CT findings. AJR Am J Roentgenol 1998;170:385-388

Laghi A, Paoolantonio P, Catalano C, et al: MR imaging of the small bowel using polyethylene glycol solution as an oral contrast agent in adults and children with celiac disease: preliminary observations. AJR Am J Roentgenol 2003;189:191-194

Marn CS, Gore RM, Ghahremani GG: Duodenal manifestations of nontropical sprue. Gastrointest Radiol 1986;11:30-35

Rickes S, Malfertheiner P: Images of interest. Gastrointestinal: sonographic features of celiac disease. J Gastroenterol Hepatol 2004;19:462

Stringer DA, Babyn PS: Pediatric Gastrointestinal Imaging and Intervention, 2nd ed. Hamilton, Ontario, Decker, 2000

Eosinophilic Enteritis

Horton KM, Fishman EK: Uncommon inflammatory diseases of the small bowel: CT findings. AJR Am J Roentgenol 1998;170:385-388

Madhotra R, Eloubeidi MA, Cunningham JT, et al: Eosinophilic gastroenteritis masquerading as ampullary adenoma. J Clin Gastroenterol 2003;34:240-242

Zollinger-Ellison Syndrome

Eire PF, Rodriguez Pereira C, Barca Rodriguez P, Varela Cives R: Uncommon case of gastrinoma in a child. Eur J Pediatr Surg 1996;6:173-174

Jensen RT, Gardner JD: Gastrinoma. *In* Go VLW, DiMagno EP, Gardner JD, et al (eds): The Pancreas: Biology, Pathology, and Disease, 2nd ed. New York, Raven Press, 1993:931-978

Norton JA, Fraker DL, Alexander HR, et al: Surgery to cure the Zollinger-Ellison syndrome. N Engl J Med 1999;341:635-644

Wilson SD: Zollinger-Ellison syndrome in children: a 25-year follow-up. Surgery 1991;110:696-702

Zollinger-Ellison syndrome. E-Medicine. http://www.emedicine.com/ped/topic2472.htm (accessed Feb 28, 2006)

Graft-versus-Host Disease

Day DL, Carpenter BL: Abdominal complications in pediatric bone marrow transplant recipients. Radiographics 1993;13:1101-1112

Donnelly LF, Morris CL: Acute graft-versus host disease in children: abdominal CT findings. Radiology 1996;1999:265-268

Lalantari BN, Mortele KJ, Cantisani V, et al: CT features with pathologic correlation of acute gastrointestinal graft-versus-host disease after bone marrow transplantation in adults. AJR Am J Roentgenol 2003;181:1621-1625

Maile CW, Frick MP, Crass JR, et al: The plain abdominal radiograph in acute gastrointestinal graft-vs-host disease. AJR Am J Roentgenol 1985;145:289-292

Stringer DA, Babyn PS: Pediatric Gastrointestinal Imaging and Intervention, 2nd ed. Hamilton, Ontario, Decker, 2000

Chronic Granulomatous Disease

Bowen A III, Gibson MD: Chronic granulomatous disease with gastric antral narrowing. Pediatr Radiol 1980;10:119-120

Granot E, Matoth I, Korman SH, et al: Functional gastrointestinal obstruction in a child with chronic granulomatous disease. J Pediatr Gastroenterol Nutr 1986;5:321-323

Griscom NT, Kirkpatrick JA, Girdany BR, et al: Gastric antral narrowing in chronic granulomatous disease of childhood. Pediatrics 1974;54:456-460

Khanna G, Kao SC, Kirby P, Sato Y: Imaging of chronic granulomatous disease in children. Radiographics 2005;25:1183-1195

Kopen PA, McAliser WH: Upper gastrointestinal and ultrasound examinations of gastric antral involvement in chronic granulomatous disease. Pediatr Radiol 1984;14:91-93

Smith FJ, Taves DH: Gastroduodenal involvement in chronic granulomatous disease of childhood. Can Assoc Radiol J 1992;43:215-217

Cystic Fibrosis

Abramson SJ, Baker DH, Amodio JB, Berdon WE: Gastrointestinal manifestations of cystic fibrosis. Semin Roentgenol 1987;22:97-113

Agrons GA, Corse WR, Markowitz RI, et al: Gastrointestinal manifestations of cystic fibrosis: radiologic-pathologic correlation. Ragiographics 1996;16:871-893

Berk RN, Lee FA: The late gastrointestinal manifestations of cystic fibrosis of the pancreas. Radiology 1973;106:337-381

Clarke LL, Stien X, Walker NM: Intestinal bicarbonate secretion in cystic fibrosis mice. JOP 2001;2:263-267

Hirokawa M, Takeuchi T, Chu S, et al: Cystic fibrosis gene mutation reduces epithelial cell acidification and injury in acid-perfused mouse duodenum. Gastroenterology 2004;127:1162-1173

Raia V, Maiuri L, De Ritis G, et al: Evidence of chronic inflammation in morphologically normal small intestine of cystic fibrosis patients. Pediatr Res 2000;47:344-350

Dermatomyositis

Schullinger JN, Jacobs JC, Berdon WE: Diagnosis and management of gastrointestinal perforations in childhood dermatomyositis with particular reference to perforations of the duodenum. J Pediatr Surg 1985;20:521-524

Wang IJ, Hsu WM, Shun CT, et al: Juvenile dermatomyositis complicated with vasculitis and duodenal perforation. J Formos Med Assoc 2001;100:844-846

136 Duodenum: Tumors and Tumor-like Conditions

ALAN E. SCHLESINGER

Neoplasms in the duodenum are, for the most part, not unique compared with those in the remainder of the small intestine. Therefore, the reader is referred to the discussion of small-bowel neoplasms (see Chapter 138). The only neoplasms that occur exclusively in the duodenum in children are those related to Brunner glands.

Brunner glands are located in the submucosa of the duodenum; their function consists of alkaline secretion to protect the duodenum from gastric acid. Hyperplasia and adenoma of Brunner glands can occur; these are differentiated on the basis of size. Lesions smaller than 1 cm are considered Brunner gland hyperplasia, and larger lesions represent adenomas. Brunner gland adenomas likely are in fact hamartomas. Malignant transformation of Brunner gland neoplasms has been rarely reported. Although this process is typically seen in adults, Brunner gland adenomas have also been reported in children. Patients with adenomas are often asymptoma-

tic but may present with abdominal pain, nausea, gastrointestinal hemorrhage, or obstruction. Obstruction may occur as the result of duodenal-jejunal intussusception when a Brunner gland hamartoma or adenoma acts as a lead point.

> **Brunner gland hyperplasia and adenoma are differentiated on the basis of size in the following manner:**
> - **Adenomas are larger than 1 cm.**
> - **Lesions smaller than 1 cm represent Brunner gland hyperplasia.**

On upper gastrointestinal examination, Brunner gland adenomas may appear as smooth-walled polypoid filling defects (Fig. 136-1). Endoscopic ultrasonography has been used to evaluate these lesions, detect involvement of adjacent structures, and diagnose metastases in the rare malignant tumor. Yadav presented a case of a giant Brunner gland imaged on computed tomography (CT).

Polypoid lesions other than those related to hyperplasia or adenomas of Brunner gland may be seen in the duodenum in children and are similar to those seen in the rest of the small bowel. Attard, in an 18-year retrospective study of patients younger than 21 years of age at The Johns Hopkins Children's Center, reported 22 duodenal polyps in 16 children. Although 33% of these polyps were related to the Brunner gland, the remainder were adenomatous polyps (42%), hamartomatous polyps (17%), and heterotopic gastric gland polyps (8%). All of the adenomatous polyps occurred in patients with familial adenomatoid polyposis syndrome, and all of the hamartomatous polyps were diagnosed in patients with Peutz-Jeghers syndrome (Fig. 136-2) (see Chapter 138). These polyps can, as in the case of duodenal polyps related to Brunner glands, result in duodeno-jejunal intussusception (Fig. 136-3). Gastroduodenal intussusception has been reported in patients with Peutz-Jeghers syndrome. Malignant transformation of periampullary adenomas with familial adenomatous polyposis syndrome is common in adults (see Chapter 143) but has not been reported in children.

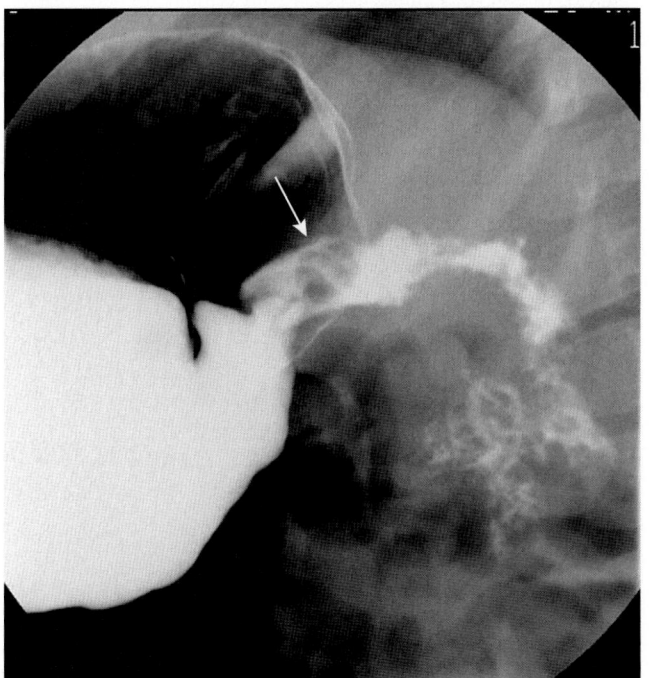

FIGURE 136-1. Brunner gland hyperplasia. Filling defect *(arrow)* in the duodenal bulb is smaller than 1 cm in diameter. (Courtesy of Kimberly Applegate, Indianapolis, IN.)

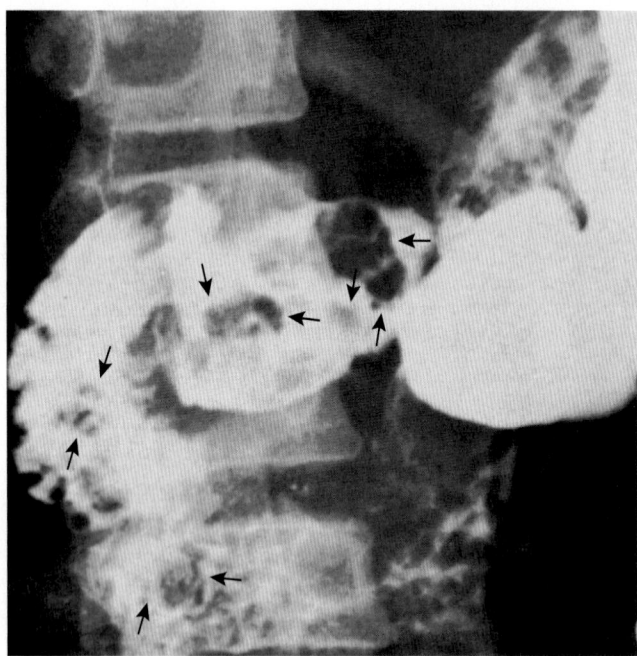

FIGURE 136-2. Multiple polyps in the duodenum *(arrows)* of a 12 year-old boy who also had polyps in the stomach, the colon, and the remainder of the small intestine. Examination of his mouth revealed the typical melanin deposits of Peutz-Jeghers syndrome.

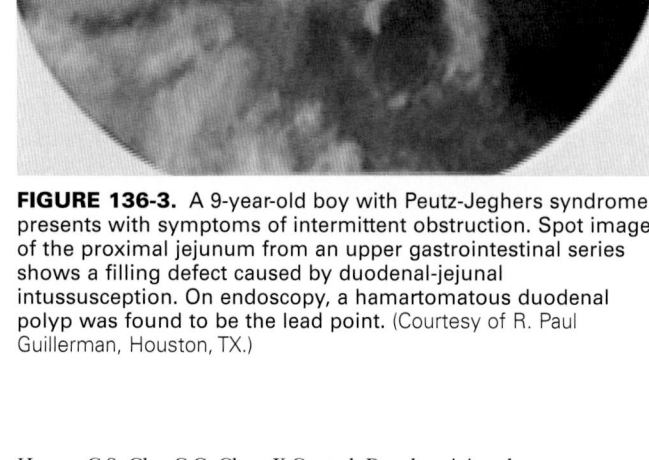

FIGURE 136-3. A 9-year-old boy with Peutz-Jeghers syndrome presents with symptoms of intermittent obstruction. Spot image of the proximal jejunum from an upper gastrointestinal series shows a filling defect caused by duodenal-jejunal intussusception. On endoscopy, a hamartomatous duodenal polyp was found to be the lead point. (Courtesy of R. Paul Guillerman, Houston, TX.)

SUGGESTED READINGS

Attard TM, Abraham SC, Cuffari C: The clinical spectrum of duodenal polyps in pediatrics. J Pediatr Gastroenterol Nutr 2003;36:116-119

Chrwastie AC: Duodenal carcinoma with neoplastic transformation of the underlying Brunner's glands. Br J Cancer 1953;7:65-67

Chuang JH, Chen WJ: Duodenojejunal intussusception secondary to hamartomatous polyp of Brunner's glands. J Pediatr Gastroenterol Nutr 1991;13:96-100

Hwang C-S, Chu C-C, Chen K-C, et al: Duodenojejunal intussusception secondary to hamartomatous polyps of duodenum surrounding the ampulla of Vater. J Pediatr Surg 2001;36:1073-1075

Stringer DA, Babyn PS: Pediatric Gastrointestinal Imaging and Intervention, 2nd ed. Hamilton, Ontario, BC Decker, 2000

Urganci N, Arapoglu M, Akyildiz B, et al: Brunner's gland adenoma: a rare cause of vomiting. Acta Pediatr 2005;94:631-633

Yadav D, Hertan H, Pitchumoni CS: A giant Brunner's gland adenoma presenting as a gastrointestinal hemorrhage. J Clin Gastroenterol 2001;32:448-450

CHAPTER 137

Small Intestine

RICHARD I. MARKOWITZ and MARTA HERNANZ-SCHULMAN

The small intestine is a long, convoluted, musculomembranous tube that begins at the pylorus and ends at the ileocecal valve. Its three major divisions are the duodenum, jejunum, and ileum. This chapter discusses normal anatomy and pathologic conditions involving the small bowel from the ligament of Treitz to the ileocecal valve. The jejunum accounts for approximately three fifths of the small bowel; the remaining two fifths is ileum. The proximal third of the small intestine commonly fills the left upper abdominal quadrant, the middle third occupies the midportion of the abdomen and the right upper quadrant, and the terminal third lies on the right side of the abdomen and pelvis. The caliber of the lumen gradually diminishes from proximal to distal, and the diameter of the terminal ileum is about one third smaller than that of the first portion of the jejunum. The external surface of the tube is smooth and devoid of permanent folds or creases. The internal surface is thrown into transverse and spiral folds, the plicae circulares of the submucosa, which are covered by villous folds of mucous membrane. These folds greatly increase the secreting and absorbing surface and facilitate digestion by retarding the passage of intestinal content.

IMAGING STUDIES

Plain radiographs are often nonspecific in patients with small intestinal disease but are extremely useful in identifying adynamic ileus, intestinal obstruction, free air produced by intestinal perforation, pathologic calcification, and masses large enough to displace normal structures.

The *contrast small intestinal series* remains the mainstay of small-bowel imaging. Barium is the most frequently used contrast agent; water-soluble nonionic agents are reserved for specific indications such as potential perforation. After the upper gastrointestinal (GI) portion of the study has been completed, radiographs are obtained at various intervals, and bowel caliber and mucosal pattern are evaluated; fluoroscopic compression and noncompression images are obtained as needed to evaluate questionable findings on radiography. Once the contrast reaches the terminal ileum, it is evaluated fluoroscopically to assess distensibility and mucosal detail, as well as any separation of bowel loops that might indicate bowel wall thickening or interloop abnormalities.

Enteroclysis is a technique that has been used in adults to obtain high-resolution, detailed images of the small intestine with uniform bowel distention. Its application in the pediatric age group is increasing, but enteroclysis is generally applied in older children and adolescents. The technique requires placement of an 8 to 10 French nasoduodenal tube to the level of the distal duodenum. A substantial amount (100-300 cc, depending on patient size) of specially formulated barium is slowly instilled into the intestine under fluoroscopic monitoring (see Fig. 140-2). To obtain a double-contrast effect, a nonopaque agent is instilled, again via a specialized pump apparatus, into the bowel. Bowel paralysis may be employed to augment bowel distention and relaxation. Thus, the entire small bowel is evaluated in detail. Drawbacks for routine use in the pediatric population include the potential need for sedation, tube placement, risk of complications, and the relatively high fluoroscopic radiation dose. The need for specialized equipment and the requirement of experienced, trained personnel are additional limitations. Nevertheless, in selected cases, under proper monitoring and supervision, the technique may be very effective in revealing difficult to find strictures, small polyps and nodules, ulcers, and other subtle mucosal abnormalities.

Although *ultrasonography* (US) is limited by intraluminal air within the intestine, when gas is scarce or compressible, US can identify thickened bowel wall and intestinal and mesenteric masses, including abscesses and intussusceptions; it also has increasing usefulness in the diagnosis of a variety of disease entities, as discussed throughout this chapter. The definition of bowel wall thickening upon US is exquisite, and colon and small bowel can often be distinguished. The terminal ileum is recognized by its termination at the ileocecal valve in the right lower quadrant, as seen when the ascending colon is followed down from the hepatic flexure. Doppler studies have proved valuable in the evaluation of inflammatory processes and in the recognition of ischemic conditions.

Computed tomography (CT) has ever-increasing usefulness in the intestinal tract. In most cases, good opacification of the bowel lumen is important for optimal CT evaluation of the intestine and mesentery. Positive contrast is the most widely used, but recently, negative contrast material has shown increasing usefulness, particularly in the evaluation of entities such as Crohn disease, because negative contrast does not obscure bowel wall enhancement. Recently, milk has been suggested as an alternative negative contrast medium. CT is useful in a wide variety of disorders, including but not limited to inflammatory bowel disease and its complications, trauma, intra-abdominal abscesses, and mass lesions. Coronal reconstructions can be extremely helpful in many cases.

Scintigraphy plays a more limited role in small bowel disease but may be useful in cases of abdominal pain or intestinal bleeding, especially where ectopic gastric mucosa is suspected. The value of scintigraphy in inflammatory disease of the intestinal tract is still debated (see discussion, Chapter 106). *Magnetic resonance imaging* (MRI) of intestinal disease has had limited utility in children. Intestinal motion and the lack of satisfactory intestinal contrast agents have severely limited the usefulness of MRI except in evaluation of mass lesions. However, newer equipment and fast sequences as well as the lack of radiation has sparked renewed interest in MRI for imaging the small bowel.

CONGENITAL ANOMALIES OF THE SMALL INTESTINE

Most congenital abnormalities of the small intestine involve intestinal atresia or meconium ileus; these are addressed in the neonatal Chapter 14. Some congenital abnormalities that present during the neonatal period, such as meconium ileus in patients with cystic fibrosis, have later equivalents that present in the older child and are discussed later. Other congenital abnormalities that are identified beyond infancy include duplication cysts, lymphangiomas or omental/mesenteric cysts, and omphalomesenteric duct remnants.

Duplication Cysts

The most frequent location for a *duplication cyst* of the intestinal tract is the region of the terminal ileum and ileocecal valve. These cysts can be located anywhere along the GI tract, but the most commonly noted areas are the esophagus, stomach, and duodenum. Multiple duplications have been reported. Duplication cysts, by definition, contain mucosal and muscular layers. They occur along the mesenteric border of the intestine and typically share a common blood supply, although each is invested with its own mucosal lining. These cysts are named by the portion of the bowel with which they share a common wall, not by the type of mucosa that they contain. Most are localized and somewhat spherical and do not communicate with the GI tract. Some duplication cysts are tubular, paralleling significant lengths of bowel, and may communicate with the normal intestinal lumen. Presenting symptoms vary with the location and size of the duplication. Many are large enough to be palpable. Obstruction can occur anywhere that a duplication cyst is present and is the most frequent cause of symptoms. Distal ileal duplication may cause intussusception, and segmental volvulus may occur at any site in the small intestine where duplication is present. Abdominal pain may be related to distention of the cyst or peptic disease if the cyst contains gastric mucosa. GI bleeding may occur from a communicating duplication that contains

gastric mucosa. Brown and colleagues described an infant with delayed diagnosis because the cyst intermittently decompressed itself by emptying its contents into the adjacent, partially communicating bowel lumen.

Plain radiographic examination is usually unrewarding unless the duplication is large enough to cause a mass effect on adjacent structures, intestinal obstruction, or secondary intussusception (Fig. 137-1), or if calcification is identified within the wall. US identifies the duplication as an anechoic, fluid-filled mass (see Fig. 137-1). Duplication cysts may act as the lead point of an intussusception, and these can be identified with sonography (see Fig. 137-1). Echogenic debris may be seen, probably produced by hemorrhage or mucosal secretions, and gut signature may help to refine the differential diagnosis (Fig. 137-2). However, this finding is not entirely specific for the diagnosis of duplication cyst; the double-layer sign can be eradicated when inflammation is noted within the cyst, and a pseudogut signature has been described in patients with cystic ovarian teratoma, mesenteric cyst, or ovarian cyst. Occasionally, cysts are multilocular. Caspi and associates described an infected duplication cyst with mixed echogenicity that mimicked a pelvic abscess. Those duplications that contain gastric mucosa may be identified by technetium-99m pertechnetate scintigraphy. CT is generally not needed once US reveals the cystic nature of the duplication, but if performed, it shows low attenuation surrounded by an enhancing wall (see Fig. 137-2). Contrast studies of the intestinal tract may show the lumina of communicating duplications but are more likely to reveal only the mass effect.

Lymphatic Malformations, Mesenteric and Omental Cysts

Lymphatic malformations have only an endothelial lining, are usually multiloculated, and may contain chyle. They typically present as painless abdominal distention with a palpable mass. Cystic structures may be adherent to small intestine, causing partial obstruction and vomiting, and surgical resection of involved bowel loops may be required. Plain radiographs show a large mass that displaces intestinal loops. Dilated loops may be seen in patients with obstruction (Fig. 137-3). GI contrast studies show displacement of bowel with no communication. US reveals the multilocular nature of the mass with fine septations (see Fig. 137-3). Most of the mass is anechoic, but some of the loculated spaces may be hypoechoic or even echogenic, depending on the chyle or blood content. Echogenic debris is commonly seen. CT usually shows septa and loculations, unless their attenuation value merges with that of the surrounding fluid. Septa may enhance with intravenous contrast injection. Attenuation values of the fluid range from near-fat to near-water, depending on its composition. Magnetic resonance imaging (MRI) studies of patients with lymphangioma show characteristics of the cyst ranging from fluid with low-intensity signal on T1-weighted images to fat with high-intensity signal.

The most common type of mesenteric or omental cyst is a lymphatic malformation; most of these tend to occur in the mesentery rather than the omentum, because of its

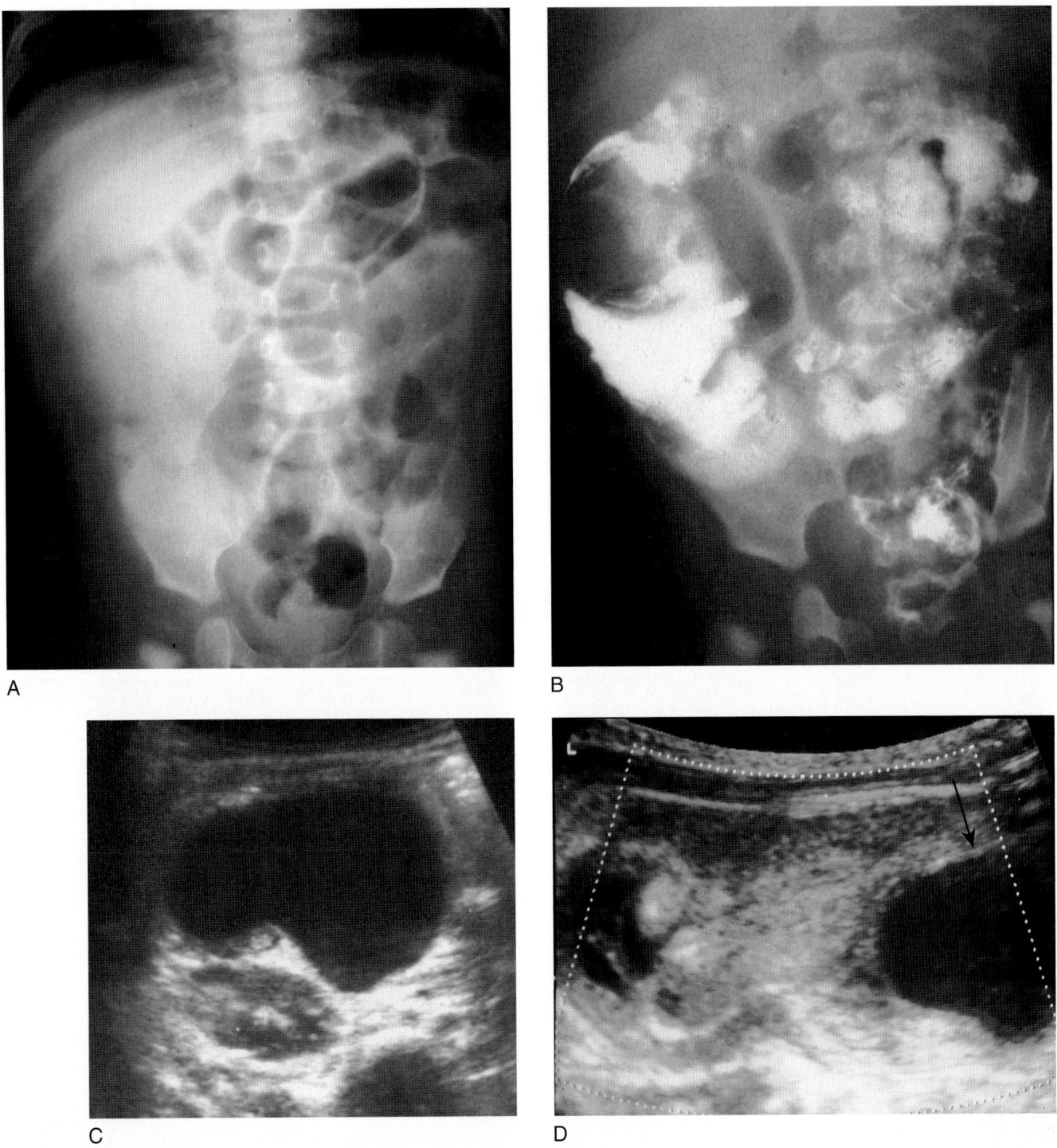

FIGURE 137-1. Ileal duplication cysts. **A,** Plain abdominal radiograph of a 4-month-old infant who presented with vomiting reveals dilated loops of small bowel and a mass effect along the right flank. **B,** An upper gastrointestinal series that was followed through to the ascending colon was performed at an outside institution. A mass effect upon the ascending colon was mistaken for an intussusception, and the child was referred to a pediatric institution for further evaluation and reduction. **C,** Ultrasonography performed upon arrival of the infant shows a large cystic mass in the right flank, with mass effect on the adjacent, empty colon. At surgery, a duplication cyst attached to the terminal ileum was identified and resected. **D,** A 3-month-old infant presented with ileocolic intussusception. Sonogram of the right lower quadrant reveals an anechoic cyst that is acting as the lead point of the intussusception (*arrow*). At surgery, an ileal duplication cyst was resected.

richer lymphatic content (Fig. 137-4). Mesothelial cysts occur in the small bowel, the mesentery, and the mesocolon. They are the result of accumulation of fluid between mesothelial layers and are therefore lined by mesothelium; they are unilocular. Nonpancreatic

pseudocysts may also occur in the mesentery or, more often, in the omentum. These are believed to result from prior trauma or infection, and although they may have a thick wall, histologically, no inner cellular lining is present. They exhibit increased echogenicity on US and

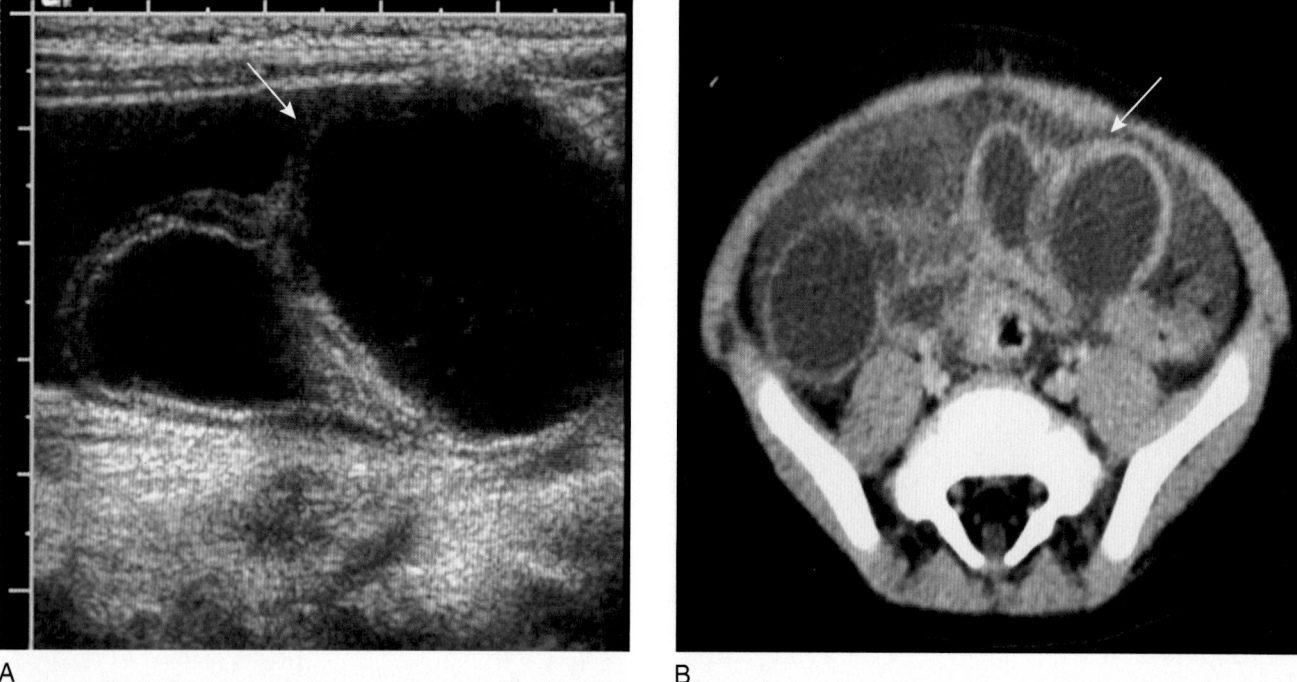

FIGURE 137-2. Ileal duplication cyst. **A,** Ultrasonography of lower abdomen reveals a duplication cyst *(arrow)* that shares a common wall with the distal ileum and contains echogenic debris. **B,** CT scan lower down in the pelvis shows an enhancing lesion *(arrow)* attached to the dilated loop of bowel. At surgery, an ileal duplication cyst was resected.

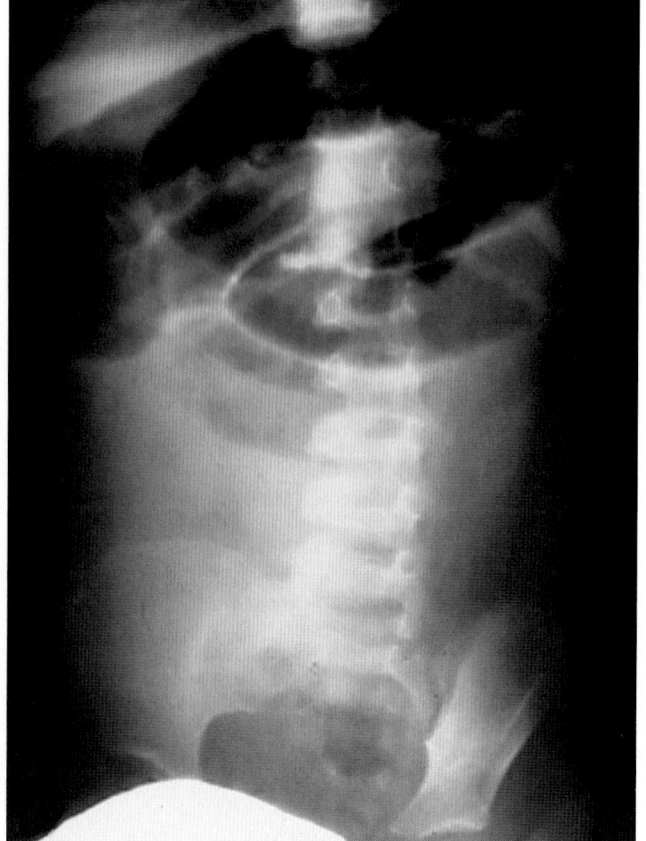

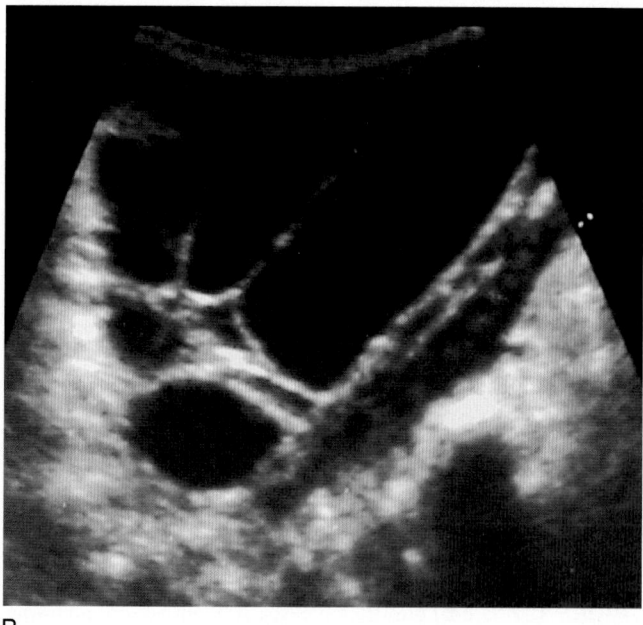

FIGURE 137-3. Lymphatic malformations. **A,** Abdominal radiograph of a patient who presented with vomiting shows dilated loops of bowel that are displaced into the upper abdomen. **B,** Longitudinal sonogram along the right flank reveals a multiseptated cystic mass occupying the lower portion of the abdomen.

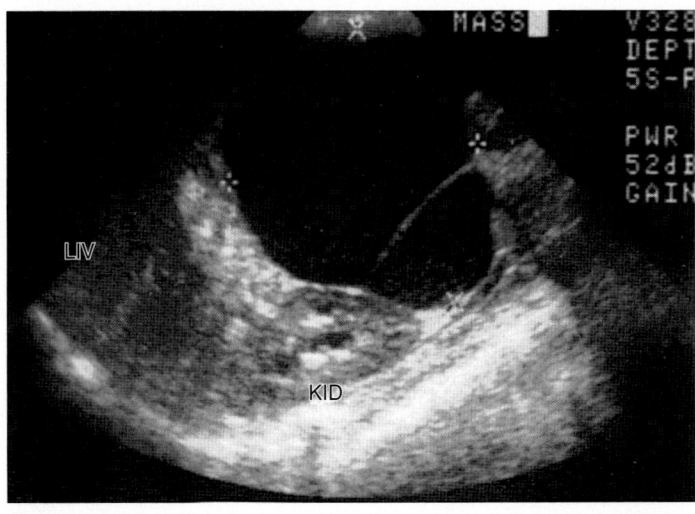

A

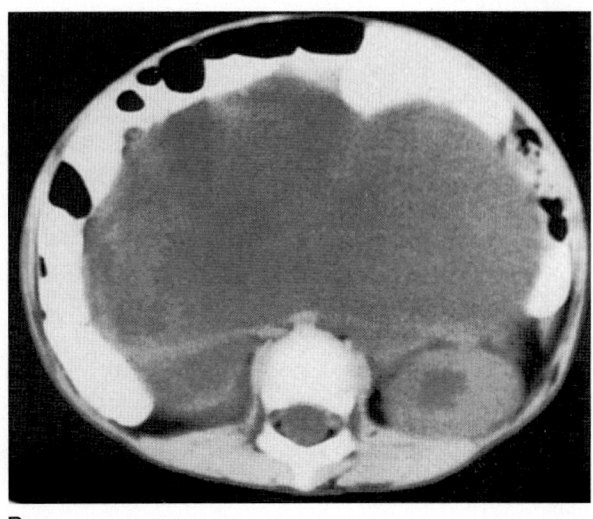

B

FIGURE 137-4. Mesenteric lymphatic malformation. **A,** Longitudinal ultrasound scan through the upper abdomen shows a septated, hypoechoic mass that is abutting the liver (LIV) and the right kidney (KID). **B,** Computed tomography scan confirms the massive fluid-filled structure that is displacing contrast-filled loops of bowel. Right-sided septation is again seen, even on unenhanced scan.

increased attenuation values on CT compared with water. Enteric cysts may also be encountered; these are lined by intestinal mucosa but differ from duplication cysts in that they lack a muscular wall and ganglion cells. In children with mesenteric cysts, the most common presenting symptoms are abdominal pain, abdominal distention, and vomiting. Teratomas may also occur in the abdominal cavity; intraperitoneal teratomas are usually identifiable by characteristics of multitissue origin, along with fat and calcifications (Fig. 137-5).

Omphalomesenteric remnants are the residua of the embryologic yolk stalk that present in several ways, depending on the type of residual omphalomesenteric abnormality and ensuing complications. (Please see also Chapter 109.) Normally, the entire attachment regresses. If the entire attachment remains patent, an umbilical sinus or omphalomesenteric fistula may ensue. The lumen may be obliterated, but a fibrous cord may persist, with or without cystic remnants within it. Persistence of the ileal portion results in a Meckel diverticulum, which can be variable in size. The clinical diagnosis of an omphalomesenteric duct remnant with a patent lumen is easily made because of the presence of bowel contents at the umbilicus. Attachment of the mid small intestine to the anterior abdominal wall via a persistent cord may lead to distal small-bowel obstruction similar to an adhesion, or the remnant may predispose to volvulus of a bowel loop about the fibrous cord.

Meckel diverticulum is the most common congenital abnormality involving the small bowel. Different from duplication cysts, which typically occur in the mesenteric border of the intestine, Meckel diverticulum nearly always occurs along the antimesenteric border. As a true diverticulum, it contains all layers of the bowel wall but may contain mucosa from any portion of the GI tract. Although Meckel diverticula are an asymptomatic incidental finding at autopsy in 1% to 4% of the population, they may cause serious problems in one of three ways: (1) GI bleeding, (2) intussusception, and (3) acute in-

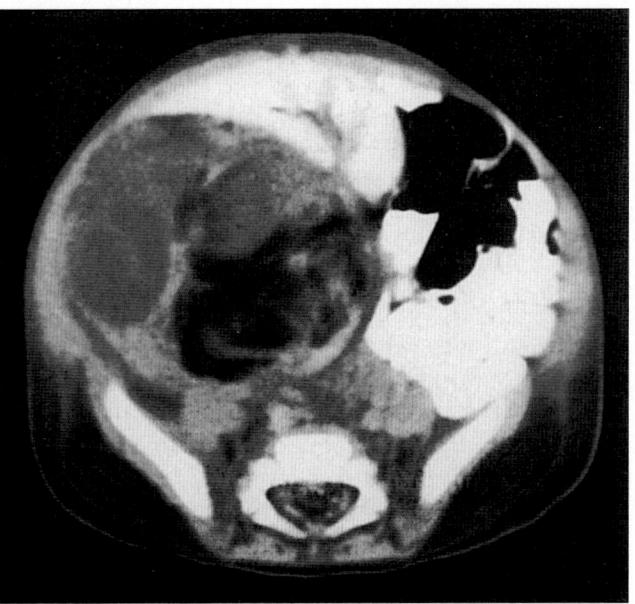

FIGURE 137-5. Intraperitoneal teratoma. Computed tomography scan shows a large intraperitoneal mass with multiple components of different attenuation values equal to those of water and of fat that are displacing bowel loops. A benign teratoma was removed at surgery.

flammation (i.e., Meckel diverticulitis). Bleeding may be associated with abdominal pain or may be painless; massive bleeding may ensue as the result of ulceration of the intestinal lining related to acid-secreting gastric mucosa within the diverticulum. Nuclear scintigraphy during active bleeding may be used to identify the site of hemorrhage. If the diverticulum contains gastric tissue, it may concentrate technetium and may be detected (see Fig. 106-13). Although most Meckel diverticula are situated in the right lower quadrant, the ileum to which they are attached can be variable in position within the abdomen, and it may be located in the midline or the left lower quadrant, which can cause confusion.

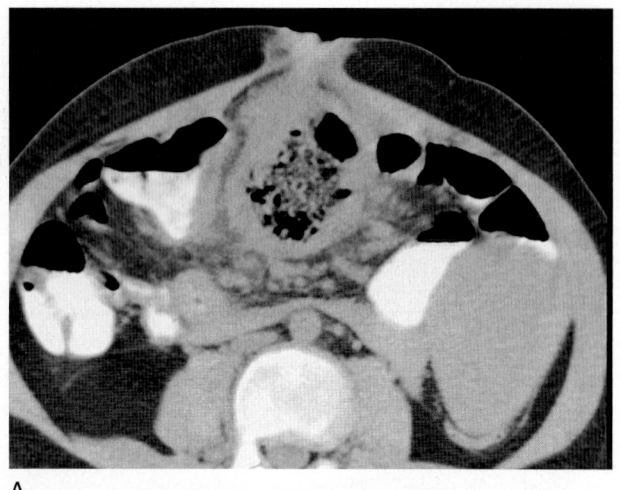
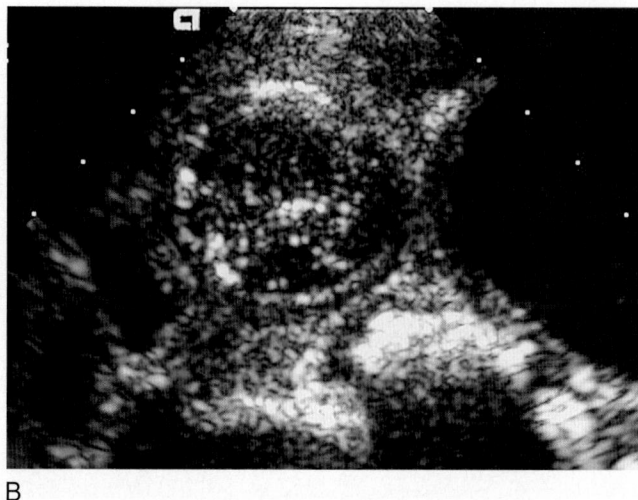

A   B

FIGURE 137-6. Meckel diverticulum. **A,** Computed tomography (CT) image in the periumbilical area reveals a large, inflamed loop of bowel in close association with the umbilicus, representing an inflamed Meckel diverticulum. **B,** Sagittal ultrasonography along the midline outlines a round structure with intestinal contents and gut signature located above the bladder fundus, with surrounding echogenicity; an inflamed Meckel diverticulum was identified at subsequent surgery.

Barium studies of the small bowel are less reliable unless careful attention is paid to separating and compressing the contrast-filled loops. Diverticula arise at right angles from the antimesenteric aspect of the intestine and have a characteristic mucosal pattern (see Fig. 109-11).

Invagination of the diverticulum with intussusception into the distal ileum is a rare complication that may cause acute or intermittent small-bowel obstruction. Acute inflammation with Meckel diverticulum may simulate acute appendicitis or may appear as an unusual structure with bowel contents and surrounding inflammation (Fig. 137-6). On sonography, gut signature that consists of an echogenic internal layer and a surrounding hypoechoic muscular layer may be identified (see Fig. 137-6).

SMALL-BOWEL OBSTRUCTION

Acquired intestinal obstruction in older children may be due to intrinsic or extrinsic abnormalities that affect the small intestine. Plain radiographic findings may reveal the level of obstruction, but in many cases, they may show less specific changes of incomplete obstruction or adynamic ileus.

Adynamic Ileus

Although adynamic (paralytic) ileus can simulate mechanical obstruction on plain radiographs, some signs, if present, are useful in distinguishing the two entities. Supine radiographs of the abdomen show dilated loops of bowel in both entities. Generalized adynamic ileus causes the small intestine and the colon to dilate, whereas mechanical obstruction usually causes proximal dilation with reduced caliber of the distal bowel. Lack of rectal gas is not a useful sign, especially in young children, because air arises from the dependent rectum on supine films. Therefore, prone radiographs, particularly prone cross-table lateral views of the rectum,

can be very helpful in differentiating obstruction from an ileus pattern. Unfortunately, for a significant number of children, differentiation is not possible. This is especially true of children with a focal ileus that affects the small intestine but not the colon. Air-fluid levels on horizontal beam films can be seen with both mechanical obstruction and adynamic ileus (Fig. 137-7). In the former condition, these are relatively short and occur at different levels in the loop of bowel, whereas in the latter condition, they are longer and scattered. Decubitus views are frequently more successful in revealing the long levels of adynamic ileus than are upright films. A prone cross-table lateral view of the rectum is helpful to the clinician in determining rectal size and often differentiating between ileus pattern and obstruction. In other children, partial small intestinal obstruction mimics adynamic ileus. CT can be helpful in revealing the level and occasionally the cause of the obstruction. Administration of oral contrast is not always necessary, but only water-soluble agents should be administered if bowel perforation is a potential complication.

Incarcerated Hernia

Incarcerated hernias are a less frequent cause of small-intestinal obstruction than they were in the past, possibly owing to the increased performance of elective outpatient herniorrhaphy. Most incarcerated hernias are inguinal; they are rarely umbilical. The diagnosis is made on clinical grounds, but plain films or US may be used to confirm the diagnosis. Erect or decubitus radiographs are helpful in ruling out bowel perforation.

Adhesions

Adhesions are a common cause of obstruction in patients who have undergone prior abdominal surgery. Adhesive bands can obstruct the small intestine, even at a site distant from the original surgical site. Plain films

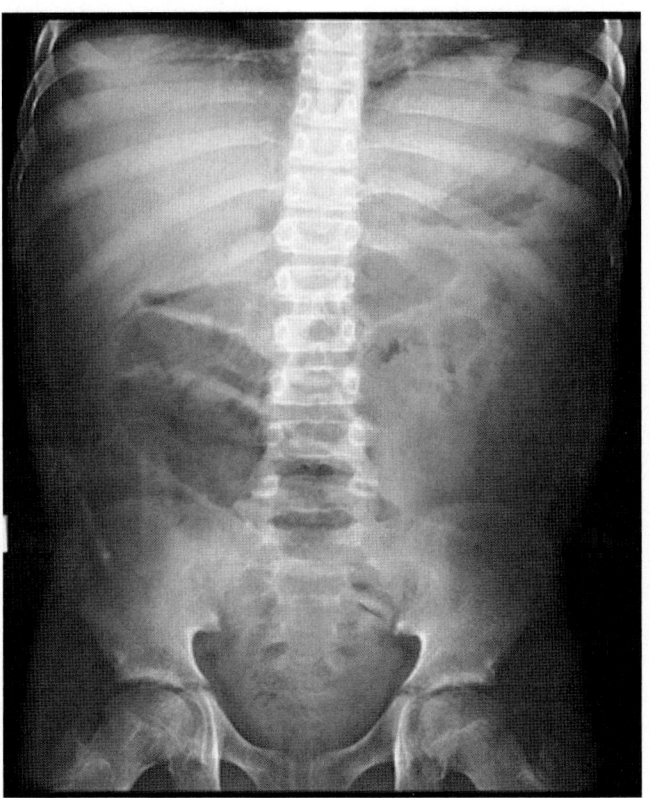 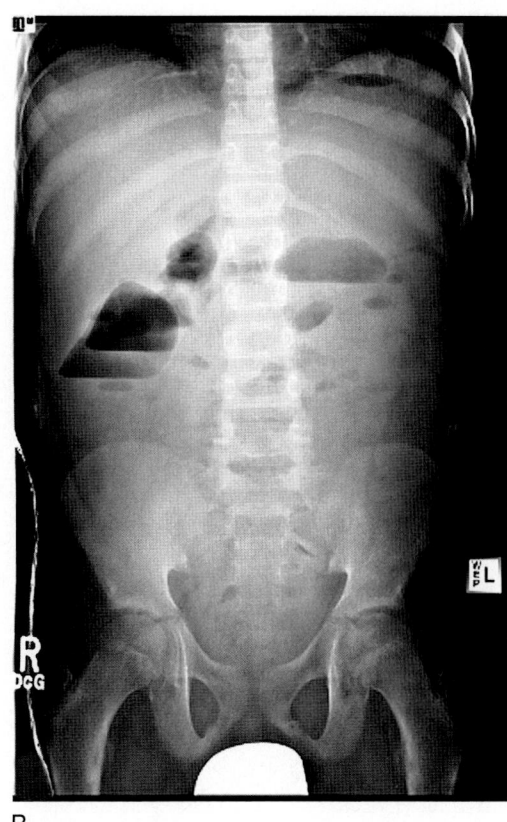

A   B

FIGURE 137-7. Small-bowel obstruction. Supine **(A)** and upright **(B)** radiographs in an adolescent boy with small-bowel obstruction related to severe Crohn disease involving the terminal ileum. Dilated loops of bowel show differential air-fluid levels on the upright image.

are useful in corroborating clinical suspicions and in ruling out intestinal perforation. Adhesions also occur in children who have had peritonitis, usually following appendicitis or inflammatory bowel disease. CT scans do not show the actual adhesions but may be helpful in indicating the level of obstruction, the presence of a mass, or the existence of a closed-loop obstruction or pneumatosis (Fig. 137-8). Collapsed bowel beyond the point of obstruction helps the clinician to pinpoint the level of obstruction.

As was discussed in the previous section, omphalomesenteric duct remnants may cause obstruction through kinking of the bowel under the fibrous remnant, closed-loop obstruction, segmental volvulus, intussusception, or inflammation of Meckel diverticulum.

ABNORMALITIES THAT MIMIC OBSTRUCTION

Dilation of various parts of the GI tract, including the small bowel, is characteristic of *intestinal pseudo-obstruction*. (This entity is discussed in Chapter 140). Another congenital abnormality that can mimic obstruction is *segmental dilation of the small bowel*. This rare disorder is characterized by segmental dilation that may appear as a single dilated loop with an air-fluid level on plain film and a focally dilated loop of bowel, usually ileum, on barium study. Transit time is normal. The lesion may be associated with other anomalies, such as omphalocele, malrotation, and Meckel diverticulum.

Patients may present with diarrhea caused by stasis and bacterial overgrowth in the dilated segment of intestine. Surgery is curative.

INFLAMMATORY CONDITIONS OF THE SMALL BOWEL

Infectious Diseases

The most common intestinal infection in children in North America and Europe is viral gastroenteritis. Parasites and bacteria, as well as viruses, are worldwide causative agents of acute gastroenteritis in children. Tragically, resultant severe diarrhea and vomiting with subsequent dehydration remains a leading cause of childhood morbidity and mortality throughout the underdeveloped countries of the world.

VIRAL GASTROENTERITIS

Viral gastroenteritis in the United States is commonly the result of rotavirus infection, although adenovirus and other enteric viruses are common seasonal pathogens. Associated upper respiratory symptoms are common and may precede the GI presentation, which usually begins with vomiting followed by severe watery diarrhea. Imaging studies are not generally indicated, but plain films are occasionally requested to rule out other potential causes of the patient's symptoms. The most common findings are fluid-filled loops of distended bowel with

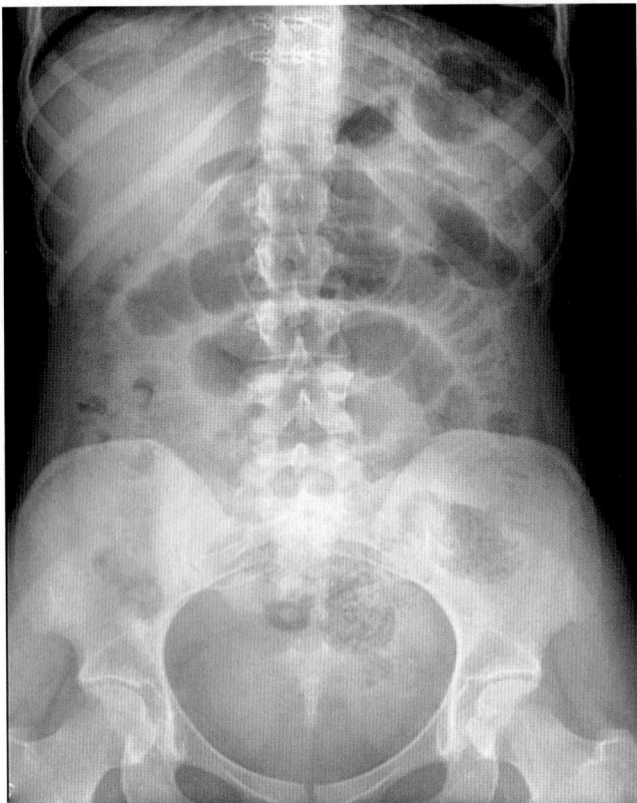

A

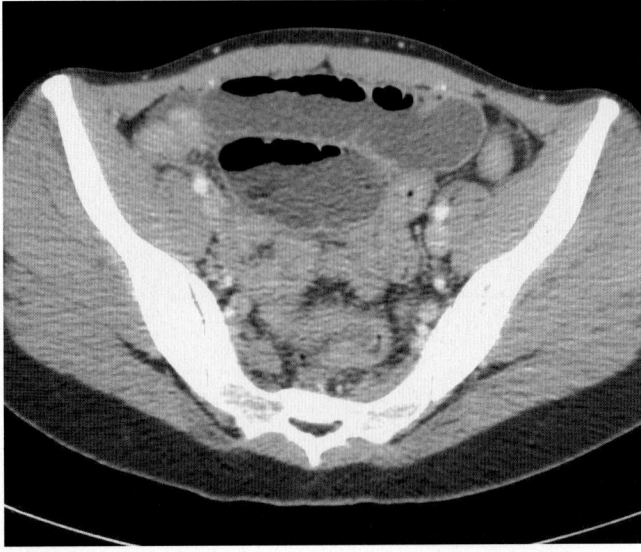

B

FIGURE 137-8. Obstruction caused by adhesions. **A,** An abdominal radiograph in an adolescent with abdominal distention and vomiting shows dilated loops of bowel in the upper abdomen. **B,** Pelvic image from a contrasted computed tomography scan performed for clinical suspicion of ruptured appendicitis reveals a small-bowel obstruction, along with collapsed distal small-bowel loops and a collapsed colon. Two parallel loops of bowel are markedly distended. Closed-loop obstruction was found at surgery and was believed to be due to adhesions resulting from surgery performed for meconium ileus during the neonatal period.

multiple scattered air-fluid levels on horizontal beam radiography. Absence of stool throughout the colon is commonly seen, along with air-fluid levels in the rectum. Depending on the time course and the degree of motility disturbance, nonobstructive dilation of bowel loops may occur. Contrast studies are not indicated; however, if they are performed for other reasons, such studies may show dilution of barium from fluid retention, minimal thickening of mucosal folds, and rapid or delayed transit time, depending on the chronicity of the disease. Disordered peristalsis is commonly seen. Capitanio and Greenberg have described pneumatosis intestinalis in two infants with rotavirus enteritis.

US is not needed in patients with clinically obvious gastroenteritis; however, if it is performed, fluid-filled distended loops of bowel and mesenteric lymph nodes may be found (Fig. 137-9). In a series published by Siegel and colleagues, viral gastroenteritis was not associated with increased bowel wall vascularity. High-resolution real-time scanning may reveal transient small-bowel intussusception during periods of hyperperistalsis.

BACTERIAL ENTEROCOLITIS

Bacterial enterocolitis is much less common than the viral form. The terminal ileum and the cecum are often involved (this is termed *infectious ileocecitis*); variable involvement of more distal portions of the colon and right lower quadrant lymphadenopathy have been noted. *Shigella, Salmonella, Escherichia coli, Yersinia enterocolitica,* and *Campylobacter fetus* are the most commonly identified bacterial agents in the United States. *Vibrio*

cholerae is the most common infectious bacterial agent in Asia. Symptoms of gastroenteritis are frequently accompanied by high fever and systemic toxicity, although clinical symptoms and host response to infection are variable. Symptoms may sometimes mimic appendicitis; therefore, it is important for the clinician to be familiar with characteristic imaging findings of these entities.

On imaging, involvement of the terminal ileum and cecum is apparent, involvement of the colon is variable, and right lower quadrant lymphadenopathy may be seen (Fig. 137-10). Matsumoto and coworkers performed US on eight children and young adults with *Yersinia* terminal ileitis. Thickening of the ileal wall was evident in all eight patients and mesenteric lymphadenopathy in six. On contrast studies, a cobblestone pattern may be seen (Fig. 137-11). Tuberculous involvement of the terminal ileum may cause small-bowel obstruction, presumably caused by adherent bowel loops. Pulmonary tuberculosis is typically the source of GI infection, and chest radiographs should always be obtained in suspected cases.

PARASITIC ENTEROCOLITIS

In the Western hemisphere, parasitic enterocolitis is most frequently caused by *Giardia lamblia* and usually results from drinking contaminated water. In the western part of the United States, virtually all of the natural mountain streams have become infested with *Giardia*. Although the protozoan easily infects otherwise normal people, it is an especially common causative agent in patients with acquired immunodeficiency syndrome (AIDS) who develop enteritis. On barium studies, giardi-

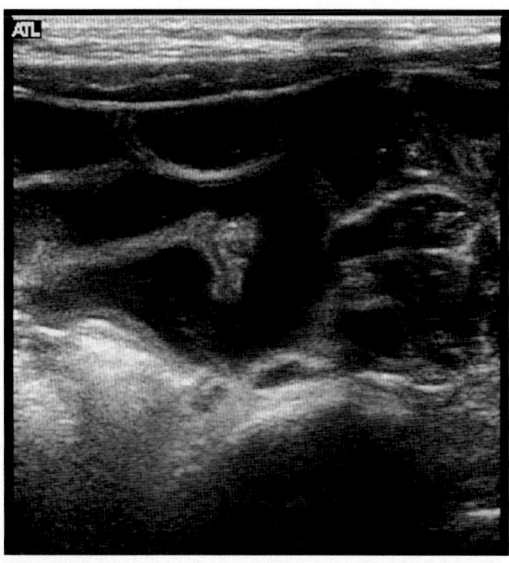
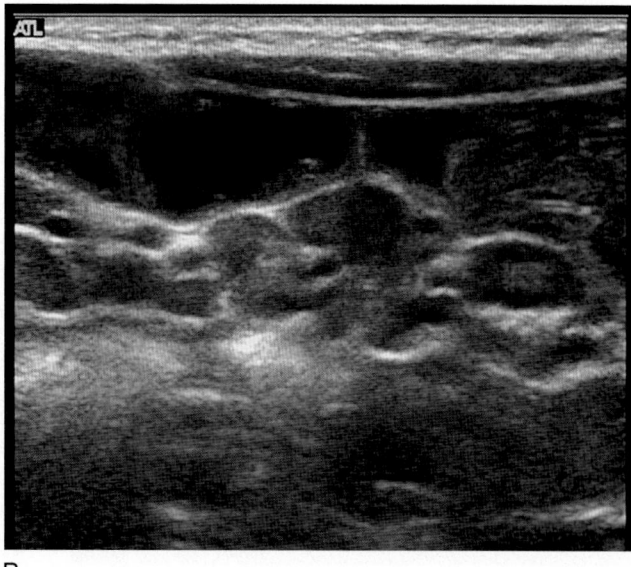

A   B

FIGURE 137-9. Gastroenteritis. A 21-month-old boy with vomiting and irritability suggestive of abdominal pain. Ultrasonography, performed to examine intussusception, reveals fluid-filled, distended, but otherwise normal loops of bowel (**A**), and right lower quadrant adenopathy (**B**) that was hyperemic on color Doppler interrogation (not shown).

asis produces thickened mucosal folds in the duodenum and jejunum that are associated with rapid transit time and dilution of contrast material (Fig. 137-12).

Helminthic enteritis can be caused by a variety of worms; *Ascaris lumbricoides* causes the most striking and diagnostic radiographic abnormalities. The disease results from swallowed larvae that grow into adult worms within the intestinal tract. Barium studies outline the characteristic vermiform organisms, which may appear singly or in clumps. The live worms may ingest barium, permitting visualization of their intestinal tracts. Infection with *Strongyloides stercoralis*, tapeworms, roundworms, and hookworms may occur.

ACQUIRED IMMUNODEFICIENCY SYNDROME

AIDS is substantially less common in children than in adults. Most early cases in children result from transmission of human immunodeficiency virus through contaminated blood products. Patients treated for hemophilia have been at particular risk. In 1989, according to Haney and associates, 80% or more of affected children acquired the virus from their mothers via transplacental passage. Currently, thanks to improvement in screening of blood products and the availability of effective antiretroviral medications, the number of children in whom AIDS is diagnosed has been declining, according to published data from the Centers for Disease Control; this trend began during the midportion of the last decade of the 20th century.

Presenting symptoms and signs are nonspecific and are related to affected organ systems. Enteritis is most frequently caused by the common pathogens described previously, but it may follow infection with opportunistic organisms such as cytomegalovirus (CMV) and *Mycobacterium avium-intracellulare,* and with ubiquitous fungi, especially *Candida albicans.* Extrapulmonic *Pneumocystis carinii* infection is reported with increasing frequency.

Candidiasis most commonly affects the esophagus, but any organism can infect any part of the GI tract. Nonspecific edema of the affected intestine is the most frequently found abnormality on barium studies. Effacement of the mucosal pattern is common, especially with *Cryptosporidium* infection. Pneumatosis intestinalis has been reported, although the cause is unclear. US and CT reveal thickening of the bowel wall, and intraabdominal and retroperitoneal lymphadenopathy is the most frequent finding. Kaposi sarcoma and lymphoma have been reported in the intestine, mesentery, and pancreas of affected children, but less frequently than in adults.

INFLAMMATORY BOWEL DISEASE

Crohn Disease

Crohn disease is commonly known as *regional enteritis;* the terms *segmental enteritis* and *terminal ileitis* are less frequently used. Peak incidence is reported in young adulthood, but 25% of patients present during childhood or adolescence. This disease has been reported in infants younger than 1 year of age. The cause remains unknown, but chronic activation of intestinal T cells has been implicated. Clinical presentation and severity of disease manifestations are highly variable. Crohn disease is characterized by segmental transmural granulomatous inflammation of the intestine. It may be localized to one segment or may involve several segments with intervening normal bowel. The terminal ileum is the most frequently involved segment, but the disease has been described everywhere in the GI tract from the mouth to the anus. The intestinal lumen is narrowed by spasm and by edematous and fibrotic thickening of the wall. The mucosal layer is extensively destroyed, and ulcers are usually present.

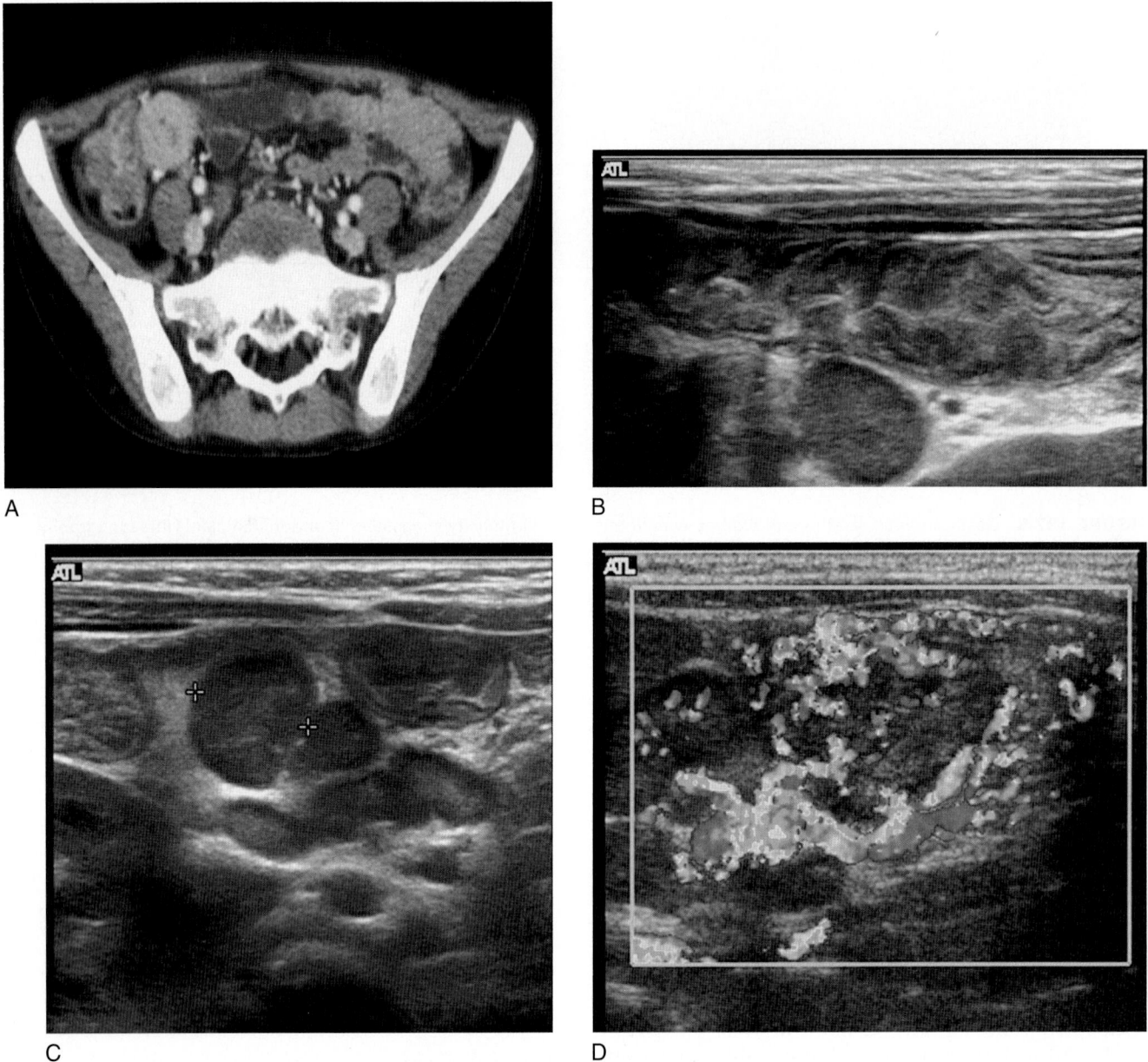

FIGURE 137-10. Bacterial enterocolitis. **A,** *Shigella* enteritis. Contrasted computed tomography scan requested to investigate appendicitis in an adolescent with abdominal pain and vomiting. Examination reveals concentric thickening and enhancement of the terminal ileum and cecum, along with a small amount of pericecal fluid. *Shigella sonnei* was cultured from the stool. **B,** In a 5-month-old with mucous diarrhea and abdominal pain, ultrasonography was requested to assess for suspected intussusception. A transverse sonogram of the right lower quadrant shows a markedly thickened terminal ileum, along with a visible transition to normal bowel more proximally. A large lymph node is seen deep to the terminal ileum. **C,** Transverse image slightly more cephalad reveals a large nodal aggregate medial to the ascending colon and anterior to the lower pole of the right kidney (calipers). **D,** Gray scale color Doppler image similar to that seen in part **B**; marked hyperemia is outlined in the thick-walled terminal ileum. (**D,** *see color plate.*)

Most children with Crohn disease present with insidious onset of GI symptoms, including diarrhea, abdominal pain, anorexia, abdominal mass, or perianal fistula. Extraintestinal manifestations of the disease may accompany or precede GI symptoms and include failure to thrive with delayed puberty, fever, aphthous stomatitis, arthralgias, arthritis, sacroiliitis, erythema nodosum, and digital clubbing. Some patients may present acutely with right lower quadrant pain and fever mimicking appendicitis.

Radiographic evaluation of the abdomen in patients with inflammatory bowel disease may be normal. The most common finding on plain abdominal radiography in patients with inflammatory bowel disease is absence of stool in involved portions of the colon. During an acute exacerbation of the disease, plain films are more likely to show abnormalities such as ileus, bowel wall thickening, or obstruction. Occasionally, a focally abnormal loop with edematous wall can be identified; this strongly suggests acute inflammation. During an acute flare-up of disease, signs of distal small-bowel obstruction lasting hours to days may occur (see Fig. 137-7).

Barium contrast small intestinal series are frequently used to evaluate jejunoileal manifestations of Crohn

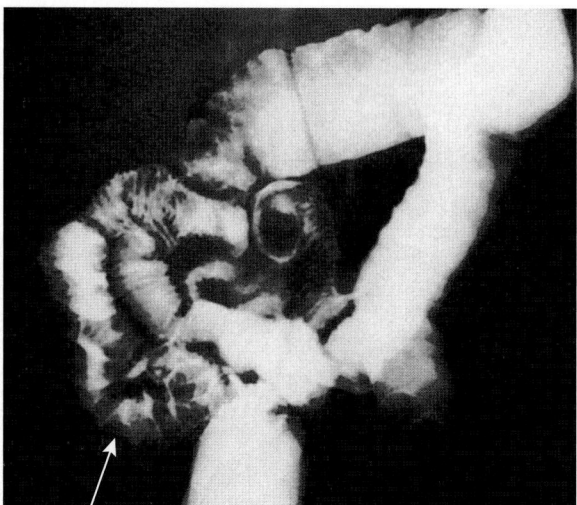

FIGURE 137-11. *Yersinia* enterocolitis. Barium enema shows "thumbprinting" *(arrow)* in the cecum and ascending colon of a 1-year-old girl. The ileum is dilated and exhibits thickened folds. *Yersinia enterocolitica* was cultured from mesenteric nodes removed at the time of exploratory laparotomy.

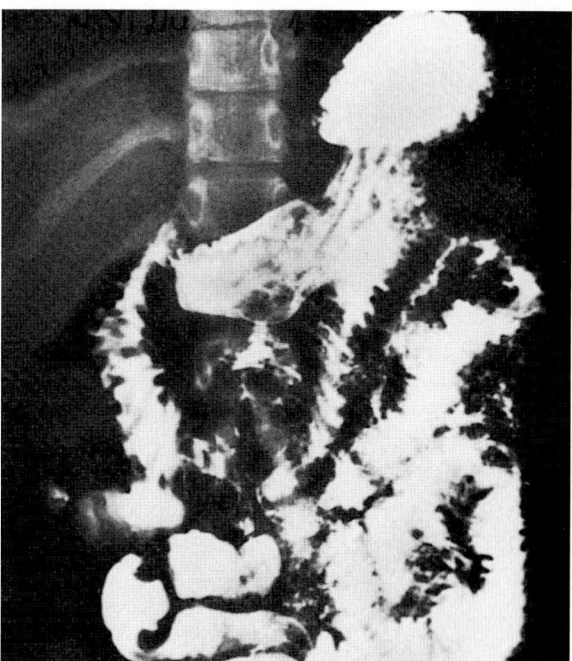

FIGURE 137-12. Giardiasis. Small intestinal barium examination in a 10-year-old girl with a history of nausea, vomiting, diarrhea, and weight loss. The mucosal folds of the duodenum and the proximal jejunum are markedly thickened. *Giardia* was identified in the stool.

disease. The terminal ileum is the most frequently involved area, but more proximal disease with sparing of the terminal ileum can occur. The earliest change is granularity, which probably reflects mucosal edema. More prominent mural edema results in thickening of mucosal folds and effacement of the mucosal pattern. Typical early findings include nodular irregularity with linear and transverse ulceration. Extensive ulceration can lead to a spiculated appearance and a "rose thorn" configuration, which results from deep ulcers extending into the thickened bowel wall, resembling thorns on a rose stem. The intersection of multiple linear and transverse ulcers leads to a cobblestone appearance also known as pseudopolyps, which represents areas of mucosa surrounded by adjacent denuded areas. Spasm of involved segments is frequently seen, and intermittent fluoroscopic observation is required to differentiate this occurrence from strictures (Fig. 137-13).

IMAGING FINDINGS IN CROHN DISEASE

RADIOGRAPHS
- Frequently normal or nonspecific; absence of normal colonic contents
- In acute exacerbations, narrowed bowel loop with edema or thickened wall may be seen

CONTRAST SMALL-BOWEL STUDY
- Mucosal edema
- Thickening of mucosal folds and effacement of mucosa ("moulage sign")
- Linear and transverse ulceration leading to cobblestone pattern
- Rose thorn ulcers
- Pseudopolyps
- Severe luminal narrowing and fibrosis
- Enteroenteric fistulas

COMPUTED TOMOGRAPHY
- Findings similar to those on small-bowel series

- More sensitive to mesenteric thickening, abscess, and fistulas

ULTRASOUND
- Thickened bowel wall
- Small nodes in surrounding mesenteric fat
- Hyperemia on Doppler evaluation

Edema, fibrosis, and spasm lead to narrowing of the intestinal lumen that may be so profound as to be labeled the "string sign" (see Fig. 137-13; Fig. 137-14). This narrowing is accompanied by persistent ulcers. The mesentery becomes inflamed, thickened, and fibrotic, causing separation and retraction of bowel loops. Enlarged mesenteric lymph nodes may cause mass effect on adjacent loops of bowel. Post-inflammation polyps may be seen. These are filiform projections of submucosa that are covered by mucosa on all sides. They represent healing of undermined mucosal and submucosal remnants and ulcers and are almost always multiple.

The diagnostic accuracy of barium studies is good. Lipson and colleagues compared barium small-bowel series with ileoscopy and biopsy results in 46 children with suspected regional enteritis of the terminal ileum. Although ileoscopy and biopsy results were consistent in all 20 positive cases, the small-bowel series had a sensitivity of 90% and a specificity of 96%. The major source of misdiagnosis was pronounced lymphoid hyperplasia on the barium study, which led to diagnostic errors in two cases.

Imaging studies other than small-bowel series are used with increasing frequency in the evaluation of patients with regional enteritis. Nuclear scintigraphy with a variety of radiopharmaceuticals can be used to identify areas of active inflammation, although success has been

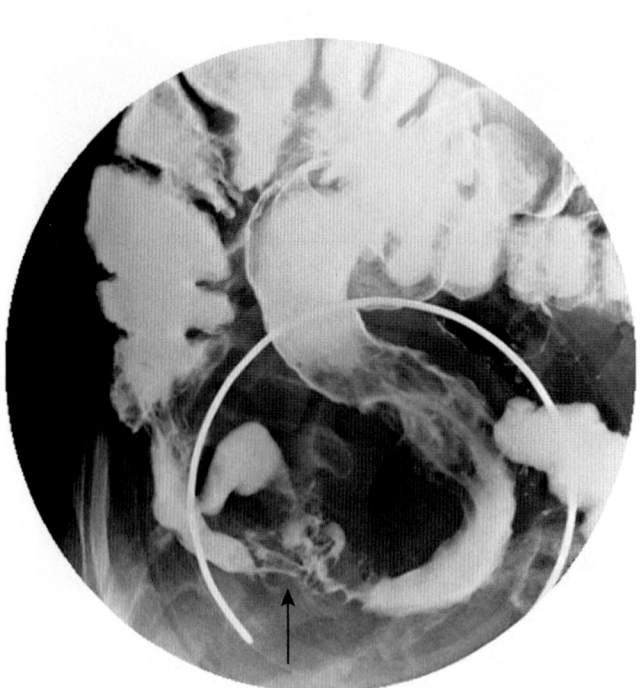

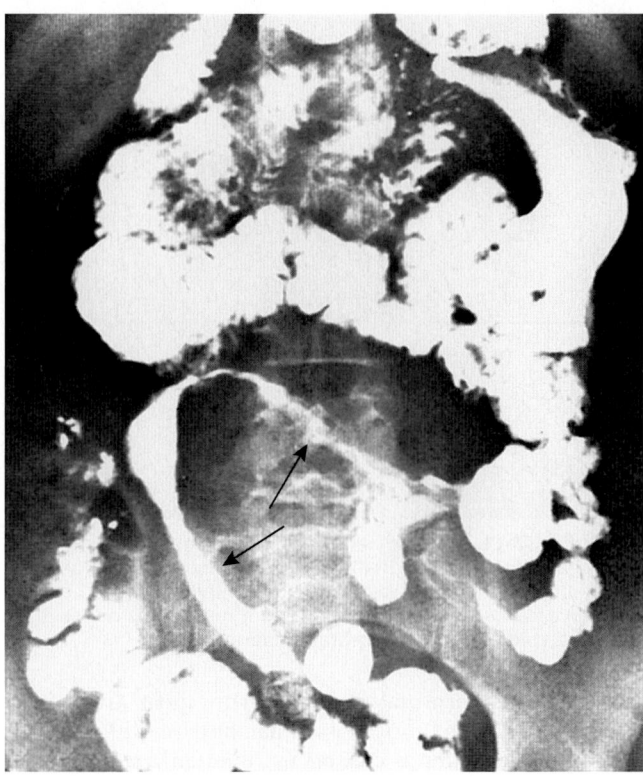

A   B

FIGURE 137-13. Crohn disease. **A,** Spot film of terminal ileum on the same patient illustrated in Figure 137-7. Examination reveals extensive involvement and ulceration of the terminal ileum, with "rose thorn" appearance and spasm. Involvement of the cecum is also apparent, and the appendix is incidentally noted at the cecal tip *(arrow).* **B,** Small-bowel series in a 14-year-old girl reveals a markedly narrowed and rigid loop of mid small bowel *(arrows).* The *upper arrow* points to a string sign, which indicates a markedly narrowed segment.

questionable in some studies; this modality has been successful in differentiating primary bowel disease from adjacent abscesses (see Chapter 106).

Ultrasound (US) is an excellent modality in the evaluation of patients with Crohn disease. The involved bowel segment shows a thickened wall with visible transition to uninvolved small bowel. Often, bowel loops are separated by intervening fat and small lymph nodes are seen within this tissue. The bowel wall is markedly hyperemic during exacerbation of disease (see Fig. 137-14); the degree of hyperemia has been noted to correlate with disease activity. A halo of submucosal edema may give a target-like appearance to the bowel wall when seen transversely, and a "double track" appearance when imaged longitudinally. Large abscesses can be identified, but small abscesses are difficult to distinguish from matted loops of inflamed bowel.

CT, which is widely used in patients with regional enteritis, readily identifies bowel wall thickening, mesenteric changes such as lymphadenopathy, fibrofatty proliferation (see Fig. 137-14), luminal narrowing and stricture formation, and phlegmon formation (see Fig. 137-14). CT enterography and enteroclysis are recently introduced imaging techniques that are used in the cross-sectional evaluation of patients with Crohn disease. CT enterography entails introduction of a negative bowel contrast such as Volumen to distend the bowel without obscuring mural enhancement. This contrast is superior to water in distention of the bowel,

but it is still important that the patient empty his or her bladder prior to the CT examination. CT enteroclysis is similar to fluoroscopic bowel enteroclysis in that a controlled positive or negative contrast volume challenge is introduced via a nasoduodenal tube. These techniques may improve identification of complications of disease, such as sinus tracts, fistulas, and strictures (Figs. 142-10 and 137-15). Recently, whole milk (4% fat) has been described as a promising small-bowel CT contrast medium, but confirmatory clinical trials have not been reported as of the time of this writing. Major intra-abdominal complications of regional enteritis include enteroenteric fistulas, sinus tracts, and abscesses. CT and MRI are the most sensitive imaging techniques for elucidation of these complications (see also Figs. 142-12, 142-13). A barium study can reveal fistulas if the examination is carefully monitored so that premature filling of a bowel loop can be seen. Sinus tracts to the skin can be injected. Water-soluble contrast is recommended for such injections in the event of an unanticipated intraperitoneal leak. Abscesses are among the most common complications of regional enteritis. CT identifies more than 90% of abscesses; CT or US can be used for guided percutaneous drainage. T1- and T2-weighted sequences in MRI, with and without fat suppression, with paramagnetic oral contrast material have been found to be highly sensitive in detection of disease activity and localization of disease, as well as in identification of fistulas beyond the GI tract, such as enterourinary and enteroretroperitoneal fistulas.

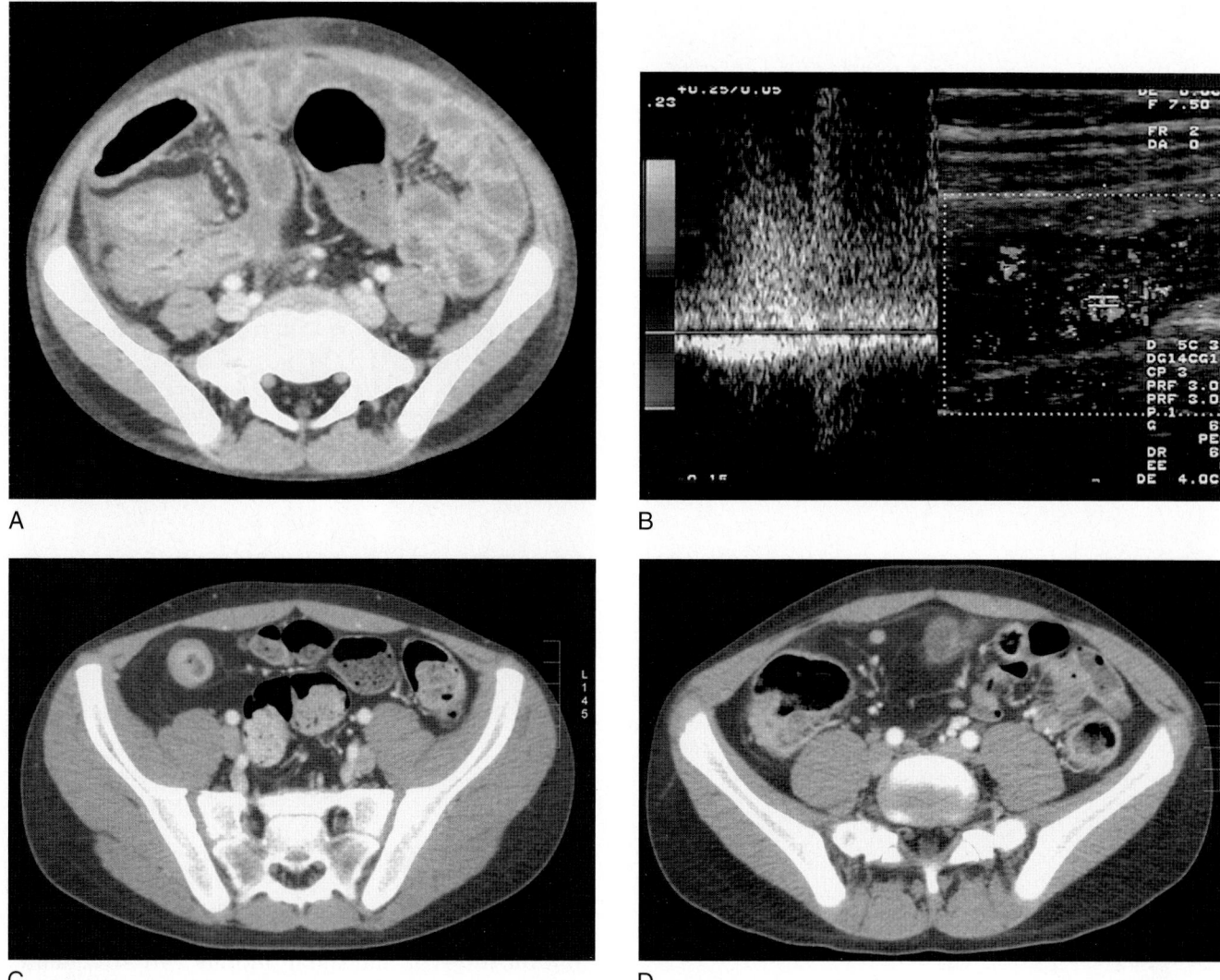

FIGURE 137-14. Crohn disease. **A,** Computed tomography (CT) scan through the pelvis of the same patient as was illustrated in Figures 137-7 and 137-13, *A.* Examination reveals marked thickening and narrowing of the terminal ileum with extensive surrounding inflammatory changes, producing more proximal partial small-bowel obstruction. The luminal narrowing resembles a string sign as seen on small-bowel examination. Surrounding inflammatory changes are identified on CT, but the fine mucosal detail noted on the small-bowel examination is lacking. **B,** Transverse image through the right lower quadrant of an adolescent with boy with Crohn disease. Gray scale rendition of color and spectral Doppler. The image shows the terminal ileum, which is markedly thickened. Flow to the wall of the terminal ileum is increased, along with venous and high diastolic arterial flow. **C,** Section through the pelvis of another adolescent boy with Crohn disease illustrates the thickened wall of the terminal ileum, hyperemic mucosa, and characteristic circumferential fat deposition, leading to increased separation of bowel loops and thin vascular channels. **D,** Section slightly more cephalad shows a milder inflammatory change in a more proximal portion of the ileum and again shows fat accumulation, along with a tiny lymph node that is located just deep to the right rectus muscle.

T2-weighted sequences, with and without fat saturation, are helpful in revealing fistulas to the perineum.

Behçet Syndrome

Findings similar to those of Crohn disease can be seen in other inflammatory diseases. Behçet syndrome is an uncommon multiorgan process that involves inflammatory changes and ulceration anywhere in the GI tract. The esophagus, the terminal ileum (Fig. 137-16), and the right colon are most commonly affected. The disease is more prevalent in Mediterranean countries, the Middle East, Japan, and countries in Southeast Asia. The central problem appears to consist of a vascular endothelial dysfunction and an excessive inflammatory response, termed *pathergy*, which occur variably as a reaction to nonspecific injury and may be an index of severity and activity of the disease. No specific diagnostic test is available for the syndrome; diagnosis is made by detection of recurrent mouth ulcers in association with at least two other major criteria, which include ocular involvement, skin lesions, recurrent genital ulcerations, and the presence of pathergy. Patients with this syndrome are at risk for thrombosis in the venous system and, less commonly, in the arterial system; complicating arterial aneurysms, including the pulmonary arterial tree, also may occur. GI ulcerations may be confused with other inflammatory bowel diseases that share extraintestinal features, such as erythema nodosum and mouth ulcers.

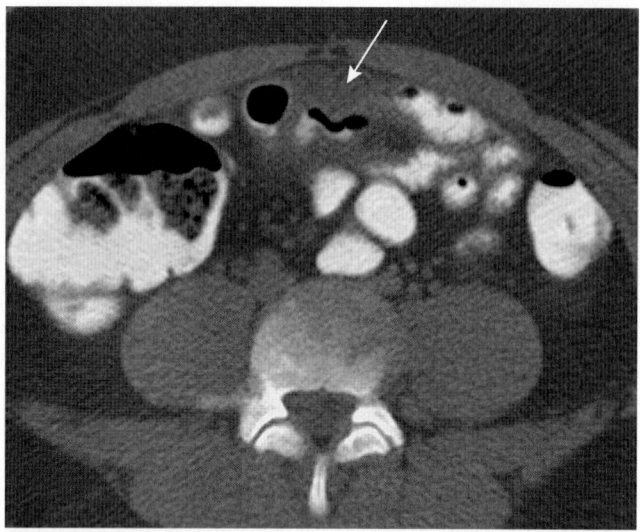

A

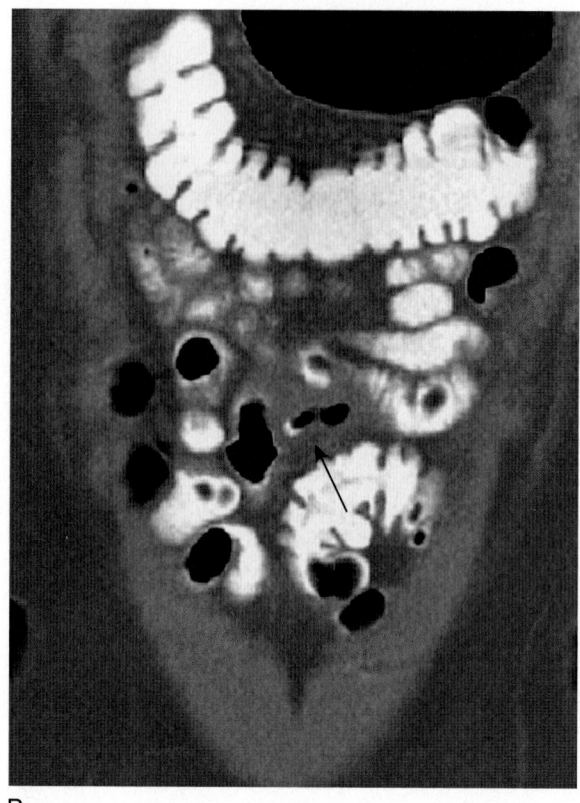

B

FIGURE 137-15. Crohn disease. Axial image **(A)** and coronal reformat **(B)** from computed tomography (CT) enteroclysis through the lower abdomen in a 15-year-old boy with Crohn disease reveal a sinus tract *(arrow)* with air and contrast extending from the small bowel and surrounded by inflammatory change. Note small nodes within the adjacent mesentery. (Courtesy Dr. Kimberly Applegate, Indianapolis, IN.)

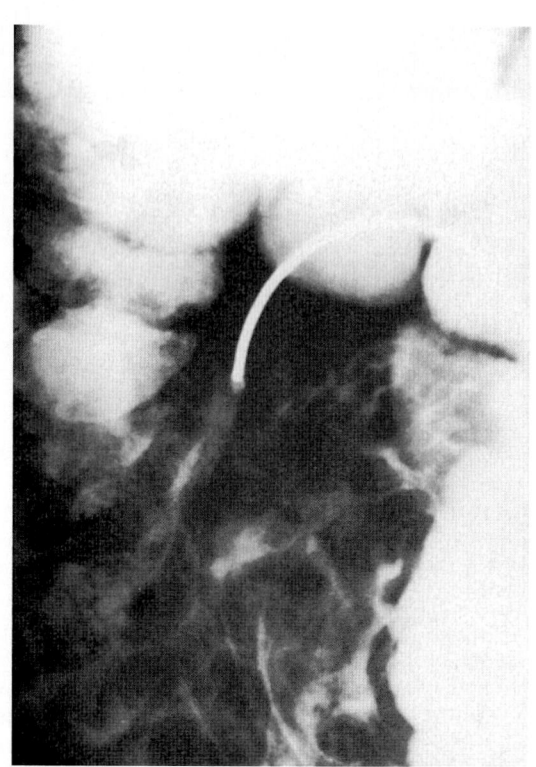

FIGURE 137-16. Behçet syndrome. Coned-down pressure spot image of the terminal ileum in a patient with known Behçet syndrome shows a cobblestone pattern similar to that seen in Crohn disease. (Courtesy Dr. P. S. Moskowitz, Los Gatos, CA.)

FUNCTIONAL AND INFILTRATIVE DISEASES

A large number of diseases of disparate origin may affect the small intestine in similar and nonspecific ways. Abnormalities of intestinal motility are frequently associated with focal or generalized intestinal dilation and with abnormalities of mucosal folds as identified on contrast examination of the small bowel.

Cystic Fibrosis

Cystic fibrosis (CF) may present during the newborn period with meconium ileus. Older children show duodenal abnormalities such as dilation, thickened folds, and filling defects that may represent abnormal collections of mucus adherent to the mucosa. As patients live longer, the most prominent intestinal abnormality is the distal intestinal obstruction syndrome (DIOS), formerly known as meconium ileus equivalent. This syndrome of intestinal obstruction occurs in 10% to 20% of patients and is more common among older children and adolescents. Patients present with colicky abdominal pain and a palpable right lower quadrant mass that represents impacted fecal material in the ileocolic region. Because mild to severe constipation is a common concomitant condition of CF, the term *DIOS* is reserved for those patients who also have signs and symptoms of small-bowel obstruction.

Radiographs show small-bowel dilation with air-fluid levels; bubbly fecal material may also be present (Fig. 137-17). If CT is performed for additional clinical

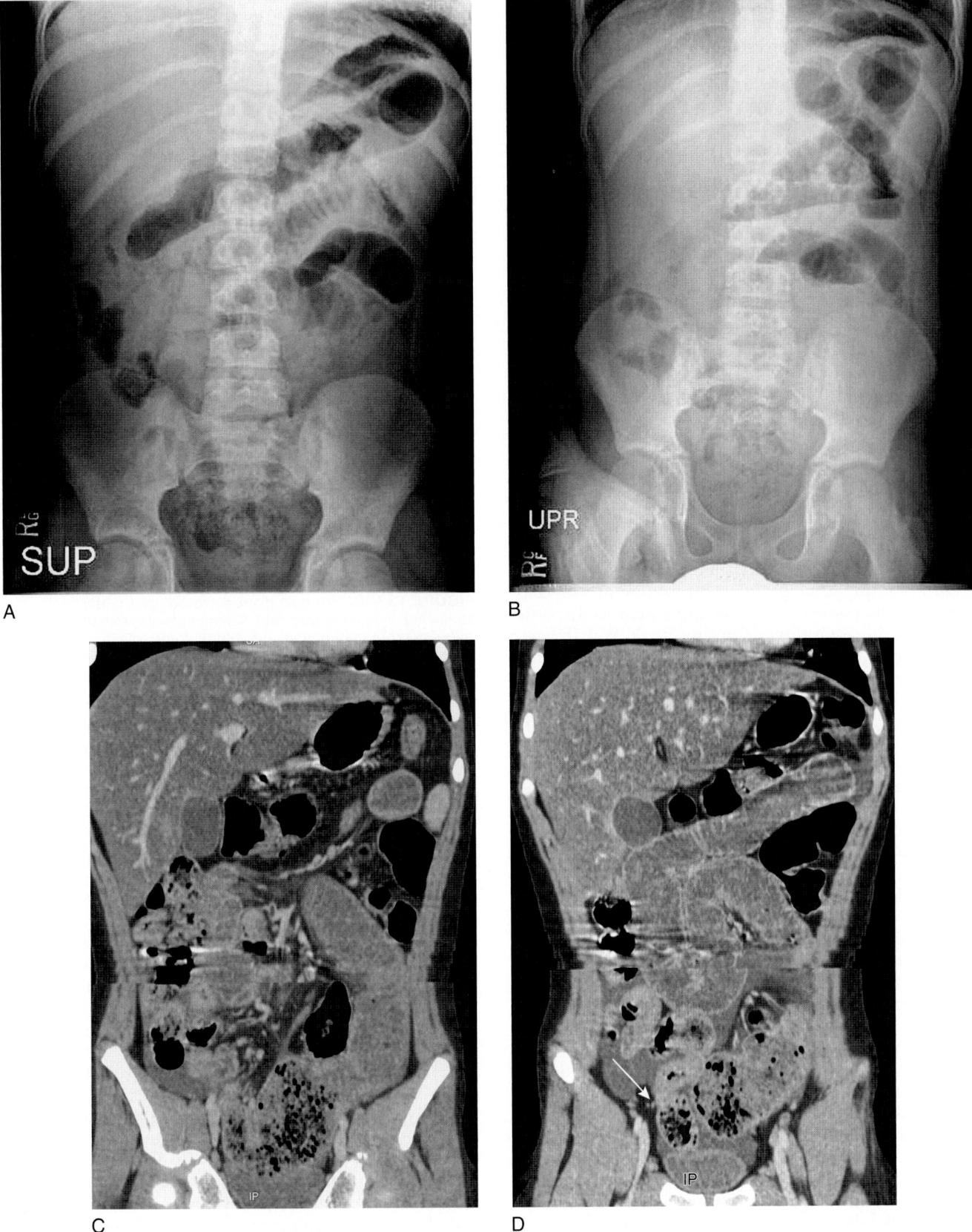

FIGURE 137-17. Distal intestinal obstructive syndrome (DIOS). Supine **(A)** and upright **(B)** radiographs of an 11-year-old boy with cystic fibrosis who presented with vomiting. Radiographs show evidence of small-bowel obstruction, along with dilated loops of small bowel and differential air-fluid levels. Bubbly fecal material is suggested in the right lower quadrant. **C, D,** Adjacent coronal reformats of computed tomography scan on the same patient outline a dilated distal small-bowel loop with fecal-appearing contents from the distal ileum to the transition point of the collapsed terminal ileum *(arrow in D)*. Free intraperitoneal fluid, hepatic steatosis, and fatty replacement of the pancreas in the left upper quadrant of **C** are also noted.

concerns, dilated small-bowel loops can be followed to the site of impaction in the distal ileum (see Fig. 137-17). Although most patients respond to enemas that include mucolytic agents, water-soluble contrast enemas given under fluoroscopic control also may be very effective. Excellent results have been achieved with a solution of powdered sodium diatrizoate in warm water. For best results, reflux into the terminal ileum is necessary. Repeated attempts over a 24- to 48-hour period may be required to completely relieve the impaction. Patients with CF may have malabsorption with dilated intestinal loops showing thickened folds. The appendix in patients with CF is normally distended, and although its contents may be expressible with compression, appendiceal diameter alone is not a reliable criterion for diagnosis of appendicitis in these patients. Patients with *Shwachman syndrome* may have malabsorption with nonspecific findings on barium studies. Ceco-colic intussusception and mucocele of the appendix are less frequent complications of CF.

Protein-Losing Enteropathies

Celiac disease is the most common cause of intestinal malabsorption in childhood. The disease is also known as nontropical sprue or gluten enteropathy because the cause is gluten intolerance. Gluten is a protein that is present in the food grains most commonly used by humans. The connection of dietary gluten to the onset of clinical disease was made during World War II, when it was noted that the prevalence of disease decreased during food shortages. Most affected children present between 4 and 24 months of age, with failure to thrive, abdominal distention, and diarrhea. Diarrhea is considered one of the hallmarks of the disease but is not present in 10% of patients with celiac disease; in fact, rarely, some children may present with constipation. Affected children may experience anemia with iron and folate deficiency, hypertransaminemia, arthritis, and behavioral disturbances. Adolescents have delayed puberty, anorexia, and clinical findings related to the hypocalcemia and hypoproteinemia of malabsorption. The disease is more prevalent in Western Europe and North America, where it may affect as many as 1 of every 120 to 300 persons. It is mediated through a T cell immune response associated with HLA-DQ2 heterodimer, and it results in denudation of villi and hyperplastic crypts. The disorder is associated with dermatitis herpetiformis and with type 1 diabetes mellitus.

Serologic tests for immunoglobulin (Ig)A antiendomysial antibody and antigliadin antibodies and trials of gluten-free diets are helpful in establishing the diagnosis; however, definitive diagnosis relies on small-bowel biopsy in the distal duodenum and the jejunum. Imaging can be helpful in suggesting the diagnosis within the appropriate clinical setting. Plain films in patients with celiac disease may show nonspecific small-bowel distention. Classic findings on barium small-bowel series consist of dilation, thickened mucosal folds, flocculation, and segmentation. The last two findings, however, are uncommonly seen with modern-day barium preparations. The mucosal folds may show reversal of the mucosal

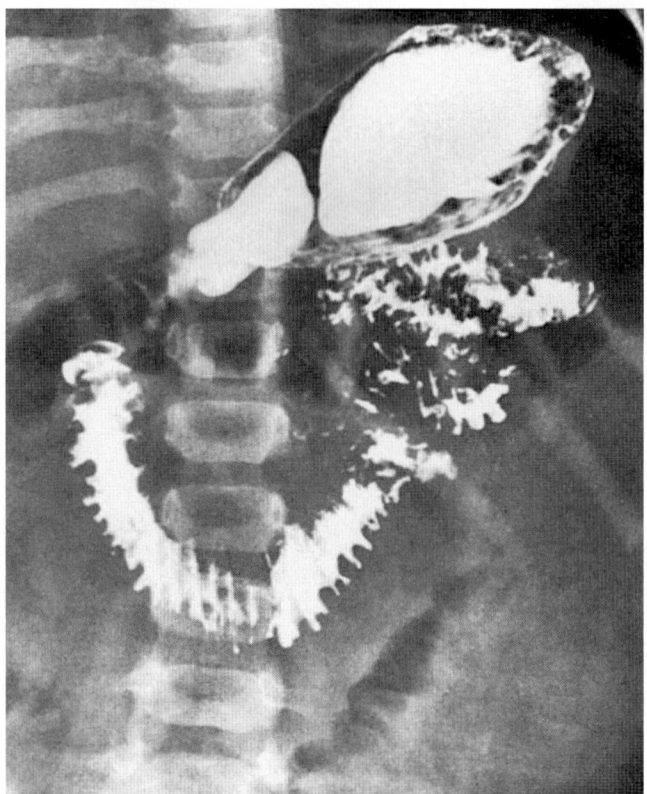

FIGURE 137-18. Whipple disease. Upper gastrointestinal series in a 2-year-old boy with Whipple disease reveals marked thickening of the duodenal and jejunal folds.

patterns of jejunum and ileum. The duodenum may exhibit mucosal erosions or thickened nodular folds. CT or US may reveal distended loops of jejunum and mesenteric or retroperitoneal lymphadenopathy, with dilution of oral contrast if given during CT examination. These findings resolve when a gluten-free diet is instituted.

Whipple disease was described in 1907 in a patient with malabsorption, lymphadenopathy, and arthritis. It is characterized by the presence of foamy macrophages containing glycoprotein granules in affected individuals. The entity is a systemic disease, and patients may present with fever and with extraintestinal manifestations, including arthritis and cardiac and neurologic involvement, sometimes in the absence of GI symptoms. The causative bacterium, *Tropheryma whipplei*, has been isolated, and its genome has been sequenced. On imaging studies, thickening of the small bowel folds is seen without dilation (Fig. 137-18). On CT, additional findings of low-density lymphadenopathy may be identified. Hepatosplenomegaly and ascites also may be present.

Intestinal lymphangiectasia is a severe protein-losing enteropathy that is characterized by dilation of intestinal lymphatics and results in protein loss as lymph leaks into the lumen of the intestine. This disease can be associated with developmental abnormalities of the intestinal lymphatics, which may be associated with abnormal lymphatics elsewhere in the body. Intestinal lymphangiectasia has been found in patients with Noonan syndrome. Lymphangiectasia also may result from diseases that cause obstruction of the intestinal lymphatics or increases in

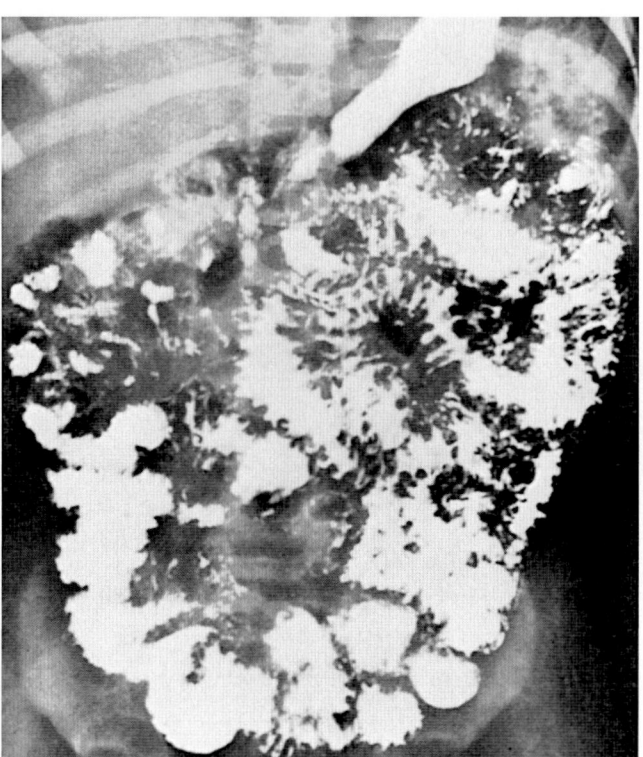

FIGURE 137-19. Intestinal lymphangiectasia. Small-bowel series in a 3-year-old girl with intestinal lymphangiectasia shows marked coarsening and thickening of the mucosal folds.

intralymphatic pressure. Such a syndrome may be found in patients with malrotation of the bowel and intermittent volvulus. Patients typically have diarrhea and hypoproteinemia. Symptoms related to malabsorption may also be present. A substantial number of affected children may have normal barium examination findings. Barium studies show mild dilation and thickened folds (Fig. 137-19) but can be definitive in patients with malrotation and chronic or intermittent volvulus as a cause of the symptoms and findings. US and CT findings are related to the edema and include thickening of the walls of the intestine and gallbladder, ascites, and a thickened mesentery. Lymphangiomas may be present, but absence of adenopathy helps to differentiate this entity from other enteropathies, such as sprue or Whipple disease.

Patients with *immunodeficiency syndromes* may have a clinical and radiographic picture similar to that seen in patients with celiac disease. Some affected patients have radiographic findings of lymphoid hyperplasia, especially prominent in the distal ileum. Small, relatively uniform polypoid mucosal filling defects are seen, characteristically with a central barium-filled umbilication. The latter is not seen uniformly, but its presence in a number of polypoid defects suggests the nature of the lesions. Reactive lymphoid hyperplasia also may be noted in patients with gastroenteritis, both infectious and allergic, and in some otherwise normal persons. Lymphoid hyperplasia of the terminal ileum may act as a lead point for ileocolic intussusception in infants.

Other causes of protein-losing enteropathy include allergic gastroenteropathy, inflammatory bowel disease, infectious mononucleosis, and polyarteritis nodosa.

Protein-losing enteropathy has been reported as a complication following the Fontan procedure and may be related to altered hemodynamics within the hepatic veins and lymphatics.

Graft-versus-Host Disease

Graft-versus-host disease (GVHD) is a reaction of donor lymphocytes against host cells. Although GVHD can be seen in patients who undergo solid organ transplantation, it is more common in patients who undergo bone marrow transplantation. Furthermore, bone marrow transplantation is more commonly performed in children than is solid organ transplantation because of its usefulness in hematologic and immunodeficiency states as well as in leukemia, lymphoma, and widespread malignancies such as metastatic neuroblastoma. Acute GVHD occurs within the first 3 months after transplantation through donor T lymphocyte–mediated epithelial damage. Patients with GI manifestations have severe diarrhea and crampy abdominal pain. Frequent accompaniments are skin rash, liver dysfunction through involvement of the biliary epithelium, and hematologic complications.

Radiographs show a pattern of adynamic ileus with separation of bowel loops, thickening of the bowel wall, and air-fluid levels. Less commonly seen are pneumatosis intestinalis and ascites. On occasion, the abdomen may be completely gasless. Contrast studies are usually not necessary but do show severe edema of the bowel wall, poor coating of the mucosa, luminal narrowing, and rapid transit time. Chronic fibrosis not unlike that seen in chronic radiation enteritis may occur. US reveals thickening of the bowel wall, sometimes with a sonolucent ring in the submucosal layer (Fig. 137-20). The bowel lumina are filled with fluid, and ascites may be detected. Thickening of the bowel wall may be evident on CT, but this is not a constant finding. The bowel is distended with fluid, and striking enhancement of the mucosa results from intravenous contrast administration. Therefore, in these patients, administration of positive oral contrast agents is not necessary and can be counterproductive (see Fig. 137-20).

Henoch-Schönlein Purpura

Henoch-Schönlein purpura is an idiopathic anaphylactoid reaction that is characterized by diffuse angiitis of small vessels in the skin, joints, GI tract, and kidneys. It is most common in children, and GI symptoms may precede other manifestations of the disease in a minority of patients. The characteristic petechial skin rash with a predilection for the lower extremities is usually diagnostic, but GI manifestations may precede its appearance. GI symptoms include nausea, vomiting, colicky abdominal pain, and hematochezia. In the small intestine, the disease manifests with bleeding into the bowel wall, which can lead to enteroenteric intussusception that often, but not invariably, reduces spontaneously (Fig. 137-21). Other findings on cross-sectional imaging studies include bowel wall thickening characterized by skip areas of abnormality; bowel dilation and mesenteric edema may also be seen. Findings on contrast studies

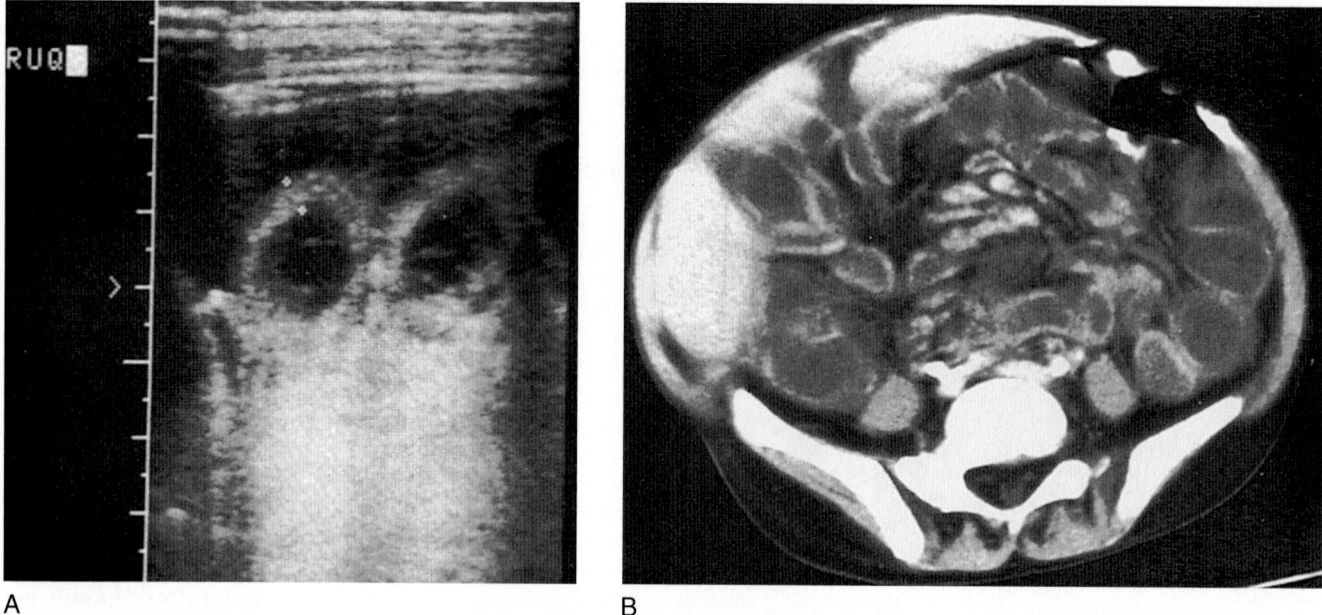

A   B

FIGURE 137-20. Graft-versus-host disease. **A,** Ultrasound examination of the right abdomen reveals ascites and a thickened small-bowel wall. **B,** Computed tomography scan with intravenous contrast shows marked edema of the bowel wall with deep mucosal enhancement.

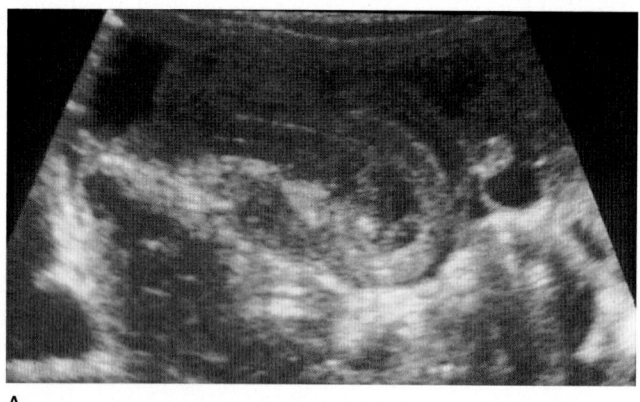

A

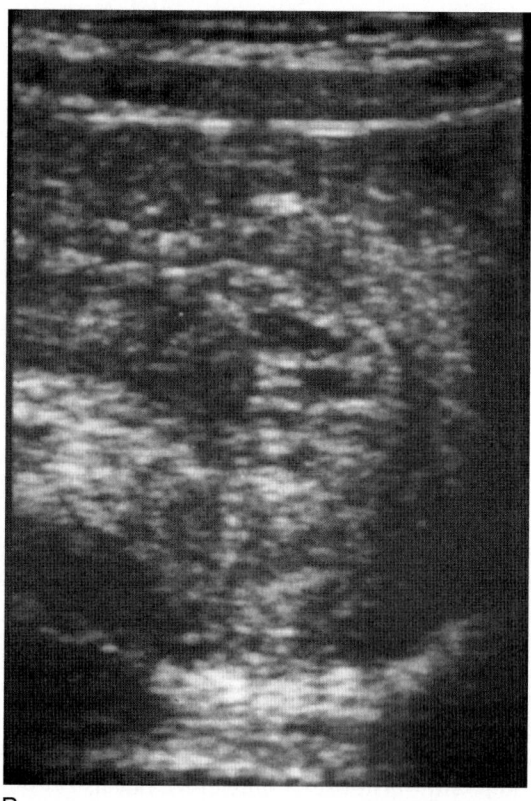

B

FIGURE 137-21. Henoch-Schönlein purpura with intussusception. **A,** Transverse sonogram of the left lower quadrant in a 6-year-old girl with acute abdominal pain reveals a thick-walled small-bowel loop with intussusception. **B,** Linear transducer image of the tip of the intussusception shows thick-walled bowel layers and sonolucent spaces in the intussuscepted mesentery, consistent with edema. At surgery several hours later, an irreducible ileo-ileal intussusception was identified; the typical petechial rash appeared on the following day.

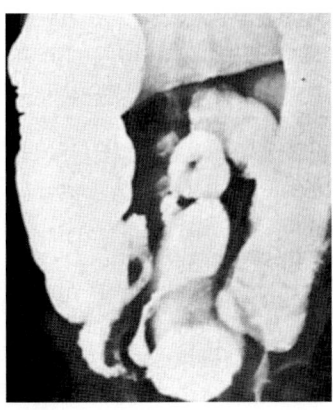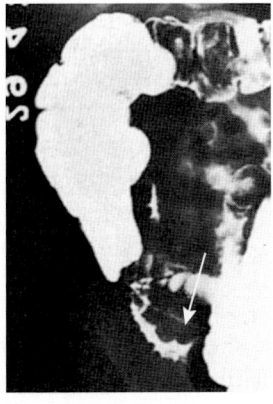

A   B

FIGURE 137-22. Henoch-Schönlein purpura. **A,** Barium enema performed in a 4-year-old boy with a 7-day history of vomiting. **B,** Postevacuation film shows marginal filling defects in the distal ileum. Henoch-Schönlein purpura was diagnosed when the characteristic rash developed during hospitalization.

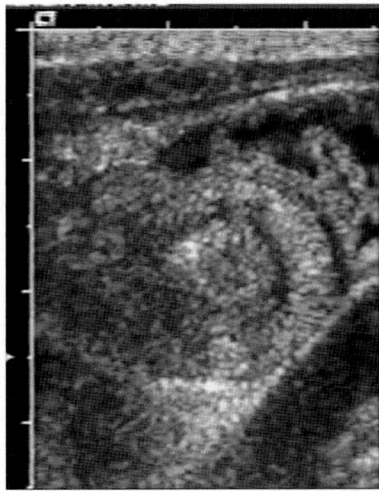

FIGURE 137-23. Short-segment intussusception. Longitudinal ultrasound image along the right flank of an infant with proven viral gastroenteritis shows short segment intussusception that occurred during the examination. Visible peristaltic activity of the intussusceptum within the intussuscipiens was visible on real time. Intussusception resolved spontaneously.

include segmental dilation and stenosis, bowel wall thickening with separation of bowel loops, filling defects, and coarsening and loss of the normal mucosal fold pattern (Fig. 137-22). Strictures may occur as a late sequela of the disease, likely associated with vasculitis and secondary focal areas of ischemia.

Small-Bowel Intussusception

Intussusceptions in the pediatric age group are typically ileocolic, or ileo-ileocolic; these are discussed in Chapter 141. Small-bowel intussusceptions occur typically with a lead point such as Meckel diverticulum, polyps in patients with such entities as Peutz-Jeghers syndrome, small-bowel hemangiomas, and lymphoma; they may be seen in patients with Henoch-Schönlein purpura, or in patients with abnormal bowel distention or motility, such as gastroenteritis; or they may occur with medications, inflammatory bowel disease, or the use of gastrojejunostomy tubes (particularly with a distal pigtail), or during the postoperative period.

Factors associated with small-bowel intussusception include the following:

- **Lead points: Meckel, polyp, hemangioma, lymphoma**
- **Mural thickening: Henoch-Schönlein purpura, nephrotic syndrome**
- **Abnormal distention of motility: gastroenteritis, medications**
- **Inflammatory conditions: Crohn**
- **Infiltrative diseases**
- **Gastrojejunostomy tubes: pigtail catheters, younger patients**
- **Postoperative condition**

Transient small-bowel intussusception is identified incidentally more frequently with increasing use of cross-sectional imaging. Findings that indicate the presence of an incidental intussusception include short length (<3 cm), thin diameter (<2.5 cm), absence of bowel obstruction at that level (dilated bowel loops proximal to the intussusception, and collapsed bowel loops distally), absence of symptoms that cannot be ascribed to presenting complaints or comorbid conditions, absence of identifiable lead point, absence of mesenteric nodes within the complex, and presence of visible bowel wall motion on sonography (Fig. 137-23). When the condition is identified, a lead point should be sought. In the absence of a lead point, the patient should be treated symptomatically, and repeat examination should be performed to document spontaneous resolution when necessary.

SUGGESTED READINGS

Cysts

Adamsbaum C, Sellier N, Helardot P: Ileocolic intussusception with enterogenous cyst: ultrasonic diagnosis. Pediatr Radiol 1989;19:325

Barr LL, Hayden CK Jr, Stansberry SD, et al: Enteric duplication cysts in children: are their ultrasonographic wall characteristics diagnostic? Pediatr Radiol 1990;20:326

Bender TM, Ledesma-Medina J, Oh KS: Radiographic manifestations of anomalies of the gastrointestinal tract. Radiol Clin North Am 1991;29:335

Bowen B, Ros PR, McCarthy MJ, et al: Gastrointestinal teratomas: CT and US appearance with pathologic correlation. Radiology 1987;162:431

Bower RJ, Sieber WKN, Kiesewetter WB: Alimentary tract duplications in children. Ann Surg 1978;188:669

Brown D, Schlesinger A, Komppa G: Ileal duplication cyst: repeated spontaneous decompression delays diagnosis. Mil Med 1989;154:553

Caspi B, Schachter M, Lancet M: Infected duplication cyst of ileum masquerading as an adnexal abscess—ultrasonographic features. J Clin Ultrasound 1989;17:431

Cheng G, Soboleski D, Danema A, et al: Sonographic pitfalls in the diagnosis of enteric duplication cysts. AJR Am J Roentgenol 2005;184:521

Egelhoff JC, Bisset GS III, Strife JL: Multiple enteric duplications in an infant. Pediatr Radiol 1986;16:160

Egozi E, Ricketts R: Mesenteric and omental cysts in children. Am Surg 1997;63:287-290

Geer LL, Mittelstaedt CA, Staab EV, et al: Mesenteric cyst: sonographic appearance with CT correlation. Pediatr Radiol 1984;14:102

Gilchrist AM, Sloan JM, Logan CJH, et al: Case report: gastrointestinal bleeding due to multiple ileal duplications diagnosed by scintigraphy and barium studies. Clin Radiol 1990;41:134

Haller JO, Schneider M, Kassner EG, et al: Sonographic evaluation of mesenteric and omental masses in children. AJR Am J Roentgenol 1978;130:269

Harvey PJ, Whitley NO: CT of benign cystic abdominal masses in children. AJR Am J Roentgenol 1984;142:1279

Hur J, Yoon C-S, Kim M-J, Kim O-H: Imaging features of gastrointestinal tract duplications in infants and children: from oesophagus to rectum. Pediatr Radiol 2007;37:691–699

Ilstad ST, Tollerud DJ, Weiss RG, et al: Duplications of the alimentary tract. Ann Surg 1988;208:184

Lamont AC, Starinsky R, Cremin BJ: Ultrasonic diagnosis of duplication cysts in children. Br J Radiol 1984;57:463

Nicolet V, Grignon A, Filiatrault D, et al: Sonographic appearance of an abdominal cystic lymphangioma. J Ultrasound Med 1984;3:85

Rifkin MD, Kurtz AB, Pasto ME: Mesenteric chylous (lymph-containing) cyst. Gastrointest Radiol 1983;8:267

Ros PR, Olmsted WW, Moser RP Jr, et al: Mesenteric and omental cysts: histologic classification with imaging correlation. Radiology 1987;164:327

Sinha A, Ojha S, Sarin YK: Completely isolated noncontiguous duplication cyst. Eur J Pediatr Surg 2006;16:127

Teele RL, Henschke CT, Tapper D: The radiographic and ultrasonographic evaluation of enteric duplication cysts. Pediatr Radiol 1980;10:9

Acquired Obstruction

Jabra A, Fishman E: Small bowel obstruction in the pediatric patient: CT evaluation. Abdom Imaging 1997;22:466-470

Ratcliffe J, Tait J, Lisle D, et al: Segmental dilatation of the small bowel: report of three cases and literature review. Radiology 1989;171:827

Infectious Diseases

Balthazar EJ, Charles HW, Megibow AJ: *Salmonella*- and *Shigella*-induced ileitis: CT findings in four patients. J Comput Assist Tomogr 1996;20:375

Bass D, Cordoba E, Dekker C, et al: Intestinal imaging of children with acute rotavirus gastroenteritis. J Pediatr Gastroenterol Nutr 2004;39:270-274

Bohrer SP: Typhoid perforation of the ileum. Br J Radiol 1966;39:37

Bradford BF, Abdenour GE Jr, Frank JL, et al: Usual and unusual radiologic manifestations of acquired immunodeficiency syndrome (AIDS) and human immunodeficiency virus (HIV) infection in children. Radiol Clin North Am 1988;26:341

Brandon J, Glick SN, Teplick SK: Intestinal giardiasis: the importance of serial filming. AJR Am J Roentgenol 1985;144:581

Brody PA, Fertig S, Aron JM: *Campylobacter* enterocolitis: radiographic features. AJR Am J Roentgenol 1982;139:1199

Capitanio MA, Greenberg SB: Pneumatosis intestinalis in two infants with rotavirus gastroenteritis. Pediatr Radiol 1991;21:361

Centers for Disease Control and Prevention (CDC): Epidemiology of HIV/AIDS—United States, 1981-2005. MMWR Morb Mortal Wkly Rep 2006;55:589

Eckberg O, Sjostrum B, Brahme F: Radiological findings in *Yersinia* ileitis. Radiology 1977;123:15

Fujii Y, Taniguchi N, Itoh K: Sonographic findings in *Shigella* colitis. J Clin Ultrasound 2001;29:48

Haney PJ, Yale-Loehr AJ, Nussbaum AR, et al: Imaging of infants and children with AIDS. AJR Am J Roentgenol 1989;152:1033

Hodes HL: Gastroenteritis with special reference to rotavirus. Adv Pediatr 1980;27:195

Jones B, Fishman EK: CT of the gut in the immunocompromised host. Radiol Clin North Am 1989;27:763

Katz M: Parasitic infections. J Pediatr 1975;87:165

Matsumoto T, Iida M, Sakai T, et al: *Yersinia* teminal ileitis: sonographic findings in eight patients. AJR Am J Roentgenol 1991;156:965

Nagi B, Duggal R, Gupta R, et al: Tuberculous peritonitis in children. Pediatr Radiol 1987;17:282

Puylaert JBCM, Kristjánsdóttir S, Golterman KL, et al: Typhoid fever: diagnosis by using sonography. AJR Am J Roentgenol 1989;153:745

Puylaert JBCM, Van der Zant FM, Mutsaers JAEM: Infectious ileocecitis caused by *Yersinia*, *Campylobacter* and *Salmonella*: clinical, radiological and US findings. Eur Radiol 1997;7:3

Robinson CG, Hernanz-Schulman M, Zhu Y, et al: Evaluation of anatomic changes in young children with natural rotavirus infection: is intussusception biologically plausible? J Infect Dis 2004;189:1382-1387

Siegel M, Friedland J, Hildebolt C: Bowel wall thickening in children: differentiation with US. Radiology 1997;203:631-635

Sivit CJ, Josephs SH, Taylor GA, et al: Pneumatosis intestinalis in children with AIDS. AJR Am J Roentgenol 1990;155:133

Sivit CJ, Taylor GA, Patterson K, et al: Bowel obstruction in an infant with AIDS. AJR Am J Roentgenol 1990;154:803

Inflammatory Bowel Disease

Balthazar EJ: CT of the gastrointestinal tract: principles and interpretation. AJR Am J Roentgenol 1991;156:23

Beets-Tan R, Beets G, van der Hoop A, et al: Preoperative MR imaging of anal fistulas: does it really help the surgeon? Radiology 2001;281:75-84

Berlinger L, Redmond P, Purow EK, et al: Computed tomography in Crohn's disease. Am J Gastroenterol 1982;77:533

Boudiaf M, Jaff A, Soyer P, et al: Small bowel diseases: prospective evaluation of multidetector row helical CT enteroclysis in 107 consecutive patients. Radiology 2004;233:338-344

Bremner AR, Griffiths M, Argent JD, et al: Sonographic evaluation of inflammatory bowel disease: a prospective, blinded, comparative study. Pediatr Radiol 2006;36:947-953

Buck JL, Dachman AH, Sobin LH: Polypoid and pseudopolypoid manifestations of inflammatory bowel disease. Radiographics 1991;11:293

Chung DJ, Park YS, Huh KC, et al: Gastrointestinal complications in an adult patient with Henoch-Schönlein purpura. AJR Am J Roentgenol 2006;187:W396

Desai RK, Tagliabue JR, Wegryn SA, et al: CT evaluation of wall thickening in the alimentary tract. Radiographics 1991;1:771

Dinker E, Dittrich M, Peters H, et al: Real-time ultrasound in Crohn's disease: characteristic features and clinical implications. Pediatr Radiol 1986;16:8

Dubois RS, Rothschild J, Silverman A, et al: The varied manifestations of Crohn's disease in children and adolescents. Am J Gastroenterol 1978;69:203

Farrell RJ, Kelly CP: Celiac sprue. N Engl J Med 2002;346:180

Gore RM: CT of inflammatory bowel disease. Radiol Clin North Am 1989;27:717

Horsthuis K, Stoker J: MRI of perianal Crohn disease. AJR Am J Roentgenol 2004;183:1309

Horton KM, Fishman EK: Uncommon inflammatory diseases of the small bowel: CT findings. AJR Am J Roentgenol 1998;170:385

Hyer W, Beattie R, Walker-Smith J, et al: Computed tomography in chronic inflammatory bowel disease. Arch Dis Child 1997;76:428-431

Jabra AA, Fishman EK, Taylor GA: Crohn disease in the pediatric patient: CT evaluation. Radiology 1991;179:495

Jones B, Fishman EK, Hamilton SR, et al: Submucosal accumulation of fat in inflammatory bowel disease: CT/pathologic correlation. J Comput Assist Tomogr 1986;10:759

Kirks DR, Currarino G: Regional enteritis in children: small bowel disease with normal terminal ileum. Pediatr Radiol 1978;7:10

Kugathasan S: Pediatric inflammatory bowel disease: clinical and therapeutic aspects. Curr Opin Gastroenterol 2001;17:350-355

Laghmari M, Karim A, Allali F, et al: Childhood Behcet's disease: clinical and evolutive aspects: about 13 cases. J Fr Opthalmol 2002;25:904

Lindquist BL, Jarnerot G, Wickbom G: Clinical and epidemiological aspects of Crohn's disease in children and adolescents. Scand J Gastroenterol 1984;19:502

Lipson A, Bartram CI, Williams CB, et al: Barium studies and ileoscopy compared in children with suspected Crohn's disease. Clin Radiol 1990;41:5

Liu YB, Liang CH, Zhang ZL, et al: Crohn disease of small bowel: multidetector row CT with CT enteroclysis, dynamic contrast enhancement, CT angiography, and 3D imaging. Abdom Imaging 2006;E Pub DOI:10.1007/s00261-006-9092-1

Loffler M, Weckesser M, Franzius C, et al: High diagnostic value of

18F-FDG-PET in pediatric patients with chronic inflammatory bowel disease. Ann NY Acad Sci 2006;1072:379-385

Maccioni F, Bruni A, Viscido A, et al: MR imaging in patients with Crohn disease: value of T2- versus T1- weighted gadolinium-enhanced MR sequences with use of an oral superparamagnetic contrast agent. Radiology 2006;238:517

Park RHR, McKillop JH, Duncan A, et al: Can [111]indium autologous mixed leucocyte scanning accurately assess disease extent and activity in Crohn's disease? Gut 1988;29:821

Pickering MC, Haskard DO: Behcet's syndrome. J R Coll Physician Lond 2000;34:169

Quillin S, Siegel M: Gastrointestinal inflammation in children: color Doppler ultrasonography. J Ultrasound Med 1994;13:751-756

Reittner P, Goritschnig T, Petritsch W, et al: Multiplanar spiral CT enterography in patients with Crohn's disease using a negative oral contrast material: initial results of a noninvasive imaging approach. Eur Radiol 2002;12:2253-2257

Riddlesberger MM Jr: CT of complicated inflammatory bowel disease in children. Pediatr Radiol 1985;15:384

Scott WW Jr, Fishman EK, Kuhlman JE, et al: Computed tomography evaluation of the sacroiliac joints in Crohn disease: radiologic/clinical correlation. Skeletal Radiol 1990;19:207

Shan-Patel LR, Koo CS, Baer JW, et al: Cost-effectiveness and patient tolerance of low attenuation oral contrast: milk versus VoLumen. Paper presented at the Radiological Society of North America 92nd Scientific Assembly and Annual Meeting Program, December 2006

Shirkhoda A: Diagnostic pitfalls in abdominal CT. Radiographics 1991;11:969

Siegel M, Friedland J, Hildebolt C: Bowel wall thickening in children: differentation with US. Radiology 1997;203:631-635

Spalinger J, Patriquin H, Miron MC, et al: Doppler US in patients with Crohn disease: vessel density in the diseased bowel reflects disease activity. Radiology 2000;217:787

Stringer DA: Imaging inflammatory bowel disease in the pediatric patient. Radiol Clin North Am 1987;25:93

Stringer DA, Cleghorn GJ, Durie PR, et al: Behcet's syndrome involving the gastrointestinal tract—a diagnostic dilemma in childhood. Pediatr Radiol 1986;16:131

Taylor GA, Nancarrow PA, Hernanz-Schulman M, et al: Plain abdominal radiographs in children with inflammatory bowel disease. Pediatr Radiol 1986;16:206

Tolia V, Kuhns LR, Chang CH, et al: Comparison of indium-111 scintigraphy and colonoscopy with histologic study in children for evaluation of colonic chronic inflammatory bowel disease. J Pediatr Gastroenterol Nutr 1991;12:336

Vlymen WJ, Moskowitz PS: Roentgenographic manifestations of esophageal and intestinal involvement in Behcet's disease in children. Pediatr Radiol 1981;10:193

Yeh H-C, Rabinowitz JG: Granulomatous enterocolitis: findings by ultrasonography and computed tomography. Radiology 1983;149:253

Functional and Infiltrative Diseases

Bartram CI, Small E: The intestinal radiological changes in older people with pancreatic cyst fibrosis. Br J Radiol 1971;44:195

Berk RN, Lee FA: The late gastrointestinal manifestations of cystic fibrosis of the pancreas. Radiology 1973;106:337

Bova JG, Friedman AC, Weser E, et al: Adaptation of the ileum in nontropical sprue: reversal of the jejunoileal fold pattern. AJR Am J Roentgenol 1985;144:299

Djurhuus MJ, Lykkegaard E, Pock-Steen OC: Gastrointestinal radiological findings in cystic fibrosis. Pediatr Radiol 1973;1:113

Donnelly LF, Morris CL: Acute graft-versus-host disease in children: abdominal CT findings. Radiology 1996;199:265

Dorne HL, Jequier S: Sonography of intestinal lymphangiectasia. J Ultrasound Med 1986;5:13

Fisk JD, Shulman HM, Greening RR, et al: Gastrointestinal radiographic features of human graft-vs-host disease. AJR Am J Roentgenol 1981;136:329

Glasier CM, Siegel MJ, McAlister WH, et al: Henoch-Schönlein syndrome in children: gastrointestinal manifestations. AJR Am J Roentgenol 1981;136:1081

Gorske K, Winchester P, Grossman H: Unusual protein-losing enteropathies in children. Am J Roentgenol Radium Ther Nucl Med 1969;92:739

Haworth EM, Hodson CJ, Pringle EM, et al: The value of radiological investigations of the alimentary tract in children with the celiac syndrome. Clin Radiol 1968;107:158

Herzog DB, Logan R, Looistra JB: The Noonan syndrome with intestinal lymphangiectasia. J Pediatr 1976;88:270

Jeong YK, Ha HK, Yoon CH, et al: Gastrointestinal involvement in Henoch-Schönlein syndrome: CT findings. AJR Am J Roentgenol 1997;168:965

Jones B, Bayless TM, Fishman EK, et al: Lymphadenopathy in celiac disease: computed tomographic observations. AJR Am J Roentgenol 1984;142:1127

Jones B, Fishman EK, Kramer SS, et al: Computed tomography of gastrointestinal inflammation after bone marrow transplantation. AJR Am J Roentgenol 1986;146:691

Koletzko S, Stringer DA, Cleghorn GJ, et al: Lavage treatment of distal intestinal obstruction syndrome in children with cystic fibrosis. Pediatrics 1989;83:727

Lanning P, Simila S, Sioramo I, et al: Lymphatic abnormalities in Noonan's syndrome. Pediatr Radiol 1978;7:106

Lardenoye SW, Puylaert JB, Smit MJ, et al: Appendix in children with cystic fibrosis: US features. Radiology 2004;232:187

Maile CW, Frick MP, Crass JR, et al: The plain abdominal radiograph in acute gastrointestinal graft-vs-host disease. AJR Am J Roentgenol 1985;145:289

Marn CS, Gore RM, Chahremani GG: Duodenal manifestations of nontropical sprue. Gastrointest Radiol 1986;11:30

Martinez-Frontanilla LA, Silverman L, Meagher DP Jr: Intussusception in Henoch-Schönlein purpura: diagnosis with ultrasound. J Pediatr Surg 1988;23:375

Mazzie JP, Maslin PI, Moy L, et al: Congenital intestinal lymphangiectasia: CT demonstration in a young child. J Clin Imaging 2003;27:330

Misbah SA, Aslam A, Costello C: Whipple's disease. The Lancet 2004;363:654

Rubinstein S, Moss RB, Lewiston NJ: Constipation and meconium ileus equivalent in patients with cystic fibrosis. Pediatrics 1986;78:473

Schimmelpenninck M, Zwaan F: Radiographic features of small intestinal injury in graft-versus-host disease. Gastrointest Radiol 1982;7:29

Taussig LM, Saldino RM, di Sant'Agnese PA: Radiographic abnormalities of the duodenum and small bowel in cystic fibrosis of the pancreas (mucoviscidosis). Radiology 1973;106:369

Weizman Z, Stringer DA, Durie PR: Radiologic manifestations of malabsorption: a nonspecific finding. Pediatrics 1984;74:530

Small Bowel Intussusception

Asai K, Tanaka S, Tanaka M, et al: Intussusception of the small bowel associated with nephrotic syndrome. Pediatr Neprol 2005;20:1818

Hughes U, Connolly B, Chait PG, et al: Further report of small bowel intussusceptions related to gastrojejunostomy tubes. Pediatr Radiol 2000;30:614

Jabra AA, Fishman EK: Small bowel obstruction in the pediatric patient: CT evaluation. Abdom Imaging 1997;22:466

Kim JH: US features of transient small bowel intussusception in pediatric patients. Korean J Radiol 2004;5:178

Knowles MC, Fishman EK, Kuhlman JE, et al: Transient intussusception in Crohn disease: CT evaluation. Radiology 1989;170:814

Kornecki A, Danema A, Navarro O, et al: Spontaneous reduction of intussusception: clinical spectrum and outcome. Pediatr Radiol 2002;30:58

Strouse PJ, DiPietro MA, Saez F: Transient small-bowel intussusception in children on CT. Pediatr Radiol 2003;33:316-320

Tyrrel RT, Baumgartner BR, Montemayor KA: Blue rubber bleb nevus syndrome: CT diagnosis of intussusception. AJR Am J Roentgenol 1990;154:105

West KW, Stephens B, Rescorla FJ, et al: Postoperative intussusception: experience with 36 cases in children. Surgery 1988;104:781

Wiersma F, Allema JH, Holscher HC: Ileoileal intussusception in children: ultrasonographic differentiation from ileocolic intussusception. Pediatr Radiol 2006;36:1177-1181

CHAPTER

138

Small Intestine: Tumors and Tumor-like Conditions

ALAN E. SCHLESINGER

Most tumors that occur in the small bowel are benign and can present in association with an underlying condition, such as neurofibromatosis, or in isolation. Intrinsic malignant small-bowel tumors are rare but can result from malignant transformation of an underlying benign lesion, such as occurs in Peutz-Jeghers syndrome.

BENIGN TUMORS

Polyps

Polyps may occur in the small intestine as part of the polyposis syndromes. These are discussed in detail in the chapter on the colon (see Chapter 143). Benign polyps involving the small intestine and related to polyposis syndromes predominantly consist of hamartomatous polyps in children with Peutz-Jeghers syndrome.

Peutz-Jeghers syndrome (PJS) is an autosomal dominant polyposis syndrome that is characterized by hamartomatous polyps and mucocutaneous pigmentation. Some patients manifest only hyperpigmentation, but others manifest polyps as well as hyperpigmentation. Brown or black pigmentation of the lips, buccal mucosa, face, palms, and soles presents during childhood, usually within the first year or two of life (often preceding the development of polyps) and typically begins to fade at adolescence. Ninety-five percent of hamartomatous polyps occur in the small intestine, typically the jejunum and ileum; therefore, these are most numerous in the small bowel. Polyps also occur in the stomach (25% of patients) and colon (30% of patients). The median age for presentation with polyps is approximately 11 years but is highly variable, and rare reports have described the presence of polyps at birth. Extraintestinal polyps have also been reported in the nares, pelvis, bladder, and lungs. An increased incidence of adenocarcinoma has been seen in the small bowel of patients with PJS, but this has not been convincingly shown to be related to malignant transformation of hamartomatous polyps. More likely, malignancies develop in coexisting adenomas in these patients. Other reported malignancies, both intestinal and extraintestinal, include those of the colon, esophagus, stomach, ovary, lung, thyroid, breast, skin, pancreas, uterus, and testis, as well as multiple myeloma. Individuals with PJS reportedly incur a 93% chance of developing cancer. Adenocarcinoma of the duodenum and stomach has been reported to occur in up to 3% of patients. In addition, an unusual benign ovarian tumor, sex cord tumor with annular tubules (SCTAT), is found in both genders and in nearly every female patient with PJS. Large cell calcifying Sertoli cell tumors of the testicle can be seen in boys with PJS and may present with gynecomastia due to elevated levels of estrogens secondary to increased aromatization of androgens.

Potential sites of malignancy associated with Peutz-Jeghers syndrome include the following:
- **Small bowel**
- **Colon**
- **Stomach**
- **Esophagus**
- **Ovary**
- **Lung**
- **Thyroid**
- **Breast**
- **Skin**
- **Pancreas**
- **Uterus**
- **Testis**
- **Multiple myeloma**

Intermittent pain, often accompanied by gastrointestinal bleeding and hemorrhage, from transient small-bowel intussusceptions is a common presentation. Small bowel–small bowel intussusceptions can be easily diagnosed on ultrasonography (US). Small-bowel follow-through is useful for identifying polyps in patients at risk.

Other Benign Neoplasms

Other benign neoplasm that occur in the small intestine of children include hemangiomas, vascular malformations, neurofibromas, telangiectasias, fibromas, lipomas, leiomyomas, gastrointestinal stromal tumors, lipomas, and lipoblastomas. Most benign small-bowel tumors manifest with gastrointestinal bleeding or intussusception.

> **Benign neoplasms of the small bowel (other than polyps) include the following:**
> - Hemangiomas
> - Vascular malformations
> - Neurofibromas
> - Telangiectasias
> - Fibromas
> - Lipomas
> - Leiomyomas
> - Gastrointestinal stromal tumors
> - Lipomas
> - Lipoblastomas

Hemangiomas can occur as isolated tumors or can be multiple. Patients with Klippel-Trenauney syndrome present with visceral and cutaneous hemangiomas. Telangiectasias (dilated superficial blood vessels) may occur in the small intestine in Osler-Weber-Rendu syndrome. Vascular malformations involving the small intestine have reportedly occurred in association with other soft tissue vascular malformations.

Neurofibromas, isolated or appearing as a manifestation of neurofibromatosis, may occur in the small intestine. Although rare, malignant degeneration of neurofibroma may occur in the intestine.

Mesenchymal spindle cell tumors, including leiomyomas or gastrointestinal stromal tumors (GISTs), rarely occur in the small intestine in children. Leiomyosarcomas are very rare in children. GISTs are spindle cell tumors that are more common in adults than in children and are more commonly seen in the stomach than in the small intestine. They have recently been recognized as a unique tumor that can be distinguished through the use of immunohistochemical techniques (expression of the overactive enzyme KIT receptor tyrosine kinase [c-KIT protein] detected as CD117 antigen). Identification of GISTs is important because these have malignant potential.

Fat-containing tumors that occur in the small intestine include lipomas and lipoblastomas. These appear primarily within the intestinal wall or in the adjacent omentum or retroperitoneum. Benign lipomas may not require surgery, but lipoblastomas may be locally invasive.

IMAGING

Benign neoplasms of the small intestine may present as polypoid or mural lesions, or they may be discovered because they act as lead points in small bowel–small bowel intussusception. Small bowel follow-through may reveal a luminal filling defect or a mural mass. If the adjacent mesentery is involved, separation of bowel loops may be noted. US is a reasonable first imaging choice if a mass is palpable, or if an intussusception is suspected. If the lesion is hyperechoic, the possibility of a lipoma should be considered. Computed tomography (CT) or magnetic resonance imaging (MRI) is often required if the lesion cannot be seen on US, or if further characterization or better delineation of the extent of the lesion is necessary. Low attenuation on CT or fat-signal characteristics on MRI may suggest a fat-containing tumor.

Intussusception associated with small-bowel tumors resembles idiopathic small bowel–small bowel intussusceptions on US and CT, with the exception that the mass that is acting as a lead point may be identified on imaging. If the lead point is a lipoma, an echogenic (on US) or low-attenuation (on CT) lesion may be seen within the intussuscipiens.

MALIGNANT TUMORS

Malignant tumors of the small intestine in children, other than lymphoma, are exceedingly rare. The benign tumors mentioned previously have their malignant counterparts. Patients with several of the polyposis syndromes can develop gastrointestinal malignancies (see discussion of PJS above and discussion of colonic polyposes in Chapter 143).

> **Malignant tumors of the small intestine in children, other than lymphoma, are rare.**

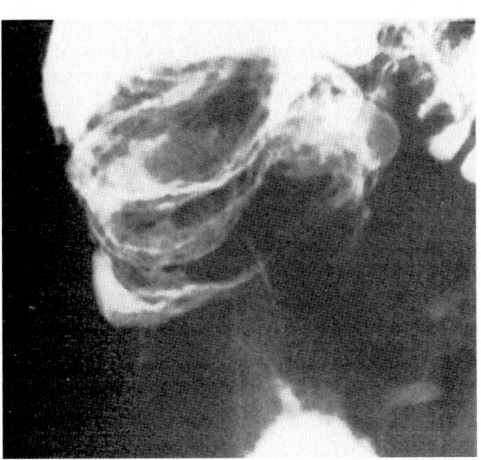

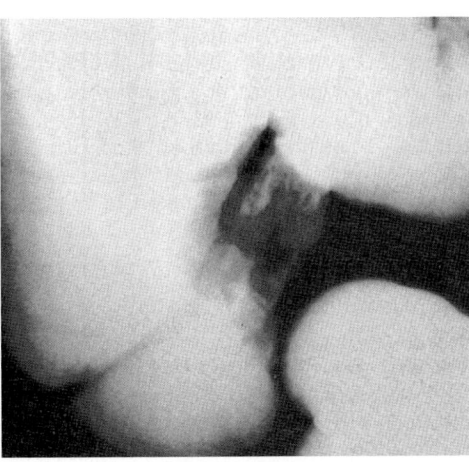

FIGURE 138-1. Burkitt lymphoma presenting as intussusception. **A,** Spot image from a barium enema shows an intussusception within the cecum. **B,** Reduction into the small intestine reveals an ileocecal mass that proved to be Burkitt lymphoma.

A   B

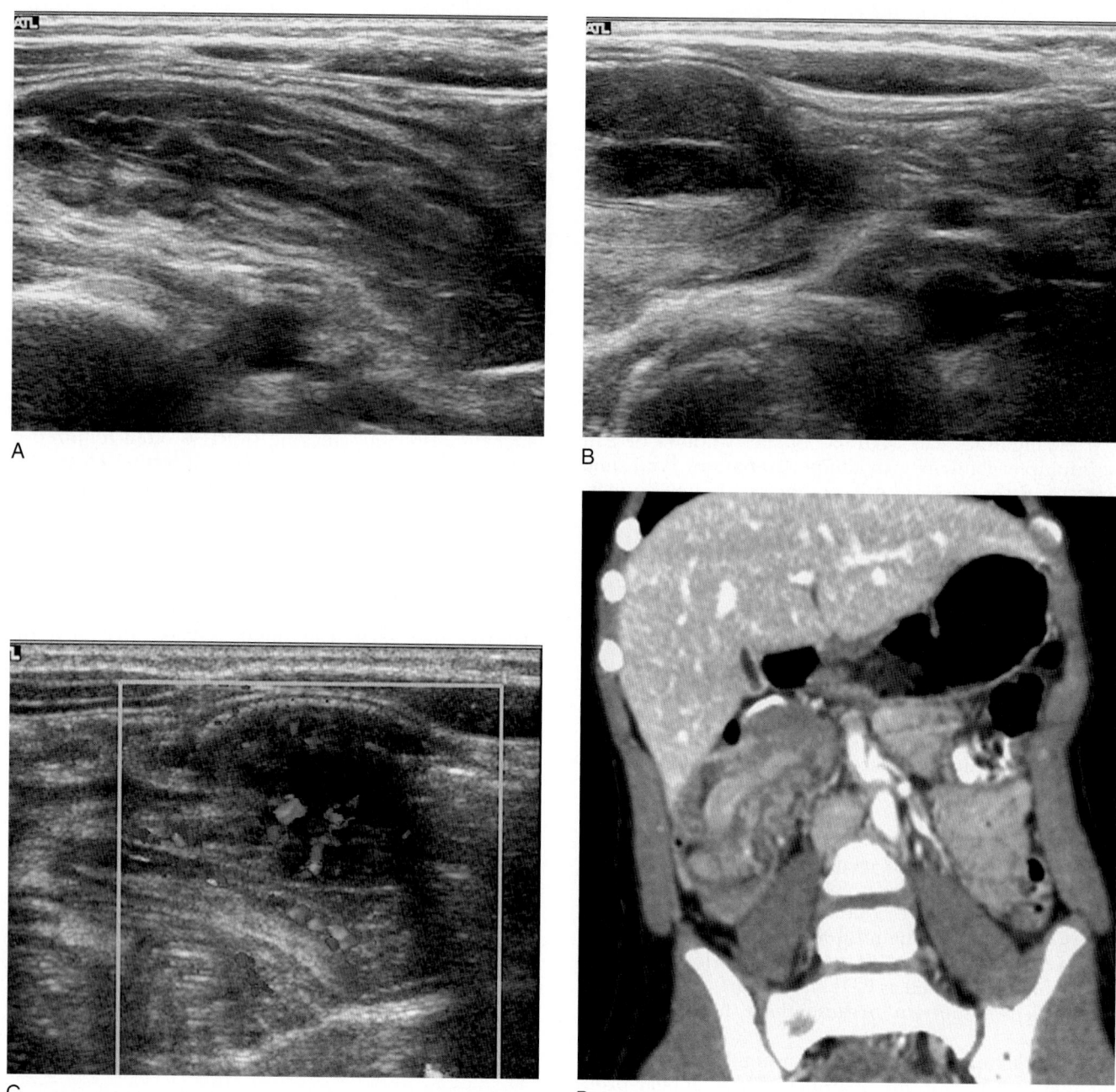

FIGURE 138-2. Burkitt lymphoma and intussusception, ultrasonography (US) and computed tomography (CT) scan. **A** through **C,** Sequential US images of the right abdomen of a 6-year-old girl with abdominal pain for 3 weeks. **A,** Thickened ileum and lymph nodes are seen within the intussusceptum complex. **B,** At the lead point in the right upper quadrant, a hypoechoic mass is identified within the hepatic flexure; note the transverse colon (intussuscipiens) distal to the mass. **C,** Color Doppler in black and white format reveals flow within the hypoechoic solid lead point, indicating that it is a solid lesion. **D,** Oblique coronal reconstruction of CT scan with intravenous contrast reveals the intussusception within the ascending colon, along with the lead point at the hepatic flexure in the right upper quadrant. (Courtesy of M. Hernanz-Schulman, MD, Nashville, TN.)

Burkitt lymphoma is a B cell lymphoma with a predilection for abdominal organs, particularly the distal ileum. It is the most common lead point in children older than 4 years of age with ileocolic intussusception (Figs. 138-1 and 138-2). Patients present with variable symptoms, including nausea, vomiting, abdominal pain, weight loss, change in bowel habits, gastrointestinal (GI) bleeding, or a right lower quadrant mass. The magnitude of symptoms tends to correlate with the degree of obstruction. A mass is frequently palpable. Half of all patients with the sporadic form of Burkitt lymphoma (formerly called *American Burkitt lymphoma*) exhibit involvement of the terminal ileum, and in 25% of patients, the disease is limited to this site. Mesenteric lymph nodes are usually involved.

Plain radiographs may be normal, may show evidence of obstruction caused by intussusception, or may show a noncalcified mass. Small-bowel follow-through study may

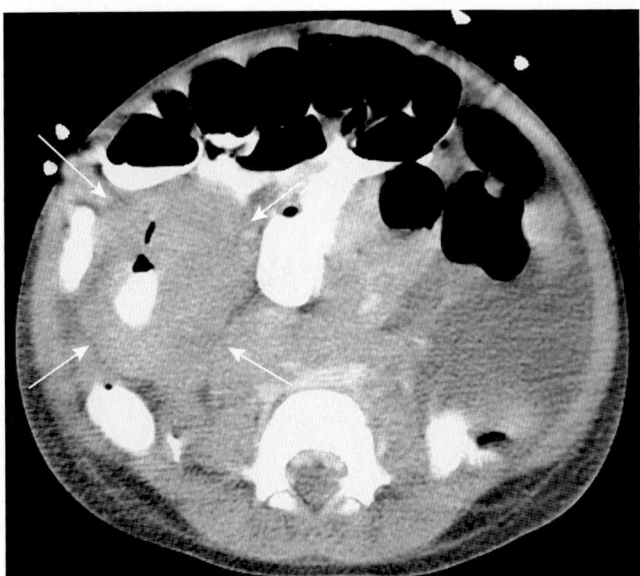

FIGURE 138-3. Axial computed tomography (CT) image of a 6-year-old boy with Burkitt lymphoma reveals a markedly thickened small-bowel wall in the right lower quadrant *(arrows)* with dilated air- and fluid-filled lumen and ascites. (Courtesy of R. Paul Guillerman, Houston, TX.)

reveal a polypoid mass, a stricture, areas of luminal narrowing that resemble inflammatory bowel disease, ulceration, or an intussusception. A large mesenteric mass may produce a mass effect on adjacent small-bowel loops.

If a mass is obvious, clinically or radiographically, US is an appropriate initial imaging study. In older patients with intussusception, a lead point is typically found and should be sought on US examination (see Fig. 138-2). US in patients with lymphoma typically reveals a mass of low or heterogeneous echogenicity. An echogenic center representing the apposed mucosal surfaces (which can be eccentrically positioned) may be seen when the lymphoma infiltrates the bowel wall. A mesenteric nodal mass also may be visible sonographically. CT shows mesenteric masses and infiltration of the bowel wall with dilation of the bowel lumen (Fig. 138-3). Siegel has shown that bowel wall thickening of 1 cm or greater or lymph nodes larger than 1 cm should raise suspicion for lymphoma. Ascites may be present and can be seen on US and CT. The tumor may involve other abdominal sites, and careful evaluation of retroperitoneal organs, liver, and spleen is mandatory.

Carcinoid tumor has been reported in children; when present in the gastrointestinal tract in children, this tumor occurs most commonly in the appendix, but it also may be found in the small bowel. Small-bowel carcinoids typically occur within the ileum and have a greater likelihood of metastasis than those occurring within the appendix. Wide resection and regional lymph node sampling are required.

SUGGESTED READINGS

Attard TM, Abraham SC, Cuffari C: The clinical spectrum of duodenal polyps in pediatrics. J Pediatr Gastroenterol Nutr 2003;36:116-119

Aziz A, Kane TD, Meza MP, et al: An unusual cause of rectal bleeding and intestinal obstruction in a child with peripheral vascular malformations. Pediatr Surg Int 2005;21:491-493

Braunstein GD: Aromatase and gynecomastia. Endocrine-Related Cancer 1999;6:315-324

Bronner MP: Gastrointestinal inherited polyposis syndromes. Mod Pathol 2003;16:359-365

Chu M-H, Lee H-C, Shen E-Y, et al: Gastro-intestinal bleeding caused by leiomyoma of the small intestine in a child with neurofibromatosis. Eur J Pediatr 1999;158:460-462

EMedicine. Gastrointestinal neoplasms. Available at: http://www.emedicine.com/PED/topic3028.htm. Accessed February 28, 2006

Harris JP, Munden MM, Minifee PK: Sonographic diagnosis of multiple small-bowel intussusceptions in Peutz-Jeghers syndrome: a case report. Pediatr Radiol 2002;32:681-683

Hughes JA, Cook JV, Said A, et al: Gastrointestinal stromal tumour of the duodenum in a 7-year-old boy. Pediatr Radiol 2004;34:1024-1027

Lowichik A, Jackson WD, Coffin CM: Gastrointestinal polyposis in childhood: clinicopathologic and genetic features. Pediatr Dev Pathol 2003;6:371-391

Schreibman IR, Baker M, Amos C, et al: The hamartomatous polyposis syndromes: a clinical and molecular review. Am J Gastroenterol 2005;100:476-490

Siegel M, Evans SJ, Balfe DM: Small bowel disease in children: diagnosis with CT. Radiology 1988;169:127-130

Spunt SL, Pratt CB, Rao BN, et al: Childhood carcinoid tumors: the St. Jude Children's Research Hospital experience. J Pediatr Surg 2000;35:1282-1286

Stringer DA, Babyn PS: Pediatric Gastrointestinal Imaging and Intervention, 2nd ed. Hamilton, Ontario, BC Decker, 2000

Vade A, Blane CE: Imaging of Burkitt lymphoma in pediatric patients. Pediatr Radiol 1985;15:123-126

CHAPTER

139 Normal Anatomy and Congenital Disorders

MARTA HERNANZ-SCHULMAN

NORMAL ANATOMY

The colon serves as a repository of ingested and secreted material, allowing accumulation and concerted elimination; its surface provides a means for absorption of water and electrolytes. The colon extends from the ileocecal valve to the anus, and it is typically divided into ascending colon, transverse colon, descending colon, sigmoid colon, and rectum, which together frame the small intestine within the peritoneal cavity (Fig. 139-1).

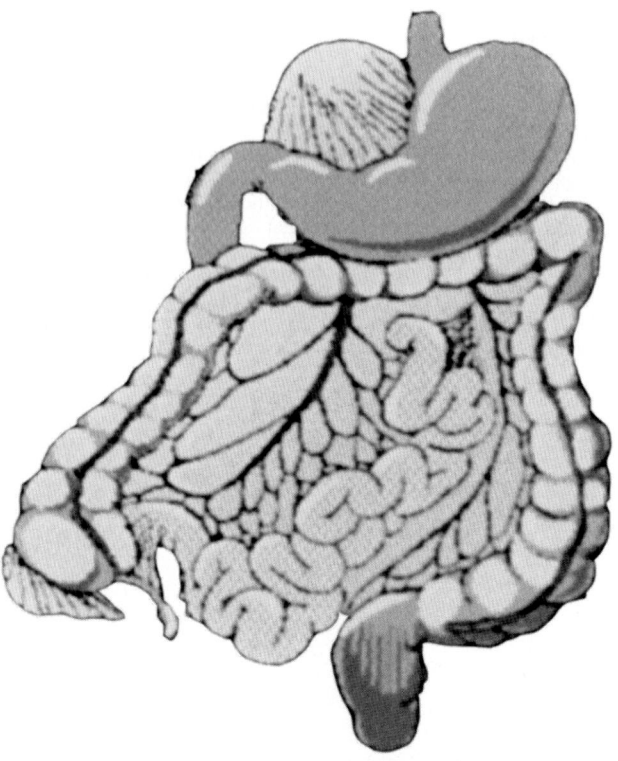

FIGURE 139-1. Schematic figure of normal colon framing the peritoneal cavity and small bowel, from cecum in right lower quadrant, through hepatic and splenic flexures, to sigmoid and rectum. (From Hernanz-Schulman M: Imaging of neonatal gastrointestinal obstruction. Radiol Clin N Am 1999;37:1163-1186.)

The cecum, or blind pouch, receives the contents of the small bowel via the ileocecal valve, and this marks the beginning of the ascending colon, which extends cephalad for a variable length to the hepatic flexure, at the undersurface of the liver, where it becomes the transverse colon. The location and shape of the cecum vary during infancy and childhood; it is typically higher in infants, in whom it may be located above the iliac crest. The shape of the cecum is conical in infants, and it may retain this outline in 2% of adults, with the appendix arising from its apex. However, in most persons, growth of the saccules, particularly the right, leads to the more typical curved apex of the cecum seen in the older child and young adult.

The transverse colon courses from right to left to its highest point in the left upper quadrant at the splenic flexure, and then it turns caudally and becomes the descending portion of the colon along the left lateral abdominal wall, forming the third border of the frame. The transverse colon is suspended by the transverse mesocolon and is thus freely mobile. The ascending and descending portions of the colon typically do not have a mesentery and are thus usually not mobile, their dorsal surface being connected by areolar tissue to the lateral surface of the kidney and the aponeuroses of the transversus abdominis and quadratus lumborum musculature. However, in some patients, these portions of the colon, particularly the cecum and to a lesser extent the ascending colon, may be suspended by a mesentery, allowing some degree of mobility.

The descending colon becomes the sigmoid colon within the pelvis; it is invested by peritoneum and is accorded considerable mobility by its mesenteric attachment. In children, the sigmoid colon tends to extend cephalad to a variable degree, and it is not unusual for the apex of the sigmoid to extend to the right upper quadrant. The distal one third of the rectum is retroperitoneal, with the peritoneal membrane reflecting off its ventral surface only.

The ascending and transverse portions of the colon derive their blood supply from the superior mesenteric artery, whereas the portions from splenic flexure to rectum are supplied by the inferior mesenteric artery.

IMAGING STUDIES

Plain films remain one of the major initial modalities for evaluation of colonic abnormalities. Air can be considered as the contrast medium in the abdominal radiograph, and gravity therefore can be used to assess the various portions of the gastrointestinal tract. In older patients, a supine or upright radiograph is ideal for assessing the transverse colon, left-side-down decubitus for assessing the ascending colon, right-side-down decubitus for the descending colon, and prone radiograph for the rectum, which is particularly well seen, when gas-filled, with the cross-table lateral prone film. The colon is outlined by stool, and stool within the rectum is often recognized on the supine radiograph routinely obtained for a view of the kidneys, ureters, and bladder (the KUB). The normal ascending and descending portions of the colon abut the properitoneal fat plane. Any separation indicates ascites, fluid within the colon, or thickened colonic wall; thickened colonic wall is best evaluated with the appropriate decubitus film, which results in air gravitating against the colonic wall, thus distinguishing fluid from true mural thickening (Fig. 139-2). The left-side-down decubitus is extremely helpful in evaluating right lower quadrant processes, such as intussusception or masses. The prone cross-table lateral view of the rectum is most useful in patients suspected of obstruction; the caliber of the colon, when obstruction is suspected in infants, is best assessed with this view. In neonates and young infants less than 1 year of age, differentiation of the colon from the small bowel cannot be made reliably, but the prone cross-table lateral view remains helpful in assessment of the rectum.

> - **Prone cross-table lateral is helpful in evaluating the size of the rectum.**
> - **Decubitus views outline air-fluid levels, free air, and the wall of the nondependent portion of the colon.**

Although other modalities are useful in specific contexts, contrast enema remains the major imaging modality for diagnostic evaluation of the colon in most conditions. The contrast agents can be air (e.g., for intussusception), barium (e.g., for evaluation of constipation or Hirschsprung disease), or water-soluble agents diluted to various osmolalities depending on the patient and condition being assessed. Barium should not be used in any case of suspected or potential perforation.

Sonography, if unimpeded by gas, is helpful in evaluating the colon, particularly its caliber, mural thickening, blood flow, and masses. The ascending colon can

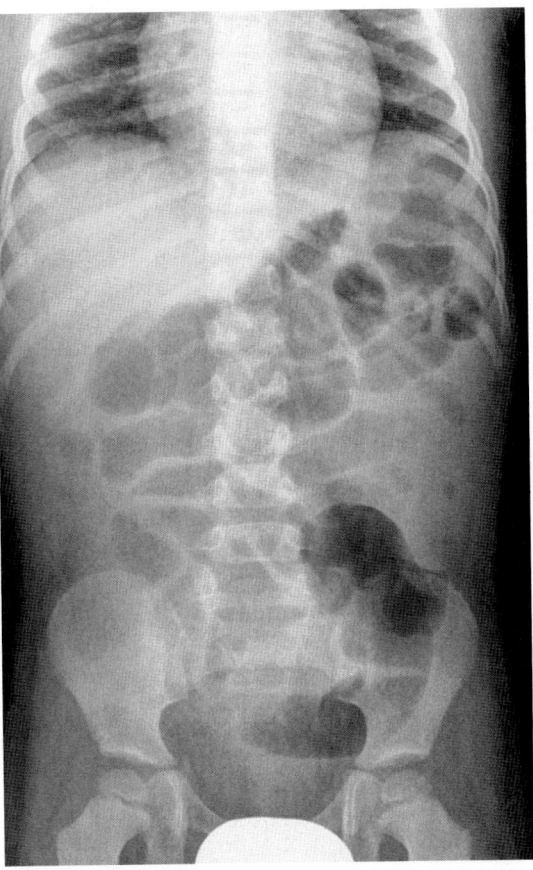
A

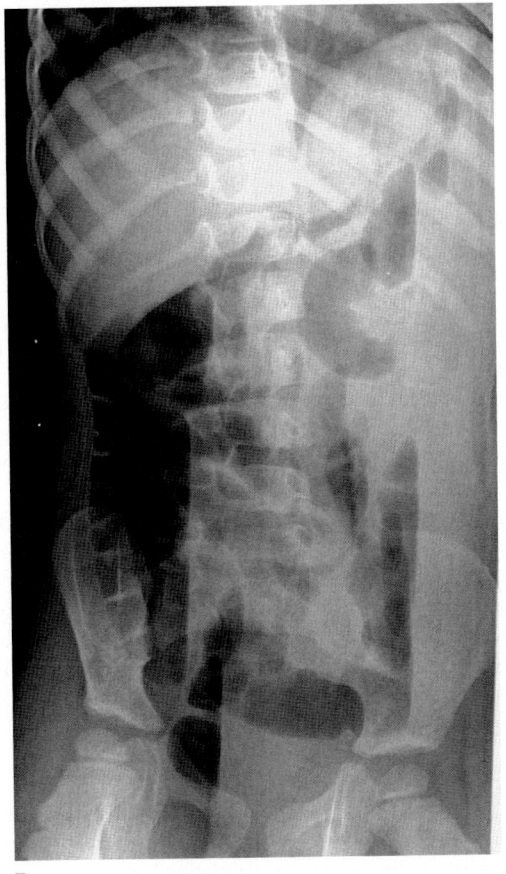
B

FIGURE 139-2. Abdominal radiograph **(A)** and decubitus film **(B)** in a child with gastroenteritis. The supine radiograph shows some distension of small-bowel loops, and fluid density along the flanks. Left-side-down decubitus film shows a long air-fluid level in the ascending colon, which has a normal-thickness wall.

be identified by finding the hepatic flexure below the liver and following it proximally to identify the terminal ileum at the ileocecal valve, and then the cecum and appendix. The splenic flexure and descending colon can be identified through coronal imaging along the left flank, with the descending colon in the plane of the left kidney. The transverse colon can be found by following the hepatic and splenic flexures along the epigastrium. Haustral markings, colonic contents, colonic caliber, mural thickening, adjacent inflammatory changes, masses such as polyps or lymphoma, duplications, intussusception, and blood flow can be identified and evaluated. The rectum is found anterior to the sacrum, behind the bladder in boys, and behind the uterus in girls. When the rectum is filled with stool or air, only the anterior wall is visible.

Computed tomography (CT), unlike sonography, is not limited by air or bone in its field of view. It does not offer the temporal resolution of fluoroscopy, nor information on fine mucosal detail. However, CT can be used to evaluate the wall of the colon and surrounding structures, as well as perfusion and vascular anatomy. Rapid acquisition and three-dimensional coronal and sagittal reconstructions with multichannel detectors render this modality particularly useful in assessing inflammatory conditions affecting the colon, such as inflammatory bowel disease, appendicitis, obstruction, and masses.

Magnetic resonance imaging (MRI) is also useful in the evaluation of masses related to the bowel, particularly pelvic lesions, and it has been used to assess inflammatory bowel disease. Although not limited by the use of ionizing radiation, MRI necessitates introduction of water or dilute gadolinium into the colonic lumen, and its requirement for patient cooperation or sedation over a relatively lengthy period does not lend it to routine use in young patients.

CONGENITAL ABNORMALITIES

Most patients with congenital abnormalities of the colon present during the neonatal period (see Chapter 14). Here, we will consider the later presentation of these primary congenital colonic abnormalities, as well as some of the complications of initial treatment and their imaging evaluation.

In the neonatal period, the presentations of congenital colonic abnormalities such as colonic atresia and Hirschsprung disease typically involve obstruction. Congenital abnormalities that can appear later in life include Hirschsprung disease, anorectal stenosis, duplication cysts, and intestinal pseudo-obstruction of various etiologies, including neuronal intestinal dysplasia (see Chapter 140).

Hirschsprung Disease

Hirschsprung disease is the result of failure of propagation of normal innervation of the bowel, due to arrest of proximal to distal migration of vagal neural crest cells, and it is therefore considered a neurocristopathy. As a result of the abnormal arrest of migration, a variable length of distal bowel lacks parasympathetic Auerbach (intermuscular) and Meissner (submucosal) plexuses, and it is unable to participate in normal peristaltic propulsion of the colonic contents, resulting in failure of relaxation and functional obstruction. Pathologic evaluation of the abnormal bowel also shows abnormal acetylcholinesterase staining and hypertrophied nerve fibers (Fig. 139-3).

Histopathology in Hirschsprung disease:
- **Absent ganglion cells**
- **Hypertrophied nerve fibers**
- **Increased acetylcholinesterase staining**

Hirschsprung disease occurs in approximately 1 per 5000 live births, and it is responsible for approximately 15% to 20% of cases of neonatal bowel obstruction, but presentation occurs after the newborn period in approximately 20% of cases. The transition point between normal and abnormal bowel can occur at any point and can extend through a variable length of the small bowel. The presence of a transition point at the rectosigmoid is termed short-segment aganglionosis, and it occurs in approximately 90% of cases. Males predominate in short-segment aganglionosis (4:1 ratio); however, male preponderance diminishes when longer segments are involved. Long-segment disease tends to occur more often in white than in black patients, with no distinction between the two races in short-segment disease. Hirschsprung disease is associated with Down syndrome, (2% to 16% of patients with Down syndrome also have Hirschsprung disease, with a boy-to-girl ratio of 5:1). Other syndromes associated with Hirschsprung disease include Waardenburg syndrome (pigmentary anomalies and sensorineural hearing loss), Goldberg-Shprintzen syndrome (mental retardation, cleft palate, and Hirschsprung disease), McKusick-Kauffman syndrome (hydrometrocolpos, polydactyly, congenital heart disease), Bardet Biedl syndrome (pigmentary retinopathy, obesity, hypogonadism), the Currarino triad, and central hypoventilation or Haddad syndrome. Between 5% and 30% of patients with Hirschsprung disease have limb, skin, central nervous system, kidney, cardiac, and other malformations. A positive family history is encountered in a minority of patients (<10%), but this increases to nearly one fourth in patients with total aganglionosis. Among the several genetic pathway abnormalities that occur in patients with Hirschsprung disease, the major mutation involves the *RET* gene, identified in 50% of familial cases and 15% to 20% of isolated cases.

Enterocolitis is a major cause of morbidity and mortality in patients with Hirschsprung disease. Clinically, it can appear insidiously, or abruptly with diarrhea, fever, abdominal distension, colicky abdominal pain, and hematochezia. The pathogenesis is unknown, but implicated mechanisms include abnormal epithelial lining, abnormal mucin production, abnormal local immune mechanisms, and viral and bacterial pathogens, notably *Clostridium difficile*. Risk factors are believed to be stasis and bowel dilation. Incidence of enterocolitis increases

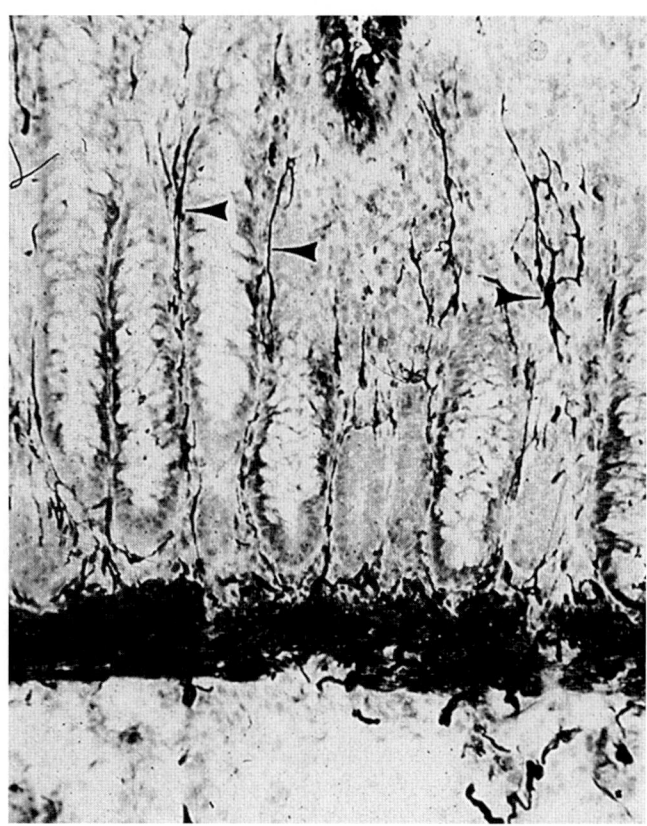

A

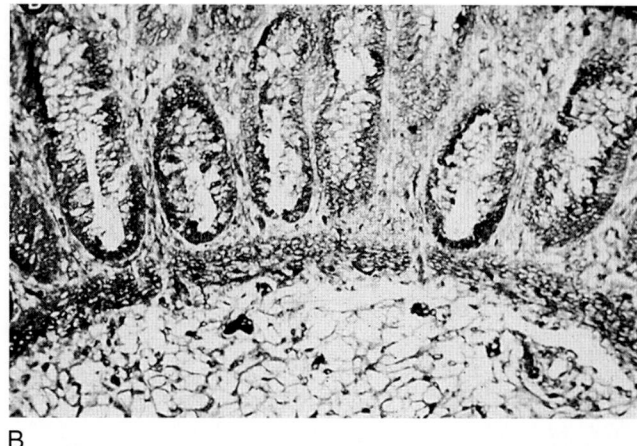

B

FIGURE 139-3. **A,** Abnormal acetylcholinesterase staining in Hirschsprung disease. Photomicrograph shows abnormally dense staining of the lamina propria, and hypertrophied nerve fibers *(arrowheads)*. **B,** Normal specimen (similarly processed) does not show the abnormal nerve fibers, and there is little staining of the lamina propria. (From Sieber WK: Hirschsprung's disease. In Welch KJ, Randolph, JG, Ravitch MM, et al (eds): Pediatric Surgery, 4th ed, Chicago, Year Book Medical, 1986:995-1016.)

with delayed diagnosis, long-segment disease, and co-morbid conditions, such as found in patients with Down syndrome. Contrast enemas are generally not indicated, but they can be performed carefully with water-soluble iso-osmolal contrast, with surgical consultation when the diagnosis is not certain (Fig. 139-4).

The clinical presentation of Hirschsprung disease in the neonate is one of distal obstruction. In older children, Hirschsprung disease presents with constipation, and with abdominal distension, vomiting, and failure to thrive in more severe cases. In late presentation, the zone of transition is nearly always the low-segment type. Plain radiographs in older children do not typically show the findings of bowel obstruction that are seen in the neonate. There is evidence of severe constipation, with at times very marked dilation of the colon, particularly in older children. In patients with functional constipation, the rectum is typically the larger portion of the colon, acting as a fecal reservoir. In patients with Hirschsprung disease, the rectum may be normal in size and filled with stool, which acts as a bougie to distend the aganglionic segment; however, unlike in patients with functional constipation, a caliber difference, with a larger diameter of the more proximal colon, is typically present (Figs. 139-5 through 139-8).

Definitive diagnosis is made by characteristic biopsy findings, as discussed earlier. Manometric studies, with failure of relaxation of the internal sphincter and with rectal distension, are helpful after the immediate neonatal period, and therefore helpful in older children.

Radiologic diagnosis is made with contrast enema, which is geared toward identification of the zone of transition (see Figs. 139-5, 139-7, and 139-8). Routine enemas before the diagnostic procedure should be avoided, but digital examination in the older age group should not affect the radiographic findings. The study is done with a small rubber catheter; we use the same catheter as in neonatal enemas, which can be placed in the rectum without effect on the zone of transition. Barium or iso-osmolal water-soluble agents can be used, but hyperosmolal media should be avoided, as it will lead to increased bowel distension. Initial images are taken in the lateral projection, as soon as the contrast begins to enter the colon, and multiple fluoro grabs are used to document the flow of contrast and the caliber of the colon. Although in adult colonic evaluation imaging is delayed until full colonic distension is achieved, this should not be done in these cases, as it could obliterate the zone of transition. The enema is terminated when the zone of transition is identified.

The distal, aganglionic colon is normal in caliber, with a sharp transition to dilated proximal colon. The aganglionic segment may exhibit a changing, serrated appearance because of aperistaltic contractions of the abnormally innervated bowel. In patients with functional constipation, there will be greater distension of the rectum, or of the rectum and sigmoid, in comparison with the more proximal colon, and this gradual caliber difference is the reverse of that encountered in patients with Hirschsprung disease. A rectosigmoid ratio of less

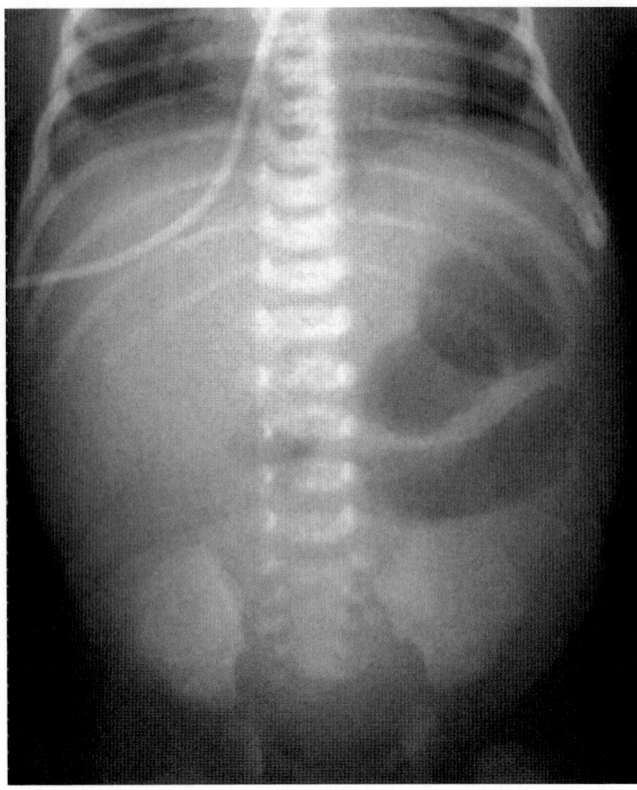

A

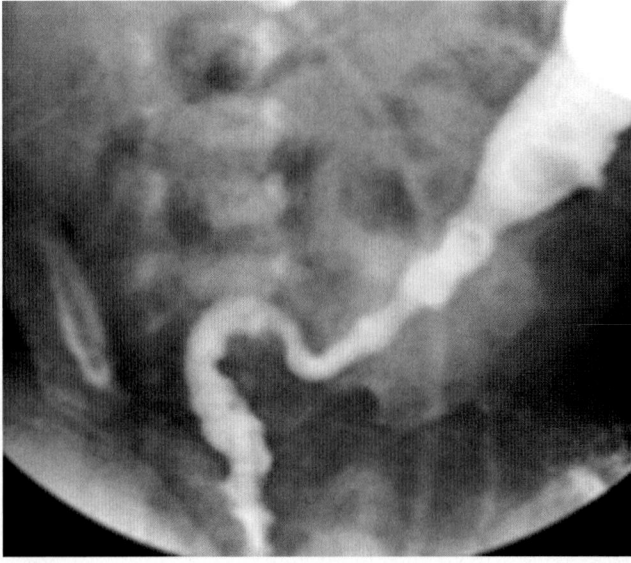

B

FIGURE 139-4. Hirschsprung enterocolitis in a 1-month-old boy. **A,** Abdominal radiograph shows distension of the flanks indicating fluid-filled distended bowel, and gaseous distension of the colon. **B,** Limited water-soluble enema shows marked colonic narrowing and mural irregularity. Histopathologic examination revealed Hirschsprung disease complicated by enterocolitis.

than 0.9 is typically seen in patients with Hirschsprung disease and is an adjunct finding. However, the recto-sigmoid ratio is rarely needed to identify the zone of transition, and it can be misleading in cases of more extensive aganglionosis. The ability of the colon to empty can be assessed by comparison of a pre-evacuation film, which can be done as a fluoro grab, followed by a post-evacuation film. Postevacuation and delayed radiographs are helpful in the neonate, particularly in patients with total colonic aganglionosis. However, in older children with constipation, they are rarely helpful.

The accuracy of the contrast enema in diagnosing Hirschsprung disease rests on the radiologist's ability to discern a transition zone. However, even when a transition zone is seen, it is often lower than the actual biopsy-proven point of transition from the ganglionic to aganglionic segment. In a study by Jamieson and colleagues, the agreement between the radiologic and pathologic level was only 62.5%, and it was much worse for long-segment Hirschsprung disease.

> *Findings of Hirschsprung disease at contrast enema:*
> - **Zone of transition between aganglionic segment and dilated proximal bowel**
> - **Irregular contractions of aganglionic segment (less uncommon)**

Surgical repair of Hirschsprung disease is effected by bringing normally innervated bowel distally toward the sphincteric mechanism through several procedures and modifications. Swenson is credited with the first description of successful surgical repair; his procedure consists of resection of the aganglionic segment, and anastomosis of normal, ganglion-containing bowel to the sphincteric mechanism. The Duhamel procedure involves leaving the anterior portion of the aganglionic rectum in place and anastomosing ganglion-containing bowel to its posterior wall (Fig. 139-9). The Soave or endorectal pull-through involves resection of the mucosa and submucosa of the aganglionic bowel, and pulling the normal ganglion-containing bowel through the muscular rectal sleeve (Fig. 139-10). The Duhamel and Soave procedures are modifications of the Swenson designed to minimize risk of injury to the sphincteric mechanism. Complications include postoperative leaks, strictures, and delayed bowel control. Residual obstruction secondary to the aganglionic internal sphincter predisposes to stasis and the consequent risk of enterocolitis. Postoperatively, some narrowing may be seen at the distal muscular sleeve, or the barium enema may appear normal, except for the double density from the retained rectal pouch in patients treated with the Duhamel procedure.

Anorectal Stenosis

Anorectal stenosis forms part of the spectrum of the anorectal malformations; anal atresia with high or low termination of the rectum, presenting in the neonatal period. Patients with anorectal stenosis may have a rectoperineal fistula or an anteriorly placed anus, and they present with constipation, sometimes in early adulthood.

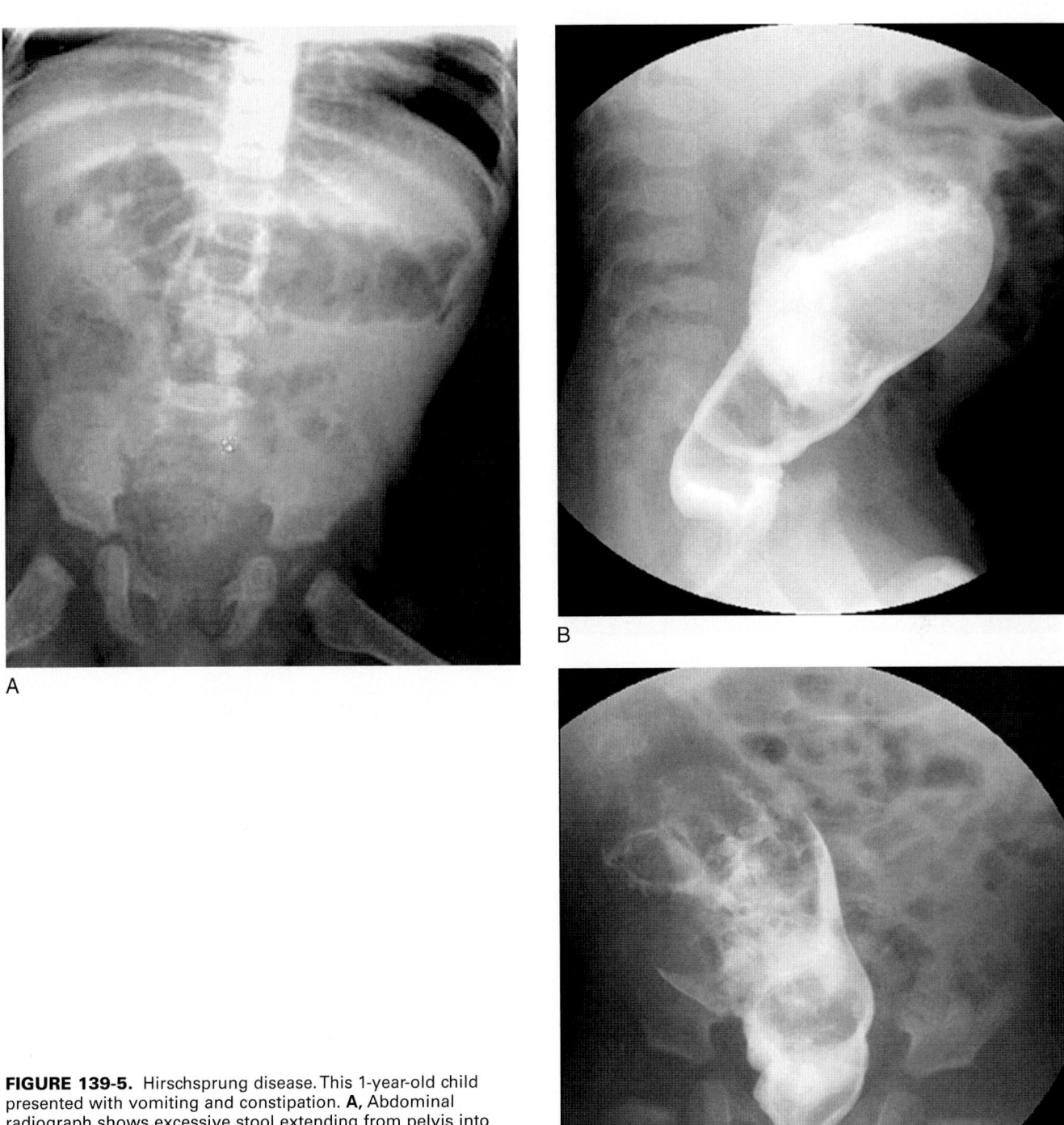

FIGURE 139-5. Hirschsprung disease. This 1-year-old child presented with vomiting and constipation. **A,** Abdominal radiograph shows excessive stool extending from pelvis into right abdomen. **B,** Lateral view of rectum during contrast enema shows zone of transition at rectosigmoid junction. **C,** Anteroposterior projection shows the dilated sigmoid colon filled with stool and extending into the right side of the abdomen.

In 1981, Currarino and colleagues described a triad of sacral anomaly, anorectal stenosis, and presacral mass, which became known as the Currarino triad. The classic sacral anomaly consists of a sickle- or scimitar-shaped hemisacrum, with partial or complete absence of a portion of the lower sacrum, which is considered pathognomonic by some authors. The condition has been associated with the *HLXB9* homeobox gene on chromosome 7q36 in a majority of patients, and several familial cases have been reported. The presacral masses originally reported by Currarino and coworkers were teratoma (most common), anterior meningocele, and enteric cyst, although others have since been reported, including dermoid, lipoma, and ectopic nephroblastoma (Fig. 139-11). However the mass is not always present, leading some authors to suggest the term *Currarino*

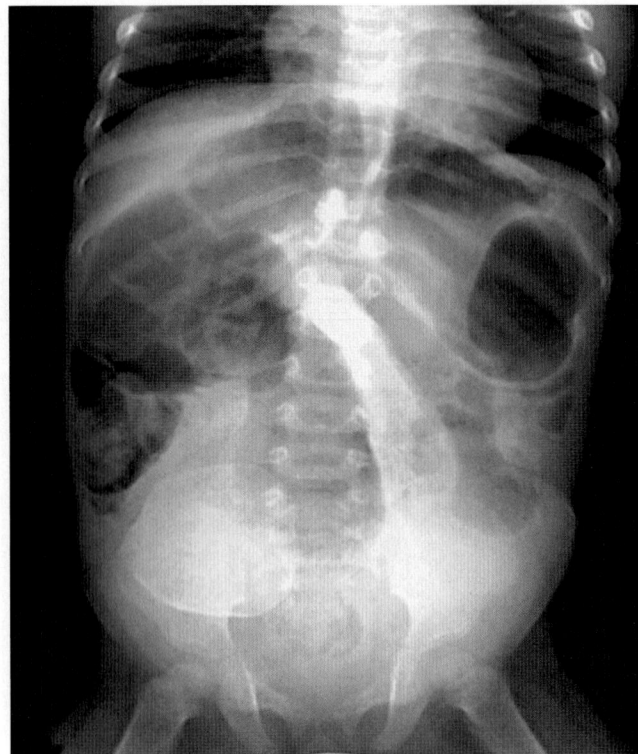

A

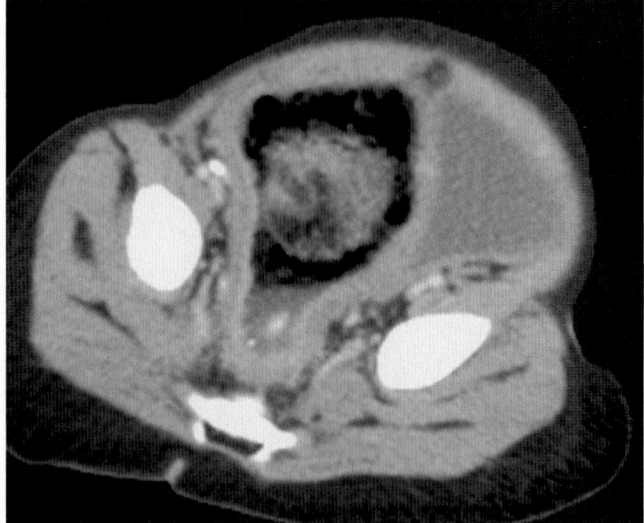

B

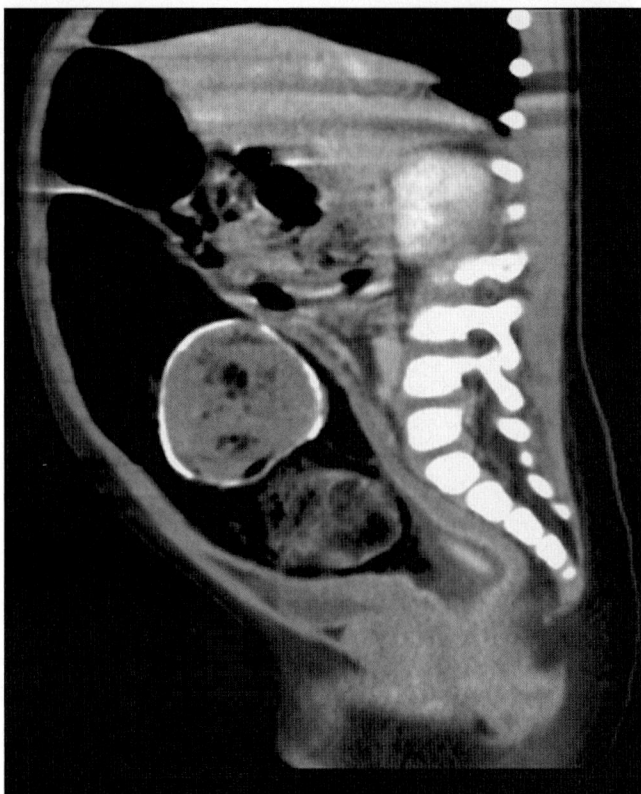

C

FIGURE 139-6. Hirschsprung disease. This 15-month-old child with a history of intermittent constipation presented to the emergency department with acute fecal retention. **A,** Abdominal radiograph shows right lower quadrant calcified mass and markedly dilated bowel. **B,** CT scan requested for concern of abdominal mass shows transition zone at rectosigmoid junction, with fecal ball in the dilated proximal sigmoid colon. **C,** Sagittal reformat shows the zone of transition and the more proximal fecal ball with calcified edges.

syndrome rather than *triad.* Other anomalies, including urologic abnormalities and Hirschsprung disease, have been reported in patients with the Currarino syndrome.

> *Currarino triad:*
> - **Scimitar sacrum**
> - **Anorectal stenosis**
> - **Presacral mass: teratoma, anterior meningocele, enteric cyst**

Colonic Duplication

Duplication cysts of the gastrointestinal (GI) tract are characterized by contiguity with and adherence to a segment of the alimentary tract for which the individual anomaly is named, by a smooth muscle coat, mucosal lining including one or more types of cells found within any portion of the alimentary canal, and a shared blood supply with native GI structures. They can occur anywhere along the length of the entire GI tract, and are most common in the terminal ileum (approximately

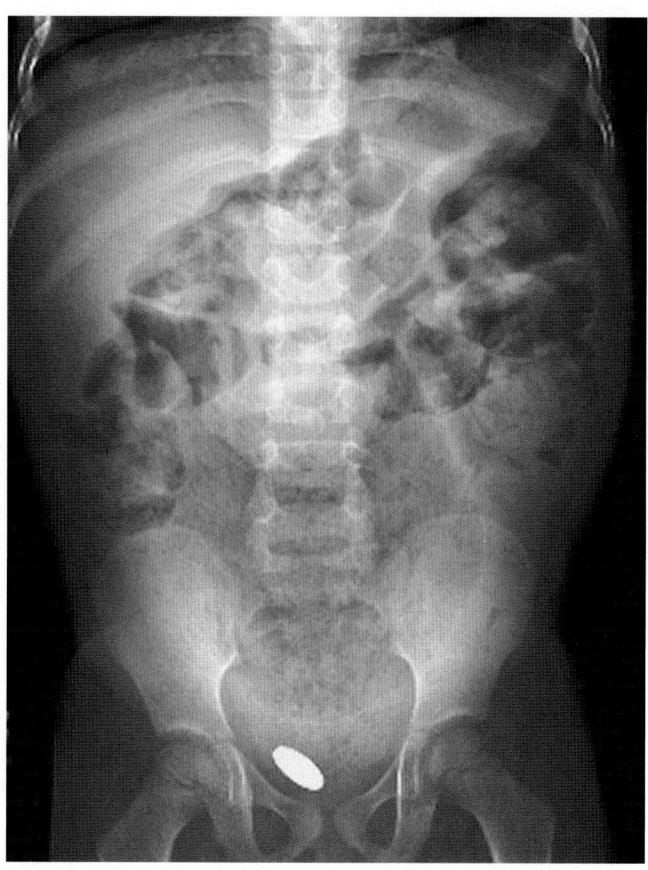

A

B

FIGURE 139-7. After repair of an interrupted aortic arch, this 4-year-old child presented with constipation and a retained coin in the rectum for several months. **A,** Abdominal radiograph shows marked fecal dilation of sigmoid, which does not extend into the rectum; the rectum contains the retained coin. **B,** Lateral early view from contrast enema clearly shows the zone of transition and the retained coin.

22%); approximately 15% of duplications are colonic, and approximately 5% are rectal.

Colonic duplications can be cystic or tubular. Cystic duplications consist of a relatively small segment of bowel duplication, typically not communicating with the adjacent lumen. The incidence of gastric mucosa within colonic duplications is reportedly less than in other types, and they can therefore remain asymptomatic and be discovered incidentally in adulthood. However, they can present with obstruction, intussusception, and volvulus.

Tubular duplications typically connect with the GI tract and often drain into the perineum via a fistula, usually located anterior to the rectum, or to a single or duplicated anus. In an extensive review of 57 cases, Yousefzadeh and coworkers defined the colon proper as that ending in a perineal anus, and the duplicated colon as that ending at a perineal fistula, at a communication with the colon proper, or blindly; however, in some cases, both colons end in a duplicated perineal anus, or in perineal fistulae. Although duplications of the GI tract are typically located on the antimesenteric side, Yousefzadeh and colleagues, using the above definition, found 12 duplicated colons to be located on the mesenteric side of the colon proper. The duplications are of variable length and can be classified as extending above or below the peritoneal reflection. If they do not extend below the peritoneal reflection and therefore do not have a perineal opening, communication with the lumen

can be at both ends or at a single end. They can extend proximally to involve the cecum, appendix, and terminal ileum. Isolated duplication of the appendix is exceedingly rare, but it has been reported. Approximately 80% of tubular colonic duplications are associated with many other anomalies, including renal anomalies, duplication of the genitourinary tract (uterus, bladder, urethra, penis), and vertebral and cord abnormalities (Fig. 139-12).

> *Tubular colonic duplications:*
> - **Are rare**
> - **May involve portions of the colon, or entire colon**
> - **Usually (but not always) connect with the GI tract**
> - **Often drain to perineum via fistula anterior to anus**
> - **Are associated with other anomalies, such as duplication of genitourinary structures**

Rectal duplications are cystic structures that are located in the presacral space (Fig. 139-13), although there have been unusual reports of rectal duplications located anterior to the rectum. Approximately half of rectal duplications drain via a fistula, which is typically, but not always, located posterior, rather than anterior, to

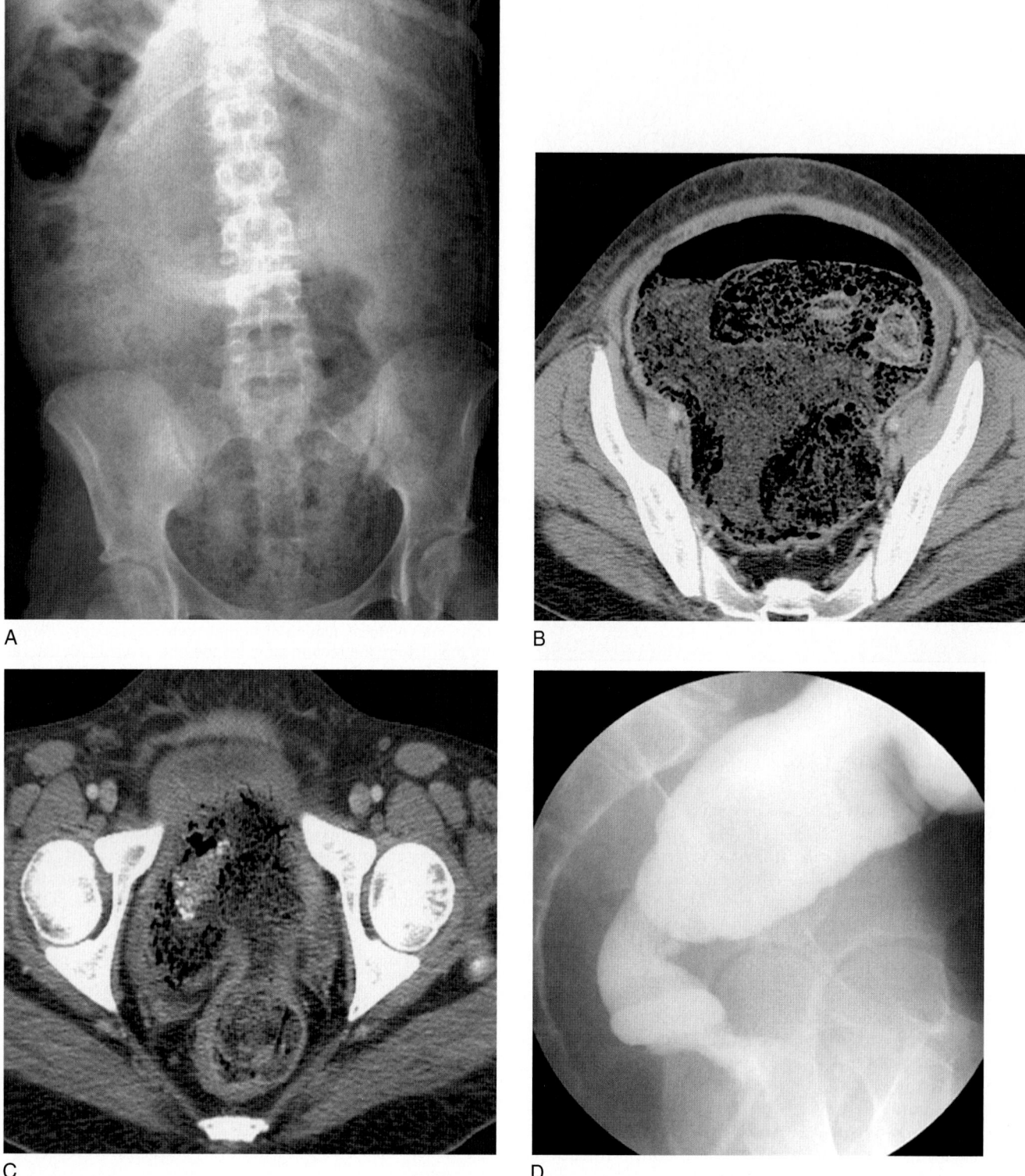

FIGURE 139-8. Hirschsprung disease. A 15-year-old girl with diabetes and a history of intermittent diarrhea presented acutely to the emergency department with increasing diarrhea and abdominal distension. CT was requested for clinical concern of appendicitis. **A,** Abdominal radiograph shows marked stool burden and colonic dilation. The sigmoid colon extends cephalad and displaces the transverse colon. **B,** CT at upper pelvis shows dilated sigmoid entering the pelvis. **C,** CT lower in the pelvis shows the zone of transition. **D,** Lateral view of contrast enema confirms the low transition zone.

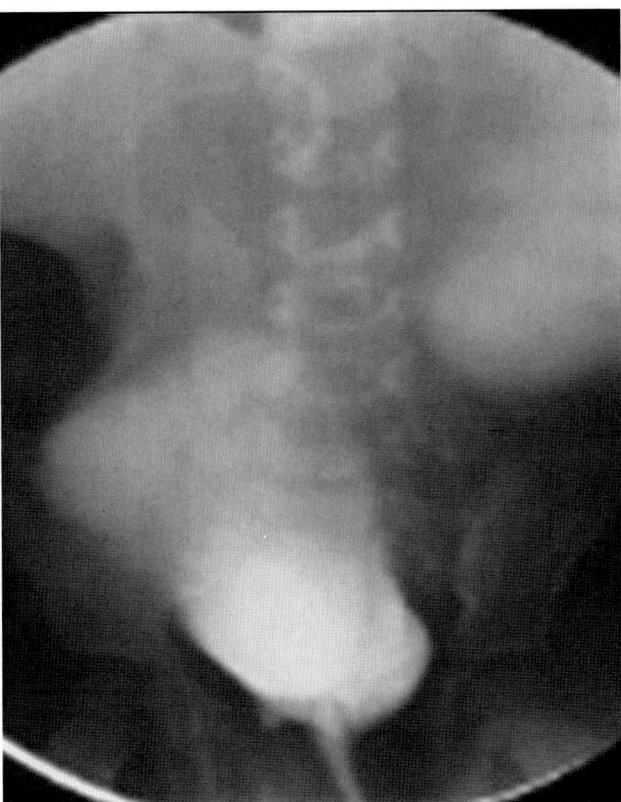

FIGURE 139-9. This 4-year-old was seen 1 year after Duhamel procedure for Hirschsprung disease. Anteroposterior image from contrast enema examination shows rectal double density from anterior pouch.

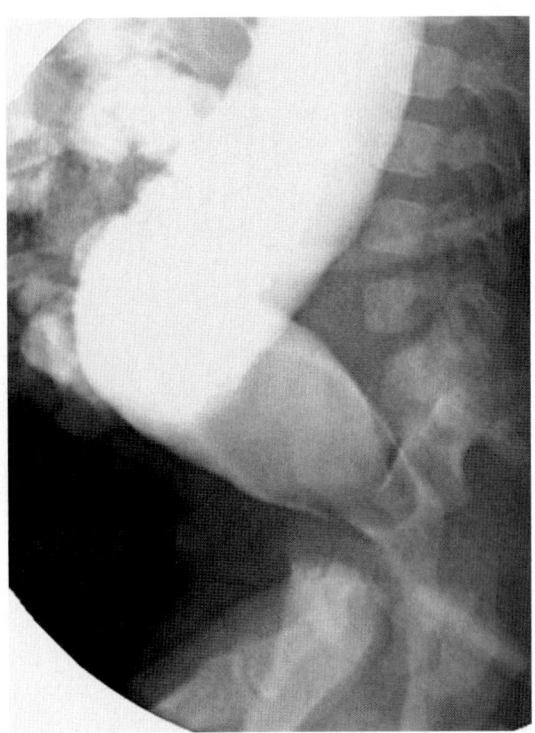

FIGURE 139-10. This 2-month-old infant was seen 1 month after an endorectal pull-through procedure for Hirschsprung disease. There is minimal narrowing at the muscular sleeve, but the examination is nearly normal.

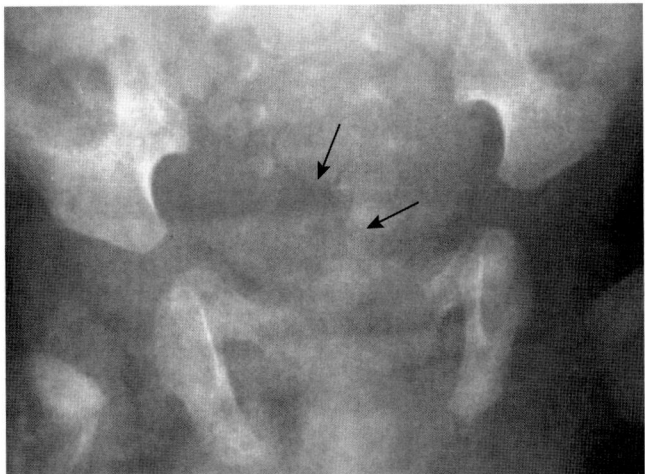

A

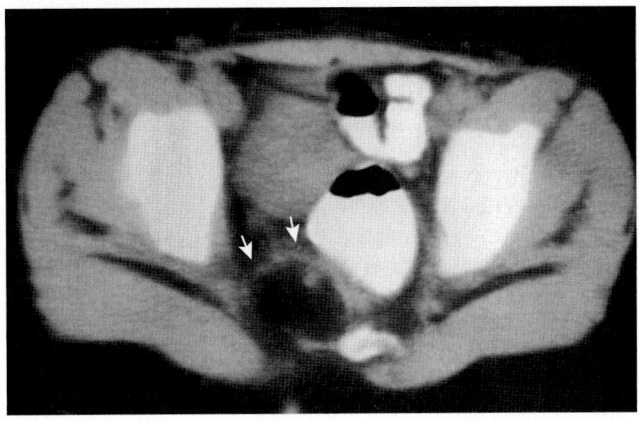

B

FIGURE 139-11. Currarino triad. **A,** Anteroposterior radiograph of the pelvis. A crescentic defect is present in the right inferior sacrum *(arrows),* producing a so-called scimitar sacrum. **B,** CT scan of the pelvis at the level of the sacral defect in a patient with anal stenosis shows a small fat-containing mass *(arrows)* at the level of the sacral defect. This was surgically removed and proved to be a teratoma.

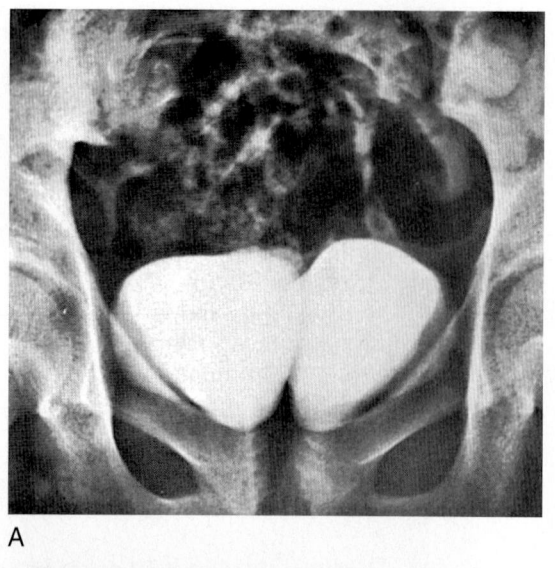

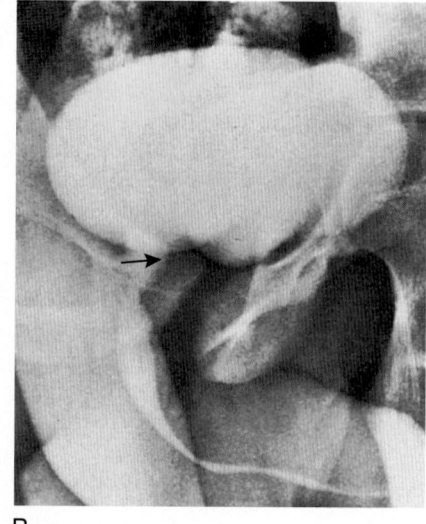

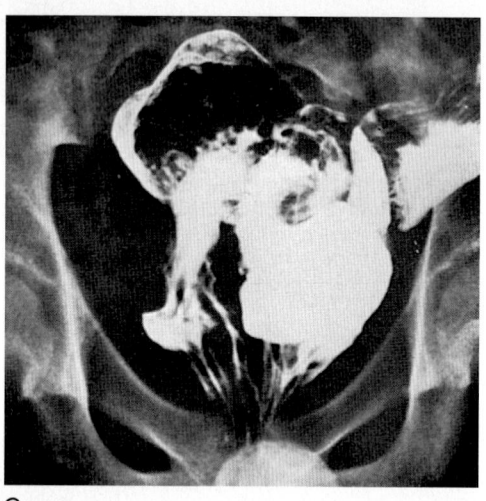

FIGURE 139-12. Duplication of the bladder and entire colon in a 15-year-old boy who had been treated in the newborn period for anal atresia. **A,** Frontal radiograph of the pelvis after excretory urography shows two bladders. Each upper urinary tract emptied into the bladder on its respective side. **B,** Voiding urethrogram. A single urethra *(arrow)* originated from the right side. **C,** Barium enema shows two rectums. Surgical exploration revealed duplication of the colon from appendix to rectum.

the anus. When not communicating with the perineum, the cysts may enlarge and exhibit mass effect on the fecal and urinary streams. Adenocarcinoma arising in rectal duplication has been reported in adult patients.

The diagnostic modality used for colonic duplication varies with the type and mode of presentation. Cystic duplications show a mass, which may be complicated by bowel obstruction as a result of volvulus or intussusception. Initial suspicion on plain films can be followed up with sonography, CT, or MRI. Tubular duplications with a perineal fistula are best diagnosed with contrast enema via both perineal orifices, outlining the bilateral lumina; antegrade contrast studies have also been shown to be diagnostic. CT with multiplanar reconstructions and

MRI will probably be diagnostic, but so far their role in the workup of these lesions is undefined. Rectal duplications can be identified in plain films and contrast enemas via a mass effect on the rectum, and on the adjacent genitourinary structures if sufficiently large. Sonography and MRI are probably the best modalities to evaluate noncommunicating cysts (see Fig. 139-13), although CT, particularly with the aid of reformats, is also useful and diagnostic if performed as the initial procedure. If the duplication communicates with the perineum, introduction of contrast is diagnostic. A search for other-system anomalies should also be undertaken with the appropriate imaging modality.

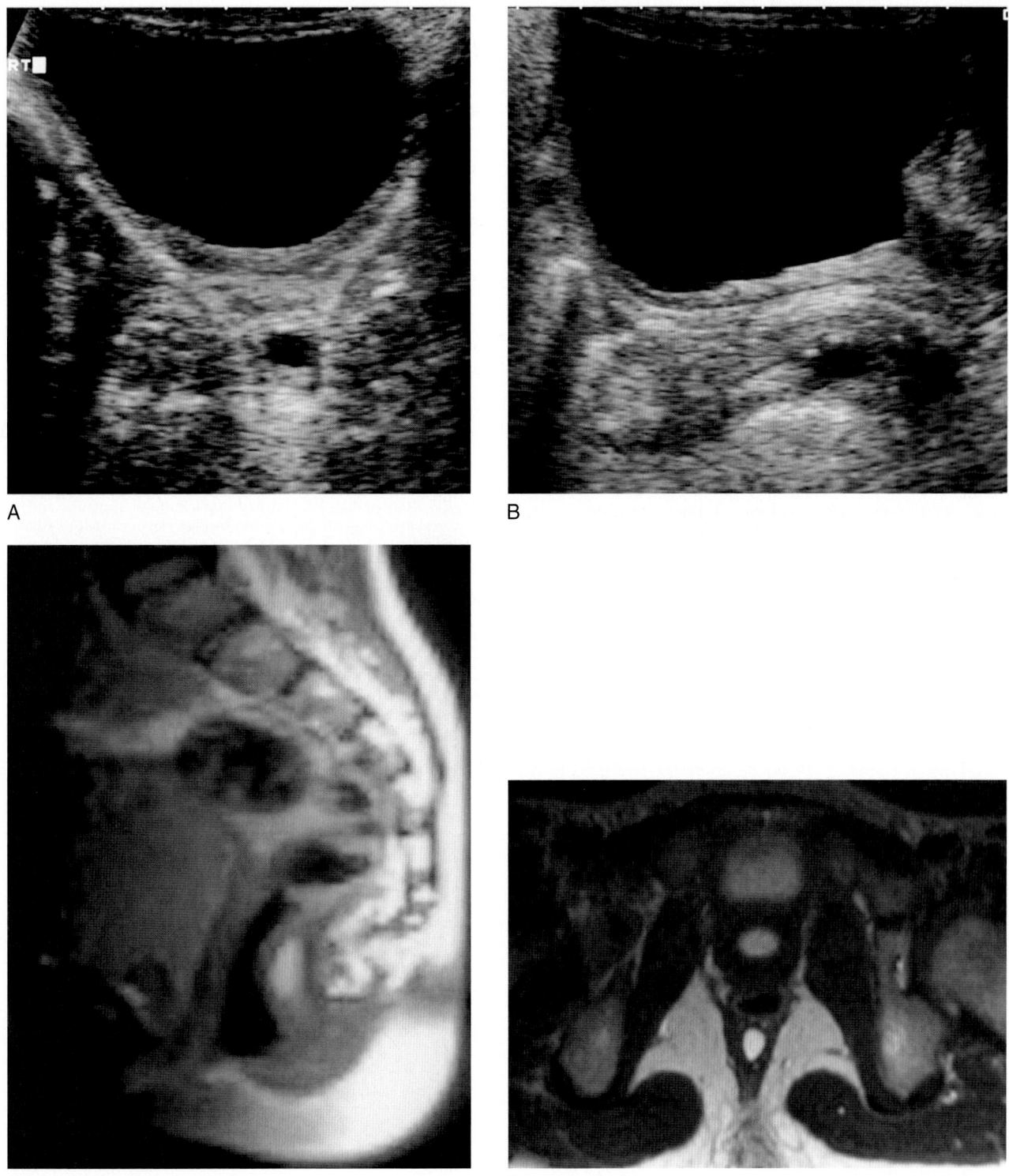

FIGURE 139-13. Rectal duplication cyst. This 6-year-old girl presented with abdominal pain and underwent sonography. A rectal duplication cyst was incidentally identified. Axial **(A)** and sagittal **(B)** midline sonographic images identify a small cyst inseparable from the posterior rectal wall. Sagittal **(C)** and axial **(D)** T2-weighted MR images demonstrate the small cystic lesion arising from the posterior rectal wall.

SUGGESTED READINGS

Hirschsprung Disease

Amiel J, Lyonnet S: Hirschsprung disease, associated syndromes, and genetics: a review. J Med Genet 2001;38:729-739

Bajaj R, Smith J, Trochet D, et al: Congenital central hypoventilation syndrome and Hirschsprung's disease in an extremely preterm infant. Pediatrics 2005;115:e737-e738

Hackam DJ, Filler RM, Pearl RH: Enterocolitis after the surgical treatment of Hirschsprung's disease: risk factors and financial impact. J Pediatr Surg 1998;33:830-833

Hackam DJ, Reblock K, Barksdale EM, et al: The influence of Down's syndrome on the management and outcome of children with Hirschsprung's disease. J Pediatr Surg 2003;38:946-949

Hackam DJ, Reblock KK, Redlinger RE, et al.: Diagnosis and outcome of Hirschsprung's disease: does age really matter? Pediatr Surg Int 2004;20:319-322

Jamieson DH, Dundas SE, Belushi SA, et al: Does the transition zone reliably delineate aganglionic bowel in Hirschsprung's disease? Pediatr Radiol 2005;34:811-815

Menezes M, Puri P: Long-term outcome of patients with enterocolitis complicating Hirschsprung's disease. Pediatr Surg Int 2006;22:316-318

Murphy F, Puri P: New insights into the pathogenesis of Hirschsprung's associated enterocolitis. Pediatr Surg Int 2005;21:773-779

Teitelbaum DH, Coran AG: Hirschsprung disease and related neuromuscular disorders. In Grosfeld J: Pediatric Surgery, 6th ed. Philadelphia, Mosby, 2006

Anorectal Stenosis

Baltogiannis N, Mavridis G, Soutis M, Keramidas D: Currarino triad associated with Hirschsprung's disease. J Pediatr Surg 2003;38:1086-1089

Currarino G, Coln D, Votteler T: Triad of anorectal, sacral, and presacral anomalies. AJR Am J Roentgenol 1981;137:395-398

Emans PJ, Kootstra G, Marcelis CL, et al: The Currarino triad: the variable expression. J Pediatr Surg 2005;40:1238-1242

Emans PJ, van Aalst J, van Heurn EL, et al: The Currarino triad: neurosurgical considerations. Neurosurgery 2006;58:924-929

Kirks DR, Merten DF, Filston HC, et al: The Currarino triad: complex of anorectal malformation, sacral bony abnormality, and presacral mass. Pediatr Radiol 1984;14:220-225

Kurosaki M, Kamitani H, Anno Y, et al: Complete familial Currarino triad: report of three cases in one family. J Neurosurg 2001;94:158-161

Lee SC, Chun YS, Jung SE, et al: Currarino triad: anorectal malformation, sacral bony abnormality, and presacral mass: a review of 11 cases. J Pediatr Surg 1997;32:58-61

Martucciello G, Torre M, Belloni E, et al: Currarino syndrome: proposal of a diagnostic and therapeutic protocol. J Pediatr Surg 2004;39:1305-1311

Mavridis G, Livaditi E, Soutis M, et al: Complete Currarino triad in all affected members of the same family. Eur J Pediatr Surg 2005;15:369-373

Colonic and Rectal Duplications

Amjadi K, Poenaru D, Soboleski D, et al: Anterior rectal duplication: a diagnostic challenge. J Pediatr Surg 2000;35:613-614

Hur J, Yoon C-S, Kim M-J, Kim O-H: Imaging features of gastrointesinal tract duplications in infants and children: from oesophagus to rectum. Pediatr Radiol 2007;37:691-699

Kaur N, Nagpal K, Sodhi P, et al: Hindgut duplication: case report and literature review. Pediatr Surg Int 2004;20:640-642

Kim EP, McClenathan JH: Unusual duplication of appendix and cecum: extension of the Cave-Wallbridge classification. J Pediatr Surg 2001;36:E18

Knudtson J, Jackson R, Grewal H: Rectal duplication. J Pediatr Surg 2003;38:1119-1120

Kuo HC, Lee HC, Shin CH, et al: Clinical spectrum of alimentary tract duplication in children. Acta Paediatr Taiwan 2004;45:85-88

Piolat C, N'Die J, Andrini P, et al: Perforated tubular duplication of the transverse colon: a rare cause of meconium peritonitis with prenatal diagnosis. Pediatr Surg Int 2005;21:110-112

Yousefzadeh DK, Bickers GH, Jackson JH Jr, et al: Tubular colonic duplication: review of 1876-1981 literature. Pediatr Radiol 1983;13:65-71

Functional Disorders

KIMBERLY E. APPLEGATE and MARTA HERNANZ-SCHULMAN

The functional disorders discussed in this chapter are entities that cause obstruction without a clearly identifiable anatomic point of obstruction. A number of poorly understood disorders (e.g., meconium plug, neonatal small left colon syndrome) cause transient, self-limited functional obstruction in neonates and are, at times, associated with Hirschsprung disease; these entities are reviewed in Chapter 14. In older children, functional disorders include pseudo-obstruction, irritable bowel syndrome, and "functional" constipation.

Intestinal pseudo-obstruction refers to a chronically recurring and at times massive dilation of the intestinal tract without an identifiable mechanical cause. The condition includes a heterogeneous group of disorders that affect the intestinal smooth muscle, resulting in failure of normal intestinal motility; the condition can be primary, neuropathic or myopathic, or secondary when associated with various underlying systemic conditions. Patients with the myopathic form tend to have involvement of other systems, particularly the urinary system, and may require vesicostomy.

Primary disease predominates in the pediatric population, with approximately 40% of patients becoming symptomatic within the first month of life and 65% within the first year. The disease is termed idiopathic when secondary disease is excluded and no other anatomic or histopathologic cause is identified. Chronicity is defined as either congenital disease persisting during the first 2 months of life or persistence for greater than 6 months. Histopathology in some of these patients may demonstrate diverse findings, such as hypoganglionosis, degenerative changes in smooth muscle fibers, additional muscle layer, collagen deposition, degeneration of neurons and axons, and proliferation of neurons, nerve fibers, or glial cells.

Children with intestinal pseudo-obstruction present with periodic vomiting, diarrhea, abdominal distention, constipation, pain, and weight loss. Bacterial overgrowth can occur secondary to stasis. Plain films demonstrate dilated loops of bowel, particularly the colon, with air-fluid levels that suggest obstruction but actually represent a severe lack of peristalsis (Figs. 140-1 and 140-2). Mega-

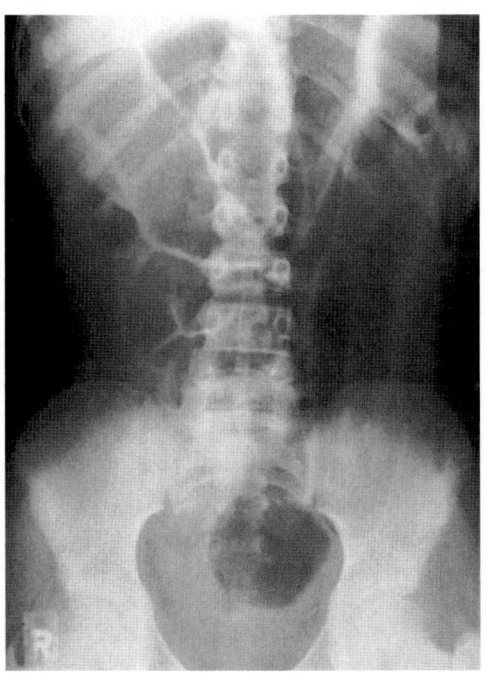

A

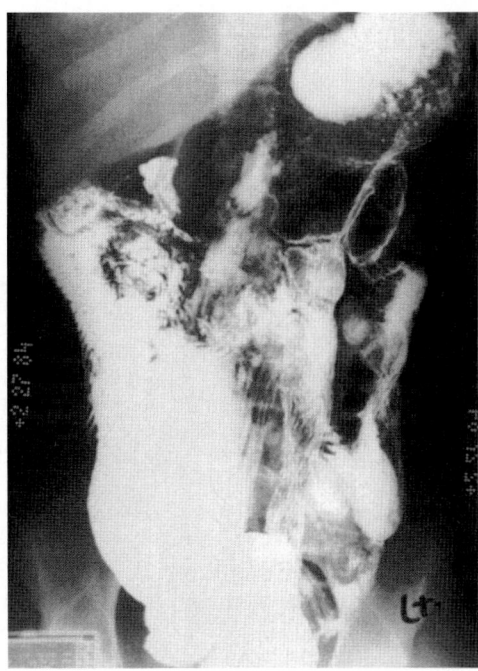

B

FIGURE 140-1. Intestinal pseudo-obstruction. **A,** Plain radiograph of the abdomen shows diffuse gaseous dilation of the small bowel. **B,** Small intestinal series reveals diffuse dilation of the bowel, with no focal obstructive lesion identified. At surgery, no mechanical obstruction was found. Ganglion cells were present in the myenteric plexus but were abnormal.

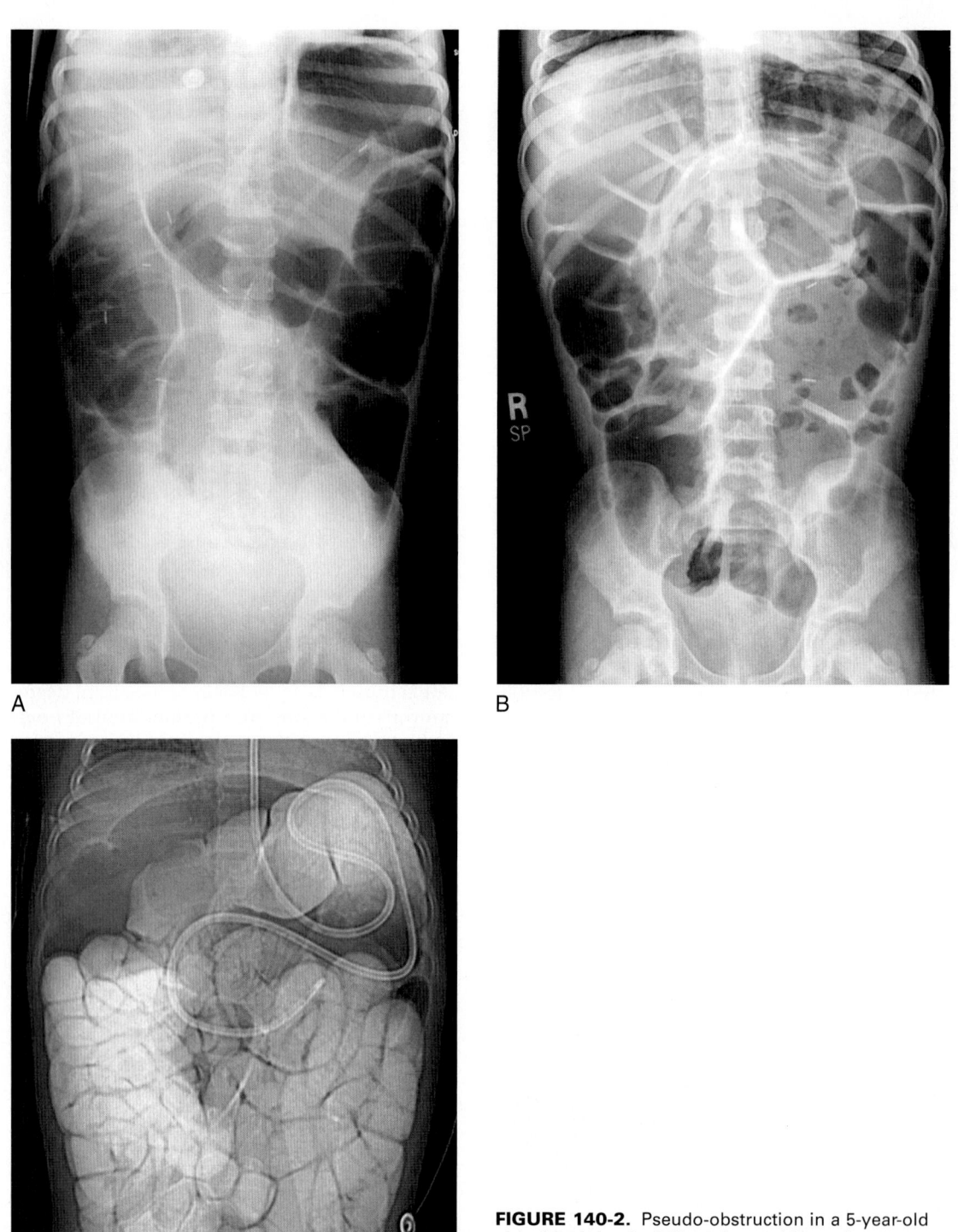

FIGURE 140-2. Pseudo-obstruction in a 5-year-old girl with abdominal distention and intermittent diarrhea. **A** and **B,** Abdominal radiographs on two different dates show different degree of diffuse colonic distention without obstruction. **C,** Enteroclysis image shows contrast material in the normal small bowel and early filling of the dilated colon. There is a duodenal tube in place.

colon is typically found with contrast enema, without the diagnostic findings of Hirschsprung disease. Contrast small bowel and enema studies show poor motor activity in affected parts of the bowel but are otherwise not specific. Gut dilation is common in the colon, stomach, and small bowel and can assume massive proportions (Fig. 140-3). Most children can be treated conservatively, although parenteral nutrition may be required. In a minority of patients, temporary diversion enterostomy or segmental resection may be warranted.

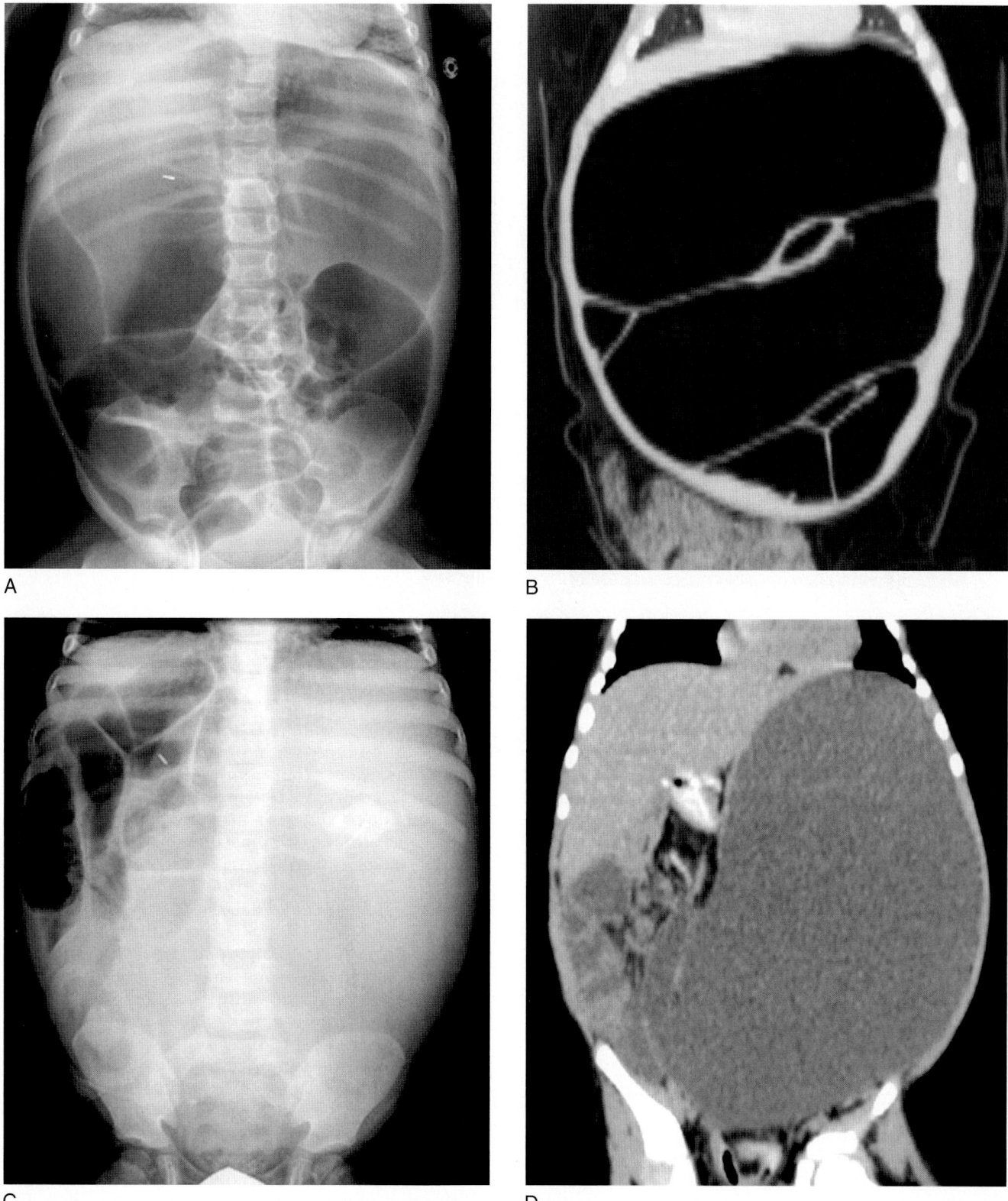

FIGURE 140-3. Five-year-old boy with myopathic pseudo-obstruction and a long history of feeding intolerance, dependent on total parenteral nutrition. **A,** Radiograph shows remarkable dilation of the colon. **B,** Coronal reformat from CT confirms colonic dilation. The small bowel was not dilated. **C,** Abdominal radiograph 6 months later shows a large mass in left abdomen, beneath the gastrostomy button. **D,** Coronal reformat from CT outlines the massively dilated stomach.

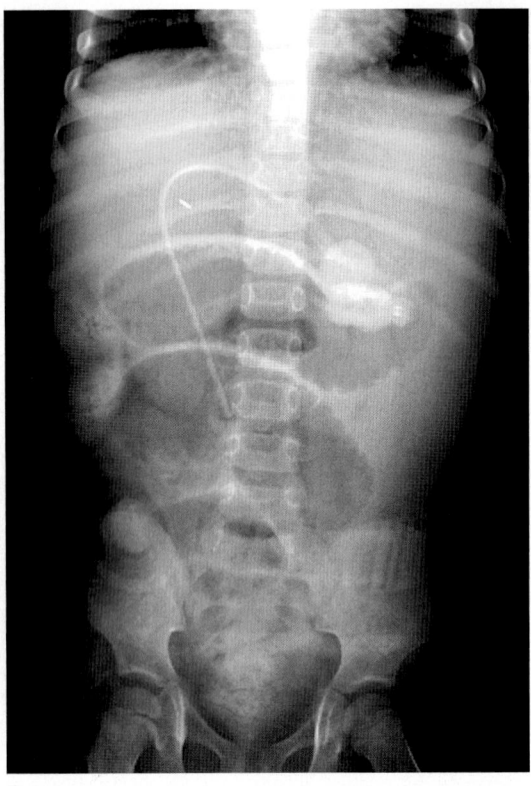

E

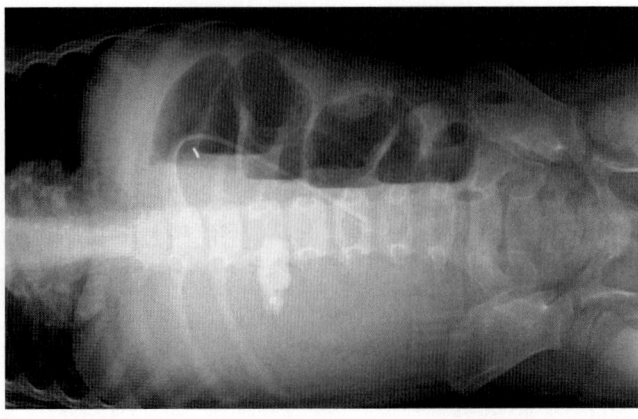

F

FIGURE 140-3, *cont'd.* Five-year-old boy with myopathic pseudo-obstruction and a long history of feeding intolerance, dependent on total parenteral nutrition. **E** and **F**, Flat radiograph **(E)** and left-side-down decubitus view **(F)** approximately 6 months later show acute small bowel dilation with air-fluid levels on the decubitus view.

Secondary disease is associated with connective tissue disorders such as scleroderma, dermatomyositis, and muscular dystrophies; infiltrative diseases such as amyloidosis; nervous system diseases such as myotonic dystrophy and familial dysautonomia; postviral syndromes such as Epstein-Barr, cytomegalovirus, herpes zoster, and rotavirus; and endocrine disease such as hypothyroidism (Fig. 140-4).

Pseudo-obstruction (or failure of normal intestinal motility) may be:

- **Primary (more common in pediatrics)**
  - **Neuropathic**
  - **Myopathic**
- **Secondary (e.g., scleroderma, dermatomyositis, myotonic dystrophy, familial dysautonomia, endocrinopathies)**

Neuronal intestinal dysplasia (NID) constitutes a form of primary disease; it is a disorder of intestinal innervation that can be diffuse or localized. Type A consists of abnormal sympathetic innervation of the intestine; type B consists of hyperplasia of the submucosal and myenteric plexus, with dysplastic and ectopic ganglion cells and increased acetylcholinesterase staining. The diagnosis of type B NID is quantitative and requires giant cells in 15% to 20% of all ganglia at submucosal biopsy. Neuronal dysplasia has been found in the proximal intestine of patients with Hirschsprung disease and can also be associated with neurofibromatosis and multiple endocrine neoplasia (MEN) type IIB. MEN type IIA can also mimic the presentation of colonic aganglionosis, but rectal biopsy shows giant ganglia.

Most children with NID present with constipation, although rectal bleeding has been described. Clinically, colonic involvement may mimic aganglionosis, but histologic examination reveals hyperplastic submucosal and myenteric plexus, giant neurons, and ganglia within the lamina propria. Contrast enema demonstrates a flaccid megacolon. Small-bowel series shows poor motor activity of the involved portions of the intestine, with focal areas of dilation and delayed passage of barium.

Irritable bowel syndrome, increasingly recognized as beginning in childhood, is a chronic, relapsing condition of abdominal pain and disturbance of bowel habits without an identified organic cause. The Rome II classification defines diagnostic criteria for children based on clinical symptoms of at least 3 months' duration. A careful history may reveal physical or sexual abuse in some cases. Symptoms consisting predominantly of constipation can be treated with serotonin agonists, whereas symptoms consisting predominantly of diarrhea can be treated with serotonin antagonists. A systematic review of treatments for chronic symptoms revealed a number of effective options, including famotidine (Pepcid), peppermint oil enteric-coated capsules, and cognitive-behavioral therapy or biofeedback. The mechanism of action of these therapeutic approaches is not fully understood.

In *functional constipation,* including irritable bowel syndrome, patients typically stool normally during the first 1 or 2 years of life, but the condition has been reported in infants. Affected children may suffer severe constipation,

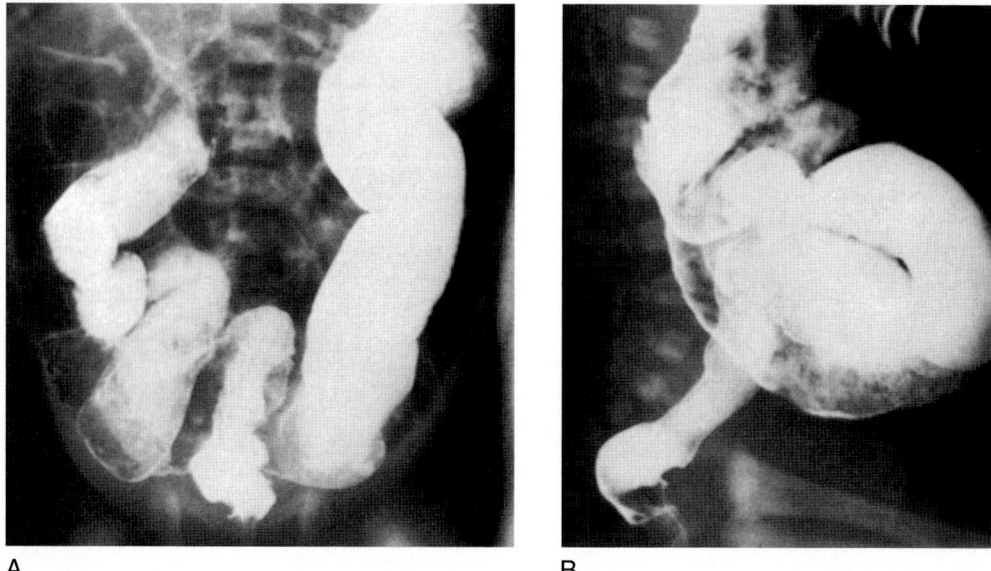

FIGURE 140-4. Frontal **(A)** and lateral **(B)** views of the abdomen following barium enema in a patient with congenital hypothyroidism. Obstipation was present before the other signs of hypothyroidism became manifest. An apparent transition from a small-caliber rectum to a dilated sigmoid mimics aganglionosis. (Courtesy of Dr. F. Lee, Pasadena, CA.)

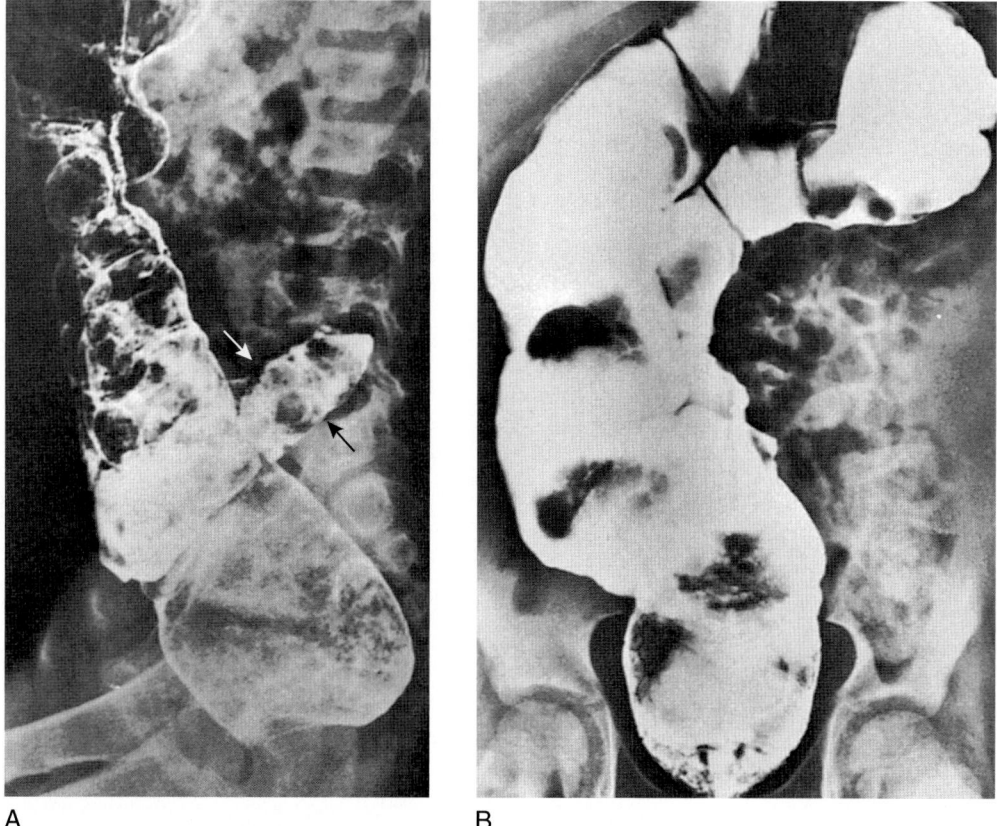

FIGURE 140-5. Functional megacolon. **A,** Lateral projection following a barium enema shows a markedly enlarged rectum that is filled with stool. *Arrows* point to the more normal-caliber proximal colon. The rectal shelf is well seen. **B,** Frontal projection during a barium enema shows fecal material throughout the distal colon down to and including the low rectum. A rectal biopsy confirmed normal ganglion cells.

which may lead to anal fissures, rectal bleeding, and painful defecation. Encopresis is common in this entity; colonic aganglionosis is much less common. Plain films demonstrate a capacious rectum filled with fecal material. Stool may back up all the way to the cecum, and secondary small bowel dilation may be seen. Contrast studies are often unnecessary, but if performed, they show a colon dilated to the anus and filled with fecal material; the rectum, and at times the sigmoid, is larger than the more proximal colon (Fig. 140-5). This appearance differs from that in Hirschsprung disease, in which the distal colon is smaller than the proximal colon. However, anal aganglionosis may not be distinguishable from functional constipation.

SUGGESTED READINGS

Borgaonkar MR, Lumb B: Acute on chronic intestinal pseudoobstruction responds to neostigmine. Dig Dis Sci 2000;45:1644-1647

Case records of the Massachusetts General Hospital: intestinal neuronal dysplasia associated with long-segment Hirschsprung's disease. N Engl J Med 1991;325:1865-1874

Glassman M, Spivak W, Mininberg D, et al: Chronic idiopathic intestinal pseudo-obstruction: a commonly misdiagnosed disease in infants and children. Pediatrics 1989;83:603

Hyman PE, Rasquin-Weber A, Fleisher DR, et al: Childhood functional gastrointestinal disorders. *In* Drossman DA, Corazziari E, Talley NJ, et al (eds): The Rome Criteria for Functional Gastrointestinal Disorders, 2nd ed. McLean, VA, Degnan Associates, 2000:533-576

Khan AH, Desjardins JG, Youssef S, et al: Gastrointestinal manifestations of Sipple syndrome in children. J Pediatr Surg 1987;22:719

Mousa H, Hyman PE, Cocjin J, et al: Long-term outcome of congenital intestinal pseudoobstruction. Dig Dis Sci 2002; 47:2298-2305

Puri P, Lake B, Nixon HH, et al: Neuronal colonic dysplasia: an unusual association of Hirschsprung's disease. J Pediatr Surg 1977;12:681

Schärli AF, Meier-Ruge W: Localized and disseminated forms of neuronal intestinal dysplasia mimicking Hirschsprung's disease. J Pediatr Surg 1981;16:164

Schuffler MD: Chronic intestinal pseudo-obstruction syndromes. Med Clin North Am 1981;65:1331-1357

Weydert JA, Ball TM, Davis MF: Systematic review of treatments for recurrent abdominal pain. Pediatrics 2003;111:e1-e11

Intussusception

KIMBERLY E. APPLEGATE

PATHOPHYSIOLOGY AND EPIDEMIOLOGY

Intussusception is an acquired invagination of the bowel into itself, usually involving both small and large bowel (Fig. 141-1). The more proximal bowel that invaginates into more distal bowel is termed the intussusceptum, whereas the recipient bowel that contains the intussusceptum is termed the intussuscipiens. Intussusception is an urgent condition, but prolonged delay in diagnosis is not uncommon, and it leads to an increased risk for obstruction, necrosis, and bowel perforation. Most cases in children between the ages of 2 months and 3 years are idiopathic—the etiology is unknown—but it is presumed that the typical childhood ileocolic intussusception results from hypertrophied lymphoid tissue in the terminal ileum (Peyer patches). Some reports suggest a viral etiology, most commonly adenovirus, but enterovirus, echovirus, and human herpes virus 6 have also been implicated. There may be an accompanying pathologic lead-point mass lesion in 5% to 6% of all children. Intestinal intussusception may occur along the entire length of the bowel from the duodenum to the colon, and intussuscepted bowel may prolapse through the rectum. However, cases of intussusception range from the classic, symptomatic, and urgent presentation, to short-segment, transient, and asymptomatic events, typically isolated to the small bowel, seen increasingly on multidetector computed tomography (CT) studies of the abdomen performed for other indications (Fig. 141-2).

The clinical signs and symptoms of intussusception are often nonspecific, and they overlap with those of gastroenteritis, malrotation with volvulus, and, in older children, Henoch-Schonlein purpura.

Intussusception, the most common cause of small bowel obstruction in children, occurs in at least 56 children per 100,000 per year in the United States. In frequency, it is second only to pyloric stenosis as a cause of gastrointestinal tract obstruction in children, occurring in boys more often than girls at a ratio of 3:2. Idiopathic intussusception occurs most commonly in infants aged between 2 months and 3 years, with a peak age of 5 to 9 months; large series report 57% to 85% of cases presenting before the age of 1 year (an average of 67% occur by age 1 year). Delay in diagnosis and treatment leads to an increase in bowel edema and ischemia, rendering enema reduction less successful, bowel resection more likely, and increasing the potential of death from bowel ischemia and perforation with supervening peritonitis.

Children with intussusception have fewer surgeries and a lower cost of care when cared for at a children's hospital, where there tends to be greater familiarity with the condition, and expertise and experience with nonoperative reduction and expedient management of

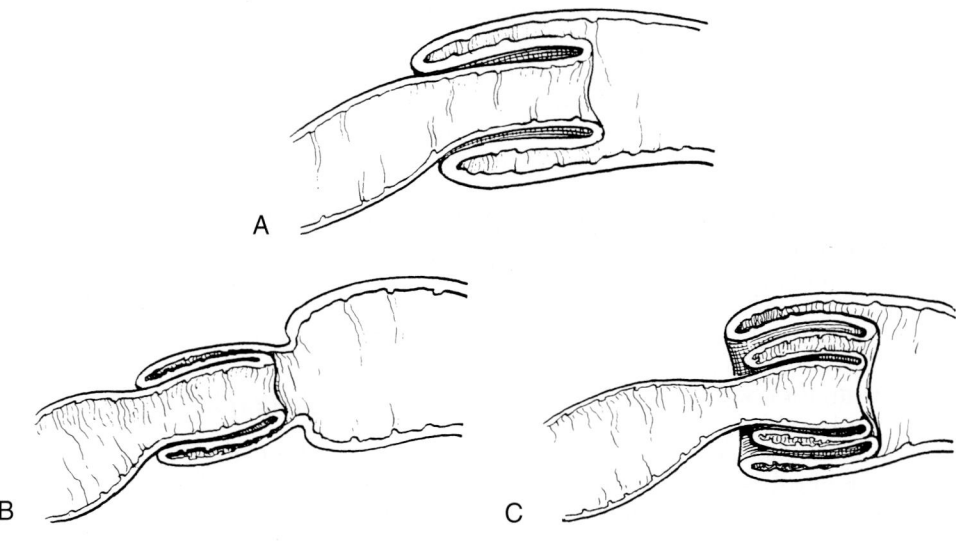

FIGURE 141-1. The common types of infantile intussusception, in longitudinal section. **A**, Ileocecal. **B**, Ileoileal. **C**, Ileoileocolic.

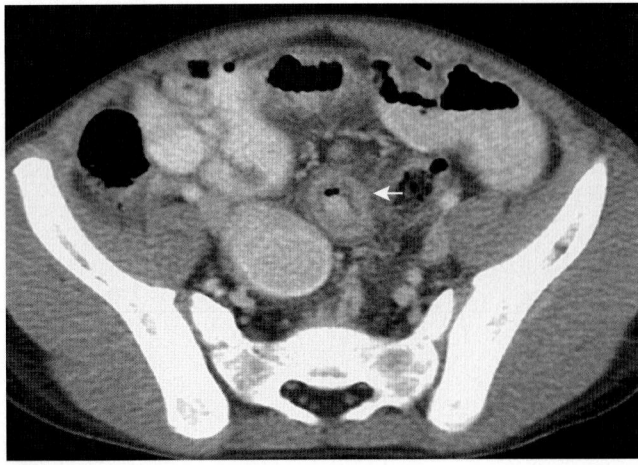
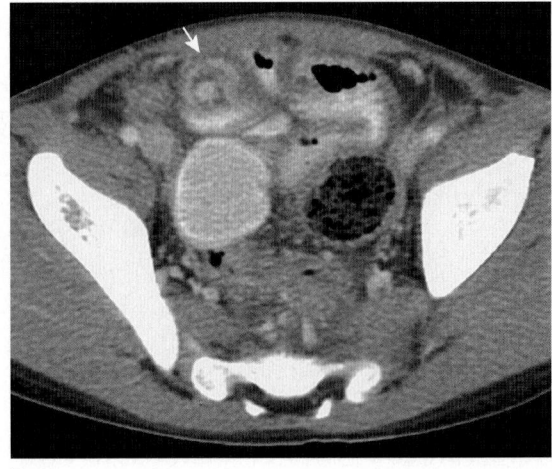

A   B

FIGURE 141-2. Transient intussusception of the small bowel in a young child undergoing abdominal CT imaging for routine follow-up of a testicular tumor. **A** and **B**, CT images of transient intussusception of the small bowel (*arrows*) that were not symptomatic and did not require treatment.

potential complications. There were 323 intussusception-associated deaths in U.S. infants reported to the Centers for Disease Control (CDC) between 1979 and 1997, with a higher rate of intussusception-related deaths among infants whose mothers were less than 20 years old, unmarried, and nonwhite, and who had less than a grade 12 education, suggesting that reduced access to specialized care, or delay in seeking care, contribute to the risk for death.

Rotavirus Vaccine

Shortly after the first rotavirus vaccine was introduced in the United States in 1998 for routine vaccination of infants at ages 2, 4, and 6 months, several reports to the CDC suggested an association between the vaccine and intussusception. The vaccine was removed from the world market in 1999. Subsequent investigations have not found a higher rate of intussusception after rotavirus vaccination, and two new vaccines have been developed.

CLINICAL PREDICTORS OF INTUSSUSCEPTION AND OF NONSURGICAL REDUCTION

The classic clinical presentation of the child with intussusception is colicky abdominal pain, vomiting, bloody stools, and a palpable abdominal mass. Children with intussusception should be diagnosed early to avoid bowel ischemia, necrosis, and surgery. However, this goal remains elusive: one report found that only 50% of children were correctly diagnosed at initial presentation to a health care provider. The classic triad of colicky abdominal pain (58% to 100% of cases), vomiting (up to 85% of cases), and bloody stools is present in less than 25% of children. There are no reliable clinical prediction models that identify all children with intussusception. Vomiting or diarrhea may lead to dehydration, which exaggerates lethargy. Venous hypertension leads to hematochezia, with a typical mixture of stool, blood, and blood clots that has been described as currant jelly stools, and this is highly suggestive of intussusception.

TABLE 141-1
Management of Intussusception

Plain radiographs have poor sensitivity and specificity for diagnosing intussusception but are useful for:
  Differential diagnosis
  Bowel obstruction
  Free air
Ultrasound is highly sensitive in detecting:
  Intussusception
  Lead point
  Diminished chance for nonoperative reduction in absence of Doppler blood flow and trapped intraperitoneal fluid
Enema is indicated for reduction in the absence of:
  Free air
  Peritoneal signs
Air is the preferred contrast agent, but water-soluble positive-contrast media may be used.

The most important factor, either alone or in combination with other factors, that predicts an unsuccessful enema reduction is a longer duration of symptoms: 48 hours is typically considered a significant delay. Other factors associated with lower rates of successful reduction include age less than 3 months, dehydration, small bowel obstruction, and intussusception encountered in the rectum (25% reduction rate).

IMAGING OF PATIENTS WITH SUSPECTED INTUSSUSCEPTION

Table 141-1 summarizes the evidence regarding imaging management of intussusception.

Diagnostic Abdominal Radiographs

Abdominal radiographs have an overall low sensitivity and specificity for the detection of intussusception (Table 141-2), even when viewed by experienced pedia-

TABLE 141-2

Sensitivity and Specificity of Diagnostic Imaging for Ileocolic Intussusception

Test	Sensitivity	Specificity
Abdominal radiograph	45%	Unknown
Ultrasound	98%-100%	88%-100%
Enema	100%	100%

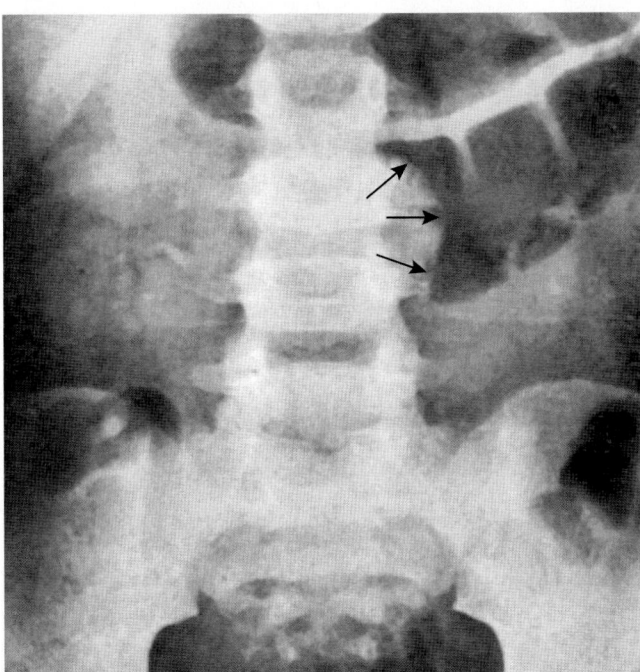

FIGURE 141-3. Ileocolic intussusception in a 4½-year-old patient. The leading edge of the intussusception is seen on this radiograph within the air column of the transverse colon *(arrows)*. No gas can be seen in the cecum or in the ascending colon. The intussusception was successfully reduced with hydrostatic pressure.

tric radiologists. Sargent and colleagues reported a sensitivity of 45% in 60 children when evaluated prospectively by pediatric radiologists, using the enema as the reference. The presence of a curvilinear mass within the course of the colon (the crescent sign), particularly in the transverse colon just beyond the hepatic flexure, is a nearly pathognomonic sign of intussusception (Fig. 141-3). The absence of stool and bowel gas in the ascending colon is one of the more suggestive signs of intussusception on radiographs. However, small bowel gas located in the right abdomen on radiographs may mimic ascending colon or cecal gas, and fluid filling the right colon in a patient with gastroenteritis may also show a similar appearance.

Abdominal radiographs may, on the other hand, serve to screen for other diagnoses suggested by a patient's symptoms, such as constipation. They are useful for assessing for the presence of small bowel obstruction and for free peritoneal air.

Diagnostic Ultrasound

Ultrasound (US) is highly sensitive in the detection of intussusception (see Table 141-2). Although the diagnosis can be confirmed at the enema procedure, US is the primary imaging modality for the initial diagnosis outside of the United States (e.g., used by 93% of European pediatric radiologists) and for a growing majority of pediatric radiologists in the United States. Initial evaluation by US circumvents the more invasive enema in patients who do not have intussusception, and it allows diagnosis of other conditions, such as mesenteric adenitis or colitis.

Intussusception can be reliably diagnosed by US when a donut, target, or "pseudokidney" sign is seen, most often in the right upper quadrant of the abdomen. This appearance arises from intussuscepted bowel and mesentery within the intussuscipiens, producing the donut or target appearance on transverse images and a hypoechoic mass with echogenic center on longitudinal images. Using a linear transducer, the bowel-within-bowel appearance can be delineated, and sometimes several concentric layers are seen on transverse images (Fig. 141-4). The optimal US technique is well described, and there are no known contraindications to or complications resulting from US for this purpose.

US also plays a role in the evaluation of the reducibility of an intussusception by Doppler assessment of blood flow. It helps to identify the presence of a lead-point mass, intussusception limited to small bowel, and alternative diagnoses. After reduction enema, US can also be helpful in determining the presence of a residual intussusception, although this can be difficult after an air enema reduction. US is the preferred screening test for children with a low clinical probability of intussusception.

US screening in children has been suggested to reduce cost, radiation exposure, and anxiety in both patients and parents over the discomfort of the enema. Its accuracy approaches 100% in experienced hands, with a sensitivity of 98% to 100% and a specificity reported at 88% to 100%. Its cost effectiveness depends on the prevalence of intussusception. One approach is for patients clinically estimated to have a high probability to be directed to enema diagnosis and reduction, whereas those patients with a lower clinical suspicion might be directed first to US. Future research is needed to further refine initial diagnostic criteria.

Ultrasound Predictors of Enema Reducibility and Bowel Necrosis

Enema reduction should be undertaken in children with intussusception after surgical consultation. The only absolute contraindications to enema reduction are signs of peritonitis on clinical examination or free air on abdominal radiographs (Table 141-3). The rate of successful overall reduction is better with air enema than with liquid enema, but the outcome depends on the experience of the radiologist. The use of delayed repeat enema for the reduction of intussusception shows promise, but data on appropriate methods and timing are limited. In patients with recurrent intussusception,

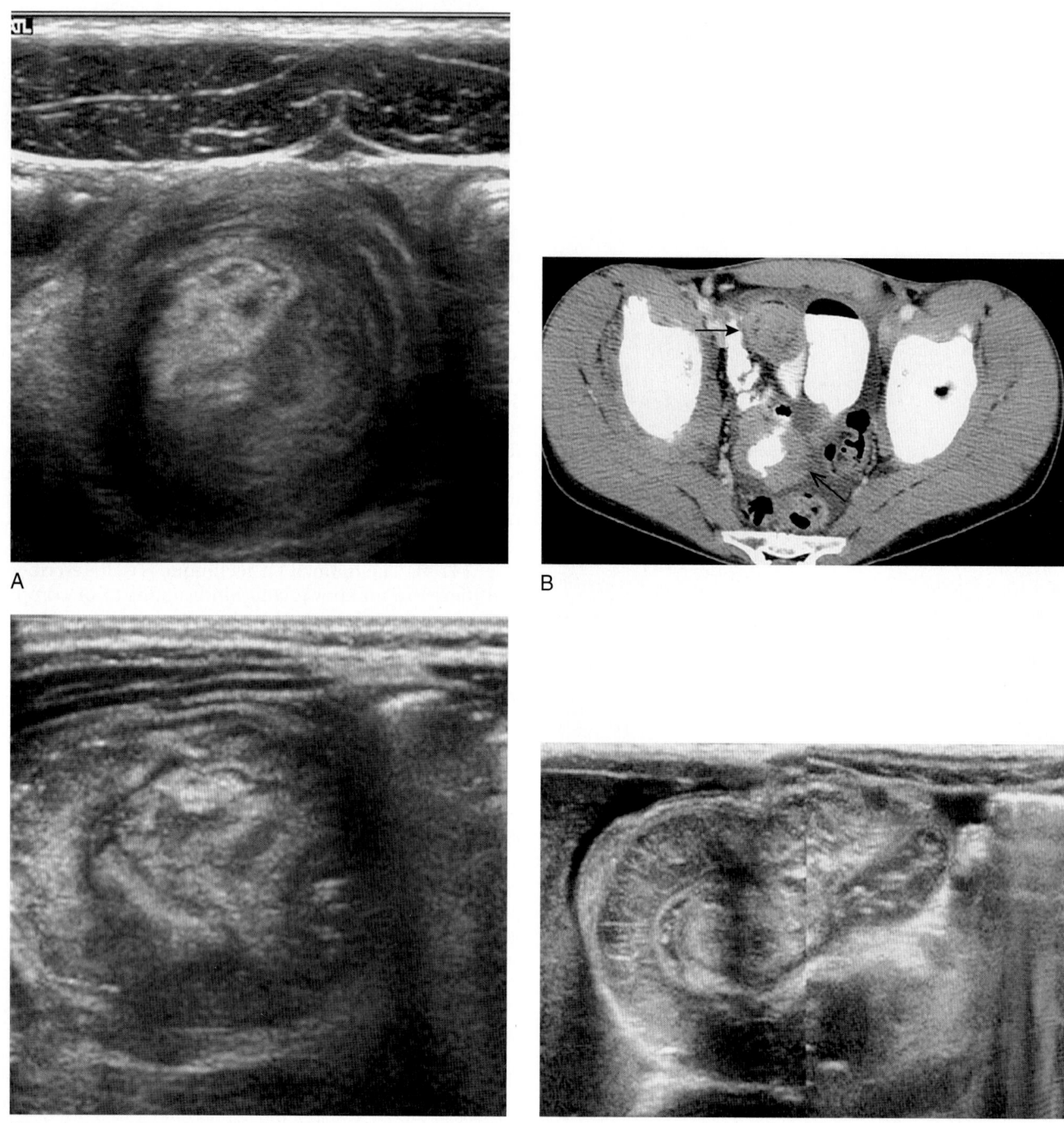

FIGURE 141-4. Burkitt lymphoma as a lead point for intussusception. Adolescent boy with Burkitt lymphoma and ileoileal intussusception. **A,** The donut sign of intussusception at US, with linear transducer. The image shows an intussusception in the midline, directly beneath the rectus muscles, with small bowel and echogenic mesentery (intussusceptum) within the lumen of the outer bowel (intussuscipiens). **B,** The CT image of the pelvis shows both the intussusception in the right lower quadrant anteriorly *(arrow)* and also ascites and tumor caking *(open arrow)* on the outer wall of a loop of ileum dorsal to the intussusception. **C,** Transverse US of right flank in a 3-year-old girl with idiopathic intussusception shows small bowel and mesentery within the intussusceptum complex. **D,** In patient shown in **C,** longitudinal image along right flank outlines the small bowel intussuscepting into the colon. The outer layer, beyond the echogenic mesentery, is composed of the returning sleeve of small bowel and the intussuscipiens. (**C** and **D,** courtesy of Marta Hernanz-Schulman, Nashville, TN.)

including multiple recurrences, enema remains the preferred method of reduction.

Lack of color Doppler signal in the wall of the intussuscepted bowel suggests bowel ischemia (Fig. 141-5). Free intraperitoneal fluid in small or moderate amounts is present in approximately half of children. There are conflicting reports that free peritoneal fluid is associated with fewer successful reductions. Similarly, some reports note that thicker bowel wall is associated with fewer successful enema reductions, but others do not find this association. Some studies report that the presence of lymph nodes trapped in the intussusception is associated

TABLE 141-3

Image-Guided Reduction of Intussusception

ABSOLUTE CONTRAINDICATIONS
Peritonitis
Free intraperitoneal air

RELATIVE CONTRAINDICATIONS
High fever, leukocytosis, abdominal tenderness (especially rebound tenderness)
Severe dehydration or profound lethargy

HYDROSTATIC REDUCTION
Be certain patient is well hydrated.
Maintain pressure head no greater than 1 m H_2O.
Make three attempts of 3 minutes each.
Be sure buttocks are well sealed.
Reduction is incomplete unless substantial amounts of small bowel are easily filled.

PNEUMATIC REDUCTION
Use available devices to control pressure.
Start at 80 mm Hg; do not exceed 120 mm Hg.
Limit each attempt to 4 minutes.
Even after small bowel is filled with air, evaluate cecum for residual mass.

with fewer successful reductions. Although some of these findings are associated with fewer successful reductions, none represents a contraindication to enema reduction. As stated earlier, the only reasons to avoid enema reduction are signs of peritonitis and free intraperitoneal air.

PATHOLOGIC LEAD POINTS

Approximately 5% to 6% of intussusceptions in children are caused by pathologic lead points, either focal masses or a diffuse bowel wall abnormality. The traditional view is that focal lead points are more common in older children. Although the absolute numbers of lead points are approximately equal in infants and in older children, the percentage of lead points in infants is lower because of the greater number of intussusceptions occurring in this age group. The most common focal lead points are (in decreasing order of incidence) Meckel diverticulum, duplication cyst, polyp, and lymphoma. In older children, lymphoma is the more likely lead point. Diffuse lead points are most commonly associated with cystic fibrosis or Henoch-Schönlein purpura.

The detection of lead points by imaging remains problematic, although US is the noninvasive standard of reference. US is reported to identify approximately 66% of lead points, and approximately 40% are identified by positive-contrast liquid enema. Air enema has a lower rate of detection (11%), leading some to suggest that US be used afterward to search for lead points. However, such an approach would be hindered by air introduced during the enema, and it seems to offer little advantage over a pre-enema diagnostic US examination. Other cross-sectional imaging modalities, such as CT, can be used for further evaluation in selected patients (see Fig. 141-4). However, CT and MRI are not part of the routine initial evaluation of suspected intussusception.

ENEMA TECHNIQUES AND REDUCTION RATES

For reduction, the air enema is considered superior to positive-contrast liquid enema for several reasons. It is cleaner, as there is no liquid or stool spillage on the table, on the patient, or on the field of view. It is considered safer, because if perforation does occur, there is less spillage of fecal material and liquid into the peritoneal cavity. Reduction is usually faster, so there is less radiation exposure. The rates of recurrence of intussusception after air or after liquid enema reductions do not differ (both are approximately 10%).

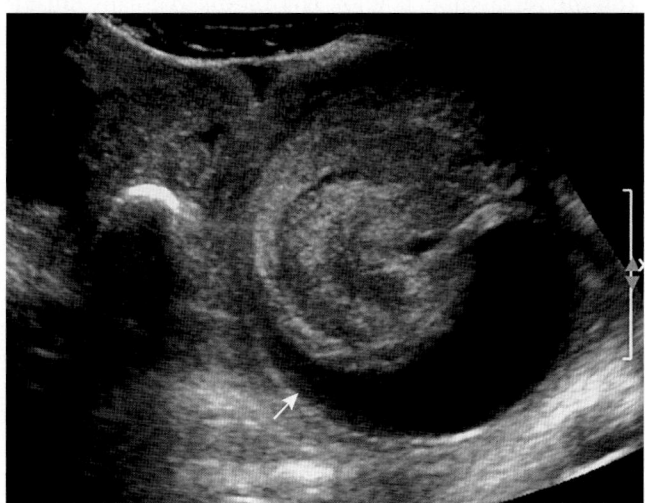

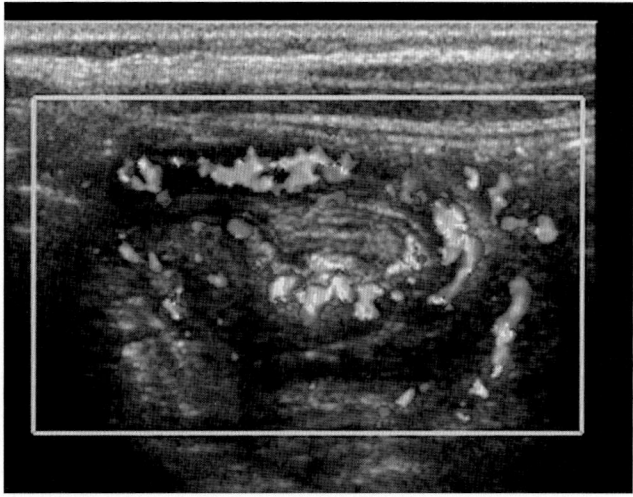

A   B

FIGURE 141-5. Intussusception. **A,** Trapped fluid in a teenage boy with Burkitt lymphoma and small bowel intussusception. US image of the intussusception shows anechoic fluid *(arrow)* trapped within the lumen of the intussuscipiens adjacent to the intussusceptum. A small amount of free intraperitoneal fluid is also noted between the intussusception and adjoining bowel loop, beneath the rectus muscle of the abdominal wall. **B,** Gray scale depiction of color Doppler transverse image of right flank in a different patient, outlining abundant flow to intussusceptum and intussuscipiens. The intussusception was successfully and rapidly reduced with air enema. (**B,** *see color plate.*) (**B,** courtesy of Dr. Marta Hernanz-Schulman, Nashville, TN.)

TABLE 141-4					
Summary of Published Studies* of Enema Reduction and Perforation Rates[†]					
		Studies (*N*)	Reduction Rate (%)	Studies (*N*)	Perforation Rate (%)
All	Simple	74	72.8 (1.8)	66	0.80 (0.16)
	Weighted	—	75.9 (0.4)	—	0.76 (0.10)
Hydrostatic	Simple	48	68.6 (2.4)	42	0.71 (0.19)
	Weighted	—	73.0 (0.5)	—	0.57 (0.10)
Pneumatic	Simple	26	81.3 (1.3)	24	0.98 (0.31)
	Weighted	—	81.5 (0.7)	—	1.02 (0.16)
p-value[‡]		—	<.001	—	.02

*Excludes two very large studies by Guo et al. (1986) and Zhang et al. (1986).
[†]All values are mean (standard error) from unweighted (simple) and weighted estimates. Weighted estimates use the sample size to adjust the reported mean reduction and perforation rates.
[‡]p-values based on logistic regression. Compare hydrostatic with pneumatic rate and perforation rate.
From Applegate KE: Intussusception in children: diagnostic imaging and treatment. *In* Blackmore CC, Medina S (eds): Evidence-Based Imaging. New York, Springer, 2006.

More than 70 published studies of enema reduction report an average reduction rate of 76% (Table 141-4). When the reduction rates are weighted by the number of children in each study, the average reduction rate for air is significantly better than liquid (82% for air and 73% for liquid). In the largest published series, Gu and colleagues used air enema in 9028 children and reported reduction rates of 95%. However, although the air enema may be preferred in experienced hands, the liquid enema is also safe and effective. There are two randomized controlled trials of the reduction rates of air versus liquid enema. One concluded that air was superior to liquid enema and the other showed no difference, although the sample size was small. The use of sedation may reduce the intra-abdominal pressure children create by the Valsalva maneuver, which is reported to increase safety during enema reduction. The superior air enema results may be due to the level of experience of those who use air reduction techniques, as well as to the presence of the higher intraluminal pressure for air compared with standard hydrostatic reduction. In 2004, 65% of pediatric radiologists in the United States reported using air enema, 33% liquid enema, and 3% liquid enema with sonographic guidance.

All children should have surgical consultation prior to enema (1) to assess for peritoneal signs precluding enema, (2) to identify children whose intussusception may not be reduced with enema or who are found to have perforation, (3) for urgent surgery in case of perforation, and (4) for management after reduction. Before enema reduction, dehydration should be treated with intravenous fluid resuscitation. Children with evidence of peritonitis, shock, sepsis, or free air on abdominal radiographs are not candidates for enema. On the basis of sonographic or enema diagnosis before surgery, the rate of spontaneous reduction is estimated to be 10%.

Air Enema Technique

In the air enema technique, the enema tip should be placed in the child's rectum and taped in place with abundant tape. The tape can be shaped into a funnel along the tube, to help form a seal. The buttocks are taped tightly together, and an assistant should also aid by holding the buttocks closed, whether the child is in a supine or a prone position. This is important because air leaking around the tube diminishes the pressure head. Air is rapidly insufflated into the colon under fluoroscopic observation, up to a constant pressure of 120 mm Hg, thus maximizing reduction and minimizing the risk for perforation. Once the intussusception is encountered, its reduction is followed fluoroscopically until it is completely reduced (Fig. 141-6). The use of pulsed fluoroscopy at a low setting, if available, is very important for reducing the radiation dosage, particularly when the reduction is lengthy. Fluoro grabs can document the progress of the reduction, without additional exposure. The radiologist should be vigilant for the appearance of free intraperitoneal air, which can be inconspicuous at first. Air should flow freely from the cecum into the distal small bowel loops to signify complete reduction. In case of perforation, it is very important to open the buttocks and the rectal tube, to allow colonic air to escape outside the patient; in addition, it is very important to have a large-gauge needle available to decompress the peritoneal cavity, as air that escapes the colon and enters the cavity can result in a tension pneumoperitoneum, elevating the diaphragm and impeding adequate breathing. Images with the intussusception reduced to the cecum can be compared with later images to help determine the distension of small bowel loops with insufflated air, thus outlining a successful reduction, particularly in potentially confusing cases that involve small bowel loops dilated from secondary small bowel obstruction.

Positive-contrast liquid enema tends to outline the small bowel loops to better advantage, and may outline the appendix at the cecal tip (Fig. 141-7). Ileoileal components may be more conspicuously identified (see Fig. 141-7). Rarely, the appendix intussuscepts into the cecum, causing abdominal pain (Fig. 141-8).

The Rule of Threes

A general guideline to the liquid enema technique, often taught to radiology residents, is the "rule of 3s": three attempts of 3 minutes' duration, with the liquid enema

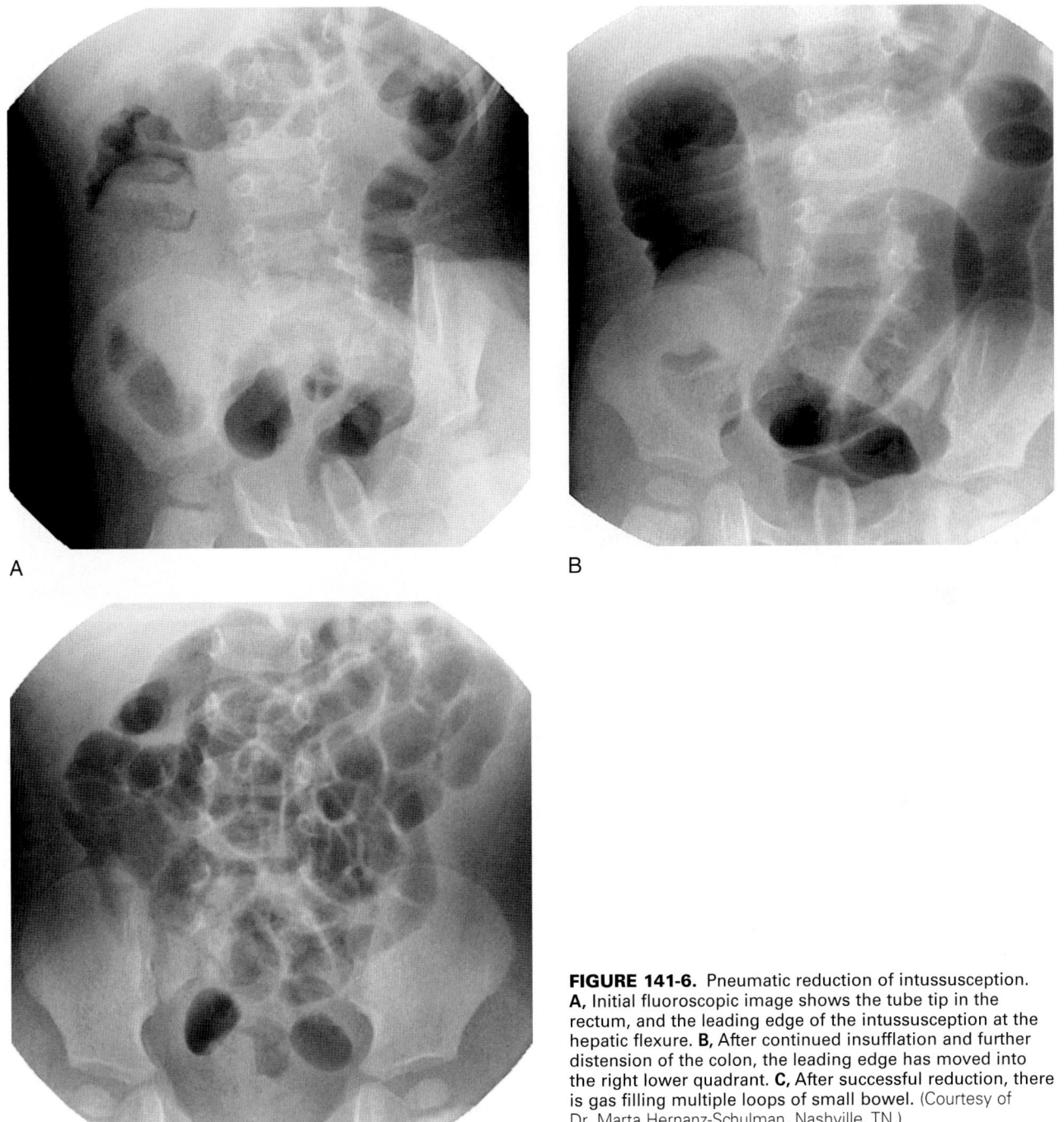

A

B

C

FIGURE 141-6. Pneumatic reduction of intussusception. **A,** Initial fluoroscopic image shows the tube tip in the rectum, and the leading edge of the intussusception at the hepatic flexure. **B,** After continued insufflation and further distension of the colon, the leading edge has moved into the right lower quadrant. **C,** After successful reduction, there is gas filling multiple loops of small bowel. (Courtesy of Dr. Marta Hernanz-Schulman, Nashville, TN.)

bag at 3 feet above the fluoroscopy table (see Table 141-3). Although there is little evidence to support this rule, particularly regarding the height of the enema bag, it serves well as a general guideline. Many experienced pediatric radiologists alter this general guide in response to the clinical status of the patient and the movement of the intussusceptum mass achieved with the initial enema, using higher pressures and more frequent attempts for longer periods of time. A study by Kuta and Benator of the pressures generated by a column of liquid media indicates that various media differ in the height at which a pressure of 120 mm Hg is generated. The air enema

allows control and documentation of the pressure used. Using the air enema technique, many pediatric radiologists suggest limiting each attempt to 4 minutes. The examination is tailored to the patient and performed in collaboration with the surgeon.

Radiation Dosage

The radiation dosage a child receives depends on a number of factors, including the type of fluoroscopy equipment, the use of pulsed fluoroscopy, the ease of reduction, the fluoroscopy time, and the contrast medium.

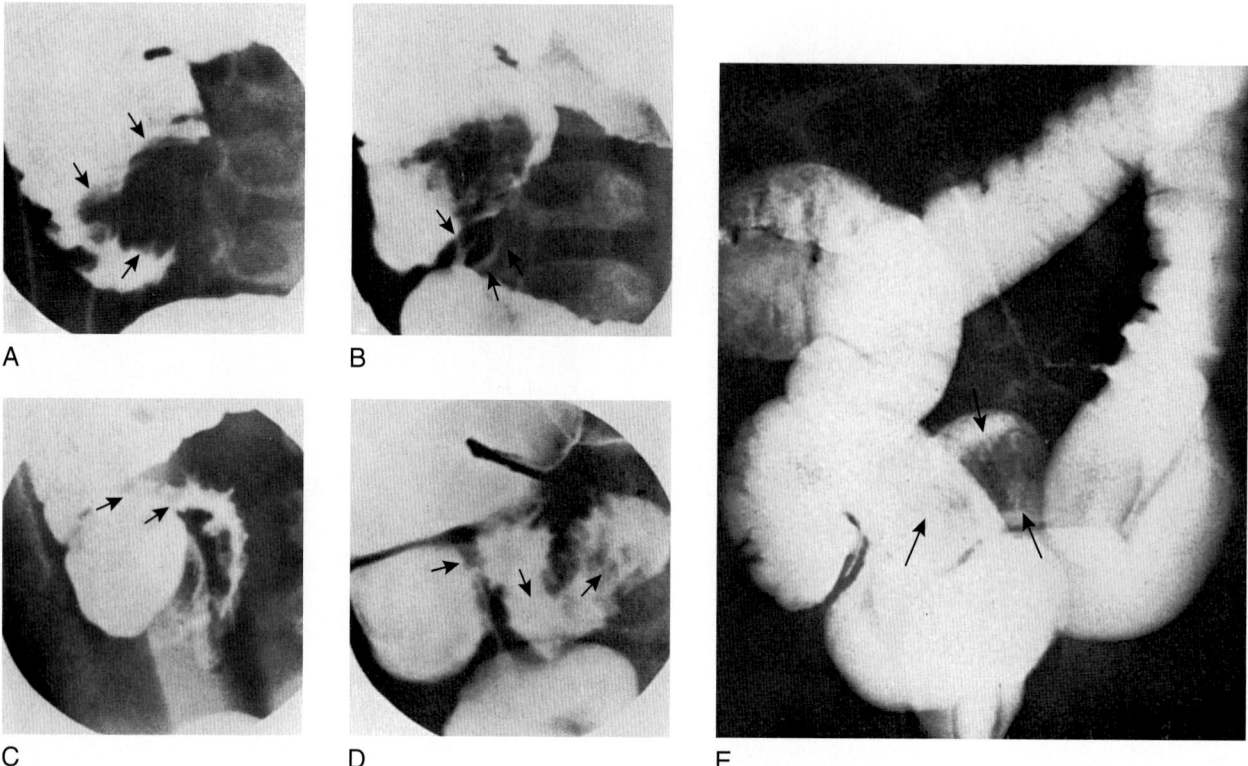

FIGURE 141-7. Hydrostatic reduction. Serial radiographic changes at the ileocecal valve during hydrostatic reduction of intussusception in an 18-month-old infant. **A,** The intussusception has moved proximally from the transverse colon into the cecum, where it causes a filling defect (*arrows*). **B,** The appendix is beginning to fill (*arrows*), and the cecal filling defect is smaller. **C,** The terminal ileum is beginning to fill (*arrows*), and the cecal filling defect has disappeared. **D,** The terminal ileum is normally dilated (*arrows*), with normal mucosal relief. **E,** In another child, residual ileoileal intussusception *(arrows)* in the terminal ileum after hydrostatic reduction of the colic component of an ileoileocolic intussusception. The leading edge was initially encountered at splenic flexure.

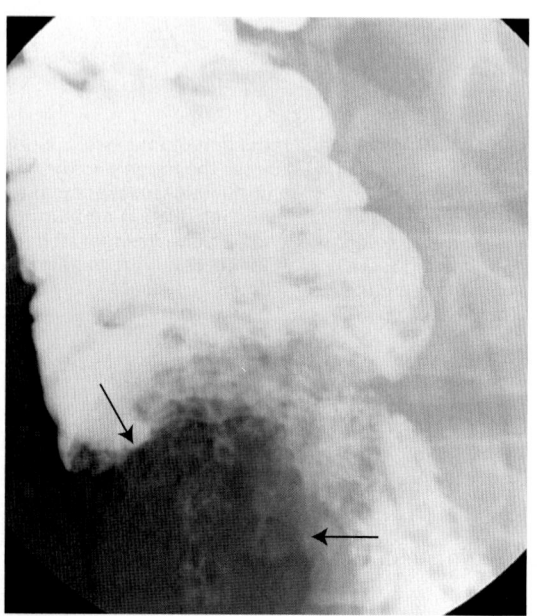

FIGURE 141-8. Ileocolic intussusception with inverted appendix in a teenage girl with recurrent abdominal pain and history of chronic constipation. Right lower quadrant image during liquid enema shows a mass *(arrows)* within the cecum. This was shown to be caused by an inverted appendix at colonoscopy on the same day.

Experienced pediatric radiologists using air enema averaged 95 seconds of fluoroscopy time to reduce an intussusception, and 42 seconds to exclude one in a child without intussusception. Air enema radiation dosages average one-third to one-half less than the dosage for liquid enema. In 2003, Henrikson and coworkers estimated that the average radiation dosage saved was 8.2 mSv (the average dosage for a negative enema) per patient.

Perforation

The most concerning potential complication of enema is bowel perforation. In a summary of over 60 studies, the mean perforation rate is less than 1% (see Table 141-4). Although the air technique tends to have higher perforation rates (1.0% versus 0.6%), the differences are not statistically significant.

The risk for perforation depends on each radiologist's patient population and technique. Although determination of clinical predictors of perforation is complicated by a lack of prospective studies, a key factor is symptom length greater than 48 hours. Several reports in both pig models and children suggest that there may be pre-existing focal perforation in the necrotic intussuscipiens or, less commonly, the intussusceptum, that are rarely radiographically apparent as free air before reduction, but are uncovered during the reduction process. The most common site is at or just proximal to the intussusception in the transverse colon.

In 1989, Campbell surveyed enema techniques and complications of North American pediatric radiologists. Respondents' combined experience was 14,000 intussusception enemas. Although they did not report enema reduction rates, the combined perforation rate was 0.39% (55 per 14,000), with only one death. This study remains the basis for the perforation risk when explained to parents to obtain consent prior to enema reduction (i.e., 1 in 250 to 1 in 300).

Barium is no longer the liquid contrast medium of choice for reduction of intussusception because of the risks for barium peritonitis, infection, and adhesions when perforation occurs during the enema. Although iodinated contrast is now preferred and is considered a safer agent than barium, it nevertheless may produce fluid and electrolyte shifts if perforation occurs, because contrast medium is absorbed from the peritoneum.

One complication unique to air enema is the tension pneumoperitoneum. In an early report, two deaths occurred from this complication, leading the proponents of air enema to advise having an 18-gauge needle readily available in the fluoroscopy room for emergent decompression. Although this is theoretically possible, there have been no reports of air embolism.

ALTERNATIVE ENEMA APPROACHES

A number of different approaches have been described to try to improve intussusception reduction via enema. These include sedation, anesthesia, use of glucagon, manual palpation, and delayed repeat enema. Except for the delayed repeat enema, none of these approaches has been proven to increase the rate of successful reduction.

Fluoroscopy versus Sonography

In North American and most European centers, fluoroscopy is almost always used during enema reduction. In the East and some European centers, sonographic guidance avoids radiation exposure. Reports on the use of sonography with either water or air reduction show rates of successful reduction as high or higher than with fluoroscopic techniques. However, the experience level required for these techniques has not been evaluated.

Delayed Repeat Enema

In children who fail an initial enema reduction attempt, delayed repeat enema may avoid the need for surgical reduction. The use of an additional (delayed) attempt, between 30 minutes and 19 hours after the initial procedure, has shown promise in increasing the success of enema reductions. Four studies report further reduction in 50% to 82% of cases that do not reduce at the initial enema. Further research to understand optimal timing and technique for delayed repeat enemas is needed. Daneman and Navarro (2004), with the largest reported experience to date, suggest a delay of 2 to 4 hours until further research yields more rigorous

guidelines. The child must remain clinically stable and be appropriately monitored during this time interval. Delayed enema should not be attempted if the initial enema does not move the intussusception at all.

SURGICAL MANAGEMENT AND COMPLICATIONS

The costs of surgical care are four to five times the costs of nonsurgical management. Depending on the patient population, approximately 20% to 40% of children who undergo surgical reduction of their intussusception will require bowel resection. The long-term risk for small bowel obstruction from adhesions is approximately 8% for neonates and 3% to 5% for children older than 1 month.

Intussusception limited to the small bowel may occur after intra-abdominal or retroperitoneal surgery in children (Fig. 141-9) and at times requires surgical reduction.

Management of Recurrent Cases

Intussusception recurrence rates average 10% in large series (range, 5% to 15%), regardless of whether the technique involved air or liquid enema. The recurrence rates are less than or equal to 5% when surgical reduction is performed, presumably because of the development of adhesions. Repeat enema is both safe and effective in recurrent intussusception, as long as the child remains clinically stable. Approximately 50% of children who develop recurrent intussusception present

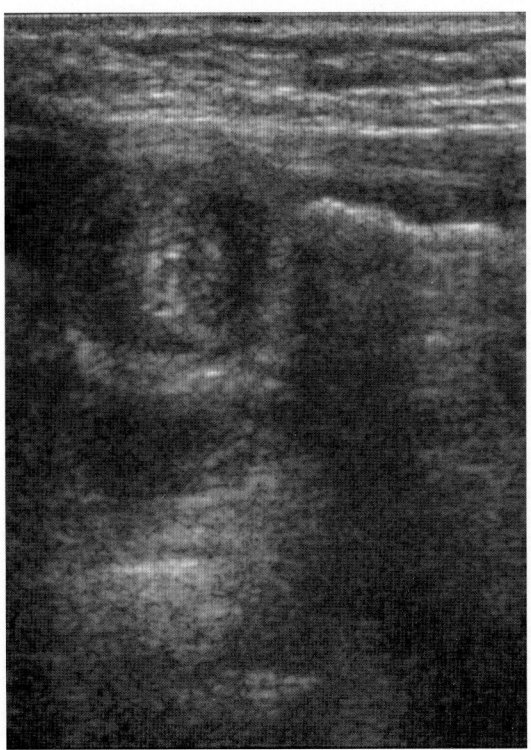

FIGURE 141-9. US scan of a patient who developed intermittent pain after a laparotomy shows an enteroenteric intussusception in the right midabdomen. This intussusception reduced spontaneously.

within 48 hours, although recurrences have been reported up to 18 months later. No clear risk factors are known to explain why some children have recurrences, although some have focal pathologic lead points. Nevertheless, the risk for lead points in children with recurrent intussusception is low. In the large series of 763 children reported by Daneman and colleagues, leads points were present in only 8% of recurrent intussusceptions, only slightly higher than the 5% to 6% incidence of lead points at first presentation of intussusception. No predictive clinical factors have been identified for the presence of lead points in children with recurrent intussusception. In children with a diffuse bowel abnormality such as cystic fibrosis, Henoch-Schönlein purpura, or celiac disease, enema reduction may be used more aggressively than in those with focal lead points who require surgery.

When there is concern for the presence of pathologic lead points, US may play an important role, detecting as many as 60%. Although US does not detect all lead points, the risk of missing a lead point without other signs or symptoms to guide management is unlikely. Ein reviewed 1200 intussusception cases over 40 years at one institution to analyze this risk. When the enema failed to detect lymphoma as a lead point, Ein noted the presence of clinical signs of illness of greater than 1 week, patient age greater than 3 years, weight loss, and palpable mass in all of these children.

In a randomized, double-blind trial comparing 144 children who received intramuscular corticosteroids with 137 who received placebo before air enema reduction, Lin and colleagues reported significantly fewer intussusception recurrences at 6 months. There were no recurrences in the children who received dexamethasone, compared with 5% in the placebo group. They hypothesized that steroids decreased the volume of mesenteric adenopathy and lymphoid hyperplasia in the terminal ileum and thus the risk for recurrence. However, further investigation of the risks and benefits of this intervention is needed.

SUGGESTED READINGS

Armstrong EA, Dunbar JS, Graviss ER, et al: Intussusception complicated by distal perforation of the colon. Radiology 1980;136:77-81

Beasley S: Intussusception. Pediatr Radiol 2004;34:302-304

Blane CE, DiPietro ME, White SJ, et al: An analysis of bowel perforation in patients with intussusception. J Can Assoc Radiol 1984;35:113-115

Bratton SL, Haberkern CM, Waldhausen JH, et al: Intussusception: hospital size and risk of surgery. Pediatrics 2001;107:299-303

Britton I, Wilkinson AG. Ultrasound features of intussusception predicting outcome of air enema. Pediatr Radiol 1999;29:705-710

Campbell JB: Contrast media in intussusception. Pediatr Radiol 1989;19:293-296

Daneman A, Alton DJ, Lobo E, et al: Patterns of recurrence of intussusception in children: a 17-year review. Pediatr Radiol 1998;28:913-919

Daneman A, Navarro O: Intussusception. Part 1: A review of diagnostic approaches. Pediatr Radiol 2003;33:79-85

Daneman A, Navarro O: Intussusception. Part 2: An update on the evolution of management. Pediatr Radiol 2004;34:97-108

Del-Pozo G, Gonzalez-Spinola J, Gomez-Anson B, et al: Intussusception: trapped peritoneal fluid detected with US: relationship to reducibility and ischemia. Radiology 1996; 201:379-383

Ein SH: Leading points in childhood intussusception. J Pediatr Surg 1976;11(2):209-211

Eklof O, Hartelius H: Reliability of the abdominal plain film diagnosis in pediatric patients with suspected intussusception. Pediatr Radiol 1980;9:199-206

Gorenstein A, Raucher A, Serour F, et al: Intussusception in children: reduction with repeated, delayed air enema. Radiology 1998;206:721-724

Gu L, Alton D, Daneman A, et al: John Caffey Award. Intussusception reduction in children by rectal insufflation of air. AJR Am J Roentgenol 1988;150:1345-1348

Gu L, Zhu H, Wang S, et al: Sonographic guidance of air enema for intussusception reduction in children. Pediatr Radiol 2000; 30:339-342

Guo JZ, Ma XY, Zhou QH: Results of air pressure enema reduction of intussusception: 6396 cases in 13 years. J Pediatr Surg 1986; 21:1201-1203

Harrington L, Connolly B, Hu X, et al: Ultrasonographic and clinical predictors of intussusception. J Pediatr 1998;132:836-839

Henrikson S, Blane CE, Koujok K, et al: The effect of screening sonography on the positive rate of enemas for intussusception. Pediatr Radiol 2003;33:190-193.

Hernanz-Schulman M, Foster C, Maxa R, et al: Experimental study of mortality and morbidity of contrast media and standardized fecal dose in the peritoneal cavity. Pediatr Radiol 2000;30:369-378

Janik JS, Ein SH, Filler RM, et al: An assessment of the surgical treatment of adhesive small bowel obstruction in infants and children. J Pediatr Surg 1981;16:225-229

Kornecki A, Daneman A, Navarro O, et al: Spontaneous reduction of intussusception: clinical spectrum, management and outcome. Pediatr Radiol 2000;30:58-63

Kuta AJ, Benator RM: Intussusception: hydrostatic pressure equivalents for barium and meglumine sodium diatrizoate. Radiology 1990;175:125-126

Lim HK, Bae SH, Lee KH, et al: Assessment of reducibility of ileocolic intussusception in children: usefulness of color Doppler sonography. Radiology 1994;191:781-785

Lin SL, Kong MS, Houng DS: Decreasing early recurrence rate of acute intussusception by the use of dexamethasone. Eur J Pediatr 2000;159:551-552

Losek JD, Fiete RL: Intussusception and the diagnostic value of testing stool for occult blood. Am J Emerg Med 1991;9:1-3

Mercer S, Carpenter B: Mechanism of perforation occurring in the intussuscipiens during hydrostatic reduction of intussusception. Can J Surg 1982;25:481-483

Meyer JS: The current radiologic management of intussusception: a survey and review. Pediatr Radiol 1992;22:323-325

Meyer JS, Dangman BS, Buonomo C, Berlin JA. Air and liquid contrast agents in the management of intussusception: a controlled, randomized trial. Radiology 1993;188:507-511

Navarro O, Daneman A: Intussusception. Part 3: Diagnosis and management of those with an identifiable or predisposing cause and those that reduce spontaneously. Pediatr Radiol 2004;34:305-312

Parashar UD, Holman RC, Cummings KC, et al: Trends in intussusception-associated hospitalizations and deaths among US infants. Pediatrics 2000;106:1413-1421

Rennels MB, Parashar UD, Holman RC, et al: Lack of an apparent association between intussusception and wild or vaccine rotavirus infection. Pediatr Infect Dis J 1998;17:924-945

Robinson CG, Hernanz-Schulman M, Zhu Y, et al: Evaluation of anatomic changes in young children with natural rotavirus infection: is intussusception biologically plausible? J Infect Dis 2004;189:1382-1387,

Sargent MA, Babyn P, Alton DJ: Plain abdominal radiography in suspected intussusception: a reassessment. Pediatr Radiol 1994;24:17-20

Sargent MA, Wilson BP: Are hydrostatic and pneumatic methods of intussusception reduction comparable? Pediatr Radiol 1991; 21:346-349

Schmit P, Rohrschneider WK, Christmann D: Intestinal intussusception survey about diagnostic and nonsurgical therapeutic procedures. Pediatr Radiol 1999;29:752-761

Shanbhogue RLK, Hussain SM, Meradji M, et al: Ultrasonography is accurate enough for the diagnosis of intussusception. J Pediatr Surg 1994;29:324-328

Shiels WE II, Kirks DR, Keller GL, et al: John Caffey Award. Colonic perforation by air and liquid enemas: comparison study in young pigs. AJR Am J Roentgenol 1993;160:931-935

Shiels WE II, Maves CK, Hedlund GL, Kirks DR: Air enema for diagnosis and reduction of intussusception: clinical experience and pressure correlates. Radiology 1991;181:169-172

Strouse PJ, DiPietro MA, Saez F: Transient small-bowel intussusception in children on CT. Pediatr Radiol 2003; 33:316-320

Swischuk LE, Hayden CK, Boulden T: Intussusception: indications for ultrasonography and an explanation of the doughnut and pseudokidney signs. Pediatr Radiol 1985;15:388-391

Verschelden P, Filiatrault D, Garel L, et al: Intussusception in children: reliability of US in diagnosis: a prospective study. Radiology 1992;184:741-744

Wang GD, Liu SJ: Enema reduction of intussusception by hydrostatic pressure under ultrasound guidance: a report of 377 cases. J Pediatr Surg 1988;23:814-818

West KW, Stephens B, Vane DW, Grosfeld JL: Intussusception: current management in infants and children. Surgery 1987;102:704-710

Zambuto D, Bramson RT, Blickman JG: Intracolonic pressure measurements during hydrostatic and air contrast barium enema studies in children. Radiology 1995;196:55-58

142 Inflammatory and Infectious Diseases

KIMBERLY E. APPLEGATE

INFLAMMATORY BOWEL DISEASE

Inflammatory bowel disease (IBD) affects 1 million Americans (Table 142-1). The incidence is equal in males and females, and the peak onset is in adolescence or early adulthood. Both ulcerative colitis (UC) and Crohn disease represent a chronic inflammatory process

TABLE 142-1

Inflammatory Diseases of the Colon

Gastroenteritis—transient
Other infectious colitides
Ulcerative colitis
Crohn disease
Pseudomembranous colitis
Hemolytic uremic syndrome
Behçet syndrome
Radiation colitis
Neutropenic colitis

without a known specific cause. UC primarily involves the colon, whereas Crohn disease involves primarily the small intestine. As many as 10% of patients defy classification as UC or Crohn disease. In children, the presentation may be nonspecific, leading to a delay in diagnosis that ranges from months to years from the onset of symptoms. The increased risk of colon carcinoma, estimated at 2%, is not limited to patients with UC and is related to both duration and severity of colonic involvement. There are inadequate clinical and laboratory markers for active disease, so repeated imaging is particularly common, especially in patients with Crohn disease.

Ulcerative Colitis

Chronic ulcerative colitis is an idiopathic inflammatory disease of the colon affecting older children and young adults. An infantile form has been described that is devastating and often fatal (Fig. 142-1). The disease is characterized by mucosal inflammation, edema, and

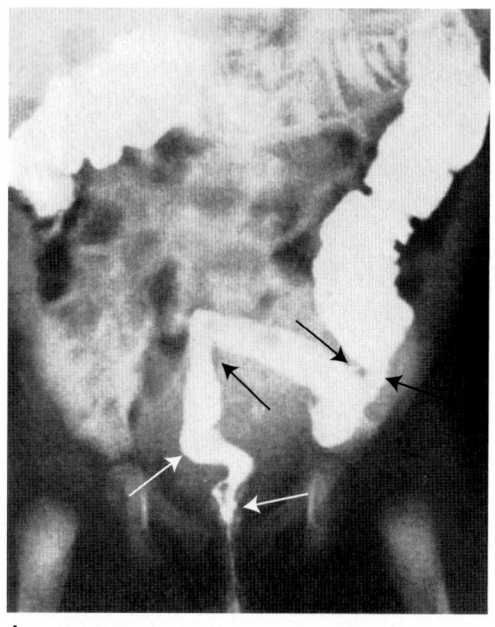 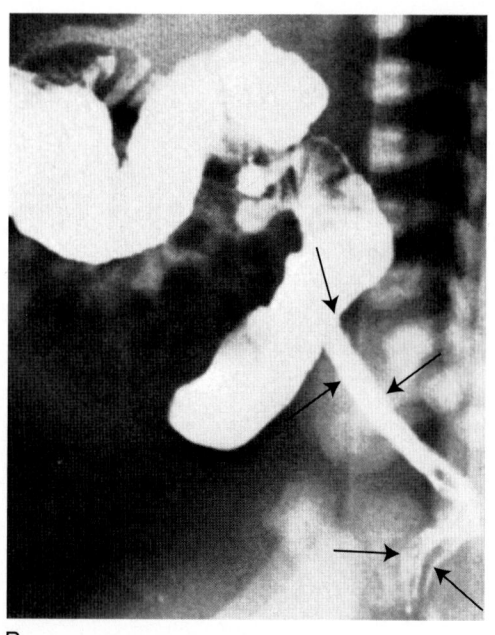

A   B

FIGURE 142-1. Infantile ulcerative colitis in a 3-week-old girl with rectal bleeding. Frontal **(A)** and lateral **(B)** projections during barium enema show tubular narrowing of the rectum and sigmoid colon *(arrows)* with an abrupt transition zone. The findings were suggestive of aganglionosis, but biopsy revealed ulcerative colitis.

ulceration. It is accompanied by submucosal edema in the early stages and fibrosis in the later stages. Transmural disease is uncommon. The disease may be localized in the distal colon or spread to involve the entire colon and the terminal ileum, but skip areas should raise the diagnostic question of Crohn disease. Fatal outcomes are less common than in years past but still occur.

Bloody diarrhea may appear explosively in as many as one third of affected patients, but the majority present with progressive chronic diarrhea. Many children present with nongastrointestinal symptoms, of which severe growth retardation is the most common and clinically striking. Arthritis may precede the colon symptoms. Typically, it is monarticular or pauciarticular, affecting large joints. Seronegative spondyloarthropathy is seen in some affected males. Skin rashes, uveitis, digital clubbing, stomal ulcers, and hepatic dysfunction (primary sclerosing cholangitis and autoimmune hepatitis) occur in variable numbers of children but less frequently than in adults. Patients with UC for 10 years or longer are at risk for colonic carcinomas, which may be multiple, as they arise in areas of dysplastic mucosa rather than in adenomatous polyps.

Plain films are most frequently nonspecific, but they typically show absence of recognizable stool from affected colonic segments and may show evidence of mucosal edema (Table 142-2 and Fig. 142-2). Occasional patients present with toxic megacolon in which marked dilation of the large bowel, primarily the transverse colon, is seen. These patients should not undergo contrast enemas because of the high risk of perforation.

Double-contrast barium enema, formerly the diagnostic imaging procedure of choice, has been virtually replaced by colonoscopy with biopsy. The disease always

TABLE 142-2

Imaging Findings in Ulcerative Colitis

PLAIN FILMS
Absence of stool from involved segments
Bowel wall edema and luminal narrowing

DOUBLE-CONTRAST ENEMAS
Mucosal granularity and edema
Ulceration
Haustral thickening
Pseudopolyposis
Colonic wall stiff, shortened, tubular
"Backwash" ileitis

COMPUTED TOMOGRAPHY
Bowel wall thickening, enhancement, fat stranding
Complications such as abscesses

affects the rectum, with contiguous proximal involvement. Skip areas do not occur, although different parts of the colon may not be equally affected. The earliest change seen with air-contrast enema is a fine granularity of the colonic mucosa. This may be accompanied by haustral thickening secondary to edema of the submucosa. The mucosa becomes progressively more irregular as the disease progresses and ulcers can be seen (see Fig. 142-2). In the early stages, the ulcers may be small enough to be confused with normal innominate grooves (Fig. 142-3), but the associated mucosal irregularity and edema should lead to the correct interpretation. They may become large, so-called collar-button ulcers. Pseudopolyposis may occur—when islands of residual mucosa are surrounded by areas of denuded mucosa—and the terminal ileum may become secondarily affected when

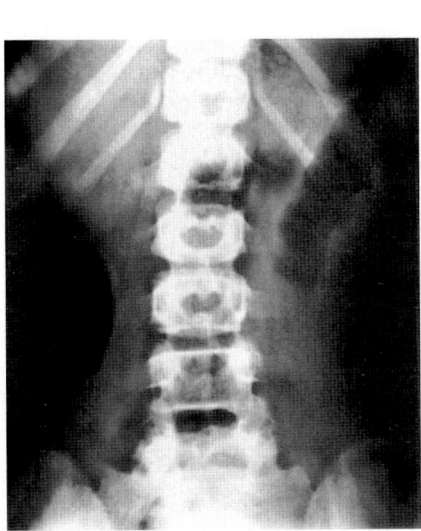 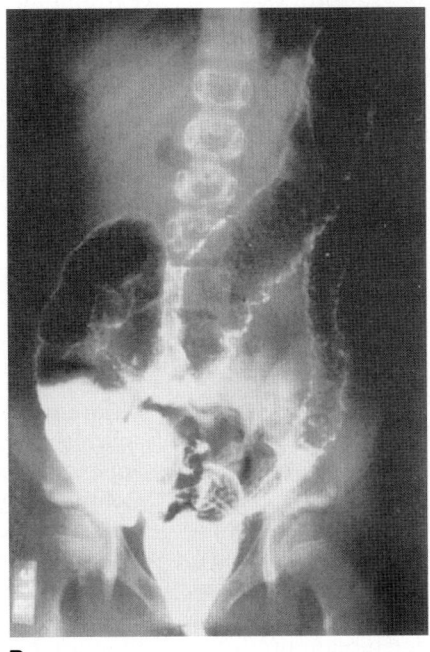 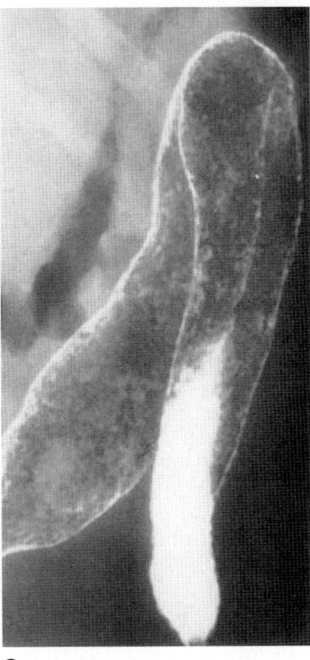

A   B   C

FIGURE 142-2. Ulcerative colitis in a 14-year-old girl. **A,** Plain radiograph shows "thumbprinting" of the distal transverse colon, suggesting mucosal and submucosal edema. **B,** Double-contrast enema shows granularity and irregularity of the colonic mucosa. Small ulcerations are seen throughout the transverse colon and the descending colon. The entire colon was involved. **C,** Coned-down view of the splenic flexure shows multiple areas of pseudopolyps.

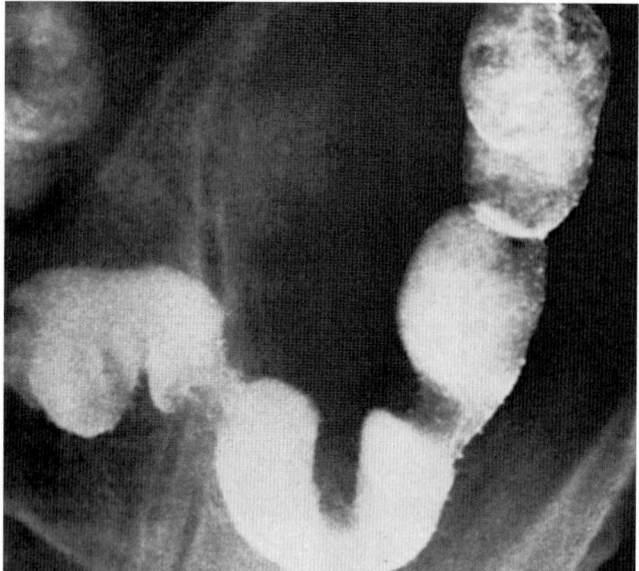

FIGURE 142-3. Innominate grooves. Coned-down view of the distal descending and proximal sigmoid colon shows regular, small spiculations that should not be confused with the ulceration of inflammatory bowel disease. The innominate grooves are less commonly seen in children than in adults.

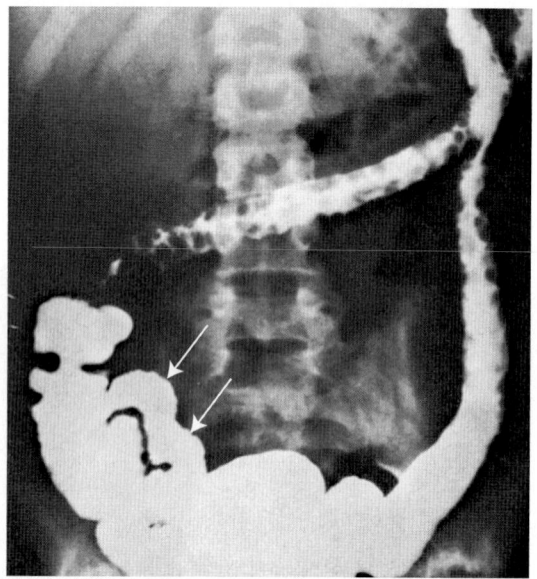

FIGURE 142-4. Ulcerative colitis with pseudopolyposis and "backwash ileitis" in a 15-year-old boy. There are multiple round marginal filling defects in the transverse and descending portions of the colon, reflecting retained islands of normal mucosa between areas of denuded mucosa. The terminal ileum *(arrows)* is rigid and lacks a normal mucosal pattern.

there is proximal colonic involvement, known as backwash ileitis (Figs. 142-4 and 142-5; see Fig. 142-2). Ultimately, the colonic wall becomes stiff, shortened, and tubular—the "lead pipe" colon—secondary to fibrosis of the submucosa (Fig. 142-6). Late-stage disease produces presacral thickening, and retroperitoneal fibrosis is a rare complication.

CT can be performed to investigate abdominal pain, fever, or other symptoms, or to investigate complications

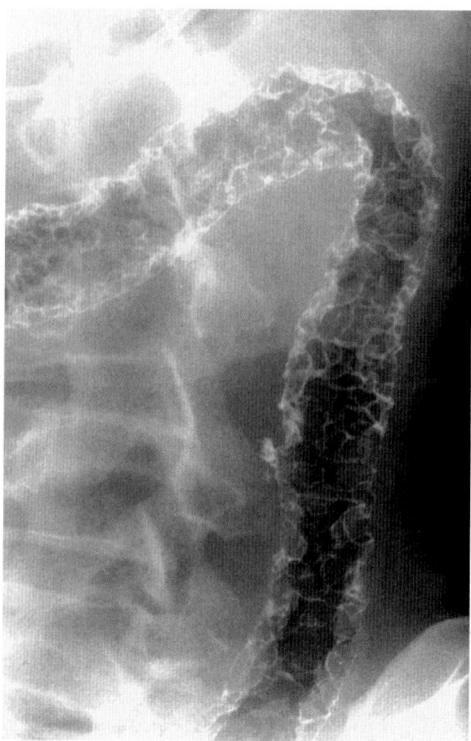

FIGURE 142-5. Active ulcerative colitis. An image of the left colon after enema shows cobblestone or pseudopolyposis appearance resulting from islands of residual mucosa surrounded by areas of denuded mucosa.

of known disease. When UC is active, CT shows colonic wall enhancement, with preservation of the smooth outer contour of the bowel (Fig. 142-7). There may be surrounding fat stranding, mesenteric adenopathy, ascites, and, when perforation occurs, abscesses, but extramural changes are much less prominent than in patients with Crohn disease. In chronic UC, fatty changes may occur in the submucosa.

Durno and colleagues reported the inability of abdominal magnetic resonance imaging (MRI) to distinguish between types of inflammatory and infectious bowel disease in children in general, although its accuracy in UC was good in a very small patient sample.

Crohn Disease

Crohn disease affecting the small bowel is discussed in Chapter 137. The disease can affect the colon as well as the small intestine. Two features that are important for differentiating Crohn disease from UC are the frequent sparing of the rectum and the presence of skip areas with adjacent involved and uninvolved colonic segments. Colonoscopy is often the initial examination in patients with suspected Crohn colitis, as colonoscopy allows visualization of earlier changes of colitis and permits biopsy for diagnosis. However, contrast enema, CT, and sonography can also be used to identify characteristic changes, to monitor exacerbation of disease, and to identify some of its complications. Repeated imaging is frequently requested in some patients to assess progression and exacerbation of the disease as well as its complications. Capsule endoscopy has diffused into adult and more

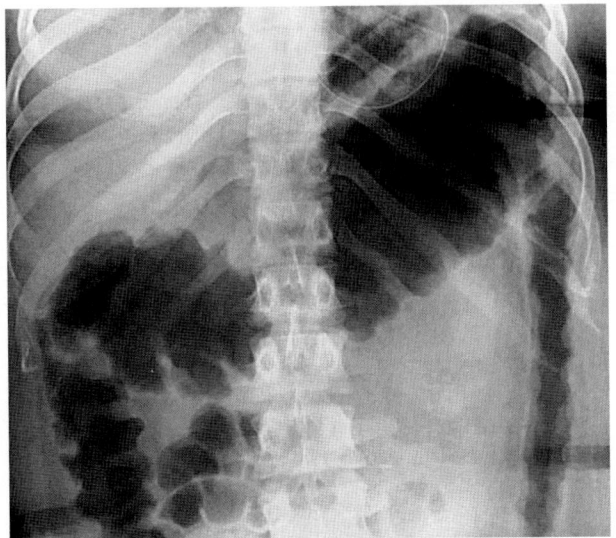

A

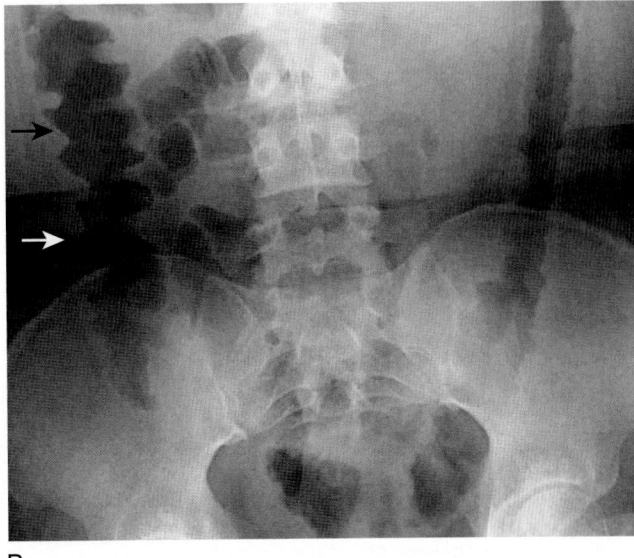

B

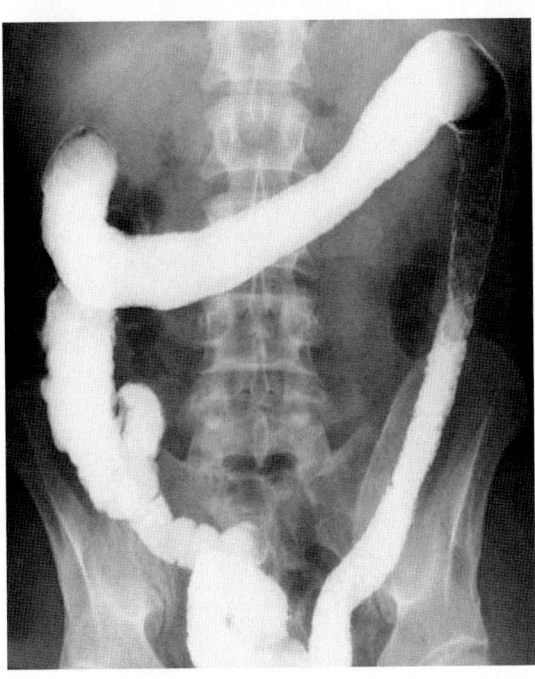

C

FIGURE 142-6. Ulcerative colitis in a teenage girl. The radiographs show both acute and chronic changes of the colon resulting from ulcerative colitis. **A,** Abdominal radiographs show that the transverse colon is very distended and the left colon has a fixed narrow ("lead pipe") appearance. **B,** In the lower abdomen, the right colon is edematous, as seen by a thumbprinting appearance *(arrows).* **C,** The enema reveals the featureless and nondistensible left colon resulting from fibrosis in chronic ulcerative colitis.

recently pediatric practice to visualize small bowel abnormalities.

Ulceration and edema are noted on air-contrast barium enemas. The ulcers are initially small and superficial (aphthous). The aphthous ulcer is characterized by an elevated edematous halo, with a central umbilication caused by barium in the shallow ulcer crater. Eventually, the inflammation becomes transmural and the characteristic "rose thorn" configuration develops, resulting from deep ulcers extending into the thickened bowel wall. A cobblestone pseudopolyposis pattern, similar to that seen in the small intestine, may be seen, resulting from areas of edematous mucosa separated by areas of denuded mucosa and deep ulcerations (Fig. 142-8). Complications of disease affecting the colon can also be identified on small bowel follow-through examinations, such as enteric fistulas (Fig. 142-9). Enteroclysis with

optimal small bowel distension via nasoduodenal intubation is helpful in unmasking focal areas of disease activity, such as strictures (Fig. 142-10).

CT is very useful in evaluation of the complications of the disease. Extent of extramural inflammatory changes and affected loops of bowel can be identified (Fig. 142-11), as well as development of colonic strictures and abscesses (Figs. 142-12 and 142-13). Crohn disease is more likely to lead to colonic strictures than is ulcerative colitis.

Other, more recently introduced imaging techniques include CT enterography and CT enteroclysis, which hold promise in improving the identification of disease activity and complications. In CT enterography, the patient drinks a negative bowel contrast agent (Volumen) that distends the lumen more than water or traditional positive contrast, and that does not mask vascular mucosal enhancement. It is important to have the patient empty

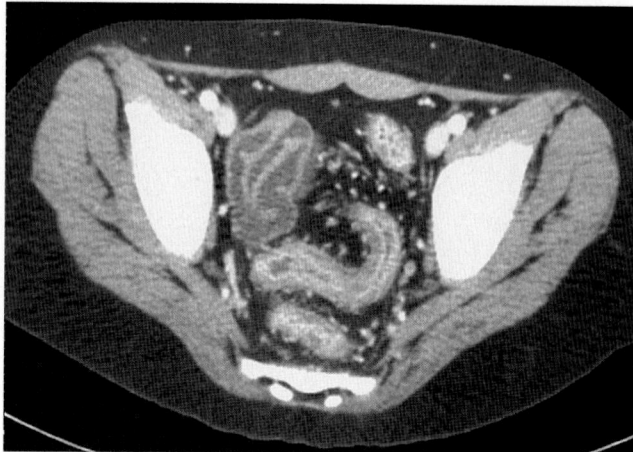

FIGURE 142-7. Ulcerative colitis. Pelvic image from abdominal-pelvic CT in a 12-year-old with known ulcerative colitis. The examination shows a smooth outer wall, with marked mucosal enhancement of the rectosigmoid colon and engorgement of pelvic vessels. (Courtesy Marta Hernanz-Schulman, Nashville, TN.)

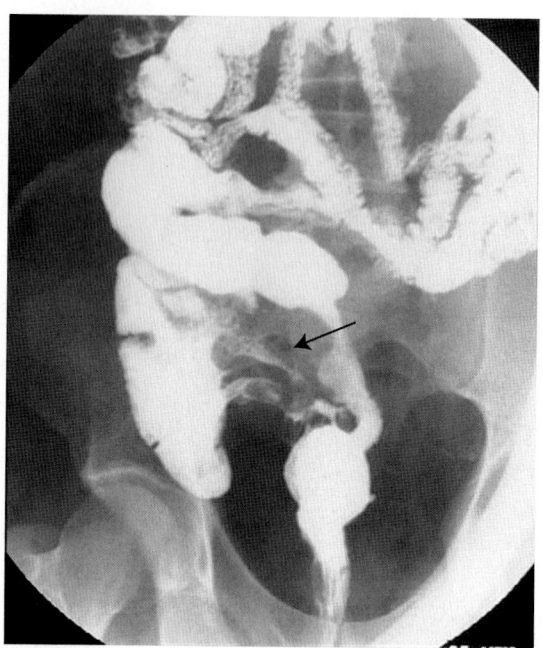

FIGURE 142-9. Active Crohn disease with fistula formation on small bowel follow-through. The fistula *(arrow)* extends between the ileum and the medial wall of the cecum.

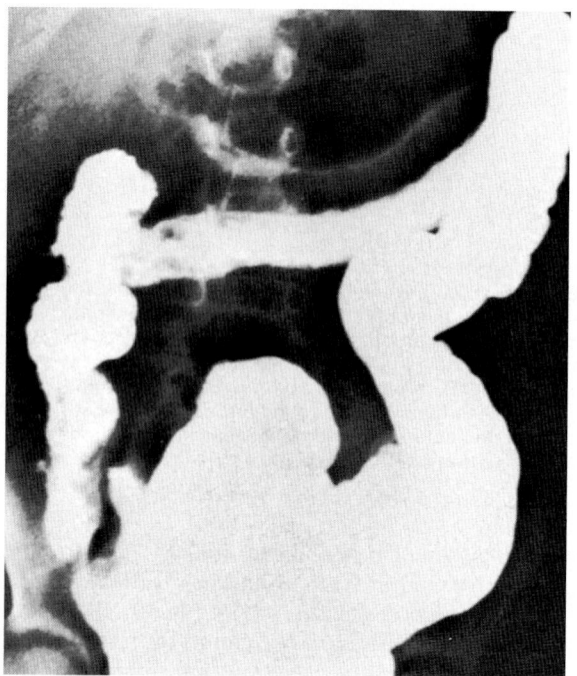

A

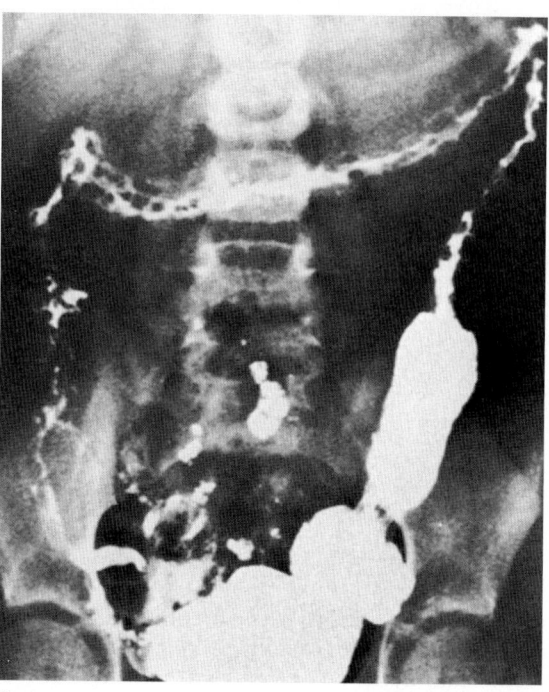

B

FIGURE 142-8. Crohn disease of the terminal ileum and colon in a 10-year-old girl with failure to thrive and vague abdominal complaints. **A,** Barium enema shows the mucosal margins of the cecum and ascending and transverse portions of the colon to be irregular, with small rounded filling defects and loss of normal haustral markings. **B,** Abdominal radiograph taken at the completion of a small-intestinal series shows a cobblestone pattern in the ascending, transverse, and proximal descending portions of the colon.

the bladder before imaging, to allow optimal evaluation of pelvic loops of bowel. CT enteroclysis, like small-bowel enteroclysis, is performed by using high-flow positive or negative contrast introduced via a nasoduodenal tube. It is more invasive than enterography, but it provides a more controlled volume challenge to the bowel. CT enterography and CT enteroclysis may better define the presence of sinus tracks and fistulae and differentiate stricture from inflammation of the bowel wall to guide specific therapies in these challenging patients. Some centers prefer MR enteroclysis to avoid radiation exposure.

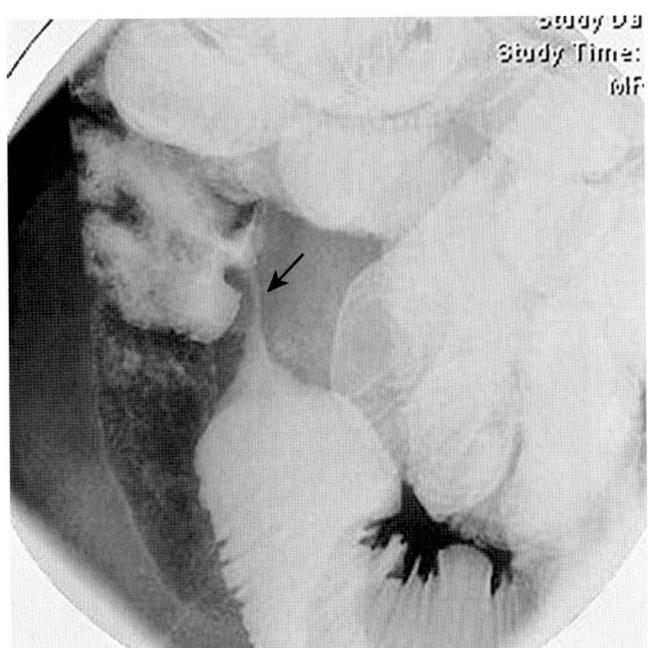

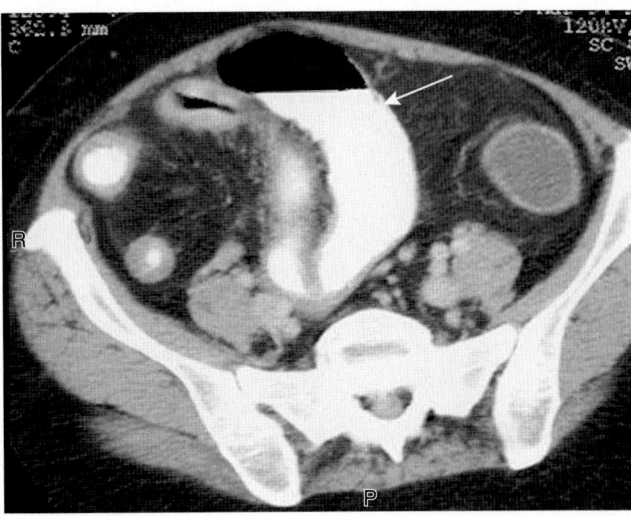

FIGURE 142-11. Active Crohn disease in a 19-year-old. CT shows the distended ileum *(arrow)* proximal to the thick walled ileal loops and mesenteric stranding and vascular engorgement resulting from active inflammation. There is mural thickening and vascular engorgement of colonic segments.

FIGURE 142-10. Crohn disease in a 12-year-old girl. The enteroclysis image shows a stricture of the terminal ileum *(arrow).* The stricture led to proximal obstruction and dilation, requiring surgical resection.

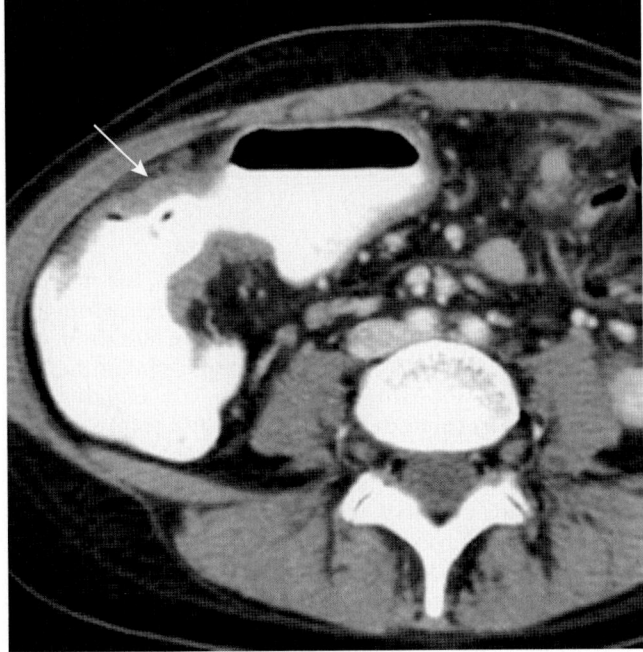

A

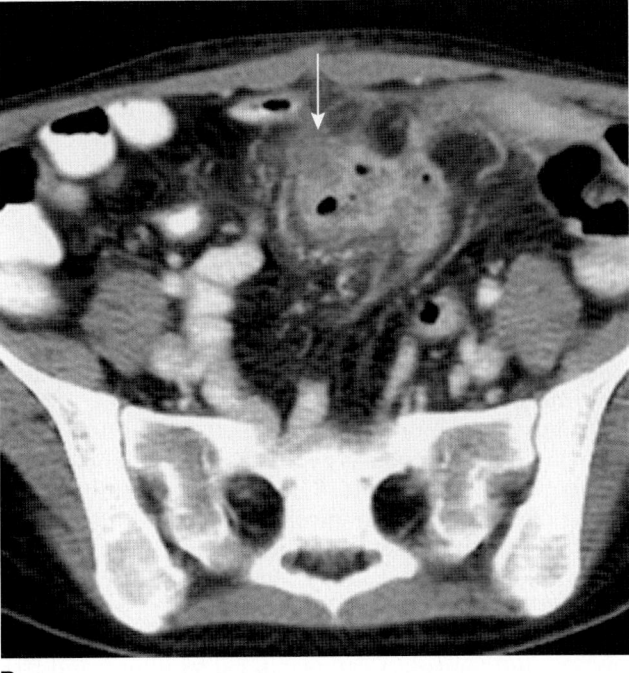

B

FIGURE 142-12. Complications of Crohn disease in a 14-year-old girl (the patient shown in Fig. 142-10), 2 years later. CT for recurrent pain and fever **A,** The right colon near the hepatic flexure is thick walled and narrowed, eventually needing resection *(arrow).* **B,** At a lower level, active colonic inflammation and small multiloculated abscesses *(arrow)* are seen.

Pseudomembranous Colitis

Pseudomembranous colitis, also known as antibiotic-associated diarrhea, is characterized by fever, diarrhea, cramping, and colonic mucositis. The condition most commonly follows antibiotic therapy (Fig. 142-14), often in debilitated or postoperative patients, but it may occur without preceding antibiotic therapy in patients in whom the gut flora has been altered, such as after weaning or surgery. The onset of diarrhea may occur within weeks after cessation of antibiotic therapy. The toxins produced by *Clostridium difficile* are the most important cause of

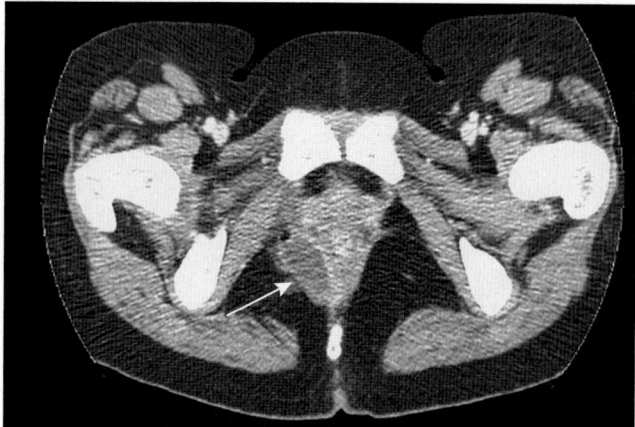

FIGURE 142-13. Crohn disease with perianal abscess. Axial CT image of a girl with active Crohn disease shows the abscess cavity *(arrow)* to the right of the distal rectal wall, with enhancing walls and small gas focus.

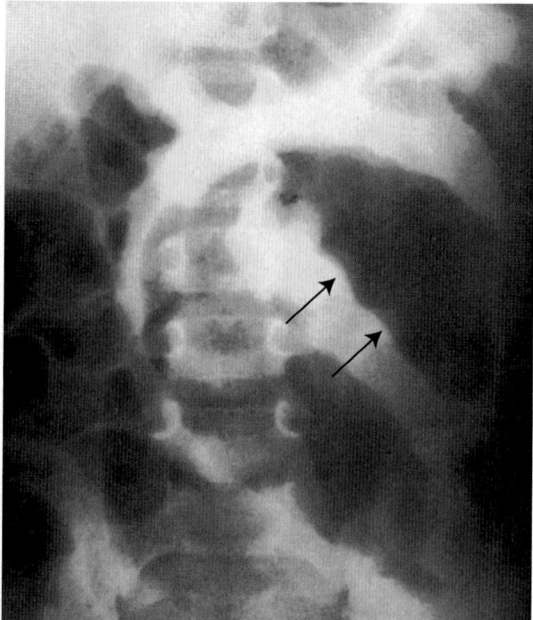

FIGURE 142-14. Pseudomembranous colitis secondary to *Clostridium* toxin. Anteroposterior view of the abdomen in a 7-year-old boy who received 1 week of antibiotic therapy for otitis media shows dilation of a loop of sigmoid colon with typical thumbprinting *(arrows)*.

antibiotic-associated pseudomembranous colitis. Other, less common toxins include those produced by *Clostridium perfringens* and *Staphylococcus aureus*. The radiographic findings are similar to those of the other colitides, and the diagnosis is a clinical one. Enema should be avoided in severe cases to avoid the risk of perforation. CT findings of pancolitis, with or without ascites, suggests the diagnosis in the appropriate clinical setting.

Hemolytic Uremic Syndrome

The hemolytic uremic syndrome (HUS) usually has a gastrointestinal prodrome of diarrhea preceding clinical evidence of acute renal failure, fever, anemia, and thrombocytopenia. This syndrome is most common during the summer months in children less than 5 years old. Most cases are caused by a toxin from *Escherichia coli* serotype 0157:H7 found in raw or incompletely cooked beef and unpasteurized dairy products. Additional toxins are produced by other bacterial agents, including *Shigella, Salmonella, Yersinia,* and *Campylobacter,* as well as by viruses.

Colitis is common, and ultrasound (US), CT, or occasionally contrast enema is generally requested before the correct diagnosis is made. The findings consist of thickening of the wall of the involved bowel segment, more typically the colon, seen as "thumbprinting" on abdominal radiographs or contrast enema (Fig. 142-15), and marked bowel wall thickening on CT or US. The involved segments are typically in continuity without skip lesions, and pancolitis can occur. Fat stranding and free fluid are often seen near the involved segments. Toxic megacolon and colonic perforation have been reported in HUS. Colonic strictures can also occur as a late complication of HUS. Renal and central nervous system complications can markedly affect the course and prognosis of this disease.

Radiation Colitis

Radiation changes occur months to years after exposure and may involve the small bowel, colon, or rectum.

Patients with radiation colitis do not usually undergo imaging examinations during the acute phase, when diarrhea and sometimes lower-intestinal bleeding are the prominent clinical features. Eventually, fibrosis may occur, leading to stiffness and loss of mobility of the affected portions of the colon, with fibrotic walls and loss of the normal mucosal pattern (Fig. 142-16).

Neutropenic Colitis

Neutropenic colitis, also known as typhlitis, is a necrotizing colitis primarily seen in children with hematopoietic malignancies, although it is also seen in children with solid tumors who undergo high-dosage chemotherapy. Development of the disease is associated with chemotherapy-related low neutrophil counts; acute lymphocytic and myelogenous leukemia are the most common underlying malignancies in pediatric patients. Abdominal pain, diarrhea, fever, and distended abdomen are the common presenting symptoms.

The disease most often affects the cecum, hence the commonly used term *typhlitis.* The appendix may be involved and may produce clinical findings that mimic acute appendicitis. Edema and inflammation of the colon, including the distal ileum, may occur, and pneumatosis, perforation, or abscess may supervene.

Radiographs are abnormal but nonspecific and may show a focal ileus in the right lower quadrant. Often, a sentinel loop of dilated terminal ileum may be seen. US shows a markedly thickened cecal wall that may be either hyperechoic or hypoechoic (Fig. 142-17). Intraluminal fluid and ascites may be identified. CT shows marked thickening of the affected portions of the colon (usually more marked in the cecum), surrounding inflammatory change, and free fluid (Fig. 142-18).

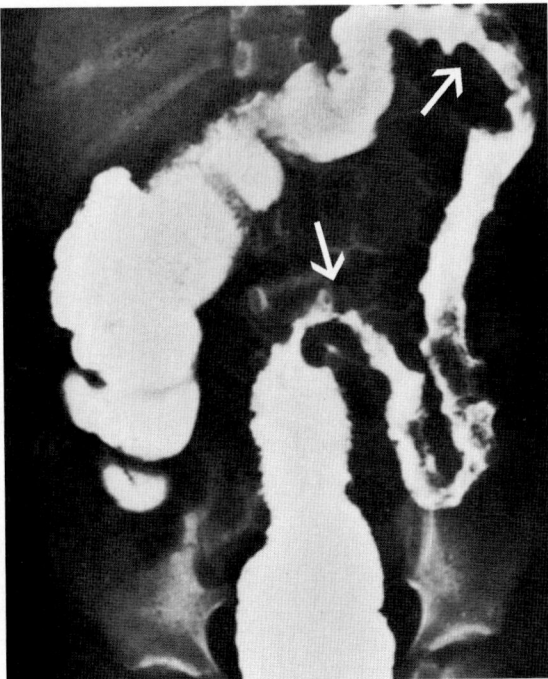
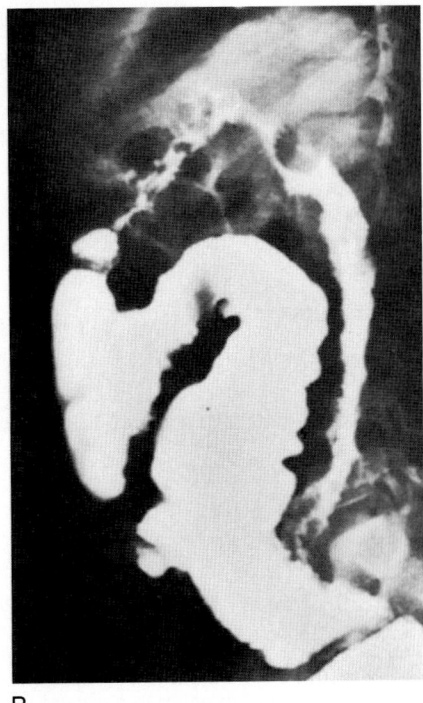

A   B

FIGURE 142-15. Hemolytic-uremic syndrome. Frontal **(A)** and lateral **(B)** radiographs after barium enema show irregular, narrow, spiculated areas from the distal transverse colon to the distal sigmoid colon (*arrows* in **A**). The clinical and radiographic gastrointestinal abnormalities preceded the renal and hematologic abnormalities.

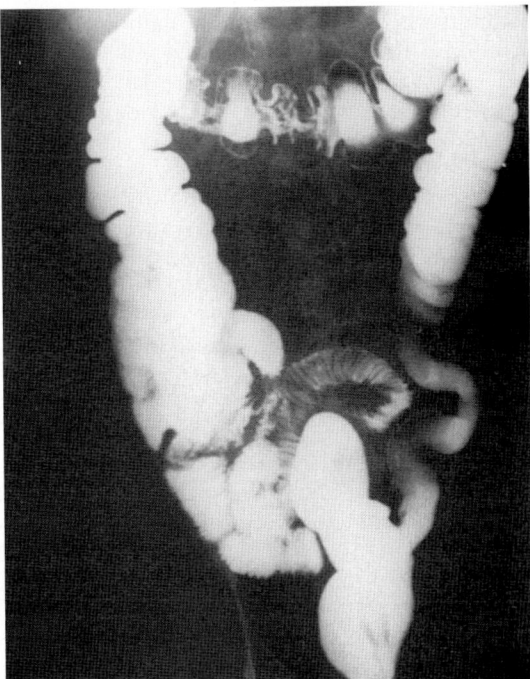

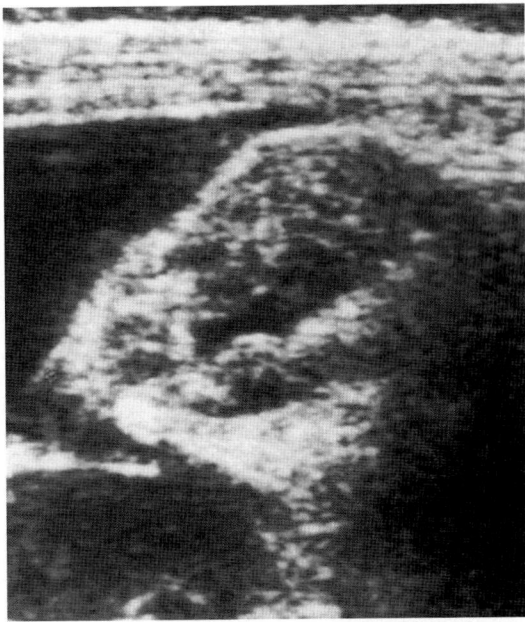

FIGURE 142-17. Neutropenic colitis. US of the right lower quadrant in an 11-year-old girl with leukemia and abdominal pain shows the cecal wall to be markedly thickened. Ascites and a small amount of fluid are seen in the cecal lumen.

FIGURE 142-16. Radiation colitis in an 8-year-old boy who had received radiation therapy for pelvic tumor 3 years earlier. Barium enema shows narrowing, rigidity, and loss of haustration in the distal descending and sigmoid portions of the colon.

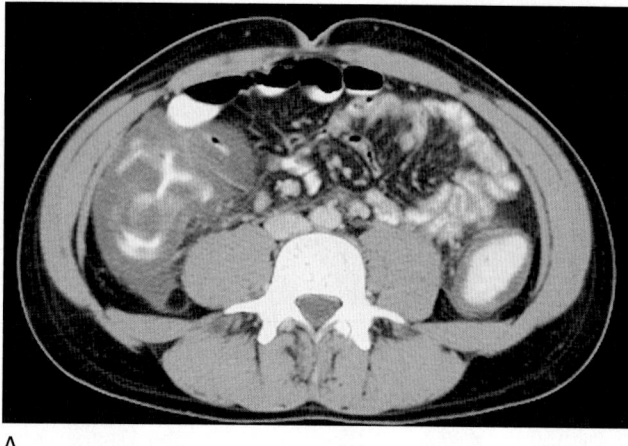

A

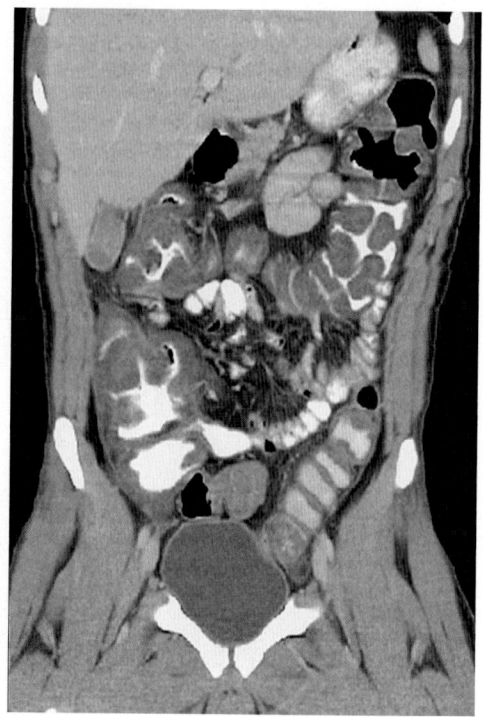

B

FIGURE 142-18. Neutropenic colitis. CT in an 18-year-old man with acute myelogenous leukemia, fever, and neutropenia. **A,** Axial CT image shows the marked thickening of the cecum and a small amount of free fluid. **B,** Coronal CT reformat shows pancolitis affecting the right colon to a greater extent.

Management most often is conservative, including antibiotics, but on occasion, resection is necessary.

Infectious Colitis

The infectious colitides are usually caused by the same agents that affect the small bowel, discussed in Chapter 137, in the section on infectious diseases. Imaging studies are rarely needed and usually show a nonspecific colitis when performed.

Fibrosing Colonopathy

Fibrosing colonopathy was first described in 1994 in patients with cystic fibrosis receiving lipase replacement therapy. The most common contrast enema findings are colonic strictures, loss of haustra, and colonic shortening. MRI has been reported to be of value in these patients, but contrast enema is still recommended as the primary imaging modality. As the doses of pancreatic enzymes are adjusted, this entity may become much less frequent.

Appendicitis

The vermiform appendix serves no significant physiologic function in humans, but inflammation of this atavistic organ is the most common reason for abdominal surgery in children. There are approximately 70,000 urgent appendectomies in children in the United States each year, at a rate of 4 per 1000 children less than 14 years old. Early diagnosis is important because morbidity is largely attributable to perforation. Death from appendicitis, even in the most complicated cases, is much less frequent in children than in adults. However, because

the history and physical findings in children with suspected appendicitis overlap with other abdominal conditions, patients without appendicitis may be sent to surgery. Only 1% to 4% of children presenting to emergency departments with acute abdominal pain do have appendicitis. Before the use of US or CT imaging, negative appendectomy rates in children were 10% to 15%. With the marked increase in use of CT and US imaging during the past decade, these unnecessary surgeries have declined in some centers to 5%.

Appendicitis occurs most frequently in the second decade of life. It is rare in children under 2 years of age, but it can occur in infancy and even in the neonate. Children under the age of 5 years are much more likely to perforate because of the overlap with more common abdominal conditions and because poor localization of pain leads to delayed diagnosis. Periumbilical abdominal pain with migration to the right lower quadrant, anorexia, vomiting, low-grade fever, and leukocytosis are common presenting signs and symptoms in nonperforated appendicitis. Initial relief of pain and/or generalized abdominal pain and fever occur after perforation. Perforation can lead to generalized peritonitis, but a local abscess adjacent to the appendix is more likely because the perforation is usually contained by the omentum. Surgery is performed without imaging studies when the diagnosis is clinically obvious. However, imaging studies can be very helpful in clinically equivocal cases.

IMAGING

Radiographs

Although radiographs are commonly used in children with suspected appendicitis, they are both insensitive and poorly specific. Cross-sectional imaging plays a more important and increasing role in the diagnosis and management of these children. Nonetheless, it is important to recognize findings that might be present on radiographs.

Pain usually leads to abdominal splinting with subsequent scoliosis of the lumbar spine, concave toward the side of pain. Dilated loops of bowel are seen, sometimes focally in the right lower quadrant but more often throughout the abdomen when perforation has occurred. When an abscess has formed, a mass effect on the air-filled cecum may be seen. On horizontal beam films, a right lower quadrant air-fluid level that has no discernible mucosal pattern is presumptive evidence of an abscess. Abscesses most commonly have a mottled appearance on supine films, but a featureless air collection may be seen as well. Perforation rarely results in free intraperitoneal air on radiographs but may lead to distal small intestinal obstruction.

Appendicoliths are calcific concretions in the appendix that are considered compelling evidence of appendicitis in symptomatic patients when seen on plain films (Fig. 142-19 and Table 142-3); many surgeons operate on these children without further imaging studies. Appendicoliths may be round or oval and uniformly calcified, or more frequently lamellated. Appendicoliths too small to visualize on plain films may be seen on cross-sectional imaging, particularly CT. The absolute criteria for appendicitis pertaining to appendicoliths large enough to be visualized on plain films do not apply to appendicoliths seen only on CT. Appendicoliths occur in up to 50% of cases, may not be seen on radiographs when visible on cross-sectional imaging, and are multiple 30% of the time.

Ultrasound

In 1986, Puylaert described the role of US in the evaluation of clinically suspected appendicitis. Numerous studies demonstrating its diagnostic accuracy have followed, with wide variability in reported results. The sensitivity of US in children ranges from 44% to 100%,

TABLE 142-3
Imaging Findings in Appendicitis

PLAIN RADIOGRAPHS
Ileus, often localized to right lower quadrant
Spinal splinting
Appendicolith
Apparent small bowel obstruction, most commonly in younger children
Abscess with mass effect and/or atypical air collection

ULTRASOUND
Appendiceal diameter >6 mm
Noncompressible appendix

INCREASED FLOW IN WALL WITH COLOR DOPPLER
Appendicolith with acoustic shadowing
Periappendiceal fluid, omentum, or abscess
Perforation may decompress the appendix
Abscess

COMPUTED TOMOGRAPHY
Dilated appendix >7 mm

WALL ENHANCEMENT AND THICKENING WITH SURROUNDING FAT STRANDING
Appendicolith(s)
Abscess(es)

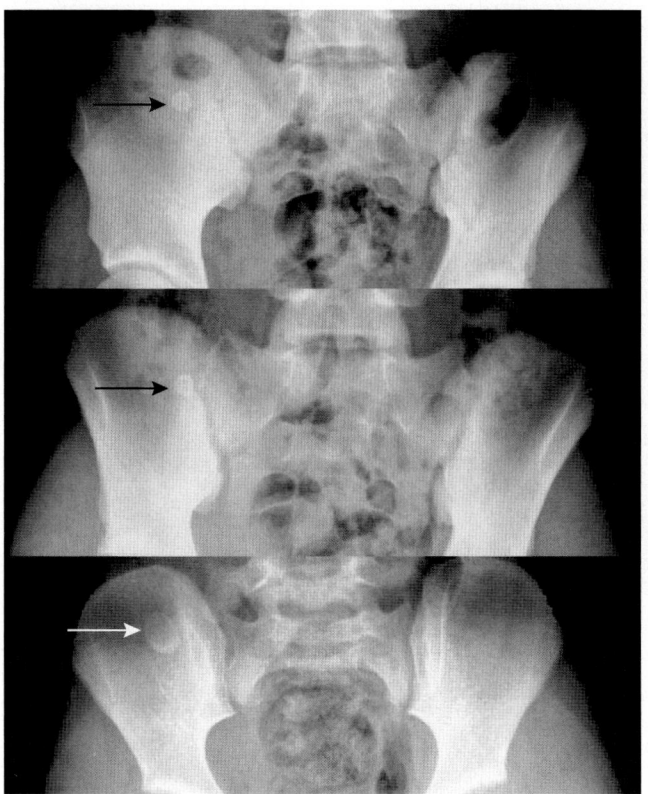

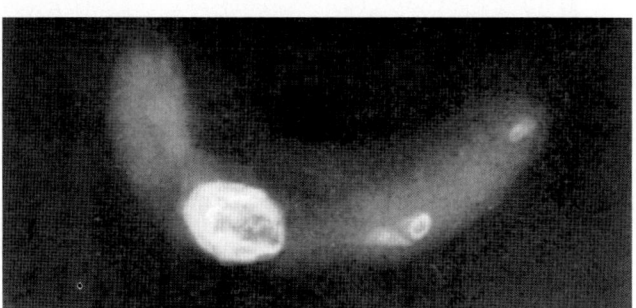

FIGURE 142-19. A, Acute appendicitis with appendicolith *(arrow)* in three different patients. **B,** Resected appendiceal specimen in another patient shows the large appendicolith obstructing the appendiceal lumen.

A

B

and the specificity from 47% to 95%, with a meta-analysis reporting overall 85% sensitivity and 92% specificity in pediatric and adult studies published between 1986 and 1994 (Table 142-4).

A high-resolution, linear array transducer is used, chosen on the basis of the size of the patient and the depth of the appendix from the abdominal wall. Transverse and longitudinal scans are performed over the point of maximal tenderness. Graded compression displaces other loops of bowel, permits higher-resolution imaging, and differentiates compressible normal bowel from the inflamed noncompressible appendix. If the appendix is not identified, a complete scan of the right abdomen and pelvis should be performed because of the variability of appendiceal position. A major advantage of US compared with CT for the diagnosis of appendicitis in children is the avoidance of ionizing radiation. How-ever, US is highly operator dependent, and visualization of the normal appendix by US is variable and may be unreliable, as the tip may not be recognized; therefore, US is more helpful in the diagnosis than in the exclusion of appendicitis.

The single most important US sign of an inflamed appendix is enlargement. It almost always measures more than 6 mm in diameter in children as well as adults, and is noncompressible. A target sign has been described with respect to the order of hypoechoic muscular and hyperechoic mucosal layers, depending on the acuity of the process. In most instances of obstructive appendicitis in children, the center of the target is hypoechoic because of fluid or pus in the lumen of the appendix (Fig. 142-20). Longitudinal images show similar findings along the length of the appendix, but they may identify abnormal findings only along the tip of the appendix (Fig. 142-21). Appendicoliths are seen more commonly by CT than on plain radiographs.

Perforation and abscess formation can be identified at sonography by the presence of periappendiceal fluid, intraperitoneal fluid, and a mass of mixed echogenicity (Fig. 142-22). The appendix may no longer be dilated if perforation occurs. Lack of visualization of a non-perforated inflamed appendix, such as one in a retro-cecal or other atypical position, appendicitis confined to the distal appendiceal tip, or perforation prior to abscess formation, may lead to false-negative US examinations. The persistence of clinical symptoms or the presence of unexplained fluid, however, should alert the examiner to the possibility, and further studies such as CT should be considered.

TABLE 142-4		
Diagnostic Performance* of US and CT for Clinically Suspected Appendicitis		
	MEAN (RANGE)	
	Ultrasound†	**Computed Tomography**
Sensitivity	85% (44%-94%)	95% (87%-100%)
Specificity	92% (47%-95%)	95% (89%-98%)

*As reported in peer-reviewed literature.
†Meta-analysis includes both adults and children, which may lower the diagnostic performance of US.

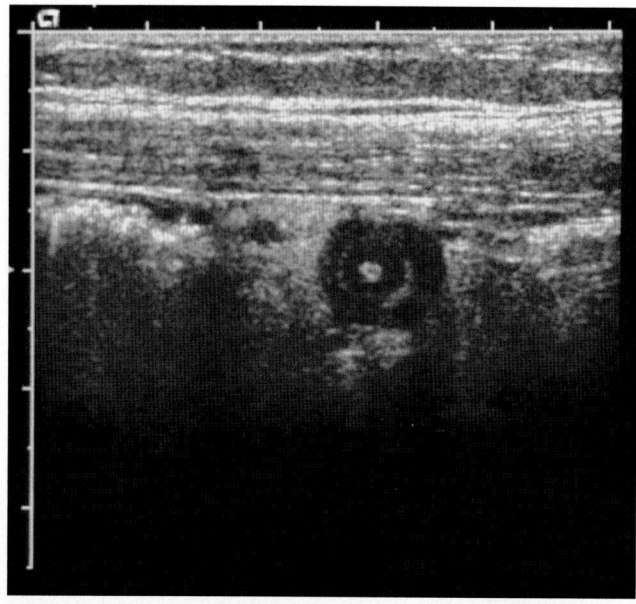

A

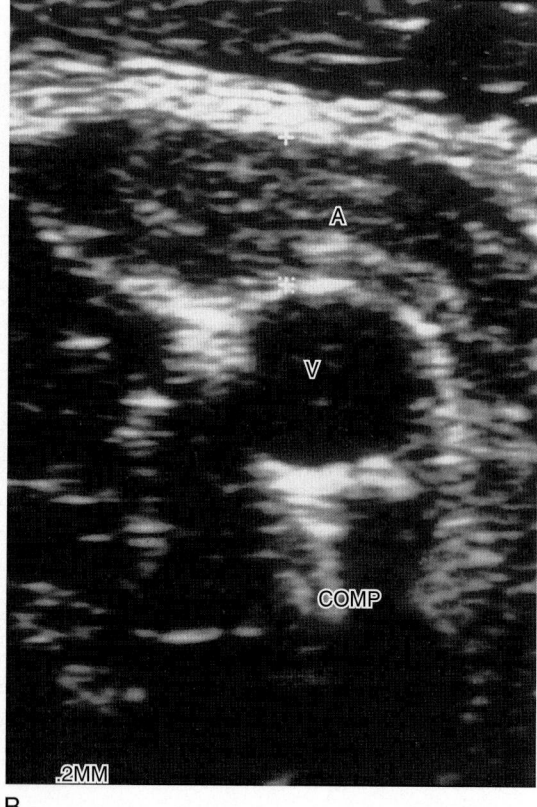

B

FIGURE 142-20. Ultrasound examination of patients with appendicitis. **A,** Transverse US scan of the appendix shows the characteristic target sign. In this case, the innermost portion is hyperechoic, compatible with an appendicolith. **B,** Transverse image through the length of appendix, which measures 7.2 mm with compression, with no appreciable change from noncompression images. A, appendix; V, vein.

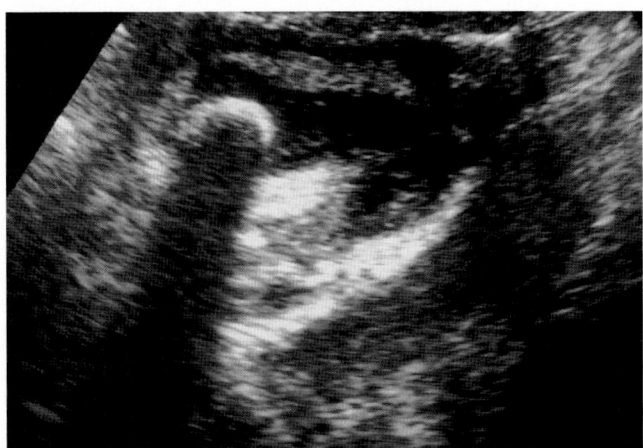

FIGURE 142-21. Appendicitis with appendicolith. US scan of the right lower quadrant shows a calcification with acoustic shadowing in a dilated appendix, which curves inferiorly in the right lower quadrant.

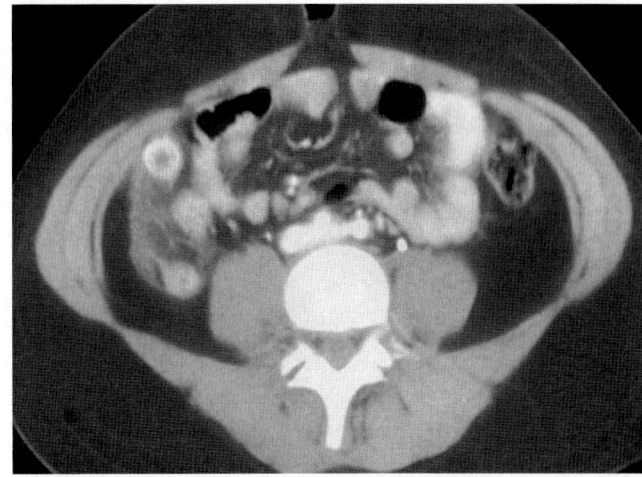

FIGURE 142-23. Appendicitis. CT shows a dilated, enhancing appendix with no evidence of abscess formation.

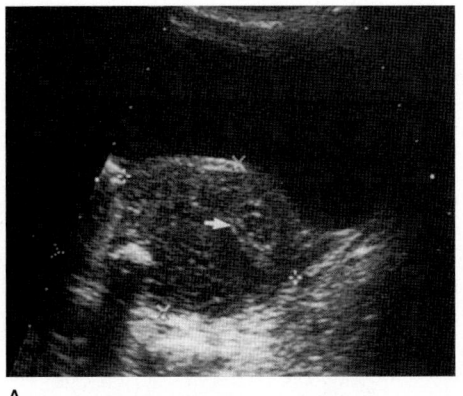

A

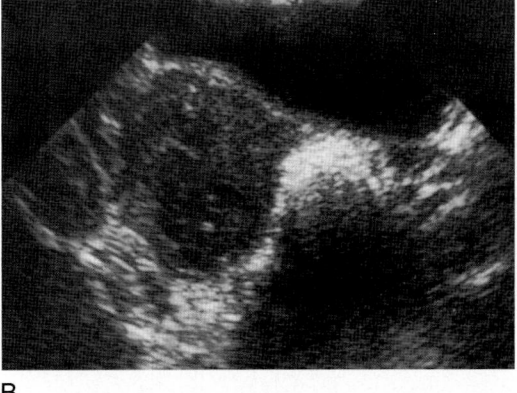

B

FIGURE 142-22. Periappendiceal abscesses. **A,** Transverse US scan of the pelvis shows a large mass of mixed echogenicity behind the bladder, with an extruded, shadowing appendicolith. The appendix *(arrow)* shows a typical target sign within the abscess collection. **B,** Longitudinal US scan in another patient shows a mass of mixed echogenicity behind the bladder. In this case, the appendix itself was not seen because of decompression secondary to perforation.

Although it is infrequent, subacute appendicitis or spontaneous resolution of acute appendicitis can occur.

CT

The use of CT has surpassed the use of US in the evaluation of appendicitis in children in the United States. Multidetector CT (MDCT) has become ubiquitous in the evaluation of abdominal pain, although techniques vary. A typical technique uses axial reconstructions of 5 mm or less and intravenous contrast with or without enteral contrast (Fig. 142-23). Some centers do only unenhanced scans, some use intravenous contrast only, and some use oral contrast, rectal contrast, or both. Many perform volumetric reconstructions in the coronal plane to improve identification of the normal or abnormal appendix.

MDCT is a highly sensitive and specific test for the diagnosis or exclusion of acute appendicitis in children (see Table 142-4). The reported CT sensitivity ranges from 87% to 100%, and the specificity from 89% to 98%, with an average of 95% for both sensitivity and specificity.

Several centers have reported a decrease in perforation and in negative appendectomy rates with the use of CT. The majority of articles show greater sensitivity and specificity for CT than for US, although in experienced hands, the accuracy of US can approach that of CT. The reasons for rapid adoption of CT for this diagnosis are multifactorial: ease in performance and availability of CT, less operator dependence compared with US, and a continuing national shortage of pediatric radiologists. Finally, clinicians may prefer CT over US to avoid false-negative results. With surgeons and emergency department physicians, Pena and colleagues have developed a multidisciplinary approach wherein US is the first imaging study used in clinically equivocal cases. If the US is negative or equivocal, CT is then performed. This protocol has reduced the negative appendectomy rate and radiation exposure in those children who did not need to go on to the second study.

Because compression is not used to express the contents of the unobstructed appendix, the diameter of the normal appendix from outer wall to outer wall overlaps the abnormal appendix at CT. A normal appendix is

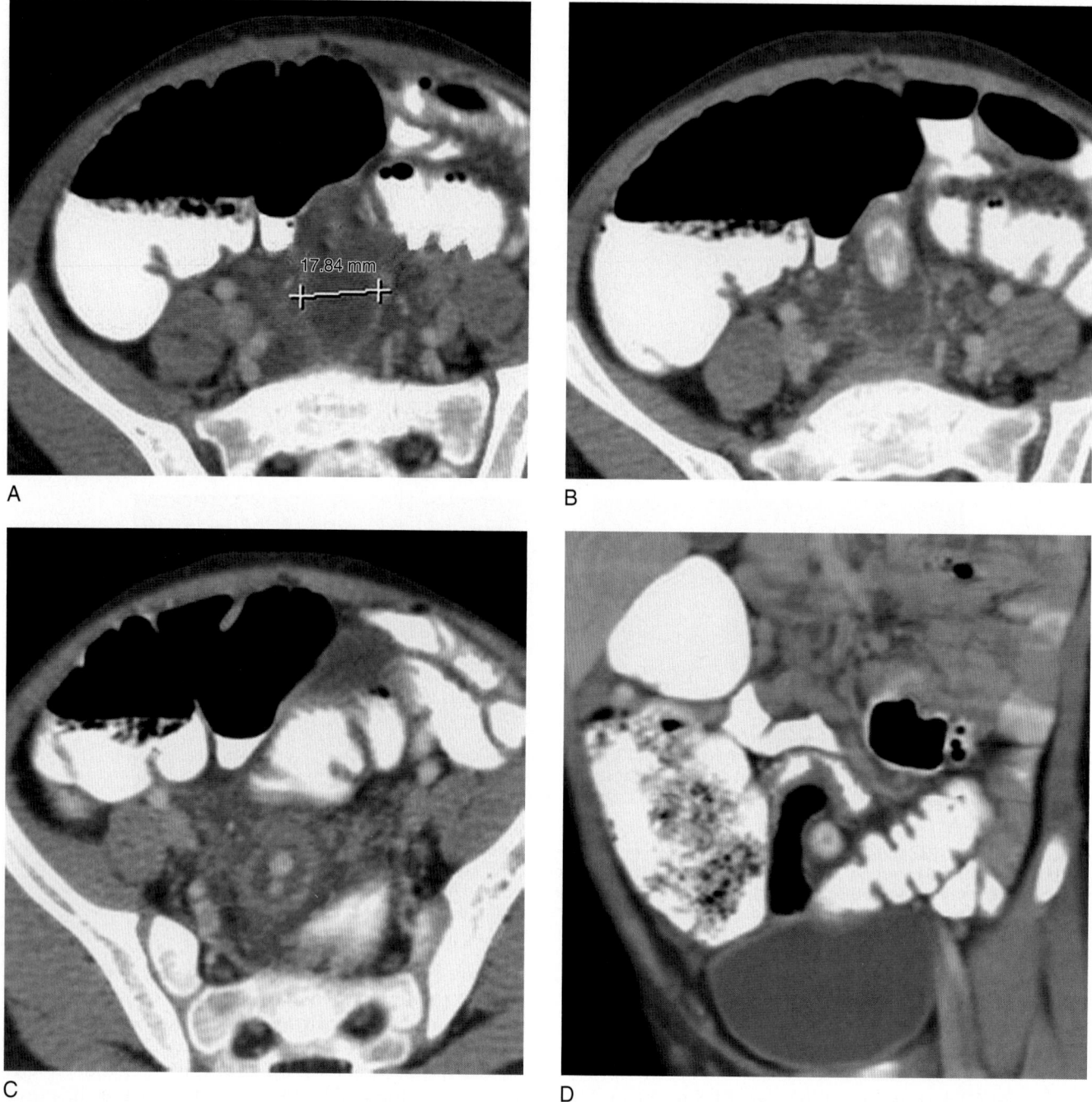

FIGURE 142-24. A-D. Acute appendicitis with multiple appendicoliths. **A,** Multidetector CT (MDCT) in a 5-year-old boy with lower abdominal pain shows a markedly dilated (1.78-cm) appendix, which at first might suggest a loop of bowel. **B** and **C,** Sequential images at adjacent levels show several appendicoliths within the dilated lumen, the larger adjacent to the cecum (seen in **B**), with smaller ones more distal (seen in **C**). **D,** Coronal reformat shows the large appendicolith in cross section, at the base of the appendix.

usually less than 7 mm, although it may be up to 11 mm when distended with gas or feces, whereas the non-perforated inflamed appendiceal diameter is usually greater than 7 mm. A large appendicolith may obstruct the appendiceal lumen, and several appendicoliths may be present more distally (Fig. 142-24). Signs of inflammation such as periappendiceal fat stranding, indistinctness of the outer appendiceal wall, and appendiceal wall thickening and enhancement are very helpful to diagnose appendicitis (see Fig. 142-23), particularly when the size is equivocal. Other common findings are adjacent cecal

wall thickening (cecal apex sign), wall thickening of the distal ileum and sigmoid colon, free fluid, ileus, and mesenteric adenopathy, although most of these signs are not specific for the diagnosis of appendicitis.

When perforated, the inflamed appendix may no longer be dilated. CT, particularly with both intravenous and enteric contrast, is very helpful in outlining the presence, location, and size of the abscess cavity (Fig. 142-25), and in detecting other potential interloop abscesses and intraperitoneal fluid or extruded fecaliths that may act as a potential source of recrudescence

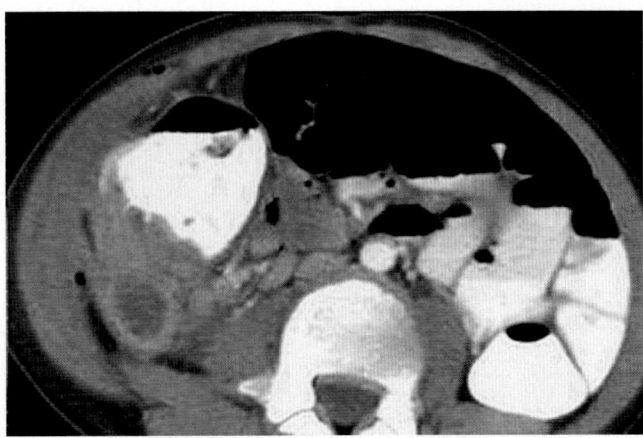

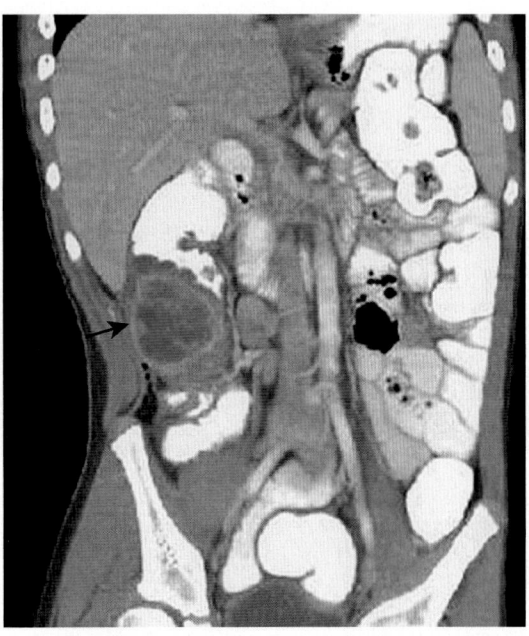

FIGURE 142-25. Perforated appendicitis in an adolescent boy. **A,** Axial CT image using intravenous, rectal, and oral contrast shows a well-defined retrocecal abscess with adjacent cecal wall thickening and mesenteric adenopathy medial to the cecum. **B,** Coronal CT reformat shows the full craniocaudal extent of the abscess *(arrow).*

of infection. Although most abscesses are adjacent to the appendix or in the pelvis, distant spread can occur. Diffuse peritonitis is more common in infants less than age 2 than in older children. Hepatic abscesses and mesenteric or portal pyelophlebitis can occur. CT also plays a major role in the imaging planning for percutaneous or surgical abscess drainage (Fig. 142-26; see Fig. 142-25).

When the appendix is normal, the radiologist must evaluate the images for alternative diagnoses. This is particularly important in young children, who are less likely to communicate their discomfort or localize their pain; many radiologists prefer to scan the entire abdomen and pelvis in children for this reason. The most common alternative diagnoses, in decreasing order of prevalence, are mesenteric adenitis, ovarian cyst, pyelonephritis, infectious or inflammatory colitis, omental infarction (Fig. 142-27), and urinary system stones.

MISCELLANEOUS DISORDERS

Colonic Volvulus

A mobile cecum is a normal variant, seen in as many as 15% of individuals. Cecal volvulus is very rare in the pediatric population, and results from dilation of a mobile cecum, typically in patients with neurologic impairment and relative immobility, resulting in severe constipation and bowel distension. On plain films, a bowel obstruction is identified, with marked dilation of the cecum, which may be present in the right lower quadrant or over the midabdomen.

Iatrogenic causes of cecal volvulus include the presence of a ventriculoperitoneal shunt (Fig. 142-28) and the Malone antegrade continence enema (MACE) procedure (Fig. 142-29). This procedure provides a catheterizable stoma for colonic enema in patients with chronic constipation, such as those with myelomeningocele, and it may provide a focal point for the bowel to twist.

Sigmoid volvulus and volvulus of the transverse colon can also rarely occur. Predisposing factors are abnormal mesenteric attachments and neurologic impairment, leading to hypomobility and severe obstipation.

Pneumatosis Coli

Pneumatosis intestinalis (PI), or pneumatosis coli (Fig. 142-30), is well known to occur in patients with underlying ischemic bowel disease, such as necrotizing enterocolitis, and in some cases of bowel obstruction. However, it is also described in a wide variety of conditions, such as Crohn disease, ulcerative colitis, trauma, acquired immunodeficiency syndrome (AIDS), and cytomegalovirus infection. It is also described as an epiphenomenon probably caused by gas dissection in cystic fibrosis, and very likely secondary to steroid therapy in patients undergoing treatment for such entities as leukemia, collagen-vascular disease, and graft-versus-host disease after bone marrow or stem cell transplants. PI has been reported in an immunocompetent adult patient with pseudomembranous colitis. Conservative management is usually successful; however, in patients with an underlying ischemic process, acidosis and portal vein gas are associated with a poor outcome.

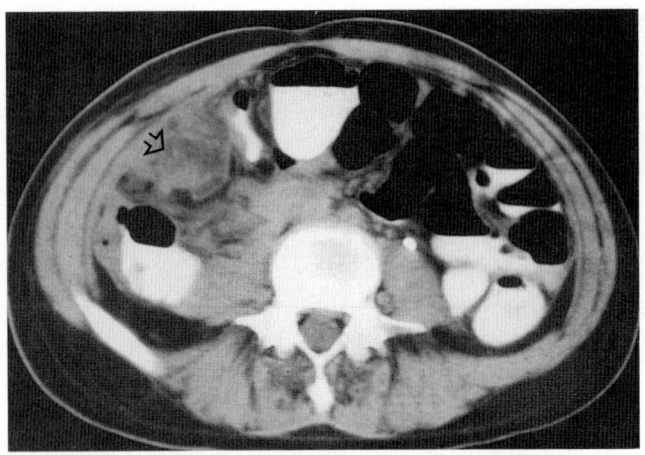

A

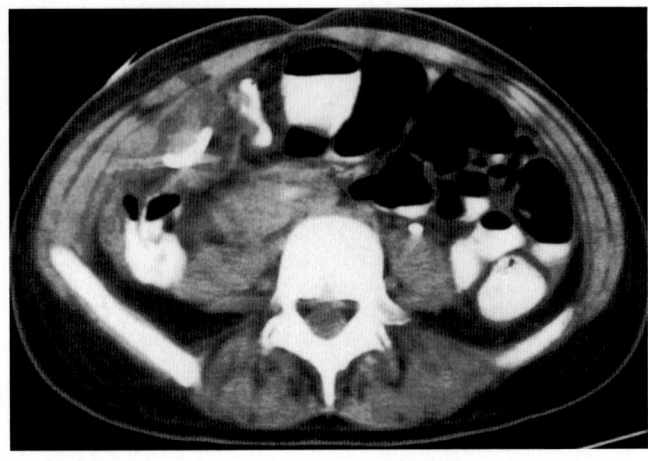

B

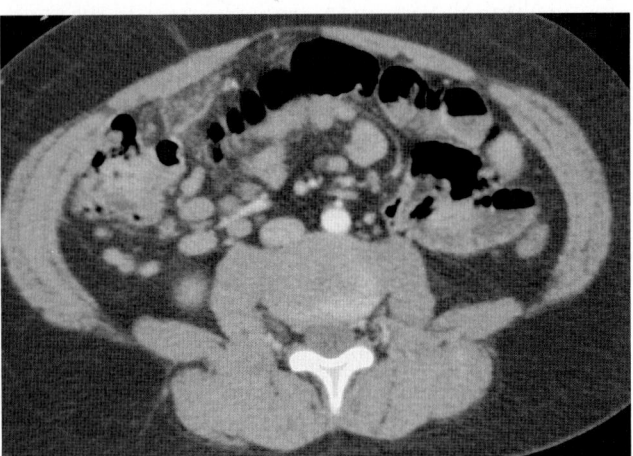

C

FIGURE 142-26. Percutaneous drainage of an appendiceal abscess. **A,** CT scan shows a mass in the right lower quadrant *(arrow)* of heterogeneously low attenuation, obliterating adjacent fat planes, characteristic of an abscess. **B,** A percutaneous drainage catheter was placed under CT control. The tip of the catheter can be seen in the center of the abscess cavity. **C,** After placement of the catheter, CT scanogram shows its course and position in the right lower quadrant.

FIGURE 142-27. Omental infarction. CT through lower abdomen in a young boy who underwent CT for clinically suspected appendicitis. Note typical location of edematous omentum anterior to the cecum, with a prominent central vein, a classic finding in omental torsion. Portions of the normal retrocecal appendix are seen, as well as several incidental mesenteric nodes medial to the cecum. The patient was managed expectantly, with resolution of the symptoms. (Courtesy Marta Hernanz-Schulman, Nashville, TN.)

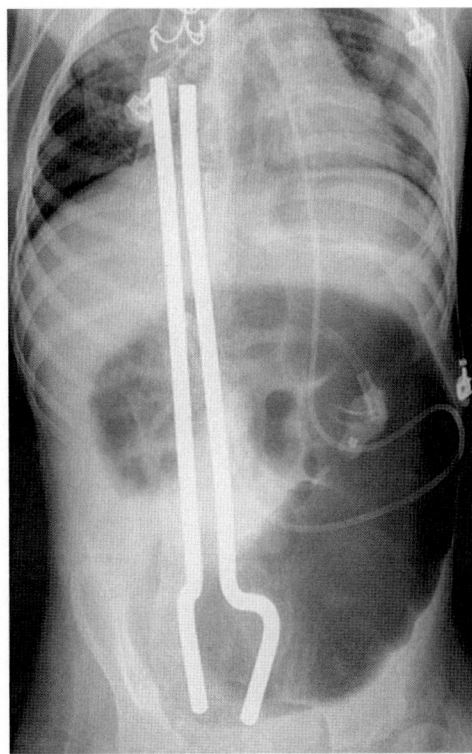

FIGURE 142-28. Acute cecal volvulus around ventriculoperitoneal shunt tubing. Frontal abdominal radiograph of a teenage boy with developmental delay and chronic constipation, who presented with acute onset of vomiting and abdominal pain. The radiograph shows marked distension of a colonic loop in the left abdomen, which was found at surgery to represent an acutely twisted cecum.

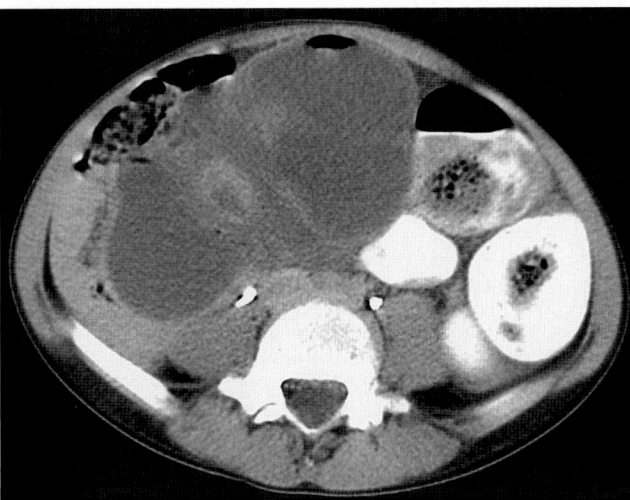

FIGURE 142-29. Acute cecal volvulus around a Malone antegrade continence enema (MACE) procedure. This 12-year-old boy presented with acute abdominal pain and vomiting without fever. He underwent rectal and IV contrast-enhanced CT, which showed a markedly dilated and nonopacified cecum. At surgery, the cecum had twisted around the MACE and was resected.

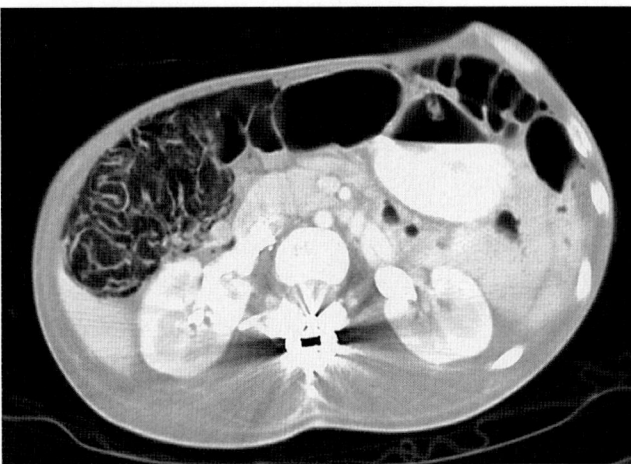

FIGURE 142-30. CT of pneumatosis coli, or pneumatosis intestinalis (PI). Young adult with Duchenne muscular dystrophy, developed PI, probably as a result of steroid therapy. On lung-windowed axial CT, the air in the wall of the right colon is clearly visualized. It resolved spontaneously.

SUGGESTED READINGS

Inflammatory and Infectious Diseases

Abramson SJ, Berdon WE, Baker DH: Childhood typhlitis: its increasing association with acute myelogenous leukemia. Radiology 1983;146:61

Aideyan UO, Smith WL: Inflammatory bowel disease in children. Radiol Clin North Am 1996;34:885-902

Ajaj WM, Lauenstein TC, Pelster G, et al: Magnetic resonance colonography for the detection of inflammatory diseases of the large bowel: quantifying the inflammatory activity. Gut 2005;54:257-263

Atkinson GO Jr, Gay BB, Ball TI Jr, et al: Yersinia enterocolitica colitis in infants: radiographic changes. Radiology 1983;146:113

Balachandran S, Hayden CK Jr, Swischuk LE: Filiform polyposis in a child with Crohn disease. Pediatr Radiol 1984;14:171

Bartlett JG: Antimicrobial agents implicated in Clostridium difficile toxin–associated diarrhea or colitis. Johns Hopkins Med J 1981;149:6

Berg DF, Bahadursingh AM, Kaminski DL, Longo WE: Acute surgical emergencies in inflammatory bowel disease. Am J Surg 2002;184:45-51

Blickman J, Boland G, Cleveland R, et al: Pseudomembranous colitis: CT findings in children. Pediatr Radiol 1995;25(Suppl 1):157

Bolandi L, Ferrentino M, Trevisani F, et al: Sonographic appearance of pseudomembranous colitis. J Ultrasound Med 1985;4:489

Cammerer RC, Anderson DL, Boyce HW Jr, Burdick GE: Clinical spectrum of pseudomembranous colitis. JAMA 1976;235:2502

Chambers WM, Warren BF, Jewell DP, et al: Cancer surveillance in ulcerative colitis. Br J Surg 2005;92:928-36

Diner WC, Barnard HJ: Toxic megacolon. Semin Roentgenol 1973;8:433

Dubinsky MC, Deslandres C, Patriquin H, Seidman EG: Pneumatosis intestinalis and colocolic intussusception complicating Crohn's disease. J Pediatr Gastroenterol Nutr 2000;30:96–98

Durno C, Sherman P, Williams T, et al: Magnetic resonance imaging to distinguish to type and severity of pediatric inflammatory bowel diseases. J Pediatr Gastroenterol Nutr 2000;30:170

Gore RM, Balthazar EJ, Ghahremani GG, Miller FH: CT features of ulcerative colitis and Crohn's disease. AJR Am J Roentgenol 1996;167:3-15

Joffe N: Diffuse mucosal granularity in double-contrast studies of Crohn's disease of the colon. Clin Radiol 1981;32:85

Karjoo M, McCarthy B: Toxic megacolon of ulcerative colitis in infancy. Pediatrics 1976;57:962

Karmali MA, Steele BT, Petric M, et al: Sporadic cases of haemolytic-uraemic syndrome associated with faecal cytotoxin and cytotoxin-producing Escherichia coli in stools. Lancet 1983;1:619

Kawamoto S, Horton KM, Fishman EK: Pseudomembranous colitis: spectrum of imaging findings with clinical and pathologic correlation. Radiographics 1999;19:887-897

Kawanami T, Bowen A, Girdany BR: Enterocolitis: prodrome of the hemolytic-uremic syndrome. Radiology 1984;151:91

Kelvin FM, Oddson TA, Rice RP, et al: Double contrast barium enema in Crohn disease and ulcerative colitis. AJR Am J Roentgenol 1978;131:207

Kirkpatrick ID, Greenberg HM: Gastrointestinal complications in the neutropenic patient: characterization and differentiation with abdominal CT. Radiology 2003;226:668-674

Kirks DR: The radiology of enteritis due to hemolytic-uremic syndrome. Pediatr Radiol 1982;12:179

Kurbekov AC, Sondheimer JM: Pneumatosis intestinalis in non-neonatal pediatric patients. Pediatrics 2001;108:402-406

Loughran CR, Tappin JA, Whitehouse GH: The plain abdominal radiograph in pseudomembranous colitis due to Clostridium difficile. Clin Radiol 1982;33:277

McNamara MJ, Chalmers AG, Morgan M, et al: Typhlitis in acute childhood leukemia: radiological features. Clin Radiol 1986;37:83

Megibow AJ, Babb JS, Hecht EM, et al: Evaluation of bowel distention and bowel wall appearance by using neutral oral contrast agent for multi-detector row CT. Radiology 2005;238:87-95

Miller FH, Ma JJ, Scholz FJ: Imaging features of enterohemorrhagic Escherichia coli colitis. AJR Am J Roentgenol 2001;177:619

Sebbag H, Lemelle JL, Moller C, Schmitt M: Colonic stenosis after hemolytic-uremic syndrome. Eur J Pediatr Surg 1999;9:119-120

Stringer DA, Sherman PM, Jakowenko N: Correlation of double-contrast high-density barium enema, colonoscopy, and histology in children with special attention to disparities. Pediatr Radiol 1986;16:298

Taylor GA, Nancarrow P, Hernanz-Schulman M, Teele RL: Plain abdominal radiographs in children with inflammatory bowel disease. Pediatr Radiol 1986;16:206

Thoeni RF, Cello JP: CT imaging of colitis. Radiology 2006;240:623-638

Tochen ML, Campbell JR: Colitis in children with the hemolytic-uremic syndrome. J Pediatr Surg 1977;12:213

Wagner ML, Rosenberg HS, Fernbach JJ, et al: Typhlitis: a complication of leukemia in childhood. Am J Roentgenol Radium Ther Nucl Med 1971;109:341

Winthrop JD, Balfe DM, Shackelford GD, et al: Ulcerative and granulomatous colitis in children. Radiology 1985;154:657

Zalis M, Singh AK: Imaging of inflammatory bowel disease in children: CT and MR. Dig Dis 2004;22:56-62

Zerin J, Kuhn-Fulton J, White S, et al: Colonic strictures in children with cystic fibrosis. Radiology 1995;194:223-226

Appendicitis

Abu-Yousef MM, Franken EA Jr: An overview of graded compression sonography in the diagnosis of acute appendicitis. Semin US CT MR 1989;10:352

Applegate KE, Sivit CJ, Salvador A, et al: Effect of cross-sectional imaging on negative appendectomy and perforation rates in children. Radiology 2001;220:103-107

Garcia Pena BM, Mandl KD, Kraus SJ, et al: Ultrasonography and limited computed tomography in the diagnosis and management of appendicitis in children. JAMA 1999;282:1041-1046

Hobson MJ, Carney DE, Molik KA, et al: Appendicitis in childhood hematologic malignancies: analysis and comparison with typhlitis. J Pediatr Surg 2005;40:214-219

Jeffrey RB Jr, Laing FC, Townsend RR: Acute appendicitis: sonographic criteria based on 250 cases. Radiology 1988;167:327

Johnson JF, Coughlin WF: Plain film diagnosis of appendiceal perforation in children. Semin US CT MR 1989;10:306

Karakas SP, Guelfguat M, Leonidas JC, et al: Acute appendicitis in children: comparison of clinical diagnosis with ultrasound and CT imaging. Pediatr Radiol 2000;30:94-98

Kharbanda AB, Taylor GA, Bachur RG: Suspected appendicitis in children: rectal and intravenous contrast-enhanced versus intravenous contrast-enhanced CT. Radiology 2007;243:520-526

Lowe L, Penney MW, Scheker LE, et al: Appendicolith revealed on CT in children with suspected appendicitis: how specific is it in the diagnosis of appendicitis? AJR Am J Roentgenol 2000;175:981

Lowe L, Penney M, Stein S, et al: Unenhanced limited CT of the abdomen in the diagnosis of appendicitis in children: comparison with sonography. AJR Am J Roentgenol 2001;176:31

Lowe L, Perez R Jr, Scheker LE, et al: Appendicitis and alternate diagnosis in children: findings on unenhanced limited helical CT. Pediatr Radiol 2001;31:569

Lund DP, Folkman J: Appendicitis. In Walker WA, Durie PR, Hamilton JR, et al (eds): Pediatric Gastrointestinal Disease: Pathophysiology, Diagnosis and Management, 2nd ed. St Louis, Mosby, 1996:907-915

Migraine S, Abri M, Bret PM, et al: Spontaneously resolving acute appendicitis: clinical and sonographic documentation. Radiology 1997;205:55-58

Pear BL: Pneumatosis intestinalis: a review. Radiology 1998; 207:13-19

Pena BM, Taylor GA, Fishman SJ, Mandl KD: Costs and effectiveness of ultrasonography and limited computed tomography for diagnosis appendicitis in children. Pediatrics 2000;106:672-676

Pena B, Taylor G, Fishman S, Mandl KD: Effect of an imaging protocol on clinical outcome among pediatric patients with appendicitis. Pediatrics 2002;110:1088

Puylaert JB: Acute appendicitis: US evaluation using graded compression. Radiology 1986;158:355

Shimkin PM: Radiology of acute appendicitis. AJR Am J Roentgenol 1978;130:1001

Siegel MJ, Carel C, Surratt S: Ultrasonography of acute abdominal pain in children. JAMA 1991;266:1987-1989

Sivit C, Applegate KE, Berlin S, et al: Evaluation of suspected appendicitis in children and young adults: helical CT. Radiology 2000;216:430

Sivit C, Applegate K, Stallion A, et al: Imaging evaluation of suspected appendicitis in a pediatric population: effectiveness of sonography versus CT. AJR Am J Roentgenol 2000;175:977

Sivit C, Newman K, Chandra R: Visualization of enlarged mesenteric lymph nodes at US examination: clinical significance. Pediatr Radiol 1993;23:471–475

Slovis TL, Haller JO, Cohen HL, et al: Complicated appendiceal inflammatory disease in children: pylephlebitis and liver abscess. Radiology 1989;171:823

Vignault F, Filiatrault D, Brandt ML, et al: Acute appendicitis in children: evaluation with US. Radiology 1990;176:501

Zerin JM: Intrathoracic appendicitis in a ten-year-old girl. Invest Radiol 1990;25:1162

Miscellaneous Disorders

Andersen JF, Eklöf O, Thomasson B: Large bowel volvulus in children. Pediatr Radiol 1981;11:129

Berger RB, Hillmeier AC, Stahl RS, et al: Volvulus of the ascending colon: an unusual complication of nonrotation of the midgut. Pediatr Radiol 1982;12:298

Campbell JR, Blank E: Sigmoid volvulus in children. Pediatrics 1974;53:702

Hernanz-Schulman M, Kirkpatrick J Jr, Schwachman H, et al: Pneumatosis intestinalis in cystic fibrosis. Radiology 1986;160:497

Kirks DR, Swischuk LE, Merten DF, et al: Cecal volvulus in children. AJR Am J Roentgenol 1981;136:419

Knight PJ, Morse TS: Splenic flexure volvulus. J Pediatr Surg 1981;16:744

Kokoska ER, Herndon CD, Carney DE, et al: Cecal volvulus: a report of two cases occurring after the antegrade colonic enema procedure. J Pediatr Surg 2004;39:916-919

Kurbekov AC, Sondheimer JM: Pneumatosis intestinalis in non-neonatal pediatric patients. Pediatrics 2001;108:402-406

Reinarz S, Smith WL, Franken EA, et al: Splenic flexure volvulus: a complication of pseudoobstruction in infancy. AJR Am J Roentgenol 1985;145:1303

Sivit CJ, Josephs SH, Taylor GA, et al: Pneumatosis intestinalis in children with AIDS. AJR Am J Roentgenol 1990;155:133

Strouse P: Disorders of intestinal rotation and fixation ("malrotation"). Ped Radiol 2004;34:837-851

Ton MN, Ruzal-Shapiro C, Stolar C, Kazlow PG: Recurrent sigmoid volvulus in a sixteen-year-old boy: case report and review of the literature. J Pediatr Surg 2004;39:1434

Vo NJ, O'Hara SM, Alonso MH: Cecal volvulus: a rare cause of bowel obstruction in a pediatric patient, diagnosed pre-operatively by conventional imaging studies. Pediatr Radiol 2005;35:1128

Yeager AM, Kanof ME, Kramer SS, et al: Pneumatosis intestinalis in children after allogeneic bone marrow transplantation. Pediatr Radiol 1987;17:18

143 Colon Tumors and Tumor-like Conditions

ALAN E. SCHLESINGER

Benign lymphoid hyperplasia, an entity identified on contrast enemas, is not a neoplasm but may be mistaken for polyposis. The filling defects seen on barium enema represent patches of lymphoid tissue in the mucosa and submucosa with an increased size and number of lymph follicles. They are uniform in size and frequently umbilicated, and they can be found along the entire colon, best seen on double-contrast enemas (Fig. 143-1). They are typically 2 to 3 mm in diameter. Larger hyperplastic lymphoid patches may be seen in patients with inflammatory bowel disease, hypogammaglobulinemia, and human immunodeficiency virus infection. Rectal bleeding has been described with benign lymphoid hyperplasia, but the association is probably fortuitous.

Characteristics of nodular lymphoid hyperplasia:
- **Uniform size (usually 2 to 3 mm)**
- **Umbilication**
- **Involving any part of the colon**
- **Better seen on double- than single-contrast enemas**

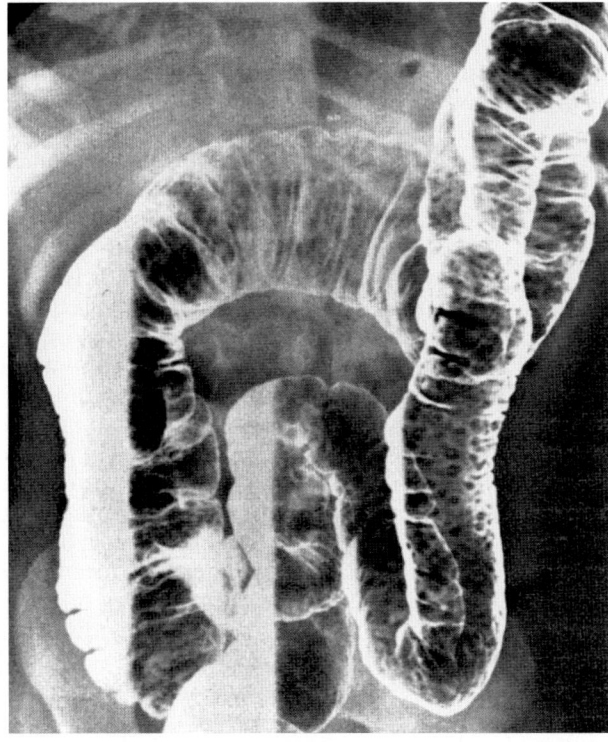
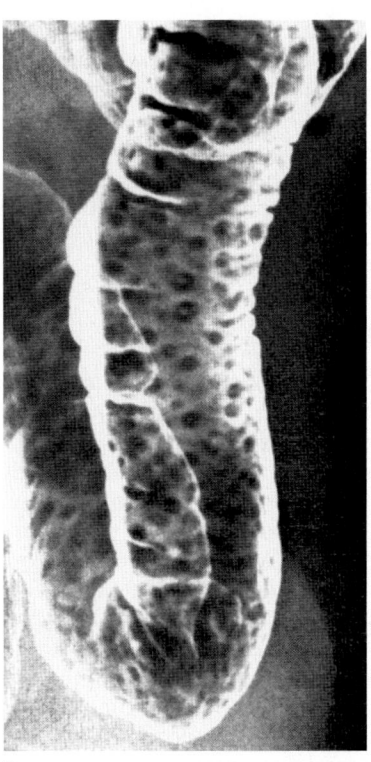

A   B

FIGURE 143-1. Nodular lymphoid hyperplasia showing multiple umbilicated polypoid filling defects throughout the colon, although more prominently seen in the left colon. Right lateral decubitus view **(A)** and close-up of the sigmoid and descending colon **(B)** show the filling defects to be relatively uniform in size, many with central umbilication. (Courtesy of Marie Capitanio, Philadelphia, PA.)

2205

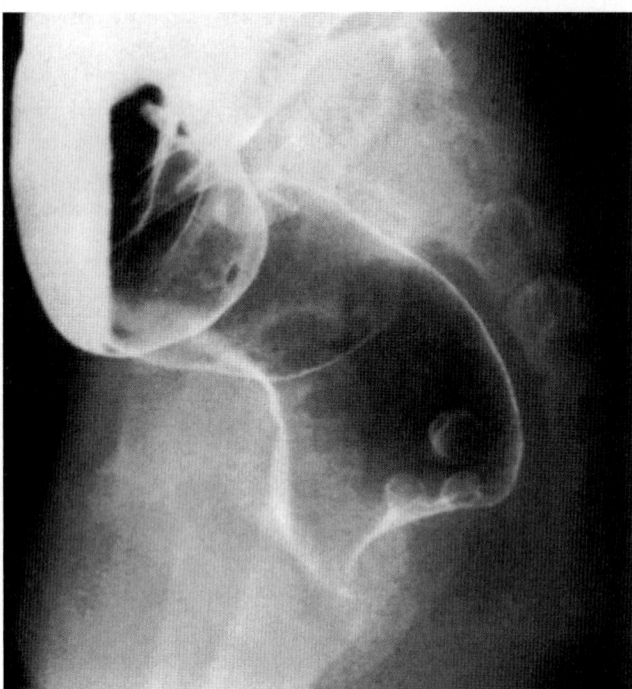

FIGURE 143-2. Prone view of the rectum after double-contrast barium enema shows multiple sessile and pedunculated polyps, all of which measured less than 2 cm in diameter. No polyps were seen in the remainder of the colon.

NEOPLASMS

Colonic neoplasms are rare in children. The majority are benign juvenile polyps. The hereditary polyposis syndromes are less common, and other primary malignancies are of great rarity. The double-contrast enema is the examination of choice in children who present with rectal bleeding or who are suspected, for any reason, of having a benign or malignant colonic neoplasm. However, these patients are increasingly evaluated with endoscopy rather than imaging.

Juvenile Polyps

Isolated juvenile polyps have been considered to be either postinflammatory or hamartomatous. They probably result from blocked hyperplastic mucus glands. They may be single or multiple, sessile or pedunculated, and they are benign with no reported tendency toward malignant degeneration. Juvenile polyps are typically diagnosed in children less than 10 years old, who present with painless bright red rectal bleeding. They are rare before 1 year of age, and the majority are found in children between the ages of 6 and 10 years. Although 75% to 85% of juvenile polyps occur in the rectosigmoid colon, they can occur anywhere in the large bowel, small bowel, or stomach. In the colon, juvenile polyps occur in the rectosigmoid, transverse, ascending, and cecal portions of the colon, in that order. They are typically smooth and less than 2 cm in diameter but may be as small as 2 to 3 mm (Fig. 143-2). Rarely, larger polyps are seen, in which case they may be irregular in contour. Polyps can also rarely cause colocolic intussusception (Fig. 143-3). Treatment is endoscopic resection.

> *Features of juvenile polyps:*
> - **Postinflammatory or hamartomatous**
> - **Single or multiple**
> - **Sessile or pedunculated**
> - **Typically diagnosed in children less than age 10 years (rare before 1 year)**
> - **Primarily occur in the rectosigmoid colon**
> - **Typically smooth, and less than 2 cm in diameter (may be as small as 2 to 3 mm)**
> - **Benign with no reported tendency to become malignant**

Polyposis Syndromes

POLYPOSIS SYNDROMES ASSOCIATED WITH HAMARTOMATOUS OR JUVENILE POLYPS

Hamartomatous polyposis syndromes occur with approximately one-tenth the frequency of adenomatous polyposis syndromes. Patients have an increased risk of colon cancer as well as gastric, small bowel, and pancreatic cancer.

Juvenile polyposis coli is an uncommon autosomal dominant syndrome consisting of hamartomatous polyps with malignant potential. The polyps occur predominantly in the rectosigmoid colon. The diagnosis can be made in a child with multiple (5 to 10) hamartomatous colonic polyps, in a child with any number of hamartomatous polyps with a positive family history of juvenile polyposis syndrome, or in a child with extracolonic hamartomatous polyps. Patients may be asymptomatic or may present with obstruction, intussusception, gastrointestinal bleeding, anemia, diarrhea, or protein-losing enteropathy. As in all the hamartomatous polyposis syndromes, patients with juvenile polyposis syndrome have an increased risk of colorectal malignancy. Associated abnormalities include midgut malrotation, amyotonia congenita, hypertelorism, hypertrophic osteoarthropathy, and hydrocephalus. Juvenile polyposis coli is a heterogeneous group of disorders, and *juvenile polyposis of infancy* is a disorder at the aggressive end of this spectrum that affects infants and has a very high mortality rate. Patients present in the first months of life with intussusception, malabsorption, and diarrhea.

Peutz-Jeghers syndrome is an autosomal dominant hamartomatous polyposis syndrome associated with intestinal (most commonly, small bowel) as well as extraintestinal polyps. There is a predilection for small bowel adenocarcinoma as well as other intestinal and extraintestinal malignancies. This disorder is discussed in greater detail in Chapter 138.

Cowden syndrome (also known as multiple hamartoma syndrome) is a rare genetic (autosomal dominant) disorder characterized by unusual facies, macrocephaly, breast lesions, thyroid tumors, skin tumors, and gastrointestinal polyps. The gastrointestinal hamartomatous polyps are indistinguishable from those in juvenile polyposis syndrome, but there may also be lipomatous polyps, inflammatory polyps, or rarely adenomatous polyps. Intestinal ganglioneuromas may also occur. These patients

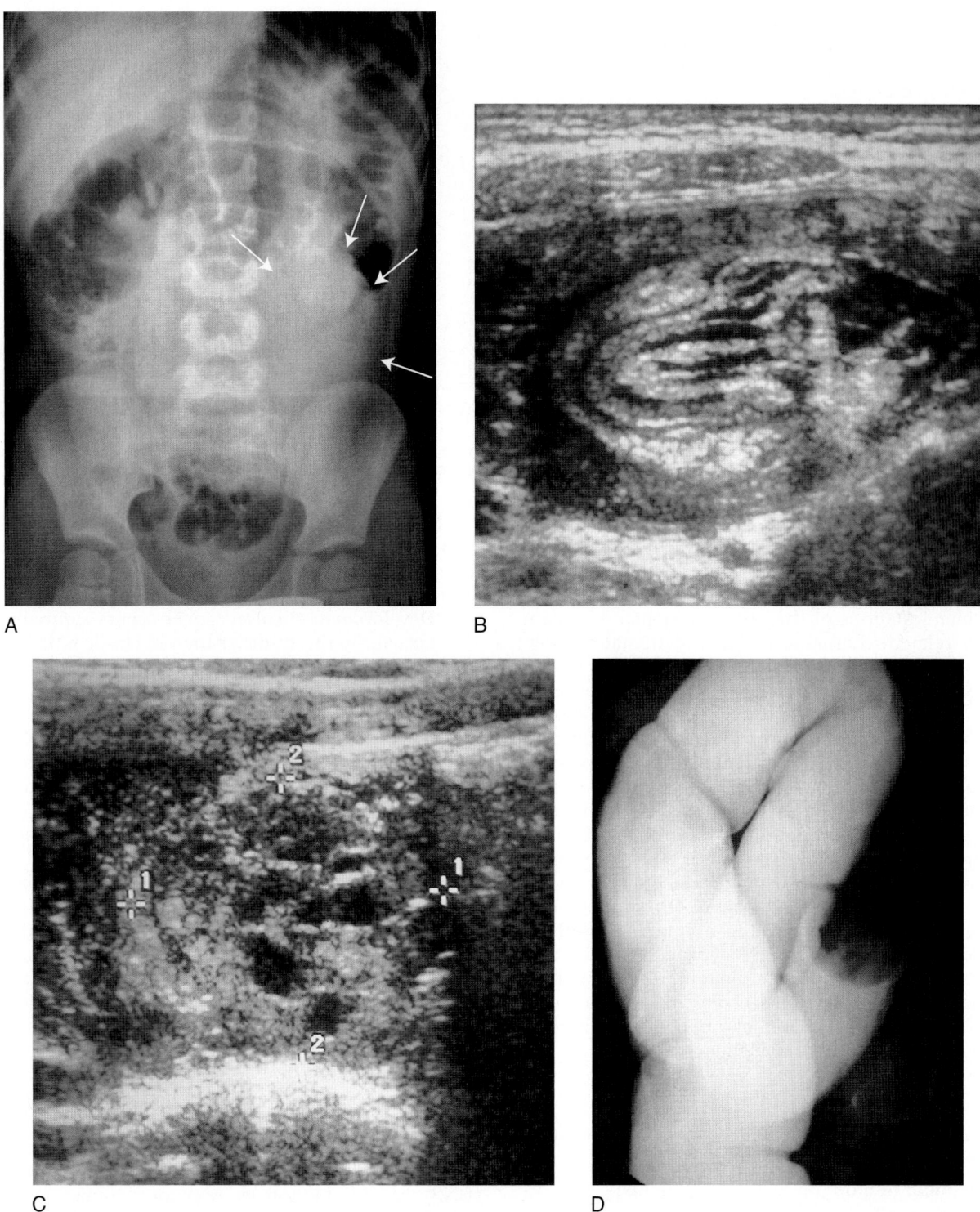

FIGURE 143-3. A 4-year-old boy with juvenile polyp in the colon. **A,** Abdominal radiograph performed for abdominal pain shows a soft tissue mass in the left midabdomen *(arrows).* **B,** US image reveals an intussusception. **C,** US image at the edge of the intussusceptum shown in **B** reveals a separate heterogeneous mass *(between calipers)* that was a surgically confirmed juvenile polyp. **D,** Contrast enema confirms intussusception in the descending portion of the colon.

are at increased risk for breast and thyroid cancer. Although these patients were previously believed to have an increased incidence of gastrointestinal cancers, this risk is now questioned.

Juvenile polyps are found in the *Cronkhite-Canada syndrome*, a disorder with a poor prognosis. However, as this syndrome does not occur in children, it will not be further discussed.

> *Hamartomatous polyposis syndromes:*
> - **Juvenile polyposis coli**
> - **Juvenile polyposis of infancy**
> - **Peutz-Jeghers syndrome**
> - **Cowden syndrome**
> - **Cronkhite-Canada syndrome (does not occur in children)**

POLYPOSIS SYNDROMES ASSOCIATED WITH ADENOMATOUS POLYPS

Classic familial adenomatous polyposis syndrome (FAP) and three variant phenotypic syndromes (attenuated FAP, Gardner syndrome, and Turcot syndrome) are all different manifestations of the same autosomal dominant disorder related to mutation in the adenomatous polyposis coli (APC) gene. Adenomatous polyps of the colon in these patients are dysplastic and predispose to adenocarcinoma. Polyps tend to develop in the second decade of life, and a majority of affected individuals have polyps by the fourth decade. If untreated, all patients develop adenocarcinoma of the colon. Other gastrointestinal adenocarcinomas may also develop in pre-existing polyps, including those involving the small intestine and, less likely, the stomach. A common location for development of adenocarcinoma in patients with FAP is the periampullary region of the duodenum (see Fig. 143-5). Extraintestinal manifestation of FAP include desmoid tumors (9% to 18% of patients) (Fig. 143-4), osteomas of the skull and mandible, fibromas, lipomas, nasopharyngeal angiofibromas, congenital hypertrophy of the retinal pigmented epithelium, dental alterations, epidermal cysts, and other malignancies.

> *Extraintestinal manifestations of familial adenomatous polyposis syndrome (FAP):*
> - **Desmoid tumors (up to 18% of patients)**
> - **Congenital hypertrophy of the retinal pigmented epithelium**
> - **Osteomas of the skull and mandible**
> - **Dental alterations**
> - **Fibromas**
> - **Epidermal cysts**
> - **Lipomas**
> - **Other malignancies**
> - **Nasopharyngeal angiofibromas**

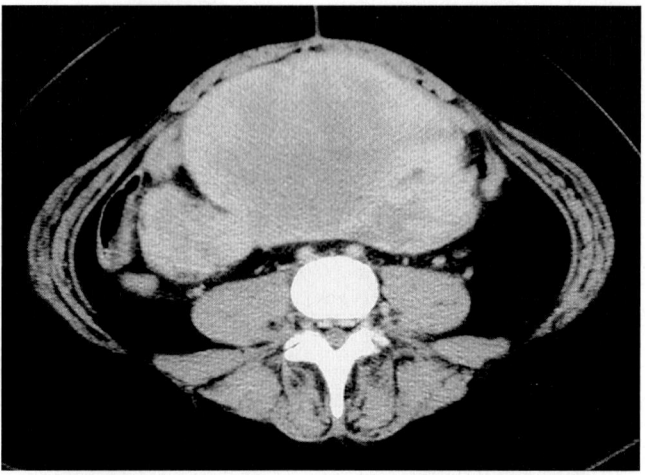

FIGURE 143-4. Axial CT image through the lower abdomen in a 15-year-old girl with familial adenomatous polyposis shows a large mass in the midabdomen that was surgically excised and pathologically confirmed to be a desmoid tumor.

Classic FAP, by definition, has over 100 colonic polyps. However, in most cases, the polyps number into the thousands. The *attenuated FAP* (AFAP) variant form has fewer polyps, averaging approximately 30 colonic adenomas. Development of colon cancer occurs approximately 12 years later in this disorder than in classic FAP. Patients with AFAP, however, are also at risk for the same upper gastrointestinal and extraintestinal lesions as patients with the classic form of the disease.

The disorder previously referred to as *Gardner syndrome* is now considered to be a variant form of FAP. Although these patients exhibit the gastrointestinal adenomatous polyps (and malignancies) seen in FAP (Fig. 143-5), the characteristic feature of Gardner syndrome is the extracolonic manifestations of FAP (often tumors). The classic extracolonic condition seen in these patients is development of desmoid tumors, a form of fibromatosis. These tumors often occur in the abdomen, can be locally aggressive, are difficult to treat, and are a major cause of morbidity and mortality in these patients (see Fig. 143-5). However, as discussed earlier, desmoid tumors also occur in 9% to 18% of patients with classic familial adenomatous polyposis syndrome (see Fig. 143-4). Other extracolonic lesions seen in Gardner syndrome include adenomas and carcinomas of the stomach, fundic gland polyps of the stomach, osteomas, fibromas, lipomas, nasopharyngeal angiofibromas, carcinomas (biliary tree, liver, and pancreas), central nervous system (CNS) medulloblastomas, hepatoblastoma, endocrine tumors (thyroid carcinoma, parathyroid adenoma, adrenal adenoma or carcinoma, pituitary adenoma) (see Fig. 143-5), abnormal dentition (supernumerary teeth, impacted teeth, odontoma, hypercementosis, excessive caries), and congenital hypertrophy of the retinal pigmented epithelium.

Turcot syndrome, another FAP variant, results either from a defect in the APC gene (the gene responsible for FAP) or in DNA mismatch repair genes (also known as HNPCC genes) and is characterized by CNS neoplasms as well as colonic polyps. The former (FAP/Turcot patients) develop cerebellar medulloblastomas, whereas

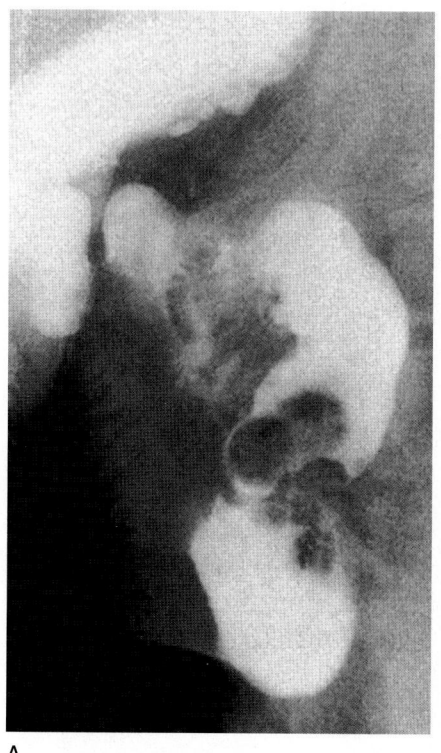

A

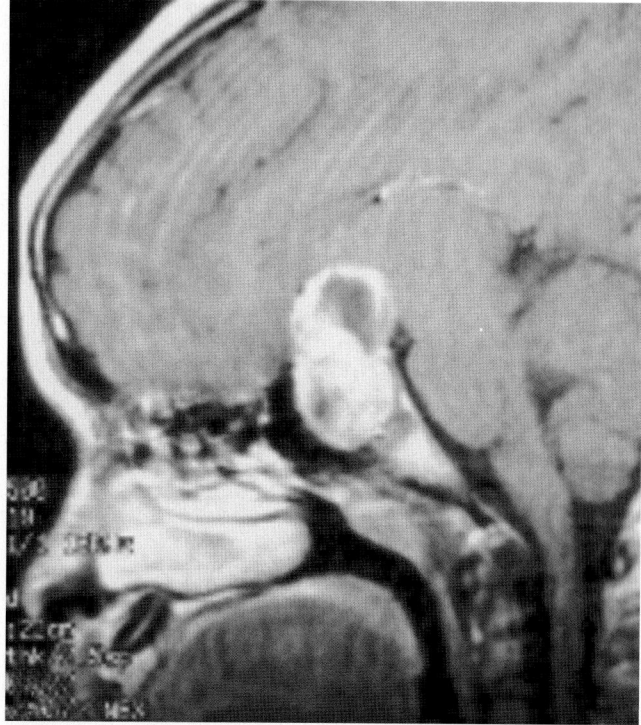

B

FIGURE 143-5. A 12-year-old boy with Gardner syndrome. **A,** Lateral view of the duodenum from an upper GI reveals filling defects from adenomas. Biopsy confirmed malignant transformation. **B,** Sagittal T2-weighted MRI image of the brain shows a heterogeneous mass originating in the sella. Biopsy confirmed a pituitary adenoma. **C,** Axial T2-weighted MR image of the abdomen reveals a heterogeneous, but predominantly hyperintense, mass in the paraspinal muscles, surgically confirmed to be a desmoid tumor. (Courtesy of Sue Kaste and Wayne Furman, Memphis, TN.)

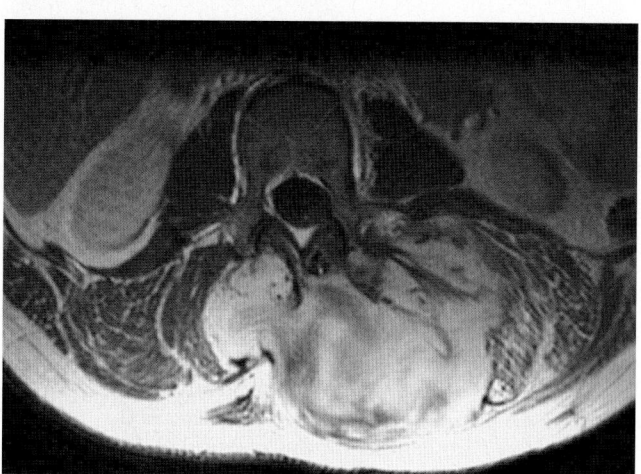

C

the latter (HNPCC/Turcot patients) develop CNS glioblastoma multiforme in addition to the manifestations of adenomatous polyposis. Sebaceous cysts, papillary thyroid carcinoma, leukemia, and spinal cord neoplasms have also been reported in Turcot syndrome.

Polyposis syndromes associated with adenomatous polyps:

- **Classic familial adenomatous polyposes (FAP)**
- **Attenuated familial adenomatous polyposes (AFAP)**
- **Gardner syndrome**
- **Turcot syndrome**

Patients with adenomatous polyps in all of the conditions described earlier can present clinically with rectal bleeding, diarrhea, and crampy abdominal pain. A family history of polyps can often be elicited. Although these patients are typically evaluated by colonoscopy, double-contrast barium enema is occasionally performed. In classic FAP, the colon is carpeted with a myriad of tiny polyps, and the appearance has been likened to a shag carpet (Fig. 143-6). The appearance can simulate lymphoid hyperplasia, but the polyps are of variable size and do not have central umbilication, whereas lymphoid hyperplasia manifests as filling defects of uniform size, many of which have central umbilication. Although the polyps affect the entire colon, they are more numerous in the left colon.

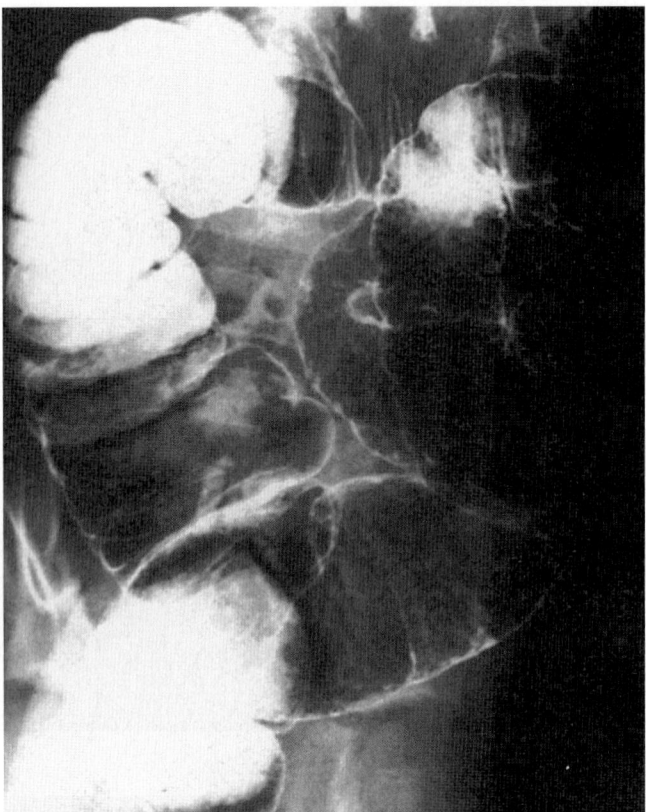

A

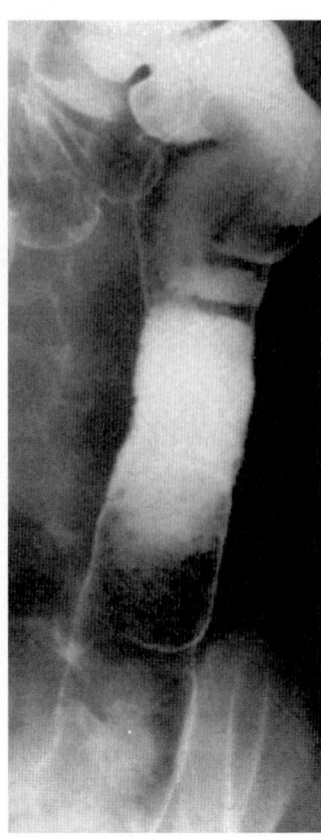

B

FIGURE 143-6. Familial adenomatous polyposis (FAP). **A,** Double-contrast barium enema in an 11-year-old boy whose father had a total colectomy for familial polyposis. Numerous mucosal filling defects of varying sizes are seen throughout the colon. None of the lesions appears umbilicated. The patient underwent total colectomy at the age of 15. **B,** Coned-down view of the descending colon during air-contrast barium enema in the patient's sister (age, 9 years). Multiple filling defects seen en face are similar to those seen in nodular lymphoid hyperplasia (compare with Fig. 143-1). Note the marginal filling defects, however, which suggest the presence of polyps. Colonoscopy confirmed the diagnosis of FAP.

Skull and facial bone lesions in Gardner syndrome are typically well seen on plain radiographs, although more detailed cross-sectional imaging may be warranted. Desmoid tumors are usually well seen by ultrasound (US), computed tomography (CT), and magnetic resonance imaging (MRI) (see Figs. 143-4 and 143-5). US typically shows a hypoechoic mass that may have scattered foci of increased echogenicity related to fat or blood vessels. On CT scans, these lesions are usually of low attenuation and show variable or heterogeneous enhancement. These lesions are hypointense or isointense relative to muscle on T1-weighted spin echo MR pulse sequences and have a heterogeneous, but somewhat hyperintense, appearance on T2-weighted images, with more frequent enhancement than on CT sections. Recent evidence suggests that high signal on T2-weighted MR may correlate with more cellular, and faster growing, desmoid tumors. The colonic polyps in Gardner syndrome have the same appearance on contrast enema studies as those in classic FAP, with carpeting of the colon. The colonic polyps in Turcot syndrome are typically less numerous than in classic FAP, with rarely more than 100 polyps. CNS lesions in these patients are best evaluated by cranial MR.

Other Colonic Neoplasms

BENIGN NEOPLASMS

Rarely, isolated benign neoplasms such as lipomas, leiomyomas, neurofibromas, and hemangiomas may occur in the colon in children, although patients with colonic hemangiomas may also have cutaneous hemangiomas.

MALIGNANT NEOPLASMS

Malignant neoplasms of the colon are also rare in children. Adenocarcinoma of the colon can occur as an isolated condition, but it is also seen in association with FAP, ulcerative colitis, Crohn disease, and Peutz-Jeghers syndrome. The risk for colon cancer in patients with ulcerative colitis is 3% in the first 10 years of the disease and an additional 10% to 15% in each subsequent decade. The risk for colon cancer in patients with Crohn disease is 20 times that of the general population.

> Risk for colon cancer in patients with Crohn disease is 20 times greater than in the general population.

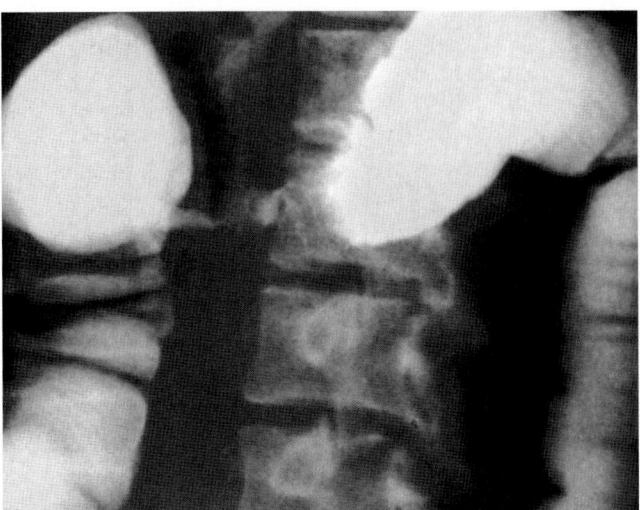

FIGURE 143-7. Carcinoma of the colon in 16-year-old boy. Oblique view from a barium enema shows a circumferential mass. There are stippled calcifications in this region that are better seen in the plain radiograph (not shown).

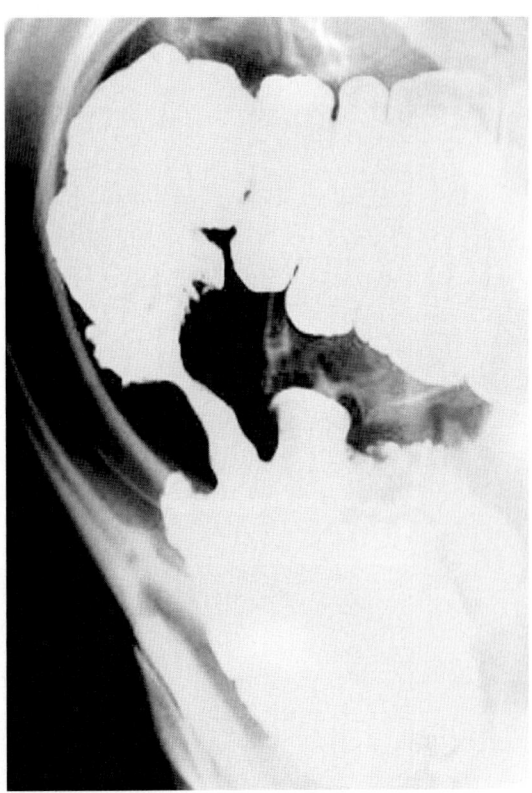

FIGURE 143-8. Spot image from a barium enema in 11-year-old girl with adenocarcinoma of the colon reveals a circumferential mass causing an "apple core" appearance.

Mucinous adenocarcinoma is the most common histologic variety of sporadic colon cancer in children. There is some evidence that environmental factors or diet may be involved in childhood colonic cancers. The most common symptoms are pain, change in bowel habits, weight loss and anorexia, anemia, rectal bleeding, and an abdominal mass. Plain radiographs can be normal but may show irregularity in the bowel gas pattern or evidence of partial obstruction. The mucinous tumors may have punctate calcification in the primary area and in metastatic deposits (Fig. 143-7). Barium enema shows findings like those described in adults, including bowel wall deformity, mucosal irregularity, and luminal narrowing (Fig. 143-8; see Fig. 143-7). CT is required for staging. Because diagnosis is often delayed as a result of a low index of suspicion on the part of physicians, the tumors tend to be larger at presentation than is frequently true in adults (Fig. 143-9). To our knowledge, cure has not been reported other than after complete surgical resection. Initial metastases are to liver, lymph nodes, and other intra-abdominal sites. Generalized carcinomatosis may occur.

Carcinoid involving the intestine in children most commonly involves the appendix and is usually considered benign. Size and depth of invasion are more important prognostic criteria than histologic features.

When the size is less than 2 cm, simple appendectomy alone is considered sufficient treatment. When larger than 2 cm, right hemicolectomy is usually advocated. Extra-appendiceal carcinoid tumors in the colon of children are rarer and have a higher likelihood of malignancy than those occurring in the appendix. Carcinoid tumors may present as a mass or as a lead point in an intussusception. Ultrasound may demonstrate a mural lesion in the colon. CT can demonstrate regional extent and distant metastases. Functioning liver metastases are rare in children.

The colon is a less frequent primary site for the development of lymphoma than the small intestine. The US characteristics are similar, with a large hypoechoic mass usually extending well beyond the bowel itself (Fig. 143-10). CT characteristics are similar to those in the small bowel (see Chapter 138) (Fig. 143-11).

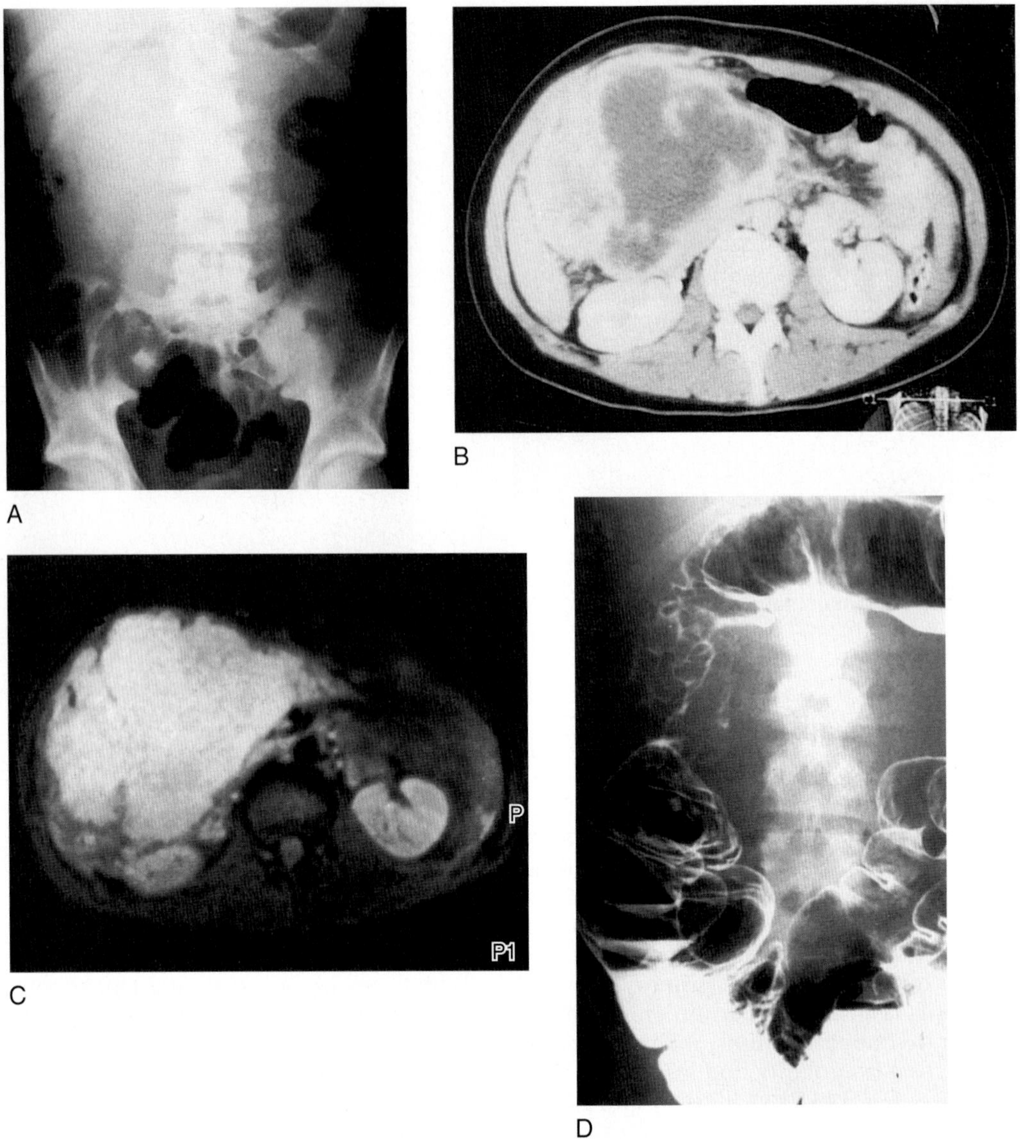

FIGURE 143-9. Mucinous adenocarcinoma of the colon. **A,** Plain radiograph of the abdomen obtained after palpation of an abdominal mass in a 14-year-old boy shows a large mass in the right upper quadrant displacing normal intra-abdominal structures. **B,** Because the presumptive diagnosis was Burkitt lymphoma, a CT scan was performed, which showed that the mass had a central area of nonenhancement that was initially believed to represent necrosis in a lymphomatous tumor. **C,** T2-weighted spin echo MR image shows marked irregularity of the mass and high signal consistent with a malignant tumor. **D,** Barium enema (performed after needle biopsy had revealed signet cells) shows a circumferential mass surrounding the lumen of the ascending colon.

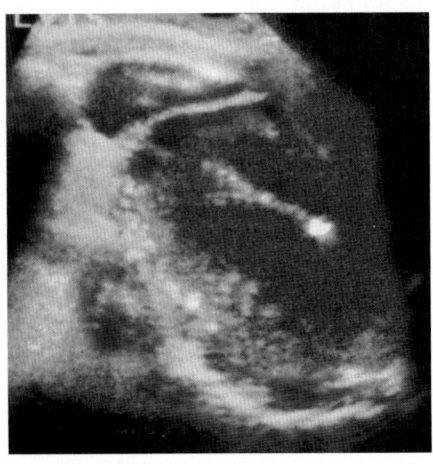
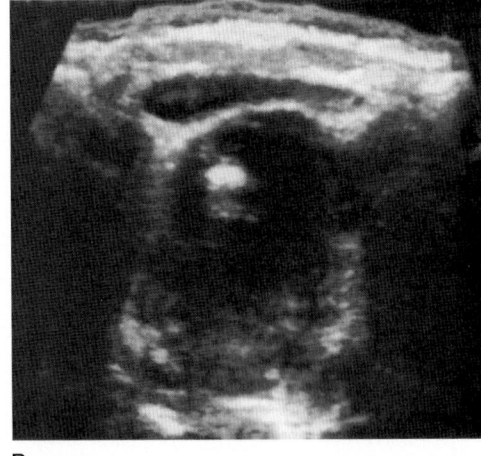

FIGURE 143-10. Perirectal lymphocytic lymphoma in a 14-year-old boy. Longitudinal **(A)** and transverse **(B)** ultrasound images of the pelvis show a large hypoechoic mass completely surrounding the rectum and displacing the bladder. The echogenic foci within the mass are related to residual intraluminal air.   *Continued*

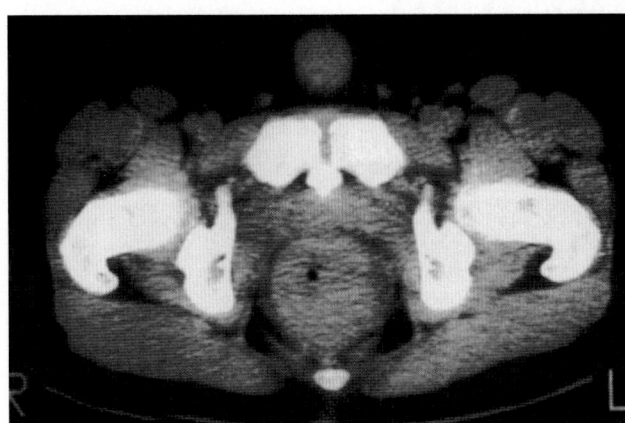

C

FIGURE 143-10, cont'd. **C,** CT image through the pelvis shows the markedly narrowed rectal lumen surrounded by the lymphomatous mass.

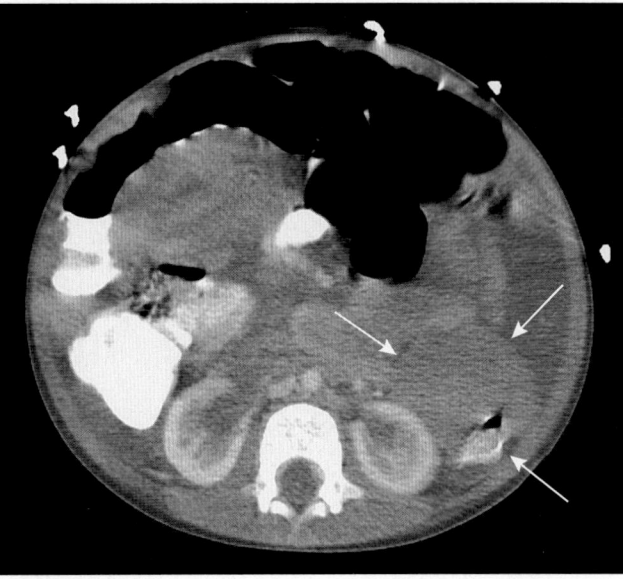

FIGURE 143-11. Axial CT image in a 6-year-old boy with Burkitt lymphoma (same patient as in Fig. 138-3) reveals asymmetrically thickened descending colonic wall in left mid-abdomen *(arrows).* (Courtesy of R. Paul Guillerman, Houston, TX.)

SUGGESTED READINGS

Aziz A, Kane TD, Meza MP, et al: An unusual cause of rectal bleeding and intestinal obstruction in a child with peripheral vascular malformations. Pediatr Surg Int 2005;21:491-493

Bethel CAI, Bhattacharyya N, Hutchinson C, et al: Alimentary tract malignancies in children. J Pediatr Surg 1997;32:1004-1009

Bronner MP: Gastrointestinal inherited polyposis syndromes. Mod Pathol 2003;16:359-365

Capitanio MA, Kirkpatrick JA: Lymphoid hyperplasia of the colon in children: roentgen observations. Radiology 1970;94:323-327

D'Aleo C, Lazzareschi I, Ruggiero A, Riccardi R: Carcinoid tumors of the appendix in children: two case reports and review of the literature. Pediatr Hematol Oncol 2001;18:347-351

EMedicine. Colon, Polyposis Syndromes. Available at http://www.emedicine.com/radio/topic567.htm. Accessed February 28, 2006

EMedicine. Gastrointestinal Neoplasms. Available at http://www.emedicine.com/PED/topic3028.htm. Accessed February 28, 2006

Erdman SH, Barnard JA: Gastrointestinal polyps and polyposis syndromes in children. Curr Opin Pediatr 2002;14:576-582

Healy JC, Reznek RH, Clark SK, et al: MR appearances of desmoid tumors in familial adenomatous polyposis. Am J Roentgenol AJR 1997;169:465-472

Laufer I, deSa D. Lymphoid follicular pattern: a normal feature of the pediatric colon. AJR Am J Roentgenol 1978;130:51-55

Levendoglu H, Rosen Y: Nodular lymphoid hyperplasia of gut in HIV infection. Am J Gastroenterol 1992;87:1200-1202

Morson BC, Dawson IMP: Gastrointestinal Pathology. Oxford, Blackwell Scientific, 1972

Okada T, Sasaki F, Ueki S, et al: Juvenile polyposis coli in a child: report of a case. Surgery Today 2004;34:609-612

Radin DR, Fortgang KC, Zee CS, et al: Turcot syndrome: a case with spinal cord and colonic neoplasms. Am J Roentgenol AJR 1984;142:475-476

Schreibman IR, Baker M, Amos C, McGarrity TJ: The hamartomatous polyposis syndromes: a clinical and molecular review. Am J Gastroenterol 2005;100:476-490

Schwartz DC, Cole CE, Sun Y, Jacoby RF: Diffuse nodular lymphoid hyperplasia of the colon: polyposis syndrome or normal variant? Gastrointest Endosc 2003;58:630-632

Spunt SL, Pratt CB, Rao BN, et al: Childhood carcinoid tumors: the St. Jude Children's Research Hospital experience. J Pediatr Surg 2000;35:1282-1286

Stoupis C, Ros PR: Imaging findings in hepatoblastoma associated with Gardner's syndrome. Am J Roentgenol AJR 1993;161:593-594

Stringer DA, Babyn PS: Pediatric Gastrointestinal Imaging and Intervention, 2nd ed. Hamilton, Ontario, BC Decker, 2000

PART 11

THE ADRENAL AND RETROPERITONEUM

The Adrenal and Retroperitoneum

ALAN DANEMAN, OSCAR NAVARRO, and JACK O. HALLER

THE ADRENAL

Normal Anatomy

The adrenal gland is composed of an outer cortex derived from fetal mesoderm and an inner medulla derived from neural crest tissue. The right adrenal gland is a triangular structure located on the superior pole of the right kidney behind and to the right of the inferior vena cava. The left adrenal gland has a semilunar shape and is located along the anteromedial surface of the superior pole of the left kidney, lateral to the aorta; it may extend above the kidney in 50% of children. Both adrenal glands are contained within the superior aspect of Gerota's fascia, to which they are firmly attached. Each adrenal gland receives blood from three separate arteries: a superior adrenal artery that originates from the inferior phrenic artery, a middle adrenal artery that comes directly from the aorta at the level of the celiac axis, and an inferior adrenal artery that arises from the main renal artery. Each gland drains through a single vein. On the right, the vein enters directly into the inferior vena cava at the T11-12 level; on the left, the adrenal vein drains either directly into the renal vein or indirectly via the inferior phrenic vein.

Imaging

The adrenal glands can be visualized on antenatal ultrasonography (US) as early as the second trimester (Fig. 144-1). During the neonatal period, the glands are relatively large because of the presence of the fetal cortex, and both adrenals can be well visualized on US (see Fig. 144-1; see also Chapter 24). Once the fetal cortex has involuted, the glands are more difficult to visualize in detail on US; therefore, computed tomography (CT) and magnetic resonance imaging (MRI) play a more important role in imaging the adrenal glands in older infants and children.

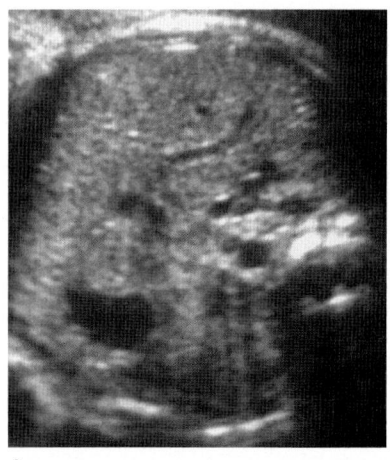
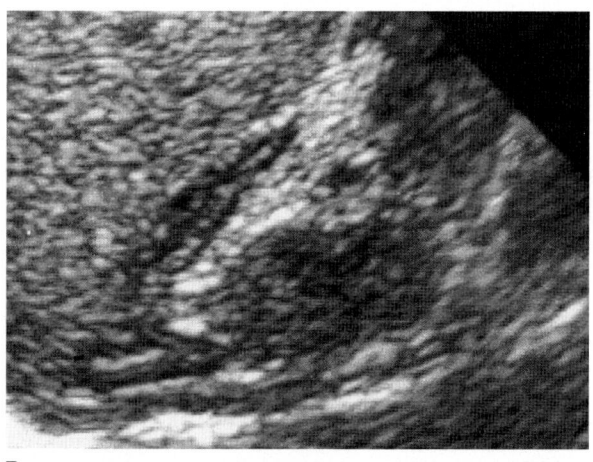

A   B

FIGURE 144-1. Antenatal and postnatal sonograms of a normal right adrenal gland. **A,** On the antenatal sonogram, the right adrenal gland has a V shape in a transverse view of the upper abdomen of the fetus. **B,** In the neonate, the longitudinal scan reveals that the right adrenal gland has a reversed Z shape.

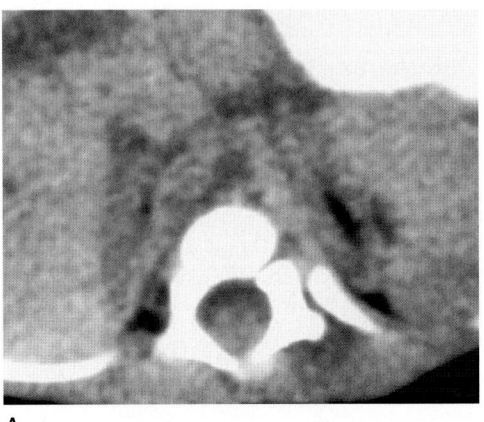
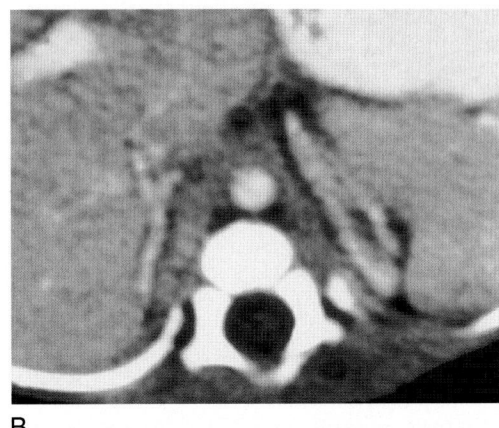

A   B

FIGURE 144-2. Normal adrenal glands. CT of the upper abdomen before **(A)** and after **(B)** intravenous injection of contrast material in a full-term neonate with normal adrenal glands. The right adrenal can be seen lying behind the inferior vena cava, lateral to the right crus of the diaphragm, and medial to the right lobe of the liver. The left adrenal lies behind the stomach, lateral to the left diaphragmatic crus, and medial to the spleen. In the postcontrast scan, the adrenals enhance dramatically, probably as a result of the large sinusoids in the fetal cortex, which persists in the neonate.

On both CT and MRI, both adrenal glands are usually easily visualized at all ages and are found anteromedial to the upper pole of the ipsilateral kidney (Fig. 144-2). The left adrenal lies lateral to the left diaphragmatic crus and aorta, posterior to the stomach and tail of the pancreas, and medial to the spleen. The right adrenal lies lateral to the right diaphragmatic crus, medial to the right lobe of the liver, and posterior to the inferior vena cava. In older infants and children, the adrenal glands are usually thinner than the adjacent diaphragmatic crura on axial CT and MR images.

Plain abdominal radiographs, excretory urography, and angiography were used extensively in the past in patients with known or suspected adrenal disease. However, these modalities cannot show subtle changes in the adrenal gland or the extent of disease as well as modern cross-sectional imaging modalities and are seldom used today.

More recently, positron emission tomography (PET) has been used to evaluate recurrent or metastatic adrenal neoplasms, mainly neuroblastoma but also adrenocortical carcinoma. Initial reports indicate that this modality is sensitive in detecting disease, sometimes more accurately than CT or MRI. The radiation exposure from PET scanning is comparable to that from other radiographic techniques and nuclear medicine studies. Based on these initial promising results, when PET becomes more widely available, it may become the standard approach to the evaluation of adrenal disease. The fusion of PET with CT or MRI may optimize the depiction and characterization of adrenal disease.

Adrenal Masses

An adrenal mass may be due to neoplasm arising from the medulla or cortex, hemorrhage, abscess, or cyst. For special consideration of masses in the neonatal period, see Chapter 24.

Medullary Neoplasms

Neoplasms arising from the medulla are of neural crest origin and may occur not only in the medulla but also in the sympathetic nerve chains. These neoplasms include neuroblastoma, ganglioneuroma, and pheochromocytoma.

NEUROBLASTOMA. Neuroblastoma is the most common extracranial solid neoplasm and accounts for almost 10% of all neoplasms seen in pediatrics (see also Chapter 24). These tumors may arise not only in the adrenal glands but also anywhere along the sympathetic nerve chains from the neck down to the pelvis. Neuroblastoma arises in the abdomen in three quarters of cases; of these, one half to two thirds of lesions occur in the adrenal gland, and the remainder occur elsewhere from sympathetic nerve tissue. Among abdominal neoplasms, neuroblastoma is the second most common after Wilms tumor.

Neuroblastoma and ganglioneuroma belong to a group of related neoplasms arising from neural crest tissue that are distinguished by their degree of cellular maturation and differentiation. Neuroblastoma accounts for the vast majority of these lesions and has the most primitive and malignant cells. It is composed of small round cells that may be characteristically arranged in rosettes. Ganglioneuroma represents the more differentiated end of the spectrum and is benign. Lesions with mixed histology are termed *ganglioneuroblastomas* and represent an intermediate group.

Most children with neuroblastoma present between 1 and 5 years of age, with a median age of almost 2 years. However, the lesion may present in the neonatal period, and it has also been detected in the fetus by antenatal US. Less commonly, it may be present in older children and teenagers. Both sexes are affected equally. Neuroblastoma has been found in association with neurofibromatosis type 1 and aganglionosis of the colon.

Most neuroblastomas present as a palpable mass. This may be an incidental finding in an apparently healthy child, or it may come to attention in a child with relatively minor abdominal trauma. More often, however, children present with symptoms and signs related to local tumor invasion, metastatic disease, or the effects of hormone production, such as catecholamines and vasoactive intestinal polypeptide (VIP). Local invasion may be into the kidneys, or there may be encasement and narrowing of the renal vessels (causing hypertension) and ureters (causing hydronephrosis). Invasion through the intervertebral foramina into the extradural intraspinal space (less common in abdominal than in thoracic neuroblastoma) may cause cord and nerve compression, leading to paraparesis, paraplegia, or bladder and bowel dysfunction. Metastatic disease is present in more than 50% of patients at presentation, and the pattern of metastatic disease is age related (see Chapter 24). The most common sites include local and distant lymph nodes (e.g., cervical nodes), bone, bone marrow, liver, and skin. Symptoms and signs thus include skeletal pain, and metastatic lesions to the metaphyses of the long bones may result in a clinical picture simulating arthritis. Metastases to the orbits may cause proptosis and periorbital ecchymoses. High levels of catecholamines may lead to hypertension, and VIP may cause diarrhea. An interesting phenomenon is presentation with the signs of opsomyoclonus, such as nystagmus and ataxia; this occurs as a result of nonmetastatic, distant paraneoplastic effects on the cerebellum.

Neuroblastoma:

- **Second most common pediatric abdominal neoplasm**
- **Arises from neural crest tissue, most commonly in the adrenal gland**
- **Most children present between ages 1 and 5 years**
- **Tends to encase vessels and may invade neuroforamina**
- **Fifty percent of patients have metastases at diagnosis**
- **Prognosis depends on age, stage, site of disease, and N-*myc* oncogene amplification**

Several classification systems have been proposed for staging neuroblastoma. The international neuroblastoma staging system is shown in Table 144-1. According to this classification, the distribution of patients at presentation is as follows: stage 1, 20%; stage 2, 10%; stage 3, 15%; stage 4, 50%; and stage 4S, 4%. The diagnosis of neuroblastoma can be made by tissue biopsy, but a combination of positive bone marrow aspirate and increased urinary catecholamine metabolites (vanillylmandelic acid and homovanillic acid) is sufficient to confirm the diagnosis. The urinary level of catecholamine metabolites is increased in almost 90% of cases of neuroblastoma.

The treatment of patients with neuroblastoma depends on several factors, including the stage of the

TABLE 144-1

International Neuroblastoma Staging System

Stage	Description
1	Localized tumor confined to area of origin; complete gross excision, with or without microscopic residual
2A	Unilateral tumor with incomplete gross excision; ipsilateral and contralateral lymph nodes negative microscopically
2B	Unilateral tumor with complete or incomplete gross excision; positive ipsilateral regional lymph node; contralateral lymph nodes negative microscopically
3	Tumor infiltrating across midline, with or without regional lymph node involvement; *or* unilateral tumor with contralateral regional lymph node involvement; *or* midline tumor with bilateral regional lymph node involvement
4	Dissemination of tumor to distant lymph nodes, bone, liver, or other organs (except as defined in stage 4S)
4S	Localized primary tumor as defined for stage 1 or 2 with dissemination limited to liver, skin, or bone marrow (<10% involvement)

disease at the time of presentation and the response to initial therapy. Surgery, chemotherapy, and radiation therapy all have a role to play. Primary surgical resection is the treatment of choice for more localized tumors, and chemotherapy is used for those that are unresectable. Radiation is used for localized disease that does not respond to chemotherapy. Delayed surgical resection may be performed for initially unresectable lesions once they have shrunk sufficiently.

The prognosis of neuroblastoma depends on the patient's age, the stage of disease at presentation, and the tumor site. A favorable prognosis is seen mainly in patients younger than 1 year with low-stage disease and with lesions that arise in extra-abdominal sites. Patients with localized disease may have an 80% 2-year survival rate, compared with 5% for those with bone metastases. Several biologic markers may also affect prognosis. A poor prognosis is seen in patients with N-*myc* oncogene amplification (>10 copies) and in those with allelic loss of chromosome 1p and diploid (decreased DNA) karyotype. In contrast, a favorable prognosis is seen with unamplified N-*myc* oncogene, well-differentiated stroma, absence of abnormalities of chromosome 1, and triploid karyotypes.

Adrenal neuroblastomas and those arising from the adjacent retroperitoneal area are usually easily identified with US, CT, or MRI because the mass is generally quite large by the time of presentation (Figs. 144-3 to 144-5). Very small masses are uncommon, and in these cases, CT and MRI play a more important role than US (Fig. 144-6). These cross-sectional imaging modalities have obviated the need for plain radiographs and urography. On US, the masses have a variety of sonographic appearances. Areas of hyperechogenicity may represent calcification, and they do not always have acoustic shadowing (see

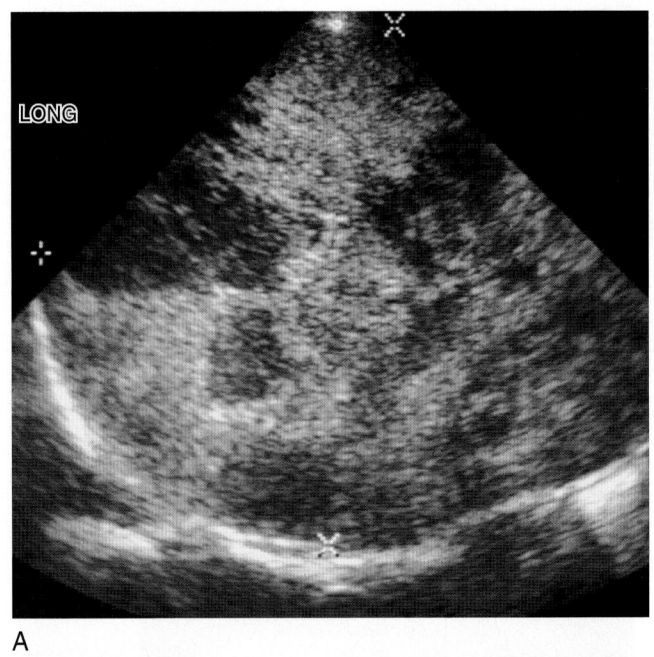

A

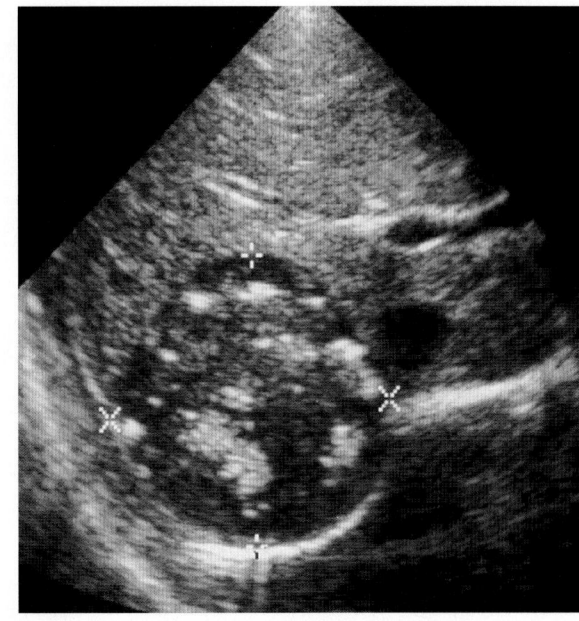

B

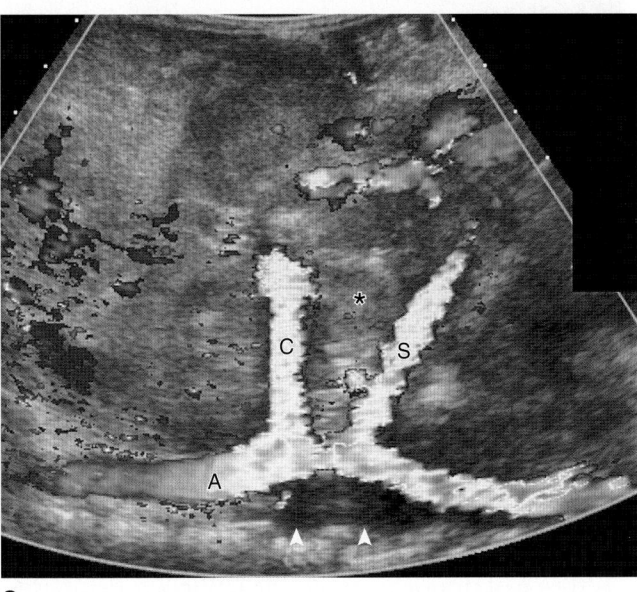

C

FIGURE 144-3. Sonograms of the right upper quadrant in three children with adrenal neuroblastoma. **A,** Longitudinal sonogram shows that the neuroblastoma has a heterogeneous echogenicity, with hyperechoic and hypoechoic areas. **B,** Transverse sonogram shows very small, globular, hyperechoic areas that represent calcification without acoustic shadowing. **C,** Longitudinal color Doppler sonogram shows a large heterogeneous soft tissue mass within the abdomen, a portion of which *(arrowheads)* extends posterior to the aorta (A), encasing it and lifting it away from the spine. A portion of the mass (*) separates and encases the celiac axis (C) and the superior mesenteric artery (S). (Courtesy of Brian D. Coley, MD.)

Fig. 144-3). Anechoic areas resulting from cystic, hemorrhagic, or necrotic changes may be present, but these are more common in Wilms tumors. Mainly cystic lesions may be present, particularly in neonates. On CT, the lesions have attenuation equal to or less than that of muscle, and calcification may be present in 85% of cases. The calcification may be coarse, globular, finely stippled, or curvilinear (see Figs. 144-4, 144-7, and 144-15). After intravenous contrast injection, the lesions enhance heterogeneously, depicting areas of vascularity more clearly than areas of necrosis, hemorrhage, and cystic change. On MRI, the lesions have low signal on T1-weighted images and high signal on T2-weighted images.

With all modalities, it is essential to assess the extent of tumor within the abdomen as accurately as possible. In this regard, US tends to underestimate the full extent of disease; for this reason, CT and MRI are required

after initial US. Local spread may be to lymph nodes (see Fig. 144-7), or there may be direct invasion into the kidneys or liver (Fig. 144-8). The ureters may be obstructed, and there may be direct or lymph node spread behind the crura into the thorax. Transverse CT scans tend to overestimate invasion into adjacent solid viscera, such as the kidneys and liver; longitudinal sagittal and coronal US or MRI scans are more helpful in this regard. Sagittal and coronal reconstruction of axial CT images with new-generation CT scanners should be used if renal or hepatic invasion is in question.

Regardless of which imaging modality is used, it should be optimized to define the anatomy of the major vessels clearly (Figs. 144-7 to 144-9). This might involve the use of color or power Doppler US, a power injector for intravenous contrast administration for CT, or magnetic resonance arteriography and venography

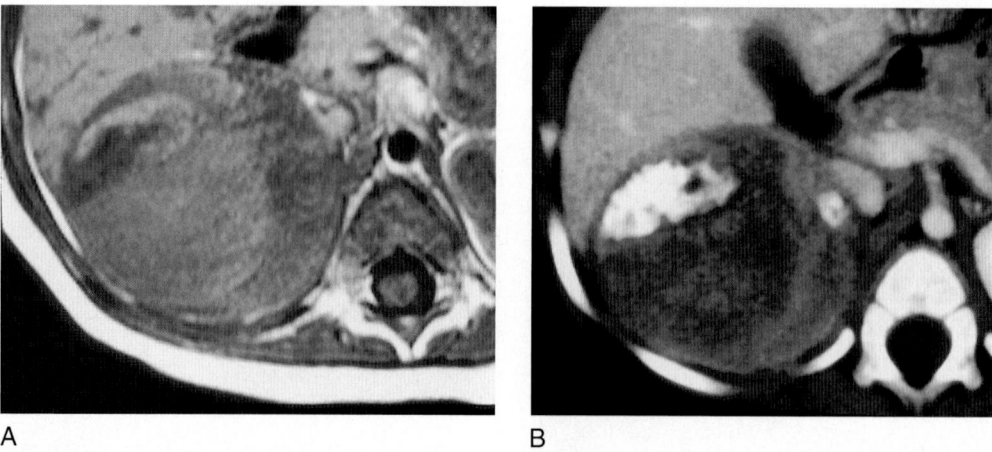

FIGURE 144-4. Neuroblastoma. MRI **(A)** and CT **(B)** of the upper abdomen in a patient with right adrenal neuroblastoma. The mass is well defined, with a large area of calcification anterolaterally. The mass displaces the inferior vena cava slightly forward. The spinal canal is uninvolved.

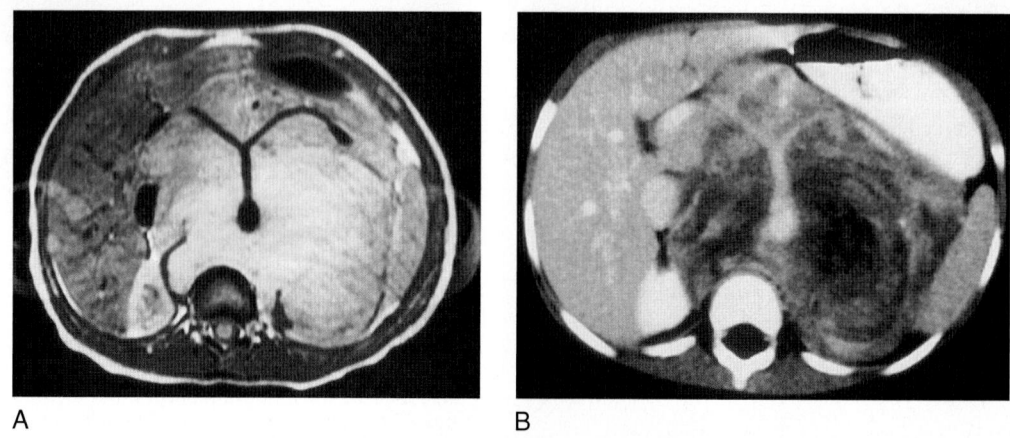

FIGURE 144-5. Neuroblastoma. T1-weighted MRI **(A)** and CT **(B)** of the upper abdomen in a patient with upper abdominal retroperitoneal neuroblastoma. In both images, the large mass crosses the midline; the aorta is displaced forward; and there is encasement of the aorta, celiac axis, and proximal portions of the splenic and hepatic arteries. The inferior vena cava is displaced anteriorly and to the right. Regardless of the imaging modality used, display of the vasculature is essential for an accurate evaluation of the extent of disease both preoperatively and during follow-up.

with gadolinium if necessary. Neuroblastoma may push major vessels aside, but more characteristically, the tumor encases the vessels (see Figs. 144-5 and 144-8). By defining the position of the vessels and determining the relationship between them and the tumor tissue, one can accurately assess the extent of tumor and determine operability. Furthermore, compression or encasement of the renal vessels may lead to renal atrophy as a result of ischemia or infarction. Neuroblastoma rarely invades the major veins, which occurs more frequently with Wilms tumor; however, in rare cases, neuroblastoma may extend up the inferior vena cava into the heart (Fig. 144-10).

Intraspinal extension occurs less commonly with abdominal neuroblastomas than with those arising in the chest, and even less commonly with those arising in the adrenal gland. However, significant intraspinal extension may be present without overt clinical symptoms or signs. Therefore, it is essential to evaluate the intraspinal contents in all children with neuroblastoma to determine the presence or absence of extradural spread, because this may affect therapy. MRI defines intraspinal spread exceptionally well, without the need for intrathecal

contrast (Fig. 144-11). The tumor is easily seen if it involves the intervertebral foramina or extradural space. Intraspinal involvement may be limited to one vertebral level, or the tumor may grow like a sheet of tissue or in a more nodular or masslike manner that involves several levels. Involvement may include sites distant from the primary intra-abdominal lesion (Fig. 144-12).

> **MRI should be used to assess the presence and extent of intraspinal involvement in all patients with neuroblastoma.**

In the past, CT was performed after the intrathecal injection of contrast material (e.g., metrizamide) to evaluate the intraspinal contents (Figs. 144-12 and 144-13). However, new-generation CT scanners can depict spinal canal details very well without the need for intrathecal contrast injection (Figs. 144-14 and 144-15). In scans done after intravenous contrast injection, the spinal cord, surrounding thecal sac, and adjacent soft tissue structures are easily identified, making visualization of

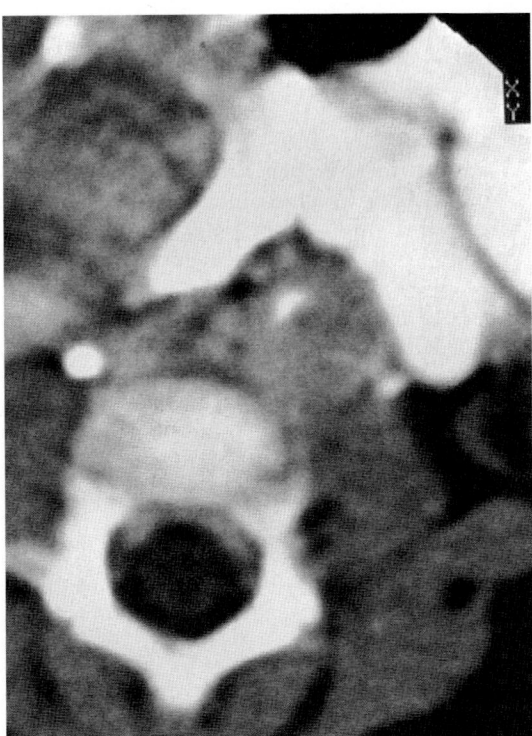

FIGURE 144-6. CT of the abdomen in a patient with retroperitoneal neuroblastoma who presented with opsomyoclonus. The small retroperitoneal mass is well defined and has a small area of calcification anteromedially. The left ureter is displaced laterally, and the contrast-filled bowel loops are displaced forward. Neuroblastomas of this size are less common than larger lesions.

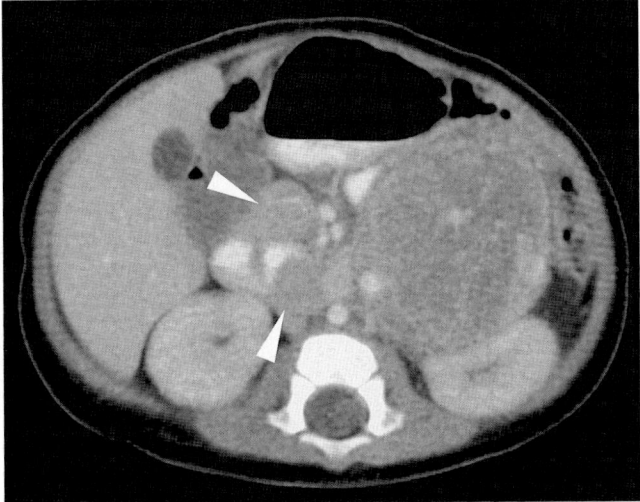

FIGURE 144-7. Neuroblastoma with metastasis. Contrast-enhanced CT shows a large left adrenal mass with calcification. Lobular masses in the retroperitoneum and mesentery *(arrowheads)* represent lymph node metastases.

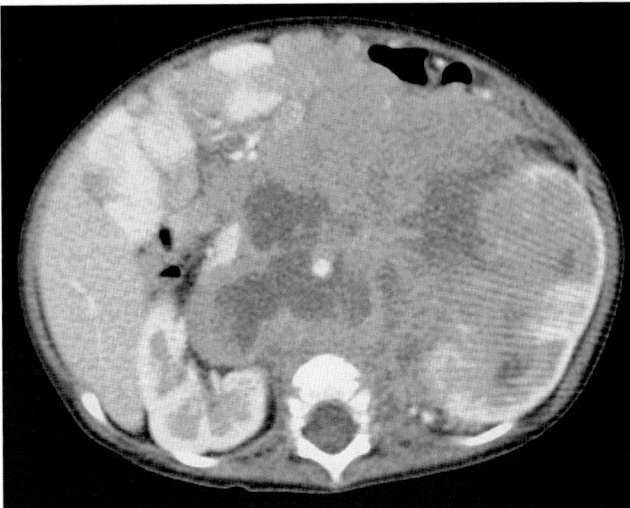

FIGURE 144-8. Neuroblastoma and renal invasion. Contrast-enhanced CT shows a large retroperitoneal neuroblastoma with an irregular, lobulated border that surrounds vessels and has displaced the right kidney. The interface with the left renal cortex is indistinct, and there is tumor invasion into the left renal hilum.

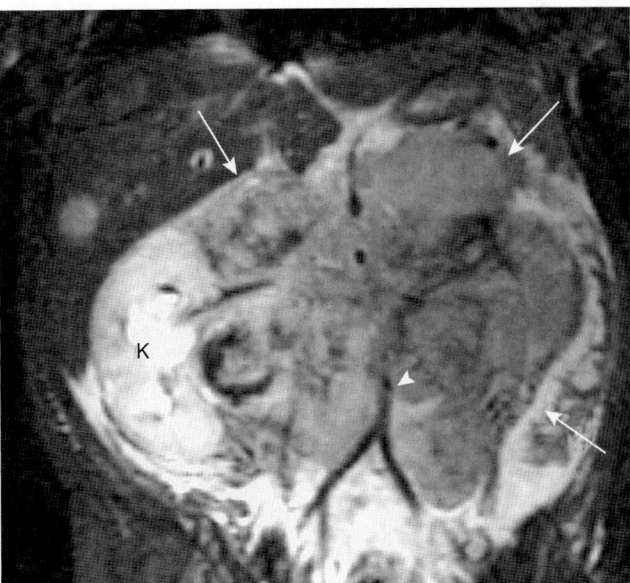

FIGURE 144-9. Neuroblastoma. Coronal T2-weighted MR image with fat saturation shows a large area of mixed signal intensity representing a large retroperitoneal neuroblastoma *(arrowhead)* encasing the aorta *(arrows)* and displacing the right kidney (K) laterally. Note also the high signal metastatic lesion in the right hepatic lobe. (Courtesy of Brian D. Coley, MD.)

any intraspinal tumor simple. In infants, US may be able to detect intraspinal extension before there is complete ossification of the posterior elements of the vertebrae.

Other features that may be present in the abdomen in patients with neuroblastoma include metastases to the liver. There may be single or multiple nodules or masses, or the metastases may be infiltrative, particularly in neonates. Rarely, peritoneal seeding with nodules and ascites may be present. Metastases to bone are best identified with radionuclide bone scans or iodine-131 metaiodobenzylguanidine (MIBG) scans. MRI has the advantage over other cross-sectional imaging techniques because it can also be used to assess the bone marrow in patients with neuroblastoma of the abdomen or other sites.

Imaging plays an important role in patient evaluation after surgery or chemotherapy. Regular follow-up is

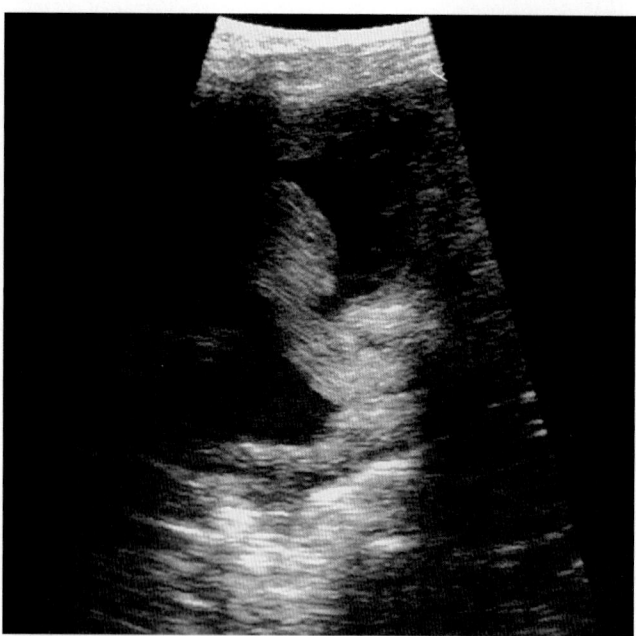

FIGURE 144-10. Longitudinal sonogram of the lower thorax shows that an echogenic tumor thrombus of abdominal neuroblastoma extends up the inferior vena cava into the right atrium and anteriorly into the right ventricle. (Courtesy of Dr. Michel Panuel, Marseilles, France.)

required after surgery to assess the tumor bed for local recurrence, and this is best achieved with CT. Similarly, follow-up is essential in patients with nonoperable tumors to assess the response to chemotherapy and determine the most appropriate time for delayed surgery. If the lesion responds to chemotherapy, there is usually a regression of the mass, which shrinks to a very small amount of soft tissue that often becomes calcified (Fig. 144-16). However, biopsy is sometimes necessary to determine whether residual tissue is fibrosis or viable tumor. Renal atrophy may also occur after treatment and may be the result of surgical trauma, chemotherapy, or radiation.

GANGLIONEUROMA. Ganglioneuroma represents the mature, benign form of neural crest neoplasm, in contrast to its malignant relative the neuroblastoma. Ganglioneuromas are composed of mature ganglion cells and nerve fibers and are usually well encapsulated. This type of neural crest tumor is far less frequent than neuroblastoma; it may develop from the maturation of a known malignant neuroblastoma, or it may be found de novo.

Most ganglioneuromas occur in the posterior mediastinum. Only one third occur in the abdomen; most are paravertebral and seldom involve the adrenal gland. They have been documented in association with neurofibromatosis. These tumors usually occur in older children, who are often asymptomatic. The tumors may be found incidentally on abdominal US or chest radiographs performed for other reasons. Occasionally, they

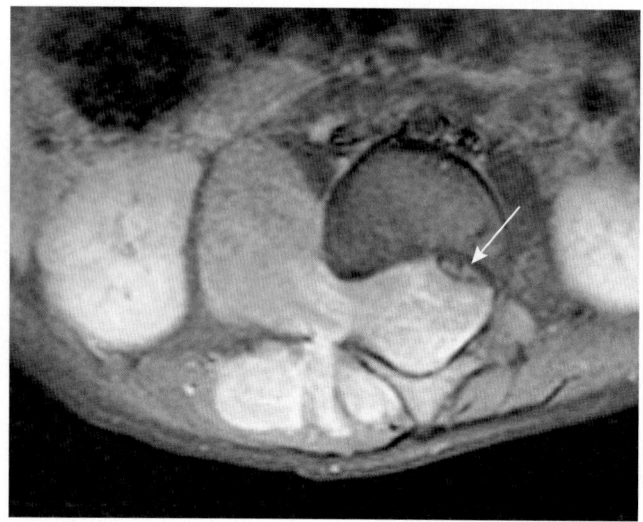

A

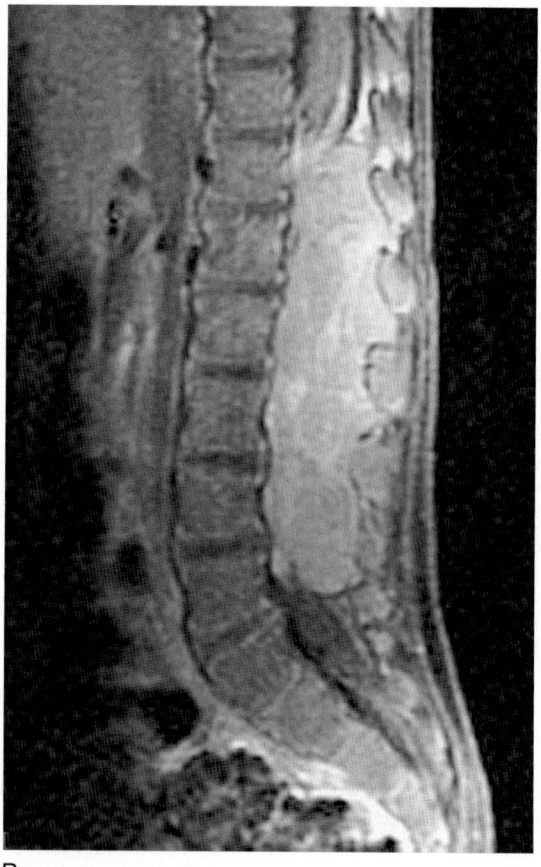

B

FIGURE 144-11. Neuroblastoma and intrathecal spread. **A,** Axial T1-weighted contrast-enhanced MR image shows a retroperitoneal tumor medial to the right kidney. It is invading the posterior paraspinal muscles and the spinal canal, displacing the spinal cord to the left *(arrow)*. **B,** Sagittal T1-weighted contrast-enhanced MR image shows tumor filling and expanding the spinal canal. (Courtesy of Brian D. Coley, MD.)

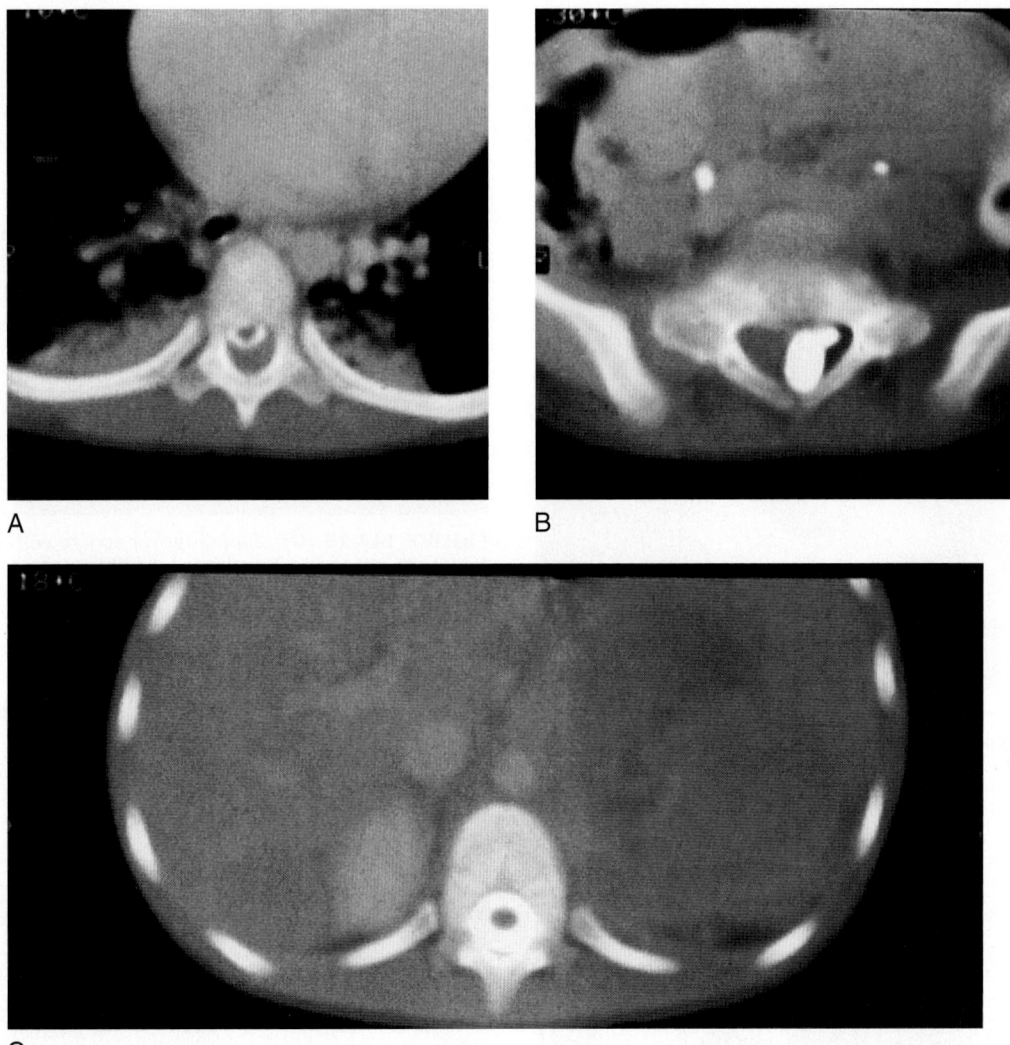

FIGURE 144-12. Adrenal neuroblastoma. CT scans through the chest (**A**), upper pelvis (**B**), and upper abdomen (**C**) in a patient with a large left adrenal neuroblastoma. This study was performed after injection of intrathecal metrizamide to outline the thecal sac. The large tumor mass is noted in the left adrenal in the upper abdomen. Displacement of the thecal sac is noted in the lower chest and in the pelvis owing to spinal canal involvement, distant from the primary tumor.

may cause symptoms resulting from growth into the intervertebral foramina, causing cord compression. Rarely, patients with ganglioneuromas present with myoclonic encephalopathy, diarrhea, or hypertension. Urinary catecholamine levels are usually normal.

The imaging appearance of ganglioneuroma is similar to that of neuroblastoma, and abdominal lesions may encase the aorta and inferior vena cava and their branches. The definitive diagnosis therefore depends on the histologic examination of tumor tissue. In some patients with abdominal ganglioneuromas, surgical removal may be difficult, particularly if the mass is large, is adjacent to vital structures, encases vessels, or extends into the intervertebral foramina. Clinicians may prefer to manage these patients nonoperatively, particularly if they are asymptomatic. In such cases, regular clinical and imaging follow-up is mandatory. There are 10 documented cases in the literature of patients with abdominal ganglioneuromas who developed malignant peripheral nerve sheath tumors in the mass many years later. Seven

of these patients had had abdominal radiation therapy for neuroblastomas that then matured into benign ganglioneuromas, but three did not. CT or MRI is essential for follow-up. Changes in the appearance of the mass or an increase in its size should alert one to the possibility of malignant degeneration, and biopsy should be performed. Patients with ganglioneuromas managed nonoperatively should probably be followed for life, but it is uncertain how often imaging should be done.

> **Imaging alone cannot reliably distinguish among neuroblastoma, ganglioneuroblastoma, and ganglioneuroma.**

PHEOCHROMOCYTOMA. Pheochromocytoma is an uncommon neoplasm in children. Five percent of all pheochromocytomas occur in children, accounting for well under 1% of all neoplasms seen in large pediatric centers. It is a potentially curable secretory tumor arising

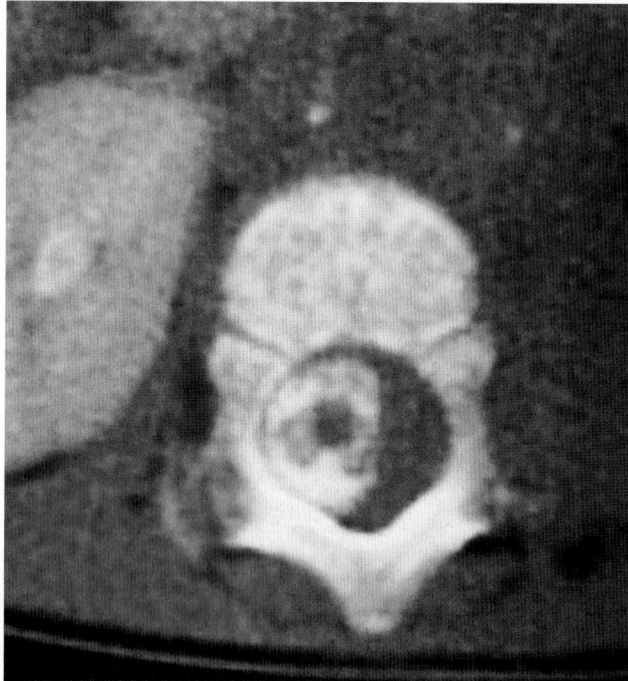

FIGURE 144-13. Intraspinal extension of neuroblastoma. CT after intrathecal injection of metrizamide. The thecal sac is compressed on the left owing to extradural, intraspinal extension from a left-sided neuroblastoma, which has caused some erosion of the vertebral body and pedicle.

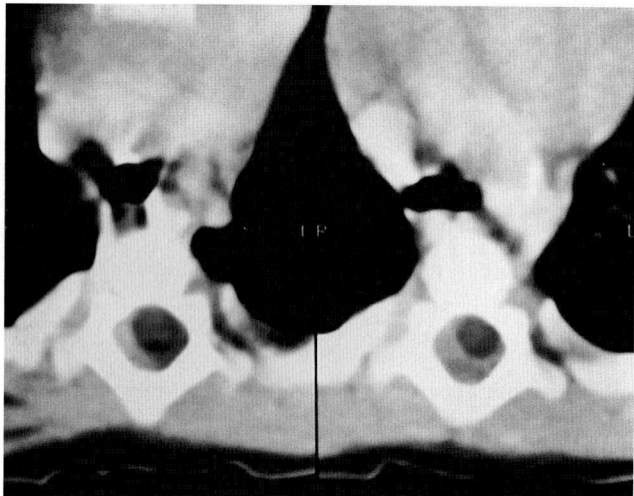

FIGURE 144-14. CT of the chest in a patient with upper abdominal neuroblastoma shows extension of the tumor sheet into the spinal canal posteriorly and on the right, displacing the thecal sac anteriorly and to the left. This tumor sheet can be seen after the intravenous injection of contrast material; intrathecal injection is not necessary.

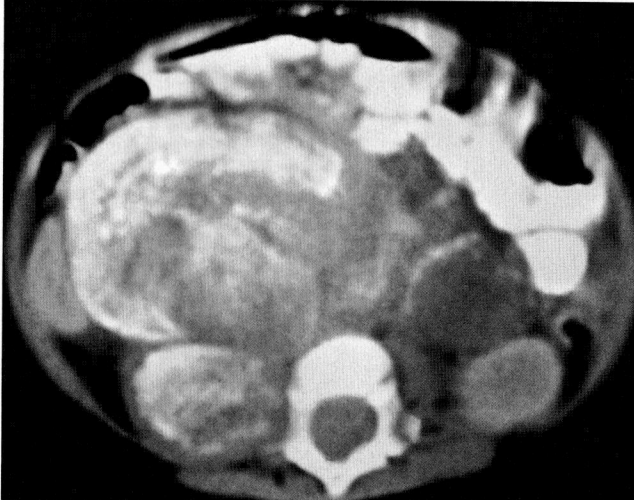

FIGURE 144-15. CT of a full-term neonate with a huge lobulated, calcified retroperitoneal right-sided neuroblastoma that crosses the midline. Contrast-filled bowel is displaced anteriorly and toward the left. Note the enlarged spinal canal as a result of tumor invasion.

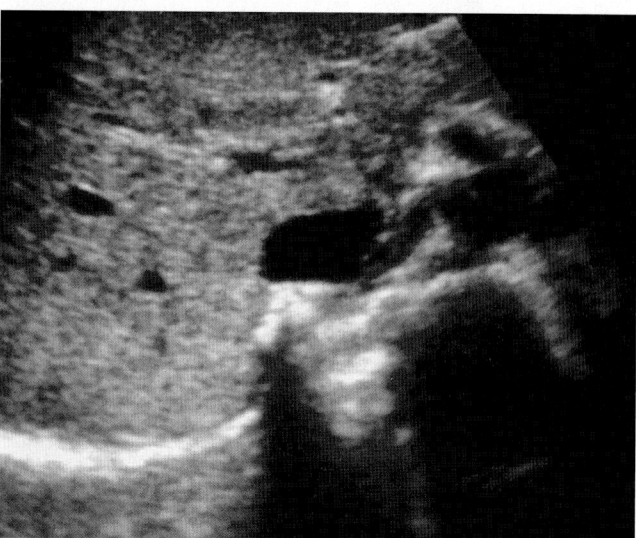

FIGURE 144-16. Adrenal neuroblastoma. Transverse sonogram of the upper abdomen shows hyperechoic foci with posterior acoustic shadowing caused by calcification lying behind the inferior vena cava. This scan was done after chemotherapy in a patient with right adrenal neuroblastoma and shows residual calcification after reduction in the size of the mass.

from chromaffin cells in the adrenal gland or in extra-adrenal sites. In children, 70% of pheochromocytomas occur in the adrenal gland, and 24% have bilateral adrenal involvement. Thirty percent of patients have extra-adrenal lesions, most of which occur in the upper abdomen. Other less common extra-adrenal sites include the sympathetic chain, anywhere from the base of the skull down to the pelvis; more rarely, they may occur in the urinary bladder, spermatic cord, or vagina. Multiple lesions are present in 30% to 70% of children and are seen mainly in those with a family history of pheochromocytoma. Malignancy is present in 10% of lesions in adults but is much less common in children. The diagnosis of malignancy is often made on the basis of metastases rather than histology.

Pheochromocytoma usually presents in older children but has been reported in infants. It is frequently familial, inherited as an autosomal dominant trait. Familial pheochromocytoma has been described in multiple endocrine neoplasia type II in association with medullary thyroid carcinoma and parathyroid hyperplasia. Pheochromocytoma may also be associated with neurofibromatosis, other neurocutaneous syndromes, and hemihypertrophy.

The clinical presentation is usually related to the secretion of catecholamines, predominantly epinephrine and norepinephrine. Patients may present with hypertension, sweating, headaches, blurred vision, papilledema, flushing, tachycardia, diarrhea, hypertensive encephalopathy, and weight loss. Chronic diarrhea may be due to the production of VIP. Rarely, patients may present with symptoms resulting from metastatic spread or from the local effects of the tumor. Although tumors may range in size from 1 to 10 cm in diameter at presentation, they are usually between 2 and 5 cm. They are well encapsulated and highly vascular and may contain some necrosis and hemorrhage.

Accurate and noninvasive localization of these tumors is required for successful surgical management. In addition, the preoperative delineation of any local invasion or metastatic disease is important, because the malignant potential of these lesions is difficult to assess on histologic grounds. In a child suspected of having pheochromocytoma, careful imaging is required to look for multiple lesions in the adrenal area as well as in extra-adrenal sites. Although US can easily depict lesions in and adjacent to the adrenal glands, it is less sensitive than CT and MRI for lesions in the mid- and lower abdomen, particularly in older children.

> **Pheochromocytoma can occur in adrenal and extra-adrenal locations.**

On US, the lesions may be homogeneously or heterogeneously echoic, with areas of decreased echogenicity caused by hemorrhage and necrosis and areas of increased echogenicity caused by hemorrhage or, less commonly, calcification (Figs. 144-17 and 144-18). On CT, the lesions have soft tissue attenuation, and enhancement may be diffuse, mottled, or rimlike. Hypertensive crises can be provoked by contrast material, which elevates the plasma catecholamine level; however, this is more often caused by angiography than by intravenous injection for CT, and angiography has been largely replaced by CT, MRI, and MIBG scans. On MRI, pheochromocytomas have low signal on T1-weighted images and high signal on T2-weighted images (Fig. 144-18), with a pattern of intense enhancement and slow washout after the administration of gadolinium. The radionuclide MIBG is also accurate in localizing these lesions but does not show the anatomy as well as CT or MRI. Evaluation of the chest is important, even though pheochromocytomas are less common in this region. Chest CT is particularly important in patients suspected of having malignant lesions.

Surgical removal of all known lesions is usually curative. However, clinical follow-up is essential, along with urinary catecholamine measurement to detect recurrence or the development of new lesions.

CORTICAL NEOPLASMS

Adrenocortical neoplasms are uncommon in children. Most occur in children older than 3 years, but they can occur rarely in neonates. Girls are affected three times more commonly than boys, and carcinomas are three times more common than adenomas. The vast majority of these tumors are functioning, and the most common endocrine abnormality is overproduction of androgens. Girls present with virilization, and boys present with pseudoprecocious puberty. Often, there is mixed endocrine dysfunction caused by the overproduction of both glucocorticoids and mineralocorticoids. In contrast, in adrenal hyperplasia, usually only one hormone type is overproduced. Less commonly, patients with adrenocortical neoplasms may present with Cushing syndrome, feminization, or hyperaldosteronism. Although cortical neoplasms are seldom nonfunctioning, when this occurs, the mass may be found incidentally. It is impossible to predict, based on the child's endocrine status, whether a lesion is carcinoma or adenoma. Only a small number of these lesions present with a palpable mass, and these are usually carcinomas. Presentation with metastatic disease is rare.

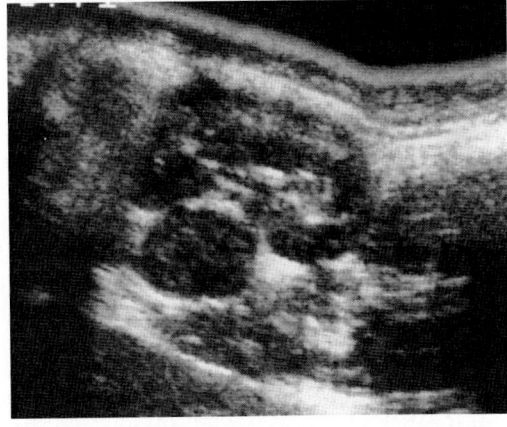
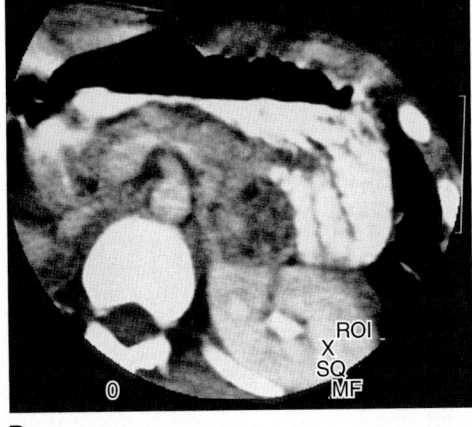

A   B

FIGURE 144-17. Pheochromocytoma. **A,** Longitudinal prone sonogram in an 8-year-old girl shows a left adrenal pheochromocytoma anterior to the left kidney. The mass is well defined and slightly heterogeneous in echogenicity, with no calcification. **B,** CT of a 17-year-old girl with left adrenal pheochromocytoma anterior to the left kidney. The mass is well defined and heterogeneous in attenuation. At age 11 years, this patient had a right adrenal pheochromocytoma removed.

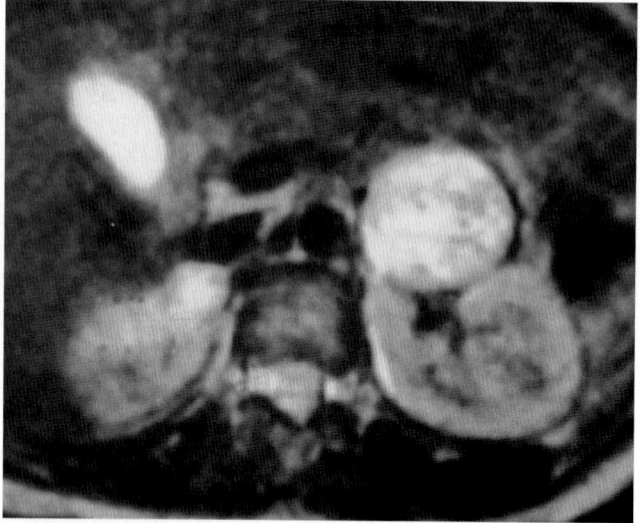

FIGURE 144-18. Bilateral pheochromocytoma. T2-weighted MR image of the upper abdomen in a 12-year-old boy with bilateral adrenal pheochromocytoma. The right adrenal lesion lies between the upper pole of the right kidney and the inferior vena cava, and the large left adrenal lesion lies in front of the kidney and to the left of the aorta. Both lesions are well defined and have high signal intensity on T2 weighting.

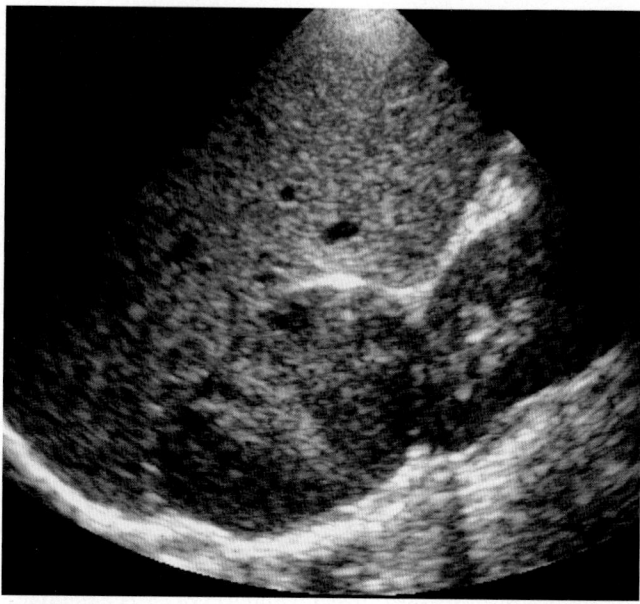

FIGURE 144-19. Adrenal adenoma. On this longitudinal sonogram in a 14-year-old girl, a nonfunctioning right adrenal adenoma was discovered incidentally. The adenoma is well defined between the liver and the right kidney and has a slightly heterogeneous echogenicity.

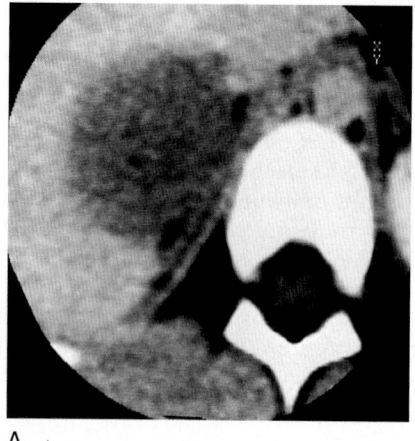
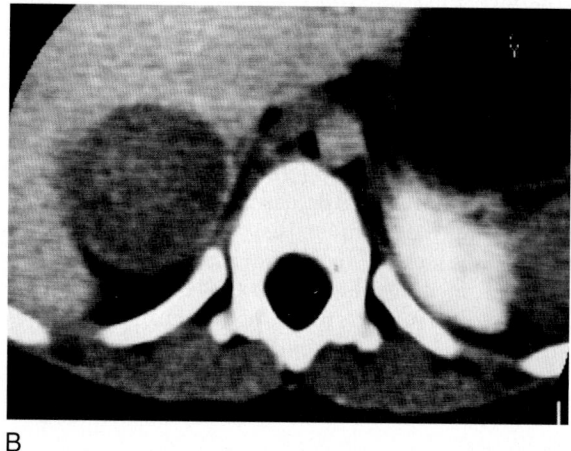

A   B

FIGURE 144-20. Adrenocortical adenoma. **A** and **B,** CT scans of the upper abdomen in a 3-year-old girl with right adrenocortical adenoma **(A)** and a 5-year-old girl with right adrenocortical carcinoma **(B).** Both lesions have low attenuation with no calcification. They are well defined, and in the child with the adenoma, part of the normal adrenal is noted posterior to the mass. With small adrenocortical lesions, it is difficult to differentiate adenoma from carcinoma, as in these two cases.

> **Most adrenocortical neoplasms are functioning tumors, producing symptoms of endocrine overproduction.**

At presentation, the masses are usually larger than 1.5 cm; it is extremely rare for adrenocortical neoplasms in children to present as smaller adrenal nodules. On occasion, the masses may be huge; these are usually carcinomas. Even smaller lesions are easily documented with US, CT, or MRI (Figs. 144-19 and 144-20). US is usually the initial modality used to evaluate the adrenals, but CT and MRI are particularly important for assessing large lesions and local invasion and spread.

On all three modalities, smaller lesions tend to have a fairly homogeneous appearance. Areas of hemorrhage, necrosis, and calcification are seen more commonly in larger lesions, usually carcinomas (Fig. 144-21). In larger lesions, there is often a central scar, with radiating linear bands that represent areas of necrosis and calcification (see Fig. 144-21). This is a characteristic appearance and may help differentiate these neoplasms from other masses in the suprarenal area. It is not always possible to predict accurately which masses are malignant unless there is local spread and invasion or metastatic disease. Initially, lesions displace the surrounding viscera, but large carcinomas may invade the kidney or grow into the inferior vena cava.

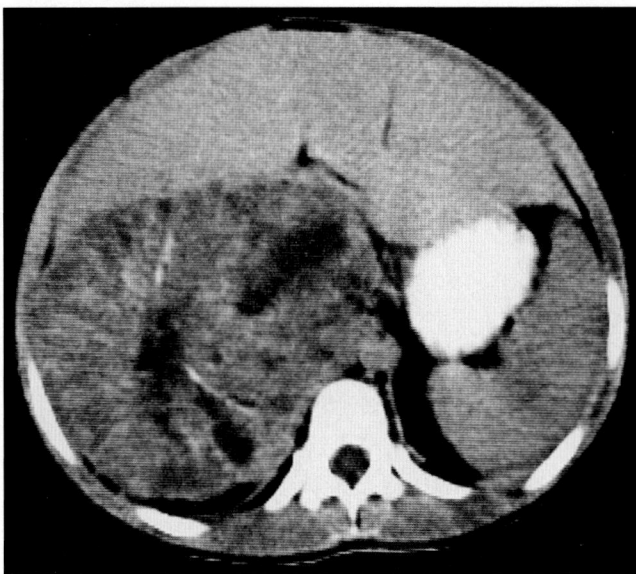

FIGURE 144-21. Adrenocortical carcinoma. CT of the upper abdomen in an 8-year-old girl with precocious puberty shows a large right adrenal mass with heterogeneous attenuation. There is a radial pattern of calcification in the mass, with adjacent areas of decreased attenuation caused by necrosis, which is characteristic of adrenocortical carcinoma. The mass is relatively well defined.

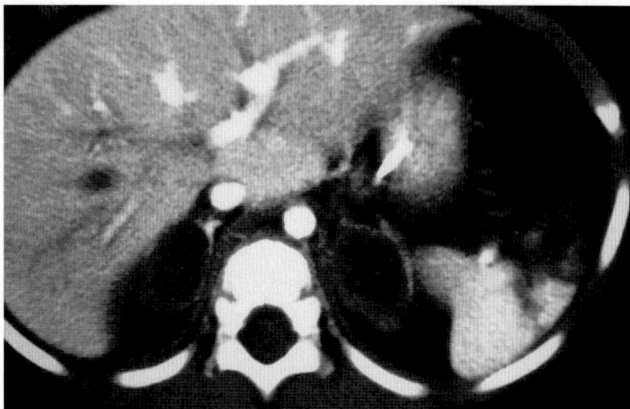

FIGURE 144-22. Adrenal hemorrhage. CT of the upper abdomen in a patient with blunt abdominal trauma shows an anterior splenic laceration and bilateral adrenal hemorrhages.

Metastatic disease from cortical neoplasms is most common in the lungs, liver, and bone, but other unusual sites have been reported. Complete resection of the primary tumor is essential for survival. Chemotherapy has had a major effect on improved outcome. Patients with larger and infiltrating tumors and those with metastatic disease do more poorly. Adenomas clearly have a good prognosis if they are removed completely, but clinical and imaging follow-up is essential, because the histologic differences between adenoma and carcinoma are not clear in all cases.

OTHER ADRENAL NEOPLASMS

Smooth muscle tumors (leiomyomas) have been described in the adrenal glands of children with acquired immunodeficiency syndrome (AIDS). More frequently, these tumors have been described in the small and large bowel in children with AIDS, and they have occasionally been reported at other sites. These tumors are usually unilateral but may be bilateral, and they may arise from the walls of adrenal vasculature. Their presence appears to be linked to the Epstein-Barr virus.

OTHER MASSES

Other adrenal mass lesions are uncommon in children beyond the neonatal period. These include hemorrhage, cyst, and infection.

Adrenal hemorrhage occurs most commonly in the neonatal period (see Chapter 24). However, it may occur in older children after blunt abdominal trauma, usually associated with traumatic lesions in other viscera (Fig. 144-22). Even if both adrenal glands are involved, there are no signs of adrenal insufficiency. Adrenal hemorrhage may also occur in bleeding diatheses, with

vasculitis, or as a complication of meningococcemia or adrenal angiography.

Large *adrenal cysts* may be found in older children. These are usually lined with endothelium and may be found incidentally (Fig. 144-23). If cross-sectional imaging reveals that they have a thin, smooth wall without any evidence of solid components, and if there is no evidence of endocrine dysfunction, hypertension, infection, or metastatic disease, they can be managed conservatively. Adrenal neoplasms seldom have large cystic components and never present as thin, smooth-walled cystic structures without solid components in older children.

Adrenal Hyperplasia

Adrenal hyperplasia usually presents in the neonatal period (see Chapter 24). However, when adrenocortical hyperplasia is seen in older children, it can be either primary or secondary. Primary hyperplasia usually results in Cushing syndrome and, much less commonly, primary aldosteronism. Secondary hyperplasia may be present in patients who produce excessive endogenous adrenocorticotropic hormone (ACTH), such as those with Cushing disease or ectopic ACTH production, or in patients receiving ACTH administration (e.g., for infantile spasms).

In older children, the adrenal glands normally are not easily visible on US, so if they are visible, one should consider the diagnosis of adrenal hyperplasia (Fig. 144-24). CT and MRI play a more important role in imaging the adrenals in older children suspected of having adrenal hyperfunction. The adrenal glands may appear bilaterally, symmetrically, and evenly enlarged (Fig. 144-25). If the adrenal limbs are thicker than the adjacent crura, adrenal hyperplasia should be considered. Enhancement of the glands on CT may be increased relative to that in normal glands. Occasionally, the adrenal enlargement is not even, and there may be one or more small nodular areas in one or both adrenal glands. However, it is important to note that finding normal-sized glands does not rule out adrenal hyperplasia. Those children with adrenal hyperplasia and no known source of ACTH should have MRI of the brain and

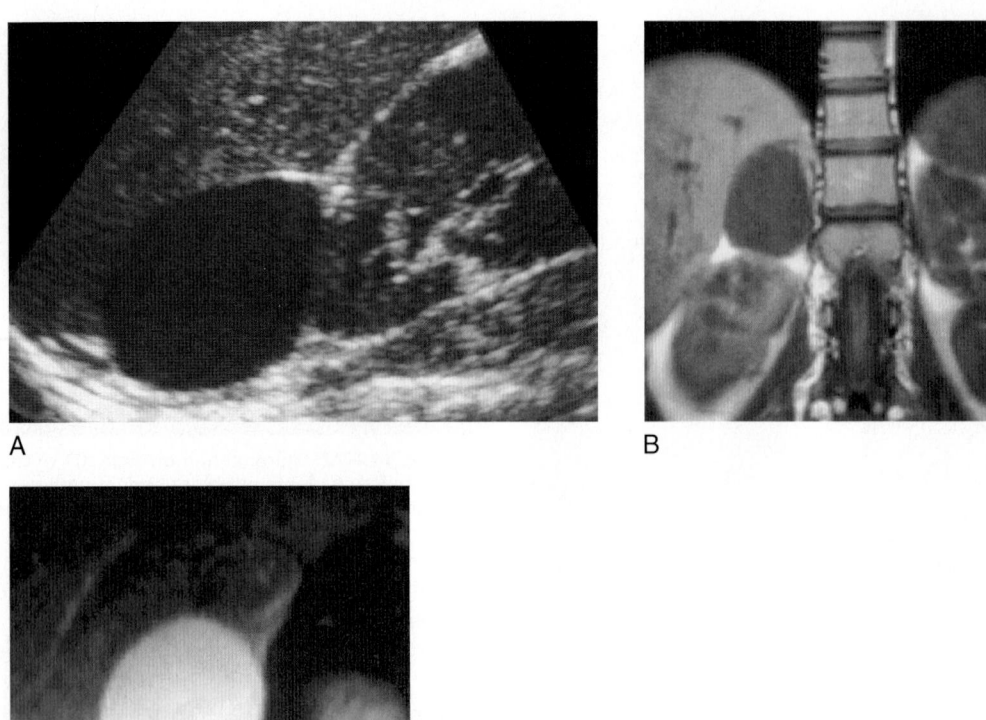

A

B

C

FIGURE 144-23. Adrenal cyst. Longitudinal sonogram of the right upper quadrant **(A)** and coronal T1-weighted **(B)** and axial T2-weighted **(C)** MR images of the upper abdomen in a teenage girl with urinary tract infection. A cyst is noted in the region of the right adrenal. The cyst is well defined, with a smooth wall and no solid components on either US or MRI.

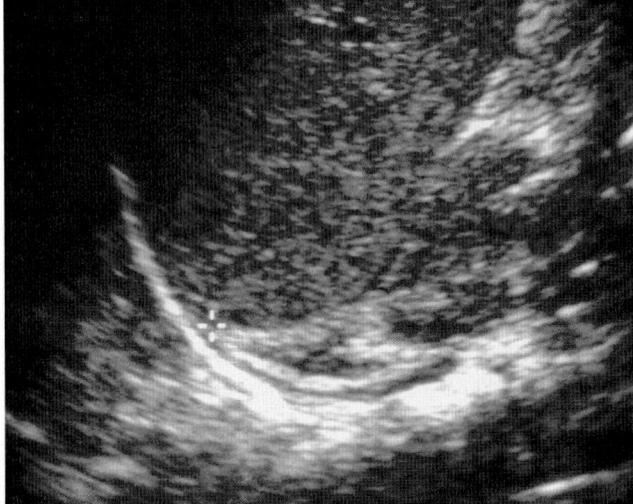

FIGURE 144-24. Adrenal hyperplasia. Longitudinal sonogram shows an enlarged right adrenal gland in a 3-year-old girl. Normally, the glands are not easily seen on US at this age.

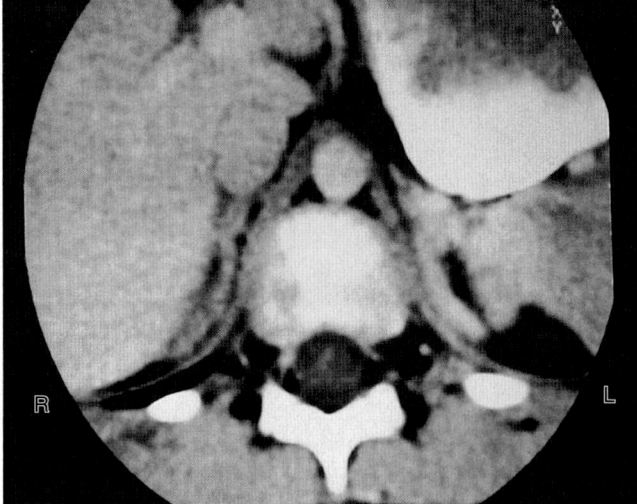

FIGURE 144-25. Cushing syndrome. CT scan of a 12-year-old girl with Cushing syndrome reveals markedly enlarged, thickened adrenal glands. The glands are symmetrically involved, with no evidence of small nodules.

pituitary to exclude pathology in this region as a source of adrenal stimulation.

THE RETROPERITONEUM

The retroperitoneum is a potential space that extends along the most posterior aspect of the abdominal cavity from the level of the diaphragms to the pelvic brim. It abuts the abdominal parietal peritoneum anteriorly. The lateral margin is formed by the lateroconal fascia, which arises from the fusion of the anterior and posterior renal fasciae. Masses located within the retroperitoneal space often arise from structures of the urinary tract and are discussed elsewhere. Those located outside the urinary tract arise from structures normally present in this space, including the adrenal glands, lymph nodes, lymphatic channels, sympathetic ganglia or other neural tissue, and iliopsoas muscle.

Retroperitoneal masses are best defined with cross-sectional imaging. US may be adequate as the initial diagnostic modality; however, its evaluation of small masses may be limited owing to obscuration by overlying bowel gas, and it may be unable to clearly define the anatomic extent of large masses. In these cases, further evaluation with CT or MRI may be required; the latter is preferred owing to the lack of radiation exposure.

Perirenal Fluid Collections

Subcapsular fluid collections around the kidney are due to renal lacerations with consequent perirenal hematoma, perirenal abscess, or urinoma from an obstructed draining system. A *subcapsular hematoma* is a collection of blood beneath the intact renal capsule following renal laceration from abdominal trauma. Most subcapsular hematomas are located along the posterolateral aspect of the kidney. The kidney parenchyma may appear flattened by the hematoma. Occasionally, persistent compression of the renal parenchyma or structures in the renal pedicle with associated fibrosis results in systemic hypertension (see Chapter 150).

A *perirenal hematoma* is a collection of blood in the perirenal space. The perirenal space is a potential space formed from the posterior and anterior renal fascia of Gerota. This space contains the adrenal gland, kidney, renal pelvis, and upper ureter. It extends inferiorly as a cone-shaped potential space to the iliac fossa. In perirenal hematoma, there is laceration or rupture of the renal parenchyma as well as the renal capsule, often from penetrating trauma. The hematoma is located posterior and inferior to the kidney and extends downward to the pelvis. Although they are often larger, perirenal hematomas produce less renal compression than subcapsular hematomas.

A *subcapsular abscess* results from contiguous spread of inflammation into the subcapsular space from an associated renal parenchymal abscess or extravasation of infected urine from an obstructed renal collecting system. *Perirenal abscesses* are extracapsular and are posterolateral and inferior in location and extend inferiorly. A *urinoma* results from spontaneous rupture of a calyceal fornix secondary to acute or chronic obstruction of the renal collecting system or from trauma. It is a rare complication of surgery and may be the result of postoperative obstruction. Perirenal urinomas that are present in utero or at birth result from fetal urinary obstruction, usually secondary to obstructed posterior urethral valves.

The presence of perirenal fluid collections and their extent are easily demonstrated by real-time US examination. CT with intravenous contrast material and delayed imaging is also helpful in identifying these abnormalities. Both methods demonstrate the nature and extent of the underlying renal parenchymal or collecting system abnormality. Chronic extravasation of urine may result in the formation of a fibrotic pseudocapsule with a

---

TABLE 144-2
Primary Retroperitoneal Tumors
NEUROECTODERMAL TUMORS OUTSIDE OF ADRENAL MEDULLA Extra-adrenal neuroblastoma Ganglioneuroblastoma Ganglioneuroma Primitive peripheral neuroectodermal tumor Neurofibroma, malignant peripheral nerve sheath tumor, schwannoma
TUMORS OF FATTY ORIGIN Lipoma Lipoblastoma Lipoblastomatosis Liposarcoma (rare)

perinephric cyst. Such cysts may surround the kidney or be located near the pelvis and proximal ureter.

> **Perirenal fluid collections are usually caused by trauma or obstruction.**

Primary Retroperitoneal Tumors

Primary tumors of the adrenal cortex and medulla were discussed earlier in this chapter. The retroperitoneum is also the site of origin of neoplasms of neuroectodermal origin, lipomatous tumors, rhabdomyosarcoma, undifferentiated sarcoma, tumors of germ cell ectodermal origin, mesenchymoma, lymphoma, and lymphangioma.

NEUROECTODERMAL TUMORS

Neuroectodermal neoplasms arising in the retroperitoneum outside of the adrenal medulla may originate from tissue of the sympathetic (autonomic) nervous system, including extra-adrenal neuroblastoma, ganglioneuroblastoma, and ganglioneuroma; alternatively, they may result from neuroectoderm, as in the case of a primitive peripheral neuroectodermal tumor (Table 144-2). Extra-adrenal pheochromocytoma also arises in the retroperitoneum. The site of origin of all these tumors is the paravertebral gutter, with resultant anterior and lateral displacement of other retroperitoneal structures, including the kidneys, ureters, and inferior vena cava. Uncommon neuroectodermal tumors are paraganglioma, neurofibroma (Fig. 144-26), malignant peripheral nerve sheath tumor (Fig. 144-27), neurilemmoma, and schwannoma (Fig. 144-28). Although they occasionally occur as isolated tumors, they are often seen as multiple tumors in patients with neurofibromatosis.

LIPOMATOUS TUMORS

Tumors of fatty origin are often quite large at the time of diagnosis and are usually benign. These include lipoma, lipoblastoma (Fig. 144-29), lipoblastomatosis, and liposarcoma (see Table 144-2). Lipoma and lipoblastoma are clearly delineated tumors; lipoblastomatosis is usually extensive and locally invasive and is difficult or impossible to remove completely.

Histologically, lipoblastoma shows adult liposarcoma-like cells. Its appearance on imaging studies may be similar to that of lipoma, but some CT scans have shown areas of relatively increased attenuation that, on pathologic examination, proved to be regions of myxoid material. Liposarcoma is extremely rare in children but is locally invasive and also metastatic to distant sites. A lipoma is easily identified on abdominal radiographs by its radiolucent appearance, with clear delineation of adjacent soft tissue structures such as the kidneys, liver margin, and psoas muscle. Abdominal US reveals a large, ill-defined mass with homogeneous hyperechogenicity. On CT, a very-low-attenuation mass, often with good delineation of its margins and diffuse displacement of surrounding structures, is characteristic. MRI also demonstrates a homogeneous mass with high signal on T1- and T2-weighted images. The boundaries of the mass are clearly delineated because of the marked contrast in signal intensity with surrounding structures.

RHABDOMYOSARCOMA AND UNDIFFERENTIATED SARCOMAS

Rhabdomyosarcoma accounts for 5% to 8% of childhood cancers and has a wide variety of histologic types

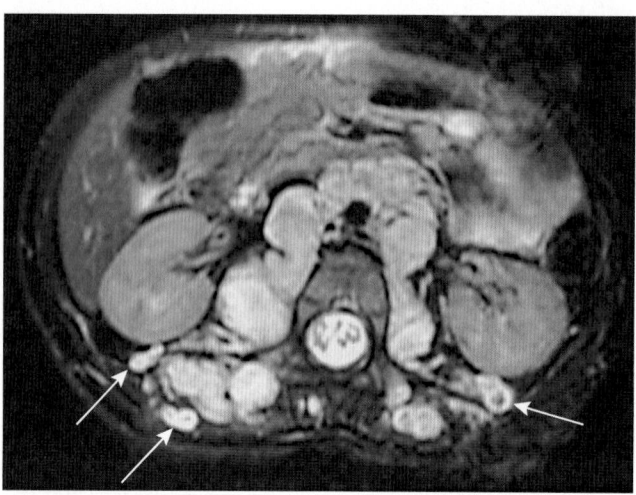

FIGURE 144-26. Plexiform neurofibroma. T2-weighted axial MR image shows a large, lobulated, hyperintense retroperitoneal mass. The mass extends along both sides of the spine, medial to the kidneys, and encases the aorta anteriorly. There is also extension into the posterior paraspinal muscles. Note the characteristic "target" sign (hyperintense rim surrounding a hypointense center) of neurofibroma *(arrows)*.

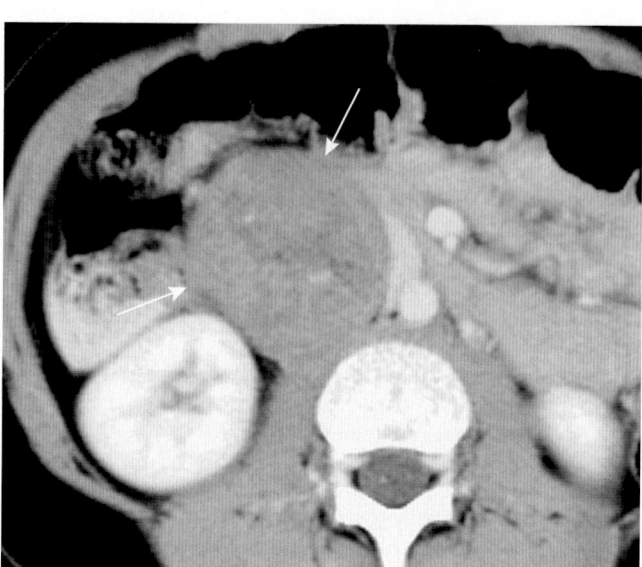

FIGURE 144-28. Schwannoma. Enhanced CT scan shows a well-defined, rounded mass *(arrows)* in the retroperitoneum between the right kidney and the inferior vena cava, which is displaced and distorted. The mass has heterogeneous enhancement owing to central necrosis.

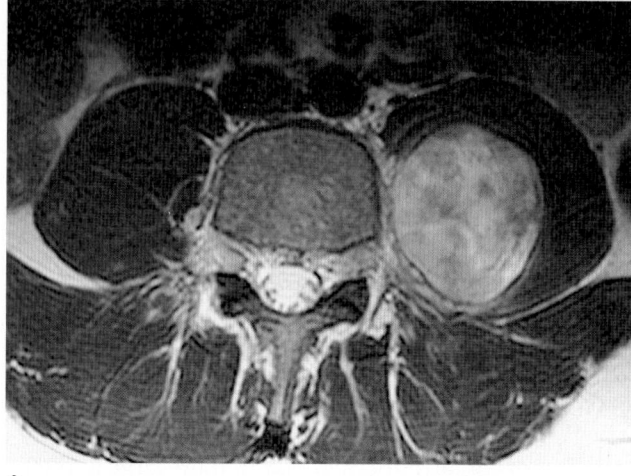

A

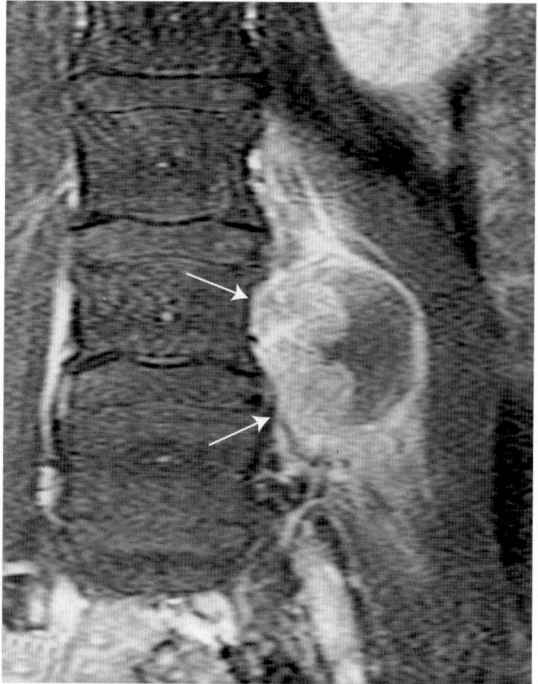

B

FIGURE 144-27. Malignant peripheral nerve sheath tumor. **A,** Axial T2-weighted MR image shows a well-defined tumor with intermediate to high signal intensity involving the left psoas muscle. **B,** Contrast-enhanced, fat-saturated, coronal T1-weighted MR image shows heterogeneous enhancement *(arrows)* with surrounding edema.

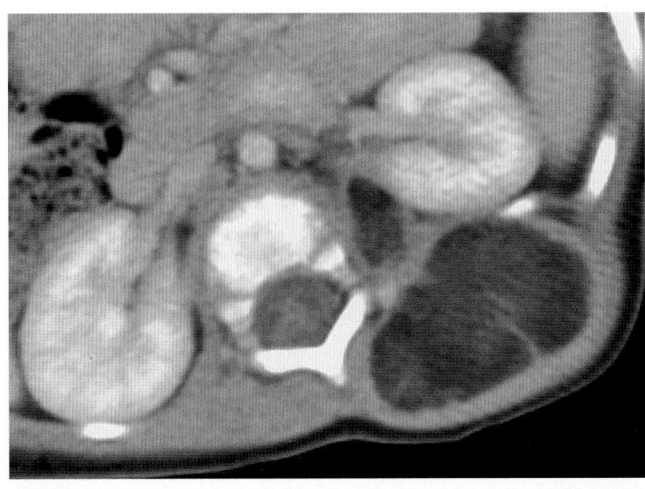
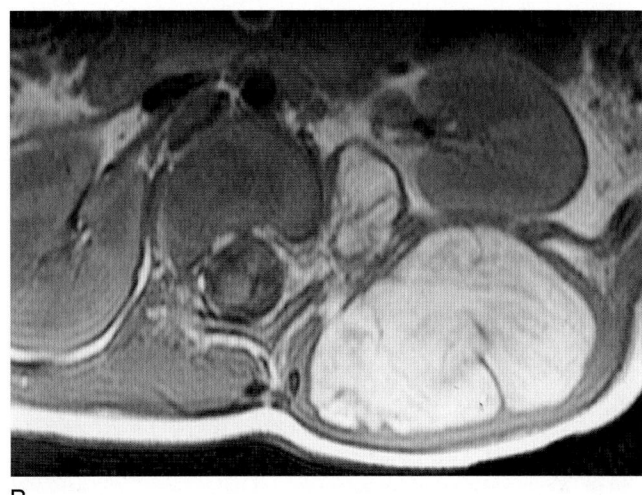

FIGURE 144-29. Lipoblastoma. Axial CT scan **(A)** and axial T1-weighted MR image **(B)** show a well-defined, bilobed mass involving the left paraspinal muscles, with extension into the retroperitoneum between the left kidney and the spine. On CT **(A)** the mass has characteristic low attenuation; on T1-weighted MRI **(B)**, it has high signal intensity, consistent with the presence of fatty tissue.

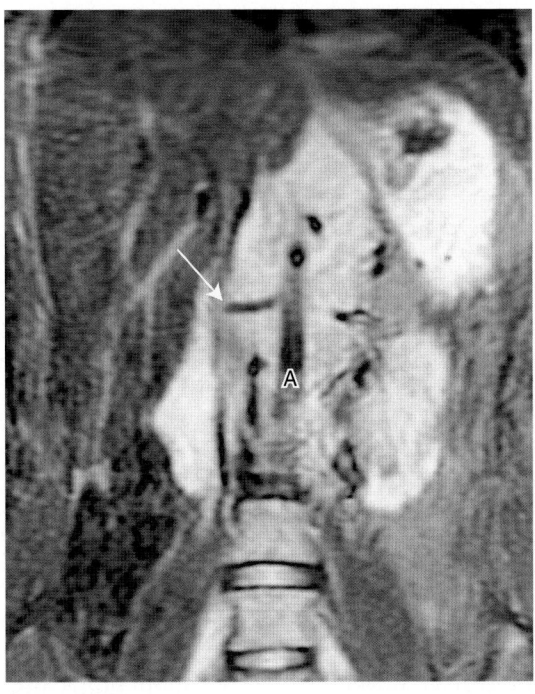
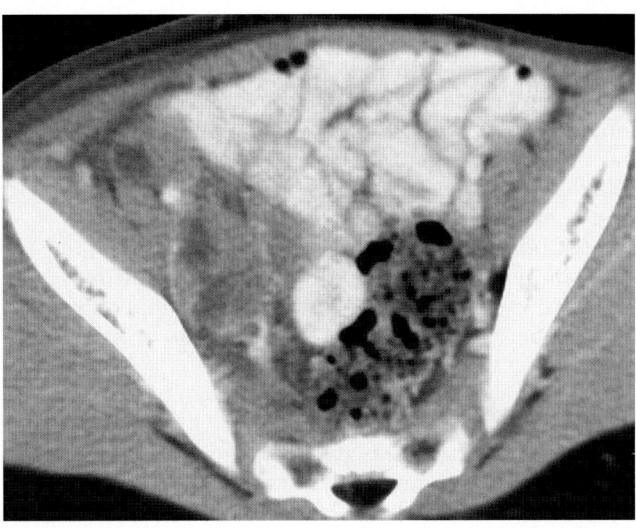

FIGURE 144-30. Rhabdomyosarcoma in two patients. **A,** Coronal, short tau inversion recovery MR image shows a lobulated, hyperintense retroperitoneal mass encasing the upper abdominal aorta (A) and the right renal artery *(arrow).* Increased signal in the vertebral bodies is due to metastatic disease. **B,** Contrast-enhanced CT scan of the pelvis in another patient shows a large, heterogeneous right pelvic mass that displaces adjacent small bowel loops and extends posteriorly, abutting the rectosigmoid.

and patterns of tumor spread (Fig. 144-30). The tumors infiltrate locally, invade lymphatics and blood vessels, and frequently present with distant hematogenous metastases to the lungs, bone marrow, and bone. The histologic appearance of rhabdomyosarcoma in young children is characterized as embryonal, alveolar, or mixed. Sarcomas of the genitourinary tract arise in the bladder and prostate and present with a polypoid appearance, hematuria, urinary obstruction, and a characteristic mass of tissue termed *sarcoma botryoides* in children younger than 4 years. Prostatic rhabdomyosarcoma presents as a large pelvic mass surrounding and

obstructing the urethra or producing constipation. It has two age peaks: 2 to 6 years and 14 to 18 years.

On imaging studies, bladder rhabdomyosarcoma exhibits bladder wall thickening or a soft tissue mass at the bladder base. If the mass is in the prostate, it elevates the bladder and elongates the urethra. MRI is the modality of choice for staging and treatment planning. It reveals a mass of equal or greater intensity than muscle (but less than fat) on T1-weighted images. The intensity increases on T2-weighted images, and there is enhancement with gadolinium contrast. Distant metastases are best evaluated with CT.

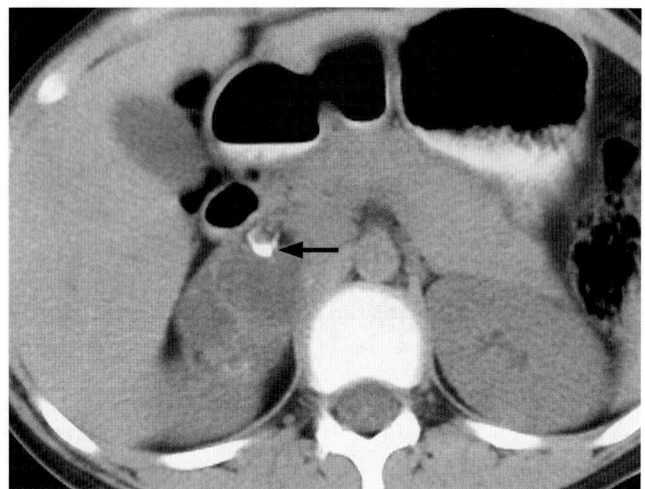
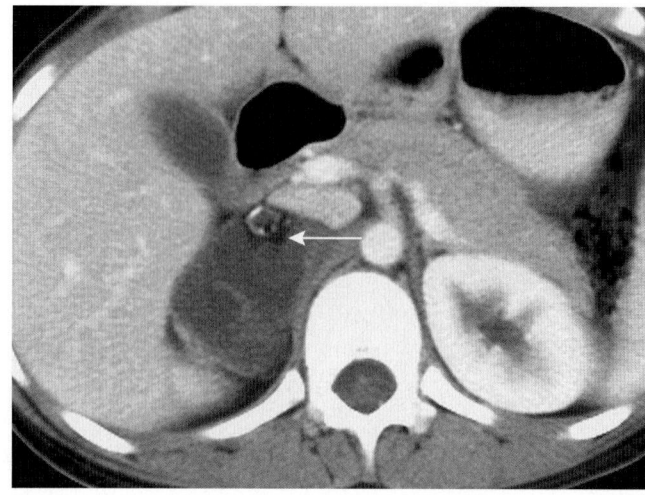

FIGURE 144-31. Retroperitoneal teratoma. Axial CT scans before **(A)** and after **(B)** intravenous contrast injection. There is a well-defined mass in the right suprarenal region, with mainly fluid attenuation and some soft tissue septa. Calcification (*black arrow* in **A**) and fatty attenuation (*white arrow* in **B**) are seen anteriorly in the mass.

Retroperitoneal pelvic tumors may be quite large at the time of diagnosis, with wide infiltration owing to the fact that they are often not well encapsulated. Their deep location within the body results in late identification of the mass and late presentation with bowel obstruction and bladder or sacral nerve root involvement. Retroperitoneal lymph node metastases, bone marrow metastases, and distant hematogenous metastases to the lungs are common at presentation. Other common sites of metastases are bone, liver, and brain. Ten percent to 20% of patients have metastases at the time of initial diagnosis.

GERM CELL TUMORS

Germ cell tumors are benign or malignant tumors derived from the primordial germinal epithelial layer cells in extragonadal or gonadal sites (see Chapters 108, 154 and 155). These tumors account for 3% of malignant tumors in children and adolescents. Two thirds of these tumors are extragonadal in origin; 41% of germ cell tumors occur in the sacrococcygeal region, and most are benign. Thoracic germ cell tumors are located in the anterior superior mediastinum. Abdominal germ cell tumors are usually located in the retroperitoneal space, though occasional involvement of the stomach, omentum, and liver is described. α-Fetoprotein is produced in immature germ cell tumors in children. Germ cell tumors with trophoblastic elements (choriocarcinomas) produce β-human chorionic gonadotropin.

Germ cell tumors include germinoma, embryonal carcinoma, endodermal sinus tumor, choriocarcinoma, polyembryoma, gonadoblastoma, and teratoma (Fig. 144-31). A teratoma arises from pluripotent cells and is composed of a variety of tissues foreign to the organ of its anatomic site of origin. The component tissues are poorly organized and in various stages of maturation, and the lesion may be solid, multicystic, or a single large cyst. Neonatal teratomas occur 80% of the time in the sacrococcygeal region. Other sites include the jaw, nasopharynx, intracranial cavity, retroperitoneum, mediastinum, and gonads.

OTHER SARCOMAS

Other sarcomas occasionally seen in children and adolescents include fibrosarcoma, malignant fibrous histiocytoma, hemangiopericytoma, and leiomyosarcoma.

LYMPHOMA AND LYMPHADENOPATHY

Malignant lymphomas are neoplasms of the cells of the immune system. Because these cells circulate through the body, lymphoma is a generalized disease from the time of origin. Lymphoma presents with a mediastinal mass 50% to 70% of the time, and in the vast majority of patients with lymphoma, the tumor is above the diaphragm in the supraclavicular region, axilla, or mediastinum. Abdominal involvement is most likely to involve only the liver and spleen; however, lymphomas with small, noncleaved cells frequently present with abdominal tumors, most often in or around the gastrointestinal tract.

Non-African Burkitt lymphoma commonly presents with an abdominal tumor. Clinical manifestations are abdominal pain or swelling, sometimes with a symptom complex characterized by intussusception, nausea and vomiting, gastrointestinal bleeding, and intestinal perforation. Palpation of a right iliac fossa mass is quite common, along with inguinal and iliac lymphadenopathy. Associated retroperitoneal adenopathy is common (Fig. 144-32). Initial presentation with a retroperitoneal mass is uncommon and is more likely to be associated with the lymphomas related to pharmacologic immune suppression, such as post-transplant lymphoproliferative disorder (see Chapter 138).

Retroperitoneal masses due to lymph node enlargement may be secondary to infection, such as tuberculosis, or metastatic spread from many neoplasms, including testicular tumors (Fig. 144-33).

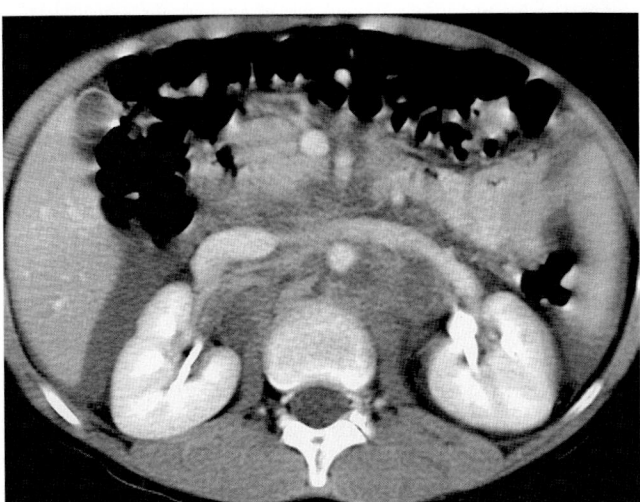

FIGURE 144-32. Retroperitoneal lymphadenopathy due to non-Hodgkin lymphoma. Contrast-enhanced CT scan shows a retroperitoneal soft tissue mass, which surrounds the vessels, due to confluent lymphadenopathy. Ascites is also seen in the right subhepatic space.

Retroperitoneal Lymphatic and Vascular Malformations

Lymphatic malformations are benign tumors of congenital lymphatic origin; they are composed of variably sized noncommunicating cysts with minimal intervening soft tissue components. The cystic spaces are lined with endothelium and contain multiple thin septa and chylous fluid. These masses are classified as macrocystic, microcystic, or mixed, depending on the size of the cystic cavities. Occasionally, adjacent congenital venous malformations coexist, and these lesions are best termed *venolymphatic malformations.* Although a lymphatic malformation may present early as a palpable abdominal mass,

its soft nature may make it difficult to identify on physical examination. Retroperitoneal lymphatic malformations may compress and displace adjacent structures, particularly the ureters.

US most commonly reveals a multilocular cystic mass containing clear or slightly turbid fluid (Fig. 144-34), with thin septations. Occasionally, the mass is unilocular. Debris levels may be seen within the cystic spaces due to complicating hemorrhage or infection. The mass is commonly large. CT and MRI also reveal the cystic nature of these masses, although the septa are not easily visible.

Hemangiomas or hemangioendotheliomas may also occur in the retroperitoneal space (Fig. 144-35). These lesions vary in size and may be well defined or ill defined with irregular margins. They have a somewhat heterogeneous appearance on US, CT, and MRI. Large lesions may displace adjacent viscera and may infiltrate extensively. Their vascularity and enhancement can be easily appreciated when evaluated with the previously mentioned modalities.

Idiopathic Retroperitoneal Fibrosis

Rarely seen in children, this abnormality is characterized by dense fibroblastic sheets of tissue, often with an inflammatory component. In adults, this abnormality results as a complication of methysergide treatment. In children, the causes of retroperitoneal fibrosis include autoimmune diseases, infection, and neoplasm; however, most cases are idiopathic. The ureters, aorta, and inferior vena cava are commonly encased by this abnormal fibrotic tissue. Clinical symptoms include flank pain, urinary tract obstruction, and lower extremity edema. Systemic hypertension secondary to renal artery involvement is noted occasionally. CT evaluation of the course of the ureters and retroperitoneum may lead to the diag-

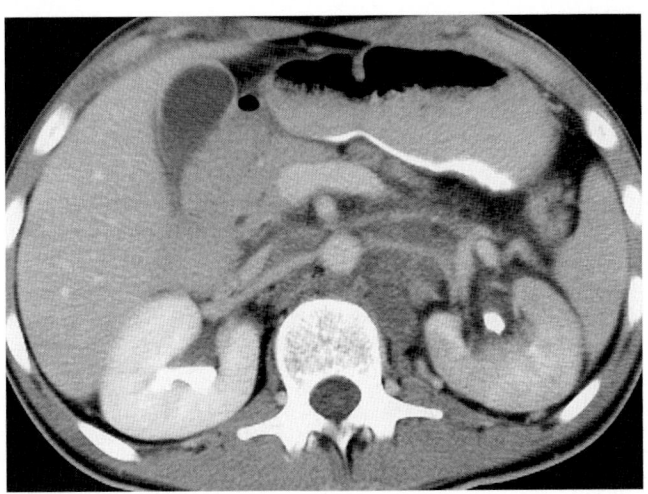

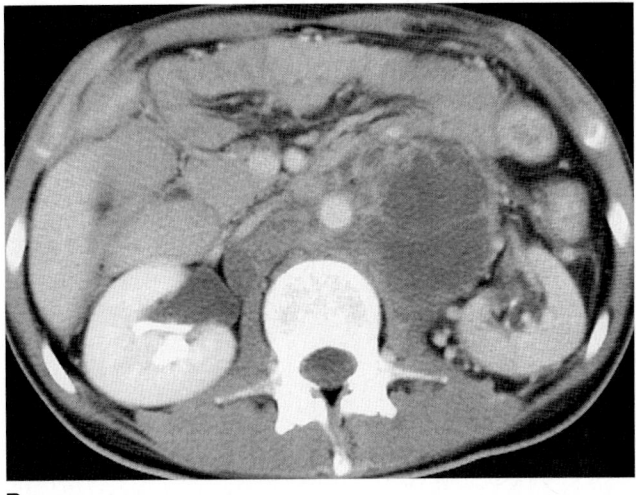

A   B

FIGURE 144-33. Retroperitoneal adenopathy from metastatic germ cell tumor of the testicle. **A** and **B,** Two contrast-enhanced axial CT scans show extensive soft tissue masses due to confluent retroperitoneal adenopathy. The lymph nodes are of low attenuation due to necrosis secondary to ongoing chemotherapy. Note how the masses displace and encase the vessels, as well as the diminished perfusion of the left kidney and the right hydronephrosis. These findings are similar to those noted in patients with lymphoma (see Fig. 144-32) or neuroblastoma (see Fig. 144-5).

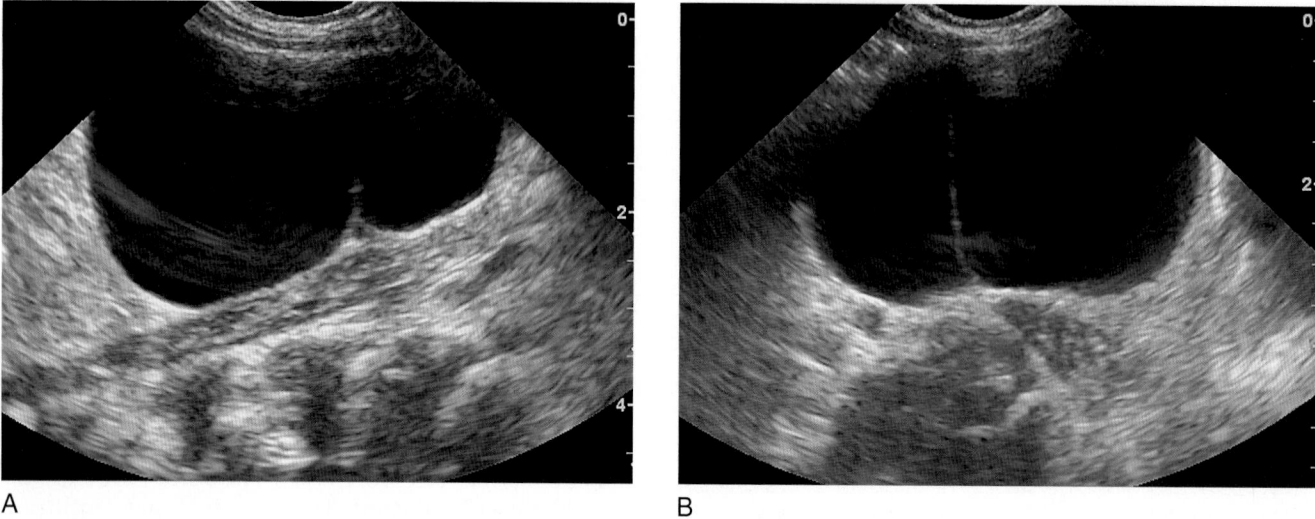

FIGURE 144-34. Lymphatic malformation. Longitudinal **(A)** and transverse **(B)** sonograms of the left lower quadrant show a well-defined cystic structure with septations anterior to the left psoas muscle and lumbar vertebrae. In this patient, the contained fluid is anechoic.

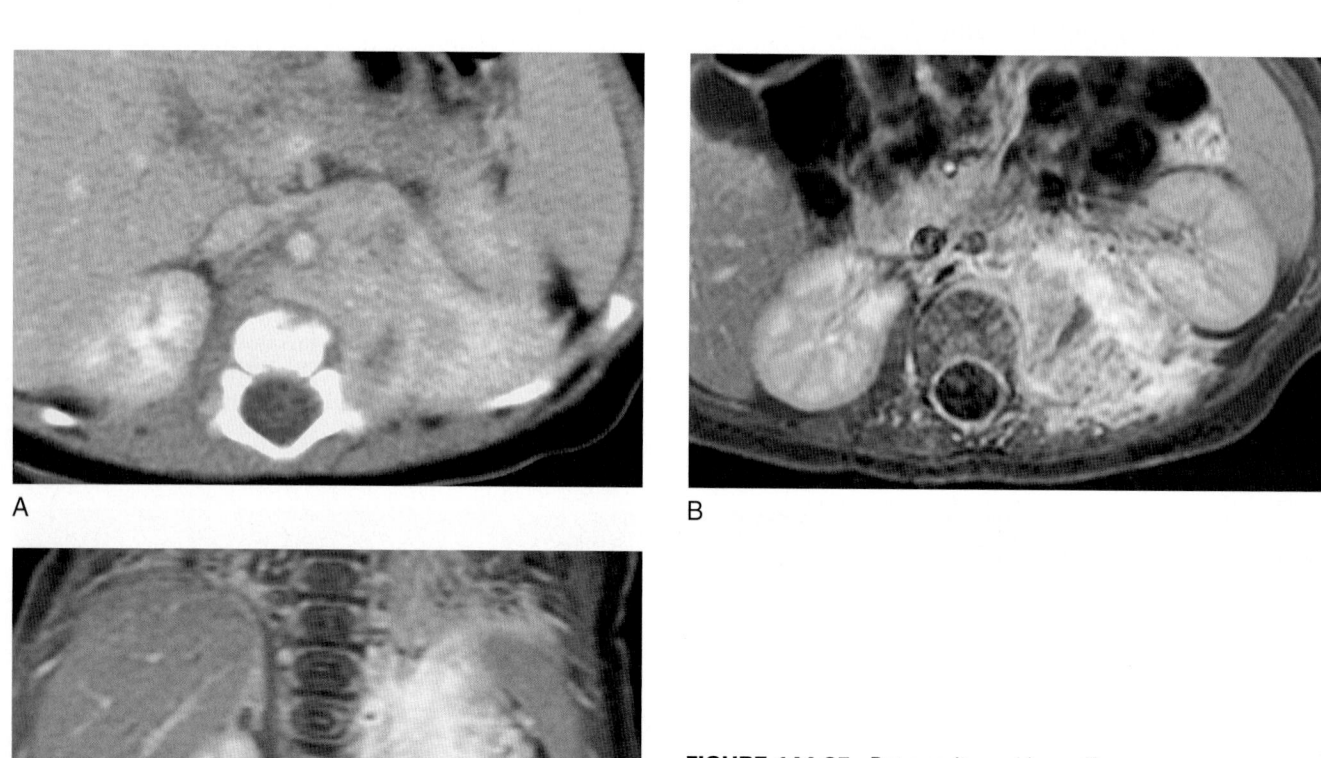

FIGURE 144-35. Retroperitoneal kaposiform hemangioendothelioma shown on contrast-enhanced CT scan **(A)**; gadolinium-enhanced axial, T1-weighted, fat-saturated MR image **(B)**; and gadolinium-enhanced coronal, T1-weighted, fat-saturated MR image **(C)**. There is an ill-defined, irregularly shaped left paravertebral mass displacing the left kidney anteriorly and laterally. There is involvement of the vertebral column, with two flattened vertebral bodies seen on the coronal image **(C)**. The mass has heterogeneous attenuation and enhancement on CT and MRI.

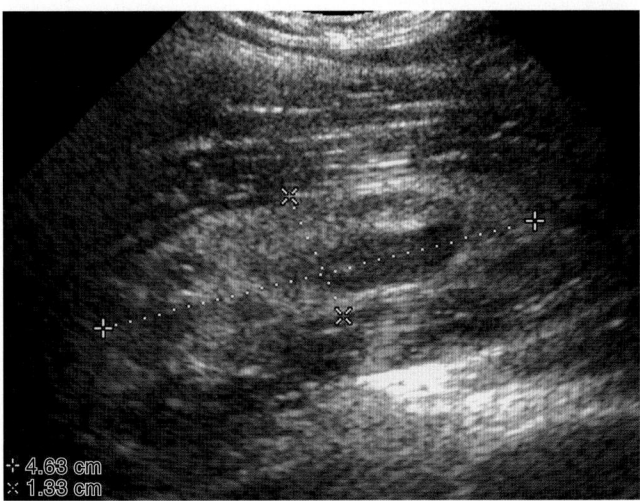

FIGURE 144-36. Hematoma of the psoas muscle in a patient with hemophilia. The cursors delineate the hematoma, which has heterogeneous echogenicity. The hematoma is primarily hyperechoic relative to the uninvolved psoas muscle, but there is a hypoechoic center due to liquefaction.

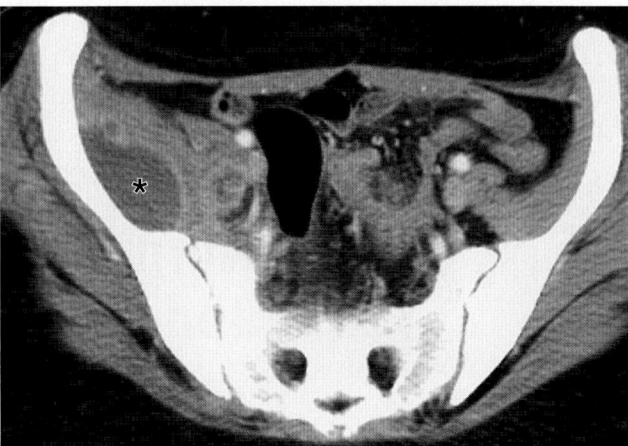

FIGURE 144-37. Abscess of the right iliopsoas muscle. Axial contrast-enhanced CT scan shows enlargement of the right iliopsoas muscle compared with the left, due to the presence of a fluid collection (*) with an enhancing rim, in keeping with an abscess.

nosis of retroperitoneal fibrosis. T2-weighted coronal MRI identifies ureteral obstruction and high-signal streaks of fibroblastic tissue. US shows homogeneous soft tissue masses involving the retroperitoneum.

Retroperitoneal Hematoma and Abscess

Hematoma of the retroperitoneum is most commonly the result of severe blunt abdominal trauma or a surgical procedure. Spontaneous retroperitoneal hematoma, usually affecting the psoas muscle, is seen in patients with hemophilia and other bleeding diatheses (Fig. 144-36). Patients receiving anticoagulant therapy may also present with this abnormality. On US examination, the psoas muscle is enlarged, with initially hyperechoic regions in the area of hemorrhage. As the blood cells break down, the area of hemorrhage becomes hypoechoic. CT examination reveals an enlarged psoas muscle with high attenuation or isoattenuation initially, which later becomes a low-attenuation region. MRI accurately identifies and documents the hemorrhage.

Retroperitoneal abscess is usually of hematogenous origin from a distant infection, such as osteomyelitis with resultant septicemia. Tuberculosis is a common cause of psoas abscess and may be associated with paraspinal abscess and extradural, intraspinal abscess extension. Osteomyelitis secondary to tuberculosis or another organism involving adjacent vertebrae is common. Gram-negative bacterial psoas abscesses are also seen in those with appendicitis or inflammatory bowel disease. Retroperitoneal abscess may be demonstrated by cross-sectional techniques or gallium and white blood cell nuclear medicine studies. US reveals a sonolucent region within the psoas muscle, with associated fluid along the margins of the psoas. US is also used to guide the therapeutic drainage of these abscesses. CT shows a low-attenuation lesion within the psoas muscle, with rim enhancement after injection of intravenous contrast material (Fig. 144-37).

SUGGESTED READINGS

Bloom DA, Schofield D, Hoffer FA: Radiologic-pathologic conference of Children's Hospital Boston: a palpable pelvic mass in an adolescent girl. Pediatr Radiol 1997;27:888

Chaudhary A, Misra S, Wakhlu A, et al: Retroperitoneal teratomas in children. Indian J Pediatr 2006;73:221

Ecklund K, Taylor GA, Schofield DH: Radiologic-pathologic conference of Children's Hospital Boston: abdominal mass in a prepubertal girl. Pediatr Radiol 1997;27:832

Groff DB: Pelvic neoplasms in children. J Surg Oncol 2001;77:65

Hussain HK, Kingston JE, Domizio P, et al: Imaging-guided core biopsy for the diagnosis of malignant tumors in pediatric patients. AJR Am J Roentgenol 2001;176:43

Iinuma Y, Iwafuchi M, Uchiyama M, et al: A case of Currarino triad with familial sacral bony deformities. Pediatr Surg Int 2000;16:134

Kim EE, Valenzuela RF, Kumar AJ, et al: Imaging and clinical spectrum of rhabdomyosarcoma in children. Clin Imaging 2000;24:257

Kocaoglu M, Frush DP: Pediatric sacral masses. Radiographics 2006;26:833

Krebs TL, Wagner BJ: MR imaging of the adrenal gland. Radiographics 1998;18:1425

Kushner BH: Neuroblastoma: a disease requiring a multitude of imaging studies. J Nucl Med 2004;45:1172

McHugh K, Pritchard J: Problems in the imaging of three common paediatric solid tumours. Eur J Radiol 2001;37:72

Miller OF, Smith LJ, Ferrara EX, et al: Presentation of idiopathic retroperitoneal fibrosis in the pediatric population. J Pediatr Surg 2003;38:1685

Navarro O, Nunez-Santos E, Daneman A, Faria P, Daltro P: Malignant peripheral nerve sheath tumor arising in previously irradiated neuroblastoma: report of 2 cases and review of the literature. Pediatr Radiol 2000;30:176

Ng WT, Ng TK, Cheng PW: Sacrococcygeal teratoma and anorectal malformation. Aust N Z J Surg 1997;67:218

Parker BR: Leukemia and lymphoma in childhood. Radiol Clin North Am 1997;35:1495

Paterson A: Adrenal pathology in childhood, a spectrum of disease. Eur Radiol 2002;12:2491

Rescorla FJ: Malignant adrenal tumors. Semin Pediatr Surg 2006;15:48

Ribeiro RC, Figueiredo B: Childhood adrenocrotical tumors. Eur J Cancer 2004;40:1117

Ruymann FB, Grovas AC: Progress in the diagnosis and treatment of rhabdomyosarcoma and related soft tissue sarcomas. Cancer Invest 2000;18:223

Shady KL, Brown JJ: MR imaging of the adrenal glands. Magn Reson Imaging Clin N Am 1995;3:73

Siegel MJ: Pelvic tumors in childhood. Radiol Clin North Am 1997;35:1455

Yang DM, Jung DH, Kim H, et al: Retroperitoneal cystic masses: CT, clinical, and pathologic findings and literature review. Radiographics 2004;24:1353

145

Normal Renal Anatomy, Variants, and Congenital Anomalies

SANDRA K. FERNBACH and KATE A. FEINSTEIN

NORMAL RENAL ANATOMY AND VARIANTS

Internal Anatomy

A coronal section of the kidney reveals that it is composed of two distinct regions: the outer cortex and the inner medulla (Fig. 145-1). Within the cortex are the nephrons. The medulla is composed of 8 to 13 pyramids that terminate in the renal papillae at the level of the calyces. Two or more pyramids may drain into the same papilla (confluent papilla), and two or more papillae may drain into a single calyx (compound calyx). Compound calyces are typically located in the poles of the kidney and produce the unusual lucency sometimes seen on ultrasonography (US). Renal cortex can extend centrally between the pyramids (column of Bertin) and may simulate a renal tumor on intravenous urography (IVU) (Fig. 145-2). US or nuclear scans using cortical

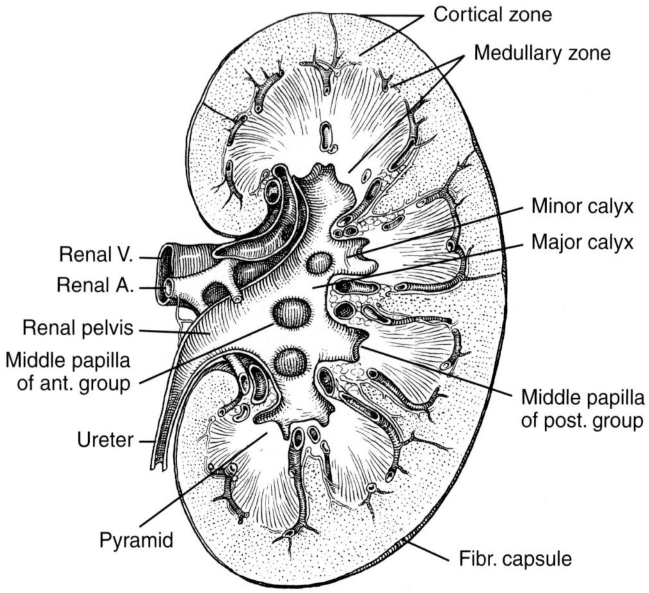

FIGURE 145-1. Macroscopic anatomy of the kidney in longitudinal section. The right kidney is seen from the back; the renal artery is posterior to the renal vein. (Redrawn from Kelly HA, Burnam CF: Diseases of the Kidneys, Ureters and Bladder, 2nd ed. New York, Appleton, 1922.)

Cortical zone
Medullary zone
Minor calyx
Major calyx
Renal V.
Renal A.
Renal pelvis
Middle papilla of ant. group
Ureter
Middle papilla of post. group
Pyramid
Fibr. capsule

agents can easily identify this variant, which occurs more often at the junction of the middle and upper group of calyces or between the two central renal echo complexes of a duplex kidney.

In newborns and infants, the kidneys have a larger medullary and a smaller cortical volume than in later life. On US, the neonatal renal cortex is moderately hyperechoic, close to the echogenicity of the adjacent liver and spleen. In newborn and premature infants, the cortical echogenicity may actually be greater than that of the liver. The pyramids are relatively hypoechoic (Fig. 145-3). This pattern can suggest hydronephrosis, especially on prenatal US studies. Between 6 months and 2 years of age, the echogenicity of the medulla and cortex resembles that of adult kidneys, making corticomedullary differentiation much less distinct on US.

> Renal echogenicity and corticomedullary differentiation are normally increased in newborns and infants.

Renal Arteries and Veins

The kidney is usually supplied by a single artery arising from the aorta. After the renal artery enters the renal hilum, posterior and slightly superior to the renal vein, it divides into anterior and posterior branches that, in turn, generally divide into superior and inferior branches (Fig. 145-4). Variations exist at all levels. About 20% to 30% of kidneys have a second or accessory renal artery that also arises from the aorta. The renal artery (or arteries) arise more distally from the aorta than normal in kidneys with ectopia (pelvic kidney and crossed renal ectopy) or fusion (horseshoe kidney).

The renal vein lies anterior and slightly inferior to the renal artery (see Fig. 145-1). The left renal vein is longer than the right, coursing anterior to the aorta, and it receives the ipsilateral suprarenal and gonadal veins before entering the inferior vena cava. The left renal vein passes between the aorta and the superior mesenteric artery, and it can become narrowed from compression between these two vessels. This so-called nutcracker ana-

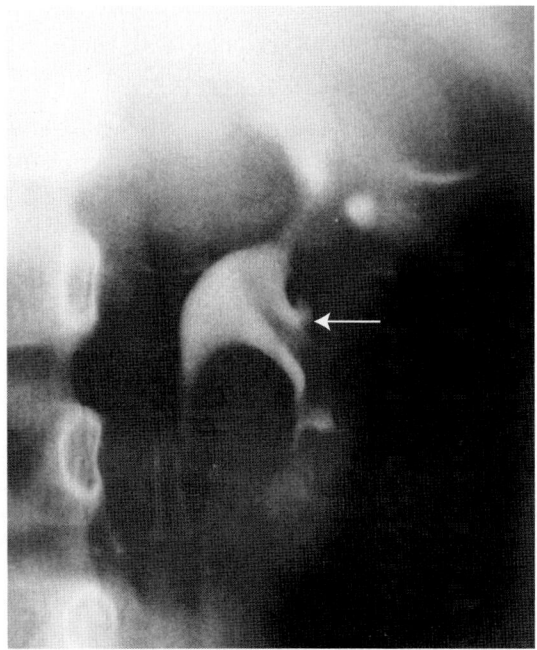

A

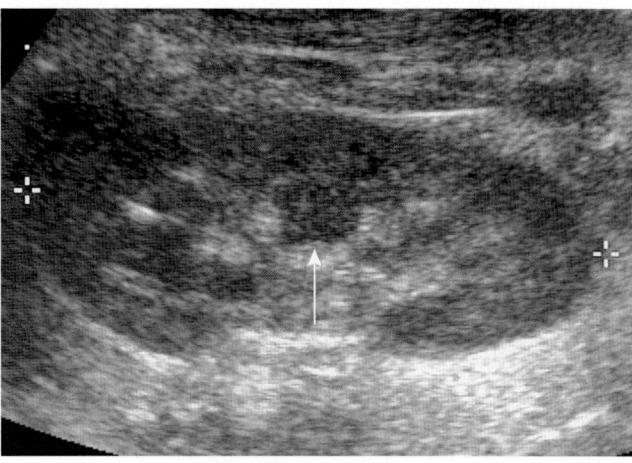

B

FIGURE 145-2. Column of Bertin. **A,** IVU shows that the column of Bertin has produced spreading of the calyces of the left kidney, simulating a renal mass. The centrally located single calyx *(arrow)* is draining this ectopic tissue. Note also the oblique vascular impression on the lower pole infundibulum (major calyx). **B,** Longitudinal sonogram in another patient shows a central column of cortical tissue *(arrow)* extending into the central sinus echoes. (**B** courtesy of Brian D. Coley, MD.)

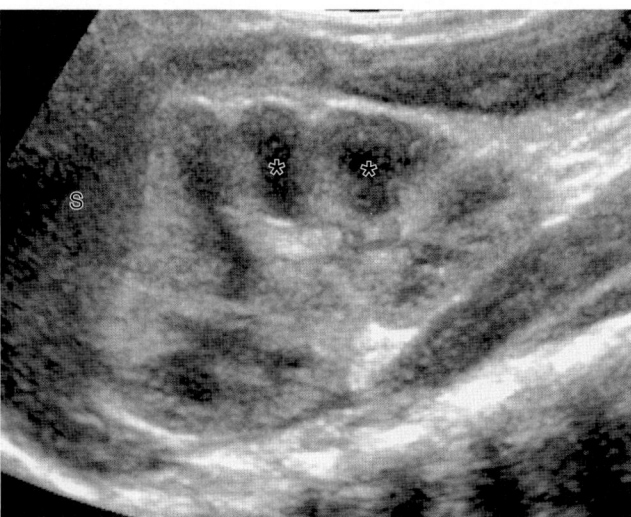

FIGURE 145-3. Normal neonatal kidney. Supine longitudinal sonogram of the left kidney shows the sharp corticomedullary differentiation common in infancy and early childhood. The hypoechoic triangular renal pyramids (*) are surrounded by cortex that is more echogenic than the adjacent spleen (S). The spleen has flattened the upper renal contour and produces the appearance of a dromedary kidney. (Courtesy of Brian D. Coley, MD.)

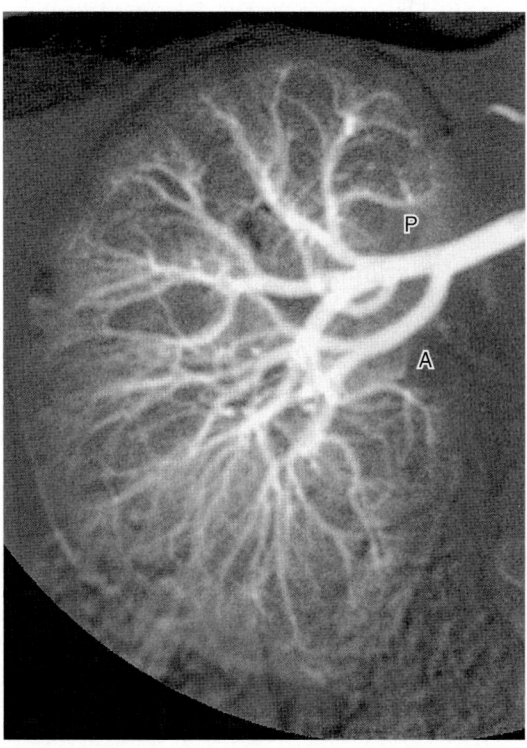

FIGURE 145-4. Normal renal arterial anatomy. Digital subtraction arteriogram of the right kidney in a 6-month-old shows a single main renal artery dividing into anterior (A) and posterior (P) branches. There is normal opacification and distribution of vessels to the level of the arcuate arteries. (Courtesy of Brian D. Coley, MD.)

tomy may predispose patients to orthostatic hematuria and proteinuria and to varicoceles. However, distention of the proximal left renal vein is not synonymous with obstruction and can be a normal variant. The main renal artery and vein can be well visualized with Doppler US, contrast-enhanced computed tomography (CT), and gadolinium-enhanced magnetic resonance imaging (MRI). Smaller intrarenal vessels can be demonstrated with all three techniques, but CT and MRI data post-processing techniques, such as maximal intensity projection reconstructions, can enhance the detection of accessory vessels.

Prominent vessels may produce nonobstructive impressions on the renal pelvis or calyceal system. Less frequently, a vessel may cause true obstruction of an infundibulum (Fig. 145-5) or even the renal pelvis. On US, echolucency of hilar vessels can simulate mild hydro-

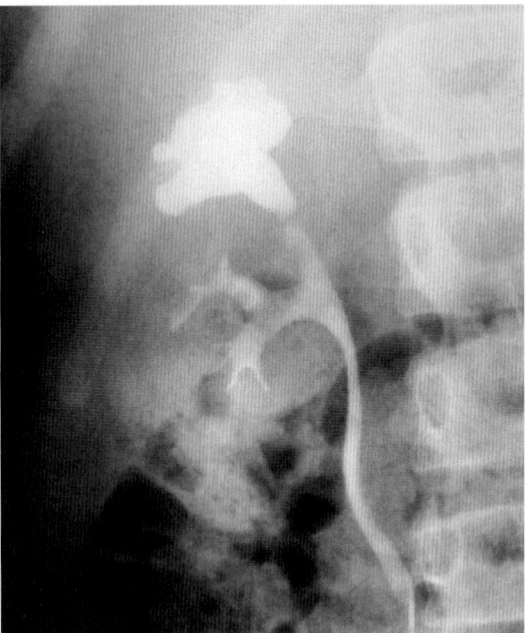

FIGURE 145-5. Extrinsic vascular compression on the upper pole infundibulum. During IVU, the upper pole infundibulum and compound calyceal system are dilated above the linear defect produced by a crossing vessel. The other calyces have a normal caliber. When this appearance is associated with persistent right upper quadrant pain (and nuclear scintigraphy documents obstruction), the process is referred to as Fraley syndrome and may require surgery.

nephrosis; the use of color Doppler US clearly differentiates vascular structures from a dilated renal pelvis.

Anatomic Relationships

Knowledge of the relationship between the kidney and adjacent structures and organs is essential for evaluating the location and spread of renal and pararenal neoplasms, infections, and fluid collections. A large portion of the posterior surface of the left kidney is in contact with the diaphragm above, along the posterior costophrenic sulcus. The renal capsule, anterior and posterior renal fascia, posterior layer of the peritoneal membrane (parietal peritoneum), and transversalis fascia delimit the following potential spaces in the region of the kidneys, respectively: subcapsular, perirenal, and anterior and posterior pararenal. The relationships between these structures and potential spaces are shown in Figure 145-6. Intraperitoneally, in front of the right kidney and the proximal descending duodenum is a posterior extension of the infrahepatic recess termed the *Morison pouch*, an important space for fluid collections. It is bordered superiorly by the right transverse colon and posteriorly by the right kidney and adrenal gland. This pouch is continuous medially with the lesser omental sac through the foramen of Winslow.

Position and Mobility

The left kidney is higher than the right in at least two thirds of people. In 5% to 10%, the left kidney is lower, and in the remainder, the kidneys are at the same height.

On supine films, the center of the renal pelvis of the left kidney is opposite the lower half of L1, whereas that of the right kidney is usually at the level of the superior half of L2.

The distance between the spine and the medial aspect of the upper calyceal system should be the same on each side. Medial deviation of the upper calyces suggests focal parenchymal scarring. Downward or lateral displacement suggests adrenal mass, left upper pole mass, or obstruction of a left upper pole ureter. On IVU, CT, and MRI, the anterior surface of the kidney projects anteriorly to the spine.

The cephalocaudal position of the kidney is determined by its relation to the underlying psoas muscle. The upper pole is medial and dorsal to the lower pole because the psoas muscle broadens as it passes inferiorly. Reversed obliquity (lower pole more medial) and increased obliquity (lower pole more lateral) are occasional normal variants. Reversed obliquity can also be seen in horseshoe kidney and in myelodysplastic children with lumbar kyphosis and psoas muscle atrophy, the so-called pseudohorseshoe kidney. An unusual orientation or position of the kidney may warrant additional imaging to exclude the presence of a flank mass or ureteral duplication with an obstructed pole.

The kidneys move slightly caudally with each inspiration and also move caudally about one vertebral body when an individual moves from the supine to the prone position. The mobility of the left kidney is greater than that of the right. In the prone position, both kidneys no longer rest on the psoas muscle. They acquire a more vertical axis and also rotate anteriorly on their long axes, causing them to appear broader.

Shape

The primitive fetal kidney comprises multiple renal lobules that fuse to form the kidney. The junction of these lobules sometimes persists and can be seen as a scalloping of the cortical border (Fig. 145-7). These fetal lobulations become increasingly effaced throughout childhood but are noted in about 10% of adults. Fetal lobulations can be differentiated from cortical scarring by their position: fetal lobulations indent between the calyces, whereas scarring occurs directly over a calyx. The junctional parenchymal defect observed with renal US (Fig. 145-8) is similarly derived from a variation in the fusion of the fetal renunculi or lobules. It appears as a thick, triangular, echogenic notch in the anterosuperior or posteroinferior aspect of the kidney (more often on the right) and mimics a cortical scar. The junctional parenchymal defect may be connected to the renal hilum by an echogenic line called the inter-renicular septum (see Fig. 145-8).

> **Fetal lobations are differentiated from cortical scars by their relationship to the calyces.**

In infants, the kidney is more rounded and relatively broader than in adults. The poles are folded into a relatively narrow renal sinus. The left kidney is apt to be

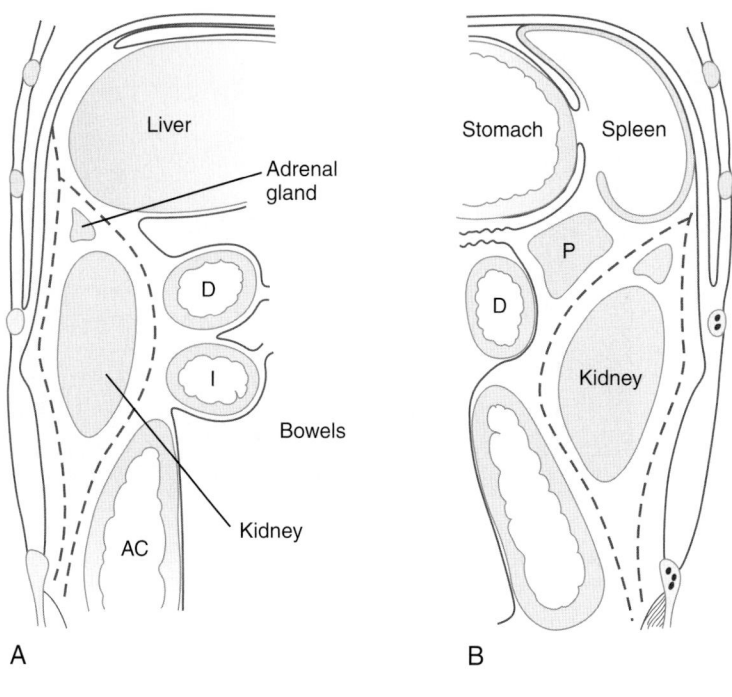

A

B

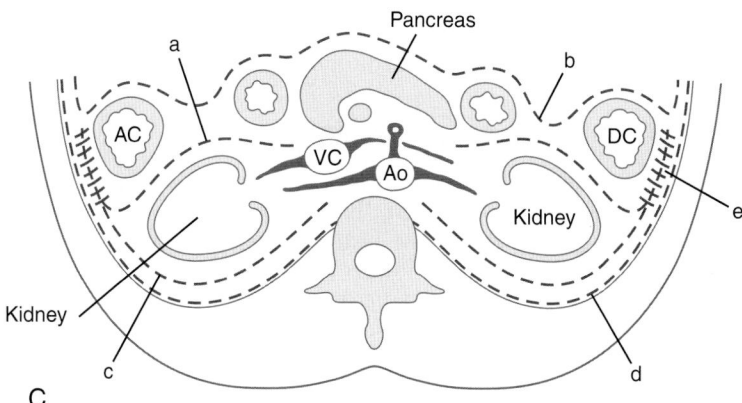

C

FIGURE 145-6. Retroperitoneal anatomy. **A** and **B,** Sagittal sections of the abdomen at the level of the right kidney **(A)** and left kidney **(B).** The liver, right adrenal gland, stomach, spleen, and left kidney are labeled, for orientation. The relationship of the right kidney to the duodenum (D), ileum (I), and ascending colon (AC) is demonstrated in **A.** In **B,** the pancreas (P) and duodenum (D) are also labeled. **C,** Axial (transverse) section of the abdomen at the level of the kidneys outlines the following spaces: the anterior perirenal space between the kidney and the anterior renal fascia *(broken line a);* the anterior pararenal space between the anterior perirenal space *(broken line a)* and the posterior peritoneal layer *(broken line b);* the posterior perirenal space between the kidney and the posterior renal fascia *(broken line c);* and the posterior pararenal space between the posterior renal fascia *(broken line c)* and the transversalis fascia *(broken line d).* The lateroconal fascia *(cross-hatched section e)* is also shown. For orientation, the pancreas (P) and kidney are labeled, as are the aorta (Ao), inferior vena cava (VC), ascending colon (AC), and descending colon (DC).

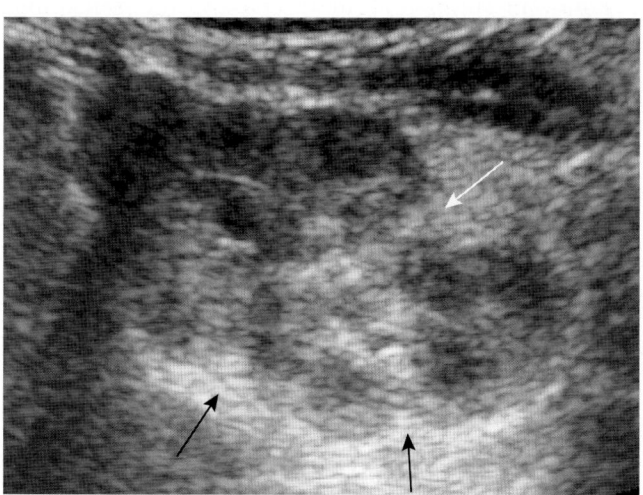

FIGURE 145-7. Fetal lobulations. Residual fetal lobulations are responsible for the scalloped border of the kidney *(black arrows)* on this sagittal sonogram. There is also a prominent junctional cortical defect *(white arrow).*

triangular in shape, with a distinct bulge along its lateral aspect, the so-called dromedary kidney (see Fig. 145-3).

Measurements

The wide range of normal findings makes sequential measurements of greater value than a single measurement. For example, a kidney studied during an acute infection may be swollen, making prior renal scarring impossible to detect. Measurements of the kidney can be made with all imaging modalities, but standards for renal size have been developed only for urography and US (Fig. 145-9). Kidney length is the most commonly measured parameter. Determinations of renal width, cortical thickness, and parenchymal area can also be made and can be used to evaluate renal growth.

On IVU, these measurements should be made only on films obtained with the child in the supine position. The length of the kidney has been correlated to age (see Fig. 145-9), body height and weight, and height of the first three or four lumbar vertebral bodies. The renal

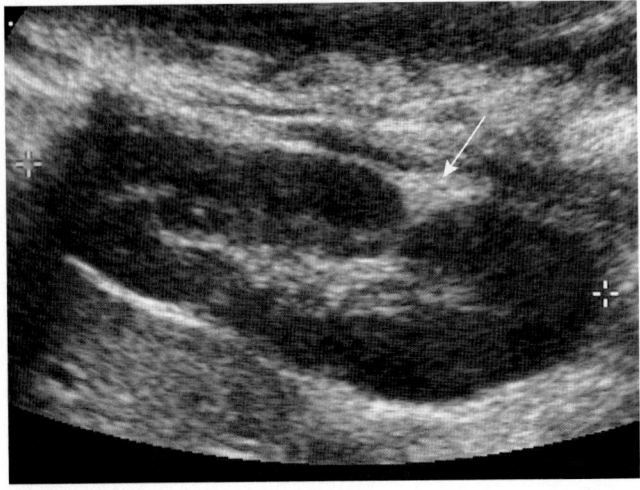
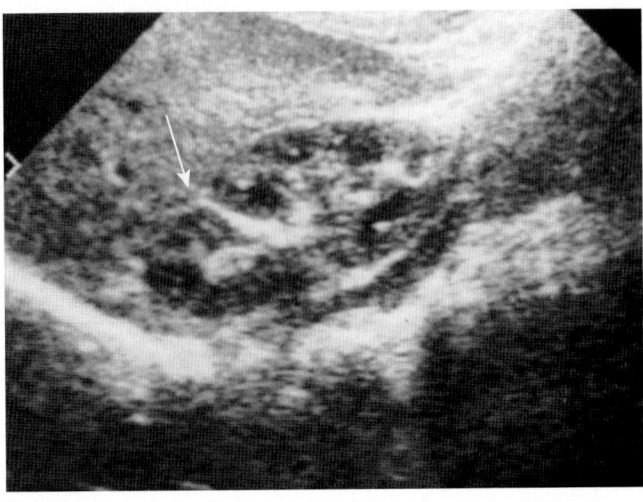

A

B

FIGURE 145-8. Junctional parenchymal defects. **A,** Longitudinal prone sonogram shows a fat-filled cleft *(arrow)* in the posterior kidney. **B,** Longitudinal supine sonogram in another patient shows a renicular septum *(arrow).* Both are normal findings, probably related to a demarcation of embryonic reniculi.

length is equal to the height of about 5 vertebral bodies (including intervening disk spaces) in newborns, 4.5 vertebral bodies in infants and children up to 1.5 years of age, and 4 vertebral bodies in older children. The left kidney may be slightly longer than the right; in adults, the difference may reach 15 mm. Kidneys with complete or partial collecting system duplication are longer than normal kidneys.

Renal length is more often measured with US than with IVU. US standards for kidney length relative to age, height, weight, and body surface have been developed (see Fig. 145-9); in addition, specific US standards have been developed for preterm infants and myelodysplastic children. The values obtained by US are generally lower than those derived from urographic films, with the difference being slightly less than 1 cm in the first 5 years of life and slightly more than 1 cm after that. Kidney volume can also be estimated by US according to the formula for a prolate ellipsoid:

$$\text{Volume} = \text{Length} \times \text{Width} \times \text{Anteroposterior diameter} \times 0.523,$$

using the maximal measurement for each parameter. The length is measured on coronal scans; the width and anteroposterior diameter are measured on transverse images. Intraobserver variation in these measurements, though generally not clinically significant, is magnified when calculating the renal volume, and in children older than 2 years, this may result in kidney volumes that deviate by 2 to 3 years' normal renal growth. Newer three-dimensional US techniques allow more accurate measurements of volume.

The width of the kidney is approximately 50% of its length and is relatively thicker in neonates than in older children. Cortical thickness is measured as that part of the renal parenchyma that lies outside a line drawn through the tips of the renal calyces on frontal IVU (Fig. 145-10). This line is roughly parallel to the outer border of the kidney. The upper pole is normally slightly thicker than the lower pole, and the renal cortex is

slightly thinner in the center of the kidney. The polar thickness is essentially the same on the two sides. Extra cortical tissue may be noted about the renal hilum and may impinge from above or below on the renal pelvis (suprahilar or infrahilar bulge; hilar lips).

Compensatory Hypertrophy

Contrary to reports in the early literature, compensatory hypertrophy can begin in utero. Children with one multicystic dysplastic kidney may be born with a contralateral kidney that is significantly larger than the norm. Lack of expected compensatory hypertrophy may indicate that the functioning kidney is compromised by a second process, such as vesicoureteral reflux. Compensatory hypertrophy is more rapid in infants than in older children and adults. It has also been described in a kidney contralateral to a severely obstructed but functioning kidney.

Following unilateral nephrectomy, the remaining normal kidney displays accelerated growth over a 2-year period. This solitary kidney reaches a length that is several standard deviations above the mean.

Pelvocalyceal System and Ureter

The renal pelvis varies in size from a small, poorly defined sac to a large, boxlike structure. The pelvis may lie entirely within (intrarenal) or almost entirely beyond (extrarenal) the renal sinus. A redundant and partially extrarenal pelvis may be flattened along its medial aspect by the psoas muscle and thus appear square instead of funnel shaped. In newborns and small infants, the pelvis is often relatively small and intrarenal and usually points medially instead of downward.

The configuration of the pelvocalyceal system is quite variable, even from side to side. In most kidneys, the pelvis branches into two major infundibula (or major calyces). The inferior infundibulum is commonly broad and short and is connected with a larger number of

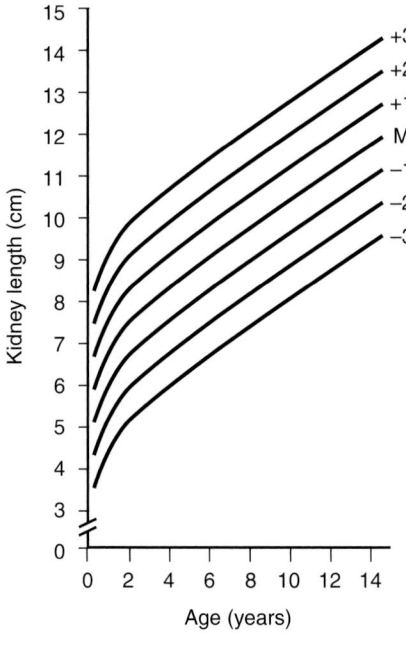

A

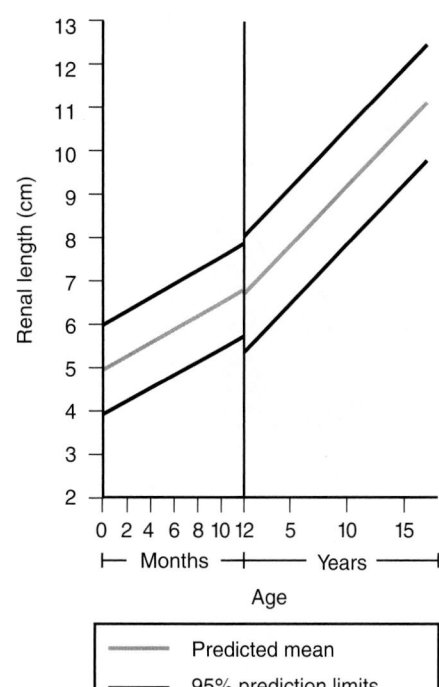

B

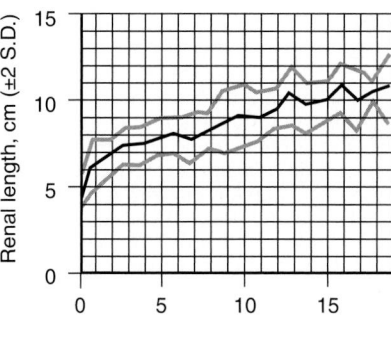

C

FIGURE 145-9. Kidney length in centimeters. **A,** Measurements obtained from supine urographic films and correlated with age, including values for 3 standard deviations (SD) above and below the mean (M). The SD is 0.75 cm. **B,** Sonographic measurements correlated with age; the values are slightly lower than those obtained from urographic films. **C,** Ultrasound measurements correlated with age, including ± 2 SD. (**A** modified from Currarino G, Williams B, Dana K: Kidney length correlated with age: normal values in children. Radiology 1984;150:703; **B** from Han BK, Babcock DS: Sonographic measurements and appearance of normal kidneys in children. AJR Am J Roentgenol 1985;145:611; **C** from Rosenbaum DM, Korngold E, Teele RL: Sonographic assessment of renal length in normal children. AJR Am J Roentgenol 1984;142:467.)

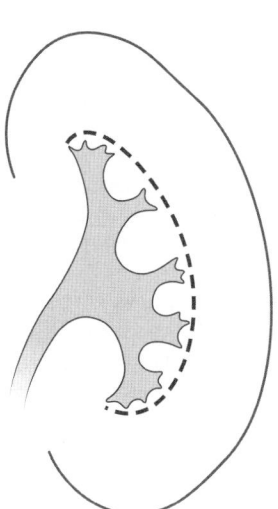

FIGURE 145-10. Renal cortical thickness. *Dashed line* at the tips of the calyces parallels the edge of the kidney. The corticomedullary junction and arcuate arteries are located approximately at the junction of the middle and outer thirds of the intervening renal parenchyma.

calyces than the upper infundibulum. In some cases, the major calyces are poorly defined, and the lesser calyces appear to originate from the renal pelvis. Also normal are the elongated, spider-like calyces that are often associated with a small or bifid renal pelvis.

Each kidney has about 8 to 13 minor calyces. These have a cup-shaped appearance that is due to protrusion of the renal papilla into the calyx. Two or more papillae may enter one calyx (compound calyx). Most calyces are directed laterally and either slightly anteriorly or posteriorly within the kidney.

The number of calyces demonstrated on IVU may change from study to study in the same child. The actual calyces that opacify may also vary; different calyces may be visualized on sequential studies.

The transition between the renal pelvis and the ureter, or the ureteropelvic junction (UPJ), may be sharply or poorly defined. Both extrinsic filling defects and local narrowing are commonly observed at the UPJ without resultant hydronephrosis. An inferior polar artery may

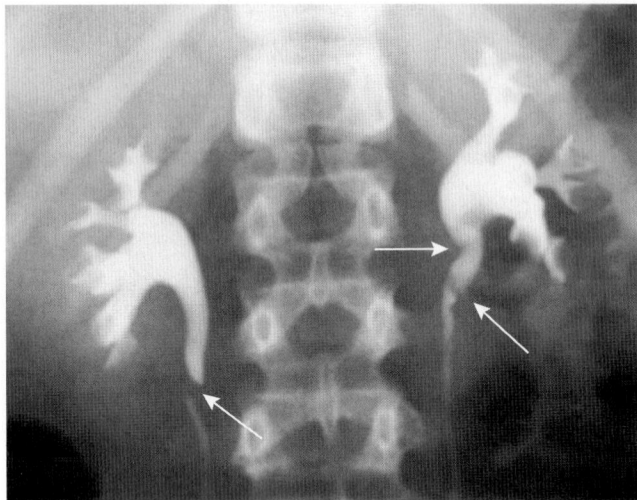

FIGURE 145-11. Renal arterial impressions. IVU in a 14-year-old girl shows several defects at the ureteropelvic junction and proximal ureter *(arrows)*, presumably caused by aberrant renal arteries.

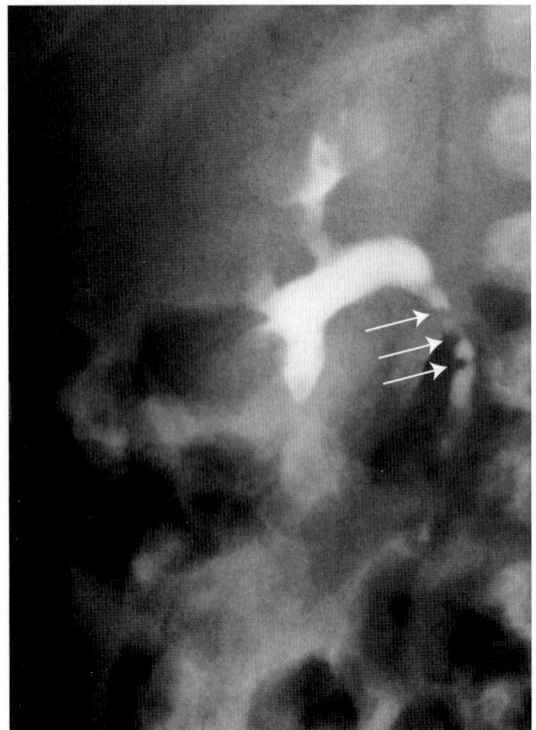

FIGURE 145-12. Retained fetal folds. IVU shows multiple nonobstructive filling defects *(arrows)* in the proximal portion of the ureter. In most children, these disappear over time.

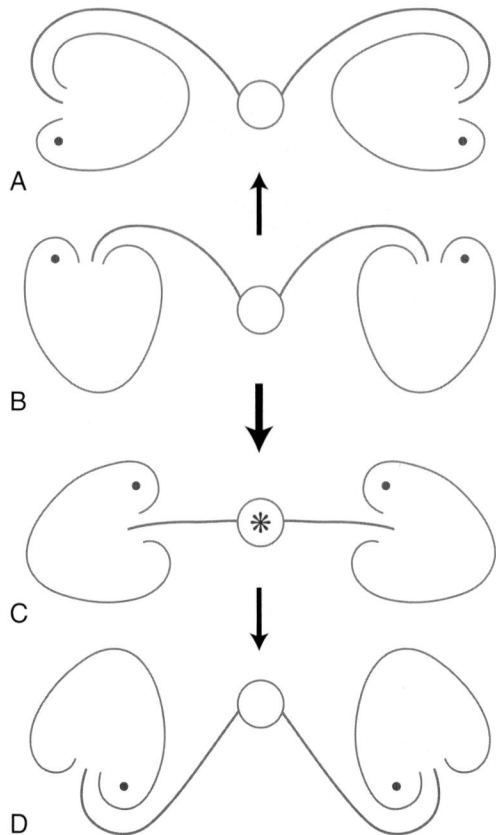

FIGURE 145-13. Normal rotation of the kidney in fetal life and various types of renal malrotation. **A,** Reversed rotation, which is rare. **B,** Primitive fetal position of the kidney with the hilum pointing forward. A persistent fetal position is referred to as an absent or incomplete rotation; this is the most common form of renal malrotation. **C,** Normal postnatal position with the hilum pointing medially and slightly forward (*, aorta). **D,** Overrotation, which is rare. All these anomalies of rotation can be unilateral or bilateral.

CONGENITAL ANOMALIES

Anomalies of Rotation

The metanephros has its origin in the fetal pelvis, and in this site, its renal pelvis is oriented anteriorly. As the kidney ascends to its normal position, the renal pelvis and hilum normally rotate 90 degrees medially (Fig. 145-13). Kidneys that fail to ascend to a normal position generally maintain some degree of the anterior orientation of the renal pelvis and are described as incompletely rotated. Such malrotation can also be observed, though much less frequently, in normally positioned kidneys. The renal pelvis of normally positioned kidneys may also be overrotated and oriented posteriorly or, even more rarely, rotated into a lateral position.

Kidneys in a normal position also have, as a rule, a normal renal axis. A line drawn from the upper calyceal system to the lower one parallels the psoas muscle, with the upper pole medial to the lower pole. The intimate relationship of the kidney to the psoas muscle results in the superior and medial portion being more dorsal than the inferior and lateral portion of the kidney, which rests on the bulkier aspect of the psoas. Incomplete ascent

produce a small extrinsic defect or notch in the ureter near the UPJ (Fig. 145-11). A sharp kink without obstruction is occasionally seen in the proximal portion of the ureter as a transient or constant finding. Folds in the upper ureter (Fig. 145-12), mild elongation and tortuosity of the ureter, and mild widening of the midureter are all seen in infant urograms. They are believed to represent a persistence of fetal characteristics and disappear in early childhood (see Chapter 151).

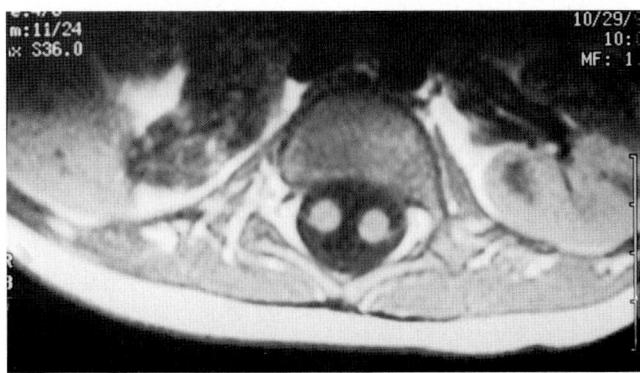

FIGURE 145-14. MRI of unilateral (right) renal agenesis. Vertebral anomalies prompted this study. The axial T1-weighted image shows a normal left kidney and a bowel loop in the right renal fossa. Note also the split spinal cord, indicating diastematomyelia. (Courtesy of Joan A. Zawin, MD.)

and fusion anomalies result in an abnormal relationship between the kidney and the psoas muscle and abnormalities of the renal axis.

Renal Ectopia and Anomalies of Fusion

Renal ectopia and agenesis and renal fusion anomalies are associated with anomalies of other organ systems. Spinal anomalies (segmentation anomalies, partial or complete sacral agenesis, and most dysraphic processes), cardiac anomalies, and limb anomalies are the most frequent associations. When specific anomalies of the gastrointestinal tract (esophageal atresia, imperforate anus) are present, the affected child is said to have the VACTERL association—a linkage of vertebral, anorectal, cardiac, tracheoesophageal, renal, and limb anomalies. The limb anomalies, originally described as affecting the radial aspect of the forearm and hand, have been extended to other lesions of the upper extremity and hand and of the lower extremities as well. Anomalies of the urethra have also been described in boys with the VACTERL association.

When MRI is used to evaluate spinal anomalies, renal anomalies should be sought (Figs. 145-14 and 145-15). Some renal anomalies described here have specific associations that are detailed in the appropriate sections.

IPSILATERAL RENAL ECTOPIA (SIMPLE UNCROSSED RENAL ECTOPIA)

PELVIC KIDNEY (INFERIOR ECTOPIA). When normal ascent to the renal fossa is incomplete, the kidney may remain in the pelvis or be located anywhere between the bony pelvis and the renal fossa. In early gestation, the kidney takes its blood supply from the middle sacral artery. As the kidney ascends, the blood supply changes; the lower vessels atrophy as vessels with a more cephalad origin develop. In turn, "renal" arteries develop from the iliac artery and then, sequentially, from higher sites on the aorta. When the kidney is in a lower than normal position, it usually retains its earlier blood supply and has some degree of abnormal rotation of the renal pelvis (Figs. 145-16 and 145-17).

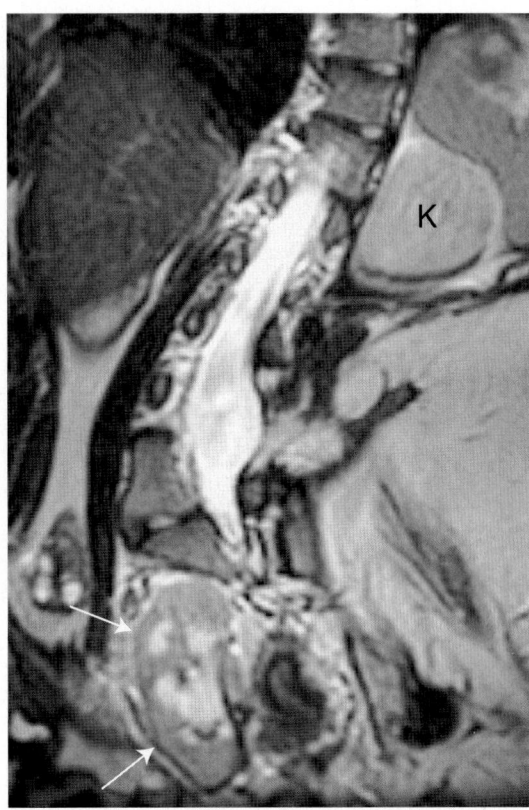

FIGURE 145-15. MRI of pelvic kidney. Coronal T2-weighted MR image in a patient with spinal dysraphism and scoliosis shows a normally positioned left kidney (K) and an unsuspected right pelvic kidney (arrows) with mild hydronephrosis. (Courtesy of Brian D. Coley, MD.)

> Anomalies of ascent are associated with variations in rotation of the pelvocalyceal system and persistence of a more primitive vascular supply.

Because the embryology of the adrenal gland is independent of that of the kidney, it is usually (in 90% of cases) in its expected position even when the kidney is absent or does not reach the renal fossa. However, the adrenal gland may develop an elongated or elliptical shape rather than its normal triangular or Y configuration. Differentiation of the adrenal cortex from the medullary tissue remains clear (Fig. 145-18). An elongated gland is easily recognized as such; an elliptical adrenal may be mistaken for a hypoplastic kidney in the renal fossa because the echogenic medulla may simulate the central renal echo complex.

The pelvic kidney is the most common type of renal ectopia (accounting for about 60% of cases). It was originally described as a poorly functioning, dysmorphic structure, but in many instances, it functions normally. It has vesicoureteral reflux more often than a normal kidney and may, in about 10% of children, be the only kidney. In some children, both kidneys are in the pelvis and may be fused into a single unit, the so-called cake kidney. Anomalies of rotation and blood supply are to be expected.

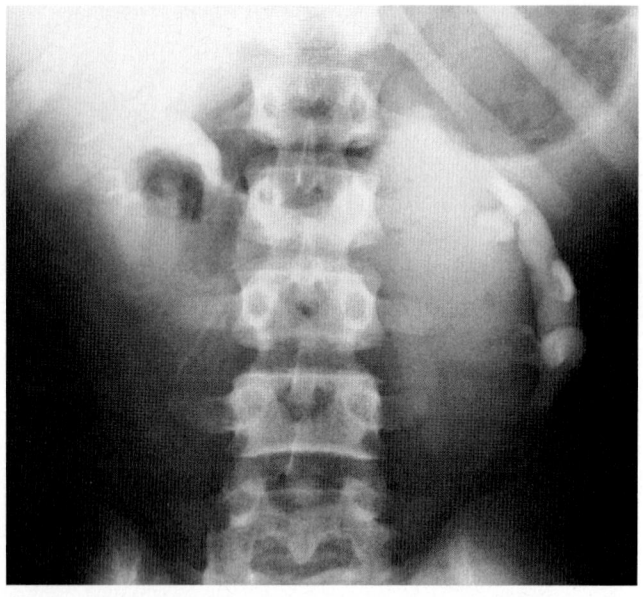

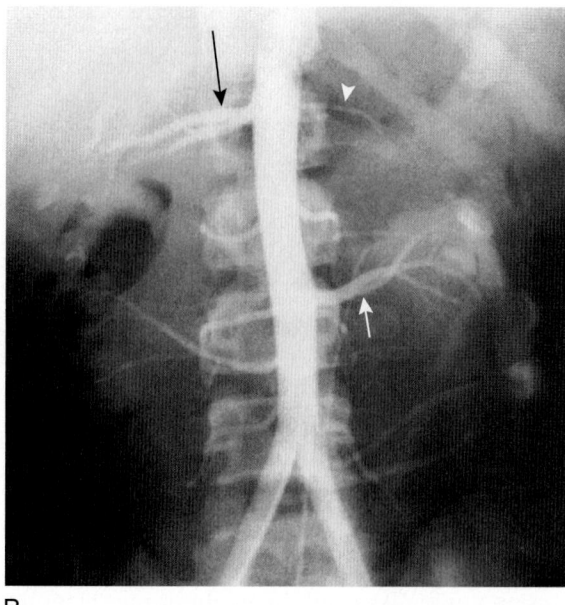

A   B

FIGURE 145-16. Failure of the kidney to ascend to a normal position. **A,** IVU shows the abnormal orientation of the left renal pelvis and calyces, typical of a kidney with inferior ectopia. The right kidney is in a normal position and is normally rotated. **B,** Arteriogram shows that the right kidney's artery has a normal origin *(black arrow).* The left kidney's blood supply arises two vertebral levels below the usual origin of the left renal artery *(white arrow).* The small vessel *(arrowhead)* is supplying the normally positioned adrenal gland.

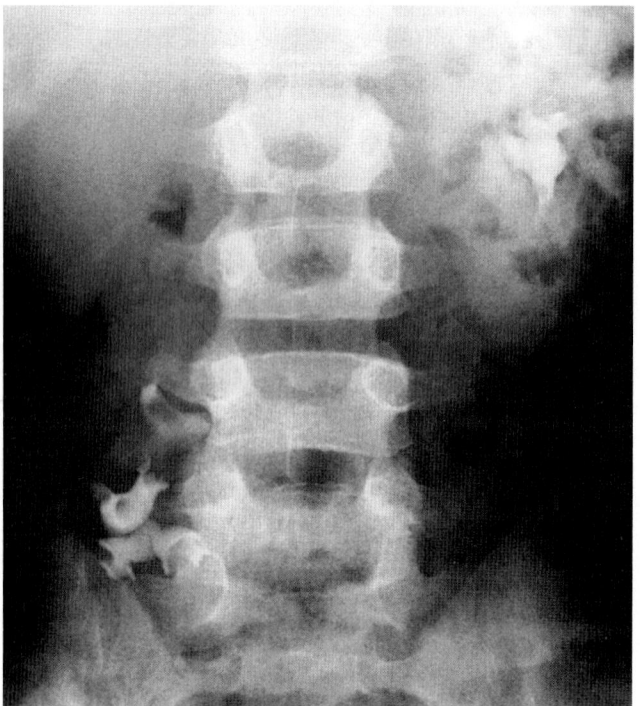

FIGURE 145-17. Iliolumbar kidney. IVU shows the left kidney in a normal position and the right kidney partially overlying the right iliac bone. Note the abnormal rotation of the right renal pelvis.

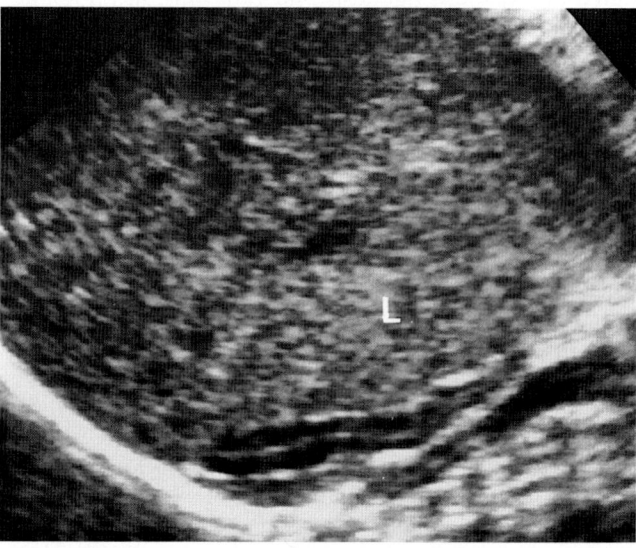

FIGURE 145-18. Appearance of the adrenal gland with renal ectopia or agenesis. Longitudinal sonogram shows an elongated adrenal gland, just beneath the liver (L). The hypoechoic tissue at the periphery is the cortex. The echogenic central stripe is the adrenal medulla.

A pelvic kidney may be discovered prenatally or incidentally when anomalies of other organ systems prompt a postnatal sonogram, or it may remain undetected until adult life. For example, a maternal pelvic kidney can interfere with normal engagement of the fetal head and precipitate a cesarean section.

On US, the pelvic kidney may have a normal appearance (Fig. 145-19), but it frequently does not (Fig. 145-20). The pelvocalyceal system may be predominantly extrarenal, resulting in images in which the kidney lacks the usual central renal echo complex. Corticomedullary differentiation may be indistinct. The extrarenal location of the pelvocalyceal system may produce hydronephrosis without obstruction, but UPJ obstruction is common in the pelvic kidney because the abnormal orientation of the ureter relative to the renal pelvis impedes drainage. Because of the high incidence of vesicoureteral reflux

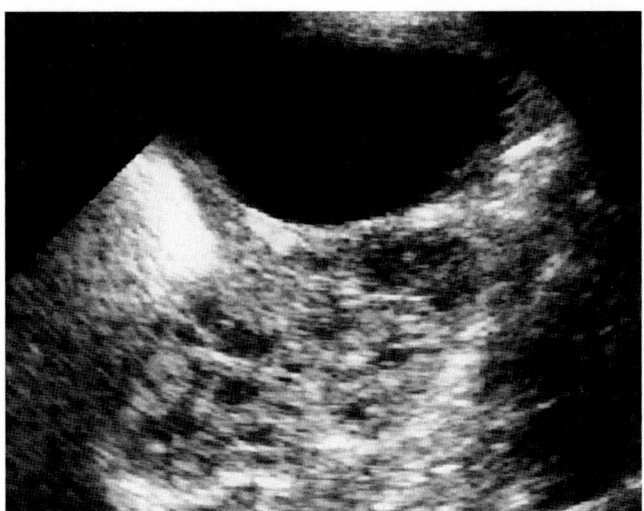

FIGURE 145-19. Normal pelvic kidney. Longitudinal sonogram shows a normal kidney adjacent to the urine-filled bladder. Normal hypoechoic medullary tissue is easily distinguished from the cortex.

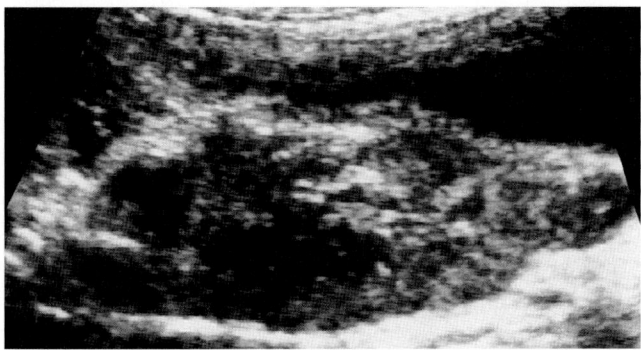

FIGURE 145-20. Abnormal pelvic kidney. Longitudinal sonogram shows an abnormal pelvic kidney; the upper and lower poles are shrunken, and the corticomedullary differentiation is indistinct.

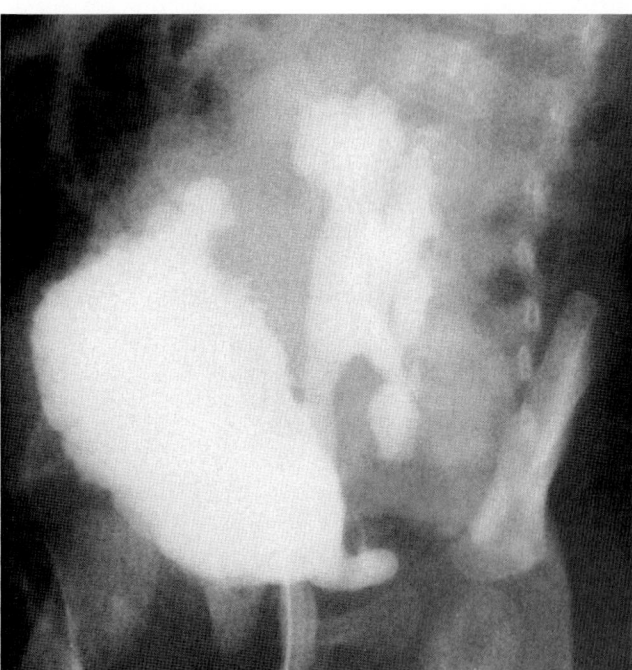

FIGURE 145-21. Vesicoureteral reflux into a pelvic kidney. Voiding cystourethrogram shows that the bladder is moderately trabeculated, a sign of a neurogenic bladder associated with a spinal cord anomaly in this child. Reflux fills and distends the ureter and pelvocalyceal system, indicating grade V reflux.

in the pelvic or contralateral kidney (up to 70%), cystography is recommended (Fig. 145-21). Renal cortical scintigraphy can be used to both locate and define the morphology of ectopic kidneys. Nuclear studies are also useful to distinguish obstructive from nonobstructive hydronephrosis when urinary tract surgery is contemplated. IVU usually provides limited information because the pelvic kidney may function poorly; even when functioning well, it may be hard to see because of the overlying shadows of the sacrum and gastrointestinal tract.

THORACIC KIDNEY (SUPERIOR ECTOPIA). The kidney may continue its ascent and enter the thorax, accounting for 20% of renal ectopia (Fig. 145-22). Superior ectopia may occur as an isolated lesion but is more often part of a larger intrathoracic herniation of subdiaphragmatic structures through the foramen of Bochdalek. Because congenital diaphragmatic hernia occurs about seven times more frequently on the left than the right, superior renal ectopia is also more frequently left-sided. The thoracic kidney tends to function well and usually receives its blood supply from a normally positioned

renal artery, although it may also have an accessory artery arising from the thoracic aorta. The ipsilateral adrenal gland is usually in a normal location.

The thoracic kidney is located in the posterior mediastinum, and on chest radiographs it may be mistaken for the usual neurogenic tumors that develop in this region: neuroblastoma, ganglioneuroblastoma, or ganglioneuroma (see Fig. 145-22). If the adjacent spine has an abnormal appearance, intrathoracic meningocele and neurenteric cyst are included in the differential diagnosis. Renal cortical scintigraphy, US, CT, or MRI can define the mass as being renal and may detect other herniated tissue or organs not appreciated with plain radiographs.

CROSSED RENAL ECTOPIA

Crossed renal ectopia occurs when both kidneys are on one side of the spine; a portion of the lower kidney—usually the one that has moved from its normal position—may extend over the spine (Fig. 145-23). This anomaly is seen in 1 in 3000 to 1 in 8000 children, with boys more often affected than girls. The ureter from the lower kidney usually crosses the midline to insert into the bladder in its normal position, contralateral to the ureter from the upper kidney. Departure from this pattern is rare but does occur (Fig. 145-24). There is also variation in the alignment of the two kidneys. Although most are oriented in a relatively vertical axis, the lower kidney may be obliquely related to the superior kidney. The absolute position of the upper kidney can also be ectopically low.

Approximately 90% of these kidneys are fused and encompassed by a common renal fascia—hence the term *crossed fused renal ectopia*. With standard imaging, it is

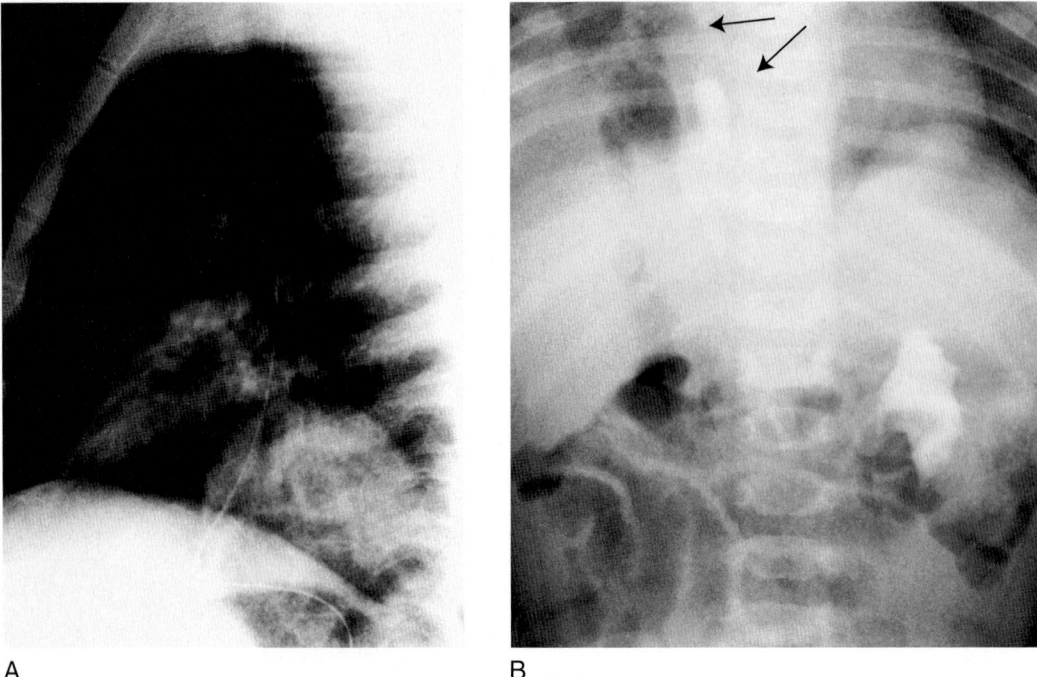

A   B

FIGURE 145-22. Thoracic kidney. **A,** Lateral chest radiograph shows an oval soft tissue mass projecting in the posterior sulcus. **B,** IVU shows that the right kidney *(arrows)* projects above the medial aspect of the right diaphragm. Also projecting above the diaphragm are several bowel loops, indicating that the kidney displacement occurred as a result of a hernia.

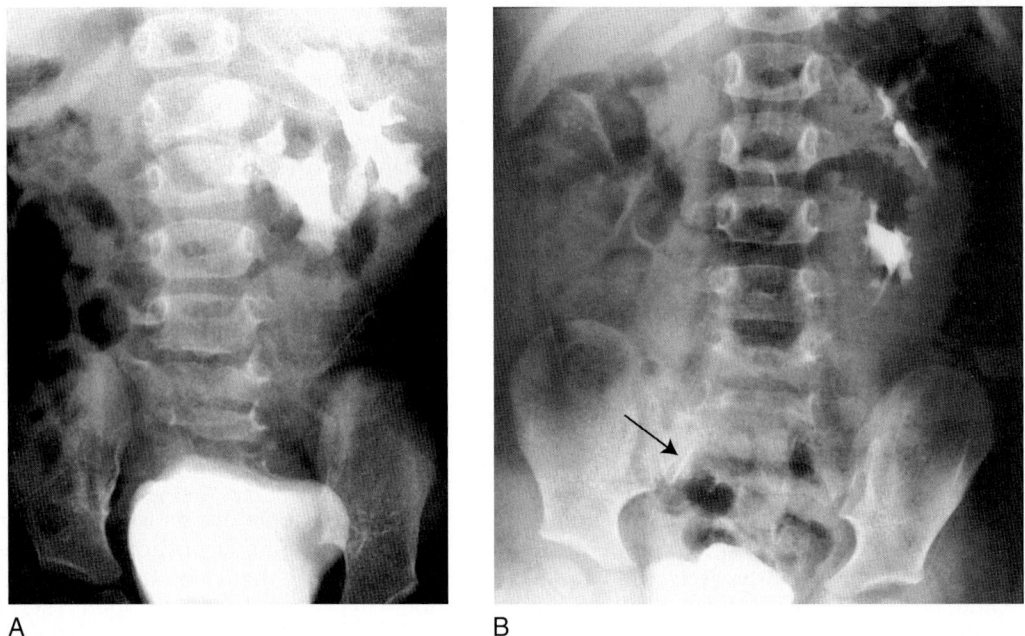

A   B

FIGURE 145-23. Crossed renal ectopia. **A,** IVU shows both renal collecting systems to the left of the spine. Segmentation anomalies of the sacrum, which are subtle in this child, are one of the skeletal anomalies associated with crossed renal ectopia. **B,** As shown in a different child, the lower kidney is usually ectopic, and its ureter *(arrow)* crosses the midline to insert into the bladder in a normal position.

impossible to differentiate kidneys that are fused from those few that are merely in close apposition. However, in most clinical settings, this information is not relevant. As expected in any type of inferior ectopia, the arterial vascularity may be anomalous, and the renal pelvis, especially of the lower kidney, may be malrotated.

Because each kidney is drained by its own ureter, multicystic dysplasia can develop in one of the kidneys. The occasional case report of unilateral crossed ectopy may be due to involution of an affected upper kidney.

Imaging demonstrates an empty renal fossa on one side (with an abnormal adrenal configuration) and an

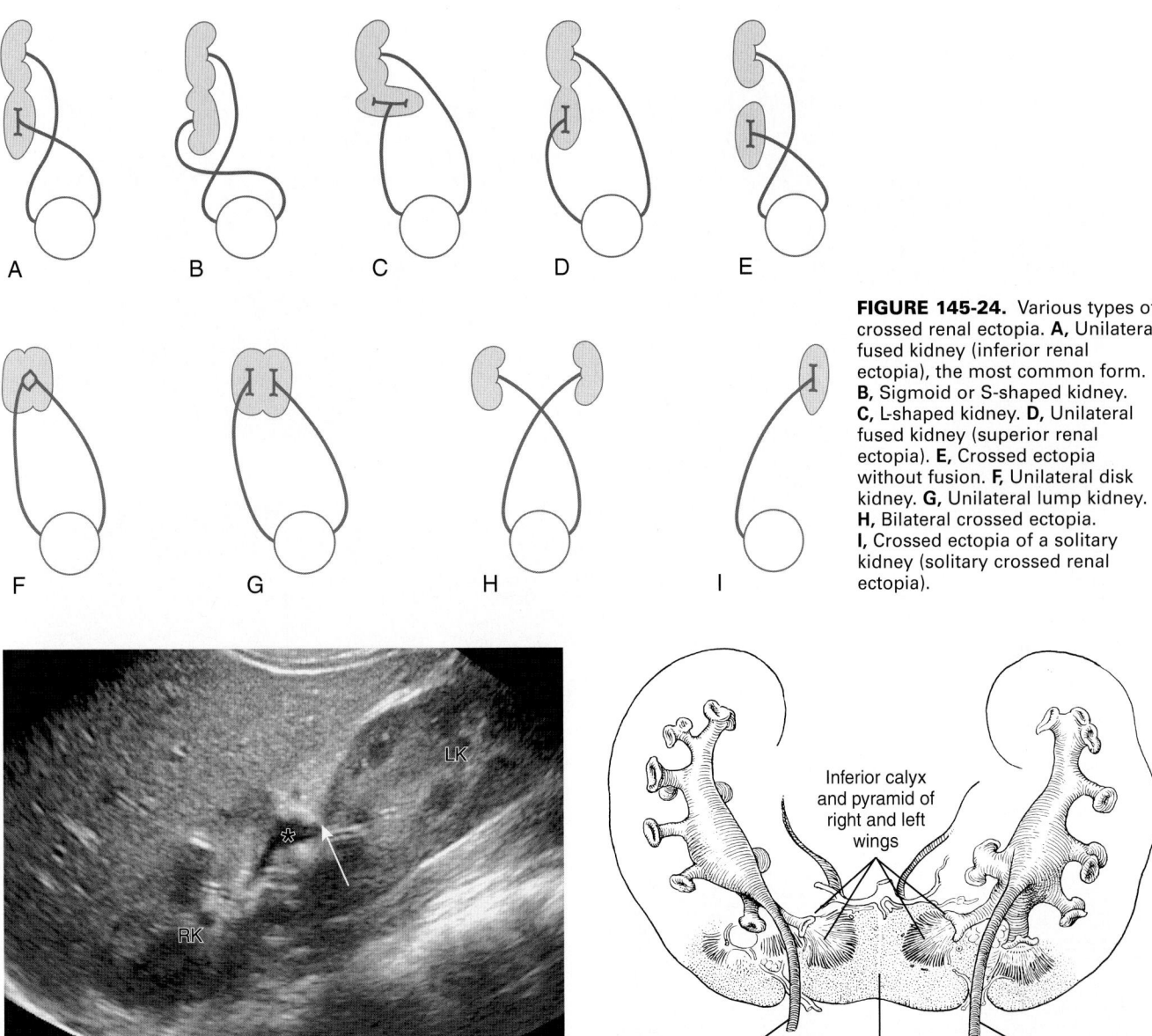

FIGURE 145-24. Various types of crossed renal ectopia. **A,** Unilateral fused kidney (inferior renal ectopia), the most common form. **B,** Sigmoid or S-shaped kidney. **C,** L-shaped kidney. **D,** Unilateral fused kidney (superior renal ectopia). **E,** Crossed ectopia without fusion. **F,** Unilateral disk kidney. **G,** Unilateral lump kidney. **H,** Bilateral crossed ectopia. **I,** Crossed ectopia of a solitary kidney (solitary crossed renal ectopia).

FIGURE 145-25. Crossed renal ectopia. Longitudinal sonogram of the right upper quadrant shows a well-defined indentation or niche *(arrow)* at the junction between the right kidney (RK) and the crossed, fused left kidney (LK). The right renal pelvis has a small amount of visible urine within it (*). (Courtesy of Brian D. Coley, MD.)

FIGURE 145-26. Horseshoe kidney with fusion of the inferior poles, spreading apart of the superior poles, and failure of rotation. The renal pelves enter the kidneys on their anterior aspect. (Redrawn from Kelly HA, Burnam CF: Diseases of the Kidneys, Ureters and Bladder, 2nd ed. New York, Appleton, 1922.)

apparently enlarged kidney on the other side. A duplex kidney rather than crossed renal ectopy may be suggested when two separate renal pelves and a larger than normal amount of renal parenchyma are detected on one side of the spine. IVU or CT shows the separate ureters, each entering its appropriate trigone. Coronal or sagittal US and renal cortical scintigraphy may allow visualization of a small indentation, or niche, between the two kidneys, even when fusion has occurred (Fig. 145-25). Doppler US may also demonstrate the jet of urine emanating from the normally positioned lower kidney. Cystography is recommended, because the lower kidney has an increased incidence of vesicoureteral reflux.

HORSESHOE KIDNEY

This common anomaly, noted in 1 in 500 to 1 in 1000 autopsies, takes its name from the U shape produced by the fusion of the lower poles of the kidneys (Fig. 145-26). The bridging tissue, known as the *isthmus,* is commonly composed of functioning parenchyma or, less commonly, fibrous tissue. Not every horseshoe kidney is symmetrically related to the spine; some are a bit more to the left or right, almost a transition to crossed renal ectopia (Fig. 145-27). In virtually all cases, the fusion occurs inferiorly; superior fusion has been reported but is rare.

There is an increased incidence of ureteral duplication, UPJ obstruction, and vesicoureteral reflux in horseshoe kidneys (Figs. 145-28 and 145-29). The UPJ

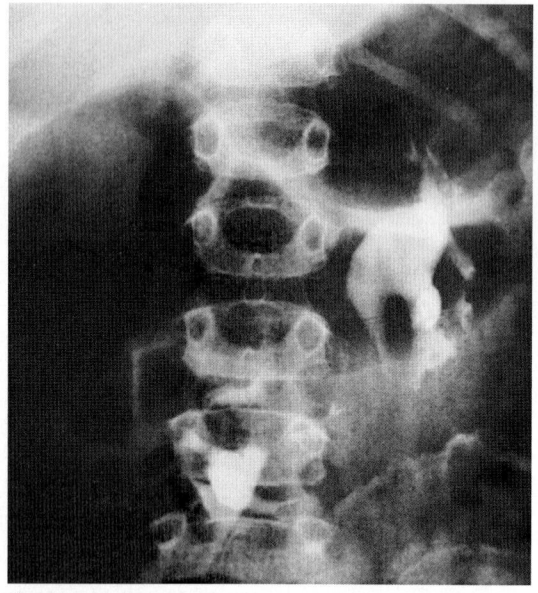

A

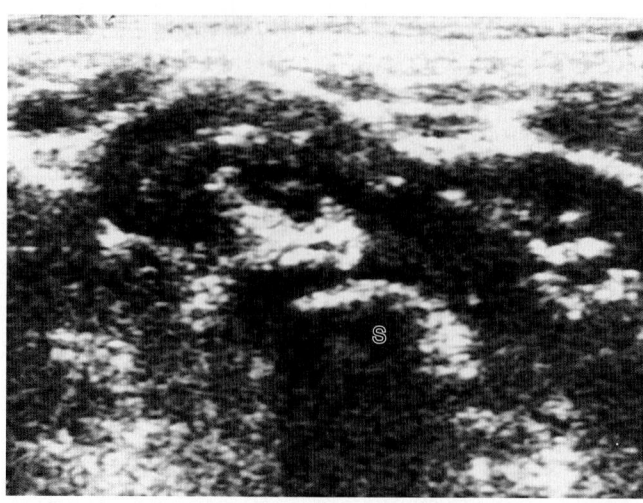

B

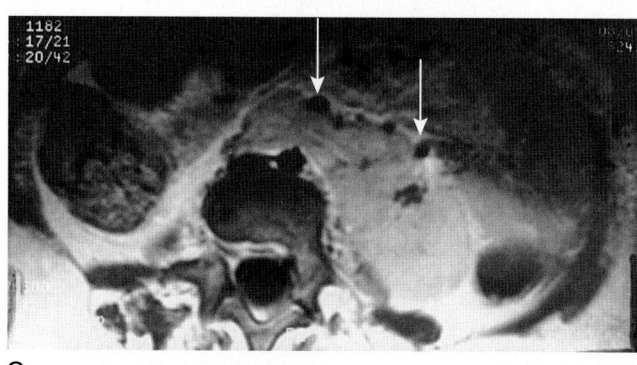

C

FIGURE 145-27. Transition between crossed renal ectopia and asymmetric horseshoe kidney. **A,** IVU shows that the axis of the left kidney is abnormal, with the lower pole directly below the upper pole. The right kidney overlies the spine. **B,** Sonogram shows that the confluence of the kidneys is anterior to the spine (S), and the kidneys are asymmetrically related to the spine. **C,** Axial T1-weighted MR image shows that the fused kidneys are anterior to and to the left of the spine. Note the multiple signal voids of the renal vessels along the anterior aspect of the kidney *(arrows).* (Courtesy of Joan A. Zawin, MD.)

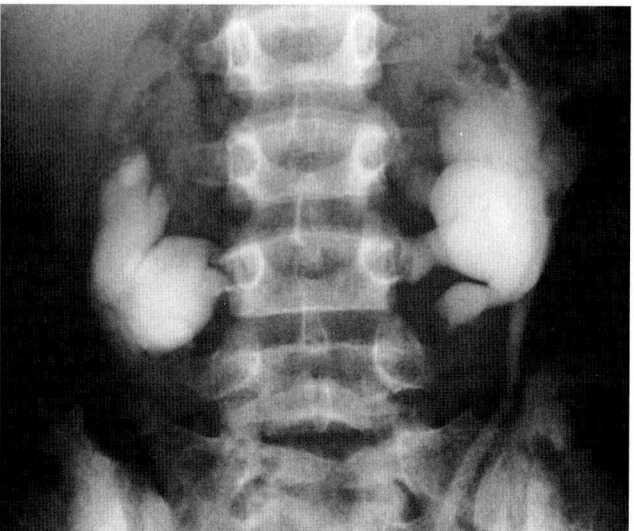

FIGURE 145-28. Horseshoe kidney with bilateral ureteropelvic junction obstruction. IVU shows the abnormal renal axes, with the lower poles medial to the upper poles—typical in horseshoe kidney. The moderate dilation of each renal pelvis suggests obstruction, which was proved with scintigraphy.

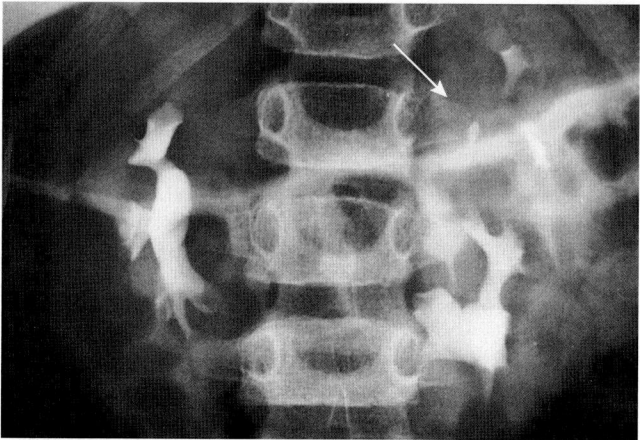

FIGURE 145-29. Horseshoe kidney with ureteral duplication. IVU shows the abnormal axis of the kidneys, pointing toward the isthmus of parenchyma anterior to the spine. The left kidney is composed of two moieties, with the upper one *(arrow)* having a more delicate appearance than the lower.

obstruction develops from the mechanical obstruction of the ureters passing over the tissue of the isthmus. However, as with pelvic kidneys, dilation of the pelvocalyceal system should not always be interpreted as obstruction, because a dilated extrarenal pelvis (also a common finding) can simulate obstruction. Multicystic dysplasia has been described in one segment of a horseshoe kidney; involution of the involved segment can produce a changing radiographic appearance of the functioning segments.

The segment of kidney that is over the spine is prone to injury from direct trauma. Wilms tumor also occurs more frequently in horseshoe kidneys than in normal

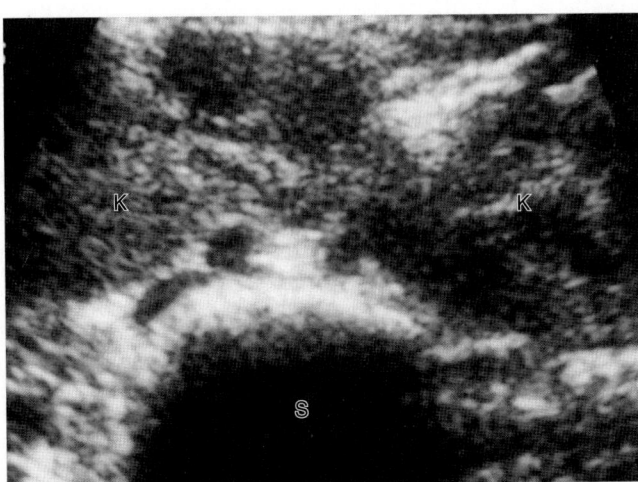

FIGURE 145-30. Horseshoe kidney. Transverse sonogram shows that the two kidneys (K) are connected in the midline, in front of the spine (S).

kidneys. In adults, stone formation and transitional cell cancer are more common in horseshoe than normal kidneys.

The fusion produces an abnormal renal axis; the lower pole of each kidney is more medial than the upper pole. The isthmus is intimately related to the inferior mesenteric artery. The kidneys are also abnormally low in the retroperitoneum. For this reason, the vascular supply of a horseshoe kidney is variable. Multiple renal arteries may arise directly from the aorta or from a single vessel that itself arises from the aorta. Unless surgery is planned, the anatomy of the vascular supply need not be defined.

Although horseshoe kidney can be an incidental finding, it occurs in association with trisomy 18, imperforate anus (more common with high imperforate anus than low), cardiac anomalies, and Turner syndrome, which itself has an increased incidence of aortic coarctation. Horseshoe kidney also occurs more frequently in infants of diabetic mothers; in this setting, it may be a forme fruste of the caudal regression syndrome, which is also more common in these infants.

Prenatal and postnatal US may demonstrate the upper portion of each kidney in a low but otherwise normal paraspinal location and the low position of the "lower pole" of the kidneys. Postnatal US, usually performed because of associated anomalies or an abnormal prenatal ultrasound examination, may demonstrate the isthmus anterior to the spine, especially when mild compression is used to displace interposed bowel loops (Fig. 145-30). The abnormal renal axis can be appreciated while scanning; the unusual orientation of the transducer when trying to obtain a sagittal view of the kidney should suggest the diagnosis. The anterior position (and possible dilation) of the renal pelvis can also be shown with US. Occasionally, horseshoe kidney is an incidental finding on MRI performed because of an obvious or suspected vertebral abnormality. Contrast studies are rarely performed for diagnosis but display the abnormal renal axis well (see Figs. 145-28 and 145-29). An abnormal renal axis should suggest a horseshoe

kidney, but in children with spinal dysraphism, the abnormal axis may be due to a secondary kyphosis of the spine and underdevelopment of the psoas muscles—known as the pseudohorseshoe kidney (Fig. 145-31). Rarely, the anatomy of an asymmetric horseshoe kidney may be difficult to demonstrate, and additional imaging may be required to differentiate it from an abdominal mass.

Renal Agenesis

BILATERAL RENAL AGENESIS

This lethal anomaly occurs in about 1 in 4000 live births. Males are affected about three times as often as females. Although the incidence is usually sporadic, renal agenesis may be an inherited trait transmitted in association with lesser degrees of renal dysplasia in some families. Bilateral renal agenesis may be an isolated finding or associated with other anomalies, especially those of the hindgut. Prenatal diagnosis is possible because the lack of urine production results in profound oligohydramnios. Also, the kidneys, which are usually seen on US in the 15th week of pregnancy, are not present in either a normal or an anomalous position. Careful US examination detects the absence of bladder filling and emptying, a phenomenon seen at regular intervals on normal prenatal studies.

> Oligohydramnios can result from a number of processes that result in diminished urine production, and US may be useful to distinguish among them.

If the diagnosis is not made until birth, the child manifests Potter sequence: pulmonary hypoplasia, abnormal facial features (micrognathia, deep folds beneath the eyes, flattening of the ears), and deformities of the limbs (tightly apposed fingers, dislocated hips, clubfeet). The pulmonary hypoplasia presents as respiratory distress; resuscitative attempts may result in pneumothorax and pneumomediastinum. Bedside US may be used to exclude other, possibly treatable causes of Potter sequence, especially if the clinical stigmata are mild.

The absence of the kidney in the renal fossa results in an unusual configuration of the adrenal gland. The entire abdomen and pelvis and the lower thorax should be evaluated before making the diagnosis of renal agenesis. With US, it may be difficult to exclude a pelvic kidney in an infant whose empty bladder precludes a full examination of the pelvic contents or one with imperforate anus and a large amount of stool or air in the pelvis. For this reason, additional imaging is occasionally warranted. Renal cortical scintigraphy can detect an obscured or dysplastic kidney or confirm the complete absence of functioning renal parenchyma. Cystography, once advocated as a way to demonstrate the tiny unused bladder, is rarely necessary today.

UNILATERAL RENAL AGENESIS

Present in about 1 in 1000 to 1 in 1500 live births, unilateral renal agenesis is sometimes detected prenatally

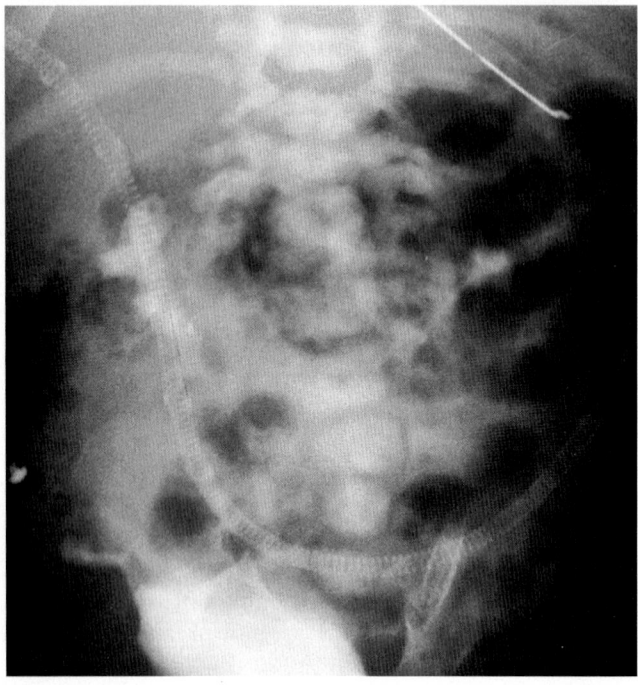

A

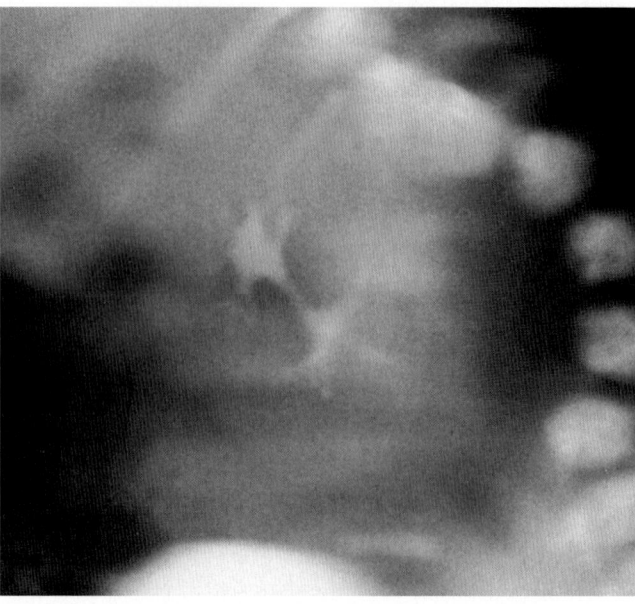

B

FIGURE 145-31. Pseudohorseshoe kidney. **A** and **B,** The abnormal renal axis shown on the anteroposterior view **(A)** from IVU is related to spinal kyphosis. The orientation of the kidney is also abnormal on the lateral view **(B),** with the upper pole anterior to the lower pole. **C,** Axial T1-weighted MR image through the lower abdomen in a different child with sacral agenesis shows that the atretic psoas musculature poorly supports the kidneys and contributes to the midline position of the nonfused kidneys. With other imaging techniques, the separation between them might not be apparent. (Courtesy of Joan A. Zawin, MD.)

C

or when postnatal US is done because of anomalies in the skeletal, gastrointestinal, or cardiovascular systems (Fig. 145-32). It is frequently seen in association with anomalies of the cervical and lumbosacral spine, with or without rectal and anal anomalies. The ipsilateral adrenal gland is present and in a normal location in about 90% of patients.

Unilateral renal agenesis may be silent until puberty, when the associated genital tract anomalies (Table 145-1) become clinically apparent, especially in females. In males, many of the anomalies are silent; occasionally, a seminal vesicle cyst can simulate a ureterocele. In females, the anomalies may present with absence of menses, increasing abdominal or pelvic mass, or pelvic pain. The association of unilateral renal agenesis with genital tract problems in females, especially absence or hypoplasia of the vagina, is called Mayer-Rokitansky-Küster-Hauser syndrome (Fig. 145-33). A more severe variation of this syndrome is the MURCS association,

consisting of müllerian anomalies, renal agenesis or ectopy, and cervicothoracic somite dysplasia.

> **Unilateral renal agenesis is associated with genital anomalies in both girls and boys. These genital anomalies may be clinically silent and difficult to detect until puberty.**

In some cases, kidneys visualized with prenatal US are absent at birth. Kidneys with multicystic dysplasia may involute so completely that the renal vasculature is no longer detectable, even at surgery. The dual pathway to unilateral renal agenesis may explain why some children have associated anomalies (those with true renal agenesis, a severe intrauterine insult) and others do not (those with involution of a multicystic dysplastic kidney, a more limited process). The dual pathway may also explain why about 80% of children with unilateral renal

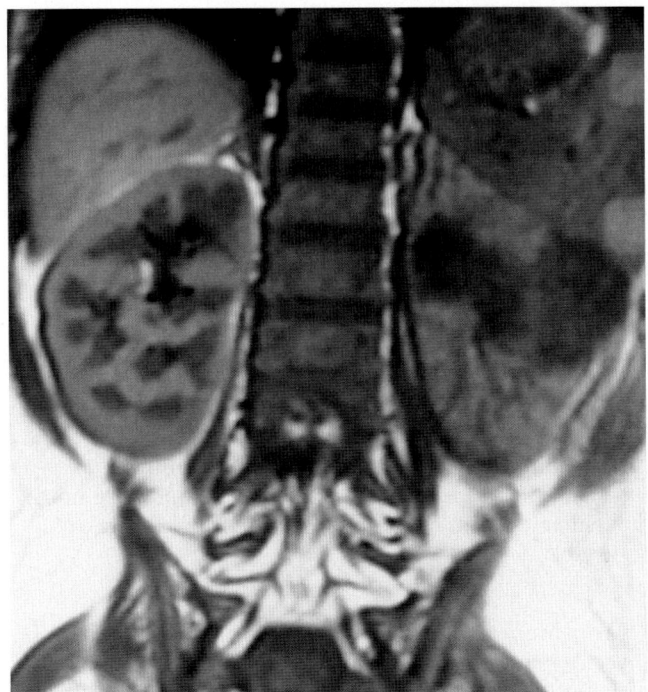

FIGURE 145-32. Solitary kidney with aberrant bowel simulating multicystic dysplastic kidney. Coronal T1-weighted MR image shows a normal right kidney. The mesentery and bowel loops in the left renal fossa could be mistaken for a multicystic dysplastic kidney. (Courtesy of Joan A. Zawin, MD.)

TABLE 145-1
Genital Anomalies Associated with Unilateral Renal Agenesis

FEMALE
Absence or hypoplasia of vagina
Absence of uterus
Failure of fusion of midline structures (müllerian derivatives)
  Bicornuate uterus, duplicated uterus
  Obstructed hemivagina and hemiuterus and hydrocolpos, hematocolpos, hematosalpinx
Gartner duct cyst (can present per vagina)
Ipsilateral absence of uterine horn and fallopian tube (unicornuate uterus)

MALE
Ipsilateral anomalies
  Absence of epididymis
  Absence of seminal vesicle
  Absence of vas deferens
  Absence or hypoplasia of testis
  Seminal vesicle cyst

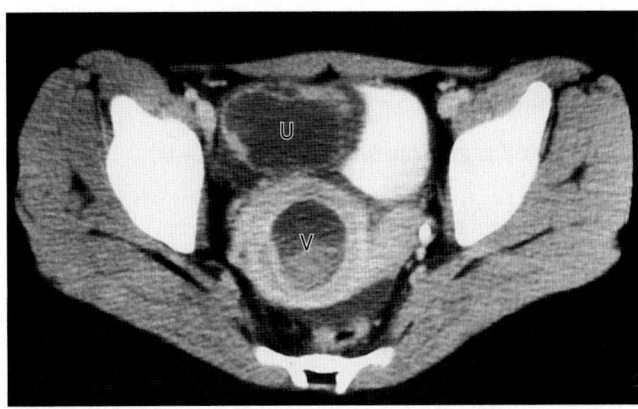

FIGURE 145-33. Mayer-Rokitansky-Küster-Hauser syndrome. Contrast-enhanced CT shows that the obstructed right hemivagina (V) is filled with menstrual debris, as is the right hemiuterus (U) above. On higher sections, the dilated fluid-filled fallopian tube could be identified. The nonobstructed system is seen to the left of the dilated vagina.

agenesis lack the ipsilateral ureter and hemitrigone of the bladder (true agenesis) and 20% have a normally developed bladder and a distal ureter of varying length (involution of multicystic dysplastic kidney). In children, cystic dysplasia of the testis is associated with only two lesions of the genitourinary tract: multicystic dysplastic kidney and unilateral renal agenesis. This may be another indication that the two processes are linked.

The plain film finding of an abnormally positioned splenic or hepatic flexure (bowel falling toward the empty fossa) is inconstant and dependent on the amount of gas in the colon and the position of the child when the film is obtained. During a contrast enema, the direction of contrast flow is reversed in the region of the splenic flexure. Neither conventional radiographs nor contrast enemas are used for the diagnosis of unilateral renal agenesis. Instead, methods that directly image the renal fossa and the remainder of the abdomen are used.

US of the affected renal fossa demonstrates the absence of the kidney and the presence of an abnormally configured adrenal gland. Renal ectopia should be excluded. Other imaging studies (nuclear studies, CT) may be necessary to differentiate a very small and poorly functioning kidney from an absent one. The contralateral kidney should be measured, because compensatory hypertrophy may be present, even in a neonate. The associated uterine and vaginal anomalies may be difficult to detect in early childhood, before these structures reach adult size. CT and MRI have been used to evaluate the associated genital anomalies (see Fig. 145-33).

Because of the increased incidence of vesicoureteral reflux into a solitary kidney and the need to protect its

parenchyma, a study to exclude reflux is recommended early in the child's life.

Congenital Renal Hypoplasia

OLIGOMEGANEPHRONIA (OLIGOMEGANEPHRONIC RENAL HYPOPLASIA)

Although a uniformly small kidney may be due to an embryologic aberration, such a kidney is rarely detected on prenatal US. It may develop when, after pre- or postnatal renal vein thrombosis, the kidney shrinks yet retains its normal morphology and some function.

Rarely, bilaterally small kidneys are noted in a child with anomalies of the central nervous system, usually microcephaly associated with some degree of mental retardation. Specific abnormalities of chromosome 4 have been noted in many of these patients. Pathologically, the small kidneys have fewer nephrons than normal, but those nephrons are much larger than normal. Oligo-meganephronia has also been diagnosed in children with a small solitary kidney or a kidney with a single papilla, again giving weight to the theory that either an embryologic insult affected the quantity of the meta-nephric blastema or the originally normal metanephric blastema did not grow and differentiate normally.

HYPOPLASIA AND DYSPLASIA WITH ECTOPIC URETERAL INSERTION

Another form of hypoplastic kidney is associated with ectopic insertion of the ureter. An abnormal origin of the ureteral bud from the wolffian duct produces an abnormal relationship between the ureter and the metanephric blastema. The ureter does not reach the greatest concentration of blastema, and the kidney is thus both hypoplastic and dysplastic. This process is much more frequent in girls than in boys, and the ectopic insertion, most commonly in the vagina, is asso-ciated with low-volume (droplet) primary incontinence. The extremely small, poorly functioning kidney may be impossible to detect with IVU or US. Nuclear scintig-raphy, contrast-enhanced CT, and magnetic resonance (MR) urography are useful when this diagnosis is being considered. Animal experiments indicate that there may be a genetic component to the anomalous origin of the ureteral bud; the presence or absence of certain proteins has been shown to affect ureteral bud location on the wolffian duct.

ASK-UPMARK KIDNEY (SEGMENTAL RENAL HYPOPLASIA)

Although segmental renal hypoplasia was initially thought to be a congenital lesion, the pattern of scarring and the pathologic changes indicate that it is likely an acquired phenomenon. More common in females, the scarring is often detected during an evaluation for hypertension. The typical thinning of the parenchyma over a clubbed calyx suggests that renal infection (pyelonephritis) with secondary scarring may cause the segmental change.

Multicystic Dysplastic Kidney

This form of cystic renal disease is often confused with the autosomal forms of renal cystic disease. It usually occurs sporadically, but in some families there appears to be autosomal linkage. Also, in contrast to the autosomal forms of renal cystic disease, this renal dysplasia is due to or associated with ureteral atresia, distal ureteral obstruction (simple ureterocele), or ectopic ureteral insertion. This condition is most often diagnosed prenatally or in the neonatal period (see Chapter 19).

> **Multicystic dysplastic kidney is a nonheritable disorder associated with obstruction of urinary drainage on the affected side. In contrast, autosomal recessive and autosomal dominant polycystic kidney disease are inherited and are not associated with obstruction of the renal pelvis or ureter.**

The numerous cysts are of varying size and may be several centimeters in diameter; they are randomly distributed within the kidney and do not communicate (Fig. 145-34). No normal parenchyma or central renal pelvis is discerned. The multicystic dysplastic kidney may also consist of only a few large cysts (see Fig. 145-34). A hydronephrotic variant of multicystic dysplastic kidney may simulate the much more common true hydroneph-rosis; it has a centrally located cyst that simulates a dilated renal pelvis, and the other cysts are of similar size and are arrayed around it. Nuclear imaging can be used to differentiate the hydronephrotic variant from a treatable obstruction; there is virtually no function in the kidney with multicystic dysplasia (Fig. 145-35). Renal scintigraphy also allows an evaluation of the contralateral kidney, which has an increased incidence of obstruction. Because reflux into the contralateral kidney (the only functioning kidney) occurs in about 25% of children,

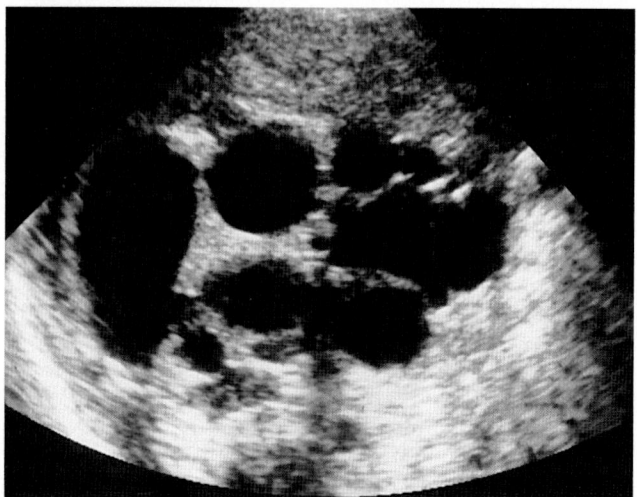
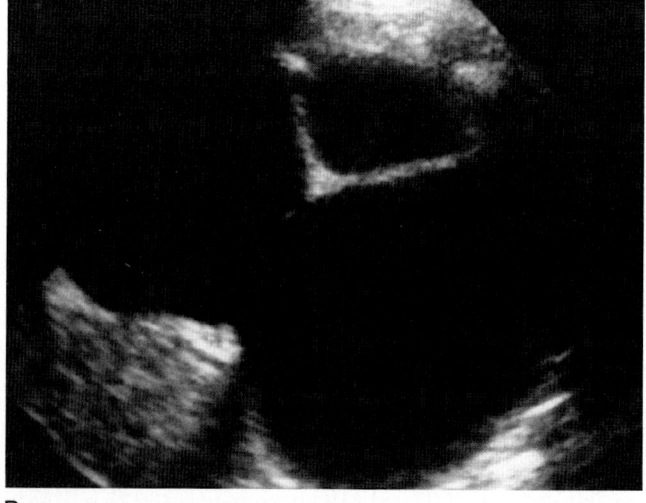

A   B

FIGURE 145-34. Multicystic dysplastic kidney. **A,** Coronal sonogram shows multiple noncommunicating cysts of varied size. No normal renal parenchyma can be identified. **B,** This multicystic dysplastic kidney is composed of a few very large cysts. At times, this appearance can mimic a hydronephrotic kidney.

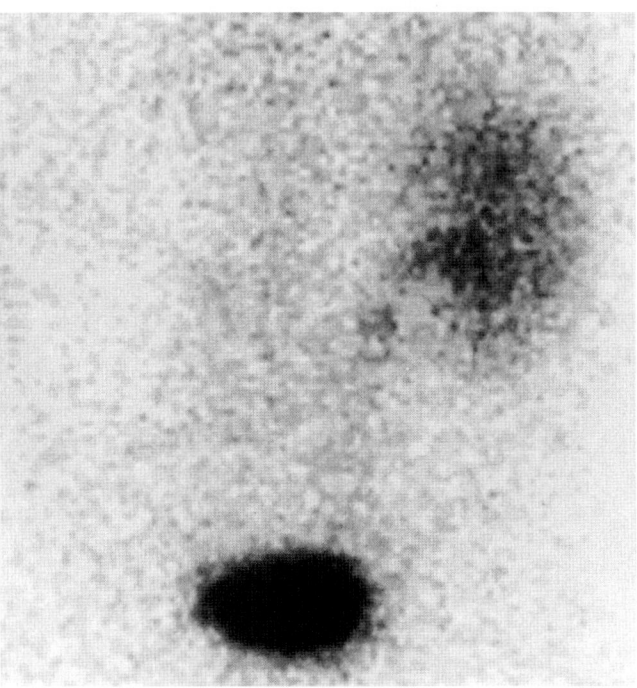

FIGURE 145-35. Renal scintigraphy of multicystic dysplastic kidney. The isotope defines the single functioning kidney. No isotope is present in the contralateral multicystic dysplastic kidney.

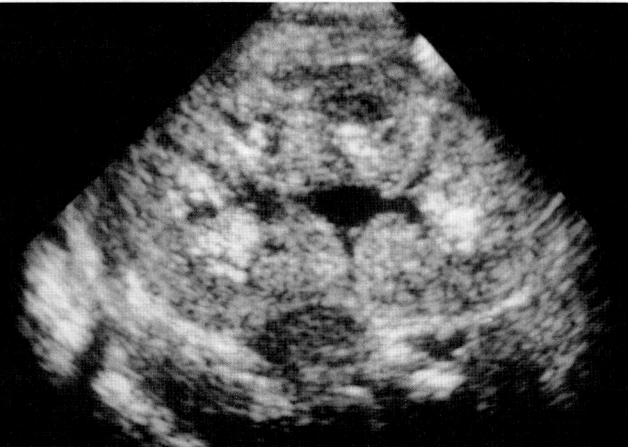

FIGURE 145-36. Autosomal recessive polycystic kidney disease. Coronal sonogram shows dilated tubules in the medulla producing numerous interfaces and, hence, the increased echogenicity of the medulla. The normal cortex, frequently seen as a lucent rim, cannot be identified in this patient.

cystography is still recommended. A few centers are beginning to question the need for these studies, however, because in about half of these children, the reflux is grade I or II; such reflux is typically outgrown without specific intervention.

At one time, the multicystic dysplastic kidney was always removed. This practice is no longer universal. The increased incidence of nephrogenic rests in the multicystic dysplastic kidney is not associated with an increased incidence of renal tumors, as was once believed.

Cystic Renal Disease

AUTOSOMAL RECESSIVE POLYCYSTIC KIDNEY DISEASE

This rare disorder (1 in 20,000 live births) affects both the kidneys and the liver with ectasia and fibrosis. In the kidneys, the ectasia involves primarily the collecting tubules; in the liver, the biliary ducts are similarly affected. Liver fibrosis is not present at birth; it develops later and may become clinically significant by the end of the first decade. The degree of fibrosis and ectasia is not parallel in the same organ, and the degree of involvement in the liver and the kidneys tends to be inversely proportional. A small number of children with autosomal recessive polycystic kidney disease (ARPKD) also have Caroli disease, or cystic dilation of the intrahepatic biliary ducts. (For information on the severe form of ARPKD, see Chapter 112.) Prenatal diagnosis can be made with US or MRI, but prenatal chromosomal analysis can provide the diagnosis even earlier than imaging studies.

In the affected neonate, the kidneys tend to be large, measuring up to 10 cm. The dilated collecting tubules create intense echogenicity within the medulla (Fig. 145-36). Because the cortex is spared, it may appear relatively hypoechoic, creating an echolucent rim at the periphery of the kidney; this is an inconstant finding, however. Occasionally, the increased medullary echogenicity defines the triangular pyramids and simulates the nephrocalcinosis of renal tubular acidosis. A "cyst" may be a true cyst or a trapped calyx. High-frequency US transducers may allow direct visualization of the dilated tubules arranged in a fanlike configuration, reminiscent of the spoke-wheel pattern noted on IVU or contrast-enhanced CT as a result of contrast pooling in the tubules (Fig. 145-37). Imaging other than US is seldom necessary. When studied with MR urography, the dilated tubules in affected kidneys demonstrate hyperintense, linear, radial patterns in the medulla, extending to the cortex. MR urography has also shown a few small cortical cysts in about half the children studied thus far.

Not all children with ARPKD present and die in infancy. In those with initially adequate (though not normal) renal function, their disease may not be detected until later in the first decade, when US is being done for nonrelated purposes; they may have little clinical renal or liver disease attributable to ARPKD at that time. Some children (20% to 45%) present in the second decade with renal failure and require dialysis or renal transplantation. Late complications include systemic hypertension and those caused by hepatic fibrosis: portal hypertension with subsequent hypersplenism and gastroesophageal varices. Intracranial aneurysms may develop, though much less commonly than in autosomal dominant kidney disease.

AUTOSOMAL DOMINANT POLYCYSTIC KIDNEY DISEASE

This common form of polycystic kidney disease (1 per 1000 live births) affects the liver and pancreas as well as the kidneys. There are two forms of autosomal dominant polycystic kidney disease (ADPKD), each with a clearly defined chromosomal mutation. The milder phenotype (PKD2) presents later, has less morbidity, and is less

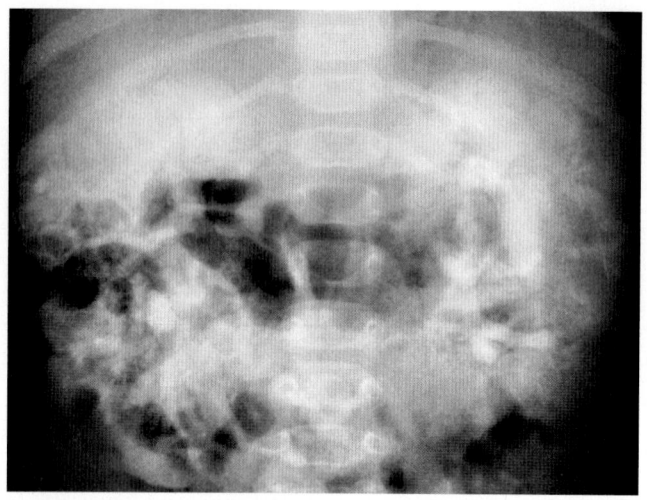

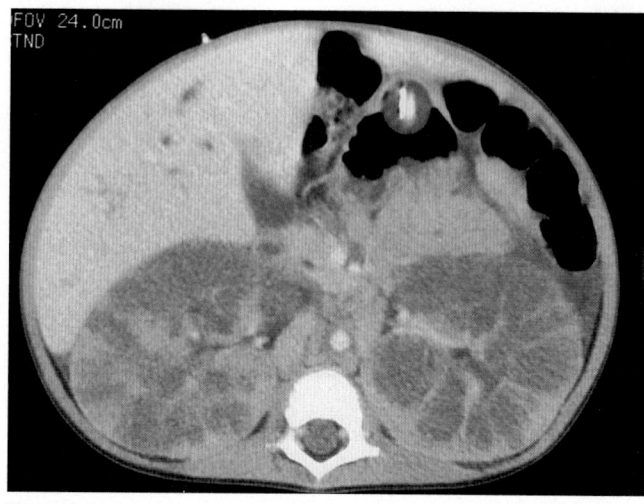

A   B

FIGURE 145-37. Autosomal recessive polycystic kidney disease. **A,** IVU shows that contrast trapped within the dilated collecting tubules gives a streaky or spoke-wheel appearance to the renal parenchyma. **B,** Noncontrast CT shows that the pathologic process is medullary. The dilated tubules have produced a linear pattern that can be clearly seen in a few regions. Cortical thinning, present along the anterior aspect of each kidney, is not a typical finding, because the cortex is usually spared.

frequent than the more severe form (PKD1), which accounts for about 85% of patients. A third form, PKD3, has been postulated; it has some clinical variation from the other two forms, it is less common, and its chromosomal mutation has not been fully localized.

Spontaneous mutations are responsible for about 10% of cases of ADPKD; thus, screening of parents and siblings of affected children, though routine, may not be positive. Screening can be done with US in adults, in whom the disease is generally more advanced. In very young children, however, screening with US may be inconclusive, because detectable cysts may not be present in the first or second decade. CT can demonstrate millimeter-size cysts but is not commonly used for screening. Affected kidneys are large, contain multiple cysts, and retain a normal renal shape. The kidneys may be asymmetrically involved and can show segmental variation within a single kidney.

Symptoms of ADPKD rarely develop in childhood; renal and liver cysts become larger and more numerous with increasing age, and patients usually present with renal failure or hypertension in the fourth or fifth decade. An association with seminal vesicle cysts has been noted. Affected adults have an increased incidence of uric acid stones.

ADPKD may be detected in a totally asymptomatic child when a urinary tract evaluation is performed for unrelated symptoms (Fig. 145-38). Occasionally, a child presents with a unilaterally enlarged kidney and hematuria. In this setting, US or CT is performed because of the presumption of neoplasm. Imaging may show conglomerate cysts, often appearing as a multicystic mass, and numerous other cysts (measuring only 1 or 2 mm) scattered through the cortex of both kidneys. If there has been bleeding into one of the cysts, causing its rapid enlargement, the child may present with flank pain. This cyst may have an atypical appearance on US or CT, making the differential diagnosis more difficult and raising the possibility of cystic neoplasm unless addi-

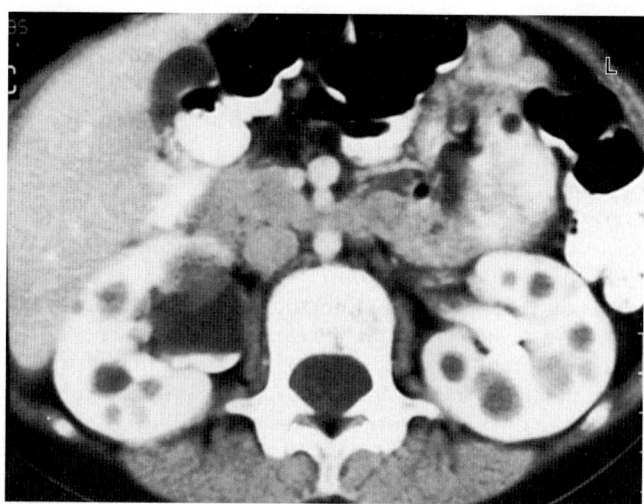

FIGURE 145-38. Autosomal dominant polycystic kidney disease (positive family history) in a 10-year-old girl. Contrast-enhanced CT shows multiple cysts throughout both kidneys. Note also the dilated right renal pelvis with a urine-contrast level due to ureteropelvic function obstruction.

tional distant cysts are identified. The cysts that affect other organs are usually absent or asymptomatic in childhood.

About 15% of patients with ADPKD have an aneurysm of the circle of Willis. Because the consequences of aneurysm rupture are so profound, screening with MR angiography is recommended in patients with ADPKD. This is usually not performed in childhood, however, because aneurysm rupture is rare in this period. The incidence of aneurysms increases with age, giving later screening studies a higher yield.

SIMPLE RENAL CYSTS

Although renal cysts are a common consequence of aging and are present in about 50% of the population

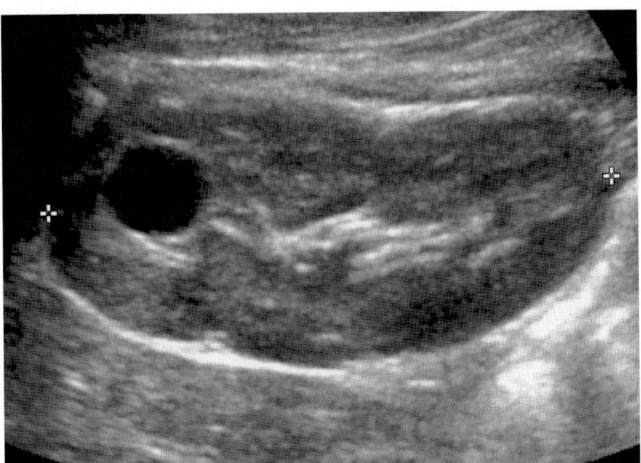

FIGURE 145-39. Simple renal cyst. Longitudinal sonogram shows a small fluid collection in the right upper pole, typical of a simple cyst: thin wall, no internal septations, and good through-transmission.

older than 50 years, they are uncommon in the pediatric population. In the past, when kidneys were evaluated primarily with IVU, renal cysts were rarely diagnosed in children. With wider use of US, simple renal cysts have become a recognized entity in the pediatric population and have even been observed on prenatal US. Most fetal renal cysts resolve, but their detection warrants additional or sequential studies to exclude cyst-associated syndromes or multicystic dysplastic kidney. Although most simple cysts are idiopathic, they can occur in

children with acquired immunodeficiency syndrome (AIDS).

If the cyst meets the ultrasound criteria of a simple cyst, no further imaging is necessary. These criteria are the same in children and adults: a thin, almost imperceptible wall; no internal echogenicity; a spherical shape; and good through-transmission (Fig. 145-39). When these criteria are not met, CT is recommended to exclude cystic Wilms tumor or cystic nephroma. Again, to be confident of the diagnosis, the CT criteria for a simple cyst must be met: density less than 15 Hounsfield units on non-contrast-enhanced CT, imperceptible wall, and no internal architecture. When more than one cyst is observed with US, CT may be necessary to exclude ADPKD. If the cyst is detected during an evaluation for urinary tract infections, and these infections continue, a contrast study may be necessary to exclude a calyceal diverticulum. This can simulate a simple cyst on US, and stasis within it can result in infection. A calyceal diverticulum fills with contrast on delayed imaging during IVU or contrast-enhanced CT. Multiple cysts may not be cysts at all but enlarged calyces in patients with infundibulopelvic stenosis (Fig. 145-40).

Most simple cysts are asymptomatic and managed conservatively. Intervention is warranted if the cyst is large and positioned such that it may contribute to pathologic fracture of the kidney or if the cyst is causing obstruction of the collecting system.

ACQUIRED RENAL CYSTS

As mentioned earlier, children with AIDS may develop renal cysts. Cysts also develop in children (and adults)

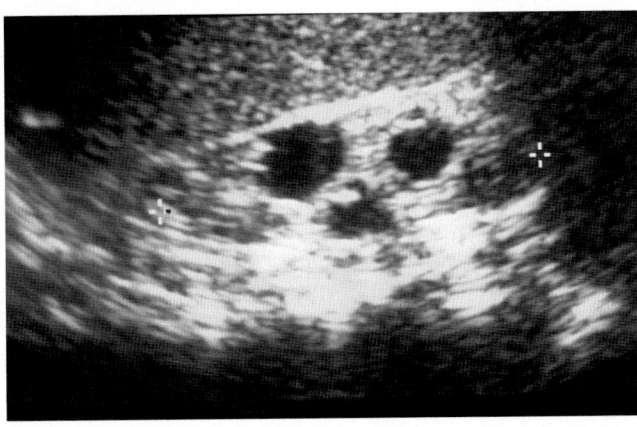

A

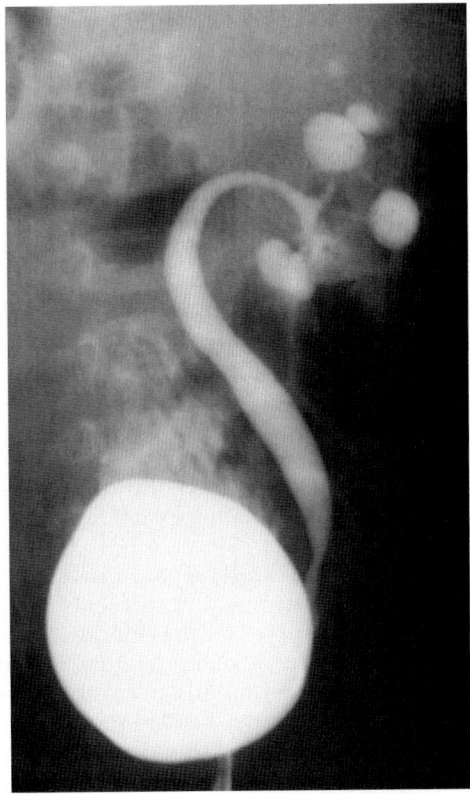

B

FIGURE 145-40. Infundibulopelvic stenosis simulating cystic kidney disease. **A,** Longitudinal sonogram shows multiple "cysts" scattered throughout the kidney in this child with the VACTERL association. **B,** Voiding cystourethrogram shows vesicoureteral reflux into the abnormal pelvocalyceal system. The ureter has a greater caliber than the renal pelvis, infundibula, and calyces. The most peripheral portion of each calyx is rounded, producing the cystic spaces seen with US.

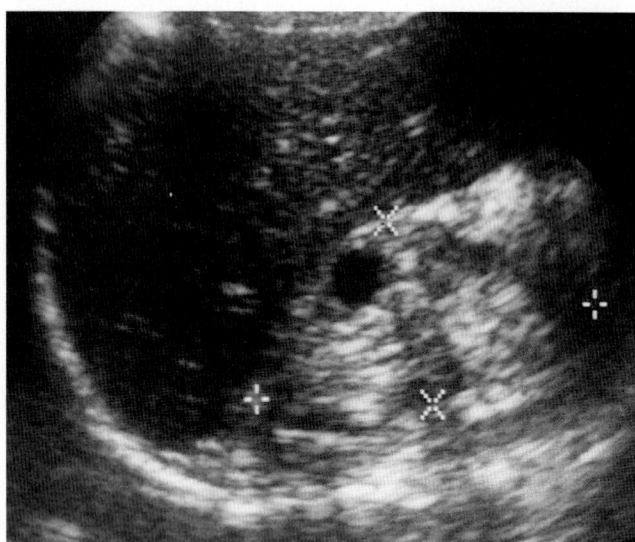

FIGURE 145-41. Acquired renal cyst in a child on dialysis. Longitudinal sonogram shows the increased echogenicity of the kidney, which is small for the child's age. A single cyst is present.

with renal failure who receive hemodialysis or peritoneal dialysis. The longer a patient is on dialysis, the greater the number of cysts. With US, the involved kidneys are generally smaller and more echogenic than normal; the cysts are scattered throughout the parenchyma and have a typical appearance of simple cysts (Fig. 145-41).

MISCELLANEOUS CYSTIC DISEASES

GLOMERULOCYSTIC DISEASE. This rare condition can be inherited as an autosomal dominant disease and is sometimes detected in children with a family history of ADPKD. The kidneys are usually of normal size but may be enlarged; they have increased echogenicity on US, regardless of size. The pathology involves cystic dilation of Bowman capsule and the proximal convoluted tubules. Children with glomerulocystic disease and small kidneys are believed to have an even rarer variant with sporadic inheritance. Glomerulocystic disease is sometimes identified in children with malformation syndromes (discussed later).

As noted, the size of the kidney is not helpful in making the diagnosis, because although most affected kidneys are normal sized, glomerulocystic disease occurs in small and large kidneys as well. Besides being increased, the echogenicity may have a specific pattern. Tiny cysts, smaller than those typical of ADPKD, have been described in the cortex. In contrast to ARPKD, the medulla has a normal appearance on US.

MICROCYSTIC RENAL DISEASE. This rare disease, inherited in an autosomal recessive pattern, presents in early life with nephrotic syndrome of the Finnish type. That is, infants have massive proteinuria that is not easily managed clinically. Renal failure, in those who survive, occurs as early as age 5 years. The kidneys are of normal size and have dilation of the proximal convoluted tubules. Initially thought to have no radiographic changes, infantile microcystic renal disease does have abnormalities on

US: small cortical cysts and increased echogenicity of the kidney, with loss of the corticomedullary junction.

JUVENILE NEPHRONOPHTHISIS AND MEDULLARY CYSTIC DISEASE. These diseases are frequently linked because of the similarities in pathology. The kidney is studded with small (<1 cm) cysts that increase in size and number over time. Because these cysts develop from dilated tubules, they occur at the corticomedullary junction. Glomerulosclerosis is also present in both diseases. The clinical symptoms—polydipsia, polyuria, and later renal failure —are noted in the first decade in those with juvenile nephronophthisis (autosomal dominant transmission) and in the third decade or beyond in those with medullary cystic disease (autosomal recessive transmission).

MEDULLARY SPONGE KIDNEY (CACCHI-RICCI DISEASE). Medullary sponge kidney is more frequently diagnosed in adults than children and is generally considered a noninherited disorder. Most often it is an incidental finding, but it may be associated with stone formation, hematuria, and urinary tract infection. It has also been described in children with the Beckwith-Wiedemann syndrome. The radiographic changes are due to the focal dilation of the collecting tubules. The number of renal pyramids involved is variable.

Plain abdominal radiographs may demonstrate multiple tiny calculi in the medulla, especially in older patients. If intravenous contrast is given, streaky linear densities (pooled contrast) develop in the affected papillae. The papillary blush noted in children receiving a bolus injection of contrast agent can simulate this process; close observation reveals that opacified tubules are normal and not dilated. US can demonstrate calcifications in the tubules before they are visible on abdominal radiographs and may also visualize the dilated tubules.

MALFORMATION SYNDROMES WITH RENAL CYSTS

Renal cysts are reported in many syndromes. In some, they are a constant and defining feature; in others, they may be present in only a percentage of patients with the syndrome. The presence of cysts is an integral part of the definition of Zellweger syndrome (cerebrohepatorenal syndrome) and Meckel syndrome. Cystic renal disease has also been reported in the following syndromes: Alagille; Bardet-Biedl; Cumming; orofaciodigital types I, II, and VI; and Joubert (especially in those with retinal dystrophy). More than 80 syndromes are associated with some form of cystic renal disease.

The most commonly recognized syndrome with renal cysts is tuberous sclerosis, an autosomal dominantly inherited phakomatosis. Like other phakomatoses, it is associated with pathology in many organ systems. Skin lesions are multiple: facial angiofibromas (incorrectly called adenoma sebaceum in the past), a depigmented area ("ash leaf") on the trunk, and a pigmented area of thickened skin in the sacral region (shagreen patch). Rhabdomyomas develop in many organs, including the heart. Characteristic brain anomalies include subependymal hamartomas, anomalies of the corpus callosum, and occasional development of subependymal giant cell astrocytoma. Clinically, the child may have seizures and mental retardation. Two different processes may develop in the kidney. The first, angiomyolipoma, is a benign neoplasm seldom seen in childhood that may grow throughout life. The second process, the development of multiple simple cortical cysts, is more common and may be present in as many as one third of children with tuberous sclerosis. Angiofibromas and renal cysts coexist in about 25% of tuberous sclerosis patients. The radiographic appearance of the affected kidneys is generally similar to that of ADPKD. Interestingly, the loci of the major genes for tuberous sclerosis and ADPKD are close to each other on chromosome 16.

Children with Beckwith-Wiedemann syndrome are usually identified at birth because of macroglossia, macrosomia, visceromegaly, and omphalocele. The increased incidence of nephrogenic rests and Wilms tumors in these children is well recognized and has resulted in surveillance radiographic studies of the kidneys. Review of these studies indicates that many other renal malformations are present in this population. Medullary renal cysts may be noted in 13% to 19%. Other processes (nephrocalcinosis, nephrolithiasis, hydronephrosis) have also been described in children with Beckwith-Wiedemann syndrome. Other syndromes associated with an increased incidence of Wilms tumor, such as Denys-Drash and WAGR (Wilms tumor, aniridia, genitourinary abnormalities or gonadoblastoma, and mental retardation) syndromes, also demonstrate changes of renal dysplasia.

Anomalies of the Pelvocalyceal System

CALYCEAL DIVERTICULUM

This focal outpouching of the calyceal system, usually in the upper pole, is believed to be developmental in origin. It is present in both pediatric and adult imaging studies with about the same frequency of 4.5 per 1000. Although it is often an incidental finding, calyceal diverticulum can be associated with stasis and, secondarily, with both infection and focal stone formation.

The calyceal diverticulum may be seen with US, appearing as a rounded fluid collection, simulating a solitary renal cyst (Fig. 145-42). The size varies from a few millimeters to several centimeters and may increase over time. On IVU and CT, the calyceal diverticulum does not fill during the early parenchymal phase, again resembling a renal cyst; however, delayed images demonstrate its thin connection to the adjacent fornix of a minor calyx when contrast fills the diverticulum (see Fig. 145-42).

When a calyceal diverticulum causes a clinical problem, it must be ablated, usually surgically. In adults, both lithotripsy of stones within the diverticulum and percutaneous ablation of the cavity have decreased the invasiveness of the treatment; these techniques have not yet been widely applied to children.

INFUNDIBULOPELVIC STENOSIS

This anomaly is thought to be very rare but may be underreported. The kidney has a specific appearance on contrast studies: the renal pelvis and infundibula are narrowed but not entirely obliterated, and the calyces become rounded (see Fig. 145-40). Despite the cystlike appearance of the calyces on contrast studies, renal sonography may be normal. The function of the kidney may be normal or severely compromised.

CONGENITAL MEGACALYCES (MEGACALYCOSIS)

This rare anomaly is associated with abnormal development of the renal medulla that causes all the calyces to be filled maximally. The ensuing stasis may produce infection and stones (Fig. 145-43). Surgery is rarely indicated, except for the removal of stones if they are serving as a nidus of secondary infection. Megacalyces can be focal, unilateral, or bilateral. Occasionally they are associated with primary megaureter. Boys are more commonly affected than girls.

Imaging findings are multiple: nephromegaly, thinning of the cortex at the expense of the medulla, visualization of a large number of calyces, calyces that are polygonal and fit close together like a mosaic, shortening of the infundibula, and mild dilation of the renal pelvis despite the absence of UPJ obstruction (see Fig. 145-43). Twenty or more calyces may be seen in each kidney. Most changes can be demonstrated with US, IVU, CT, or MRI. Nuclear diuretic renography may be useful to exclude mild, intermittent but significant obstruction as a cause of the dilated pelvocalyceal system.

URETEROPELVIC JUNCTION OBSTRUCTION

UPJ obstruction occurs in about 3 in 1000 live births, more often in boys than in girls. It is more common on the left than the right, is bilateral in 10% to 20% of cases, and is seen in association with inferior ectopia and lower pole duplication, both incomplete and complete. Like adults, older children who first present with UPJ obstruction are likely to have extrinsic compression from crossing vessels.

UPJ obstruction is frequently suggested by prenatal US showing hydronephrosis (see Chapter 12). Postnatal US is usually performed after a 3- to 5-day wait, but earlier imaging may detect those with significant obstruction (see Chapter 19). Most centers evaluate postnatal hydronephrosis using the grading system of the Society of Fetal Urology, because this has prognostic significance. Long-term follow-up of children with prenatally diagnosed hydronephrosis indicates that about 50% undergo surgical correction of the obstruction. Those with higher grades of hydronephrosis are more likely to undergo surgery. However, recent experience suggests that surgical correction may not be necessary as often as was previously believed.

When UPJ obstruction is not detected prenatally, the child usually presents with a palpable abdominal mass. In fact, UPJ obstruction is the most frequent cause of neonatal abdominal mass. Plain abdominal radiographs show soft tissue fullness, bulging of the ipsilateral flank, and displacement of bowel loops from the affected side. IVU is no longer performed for diagnosis, but the obstructed kidney has delayed opacification and delayed excretion of contrast material. Contrast pools in the obstructed tubules adjacent to the dilated calyces, producing calyceal crescents (Fig. 145-44). Delayed films help visualize the renal pelvis (see Fig. 145-44); prone

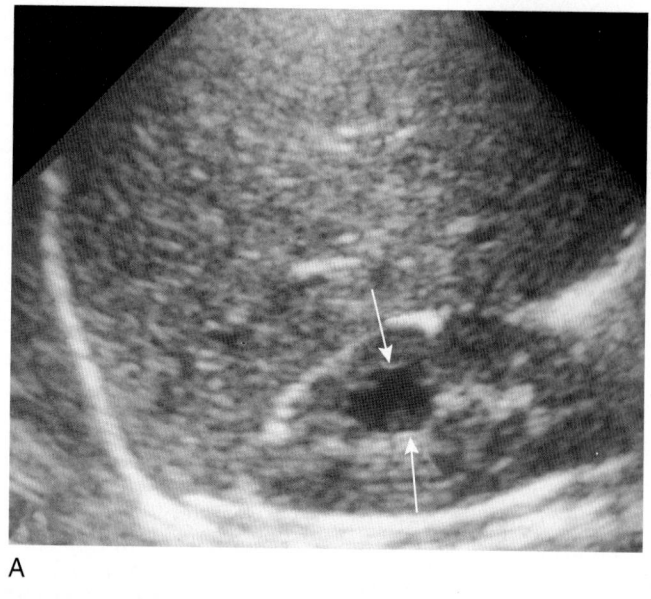

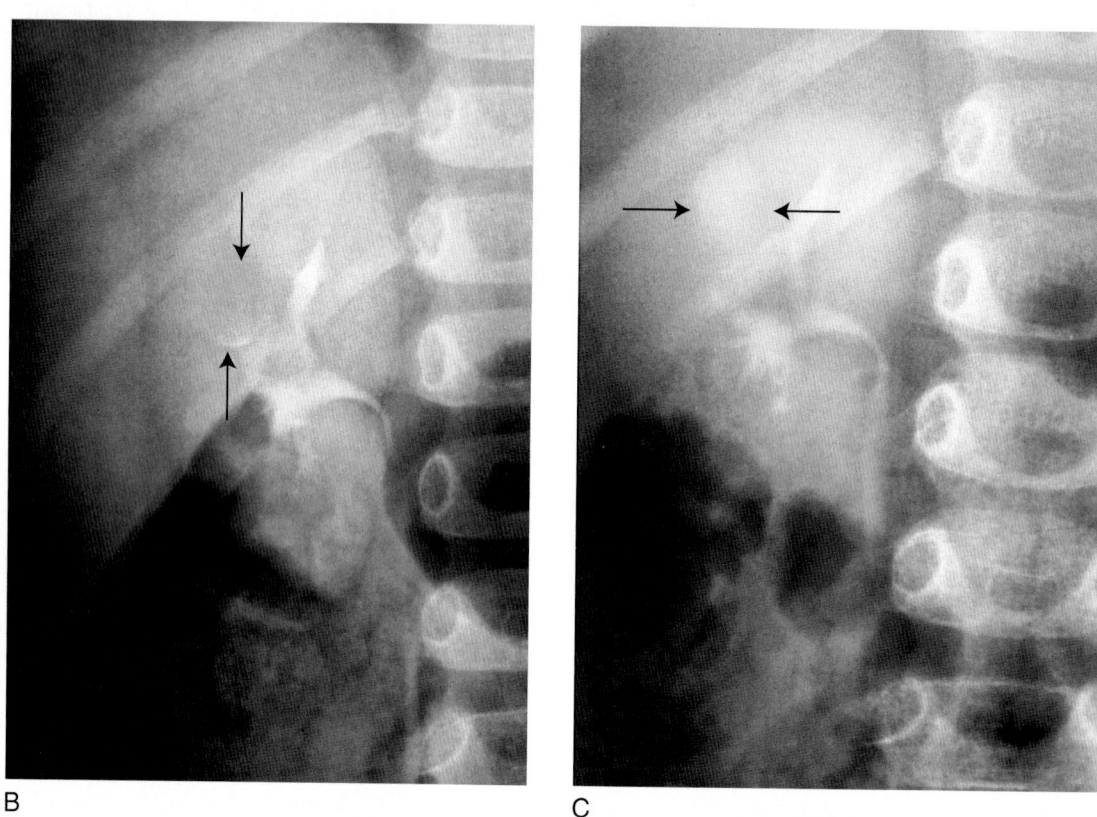

FIGURE 145-42. Calyceal diverticulum. **A,** Longitudinal sonogram reveals a medullary cyst *(arrows)*. **B,** IVU, early image. As the parenchyma opacifies, a nonenhancing region is noted adjacent to the calyces *(arrows)*. A tiny amount of contrast material has entered the diverticulum, creating a semilunar density along its inferior aspect. **C,** IVU, late image from another patient. Contrast material is seen in the calyceal system and has filled and opacified a large diverticulum *(arrows)*.

films are useful because, with the child in this position, contrast material moves from the calyces to the anteriorly located renal pelvis. Prone positioning also promotes filling of the ureter, allowing differentiation between UPJ obstruction and ureterovesical junction obstruction. Similar changes may be noted on contrast-enhanced CT. Preoperative retrograde ureterography is not routinely performed, because newer imaging

techniques are sufficient to make the diagnosis; however, it may be helpful in unusual cases (Fig. 145-45). Diuretic renography is commonly used to evaluate possible UPJ obstruction; both renal function and drainage are evaluated. Diuretic-enhanced US improves detection of the obstructed renal pelvis. MR urography is an increasingly important tool in the diagnosis of UPJ obstruction but is not yet widely used (Fig. 145-46).

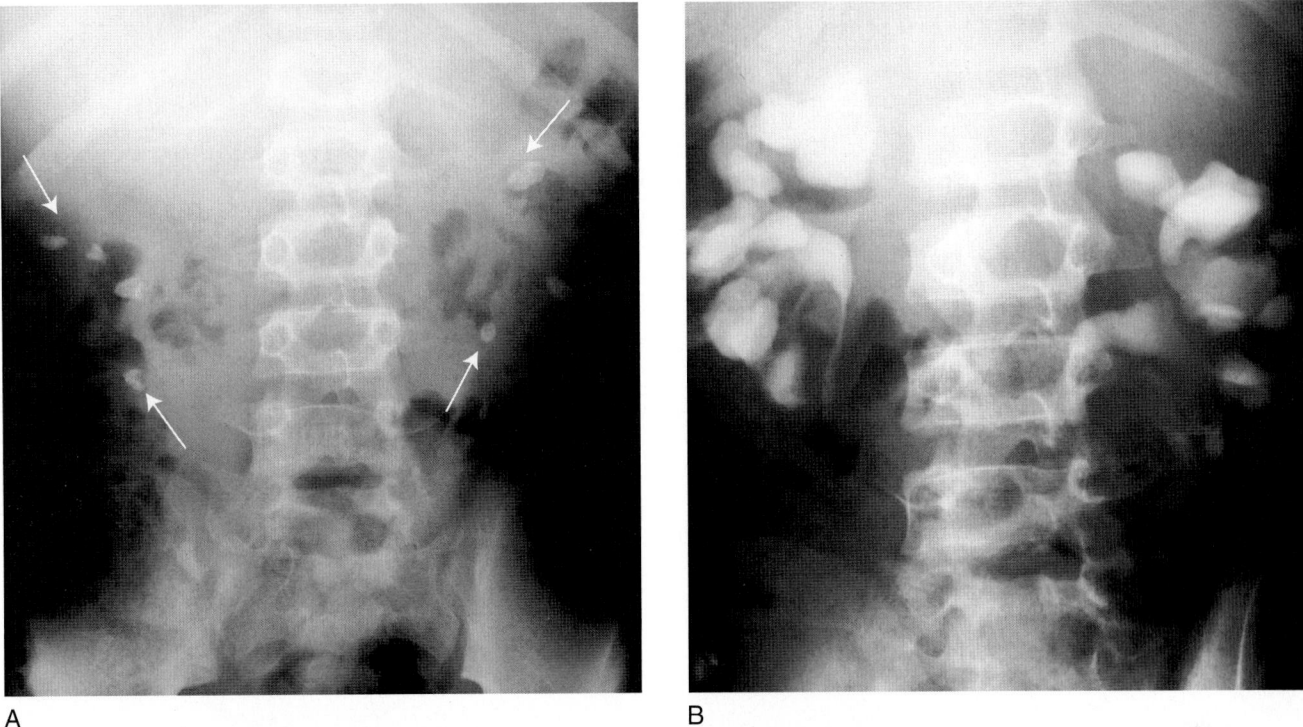

FIGURE 145-43. Congenital megacalyces. **A,** Abdominal radiograph shows multiple calculi present in each kidney *(arrows).* **B,** IVU shows contrast material filling the many polygon-shaped calyces. Note the relative nephromegaly despite the thinning of the tissue over the calyces. The renal pelvis is not dilated.

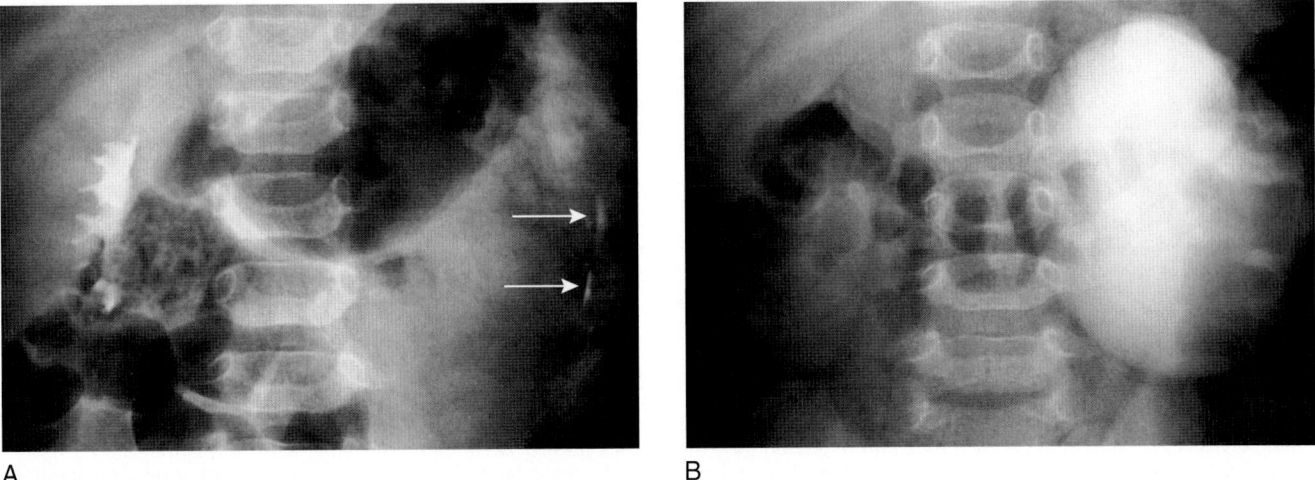

FIGURE 145-44. Ureteropelvic junction obstruction. **A,** On this 10-minute IVU image, the right kidney appears normal, with contrast material in the normal pelvocalyceal system. On the left, a few calyceal crescents are present at a great distance from the spine *(arrows).* **B,** On the 1-hour prone film, the dilated left renal pelvis is seen extending from the spine to the lateral abdominal wall. It is obscuring the calyces.

> **Ureteropelvic junction obstruction is the most common cause of abdominal masses in neonates.**

Postoperative evaluation has changed over the years, with IVU being supplanted by other tests. The dilation of pelvocalyceal system and overlying parenchymal thickness can be assessed with US if a preoperative examination is available for comparison. A good test of differential renal function is the nuclear renogram. This, too, can be compared with preoperative studies. Interestingly, some authors report a definite improvement in function in the majority of their patients, whereas others describe only a stabilization of renal function.

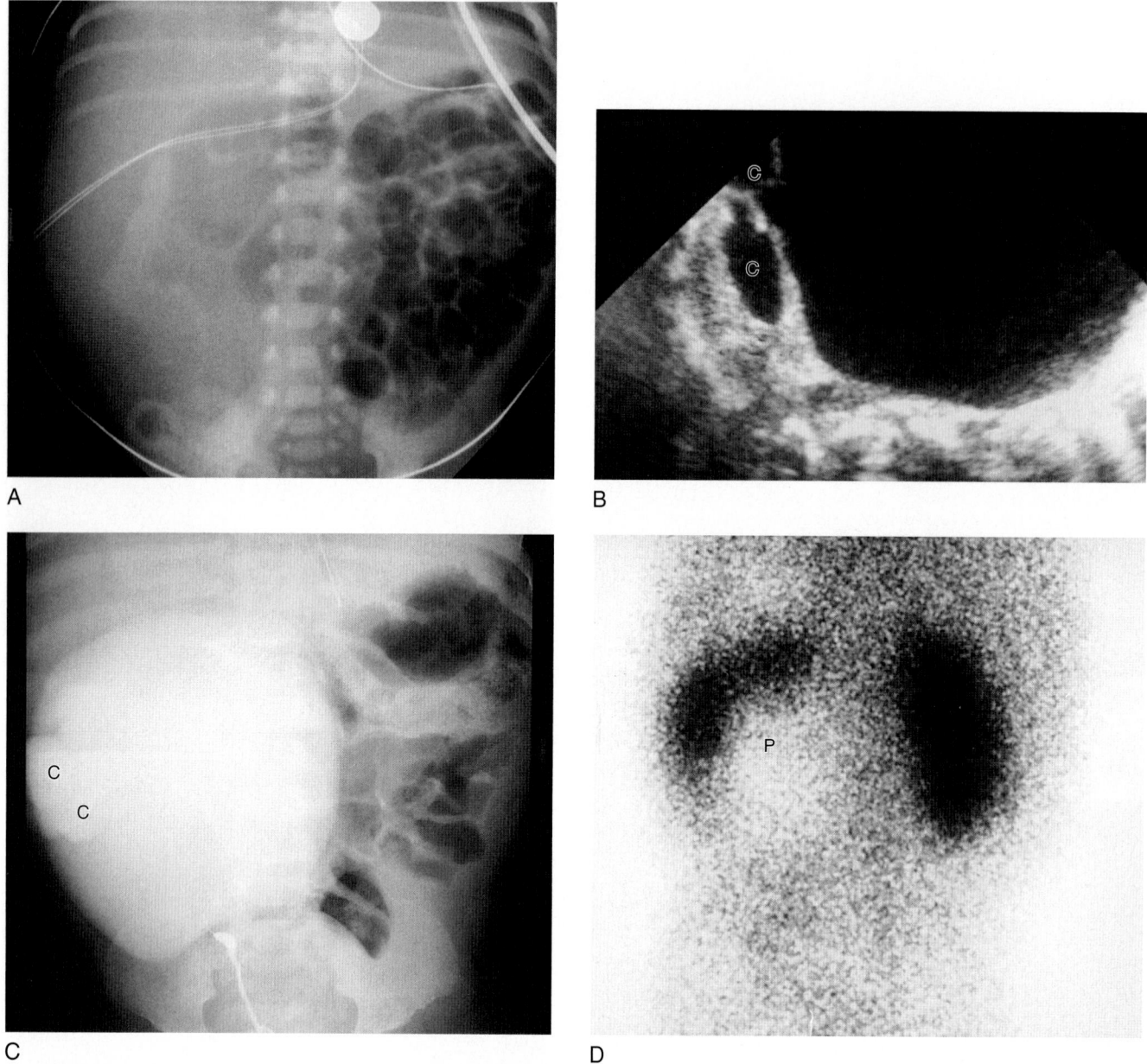

FIGURE 145-45. Ureteropelvic junction obstruction. **A,** Plain radiograph in a newborn (note the umbilical clamp) shows bowel loops displaced from right to left by a soft tissue mass. **B,** Transverse sonogram shows that the soft tissue mass is a markedly dilated renal pelvis associated with dilated calyces (C). **C,** Ureteral retrograde contrast injection confirms that the obstruction is at the level of the renal pelvis. Again, the renal pelvis is much more dilated than the calyces (C) are. **D,** Renal scintigraphy with technetium-99m mercaptotriglycylglycine shows a normal left kidney. On the right, the thinned renal parenchyma is displaced superiorly and laterally by the dilated renal pelvis, seen as the photopenic region (P).

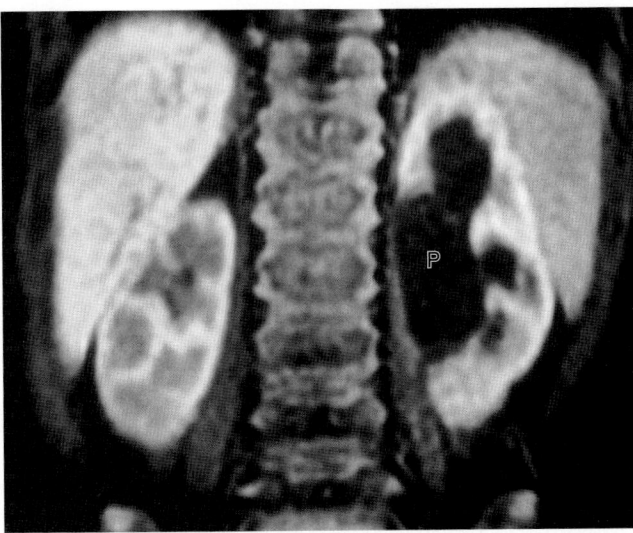

FIGURE 145-46. Ureteropelvic junction obstruction. Coronal contrast-enhanced T1-weighted MR image shows a normal right kidney with a well-defined corticomedullary junction. On the left, the corticomedullary junction is poorly seen. The pelvis (P) and the calyceal system are dilated.

SUGGESTED READINGS

Normal Renal Anatomy and Variants

Auh YH, Rubinstein WA, Markisz JA, et al: Extraperitoneal paravesical spaces: CT delineation with US correlation. Radiology 1986;159:319

Auh YH, Rubinstein WA, Markisz JA, et al: Intraperitoneal paravesical spaces: CT delineation with US correlation. Radiology 1986;159:311

Currarino G, Williams B, Dana K: Kidney length correlated with age: normal values in children. Radiology 1984;150:703

Dodds WJ, Darweesh RM, Lawson TL, et al: The retroperitoneal spaces revisited. AJR Am J Roentgenol 1986;147:1155

Erwin BC, Carroll BA, Muller H: A sonographic assessment of neonatal renal parameters. J Ultrasound Med 1985;4:217

Fernbach SK, Davis TM: The abnormal renal axis in children with spina bifida and gibbus deformity—the pseudohorseshoe kidney. J Urol 1986;136:1258

Gross GW, Boal DK: Sonographic assessment of normal renal size in children with myelodysplasia. J Urol 1988;140:784

Haller JO, Berdon WE, Friedman AP: Increased renal cortical echogenicity: a normal finding in neonates and infants. Radiology 1982;142:173

Han BK, Babcock DS: Sonographic measurements and appearance of normal kidneys in children. AJR Am J Roentgenol 1985;145:611

Hill LM, Nowak A, Hartle R, et al: Fetal compensatory hypertrophy with a unilateral functioning kidney. Ultrasound Obstet Gynecol 2000;15:191

Hoffer FA, Hanabergh AM, Teele RL: The interrenicular junction: a mimic of renal scarring on normal pediatric sonograms. AJR Am J Roentgenol 1985;145:1075

Jequier S, Paltiel H, Lafortune M: Ureterovesical jets in infants and children: duplex and color Doppler US studies. Radiology 1990;175:349

Kaufman RA, Dunbar JS, Gole DE: Normal dilatation of the proximal ureters in children. AJR Am J Roentgenol 1981;137:945

Kenney IJ, Wild SR: Renal parenchymal junctional line in children: ultrasonic frequency and appearance. Br J Radiol 1987;60:865

Lafortune M, Constantin A, Breton G, et al: Sonography of hypertrophied column of Bertin. AJR Am J Roentgenol 1986;146:53

McClennan BL, Lee JKT, Peterson RR: Anatomy of the perirenal area. Radiology 1986;158:555

Rosenbaum DM, Korngold E, Teele R: Sonographic assessment of renal length in normal children. AJR Am J Roentgenol 1984;142:467

Rottenberg GT, De Bruyn R, Gordon I: Sonographic standards for a single functioning kidney in children. AJR Am J Roentgenol 1996;167:1255

Schlesinger AE, Hedlund GL, Pierson WP, et al: Normal standards for kidney length in premature infants: determination with US. Work in progress. Radiology 1987;164:127

Schlesinger AE, Hernandez RJ, Zerin JM, et al: Interobserver and intraobserver variations in sonographic renal length measurements in children. AJR Am J Roentgenol 1991;156:1029

Vade A, Lau P, Smick J, et al: Sonographic renal parameters as related to age. Pediatr Radiol 1987;17:212

Zerin JM, Meyer RD: Sonographic assessment of renal length in the first year of life: the problem of "spurious nephromegaly." Pediatr Radiol 2000;30:52

Renal Ectopia and Anomalies of Fusion

Renal Ectopia

Barnewolt CE, Lebowitz RL: Absence of a renal sinus complex in the ectopic kidney of a child: a normal finding. Pediatr Radiol 1996;26:318

Barwick TD, Malhotra A, Webb JAW, et al: Embryology of the adrenal glands and its relevance to diagnostic imaging. Clin Radiol 1005;60:953

Chow JS, Benson CB, Lebowitz RL: The clinical significance of an empty renal fossa on prenatal sonography. J Ultrasound Med 2005;24:1049

Fernbach SK: Urethral abnormalities in male neonates with VATER association. AJR Am J Roentgenol 1991;156:137

Guarino N, Casamassima MG, Tadini B, et al: Natural history of vesicoureteral reflux associated with kidney anomalies. Urology 2005;65:120

Hertz M, Rubenstein ZJ, Shahin N, et al: Crossed renal ectopia: clinical and radiological findings in 22 cases. Clin Radiol 1977;289:339

Hoffman CK, Filly RA, Callen PW: The "lying down" adrenal sign: a sonographic indicator of renal agenesis or ectopia in fetuses and neonates. J Ultrasound Med 1992;11:533

Jimenez-Hefferman A, Rebollo AC, Garcia-Martin M, et al: Tc-99m DMSA and Tc-99m MAG3 findings in crossed renal ectopia. Clin Nucl Med 1998;239:255

Kenney PJ, Robbins GL, Ellis DA, et al: Adrenal glands in patients with congenital renal anomalies: CT appearance. Radiology 1985;155:181

N'Guessen G, Stephens FD, Pick J: Congenital superior ectopic (thoracic) kidney. Urology 1984;24:219

Nussbaum AR, Hartman DS, Whitley N, et al: Multicystic dysplasia and crossed renal ectopia. AJR Am J Roentgenol 1987;149:407

Yuksel A, Batukan C: Sonographic findings of fetuses with an empty renal fossa and normal amniotic fluid volume. Fetal Diagn Ther 2004;19:525

Horseshoe Kidney

Cascio S, Sweeney B, Granata C, et al: Vesicoreteral reflux and ureteropelvic junction obstruction in children with horseshoe kidney: treatment and outcome. J Urol 2002;167:2566

Fernbach SK, Davis TM: The abnormal renal axis in children with spina bifida and gibbus deformity—the pseudohorseshoe kidney. J Urol 1986;136:1258

Huang EY, Mahour GH: Wilms' tumor and horseshoe kidneys: a case report and review of the literature. J Pediatr Surg 2004;39:207

Mandell GA, Maloney K, Sherman NH, et al: The renal axes in spina bifida: issues of confusion and fusion. Abdom Imaging 1996;21:541

Neville H, Ritchey ML. Shamberger RC, et al: The occurrence of Wilms tumor in horseshoe kidneys: a report from the National Wilms Tumor Study Group (NWTSG). J Pediatr Surg 2002;37:1134

Strauss S, Dushnitsky T, Peer A, et al: Sonographic features of horseshoe kidney: a review of 34 patients. J Ultrasound Med 2000;19:27

Unilateral and Bilateral Renal Agenesis

Cascio S, Paran S, Puri P: Associated urological anomalies in children with unilateral renal agenesis. J Urol 1999;162:1081

Cassart M, Massez A, Metens T, et al: Complementary role of MRI after sonography in assessing bilateral urinary tract anomalies in the fetus. AJR Am J Roentgenol 2004;182:1823

Daneman A, Alton DJ: Radiographic manifestations of renal anomalies. Radiol Clin North Am 1991;29:351

Fedele L, Bianchi S, Agnoli B, et al: Urinary tract anomalies associated with unicornuate uterus. J Urol 1996;155:847

Guarino N, Casamassima MGS, Tadini B, et al: Natural history of vesicoureteral reflux associated with kidney anomalies. Urology 2005;67:1208

McGahan JP, Myracle MR: Adrenal hypertrophy: possible pitfall in the sonographic diagnosis of renal agenesis. J Ultrasound Med 1986;5:265

O'Neill MJ, Yoder IC, Connolly SA, et al: Imaging evaluation and classification of developmental anomalies of the female reproductive system with an emphasis on MR imaging. AJR Am J Roentgenol 1999;173:407

Oppelt P, Renner SP, Kellerman A, et al: Clinical aspects of Mayer-Rokitansky-Küster-Hauser syndrome: recommendations for clinical diagnosis and staging. Hum Reprod 2005;21:792

Palmer LS, Andros GJ, Maizels M, et al: Management considerations for treating vesicoureteral reflux in children with solitary kidneys. Urology 1997;49:604

Schlegel PN, Shin D, Goldstein M: Urogenital anomalies in men with congenital absence of the vas deferens. J Urol 1996;155:1644

Song JT, Ritchey ML, Zerin JM, et al: Incidence of vesicoureteral reflux in children with unilateral renal agenesis. J Urol 1995;153:1249

Tanaka YO, Kurosaki Y, Kobayashi T, et al: Uterus didelphys associated with obstructed hemivagina and ipsilateral renal agenesis: MR findings in seven cases. Abdom Imaging 1998;23:437

Tarry WF, Duckett JW, Stephens FD: The Mayer-Rokitansky syndrome: pathogenesis, classification, and management. J Urol 1986;136:648

Valenzano M, Paoletti R, Rossi A, et al: Sirenomelia: pathological features, antenatal ultrasonographic clues, and a review of current embryogenic theories. Hum Reprod Update 1999;5:82

van den Ouden D, Blom JH, Bangma C, et al: Diagnosis and management of seminal vesicle cysts associated with ipsilateral renal agenesis: a pooled analysis of 52 cases. Eur Urol 1998;33:433

Wojcik LJ, Hansen K, Diamond DA, et al: Cystic dysplasia of the rete testis: a benign congenital lesion associated with ipsilateral urological anomalies. J Urol 1997;158:600

Renal Hypoplasia and Dysplasia

Ansari MS, Hemal AK, Gupta NP, et al: Laparoscopy for the diagnosis and treatment of radiologically occult but symptomatic hypoplastic kidneys. Urology 2003;64:627

Dziarmaga A, Quinlan J, Goodyer P: Renal hypoplasia: lessons from Pax2. Pediatr Nephrol 2006;21:26

Salomon R, Tellier AL, Attie-Bitach T, et al: PAX2 mutations in oligomeganephronia. Kidney Int 2001;59:457

Wood AS, Price KL, Scambler PJ, et al: Evolving concepts in human renal dysplasia. J Am Soc Nephrol 2004;15:998

Yan YJ, Feng ZX, Min ZH, et al: Single-system ectopic ureters associated with renal dysplasia. Pediatr Surg Int 2004;20:851

Multicystic Dysplastic Kidney

Armando E, Oliveira EA, Silva GS, et al: Predictive factors of ultrasonographic involution of prenatally detected multicystic dysplastic kidney. BJU Int 2005;95:868

Belk RA, Thomas FM, Mueller RF, et al: A family study and the natural history of prenatally detected unilateral multicystic dysplastic kidney. J Urol 2002;167:666

Blane CE, Ritchey ML, DiPietro MA, et al: Single system ectopic ureters and ureteroceles associated with dysplastic kidney. Pediatr Radiol 1992;22:217

Gordon AC, Thomas DF, Arthur RJ, et al: Multicystic dysplastic kidney: is nephrectomy still appropriate? J Urol 1998;140:1231

Heymans C, Breysem L, Proesman W: Multicystic kidney dysplasia: a prospective study on the natural history of the affected and the contralateral kidney. Eur J Pediatr 1998;157:673

Ismali K, Avni FE, Alexander M, et al: Routine voiding cystourethrography is of no value in neonates with unilateral multicystic dysplastic kidney. J Pediatr 2005;146:759

John U, Rudnik-Schoneborn S, Zerres K, et al: Kidney growth and renal function in unilateral multicystic dysplastic kidney. Pediatr Nephrol 1998;12:567

Karmazyn B, Zerin JM: Lower urinary tract abnormalities in children with multicystic dysplastic kidney. Radiology 1997;203:223

Kuwertz-Broeking E, Brinkman OA, Von Lengerke HJ, et al: Unilateral multicystic dysplastic kidney: experience in children. BJU Int 2004;93:388

Lazebnik N, Bellinger MF, Ferguson JE 2nd, et al: Insights into the pathogenesis and natural history of fetuses with multicystic dysplastic kidney disease. Prenat Diagn 1999;19:418

Miller DC, Rumohr JA, Dunn RL, et al: What is the fate of the refluxing contralateral kidney in children with multicystic dysplastic kidney? J Urol 2004;172:1630

Okada T, Yoshida H, Matsunga T, et al; Multicystic dysplastic kidney detected by prenatal ultrasonography: natural history and conservative management. Pediatr Surg Int 2003;19:207

Perez LM, Naidu SI, Joseph DB: Outcome and cost analysis of operative versus nonoperative management of neonatal multicystic dysplastic kidneys. J Urol 1998;160:1207

Rottenberg GT, De Bruyn R, Gordon I: Sonographic standards for a single functioning kidney in children. AJR Am J Roentgenol 1996;167:1255

Rottenberg GT, De Bruyn R, Gordon I: The natural history of the multicystic dysplastic kidney in children. Br J Radiol 1997;70:347

Simoneaux SF, Atkinson GO, Ball TI: Cystic dysplasia of the testis associated with multicystic dysplastic kidney. Pediatr Radiol 1995;25:379

Snodgrass WT: Hypertension associated with multicystic dysplastic kidney in children. J Urol 2000;164:472

Strife JL, Souza AS, Kirks DR, et al: Multicystic dysplastic kidney in children: US follow-up. Radiology 1993;186:785

Truong LD, Choi Y-J, King BF, et al: Renal cystic neoplasms and renal neoplasms associated with cystic renal disease: pathogenetic and molecular links. Adv Anat Pathol 2003;10:135

Vinocur L, Slovis TL, Perlmutter AD, et al: Follow-up studies of multicystic dysplastic kidneys. Radiology 1988;167:311

Wiesel A, Queisser-Luft A, Clementi M, et al: Prenatal detection of congenital renal malformations by fetal ultrasonographic examination: an analysis of 709,030 births in 12 European countries. Eur J Med Genet 2005;48:131

Zerin JM, Baker DR, Casale JA: Single-system ureteroceles in infants and children: imaging features. Pediatr Radiol 2000;30:139

Zerin JM, Leiser J: The impact of vesicoureteral reflux on contralateral renal length in infants with multicystic dysplastic kidney. Pediatr Radiol 1998;28:683

Cystic Renal Disease

Autosomal Recessive Polycystic Kidney Disease

Avni FE, Garel L, Cassart M, et al: Perinatal assessment of hereditary cystic renal diseases: the contribution of sonography. Pediatr Radiol 2006;36:405

Avni FE, Guissade G, Hall M, et al: Hereditary polycystic kidney disease in children: changing sonographic patterns throughout childhood. Pediatr Radiol 2002;32:169

Guay-Woodford LM, Desmond RA: Autosomal recessive polycystic kidney disease: the clinical experience in North America. Pediatrics 2003;111:1072

Herman TE, Siegel MJ: Pyramidal hyperechogenicity in autosomal recessive polycystic kidney disease resembling nephrocalcinosis. Pediatr Radiol 1991;20:270

Jung G, Benz-Bohm G, Kugel H, et al: MR cholangiography in children with autosomal recessive polycystic kidney disease. Pediatr Radiol 1999;29:463

Kern S, Zimmerhackl LB, Hildebrandt F, et al: RARE-MR-urography—a new diagnostic method in autosomal recessive polycystic kidney disease. Acta Radiol 1999;40:543

Lonergan GJ, Rice RR, Suarez ES: Autosomal recessive polycystic kidney disease: radiologic-pathologic correlation. Radiographics 2000;20:837

Roy S, Dillon MJ, Trompeter RS, et al: Autosomal recessive polycystic kidney disease: long term outcome of neonatal survivors. Pediatr Nephrol 1997;11:302

Traubici J, Daneman A: High-resolution renal sonography in children with autosomal recessive polycystic kidney disease. AJR Am J Roentgenol 2005;184:1630

Wisser J, Hebisch G, Froster U, et al: Prenatal sonographic diagnosis of autosomal recessive polycystic kidney disease (ARPKD) during the early second trimester. Prenat Diagn 1995;15:868

Zerres K, Senderek J, Rudnik-Schoneborn S, et al: New options for prenatal diagnosis in autosomal recessive polycystic kidney disease by mutation analysis of the PKHD1 gene. Clin Genet 2004;66:53

Autosomal Dominant Polycystic Kidney Disease

Butler WE, Barker FG 2nd, Crowell RM: Patients with polycystic kidney disease would benefit from routine magnetic resonance angiographic screening for intracerebral aneurysms: a decision analysis. Neurosurgery 1996;38:506

Danaci M, Akpolat T, Bastemir M, et al: The prevalence of seminal vesicle cysts in autosomal dominant polycystic kidney disease. Nephrol Dial Transplant 1998;13:2825

Hateboer N, van Dijk MA, Bogdanova N, et al: Comparison of phenotypes of polycystic kidney disease types 1 and 2. European PKD1-PKD2 Study Group. Lancet 1999;353:103

Jain M, LeQuesne GW, Bourne AJ, et al: High-resolution ultrasonography in the differential diagnosis of cystic diseases of the kidney in infancy and childhood: preliminary experience. J Ultrasound Med 1997;16:235

MacDermot KD, Saggar-Malik AK, Economides DL, et al: Prenatal diagnosis of autosomal dominant polycystic kidney disease (PKD1) presenting in utero and prognosis for very early onset disease. J Med Genet 1998;35:13

Nakajima F, Shibahara N, Arai M, et al: Intracranial aneurysms and autosomal dominant polycystic kidney disease: followup study by magnetic resonance angiography. J Urol 2000;164:331

Schrier RW, Belz MM, Johnson AM, et al: Repeat imaging for intracranial aneurysms in patients with autosomal dominant polycystic kidney disease with initially negative studies: a prospective ten-year follow-up. J Am Soc Nephrol 2004;15:1023

Simple and Acquired Renal Cysts

Acquired cystic kidney disease in children undergoing continuous ambulatory peritoneal dialysis. Kyushu Pediatric Nephrology Group. Am J Kidney Dis 1999;34:242

Bisceglia M, Galliani CA, Senger S, et al: Renal cystic diseases: a review. Adv Anat Pathol 2006;13:26

Blazer S, Zimmer EZ, Blumenfeld Z, et al: Natural history of fetal simple renal cysts detected in early pregnancy. J Urol 1999;162:812

Leichter HE, Dietrich R, Salusky IB, et al: Acquired cystic renal disease in children undergoing long-term dialysis. Pediatr Nephrol 1988;2:8

Zinn HL, Rosberger ST, Haller JO, et al: Simple renal cysts in children with AIDS. Pediatr Radiol 1997;27:827

Miscellaneous Cystic Diseases

Ala-Mello S, Jaaskelainen J, Koskimies O: Familial juvenile nephronophthisis: an ultrasonographic follow-up of seven patients. Acta Radiol 1998;39:84

Bernstein J: Glomerulocystic kidney disease—nosologic considerations. Pediatr Nephrol 1993;7:464

Blowey DL, Querfeld U, Geary D, et al: Ultrasound findings in juvenile nephronophthisis. Pediatr Nephrol 1996;10:22

Caridi G, Dagnino M, Miglietti N, et al: Juvenile nephronophthisis and related clinical variants: clinical features and molecular approach. Contrib Nephrol 2001;136:57

Chuang YF, Tsai TC: Sonographic findings in familial juvenile nephronophthisis-medullary cystic disease complex. J Clin Ultrasound 1998;26:203

Dedeoglu IO, Fisher JE, Springate JE, et al: Spectrum of glomerulocystic kidneys: a case report and review of the literature. Pediatr Pathol Lab Med 1996;16:941

Fitch SJ, Stapleton FB: Ultrasonographic features of glomerulocystic disease in infancy: similarity to infantile polycystic kidney disease. Pediatr Radiol 1986;16:400

Jain M, LeQuesne GW, Bourne AJ, et al: High-resolution ultrasonography in the differential diagnosis of cystic diseases of the kidney in infancy and childhood: preliminary experience. J Ultrasound Med 1997;16:235

Kumada S, Hayashi M, Arima K, et al: Renal disease is Arima syndrome is nephronophthisis as in other Joubert-related cerebello-oculo-renal syndromes. Am J Med Genet 2044;131A:71

Parisi MA, Bennett CL, Eckert ML et al: The NPHP1 gene deletion associated with juvenile nephronophthisis is present in a subset of individuals with Joubert syndrome. Am J Hum Genet 2004;75:82

Patriquin HB, O'Regan S: Medullary sponge kidney in childhood. AJR Am J Roentgenol 1985;145:315

Sharp CK, Bergman SM, Stockwin JM, et al: Dominantly transmitted glomerulocystic kidney disease: a distinct genetic entity. J Am Soc Nephrol 1997;8:77

Malformation Syndromes with Renal Cysts

Borer JG, Kaefer M, Barnewolt CE, et al: Renal findings on followup of patients with Beckwith-Wiedemann syndrome. J Urol 1999;161:235

Choyke PL, Siegel MJ, Craft AW, et al: Screening for Wilms tumor in children with Beckwith-Wiedemann syndrome or idiopathic hemihypertrophy. Med Pediatr Oncol 1999;32:196

Choyke PL, Siegel MJ, Oz O, et al: Nonmalignant renal disease in pediatric patients with Beckwith-Wiedemann syndrome. AJR Am J Roentgenol 1998;17:733

Cook JA, Oliver K, Mueller RF, et al: A cross sectional study of renal involvement in tuberous sclerosis. J Med Genet 1996;33:480

Dibbern KM, Graham JM, Lachman RS, et al: Cumming syndrome: report of two additional cases. Pediatr Radiol 1998;28:798

Dippell J, Varlam DE: Early sonographic aspects of kidney morphology in Bardet-Biedl syndrome. Pediatr Nephrol 1998;12:559

Ewalt DH, Sheffield E, Sparagana SP, et al: Renal lesion growth in children with tuberous sclerosis complex. J Urol 1998;160:141

Fitzpatrick DR: Zellweger syndrome and associated phenotypes. J Med Genet 1996;33:863

Gershoni-Baruch R, Nachieli T, Leibo R, et al: Cystic kidney dysplasia and polydactyly in 3 sibs with Bardet-Biedl syndrome. Am J Med Genet 1992;44:269

Haug K, Khan S, Fuchs S, et al: OFD II, OFD VI, and Joubert syndrome manifestations in 2 sibs. Am J Med Genet 2000; 91:135

Martin SR, Garel L, Alvarez F: Alagille's syndrome associated with cystic renal disease. Arch Dis Child 1996;74:232

O'Dea D, Parfrey PS, Harnett JD, et al: The importance of renal impairment in the natural history of Bardet-Biedl syndrome. Am J Kidney Dis 1996;27:776

Odent S, Le Marec B, Toutain A, et al: Central nervous system malformations and early end-stage renal disease in oro-facio-digital syndrome type I: a review. Am J Med Genet 1998;75:389

O'Hagan AR, Ellsworth R, Secic M, et al: Renal manifestations of tuberous sclerosis complex. Clin Pediatr 1996;35:483

Puechel SM, Oyer CE: Cerebrohepatorenal (Zellweger) syndrome: clinical, neuropathological, and biochemical findings. Childs Nerv Syst 1995;11:639

Sampson JR, Maheshwar MM, Aspinwall R, et al: Renal cystic disease in tuberous sclerosis: the role of the polycystic kidney disease 1 gene. Am J Hum Genet 1997;61:843

Sepulveda W, Sebire NJ, Souka A, et al: Diagnosis of the Meckel-Gruber syndrome at eleven to fourteen weeks' gestation. Am J Obstet Gynecol 1997;176:316

Whitfield J, Hurst D, Bennett MJ, et al: Fetal polycystic kidney disease associated with glutaric aciduria type II: an inborn error of metabolism. Am J Perinatol 1996;13:131

Wright C, Healicon R, English C, et al: Meckel syndrome: what are the minimum diagnostic criteria? J Med Genet 1994;31:482

Anomalies of the Pelvocalyceal System

Calyceal Diverticulum

Kavukcu S, Cakmakci H, Babayigit A: Diagnosis of caliceal diverticulum in two pediatric patients: a comparison of sonography, CT, and urography. J Clin Ultrasound 2003;31:218

Monga M, Smith R, Ferral H, et al: Percutaneous ablation of caliceal diverticulum: long-term follow up. J Urol 2000;163:28

Patriquin H, Lafortune M, Filiatrault D: Urinary milk of calcium in children and adults: use of gravity-dependent sonography. AJR Am J Roentgenol 1985;144:407

Timmons JW, Malek RS, Hattery RR, et al: Caliceal diverticulum. J Urol 1975;114:6

Congenital Megacalyces (Megacalycosis)

Hill LM, Macpherson T, Roman L, et al: Prenatal sonographic findings of fetal megacalycosis. J Ultrasound Med 2002;21:1179

Kasao B, Kavukcu S, Soylu A, et al: Megacalycosis: report of two cases. Pediatr Nephrol 2005;20:828

Sethi R, Yang DC, Mittal P, et al: Congenital megacalyces: studies with different imaging modalities. Clin Nucl Med 1997;22:653

Vargas B, Lebowitz RL: The coexistence of congenital megacalyces and primary megaureter. AJR Am J Roentgenol 1986;147:313

Ureteropelvic Junction Obstruction

Anderson N, Clautice-Engle T, Allan R, et al: Detection of obstructive uropathy in the fetus: predictive value of sonographic measurements of renal pelvic diameter at various gestational ages. AJR Am J Roentgenol 1995;164:719

Cain MP, Rink RC, Thomas AC, et al: Symptomatic ureteropelvic junction obstruction in children in the era of prenatal sonography: is there a higher incidence of crossing vessels? Urology 2001;57:338

Chertin B, Pollack A, Koulikov D, et al: Conservative treatment of ureteropelvic junction obstruction in children with antenatal diagnosis: lessons learned after 16 years of follow-up. Eur Urol 2006;49:734

Conway JJ, Maizels M: The "well tempered" diuretic renogram: a standard method to examine the asymptomatic neonate with hydronephrosis or hydroureteronephrosis. A report from combined meetings of the Society for Fetal Urology and members of the Pediatric Nuclear Medicine Council—the Society of Nuclear Medicine. J Nucl Med 1992;33:2047

Docimo SG, Silver RI: Renal ultrasonography in newborns with prenatally detected hydronephrosis: why wait? J Urol 1997;156:1387

Dremsek PA, Gindl K, Voitl P, et al: Renal pyelectasis in fetuses and neonates: diagnostic value of renal pelvis diameter in pre- and postnatal sonographic screening AJR Am J Roentgenol 1997;168:1017

Fernbach SK, Maizels M, Conway JJ: Ultrasound grading of hydronephrosis: introduction to the system used by the Society for Fetal Urology. Pediatr Radiol 1993;23:478

Fernbach SK, Zawin JK, Lebowitz RL: Complete duplication of the ureter with ureteropelvic junction obstruction of the lower pole of the kidney: imaging findings. AJR Am J Roentgenol 1995;164:701

Frauscher F: Value of contrast-enhanced color Doppler imaging for detection of crossing vessels in patients with ureteropelvic junction obstruction. Radiology 2000;217:916

Gonzalez R, Schimke CM: Ureteropelvic junction obstruction in infants and children. Pediatr Clin North Am 2001;48:1505

Herndon CD, McKenna PH, Kolon TF, et al: A multicenter outcomes analysis of patients with neonatal reflux presenting with prenatal hydronephrosis. J Urol 1999;162:1203

Houben CH, Wischermann A, Bomer G, et al: Outcome analysis of pyeloplasty in infants. Pediatr Surg Int 2000;16:189

Joseph DB, Bauer SB, Colodny AH, et al: Lower pole ureteropelvic junction obstruction and incomplete renal duplication. J Urol 1989;141:896

McDaniel BB, Jones RA, Scherz H, et al: Dynamic contrast-enhanced MR urography in the evaluation of pediatric hydronephrosis. Part 2. Anatomic and functional assessment of ureteropelvic junction obstruction. AJR Am J Roentgenol 2005;185:1608

McGrath MA, Estroff J, Lebowitz RL: The coexistence of obstruction at the ureteropelvic and ureterovesical junctions. AJR Am J Roentgenol 1987;149:403

Mitsumori A, Yasui K, Akaki S, et al: Evaluation of crossing vessels in patients with ureteropelvic junction obstruction by means of helical CT. Radiographics 2000;20:1383

Perez-Brayfield MR, Kirsch A, Jones RA, et al: A prospective study comparing ultrasound, nuclear scintigraphy and dynamic contrast enhanced magnetic resonance imaging in the evaluation of hydronephrosis. J Urol 2003;170:1330

Ross JH, Kay R, Knipper NS, et al: The absence of crossing vessels in association with ureteropelvic junction obstruction detected by prenatal sonography. J Urol 1998;160:973

Rossleigh MA: Renal cortical scintigraphy and diuresis renography in infants and children. J Nucl Med 2001;42:91

Rushton HG, Salem Y, Belman AB, et al: Pediatric pyeloplasty: is routine retrograde pyelography necessary? J Urol 1994;152:604

Strauss J, Connolly LP, Connolly SA, et al: Dynamic renal scintigraphy in children with vesicoureteral reflux and suspected coexisting ureteropelvic junction obstruction. J Urol 2003;170:1966

Takla NV, Hamilton BD, Cartwright PC, et al: Apparent unilateral ureteropelvic junction obstruction in the newborn: expectation for resolution. J Urol 1998;160:2175

Yerkes EB, Adams MC, Pope JC 4th, et al: Does every patient with prenatal hydronephrosis need voiding cystourethrography? J Urol 1999;162:1218

CHAPTER 146

Infections

SANDRA K. FERNBACH

URINARY TRACT INFECTION

Urinary tract infection (UTI) is very common in pediatric practice, affecting up to 3% of school-age girls and less than 1% of school-age boys. Factors that predispose one to UTI include young age, gender (male at younger than 1 year, female at all other ages), voiding dysfunction, family history, anatomic abnormalities, host immunocompetence, and virulence of organisms. In very young children, the diagnosis of UTI can be difficult because symptoms often are not very specific, and urinalysis and urine culture are required. Similarly, the distinction between lower UTI and upper UTI (pyelonephritis, discussed later) can be difficult, although children with upper urinary involvement generally have higher fevers.

Once a UTI has been diagnosed, imaging is often undertaken to guide patient treatment. Although this is one of the more common problems in clinical pediatrics, the appropriate examinations to be performed in various clinical scenarios remain a matter of debate and research. Imaging options include anatomic evaluation of the urinary tract (ultrasonography [US], computed tomography [CT], magnetic resonance imaging [MRI]), evaluation of renal infection (DMSA cortical scintigraphy, Doppler US, MR, CT), evaluation of renal function (nuclear renography, magnetic resonance urography [MRU]), and evaluation of vesicoureteral reflux (voiding cystourethrogram [VCUG], nuclear medicine cystogram, contrast-enhanced cystosonography). In general, at least two tests are required: one for anatomy or renal infection, and one for reflux. Although some recent studies suggest that renal US may not be necessary (especially if a fetal examination was performed during the third trimester), and that reflux may not be as important as was once thought, most professional societies in North America still recommend for a US and voiding study in the evaluation of UTI in the young child, with the philosophy that identification of reflux is a key factor in management. European practitioners tend to perform a greater number of scintigraphic DMSA scans acutely (for evaluation of pyelonephritis) and on a delayed basis (for scarring), because it is well known that upper UTI can occur in the absence of reflux, especially in younger children. Data are available to support many different practices, and imaging approaches must be tailored to patient age, gender, and clinical variables. A suggested approach, based on current North American practice, is given in Table 146-1. With ongoing research into the natural history of UTI and its consequences, one must remain open to new developments; recommendations are likely to change in the future.

ACUTE BACTERIAL PYELONEPHRITIS (ACUTE PYELONEPHRITIS, RENAL OR PERIRENAL ABSCESS)

The terminology of acute kidney infection was revised in the early 1990s, when US and CT showed that focal infections frequently occurred in a non-lobar distribution. The term *acute bacterial pyelonephritis* was used to encompass focal and diffuse acute bacterial inflammation, and it was extended to include severe or complicated infections, including renal abscess.

Children with UTI present a unique challenge to the clinician and the radiologist. The usual signs, symptoms, and laboratory test results that allow distinction between kidney infections and lower UTIs are less reliable in children than in adults. Because UTIs of the upper urinary tract are treated differently from those of the lower urinary tract, these must be differentiated from each other as quickly and precisely as possible. Imaging can reveal whether a kidney infection is present, how much of the kidney is involved, and whether antibiotic treatment alone will suffice. Imaging can be used to detect structural abnormalities that increase the likelihood of infection or reduce the effectiveness of standard treatment.

TABLE 146-1
Urinary Tract Infection Evaluation

Child younger than 5 years of age
- Renal ultrasonography (US)
- Voiding cystourethrogram (VCUG)—boys; VCUG or radionuclide cystogram (RNC)—girls
- If high fevers and normal US, consider DMSA cortical scan or magnetic resonance imaging (MRI)

Child older than 5 years of age
- Renal US
- If high fevers and normal US, consider DMSA cortical scan or MRI
- Consider reflux study, particularly if recurrent urinary tract infection or abnormal US

> **Pyelonephritis may be difficult to diagnose in children, may occur without vesicoureteral reflux (VUR), and may occur without pyuria.**

These two questions are frequently put to the radiologist: (1) When do we image a child with UTI? (2) What modalities should we use to evaluate the child with febrile (or afebrile) UTI?

Some form of cystography is usually performed after an acute UTI, even though as many as two thirds of these studies are normal, and children with known pyelonephritis or renal scarring may not have vesicoureteral reflux (VUR). Cystography can be done subacutely (during hospitalization) or after a short period (about a month), during which the child receives prophylactic antibiotics. Techniques, indications, value, and problems of voiding cystourethrography and nuclear cystography are addressed in Chapters 107 and 151. Alternatively, sonicated material placed into the bladder via catheter can be used in combination with US to diagnose reflux, but this technique remains in limited clinical use in North America. Renal US, once routinely used to detect obstructive lesions in children with UTI, might be more appropriately performed only in those without documentation of renal status on prenatal US. Some authors, but not the American Academy of Pediatrics, have suggested that renal US can be eliminated in children with acute UTI who are responding appropriately to antibiotics. When a child is not responding appropriately to antibiotics, renal US may be used to exclude the rare parenchymal abscess or collecting system obstruction that needs drainage.

Pyelonephritis can be observed with many imaging modalities. Specific signs on US of acute pyelonephritis consist of diffuse or local parenchymal swelling, loss of definition of the corticomedullary junction, thickening of the walls of the upper urinary tract, renal sinus hyper-echogenicity, and focal area(s) of abnormal echogenicity. During an acute infection, the parenchyma may develop small anechoic regions that are not true abscesses; response of these to conservative treatment can be monitored through serial US examinations. Despite the numerous potential findings on US produced by infection, gray scale US is not particularly sensitive to pyelonephritis; an infected kidney frequently appears normal.

Renal abscess is a rare complication that is more often seen in children who are immunocompromised or have diabetes mellitus or sickle cell disease. On US, a true abscess appears as a round hypoechoic region with good through-transmission (Fig. 146-1). The abscess wall becomes thicker as the process progresses. Contrast-enhanced CT (CECT) shows a renal abscess as a round lesion that fails to enhance when contrast is given; this appearance differentiates it from the wedge-shaped, poorly enhancing regions of pyelonephritis (Fig. 146-2). A thick abscess wall is an inconstant finding. CT use is limited in pediatrics by concern about radiation-induced malignancy; CT may be withheld until a renal abscess is strongly suspected. An enlarging abscess can be drained under guidance of US or CT.

Acute infection produces wedge-shaped areas with decreased perfusion on Doppler US. These can be seen with color Doppler US but are better shown with power Doppler. However, power Doppler US is not as sensitive to pyelonephritis as is renal cortical scintigraphy, and it may detect only about 80% of lesions seen with CECT.

Renal cortical scintigraphy, CECT, and MRI are all used to detect focal areas of pyelonephritis (see Fig. 146-2; Figs. 146-3, 146-4). Pyelonephritis-induced areas of ischemia and tubular dysfunction become evident after intravenous injection of isotope, iodinated contrast material, or gadolinium, respectively. In each instance, the injected material does not enter the abnormal parenchyma as readily as it enters the normal area. CECT changes of acute pyelonephritis (see Fig. 146-2) include

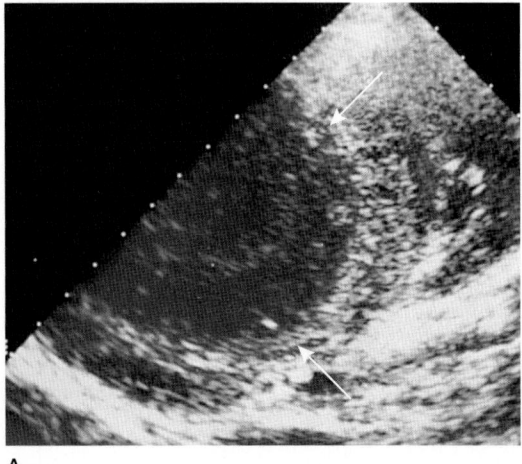
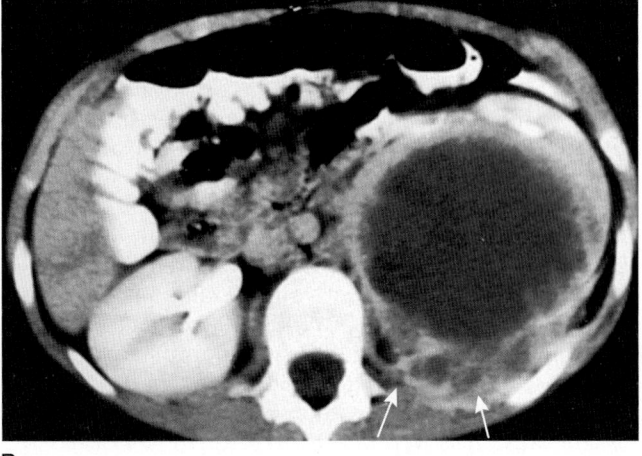

A   B

FIGURE 146-1. Renal abscess. **A,** Longitudinal sonogram shows a large hypoechoic mass *(arrows)* with good through-transmission. A few scattered echoes within the center of the mass suggest that the contents consist of a thickened fluid, or that septations are poorly seen. The wall of the mass is thickened and is more echogenic than the central portion of the mass. **B,** Contrast-enhanced computed tomography shows the large intrarenal abscess collection, with poor contrast enhancement and excretion of the adjacent renal parenchyma *(arrows)*. (Courtesy of Dr. A'Delbert Bowen, Pittsburgh, PA.)

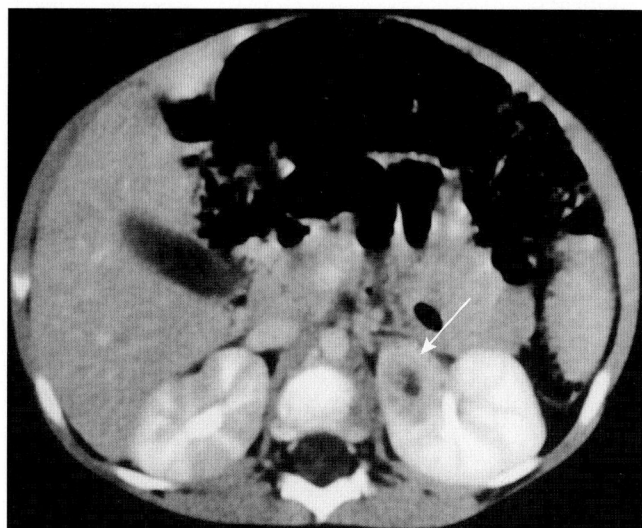

FIGURE 146-2. Acute pyelonephritis. Contrast-enhanced computed tomography scan shows swelling of the left kidney that causes it to appear diffusely larger than the right. Along the anteromedial aspect of the left kidney is a small abscess *(arrow)*, which is seen as a low-density region surrounded by poorly enhancing parenchyma. On the right, multiple poorly enhancing, wedge-shaped regions extend from the renal pelvis to the periphery—another sign of acute pyelonephritis.

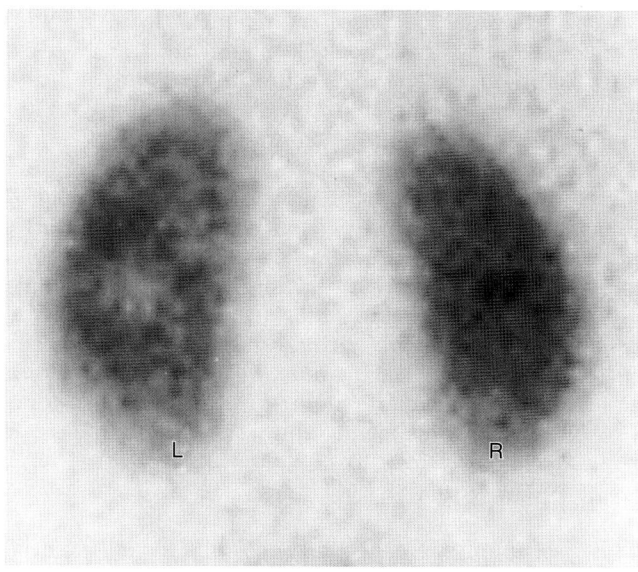

FIGURE 146-3. Acute pyelonephritis. Technetium-99m glucoheptonate study shows a normal right kidney. The infected left kidney exhibits diffusely less isotope uptake than the right and has some focal photopenic areas—an indication of tubulointerstitial edema and diminished blood flow.

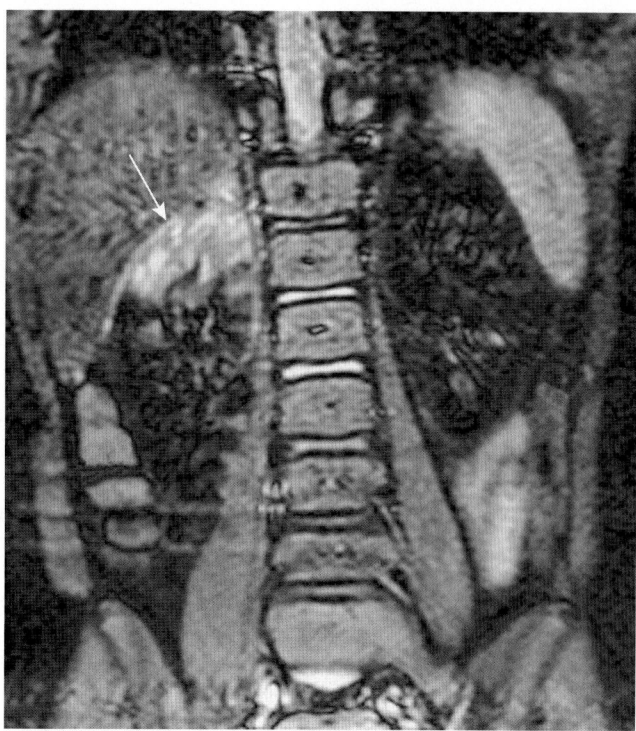

FIGURE 146-4. Acute pyelonephritis. Coronal contrast-enhanced short tau inversion recovery magnetic resonance image shows abnormal increased signal in the upper pole of the right kidney *(arrow)*. Normal portions of the right kidney and the left kidney have very low signal. (Courtesy of Damien Grattan-Smith, MD, Atlanta, GA.)

focal or diffuse swelling, loss of definition of the corticomedullary junction, and wedge-shaped, poorly enhancing regions (broadening from renal sinus to periphery). CECT is rarely used for the diagnosis of UTI, but when it is performed in children with a clinically acute abdomen, changes may be evident. Because pyelonephritis can be present despite a normal urine culture, these children are not suspected of having a renal infection until CECT is performed. Gadolinium-enhanced MRI,

with the use of inversion recovery sequences, shows infected parenchyma as bright regions (see Fig. 146-4). MRI is as successful as renal cortical scintigraphy in detecting abnormal regions, and it eliminates the radiation associated with CT studies. Furthermore, MRI has a high rate of interobserver agreement regarding lesions, thus eliminating a potential pitfall of renal cortical scintigraphy. However, the limited accessibility and high cost of MRI have restricted its clinical use for this purpose.

Renal cortical scintigraphy can be performed by tagging technetium-99m (^{99m}Tc) with dimercaptosuccinic acid (DMSA) or, less frequently, glucoheptonate (GHA). Imaging with mercaptoacetyltriglycine (MAG3) tagged to ^{99m}Tc can reveal infection-produced cortical defects, but this isotope is not routinely used for this purpose. The sensitivity of renal scintigraphy is enhanced when pinhole collimation or single-photon emission CT (SPECT) imaging is added. Gallium-67 SPECT imaging is sensitive and specific for pyelonephritis and can readily differentiate scars from active infection, but this technique is uncommonly used because of the relatively large radiation dose, especially to growth plates, associated with this isotope.

Intravenous urography (IVU) is rarely performed for diagnosis of UTI. In most instances, the study is normal even when renal infection is present; when abnormal, the extent of the infection is poorly displayed. IVU findings of renal infection include focal or diffuse renal enlargement, poor uptake and poor excretion of contrast material, and narrowing of the pelvicalyceal system as a result of parenchymal edema.

XANTHOGRANULOMATOUS PYELONEPHRITIS

Xanthogranulomatous pyelonephritis (XGP) is a chronic type of pyelonephritis that is rare in childhood; it typically occurs in females during their fifth through seventh decades. However, XGP can develop in childhood and can even affect infants. The process, which is virtually always unilateral, often involves the entire kidney but may affect only a segment. Contralateral renal hypertrophy, which is identified in about half of patients, indicates loss of function in the affected kidney and the chronicity of the process. The infection, usually caused by *Proteus mirabilis* and, less commmonly, *Escherichia coli* or *Staphylococcus aureus*, results in necrotic loss of renal parenchyma. In about 80% of cases, the process dissects into the perirenal space and produces focal adhesions. Further extension of the infection is responsible for some of the less common presentations, including fistulous tracts to the skin, psoas muscle, colon, and even the bronchi. The infected region is composed of multiple abscesses. Grossly, infected areas have a nodular yellow appearance. Microscopically, inflammatory cells are interspersed within fibrogranulomatous tissue; nodules of lipid-filled macrophages (foam or xanthoma cells) and areas of necrotic parenchyma are identified.

Diffuse and segmental forms have been reported in association with anatomic renal anomalies such as ureteropelvic junction obstruction (more often diffuse) or an obstructed infundibulum or upper moiety within a duplex system (segmental). An association with vesicoureteric reflux has also been noted. A staghorn calculus may be the cause of or may result from an obstruction at the renal pelvis; smaller renal calculi may also be present.

Focal and diffuse forms may be tumefactive and can simulate other renal masses; in childhood, Wilms tumor may be simulated. The child may have flank pain or a palpable renal mass. Although few children have hematuria, most are anemic at presentation. Weight loss or failure to thrive may occur. Most affected children have pyuria, a finding not typically associated with a Wilms tumor. Typical symptoms and signs of acute UTI may be absent. Some children have a history of repeated UTIs with poor response to antibiotic therapy.

The radiologic findings of XGP are multiple. Plain abdominal radiographs may show a flank mass with calculi. The kidney is initially enlarged but may decrease in size with longer infections. IVU, no longer a primary modality in this setting, shows focal or diffuse renal enlargement and focal or diffuse nonfunction or diminished function. US is usually performed as the first study in children with UTI, hematuria, or flank mass. On US, diffuse XGP has been reported to show a massively enlarged but reniform kidney; the parenchyma may have increased echogenicity. As the process progresses, the kidney is replaced by necrotic tissue and may appear filled with fluid and debris; the appearance may overlap with that of pyonephrosis. Occasionally, echogenic calculi are evident within the calyces, but it may be difficult to appreciate a large calculus in the renal pelvis. In the focal form of XGP, the abnormal segment is adjacent to normal-appearing parenchyma. Extension of the process

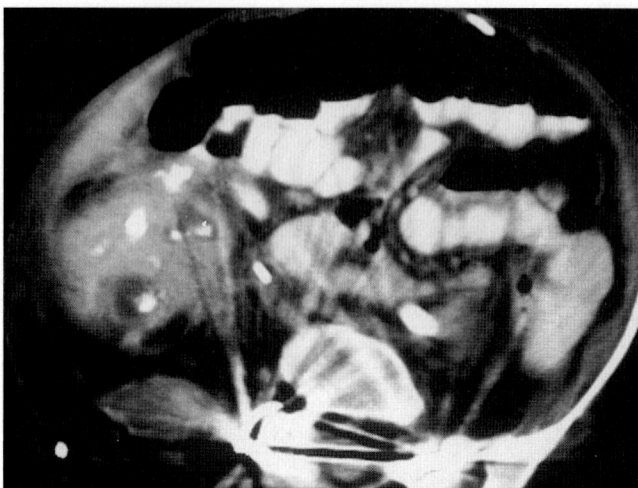

FIGURE 146-5. Xanthogranulomatous pyelonephritis. Contrast-enhanced computed tomography shows a right kidney with multiple stones surrounded by low-density regions of abscess or necrosis. The process has extended into the perirenal tissues, which are edematous and poorly defined, and into the soft tissues beneath the right abdominal wall, which are thickened. Metal-induced artifacts are produced by spinal fixation hardware in this child with dysraphism.

into the perirenal space or adjacent structures may be shown on US but is easier to see with CECT. CECT also reveals intrarenal calcifications, necrotic tissue, nodules of granulation tissue, and lack of function (Fig. 146-5). MRI findings, reported in a few adult patients, indicate that MRI clearly depicts extrarenal extension but has not proved diagnostically more accurate than CT.

Increased recognition of the process in children and increased familiarity with imaging findings have reduced the need for previously used aggressive diagnostic procedures such as retrograde pyelography and renal angiography. If the diagnosis is uncertain, fine-needle aspiration can be used to differentiate XGP from a true renal tumor. When the entire kidney is involved, nephrectomy is performed. Focal disease may be treated with resection of the affected parenchyma or by nephrostomy (for drainage) with systemic antibiotics.

PYONEPHROSIS

This term applies to the presence of infected material (pus) in the pelvocalyceal system, most often associated with an obstruction. In children, pyonephrosis is frequently caused by a congenital ureteropelvic junction obstruction. Prompt diagnosis and treatment (drainage) preserves renal function. Delayed diagnosis may result in severe or chronic renal parenchymal infection and has been implicated in the development of XGP. The organisms most frequently cultured when pyonephrosis is drained are *E. coli* and *P. mirabilis,* which are also the most common organisms cultured in children with XGP.

The affected child presents with the usual signs and symptoms of UTI. Urine culture is positive. Hematuria frequently accompanies the infection.

Pyonephrosis cannot be diagnosed with plain films or IVU. However, plain films may show a calculus in the renal pelvis that is contributing to or is caused by the obstruction. The inability of the kidney to concentrate contrast results in poor visualization or nonvisualization on IVU, a nonspecific finding. US successfully depicts pyonephrosis when the fluid within the dilated pelvo-calyceal system contains gravity-dependent echogenic debris, that is, the pus and particulate matter (crystals) that develop above an obstruction (Fig. 146-6). In some children, the fluid may have few internal echoes and the findings may suggest an uncomplicated hydronephrosis. The renal parenchyma must be carefully assessed for exclusion of an abscess.

> **Pyonephrosis occurs when urine above an obstruction becomes infected. US is the best method for diagnosis.**

CT can show the hydronephrotic pelvocalyceal system with gravity-dependent debris below the urine and may be used to evaluate the parenchyma, especially to exclude the presence of abscesses. Parenchymal loss and calculi may be better seen with CT than with US.

Immediate treatment consists of drainage of the obstructed system, usually under US or CT guidance, and administration of organism-specific antibiotics. If calculi are present, they must be removed surgically or through extracorporeal shock wave lithotripsy. To prevent recurrence, the site and cause of the obstruction must be identified and corrected.

FUNGAL INFECTIONS

Fungal infections rarely occur in a normal host. In pediatrics, premature neonates are the most commonly affected. Fungal infections also may develop in those who are immunocompromised by a malignancy or its treatment, by human immunodeficiency virus (HIV)-induced disease, or in those who are on immunosuppressive medications. Open wounds (burns, surgery) and central vascular catheters also predispose to fungal infection.

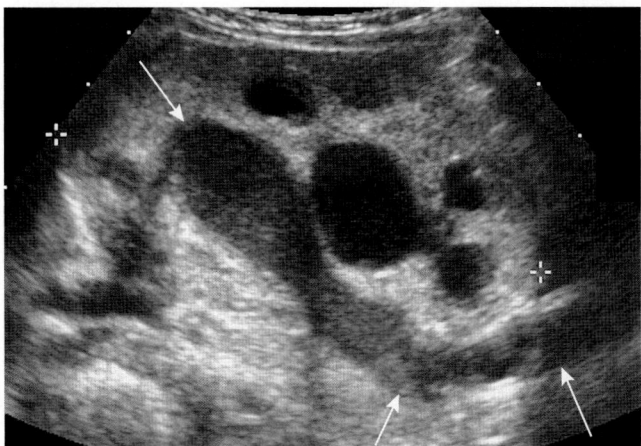

FIGURE 146-6. Pyonephrosis. Longitudinal sonogram shows a duplex collecting system with dilation of the upper and lower poles. Debris is seen within the upper pole collecting system and the ureter (arrows). Lesser debris is observed within the lower pole collecting system.

The most common fungal disease involving the urinary tract is *candidiasis*, which is most often caused by *Candida albicans. Candida* is responsible for about 80% of renal fungal infections. At one time, up to 10% of extremely premature infants (gestational age less than 32 weeks) had a candidal infection during their initial hospitalization; however, currently, the risk for candidemia is much lower, at about 1% or 2%. In many infants, thrush or other colonization of the gastrointestinal tract precedes candidemia; hematogenous spread is the presumed route of renal involvement. Significant other risk factors for candidemia include a 5-minute Apgar score less than 5, shock, disseminated intravascular coagulopathy, prior use of intralipid and parenteral nutrition, and treatment with histamine-2 blockers.

> ***Candida albicans*** **is the most common causative agent in renal fungal infection; it most commonly occurs in premature infants and immunocompromised patients.**

Candida species are the most frequently detected fungal infections in the neonatal nursery. *Candida* infections can manifest as a septic process, or focally, they may infect the brain, the globe, or the urinary tract. Ascending infection occurs when the perineal skin is colonized and the bladder becomes infected via the urethra. Hematogenous seeding produces renal parenchymal disease that may enter the pelvocalyceal system and, secondarily, the bladder. Neonates with urinary tract candidiasis may present with hypertension, oliguria, or anuria; these symptoms may mistakenly be attributed to a catheter-induced vascular clot. Diagnosis of renal candidiasis is made when a properly obtained urine culture contains *Candida;* when urine and an otherwise sterile body fluid contain *Candida;* or when urine contains *Candida* and changes of candidiasis are apparent on renal US.

In general, premature neonates are an unusual subpopulation of those who present with UTI. Boys are more frequently involved than girls; the ratio is as high as 10:1 in those with extremely low birth weight (BW <1000 g). In this population, the most commonly cultured organism is *Klebsiella,* but *C. albicans* accounts for about 15% of UTIs.

These fragile neonates are usually studied with bedside US. Kidneys infected with *Candida* may be enlarged or may have small fluid collections thought to represent abscesses. Increased cortical echogenicity may develop but can be difficult to differentiate from the increased cortical echogenicity typical of premature neonates. Fungus balls (mycetomas, fungal bezoars) within the pelvocalyceal system appear as echogenic, non-shadowing structures (Fig. 146-7) that may cause upper urinary tract obstruction. Initial US is likely to show the mycetoma in those with candiduria, but in a few infants, serial studies are needed before it can be identified. With treatment, fungus balls may slowly resolve or calcify. US shows parenchymal disease or fungus balls in about 40% of neonates with candiduria. Infections limited to the bladder may produce bladder wall thickening or gravity-dependent debris within the bladder lumen. Doppler

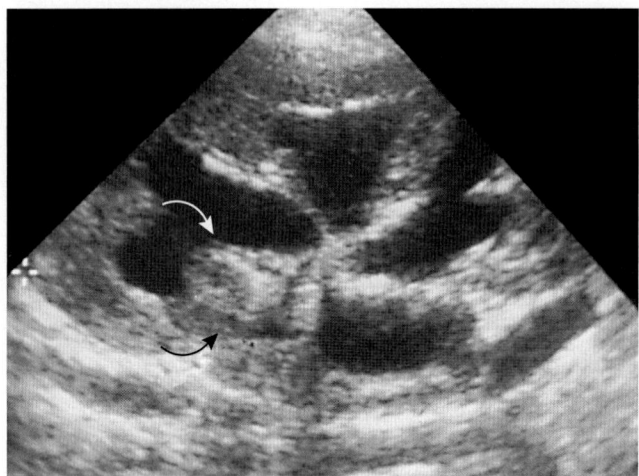

FIGURE 146-7. Candidiasis. Longitudinal sonogram of the left kidney in a premature infant with urinary candidiasis shows hydronephrosis and a small fungus ball in the right upper collecting system *(arrows)*. (Courtesy of Dr. Beverly Wood, Los Angeles, CA.)

US is a complementary part of the examination; it can document normal blood flow, thereby excluding a vascular cause of the oliguria or anuria.

In older children, the presentation of urinary tract *Candida* infection is that of a typical UTI: fever, chills, dysuria, and flank pain. Most affected children have one or more of the risk factors described earlier.

Medical treatment is successful in almost all cases of renal involvement; rarely is nephrectomy needed. Systemic antifungal medication may be augmented by percutaneous drainage and instillation of antifungal medication.

The second most common fungal infection that involves the urinary tract, *aspergillosis,* occurs as the result of disease elsewhere, usually in the lungs. The affected population is slightly different from those who develop renal candidiasis and includes few premature neonates. Instead, the other immunosuppressive states that are associated with renal candidiasis (see earlier) underlie *Aspergillus* infection of the urinary tract. Diagnosis is usually made with US, which shows a focal renal abscess or collecting system or a bladder fungal ball. In adults, rare instances of associated ureteral disease have been reported and may result in hydronephrosis.

Blastomycosis is a rare fungal infection that can involve the urinary tract but more commonly involves (in decreasing frequency) the lungs, the skin, the bones, and the central nervous system. Pulmonary disease is seen in more than 80% of patients and is the source from which other sites become infected (hematogenous spread). *Cryptococcosis* usually involves the central nervous system (meninges and parenchyma) in immunocompromised patients. A few reports describe renal changes, including papillary necrosis and abscess formation, but no reports have emerged of imaging in an affected pediatric population.

TUBERCULOSIS OF THE URINARY TRACT

Although genitourinary tract tuberculosis is a major cause of infertility in Third World nations, involvement of the genital tract is rarely encountered in the pediatric population, especially in North America, where UTI occurs instead. A rise in the number of tuberculosis cases has been documented to parallel the spread of HIV-related illness.

Primary pulmonary tuberculosis usually precedes hematogenous spread to other organs. Although the kidney is the most commonly seeded site, accounting for as much as 30% of extrapulmonary disease, urinary tract tuberculosis remains a rare and perhaps underdiagnosed clinical problem in childhood. The lower urinary tract is infected by antegrade seeding (submucosal, lymphatic) from the infected upper tract. Urinary tract disease may become apparent years after the initial infection occurs, as a result of reactivation of original deposits of the bacterium; the lungs, mediastinum, and pleura have frequently healed without scarring by the time the renal disease is detected. Usual urinary tract symptoms at presentation include frequency and dysuria. Abdominal and flank pain more commonly occurs in affected children than in adults. Sterile pyuria is noted in about 25% of cases and may be accompanied by microscopic hematuria or urine with an acid pH. Diagnosis is made by urine culture and specific staining of the urine for *Mycobacterium tuberculosis*; this is augmented by skin testing and, when applicable, biopsy of affected tissue.

The bacterium is preferentially deposited at the corticomedullary junction; tubercles form, enlarge, coalesce, and spread the infection to the cortex and the medulla. Early treatment may prevent irreversible changes of parenchymal loss and fibrosis. The radiographic appearance of the affected kidney reflects the stage of disease at the time of detection. No change may be noted in the acute phase. Although hematogenous spread infects both kidneys, unilateral disease is usually evident. Parenchymal necrosis is associated with loss of renal parenchyma and, later, dystrophic calcification. Calcifications may take the form of small, poorly seen nodules, or the markedly calcified kidney may have undergone autonephrectomy. Focal disease with secondary stricture in the pelvocalyceal system may result in dilation of a calyx or calyces.

Plain films may reveal calcifications. IVU or CT shows changes related to the stage of the evolving pathologic process. Acutely, edema or large tubercles can compress and distort the calyceal system. Later, poor or delayed renal function may be noted. As tubercles coalesce and cavitation develops, contrast may pool in the parenchyma. The classical moth-eaten appearance of a calyx is caused by focal edema and usually precedes adjacent papillary necrosis. Strictures of a calyx, infundibulum, or renal pelvis occur late and cause obstruction with focal dilation or hydronephrosis.

Ureteral changes rarely occur without visible renal disease, and ureteral disease changes over time. Acute inflammation produces mucosal irregularity; later granuloma formation results in ureteral nodularity or notching. The normal undulant course of the ureter may be lost as it becomes narrowed and straightened or beaded by fibrosis. Lower ureteral strictures may form with consequent hydroureteronephrosis.

Involvement of the bladder similarly progresses from the mucosa to bladder wall. Initial mucosal irregularity is followed by bladder wall thickening. Eventual fibrosis and contraction of the bladder produces voiding abnormalities and a small-volume bladder on imaging. Vesicoureteral reflux is a frequent result of tuberculosis of the bladder. Bladder wall calcification can occur but is rare in childhood.

On CT, the infection may be difficult to differentiate from other infections that produce parenchymal thinning, necrosis, and calcification, such as XGP and pyonephrosis.

Multiple-drug antituberculous therapy is routinely given when genitourinary tuberculosis is diagnosed. Surgery is needed to treat strictures of the upper and lower urinary tract but should not be performed hastily, because some apparent strictures are areas of edema that will regress during treatment, and because all developing strictures may not be clinically apparent for several months. Bladder augmentation may be needed if the bladder is contracted, or if reflux persists.

SCHISTOSOMIASIS (BILHARZIASIS)

Humans are an intermediate host in the life cycle of any flatworm of the *Schistosoma* species. Of the five species that affect humans (*japonicum, mansoni, haematobium, intercalatum, mekongi*), only *S. haematobium* produces changes in the urinary tract.

Also referred to as bilharziasis, primary infection with *S. haematobium* is rare in North America and Europe but is common in parts of Africa and the Middle East. Increased immigration from and travel to and from these regions have extended the infected population beyond endemic regions. Boys and men are consistently affected more often than female patients.

At the cercaria stage, the parasite lives in fresh water. It enters the bodies of bathers, and there, it goes through its life cycle. An acute flulike illness associated with lymphadenopathy, sun sensitivity, and eosinophilia (Katayama syndrome) may develop.

The fluke migrates and establishes itself in the venules of the bladder wall, just beneath the mucosa. At this site, it produces large quantities of ova that break out of the venules and pass into the surrounding tissues (both bladder and adjacent ureter) or into the bladder lumen directly or via the ureter. This process is associated with microscopic or gross hematuria. Protein and eosinophils may also be detected in the urine. Urine samples can be tested for ova, but only about 45% of those with infection proven by other techniques, including serology, are found to have ova in their urine. Clinical and radiographic changes are due to the ova and the host response to them.

As many as 50% of those proven to have schistosomiasis are asymptomatic. About 50% show changes on US, the technique most frequently used to assess the urinary tract in endemic regions. It is not surprising that the bladder is more likely to exhibit changes than is the upper tract. Acutely, the bladder may appear normal. The subacute inflammatory response manifests as bladder wall thickening (most common in children younger than 10 years) and mucosal irregularity that can progress to polyp or pseudopolyp formation (most common in

children 10 to 14 years of age). Fewer subacute changes are seen in adults, but bladder wall fibrosis may develop later in the course of the disease. Calcification of the bladder wall occurs when large amounts of ova are deposited into it; this is seen almost exclusively in adults.

US can be used to evaluate the response of the bladder to treatment. Severe bladder changes regress more quickly and dramatically than minor ones. Recurrence of early bladder changes, sometimes referred to as *resurgence*, is more common among those whose initial studies revealed pronounced disease and in those who have ongoing exposure to the parasite.

The lower ureter, especially the perivesical segment, shows pathologic changes that parallel those noted in the bladder. Bilateral disease is the rule, although changes usually are not symmetric. The ureters have diminished numbers of peristaltic waves and may appear dilated as a result of obstruction produced by distal ureteral edema. Later, distal ureteral strictures develop, especially in the intravesical portion, and ureteral dilation above may persist. Dilation of the pelvocalyceal system may follow. Ureteral changes may ascend and take the form of multiple stenoses or granulomas. Such changes are more frequently seen in those 10 to 19 years of age. Ureteral abnormalities may regress when antiparasitic medications are given, but they do so less often and less completely than abnormalities within the bladder.

IVU is uncommonly performed in affected children, in part because of the medical circumstances in endemic regions, and in part because it does not clearly demonstrate changes. Genital pathology can develop but is rarely encountered in a pediatric population. Reproductive problems (infertility/ectopic pregnancy) follow schistosome-induced adnexal inflammation. Prostatic fibrosis has been described in adult males.

SUGGESTED READINGS

Urinary Tract Infection

American Academy of Pediatrics, Committee on Quality Improvement, Subcommittee on Urinary Tract Infection: Practice parameter: the diagnosis, treatment, and evaluation of the initial urinary tract infection in febrile infants and young children. Pediatrics 1999;103(4 Pt 1):843

Chang SL, Shortliffe LD: Pediatric urinary tract infections. Pediatr Clin N Am 2006;53:379

Conway PH, Cnaan A, Zaoutis T, et al: Recurrent urinary tract infections in children. Risk factors and association with prophylactic antimicrobials. JAMA 2007;298:179-186

Dacher JN, Hitzel A, Avni FE, et al: Imaging strategies in pediatric urinary tract infection. Eur Radiol 2005;15:1283

Giordano M, Marzolla R, Puteo F, et al: Voiding urosonography as first step in the diagnosis of vesicoereteral reflux in children: a clinical experience. Pediatr Radiol 2007;37:674-677

Leroy S, Romanello C, Galetto-Lacour A, et al: Procalcitonin to reduce the number of unnecessary cystographies in children with a urinary tract infection: a European validation study. J Pediatr 2007;150:89-95

Lindert KA, Shortliffe LMD: Evaluation and management of pediatric urinary tract infections. Urologic Clin N Am 1999;26:719

Nickel JC: Management of urinary tract infections in children: simplifying the controversies? Rev Urol 2003;5:132

Riccabona M, Fotter R: Urinary tract infection in infants and children: an update with special regard to the changing role of reflux. Eur Radiol 2004;14:L78

Tseng M-H, Lin W-J, Lo W-T, et al: Does a normal DMSA obviate the performance of voiding cystourethrography in evaluation of young children after their first urinary tract infection? J Pediatr 2007;150:96-99

Wan K-S, Liu C-K, Chen L-H: Primary urinary tract infection in infants: prophylaxis for uncomplicated pyelonephritis. Nephrology 2007;12:178-181

Zier JL, Kvam KA, Kurachek SC, Finkelstein M: Sedation with nitrous oxide compared with no sedation during catheterization for urologic imaging in children. Pediatr Radiol 2007;37:678-684

Acute Pyelonephritis

Alon US, Ganapathy S: Should renal ultrasonography be done routinely in children with first urinary tract infection? Clin Pediatr (Phila) 1999;38:21

American Academy of Pediatrics, Committee on Quality Improvement, Subcommittee on Urinary Tract Infection: Practice parameter: the diagnosis, treatment, and evaluation of the initial urinary tract infection in febrile infants and young children. Pediatrics 1999;103(4 Pt 1):843

Chan YL, Chan KW, Yeung CK, et al: Potential utility of MRI in the evaluation of children at risk of renal scarring. Pediatr Radiol 1999;29:856

Dacher JN, Pfister C, Monroc M, et al: Power Doppler sonographic pattern of acute pyelonephritis in children: comparison with CT. AJR Am J Roentgenol 1996;166:1451

Darge K: Diagnosis of vesicoureteral reflux with ultrasonography. Pediatr Nephrol 2002;17:52

Dascher JN, Avni F, Francois A, et al: Renal sinus hyperechogenicity in acute pyelonephritis: description and pathological correlation. Pediatr Radiol 1999;29:179

Ditchfield MR, Gromwood K, Cook DJ, et al: Persistent renal cortical scintigram defects in children 2 years after urinary tract infection. Pediatr Radiol 2004;34:465

Giorgi LJ, Bratslavsky G, Kogan BA: Febrile urinary tract infections in infants: renal ultrasound remains necessary. J Urol 2005;173:568

Hoberman A, Charron M, Hickey RW, et al: Imaging studies after a first urinary tract infection in young children. N Engl J Med 2003;348:195

Ilyas M, Mastin ST, Richard GA: Age-related radiological imaging in children with acute pyelonephritis. Pediatr Nephrol 2002;17:30

Kanellopoulos TA, Vassilakos PJ, Kamtzis M, et al: Low bacterial count urinary tract infection in infants and young children. Eur J Pediatr 2005;164:355

Laguna R, Silva F, Orduna E, et al: Technetium-99m MAG3 in early identification of pyelonephritis in children. J Nucl Med 1998;39:1254

Lonergan GJ, Pennington DJ, Morrison JC, et al: Childhood pyelonephritis: comparison of gadolinium-enhanced MR imaging and renal cortical scintigraphy for diagnosis. Radiology 1998;207:377

Paterson A, Frush DP, Donnelly LF: Helical CT of the body: are settings adjusted for pediatric patients? AJR Am J Roentgenol 2001;176:297

Piepsz A, Blaufox MD, Gordon I, et al: Consensus on renal cortical scintigraphy in children with urinary tract infection. Semin Nucl Med 1999;29:160

Rodriguez LV, Spielman D, Herfkens RJ, et al: Magnetic resonance imaging for the evaluation of hydronephrosis, reflux and renal scarring in children. J Urol 2001;166:1023

Sorantin E, Fotter R, Aigner R, et al: The sonographically thickened wall of the upper urinary tract system: correlation with other imaging methods. Pediatr Radiol 1997;27:667

Stokland E, Hellstrom M, Jacobsson B, et al: Evaluation of DMSA scintigraphy and urography in assessing acute and permanent renal damage in children. Acta Radiol 1998;39:447

Yen TC, Tzen KY, Chen WP, et al: The value of Ga-67 renal SPECT in diagnosing and monitoring complete and incomplete treatment in children with acute pyelonephritis. Clin Nucl Med 1999;24:669

Xanthogranulomatous Pyelonephritis and Pyonephrosis

Bingol-Kologlu M, Ciftci AO, Senocak ME, et al: Xanthogranulomatous pyelonephritis in children: diagnostic and therapeutic aspects. Eur J Pediatr Surg 2002;12:42

Chen HJ, Tsai JD, Lee HC, et al: Diffuse xanthogranulomatous pyelonephritis in a child with severe complications. Pediatr Nephrol 2004;19:1408

Kim J: Ultrasonographic features of focal xanthogranulomatous pyelonephritis. J Ultrasound Med 2004;23:409

Levy M, Baumal R, Eddy AA: Xanthogranulomatous pyelonephritis in

children: etiology, pathogenesis, clinical and radiologic features and management. Clin Pediatr 1994;33:360

Matthews GJ, McLorie GA, Churchill BA, et al: Xanthogranulomatous pyelonephritis in pediatric patients. J Urol 1995;153:1958

Perez LM, Netto JM, Induhara R, et al: Xanthogranulomatous pyelonephritis in an infant with an obstructed upper pole renal moiety. Urology 1999;54:744

Quinn FM, Dick AC, Corbally MT, et al: Xanthogranulomatous pyelonephritis in childhood. Arch Dis Child 1999;81:483

Samuel M, Duffy S, Capps S, et al: Xanthogranulomatous pyelonephritis in childhood. J Pediatr Surg 2001;36:598

Schneider K, Helmig FJ, Eife R, et al: Pyonephrosis in childhood—is ultrasound sufficient for diagnosis? Pediatr Radiol 1989;19:302

Takamizawa S, Yamataka A, Kaneko K, et al: Xanthogranulomatous pyelonephritis in childhood: a rare but important clinical entity. J Pediatr Surg 2000;35:1554

Fungal Infections

Benjamin DK Jr, Fisher RG, McKinney RE Jr, et al: Candidal mycetoma in the neonatal kidney. Pediatrics 1999;104(5 Pt 1):1126

Bryant K, Maxfield C, Rabalais G: Renal candidiasis in neonates with candiduria. Pediatr Infect Dis J 1999;18:959

Chapman RL: *Candida* infections in the neonate. Curr Opin Pediatr 2003;15:97

Eliakim A, Dolfin T, Korzets Z, et al: Urinary tract infection in premature infants: the role of imaging studies and prophylactic therapy. J Perinatol 1997;17:305

Grobskopf LA, Sinkowitz-Cohen RL, Garrett DO, et al: A national point prevalence survey of pediatric intensive care unit–acquired infection in the United States. J Pediatr 2002;140:432

Hitchcock RJ, Pallett A, Hall MA, et al: Urinary tract candidiasis in neonates and infants. Br J Urol 1995;76:252

Khoory BJ, Vino L, Dall'Agnola A, et al: Candida infections in newborns: a review. J Chemother 1999;11:367

Saiman L, Ludlington E, Pfaller M, et al: Risk factors for candidemia in neonatal intensive care unit patients. The National Epidemiology of Mycosis Survey Study Group. Pediatr Infect Dis J 2000;19:319

Wise GJ, Talluri GS, Marella VK: Fungal infections of the genitourinary system: manifestations, diagnosis, and treatment. Urol Clin North Am 1999;26:701

Tuberculosis of the Urinary Tract

Chattopadhyay A, Bhatnagar V, Agarwala S, et al: Genitourinary tuberculosis in pediatric surgical practice. J Pediatr Surg 1997;32:1283

Eastwood JB, Corbishley CM, Grange JM: Tuberculosis and the kidney. J Am Soc Nephrol 2001;12:1307

Engin G, Acuna B, Acuna G, et al: Imaging of extrapulmonary tuberculosis. Radiographics 2000;20:471

Ferrie BG, Rundle JS: Genitourinary tuberculosis in patients under twenty-five years of age. Urology 1985;25:576

Fonseca-Santos J: Tuberculosis in children. Eur J Radiol 2005;55:202

Harisinghani MG, McLoud T, Shepard JO, et al: Tuberculosis from head to toe. Radiographics 2000;20:449

Schistosomiasis

Brouwer KC, Ndhlovu PD, Wagatsuma Y, et al: Epidemiological assessment of *Schistosoma haematobium*–induced kidney and bladder pathology in rural Zimbabwe. Acta Trop 2003;85:339

Hatz CF: The use of ultrasound in schistosomiasis. Adv Parasitol 2001;48:225

Palmer PE: Schistosomiasis. Semin Roentgenol 1998;33:6

Richter J: Evolution of schistosomiasis-induced pathology after therapy and interruption of exposure to schistosomes: a review of ultrasonographic studies. Acta Trop 2000;77:111

Summer AP, Satuffer W, Maroushek SR, et al: Hematuria in children due to schistosomiasis in a nonendemic setting. Clin Pediatr 2006;45:177-181

Wagatsuma Y, Aryeetey ME, Sack DA, et al: Resolution and resurgence of *Schistosoma haematobium*–induced pathology after community-based chemotherapy in Ghana, as detected by ultrasound. J Infect Dis 1999;179:1515

Whitty CJ, Mabey DC, Armstrong M, et al: Presentation and outcome of 1107 cases of schistosomiasis from Africa diagnosed in a non-endemic country. Trans R Soc Trop Med Hyg 2000;94:531

147

Urolithiasis and Nephrocalcinosis

ROBERT WELLS

Urinary tract calcifications can occur within the kidneys, ureters, bladder, or urethra. Intraluminal stones represent *urolithiasis*; the term *nephrolithiasis* indicates calculi within the pelvicalyceal system. Urolithiasis can be divided into upper tract (pelvicalyceal system and ureter) and lower tract (bladder and urethra) varieties. The term *nephrocalcinosis* indicates the presence of intraparenchymal renal calcifications, either medullary or cortical. Medullary nephrocalcinosis is an important source of upper tract urolithiasis that is due to erosion of a stone into a calyx. *Dystrophic calcification* is the third major category of calculus disease of the urinary tract. This refers to calcification of abnormal tissue, such as the wall of a renal cyst, inflammatory tissue, or neoplasm.

NEPHROCALCINOSIS

Nephrocalcinosis is uncommon in children. The pattern of nephrocalcinosis can be cortical, medullary, or both. The most common sites of calcium deposition are the tubules, tubular epithelium, and interstitial tissue. Most often, the calcification is multifocal and bilateral. Bilateral renal involvement, when present, helps distinguish nephrocalcinosis from focal dystrophic calcification.

Medullary Nephrocalcinosis

Medullary nephrocalcinosis accounts for more than 90% of nephrocalcinosis in children. The most common causes of medullary renal calcification in children are metabolic conditions that result in hypercalcemia and hypercalciuria (Table 147-1).

Type 1 renal tubular acidosis (RTA) is the most common metabolic condition associated with nephrocalcinosis in children. With type 1 RTA, appropriate hydrogen ion secretion does not occur in the distal renal tubules; thus, the kidneys are prevented from excreting acidic urine. This leads to bicarbonate loss, reduced acid excretion, secondary aldosteronism, and hypokalemia. Major factors that predispose these patients to renal calcification include hypercalciuria, alkaline urine, and diminished citrate elimination. Nephrocalcinosis occurs in about three quarters of patients with type 1 RTA and may progress to urolithiasis.

The long-term administration of *loop diuretics*, such as furosemide, is an important factor in nephrocalcinosis of neonates. Loop diuretics impair the reabsorption of magnesium and calcium, thereby producing hyper-

calciuria. Neonates are particular susceptible because of their low baseline rates of calcium absorption related to tubular immaturity (see Chapter 22). An inverse relationship has been observed between the prevalence of nephrocalcinosis in neonates receiving furosemide and the gestational age and birth weight. The typical time course to the earliest manifestations of stone formation is approximately 30 days after the start of diuretic therapy. Spontaneous resolution occurs in most, but not all, of these children within several months.

> The most common causes of medullary nephrocalcinosis are renal tubular acidosis, diuretic use, and metabolic conditions that produce hypercalcemia and hypercalciuria.

TABLE 147-1

Causes of Medullary Nephrocalcinosis

Hypercalciuria
  Endocrine
    Hyperparathyroidism
    Cushing syndrome
    Diabetes insipidus
    Hyperthyroidism
  Renal
    Renal tubular acidosis
  Alimentary
    Milk alkali syndrome
    Hypervitaminosis D
  Skeletal
    Immobilization
    Metastatic disease
  Drugs
    Furosemide
    Steroids
  Miscellaneous
    Idiopathic hypercalciuria
    Idiopathic hypercalcemia
    Nephropathic cystinosis
Urinary stasis
  Obstructive uropathy
  Medullary sponge kidney
Hyperoxaluria
  Primary
Hyperuricosuria
  Secondary

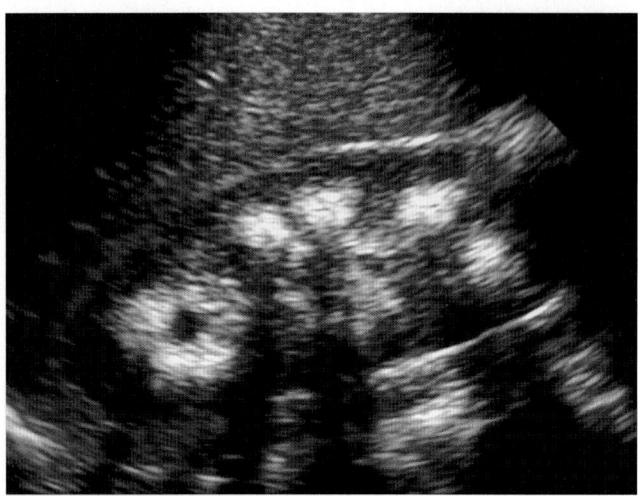

FIGURE 147-1. Medullary nephrocalcinosis. Longitudinal sonographic image of a child with type 1 renal tubular acidosis and medullary nephrocalcinosis shows markedly echogenic renal pyramids, some of which produce acoustic shadowing.

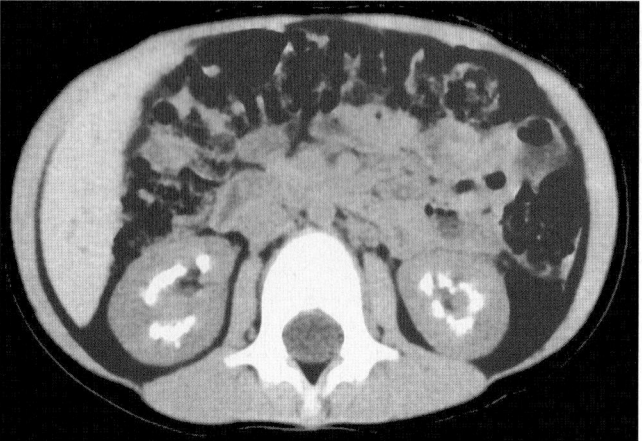

FIGURE 147-2. Medullary nephrocalcinosis. Unenhanced computed tomography shows dense renal pyramid calcifications in a child with type 1 renal tubular acidosis.

TABLE 147-2
Causes of Cortical Nephrocalcinosis
Renal cortical necrosis
Chronic glomerulonephritis
Renal transplant rejection
Alport syndrome
Ethylene glycol poisoning
Hyperoxaluria
AIDS-associated infections

AIDS, acquired immunodeficiency syndrome.

Medullary sponge kidney is an idiopathic developmental abnormality in which collecting tubule dilation occurs in one or more renal pyramids. Involvement is usually diffuse and bilateral but can be unilateral or segmental. Calcifications can form within the dilated collecting tubules; the pathogenesis apparently involves urinary stasis, hypercalciuria, and RTA. These calcifications can migrate into the pelvicalyceal system. Macroscopic renal calcifications are present in about 15% of patients with medullary sponge kidney.

The major sonographic feature of medullary nephrocalcinosis is hyperechogenicity of one or more renal pyramids (Fig. 147-1). With macroscopic calcification, acoustic shadowing is usually noted. The earliest sonographic sign of medullary nephrocalcinosis is loss of normal papillary hypoechogenicity. In some instances, hyperechogenicity is confined to the tips of the pyramids.

With extensive nephrocalcinosis, medullary calcifications are visible on standard radiographs. With most forms of medullary nephrocalcinosis, diffuse or uniform calcifications are seen within the medullary pyramids, resulting in a triangular pattern. Renal calcification in patients with type 1 RTA typically involves all the medullary pyramids in a uniform fashion, with extensive dense calcification. Calcifications associated with medullary sponge kidney tend to be asymmetric. Intravenous urography of patients with medullary sponge kidney reveals contrast-filled ectatic tubules, in addition to the calcifications.

Computed tomography (CT) is a sensitive imaging technique for the detection of renal calcifications that allows definitive localization to the medullary or cortical region (Fig. 147-2). With medullary sponge kidney, medullary calculi typically occur in clusters within the renal pyramids. Stagnation of contrast is evident within the dilated collecting tubules on enhanced CT. With mild disease, this appears as linear papillary opacities; small cystic components may be visible with more advanced disease. Contrast within the collecting tubules surrounds calculi. In patients with RTA, the contrast does not uniformly surround calcific deposits because calcification occurs within the medullary interstitium and within the tubular lumina.

The Anderson-Carr-Randall progression theory of urolithiasis suggests that microscopic calcifications within a renal pyramid can coalesce to form a plaque that migrates toward the calyx to form a stone nidus. These microscopic calcifications arise as the result of high calcium concentrations in the peritubular fluid spaces when the amount of calcium exceeds the capacity of lymphatic clearance. High-resolution ultrasonography in young children may reveal papillary hyperechogenicity caused by these microscopic calcifications despite normal findings on other imaging studies; hyperechoic pyramids are present in about 50% of children with diseases that predispose to nephrocalcinosis. Subepithelial calcium phosphate plaques sometimes are visible on radiographs or CT as slivers of calcification adjacent to the papillary tip.

Cortical Nephrocalcinosis

Cortical nephrocalcinosis involves the periphery of the kidney and the central septa of Bertin. In the pure forms of cortical nephrocalcinosis, the medullary pyramids are not involved. The most common causes of cortical nephrocalcinosis are chronic glomerulonephritis, acute cortical necrosis, and oxalosis (Table 147-2). Standard abdominal radiographs may show thin linear peripheral calcifications, diffuse homogeneous renal calcification, or diffuse punctate calcifications. On sonography, the involved cortex is echogenic, but acoustic shadowing does not occur unless conglomerate calcifications are present. CT accurately reveals the cortical location of calcification.

Hyperoxaluria can cause cortical nephrocalcinosis, mixed medullary and cortical nephrocalcinosis, or nephrolithiasis. Calcium oxalate crystal deposition usually occurs in various extrarenal tissues as well. Renal calcifications in these patients are often predominantly cortical and may be patchy or homogeneous. Occasionally, calcification occurs throughout the cortical and medullary regions. During infancy, sonography may reveal enlarged hyperechoic kidneys, without acoustic shadowing. Eventually, parenchymal thickness decreases. In addition to nephrocalcinosis, radiographic studies of children with hyperoxaluria may show skeletal manifestations of renal osteodystrophy and deposition of oxalate within bone.

Acute renal cortical necrosis is a potential consequence of severe, prolonged shock. Renal ischemia leads to necrosis of the renal cortex, with relative sparing of the medulla. The pathophysiology may involve selective spasm of the small intracortical arteries. Parenchymal involvement can be diffuse, multifocal, or focal. Sparing of a subcapsular rim of cortex often occurs as the result of collateral circulation.

The earliest sonographic feature of acute renal cortical necrosis is loss of normal cortical-medullary differentiation. A hypoechoic rim may be seen at the outer margin of the cortex. CT during this acute phase shows lack of enhancement of most of the renal cortex, with preserved enhancement of the medulla and a thin subcapsular rim (the "cortical rim sign"). Within a few weeks of the injury, sonography may show prominent cortical echogenicity due to early calcification. Calcifications become more obvious sonographically and radiographically over time. Progressive renal atrophy also occurs.

Various potential patterns of nephrocalcinosis are associated with renal cortical necrosis. In some patients, punctate calcifications predominate, representing necrotic cortical glomeruli and tubules. An additional potential pattern is bandlike peripheral calcification with perpendicular extensions into the columns of Bertin. Thin, parallel curvilinear calcifications (continuous or interrupted) may be noted at the interface between the necrotic cortex and the viable subcapsular cortex (i.e., the "tram-track" pattern).

UROLITHIASIS

Epidemiology

The prevalence of urolithiasis varies according to geographic area, age, sex, and race. The prevalence of urolithiasis in children in the United States is approximately 1 in 1000. About 7000 hospital admissions per year involve pediatric patients with urinary tract stones. Urolithiasis is slightly more common in Europe than in North America and is considerably more common in Asia. In American children, the prevalence of urolithiasis is greatest in southern California and in the southeastern states.

The predominant mechanisms of stone formation and stone types also vary with geographic region. Bladder stones are endemic in most developing countries, at least in part because of the predominantly cereal-based low-protein diets that children in these areas consume. In contrast, upper tract stones predominate in the developed countries of Europe and North America. As living standards improve in a geographic area, a shift from lower tract to upper tract stones tends to occur. In the United Kingdom and some European countries, many calculi are due to urinary tract infections, whereas metabolic disorders are the most common causes of kidney stones in the United States and Scandinavia.

In contrast to the marked male predominance of urolithiasis in adults, only minimal male prominence is reported in children; the male-to-female ratio is approximately 1.4:1. Urolithiasis is more common in whites than in African Americans. Reported recurrence rates for urinary stones in children range from 6% to 50%, and the mean interval to recurrence is 3 to 5 years.

Mechanism

Urinary tract stone disease involves the formation of a crystal lattice in urine (nucleation) and retention of the growing stone within the urinary tract. Three major factors affect the propensity for stone formation: (1) concentrations of the precipitating substances (i.e., the crystallizing salts) and the solubilities of these substances in urine, (2) the presence of promoters of crystallization and aggregation, and (3) levels of inhibitors of crystallization and aggregation. Supersaturation refers to urinary concentrations of a substance at which crystal formation occurs in the presence of pre-existing nuclei, such as other crystals, cellular debris, or hyaline urinary casts. Spontaneous crystal formation occurs only at higher concentrations of the substance (i.e., concentrations above the formation product). Urine pH is an important ancillary factor that affects the solubility of some stone-forming substances. An increase in urine pH increases the solubility of uric acid, but a high pH decreases calcium phosphate solubility. The pH also affects the availability of inhibitors of crystal formation, thereby influencing the state of saturation of some stone-forming salts.

Crystallization inhibitors in urine include magnesium, pyrophosphate, and citrate. Inhibitors of crystallization act by binding particular lithogenic ions, thereby decreasing their concentration in the urine. Complexes formed by this process are more soluble than are free ions. Citrate and pyrophosphate act by binding to calcium, and magnesium and sodium bind oxalate. Other inhibitors include glycosaminoglycans, uropontin, and Tamm-Horsfall mucoprotein. In some stone-forming patients, an organic matrix in the urine may promote crystallization. As was noted earlier, some urinary tract calculi arise in the renal pyramids and migrate into the collecting system, where further deposition of crystallizing salts can occur (i.e., the Anderson-Carr-Randall progression theory). Many of the medical conditions that are associated with nephrocalcinosis also impart a propensity for urolithiasis.

The predominant cation of most urinary tract calculi is calcium; calcium-containing stones account for at least 75% to 80% of urinary calculi in North American children. Most of these stones contain combinations of calcium, oxalate, and phosphate salts. Infection-related stones include struvite (magnesium ammonium phosphate) and carbonate apatite (calcium carbonate and calcium phosphate); these account for 10% to 15% of pediatric stones. Calcium and apatite stones are moderately to markedly radiopaque. Uric acid stones account for less than 5% of urinary stones. They are radiolucent in pure form but relatively radiopaque when mixed with calcium salts or struvite. Cystine stones are rare and are moderately radiopaque because of their physical density and higher effective atomic number compared with adjacent fluid and tissue. They may occur in mixed form with calcium oxalate or calcium phosphate. Xanthine stones that occur in pure form are radiolucent. Matrix stones consist of nonradiopaque inspissated mucoproteins, usually in conjunction with laminated or scattered calcific components (Table 147-3).

Pediatric urinary tract calculi:

- **75% to 80% calcium oxalate and calcium phosphate**
- **10% to 15% magnesium ammonium phosphate, calcium carbonate, calcium phosphate (infection related)**
- **<5% uric acid**
- **Rare: cystine and xanthine**

Idiopathic Stones

About 30% of pediatric urolithiasis is idiopathic (i.e., it has no known predisposing condition). Calcium phosphate or calcium oxalate represents the usual composition. Idiopathic calcium stones may have a nucleus of urate, indicating that the primary disease is uric acid lithiasis rather than primary calcium stone disease.

Stones Related to Urinary Stasis, Foreign Body, or Urinary Tract Infection

Stasis of urine is associated with a propensity for urolithiasis. Urinary stasis results in diminished flushing of microcrystals from the urinary tract, thereby allowing aggregation into macroscopic stones. Stasis may result in elevated concentrations of crystallizing salts. Other potential consequences of urinary stasis that result in a favorable environment for stone formation include chronic or recurrent infection, endothelial damage that leads to defective distal tubular acidification, and elevation of urine pH. Obstructing lesions of the urinary tract cause urinary stasis and can impede passage of a small stone. About 30% of children with urolithiasis have myelodysplasia, and 26% have some other structural abnormality of the urinary tract. The most common causes of urinary stasis in children are neurogenic bladder and congenital urinary tract anomalies such as ureteropelvic junction obstruction and obstructed megaureter (Fig. 147-3). Pyelocalyceal diverticulum is a developmental lesion of the intrarenal collecting system that is characterized by a localized form of urinary stasis; stones are relatively common in these diverticula. Surgical urinary diversions, such as an ileal loop, may lead to urinary stasis and stone disease.

Urinary tract stones containing magnesium ammonium phosphate form when urine pH is greater than 7.2, and they commonly occur in the setting of a urinary tract infection with a urea-splitting gram-negative enteric organism such as *Proteus mirabilis*, *Klebsiella*, *Proteus vulgaris*, and *Pseudomonas aeruginosa*. These calculi are commonly termed *infection stones*. Pure magnesium ammonium phosphate (struvite) stones are rare. Most often, calcium phosphate (apatite) is also present; this mixture of struvite and apatite represents the "triple phosphate stone," which is the most common type of infection stone. Nonstruvite stones can also occur in association with urinary tract infections; these are termed *infection-associated stones*. Matrix calculi are rare stones that can occur in association with chronic urinary tract infections.

TABLE 147-3		
Radiopacity of Urinary Stones		
	Mineral Composition	**Opacity**
Calcium stones		
	Calcium oxalate	+++
	Calcium phosphate	+++
	Calcium hydrogen phosphate	+++
Struvite	Magnesium ammonium phosphate	−
Triple phosphate		++
Cystine		+
Uric acid		−
Xanthine		−
Matrix		−

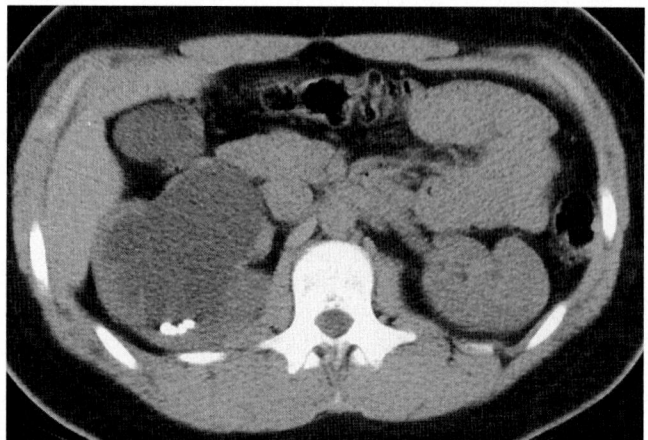

FIGURE 147-3. Urolithiasis. Unenhanced computed tomography scan shows multiple small stones in the dependent portion of a dilated right renal collecting system.

About 30% of patients with infection-induced stones have an anatomic lesion that probably contributes to stone formation. These include ureteropelvic junction obstruction, neurogenic bladder, obstructed megaureter, and surgical urinary diversion. Vesicoureteral reflux is present in 10% of patients with infection stones. Infection stones compromise approximately 25% of the total number of urolithiasis cases in North American children, and 50% of cases in European children. Two thirds of patients with infection stones are younger than 5 years of age. This type of stone is located in the pelvicalyceal system in about 70% of cases.

The injured uroepithelial lining in the presence of urinary tract infection can serve as a nidus for crystal aggregation. Infection-induced bacterial and inflammatory cellular debris represents an additional potential nidus. These factors allow stone growth at lower solute concentrations through the process of heterogeneous nucleation. Infections with urea-splitting gram-negative organisms cause the release of ammonia into the urine, where urease from the bacteria acts on urea in the urine. This increases urine pH and urine ammonium; the ammonium substantially binds with phosphate and magnesium ions, thereby facilitating the formation of struvite stones. These stones often achieve a large size; about 70% of staghorn calculi are infection-related struvite stones (Fig. 147-4). Surgical removal is often required for effective treatment of infection stones. Bacteria interspersed within the structure of the stone interfere with antibiotic penetration, leading to recurrence or persistence of the infection. Therefore, treatment of infection stones usually consists of aggressive antibiotic therapy and complete removal of all stone fragments. The recurrence rate after initial management is higher than 10%, and in those cases associated with anatomic abnormalities, the median interval to recurrence after initial surgery is approximately 1 year.

Foreign material in the urinary tract can serve as an initiator for stone formation. The surface of an indwelling urinary catheter can act as a nidus for stone formation. In addition, most patients with a long-standing urinary catheter have an underlying obstruction or other condition that is associated with stasis of urine. Indwelling catheters also may become colonized with bacteria. Therefore, patients with medically introduced foreign material often have multiple risk factors for stone disease (Fig. 147-5).

Hypercalciuria

Hypercalciuria is the most common biochemical abnormality in children with urolithiasis. Patients with hypercalciuria are at risk for the formation of calcium-containing stones, most often calcium oxalate. The three basic mechanisms of hypercalciuria are increased intestinal absorption of calcium, excessive calcium mobilization from bone, and decreased renal tubular reabsorption of calcium (Table 147-4). Although some of these disorders are associated with elevated blood calcium levels (e.g., sarcoidosis), 98% of pediatric urinary tract stone disease occurs in the presence of normocalcemia. Many of the disorders associated with urolithiasis also can lead to nephrocalcinosis (see earlier).

Idiopathic hypercalciuria is the most common form of

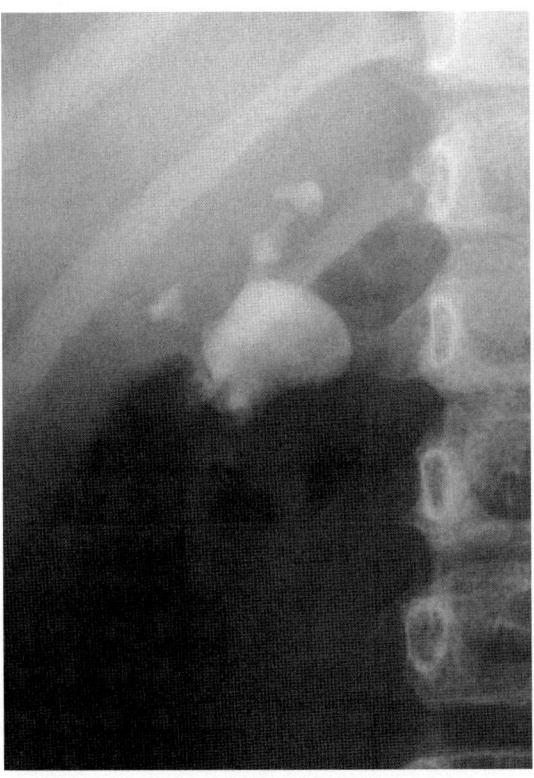

FIGURE 147-4. Staghorn calculus. Radiograph reveals a triple phosphate infection stone with a staghorn configuration.

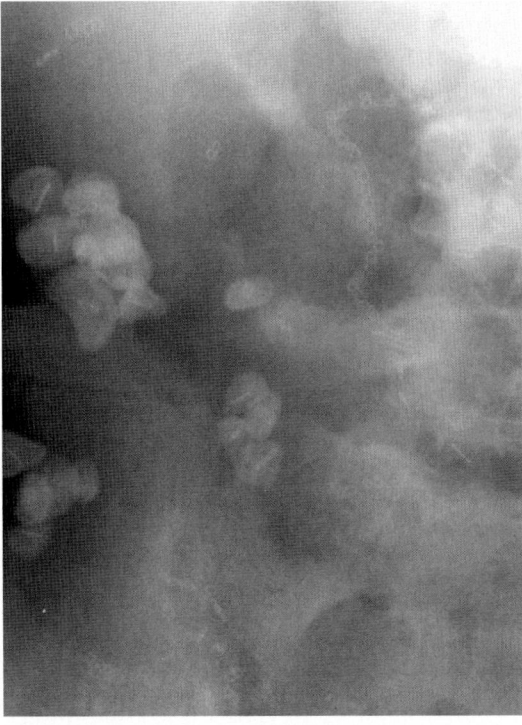

FIGURE 147-5. Bladder calculi. Radiograph shows multiple calculi within a bladder augmentation. A surgical clip serves as the nidus for each of the stones.

TABLE 147-4
Causes of Hypercalciuria

Increased absorption
    Idiopathic hypercalciuria
    Hypervitaminosis D
    Sarcoidosis
    Idiopathic infantile hypercalcemia
Increased mobilization
    Immobilization
    Hyperparathyroidism
    Prolonged corticosteroid therapy
    Hyperthyroidism
    Bone metastasis
    Juvenile rheumatoid arthritis
Decreased tubular resorption
    Type 1 renal tubular acidosis
    Long-term diuretic use
    Fanconi syndrome

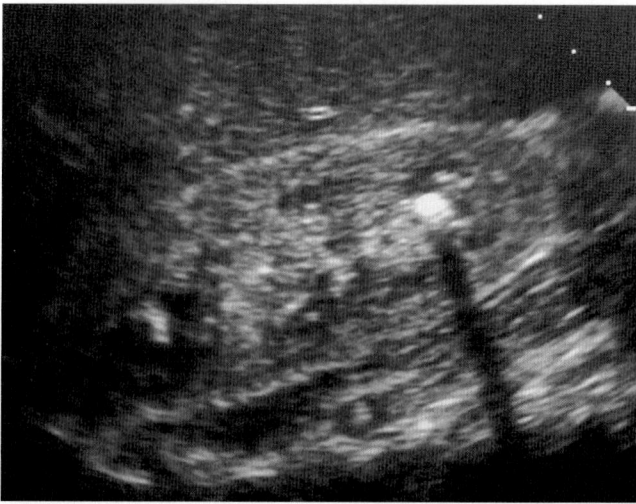

FIGURE 147-6. Nephrolithiasis. Longitudinal sonographic image of an infant with hypercalcemia and Williams syndrome reveals an echogenic calculus in a right lower pole calyx.

elevated urinary calcium. This term encompasses various idiopathic disorders. Patients have elevated levels of urinary calcium while consuming a regular diet; by definition, this medical condition has no known cause. Most commonly, idiopathic hypercalciuria behaves as an autosomal dominant disorder with incomplete penetrance. Therefore, a family history of urolithiasis is often reported. The mechanism may involve an alteration in intestinal response to vitamin D, resulting in increased absorption of calcium and suppression of parathyroid function. The most common clinical feature of idiopathic hypercalciuria is hematuria, usually microscopic. Patients may develop flank pain, dysuria, frequency, or enuresis. Without therapy, approximately 20% of children with idiopathic hypercalciuria develop symptomatic urolithiasis within 5 years of onset of hematuria.

Idiopathic infantile hypercalcemia is a rare disorder that is apparently caused by mutations in the elastin gene on the long arm of chromosome 7. It can occur in association with Williams syndrome (Fig. 147-6). Other causes of hypercalcemia in infants include dietary deficiency of phosphate, excessive administration of calcium or vitamin D, neonatal hyperparathyroidism, and Murk Jansen syndrome.

Hyperparathyroidism accounts for up to 10% of calcium stone disease in adults, but is uncommon in children. Patients may form calcium oxalate or calcium phosphate stones. Elevated serum parathyroid hormone concentrations lead to increased intestinal absorption of calcium and bone resorption of calcium. Although it is most often a sporadic disorder, primary hyperparathyroidism occasionally occurs as an isolated autosomal dominant disorder or as a component of a multiple endocrine neoplasia (MEN) syndrome. Hyperparathyroidism occurs in 95% of patients with MEN 1.

Sarcoidosis is a chronic granulomatous disorder. Although it is predominantly a disease of adults, sarcoidosis can occur in children of all ages. An increased prevalence has been observed in African Americans and Hispanic children. Granulomatous pulmonary disease results in the major clinical manifestations of sarcoidosis.

Urolithiasis is most common in those with extensive active disease or a coexistent risk factor such as high dietary calcium and vitamin D. The pathogenesis of urinary tract stone disease in patients with sarcoidosis predominantly involves excessive intestinal absorption of calcium due to abnormal production of activated vitamin D by macrophages. Renal damage may be caused by granulomas. Most urinary tract stones in patients with sarcoidosis are composed of pure calcium oxalate.

Type 1 (distal) renal tubular acidosis (RTA), in its primary and secondary forms, leads to hypercalciuria. An alkaline urine, hyperphosphaturia, and low urine citrate also facilitate stone formation. Most urinary tract stones in patients with RTA are composed of calcium phosphate or calcium carbonate; calcium oxalate stones also occur.

Immobilization for as short as several weeks can lead to hypercalciuria. This is predominantly the result of increased mobilization of calcium from bone. Long-term diuretic use (especially furosemide) can lead to urolithiasis; premature infants with chronic lung disease and young children with congestive heart failure are most susceptible. Other potential causes of calcium urolithiasis in children include excess exogenous vitamin D, malignancies with metastatic bone disease, and juvenile rheumatoid arthritis.

Hyperoxaluria

Because most calcium-containing stones in the urinary tract occur as calcium oxalate compounds, excess levels of urinary oxalate can lead to urolithiasis. *Hyperoxaluria* indicates an abnormally increased concentration of oxalate in the urine. *Oxalosis* refers to precipitation of oxalate crystals in extrarenal tissues, such as myocardium, lung, or spleen. Oxalate is an end product of normal metabolism. Excretion occurs primarily via the kidneys. Most urine oxalate derives from endogenous metabolism; ascorbic acid and glyoxylic acid represent the main precursors. Normally, about 10% of urine oxalate derives from diet. Patients with hyperoxaluria may develop nephrocalcinosis (cortical more commonly than medullary) or urolithiasis. Hyperoxaluria accounts for about 2% of calcium urolithiasis in children.

Hyperoxaluria and oxalosis occur in primary and secondary forms. *Primary oxaluria* is a rare autosomal recessive disorder of glyoxylate metabolism. Urolithiasis and nephrocalcinosis are common in these children. This disorder may account for up to 50% of oxalate stones in children. Two types of primary hyperoxaluria have been identified: Type I (80%) is due to a deficiency in the hepatic peroxisomal enzyme alanine-glyoxylate aminotransferase; type II is due to a deficiency of the enzyme D-glycerate dehydrogenase. Type I, the more clinically severe of the two forms, usually presents early in childhood with manifestations of nephrolithiasis and urolithiasis; progression to renal failure is typical.

The most common secondary form of hyperoxaluria and oxalosis is due to small-bowel disease, such as Crohn disease or extensive small bowel resection. Fat malabsorption in these patients causes complexing of calcium by fatty acids within the intestinal lumen, which allows absorption of a greater quantity of free oxalate (i.e., increased solubility of oxalate). Increased permeability of the colon accentuates oxalate absorption. A high dietary consumption of oxalate-containing foods appears to be a rare factor in oxalate urolithiasis; foods with high oxalate content include rhubarb, peanuts, spinach, and collard greens. Hyperoxaluria can occur with overconsumption of vitamin C supplements.

Hyperuricosuria

In North America, uric acid stones account for about 5% of urolithiasis in children. As with other forms of urolithiasis, considerable geographic variation has been noted in the prevalence of uric acid stones; about three quarters of urinary tract calculi in Israel are composed of uric acid. Most patients with uric acid stones have hyperuricosuria, but they do not necessarily have hyperuricemia. Low urine pH and low urine volume facilitate uric acid stone formation. These stones can also occur in the presence of elevated urine ammonium concentration caused by urinary tract infection, dehydration, or starvation. Uric acid is the end product of purine metabolism. In the urine, uric acid occurs as free or as relatively soluble sodium urate; in acidic urine, a greater proportion of the less soluble free form is found. Persistently low urine pH can occur in patients with chronic diarrhea or who have undergone an ileostomy, and in those taking medications to acidify their urine.

A relatively common cause of hyperuricosuria is elevated purine biosynthesis, as occurs in lymphoproliferative and myeloproliferative disorders. During the active stage of tumor reduction after chemotherapy or radiation therapy, precipitation of uric acid crystals within the collecting tubules can lead to intrarenal urinary obstruction, oliguria, and anuria. Uric acid stones can also occur in patients with polycythemia. Other causes of hyperuricosuria include a high purine diet, various medications (e.g., salicylates, probenecid), obesity, and alcohol abuse. Hyperuricemia and hyperuricosuria are common in patients with Lesch-Nyhan syndrome.

Cystinuria

Cystinuria is a rare autosomal recessive genetic disorder that is characterized by abnormal transport of the dibasic amino acids cystine, lysine, ornithine, and arginine into the proximal renal tubules and the gastrointestinal tract. The responsible gene is *SLC3A1*. Three genetically distinct forms of cystinuria have been identified. Type I is the most common and severe, and types II and III are homozygous variants. Although increased levels of all four dibasic amino acids occur, stone formation involves only cystine because of its poor solubility. Other clinical disorders associated with cystinuria include hemophilia, retinitis pigmentosa, Down syndrome, muscular dystrophy, and hereditary pancreatitis.

Cystinuria accounts for about 5% of urolithiasis in North American children. Urinary tract stone disease is the only important clinical consequence of cystinuria. The clinical presentation of stone disease in these patients can occur at any time from infancy through adulthood; the peak age of presentation is during the second and third decades of life. Recurrent stone disease can lead to progressive renal damage.

Xanthinuria

Xanthine stones are rare. They may occur with hereditary xanthinuria and in patients treated with allopurinol. Hereditary xanthinuria is an autosomal recessive disorder of purine metabolism that is characterized by diminished conversion of hypoxanthine and xanthine to uric acid. Many patients with xanthinuria are asymptomatic. Xanthine urolithiasis occurs in about 25% to 30% of affected patients.

Location of Stones

About half of urinary system stones are located only in the kidney and 15% are located in the kidney and the ureter. Stones in the pelvicalyceal system may be single or multiple and range in size from tiny, sandlike densities to large, conglomerate masses. A staghorn calculus refers to a stone that produces a cast of the pelvicalyceal system. A staghorn calculus is usually a struvite stone, but occasionally, it consists of uric acid, cystine, or calcium oxalate. Most patients with a staghorn calculus have preexisting obstructive hydronephrosis. Renal urolithiasis can also occur within a congenital calyceal diverticulum, congenitally obstructed calyces, or dilated tubules of medullary sponge kidney. A genitourinary anomaly is present in at least one third of children with nephrocalcinosis and in nearly all patients with renal calculi related to infection.

Ureteral calculi typically originate in the pelvicalyceal system; rarely, primary stone formation occurs within the ureter, proximal to an obstruction or on the surface of a foreign object. Most symptomatic ureteral stones are located in the distal portion of the ureter and are associated with some degree of obstruction. A stone may also lodge at the ureteropelvic junction.

Stones within the urinary bladder may originate from the upper urinary tract or may form within the bladder

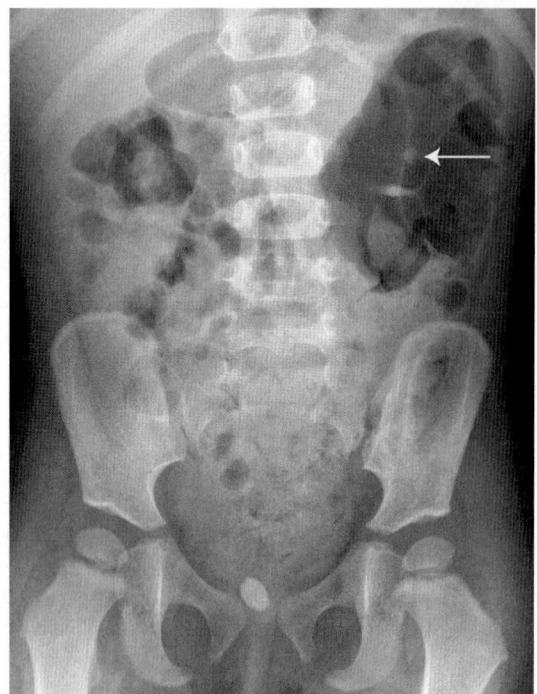

FIGURE 147-7. Calculi. Abdominal radiograph reveals an oval bladder calculus and a smaller stone in the left kidney *(arrow)*.

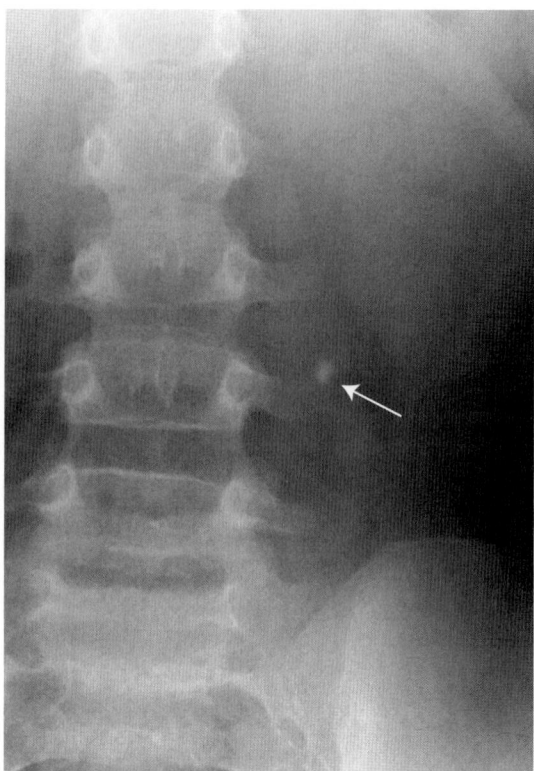

FIGURE 147-9. Ureteral calculus. Radiograph shows a calcium oxalate stone *(arrow)* in the left ureter.

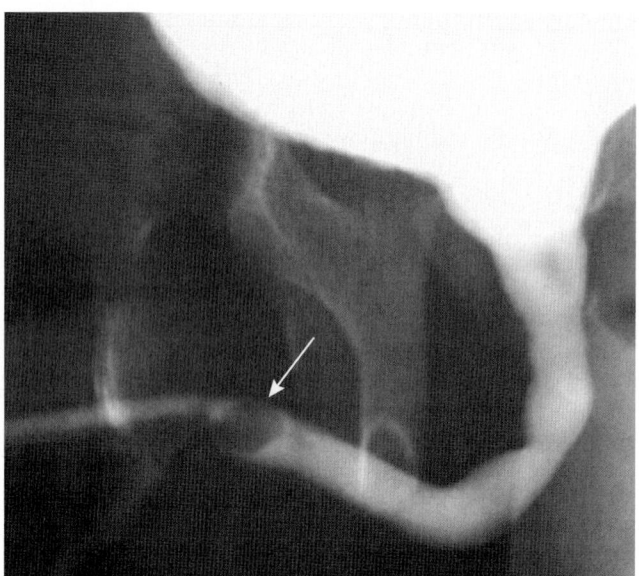

FIGURE 147-8. Urethral calculus. Urethrogram shows a partially obstructing urethral calculus as a filling defect *(arrow)* in the contrast column.

(Fig. 147-7). Stones that form in the bladder may occur in association with chronic bladder infection, neurogenic bladder, hypotonic bladder, or an intravesical foreign body. Bladder stones are often laminated and sometimes reach a very large size. Bladder stones can form in a bladder diverticulum, surgical pouch, or urachal remnant.

Urethral calculi are rare and only occur in males (Fig. 147-8). They may originate from a more proximal portion of the urinary tract or may form locally. Stasis and infection are important factors in the development of primary urethral calculi. These may develop in association with prolonged obstruction or may form within a urethral diverticulum or the prostatic utricle.

Clinical Presentation

The most common clinical manifestation of urolithiasis is pain, which is present in 50% to 75% of children at the time of diagnosis. The pain often has a nonspecific character and can be vague, dull, or sharp. Pain may localize to the abdomen or flank and may or may not radiate. The classical adult pattern of renal colic with intermittent excruciating pain that radiates to the groin is rare in children. Hematuria occurs in 50% to 90% of children with urolithiasis. Additional potential clinical manifestations include urgency, dysuria, frequency, fever, pyuria, and bacteriuria. Pain tends to be the most frequent presenting symptom in older children with urolithiasis; younger patients often are asymptomatic or have findings of a urinary tract infection. Urinary retention may occur with bladder and urethral stones.

In the acute setting, medical management of urolithiasis involves analgesia, treatment of concurrent infection, and increased hydration to promote passage of the stone. Calculi smaller than 6 mm in greatest dimension usually pass spontaneously. Maintenance of adequate fluid intake is an important long-term treatment for prevention of further stone formation. Disease-specific measures may be helpful when an underlying cause of urolithiasis, such as a metabolic disorder, is discernible.

Diagnostic Imaging

About 90% of urinary tract calculi are sufficiently radiopaque for visualization on standard radiographs (Fig. 147-9). From a classification standpoint, a radiopaque versus nonopaque (or radiolucent) stone refers to its appearance on standard radiographs; most nonopaque stones are hyperattenuating on CT. Important influences regarding the radiographic detectability of a urinary tract stone are the size and composition of the stone, the radiographic technique used, and the nature of overlying structures. In general, calcium stones are radiopaque. Stones composed of pure uric acid, xanthine, or struvite are usually nonopaque. Cystine stones are moderately radiopaque (see Table 147-3).

Bowel and skeletal structures can obscure a small urinary tract calculus on standard radiographs. In addition, ingested material and various non–urinary tract calcifications in the abdomen and pelvis can mimic the appearance of urolithiasis. Gallstones can project over the right kidney. Costal cartilage calcifications sometimes overlie the kidneys as well. The most common mimicking structure in the pelvis is a phlebolith. Phleboliths are usually round, have a central lucency, and are located in the inferior aspect of the true pelvis.

In current practice, excretory urography is not part of the standard evaluation of the patient with suspected stone disease. A preliminary radiograph should always be obtained because contrast can obscure a small stone. With acute obstruction due to urolithiasis, excretory urography shows delayed opacification of the involved collecting system. Delay is noted in the ipsilateral nephrogram, along with subsequent persistence of a dense nephrogram. In patients with no underlying anatomic abnormalities, the most common sites of a symptomatic stone are the ureteropelvic junction, the point at which the ureter crosses the iliac vessels, and the ureterovesical junction.

Both radiopaque and nonopaque urinary tract stones appear echogenic on sonography and produce acoustic shadowing (Fig. 147-6). Sonography is sensitive for the detection of nephrolithiasis but is of limited use for visualizing calculi in the ureters. An obstructing ureteral calculus usually is associated with some degree of ureteropelvocalyectasis, however. The sonographic appearance of acoustic shadowing aids in the differentiation of a bladder calculus from blood clot, debris, or tumor.

Helical CT is the most sensitive imaging technique used for the detection of urolithiasis (Fig. 147-10). Regardless of composition, nearly all urinary tract stones are hyperattenuating on CT. Calcium oxalate stones generally have attenuation values in the 800 to 1000 HU range, infection stones are in the 300 to 900 HU range, and uric acid stones usually measure between 150 to 500 HU. Secondary CT signs of an obstructing urinary tract stone include hydronephrosis, hydroureter, nephromegaly, periureteral edema, and perinephric stranding or fluid. As with standard radiography, non–urinary tract calcifications sometimes mimic a ureteral calculus on CT. Usually, the portion of the ureteral wall that surrounds a calculus thickens (i.e., the "rim sign"); this sign is typically lacking with a phlebolith or other mimicking calcification. A linear soft tissue density (the involved pelvic vein) often extends from a phlebolith; this is the "comet tail sign." Supplemental CT images obtained in the prone or decubitus position can be helpful in differentiating a calculus in the bladder from a distal ureteral stone.

SUGGESTED READINGS

Abrahams HM, Stoller ML: Infection and urinary stones. Curr Opin Urol 2003;13:63-67

Alon US: Nephrocalcinosis. Curr Opin Pediatr 1997;9:160-165

Bartosh SM: Medical management of pediatric stone disease. Urol Clin North Am 2004;31:575-587, x-xi

Cameron MA, Sakhaee K, Moe OW: Nephrolithiasis in children. Pediatr Nephrol 2005;20:1587-1592

Coward RJ, Peters CJ, Duffy PG, et al: Epidemiology of paediatric renal stone disease in the UK. Arch Dis Child 2003;88:962-965

Diallo O, Janssens F, Hall M, et al: Type 1 primary hyperoxaluria in pediatric patients: renal sonographic patterns. AJR Am J Roentgenol 2004;183:1767-1770

Dick PT, Shuckett BM, Tang B, et al: Observer reliability in grading nephrocalcinosis on ultrasound examinations in children. Pediatr Radiol 1999;29:68-72

Downing GJ, Egelhoff JC, Daily DK, et al: Furosemide-related renal calcifications in the premature infant: a longitudinal ultrasonographic study. Pediatr Radiol 1991;21:563-565

Faerber GJ: Pediatric urolithiasis. Curr Opin Urol 2001;11:385-389

Francois M, Tostivint I, Mercadal L, et al: MR imaging features of acute bilateral renal cortical necrosis. Am J Kidney Dis 2000; 35:745-748

Gillespie RS, Stapleton FB: Nephrolithiasis in children. Pediatr Rev 2004;25:131-139

Kimme-Smith C, Perrella RR, Kaveggia LP, et al: Detection of renal stones with real-time sonography: effect of transducers and scanning parameters. AJR Am J Roentgenol 1991;157:975-980

Knoll T, Zollner A, Wendt-Nordahl G, et al: Cystinuria in childhood and adolescence: recommendations for diagnosis, treatment, and follow-up. Pediatr Nephrol 2005;20:19-24

Kraus SJ, Lebowitz RL, Royal SA: Renal calculi in children: imaging features that lead to diagnoses: a pictorial essay. Pediatr Radiol 1999;29:624-630

Laing CM, Toye AM, Capasso G, et al: Renal tubular acidosis: developments in our understanding of the molecular basis. Int J Biochem Cell Biol 2005;37:1151-1161

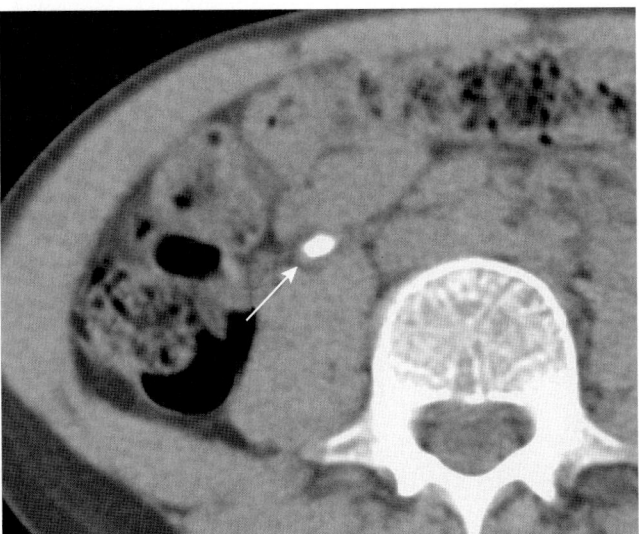

FIGURE 147-10. Ureteral calculus. Unenhanced computed tomography shows a right ureteral calculus with a surrounding thickened ureteral rim *(arrow)*.

Lieske JC, Monico CG, Holmes WS, et al: International registry for primary hyperoxaluria. Am J Nephrol 2005;25:290-296

Memarsadeghi M, Heinz-Peer G, Helbich TH, et al: Unenhanced multi-detector row CT in patients suspected of having urinary stone disease: effect of section width on diagnosis. Radiology 2005;235:530-536

Palmer JS, Donaher ER, O'Riordan MA, et al: Diagnosis of pediatric urolithiasis: role of ultrasound and computerized tomography. J Urol 2005;174(4 Pt 1):1413-1416

Patriquin H, Robitaille P: Renal calcium deposition in children: sonographic demonstration of the Anderson-Carr progression. AJR Am J Roentgenol 1986;146:1253-1256

Schwartz BF, Stoller ML: The vesical calculus. Urol Clin North Am 2000;27:333-346

Stapleton FB: Childhood stones. Endocrinol Metab Clin North Am 2002;31:1001-1015, ix

Strouse PJ, Bates DG, Bloom DA, et al: Non-contrast thin-section helical CT of urinary tract calculi in children. Pediatr Radiol 2002;32:326-332

Renal Neoplasms

KATE A. FEINSTEIN

NEPHROBLASTOMATOSIS COMPLEX

Nephrogenesis is completed by the 36th gestational week. A focus of fetal metanephric blastema or embryonal renal tissue that persists into infancy is called a *nephrogenic rest*. Multiple foci or diffuse nephrogenic rests are termed *nephroblastomatosis*. Nephroblastomatosis is identified in about 1% of neonatal autopsies, but these areas are usually no longer found after 4 months of age. Genetic abnormalities and syndromes may be associated with nephroblastomatosis; however, most patients with nephroblastomatosis do not have these abnormalities. Malignant transformation of the fetal metanephric blastema may occur, along with development of Wilms tumor (nephroblastoma), or nephroblastomatosis may resolve spontaneously.

> **Nephroblastomatosis commonly regresses and resolves spontaneously; however, it may degenerate into Wilms tumor.**

Nephrogenic rests can occur anywhere in the kidney, depending on when nephrogenesis is interrupted. These may be located in the renal lobe (intralobar) or in the cortex that envelops the renal lobe (perilobar). The two types of nephrogenic rests have different appearances, malignant potential, and associated genetic abnormalities. Nephrogenic rests are also classified according to histologic features of development; hyperplastic rests are thought to be active and to have malignant potential. Regressing or sclerosing nephrogenic rests are considered inactive.

Intralobar nephrogenic rests are less common than perilobar nephrogenic rests. Intralobar nephrogenic rests are more likely to degenerate into Wilms tumor. These tend to be few and are located randomly in the renal lobe. Intralobar nephrogenic rests are seen in patients with sporadic aniridia, Drash syndrome (male pseudophermaphrodism and nephritis), and WAGR syndrome (Wilms tumor, aniridia, genital anomalies, and mental retardation). Patients with sporadic aniridia have a 30% to 40% risk of developing Wilms tumor; this represents the greatest likelihood of all of the genetic and syndromic abnormalities associated with nephroblastomatosis.

> **Intralobar nephrogenic rests in association with genetic and syndromic abnormalities have the greatest increased risk of malignant transformation into Wilms tumor.**

Perilobar nephrogenic rests are multiple and are located at the corticomedullary junction or in the cortex. Also called *diffuse perilobar nephrogenic rests* or *diffuse perilobar nephroblastomatosis*, these are found in hemihypertrophy and in Beckwith-Wiedemann (macroglossia, macrosomia, and omphalocele), Perlman (fetal gigantism and multiple congenital anomalies), and trisomy 18 syndromes. Patients with hemihypertrophy and Beckwith-Wiedemann syndrome have about a 5% risk of developing Wilms tumor.

> **Perilobar nephrogenic rests associated with hemihypertrophy and Beckwith-Wiedemann syndrome have an increased risk of malignant transformation into Wilms tumor.**

Microscopic nephrogenic rests cannot be identified radiologically. Diffuse perilobar nephroblastomatosis and multifocal nephroblastomatosis can be evaluated through ultrasonography (US), computed tomography (CT), and magnetic resonance imaging (MRI). In diffuse perilobar nephroblastomatosis, the affected kidney may be enlarged. On sonography, corticomedullary differentiation is absent. Regions of nephroblastomatosis may be hypoechoic or isoechoic with respect to normal renal cortex (Fig. 148-1). Multifocal nephroblastomatosis is more difficult to identify on sonography.

CT is more sensitive than US for the evaluation of nephroblastomatosis. On CT, areas of nephroblastomatosis are well defined because they enhance to a lesser extent than normal renal cortex (Fig. 148-2). Bulky masses of nephroblastomatosis may distort the pelvicalyceal system. Involvement may be symmetric or asymmetric (Fig. 148-3). In diffuse perilobar nephroblastomatosis, a thick rind of lower attenuation tissue encases normally enhancing but architecturally distorted parenchyma. In multifocal nephroblastomatosis, multiple round masses of low attenuation are present. Flat or plaquelike areas of involvement may be difficult to identify on CT.

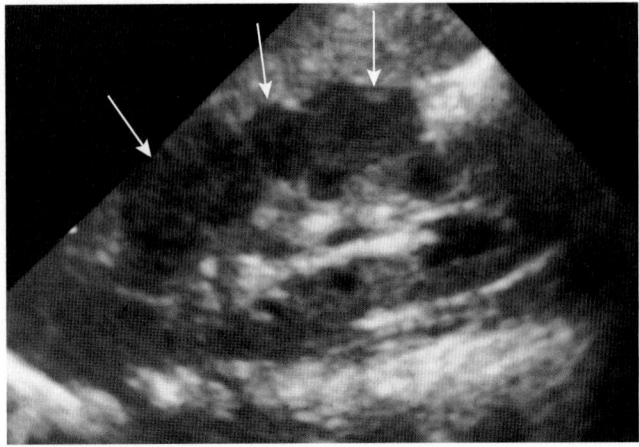

A

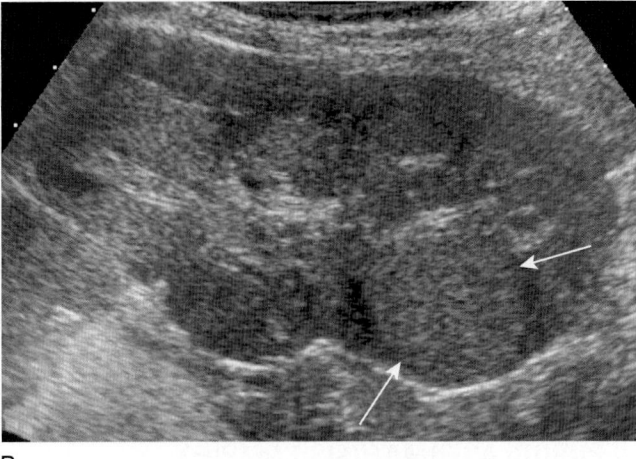

B

FIGURE 148-1. Nephroblastomatosis. **A,** Diffuse perilobar form. Longitudinal sonogram shows an enlarged right kidney with lobulated contour and hypoechoic cortical masses *(arrows)*. **B,** Focal intralobar form. Longitudinal sonogram shows a lower pole mass *(arrows)* that is isoechoic with renal cortex.

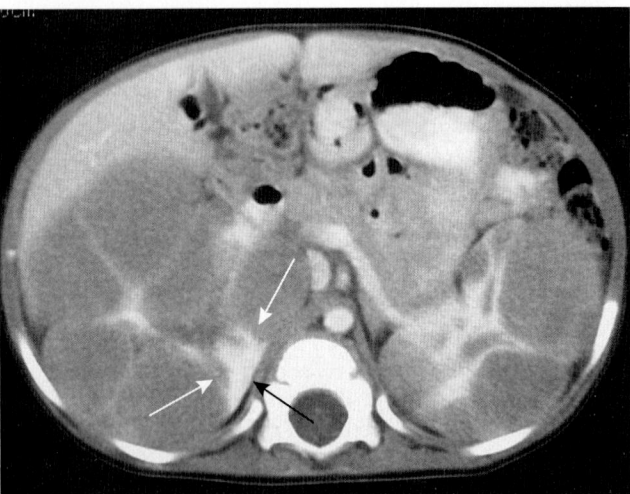

FIGURE 148-2. Diffuse perilobar nephroblastomatosis with symmetric involvement. On contrast-enhanced computed tomography scan, the kidneys are enlarged and multiple, round, peripheral masses of low attenuation are present. Architectural distortion at this level is pronounced; in the medial portion of the right kidney, only a peripheral area of normally enhancing kidney *(arrows)* is present.

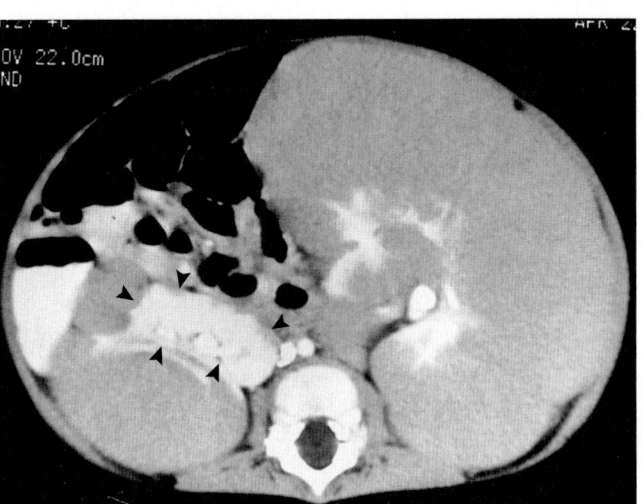

FIGURE 148-3. Diffuse perilobar nephroblastomatosis with asymmetric involvement. On contrast-enhanced computed tomography scan, the left kidney is much larger than the right. The architecture of the kidneys is distorted. A portion *(arrowheads)* of normally enhancing right kidney consists of parenchyma and calyces.

On MRI, nephroblastomatosis cannot be distinguished from normal renal parenchyma on T1-weighted sequences and is isointense or hyperintense on T2-weighted sequences. It appears hypointense relative to normal renal parenchyma after contrast administration on T1-weighted sequences, which are the most sensitive for detection. Active areas of nephroblastomatosis may be hyperintense on T2-weighted sequences and inactive areas hypointense. The signal intensity of nephroblastomatosis is homogeneous, whereas foci of Wilms tumor tend to be heterogeneous.

Children with genetic abnormalities or syndromes associated with nephroblastomatosis should be monitored to detect Wilms tumor development because the prognosis for Wilms tumor is best with small lesions. Children with hemihypertrophy or Beckwith-Wiedemann syndrome are at risk for developing other embryonal tumors such as hepatoblastoma and adrenal cell carcinoma. No large studies have been performed to establish the optimal screening interval for Wilms tumor surveillance; however, large tumors with metastases that develop over a 6-month period are reported. A baseline CT of nephroblastomatosis-related genetic abnormalities or syndromes at 6 months of age (or at diagnosis if the patient is older than 6 months), followed by US examinations every 3 to 4 months until the child is 8 years of age, is recommended on the basis of results from the National Wilms Tumor Studies. An area of nephroblastomatosis that grows larger and rounder is suspicious for malignant degeneration.

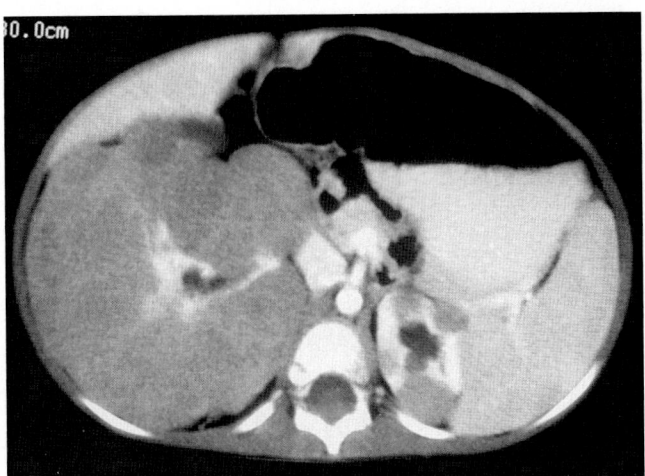

FIGURE 148-4. Diffuse perilobar nephroblastomatosis and right Wilms tumor. Contrast-enhanced computed tomography scan shows round, peripheral masses that enhance to a lesser extent than normal renal parenchyma in the upper pole of the left kidney. The right kidney has a thick rind of lobulated, hypoattenuating tissue without a discreet mass. Biopsy showed Wilms tumor on the right, and a nephrectomy was performed.

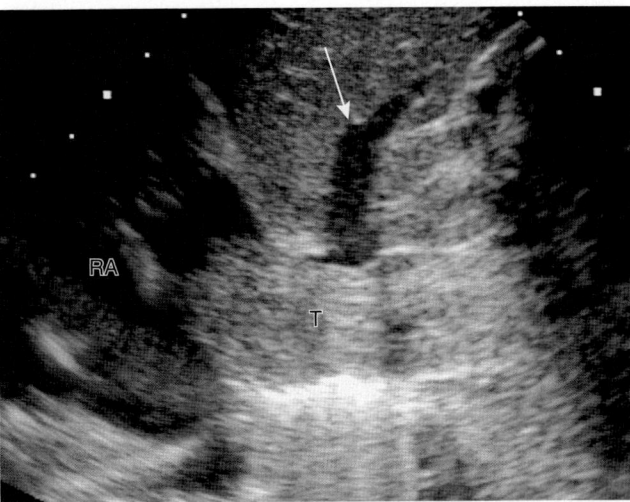

FIGURE 148-5. Wilms tumor extending into the inferior vena cava and the right atrium. Longitudinal sonogram shows tumor thrombus (T) expanding the inferior vena cava and extending into the right atrium (RA). The tumor partially occludes drainage from one of the hepatic veins (arrow).

> Children with genetic and syndromic abnormalities associated with nephroblastomatosis should be screened for Wilms tumor with the use of US at 3- to 4-month intervals.

WILMS TUMOR

Wilms tumor is the most common abdominal malignancy of childhood. It occurs predominantly in the toddler but has been described in teenaged children and adults. The most common renal tumor in the neonatal period is congenital mesoblastic nephroma; however, Wilms tumor has been reported in neonates, as well as in fetuses. As discussed in the Nephroblastomatosis Complex section, certain syndromes and genetic abnormalities predispose to development of Wilms tumor (Fig. 148-4). Bilateral Wilms tumors almost exclusively occur in patients with nephroblastomatosis. Most Wilms tumors arise from the renal parenchyma; however, extrarenal Wilms tumors may develop rarely in the abdomen or at distant sites.

In the United States, tumor stage is determined operatively, and the grade is established on pathologic examination. The classical triphasic Wilms tumor contains blastemal, stromal, and epithelial elements. Tumors with favorable histology do not contain any anaplastic changes. The prognosis for tumors with favorable histology is excellent, even for those at higher stages. In Europe, the staging system is based completely on radiologic findings. Tumors are classified on the basis of their imaging appearance, and chemotherapy is given before definitive surgery is performed. Tumors with extension into the inferior vena cava or invasion through the renal capsule are easier to resect after tumor shrinkage produced by chemotherapy.

Radiologic evaluation of Wilms tumor is focused on identifying the site(s) of involvement, extension, and metastases to assist in surgical planning. Preoperative imaging includes conventional chest radiography, abdominal and pelvic sonography, and thoracic, abdominal, and pelvic CT. In some centers, MRI is also employed.

On sonography, Wilms tumor is an intrarenal mass of heterogeneous echogenicity. Some Wilms tumors may contain cystic components, portions of obstructed and entrapped pelvicalyceal systems, or hemorrhagic and necrotic tumor. Extension into the inferior vena cava and the right atrium are characteristic routes of tumor growth and can be well visualized on US (Fig. 148-5), CT (Fig. 148-6), and MRI. The tumor typically forms a pseudocapsule but may invade the renal capsule, seed the peritoneal space, or grow directly into the mesentery and omentum. Hepatic metastases are also possible. The contralateral kidney may contain a smaller Wilms tumor or nephroblastomatosis. Synchronous or metachronous bilateral Wilms tumor may occur in up to 10% of patients.

> US may be better than CT for evaluation of Wilms tumor extension into the inferior vena cava via the renal vein.

On CT, Wilms tumor is generally spherical and intrarenal. It may contain small amounts of fat or fine calcification (Figs. 148-7 and 148-8) because the metanephric blastema cell is a pleuripotential embryonal cell. Dystrophic calcifications are seen in about 9% of Wilms tumors. The tumor enhances to a lesser extent than does renal parenchyma. In patients who have been screened ultrasonographically because of genetic or syndromic conditions, the tumor is usually smaller than 4 cm in diameter. Children who are evaluated because of physical examination abnormalities generally have tumors larger than 10 cm in diameter. CT and conventional radiographs of the chest are used to identify pulmonary metastases. On MRI, Wilms tumor is isointense with

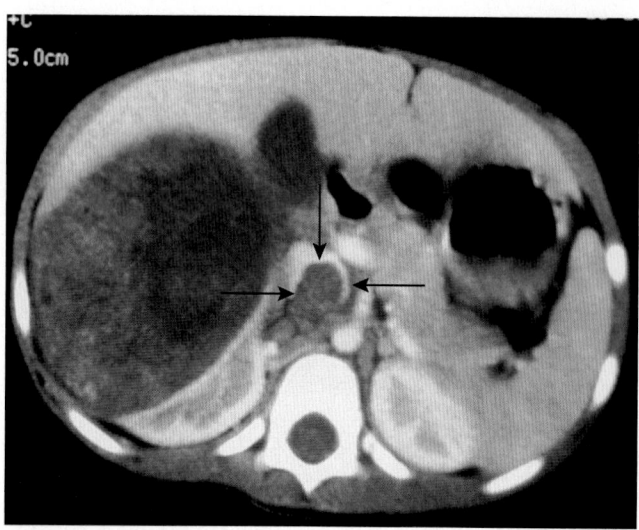

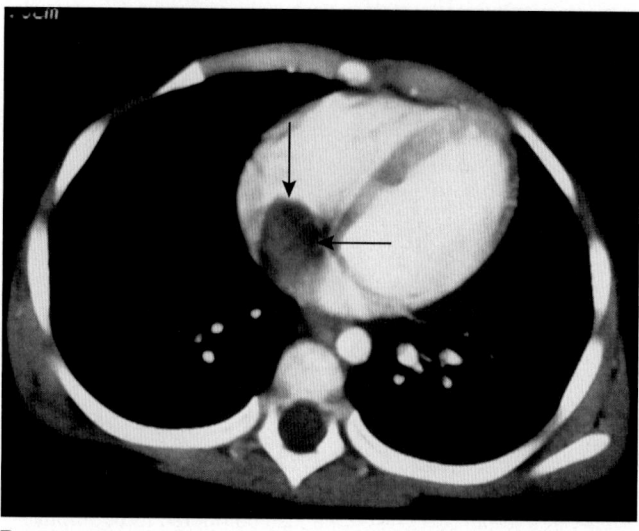

A   B

FIGURE 148-6. Wilms tumor extending into the inferior vena cava and right atrium. **A,** Contrast-enhanced computed tomography scan reveals a large, round, heterogeneous mass in the right kidney that enhances to a lesser extent than normal renal parenchyma. Contrast material opacifies the lateral and anterior margins of the inferior vena cava that contain hypoattenuating tumor *(arrows)*. **B,** The tumor *(arrows)* extends into the right atrium.

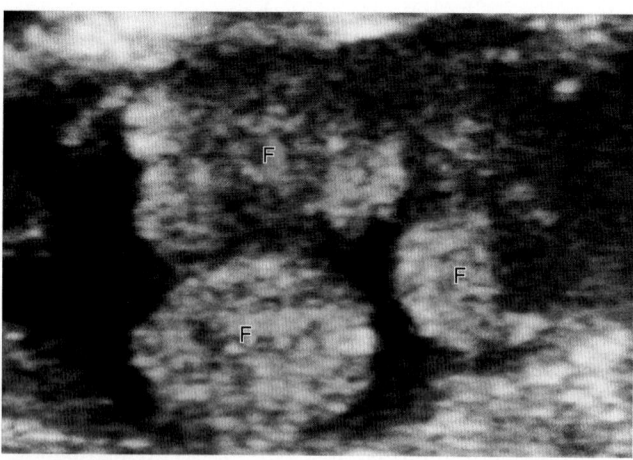

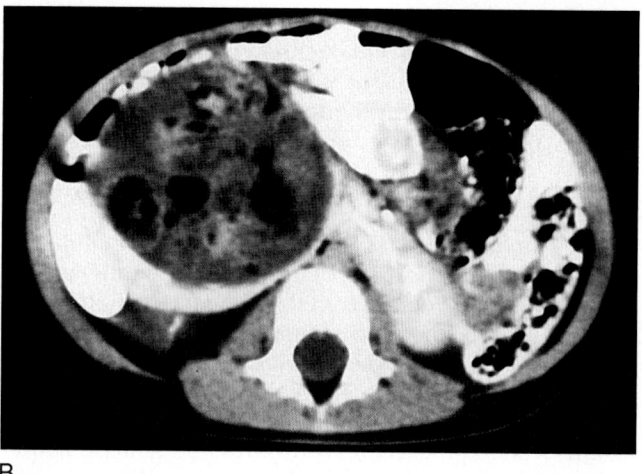

A   B

FIGURE 148-7. Wilms tumor containing fat in a horseshoe kidney. **A,** Axial sonogram of part of the Wilms tumor reveals hyperechoic fat-containing lobules (F). **B,** Contrast-enhanced computed tomography scan shows areas of fat within the mass. The isthmus of the renal parenchyma extends across the midline.

respect to normal renal parenchyma on T1-weighted sequences and hyperintense with respect to normal renal parenchyma on T2-weighted sequences. After contrast administration, Wilms tumor is hypointense relative to normal renal parenchyma and has inhomogeneous signal intensity (Fig. 148-9). Effectively treated Wilms tumor may be hypointense on T2-weighted sequences.

> **Wilms tumor may contain soft tissue, fluid, fat, and calcific elements.**

Surgery for Wilms tumor typically begins with a complete abdominal exploration before attention is given to the kidneys. The unaffected kidney is initially visualized and palpated to assess for masses or areas of superficial nephroblastomatosis before en bloc resection of the affected kidney is performed. Excisional biopsy of lung nodules is done to ensure that the stage of the tumor is correctly assigned. Patients with bilateral disease undergo staging surgery as well. Results of the surgical staging and the histologic examination determine selection of therapy. In patients with bilateral disease, treatment is provided according to the tumor histology of the higher stage side, along with later nephron-sparing surgery. When the tumor is very large, or when the tumor extends into the right atrium via the inferior vena cava, the surgeon may defer surgery until several courses of chemotherapy have reduced the tumor size or extension.

CLEAR CELL SARCOMA OF THE KIDNEY

Clear cell sarcoma of the kidney was considered a sarcomatous subtype of Wilms tumor before 1978, when

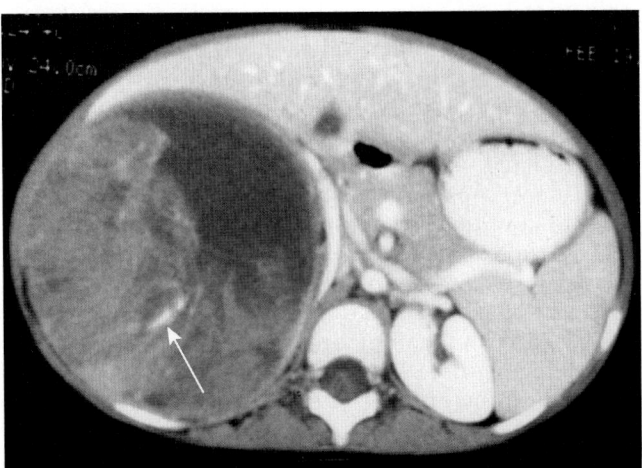

FIGURE 148-8. Wilms tumor containing calcification. Contrast-enhanced computed tomography scan reveals fluid-attenuating material anteromedially, most likely hemorrhage, within the large heterogeneous mass. Linear calcification is present posteriorly *(arrow)*.

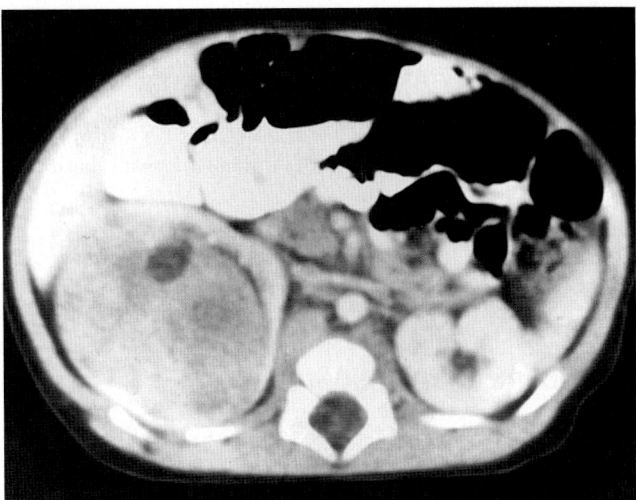

FIGURE 148-10. Clear cell sarcoma of the kidney. Contrast-enhanced computed tomography (CT) scan shows a large, round heterogeneous right renal mass. The mass was identified on antenatal sonography, and CT was performed on the second day of life.

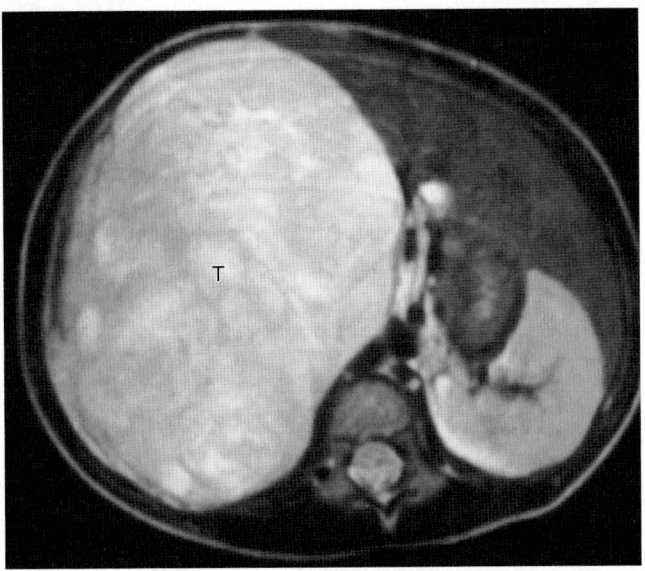

A

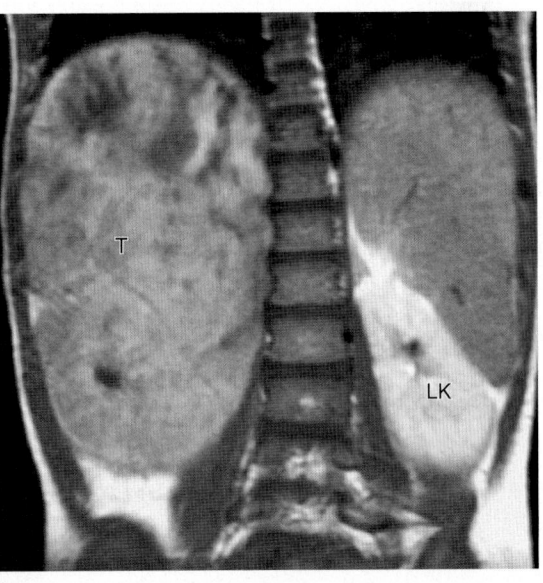

B

FIGURE 148-9. Wilms tumor. **A,** Axial T2-weighted magnetic resonance imaging shows a large tumor (T) replacing the right kidney which is hyperintense to other soft tissue structures. **B,** Coronal T1-weighted MRI after gadolinium in the same patient shows that the large tumor (T) is hypointense relative to the normally enhancing left kidney (LK).

it was reclassified as a separate entity from Wilms tumor. Formerly, it was called *bone metastasizing renal tumor of childhood*. It occurs in an age group similar to that affected by Wilms tumor, and its imaging features are not distinct from those of Wilms tumor (Fig. 148-10). Clear cell sarcoma has a predilection for bone metastases. These may occur at presentation or relapse. A pathologic diagnosis of clear cell sarcoma necessitates an evaluation of the skeletal system. Bone scintigraphy or conventional radiographic skeletal survey may be used. The prognosis is poor because of the aggressive behavior of the tumor.

> The imaging features of clear cell sarcoma of the kidney are similar to those of Wilms tumor.

RHABDOID TUMOR OF THE KIDNEY

Rhabdoid tumor of the kidney was also considered a sarcomatous variant of Wilms tumor before 1978, when it was reclassified as a separate entity from Wilms tumor. As is seen with clear cell sarcoma of the kidney, rhabdoid tumor of the kidney has imaging features similar to those of Wilms tumor, but it occurs in a slightly younger age group. Rhabdoid tumor of the kidney has a distinct metastatic pattern: it is frequently associated with primary or metastatic central nervous system lesions. After tissue diagnosis, MRI of the brain is recommended. Rhabdoid tumor has the worst prognosis of all of the childhood renal tumors.

> **Rhabdoid tumor of the kidney has a bleak prognosis.**

MESOBLASTIC NEPHROMA

Formerly, mesoblastic nephroma was thought to be an infantile type of Wilms tumor; however, patients with this diagnosis had excellent outcomes. The tumor is composed of spindle cells and does not have the typical histology of Wilms tumor. Although it is most common in the neonatal period, mesoblastic nephroma has been reported in adults, older children, and fetuses. On sonography, mesoblastic nephroma is predominantly solid and may contain cystic components (Fig. 148-11). The mass may distort and displace the pelvicalyceal system. On CT, congenital mesoblastic nephroma may be homogeneous or heterogeneous. Enhancement patterns are variable. The tumor, although benign, has been known to metastasize.

> **Mesoblastic nephroma has a predilection for the neonatal period; this distinguishes it from Wilms tumor, even though many of the imaging features are similar.**

MULTILOCULAR CYSTIC RENAL TUMOR

Multilocular cystic renal tumor occurs predominantly in boys during infancy and toddler stages and in women during their seventh and eighth decades. When the cystic mass has blastemal elements within its septa, it is called *cystic partially differentiated nephroblastoma.* Multilocular cystic tumors with septa that contain completely differentiated tissue are called cystic nephroma. Partially differentiated cystic nephroblastoma is found in the child more commonly than is cystic nephroma. Cystic nephroma is more commonly identified in women. This benign tumor may recur locally if it is incompletely excised.

Partially differentiated cystic nephroblastoma and cystic nephroma cannot be distinguished on the basis of imaging features. The multilocular cystic renal tumor may involve the entire kidney or a small portion. US is more sensitive than CT for identification of septa (Fig. 148-12). The septa may appear thin or thick. The pelvicalyceal system may be distorted and displaced.

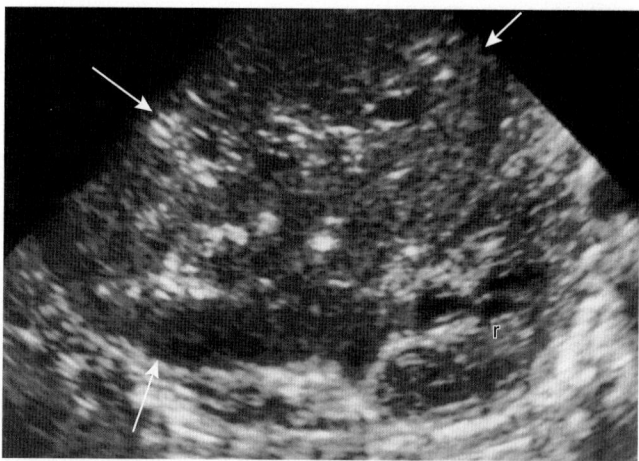

FIGURE 148-11. Congenital mesoblastic nephroma. On coronal sonography, the large, round mass *(arrows)* is predominantly solid, with foci of hyperechogenicity. A portion of the normal kidney (r) is present inferomedially.

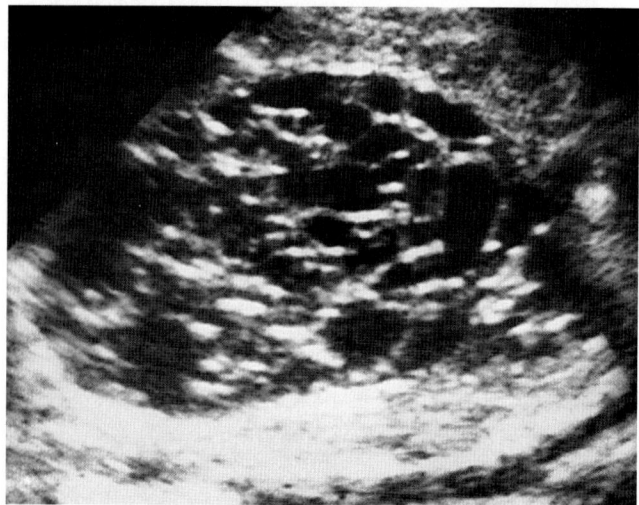

A

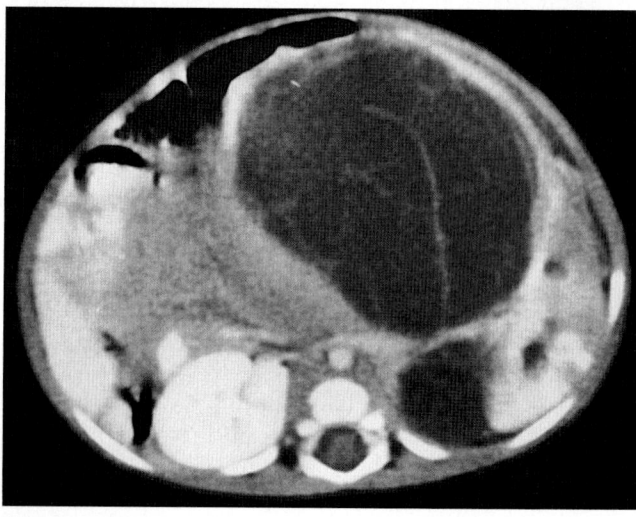

B

FIGURE 148-12. Partially differentiated cystic nephroblastoma. **A,** Sagittal sonogram of the left kidney reveals a cystic mass that contains many septa and locules of varying sizes. **B,** Contrast-enhanced CT scan reveals the hypoattenuating mass with very delicate-appearing septa.

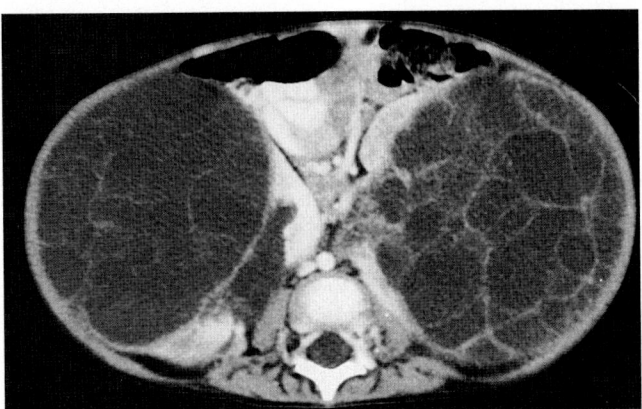

FIGURE 148-13. Bilateral partially differentiated cystic nephroblastoma. Contrast-enhanced computed tomography scan shows the septa, with similar attenuation to renal parenchyma, coursing through low-density masses.

On CT, the septa enhance but the locules do not (Fig. 148-13).

> Multilocular cystic renal tumor occurs in two distinct groups: young boys and elderly women.

RENAL CELL CARCINOMA

Renal cell carcinoma, which is rare in childhood, has been reported as a secondary malignant neoplasm after chemotherapy or radiation therapy. Children with tuberous sclerosis complex appear to be at increased risk for developing renal cell carcinoma. Calcification and ossification occur more commonly in children than in adults. During the second decade of life, a solid renal mass is equally likely to be a renal cell carcinoma or a Wilms tumor. During the first decade of life, a solid renal mass is much more likely to be a Wilms tumor.

Well-defined intrarenal lesions have been described on US and CT (Fig. 148-14). In some case reports, the tumor has been of increased attenuation relative to renal parenchyma. About 25% of renal cell carcinomas contain calcifications. Renal cell carcinoma enhances to a lesser extent than does normal renal parenchyma.

MEDULLARY CARCINOMA OF THE KIDNEY

Medullary carcinoma of the kidney was described as a distinct entity in 1995. It has been identified almost exclusively in patients of African descent with sickle cell trait or hemoglobin SC disease. The tumor develops in the renal medulla, infiltrates the cortex, and encases the renal pelvis, causing calyectasis while reniform shape is maintained (Fig. 148-15). Medullary carcinoma metastasizes rapidly to regional lymph nodes and lung.

RENAL ANGIOMYOLIPOMA

Angiomyolipomas and cysts are hamartomatous renal lesions that are seen in children with tuberous sclerosis. Most children with tuberous sclerosis have angiomyo-

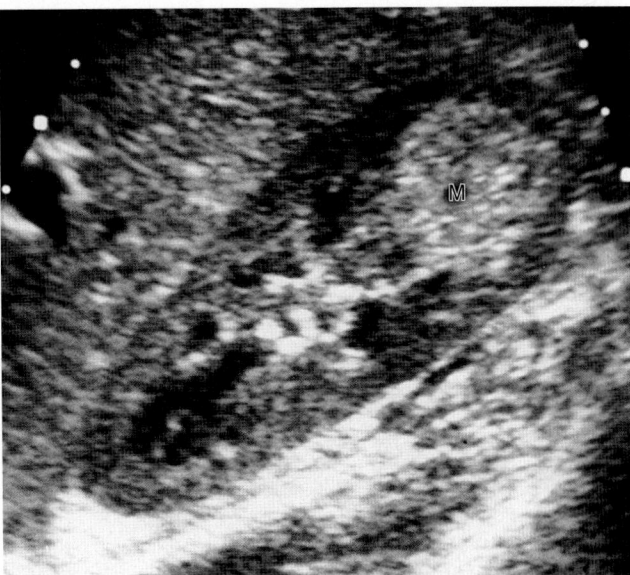

FIGURE 148-14. Renal cell carcinoma. Sagittal sonogram of the right kidney shows a round, hyperechoic mass (M) in the lower pole.

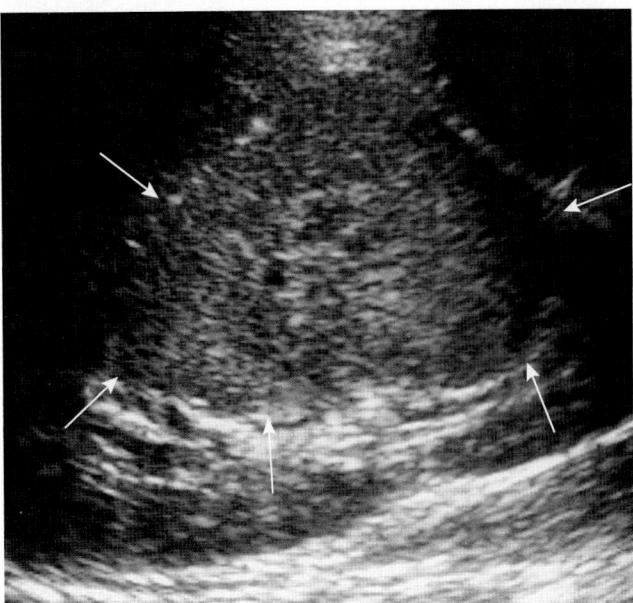

FIGURE 148-15. Medullary carcinoma of the kidney. Sagittal sonogram of the right kidney shows a mass (arrows) that is isoechoic to parenchyma effacing and abutting the renal pelvis.

lipoma by 10 years of age. Angiomyolipoma occurs in at least 50% of patients with tuberous sclerosis and may be the only manifestation of the disease.

Angiomyolipomas contain a variable amount of fat and can be mistaken for Wilms tumor or renal cell carcinoma. Bilateral lesions are often seen in tuberous sclerosis (Fig. 148-16). The vascular supply for angiomyolipoma is characteristic and consists of tortuous, dilated vessels with aneurysm formation.

On sonography, an angiomyolipoma is hyperechoic. Lesions larger than 4 cm may be selectively embolized or surgically removed to prevent life-threatening hemor-

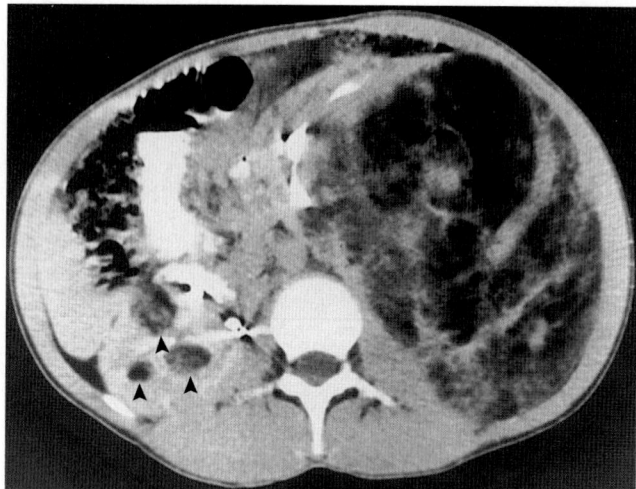

FIGURE 148-16. Angiomyolipomas of the kidneys. Contrast-enhanced computed tomography scan depicts a huge angiomyolipoma in the left kidney and three smaller ones *(arrowheads)* in the right kidney.

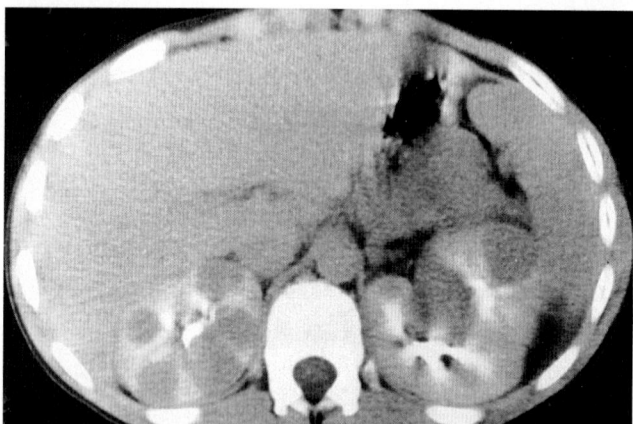

FIGURE 148-17. Non-Hodgkin lymphoma of the kidneys. Delayed contrast-enhanced computed tomography image reveals multiple, round hypoattenuating cortical masses.

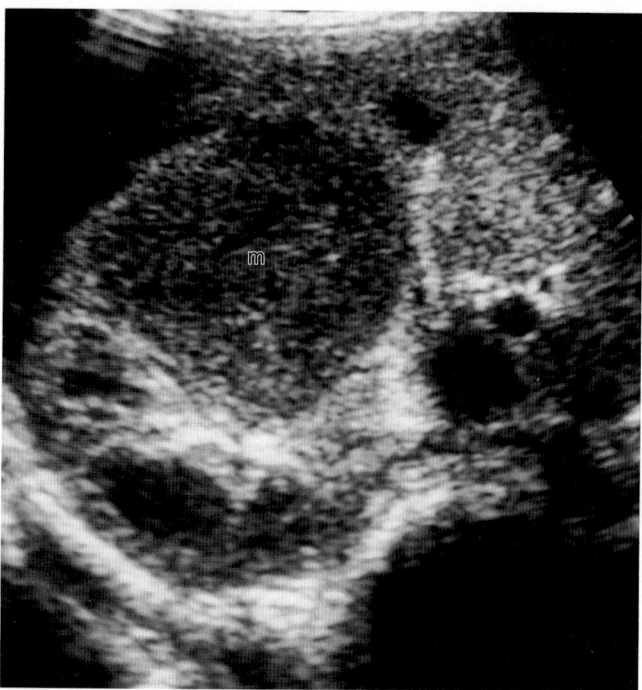

FIGURE 148-18. Non-Hodgkin lymphoma of the kidney. Axial sonogram of the right kidney shows a hypoechoic mass (m) that is replacing the anteromedial portion of the kidney.

rhage. US screening to monitor angiomyolipoma size is recommended every 2 to 3 years before puberty and then annually after puberty.

> Life-threatening retroperitoneal hemorrhage is a complication of angiomyolipomas that are larger than 4 cm.

RENAL LYMPHOMA

Lymphoma of the kidney is due to hematogenous spread or extension from retroperitoneal sites; the kidney does not normally contain lymphoid tissue, a fact that makes primary renal lymphoma rare. Non-Hodgkin lymphoma involving the kidneys is more common than Hodgkin lymphoma; however, it occurs seldom.

CT is better than sonography for locating renal lesions. On CT, multiple round masses enhance to a lesser extent than normal renal parenchyma (Fig. 148-17). On

sonography, the mass(es) may be occult. The kidney may be normal in appearance. Nephromegaly due to diffuse tumor infiltration may be the only finding. Hypoechoic, isoechoic, and hyperechoic subcortical masses have been described (Fig. 148-18).

SUGGESTED READINGS

Nephroblastomatosis Complex

Beckwith JB: Questions and answers: Wilms' tumor screening. AJR Am J Roentgenol 1995;164:1294

Borer JG, Kaefer M, Barnewolt CE, et al: Renal findings on radiological follow-up of patients with Beckwith-Wiedemann syndrome. J Urol 1999;161:235

Choyke PL, Siegel MJ, Craft AW, et al: Screening for Wilms' tumor in children with Beckwith-Wiedemann syndrome or idiopathic hemihypertrophy. Med Pediatr Oncol 1999;32:196

Gylys-Morin V, Hoffer FA, Kozakewich H, et al: Wilms' tumor and nephroblastomatosis: imaging characteristics at gadolinium-enhanced MR imaging. Radiology 1993;188:517

Hennigar RA, O'Shea PA, Grattan-Smith JD: Clinicopathologic features of nephrogenic rests and nephroblastomatosis. Adv Anat Pathol 2001;8:276

Hoyme HE, Seaver LH, Jones KL, et al: Isolated hemihyperplasia (hemihypertrophy): report of a prospective multicenter study of the incidence of neoplasia and review. Am J Med Genet 1998;79:274

Lonergan GJ, Martinez-Leon MI, Agrons GA, et al: Nephrogenic rests, nephroblastomatosis, and associated lesions of the kidney. RadioGraphics 1998;18:947

Perlman EJ, Faria P, Soares A, et al: Hyperplastic perilobar nephroblastomatosis: long-term survival of 52 patients. Pediatr Blood Cancer 2006;46:203

Rohrschneider WK, Weirich A, Rieden K, et al: US, CT, and MR imaging characteristics of nephroblastomatosis. Pediatr Radiol 1998;28:435

White KS, Kirks DB, Bove KE: Imaging of nephroblastomatosis: an overview. Radiology 1992;182:1

Wilms Tumor

Andrews MA, Amparo EG: Wilms' tumor in a patient with Beckwith-Wiedemann syndrome: onset detected with 3-month serial sonography. AJR Am J Roentgenol 1992;159:835

Applegate KE, Ghei M, Perez-Atayde AR: Prenatal detection of a Wilms' tumor. Pediatr Radiol 1999;29:64

Carrico CWT, Cohen MD, Zerin JM, et al: Wilms' tumor imaging: patient costs and protocol compliance. Radiology 1997;204:627

Cohen MD: Commentary: imaging and staging of Wilms' tumors: problems and controversies. Pediatr Radiol 1996;26:307

De Kraker J, Delemarre JF, Lilien MR, et al: Misstaging in nephroblastoma: causes and consequences: a report of the Sixth Nephroblastoma Trial and Study of the International Society of Paediatric Oncology. Eur J Pediatr Surg 1999;9:153

Ehrlich PF, Hamilton TE, Grundy P, et al: The value of surgery in directing therapy for patients with Wilms' tumor with pulmonary disease: a report from the National Wilms' Tumor Study Group (National Wilms' Tumor Study 5). J Pediatr Surg 2006;41:162

Geller E, Smergel EM, Lowry PA: Renal neoplasms of childhood. Radiol Clin North Am 1997;35:1391

Godzinski J, Tournade MF, de Kraker J, et al: The role of preoperative chemotherapy in the treatment of nephroblastoma: the SIOP experience. Societe Internationale d'Oncologie Pediatrique. Semin Urol Oncol 1999;17:28

Goske MJ, Mitchell C, Reslan WA: Imaging of patients with Wilms' tumor. Semin Urol Oncol 1999;17:11

Hoffer FA: Magnetic resonance imaging of abdominal masses in the pediatric patient. Semin Ultrasound CT MR 2006;26:212

Kullendorff C-M, Wiebe T: Wilms' tumour in infancy. Acta Paediatr 1998;87:747

Lowe LH, Isuani BH, Heller RM, et al: Pediatric renal masses: Wilms' tumor and beyond. Radiographics 2000;20:1585

Meisel JA, Guthrie KA, Breslow NE, et al: Significance and management of computed tomography detected pulmonary nodules: a report from the National Wilms' Tumor Study Group. Int J Radiat Oncol Biol Physics 1999;44:579

Neville HL, Ritchey ML: Wilms' tumor: overview of National Wilms' Tumor Study Group results. Urol Clin N Am 2000;27:435

Olsen OE, Jeanes AC, Sebire NJ, et al: Changes in computed tomography features following preoperative chemotherapy for nephroblastoma: relation to histopathological classification. Eur Radiol 2004;14:990

Porteus MH, Narkool P, Neuberg D, et al: Characteristics and outcome of children with Beckwith-Wiedemann syndrome and Wilms' tumor: a report from the National Wilms' Tumor Study Group. J Clin Oncol 2000;18:2026

Scott DJ, Wallace WHB, Hendry GMA: With advances in medical imaging can the radiologist reliably diagnose Wilms' tumours? Clin Radiol 1999;54:3217

Slasky BS, Bar-Ziv J, Freeman AI, et al: CT appearance of involvement of the peritoneum, mesentery and omentum in Wilms' tumor. Pediatr Radiol 1997;27:14

Suzuki K, Miyake H, Tashiro M, et al: Extrarenal Wilms' tumor. Pediatr Radiol 1993;23:149

Wootton-Gorges SL, Albano EA, Riggs JM, et al: Chest radiography versus chest CT in the evaluation for pulmonary metastases in patients with Wilms' tumor: a retrospective review. Pediatr Radiol 2000;30:533

Clear Cell Sarcoma of the Kidney

Argani P, Perlman EJ, Breslow NE, et al: Clear cell sarcoma of the kidney: a review of 351 cases from the National Wilms' Tumor Study Group Pathology Center. Am J Surg Pathol 2000;24:4

Glass RBJ, Davidson AJ, Fernbach SK: Clear cell sarcoma of the kidney: CT, sonographic, and pathological correlation. Radiology 1991;180:715

Khalil RM, Aubel S: Clear cell sarcoma of the kidney: a case report. Pediatr Radiol 1993;23:407

Rhabdoid Tumor of the Kidney

Agrons GA, Kingsman KD, Wagner BJ, et al: Rhabdoid tumor of the kidney in children: a comparative study of 21 cases. AJR Am J Roentgenol 1997;168:447

Chung CJ, Lorenzo R, Rayder S, et al: Rhabdoid tumors of the kidney in children: CT findings. AJR Am J Roentgenol 1995;164:697

Tomlinson GE, Breslow NE, Dome J, et al: Rhabdoid tumor of the kidney in The National Wilms' tumor study: age at diagnosis as a prognostic factor. J Clin Oncol 2005;23:7641

Mesoblastic Nephroma

Goldberg J, Liu P, Smith C: Congenital mesoblastic nephroma presenting with hemoperitoneum and shock. Pediatr Radiol 1994;24:54

Hartman DS, Lim Lesar MS, Madewell JE, et al: Mesoblastic nephroma: radiologic-pathologic correlation of 20 cases. AJR Am J Roentgenol 1981;136:69

Schlesinger AE, Rosenfield NS, Castle VP, et al: Congenital mesoblastic nephroma metastatic to the brain: a report of two cases. Pediatr Radiol 1995;25:S73

Willert JR, Feuser J, Beckwith JB: Congenital mesoblastic nephroma: a rare cause of perinatal anemia. J Pediatr 1999;134:248

Multilocular Cystic Renal Tumor

Agrons GA, Wagner BJ, Davidson AJ, et al: Multilocular cystic renal tumor in children: radiologic-pathologic correlation. RadioGraphics 1995;15:653

Hartman DS, Davis CJ, Sanders RC, et al: The multiloculated renal mass: considerations and differential features. Radiographics 1987;7:29

Madewell JE, Goldman SM, Davis CJ, et al: Multilocular cystic nephroma: a radiographic-pathologic correlation of 58 patients. Radiology 1983;146:309

Renal Cell Carcinoma

Allison JW, James CA, Figarola MS: Pediatric case of the day: renal cell carcinoma in a child with tuberous sclerosis. Radiographics 1999;19:1388

Donnelly LF, Rencken IO, Shardell K, et al: Renal cell carcinoma after therapy for neuroblastoma. AJR Am J Roentgenol 1996;167:915

Fenton DS, Taub JW, Amundson GM, et al: Renal cell carcinoma occurring in a child 2 years after chemotherapy for neuroblastoma. AJR Am J Roentgenol 1993;161:165

Kabala JE, Shield J, Duncan A: Renal cell carcinoma in childhood. Pediatr Radiol 1992;22:203

Pursner M, Petchprapa C, Haller JO, et al: Renal carcinoma: bilateral breast metastases in a child. Pediatr Radiol 1997;27:242

Sostre G, Johnson JF, Cho M: Ossifying renal cell carcinoma. Pediatr Radiol 1998;28:458

Medullary Carcinoma of the Kidney

Davidson AJ, Choyke PL, Hartman DS, et al: Renal medullary carcinoma associated with sickle cell trait: radiologic findings. Radiology 1995;195:83

Davis CJ, Mostofi FK, Sesterhenn IA: Renal medullary carcinoma: the seventh sickle cell nephropathy. Am J Surg Pathol 1995;19:1

Kalyanpur A, Schwartz DS, Fields JM, et al: Renal medulla carcinoma in a white adolescent. AJR Am J Roentgenol 1997;169:1037

Pickhardt PJ: Renal medullary carcinoma: an aggressive neoplasm in patients with sickle cell trait. Abdom Imaging 1998;23:531

Renal Angiomyolipoma

Carter TC, Angtuaco TL, Shah HR: Ultrasound case of the day: large, bilateral angiomyolipomas of the kidneys with tuberous sclerosis. Radiographics 1999;19:555

Ewalt DH, Sheffield E, Sparagana SP, et al: Renal lesion growth in children with tuberous sclerosis complex. J Urol 1998;160:141

Henske EP: Tuberous sclerosis and the kidney: from mesenchyme to epithelium, and beyond. Pediatr Nephrol 2005;20:854

Kim JK, Park SY, Shon JH, et al: Angiomyolipoma with minimal fat: differentiation from renal cell carcinoma at biphasic helical CT. Radiology 2004;230:677

Tchaprassian Z, Mognato G, Paradias G, et al: Renal angiomyolipoma in children: diagnostic difficulty in 3 patients. J Urol 1998;159:1654

Renal Lymphoma

Fernbach SK, Glass RBJ: Uroradiographic manifestations of Burkitt's lymphoma in children. J Urol 1986;135:986

Hartman DS, Davis CJ, Goldman SM, et al: Renal lymphoma: radiologic-pathologic correlation of 21 cases. Radiology 1982;144:759

Weinberger E, Rosenbaum DM, Pendergrass TW: Renal involvement in children with lymphoma: comparison of CT with sonography. AJR Am J Roentgenol 1990;155:347

RENAL FAILURE

Acute Renal Failure

Acute renal failure (ARF) represents a sudden decrease in and even cessation of renal function, such that the kidneys can no longer support normal fluid, electrolyte, and acid-base homeostasis. The normal full-term infant produces between 15 and 50 ml of urine per 24 hours during the first 48 hours of life and 50 to 100 ml/kg/day during the next month. The term *oliguria* indicates urine output of less than 1 ml/hr. An increase in serum creatinine of 50% from baseline or normal values, along with an increase in blood urea nitrogen, is considered indicative of renal failure. Although a decreased urine output of less than 0.5 to 1.0 ml/kg/hr is regarded as renal failure, as many as 60% of neonates with renal insufficiency will not have oliguria. Patients with nonoliguric renal failure have markedly less morbidity and mortality than those with oliguria.

The actual incidence of pediatric ARF is not precisely known, but it is estimated to be about 20% of the adult incidence of 209 per million people. Among children, however, the incidence of ARF is highest among neonates and infants, with up to 24% of neonates requiring intensive care unit admission after developing renal failure. Nephrogenesis continues until the 36th week of gestation, so renal injury and failure in premature neonates may produce short- and long-term problems through disruption of normal renal development. Cardiac surgery is a strong risk factor in neonates, as is hypoxia or ischemia. Other predisposing factors in children include sepsis, infection, hematologic-oncologic complications, trauma, and gastrointestinal disease. Mortality depends on the severity of renal failure and on the underlying cause. Children younger than 1 year of age have increased mortality; those with multiorgan dysfunction and failure of three or more organ systems have a greater than 50% mortality rate.

The causes of ARF are generally divided into prerenal, intrinsic renal, and postrenal causes. However, as is discussed later, prerenal and postrenal abnormalities can produce renal injury and subsequent intrinsic renal dysfunction. Prerenal conditions are the most common

cause of ARF in children. Primary renal disease accounts for less than 10% of cases but is the causative factor among most patients who require long-term renal replacement therapy.

Sonography is the primary modality used for evaluating ARF. Morphologic information about underlying renal dysplasia, obstruction, and parenchymal echogenicity is readily obtained. Doppler techniques provide information about renal perfusion and vascular abnormalities. Combined with laboratory data and the clinical setting, ultrasonography (US) is often sufficient for the imaging evaluation. However, more precise functional information requires nuclear medicine studies, which can help to differentiate prerenal, renal, and postrenal causes of ARF in unclear cases. Functional evaluation requires measurement of effective renal plasma flow (ERPF) with ^{131}I-orthoiodohippurate (^{131}I-OIH), assessment of glomerular filtration rate (GFR) with technetium-99m diethylenetriaminepenta-acetic acid (^{99m}Tc-DTPA), and determination of the filtration fraction (or ratio of GFR to ERPF). Specific findings for the various causes of ARF are discussed later.

> Prerenal conditions are the most common cause of acute renal failure (ARF) in children.

PRERENAL ACUTE RENAL FAILURE

Prerenal ARF results from hypoperfusion of an otherwise normal kidney. Most common in neonates and infants, this condition may result from hypoxia/ischemia, dehydration, hemorrhage, shock, cardiac failure, or other organ system dysfunction. If perfusion is restored, then renal function rapidly returns. The kidney responds to hypoperfusion through activation of the renin-angiotensin system to produce afferent arteriolar dilation and efferent arteriolar constriction to maintain glomerular filtration pressure. Intrarenal production of prostaglandins causes renal vascular dilation to help maintain perfusion. However, if perfusion remains compromised for longer than the compensatory mechanisms can tolerate, or if it is too severe, then renal damage may occur and intrinsic renal dysfunction develops (as in acute tubular necrosis).

The infant kidney is vulnerable to hypoperfusion because renal blood flow is proportionately lower in

*The authors wish to acknowledge the contribution of John R. Sty, MD, from prior editions of this book.

neonates and infants and glomerular filtration is low, especially in infants with respiratory abnormalities. Administration of nonsteroidal anti-inflammatory drugs (such as indomethacin for treatment of a patent ductus arteriosus) interrupts the production of prostaglandins and may compromise renal function. Forty percent of newborns receiving indomethacin have a decrease in renal function, with up to 27% reduction in GFR and 56% reduction in urine flow. In most infants, fortunately, these alterations are transient and reversible.

> **Sonography is the primary imaging modality for evaluating ARF.**

Imaging in ARF is performed primarily to exclude other causes of acute renal failure, such as vascular occlusion (see Chapter 150) or bilateral obstructive uropathy (see Chapters 19 and 145). Acutely, renal sonography is often completely normal, or it may show an increase in cortical echogenicity. Unfortunately, this is a nonspecific finding that is seen in many causes of renal dysfunction. Doppler examination may reveal tachycardia and diminution of diastolic flow compatible with hypovolemia, as well as poor peripheral color Doppler perfusion. Again, these changes are not specific for prerenal ARF because any decrease in the size of the lumen of small intrarenal arteries or arterioles leads to increased resistance to flow. Compression of small vessels by intrarenal edema (as in renal vein thrombosis), inflammation (as in glomerulonephritis), or urinary tract obstruction may result in an identical arterial Doppler pattern. Although they are not generally required for evaluation of prerenal ARF, nuclear medicine studies show a delayed ^{131}I-OIH uptake peak and a decreased ERPF and filtration fraction.

INTRINSIC ACUTE RENAL FAILURE

This category of renal failure is associated with an insult to the renal parenchyma. Conditions responsible for prerenal ARF may result in intrinsic ARF if the ischemic event is severe and prolonged. Renal cortical and renal medullary necrosis, hemolytic-uremic syndrome, acute immune-related nephropathies, rhabdomyolysis, and Tamm-Horsfall proteinuria may result in intrinsic ARF. Renal artery or renal vein thrombosis frequently produces ARF in the neonate (see Chapter 150). Intrinsic renal dysfunction may also be an end result of obstructive uropathies (such as posterior urethral valves; see Chapter 19) and of abnormalities of nephrogenesis and resultant renal hypodysplasia.

ACUTE TUBULAR NECROSIS. Acute tubular necrosis (ATN), the most common form of intrinsic ARF, proceeds from prerenal causes. Hypoxia/ischemia, the most common cause, leads to intrarenal vasoconstriction and resultant tubular necrosis. If prolonged or severe, thrombosis of intrarenal vessels may lead to irreversible tubular injury and even to necrosis of the renal cortex. Although ATN is generally reversible and has a good prognosis, if it leads to medullary or cortical necrosis, damage to renal function may be severe and permanent.

Clinically, severe ATN is associated with oliguria or anuria, whereas more moderate insults often produce no decrease in renal urine output. Urinalysis may show mild proteinuria and granular casts. Because the relatively poorly perfused medullary tubules are affected most often, renal concentrating ability is impaired with demonstrable abnormalities in sodium and water conservation. The creatinine rises sharply, and the extent of increase correlates with the severity of renal insult.

Imaging findings depend on the severity of parenchymal injury. In the very earliest stages of ATN, or with very mild disease, the kidneys may appear normal or may have only mildly increased cortical parenchymal echogenicity; corticomedullary differentiation may be poor. Doppler shows nonspecific poor peripheral perfusion and elevated resistance to diastolic flow caused by increased intrarenal vascular impedance (Fig. 149-1). In renal cortical necrosis, the cortex of both kidneys is affected in a similar manner with a similar distribution. Frequently, early in the course of the disease, sonography is normal except for slight nephromegaly. Renal sonography characteristically shows the pattern of increased cortical echogenicity and accentuation of the corticomedullary junction. The renal pyramids usually are not affected and remain hypoechoic. US is useful in showing the severity of changes and excluding other causes of ARF such as renal arterial or venous occlusion and urinary tract obstruction. Normalization of Doppler flow to the kidneys suggests improvement in the disease.

Nuclear medicine studies are seldom currently performed for ATN, but nuclear medicine DTPA or

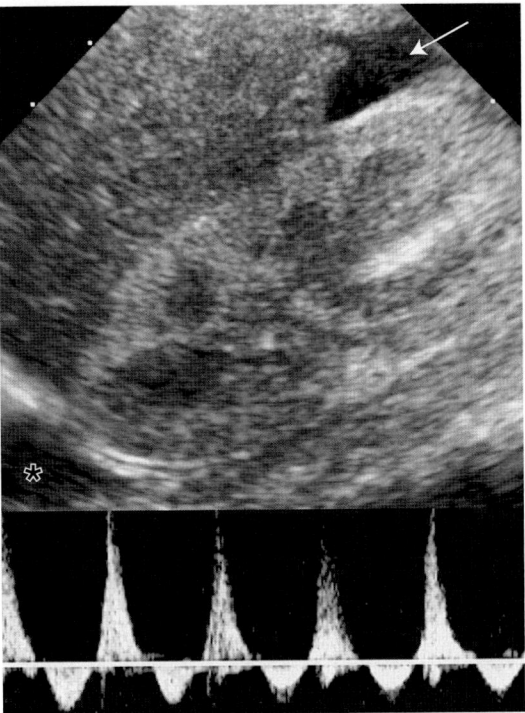

FIGURE 149-1. Acute tubular necrosis. Longitudinal sonogram of the right kidney in a child with poor urine output after cardiac surgery shows echogenic renal cortex, fluid below the liver *(arrow)*, and a small right pleural effusion *(asterisk)*. The corresponding main renal artery Doppler waveform shows very high resistance flow with reversal of flow in diastole.

MAG3 studies show delayed renal uptake and excretion, with normal or slightly diminished blood flow. ATN is characterized by delayed ^{131}I-OIH uptake, along with a generally high filtration fraction. The uptake of radiopharmaceutical in the later phase of the study is related to prognosis, although the time taken for eventual return to normal function cannot be predicted.

HEMOLYTIC-UREMIC SYNDROME. Hemolytic-uremic syndrome (HUS) is one of the most common causes of pediatric ARF. The disease is most commonly associated with infection by *Escherichia coli* 0157:H7 and is characterized by fever, vomiting, bloody diarrhea, and abdominal discomfort. The disease is caused by a microvascular vasculitis (see also Chapter 150) that involves many organ systems and commonly results in varying degrees of ARF that last up to a month. Almost all patients with HUS survive, and mortality rates have declined with improvements in care. However, up to 57% of patients require dialysis during the course of their treatment. Recovery of renal function tends to be complete, but some children have permanent injury that even progresses to chronic renal failure.

US may initially show normal kidneys, perhaps with minimal nephromegaly. By the time renal failure manifests, however, the kidneys show a nonspecific increase in parenchymal echogenicity (Fig. 149-2). Doppler shows reduction in diastolic flow (increased resistive index) caused by increased intrarenal arterial impedance, which is again not specific to any single cause. However, in patients with HUS, improvement in renal diastolic flow has been shown to precede the return of renal function by 24 to 48 hours; this management information may be useful in those patients who require renal replacement therapy.

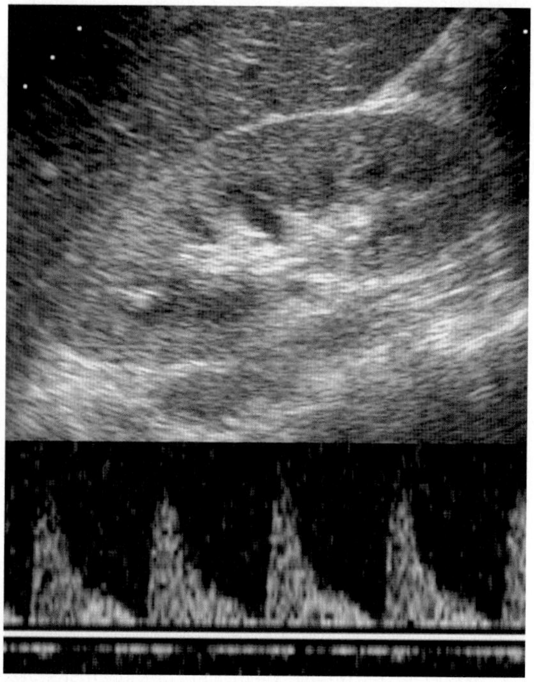

TUBULAR DYSFUNCTION. Tamm-Horsfall protein, a normal protein found in the luminal side of the distal tubule, has been identified in the interstitial tissue of kidneys in patients with vesicoureteral reflux (VUR) and reflux nephropathy (see Chapter 19). It has also been identified as a causative agent of tubular obstruction in patients with proteinuria caused by asphyxia, sepsis, contrast nephrotoxicity, or other causes of ARF. This protein probably elicits a cellular immune response from the lymphocytes of individuals with renal damage; this is thought to be a humoral response to a foreign antigen within the kidney. In neonates, Tamm-Horsfall proteinuria commonly occurs during the first week of life. This is usually an incidental finding that spontaneously resolves as urine output increases during the first few days of life, although some believe that decreased urine output may be causative. On sonography, Tamm-Horsfall proteinuria is characterized by normal-appearing renal cortex and hyperechoic medullary pyramids, especially at the tips (Fig. 149-3). With resolution, the medullary pyramids become normally hypoechoic.

Hemolysis and rhabdomyolysis release the proteins hemoglobin and myoglobin that are normally cleared by the kidneys. Underlying risk factors include immunologic abnormalities, dehydration, sepsis, electrical and crush injuries, medications, and exercise-induced muscle damage. Large amounts of hemoglobin and myoglobin, however, can lead to tubular dysfunction and renal failure, probably resulting from a combination of tubular obstruction, perfusion alterations, and inflammatory reaction to precipitated proteins. Clinically, hemoglobinuria or myoglobinuria occurs with decreased urine output. Serum creatinine rises and serum myoglobin and creatine phosphokinase are increased, reflecting muscle

FIGURE 149-2. Hemolytic-uremic syndrome. Longitudinal sonogram shows an echogenic right kidney with some preservation of corticomedullary differentiation. The corresponding main renal artery Doppler waveform shows diminished diastolic flow with a resistive index of 1.

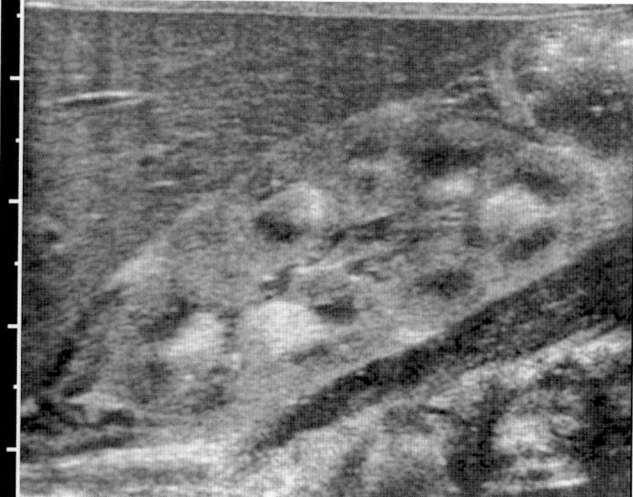

FIGURE 149-3. Tamm-Horsfall proteinuria on ultrasonography. Longitudinal sonogram of a 3-day-old with mildly reduced renal function shows increased echogenicity at the papillary tips. Follow-up US 1 week later was normal.

injury. US usually shows normal to slightly enlarged kidneys with markedly increased echoes throughout. If patients are imaged with bone-seeking radiopharmaceuticals, the kidneys are enlarged and show intense uptake.

Oncologic events are an important cause of ARF in children. The most common of these, tumor lysis syndrome, results not from direct neoplastic involvement of the kidneys, but from the death and breakdown of neoplastic cells. Tumor lysis syndrome is most common with acute leukemias and Burkitt lymphoma. Although it may occur even prior to the start of chemotherapy in these rapidly proliferating tumors, it usually appears during the first few days after initiation of chemotherapy. Lysis of tumor cells results in hyperkalemia, hyperuricemia, and hyperphosphatemia. High levels of these cell breakdown products overwhelm the kidneys' excretory ability, and oliguric or anuric ARF ensues. The acidic environment of the renal tubule causes uric acid and calcium phosphate crystal deposition within the tubules and further renal dysfunction, which is exacerbated by intravascular volume depletion. Ensurance of adequate hydration and urine output, pretreatment with allopurinol, and urine alkalinization have reduced this complication in current practice. Uric acid nephropathy may be noted at the time of diagnosis and may progress with treatment as a result of cell lysis. Sonographic findings include nephromegaly, a thickened and echogenic cortex, and loss of normal corticomedullary demarcation. Chronic changes associated with uric acid nephropathy include renal cortical thinning and increased renal sinus echoes (resulting from deposition of fat). In general, however, imaging has little usefulness in this condition. Neoplastic renal involvement (see Chapter 148), collecting system obstruction, and pre-existing renal dysfunction are all risk factors for tumor lysis syndrome that can be documented with the use of imaging.

> **Oncologic events are an important cause of ARF in children.**

Renal medullary necrosis (papillary necrosis) results from an ischemic event that occurs predominantly in the interstitium of the renal pyramids. Ischemic necrosis of the medulla (loops of Henle and vasa recta) occurs as the result of interstitial edema or intrinsic vascular obstruction. Causes include pyelonephritis, obstruction, sickle cell disease, nephrotoxic chemicals, and renal vein thrombosis. The condition occasionally follows or is associated with dehydration, hemophilia, severe infantile diarrhea, and high-dose intravenous contrast. Necrosis in situ occurs when the necrotic papilla detaches but remains unextruded within its bed. In the medullary form, partial sloughing of the papilla results in a single irregular cavity located concentrically or eccentrically within the papilla, and the long axis parallels the long axis of the papilla and communicates with the calyx. The papillary form occurs when the entire papilla is sloughed. This process can be localized or diffuse. ARF is uncommon but may occur if both kidneys become obstructed by sloughed papillary material.

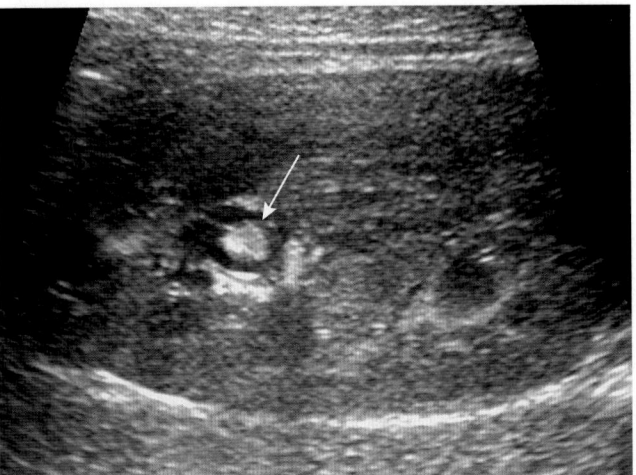

FIGURE 149-4. Papillary necrosis. Longitudinal sonogram shows an echogenic sloughed papillary tip *(arrow)* with enlargement of the adjacent calyx *(arrow)*.

Imaging findings are variable. The kidneys may be large or small, as may be seen in analgesic nephropathy. Bilateral renal enlargement may occur during the acute stage. The margins of the kidney are usually reniform and smooth. US shows highly echogenic papillae. In the medullary form of necrosis, the process is limited to the center of the papilla, whereas in the papillary type, the entire papilla becomes necrotic. When contrast is used in evaluation of the urinary tract, diminished density is frequently noted in the nephrogram phase. The fornices widen as a result of necrotic shrinkage, and the calyces may be club shaped when the papilla detaches. Intraluminal filling defects occur when sloughed papillae are contained (Fig. 149-4). On occasion, calcifications can be seen in the papillae that may be ringlike if attached to the papillae. When the papillae slough completely, clublike calyces remain. With severe combined necrosis (cortical and medullary), the affected kidney becomes smaller as the result of diffuse or focal scarring. Similar imaging findings are seen with reflux nephropathy.

ACUTE CORTICAL NECROSIS. Acute cortical necrosis is a very uncommon disorder that involves patchy or complete necrosis of the renal cortex. Also involved are proximal convoluted tubules in the medulla that result from distention of the glomerular capillaries, with 1 to 2 mm of peripheral cortical sparing. This disorder occurs in patients with severe dehydration, fever and infection, HUS, transfusion reactions, heart failure, burns, snakebites, and hyperacute renal transplant rejection. Imaging findings vary with stage and severity of the disease. Diffusely enlarged smooth kidneys are apparent early. Sonography shows a hyperechoic cortex, and radionuclide studies reveal impaired renal perfusion. Contrast studies reveal an absent or faint nephrogram phase (Fig. 149-5). Late in the disease, usually after 1 month, the kidneys become small with a scarred, often calcified parenchyma. Sonography at this stage shows a hyperechoic cortex with acoustic shadowing.

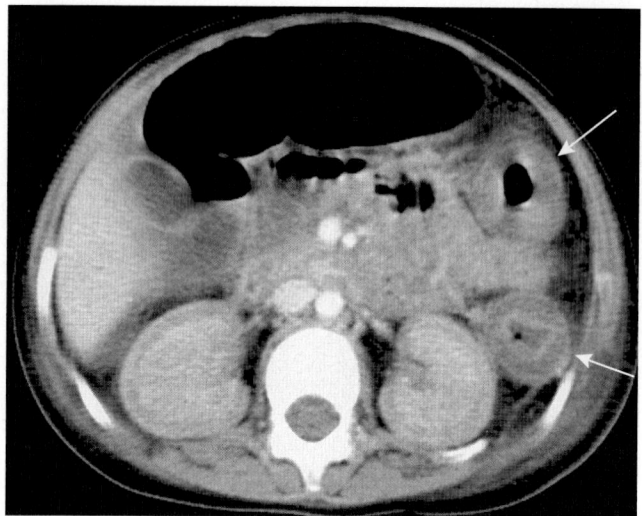

FIGURE 149-5. Acute cortical necrosis. Contrast-enhanced computed tomography of a 6-year-old girl with hemolytic-uremic syndrome shows very poor renal cortical enhancement despite excellent vascular contrast enhancement. Note the associated colitis *(arrows)*. (Courtesy of Harriet J. Paltiel, MD, Boston, MA.)

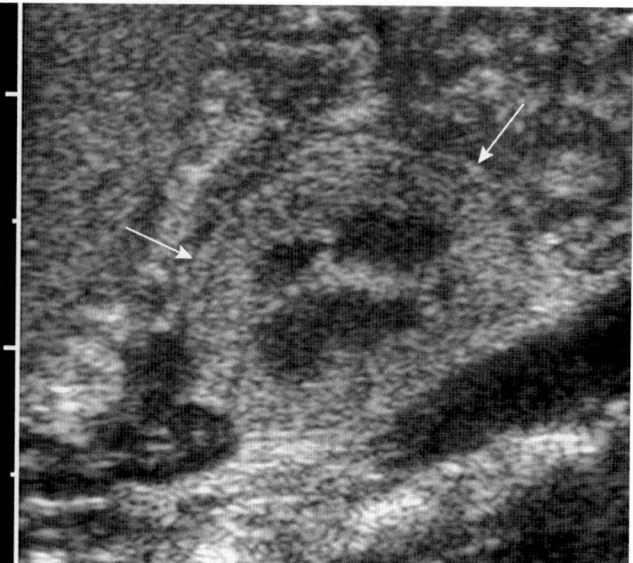

FIGURE 149-6. Renal hypodysplasia. Longitudinal sonogram of the left kidney in a newborn with multiple anomalies and renal insufficiency shows a severely hypoplastic kidney *(arrows)*. The right kidney looked the same.

OTHER CAUSES. Nephrotoxicity and ARF can be caused by many different medications. The most common of these are amphotericin B and aminoglycoside antibiotics, nonsteroidal anti-inflammatory drugs, chemotherapeutic agents, and radiographic contrast media. Aminoglycoside nephrotoxicity is related to dose and duration of therapy, usually produces nonoliguric renal failure, and is typically reversible once the medication has been stopped. Nonsteroidal anti-inflammatory drugs (as discussed earlier) interrupt the production of prostaglandins that help support renal blood flow; this may eventually lead to intrinsic renal abnormalities. As was discussed in Chapter 107, radiographic contrast agents may produce alterations in renal blood flow or proteinuria, and they may be nephrotoxic. In an otherwise healthy child, the use of low osmolar contrast media for diagnostic studies poses very little risk of renal injury. However, in the setting of pre-existing illness, hypovolemia, renal disease, or use of high-contrast doses for interventional radiologic or cardiologic procedures, nephrotoxicity may occur.

Acute glomerulonephritis usually affects children from ages 5 to 15 years, although it may occur at any age. Boys are more commonly affected. Underlying causes, all of which incite glomerular inflammation, are variable. Postinfectious glomerulonephritis is most commonly seen after streptococcal infection, although other bacterial, parasitic, fungal, and viral agents have been implicated. Other, more generalized autoimmune disorders (such as Wegener granulomatosis, systemic lupus erythematosus) are associated with glomerulonephritis, as are disorders that are more limited to the kidney (such as membranoproliferative glomerulonephritis and immunoglobulin [Ig]A nephropathy) Immune complexes are deposited or formed in the glomeruli, producing swelling and an inflammatory reaction with complement deposition. Patients present acutely with generalized systemic complaints, along with edema, decreased urine output, hematuria, flank pain, and hypertension. Mortality is low, but as many as 10% of pediatric patients show progression to chronic renal failure. As with many causes of ARF, imaging is nonspecific. US shows enlarged echogenic kidneys with variable preservation of corticomedullary differentiation, along with poor renal perfusion and an elevated resistive index on Doppler. Definitive diagnosis may require renal biopsy.

Renal hypodysplasia may occur as a primary abnormality of renal development, or as the result of prenatal urinary tract obstruction. When unilateral, renal function may be normal and the abnormal kidney detected incidentally. When bilateral, renal failure occurs in the neonatal period or during early childhood. Common causes include bilateral multicystic dysplastic kidneys (MCDK; as may occur with Meckel-Gruber syndrome), autosomal recessive polycystic kidney disease, and in utero obstructive uropathy. Imaging findings are variable, reflecting the underlying disease process (Fig. 149-6).

Vasculitides that may cause ARF, such as Henoch-Schönlein purpura and polyarteritis nodosa, are discussed in Chapter 150.

POSTRENAL ACUTE RENAL FAILURE

Postrenal ARF results from obstruction to the flow of urine from the collecting system. This can occur with bladder outlet obstruction, bilateral ureteric obstruction caused by stones or retroperitoneal tumor (see Chapter 151), or obstruction of a solitary kidney. Prenatal urinary tract obstruction produces renal failure in the newborn that is sometimes complicated by respiratory insufficiency from in utero oligohydramnios. Frequently, bilateral hydronephrosis and hydroureter are caused by obstruction at the level of the bladder or bladder outlet (see Chapter 19). The most common cause is posterior urethral valves, although urethral polyps and pelvic masses may also produce obstruction (see Chapters 19 and 152).

Imaging begins with US, which readily reveals dilation of the collecting system. Posterior urethral valves may be diagnosed by sonography with evidence of a dilated posterior urethra. Voiding cystourethrograms should be performed for optimal visualization of the urethra and the posterior urethral valve. A pelvic mass such as a sacrococcygeal teratoma or hydrometrocolpos may produce extrinsic obstruction of the bladder outlet. These entities can be diagnosed readily with the use of US, CT, and MRI (Fig. 149-7). VUR commonly coexists with bladder outlet obstruction, no matter the cause.

Chronic Renal Failure

The diagnosis of chronic renal failure (CRF) is rarely suspected on clinical grounds alone until the GFR has fallen to below 20 to 25 ml/min/1.73 m^2. Up to this level, remaining functioning nephrons are capable of regulating body chemistry through adaptive alterations in tubular function.

Obstructive uropathy may lead to CRF years after obstruction has been relieved. The number of nephrons is reduced and nephrons that exist may be abnormal because of in utero obstruction. The fact that in utero surgical relief of obstruction does not appear to prevent renal damage indicates that the effects of obstruction on nephrogenesis are likely more complex than was initially believed. Severe VUR may also produce enough renal parenchymal damage (with associated infection) to adversely affect renal function. In both of these conditions, remaining nephrons are often able to maintain sufficient function until puberty because of progressive glomerulosclerosis caused by chronic hyperfiltration and the increasing metabolic demands of a larger body.

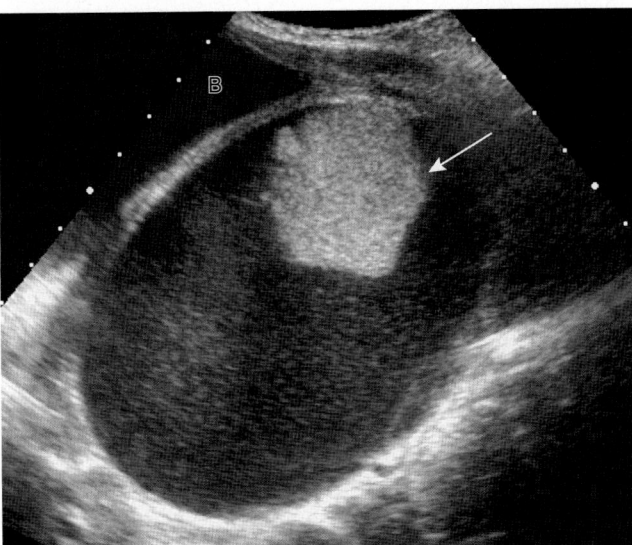

FIGURE 149-7. Sacrococcygeal teratoma causing bladder outlet obstruction. Longitudinal midline sonogram of the pelvis in a 3-month-old girl with poor urine output and abdominal distention shows a large complex mass with solid (*arrow*) and cystic components arising from the pelvis. The bladder (B) is displaced superiorly. Severe bilateral hydroureteronephrosis is seen on other images.

> **Obstructive uropathy may lead to CRF years after obstruction has been relieved.**

Renal hypodysplasia and inherited renal abnormalities are major causes of CRF. Even if they involve only one kidney (as with MCDK), the child has a reduced total number of nephrons and is thus more susceptible to renal damage or injury. Cystic renal disease may produce CRF early or later in life, depending on the inherited type. Other inherited diseases that may lead to renal failure include Alport syndrome, cystinosis, and primary oxalosis.

Any of the causes of ARF may lead to secondary CRF, even many years after the initial event. Up to 10% of patients with acute glomerulonephritis develop CRF. Newborns with substantial hypoxic/ischemic renal injury have been shown to have a high incidence of CRF. Hypertension may result from CRF and may lead to further injury of already impaired kidneys. For this reason, any child who has experienced ARF must be followed carefully for signs of worsening renal function.

Because of the slow evolution of chronic renal disease in most children, they are much more susceptible to the deleterious effects of CRF on nutritional status and growth, and the manifestations that bring children to medical attention are frequently nonspecific. CRF may be detected in the course of evaluation of a child for failure to thrive, urinary tract infection, hypertension, abdominal masses, or urinary abnormalities such as hematuria or proteinuria. Cardiomegaly, uremic myocarditis and pericarditis, congestive heart failure, pleural effusion and pulmonary edema, peripheral edema, and hypertension are common systemic manifestations of CRF. Peptic ulcers, ulcerated necrotic lesions of the large and small bowel, uremic colitis, pancreatitis, malabsorption syndrome, and ascites are gastrointestinal manifestations. Esophageal varices occur in older patients with autosomal recessive polycystic kidney disease and hepatic fibrosis.

As with ARF, imaging is often nonspecific about the cause of CRF. However, some findings can be predictive of certain conditions. US is the most useful approach because it can reveal the size and configuration of the kidney, along with information about its vascular supply, independent of renal function. A dilated collecting system directs the evaluation toward obstructive uropathy or severe reflux. Renal cystic disease is apparent and should prompt evaluation of other family members. Dense calcification of the renal cortex suggests prior cortical necrosis or primary oxalosis (Fig. 149-8). In general, however, the kidneys of patients with CRF are small and echogenic, indicating an irreversible loss or maldevelopment of renal parenchyma (Fig. 149-9). This increased echogenicity is frequently the result of fibrosis and collagen deposition, and even calcification.

Radionuclide imaging has helped in assessment of the relative amount of renal tissue in each kidney, detection of urinary tract obstruction, and quantification of GFR. Excretory urography is rarely useful because low GFR does not allow adequate visualization of the urinary tract. Voiding cystourethrography (VCUG) is required if a

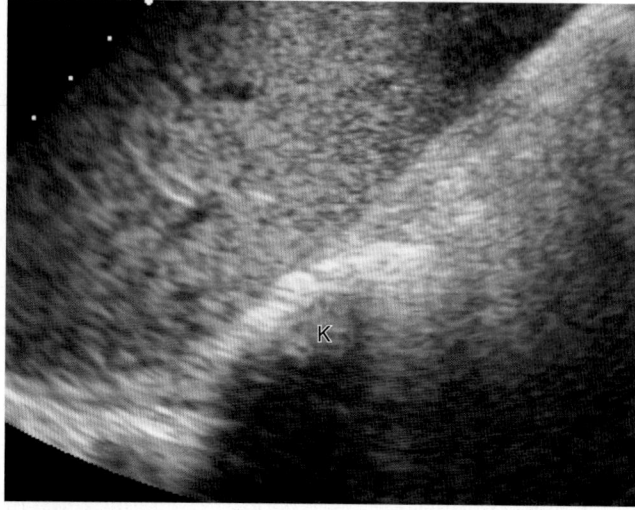

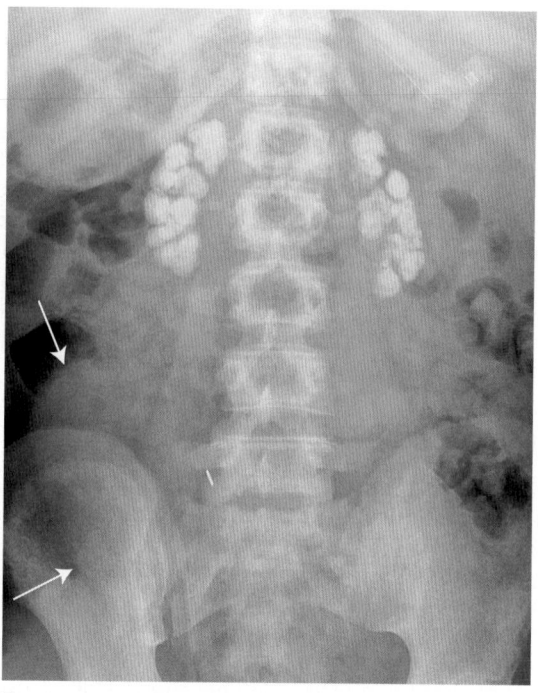

FIGURE 149-8. Primary oxalosis. **A,** Longitudinal sonogram of the right kidney shows a brightly echogenic structure with posterior acoustic shadowing (K). **B,** Plain radiograph after renal transplantation *(arrows)* shows small, densely calcified native kidneys. Note bony changes of renal osteodystrophy.

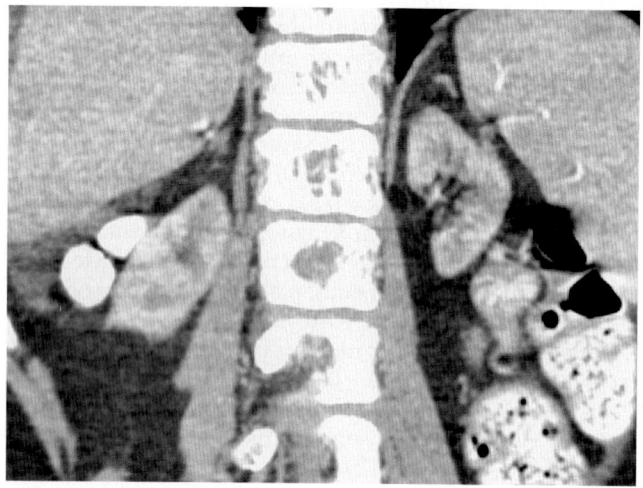

FIGURE 149-9. Chronic renal failure. Coronal reformatted computed tomography image in a teenager with multiple medical problems and chronic renal insufficiency shows very small kidneys. At sonography, these kidneys were echogenic with poor corticomedullary differentiation.

history of prior urinary tract infections is reported, or an abnormal voiding pattern or abnormalities of the urinary tract are detected on sonography. VCUG assesses for bladder outlet obstruction and bladder morphology and is used to detect VUR. However, in cases of reflux nephropathy, the VCUG may be normal because VUR will have resolved by the time CRF becomes apparent.

> **Radionuclide imaging helps in the assessment of relative amounts of renal tissue in each kidney.**

Secondary radiographic signs may be apparent in children with CRF. Renal osteodystrophy is a frequent complication that produces a generalized increase in bone density. The vertebral body shows sclerosis of the upper and lower thirds (rugger jersey vertebrae) in some severely affected and untreated patients. Secondary hyperparathyroidism produces cortical and subligamentous erosions (see Chapters 167 and 168). Metaphyseal changes, also in part the result of hyperparathyroidism, may be indistinguishable from typical rickets, and the growing ends of long bones are irregularly mineralized and markedly disorganized. Metaphyseal fracture may occur, as may slipping of weight-bearing epiphyses, genu valgum, and bowing of the long bones. Brown tumors rarely occur in childhood. Arterial and periarticular soft tissue calcifications may be small, linear, or masslike.

RENAL REPLACEMENT THERAPY

Management of ARF consists of supportive care until the kidney recovers from the acute insult. CRF is managed medically in most cases. However, when renal insufficiency is so severe that metabolic and volume homeostasis cannot be maintained, renal replacement therapy must be instituted. This can take the form of peritoneal dialysis, hemodialysis, and hemofiltration.

Peritoneal dialysis used to be the preferred method in pediatric ARF and even in some patients with CRF, and it is preferred for use in neonates and small children in whom adequate vascular access may not be possible. A catheter is surgically inserted into the peritoneal cavity and sterile dialysate fluid instilled. The peritoneum itself acts as a semipermeable membrane that allows the removal of excess solutes and water. Peritoneal dialysis can be performed at home, although this is time consuming. Many complications, among them peritonitis, hernias, and obstruction, may occur. Plain radiographs obtained after peritoneal catheter placement should show the catheter directed toward the dependent part of the pelvis because this allows better fluid drainage. Catheter dysfunction may be seen with catheter migration out of the pelvis (Fig. 149-10) or with peritoneal loculations after peritonitis (that may be documented by CT).

Hemofiltration reproduces the glomerular filtration function of the kidney; it allows rapid fluid removal and has become the preferred method of treatment of patients with ARF. In hemofiltration, waste products are removed by convective transport; this occurs independent of their molecular weight but depends on the molecular weight of solute and the rate of flow of the filtrate. A dialysis filter may be added to the circuit to facilitate solute removal in accordance with the patient's metabolic abnormalities. Hemofiltration may be arteriovenous or venovenous, and access is usually gained via large-bore vascular catheters, often inserted by interventional radiologists. Hemodynamic instability in the acute setting is generally less pronounced than with hemodialysis. Patients often require heparinization while on therapy, and they may experience fluid and electrolyte imbalances.

Hemodialysis allows the rapid correction of metabolic abnormalities and hypervolemia, and it is commonly used for the treatment of patients with end-stage renal disease (ESRD).

With hemodialysis, solute transport occurs by diffusion along with elimination of uremic substances according to their molecular weight. The patient's arterial blood is brought into contact with a dialysis solution across a series of semipermeable membranes within the dialyzer and is returned as dialyzed blood to the patient's venous

system. Temporary hemodialysis may be achieved with insertion of special large-caliber double-lumen catheters into the right internal jugular vein. For long-term access, a synthetic arteriovenous graft or an arteriovenous fistula between native artery and vein is created to allow ready access to the patient's arterial and venous circulation. In patients with prior central venous access, imaging should be done to evaluate proximal stenoses and occlusions prior to graft or fistula creation (Fig. 149-11). Complica-

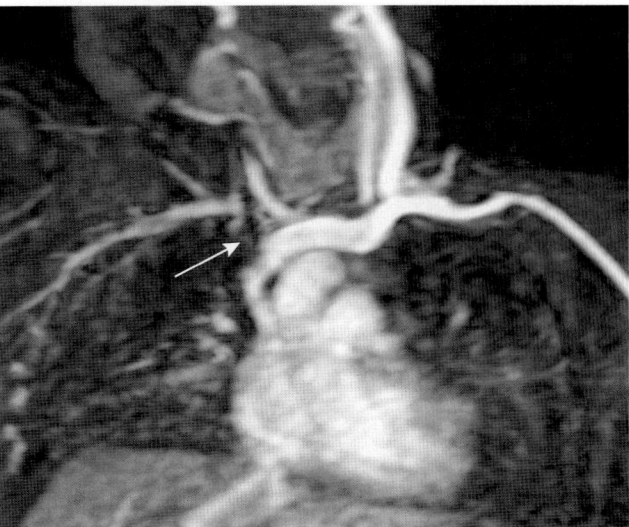

FIGURE 149-11. Central venous stenosis. Contrast-enhanced magnetic resonance venogram in a child with multiple vascular access procedures shows occlusion of the medial subclavian vein, an occluded right brachiocephalic vein *(arrow)*, and lack of flow in the right internal carotid vein. Collateral channels are seen over the right shoulder. The left venous system is patent.

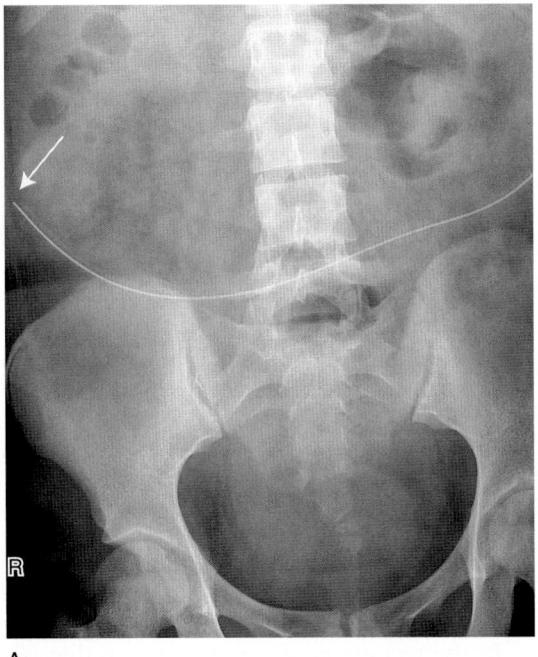
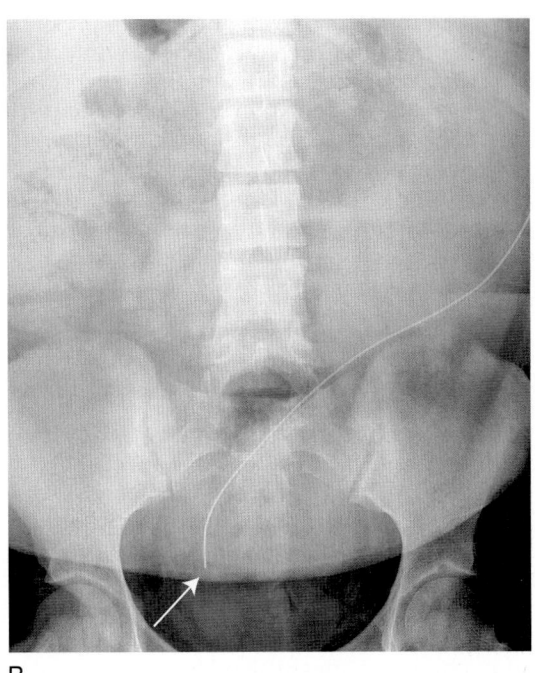

A   B

FIGURE 149-10. Peritoneal dialysis catheter. **A,** Plain radiograph taken because of decreased effectiveness shows a peritoneal dialysis catheter tip in the right flank *(arrow)*. **B,** After interventional radiologic manipulation, the catheter tip *(arrow)* is appropriately positioned within the dependent portion of the pelvis.

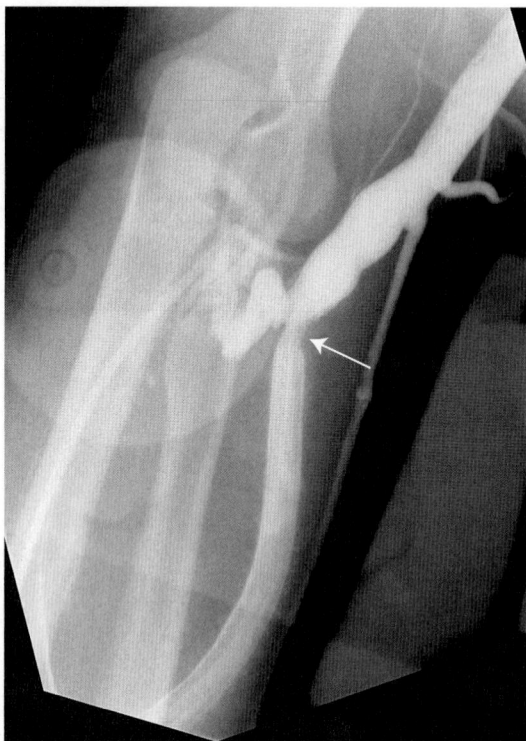

FIGURE 149-12. Dialysis graft venous outflow stenosis. Venogram of a forearm dialysis graft with increasing venous pressures shows narrowing of venous outflow *(arrow)* just distal to the end of the synthetic graft. Pressures returned to normal after angioplasty was performed.

TABLE 149-1			
Renal Failure Recurrence and Graft Loss			
Disease*	Recurrence Rate, %	Severity	Graft Failure, %
FSGS	25-30	High	50
MPGN type I	70	Mild	25
MPGN type II	100	Low	10
SLE	5-50	Low	5
HSP	50-75	Mild	10
HUS	10-20	Moderate	5

*FSGS, focal segmental glomerulosclerosis; HSP, Henoch-Schönlein purpura; HUS, hemolytic-uremic syndrome; MPGN, membranoproliferative glomerulonephritis; SLE, systemic lupus erythematosus.

tions that most commonly result in access site failure include thrombosis of the graft or fistula and stenosis in the proximal venous drainage. Venous obstruction and thrombosis are evident on US or magnetic resonance (MR) venography, or with injection of contrast material (Fig. 149-12). Venous injection with an inflated pressure cuff allows opacification of the graft or fistula. Injection should be forceful enough to allow reflux of contrast into the artery to allow evaluation for inflow stenosis. Aneurysms at the site of anastomosis or within the graft, excessive arterial-venous shunting, and distal arterial insufficiency are other types of complications.

Patients on long-term hemodialysis may develop cortical renal cysts. Single or multiple neoplasms, usually adenomas or carcinomas, may occur in association with cysts.

RENAL TRANSPLANTATION

Despite advances in renal replacement therapy, no substitute for a functioning kidney has been found. Children with ESRD have only approximately one-quarter the life span of their contemporaries who have normal renal function. Renal transplantation is the preferred method of treatment for children with ESRD. Transplant recipients have a lower rate of mortality compared with patients on hemodialysis; the greatest benefit is perceived in children younger than 4 years of age.

The primary renal disease that has resulted in end-stage renal failure is an important consideration prior to transplantation because the pathologic process that affects the native kidneys can reoccur within the allograft (Table 149-1). Renal biopsy may be required. Focal glomerulosclerosis is the most common specific glomerular disease that causes ESRD during childhood. It is also the most common glomerular disease with the potential for recurrence in the allograft. Two metabolic diseases that may cause ESRD in children are cystinosis and oxalosis. Cystine crystals are identifiable in the allografts of transplant recipients who have cystinosis; these apparently have little effect on allograft function. A poor outcome of renal transplantation is seen in patients with primary oxalosis as the metabolic defect involves hepatic metabolism. These patients have a high incidence of recurrence of oxalate deposition in the transplanted kidney, unless the liver is transplanted as well.

In preparation for renal transplantation, it is necessary to minimize the risk of rejection. Mechanisms of rejection are based on T cell–mediated (cellular) and B cell–mediated (humoral) immune mechanisms, as well as genetically related cell surface antigens represented in the human leukocyte antigen (HLA) system. The HLA system is the major antigen-matching technique used in evaluation of donor sources. Presensitization of the recipient may have occurred during previous organ transplantations or blood transfusions. It has been observed, however, that graft survival is enhanced in patients who receive more than 10 blood transfusions, and a program of donor-specific transfusions is sometimes undertaken to decrease the risk of presensitization. Nephrectomy of native dysfunctional kidneys is indicated only in patients with hydronephrosis in whom post-transplant urinary tract infections may continue to occur, or in those with severe hypertension or massive proteinuria. It is important that the bladder and the urethra be adequate for effective urine collection and voiding to completion. Patients with dysfunctional voiding and bladder abnormalities have a much higher rate of transplant graft failure. If the urinary tract has previously been diverted, reversal of the diversion is required.

In the technique of transplantation that is commonly used, the aorta or the iliac artery is the site of arterial anastomosis, and the renal vein enters the inferior vena cava or the common iliac artery. The transplanted kidney is placed in the retroperitoneum or preperitoneal space in older children, and intraperitoneally in very small children. The ureter is reimplanted via transvesical or intravesical antirefluxing techniques. Once perfusion has been re-established, the transplanted kidney should begin to function immediately.

Factors that influence graft survival include severity and type of underlying disease; the high incidence of urologic abnormalities, which must be corrected in children; donor–recipient organ size discrepancy with necessary alterations in recipient graft sites; small recipient vessel size; and the need for larger, more proximal recipient vessels, including aorta, vena cava, and iliac arteries. Recipient survival is improved in children older than 5 years of age because of the decreased incidence of vascular thrombosis when compared with the younger age group.

The introduction of cyclosporine therapy has markedly improved allograft survival but has also introduced cyclosporine nephrotoxicity into the differential diagnosis of graft dysfunction. Cyclosporine nephrotoxicity does not primarily affect tubular cells: rather, it has a vasoconstrictive effect that decreases ERPF and perfusion indices of the kidney.

Renal allografts result in better survival in children with normal bladder function compared with those in whom urinary transport is impaired and higher bladder pressures are maintained. It is postulated that diuresis and reduced concentrating ability of the renal allograft diminish the effectiveness of the transplant ureter. Inefficient ureteral urine transport leads to diminished renal blood flow and diminished glomerular filtration and eventual ischemia, necrosis, and graft loss, particularly when combined with the effects of rejection. Survival is better in children with primary reflux or pyelonephritis compared with children with posterior urethral valves or other severe, long-standing obstructive uropathies.

Renal Transplantation Complications

Immediate complications from pediatric renal transplantation may result from physiologic alterations from the donor kidney. Because an adult kidney sequesters a volume of between 250 and 300 ml of blood, a substantial percentage of the blood volume and cardiac output of a small child will enter the kidney. Thus, hypotension, renal ischemia, and vascular thrombosis can occur. The transplanted kidney may excrete a large volume of fluid, approaching the blood volume of a young infant on an hourly basis. This requires careful maintenance of an expanded blood volume and good cardiac output while normal glucose and electrolyte balance are maintained and hypertension is avoided.

Surgical complications usually present early after transplantation. Urologic complications of transplantation may be as high as 30% in pediatric patients. Urinary fistulas at the site of bladder reimplantation can lead to urine leaks and urinoma formation. Wound infection and wound abscesses occur early in the postoperative period. Injury during surgery to the lymphatics of the recipient can cause lymphocele formation. This frequently is noted during the second or third month after transplan-

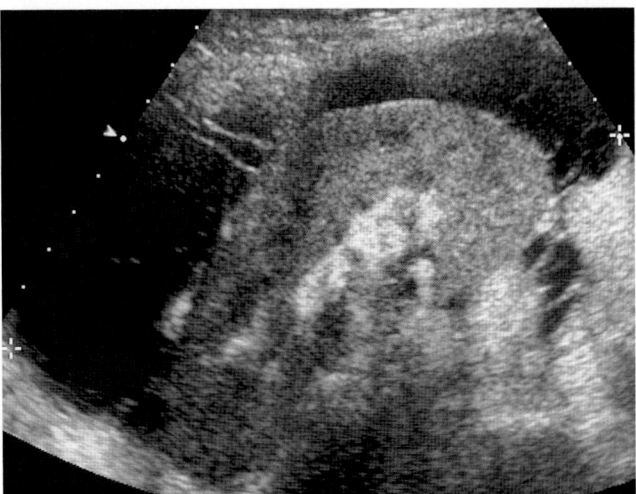

FIGURE 149-13. Peritransplant lymphocele. Longitudinal sonogram 3 weeks after right lower quadrant renal transplantation shows septated fluid collection surrounding the kidney.

tation. Hematomas are identified in the immediate postoperative period. Lesions, if of sufficient size, can put pressure on the graft, its collecting system, or the urinary bladder; this results in obstruction. Intrinsic obstruction may be caused by ureteral stenosis, blood clots, or early formation of calculi. US, the method of choice for imaging the transplanted kidney, readily shows perinephric collections (Fig. 149-13) and collecting system dilation, and it can be used to guide percutaneous therapy (see Chapter 192). Radionuclide imaging may be useful for documenting urinary leaks.

Vascular complications of transplantation include thrombosis, renal vascular hypertension related to anastomotic or postanastomotic renal artery narrowing, and peripheral thromboembolic disease. Other causes of malfunction of a renal allograft after surgery include dehydration, ATN, hyperacute or accelerated rejection, cyclosporine toxicity, and infection. Radionuclide imaging used to be routine after renal transplantation for evaluation of function and any subsequent complications. Currently, however, US performed with Doppler is the best method available for evaluating transplant vasculature and perfusion. Doppler examination is a reliable indicator of the patency of newly anastomosed vessels and of flow in the intrarenal arteries and veins. The renal artery is followed from the hilum to the iliac anastomosis, and detection of renal artery stenosis in a graft is much easier than in a native kidney. Doppler waveform changes from low-resistance flow in the renal artery to the typical high-resistance triphasic pattern in the iliac artery distal to the graft. Arterial stenosis is identified by high-frequency Doppler shift (Fig. 149-14). Doppler waveforms distal to a hemodynamically significant stenosis show delayed acceleration times and loss of the normal early systolic peak.

> **Sonography is the method of choice for detecting complications of renal transplantation.**

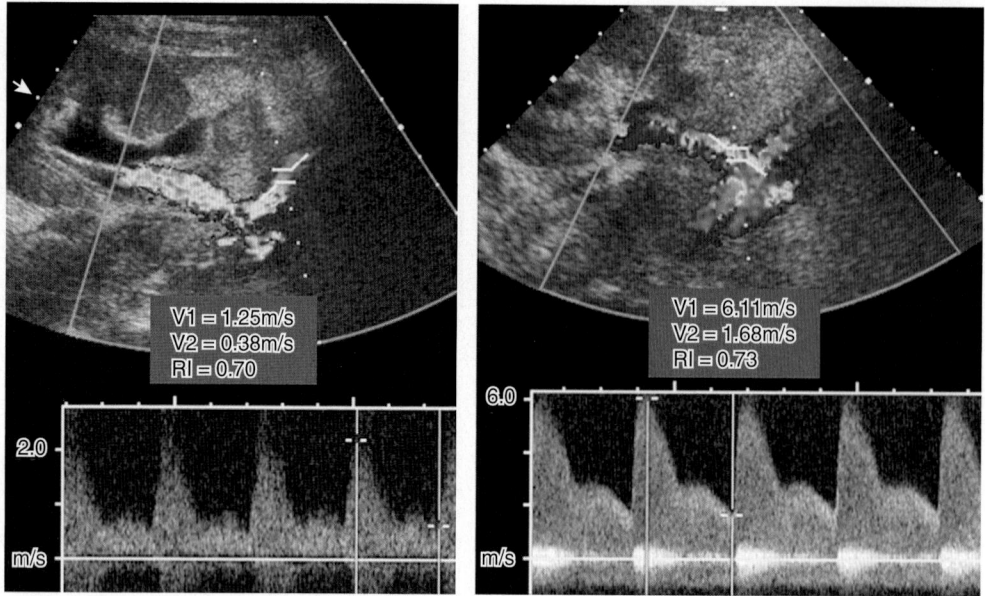

FIGURE 149-14. Transplant renal arterial stenosis. Doppler sonogram of a patient with rising creatinine shows a nearly fivefold increase in renal arterial peak systolic velocity *(right image)* compared with the supplying external iliac artery *(left image),* indicating hemodynamically significant stenosis.

Graft Rejection

Graft rejection is the recipient's response to an allograft that is related to antigenic stimulation of cytotoxic T lymphocytes to develop interleukin-2 receptors and promote interleukin-1 release from macrophages. Rejection is classified as hyperacute, accelerated acute, acute, and chronic. Hyperacute rejection may be seen within hours of transplantation and is the result of antibodies against the graft tissue that are already present in the host prior to transplantation. Hyperacute rejections are rare with modern assays for presensitization. Accelerated acute rejection occurs during the initial week of transplantation in poorly matched living donor grafts. It can also be caused by presensitization. It is characterized by fever, pain, hypertension, and oliguria. Acute rejection occurs within the first year, usually within several months of the transplantation, and presents with pain, fever, and oliguria.

Other causes of graft dysfunction have been noted during the first days or week after transplantation. These include ATN, obstructive uropathy, perirenal fluid collection, cyclosporine toxicity, acute renal vein thrombosis, and renal infection. The clinical spectrum of findings in all cases is similar and includes decreased urine output, elevated serum creatinine, pain, fever, and leukocytosis.

US is considered the most valuable diagnostic aid in the evaluation of postoperative renal transplant failure; it is used during initial investigation of a failing graft. During acute rejection, enlarged and sonolucent pyramids may become evident, and areas of decreased parenchymal echogenicity, alteration in sharpness of the corticomedullary junction, and increased corticomedullary ratio are apparent. Wall thickening of the renal collecting system can be seen, but it is nonspecific and may be noted in urinary tract infection, reflux, or obstruction. Diagnosis of acute rejection may require renal biopsy.

> **Diagnosis of rejection may require renal biopsy.**

Doppler sonography is extremely sensitive for evaluating the increasing intrarenal impedance that is associated with acute vascular rejection. If serial measurements can be obtained through a baseline study performed after the operation, then the patient's resistive index (RI) can be compared against his or her own baseline value rather than versus population norms. A single measurement of intrarenal impedance is of little value, although patients with increased RI immediately after transplantation have been shown to have a greater number of graft complications. To evaluate alterations in intrarenal arterial resistance commonly found in the transplanted kidney, an anatomic study and pulsed Doppler are needed. In patients with ATN, RIs become elevated immediately after surgery and typically return to baseline after 2 weeks. Renal volume increases slightly. With cyclosporine toxicity, frequently, little change occurs in RI or renal volume. With acute rejection, the RI shows an initial slight decrease followed in a few days by a rapid and progressive rise. Renal volume increases during this time. When acute vascular rejection is effectively treated, T cell–mediated graft inflammation is reduced; the resultant decrease in intrarenal resistance is dramatic and is well identified with Doppler.

Long-term living related donor graft survival rates generally are higher than those for cadaveric donor grafts. Long-term survival rates are better in pediatric patients than in adult patients. Graft loss after 10 years continues to be a problem despite low mortality rates. Major detriments to graft survival include episodes of rejection and progressive renal failure caused by chronic rejection or intrinsic disease. Systemic hypertension,

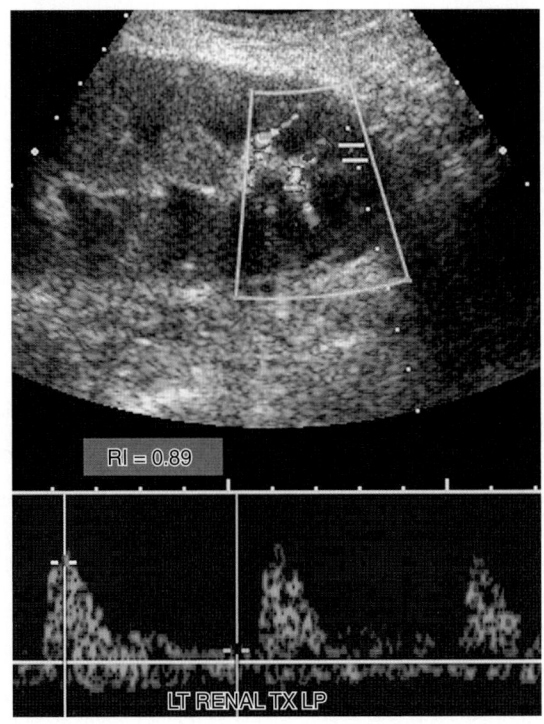

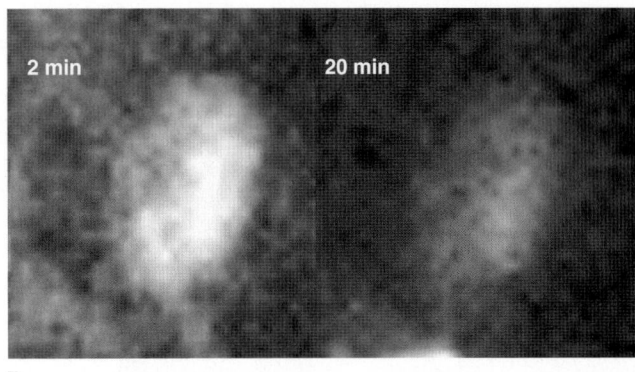

FIGURE 149-15. Chronic renal transplant rejection. **A,** Duplex Doppler sonogram from a 16-year-old girl with biopsy-proven chronic rejection shows poor peripheral color Doppler flow to the renal periphery. The resistive index is elevated, at 0.89. **B,** Radionuclide MAG3 renogram shows patchy uptake and poor radiopharmaceutical clearance—a nonspecific indicator of renal dysfunction. (Courtesy of Harriet J. Paltiel, MD, Boston, MA.)

glomerular hyperfiltration, and hypercholesterolemia may cause glomerular sclerosis and interstitial fibrosis, resulting in progressive loss of renal function. Dietary effects on glomerular perfusion and optimal measures to improve long-term function of pediatric recipients remain to be determined.

Chronic rejection is insidious and asymptomatic and results in loss of graft function months to years after transplantation. It seems to result from multiple episodes of unsuccessfully treated acute rejection. It is characterized histologically by an arteritis and tubular atrophy. The glomeruli are smaller than normal and may become hyalinized. With chronic rejection, vascular intimal proliferation is noted in the interlobar and arcuate arteries. This decreases the diameter of small vessels, which increases vascular impedance, and causes decreased or absent diastolic arterial flow on Doppler interrogation. Color Doppler may show diminished peripheral perfusion in the transplant renal cortex (Fig. 149-15). US may show increased parenchymal echogenicity, diminished corticomedullary differentiation, and volume loss.

Other Complications

Transplantation and immunosuppressant therapy have been associated with increased incidence of malignancy. Post-transplant lymphoproliferative disorder (PTLD) occurs in from 1% to 10% of pediatric renal transplant recipients and is more common in children than in adults. The mildest form of PTLD is benign hyperplasia with normal and preserved lymph node architecture. The polymorphic form is of an intermediate grade and is characterized by altered nodal histology and polyclonal proliferation. Monomorphic PTLD represents transfor-

mation into lymphoma. PTLD is associated with Epstein-Barr virus (EBV) infection. In healthy individuals and in patients previously exposed to EBV, T cell immune responses to EBV-carrying B cells keep proliferation under control. However, children are often not exposed to EBV at the time of transplantation, after which they are intentionally immunosuppressed. If they are subsequently exposed to EBV, these children cannot adequately suppress the infected B cells, and this may eventually lead to neoplastic transformation. EBV recipient sero-negativity and severe immunosuppression are the two primary factors that predispose to PTLD. Mean time to diagnosis is just under 2 years from transplantation, but it may occur from weeks to years later.

Imaging findings of PTLD resemble those of lymphoma, although extranodal sites of disease are more common. Abdominal involvement occurs in one half of affected renal transplant recipients and may involve the liver, spleen, gastrointestinal tract, and even the renal graft itself. Appearance on US and computed tomography (CT) is usually that of focal hypoechoic masses, although more diffuse infiltration may occur (Fig. 149-16). Involvement of the thorax, head and neck, and central nervous system is uncommon in renal transplant recipients. Imaging may provide guidance for confirmatory tissue sampling.

The principal treatment of PTLD involves reduction of immunosuppression, which may reverse the disease in up to one half of patients. Rituximab halts B cell proliferation but is associated with a high rate of infectious complications. The use of interferon-alpha stimulates the host immune response, halting PTLD, but it may also lead to graft loss. Lastly, standard chemotherapeutic approaches and even removal of the graft may be effec-

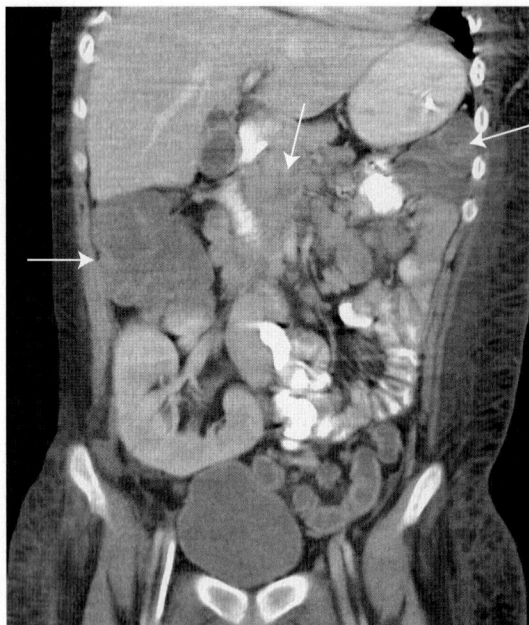

FIGURE 149-16. Post-transplant lymphoproliferative disorder. Coronal reformatted image from contrast-enhanced computed tomography in a 17-year-old boy shows a right lower quadrant renal transplant. Multiple low-density conglomerate masses within the abdomen represent lymphoproliferative tissue *(arrow)*. (Courtesy of Harriet J. Paltiel, MD, Boston, MA.)

tive. Regardless of the treatment used, results remain disappointing, with survival at around 50%, depending on the extent and number of organs involved.

> **Post-transplant lymphoproliferative disease (PTLD) occurs in from 1% to 10% of pediatric renal transplant recipients.**

Avascular necrosis has been reported to occur in 10% to 20% of pediatric allograft recipients. The most commonly involved bones are the femoral head and the femoral condyles, but multiple bone involvement is not unusual. Pain is the initial clinical manifestation. The exact cause is unclear, but corticosteroid therapy and secondary hyperparathyroidism have been postulated in the pathogenesis.

Immunosuppressive treatment used for the prevention of rejection renders transplant patients susceptible to infection. Infections of the urinary tract and surgical wounds with *Staphylococcus aureus* and *Escherichia coli* are common during the first few weeks post transplant; after this time, opportunistic infections increase. The most common viral infections are caused by cytomegalovirus, herpesvirus, and varicella-zoster. Cytomegalic infection results in significant morbidity and mortality in immunocompromised children.

SUGGESTED READINGS

Renal Failure

Alwaidh MH, Cooke RW, Judd BA: Renal blood flow velocity in acute renal failure following cardiopulmonary bypass surgery. Acta Paediatr 1998;87:644-649

Andreoli SP: Acute renal failure. Curr Opin Pediatr 2002;14:183-188

Andreoli SP: Acute renal failure in the newborn. Semin Perinatol 2004;28:112-123

Balinsky W: Pediatric end-stage renal disease: incidence, management, and prevention. J Pediatr Health Care 2000;14:304-308

Barletta GM, Bunchman TE: Acute renal failure in infants and children. Curr Opin Crit Care 2004;10:499-504

Choyke PL, Grant EG, Hoffer FA, et al: Cortical echogenicity in the hemolytic uremic syndrome: clinical correlation. J Ultrasound Med 1988;7:439-442

Filiatrault D, Perreault G: Transient acute tubular disease in a newborn and a young infant: sonographic findings. J Ultrasound Med 1985;4:257-258

Flynn JT: Causes, management approaches, and outcome of acute renal failure in children. Curr Opin Pediatr 1998;10:184-189

Galesic K, Sabljar-Matovinovic M, Tomic M, et al: Renal vascular resistance in glomerular diseases: correlation of resistance index with biopsy findings. Coll Antropol 2004;28:667-674

Groothoff JW: Long-term outcomes of children with end-stage renal disease. Pediatr Nephrol 2005;20:849-853

Kaplan BS, Meyers KE, Schulman SL: The pathogenesis and treatment of hemolytic uremic syndrome. J Am Soc Nephrol 1998;9:1126-1133

Kazzi AA, Tehranzadeh AD. Glomerulonephritis, acute. Available at: www.emedicine.com/EMERG/topic219.htm.accessed February 25, 2007

Khati NJ, Hill MC, Kimmel PL: The role of ultrasound in renal insufficiency: the essentials. Ultrasound Q 2005;21:227-244

Kozlowski K, Brown RW: Renal medullary necrosis in infants and children. Pediatr Radiol 1978;7:85-89

Luciano R, Gallini F, Romagnoli C, et al: Doppler evaluation of renal blood flow velocity as a predictive index of acute renal failure in perinatal asphyxia. Eur J Pediatr 1998;157:656-660

Maxvold NJ, Smoyer WE, Gardner JJ, et al: Management of acute renal failure in the pediatric patient: hemofiltration versus hemodialysis. Am J Kidney Dis 1997;30:S84-S88

Moghal NE, Brocklebank JT, Meadow SR: A review of acute renal failure in children: incidence, etiology and outcome. Clin Nephrol 1998;49:91-95

Patriquin HB, O'Regan S, Robitaille P, et al: Hemolytic-uremic syndrome: intrarenal arterial Doppler patterns as a useful guide to therapy. Radiology 1989;172:625-628

Polito C, Papale MR, La Manna A: Long-term prognosis of acute renal failure in the full-term neonate. Clin Pediatr 1998;37:381-385

Roth KS, Koo HP, Spottswood SE, et al: Obstructive uropathy: an important cause of chronic renal failure in children. Clin Pediatr 2002;41:309-314

Siegel MJ, Van Why SK, Devarajan P, et al: Pathogenesis of acute renal failure. In Barrat TM, Avner ED, Harmon WE (eds): Pediatric Nephrology. Baltimore, Lippincott Williams & Wilkins, 1999:1109-1118

Vergesslich KA, Sommer G, Wittich GR, et al: Acute renal failure in children: an ultrasonographic-clinical study. Eur J Radiol 1987;7:263-265

Williams DM, Sreedhar SS, Mickell JJ, et al: Acute kidney failure: a pediatric experience over 20 years. Arch Pediatr Adolesc Med 2002;157:893-900

Wong SN, Lo RN, Yu EC: Renal blood flow pattern by noninvasive Doppler ultrasound in normal children and acute renal failure patients. J Ultrasound Med 1989;8:135-141

Renal Replacement Therapy

Bay WH, Henry ML, Lazarus JM, et al: Predicting hemodialysis access failure with color flow Doppler ultrasound. Am J Nephrol 1998;18:296-304

Dittrich S, Dahnert I, Vogel M, et al: Peritoneal dialysis after infant open heart surgery: observations in 27 patients. Ann Thorac Surg 1999;68:160-163

Litherland J, Lupton EW, Ackrill PA, et al: Computed tomographic peritoneography: CT manifestations in the investigation of leaks and abnormal collections in patients on CAPD. Nephrol Dial Transplant 1994;9:1449-1452

Robbin ML, Oser RF, Allon M, et al: Hemodialysis accesses graft stenosis: US detection. Radiology 1998;208:655-661

Stafford-Johnson DB, Wilson TE, Francis IR, et al: CT appearance of sclerosing peritonitis in patients on chronic ambulatory peritoneal dialysis. J Comput Assist Tomogr 1998;22:295-299

Renal Transplantation and Complications

Adams J, Mehls O, Wiesel M: Pediatric renal transplantation and the dysfunctional bladder. Transpl Int 2004;17:596-602

Babcock DS, Slovis TL, Han BK, et al: Renal transplants in children: long-term follow-up using sonography. Radiology 1985;156:165-167

Bereket G, Fine RN: Pediatric renal transplantation. Pediatr Clin North Am 1995;42:1603-1628

De Morais RH, Muglia VF, Mamere AE, et al: Duplex Doppler sonography of transplant renal artery stenosis. J Clin Ultrasound 2003;31:135-141

Gottlieb RH, Voci SL, Cholewinski SP, et al: Sonography: a useful tool to detect the mechanical causes of renal transplant dysfunction. J Clin Ultrasound 1999;27:325-333

Hoyer PF, Schmid R, Wunsch L, et al: Color Doppler energy—a new technique to study tissue perfusion in renal transplants. Pediatr Nephrol 1999;13:559-563

Isiklar I, Aktas A, Uzuner O, et al: Power Doppler ultrasonography compared with scintigraphy in the diagnosis of renal allograft dysfunction. Transpl Proc 1999;31:3330-3331

Mutze S, Turk I, Schonberger B, et al: Colour-coded duplex sonography in the diagnostic assessment of vascular complications after kidney transplantation in children. Pediatr Radiol 1997;27:898-902

Nathason S, Debray D, Delarue A, et al: Long-term survival after post-transplant lymphoproliferative disease in children. Pediatr Nephrol 2002;17:668-672

Nuininga JE, Feitz WFJ, van Dael KCML, et al: Urological complications in pediatric renal transplantation. Eur Urol 2001;39:598-602

Pickhardt PJ, Siegel MJ, Hayashi RJ, et al: Posttransplantation lymphoproliferative disorder in children: clinical, histopathologic, and imaging features. Radiology 2000;217:16-25

Raiteri M, Ferraresso M, Pozzoli E, et al: Value of intraoperative resistive index in kidney transplant. Transpl Proc 2005;37:2472-2473

Salgado O, Garcia R, Rincon O, et al: Acute tubular necrosis in renal transplantation evaluated by color duplex sonography. Transplant Proc 1996;28:3337-3339

Shroff R, Rees L: The post-transplant lymphoproliferative disorder—a literature review. Pediatr Nephrol 2004;19:369-377

Stringer DA, O'Halpin D, Daneman A, et al: Duplex Doppler sonography for renal artery stenosis in the post-transplant pediatric patient. Pediatr Radiol 1989;19:187-192

Surratt JT, Siegel MJ, Middleton WD: Sonography of complications in pediatric renal allografts. Radiographics 1990;10:687-699

Townsend RR, Tomlanovich SJ, Goldstein RB, et al: Combined Doppler and morphologic sonographic evaluation of renal transplant rejection. J Ultrasound Med 1990;9:199-206

Vergesslich KA, Khoss AE, Balzar E, et al: Acute renal transplant rejection in children: assessment by duplex Doppler sonography. Pediatr Radiol 1988;18:474-478

ROBERT WELLS

HYPERTENSION

The prevalence of hypertension in the pediatric age group is approximately 2% to 4%. Severe hypertension occurs in at least 10% of these individuals. Although the overall prevalence of hypertension in children is much lower than in adults, clinically identifiable causes of hypertension are much more common; approximately 90% of hypertensive children younger than 10 years of age have a secondary form, as compared with 10% of adults. In addition, the underlying causes of clinically significant hypertension in the pediatric population differ considerably from those of adults. In children, secondary hypertension is most often related to renal disease, whereas endocrine and renal vascular disorders account for a greater proportion of secondary hypertension in adults. In general, the higher the blood pressure and the younger the child, the more likely it is that a secondary cause underlies the hypertension. Appropriate clinical and radiographic evaluation is essential for all children with substantial hypertension, to detect a potentially correctable underlying cause (Table 150-1).

The prevalence and most common causes of pediatric hypertension vary with patient age. Hypertension is uncommon in neonates. Some infants, however, are at increased risk. These include premature infants hospitalized in neonatal intensive care units, infants with a history of umbilical catheterization, and those with bronchopulmonary dysplasia. The most frequent causes of neonatal hypertension include renal artery thrombosis, renal artery stenosis, congenital renal malformations, coarctation of the aorta, and bronchopulmonary dysplasia. From infancy to 6 years of age, renal parenchymal disease, renal artery stenosis, and coarctation are the most common causes of hypertension. From 6 to 10 years of age, renal parenchymal disease and renal artery stenosis are the most common causes of hypertension. Onset of primary, or essential, hypertension occasionally occurs during adolescence or late childhood, often with relatively mild elevations in blood pressure. The incidence of childhood-onset essential hypertension increases with age. Other relatively common causes of late-onset childhood hypertension include renal parenchymal disease and obesity.

All children with sustained hypertension require a thorough clinical examination. Clinical findings and the presence or absence of various risk factors determine the need for a diagnostic imaging evaluation. In general, the adolescent with mild labile hypertension and no laboratory abnormalities most likely has essential hypertension and may not require imaging studies. Imaging is indicated, however, for any patient with clinical or laboratory findings suggestive of pheochromocytoma or renal vascular disease. The severity of hypertension, the age of the child at presentation, and a history of a predisposing medical condition (e.g., neuroectodermal disorder) are other important considerations.

Sonography is the initial diagnostic imaging procedure of choice for use in most hypertensive children who

TABLE 150-1

Causes of Hypertension

Essential hypertension	
Obesity	
Cardiovascular	Coarctation
	Renal artery stenosis
	Renal artery thrombosis
	Systemic arteritis
	Middle aortic syndrome
Renal	Structural abnormalities (obstruction, reflux)
	Glomerulonephritis
	Nephritis
	Chronic renal failure
	Diabetic nephropathy
	Renal trauma
	Renal vein thrombosis
	Segmental hypoplasia
Endocrine	Hyperthyroidism
	Congenital adrenal hyperplasia
	Primary aldosteronism
	Hyperparathyroidism
Neurologic	Intracranial hypertension
	Guillain-Barré syndrome
	Familial dysautonomia
Neoplasm	Neuroblastoma
	Pheochromocytoma
	Adrenal adenocarcinoma
	Juxtaglomerular tumor (reninoma)
Drug ingestion	Corticosteroids
	Oral contraceptives
	Cocaine
	Sympathomimetics
	Phencyclidine

require radiologic evaluation. Sonography may or may not indicate a specific cause for the hypertension, but it generally narrows the differential diagnosis and helps guide the selection of additional imaging procedures. It is important to recognize that a normal ultrasound examination does not exclude a renal cause of hypertension. Sonography may reveal a specific underlying renal abnormality, such as cystic disease or hydronephrosis. Vascular lesions of the aorta or renal arteries are sometimes detectable by this technique. If sonography shows unilateral or bilateral renal hypoplasia or atrophy, careful correlation with clinical and laboratory findings helps the clinician to determine whether this is due to renovascular disease or parenchymal disease. Supplemental imaging techniques helpful for the evaluation of suspected renovascular disease include captopril renal scintigraphy, computed tomographic angiography (CTA), magnetic resonance angiographic (MRA), and conventional angiography. Computed tomography evaluation is usually indicated for patients with evidence of adrenal pathology or neoplasia.

Renal Parenchymal Hypertension

Renal disease is the most common cause of hypertension in children. The two major categories of underlying renal pathology consist of disorders that predominantly involve the parenchyma and those that involve the major renal arteries. Parenchymal disorders account for about 80% of cases of secondary renal hypertension in the pediatric age group. Renal parenchymal and vascular disorders can lead to hypertension through multiple potential mechanisms. The kidneys influence systemic blood pressure through two primary mechanisms and multiple secondary mechanisms. Primary mechanisms are those by which the kidney directly responds to changes in arterial blood pressure by way of a feedback phenomenon. The two important primary mechanisms are the renal blood volume pressure control mechanism and the renin-angiotensin system. Secondary mechanisms include the effects of various extrinsic factors that act on the two primary renal blood pressure control mechanisms. For example, aldosterone released by the adrenal glands influences renal water and sodium retention. Antidiuretic hormone and the nervous system also secondarily affect renal blood pressure control functions.

Acute glomerulonephritis is the most common cause of acute hypertension in children. Glomerulonephritis includes various disorders characterized by disruption of the normal glomerular filtration mechanism. Acute glomerulonephritis is usually an immunologically mediated inflammation of glomerular capillaries. Acute glomerulonephritis may occur as part of a systemic disease, or it can follow infection with various bacteria or viruses. Hypertension occurs in 60% to 80% of patients with acute glomerulonephritis and is usually mild to moderate in severity. The mechanism of hypertension in these patients is incompletely elucidated but apparently involves intracellular volume expansion and generalized vasospasm. Hypertension usually spontaneously resolves, beginning within a few weeks of onset.

> **Glomerulonephritis is the most common cause of acute hypertension in children.**

Chronic glomerulonephritis, which is uncommon in children, usually involves an immune response that leads to excessive inflammation and progression to interstitial fibrosis in the kidneys. In those patients with renal failure, hypertension is common. Hypertension does not usually occur, however, in conjunction with mild disease and relatively preserved renal function.

Hypertension can occur in association with other various forms of nephritis. In some instances, hypertension due to renal pathology precedes the other clinical manifestations of these disorders. Nephritis can occur in patients with systemic lupus erythematosus, dermatomyositis, scleroderma, and polyarteritis nodosa.

Various chronic diseases that destroy renal tissue through inflammation or scarring can lead to hypertension. Examples include chronic pyelonephritis, reflux nephropathy, radiation nephritis, end-stage cystinosis, and chemical nephrotoxicity. Reflux nephropathy is a relatively common cause of hypertension in children.

Sonography of the patient with hypertension related to renal parenchymal disease reveals renal volume, collecting system anatomy, focal lesions, and general parenchymal integrity. Many of the parenchymal diseases lead to diffuse parenchymal hyperechogenicity and lack of normal corticomedullary differentiation. Ultrasonography is helpful for detecting congenital renal abnormalities and scarring from prior insults. Cortical echogenicity in patients with acute glomerulonephritis ranges from normal to moderately increased; global enlargement of the kidneys is often observed. The most common sonographic appearance of chronic glomerulonephritis consists of prominent cortical echogenicity and preservation of cortical medullary differentiation; the kidneys may be atrophic.

Renovascular Hypertension

Renovascular hypertension refers to elevation of blood pressure due to narrowing of the main renal artery or one of its branches. Physiologically significant renal artery stenosis diminishes renal perfusion pressure, leading to a multistep compensatory mechanism that serves to maintain renal perfusion pressure and glomerular filtration. In response to reduced perfusion pressure, the juxtaglomerular apparatus releases the proteolytic enzyme renin, which, in turn, converts angiotensinogen to angiotensin I. Angiotensin-converting enzyme converts angiotensin I to angiotensin II. Angiotensin II is a potent vasoconstrictor that also increases blood pressure by stimulating adrenal gland release of aldosterone, which promotes retention of sodium and water.

Approximately 5% to 10% of children and adolescents with severe hypertension have an underlying renal vascular lesion. In infants, up to 70% of clinically significant hypertension is due to renovascular disease. Potential causes of renovascular hypertension include (1) developmental arterial abnormalities (e.g., hypoplasia, aneurysm),

TABLE 150-2

Causes of Renovascular Hypertension

Fibrous dysplasia	
Inflammatory disease	Takayasu arteritis
	Kawasaki disease
	Moyamoya disease
	Irradiation
Genetic disorders	Williams syndrome
	Neurofibromatosis
	Klippel-Trenaunay-Weber syndrome
	Feuerstein-Mims syndrome
	Rett syndrome
	Degos-Köhlmeier disease
	Marfan syndrome
Atherosclerosis	Hyperlipidemias
Vascular anomaly	Renal arteriovenous malformation
	Renal artery aneurysm
	Renal artery hypoplasia
Thromboembolism	Umbilical artery catheterization
	Neonate of diabetic mother
Renal transplantation	Rejection
	Arterial narrowing
Other	Congenital rubella
	Compression by mass
	Congenital fibrous band
	Post-traumatic causes
	Retroperitoneal fibrosis

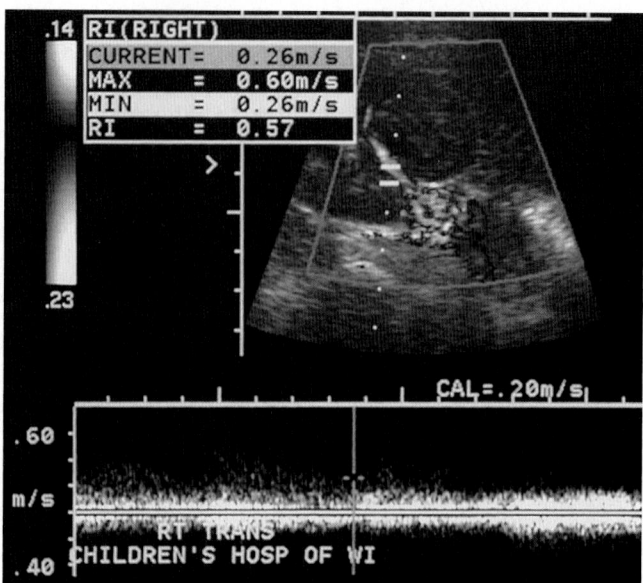

FIGURE 150-1. Renal artery stenosis. Doppler evaluation of the renal artery distal to severe stenosis in a child with renal arterial fibrous dysplasia shows a low-velocity monophasic arterial waveform.

(2) localized muscular or fibrous thickening of the renal arterial wall (e.g., fibrous dysplasia), (3) thrombosis, (4) trauma, (5) extrinsic compression (e.g., neoplasm, hematoma), (6) diseases of small intrarenal vessels, and (7) radiation vasculopathy (Table 150-2).

A complication related to umbilical artery catheterization is the most common cause of renovascular hypertension in neonates (see Chapter 21). This typically involves embolization or extension of thrombus from the abdominal aorta into the renal vessels. In older children, renal vascular fibrous dysplasia is the most common cause of renovascular hypertension. Other potential underlying conditions include neurofibromatosis type 1, aortic coarctation, middle aortic syndrome, Williams syndrome, arteritis, neoplasm, and trauma.

Asymmetry of the kidneys is an important sign of possible renovascular hypertension on noninvasive imaging studies such as sonography. The affected kidney is often small and may show manifestations of scarring. Evaluation of the aorta is also an important component of the examination. Direct visualization of a stenotic renal arterial lesion is uncommon with sonography, however. With Doppler evaluation, a renal artery-to-aorta peak systolic velocity ratio of greater than 3.5 carries a strong association with renal arterial stenosis. A peak velocity in the renal artery of greater than 100 cm per second is also suggestive of renal artery stenosis. Distal to the stenotic lesion, the systolic peak of the renal arterial waveform often appears flattened (Fig. 150-1). With severe stenosis, Doppler evaluation of distal arteries shows a tardus-parvus pattern, with slow systolic acceleration and diminished peak systolic velocity. Diastolic flow in the main renal artery is sometimes elevated.

The most useful scintigraphic technique for detection of renovascular hypertension involves the evaluation of renal function without and with the use of an angiotensin-converting enzyme inhibitor, usually captopril or enalaprilat. Tc-99m mercaptoacetyltriglycine (MAG3) is the preferred imaging agent for this study, although technetium-99m diethylenetriaminepentaacetic acid (^{99m}Tc-DTPA) and ^{123}I-orthoiodohippurate (^{123}I-OIH) can also be used. The technique involves scintigraphy performed on two dates, one with angiotensin-converting enzyme antihypertensive therapy and one without. In the presence of renovascular disease, imaging in conjunction with angiotensin-converting enzyme inhibitor therapy typically shows diminished function in the affected kidney (or in the affected portion of the kidney) (Fig. 150-2). The findings include diminished perfusion, diminished initial uptake, and poor parenchyma clearance. Comparative imaging in the absence of antihypertensive therapy shows a greater degree of function in the involved kidney. The sensitivity of this technique for the detection of renovascular hypertension is approximately 85% to 90%. Bilateral renal artery stenosis or markedly compromised renal function can lead to false-negative examinations.

Transcatheter angiography is the most sensitive and specific technique for the detection and identification of small-vessel disease. CTA and MRA represent important noninvasive techniques for visualization of renal vascular anatomy. With contrast administration, global and regional alterations in kidney perfusion and function can also be assessed with CT and magnetic resonance imaging (MRI). In general, narrowing of the renal arterial diameter of greater than 50% is hemodynamically significant. The presence of enlarged collateral pathways is an additional indicator of significant renal artery stenosis.

Transcatheter renal vein renin sampling is useful in selected cases of suspected renal hypertension. This

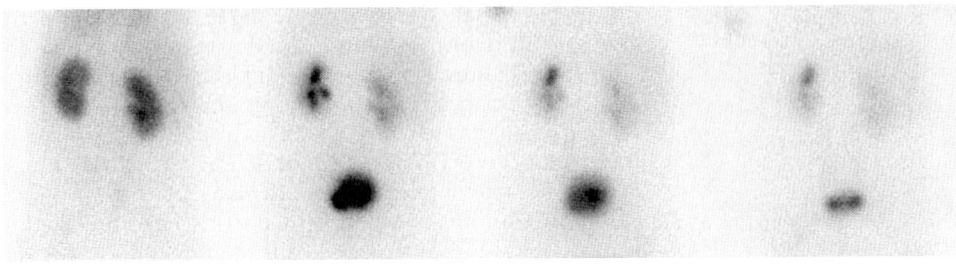

A

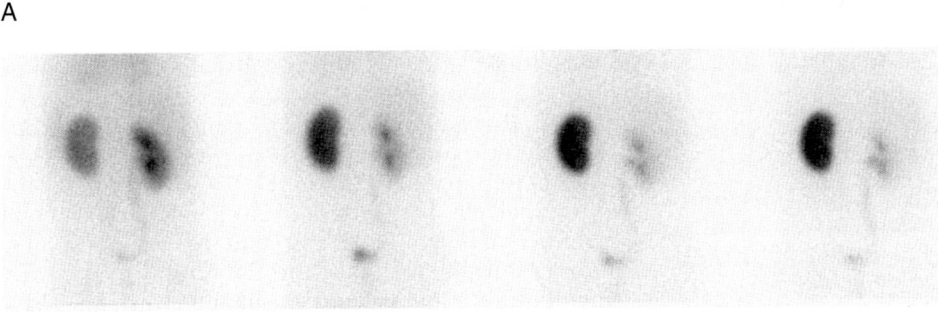

B

FIGURE 150-2. Renovascular hypertension and angiotensin-converting enzyme (ACE) inhibition scintigraphy. **A,** Renogram shows normal uptake and excretion from both kidneys. **B,** Renogram after administration of an ACE inhibitor shows marked radiopharmaceutical retention in the left kidney, indicating renal artery stenosis. (Courtesy of Douglas F. Eggli, MD, Hershey, PA.)

involves measurement of renin levels within blood sampled from the renal veins and the infrarenal and suprarenal portions of the inferior vena cava; branch renal vein sampling is occasionally indicated. In patients with renovascular hypertension due to unilateral kidney involvement, plasma renin activity is elevated in venous drainage from the underperfused kidney. Renin excretion from the normal kidney is suppressed. The most commonly applied standard for clinically significant lateralization is an ipsilateral/contralateral renal vein–to–renin ratio of 1.5 or greater. This lateralization may not be present in patients with substantial aortic disease or with bilateral renal artery stenosis. In addition, the formation of collateral vessels may affect the degree of lateralization in patients with bilateral disease.

Endocrine Causes of Hypertension

The most common endocrine form of hypertension in childhood is iatrogenic and is due to the exogenous administration of adrenocortical steroids or related synthetic steroid derivatives. Intrinsic causes include pheochromocytoma, adrenal adenoma, adrenocortical carcinoma, adrenogenital syndrome, and primary aldosteronism. Hypertension occasionally occurs in association with neuroblastoma as the result of tumor secretion of endocrinologically active substances.

Pheochromocytoma is an endocrinologically active neoplasm that secretes catecholamines (see Chapter 144). About 80% of children with this tumor have clinically significant hypertension. Hypertension in these patients is usually (90%) sustained, but paroxysmal hypertensive crises can be life threatening. Pheochromocytoma arises from neural crest derivatives. About 70% arise in the adrenal gland; other potential sites of origin include the thoracic and abdominal sympathetic chains, the organ of Zuckerkandl, the bladder wall, and the periureteral region.

Three distinct clinical forms of pheochromocytoma have been identified: primary sporadic, malignant metastatic, and familial. About 85% of pediatric cases are of the primary sporadic benign type and usually occur as an isolated adrenal lesion. Metastatic malignant pheochromocytoma accounts for about 5% of pediatric pheochromocytomas. The familial form occurs in about 10% of children with pheochromocytoma; these children often have multiple lesions. Syndromes that are associated with pheochromocytoma include neurofibromatosis type 1, von Hippel–Lindau disease, tuberous sclerosis, and multiple endocrine neoplasia types IIA, IIB, and III.

Pheochromocytomas are heterogeneous lesions that may contain cysts, necrosis, calcification, fibrosis, fat, and hemorrhage. Calcification within an adrenal pheochromocytoma is occasionally visible on standard radiographs. Sonography is of reasonable sensitivity for the detection of an adrenal lesion. However, the most appropriate initial imaging technique for the child with clinical findings that suggest the presence of a pheochromocytoma is CT or MRI. Intra-arterial or intravenous injection of iodinated contrast material can precipitate catecholamine release from a pheochromocytoma that leads to a hypertensive crisis. Alpha-adrenergic blockade blunts this effect; the use of low osmolar nonionic contrast also diminishes the release of catecholamines.

Cross-sectional imaging studies show pheochromocytoma as a well-defined mass, often with a round configuration. Large lesions tend to be heterogeneous in composition. Prominent contrast enhancement is evident on CT. Pheochromocytoma typically is hypointense to liver on T1-weighted magnetic resonance (MR) images and markedly hyperintense on T2-weighted images. As with CT, contrast enhancement is striking. Pheochromocytoma accumulates ^{131}I-metaiodobenzylguanidine and ^{111}In-DTPA-D-Phe-pentetreotide (octreotide).

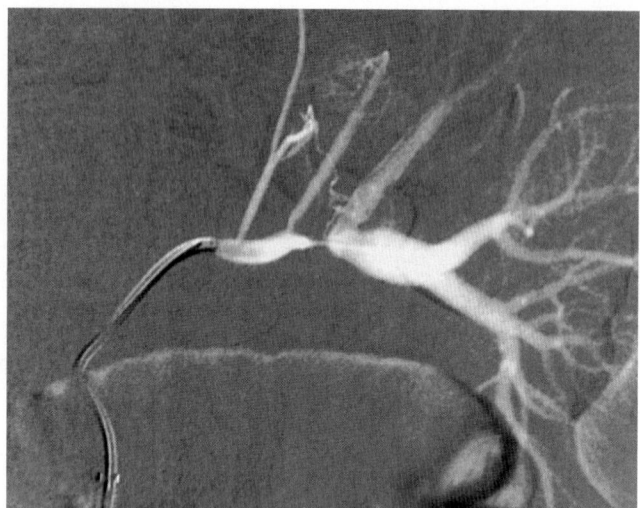

FIGURE 150-3. Renal artery stenosis. Selective renal arteriogram of a 12-year-old female with hypertension due to primary intimal fibroplasia shows severe stenosis of the main renal artery. Poststenotic dilation is present.

RENAL ARTERIAL FIBROUS DYSPLASIA

Renal arterial fibrous dysplasia (fibromuscular dysplasia, fibrodysplasia) is the most common cause of renal artery stenosis in children. Various forms of this disorder include congenital vascular dysplasias with maldevelopment of the fibrous muscular and elastic tissues of the renal arteries. Subcategorization of fibrous dysplasia is based on the layer of the arterial wall that is involved. This classification is important because each type of fibrous dysplasia has distinct histologic and angiographic features and occurs in a different clinical setting.

> **Fibromuscular dysplasia is the most common cause of renal arterial stenosis in children.**

Primary intimal fibroplasia is characterized by circumferential accumulation of collagen subintimally and within the internal elastic membrane. This form of fibrous dysplasia is more common in children than in adults and is the most common cause of renal artery stenosis during childhood. Angiographically, a smooth, localized stenosis usually involves the distal two thirds of the renal artery or a branch vessel. The nature of stenotic lesions varies between patients; they may be bandlike, tubular, or funnel shaped (Fig. 150-3). Although this disease most often involves the renal arteries alone, it sometimes occurs as a generalized disorder with involvement of the vessels of the aortic arch, upper and lower extremities, and viscera.

Perimedial or *subadventitial fibrodysplasia* is another of the fibrous dysplasias that tends to occur in childhood. Collagen is deposited in the outer border of the media over a variable length of the renal artery. Thickness of the collagen varies along the involved segment of the vessel. Angiography typically shows severe long-segment narrowing of the renal artery, with a beaded appearance. Enlarged collateral vessels are often present. This disease

occurs almost exclusively in girls older than 10 years of age, and it involves only the renal arteries or branches. The right kidney is involved more commonly than the left; approximately 15% of cases are bilateral.

Fibromuscular hyperplasia is an extremely rare vasculopathy that can occur in childhood. This is the only renal arterial obstructive lesion that displays true hyperplasia of the smooth muscle cells. Concentric thickening of the renal arterial wall is due to proliferating smooth muscle and fibrous tissue. Angiographically, this lesion appears as a smooth stenosis of the renal artery or its branches; its appearance may be indistinguishable from that of intimal fibroplasia.

Medial fibroplasia is the most common cause of nonarteriosclerotic renovascular disease in adults, but it is rare in children. Alternating areas of focal thinning of the internal elastic membrane and focal collagenous thickening of the medial muscular layer are present. Angiographically, medial fibrodysplasia produces a string-of-beads appearance, typically involving the distal two thirds of the main renal artery and its branches. Areas of dilation between stenoses are usually greater in caliber than the normal renal artery. Prominent collateral circulation is usually absent. These features are important in differentiating medial fibroplasia from perimedial fibroplasia.

NEUROFIBROMATOSIS

The most common vascular pathology in patients with neurofibromatosis 1 (NF1) involves stenosis of the aorta or a large branch vessel that is due to intimal changes associated with proliferation of neural tissue in the arterial wall and perivascular nodular proliferations; an aneurysm occasionally occurs. In the kidney, a small-vessel mesodermal dysplasia can also occur. Both of these mechanisms can cause hypertension. Renal artery stenosis is the most common vascular abnormality that is responsible for hypertension in patients with NF1. Other potential causes of hypertension in NF1 patients include coarctation of the aorta and pheochromocytoma. In the kidney, arterial stenosis usually occurs at the vessel origin or in the proximal third of the main renal artery. Angiographic features of renal artery stenosis due to neurofibromatous vasculopathy are similar to those of intimal fibroplasia. However, aortic narrowing often accompanies visceral artery stenoses in patients with NF1.

TAKAYASU ARTERITIS

Takayasu arteritis is a rare idiopathic chronic inflammatory arteritis that causes thrombosis, stenosis, dilation, and aneurysm formation in the pulmonary arteries, aorta, and major aortic branch vessels. Involved vessels are narrowed as the result of concentric mural thickening and calcification; aneurysms can also occur. Takayasu arteritis most often affects young adult women; pediatric cases usually present during the second decade of life. Hypertension due to renal arterial stenosis or abdominal aortic narrowing is common. Other potential clinical features include dyspnea, hemoptysis, and neurologic symptoms.

CT and MRI features of Takayasu arteritis include narrowing, mural thickening, adherent thrombus, and mural calcification of the aorta, pulmonary arteries, and major aortic branch vessels. With active disease, the thickened vascular wall has prominent contrast enhancement. Angiographic studies usually show one or more long stenotic vascular lesions. Vessel wall irregularity and poststenotic dilation may be evident. Ectatic vessels or true aneurysms are present in some patients.

MIDDLE AORTIC SYNDROME

Middle aortic syndrome (midaortic dysplastic syndrome) is an acquired, progressive vascular disorder that involves the midthoracic through abdominal segments of the aorta and is usually accompanied by narrowing of major visceral branches, including the renal arteries. Middle aortic syndrome most often presents during the second decade of life with hypertension, lower extremity weakness, and weak or absent lower extremity pulses. Often, an abdominal bruit is noted. Manifestations of arteritis, such as fever and sedimentation rate elevation, are lacking in patients with middle aortic syndrome.

Imaging studies of middle aortic syndrome show diffuse narrowing of the thoracoabdominal segment of the aorta and the major branch vessels (Fig. 150-4). The aorta usually appears smoothly tapered; narrowing often is most marked in the infrarenal portion. Renal artery involvement typically occurs as long stenoses. If renal artery narrowing is severe, collateral flow to the kidneys usually moves from ureteral, adrenal, and gonadal

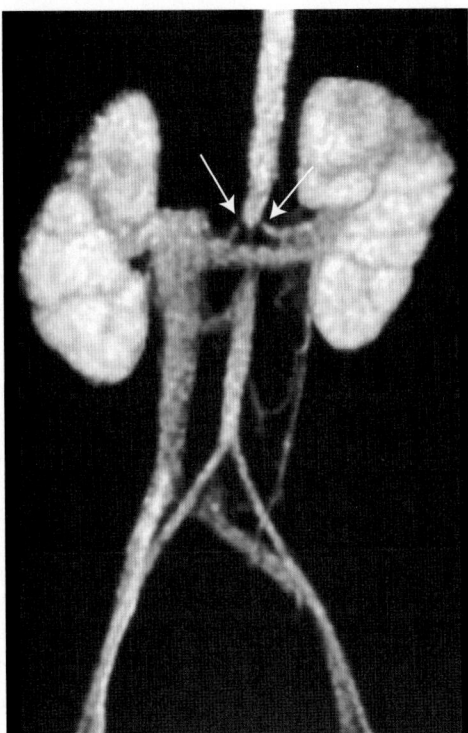

FIGURE 150-4. Middle aortic syndrome. Computed tomography (CT) angiography of a child with middle aortic syndrome reveals severe narrowing of the infrarenal portion of the abdominal aorta. The main renal arteries are also involved *(arrows)*.

arteries that fill from lower intercostal vessels. Because no active inflammation occurs with middle aortic syndrome, abnormal vessel wall enhancement is not present on CT and MRI. In contrast to Takayasu disease, the great vessels of the thorax are not involved in patients with middle aortic syndrome.

COARCTATION OF THE AORTA

Coarctation of the aorta typically occurs within the aortic arch. Although the renal arteries are not directly involved in these patients, diminished distal flow may lead to renin-mediated hypertension. Atypical coarctation can occur within the abdominal aorta; further classification of this variety differentiates it into suprarenal, interrenal, and infrarenal types. In some instances, narrowing of one or both renal arteries is apparent. Hypertension is common in patients with abdominal aortic coarctation.

TRAUMA

Potential renal arterial injuries include intimal disruption, main renal artery avulsion, branch vessel transection, false aneurysm, and arteriovenous fistula. Most renal injuries in children are related to blunt trauma; penetrating injuries are uncommon. Injuries of the major renal vessels can also occur in association with major deceleration forces, as the result of stretching as the kidney moves relative to the more securely fixed aorta. The intima is most susceptible to stretching injury because it is less elastic than the media and the adventitia. An intimal tear can precipitate dissection, luminal occlusion, or thrombosis. Stretching injury can also cause spasm of the renal artery without a tear. With severe, rapid motion of the kidney, vascular avulsion can occur. Penetrating injuries and iatrogenic mechanisms, such as needle biopsy, can lead to an intrarenal arteriovenous fistula.

Globally deficient parenchymal contrast enhancement is an important CT indicator of possible main renal artery injury. This pattern can occur with disruption, thrombosis, or spasm of the main renal artery; CT angiography provides additional characterization of the vascular anatomy. The "cortical rim sign" is a radiographic finding that is associated with acute renal arterial occlusion. This refers to contrast enhancement in the periphery of an ischemic kidney; the mechanism apparently involves collateral perfusion. The cortical rim sign does not develop until at least 8 hours after the onset of ischemia, and in many patients, it is not present until a few days after the injury. This sign generally indicates that renal salvage is not possible because of the prolonged nature of the ischemia.

With complete traumatic disruption of the main renal artery, CT shows a large adjacent hematoma. The compartmentalized nature of the retroperitoneum (e.g., Gerota fascia) limits the bleeding, however, and exsanguination is uncommon. A localized renal infarction due to traumatic occlusion of an intrarenal vessel results in a wedge-shaped or rounded area of absent enhancement, often with sharp margins. With partial main renal artery occlusion, the intensity of the nephrogram is diminished. In the nonacute setting, renal scintigraphy can be used to assess regional and global kidney function after trauma.

ANEURYSM

Renal artery aneurysms are rare in childhood. Major features used for classification of these lesions include location (extraparenchymal and intraparenchymal) and morphology (saccular, fusiform, dissecting, and false). Some pediatric renal artery aneurysms are idiopathic; others are due to infection (i.e., mycotic aneurysms), renal artery stenosis (often related to neurofibromatosis type 1 or fibromuscular dysplasia), or autoimmune vasculitis (e.g., polyarteritis nodosa). Aneurysms of the renal artery can occur in patients with Kawasaki disease and Ehlers-Danlos syndrome.

Renal artery aneurysms may be single or multiple; most are saccular. Clot or calcification is occasionally present within the aneurysm (Fig. 150-5). Aneurysms that occur in patients with polyarteritis nodosa tend to be small, multiple, and intraparenchymal. The most common clinical manifestations of a renal artery aneurysm are hematuria and flank pain. Most are detectable with sonography, CTA, or MRA; Doppler sonography is helpful in differentiating a cyst from an aneurysm. Conventional angiography is sometimes required for the detection and characterization of small lesions.

ARTERIOVENOUS MALFORMATION AND FISTULA

About three quarters of renal arteriovenous fistulas are iatrogenic (e.g., biopsy, surgery) or related to trauma. The kidney is a rare site for congenital arteriovenous

malformations. Rarely, an arteriovenous lesion is associated with a primary renal neoplasm. Hematuria is common in patients with a renal arteriovenous malformation or fistula. Physical examination may reveal a bruit. A large arteriovenous fistula can cause congestive heart failure. Imaging studies show a renal arteriovenous fistula as a focus of abnormal communication between an artery and a vein. Supplying and draining vessels become enlarged. Doppler analysis shows turbulent flow with arterial characteristics in the draining veins. Conventional angiography shows rapid flow through the lesion. With a congenital arteriovenous malformation, arteriovenous shunting occurs at a variably sized vascular mass, the nidus.

> **Most arteriovenous fistulas are iatrogenic.**

THROMBOSIS, EMBOLISM, AND INFARCTION

Thromboembolic disease of the renal arteries is uncommon in children. Predisposing conditions include sepsis, prolonged hypotension, severe dehydration, congenital heart disease, trauma, and hypercoagulable disorders. In neonates, the most common cause is umbilical arterial catheters, particularly when the catheter tip is located near the origins of the renal arteries. Infants of diabetic mothers are at increased risk for renal arterial thrombosis.

In older children, acute occlusion of a major renal artery may lead to flank pain, nausea, vomiting, fever, and hematuria. Small emboli or minor thrombosis may be asymptomatic; hypertension often develops as the result of renin secretion from ischemic tissue. In the acute phase of renal artery thromboembolism, sonography may be normal or may show nonspecific renal enlargement and cortical hyperechogenicity. Doppler evaluation sometimes reveals global, focal, or multifocal perfusion deficits. Flow within the capsule may be increased. Careful evaluation of the main renal artery may show echogenic clot, as well as abnormal arterial waveforms. If the main renal artery is patent, the resistive index is often elevated in the presence of substantial renal infarction.

CT and CTA in patients with renal arterial thromboembolic disease may reveal filling defects or narrowing of the renal artery. With global renal infarction, renal parenchymal enhancement and contrast media excretion are lacking. One or more wedge-shaped enhancement defects may occur in the presence of segmental renal infarction. In about 50% of patients with renal infarction, a thin, prominently enhancing rim is seen at the peripheral margin of an infarction. Renal scintigraphy in the presence of thromboembolic disease shows global or multifocal deficiency of renal function.

DISEASES OF INTRARENAL ARTERIES

Renal Vasculitis

The kidney is a relatively common site of involvement in various forms of vasculitis. The most widely used

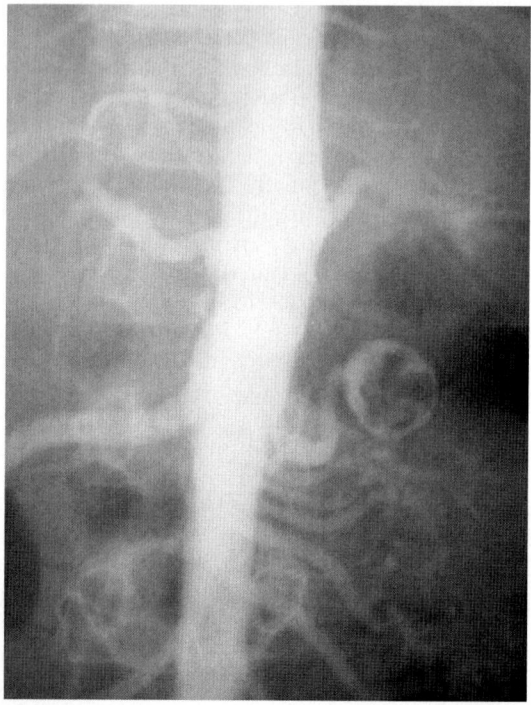

FIGURE 150-5. Renal artery aneurysm. Abdominal aortogram shows a partially thrombosed saccular aneurysm of the left renal artery.

classification of vasculitis is based on the size of the predominantly involved vessels. Takayasu arteritis is an example of large-vessel vasculitis. Polyarteritis nodosa and Kawasaki disease predominantly involve medium-sized vessels. The presence or absence of antineutrophil cytoplasmic antibodies (ANCAs) allows subcategorization of the small-vessel vasculitides. Henoch-Schönlein purpura is ANCA negative; ANCA-positive vasculitides that can affect the kidney include Wegener granulomatosis and microscopic polyarteritis. Small-vessel vasculitis can also occur in association with various infectious diseases, such as Rocky Mountain spotted fever, human immunodeficiency virus, hepatitis B, and tuberculosis.

Polyarteritis Nodosa

Polyarteritis nodosa is a rare idiopathic focal segmental necrotizing vasculitis that can occur in children of any age. Renal involvement occurs in slightly more than half of affected children. Potential clinical manifestations of kidney involvement include hematuria, proteinuria, and hypertension. The major pathologic consequence of polyarteritis nodosa is the development of small aneurysms along the walls of medium-sized arteries. Imaging studies of the kidneys may show manifestations of focal or multifocal renal ischemia. Intraparenchymal or peri-renal hemorrhage can occur as the result of aneurysm rupture. Arteriography reveals small aneurysms, typically located at the bifurcations of interlobular or arcuate arteries. Small intrarenal vessels are irregular and tortuous because of vascular and perivascular inflammation.

Wegener Granulomatosis and Microscopic Polyarteritis

Wegener granulomatosis is a rare necrotizing vasculitis that predominantly affects the respiratory tract. Up to 80% of patients have evidence of renal involvement, as manifested in hematuria, proteinuria, and (in many patients) diminished glomerular filtration rate (GFR). Similar clinical findings occur in patients with microscopic polyarteritis, although respiratory system involvement is lacking with this disorder. Diagnostic imaging findings of kidney involvement with these two vasculitides are nonspecific. Foci of parenchymal scarring may occur as the result of ischemia. Parenchymal or perirenal hemorrhage can occur because of rupture of a small-vessel aneurysm. Imaging findings are similar to those of polyarteritis nodosa.

Systemic Lupus Erythematosus

Systemic lupus erythematosus is a systemic autoimmune disease that frequently involves the kidneys; 50% to 75% of children with this disorder have clinical manifestations of renal involvement. A clinical spectrum ranges from mild asymptomatic disease to severe forms that lead to end-stage renal disease or death. The major pathologic manifestation is thickening of the basement membrane due to focal glomerulonephritis; inflammatory narrowing of interlobular arteries may also be evident. Imaging findings roughly correlate with the clinical severity of kidney involvement. In the absence of renal failure, the kidneys may appear normal. In some instances, mild nephromegaly is noted. Diffuse or multifocal hyperechogenicity of the renal parenchyma may be present on sonography. Elevation of the resistive index on Doppler ultrasonography may be predictive of worsening renal function.

Hemolytic-Uremic Syndrome

Hemolytic-uremic syndrome is the most common cause of acute renal failure in early childhood. The pathogenesis involves endothelial cell damage within glomeruli and renal arterioles, which diminishes the GFR. The kidney is the main target of this microangiopathy, although the intestines, lung, and brain may be affected. Typically, a prodromal viral respiratory or gastrointestinal (diarrheal) infection may occur. In most cases of hemolytic-uremic syndrome, an otherwise healthy infant develops fever, vomiting, bloody diarrhea, and abdominal discomfort. The child, usually around 3 years of age, may become critically ill with signs and symptoms that include pallor, irritability, seizures, heart failure, hypertension, gastrointestinal bleeding, and oliguria. Individual variation in disease severity is noted, and some patients have only a transient decrease in the volume of urine output. Acute renal failure usually lasts for 1 to 4 weeks, with subsequent slow improvement. Clinical recovery is complete in most patients, but some children have permanent neurologic or renal damage. In approximately 20% of patients, progressive deterioration of renal function leads to chronic uremia.

> **Hemolytic-uremic syndrome is the most common cause of acute renal failure in childhood.**

During the acute phase of hemolytic-uremic syndrome, radiographs of the abdomen may show renal enlargement. Frequently, the colon is distended with air. Thumbprinting may be present in the colon wall. In most patients, renal size returns to normal as the disease resolves, but more severe injury is associated with eventual kidney atrophy; calcification may occur in the cortex. Sonography is useful in hemolytic-uremic syndrome for estimating renal size and assessing changes in the renal parenchyma. Early in the disease, sonography is normal or shows minimal nephromegaly. Subsequent abnormally increased parenchymal echogenicity is usually most prominent in the glomerular and subcortical regions. The degree of cortical echogenicity correlates with the severity of the illness.

Peripheral renal arterial narrowing that occurs in hemolytic-uremic syndrome causes resistance to blood flow that is demonstrable through Doppler examination. With severe disease, intrarenal arterial flow may not be detectable, or systolic Doppler signals may be identified and diastolic Doppler shifts may be absent or reversed (elevated resistive index). With clinical improvement, early diastolic flow reappears and Doppler signal is absent at the end of diastole. With complete regression of arterial obstruction, the Doppler signal pattern returns to normal. Doppler studies in these children reveal the severity of the illness and guide the clinician in predicting the course of recovery.

Henoch-Schönlein Purpura

Henoch-Schönlein purpura is a hypersensitivity vasculitis that affects small vessels and is an important cause of nephritis in children. The clinical tetrad includes a purpuric rash, arthralgias, abdominal pain, and glomerulonephritis. Renal involvement of variable degree occurs in most patients. In some patients, no overt symptoms of renal disease are reported; others have findings similar to those of acute poststreptococcal glomerulonephritis. Between 20% and 30% of patients with Henoch-Schönlein purpura have hematuria, and 30% to 70% have proteinuria. In those patients with profound proteinuria, nephrotic syndrome and renal insufficiency may occur. Clinical signs of renal involvement may follow or coincide with the appearance of purpura, but they rarely antedate skin findings. Renal involvement is particularly common in patients with recurrent attacks of purpura and in those with abdominal manifestations of the disease. Henoch-Schönlein purpura is usually a self-limited disorder, but it can be complicated by hypertension or chronic renal failure. Long-term renal disease occurs in up to 20% of children with Henoch-Schönlein purpura.

As with the clinical presentation, the imaging features of Henoch-Schönlein purpura are similar to those of acute glomerulonephritis. Sonography may show normal or bilaterally enlarged kidneys. Hyperechogenicity of the renal cortex is usually diffuse, and the medullary pyramids remain hypoechoic. Renal cortical hyperechogenicity diminishes as the acute disease regresses. Occasionally, cross-sectional imaging studies show findings of an intramural hematoma within the bladder wall or ureter. Ureteral fibrosis is a rare complication; intravenous urography in this instance shows a beaded appearance of the ureter, often in association with hydronephrosis. Up to 3% of males with Henoch-Schönlein purpura have scrotal involvement that can clinically mimic testicular torsion; sonography may reveal scrotal wall hemorrhage or edema, as well as epididymal and testicular enlargement and hyperemia.

Sickle Cell Disease

Various structural and functional abnormalities of the kidneys occur in patients with sickle cell disease. Sludging of red blood cells within the medulla is common in these patients because of the high osmolality and the low oxygen tension found in this region. Recurrent episodes of medullary ischemia lead to alterations in papillary morphology. Cortical hypertrophy may occur. Papillary necrosis develops when medullary ischemia is severe. Nephropathy of sickle cell anemia involves the entire renal parenchyma. Histologic features include dilation and engorgement of cortical capillary tufts, glomerulosclerosis, increased mesangial matrix, and iron deposition in the glomerular epithelium and glomerular basement membrane. Sickled erythrocytes

may be present within engorged glomerular, cortical, and medullary capillaries. Occasionally, glomerular sclerosis progresses to complete obliteration of glomerular tufts.

The kidneys in patients with sickle cell disease may have a defect in their ability to concentrate urine. Defective hydrogen ion production can lead to deterioration of normal metabolic homeostatic mechanisms. Abnormally elevated GFR, effective renal plasma flow (ERPF), and tubular excretion of *para*-iminohippuric acid may be noted. These functional alterations are most prominent during childhood and tend to decrease until about the age of 40. Glomerular disease can lead to subnormal creatinine clearance.

Recurrent ischemia in patients with sickle cell disease leads to various alterations in renal morphology on imaging studies. The characteristic imaging finding of the infundibular collecting system is termed *sickle cell calyectasis*. Intravenous urography may show calyceal blunting and prominent papillae, with broad, deep calyces. The collecting system is often distorted as the result of cortical hypertrophy (Fig. 150-6). In some patients, papillary necrosis is evident. Nephromegaly, usually bilateral, is common in sickle cell disease. Enlarged kidneys with a bizarre-looking collecting system may suggest this disorder. Recurrent infarction and subsequent fibrosis may eventually lead to scarring and atrophy.

Renal sonography in patients with sickle cell disease typically shows mild diffuse enlargement, hyperechogenicity, and loss of corticomedullary differentiation

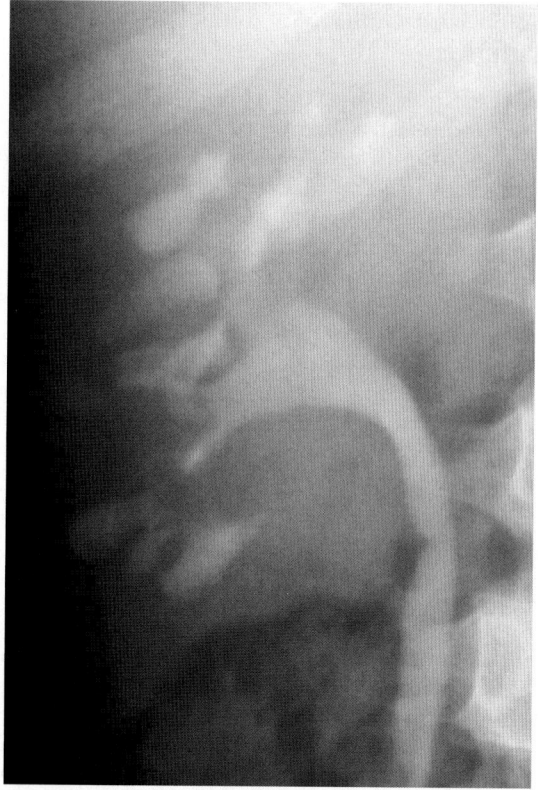

FIGURE 150-6. Sickle cell disease. Intravenous urogram of a 13-year-old child with sickle cell disease shows calyceal dilation and collecting system distortion.

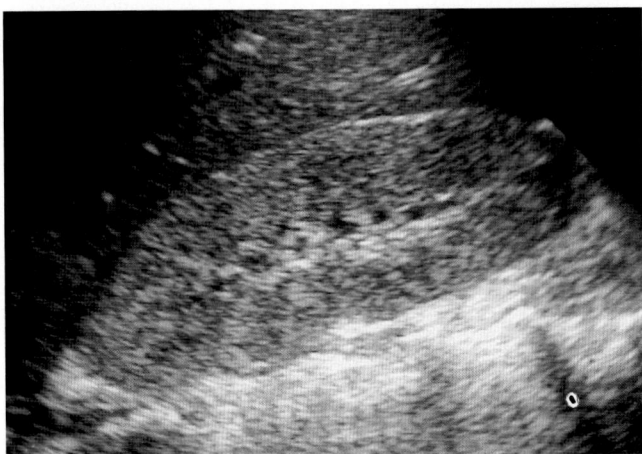

FIGURE 150-7. Sickle cell disease. Longitudinal sonographic image of a 15-year-old male with sickle cell disease shows hyperechogenicity of the kidney and absent corticomedullary differentiation.

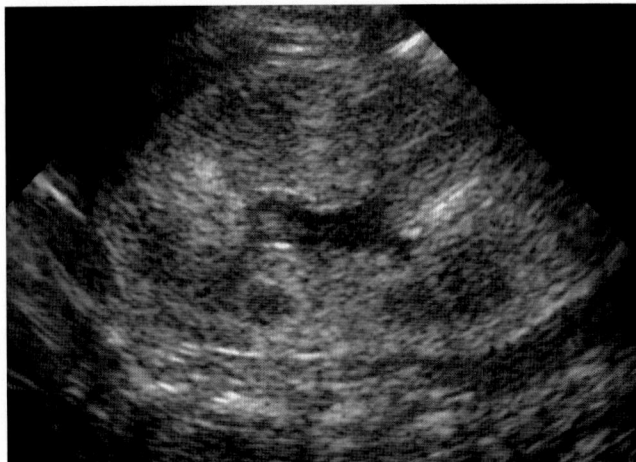

FIGURE 150-8. Renal vein thrombosis. Sonography of an infant with renal vein thrombosis shows an enlarged, echogenic kidney, with loss of corticomedullary differentiation.

(Fig. 150-7). A perirenal hematoma can occur as a complication of renal infarction. MRI shows changes peculiar to sickle cell disease, with decreased cortical signal relative to the medulla on T1-weighted and T2-weighted images. These findings are due to iron deposition in the renal cortex.

Sickle cell trait is sometimes associated with prominent renal papillae. Excretory urography may show broad, deep calyces, without forniceal blunting. Occasionally, cortical hypertrophy in these patients leads to distortion of the collecting system. Medullary carcinoma of the kidney is a rare neoplasm that almost exclusively occurs in patients with sickle cell trait, or SC disease.

Renal Vein Thrombosis

Renal vein thrombosis is the most common renal vascular abnormality in the neonatal age group. Most affected neonates have a predisposing systemic abnormality, such as dehydration, sepsis, or maternal diabetes mellitus. Small intrarenal vessels are the initial or only site of thrombosis in these infants; bilateral renal involvement can occur. Propagation of a central venous catheter–related inferior vena cava (IVC) clot is an additional potential mechanism. Renal vein thrombosis in older patients can occur as the result of nephrotic syndrome, glomerulonephritis, hypercoagulable state, trauma, or a retroperitoneal tumor. Typical clinical manifestations of renal vein thrombosis include nephromegaly, signs of renal insufficiency, hematuria, and hypertension.

> **Renal vein thrombosis is the most common neonatal renovascular abnormality.**

Sonography of the kidney with venous thrombosis shows abnormal parenchymal echogenicity and loss of corticomedullary differentiation; in some cases, interlobular echogenic streaks are apparent (Fig. 150-8). Doppler evaluation shows elevation of the arterial resistive index; diminution of renal arterial flow occurs because of

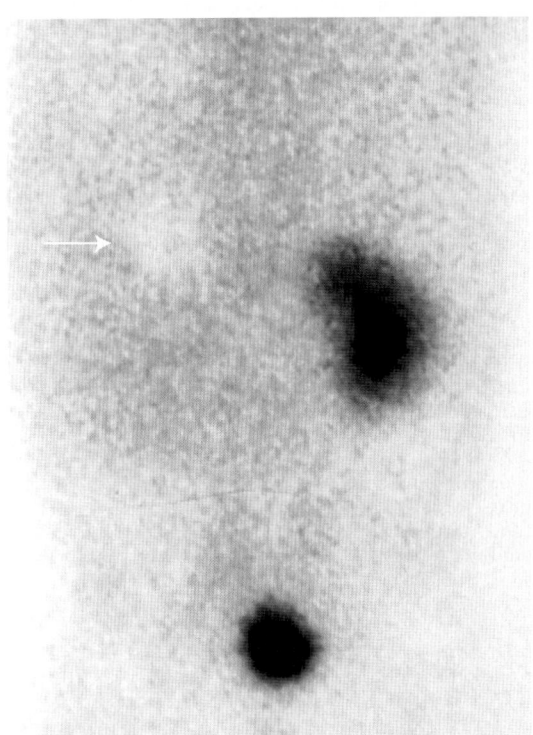

FIGURE 150-9. Renal vein thrombosis. Posterior technetium-99m diethylenetriaminepenta-acetic acid (^{99m}Tc-DTPA) scintigraphic image of an infant with left renal vein thrombosis shows absent left renal function. An oval suprarenal photopenic focus (arrow) is due to concomitant adrenal hemorrhage.

venous outflow obstruction. Narrowing of the systolic peak is also common. Careful sonographic evaluation of the renal veins sometimes reveals echogenic clot; however, absence of clot within the major renal veins does not exclude the diagnosis of renal vein thrombosis. With severe involvement, Doppler evaluation may show absence of flow within the main renal vein. In other patients, renal vein flow is monophasic. In neonates with renal vein thrombosis, coexistent adrenal hemorrhage may be noted.

Renal scintigraphy during the acute phase of renal vein thrombosis provides prognostic information; mild compromise of uptake and excretion indicates a good prognosis (Fig. 150-9). Within a few weeks of onset of renal vein thrombosis, the affected kidney shows a decrease in size on imaging studies. In some patients, progression to global atrophy occurs; this is usually mild. In most circumstances, substantial return of clinical renal function is evident. In a small number of cases, a radiographically identifiable reticular pattern of calcification develops in the intrarenal veins. These calcifications are particularly well exhibited on CT, and this finding is essentially pathognomonic of previous renal vein thrombosis.

SELECTED READINGS

Aasarod K, Iversen BM, Hammerstrom J, et al: Wegener's granulomatosis: clinical course in 108 patients with renal involvement. Nephrol Dial Transplant 2000;15:611-618

Abernethy LJ, Hendry GM, Reid JH: Fibromuscular dysplasia of the renal artery in a child: detection by Doppler ultrasound and correction by percutaneous transluminal angioplasty. Pediatr Radiol 1989;19:539-540

Adams WM, John PR: US demonstration and diagnosis of the midaortic syndrome. Pediatr Radiol 1998;28:461-463

Adelman RD, Karlowicz MG: What is the appropriate workup and treatment for an infant with an umbilical artery catheter-related thrombosis? Semin Nephrol 1998;18:362-364

Alexander AA, Merton DA, Mitchell DG, et al: Rapid diagnosis of neonatal renal vein thrombosis using color Doppler imaging. J Clin Ultrasound 1993;21:468-471

Bakkaloglu A, Ozen S, Baskin E, et al: The significance of antineutrophil cytoplasmic antibody in microscopic polyangitis and classic polyarteritis nodosa. Arch Dis Child 2001;85:427-430

Bartosh SM, Aronson AJ: Childhood hypertension: an update on etiology, diagnosis, and treatment. Pediatr Clin North Am 1999;46:235-252

Bogdanovic R, Nikolic V, Pasic S, et al: Lupus nephritis in childhood: a review of 53 patients followed at a single center. Pediatr Nephrol 2004;19:36-44

Brogan PA, Davies R, Gordon I, et al: Renal angiography in children with polyarteritis nodosa. Pediatr Nephrol 2002;17:277-283

Callicutt CS, Rush B, Eubanks T, et al: Idiopathic renal artery and infrarenal aortic aneurysms in a 6-year-old child: case report and literature review. J Vasc Surg 2005;41:893-896

Chandar JJ, Sfakianakis GN, Zilleruelo GE, et al: ACE inhibition scintigraphy in the management of hypertension in children. Pediatr Nephrol 1999;13:493-500

Daniels SR: Consultation with the specialist: the diagnosis of hypertension in children: an update. Pediatr Rev 1997;18:131-135

Ein SH, Pullerits J, Creighton R, et al: Pediatric pheochromocytoma: a 36-year review. Pediatr Surg Int 1997;12:595-598

Fernandes E, McCrindle BW: Diagnosis and treatment of hypertension in children and adolescents. Can J Cardiol 2000;16:801-811

Ford KT, Teplick SK, Clark RE: Renal artery embolism causing neonatal hypertension: a complication of umbilical artery catheterization. Radiology 1974;113:169-170

Fossali E, Signorini E, Intermite RC, et al: Renovascular disease and hypertension in children with neurofibromatosis. Pediatr Nephrol 2000;14:806-810

Goonasekera CD, Dillon MJ: Reflux nephropathy and hypertension. J Hum Hypertens 1998;12:497-504

Hibbert J, Howlett DC, Greenwood KL, et al: The ultrasound appearances of neonatal renal vein thrombosis. Br J Radiol 1997;70:1191-1194

Hiner LB, Falkner B: Renovascular hypertension in children. Pediatr Clin North Am 1993;40:123-140

Kavaler E, Hensle TW: Renal artery thrombosis in the newborn infant. Urology 1997;50:282-284

Knudson MM, Harrison PB, Hoyt DB, et al: Outcome after major renovascular injuries: a Western trauma association multicenter report. J Trauma 2000;49:1116-1122

Lande IM, Glazer GM, Sarniak S, et al: Sickle-cell nephropathy: MR imaging. Radiology 1986;158:379-383

Loges RJ, Tulchinsky M, Boal DK, et al: Tc-99m MAG3 renography in renal vein thrombosis secondary to Finnish-type congenital nephrotic syndrome. Clin Nucl Med 1994;19:888-891

Makker SP, Moorthy B: Fibromuscular dysplasia of renal arteries: an important cause of renovascular hypertension in children. J Pediatr 1979;95:940-945

McCulloch M, Andronikou S, Goddard E, et al: Angiographic features of 26 children with Takayasu's arteritis. Pediatr Radiol 2003;33:230-235

Mittal BR, Kumar P, Arora P, et al: Role of captopril renography in the diagnosis of renovascular hypertension. Am J Kidney Dis 1996;28:209-213

Nastri MV, Baptista LP, Baroni RH, et al: Gadolinium-enhanced three-dimensional MR angiography of Takayasu arteritis. Radiographics 2004;24:773-786

Pandya KK, Koshy M, Brown N, et al: Renal papillary necrosis in sickle cell hemoglobinopathies. J Urol 1976;115:497-501

Riccabona M, Schwinger W, Ring E: Arteriovenous fistula after renal biopsy in children. J Ultrasound Med 1998;17:505-508

Sarkar R, Coran AG, Cilley RE, et al: Arterial aneurysms in children: clinicopathologic classification. J Vasc Surg 1991;13:47-56; discussion 56-57

Sfakianakis GN, Bourgoignie JJ, Georgiou M, et al: Diagnosis of renovascular hypertension with ACE inhibition scintigraphy. Radiol Clin North Am 1993;31:831-848

Siegel MJ, St Amour TE, Siegel BA: Imaging techniques in the evaluation of pediatric hypertension. Pediatr Nephrol 1987;1:76-88

Siegler R, Oakes R: Hemolytic uremic syndrome: pathogenesis, treatment, and outcome. Curr Opin Pediatr 2005;17:200-204

Sinaiko AR: Hypertension in children. N Engl J Med 1996;335:1968-1973

Tenenbaum F, Lumbroso J, Schlumberger M, et al: Comparison of radiolabeled octreotide and meta-iodobenzylguanidine (MIBG) scintigraphy in malignant pheochromocytoma. J Nucl Med 1995;36:1-6

Ting TV, Hashkes PJ: Update on childhood vasculitides. Curr Opin Rheumatol 2004;16:560-565

Trapani S, Micheli A, Grisolia F, et al: Henoch-Schönlein purpura in childhood: epidemiological and clinical analysis of 150 cases over a 5-year period and review of literature. Semin Arthritis Rheum 2005;35:143-153

Wells TG, Belsha CW: Pediatric renovascular hypertension. Curr Opin Pediatr 1996;8:128-134

Zerin JM, Hernandez RJ: Renal imaging in children with persistent hypertension. Pediatr Clin North Am 1993;40:165-178

151 The Ureter and Vesicoureteral Reflux

MICHAEL RICCABONA

EMBRYOLOGY, NORMAL ANATOMY, AND VARIANTS

Embryology

Embryonic development of the urinary and the genital system is closely related. The urogenital breach forms from the intermediate mesoderm and develops into the nephrogenic cord, which forms the urinary system. The ureter develops from a branch of the mesonephric duct called the ureteric bud. It arises during the fourth to fifth week of pregnancy and grows dorsally and upward until it contacts the nephrogenic cord. This contact of the ureteric bud with the metanephric blastema then induces normal kidney development. The ureterovesical junction (UVJ) develops as the distal parts of the mesonephric duct are incorporated into the enlarging bladder originating from the urogenital sinus. As the mesonephric ducts are absorbed, the ureters come to open separately into the urinary bladder with the orifice moving superolaterally and the distal ureteral segments entering obliquely through the base of the bladder. During this complex course of development numerous variations concerning the position of the kidney, the course of the ureter, and the anatomy of the UVJ, as well as the ureteropelvic junction (UPJ), may arise. Knowledge about the embryologic development of the ureter is crucial for understanding ureteral malformations, for proper recognition and diagnosis, and for therapeutic decision making, particularly in duplicated systems and vesicoureteral reflux (VUR).

Normal Anatomy

In the fetus the ureter is characterized by elongation and tortuosity with mild widening of the midureter and short kinks or intraluminal mucosal folds at the proximal ureter. This situation may persist in early infancy as a transient condition. Until late in childhood the ureters may be highly mobile and can be displaced by other abdominal structures, such as distended bowel loops. In the fetus, because of little urine production, the normal ureters usually are not well filled and therefore not visible by present imaging methods. Thus, a visible ureter in a fetus usually implies ureteral pathology, either refluxive or obstructive.

The ureter is a tubular structure that courses retroperitoneally from the bladder to the kidney and has three major components—the upper ureter and UPJ, the midureter, and the lower ureter and UVJ (including the transmural ureter and the ureteral orifice). The abdominal or upper ureter starts at the UPJ with a smooth tapering from the renal pelvis. Histologically it consists of a central mucosal epithelium (urothelium) that has longitudinal folds and appears star-like on cross section. Three muscular layers constitute the ureteral wall, with a thin outer adventitial covering that contains a rich vascular and lymphatic plexus. The abdominal ureter lies adjacent to the psoas muscle, being crossed by the testicular vessels before passing behind the iliac vessels. The small bowel mesentery (on the right side) and the sigmoid mesocolon (on the left side) are anterior to the middle ureters. The pelvic or lower ureter lies along the lateral pelvic wall, coursing downward behind the bladder. As the ureter enters the bladder wall, it takes an oblique course from a superolateral entry point to an inferomedial ostium and eventually opens into the bladder. Its course through the bladder wall can be seen (called the plica ureterica at cystoscopy) and constitutes the lateral border of the bladder trigone. Vascular supply of the ureter is from bladder vessels (inferior vesical artery), gonadal arteries (testicular artery), and the renal artery superiorly. Note that the ureter has no dedicated vascular supply; thus, the ureter is prone to vascular injuries, particularly the midportion. Nerves supplying the ureter follow the same course as the arteries.

The purpose of the ureter is to transport urine from the renal pelvis into the urinary bladder. This is performed by rhythmic peristaltic contractions that occur two to seven times per minute, starting at the renal pelvis and propagating down to the bladder. Focal disruption of anatomy, dysplasia of the wall with less muscle and more fibrous tissue, as well as dysplastic segments with altered innervation can cause impairment to this peristalsis, with consequent deterioration of urine transport and ureteral dilatation.

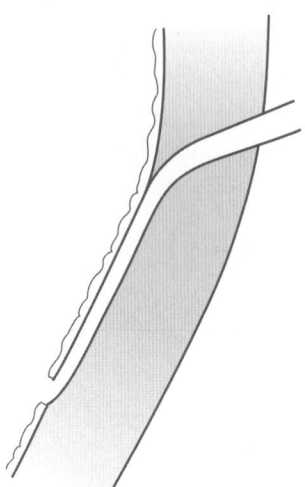

FIGURE 151-1. Course of the distal segment of ureter within the bladder wall. The ureter at first traverses the bladder musculature almost perpendicularly and then descends submucosally for a much longer segment (submucosal tunnel).

An important anatomic region is the UVJ, because the anatomic relationship of the distal ureter to the bladder wall is important in preventing VUR (Fig. 151-1). Normally, the distal ureter courses through the bladder musculature at an oblique angle and then continues submucosally to end in the lateral corner of the trigone. The submucosal ureteral tunnel contains only longitudinal muscular fibers, in contrast to the extravesical ureter, which contains both longitudinal and circular fibers. Some longitudinal fibers continue to the opposite ureteral orifice along the trigonal ridge whereas others fan out to the trigone or are in continuity with the musculature of the proximal urethra. The UVJ acts as a passive flap valve. Continence is ensured by apposition of the roof and floor of the submucosal tunnel when intravesical pressure increases and is enhanced by the action of the intrinsic local musculature. Size of the ureteral orifice, proper obliquity, length, diameter, and flexibility of the tunnel, and adequate support of the tunnel by the bladder musculature are also important in preventing VUR. The normal submucosal ureter measures 0.5 cm long in the newborn, is approximately 1 cm long at 12 years, and is 2 cm long in adults, with a ureteral tunnel length to ureteral diameter ratio in children of 5:1. A ratio of at least 3:1 is necessary for UVJ competence. In patients with VUR, the ratio may be as low as 1.5:1. The ostium itself usually has a slit-like opening; variation of this shape may be associated with ostium dysfunction, causing obstruction or VUR. In general, one may assume that the larger the ureteral orifice, the more lateralized the ostium position, and the shorter the submucosal tunnel, the more severe the VUR.

IMAGING OF THE URETER

Ultrasonography (US) has become the first-line imaging tool in the pediatric urinary tract. Using modern sonographic capabilities it reveals valuable information about the ureteral orifice, the transmural and distal ureter, the UPJ and proximal ureter (particularly if dilated), and ureteral peristalsis. The ureter is much more difficult to image than other parts of the urinary tract, such as the bladder and the kidneys. On US the ureter can only be visualized when sufficiently filled with urine. For visualizing the distal ureter a sufficiently distended urinary bladder is mandatory because it serves as a window to the retrovesical space. With sufficient bladder filling the normal ureter can be detected and followed superiorly for several centimeters. Further visualization up to the iliac vessels or higher is only possible in cases with a significantly dilated ureter and sufficient sonographic access. Because ureteral dilatation is a key feature of most ureteral pathologic processes, an attempt to find and visualize the ureter can be rewarding more often than expected but needs meticulous scanning techniques.

> **The ureter is much more difficult to image than other parts of the urinary system.**

The patency of the ureteral orifice can sonographically be assessed by observing the urine inflow jet into the urinary bladder. This ureteral jet can sometimes be seen on gray scale as a rush of pseudoechoes from the ureteral ostium into the bladder lumen (particularly if there are some particles in the urine), but it is more easily seen with color Doppler ultrasonography. Color Doppler imaging allows not only visualization of ureteral patency and osteal position but also evaluation of the frequency of the inflow jet indicating ureteric peristaltic activity. M-mode is another useful US technique allowing for semi-quantitative assessment of ureteral peristalsis that may prove helpful during follow-up in patients with megaureter as well as for documentation of impaired peristalsis in dysplastic or decompensated ureters. Three-dimensional US–based virtual cystoscopy allows for bladder surface visualization and potential demonstration of particularly pathologically shaped ostia. Thus, asymmetric jets, atypical direction of the ureteral jet, or a lateralized orifice position, as well as unusual ostial shape and impaired ureteral peristalsis, may be used as indirect signs for ureteral pathology or dysfunction such as obstruction or VUR. The UPJ can usually be sonographically visualized only in well-hydrated patients with a tapering of the pelvis toward the proximal ureter, using the kidney as an acoustic window from a dorsal or lateral approach. Particularly in cases with suspected higher ureteral obstruction or duplex systems, a sincere effort to find and visualize the proximal ureter may be beneficial.

Historically the method of choice of visualizing the ureter was intravenous urography (IVU). Provided there is sufficient renal function and contrast excretion, the ureter can at least be partially visualized. Visualization of the entire ureter throughout its course is unusual in children and often associated with ureteral disease, such as obstruction or laxity and inflammation. In some instances an oblique view can be helpful to assess for focal compression and indention of the ureter (e.g., with retrocaval or retroiliac ureter). The visualization of the distal ureter is only possible on postvoid films. IVU additionally allows for functional information by taking serial films demonstrating urinary drainage dynamics. Today, with improved US capabilities, changes in imaging paradigms and algorithms, and the advent of CT and MR urography, IVU is used much less frequently. If required, an adapted protocol with individually timed and selected films should be performed. The other historically important method of ureteral visualization was retrograde or antegrade ureterography with intubation of the ureter either via nephrostomy or cystoscopy for contrast instillation. This invasive method remains the gold standard for assessment of complicated anatomic conditions as well as for image-guided treatment and interventions (see Chapter 192); however, it is restricted to rare selected cases and often is performed in a perioperative or peri-interventional setting only.

Voiding cystourethrography (VCUG) can be used to visualize the ureter in cases of VUR. Oblique views are necessary to properly delineate the anatomy of the distal ureter and the UVJ, as well as the UPJ. Modern multislice CT is an additional powerful imaging tool that provides high spatial and anatomic resolution. Unenhanced acquisitions have become standard for ureteral stone detection in adults. This approach, however, may impose a significant radiation burden even using low-dose pediatric protocols. Thus, in pediatric uroradiology, CT should be restricted to uncommon and complicated cases and less generously used. Contrast-enhanced CT allows for excellent delineation of the entire ureter. By using three-dimensional reformatting and viewing techniques an IVU-like comprehensive overview over the entire ureter can be achieved. This technique is usually applied in rare or difficult cases, such as for assessment of a retrocaval ureter, ureteral tumors, and paraureteral pathology compressing or displacing the ureter.

With the advent of MR urography (MRU) a new powerful imaging tool has become available for imaging the ureter. By applying heavily T2-weighted sequences, a sufficiently distended or dilated ureter can be visualized in its entire course without administration of a contrast agent. However, diuretic stimulation before the investigation is helpful and mandatory in many cases. With dynamic techniques, ureteral peristalsis can be assessed and documented and the relationship of the ureter to surrounding structures can be assessed. Diuretic contrast-enhanced MRU additionally allows for functional assessment by using fast T1-weighted sequences (usually three-dimensional gradient-echo or turbo-flash) that give a good gadolinium signal. The spatial resolution of MRU is less than on IVU or CT, so small folds or tiny stones can be overlooked or only depicted by indirect signs. In the lower parts of the ureter, where motion from breathing is less likely, high-resolution MR sequences can improve spatial resolution for depiction of small structures, such as an unusual course or site of drainage of an ectopically inserting ureter.

> **MR urography is a new powerful tool for imaging the ureter.**

The best method for assessment of ureteral function and drainage at present is the readily available dynamic nuclear scintigraphy. Using serial acquisition after intravenous injection of technetium-99m–labeled mercapto-acetyltriglycine (MAG3) and diuretic stimulation, ureteral drainage can be visualized and quantified in a standardized fashion. However, the normal ureter usually is difficult to assess by this method and, despite its excellent functional information, anatomic resolution is poor.

> **Diuretic scintigraphy is the current best assessment of ureteral drainage, although MR urography is developing rapidly and also allows anatomic assessment of the kidney and ureter.**

In summary, IVU and CT as well as antegrade or retrograde ureterography are today rarely used for assessment of the ureter in pediatric uroradiology. US is the first-line imaging tool, and VCUG demonstrates ureteral anatomy in patients with VUR. Increasingly, diuretic MRU is becoming utilized for anatomic queries whereas MAG3 scintigraphy is used for assessment of ureteral function.

VARIANTS OF THE URETER

Ureteral duplication (duplication of the renal pelvis and ureter) is one of the most common anomalies of the urinary tract (Fig. 151-2). It may be partial or complete. Incomplete duplication ranges from a bifid renal pelvis to two ureters joining anywhere along their course and continuing inferiorly as a single structure. In completely duplicated systems, the two ureters are separate throughout their entire course. The ureter draining the upper pole of the kidney normally inserts into the bladder more caudad and more medially than the lower pole ureter (Weigert-Meyer rule) and has a longer submucosal tunnel than the lower pole ureter. Embryologically, the more cranial of the two ureteric buds from the mesonephric duct separates from the duct later and is thus carried caudad and medially, yet the more cranial ureteral portion of the metanephros unites with the more cranial ureteric bud. This renders the inferior and medially inserting ureter the drain for the upper pole. In all types of duplication, the affected kidney is often longer than the opposite organ and the lower pelvo-calyceal system is usually larger and has more calyces and a better-defined pelvis than the upper one. Ureteral duplication commonly is unilateral, although it may be bilateral. In completely duplicated systems VUR may involve both ureters; more often VUR is limited to the lower pole ureter, and VUR limited to the upper pole ureter is rare. Ureteroureteral reflux ("yo-yo phenomenon") may occur in double ureters joining in the lumbar area ("Y-ureters"), when urine flowing from one limb of the Y ascends into the other limb rather than passing down the common stem. Ureteral duplication is of no clinical importance unless it is complicated by another congenital lesion or an acquired process. These conditions, such as ureteral ectopia, VUR and urinary tract infection (UTI), and congenital UPJ obstruction, are addressed subsequently.

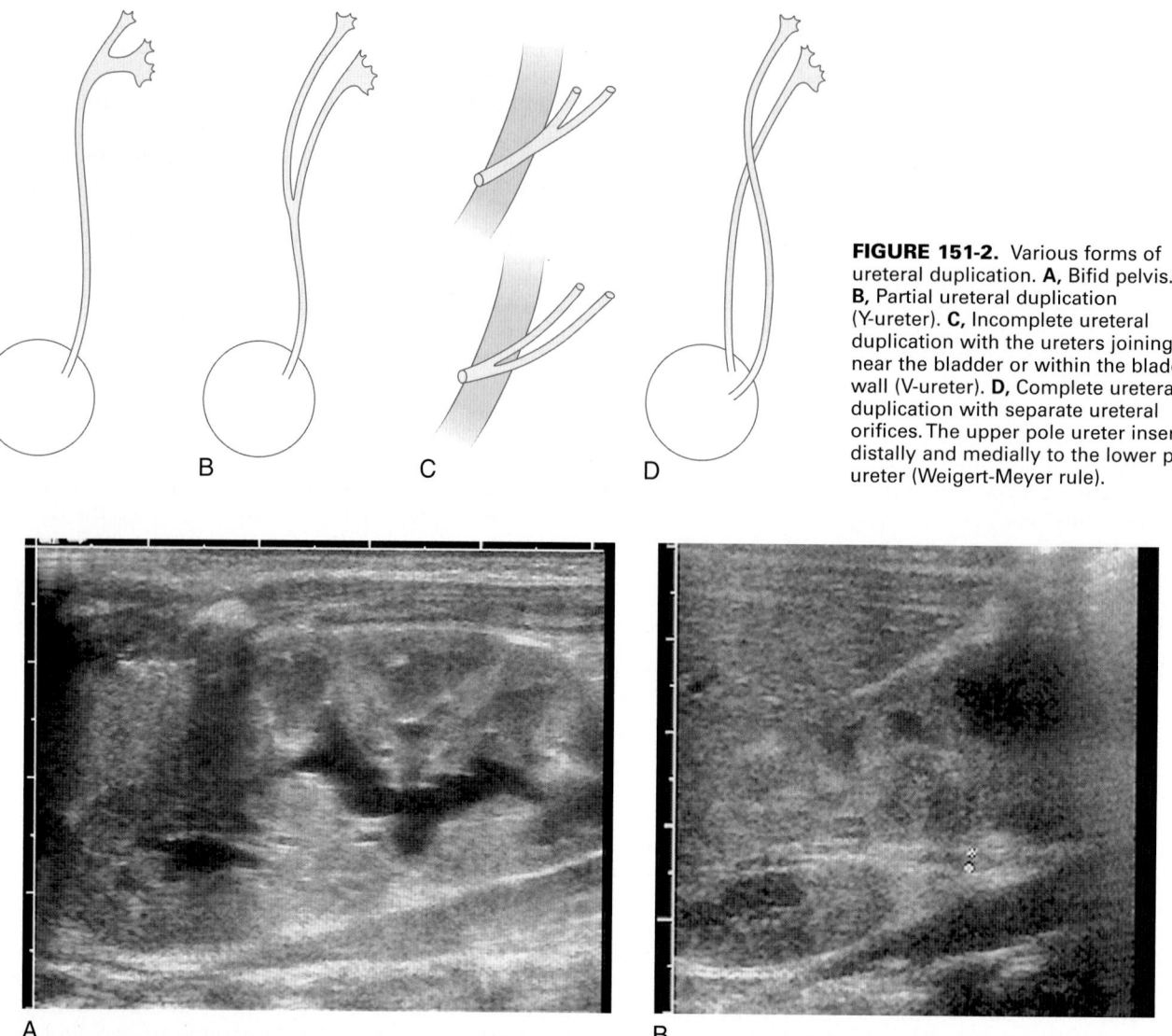

FIGURE 151-2. Various forms of ureteral duplication. **A,** Bifid pelvis. **B,** Partial ureteral duplication (Y-ureter). **C,** Incomplete ureteral duplication with the ureters joining near the bladder or within the bladder wall (V-ureter). **D,** Complete ureteral duplication with separate ureteral orifices. The upper pole ureter inserts distally and medially to the lower pole ureter (Weigert-Meyer rule).

FIGURE 151-3. Duplex collecting system. **A,** Longitudinal sonogram in a neonate demonstrates two separate collecting systems with disproportional dilatation of the lower moiety and the central "parenchymal bridge" separating them. **B,** Longitudinal sonogram more medially shows the separate nondilated ureter originating from the upper calyx *(cursors).*

> *Weigert-Meyer rule:* **In duplicated collecting systems, the upper pole ureter inserts distally and medially whereas the lower pole ureter inserts more cranially and laterally, often in a nearly normal position.**

Duplication of the pelvocalyceal system and ureter is often visible on US in well-hydrated infants and children. Signs are a prominent segment of renal cortex (column of Bertin) between the two pelvocalyceal systems or two renal pelves with two separate proximal ureters (Fig. 151-3). When renal function is adequate, IVU confirms the diagnosis; however, it may sometimes be difficult to determine whether the duplication is partial or complete without visualization of the ureters (Fig. 151-4). In these cases, retrograde studies or contrast enhanced MRU may be more helpful. Diagnosis of duplication may be clearly established by CT (demonstration of two separate pelvo-

calyceal systems and two ureters). However, these variations uncommonly cause any disease or symptoms and the diagnosis rarely alters clinical management, so imaging with ionizing radiation methods should be avoided.

When the superior moiety of a duplicated system is not visualized on an IVU, as is frequently the case in patients with ureteral ectopia (with or without ureterocele) or associated renal dysplasia, the diagnosis can be suspected from the appearance of the opacified lower collecting system (Fig. 151-5). In such cases the visualized calyces are fewer than usual and the proximal calyces may be short and broad. The distance between the uppermost medial calyx and the spine is increased compared with the opposite side. The longitudinal axis of the kidney tends to be perpendicular or is reversed, and the visualized calyces and pelvis are displaced laterally and downward by the nonvisualized upper pelvocalyceal system ("drooping lily" appearance). The opacified ipsi-

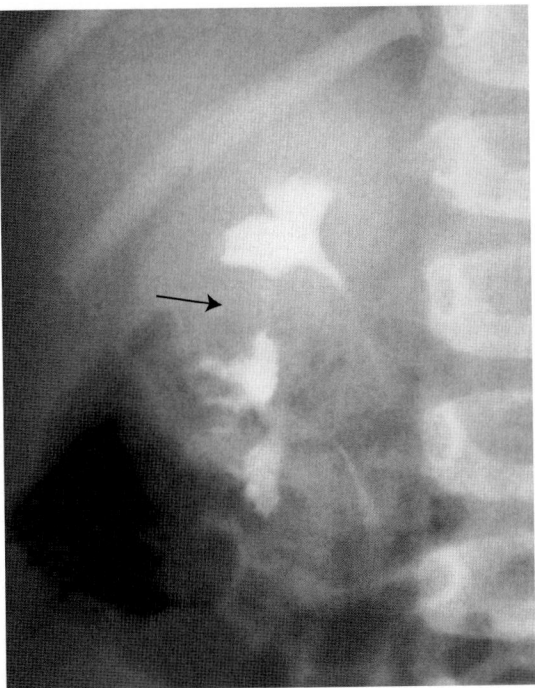

FIGURE 151-4. Collecting system duplication. IVU in an infant shows renal parenchyma *(arrow)* separating the upper and lower pole pelvocalyceal systems.

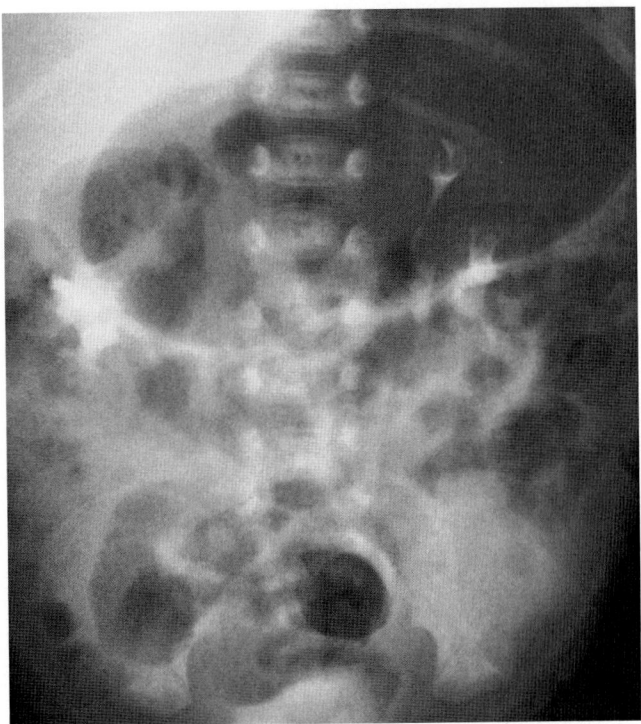

FIGURE 151-5. Right upper pole obstruction from ureterocele. IVU image shows a normal duplicated left collecting system. On the right, the lower pole is opacified but not the upper pole.

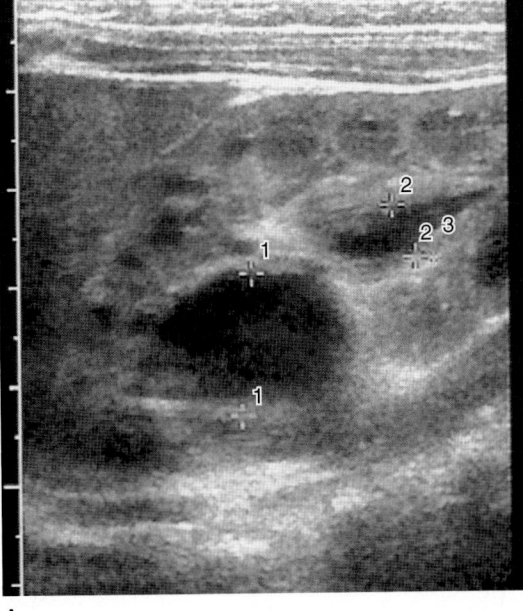

A

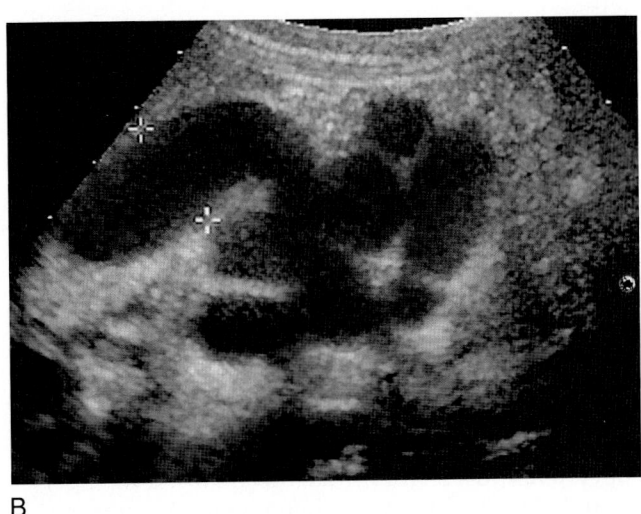

B

FIGURE 151-6. Duplex collecting system. **A,** Longitudinal sonogram shows a dilated upper pole system *(1 cursors)* with wall thickening and a minimally dilated lower system *(2 cursors)*. Note the thickening of the urothelium *(3)*. **B,** Longitudinal sonogram inferiorly shows corresponding megaureter *(cursors)*.

lateral ureter frequently is displaced laterally by a dilated, nonvisualized upper pole ureter. This unopacified, poorly functioning, dilated upper pole pelvis with thin and often dysplastic renal parenchyma, and the corresponding dilated unopacified ureter are easily identified on US (Fig. 151-6), demonstrating the complementary role of various imaging modalities in the urinary tract.

However, urographic findings may be very subtle when the nonvisualized system is not dilated, and in some cases the IVU and US are entirely normal. MRU or CT may be diagnostic in these cases.

Supernumerary kidneys are another rare anomaly in which there is an accessory third kidney that is separate from or very loosely attached to a normal kidney. In the

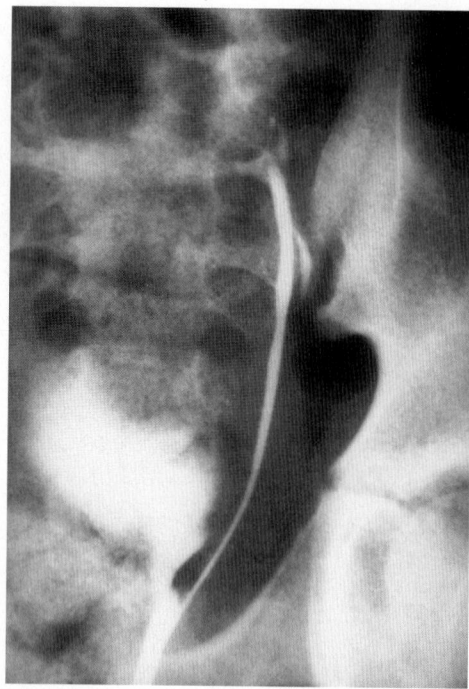
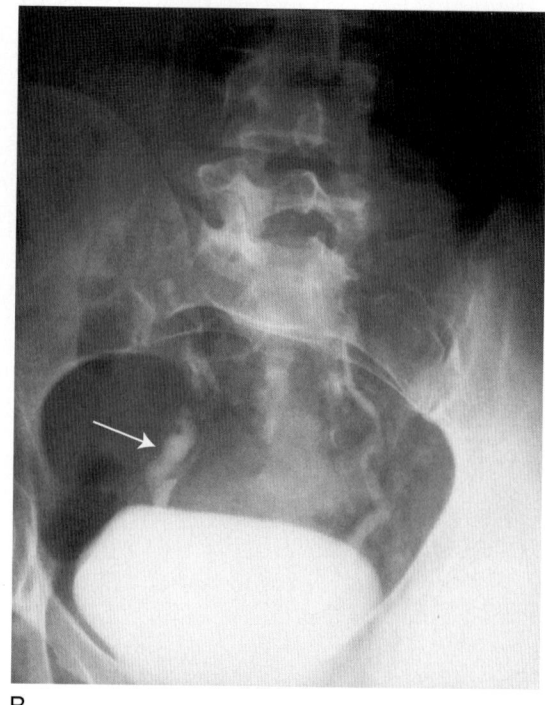

A   B

FIGURE 151-7. Rare forms of ureteral duplication. **A,** Retrograde ureterogram demonstrates a blind-ending accessory ureter. **B,** VCUG demonstrates vesicoureteral reflux into normal right and left ureters and a blind-ending right ureteral stump *(arrow)*.

first type, the accessory and the adjacent normal kidneys are drained by a common Y-shaped ureter. In the second type, the accessory kidney has a separate ureter that drains usually into the bladder but sometimes drains into the urethra or vagina.

Other variants of ureteral duplications include the *accessory ureter* or a *ureteral stump*. These entities are probably related to ureteral duplication. The accessory ureter is a tubular structure originating from the distal segment of a normal ureter and extending cephalad along the normal ureter to end blindly proximally, without connection to a pelvocalyceal system or renal parenchyma. The ureteral stump varies in length from a few centimeters to a narrow but patent cord that extends almost to the kidney. The anomaly is difficult to diagnose on US but may be demonstrated by IVU, MRU, or VCUG (if refluxing) and is further delineated by retrograde ureterography (Fig. 151-7).

Ureteral triplication (Fig. 151-8) is another rare anomaly in which three ureters arise from the kidney, one from the upper pole, the second from the midzone of the kidney, and the third from the lower pole. The three ureters may drain separately into the bladder or one may end ectopically; the parenchyma drained by the ectopic ureter is usually small and poorly functioning. In a second type, two of the three ureters may join in the lumbar area to form a single Y-shaped ureter that drains usually into the bladder, together with a normal upper pole ureter. In a third type, the three ureters join in the lumbar area to form a common distal ureter that drains into the bladder. More than half the cases of ureteral triplication defy the Weigert-Meyer rule. Four ureters emanating from a single kidney have been described.

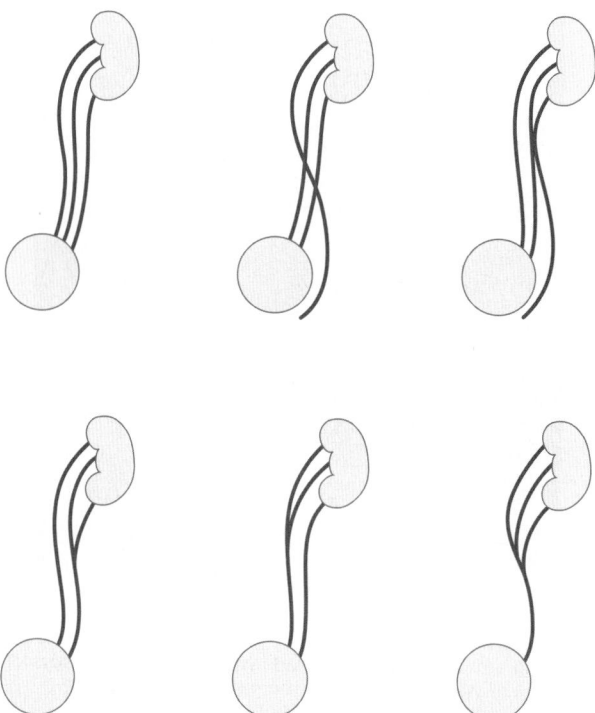

FIGURE 151-8. Types of ureteral triplication. **Top,** Complete triplication: all three ureters enter the bladder separately, or one may insert ectopically. **Bottom,** Incomplete triplication: varying degrees of communication with one or two separate ureteral orifices into the bladder.

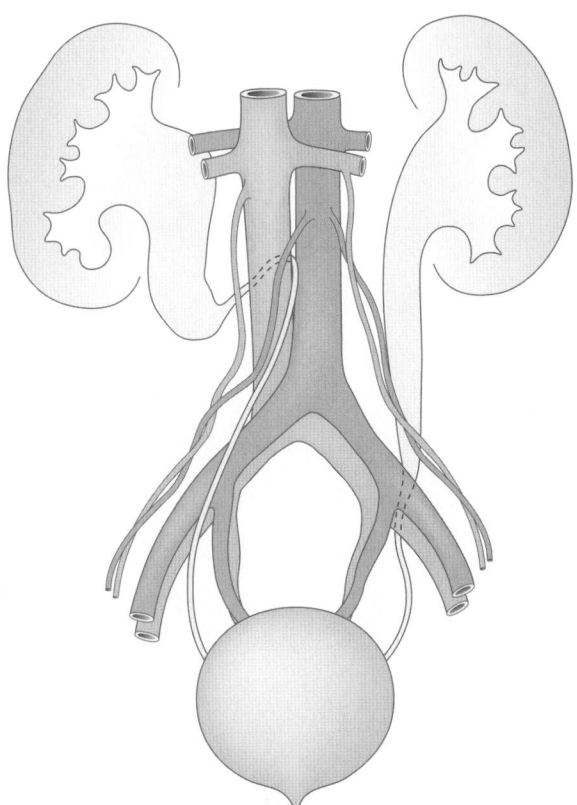

FIGURE 151-9. Abnormal ureteral course. Anatomic diagram shows a right retrocaval ureter and a left retroiliac ureter.

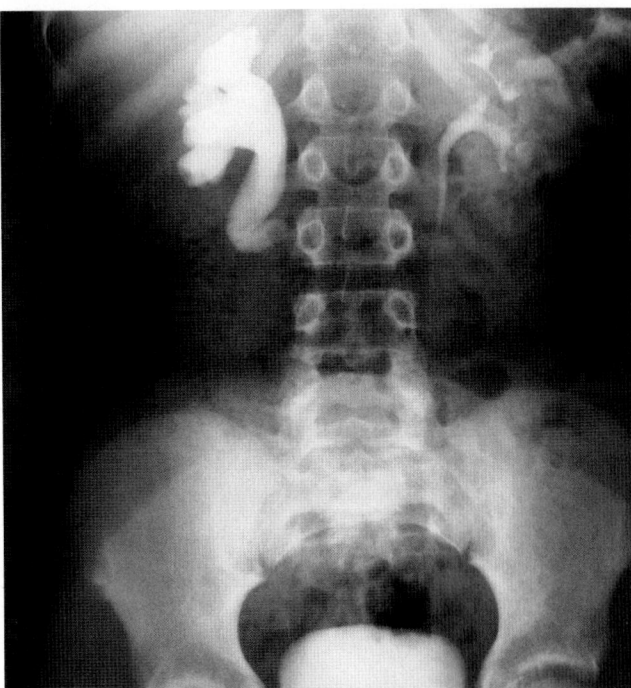

FIGURE 151-10. Retrocaval ureter. IVU image shows right hydronephrosis. The dilated right ureter passes behind the inferior vena cava in front of the L3 pedicle.

Knowledge about the embryologic development of the ureter is a key factor for understanding of ureteral anatomy, variations, and malformations. Ureteral duplications are the most common variants and may sometimes be difficult to diagnose. However, invasive diagnostic efforts are only indicated in patients with clinical symptoms and potential therapeutic consequences of such a diagnosis.

OBSTRUCTION OF THE URETER

Definition

Ureteral obstruction is defined as impaired ureteral drainage due to some hindering phenomenon. Obstruction may be severe, threatening renal function and urine drainage, or partial and minor without any clinical consequence. Note that ureteral dilatation does not equal obstruction. Most ureteral obstructions occur at the UPJ or UVJ. Obstructive lesions between these two points are uncommon and include retrocaval ureter, retroiliac ureter, ureteral obstruction caused by other vessels, ureteral valves, acquired ureteral strictures, ureteral urolithiasis, ureteral neoplasms, and extrinsic lesions affecting the ureter.

Vascular Obstruction

Retrocaval or *circumcaval ureter* (Fig. 151-9) is an uncommon anomaly in which the right ureter, in its course

to the bladder, passes behind the inferior vena cava, emerges between the cava and the aorta, and then curves around and in front of the cava to return to its normal position in the pelvis. This anomaly results from abnormal persistence of the subcardinal vein in the definitive inferior vena cava. Two types are described. In the first type (low loop), the ureter descends from the renal pelvis and crosses behind the inferior vena cava near its bifurcation. It then curves medially and upward, forming a reversed-J appearance (Fig. 151-10). Ureteral obstruction at this level is common. In the second type (high loop) the renal pelvis and upper ureter lie nearly horizontally so that the retrocaval element of the ureter is at the level of the renal pelvis. A variable degree of ureteral obstruction at this level may be present but is less often seen than in the low loop type. In both types, dilatation of the upper tract above the lesion is caused in part by compression of the ureter by the vena cava but a kink of the ureter at this level, local adhesions, an intrinsic ureteral stricture, or an adynamic ureteral segment may be the principal cause of the obstruction. Retrocaval ureter is more common in males than in females and usually manifests in adult life, perhaps because the hydronephrosis is slow to develop. Often the lesion is asymptomatic and is discovered as an incidental finding; it may be associated with Turner syndrome. The diagnosis is difficult to make on US. Historically, the diagnosis was usually suspected on IVU and confirmed by retrograde ureterography and an inferior vena cavogram. The anomaly may be demonstrated with contrast-enhanced MDCT, but MRU (with or without contrast) provides a less invasive and nonionizing imaging option.

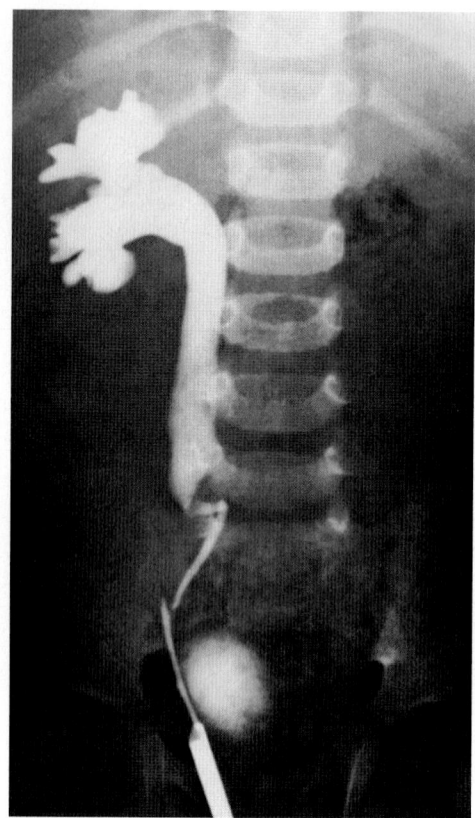

FIGURE 151-11. Ureteral obstruction from crossing vessel. Retrograde study in a child with partial ureteral obstruction, secondary to an overlying hypogastric artery.

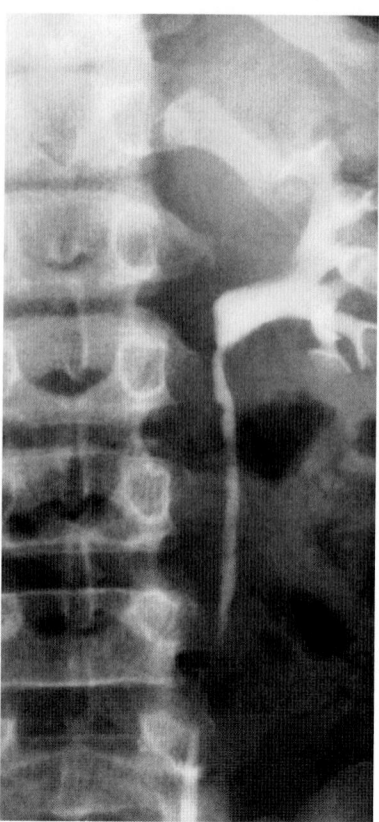

FIGURE 151-12. Vascular impressions. IVU image shows sharply defined rounded filling defects along the ureter.

Retroiliac ureter is very rare. The affected ureter courses behind one or both iliac vessels rather than in front of them (Fig. 151-11). The proximal ureter and the pelvocalyceal system are variably dilated. In the lateral or steep oblique IVU or ureterography projection, an anterior defect of the ureter at the level of the iliac vessels may be recognized. The anomaly may be corrected surgically by excision of the involved ureteral segment and reanastomosis. The lesion should be differentiated from the defect in the posterior aspect of the ureter normally caused by the iliac vessels. This is sometimes associated with slight dilatation of the proximal ureter; with the patient upright or prone, these ureters drain without residual dilatation.

Ureteral obstructions caused by other vessels are also rare. The vessels most often involved are accessory renal arteries, the ovarian artery, and the hypogastric artery or one of its branches (Fig. 151-12). Usually the obstruction is in the lower third of the ureter, and in many instances an intrinsic ureteral stricture coexists. Vascular impressions are occasionally seen on imaging and often may be normal (Fig. 151-13).

Ureteral Valves and Striations

Only a few cases of *ureteral valves* have been reported. These valves are said to consist of a cusp-like fold or an iris diaphragm composed of ureteral mucosa and smooth muscle fibers. They are commonly found in the

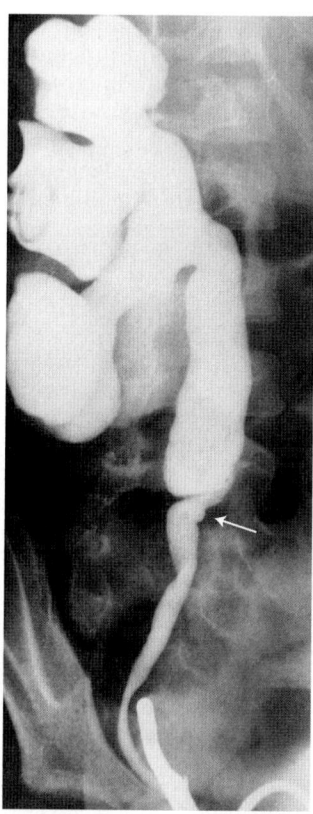

FIGURE 151-13. Ureteral mucosal fold. Retrograde study shows midureteral obstruction and hydronephrosis caused by a congenital valvelike mucosal fold *(arrow)*.

lower third of the ureter but have been reported in the middle or upper third of the ureter as well. In neonates and infants, they may be difficult to differentiate from physiologic ureteral folds, which are immature remnants that disappear during the first years of life. *Ureteral striations* are longitudinal mucosal folds that may be seen in normal ureters but are often a sign of inflammatory disease, VUR, or previous obstruction. They must be distinguished from submucosal hemorrhage and collateral circulation from compensated renal vein or IVC thrombosis.

Distal Ureteral Obstructions

Obstructions of the distal end of the ureter are relatively common. They are characterized by dilatation of the ureter (megaloureter or megaureter) as seen on US and by failure of the ureter to empty normally on postvoid films of an IVU (or VCUG if refluxing) or on delayed films of a retrograde ureterogram (Fig. 151-14). Megaureter can be assessed by diuretic MRU and diuretic renography (both of which require an empty bladder) and in difficult cases by pressure-flow studies (Whitaker test). Two types of distal ureteral obstruction are described: (1) megaureter resulting from an organic lesion and (2) primary megaureter, which is mostly functional in origin. Obstruction of the distal end of a refluxing ureter may also occur.

Megaureter may arise from organic causes. Atresia of the distal end of the ureter with marked ureteral dilatation presenting as an abdominal mass has been reported. Primary organic obstructions in the distal end of the ureter or at the UVJ caused by congenital narrowing or fibrosis also exist, but their incidence is not known (Fig. 151-15). Extravesical ectopic ureters without ureterocele occurring in a duplicated or unduplicated upper tract are often partially obstructed at their distal end. Ureters associated with an intravesical or an ectopic ureterocele are obstructed to varying degrees at their termination. UVJ obstruction may also be observed in cases of posterior urethral valves or neurogenic bladder caused by markedly thickened, stiff, and poorly functioning bladder wall musculature. Acquired distal ureteral obstruction may also be caused by a calculus, blood clot, polyp, or fungus ball; may be a complication of a surgical procedure (usually ureteral reimplantation); or may result from severe local infection or from compression by an extrinsic mass, such as a tumor or intestinal disease (e.g., Crohn disease) (Table 151-1; Fig. 151-16).

The *coexistence of VUR and obstruction* of the distal end of the refluxing ureter is not uncommon (Fig. 151-17). VUR may be primary and caused by a congenital anomaly of the UVJ, or it may be secondary to a lower urinary tract obstruction, neurogenic bladder, or other functional voiding disorder. Extravesiculation of the intramural portion of the ureter has been suggested as a possible cause of obstruction in some cases. This segment of the ureter is composed of only circular muscle fibers, which would prevent normal progress of ureteral peristalsis and cause a functional obstruction. VUR may also be observed in patients with primary megaureter (see later).

> **Distal ureteral obstruction and VUR may coexist.**

Ureteral Ectopia

An ectopic ureter is one that drains in an abnormal location (outside the posterolateral angle of the trigone) either within the bladder or extravesically. Extravesical ureteral ectopia is more common and clinically more important than the intravesical type. It is also more common in girls than in boys, with some anatomic and functional differences between the two sexes (Table 151-2). It is more common in ureteral duplication anomalies (up to 80%).

Two types of *intravesical ureteral ectopia* are recognized: lateral and caudal. In lateral ectopia, the more common of the two, one or both ureters (the lower pole ureter in a duplicated system) drain into the bladder more laterally and craniad than normal. The intramural submucosal tunnel of the affected ureter tends to be short or otherwise defective, leading to VUR in many cases. In the second type, one or both ureters (the upper pole ureter in a duplicated system) drain caudad and medial to the usual site along a line extending from the normal lateral corner of the trigone to the bladder neck. These ureters are less prone to VUR than the lateral type.

Extravesical ureteral ectopia in girls (Fig. 151-18) is associated with a duplicated system in at least 85% of the cases and affects the upper pole ureter in practically all cases. Partial or complete duplication of the opposite system is common, and sometimes the anomaly is bilateral. The ectopic ureter may end in the urethra or in the vestibule or, less commonly, in the vagina (Fig. 151-19). A common presenting complaint is continuous leakage of urine in the context of an otherwise normal voiding pattern. Leakage of urine is observed even if the anomalous ureter ends in the proximal urethra, owing to relative weakness of the external urethral sphincter in girls. The ectopic-ending ureter is frequently dilated and tortuous but may be normal and sometimes it ends superiorly in a minute collecting system and a diminutive upper pole. The renal parenchyma drained by the ectopic ureter is often dysplastic with decreased or absent function. The ipsilateral lower pole ureter may be normal or dilated and is frequently the site of reflux. Its dilatation and tortuosity is partially aggravated by its path meandering around the dilated and obstructed upper pole ureter and spontaneously improves after treatment of this underlying conditions; thus, initial assessment tends to overestimate the degree of disease of the lower pole ureter.

> **A history of constant urine leakage in a girl with otherwise normal voiding should suggest extravesical ureteral ectopia.**

US is the initial imaging method of choice and is often diagnostic, particularly when the anomalous ureter is dilated and sufficient renal parenchyma or even cysts of the corresponding renal moiety are present. The course of this ureter may often be followed down to and beyond

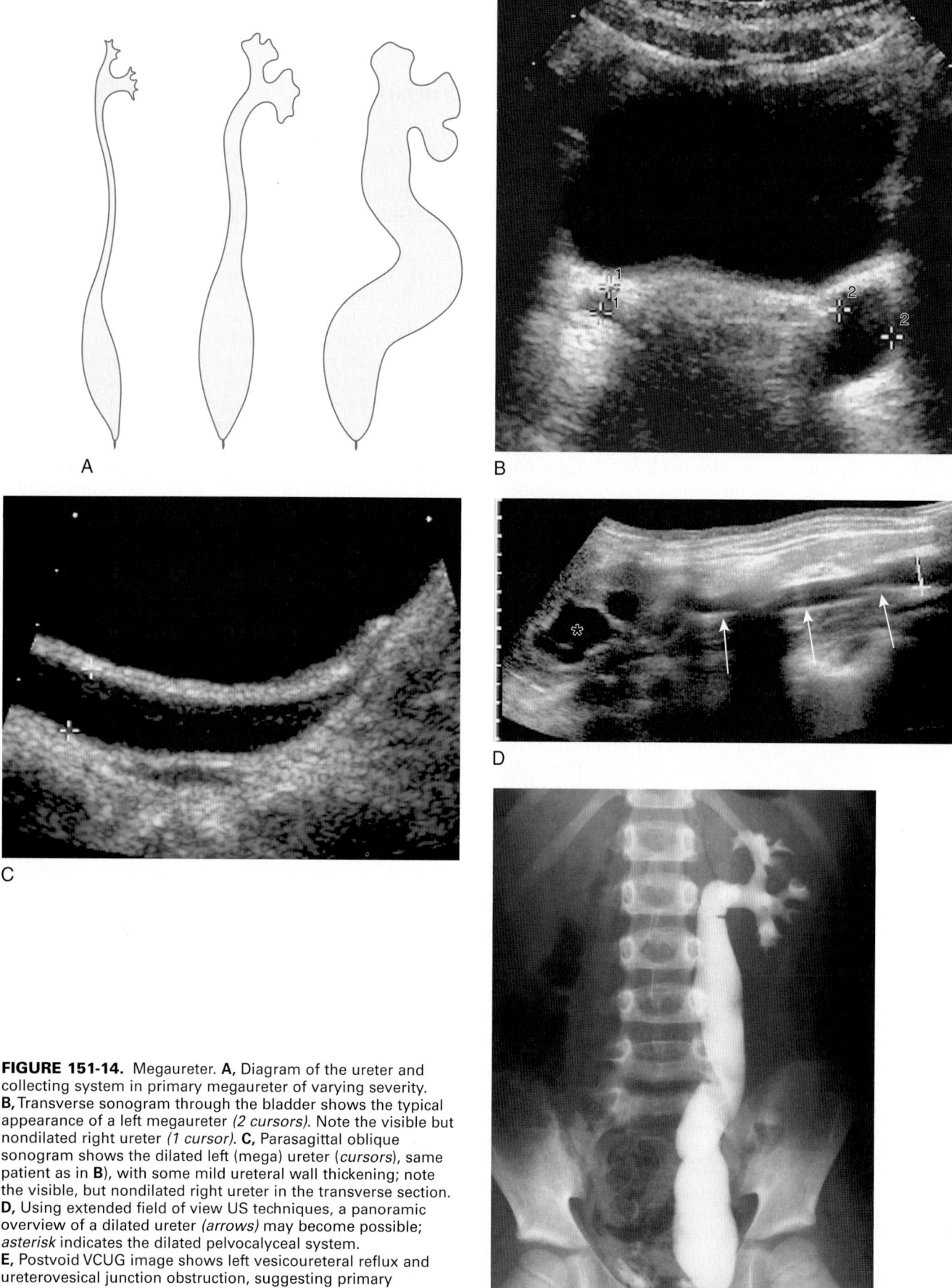

FIGURE 151-14. Megaureter. **A,** Diagram of the ureter and collecting system in primary megaureter of varying severity. **B,** Transverse sonogram through the bladder shows the typical appearance of a left megaureter *(2 cursors)*. Note the visible but nondilated right ureter *(1 cursor)*. **C,** Parasagittal oblique sonogram shows the dilated left (mega) ureter *(cursors)*, same patient as in **B**), with some mild ureteral wall thickening; note the visible, but nondilated right ureter in the transverse section. **D,** Using extended field of view US techniques, a panoramic overview of a dilated ureter *(arrows)* may become possible; *asterisk* indicates the dilated pelvocalyceal system. **E,** Postvoid VCUG image shows left vesicoureteral reflux and ureterovesical junction obstruction, suggesting primary megaureter. The ureteral dilatation is most pronounced in the lower ureter, and the renal pelvis and calyces are little affected.

the bladder. A vaginal ectopic ureter may be shown by US to be connected with a urine-filled vagina (Fig. 151-20). Cases with sufficient function of the ectopically draining system may be visualized on IVU, often only on delayed films. A nonfunctioning system is visualized best by MRU (or CT) (Fig. 151-21). When the aberrant ureter empties in the urethra, VUR into the ectopic ureter is occa-

sionally demonstrated by VCUG (Fig. 151-22). A vaginogram or genitogram may show reflux in the affected ureter if it terminates in the vagina. A dynamic nuclear renogram may show essentially the same findings as the IVU, and a static cortical scintigram (with dimercaptosuccinic acid [DMSA]) may be useful in evaluation of the renal parenchyma and function, depicting parenchymal uptake even in units with no apparent function on other imaging.

Single (unduplicated) ureteral ectopia in girls is uncommon and usually unilateral. The corresponding kidney is frequently small and dysplastic and may be ectopic. Sometimes the ectopic ureter is connected with a minute dysplastic kidney (renal aplasia, MCDK), or ends blindly superiorly without renal tissue (renal

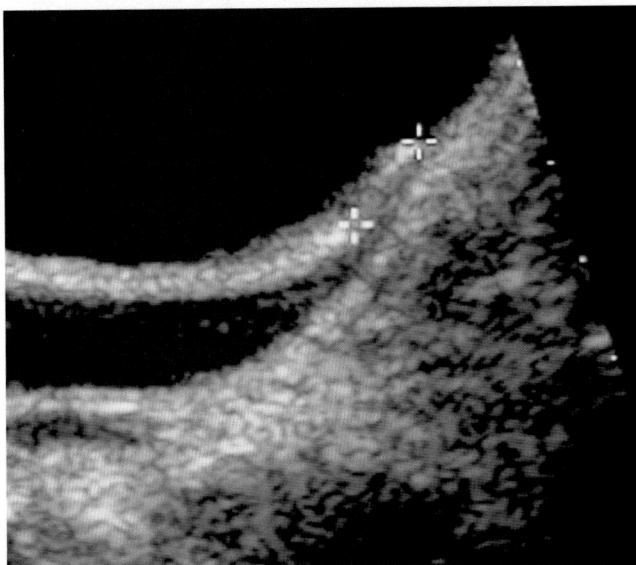

FIGURE 151-15. Megaureter. Longitudinal sonogram demonstrates a distal stenotic segment of a megaureter with ureterovesical junction obstruction *(cursors)*.

TABLE 151-1
Types of Megaureter
Primary megaureter
Congenital ureterovesical junction obstruction
Retrocaval or retroiliac megaureter
Prune-belly syndrome
Refluxing megaureter
Megaureter caused by stone, fungus balls, polyps, valves and folds, or other intrinsic lesions
Bladder outlet obstruction
Megaureter caused by extrinsic compression (masses)
Postoperative megaureter, or secondary to other acquired strictures

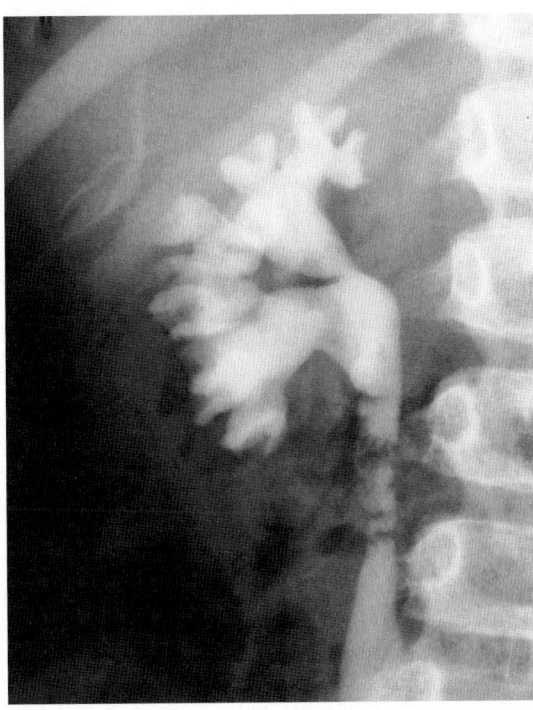
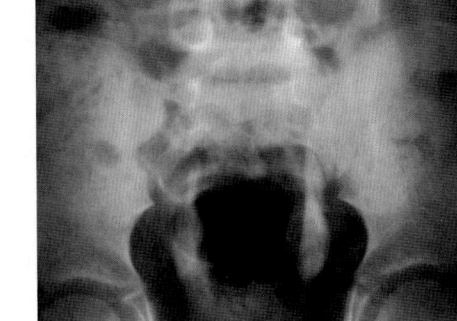

A   B

FIGURE 151-16. Ureteral obstruction. **A,** Ureteral polyps. IVU image shows mild hydronephrosis and proximal ureteral filling defects surgically proven to be polyps. **B,** Megaureter and neuroblastoma. IVU image in a child being evaluated for primary megaureter shows lateral deviation of the left kidney and proximal ureter from an unsuspected retroperitoneal mass, later shown to be a neuroblastoma.

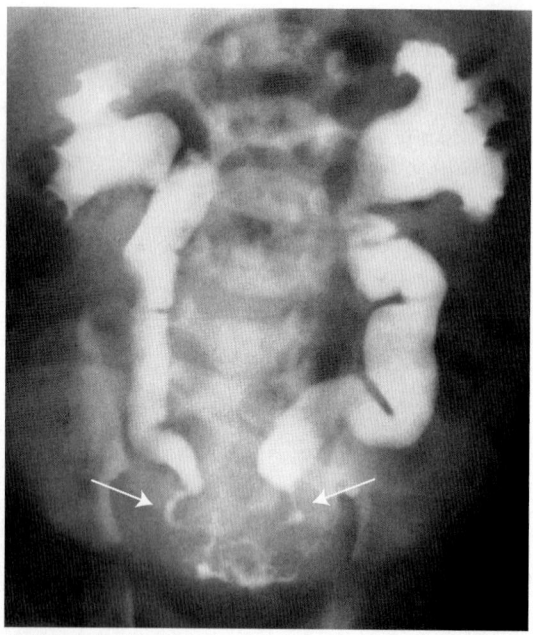

FIGURE 151-17. Megaureter and vesicoureteral reflux. Postvoid image from a VCUG shows bilateral vesicoureteral reflux and bilateral ureterovesical junction obstruction caused by stenosis of the distal ureters (arrows).

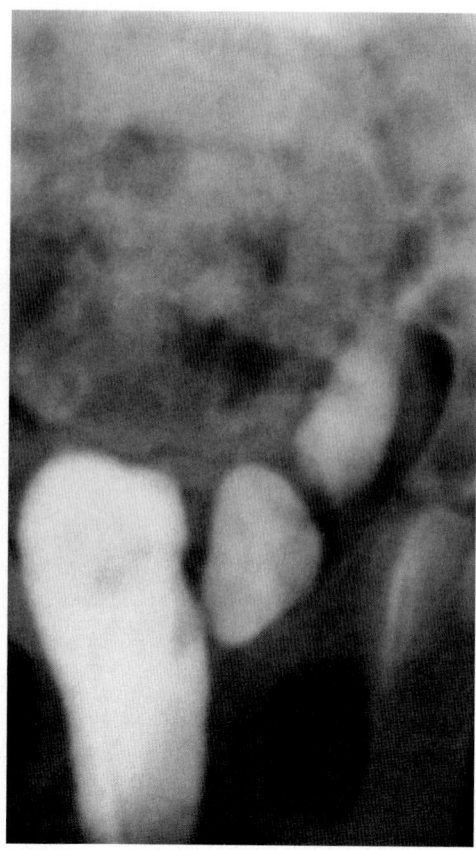

FIGURE 151-19. Ureteral ectopia. Contrast medium injected into the vagina is seen filling the distal left ureter.

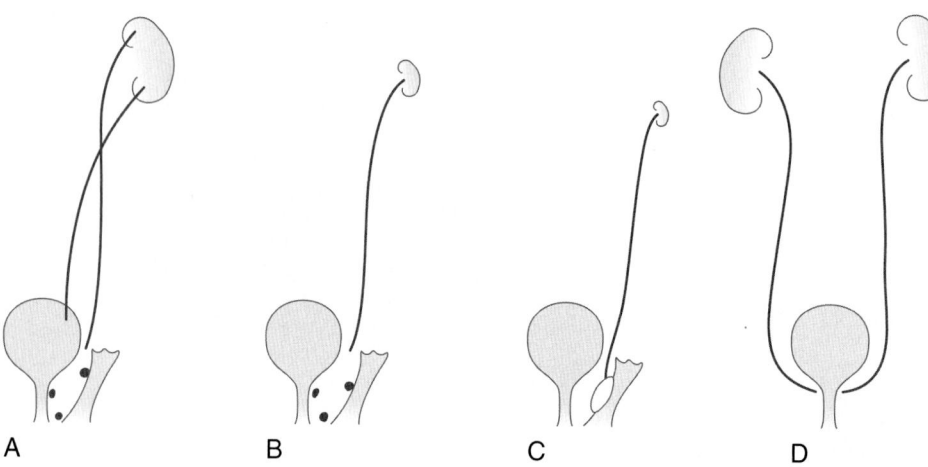

A   B   C   D

FIGURE 151-18. Types of ureteral ectopia in females. **A,** In the most common variant there is ureteral duplication with the upper pole ureter draining into the urethra, into the perineum near the urethral meatus, or into the vagina. **B,** Ectopic ureteral drainage as in **A,** but from a single collecting system. The kidney may be small and dysplastic. **C,** Ectopic drainage from a single system into a Gartner duct cyst in the wall of the vagina. The ipsilateral kidney may not be identifiable. **D,** Bilateral single-system ectopic drainage into the bladder neck or proximal urethra. This uncommon form is found almost exclusively in females and is usually associated with a wide bladder neck, a defective internal sphincter, sometimes a malformed urethra, and urinary incontinence.

agenesis). The anomalous ureter may terminate in the urethra, vestibule, or vagina. Occasionally, a single ectopic ureter ends in a blind cystic structure in the lateral wall of the vagina (Gartner duct cyst) (Fig. 151-23). In these cases the ipsilateral kidney is usually nonfunctioning or may be absent. Sometimes a Gartner duct cyst is found in the wall of the vagina without a demonstrable ureter or kidney on that side. Note that many of these anomalies are accompanied by ipsilateral malformations of the genitalia. A thorough investigation of the vagina, the uterus, and the ovaries by US or MRI is recommended.

Bilateral unduplicated ureteral ectopia (no ureter entering the bladder) is a rare anomaly affecting females almost exclusively. The two ureters terminate at the bladder neck or in the proximal urethra. This form of ureteral ectopia is usually accompanied by defective formation of the trigone and bladder base, a wide bladder neck, a deformed internal sphincter, and, in

TABLE 151-2

Extravesical Ureteral Ectopia

	Girls	Boys
DUPLICATED SYSTEM	More common	Less common
	Inserts into urethra, vestibule, vagina	Inserts into prostatic urethra, bladder neck, genital ducts
	Urethral-ending ureter refluxes	Same
	Ectopic ureter normal	Same
	Drains atrophic nubbin	Same
	Lower pole refluxes	Same
	Chief complaint: continuous urine leakage	Chief complaint: infection
SINGLE SYSTEM	Uncommon	Uncommon
	Associated with small, often ectopic kidney	Associated with dysplastic kidney
	May insert in urethra, vestibule, vagina	May insert in seminal vesicle
	Gartner duct cyst	Ejaculatory duct wolffian tissue posterior to bladder

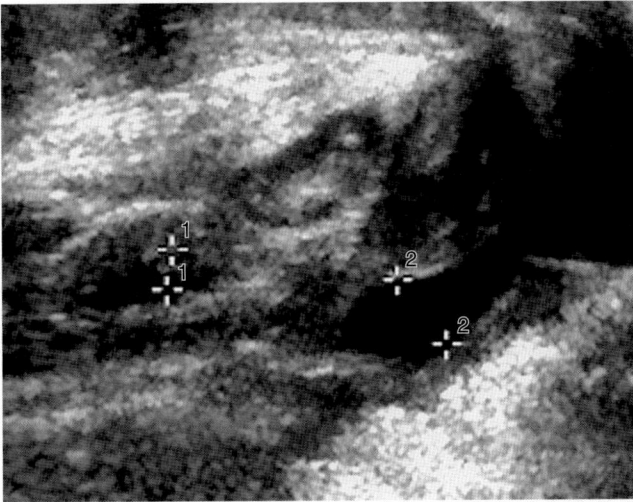

FIGURE 151-20. Ectopic ureteral insertion. Longitudinal sonogram demonstrates a urine-filled vagina *(2 cursors)* with a nearly empty bladder *(1 cursors)* in a girl with ectopic vaginal ureteral insertion.

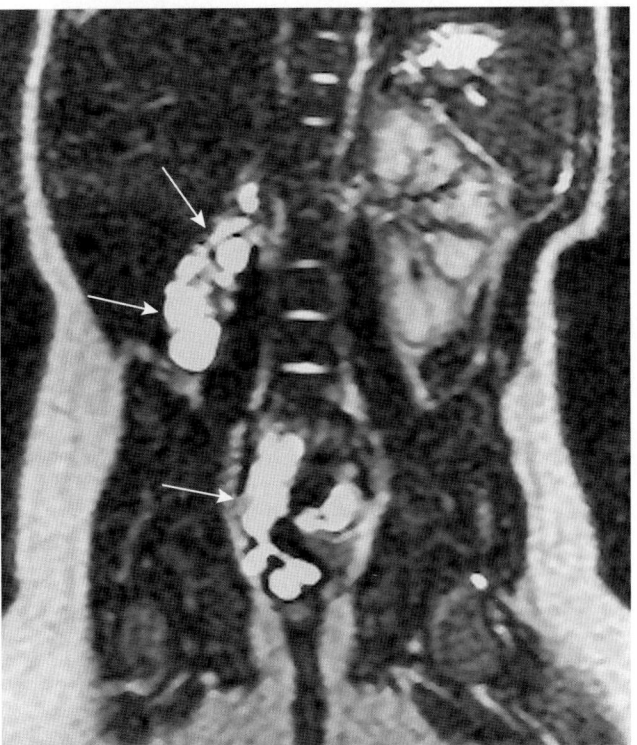

FIGURE 151-21. Ectopic ureteral insertion. MRU demonstrating cystic remnant of an ectopic renal bud *(top arrows)* with only minimal residual function and a dilated and tortuous dysplastic ureter *(bottom arrow)* ectopically inserting into the vagina.

some cases, a short and broad urethra. Incontinence is the rule even after ureteral reimplantation.

Extravesical ureteral ectopia in boys occurs much less commonly than in girls. The anomaly commonly involves the upper pole ureter in a duplex system but also may occur in a single, unduplicated ureter. The anomalous ureter may insert in the prostatic urethra, sometimes near the bladder neck, and much less often in the genital ducts (Fig. 151-24). Ureteral ectopia to the posterior urethra usually ends slightly above or at the level of the verumontanum or in the utricle (Fig. 151-25). The renal parenchyma drained by the ectopic ureter is commonly small and dysplastic and often nonfunctioning. The opposite upper tract may be duplicated. UTI is the most common clinical manifestation. Urinary incontinence rarely is a problem in boys because the ectopic ureter drains above the strongly developed external urethral sphincter. The urographic and sonographic features are similar to those described in girls.

In ureteral ectopia to the genital tract in males, the affected ureter is almost always single (unduplicated)

and ends in a markedly dilated seminal vesicle, the vas deferens, the ejaculatory duct, or a mass of ill-defined, tortuous tubular structures located behind the trigone of the bladder. Some of these structures probably represent a persistent and markedly dilated and distorted embryonic common distal duct for the wolffian (spermatic) duct and primitive ureter. The ipsilateral kidney is usually severely dysplastic or absent, and the affected ureter may be atretic. Cryptorchidism or testicular hypoplasia on the side of the lesion is common. Pain on voiding and straining to void are common clinical manifestations. Epididymo-orchitis is a common complication.

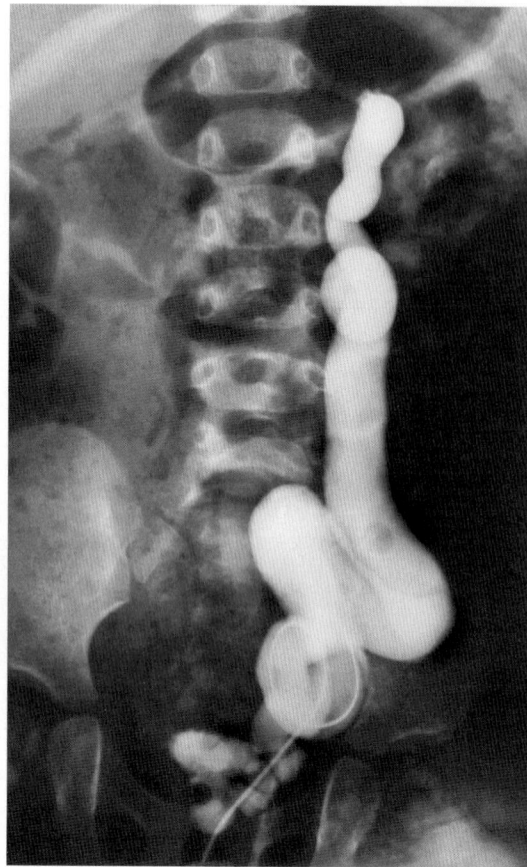

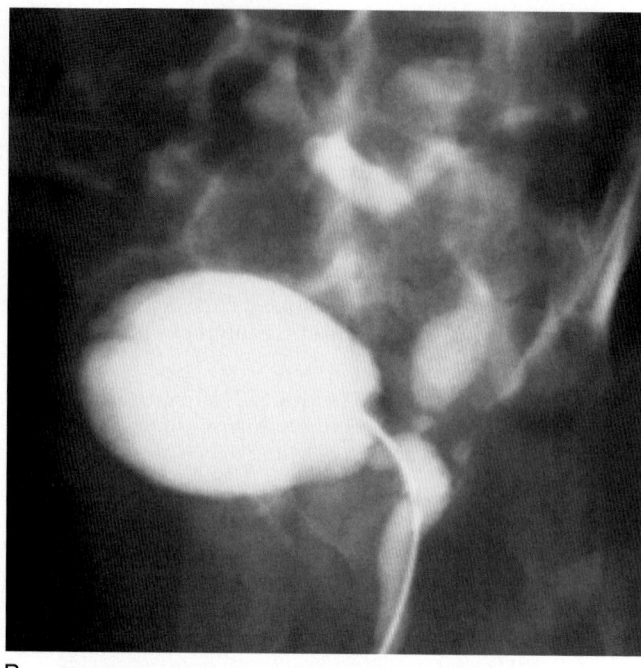

B

A

FIGURE 151-22. Ureteral ectopia into urethra. **A,** VCUG image shows that the catheter has passed from the urethra directly into the ureter, which drains an atrophic upper pole. **B,** VCUG image during voiding shows vesicoureteral reflux into the ureter, which drains into the posterior urethra.

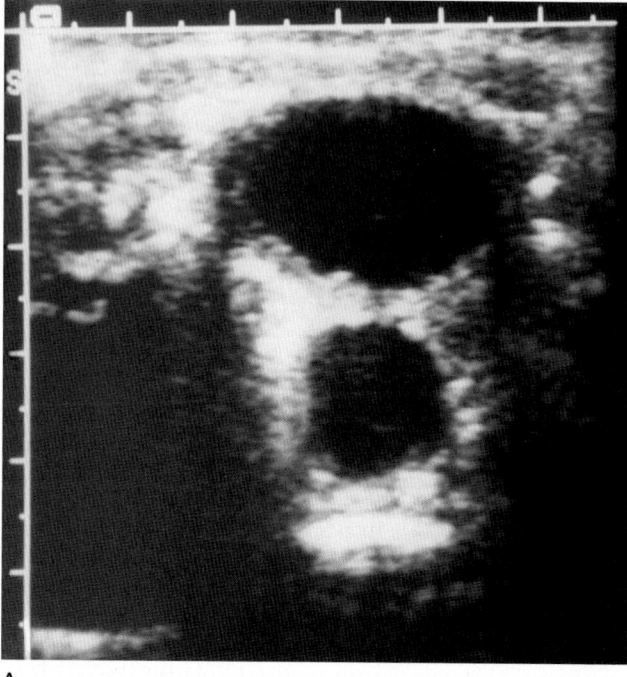

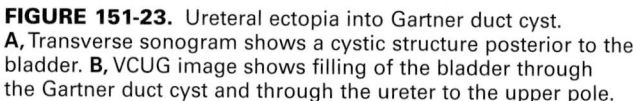

A

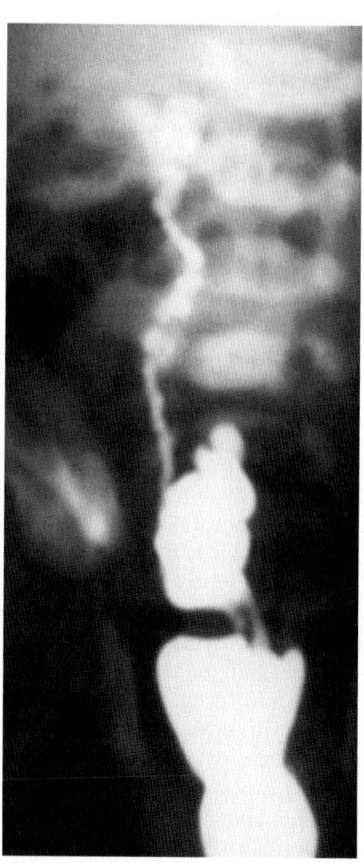

FIGURE 151-23. Ureteral ectopia into Gartner duct cyst. **A,** Transverse sonogram shows a cystic structure posterior to the bladder. **B,** VCUG image shows filling of the bladder through the Gartner duct cyst and through the pelvis ureter to the upper pole.

B

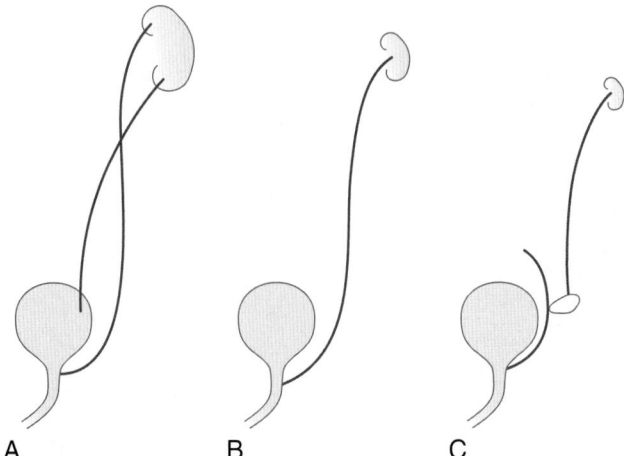

A   B   C

FIGURE 151-24. Types of ureteral ectopia in males. **A,** In the most common variant there is ureteral duplication with the upper pole ureter draining into the posterior urethra. **B,** Ectopic ureteral drainage as in **A** but from a single collecting system. The kidney may be small and dysplastic. **C,** Ectopic drainage from a single system into a seminal vesicle, vas deferens, or ejaculatory duct. The ipsilateral kidney may not be identifiable.

A mass may be felt between the rectum and the bladder on rectal examination. IVU almost invariably reveals no renal function on the affected side and commonly shows an extrinsic mass deforming the base of the bladder posterolaterally. The DMSA scan may, however, still demonstrate some residual renal parenchyma. The VCUG often shows an extrinsic deformity of the posterior wall of the bladder and may reveal reflux of contrast material in the ipsilateral ejaculatory duct. The cystic nature of the mass may be demonstrated by US. Additionally, US (particularly using harmonic imaging, image compounding, and the perineal approach) may visualize the anatomy of the complex cystic structure behind the urinary bladder and may depict the dysplastic or ectopic residual renal parenchyma. The pathology and pelvic anatomy may also be demonstrated by MRU (and CT), particularly for small ectopic kidneys.

Ureterocele

A ureterocele is a cyst-like expansion of the terminal segment of the ureter projecting into the lumen of the urinary bladder. The anomaly is relatively common and has two subtypes: (1) intravesical ureterocele, which is located entirely within the bladder, and (2) ectopic ureterocele, which is usually large and extends to the bladder neck area or proximal urethra. Both forms may be associated with a duplicated or an unduplicated system. This differentiation, except for different clinical presentations, has only minor implications on imaging and therapy. Treatment consists of cystoscopic fenestration of the ureterocele and/or resection and reimplantation of the ureter, especially if the ureterocele causes VUR or bladder outlet obstruction. There are varied theories about ureterocele origins (applicable to both forms of ureterocele) produced by a herniation of the very distal end of the ureter into the bladder. Embryologically, it may be due to persistence of the Chwalla membrane that initially separates the ureteric bud from the bladder lumen. Others have theorized an abnormal musculature of the transmural ureter, leading to a ballooning of this ureteral segment, which then protrudes into the bladder. Other hypotheses include a developmental stimulus that induces bladder expansion and by error also affects the intravesical ureter.

US is the modality of choice for initial imaging diagnosis and is diagnostically definitive in many cases. The main findings include the demonstration of an intravesical cystic lesion of variable size attached to the posterolateral wall of the bladder and protruding into the lumen of the bladder ("cyst within cyst"), often associated with a cystic structure in the upper pole of the ipsilateral kidney (in duplicated systems) (Fig. 151-26). The dilated ureter connecting with the ureterocele may be demonstrated, as well as the corresponding renal unit. In duplex systems both ureters on the side of the ureterocele may be dilated. Ureteral peristalsis can be assessed, and the urine inflow into the bladder can be demonstrated, differentiating an either central ostium at the top of the ureterocele or a more mediocaudal orifice position at the base of the ureterocele close to the bladder wall (see Fig. 151-26).

Although IVU is rarely currently used for diagnosis, it reveals characteristic findings. The affected ureter is variously dilated. In simple ureteroceles, the dilatation involves predominantly the lower half of the ureter, but the entire ureter, pelvocalyceal system, and renal parenchyma may also be affected in more severely obstructed cases. On early images, the lesion generally presents as a round, radiolucent defect at the trigone. As contrast material collects within the bladder and in the ureterocele, it outlines a rounded mass surrounded by a radiolucent halo representing the nonopacified wall of the ureterocele. This is the well-known "cobra head" or "spring onion" formation characteristic of the lesion (Fig. 151-27). In ectopic ureteroceles, the IVU shows no function of the renal parenchyma drained by the ureterocele-bearing ureter in 90% of the cases and poor function in 10%; therefore, the affected ureter is very seldom visualized. In the usual type of ureterocele associated with a duplex system, the visualized lower pelvocalyceal system is displaced downward and laterally and the ureter is frequently displaced laterally by the dilated, nonvisualized upper tract (Table 151-3). The IVU in patients with ectopic ureterocele in a single ureter usually shows no function on the side of the lesion. Still, in most cases when the ureterocele is mostly intravesical and sufficiently large, the ureterocele is clearly delineated by the excreted contrast material accumulated in the bladder as a rounded and usually eccentrically placed filling defect. Occasionally, the defect is lobulated. A double ureterocele, one on each side of the midline, is seen in bilateral cases. The outline of simple or intravesical ureteroceles is usually clearly defined by contrast material, but the lower margin of ectopic ureteroceles may be poorly seen when they are confluent with the base of the bladder and bladder neck. This is in contrast to intravesical or simple ureteroceles, which are usually completely outlined. In current imaging practice, IVU has been replaced by methods such as dynamic MRU as

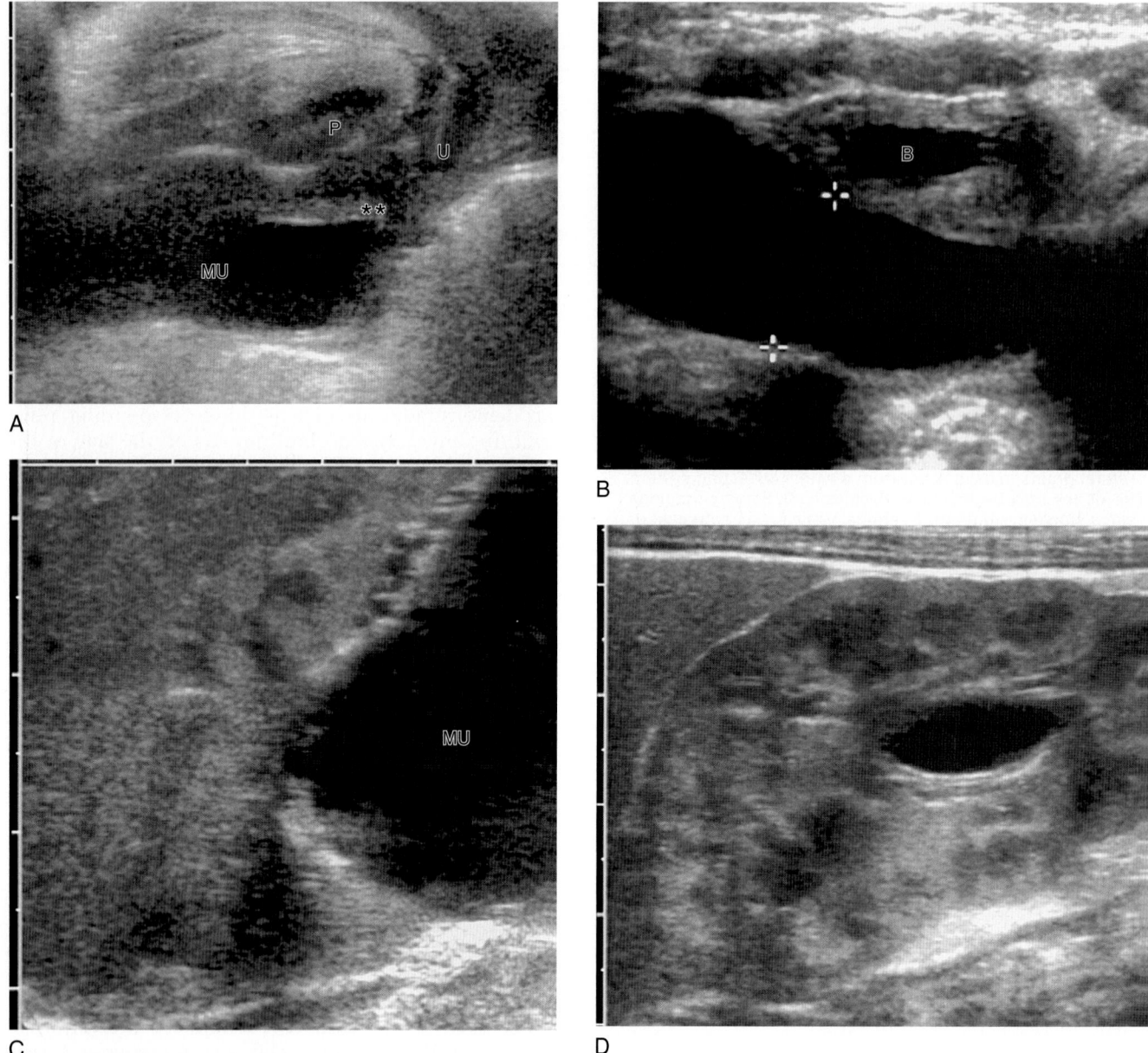

FIGURE 151-25. US and VCUG in two patients with an ectopic ureter inserting into the urethra. **A,** Perineal US of the urethra and the distal megaureter (MU) inserting ectopically *(asterisks).* U, urethra, P, pubis. **B,** Megaureter *(cursors)* behind the urinary bladder (B). **C,** Longitudinal sonogram shows the upper dysplastic moiety of the kidney draining into the megaureter (MU). **D,** Longitudinal sonogram shows some dilatation of the lower moiety of the duplex kidney due to compression of the ureteropelvic junction by the upper pole megaureter.   *Continued*

the modality of choice for preoperative imaging, because it provides all the functional information as well as superior anatomic detail and can reveal associated renal abnormalities and genital malformations (Fig. 151-28).

A radiolucent filling defect is usually the only finding on VCUG, unless the corresponding ureter is refluxing or part of a duplex system, with VUR into the lower pole moiety (Fig. 151-29). The negative filling defect of the ureterocele may be obscured by the concentrated contrast material later in the study when bladder volume is high; thus, imaging during early filling of the bladder is essential. If the bladder is overdistended by contrast material or when bladder pressure increases during voiding, the ureterocele may be compressed and flattened

against the bladder wall and can even evert, simulating a paraureteral diverticulum. During voiding the VCUG may show prolapse of the ureterocele into the urethra, where it may produce bladder outlet obstruction. VUR into an ureterocele is rare initially but common after endoscopic incision (Fig. 151-30).

> **Ureteroceles are best seen with US, which also evaluates the ureter and kidney. Early filling VCUG images are essential in demonstrating ureteroceles.**

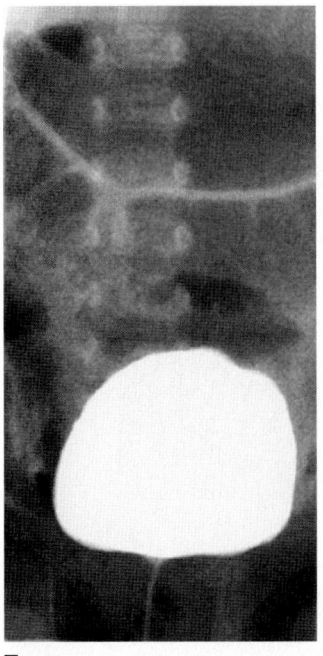 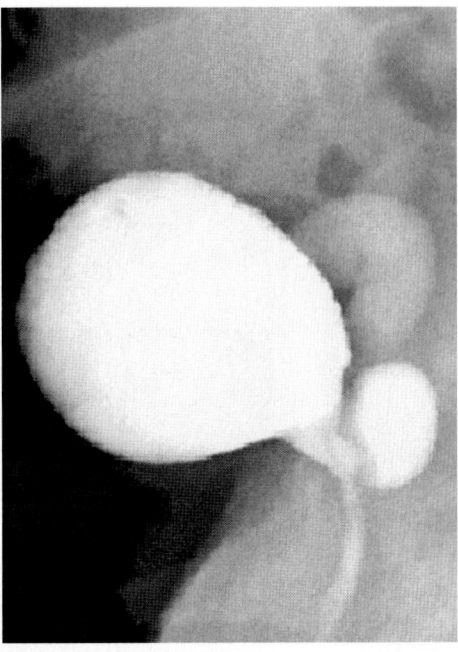 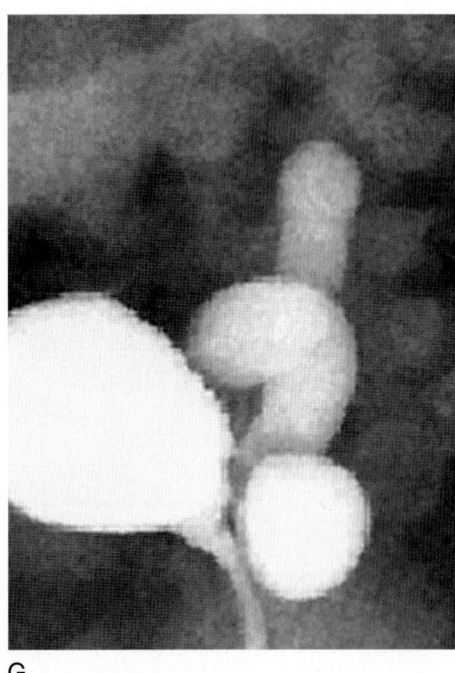

E   F   G

FIGURE 151-25, _cont'd._ US and VCUG in two patients with an ectopic ureter inserting into the urethra. **E-G,** VCUG image series in a girl with a refluxing ectopic ureterocele inserting into the urethra: no VUR during filling (**E**) and filling of a diverticula-shaped ureterocele connected to the posterior urethra during voiding (**F**) with consecutive slow vesicoureteral reflux into the fluid-filled corresponding megaureter (**G**).

TABLE 151-3

Imaging Findings In Ectopic Ureterocele

- Poor or nonfunctioning upper pole, with dysplasia, dilatation, and poor vascularization on US
- "Drooping lily" appearance on IVU or VCUG (if refluxing lower moiety)
- Filling defect in bladder, often double filling defect (IVU+ VCUG, on early filling of bladder)
- Cystic structure in or adjacent to the bladder on US
- Seldom refluxes, but may after injury by instrumentation or catheterization
- May evert, simulating diverticulum
- May show as urethral mass, and may cause bladder outlet obstruction
- Nuclear medicine studies show decreased function in upper pole, photon-deficient area in bladder
- MR: "cyst in cyst" often poorly visualized on non-enhanced acquisitions; becomes obvious on contrast enhanced diuretic T1-weighted MRU

Renal scintigraphy reveals similar changes as IVU, including decreased function at the superior pole of the kidney and often a photopenic area in the bladder corresponding to the ureterocele. Sometimes scintigraphy shows function in parts of the kidney connected with the ureterocele that are not visualized by IVU but usually are associated with residual vascularity on color Doppler imaging (Fig. 151-31).

The _intravesical ureterocele_ (also called stenotic, orthotopic, simple, or adult-type ureterocele) is more common in adults than in children, suggesting that it may be acquired in many cases. In children, it is more frequently associated with significant hydroureteronephrosis. The ureterocele is located at the orthotopic ureteric ostium position (i.e., at the lateral angle of the trigone) and is entirely within the bladder (Fig. 151-32). The ureteral orifice is on the surface of the ureterocele and is variously stenotic, a feature that may be responsible in part for the anomaly. Intravesical ureteroceles may be bilateral and, although commonly seen in single (unduplicated) ureters, may involve the upper and sometimes the lower pole ureter of a duplicated system. Intravesical ureteroceles may be discovered as an incidental asymptomatic finding but when large may be associated with a more severe degree of ureteral obstruction and can even obstruct the bladder outlet. Stone formation within the ureterocele has been reported. VUR into the ureter may occur.

The _ectopic or infantile ureterocele_ is one of the most important urologic disorders in children and is the most common cause of bladder outlet obstruction in girls. In children it is more common than the intravesical type and is five to seven times more frequent in females than males. It is unilateral in 90% of the cases and bilateral in 10%. Its anatomy differs from that of an intravesical ureterocele in several respects. Ectopic ureteroceles most often occur in a duplicated system and almost always are connected with the upper pole ureter. An ectopic ureterocele of a similar configuration also occurs in unduplicated ureter, more commonly in boys than in girls. In both types, the ureter connected with the ureterocele enters the bladder wall at the normal site, descends toward the bladder neck submucosally, passes through the internal urethral sphincter, and terminates ectopically in the proximal urethra. In contrast to simple ureterocele, in which the "cyst" is formed by herniation of the distal end of the ureter, the ectopic ureterocele represents

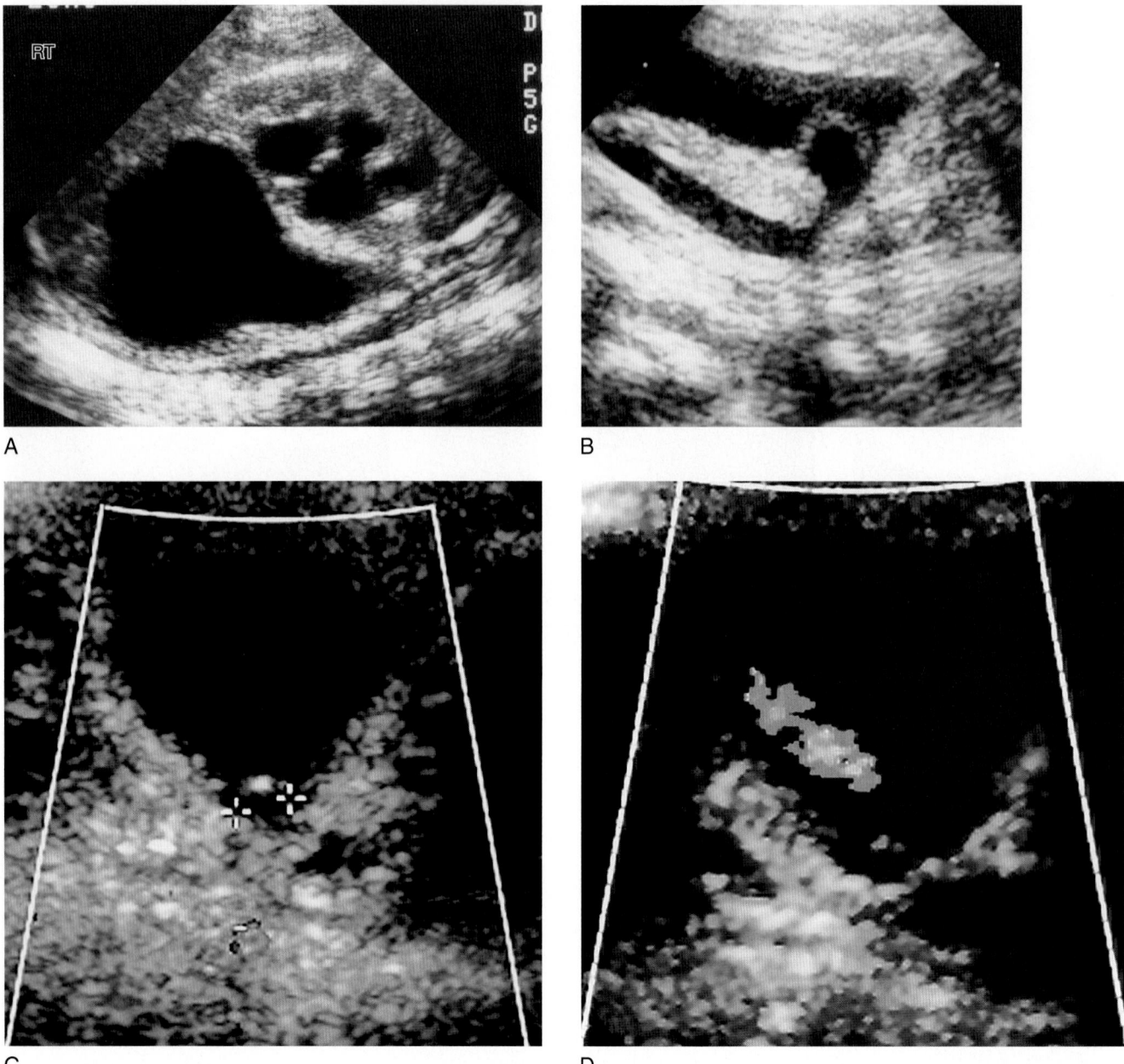

FIGURE 151-26. Ureterocele. **A,** Longitudinal sonogram of the right kidney shows marked upper pole hydronephrosis and parenchymal thinning along with mild lower pole hydronephrosis. **B,** Longitudinal sonogram of the right pelvis shows a dilated right ureter ending in a ureterocele that protrudes into the bladder. **C,** Sonogram shows a tiny ureterocele *(cursors).* **D,** Color Doppler sonogram demonstrating the inflow jet. Note that small ureteroceles can be missed if the bladder is overdistended or empty, or in nonhydrated patients, as they collapse due to poor diuresis.

a dilatation and protrusion of the entire submucosal segment of the ureter into the lumen of the bladder and at the bladder neck. The ectopic ureterocele has a broad base and tends to be larger than the simple intravesical type and characteristically is located more inferiorly in the bladder and may extend to the bladder neck area and proximal urethra. Its orifice is almost always in or close to the posterior urethra and may be stenotic, but more often it is patent. The ureterocele may additionally be obstructed by the sphincteric action of the bladder neck. In rare instances, the ureterocele has a patulous orifice in the bladder, even though the dilated submucosal ureter extends downward through the bladder neck to end blindly in the urethra. This anatomic arrangement is termed a *cecoureterocele.* A typical ureterocele with an acquired perforation resulting from infection or previous bladder instrumentation may acquire a similar configuration. The ureterocele may obstruct the bladder neck or the opposite ureteral orifice, and in patients with ureteral duplication it may deform the musculature or position and course of the adjacent ureter so that VUR into the lower pole ureter occurs (40% to 50% of cases). VUR may also occur on the opposite side (15%), where a partial or complete duplication of the renal collecting system is common (35% to 50% of cases). VUR into the ureter connected with the ureterocele is very unusual.

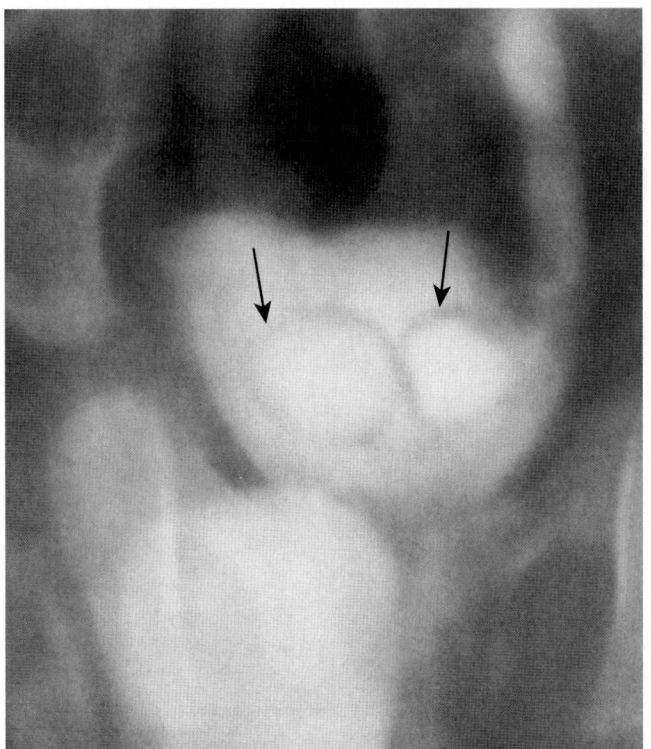
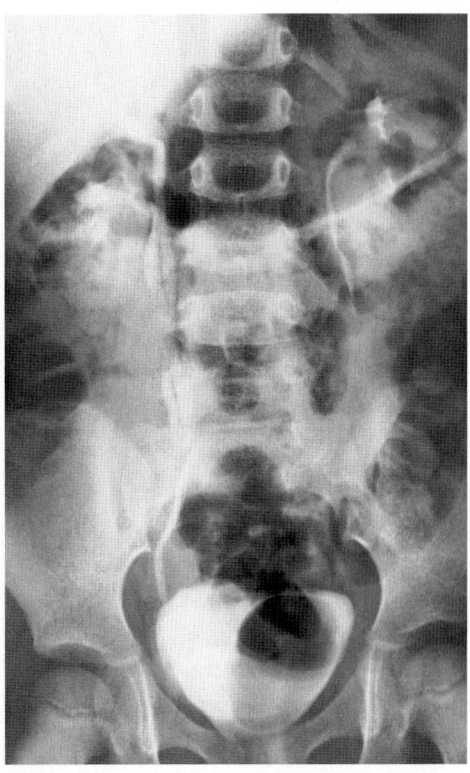

A   B

FIGURE 151-27. Single-system ureteroceles. **A,** IVU image of the bladder shows two "cobra heads" *(black arrows),* one from each ureter. **B,** IVU image shows a left ureterocele from a nonduplicated left collecting system as a bladder filling defect. The right collecting system is duplicated.

Occasionally, the ureterocele herniates into the urethra, causing urethral obstruction, or may evert, appearing as a diverticulum (Fig. 151-33); in females, it may present as a fleshy mass at the external urethral meatus resembling a prolapsed urethra. The ureter connected with the ureterocele is often dilated and tortuous. Its proximal segment and the corresponding pelvocalyceal system may also be very large but sometimes are only mildly dilated. Sometimes the entire ureter is of normal size and ends in a point at the level of the kidney. The adjacent ureter and the opposite ureter(s) are commonly dilated. In the majority of cases, the proximal moiety of the kidney on the affected side (the entire kidney in an unduplicated ureter) is hypodysplastic and may be further reduced in size by atrophy and infection.

More than 90% of the cases are discovered in children younger than 3 years of age, and the majority is diagnosed prenatally or in the newborn period. UTI is the most common presenting clinical manifestation. Failure to thrive, difficulty in voiding, urinary retention, flank pain, and sometimes chronic renal failure are prominent manifestations of the anomaly in older infants and in children. Dribbling of urine is not a feature of the disorder.

Acquired Ureteral Obstruction

Acquired strictures of the body of the ureter are uncommon. They may be due to a local surgical procedure, instrumentation, ureteral wall inflammation, or peri-ureteral infection; may be a complication of Henoch-Schönlein purpura, periarteritis nodosa, tuberculosis, or granulomatous disease of childhood (e.g., Crohn disease); may be the result of trauma or submucosal hemorrhage in patients on anticoagulant medication; or may follow local radiation. Other acquired intrinsic ureteral obstructions include sludge balls, blood clots, various calculi (see Chapter 147), and fungus balls. Note that acute obstructions may exhibit only minor collecting system dilatation but patients will have severe pain and renal colic.

Imaging usually starts with US, assessing the distal ureter and the ureteral inflow jet through a sufficiently distended urinary bladder. The upper ureter and pelvocalyceal system are then evaluated, before looking at the renal parenchyma and renal blood flow and Doppler changes. US is usually supplemented by an abdominal radiograph. Although rarely used in Europe, CT (with or without contrast medium enhancement) is commonly used in North America. Limited IVU with individually timed films may be useful. Advanced imaging such as MRU is rarely necessary.

Primary Ureteral Neoplasms

Primary neoplasms of the renal pelvis and ureters, such as *rhabdomyosarcoma* or *urothelial cell carcinoma,* are extremely rare in children. Secondary involvement of the pelvocalyceal system by Wilms tumor, and Wilms tumor implants in the ureter, may occur. The ureter may

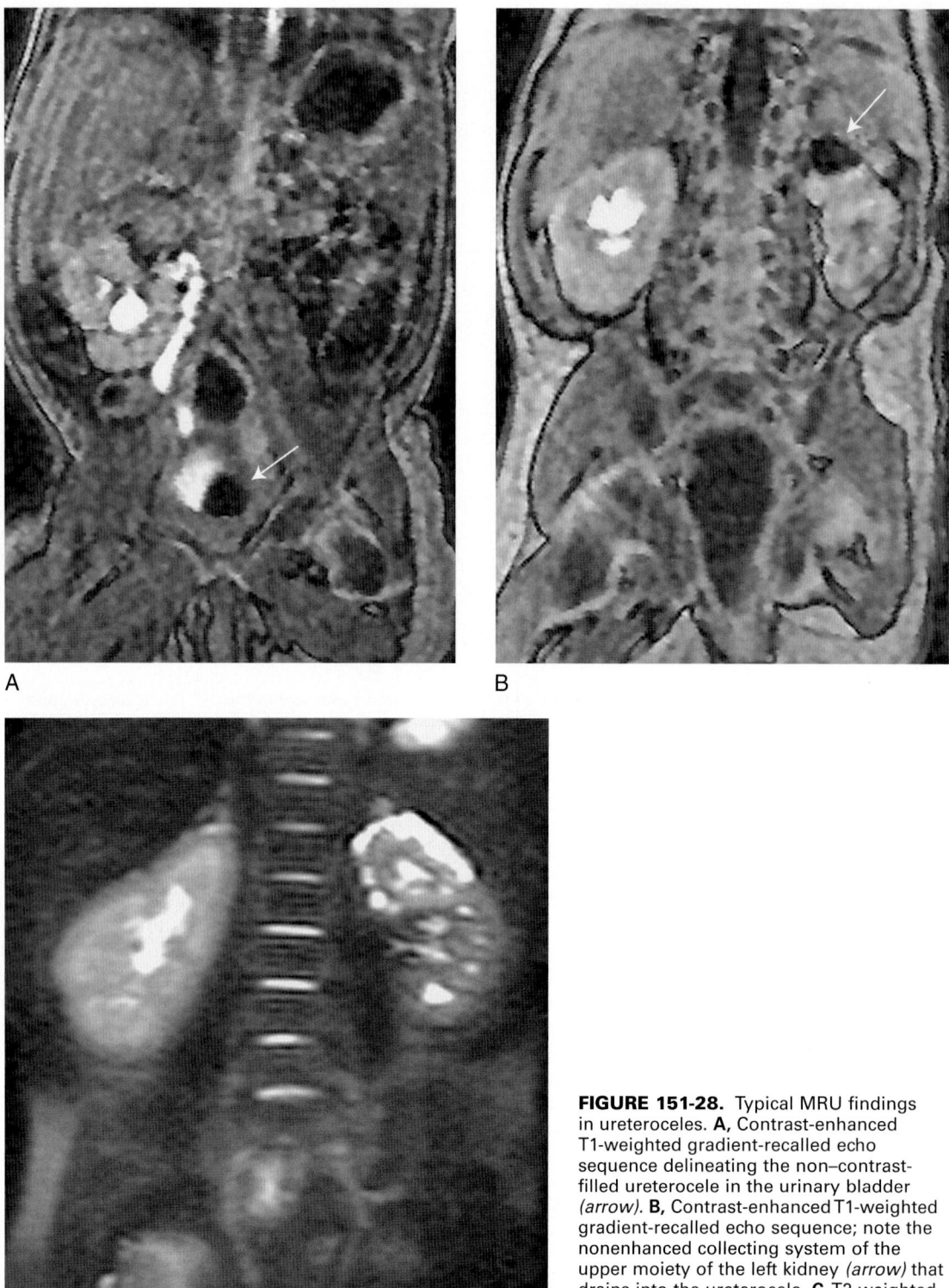

FIGURE 151-28. Typical MRU findings in ureteroceles. **A,** Contrast-enhanced T1-weighted gradient-recalled echo sequence delineating the non–contrast-filled ureterocele in the urinary bladder *(arrow).* **B,** Contrast-enhanced T1-weighted gradient-recalled echo sequence; note the nonenhanced collecting system of the upper moiety of the left kidney *(arrow)* that drains into the ureterocele. **C,** T2-weighted, nonenhanced image demonstrates the cystic/dysplastic nature of the left upper pole parenchyma.

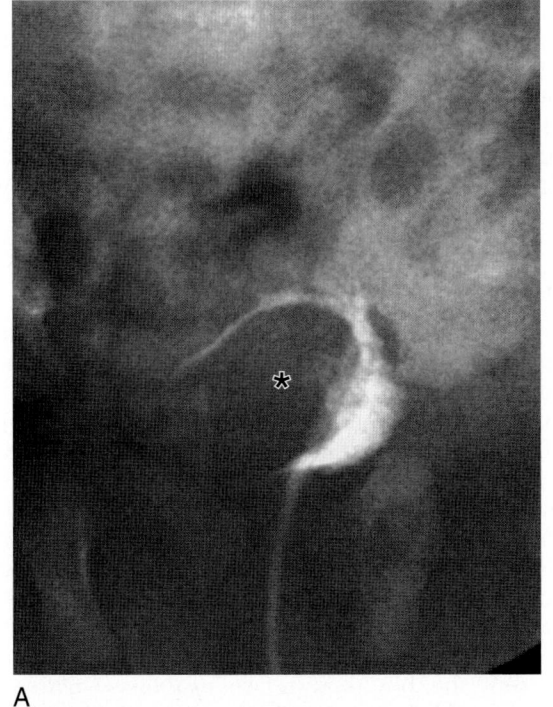

A

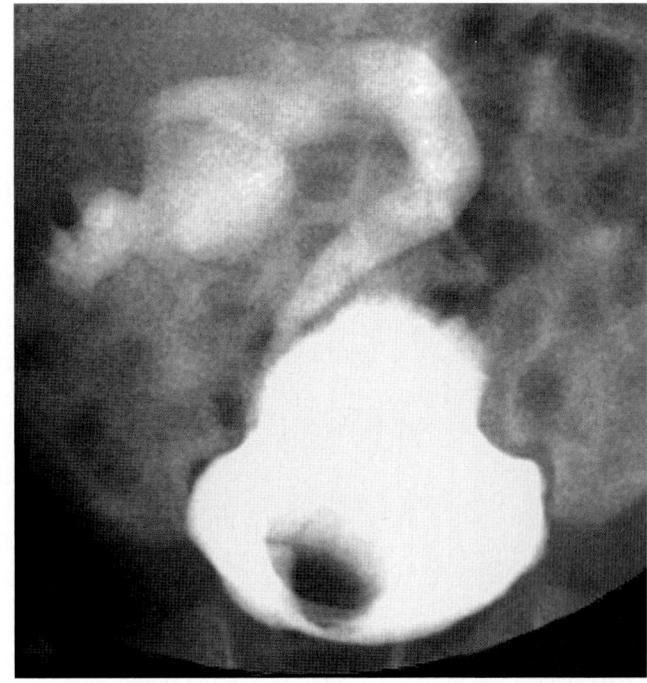

B

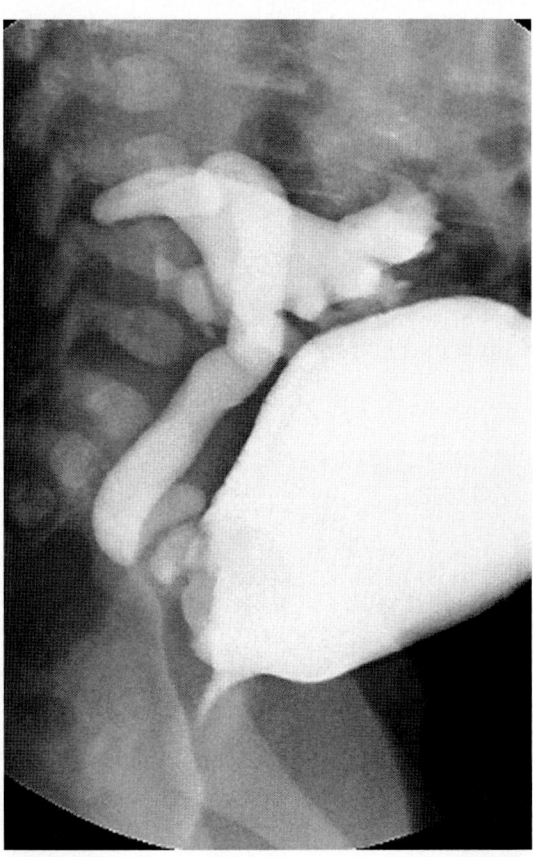

C

FIGURE 151-29. Ureterocele and vesicoureteral reflux. VCUG series demonstrating the defect caused by the ureterocele *(asterisk)* during early bladder filling (**A**), as well as high-grade low-pressure vesicoureteral reflux into the lower pole system ("drooping lily" appearance) during later filling (**B**) and effacement of the ureterocele during late filling (**C**).

be infiltrated or secondarily involved by other retroperitoneal tumors of infancy and childhood, such as *neuroblastoma, rhabdomyosarcoma, peripheral neuroectodermal tumor,* or *malignant teratoma.* Instances of benign and

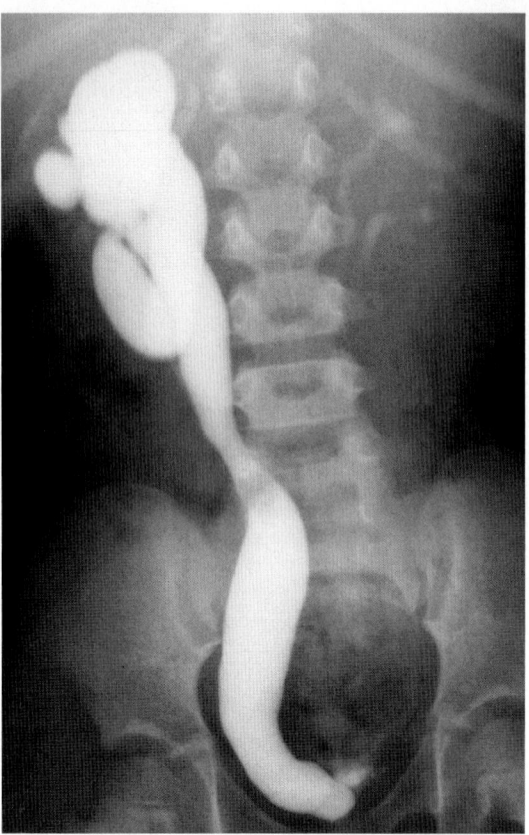

FIGURE 151-30. Ureterocele and vesicoureteral reflux. VCUG image shows reflux into the right-sided ureterocele and distorted right upper pole collecting system. There is grade II vesicoureteral reflux on the left as well.

usually pedunculated *fibrous polyps* in the upper third of the ureter (occasionally bilateral) have been reported. They may cause hematuria or, rarely, obstruction and have no malignant potential. They are more common in adults. US is only useful to detect large tumors with a significant extraureteral component or to visualize indirect signs caused by the obstruction. Otherwise, imaging relies on CT, MRI, or even ureterography.

Extrinsic Lesions

Extrinsic lesions causing ureteral displacement or obstruction include many of the primary or secondary retroperitoneal processes as described in Chapter 144. *Extra-adrenal paraspinal neuroblastoma* and *ganglioneuromas* are the most common primary retroperitoneal neoplasms that may affect the ureter extrinsically (Fig. 151-34). Other primary neoplasms of the area include *teratoma, rhabdomyosarcoma, lipomatous tumors,* and *lymphangiomas.* Additionally, the ureters are commonly displaced by enlarged retroperitoneal lymph nodes from *lymphoma, leukemia, Wilms tumor, neuroblastoma,* and *gonadal neoplasms.* Of the acquired non-neoplastic retroperitoneal processes, the best known are *appendiceal abscess* and *retroperitoneal hematoma* or *fibrosis.*

In the differential diagnosis of ureteral displacement, certain anatomic variants should be kept in mind, particularly congenital malpositions of the kidney, normal meandering of the ureter over the psoas muscle, displacement of the ureter by asymmetric enlargement of the psoas muscle, displacement of the ureters by distended bowel (especially a large colon in patients with severe constipation), or by upper pole megaureter, with the lower pole ureter meandering around during its course. US and MRI (as well as in some instances contrast-enhanced CT) scans may be helpful when the diagnosis is in doubt.

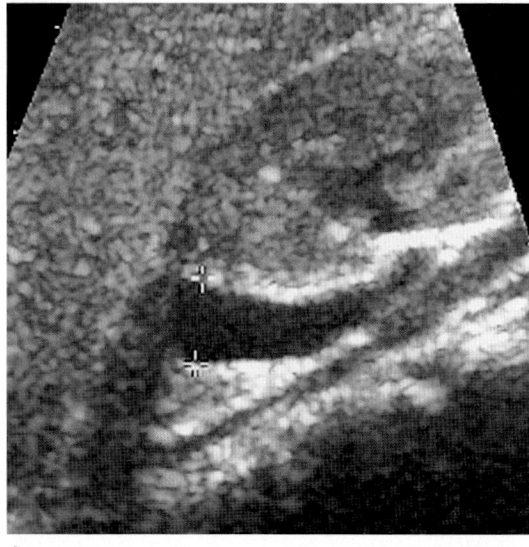

A

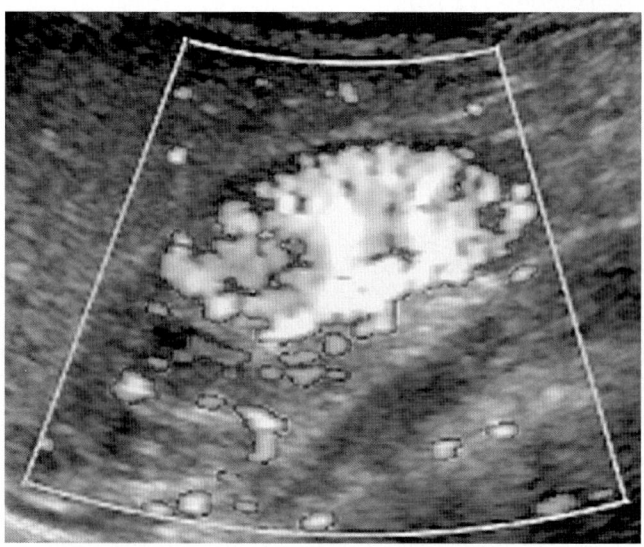

B

FIGURE 151-31. Duplex collecting system. **A,** Longitudinal sonogram shows enlargement of the upper pole collecting system *(cursors)* due to obstruction by a distal ureterocele. **B,** Longitudinal color Doppler image shows reduced vascularity and perfusion of the upper pole parenchyma compared with the lower moiety. (**B,** *see color plate.*)

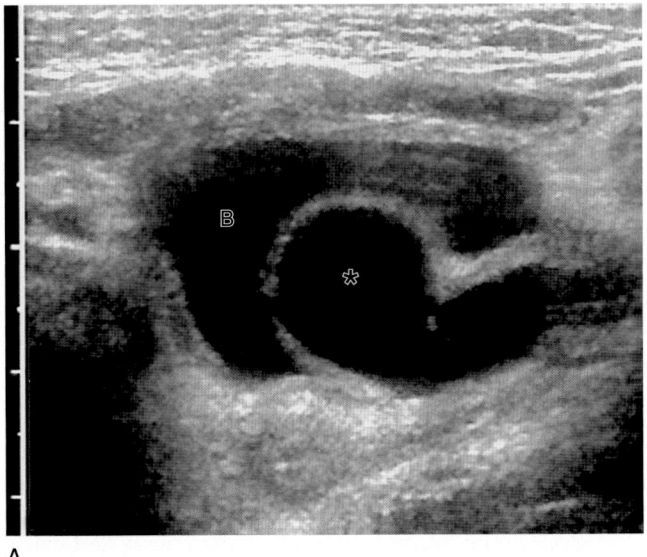

A

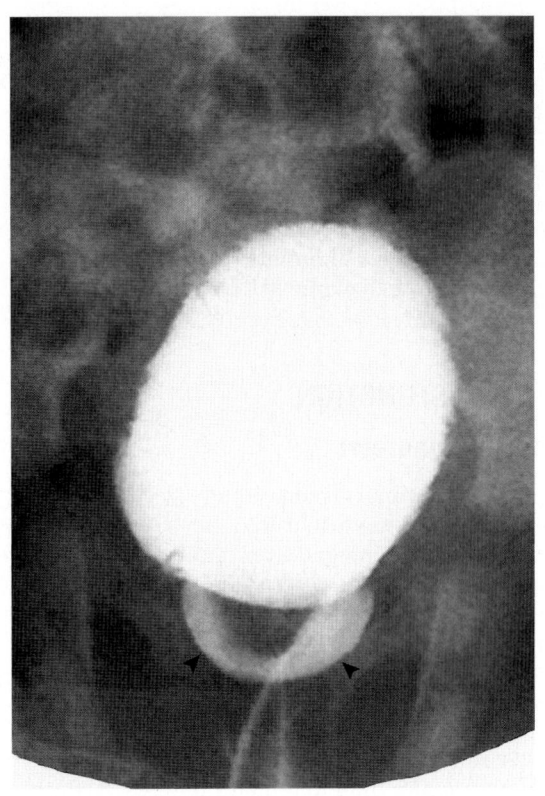

B

FIGURE 151-32. Ureterocele. **A,** Typical sonogram of a large ureterocele *(asterisk)* protruding into the bladder (B) lumen. **B,** Corresponding VCUG demonstrates inferior herniation of the ureterocele *(arrowheads)* into the bladder neck.

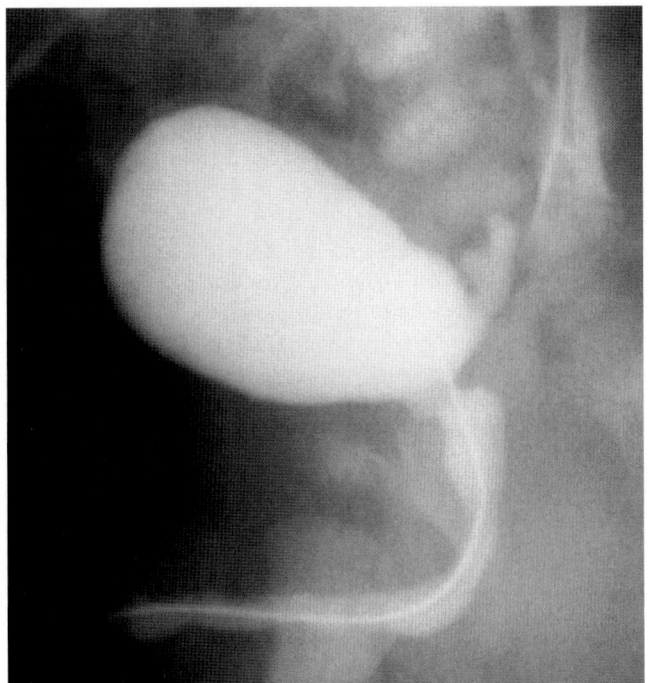

FIGURE 151-33. Everting ureterocele. VCUG image during voiding shows a diverticulum-like structure from the posterior bladder.

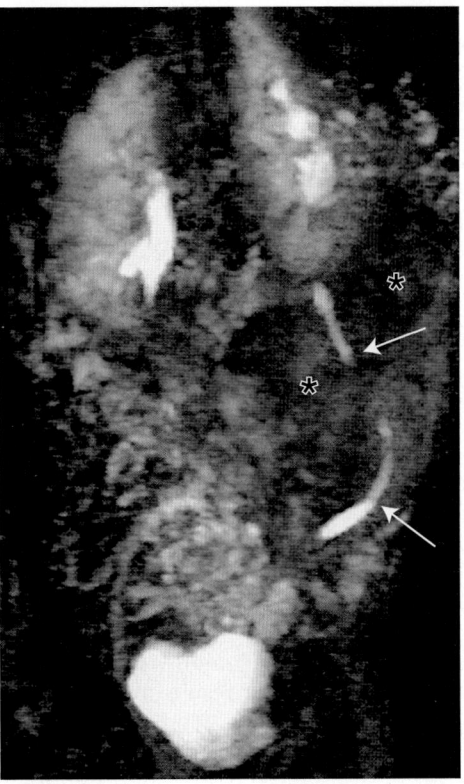

FIGURE 151-34. Ureteral displacement due to neuroblastoma. Heavily T2-weighted three-dimensional–reconstructed image demonstrates ureteral displacement *(arrows)* and encasement by tumor *(asterisks)*.

> There are many causes for ureteral obstruction and dilatation. Imaging, usually based on US, VCUG, IVU, and MRU, should help establish the diagnosis, reveal detailed anatomic information on the underlying condition (ectopic insertion, duplex system, associated genital anomalies), and grade obstruction as well as assess function of the corresponding renal moiety (often achieved by scintigraphy or dynamic MRU).

URETER DYSFUNCTION

Primary Megaureter

This type of primary megaureter (see Fig. 151-14) (a condition sometimes also called the *"Hirschsprungs" of the ureter*, obstructive megaureter, functional megaureter, ureteral achalasia, and aperistaltic, adynamic, or atonic ureter) is an uncommon nonhereditary lesion that is probably congenital. It is caused by an adynamic distal ureteral segment, usually 0.5 to 4 cm in length (but may involve longer segments of the ureter), that prevents normal caudal propagation of ureteral peristalsis. The disorder is discovered in patients of any age and is more common in males than in females. Three fourths of cases are unilateral, with the left ureter being involved more often than the right. Bilateral cases are more common in children younger than than 1 year of age. The affected ureter is variously dilated but tapers down rather abruptly to a curved, short distal segment that appears normal in caliber or slightly narrowed on US, IVU, or MRU. The dilatation is often limited to (or is most marked in) the lower half of the ureter. Diffuse dilatation with involvement of the pelvocalyceal system also occurs, but even in these cases the dilatation is more severe in the lower ureter, particularly in older children. The ureter is usually straight or only mildly tortuous, in contrast to megaureter resulting from VUR, lower urinary tract obstruction, or prune-belly syndrome, in which the ureters tend to be elongated and tortuous. The renal parenchyma is usually of normal thickness, but in more severe cases it is variously thinned or even dysplastic and atrophic.

At gross pathology, the distal segment of the ureter appears normal, without evidence of organic narrowing on probing with ureteral catheters. Histologically, however, the ureter shows normal ganglion cells (which may be reduced in number), hypoplasia and atrophy of muscle fibers, and an increase in collagen tissue. The remaining muscle fibers are predominantly circular, and in severe cases there is little or no muscle tissue present. The proximal dilated segment of the ureter shows muscular hypertrophy that results from hyperperistalsis. The ureteral orifices are cystoscopically normal.

The symptoms of primary megaureter include recurrent UTI, abdominal pain (and distention if severe and bilateral), and hematuria. Ureteral stone formation has been reported. However, this condition is often discovered as an incidental finding in asymptomatic patients. The findings on imaging reflect the pathologic changes in the ureter and kidney. A short, nondilated distal segment of the ureter can be seen best on postvoid IVU images. The VCUG shows no organic or functional abnormalities of the bladder or urethra. VUR is not a typical feature of the disorder but does occur in some children. As seen fluoroscopically on ureterography, or by US and dynamic MRU, the ureter shows normal or hyperactive peristalsis with waves starting in the proximal ureter and increasing in amplitude and fading distally into the dilated portion of the ureter. Antiperistaltic waves may be observed. Renal agenesis and other contralateral abnormalities have been described, and ipsilateral megacalycosis and hydronephrosis may occur.

Hypotonia, Hypomotility, and Dyskinesia

These are disturbances of the ureter primarily affecting motility and function. An *adynamic or dysplastic ureteral segment* may cause functional impairment and cause segmental ureteral dilatation, with urine drainage relying on gravity. Furthermore, *peristalsis and tension alteration* may be seen during and shortly after UTI, as well as after instrumentation, operations, or with in situ foreign bodies such as nephroureteral stents, causing *reactive hypotonia* with an adynamic or hypoperistaltic ureter. Finally, *transient hypomotility* of the ureter may be observed in postoperative settings and due to medications that affect the smooth muscles. Ureteral peristalsis may be assessed and documented using M-mode US or US cine-loop clips (Fig. 151-35); ureteral drainage and function is evaluated by MAG3 scintigraphy or dynamic MRU.

> Ureteral dysfunctions can be a secondary or a congenital condition; differentiation between a transient problem and evolving disease is crucial for patient management, and assessment of functional impairment is heavily based on imaging.

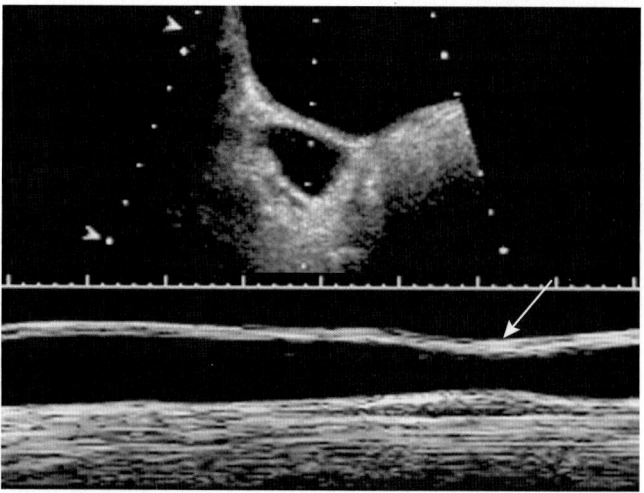

FIGURE 151-35. Megaureter peristalsis. M-mode sonogram shows peristalsis *(arrow)* in a megaureter.

TABLE 151-4

Findings in Patients with Vesicoureteral Reflux

- African Americans have lower VUR incidence.
- Hispanics have questionable lower VUR incidence.
- There is a family history to VUR: parent-child or sibling-sibling.
- Children with VUR have twice the incidence of pyelonephritis.
- Fifty percent of children with postinfectious nephropathy do not have VUR.
- Cyclic voiding studies increase VUR detection.
- For VUR assessment VCUG, radionuclide cystogram and echo-enhanced urosonography can be used.
- Filling the initially empty bladder to capacity increases VUR detection, with assessment also during and after voiding as well as in early filling phase.
- The prevalence of VUR in children without UTI is almost equal to that in children with UTI.
- Bladder infections do not cause VUR.
- UTI is independent of the presence of VUR.
- Sterile VUR does not produce renal scars or other damage, in the absence of increased voiding pressures, as in bladder dysfunction or bladder outlet obstruction particularly in fetal life).

- New scars rarely develop after puberty; the kidney is most vulnerable during first years of life.
- Despite the initial severity or persistence of VUR, renal growth rates remain unaffected, except for associated congenital dysplasia.
- VUR and asymptomatic bacteriuria does not result in scars.
- In the treatment of VUR, there is no difference between continuous antibiotic prophylaxis or just treating episodes of UTI in terms of renal scar development.
- Most patients with VUR do not demonstrate defects at DMSA scintigraphy, and those children with defects often do not have VUR.
- Symptomatic and asymptomatic VUR have the same natural history and resolution.
- Bladder urodynamics are related to the presence and resolution of VUR.
- UTI per se does not result in end-stage kidney disease.
- Breakthrough infections, changes in renal function or growth, and new or progressive scarring are seen with similar frequency in both medical and surgical treatment of VUR.

VESICOURETERAL REFLUX

Definition

Vesicoureteral reflux refers to the retrograde passage of urine from the urinary bladder into the ureter and often to the calyces. It is a common and potentially important childhood problem that is generally regarded as abnormal at all ages. Owing to recent insights into the natural history of fetal and neonatal urinary tract development, this judgment is increasingly under discussion and review. VUR itself causes neither UTI nor renal damage, but it may be associated with bladder dysfunction. However, VUR is a risk factor for the development of upper UTI and pyelonephritis, with consequent renal scarring and potential long-term sequelae (Table 151-4).

Imaging Studies

The major objective in the evaluation of children with UTI has traditionally been to diagnose or exclude VUR. Today, the focus of imaging in UTI has shifted to evaluation of renal inflammatory involvement or existing renal scarring and to assessment of structural or functional abnormalities of the urinary tract that may predispose to renal damage, complicated UTI, and VUR, particularly early depiction of anomalies that may require prompt interventional or surgical treatment to prevent renal damage. The other major task in pediatric uroradiology is to evaluate those infants who have been prenatally diagnosed as having some sort of urinary tract malformation, especially "hydronephrosis." This is a constantly increasing number of patients due to prenatal US screening. Besides confirmation of prenatal findings and establishing a definite diagnosis, imaging is asked to find or exclude VUR.

The diagnostic imaging modalities available for the evaluation of VUR include US, VCUG, and nuclear

---

TABLE 151-5

Imaging Studies for Vesicoureteral Reflux

VOIDING CYSTOURETHROGRAM
Defines anatomy (urethra in males)
Accurate grading of VUR, good comparability on follow-up
Visualization of diverticula, and (if refluxing) ureterovesical junction + ureteral anatomy

NUCLEAR STUDIES
Decreased ability to see urethra in males
Continuous imaging
Less accurate VUR grading
Don't need to see urethra in girls: can be used as initial study in girls
Decreased gonadal radiation dose: good for screening familial VUR and follow-up examinations

ECHO-ENHANCED UROSONOGRAPHY
No radiation, therefore ideal for screening, follow-up, and in girls
Longer observation period than on VCUG, similar or higher VUR incidence/detection rate
Tends to grade low degree VUR slightly higher than VCUG
Fewer anatomic details (urethra, ureters, diverticula) and less panoramic display
Information on renal parenchyma, prefilling anatomy, and non-refluxing systems
Contrast material not available for pediatric use in many countries; economics often unfavorable

---

cystography (Table 151-5). On US, either indirect signs such as a gaping ostium, ureteral dilatation and ureteral wall thickening, changing dilatation of the pelvocalyceal system, direct VUR visualization using color Doppler imaging (if reflecting particles are present in the urine), as well as increasing ureteral and pelvocalyceal dilatation with increasing bladder filling or after voiding are used

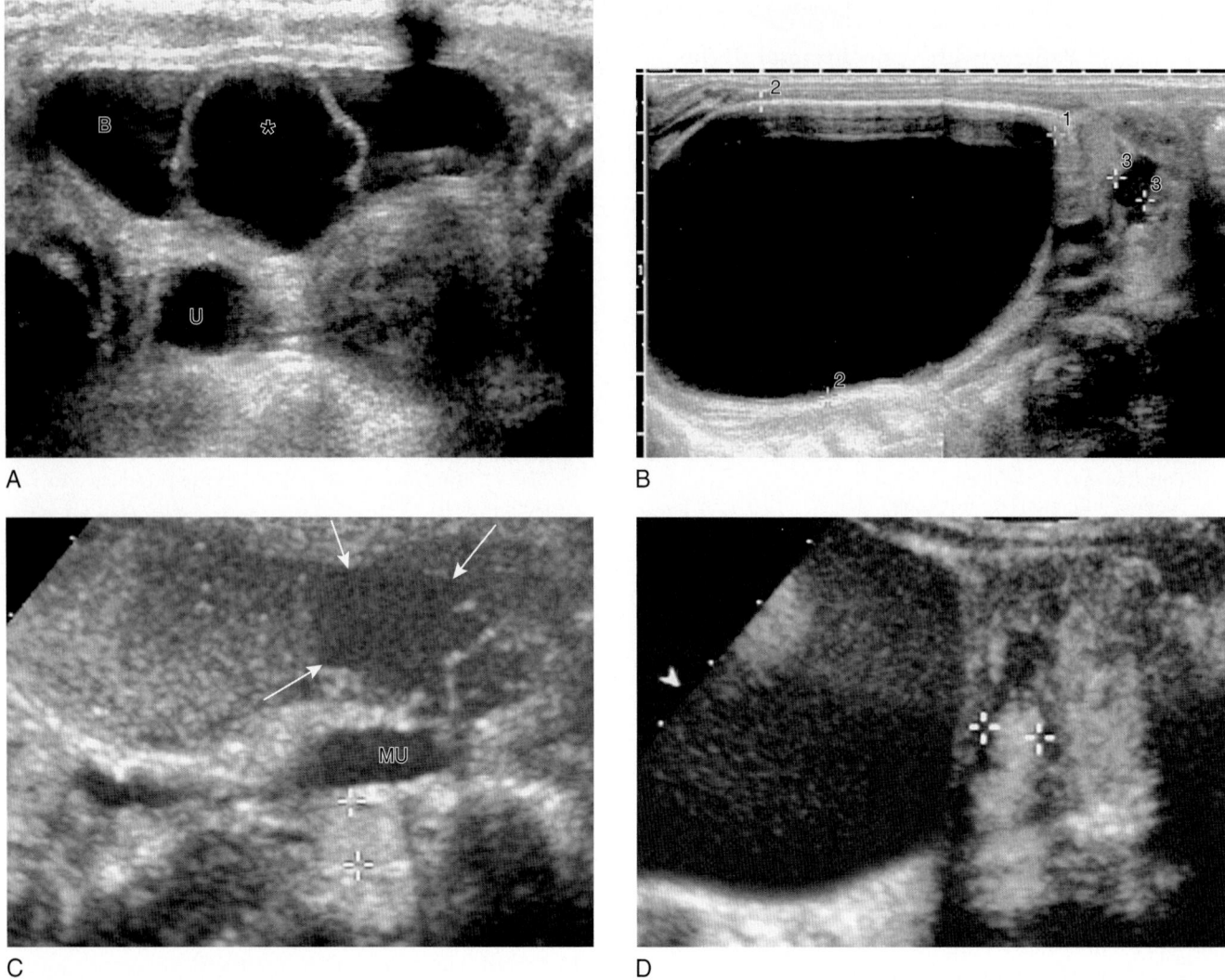

FIGURE 151-36. Vesicoureteral reflux demonstrated by ee-US. **A,** Transverse unenhanced bladder sonogram reveals a ureterocele *(asterisk)* within and a dilated ureter (U) behind the urinary bladder (B). **B,** Longitudinal sonogram of the duplex right kidney shows a markedly dilated upper moiety and only mild dilatation of the lower pole moiety. **C,** Longitudinal sonogram after contrast instillation (Levovist) into the urinary bladder shows the nonrefluxing ureterocele *(arrows)* and corresponding megaureter (MU) and echogenic contrast material within the refluxing lower pole ureter *(cursors)*. **D,** Longitudinal renal sonogram shows echogenic contrast in the dilated pelvocalyceal system of the lower pole moiety *(cursors)*, thus diagnosing high-grade vesicoureteral reflux.

for establishing a diagnosis (Fig. 151-36). A new method for VUR assessment is echo-enhanced urosonography (ee-US). This method uses US contrast material (e.g. shaken saline, air, or commercially available contrast agents) instilled into the urinary bladder via suprapubic or transurethral catheterization and bladder filling. The reflux of contrast into the upper tracts can be readily appreciated by alternately scanning both kidneys as well as the retrovesical space during filling and before and after voiding. US techniques such as harmonic imaging, stimulated acoustic emission, or other contrast-specific techniques have further enhanced ee-US potential for VUR depiction and grading, resulting in a reported equal sensitivity and specificity as VCUG (Fig. 151-37).

> **The role of VUR in pediatric urinary tract disease is decreasing and is being discussed and reviewed.**

VCUG is and remains the basic imaging technique for VUR assessment. It uses radiopaque contrast material instilled into the catheterized and emptied urinary bladder for detection of VUR into the upper urinary tract. Fluoroscopic observation of the (early) filling phase, the distal ureters (in oblique projections), the renal collecting system, and the urethra during voiding (lateral projection, particularly in boys) enables obtaining focused images of critical areas and conditions such as of intrarenal VUR or UVJ anatomy. Cyclic VCUG should be performed in infants to avoid missing significant VUR. A modified VCUG protocol using a slow low-pressure contrast infusion as a sort of manometer to monitor intravesical pressure allows for functional evaluation and improved assessment of VUR; changes in infusion speed or infusion stops may guide fluoroscopy to moments of increased intravesical pressure with transient high-pressure VUR or sphincter-detrusor dyscoordination.

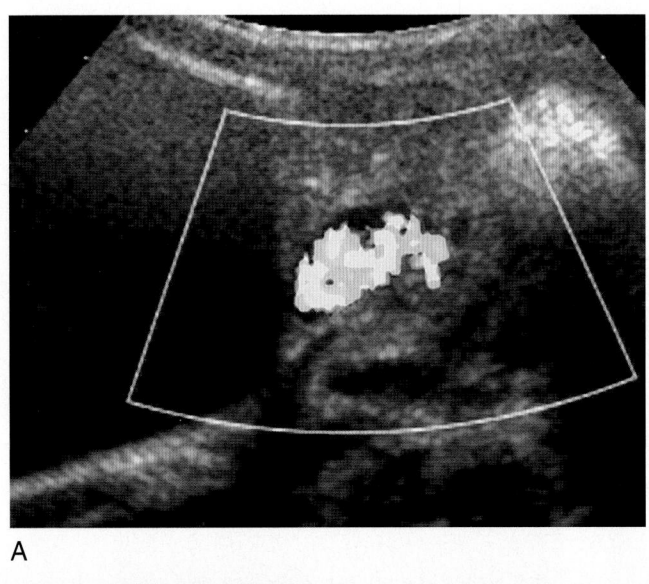

A

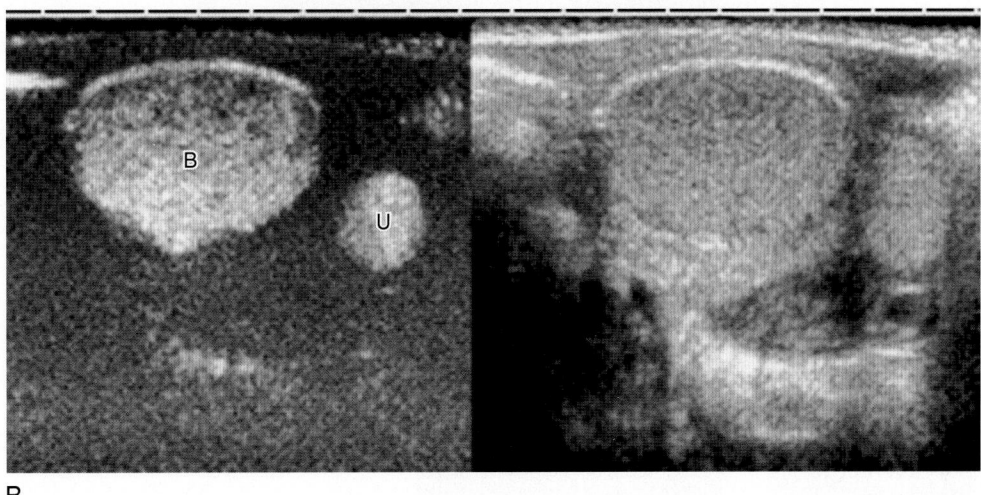

B

FIGURE 151-37. Improved detection of vesicoureteral reflux using contrast-specific techniques. **A,** Same patient as in Figure 151-36, with reflux into the right lower moiety. Reflux is now depicted using stimulated acoustic emission with high US power (high mechanical index) to burst the contrast bubbles, thus creating strong color signals. (*See color plate.*) **B,** Contrast-specific imaging techniques (CDI, Siemens, Mountain View, CA) provide exquisite contrast delineation in a patient with refluxing megaureter, using double-image technique for visualization (*left* = contrast image, *right* = generic image with simultaneous contrast and harmonic imaging gray scale information) B, bladder; U, ureter.

For studying the renal parenchyma, US and DMSA scintigraphy are commonly used. Other methods for the evaluation of the upper tract are contrast-enhanced CT and MRI, which may become indicated for assessment of complicated disease. IVU has been an important imaging tool in the past, but today its role is very restricted. The choice of imaging method for VUR assessment depends in large part on individual preference, availability, and the experience of the examiner. Other variables include the age, sex, and race of the patient; whether an initial or a follow-up examination is being done; and the cost of and time required to perform the procedure. All male infants and all patients before surgery should have a conventional VCUG performed for detailed anatomic assessment.

It is generally agreed that an imaging investigation is indicated in all patients with significant prenatal hydronephrosis and those after the first documented UTI, particularly infants and young children after febrile infections in whom early detection of VUR and treatment of infection are critical for the prevention of renal scarring. An initial US is the accepted procedure in most of these cases, complemented (at least in the first 2 years of life) by a conventional VCUG (in boys; other methods for VUR detection may be used in girls). A late DMSA scan is often warranted if there were clinical or sonographic signs for upper UTI with renal involvement. In the investigation of asymptomatic patients who may have VUR (e.g., siblings of patients with the disorder), a baseline urinary tract US and a nuclear cystogram or ee-US may be sufficient as the initial study, followed by other procedures when necessary. School-age patients with UTI should undergo an initial US, potentially a urodynamic assessment, and a late DMSA scan; VUR assessment

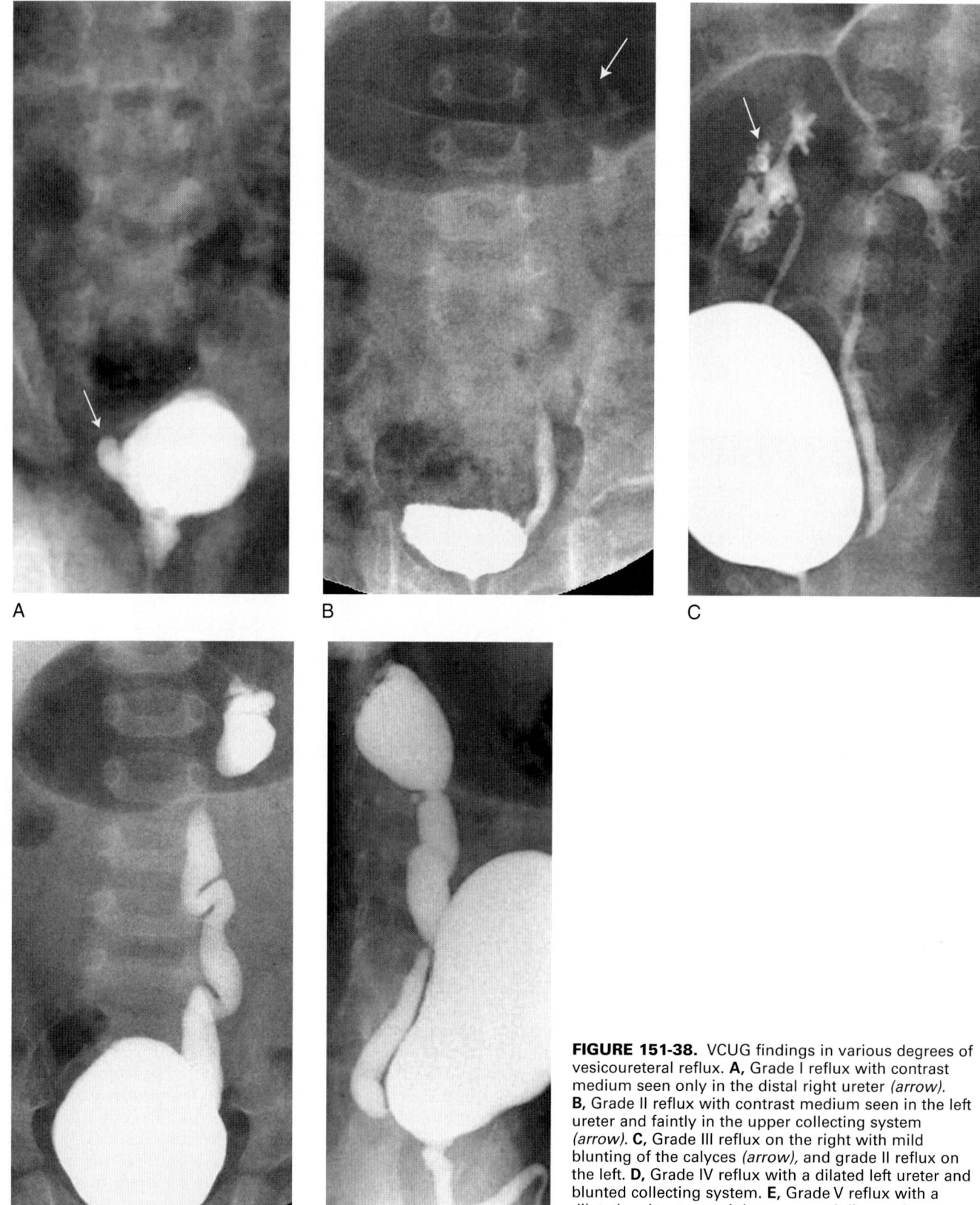

FIGURE 151-38. VCUG findings in various degrees of vesicoureteral reflux. **A,** Grade I reflux with contrast medium seen only in the distal right ureter *(arrow)*. **B,** Grade II reflux with contrast medium seen in the left ureter and faintly in the upper collecting system *(arrow)*. **C,** Grade III reflux on the right with mild blunting of the calyces *(arrow),* and grade II reflux on the left. **D,** Grade IV reflux with a dilated left ureter and blunted collecting system. **E,** Grade V reflux with a dilated and tortuous right ureter and distorted upper collecting system.

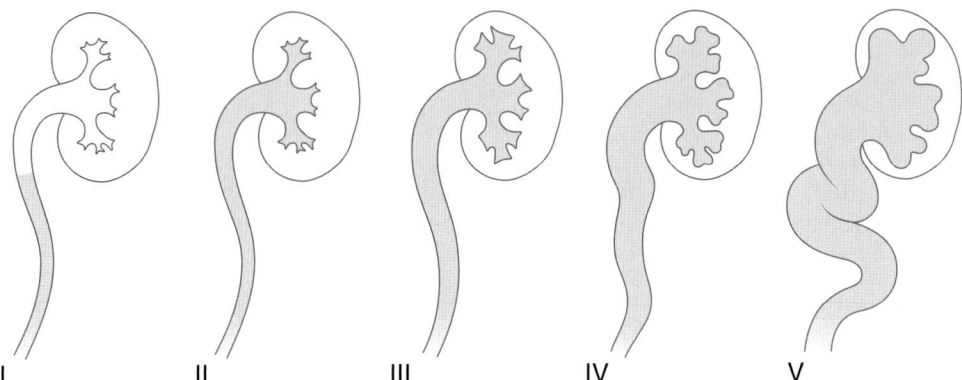

FIGURE 151-39. Schematic drawing demonstrating vesicoureteral reflux grading system on VCUG. (From Lebowitz RL, Olbing H, Parkkulainen KV, et al: International reflux study in children: International system of radiographic grading of vesicoureteral reflux: International Reflux Study in Children. Pediatr Radiol 1985;15:105.)

is only promoted in those with renal scarring, severe functional disorders, and recurrent infections. In teenage girls with afebrile UTI, no previous history of urinary tract disease, and clinical signs of cystitis, US of the upper tracts may be the only procedure necessary. In follow-up examinations and in postimplantation studies, a nuclear cystogram (or ee-US) may replace VCUG for evaluation of VUR, and US and DMSA scans may be used to monitor the upper tracts.

Grading

The severity of VUR is commonly judged according to the degree of upper tract dilatation and ureteral tortuosity on the VCUG or ee-US. International criteria for grading VUR (based on VCUG) are shown and described in clinical example in Figure 151-38 and diagrammatically in Figure 151-39. Similar comparable grading scales exist for ee-US and nuclear cystography. Although simple and easy to use, this and other similar classifications reflect only the appearance of the upper tracts and do not take into consideration other important factors such as the age and sex of the patient, the presence of intrarenal reflux or urinary tract obstruction, renal function and scarring, high- or low-pressure VUR, early or late VUR, slow or quick clearance from the upper collecting system, cystoscopic findings, and the presence or absence of associated disorders (e.g., ureteral duplication, ureteral ectopia, ureterocele, bladder diverticula, prune-belly syndrome, urethral obstruction, megacystis-megaureter association, or neurogenic bladder). This additional information is sometimes essential for making decisions about therapy.

Causes

The most common cause of VUR is a developmental anomaly of the UVJ in which the ureteral orifice may be lateralized or too large ("golf hole ostium") or the submucosal ureter is too short and/or deficient in longitudinal muscle fibers. VUR is often seen in patients with other urinary tract anomalies, such as duplex systems, UPJ obstruction, MCDK, renal or ureteral ectopia, and megaureter, or it may be secondary to an underlying urinary tract condition (Table 151-6). Additionally, some sort of immaturity of the UVJ may play a role in fetal and neonatal VUR, as a large percentage of congenital VUR

TABLE 151-6
Causes and Associations of Vesicoureteral Reflux

PRIMARY
Developmental, idiopathic, and immaturity
Anomalous development at the ureterovesical junction
Prune-belly syndrome
Diverticula

SECONDARY
Bladder outlet obstruction, particularly posterior urethral valves
Neurogenic bladder/myelomeningocele
Bladder dys-synergia and dysfunctional voiding
Postoperative bladder
Indwelling catheter
Foreign body
Bladder calculi
Iatrogenic
Ureterocele surgery

decreases spontaneously within the first years of life. This type of VUR, often referred to as *primary* or *congenital VUR*, is seen more frequently in girls than in boys. It is rarely seen in African Americans. Numerous familial cases have been reported, including siblings, twins, and members of consecutive generations. The high-grade congenital VUR in male infants, often with severe congenital renal dysplasia ("congenital reflux nephropathy") constitutes a different entity with a far more serious prognosis (see later).

A much less common type of primary VUR is that caused by an anatomically or histologically abnormally formed bladder wall with an inadequate detrusor musculature and diminished support of the ureteric submucosal tunnel. Prune-belly syndrome, a large smooth-walled bladder from other causes, and primary paraureteral or Hutch diverticula are examples.

Secondary VUR is seen in patients with bladder outlet obstruction (e.g., posterior urethral valves) or with neurogenic bladder disease (e.g., myelomeningocele). It is in part caused by thinning and weakening of the UVJ musculature precipitated by chronically increased intravesical pressure. However, the fact that VUR in these disorders may be absent and is frequently unilateral suggests the possibility of an associated congenital weakness of the UVJ or a protective measure of a potentially thickened bladder wall that may otherwise lead to ureteral obstruction. Many girls who have VUR have signs of bladder instability both clinically and on urodynamic studies. In some cases, VUR and UTI may improve or resolve when bladder instability is treated, and even successfully treated VUR may recur in patients with functional bladder disorders. Although lesser degrees of lower urinary tract obstruction per se do not seem to cause VUR in patients with a completely normal UVJ, they may precipitate VUR (with spreading of infection to the upper tracts and kidneys) in people with ostia of borderline competence, as the result of local edema and cellular infiltration, causing further weakening of the UVJ. Recent bladder surgery, indwelling catheters, foreign bodies, bladder calculi, and other local irritants may also cause VUR in a marginally competent UVJ.

On rare occasions, VUR is *iatrogenic* after surgery or instrumentation on the UVJ, particularly in unsuccessful ureteral reimplantations or after unroofing of a ureterocele.

Association with Ureteral Duplication

Vesicoureteral reflux is more common in children (mostly girls) with complete ureteral duplication than in those with single unduplicated ureters. VUR may affect both ureters but is more often limited to the ureter draining the lower pole. The corresponding renal parenchyma (usually the lower renal pole) is especially prone to secondary changes. This variant of primary VUR is probably caused by a defective UVJ accompanying lateral ureteral ectopia (see earlier). VUR limited to the upper pole ureter in complete ureteral duplication is quite rare.

Natural History

Vesicoureteral reflux has a tendency to improve and to disappear spontaneously during the first decade of life, often during the preschool years. This tendency is attributed to a maturation process of the UVJ with age, with an increase in the length of the intramural ureter and strengthening of its musculature. Mild VUR (grades I and II) with normal-sized ureters and ureteral orifices has a favorable prognosis and disappears with time in more than 80% of the cases, whereas more severe forms of VUR with dilated ureters have a lower incidence of spontaneous recovery (grade III, about 50%; grade IV, 30%; grade V, rarely). VUR associated with anatomic anomalies such as a large ureteral orifice and short submucosal tunnel at cystoscopy is not likely to resolve. VUR occurring in an ectopically ending ureter or associated with a large paraureteral diverticulum also tends to persist, especially if the ureter ends in the diverticulum; in these circumstances VUR is often only seen when the diverticula unfolds and thus impairs the ostial valve mechanism. VUR occurring in patients with lower urinary tract obstruction may disappear after correction of the lesion but is considered uncured if it is still present 1 year postoperatively. VUR occurring in neurogenic bladder disease or bladder dysfunction also tends to

persist until the functional disturbance is successfully treated.

Effects on the Kidney

There are various potential changes in affected upper urinary tracts. The appearance of refluxing ureters and pelvocalyceal systems on VCUG is quite variable, ranging from normal-sized upper tracts to extreme upper tract dilatation and marked ureteral tortuosity (Fig. 151-40). These changes may reflect only an increased volume and decreased motility of the ureters, but in some cases a developmental defect of the ureter related either to in-utero VUR or to an inadequate development of the ureteral musculature is suspected (e.g., prune-belly syndrome). In some patients, VUR is accompanied by marked ballooning of the pelvocalyceal system without evidence of UPJ obstruction (Fig. 151-41). The phenomenon may be transient, with a prompt emptying of renal pelvis afterward and no discrepancy between the size of the pelvis and that of the ureter. This finding reflects an increased elasticity of unknown cause in the upper collecting system. Sometimes VUR may induce a kink at the UPJ, with a valve-like mechanism that may even deteriorate after antireflux procedures, producing a functional UPJ obstruction with similar distention and delayed emptying of the pelvocalyceal system as seen with an organic UPJ obstruction, and may potentially be associated with other urinary tract anomalies (Fig. 151-42). The obstruction may be related to local scarring from infection, to anatomic kinks in the ureter, or to overlying aberrant vessels or fibrous bands. Thus, a primary congenital UPJ obstruction and primary VUR may coexist as associated anomalies. Some patients with VUR develop an obstruction at the UVJ over time. Despite this obstruction, VUR usually continues. On direct inspection and catheterization at cystoscopy, the ureteral orifice and distal ureter are not stenotic, suggesting a functional rather than an organic cause.

On US and in IVU, the ureters and pelvocalyceal systems of patients with VUR often appear normal even if they appear dilated on VCUG (particularly when the bladder is empty or catheterized). Minor urographic changes observed in patients with VUR include mild dilatation of the lower ureter, fullness of the entire ureter, and visualization of the entire ureter in more than one film. Longitudinal striations of the pelvis and proximal ureter on the side of the VUR are not uncommon (Fig. 151-43). They probably represent mucosal wrinkles that occur when a dilated pelvis and proximal ureter are seen in a partially collapsed state. Indirect sonographic signs for VUR are uroepithelial thickening of the ureter or renal pelvis, changing diameter of the pelvocalyceal system and ureter, quick refilling of the bladder after voiding, asymmetric ureteral inflow jets, and a lateralized position or unusual shape of the ostium (Fig. 151-44). In more severe cases, the refluxing upper tracts are grossly dilated, with clubbing of the calyces and elongated and tortuous ureters (Fig. 151-45). Ureteral peristalsis is generally poor, especially in the presence of urinary infection and high-grade VUR. Kinks in the proximal ureter or distal segment of the ureter are common.

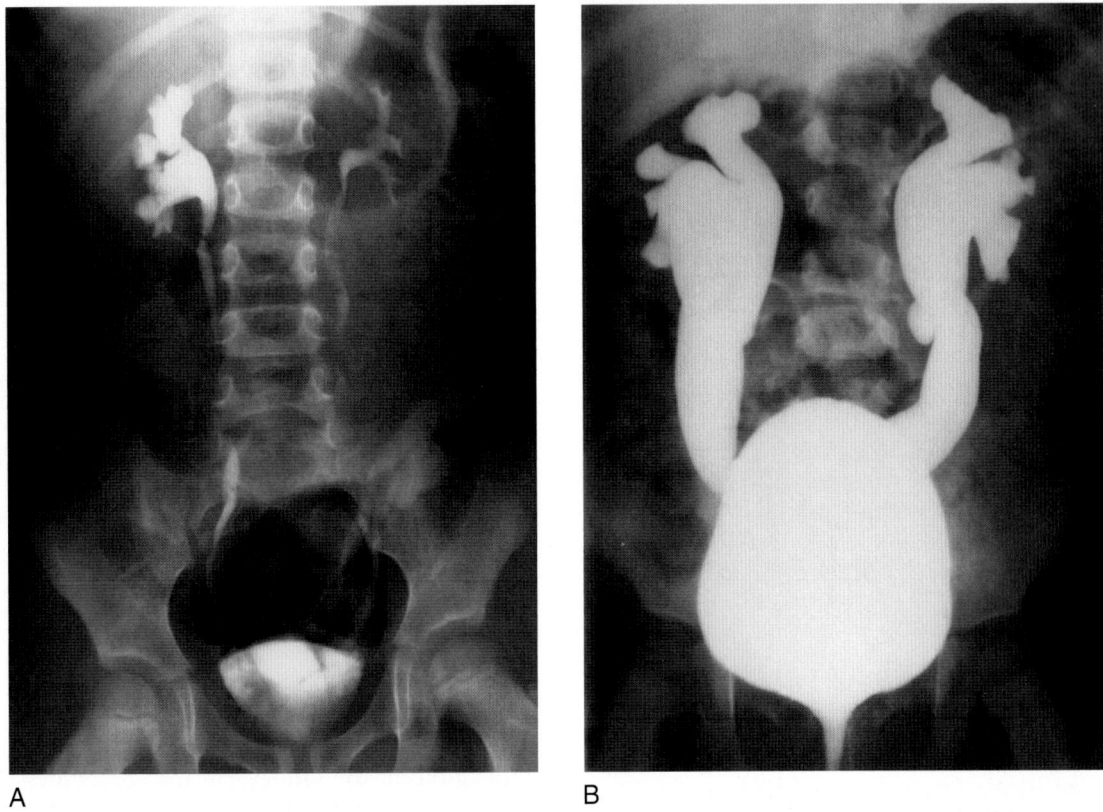

A   B

FIGURE 151-40. Vesicoureteral reflux. **A,** VCUG image shows left grade II vesicoureteral reflux with thin and delicate calyces and right grade III reflux where the calyces are dilated and blunted. **B,** VCUG image shows bilateral grade IV vesicoureteral reflux.

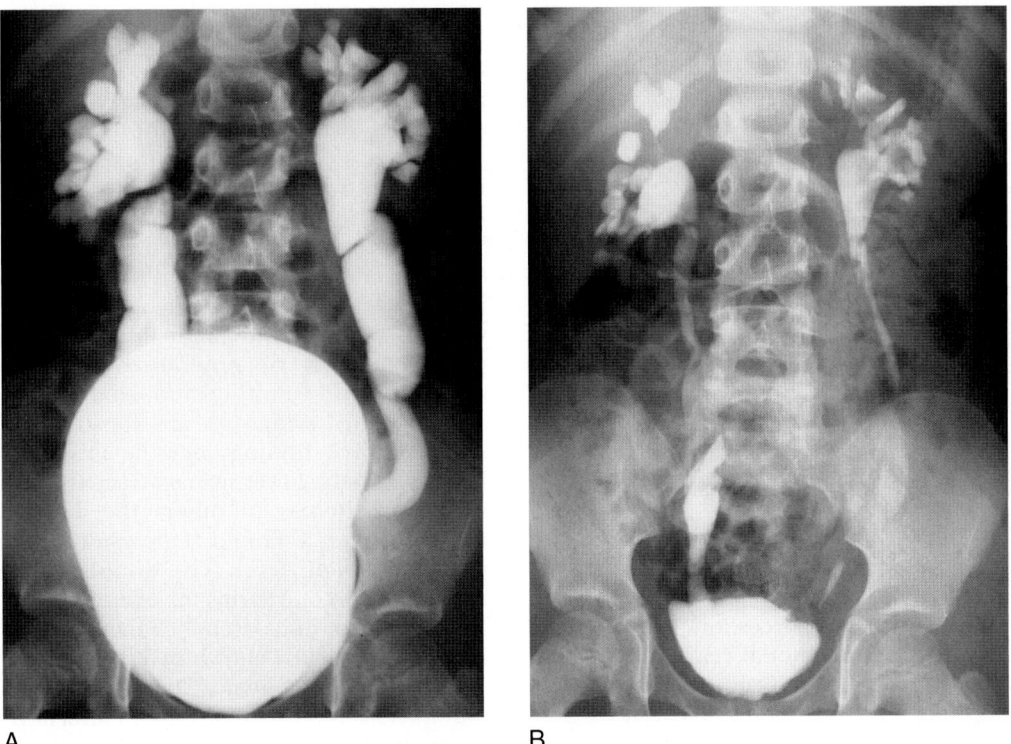

A   B

FIGURE 151-41. Vesicoureteral reflux. **A,** VCUG in a 5-year-old girl with recurrent urinary tract infection shows a large smooth-walled bladder and bilateral grade V vesicoureteral reflux. **B,** Postvoid image shows only mild hydroureteronephrosis, along with bilateral renal parenchymal loss.

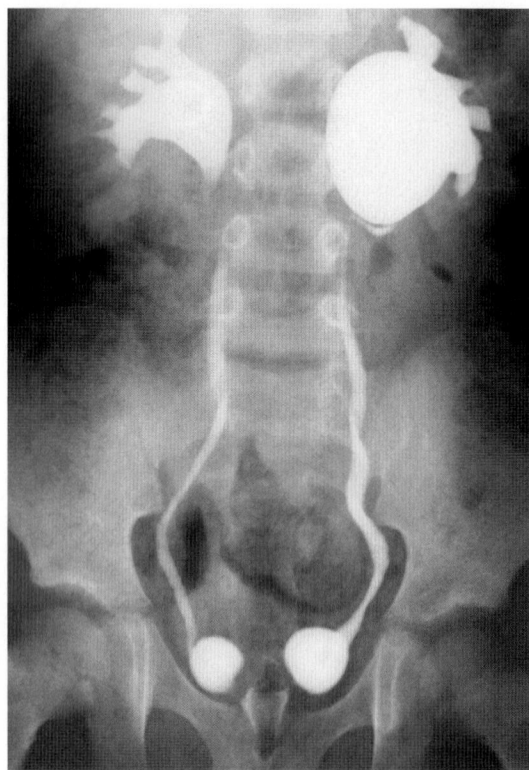

FIGURE 151-42. Vesicoureteral reflux and functional ureteropelvic junction obstruction. Postvoid VCUG image shows bilateral vesicoureteral reflux and ballooning of the left renal pelvis. The IVU (not shown) was entirely normal. There are also bilateral paraureteral (Hutch) diverticula.

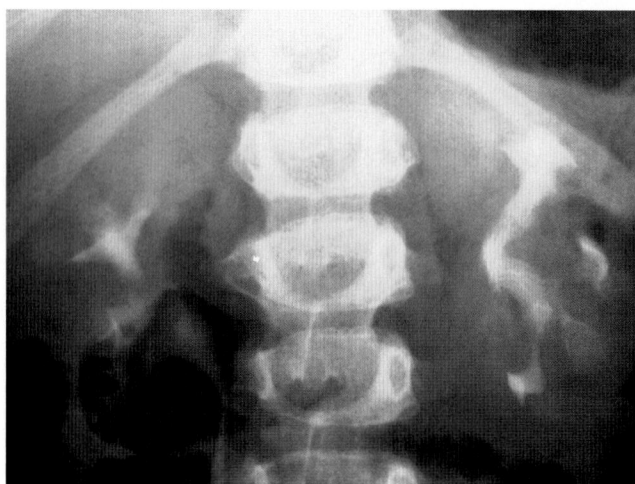

FIGURE 151-43. Pelvic striations. IVU image shows linear striations in the left renal pelvis.

In patients with VUR to the calyces, one may observe transient pyelotubular and interstitial reflux of contrast material extending outward in a wedge-shaped pattern from one or more papillae to the renal cortical surface (Fig. 151-46). This *intrarenal reflux* is generally seen in children younger than 4 years of age and occurs most often in infants. It is seen in less than 10% of patients with VUR in these age ranges and most often when VUR is severe or when it occurs at high intravesical pressure.

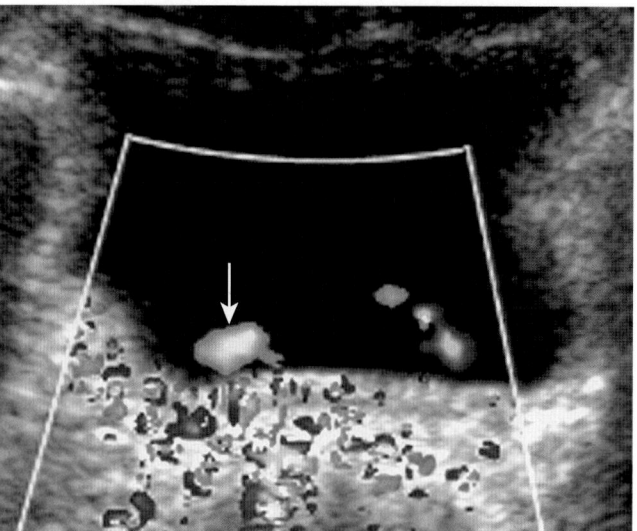

FIGURE 151-44. Lateralized ureteral orifice. Transverse color Doppler image shows laterally positioned and abnormally oriented right ureteral jet (*arrow*). Such indirect signs may help US diagnosis of vesicoureteral reflux. (*See color plate.*)

Intrarenal reflux is an important finding because of its association with renal scarring. It is often limited to the upper pole of the kidney but may occur in other areas of the kidney. It is believed that the morphology of the opening of the collecting ducts of Bellini on the renal papilla is partly responsible for intrarenal reflux. The opening of these ducts on compound, flat-topped papillae (more common at the poles) are round and therefore less resistant to retrograde flow than the slit-like openings of the ducts of simple or conical papillae. The fact that intrarenal reflux does not occur in all infants and that it is rarely seen after age 4 years suggests an additional local defect that improves with age.

UTIs are a common pediatric problem, affecting especially infants and children of preschool years, with a tendency to recur and to damage the kidney. UTI, like VUR, decreases with age and is less common in older children and adolescents, with a strong female predominance after 3 to 6 months of age. In infancy, UTIs occur with an equal frequency in both sexes and are often present as part of generalized sepsis. They may be associated with vomiting, anorexia, and failure to thrive; often, clinical symptoms are very unspecific and even urine dipstick findings may be misleading. Symptoms referable to the lower urinary tract are common in some children, whereas in others the clinical features are those of upper UTI and acute pyelonephritis with flank pain, chills, and fever. The distinction between cystitis and acute pyelonephritis may be difficult by clinical and laboratory methods. Renal changes of acute pyelonephritis may be clearly shown by US using meticulous scanning technique and color Doppler imaging, which shows diminished flow to areas of renal infection (Fig. 151-47); alternatively, DMSA renal scintigraphy may serve for diagnosis of upper UTI with renal involvement (see also Chapters 107 and 146). The diagnosis of UTI depends on laboratory confirmation of significant bacterial counts in cultures of properly collected urine specimens.

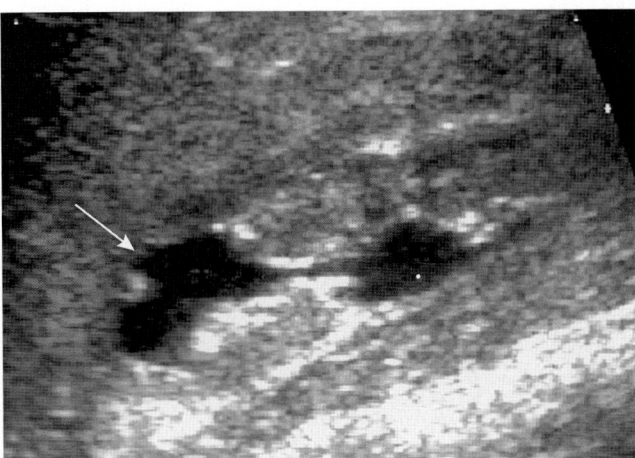

A

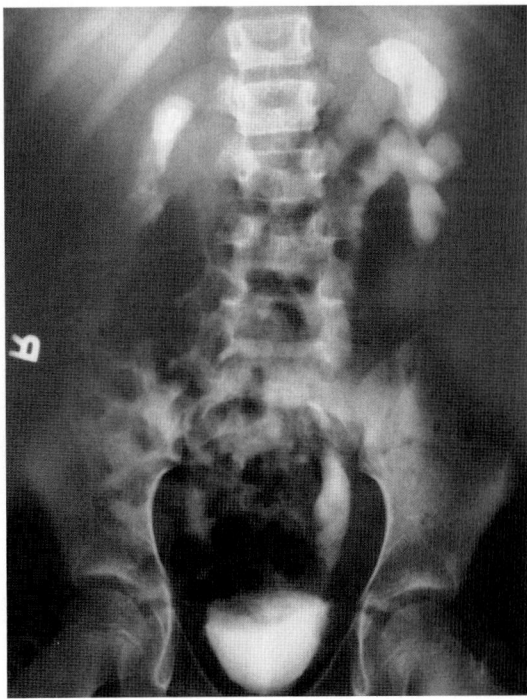

B

FIGURE 151-45. Reflux nephropathy. **A,** Longitudinal sonogram shows features of a scarred kidney from severe vesicoureteral reflux with recurrent urinary tract infection: dilated and clubbed calyces, with focal overlying parenchymal narrowing *(arrow)* and echogenic nondifferentiated parenchyma with irregular contours. **B,** IVU image shows a small and atrophic functioning right kidney with markedly thinned parenchyma. The left kidney collecting system is distorted as well.

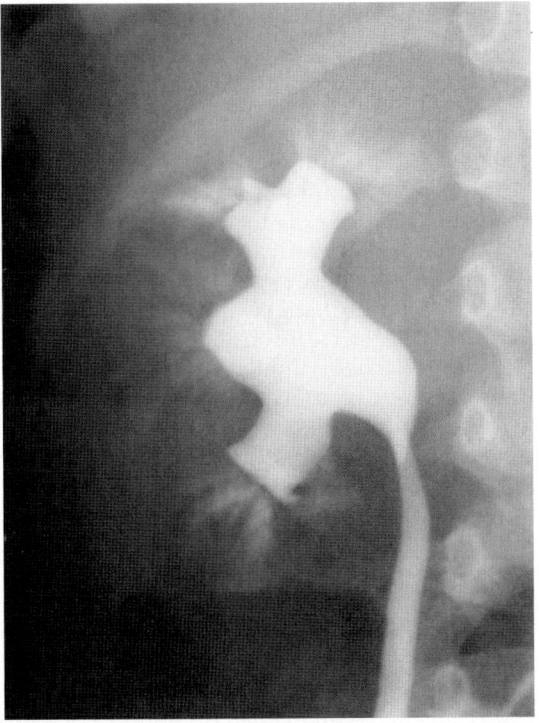

FIGURE 151-46. Intrarenal reflux. VCUG image in a 2-year-old girl shows right vesicoureteral reflux and diffuse intrarenal reflux.

The infecting organisms are most often gram-negative bacteria of fecal flora, especially *Escherichia coli.*

In infants, UTI often originates hematogenously. In girls, the infection usually originates in the perineum and ascends to the bladder via the short urethra. The port of entry of infection in males is more difficult to explain; however, it is known that noncircumcised male infants have a higher UTI incidence. Stasis of urine in the bladder as a result of an obstruction or a functional abnormality of the bladder may foster growth of bacteria that would otherwise be eliminated by complete emptying of the bladder. The resistance of the bladder mucosa to infection may also be altered by increased intravesical pressure, intravesical catheters, calculi, or local irritants. Other factors, less well understood, may predispose to or aggravate UTIs, with some related to an increased bacterial virulence and others to a decrease in host resistance. One of the factors enhancing bacterial activity is the ability of certain bacteria, particularly strains of P-fimbriated *Escherichia coli,* to adhere to the urothelium. This property enhances bacterial colonization and invasiveness, in part by increasing the resistance to the normal clearing of bacteria during bladder emptying.

Propagation of infection from the bladder to the upper tracts and to the kidneys is supported by VUR, which can be demonstrated in many patients with recurrent UTI (70% of patients aged younger than 1 year, 25% at 1 year, 10% at 12 years, and 5% in adults). In the presence of VUR, bacteria require less virulence to produce upper UTI. The view that VUR is an important factor in the origin of renal infection is supported by the frequent cessation of renal infections after a successful antireflux procedure; the procedure, however, does not seem to prevent recurrent cystitis (in girls). As already indicated, bladder infection may precipitate VUR by weakening a marginally competent UVJ with propagation of infection to the kidney. The decreased incidence of renal infections with age is potentially related to a decreased incidence of VUR secondary to normal maturation of the UVJ.

Renal scarring is a common and potentially serious problem in patients with VUR and upper UTI (acute

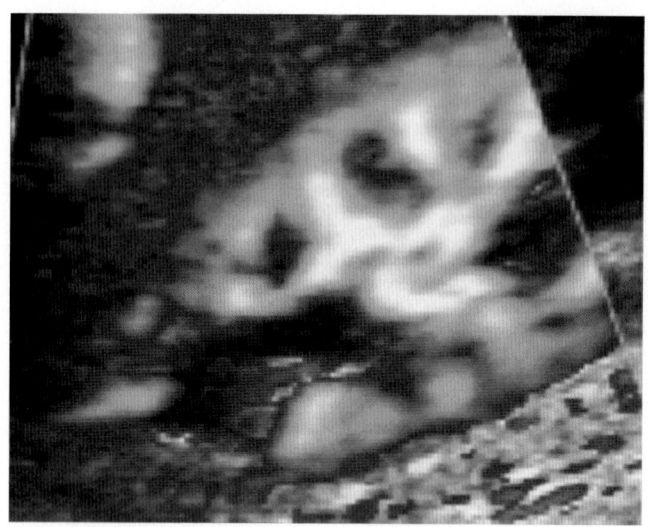
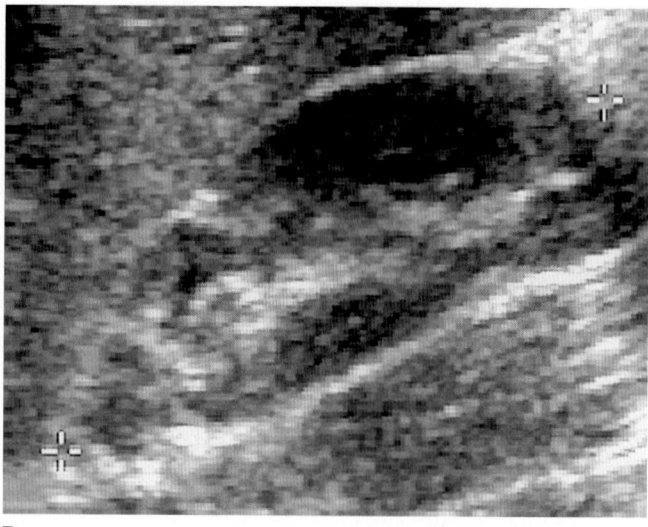

A
B

FIGURE 151-47. Acute pyelonephritis. **A,** Longitudinal color Doppler image shows a focal perfusion defect in the upper pole associated with a dilated calyx in an infant with acute febrile upper urinary tract infection. Evaluation found grade III vesicoureteral reflux. **B,** Follow-up longitudinal sonogram shows the development of upper pole scarring. (**A,** *see color plate.*)

pyelonephritis). Renal scarring is characterized by one or more areas of renal cortical atrophy that is almost always associated with blunting or distortion of the underlying calyx or group of calyces, retraction of the papillae, and reduction of the medullary zone. Histologically, the affected kidneys show areas of cortical loss with tubular destruction and atrophy and interstitial fibrosis. Obliteration of glomeruli, arteriolar changes, and minor signs of interstitial inflammation may also be observed. The scarring characteristically has a focal or segmental pattern with a predisposition for the upper pole (38%) and less frequently for the lower pole. Multiple areas of scarring may also be seen in other parts of the kidney, and in some cases the process affects the whole kidney diffusely. The areas of scarring result in one or more clefts or depressions of various sizes in the outline of the kidney. They are sharply demarcated from the adjacent normal renal parenchyma and are usually wedge shaped, with the apex at a calyx or group of calyces. The calyces of the affected area of the kidney are close to the surface of the kidney and closer together than normal. The unaffected renal parenchyma may be hypertrophied, sometimes simulating a renal mass (pseudotumor). When the process is diffuse and severe, it results in global renal atrophy. The parenchymal changes may be directly depicted by US as areas of depression in the outline of the kidney with increased echogenicity of the nondifferentiated parenchyma at the dilated and distorted calyx; color Doppler imaging reveals focally reduced peripheral vascularity (see Fig. 151-47). Nuclear scintigraphy, using a cortical agent such as DMSA, is especially sensitive in detecting renal cortical scars and is considered the gold standard. MRU has been shown to hold great potential for diagnosis of renal involvement in UTI and renal scarring but, because of its restricted availability, high costs, and need for sedation, is seldom used. Parenchymal changes are also visualized in the early phase of the IVU, or on contrast-enhanced CT, but these studies are not indicated for the evaluation of renal scarring.

Like UTI, renal scarring is much more common in girls than in boys and is uncommon in African Americans. In early life, it is often associated with VUR and is seen in about one third of patients who have both UTI and VUR. However, VUR may be absent in patients with renal scarring. In older children and adolescents this may be explained by VUR maturation and disappearance with age. VUR is of paramount importance in the transport of bacteria from the bladder to the upper tract. But, because scarring may be seen in refluxers and nonrefluxers, VUR is not necessary to develop scars. The observation that scars are located preferentially in the renal poles, where compound papillae and intrarenal reflux predominate, has suggested the theory that intrarenal reflux may play an important role in the development of renal scars. Although sterile intrarenal reflux does not seem to cause parenchymal scarring (except perhaps prenatally in some severe cases) there is evidence both clinically and from animal experiments that renal scars may partially result from the intrarenal reflux of infected urine.

Renal scarring has been interpreted as an event that occurs in the first few months of life, perhaps after the first episode of infantile acute pyelonephritis, and usually remains stable thereafter. It has also been suggested that all the areas of the kidneys that are susceptible to intrarenal reflux (i.e., all the refluxing or compound papillae) are affected simultaneously ("big bang theory"), whereas all the unaffected areas of the kidney drained by a single conical papilla (and therefore more resistant to intrarenal reflux) are spared. According to this theory, infants with UTI and VUR are at greater risk of developing renal scars than older children with VUR and UTI. However, this theory explains only some scars; many additional aspects need to be considered such as early and correct diagnosis and treatment of UTI, development of bacterial resistance to certain antibiotics, and the individual immunology as well as probable genetic aspects. Additionally, renal scarring also occurs with hematogenous UTI without VUR or compound papillae.

It may take a few weeks to several months for a scar to become apparent on imaging. Some apparently new renal scars that are seen in follow-up examinations may represent the end stage of an old insult to the kidney that was not previously apparent or may be secondary to intercurrent infections. Also, what appears to be a progression of a previously demonstrated scar on follow-up may only reflect continuing growth and hypertrophy of adjacent normal renal tissue contrasting to a fixed atrophic area, creating an increasing mismatch during physiologic growth.

Renal scarring may lead to hypertension and end-stage renal disease (ESRD). Systemic arterial hypertension is a relatively common complication, occurring probably in 10% to 20% of children with unilateral or bilateral renal scarring, with an increased risk after 15 years of age. Hypertension may develop 10 or more years after VUR treatment, as well as in patients in whom VUR has subsided spontaneously; in fact, older children and young adults with hypertension and scarred kidneys often fail to show VUR when the hypertension is first noted. The plasma renin level is elevated as seen in patients with vascular origin of hypertension (see Chapter 150), but an elevated renin value may also be found in patients with "reflux nephropathy" who do not have hypertension. Women with significant renal scarring bear a higher risk for complications during pregnancy such as premature labor and gestosis (edema, proteinuria, and hypertension). Severe renal scarring is also associated with decreased renal function of varying severity and is a relatively common cause of ESRD leading to dialysis and renal transplantation. It is responsible for 8% of all cases of ESRD, but how many children with scarred kidneys eventually develop this complication is difficult to establish, because VUR may not be demonstrated at the time of diagnosis (because of previous ureteral reimplantation or because of spontaneous resolution of the VUR). ESRD resulting from scarring is seen most commonly in older children, adolescents, and young adults, with an increased risk in patients with hypertension. The ESRD of these patients is probably the result of a decrease in the number of nephrons, a limited growth potential of the unaffected nephrons, plus an acquired glomerulosclerosis caused by an increased workload (hyperperfusion) of these unaffected glomeruli, similar to patients with a posterior urethral valve who additionally suffer from congenital renal hypodysplasia.

Other effects of VUR on the kidney need to be briefly considered. Clinical observations of patients with long-standing VUR suggest that sterile VUR is usually well tolerated. Males with primary VUR (not associated with lower urinary tract obstruction or neurogenic bladder) are not as prone to develop UTI as are females and can tolerate VUR without complications for many years. However, some of them exhibit already severe renal damage and dysplasia at birth ("congenital reflux nephropathy") and often eventually develop ESRD. VUR in patients with UTI may cause a decreased growth rate of the affected kidney, potentially followed by resumption

of the normal growth rate when the infection is fully under control. During an episode of acute pyelonephritis, the affected kidney may be significantly enlarged, a phenomenon that should be kept in mind when interpreting serial measurements of kidney size in patients with reflux.

Treatment

Eradication or early treatment of UTI and prevention of recurrences are the main therapeutic objectives in children with VUR, with emphasis on infants and small children who are at particularly high risk of developing renal scars. These objectives may be attained by long-term suppressive medication with antibiotics until the patient is 4 to 5 years of age or until VUR ceases. This medical treatment is thought to be often sufficient in patients with low-grade VUR. However, with the new knowledge of the natural history of VUR and the increasing number of resistant bacteria causing breakthrough infections, this strategy is increasingly under discussion, particularly in low-grade VUR. An antireflux procedure may become necessary in many patients with symptomatic and persisting high-grade VUR and is usually indicated in grade V VUR, the latter sometimes after temporary urinary diversion via ureterostomy. The success rate of ureteral reimplantation is high (up to 95%) in patients with grade I and II VUR but decreases as the size of the affected ureter increases (a 60% success rate in grade V has been reported). Endoscopic intravesical injection of a small amount of some material (e.g., Silicon, Teflon paste, dextranomer/hyaluronic acid [Deflux]) into the bladder wall behind the submucosal ureteral tunnel offers an alternative to the surgical procedures (Fig. 151-48). The injected material elevates and narrows the ureteral tunnel and causes a localized protrusion of the bladder wall at the lateral angle of the trigone containing the ureteral orifice. The injected material is well seen by US as a rounded echogenic focus (Fig. 151-49). UTI may still occur after a successful antireflux procedure, but it is mostly limited to the bladder. In patients with voiding or functional bladder disorders, VUR may recur in up to

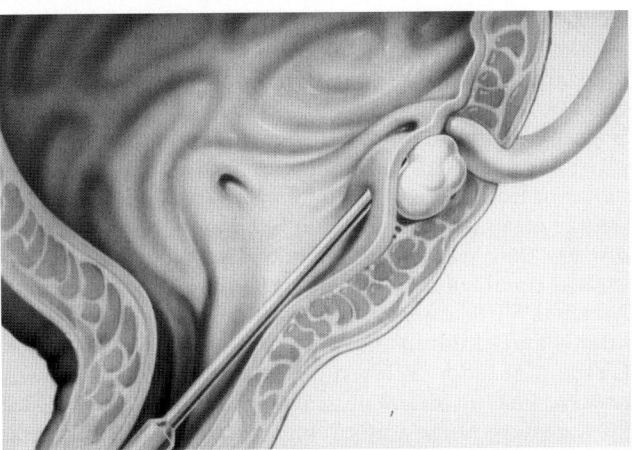

FIGURE 151-48. Subureteric injection. Diagrammatic representation of injection of material under the entrance of the ureter into the bladder to eliminate vesicoureteral reflux.

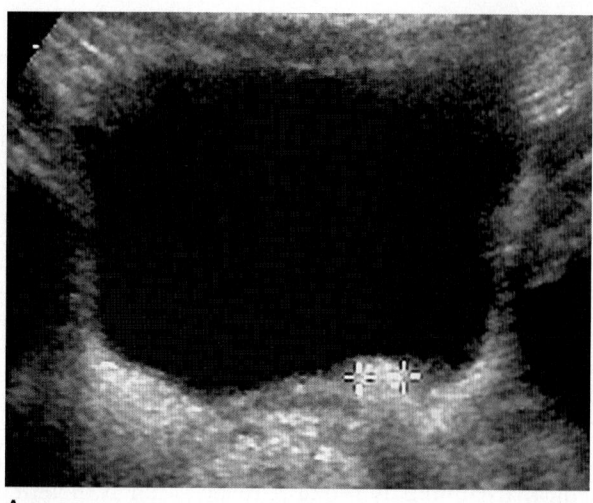
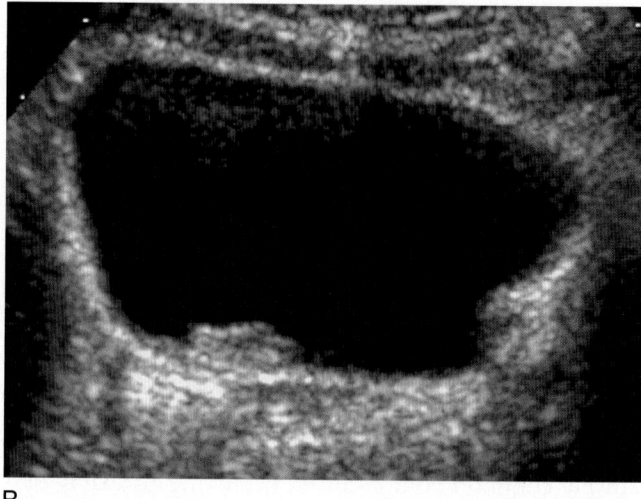

A

B

FIGURE 151-49. Postoperative imaging for vesicoureteral reflux. **A,** Transverse bladder sonogram after cystoscopic injection shows echogenic material at the left ureterovesical junction *(cursors).* **B,** Parasagittal bladder sonogram shows nodularity at the site of ureteral reimplantation.

50% if this condition is not successfully diagnosed and treated. The main objective of an antireflux procedure is to prevent propagation of infection from the bladder to the upper tract and kidney and thus to prevent progression of renal scarring with consecutive long-term sequelae. Another justification for cystoscopic treatment is "bridging" until normal maturation has occurred, thus making antibiotic prophylaxis or further surgery for renal protection unnecessary.

Imaging Algorithms for Evaluation and Follow-Up

There are different recommendations for VUR imaging and imaging during or after UTI in different parts of the world. The differences are variations in the methods used and in indications for VUR assessment as well as the intensity of imaging in various scenarios. With the new knowledge and insight into the nature and pathophysiology of VUR and renal damage, many of these imaging algorithms are undergoing changes. Imaging is increasingly focused on phenomena that define prognosis and risk for long-term sequelae, such as the kidney with potential renal scars and bladder function disturbances. We want to avoid diagnostic over-imaging, not only for economic reasons but also for patient concerns. Catheterization is an uncomfortable procedure with a potential negative physiologic and psychologic impact on children, and methods using ionizing radiation pose an additional risk. On the other hand, one would like not to miss significant disease that eventually may lead to severe sequelae such as renal failure. In large parts of Europe and North America, VUR assessment is considered indicated in all infants and children up to 2 years of age after the first UTI and in older children if there has been a UTI with proven renal involvement, scars, or recurrent upper UTI. Furthermore, some sort of cystogram is considered indicated in all neonates with significant hydronephrosis, and in all patients with significant urinary tract malformations, particularly preoperatively. Patients with a

TABLE 151-7
Imaging Objectives and Imaging Algorithms in Urinary Tract Infections

1. Differentiate between lower and upper UTI (renal involvement).
2. Assess for renal scarring and growth after UTI.
3. Find pre-existing urinary tract malformations.
4. Find signs for complicated or atypical infection.
5. Find complications in patients with a protracted clinical course, and help with differential diagnosis.
6. Assess for VUR, particularly in patients with upper UTI and renal scars.

family risk can undergo US and cystography, with ee-US and nuclear cystogram being preferred in this patient group to minimize radiation exposure. In UTI, imaging is increasingly being focused on the kidney; thus, an early US or DMSA study is considered compulsory in any febrile patient with an upper UTI. To differentiate acute renal inflammatory changes from persisting scars, a DMSA study 6 to 12 months after the infection is recommended. Indication for VUR assessment in these patients varies with age and gender as well as country (Table 151-7, Fig. 151-50).

> VUR is a potentially serious condition; however, its importance is presently undergoing re-estimation based on new insights into natural history and new management strategies. Considering the relative invasiveness of VUR imaging, indications for the various forms of cystography are undergoing changes, with increasing focus on potential renal sequelae, particularly in conjunction with UTI.

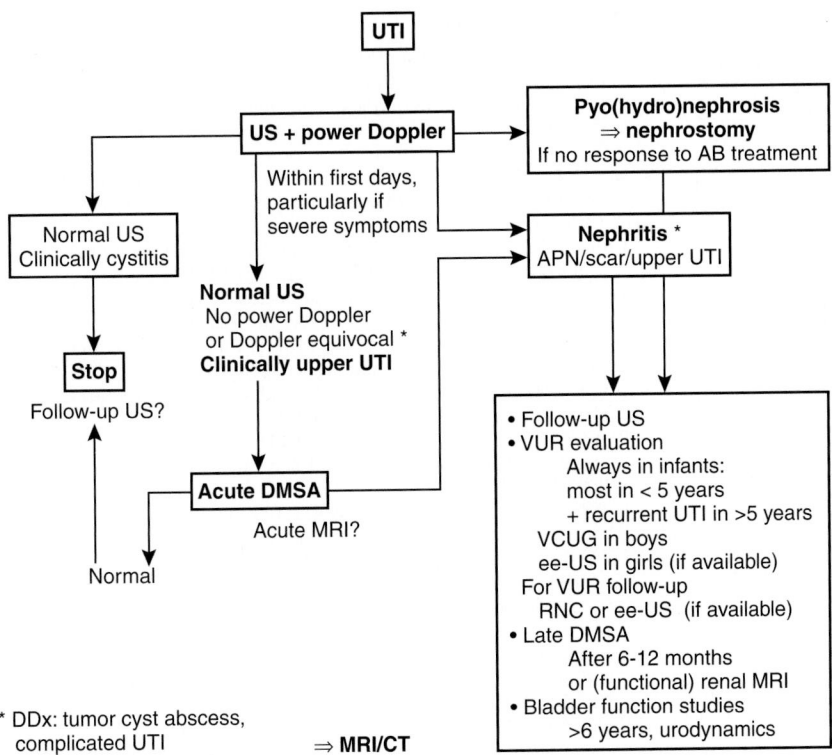

* DDx: tumor cyst abscess,
  complicated UTI   ⇒ **MRI/CT**

CT indications: complicated stone disease (unenhanced scan)

UTI criteria:
Urine sample and blood count, leukocyturia, positive nitrite, positive culture
(10^4 - catheter sample, 10^6 normal voiding), leukocytosis, elevated C = reactive protein

Reliable clinical diagnosis is essential and the most important entry criteria for imaging!

FIGURE 151-50. Imaging algorithm. AB, antibiotic; APN, acute pyelonephritis. (Adapted from Riccabona M, Fotter R: Reorientation and future trends in paediatric uroradiology. Minutes of a symposium held in Graz, 5-6 September, 2002. Pediatr Radiol 2004;34:295.)

MISCELLANEOUS CONDITIONS

Preoperative imaging needs to reveal all relevant information the surgeon needs for either planning or performing the operation. Because a comprehensive overview and display may be crucial, US alone is often considered insufficient, particularly regarding its limited potential to visualize the entire ureter. Therefore, VCUG (in refluxing units) and MRU (or IVU) are usually integrated in a standard preoperative imaging workup; more invasive procedures such as ureterography may be performed at the beginning of or during surgery in the course of the same anesthesia. *Postoperative imaging* is heavily based on US. However, US is poor in assessment and grading of urinary drainage; therefore, an adapted limited IVU or a functional scintigraphic study, as well as MRU (or CT), may sometimes prove helpful. If *postoperative complications* occur (e.g., ureteral obstruction after antireflux procedures, ureteral obstruction due to blood clots, manifestation of UPJ obstruction after ureteral surgery, ureteral fibrosis, stenosis, and compression), imaging not only may detect them but also may offer treatment options. These *image-guided interventions* and treatment strategies consist of ureteral recanalization, balloon dilatation of fibrous stenoses and ureteral stenting for keeping a compressed or recanalized ureter patent, and percutaneous nephrostomy. They are indicated not only for postoperative complications but also for the primary treatment of many urinary tract conditions (see Chapter 192).

SUGGESTED READINGS

General

Avni F, Bali MA, Regnault M, et al: MR urography in children. Eur J Radiol 2002;43:154

Avni FE, Nicaise N, Hall M, et al: The role of MR imaging for the assessment of complicated duplex kidneys in children: preliminary report. Pediatr Radiol 2001;31:215

Berdon WE: Contemporary imaging approach to pediatric urologic problems. Radiol Clin North Am 1991;29:605

Blair D, Rigsby C, Rosenfield AT: The nubbin sign on computed tomography and sonography. Urol Radiol 1987;9:149

Borthne A, Nordshus T, Reiseter T, et al: MR urography: the future gold standard in pediatric urogenital imaging? Pediatr Radiol 1999;29:694

Fernbach SK, Feinstein KA: Abnormalities of the bladder in children: imaging findings. AJR Am J Roentgenol 1994;162:1143

Fernbach SK, Feinstein KA, Schmidt MB: Pediatric voiding cystourethrography: a pictorial guide. Radiographics 2000;20:155

Fotter R: Neurogenic bladder in infants and children—a challenge for the radiologist. Abdom Imaging 1996;21:534

Fotter R: Functional disorders of the lower urinary tract and neurogenic bladder in infants and children. *In* Fotter R (ed): Pediatric Uroradiology. Berlin, Springer, 2001:185

Giordano M, Marzolla R, Puteo F, et al: Voiding urosonography as first step in diagnosis of vesicoureteral reflux in children: a clinical experience. Pediatr Radiol 2007;37:674-677

Gordon I, Riccabona M: Investigating the newborn kidney—update on imaging techniques Seminar Neonatol 2003;8:269-278

Gunn T, Mora D, Pease P: Antenatal diagnosis of urinary tract abnormalities by ultrasound after 28 weeks. Am J Obstet Gynecol 1995;172:476

Hernandez RH, Goodsitt M: Reduction of radiation dose in pediatric patients using pulsed fluoroscopy. AJR Am J Roentgenol 1996;167:1247

Maudgil DD, McHugh K: The role of CT in modern pediatric uroradiology. Eur J Radiol 2002;43:129

Riccabona M: Potential of modern sonographic techniques in paediatric uroradiology. Eur J Radiol 2002;43:110-121

Riccabona M: VUR. In Carty H, Brunelle F, Shaw D, Kendal B (eds): Imaging Children, 2nd ed. Edinburgh, Churchill Livingstone, 2006

Riccabona M, Fotter R: Reorientation and future trends in paediatric uroradiology: minutes of a symposium. Pediatr Radiol 2004;34:295

Riccabona M, Fotter R: Radiographic studies in children with kidney disorders: what to do and when. In Hogg R (ed): Kidney Disorders in Children and Adolescents. Birmingham, Taylor & Francis, 2006:15-34

Riccabona M, Fritz G, Ring E: Potential applications of three-dimensional ultrasound in the pediatric urinary tract: pictorial demonstration based on preliminary results. Eur Radiol 2003;13:2680-268

Riccabona M, Lindbichler F, Sinzig M: Conventional imaging in paediatric uroradiology. Eur J Radiol 2002;43:100

Riccabona M, Ruppert-Kohlmeier A, Ring E, et al: Potential impact of pediatric mr-urography on the imaging algorithm in patients with a functional single kidney? AJR Am J Roentgenol 2004;183:795

Riccabona M, Schwinger W, Ring E, Aigner R: Amplitude coded color Doppler sonography in pediatric renal disease. Eur Radiol 2001;11:861

Riccabona M, Simbrunner J, Ring E, et al: Feasibility of MR-urography in neonates and infants with anomalies of the upper urinary tract. Eur Radiol 2002;12:1442

Riccabona M, Sorantin E, Hausegger K: Imaging guided interventional procedures in paediatric uroradiology—a case-based overview. Eur J Radiol 2002;43:167

Riccabona M, Uggowitzer M, Klein E, et al. Contrast enhanced color Doppler sonography in children and adolescents. J Ultrasound Med 2000;19:783

Schöllnast H, Lindbichler F, Riccabona M: Ultrasound (US) of the urethra in infants: comparison US versus VCUG. J Ultrasound Med 2004;23:769

Teele RL, Share JC: Transperineal sonography in children. AJR Am J Roentgenol 1997;168:1263

Zier JL, Kvam KA, Kurachek SC, Finkelstein M: Sedation with nitrous oxide compared with no sedation during catheterization for urologic imaging in children. Pediatr Radiol 2007;37:678-684

Embryology, Normal Anatomy, and Variants

Bloom RA, Crooks EK, Wise HA: Complete ureteral triplication with ectopia. Urology 1984;25:176

Caldamone AA: Duplication anomalies of the upper tract in infants and children. Urol Clin North Am 1991;12:75

Gosalbez R Jr, Gosalbez R, Piro C, et al: Ureteral triplication and ureterocele: report of 3 cases and review of the literature. J Urol 1991;145:105

Hawas N, Noah M, Pattel PJ: Blind-ending ureter: clinical significance? An analysis of 13 cases with review of the literature. Eur Urol 1987;13:39

Herman TE, McAlister OH: Radiographic manifestations of congenital anomalies of the lower urinary tract. Radiol Clin North Am 1991;29:365

Hulnick DH, Bosniak MA: Faceless kidney: CT sign of renal duplicity. J Comput Assist Tomogr 1986;10:771

King BF, Hattery RR, Lieber MM, et al: Congenital cystic disease of the seminal vesicle. Radiology 1991;178:207

N'Guessan G, Stephens FD: Supernumerary kidney. J Urol 1983;130:649

Tilley EA, Dow CJ: Cranial blind-ending branch of a bifid ureter: report of 3 cases. Br J Urol 1988;62:127

Zaontz MR, Kass EJ: Ectopic ureter opening into seminal vesicle cyst associated with ipsilateral renal agenesis. Urology 1987;24:523

Ureteral Obstruction

Amis ES, Cronan JJ, Pfister RC: Lower moiety hydronephrosis in duplicated kidneys. Urology 1985;26:82

Bisset GS, Strife JL: The duplex collecting system in girls with urinary tract infection: prevalence and significance. AJR Am J Roentgenol 1987;148:497

Braverman RM, Lebowitz RL: Occult ectopic ureter in girls with urinary incontinence: diagnosis using CT. AJR Am J Roentgenol 1991;156:365

Churchill BM, Abara EO, McLorie GA: Ureteral duplication, ectopy and ureteroceles. Pediatr Clin North Am 1987;34:1273

Cremin BJ: A review of ultrasonic appearances of posterior urethral valves and ureteroceles. Pediatr Radiol 1986;16:357

Currarino G: Single vaginal ectopic ureter and Gartner's duct cyst with ipsilateral renal hypoplasia (or agenesis). J Urol 1982;128:988

Docimo SG, Lebowitz RL, Retik AB, et al: Congenital midureteral obstruction. Urol Radiol 1989;11:156

Gylys-Morin VM, Minevich E, Tackett LD, et al: Magnetic resonance imaging of the dysplastic renal moiety and ectopic ureter. J Urol 2000;164:2034

Horgan JG, Rosenfield NS, Weiss RM, Rosenfield AT: Is renal ultrasound a reliable indicator of a nonobstructed duplication anomaly? Pediatr Radiol 1984;14:388

Kaefer M, Barnewolt C, Retik AB, et al: The ultrasound diagnosis of infravesical obstruction in children: evaluation of bladder wall thickness indexed to bladder filling. J Urol 1997;157:989

Kass EJ, Fink-Bennett D: Contemporary techniques for the radioisotopic evaluation of the dilated urinary tract. Urol Clin North Am 1990;17:273

Keating MA, Retik AB: Management of dilated obstructed ureter. Urol Clin North Am 1990;17:291

Korogi Y, Takahashi M, Fujimura N, et al: Computed tomography demonstration of renal dysplasia with a vaginal ectopic ureter. J Comput Tomogr 1986;10:273

Kraus SJ, Lebowitz RL, Royal SA: Renal calculi in children: imaging features that led to diagnoses: a pictorial essay. Pediatr Radiol 1999;29:624

Leighton DM, Mayne V: Obstruction in the refluxing urinary tract: a common phenomenon. Clin Radiol 1989;40:271

MacDonald GR: The ectopic ureter in men. J Urol 1986;135:1269

Lautin EM, Haramati N, Frager D, et al: CT diagnosis of circumcaval ureter. AJR Am J Roentgenol 1988;150:591

Matsumoto J: Acquired lesions involving the ureter in childhood. Semin Roentgenol 1986;21:166

Nussbaum AR, Dorst JP, Jeffs RD, et al: Ectopic ureter and ureterocele: their varied radiographic manifestations. Radiology 1986;159:227

Reinberg Y, Alaibadi H, Johnson P, Gonzalez R: Congenital ureteral valves in children: case report and review of the literature. J Pediatr Surg 1987;22:379

Reitelman C, Perlmutter AD: Management of obstructing ectopic ureterocele. Urol Clin North Am 1990;17:318

Sen S, Ahmed S: Single system ureteroceles in childhood. Aust N Z J Surg 1988;58:903

Share JC, Lebowitz RL: Ectopic ureterocele without ureteral and calyceal dilatation (ureterocele disproportion): findings on urography and sonography. AJR Am J Roentgenol 1989;152:567

Sorantin E, Fotter R, Aigner R, et al: The sonographically thickened wall of the upper urinary tract: correlation with other imaging methods. Pediatr Radiol 1997;27:667

Strehlau J, Winkler P, de la Roche J: The ureterovesical jet as a functional diagnostic tool in childhood hydronephrosis. Pediatr Nephrol 1997;11:460

Wasserman NF: Inflammatory disease of the ureter. Radiol Clin North Am 1996;34:1131

Ureteral Dysfunction

Peters CA, Mandell J, Lebowitz RL, et al: Congenital obstructed megaureters in early infancy: diagnosis and treatment. J Urol 1989;142:641

Pfister RC, Hendren WH: Primary megaureter in children and adults: clinical and pathophysiologic features of 150 ureters. Urology 1978;12:160

Riccabona M, Sorrantin E, Fotter R: Application of functional m-mode sonography in pediatric patients. Eur Radiol 1998; 8:1457

Vesicoureteral Reflux

Alon U, Berant M, Pery M: Intravenous pyelography in children with urinary tract infection and vesicoureteral reflux. Pediatrics 1989;83:332

Alton DJ, Lequesne GW, Gent R, et al: Sonographically demonstrated thickening of the renal pelvis in children. Pediatr Radiol 1992;22:426

American Academy of Pediatrics Committee on quality improvement. Subcommittee on UTI: Practice parameter: The diagnosis, treatment and evaluation of the initial UTI in febrile infants and young children. Pediatrics 1999;103:843

Anderson PAM, Rickwood AMK: Features of primary vesicoureteral reflux detected by prenatal ultrasound. Br J Urol 1991;67:267

Andriole VT: Urinary tract infections: recent developments. J Infect Dis 1987;156:865

Arant BS: Vesicoureteral reflux and renal injury. Am J Kidney Dis 1991;17:491

Arant BS: Medical management of mild and moderate vesicoureteral reflux: follow-up studies of infants and young children—a preliminary report of the Southwest Pediatric Nephrology Group. J Urol 1992;148:1683

Arnold AJ, Brownless SM, Carty HM, Rickwood AM: Detection of renal scarring by DMSA scanning: an experimental study. J Pediatr Surg 1990;25:391

Ascenti G, Chimenz R, Zimbaro G, et al: Potential role of colour-Doppler cysto-sonography with echocontrast in the screening and follow-up of vesicoureteral reflux. Acta Pediatr 2000;89:1336

Assael BM, Guez S, Marra G, et al: Congenital reflux nephropathy: a follow-up of 108 cases diagnosed perinatally. Br J Urol 1998;82:252

Atala A, Wible JH, Share LC, et al: Sonography with sonicated albumin in the detection of vesico-ureteral reflux. J Urol 1993;150:756

Auringer ST: Pediatric uroradiology update. Urol Clin North Am 1997;24:673

Avni EF, Vandemerckt C, Braude P, et al: US evaluation of renal inflammatory diseases in children. J Urol 1988;6:18

Avni EF, VanGansbeke D, Thoua Y, et al: Ultrasound demonstration of pyelitis and ureteritis in children. Pediatr Radiol 1988;18:134

Avni FE, Ayadi K, Rypens F, et al: Can careful ultrasound examination of the urinary tract exclude vesico-ureteric reflux in the neonate. Br J Radiol 1997;70:977

Avni FE, Hall M, Janssens F: Urinary tract infection. In Fotter R (ed): Pediatric Uroradiology. Berlin, Springer, 2001:145

Bates CP, Whiteside CG, Turner-Warwick RT: Synchronous cine pressure flow cysto-urethrography, with special reference to stress and urge incontinence. Br J Urol 1970;42:714

Benador D, Benador N, Slosman DO, et al: Cortical scintigraphy in the evaluation of renal parenchymal changes in children with pyelonephritis. J Pediatr 1994;124:17

Ben-Ami T, Gayer G, Hertz M, et al: Natural history of reflux in the lower pole of duplicated collecting systems: a controlled study. Pediatr Radiol 1989;19:308

Ben-Ami T, Sinai L, Hertz M, Boichis H: Vesicoureteral reflux in boys: review of 196 cases. Radiology 1989;173:681

Berg UB: Long term follow-up of renal morphology and function in children with recurrent pyelonephritis. J Urol 1992;148:1715

Bernstein J, Arant BS: Morphological characteristics of segmental scarring in vesicoureteral reflux. J Urol 1992;148:1712

Berrocal T, Gaya F, Arjonilla A, Lonergan GJ: Vesicoureteral reflux: diagnosis and grading with echoenhanced cystosonography versus voiding cystourethrography. Radiology 2001;221:359

Biggi A, Dardanelli L, Pomero G, et al: Acute renal cortical scintigraphy in children with a first urinary tract infection. Pediatr Nephrol 2001;16:733

Björgvinsson E, Majd M, Eggli KD: Diagnosis of APN in children: comparison of US and Tc-DMSA scintigraphy. AJR 1991;157:539

Blake NS, O'Connell E: Endoscopic connection of vesico-ureteric reflux by subureteric Teflon injection: follow-up ultrasound and voiding cystography. Br J Radiol 1989;62:443

Blickman J, Taylor G, Lebowitz R: Voiding cystourethrography: the initial study in children with UTI. Radiology 1985;156:659

Bollgren I: Antibacterial prophylaxis in children with UTI. Acta Pediatr Scand 1999;431(S):48

Bosio M: Cystosonography with echocontrast: a new imaging modality to detect vesico-ureteric reflux in children. Pediatr Radiol 1998;28:250

Burge D, Griffith M, Malone P, et al: Fetal vesicoureteral reflux: outcome following conservative management. J Urol 1992;148:1743

Chambers T: An essay on the consequences of childhood urinary tract infection. Pediatr Nephrol 1997;11:178

Chan Y, Chan K, Roebuck D, et al: Potential utility of MRI in the evaluation of children at risk of renal scarring. Pediatr Radiol 1999;29:856

Chapman SJ, Chandler C, Haycock GB, et al: Radionuclide cystography in vesico-ureteral reflux. Arch Dis Child 1988;63:650

Connolly LP, Treves ST, Zurakowski D, Bauer SB: Natural history of vesicoureteral reflux in siblings. J Urol 1996;156:1805

Dacher JN, Boillot B, Eurin D, et al : Rational use of CT in acute pyelonephritis: findings and relationships with vesico-ureteral reflux. Pediatr Radiol 1993;23:281

Dacher JN, Avni FE, Arnaud F, et al: Renal sinus hyperechogenicity in acute pyelonephritis; description and pathological correlation. Pediatr Radiol 1999;29:179

Dacher JN, Pfister C, Monroc M, et al: Power Doppler sonographic pattern of acute pyelonephritis in children: comparison with CT. AJR Am J Roentgenol 1996;166:1451

Darge K, Tröger J, Duetting T, et al: Reflux in young patients: Comparison of voiding ultrasound of the bladder and the retrovesical space with echo-enhancement versus voiding cystourethrography for diagnosis. Radiology 1999;210:201

Darge K, Zieger B, Rohrschneider W, et al: Contrast-enhanced harmonic imaging for the diagnosis of vesicoureteral reflux in pediatric patients. AJR Am J Roentgenol 2001;177:1411

Decter RM, Roth DR, Gonzales ET Jr: Vesicoureteral reflux in boys. J Urol 1988;140:1089

Diard F, Nicolau A, Bernard S: Intra-renal reflux: a new cause of medullary hyperechogenicity? Pediatr Radiol 1987;17:154

Dick PT, Feldman W: Routine diagnostic imaging for childhood urinary tract infection: a systematic overview. J Pediatr 1996;128:15

Dillon MJ, Goonasekera CDA: Reflux nephropathy. J Am Soc Nephrol 1998;9:2377

Dinkel E, Orth S, Dittrich M, et al: Renal ultrasound in the differentiation of upper from lower urinary tract infection. AJR Am J Roentgenol 1986;146:775

Ditchfield MR, DeCampo JF, Cook DJ, et al: Vesico-ureteric reflux: an accurate predictor of acute pyelonephritis in childhood urinary tract infection? Radiology 1994;190:413

Ditchfield MR, DeCampo JF, Nolan TM, et al: Risk factors in the development of early renal cortical defects in children with UTI. AJR Am J Roentgenol 1994;152:1393

Eggli KD, Eggli D: Color Doppler US in pyelonephritis. Pediatr Radiol 1992;22:422

Farkas A, Moriel EZ, Lupa S: Endoscopic correction of vesicoureteral reflux: our experience with 115 ureters. J Urol 1990;144:534

Farnsworth RH, Rossleigh MA, Leighton DM, et al: The detection of reflux nephropathy in infants by Tc DMSA studies. J Urol 1991;145:542

Fotter R, Kopp W, Klein E, et al: Unstable bladder in children: functional evaluation by modified voiding cystourethrography. Radiology 1986;161:811

Garin EH, Campos A, Homsy Y: Primary vesicoureteral reflux: review of current concepts. Pediatr Nephrol 1998;12:249

Gedroye WMW, Chaudhuri R, Saxton HM: Normal and near-normal calyceal pattern in reflux nephropathy. Clin Radiol 1988;39:615

Gelfand MJ, Koch BL, Elgazzar AH, et al: Cyclic cystography: diagnostic yield in selected pediatric populations. Radiology 1999;213:118

Ginalski J-M, Michaud A, Genton N: Renal growth retardation in children: sign suggestive of vesicoureteral reflux. AJR Am J Roentgenol 1985;145:617

Godley ML, Ransley PG, Parkhouse HF, et al: Quantitation of vesico-ureteral reflux by radionuclide cystography and urodynamics. Pediatr Nephrol Sem 1990;4:485

Goldman M, Lahat E, Strauss S, et al: Imaging after urinary tract infection in male neonates. Pediatrics 2000;195:1232

Goldraich NP, Goldraich IJ: Follow-up of conservatively treated children with high and low grade vesicoureteral reflux: a prospective study. J Urol 1992;148:1688

Goldraich NP, Ramos OL, Goldraich IH: Urography versus DMSA scan in children with vesicoureteric reflux. Pediatr Nephrol 1989;3:1

Good CD, Vinnicombe SJ, Minty IL, et al: Posterior urethral valves in male infants and newborns: detection with ultrasound of the urethra before and during voiding. Radiology 1993;198:387

Goonasekera C, Dillon MJ: Hypertension in reflux nephropathy. Br J Urol 1999;83:1

Gordon I: Vesicoureteral reflux, urinary tract infection and renal damage in children. Lancet 1995;346:489

Gore MD, Fernbach SK, Donaldson JS, et al: Radiographic evaluation of suburetic injection of Teflon to correct VUR. AJR Am J Roentgenol 1989;152:115

Gross GW, Lebowitz RL: Infection does not cause reflux. AJR 1981;137:929

Haberlik A: Detection of low-grade vesicoureteral reflux in children by color Doppler imaging mode. Pediatr Surg Int 1998;12:38

Hanbury DC, Coulden RA, Farman P, et al: Ultrasound cystography in the diagnosis of vesico-ureteral reflux. Br J Urol 1990;65:250

Hanson S, Jodal U, Noren L, Bjure J: Untreated bacteriuria in asymptomatic girls with renal scarring. Pediatrics 1998;84:964

Hellerstein S: Urinary tract infection: old and new concepts. Pediatr Clin North Am 1995;42:1433

Hellström M, Jacobsson B, Marild S, Jodal U: Voiding cystourethrography as a predictor of reflux nephropathy in children with urinary-tract infections. AJR Am J Roentgenol 1989;152:801

Hiraoka M, Hashimoto G, Hori C, et al: Use of ultrasound in the detection of vesico-ureteral reflux in children suspected of having urinary tract infection. J Clin Ultrasound 1997;25:195

Hiraoka M, Kasuga K, Hori C, et al: Ultrasound indicators of vesico-ureteral reflux in the newborn. Lancet 1994;343:519

Hollowell JG, Altman HG, Snyder HM 3rd, Duckett JW: Coexisting ureteropelvic junction obstruction and vesicoureteral reflux: diagnosis and therapeutic implications. J Urol 1989;142:490

International Reflux Study Committee: Medical versus surgical treatment of primary vesicoureteral reflux: a prospective international reflux study in children. J Urol 1981;125:277

Jakobsson B, Berg U, Svensson L: Renal scarring after acute pyelonephritis. Arch Dis Child 1994;70:111

Jakobsson B, Esbjorner E, Hansson S: Minimum incidence and diagnostic rate of first urinary tract infection. Pediatrics 1999;104:222

Jakobsson B, Nolstedt L, Svensson L, et al: ^{99m}Tc-dimercapto-succinic acid (DMSA) in the diagnosis of acute pyelonephritis in children: relation to clinical and radiological findings. Pediatr Nephrol 1992;6:328

Jecquier S, Jecquier JC: Reliability of voiding cystourethrography to detect vesico-ureteral reflux. AJR Am J Roentgenol 1989;153:807

Jecquier S, Paltiel H, Lafortune M: Ureterovesical jets in children and infants: duplex and color Doppler US studies. Radiology 1990;175:349

Jequier S, Forbest PA, Nogrady MB: The value of ultrasonography as a screening procedure in a first documented urinary tract infection in children. J Ultrasound Med 1985;4:393

Jequier S, Jequier JC: Reliability of voiding cystourethrography to detect reflux. AJR Am J Roentgenol 1989;153:807

Jodal U: Urinary tract infections (UTI): significance, pathogenesis, clinical features and diagnosis. In Postelstwaite RJ (ed): Butterworth and Heinneman Clinical Pediatric Nephrology, 2nd ed. Cambridge, Oxford, 1994:151-159

Kass EJ, Fisk-Bennett D, Cacciarelli AA: The sensitivity of renal scintigraphy and ultrasound in detecting nonobstructive acute pyelonephritis. J Urol 1992;148:606

Kenda RB, Novljan G, Kenig A, et al: Echo-enhanced ultrasound voiding cystography in children: a new approach. Pediatr Nephrol 2000;14:297

Kenny PJ: Imaging of chronic renal infections. AJR Am J Roentgenol 1990;155:485

Kim B, Lim HK, Choi MH, et al: Detection of parenchymal abnormalities in acute pyelonephritis by pulse inversion harmonic imaging with or without microbubble ultrasonographic contrast agent: correlation with computed tomography. J Ultrasound Med 2001;20:5

Kleinman PK, Diamond DA, Karellas A, et al: Tailored low dose fluoroscopic voiding cystourethrography for the reevaluation of vesicoureteral reflux in girls. AJR 1994;162:1151; discussion 1154

Koff S, Wagner T, Jayanthi V: The relationship among dysfunctional elimination syndromes, primary vesicoureteral reflux and urinary tract infections in children. J Urol 1998;160:1019

Larcombe J: Urinary tract infection in children. BMJ 1999;319:1173

Lebowitz RL, Mandell J: Urinary tract infection in children: putting radiology in its place. Radiology 1987;165:1

Lebowitz RL, Olbing H, Parkkulainen KV, et al: International Reflux Study in children: International system of radiographic grading of vesico-ureteral reflux. Pediatr Radiol 1985;15:105

Lebowitz RL: The detection and characterization of vesicoureteral reflux in the child. J Urol 1992;148:1640

Lenaghan D, Whitaker JG, Jensen F, Stephens FD: The natural history of reflux and long-term effects of reflux on the kidney. J Urol 1976;115:728

Lerner GR, Fleischmann LE, Perlmutter AD: Reflux nephropathy. Pediatr Clin North Am 1987;34:747

Lonergan GJ, Pennington DJ, Morrison JC, et al: Childhood pyelonephritis: comparison of gadolinium-enhanced MR imaging and renal cortical scintigraphy for diagnosis. Radiology 1998;207:377

MacKenzie JR, Fowler K, Hollman AS, et al: The value of ultrasound in the child with an acute urinary tract infection. Br J Urol 1994;74:240

Mahant S, To T, Friedman J: Timing of voiding cystourethrogram in the investigation of urinary tract infections in children. J Pediatr 2001;139:568

Majd M, Nussbaum Blask AR, Markle BM, et al: Acute pyelonephritis: comparison of diagnosis with ^{99m}Tc-DMSA SPECT, spiral CT, MR imaging, and power Doppler ultrasound in an experimental pig model. Radiology 2001;218:101

Mandel GA, Eggli DF, Gilday DL, et al: Procedure guideline for radionuclide cystography in children. J Nucl Med 1997;38:1650

Martinelli J, Claesson I, Lidin-Janson G, et al: Urinary infection, reflux and renal scarring in females continuously followed for 13-18 years. Pediatr Nephrol 1995;9:131

Mason WG Jr: Urinary tract infections in children: renal ultrasound evaluation. Radiology 1989;153:109

Matsumo T, Fukushima Motoyama H, Higushi E, et al: Color flow imaging for detection of vesico-ureteral reflux. Lancet 1996;347:757

Matsuoka H, Oshima K, Sakamoto K, et al: Renal pathology in patients with reflux nephropathy. Eur Urol 1994;26:153

McLorie GA, Alaibadi H, Churchill BM, et al: ^{99m}Technetium-dimercapto-succinic acid renal scanning and excretory urography in diagnosis of focal renal scans in children. J Urol 1989;142:790

McLorie GA, McKenna PH, Jumper BM, et al: High grade vesicoureteral reflux: analysis of observational therapy. J Urol 1990;144:537

Mentzel HJ, Vogt S, Patzer L, et al: Contrast enhanced sonography of vesico-ureteral reflux in children: primary results. AJR Am J Roentgenol 1999;173:737

Merguerian PA, Jamal MA, Agarwal SK, et al: Utility of DMSA scanning in the evaluation of children with primary vesico-ureteral reflux. Urology 1999;53:1024

Merrick MC, Notghi A, Chalmers N, et al: Long term follow-up to determine the prognostic value of imaging after urinary tract infection: II. Scarring. Arch Dis Child 1995;72:393

Morin D, Veyrac C, Kotzki PO, et al: Comparison of ultrasound and DMSA scintigraphy changes in acute pyelonephritis. Pediatr Nephrol 1999;13:219

Mozley D, Heyman S, Duckett J, et al: Direct vesicoureteral scintigraphy: quantifying early outcome predictors in children with primary reflux. J Nucl Med 1994;35:1602

Najmalin A, Burge DM, Arwell JD: Fetal vesico-ureteral reflux. Br J Urol 1990;65:403

Najmalin A, Burge DM, Atwell JD: Reflux nephropathy secondary to intra-uterine vesico-ureteral reflux. J Pediatr Surg 1990;25:387

Nancarrow PA, Lebowitz RL: Primary vesicoureteral reflux in blacks with posterior urethral valves: does it occur? Pediatr Radiol 1988;19:31

Oswald J, Brenner E. Schwentner C, et al: The intravesical ureter in children with vesicoureteral reflux: a morphological and immunohistochemical characterization. J Urol 2003;170:2423

Paltiel H, Rupich R, Kiruluta G: Enhanced detection of VUR in infants and children with use of cycling VCUG. Radiology 1992;184:753

Parker MD, Clark RL: Urothelial striations revisited. Radiology 1996;198:89

Pennington DJ, Lonergan GL, Flack CE, et al: Experimental pyelonephritis in piglets: diagnosis with MR imaging. Radiology 1998;207:377

Pennington DJ, Zerin MJ: Imaging of the urinary tract infection. Pediatr Ann 1999;28:678

Pickworth FE, Carlin JB, Ditchfeld MR, et al: Ultrasound measurements of renal enlargement in children with acute pyelonephritis and time needed for resolution: implications for renal growth assessment. AJR Am J Roentgenol 1995;165:405

Poli-Merol M, Francois S, Pfliger F, et al: Interest of direct radionuclide cystography in repeated urinary tract infection exploration in children. Eur J Pediatr Surg 1998;8:339

Poustchi-Amin M, Leonidas JC, Palestro C, et al: Magnetic resonance imaging in acute pyelonephritis. Pediatr Nephrol 1998;12:579

Radmayr C, Klauser A, Pallwein L, et al: Contrast enhanced reflux sonography in children: a comparison to standard radiological imaging. J Urol 2002;167:1428

Reid BS, Bender TM: Radiographic evaluation of children with urinary tract infections. Radiol Clin North Am 1988;26:393

Riccabona M: Cystography in infants and children—a critical appraisal of the many forms, with special regard to voiding cystourethrography. Eur Radiol 2002;12:2910

Riccabona M: Vesico-ureteral reflux (VUR). In Carty H, Brunelle F, Stringer D, Kao SC (eds): Imaging Children, 2nd ed, vol I. Philadelphia, Elsevier Science, 2005:671-690

Riccabona M: Urinary tract infection. In Carty H, Brunelle F, Stringer D, Kao SC (eds). Imaging Children, 2nd ed, vol I. Philadelphia, Elsevier Science, 2005:691-712

Riccabona M, Haberlik A, Ring E: Virtual cystoscopy in children, based on three-dimensional ultrasound (3DUS) data: preliminary results. Eur Radiol 2006;16(Supp 1):284

Riccabona M, Mache CJ, Lindbichler F: Echoenhanced Color Doppler cystosonography of vesico-ureteral reflux in children: improvement by stimulated acoustic emission. Acta Radiol 2003;44:18

Riccabona M, Ring E, Maurer U, et al: Scintigraphy and sonography in reflux nephropathy: a comparison. Nucl Med Com 1993;14:339

Robben GF, Boesten M, Linmans J, et al: Significance of thickening of the wall of the renal collecting system in children: an ultrasound study. Pediatr Radiol 1999;29:736

Rushton HG: The evaluation of acute pyelonephritis and renal scarring with Tc DMSA scintigraphy: evolving concepts and future directions. Pediatr Nephrol 1997;11:108

Rushton HG, Majd M, Jantausch B, et al: Renal scarring following vesico-ureteral reflux and non-reflux pyelonephritis in children: evaluation with Tc-DMSA. J Urol 1992;147:1327

Salih M, Baltaci S, Kilic S, et al: Color flow Doppler ultrasound in the diagnosis of vesico-ureteral reflux. Eur Urol 1994;26:93

Sargent MA: What is the normal prevalence of vesicoureteral reflux? Pediatr Radiol 2000;30:723

Schneider K, Jablonski C, Wiessner M, et al: Screening for vesicoureteral reflux in children using real-time sonography. Pediatr Radiol 1984;14:400

Seruca H: Vesicoureteral reflux and voiding dysfunction: a prospective study. J Urol 1989;142:494

Shanon A, Feldman W, McDonald P, et al: Evaluation of renal scars by Tc-DMSA scan, intravenous urography and ultrasound: a comparative study. J Pediatr 1992;120:399

Shanon A, Feldman W: Methodologic limitations in the literature on vesicoureteral reflux: a critical review. J Pediatr 1990;117:171

Shapiro E, Elder J: The office management of recurrent urinary tract infection and vesico-ureteral reflux in children. Urol Clin 1998;4:725

Shimada K, Matsui T, Ogino T, et al: Renal growth and progression of reflux nephropathy in children with vesicoureteral reflux. J Urol 1988;140:1097

Sillen U: Vesicoureteral reflux in infants. Pediatr Nephrol 1999;13:355

Skoog SJ, Belman AB: Primary vesicoureteral reflux in the black child. Pediatrics 1991;87:538

Smellie JM, Poulton A, Prescod NP: Retrospective study of children with renal scarring associated with urinary infection. BMJ 1994;308:1193

Smellie JM, Prescod NP, Shaw PJ, et al: Childhood reflux and urinary infection: a follow-up of 10-41 years in 226 adults. Pediatr Nephrol 1998;12:727

Smellie JM, Shaw PJ, Prescod NP, Bantock HM: ^{99m}Tc dimercaptosuccinic acid (DMSA) scan in patients with established radiological renal scarring. Arch Dis Child 1988;63:1315

Smellie LM, Rigden SPA, Prescod NP, et al: Urinary tract infection: a comparison of four methods of investigation. Arch Dis Child 1995;72:247

Sobel JD: Pathogenesis of urinary tract infection. Infect Dis Clin North Am 1997;11:531

Sreenarasimhalah S, Hellerstein S: Urinary tract infections per se do not cause end-stage kidney disease. Pediatr Nephrol 1998;12:210

Stark H: Urinary tract infection in girls: the cost-effectiveness of currently recommended investigative routines. Pediatr Nephrol 1997;11:174

Stock JA, Wilson D, Hanna MN: Congenital reflux nephropathy and severe unilateral reflux. J Urol 1998;160:1017

Stokland E, Hellström M, Jacobsson B, et al: Early ^{99m}Tc dimercaptosuccinic acid (DMSA) scintigraphy in symptomatic first-time urinary tract infection. Acta Paediatr 1996;85:430

Stokland E, Hellström M, Hansson S, et al: Reliability of ultrasound in identification of reflux nephropathy in children. BMJ 1994;309:235

Stokland E, Hellström M, Jacobsson B, et al: Renal damage one year after first urinary tract infection: role of DMSA scintigraphy. J Pediatr 1996;129:815

Tamminen-Mobius T, Brunier E, Ebel KD, et al: Cessation of vesicoureteral reflux for five years in infants and children allocated to medical treatment. J Urol 1992;148:1662

Tsai JD, Huang FY, Tsai TC: Asymptomatic vesicoureteral reflux detected by neonatal ultrasound screening. Pediatr Nephrol 1998;12:206

Valenti AL, Salvaggio E, Manzoni C, et al: Contrast-enhanced gray-scale and color Doppler voiding urosonography versus voiding cystourethrography in the diagnosis and grading of vesicoureteral reflux. J Clin Ultrasound 2001;29:65

Walsh G, Dubbins PA: Antenatal renal pelvis dilatation: a predictor of vesico-ureteral reflux? AJR Am J Roentgenol 1996;167:897

Wennerstrom M, Hansson S, Jodal U, et al: Primary and acquired renal scarring in boys and girls with urinary tract infection. J Pediatr 2000;136:30

White RHR: Vesicoureteric reflux and renal scarring. Arch Dis Child 1989;64:407

Winter DW: Power Doppler sonographic evaluation of acute pyelonephritis in children. J Ultrasound Med 1996;15:91

Miscellaneous Conditions

Rypens F, Avni F, Bank WO, et al: The uretero-vesical junction in children: ultrasound findings after surgical or endoscopic treatment. AJR Am J Roentgenol 1992;158:837

CHAPTER

152 The Bladder and Urethra

D. GREGORY BATES

DEVELOPMENT AND EMBRYOLOGY

The Bladder and Trigone

In the developing embryo, the terminus of the hindgut develops into an endodermal-lined chamber called the cloaca. Progressive lateral and cranial mesenchymal ingrowths around the cloaca elevate the surrounding ectoderm into labial scrotal swellings and the genital tubercle, the primordium of the phallus or clitoris. Beginning at about 28 days, the cloaca is divided in the coronal plane by the descending urorectal septum (the Tourneux fold). By the seventh week, the cloaca is divided into a separate dorsal rectum and primitive ventral urogenital sinus (Fig. 152-1). Following communication with the mesonephric ducts (wolffian derivatives), the cranial portion of the primitive urogenital sinus develops into the vesicourethral canal and the caudal portion becomes the urogenital sinus. Paramesonephric ducts (müllerian derivatives) communicate with the posterior vesicourethral canal to form the Müller's tubercle. The perineal body represents the distal apposition of the urorectal septum and cloacal membrane.

After mesonephric duct (mesoderm) fusion with the urogenital sinus (endoderm), the ureteric bud branches from the mesonephric duct. By day 33, the segment of mesonephric duct below the ureteric bud dilates as the common excretory duct forming the precursor of the hemitrigone. The right and left common excretory ducts are absorbed into the urogenital sinus and migrate toward the midline. The epithelia of both ducts fuse as a triangular region, the primitive trigone. The mesonephric ducts extend caudad, along with the medially paired paramesonephric ducts, to form the site of the verumontanum in the male and the cervix in the female (Fig. 152-2). Continued growth of the epithelium and mesoderm of the common excretory ducts separates the ureteral orifices laterally at the trigone. By day 37, the ureter enters the bladder directly. Abnormal formation and/or separation of the common excretory duct from the ureter helps to explain a variety of congenital anomalies

to include the insertion of the vas deferens (derived from the mesonephric duct) into the ureter rather than the verumontanum, ureteric budding from the paramesonephric duct, ureteral insertion into the vas deferens or seminal vesicle cyst with ipsilateral renal agenesis (Fig. 152-3), and abortive development of the wolffian duct derivatives to include the vas deferens and body and tail of the epididymis (the head of the epididymis is derived from the gonadal ridge).

The bladder forms from the superior extent of the urogenital sinus (vesicourethral canal) and is lined with connective tissue by 10 weeks' gestation. The apex of the canal tapers as the urachus. The urachus is in continuity with the allantois at the umbilicus and allows drainage of urine produced by the kidneys (beginning at 6 weeks' gestation). By 12 weeks' gestation the connection between the bladder and allantois involutes. Progressive fibrosis of the urachus results in formation of the median umbilical ligament. By 13 weeks' gestation bladder mesenchyme has developed into interlacing circular and longitudinal strands of smooth muscle. By 16 weeks' gestation the entire bladder has discrete inner and outer longitudinal layers and a middle circular layer. The muscle fibers of the trigone are contiguous with the developing ureter and are separate from the bladder musculature. Muscularization is preferential at the bladder base, stimulating thickening of the trigone and narrowing of the bladder lumen at the internal bladder sphincter. The outer longitudinal layer extends from the bladder apex to insert into the posterior upper prostate in the male and the anterior wall of the vagina in the female. The middle circular muscle forms the internal sphincter at the bladder neck (Fig. 152-4). By term, the inner longitudinal layer is complete on the anterior bladder wall but posteriorly is evident only in the region of the trigone, where it extends distally to become continuous with the longitudinal smooth muscle layer in the urethra. The outer striated muscle of the external sphincter is believed to originate from myogenic stem cell precursors invading the urethral wall from the anterior surface of the rectum (puborectalis muscle) and insert at the

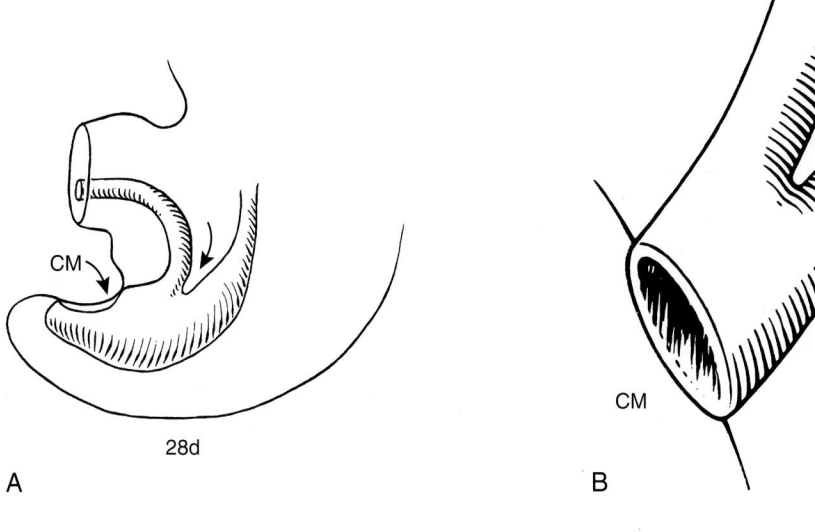

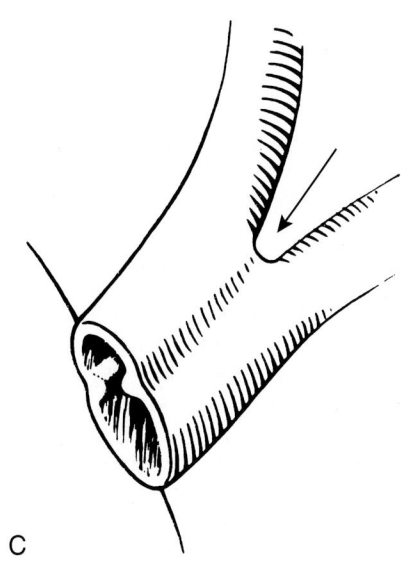

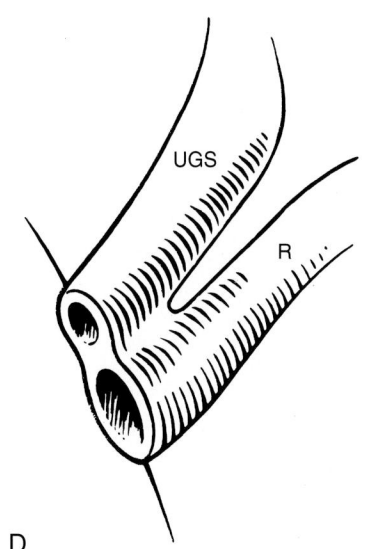

FIGURE 152-1. Septation of the cloaca. **A,** Lateral view of the caudal embryo (CM, cloacal membrane). Septation of the cloaca occurs in a coronal plane as a Tourneux fold (**B**) extends to the cloacal membrane from above and (**C**) as Rathke's plicae extend toward each other from the sides. **D,** Septation establishes the primitive urogenital sinus (UGS) and rectum (R). (From Stephens FD, Smith ED: Anorectal Malformations in Children. Chicago, Year Book Medical Publishers, 1971.)

junction of the membranous and bulbous urethra. Complete formation of the external muscular sphincteric ring occurs postnatally in the male by 13 years of age and in the female by 10 years of age.

In early gestation, bladder compliance is low and the bladder functions as a conduit rather than a storage organ. As the ultrastructure of the bladder changes throughout gestation (decreased ratio of type I to type III collagen and increased elastic fibers), compliance increases. As urine production increases and a functioning sphincter mechanism develops, mechanical distention of the bladder occurs. Normal cycles of bladder filling and emptying promote normal trigonal development and muscularization of the bladder. Bladder dysfunction at this stage may result in anomalous development of the trigone and ureterovesical junction.

The Urethra

In the male, the urogenital sinus develops into a narrow proximal (pelvic urethra) and expanded distal (phallic urethra) segments. The pelvic urethra forms the prostatic and membranous portions of the urethra, while the phallic urethra forms the bulbar and penile urethra. The phallic urethra develops from a plate of thickened endodermal cells within the inner portion of the distal urogenital membrane at the genital tubercle. Mesenchyme expands to raise the lateral ectodermal surface to form the urethral folds. Between 8 and 12 weeks' gestation the urethral plate degenerates and the urethral folds fuse ventrally. Fusion progresses distally along the median raphe to form the tubularized phallic urethra. Concomitantly, the external genitalia begin to masculinize by the 10th week. The genital tubercle elongates into a cylindrical phallus. Mesenchyme in the tubercle condenses to form the cavernous tissue. The scrotal swellings become round and migrate inferiorly and medially to form the scrotum at the base of the penis (Fig. 152-5). Distal glandular urethra patency appears during the 16th week, likely owing to a combination of progressive ventral fusion of the urethral folds and primary canalization of the glans. Prostatic development occurs following epithelial outgrowths from the pelvic urethra into the surrounding mesenchyme. By 12 weeks' gestation, five groups of tubules have formed the lobes of the prostate. Similarly, Cowper glands develop as endodermal buds and penetrate the adjacent mesenchyme to the level of the membranous urethra. The buds enlarge and develop glandular epithelium by 18 weeks' gestation.

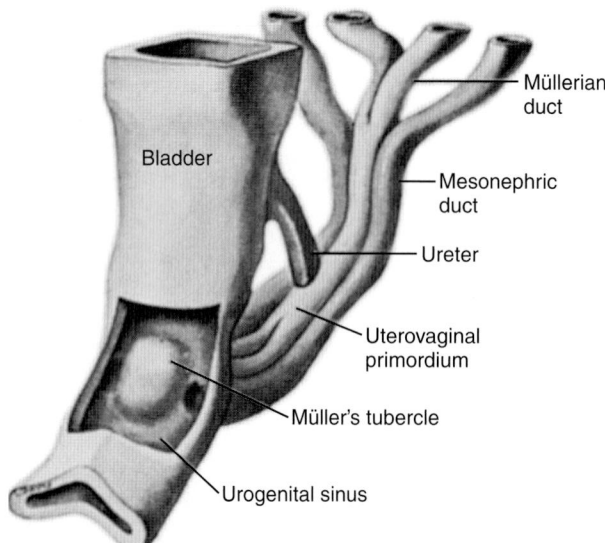

FIGURE 152-2. Diagrammatic view of the development of the ducts of the genitalia. The paramesonephric ducts descend toward the pelvis medial to the mesonephric ducts. After the mesonephric ducts are absorbed into the trigone, they migrate medially and caudally, flanking the paramesonephric ducts. The termini of these four ducts are the site of the verumontanum in the male and the cervix in the female. (From Arey. After Broman, Arey LB: Developmental Anatomy, 7th ed. Philadelphia, WB Saunders, 1974.)

In the female, the pelvic portion of urogenital sinus develops into the lower portion of the definitive urethra and vagina. Epithelial-lined tubules branch from the urethra at approximately 11 weeks to form the paraurethral glands of Skene, the female homologs of the prostate. In the absence of androgen, the external genitalia begin to slowly feminize at 10 to 12 weeks' gestation. The genital swellings grow superiorly and laterally to cover the clitoris. A single perineal opening serves as the urethra and vagina at this stage. After production of fetal pituitary follicle-stimulating hormone, there is ventral outgrowth of the perineum separating the urethral and vaginal openings. The labia minora and majora progressively enlarge. The female phenotype is complete by 26 weeks' gestation (Fig. 152-6). Masculinization, on the other hand, is complete by 14 weeks' gestation.

URACHAL ANOMALIES

During early fetal development, the bladder communicates with the allantois via the urachus, which is an elongated fibromuscular tube lying between the peritoneum and the transversalis fascia of the anterior abdominal wall. The urachus contains three layers: an inner layer of transitional epithelium, an intermediate layer of fibroconnective tissue, and an outer layer of external smooth muscle continuous with the detrusor muscle. Based on this histology, the origin of the urachus is thus likely from the bladder, as opposed to the allantois. Debate exists as to the actual timing of functional closure of the urachus. Considerations include obliteration between the 6th and 12th weeks of gestation coinciding with urethral development, obliteration during the fourth to fifth months of gestation at the time of descent of the bladder into the pelvis, and postnatally based on the ultrasonographic and histologic identification of a persistent narrow lumen within the urachus in the

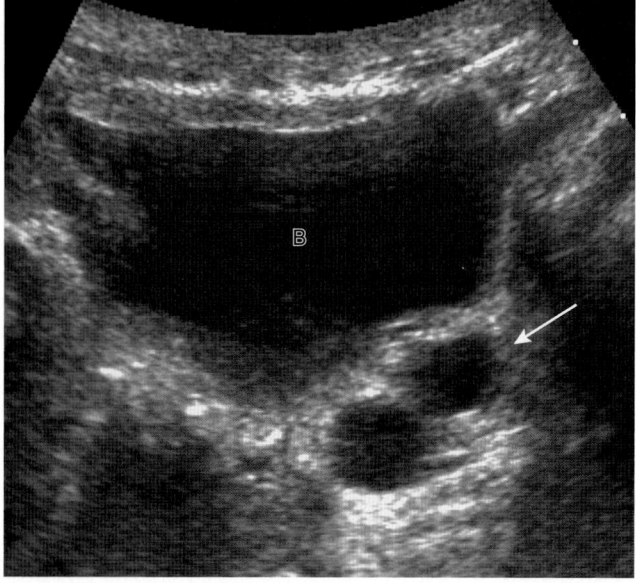

A

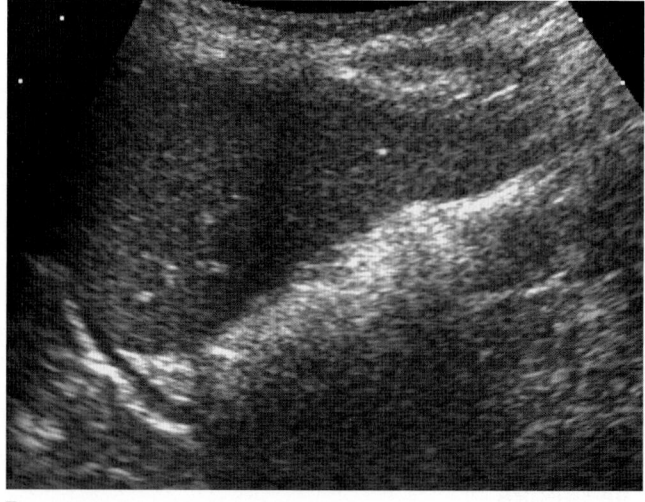

B

FIGURE 152-3. Seminal vesicle cyst. **A,** Transverse ultrasound of the pelvis shows a left-sided bilobed cyst (arrow) adjacent to the floor of the bladder (B). **B,** Longitudinal image of the left upper quadrant shows absence of the left kidney.

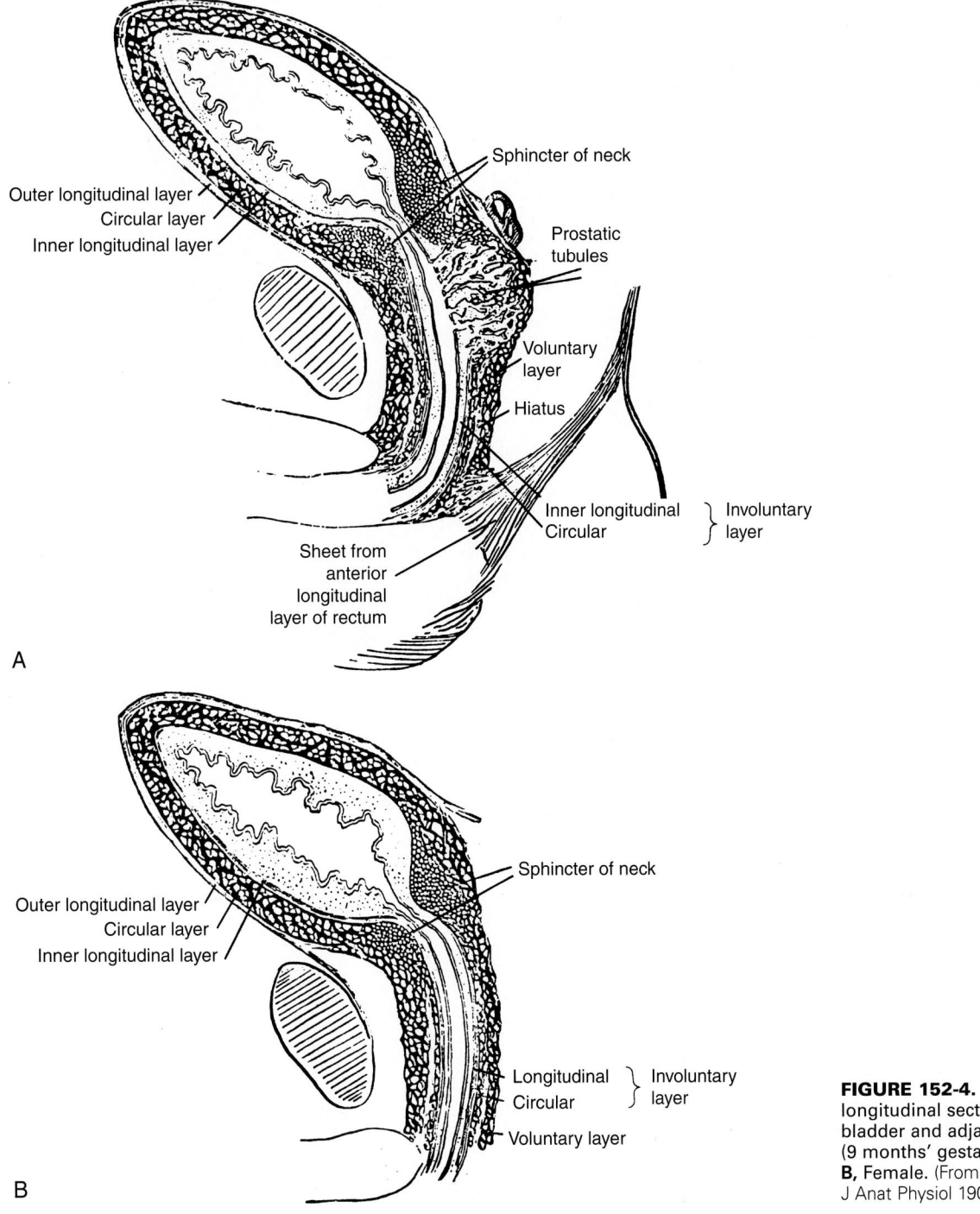

FIGURE 152-4. Semidiagrammatic longitudinal section of a human bladder and adjacent urethra (9 months' gestation). **A,** Male. **B,** Female. (From Wood-Jones F: J Anat Physiol 1901-1902;36:51.)

neonatal period. Regression of the urachus typically extends from the umbilicus toward the bladder. The urachus may lose its umbilical attachment and becomes attached in the infraumbilical midline.

Failure of the urachus to normally regress results in one of four disorders: patent urachus, urachal sinus, urachal diverticulum, and urachal cyst (Fig. 152-7). In patent urachus, the urachus develops normally but fails to obliterate, resulting in a vesicoumbilical fistula (Fig. 152-8). In urachal sinus, the urachus is closed at the level of the bladder but remains patent at the umbilicus (Fig. 152-9). In urachal diverticulum, the urachus is obli-

terated at the level of the umbilicus but communicates with the bladder (Fig. 152-10). In urachal cyst, the urachus is obliterated at both ends but remains patent in its midportion; there may be multiple small urachal cysts as a result of segmental obliteration of the urachus.

Failure of urachal regression can result in a patent urachus, urachal sinus, urachal diverticulum, or urachal cyst.

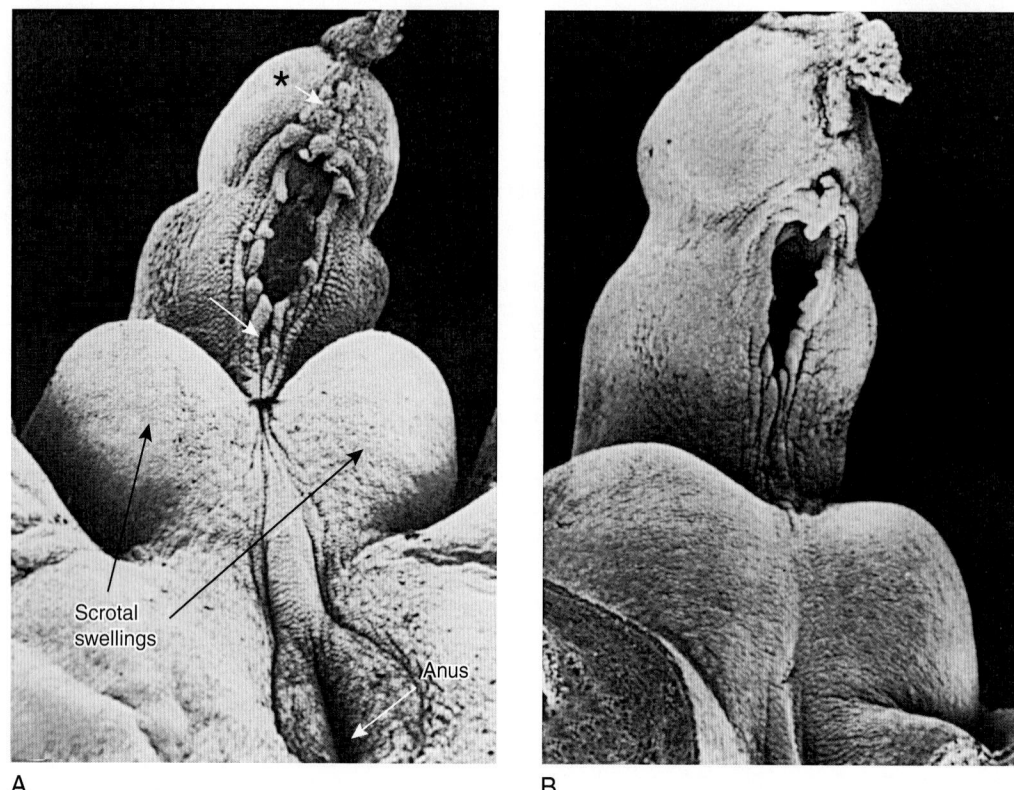

FIGURE 152-5. Development of the male human genitalia (10 weeks old). Scanning electron micrographs of the ventrum of the genitalia. **A,** The urethral folds are fusing to form the penile urethra. The paired scrotal swellings are converging toward each other *(arrows).* The *asterisk* marks the urethral plate. The fossa will come to be filled with squames, and the process of fusion of the urethral folds will continue on the glans to complete the glandular urethra during the 4th month. **B,** The urethral folds have fused further to form the penile urethra. The fusion is complete by the end of the 12th week. A sulcus separates the glans from the shaft of the phallus. (From Waterman RE: Human embryo and fetus. *In* Hafez ESE, Kenemans P [eds]: Atlas of Human Reproduction. Hinghan, MA, Kluwer Boston, 1982.)

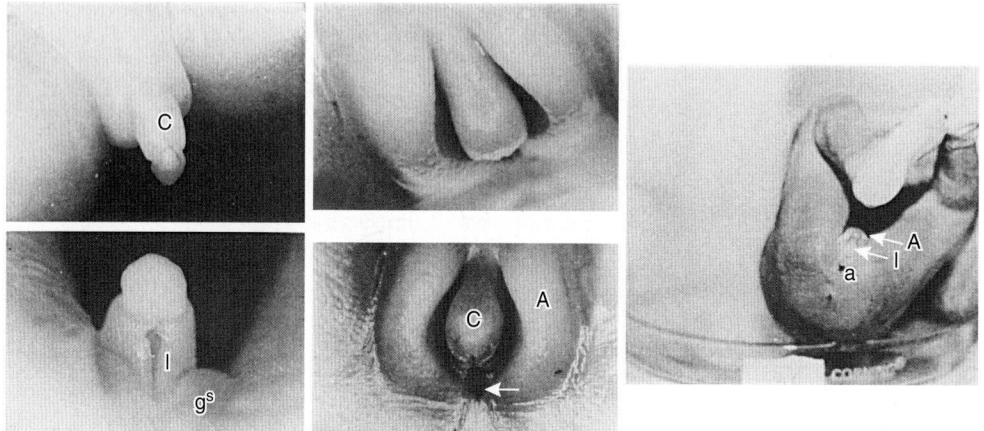

FIGURE 152-6. Feminization of the external genitalia. **Left,** At 12 weeks' gestation, the clitoris (c) is phallus-like, the urethral folds (l) are separate up to the base of the clitoris, and the genital swellings (gs) are separate. The urethral folds do not fuse. **Right,** At 22 weeks' gestation the clitoris (c) is prominent and the genital swellings have migrated up to structure the labia majora (A). a, anus. (**Left image** from Jirasek JE: Morphogenesis of the genital system in the human. Birth Defects 1977;15:13; **Right image** from Ammini AC, Pandey J, Vijyaraghavan M, Sabherwal U: Human female phenotypic development: role of the fetal ovaries. J Clin Endocrinol Metab 1994;79:604-608.)

All these abnormal structures are related to the anterior abdominal wall, are extraperitoneal (space of Retzius), and are midline in location. They frequently occur as isolated lesions, but they may be seen in association with other anomalies. A patent urachus may be seen in patients with severe congenital lower urinary tract obstructions but is unusual even in the most severe posterior urethral valves. It is unlikely that primary urethral obstruction is responsible for persistence of the urachus. A patent urachus and urachal diverticula are

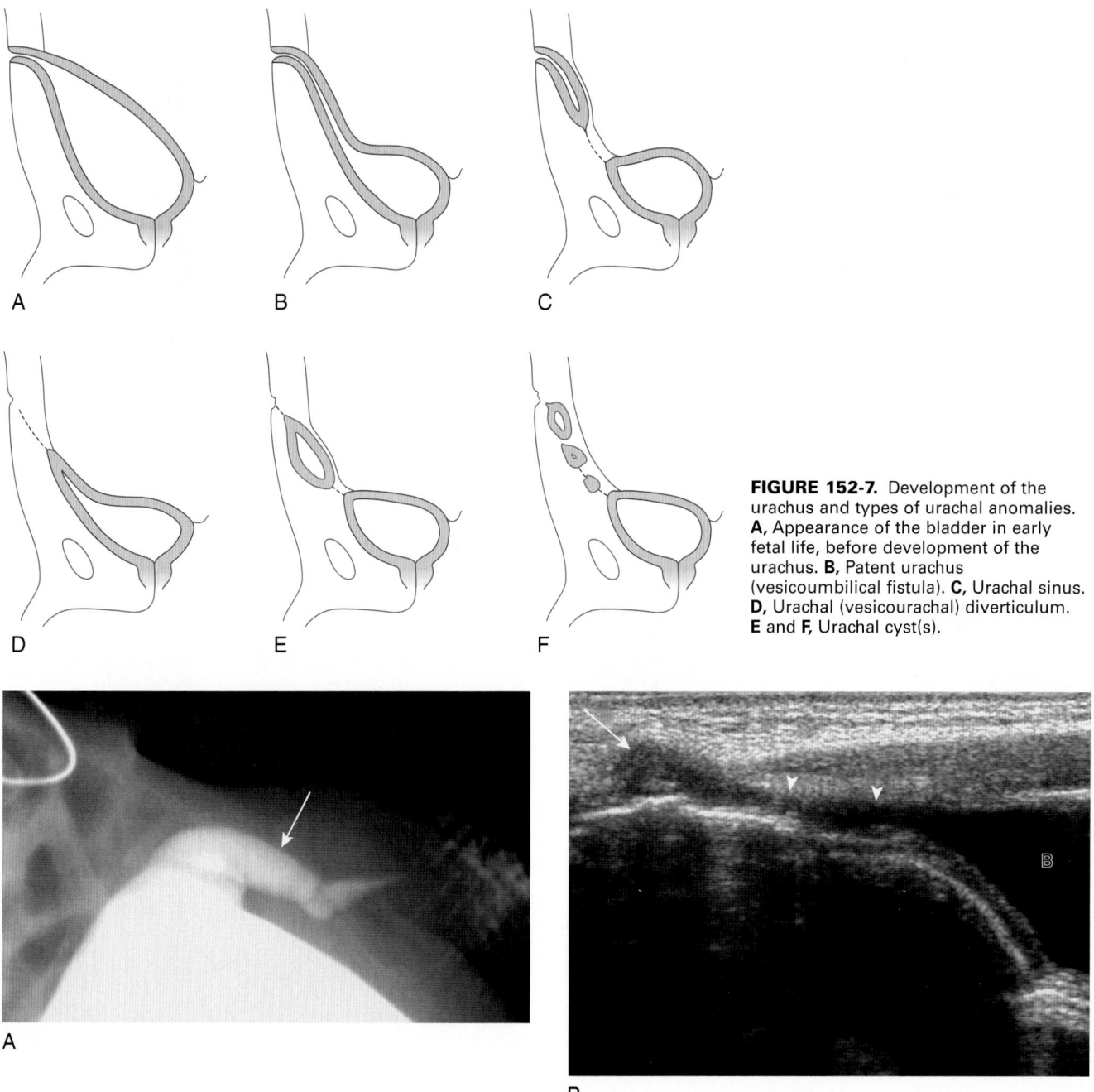

FIGURE 152-7. Development of the urachus and types of urachal anomalies. **A,** Appearance of the bladder in early fetal life, before development of the urachus. **B,** Patent urachus (vesicoumbilical fistula). **C,** Urachal sinus. **D,** Urachal (vesicourachal) diverticulum. **E** and **F,** Urachal cyst(s).

FIGURE 152-8. Patent urachus. **A,** Lateral view during a VCUG shows a fistulous tract *(arrow)* leading from the dome of the bladder to the umbilicus. **B,** Longitudinal sonogram shows a urine-filled patent urachus *(arrowheads)* extending from the dome of bladder (B) to the umbilicus *(arrow)*.

frequent findings in prune-belly syndrome. Small diverticula are generally of no clinical significance. However, large diverticula may be poorly contractile, expanded paradoxically during voiding, and contain calculi (Fig. 152-11). Urachal sinuses and cysts often become infected. Urachal cysts likely maintain a communication with the bladder or umbilicus through which infection may occur (Fig. 152-12). Abscess formation may progress to rupture within the abdominal wall or into the peritoneal cavity. Malignant degeneration within urachal remnants is reported in adults and accounts for one third of all bladder adenocarcinomas. The change from transitional to glandular epithelium may result from

metaplasia secondary to chronic irritation from trapped debris, chronic infection, or lack of normal contact with urine. Cloacal remnants or enteric rests are also considered as possible causes.

Leakage of urine at the umbilicus suggests the presence of a patent urachus. The diagnosis is confirmed by catheterization of the bladder through the umbilicus (Fig. 152-13) or by voiding cystourethrography (VCUG) with films in the lateral projection. The differential diagnosis of a wet umbilicus in the infant includes patent urachus, urachal sinus, omphalitis, granulation tissue of the healing umbilical stump, and patent omphalomesenteric duct. The diagnosis of urachal sinus can be made

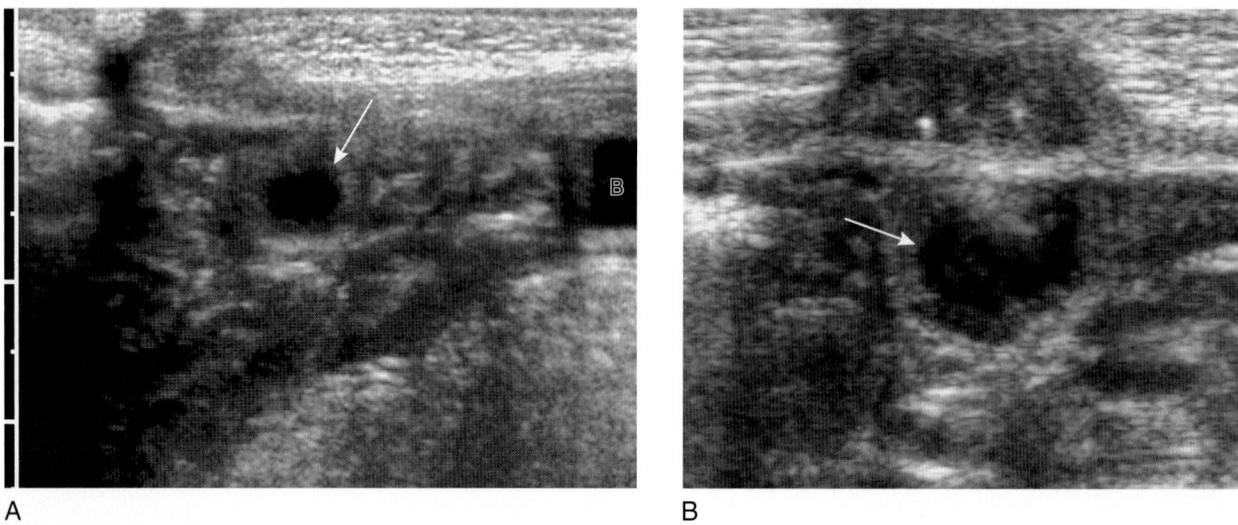

FIGURE 152-9. Urachal sinus. Longitudinal (**A**) and transverse (**B**) linear sonograms show an anechoic cyst in the infraumbilical region (arrows). B, Bladder.

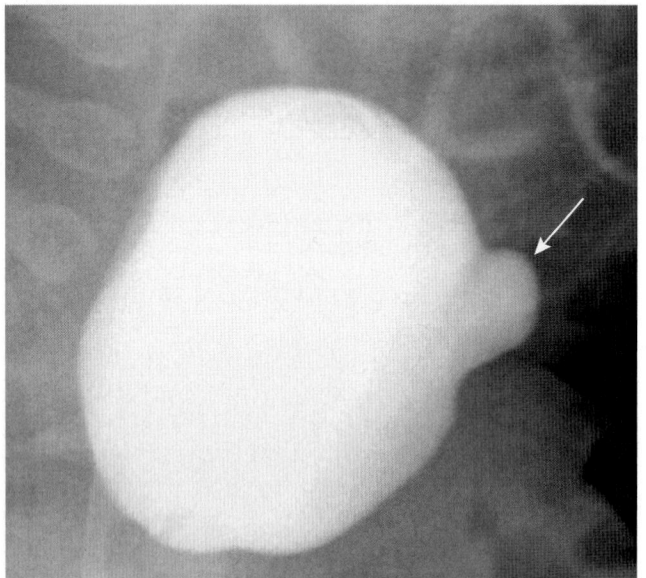

FIGURE 152-10. Urachal diverticulum. Lateral view during a VCUG shows a urachal diverticulum extending from the bladder dome (arrow).

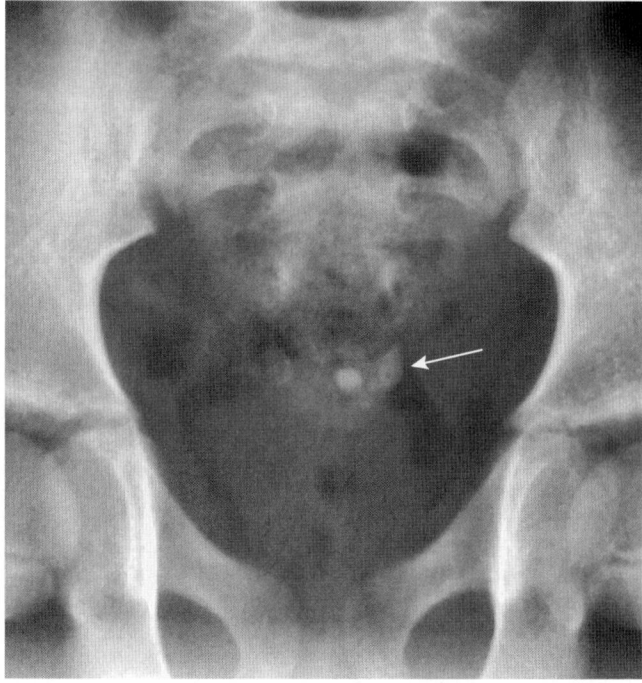

FIGURE 152-11. Calcification in urachal remnant. Supine radiograph of the pelvis shows a cluster of calcifications in the midline pelvis (arrow).

only by catheterization and opacification of the umbilical fistula, which demonstrates an inferior course of the tract toward the bladder. Urachal diverticula are best shown on a cystogram in the lateral projection. The diagnosis of urachal cyst is more difficult (Fig. 152-14). The cystogram may show only an extrinsic compression defect on the dome of the bladder in the midline or slightly to one side. Ultrasound (US), computed tomography (CT), or magnetic resonance imaging (MRI) show this lesion more effectively. Percutaneous catheter drainage of an infected urachal cyst under US guidance may be carried out before excision (Fig. 152-15).

BLADDER DIVERTICULA

Most bladder diverticula are localized outpouchings of the bladder mucosa between fibers of the detrusor muscles (pseudodiverticula), resulting from a congenital or acquired defect in the bladder wall. The neck of the diverticulum varies greatly from a few millimeters in diameter to very large. Small diverticula, less than 2 cm in diameter, are sometimes called saccules. Bladder diverticula may be primary (idiopathic), secondary, or iatrogenic (postoperative) (Table 152-1). In infants and young children, the incompletely full bladder may transiently herniate a portion inferolaterally into the internal inguinal ring producing so-called bladder ears (Fig. 152-16). Although there may be an associated inguinal hernia, this is a normal finding and disappears with increased bladder distention and should not be confused with a diverticulum.

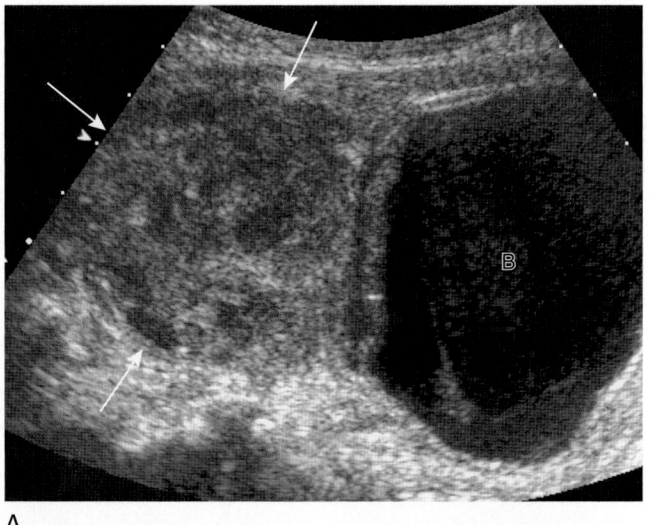

A

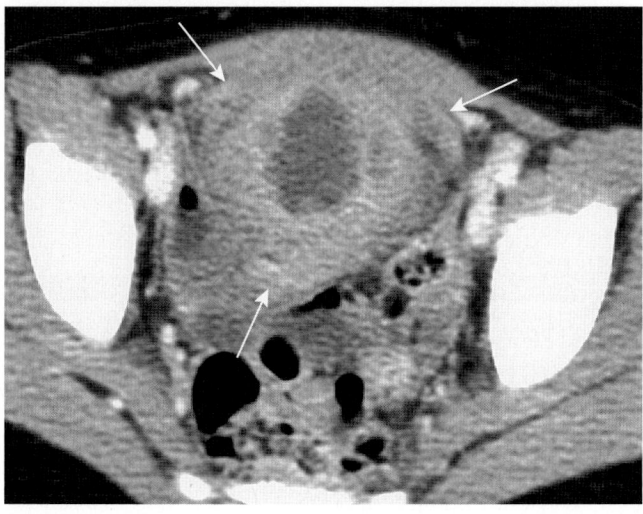

C

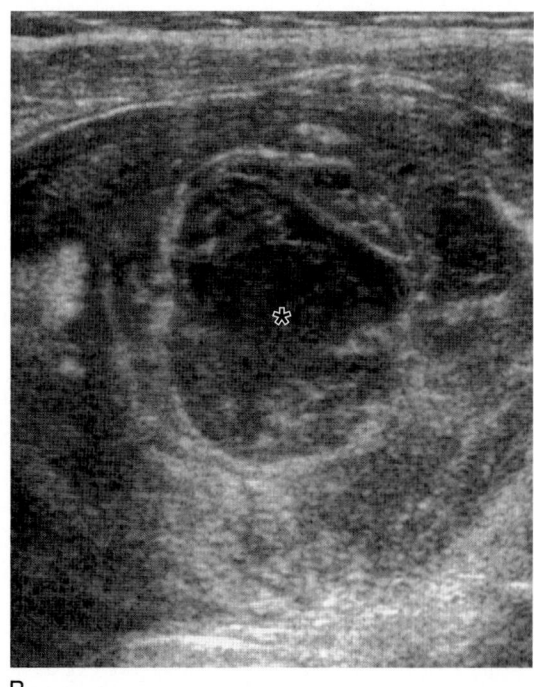

B

FIGURE 152-12. Urachal abscess. **A,** Longitudinal midline sonogram of the pelvis shows a large complex echoic mass *(arrows)* atop the bladder (B). **B,** Transverse sonogram of the mass shows complex hypoechoic center *(asterisk).* **C,** Contrast-enhanced CT image through the pelvis shows enhancing thick wall mass with low density center consistent with abscess *(arrows).*

Primary or idiopathic diverticula are the most common, are seen more often in males than in females, and may be single or multiple. They occur anywhere in the bladder but most frequently appear in the trigonal area. A common type of bladder diverticulum, referred to as paraureteral diverticulum or Hutch diverticulum (after the author who first described it), is located laterally and cephalad to the ureteral orifice (Fig. 152-17). The ureter enters the bladder near the base of the diverticulum, but, if the diverticulum is large, it may engulf the ureteral meatus and the ureter may empty into the diverticulum. Associated vesicoureteral reflux is present in about half of the cases and may be expected to occur when the ureter terminates in the diverticulum (Fig. 152-18). A large diverticulum originating from the trigonal area of the bladder may expand posteriorly and caudad below the bladder neck and compress the urethra, causing bladder outlet obstruction. Primary bladder diverticula, often multiple, may be seen in several syndromes, including cutis laxa, Ehlers-Danlos syndrome, fetal alcohol syndrome, Menkes syndrome, and Williams syndrome.

Secondary bladder diverticula are the result of chronically increased intravesical pressure with hypertrophy of bladder musculature. They may occur anywhere in the bladder but are most common in the paraureteral area. Secondary diverticula are seen mostly in patients with severe lower urinary tract obstruction (e.g., posterior urethral valves) and in patients with neurogenic bladder disease. Iatrogenic diverticula are seen most often in the anterior wall of the bladder at the site of a previous vesicostomy or suprapubic drainage catheter and at the ureterovesical junction (UVJ) after ureteral reimplantation.

Bladder diverticula may become visible only during voiding when contractions of the bladder force urine into the diverticulum (Fig. 152-19). Diverticula with a narrow neck empty much slower than those with a large neck and are best seen when the bladder is empty. Those located in the anterior or posterior wall of the bladder may be visible only in lateral or steep oblique views. The size of the diverticulum and the width of its neck are best judged on films obtained with the x-ray beam angled tangentially to the area. Bladder diverticula may also be demonstrated and evaluated by US.

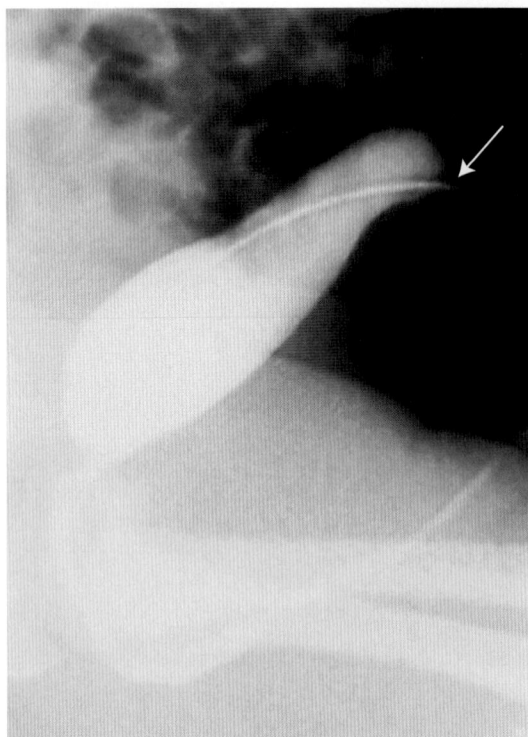

FIGURE 152-13. Patent urachus. Lateral view during VCUG performed after catheterization of the bladder through the umbilicus *(arrow).*

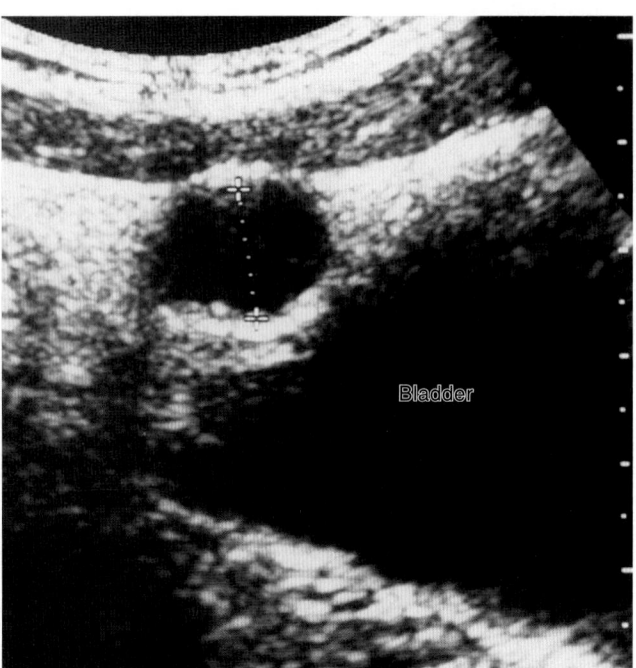

FIGURE 152-14. Urachal cyst. Longitudinal sonogram of the pelvis shows a cystic mass at the dome of the bladder *(cursors).*

> **Primary bladder diverticula are more common than secondary diverticula. Diverticula may be seen on VCUG only during voiding.**

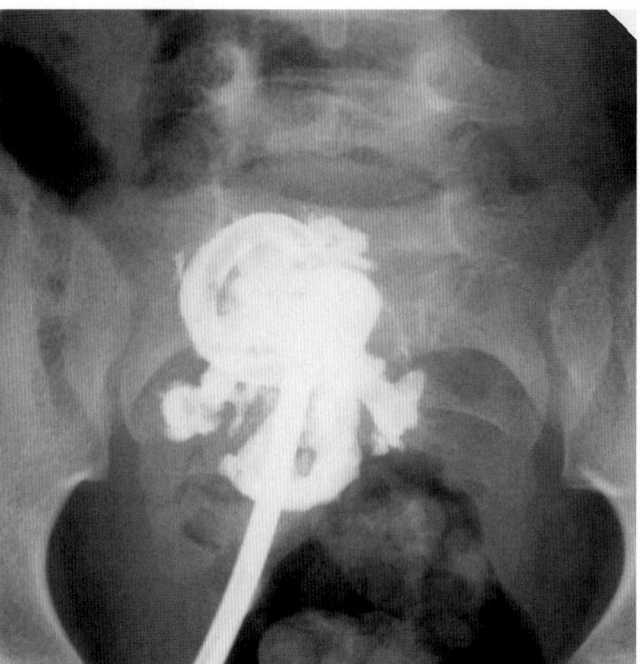

FIGURE 152-15. Catheter drainage of urachal abscess. Anterior image acquired after pigtail catheter drainage of urachal abscess (same patient as shown in Fig. 152-12). Contrast medium partially distends the irregular residual cavity.

TABLE 152-1
Types and Causes of Bladder Diverticula
PRIMARY (Congenital, Idiopathic) Multiple syndromes: cutis laxa, Ehlers-Danlos, fetal alcohol, Menkes, Williams **SECONDARY** Posterior urethral valves Urethral obstruction Neurogenic bladder **IATROGENIC** Vesicostomy site Suprapubic drainage site Urethral reimplantation site

MEGACYSTIS

Megacystis is a descriptive term for a large, smooth-walled bladder. The finding may be a normal variant or a congenital anomaly of little clinical significance. A large, smooth-walled bladder is common with prune-belly syndrome and may also be seen in patients who produce an excessive amount of urine chronically (e.g., patients with diabetes insipidus) or in patients with severe vesicoureteral reflux. The ureters in these patients may be dilated as well. Other causes include bladder atony after infection, megacystis/microcolon/intestinal hypoperistalsis syndrome (Fig. 152-20), and metabolic abnormalities. Although megacystis may also be seen in true neurogenic disease, this is quite uncommon in children; in most pediatric cases, true neurogenic disease is associated with a hypertonic, trabeculated bladder.

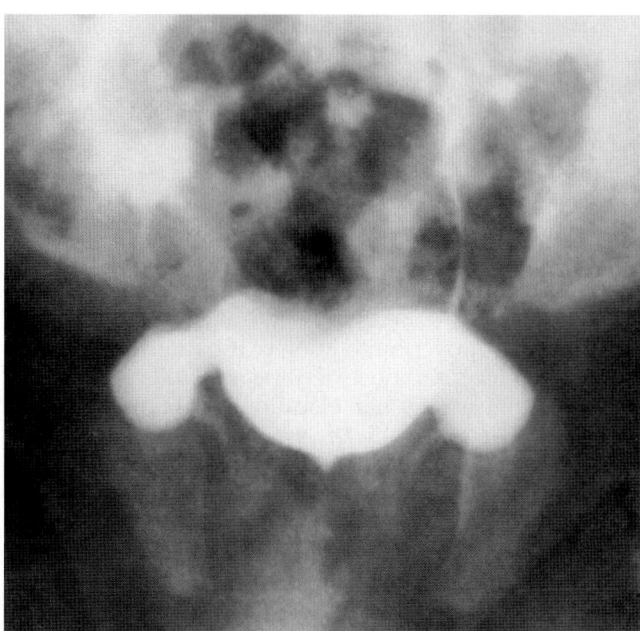

FIGURE 152-16. Bladder ears. VCUG shows transient lateral herniations of the bladder ("bladder ears") in a normal infant. (Courtesy of Sandra K. Fernbach, MD, and Kate A. Feinstein, MD.)

CYSTITIS

Acute hemorrhagic cystitis, cyclophosphamide (Cytoxan) cystitis, pseudotumoral cystitis, and eosinophilic cystitis are the most important forms of pediatric cystitis of radiologic interest seen in North America (Table 152-2).

Acute idiopathic hemorrhagic cystitis is one of the most common causes of gross hematuria in children. Dysuria and frequent urination of relatively sudden onset are associated symptoms. The disorder may occur throughout childhood but most often is in children 5 to 7 years of age. It is a self-limited disease that generally subsides in a few days to 2 or 3 weeks without sequelae. Adenovirus and *Escherichia coli* have been cultured in more than one third of the cases. On cystography and US, the bladder may be rounded, spastic, and small and may show contour irregularities, thickening of the mucosal folds, or a cobblestone pattern. These findings may be diffuse (Fig. 152-21) or limited to the base of the bladder or bladder trigone (Fig. 152-22). Mild ureterectasis may be present, and reflux is sometimes demonstrated.

Cyclophosphamide cystitis is a sterile inflammatory reaction of the bladder mucosa occurring primarily in oncologic patients undergoing preparative therapy for bone marrow transplantation. Cyclophosphamide is converted by the liver to the active metabolite acrolein, which is excreted in the urine and results in sloughing, thinning, and inflammation of the bladder urothelium. Exposure and rupture of the submucosal blood vessels leads to gross hematuria, clot retention, and occasional life-threatening hemorrhage. As a result, patients may have a prolonged hospital course, protracted need for blood products, and impaired bladder and renal function. An acute and a chronic form of cyclophosphamide cystitis are described. The acute form usually develops a few

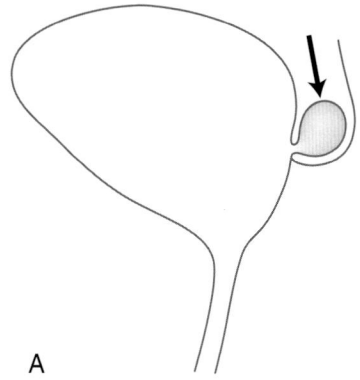

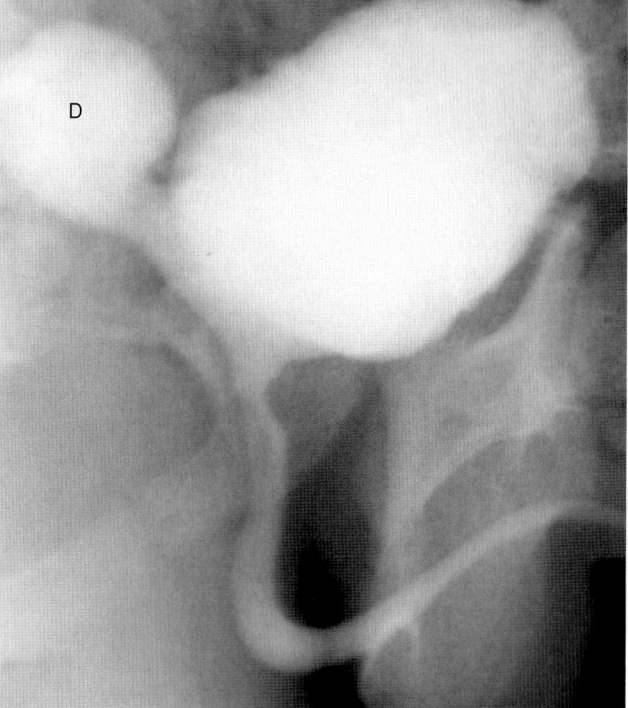

B

FIGURE 152-17. Hutch diverticulum. **A,** Diagram of a paraureteral bladder diverticulum (Hutch diverticulum) (*arrow*) located immediately above the ureterovesical junction. **B,** Left lateral oblique view during VCUG shows a right-sided diverticulum (D) originating at the trigone.

days or weeks after initiation of treatment, occasionally after the first dose. Patients develop urgency, frequency, suprapubic pain, and passage of blood clots. Ultrasonography (US) identifies focal or diffuse bladder wall thickening; color Doppler imaging demonstrates hypervascularity of the bladder wall and may identify the site of active bleeding. Cystoscopy shows diffuse mucosal edema, inflammation, submucosal hemorrhages, engorged vessels, and occasionally areas of necrosis. The cystogram reveals a small spastic bladder with nodular mucosal irregularities, especially at the level of the bladder trigone. The process generally clears after withdrawal of the drug, increased hydration, and a period of bladder drainage. If hemorrhage persists, intravesical sclerotherapy may be needed. A VCUG is required in these cases to determine bladder volume and the presence of vesicoureteral reflux. If reflux is present, ureteral orifice occlusion with a Fogarty balloon before instillation of the sclerosing agents prevents ureteral and kidney damage. Color Doppler imaging demonstrates diminished blood flow to the bladder wall after therapy. The chronic form of cyclophosphamide cystitis is a much more serious problem. It presents as continuous or intermittent painless hematuria, usually developing 2 to 3 months after initiation of therapy, sometimes only after its completion. The bladder becomes contracted and fibrotic, with diffuse mucosal telangiectasia. The cystogram shows a markedly contracted bladder with elevation and deformity of the bladder base and occasionally UVJ obstruction or vesicoureteral reflux.

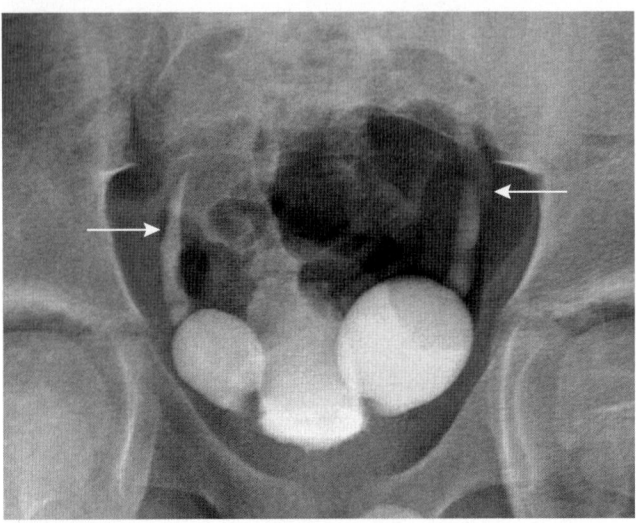

FIGURE 152-18. Bilateral hutch diverticula. Anterior image during a VCUG shows bilateral diverticula associated with bilateral vesicoureteral reflux (arrows).

Pseudotumoral cystitis is an uncommon inflammatory process of the bladder, usually presenting with clinical symptoms of dysuria, hematuria, and suprapubic pain and characterized by a nodular inflammatory mass (or masses) of the bladder, often mimicking a bladder neoplasm (Fig. 152-23). The process has a predilection for the base of the bladder and bladder trigone and may cause ureteral obstruction. The gross appearance and the histologic features are quite variable, with changes classified descriptively as bullous cystitis, cystitis cystica, cystitis follicularis, and cystitis granularis. Edema within the lamina propria, proliferation of the transitional epithelium, and proliferation of mucosal and submucosal glands produces mass-like elevations of the mucosal surface. A hypoechoic or hyperechoic mass appears smooth or lobulated on US. The cause of this disorder or group of disorders is not clear. In some instances, the changes may be the sequelae of bacterial or viral infection. Cystoscopy and biopsy may be necessary for diagnosis.

Eosinophilic cystitis is an inflammatory process that is more frequent in males and presents as irritative symptoms that include dysuria, hematuria, frequency, and pain. The cause is believed to be a hypersensitivity reaction to an antigenic stimulus that promotes an IgE-mediated attraction of eosinophils throughout the bladder wall with subsequent mast cell degranulation. This process leads to lysosomal membrane rupture and release of inflammatory mediators. Some have associated it with injury, medications, parasitic infections, food reactions, and other allergens. Medical conditions associated with eosinophilic cystitis include hyperimmunoglobulinemia E and chronic granulomatous disease. It may present as a focal mass simulating a rhabdomyosarcoma or appear as diffuse or localized bladder wall thickening. If suggested by eosinophils in the urine and/or peripheral blood, the diagnosis is confirmed by

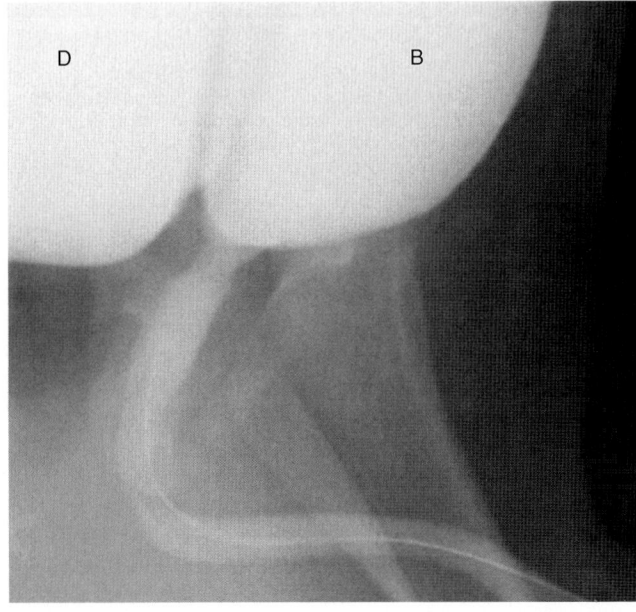

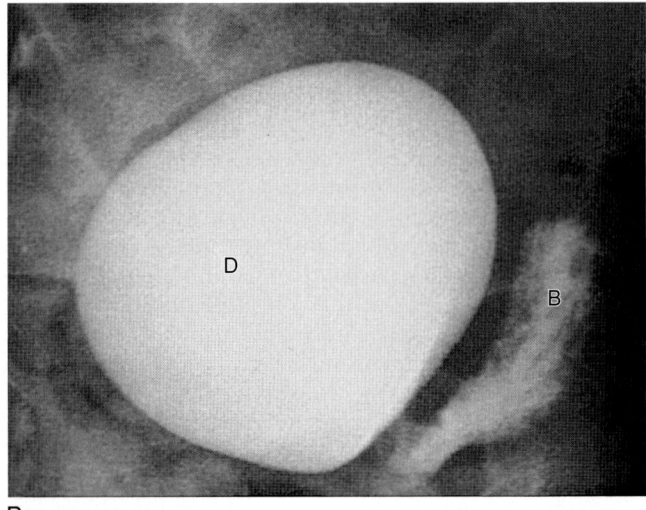

A   B

FIGURE 152-19. Expanding diverticulum. A, Oblique view during VCUG shows an expanding right bladder diverticulum during voiding (D). B, Bladder. B, At the end of voiding, a large contrast medium–filled diverticulum remains (D) with an empty bladder (B).

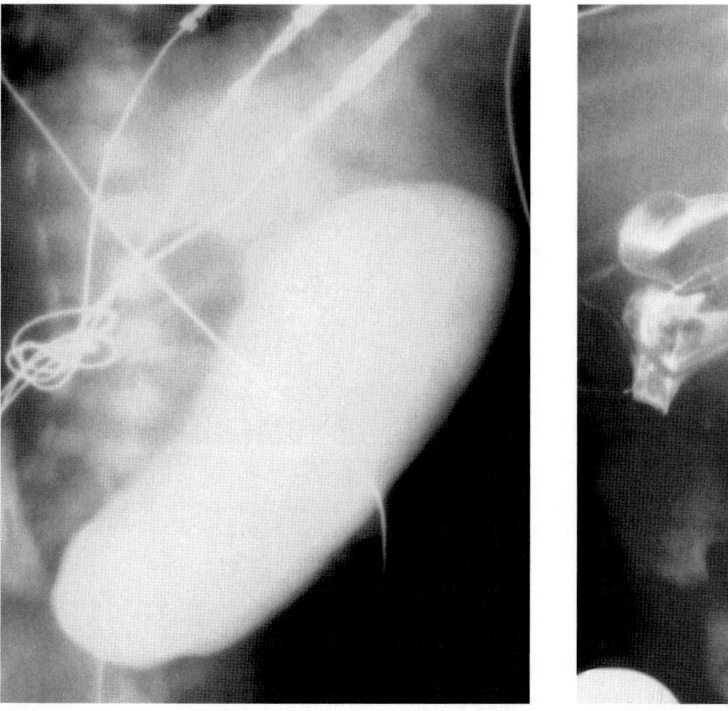
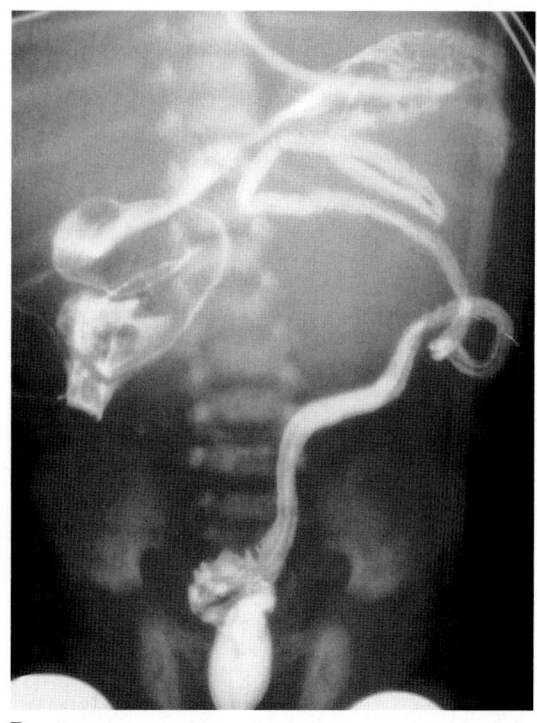

A   B

FIGURE 152-20. Megacystis-microcolon. **A,** Oblique view during a VCUG shows a large urinary bladder. **B,** Anterior view from a contrast enema showing a severe microcolon.

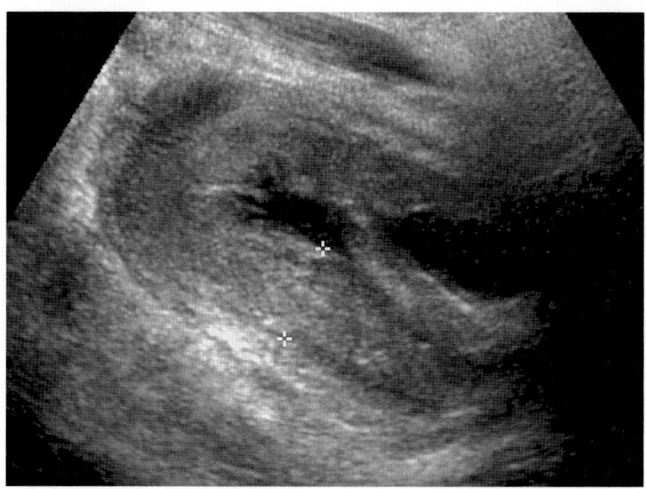
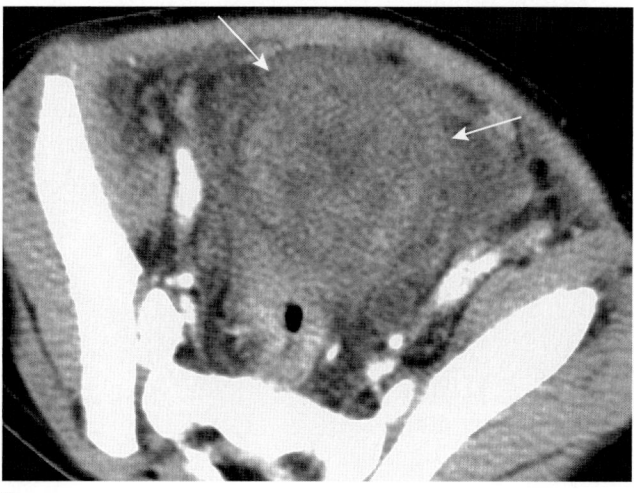

A   B

FIGURE 152-21. Hemorrhagic cystitis. **A,** Longitudinal sonogram of the pelvis shows marked circumferential bladder wall thickening (cursors). **B,** Contrast-enhanced CT image through the pelvis shows a hyperdense thick-walled bladder (arrows).

TABLE 152-2

Cystitis

FORMS OF CYSTITIS
Hemorrhagic
Cyclophosphamide
Tumoral
Eosinophilic

IMAGING FINDINGS (All enhance on CT and MRI)
Thick-walled, irregular bladder
Localized bladder wall thickening
Tumoral mass

biopsy. Treatment combines corticosteroids and antihistamines with avoidance of all possible allergens, inciting medications, or irritating foods. Eosinophilic cystitis is generally a self-limited process, with the bladder returning to normal in weeks to months.

NEOPLASMS OF THE BLADDER

Neoplasms of the bladder, urethra, and prostate are uncommon in children. Hematuria and urinary retention are the most frequent clinical manifestations. An abdominal mass may be palpated in some cases. The Intergroup

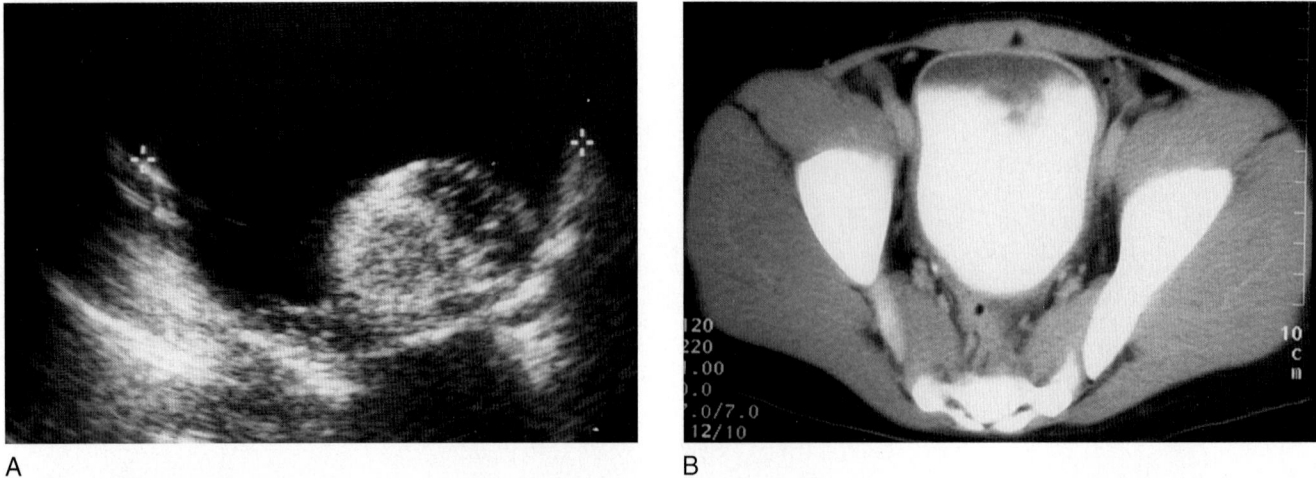

A   B

FIGURE 152-22. Hemorrhagic cystitis. **A,** Transverse sonogram of the bladder shows an echogenic blood clot. **B,** Contrast-enhanced CT of the bladder shows bladder wall enhancement indicating inflammation, and intraluminal filling defects representing blood clots.

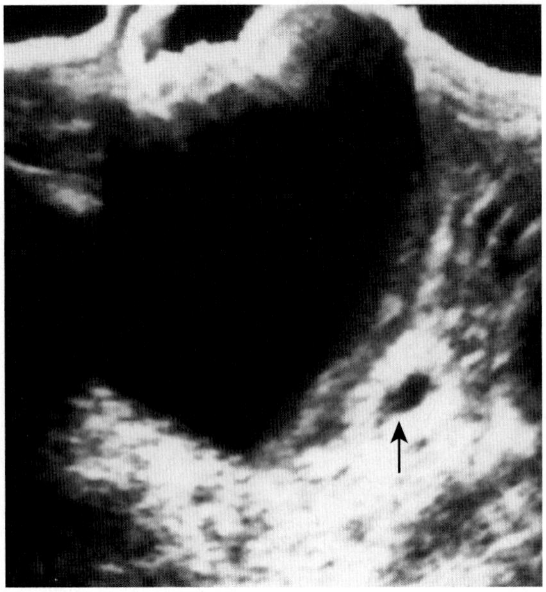

A 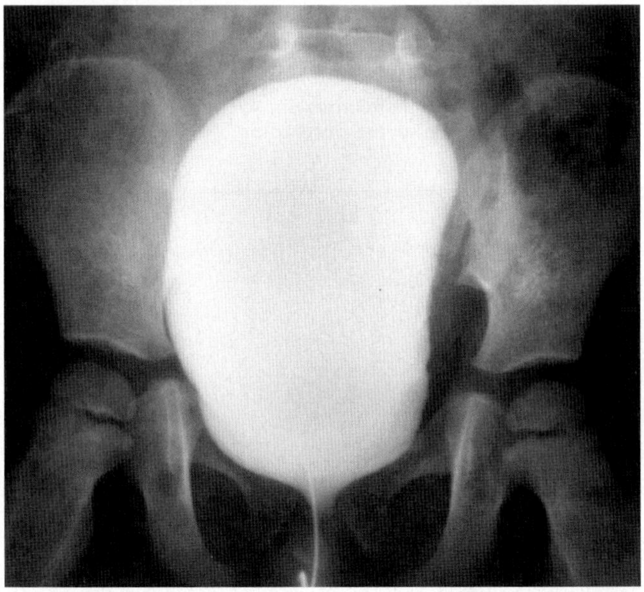   B

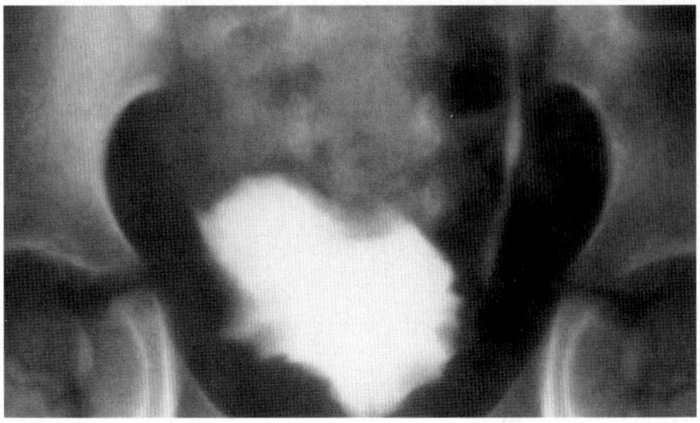

                                               C

FIGURE 152-23. Cystitis. **A,** Bladder sonogram in a 2-year-old boy with chronic granulomatous disease and pyuria shows focal posterior bladder wall thickening with a central hypoechoic area (*arrow*) representing an abscess. **B,** VCUG shows straightening and mass effect on the left side of the bladder. **C,** IVU image in a patient with bullous cystitis shows bladder wall lobulation, which cleared after antibiotic treatment.

TABLE 152-3

Intergroup Rhabdomyosarcoma Study Staging System for Neoplasms of the Bladder

Stage	Description
I	Localized tumor, completely resected
IIA	Localized tumor, grossly resected with microscopic residual
IIB	Tumor with regional disease or lymph node involvement, completely resected
IIC	Tumor with regional disease or involved lymph nodes, grossly resected with microscopic residual
IIIA	Gross residual tumor after biopsy only
IIIB	Distant metastases present at diagnosis

Rhabdomyosarcoma Study staging system for neoplasms of the bladder is given in Table 152-3.

Rhabdomyosarcoma is the most common and important neoplasm of the lower genitourinary tract and accounts for about 10% of all rhabdomyosarcomas seen in children. It is the most frequent bladder neoplasm in children in the first decade of life. The tumor is discovered most often during the first 2 or 3 years of life, occasionally at birth, and has a slight male predominance. In more than half of the cases, the neoplasm arises from the prostate. In the rest of the cases, it originates in the bladder, frequently from the area of the trigone, and occasionally from the dome (Fig. 152-24). The tumor is locally invasive and frequently extends toward the bladder outlet, causing urethral obstruction. In females, rhabdomyosarcoma may also arise from the vagina and uterine cervix and invade the same areas of the bladder. When local extension is present, it may not be possible to determine the site of origin. Symptoms usually include hematuria, frequency, urinary retention, and obstruction (i.e., hydronephrosis).

Histologically, the tumor is divided into three subtypes: embryonal, alveolar, or polymorphic. Embryonal rhabdomyosarcoma is further subdivided into three categories: classic embryonal, botryoid, and spindle cell. The embryonal form is by far the most common, accounting for approximately two thirds of all rhabdomyosarcomas. The embryonal botryoid subtype accounts for one fourth of the cases and has a lobulated, polypoid appearance resembling a bunch of grapes, hence the name *sarcoma botryoides* often used for this variant. The alveolar subtype accounts for approximately a third of cases and the pleomorphic rhabdomyosarcoma is rare, almost exclusively seen in adults.

> **Rhabdomyosarcoma is the most common pediatric bladder tumor and is divided into embryonal, alveolar, and polymorphic subtypes.**

The growth pattern of the tumor is important for prognosis. A polypoid (exophytic) tumor with superficial tumor cells and a myxoid center and base is exclusive to the botryoid form. A polypoid (exophytic) tumor with more evenly distributed tumor cells characterizes both the botryoid and classic embryonal forms. Diffusely growing tumors with evenly distributed tumor cells predominately within the wall of the organ of origin are seen in the classic embryonal and alveolar forms and spindle cell variants. The polypoid forms are less aggressive and have a better prognosis. Both the bladder and vagina have a relatively high incidence of the botryoid subtype. This is thought to occur because of the relative loose subepithelial tissue in these organs allowing the tumor to expand into the lumen. Rhabdomyosarcoma spreads by local extension from the bladder, prostate, and vagina into regional and retroperitoneal lymph nodes and muscle. Lymph node involvement or distant tumor spread is found at initial diagnosis in 10% to 20% of patients.

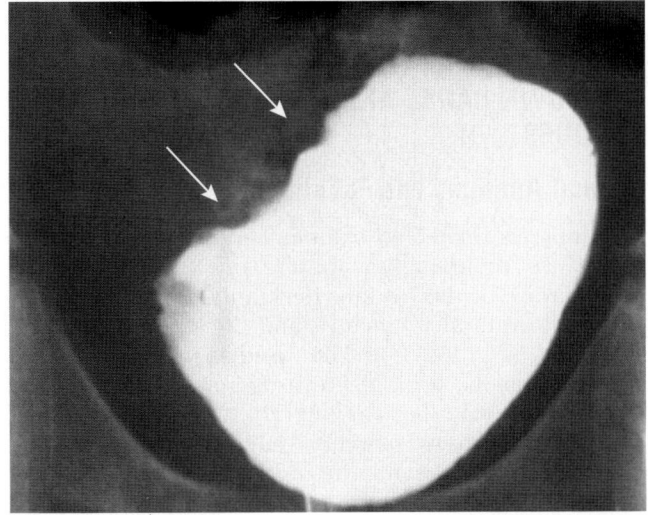
A

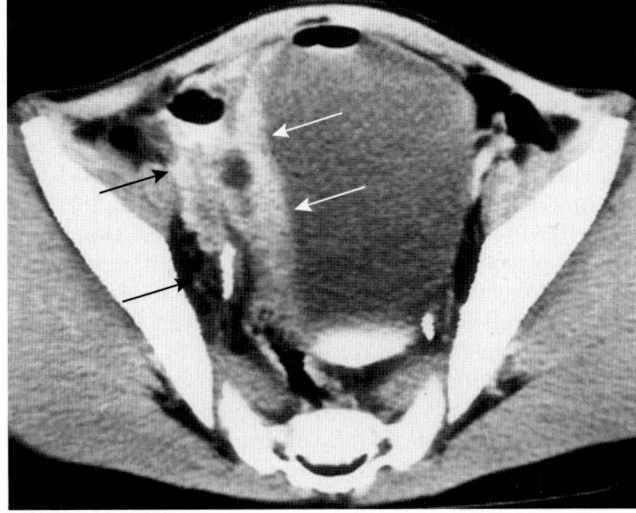
B

FIGURE 152-24. Rhabdomyosarcoma. **A,** Cystogram from a 9-year-old boy with hematuria shows a lobular mass involving the right bladder *(arrows).* **B,** Contrast–enhanced CT scan shows thickening and enhancement of the right bladder wall *(white arrows)* and extension toward the right pelvic sidewall *(black arrows).*

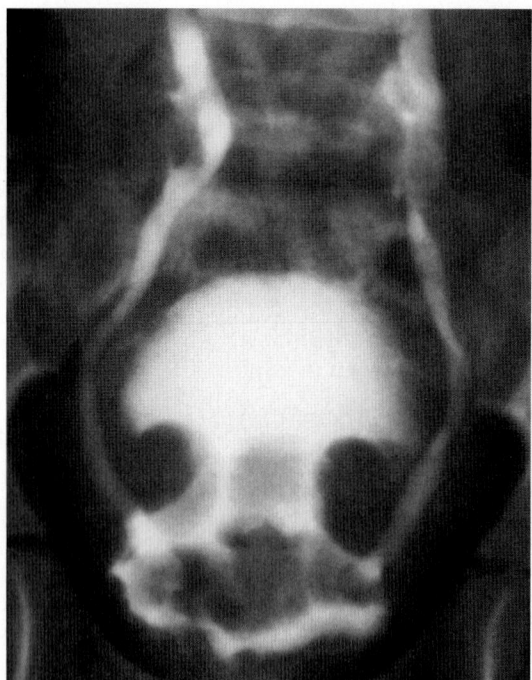

FIGURE 152-25. Bladder rhabdomyosarcoma. Anterior image from an intravenous pyelogram showing multiple lobular filling defects in the bladder.

Survival rate is also dependent on the site of origin. Tumors of the urinary bladder and prostate have an overall 5-year survival rate of approximately 70%. Tumors originating in nonbladder/prostate sites (paratesticular, vagina, and cervix) have a better 5-year survival rate, between 84% and 89%. The prognosis is generally worse when the tumor occurs in the first year of life. Urogenital rhabdomyosarcomas overall have a more favorable prognosis than tumors in retroperitoneum, extremities, or parameningeal sites. Treatment combines surgical removal of as much of the tumor as possible, chemotherapy, and radiation therapy.

When rhabdomyosarcoma originates in the bladder, intravenous urography (IVU) (Fig. 152-25) and voiding cystourethrography (VCUG) show a large and often lobulated filling defect in the posteroinferior aspect of the bladder. When originating in the prostate (Fig. 152-26), the cystogram usually shows an upward displacement of the bladder floor or a smooth, lobulated mass at the base of the bladder and the urethrogram may reveal elongation and displacement of the posterior urethra, sometimes with a lobulated filling defect. The bladder may be enlarged and the ureters may be obstructed. Whereas the initial diagnosis is often made with US, CT and MRI are required for evaluating extent of disease and presence of metastases. T1-weighted MRI is used for evaluating fat invasion and lymph node spread, whereas T2-weighted images document soft tissue invasion (especially with fat-suppression techniques). Distant metastases, particularly to the lungs, bones, and liver, also occur but usually only late in the disease. CT is less time consuming and less expensive than MRI and is superior for imaging lung metastases. CT and MRI are comparable for detecting liver metastases, with MRI having the advantage of avoiding radiation.

Other primary malignant neoplasms of the lower urinary tracts are very rare. Instances have been reported of papillary epithelial bladder tumors, leiomyosarcoma and primary lymphoma of the bladder, malignant neoplasms of the urachus, pheochromocytoma, and rhabdoid tumors. The bladder may also be involved secondarily by leukemia and lymphoma.

Among the benign neoplasms, hemangioma of the bladder is probably the most common. It presents as a discrete solitary mass of variable size, usually projecting from the dome of the bladder. Hematuria is the most common clinical finding. Coexistent hemangiomas of the skin may be observed in 20% to 30% of the cases. US and CT demonstrate bladder wall thickening, intramural anechoic spaces, and occasional calcification associated with these lesions. Inflammatory pseudotumor (inflammatory pseudosarcoma, pseudosarcomatous myofibroblastic tumor, pseudomalignant spindle cell proliferation, plasma cell tumor, histiocytoma) is a rare benign tumor of the bladder in children. The etiology of this lesion remains unclear. There is no sex predilection, with most cases diagnosed in the first decade (35% in the first 5 years of life). Histologic examination demonstrates spindle cell myofibroblastic and fibroblastic proliferation with a prominent inflammatory cell infiltrate composed of plasma cells, lymphocytes, and histiocytes, and occasionally neutrophils and eosinophils. They do not metastasize or undergo malignant transformation. Radiologic imaging and cystoscopy identify a polypoid or submucosal mass indistinguishable from embryonal rhabdomyosarcoma. Neurofibromas of the bladder may occur as part of systemic neurofibromatosis or as an isolated lesion (Fig. 152-27). Other reported benign neoplasms of the bladder include fibromas, fibromatous polyps, hematoma (Fig. 152-28), inverted papilloma (Fig. 152-29), and nephrogenic adenoma of the bladder. Isolated instances of benign neurofibroma and leiomyoma of the prostate have been reported.

DYSFUNCTIONAL VOIDING DISORDERS OF UNKNOWN CAUSE AND CLASSIC NEUROGENIC BLADDER

Normal Anatomy and Function

The muscles related to bladder continence and micturition are the detrusor muscle of the bladder, the musculature of the bladder neck and proximal urethra (internal urethral sphincter), and the external urethral sphincter (Fig. 152-30). The urethra is also affected indirectly, at the level of the urogenital diaphragm, by the striated voluntary muscles of the pelvic floor; a contraction of these muscles results in elevation of the pelvic floor, compressing the urethra.

The muscles of micturition are under the control of the autonomic nervous system (parasympathetic with center at S2 to S4 and sympathetic with center at T10 to L2) and of the voluntary somatic nerves (via the pudendal nerves with center at S2 to S4). The various

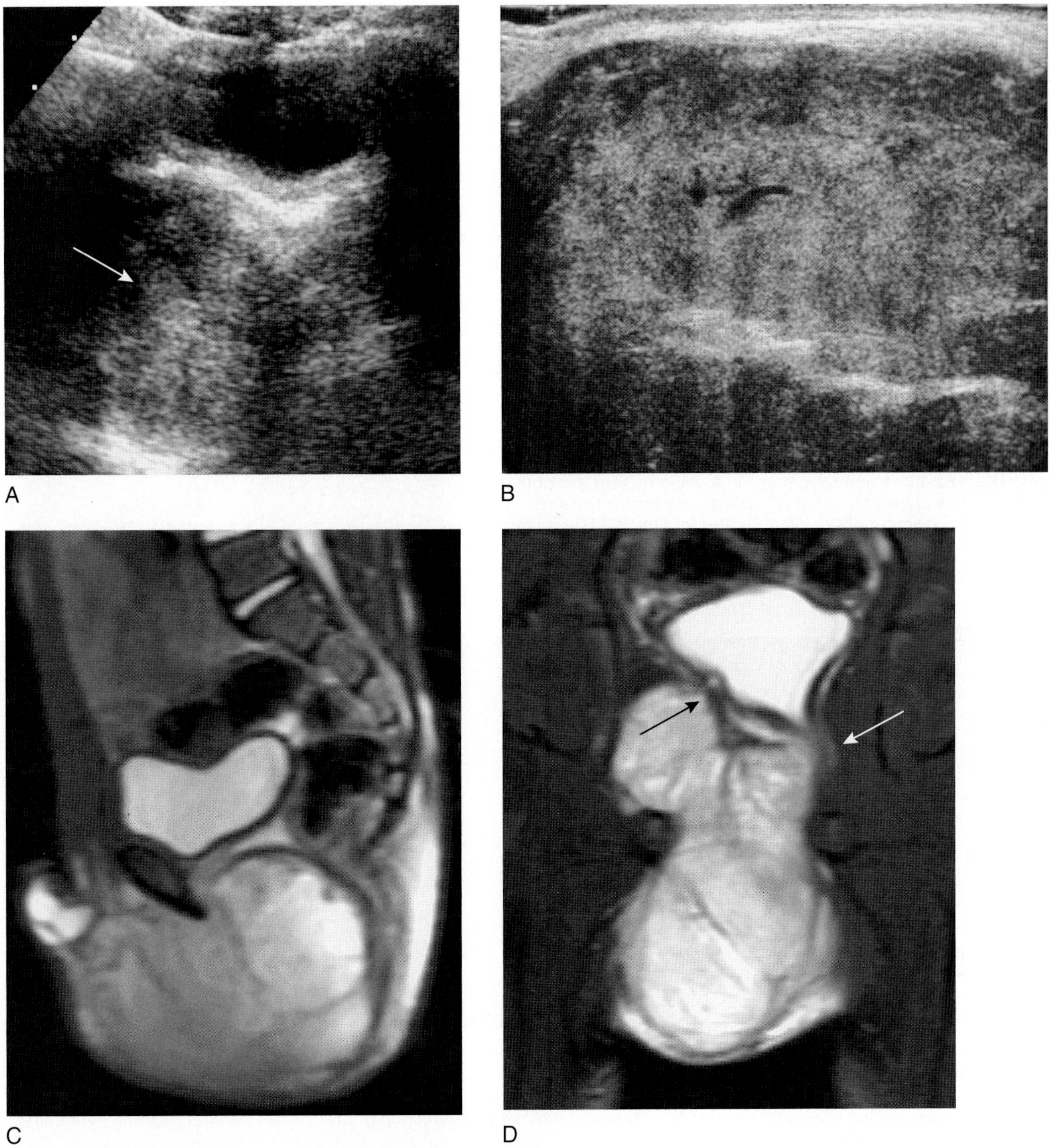

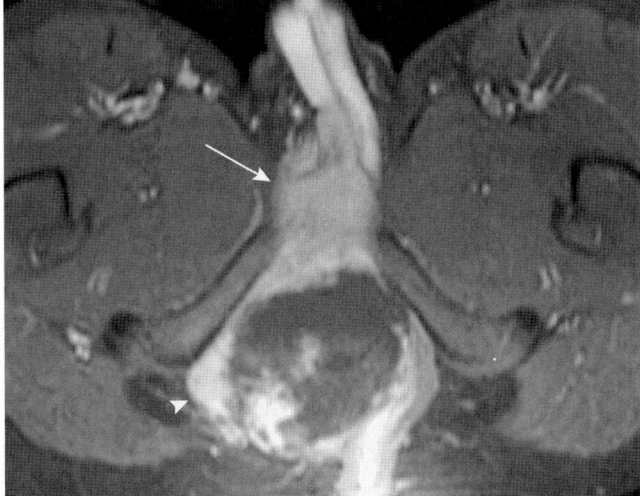

FIGURE 152-26. Prostatic rhabdomyosarcoma.
A, Transverse sonogram of the pelvis in a 5-year-old boy shows a large predominately isoechoic mass below the bladder base *(arrow).* **B,** Longitudinal transperineal sonogram better demonstrates the large solid mass. **C,** Sagittal T2-weighted MR image shows a large, lobulated, bright, and heterogeneous mass extending from the bladder base to the perineum. **D,** Coronal T2-weighted MR image shows the bladder base displaced to the left *(black arrow),* and the rectum displaced to the left and partially encased *(white arrow).* **E,** Axial, T1-weighted, fat-saturated MR image shows the mass extends through the right obturator foramen *(arrowhead)* and there is direct invasion of the base of the penis *(arrow).*

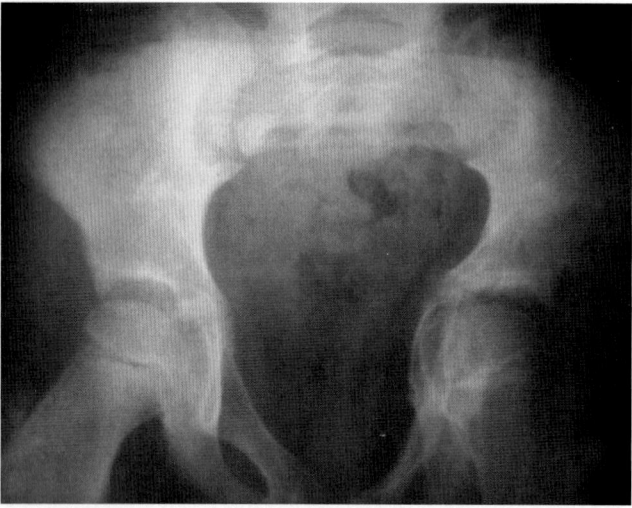

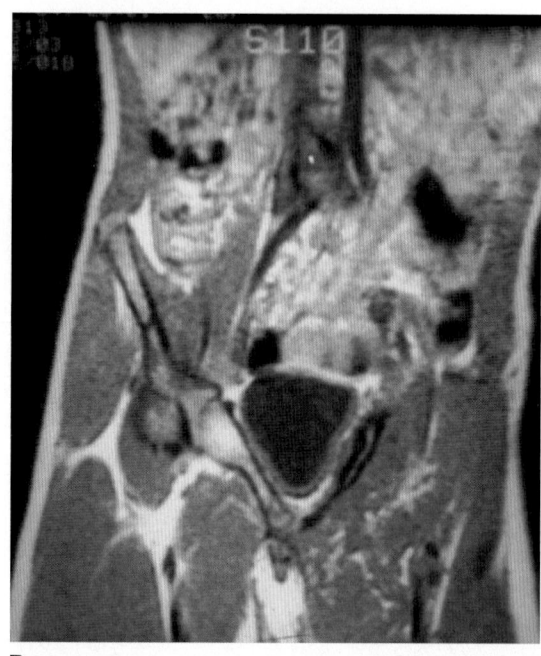

FIGURE 152-27. Neurofibromatosis. **A,** Plain radiograph of the pelvis shows distortion of the left pelvic bony structures and medial displacement of the left obturator fat line. **B,** T1-weighted, coronal MR image shows a mass extending from the pelvic inlet inferiorly through the obturator foramen to the leg.

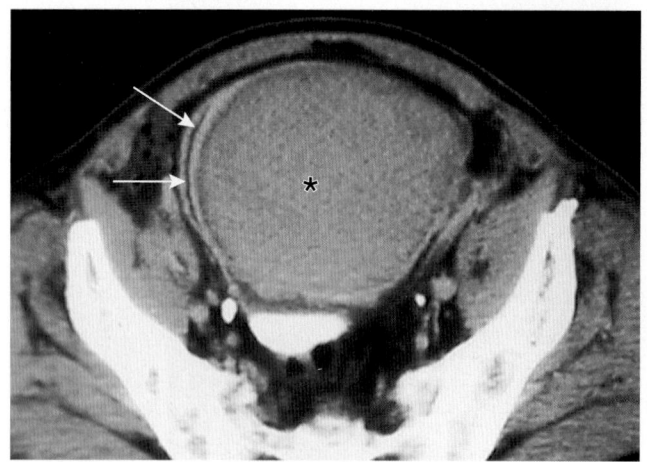

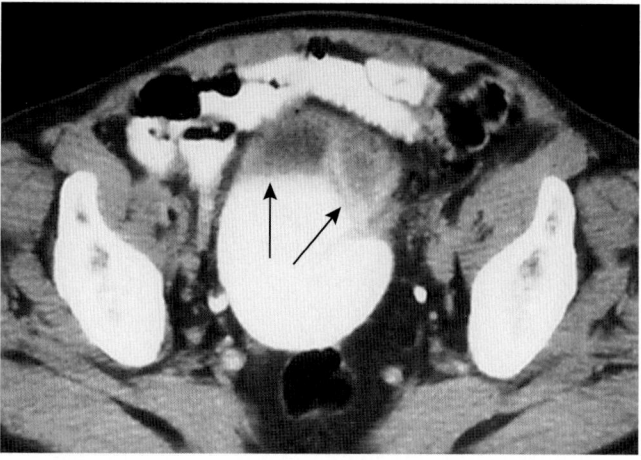

FIGURE 152-28. Bladder wall hematoma. **A,** Contrast-enhanced CT image through the pelvis demonstrates a large, mildly hyperdense mass *(asterisk)* within the wall of the bladder. The mass nearly obliterates the bladder lumen, with a only small crescentic collection of urine separating the walls *(arrows)*. **B,** Follow-up study shows reduction of the hematoma with residual hypodense clot *(arrows)* outlined by contrast medium.

nerves and muscles involved in bladder control and normal bladder filling and emptying are closely interrelated. Parasympathetic stimulation results in increased tone of the detrusor and, as a secondary phenomenon, in relaxation of the bladder neck and relaxation of urethral smooth muscle. Sympathetic stimulation results in a contraction of the bladder neck and urethral smooth muscle and a decrease in the tone of the detrusor. A voluntary contraction of the external sphincter and perineal muscles narrows the urethra and, indirectly, causes an increase in the tone of the bladder neck and relaxation of the detrusor.

The activity of the sacral (parasympathetic) micturition center (S2 to S4) is modulated by impulses from a micturition center in the rostral pons (locus coeruleus) that is under the voluntary control of cortical areas of the brain (perirolandic region). During normal bladder filling, intravesical pressure remains relatively low until a certain point of detrusor stretch is reached, when reflex activity causes increased tone of the detrusor and an urge to void. If the conditions for micturition are not favorable (or during voluntary interruption of micturition), bladder emptying can be prevented (up to a certain bladder volume and pressure) by voluntary cortical inhibition of the sacral micturition center (which depresses detrusor tone), and by voluntary impulses from the motor cortex to the sacral nuclei of the pudendal nerves (which cause external sphincter contraction and, secondarily, increased internal sphincter tone and detrusor relaxation).

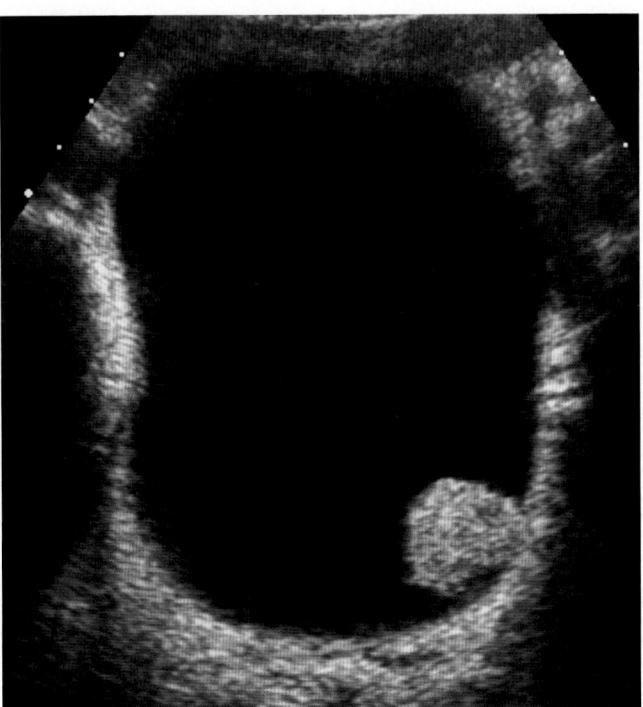

FIGURE 152-29. Inverted papilloma. Transverse sonogram through the bladder shows an echogenic polypoid mass arising from the left side of the bladder floor.

> **Voiding is controlled by a complex interaction of sympathetic and parasympathetic innervation coordinating detrusor, internal sphincter, and external sphincter actions.**

The act of micturition is a complex function requiring several years to develop, from a single spinal cord reflex action in infancy (infantile bladder) to complete bladder control, both conscious and subconscious, which is

attained in the vast majority of children during the fourth year. The remaining children acquire full bladder control in the subsequent years, with only 2% to 3% still showing some nocturnal enuresis or daytime frequency at puberty.

Dysfunctional Voiding Disorders

Under this heading are included functional disorders of the bladder and urethral musculature manifested in some patients by a delay in maturation of bladder control, in others by a hyperreflexia of the detrusor muscle with normal external sphincter activity, and in still others by a lack of coordination of the detrusor and the external sphincter. The so-called lazy bladder syndrome of infrequent voiders is also included in this group. The causes of these disorders are not certain. There are no demonstrable neurogenic organic lesions, and there are no abnormalities of the spine or spinal cord demonstrable by imaging methods.

ENURESIS

Urinary incontinence in children is the result of a variety of functional and organic disorders. Confusion arises due to the various terms and definitions commonly used when classifying incontinence (Table 152-4). Incontinence is the leakage of at least 1 ml of urine, at least once a week, in a child of at least 5 years of age. Enuresis is normal voiding that occurs at an inappropriate time or social setting and is involuntary in the setting of normal anatomic and neurologic findings. It typically is used to define night-time (nocturnal) wetting. A child with night-time wetting at age 5 years or older is considered a "bedwetter" by the American Psychiatric Association. Urodynamic studies in these children are often normal and are usually reserved for treatment nonresponders.

Some of the commonly accepted facts about children with enuresis are presented in Table 152-5. Most children are toilet trained by 3 to 4 years of age, with girls achieving

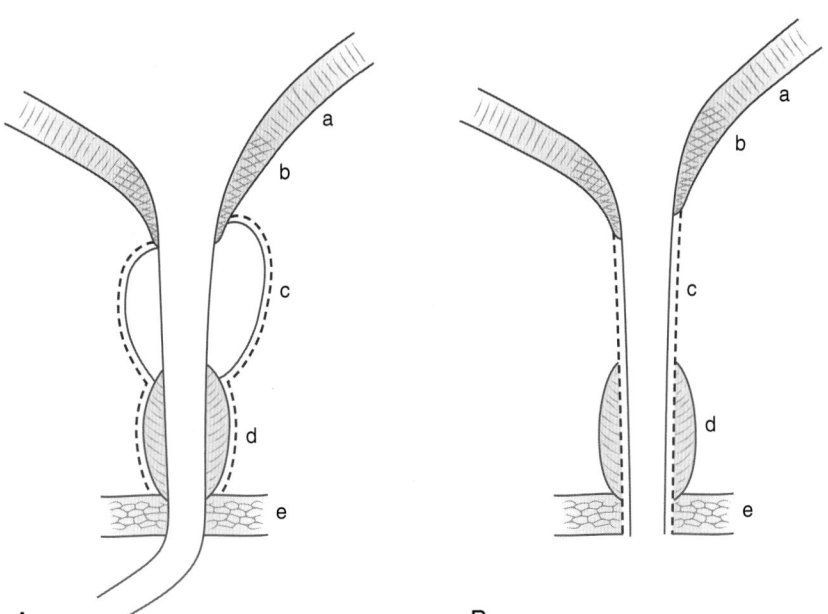

FIGURE 152-30. Diagram of the muscles of micturition in the male (**A**) and in the female (**B**). These muscles include a, detrusor of the bladder (smooth muscle fibers, autonomic innervation); b, bladder neck musculature (smooth muscle fibers, autonomic innervation); c, fibers of the detrusor of the bladder extending to the capsule of the prostate and eternal urethral sphincter in the male, and to the entire urethra underneath the external sphincter in the female; d, external urethral sphincter (striated muscles, somatic innervation); and e, muscles of the pelvic floor (striated muscles, somatic innervation).

A   B

TABLE 152-4

Bladder Control Terminology

Primary nocturnal enuresis	The child who has never been dry at night for more than 6 months. This is more common than secondary enuresis.
Secondary nocturnal enuresis	Bedwetting after a period of at least 6 months of night-time dryness. This is associated with an underlying psychological or organic cause.
Monosymptomatic nocturnal enuresis	Bedwetting with daytime continence. This is the most common form of enuresis.
Non-monosymptomatic nocturnal enuresis	Bedwetting with daytime voiding symptoms of urgency and frequency with or without daytime incontinence. This suggests underlying bladder dysfunction.
Urinary incontinence	Daytime wetting without bedwetting.
Organic incontinence	Urinary leakage due to a known or suspected cause. This includes neurogenic bladder secondary to myelodysplasia, central nervous system disorders, anorectal malformations and spinal cord injury, and anatomic abnormalities such as ectopic ureters, posterior urethral valves, and fistulous disease.

TABLE 152-5

Common Observations of Childhood Enuresis

- Daytime control precedes night-time control.
- 15%-20% of 5-year-old children wet the bed.
- 10% have enuresis when older than age 10 years.
- 1% have enuresis when older than age 15 years.
- 15% of children become spontaneously continent each year.
- Diurnal (day and night) wetters = 20%.
- Positive family history is frequent.
- Autosomal dominant inheritance is linked to chromosomes 8, 12, 13, and 22.
- Cystic fibrosis, sickle cell disease, attention deficit hyperactivity disorder, obstructive sleep apnea, and constipation are associated with nocturnal enuresis.

continence at an earlier age than boys, and daytime control precedes nocturnal continence. Nocturnal enuresis appears to be dependent on three factors: (1) nocturnal urine production, (2) nocturnal bladder function, and (3) sleep and arousal mechanisms. Urine production follows a circadian rhythm that is established between the ages of 2 and 5 years, with daytime urine production two to three times that of the night-time period. In two thirds of children with bedwetting there is loss of the circadian rhythm of vasopressin release and the development of nocturnal polyuria. One third of children have frequent uninhibited detrusor contractions and reduced functional capacity of the bladder. These children have normal detrusor activity and functional bladder capacity while awake. Defects in sleep arousal are also common in enuritic children, despite both detrusor contractions and bladder overdistention being arousal stimuli. Patients can be categorized into those with diuresis-dependent enuresis and detrusor-dependent enuresis. Those in the former group have full but stable bladders at night and respond favorably to desmopressin (an antidiuretic hormone analog) treatment. The latter group voids secondary to failed suppression of detrusor contractions and are poor responders to desmopressin therapy. Anticholinergics can be tried, often with success in these children. Combination therapy with the enuresis alarm and behavioral interventions

(regular waking of the child at night) are used to awaken the child at the moment of enuresis and recognize imminent bladder voiding.

URGE SYNDROME (UNSTABLE BLADDER) IN CHILDREN

This relatively common disorder, also called detrusor instability and idiopathic detrusor hyperreflexia, is characterized by phasic uninhibited (involuntary) detrusor contractions early in the bladder filling phase and normal external sphincter activity. It is seen usually in children between 3 and 14 years (median, 6 to 8 years) and is more common in girls than in boys. The clinical manifestations include frequent daytime voiding and urge to void (peaking in the afternoon) that may result in episodes of incontinence. Nocturnal enuresis is common. The patients may react to detrusor contractions by increasing the external sphincter and perineal muscular activity and frequently assume characteristic postures or develop special maneuvers to prevent urine loss. Vesicoureteral reflux and urinary tract infections are not uncommon. The increased pelvic floor activity contributes to the development of chronic constipation and soiling. The combination of urinary tract and bowel dysfunction may be referred to as the dysfunctional elimination syndrome. The patient can void on command, and the act of voiding is usually well coordinated.

Increased thickness of the bladder wall is demonstrated by US (Fig. 152-31). On VCUG, the bladder is commonly smaller than normal and hypertonic, and it may be smooth in outline or slightly trabeculated. Vesicourethral reflux may be observed. The urethra may show transient narrowing at the level of the external sphincter with proximal urethral dilatation (the "spinning top" urethra in females, see later). The patient can void with a sustained flow without residual urine in the bladder at the end of voiding. Signs and symptoms of transient detrusor contractions may be noted during the examination, including the urge to void at low bladder volumes, intermittent slowing or cessation or even reversal of the flow of contrast material in the tubing, and intermittent widening of the bladder neck and proximal urethra during bladder filling. The upper urinary tracts are usually normal. Bladder instability is a generally benign disorder that tends to resolve spontaneously with age.

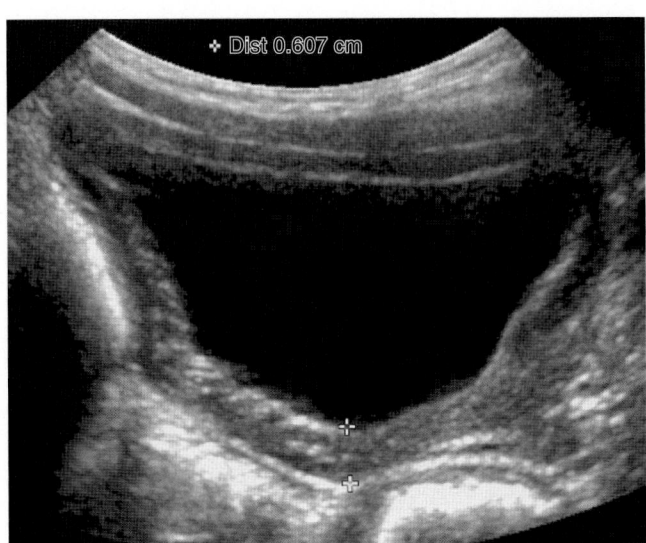
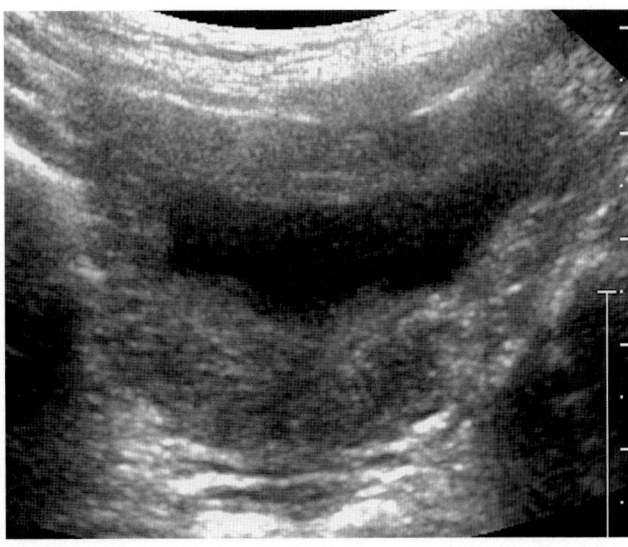

FIGURE 152-31. Bladder wall thickening. Prevoid transverse (**A**) and postvoid transverse (**B**) sonograms of the bladder in a patient with dysfunctional voiding show circumferential smooth bladder wall thickening (**A**, *cursors*).

DETRUSOR/EXTERNAL SPHINCTERIC DYSSYNERGIA

This relatively uncommon type of voiding dysfunction, also called non-neurogenic neurogenic bladder, syndrome of vesicoureteral incoordination, and Hinman syndrome, is the most severe of the group. It is characterized by an incoordination, or dyscoordination, in the activity of the detrusor muscle and that of the external sphincter. The two muscles tend to contract at the same time, preventing efficient emptying of the bladder and leading to a chronically increased intravesical pressure and obstructive changes in the bladder and upper urinary tracts similar to those seen in classic neurogenic bladder (see later).

The condition occurs with equal frequency in boys and girls and is commonly encountered between ages 2 and 13 years. Recurrent urinary infections, night-time wetting, and daytime urgency and frequency are common manifestations. Episodes of urinary retention may occur, and an occasional patient presents with clinical signs of chronic uremia. Dribbling between voidings, possibly an overflow phenomenon, may be observed. Voluntary initiation of voiding may be difficult, requiring much straining. The distended and firm bladder is sometimes present on physical examination. Many children with this disorder also have bowel dysfunction manifested by chronic constipation and soiling. A wide range of behavioral or psychological disturbances is common and may contribute to the severity of the symptoms and impact the response to therapy.

US shows an increased thickness of the bladder wall, and on VCUG the scout film may show a large amount of feces in the colon. The bladder is commonly enlarged, hypertonic, and variably trabeculated and may point upward and to the right, as in classic neurogenic bladder. Unilateral or bilateral vesicoureteral reflux is also common, occurring in about 50% of the patients, and the refluxing upper tracts are frequently dilated. The bladder neck and urethra appear normal, but the area of the external sphincter may show a constant or intermittent narrowing (spasm) of the urethra at that level with dilatation proximally. In girls, the urethra may assume a "spinning top" configuration (Fig. 152-32). A large postvoid residual is very common.

US and IVU may show unilateral or bilateral upper tract dilatation that is sometimes severe. Atrophy of the renal parenchyma may be present, and renal function may be decreased. The more severe upper tract changes are seen in patients with reflux and urinary tract infections. In some cases, the urinary tract changes are already developed at the time of the first examination. VCUG performed in early life may show that the bladder was originally smooth, indicating that the trabeculation is an acquired and progressive phenomenon.

The uncoordinated activity of the detrusor and external sphincter muscles tends to improve in late childhood or early adolescence, but by this time secondary changes in the upper tracts may have progressed to renal insufficiency. Current treatment consists of biofeedback training and an intensive and prolonged bladder retraining program, including frequent and "relaxed" voiding with complete emptying of the bladder and other forms of behavior modification.

LAZY BLADDER SYNDROME

The lazy bladder syndrome, characterized by a dilated hypotonic and hyporeflexic bladder, is seen predominantly in girls and usually becomes manifest between 2 and 6 years of age with recurrent urinary tract infections, infrequent voiding, passage of small amounts of urine, and sometimes overflow or stress incontinence. The child may delay voiding for long periods of time and usually voids only once or twice a day. Constipation and soiling are common. VCUG demonstrates a large, smooth-walled bladder with a decreased sensation of fullness (Fig. 152-33). Initiation of voiding may be difficult and require much straining and coaxing. Urine flow may be interrupted (fractionated voiding). The bladder neck

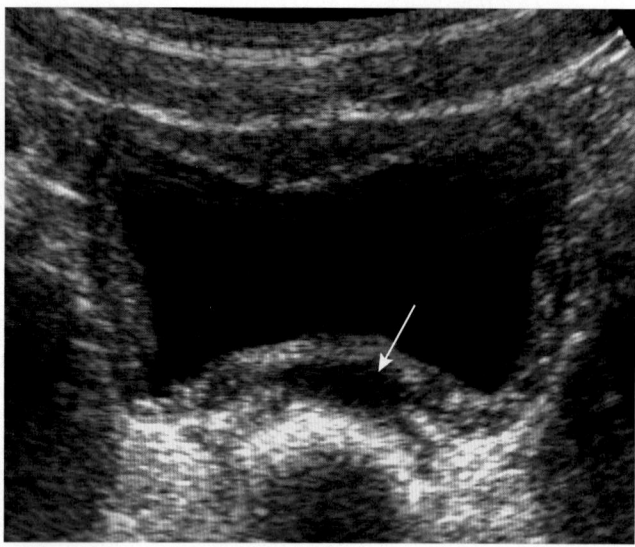

A

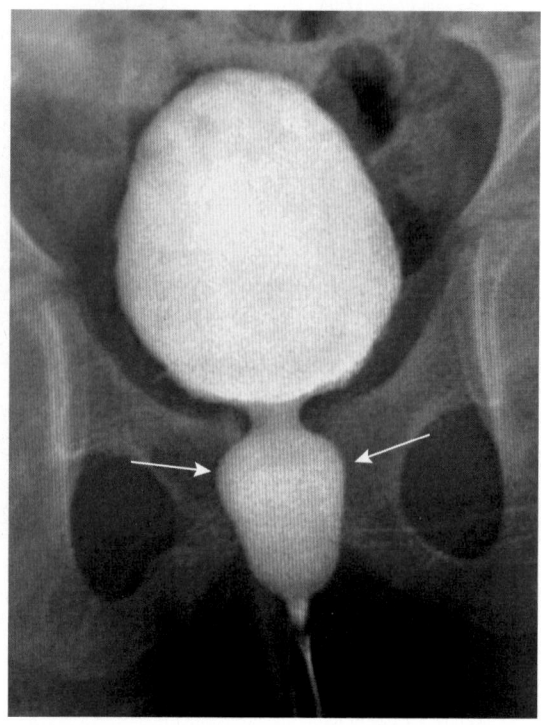

B

FIGURE 152-32. Spinning top urethra. **A,** Transverse ultrasound image of the bladder base shows anechoic fluid in the proximal urethra *(arrow)*. **B,** Anterior image during voiding phase of VCUG shows dilation of the posterior urethra *(arrows, "spinning top")* in this girl with voiding dyssynergia.

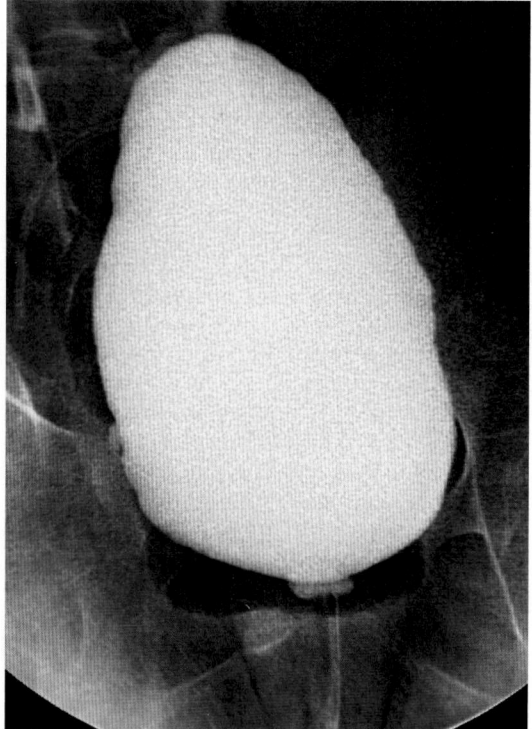

FIGURE 152-33. Megacystis. Anterior image obtained during VCUG shows a large capacity (800 ml) bladder in this patient with difficulty voiding.

and urethra appear normal during voiding, but postvoiding bladder residual is common. Reflux is not present or is very mild. Urodynamic studies show a hypotonic large-capacity bladder with elevation of intravesical pressure during filling occurring well beyond the level when the urge to void is normally expected. The detrusor contractions are small, ineffective, unsustained, or absent, with normal electromyelographic activity of the external sphincter. Voiding occurs by increased abdominal pressure. Environmental or psychological factors and urinary retention from habitual neglect may play a role in the etiology of the condition. These lazy bladders should be distinguished from the large, smooth, and thin-walled bladders (megacystis) seen in some patients with severe vesicoureteral reflux that are probably caused by a myogenic failure resulting from the constant passage of urine from the bladder to the ureters and back to the bladder.

Classic Neurogenic Bladder

CAUSES

In contrast to adult patients, in whom neurogenic bladder is most often due to an acquired, usually traumatic spinal cord lesion, the vast majority of children affected with this disorder have myelodysplasia (myelomeningocele, occult spinal dysraphism, sacral agenesis). Plain radiographs or fluoroscopic images may show widening of the neural canal, defective posterior neural arches, absence of the posterior spinous processes, and a widened interpedicular distance involving several segments with elongated and flattened or defective pedicles. Additional findings include vertebral body segmentation abnormalities and sacral malformations.

Neurologic injury and subsequent bladder dysfunction after relatively minor trauma may occur in patients with hemophilia (intraspinal hematoma) or achondroplasia (narrow spinal canal). Neurogenic bladder may also be caused by injury to the nerve supply of the bladder during surgical correction of congenital anorectal anomalies or Hirschsprung disease, excision of a pelvic tumor, or extensive pelvic dissection for other reasons. Other causes of neurogenic bladder include multiple sclerosis, cerebral vasculopathies and stroke, epidural abscesses, primary or secondary intraspinal neoplasms, paravertebral neoplasms extending into the neural canal, vertebral neoplasms or osteomyelitis, transverse myelitis, and peripheral neuropathies.

FUNCTIONAL CHANGES

Based on the level of the causative lesion and the functional aspects of voiding, several types of neurogenic bladder have been observed in experimental animals and are sometimes found in pure forms in people. The best-known types include:

- Uninhibited hyperreflexic bladder resulting from an acquired disease of the cerebral cortex
- Uninhibited hyperreflexic bladder resulting from a congenital or acquired lesion of the spinal cord above the sacral centers, resulting in an interruption of the inhibitory impulses from higher centers and a purely reflex bladder
- Autonomic bladder resulting from a lesion affecting the sacral center or the neural pathways connecting the sacral center with the bladder, causing separation of the bladder from the spine and loss of the sacral micturition reflex

Although well-defined clinical and radiographic features have been attributed to these and other postulated forms of neurogenic bladder, these classifications are often impractical because the primary lesion may be incomplete or not sharply limited and because motor and sensory nerve fibers may be involved in different degrees. Also, the clinical and radiographic features may be greatly modified by the duration of the disease and previous urinary tract infections. Furthermore, the vast majority of cases of neurogenic bladder in pediatrics fall in the large, heterogeneous group of hyperreflexic bladders caused by sacral and suprasacral lesions and are

frequently complicated by detrusor/external sphincter dyssynergia.

CLINICAL MANIFESTATIONS

The principal clinical manifestation in most children with a neurogenic bladder results from a dysfunction of the detrusor, usually associated with a dysfunction of the external sphincter. In mild or early cases there may be only night and day wetting and urinary urgency and frequency. In severe advanced cases, there is total loss of bladder sensation and urinary control, with constant dribbling of urine, urine retention, and overflow incontinence. The urethral resistance is usually increased, and it may not be possible to empty the bladder by manual compression. Between these two extremes are all grades of severity and combinations of symptoms. Urinary tract infections with episodes of sepsis and pyelonephritis are common complications, and in some patients there is a deterioration of renal function that may lead to renal insufficiency. Urinary tract calculi are common.

IMAGING

Ultrasonography provides information on both the lower and upper urinary tract. The upper tract evaluation may be entirely normal in early cases of neurogenic bladder, and dilatation of the upper tracts may not be observed until after repair of a myelomeningocele (Fig. 152-34). One or both upper urinary tracts may be dilated, even in the absence of reflux. UVJ obstruction attributed to a thickened, heavily trabeculated bladder may be observed. Often, in the resting state, the bladder neck area has a funnel-like configuration, with contrast material in the bladder extending downward into the proximal urethra. In patients with long-standing neurogenic bladder, US of the kidneys may show loss of renal parenchyma. Nuclear medicine studies with dimercaptosuccinic acid (DMSA) are useful to detect more subtle parenchymal injury, and studies with diethylenetetraaminepentaacetic acid (DTPA) or mercaptoacetylglycine (MAG3) are useful to evaluate renal function and to

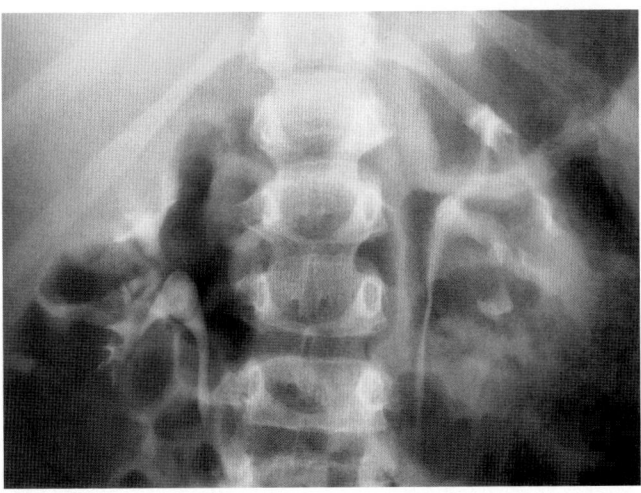

A

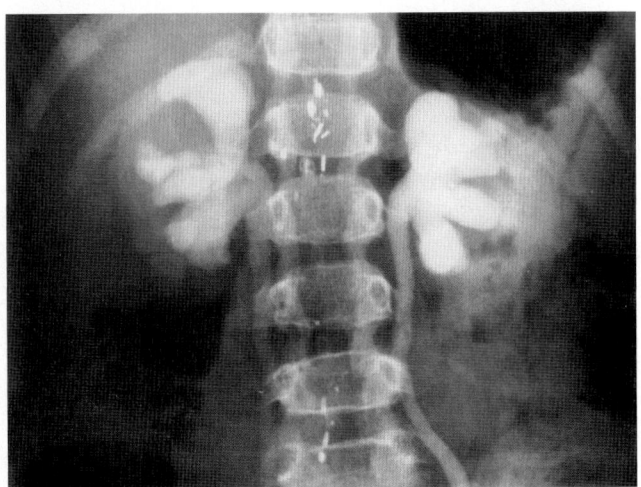

B

FIGURE 152-34. Renal effects of neurogenic bladder. **A,** IVU before resection of a spinal cord tumor shows normal parenchymal thickness and collecting systems. **B,** Two years after surgery, IVU shows renal parenchymal loss and calyceal blunting.

separate obstructive from nonobstructive collecting system dilatation.

VCUG is used to evaluate the anatomy of the bladder, bladder neck, urethra, and to demonstrate vesicoureteral reflux. As a functional study, it complements the urodynamic investigation and contributes information regarding the amount of urine at the time of catheterization, bladder capacity, sensation of bladder fullness, behavior of the detrusor muscle and urethral sphincter during bladder filling and voiding, ability to stop and start micturition voluntarily, the voiding pattern, the effect of the Credé maneuver on bladder emptying, and the amount of residual urine on postvoid films. When VCUG recorded on videotape is combined with a synchronous multichannel urodynamic study, continuously recording flow rates, intravesical and rectal pressures, and the electromyographic findings (synchronous, cine, or pressure-flow cystometrography, or videocystourodynamic study), it may be possible to compare and correlate more precisely the various phases of filling and emptying and the behavior of the bladder, bladder neck, and external sphincter with a corresponding display of the urodynamic changes at each level.

In early and mild cases of neurogenic bladder, the VCUG may show no abnormalities or only minor changes (Fig. 152-35). In more advanced cases, residual urine at the time of catheterization is common. Full distention of the bladder or retrograde filling is often impossible. The bladder is usually hypertonic and may be round, smooth, or trabeculated (Fig. 152-36). Paraureteral diverticula may be demonstrated. The bladder may become elongated, pointing upward and often to the right. Whether hypertonic or relatively smooth, the bladder may be small, of normal size, or large, depending on the status of the urethral resistance and previous or current infections. A purely atonic, large, and smooth-walled bladder of the type seen in adults with isolated sensory nerve root disease is uncommon in children. In patients with gross incontinence, voiding may occur during filling of the bladder. Once the bladder is filled, voiding may be initiated spontaneously or may be obtained only with a Credé maneuver. Sometimes voiding continues in an uncontrolled fashion with a good and sustained stream or is intermittent. The patient may or may not be able to stop and start micturition voluntarily.

During voiding, the bladder neck and proximal urethra are frequently dilated. At the level of the external sphincter, the urethra is usually narrowed intermittently or constantly as a result of external sphincter hyperactivity, sometimes from local denervation, muscle atrophy, and fibrosis. The urethra above the narrow sphincter area is dilated, sometimes resembling posterior urethral valves in males. Reflux of contrast material into the prostatic ducts may be observed (Fig. 152-37). In males, the bulbocavernosus muscle may be spastic, causing a constant or intermittent narrowing of the bulbar urethra. Abnormal function of the pelvic floor musculature is observed in some cases and is characterized by an exaggerated relaxation of these muscles with a marked descent of the pelvic floor during urination and an incomplete ascent at the end of micturition. Vesicoureteral reflux is frequent, may be bilateral, and is associated with variable ureterectasis. Residual contrast in the bladder at the end of the procedure is a common finding.

> Radiographic evaluation of neurogenic bladder must involve the upper and lower urinary tract. Findings are determined by the severity of disease, duration of involvement, and complications.

EVALUATION OF THE ARTIFICIAL URINARY SPHINCTER

Artificial urinary sphincters are designed to alleviate urinary incontinence in patients with low urethral resistance, normal or near-normal detrusor function and

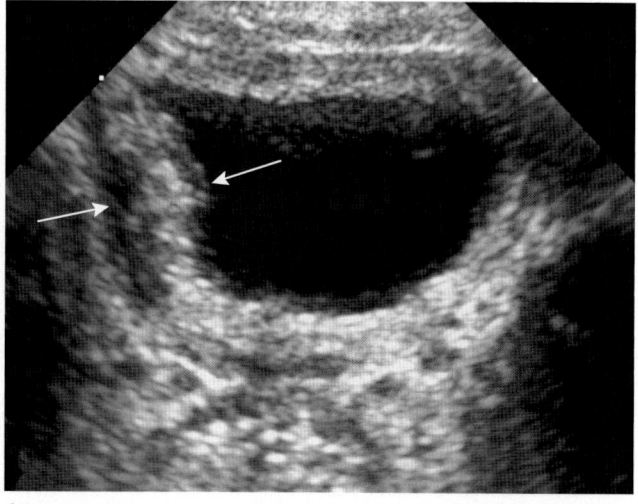
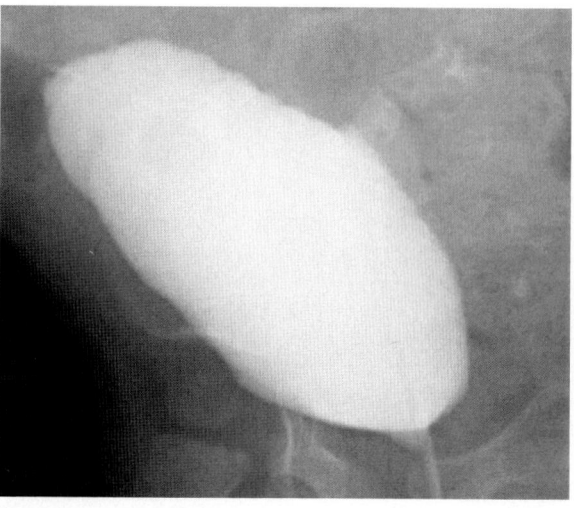

A   B

FIGURE 152-35. Neurogenic bladder. **A,** Transverse sonogram of the bladder shows irregular circumferential bladder wall thickening *(arrows).* **B,** Right posterior oblique image obtained during VCUG shows an elongated bladder with mild irregularity of the wall.

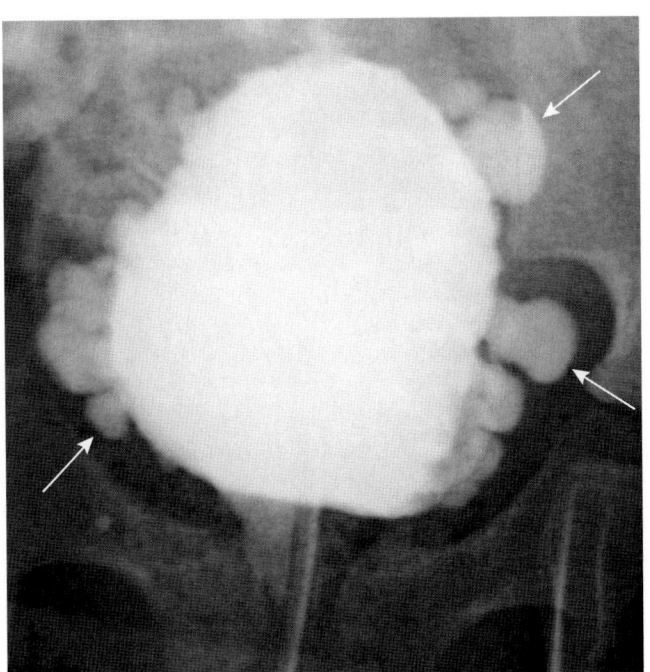

A

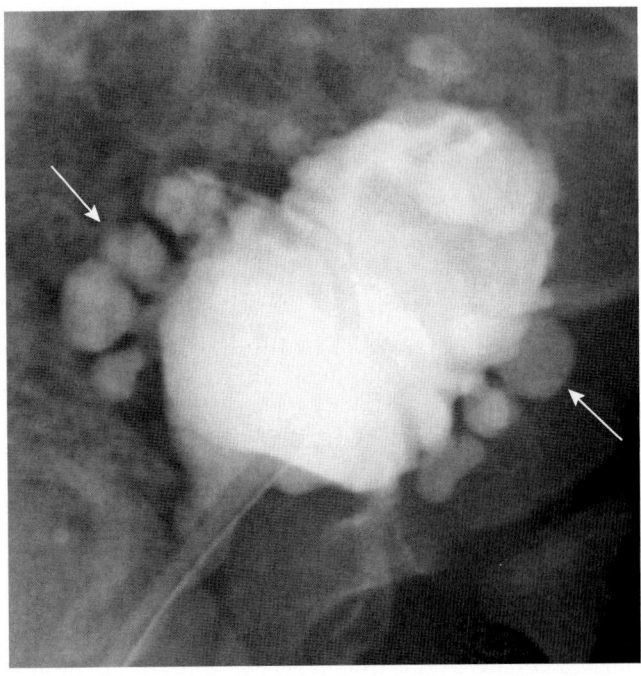

B

FIGURE 152-36. Neurogenic bladder. Anterior (**A**) and oblique (**B**) images during VCUG show a small, trabeculated bladder with multiple cellules *(arrows)*.

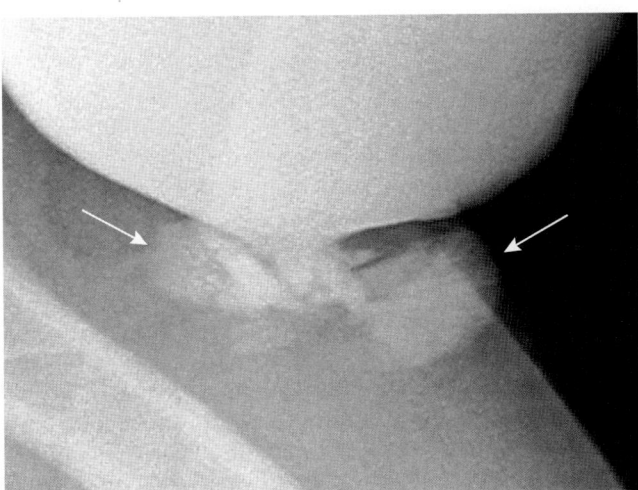

FIGURE 152-37. Prostatic duct reflux. Oblique image during VCUG shows marked prostatic duct reflux *(arrows)* with inability to spontaneously void.

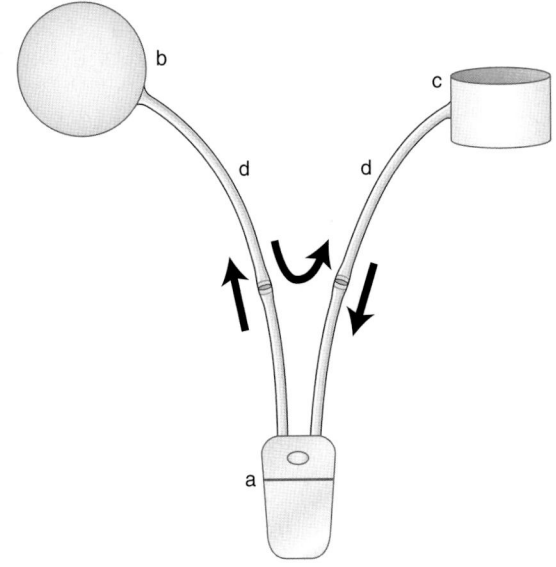

FIGURE 152-38. Diagram of artificial urinary sphincter. The device is composed of a combined pump and control assembly with an on/off button (a), a regulator pressure balloon or balloon reservoir (b), an inflatable cuff (c), and tubing connecting the components (d). *Arrows* indicate the possible direction of fluid flow within the system, controlled by one-way valves and a resistor circuit in the control assembly.

bladder compliance, and absence of significant bladder diverticula or vesicoureteral reflux. Reflux, when present, can be corrected before the implantation of the sphincter.

The artificial sphincter most commonly used at this time is the AMS 800 (American Medical Systems, Minnetonka, Minnesota). The device, shown diagrammatically in Figure 152-38, is composed of a pump or bulb with a control assembly, a regulator pressure balloon or reservoir, an inflatable cuff, and connecting tubes. The pump with the attached control assembly is implanted in the scrotum above the testis or in one of the labia majora, the balloon reservoir is placed beneath the fascia of the anterior abdominal wall near the bladder, and the

inflatable cuff is implanted around the bladder neck. An isotonic solution of iodinated contrast material is used as hydrostatic fluid to fill the system. The cuff may be deflated manually by squeezing the pump. With this maneuver, the content of the pump is forced into the reservoir through a one-way valve in the control assembly; the pump refills promptly by withdrawing fluid from the cuff through another one-way valve in the control assembly, thus deflating the cuff and allowing emptying of the bladder; a resistor in the control assembly causes a slow refilling of the cuff from the reservoir.

A functional failure of the device is manifested most commonly by recurrence of urinary incontinence, sometimes by urinary retention (and overflow incontinence), and is caused most often by loss of fluid from the system. Although the site of leakage (most often the cuff) cannot be recognized in abdominal radiographs, it may be possible to determine in most cases that loss of fluid from the system has occurred. When the fluid loss is complete, the entire system is empty and invisible radiographically; in less severe cases, the system is partially collapsed with a decrease in the thickness of the cuff sleeve and a decrease in diameter or loss of the spherical shape of the balloon reservoir. These changes may be subtle, because even a significant fluid loss from the device may be associated with a difference of only a few millimeters in balloon diameter compared with the baseline study.

Urinary retention, frequently associated with overflow incontinence, is most often the result of failure of the bulb to deflate, and is usually due to kinks in the tubing that may be apparent only on lateral or oblique views or fluoroscopically. Migration of the deflated pump into the inguinal canal with failure to palpate the pump is an uncommon cause of sphincteric failure. Erosion of the bladder neck and proximal urethra by the cuff is an infrequent but serious complication resulting in bladder neck obstruction, urinary retention, detrusor hyperreflexia, and sometimes incontinence. Hematuria, dysuria, and pain when the pump is activated are common manifestations. Local erosion caused by the cuff may result in contour irregularities of the area and local extravasation of contrast material demonstrable by cystourethrography, retrograde urethrography, and cystourethroscopy.

Other causes of malfunction of the device include decreased bladder compliance, worsening of the existing abnormalities such as vesicoureteral reflux or bladder diverticula, and development of inhibited bladder contractions or hypertonicity leading to increased intravesical pressure relative to the pressure within the cuff. Some of these complications can be demonstrated by cystourethrography or other urographic procedures, but in others the underlying abnormality can be diagnosed only by urodynamic studies.

POSTERIOR URETHRAL VALVES

Posterior urethral valves (PUV), more recently considered congenital obstructive posterior urethral membranes (COPUM), are the most common cause of congenital bladder outlet obstruction (Fig. 152-39). The degree of urethral obstruction, however, is variable. Antenatal ultrasound findings of megacystis, thickened bladder wall, dilated posterior urethra (keyhole sign), hydroureteronephrosis, and oligohydramnios represent severe urethral obstruction with the poorest postnatal prognosis. Those children who escape antenatal detection and are not apparent clinically in the newborn period represent milder degrees of urethral obstruction. These

TABLE 152-6
Imaging Findings in Patients with Posterior Urethral Valves

ULTRASONOGRAPHY
Renal cysts
Bilateral (unilateral) hydronephrosis
Thick-walled bladder
Actual valves

VOIDING CYSTOURETHROGRAPHY
Dilated posterior urethra
Actual valves
Reflux into prostatic and/or ejaculatory ducts
Thick bladder neck
Trabeculated bladder
Reflux (50% of cases)

children may present in the first months or years of life with urinary tract infections, sepsis, voiding disorders, hematuria, vomiting, failure to thrive, urinary retention, hydronephrosis, ascites, and congestive heart failure. In some of these patients, there may be a history of respiratory distress in the newborn period that gradually subsided. There are still other patients with PUV that have caused little or no change in the urinary tract and who may present during childhood or adolescence with only functional voiding disorders or urinary tract infections. The diagnosis can be made on the basis of imaging findings (Table 152-6).

Age at detection of posterior urethral obstruction is critical. When detected prenatally, severe obstructive urethral valve disease significantly influences renal and pulmonary development. Increased intravesical pressure is diverted to the upper urinary tract when associated with incompetent refluxing ureterovesical junctions. Varying degrees of renal dysplasia result from pressure damage to the developing renal pelvis, collecting ducts, and parenchyma. Organogenesis of the kidney is complete at the 12th gestational week, and renal damage is irreversible at the 20th gestational week. Subsequent development of oligohydramnios with resultant pulmonary hypoplasia represents the immediate life-limiting factor for these children. If the fetus survives, up to 45% will develop renal insufficiency or end-stage renal disease requiring renal dialysis or transplantation before 5 years of age. At the other end of the spectrum are patients with late presentation of PUV. These patients have a mild form of disease whose detection may be delayed as late as adolescence. The most common reported presenting symptoms are voiding dysfunction, including nocturnal enuresis and urinary frequency. Associated findings include urinary tract infection, microhematuria, and mild age-corrected hypertension. Findings on US may range from normal to demonstrating varying degrees of hydronephrosis and postvoid residual bladder volume.

The degree of urethral obstruction and its initial effects on bladder and renal function are the main determinants of long-term outcome in these patients. Despite early detection and relief of urethral obstruction, late renal insufficiency or failure may develop in 25% to 40% of patients throughout adolescence and into adulthood,

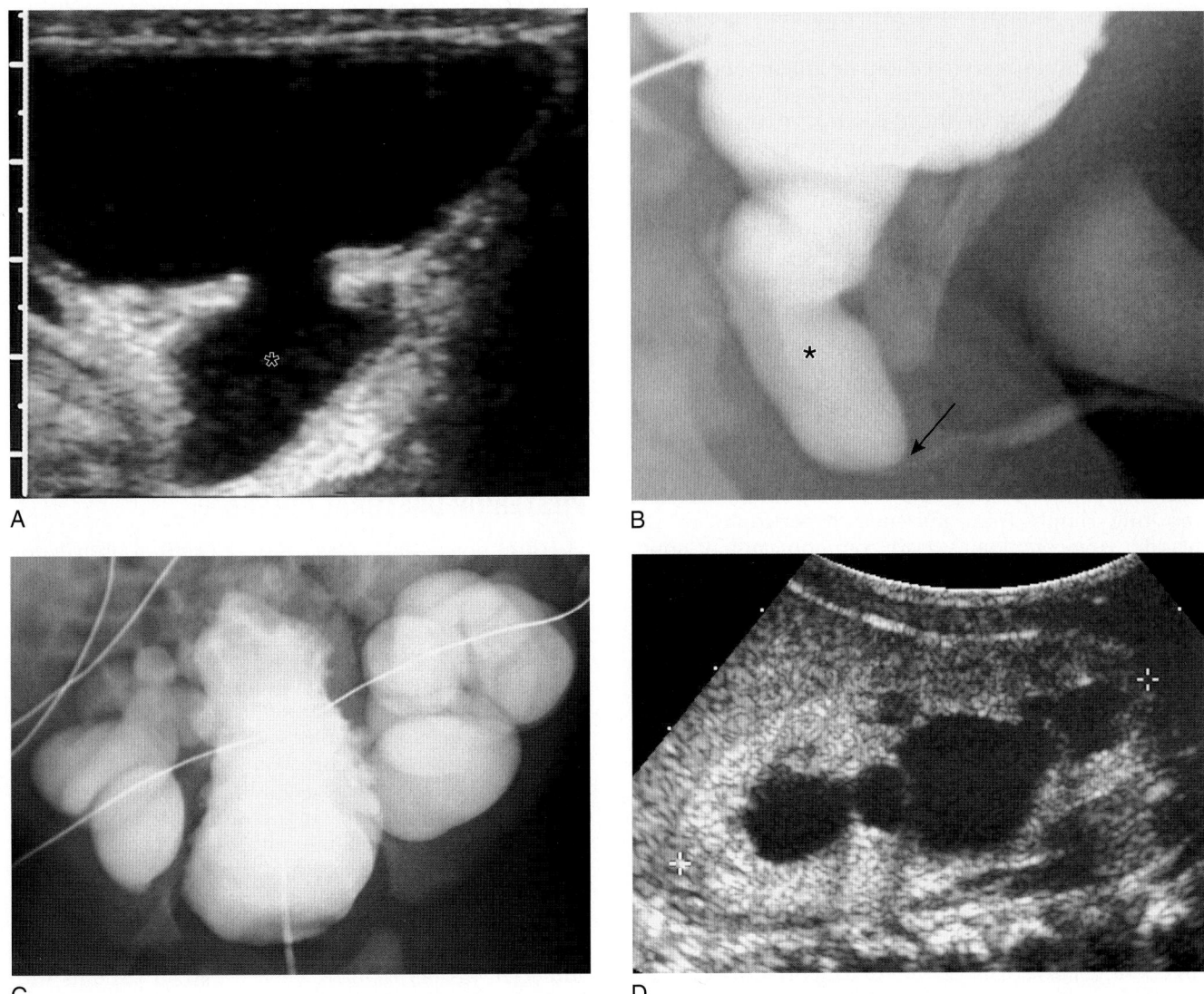

FIGURE 152-39. Posterior urethral valves. **A,** Transverse ultrasound image of the bladder shows dilated posterior urethra *(asterisk)*, representing the "keyhole" sign. **B,** Oblique image during VCUG shows a dilated posterior urethra *(asterisk)* with abrupt transition at level of valves to narrow anterior urethra *(arrow)*. **C,** Anterior image of same patient demonstrates a heavily trabeculated bladder with severe bilateral vesicoureteral reflux. **D,** Longitudinal sonogram of the same patient demonstrates an echogenic right kidney with absent corticomedullary differentiation and hydronephrosis.

even in the setting of initially normal renal function in infancy. Prognostic factors related to long-term outcome in PUV patients include age at diagnosis, degree of bladder dysfunction, serum creatinine level, glomerular filtration rate, the presence or absence of vesicoureteral reflux at diagnosis, the appearance of proteinuria, hypertension, urinary tract infection, daytime urinary incontinence after 5 years of age, and altered renal echogenicity.

Bladder dysfunction is now recognized as playing a critical role in progressive development of renal insufficiency despite initial relief of obstructing valvular tissue. Urodynamic studies demonstrate bladder dysfunction in as many as 75% of patients. Structural, biochemical, and functional changes in the bladder occur early in fetal development and may be irreversible. The so-called valve bladder syndrome describes a group of associated findings to include persistent upper tract dilation, noncompliant

thick-walled bladder, incontinence, and nephrogenic diabetes insipidus. Histologic bladder examinations of experimentally induced urethral obstruction in animals and in autopsied human fetuses with PUV demonstrate increased muscarinic cholinergic receptor density, altered myosin content, reversed collagen subtype ratio, and increased elastin fibers. As a consequence, the bladder loses contractile strength and compliance with subsequent development of high filling pressures. Distortion of the anatomy of the trigone and UVJ may lead to obstruction and/or vesicoureteral reflux. Combined with polyuria secondary to impaired renal concentrating ability, the upper tracts remain dilated, and persistent increased hydrostatic pressure on the kidneys leads to progressive renal injury. As opposed to early childhood when renal insufficiency is more likely the result of renal dysplasia, late renal insufficiency is likely the combination of abnormal bladder function, increased metabolic demands of puberty, and hyperfiltration glomerular injury.

After transurethral resection or fulguration of the obstructing valvular structures, VCUG commonly shows a prompt decrease in the dilatation of the posterior urethra, but in about one fourth of the patients the dilatation persists despite a widely patent, unobstructed urethra, possibly as the result of prostatic gland hypoplasia. Residual valve tissue with obstruction is not uncommon, and stricture formation at the site of the previous urethral valves, or in the membranous urethra as a complication of surgery, may occur. Urethroscopy is usually more reliable than the urethrogram in the diagnosis of these lesions.

Upper urinary tract dilatation generally improves after surgery and sometimes disappears. Persisting dilatation may be due to a residual or acquired ureteral obstruction, continuing vesicoureteral reflux, or poor ureteral peristalsis. Ureteral obstruction at the UVJ resulting simply from muscular hypertrophy of the bladder is uncommon. A more common cause of upper tract dilatation and apparent UVJ obstruction is the so-called valve-bladder syndrome as discussed earlier. Patients with residual upper tract dilatation or recurrent urinary tract infections and deterioration of renal function are investigated by VCUG for evidence of reflux or urethral stricture, to determine the size and shape of the bladder and, to some extent, the function of the bladder during voiding. Urodynamic studies may be indicated if a functional disorder of the bladder is suspected. The upper tracts are best evaluated by US. Diuretic DTPA renal scintigraphy and sometimes a Whitaker test may be necessary to differentiate a functional from an obstructive ureterectasis. The renal parenchyma is best followed by DMSA renal scans.

Refinements in surgical approach and in preoperative and postoperative management of patients with PUV have resulted in a significant improvement in initial results. However, long-term results continue to be disappointing. A large percentage of patients with PUV show progressive deterioration of renal function to chronic renal insufficiency with growth failure, systemic arterial hypertension, renal osteodystrophy, and other complications of chronic renal failure, and in many cases end-stage renal disease requiring dialysis and renal transplantation. End-stage renal disease may be reached within a few months to 15 or more years after the diagnosis of PUV. It is important to recognize that renal function can be damaged during prenatal or postnatal life and that urethral valve ablation does not prevent progressive renal injury. Renal and bladder function must be monitored throughout childhood and into adult life. Early recognition and aggressive therapy of bladder dysfunction with anticholinergic medications, double voiding, clean intermittent catheterization, and bladder augmentation may slow or improve the long-term prognosis.

Renal failure is common in boys with PUV and may occur months to decades after diagnosis.

TABLE 152-7

Characteristics of Posterior Urethral Polyps

Originate at verumontanum
Usually found at 3-6 years of age
Hamartoma with muscle, neural, and vascular tissue
Stalk present
Signs/symptoms
    Intermittent urethral obstruction
    Urinary retention
    Hematuria
    Infections
    Bladder tics
Imaging findings
    Filling defect at bladder neck-midurethra
    Vesicoureteral reflux
    Dilatation of upper tracts

POSTERIOR URETHRAL POLYPS

Urethral polyps are a rare cause of urethral obstruction in boys. In males the lesion typically arises from the posterior urethra (also called congenital polyp of the verumontanum) and consists of an elongated, freely movable polypoid mass on a long stalk originating from the region of the verumontanum (Table 152-7). It is a benign hamartomatous lesion, thought to represent a persistence of the Müller's tubercle, composed of a fibroconnective tissue core containing smooth muscle elements, blood vessels, nests of glandular cells, and sometimes neural tissue. It is covered by a transitional cell epithelium, sometimes with glandular metaplastic changes. An inflammatory infiltrate has not been identified in any male urethral polyp. The lesion is typically diagnosed in the first decade of life at a mean age of 8 to 10 years, although it has been reported in infants and adults. It has occasionally been found in patients with Beckwith-Wiedemann syndrome and hepatoblastoma.

Female urethral polyps are exceedingly rare, with only 11 reported cases in the English language literature. As opposed to the urethral polyp in males, polyps in the female urethra appear to originate from chronic prolapsing urothelium and can be found in the proximal, mid, or distal urethra. The histology is also different, being composed of a central core of inflammatory cells with congested and edematous soft tissue elements, congested blood vessels, and focal areas of squamous epithelium. The age presentation ranges from the neonate to 10 years.

The classic symptoms in the male are those of intermittent urethral obstruction with straining on voiding, abnormal voiding pattern, and urinary retention. Hematuria and urinary tract infections may also be observed. In the female, vaginal bleeding is the most common reported symptom.

VCUG remains the imaging gold standard in males. Before voiding, the tip of the polyp is frequently located at the level of the bladder neck, causing a small rounded filling defect at that level (Fig. 152-40). In the voiding phase, the polyp moves downward into the distal posterior urethra and occasionally into the bulbar urethra. Sometimes the polyp becomes impacted in the posterior

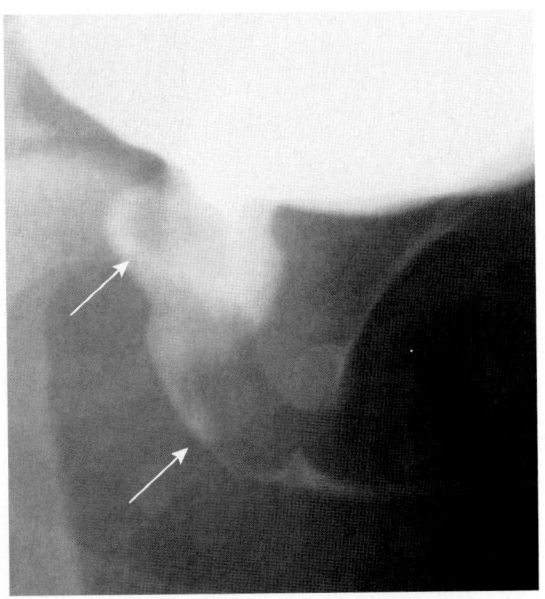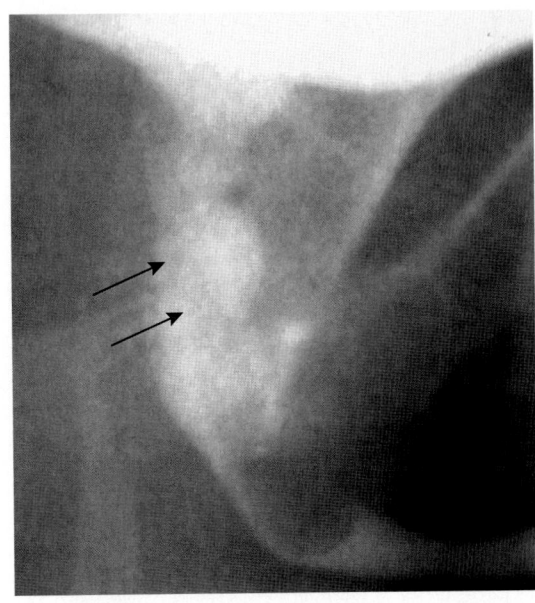

A   B

FIGURE 152-40. Urethral polyp. **A,** Oblique image during VCUG shows a lobular filling defect in the posterior urethra representing a polyp on a stalk *(arrows).* **B,** With voiding, the polyp moves distally into the urethra and the stalk is better appreciated *(arrows)* with the attachment at the verumontanum.

urethra, obstructing urine flow. At the end of voiding, the polyp is displaced backward to the level of the bladder outlet by the contraction of the external urethral sphincter. Bladder trabeculations, vesicoureteral reflux, and upper tract dilatation may be present. US may demonstrate a mobile pedunculated mass with medium-level echogenicity at the bladder base and indirect signs of bladder outlet obstruction (hydronephrosis and large bladder with or without bladder wall hypertrophy). In females, diagnosis is made by direct observation of an interlabial mass. Endoscopic laser excision is the current treatment of choice, with recurrence reported only with incomplete initial removal.

PROSTATIC UTRICLE AND MÜLLERIAN DUCT CYSTS

The *prostatic utricle* is a small, epithelium-lined diverticulum of the prostatic urethra. It is located in the verumontanum between the openings of the two ejaculatory ducts and extends backward and slightly upward for a very short distance within the medial lobe of the prostate. It is a normal anatomic variant representing the remnant of the fused caudal ends of the müllerian ducts, and thus is the homolog of the female vagina and uterine cervix.

When there is deficient secretion or resistance to müllerian inhibitory factor (MIF), normally produced by functioning testes beginning at approximately the 8th week of gestation, there is failure of normal fusion of the urogenital folds resulting in hypospadias. The urethral orifice opens proximal to the normal meatus on the ventral surface of the penis; in mild cases at the glans and in severe cases on the perineum. Hypospadias has the most common association with prostatic utricles, with an estimated incidence of 14% to 47%. In the absence of other müllerian duct derivatives (fallopian tubes, uterus,

and upper vagina), hypospadias and utricular enlargement are not indicative of an intersex condition. The increasing severity of the hypospadias correlates with increasing size of the utricle. Utricles are not uncommon in prune-belly syndrome and may be seen in patients with imperforate anus and rectourethral fistula and in patients with Down syndrome. The prostatic utricle distends with urine during voiding and then passively drains. Poor emptying leads to urine retention and stasis. Patients present clinically with chronic urinary tract infection, epididymitis, and voiding dysfunction.

The normal prostatic utricle is occasionally seen as an incidental finding on routine VCUG as a tiny diverticulum of a few millimeters in length or on rare occasions measuring up to 1 cm or more (Fig. 152-41). Large prostatic utricles are more often associated with male hypospadias (Fig. 152-42). VCUG and retrograde urethrography (RUG) define the utricular size and its origin from the prostatic urethra. Occasionally, a prostatic utricle is bifid, reflecting the bifid nature of its precursors, the paired müllerian ducts. In patients with large prostatic utricles, direct catheterization of the bladder during VCUG may be difficult secondary to preferential passage into the utricle (Fig. 152-43). Facilitation of catheter placement into the bladder can be accomplished with use of a Coudé catheter with the tip directed anteriorly, direct perineal pressure, and/or insertion of a finger in the rectum with upward pressure during catheter placement.

> Large prostatic utricles are often associated with hypospadias.

A *müllerian duct cyst,* or cyst of the prostatic utricle, is a cystic dilatation of an obstructed utricle occurring in

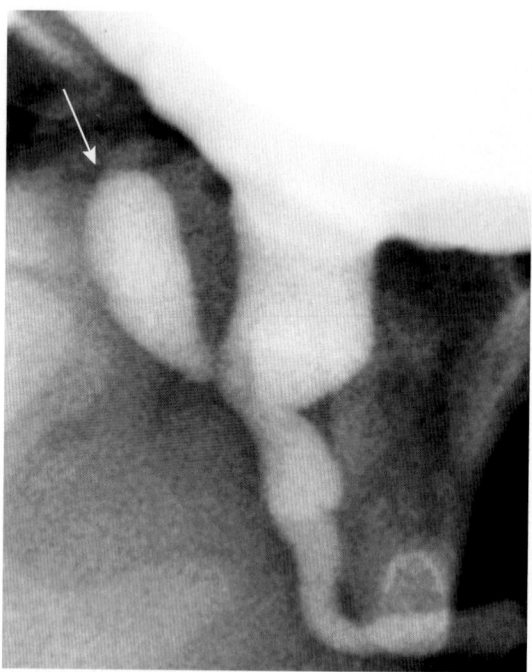

FIGURE 152-41. Utricle. Oblique image during VCUG in a patient without hypospadias showing a utricle *(arrow)* arising from the ventral prostatic urethra.

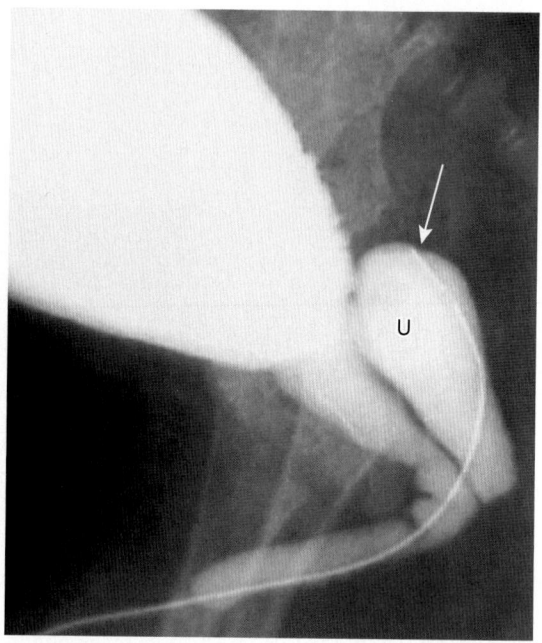

FIGURE 152-43. Catheter in utricle. Oblique image from VCUG shows catheter *(arrow)* positioned in utricle (U). Bladder filling and voiding were achieved without repositioning of catheter.

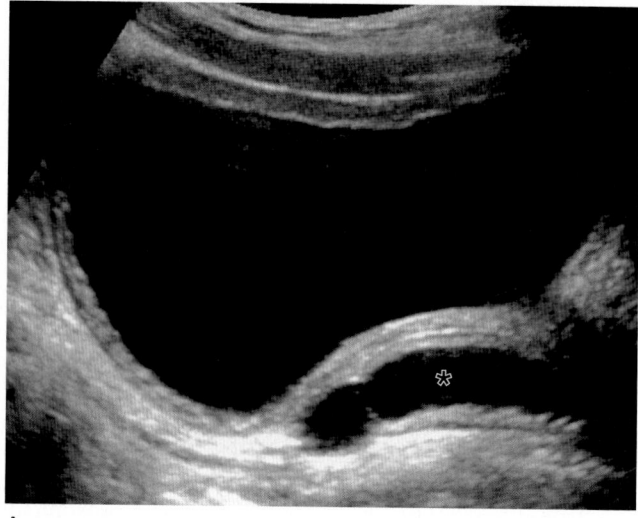

A

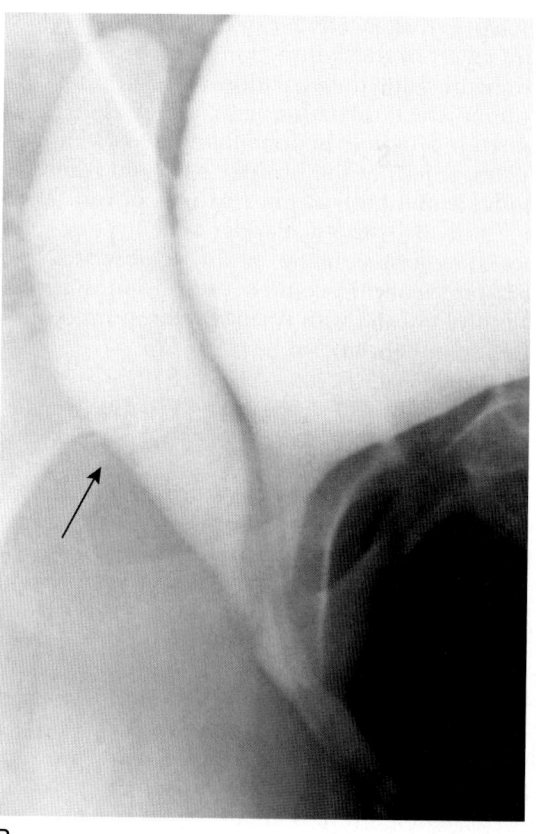

B

FIGURE 152-42. Utricle. **A,** Longitudinal ultrasound image of the bladder in patient with hypospadias shows a blind-ending anechoic tubular structure *(asterisk)* posterior to the bladder. **B,** Corresponding oblique view from a VCUG shows a large utricle *(arrow)* extending posterior to the bladder.

patients with an otherwise normal lower urinary tract and external genitalia. The obstruction has been attributed to congenital valves or mucosal folds, local infection, or desquamation of the epithelium. Müllerian cysts are rare and are most often discovered in adults. They vary greatly in size from a few centimeters in diameter to a large pelvic mass displacing the bladder upward and forward and sometimes obstructing the urethra. Stone formation within these cysts has been reported. Sometimes these cysts are found to communicate with the

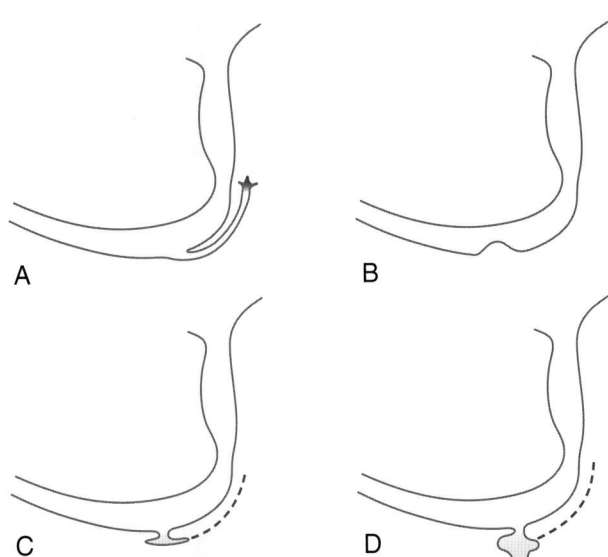

FIGURE 152-44. Various configurations of cowperian ducts and Cowper's glands on urethrography. **A,** Filling of the duct up to the gland. **B,** Opening of the duct is obliterated, causing a small mass on the floor of the bulbar urethra. **C** and **D,** Diverticula originating from the floor of the bulbar urethra; the duct is not usually opacified in these cases.

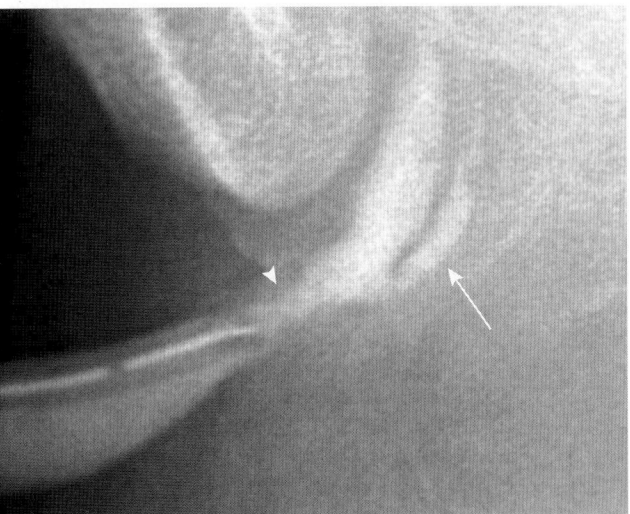

FIGURE 152-45. Cowper's duct. Oblique image from retrograde urethrogram in a patient with a bulbar urethral stricture *(arrowhead)* shows retrograde filling of a ventral tubular structure *(arrow)* paralleling the urethra.

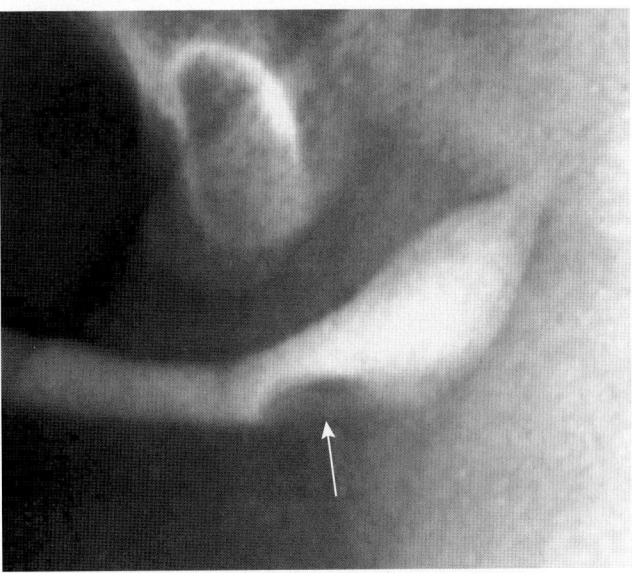

FIGURE 152-46. Cowper's duct cyst (syringocele). Oblique image from a retrograde urethrogram shows lobular filling defect *(arrow)* along the ventral surface of the bulbous urethra.

urethra by a minute tract, which may only be identified after insertion of a small catheter into the utricle at urethroscopy. The cystic nature and location of the pelvic mass is readily determined by US, CT, or MRI.

ABNORMALITIES OF COWPER'S GLANDS

The bulbourethral (Cowper's) glands are two pea-sized bodies on either side of the membranous urethra between the two layers of the urogenital diaphragm (Fig. 152-44). They are the homolog of the Bartholin glands of the female. Their ducts are 2 to 3 cm in length and are directed forward through the bulb of the corpus spongiosum to end in the ventral aspect of the bulbar urethra. The ducts may occasionally fuse proximally and enter the urethra as a single opening. These accessory sexual organs secrete a clear mucous substance that acts as a lubricant for spermatozoa. Both the ducts and glands may opacify during VCUG when the distal orifice is patulous. A contrast medium–filled tubular structure is seen paralleling the undersurface of the bulbous urethra (Fig. 152-45). This finding, as a rule, is of no clinical significance. Recognition of the characteristic location and course of the Cowper duct prevents misinterpretation of this finding as a urethral duplication, ectopic ureter, or fistula.

When a dilated duct forms a globular cavity on the ventral surface of the bulbar urethra, a urethral diverticulum might be considered. It is suspected that many diverticula of the bulbar urethra reported in the earlier literature were, in fact, dilated Cowper ducts. When the ductal orifice becomes stenotic, a dilated Cowper gland (syringocele) and duct are formed. The diagnosis can be made at VCUG by demonstrating a smooth extrinsic mass effect along the ventral surface of the bulbous urethra (Fig. 152-46). At urethroscopy, these lesions appear cystic.

Transurethral marsupialization or incision demonstrates these lesions to be filled with clear or blood-tinged fluid. Instances have been reported of very large congenital retention cysts of these ducts causing urethral obstruction. US and MRI may be used as alternative imaging methods when the diagnosis is uncertain.

MEGALOURETHRA, ANTERIOR URETHRAL DIVERTICULA, AND ANTERIOR URETHRAL VALVE

These uncommon anomalies of the male urethra are considered together because of common features and transitional forms suggesting a spectrum of related deformities. Their causes and modes of development are still debated.

Fusiform megalourethra, the rarest of the group, is characterized by a diffuse ectasia of the penile urethra secondary to an absence or partial deficiency of the corpus spongiosum and corpora cavernosa without distal obstruction. The penis is large, misshapen, and flabby, with redundant and wrinkled skin. Erections are not possible owing to the defective corpora cavernosa. During voiding, the urethra and penis become markedly distended. The patient voids with a poor urinary stream. On VCUG or RUG, the penile urethra is markedly dilated and fusiform, tapering both distally and proximally into a relatively normal urethra (Fig. 152-47). The proximal urethra may be dilated. Sometimes the anomaly affects only a small portion of the urethra (Fig. 152-48). The anomaly may occur as an isolated lesion but is seen more commonly in patients with prune-belly syndrome. The clinical symptoms and prognosis vary with the severity of the associated anomalies.

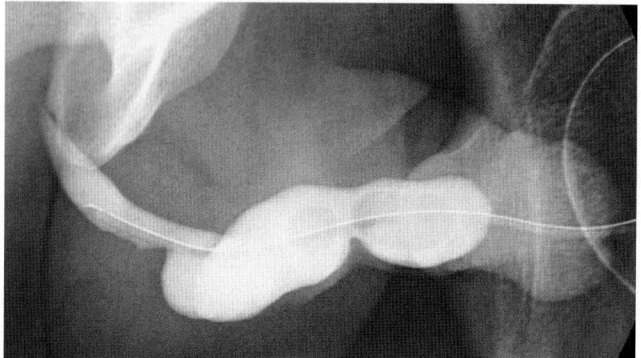

FIGURE 152-47. Megalourethra. Oblique image from a retrograde urethrogram shows fusiform dilation of the penile urethra.

Scaphoid megalourethra is much more common than the fusiform type. It consists of a localized saccular dilatation of the penile urethra, apparently caused by a localized absence or underdevelopment of the corpus spongiosum. The corpora cavernosa are intact. The penis is of normal size or somewhat enlarged and appears shorter dorsally than ventrally, causing a mild dorsal chordee. Ventrally, the penis is soft and baggy with redundant skin. During voiding, the affected part of the urethra balloons markedly, causing a large, smooth bulge in the ventral surface of the penis. The patient voids with a poor stream. During voiding or during an erection, the penis and pendulous urethra assume a scaphoid configuration. On VCUG, the dilated segment of the urethra blends gradually with a normal urethra distally and proximally. The proximal urethra may be slightly dilated. Associated anomalies in the rest of the urinary tract are much less common than in fusiform megalourethra. Scaphoid megalourethra may also occur in association with prune-belly syndrome.

Anterior urethral diverticulum is a saccular outpouching of the ventral aspect of the anterior urethra into the corpus spongiosum, usually near the penoscrotal junction. Proposed theories for diverticular development include dilation of periurethral glands, incomplete urethral duplication, defective fusion of the ventral folds over the urethral groove, and faulty development of the corpus spongiosum. Circumferential thinning or deficiency and local fibrosis of the corpus spongiosum is often present. The corpora cavernosa are intact. Anterior urethral diverticula are classified into the more common saccular versus globular forms. The communication of the urethra with the diverticulum is usually wide and centrally placed. The diverticulum has a well-defined, valve-like anterior lip, and a less well-defined posterior

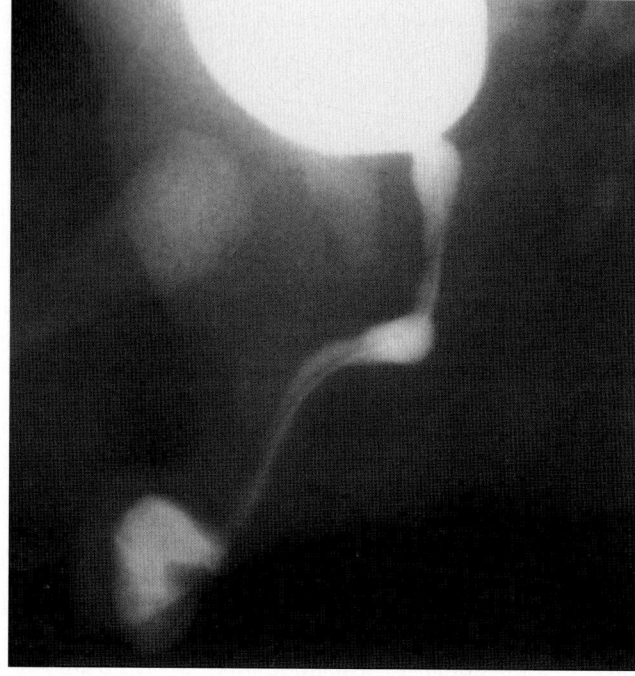

A

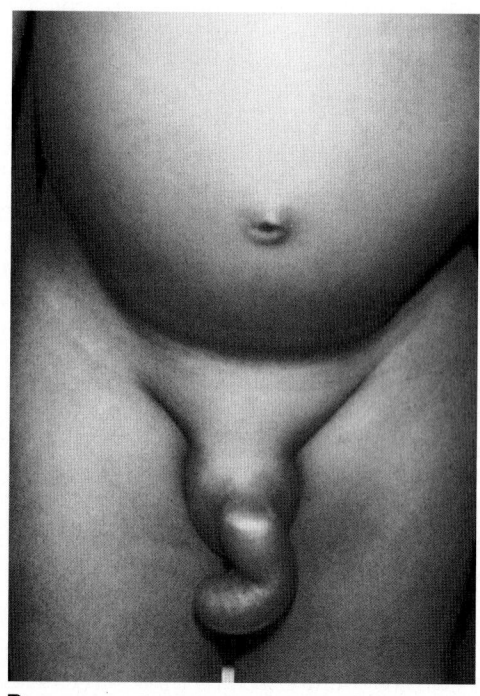

B

FIGURE 152-48. Megalourethra. **A,** VCUG shows dilatation of the anterior penile urethra. **B,** Postvoid photograph of the same child.

lip. During voiding, urine distends the diverticulum and displaces the anterior lip of the diverticulum forward and against the dorsal wall of the urethra, obstructing the flow of urine. A tense bulge on the ventral aspect of the penis at the level of the diverticulum is observed during voiding. The clinical symptoms depend on the degree of obstruction and include urinary retention, poor urinary stream, urinary tract infection, incontinence, and enuresis. Rare cases may present with uremia secondary to end-stage renal disease. Stone formation within the diverticulum is uncommon.

VCUG shows that the urethra proximal to the diverticulum is dilated, with a sharp demarcation with the unobstructed distal urethra (Fig. 152-49). The lateral edges of the roof of the diverticulum may be seen on the lateral projection as two thin horizontal lines. The posterior lip is usually not well delineated. The lesion is not well shown on a retrograde urethrogram, because it tends to fill poorly with retrograde contrast injection. Bladder trabeculations, bladder diverticula, and vesico-

ureteral reflux may be present. On US the upper tracts may be dilated, and there may be evidence of parenchymal scarring.

An *anterior urethral valve* is a semilunar fold very much like the anterior lip of a urethral diverticulum. It originates in the floor of the urethra near the penoscrotal junction. It is directed backward and is anchored laterally in such a way as to be raised up against the dorsal aspect of the urethra during voiding, obstructing the flow of urine (Fig. 152-50). It differs from a urethral diverticulum in that it lacks a posterior lip and usually causes a lesser degree of localized swelling of the ventral aspect of the penis during micturition. No abnormalities of the corpus spongiosum or corpora cavernosa are present. It is possible that an anterior urethral valve originates from an anterior urethral diverticulum with loss of the posterior lip. The clinical manifestations, complications, and radiographic appearance are the same as those described for anterior urethral diverticula but are often milder. The differential diagnosis from urethral diverticulum may be possible only at endoscopy or at the time of surgery.

URETHRAL DUPLICATION

Duplication of the urethra is an uncommon congenital anomaly that is more frequent in males than in females. There is no single unifying theory to explain all the various forms of duplication, and more than one classification scheme exists in the literature. These developmental anomalies are characterized by the presence of a complete or partial accessory urethral channel arising from the bladder to the distal urethra (Fig. 152-51). Incomplete duplications arise from the penile surface or from the urethral channel but end blindly in the periurethral tissue. Sagittal plane duplication is most common with a ventral and dorsal urethra (one urethra atop the other). It is important to remember that in almost all cases the ventral urethra is the functioning channel and contains the urethral sphincter and veru-

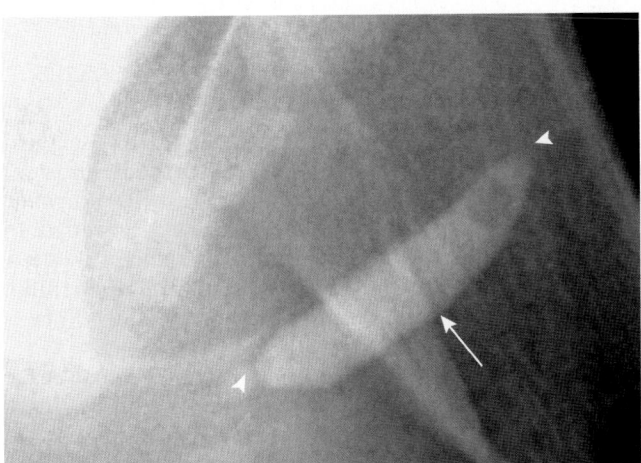

FIGURE 152-49. Urethral diverticulum. Oblique image during VCUG shows saccular outpouching *(arrow)* along the ventral urethra. Acute angles are formed at the junction of the anterior and posterior lips with the urethra *(arrowheads)*.

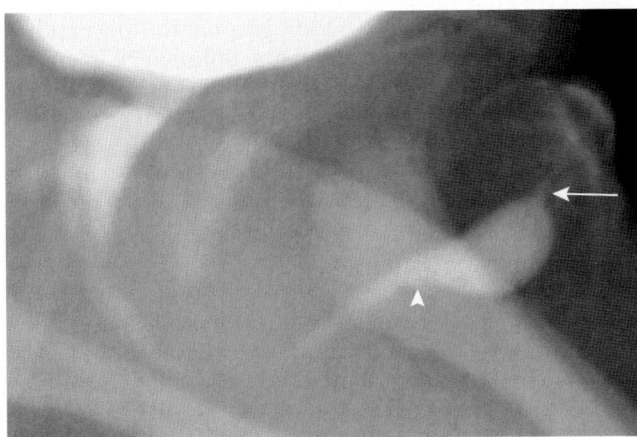

A

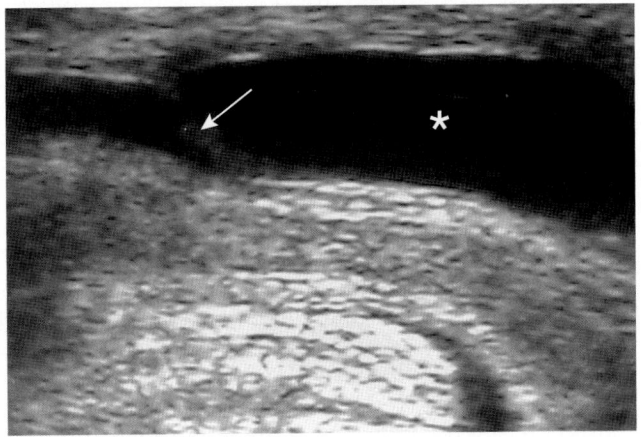

B

FIGURE 152-50. Anterior urethral valve. **A,** Oblique image during VCUG shows a focal saccular dilation of the distal anterior urethra. Distally, an acute angle is formed at the junction with the narrowed urethra *(arrow)*. Proximally, an obtuse angle is present *(arrowhead)*. **B,** Longitudinal ultrasound image of the urethra during voiding shows thin echogenic valve traversing the urethra *(arrow)*. Proximal to the valve, urethral dilation is seen *(asterisk)*. (From Bates DG, Coley BD: Ultrasound diagnosis of the anterior urethral valve. Pediatr Radiol 2001;31:634-636.)

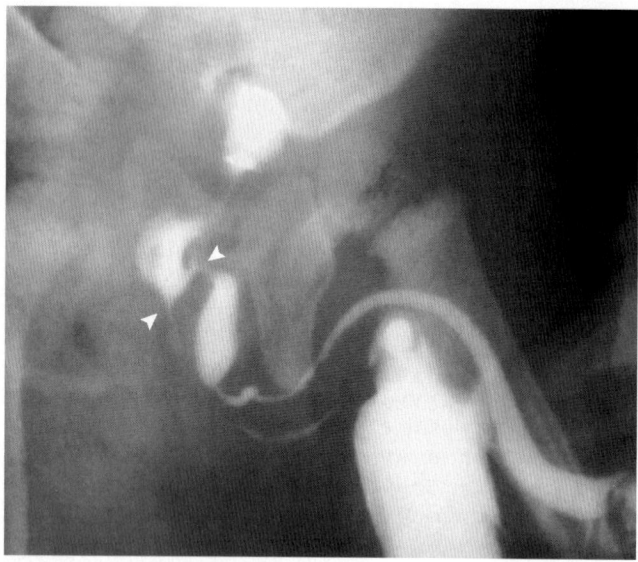 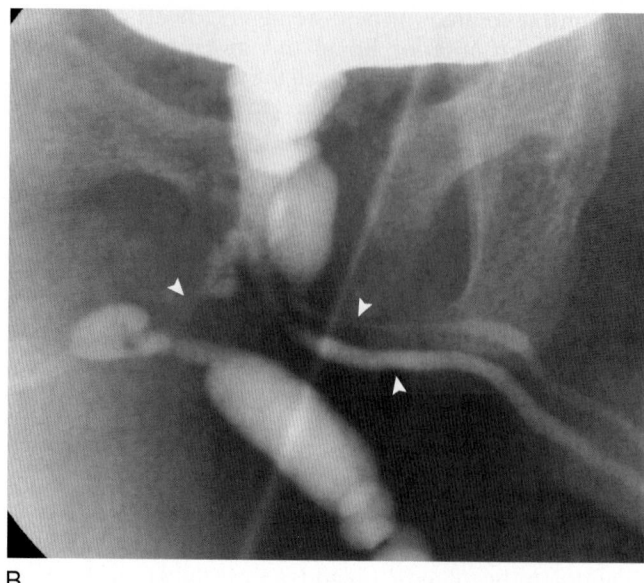

A   B

FIGURE 152-51. Urethral duplications. **A,** Oblique image from retrograde urethrogram after simultaneous injection of both the glandular and ventral penile openings shows partial duplication of the urethra originating at the prostatic urethra *(arrowheads)*. **B,** Oblique imaging during VCUG shows triplication of the urethra *(arrowheads)* originating from the prostatic urethra.

montanum. According to the location of the accessory urethral opening on the dorsal or ventral aspect of the penis, urethral duplications are divided into epispadic (the most common type) and hypospadic types, respectively. Coronal plane urethral duplication is far less common and frequently combined with duplication of the phallus and bladder.

In the *epispadic type* an incomplete accessory channel has a dorsal opening in the phallus and ends blindly. The complete or partial forms originate from the bladder or proximal urethra and course through the dorsal aspect of the penis to end in an epispadic position anywhere between the glans and the root of the penis (often associated with dorsal penile chordee and absent fusion of the dorsal foreskin), or rarely they originate from a minute cavity (nonfunctional sagittal plane duplicated bladder) located behind the pubic symphysis and in front of the normal bladder. The ventral urethra is normally positioned and ends in the glandular meatus (in rare cases the normal urethra ends in a hypospadic location).

In the *hypospadic type* an incomplete accessory channel has a ventral opening in the phallus and ends blindly or originates from the normal proximal urethra and ends blindly in the periurethral tissue similar in appearance to a urethral diverticulum or Cowper duct. Complete or partial duplications arise from the bladder or proximal urethra and course through the ventral aspect of the penis to end in a hypospadic position along the shaft. An important form of urethral duplication of the hypospadic type is referred to as Y-type duplication. The ventral urethra originates from the midprostatic urethra and terminates in the anal canal or in the perineum along the anterior anal margin. Urine flows preferentially through this ventral channel and is considered the normal urethra as it traverses the sphincter mechanism. A normally positioned dorsal urethra is usually stenotic

or partially atretic. The congenital urethroperineal fistula has a similar location but is a distinctly different developmental anomaly (Fig. 152-52). The normally positioned dorsal channel is the functioning urethra in this case, and micturition is normal. Clinically, only a few drops of urine are present at the perineal opening. Ventral channel excision in urethroperineal fistula is curative.

Accessory urethras may be asymptomatic or may cause a double urinary stream, urinary incontinence, urinary tract infections, and urinary retention. Appropriate evaluation of urethral duplication includes anatomic delineation of all channels, recognition of the functional urethra, and identification of associated anomalies. VCUG is adequate if both urethral channels can be clearly identified. RUG may be necessary for hypoplastic channels not visualized on VCUG. Cystoscopy may be performed to confirm the radiographic findings and to ensure which urethra contains the sphincteric mechanism and normal verumontanum. Upper tract anomalies are evaluated by US or cross-sectional imaging. MRI can identify associated spinal or internal genital organ anomalies. Preservation and reconstruction of the functional urethral channel is the primary goal of treatment.

URETHRAL STRICTURES

Urethral strictures are almost entirely limited to males. They are relatively uncommon but constitute an important and often serious problem that may be difficult to treat. In most cases, the stricture is iatrogenic or is secondary to external trauma or infection (Fig. 152-53). Sometimes the cause of the stricture is unknown.

Iatrogenic strictures account for about two thirds of the cases. Urethral strictures occurring after urethral instrumentation are located predominantly near the penoscrotal junction, an area that is particularly vulner-

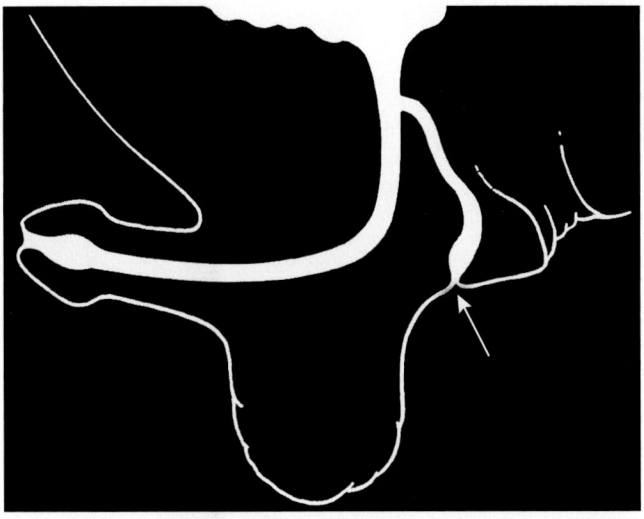

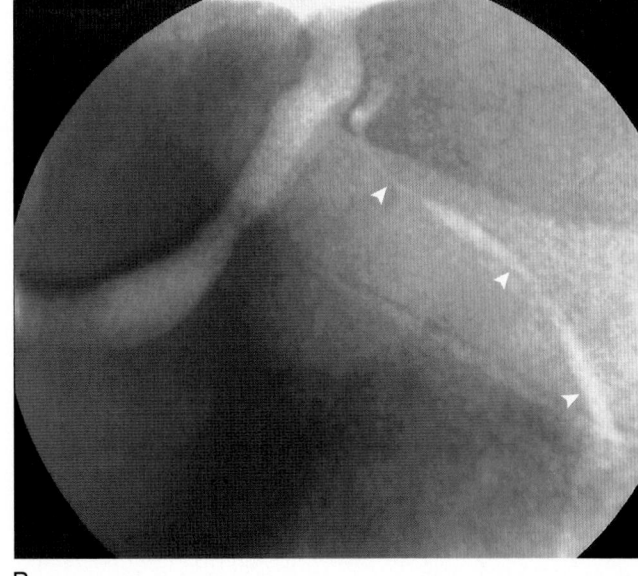

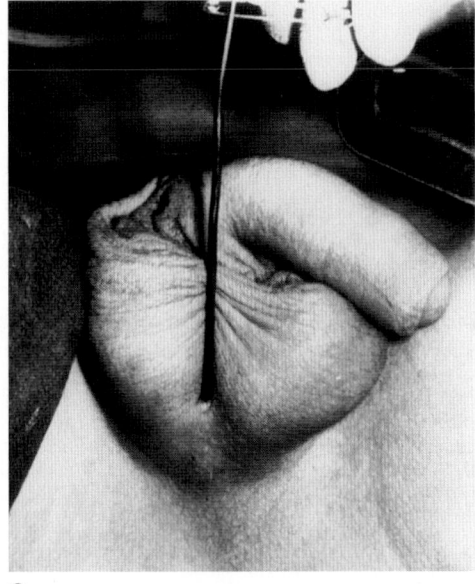

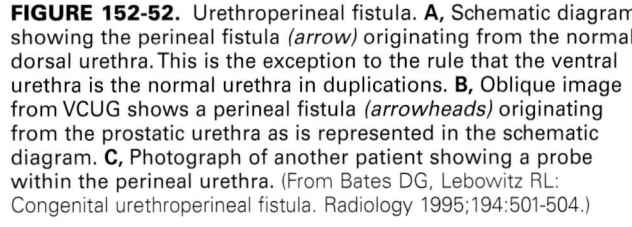

FIGURE 152-52. Urethroperineal fistula. **A,** Schematic diagram showing the perineal fistula *(arrow)* originating from the normal dorsal urethra. This is the exception to the rule that the ventral urethra is the normal urethra in duplications. **B,** Oblique image from VCUG shows a perineal fistula *(arrowheads)* originating from the prostatic urethra as is represented in the schematic diagram. **C,** Photograph of another patient showing a probe within the perineal urethra. (From Bates DG, Lebowitz RL: Congenital urethroperineal fistula. Radiology 1995;194:501-504.)

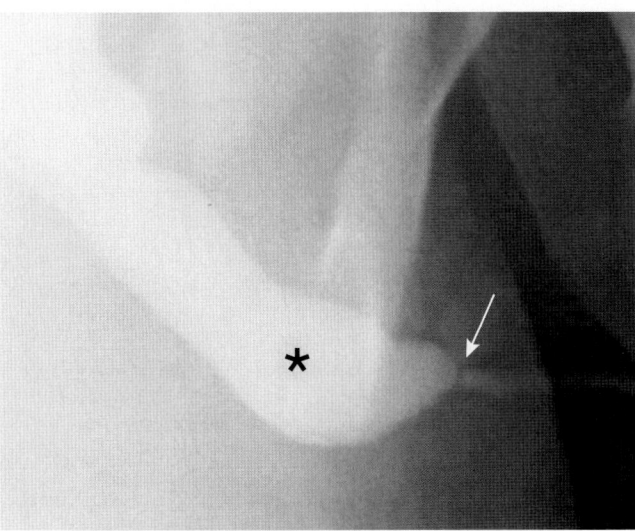

FIGURE 152-53. Urethral stricture. Oblique image during VCUG shows tight focal stricture *(arrow)* in the bulbous urethra with posterior urethral dilation *(asterisk).*

able to internal trauma. Pelvic fractures, penetrating injuries, direct blows to the perineum, and straddle injuries are the most common forms of external trauma. The membranous urethra is the area most often injured, owing to its fixation by the urogenital diaphragm. Strictures from straddle injuries are usually located in the bulbar urethra (Fig. 152-54). Urethral infections are uncommon causes of urethral strictures in children as opposed to young adults, in whom urethral strictures are often due to *Neisseria gonorrhoeae* infection. The strictures caused by *Neisseria* predominate in the bulbar urethra and are usually multiple. Urethral strictures of unknown cause in symptomatic boys are not rare. They are located most often in the bulbar urethra and are usually very short and diaphragm-like. They may be the result of unrecognized external trauma or urethritis, Cowper's duct infection, or rupture of a Cowper's duct cyst or may be secondary to incomplete dissolution of the urogenital membrane at the junction of the cloaca and genital groove (Cobb's collar). The possibility of a congenital

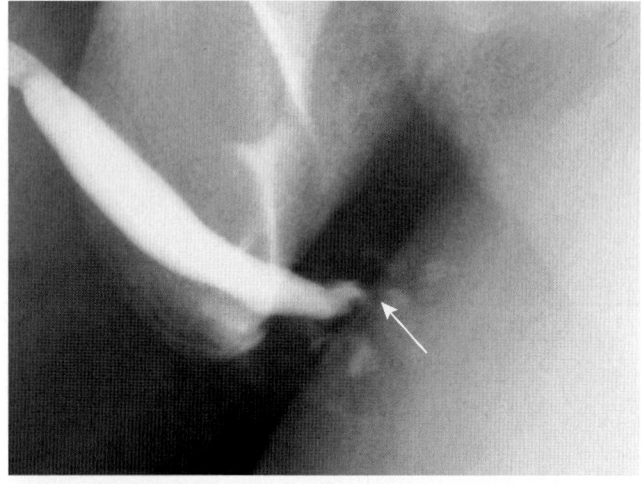

A

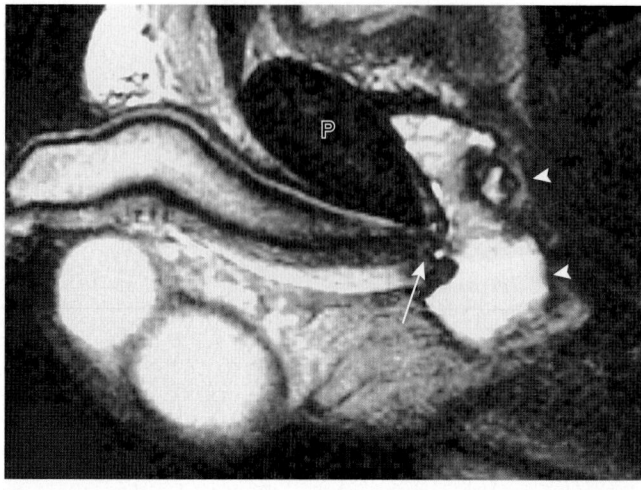

B

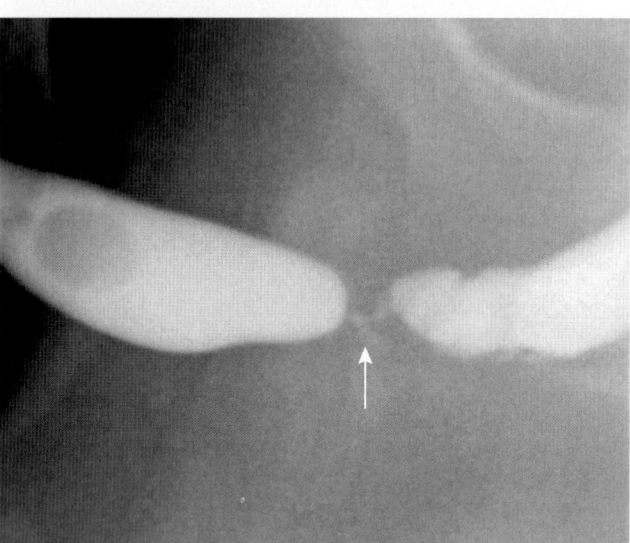

C

FIGURE 152-54. Straddle injury. **A,** Retrograde urethrogram shows bulbar urethral disruption *(arrow)* and contrast extravasation. **B,** Sagittal T2-weighted magnetic resonance image in the same patient shows urethral disruption *(arrow)* directly beneath the pubis (P). The urethral fragments are separated by an intervening hematoma *(arrowheads).* **C,** Follow-up retrograde urethrogram after repair shows high-grade urethral stricture *(arrow).*

stricture is suggested in some cases, particularly when there is a family history of a similar lesion (Fig. 152-55).

> **Urethral strictures are usually secondary to iatrogenic or traumatic injury and often occur at the penoscrotal junction.**

The clinical manifestations of urethral strictures include poor urinary stream, straining to void, urinary retention, painful urination, hematuria, urinary infections, and recurrent epididymitis. The diagnosis is readily established by VCUG when the bladder can be catheterized. Compression of the distal penis during voiding (choke urethrogram) or RUG results in distention of the normal urethra and a better delineation of the true extent of the stricture. A voiding urethrogram using the contrast material accumulated in the bladder at the end of an IVU may be the only radiographic procedure available to study the urethra when catheterization of the bladder or a retrograde urethrogram is not possible. An alternative to fluoroscopic evaluation is US of the

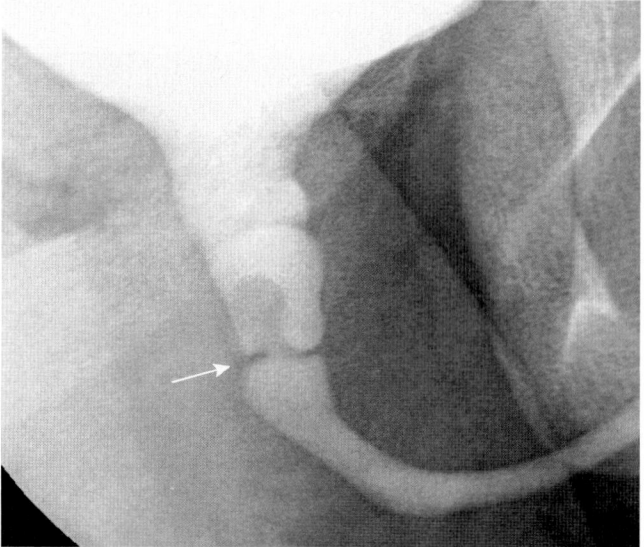

FIGURE 152-55. Congenital urethral diaphragm. Oblique image during VCUG shows a linear filling defect in the posterior urethra at the base of the verumontanum *(arrow).* There is mild posterior urethra dilation.

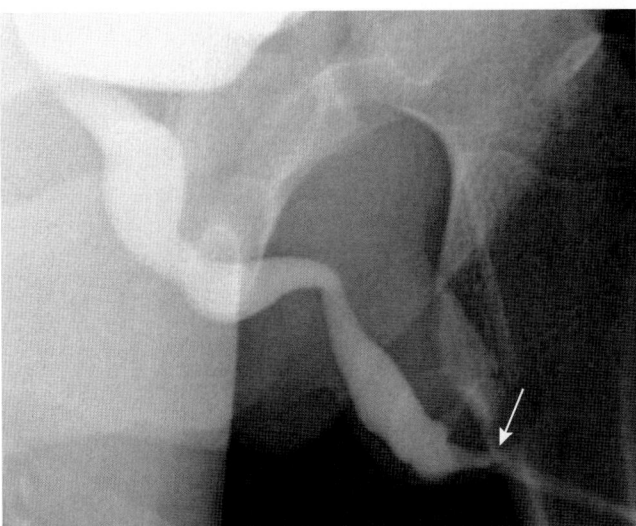

FIGURE 152-56. Meatal stenosis. Oblique image during VCUG shows a dilated urethra to the meatus *(arrow),* where the exiting urinary stream becomes attenuated.

urethra, which provides information about the urethra as well as periurethral tissues. The urethra proximal to the stricture may be dilated. Bladder trabeculation, vesicoureteral reflux, and upper tract dilatation may coexist. In the interpretation of the urethrogram, it is important to keep in mind that normal areas of narrowing at the level of the urogenital diaphragm or narrowing caused by spasm of the bulbocavernosus or external sphincter muscles may simulate a stricture.

MEATAL STENOSIS IN BOYS AND DISTAL URETHRAL STENOSIS IN GIRLS

Meatal stenosis in males is seen most frequently in patients with hypospadias and as an acquired process in circumcised boys. Except for severe cases, meatal stenosis is not believed to be as important as was once suggested. On the voiding cystogram, the urethra is generally dilated throughout, in contrast with the thin urinary stream outside the penis (Fig. 152-56). Narrowing of the distal female urethra as a result of spasm of the external sphincter with proximal urethral dilatation ("spinning top" urethra) is common on routine VCUGs in young girls. Initially believed to be secondary to urethral stenosis, transient dilation of the proximal urethra during voiding is now considered to be a normal variant, but it can also be observed in some girls with unstable bladders (bladder dyssynergia), discussed earlier.

SUGGESTED READINGS

General

Berrocal T, Lopez-Pereira P, Arjonilla A, et al: Anomalies of the distal ureter, bladder, and urethra in children: embryologic, radiologic, and pathologic features. Radiographics 2002; 22:1139-1164

Herman TE, McAllister WH: Radiographic manifestations of the lower urinary tract. Radiol Clin North Am 1991;29:365

Kawashima A, Sandler CM, Wasserman NF, et al: Imaging of urethral disease: a pictorial review. Radiographics 2004; 24(Suppl 1):S195-S216

Koff SA: Evaluation and management of voiding disorders in children. Urol Clin North Am 1988;15:769

Lo WC, Wang CR, Lim KE: Diagnosis of the congenital urethral anomalies of male child by voiding cystourethrography. Acta Paediatr Taiwan 1999;40:152-156

Pavlica P, Barozzi L, Menchi I: Imaging of the male urethra. Eur Radiol 2003;13:1583-1596

Embryology and Development

Cohen HL, Kravets F, Zucconi W, et al: Congenital abnormalities of the genitourinary system. Semin Roentgenol 2004;39:282-303

Klimberg I: The development of voiding control. Am Urol Assoc Update Series 1988;7:161

Ludwikowski B, Oesch Hayward I, Brenner E, et al: The development of the external urethral sphincter in humans. BJU Int 2001;87:565-568

Sebe P, Fritsch H, Oswald J, et al: Fetal development of the female external urinary sphincter complex: an anatomical and histological study. J Urol 2005;173:1738-1742

Volmar KE, Fritsch MK, Perlman EJ, et al: Patterns of congenital lower urinary tract obstructive uropathy: relation to abnormal prostate and bladder development and the prune belly syndrome. Pediatr Dev Pathol 2001;4:467-472

Urachal Anomalies

Avni FE, Matos C, Diard F, Schulman CC: Midline omphalovesical anomalies in children: contributions of ultrasound imaging. Urol Radiol 1988;10:189

Leicher-Duber A, Schumacher R: Urachal remnants in asymptomatic children: sonographic morphology. Pediatr Radiol 1991;21:200

Little DC, Shah SR, St Peter SD, et al: Urachal anomalies in children: the vanishing relevance of the preoperative voiding cystourethrogram. J Pediatr Surg 2005;40:1874-1876

Ozbek SS, Pourbagher MA, Pourbagher A: Urachal remnants in asymptomatic children: gray scale and color Doppler. J Clin Ultrasound 2001;29:218

Pomeranz A: Anomalies, abnormalities, and care of the umbilicus. Pediatr Clin North Am 2004;51:819-827

Rafal RV, Markicz JA: Urachal carcinoma: the role of magnetic resonance imaging. Urol Radiol 1991;12:184

Ueno T, Hashimoto H, Yokoyama H, et al: Urachal anomalies: ultrasonography and management. J Pediatr Surg 2003; 38:1203-1207

Yu JS, Kim KW, Lee HJ, et al: Urachal remnant diseases: spectrum of CT and US findings. Radiographics 2001;21:451-461

Bladder Diverticula

Evangelidis A, Castle EP, Ostlie DJ, et al: Surgical management of primary bladder diverticula in children. J Pediatr Surg 2005; 40:701-703

Hernanz-Schulman M, Lebowitz FL: The elusiveness and importance of bladder diverticula in children. Pediatr Radiol 1985;15:399

Levine PM, Gonzales ET Jr: Congenital bladder diverticula causing ureteral obstruction. Urology 1985;25:273

Shukla AR, Bellah RA, Canning DA, et al: Giant bladder diverticula causing bladder outlet obstruction in children. J Urol 2004; 172(5 pt 1):1977-1979

Megacystis

Burbige KA, Lebowitz RL, Colodny AH, et al: The megacystis-megaureter syndrome. J Urol 1984;131:1133

Ghavamian R, Wilcox DT, Duffy PG, et al: The urological manifestations of hollow visceral myopathy in children. J Urol 1997;158(3 pt 2):1286-1290

Levin TL, Soghier L, Blitman NM, et al: Megacystis-microcolon-intestinal hypoperistalsis syndrome and prune belly: overlapping syndromes. Pediatr Radiol 2004;34:995-998

Cystitis

Allen CW, Alexander SI: Adenovirus associated hematuria. Arch Dis Child 2005;90:305-306

Friedman EP, de Bruyn R, Mather S: Pseudotumoral cystitis in children: a review of the ultrasound features in four cases. Br J Radiol 1993;66:605-608

Kumar A, Aggarwal S: Case report: the sonographic appearance of cyclophosphamide-induced acute haemorrhagic cystitis. Clin Radiol 1990;41:289

Mattox TF: Interstitial cystitis in adolescents and children: a review. J Pediatr Adolesc Gynecol 2004;17:7-11

McCarville MB, Hoffer FA, Gingrich JR, et al: Imaging findings of hemorrhagic cystitis in pediatric oncology patients. Pediatr Radiol 2000;30:131-138

Rosenberg HK, Eggli KD, Zerin JM, et al: Benign cystitis in children mimicking rhabdomyosarcoma. J Ultrasound Med 1994;13:921-932

Thompson RH, Dicks D, Kramer SA: Clinical manifestations and functional outcomes in children with eosinophilic cystitis. J Urol 2005;174:2347-2349

Verhagen PC, Nikkels PG, de Jong T: Eosinophilic cystitis. Arch Dis Child 2001;84:344

Bladder Neoplasms

Asanuma H, Nakai H, Shishido S, et al: Inflammatory pseudotumor of the bladder in neonates. Int J Urol 2000;7:421-424

Dennery MP, Rushton HG, Belman AB: Sonography for the detection and follow-up of primary nonsarcomatous bladder tumors in children. Urology 2002;59:119-121

Leuschner I, Harms D, Mattke A, et al: Rhabdomyosarcoma of the urinary bladder and vagina: a clinicopathologic study with emphasis on recurrent disease: a report from the Kiel Pediatric Tumor Registry and the German CWS Study. Am J Surg Pathol 2001;25:856-864

McCarville MB, Hoffer FA, Gingrich JR, et al: Imaging findings of hemorrhagic cystitis in pediatric oncology patients. Pediatr Radiol 2000;30:131-138

Poggiani C, Teani M, Auriemma A, et al: Sonographic detection of rhabdomyosarcoma of the urinary bladder. Eur J Ultrasound 2001;13:35

Schneider G, Ahlhelm F, Altmeyer K, et al: Rare pseudotumors of the urinary bladder in childhood. Eur Radiol 2001;11:1024-1029

Siegel MJ: Pelvic tumors in childhood. Radiol Clin North Am 1997;75:1455

Wu HY, Snyder HM 3rd: Pediatric urologic oncology: bladder, prostate, testis. Urol Clin North Am 2004;31:619-627

Dysfunctional Voiding Disorders

Amis ES, Blaivas JG: The role of the radiologist in evaluation voiding dysfunction. Radiology 1990;175:317

Caldwell PH, Edgar D, Hodson E, Craig JC: Bedwetting and toileting problems in children. Med J Aust 2005;182:190-195

Chiozza ML: Dysfunctional voiding. Pediatr Med Chir 2002; 24:137-140

Cvitkovic-Kuzmic A, Brkljacic B, Ivankovic D, et al: Ultrasound assessment of detrusor muscle thickness in children with non-neuropathic bladder/sphincter dysfunction. Eur Urol 2002;41:214-218

Dacher JN, Savoye-Collet C: Urinary tract infection and functional bladder sphincter disorders in children. Eur Radiol 2004; 14(Suppl 4):L101-L106

Feldman AS, Bauer SB: Diagnosis and management of dysfunctional voiding. Curr Opin Pediatr 2006;18:139-147

Fotter R, Kopp W, Klein E, et al: Unstable bladder in children: functional evaluation by modified cystourethrography. Radiology 1986;161:811

Hoebeke P, Van Laecke E, Van Camp C, et al: One thousand video-urodynamic studies in children with non-neurogenic bladder sphincter dysfunction. BJU Int 2001;87:575-580

Kajiwara M, Inoe K, Kato M, et al: Nocturnal enuresis and overactive bladder in children: an epidemiological study. Int J Urol 2006;13:36-41

Kindo A: Cystourethrogram characteristics of bladder instability in children. Urology 1990;35:242

Kuo HC, Liu HT: Investigation of dysfunctional voiding in children with urgency frequency syndrome and urinary incontinence. Urol Int 2006;76:72-76

Mundy AR: Detrusor instability. Br J Urol 1988;62:393

Neveus T, Lackgren G, Tuvemo T, et al: Enuresis—background and treatment. Scand J Urol Nephrol Suppl 2000;(206):1-44

Noe HN: The role of dysfunctional voiding in failure or complication of ureteral reimplantation for primary reflux. J Urol 1985; 134:1172

Schulman SL, Quinn CK, Plachter N, Kodman-Jones C: Comprehensive management of dysfunctional voiding. Pediatrics 1999;103:E31

Van Gool JD: Enuresis and incontinence in children. Semin Pediatr Surg 2002;11:100-107

Wan J, Greenfield S: Enuresis and common voiding abnormalities. Pediatr Clin North Am 1997;44:117

Neurogenic Bladder

Batista J, Bauer S, Shefner J, et al: Urodynamic findings in children with spinal cord ischemia. J Urol 1995;154:1183

Bauer SB: Neurogenic bladder dysfunction. Pediatr Clin North Am 1987;34:1121

Boemers T, van Gool J, de Jong T, et al: Urodynamic evaluation of children with caudal regression syndrome (caudal dysplasia sequence). J Urol 1994;151:1041

Campioni P, Goletti S, Nannni M, et al: Diagnostic imaging of neurogenic bladder. Rays 2002;27:121-125

Campioni P, Goletti S, Palladino F, et al: The neurogenic bladder: anatomy and neurophysiology. Rays 2002;27:107-114

Erickson D, Bartholomew T, Marlin A: Sonographic evaluation and conservative management of newborns with myelomeningocele and hydronephrosis. J Urol 1989;142:592

Flood HD, Ritchey ML, Bloom DA, et al: Outcome of reflux in children with myelodysplasia managed by bladder pressure monitoring. J Urol 1994;152:1574

Artificial Urinary Sphincter

Gonzalez R, Jednak R, Franc-Guimond J, et al: Treating neuropathic incontinence in children with seromuscular colocystoplasty and an artificial urinary sphincter. BJU Int 2002;90:909-911

Petrou SP, William HJ, Young PR: Radiographic imaging of the artificial urinary sphincter pressure regulating balloon. J Urol 2001;165:1773-1775

Taylor GA, Lebowitz RL: Artificial urinary sphincters in children: radiographic evaluation. Radiology 1985;155:91

Posterior Urethral Valves

Ghanem MA, Wolffenbuttel KP, DeVylder A, et al: Long-term bladder dysfunction and renal function in boys with posterior urethral valves based on urodynamic findings. J Urol 2004; 171(6 pt 1):2409-2412

Gordon I, Ransley PG, Hubbard CS: ^{99}mTc DTPA scintigraphy compared with intravenous urography in followup of posterior urethral valves. Br J Urol 1987;60:447

Eckoldt F, Heling KS, Woderich R, et al: Posterior urethral valves: prenatal diagnostic signs and outcome. Urol Int 2004;73:296-301

Holmdahl G, Sillen U: Boys with posterior urethral valves: outcome concerning renal function, bladder function and paternity at ages 31 to 44 years. J Urol 2005;174:1031-1034

Jaureguizar E, Lopez-Pereira P, Martinez-Urrutia MJ: The valve bladder: etiology and outcome. Curr Urol Rep 2002;3:115-120

Krishnan A, deSouza A, Konijeti R, et al: The anatomy and embryology of posterior urethral valves. J Urol 2006;175:1214-1220

Lal R, Bhatanger V, Mitra DK: Upper-tract changes after treatment of posterior urethral valves. Pediatr Surg Int 1998;13:396-399

Lopez Pereira P, Martinez Urrutia MJ, Jaureguizar E: Initial and long-term management of posterior urethral valves. World J Urol 2004;22:418-424

Lopez Pereira P, Espinosa L, Martinez Urrutina MJ: Posterior urethral valves: prognostic factors. BJU Int 2003;91:687-690

Narasimham KL, Mahajan JK, Kaur B: The vesicoureteral reflux dysplasia syndrome in patients with posterior urethral valves. J Urol 2005;174(4 pt 1):1433-1435

Parkhouse HF, Barratt TM, Dillon MJ, et al: Long-term outcome of boys with posterior urethral valves. Br J Urol 1988;62:59

Rittenberg MH, Hulbert WC, Snyder HM 3rd, Duckett JW: Protective factors in posterior urethral valves. J Urol 1988;140:993

Schober JM, Dulabon LM, Woodhouse CR: Outcome of valve ablation in late-presenting posterior urethral valves. BJU Int 2004;94:616-619

Tejani A, Butt K, Glassberg K, et al: Predictors of eventual end stage renal disease in children with posterior urethral valves. J Urol 1986;136:857

Posterior Urethral Polyps

Ben-Meir D, Yin M, Chow CW: Urethral polyps in prepubertal girls. J Urol 2005;174(4 pt 1):1443-1444

Caro P, Rosenberg H, Snyder HM: Congenital urethral polyp. AJR Am J Roentgenol 1986;147:1041

Gleason PE, Kramer SA: Genitourinary polyps in children. Urology 1994;44:106-109

Maddeen NP, Turnock RR, Rickwood AMK: Congenital polyps of the posterior urethra in neonates. J Pediatr Surg 1986;21:193

Musselman P, Kay R: The spectrum of urinary tract fibroepithelial polyps in children. J Urol 1986;136:476

Utricle and Müllerian Duct Cysts

Currarino G: Large prostatic utricles and related structures, urogenital sinus and other forms of urethrovaginal confluence. J Urol 1986;136:1270

Devine CJ Jr, Gonzalez-Serva L, Strecker JF Jr, et al: Utricular configuration in hypospadias and intersex. J Urol 1980;123:407

Higashi TS, Takizawa K, Suzuki S, et al: Mullerian duct cyst: ultrasonographic and computed tomographic spectrum. Urol Radiol 1990;12:39

Ikoma F, Shima H, Yabumoto H: Classification of enlarged prostatic utricle in patients with hypospadias. Br J Urol 1985;57:334

Lopatina OA, Berry TT, Spottswood SE: Giant prostatic utricle (utriculus masculinis): diagnostic imaging and surgical implications. Pediatr Radiol 2004;34:156-159

Thurnher S, Hricak H, Tanagho EA: Müllerian duct cyst: diagnosis with MR images. Radiology 1988;168:25

Troiano RN, McCarthy SM: Müllerian duct anomalies: imaging and clinical issues. Radiology 2004;233:19-34

Cowper Glands

Colodny AH, Lebowitz RL: Lesions of the Cowper's ducts and glands in infants and children. Urology 1978;11:321

Currarino G, Fugua F: Cowper's glands in the urethrogram. Am J Roentgenol Radium Ther Nucl Med 1972;116:838

Kickuth R, Laufer U, Pannek J: Cowper's syringocele: diagnosis based on MRI findings. Pediatr Radiol 2002;32:56-58

Maizels M, Stephens FD, King LR, Firlit CF: Cowper's syringocele: a classification of dilatations of Cowper's gland duct based upon clinical characteristics of eight boys. J Urol 1983;129:111

Moskowitz PS, Newton NA, Lebowitz RL: Retention cysts of the Cowper's duct. Radiology 1976;120:377

Megalourethra, Anterior Urethral Diverticulum, and Anterior Urethral Valve

Appel RA, Kaplan GW, Brock WA, Streit D: Megalourethra. J Urol 1986;135:747

Baker AR, Neoptolemos JP, Wood KF: Congenital anterior urethral diverticulum: a rare cause of lower urinary tract obstruction in childhood. J Urol 1985;34:751

Bates DG, Coley BD: Ultrasound diagnosis of the anterior urethral valve. Pediatr Radiol 2001;31:634-636

Brown WC, Dillon PW, Hensle TW: Congenital urethral-perineal fistula: diagnosis and new surgical management. Urology 1990;36:157

Gupta DK, Srinivas M: Congenital anterior urethral diverticulum in children. Pediatr Surg Int 2000;16:565-568

Jones EA, Freedman AL, Ehrlich RM: Megalourethra and urethral diverticula. Urol Clin North Am 2002;29:341-348

Karnak I, Senocak ME, Buyukpamukcu N, Hicsonmez A: Rare congenital anomalies of the anterior urethra. Pediatr Surg Int 1997;12:407

Kolte SP, Joharapurkar SR: Anterior urethral valves, a rare cause of obstruction. Indian J Pediatr 2001;68:83

McLellan DL, Gaston MV, Diamond DA, et al: Anterior urethral valves and diverticula in children: a result of ruptured Cowper's duct cyst. BJU Int 2004;94:375-378

Mortensen PHG, Johnson HW, Coleman GU: Megalourethra. J Urol 1985;134:358

Netto NR, Lemos GC, Claro JF, Hering FL: Congenital diverticulum of male urethra. Urology 1984;24:239

Ozokutan BH, Kucukaydin M, Ceylan H: Congenital scaphoid megalourethra: a report of two cases. Int J Urol 2005;12:419-421

Sharma AK, Shekhawat NS, Agarwal R: Megalourethra: a report of four cases and review of literature. Pediatr Surg Int 1997;12:458-460

Tank ES: Anterior urethral valves resulting from congenital urethral diverticula. Urology 1987;30:467

Urethral Duplication

Bae KS, Jeon SH, Lee SJ: Complete duplication of bladder and urethra in coronal plane with no other anomalies: case report with review of the literature. Urology 2005;65:388

Bruce R, Alton D: Duplication of urethra with communication to the rectum. Pediatr Radiol 1986;16:79

Kumaravel S, Senthilnathan R, Sankkarabarathi C: Y-type urethral duplication: an unusual variant of a rare anomaly. Pediatr Surg Int 2004;20:866-868

Ortolano V, Nasrallah FP: Urethral duplication. J Urol 1986;136:909

Podesta ML, Medel R, Castera R, Ruarte AC: Urethral duplication in children: surgical treatment and results. J Urol 1998;160:1830

Prasad N, Vivekandhan KG, Ilangovan G, Prabakaran S: Duplication of the urethra. Pediatr Surg Int 1999;15:419

Psihramis KE, Colodny AH, Lebowitz RL, et al: Complete patent duplication of the urethra. J Urol 1986;136:63

Salle JL, Sibai H, Rosenstein D, et al: Urethral duplication in the male: review of 16 cases. J Urol 2000;163:1936

Urethral Strictures

Currarino G, Stephens FD: An uncommon type of bulbar urethral stricture, sometimes familial, of unknown cause: congenital versus acquired. J Urol 1981;126:658

Gallentine ML, Morey AF: Imaging of the male urethra for stricture disease. Urol Clin North Am 2002;29:361-372

Morey AF, McAninch JW: Ultrasound evaluation of the male urethra for assessment of urethral stricture. J Clin Ultrasound 1996;24:473-479

Saxton HM, Borzyskowski M, Mundy AR, Vivian GC: Spinning top urethra: not a normal variant. Radiology 1988;168:147

Sugimoto M, Kakehi Y, Yamashita M, et al: Ten cases of congenital urethral stricture in childhood with enuresis. Int J Urol 2005;12:558-562

Meatal Stenosis

Bueschen AJ, Royal SA: Urethral meatal stenosis in a girl causing severe hydronephrosis. J Urol 1986;136:1302

Levitt SB, Reda EF: Hypospadias. Pediatr Ann 1988;17:48

Nuininga JE, DeGier RP, Verschuren R, et al: Long-term outcome of different types of 1-stage hypospadias repair. J Urol 2005;174(4 pt 2):1544-1548

Van Howe RS: Incidence of meatal stenosis following neonatal circumcision in a primary care setting. Clin Pediatr 2006;45:49-54

CHAPTER

153   Anomalies of Sex Differentiation

HARRIS L. COHEN

There are various conditions and etiologies that result in abnormalities or confusion with regard to a patient's sex differentiation. In some cases, excessive androgen stimulation of the female fetus in early gestation may lead to anatomic findings that can confuse sexual identification by phenotype. The same is true in males when there is either deficient synthesis or metabolism of testosterone or deficient end-organ sensitivity to normal testosterone. Other conditions that lead to abnormal sex differentiation are due to abnormalities of the sex chromosomes or gonads themselves. The external genitalia of such patients range from deformed to ambiguous to normal. Problems of sex differentiation may be noted in patients whose genitalia are consistent with their genetic (chromosomal) and gonadal (ovary or testis) sex or in patients with discordance between their external genitalia and their genetic or gonadal sex (e.g., a female phenotype in a patient who has a 46,XY chromosome make-up).

> Abnormal sexual differentiation may be caused by abnormalities of hormone production, end-organ response, chromosomes, or gonads.

EMBRYOLOGY, SEX DIFFERENTIATION, AND GONAD DIFFERENTIATION

A person's genetic sex is determined at the time of fertilization. The development of a male genital system occurs as an "active" process requiring the presence of testes and their production of müllerian inhibiting factor (MIF), which in turn causes müllerian duct system involution. The enzyme 5α-reductase converts testosterone intracellularly within the target tissues into the powerful androgen dihydrotestosterone (DHT). DHT allows the wolffian duct system to develop into the epididymis, vas deferens, and seminal vesicles. Differentiation of the primitive gonad into a testis begins at 7 weeks of fetal life in the presence of H-Y antigens, which are found in the cell membranes of normal XY males. If there is no Y

chromosome or there is abnormal H-Y antigen expression, the gonad will passively differentiate into an ovary by as early as 12 weeks' to as late as 17 weeks' gestation when in the presence of *two* X chromosomes. Absence of two X chromosomes may lead to abnormal or streak ovaries. The ovaries, however, are thought to have no apparent role in sex differentiation of the female genital tract.

> The development of a male genital system occurs as an "active" process requiring the presence of testes and their production of müllerian inhibiting factor (MIF).

SEX DIFFERENTIATION DISORDERS WITHOUT AMBIGUITY OF EXTERNAL GENITALIA

Phenotypic Females

The best-known sex differentiation disorders that occur without ambiguity of external genitalia in phenotypic females are the classic XO Turner syndrome, the chromatin-positive variant of Turner syndrome, and XX and XY gonadal dysgenesis.

TURNER SYNDROME (XO GONADAL DYSGENESIS)

Turner syndrome is the most common gonadal dysgenesis associated with an abnormal karyotype in girls. It is relatively common and nonfamilial. It is characterized by an abnormal sex chromosome, gonadal dysgenesis, and a number of somatic anomalies. At least half of affected patients have classic Turner syndrome with an isochromatous 45,XO karyotype pattern. The second X chromosome is absent. In the case of classic Turner syndrome, the presence of only a single X chromosome is the probable cause for the presence of streak ovaries (streaks or ridges of connective tissue in the mesosalpinges parallel to the fallopian tubes), rather than normal ovaries. Some functional ovarian elements are present in a few cases. Fallopian tubes, a uterus, and a vagina are present, and no wolffian duct derivatives are found.

> **Turner syndrome is the most common gonadal dysgenesis associated with an abnormal karyotype in girls.**

Patients with classic Turner syndrome have several somatic findings, some more common than others. Affected patients are short in stature (usually no greater than 58 inches), with a distinctive facies that includes low-set ears, a low hairline, and a high, arched palate. They have a short, broad, and webbed neck, widely spaced nipples, and a shield chest. Skeletal abnormalities, which are common, include cubitus valgus, short fourth and/or fifth metacarpals, and osteoporosis of hands, feet, elbows, and upper femora. Bone age is normal to slightly delayed during childhood. Steroid deficiency is considered the cause of typically delayed postpubertal bone age. Lymphedema of the extremities, particularly the hands and feet, as well as pleural effusions and ascites seen at birth may be linked to the cystic hygromas of the neck area noted in fetal life, of which the webbed neck is thought to be a residuum. Other variably seen findings include large aortic roots, coarctation of the aorta (particularly in those patients with webbed necks), and multiple pigmented nevi. One fourth of patients with Turner syndrome have renal anomalies, usually horseshoe kidneys but also including malrotation, duplication anomalies, and ureteropelvic junction obstruction. Systemic arterial hypertension is not uncommon and is thought to be of renovascular origin. However, a proven causative vascular lesion has not been imaged. Patients with Turner syndrome have an increased incidence of autoimmune disorders, particularly Hashimoto thyroiditis.

Patients with Turner syndrome have a history of delayed onset of puberty, infantile internal and external genitalia, and primary amenorrhea. Young adolescents have sparse axillary and pubic hair. Ultrasound (US) evaluation typically shows a prepubertal uterus (Fig. 153-1). The prepubertal uterus and vagina are normally formed and will respond to exogenous hormone stimulation. The dysgenetic or streak gonads are difficult to image. According to some sources, the gonads contain a normal amount of oocytes in early fetal/neonatal life, but accelerated oocyte loss leads to their depletion within the first years of life. When the adnexa are measurable, they are typically less than 1 cm^3 in volume. In older adolescence, many patients with Turner syndrome will have pubic and axillary hair but no breast development or vaginal mucosal estrogenization.

Mosaic Turner Syndrome

As many as one fourth of patients with 45,XO Turner syndrome have a so-called chromatin-positive pattern. Their karyotype is a mosaic consisting most often of a mixture of 45,XO and 46,XX chromosomes. Less often, there are other mosaic patterns without a Y cell line (e.g., XO/XXX or XO/XX/XXX) or 46,XX with an abnormal X chromosome. In such cases, the gonads may consist of a streak ovary on one side and a hypoplastic or normal ovary on the other side, bilateral hypoplastic ovaries, or essentially normal ovaries. External and internal geni-

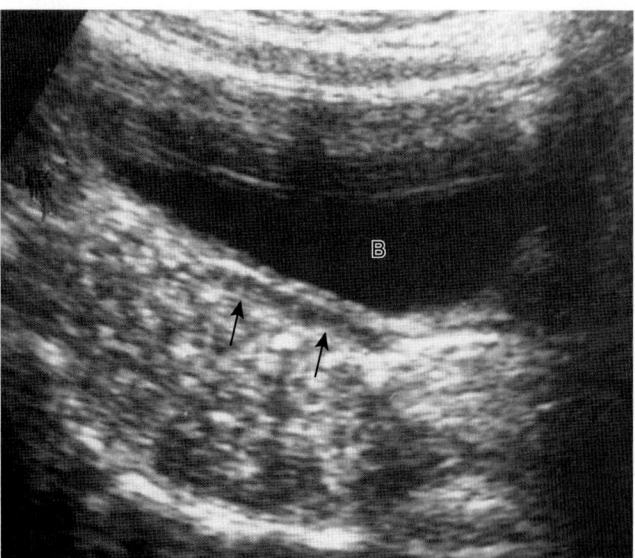

FIGURE 153-1. Turner syndrome. Longitudinal sonogram of the pelvis shows a small tubular uterus *(arrows)* in this 16-year-old with primary amenorrhea. She was a 45,XO Turner syndrome patient. Her ovaries could not be definitively identified. B, bladder.

talia are entirely female, without wolffian duct remnants. These patients usually do not have the somatic abnormalities typically attributed to classic Turner syndrome, but many will still be short.

> **When a Turner syndrome patient's karyotype is a mosaic pattern there may be normal gonadal development.**

It is these patients with mosaic Turner syndrome who have only partial ovarian failure, who may develop secondary sex characteristics at puberty (found to occur in about 50%), and who may in some cases menstruate regularly. Instances of pregnancy have been reported. Although some (typically mosaic) Turner syndrome patients can have estrogen production, such production requires the clinician to rule out the possibility of estrogen production from an associated theca-lutein cyst or a germ cell tumor. US is an excellent tool for this analysis.

Amenorrhea Caused by Hypergonadotropic Hypogonadism

Amenorrhea is an important indication for US of the adolescent pelvis. Primary amenorrhea is defined as a lack of menses by age 16. There are many causes of primary amenorrhea. Many of these causes may also be linked to causes of delayed or retarded sexual development, as well as causes of secondary amenorrhea, defined as the cessation of menses at any point in time after menarche and before menopause.

> **Primary amenorrhea is defined as a lack of menses by age 16. Many of the causes may also be linked to causes of delayed sexual development.**

Turner syndrome is the primary example of the hypergonadotropic hypogonadism group of patients with primary amenorrhea. Such adolescents, who have high levels of follicle-stimulating hormone and luteinizing hormone by serum assays and yet do not have menses, are amenorrheic because of ovarian failure in which their gonadal tissues fail to respond to endogenous gonadotropins. In the pure form of the diseases that make up this group, secondary sex characteristics fail to develop and menses does not occur. Other karyotype abnormalities placed under a broad heading of gonadal dysgenesis, including 46,XY and familial 46,XX gonadal dysgenesis, are also associated with failure of affected patients to develop secondary sexual characteristics or menses as a result of hypergonadotropic hypogonadism.

There are other causes of hypergonadotropic hypogonadism that can lead to amenorrhea. Patients may have secondary ovarian failure as a result of radiation (usually 800 cGy or greater to the pelvis) or chemotherapy (at least transient amenorrhea occurs in 50% of women who undergo chemotherapy), or on an autoimmune basis (autoimmune oophoritis). Premature menopause, as a complication of chemotherapy or radiotherapy, is usually seen in those patients who are treated when 25 years of age or older and is unusual among those first treated as adolescents. Adolescents with secondary causes of hypergonadotropic hypogonadism may have varying degrees of pubertal development.

46,XY GONADAL DYSGENESIS

The typical patient with 46,XY gonadal dysgenesis is phenotypically female, with streak gonads and infantile internal and external female genitalia, but is neither typically short nor has the somatic findings of patients with Turner syndrome. Patients are usually first diagnosed as abnormal in adolescence. As with other forms of gonadal dysgenesis, such patients may not have an absent sex chromosome but rather have abnormality of the sex chromosome that *is* present. One tenth of patients with XY gonadal dysgenesis have a deletion of the small arm of the Y chromosome linked to a testis-determining factor (and perhaps to MIF). Mosaicism may lead to the development of ovaries. If a Y chromosome is a component of the karyotype of a patient with gonadal dysgenesis and ovaries, the patient has an increased risk of developing a gonadoblastoma within a dysgenetic ovary. Imaging asymmetrically sized adnexa, especially if the larger adnexa is a solid mass, suggests the possibility of gonadoblastoma. Seminomas also occur in these patients. Inheritance of this condition is thought to be X-linked recessive or sex-limited autosomal dominant.

> **Patients with 46,XY gonadal dysgenesis are phenotypically female. They are at increased risk for developing gonadoblastomas.**

FAMILIAL 46,XX GONADAL DYSGENESIS

Familial 46,XX gonadal dysgenesis may be sporadic or inherited as an autosomal recessive trait. In some familial cases there is associated sensorineural deafness. The gonads consist of bilateral streaks in some cases, whereas in others there may be hypoplastic ovaries or a hypoplastic ovary on one side and a streak gonad on the other. The internal and external genitalia are entirely female, without wolffian duct derivatives. Incomplete puberty may be observed in patients with residual ovarian tissue. Sexual infantilism and primary amenorrhea are typical findings in those patients with bilateral streak gonads.

Phenotypic Males

KLINEFELTER SYNDROME (47,XXY SEMINIFEROUS TUBULAR DYSGENESIS)

Seminiferous tubular dysgenesis (Klinefelter syndrome) is the most common human sex chromosome aberration. The typical 47,XXY karyotype is found in phenotypic males with primary hypogonadism. It is nonfamilial, occurring in 1 in every 750 to 1000 males. Variants have been described with less common chromosomal abnormalities, including XX/XXY or XY/XXY mosaicism, as well as XXXY, XXXXY, XXYY, or XXXYY sex chromosomal karyotypes. The external genitalia, especially the testes, are small. The testes are usually less than 3 cm in length and firm. Cryptorchidism and hypospadias are common. Progressive fibrosis of the seminiferous tubules occurs, especially after puberty, leading to azoospermia and sterility in most patients. Patients are often long legged. They are often mentally retarded or have psychological problems. The diagnosis is usually not made until after puberty. Gynecomastia develops in almost half of the older patients, and affected patients (particularly those with the classic 47,XXY karyotype) are at an increased risk for breast cancer. Testicular and extragonadal germ cell neoplasms have been uncommonly reported.

> **Seminiferous tubular dysgenesis (Klinefelter syndrome) is the most common human sex chromosome aberration.**

A variant form (49,XXXY) of Klinefelter syndrome has somatic findings including radioulnar synostosis, coxa valga, abnormal facies, short neck, delayed bone age, hypertonia, small external genitalia, and severe mental retardation. These findings may allow diagnosis earlier than puberty.

PERSISTENT MÜLLERIAN DUCT SYNDROME

Persistent müllerian duct syndrome (also known as uterine hernia syndrome and hernia uteri inguinalis) is a rare type of sexual differentiation abnormality of males caused by deficiency of MIF, the testicular hormone that causes normal regression of the müllerian duct system in the male fetus. The patients usually have a normal 46,XY karyotype and are phenotypically male, but they have a small uterus and fallopian tubes and a small vagina connected to the posterior urethra at the level of the verumontanum. Unilateral or bilateral cryptorchidism is common. If the undescended testis is underdeveloped, the ipsilateral vas may be absent. Unilateral or bilateral inguinal hernias are common. A uterus (uteri hernia syndrome), fallopian tubes, or sometimes a testis may be found in the hernia. Uncommonly, gonadal neoplasia may occur. The disorder, typically sporadic, has been reported in siblings. The voiding or retrograde urethrogram is usually normal. In these patients, direct catheterization and injection of the utricle (noted on US as a cystic area in the region of the prostate, extending from the seminal colliculus and said to be the male analog of the uterus and vagina and residua of the fused posterior ends of the müllerian ductal system; see Chapter 152) with contrast material at urethroscopy may demonstrate a uterus and/or fallopian tubes. Patients may present with renal stones, infections, or other problems related to an associated abnormal urinary tract.

DISORDERS OF SEX DIFFERENTIATION WITH AMBIGUOUS EXTERNAL GENITALIA

The four main groups with ambiguous external genitalia and problems of sex differentiation are female intersex (pseudohermaphroditism), male intersex, gonadal dysgenesis, and true hermaphrodites.

Pseudohermaphroditism (Intersex)

Pseudohermaphroditism or intersex problems are abnormalities in which there is nonaccord of chromosomal, gonadal, and genital sex. Unlike true hermaphroditism, in which two types of gonadal tissue is present, pseudohermaphroditism has nonaccord but only one gender's gonads are present. By definition, male intersex patients have testes and female intersex patients have ovaries or ovarian tissue.

> Pseudohermaphroditism or intersex problems are abnormalities in which there is nonaccord of chromosomal, gonadal, and genital sex and the presence of only one type of gonad. Male intersex patients have testes and female intersex patients have ovarian tissue.

Female Intersex

Female intersex is usually diagnosed in neonatal life in chromosomally normal females (46,XX) with masculinized external genitalia. The cause is usually increased fetal adrenal androgen production, most commonly from congenital adrenal hyperplasia or adrenogenital syndrome. Congenital adrenal hyperplasia is by far the most common cause of abnormal sex differentiation in females, occurring in 1 in 15,000 live births worldwide (see Chapters 24 and 144). It is due to an inherited deficiency of enzymes involved in adrenocortical hormone biosynthesis. Other cases may be due to maternal causes such as androgen ingestion in early pregnancy or, rarely, to a masculinizing ovarian tumor in the mother. Excess androgen exposure leading to female intersex is thought to usually occur in the first trimester. Affected patients have normal ovaries, uterus, and fallopian tubes. They have no testicular tissue or internal wolffian duct derivatives. In most cases the external genitalia are ambiguous

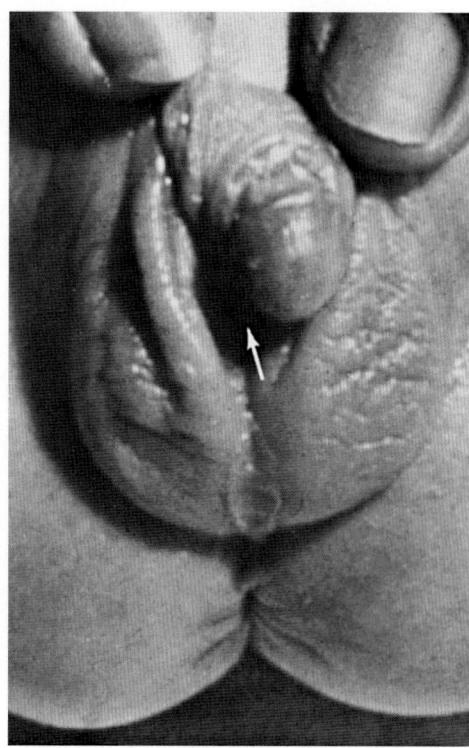

FIGURE 153-2. Ambiguous external genitalia in a 1-month-old infant. A phallus and scrotum are present, but no gonads are palpable. A single perineal opening was found at the base of the phallus *(arrow).*

(Fig. 153-2), with a prominent phallus or partially fused labial scrotal folds. There is a variously sized vagina connected with the posterior urethra and forming a urogenital sinus, which commonly empties at the base of the phallus (Fig. 153-3). There is a spectrum of possible external genital findings ranging from mild virilization manifested by clitoral hypertrophy to rare patients with an advanced degree of virilization and a normal-appearing but empty "scrotum," a large phallus resembling a penis, and a penile (phallic) urethra usually associated with hypospadias. No gonads can be palpated in the labioscrotal folds or in the inguinal canal of such patients because they are within the pelvis. US can assess enlarged adrenal glands as well as normal uterine development in patients suspected of having this problem. Voiding cystourethrography often shows a male-type elongated urethra (Fig. 153-4). These patients are potentially fertile with external genital reconstruction and correct sex assignment.

> Female intersex occurs in chromosomally normal females, usually due to increased fetal adrenal androgen production.

Male Intersex

Male intersex patients are true males with a normal 46,XY male karyotype, present H-Y antigens, normal or mildly defective (and usually undescended) testes, but incomplete masculinization or frank ambiguity of their

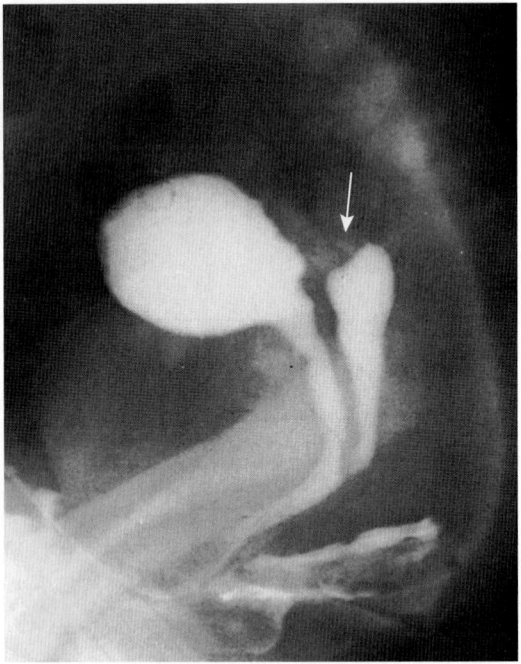 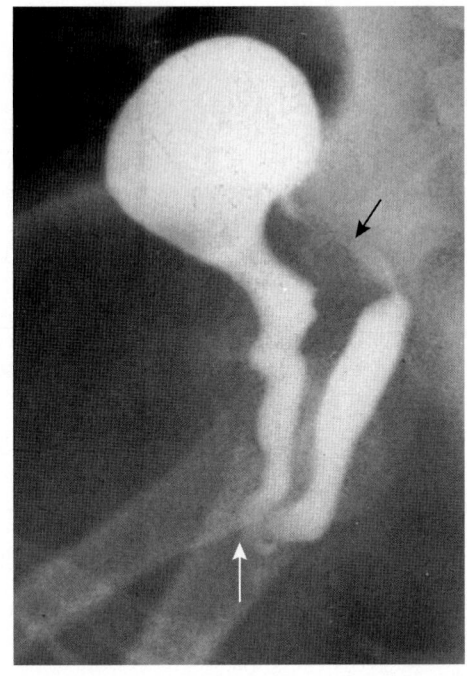

A   B

FIGURE 153-3. Adrenogenital syndrome showing different degrees of masculinization of the lower urogenital tract as seen on VCUG. **A,** Urogenital sinus, the most common appearance of the lower urogenital tract in adrenogenital syndrome. A well-developed vagina with a well-defined impression of the uterine cervix on the vaginal vault *(arrow)* joins the distal end of the urethra to form a long common sinus tract (urogenital sinus) that ends in the perineum at the base of a prominent phallus. Barium paste was applied on the perineum to show the distance between the vagina and perineum. **B,** VCUG of a second infant shows a well-developed vagina with opacification of the uterine canal *(black arrow)* that joins the urethra very near the perineum to form an ultrashort urogenital sinus *(white arrow)*. An enlarged clitoris, posterior fusion of the labia, and a single perineal opening were the only external signs of the disorder, which caused only mild virilization.

external genitalia. Cases of pure male intersex (pseudo-hermaphroditism) are usually not diagnosed until after puberty. These patients are thought to be female and may present with the clinical concern of primary amenor-rhea. Other cases of male intersex have either in-complete testosterone production or early destruction or dysgenesis of the testes and do not produce testosterone. Decreased testosterone production and a lack of MIF production results in a karyotypically normal male with a female phenotype (except for partial masculinization of the external genitalia), and incomplete inhibition of the development of müllerian elements such as the uterus, vagina, and fallopian tubes (Fig. 153-5). Such patients usually have no secondary sexual development at puberty and may have an infantile uterus on US. If production of MIF by the testes is not affected, no internal müllerian system structures (uterus and fallopian tubes) will devel-op. The underlying defect in these cases is an abnor-mality of metabolism of testosterone by the fetal testes. The biochemical defect may be decreased androgen synthesis, decreased DHT production as a result of defi-ciency of 5α-reductase, or a defect in the androgen recep-tors. In many cases the exact etiology remains unknown.

> Male intersex patients are karyotypic males with varying degrees of phenotypic genital ambiguity due to abnormal androgen synthesis or end-organ response.

There are a variety of rarer forms of male intersex caused by deficiency of various enzymes necessary to produce testosterone. Manifestations are variable. Deficiency of enzymes affecting the synthesis of both corticosteroids and testosterone (e.g., 20,22-desmolase, 3β-hydroxysteroid dehydrogenase) or affecting only the synthesis of testosterone by the testis (17β-ketosteroid reductase) may produce infants with an entirely female phenotype with a blind-ending vaginal pouch emptying in the perineum who may be partially masculinized with varying degrees of genital ambiguity similar to that seen in congenital adrenal hyperplasia. The testes are undescended. Defects involving the synthesis of both testosterone and corticosteroids are considered variants of congenital adrenal hyperplasia and are complicated by severe salt wasting or hypertension. At puberty, patients with decreased testosterone synthesis by the testes often show some virilization and may develop gynecomastia. Gonadal neoplasia has not been reported in these cases.

Another form of male intersex, caused by a deficiency in 5α-reductase (see Fig. 153-5), results in pseudovaginal perineal hypospadias. Production of testosterone and MIF is not affected. The testes are well developed and normal histologically. They may be located intra-abdominally, in the inguinal canals, or in the scrotal folds. The external genitalia are poorly masculinized, with a phallus of inter-mediate size resembling a clitoris more than a penis. The urethra opens at the base of the phallus (perineoscrotal hypospadias), and the vagina is a blind-ending structure of variable size emptying onto the perineum behind the

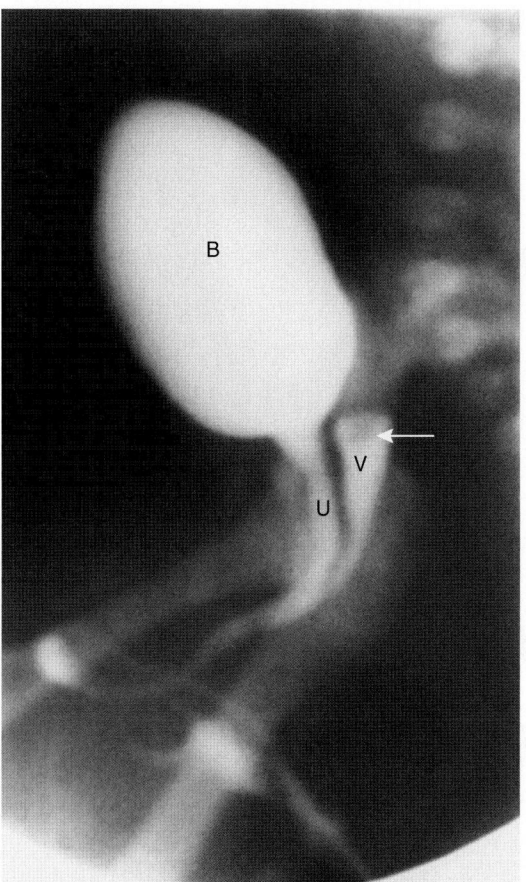

FIGURE 153-4. Congenital adrenal hyperplasia. Lateral VCUG image shows a bladder (B) with an elongated male-type urethra (U). Posterior to it is a vagina (V) with a subtle impression *(arrow)* of a cervix superiorly. The patient was a 46,XX neonate from an area in Puerto Rico where congenital adrenal hyperplasia is common. (From Cohen H, Haller J: Pediatric and adolescent genital abnormalities. Clin Diagn Ultrasound 1988; 24:187-216, with permission. Copyright Elsevier Science [USA].)

urethral opening (pseudovagina), or occasionally in the urethra (urogenital sinus) (see Fig. 153-5). There are no internal müllerian derivatives (uterus and tubes), and the epididymis, vas deferens, seminal vesicles, and ejaculatory ducts are present and empty into the vagina. There is an underdeveloped prostate. At puberty there is variable, sometimes remarkable, masculinization of the patient, with descent of the testes, increased phallus size, development of normal axillary and pubic hair, deepening of the voice, and increased muscle mass. Spermatogenesis has been reported. Gynecomastia does not develop. Gonadal neoplasms may occur but are uncommon.

TESTICULAR FEMINIZATION SYNDROME (ANDROGEN RECEPTOR DEFECT)

Testicular feminization syndrome (Fig. 153-6) is a form of intersex in which 46,XY patients have well-formed testes (usually undescended within the abdomen or inguinal region) that produce androgens and MIF. The patients, however, do not have an end-organ response to the androgens. Müllerian system development is inhibited, and patients do not develop a uterus, fallopian tubes, or the upper two thirds of the vagina. They do develop secondary female sexual characteristics via circulating

estrogens (produced from the breakdown of testosterone and adrenal steroids as well as from direct production by the testes). Because there is no turnoff mechanism for testosterone, there are, at times, higher than normal amounts of testosterone converted to estrogen. Patients with the complete form of the abnormality appear as phenotypically normal females, although they may have inguinal or labial masses resulting from the undescended testes (see Fig. 153-6). They have normal breast development, but pubic and axillary hair is scant. They do not suffer from acne. They may or may not have a short, blind-ending vagina behind the urethral opening. They often first present with amenorrhea. US will show no uterus (see Fig. 153-6) and no ovaries. This inherited end-organ unresponsiveness to the action of endogenous or exogenous androgen (androgen resistance) is caused by a defect in a specific cytoplasmic receptor protein (cytosol receptor) that normally binds DHT to the plasma membrane and transports it to the nuclear chromatin.

The complete form of testicular feminization syndrome is seen in 1 in every 20,000 to 60,000 apparent females. It is inherited as an X-linked recessive trait, affecting 50% of the karyotypic males within families. Affected females are carriers. After puberty, many such patients undergo gonadectomy because of the risk of neoplasia in undescended testes. These patients are treated with substitutional estrogen therapy.

INCOMPLETE FORMS OF TESTICULAR FEMINIZATION SYNDROME

There is an incomplete form (10% to 20% of cases) of testicular feminization that can present earlier in life than the complete form and in which the affected patient has ambiguous genitalia. Affected patients may have a predominantly female phenotype (incomplete testicular feminization) or a predominantly male phenotype (Reifenstein syndrome). These patients have an incomplete androgen receptor defect. Those with a predominantly female phenotype have the same anatomic abnormalities as patients with complete testicular feminization except for the presence of mild virilization of the external genitalia in some cases (clitoromegaly and partial labial fusion) and the presence of wolffian duct derivatives that empty into the vagina (see Fig. 153-5). A varying degree of virilization or feminization is observed at puberty, but menses does not occur. Those patients with Reifenstein syndrome have a more advanced degree of virilization. The degree of masculinization may vary greatly even in the same family. In the most severely affected (poorly virilized) patients, there is a small phallus and an incomplete fusion of the labial scrotal folds or a bifid scrotum. The urethra empties at the base of the phallus, and there may be a separate vaginal pouch ending in the perineum behind the urethra (pseudovagina). More commonly, however, the patient is less severely affected (more virilized) and has a better developed penis and scrotum.

Hypospadias is a usual finding and ranges from perineoscrotal to penile. A large prostatic utricle (Fig. 153-7) or a blind vaginal pouch connected to the posterior urethra may be present. The testes tend to be smaller than normal and are often undescended. The prostate is

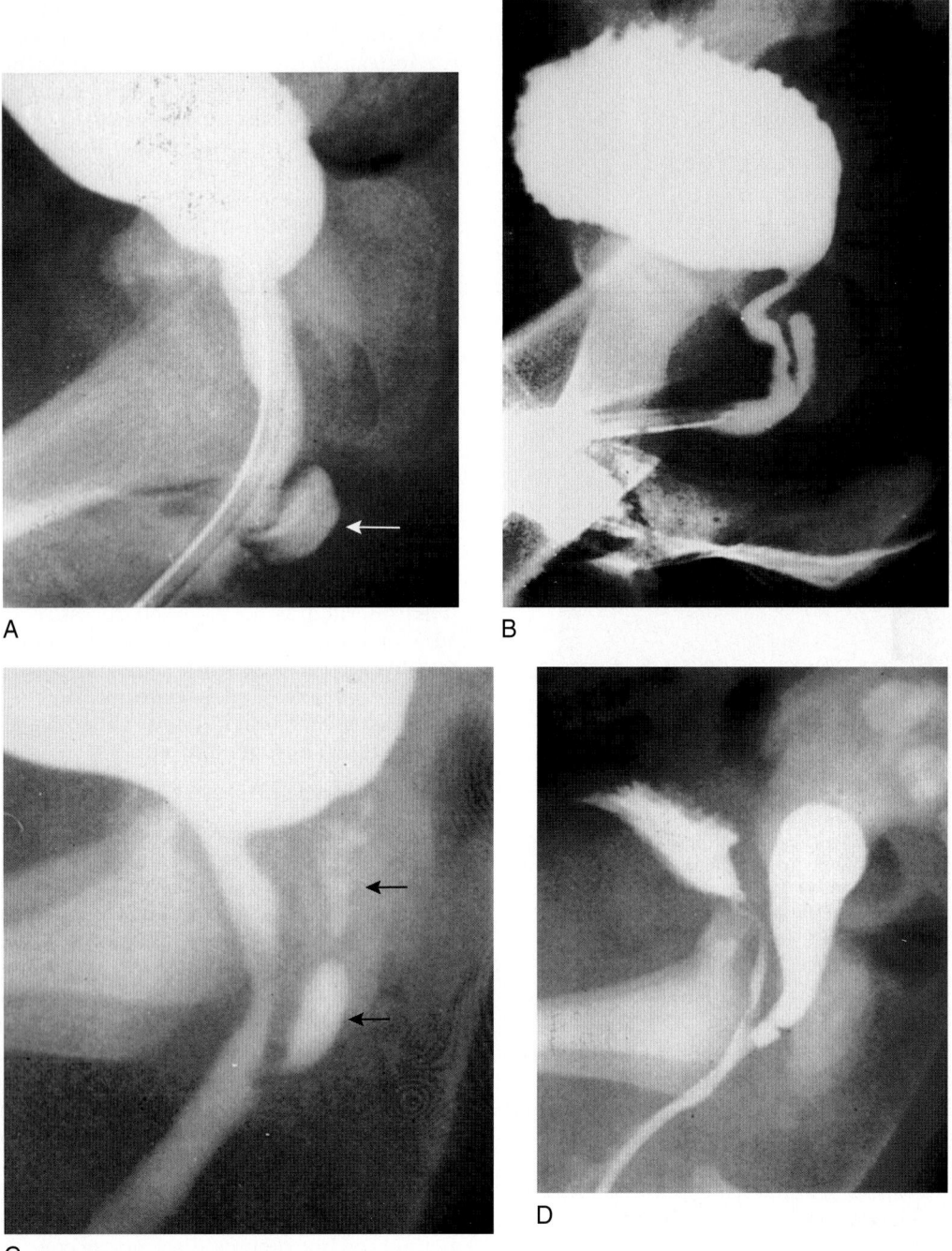

FIGURE 153-5. Four cases of male pseudohermaphroditism. **A,** Incomplete testicular feminization syndrome in a patient with a predominantly female phenotype. VCUG shows a mildly elongated urethra and retrograde opacification of a short, blind-ending vaginal pouch *(arrow)* in the perineum behind the urethra. Seminal ducts may end in a vaginal pouch such as this. A similar configuration can be seen in patients with complete testicular feminization syndrome and in patients with 5α-reductase deficiency. **B,** Three-year-old child with ambiguous external genitalia and 5α-reductase deficiency. A retrograde urethrogram shows a urogenital sinus and a small vagina without a cervical imprint. A more common pattern in 5α-reductase deficiency is that shown in **A. C,** A male infant with severe hypospadias (perineal and scrotoperineal), bilateral cryptorchidism, small penis, and unfused scrotal folds shows a utricle or blind vaginal pouch that is very short and extending off the distal aspect of the posterior urethra. *Arrows* show spermatic ducts emptying into the utricle. The male urethra is somewhat short. **D,** Infant with severe hypospadias. Retrograde urethrogram shows a somewhat longer utricle connected with the distal end of the posterior urethra. The male urethra is somewhat short.

absent. Wolffian duct derivatives are usually present but may be incompletely developed and may empty in the utricle or vaginal pouch. There is no uterus or fallopian tubes. The body habitus is generally masculine, and most patients are reared as males. At puberty, there is some development of axillary and pubic hair but no chest or facial hair or voice changes. Postpubertal gynecomastia, azoospermia, and infertility are typical. In both types of incomplete testicular feminization, gonadal neoplasms have been reported uncommonly.

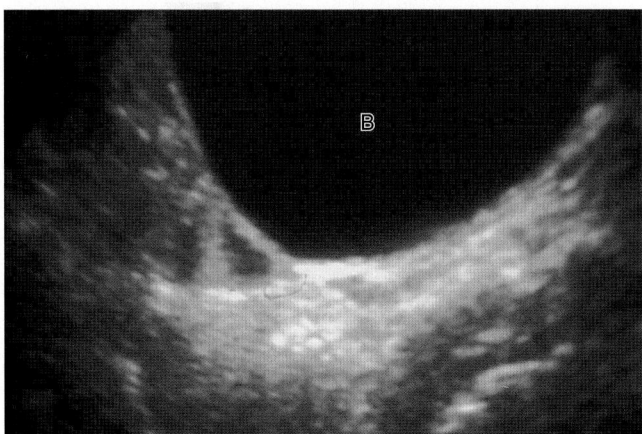

A

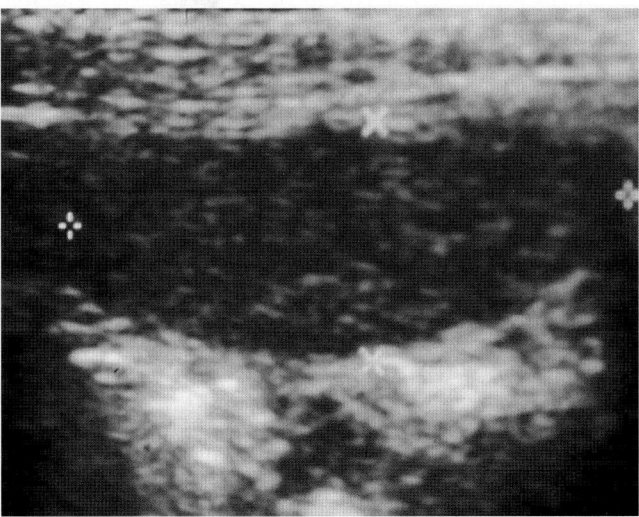

B

FIGURE 153-6. Testicular feminization syndrome. **A,** A phenotypically normal 16-year-old girl presented with primary amenorrhea. Longitudinal midline sonogram showed no uterus posterior to the bladder (B). Ovaries were not seen. Karyotyping showed 46,XY, and the patient was proven to have testicular feminization syndrome. **B,** On examination for primary amenorrhea, this patient was noted to have bilateral inguinal masses. An oval structure *(cursors)* without contained cysts was found in the patient's left inguinal region on sonography that proved to be an undescended testis. (Courtesy of Joseph Yee, MD.)

Gonadal Dysgenesis

MIXED GONADAL DYSGENESIS (DYSGENETIC MALE PSEUDOHERMAPHRODITISM)

Mixed or asymmetric gonadal dysgenesis (also known as XO/XY gonadal dysgenesis) is a relatively common form of abnormal sexual differentiation, usually occurring sporadically. Affected patient karyotypes are most often a mosaic of 45,XO and 46,XX. At times, XO/XYY or other mosaicisms are seen. These patients often have a streak gonad similar to that seen in Turner syndrome on one side and a usually dysgenetic (but occasionally normal) testis on the other. A fallopian tube is often present on the side of the streak gonad, and a vas deferens may be

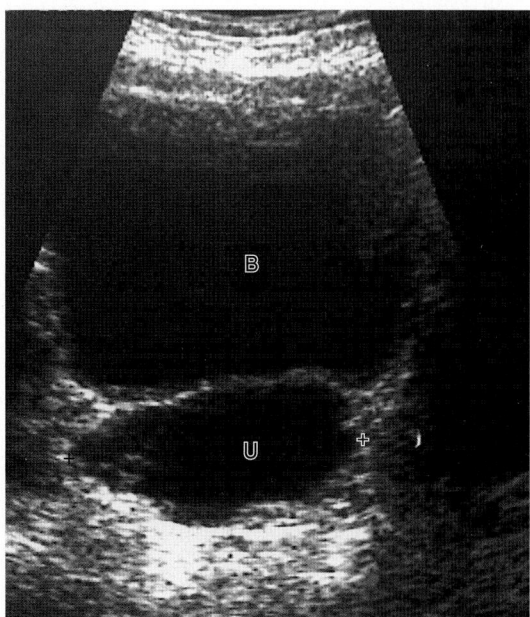

FIGURE 153-7. Utricle. Transverse sonogram of the pelvis shows a cystic mass (U) posterior to the bladder (B) of a boy with significant hypospadias and incomplete testicular feminization syndrome. (From Cohen HL, Bober S, Bow S: Imaging the pediatric pelvis: the normal and abnormal genital tract and simulators of its diseases. Urol Radiol 1992;14:273–283.)

present on the side of the testis. The testis is usually intra-abdominal but can be partially or completely descended. The external genitalia cover a wide spectrum of appearances from that of an almost normal female to that of an essentially normal male with hypospadias. Most patients have ambiguous external genitalia (as seen in other intersex situations), with a phallus/clitoris of variable size, unfused labioscrotal folds, and a variously sized vagina connected with the urethra (urogenital sinus) and commonly emptying at the base of the phallus (Fig. 153-8). A uterus, said to be present in all cases, is usually small or rudimentary. Most patients are raised as females, but at puberty some virilization may take place (usually without gynecomastia).

Mixed gonadal dysgenesis patients, as already noted, are at a high risk for developing gonadal neoplasia. The risk increases with increasing patient age. Gonadectomy is recommended at the time of diagnosis. Although gonadal neoplasia is common in XO/XY mosaicism, cases may also occur in 46,XY males with a structurally abnormal Y chromosome or in patients with the 46,XY variant of gonadal dysgenesis.

> **Patients with mixed gonadal dysgenesis are at a high risk for developing gonadal neoplasia.**

FAMILIAL 46,XY GONADAL DYSGENESIS

Familial 46,XY gonadal dysgenesis is an X-linked autosomal dominant trait associated with camptomelic dwarfism. The gonads are variable and may be bilateral streaks, bilateral dysgenetic testes, or a streak on one side and a dysgenetic testis on the other (mixed gonadal

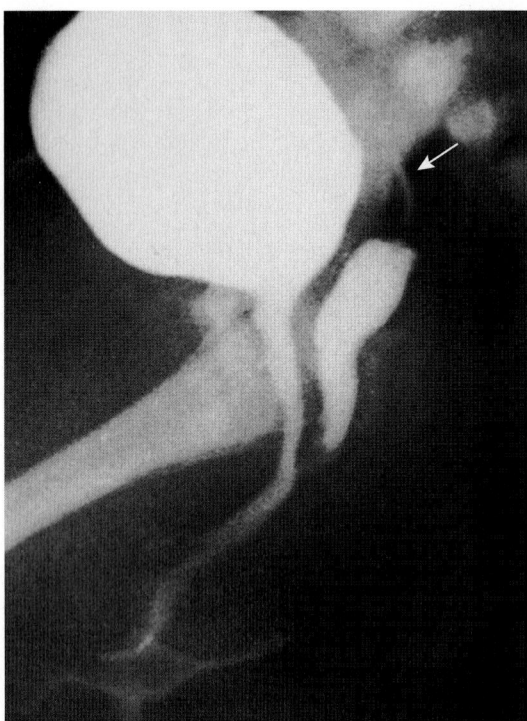

FIGURE 153-8. Mixed gonadal dysgenesis. Lateral VCUG image shows a urogenital sinus with a well-developed vagina in an 11-day-old with ambiguous external genitalia. There is a cervical imprint, and contrast material opacifies the uterine canal *(arrow)*.

dysgenesis). Cases with different gonadal anatomy may be observed in the same family.

Patients with bilateral streak gonads have a female phenotype with normal fallopian tubes, uterus, and vagina, usually clitoromegaly, and absence of wolffian duct derivatives. Sexual infantilism and amenorrhea are expected at puberty. Somatic features similar to those of Turner syndrome may be observed. Patients with bilateral dysgenetic testes or with a mixed form of gonadal dysgenesis typically have ambiguous or incompletely masculinized external genitalia. Müllerian and wolffian duct derivatives are present but may be hypoplastic or rudimentary. At puberty, various degrees of virilization usually take place. Patients with this form of gonadal dysgenesis have the same high risk of developing gonadal tumors as those with XO/XY gonadal dysgenesis.

DRASH SYNDROME—GONADAL DYSGENESIS, NEPHROPATHY, AND WILMS TUMOR

Drash syndrome is an uncommon form of gonadal dysgenesis and male intersex. Patients most often have a 46,XY karyotype, bilateral gonadal dysgenesis with a variable histologic pattern, ambiguous external genitalia, and intra-abdominal testes. They have chronic glomerulonephritis with histologic features similar to those of congenital nephrosis. They develop end-stage renal disease in early life. More than half of these patients develop a Wilms tumor at a young age, purportedly occurring only in those patients with a female phenotype. Twenty percent to 30% of patients with Drash syndrome develop gonadal neoplasia.

> Drash syndrome is an uncommon form of male intersex and gonadal dysgenesis, associated with renal failure and Wilms tumor.

46,XY GONADAL AGENESIS (VANISHING TESTES SYNDROME)

Patients with this condition are male with a 46,XY karyotype. No gonads are present, and there is absent or incomplete male sex differentiation as a result of testicular resorption of unknown cause in early fetal life (first trimester). The external genitalia are ambiguous, and there is usually complete absence of both müllerian and wolffian duct derivatives. Occasional cases may have partial development of both systems. This vanishing testes syndrome is differentiated from cases of bilateral anorchia (congenital absence of the testes), which are presumably due to resorption of the testes after the first trimester (i.e., beyond 13 to 14 weeks' gestational age). Patients with bilateral anorchia have normal male sex development and no residual müllerian structures. However, some families have individuals with 46,XY gonadal agenesis as well as individuals with bilateral anorchia, suggesting some link between the two conditions.

True Hermaphroditism

True hermaphroditism is a rare condition. It is a sporadic disorder in which the affected patient has both testicular and ovarian tissue in the same or contralateral gonads. More than half such patients have a 46,XX karyotype. Mosaic karyotype patterns with at least one line with a Y chromosome do exist, including XO/XY, XX/XXY, or XX/XY chimerism (30%). Fifteen percent of patients are 46,XY. All true hermaphrodites are H-Y antigen positive regardless of karyotype. In 45,XX patients, undetected Y chromosomal material is probably present and transferred to another chromosome. Half of the cases have a testis (or an ovary) on one side and an ovotestis on the other, 30% have a testis on one side and an ovary on the other, and 20% of the time there are bilateral ovotestes. The testes or ovotestes may be intra-abdominal, in the inguinal region, in the scrotal area, or in the labia majora. The ovaries of hermaphrodites are almost always intra-abdominal. The testis or the testicular portion of an ovotestis is usually dysgenetic, and spermatogenesis after puberty is rare. Ovulation occurs more commonly. Internal gonadal ducts are usually consistent with the ipsilateral gonad (i.e., a vas on the side of a testis and a fallopian tube on the side of an ovary). In the case of ovotestes, the associated internal gonadal duct is usually a fallopian tube. A uterus is found in almost all cases but is most often hypoplastic and may be bicornuate.

> True hermaphroditism is a rare condition. It is a sporadic disorder in which the affected patient has both testicular and ovarian tissue in the same or contralateral gonads.

There is a wide spectrum of external genitalia ranging from normal male to ambiguous to female. Cryptorchidism is common. Inguinal hernias are common and, as with normal patients, can contain a gonad with its internal gonadal duct or even a uterus. About 75% of hermaphrodites are brought up as males. At puberty, there is usually some virilization as well as gynecomastia. Fertility and childbearing have been described in some 46,XX patients. Gonadal neoplasms are uncommon.

GONADAL NEOPLASIA OF PATIENTS WITH DISORDERS OF SEX DIFFERENTIATION

As discussed, the gonads in several intersex disorders (with or without ambiguous genitalia) are at an increased risk for developing neoplasms. Neoplasms are almost always germ cell in type, including seminoma or dysgerminoma and gonadoblastoma. Less commonly, patients may develop a gonadal teratoma, teratocarcinoma, yolk sac tumor, embryonal carcinoma of the adult type, or choriocarcinoma. These neoplasms are rare in patients who do not have a Y chromosome as part of their karyotype. The risk is apparently related to the H-Y antigen. One must be aware that because the gonad may be in an unusual location (i.e., inguinal area, labia, abdomen) that is also where the neoplasm may be discovered. This is especially true for intra-abdominal gonads. The fact that in some intersex disorders the incidence of gonadal neoplasia is higher than in males with simple cryptorchidism suggests that there is an additional causative factor of unknown etiology.

> **Patients with several of the intersex disorders are at an increased risk for developing gonadal germ cell neoplasms.**

Patients with the highest risk of developing gonadal neoplasia are those with XO/XY mixed gonadal dysgenesis and those with 46,XY gonadal dysgenesis. The incidence of a gonadal tumor in both these conditions increases from 3% to 4% by age 10 years to 10% to 20% within the second decade of life and to 70% or more in older patients. Gonadal neoplasms are less frequent in patients with complete testicular feminization syndrome but still more common than in simple cryptorchidism. One fifth of those patients develop a gonadal tumor after 25 years of age but have little risk of such a tumor in childhood.

Gonadal neoplasms also occur in Klinefelter syndrome, persistent müllerian duct syndrome, incomplete testicular feminization, 5α-reductase deficiency, and true hermaphroditism, but with a risk equal to or lower than that in simple cryptorchidism.

DIAGNOSTIC EVALUATION OF PATIENTS WITH AMBIGUOUS GENITALIA

The discovery of anomalous or ambiguous genitalia in a newborn has been described as an emergency from a social perspective (although some patient advocate groups have disagreed) and, hence, to many from a clinical perspective as well. Of the seven components of sexual identity described by Hanson (chromosomes, gonads, external genital anatomy, internal genital anatomy, hormones, rearing, and psychosexual orientation), rearing has been considered key and perhaps the most important factor. Paramount in the decision on how to rear a child is the identification of the uterus, vagina, or urogenital sinus by US, contrast fistulogram, or vaginogram. These findings can then be correlated and sexual identification aided by current laboratory methods used in the treating institution. The key method of laboratory diagnosis is karyotyping. Hormone assays beginning after the third day of life, analysis of blood electrolytes and metabolites, fluorescent studies for Y chromosomes, and more specific analysis of the Y chromosome for the testis-determining gene may be performed. Other laboratory analyses include the culture of genital skin fibroblasts for androgen receptor binding and tests for androgen responsiveness (Wilson TA: personal communication, 2006). Sometimes the definitive anatomic diagnosis is made only at laparoscopy or laparotomy and on the basis of gonadal biopsy. The main role of US is identification of the uterus, a relatively easy task in the newborn female.

Important diagnostic clues as to sexual identity and causes of gender identification confusion may be obtained from clinical history (particularly the history of maternal exposure to androgens or progestins during the first trimester of pregnancy) or the history of similar findings in other members of the newborn's family. The appearance of the external genitalia is seldom diagnostic of a specific intersex disorder, but palpable gonads in the inguinal canal, labioscrotal folds, or scrotum can exclude female pseudohermaphroditism in most cases. There are females with inguinal hernias who may have an ovary, perhaps with the fallopian tube, in the inguinal region or the labia.

A detailed radiographic study of the lower genitourinary tract (genitography) is important for diagnosis and as a guide in surgical reconstructive procedures. Patients usually have a urogenital sinus, a common terminal channel for the anterior urethra and posterior vaginal pouch. This sinus usually empties at the base of the phallus. A urogenital sinus anomaly should be suspected whenever there is a single perineal opening and any degree of ambiguity of the external genitalia. A voiding cystourethrogram (VCUG), particularly on lateral view, may outline the entire anatomy needed for evaluation. If the urethral catheter can be advanced only to the vagina, an injection with the catheter in that position may opacify the vagina, the urogenital sinus, and often the proximal urethra. If there is still confusion about the anatomy during the VCUG examination, a retrograde injection of contrast material may be attempted through a catheter whose tip is placed just inside the "urethral" meatus. At times, a firmer catheter (with a curved tip) manipulated under fluoroscopic control into the urethra and bladder or into the vagina may improve contrast study of the area. At times, it may be impossible to opacify all the components of the urogenital sinus anomaly at the same time. An effort should be made on the VCUG/vaginogram to determine if a uterine cervix is present. Often, if a uterus (especially if normal) is present, there is a mass impression of the cervix on the contrast medium–filled vagina (see Fig. 153-4). A cervi-

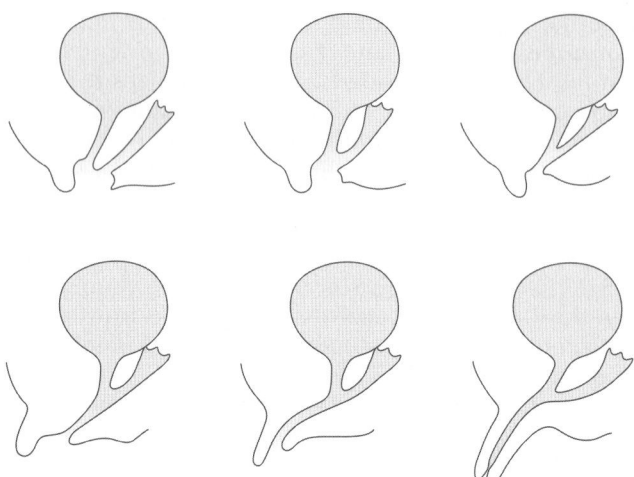

FIGURE 153-9. Different types of urogenital sinus are arranged in order of increasing masculinization, from an almost normal female pattern to a penile urethra. The urogenital sinus is of variable length, and the vagina may enter the urogenital sinus at various levels.

cal imprint, however, may not be apparent if the vagina is not sufficiently distended or if the uterus is hypoplastic.

In some patients evaluated by VCUG/contrast vaginogram, the urogenital sinus is quite short and joined by the vagina very close to the perineal surface (Fig. 153-9). In other patients it is a much longer channel, joined by the vagina at a much higher level, occasionally near the bladder neck. A very high insertion of the vagina in the urogenital sinus may pose a problem at the time of vaginal reconstruction because of the danger of injuring the external urethral sphincter. In patients evaluated for abnormalities of sex differentiation/ambiguous genitalia, the vagina may vary in size from a small cavity to an organ of normal size for the patient's age. Occasionally its distal end is stenosed or is completely obliterated, resulting in hydrocolpos at birth or hematocolpos at puberty (Fig. 153-10).

The length of the urogenital sinus and the level of insertion of the vagina into the urogenital sinus are good indicators of the degree of virilization that has taken place, but the findings are nonspecific regarding the true sex of the patient or the type of underlying disorder. For this purpose, the presence or absence of a cervical imprint on the vaginogram is more important. A uterine cervix is present in all female intersex patients. It is a common finding among many patients with mixed gonadal dysgenesis or true hermaphroditism as well. All members of

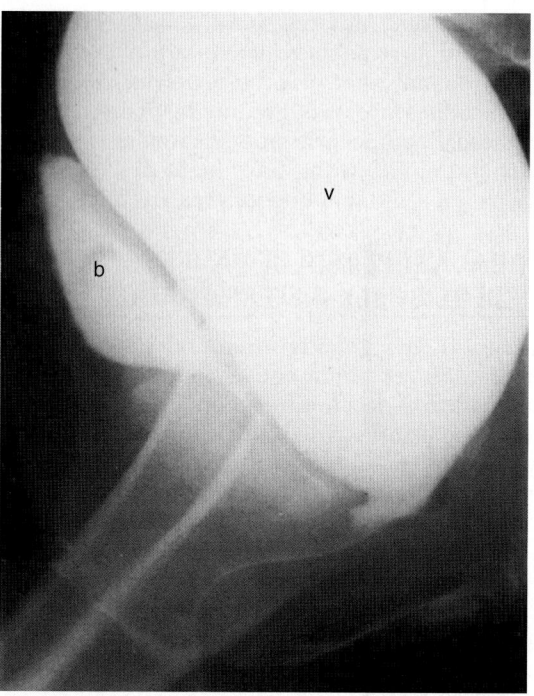

FIGURE 153-10. Hydrocolpos in adrenogenital syndrome. Lateral view from a retrograde vaginogram of a 14-year-old girl with adrenogenital syndrome and urogenital sinus shows a catheter within a large obstructed vagina. She had presented with abdominal pain and a pelvic mass. v, vagina; b, bladder.

these groups may have a hypoplastic or rudimentary uterus that may not be noted radiographically. Cervical imprints are not seen in male pseudohermaphroditism or male hypospadias.

Pelvic US is valuable in evaluating infants with ambiguous genitalia. US is an excellent imaging tool for identification of uterine tissue, although may be difficult with hypoplastic uteri. The proximal vagina may also be demonstrated, particularly if it contains urine, but the urethra and urogenital sinus cannot be studied by this method. US does not replace genitography but is of particular value when genitography is unsuccessful. Instillation of fluid in the rectum may be helpful in separating stool from a retrovesical mass. Ovaries are often seen. Fallopian tubes, unless obstructed, are more difficult to image. US is an excellent tool for the identification of the adrenal gland in the newborn as well as the older child. Some enlargement of the adrenal glands may be seen in congenital adrenal hyperplasia, but the occurrence of normal-sized adrenal glands does not rule out this diagnosis. In addition, the adrenal glands of newborns are usually prominent. Pelvic MRI is of great value (Fig. 153-11) in evaluating patients with complex anatomy, particularly those with complex müllerian duct system abnormalities, in whom US and genitography do not provide sufficient information.

> The length of the urogenital sinus and the level of insertion of the vagina are indicators of the degree of virilization but are nonspecific regarding the type of underlying disorder. For this purpose, the presence or absence of a cervical imprint on the vaginogram is more important. A uterine cervix is present in all female intersex patients.

> Pelvic MRI is of great value in evaluating complex genital anatomy when US and genitography do not suffice.

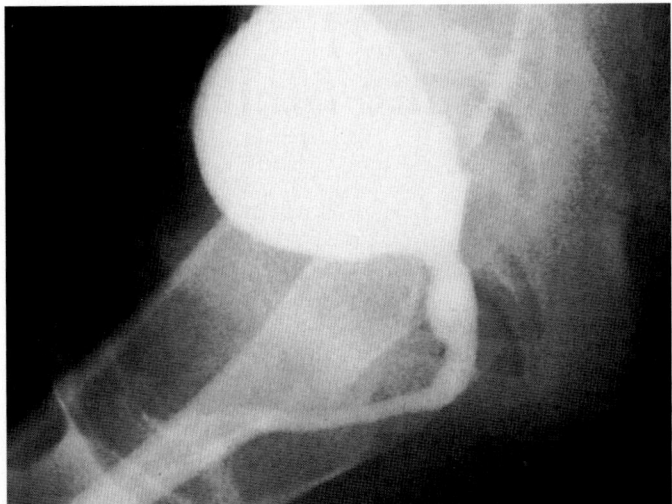

A

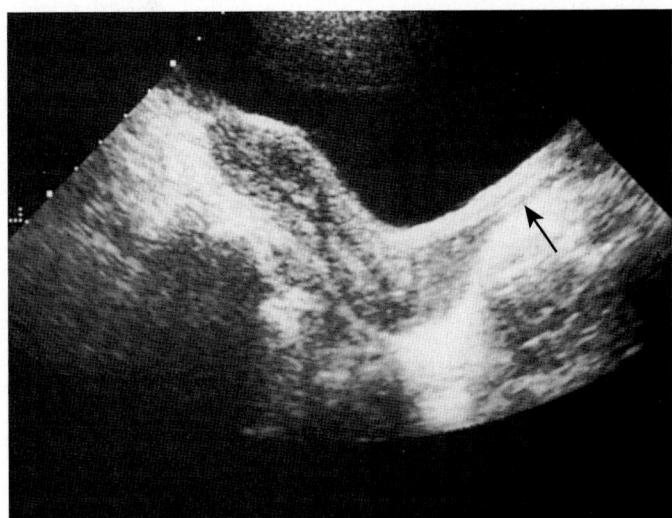

B

FIGURE 153-11. Anatomic evaluation of a 13-year-old with known adrenogenital syndrome being evaluated before surgical vaginoplasty. **A,** VCUG shows a phallic urethra. A vagina is not seen. **B,** Sagittal sonogram shows a normal adult uterus. The proximal two thirds of the vagina *(arrow)* are noted and appear normal. **C,** Sagittal T1-weighted MR image shows the vagina (V) throughout its course posterior to the bladder and anterior to rectum. Uterine tissue *(arrow)* is seen anterosuperior to it.

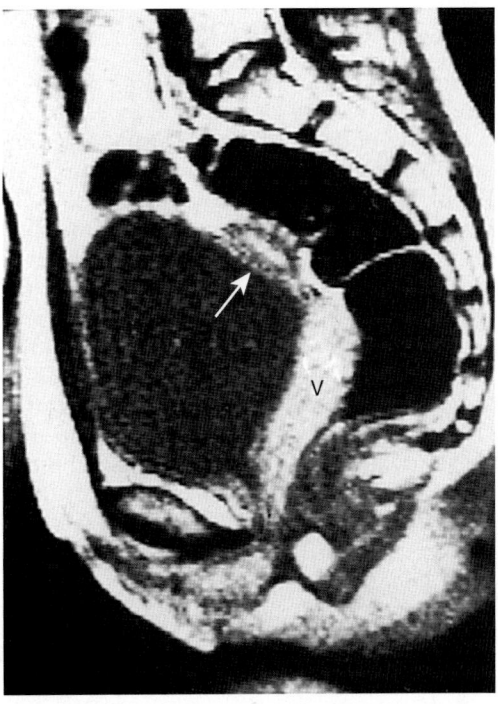

C

SUGGESTED READINGS

Boechat MI, Westra SJ, Lippe B: Normal US appearance of ovaries and uterus in four patients with Turner's syndrome and 45,X karyotype. Pediatr Radiol 1996;26:37

Cohen HL: Evaluation of the adolescent and young adult with amenorrhea: role of US. *In* Bluth E, Arger P, Hertzberg B, Middleton W (eds): Syllabus: A Special Course in Ultrasound: Clinical Questions, Practical Answers. Oak Brook, IL, RSNA Publications, 1996:171

Cohen HL, Bober S, Bow S: Imaging the pediatric pelvis: the normal and abnormal genital tract and simulators of its diseases. Urol Radiol 1992;14:273

Cohen HL, Haller JO: Pediatric and adolescent genital abnormalities. Clin Diagn Ultrasound 1988;24:187

Conte F, Grumbach MM: Pathogenesis, classification, and treatment of anomalies of sex. *In* DeGroot LJ (ed): Endocrinology. Philadelphia, WB Saunders, 1989:1810

Coran AG, Polley TZ Jr: Surgical management of ambiguous genitalia in the infant and child. J Pediatr Surg 1991;26:812

Currarino G, Wood B, Majd M: Abnormalities of the genital tract. *In* Silverman F, Kuhn J (eds): Caffey's Pediatric X-Ray Diagnosis, 9th ed. St. Louis, Mosby–Year Book, 1993:1375

Fernandes E, Fernandes E, Hollabaugh S, et al: Persistent müllerian duct syndrome. Urology 1990;36:516

Ganong W (ed): The gonads: development and function of the reproductive system. *In* Review of Medical Physiology, 17th ed. Norwalk, CT, Appleton & Lange, 1995:399

Guyton AC, Hall JE: Textbook of Medical Physiology, 11th ed. Philadelphia, Elsevier Saunders, 2006:996

Halbertsma F, Otten B, Wijnen R, Feitz W. [A baby boy with cryptorchism, inguinal hernia and internal female genitalia: the persistent Müllerian duct syndrome]. Ned Tijdschr Geneeskd 2004;148:484

Hall JG, Gilchrist DM: Turner syndrome and its variants. Pediatr Clin North Am 1990;37:1421

Marcantonio SM, Fechner PY, Migeon CJ, et al: Embryonic testicular regression sequence: a part of the clinical spectrum of 46,XY gonadal dysgenesis. Am J Med Genet 1994;49:1

Nidecker A, Cohen HL, Zinn HL: Amenorrhea in the adolescent or young adult. *In* Bluth E, Arger P, Benson C, et al (eds): Ultrasound. A Practical Approach to Clinical Problems, 2nd ed. New York, Thieme (in press)

Ratani R, Cohen HL, Fiore E: Pediatric gynecologic ultrasound. Ultrasound Q 2004;20:127

Rosenberg HK: Pediatric pelvic sonography. *In* Rumack C, Wilson S, Charboneau J (eds): Diagnostic Ultrasound, 3rd ed. St. Louis, Elsevier Mosby, 2005:1997

Sivit CJ, Hung W, Taylor G, et al: Sonography in neonatal congenital adrenal hyperplasia. AJR Am J Roentgenol 1991;156:141

Speiser P: Prenatal treatment of congenital adrenal hyperplasia. J Urol 1999;162:534

CHAPTER 154

Abnormalities of the Male Genital Tract

HARRIS L. COHEN

NORMAL SCROTAL ANATOMY

The normal infant testis is about 1.0 cm long. In early childhood, the testis is largest at 2 to 3 months of age, with a volume of 2 cm³. This somewhat more prominent size is probably related to the androgen surge of the first months of life that subsequently declines. By 6 months of age, the average pediatric testis is somewhat smaller than it is at 2 months of age. Testicular volume increases slowly until pubescence, when a greater degree of enlargement usually occurs with a rise in gonadotropins. In a 1966 Swiss study of 300 healthy boys and 300 healthy men, Prader found a 2- to 5-cm³ testicular volume at age 12, a 5- to 10-cm³ volume at the beginning of testicular growth at age 13, and a 15- to 25-cm³ volume after a rapid growth spurt at about 15 years of age. These measurements are obviously related to the ages of puberty in a given population. Testicular growth ceased at about 18 years of age. At that time the average testicular volume was 15 to 25 cm³.

> **Normal testicular volume is 2 to 5 ml at age 12, 5 to 10 ml at age 13, and 1 to 25 ml at age 15. Testicular growth ceases at about 18 years of age.**

The development of secondary sexual characteristics in males is a good indicator of testosterone production by the Leydig cells of the testis. Testicular size is a good indicator of tubular function and spermatogenesis. In the adolescent, the left testis is marginally smaller than the right. The mature postpubescent testis measures 2.5 × 3.0 × 4.0 cm. The normal testes should be ovoid and symmetric on physical examination as well as all imaging examinations.

> **The development of secondary sexual characteristics indicates testosterone production by Leydig cells. Testicular size is an indicator of tubular function and spermatogenesis.**

IMAGING MODALITIES

Ultrasound (US), including Doppler imaging in all its forms (i.e., duplex, color, and power Doppler), is the main diagnostic imaging tool for evaluating the scrotum.

Computed tomography (CT) may be used for the analysis of intrapelvic or intra-abdominal extension of intrascrotal masses but is predominantly used to denote metastatic spread of testicular or other intrascrotal tumors. Magnetic resonance imaging (MRI) has been used in the search for undescended testes that remain in an intra-abdominal position. MRI, like CT, can be used to analyze metastatic spread of testicular tumor. Its uses in intra-abdominal, intrapelvic, and intrascrotal imaging are evolving.

Scrotal US has developed into a highly accurate imaging modality for determining the presence of testes within the scrotum, evaluating echogenicity patterns of the testes to identify normal versus abnormal testes, and evaluating the testicular adnexa, particularly each epididymis. US is highly accurate in determining whether an intrascrotal abnormality is testicular or extratesticular and whether it is cystic or solid.

Scrotal Ultrasound Technique

Scrotal US is performed using a high-frequency transducer. As with other body areas, the choice of an US transducer is a compromise between the better near-field resolution obtained with a high-frequency (e.g., 7.5 or 10 MHz) transducer and the better penetration afforded by lower frequency transducers (e.g., 3.5 MHz). The superficial position of testes in the normally thin-walled scrotum allows excellent imaging with a transducer of 7.5 MHz or higher. Some authors limit their examinations to linear array transducers only. Others include views obtained with a sector, vector, or convex array transducer so that both testes can be examined, in full, side by side. A sector or convex array transducer in addition to a linear array may allow better side-by-side testicular morphologic and vascular flow comparison. This allows better analysis of differences in echogenicity, which is an important point in analyzing patients for testicular torsion, particularly when the torsion is subacute. At times, a lower-frequency transducer may be necessary to analyze the scrotum and its contents when it is enlarged by, for example, a large amount of hydrocele (Fig. 154-1) or its wall is thickened by edema or trauma. This is more often a problem in adult imaging, but the technique can be helpful for evaluation of the postpubertal adolescent.

More often, in children, the technical difficulties for US imaging relate to the small size of the scrotum and its

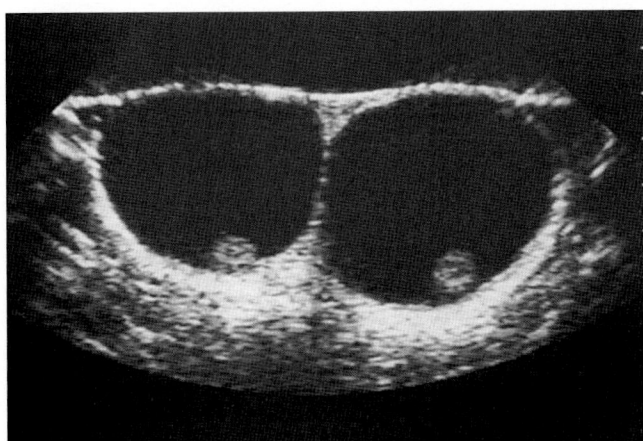

FIGURE 154-1. Hydroceles. On transverse plane ultrasound, two normal testes are seen as small echogenic structures within a very enlarged scrotum of a young child with large hydroceles. Typically, high-frequency transducers (e.g., 7.5 MHz and greater) are used for improved near-field resolution of superficial structures such as the testes. In cases, such as this one, with large hydroceles, a lower-frequency transducer may be needed to better penetrate the greater distance between the anterior and posterior scrotal walls to image the testes.

contents. Examiner persistence will often prove rewarding. Some examiners cup the scrotum with one hand while holding the transducer in the other. A small palpated lesion may be more easily positioned for US evaluation by having the sonologist or the older or more cooperative patient hold the area of concern between two fingers while the examiner places the transducer directly on it.

> Imaging of a palpable testicular mass may be aided by the patient holding the mass between 2 fingers during the US examination.

Longitudinal (Fig. 154-2), transverse (Fig. 154-3), and coronal US views are taken of each hemiscrotum. Transverse views, particularly with a convex array transducer (see Fig. 154-3), allow the best side-by-side comparison of both testes and their adnexae, especially when checking for differences in size and echogenicity. Occasionally, one

may accomplish the same with a linear-array transducer with a footprint that encompasses the entire scrotum. Coronal views using the near-field testis as an ultrasonic window may help in evaluating the contralateral testis. However, because of differences in depth of beam penetration for each testis, coronal views are not optimal for echogenicity comparisons between testes.

The adolescent scrotum is examined in a manner similar to that used with the adult scrotum. A folded towel is used as a bridge to lift the scrotum off the thighs. By holding the ends of the towel, the patient can control positioning, thus alleviating some of the discomfort of inadvertent motion during the examination of the painful scrotum. The bridge helps cup the scrotum, decreasing the size of the area to be examined. Furthermore, both testes can be seen better for side-by-side comparison when they are placed closer to each other.

Imaging Findings on Scrotal Ultrasonography

On US examination, the testes should be homogeneously echogenic. A highly echogenic linear density (seen posteriorly and superiorly) represents the mediastinum testis (Fig. 154-4), which is the inward extension of the tightly adherent covering of the testis, the tunica albuginea (Fig. 154-5). The mediastinum tends not to be

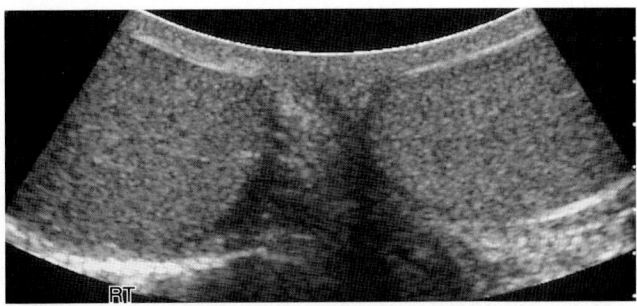

FIGURE 154-3. Normal testes. The testes of a teenager are seen as homogeneously echogenic on ultrasound in the transverse plane. This image was obtained using a convex linear array probe that allowed imaging of most of both testes. These transducers can show both testes in their entirety in most cases and are therefore an improvement over linear array transducers (which are limited by the size of their footprint) for side-by-side comparisons of testes.

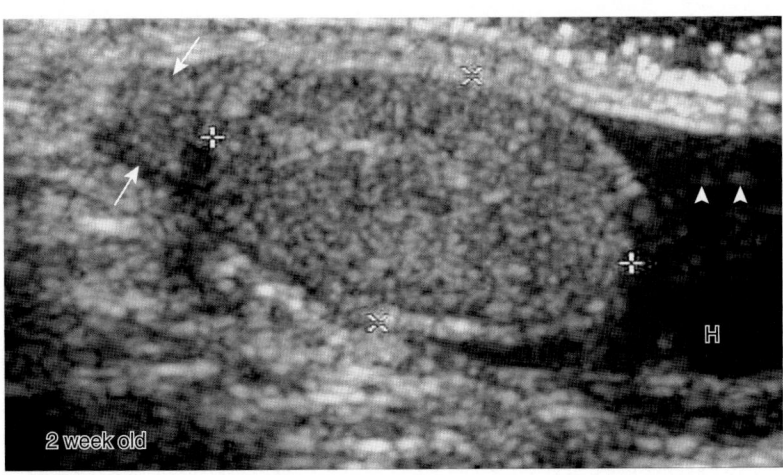

FIGURE 154-2. Hydrocele with some contained meconium in the normal testis of a 2-week-old boy as seen on a longitudinal sonogram. *Cursors* mark off the right testis. The triangular structure *(arrows)* superior to it is the head of the epididymis. The relatively echoless area inferior to it is part of a hydrocele (H). This hydrocele has echogenic debris *(arrowheads)* within it consistent with some meconium. The walls of the scrotum are seen surrounding the testis and can best be individually identified anterior and posterior to the hydrocele.

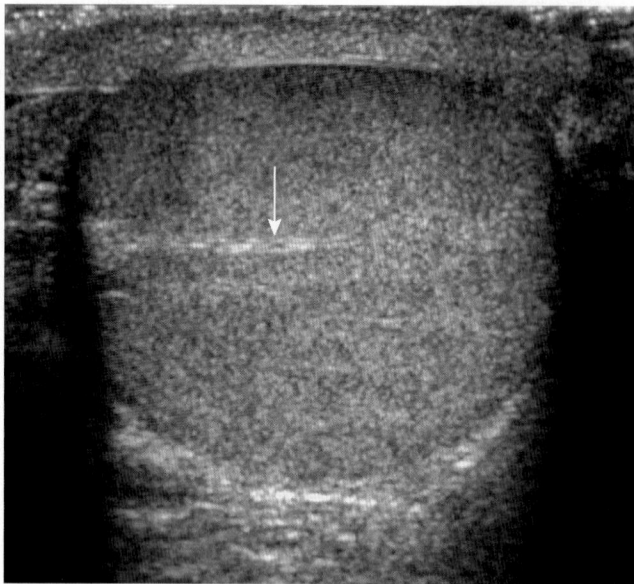

FIGURE 154-4. Mediastinum testis. Transverse sonogram shows a linear echogenicity *(arrow)* within a normal testis that is the mediastinum testis.

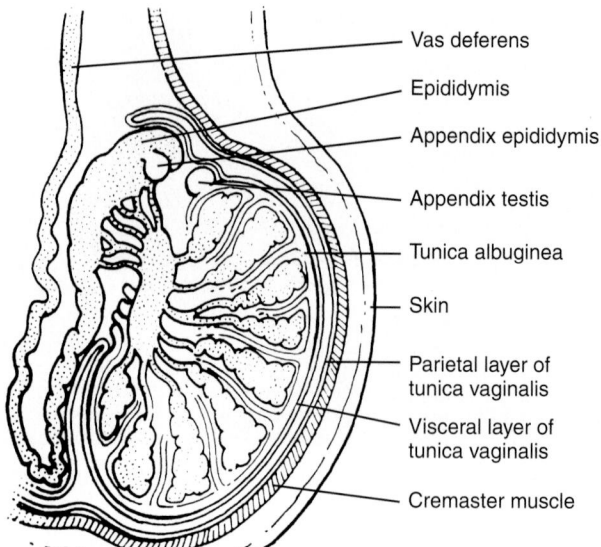

FIGURE 154-5. Schematic drawing of the scrotum and its contents as seen in the longitudinal plane through a single testis. Note the tunica albuginea surrounding the lobules of the testes. The tunica albuginea, in turn, is surrounded by the visceral layer of the tunica vaginalis and the more superficial parietal layer of the tunica vaginalis. (From Cohen HL, Sivit C [eds]: Fetal and Pediatric Ultrasound: A Casebook Approach. New York, McGraw-Hill, 2001. Reproduced with permission of McGraw-Hill Companies.)

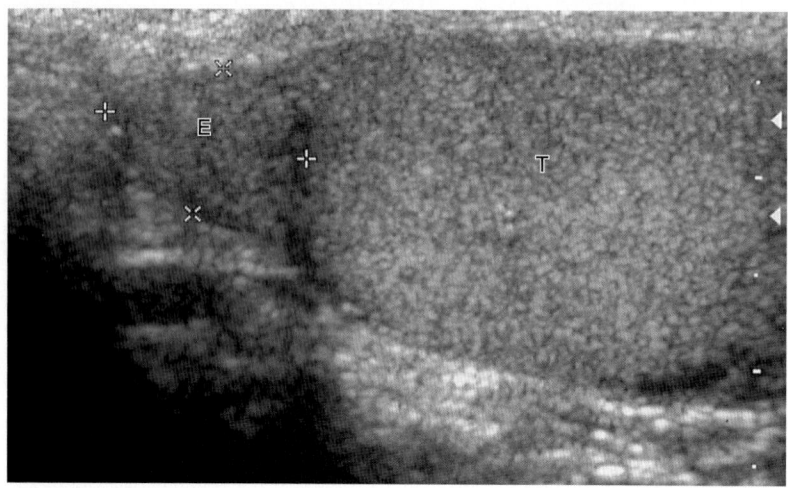

FIGURE 154-6. Normal epididymis. *Cursors* mark off the head of the epididymis (E), which sits atop the superior testis (T), in this longitudinal sonogram. The normal epididymal body and tail, which travel along the side of the testis, are more difficult to separate from normal testis.

well seen until after pubescence. Fibrous septa extending from the mediastinum testes, which are not typically seen on US examination, divide the testes into more than 250 lobules. The spermatic cord, draining veins, lymphatics, nerves, vas deferens, and a single testicular artery run within the mediastinum testis.

> **The spermatic cord, draining veins, lymphatics, nerves, vas deferens, and a single testicular artery run within the mediastinum testis.**

The head of the epididymis (Fig. 154-6) sits atop the superior pole of each testis. The head is continuous with the epididymal body and tail, which travel inferiorly along the posterolateral margin of the testis. The epididymal head is about three to four times the diameter of the epididymal body and tail. It is more readily imaged as a structure separate from the testes as compared with the epididymal body or tail. The echogenicity of the epididymis is normally homogeneous. It may be of equal or of slightly greater or lesser echogenicity than that of the testes.

The scrotal wall should be between 3 and 6 mm thick. Beneath the scrotal wall are the two layers of the tunica vaginalis (see Fig. 154-5), the outer (parietal) and the inner (visceral) layers that are the residua of the processus vaginalis (peritoneum that descended with the testis from the abdomen). The visceral layer covers the testis on its anterior border and is attached to the tunica albuginea. Between the tunica's two layers is a potential space that may contain as much as 1 to 2 ml of fluid in normal patients. It is here that the fluid of hematocele or hydrocele may accumulate.

> The two layers of the tunica vaginalis are the residua of the processus vaginalis, which is peritoneum that descended with the testis from the fetal abdomen.

Three small, persistent, vestigial remnants of the mesonephric and müllerian duct systems may occasionally be seen, usually only when a normal testis is surrounded by hydrocele fluid. These are the appendix testis (Fig. 154-7) (a remnant of the müllerian duct), attached to the upper pole of the testis (and the most common one to potentially torse); the appendix epididymis (a remnant of the mesonephron), attached to the head of the epididymis; and the vas aberrans (a remnant of the mesonephron), attached to the epididymis at the junction of its body and tail. Torsion of any of these remnants can result in scrotal pain, swelling, local erythema, and clinical complaints similar to those of testicular torsion. The torsed remnant may be visualized, but it may be difficult to distinguish which of the three remnants is the torsed one.

> There are three appendices off the testis or epididymis that may torse and simulate testicular torsion: the appendix testis at the upper pole, the appendix epididymis at the head of the epididymis, and the vas aberrans at the junction of the epididymal body and tail.

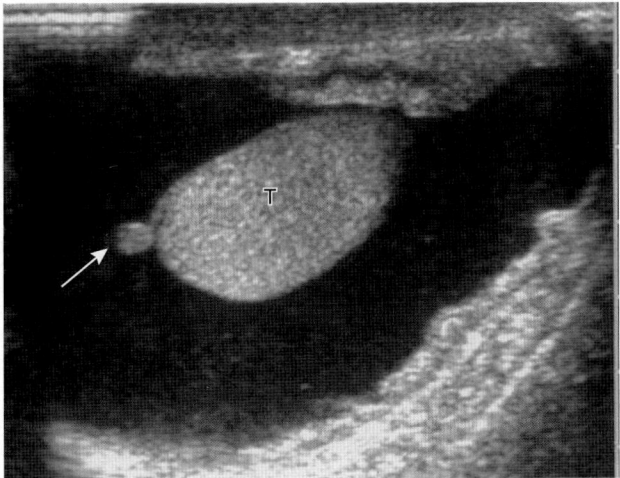

FIGURE 154-7. Appendix testis. Longitudinal sonogram shows a small circular structure *(arrow)* extending off the testis (T) that is a normal appendix testis. It was readily seen on this image because of the presence of a large hydrocele. It would otherwise probably not have been imaged.

CONGENITAL ABNORMALITIES OF THE TESTES

Monorchidism and Anorchidism

Monorchidism, the presence of a single testis, occurs in 1 of every 5000 males. It is four times more common than anorchidism. US, MRI, CT, or laparoscopy may be used to prove that there is no undescended testis or testes (cryptorchidism) simulating monorchidism or anorchidism. When a blind-ending spermatic vessel is found at surgery, it suggests anorchidism, probably on the basis of an intrauterine vascular insult. With that knowledge, no further ipsilateral exploration for an undescended testis is necessary.

Cryptorchidism

By 32 weeks' gestational age, the testes have descended into the scrotum via the inguinal canal in 93% of all male fetuses. By 6 weeks of age, only 4% of term infants have a nonpalpable testis. Of these, 20% have true cryptorchidism (undescended testes). Cryptorchidism occurs bilaterally in 10% to 33% of cases. It is more common on the right (70%). It may be familial. Beyond the age of 1 year, the prevalence of true cryptorchidism in the male population remains unchanged at 0.7% to 1%.

> By 6 weeks of age, only 4% of term infants have a nonpalpable testis. Of these, 20% have true cryptorchidism.

Most cases of nonpalpable testes are related to testicular agenesis or dysgenesis. The determination of serum levels of müllerian inhibiting substance (MIS) (also known as anti-müllerian hormone) can detect the presence of any functioning testicular tissue in the prepubertal patient. The disruption of testicular descent, in cases of cryptorchidism, usually occurs within or just above the external inguinal ring. Occasionally, the testis may be intra-abdominal. In rare cases, an undescended testis may be in a femoral location. The undescended testis that remains within the abdomen is at 10 to 40 times greater risk for developing a future malignancy than either of a pair of normally descended testes. Seminoma is the most common tumor that develops, but other germ cell–type tumors, such as embryonal carcinoma or teratocarcinoma, may occur. The risk of malignancy in the contralateral, normally descended testis is also increased as compared with the risk of malignancy in a testis of someone with two normally descended gonads. Patients with bilateral nondescent in which one testis develops a neoplasm have a 25% chance that a neoplasm will occur in the remaining testis.

> The undescended testis that remains within the abdomen has a 10 to 40 times greater risk for a future malignancy. There is a somewhat increased risk for malignancy in the descended contralateral testis.

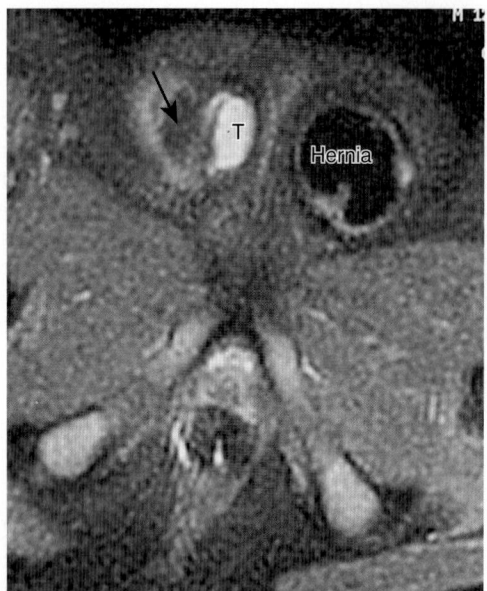

FIGURE 154-8. Inguinal hernia. T2-weighted MRI study with fat suppression in the axial plane. A child with a history of cryptorchidism and growth hormone therapy that allowed the right testis to descend is noted to have a normal-appearing testis (T) within the scrotum, seen as a homogeneously intense area, medial to a right inguinal hernia *(arrow)*. On the left side of the scrotum, a testis was neither palpated nor imaged. Bowel from a left inguinal hernia is noted *(hernia)*. (Courtesy of Dr. David Bluemke.)

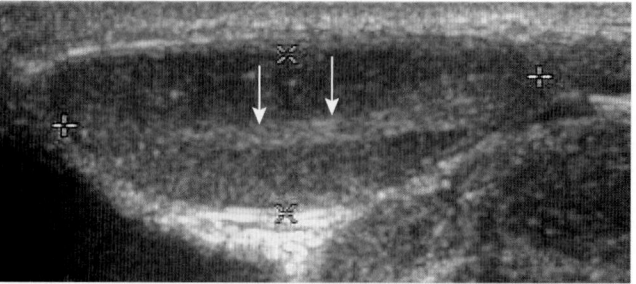

A

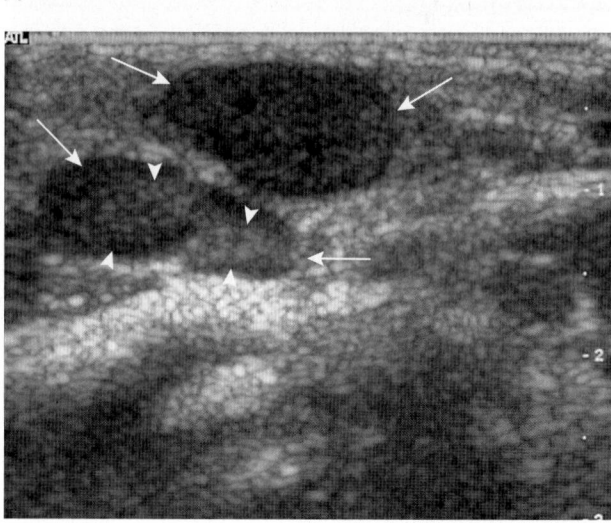

B

FIGURE 154-9. Analysis of groin for undescended testes. **A,** Sonogram of inguinal region. *Cursors* mark off the borders of a normal undescended testis found in the right groin of a child. *Arrows* point to the mediastinum of the testis. Color Doppler imaging denoted normal flow to the testis, which appeared homogeneous and normal. Its superficial position required a high-frequency transducer (10 MHz). **B,** Lymph nodes in groin on ultrasound in the transverse plane. Two oval structures *(arrows)* are noted in the right groin of a child with undescended testes. The presence of two similar structures goes against the possibility that either is a testis. The fact that each is somewhat lobular rather than smooth goes against either being a typical normal testis. The contained brighter echogenicity *(arrowheads)* within the inner three fourths of the more inferior mass is typical of the fat noted in benign nodes and not a testis.

Men with unilateral cryptorchidism are less fertile than men after unilateral orchiectomy. The cause is thought to be due to immobilizing antibodies that develop to the patient's sperm. This was noted in one third of a group of 33 infertile men with cryptorchidism.

The occurrence of an inguinal hernia (Fig. 154-8) ipsilateral to an undescended testis is common. Ten percent to 20% of affected patients have an associated genitourinary abnormality, such as vesicoureteral reflux, hydronephrosis, horseshoe kidney, renal ectopia, or renal agenesis. Rare and unusual cases of testicular absence in association with ipsilateral absence of the spermatic duct and the kidney point to a developmental abnormality of the entire urogenital ridge.

The cause of cryptorchidism is not clear; it may be hormonal or mechanical (lack of proper fixation of the testis or an abnormal gubernaculum), or a combination of the two. Cryptorchidism is the rule in cases of male pseudohermaphroditism, gonadal dysgenesis, and true hermaphroditism. It occurs with some frequency in males with hypospadias.

IMAGING EVALUATION

US is commonly the initial procedure for localization of a testis not palpable within the scrotum and is excellent for denoting a testis or nubbin of testis in the high scrotum or inguinal area (Fig. 154-9). It can usually differentiate between testis and node when imaging a mass in the inguinal area. Lymph nodes (see Fig. 154-9) (which are common in the inguinal region of children) often have echogenic fat in their central hilar areas and a relatively specific blood flow pattern into the central hilum that

extends outward to the periphery of the node. The undescended testes are usually small and hypoplastic, although usually of equal echogenicity compared with the normal testis. The descended testis may demonstrate hypertrophy, simulating a scrotal mass.

MRI is generally more effective than CT for intra-abdominal testes because of its ability to provide multi-planar images and the fact that it may also give more information about the texture of the testis. Normal testes have homogeneous high signal on T2-weighted images (see Fig. 154-8). Finding normal testes on MRI is aided by fat-suppression techniques. Despite improvements in imaging capabilities, many urologists now favor going directly to laparoscopy in cases in which US or other analysis fails to discover an undescended testis between the groin and the scrotum.

SURGICAL TREATMENT

Surgical treatment for undescended testes consists of orchiopexy whenever possible. It is performed, especially in cases of intra-abdominal testes, because of the great risk for developing testicular neoplasia. In light of the occasional occurrence and therefore possibility of spontaneous descent during the first year of life (from an endogenous surge of luteinizing hormone [LH]), surgical correction is typically delayed until early in the second year of life. Although orchiopexy may not reduce the risk for malignant degeneration, the exteriorized testis is more easily followed both clinically and by US.

It is hoped that early orchiopexy also aids the fertility potential of affected patients. Undescended testes are said to be normal histologically until the second year of life, when progressive tubular changes may develop. Somewhat problematic for this concept is the fact that these histologic findings may be noted in the contra-lateral descended testis as well. A review by Giwercman and associates of the US and Doppler imaging findings of 75 maldescended testes studied 2 to 11 years after orchiopexy showed 53% of the testes to be abnormal by either position, volume, structure, or perfusion. Of interest is the fact that in 19 cases surgery was done within the first 2 years of life, but 49 of the testes had operative intervention at a later time. There was no correlation between abnormal US findings and the time of the surgical intervention.

Polyorchidism

Polyorchidism is a rare condition that is most often discovered at puberty because of a scrotal mass. Usually the mass consists only of a small accessory testis in addition to two normal testes or two unequal testes, both smaller than the contralateral normal one, each with an individual epididymis and a shared vas deferens allowing spermatogenesis from each.

HYDROCELE

A hydrocele (see Fig. 154-7) is the most common scrotal mass in a child. Figure 154-10 is a schematic drawing of several types of hydrocele. The most common type after the first year of life is the scrotal hydrocele. Hydroceles represent fluid accumulated within the layers of the tunica vaginalis, which, although predominantly anterior to each testis, appear to surround the testis except for the area of the epididymal head. The proximal portion of the processus vaginalis typically closes before 18 months of age. This prevents abdominal contents from entering the scrotum and the tunica vaginalis. Residual fluid from testicular descent is responsible for non-communicating hydroceles reported in at least 15% of male fetuses beyond 28 weeks of life. Such physiologic hydroceles occur in at least 16 of every 1000 newborns and tend to resolve spontaneously by fluid resorption by 6 to 9 months of age. The processus vaginalis is closed in 50% to 75% of individuals by the time they are born and in most of the remainder of children by the end of the first year of life. If the processus fails to close, there will be communication between the peritoneal cavity and

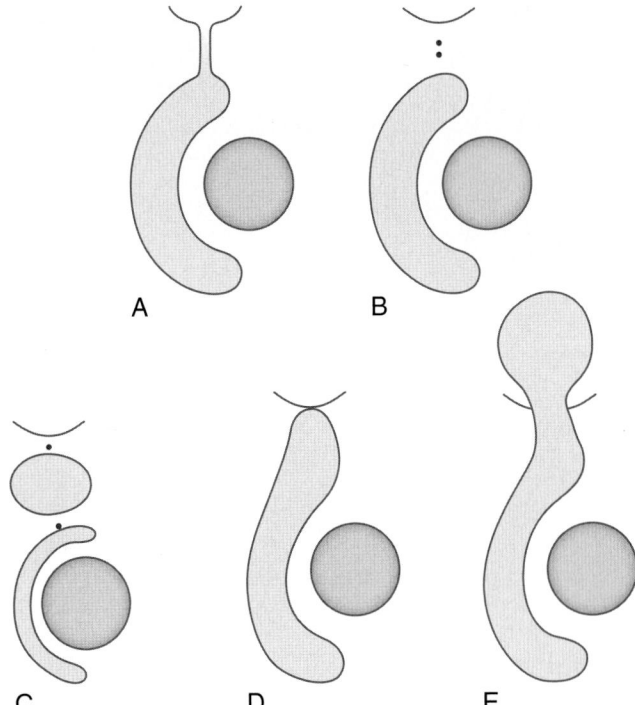

FIGURE 154-10. Hydrocele types. **A,** Congenital or intermittent hydrocele. **B,** Scrotal hydrocele. **C,** Hydrocele of the cord. **D,** Inguinoscrotal hydrocele. **E,** Abdominoscrotal hydrocele.

the scrotum. A communicating hydrocele can develop in such patients. Enlarging hydroceles may be due to an intrascrotal cause such as neoplasm, infection, or torsion. Increasing hydrocele without an intrascrotal cause suggests a patent processus vaginalis and the presence of an associated inguinal hernia. At times, a hernia, denoted by the presence of bowel within the scrotum, can be diagnosed by US, particularly if the bowel is surrounded by fluid (Fig. 154-11). However, air-filled bowel may obscure US analysis of the scrotum.

> A hydrocele is the most common scrotal mass in a child, representing accumulated fluid between the layers of the tunica vaginalis. The processus vaginalis is closed in 50% to 75% of individuals by the time they are born and in most children by the end of the first year of life.

It is well known that the patent processus of fetal life allows the possible descent of meconium into the scrotum in cases of meconium peritonitis. This meconium can calcify within the scrotum as it can within the abdomen. US may image the calcified meconium as one or several small echogenic masses within the scrotum but not within the testis. Pus, air, urine, or cerebrospinal fluid (in patients with ventriculoperitoneal shunts), or even blood from blunt trauma, may also enter the scrotum from the peritoneal cavity as long as the processus vaginalis remains patent.

In most cases a hydrocele found in the child or adolescent is idiopathic in etiology. Acquired hydroceles occur mostly in patients with a normally closed processus

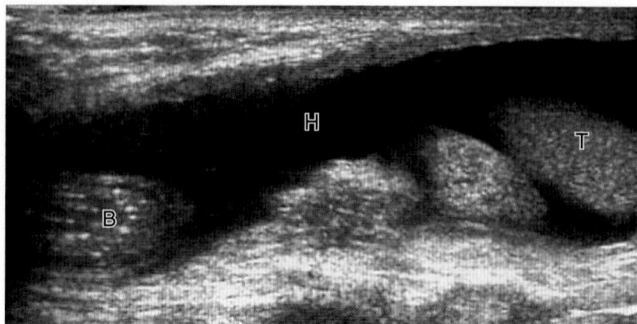

FIGURE 154-11. Hernia. Longitudinal sonogram shows bowel herniated into the scrotum. This teenager had an enlarged scrotum as a result of a contained hydrocele (H). Within the hydrocele were several loops of bowel, with the largest denoted (B). The testis (T) is seen inferiorly within the enlarged scrotum.

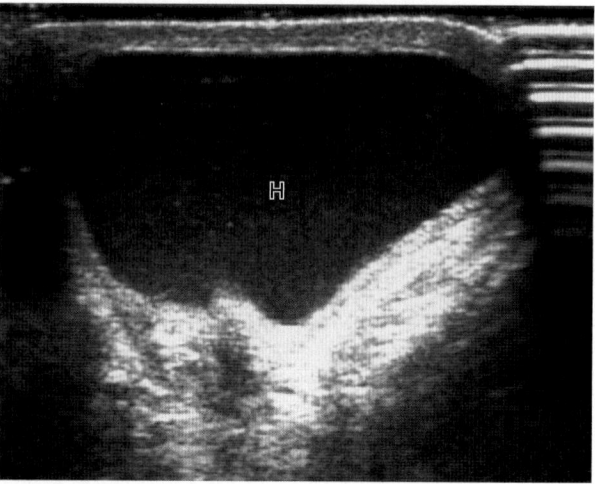

FIGURE 154-12. Chronic hydrocele. Transverse sonogram shows echogenic debris-filled fluid in a large chronic hydrocele (H) in an older teenager. The normal testis was seen elsewhere in the scrotum. In an infant, the contained debris may be related to meconium. In an older patient, such as this one, it is most often due to contained cholesterol crystals, often found in the fluid of chronic hydroceles. Proteinaceous, hemorrhagic, or infectious material may also be considered as less likely possibilities.

vaginalis after scrotal trauma or as a complication of epididymitis or orchitis, testicular torsion, or intrascrotal neoplasm (reactive hydrocele).

A hydrocele may vary in size according to the amount of contained fluid. There may be small amounts of fluid, not detectable clinically, to moderate or larger amounts contained within the scrotum. Scrotal US shows the cystic nature of the hydrocele as it appears to surround the normal homogeneously echogenic testes. Septations and debris may be present in a hydrocele, particularly if the hydrocele is infected or hemorrhagic. Echogenic debris (Fig. 154-12) is often seen in the fluid of chronic hydroceles. The exact etiology for this is unknown, although cholesterol crystals have been shown to be the cause of this in some adults with chronic hydrocele. Calcifications may occasionally develop within the scrotum of patients with chronic hydroceles and chronic inflammation, purportedly from shed cells and disturbed hydrocele resorption. Nuclear medicine scintigraphy with technetium pertechnetate, once a popular imaging method, shows a hydrocele as a photon-deficient area that may mimic the lack of flow to a testis in cases of testicular torsion, a space-occupying mass such as bowel in a patient with an intrascrotal hernia, or intrascrotal hematoma in a patient after trauma. The evolution of scrotal imaging away from nuclear medicine examinations and toward US examination has helped avoid this potential diagnostic confusion.

> **Septations and debris may be present in a hydrocele, particularly if the hydrocele is infected, hemorrhagic, or chronic.**

Less common types of hydroceles (see Fig. 154-10) of congenital origin include hydrocele of the cord, inguinoscrotal hydrocele, and abdominoscrotal hydrocele. In hydrocele of the cord, or funicular hydrocele, the processus vaginalis is obliterated in its proximal and distal end and the hydrocele is contained in the patent space between these two points. In inguinoscrotal hydrocele, the processus vaginalis is obliterated only at the internal inguinal ring and the hydrocele extends cephalad from the scrotum into the inguinal canal. In abdominoscrotal hydrocele (Fig. 154-13) there is also closure of the funicular process at the internal inguinal ring and the hydrocele is very large and forms a dumbbell-shaped cystic mass that protrudes into the extraperitoneal space of the anterior abdominal wall above the inguinal area. The inguinal mass can be made to vary in size depending on the pressure placed on either the inguinal or the scrotal end of the abdominoscrotal hydrocele. The abdominoscrotal hydrocele presents as an inguinal or intra-abdominal mass and must be considered when evaluating lower abdominal masses occurring in the first year of life. They are discovered at abdominal palpation in children with scrotal hydroceles or by noting that a hydrocele evaluated by US extends above the scrotum and into the inguinal region and/or abdomen. They are treated by total excision of the mass through an extensive inguinal incision.

> **In an abdominoscrotal hydrocele the hydrocele is very large and forms a dumbbell-shaped cystic mass that protrudes above the inguinal area.**

HEMATOCELES

Hematoceles (Fig. 154-14) are complex extratesticular fluid collections containing hemorrhagic material separating the layers of the tunica vaginalis. Acutely, after fibrin deposition, hemorrhage is echogenic on US examination. With time, the contained hemorrhage becomes less echogenic and the fluid may become more typical of hydrocele. Such hematoceles may contain low-level echoes similar to chronic hydroceles or septations seen more often in cases of infected hydroceles.

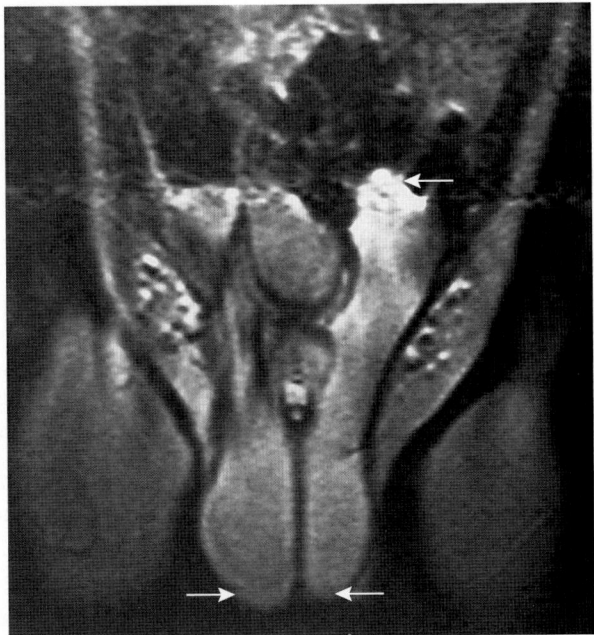

A

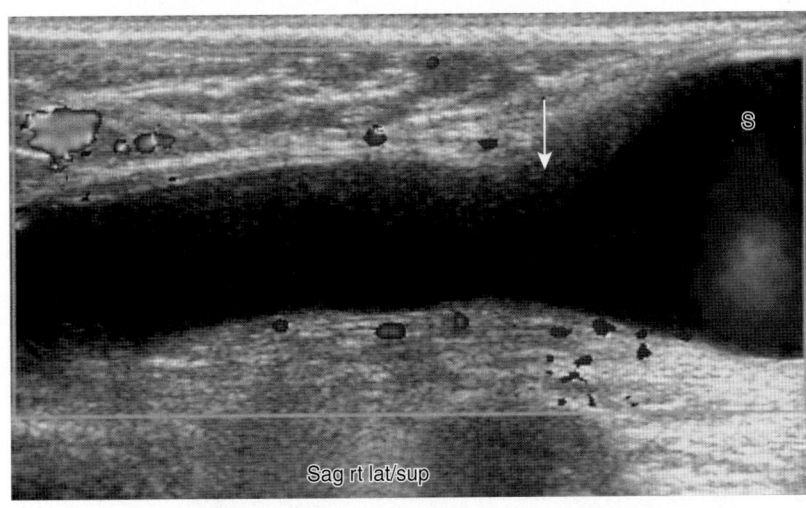

Sag rt lat/sup

B

FIGURE 154-13. Abdominoscrotal hydrocele. **A,** Tubular structures *(arrows)* are seen extending from each side of the scrotum superiorly into the abdominal cavity on a coronal T1-weighted MR image. This child had bilateral abdominoscrotal hydroceles; the superior extent on the right is not well seen on this image. He presented with an enlarged scrotum and palpable inguinal area masses whose size changed with scrotal compression. **B,** Longitudinal sonogram in another patient shows a right-sided tubular, fluid-filled structure extended from the scrotum (S) to above the inguinal area *(arrow).* (**A** from Cohen HL, Sivit C [eds]: Fetal and Pediatric Ultrasound: A Casebook Approach. New York, McGraw-Hill, 2001. Reproduced with permission of McGraw-Hill Companies.)

Hematoceles may develop from scrotal trauma but may also accumulate from distant trauma (e.g., bleeding from an injured spleen) if there is a patent processus vaginalis. In cases of scrotal trauma, unless there is an associated break in the tunica albuginea of the testis or testicular blood flow is compromised, the presence of a hematocele and even a testicular fracture is not a definitive indication for surgery.

Various US findings may be seen in patients who have had scrotal trauma. In one study by Anderson and colleagues of 19 blunt traumas, the authors noted four hematoceles, two epididymal hematomas, two cases of post-traumatic epididymitis, two cases of post-traumatic hydrocele, and seven cases of testicular rupture.

Testicular rupture (Fig. 154-15) is thought to be uncommon, occurring mostly in athletes or in victims of vehicular or industrial accidents. It is usually caused by a nonpenetrating crush injury in which the testis is trapped between the pubic ramus and the crushing object. A tear develops in the tunica albuginea, with subsequent hemorrhage and extravasation of seminiferous tubules and other testicular contents into the potential space of the tunica vaginalis. On US there is often bizarre heterogeneous echogenicity to the testicular parenchyma, caused by infarction and hemorrhage; irregularity of the normally smooth testicular border; and, on occasion, nonvisualization of any normal testicular parenchyma. The testes may be displaced into the inguinal canal. A reactive hydrocele or hematocele (because of concomitant bleeding) may occur. Discrete fracture lines are unusual. Testicular tumors may predispose a testis to rupture. One must be wary of the possibility that a bizarre heterogeneous echogenicity in a traumatized scrotum may actually be a hematoma that has displaced a normal testis (Fig. 154-16), often superiorly.

One must be wary of the possibility that a heterogeneous mass image in a traumatized scrotum may actually be a hematoma that has displaced a normal testis.

SCROTAL WALL THICKENING

Not all scrotal enlargement is due to contained fluid. In older adults, massive scrotal enlargement often has

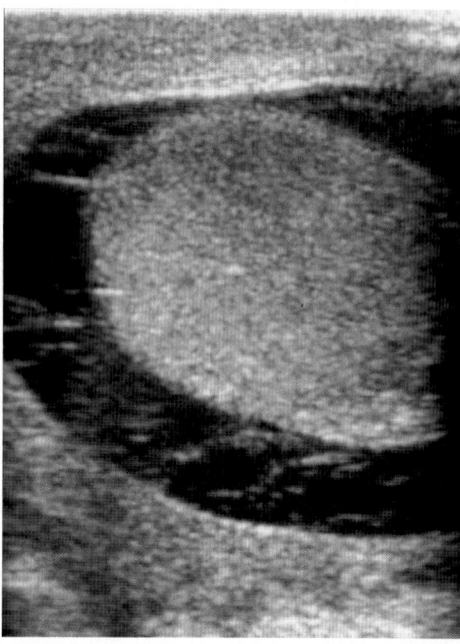

FIGURE 154-14. Hematocele. Longitudinal sonogram shows fluid with contained echogenic material that surrounds the normal testis of a 14-year-old who was kicked in the scrotum several days before imaging.

a component of scrotal wall thickening. This is less common in children. Certainly in either age group the scrotal wall may be thickened by contained infection or hemorrhage. Occasionally, a child with nephrotic syndrome may present with an enlarged scrotum made up predominantly of an edematous, and therefore thickened, scrotal wall (Fig. 154-17).

TESTICULAR TORSION

Testicular torsion is a relatively common clinical problem that, if left uncorrected, leads to ischemic necrosis of the testis and loss of testicular function. Torsion may occur at any age but is seen most often in adolescent boys between 11 and 18 years of age, perhaps because of the increase in testicular growth and weight during this time. Torsion may also be seen with some frequency in the newborn period, often as a result of a torsion that occurred antenatally.

Testicular torsion is seen most often between 11 and 18 years of age.

Clinical Findings

Testicular torsion represents 20% of cases of acute scrotal pathology in the postpubertal male. The normal testis is strongly attached to the epididymis, which in turn is applied to the posterior scrotal wall. If these attachments fail to develop properly, the testis, suspended within the tunica vaginalis, may rotate and the spermatic cord undergo torsion (the clapper-in-a-bell phenomenon), with compromise of blood flow to the testis and epididymis. After 2 hours, the cells of spermatogenesis are damaged and are said to be destroyed by 6 hours.

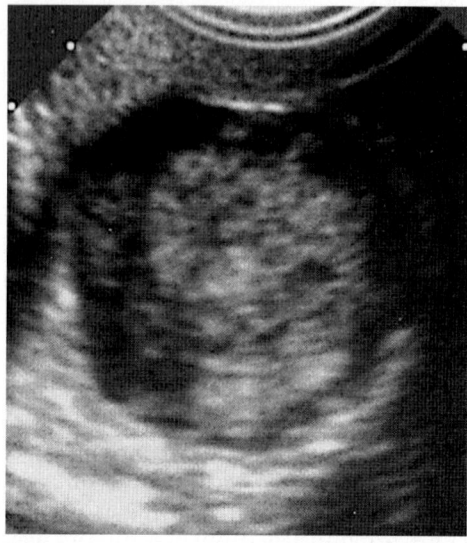
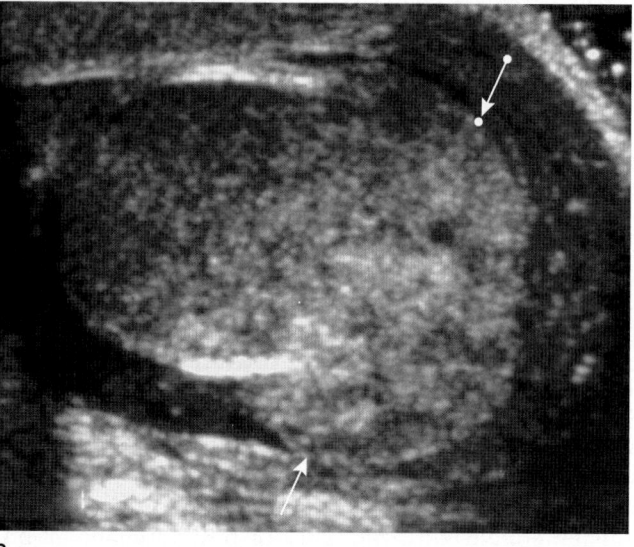

A   B

FIGURE 154-15. Testicular trauma. **A,** On a transverse plane ultrasound image, a small amount of hydrocele surrounds an irregularly shaped and heterogeneously echogenic mass that is a fractured testis. The fracture occurred from a direct blow with a hammer. **B,** Longitudinal sonogram in another patient shows that the inferior third of the testis (*arrows*) has lost its smooth contour due to a fracture. The parenchyma in the distal one third extended through a traumatic tear in the tunica albuginea. (Courtesy of Robert Wasnick, MD.)

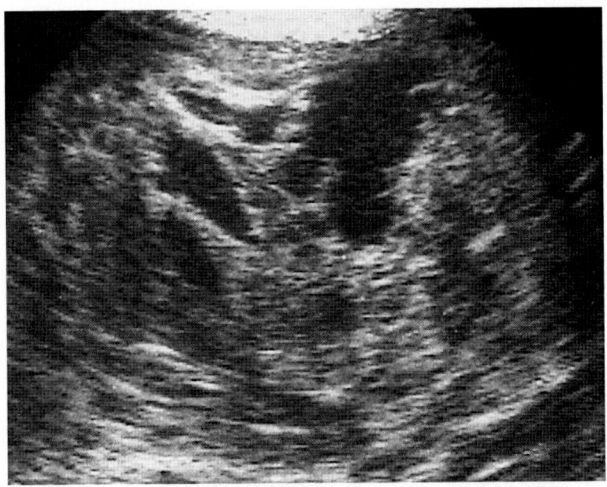

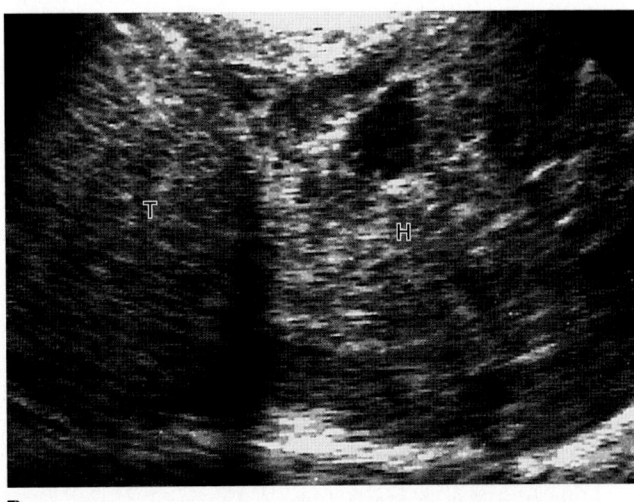

A   B

FIGURE 154-16. Scrotal hematoma simulating testicular fracture. **A,** Transverse sonogram shows a solid mass with irregular borders and heterogeneous echogenicity that was thought to be a testicular fracture in the lower half of the scrotum by a covering house officer. Irregular borders suggesting a tunica albuginea fracture would have required surgical intervention. **B,** An orthogonal view in the longitudinal plane of the hemiscrotum in **A** shows the mass of concern to be not the testis but rather a hematoma (H). A normal testis (T) was imaged in a more superior portion of the scrotum, where it had been pushed by the hematoma. The ultrasound examination was performed 6 days after trauma to the patient's scrotum.

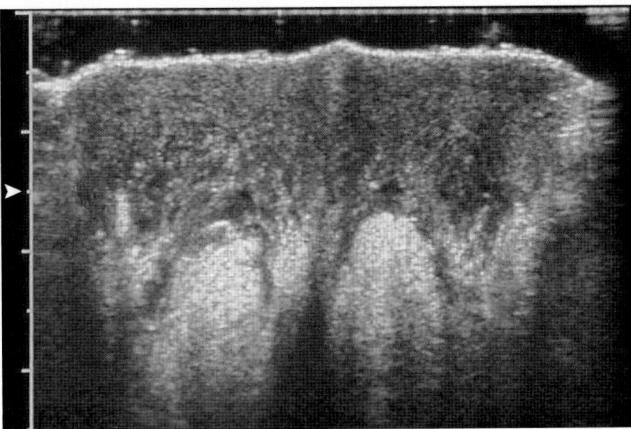

FIGURE 154-17. Scrotal edema. Transverse sonogram in a 5-year-old with an enlarged scrotum shows normal testes deep to the thick, soft tissues of the scrotum. This thickening was due to scrotal wall edema in this patient with nephrotic syndrome that had not been diagnosed before the ultrasound examination.

Testicular torsion represents 20% of cases of acute scrotal pathology in the postpubertal male. Viable torsed testes undergo orchiopexy; nonviable testes are removed. Preventive orchiopexy is performed on the contralateral nontorsed testis.

The patient with acute torsion develops sudden acute scrotal pain. The pain may waken him or develop suddenly during the daytime waking hours. The pain may radiate to the groin or abdomen. Nausea or vomiting occurs occasionally. Dysuria is not present, and urinalysis results are negative. Patients may occasionally have fever, and leukocytosis may be present. In some cases there is a history of previous episodes of scrotal pain and tenderness, suggesting previous episodes of torsion with spontaneous detorsion. A history of recent trauma to the testis or strenuous physical exercise is occasionally elicited. An important finding on physical examination that helps make the diagnosis is noting a change in testicular axis from the normal vertical positioning of the testis in the scrotum to a more horizontal one. Within hours of torsion, the patient develops a reddened scrotum, with or without enlargement. The differential diagnostic possibilities include acute idiopathic scrotal edema, hemorrhage into a testicular tumor, and torsion of an intrascrotal hernia sac. Most common in the sexually active male, epididymitis and epididymo-orchitis must be considered. Torsion of appendages of the testis or epididymis may also simulate testicular torsion.

Detorsion is necessary for testicular viability. Surgery within 24 hours leads to 60% to 70% testicular salvage, but after 24 hours salvage is only 20%. Because abnormal testicular fixation is considered a bilateral phenomenon, preventive orchiopexy is often performed on the contralateral nontorsed testis. Hadziselimovic found preexisting contralateral testicular abnormality in 58% of 38 boys with acute torsion who underwent contralateral testicular biopsy at the time of surgery. This finding gives credence to the concept that torsion is a bilateral phenomenon and supports the current clinical approach of saving viable twisted testes and removing nonviable testes.

Acute testicular torsion may be suggested by the discovery of a change in testicular axis from the normal vertical orientation within the scrotum to a more horizontal one.

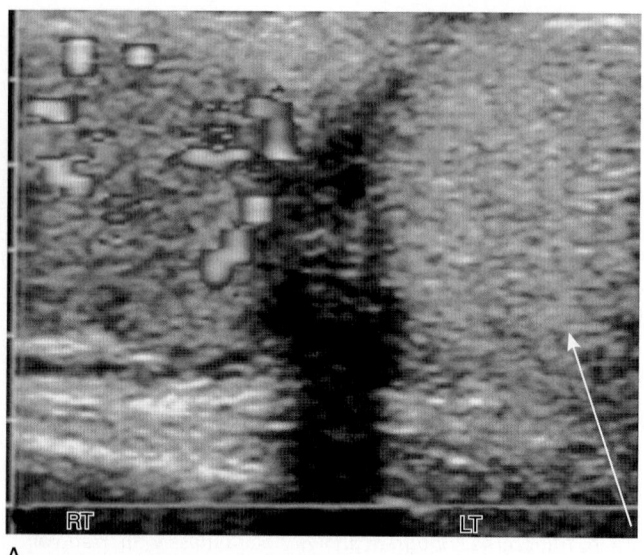
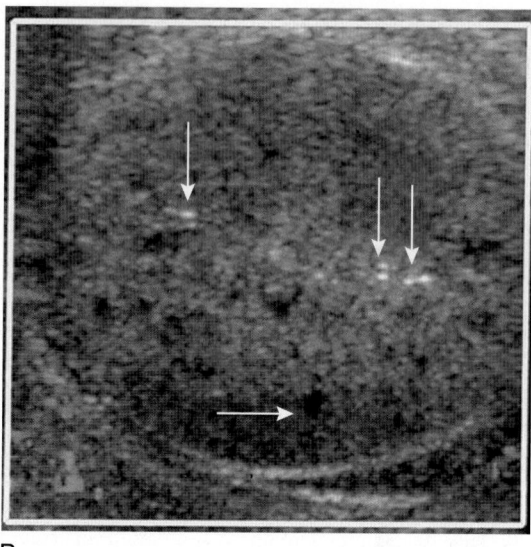

A   B

FIGURE 154-18. Testicular torsion. **A,** Transverse sonogram of acute left testicular torsion shows that the right testis is more echopenic than the left testis. Often the acutely torsed testis is more echopenic than the normal one. However, in this case, color flow is seen only in the right testis. The left testis, despite having the more normal echogenicity pattern, has no color flow and is, therefore, torsed. Note that the high-frequency linear array transducer image used does not allow complete imaging of the lateral aspects of each testis. **B,** Longitudinal Doppler sonogram of a delayed diagnosis of testicular torsion shows an enlarged testis with heterogeneous echogenicity and no contained color flow in this teenager whose testis had by history torsed 4 days before his seeking medical care. Echoless areas (*horizontal arrow* points to one) are consistent with destroyed areas of testicular parenchyma. A few bright echoes (*vertical arrows*) were consistent with areas of hemorrhage.

Imaging Findings

Ultrasonography is the key initial imaging tool and often the only diagnostic tool necessary to make the diagnosis of torsion and suggest surgical exploration. The typical image of a testis that has undergone acute torsion is one of a normal-sized to enlarged testis of normal to decreased echogenicity. Enlargement and hypoechogenicity are thought to be due to venous congestion. The echogenicity pattern is usually homogeneous. Comparing the echogenicity of the affected testis with that of the contralateral normal testis (Fig. 154-18) can be of great help. This is best seen on transverse images. Many high-frequency linear-array transducers with small footpads are able to show only the medial portions of each testis for side-by-side comparison. Additional imaging with a high-frequency curved-array transducer will allow more complete imaging of both testes in the transverse plane, if they have not been completely imaged with the linear-array transducer.

> Comparing the echogenicity of a possibly torsed testis with that of the contralateral normal testis is best made using transverse images.

Epididymal enlargement may be an early finding in some cases of torsion. At least 10% of cases of torsion have associated reactive hydroceles. A torsion for which US examination is not performed for more than 48 hours after symptomatology, and the diagnosis of which is therefore delayed (the pejorative term *missed torsion* is often incorrect) (see Fig. 154-18), may show heterogeneous or increased echogenicity because of contained hemorrhage or hemorrhagic necrosis.

The key element in the US diagnosis of testicular torsion is Doppler imaging, which allows rapid evaluation of testicular blood flow. Earlier conventional duplex Doppler could listen for absent or decreased arterial flow in the spermatic cord, but intratesticular flow was, at times, difficult to evaluate by this method, owing to the smallness of the intratesticular vessels and the necessity to image an individual vessel before insonating it. The lesser sensitivity of Doppler imaging at that time made nuclear medicine studies the gold standard for analysis of patients with possible testicular torsion. The development of color Doppler US provided a more sensitive tool that was easier to use and that has improved over subsequent years. It allowed a triplex display of gray-scale real-time images of the testes with simultaneous display of vascular flow as a color signal that could be insonated for its spectral pattern. Subsequent experimental and clinical studies have shown color Doppler imaging to be at least as sensitive (if not more) as scintigraphy in the evaluation of testicular torsion, particularly cases of incomplete or partial torsion in which some residual blood flow persists.

Color Doppler imaging of a testis without torsion (Fig. 154-19) shows readily evident vascular color flow within the testis. Insonation of the vessels proves them to be arterial or venous. Classically, color Doppler of a case of testicular torsion shows no arterial signals from the testis or the spermatic cord. The sonologist, however, is warned to be wary not only of a lack of flow but also of reductions in flow when comparing a testis of concern with the opposite normal testis.

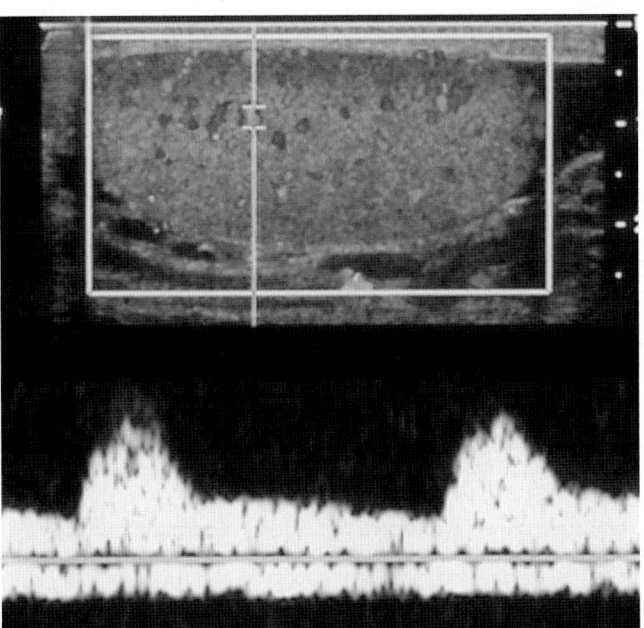

FIGURE 154-19. Normal Doppler flow in a testis. The *upper half of the image* shows the normal testis, with color filling vessels with moving blood. Insonation of a point in the upper third of the testis provides a spectral pattern *(lower half of the image)* that shows classic arterial signal with its systolic and diastolic components above the baseline and relatively unchanging and continuous venous signal below it.

> In assessing for testicular torsion, the examiner should be wary not only of a lack of intratesticular flow but also of evident reductions in flow when comparing the testis of concern to the contralateral normal testis.

Color Doppler imaging is also a convenient and reliable procedure for evaluating patients with known or suspected testicular torsion after manual or spontaneous detorsion to determine if the therapy has been successful and vascular flow restored.

Power Doppler imaging has historically been a more sensitive form of Doppler US that can detect more subtle (10 to 15 dB) vascular flow and show it as a bright color US image. It has helped make nondiagnostic US studies much rarer. The fact that power Doppler imaging, unlike color Doppler imaging, does not provide information on flow direction is irrelevant in the analysis of flow in the testis. Recent improvements in color Doppler imaging sensitivity, however, have made the need for power Doppler US uncommon in most clinical situations.

State-of-the-art color or power Doppler imaging methods have made US the gold standard for the imaging and preoperative diagnosis of testicular torsion. Identification by Doppler imaging of arterial (and venous) flow in the center of a testis goes against the diagnosis of torsion. The spermatic cord should be always seen and be straight versus circuitous. The latter may be seen in torsion/detorsion. Venous flow is lost

before arterial flow ceases. Flow may be normal in a torsed testis that spontaneously detorsed. Color flow comparison to the contralateral testis is helpful and necessary, particularly when torsion may be less than complete, in which case the diagnosis may be suggested not by a lack of flow but by an asymmetry of blood flow.

Testicular torsion can occur in undescended testes as well. If a torsed undescended testis is present in the inguinal canal, one may observe pain, swelling, redness, and tenderness in the affected groin. Torsion of an intra-abdominal testis in postnatal life may present as abdominal pain and other findings suggesting acute appendicitis.

Testicular Torsion in the Fetus and Newborn

Infants can be born with torsed testes. The torsion that occurs or is first diagnosed in the newborn period usually presents as a painless, firm scrotal mass often associated with bluish red discoloration of the scrotum. It may present as scrotal enlargement that may simulate hydrocele. The affected testis is generally nonviable. If the torsion occurred in intrauterine life, one is imaging the neonatal equivalent of a temporally older (delayed diagnosis) torsion.

> Testicular torsion diagnosed in the newborn period usually presents as a painless, firm scrotal mass often associated with bluish red discoloration of the scrotum.

Antenatal torsion may be diagnosed on fetal US examination. It must be considered if the fetal testis or testes are heterogeneous in echogenicity or of asymmetric size (Fig. 154-20). Diagnosis in the newborn is also made by noting similar imaging findings. Imaging homogeneous testes that are symmetric and of normal echogenicity and denoting central arterial flow goes against torsion. The antenatal US analysis may be limited by fetal lie, fetal positioning in that lie, and maternal size. Neonatal US analysis may be difficult because the small scrotum is difficult to image. The presence of hydrocele seen in many newborns actually aids diagnosis by allowing easier imaging of the testis.

Torsion of Testicular and Epididymal Appendages—Simulators of Testicular Torsion

Testicular (and epididymal) appendages may torse. This condition occurs most typically in the 6- to 12-year-old age group and represents 5% of cases of acute scrotal pathology in the child and young adolescent. Early in the course of testicular appendix torsion, patients may have localized pain, a pea-sized mass in the area of the upper pole of the testis suggesting the diagnosis, and, at times, a pinpoint discoloration ("blue dot" sign) seen through the overlying scrotal skin. However, within hours the clinical picture may become indistinguishable from that of classic testicular torsion, albeit in a somewhat younger age group. In such cases, US will show normal testicular echogenicity and normal testicular vascular flow. Normal testicular/epididymal appendages are not seen unless

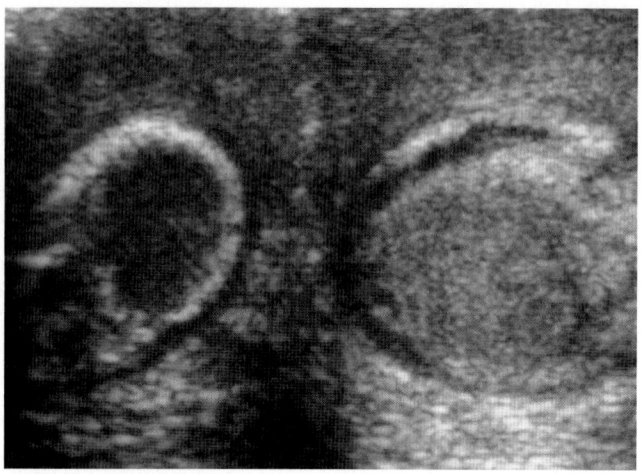
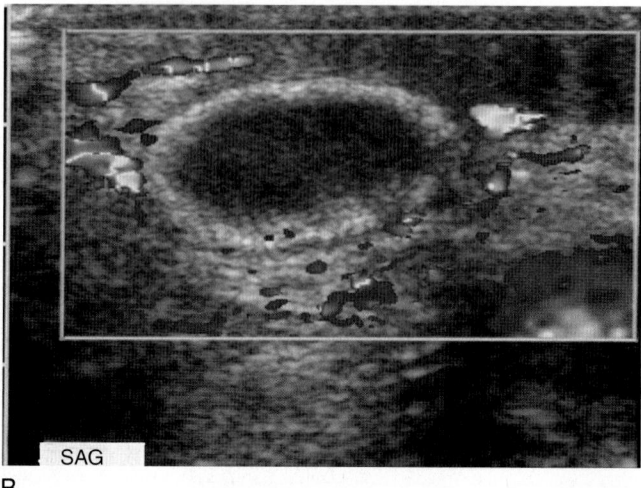

A   **B**

FIGURE 154-20. Bilateral antenatal testicular torsion. **A,** Transverse sonogram shows two testes with torsion of different ages in a newborn with scrotal swelling. The testes are seen deep to a more superficial thickened scrotal wall. The right testis is echopenic with a somewhat echogenic periphery, suggesting an old torsion. The grayer left testis does not appear particularly abnormal on this image, although its periphery is more echogenic than the remainder of its parenchyma. Color Doppler imaging showed no flow in either testis. Both testes were proved to be torsed at surgery. The torsion of the left testis probably occurred later in fetal life. There are tiny hydroceles bilaterally. The small scrotum of this newborn allowed it to be seen completely by the high-frequency (14 MHz) linear array probe despite its small footpad. **B,** Longitudinal sonogram of the torsed right testis. No color flow is seen within the echopenic parenchyma or the surrounding echogenic periphery of this neonate's testis, which torsed during fetal life.

there is significant hydrocele surrounding a testis (see Fig. 154-7). They are usually small and circular or comma shaped. Often, US can image the enlarged torsed appendage as a small circular mass (Fig. 154-21) of variable echogenicity (sometimes with increased echogenicity, sometimes echopenic with increased echogenicity peripherally) near the testis or epididymis of the affected side. This mass represents the twisted and edematous appendage. Some authors have noted associated epididymal swelling. Although the ability to denote vascular flow to these enlarged appendices via color Doppler imaging is not consistent or helpful, color Doppler imaging certainly allows rapid identification of color flow in the testis, so as to negate the possibility of testicular torsion.

> Testicular (and epididymal) appendages may torse, most typically in the 6- to 12-year-old age group, and may mimic testicular torsion.

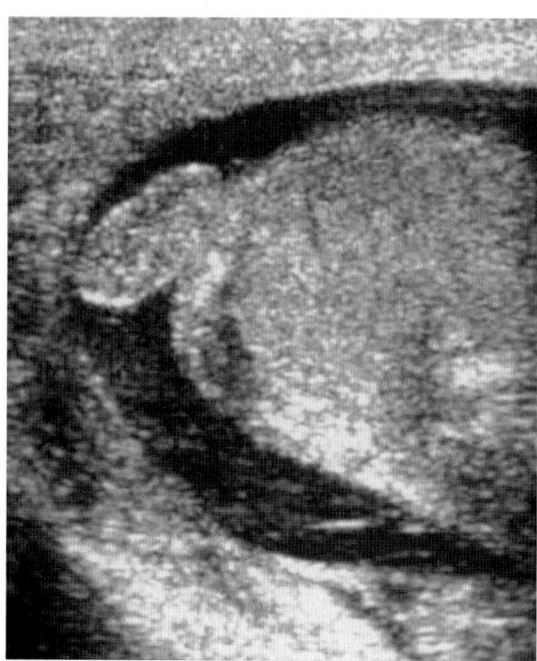

FIGURE 154-21. Torsed appendix testis. Longitudinal sonogram of the superior portion of the scrotum shows a prominent oval structure superior to the testis of a child who presented with sudden testicular pain. The oval structure is of equal echogenicity to the testis and is an enlarged torsed testicular appendage. Color flow of the testis was normal, proving there was no testicular torsion. There is some debris in a small surrounding hydrocele.

EPIDIDYMITIS

Epididymitis is the most common cause of an acute painful scrotum in the postpubescent male. The cause is usually bacterial, although in pediatric and some adolescent patients epididymitis may be viral (e.g., mumps). Although common in adolescents who are active sexually, it is important to distinguish between scrotal swelling and testicular pain resulting from epididymitis, requiring antibiotics for treatment, and that resulting from testicular torsion, requiring urgent surgical exploration. In the adolescent (younger than 20 years of age), the ratio of epididymitis to torsion cases has been reported as 3:2. After age 20 the ratio is 9:1. These ratios

may become somewhat different as sexually transmitted disease becomes more epidemic in the adolescent population. Epididymitis may be seen at an earlier age than adolescence and even, occasionally, in newborns, essentially always on a nonsexual basis.

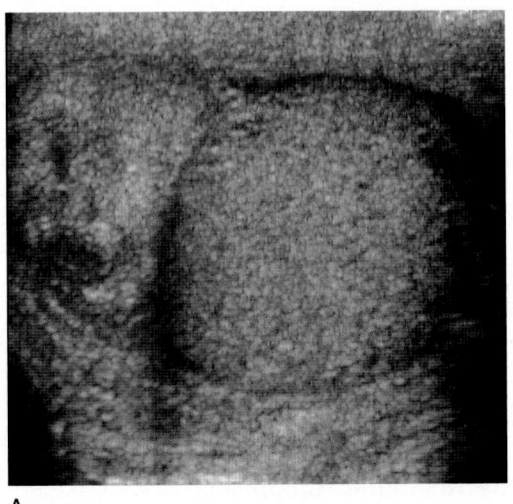
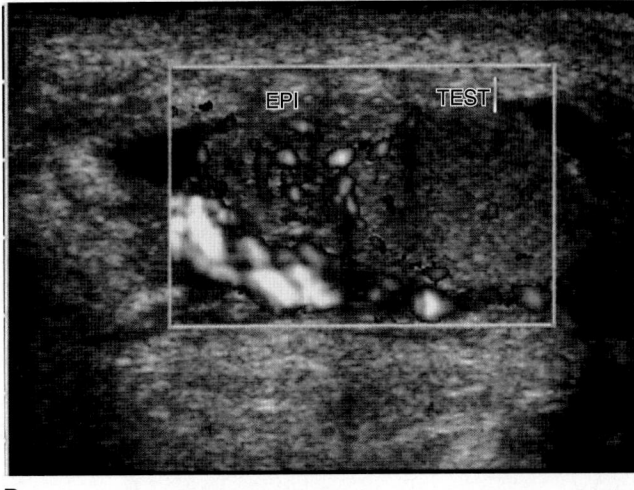

A   B

FIGURE 154-22. Epididymitis. **A,** Longitudinal sonogram shows that the left epididymis of this teenager is very large compared with the normal testis. **B,** Longitudinal color Doppler sonogram shows that flow to the prominent right epididymis (EPI) of this 10-year-old is greater than that to the testis (TEST). (**B,** *see color plate.*)

> **Epididymitis is the most common cause of an acute painful scrotum in the postpubescent male.**

Although the pain of epididymitis usually develops more gradually than in classic cases of testicular torsion (i.e., over a 1- to 2-day period), the clinical picture may simulate torsion. Unlike patients with torsion, patients with epididymitis are often febrile and at least half complain of dysuria. There is often scrotal edema, testicular tenderness, and a reactive hydrocele. An enlarged epididymis may be palpated. Pyuria is common, and nausea, vomiting, and leukocytosis may be present.

The infection usually responds to antibiotics. The infecting agents include *Staphylococcus, Streptococcus, Proteus mirabilis, Escherichia coli, Klebsiella, Pseudomonas,* and in adolescents also *Neisseria gonorrhoeae* and *Chlamydia trachomatis. E. coli* and *Proteus* are the most common cause of infection in prepubescent males and males older than 35 years of age. Often no organism can be demonstrated. The infection usually reaches the epididymis through the spermatic ducts. Occasionally, infection is via a hematogenous or lymphatic route. Causative factors include urinary tract infections, urethral instrumentation and indwelling catheters, distal urethral obstruction, and reflux of urine from the urethra into the seminal ducts as a result of a congenitally patulous orifice, an ectopic ureter draining into the vas deferens, and an ectopic vas draining into the bladder or ureter. Epididymitis has also been reported in patients with a rectourethral fistula, in patients after scrotal trauma, and in association with sepsis, Kawasaki disease, and Henoch-Schönlein purpura.

Complications of epididymitis include direct spread of the infection to the testis (i.e., epididymo-orchitis), which can be seen in as many as 20% of cases. Although an uncommon complication, an abscess may develop within the scrotum or testes and require drainage. In unusual cases, acute epididymitis may impede testicular blood flow, resulting in focal or diffuse infarction of the testis or epididymis even in the absence of torsion.

> **Complications of epididymitis include direct spread of the infection to the testis, which can be seen in as many as 20% of cases.**

Epididymitis evaluated by gray-scale US shows enlargement of the epididymis (Fig. 154-22) and commonly a reactive hydrocele or pyocele. There may be scrotal wall thickening. A common area of involvement is the head of the epididymis, just superior to the testis. Enlargement indicating involvement also occurs in other areas such as the epididymal body or tail. The echogenicity of the enlarged epididymis may be normal, slightly decreased, or slightly increased. In chronic cases, the epididymis is typically hyperechoic. The affected area of epididymis, although enlarged, usually maintains its normal shape. The diagnosis is supported by color Doppler imaging showing increased flow to the affected epididymis (see Fig. 154-22)

In most cases of epididymitis, the adjacent testis is usually normal in appearance. With spreading of the infection to the testis, the homogeneous echogenicity pattern of the testis is lost. Most often, an echopenic area of involvement is seen within the testis directly adjacent to the area of involved epididymis, suggesting the diagnosis of epididymo-orchitis (Fig. 154-23). Although possibly caused by lymphatic or bloodborne organisms, this hypoechoic area is usually caused by direct spread from the epididymis. Color Doppler imaging usually shows increased flow to the involved portion of adjacent testis as well as the epididymis.

Testicular ischemia may play a role in the development of the associated orchitis, because the inflamed and edematous epididymis compresses terminal branches of the spermatic vessels (making this ischemic peripheral area more susceptible to bacterial invasion). The testicular mass of focal orchitis may simulate tumor on US examinations, but the clinical presentation, its association with an enlarged epididymis, and its resolution within weeks with appropriate antibiotic therapy and

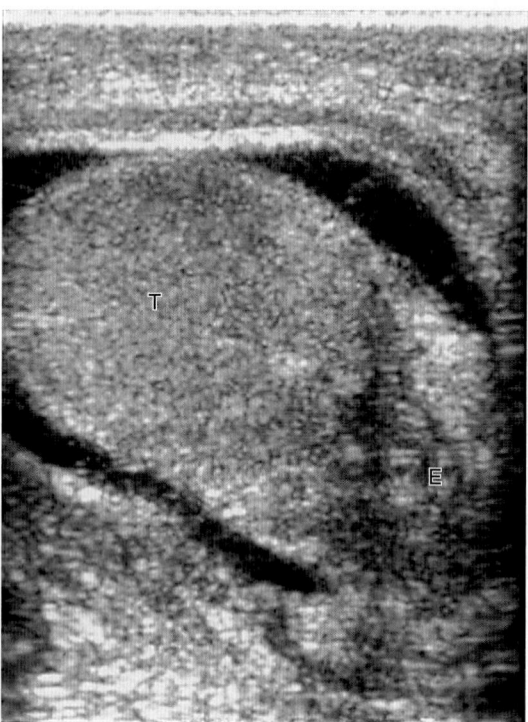

FIGURE 154-23. Epididymo-orchitis. Longitudinal sonogram of the left testis shows that the scrotum is somewhat thickened, and there is a hydrocele. An enlarged and echopenic portion of the epididymis (E) is seen inferiorly and is difficult to separate from the testis (T). The testis is echopenic where it is in contact with the inflamed epididymis. The findings are consistent with extension of the infection into the testis.

"tincture of time" helps confirm the infectious etiology and the diagnosis of epididymo-orchitis.

Testicular scintigraphy is not often used today. In cases of epididymitis, it can show increased blood flow with increased uptake of the radionuclide in the scrotum both during perfusion and in the tissue phase of the nuclear medicine examination. In the younger patient when epididymitis may be secondary to a congenital anomaly, a voiding cystourethrogram may be performed. Abnormalities such as reflux of contrast agent into a vas deferens may be imaged.

SCROTAL COMPLICATIONS OF HENOCH-SCHÖNLEIN PURPURA

Henoch-Schönlein purpura is a generalized vasculitis of unknown cause characterized clinically by a purpuric rash, abdominal pain, joint manifestations, and often hematuria. Severe vasculitis of the testis and epididymis may result in scrotal swelling and tenderness. Sometimes the process is complicated by testicular torsion. Not uncommonly, the scrotum alone is involved by severe purpura and swelling, simulating an intrascrotal problem. Imaging may be indicated to exclude testicular torsion. A stand-off pad of water-equivalent material can help US imaging of the superficial scrotal wall by placing it somewhat distant to the transducer surface. Some of the newer higher-frequency linear-array probes (e.g., 10 MHz) can at times help image the superficial scrotal wall without the necessity of a stand-off pad.

TESTICULAR MASSES

Asymptomatic testicular enlargement may be idiopathic or be caused by such conditions as juvenile hypothyroidism with precocious puberty, X-linked megalotestis syndrome, congenital adrenal hyperplasia, and metastatic tumor. Patients with unilateral cryptorchidism may develop compensatory enlargement of the intrascrotal testes. Testicular US is the primary imaging modality used to rule out neoplasm. The finding of homogeneous normal testicular echogenicity makes a tumor an unlikely possibility, although follow-up examination may aid in assuring the absence of an isoechoic lesion.

TESTICULAR AND PARATESTICULAR NEOPLASMS

Primary Testicular Neoplasms

Testicular neoplasms are usually a problem of young adults, representing the most common solid tumors of 20- to 35-year-old men. They are uncommon in infants and children, representing 1% to 1.5% of all childhood malignancies. When they do occur in children, they tend to occur in the very young, with a peak incidence at 2 years of age and with 60% of the cases occurring in those younger than 2 years of age. Such tumors usually present as a painless, nontender, and firm scrotal mass often of weeks' to months' duration. Scrotal pain and tenderness may occur if associated torsion of the testis occurs. The increased weight of the testis containing a tumor may be responsible for the torsion. Testicular tumors are occasionally bilateral. Signs of precocious puberty or gynecomastia may be present in some cases.

> Testicular neoplasms are uncommon in infants and children, representing 1% to 1.5% of all childhood malignancies. Sixty percent of those that do occur are seen in children younger than 2 years of age.

Imaging

The predominant imaging tool for the search for and evaluation of tumors of the scrotum and its contents is US. Abdominal US, CT, or MRI is often performed for detection of pelvic or retroperitoneal lymph node enlargement and is used as well in the search for solid organ metastases. Chest radiographs and CT are used to search for pulmonary metastases. Laboratory serum analysis for testicular tumor markers such as serum α-fetoprotein and human chorionic gonadotropin (hCG) can help suggest the primary diagnosis but are more often used to identify recurrences and analyze effectiveness of therapy.

Scrotal US shows most testicular neoplasms to be hypoechoic (Fig. 154-24). The image is nonspecific and may be simulated by infarcts, granulomas, and focal orchitis. Contained anechoic areas within such tumors either represent cystic components or more often are evidence of focal necrosis as the tumor outstrips its blood supply. Acute hemorrhage appears echogenic; older

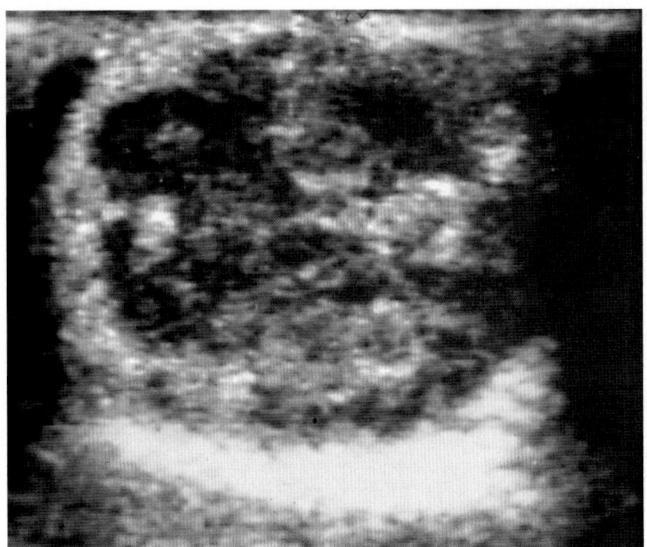

FIGURE 154-24. Seminoma. Transverse sonogram shows a predominantly echopenic mass taking up almost the entirety of this patient's left testis. There is some residual normal tissue at the periphery seen predominantly to the reader's left.

hemorrhage evolves from echogenic to echoless areas as fibrin is deposited and then dissolves. Testicular teratomas, the second most common testicular tumor in prepubertal boys, are usually less homogeneous than other testicular neoplasms. Just as in other areas of the body, teratomas show cystic areas, echogenic fat-containing areas, and echogenic foci with posterior shadowing corresponding to intratumoral calcifications or bony/dental structures. Reactive hydroceles are seen in association with testicular tumors in at least 15% to 20% of cases. Color Doppler and power Doppler US demonstrate increased vascularity in the majority of malignant tumors and may help define the mass itself.

Classification of Primary Neoplasms

Primary testicular tumors are classified according to their tissue of origin:
1. Germ cell tumors (yolk sac carcinoma, teratoma, teratocarcinoma, choriocarcinoma, seminoma) occurring as pure histologic patterns or in various combinations (mixed germ cell tumors)
2. Gonadal stromal tumors (Sertoli–granulosa cell, Leydig cell, or granulosa cell tumors)
3. Germ cell plus stromal cell tumors (gonadoblastoma)
4. Tumors of supporting tissues (fibroma, leiomyoma, hemangioma)

Germ Cell Tumors

The majority (65% to 75%) of childhood testicular tumors are germ cell in origin. This is in contrast to adults, in whom almost all (95%) testicular tumors are germ cell in type. Among adults, these are typically choriocarcinoma, seminoma, teratocarcinoma, and embryonal carcinoma, which are rare in children.

Yolk sac tumor (also known as yolk sac carcinoma, orchioblastoma, endodermal sinus tumor, or embryonal carcinoma of infancy) is by far the most common germ cell tumor (80% to 90%) in children and therefore the most common testicular neoplasm in children. Three fourths of yolk sac tumors are diagnosed by 24 months of age. They may be aggressive and invade the tunica, distorting the testicular contour. Frequently hemorrhage, particularly after clot dissolution, causes echo-free areas within this typically echopenic, somewhat well-circumscribed mass. An elevated serum α-fetoprotein level is a tumor marker in approximately 90% of affected patients.

> Yolk sac tumor is by far the most common germ cell tumor in children and therefore the most common testicular neoplasm in children.

Testicular teratoma represents 10% to 15% of childhood germ cell tumors, usually developing in children between 3 months and 5 years of age. The mean age of diagnosis is 18 months, with 65% of cases diagnosed before 2 years of age. As noted, they appear on US as complex masses with cystic and solid components (Fig. 154-25). They are made up of elements derived from all three germ cell layers and may contain cartilage, bony spicules, and epidermal elements such as keratin, fibrous tissue, smooth muscle, and adipose tissue. Many of these tumors contain glial tissue. Contained calcifications and bony or dental structures are often visible on plain radiographs (see Fig. 154-25). Bony and dental elements are echogenic with posterior shadowing on US, whereas the adipose component appears echogenic but without shadowing. Once thought universally benign, at least one third will show metastases within 5 years of diagnosis. Prepubertal teratomas are said to almost always follow a benign course even if they contain islands of malignant germ cells (15%). Postpubertal teratomas, in contrast, are frequently malignant or are potentially malignant owing to their propensity to develop components of other germ cell tumors, resulting in teratocarcinomas. The serum hCG level in these cases is usually elevated.

It is known that an undifferentiated testicular teratoma may undergo conversion ("retroconversion") to a mature differentiated teratoma after chemotherapy. One report showed conversion of liver metastases in such a patient to benign fatty and cystic liver masses after chemotherapy.

Some pathologists support the separate categorization of dermoid cyst of the testis from teratoma because the dermoid cyst does not have a propensity to develop malignancy (see later section on epidermoid cyst).

Both *choriocarcinoma* and *seminoma* (the most common tumor in adults) are extremely rare testicular tumors in children but may occur as histologic components of mixed germ cell tumors.

Gonadal Stromal Tumors

Non–germ cell testicular tumor types represent only 25% to 30% of pediatric testicular tumors. *Leydig cell* tumors and *Sertoli–granulosa cell* tumors are very uncommon but

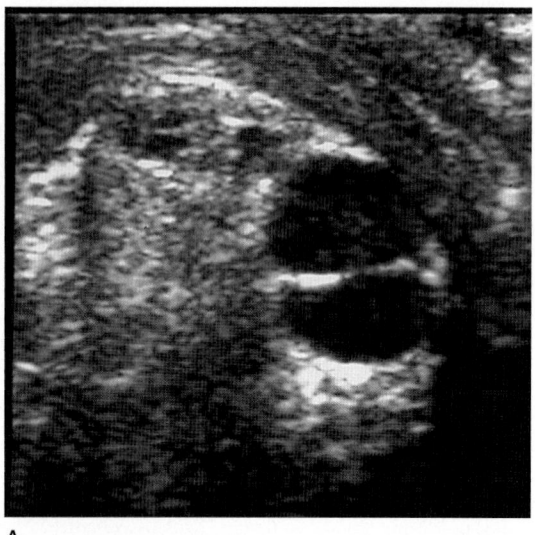
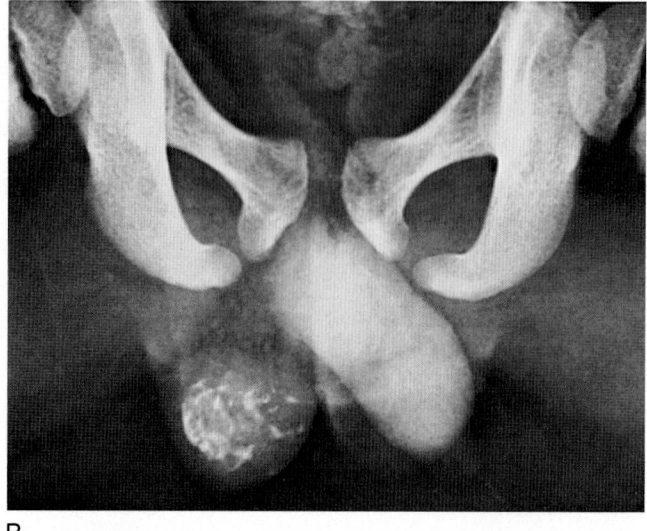

A   B

FIGURE 154-25. Testicular teratoma. **A,** Transverse sonogram shows a testicular mass with cystic, debris-filled, and echogenic areas. **B,** On plain radiograph, calcification within the scrotum of this child proved to be from a teratoma of the right testis. (Courtesy of Dr. Leslie E. Grissom.)

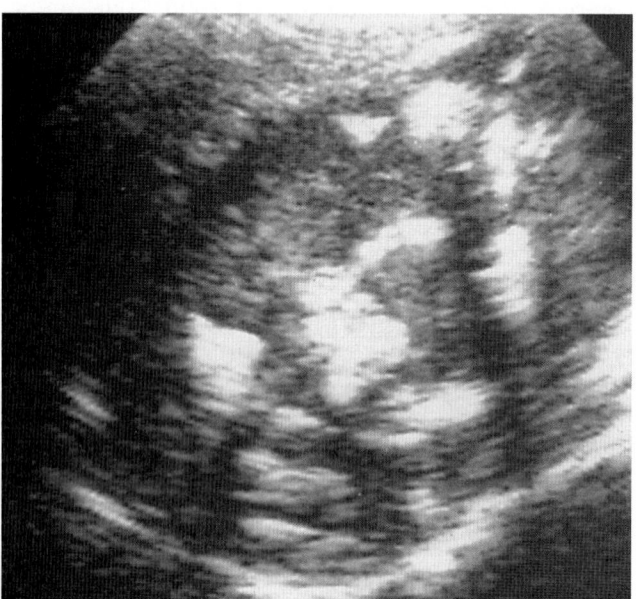

FIGURE 154-26. Leydig cell tumor. Longitudinal sonogram in an African American with precocious puberty (i.e., early virilization) shows multiple calcifications (bright echogenicities) scattered in the testicular parenchyma. There is shadowing beyond one or two of the calcifications. (Courtesy of Dr. Kenneth Glassberg.)

represent the most common gonadal stromal tumors of childhood. They are almost always benign adenomas. Almost half (45%) are Leydig cell tumors, which have a peak incidence at 4 years of age and are the most common testicular neoplasm in African American children. Usually diagnosed between the ages of 2 and 9 years, Leydig cell tumors are painless but may be associated with hormone production. Patients may develop premature virilization (Fig. 154-26) if androgen is produced or gynecomastia if estrogen is produced. Sertoli cell tumors represent 20% of the non–germ cell

tumors. Half are diagnosed in the first year of life. Gynecomastia caused by estrogen production may occur. Tumors containing a mixture of non–germ cell histologic patterns may occur.

Germ Cell Plus Stromal Cell Tumors

Gonadoblastomas are composed of germ cells and gonadal stromal cell elements. They are very uncommon and most often seen in older children and adolescents. Punctate dystrophic calcifications within the tumor are common and may be detected roentgenographically. Gonadoblastomas are frequently bilateral and generally benign. One tenth of cases, however, are associated with or develop germ cell tumors, including embryonal carcinoma, yolk sac tumor, and choriocarcinoma. Pure germ cells tumors and mixed germ cell tumors, particularly containing seminoma and gonadoblastoma, occur with some frequency in mostly adult patients born with certain disorders of sex differentiation, particularly in patients born with a Y chromosome, dysgenetic gonads, and ambiguous external genitalia.

Epidermoid Cyst

The epidermoid cyst (Fig. 154-27), also known as a keratocyst, is a benign tumor of germ cell origin representing less than 1% of all testis tumors. It is most commonly found in the third to fifth decades of life. It typically consists of a simple squamous cell–lined echopenic area located within the testicular parenchyma usually just below the tunica albuginea. The wall is made up of fibrous tissue, and its lumen contains cheesy keratinized material or amorphous debris. Patients usually present with a painless 0.5- to 4-cm nodule often picked up incidentally on routine physical examination. Occasionally, patients may present with diffuse testicular enlargement. US examination shows an echopenic mass with an echogenic wall. The "cyst" contents prevent the description as

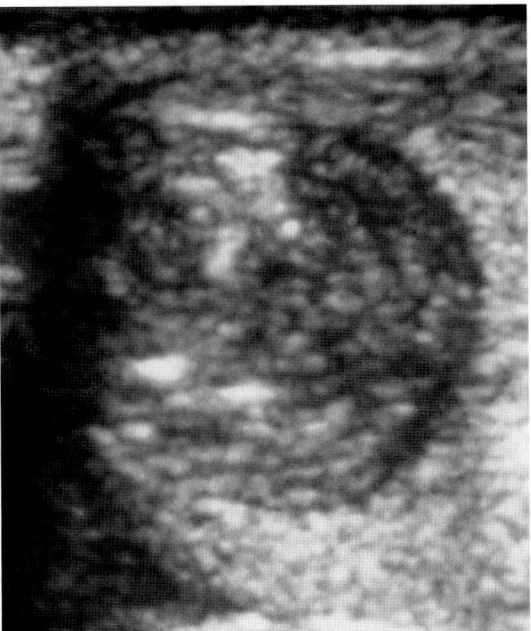

FIGURE 154-27. Epidermoid. Transverse sonogram shows an echopenic mass with some echogenic (onion skin) layering in the testis of this young adult. (Courtesy of Dr. Sheila Sheth.)

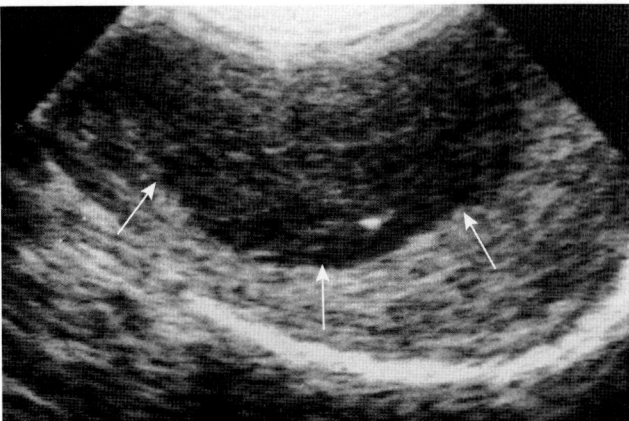

FIGURE 154-28. Leukemia. Longitudinal sonogram of an enlarged right testis of this teenager with leukemia who was thought to be in remission shows a hypoechoic mass *(arrows)*. The echopenic area proved to be due to leukemic involvement of the testis. (From Cohen HL, Sivit C [eds]: Fetal and Pediatric Ultrasound: A Casebook Approach. New York, McGraw-Hill, 2001. Reproduced with permission of McGraw-Hill Companies.)

a classic cyst on US. Occasionally the wall may calcify. There are four basic US appearances, including a halo with central increased echogenicity, a sharply defined mass with peripheral calcification, and a solid mass with an echogenic rim. The classic appearance is an onion-ring pattern with alternating hyperechoic and hypoechoic rings that is typically avascular. These tumors do not contain elements such as sebaceous material or hair that would suggest testicular teratoma and therefore the possibility of premalignancy. However, often one cannot definitively differentiate the US image of this mass from that of a teratoma and histologic analysis is necessary before making a definitive diagnosis and resultant therapeutic decisions.

> The classic appearance of an epidermoid cyst is an onion-ring pattern with alternating hyperechoic and hypoechoic rings.

Testicular Tumors Originating from Testicular Supporting Tissues

Testicular tumors originating from testicular supporting tissues are rare and mostly benign. They include leiomyoma, fibroma, hemangioma, and lymphangioma. Isolated and rare cases of leiomyosarcoma and fibrosarcoma can occur in childhood. Their US images are similar to those of connective tissue tumors elsewhere in the body. They appear solid. Many originate from the cells of the tunica albuginea.

Secondary Testicular Neoplasms

Testicular metastases are rare in children, representing far less than 1% of testicular tumors. Leukemia and lymphoma are the most common causes. Enlarged testes caused by leukemic or lymphomatous infiltration are uncommon but may be the primary manifestation of these diseases.

> Testicular metastases are rare in children. Leukemia and lymphoma are the most common causes.

Acute lymphocytic (lymphoblastic) leukemia (ALL) is the most common secondary testicular neoplasm in children. The lesion is often bilateral. The affected testis may be normal or enlarged. At least 8% of ALL patients have testicular involvement at some point during the course of their disease. There is an incidence among autopsy specimens of 92%. These enlarged testes have focal (Fig. 154-28) or diffuse areas of decreased echogenicity. Areas of hemorrhage appear echogenic, and lymphatic obstruction may lead to hydrocele. Color Doppler imaging often shows significant increases in flow, often in an asymmetric pattern related to the position of the infiltrating masses within the testis.

Testicular involvement is a key diagnostic consideration when analyzing patients with intrascrotal symptomatology who have undergone treatment for leukemia in the past and are in remission. With more aggressive treatment to prevent the central nervous system of patients with leukemia from becoming a sanctuary site for leukemic cells, the testes are now the main potential sanctuary site in boys and therefore a key area to evaluate for recurrence of leukemia. Unilateral or bilateral testicular enlargement seen in the first 2 years after bone marrow remission can be a first sign of relapse. This may be followed by bone marrow relapse and widespread metastatic disease because chemotherapy is less effective in dealing with leukemic cells in the testis as compared with other organs.

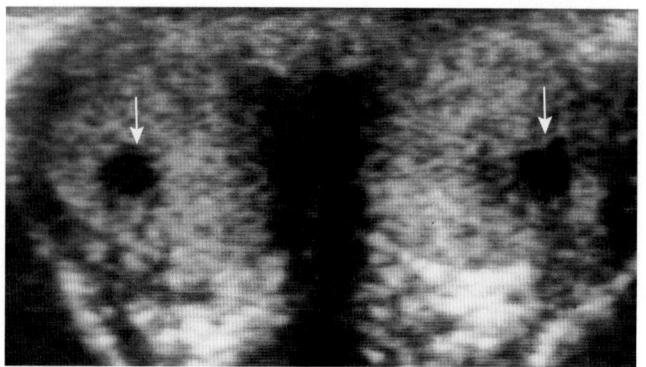

FIGURE 154-29. Adrenal rests. Transverse sonogram shows single echopenic masses *(arrows)* in both the right and left testes of this boy with congenital adrenal hyperplasia. (Courtesy of Dr. Carlos Sivit, Cleveland, OH.)

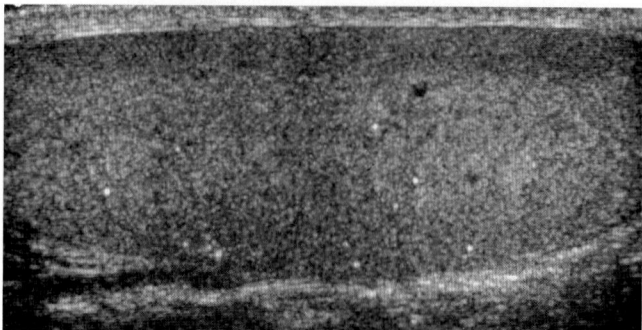

FIGURE 154-30. Testicular microlithiasis. Longitudinal sonogram shows several tiny, bright echoes within the otherwise normal right testis of this teenager. This was an incidental finding in both his testes.

> In patients with leukemia histories, testicular enlargement seen in the first 2 years after bone marrow remission can be a first sign of relapse.

Adrenal Rests

Adrenal rests are simulators of intratesticular tumors. At times aberrant cells from the adrenal cortex may travel with gonadal tissue and be incorporated into the testis during fetal life. With high levels of adrenocorticotropic hormone and associated cortical cell stimulation, these rests may enlarge and appear masslike (Fig. 154-29). This stimulation occurs in patients with congenital adrenal hyperplasia, whether early in life as infants or later as adolescents or young adults. It can also occur in patients with Cushing syndrome. Patients present with testicular mass or enlargement. On US, one usually sees several echopenic masses, usually in both testes. They can be echogenic. A typical color Doppler US pattern has been described in which multiple peripheral vessels radiate in a spokelike fashion from the centers of individual rest masses. Similar rests may be found in the epididymis or spermatic cord.

Testicular Microlithiasis and Its Association with Testicular Tumors

Testicular microlithiasis is an uncommon condition characterized by calcifications within the lumina of seminiferous tubules. It is denoted on US by individual tiny (2-3 mm), bright echogenicities without shadowing (Fig. 154-30) within the testicular parenchyma. Some reserve the diagnosis for cases in which more than five microliths are noted on a single US image. It is usually an incidental finding. However, there is a debated association between the presence of testicular microlithiasis and the presence or development of testicular neoplasm, particularly germ cell neoplasia. Although usually seen in young adults, the finding may be made in children, particularly adolescents. Testicular microlithiasis has been associated with cryptorchidism, infertility, male intersex, Klinefelter syndrome, and pulmonary alveolar microlithiasis.

According to two major studies of prevalence of testicular microlithiasis and tumor risk by Cast and coworkers and Skyrme and associates there is a 0.68% to 1.1% prevalence and a 13 to 21.6 times greater risk for the presence of a testicular neoplasm. Among the 54 tumors noted by these studies, there were 28 seminomas, 14 teratomas, 8 mixed germ cell tumors, 2 Leydig cell tumors, and 2 non-Hodgkin lymphomas. Because of the association of microlithiasis and tumors, patients with testicular microlithiasis alone are followed closely both clinically and by US (follow-up by 6 months to 1 year) for possible tumor development over time.

> Testicular microlithiasis may predispose individuals to the development of testicular neoplasia.

INTRASCROTAL EXTRATESTICULAR MASSES

PARATESTICULAR RHABDOMYOSARCOMA

Primary extratesticular neoplasms are rare; 70% are benign spermatic cord tumors. Paratesticular neuroblastomas have been reported. Rhabdomyosarcoma is the most common malignant paratesticular mass in the child, representing 10% of intrascrotal tumors of childhood. It originates from the supporting stroma of the spermatic cord, testicular appendages, and paratesticular tunics and is often located superior to the testis. It often presents as a painless mass in the scrotum of a young boy. There are two incidence peaks for intrascrotal rhabdomyosarcoma, one at 2 to 4 years of age and the other between 15 and 17 years. Rhabdomyosarcomas grow rapidly and are frequently large at presentation. They spread early to regional and retroperitoneal lymph nodes. Venous invasion and distant metastases, especially to the lungs, are not uncommon. There are three types of rhabdomyosarcomas: (1) the anaplastic type, (2) a type composed of round cells of uniform size, and (3) a mixed type. The mixed type is the most common (80%) and has a more favorable prognosis. Prognosis is related to the extent of the tumor at diagnosis. On US examination, the mass is predominantly echogenic with focal anechoic areas caused by necrosis. As with all extratesticular masses, if the testes are invaded, differentiating the lesion from a mass of testicular origin may be difficult.

> **Rhabdomyosarcoma is the most common malignant paratesticular mass in children.**

Varicoceles

A common mass found within the scrotum of adults or teenagers is a varicocele, which is made up of dilated veins of the pampiniform plexus. Varicoceles are usually thought to develop because of incompetence of the internal spermatic vein. They are graded according to their size. Approximately 65% are grade I, which are defined as small varicoceles palpated with difficulty, and usually appearing as only mild thickening of the cord on physical examination. One fourth (24%) are grade II, defined as moderate in size, easily discovered on physical examination, and consisting of a mass of veins up to 2 mm in diameter. Ten percent of cases are grade III, with the varicocele made up of individual veins greater than 2 mm in diameter. The scrotum of such affected individuals is said to look like a "bag of worms."

When unilateral, 99% of varicoceles are left sided. Theoretically, this is a result of increased pressure on the left renal vein with concomitant increased pressure and retrograde flow into its branch (the left spermatic vein) caused either by compression between the aorta and the superior mesenteric artery (the "nutcracker" phenomenon) or by incompetent or absent valves in the internal spermatic vein. Varicoceles most often develop on the left side of the body where the spermatic vein enters the renal vein at a right angle. This anatomic situation is linked to a far greater incidence of venous incompetence compared with that of the right side, where the right spermatic vein enters the inferior vena cava directly at an oblique angle. The occurrence of bilateral varicoceles is common. Because of the aforementioned facts regarding normal anatomy that seem to protect the right side, finding a solitary right-sided varicocele is extremely uncommon. If noted, the examiner must rule out intra-abdominal neoplasm or another mass as a cause. Varicoceles are painless and may disappear on supine examination. Therefore, physical examination with the patient standing and, if necessary, bearing down, may be required to make the diagnosis.

> **When unilateral, 99% of varicoceles are left sided. Unilateral right-sided varicoceles raise concern for a possible obstructing mass.**

The major imaging method for varicocele analysis is US. On US examination, varicoceles are tortuous, tubular, echo-free structures (Fig. 154-31) that may be situated superior, lateral, and/or posterior to the testis. Doppler examination (especially color Doppler imaging) can confirm the vascular nature of these structures. More often the diagnosis is confirmed by having the patient perform a Valsalva maneuver, sometimes standing but even supine, and noting via color Doppler imaging that the tubular vessels, which may not show evident intra-luminal flow before the maneuver, will fill with color (see Fig. 154-31). Flow can be proved as venous by spectral

A

B

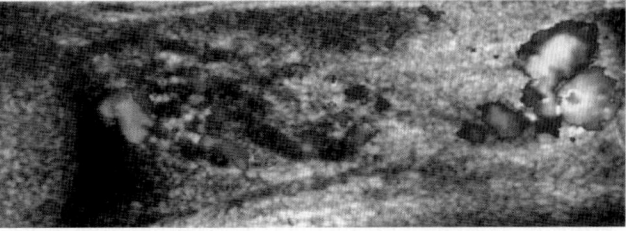

C

FIGURE 154-31. Varicocele. **A,** Transverse sonogram shows tubular echoless structures lateral to a teenager's left testis. One *(cursors)* is noted to be 2.7 mm wide. **B,** Color Doppler image during straining by the patient. Color fills several of the tubular structures. A venous spectral pattern was obtained to prove them to be varicoceles. The normal testis is seen to the reader's left. **C,** In another teen, the top image of a triplex Doppler shows tubular structures in the scrotum. The lower half of the image shows the spectral pattern over time. *Arrows* point out when the patient strained. The strain resulted in significant venous-type flow increase, proving the structures to be due to a varicocele. (**B,** *see color plate.*)

Doppler analysis. Having the patient strain or perform a Valsalva maneuver may show the spectral pattern change (see Fig. 154-31) from no or little flow to a significant increase in spectral flow that is equivalent to the change seen with strain and color Doppler flow imaging.

Intratesticular varicocele is considered a rare form of varicocele found within the testicular substance, usually associated with an extratesticular varicocele. Echoless tubular vessels similar to those seen with extratesticular varicocele can be seen in part or throughout the testicular parenchyma. There are rare instances of intratesticular varicoceles that appear as cystic areas with venous flow patterns replacing the testicular parenchyma. Vascular flow is either readily noted on Doppler evaluation or can be elicited with straining. The clinical significance of this lesion is currently unknown.

The diagnosis of varicoceles is of significance because of the association with infertility in the adult male (39% of infertile men have varicoceles) and the possible gonadotoxic effect on the testes over time. Surgical ligation of the varicocele is therapeutically recommended in cases when there is ipsilateral testicular volume loss of 2 ml or greater. Histologic analysis of such testes has shown various degrees of tubal hypoplasia, decreased spermatogenesis, focal fibrosis, or arrest of germ cell maturation. Kass and colleagues operated on 20 patients with grade II to III disease with left varicocele and testicular volume loss and showed that 16 had increases in left testicular volume on follow-up after ligation of the varicoceles.

> **Surgical ligation of a varicocele is recommended when there is ipsilateral testicular volume loss of 2 ml or more.**

Other Extratesticular Masses

Cystic masses in the epididymis may either be *spermatoceles* or *epididymal cysts*. They both represent a confluence of dilated efferent ductules of the testis. Most are of idiopathic origin. They are not uncommon. Cysts contain serous fluid. Spermatoceles contain spermatozoa as well as fatty and cellular debris. They can occur in patients with chronic epididymitis and have been reported in patients whose mothers were exposed to diethylstilbestrol. On US examination, a spermatocele typically appears as a solitary echo-free mass (Fig. 154-32) that on occasion may appear septated.

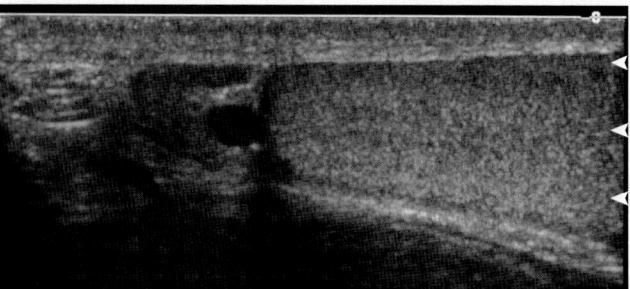

FIGURE 154-32. Spermatocele. Longitudinal sonogram of this teenager's epididymis shows a small cystic area.

Epididymal sperm cell granulomas may simulate neoplasm. This typically hypoechoic solid mass with echogenicity caused by contained fibrous connective tissue is the result of an inflammatory response to the extravasation of spermatozoa. Epididymal sperm cell granulomas may present as a painless intratesticular or extratesticular mass.

SUGGESTED READINGS

Akin, EA, Khati NJ, Hill MC: Ultrasound of the scrotum. Ultrasound Q 2004;20:181-200

Anderson K, McAninch J, Jeffrey RB, Laing F: Ultrasonography for the diagnosis and staging of blunt scrotal trauma. J Urol 1983;130:933

Avila N, Premkumar A, Shawker T, et al: Testicular adrenal rest tissue in congenital adrenal hyperplasia: findings at gray-scale and color Doppler US. Radiology 1996;198:99

Bach A, Hann L, Shi W et al: Is there an increased incidence of contralateral testicular cancer in patients with intratesticular microlithiasis. AJR Am J Roentgenol 2003;180:497

Benson CB, Doubilet PM, Richie JP: Sonography of the male genital tract. AJR Am J Roentgenol 1989;153:705

Brown SM, Casillas V, Montalvo B, Aldores-Saavedra J: Intrauterine spermatic cord torsion in the newborn with sonographic and pathologic correlation. Radiology 1990;177:755

Burks DD, Markey B, Burkhard T, et al: Suspected testicular torsion and ischemia: evaluation with color Doppler sonography. Radiology 1990;175:815

Cast J, Nelson W, Early A, et al: Testicular microlithiasis: prevalence and tumor risk in a population referred for scrotal sonography. AJR Am J Roentgenol 2000;175:1703

Cohen HL, Haller J: Scrotal ultrasound in the pediatric and adolescent patient. Radiol Rep 1990;2:276

Cohen HL, Moore W. Commemoration: History of emergency US. J Ultrasound Med 2004;23:451

Cohen HL, Shapiro M, Haller J, Glassberg K: Sonography of intrascrotal hematomas simulating testicular rupture in adolescents. Pediatr Radiol 1992;2:296

Cohen HL, Shapiro M, Haller J, Glassberg K: Torsion of the testicular appendage. J Ultrasound Med 1992;11:81

Cohen HL, Sivit C (eds): Fetal and Pediatric Ultrasound: A Casebook Approach. New York, McGraw-Hill, 2001

Connor S, Guest P: Conversion of multiple solid testicular teratoma metastases to fatty and cystic liver masses following chemotherapy: CT evidence of "maturation." Br J Radiol 1999;72:111

Dogra VS, Gottlieb RH, Oka M, Rubens D: Sonography of the scrotum. Radiology 2003;227:18

Dambro T, Stewart R, Carroll B: The scrotum. In Rumack C, Wilson S, Charboneau J (eds): Diagnostic Ultrasound, 2nd ed. St. Louis, Mosby, 2001:791

Danrad R, Ashker L, Smith W: Polyorchidism: imaging may denote reproductive potential of accessory testicle. Pediatr Radiol 2004;34:492-494

Ganem J: Testicular microlithiasis. Curr Opin Urol 2000;10:99

Giwercman A, Grindsted J, Hansen B, et al: Testicular cancer risk in boys with maldescended testis: a cohort study. J Urol 1987; 138:1214

Gross B, Cohen HL, Schlessel J: Perinatal diagnosis of bilateral testicular torsions: beware of torsions simulating hydroceles. J Ultrasound Med 1993;12:479

Hadziselimovic F: Treatment of cryptorchidism with GnRH. Urol Clin North Am 1982;9:413

Hamper UM: Testicular microlithiasis with germ cell tumor. In Herzberg BS, Hill MC, Cohen HL (eds): Ultrasound (third series). Reston, ACR, 2005:155

Horstman W, Middleton W, Melson G, Siegel B: Color Doppler US of the scrotum. Radiographics 1991;6:941

Jensen MC, Lee K, Halls J, Ralls P: Color Doppler sonography in testicular torsion. J Clin Ultrasound 1990;18:446

Josso N, Picard J, Rey R, di Clemente N: Testicular anti-Müllerian hormone: history, genetics, regulation and clinical applications. Pediatr Endocrinol Rev 2006;3:347

Karmazyn B, Steinberg R, Kornreich L, et al: Clinical and sonographic criteria of acute scrotum in children: a retrospective study of 172 boys. Pediatr Radiol 2005;35:302-310

Kass E, Chandra R, Belman A: Testicular histology in the adolescent with a varicocele. Pediatrics 1987;79:996

Kessler A, Meirsdorf S, Graif M, et al: Intratesticular varicocele: gray scale and color Doppler sonographic appearance. J Ultrasound Med 2005;24:1711

Kirsch A, Bastian W, Cohen HL, Glassberg K: Precocious puberty in a child with unilateral Leydig cell tumor of the testis following orchiopexy. J Urol 1993;150:1483-1485

Koff WJ, Scaletscky R: Malformations of the epididymis in undescended testes. J Urol 1990;143:340

Kravets F, Cohen HL, Sheynkin Y, Sukkarieh T: Intraoperative sonographically guided needle localization of nonpalpable testicular tumors. AJR Am J Roentgenol 2006;186:141

Kurtz A, Middleton W: Ultrasound: The Requisites. St. Louis, Mosby, 1996:446

Lerner RM, Mevorach RA, Hulbert WC, Rabinowitz R: Color Doppler US in the evaluation of acute scrotal disease. Radiology 1990;176:355

McAlister WH, Sisler CL: Scrotal sonography in infants and children. Curr Probl Diagn Radiol 1990;19:207

Middleton WD, Siegel B, Melson G, et al: Acute scrotal disorders: prospective comparison of color Doppler US and testicular scintigraphy. Radiology 1990;177:177

Moore CCM: The role of routine radiographic screening of boys with hypospadias: a prospective study. J Pediatr Surg 1990;25:339

Musmanno ML, White JM: Scrotal ultrasonography as adjunct to testis biopsy in leukemia. Urology 1990;35:239

Ozcan H, Aytac S, Yagci C, et al: Color Doppler ultrasonographic findings in intratesticular varicocele. J Clin Ultrasound 1997;25:325

Prader A: Testicular size: assessment and clinical importance. Triangle 1966;7:240-243

Ralls PW: Acute epididymo-orchitis. In Herzberg BS, Hill MC, Cohen HL (eds): Ultrasound (third series). Reston, ACR, 2005:2

Ralls PW, Larsen D, Johnson M, Lee K: Color Doppler sonography of the scrotum. Semin Ultrasound CT MR 1991;12:109

Riebel T, Herrmann C, Wit J, Sellin S: Ultrasonographic late results after surgically treated crytorchidism. Pediatr Radiol 2000;30:151

Siegel M (ed): Male genital tract. In Pediatric Sonography, 2nd ed. New York, Raven Press, 1995:479

Skyrme R, Fenn N, Jones A, Bowsher W: Testicular microlithiasis in a UK population: its incidence, association and follow-up. BJU Int 2000;86:482

Trambert MA, Mattrey R, Levine D, Berthoty D: Subacute scrotal pain: Evaluation of torsion versus epididymitis with MR imaging. Radiology 1990;175:53

Troughton AH, Waring J, Longstaff A, Goddard P: Role of magnetic resonance imaging in the investigation of undescended testes. Clin Radiol 1990;41:178

Ulbright T, Srigley J: Dermoid cyst of the testis: a study of five postpubertal cases, including a pilomatrixoma-like variant, with evidence supporting its separate classification from mature testicular teratoma. Am J Surg Pathol 2001;25:788

Vanzulli A, DelMaschio A, Paesano P, et al: Testicular masses in association with adrenogenital syndrome: US findings. Radiology 1992;183:425

Woodward P: Case 70: Seminoma in an undescended testis. Radiology 2004;231:388

Zerin JM, DiPietro MA: Testicular infarction in a newborn: ultrasound findings. Pediatr Radiol 1990;20:329

CHAPTER 155

Abnormalities of the Female Genital Tract

HARRIS L. COHEN

IMAGING TECHNIQUES

The key technique in the analysis of the pediatric gynecologic tract, its diseases, and the simulators of those diseases is ultrasound (US). It provides quick analysis of the uterus, ovaries, and cul-de-sac. Real-time examinations allow for rapid shifting of transducer position and the subsequent assessment of other organs (e.g., kidney for renal stones) or organ systems (e.g., the gastrointestinal tract to rule out nonperforated appendicitis), when necessary. This allows the examiner to complete the analysis of an apparent gynecologic complaint that may have a nongynecologic cause. US performs these assessments without the use of radiation, an important issue, particularly in the young.

> US is the key technique in the analysis of the pediatric gynecologic tract, its diseases, and the simulators of those diseases.

Computed tomography (CT) allows excellent analysis of the global contents of the pelvis in an axial plane. It is most helpful in cases in which the US examination is inconclusive, usually because of bowel gas interference. When additional information is needed, CT is particularly useful regarding localization of a pelvic mass and the assessment of its resectability. Despite this ability, once a mass is very large, the analysis of its borders and determination of its organ of origin may be limited or impossible. CT is extremely sensitive in denoting density differences among imaged structures and can note the presence of subtle areas of calcium or fat within pelvic masses. It is of major help in the analysis of the bony pelvis. Use of the technique has been limited in children because of the need to sedate (now less necessary because of faster multislice spiral and volume CT scanning) as well as the child's paucity of intrapelvic and intra-abdominal fat, which obscures the exact identification of visceral borders. CT is far less helpful than US for the analysis of the normal and anomalous gynecologic tract because it does not image the ovaries (particularly normal ones) as well, uses radiation, and provides initial imaging in only one plane. Quicker two- and three-dimensional reconstruction programs for picture archiving and communications system (PACS) workstations are making the last comment of lesser concern. US surpasses CT in the ability to analyze small cysts and cystic structures, including ovarian follicles and cysts.

> The use of CT in young children is limited by the paucity of intrapelvic and intra-abdominal fat, which inhibits the exact identification of visceral borders.

Magnetic resonance imaging (MRI) provides multiplanar analysis without radiation and with superior tissue resolution. These examinations have poorer spatial resolution than CT and difficulty in imaging calcium. MRI continues to make progress in providing improved analysis of uterine and other müllerian duct anomalies. It remains a secondary examination because of its cost and the need to sedate the uncooperative or younger patient because study times are far longer than those of CT and usually US. The prolonged positioning of patients undergoing MRI in a confined and noisy space also hinders its use in the young or uncooperative patient without sedation.

CT and MRI provide a more global view of the pelvis and abdomen than does US and are preferred for the analysis of tumor extent and metastases. They are particularly helpful and better than US in the assessment of the mesentery and peritoneum.

The aforementioned cross-sectional imaging modalities, as well as plain radiography, nuclear medicine, genitourinary and gastrointestinal contrast examinations, and angiography, are the imager's tools in the evaluation of the pediatric pelvis. Each has its limitations and drawbacks. The drawbacks of radiation exposure, less than optimal control of the patient's environment (e.g., the need to be removed from an isolette), and the need to sedate are of particular relevance in the pediatric patient (although they become less so with increasing patient age) and are the reason that US continues to remain the screening examination of choice in these assessments.

Diagnostic Ultrasound: Technique and Technical Factors

US examinations of the pelvis are hindered by air-containing bowel. Fluid in the bladder from ingestion or from instillation via a Foley catheter lifts loops of small bowel superiorly and out of the pelvis. The fluid-filled bladder is an excellent US window for analysis of the gynecologic structures posterior and posterolateral to it. Little of the US beam is lost to scatter. Avoiding bladder overdistention is important to limit patient discomfort. Imaging should be performed with the highest-frequency transducer capable of adequate depth penetration. Newer multifrequency transducers have expanded the sonographer's choices. These transducers have a range of megahertz capability, allowing the examiner to penetrate to deeper structures requiring lower settings (e.g., 3.5 MHz) and then change the same transducer's setting to a higher frequency (e.g., 7.5 MHz). Transducer choices are always a compromise between the better near-field resolution of high-frequency transducers and the better penetration of low-frequency transducers.

Transvaginal (TV) transducers have been a boon in the diagnosis of ectopic pregnancy, pelvic inflammatory disease (PID), and other intrauterine and adnexal assessments. The TV or endovaginal transducer allows improved resolution of structures within its field of view (i.e., the uterus and the ovaries) when present in the lower pelvis. It can be placed endovaginally in sexually active teenagers, after being placed in a probe cover containing some couplant gel. Transducer gel is also used on the outside of the probe and cover for proper imaging, because air between the transducer and the examined part may hinder proper imaging. A full bladder is not necessary for TV imaging. However, because of the limitation of the far-field view with the higher megahertz TV transducer, many radiologists will examine a patient with routine transvesicle (through a filled bladder) technique to assess the pelvis globally, have the patient void, and then perform a transvaginal examination for additional information that may be needed. Some physicians will begin a study with the TV probe and then wait for the patient's bladder to fill or fill the bladder with a Foley catheter if an answer is not obtained or transabdominal (TA) images are needed. In the virginal patient, one can obtain some of the benefits of TV scanning by transperineal (translabial) scanning. The covered TV or other probe is placed at the introitus. Images in longitudinal and transverse planes are typically obtained. This method has been successfully used for the assessment of vaginal stenosis and vaginal obstruction.

> **In the virginal patient, one can obtain some of the benefits of TV scanning by transperineal (translabial) scanning.**

Some recent work with three-dimensional US software, which has proved helpful in fetal anatomy analysis, has shown usefulness with regard to uterine anatomy, particularly for müllerian duct anomalies.

THE PEDIATRIC AND ADOLESCENT GYNECOLOGIC TRACT: WHAT IS NORMAL?

The Normal Ovary

The normal ovary is an ovoid structure located in the mesovarium of the broad ligament. The two ovaries are

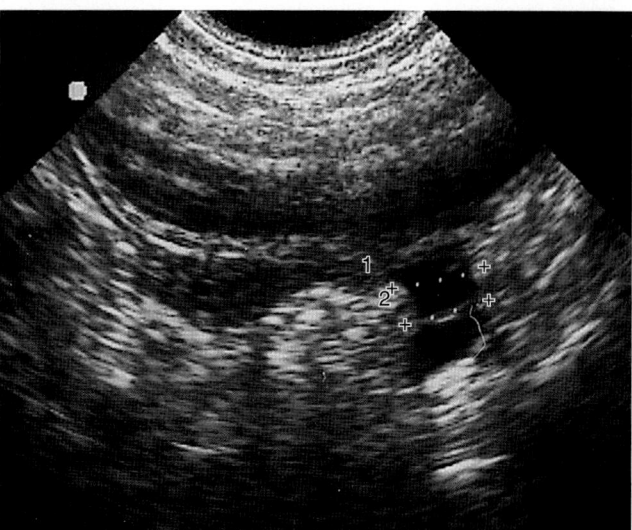

FIGURE 155-1. Normal prepubertal ovary. Transverse sonogram in a prepubertal 6-year-old shows two cysts (cursors) in an ovary lateral to the uterus. Bladder fluid is filled in by near-field artifact.

generally located posterior or lateral (Fig. 155-1) to the uterus, medial and anterior to their ipsilateral iliac vessels, and adjacent to the ipsilateral obturator internus muscle. They can often be found alongside the uterus when it is examined in the axial plane while the transducer is angled in a superoinferior direction. One can occasionally follow the fallopian tube from the cornu of the uterus laterally to find them. Contained follicles help one avoid confusing the ovary with nearby collapsed small bowel. Ovaries may be located anywhere along their embryologic course from the inferior border of the kidney to the broad ligament. The true absence of an ovary is rare. The discovery at surgery of an absent ovary and ipsilateral fallopian tube suggests antenatal torsion with secondary necrosis. Ovaries may be involved in indirect inguinal hernias, 15% of which occur in females. Herniated ovaries can extend as low as the labia, the female equivalent of the scrotum.

> **The discovery at surgery of an absent ovary and ipsilateral fallopian tube suggests antenatal torsion with secondary necrosis. Herniated ovaries can extend as low as the labia, the female equivalent of the scrotum.**

Despite what has been stated in older articles, the ovaries of pediatric patients are regularly imaged by US. Cohen and coworkers were able to image in three dimensions 64% of the ovaries of 77 patients between newborn and 2 years of age and 78% of the ovaries of 101 premenarchal children between 2 and 12 years of age.

Adnexal volume is determined by US using the formula for a modified prolate ellipse: $\pi/6$ (or 0.523) $\times$ L $\times$ W $\times$ D, a formula often simplified as L $\times$ W $\times$ D divided by 2. Length (L) and depth (D) are usually measured on a longitudinal (parasagittal) image (Fig. 155-2) and width (W) is measured on a transverse view. Concepts of normal ovarian volumes and echogenicity have changed

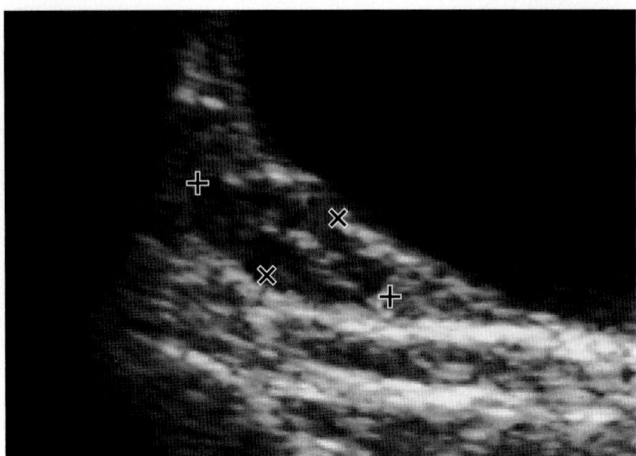

FIGURE 155-2. Normal prepubertal ovary. Longitudinal sonogram shows a normal left ovary *(cursors).* A few echoless follicles are seen within the ovary.

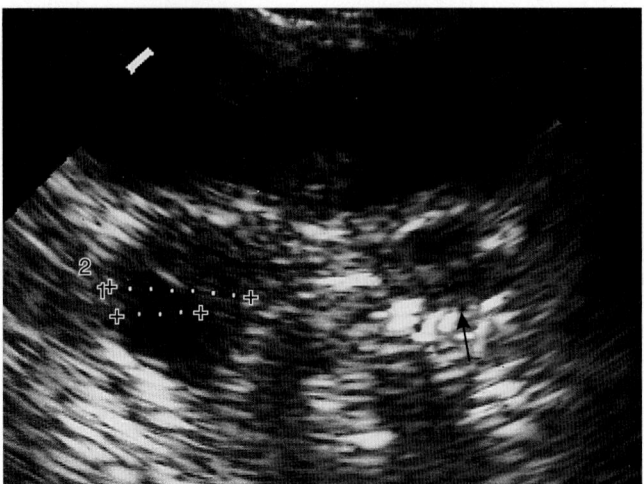

FIGURE 155-3. Normal infant ovary. Transverse sonogram shows *cursors* marking the width of an ovary (2) and a contained follicle (1), common in infants such as this 2-month-old. The left adnexum *(arrow)* can also be seen with contained follicles.

significantly over the past decade for adults as well as children. For example, the often-repeated but incorrect "3 × 2 × 1 cm" (3 cm^3 volume) ovarian measurements ascribed to normal adults and older adolescents underestimate the 6 to 9.8 cm^3 mean volumes for menstruating females noted in more recent studies.

What are considered correct ovarian measurements in neonates and children have also changed in recent years. Whereas at one time imaging ovaries in the neonatal group was considered uncommon, it is now considered the norm. Whereas once a measurement of 1 cm^3 was considered the high end of normal for all children, this, too, has changed. In the first 3 months of life, when gonadotropin levels are highest in children (as a consequence of the decrease in neonatal estrogen and progesterone levels caused by separation from the placenta) ovarian volumes average 1.06 cm^3 but have a range of normal as high as 3.6 cm^3. The high end of the range of normal is 2.7 cm^3 for 4- to 12-month-olds and 1.7 cm^3 for 13- to 24-month-olds. The mean ovarian volume reported by Herter and colleagues for children older than 2 years of age who have not undergone puberty is 1 cm^3.

> **In the first 3 months of life ovarian volumes average 1 cm^3 but have a range of normal as high as 3.6 cm^3.**

Salardi and Orsini and colleagues noted mean volumes ranging between 0.75 and 4.18 cm^3 for 101 premenarchal girls. However, they suggested that the normal pediatric ovary was homogeneous in echogenicity (i.e., without follicles/cysts). Using older equipment, they stated that the typical ovary in a child of 6 or younger had no imaged follicles and that cysts and particularly macrocysts (defined by them as >9 mm in largest diameter) were uncommon before 11 years of age. Cohen and coworkers' more recent work showed follicles or cysts in the majority of children of all ages. Cysts were noted in 80% of the imaged ovaries of a group

of healthy newborns to 2-year-olds (Fig. 155-3), 72% of a 2- to 6-year-old group, and 68% of a 7- to 10-year-old group. Macrocysts were occasionally seen in all age groups. These more recent US findings are consistent with Rokitansky's 1861 report in the pathology literature that noted the presence of cystic follicles in the ovaries of fetuses, neonates, and children. The ovary is not a quiescent organ in childhood but rather a dynamic organ undergoing constant internal change.

> **Follicles/cysts exist in the ovaries of the majority of children.**

The fact that ovarian cysts are common findings in children has helped in other aspects of US diagnosis. Imaging the follicle/cysts in a labial or inguinal mass in a girl with ambiguous genitalia or herniated ovary suggests that the mass is an ovary. Finding follicles in otherwise normal-appearing ovaries of a child with precocious puberty should not concern the sonologist or endocrinologist. The presence of cysts, therefore, does not help to differentiate the healthy child and the child with isosexual precocious puberty.

The Normal Uterus

Uterine shape and size change during pediatric life. In the first months of life, the high circulating gonadotropin levels that develop with the decline of maternal estrogen and progesterone after separation of the neonate from the placenta influence uterine shape and size. The uterus of the newborn has a mean length of 3.5 cm, which decreases to 2.6 to 3 cm by the fourth month of life as the gonadotropin levels decrease. It is not uncommon to find on the US examination of the newborn's uterus either a hypoechoic halo around an imaged echogenic endometrial cavity stripe (Fig. 155-4), seen in 29% of the patients of Nussbaum's study, or endometrial

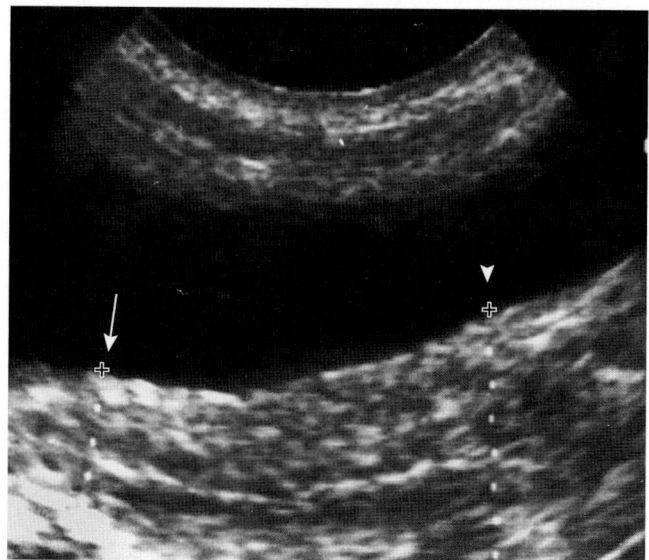

FIGURE 155-4. Normal neonatal uterus. Longitudinal sonogram shows a spade-shaped uterus posterior to the echoless bladder. *Cursors (arrow)* show a relatively narrow uterine fundus, compared with the far wider cervical region *(arrowhead)* of the newborn's uterus. Note the central echogenic line, which is the endometrial cavity. (From Cohen HL: The female pelvis. *In* Siebert J [ed]: Syllabus: Current Concepts: A Categorical Course in Pediatric Radiology. Chicago, RSNA Publications, 1994:65-72.)

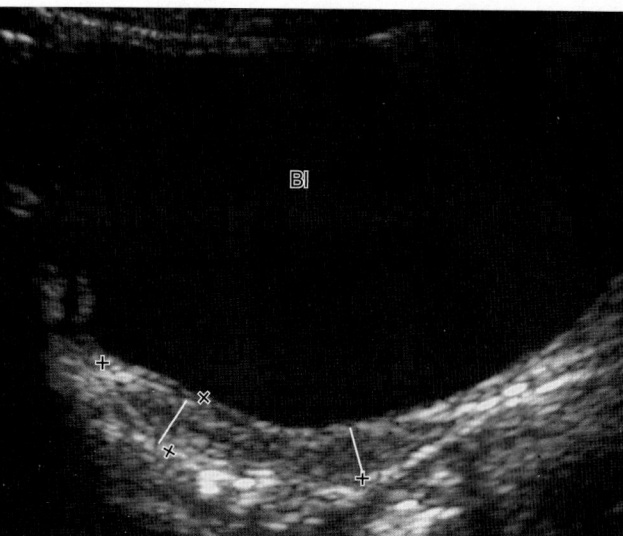

FIGURE 155-5. Normal prepubertal uterus. Longitudinal sonogram of a 6-year-old child. Lines mark off the widths of the cervical area and fundal area, which are similar. Bl, bladder.

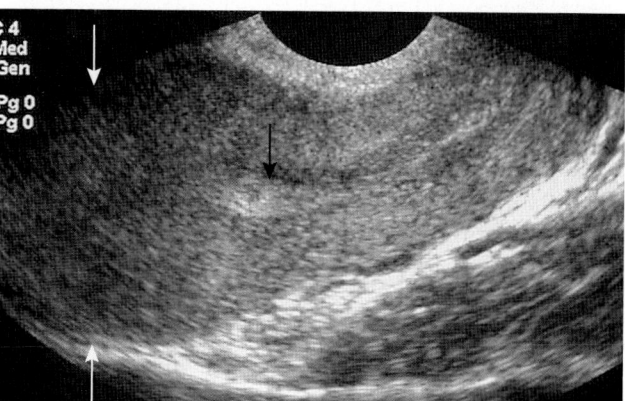

FIGURE 155-6. Normal postmenarchal uterus. On this transvaginal sagittal sonogram of a sexually active teenager, *white arrows* mark off the widest part of the uterus, the fundus. The cervix, to the right, is far less wide. A *black arrow* points to the patient's normal endometrial cavity echogenicity.

cavity fluid (23%), both of which are findings far more typical of an adolescent or adult uterus under the cyclical hormonal influences of postmenarchal life.

The typical newborn's uterus is shaped like a spade (see Fig. 155-4), with the anteroposterior diameter of the cervix as much as twice that of its fundus. The newborn's cervix is also longer than the fundus. A small number of patients may show a tube-shaped (anteroposterior diameter of cervix equal to fundus) or even adult pear-shaped (fundus wider than cervix) uterus. After the first year of life, the typical uterus is tube shaped (Fig. 155-5) and remains that way for at least several years.

> The typical newborn's uterus is shaped like a spade, with the anteroposterior diameter of the cervix twice as wide as that of the fundus.

Identification of the uterus is important information for several clinical diagnostic workups, most notably evaluations of children with ambiguous genitalia. The easiest time to image the child's uterus is in the first few months of life. However, it can be imaged posterior to a fluid-filled bladder at all ages.

Uterine length increases gradually between 3 and 8 years of age. The mean perimenarchal measurement is 4.3 cm. Salardi and associates believe that changes in uterine length and change into the adult pear shape are not solely a matter of increasing estradiol levels but also a function of two other independent variables: age and size of the girl. There is a moderate ($r = .69$) correlation between uterine length and weight in childhood.

After puberty, the typical pear-shaped (Fig. 155-6) uterus measures 5 to 8 cm in length. It is said to descend deeper in the pelvis and no longer maintains the typical neutral position of premenarchal life but instead may be anteverted or retroverted.

MRI and its multiplanar capability can help in the analysis of the uterus, particularly if a müllerian duct anomaly is suspected. MRI can help identify the tissue composition of an intrauterine septum, thereby allowing differentiation between a bicornuate uterus (Fig. 155-7) whose septum contains myometrium and a septate uterus whose septum does not contain myometrium.

EMBRYOLOGY OF THE (MALE AND) FEMALE GENITAL SYSTEM

Differentiation of the primitive gonad into a testis begins at 7 weeks of fetal life in the presence of the H-Y antigen found on the Y chromosome. If there is no Y chromosome, ovarian differentiation begins at 17 weeks' gestation in the presence of two X chromosomes.

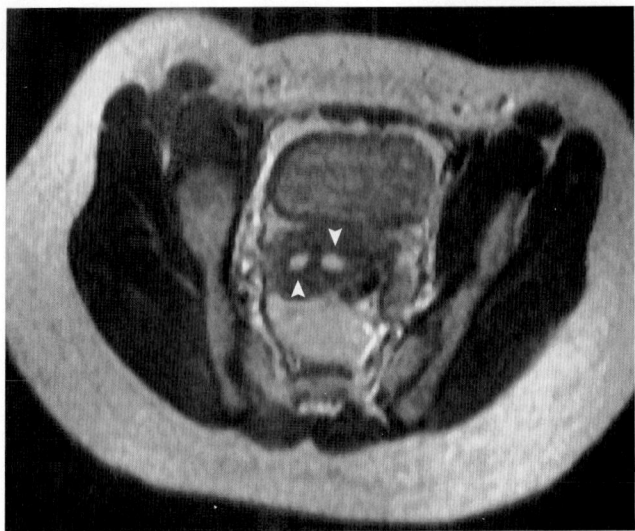

FIGURE 155-7. Bicornuate uterus. Axial T1-weighted MR image demonstrates a gray structure containing two bright echoes representing the two endometrial cavities *(arrowheads).* The intensity of the tissue between the cavities is the same as that of the surrounding uterus, making it consistent with uterine tissue. (From Cohen HL, Bober S, Bow S: Imaging the pediatric pelvis: the normal and abnormal genital tract and simulators of its diseases. Urol Radiol 1992;14:273-283.)

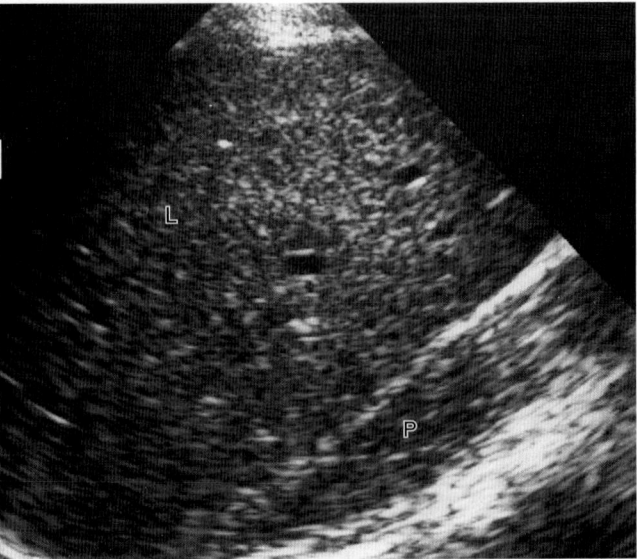

FIGURE 155-8. Renal agenesis and MDS anomaly. Longitudinal sonogram right upper quadrant shows the liver (L) and right psoas muscle (P). No kidney is seen between them, suggesting renal agenesis or ectopia. Nuclear medicine examination proved that there was no right renal ectopia. On the basis of right renal agenesis, the gynecologic tract was assessed in this teenager. The patient had an associated müllerian duct system abnormality—a bicornuate uterus.

> **Differentiation of the primitive gonad into a testis begins at 7 weeks of fetal life, and ovarian differentiation begins at 17 weeks' gestation.**

Development of the urinary system and genital system are closely associated. Urogenital ridges develop from the intermediate mesoderm and are situated on each side of the primitive aorta and give rise to parts of the genital and urinary systems.

The association of uterine and renal abnormalities is quite common, and, when there is a gynecologic anomaly, one should evaluate the renal bed to rule out ectopia or agenesis (Fig. 155-8) and vice versa. Both sexes develop two different pairs of genital ducts. Components of the wolffian (mesonephric) duct system develop into the epididymis, vas deferens, and seminal vesicles under the influence of testosterone. By 6 weeks, a müllerian (paramesonephric) duct has developed lateral to each ipsilateral wolffian duct. In the female, the müllerian duct system (MDS) develops into the fallopian tubes, uterus, and upper two thirds of the vagina, and the wolffian system degenerates. External genital development proceeds along female lines except in the presence of androgens.

> **In girls, the müllerian duct system develops into the fallopian tubes, uterus, and upper two thirds of the vagina. The association of uterine and renal abnormalities is common.**

By 11 weeks, a Y-shaped uterovaginal primordium has developed into the two fallopian tubes and, with fusion of a large portion of the MDS of both sides, a single uterus and a single upper two thirds of the vagina. This occurs "passively" (i.e., with or without the presence of ovaries), as long as there are no testes or high levels of androgens present. The testes produce testosterone, a masculinizing hormone, and müllerian inhibiting factor, which suppresses the further development of the paramesonephric ducts. In females, nonfusion or variably incomplete fusion of the MDS can lead to a wide spectrum of anomalies (Fig. 155-9). Complete nonfusion results in a didelphys uterus, in which there are two vaginas, two cervices, and two uterine bodies. Various anomalies are associated with incomplete müllerian duct fusion. Partial fusions of only the caudal ends of the MDS result in a bicornuate uterus, in which there is variable nonfusion of the cranial portion of the uterus resulting in paired and variably separated uterine horns at the fundus that communicate with a correctly fused single uterine body, cervix, and vagina. The bicornuate uterus results in a wider than normal uterus that may be diagnosed on physical examination (usually when a patient is pregnant) by an anterior uterine depression or by US when two endometrial cavity echogenicities (Fig. 155-10) are imaged. This is usually most readily imaged during the luteal phase of the menstrual cycle or during pregnancy.

Where the MDS joins the urogenital sinus, the lower one third of the vagina develops by elongation of the primitive vaginal plate into a core of tissue that canalizes by week 20. Until late fetal life, the lumen of the vagina is separated from the vestibule of the vagina by a hymenal membrane. The hymen usually ruptures in the perinatal period, remaining as a thin fold of mucous membrane around the vaginal entry.

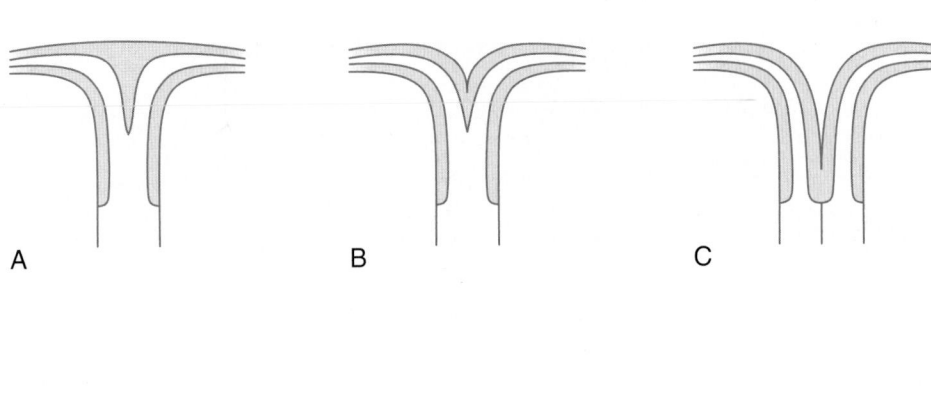

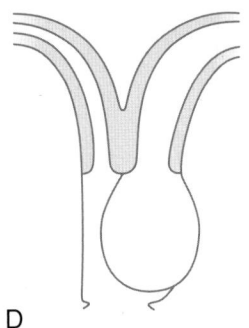
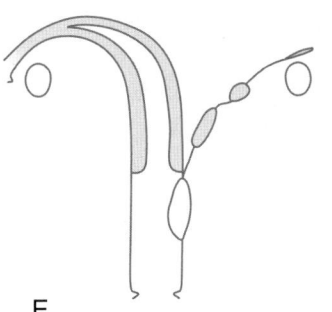
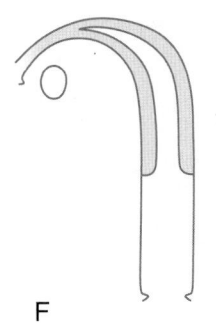

FIGURE 155-9. Fusion defects of the müllerian ducts (septate vagina with normal uterus not included). **A,** Uterus subseptus (uterus septus if septum extends to cervix). **B,** Uterus bicornis unicollis. **C,** Uterus duplex bicornis bicollis and uterus didelphys with septate vagina. **D,** Uterus didelphys with congenital occlusion of one hemivagina. **E** and **F,** Rudimentary hemiuterus and unicornuate uterus.

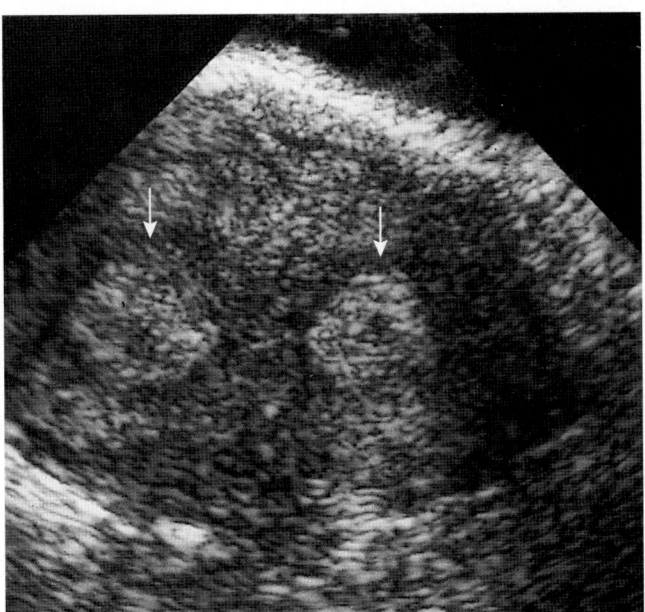

FIGURE 155-10. Bicornuate uterus. Transverse sonogram shows two endometrial cavity echogenicities in the uterus of a teenager. Their presence suggests a bicornuate uterus, which was confirmed. The findings are similar to those on the MR image in Figure 155-7. The patient was in the second half of her menstrual cycle, an easier time to see the two endometrial cavity echogenicities *(arrows),* which tend to be wider and more echogenic closer to the time of menses.

Where the MDS joins the urogenital sinus, the lower one third of the vagina develops by elongation of the primitive vaginal plate into tissue that canalizes by week 20.

Male genital system development is "active," requiring the presence of testes and their production of müllerian inhibiting factor, which causes MDS involution. The enzyme 5α-reductase converts testosterone intracellularly within the target tissues into the powerful dihydrotestosterone. Dihydrotestosterone, acting locally, allows the wolffian duct system to develop into the epididymis, vas deferens, and seminal vesicles.

CLINICAL PROBLEMS IN THE PELVIS OF THE FEMALE CHILD AND ADOLESCENT

Uterine Masses Caused by Vaginal and/or Vaginal-Uterine Obstruction

Uterine masses are uncommon in childhood. The predominant pelvic mass found in neonates and infants is a distended vagina (colpos) or uterus (metros) filled with secretions (muco), fluid (hydro), or blood (hemato). For example, *hematometrocolpos* is defined as hemorrhagic material filling a distended vagina and uterus. US images are similar in appearance whether the affected individual is a neonate or a menarchal teenager. On US, the distended vagina appears as a tubular mass that is usually midline (Fig. 155-11), often with contained echogenicities either from accumulated cervical mucus secretions or hemorrhage from sloughing of a hormonally stimulated endometrial lining. The uterus can be identified separately from the vagina because the muscular uterine wall surrounding the debris- or heme-filled endometrial cavity is thick, whereas the vaginal wall is thin (Fig. 155-12).

The predominant pelvic mass found in neonates and infants is a distended vagina or uterus filled with secretions, fluid, or blood.

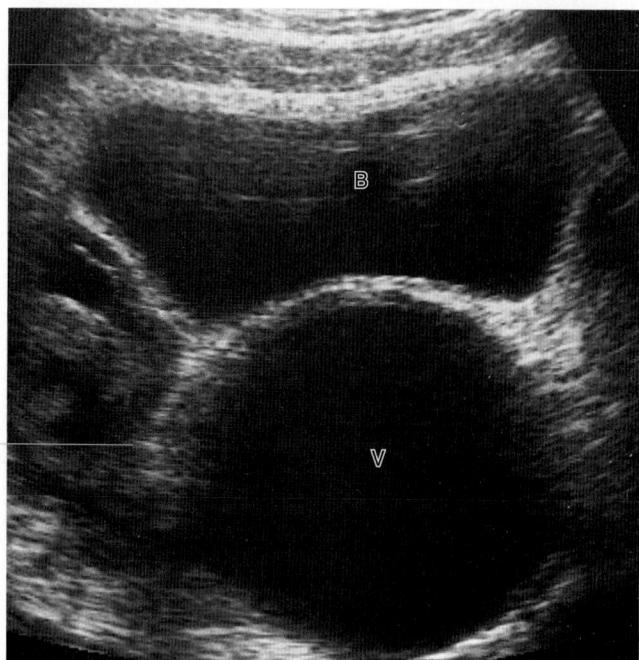

FIGURE 155-11. Hydrocolpos. Transverse sonogram shows a large midline circular cystic structure behind the bladder (B) due to a fluid-filled, dilated vagina (V) in a teenager with an imperforate hymen.

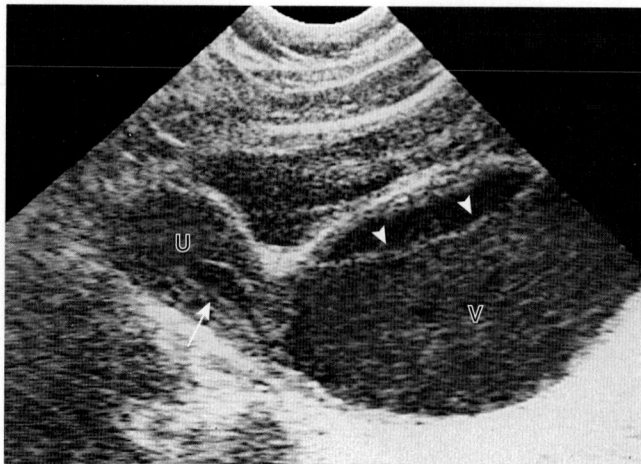

FIGURE 155-12. Hematometrocolpos. Longitudinal sonogram in this patient with pelvic pain and amenorrhea shows a dilated vagina (V). It contains debris with a fluid-debris level *(arrowheads)* seen in its anterior portion. The uterus (U) has a smaller amount of contained fluid *(arrow).* The uterus can be distinguished from the vagina by its thick muscular wall. Dilatation of the uterus and vagina with contained debris indicates hematometrocolpos, which this patient had because of menses and an imperforate hymen. (From Cohen H, Haller J: Pediatric and adolescent genital abnormalities. Clin Diagn Ultrasound 1988;24:187–216.)

An obstructed uterus and vagina discovered in neonatal life is usually suggested clinically by either seeing an interlabial mass or palpating a uterine mass. Pelvic US is used to confirm these findings. The mass develops in the neonate because of the influence of the high gonadotropin levels on a normal endometrial lining. If the uterus, cervix, and vagina are present and not obstructed, the neonate will soon pass cellular debris, mucoid material, or blood, the equivalent of withdrawal bleeding. If the uterus is obstructed, hydrometra, mucometra, or hematometra will develop. If the uterus and cervix are patent but the vagina is obstructed, hydro-, muco-, or hematometrocolpos may develop. The obstructed material may, at times, also be noted in dilated fallopian tubes. At times, the amount accumulated will only fill the vagina. If this obstructive phenomenon is not discovered in neonatal life, the endometrial effluvia will be resorbed and the obstruction will not be discovered until postmenarchal life.

Patients with neonatal hydro/hematometrocolpos can be divided into two groups: those with and those without associated cloacal (single perineal opening for bladder, vagina, and rectum) or urogenital sinus (single perineal opening for bladder and vagina) malformations.

Only a few patients with a congenital vaginal obstruction present at birth with hydrocolpos. Most patients are asymptomatic at birth and during childhood but present in the early postpubertal years because of failure of menstruation despite normal development of secondary sex characteristics. Clinical presentations include amenorrhea and cyclic crampy abdominal pains or a pelvic mass resulting from accumulation of menstrual blood in the proximal vagina (and uterus and tubes). The degree of vaginal and uterine dilatation is related to the degree of obstruction (usually complete) and the time lapse between true menarche and the diagnosis. Patients with an imperforate hymen may present with a bulging, bluish cystic mass protruding from the introitus. In others, only a cystic pelvic mass is diagnosed clinically, by US, or by MRI. A vaginogram may show a shallow, blind-ending vagina in such patients.

> Only a few patients with a congenital vaginal obstruction present at birth. Most patients present in the postpubertal years because of amenorrhea despite normal development of secondary sex characteristics.

The diagnosis of hydro/hematometrocolpos is more common among teenagers, occurring in 1 in every 1000 to 2000 adolescent females. Such masses may become large enough to result in reported cases of lymphatic or venous flow obstruction or cause hydronephrosis from mass effect on the bladder and ureters. Occasional patients will complain of a relatively recent history of difficulty with micturition.

Complete or partial vaginal and/or uterine obstructions may occur in association with various MDS anomalies. These may include vaginal agenesis associated with uterine cervix atresia, isolated atresia of the uterine cervix, and cases of absence of the vagina in the presence of an entirely normal uterus. As stated, hematocolpos or hematometrocolpos usually suggests an imperforate hymen or transverse vaginal septum. Hematometra alone, however, suggests a more unusual abnormality, such as cervical dysgenesis or a partial obstruction of the uterus (e.g., only one horn of a bicornuate system).

Syndrome of Vaginal Agenesis with Rudimentary Uterus (Mayer-Rokitansky-Küster-Hauser Syndrome)

A patient with a dysgenetic MDS may have an absent or rudimentary vagina or uterus as in the Mayer-Rokitansky-Küster-Hauser syndrome. Such patients have normal karyotypes and normal secondary sex development but have associated renal (33% to 50%) and skeletal (12%) anomalies.

> **Mayer-Rokitansky-Küster-Hauser syndrome patients have an absent or rudimentary vagina and uterus and associated renal and skeletal anomalies.**

Vaginal agenesis, the failure of vaginal development in otherwise normal females, occurs in 1 in 4000 to 5000 female births. It is the most frequent cause of primary amenorrhea (no menses by age 16) after Turner syndrome. The proximal two thirds of the vagina and sometimes the entire vagina is absent. The uterus is usually rudimentary and is often bicornuate (rudimentary uterus duplex). At times, one of the two uterine anlagen will contain some functioning endometrium. Fallopian tubes are usually normal but may be hypoplastic or absent. Ovaries are almost always present and are usually anatomically and functionally normal. The external genitalia are also normal except for an absent introitus in some cases.

Vaginal agenesis may be familial. There is frequent association with congenital anomalies (more so than in cases of vaginal obstruction) of other organ systems. Typical malformations are those of the upper urinary tract, including solitary kidney, renal fusion, unilateral renal ectopia, and especially pelvic kidney. Anomalies of the renal pelves and ureters as well as the occurrence of vesicoureteral reflux have been reported in these patients. Skeletal abnormalities (12%) are often vertebral, including the Klippel-Feil anomaly, but may also encompass rib anomalies, congenital hip dislocation, pectus deformity, and syndactyly. Cardiac malformations and deafness resulting from middle ear defects occur. An association of absent vagina with middle ear conductive deafness and Klippel-Feil anomaly has been described, as has another entity consisting of müllerian duct aplasia, renal aplasia, and cervicothoracic somite dysplasia (MURCS).

Vaginal Obstructions

TRANSVERSE VAGINAL SEPTUM

In transverse vaginal septum, the vagina is obliterated by fibrous connective tissue with vascular and muscular elements lined by squamous epithelium. The area of obliteration may be a thin membrane, but more commonly it involves a segment of the vagina (segmental vaginal atresia). Vaginal septa are most common in the midportion of the vagina but may affect the proximal third of the vagina near the cervix and occasionally the distal vagina near the hymen.

An association of transverse vaginal septum or segmental atresia of the vagina with postaxial polydactyly has been described as a separate entity occurring as an autosomal recessive trait (McKusick-Kauffman syndrome). Other commonly occurring anomalies in this syndrome are those of the gastrointestinal tract, including imperforate anus and Hirschsprung disease. Other reported anomalies include those of the eyes, the cardiovascular system, the limbs, the urinary tract (especially dilated pyelocalyceal systems), and the genital system, including displacement of the urethral meatus into the distal vaginal wall (female hypospadias) and duplication of the vagina and uterus. Female members of affected families may show only polydactyly and/or congenital heart disease. Male relatives may be affected by polydactyly and/or hypospadias.

IMPERFORATE HYMEN

An imperforate hymen is the simplest and most easily correctable cause of vaginal obstruction. In such cases, the vagina is obliterated by a thin membrane, the hymen, which forms at the junction of the caudal end of the müllerian ducts and the cranial end of the urogenital sinus. The imperforate hymen is not considered a müllerian anomaly because it originates from the urogenital sinus. A transperineal US approach (placing a transducer on the perineum) may more readily denote vaginal obstruction by an imperforate hymen (Fig. 155-13). Patients with imperforate hymen or vaginal membrane have normal external genitalia, ovaries, fallopian tubes, and uterus.

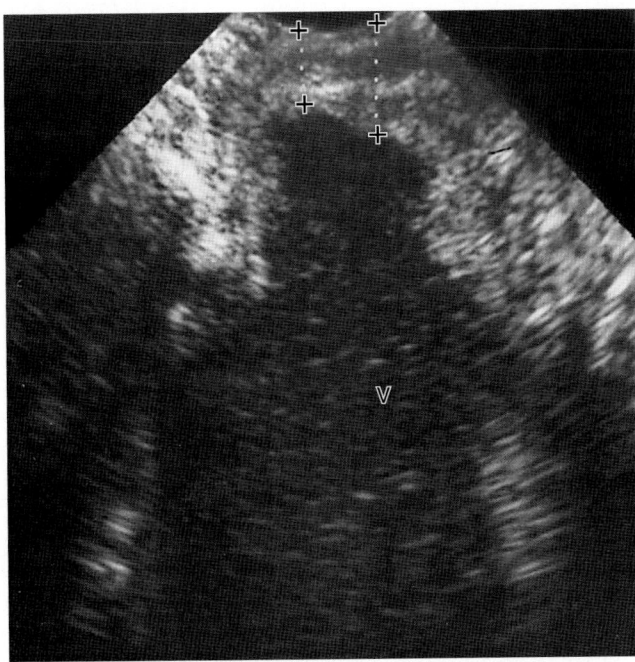

FIGURE 155-13. Imperforate hymen. Transverse transperineal sonogram shows a somewhat asymmetric soft tissue structure *(cursors)* that is obstructing the vagina in this 13-year-old who presented with abdominal pain and fever. The distended vagina (V) deep to the superficial hymen has contained debris from hemorrhagic material. The uterus is too distant to be seen on this image.

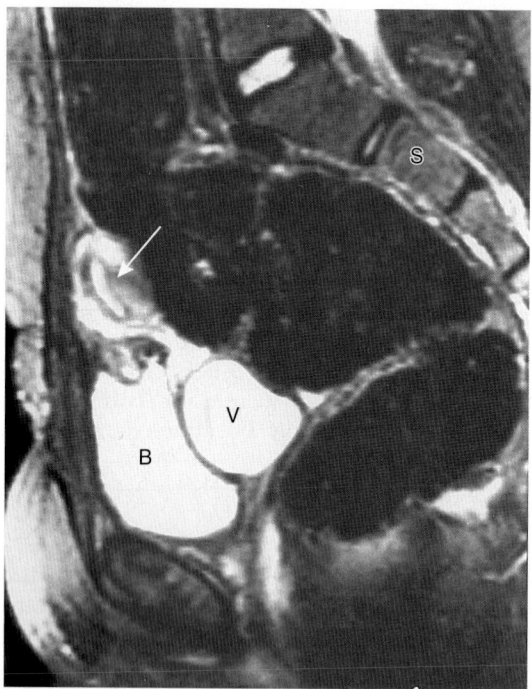

FIGURE 155-14. Hydrometrocolpos. Sagittal T2-weighted MRI shows a dilated, fluid-filled vagina (V) posterior to the bladder (B). High signal fluid filling the bladder, vagina, and endometrial cavity *(arrow)* all appears of similar intensity. S, sacrum. (From Cohen HL: Evaluation of the adolescent and young adult with amenorrhea: role of US. *In* Bluth E, Arger P, Hertzberg B, Middleton W [eds]: Syllabus: A Special Course in Ultrasound: Clinical Questions, Practical Answers. Oak Brook, IL, RSNA Publications, 1996:171-184, with permission.)

> An imperforate hymen is the simplest and most easily correctable cause of vaginal obstruction. It forms at the junction of the caudal end of the müllerian ducts and the cranial end of the urogenital sinus.

IMAGING VAGINAL OBSTRUCTIONS

Ultrasonography is the most important and initial diagnostic tool in neonatal life. Scattered internal echoes representing cellular and mucous debris and fluid–debris levels may be observed in the dilated obstructed vagina (see Fig. 155-12). US can denote the linear echogenicity of the nonobstructed coapted vagina. Pelvic MRI in the sagittal or coronal plane can show the dilated vagina (Fig. 155-14) as well. Although vaginal obstruction may also be noted by CT, that modality has historically been limited to the axial plane. If a diagnosis is still not certain, a contrast vaginogram can be helpful in showing obstruction or narrowing on fluoroscopy. In cases in which an obstructed vaginal lesion exists at a high level, a vaginogram may demonstrate a short, blind-ending vagina. A congenital fistula between the urethra and vagina proximal to a vaginal obstruction may be present, which may fill the obstructed vagina during voiding on voiding cystourethrography.

DIFFERENTIAL DIAGNOSTIC CONSIDERATIONS FOR A BULGING MASS AT THE INTROITUS

Although a bulging cystic mass at the introitus associated with a cystic pelvic mass detectable by US in a newborn or at puberty in an amenorrheic girl is characteristic of neonatal hydrocolpos or pubertal hematocolpos caused by an imperforate hymen, there is a differential diagnosis. The main other possibilities are complex MDS anomalies with obstructions of only a portion of the uterus (e.g., one horn) or a portion of a vagina in cases of duplication and distal obstruction of one hemivagina.

TREATMENT OF VAGINAL OBSTRUCTIONS

The vaginal obstruction in patients with congenital hydrocolpos is corrected in the newborn period. In patients presenting with hematometrocolpos at puberty, the obstruction should be corrected as promptly as possible. This is done, in part, to avoid endometriosis as a result of distal obstruction and repeated reverse spillage of menstrual blood into the peritoneal cavity through the fallopian tubes. Chronic hematosalpinx can also lead to chronic epithelial changes in the fallopian tubes, placing fertility at risk and increasing the possibility of ectopic pregnancy. Hysterectomy is indicated in patients with vaginal agenesis with rudimentary uterus and a functional endometrium and in patients with cervical atresia occurring as an isolated lesion or in association with vaginal agenesis. A detailed evaluation of the uterus, uterine cervix, and vagina by US and/or by MRI is indicated before any surgery (Figs. 155-15 and 155-16). At times, however, the true anatomy of the lesion will only be discovered at surgical exploration.

> When a patient presents with hematometrocolpos at puberty, the obstruction should be corrected as promptly as possible to prevent endometriosis and to improve fertility.

Müllerian Duct System Anomalies and Unilateral Hydro/Hematometrocolpos

The MDS undergoes a series of complex and significant changes to develop from a bifid system into a single uterus, a single cervix, a single vagina (upper two thirds), and two fallopian tubes. Many potential errors may occur in this embryologic process. MDS anomalies are common, occurring in at least 0.1% to 0.5% of females, with some reports indicating an incidence as high as 12%. An incomplete fusion of the distal segment of the two müllerian ducts can result in various degrees of bifidity of the uterus or vagina or both (see Fig. 155-9). Abnormalities may range (in order of increasing complexity) from a septate uterus (with merely a septum separating a variable portion of the uterine endometrial cavity) to a bicornuate uterus to the more complex anomalies. Most simple abnormalities may never be discovered unless there is a problem with fertility or the ability to carry an infant to term. As an example, the bicornuate uterus is usually not discovered until later pregnancy, when the growth of the uterus allows the clinician to feel the typical anterior depression in the upper

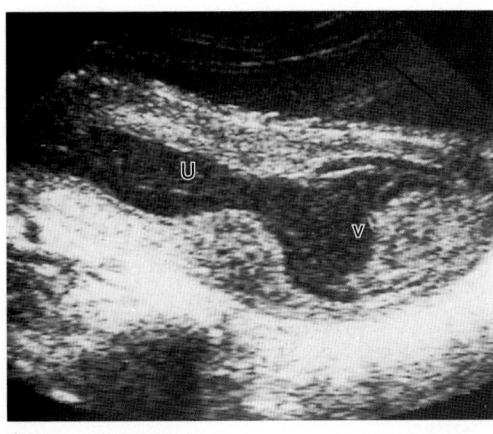
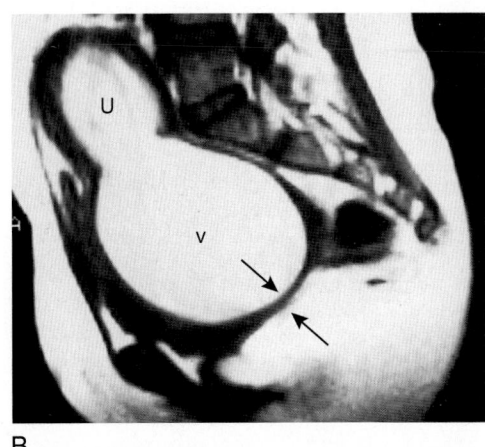

A   B

FIGURE 155-15. Hematometrocolpos from imperforate hymen. **A,** Longitudinal sonogram shows a large midline cystic structure consistent with a distended vagina (v) and uterus (U). The lower part of the vagina contains echogenic material. The patient is a 13-year-old girl who was evaluated because of crampy abdominal pain and a pelvic mass. The external genitalia appeared normal on inspection. **B,** Midline sagittal T2-weighted MRI obtained for presurgical planning shows an enlarged vagina (v) and uterus (U) filled with material consistent with old blood. The obstruction is in the distal vagina and measures 0.5 cm in thickness *(arrows)*. At surgery, this was either a very low vaginal septum or a very thick imperforate hymen.

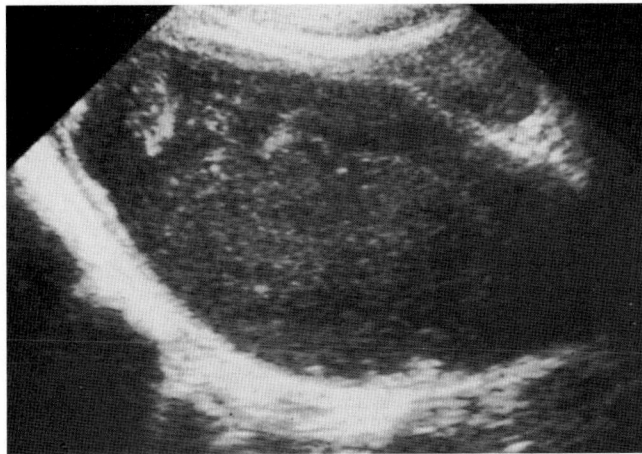

A

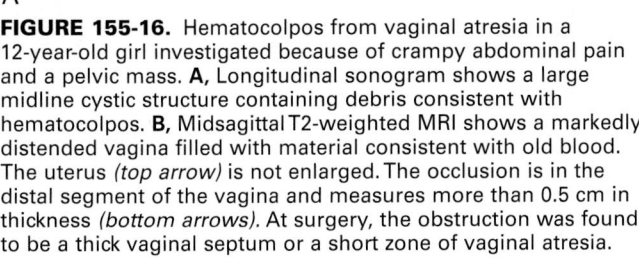

FIGURE 155-16. Hematocolpos from vaginal atresia in a 12-year-old girl investigated because of crampy abdominal pain and a pelvic mass. **A,** Longitudinal sonogram shows a large midline cystic structure containing debris consistent with hematocolpos. **B,** Midsagittal T2-weighted MRI shows a markedly distended vagina filled with material consistent with old blood. The uterus *(top arrow)* is not enlarged. The occlusion is in the distal segment of the vagina and measures more than 0.5 cm in thickness *(bottom arrows)*. At surgery, the obstruction was found to be a thick vaginal septum or a short zone of vaginal atresia.

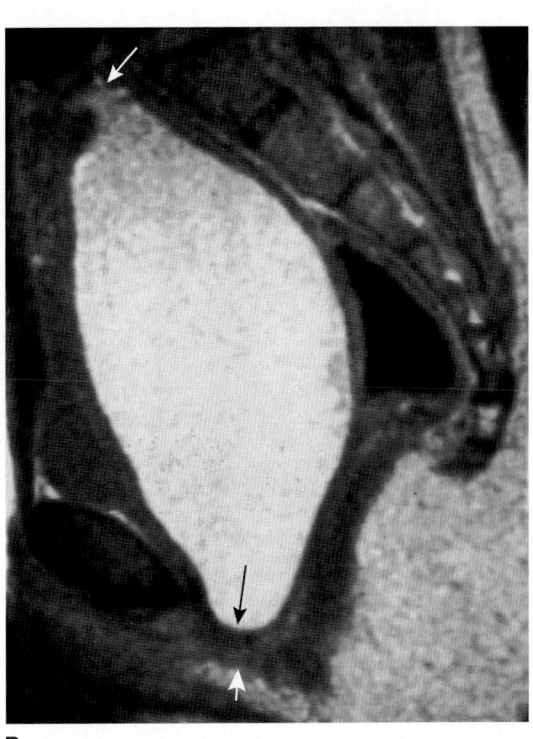

B

uterus from variable separation of the upper uterus into two horns. It is the more abnormal cases that may be more difficult to diagnose, such as uterus didelphys with unilateral vaginal obstruction and unicornuate uterus (syndrome), that may act as potential simulators of simple hydrocolpos.

> **MDS anomalies are very common, occurring in at least 0.1% to 0.5% of females.**

A didelphys uterus refers to the presence of two hemi-uteri, each connected with a separate fallopian tube and with a separate cervix, and often associated with a sagittal vaginal septum. This septum originates at the junction of the two cervices and ends caudad at or near the hymen. In some instances of duplex uterus with a vaginal septum, the caudal end of one hemivagina, more often the one on the left, is congenitally obstructed (uterus didelphys with septate vagina and unilateral vaginal obstruction) (Fig. 155-17). No hymenal tissue is found on the obstructed side. Renal agenesis, or severe renal dysplasia (and ectopic ureter), is almost always noted on the side of the vaginal obstruction. The disorder may be familial. It may present at birth with a pelvic mass caused by an accumulation of vaginal and cervical secretions within

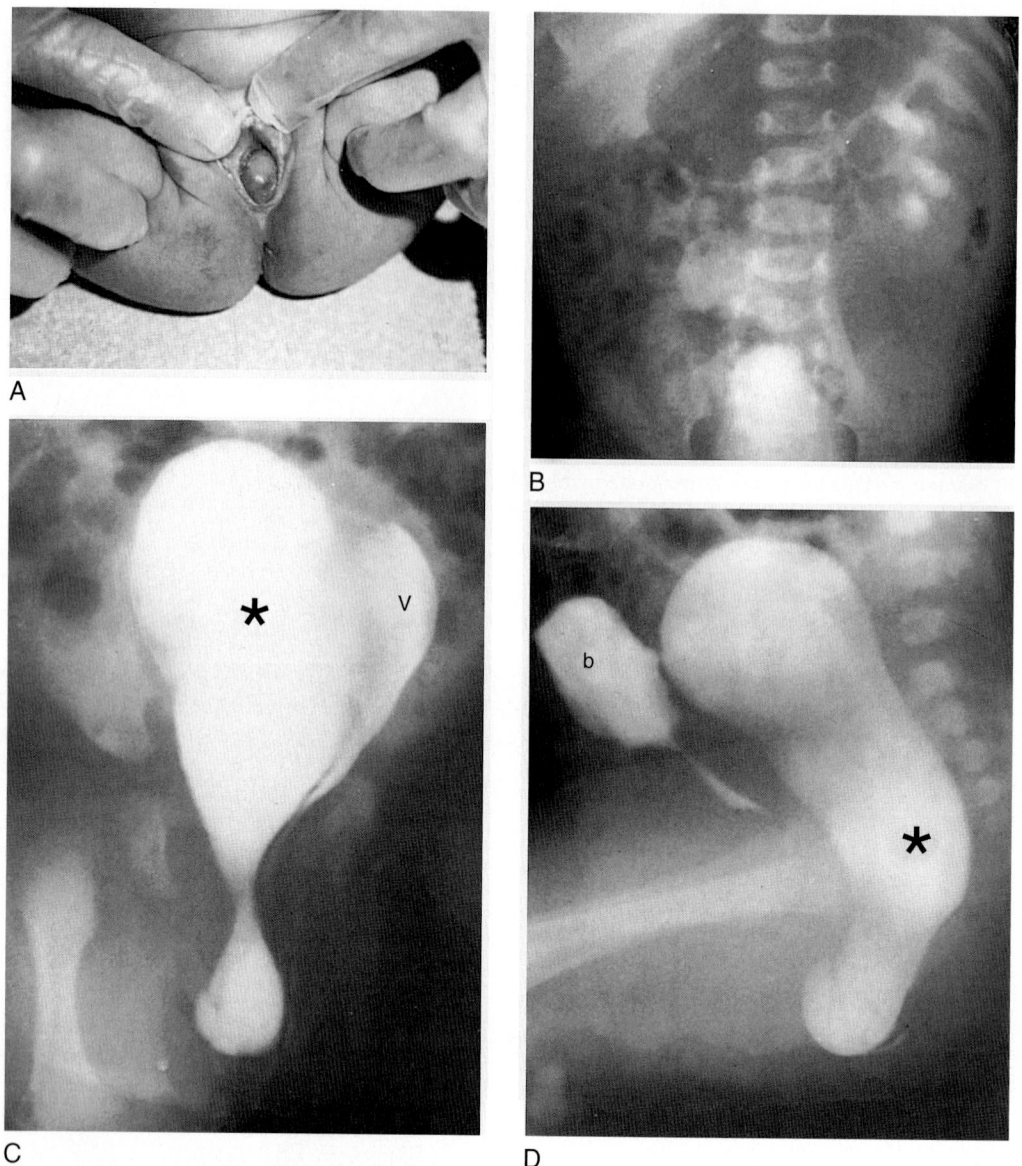

FIGURE 155-17. Occluded right hemivagina. **A,** A 2-day-old girl presented with a gray cystic mass at the vaginal introitus. **B,** IVU shows no right renal function (probably absent kidney). In a cystogram (not shown), the bladder was displaced forward by the mass. The patent left hemivagina could be catheterized and was found to be markedly displaced to the left. On frontal (**C**) and lateral (**D**) vaginograms, contrast material introduced through a needle inserted in the cystic mass at the introitus opacifies a markedly distended right hemivagina and uterus (unilateral hydrometrocolpos) *(asterisks).* Contrast material from previous studies is still present in the patent vagina (V) and bladder (b).

the obstructed hemivagina and hemiuterus. The ipsilateral fallopian tube may also be enlarged. More commonly, as with simpler hymenal membrane obstruction, the patient may present at puberty with cyclic abdominal pain and/or a pelvic mass or on physical examination with a cystic mass protruding from her introitus. A vaginogram may show lateral displacement of the normal patent hemivagina toward the contralateral side.

Unicornuate uterus, or rudimentary uterine horn syndrome, is at the extreme end of the spectrum of müllerian duct anomalies. One of the two müllerian ducts fails to develop or is resorbed, resulting in an absent or rudimentary ipsilateral tube, hemiuterus, and hemivagina. Affected patients therefore have two ovaries and only one tube, uterus, and vagina. The kidney on the side of the missing or malformed hemiuterus is almost

always absent. If a rudimentary hemiuterus contains functioning endometrium, the patient may develop an accumulation of blood within this structure at the time of puberty. If the hemiuterus does not communicate with the rest of the uterus, it may appear as a cystic mass or a debris-filled one.

A minor and relatively common form of müllerian fusion defect is the simple septate vagina, in which the vagina is divided in two lateral compartments by a midline sagittal septum, without any associated uterine anomalies.

Cloacal Malformation

Cloacal malformation is an uncommon anomaly in which the rectum, vagina, and urethra end in a common terminal channel as the only outlet for the gastrointestinal, genital, and urinary systems. The anomaly represents a persistence of the primitive fetal cloaca with failure of the urogenital and the urorectal septa to develop and separate the three structures. The presence of cloacal malformation should be suspected in a newborn girl with imperforate anus and a single perineal opening (see also Chapter 25).

> **In cloacal malformation, the rectum, vagina, and urethra end in a common terminal channel as the only outlet for the gastrointestinal, genital, and urinary systems.**

Interlabial Masses in Young Girls

Several abnormalities may present as interlabial masses in female infants and young girls. They may be related to problems originating at the level of the urethral meatus or problems originating at the level of the vaginal introitus.

INTERLABIAL MASSES ASSOCIATED WITH THE URETHRAL ORIFICE

Prolapse of an ectopic ureterocele may protrude from the urethral orifice as a small cystic mass. The prolapse may be noted only during voiding. Prolapse of urethral mucosa may be noted as a small, reddened, doughnut-like mass with its central opening being the urethral meatus itself. This abnormality is most often seen in African Americans. Cystic dilatation of an obstructed paraurethral (Skene) gland may present as an interlabial mass located on either side of the urethral meatus, which is itself displaced in the opposite direction by the mass.

INTERLABIAL MASSES ASSOCIATED WITH THE VAGINAL INTROITUS

Newborns with prolapse of a vaginal cyst may present with an interlabial mass arising from the vagina. These cysts arise from rests of the wolffian or müllerian duct systems or may represent epithelial inclusions originating from elements of the urogenital sinus. As previously discussed, patients with an imperforate hymen may present at birth with hydrocolpos but more often present at puberty or beyond because of hematocolpos with a smooth cystic mass extending from the vaginal introitus. Patients with a didelphys uterus with a septate vagina may present with a similar mass because of congenital obstruction of one of the hemivaginas (see Fig. 155-17). Cystic dilatation of an obstructed greater vestibular or Bartholin gland may result in a mass that may be found posterolaterally on either side of the vaginal introitus. The vaginal opening may be displaced to the opposite side by the mass. An important differential possibility is the prolapse of a sarcoma botryoides or rhabdomyosarcoma of the vagina. Such a tumor is often seen as a lobulated and grapelike mass protruding from the vaginal introitus.

> **Rhabdomyosarcoma of the vagina is often seen as a lobulated mass protruding from the vaginal introitus.**

DIFFERENTIAL DIAGNOSIS

The differential diagnoses of interlabial masses are usually made on visual inspection based on the location and external appearance of the mass. Diagnosis is more difficult when the mass is very large, filling the entire vulvar area. Catheterization of the urethra and a cystogram and catheterization of the vagina and a vaginogram, as well as US of the bladder and upper genitourinary tract, may be necessary to further define the lesion. CT, MRI, or excretory urography may help if continued anatomic questions remain. At times, only surgery is conclusive.

Vaginal Foreign Bodies

All kinds of foreign bodies have been found in the vagina in children. Foreign bodies in the vagina of long standing may cause local inflammation, a foul-smelling discharge, and sometimes a bloody discharge. Foreign bodies are the most common cause of nonphysiologic vaginal bleeding in the prepubertal child. The most common foreign body is toilet paper. The diagnosis of a vaginal foreign body may be markedly delayed. Some foreign bodies are opaque and are easily recognized in frontal and lateral radiographs, but a vaginogram may be indicated for confirmation of a radiopaque foreign body or discovery of a radiolucent one (Fig. 155-18). US, usually performed with downward angulation through a fluid-filled bladder, can show the normal coapted vaginal mucosa as an echogenic line without shadowing (Fig. 155-19). Foreign bodies in the vagina will create a change to that image. Attempts at distal vaginal analysis by US may be better made by a transperineal US approach. Obviously, direct inspection, when possible, may make a definitive diagnosis of a vaginal foreign body. General anesthesia may be required for direct inspection of the vagina and for removal of the foreign body.

> **Foreign bodies are the most common cause of nonphysiologic vaginal bleeding in the prepubertal child. The most common foreign body is toilet paper.**

Pelvic Inflammatory Disease

The sexually active teenager is at particularly high risk for sexually transmitted diseases. Increased sexual activity among adolescents in the past decades has resulted in a markedly increased incidence of sexually transmitted diseases, particularly among girls.

Pelvic inflammatory disease (PID) is the most serious complication of sexually transmitted diseases. The infection ascends from the vagina into the "higher" portions of the gynecologic tract, the uterus, and then the fallopian tubes and the ovaries. PID includes a spectrum of abnormality that ranges from isolated endometritis to extension of infection into the tubes (salpingitis) and ovaries (oophoritis), potentially resulting in a tubo-ovarian abscess (TOA), and even extension into the peritoneum as disseminated peritonitis. *Neisseria gonorrhoeae* and *Chlamydia trachomatis* are the most common etiologic agents. Involvement of the fallopian tubes (and ovaries)

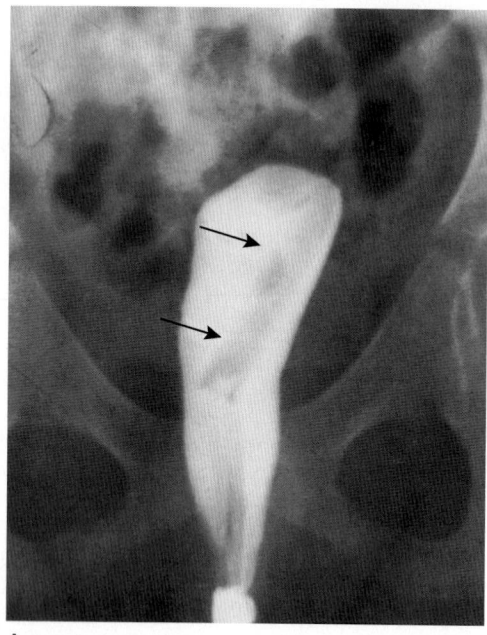
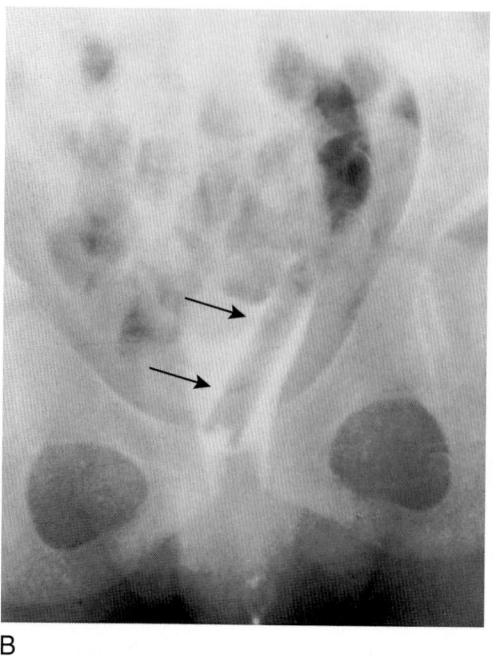

A   B

FIGURE 155-18. Vaginal foreign body. **A** and **B,** Foreign body that was not apparent on plain radiographs of the abdomen is by contrast vaginography noted in the vagina *(arrows)* of a 3-year-old girl. (From Jaramillo D, Lebowitz RL, Hendren WH: The cloacal malformation: radiologic findings and imaging recommendations. Radiology 1990;177:441–448.)

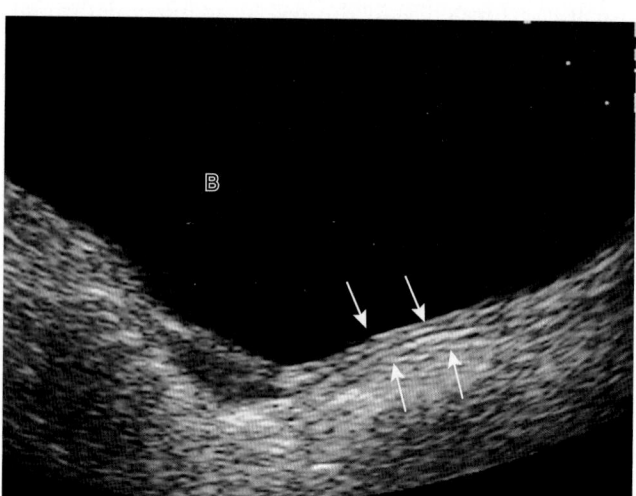

FIGURE 155-19. Normal vagina. Longitudinal sonogram shows the normal coapted vaginal walls *(arrows)* of this child as a long linear area with echogenic lines representing the outer walls and the coapted inner wall. If the vagina were obstructed, the walls would be separated and filled with material. The vagina is seen distal (inferior) to the uterus and cervix and posterior to the fluid-filled bladder (B). (From Cohen HL: Evaluation of the adolescent and young adult with amenorrhea: role of US. In Bluth E, Arger P, Hertzberg B, Middleton W [eds]: Syllabus: A Special Course in Ultrasound: Clinical Questions, Practical Answers. Oak Brook, IL, RSNA Publications, 1996:171-184.)

can lead to decreased fertility and increased chances for a future ectopic pregnancy. As far back as 1985, Weckstein reported the annual incidence of PID among 15- to 19-year-olds as 2%. The risk of PID for a sexually active 15-year-old girl was 1 in 8 as compared with the far lesser 1 in 80 for a 24-year-old woman. This risk of PID is particularly high in adolescents because of the high

incidence of multiple sexual partners and the prevalence of chlamydia and gonorrhea in this age group.

> **The increased risk of pelvic inflammatory disease among adolescents has been linked to the high incidence of multiple sexual partners and the greater prevalence of chlamydia and gonorrhea in this age group.**

Infected fallopian tubes may become edematous and bulky. Spread of purulent exudate from tubal openings to adjacent pelvic surfaces may result in dense adhesions and distortion of local structures. If the fimbriated ends of the fallopian tubes (salpinges) become adherent to the ovaries, the tubes may obstruct and distend with fluid (resulting in a hydrosalpinx) or with pus (resulting in a pyosalpinx) (Fig. 155-20). The infection may extend to the ovaries, resulting in a TOA (Fig. 155-21) with further adhesions or distortions of pelvic structures and an increase in the pelvic mass. Rupture of a TOA is an uncommon but serious complication of the disease. After adequate antibiotic therapy, acute PID may resolve, but residual chronic changes are not uncommon, including adhesions and hydrosalpinx. It also may be difficult to know whether the finding of prominent size and/or adherence of ovaries to the uterus is of acute or chronic cause without correlation with clinical and historical information. Previous bouts of PID predispose to recurrent episodes of the same process. The long-term sequelae of PID are infertility, ectopic pregnancy, and chronic pelvic pain.

A high index of suspicion is important for the diagnosis of acute PID, because symptoms and findings are often variable and nonspecific. Patients may present

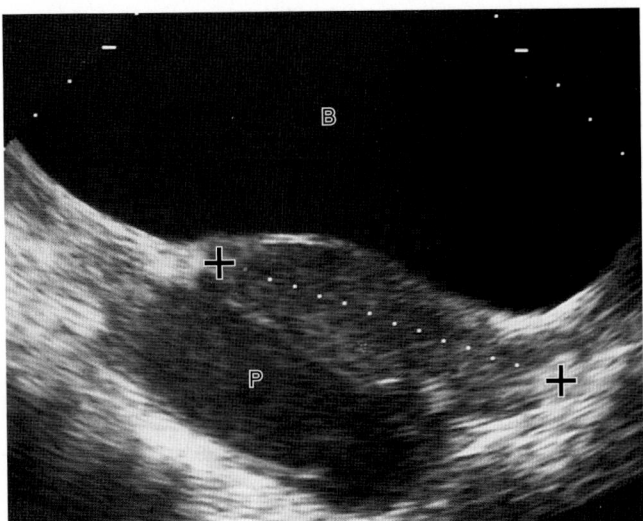

FIGURE 155-20. Pyosalpinx. Midline longitudinal sonogram shows a fluid-filled tubular structure (P), allowing good through-transmission of sound, located posterior to the uterus *(cursors).* It contains debris and was determined to be a pyosalpinx. B, bladder.

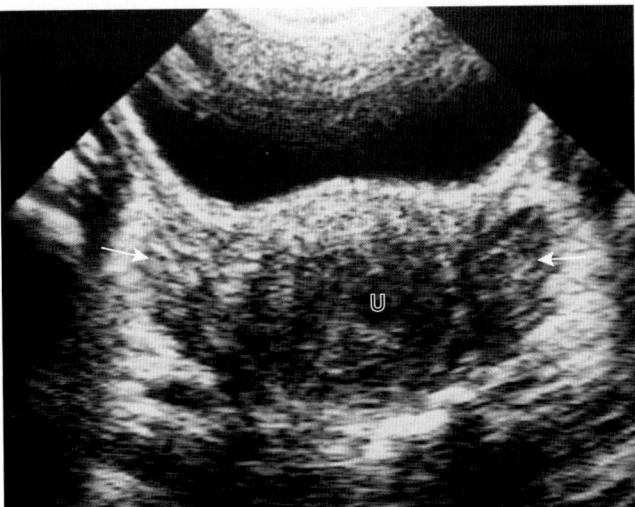

FIGURE 155-22. Salpingo-oophoritis. Transverse sonogram shows prominent adnexa *(arrows)* hugging the uterus (U), suggesting they are adherent to the uterus. A triangular echogenic area within the uterus was consistent with a prominent endometrial echo, which may be related to menstrual cycle stage or pelvic inflammatory disease. We have likened this image to a koala bear's head and have called it the "koala bear" sign.

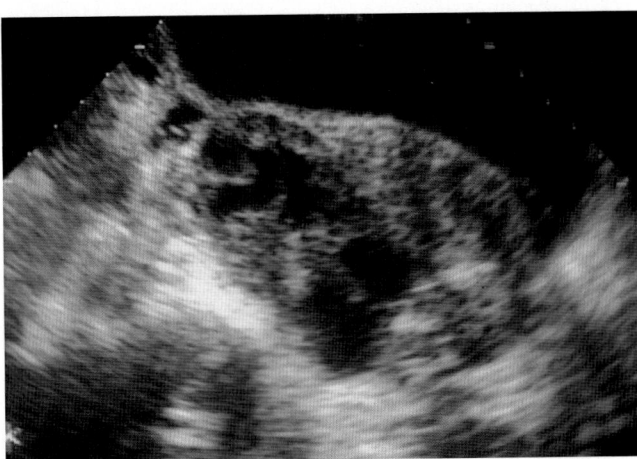

FIGURE 155-21. Tubo-ovarian abscess. Oblique transverse sonogram of the right adnexa shows a large, heterogeneous oval structure with contained echoless circular and tubular structures that were not typical of normal follicles or cysts on transverse or longitudinal images. This abscess was in a teenager with a history of pelvic inflammatory disease. At times a dilated fallopian tube arising from a tubo-ovarian abscess accounts for part of the contained cystic structure. This is most likely when the structure appears tubular in at least one of the imaged planes.

with lower abdominal/pelvic pain. Most patients have cervical motion tenderness, fever, and leukocytosis and an elevated erythrocyte sedimentation rate. Many will have a purulent vaginal discharge, cultures of which may yield *N. gonorrhoeae* and *C. trachomatis.* Occasionally, patients may complain of right upper quadrant pain and tenderness thought to be due to perihepatitis (Fitz-Hugh–Curtis syndrome). This uncommon abnormality is rarely diagnosed by imaging, although seeing septations within fluid surrounding liver parenchyma may suggest it. A pelvic mass may be detected on physical examina-

tion. Adnexal tenderness, generally bilateral, and cervical motion tenderness, hallmarks for the clinical diagnosis, may be elicited on bimanual examination.

ULTRASOUND FINDINGS IN PELVIC INFLAMMATORY DISEASE

Pelvic US is an important tool in the analysis of teenagers with clinical complaints that may suggest PID or one of its simulators. The sonographic findings vary with the extent of the disease. In early PID, or salpingitis, there may be no abnormal US findings and the diagnosis will be based solely on clinical and laboratory evaluation. A helpful US finding in somewhat more advanced cases (i.e., salpingo-oophoritis) is prominent ovaries that may be adherent to the uterus. Ovarian findings are most often bilateral and symmetric. We have labeled this image the "koala bear" sign (Fig. 155-22) because the ovaries resemble the ears of a koala, with the koala's face represented by the uterus. A prominent endometrial cavity echo that may be physiologic, particularly in the second half of the menstrual cycle, or prominent on the basis of infection, represents the koala bear's nose. Adherence of the ovaries does not indicate acuity of the infection (unless old US studies are available and are normal) because it can be seen as a consequence of prior pelvic infection. An ovary of greater than 20 cm^3 volume in a postmenarchal female is enlarged (despite the fact that some normal patients may fit into that group). A volume of 15 to 20 cm^3 is a gray zone for adnexal enlargement. Patients with greater than 15-cm^3 ovaries may be monitored, at the very least, with a 6-week follow-up examination (at a different phase of the next menstrual cycle). One must be careful to remember that the presence of physiologic cysts may falsely elevate an ovarian volume. Patients with salpingo-oophoritis usually do well on antibiotic therapy.

> **The imaging of prominent ovaries adherent to the uterus is indicative of salpingo-oophoritis.**

More advanced cases of acute or, more often, chronic PID may demonstrate evidence of hydrosalpinx or pyosalpinx or TOA. Although it would be convenient if echoless dilated tubes were always hydrosalpinges and echo-filled fluid within dilated tubes were indicative of infection (i.e., pyosalpinx); this is *not* always true. The echogenicity of the fluid is not a reliable indicator of the presence or absence of infection. The affected tubal walls may be thickened and linear echoes may extend from them into the tubal lumen.

An important imaging finding to be made is that of TOA (see Fig. 155-21), which is said to be seen in 14% to 38% of patients hospitalized for PID. TOA appears on US as partial or complete replacement of the normal ovarian tissue by a heterogeneous mass or an echopenic area with contained debris. When they represent only part of the imaged ovary, they may be hard to differentiate from physiologic cysts with hemorrhage. Complete replacement of ovarian tissue allows a readier diagnosis. Cystic components of a TOA, the usual cause of its heterogeneous image, may be due to portions of a dilated fallopian tube. An orthogonal projection may help prove the presence of a true tubular structure extending beyond the confines of the ovary. The contents (debris filled) of the echopenic areas of a TOA can often be better seen by TV examination. It is important to diagnose a TOA, because they are usually treated aggressively with intravenous antibiotic regimens and, if necessary, percutaneous drainage or surgery.

A hemorrhagic cyst or an endometrioma can also appear as a complex debris-filled cyst and can therefore simulate the US image of the TOA. The images of these entities may all look alike. It is the patient's history and clinical and laboratory findings that may be necessary to differentiate between these three possibilities.

> **History, clinical, and laboratory findings may be necessary to differentiate among TOA, hemorrhagic cyst, and endometrioma, which may look alike on US.**

The US finding of echoless fluid in the cul-de-sac can be seen in patients with PID but also in normal patients, usually because of physiologic rupture of a cyst. It is a nonspecific finding. Echogenic fluid in the cul-de-sac is of greater concern because of the possibility that the fluid is proteinaceous, infected, or hemorrhagic. Hemorrhagic cul-de-sac fluid is of particular concern when considering ectopic pregnancy. Other causes for complex fluid in the cul-de-sac, such as perforated appendicitis, should be considered. Be aware that patients with ventriculoperitoneal shunts and patients undergoing peritoneal dialysis will often have cul-de-sac fluid and more significant amounts of free intraperitoneal fluid.

Normal Pregnancy/Ectopic Pregnancy

Pregnancy is a relatively common cause of pelvic mass and/or pelvic pain in postpubertal girls. It is the most common physiologic cause of secondary amenorrhea in girls older than 9 years of age. It therefore must be considered in any girl after menarche, particularly (but not exclusively) if she discloses a sexual history. Most pregnancies in adolescents are not intended and occur within 1 to 2 years of becoming sexually active. Such adolescents often deny the possibility of pregnancy and ascribe symptoms of pregnancy to other physical causes. The examining physician should be aware of the possibility of a normal or abnormal pregnancy even with a noncontributory history. Pregnancy can be confirmed or ruled out by the appropriate laboratory tests. US can prove the presence of an intrauterine pregnancy by imaging a gestational sac within the uterus (Fig. 155-23), and a viable pregnancy by denoting a gestational sac with a contained embryo with normal cardiac motion.

> **Pregnancy is the most common physiologic cause of secondary amenorrhea in girls older than 9 years of age. It therefore must be considered in any girl after menarche.**

Ectopic pregnancy is a pregnancy in a location other than the uterus. It is the cause of 6% to 11% of all maternal deaths and is the leading cause of first-trimester maternal mortality. The incidence of ectopic pregnancy in teenage girls has increased in recent years coincident with an increase of sexually transmitted diseases in this group. The incidence is particularly increased in individuals with a prior history of PID. Antibiotic therapy for PID has been thought responsible for maintaining fertility in those patients who would otherwise have developed obstructed fallopian tubes preventing pregnancy, but instead have patent tubes, with abnormal cilia that can limit the speed and transit of a fertilized egg to an implantation site in the uterus. Most (95% to 97%) ectopic pregnancies occur at the ampullary end of the fallopian tube or the more proximal isthmus. When the pregnancy grows beyond the ability of the fallopian tube to contain it (8 to 12 weeks' gestational age), the tube may rupture and an abdominal crisis may occur, with patients presenting with severe hypotension or shock, possibly leading to death. Two percent to 5% of cases are cornual ectopic pregnancies, occurring at the cornua of the uterus, with the embryo able to grow larger and for a longer time owing to the greater expandability of the cornua because of its contained myometrium. Rare sites of ectopic pregnancy include the ovary (0.5% to 1%) and the cervix (0.1%).

> **Most ectopic pregnancies occur at the ampullary end of the fallopian tube or the more proximal isthmus.**

The diagnosis of ectopic pregnancy is easy when a viable extrauterine gestational sac (Fig. 155-24) is seen

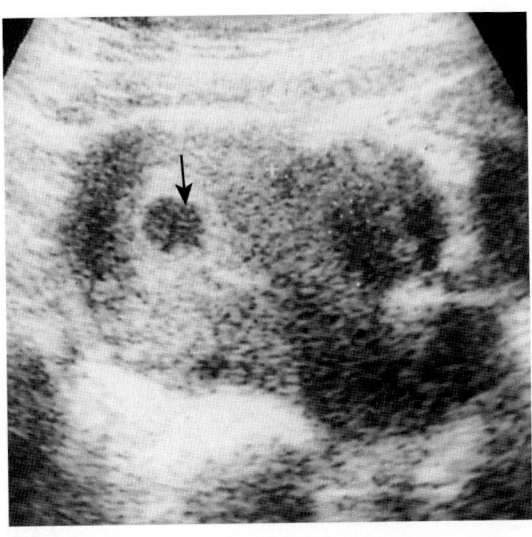
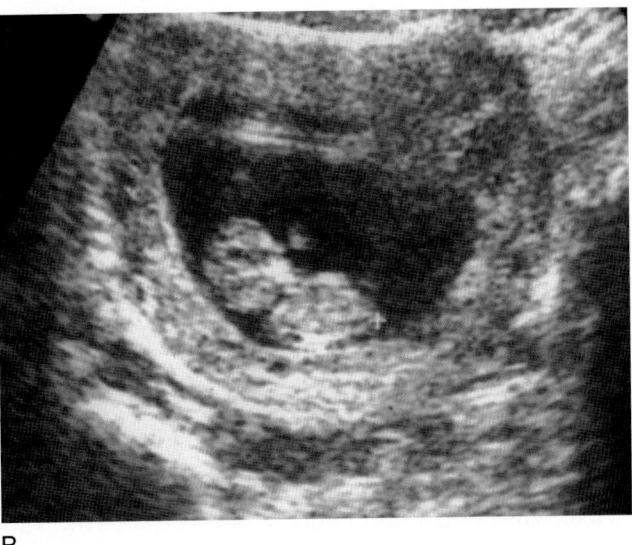

A   B

FIGURE 155-23. Normal intrauterine pregnancy. **A,** Early pregnancy. A small, circular echoless area *(arrow)* consistent with a gestational sac is seen within the uterus of this teenager with a several-week history of secondary amenorrhea. Immediate surrounding echogenicity is consistent with trophoblastic tissue. The gestational sac is completely surrounded by the uterus, denoting an intrauterine pregnancy and excluding it as being an ectopic pregnancy. **B,** Older first-trimester pregnancy. A fetal pole *(cursors)* is seen in the gestational sac, which is completely surrounded by uterine muscle. Fetal heart motion was noted. This proved it to be a viable intrauterine pregnancy. This fetus was 10 weeks by measurement of crown–rump length. Modern equipment aided by endovaginal transducers will usually denote fetal heart motion and a yolk sac by 4 to 5 weeks' gestational age.

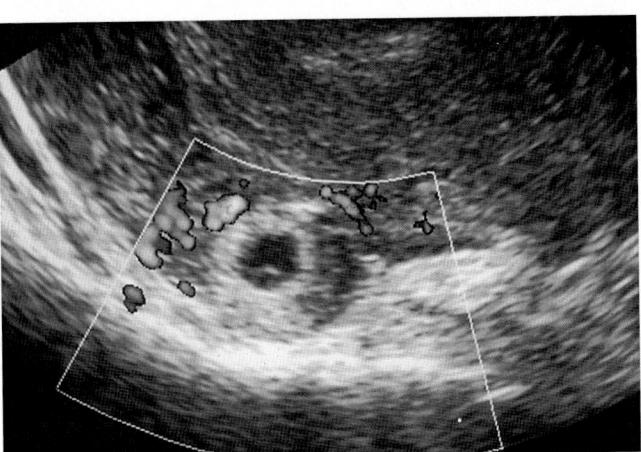

FIGURE 155-24. Ectopic pregnancy. Longitudinal oblique sonogram shows a color Doppler imaging box around a fluid-filled circular structure with an echogenic periphery made up of trophoblastic tissue. It contains a small circular echogenic structure that proved to be a yolk sac of an early pregnancy. The fact that the circular structure is not surrounded by uterine tissue suggests that it is an ectopic gestational sac. The uterus of this teenager is superficial to the gestational sac. Of note is the fact that color Doppler flow about the ectopic gestational sac is only limited in amount. It was once hoped that reports of significant color flow around ectopic pregnancies would help make the diagnosis easier. In reality, flow is variable and equivalent flow can be seen around physiologic corpora lutea cysts.

with its contained embryo and heartbeat. Any time there is an ectopic pregnancy, no matter what its US image, a pseudogestational sac (i.e., some associated fluid within the endometrial cavity) may falsely simulate an intra-uterine gestational sac. A normal pregnancy is never within the endometrial cavity but, rather, implanted within one of the walls deep to the endometrial cavity. A common finding of concern for ectopic pregnancy is a complex or solid adnexal mass that is separate from the ipsilateral ovary. Ectopic pregnancies often have associated cul-de-sac fluid collections. One must consider an ectopic pregnancy if there is a positive pregnancy test and no intrauterine pregnancy, even if an extrauterine pregnancy or mass cannot be directly observed.

> Finding a complex or solid adnexal mass that is separate from the ipsilateral ovary is suggestive of ectopic pregnancy.

Ovarian Torsion

Ovarian torsion is an uncommon but important cause of abdominal pain in the first 3 decades of life. It is caused by partial or complete rotation of the ovary on its pedicle, compromising first lymphatic, then venous, and finally arterial flow, leading to hemorrhagic infarction. Torsion of the ovary is most often seen among children in peripubertal or older girls. It may occur in patients of all ages, including newborns, and has been shown to occur also in utero. It is said that if an ovary and its ipsilateral fallopian tube are not found at surgery, the cause is not agenesis of the ovary but antenatal torsion of the ovary and fallopian tube (tubo-ovarian torsion). Ovarian torsion usually occurs in anatomically normal ovaries (perhaps having had a recent size or weight increase with, for example, puberty or a large physiologic cyst). Many cases, however, occur in ovaries with an associated ovarian or paraovarian mass or neoplasm. Bilateral, asynchronous ovarian torsion has been reported. Historically, the diagnosis of ovarian torsion has been made at surgery. More recently, US has proved a helpful tool for the diagnosis. A prompt diagnosis is important because surgical detorsion can help avoid irreversible damage to the ovary.

Clinically, affected pediatric patients may have symptoms that simulate gastroenteritis, appendicitis, intussusception, or any other acute abdominal condition affecting the child or adolescent. The classic ovarian torsion pain is sudden and acute. A subacute course of several days, however, can occur. Patients may report being awakened from sleep by their pain. Associated complaints of nausea, vomiting, or constipation may occur and mislead the clinician. Fever is rare. This fact can help differentiate right-sided torsion from classic cases of appendicitis. In contrast to appendicitis, the pain is sharp and localized immediately. At least half of patients with ovarian torsion claim prior bouts of such pain. This suggests previous bouts of torsion and detorsion. Leukocytosis with a shift to the left may be present.

> The classic pain of ovarian torsion is sudden and acute. A subacute course of several days, however, can occur.

Diagnostic US is the most important first imaging tool for the analysis of ovarian torsion. Ovaries involved in torsion have a variable appearance related to the degree of internal hemorrhage, stromal edema, and infarction that has occurred by the time they are imaged. The ovaries may appear cystic, cystic with septations, cystic with a debris layer, or complex with mixed solid and cystic components, as well as solid. Each of these images may suggest its own list of differential diagnostic considerations. One relatively specific US image was reported by Graif and Itzchak, who noted in 7 of 11 cases of ovarian torsion a unilaterally enlarged solid ovary with multiple peripheral (i.e., cortical zone) follicles (Fig. 155-25). Similar images of a large ovary with peripheral follicles can be seen with CT or MRI. The acute torsed ovary is larger than a normal ovary. Ovarian volumes of 150 cm^3 or greater are often measured in the postmenarchal patient. None of our cases among teen or adult patients has been less than 57 cm^3 in volume. Graif and Itzchak noted volumes of the torsed ovaries in their study to be at least 34 times larger among prepubertal and 15 times larger among postpubertal unaffected ovaries. Others have reported volumes of only 3.2 to 24 times normal. Comparison with the volume and morphology of the contralateral ovary may help make the diagnosis under the appropriate clinical circumstances. One must know what is normal for a given age group to determine what constitutes ovarian enlargement. Cul-de-sac fluid may be noted in patients with a torsed ovary but is also commonly seen in normal postpubertal females.

> Torsed ovaries have a variable appearance related to the degree of internal hemorrhage, stromal edema, and infarction that has occurred by the time they are imaged. The acute torsed ovary is larger than a normal ovary.

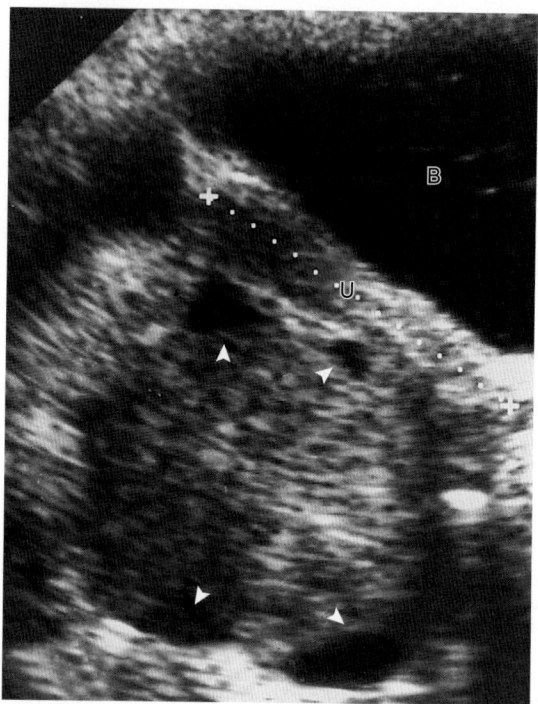

FIGURE 155-25. Ovarian torsion. Longitudinal sonogram shows a tubular uterus (cursors) that is posterior to the bladder (B) and anterior to a large solid mass with a few peripheral cysts (arrowheads). This is a relatively classic image of early torsion. Infarction or acute hemorrhage would make the internal contents of the torsed ovary more heterogeneous. (From Cohen HL, Safriel YI: Ovarian torsion. In Cohen HL, Sivit C [eds]: Fetal and Pediatric Ultrasound: A Casebook Approach. New York, McGraw-Hill, 2001:516.)

Reviews of color Doppler imaging used in the analysis of cases of ovarian torsion are confusing with regard to its reliability. This is in part because the Doppler signal may be difficult to obtain even in normal ovaries, particularly using the transvesicle technique. In addition, there are well-documented cases of surgically proven torsed ovaries that color Doppler imaging evaluation showed having peripheral and even central arterial flow. Other groups have reported success with color Doppler imaging, particularly for determining viable versus infarcted torsed ovaries. Fleischer and Brader noted that an assurance of viability can only be made by imaging central venous flow in a torsed ovary. Lee and colleagues reported an 87% diagnostic accuracy for determining viability by verifying blood flow changes at the twisted vascular pedicle itself. Their patients with no blood flow at the twisted pedicle had necrotic ovaries.

It is hoped that detorsion and, if necessary, removal of a mass causing torsion will save the gonad and preserve its function. The time from clinical complaint to diagnosis and therapy plays a large role in preserving ovarian function. US (with or without Doppler) is certainly a time-efficient way of making this analysis. Doppler imaging may have a role in assessing the recovery of a torsed ovary in follow-up studies after surgical treatment.

Several case reports of adults, children, and even infants have discussed finding a detached and often freely movable and usually calcified ovary in the pelvis at some distance from the normal ovarian site. The lesion is believed to be the result of a prior episode of prenatal or postnatal torsion. Such a detached ovary may parasitize the blood supply from a bowel loop, liver, or other abdominal structure, resulting in a partially calcified cystic mass with a long vascular pedicle that may be located anywhere in the abdomen.

Ovarian Masses

OVARIAN CYSTS IN CHILDREN AND ADOLESCENTS

The normal pediatric ovary and its adnexa are not felt on physical examination. Non-neoplastic cysts of follicular origin (i.e., functional ovarian cysts) are the most common cause of enlargement. Follicles are seen routinely throughout childhood and are part of normal ovaries. It is a noninvoluted follicle that may become an enlarged cyst.

The increased use of US and the improvements in its technology have made possible the detection of small follicles in normal ovaries occurring as normal functional variants. This has also resulted in a more frequent diagnosis of ovarian cysts in children and in a better understanding of their natural history. The majority of ovaries in girls from birth to 12 years of age are able to be visualized by US. Follicles are routinely visualized in prepubertal ovaries and should not necessarily be considered abnormal.

Beyond puberty the adolescent ovary is similar to that of the adult, developing several follicles early in the menstrual cycle until a dominant follicle develops, rupturing at midcycle while the others atrophy and resorb. Occasionally one or more of these follicles fails to resorb and instead enlarges as a functional cyst or as a retention cyst. These cysts can reach a large size but are usually no greater than 3 cm. The majority of functional ovarian cysts are treated conservatively (i.e., watched clinically and sonographically) and resolve spontaneously. Rarely, there is a complication, the most common being ovarian torsion, which occurs often in ovaries with large cysts or masses. Functional cysts may rupture and result in free cul-de-sac fluid that is usually echoless but may be echogenic. Occasionally a ruptured cyst may result in more significant amounts of peritoneal fluid. A 6-week follow-up allows analysis of the possible ovarian cyst in the other half of a different menstrual cycle so as to document resolution or diminution and thereby help prove it to be a physiologic cyst and to disprove the far less likely diagnosis of a cystic neoplasm. The classic cyst on US examination is echoless with a sharp back wall and excellent through-transmission.

Occasionally, a cystic mass is seen near the bladder of a female fetus. This is usually due to an enlarged ovarian cyst, perhaps developing because of increased sensitivity to maternal hormone stimulation. Less likely possibilities include a duplicated portion of bowel or a diverticulum of the bladder. These possibilities may be considered and analyzed for during follow-up pelvic US evaluation of the newborn.

HEMORRHAGIC OVARIAN CYSTS

Hemorrhagic ovarian cysts represent a complication that occurs to physiologic/functional ovarian cysts. Functional ovarian cysts result from failure of a normal maturing follicle to involute. The follicle/cyst continues to enlarge, usually because of a temporary or persistent hormonal imbalance. Functional cysts may develop internal hemorrhage. This occurs when theca interna vessels rupture into the cyst cavity. Such hemorrhagic ovarian cysts can arise from ovarian follicles at any stage in their maturation, even as they involute. They may develop in the corpus luteum, which develops from the dominant or graafian follicle, after ovulation.

The typical clinical presentation of a hemorrhagic ovarian cyst is either that of sudden, severe, transient lower abdominal pain of 1 to 3 hours' duration or that of lower abdominal pain and a palpable mass. The pain is thought to result from sudden distention of the ovarian cyst by the hemorrhage. The finding can be incidental. Among 70 adolescent and adult patients with these cysts studied by Baltarowich and colleagues, only 4% were asymptomatic. Slightly more than one fourth (26%) of the patients in that series had prior, concurrent, or subsequent simple or hemorrhagic cysts. Because some individuals have a greater tendency to produce functional cysts, some may also have a greater tendency to develop hemorrhagic ovarian cysts when in a particular hormonal milieu. In the majority of cases, the clot hemolyzes and is gradually resorbed.

Hemorrhagic ovarian cysts are a common reason for a teenager to present with lower abdominal or pelvic pain that may mimic appendicitis. Once the patient is diagnosed with this type of cyst, resolution of pain and confirmation of a stable hematocrit allow conservative management with follow-up of the cyst by US to resolution. Such resolution includes the disappearance of the cyst altogether or a change in the cyst's echogenic hemorrhagic contents as a result of clot lysis.

ULTRASONOGRAPHIC FINDINGS. The US diagnosis of any complicated cyst becomes more difficult when the classic US characteristics (echoless, sharp posterior wall, and strong posterior acoustic enhancement) are lost. The majority of hemorrhagic ovarian cysts are heterogeneous in echogenicity. In one study of 15 hemorrhagic ovarian cysts, Baltarowich and coworkers reported 93% to have hypoechoic or hyperechoic areas separated by thin or thick linear echoes or to be hypoechoic with contained thin (Fig. 155-26) or thick linear echoes in various orientations. However, hemorrhagic ovarian cysts may also be essentially echoless or echoless with a contained round echogenicity of variable size indicating clot. They may contain fluid–debris levels. When clot fills the hemorrhagic ovarian cyst cavity or there is decreased posterior enhancement (through-transmission), it can be confused with a solid mass, including neoplasm.

Hemorrhagic ovarian cysts tend to be clearly separable from the uterus. Their size ranges widely, with Baltarowich and coworkers noting a size range of 2.5 to 14 cm in longest length. Most of these cysts are between 2 and 3 cm. A changing US appearance over time can help confirm the diagnosis. Image change is expected because hemorrhage changes its US appearance with time. The initial bright echogenicity of acute hemorrhage, caused by fibrin deposition, becomes less echogenic and

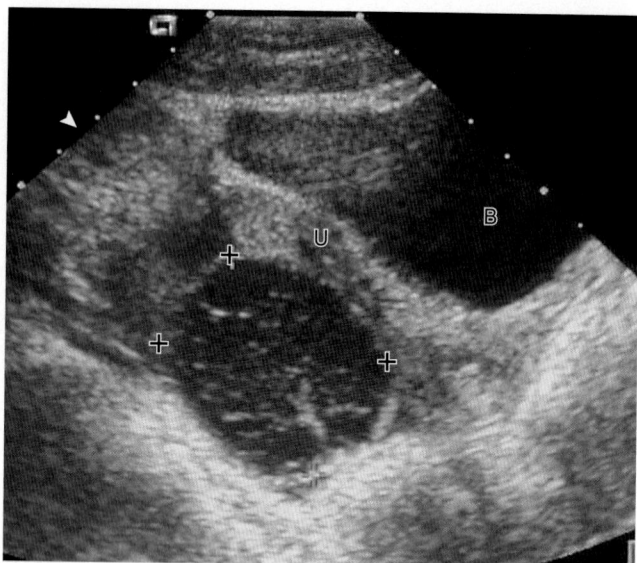

FIGURE 155-26. Hemorrhagic ovarian cyst. Longitudinal sonogram shows an echopenic mass *(cursors)* containing criss-crossing linear echogenicities in the adnexal area of a 12-year-old with acute abdominal pain. Tubo-ovarian abscess and endometrioma may look similar but present with different clinical scenarios. B, bladder; U, uterus.

eventually fluidlike as the fibrin dissolves and the clot lyses. Technically, a TV examination using a higher frequency transducer (e.g., 6.5 MHz) can help improve evaluation of the contents of any complex cystic mass lying in the low pelvis and close to the transducer.

> A changing US appearance over time can help confirm the diagnosis of hemorrhagic ovarian cyst.

DIFFERENTIAL DIAGNOSIS. Hemorrhagic cysts may look very similar to TOAs or endometriomas. The associated clinical stories vary significantly. Patients with TOAs have a history or a clinical picture of PID. Patients with endometriomas have a history of very painful periods and perhaps already diagnosed endometriosis. Beyond these two imaging simulators, the differential diagnosis of the hemorrhagic ovarian cyst would include other complex ovarian masses. One may consider a benign cystic teratoma (if it does not have a significant solid component), an ectopic pregnancy (but it would have to be chronic or complicated so as not to look like a gestational sac with a contained fetal pole), a torsed ovary (torsed ovaries are usually very large), or an appendiceal abscess (but an ipsilateral adnexa could be imaged in such a case).

OVARIAN CYSTS AND HYPOTHYROIDISM

Bilateral ovarian cysts have been observed in older girls with long-standing, untreated hypothyroidism, possibly on the basis of a secondary hypothalamic-pituitary hyperfunction. Precocious puberty and galactorrhea may be present. Rapid regression of the cysts has been demonstrated after the initiation of thyroid hormone replacement. Ovarian cysts have also been recognized prenatally in infants who postnatally were shown to have hypothyroidism.

OVARIAN CYSTS AND CYSTIC FIBROSIS

Bilateral multifollicular cysts were noted by Galli-Tsinopoulou and colleagues among female adolescents with cystic fibrosis (CF). Luteinizing hormone (LH) and LH/follicle stimulating hormone (FSH) levels were significantly higher among 18 CF patients compared with controls. Levels of sex hormone-binding globulin were significantly lower. Hormone changes were said to be similar to those of polycystic ovary syndrome but with absent acne or hirsutism, perhaps on the basis of decreased body fat or other causes.

POLYCYSTIC OVARY SYNDROME

Polycystic ovary syndrome (PCOS; also known as Stein-Leventhal syndrome) is a hyperandrogenic state with resultant peripheral conversion of larger than normal amounts of estrogen. The chronic hyperestrogenic hyperandrogenic stimulation leads to chronic anovulation and is responsible for the classic bilaterally enlarged ovaries, which may be asymmetric but usually contain multiple small follicles/cysts. PCOS is the most common pathologic cause of amenorrhea, usually secondary, in the adolescent and young adult. Patients often, but far from always, suffer from the classic triad of obesity (31%), hirsutism (62%), and menstrual abnormalities (80%), including amenorrhea, irregular menses, and prolonged uterine bleeding. Laboratory diagnosis is made by noting increased LH:FSH ratios and elevated androstenedione levels. The syndrome is usually first noted at or shortly beyond puberty.

> Polycystic ovary syndrome is a hyperandrogenic state with resultant peripheral conversion of larger than normal amounts of estrogen. It is the most common pathologic cause of amenorrhea, usually secondary, in the adolescent and young adult.

IMAGING FINDINGS. There are some confusing data in the literature on the diagnosis of PCOS by imaging. Part of the problem is that there is an overlap between normal US findings and the US findings reported in patients with PCOS. This is true whether patients are examined with TA or TV US. One must be aware of the fact that TV US will show increased numbers of ovarian follicles/cysts in both normal and PCOS patients compared with TA examinations. PCOS patients have high numbers of subcapsular follicles in their ovaries. These follicles are hyperstimulated but do not reach maturity. A dominant follicle does not develop. Typically, there are at least five cysts of 5 to 8 mm in diameter noted on TA evaluation of each ovary (Fig. 155-27). Follicles of classic cases should not be greater than 10 mm in diameter. Larger follicles or the presence of a single large (dominant) cyst goes against the diagnosis of PCOS. PCOS ovaries are larger and more echogenic than normal. Takahashi and coworkers noted mean ovarian volumes of 10.3 cm³ in 47 affected patients, a volume significantly greater than the mean for their control group. Among their PCOS patients, 94% had either an ovarian volume greater than 6.2 cm³ or more than 10 follicles of 2 to 8 mm in diameter. Six percent of their patients had normal

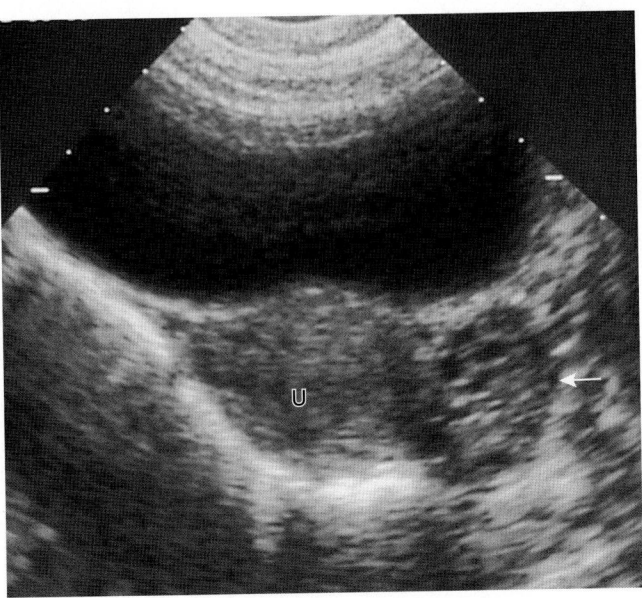

A

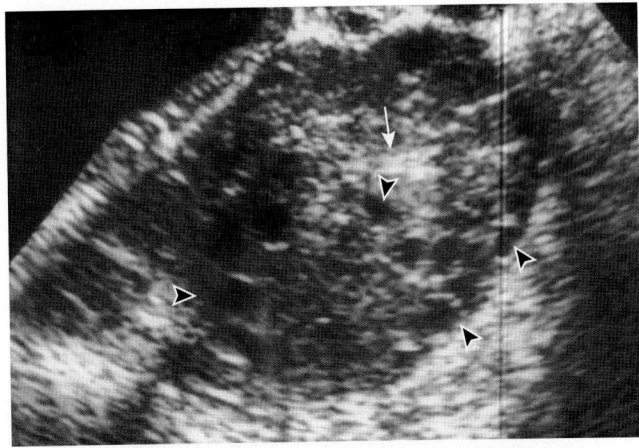

B

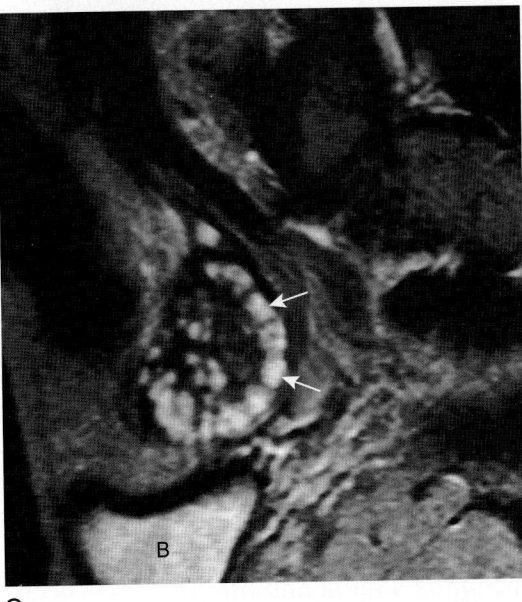

C

FIGURE 155-27. Polycystic ovarian disease. **A,** Transverse sonogram shows an enlarged left ovary *(arrow)* containing multiple small follicles is seen adjacent to the uterus (U). A similar right ovary was seen in another plane. The echogenicity of the ovarian stroma is increased. **B,** Transvaginal sagittal sonogram shows many small follicles *(arrowheads)* seen within the ovary of a teen with polycystic ovary syndrome. Some bright echogenicity *(arrow),* not seen in normal ovaries, is noted in the superior third of this imaged ovary. **C,** Sagittal T2-weighted MR image shows multiple cortical cysts particularly at the periphery of the right ovary of a teenager proved to have polycystic ovary syndrome. The ovary is superior to the bladder (B), and its follicles/cysts *(arrows)* have similar high signal intensity. (**A** and **B** from Cohen HL, Ruggiero-Delliturri M: Polycystic ovary syndrome. *In* Cohen HL, Sivit C [eds]: Fetal and Pediatric Ultrasound: A Casebook Approach. New York, McGraw-Hill, 2001:496; **C** courtesy of Mark Flyer, MD.)

ovarian volumes and normal numbers of follicles. As we know, however, many normal adolescent have ovarian volumes greater than 6.2 cm^3. As previously noted, our US laboratory uses 15 cm^3 to less than 20 cm^3 as a gray zone for ovarian enlargement and a figure of 20 cm^3 or greater as evidence of definitive enlargement of the ovary in adults and older adolescents.

A helpful indicator of PCOS is increased ovarian echogenicity (Fig. 155-27). This is thought to be due to ovarian stromal hypertrophy, which is considered to be evidence of hyperandrogenism. Battaglia and colleagues found some PCOS ovaries to have lower ovarian arterial resistance. High androstenedione levels are linked to high uterine artery resistance. Pinkas and coworkers did not see differences in the resistances between PCOS patients and controls.

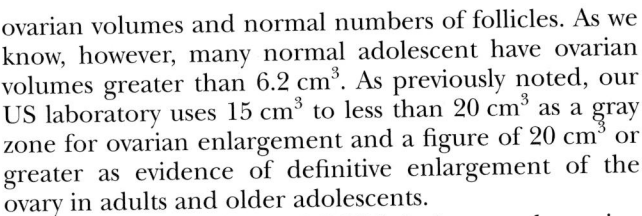

PCOS ovaries show increased ovarian echogenicity and typically at least five cysts of 5 to 8 mm on TA US.

OTHER CLINICAL CONSIDERATIONS IN CASES OF POSSIBLE POLYCYSTIC OVARY SYNDROME. The symptoms of obesity, menstrual irregularity, and hirsutism, individually or in combination, can be observed in normal patients as well as in those with other abnormalities. There are patients with familial hirsutism. Many young teenagers take a while for their cycles to become regular. Many individuals are obese. If signs of virilization are found, a workup to rule out a virilizing adrenal or ovarian tumor is required. Certainly, if a unilateral ovarian mass is imaged an endocrinologically active ovarian tumor must be considered. Androgen excess may also occur in cases of idiopathic hirsutism, late-onset forms of congenital adrenal hyperplasia, exaggerated adrenarche, Cushing disease, hyperprolactinemia, and acromegaly. Most hyperandrogenic adolescents are found to have PCOS.

OTHER CAUSES OF POLYCYSTIC OVARIES. Not all polycystic ovaries are due to hyperandrogenism. Unopposed estrogen stimulation from any source can result in polycystic ovaries. Genetic deficiencies of the enzymes 21-hydroxylase, 3α-hydroxysteroid dehydrogenase, or

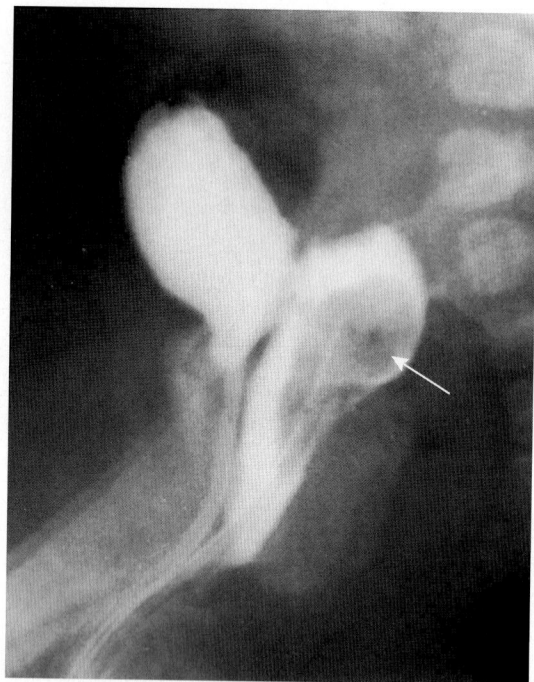

FIGURE 155-28. Endodermal sinus tumor of the vagina. Lateral vaginogram shows a mass *(arrow)* within the contrast-filled vagina of a 6-month-old girl, originating from the vagina's posterior wall. The contrast-filled bladder seen anterior to the vagina was filled by a separate injection.

11α-hydroxylase have all been associated with polycystic ovary development.

NEOPLASMS OF THE GYNECOLOGIC TRACT IN CHILDREN AND ADOLESCENTS

Neoplasms of the Vagina and Uterus

Tumors of the vagina and uterus are rare in childhood. They are usually malignant. They often present as a bloody vaginal discharge and may protrude from the introitus. Pelvic US performed using a fluid-filled bladder or a transperineal approach with the transducer placed on the labia can help define the extent of the lesion and dismiss the possibility of simulation by hemato/hydrocolpos from an obstructed vagina. Better definition of the origin, extent, and internal characteristics of the tumor can be obtained by CT, but particularly by multiplanar MRI. The most common neoplasms of the vagina and uterus in children are embryonal rhabdomyosarcoma, endodermal sinus tumor, and clear cell adenocarcinoma.

> **The most common neoplasms of the vagina and uterus in children are embryonal rhabdomyosarcoma, endodermal sinus tumor, and clear cell adenocarcinoma.**

Embryonal rhabdomyosarcoma is the most common genital neoplasm in children of both sexes. It is generally seen before the age of 3 years but rarely at birth. It is rare in older patients. Urogenital sinus remnants are thought to be the origin of some rhabdomyosarcomas (sarcoma botryoides) usually originating from the anterior vagina near the cervix. They may occasionally arise from the cervix. The mass may protrude from the vaginal introitus, often with a polypoid or cluster-of-grapes appearance (botryoid variant). These rhabdomyosarcomas are aggressive tumors that spread rapidly by direct invasion of the vaginal wall and pelvic structures. The tumor may extend to the uterus, bladder, ureters, or rectum. Metastases to regional lymph nodes, the lungs, and other organs may occur. Local recurrence is common.

> *Embryonal rhabdomyosarcoma* **is the most common genital neoplasm in children of both sexes.**

Endodermal sinus tumor of the vagina, also known as yolk sac carcinoma or adenocarcinoma of the infant vagina, is seen usually in infants between 8 and 15 months and rarely after the second year. It often originates in the posterior wall of the vagina (Fig. 155-28) and may have a polypoid appearance very similar to that of sarcoma botryoides. The tumor spreads to pelvic soft tissues, para-aortic nodes, liver, and lungs.

Clear cell (or mesonephric) *adenocarcinoma* usually originates from the vagina and uncommonly from the cervix. It is usually seen after menarche. In the past few decades, about two thirds of patients with this tumor had a history of maternal exposure to diethylstilbestrol or related substances during the first 3 months of pregnancy. These tumors can become quite large, filling the entire vagina by the time of diagnosis. Tumor spread is via the lymphatics and to pelvic nodes. Local recurrence is common. Pulmonary metastases can occur.

Ovarian Neoplasms

Ovarian neoplasms are uncommon in children. Despite this fact, they may be seen among all the age groups of pediatric life, from newborn to adolescence. Neoplasms are not the most common cause of noncystic ovarian masses in children and adolescents. Wu and Siegel's review of 70 such masses in girls ranging in age from neonate to late adolescence found 18 complex masses; 7 were hemorrhagic cysts, 5 were TOAs, 5 were teratomas, and there was only 1 malignant dysgerminoma. Of the solid-appearing adnexal masses, 2 were torsed ovaries, 3 were echo-filled hemorrhagic cysts, and only 3 were neoplasms.

Ovarian neoplasms are commonly divided into groups based on the apparent origin of their cellular components: germ cell tumors, sex cord/stromal tumors, and surface epithelial tumors. Unlike adults, in whom epithelial cell tumors are the most common ovarian tumor type, in children germ cell tumors are the most common. Sixty percent of all pediatric ovarian neoplasms are of germ cell origin. Of the germ cell tumors, 70% are teratomas, 25% are dysgerminomas, and 5% are endodermal sinus or yolk sac tumors. Only one fifth of pediatric ovarian tumors are epithelial cell in origin, including cystadenoma (80%) and cystadenocarcinoma (10%).

The final 10% of pediatric ovarian tumors are sex cord tumors or tumors of stromal/mesenchymal origin. Fifteen percent of those are arrhenoblastomas and 75% are granulosa/theca cell tumors. Granulosa/theca cell tumors are the most common ovarian cause of isosexual precocious puberty in children.

> **Most pediatric ovarian tumors are of germ cell origin: 70% are teratomas, 25% are dysgerminomas, and 5% are endodermal sinus or yolk sac tumors.**

Greater than half of childhood ovarian tumors are diagnosed in girls between 10 and 14 years of age. The majority are teratomas, usually picked up incidentally on plain radiographs or US examination. Ovarian tumors have variable presentations; some present with abdominal pain and some because of a mass felt on physical examination. Ovarian neoplasms are usually unilateral, but bilateral involvement may occur, particularly in the case of teratomas.

Overall, one third of ovarian neoplasms are malignant. This percentage decreases with increasing age. As many as half of hormonally active tumors are malignant. Of the malignant lesions, 85% are germ cell tumors (dysgerminomas, immature teratomas, endodermal sinus tumor, embryonal cell carcinoma, and choriocarcinoma); 10% are stromal (Sertoli–Leydig cell, granulosa/theca cell, and undifferentiated neoplasms); and 5% are epithelial cell tumors (serous and mucinous adenocarcinoma). Malignant neoplasms tend to break through the ovary's capsule and invade adjacent organs. Metastases are most often to the peritoneum, opposite ovary, pelvic and retroperitoneal lymph nodes, omentum, liver, and abdominal organs. Involvement of peritoneal and pleural linings may lead to ascites or pleural effusions.

> **One third of all ovarian neoplasms are malignant. As many as half of hormonally active tumors are malignant.**

IMAGING

Abdominal plain radiographs may show a soft tissue density suggesting an abdominal or pelvic mass. Occasionally fat from a teratoma can be seen as a circular or oval radiolucency. This can readily be confirmed by denoting an area of homogeneous increased echogenicity without shadowing on US or a low-density area with negative Hounsfield units (e.g., –100 HU) on CT. Intrinsic tumor calcifications, often seen in teratomas, may be noted as radiodensity on plain radiographs (see Fig. 155-30), increased echogenicity with posterior shadowing on US, or high-density areas (e.g., +100 HU or greater) on CT examination. Extrinsic compression of the bladder and bowel by ovarian masses has been reported to occasionally cause bowel obstruction or urinary complaints. Intravenous urography and barium studies have been replaced by cross-sectional imaging methods in most of these evaluations. Pelvic US is the

TABLE 155-1

Staging for Ovarian Neoplasms

Stage	Characteristics
I	Tumor limited to one or both ovaries (with subgroups)
II	Tumor involving one or both ovaries with extension to uterus, tubes, or other pelvic areas
III	Tumor involving one or both ovaries with widespread intraperitoneal involvement
IV	Tumor involving one or both ovaries with distant metastases outside the peritoneal cavity

Adapted from Eman S, Goldstein D (eds): Pediatric and Adolescent Gynecology, 3rd ed. Boston, Little Brown, 1990:149.

initial procedure of choice to investigate patients with a possible ovarian tumor. It may provide information as to the location and origin of the mass and readily differentiates a cystic from a mixed or solid lesion. Once a mass is large, its analysis by US or any other method for organ of origin becomes difficult. CT or MRI studies may provide further information and may help elucidate US findings. CT is used particularly for a more global view of tumoral and metastatic involvement. CT and/or MRI are more valuable for staging tumors than is US. Table 155-1 shows a commonly used staging.

Malignant tumors in postpubertal girls are usually large, often 15 cm or greater by the time they are discovered. On US, they are predominantly solid with contained areas of necrosis. Whereas coarse calcifications are typical of malignant teratoma, stippled calcifications can be seen in dysgerminoma. Endodermal sinus tumors typically have both echogenic and hypoechoic components. They grow rapidly, and patients often present because of abdominal pain, occasionally resulting from torsion or rupture of the tumor. When imaging predominantly cystic masses, the presence of contained papillary projections or evidence of capsular invasion is suggestive of malignancy. This is the case with the serous cystadenocarcinoma, a common adult malignant neoplasm that is uncommon in adolescents and rarely noted before puberty. Malignant ovarian tumors may metastasize by direct extension to adjacent structures or by hematogenous or lymphangitic spread to more distant locations. Findings beyond the ovary (i.e., significant ascites, pelvic fixation, or distant metastases) can underline concern that an ovarian mass is malignant and probably metastatic. Again, CT and MRI will allow a more global analysis of a mass and its relationship to surrounding tissues. Within the abdomen, these modalities are particularly helpful in diagnosing omental involvement ("caking") and peritoneal implants (Fig. 155-29), as well as lymphadenopathy. Common sites for distal parenchymal metastases are the liver and lung.

> **US is the initial imaging modality of choice for suspected ovarian neoplasm. CT and MRI are more useful for very large tumors and for assessing possible disease extension or metastasis.**

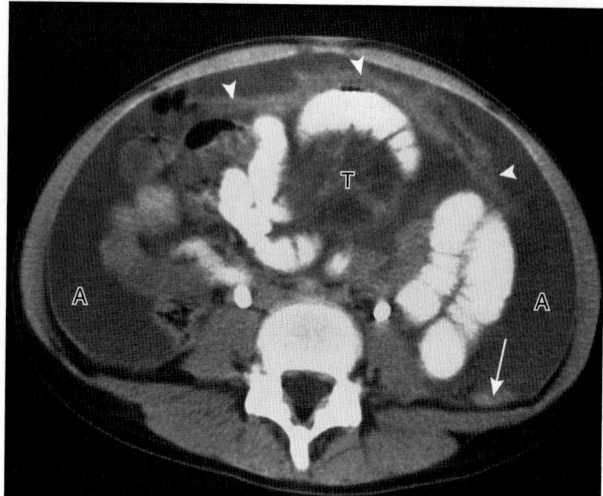

FIGURE 155-29. Endodermal sinus tumor with omental "caking" and peritoneal implants. Contrast-enhanced CT shows malignant omental spread ("caking") *(arrowheads)* in this 13-year-old with malignant endodermal sinus tumor of the ovary. There is moderate ascites (A). An *arrow* points to a posterior left-sided peritoneal metastasis. T, the most superior portion of the ovarian tumor. (From Cohen HL, Bober S, Bow S: Imaging the pediatric pelvis: the normal and abnormal genital tract and simulators of its diseases. Urol Radiol 1992;14:273-283.)

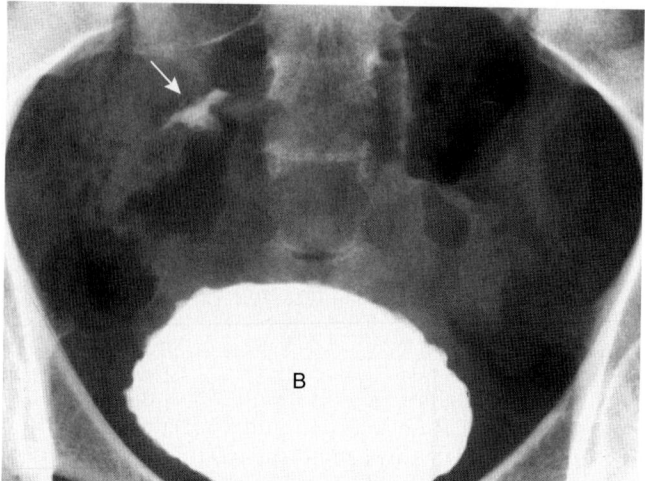

FIGURE 155-30. Ovarian teratoma. Plain radiograph of the pelvis shows a triangular calcification *(arrow)* in the right side of the pelvis. It proved to be within a right ovarian teratoma. The finding was made incidentally during IVU. B, bladder.

OVARIAN TUMORS OF GERM CELL ORIGIN

Germ cell tumors represent the majority of pediatric ovarian neoplasms. They include mature and immature teratomas, dysgerminoma, endodermal sinus tumor, embryonal carcinoma, choriocarcinoma, and gonado-blastoma. About 20% of these tumors contain islands of different germ cell neoplasms and are therefore known as mixed germ cell tumors. Endodermal sinus tumor, embryonal carcinoma, and some immature teratomas are associated with elevated serum α-fetoprotein levels, a finding that may be of value in the initial diagnosis but more so in the detection of residual tumor or recurrences on follow-up. Germ cell tumors are generally unilateral, but bilateral involvement by the same or a different germ cell neoplasm may occur.

OVARIAN TERATOMAS. Mature ovarian teratomas (or dermoid cysts) are the most common ovarian neoplasm in pediatric patients. They are less common in children and therefore more typically found in the adolescent. Although teratomas and dermoid cysts are talked about almost interchangeably, dermoids by definition contain two cell layers—mesoderm and ectoderm—whereas teratomas are made up of elements from all three germ cell layers, including the endoderm. Almost all dermoids and teratomas are benign. Malignancy is found in 2% to 10% of cases or less.

> Mature ovarian teratomas and dermoid cysts are the most common ovarian neoplasm in pediatric patients.

Teratomas are usually asymptomatic, so their true incidence may be underestimated. One third of cases are thought to present with symptomatology. Of teratomas diagnosed in children because of symptoms, the usual history is that of a 6- to 11-year-old with an abdominal mass (65% to 70% of cases) or pain secondary to torsion of or hemorrhage within the cyst. Teratomas are most often discovered by chance during pelvic US examinations performed on adolescents for other reasons. They may occasionally be diagnosed by the incidental discovery of calcifications (particularly teeth or bone) in the adnexal area on plain radiograph examination (Fig. 155-30). One fourth of ovarian teratomas are bilateral. The tumors may vary in size from those contained solely within the ovary itself to those that extend 5 to 10 cm beyond the ovary.

The US appearance of teratomas is highly variable because of the varied contents of these masses. The classic US appearance shows a prominent cystic component and at least one contained mural nodule (dermoid plug, Rokitansky projection) (Fig. 155-31) that is often echogenic as a result of either contained fat, hair, sebum, or calcium (e.g., teeth or bone). The contained teeth and bone and perhaps other components may cause posterior shadowing of the US beam. The shadowing may obscure deeper portions of the mass, a phenomenon called the "tip of the iceberg" sign. The anechoic component of teratomas is made up of serous fluid or sebum, which is in a fluid state when at body temperature. Fat–fluid levels and hair–fluid levels may be seen as part of the cystic component. Echogenic fat may float on top of the cystic component, or echogenic particulate matter may be the dependent component of a fluid–debris level.

Two thirds of teratomas are sonographically complex cysts with anechoic, hypoechoic, and echogenic components. One third of cases are claimed to be either purely echoless (perhaps because the solid component is at the mass's periphery and not imaged) or purely echogenic. Purely cystic tumors are rare. Occasionally, the cystic component of a teratoma may be so large or so positioned that it may simulate the bladder or extend beyond the pelvis and have its size underestimated or its

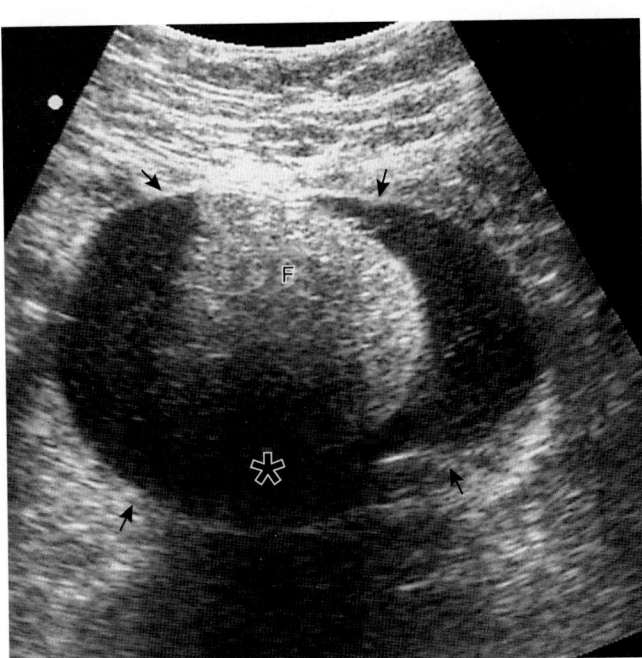

FIGURE 155-31. Ovarian teratoma. Transverse sonogram shows a large left adnexal mass *(arrows)* with a highly echogenic component (F). There is shadowing *(asterisk)* distal to the central portion that represents a dermoid plug. The echogenicity is predominantly due to fat. Some calcification, which is not evident in this plane, was responsible for the shadowing. The periphery of the mass is fluid with contained debris. (From Ruggierro M, Awobuluyi M, Cohen H, Zinn D: Imaging the pediatric pelvis: role of ultrasound. Radiologist 1997;4:155–170.)

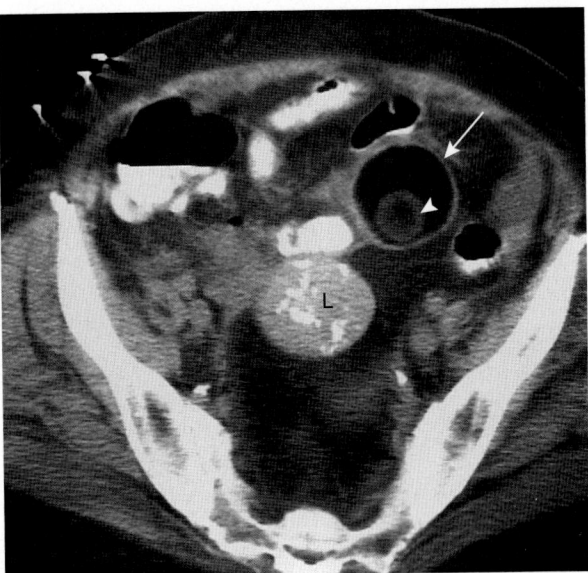

FIGURE 155-32. Ovarian teratoma. Contrast-enhanced CT shows a circular low-Hounsfield-unit mass *(arrow)* in the anterior left pelvis. The CT technique used makes its predominant component appear to be of the same low density as the air seen within nearby bowel or the fat seen in the posterior pelvis anterior to the sacrum. Its actual Hounsfield measurements were consistent with fat. It contains a mural nodule *(arrowhead)* that has no contained calcification. Incidentally noted is a midpelvic mass (L) with calcifications that was a leiomyoma. (From Cohen HL, Safriel YI: Benign cystic teratomas of the ovaries. *In* Cohen HL, Sivit C [eds]: Fetal and Pediatric Ultrasound: A Casebook Approach. New York, McGraw-Hill, 2001:516.)

contained echogenic components missed. Septations or fluid–fluid levels within the cyst may be seen. These findings may also be demonstrated by abdominal CT (Fig. 155-32) or MRI. CT may show calcifications that are not seen by other methods. MRI is particularly valuable in demonstrating the fatty components of the mass. Signal characteristics on MRI reflect the composition of a teratoma. Calcium, bone, and hair have low signal intensity on both T1- and T2-weighted images. Fat has a high signal on T1-weighted studies. Fluid has a high signal on T2-weighted studies.

In a large Turkish study, Ekici and associates found US to be 94% sensitive, 98% accurate, and 99% specific for differentiating mature and benign teratomas from other adnexal masses. The findings used for the diagnosis were an echogenic mass with or without acoustic enhancement, a dermoid plug, layered lines, a fat–fluid level, isolated bright echoes with acoustic shadowing within a complex mass, linear echogenicities (hair) in low-viscosity fluid, contained teeth or bone fragments, or an intraovarian echogenic mass (Fig. 155-33) with or without shadowing or enhancement (evidence of an intraovarian dermoid cyst).

> The classic US appearance of a benign teratoma shows a prominent cystic component and at least one echogenic mural nodule. Malignant teratomas are generally solid masses.

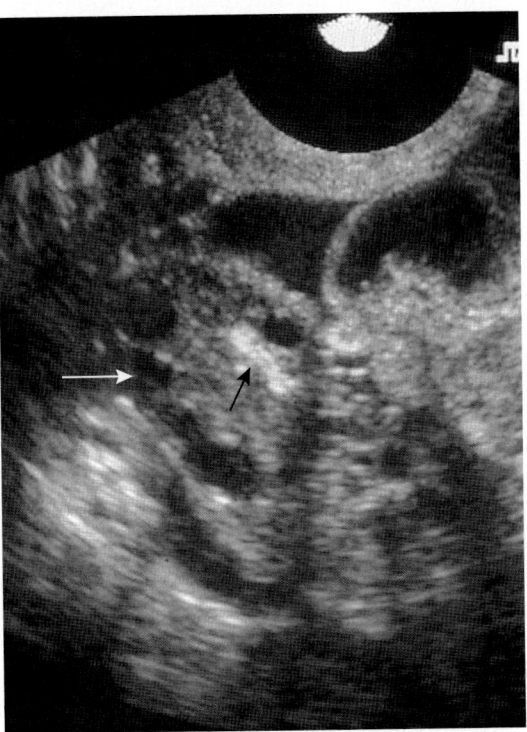

FIGURE 155-33. Intraovarian teratoma. Endovaginal ultrasound shows an echogenic area consistent with the fat of a small intraovarian teratoma *(black arrow)* within the right ovary *(white arrow)*. This was noted after discovery of a large left ovarian cystic teratoma.

Classic benign teratomas do not look like malignant teratomas. In analyzing ovarian masses for malignancy, noting a purely cystic ovarian mass or a mixed mass with well-differentiated epithelial elements such as hair, sebum, or teeth suggests that it is benign. A lack of ascites helps assure this. Immature, partially differentiated malignant teratomas are uncommon and are generally solid. Well-differentiated teratomas with foci of embryonal carcinoma, endodermal sinus tumor, or other malignant germ cell neoplasms are included in this subgroup. Some immature teratomas are hormonally active and can cause precocious puberty. Immature teratomas are almost universally unilateral, but a mature teratoma may be seen in the contralateral ovary in 5% to 10% or more of cases.

OVARIAN DYSGERMINOMA. Dysgerminoma is the second most common ovarian neoplasm in children and adolescents after mature teratoma. It is the most common malignant ovarian tumor of pediatric life but is considered a low-grade malignancy. It is said to be the histologic counterpart to the testicular seminoma of boys. Imaging or inspection shows it to be solid, smooth, and well encapsulated. These tumors are often large when first diagnosed. One fifth of cases have bilateral involvement. Dysgerminoma may arise in dysgenetic gonads but much less commonly than gonadoblastoma. Pure dysgerminomas are nonfunctioning tumors, but function may be observed in germinomas that contain islands of cells of other germ cell tumors. These tumors can spread locally and to retroperitoneal nodes. These tumors are very radiosensitive, and prognosis with treatment is generally good, with an overall survival of more than 90%.

> Dysgerminoma is the second most common ovarian neoplasm in children and adolescents after mature teratoma. One fifth show bilateral involvement.

ENDODERMAL SINUS TUMOR. Endodermal sinus tumor (yolk sac tumor, yolk sac carcinoma, Teilum tumor) is an uncommon malignant neoplasm that can occur at any age. It is often bulky at the time of diagnosis. Its US image (Fig. 155-34) is predominantly solid but may contain cystic spaces within the tumor. In most cases serum α_1-fetoprotein levels are increased. Some endodermal sinus tumors secrete human chorionic gonadotropin, causing incomplete precocious puberty by stimulating estrogen production by the ovary. This can cause menstrual irregularities in postpubertal girls. The tumor is very radiosensitive, but there is a high incidence of recurrences. There is a high survival rate among treated patients.

CHORIOCARCINOMA. Choriocarcinoma of the ovary is very uncommon but is sometimes seen as a component of mixed germ cell tumors. It may secrete human chorionic gonadotropin.

GONADOBLASTOMA. Gonadoblastomas are composed of both germ cells plus sex cord/stromal cells. They usually

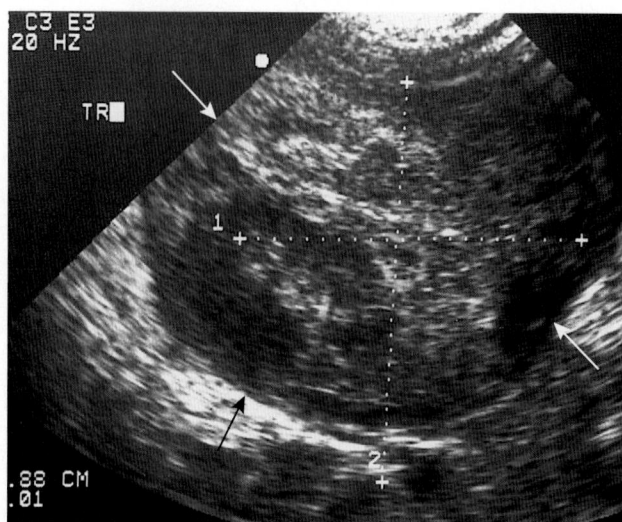

FIGURE 155-34. Endodermal sinus tumor. Transverse sonogram shows a large solid mass *(arrows)* extending beyond the measurement cursors in this 13-year-old who presented with a distended abdomen. CT showed significant metastatic disease (see Fig. 155-30).

are seen in postpubertal patients. They are considered potentially malignant because about 10% give rise to dysgerminomas and other malignant germ cell tumors. These tumors may have punctate calcifications that may be seen on plain radiographs.

MIXED GERM CELL NEOPLASMS. Mixed germ cell neoplasms containing seminoma, dysgerminoma, or gonadoblastoma, may be seen in some patients with intersex disorders and a Y chromosome.

OVARIAN TUMORS OF (SURFACE) EPITHELIAL ORIGIN

Surface epithelial tumors in children are similar to those in adults and consist predominantly of cystadenoma and cystadenocarcinoma. Cystadenomas are very uncommon before puberty and are usually unilateral. They vary in size from 3 to 30 cm. Of the two types of cystadenomas, serous cystadenomas contain clear watery fluid and the less common mucinous cystadenomas contain mucin, a jelly-like material. Most of these tumors are multiseptated cystic masses (Fig. 155-35) when imaged by US. Cystadenomas are benign neoplasms, but a serous papillary form is reported to be prone to rupture, with spillage of tumor material into the peritoneal cavity causing a serous papillomatosis.

Cystadenocarcinomas are much less common than their benign counterparts. They may appear similar to cystadenomas. The presence of irregular margins, thick septations, and papillary projections suggests malignancy. Ascites, omental or peritoneal implants, lymphadenopathy, and hepatic metastases suggest malignant spread.

OVARIAN TUMORS OF SEX CORD OR MESENCHYMAL ORIGIN

Sex cord (gonadal stromal) tumors are uncommon. They include granulosa/theca cell tumors (75%) and arrhenoblastoma (15%).

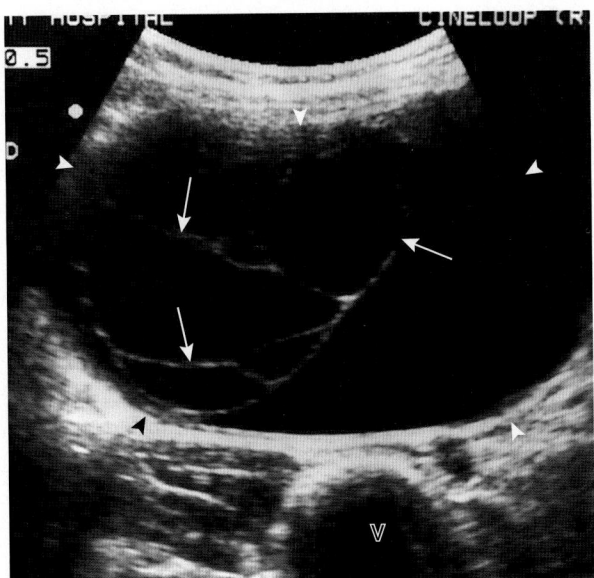

FIGURE 155-35. Ovarian cystadenoma. Transverse sonogram in a teenager shows a large cystic mass *(arrowheads)* with several intersecting septations *(arrows)*. These are much more common tumors of the adult ovary than of the child's ovary. V, vertebral body. (From Ruggierro M, Awobuluyi M, Cohen H, Zinn D: Imaging the pediatric pelvis: role of ultrasound. Radiologist 1997;4:155-170.)

GRANULOSA/THECA CELL TUMORS. Granulosa/theca cell tumors are generally large at the time of diagnosis. They are predominantly solid, but mixed solid and cystic patterns or a predominantly cystic type are also seen. Three fourths of juvenile granulosa cell tumors produce estrogen, which causes isosexual precocious puberty. Postpubertal girls with these tumors may develop abnormal menses. As already noted, greater than 50% of hormonally active childhood ovarian tumors are malignant. Nonfunctioning granulosa cell tumors may be discovered incidentally as a mass on physical examination or US. The vast majority of nonfunctioning granulosa cell tumors are benign, with recurrences and metastases a rarity.

> Granulosa/theca cell tumors are the most common ovarian cause of isosexual precocious puberty.

ARRHENOBLASTOMAS. Arrhenoblastomas (Leydig cell tumors) are usually large and unilateral. They may be solid or cystic. They are usually well differentiated and benign, but a poorly differentiated form also occurs. Most arrhenoblastomas produce androgenic substances, causing virilization in prepubertal girls and signs of virilization, hirsutism, and oligomenorrhea or amenorrhea after puberty.

> Arrhenoblastomas (Leydig cell tumors) may produce androgens, causing virilization and menstrual disturbances.

OVARIAN INVOLVEMENT IN LEUKEMIA

Ovarian involvement in cases of acute leukemia is a common microscopic finding, noted incidentally in 35% to 50% of autopsies performed on girls dying of acute lymphoblastic leukemia. By contrast, leukemia infiltrating the ovary, occurring as the primary site of leukemia relapse after completion of chemotherapy, is rarely identified during life. This is probably because more intensive chemotherapy has been used in recent protocols to avoid this problem. Ovarian relapse in acute lymphoblastic leukemia is about 50 times less common than testicular relapse. It should be considered, however, if there is asymmetric (solid) enlargement of the adnexa in such a patient. Leukemic infiltration of the ovary may present with abdominal pain and a lower abdominal mass resulting from ovarian enlargement. Involvement is usually bilateral. Patients may develop hydronephrosis.

US examination of ovaries with leukemic infiltration reveals them to be solid and usually more hypoechoic than normal because of the ready penetration by US of areas containing homogeneous arrays of infiltrating small cells. The response to chemotherapy, radiotherapy, and surgical resection of ovarian leukemic infiltration is generally poor.

OTHER OVARIAN TUMORS

Rare solid ovarian fibromas have been reported in prepubertal and postpubertal females. They have been associated with ascites and/or pleural effusion in Meig syndrome. These typically benign ovarian tumors range in US appearance from anechoic to solid to calcified. If they are bilateral and calcified, one should consider basal cell nevus syndrome and its associated multiple basal cell carcinomas, as well as mandibular cysts and rib anomalies.

DIFFERENTIAL DIAGNOSIS OF OVARIAN NEOPLASMS

Neoplasms that may simulate solid and complex gynecologic adnexal masses include sacral and pelvic girdle tumors, retroperitoneal or pelvic soft tissue sarcomas (particularly rhabdomyosarcoma), neuroblastomas, and bowel tumors. Non-neoplastic simulators of adnexal masses include adenopathy, gynecologic (tubo-ovarian) and gastrointestinal (appendicitis, inflammatory bowel disease) inflammatory masses, endometriomas, and uterine (müllerian duct) anomalies.

SUGGESTED READINGS

Atiomo W, Pearson S, Shaw S, et al: Ultrasound criteria in the diagnosis of polycystic ovary syndrome (PCOS). Ultrasound Med Biol 2000;26:977

Baltarowich OH, Kurtz A, Pasto M, et al: The spectrum of sonographic findings in hemorrhagic ovarian cysts. AJR Am J Roentgenol 1987;148:901

Battaglia C, Artini P, Genazzani A, et al: Color Doppler analysis in oligo- and amenorrheic women with polycystic ovary syndrome. Gynecol Endocrinol 1997;11:105

Boechat M: Magnetic resonance imaging of abdominal and pelvic masses in children. Top Magn Reson Imaging 1990;3:25

Bulas D, Ahlstrom P, Sivit C, et al: Pelvic inflammatory disease in the adolescent: comparison of transabdominal and transvaginal sonographic evaluation. Radiology 1992;183:435

Caloia D, Morris H, Rahmani M: Congenital transverse vaginal septum: vaginal hydrosonographic diagnosis. J Ultrasound Med 1998;17:261

Carrington B, Hricak H, Nuruddin R, et al: Mullerian duct anomalies: MR imaging evaluation. Radiology 1990;176:715

Cil A, Akgul M, Tulunay G, Atayar Y: Recovery of ovarian function after detorsion: Doppler findings. Acta Radiol 2006;47:618

Cohen HL: Evaluation of the adolescent and young adult with amenorrhea: role of US. In Bluth E, Arger P, Hertzberg B, Middleton W (eds): Syllabus: A Special Course in Ultrasound: Clinical Questions, Practical Answers. Oak Brook, IL, RSNA Publications, 1996:171

Cohen HL: The female pelvis. In Siebert J (ed): Current Concepts: A Categorical Course in Pediatric Radiology. Chicago, RSNA Publications, 1994:65

Cohen HL: History of emergency US—reply [letter to the editor]. J Ultrasound Med 2004;23:1130-1133

Cohen HL: Physiologic ovarian cysts in a newborn. In Hertzberg B, Hill M, Cohen HL (eds): Ultrasound (third series): Test and Syllabus. Baltimore, ACR Publications, 2005:248-256.

Cohen HL, Bober S, Bow S: Imaging the pediatric pelvis: the normal and abnormal genital tract and simulators of its diseases. Urol Radiol 1992;14:273

Cohen HL, Eisenberg P, Mandel F, Haller J: Ovarian cysts are common in premenarchal girls: a sonographic study of 101 children 2 to 12 years of age. AJR Am J Roentgenol 1992;159:89

Cohen HL, Shapiro MA, Mandel FS, Shapiro ML: Normal ovaries in neonates and infants: a sonographic study of 77 patients 1 day to 24 months old. AJR Am J Roentgenol 1993;160:583

Cohen HL, Sivit CJ (eds): Fetal and pediatric ultrasound: a casebook approach. New York, McGraw-Hill, 2001

Cohen HL, Smith W, Kushner D, et al: Imaging evaluation of acute right lower quadrant and pelvic pain in adolescent girls (ACR Appropriateness Criteria). Radiology 2000;215S:833–840

Cohen HL, Tice H, Mandel F: Ovarian volumes measured by US: bigger than we think. Radiology 1990;177:189

Currarino G, Wood B, Majd M: Abnormalities of the genital tract. In Silverman F, Kuhn J (eds): Caffey's Pediatric X-Ray Diagnosis, 9th ed. St. Louis, Mosby–Year Book, 1993:1375

Davis AJ, Fein NR: Subsequent asynchronous torsion of normal adnexa in children. J Pediatr Surg 1990;25:687

Eberenz W, Rosenberg H, Moshang T, et al: True hermaphroditism: sonographic identification of ovotestes. Radiology 1991;179:429

Eisenberg P, Cohen H, Mandel F, et al: US analysis of premenarchal gynecological structures. J Ultrasound Med 1991;10:S30

Ekici E, Soysal M, Kara S, et al: The efficiency of ultrasonography in the diagnosis of dermoid cysts. Zentralbl Gynakol 1996;118:136

Emans S, Goldstein D (eds): Delayed puberty and menstrual irregularities. In Pediatric & Adolescent Gynecology, 3rd ed. Boston, Little Brown, 1990:149

Emans S, Goldstein D (eds): The physiology of puberty. In Pediatric & Adolescent Gynecology, 3rd ed. Boston, Little Brown, 1990:95

Fedele L, Dorta M, Brioschi D, et al: Magnetic resonance imaging in Mayer-Rokitansky-Küster-Hauser syndrome. Obstet Gynecol 1990;76:593

Fleischer AC, Brader KR: Sonographic depiction of ovarian vascularity and flow: current improvements and future applications. J Ultrasound Med 2001;20:241

Galli-Tsinopoulou A, Moudiou T, Mamopoulos A, et al: Multifollicular ovaries in female adolescents with cystic fibrosis. Fertil Steril 2006;85:1484

Garel L, Filiatrault D, Brandt M, et al: Antenatal diagnosis of ovarian cysts: natural history and therapeutic implications. Pediatr Radiol 1991;21:182

Graif M, Itzchak Y: Sonographic evaluation of ovarian torsion in childhood and adolescence. AJR Am J Roentgenol 1988;150:647

Herter L, Magalnaes J, Spritzer P: Association of ovarian volume and serum LH levels in adolescent patients with menstrual disorders and/or hirsutism. Braz J Med Biol Res 1993;26:1041

Herter L, Golendziner E, Flores J, et al: Ovarian and uterine sonography in healthy girls between 1 and 13 years old: correlation of findings with age and pubertal status. AJR Am J Roentgenol 2002;178:1531

Herter L, Golendziner E, Flores J, et al: Ovarian and uterine findings in pelvic sonography: comparison between prepubertal girls, girls with isolated thelarche, and girls with central precocious puberty. J Ultrasound Med 2002;21:1237

Hugosson C, Jorulf H, Bakri Y: MRI in distal vaginal atresia. Pediatr Radiol 1991;21:281

Jaramillo D, Lebowitz RL, Hendren WH: The cloacal malformation: radiologic findings and imaging recommendations. Radiology 1990;177:441

Kurtz AB, Middleton WD: Ultrasound: The Requisites. St. Louis, Mosby–Year Book, 1996:202

Larsen W, Felmar E, Wallace M, Frieder R: Sertoli-Leydig cell tumor of the ovary: a rare cause of amenorrhea. Obstet Gynecol 1992;79:831

Lee E, Kwon H, Joo H, et al: Diagnosis of ovarian torsion with color Doppler sonography: depiction of twisted vascular pedicle. J Ultrasound Med 1998;17:83

Levitin A, Haller K, Cohen HL, et al: Endodermal sinus tumor of the ovary: imaging evaluation. AJR Am J Roentgenol 1996;167:791

Linam LE, Darolia R, Naffaa LN, et al: US findings of adnexal torsion in the pediatric and adolescent population: size really does matter. Pediatr Radiol 2007; in press

Nussbaum A, Sanders R, Jones M: Neonatal uterine morphology as seen on real-time US. Radiology 1986;160:641

Nussbaum Blask AR, Sanders RC, Gearhart JP: Obstructed ureterovaginal anomalies: demonstration with sonography: I. Neonates and infants. Radiology 1991;179:79

Orsini L, Salardi S, Pilu G, et al: Pelvic organs in premenarchal girls: real-time ultrasonography. Radiology 1984;153:113

Pais RC, Kim T, Zwiren G, Ragab A: Ovarian tumors in relapsing acute lymphoblastic leukemia: a review of 23 cases. J Pediatr Surg 1991;26:70

Pinkas H, Mashiach R, Rabinerson D, et al: Doppler parameters of uterine and ovarian stromal blood flow in women with polycystic ovary syndrome and normally ovulating women undergoing controlled ovarian stimulation. Ultrasound Obstet Gynecol 1998;12:197

Quillin S, Siegel M: Color Doppler ultrasound of children with acute lower abdominal pain. Radiographics 1993;13:293

Ratani R, Cohen HL, Firoe E: Pediatric gynecologic ultrasound. Ultrasound Q 2004;20:127-139

Reed M, Griscom N: Hydrometrocolpos in infancy. Am J Roentgenol Radium Ther Nucl Med 1973;118:1

Reid R: Amenorrhea. In Copeland L (ed): Textbook of Gynecology. Philadelphia, WB Saunders, 1993:367

Reinhold C, Hricak H, Forstner R, et al: Primary amenorrhea: evaluation with MR imaging. Radiology 1997;203:383

Rosenblatt M, Rosenblatt R, Kutcher R, et al: Utero-vaginal hypoplasia: sonographic, embryologic and clinical considerations. Pediatr Radiol 1991;21:536

Rosenfield R: Hyperandrogenism in peripubertal girls. Pediatr Clin North Am 1990;37:1333

Ruggierro M, Awobuluyi M, Cohen H, Zinn D: Imaging the pediatric pelvis: role of ultrasound. Radiologist 1997;4:155

Salardi S, Orsini L, Cacciari E, et al: Pelvic ultrasonography in premenarchal girls: relation to puberty and sex hormone concentrations. Arch Dis Child 1985;60:120

Scanlan KA, Pozniak M, Fagerholm M, Shapiro S: Value of transperineal sonography in the assessment of vaginal atresia. AJR Am J Roentgenol 1990;154:545

Servaes S, Zurakowski D, Laufer MR, et al: Sonographic findings of ovarian torsion in children. Pediatr Radiol 2007;37:446-451

Shah R, Woolley M, Costin G: Testicular feminization syndrome: the androgen insensitivity syndrome. J Pediatr Surg 1992;27:757

Sherer D, Shah Y, Eggers P, Woods J: Prenatal sonographic diagnosis and subsequent management of fetal adnexal torsion. J Ultrasound Med 1990;9:161

Siegel MJ: Pediatric gynecologic sonography. Radiology 1991;179:593

Sisler CL, Siegel MJ: Ovarian teratomas: a comparison of the sonographic appearance in prepubertal and postpubertal girls. AJR Am J Roentgenol 1990;154:139

Steele GS, Clancy T, Datta M, et al: Angiosarcoma arising in a testicular teratoma. J Urol 2000;163:1872

Surratt J, Siegel M: Imaging of pediatric ovarian masses. Radiographics 1991;11:533

Takahashi K, Okada M, Ozaki T, et al: Transvaginal ultrasonographic morphology in polycystic ovarian syndrome. Gynecol Obstet Invest 1995;39:201

Ulbright T, Srigley J: Dermoid cyst of the testis: a study of five postpubertal cases, including a pilomatrixoma-like variant, with evidence supporting its separate classification from mature testicular teratoma. Am J Surg Pathol 2001;25:788

Weckstein L: Current perspective on ectopic pregnancy. Obstet Gynecol Surg 1985;40:259

Westrom L: Incidence, prevalence and trends of acute pelvic inflammatory disease and its consequences in industrialized countries. Am J Obstet Gynecol 1980;138:880

White M, Stella J: Ovarian torsion: 10-year perspective. Emerg Med Australas 2005;17:231

Woodward P, Sohaey R, Wagner B: Congenital uterine malformations. Curr Probl Diagn Radiol 1995;24:177

Wu A, Siegel MJ: Sonography of pelvic masses in children: diagnostic predictability. AJR Am J Roentgenol 1987;148:1199

CHAPTER 156

Abnormalities of Puberty and Amenorrhea

HARRIS L. COHEN

Indications for the evaluation of the adolescent pelvis are most often complaints of abdominal pain, pelvic pain, or mass. Much of the differential diagnosis for these complaints has been reviewed in Chapter 155. Other key clinical complaints resulting in ultrasonography (US) and other imaging evaluations in females relate to abnormalities of development of the secondary sexual characteristics of puberty. These changes may be seen earlier than normal (precocious puberty), may be delayed (delayed puberty), or may fail to develop (hypogonadism, sexual infantilism) in adolescents. The other key reason for adolescent gynecologic evaluations is amenorrhea (lack of menses), whether primary or secondary. Much of what causes pubertal delay may also cause primary or secondary amenorrhea.

PUBERTY

Puberty among girls is the stage of development in between childhood and adulthood when activation of the hypothalamic-pituitary-ovarian-uterine (H-P-O-U) axis produces maturation of the gonads, resulting in an increased production of sex hormones, development of secondary sex characteristics, a growth spurt, and development of reproductive capability. The earliest signs of puberty among girls are breast development (usually occurring between ages 8 and 13 years) and pubic hair growth (at age 8 to 14 years). This is followed by a growth spurt (at age 9.5 to 14.5 years), axillary hair development, and menarche (at age 10 to 16 years). Puberty is usually completed within about 4 years.

Puberty among males begins between 9 and 14 years of age and is completed in 3.5 to 4 years. It begins with testicular enlargement (usually occurring between age 9 and 13.5 years), followed by the appearance of pubic hair (at age 10 to 15 years), enlargement of the penis (at age 11 to 12.5 years), and development of axillary and facial hair as well as a growth spurt (at age 10.5 to 16 years).

PHYSIOLOGIC CHANGES AT PUBERTY AND THE NORMAL OVULATORY MENSTRUAL CYCLE

All the components necessary for menstruation can be found in the normal female at the time of birth. This is evidenced by the occasional neonatal withdrawal bleeding that may result from decreasing estrogen and progesterone levels after separation from the placenta.

Ordinarily, until the age of at least 8 years, an unknown "central restraining mechanism" prevents the pulsatile release of gonadotropin-releasing hormone (GnRH) from the arcuate nucleus of the hypothalamus. Pulsatile release of GnRH appears necessary for ovulation and development of corpus luteum. Evidence of this central control (rather than a negative feedback mechanism from ovarian hormone production) can be shown by the inhibition of GnRH production even in patients with Turner syndrome who have no apparent functioning gonadal tissue. In early puberty the pulsatile GnRH release is maximal only at night, but with time the typical adult pattern of continuous pulsatile GnRH secretion develops.

With the earliest activation of GnRH, most individuals undergo ovarian folliculogenesis without ovulation. Unopposed estrogen production leads to progressive uterine growth and endometrial proliferation. There is breast budding, physiologic leukorrhea, and accelerated linear growth of the girl. The H-P-O-U axis continues to mature. Over an approximately 2-year span, cycles with subnormal progesterone production and shortened intermenstrual intervals are replaced by normal corpus luteum function and fertile cycles.

> Unopposed estrogen production leads to progressive uterine growth and endometrial proliferation. Axillary and pubic hair development are the result of ovarian and adrenal gland androgen production.

The typical ovulatory cycle has a 24- to 35-day intermenstrual interval and usually a premenstrual molimina. Longer intervals are often associated with anovulation, although the eventual menses is often associated with some corpus luteum activity. Improved nutrition and living conditions are thought to be responsible for the gradual fall in mean menarchal age over the past century. In North America, it is currently 12.4 years with a range of 9 to 17 years. Menarche usually occurs 2 to 5 years after breast bud development.

> In North America, mean menarchal age is 12.4 years, with a range of 9 to 17 years.

PREMATURE THELARCHE AND PREMATURE ADRENARCHE

Premature thelarche and adrenarche are relatively common, self-limited variants of normal pubertal development in girls. Premature thelarche refers to premature breast development without other signs of precocious sexual maturation in girls younger than 8 years of age. It usually is seen between 1 and 4 years of age. A third of the cases resolve spontaneously. At puberty, breast development is normal. Premature adrenarche refers to the appearance of pubic and axillary hair without other signs of precocious sexual maturity. In both premature thelarche and premature adrenarche, bone age and patient height are normal to only slightly increased. The cause of premature thelarche or adrenarche is not certain. The levels of circulating sex hormones are usually normal. Increased end-organ sensitivity to normal levels of estrogen or androgen has been suggested as a possible cause.

In boys, premature appearance of pubic and axillary hair without other signs or only minor signs of precocious puberty is a relatively common variant of normal development that may be due to an increase in circulating androgens from premature maturation of the adrenal glands of unknown cause. There is no penile enlargement, presumably because the levels of circulating androgens are not sufficiently elevated. The bone age and growth rate are slightly increased. The rest of pubertal development occurs at a normal age.

PRECOCIOUS PUBERTY

Precocious puberty refers to the appearance of external signs of adolescence (secondary sex characteristics) before 8 years of age in girls and before 9 years of age in boys. Precocious puberty and its clinical problems are more common in girls than in boys. In girls, precocious breast development (thelarche), axillary or pubic hair development (adrenarche), or menses (menarche) may occur.

> **Precocious puberty refers to the appearance of external signs of adolescence before 8 years of age in girls and before 9 years of age in boys.**

Precocious puberty is divided into two main types: (1) complete, central, gonadotropin-dependent, or *true* precocious puberty and (2) incomplete, peripheral, gonadotropin-independent, *pseudo*precocious puberty, or precocious pseudopuberty. Whereas the complete form is characteristically isosexual, with development of secondary sex characteristics that are appropriate for the patient's gender, the incomplete form may be either isosexual or heterosexual. Incomplete heterosexual precocious puberty is manifested by signs of virilization in girls and by gynecomastia or other signs of feminization in boys.

Complete or Central Isosexual Precocious Puberty

This form of precocious puberty results from premature activation of the hypothalamic-pituitary-gonadal complex, with increased production of gonadotropic and sex hormones and an early onset of ovulation or spermatogenesis. Complete precocious puberty may be idiopathic or secondary to organic central nervous system (CNS) lesions.

The cause of precocious puberty in girls is idiopathic in at least 80% of cases. Early menarche results from an idiopathic increase in the activity of the hypothalamic-pituitary-gonadal axis. About 20% of affected girls have a hypothalamic or pituitary lesion. These can be defined by CT or MRI. Pelvic US helps assess the presence of normal or abnormal uterus and ovaries. Less than 10% of cases of true precocious puberty in boys have an idiopathic cause. A familial tendency to early pubertal development of the idiopathic type is observed in some cases (constitutional or genetic precocious puberty).

> **The cause of precocious puberty is idiopathic in at least 80% of girls but in less than 10% of boys.**

Possible causes of precocious puberty in either sex include intracranial tumors or cysts, hydrocephalus, sequelae of intracranial inflammatory processes or trauma, and other intracranial lesions that may activate the hypothalamus by pressure or invasion. Of the CNS neoplasms that may cause true precocious puberty, hamartoma of the tuber cinereum (Fig. 156-1), or hypothalamic hamartoma, is the most common. This usually small CNS tumor is more common in boys than in girls, is generally benign, and is nonprogressive. The associated symptoms usually cannot be surgically corrected. The tumor may be pedunculated and appear as an excrescence on the tuber cinereum below the mammillary body. It secretes GnRH. The onset of puberty in patients with this lesion is usually at a younger age (2 years) than in patients with idiopathic precocious puberty. Use of MRI has increased the frequency of the diagnosis.

> **Hypothalamic hamartoma is the most common CNS neoplasm to cause true precocious puberty.**

Other CNS neoplasms that may cause true precocious puberty in either sex are usually located in or near the hypothalamus and include hypothalamic or optic gliomas, astrocytoma, ependymoma, dysgerminoma, and prolactinoma. Suprasellar dysgerminoma (ectopic pinealoma) in boys may also cause incomplete precocious puberty through secretion of human chorionic gonadotropin (hCG) by the tumor.

True precocious puberty may be observed in some children with long-standing untreated hypothyroidism. It is often accompanied by galactorrhea. Affected patients show little, if any, development of secondary sexual characteristics, especially pubic hair. These patients have arrested linear growth, and bone age is not advanced. All of these changes regress with treatment of the hypothyroidism. The increased production of gonadotropic hormones and prolactin seen in these patients may be due to a hormonal overlap in the pituitary response to thyroid deficiency.

Premature maturation of the hypothalamic-pituitary complex, increased gonadotropin secretion, and true precocious puberty may also occur after chronic exposure to endogenous or exogenous androgens, and sometimes also estrogens. This is especially true when the source of the sex hormone is removed, such as after ending therapy for congenital adrenal hyperplasia (CAH) or after surgical removal of an androgen-secreting neoplasm or an estrogen-secreting ovarian tumor or cyst.

Incomplete (Pseudosexual) Precocious Puberty in Girls

Pseudosexual (or incomplete) precocious puberty in girls usually presents before 5 years of age. Excess circulating estrogens or related substances develop independent of stimulus by the hypothalamus and pituitary gland. These estrogens are usually produced by the ovaries or adrenal glands. They may be from an exogenous source, such as food, parenteral or oral medications, creams, lotions, or other substances.

Gonadotropin levels are not high, but rather low, and the gonads remain immature. The most common ovarian source is an autonomous estrogen-secreting follicular (granulosa-thecal) cyst (Fig. 156-2). The cyst (or cysts) may rupture or regress spontaneously, resulting in a decreased estrogen level and vaginal withdrawal bleeding. They may redevelop, and symptoms may recur. Other causes are estrogen-producing ovarian neoplasms, particularly granulosa cell (or granulosa-theca cell) tumors (Fig. 156-3), and rare estrogen-secreting adrenal neoplasms (adenomas or carcinomas).

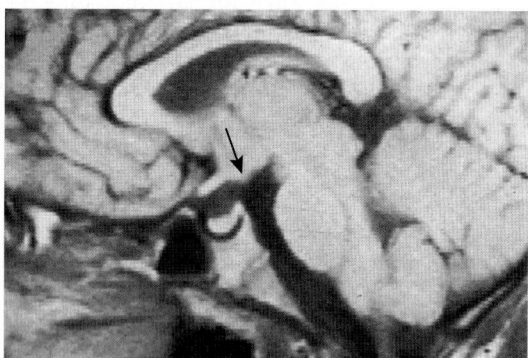
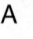
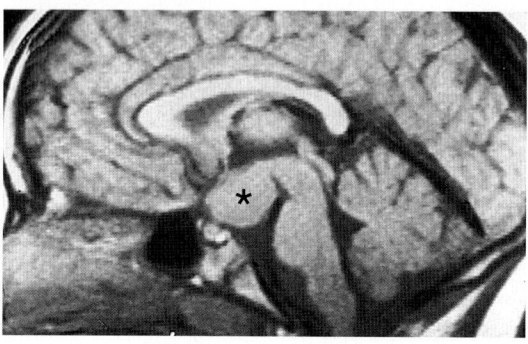

FIGURE 156-1. Precocious puberty caused by hamartoma of the tuber cinereum. **A** and **B,** On midline sagittal T1-weighted MR images of the brain, an *arrow* points to a small hamartoma in the brain of an 8-year-old and an *asterisk* indicates an unusually large hamartoma in a 7-year-old, both of whom had a long-standing history of precocious puberty.

> Pseudosexual precocious puberty in girls usually presents before 5 years of age. Excess circulating estrogens or related substances develop independent of central stimulation. The most common source is an autonomous estrogen-secreting ovarian follicular cyst.

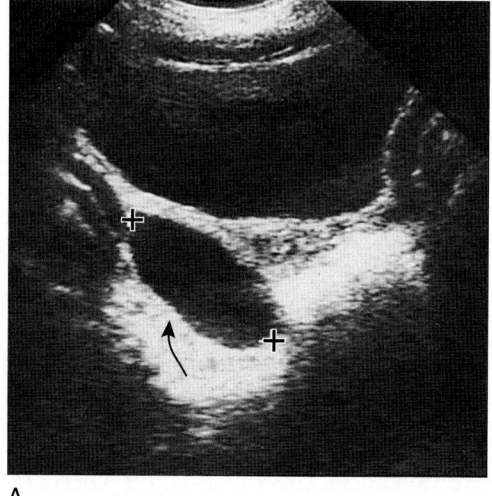
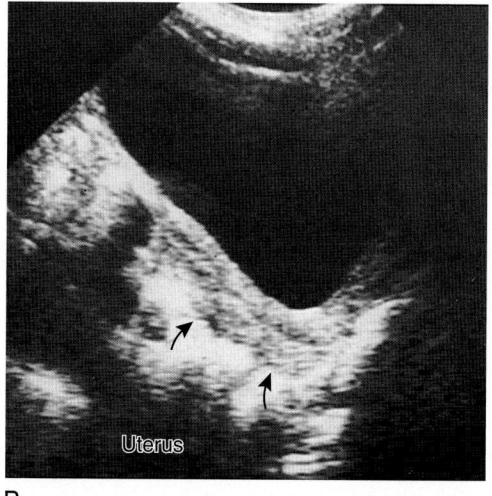

A   B

FIGURE 156-2. Precocious puberty due to autonomous estrogen-secreting ovarian cyst. **A,** Parasagittal sonogram of the right adnexa *(arrow)* of a 3-year-old with precocious puberty shows a large cyst *(cursors).* This cyst was proved to autonomously secrete estrogen. The left adnexa was normal. **B,** Midline longitudinal sonogram shows that the child's uterus *(arrows)* is longer than normal for her age. It is not the tubular shape typical of childhood but appears almost pear shaped, with an evident echogenic central endometrial cavity suggesting estrogenization.

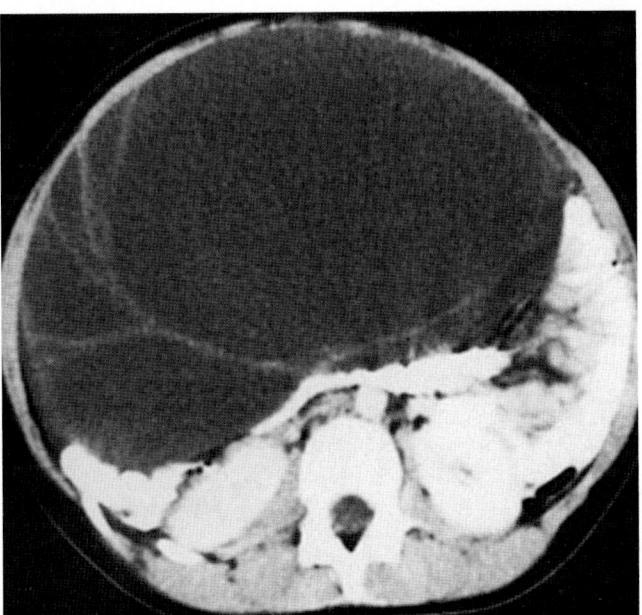

FIGURE 156-3. Precocious puberty caused by granulosa cell tumor. Contrast-enhanced CT at the level of the kidneys shows a large, cystic, septated mass occupying most of the abdomen in a 10-year-old girl. The mass proved to be a juvenile granulosa cell tumor that produced estrogen and caused precocious puberty.

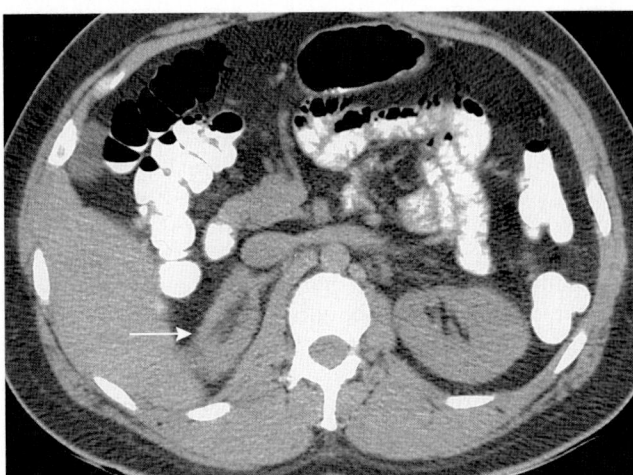

FIGURE 156-4. Congenital adrenal hyperplasia. CT scan at the level of right adrenal and left kidney. The right adrenal gland *(arrow)* is thicker than normal in this 24-year-old with simple virilizing congenital adrenal hyperplasia. As is typical with this disorder, the adrenal gland maintains its normal shape.

McCune-Albright syndrome consists of polyostotic fibrous dysplasia, cutaneous café au lait spots, and precocious puberty. The syndrome is predominantly found in females. Vaginal bleeding is often the first sign of precocious puberty, which is usually pseudoprecocious in type. Autonomously functioning ovarian cysts are seen in some cases. In others, no anatomic cause is noted. McCune-Albright syndrome occasionally presents as complete or true precocious puberty. It has been suggested that the initially partial or incomplete precocious puberty in these patients becomes complete (gonadotropin dependent) as the result of an early maturation of the hypothalamic-pituitary-gonadal complex caused by a long-standing exposure to estrogen.

Virilizing Disorders (Heterosexual Precocious Puberty)

Testosterone, as already noted, is the most potent of the circulating androgens. It is produced in normal females by the adrenal (25%), by the ovary (25%), and by peripheral conversion of Δ4-androstenedione (50%), with only 1% typically free and biologically active. A form of pseudosexual precocity may occur in girls when either androgen levels are excessive or end organs become excessively sensitive to normal amounts of circulating androgens. In either case, this may lead to heterosexual pseudoprecocious puberty as the girls undergo virilization and develop secondary sexual characteristics of males. Clinical findings include increases in body and facial hair (hirsutism), acne, deepening of the voice, clitoromegaly, increased muscle mass, and temporal balding. Menstrual abnormalities are common among affected adolescents. Postpubertal virilized girls may become defeminized, with decreases in breast size and the development of vaginal atrophy.

CONGENITAL ADRENAL HYPERPLASIA

Congenital adrenal hyperplasia is the most common form of hyperandrogenism. The increased production of androgenic substance is due in most cases to a deficiency of 21-hydroxylase and, far less commonly, to deficiencies in 11β-hydroxylase, 3β-hydroxysteroid dehydrogenase, or other enzymes involved in cortisol and/or aldosterone synthesis. These are typically autosomal recessive disorders.

Imaging of the adrenal gland will show enlargement (Fig. 156-4) that is usually bilateral and diffuse. The normal adrenal shape is maintained.

> **Congenital adrenal hyperplasia is the most common form of hyperandrogenism, due in most cases to 21-hydroxylase deficiency.**

OTHER CAUSES OF VIRILIZATION IN GIRLS

Adrenal adenomas or adrenal carcinomas may produce increased androgens and virilization. Signs of Cushing syndrome may be seen in such patients as a result of associated secretion of glucocorticoid hormones by the tumor.

Some ovarian neoplasms may secrete androgens and cause virilization, including Sertoli–Leydig cell tumors (once known as an androblastoma or arrhenoblastoma), thecoma (luteoma; a virilizing dysgerminoma containing theca cells), or a gonadoblastoma (occurring mostly in dysgenetic gonads). Exogenous exposure to androgens or androgen-like substances may cause virilization at all ages. Again, some girls with rare anomalies of sex differentiation, such as 46,XY gonadal dysgenesis, may develop virilization at puberty, despite being phenotypically normal females at birth.

Idiopathic hirsutism and polycystic ovarian disease are also considered among the virilizing disorders of females. Idiopathic hirsutism consists of an increase in body and facial hair (hirsutism, hypertrichosis) occurring as the sole or predominant abnormality and is a relatively common problem in otherwise normal pubertal and postpubertal girls. It may be precipitated by any of the causes of virilization. It may be seen in families or as a result of polycystic ovary syndrome (PCOS). The cause is usually idiopathic and believed to be a result of an altered response of the end organ (hair follicle) to normal levels of circulating androgens. In PCOS (see Chapter 155), both ovaries are larger and more echogenic than normal. They contain many small follicular cysts. The hirsutism seen in these cases may result from an increased androgen production by the ovarian cysts.

Incomplete Isosexual (Pseudoprecocious) Puberty in Boys

Isosexual pseudoprecocity of sexual development in boys is due to an increase in circulating androgen or androgen-like substances either because of their production by adrenal glands or testes or by their addition to the bloodstream from an exogenous source. CAH is the most common cause for excessive androgen production by the adrenal gland of either sex. Affected males are born with normal external genitalia, but if the CAH is untreated they soon develop signs of sexual precocity. Isosexual pseudoprecocious puberty in males, sometimes associated with signs of glucocorticoid excess, can also occur because of androgen-secreting neoplasms of the adrenal cortex (adenocarcinoma, benign adenoma). A rare cause of isosexual precocity in boys is an androgen-secreting Leydig cell tumor of the testis (benign or malignant) (see Chapter 154). Several extrapituitary hCG-secreting tumors can also result in an incomplete form of isosexual precocious puberty by stimulating testosterone production by the Leydig cells of the testis. These tumors include some hepatomas, hepatoblastomas, and some teratomas or chorioepitheliomas of the mediastinum and retroperitoneum. A suprasellar germinoma or ectopic pinealoma may secrete hCG and cause pseudoprecocious puberty in males through the same mechanism. A familial form of gonadotropin-independent precocious puberty in boys is caused by premature maturation and sometimes hyperplasia of the Leydig cells of the testis, with production of testosterone. Exposure to exogenous androgens or the administration of hCG for undescended testes may be further causes of incomplete virilization in males.

Adolescent Gynecomastia and Feminizing Disorders in Boys

Mild breast development may occur transiently in adolescent boys between 13 and 15 years of age. The gynecomastia, although sometimes pronounced, is seldom severe enough to require surgical correction. It is usually bilateral, is idiopathic, and may be familial. Usually, no source of excessive androgen is found. The gynecomastia generally regresses in 2 or 3 years, but in a few cases it may persist into adult life. Pathologic causes of gynecomastia in boys, sometimes associated with other signs of feminization, may be due to exposure to exogenous estrogens, as well as to the presence of an estrogen-secreting neoplasm of the testis or adrenal cortex or a prolactin-secreting neoplasm of the pituitary gland. Gynecomastia may also be noted in Klinefelter syndrome, congenital bilateral anorchia, acquired testicular failure, and in other conditions with some biochemical defect in testosterone production or androgen end-organ receptor.

Clinical and Laboratory Evaluation of Precocious Puberty

A detailed medical history and physical examination can help make the correct diagnosis. A history of previous exposure to estrogen or androgenic substances should be questioned. Physical examination should denote the type and degree of pubertal development as well as the size, shape, and firmness of the testes. In complete precocious puberty, both testes are enlarged; in partial sexual precocity they are often of normal size. Unilateral testicular enlargement suggests a testicular neoplasm. The abdomen should be evaluated for a flank or pelvic mass. A detailed neurologic evaluation should be obtained, including funduscopic examination. The presence of café au lait spots should suggest the diagnosis of fibrous dysplasia or neurofibromatosis. The latter may be associated with intracranial neoplasms, mostly gliomas, in or around the hypothalamus, which may lead to increased pituitary function and precocious puberty. Laboratory studies may include luteinizing hormone, follicle-stimulating hormone, and estradiol levels; gonadotropin response to GnRH; thyroid studies; and vaginal smear in girls as well as plasma and urinary testosterone levels.

Imaging Workup of Precocious Puberty

An anteroposterior film of the left hand, including carpal bones and distal forearm, is used for bone age determination. Bone age is commonly advanced in patients with true precocious puberty and in patients with androgenic stimulation but may be normal or only slightly increased in patients with premature thelarche or adrenarche. Normal bone ages are followed at 6-month intervals. The skeletal length is often increased early in cases with advanced bone age. However, if the precocious puberty is not treated, premature fusion of the epiphyses may develop and result in a decrease in the patient's potential height.

Imaging studies may be used to search for a possible causative intra-abdominal mass. Abdominal US, with emphasis on the adrenals and the ovaries, has become, together with bone age determination, the primary radiologic study in the initial evaluation of patients with precocious puberty. In girls with true precocious puberty, pelvic US may show some bilateral enlargement of the ovaries and prominence of the uterus. In rare cases, a large estrogen-secreting ovarian cyst has resulted in stimulation of the hypothalamic-pituitary complex, causing true precocious puberty as described earlier. Small and multiple ovarian cysts/follicles may be seen in girls with true precocious puberty because of high gonadotropin levels, but may also be seen in those with isosexual pseudoprecocity. These cystic ovaries may look and be similar to those seen normally throughout childhood. Pseudoprecocity caused by the autonomous estrogen secretion of an ovarian cyst or tumor will be denoted by asymmetry of the ovaries of the child, with the autonomous mass being found in the larger ovary (see Fig. 156-2). The finding in prepubertal girls of an increased uterine size and a well-defined central endometrial echo indicates an increase in circulating estrogen from any cause. A skeletal survey is indicated when fibrous dysplasia is suspected.

Patients with isosexual precocious puberty that is suspected to be of the complete or central type should have MRI of the brain with special attention to the tuber cinereum. Skull radiographs are of limited diagnostic value but may show intracranial calcifications, enlargement of the sella turcica, signs of increased intracranial pressure, or skull changes of fibrous dysplasia.

DELAYED OR ABSENT PUBERTAL DEVELOPMENT

Puberty is considered to be delayed and should be investigated in girls when secondary sex characteristics fail to appear by 13 years of age, considered two standard deviations beyond the norm. Causes of pubertal delay in girls are also causes for primary amenorrhea. Evaluations for pubertal delays in boys are suggested when pubic and axillary hair or other external secondary characteristics, particularly enlargement of the testes and penis, fail to appear by age 14. Delayed puberty or failure of puberty to develop may be idiopathic (constitutional) or due to chronic systemic disorders, disorders of the hypothalamic-pituitary complex causing decreased gonadotropin secretion (secondary or hypogonadotropic hypogonadism), or primary disorders of the gonads with a secondary elevation of gonadotropic hormone secretion (primary or hypergonadotropic hypogonadism).

> **Puberty is considered to be delayed when secondary sex characteristics fail to appear by 13 years of age in girls and 14 years of age in boys.**

Idiopathic (Constitutional) Pubertal Delay

In some otherwise normal children, the onset of puberty is delayed for up to several years. When puberty eventually starts, it usually continues to completely normal secondary sexual development. These occurrences underline the fact that there may be constitutional or genetic causes for delay in the maturation of the hypothalamic-pituitary complex. Often, such children may have delay in bone age and height development. The ability to differentiate between constitutional pubertal delays in otherwise normal children and true disorders of the hypothalamic-pituitary axis may not be simple and make take years of clinical and laboratory observation.

Delayed Puberty in Chronic Systemic Disorders

Delayed puberty may occur on a physiologic basis in patients with chronic disease such as inflammatory bowel disease (Fig. 156-5) or long-term disorders of cardiac, pulmonary, renal, or other body systems. Patients with other long-term debilitating processes as well as anorexia nervosa may have delays in pubertal development. Such delays may also be noted in children or adolescents who undergo prolonged and vigorous physical exertion, such as long-distance running or ballet. All these possibilities must be considered in evaluating patients with amenorrhea as well, and may justify delaying a full endocrinologic evaluation. Puberty may develop or proceed normally in some of these patients after improvement or removal of the precipitating cause. Any halt, however, in the pubertal development of a patient is a cause for concern and immediate endocrinologic workup.

> **Delayed puberty may occur on a physiologic basis in patients with chronic or debilitating disease, extreme or prolonged exercise, as well as anorexia nervosa.**

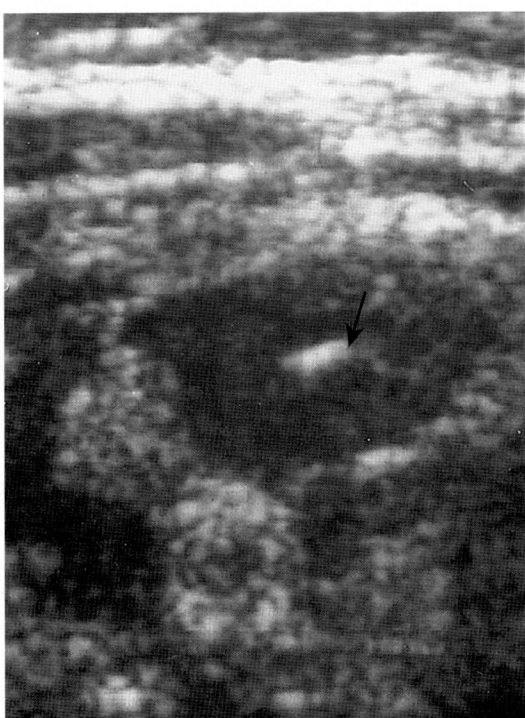

FIGURE 156-5. Crohn disease as a cause of delayed puberty or primary amenorrhea. A transverse sonogram through the right lower quadrant shows an abnormally thick bowel wall about a central echogenic linear area *(arrow)* representing air in the small bowel lumen. The area did not compress well. This teenager presented for a workup for amenorrhea/delayed puberty. Ultrasonography showed an infantile uterus. After noting the abnormal small bowel, the history of chronic disease (i.e., long-term Crohn disease) was elicited.

Hypogonadism Caused by Hypothalamic-Pituitary Disorders (Hypogonadotropic Hypogonadism)

Several disorders of the hypothalamic-pituitary complex result in decreased gonadotropin production and, secondarily, a decrease in gonadal sex steroids. Impaired or absent gonadal function causes an absence of pubertal development. In girls, the uterus remains infantile, menses does not occur, and breast budding and other secondary sexual characteristics do not develop. In boys, the penis and scrotum are infantile and the testes remain immature and smaller than expected for age. Pubic and axillary hair is scanty or absent, the voice remains high pitched, and there is often increased fat deposition, particularly at the hips, pelvis, abdomen, and breast. Delayed closure of the epiphyses with elongation of the limbs is observed unless there is an associated growth hormone deficiency.

Causative abnormalities include intracranial tumors such as craniopharyngioma, hypothalamic and optic gliomas, dysgerminoma, as well as other tumors of the pituitary gland and hypothalamus or adjacent areas. Other manifestations of pituitary insufficiency, such as diabetes insipidus and short stature, may be present. Primary or secondary hypogonadotropic hypogonadism may also be seen in patients with Langerhans cell histiocytosis and in patients with certain congenital midline defects of the face, the base of the skull, and the CNS (e.g., septo-optic dysplasia or holoprosencephaly), which may be associated with developmental anomalies of the hypothalamus and pituitary gland resulting in hypogonadism.

> **Primary or secondary hypogonadotropic hypogonadism may be seen in patients with histiocytosis, congenital midline CNS defects, CNS neoplasms, and primary gonadotropin deficiencies.**

Functional causes of hypogonadism include idiopathic hypopituitarism characterized by short stature resulting from growth hormone deficiency and sometimes other findings associated with deficiencies of other pituitary hormones. Cases of isolated gonadotropic deficiency, sporadic or familial, may occur in association with anosmia or hyposmia and other abnormalities that characterize Kallmann syndrome. Isolated LH deficiency in males, sometimes familial, results in failure of pubertal development, usually associated with gynecomastia but with the preservation of spermatogenesis (fertile eunuch syndrome). Hypogonadism, probably also related to abnormalities of hypothalamic function, can be observed in Prader-Willi and Laurence-Moon-Biedl syndromes.

Hypogonadism Caused by Gonadal Lesions (Hypergonadotropic Hypogonadism)

Certain congenital or acquired lesions of the gonads may result in hypogonadism and failure of pubertal development. Gonadal sex steroids are decreased, and because of this there is an increased secretion of gonadotropins by the pituitary, hence the term *hypergonadotropic hypogonadism*. Just as in hypogonadotropic hypogonadism, there is absent pubertal development in girls or boys. The key gonadal lesions in girls include Turner syndrome, XX gonadal dysgenesis, XY gonadal dysgenesis, and a gonadal dysgenesis with galactosemia and immune oophoritis (often associated with Hashimoto thyroiditis, hypoparathyroidism, adrenal insufficiency, pernicious anemia, chronic active hepatitis, and candidiasis). Hypergonadotropic hypogonadism can also occur among patients with normal karyotypes who develop secondary ovarian failure either by infarction, as with cases of bilateral ovarian torsion, surgical removal of both ovaries, radiation therapy (usually of 800 cGy or greater) to the pelvis, chemotherapy, or autoimmune oophoritis.

Gonadal lesions in boys leading to hypogonadism include congenital bilateral anorchia with otherwise normal external genitalia, caused by resorption of the testes after the 13th week of gestation (vanishing testes and functional prepubertal castrate syndromes) and acquired testicular atrophy resulting from bilateral testicular torsion, surgical injury during bilateral orchiopexy, radiation, or other causes. Absence of puberty is also observed in some genetic males born with an entirely female phenotype, including those with XY gonadal dysgenesis, and some forms of male pseudohermaphroditism with impaired biosynthesis of active sex steroids as a result of an inherited enzymatic deficiency.

DIAGNOSTIC AND HISTORICAL CONSIDERATIONS

Important information may be obtained from the patient's family history, past medical history, associated medical disorders, and physical examination. On physical examination, special emphasis should be placed on pubertal staging (Tanner classification), on assessment of general growth and maturation, on detection of signs and symptoms of CNS disease, and on systemic diseases or syndromes that may be chronic and or debilitating and therefore associated with abnormal pubertal development. Visual fields testing, gynecologic evaluation, and chromosomal analysis should be carried out as indicated. The hormonal studies include measurements of serum testosterone, estradiol, and gonadotropins; gonadotropic response to GnRH stimulation; and testosterone response to hCG stimulation. Measurements of circulating prolactin and growth hormone, as well as thyroid function tests, may be undertaken in special cases. The radiologic procedures include bone age determination, head CT or MRI, pelvic US to evaluate the size of the ovaries and uterus, and other studies as indicated.

ANALYSIS OF PATIENTS WITH AMENORRHEA

Causes of pubertal delay in girls may be similar to causes of primary or secondary amenorrhea. Primary amenorrhea is defined as a lack of menses by age 16. Secondary amenorrhea is defined as a cessation of menses at any point in time after menarche and before menopause.

> **Primary amenorrhea is defined as a lack of menses by age 16. Secondary amenorrhea is defined as a cessation of menses at any time after menarche and before menopause.**

TABLE 156-1

Etiology of Primary Amenorrhea

Hypothalamus
  Systemic illness
  Chronic disease
  Familial
  Stress
  Competitive athletics
  Eating disorders
  Obesity
  Drugs
Pituitary
  Idiopathic hypopituitarism
  Tumor
  Hemochromatosis
Thyroid gland
  Hypothyroidism
  Hyperthyroidism
Adrenal glands
  Congenital adrenocortical hyperplasia
  Adrenal tumor
Ovaries
  Gonadal dysgenesis
  Ovarian failure
  Polycystic ovary syndrome
  Ovarian tumor
Cervix: agenesis
Vagina
  Agenesis
  Transverse septum
Hymen: imperforate

Adapted from Emans S, Goldstein D (eds): Delayed puberty and menstrual irregularities. *In* Pediatric and Adolescent Gynecology, 3rd ed. Boston, Little Brown, 1990:149.

Primary amenorrhea has many causes and involves several organ systems (Table 156-1). It may be seen in adolescents with normal pubertal development as well as those with delayed sexual development, delayed menarche with some pubertal development, and delayed menarche plus virilization. We have already reviewed many of its causes. They include hypogonadotropic hypogonadism, hypergonadotropic hypogonadism, pseudo-hermaphroditism, female adolescents with virilization, PCOS, eugonadism estrogenization with genital obstruction (e.g., hematometra/hematometrocolpos), and uterine aplasia or hypoplasia. Secondary amenorrhea is often due physiologically to pregnancy and pathologically to PCOS.

SUGGESTED READINGS

Argyropoulos M, Kiortsis D: MRI of the hypothalamic-pituitary axis in children. Pediatr Radiol 2005;35:1045

Bajpai A, Sharma J, Kabra M, et al: Precocious puberty: clinical and endocrine profile and factors indicating neurogenic precocity in Indian children. J Pediatr Endocrinol Metab 2002;15:1173

Battaglia C, Artini P, D'Ambrogio G, et al: The role of color Doppler imaging in the diagnosis of polycystic ovary syndrome. Am J Obstet Gynecol 1995;172:108

Cohen HL: Evaluation of the adolescent and young adult with amenorrhea: role of US. *In* Bluth E, Arger P, Hertzberg B, Middleton W (eds): Syllabus: A Special Course in Ultrasound: Clinical Questions, Practical Answers. Oak Brook, IL, RSNA Publications 1996:171

Cohen HL, Bober S, Bow S: Imaging the pediatric pelvis: the normal and abnormal genital system and simulators of its diseases. Urol Radiol 1992;14:273

Cohen HL, Eisenberg P, Mandel F, Haller J: Ovarian cysts are common in premenarchal girls: a sonographic study of 101 children 2–12 years old. AJR Am J Roentgenol 1992;159:89

Cohen HL, Shapiro MA, Mandel FS, Shapiro ML: Normal ovaries in neonates and infants: a sonographic study of 77 patients 1 day to 24 months old. AJR Am J Roentgenol 1993;160:583

Currarino G, Wood B, Majd M: Abnormalities of the genital tract. *In* Silverman F, Kuhn J (eds): Caffey's Pediatric X-Ray Diagnosis, 9th ed. St. Louis, Mosby–Year Book, 1993:1375

Daya S: Habitual abortion. *In* Copeland L (ed): Textbook of Gynecology. Philadelphia, WB Saunders, 1993:204

Emans S, Goldstein D (eds): Delayed puberty and menstrual irregularities. *In* Pediatric and Adolescent Gynecology, 3rd ed. Boston, Little Brown, 1990:149

Emans S, Goldstein D (eds): The physiology of puberty. *In* Pediatric and Adolescent Gynecology, 3rd ed. Boston, Little Brown, 1990:95

Falsetti L, Pasinetti E, Mazzani M, Gastaldi A: Weight loss and menstrual cycle: clinical and endocrinological evaluation. Gynecol Endocrinol 1992;6:49

Ganong W (ed): The gonads: development and function of the reproductive system. *In* Review of Medical Physiology, 17th ed. Norwalk, CT, Appleton & Lange, 1995:399

Herter L, Magalnaes J, Spritzer P: Association of ovarian volume and serum LH levels in adolescent patients with menstrual disorders and/or hirsutism. Braz J Med Biol Res 1993;26:1041

Kawashima A, Sandler C, Fishman E, et al: Spectrum of CT findings in nonmalignant disease of the adrenal gland. Radiographics 1998;18:393

Larsen W, Felmar E, Wallace M, Frieder R: Sertoli-Leydig cell tumor of the ovary: a rare cause of amenorrhea. Obstet Gynecol 1992;79:831

Lee PA: Neuroendocrinology of puberty. Semin Reprod Endocrinol 1988;6:13

Lee PA: Physiology of puberty. *In* Principles and Practice of Endocrinology and Metabolism. Philadelphia, JB Lippincott, 1990:740

Lee PA, O'Dea L: Primary and secondary testicular insufficiency. Pediatr Clin North Am 1990;37:1359

Mahoney CP: Adolescent gynecomastia: differential diagnosis and management. Pediatr Clin North Am 1990;37:1389

Polk D: Abnormalities of sexual differentiation. *In* Taeush H, Ballard R, Avery M (eds): Schaeffer & Avery's Diseases of the Newborn, 6th ed. Philadelphia, WB Saunders, 1991:946

Reid R: Amenorrhea. *In* Copeland L (ed): Textbook of Gynecology. Philadelphia, WB Saunders, 1993:367

Rosenfeld RL: Clinical Review 6: Diagnosis and management of delayed puberty. J Clin Endocrinol Metab 1990;70:559

Rosenfeld RL: Hyperandrogenism in peripubertal girls. Pediatr Clin North Am 1990;37:1333

Schwartz ID, Root AW: Puberty in girls: early, incomplete or precocious? Contemp Pediatr 1990;7:147

Shah R, Woolley M, Costin G: Testicular feminization syndrome: the androgen insensitivity syndrome. J Pediatr Surg 1992;27:757

Starceski PJ: Hypothalamic hamartomas and sexual precocity. Am J Dis Child 1990;144:225

Takahashi K, Okada M, Ozaki T, et al: Transvaginal ultrasonographic morphology in polycystic ovarian syndrome. Gynecol Obstet Invest 1995;39:201

Tarani L, Lampariello S, Raguso G, et al: Pregnancy in patients with Turner's syndrome: six new cases and review of literature. Gynecol Endocrinol 1998;12:83

Wheeler MD, Styne DM: Diagnosis and management of precocious puberty. Pediatr Clin North Am 1990;37:1255

CHAPTER

157 Abdominal Trauma

CARLOS J. SIVIT

Trauma accounts for more than 500,000 hospital admissions and 20,000 deaths per year in children. Following the head, the abdomen is the second most common site of injury, and approximately 80% of abdominal injuries are due to blunt force trauma. The most common reported mechanism is motor vehicle crashes, followed by automobile–pedestrian injuries. Other common injuries are related to falls from a height and bicycle injuries. In young children, injuries may also result from intentional trauma.

Computed tomography (CT) is the imaging method of choice in the evaluation of abdominal and pelvic injury after blunt trauma in hemodynamically stable children. Evaluation with CT allows for accurate detection and quantification of injury to solid and hollow viscera. CT also identifies and quantifies intraperitoneal and extraperitoneal fluid and blood and can detect active bleeding. Additionally, CT reveals associated bony injury to ribs, spine, and pelvis. The roles of CT in the assessment of injured children include establishing the presence or absence of visceral and bony injury, identifying injury that requires close monitoring and operative intervention, detecting active bleeding, and estimating associated blood loss. A normal CT also serves an important function in management of injury and in exclusion of an intra-abdominal or pelvic source of blood loss.

The rapid and accurate evaluation of injured children with CT has resulted in improved triage and has contributed to reduced morbidity and mortality. CT findings have been shown to change the initial management plan after clinical assessment in nearly one half of children assessed after blunt abdominal trauma. In most of these cases, the use of CT resulted in a decision to reduce the intensity of care. Thus, the use of CT as the primary screening modality in the assessment of injured children, along with improvements in supportive care, has played a critical role in the success of nonoperative management of solid viscus injuries.

INDICATIONS

Indications for imaging after blunt trauma include physical examination or laboratory findings suggestive of abdominal injury. These include abdominal bruising or ecchymosis, abdominal distention, abdominal pain, absence of bowel sounds, vomiting, decreased hematocrit, hematuria, and blood per rectum or nasopharyngeal tube aspirate. Children should be hemodynamically stable prior to CT. An unstable patient must be stabilized or should proceed directly to surgery for evaluation.

Clinical variables that have been associated with a high risk of injury include gross hematuria, abdominal tenderness, lap belt ecchymoses, and a low trauma score. Lap belt ecchymoses represent an important high-risk marker for injury. These linear ecchymoses across the lower abdomen or flank are seen in passengers wearing a lap belt, who are involved in motor vehicle crashes. The ecchymoses show the pattern of the lap belt. Such ecchymoses are associated with a complex of injury to the lumbar spine, bowel, and bladder that accounts for most injuries to belted motor vehicle passengers.

Two clinical findings that are frequently used as indications for CT but have a low diagnostic yield in predicting injury are asymptomatic hematuria and neurologic impairment in the absence of abdominal signs and symptoms. Abdominal injuries in both of these groups have been shown to be uncommon and minor in significance. Several points to be noted regarding hematuria and abdominal injury include the following: (1) Most children with hematuria do not have urinary tract injury, (2) non–urinary tract injury is observed more frequently than urinary tract injury in children with hematuria, and (3) asymptomatic hematuria is a low-risk indicator for abdominal injury.

> **Indications for CT scanning after blunt abdominal trauma include gross hematuria, abdominal tenderness, lap belt ecchymoses, and a low trauma score.**

TECHNIQUE

A precise protocol is critical in minimizing the length of the examination and maximizing the information obtained. Monitoring devices and metallic leads should be moved from the scanning plane because they yield streak artifacts. Gastric distention should be relieved because artifacts may arise from air-fluid interfaces. Sedation is rarely required prior to CT. However, excessive patient motion results in image degradation. Therefore, in select instances, a short-acting sedative may be necessary if diagnostic images are to be obtained.

The use of intravenous (IV) contrast by rapid bolus injection is essential for maximizing opacification of solid viscera and ensuring adequate injury detection. We administer 2 ml/kg to a maximum amount of 120 ml. Without appropriate IV contrast administration, solid viscus laceration or hematoma may be relatively isodense to unenhanced or poorly enhanced solid viscera. Additionally, the use of IV contrast allows for the detection of active hemorrhage. Scanning of the pelvis may be delayed by several minutes after IV contrast injection to optimize bladder distention by IV contrast. If a renal parenchymal injury is noted at initial scanning, delayed scanning through the kidneys is helpful in the detection of renal collecting system injury.

Controversy surrounds the use of oral contrast after blunt trauma. Potential advantages to the use of oral contrast include (1) enhanced detection of small intramural or mesenteric hematomas, (2) improved delineation of the pancreas from surrounding bowel, and (3) detection of oral contrast extravasation as a sign of bowel rupture. Potential disadvantages include (1) time constraints and decreased bowel motility in injured children, which limit the possibility of opacification much beyond the proximal small bowel, (2) creation of artifacts from air-contrast interfaces in the stomach, and (3) the possibility of vomiting with resultant aspiration. If oral contrast is used, dilute (2%) water-soluble contrast material should be administered at least 30 minutes prior to scanning.

COMPUTED TOMOGRAPHIC FINDINGS IN ABDOMINAL TRAUMA

Hepatic Injury

The liver is the most frequently injured viscus after blunt trauma. Most hepatic injury occurs in the posterior segment of the right lobe. The effects of blunt force are maximized in this location because the posterior right lobe is fixed by the coronary ligaments, which limit its movement while the rest of the liver is free to move; resultant shearing forces are centered in the posterior segment of the right lobe. A hepatic laceration appears as a non-enhancing region of varying configuration (Fig. 157-1) that may be linear or branching. Lacerations may be associated with a parenchymal or a subcapsular hematoma.

The liver is surrounded by a thin capsule that in turn is covered by peritoneal reflection of thin connective tissue. The presence of hemoperitoneum associated with hepatic injury principally relates to violation of the liver capsule at the site of injury. In several large series, hepatic injury was associated with hemoperitoneum in approximately two thirds of cases. Associated hemoperitoneum may be seen throughout the greater peritoneal cavity. Often the largest fluid pockets are located in the pelvis.

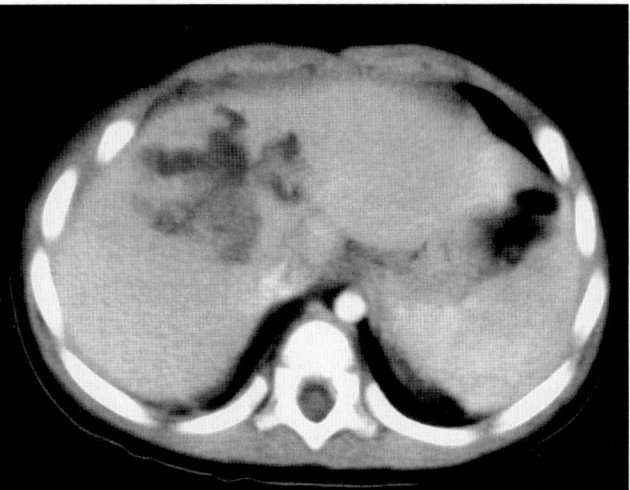

FIGURE 157-1. Hepatic laceration. Contrast-enhanced CT scan through the upper abdomen reveals a complex hepatic laceration.

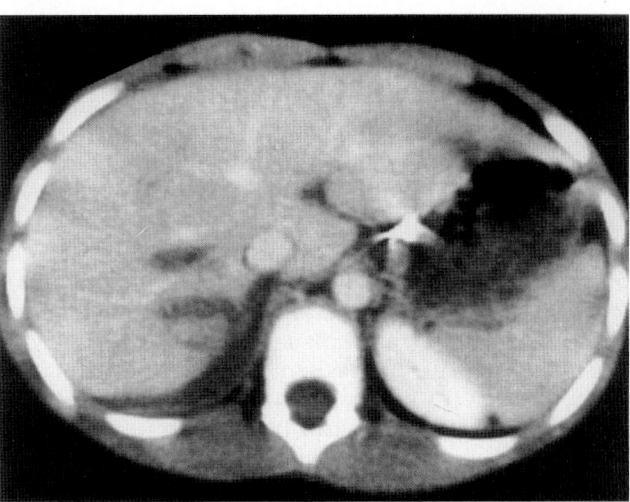

FIGURE 157-2. Hepatic laceration through the bare area. Contrast-enhanced CT scan through the upper abdomen reveals a laceration that extends into the bare area of the liver.

Hepatic injury may not be associated with intraperitoneal hemorrhage if the injury does not extend to the surface of the liver, if the hepatic capsule is not disrupted, or if the injury extends to the liver surface in the bare area of the liver, which is devoid of peritoneal reflection (Fig. 157-2). The bare area is the site of insertion of the coronary ligaments. Injury that extends to the bare area may lead to associated retroperitoneal hemorrhage, with blood often surrounding the right adrenal gland or extending into the anterior pararenal space.

Circumferential zones of periportal low attenuation may be seen in the liver after trauma (Fig. 157-3). The presence of these low attenuation zones does not indicate hepatic injury. They are likely due to intravascular third-space fluid losses that occur after fluid resuscitation. The fluid extends to the periportal lymphatics, which are located within the portal triad. Thus, the periportal zones of low attenuation result from distention of these lymphatics.

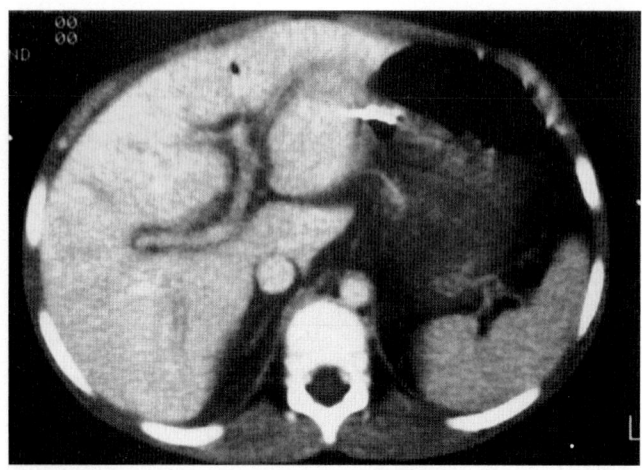

A

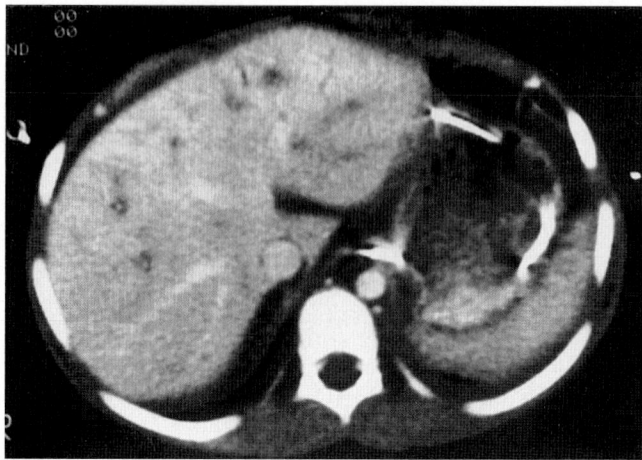

B

FIGURE 157-3. Periportal low attenuation zones. Contrast-enhanced CT scan through the liver reveals circumferential periportal low attenuation zones surrounding the right and left main portal veins **(A)** and surrounding the peripheral portal venules **(B)**.

A number of grading scales have been proposed to quantify the severity of hepatic injury. These scales emphasize the anatomic extent of the injury, including capsular integrity, extent of subcapsular collection, extent of parenchymal disruption, and state of the vascular pedicle. The most widely used grading scale was developed by the American Association for the Surgery of Trauma. It was initially devised to reflect surgical findings but is commonly used to report organ injury severity at CT. In children, these scales are not predictive of the need for operative management because the vast majority of hepatic injuries can be successfully managed nonoperatively regardless of severity, in that bleeding typically stops spontaneously. It has been reported that between 1% and 3% of children with hepatic injury require surgical hemostasis. This is likely a result of the relatively smaller size of blood vessels and enhanced vasoconstrictive response in children relative to adults. However, injury grading scales are often used in patient management decision making regarding duration and intensity of hospitalization and activity restriction.

> The liver is the most commonly injured viscus after blunt trauma in children.

Splenic Injury

Splenic injury is also common after blunt trauma. It is frequently associated with other organ injuries. Splenic lacerations have a variable appearance ranging from a linear to a branching pattern. Because the spleen is much smaller than the liver, complex injury results in shattering or fragmentation of the organ (Fig. 157-4). Associated intraparenchymal or subcapsular hematoma may be present (Fig. 157-5). As with hepatic injury, associated intraperitoneal hemorrhage is not always present. If the splenic capsule remains intact, no hemoperitoneum is associated. Absence of hemoperitoneum is observed in approximately 25% of splenic injuries. Blood can

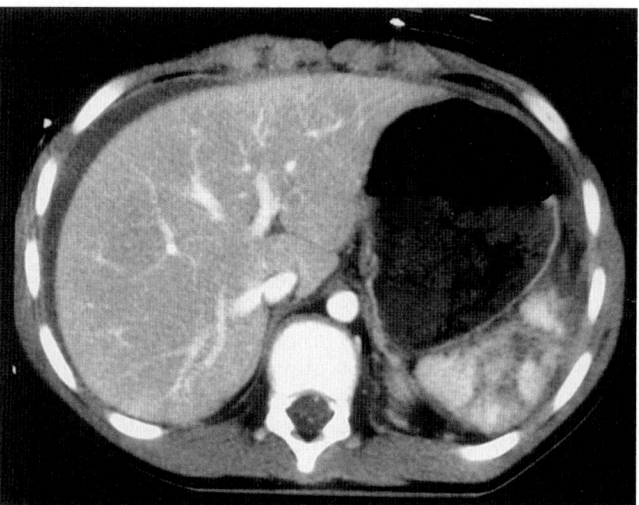

FIGURE 157-4. Shattered spleen. Contrast-enhanced CT scan through the upper abdomen shows a shattered spleen.

track into the retroperitoneum after splenic injury. This typically occurs with injury that extends to the splenic hilum. In these instances, blood extends along the splenorenal ligament into the anterior pararenal space surrounding the pancreas (Fig. 157-6).

Various injury grading scales have been described for quantifying injury to the spleen. As is true for hepatic injury, these scales are not predictive of surgical treatment in children because bleeding typically stops spontaneously, and nonoperative management is successful in most splenic injuries. Grade of injury is often used for clinical decision making, similar to the use of grading in hepatic injury.

Pitfalls that may result in false-positive diagnosis of splenic injury include heterogeneous early splenic enhancement and splenic lobulations and clefts that mimic a laceration. The heterogeneous splenic enhancement is due to differences in enhancement between red

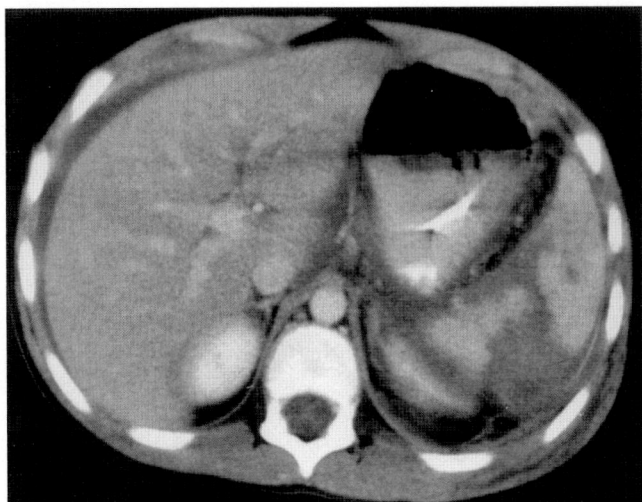

FIGURE 157-5. Splenic laceration with associated intraparenchymal hematoma. Contrast-enhanced CT scan through the upper abdomen reveals a splenic laceration with associated intraparenchymal hematoma posteriorly.

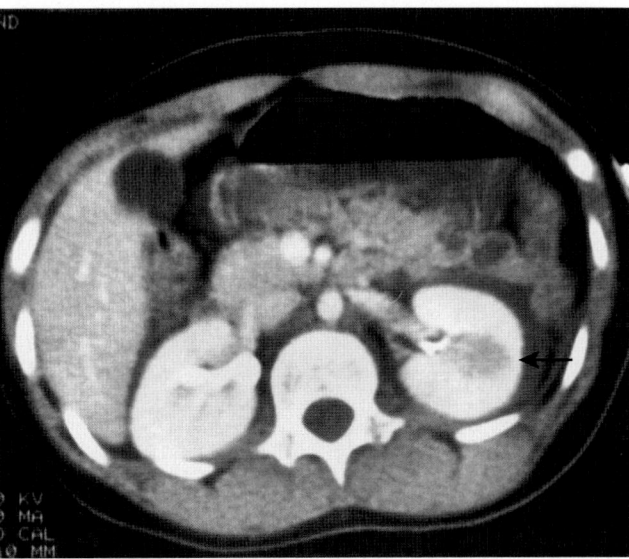

FIGURE 157-7. Left renal contusion. Contrast-enhanced CT scan through the midabdomen shows a rounded focus of low attenuation in the midpole of the left kidney *(arrow)* indicative of contusion.

Renal Injury

The kidney is the third most frequently injured abdominal viscus in children. Renal parenchymal injury typically results from direct impact, whereas vascular and collecting system injury usually results from deceleration. The most common type of renal injury is the parenchymal contusion, which manifests on CT as a focal or diffuse region of delayed contrast enhancement (Fig. 157-7). The contusion, which represents an organ bruise, is characterized by microscopic areas of hemorrhage and surrounding edema. The involved kidney may also appear larger on CT as a result of the associated edema.

Renal injury may be complicated by perirenal hematoma, which may be subcapsular or perinephric. These two types of hematoma can be differentiated on the basis of CT features: A subcapsular hematoma is limited in its extension by the renal capsule and therefore exerts greater mass effect on the renal parenchyma (Fig. 157-8), whereas a perinephric hematoma is distributed throughout the perirenal space and typically exhibits less mass effect on the renal parenchyma.

Renal collecting system injury results in urinary extravasation of IV contrast medium (Fig. 157-9). Delayed scanning CT is useful in detecting such extravasation. Urine leakage that remains encapsulated in the perirenal space is termed a *urinoma*. Occasionally, hemorrhage or urinary extravasation may extend into the pelvis owing to direct communication between the perirenal space in the abdomen and the prevesical extraperitoneal space in the pelvis. Renal collecting system injury is typically managed nonoperatively, particularly if the leak is confined to the perirenal space.

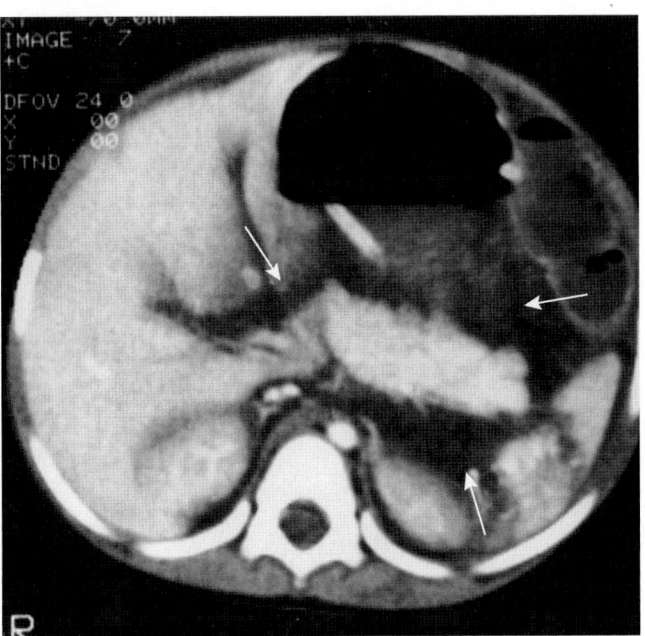

FIGURE 157-6. Splenic injury with retroperitoneal extension of hemorrhage. Contrast-enhanced CT scan through the upper abdomen shows a splenic laceration associated with blood in the anterior pararenal space *(arrows)* surrounding the pancreas.

and white pulp in the spleen. This artifact can be avoided by instituting a delay of at least 70 seconds prior to scanning after administration of IV contrast. Splenic clefts and lobulations typically have smooth contours and thus can be differentiated from lacerations, which typically have irregular contours.

> **Avoid the pitfall of heterogeneous splenic enhancement.**

Pancreatic Injury

Pancreatic injury is relatively uncommon in children. Injury to the body of the pancreas typically results from

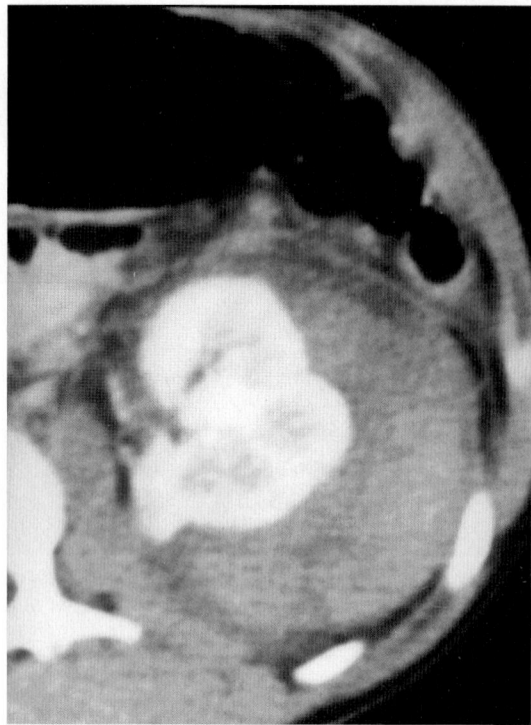

FIGURE 157-8. Subcapsular renal hematoma. Contrast-enhanced CT through the midabdomen shows a large, left-sided subcapsular hematoma compressing the left renal parenchyma.

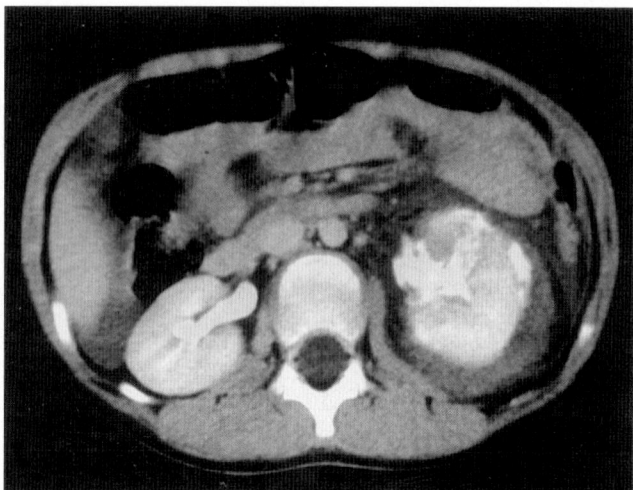

FIGURE 157-9. Renal collecting system injury. Contrast-enhanced CT scan through the midabdomen shows a left renal laceration with extravasation of intravenous contrast into the perirenal space. Also note low attenuation perinephric fluid.

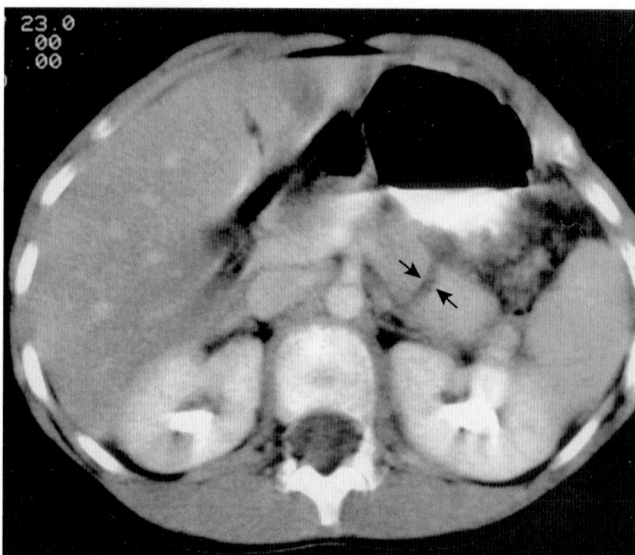

FIGURE 157-10. Pancreatic injury. Contrast-enhanced CT scan through the upper abdomen shows a laceration through the junction of the body and the tail of the pancreas (arrows).

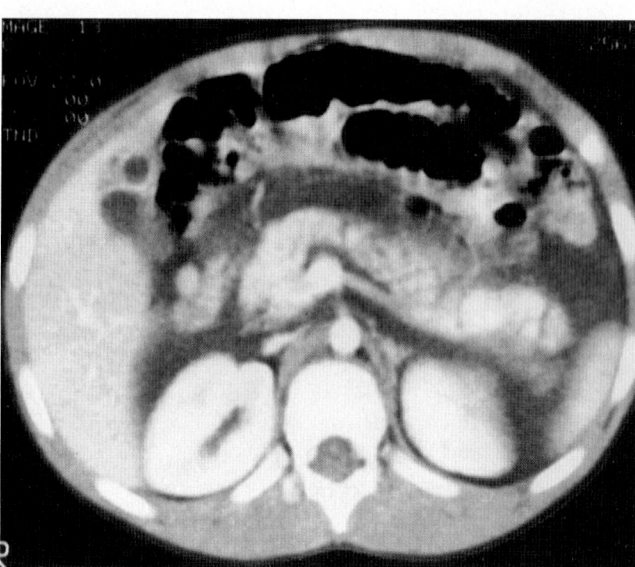

FIGURE 157-11. Pancreatic injury with associated peripancreatic fluid. Contrast-enhanced CT scan through the upper abdomen shows fluid in the anterior pararenal space surrounding the pancreas. Also note fluid dissecting between the splenic vein and the pancreas.

direct compression of the gland against the vertebral column. The most common cause is a bicycle handlebar injury. Injury to the head or tail of the pancreas results from a blow to the flank. Direct signs of injury may be difficult to identify because of the small size of the gland, the paucity of surrounding fat, and the minimal separation of fracture fragments (Fig. 157-10).

The best indicator of pancreatic injury at CT is unexplained peripancreatic fluid (fluid in the anterior pararenal space or lesser sac) (Fig. 157-11). This finding may be seen more often than the actual laceration. When fluid collects in the anterior pararenal space, it also may dissect between the pancreas and the splenic vein. Pancreatic injury is only one cause of fluid in the anterior pararenal space. Other causes include third-space intravascular fluid loss, blood that extends from injury to the spleen or to the bare area of the liver, blood or bowel contents from a duodenal injury, and blood or urine that exudes from a renal injury after disruption of the renal fascia.

Additional CT signs of pancreatic injury include focal or diffuse gland enlargement, stranding of peripancreatic and/or mesenteric fat, thickening of the anterior renal fascia, and free peritoneal fluid. These findings are typically due to a secondary pancreatitis that develops after injury. Trauma is the leading cause of pancreatitis in children.

A false-positive diagnosis of pancreatic injury may result from the partial volume effect caused by the gland's small size and undulating nature. This pitfall may be avoided by obtaining repeat sections through the pancreas with the use of thinner collimation and by creating coronal reformatted images that reflect overlapping data.

> **The best indicator of pancreatic injury on CT is unexplained peripancreatic fluid.**

Pancreatic injury may be complicated by peripancreatic fluid collections, which may evolve into pancreatic pseudocysts. Approximately one half of focal fluid collections that develop after pancreatic injury spontaneously resolve, and one half evolve into pseudocysts. The most common locations for pseudocyst formation is the intrapancreatic or peripancreatic anterior pararenal space, or lesser sac (Fig. 157-12). However, pseudocysts may develop anywhere in the abdomen or pelvis. Approximately one half of pseudocysts resolve spontaneously. The others require percutaneous or surgical drainage.

Currently, divergent opinions have been expressed regarding the management of pancreatic injury. Some workers have shown that nonoperative management of most pancreatic injury is successful, even when the pancreatic duct is involved. Others believe that distal pancreatectomy for transection to the left of the spine is the treatment of choice because it is definitive and is accompanied by an acceptable level of morbidity.

PERITONEAL FLUID AND HEMORRHAGE

Attenuation values of blood in the peritoneal cavity vary widely, depending on whether it is unclotted blood (hemoperitoneum), clotted blood, or active hemorrhage. Furthermore, several factors affect measured attenuation values for peritoneal fluid on CT, including measurement technique, fluid location within the field, artifacts, and delayed fluid enhancement after IV contrast administration. Unclotted hemoperitoneum has attenuation values that range from 20 to 60 Hounsfield units (H.U.). Approximately one third of fluid pockets exhibit attenuation values lower than 30 H.U. Low attenuation fluid (<60 H.U.) in the acutely injured child may also represent bile, urine, bowel contents, third-space fluid losses, or pre-existing ascites.

Clotted blood has higher attenuation values (60 to 90 H.U.) than free-flowing blood because of its greater density and hemoglobin content. Because clotted blood is typically seen adjacent to the site of injury, the presence of focal, higher attenuation clotted blood has been described as the "sentinel clot" sign; it is a marker for the principal site of hemorrhage and may occasionally be useful in localizing the site of injury.

Children are typically excluded from CT when ongoing bleeding is clinically evident. Occasionally, CT may reveal active hemorrhage in children who appear hemodynamically stable. The amount of hemoperitoneum noted on CT is not a measure of ongoing hemorrhage; rather, it reflects the cumulative amount of bleeding that occurred between the time of injury and the time that CT was obtained. The only sign of active hemorrhage on CT is the presence of focal or high attenuation areas (>90 H.U.) (Fig. 157-13). This finding has also been referred to in the literature as a contrast blush. The rate of active bleeding required for detection on CT is unclear. However, CT is useful not only in identifying active bleeding but in localizing the site of hemorrhage. Occasionally, this finding may be observed only on delayed scanning.

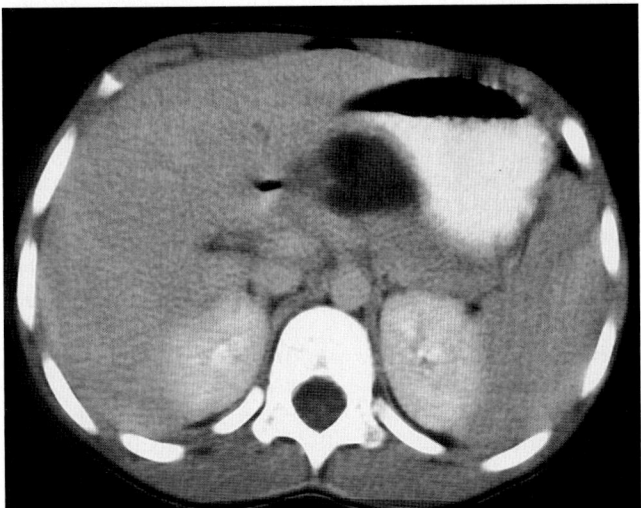

FIGURE 157-12. Pancreatic pseudocyst. Contrast-enhanced CT scan through the upper abdomen shows a focal fluid collection representing a pancreatic pseudocyst in the anterior pararenal space.

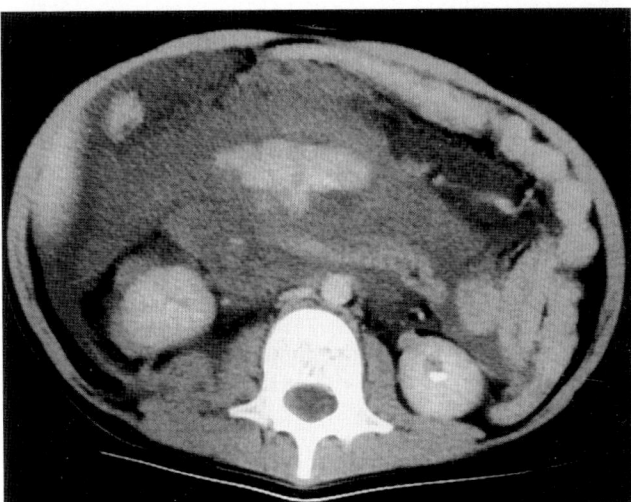

FIGURE 157-13. Active hemorrhage. Contrast-enhanced CT scan through the midabdomen shows a focal high attenuation collection representing intravenous contrast extravasation from a mesenteric arterial tear.

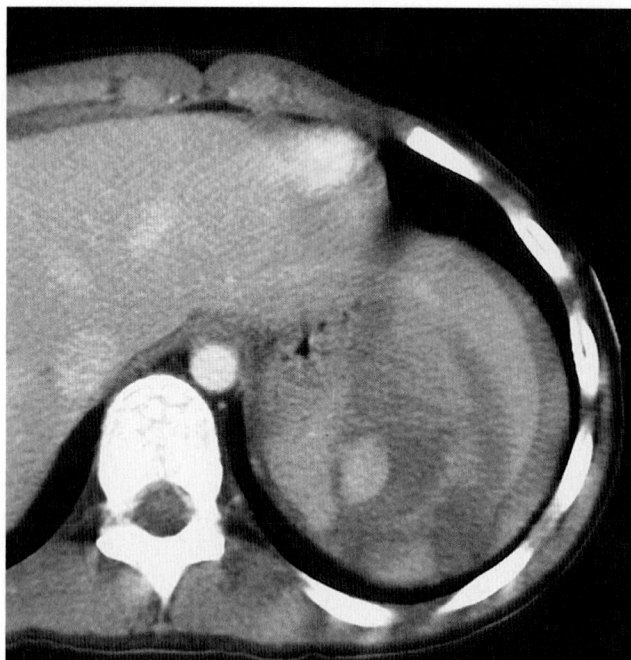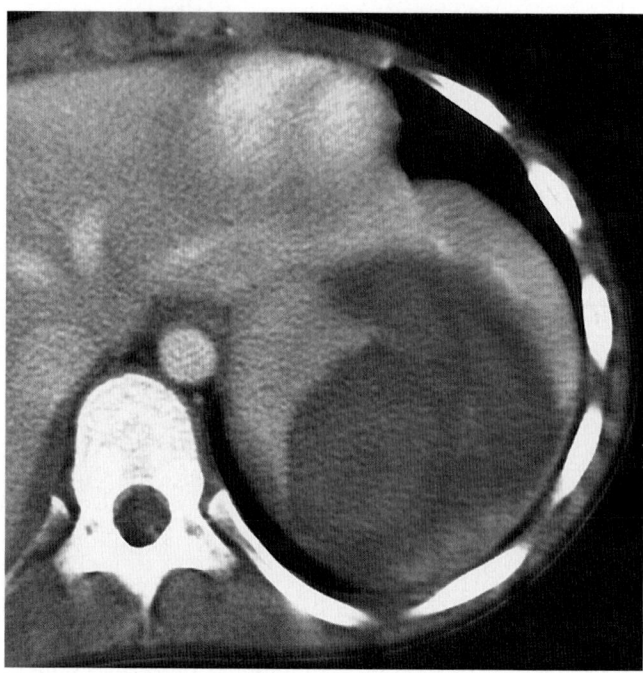

A   B

FIGURE 157-14. Active splenic hemorrhage that did not require laparotomy. **A,** Contrast-enhanced CT scan through the upper abdomen shows a complex splenic laceration with a focal area of increased attenuation within the spleen representing active hemorrhage. The patient was managed nonoperatively. **B,** Follow-up scan 1 week later shows resolving low attenuation hematoma within the spleen.

Most children with active hemorrhage detected on CT do not require operative intervention. It has been reported that 20% or less of children with hepatic or splenic injury and active hemorrhage have required operative hemostasis (Fig. 157-14).

The absence of peritoneal fluid or blood does not exclude the presence of hepatic or splenic injury. More than one third of hepatic injuries and one fourth of splenic injuries in children have no associated peritoneal fluid. The relatively high prevalence of hepatic and splenic injury without associated peritoneal fluid has significant implications for imaging strategies in the assessment of injured children. Sonography is highly sensitive in the detection of peritoneal fluid. However, the sensitivity of sonography in the detection of solid viscus injury has not been as good; more than one third of injuries have been missed in some studies. Further, the sole identification of fluid does not necessarily reveal the cause or the site of injury. Thus, if one relies on identification of peritoneal fluid as a marker for hepatic and splenic injury, one will miss a significant number of injuries.

> **Most children with active hemorrhage on CT do not require operative intervention.**

BOWEL INJURY

Bowel injury is uncommon after blunt trauma in children. However, partial-thickness injury can result in intramural hematoma, and full-thickness injury may cause bowel rupture. Associated mesenteric injury is often present. Most injuries are noted in children who have been involved in motor vehicle crashes and who display lap belt ecchymoses. These injuries may be seen even in children who are wearing three-point restraints. However, one must always suspect nonaccidental injury in a child with a history of minor, blunt trauma who has a bowel perforation. The clinical diagnosis of bowel injury may be challenging. Clinical signs and symptoms may be absent, minimal, or delayed. Therefore, CT plays an important role in the diagnosis. Increased morbidity and mortality are associated with delayed diagnosis because of the increased severity of associated peritonitis.

Intramural hematoma results from hemorrhage into the bowel wall after a partial-thickness tear has occurred. The most common location is the duodenum. The injury can usually be managed nonoperatively. Large hematomas can result in obstruction of the bowel proximal to the injury. The CT appearance is that of focal bowel wall thickening that is often eccentric. Large duodenal hematomas may appear dumbbell shaped (Fig. 157-15). No extraluminal air or extravasated contrast material should be present.

Bowel rupture most commonly occurs in the mid to distal small intestine. The most common site is the jejunum. Extraluminal air is noted on CT in only approximately one third of cases. Review of the examination at a wide window setting is helpful in the detection of small amounts of extraluminal air (Fig. 157-16). The prevalence of extravasation of oral contrast material is even lower, ranging from 0% to 12% in published series. The most frequent CT finding associated with bowel rupture is "unexplained" peritoneal fluid (moderate to large

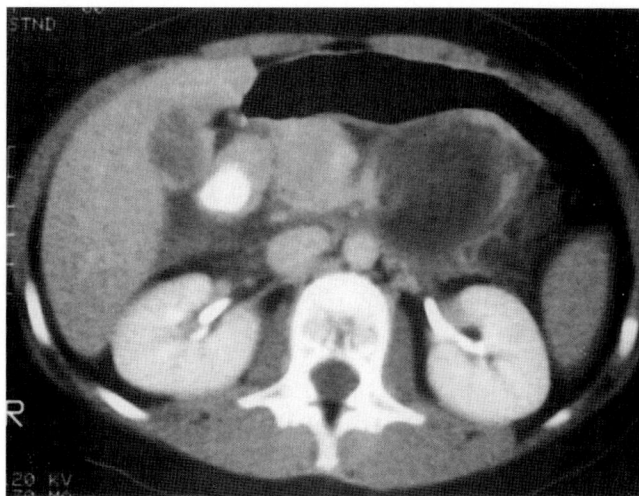

FIGURE 157-15. Duodenal hematoma. Contrast-enhanced CT scan through the upper abdomen shows a rounded duodenal hematoma to the left of midline. Oral contrast material is present within the lumen of the descending duodenum.

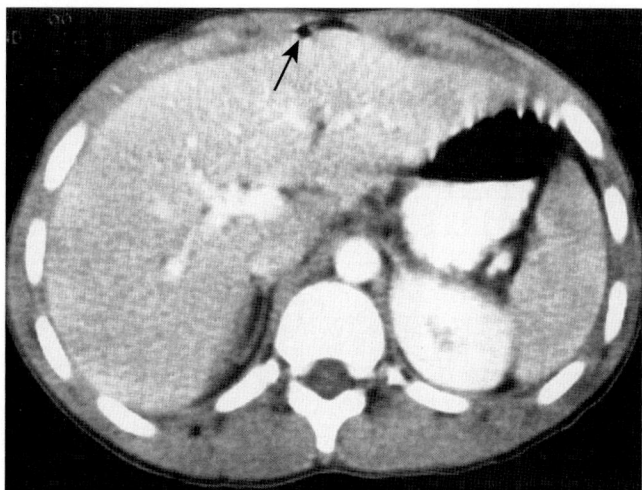

FIGURE 157-16. Bowel rupture with associated extraluminal air. Contrast-enhanced CT scan through the upper abdomen shows a small collection of extraluminal air *(arrow)* anterior to the left lobe of the liver.

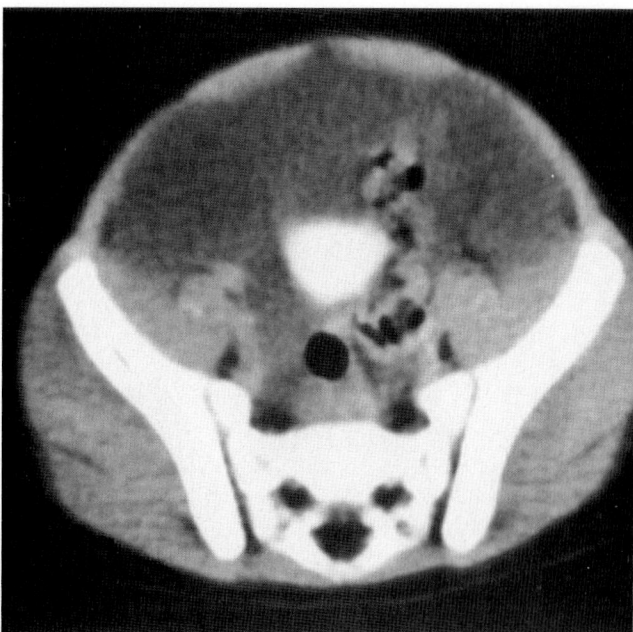

FIGURE 157-17. Bowel rupture with large amount of "unexplained" peritoneal fluid. Contrast-enhanced CT scan through the upper pelvis shows a large amount of peritoneal fluid. No other abnormalities were noted on CT. At surgery, a jejunal rupture was noted.

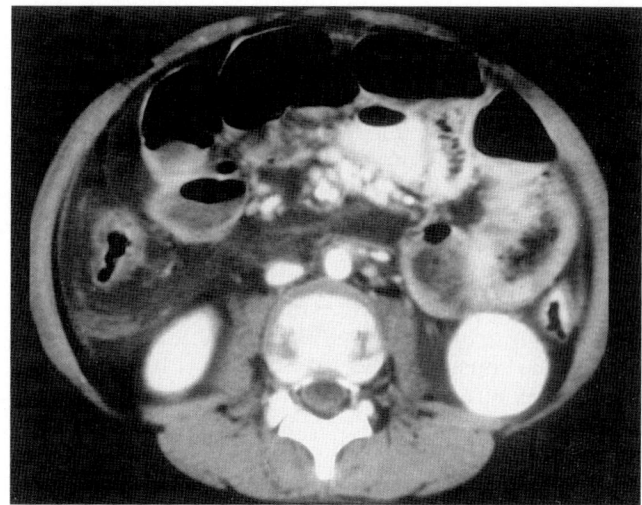

FIGURE 157-18. Bowel rupture with abnormally intense bowel wall enhancement and bowel wall thickening. Contrast-enhanced CT scan through the midabdomen shows focally thick-walled bowel loops anterior to the left kidney. Note the associated intense bowel wall enhancement. At surgery, jejunal rupture was noted.

amounts of fluid in the absence of solid viscus injury or bony pelvic fracture) (Fig. 157-17). Approximately one half of children with moderate to large amounts of peritoneal fluid as the only finding on CT after blunt trauma have a bowel injury. Additional CT findings associated with bowel rupture include abnormally intense bowel wall enhancement (Fig. 157-18), focal bowel wall discontinuity (Fig. 157-19), bowel dilation, bowel wall thickening, and streaky infiltration of mesenteric fat. The latter finding may result from associated mesenteric injury or chemical irritation of the mesentery caused by spilled intestinal contents.

BLADDER INJURY

Bladder injury is also uncommon in children. Bladder rupture can be intraperitoneal or extraperitoneal.

Combined injuries may occur. Extraperitoneal bladder rupture occurs more frequently than intraperitoneal rupture in children; approximately two thirds of post-traumatic bladder ruptures are extraperitoneal in location. Intraperitoneal rupture typically results from shearing of the distended bladder by a lap belt, whereas extraperitoneal rupture often is produced by laceration caused by a bony spicule from a pelvic fracture.

Bladder distention is essential in the detection of bladder injury on CT, for revealing extravasation of IV

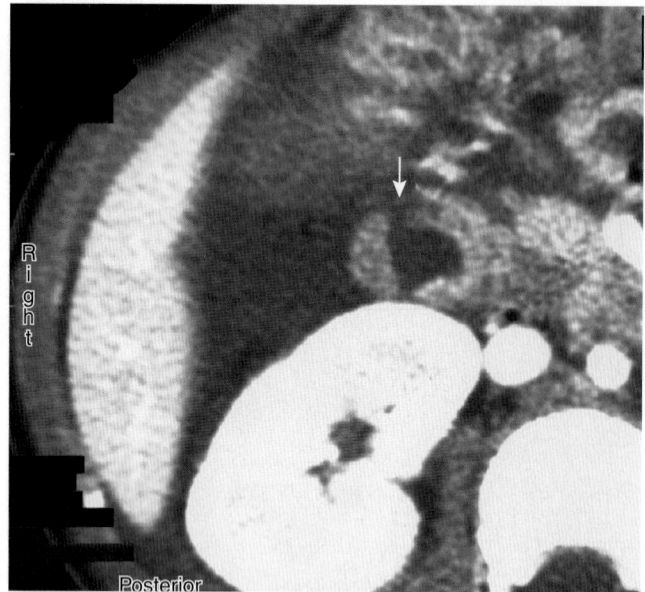

FIGURE 157-19. Bowel rupture with bowel wall discontinuity. Contrast-enhanced CT scan through the upper abdomen shows discontinuity in the wall of the duodenum *(arrow)* indicative of bowel wall rupture.

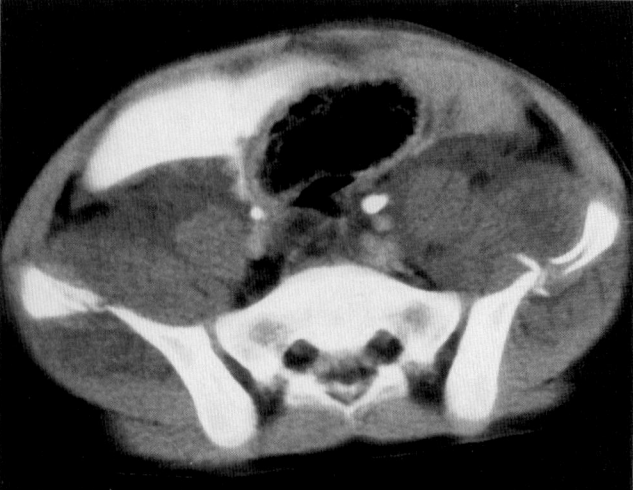

FIGURE 157-20. Intraperitoneal bladder rupture. Contrast-enhanced CT scan through the upper pelvis shows high attenuation fluid in the right lateral pelvic recess related to intraperitoneal bladder rupture. Note contrast within the ureters, bilateral pelvic fractures, and hematomas.

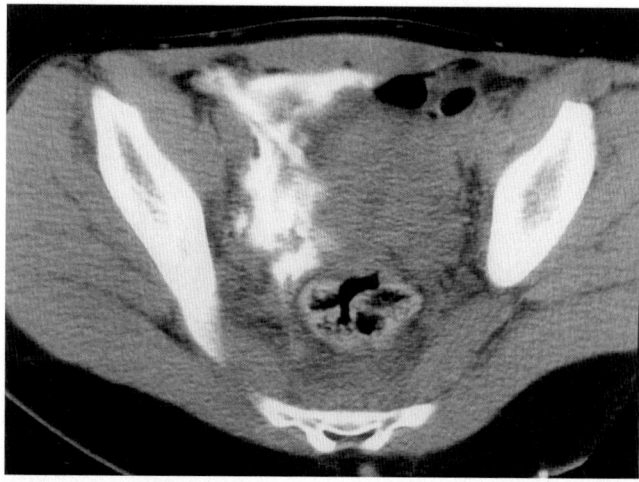

FIGURE 157-21. Extraperitoneal bladder rupture. Contrast-enhanced CT scan through the pelvis shows high attenuation fluid adjacent to the pelvic side walls and low attenuation fluid posterior to the rectum. These fluid collections are extraperitoneal in location, consistent with extraperitoneal bladder rupture.

contrast material. This can be achieved with the use of a scanning delay before the pelvis is imaged or by CT cystogram (Fig. 157-20). When the bladder is being evaluated after examination of the abdomen, the Foley catheter should be clamped prior to IV contrast administration. CT cystography is performed by instilling dilute iodinated contrast into the bladder in a retrograde fashion, which is followed by clamping of the Foley catheter. Images are then obtained through the pelvis over several minutes.

The location of extravasated IV contrast material on CT is useful in differentiating intraperitoneal from extraperitoneal bladder rupture. This distinction is important because an extraperitoneal bladder rupture is typically managed nonsurgically, whereas an intraperitoneal rupture requires immediate surgical repair. Intraperitoneal fluid in the pelvis is located in the lateral perivesical spaces superior to the bladder and anterior to the rectosigmoid colon. Extraperitoneal pelvic fluid is found in the perivesical space that surrounds the bladder superior and anterior to the umbilicus, and posteriorly behind the rectum. Thus, if pelvic fluid is noted lateral to the bladder or behind the rectum, it is extraperitoneal in location (Fig. 157-21). Fluid superior and anterior to the bladder may be intraperitoneal or extraperitoneal. If fluid superior to the bladder is extraperitoneal, it extends superiorly and anteriorly to the level of the umbilicus. If fluid superior to the bladder is intraperitoneal, it is found in a more lateral location (see Fig. 157-20) and typically is contiguous with fluid in the lateral pericolic spaces.

HYPOPERFUSION COMPLEX

A characteristic complex of findings on CT associated with hypovolemic shock in severely injured children has been characterized as the "hypoperfusion complex." Most of these children have had arterial hypotension on admission. The hypotension may be transiently corrected, and it may be believed that the child is hemodynamically stable enough to undergo CT, but the child may subsequently develop rapid hemodynamic decompensation.

CT findings in all children with the hypoperfusion complex include diffuse intestinal dilation with fluid; abnormally intense contrast enhancement of bowel wall, mesentery, kidneys, aorta, and inferior vena cava; and diminished caliber of the aorta and inferior vena cava (Fig. 157-22). Variable findings include periportal low attenuation zones; intense adrenal, pancreatic, and mesenteric enhancement; decreased pancreatic and splenic enhancement; peritoneal and retroperitoneal fluid; and bowel wall thickening (Fig. 157-23).

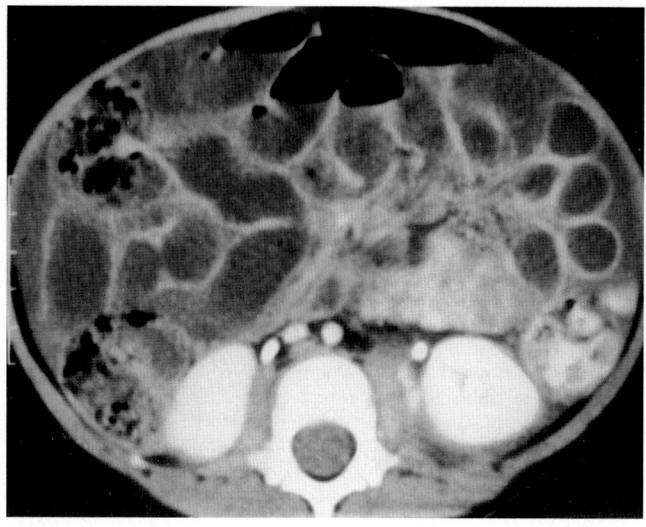
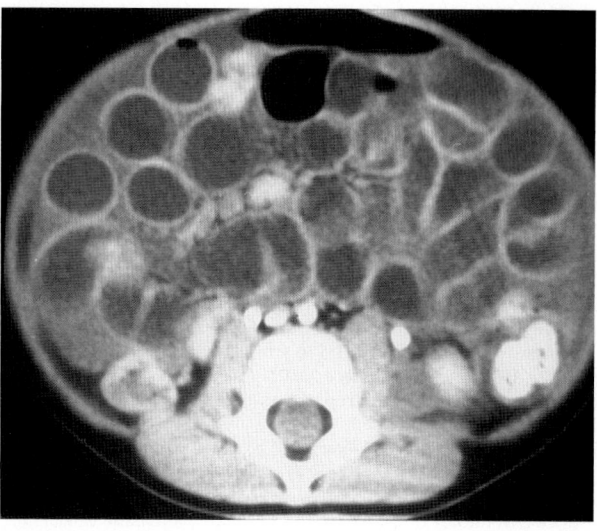

A   B

FIGURE 157-22. Hypoperfusion complex. Contrast-enhanced CT scans through the upper **(A)** and mid- **(B)** abdomen show diffuse intestinal dilation with fluid, intense contrast enhancement of the bowel wall, and diminished caliber of the great vessels indicative of systemic hypoperfusion.

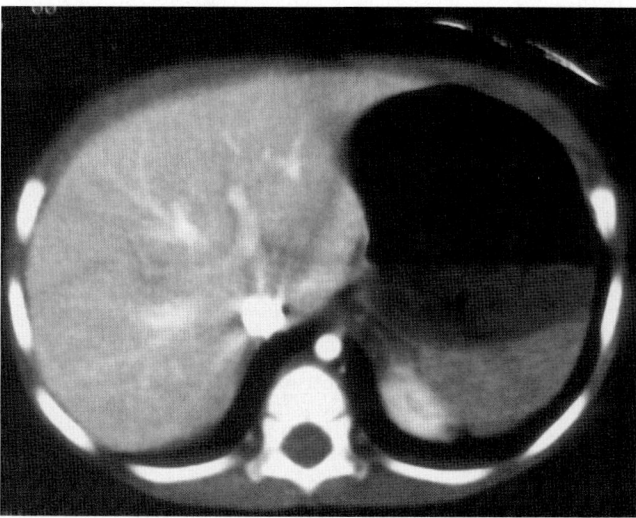

FIGURE 157-23. Hypoperfusion complex. Contrast-enhanced CT scans through the upper abdomen show absence of splenic enhancement. The spleen appeared normal at surgery. Findings were believed to be related to systemic hypoperfusion.

The hypoperfusion complex is a marker for a tenuous hemodynamic state and a predictor of a poor outcome. The mortality rate in children with this constellation of findings on CT is higher than 80%.

INTENTIONAL TRAUMA

Most abdominal injury in children is nonintentional, and the mechanism of injury is clear. However, abdominal injury may also be intentional. This is most often noted in younger children. Obviously, in these children, clinical information directing caregivers toward the possible diagnosis may be limited. Abdominal injury in battered children is often seen in the absence of skeletal and head injury. In one series, the abdomen was the only site of injury in one half of children. The spectrum of abdominal injury associated with intentional trauma is similar to that associated with unintentional trauma; the liver, spleen, duodenum, and adrenal gland are usually involved. The management of visceral injury in these children is similar to that in children with unintentional trauma; most cases are managed nonoperatively.

SONOGRAPHY IN THE ASSESSMENT OF ABDOMINAL TRAUMA

Sonography remains widely used in the screening of injured children and adults, although it appears to have limited usefulness. Sonography has been shown to have high sensitivity and specificity in the detection of hemo-peritoneum. However, the presence of hemoperitoneum in the hemodynamically stable child typically does not affect clinical management decisions. Furthermore, sonography has important limitations in evaluation of the abdomen in injured children. First, it provides no diagnostic information regarding injury to the bony pelvis or lumbar spine. Additionally, sonography cannot be used in the diagnosis of hollow viscus injury. Finally, sonography has been shown to miss approximately one fourth to one third of solid viscus injuries. An important issue that should not be overlooked when the impact of CT is evaluated as the primary screening modality for children after abdominal trauma relates to the value of a normal examination. A normal CT examination may prevent unnecessary surgical exploration because it can provide a comprehensive evaluation of the abdomen and pelvis. It would be difficult to attain such a comprehensive assessment with sonography. As a result, in North America, CT remains the primary imaging modality for evaluation of pediatric abdominal injury. Nevertheless, sonography has a potential role in the hemodynamically unstable patient because it can be performed rapidly at the bedside before the patient is taken to the operating room. In this role, it serves as a fast, noninvasive replacement for diagnostic peritoneal lavage.

SUGGESTED READINGS

Basile KE, Sivit CJ, O'Riordan MA, et al: Acute hemoperitoneum in children: prevalence of low-attenuation fluid. Pediatr Radiol 2000;30:168

Bensard DB, Beaver BL, Besner GE, et al: Small bowel injury in children after blunt abdominal trauma: is diagnostic delay important? J Trauma 1996;41:476

Benya EC, Bulas DI, Eichelberger MR, et al: Splenic injury from blunt abdominal trauma in children: follow-up evaluation with CT. Radiology 1995;195:685

Bond SJ, Eichelberger MR, Gotschall CS, et al: Nonoperative management of blunt hepatic and splenic injury in children. Ann Surg 1996;223:286

Canty TG, Weinman D: Management of major pancreatic duct injuries in children. J Trauma 2001;50:1001

Cloutier DR, Baird TB, Gormley P, et al: Pediatric splenic injuries with a contrast blush: successful nonoperative management without angiography and embolization. J Pediatr Surg 2004;39:969

Coley BD, Mutabagani KH, Martin LC, et al: Focused abdominal sonography for trauma (FAST) in children with blunt abdominal trauma. J Trauma 2000;48:902

Cooper C, Silverman PM, Davros WJ, et al: Delayed contrast enhancement of ascitic fluid on CT: frequency and significance. AJR Am J Roentgenol 1993;161:787

Federle MP, Yagan N, Peitzman AB, et al: Abdominal trauma: use of oral contrast material for CT is safe. Radiology 1997;205:91

Hollingsworth CL, Bisset GS: CT evaluation of pediatric abdominal trauma: pitfalls and quandaries. Emerg Radiol 2001;8:67

Hulka F, Mullins RJ, Leonardo V, et al: Significance of peritoneal fluid as an isolated finding on abdominal computed tomographic scans in pediatric trauma patients. J Trauma 1998;44:1069

Jamieson DH, Babyn PS, Pearl R: Imaging gastrointestinal perforation in pediatric blunt abdominal trauma. Pediatr Radiol 1996;26:188

Levine CD, Patel US, Silverman PM, et al: Low attenuation of acute traumatic hemoperitoneum on CT scans. AJR Am J Roentgenol 1996;166:1089

Luks F, Lemire A, St-Vil D, et al: Blunt abdominal trauma in children: the practical value of sonography. J Trauma 1993;34:607

Lutz N, Mahboubi S, Nance ML, et al: The significance of contrast blush on computed tomography in children with splenic injuries. J Pediatr Surg 2004;39:491

McGahan JP, Richards JR: Blunt abdominal trauma: the role of emergent sonography and a review of the literature. AJR Am J Roentgenol 1999;172:897

Miller K, Kou D, Sivit CJ, et al: Pediatric hepatic trauma: does clinical course support intensive care unit stay? J Pediatr Surg 1998;33:1459

Morgan DE, Nallamala LK, Kenny PJ, et al: CT cystography: radiographic and clinical predictors of bladder rupture. AJR Am J Roentgenol 2000;174:89

Neisch AS, Taylor GA, Lund DP, et al: Effect of CT information on the diagnosis and management of acute abdominal injury in children. Radiology 1998;206:327

Nwomeh BC, Nadler EP, Meza MP, et al: Contrast extravasation predicts the need for operative intervention in children with blunt splenic trauma. J Trauma 2004;56:537

Orwig D, Federle MP: Localized clotted blood as evidence of visceral trauma on CT: the sentinel clot sign. AJR Am J Roentgenol 1989;153:747

Patrick LE, Ball TI, Atkinson GO, et al: Pediatric blunt abdominal trauma: periportal tracking at CT. Radiology 1992;183:689

Patten RM, Spear RP, Vincent LM, et al: Traumatic laceration of the liver limited to the bare area: CT findings in 25 patients. AJR Am J Roentgenol 1993;160:1019

Ruess L, Sivit CJ, Eichelberger MR, et al: Blunt hepatic and splenic trauma in children: correlation of a CT injury severity scale with clinical outcome. Pediatr Radiol 1995;25:321

Ruess L, Sivit CJ, Eichelberger MR, et al: Blunt abdominal trauma in children: impact of CT on operative and nonoperative management. AJR Am J Roentgenol 1997;169:1011

Shankar KR, Lloyd DA, Kitteringham L, et al: Oral contrast with computed tomography in the evaluation of abdominal trauma in children. Br J Surg 1999;86:1073

Shilyansky J, Sena LM, Kreller M, et al: Nonoperative management of pancreatic injuries in children. J Pediatr Surg 1998;33:343

Sievers EM, Murray JM, Chen D, et al: Abdominal computed tomography scan in pediatric blunt abdominal trauma. Am Surg 1999;65:968

Sivit CJ, Cutting JP, Eichelberger MR: CT diagnosis and localization of rupture of the bladder in children with blunt abdominal trauma: significance of contrast material in the pelvis. AJR Am J Roentgenol 1995;164:1243

Sivit CJ, Eichelberger MR: CT diagnosis of pancreatic injury in children: significance of fluid separating the splenic vein and pancreas. AJR Am J Roentgenol 1995;165:921

Sivit CJ, Eichelberger MR, Taylor GA: CT in children with rupture of the bowel caused by blunt trauma: diagnostic efficacy and comparison with hypoperfusion complex. AJR Am J Roentgenol 1994;163:1195

Sivit CJ, Eichelberger MR, Taylor GA, et al: Blunt pancreatic trauma in children: CT diagnosis. AJR Am J Roentgenol 1992;158:1097

Sivit CJ, Frazier AA, Eichelberger MR: Prevalence and distribution of hemorrhage associated with splenic injury in children. Radiology 1995;197:298

Sivit CJ, Peclet MH, Taylor GA: Life-threatening intraperitoneal bleeding: demonstration with CT. Radiology 1989;171:430

Sivit CJ, Taylor GA, Bulas DI, et al: Post-traumatic shock in children: CT findings associated with hemodynamic instability. Radiology 1992;182:723

Sivit CJ, Taylor GA, Eichelberger MR: Visceral injury in battered children: a changing perspective. Radiology 1989;173:659

Sivit CJ, Taylor GA, Eichelberger MR, et al: Significance of periportal low-attenuation zones following blunt trauma in children. Pediatr Radiol 1993;23:388

Sivit CJ, Taylor GA, Newman KD, et al: Safety-belt injuries in children with lap-belt ecchymosis: CT findings in 61 patients. AJR Am J Roentgenol 1991;157:111

Strouse PJ, Bradley JC, Marshall KW, et al: CT of bowel and mesenteric trauma in children. Radiographics 1999;19:1237

Stylianos S: Compliance with evidence-based guidelines in children with isolated spleen or liver injury: a prospective study. J Pediatr Surg 2002;37:453

Stylianos S: Outcomes from pediatric solid organ injury: role of standardized care guidelines. Curr Opin Pediatr 2005;17:402

Stylianos S, APSA Liver/Spleen Trauma Study Group: Evidence-based guidelines for resource utilization in children with isolated spleen or liver injury. J Pediatr Surg 2000;35:164

Taylor GA, Eichelberger MR: Abdominal CT in children with neurologic impairment following blunt trauma. Ann Surg 1989;210:229

Taylor GA, Eichelberger MR, O'Donnell R: Indications for computed tomography in children with blunt abdominal trauma. Ann Surg 1991;213:212

Taylor GA, Eichelberger MR, Potter BM: Hematuria: a marker of abdominal injury in children after blunt trauma. Ann Surg 1988;208:688

Taylor GA, Fallat ME, Eichelberger MR: Hypovolemic shock in children: abdominal CT manifestations. Radiology 1987;164:479

Taylor GA, Kaufman RA, Sivit CJ: Active hemorrhage in children after thoracoabdominal trauma: clinical and CT features. AJR Am J Roentgenol 1994;162:401

Taylor GA, O'Donnell BA, Sivit CJ, et al: Abdominal injury score: a clinical score for the assignment of risk in children after blunt trauma. Radiology 1994;190:689

Taylor GA, Sivit CJ: Posttraumatic peritoneal fluid: is it a reliable indicator of intraabdominal injury in children? J Pediatr Surg 1995;30:1644

Wales PW, Shuckett B, Kim PCW: Long-term outcome after nonoperative management of complete traumatic pancreatic transection in children. J Pediatr Surg 2001;36:823

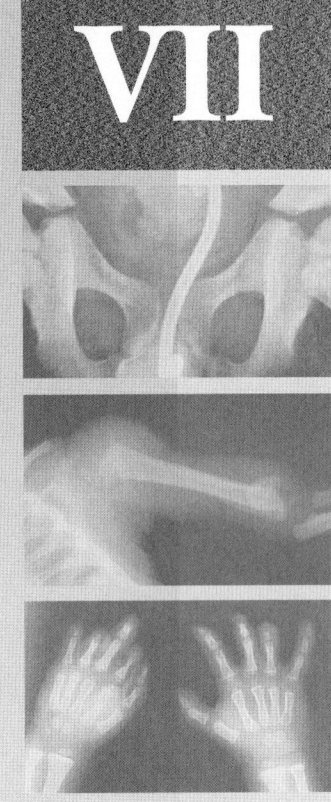

MUSCULOSKELETAL SYSTEM

PETER J. STROUSE

PART 1 OVERVIEW OF MUSCULOSKELETAL IMAGING

CHAPTER 158

Overview

PETER J. STROUSE

The practice of pediatric musculoskeletal radiology demands specialized knowledge of normal growth, development, and morphology needed for one to recognize and understand the diverse injuries, diseases, syndromes, and malformations that are peculiar to infancy, childhood, and adolescence. In the past, much of this knowledge was acquired through observations of plain radiographs. Indeed, readers of older editions of this book will remember the superb descriptions of musculoskeletal disorders that were based on Dr. Caffey's original observations and were later expanded on by Dr. Frederic N. Silverman. In recent years, growing use of other imaging modalities such as ultrasonography, computed tomography (CT), magnetic resonance imaging (MRI), and nuclear scintigraphy (Table 158-1) has added significantly to the knowledge base. Shepherded by Dr. Barry D. Fletcher, the musculoskeletal section of the 10th edition of this text reflected a remarkable expansion of our ability to image pediatric musculoskeletal disorders. Newer technologies provided richness of anatomic and pathologic detail. Technology continues to improve and evolve at a rapid pace. Through imaging and other advances in medicine, our understanding of pediatric disease improves. Pediatric disease, itself, also evolves.

This, the musculoskeletal section of the 11th edition of *Caffey's Pediatric Diagnostic Imaging*, builds upon the foundation laid by the previous 10 editions. This section comprises the combined specialized expertise of more than two dozen authors. Old focuses remain; however, new ones have arisen. Three new chapters address the imaging of vascular lesions of soft tissues, bone mineral density assessment, and sports injury. Each of these subjects represents an area of rapidly advancing clinical knowledge that is compounded by advancing imaging techniques.

Our overriding goal remains to provide the reader with the most up-to-date information on disorders of the pediatric musculoskeletal system. We strive to provide a cogent, balanced, and practical discussion of the application of our expanding array of imaging techniques.

RADIOGRAPHY

Radiography remains the primary method of detecting and analyzing skeletal abnormalities. In many patients, plain radiographs may be the only medium needed to portray a disorder. The spatial resolution of radiography is superior to that of all other modalities. Radiation exposure to the patient is minimal, and the monetary cost is low. Most fractures and congenital deformities are sufficiently imaged with radiography without the need for additional imaging.

Rapid advances in genetics have improved the clinical diagnosis of children with suspected genetic disorders and skeletal dysplasias. Nevertheless, the radiographic

TABLE 158-1

Frequent Application of Imaging Modalities for the Evaluation of Pediatric Musculoskeletal Disorders

	IMAGING MODALITY				
	RAD	US	CT	MR	NM
Congenital disorders	√	√		√	
Metabolic disorders	√				
Infection	√	√	√	√	Tc, Ga, Ind
Osseous trauma	√		√	√	Tc
Soft tissue trauma		√		√	
Arthropathy	√	√		√	
Bone tumors	√		√	√	Tc, Ga, MIBG, PET
Soft tissue tumors		√		√	PET

√ indicates frequent applications; CT, computed tomography; Ga, gallium-67 citrate; Ind, indium-111–labeled white blood cells; MIBG, iodine-131 or iodine-123 *meta*-iodobenzylguanidine (for neuroblastoma bone metastases); MR, magnetic resonance imaging; NM, nuclear imaging; PET, positron emission tomography; RAD, radiography; Tc, technetium-99m methylene diphosphonate (MDP); US, ultrasound.

skeletal survey remains an important component in the evaluation of many patients with a skeletal dysplasia or syndrome. Skeletal surveys continue to be of paramount importance in the diagnosis and evaluation of suspected victims of child abuse. However, these surveys have largely been replaced by technetium-99m methylene diphosphonate (MDP) nuclear scintigraphy for the detection of metastatic disease to the skeleton. Positron emission tomography (PET) and/or whole body MRI may soon supplant scintigraphy for this function.

Radiographs often guide the selection of additional imaging modalities. Even when more detailed investigation is required with the use of other modalities, radiographs are frequently used to follow the clinical course and response to treatment for such entities as arthritis, infection, metabolic disorders, and growth disorders.

Radiographs are less relevant to the study of soft tissues because of their narrow contrast range, but plain radiographs can improve the diagnostic specificity of soft tissue lesions by depicting calcifications, fat, gas, or foreign material within the lesion or by showing the extent of secondary involvement of adjacent bone.

ULTRASONOGRAPHY

The role of diagnostic ultrasonography in the management of musculoskeletal disorders is somewhat limited by its narrow field of view, operator dependence, and the physical constraints of sonic transmission through bone. However, ultrasonography is inexpensive, accessible, and versatile and does not require ionizing radiation, thus making it one of the most valuable tools in the pediatric imaging armamentarium. The real-time "hands-on" capabilities of ultrasonography make it an ideal modality for evaluation of soft tissues and joints of the pediatric musculoskeletal system. Processes that originate from bone and extend into soft tissues, such as subperiosteal abscesses and tumor, can be detected on ultrasonography.

Soft tissue neoplasms and vascular malformations are frequent causes of soft tissue masses in children. Spectral, color, and power Doppler ultrasonographic techniques allow for assessment of blood flow rates and delineation of the vascular components of soft tissue lesions. For example, fast flow suggests a diagnosis of hemangioma, arteriovenous malformation, or fistula, whereas a compressible slow-flow lesion indicates the presence of a venous malformation. A growing cystic lesion that lacks flow is highly suggestive of a lymphatic malformation. In the presence of characteristic clinical and sonographic findings of vascular malformation, the need for additional more complex or invasive procedures may be avoided.

Ultrasonography is helpful to the clinician in determining whether a mass is cystic and fluid filled or solid in composition. Occasionally, the ultrasonographic appearance of a lesion is sufficiently specific to suggest the diagnosis of a specific benign lesion such as hematoma, hemangioma, or lipoma. Conversely, disordered, complex echoes from within a mass may point to the possibility of soft tissue sarcoma—a rare diagnosis in children—and the need for further imaging and clinical investigation. However, the usefulness of ultrasonography for distin-guishing types of tissue within a mass is limited. MRI is often the next step when further definition of tissue composition or anatomy of soft tissue mass is desired.

Unossified cartilage of the immature skeleton is well seen on ultrasonography. For example, the capability of imaging the morphology and location of the unossified proximal femoral epiphysis in infants made ultrasonography integral to the diagnosis and management of developmental dysplasia of the hip. Real-time, dynamic evaluation of the infant hip provides valuable diagnostic information. Ultrasonography can detect injuries to muscles or tendons that are occult on radiography. Ultrasonography is also used to detect cartilaginous epiphyseal fractures that are not visible on radiography. Ultrasonography is highly sensitive to the presence of excess intra-articular fluid. Therefore, it serves as the primary method of identifying joint fluid and possible septic arthritis at the hip; in patients with juvenile rheumatoid arthritis, ultrasonography is used to detect joint effusion and to differentiate it from synovial hypertrophy.

COMPUTED TOMOGRAPHY

CT images achieve greater contrast resolution than is attained by plain radiographs; they are therefore more sensitive than radiographs to variations in bone and soft tissue density. CT is a powerful tool for evaluating bone. Although the administration of contrast material further improves the soft tissue contrast resolution of CT, ultrasonography and MRI are usually preferred to CT for delineation of soft tissue processes.

CT is a very sensitive method of detecting cortical disruption, periosteal reaction, and other osseous changes associated with infection, trauma, and neoplasia. Some tumors (e.g., osteoid osteoma) may be more readily detected by CT than by other modalities. CT is superior to MRI for detecting bony sequestra associated with osteomyelitis. Although CT is not as sensitive as MRI to differences in soft tissue contrast, subtle increases in the normally hypodense marrow of older children can be seen on CT images. CT is also more sensitive than radiographs to the presence of abnormal calcifications, fat, and air within soft tissues. CT angiography is occasionally useful for delineation of vasculature relative to a tumor or in the setting of trauma with suspected vascular compromise.

In the past, CT scanning has been generally limited to the axial plane. This is no longer true. Modern multidetector CT scanners allow for acquisition of axial images at sub-millimeter slice thickness. The CT data set can be reformatted into any plane with isotropic or near-isotropic resolution. Volume-rendered images yield spectacular displays of osseous pathology. The modern pediatric musculoskeletal radiologist must be increasingly adept in post processing to efficiently use CT data sets.

Even with the recent increase in attention paid to limiting radiation exposure in children during CT scans, CT remains the major source of radiation exposure to the pediatric population in medical imaging. The use of CT in the pediatric musculoskeletal system should be restricted to clinical situations with clearly defined imaging goals. Scanning should be limited to regions of interest; this minimizes unnecessary exposure to adjacent tissues. Radiation dose is minimized by reducing milliamperage to levels well below those of standard protocols used for imaging adults. The density and inherent contrast of ossified bone allow for further lowering of milliamperage. Kilovoltage potential (kVp) can also be lowered because of the high contrast of bone. CT techniques routinely used for imaging of the bones of children thus have a lower radiation dose as compared with CT techniques for imaging other organ systems.

MAGNETIC RESONANCE IMAGING

MRI has had a major impact on musculoskeletal imaging because of its capability of producing high-contrast images of structures that are invisible or that are poorly visualized with x-ray–based modalities. This feature is especially important in children because the immature skeleton contains a high proportion of radiolucent cartilage. With the use of high-field imaging systems, specialized pulse sequences, and dedicated surface coils, multiplanar images with excellent spatial and contrast resolution can be obtained. Lack of ionizing radiation and the relative safety of gadolinium-based contrast agents have enhanced the usefulness of this modality in the investigation of pediatric musculoskeletal disorders. Indications continue to expand.

One disadvantage of MRI that persists is the relatively long imaging time required. Although newer imaging sequences have faster acquisition times than in the past with similar or improved image quality, the overall duration of an MRI study remains long relative to that of other modalities and long relative to the ability of a young child to hold still. Sedation or anesthesia is required in young children.

MRI tissue contrast is dependent on the concentration of protons in tissue, the T1 and T2 relaxation rates of tissue, and the imaging sequence employed (Table 158-2). In general, combinations of conventional spin echo, fast spin echo, and gradient echo sequences are employed to achieve the clinical goals of each examination. Chemical fat saturation and inversion recovery techniques can be used to diminish signal from fat and increase the conspicuity of pathologic processes. Gadolinium-based paramagnetic contrast agents increase the signal intensity of tissues on T1-weighted images. Pathologic processes such as tumor and inflammation tend to show greater enhancement than normal tissues. Accumulated experience has shown that gadolinium is very safe for administration in children. Gadolinium, which is instrumental in the imaging of musculoskeletal tumors and infections, is not needed for many orthopedic MRI indications. Magnetic resonance (MR) arthrography with dilute gadolinium is now commonly used in the diagnosis of some joint disorders, most notably labral abnormalities in the shoulder and hip.

The strengths of MRI lie in its multiplanar capability and inherent tissue contrast. A good musculoskeletal MRI protocol uses complementary imaging planes and imaging sequences to fully delineate and characterize anatomy and pathology. Standard protocols are warranted for common indications; however, novel protocols or modifications of standard protocols are often needed for the varied pathologies encountered in children.

On MRI, bone and other dense tissues, including intact ligaments and tendons, show lack of signal. This characteristic absence of signal provides negative contrast in comparison with muscle, which is of intermediate intensity, and yellow marrow, which is hyperintense on T1-weighted images. Accumulations of fluid within joints and bursae are hyperintense on T2-weighted images, as are fluid-containing lesions such as abscesses and cysts. The use of gadolinium with T1-weighted imaging sequences can help to differentiate joint effusions, which show only very slow enhancement, from rapidly enhancing vascularized tissues such as hypertrophied synovium or juxta-articular tumors. Proton density and gradient echo sequences with fat saturation are very useful for displaying cartilage, which appears intense on these images.

Bone marrow edema, indicated by alterations in marrow signal (decreased on T1 weighting, increased on T2 weighting), may indicate the presence of subtle or radiographically undetectable microfractures. Patterns of bone marrow edema may predict a particular soft tissue injury, such as tear of the anterior cruciate ligament.

TABLE 158-2

Relative Magnetic Resonance Imaging Signal Intensities of Normal and Pathologic Tissues

	IMAGING SEQUENCE				
	T1 Weighted	T2 Weighted	T2 Weighted with Fat Saturation	Inversion Recovery	T1 Weighted with Fat Saturation and Gadolinium
Muscle	++	++	++	++	++
Bone	+	+	+	+	+
Fat	+++	+++	–	–	–
Yellow marrow	+++	+++	–	–	–
Red marrow	++	++	++	++	++
Tendons, ligaments	+	+	+	+	+
Cartilage	++	++ to +++	++ to +++	+++	++
Joint effusion	+	+++	+++	+	+
Pathologic tissues	++	+++	+++	+++	+++

Scoring: + to +++, least to most intense signal; –, nulled fat signal.

MRI has proved sensitive to injuries and malformations involving the physis and epiphysis. This permits diagnosis of radiographically occult fractures and allows for early detection and delineation of post-traumatic bony physeal bridges. MRI is also useful during the course of inflammatory conditions such as juvenile rheumatoid arthritis, hemarthroses associated with blood coagulation disorders, and internal articular derangements from trauma or sports injury.

Before the advent of MRI, detection and diagnosis of soft tissue lesions by radiologic means was limited. MRI may provide a specific diagnosis for lesions that contain fat and vascular elements. However, the MR signal characteristics of most soft tissue tumors are nonspecific, that is, isointense to muscle on T1-weighted images, hyperintense on T2-weighted images, and enhanced with gadolinium. Although not diagnostic, these characteristics permit precise evaluation of tumor size, configuration, and location.

The advantage of MRI over radiography and CT for bone tumors lies in its superior tissue contrast that allows delineation of tumor anatomy in multiple planes. The extent of medullary involvement, adjacent soft tissue extension, and joint involvement is readily defined. MR angiography can be used to map the relationship of major blood vessels to tumors to help plan surgery and determine resectability. Dynamic contrast-enhanced MRI, diffusion imaging, and MR spectroscopy are all techniques that have been applied to imaging of pediatric musculoskeletal tumors. Further sequence development and research will determine whether these techniques are truly beneficial in the diagnosis, delineation, and follow-up of pediatric musculoskeletal tumors.

MRI remains the only modality that permits direct visualization of normal bone marrow. The signal characteristics of normal marrow vary depending on the age of the child and the location of bone marrow within the skeleton. An array of pathologic processes can affect the bone marrow. MRI is a powerful tool that is used to identify marrow pathology, thus guiding diagnostic procedures and therapy. Currently, whole body MRI techniques that employ fast inversion recovery sequences are under investigation for the detection of metastases or lymphoma within the bone marrow. Such techniques will also likely prove valuable in assessing the skeleton for infection or occult trauma.

NUCLEAR IMAGING

Skeletal scintigraphy performed with the use of technetium-labeled phosphates was introduced more than three decades ago. The "bone scan" remains the most frequently performed pediatric nuclear medicine imaging study. Bone scans have a higher sensitivity relative to skeletal radiography. The radiopharmaceutical most commonly used is technetium-99m MDP. Images obtained after injection of this compound reflect a combination of pathophysiologic functions (blood flow and bone turnover) but are nonspecific and do not provide exceptional anatomic detail. Images should therefore be interpreted in the context of the patient's clinical presentation and relevant radiologic findings. Indeed, a reasonable dictum holds that bone scans of pediatric patients should be viewed along with the appropriate bone radiographs to avoid common pitfalls in interpretation caused by the normally nonuniform distribution of radiotracer in the growing skeleton. The anatomic areas that are most difficult to image and interpret accurately are the growth centers. Before closure of the physes, these rapidly growing areas display especially high uptake that may mask the activity associated with an adjacent pathologic lesion. Proper performance of bone scans in children requires meticulous attention to technique.

The addition of single-photon emission CT (SPECT) helps in localization of such lesions because it improves the spatial resolution of activity in contiguous and overlapping structures. The newest platform of SPECT allows fusion of three-dimensional bone scan data with CT images. Restraint is necessary to avoid overuse of the CT component in children.

Indications for skeletal scintigraphy are varied and include investigation of bone pain and diagnosis of early and chronic osteomyelitis, avascular necrosis, and occult trauma, including nonaccidental trauma and stress fractures. Improvements in the diagnostic accuracy of CT and MRI have usurped skeletal scintigraphy in many clinical settings; however, bone scanning remains a very useful imaging tool.

Other scintigraphic techniques may be used in evaluating the pediatric musculoskeletal system. Indium-111–labeled white blood cells may be valuable in assessing for infection. Gallium-67 citrate can be used to identify sites of inflammation for tumor imaging. Other scintigraphic agents are being developed that will identify infection or inflammation. The problem of differentiating infarction from osteomyelitis in patients with sickle cell anemia has been addressed with some success by the use of dual, sequential bone and bone marrow scans, the latter employing technetium-99m–sulfur colloid. In patients with neuroblastoma, *meta*-iodobenzylguanidine (MIBG) tagged with ^{123}I or ^{131}I is used in an effort to enhance specificity and sensitivity in the diagnosis of metastatic disease. Thallium-201 has been used in the evaluation of osteosarcoma.

Positron emission tomography (PET) imaging is now a standard part of the imaging armamentarium. PET imaging with 2-[^{18}F]fluoro-2-deoxyglucose (FDG) offers improved spatial resolution and greater sensitivity for detection of aggressive bone neoplasms. FDG-PET is particularly effective in detecting active tumor. Because of its high sensitivity, increased signal on PET is nonspecific. Fusion of PET with CT (PET-CT) allows for better spatial localization of lesions and improves the characterization of lesions. PET is also an effective method of determining response of malignant bone tumors to therapy. Direct fusion of PET with MRI (PET-MRI) is on the near horizon and will further improve the clinical usefulness and specificity of PET.

MOLECULAR IMAGING

As this edition takes form, molecular imaging techniques are in their infancy, but it would be shortsighted to neglect to acknowledge that molecular imaging has the potential to revolutionize the imaging of many disorders of the pediatric musculoskeletal system. PET and MRI will likely benefit from advances in molecular imaging.

CONCLUSION

Expanding knowledge, changing pathology, evolving therapies, and a wider array of imaging modalities continually increase the challenge of pediatric musculoskeletal imaging. Radiologists must be able to interpret images, but they also must be prepared to advise clinical colleagues on the appropriate selection and application of imaging techniques. The following chapters provide fundamental information on the musculoskeletal disease processes that commonly occur in pediatric patients and guidance regarding the appropriate use of imaging modalities.

CHAPTER

159

The Soft Tissues

KATHLEEN H. EMERY

OVERVIEW

Alterations in the soft tissues are a problem for which pediatric patients frequently seek medical attention. Soft tissues cover all areas of the body but are largely ignored in many radiology texts, even though they are present on virtually all imaging studies. The skin is the largest single organ, and it is most efficiently evaluated by direct visual inspection. Suspected pathology in the deeper soft tissues, including subcutaneous fat, muscles, fascia, blood and lymphatic vessels, nerves, and lymph nodes, which are not amenable to direct visual inspection, may require imaging evaluation. At times visual inspection of the skin itself provides important clues to underlying pathology in the deeper soft tissues. For example, bluish discoloration over a hemangioma may trigger the need for imaging to define the lesion and determine its extent.

A variety of modalities for soft tissue evaluation are currently available. Conventional radiography is widely available, easily performed, and economical and does not require sedation. Radiographs have relatively narrow density latitude, which limits their usefulness. Most soft tissues, with the exception of fat, are of the same density on conventional radiographs. However, radiographs may provide important information about amount of soft tissue (too much or too little), presence or absence of abnormal radiopaque or radiolucent structures (such as calcification or air), and the integrity of underlying skeletal structures. For soft tissue evaluation in children, radiographs are best used to search for a suspected foreign body and to screen soft tissues before more advanced imaging is performed.

Computed tomography (CT) provides broader density latitude than radiography, and its cross-sectional capability allows more precise localization of disease. However, the soft tissue contrast of CT is limited (particularly without intravenous [IV] contrast), and the relative radiation dose is high; therefore, the value of CT in soft tissue evaluation is limited.

Sonography brings unique capabilities to soft tissue evaluation. Primarily, the absence of ionizing radiation,

the lack of need for sedation to obtain a diagnostic study, and the wide availability of high-resolution transducers to visualize superficial structures (7, 10, and even 15 MHz) make this type of imaging very attractive for use in the pediatric population. Determination of cystic or solid contents and evaluation of vascularity with Doppler are distinct roles of sonography in assessment of soft tissue lesions. The soft tissue contrast of ultrasonography is somewhat limited as is field of view; thus, the role of sonography is limited as well. Newer ultrasound technologies allow for a broader field of view and may improve the usefulness of this modality.

Magnetic resonance imaging (MRI) provides the most exquisite soft tissue contrast available along with the added benefit of no ionizing radiation and a wide range of flexibility for field-of-view coverage, as seen in the variety of coils at one's disposal. Even though magnetic resonance (MR) images may be degraded by ferromagnetic structures in the field of interest and small foreign bodies that emit no signal may be difficult to recognize, this modality has revolutionized the radiologist's ability to diagnose soft tissue abnormalities. A normal MRI may help the clinician to confidently exclude pathology. The cost of MRI remains high, and reliance on sedation is common in the vast majority of patients younger than 8 years of age. Nonetheless, MRI has proved to be a powerful tool for evaluating focal and diffuse soft tissue disease.

A wide variety of pathologic conditions may involve the soft tissues. Many of these, including congenital malformations, vascular lesions, and neoplastic conditions, are addressed in subsequent chapters. This chapter focuses on soft tissue foreign body evaluation; conditions that may cause abnormal focal or diffuse soft tissue radiodensity, calcification, or ossification (Table 159-1); soft tissue infections and disorders that result in abnormal soft tissue excess or deficiency (i.e., neuromuscular disorders).

CUTANEOUS CALCIFICATION/OSSIFICATION

Calcification or ossification normally occurs in the teeth and bones but may develop in the skin in a variety of

TABLE 159-1

Differential Diagnosis of Soft Tissue Calcification

TRAUMA
Myositis ossificans
Hematoma
Subcutaneous fat necrosis

INFLAMMATION
Dermatomyositis
Scleroderma
Lupus
Ehlers-Danlos syndrome
Acne vulgaris (treated with tetracyclines)
Parasitic infection (i.e., *Taenia solium*—pork tapeworm)

NEOPLASM
Pilomatrixoma
Epidermal cyst
Lipoma
Synovial sarcoma

CONGENITAL DISORDERS
Fibrodysplasia ossificans progressiva
Venous malformation (phleboliths)
Albright hereditary osteodystrophy

METABOLIC DISORDERS
Tumoral calcinosis
Chronic renal failure
Milk alkali syndrome
Vitamin D intoxication
Parathyroid neoplasms

MISCELLANEOUS
Injection sites
Multiple heelsticks
Immobilization
Electroencephalogram electrodes (scalp)

pathologic conditions. It may be focal or diffuse and symptomatic or asymptomatic.

Calcinosis Cutis

Precipitation or deposition of hydroxyapatite crystals of calcium phosphate within cutaneous tissues is a pathologic condition known under the general term *calcinosis cutis.* Most forms of this disorder fall into one of three categories—dystrophic, metastatic, or idiopathic—depending on the underlying disease process.

Dystrophic calcinosis cutis occurs in previously damaged tissue without an associated metabolic disturbance of the calcium-to-phosphorus ratio. Localized forms occur in inflammatory and traumatic lesions, including acne, ulcers, and foreign body granulomas and after heelsticks for blood drawing in neonates. Neoplastic conditions, including epidermal cysts, lipomas, and pilomatrixomas (benign tumors of hair matrix cell origin), are known to cause localized dystrophic calcification. More widespread dystrophic cutaneous calcification (calcinosis universalis) may be seen in dermatomyositis, scleroderma, pseudoxanthoma elasticum, Ehlers-Danlos syndrome, and systemic lupus erythematosus.

Metastatic calcinosis cutis occurs in undamaged tissue in conditions with an abnormality of calcium and/or phosphorus metabolism. Examples include chronic renal failure, milk alkali syndrome, vitamin D intoxication, parathyroid neoplasms, and sarcoidosis.

Idiopathic calcinosis cutis occurs without a metabolic abnormality or regional soft tissue defect. Usually, these are localized tiny nodules in the skin found on the face or ears of neonates and small children. Idiopathic calcinosis of the skin of the scrotum or labia may also occur.

Osteoma Cutis

Spontaneous new bone formation may occur in the skin and is termed *osteoma cutis* (Fig. 159-1). This condition may be primary or secondary. Primary osteoma cutis occurs without an underlying skin lesion and is an isolated condition or is seen with Albright hereditary osteodystrophy and the associated pseudohypoparathyroidism or pseudo-pseudohypoparathyroidism. Secondary osteoma cutis arises in cutaneous neoplasms (similar to calcinosis cutis) or areas of inflammation, most notably in cases of acne vulgaris treated with tetracycline compounds.

Osteoma cutis may occur at any age. Isolated or multiple hard, raised nodules that measure 1 to 5 mm are found, most commonly on the face. The lesions may be painful. Overlying skin varies from normal to ulcerated. Laboratory values are typically normal, unless the patient has pseudohypoparathyroidism with decreased serum calcium and elevated serum phosphorus. The treatment of choice is surgical excision.

FOREIGN BODY

Suspected foreign body is a relatively common indication for imaging evaluation of the soft tissues in children. Foreign bodies include any substances that may penetrate the skin. These vary from inert materials such as glass and metal to organic materials such as thorns, cactus needles, and sea urchin spines. Once present, a significant foreign body reaction may occur in the surrounding soft tissues along with a local inflammatory response, particularly with organic materials. Some foreign bodies are clinically obvious, and others are occult. The occult foreign body with surrounding soft tissue granuloma may produce adjacent bone changes and simulate a neoplasm. More severe reactions can occur if the offending agent enters a joint.

Evaluation of any suspected foreign body should begin with conventional radiography of the area of concern through the soft tissue technique (lower kilovolt peak [kVp]). Two views obtained in planes at 90 degrees to each other with the entry site indicated are usually adequate to screen for radiopaque or radiolucent foreign bodies. Any foreign body that contains gas will produce a radiolucent appearance. The most common example is a lead pencil in which the "lead" is actually water-density graphite. The surrounding soft wood has a higher gas content that casts a radiolucent shadow around the graphite core in the acute stage, making it visible on radiography (Fig. 159-2). As the gas is resorbed and soft tissue reaction occurs, the pencil fragment

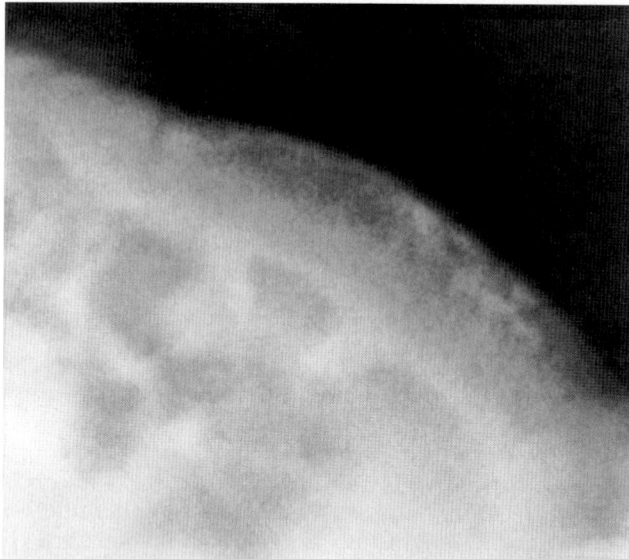

A

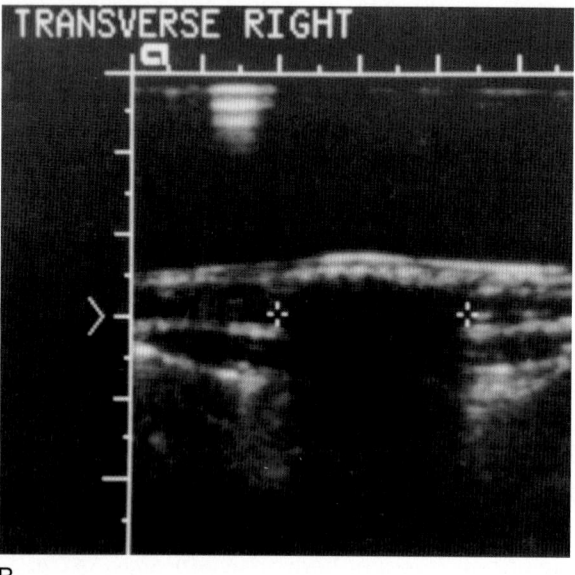

B

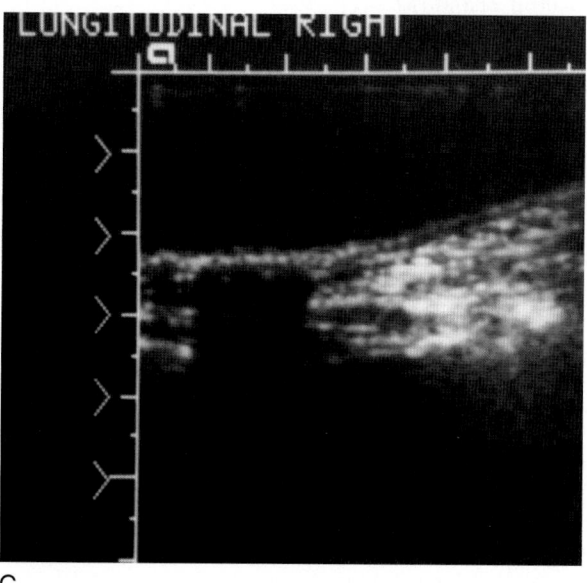

C

FIGURE 159-1. Osteoma cutis. Localized firm plaque was observed on the lower abdomen at 1 month; no birth trauma or hypothermia had occurred, and calcium and phosphorus concentrations were normal. The plaque increased in size, and a biopsy was obtained at 4 months. **A,** Radiograph at 4 months shows low anterior abdominal wall calcification. **B,** On transverse ultrasound scan through the area of abnormality, the calcification is superficial to the rectus muscles and acoustic shadowing is seen. **C,** A longitudinal midline ultrasound scan also shows shadowing; the urinary bladder below is partially distended. Sonograms were performed with a "water bath" to improve the image of superficial skin. (Courtesy of Dr. Diane Babcock, Cincinnati, OH.)

becomes invisible on radiographs, as are most organic foreign bodies.

Most published studies find that sonography is valuable for reliably detecting radiographically occult foreign bodies as small as 2.5 mm in live patients and cadaveric specimens. Detection of a foreign body on sonography requires meticulous attention to detail with high-resolution transducers, stand-off pads as necessary, and methodical scanning of the area in question. Most foreign bodies appear as hyperechoic foci with varying degrees of posterior acoustic shadowing depending on the composition of the foreign substance (Fig. 159-3). Sonography has also proved valuable in guiding foreign body removal. However, attempts to localize a nonradiopaque foreign body for removal may be compromised if a large amount of air is introduced into the surrounding soft tissue by extensive dissection prior to scanning.

In cases where foreign body penetration is not recognized, the clinical picture is more puzzling. If the foreign body is not removed, it becomes surrounded by fibrous tissue, forming a localized granuloma. The child may present with a new soft tissue mass with or without systemic findings of infection. Radiographs may demonstrate the foreign body if radiopaque. Often, foreign bodies are not visible, and radiographs may present a confusing picture of reactive changes in adjacent bone that could mimic neoplasm. In this setting, MRI becomes the study most frequently requested for evaluation. CT might be useful in localizing some foreign bodies (Fig. 159-4), but it does not offer the soft tissue contrast and marrow evaluation necessary in these confusing cases, in which bone and soft tissue tumors are under diagnostic consideration. MRI provides this type of evaluation and may well demonstrate the foreign body as an area of signal void often surrounded by a high T2-signal mass or fluid collection with varying degrees of contrast enhancement (Fig. 159-5). Histologically, foreign body giant cells with an inflammatory reaction

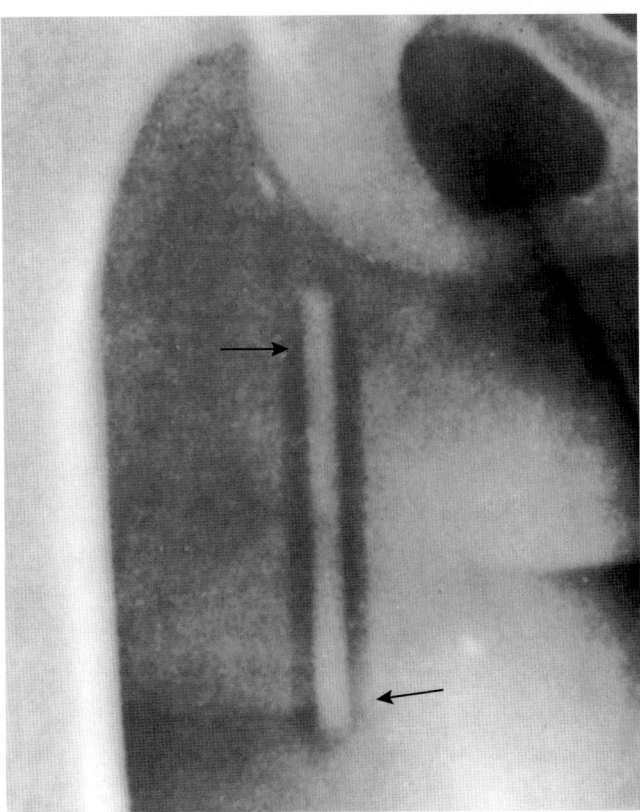

FIGURE 159-2. Fragment of a standard lead pencil in the right buttock of a 6-year-old boy said to have "sat down on a sharp pencil" that penetrated the skin, leaving this fragment *(arrows)*. Because of its high gas content, the soft wood of the pencil casts a radiolucent tubular image around the central core of the graphite cylinder, which approximates the density of water. "Lead" pencils, of course, contain no lead.

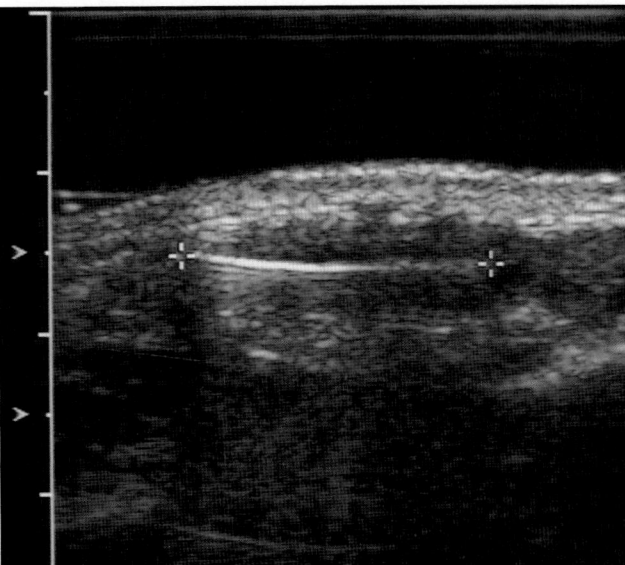

FIGURE 159-3. Foreign body (glass) in the cheek of a 15-year-old struck in the face with a bottle. Calipers on this sonogram mark the 2-cm echogenic foreign body in the subcutaneous tissues.

are seen. Most fluid collections are sterile. In cases where a foreign body is discovered in close proximity to a joint, MRI might be useful for preoperative joint evaluation. Foreign body removal with antibiotic therapy as needed is usually curative.

> On ultrasound, most foreign bodies are hyperechoic with varying posterior acoustic shadowing depending on the composition of the foreign body.

SUBCUTANEOUS GRANULOMA ANNULARE

Subcutaneous granuloma annulare (SGA) is a benign, self-limited inflammatory skin lesion. Unlike the other subtypes of granuloma annulare (localized, generalized, and perforating), SGA occurs exclusively in children. It is seen most frequently in children 2 to 5 years of age; the typical presentation is that of a nontender deep dermal or subcutaneous nodule. SGA has been identified in a variety of locations, including the hand and scalp; the lower extremity is the most common site, especially in pretibial locations (Fig. 159-6). Histologically, SGA is characterized by foci of collagen and degeneration with peripheral histiocytes and a surrounding zone of reactive inflammation and fibrosis. It resembles the nodules seen

in adults with rheumatoid arthritis and skin lesions in adult patients with diabetes patients (necrobiosis lipoidica diabeticorum). Different from its occurrence in adults, in whom granuloma annulare variants are associated with connective tissue disease, SGA is not a feature of connective tissue disorders in children. One report suggests a possible association with diabetes in children.

Children with SGA often present to a physician who is unfamiliar with this characteristic dermatologic lesion. Not uncommonly, imaging is then requested to evaluate a soft tissue mass. On conventional radiography, SGA may appear as a soft tissue mass without calcifications. On MRI, a poorly defined subcutaneous soft tissue mass is seen that is isointense to hyperintense relative to muscle on T1-weighted images, with variable increased signal on T2-weighted images. After intravenous gadolinium has been administered, a propensity for relatively diffuse enhancement of the lesion has been noted. Local recurrence is common but does not warrant additional biopsy because this is a self-limited condition.

> Subcutaneous granuloma annulare most commonly presents in children 2 to 5 years of age and most often occurs in the pretibial subcutaneous tissues.

INFLAMMATORY MUSCLE DISEASES

Inflammatory muscle disorders in children are either acute or chronic. Acute muscular symptoms beyond trauma or overuse are most commonly associated with an infectious agent that may be bacterial, viral, or parasitic. Other environmental triggers of myositis include drugs, vaccines, growth hormone, and bone marrow transplants that may induce graft-versus-host myositis. The subgroup of chronic myositis is a diverse collection of rare syn-

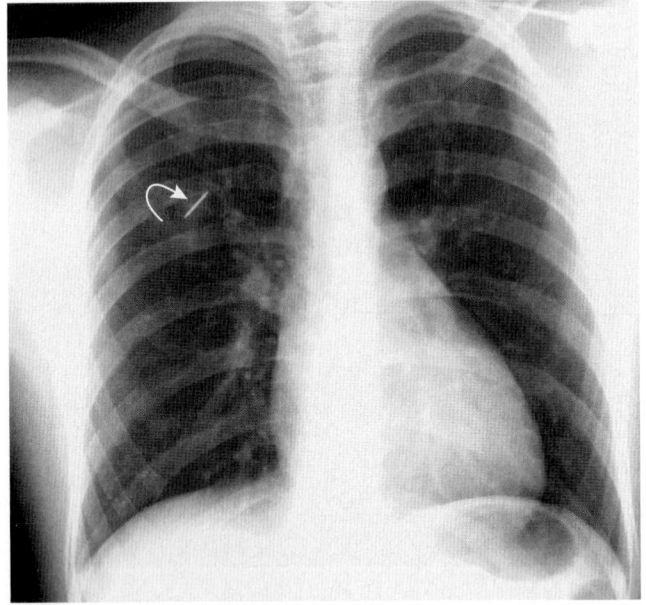

A

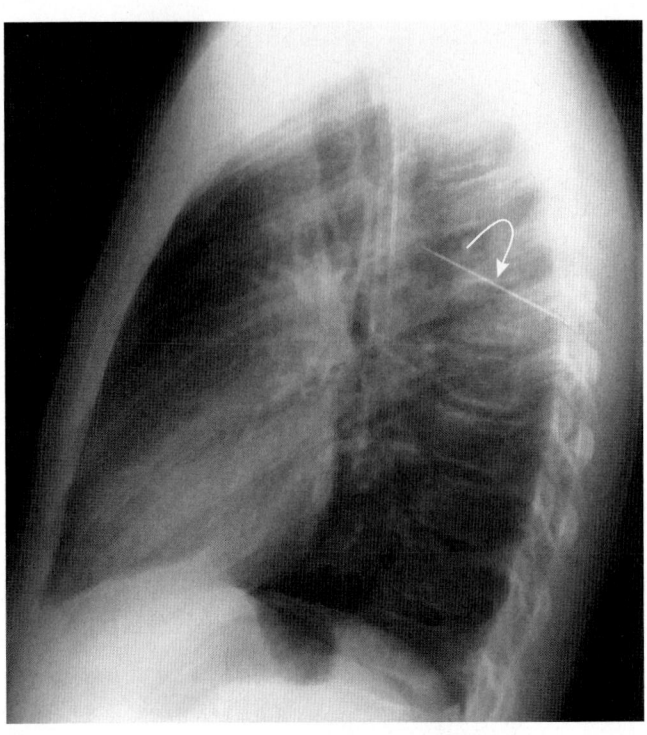

B

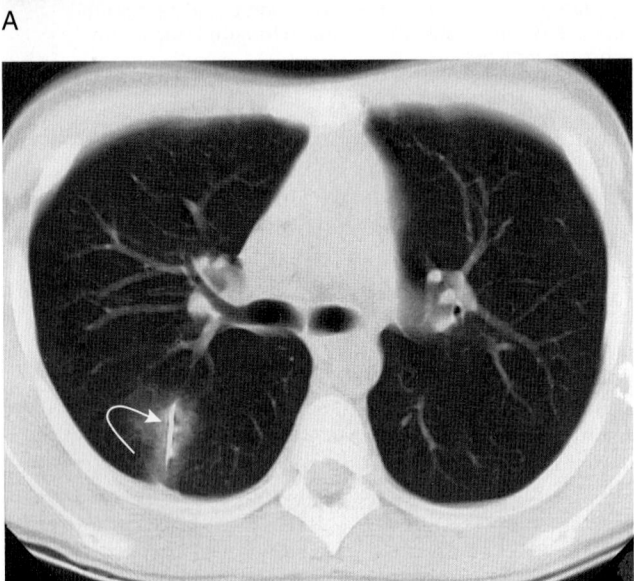

C

FIGURE 159-4. Foreign body (needle). This 10-year-old presented with shoulder pain and unequal breath sounds. **A** and **B,** Chest radiographs show a needle in the posterior right chest *(curved arrow).* **C,** Chest computed tomography better reveals the soft tissue reaction surrounding the needle *(curved arrow)* and lack of major vessel injury or pneumothorax.

dromes that share the common finding of chronic muscle inflammation of as yet undetermined patho-physiology, leading to damaged function of smooth and striated muscle. The juvenile idiopathic inflammatory myopathies include a variety of syndromes, the most common of which are dermatomyositis, polymyositis, and overlap myositis (myositis with another connective tissue disease in which vasculitis is a component, such as lupus or mixed connective tissue disease).

Dermatomyositis

Juvenile dermatomyositis is the most common form of idiopathic inflammatory myopathy in childhood; it has a more prominent vasculitis component than do other myopathic syndromes. It occurs 10 to 20 times more frequently than polymyositis and has a peak age distribution

between 5 and 14 years of age. No definite genetic link has been documented, although various genetic components may be associated with disease expression and susceptibility. Children typically present with the symptom of persistent and progressive symmetric proximal muscle weakness that may be insidious in onset. The characteristic rash is violaceous, involves the eyelids and nasal bridge, and is photosensitive (heliotropic), perhaps accounting in part for its increased occurrence in the springtime. Scaly erythematous papules (Gottron papules) are another common cutaneous finding that is most frequently seen over the small joints on the dorsum of the hands. One or more of the muscle-associated enzymes, including creatine phosphokinase (CPK), aldolase, lactate dehydrogenase (LDH), and the transaminases, are typically elevated. Evidence of inflammatory myopathy is sought on electromyography (EMG) and

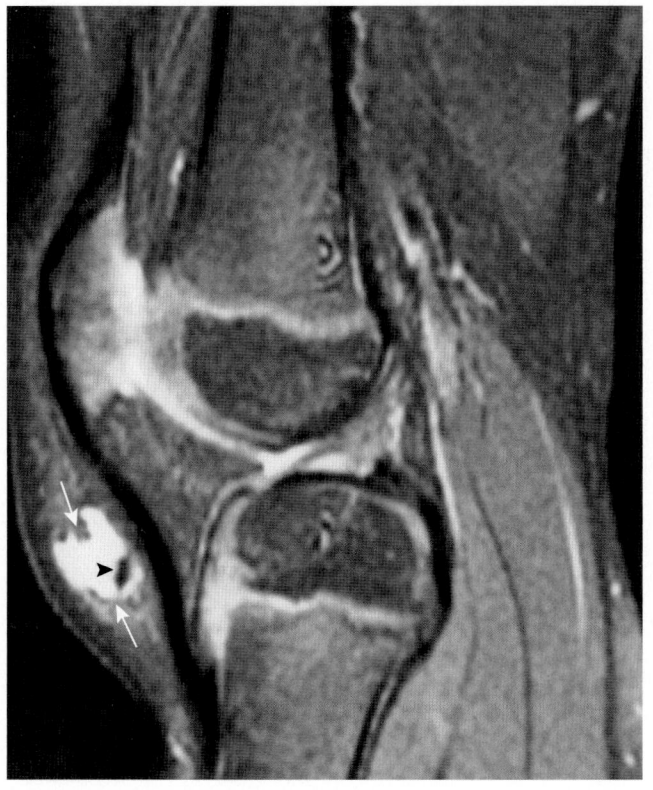

A

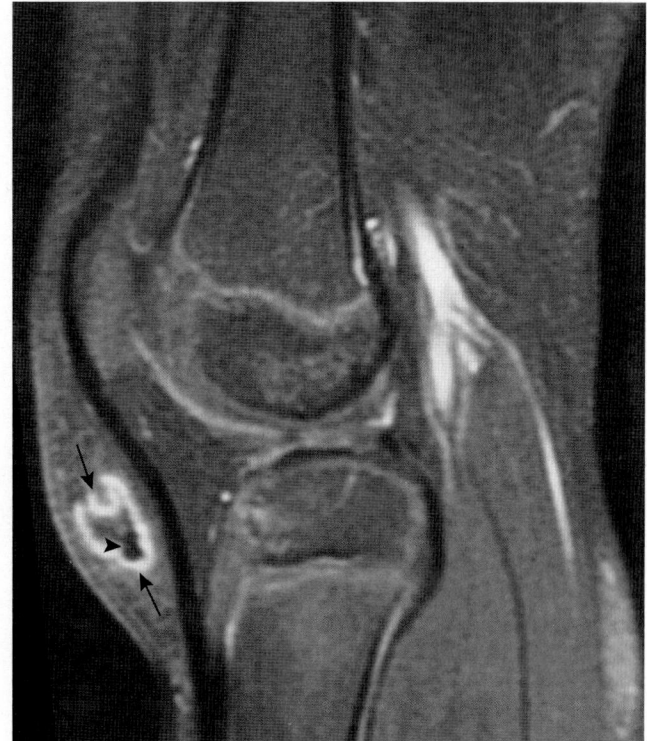

B

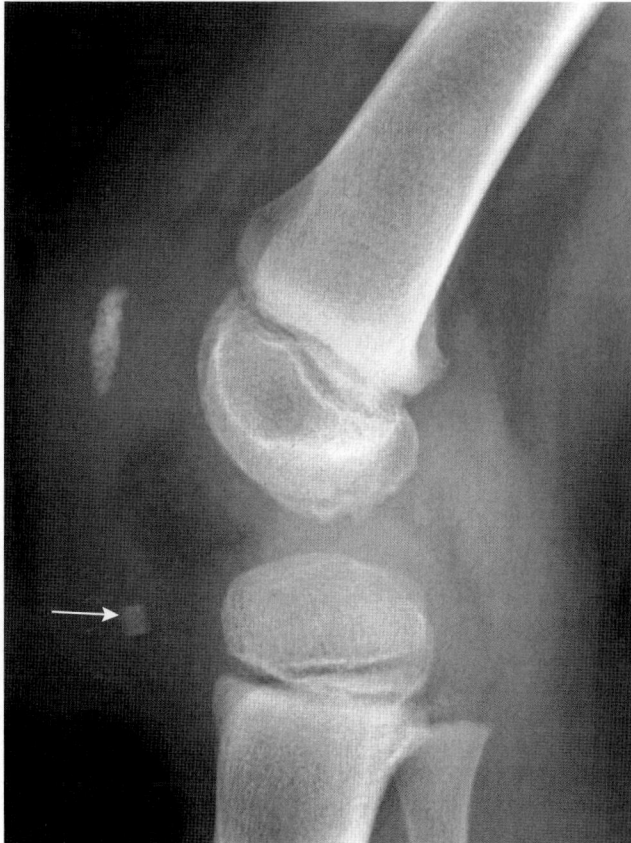

C

FIGURE 159-5. Foreign body reaction. This 5-year-old had a palpable infrapatellar mass without a history of trauma. On magnetic resonance imaging, sagittal T2-weighted fast spin echo **(A)** and gadolinium-enhanced T1-weighted **(B)** images, both with fat suppression, show a high T2 signal mass *(arrows)* with peripheral enhancement and a focal area of persistent signal void inferiorly *(arrowhead)*. **C,** This proved on radiography to represent a radiopaque foreign body *(arrow)*.

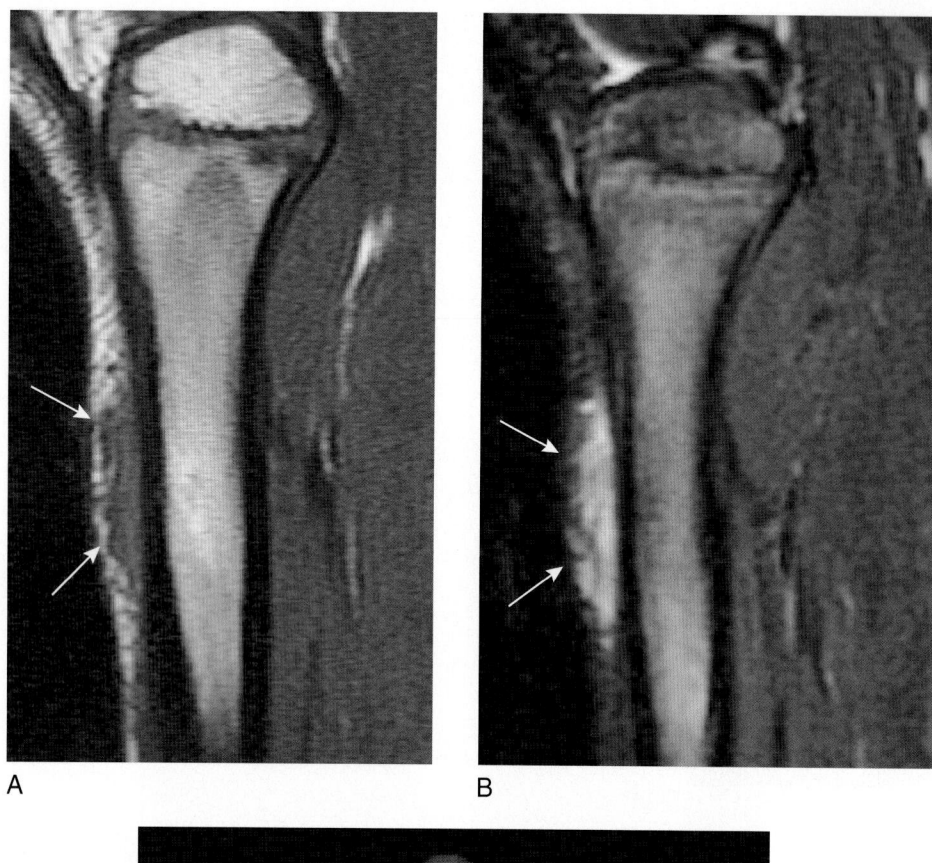

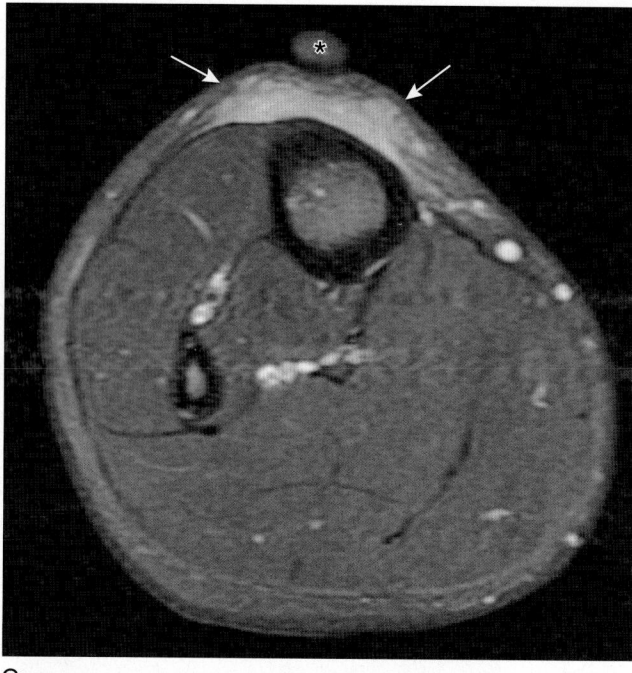

FIGURE 159-6. Subcutaneous granuloma annulare. This 8-year-old boy presented with a painless pretibial mass. On magnetic resonance imaging, sagittal T1-weighted **(A)** and short tau inversion recovery **(B)** images show a poorly defined, plaquelike subcutaneous pretibial mass *(arrows)* that enhances diffusely on the postgadolinium fat-suppressed T1-weighted sequence **(C)**. Asterisk, vitamin E capsule.

histopathology. Muscle biopsy shows chronic inflammatory infiltrates of perivascular or interstitial mononuclear cells with myocyte degeneration, necrosis, and regeneration. Evidence of the characteristic rash observed as meeting three of the other four criteria (proximal muscle weakness, elevated muscle-associated enzymes, EMG findings of inflammatory myopathy, and/or characteristic muscle biopsy findings) is necessary for diagnosis. Polymyositis is similar but lacks cutaneous involvement

and has a different histologic picture. The vasculopathy that characterizes dermatomyositis may also cause gastrointestinal (GI) dysfunction (mainly swallowing and esophageal abnormalities), pulmonary fibrosis, and reversible cardiac conduction abnormalities.

MRI has proved very helpful in the diagnosis and management of adult and pediatric patients with dermatomyositis. Inflammatory changes in skin, subcutaneous tissue, muscle, and fascia, although not visible on T1-

weighted images, are exquisitely revealed as high signal areas on fat-saturated T2-weighted and short tau inversion recovery (STIR) sequences (Fig. 159-7). Although they are highly sensitive, MRI findings are not specific and may be seen after traumatic denervation or with rhabdomyolysis, infection, or necrotizing fasciitis. Exercise for approximately 30 minutes in patients with known inflammatory myopathy has been shown to visibly increase the muscle signal intensity on STIR sequences. Fat suppression is strongly recommended with T2 weighting to avoid a pronounced chemical shift artifact

that is seen as a high signal band along the frequency encoding gradient at the muscle–fat interface of involved regions. This artifact will be more pronounced at high field strength (3 T and above) because fat and water resonance peaks are farther separated than at lower field strength. Reticulated areas of increased T2 signal are frequently seen in the subcutaneous fat in patients with skin involvement and are helpful for non-invasively evaluating disease activity. They may also be the precursor for development of calcinosis, one of the more incapacitating features of juvenile dermatomyositis.

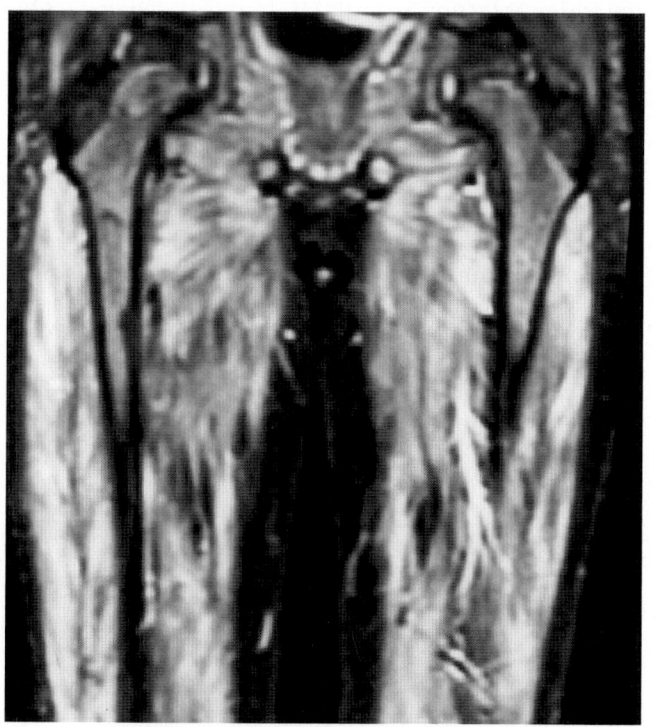

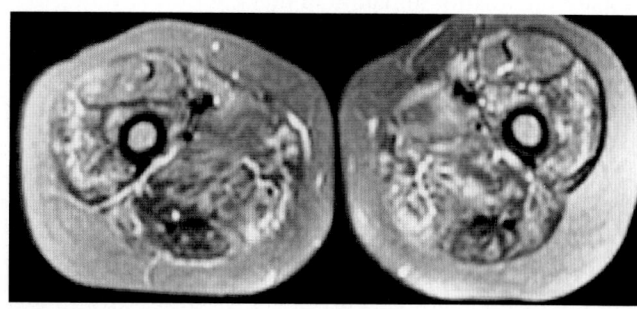

FIGURE 159-7. Dermatomyositis in an 8-year-old boy. T2-weighted fast spin echo magnetic resonance images with fat suppression in the coronal (**A**) and axial (**B**) planes at diagnosis show diffusely abnormal increased signal intensity throughout the muscles of both thighs. **C** and **D**, Same sequence of images after 10 months of therapy now shows normal muscle signal intensity.

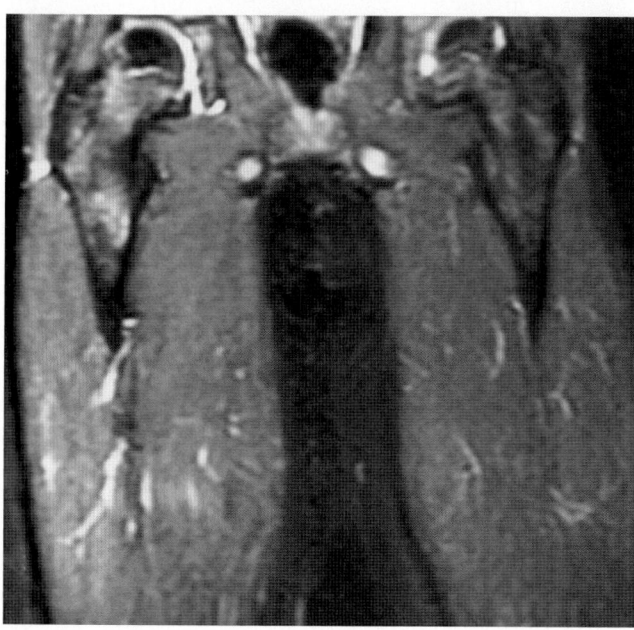

A

C

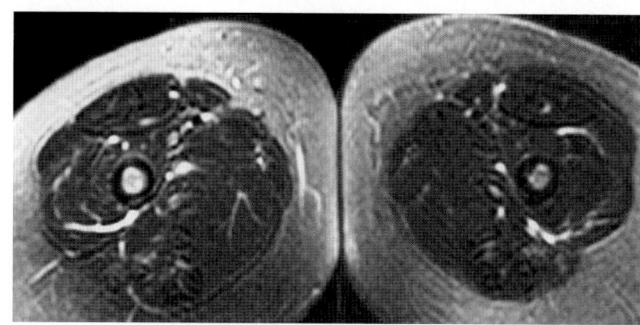

B

D

Soft tissue calcification is reported to occur in 30% to 70% of patients with juvenile dermatomyositis and may be related to disease duration and severity. Calcium deposition in the soft tissues typically occurs at sites exposed to trauma (e.g., buttocks, elbows, knees). The calcinosis is dystrophic and is believed to be the end result of scarring from microvascular destruction and tissue necrosis. The following five patterns have been described: (1) superficial plaques on the extremities (calcinosis cutis), (2) deep tumorous deposits within proximal muscles (calcinosis circumscripta), (3) intermuscular fascial plane deposits (calcinosis universalis), (4) subcutaneous reticular exoskeleton-like deposits, and (5) mixed forms. In patients with severe forms of calcinosis, milk of calcium fluid collections have been described within soft tissues. Although they are readily visible on radiography and CT, areas of calcinosis are much less conspicuous on MR images (Fig. 159-8). They appear as areas of signal void on T1- and T2-weighted images that may be enhanced on gradient echo sequences. When chronic muscle atrophy develops, fatty muscle infiltration will be apparent on T1-weighted images.

The distribution of muscle involvement is often symmetric and may be patchy. Because of the patchy distribution, EMG and muscle biopsy may be falsely negative owing to sampling error. Occasionally, muscle enzymes are deceptively normal, as they may be at disease onset, after initiation of therapy, during remission, or with severe muscle atrophy. MRI is very helpful in non-invasively confirming or excluding muscle abnormality, particularly in patients with atypical clinical and laboratory findings (Fig. 159-9). The results of MRI are useful for optimizing biopsy location or EMG lead placement. In one study in adults, Schweitzer and Fort showed MRI to be cost-effective for patients with polymyositis because it reduces the number of false-negative biopsy results. For patients who are difficult to assess clinically, MRI may be useful for monitoring disease progress or return to normalcy after steroid or other immunosuppressive therapy. Whether the use of intravenous gadolinium is warranted remains unanswered by any controlled study. It may be helpful to exclude abscess formation in patients for whom infection is in the differential diagnosis. Our clinicians use gadolinium enhancement to confirm areas of active inflammation prior to biopsy.

MR spectroscopy (MRS) with the use of phosphorus-31 and quantitative T2 mapping may provide a quantitative assessment of metabolic abnormalities in dermatomyositis and can be performed at the time of the MRI study. Studies in adults and children have shown lower than normal levels of adenosine triphosphate (ATP) and phosphocreatine (PCr) at P-31 spectroscopy in involved muscles at rest; these levels correlate with weakness and fatigue. Changes may be accentuated with exercise. Quantitative T2 mapping has shown significantly increased T2 relaxation in actively inflamed muscle as compared with inactive dermatomyositis and normal muscle. Additional studies will be needed to identify the

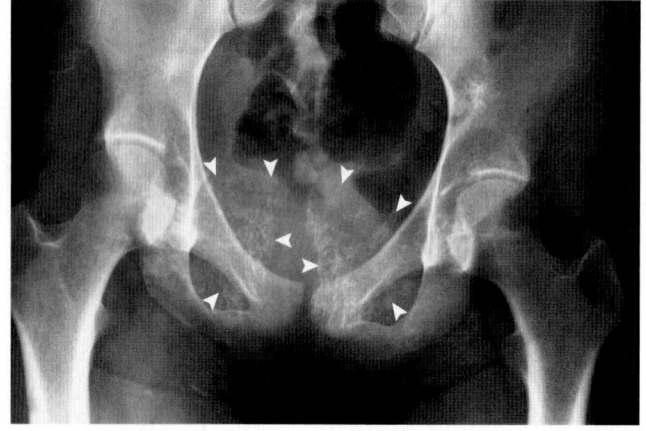

A

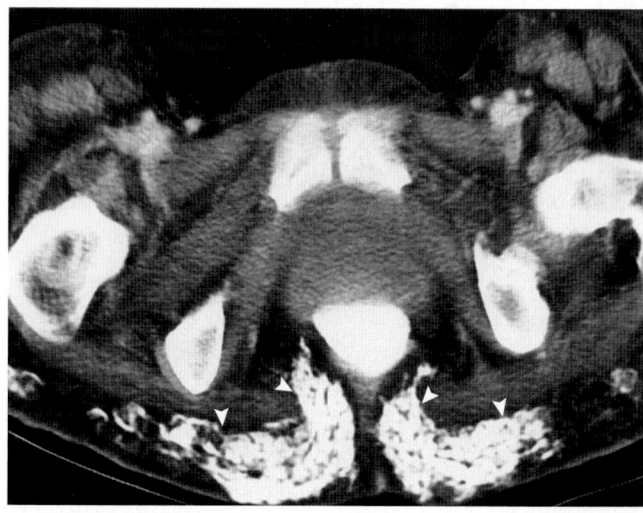

B

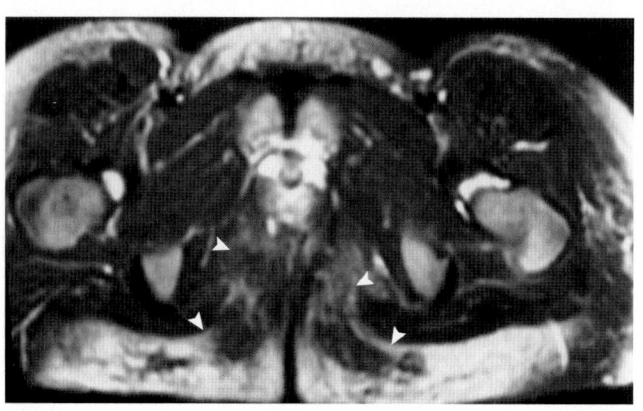

C

FIGURE 159-8. Dermatomyositis. Extensive soft tissue calcifications, predominantly in the subcutaneous gluteal fat *(arrowheads)* in this 19-year-old female with severe multisystemic involvement, are much more conspicuous on radiography **(A)** and computed tomography **(B)** than on T2-weighted magnetic resonance imaging **(C)**.

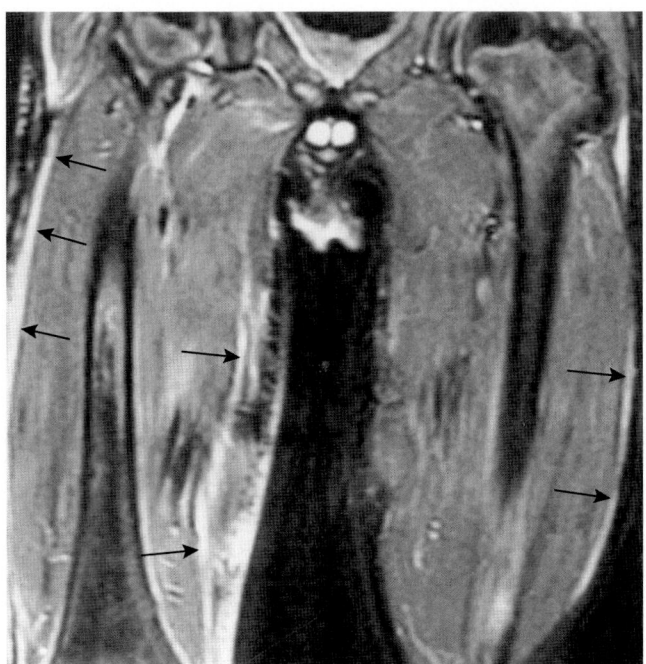

A

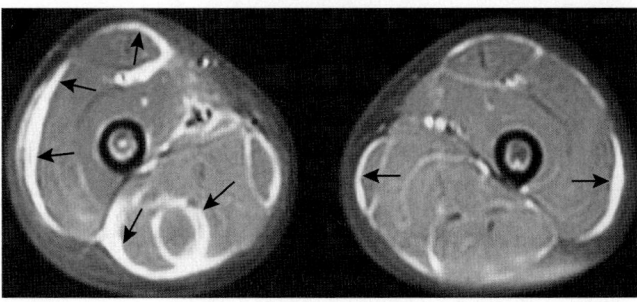

B

FIGURE 159-9. Eosinophilic fasciitis. This 3-year-old boy presented with pain and swelling in the lower extremities with joint contractures. On magnetic resonance imaging coronal T2-weighted fast spin echo **(A)** and axial postgadolinium T1-weighted **(B)** images, both with chemical fat suppression, the abnormal increased signal and enhancement are limited to the superficial and deep fascial planes of both thighs *(arrows)*, right worse than left, with sparing of the adjacent muscles.

role of these novel noninvasive approaches in monitoring disease status and guiding therapy.

> **In patients with juvenile dermatomyositis, MRI is useful for optimizing biopsy location.**

Pyomyositis

Pyomyositis is a localized primary infection of muscle characterized by progression to abscess formation that can mimic tumor, trauma (hematoma), osteomyelitis, septic arthritis, cellulitis, or thrombophlebitis. This disorder is endemic in Africa, South America, southeastern Asia, and the South Pacific. Pyomyositis is increasingly reported in temperate climates, including northern United States. Pyomyositis occurs in otherwise healthy children and in those predisposed to infection by debilitating diseases, including human immunodeficiency virus infection. *Staphylococcus aureus* is the causative organism in 95% of cases. Multifocal pyomyositis may be seen as a complication of bacterial endocarditis. Secondary pyomyositis may also occur as the result of extension from adjacent osteomyelitis, particularly in the pelvis. Damaged muscle with some degree of underlying immune suppression and a source of bacteremia are the key elements involved in the development of pyomyositis. Underlying muscle damage is important in that normal muscle is resistant to suppuration.

Clinically, the gluteal muscles, thighs, and calves are more commonly affected than the upper extremities, trunk, and chest wall. Usually, only a single muscle is involved. Early in the course of illness, patients experience localized pain and tenderness, often in the absence of fever. The involved area lacks cutaneous erythema, which is usually evident with cellulitis, and has a "woody" nonfluctuant feel. Fever usually occurs as infection advances. Infections of the pelvic musculature may clinically mimic osteomyelitis or septic arthritis by producing hip or groin pain. Infection of the piriformis muscle may irritate the adjacent sciatic nerve and produce pain that extends into the ipsilateral lower extremity. Pyomyositis is usually accompanied by elevations in white blood cell count, erythrocyte sedimentation rate, and C-reactive protein level.

Early in the development of pyomyositis, the affected muscle is enlarged and edematous without a frank abscess. Without treatment, the process progresses to form an intramuscular abscess. Ultrasonography may be helpful in localizing relatively superficial sites of pyomyositis (Fig. 159-10). Infections at deeper sites and infections that have not yet formed an intramuscular abscess are less readily detected on ultrasonography. If infection is suspected, CT is not the modality of choice; however, most intramuscular abscesses are readily seen at all locations. CT findings indicative of abscess include enlargement of the involved muscle, central low attenuation fluid collection, and a peripheral rim that enhances upon administration of intravenous contrast (Fig. 159-11).

MRI is the preferred modality for imaging of suspected pyomyositis in children. MRI is also preferred if infection is suspected and symptoms are relatively localized and is particularly valuable in cases of pelvic pyomyositis. On MRI, the involved muscle appears enlarged and edematous with increased signal on T2 weighting and inversion recovery sequences. On T1-weighted images, the signal intensity of some abscesses is homogeneously greater than that of the involved muscle. On T2-weighted images, the abscess is seen as high signal with a hypointense rim and less well-defined hyperintensity of the adjacent muscle (see Fig. 159-10). Postgadolinium T1-weighted images best reveal the abscess, and the abscess wall densely enhances (see Fig. 159-10). Changes may result from associated cellulitis and include skin thickening, stranding of the subcutaneous fat, and swelling of fascial planes; these findings are best seen on fat saturation T2-weighted and inversion recovery images. A sympathetic effusion may

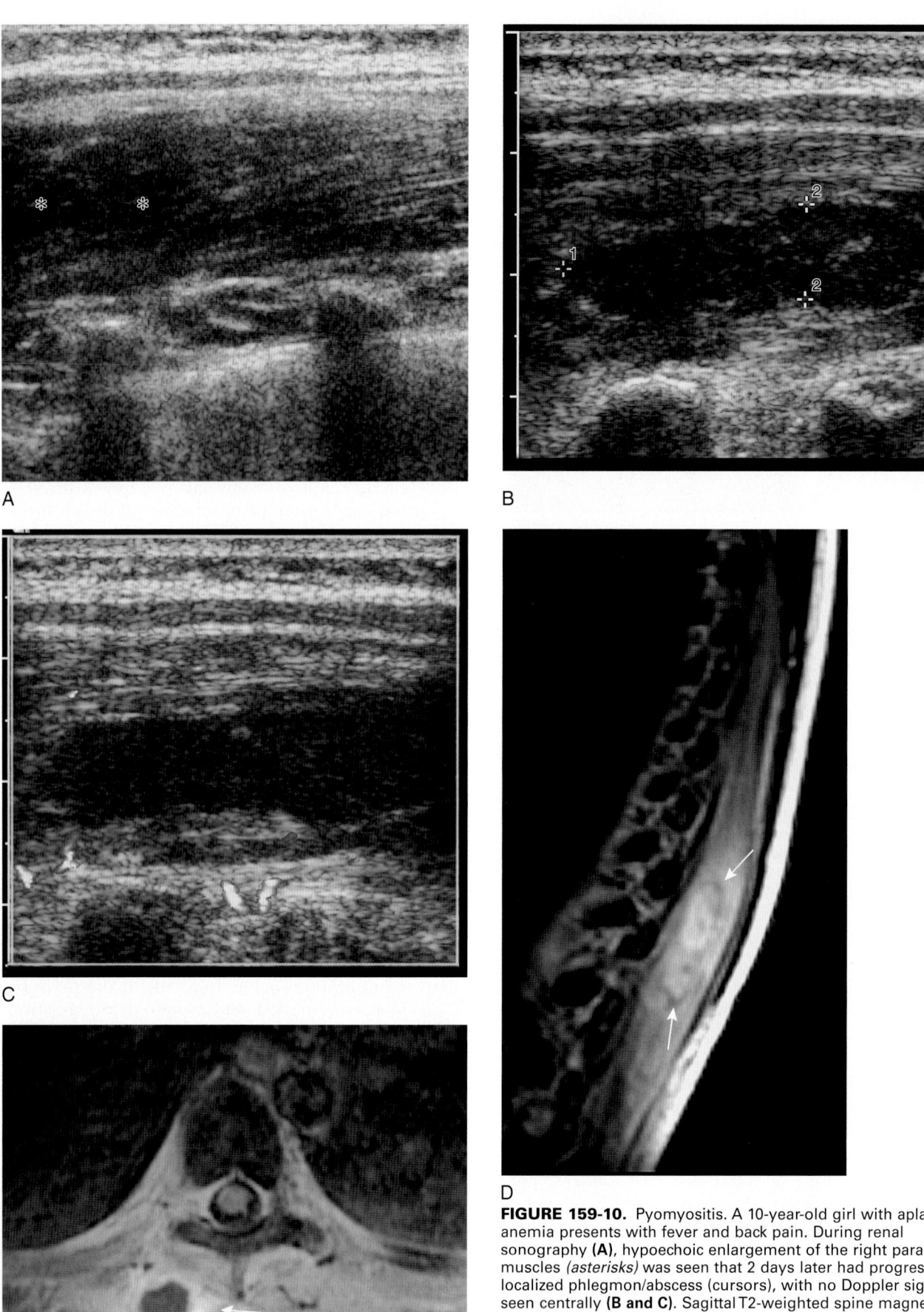

A

B

C

D

FIGURE 159-10. Pyomyositis. A 10-year-old girl with aplastic anemia presents with fever and back pain. During renal sonography (**A**), hypoechoic enlargement of the right paraspinal muscles *(asterisks)* was seen that 2 days later had progressed to localized phlegmon/abscess (cursors), with no Doppler signal seen centrally (**B and C**). Sagittal T2-weighted spine magnetic resonance imaging shows right paraspinal muscle edema with a central higher signal intensity collection surrounded by a lower signal intensity rim *(arrows)* (**D**). On axial fat-suppressed T1-weighted images after gadolinium administration (**E**), the collection *(arrows)* is characterized by an irregular rim of enhancement and lack of contrast enhancement centrally. Note low signal intensity marrow, likely due to iron deposition from multiple transfusions.

E

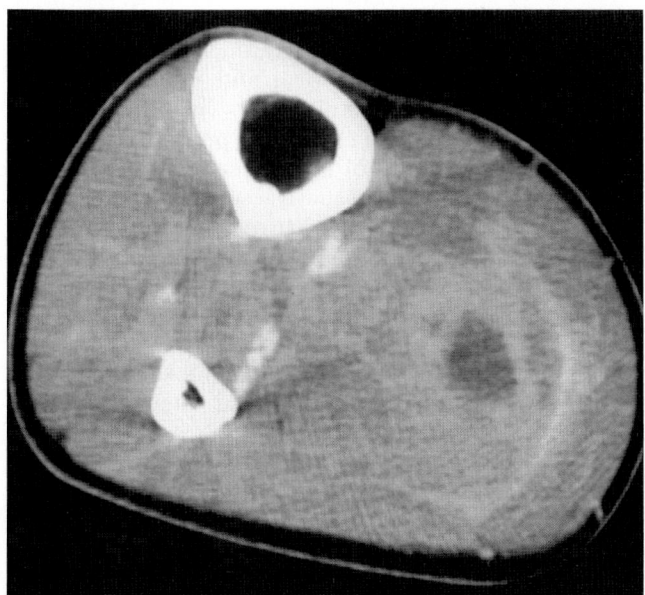

FIGURE 159-11. Pyomyositis. An abscess in the lower leg of a 16-year-old boy with leukemia. A contrast-enhanced computed tomography scan image shows a central low attenuation collection with an ill-defined enhancing peripheral rim.

be present if infection is found near a joint. Often, the chief clinical differential diagnosis is osteomyelitis. In pyomyositis, underlying bones usually appear normal, and the process is displaced or eccentric to underlying bone, whereas in osteomyelitis, signal abnormality is seen within the medullary space, and the process is centered on involved bone.

Muscle abscesses show avidity for gallium-67 and indium-labeled leukocytes; however, these techniques are usually reserved for patients in whom the site of infection is not localized or in whom multifocal disease is suspected.

Drainage of abscesses and appropriate antibiotic therapy are usually curative of pyomyositis. More aggressive abscesses may require greater debridement of muscle.

Imaging may be used to guide percutaneous aspiration or drainage of larger collections.

NECROTIZING FASCIITIS/CELLULITIS

Necrotizing fasciitis is a rapidly progressive, sometimes fatal soft tissue infection that characteristically involves deep fascia of the extremities and trunk. The disease tends to affect the elderly and those with impaired immunity, but it can occur in immune competent patients of any age. Underlying skin infection related to lesions such as furuncles, insect bites, and even minor trauma or surgery has been associated with this condition. It is most commonly a polymicrobial infection with both aerobic and anaerobic organisms. In children with chicken pox, secondary infection of vesicular skin lesions with *S. aureus* or group A *Streptococcus* has been linked to development of cellulitis and, less frequently, necrotizing fasciitis.

Cellulitis is amenable to medical therapy with IV antibiotics; necrotizing fasciitis is a life-threatening emergency that requires additional urgent surgical debridement of necrotic tissue. Therefore, distinction between these two entities is critical for patient management. The early clinical presentation of necrotizing fasciitis is nonspecific with vague systemic complaints of fever and malaise and rapid progression to sepsis and acute renal failure. Initial soft tissue findings are those of warmth and induration. The infection does not wall off, as would an abscess; therefore, it spreads rapidly and localization is difficult. A high index of suspicion is paramount for early diagnosis.

Imaging can facilitate the diagnosis. Radiographs are insensitive to changes of necrotizing fasciitis, until they are advanced, at which time gas can be seen in the soft tissues. Characteristic CT findings include soft tissue air, deep fascial fluid collections, and fascial enhancement, although these findings are not consistently seen (Fig. 159-12). Ultrasonography may depict deep soft tissue changes and fluid collections, offering the benefits of portability, lack of ionizing radiation, and no need for

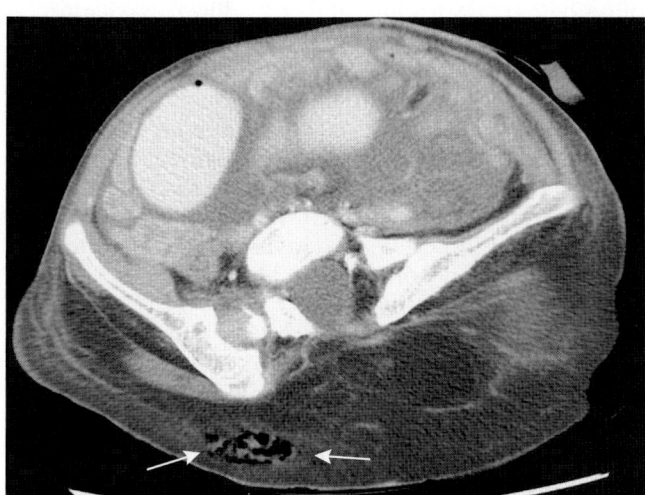

A

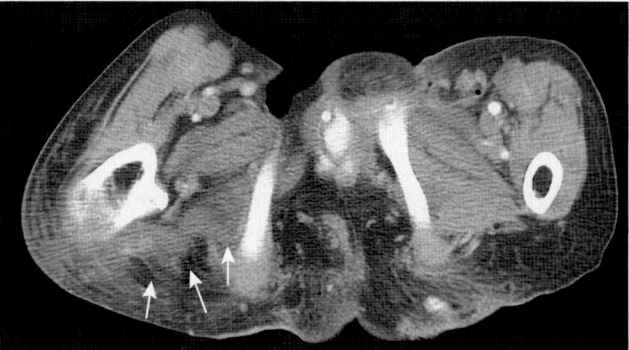

B

FIGURE 159-12. Necrotizing fasciitis. This female patient with spinal dysraphism and cloacal exstrophy status post bladder augmentation presented with sepsis. Contrast-enhanced computed tomography **(A and B)** shows gas in the soft tissues of the right buttock (*arrows* in **A**) and diffuse deep fascial thickening with low attenuation (*arrows* in **B**).

sedation, along with the ability to guide for diagnostic aspiration.

However, pathologic changes and extent of necrotizing fasciitis and cellulitis are detected most sensitively on MRI with fat-suppressed T2, STIR, and post-IV gadolinium fat–suppressed T1-weighted imaging (Fig. 159-13). Cellulitis is characterized by high T2 signal thickening and gadolinium enhancement with or without fluid collection in the subcutaneous tissue and superficial fascia (Fig. 159-14). Necrotizing fasciitis should be considered when these changes extend to the deep fascia. High T2 signal regions with only peripheral gadolinium enhancement suggest necrosis or abscess formation. Soft tissue gas appears as areas of signal absence with susceptibility artifact. Although these findings are sensitive, they overlap with those of other pathologic conditions, including dermatomyositis, pyomyositis, and lymphedema. Additionally, in the very early stages of necrotizing fasciitis, deep fascial involvement may be minimal or lacking. Therefore, even though exclusion of deep fascial involvement on MRI is fairly reliable for exclusion of necrotizing fasciitis, ultimate patient management relies on a combination of imaging and clinical findings.

> The diagnosis of necrotizing fasciitis relies on clinical findings in conjunction with MRI findings.

FIBRODYSPLASIA OSSIFICANS PROGRESSIVA

Fibrodysplasia ossificans progressiva is a rare inheritable disorder that is characterized by shortening of the great toe and thumb, which is associated with progressive development of heterotopic ossification in connective tissue and striated muscle and results in disabling ankylosis and muscle fixation.

Most cases of this disease represent spontaneous mutations, although an autosomal dominant mode of inheritance has been confirmed. Affected individuals are normal at birth with the exception of digital abnormalities, most commonly, microdactyly of the great toe with hallux valgus. At some time during infancy or young childhood, patients develop soft tissue nodules or masses—often painful and erythematous—typically over the upper trunk or neck, which may be associated with trauma. Swellings resolve or ossify (Fig. 159-15). Heterotopic ossification begins at a mean age of 5 years, and the course of the disease follows that of exacerbations of nodular swellings, with progressive ossification of muscle and connective tissue that proceeds from the posterior neck and shoulder girdle distally, caudally, and anteriorly. Involvement of the chest wall and muscles of mastication contributes to nutritional deficiencies, restrictive pulmonary disease, and pneumonia, which commonly lead to death in adulthood.

Prior to ossification, cross-sectional imaging may simply reveal nonspecific soft tissue masses on CT that exhibit high T2 signal on MRI (Fig. 159-16). Recognition of characteristic digital changes can help avert biopsy, which is known to aggravate the condition. Once lesions begin to ossify, they may be recognized on CT and by radionuclide bone scan, even before bandlike areas of heterotopic bone formation are visible on conventional radiographs. Additional radiographic findings include narrow anteroposterior cervical and lumbar vertebral body diameter (possibly explained by hypotonia).

Biopsy of fibrodysplasia ossificans progressiva typically reveals different phases of normal endochondral osteogenesis at heterotopic sites. Early lesions show infiltrating loose myxoid fibrous tissue that may be misinterpreted as fibromatosis or sarcoma, hence the importance of recognizing characteristic findings in the great toe—as seen in nearly all patients—that obviate the need for biopsy. The coexistence of pathologic changes with congenital malformations of the great toes implies that defective induction of endochondral osteogenesis may underlie this disorder.

Surgical therapy is not indicated in this disease. Diphosphonate may be given to inhibit the ossification process, possibly with steroids to diminish inflammation, although results are inconsistent. Nutritional supplementation, prevention of pressure sores, and use of devices to assist with mobility are often necessary.

> A characteristic deformity of the great toes with hallux valgus and short, deformed first metacarpal is seen in nearly all patients with fibrodysplasia ossificans progressiva.

TUMORAL CALCINOSIS

Tumoral calcinosis is a relatively rare, benign condition that is characterized by masslike calcific deposits of hydroxyapatite crystals in the soft tissues near major joints. The idiopathic variety tends to occur in otherwise healthy adolescents and young adults. A number of cases of tumoral calcinosis have been reported in infants. Secondary tumoral calcinosis is a variation that occurs in patients with a high calcium–phosphorus product and metastatic calcification (as in renal failure and secondary hyperparathyroidism).

Although the precise pathogenesis of the idiopathic form is unknown, an inborn error of phosphorus metabolism is considered likely to be related to abnormal phosphate reabsorption and 1,25-dihydroxyvitamin D formation in the proximal renal tubule. An autosomal dominant mode of genetic transmission has been identified in this condition, which occurs more frequently in African Americans. Serum calcium levels are normal, but hyperphosphatemia and elevated serum 1,25-dihydroxyvitamin D may be found. Despite these abnormalities in some individuals, normal serum phosphorus and vitamin D levels in others and juxta-articular predilection and morphology of these calcific masses remain unexplained.

Patients typically present with a painless mass or masses in a juxta-articular location. The most common sites of involvement include the shoulder, hip, and elbow, although the knee, hands, and feet may be involved. On conventional radiographs, tumoral calcinosis is usually seen as a well-defined mass with a lobulated appearance and fibrous septa that give a cobblestone or "chicken wire" appearance (Fig. 159-17). If semifluid calcific

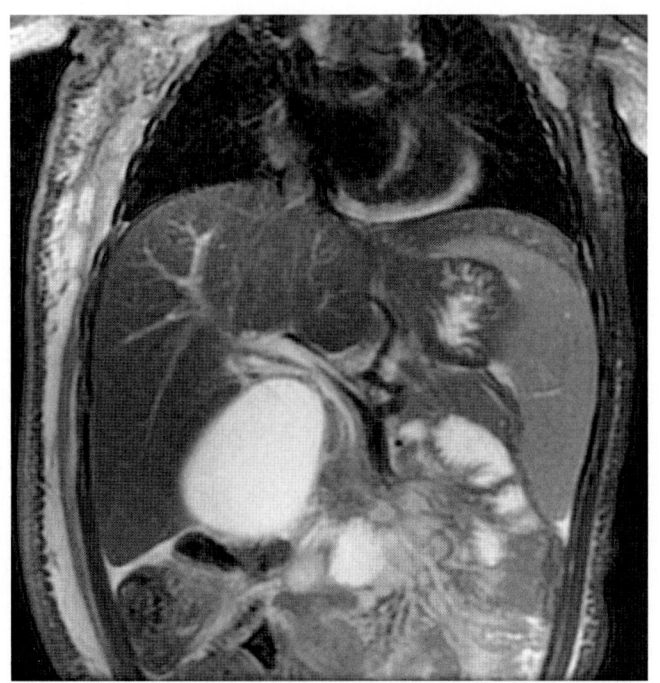

A

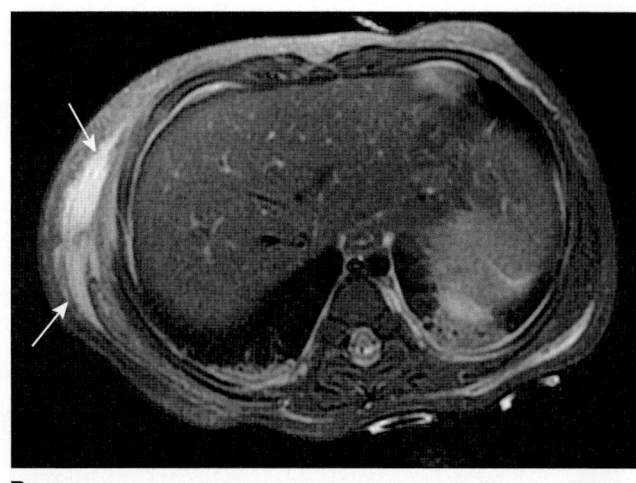

B

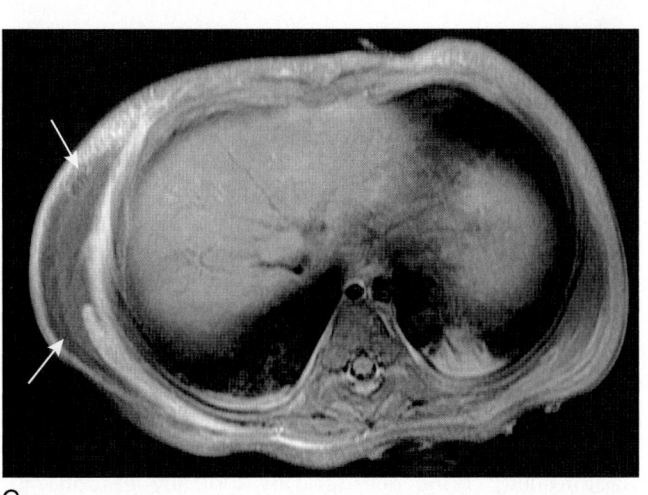

C

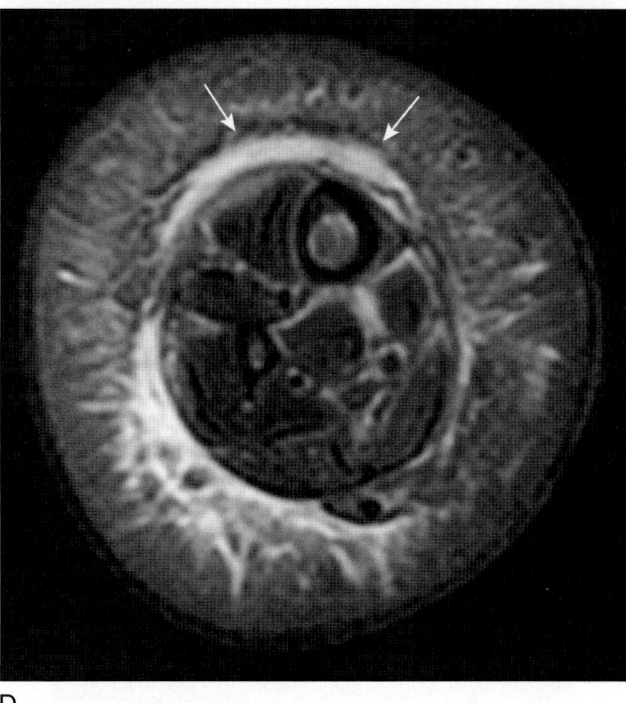

D

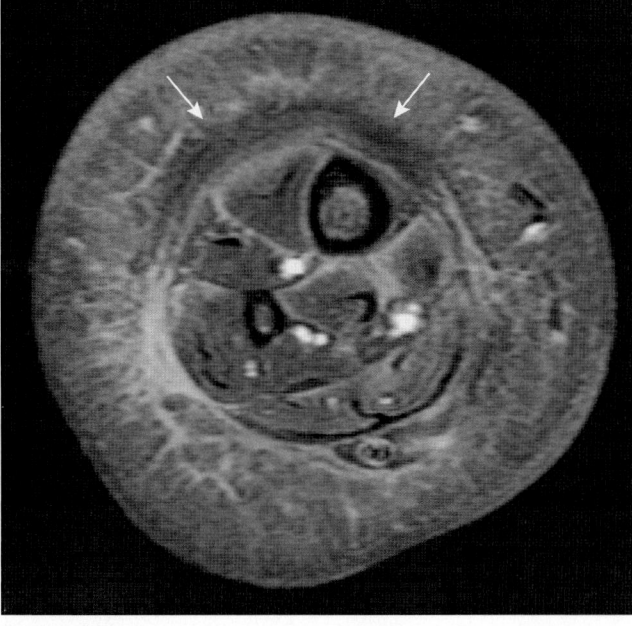

E

FIGURE 159-13. Necrotizing fasciitis. A 1-year-old girl with a 2-week history of progressive fever, leukocytosis, and swelling of the right side of the chest wall and right calf. Coronal **(A)** and axial **(B)** T2-weighted magnetic resonance images show asymmetric high signal in the muscle and superficial and deep fascial layers of the right chest and abdominal wall *(arrows)*. Axial fat-suppressed T1 sequence **(C)** after intravenous gadolinium shows enhancement of these areas with more superficial nonenhancing fluid lacking rim enhancement *(arrows)*. Similar changes *(arrows)* are seen in the right lower leg on axial T2-weighted **(D)** and postcontrast fat-suppressed T1-weighted images **(E)**. Biopsy of both sites showed acute inflammation with coagulative necrosis. Cultures were negative, but dramatic clinical improvement was noted with intravenous antibiotic therapy.

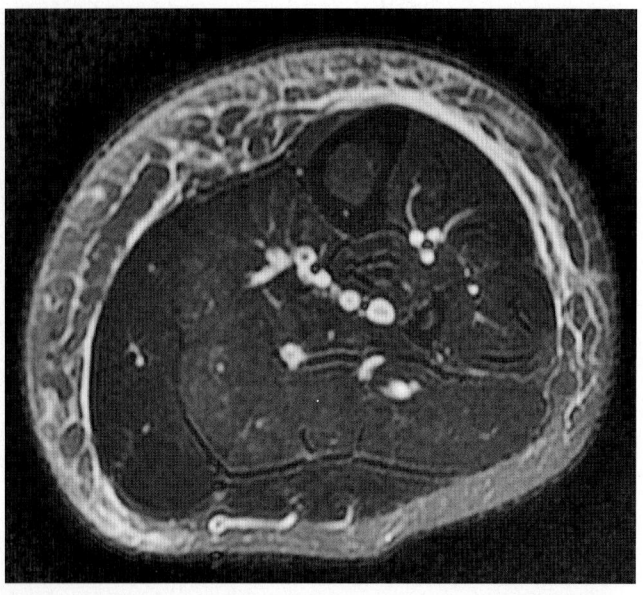 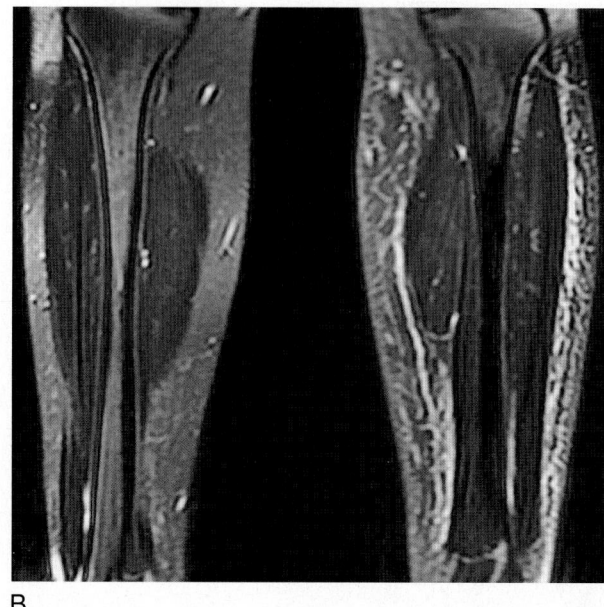

A   B

FIGURE 159-14. Cellulitis. This 16-year-old girl presented with left leg swelling, fever, and rash. Axial **(A)** and coronal **(B)** T2-weighted magnetic resonance images show reticulated high signal in the subcutaneous fat and superficial fascia without deep involvement.

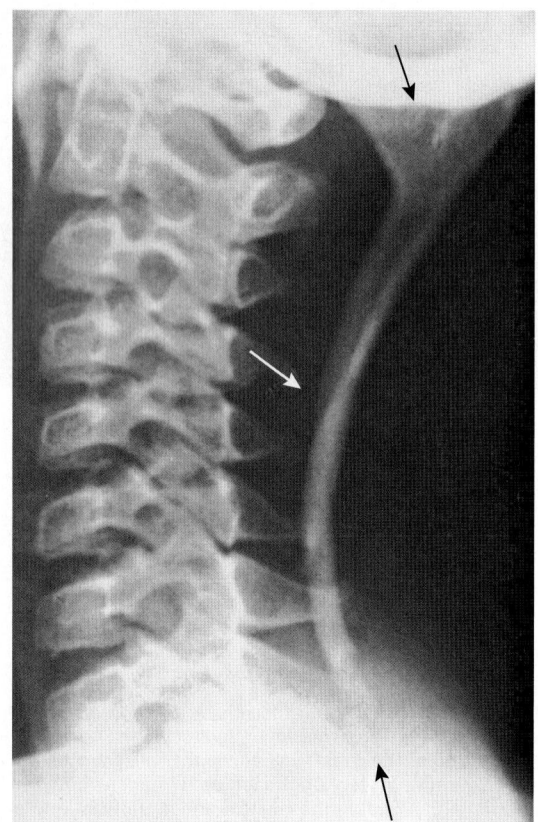

FIGURE 159-15. Juvenile progressive fibrodysplasia ossificans in a 9-year-old girl who had a history of swellings in the neck and back since age 4. A tubular mass of calcium density is seen in the position of the ligamentum nuchae *(arrows)* on this radiograph. The texture and shape of the ossified mass resemble those of a tubular bone with cortex and medullary cavity.

material is present within, the mineral portion will pool dependently, creating fluid-calcium levels (the "sedimentation sign") on radiographs, CT, or MRI. Other entities that may present with individual lesions with calcifications include hyperparathyroidism, hypervitaminosis D, chronic renal disease, milk alkali syndrome, and soft tissue chondromas.

Uncommonly, patchy areas of marrow calcification (calcific myelitis) may be seen in the diaphyses of long bones with associated periostitis that may resemble bone marrow infarcts, osteomyelitis, or neoplasm. Despite the calcified appearance of marrow lesions, high signal on T2-weighted images is present and is likely attributable to an inflammatory response to the pathologic calcification. Radionuclide bone scintigraphy typically exhibits increased uptake in the soft tissue masses and the marrow lesions.

Pathologically, multiple irregular cysts separated by dense fibrous tissue are present that contain pasty white to yellow material sometimes mistaken for pus, although no organisms are present. Chronic inflammatory changes surrounding calcified central material in the active phase are lacking in the inactive phase. The exact anatomic origin of these calcific masses remains unclear. On the basis of their locations on CT and the early pattern of calcification resembling bursitis, some authors believe that these masses occur in synovial bursae around joints. However, conspicuous absence of bursal or synovial tissue is noted on histologic examination; this is attributed by some to destruction of synovial tissue in the bursa by progressive growth of the masses.

Appropriate therapy in the skeletally immature patient remains unclear. Phosphate restrictions imposed on adults may, in theory, be rachitogenic in children, although this approach might be attempted. Resection of symptomatic lesions is sometimes necessary and

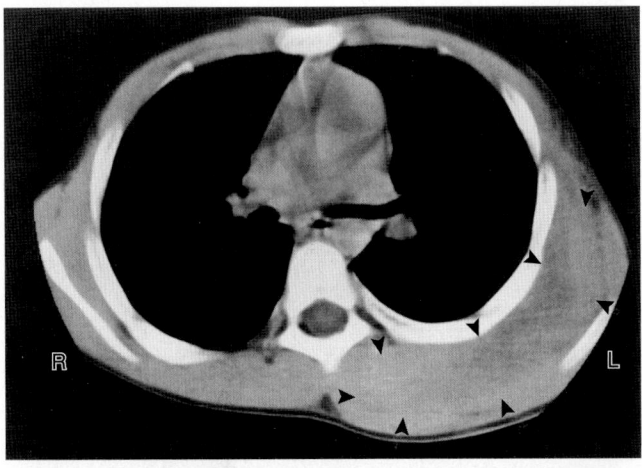

A

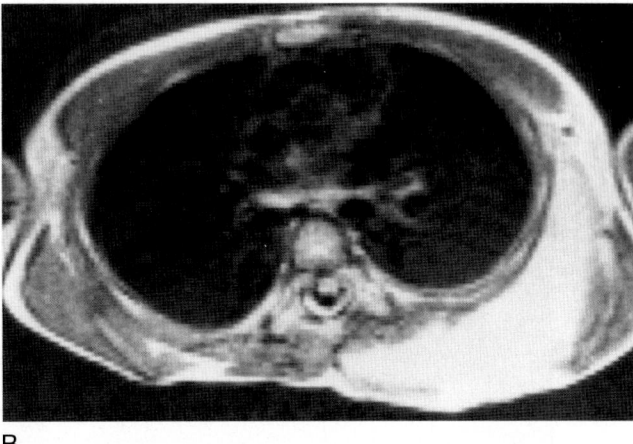

B

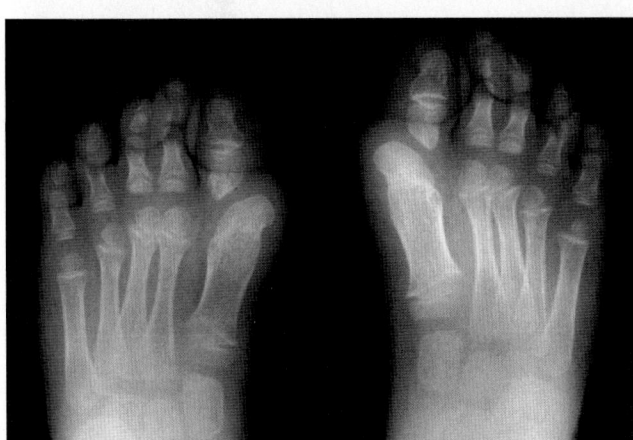

C

FIGURE 159-16. Fibrodysplasia ossificans progressiva prior to calcification in a 5-year-old boy. **A,** A nonenhanced computed tomography scan of the chest shows a noncalcified soft tissue mass in the left posterior chest wall *(arrowheads).* **B,** T2-weighted magnetic resonance image shows diffuse high signal throughout the mass, possibly representing neoplasm. Skeletal survey revealed short first metacarpals and **(C)** hallux valgus deformity bilaterally. Biopsy findings of a fibrous lesion in association with these characteristic skeletal findings were diagnostic of the disorder and directed conservative management. (From Caron KH, DiPietro MA, Aisen AM, et al: MR imaging of early fibrodysplasia ossificans progressiva. J Comput Assist Tomogr 1990;14:318-321.)

curative but may lead to skin ulceration and infection if excision is incomplete.

SUBCUTANEOUS FAT NECROSIS

Fat necrosis of the subcutaneous tissues is an uncommon entity that may result in soft tissue calcification. It has been described in association with local trauma and in newborns who have suffered difficult deliveries.

Subcutaneous fat necrosis of the newborn presents 1 to 6 weeks after birth in a full-term or post-term neonate as firm, red to violaceous nodules that appear on the cheeks, shoulders, back, buttocks, or thighs and measure several millimeters to centimeters. It is usually associated with stressful delivery and hypothermia, but the exact origin is not known. Newborns with subcutaneous fat necrosis can develop potentially fatal hypercalcemia, and their serum calcium levels should be monitored. Although the reason for this association is not completely clear, unregulated production of 1,25-dihydroxyvitamin D by granulomatous cells involved in fat necrosis may be causative. Elevated prostaglandin E levels may also be identified in some hypercalcemic infants with fat necrosis.

On histology, lobular panniculitis with fat crystallization and possibly deposits of calcium may be seen. Calcification may be visible on radiographs (Fig. 159-18). Infants might undergo MRI if the diagnosis is not recognized clinically and concern arises regarding other soft tissue masses or malignancy. Linear areas of increased T2 signal in the subcutaneous fat without a discrete mass have been seen in traumatic and neonatal forms of subcutaneous fat necrosis (Fig. 159-19). CT may reveal nonspecific subcutaneous nodules or fullness. With hypercalcemia, venous calcifications may be identified; nephrocalcinosis and nephrolithiasis have been observed on sonography.

Lesions typically resolve without specific therapy during the first few months of life. If calcified, nodules may persist. Complicating hypercalcemia must be actively treated if a potentially fatal outcome is to be avoided.

NEUROMUSCULAR DISORDERS

The size, shape, and density of muscle groups may be altered by a wide range of neuromuscular disorders, most commonly cerebral palsy and myelodysplasia.

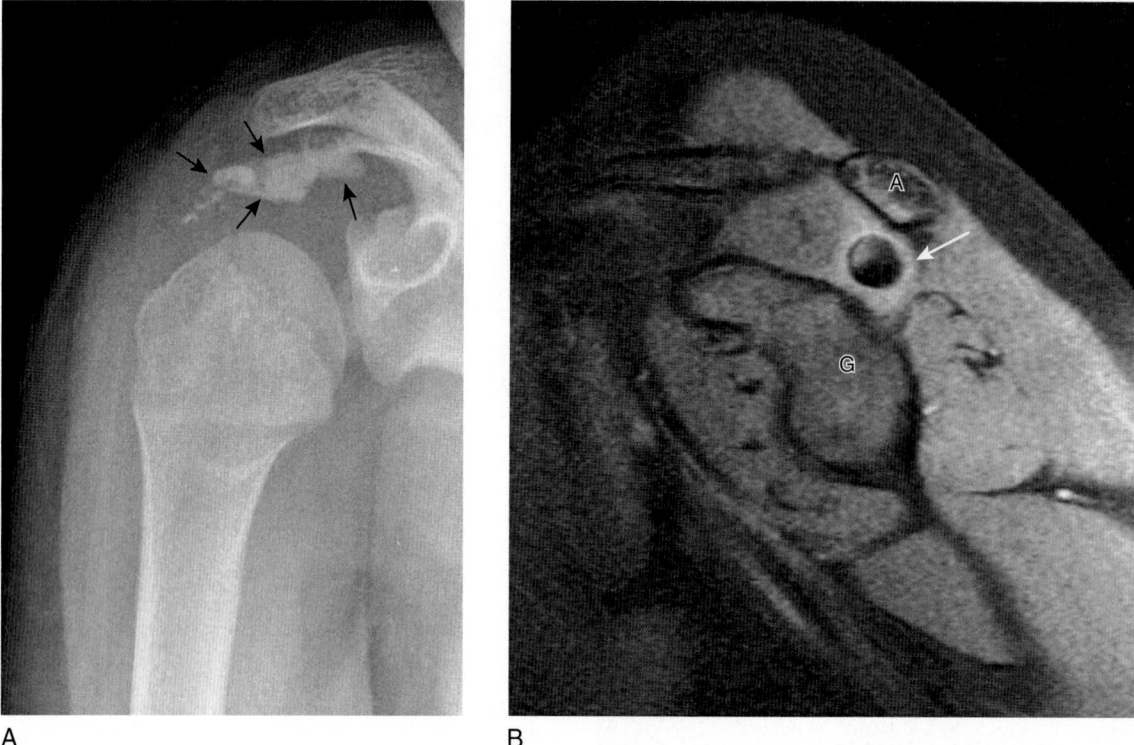

FIGURE 159-17. Tumoral calcinosis. Radiograph of the right shoulder **(A)** in a 7-year-old boy with pain and stiffness shows a lobulated calcified mass *(arrows)* in the subacromial space. Magnetic resonance imaging shows a dark mass with a thin peripheral high signal rim *(arrow)* on sagittal proton density **(B)**, coronal T2 **(C)**, and axial gradient echo **(D)** sequences. The rim enhances on fat-suppressed sagittal T1-weighted imaging **(E)** postgadolinium administration. A, acromion; C, clavicle; G, glenoid; H, humeral head.   *Continued*

Other less common neuromuscular abnormalities that cause muscle atrophy include the muscular dystrophies, spinal muscular atrophy, Friedreich ataxia, hereditary motor sensory neuropathies, and poliomyelitis.

The muscular dystrophies are a group of inherited disorders that cause progressive degeneration and weakness of skeletal muscle. They are not associated with inflammation, and no central or peripheral nervous system cause is present. Duchenne muscular dystrophy, a sex-linked recessive trait, is the most common form. In spinal muscular atrophy, muscular weakness and atrophy are the result of degeneration of the anterior horn cells of the spinal cord. These disorders are classified by age of onset and severity, although considerable overlap is seen with acute Werdnig-Hoffman disease, the most recognizable and severe form. Friedreich ataxia is the most common form of the group of spinocerebellar degenerative diseases with autosomal dominant inheritance. Hereditary motor sensory neuropathies, of which Charcot-Marie-Tooth disease is the prototype, are a group of variably inherited peripheral neuropathic disorders that cause skeletal muscle weakness and atrophy. Poliomyelitis, although it has been largely eradicated by routine vaccination in this country, remains a health problem in developing nations. The poliovirus enters via the gastrointestinal tract and settles in the anterior horn cells of the spinal cord and several brainstem nuclei, resulting in denervation atrophy and fatty infiltration, most commonly of muscles supplied by the cervical and lumbar segments.

All of these disorders result in varying degrees of skeletal muscle atrophy and fatty infiltration that can be observed on conventional radiographs but are more readily detected on CT and MRI scans (Fig. 159-20). Proton MRS may be helpful in detecting and quantifying intramyocellular and extramyocellular lipid deposition. Acquired muscular atrophy, such as trauma caused by rotator cuff tear or immobilization in a cast, may exhibit similar findings. Associated scoliosis, contractures, and foot deformities are common with the neuromuscular disorders and are the major reasons for therapeutic intervention.

SUBCUTANEOUS FAT EXCESS/DEFICIENCY

Childhood obesity has become a recognized problem in the United States and other industrialized countries around the world and may cause multiple health problems. It is also the focus of much research. A number of syndromes aside from excessive caloric intake and limited physical activity may cause obesity and excessive adipose tissue that is evident on imaging studies. Examples include endogenous and exogenous Cushing syndrome, Prader-Willi syndrome, Stein-Leventhal syndrome (polycystic ovaries), Bardet-Biedl syndrome, and pickwickian syndrome. Newborn infants of diabetic

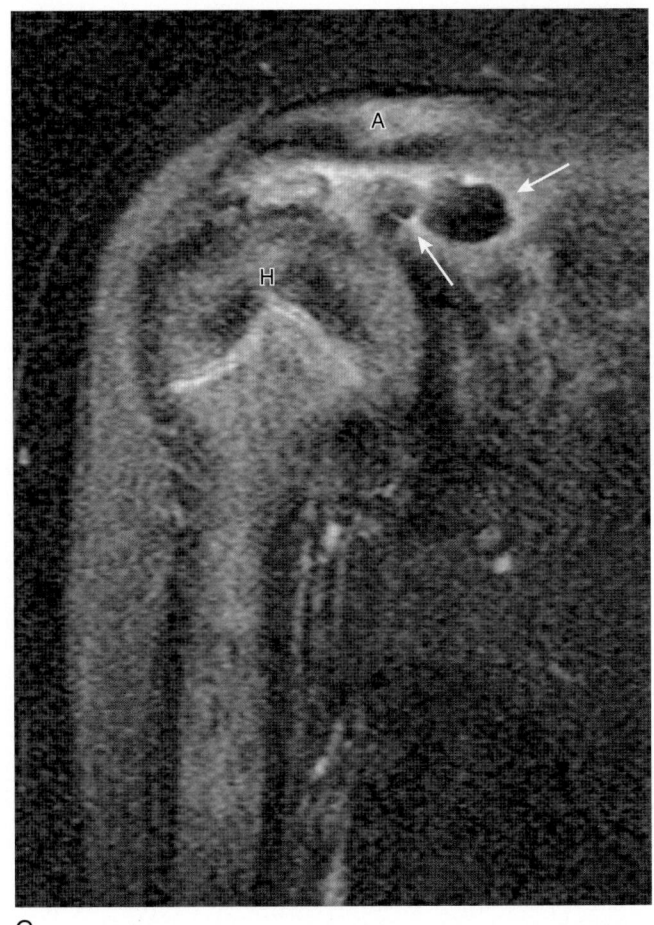

C

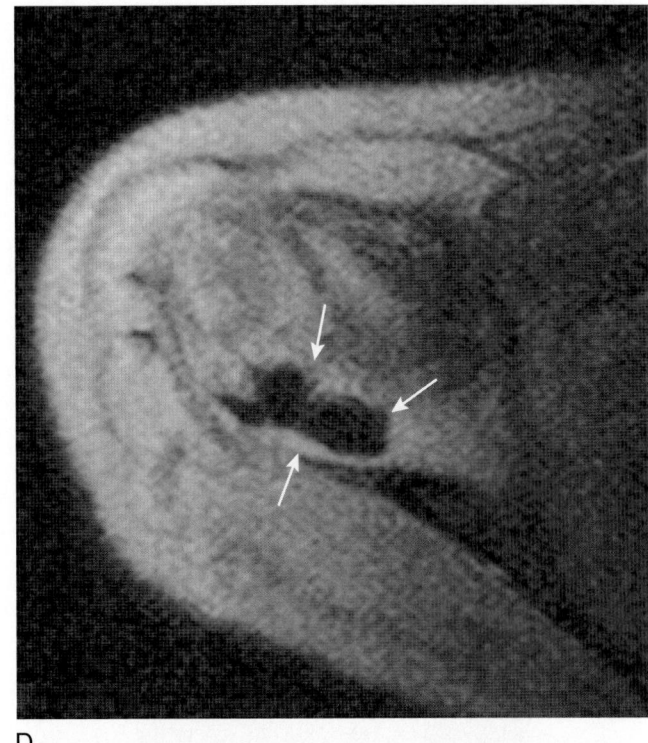

D

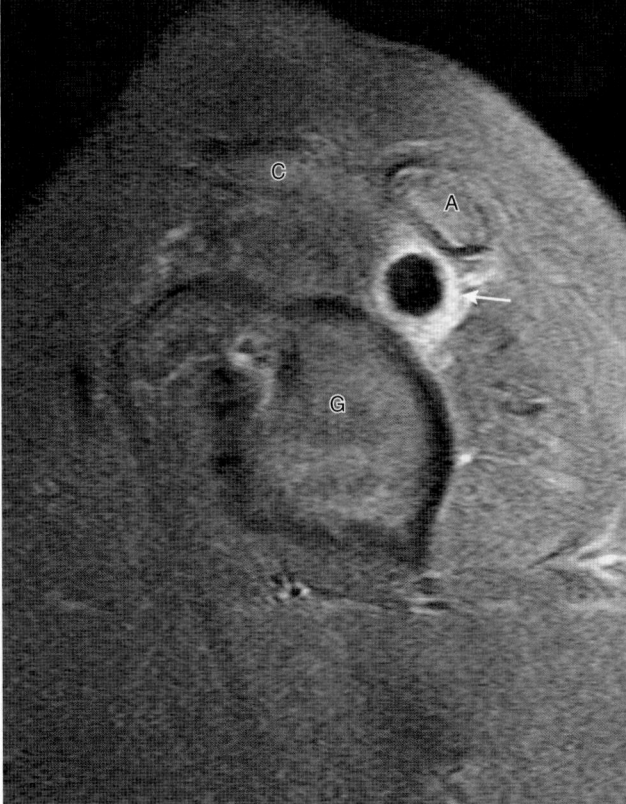

E

FIGURE 159-17, *cont'd.*

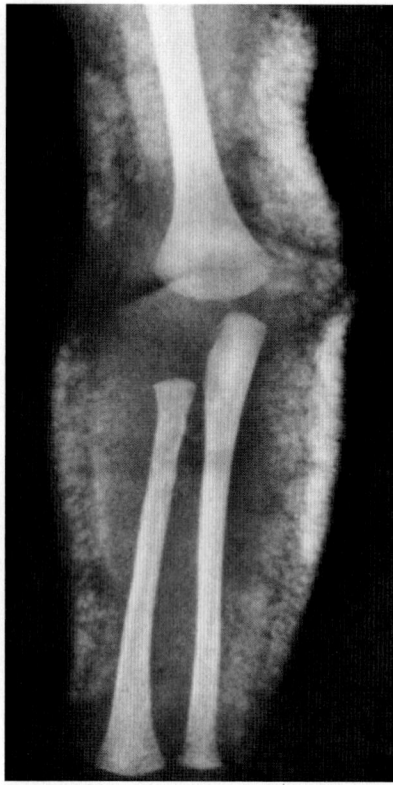

FIGURE 159-18. Generalized subcutaneous fat necrosis in an infant 5 months of age who was thriving otherwise. Subcutaneous fat of the right arm and forearm is extensively calcified in a diagnostically lobulated pattern on this radiograph. Similar changes were present in the skin of both arms, both legs, and the abdomen and pelvis. (Courtesy of Dr. R. Parker Allen, Denver, CO.)

mothers often demonstrate excess subcutaneous fat, especially over the shoulders. Excessive fat may also accumulate in patients with neuromuscular disorders who have limited physical activity and progressive muscular atrophy.

Subcutaneous fat deficiency is encountered less frequently. It is seen in infants with insufficient fat stores, most commonly premature infants or, less commonly, in markedly postmature infants who have consumed their fat stores. Malnourished children may have severely depleted subcutaneous fat. Syndromic forms of lipodystrophy or lipoatrophy are associated with diffuse and localized absence of subcutaneous fat. Congenital total lipodystrophy (Berardinelli-Seip syndrome) is associated with total absence of subcutaneous fat, prominent musculature, hirsutism, and insulin-resistant diabetes mellitus. Localized forms of lipodystrophy are seen at insulin injection sites in patients with diabetes mellitus.

Macrodystrophia Lipomatosa

Macrodystrophia lipomatosa is a congenital, nonhereditary disorder that results in localized limb enlargement and is usually recognized at birth. It is characterized by an increase in all of the mesenchymal elements and proportionately more fibroadipose tissue. Upper and lower extremities may be involved. Unilateral enlargement of one or two digits, most often the second and third digits, may occur (Fig. 159-21). Enlargement of the digits follows the distribution of a nerve. The median nerve in the upper extremity and plantar nerves in the lower extremity are commonly affected. Infiltration of the nerve sheath by fibroadipose tissue can result in neural enlargement. It may be difficult to distinguish between

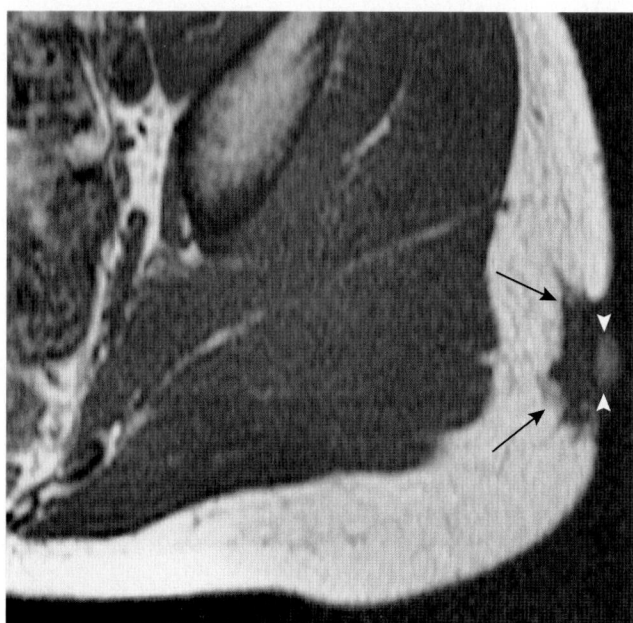
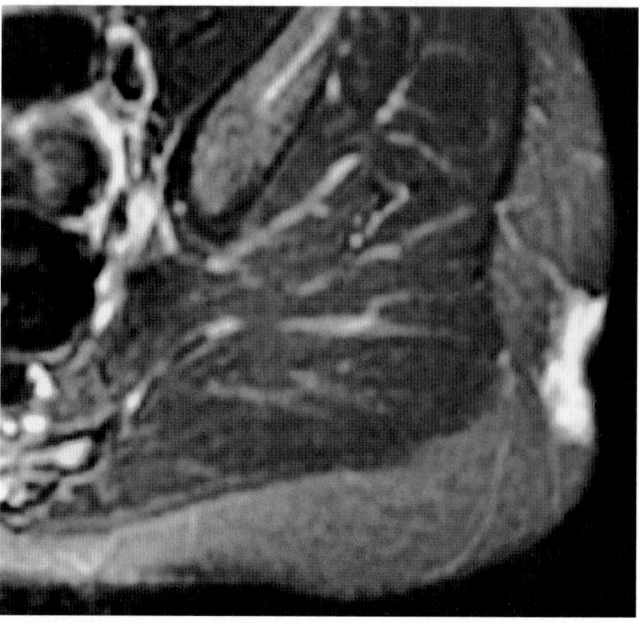

A

B

FIGURE 159-19. Subcutaneous fat necrosis in an 8-year-old boy as seen on MRI. **A,** T1-weighted image shows a stellate area of low signal limited to the subcutaneous fat of the left buttock *(arrows)* *(arrowheads* indicate a vitamin E capsule). **B,** T2-weighted fast spin echo image with fat suppression shows the mass to be of high signal. No significant enhancement occurred after gadolinium administration (not pictured).

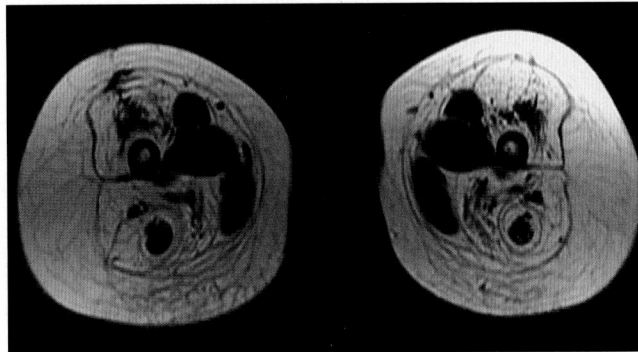
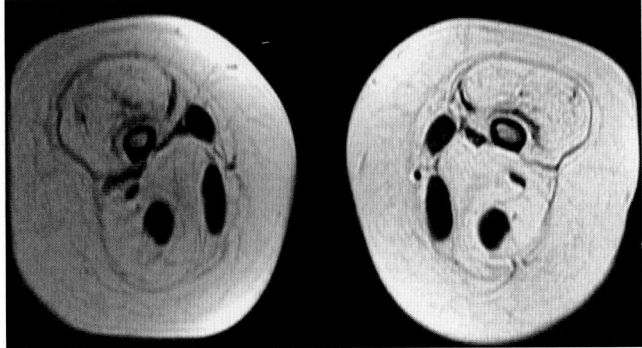
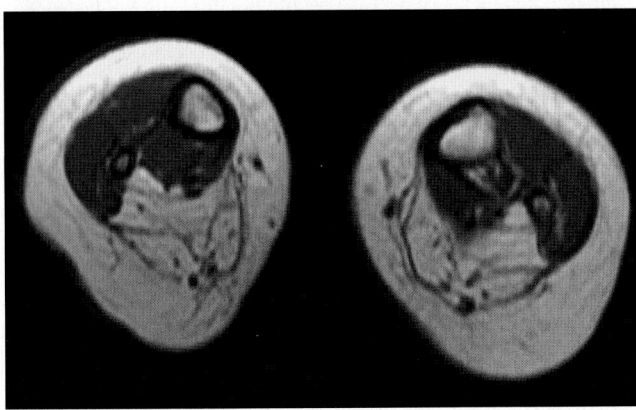

FIGURE 159-20. Fatty replacement of muscle on magnetic resonance imaging in a 3-year-old girl with glycogen storage disease. Axial T1-weighted images through the thighs **(A and B)** and lower legs **(C)** exquisitely depict the marked fatty replacement of quadriceps and lateral muscle groups in the thighs and posterior muscles of the lower legs.

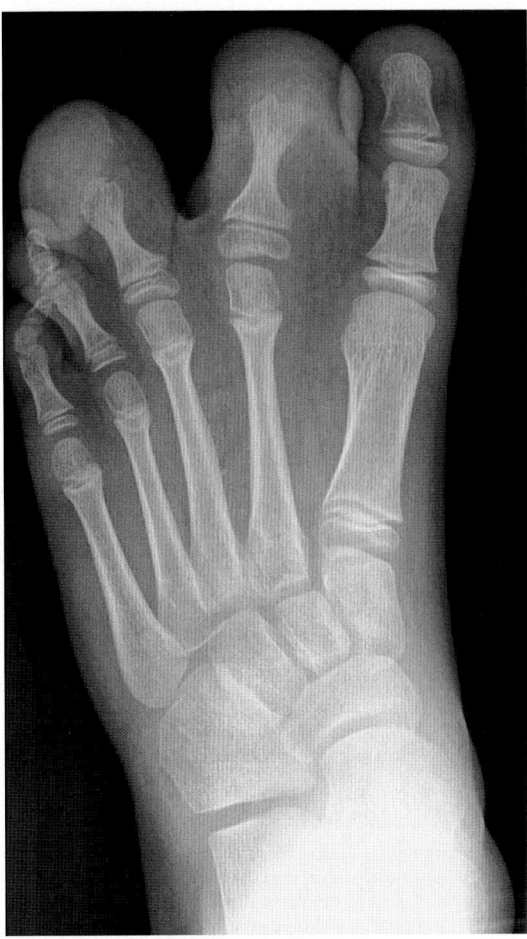

FIGURE 159-21. Macrodystrophia lipomatosa. Radiograph of the left foot in an 8-year-old boy shows overgrowth of the second and third rays with predominant overgrowth of the soft tissues characterized mainly by marked increase in fatty low attenuation tissue. (The middle and distal phalanges of these toes had been resected previously.)

macrodystrophia lipomatosa and neurofibromatosis on the basis of clinical evaluation alone because neurofibromatosis can also affect mesenchymal elements in a neural distribution, resulting in limb enlargement. The cause of localized hypertrophy can be determined on the basis of signal characteristics on MRI. Proliferation of fat (high T1 signal intensity), which is characteristic of macrodystrophia lipomatosa, can be differentiated from the high T2 signal intensity of a neurofibroma or lymphatic malformation.

SUGGESTED READINGS

Cutaneous Calcification/Ossification

Bernardo BD, Huettner PC, Merritt DF, et al: Idiopathic calcinosis cutis presenting as labial lesions in children: report of two cases with literature review. J Pediatr Adolesc Gynecol 1999;12:157-160
Dehner L, Kaye V: The skin. In Stocker J, Dehner LP (eds): Pediatric Pathology, 2nd ed. Philadelphia, JB Lippincott, 1992:1157-1158
Evans MJ, Blessing K, Gray ES: Subepidermal calcified nodule in children: a clinicopathologic study of 21 cases. Pediatr Dermatol 1995;12:307-310
Mallory SB: Infiltrative diseases. In Schachner LA, Hansen RC (eds): Pediatric Dermatology, 2nd ed. New York, Churchill Livingstone, 1995:848-851
Moritz DL, Elewski B: Pigmented postacne osteoma cutis in a patient treated with minocycline: report and review of the literature. J Am Acad Dermatol 1991;24:851-853
Prendiville JS, Lucky AW, Mallory SB, et al: Osteoma cutis as a presenting sign of pseudohypoparathyroidism. Pediatr Dermatol 1992;9:11-18
Rodriguez-Cano L, Garcia-Patos V, Creus M, et al: Childhood calcinosis cutis. Pediatr Dermatol 1996;13:114-117
Sell EJ, Hansen RC, Struck-Pierce S: Calcified nodules on the heel: a complication of neonatal intensive care. J Pediatr 1980;96:473-475
Wright S, Navsaria H, Leigh IM: Idiopathic scrotal calcinosis is idiopathic. J Am Acad Dermatol 1991;24:727-730

Foreign Body

Bodne D, Quinn SF, Cochran CF: Imaging foreign glass and wooden bodies of the extremities with CT and MR. J Comput Assist Tomogr 1988;12:608-611

Borgia CA: An unusual bone reaction to an organic foreign body in the hand. Clin Orthop Relat Res 1963;30:188-193

Butler WP: Plant thorn granuloma. Mil Med 1995;160:39

Jacobson JA, Powell A, Craig JG, et al: Wooden foreign bodies in soft tissue: detection at US. Radiology 1998;206:45-48

Laor T, Barnewolt CE: Nonradiopaque penetrating foreign body: "a sticky situation." Pediatr Radiol 1999;29:702-704

Leung A, Patton A, Navoy J, et al: Intraoperative sonography-guided removal of radiolucent foreign bodies. J Pediatr Orthop 1998;18:259-261

Maylahn D: Thorn-induced "tumors" of bone. J Bone Joint Surg Am 1952;34:386-388

Shiels WED, Babcock DS, Wilson JL, et al: Localization and guided removal of soft-tissue foreign bodies with sonography. AJR Am J Roentgenol 1990;155:1277-1281

Subcutaneous Granuloma Annulare

Chung S, Frush DP, Prose NS, et al: Subcutaneous granuloma annulare: MR imaging features in six children and literature review. Radiology 1999;210:845-849

Grogg KL, Nascimento AG: Subcutaneous granuloma annulare in childhood: clinicopathologic features in 34 cases. Pediatrics 2001;107:E42

Kransdorf MJ, Murphey MD, Temple HT: Subcutaneous granuloma annulare: radiologic appearance. Skeletal Radiol 1998;27:266-270

Letts M, Carpenter B, Soucy P, et al: Subcutaneous granuloma annulare of the extremities in children. Can J Surg 2000;43:425-430

Inflammatory Muscle Diseases

Bowyer SL, Blane CE, Sullivan DB, et al: Childhood dermatomyositis: factors predicting functional outcome and development of dystrophic calcification. J Pediatr 1983;103:882-888

Brown VE, Pilkington CA, Feldman BM, et al: An international consensus survey of the diagnostic criteria for juvenile dermatomyositis (JDM). Rheumatology (Oxford) 2006;45:990-993

Fleckenstein JL, Watumull D, Connor KE: Denervated human skeletal muscle: MR imaging evaluation. Radiology 1993;187:213-218

Hernandez RJ, Keim DR, Chenevert TL, et al: Fat-suppressed MR imaging of myositis. Radiology 1992;182:217-219

Hernandez RJ, Sullivan DB, Chenevert TL, et al: MR imaging in children with dermatomyositis: musculoskeletal findings and correlation with clinical and laboratory findings. AJR Am J Roentgenol 1993;161:359-366

Kimball AB, Summers RM, Turner M, et al: Magnetic resonance imaging detection of occult skin and subcutaneous abnormalities in juvenile dermatomyositis: implications for diagnosis and therapy. Arthritis Rheum 2000;43:1866-1873

Maillard SM, Jones R, Owens C, et al: Quantitative assessment of MRI T2 relaxation time of thigh muscles in juvenile dermatomyositis. Rheumatology 2004;43:603-608

Pachman LM: Juvenile dermatomyositis: pathophysiology and disease expression. Pediatr Clin North Am 1995;42:1071-1098

Park JH, Niermann KJ, Ryder NM, et al: Muscle abnormalities in juvenile dermatomyositis patients: P-31 magnetic resonance spectroscopy studies. Arthritis Rheum 2000;43:2359-2367

Park JH, Olsen NJ, King J Jr, et al: Use of magnetic resonance imaging and P-31 magnetic resonance spectroscopy to detect and quantify muscle dysfunction in the amyopathic and myopathic variants of dermatomyositis. Arthritis Rheum 1995;38:68-77

Rider LG, Miller FW: Classification and treatment of the juvenile idiopathic inflammatory myopathies. Rheum Dis Clin North Am 1997;23:619-655

Samson C, Soulen RL, Gursel E: Milk of calcium fluid collections in juvenile dermatomyositis: MR characteristics. Pediatr Radiol 2000;30:28-29

Schweitzer ME, Fort J: Cost-effectiveness of MR imaging in evaluating polymyositis. AJR Am J Roentgenol 1995;165:1469-1471

Steinbach LS, Tehranzadeh J, Fleckenstein JL, et al: Human immunodeficiency virus infection: musculoskeletal manifestations. Radiology 1993;186:833-838

Stock KW, Helwig A: MRI of acute exertional rhabdomyolysis—in the paraspinal compartment. J Comput Assist Tomogr 1996;20:834-836

Summers RM, Brune AM, Choyke PL, et al: Juvenile idiopathic inflammatory myopathy: exercise-induced changes in muscle at short inversion time inversion-recovery MR imaging. Radiology 1998;209:191-196

Pyomyositis

Gordon BA, Matinez S, Collins AJ: Pyomyositis: characteristics at CT and MR imaging. Radiology 1995;197:279-286

Hernandez RH, Strouse PJ, Craig CL, et al: Focal pyomyositis of the periosciatic muscles in children. AJR Am J Roentgenol 2002;179:1267-1271

Karmazyn B, Kleiman MB, Buckwater K, et al: Acute pyomyositis of the pelvis: the spectrum of clinical presentations and MR findings. Pediatr Radiol 2006;36:338-343

Pannaraj PS, Hulton KG, Gonzalez BE, et al: Infective pyomyositis and myositis in children in the era of community-acquired methicillin-resistant Staphylococcus aureus infection. Clin Infect Dis 2006;43:953-960

Spiegel DA, Meyer JS, Dormans JP, et al: Pyomyositis in children and adolescents: report of 12 cases and review of the literature. J Pediatr Orthop 1999;19:143-150

Trusen A, Beissert M, Schulz G, et al: Ultrasound and MRI features of pyomyositis in children. Eur Radiol 2003;13:1050-1055

Yu CW, Hsaio JK, Hsu CY, et al: Bacterial pyomyositis: MRI and clinical correlation. Magn Reson Imaging 2004;22:1233-1241

Necrotizing Fasciitis/Cellulitis

Arslan A, Pierre-Jerome C, Borthne A: Necrotizing fasciitis: unreliable MRI findings in the preoperative diagnosis. Eur J Radiol 2000;36:139-143

Brothers TE, Tagge DU, Stutley JE, et al: Magnetic resonance imaging differentiates between necrotizing and non-necrotizing fasciitis of the lower extremity. J Am Coll Surg 1998;187:416-421

Clark P, Davidson D, Letts M, et al: Necrotizing fasciitis secondary to chickenpox infection in children. Can J Surg 2003;46:9-14

Fugitt JB, Puckett ML, Quigley MM, et al: Necrotizing fasciitis. Radiographics 2004;24:1472-1476

Headley AJ: Necrotizing soft tissue infections: a primary care review. Am Fam Physician 2003;68:323-328

Lesko SM, O'Brien KL, Schwartz B, et al: Invasive group A streptococcal infection and nonsteroidal antiinflammatory drug use among children with primary varicella. Pediatrics 2001;107:1108-1115

Robben SG: Ultrasonography of musculoskeletal infections in children. Eur Radiol 2004;14(Suppl 4):L65-L77

Schmid MR, Kossmann T, Duewell S: Differentiation of necrotizing fasciitis and cellulitis using MR imaging. AJR Am J Roentgenol 1998;170:615-620

Fibrodysplasia Ossificans Progressiva

Brantus JF, Meunier PJ: Effects of intravenous etidronate and oral corticosteroids in fibrodysplasia ossificans progressiva. Clin Orthop Relat Res 1998;346:117-120

Caron KH, DiPietro MA, Aisen AM: MR imaging of early fibrodysplasia ossificans progressiva. J Comput Assist Tomogr 1990;14:318-321

Cohen RB, Hahn GV, Tabas JA, et al: The natural history of heterotopic ossification in patients who have fibrodysplasia ossificans progressiva: a study of forty-four patients. J Bone Joint Surg Am 1993;75:215-219

Fang MA, Reinig JW, Hill SC, et al: Technetium-99m MDP demonstration of heterotopic ossification in fibrodysplasia ossificans progressiva. Clin Nucl Med 1986;11:8-9

Kaplan FS, McCluskey W, Hahn G, et al: Genetic transmission of fibrodysplasia ossificans progressiva: report of a family. J Bone Joint Surg Am 1993;75:1214-1220

Kaplan FS, Tabas JA, Gannon FH, et al: The histopathology of fibrodysplasia ossificans progressiva: an endochondral process. J Bone Joint Surg Am 1993;75:220-230

Reinig JW, Hill SC, Fang M, et al: Fibrodysplasia ossificans progressiva: CT appearance. Radiology 1986;159:153-157

Sponseller P: Localized disorders of bone and soft tissue. In Morrissy RT, Winstein SL (eds): Lovell & Winter's Pediatric Orthopaedics, 4th ed. Philadelphia, Lippincott-Raven, 1996:332-334

Thickman D, Bonakdar-pour A, Clancy M, et al: Fibrodysplasia ossificans progressiva. AJR Am J Roentgenol 1982;139:935-941

Tumoral Calcinosis

Ballina-Garcia FJ, Queiro-Silva R, Fernadex-Vega F, et al: Diaphysitis in tumoral calcinosis syndrome. J Rheumatol 1996;23:2148-2151

Clarke E, Swischuk LE, Hayden CK Jr: Tumoral calcinosis, diaphysitis, and hyperphosphatemia. Radiology 1984;151:643-646

Cofan F, Garcia S, Combalia A, et al: Uremic tumoral calcinosis in patients receiving longterm hemodialysis therapy. J Rheumatol 1999;26:379-385

Greenberg SB: Tumoral calcinosis in an infant. Pediatr Radiol 1990;20:206-207

Heydemann JS, McCarthy RE: Tumoral calcinosis in a child. J Pediatr Orthop 1988;8:474-477

Kolawole TM, Bohrer SP: Tumoral calcinosis with "fluid levels" in the tumoral masses. Am J Roentgenol Radium Ther Nucl Med 1974;120:461-465

Kozlowski K, Barylak A, Campbell J, et al: Tumoral calcinosis in children (report of 13 cases). Australas Radiol 1988;32:448-457

Lyles KW, Burkes EJ, Ellis GJ, et al: Genetic transmission of tumoral calcinosis: autosomal dominant with variable clinical expressivity. J Clin Endocrinol Metab 1985;60:1093-1096

Pakasa NM, Kalengayi RM: Tumoral calcinosis: a clinicopathological study of 111 cases with emphasis on the earliest changes. Histopathology 1997;31:18-24

Prince MJ, Schaeffer PC, Goldsmith RS, et al: Hyperphosphatemic tumoral calcinosis: association with elevation of serum 1,25-dihydroxycholecalciferol concentrations. Ann Intern Med 1982;96:586-591

Richardson PH, Yang YM, Nimityongskul P, et al: Tumoral calcinosis in an infant. Skeletal Radiol 1996;25:481-484

Rodriguez-Peralto JL, Lopez-Barea F, Torres A, et al: Tumoral calcinosis in two infants. Clin Orthop Relat Res 1989;242:272-276

Steinbach LS, Johnston JO, Tepper EF, et al: Tumoral calcinosis: radiologic-pathologic correlation. Skeletal Radiol 1995;24:573-578

Zaleske DJ: Metabolic and endocrine abnormalities. In Morrissy RT, Winstein SL (eds): Lovell & Winter's Pediatric Orthopaedics, 4th ed. Philadelphia, Lippincott-Raven, 1996:178

Subcutaneous Fat Necrosis

Anderson DR, Narla LD, Dunn NL: Subcutaneous fat necrosis of the newborn. Pediatr Radiol 1999;29:794-796

Burden AD, Krafchik BR: Subcutaneous fat necrosis of the newborn: a review of 11 cases. Pediatr Dermatol 1999;16:384-387

Cunningham K, Atkinson SA, Paes BA: Subcutaneous fat necrosis with hypercalcemia. Can Assoc Radiol J 1990;41:158-159

Fretzin DF, Arias AM: Sclerema neonatorum and subcutaneous fat necrosis of the newborn. Pediatr Dermatol 1987;4:112-122

Gu LL, Daneman A, Binet A, Kooh SW: Nephrocalcinosis and nephrolithiasis due to subcutaneous fat necrosis with hypercalcemia in two full-term asphyxiated neonates: sonographic findings. Pediatr Radiol 1995;25:142-144

Kruse K, Irle U, Uhlig R: Elevated 1,25-dihydroxyvitamin D serum concentrations in infants with subcutaneous fat necrosis. J Pediatr 1993;122:460-463

Norton KI, Som PM, Shugar JM, et al: Subcutaneous fat necrosis of the newborn: CT findings of head and neck involvement. AJNR Am J Neuroradiol 1997;18:547-550

Prendiville JS: Diseases of the dermis and subcutaneous tissues: nodular diseases. In Schachner LA, Hansen RC (eds): Pediatric Dermatology, 2nd ed. New York, Churchill Livingstone, 1995:821-822

Sharata H, Postellon DC, Hashimoto K: Subcutaneous fat necrosis, hypercalcemia, and prostaglandin E. Pediatr Dermatol 1995;12:43-47

Tsai TS, Evans HA, Donnelly LF, et al: Fat necrosis after trauma: a benign cause of palpable lumps in children. AJR Am J Roentgenol 1997;169:1623-1626

Neuromuscular Disorders

Hawley RJ Jr, Schellinger D, O'Doherty DS: Computed tomographic patterns of muscles in neuromuscular diseases. Arch Neurol 1984;41:383-387

Iannaccone ST, Browne RH, Samaha FJ, et al: Prospective study of spinal muscular atrophy before age 6 years. DCN/SMA Group. Pediatr Neurol 1993;9:187-193

Misra A, Sinha S, Kumar M, et al: Proton magnetic resonance spectroscopy study of soleus muscle in non-obese healthy and Type 2 diabetic Asian Northern Indian males: high intramyocellular lipid content correlates with excess body fat and abdominal obesity. Diabet Med 2003;20:361-367

Murphy WA, Totty WG, Carroll JE: MRI of normal and pathologic skeletal muscle. AJR Am J Roentgenol 1986;146:565-574

Pearn J: Classification of spinal muscular atrophies. Lancet 1980;1:919-922

Pfirrmann CW, Schmid MR, Zanetti M, et al: Assessment of fat content in supraspinatus muscle with proton MR spectroscopy in asymptomatic volunteers and patients with supraspinatus tendon lesions. Radiology 2004;232:709-715

Serratrice G, Salamon G, Jiddane M, et al: Results of muscular x-ray computed tomography in 145 cases of neuromuscular disease. Rev Neurol (Paris) 1985;141:404-412

Sinha R, Dufour S, Petersen KF, et al: Assessment of skeletal muscle triglyceride content by (1)H nuclear magnetic resonance spectroscopy in lean and obese adolescents: relationships to insulin sensitivity, total body fat, and central adiposity. Diabetes 2002;51:1022-1027

Stern LM, Caudrey DJ, Clark MS, et al: Carrier detection in Duchenne muscular dystrophy using computed tomography. Clin Genet 1985;27:392-397

Strebel PM, Sutter RW, Cochi SL, et al: Epidemiology of poliomyelitis in the United States one decade after the last reported case of indigenous wild virus-associated disease. Clin Infect Dis 1992;14:568-579

Thompson G: Neuromuscular disorders. In Morrissy RT, Weinstein SL (eds): Lovell and Winter's Pediatric Orthopaedics, 4th ed. Philadelphia, Lippincott-Raven, 1996:537-577

Subcutaneous Fat Excess/Deficiency

Kakourou T, Dacou-Voutetakis C, Kavadias G, et al: Limited joint mobility and lipodystrophy in children and adolescents with insulin-dependent diabetes mellitus. Pediatr Dermatol 1994;11:310-314

Kuhns LR, Berger PE, Roloff DW, et al: Fat thickness in the newborn infant of a diabetic mother. Radiology 1974;111:665-671

Must A, Strauss RS: Risks and consequences of childhood and adolescent obesity. Int J Obes Relat Metab Disord 1999;23(Suppl 2):S2-S11

Smevik B, Swensen T, Kolbenstvedt A: Computed tomography and ultrasonography of the abdomen in congenital generalized lipodystrophy. Radiology 1982;142:687-689

Strauss R: Childhood obesity. Curr Probl Pediatr 1999;29:1-29

Taybi HL, Lachman RS: Radiology of Syndromes, Metabolic Disorders, and Skeletal Dysplasias, 3rd ed. Chicago, Year Book Medical Publishers, 1990

Macrodystrophia Lipomatosa

Blacksin M, Barnes FJ, Lyons MM: MR diagnosis of macrodystrophia lipomatosa. AJR Am J Roentgenol 1992;158:1295-1297

Goldman AB, Kaye JJ: Macrodystrophia lipomatosa: radiographic diagnosis. AJR Am J Roentgenol 1977;128:101-105

Gupta SK, Sharma OP, Sharma SV, et al: Macrodystrophia lipomatosa: radiographic observations. Br J Radiol 1992;65:769-773

Levine C: The imaging of body asymmetry and hemihypertrophy. Crit Rev Diagn Imaging 1990;31:1-80

Wang YC, Jeng CM, Mercantonio DR, et al: Macrodystrophia lipomatosa: MR imaging in three patients. Clin Imaging 1997;21:323-327

160 Soft Tissue Neoplasms

JAMES S. MEYER and BARRY D. FLETCHER

Diagnostic imaging in the assessment of soft tissue neoplasms is generally guided by the patient's clinical presentation. In children with subtle masses, the primary objective of imaging is to confirm or exclude the presence of a mass. In most children, however, the mass is clinically obvious, and imaging is performed to assess the local extent of the tumor and provide information that results in a specific diagnosis or, more often, characterizes the lesion in a manner that helps the clinician to determine whether biopsy is needed.

In children with a hard, fixed mass, conventional radiographs are often performed to determine whether an underlying bone lesion is present (Fig. 160-1) that is simulating or is associated with a soft tissue mass. When a soft tissue mass is clearly present, conventional radiographs are sometimes performed and may show secondary changes in the configuration of adjacent bones

and/or the presence of cortical bone erosion, periosteal reaction, and soft tissue calcifications. Occasionally, radiolucency indicates the presence of a fat-containing tumor.

Superficial masses are often assessed by ultrasonography, which can reveal whether a mass is solid, complex, or purely cystic, and therefore benign. Ultrasonography has the advantages of easy accessibility and no ionizing radiation, and sedation is rarely required to obtain high-quality images. In addition, color and spectral Doppler ultrasonography can provide information on the vascularity of a mass. This information can be particularly valuable in children in whom enlarged lymph nodes may

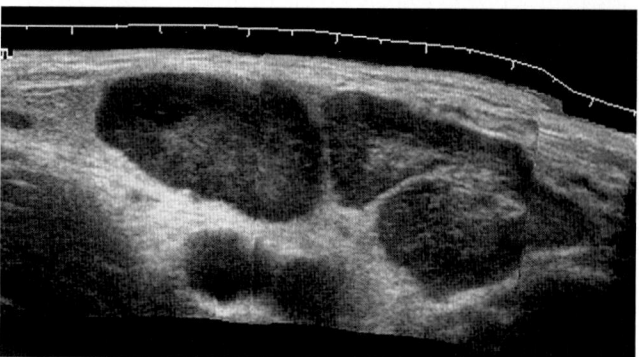

A

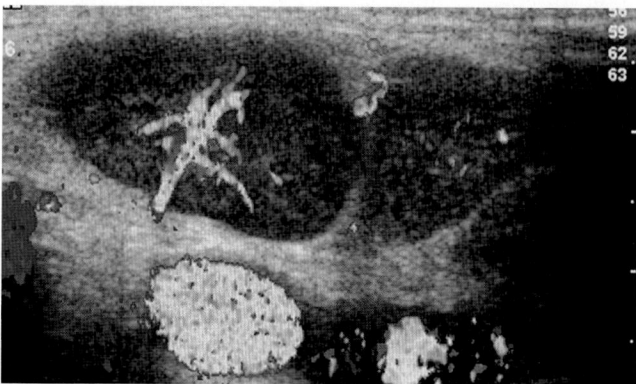

B

FIGURE 160-2. A, Ultrasound image shows masses with central increased echogenicity typical of lymph nodes. **B,** Color Doppler image shows central hilar flow pattern that is also characteristic of a lymph node. (**B,** *see color plate.*)

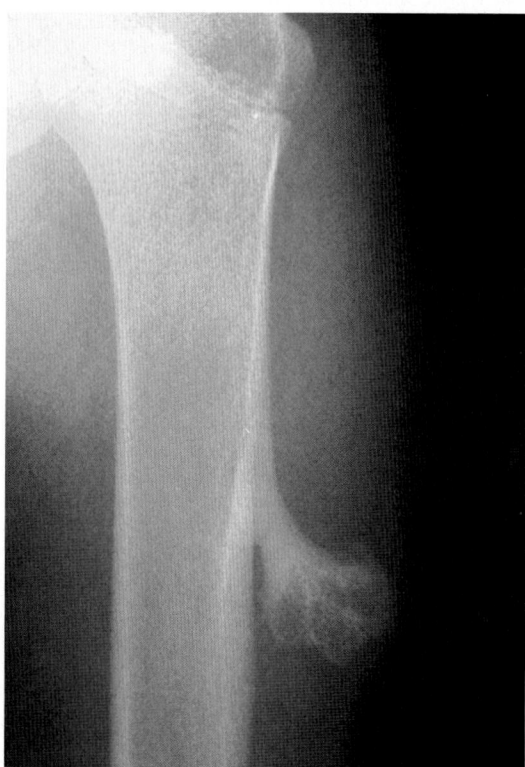

FIGURE 160-1. Conventional radiograph shows an osteochondroma of the proximal humerus.

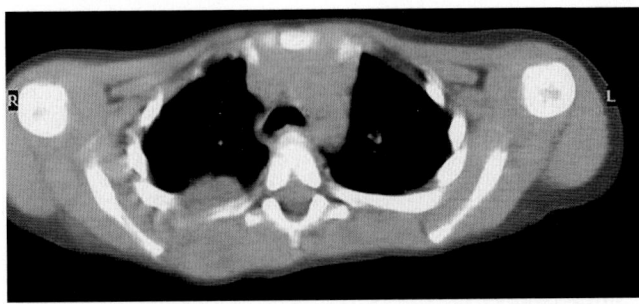

A

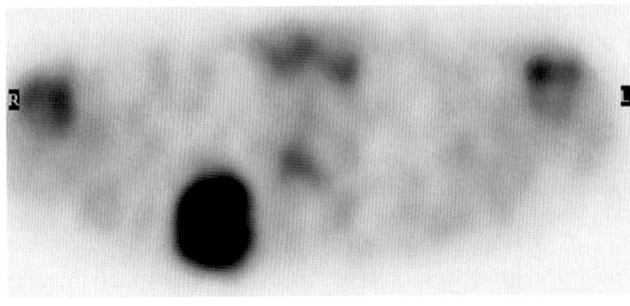

B

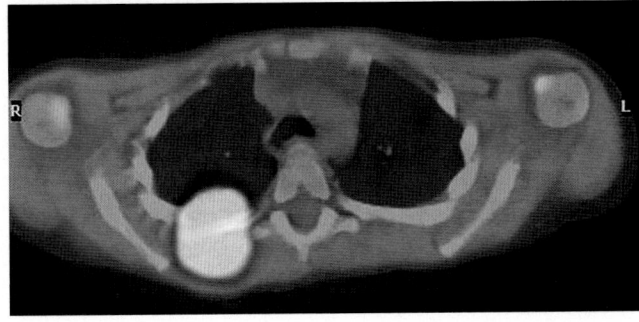

C

FIGURE 160-3. Embryonal rhabdomyosarcoma in a 4-year-old boy. Computed tomography (CT) scan (**A**), positron emission tomography (PET) scan (**B**), and PET/CT scan (**C**) show the tumor. (Images courtesy of Barry L. Shulkin, MD, St. Jude Children's Research Hospital, Memphis, TN.) (**C,** *see color plate.*)

simulate a mass. In these cases, the typical color Doppler appearance of the vascularized hilum confirms that the mass is an enlarged lymph node (Fig. 160-2).

Nuclear medicine also plays a significant role in the assessment of soft tissue tumors. Many soft tissue sarcomas are detected by gallium-67 and thallium-201 scintigraphy. Technetium-99m–methylene diphosphonate (MDP) bone scintigraphy may be performed to identify local bone involvement and distant skeletal metastases. In addition, positron emission tomography (PET) and PET/CT (computed tomography) (Fig. 160-3) are playing an increasing role in assessment of pediatric tumors at presentation and in evaluation of tumor response and recurrence.

CT provides similar but more detailed information than is provided by conventional radiographs. CT is superior to magnetic resonance imaging (MRI) in the detection of calcification or gas within soft tissues, and CT is the imaging study of choice for masses in which myositis ossificans is a diagnostic possibility. CT of the lungs is usually performed for assessment of metastatic disease in children with malignant soft tissue tumors. In children with malignant tumors involving the lower extremities, CT of the abdomen and pelvis is often performed to assess inguinal and retroperitoneal lymph node involvement. The use of CT to assess the primary soft tissue mass, however, is limited; often CT is performed only when MRI is unavailable or is contraindicated.

MRI is the imaging study of choice for the assessment of most soft tissue tumors. The superb soft tissue contrast and multiplanar images provide details on the tumor's extent and relationship to underlying anatomic structures. Although MRI technology continues to evolve, the basic tenets of the MRI examination of a child with a soft tissue tumor have remained constant.

> Conventional radiography, ultrasonography, CT, and nuclear medicine studies are useful for the assessment of soft tissue tumors. MRI, however, is the imaging study of choice for the assessment of most soft tissue tumors.

First, magnetic resonance (MR) images should reveal the entire tumor so as to delineate its margins, and they should include any needle biopsy tracks that may have to be excised at the time of surgical resection. Care must be taken to use the smallest coil and/or other methods to ensure quality images and coverage of the entire lesion and important adjacent structures.

The area that contains the tumor should be imaged in at least two orthogonal planes. T1-weighted and T2-weighted images should be obtained. Fat saturation is often added to confirm the presence of fat in a lesion and/or to highlight the presence of enhancement after intravenous gadolinium administration. In cases of fatty tumors, a T1-weighted sequence without fat saturation is also performed. Short tau inversion recovery (STIR) sequences are useful because they inherently suppress signal from fat and do not require a homogeneous magnetic field. However, STIR images tend to overestimate tumor margins because they also accentuate the signal of adjacent edema. Gadolinium-enhanced T1-weighted images add information about tumor vascularity and are helpful in guiding percutaneous biopsy in that viable tumor can be differentiated from areas of necrosis. Furthermore, cystic lesions may be identified by their lack of central enhancement. MR angiography is useful for detecting the presence of blood flow within the tumor and for planning the optimal surgical approach when large vessels may be involved.

Most soft tissue tumors have low signal intensity, similar to muscle on T1-weighted images, and heterogeneous high signal intensity, which is greater than that of fat on T2-weighted images. Tumors that produce high-intensity signals on T1-weighted images are likely to contain fat, methemoglobin blood products, or abundant proteinaceous material. Tumor hypointensity on T2-weighted images suggests relative acellularity and abundant collagen formation. Hemosiderin that results from previous hemorrhage is hypointense to muscle on T1- and T2-weighted images, and calcifications are usually hypointense.

> MRI examination should cover the entire soft tissue mass, should use at least T1- and T2-weighted sequences, and should include fat-saturated, angiographic, and postgadolinium sequences as needed to better characterize the tumor.

The MR signal characteristics of most soft tissue tumors are nonspecific and usually cannot predict histology, nor can they differentiate between benign and malignant neoplasms. Although some MRI characteristics and associated findings (Table 160-1) are helpful in suggesting the underlying malignant nature of a mass, biopsy is necessary for histologic diagnosis. Nonetheless, familiarity with MRI characteristics of soft tissue masses, especially in conjunction with the patient's clinical presentation, often yields a focused differential diagnosis (Tables 160-2 and 160-3).

> MRI characteristics of most soft tissue tumors are nonspecific.

BENIGN SOFT TISSUE TUMORS

Most soft tissue neoplasms in children are benign and vascular in origin. These vascular tumors include infantile hemangiomas and vascular malformations, which are covered in Chapter 161. In this section, we review the clinical and imaging presentations of a variety of other benign soft tissue tumors.

> Most soft tissue tumors in children are benign.

Desmoid Tumors

Desmoid tumors are rare quasi-neoplastic lesions that are included in the fibroblastic/myofibroblastic section of the 2002 World Health Organization (WHO) Soft Tissue Tumor Classification. These tumors are more prevalent in adults than in children and have been categorized by Enzinger into superficial and deep groups. Superficial tumors are usually small and slow growing. Deep lesions may occur in the abdomen or extra-abdominally. Most desmoid tumors in patients with

TABLE 160-1

Musculoskeletal Soft Tissue Tumors: Magnetic Resonance Imaging Features of Malignancy

Neurovascular encasement	Highly suggestive
Adjacent bone/joint involvement	Highly suggestive
Marrow abnormality	Highly suggestive
Homogeneous T1W, heterogeneous T2W pattern	Suggestive
Necrosis	Suggestive
Poorly defined, irregular margins	Suggestive
Peritumoral edema	Not helpful

From Hanna SL, Fletcher BD: MR imaging of malignant soft tissue tumors. Magn Imaging Clin N Am 1995;3:629-650.
T1W, T1-weighted; T2W, T2-weighted.

TABLE 160-2

Imaging Features of Benign Soft Tissue Tumors

Benign	Common Location	X-ray/CT	MRI*	Other
Desmoid tumor	Deep tissue, head and neck, trunk, extremities	Mild hyperattenuation	1. Variable signal 2. Homogeneous or heterogeneous 3. Signal intensities correlate with histology	Extra-abdominal desmoids also called aggressive fibromatosis
Peripheral nerve sheath tumor	Peripheral nerve	1. Calcification in degenerating schwannomas 2. Hypoattenuating on CT	1. Hypointense on T1W images 2. Hyperintense on T2W images with target-like appearance	1. Associated with muscle atrophy 2. NF1 present in 10% with diffuse neurofibromas
Lipoblastoma and lipoblastomatosis	Extremities, head and neck, trunk	Mixed attenuation; fat, myxoid tissue	Fatty components: hyperintense on T1W images and isointense on T2W images	Lipoblastomatosis often infiltrates deep tissues; tends to recur locally

CT, computed tomography; MRI, magnetic resonance imaging; NF1, neurofibromatosis type 1; T1W, T1-weighted; T2W, T2-weighted.
*T1-weighted signal intensity relative to that of muscle; T2-weighted signal intensity relative to that of subcutaneous fat.

TABLE 160-3

Imaging Features of Malignant Soft Tissue Tumors

Malignant	Common Location	Radiograph/CT	MRI*	Other
Rhabdomyosarcoma	About 20% occur in extremities	May erode bone	Nonspecific	15% to 20% with detectable metastases at presentation
Peripheral primitive neuroectodermal tumor (PPNET) and extraosseous Ewing sarcoma	Trunk, paravertebral space, extremities	May erode bone; no calcification	Nonspecific	Askin tumor involves chest wall
Synovial sarcoma	Near joints; lower extremities more common than upper	Calcification in 30%; may erode bone	Nonspecific; may contain hemorrhage; may have triple signal pattern	May involve vessels
Malignant peripheral nerve sheath tumor (MPNST)	Lower extremity (thigh)	Nonspecific	Nonspecific	Gallium-avid; associated with NF1
Infantile fibrosarcoma	Most in extremities	May erode bone	Nonspecific	Low-grade malignancy; 5% metastases
Dermatofibrosarcoma protuberans	Dermis; may extend into underlying soft tissues	—	Nonspecific	May be congenital; red-blue or pink plaque; may be depressed
Liposarcoma	Lower extremity (thigh)	Well differentiated: low attenuation	Well-differentiated: hyperintense on T1W images; isointense on T2W images. Myxoid: nonspecific with small fatty components	More fat in well-differentiated tumors
Alveolar soft part sarcoma (ASPS)	Lower extremity (thigh)	Marked CT enhancement; necrotic center; draining veins	Hyperintense on T1W and T2W images	Highly vascular; draining veins
Epithelioid sarcoma	Upper extremity (forearm)	Rare calcification	Nonspecific; may contain hemorrhage	Subcutaneous lymphatic spread
Lymphoma	Muscle, skin	Diffuse muscle enlargement; density similar to that of muscle	Nonspecific	Gallium and FDG avid
Granulocytic sarcoma	Orbits, subcutaneous tissue	Isoattenuating to slightly hyperattenuating to muscle on noncontrast CT; hyperattenuating to muscle on contrast CT	Nonspecific	Also known as chloroma; children more often affected than adults

CT, computed tomography; FDG, fluorodeoxyglucose; MRI, magnetic resonance imaging; NF1, neurofibromatosis type 1; T1W, T1-weighted; T2W, T2-weighted.
*T1-weighted signal intensity relative to muscle; T2-weighted signal intensity relative to subcutaneous fat.

Gardner syndrome are found in the abdomen. Extra-abdominal desmoid tumors, which are also referred to as *aggressive fibromatosis*, are usually solitary and arise from the fascial sheaths and aponeuroses of striated muscle. Histologically, they consist of benign fibrous tissues that contain spindle cells and abundant collagen. Although they do not metastasize, they can infiltrate contiguous structures, including bone. In children, extra-abdominal

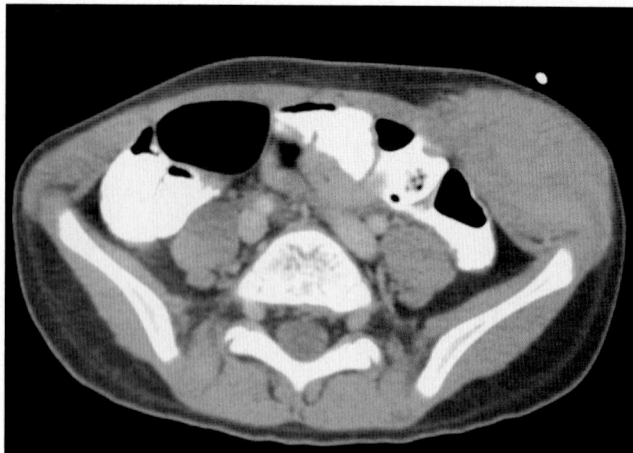

FIGURE 160-4. Extra-abdominal desmoid tumor (Gardner fibroma) in a 5-year-old girl. Axial, contrast-enhanced computed tomography image shows a large lenticular-shaped mass originating in the anterior abdominal wall musculature.

desmoid tumors are more common than the abdominal type.

Extra-abdominal desmoid tumors are deep seated. In a series of tumors studied at St. Jude Children's Research Hospital, head and neck, truncal, and extremity involvement was seen with approximately equal frequency. These tumors are variably echogenic on ultrasonography, and their borders may be smooth or irregular. On contrast-enhanced CT images, most desmoid tumors appear more attenuated than does striated muscle (Fig. 160-4). On MRI, these tumors may be nodular with infiltrative or well-defined margins. Tumors may be homogeneous or heterogeneous with varying signal characteristics. Some lesions are low signal on T1- and T2-weighted images. More often, tumors are heterogeneous and contain areas that are hyperintense to fat on T2-weighted images. On T1-weighted images, these masses contain areas that are hypointense, isointense, or slightly hyperintense when compared with muscle (Fig. 160-5). This variability in signal reflects differences in the relative proportions of collagen, spindle cells, and mucopolysaccharides within the lesion. On T2-weighted images, low signal generally reflects collagen, and high signal is seen in tumors with a greater quantity of cellular tissue (Fig. 160-6). Tumors with high signal on T1-weighted images have been found to contain fat or myxoid material. Enhancement after gadolinium injection may be homogeneous, heterogeneous, or absent and does not correlate with clinical outcome.

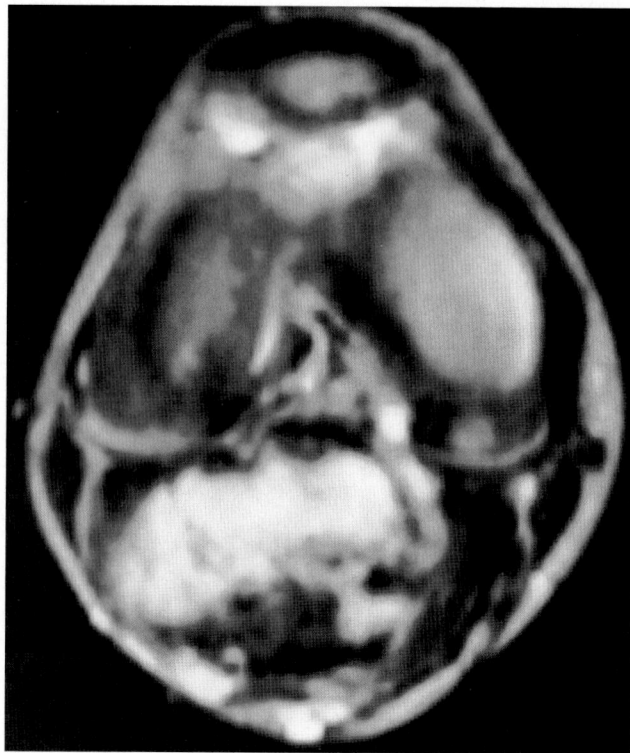
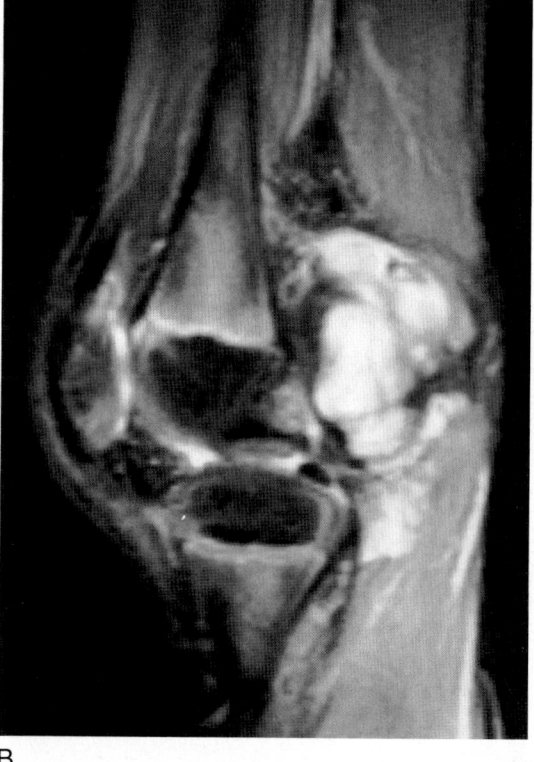

A   B

FIGURE 160-5. Desmoid tumor in a 6-year-old boy. On magnetic resonance imaging, transverse T2-weighted (**A**) and sagittal short tau inversion recovery (**B**) images of the knee show heterogeneously high signal intensity with peripheral ill-defined hypointense foci.

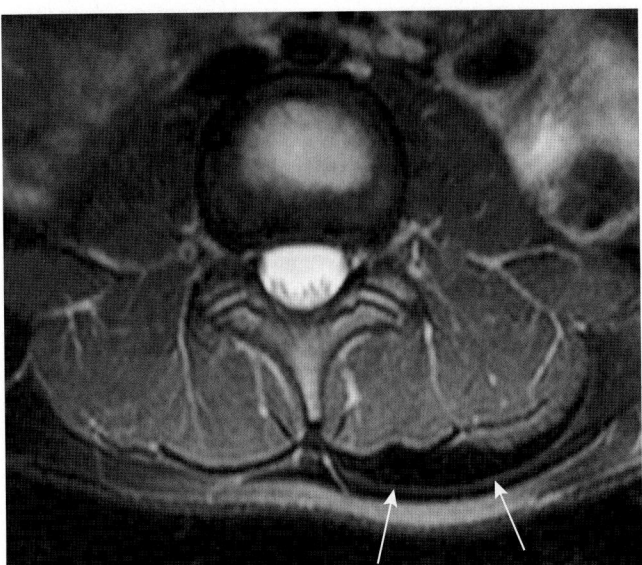

FIGURE 160-6. Extra-abdominal desmoid tumor (Gardner fibroma) in a 5-year-old boy. Axial T2-weighted with fat saturation magnetic resonance image shows a low-signal plaquelike mass along the posterior margin of the left paraspinal musculature *(arrows)*.

> **MRI signal characteristics of desmoid tumors reflect differences in the relative proportions of collagen, spindle cells, and mucopolysaccharides within the lesions.**

Desmoid tumors are related histologically to generalized fibromatosis (congenital fibromatosis, juvenile fibromatosis, infantile myofibromatosis), and some have histologic features that suggest hemangiopericytoma. Other fibrous tumors of infants and children include fibrous hamartoma, fibromatosis coli, digital fibromatosis, calcifying aponeurotic fibroma, and hyaline fibromatosis.

Infantile Myofibromatosis

Infantile myofibromatosis is the most common fibrous tumor of infancy. Tumors may involve skin, muscle, bone, or viscera and may be solitary (myofibroma) or multiple (myofibromatosis). Myofibromatosis occurs in children younger than 2 years of age. The prognosis of musculoskeletal lesions is excellent, and spontaneous resolution usually occurs. Visceral involvement may portend a poorer prognosis. Lesions have a variable appearance on ultrasonography, ranging from solid to anechoic centrally with a thick wall. On CT, myofibromas enhance to a lesser extent than or similarly to muscle and often exhibit a peripheral rim of enhancement. On MRI, lesions are low signal on T1 weighting and usually high signal on T2 weighting. Some masses show decreased central signal on T2 weighting. Peripheral enhancement is seen with gadolinium administration (Fig. 160-7).

Benign Peripheral Nerve Sheath Tumors

Benign peripheral nerve sheath tumors are divided into schwannomas (also known as neurinomas and neuri-

lemomas) and neurofibromas. Benign neurofibromas and, less commonly, schwannomas are frequently multiple and are associated with neurofibromatosis type 1 (NF1). However, both tumors may be solitary and may occur sporadically. They are similar histologically and are composed primarily of Schwann cells; therefore, they exhibit similar imaging characteristics. Microscopic examination reveals a dense central core of Schwann cells surrounded by a peripheral zone of myxoid tissue. Peripheral nerve sheath tumors have a low incidence of malignant degeneration.

> **Neurofibromas and schwannomas are often associated with neurofibromatosis type 1 (NF1), but they may occur sporadically.**

A tumor can be suspected to have a neurogenic origin if it is located along the distribution of a peripheral nerve. Calcification in degenerating ("ancient") schwannomas may be visible radiographically; on bone scintigrams, these tumors have been observed to take up technetium-99m MDP. Peripheral nerve sheath tumors may be accompanied by subtle atrophy of surrounding or distally innervated muscle. Most of these tumors are well-defined spherical or fusiform masses. On CT images, they tend to be hypoattenuated, possibly because of lipids in their Schwann cells, adipocytes, and perineural tissues. On MRI, the bulk of the tumor is low in intensity on T1-weighted sequences and high in intensity on T2-weighted sequences. Typically, the central zone consists of collagen and neurofibroma cells and is hypointense on T2-weighted images, lending a "target" appearance to the lesion. This target appearance can also be seen on contrast-enhanced T1-weighted images and is more easily appreciated when wide window settings are used to view the images. The presence of a target sign helps to distinguish these benign tumors from their less well-organized malignant counterparts (see Fig. 160-12).

> **The "target" appearance of peripheral nerve sheath tumors on T2-weighted images is due to a hypointense central zone that consists of collagen and neurofibroma cells. Loss or absence of the "target" appearance heightens concern regarding malignancy.**

On MRI, differentiating a schwannoma from a neurofibroma can be difficult. Schwannomas, however, may contain more prominent areas of hemorrhage, cystic change, and necrosis, with resultant heterogeneous signal intensities. In addition, neurofibromas intimately involve and are inseparable from the normal nerve. Schwannomas are eccentric to the nerve, and this may be apparent on MRI in tumors that involve larger nerves. When smaller nerves are involved, schwannomas may obliterate the nerve of origin, and the MRI appearance is indistinguishable from that of a neurofibroma.

Plexiform neurofibromas arise from the axis of a primary nerve and form tortuous cordlike tumors along its axis. They are regarded as indicators of neurofibro-

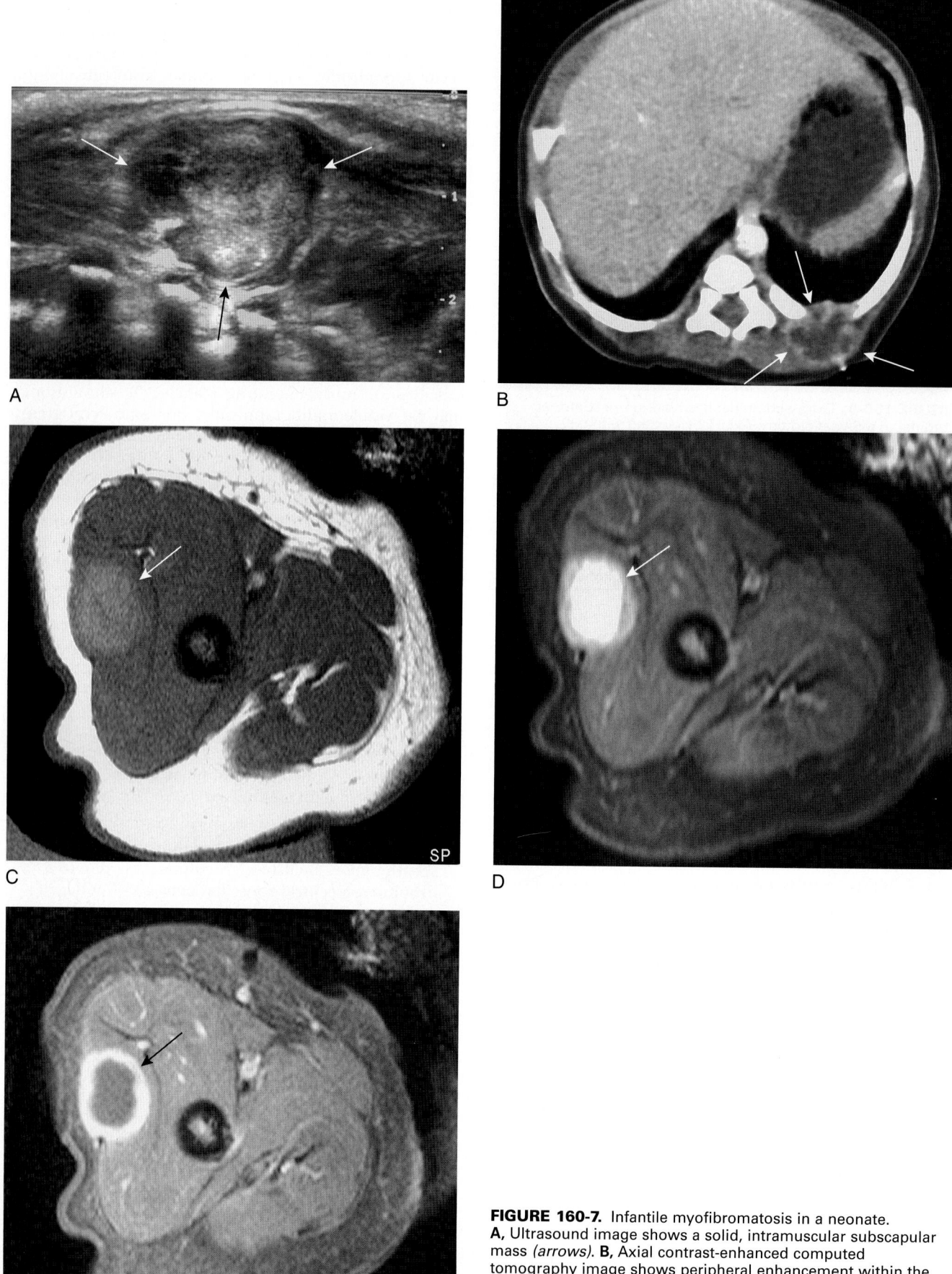

FIGURE 160-7. Infantile myofibromatosis in a neonate.
A, Ultrasound image shows a solid, intramuscular subscapular mass *(arrows)*. **B,** Axial contrast-enhanced computed tomography image shows peripheral enhancement within the mass *(arrows)*. Another lesion in the same patient is shown on T1-weighted (**C**), T2-weighted with fat saturation (**D**), and postgadolinium T1-weighted with fat saturation (**E**) magnetic resonance images.

matosis, even when they are the sole manifestation of this disease. Tumors tend to appear as lobulated, amorphous masses with ill-defined borders. Similar to solitary neurofibromas, these tumors are usually hyperintense on T2-weighted imaging and often have well-defined, central, tubular, hypointense structures, or they may form large masses that resemble a "bag of worms" on transverse images.

A particularly uncommon form of neurofibroma is the diffuse type. These lesions occur primarily in children and young adults and most commonly involve the head and neck regions. These ill-defined, infiltrative lesions tend to be located in the skin and subcutaneous tissues. They appear as linear or reticular strands of intermediate signal on T1-weighted images and of high signal intensity on T2-weighted images, with linear areas of enhancement after gadolinium administration. NF1 is present in about 10% of patients with diffuse neurofibroma.

Benign Fatty Tumors

The 2002 WHO Soft Tissue Tumor Classification includes nine types of benign fatty tumor: lipoma, lipomatosis, lipomatosis of nerve, lipoblastoma/lipoblastomatosis, angiomyolipoma, myolipoma of soft tissue, chondroid lipoma, spindle cell lipoma/pleomorphic lipoma, and hibernoma. Except for lipoblastoma, all of these tumors are more common in adults than in children.

Lipoblastoma and lipoblastomatosis are benign mesenchymal tumors of immature fat that occur primarily in infants and young children, most often in boys younger than 8 years of age. Collins and Chatten reported that the average age of patients at the time of presentation is 3.6 years. Lipoblastomas are usually painless superficial tumors that are most commonly located in the extremities and the head and neck region, but they may also involve the trunk and deeper structures such as the mediastinum and retroperitoneum. The tumor consists of lobules of immature adipose tissue with a variable amount of myxoid stroma separated by richly vascularized septa composed of connective tissue. The discrete form, lipoblastoma, is a well-circumscribed lesion that occurs in approximately 70% of cases and involves the superficial soft tissues. Lipoblastomas eventually evolve into mature lipomas. Lipoblastomatosis refers to the diffuse type that often infiltrates adjacent deeper tissues such as muscle and has a tendency to recur locally. Lipoblastomatosis has been reported to resolve spontaneously.

Imaging features reflect the amount of fatty tissue present. On ultrasound images, hyperechoic fat can be clearly delineated from the myxoid component, and CT images show a similar combination of hypoattenuated fat and denser myxoid tissue (Fig. 160-8). On MR images, the signal is often heterogeneous (see Fig. 160-8), and lipomatous elements appear hyperintense to muscle on T1-weighted images and isointense to subcutaneous fat on T2-weighted images, whereas nonfatty tissues produce lower signal intensity than fat on T1-weighted images and are more intense than fat on T2-weighted

images. In addition to low T1 signal myxoid components, the fatty mass may contain low signal fibrous septa that enhance with gadolinium on T1-weighted images.

The differential diagnosis includes lipoma, which is much more prevalent in adults than in children; hibernoma, a rare tumor analogous to brown fat; and myxoid liposarcoma. Liposarcoma is rare in children younger than 5 years of age. Thus, a fat-containing tumor, even with nonlipomatous components, that occurs in a child younger than 2 years of age is almost invariably a lipoblastoma.

> Lipoblastoma occurs most often in young children; it may contain myxoid tissue and enhancing fibrous septations.

MALIGNANT SOFT TISSUE TUMORS

Soft tissue sarcomas (STSs) are a heterogeneous group of malignant tumors that arise from primitive mesenchymal cells and account for about 7% of malignant tumors in children. Rhabdomyosarcomas (RMSs) occur predominantly in children and account for slightly more than half of pediatric soft tissue sarcomas. In contrast to RMS, nonrhabdomyosarcoma soft tissue tumors (NRSTSs) of the musculoskeletal system are more common in adults. NRSTSs include fibrosarcoma, neurofibrosarcoma, malignant fibrous histiocytoma (MFH), synovial sarcoma, alveolar soft part sarcoma (ASPS), and liposarcoma, as well as peripheral primitive neuroectodermal tumors (PPNETs), which are histologically and cytogenetically related to Ewing sarcoma.

Diagnosis of STS is complex and depends on histologic, cytologic, histochemical, and molecular genetic studies. Imaging is usually nonspecific but essential for staging and surgical management. MRI has superseded CT and ultrasonography in this clinical setting. MRI can define the anatomic location of the tumor, indicate its relationship to important nerves and blood vessels, and reveal local involvement of bone or lymph nodes.

Most STSs are isointense or hypointense to muscle on T1-weighted images, hyperintense to fat and muscle on T2-weighted and STIR images, and are enhanced after gadolinium administration. MRI should be performed prior to biopsy so that postbiopsy edema and blood do not obscure the tumor mass, thereby simulating more extensive local involvement. Coronal and sagittal MR images are particularly helpful because the surgical approach to STS of the extremities is usually longitudinal rather than transverse.

In the following sections, we review the clinical and imaging presentations of a variety of STSs. Clinical and imaging features of STS are shown in Table 160-3.

Rhabdomyosarcoma

RMSs contain a mixture of rhabdomyoblasts, which are recognized by their typical cross striations, and undifferentiated cells. These tumors are thought to arise from progenitor cells for striated muscle and can occur anywhere in the body, even in areas with no striated muscle.

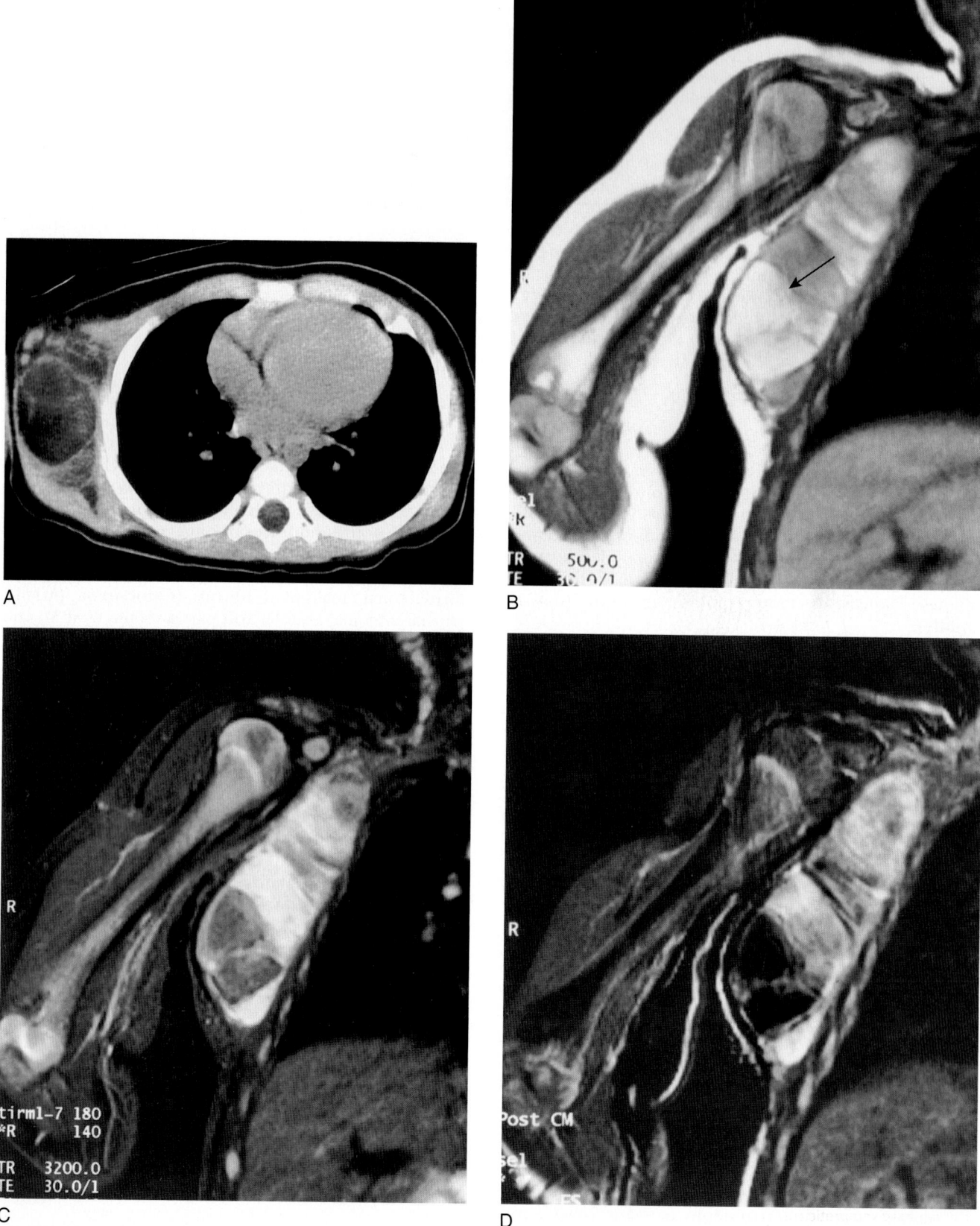

FIGURE 160-8. A, Computed tomography scan section of the chest of a 5-month-old patient with a lipoblastoma arising from the right axilla shows a low attenuation mass. **B,** On a coronal T1-weighted magnetic resonance image, the inferior portion of the mass *(arrow)* is markedly hyperintense as a result of adipose tissue. The low signal in this portion of the mass shown in short tau inversion recovery **(C)** and fat-suppressed contrast-enhanced T1-weighted **(D)** images is also characteristic of fat.

RMSs account for more than 60% of STSs in children younger than 5 years of age but only 25% of STSs in 15- to 19-year-olds.

> **Rhabdomyosarcomas constitute more than half of pediatric soft tissue sarcomas.**

The head and neck and genitourinary tract are the most frequent locations of RMS. About 20% of these tumors occur in the extremities. Most extremity RMSs are alveolar or undifferentiated histologic types, as opposed to the embryonal or botryoid types that are found in the face and neck and in the genitourinary system. Prognosis is less favorable for patients with RMSs of the extremities than for those with tumors arising from the genitourinary system or the head and neck region. In the extremities, tumors tend to be deep and to spread along fascial planes. RMSs may cause erosion of adjacent bone. MR imaging characteristics are nonspecific, and most tumors are predominantly low signal on T1-weighted images and high signal on T2-weighted images.

> **In all, 20% of rhabdomyosarcomas occur in the extremities; these tumors are usually of the alveolar type, and they have a less favorable prognosis than the embryonal type.**

Only 15% to 20% of patients with RMS have clinically detectable metastases at presentation. All patients, however, are considered to have micrometastatic disease; this has resulted in the universal use of chemotherapy. The lungs, bone marrow, and bone are the most common sites of distant metastases. Metastatic lymph nodes may also be involved (Fig. 160-9). Bone metastases resemble those that occur with neuroblastoma; they have been reported even in the absence of detectable primary tumor. The 5-year survival rate for children with RMS has improved from 55% in the 1970s to more than 70% currently.

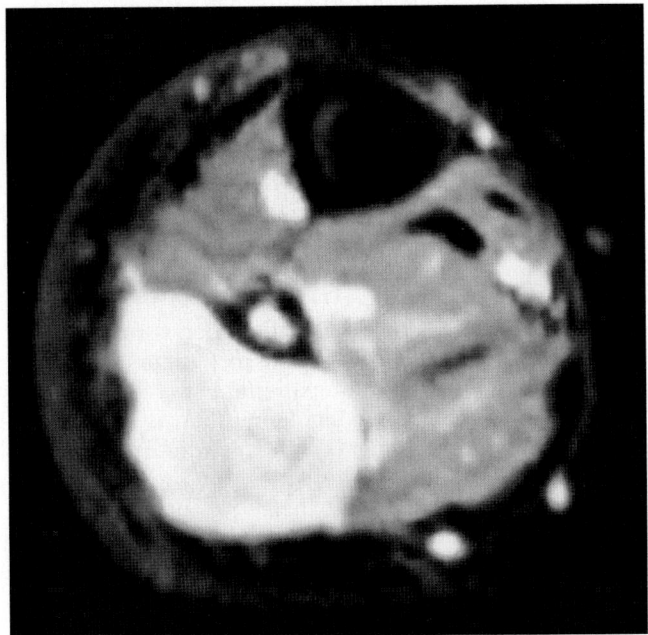
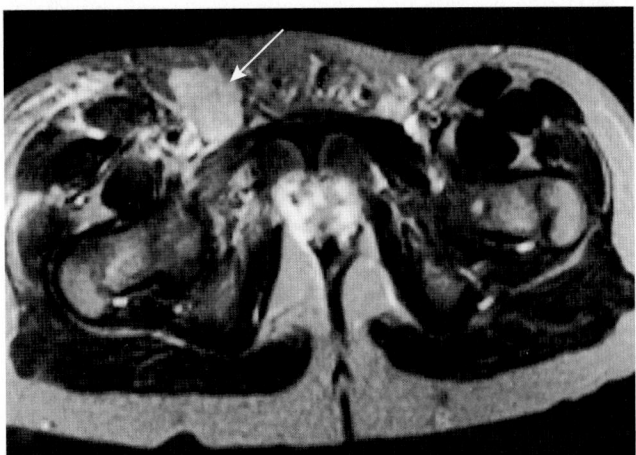
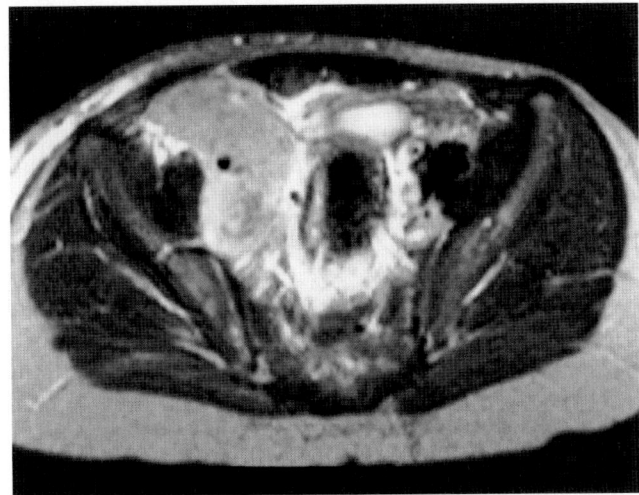

FIGURE 160-9. Rhabdomyosarcoma. **A,** A transverse T2-weighted magnetic resonance image of the right leg of a 12-year-old boy with rhabdomyosarcoma shows a hyperintense soft tissue tumor and abnormally high signal in the adjacent fibular bone marrow consistent with metastases. Transverse T2-weighted images of the hips (**B**) and pelvis (**C**) show right inguinal (*arrow*) and right parailiac lymph node involvement.

2514 SECTION VII — MUSCULOSKELETAL SYSTEM

Primitive Peripheral Neuroectodermal Tumor and Extraosseous Ewing Sarcoma

PPNET and extraosseous Ewing sarcoma (EOES) are small round cell neoplasms that belong to the Ewing sarcoma family of tumors; they can arise in soft tissue or bone. These neoplasms are related histogenically and share a common cytogenetic characteristic—the translocation of bands 24 and 12 of the short arms of chromosomes 11 and 22—but are often indistinguishable histologically. PPNETs, also known as peripheral neuroepithelioma, have a higher degree of neural differentiation than is seen with Ewing sarcoma; thus, these two tumors can be distinguished on the basis of immunohistochemical markers. This distinction is important because disease-free survival is poorer for patients with PPNET than for those with EOES.

Both tumors occur most commonly in truncal and paravertebral soft tissues (50% to 60% of cases) and in the extremities (25% of cases), although PPNET occurs less commonly in the extremities than does EOES, and patients with EOES are generally younger. Askin tumors are thoracic PPNETs that involve the chest wall (see Chapter 80). These tumors can be very large at the time of presentation and tend to be poorly circumscribed. The soft tissue mass does not calcify but may erode adjaent bone. On MRI, these tumors are typically isointense to muscle on T1-weighted images and inhomogeneously hyperintense on T2-weighted and STIR images; they show variable enhancement after gadolinium administration. Distant spread occurs to bone, lung, liver, and brain. Distant metastases, however, are uncommon with Askin tumors.

> **PPNET and Ewing sarcoma are small round cell sarcomas that may erode adjacent bone.**

Synovial Sarcoma

Synovial sarcomas predominantly occur in adults younger than 50 years of age, but they account for about 10% of pediatric STSs. These tumors are not derived from true synovial cells; they arise from undifferentiated mesenchymal cells. A monophasic variety comprises spindle cells, and a biphasic variety consists of spindle cells and epithelial elements. Although synovial sarcomas often occur close to joints, tendons, and bursae, they are rarely intra-articular. About 80% of synovial sarcomas occur in the extremities; considerably more lower than upper extremity involvement has been noted. Synovial sarcomas may spread to regional lymph nodes; the lungs are the most common site of distant metastasis.

Radiographically visible calcifications are present in 30% of cases. On MRI, synovial sarcomas are often lobulated, well-defined, deep-seated lesions, although they may be infiltrative and can encase major blood vessels. Femoral vein invasion has been described, and erosion of the cortex of adjacent bones is present in up to 20% of patients (Fig. 160-10).

MRI signal characteristics are nonspecific. Synovial sarcomas are usually isointense to muscle on T1-weighted images. Foci of high T1-weighted signal may be present (see Fig. 160-10), and fluid-fluid levels (Fig. 160-11) are caused by hemorrhage. The tumors generally have heterogeneous signal with areas of high intensity on T2-weighted images (see Fig. 160-10). In a large series by Jones and associates of patients with synovial sarcoma from the Armed Forces Institute of Pathology, 35% of tumors showed a triple signal pattern on T2-weighted images; these findings are consistent with high (fluid) signal intensity, intermediate signal intensity similar to that of fat, and low signal intensity resembling that of fibrous tissue. Some synovial sarcomas simulate cysts through their homogeneous signal intensity on T1- and T2-weighted images and their well-defined borders. A multilocular appearance with fluid-fluid levels may be seen in 18% to 25% of these tumors.

> **Synovial cell sarcomas are rarely intra-articular, but they do arise close to joints. In all, 30% contain radiographically visible calcifications. Hemorrhagic material may be seen on MRI.**

Malignant Peripheral Nerve Sheath Tumor

Malignant peripheral nerve sheath tumor (MPNST) is the accepted name for a spindle cell sarcoma that arises from a nerve or a neurofibroma. In contrast to other STSs that are of mesenchymal cell origin, MPNSTs are of neuroectodermal origin. *MPNST* has replaced many formerly used terms, including *malignant schwannoma, neurofibrosarcoma, neurogenic sarcoma,* and *malignant neural neoplasm.* A variant of MPNST is the "triton" tumor, which contains neural and rhabdomyosarcomatous elements; this tumor was named after a salamander in which transplantation of the sciatic nerve induces growth of a supernumerary limb.

MPNSTs, which account for about 4% to 10% of STSs, are the most common malignancy associated with NF1. Half of these tumors occur in patients with NF1; conversely, 2% to 29% of patients with NF1 develop MPNST—a much higher incidence than is seen in the general population. Patients with NF1 who have MPNSTs are usually younger than those in whom the tumor arises without associated NF1. Furthermore, in patients with NF1, MPNSTs tend to arise in pre-existing benign neurofibromas; they are high-grade tumors that have a tendency to local recurrence and metastasis. MPNSTs also may arise at previously irradiated sites.

Similar to benign neurofibromas, MPNSTs are deep soft tissue lesions that are often associated with primary nerves, especially those of the thigh and the lower extremities. The appearance of these tumors on CT and MR images is nonspecific. They may be well or poorly defined or homogeneous or inhomogeneous, and they occasionally erode bone. Malignant transformation of benign neurofibromas should be considered in patients in whom the mass is painful or enlarging, or when the typical target appearance of a benign neurofibroma is absent (Fig. 160-12). Tumor uptake on gallium scintigrams may indicate malignant transformation or progressive growth of neurofibromas. However, biopsy is usually necessary to confirm malignancy.

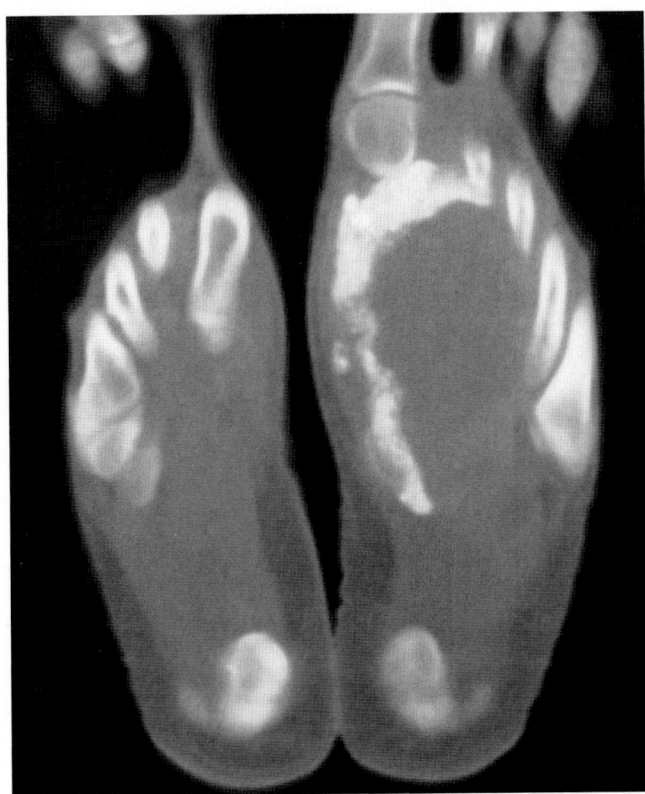

A

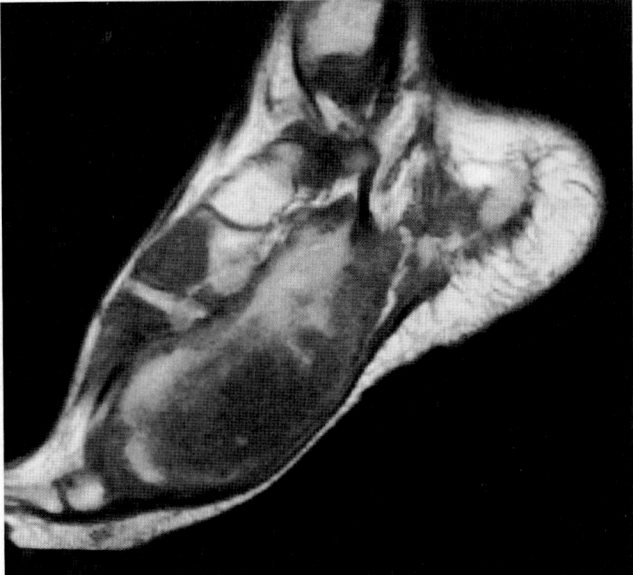

B

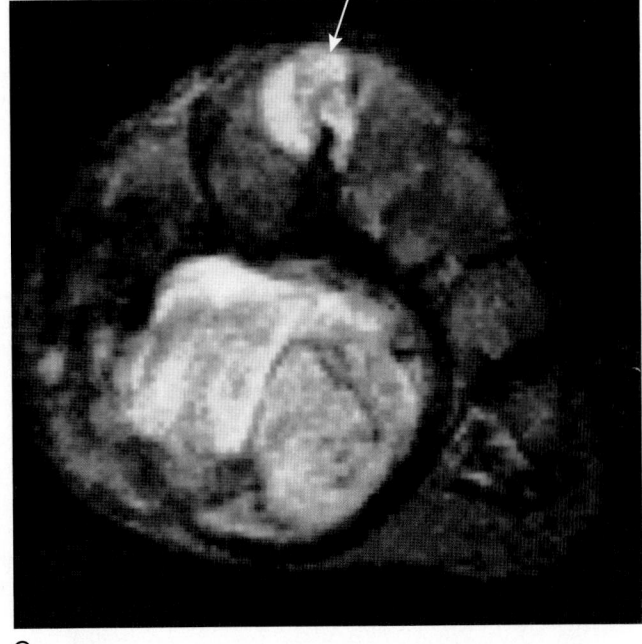

C

FIGURE 160-10. Synovial sarcoma of the foot of a 19-year-old young man. **A,** Computed tomography scan section shows peripheral tumoral calcification and deformity of the metatarsals. **B,** A sagittal T1-weighted magnetic resonance image of the foot shows an inhomogeneous plantar mass that contains areas of high signal intensity caused by hemorrhage. **C,** The signal is predominantly hyperintense on a T2-weighted transverse image. A metastasis is present in the cuneiform bone *(arrow).* (**A** and **B** from Fletcher BD: MRI of musculoskeletal tumors in children. *In* Thrall JD [ed]: Current Practice of Radiology. St. Louis, Mosby, 1993:783.)

> Malignant transformation of benign neurofibroma should be considered when the mass is painful or growing, and when the typical target appearance of a benign neurofibroma is not observed.

Infantile Fibrosarcoma

Infantile fibrosarcoma is an uncommon tumor that contains fibroblasts and myoblasts and occurs in young children, especially during the first 3 months of life. This tumor is now considered a low-grade malignancy, in distinction from an adult fibrosarcoma, which occurs in older children (10 to 15 years of age) and is a more aggressive tumor.

Clinically, infantile fibrosarcomas present as enlarging, sometimes painful, masses. Tumors often occur in the distal ends of the extremities and occasionally in the head and neck and trunk. Because of their high degree of vascularization, they may be confused with hemangiomas on physical and imaging examinations. These tumors may rarely erode adjacent bone, and angiographic studies may reveal tumor vasculature. MR imaging characteristics are nonspecific (Fig. 160-13). Fibrosarcomas are usually isointense to muscle on T1-weighted images and hyperintense on T2-weighted images. They may contain hypointense foci, which correlate with fibrosis. These

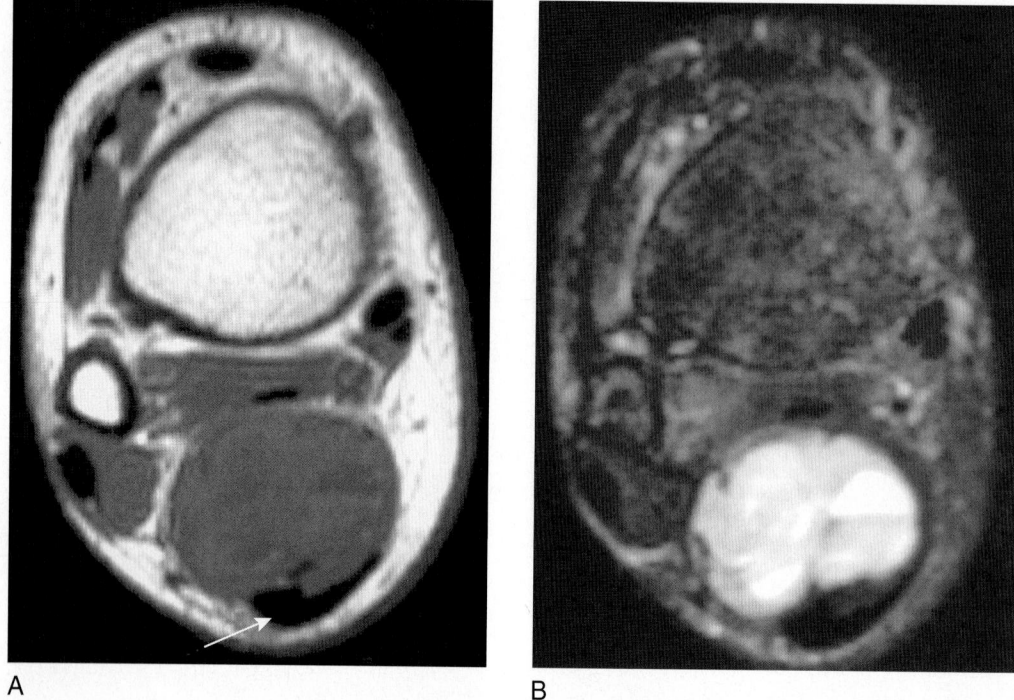

A B

FIGURE 160-11. Synovial sarcoma adjacent to the Achilles tendon. **A,** A transverse T1-weighted magnetic resonance image shows mixed intermediate and low signal in the mass. *Arrow,* Achilles tendon. **B,** A transverse fat-saturated T2-weighted magnetic resonance image at the same level shows fluid-fluid level typical of hemorrhage.

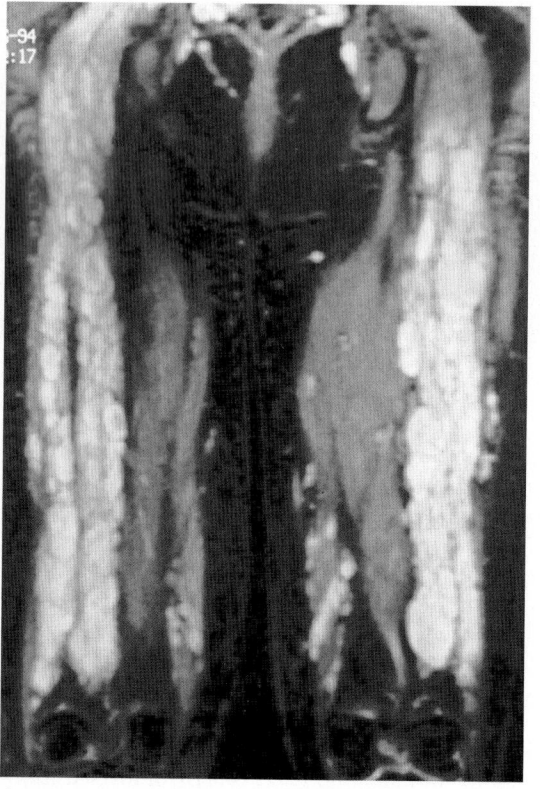

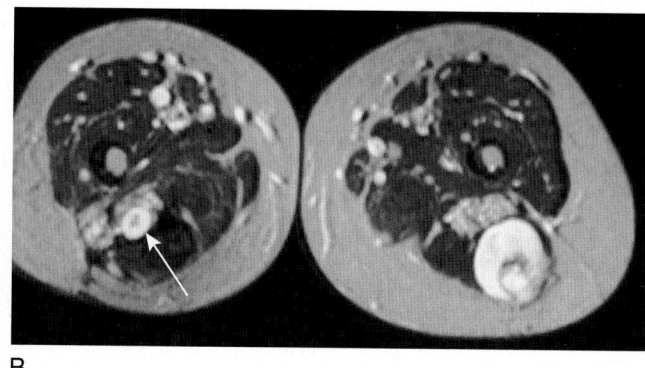

B

A

FIGURE 160-12. A, A coronal short tau inversion recovery magnetic resonance image of the thighs shows multiple neurofibromas distributed along the sciatic nerves of a young woman first seen at the age of 16 with a malignant peripheral nerve sheath tumor. **B,** Transverse T2-weighted images show multiple discrete high-intensity neurofibromas. A characteristic target sign is present *(arrow).* The larger lesion in the posterior left thigh, which had shown recent growth, was a low-grade malignant peripheral nerve sheath tumor.

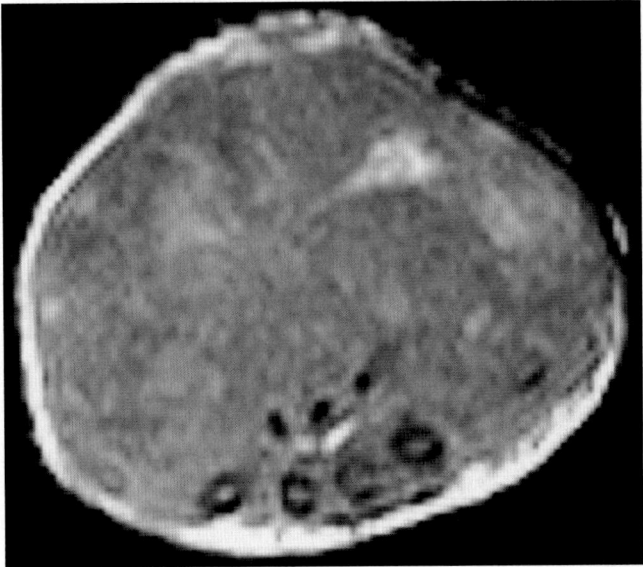

A

FIGURE 160-13. Infantile fibrosarcoma of the distal arm that was present at birth. **A,** A transverse T1-weighted magnetic resonance image shows mixed intermediate and low signal. **B,** Coronal fat-saturated T2-weighted magnetic resonance image shows mixed high and low signal intensity in the mass. **C,** Coronal fat-saturated T1-weighted magnetic resonance image obtained after intravenous gadolinium–diethylenetriaminepenta-acetic acid (DTPA) shows minimal enhancement in the mass.

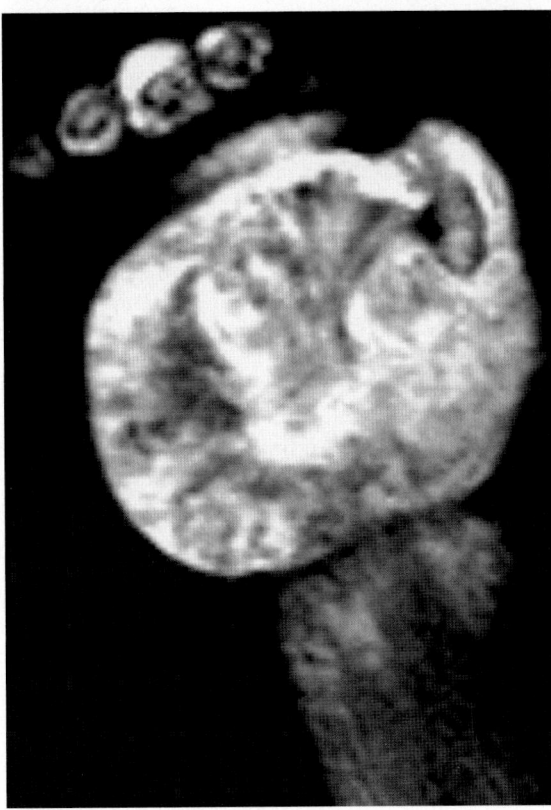

B

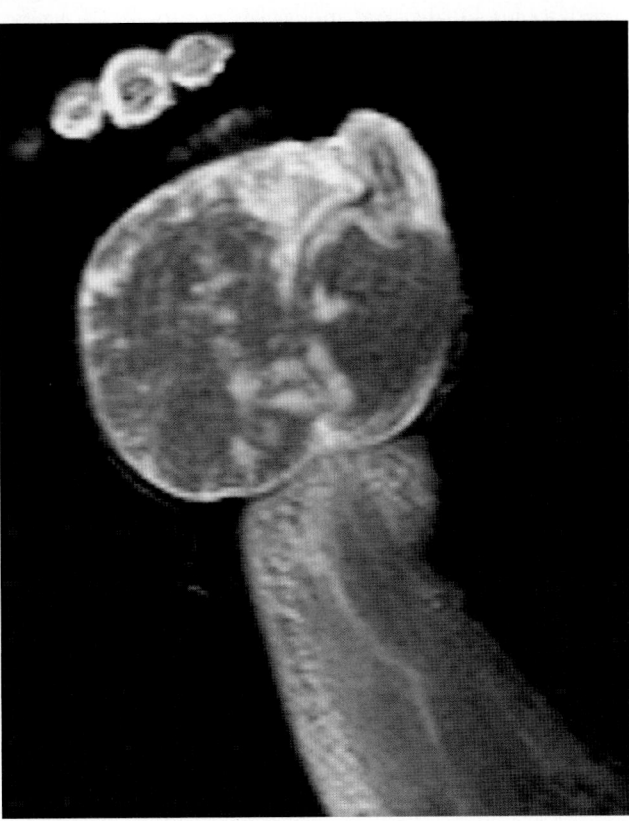

C

tumors recur in up to 30% of cases, and metastases occur in about 5%. Prognosis is good, with 5-year survival up to 94%.

> **Infantile fibrosarcoma is a low-grade malignancy that has a favorable prognosis, in contrast to adult fibrosarcoma.**

Dermatofibrosarcoma Protuberans

Dermatofibrosarcoma protuberans is an intermediate-grade malignancy that involves the dermis (Fig. 160-14). This tumor is most often seen in adults; it occurs rarely in children but may be seen at birth. The tumor most commonly presents as a red-blue or pink plaque that grows slowly and may become nodular. A less common atrophic variant presents as a depressed plaque. Lesions

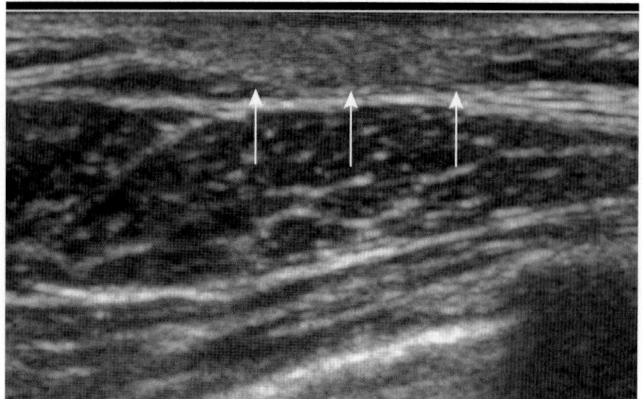

FIGURE 160-14. Dermatofibrosarcoma presenting as a small soft tissue mass adjacent to the clavicle in a 1-month-old boy. Ultrasonography shows an area of increased echogenicity *(arrows)* in the skin and subcutaneous tissues.

are typically fixed to the dermis but may extend into the underlying tissues in time or upon recurrence. Lesions frequently recur locally, and metastasis occurs in 1% to 6% of patients. Seventy-five percent of metastases occur in the lungs.

> Dermatofibrosarcoma protuberans, which involves the dermis, may be seen as a raised nodule or a depressed plaque.

MR imaging is useful for determining the extent of disease, especially with deep tumor invasion. MRI characteristics are nonspecific. On T1-weighted images, lesions are hypointense to fat, and may be isointense, hyperintense, or slightly hypointense to muscle. On T2-weighted images, lesions are isointense or hyperintense to fat. Lesions can enhance after gadolinium administration. On MRI, these tumors may be confused with subcutaneous granuloma annulare, a benign inflammatory dermatosis that may be localized and occurs in children.

Liposarcoma

Liposarcoma is one of the more common soft tissue tumors of adults. Liposarcoma is rare in children, especially those younger than 5 years of age, in whom lipoblastoma is prevalent. The lower extremities, particularly the thigh, are the most common sites of liposarcoma. These tumors may also involve the retroperitoneum, mediastinum, neck, back, axilla, buttocks, and forearm. In the extremities, tumors can be subcutaneous or intramuscular, and they may involve fascial planes.

The 2002 WHO Classification lists five distinct histologic subtypes of liposarcoma: well differentiated, dedifferentiated, myxoid, pleomorphic, and mixed. Well differentiated and myxoid are the two most common subtypes. Myxoid liposarcomas are by far the more common type in children, accounting for 76% of 17 cases studied by Shmookler and Enzinger. These lobular, partially encapsulated neoplasms contain primitive mesenchymal cells, lipoblasts, and capillaries in a myxoid matrix.

Distinguishing a well-differentiated liposarcoma from a lipoblastoma or a lipoma can be difficult. Well-differentiated liposarcomas have imaging characteristics similar to those of fat, with high T1-weighted signal and intermediate intensity on T2-weighted images. Enhancement is slight and is best shown on subtraction or fat-suppressed images. An intramuscular location, large size (>10 cm), and the presence of high signal intensity septations or nodular areas on T2-weighted images favor a well-differentiated liposarcoma. Myxoid liposarcomas are typically large, well-defined, multilobular, intramuscular masses that are isointense to muscle on T1-weighted images and have high signal intensity on T2-weighted images. In the myxoid subtype, the fat component is typically less than 10% of the overall tumor volume and is often seen as small fatty nodules or septations. In children, well-differentiated and myxoid types appear to have only low-grade malignant potential, but local recurrence is possible.

> Distinguishing a well-differentiated liposarcoma from a lipoblastoma or a lipoma can be difficult. A lipoma can be diagnosed only when a purely fatty lesion has well-defined margins and has no septations, nonfatty components, or muscle invasion. Liposarcomas are very rare in children.

Alveolar Soft Part Sarcoma

ASPS is a very rare tumor; it accounts for only 0.5% to 1.0% of all soft tissue sarcomas, and the highest incidence is reported in adolescents and young adults. It has no benign counterpart, and its possibly myogenic histogenesis remains unproven. The tumor is usually found in the muscles of the lower extremities, especially those of the thigh, although isolated cases have involved many other sites. Destruction of adjacent bone may occur. Despite slow growth, ASPS is highly malignant, and metastasis to lymph nodes, lungs, bones, and brain can occur early or late in the disease course.

The tumor consists of alveolar arrangements of large granular cells separated by vascular channels. Because of its high vascularity, ASPS may present as a pulsatile mass with a bruit that may lead to an erroneous diagnosis of vascular malformation.

On noncontrast CT images, the tumor is less attenuating than muscle, and punctate calcification may be visible. As with hemangiomas, marked enhancement may be noted with contrast. However, different from most hemangiomas, ASPS is low in attenuation at its center; this finding is consistent with necrosis. CT may exhibit bone erosion. The highly vascular nature of ASPS may account for an appearance on MRI that is similar to that of hemangioma but different from that of other soft tissue sarcomas in that the signal intensity of ASPS is usually higher than that of muscle on T1-weighted images. Intensity on T2-weighted images may be very high. Tubular flow voids at the margins and in the substance of tumors are consistent with enlarged vessels.

Despite the vascularity of the tumor, flow within it is slow, and angiographic presentation of delayed contrast washout can help distinguish ASPS from arteriovenous malformation. Prominent draining veins may be seen angiographically and on CT or MRI (Fig. 160-15).

> **Alveolar soft part sarcoma is a highly vascular tumor that must be differentiated from hemangioma.**

Malignant Fibrous Histiocytoma

Until recently, MFH was considered the most common STS in adults and a tumor that occurred occasionally in children. However, the 2002 WHO Soft Tissue Tumor Classification has changed the designation of MFH. Pleomorphic MFH is no longer considered a definable or reproducible entity. As a result, many lesions that had been regarded as MFH will be classified as other entities.

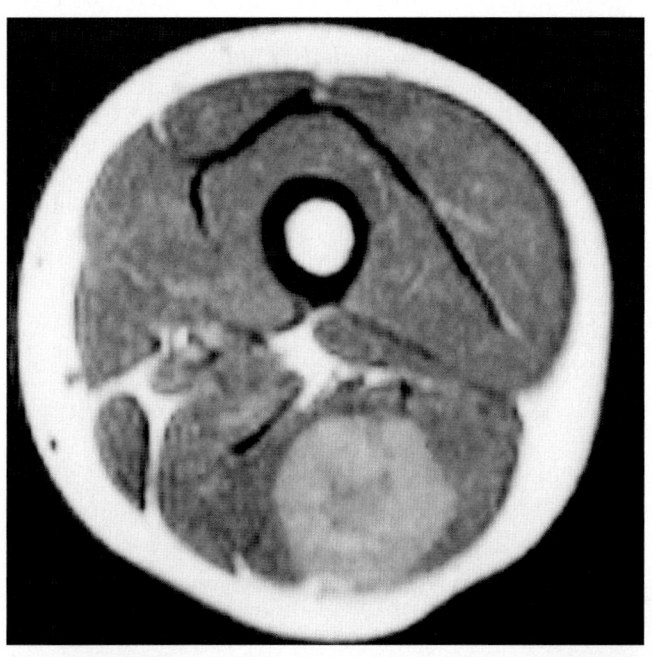

A

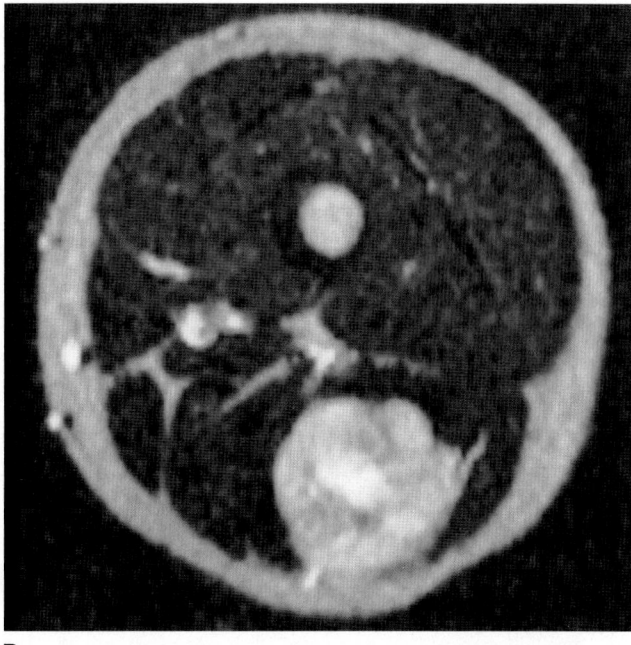

B

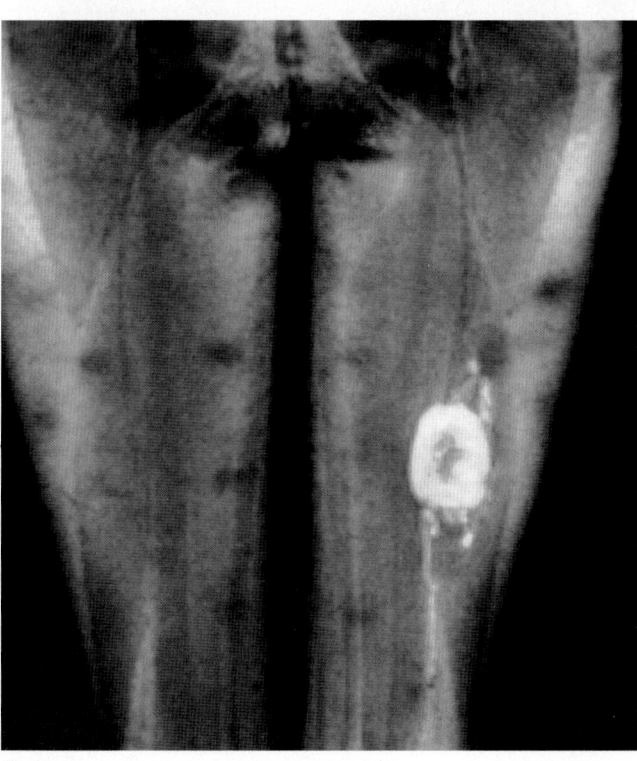

C

FIGURE 160-15. Typical findings of alveolar soft part sarcoma in the thigh of a 9-year-old girl. The tumor is hyperintense to muscle on T1-weighted (**A**) and T2-weighted (**B**) magnetic resonance images. Note that the necrotic, slightly hypointense center on the T1-weighted image becomes hyperintense on the T2-weighted image. **C,** A contrast-enhanced T1-weighted gradient echo coronal image shows peripheral draining veins and a necrotic, nonenhancing center.

The term *pleomorphic MFH* is now synonymous with *undifferentiated pleomorphic sarcoma*, which is essentially a diagnosis of exclusion that should account for approximately 5% of adult STS. It seems that MFH was included in the 2002 classification so that this conceptual shift could be explained; it is likely that the term *MFH* will be dropped from future classifications.

Epithelioid Sarcoma

Epithelioid sarcoma is a soft tissue tumor of uncertain histogenesis that is characterized by epithelial differentiation. This tumor is sometimes difficult to differentiate from chronic inflammation, necrotizing granuloma, and squamous cell carcinoma. This neoplasm accounted for only 7% of 112 nonrhabdomyosarcomatous soft tissue sarcomas treated at St. Jude Children's Research Hospital during an 11-year period, as reported by Gross and colleagues. Two of eight children with epithelioid sarcoma died of early progressive disease. About half of these sarcomas involve the upper extremity; the volar aspect of the forearm is a typical location (Fig. 160-16). Epithelioid sarcoma may be subcutaneous, presenting as single or multiple firm, sometimes ulcerating nodules, or it may be deep-seated, involving muscle, tendons, tendon sheaths, and fascia. The tumor spreads along neurovascular bundles and may invade vascular structures, but it rarely involves bone. Involvement of regional lymph nodes is occasionally seen. Metastases, which may be late, occur most often to the lung.

> **Epithelioid sarcoma may involve subcutaneous tissues, as when it presents as an ulcerating nodule, or it may occur in muscle, tendons, tendon sheaths, or fascia.**

Epithelioid sarcomas rarely calcify, but one tumor with radiographically visible bone formation has been reported. Various MRI patterns have been observed. Nonhemorrhagic lesions are typically isointense to muscle on T1-weighted images and hyperintense to muscle on T2-weighted images. Hemorrhagic lesions can be hyperintense on T1- and T2-weighted images and may contain hemorrhagic fluid-fluid levels. An unusual MRI presentation exhibits honeycombing of subcutaneous fat as the result of lymphatic involvement and denervation-induced muscle atrophy; high T2-weighted signal is seen in the large muscles of the arm.

DISSEMINATED DISEASE OF SOFT TISSUES
Lymphoma

Muscle involvement by non-Hodgkin lymphoma is usually due to metastatic spread via lymphatic and hematogenous routes; however, it may be the result of

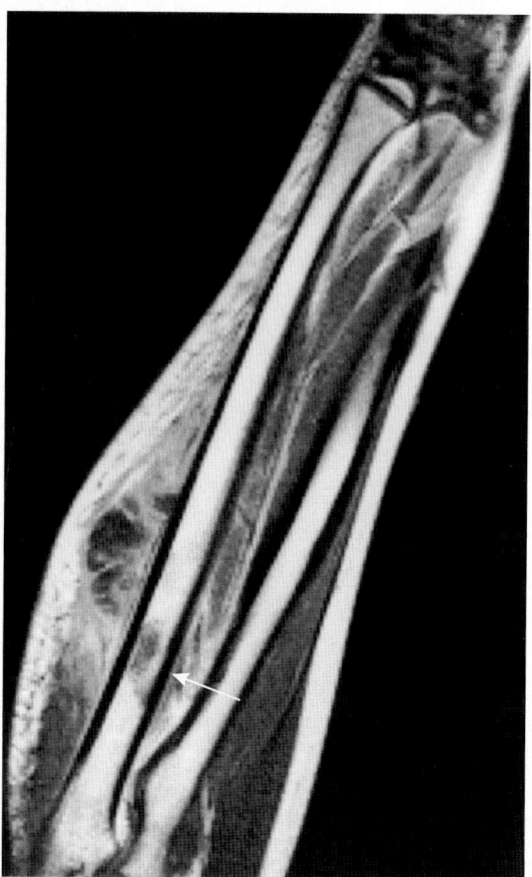

A

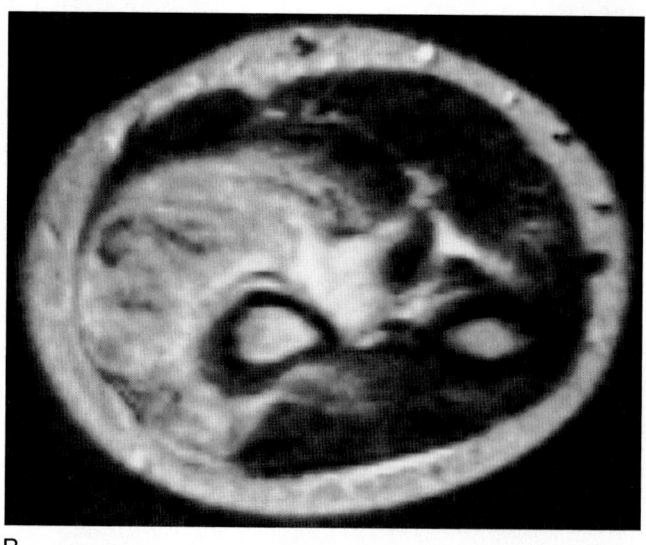

B

FIGURE 160-16. Epithelioid sarcoma. Coronal contrast-enhanced T1-weighted (**A**) and transverse T2-weighted (**B**) magnetic resonance images of the forearm of an 11-year-old boy show an epithelioid sarcoma in a typical location. The unenhanced, hypointense areas in **A** are consistent with necrosis. Note involvement of the marrow of the proximal ulna *(arrow)*. (From Hanna SL, Kaste S, Jenkins JJ, et al: Epithelioid sarcoma: clinical, MR imaging and pathologic findings. Skeletal Radiol 2002;31:403.)

direct extension from primary bone lymphoma. Much less commonly, muscle lymphoma occurs as a primary extranodal tumor. Muscle involvement results in solitary or multiple masses that are detectable on CT and MRI and with the use of gallium-67 scintigraphy and 2-[^{18}F]fluoro-2-deoxy-D-glucose (FDG) PET. The disease can cross compartmental boundaries, or it may invade subcutaneous tissues. Involvement of adjacent bone and bone marrow may also be noted. Primary T cell lymphoma of the skin is referred to as *mycosis fungoides*. Typical findings include focal thickening caused by dermal and epidural infiltrates and lymphadenopathy in advanced-stage disease.

> **Lymphoma may involve the skin or the muscles.**

On CT, muscles affected by lymphoma appear diffusely enlarged with or without obliteration of normal fat planes. The tumor may be poorly defined, and its attenuation is equal to or slightly less than that of normal muscle on contrast-enhanced and noncontrast CT images.

On MRI, masses are isointense or slightly hypointense to normal muscle on T1-weighted images and hyperintense on T2-weighted images. They are markedly hyperintense on STIR images and enhance homogeneously with gadolinium. Abnormal activity as seen in the masses on gallium-67 and FDG PET scintigrams correlates well with MRI findings.

Granulocytic Sarcoma

Granulocytic sarcoma is a rare solid tumor of primitive precursors of white blood cells. This tumor is also known as *chloroma* and *extramedullary myeloblastoma*, and it occurs in patients with acute and chronic myelogenous leukemia and other myeloproliferative diseases. Children are more often affected than adults; 60% of these tumors occur in children younger than 15 years of age.

> **Granulocytic sarcoma is also known as *chloroma* and *extramedullary myeloblastoma*; it occurs in patients with acute or chronic myelogenous leukemia and those with other myeloproliferative diseases.**

Chloromas may be solitary or multiple, and they can involve any part of the body, including the brain and muscles. Orbits and subcutaneous tissues, however, are the most common sites. These tumors are typically isoattenuating to slightly hyperattenuating to muscle on noncontrast CT and hyperattenuating to muscle on contrast CT. On MRI, lesions are typically isointense to muscle on T1-weighted images and hyperintense to muscle on T2-weighted images. Tumors usually enhance after gadolinium administration.

Metastases

Subcutaneous tissues and muscles may be involved in metastatic lesions. Neuroblastoma, in particular, may

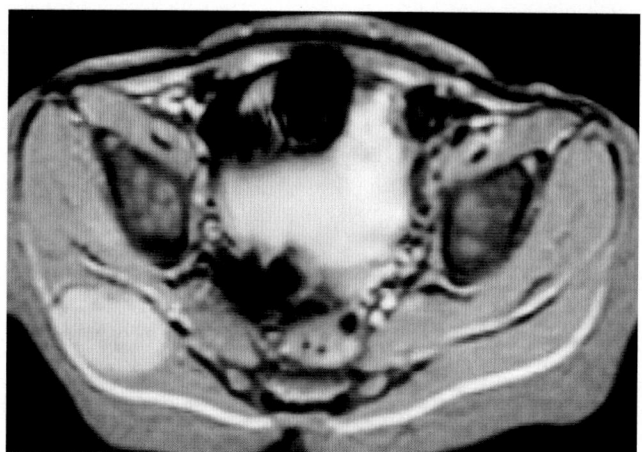

FIGURE 160-17. Neuroblastoma. A transverse T2-weighted magnetic resonance image of the pelvis of a 2-year-old girl with stage IV neuroblastoma shows a large metastasis in the right gluteal muscle.

metastasize to the skin, subcutaneous tissue, or muscle (Fig. 160-17). Despite its proportionately large mass, muscle is not a frequent site for metastatic disease. On CT, muscle metastases produce low attenuation masses with loss of normal muscle planes. On MRI, metastases are similar in intensity to muscle on T1-weighted images and are hyperintense on T2-weighted images. Contrast-enhanced T1-weighted images show high signal intensity masses. Focal necrosis may occur.

> **Metastatic lesions may involve the skin or the muscles.**

CONCLUSION

Soft tissue tumors occur commonly in children. Most are benign. Clinical presentation guides the imaging assessment of these masses. Imaging findings are often nonspecific; when indicated, biopsy is required to confirm histologic diagnosis.

SUGGESTED READINGS

Soft Tissue Tumors—General

Albritton KH: Sarcomas in adolescents and young adults. Hematol Oncol Clin N Am 2005;19:527-546

Bitran JD, Bekerman C, Golomb HM, Simon MA: Scintigraphic evaluation of sarcomata in children and adults by Ga^{67} citrate. Cancer 1978;42:1760-1765

Brisse H, Orbach D, Klijanienko J, et al: Imaging and diagnostic strategy of soft tissue tumors in children. Eur Radiol 2006; 16:1147-1164

Dwyer AJ, Frank JA, Sank VJ, et al: Short-TI inversion-recovery pulse sequence: analysis and initial experience in cancer imaging. Radiology 1988;168:827-836

Enzinger FM, Weiss SW: Soft Tissue Tumors, 3rd ed. St. Louis, Mosby–Year Book, 1995

Finlay K, Probyn L: Ultrasonography of lumps and bumps. Can Assoc Radiol 2002;53:39-49

Fletcher CD: The evolving classification of soft tissue tumours: an update based on the new WHO classification. Histopathology 2006;48:3-12

Gielen JLMA, De Schepper AM, Vanhoenacker F, et al: Accuracy of MRI in characterization of soft tissue tumors and tumor-like lesions: a prospective study in 548 patients. Eur Radiol 2004;14:2320-2330

Hanna SL, Fletcher BD: MR imaging of malignant soft-tissue tumors. Magn Reson Imaging Clin N Am 1995;3:629-650

Howman-Giles R, Uren RF, Shaw PJ: Thallium-201 scintigraphy in pediatric soft-tissue tumors. J Nucl Med 1995;36:1372-1376

Kransdorf MJ, Jelinek JS, Moser RP Jr, et al: Soft-tissue masses: diagnosis using MR imaging. AJR Am J Roentgenol 1989;153:541-554

Laor T: MR imaging of soft tissue tumors and tumor-like lesions. Pediatr Radiol 2004;34:24-37

May DA, Good RB, Smith DK, et al: MR imaging of musculoskeletal tumors and tumor mimickers with intravenous gadolinium: experience with 242 patients. Skeletal Radiol 1997;26:2-15

Meyer JS, Dormans JP: Differential diagnosis of pediatric soft tissue musculoskeletal masses. Magn Reson Imaging Clin N Am 1998;6:561-577

Meyer WH, Spunt SL: Soft tissue sarcomas of childhood. Cancer Treat Rev 2004;30:269-280

Petasnick JP, Turner DA, Charters JR, et al: Soft-tissue masses of the locomotor system: comparison of MR imaging with CT. Radiology 1986;160:125-133

Pizzo PA, Poplack DG: Principles and Practice of Pediatric Oncology, 2nd ed. Philadelphia, JB Lippincott, 1993

Sundaram M, McGuire MH, Herbold DR, et al: High signal intensity soft tissue masses on T1-weighted pulsing sequences. Skeletal Radiol 1987;16:30-36

Sundaram M, McGuire MH, Schajowicz F: Soft-tissue masses: histologic basis for decreased signal (short T2) on T2-weighted MR images. AJR Am J Roentgenol 1987;148:1247-1250

Van Rijswijk CSP, Geirnaerdt MJA, Hogendoorn PCW, et al: Soft-tissue tumors: value of static and dynamic gadopentetate dimeglumine-enhanced MR imaging in prediction of malignancy. Radiology 2004;233:493-502

Vilanova JC, Woertler K, Narvaez JA, et al: Soft-tissue tumors update: MR imaging features according to the WHO classification. Eur Radiol 2007;17:125-138

Weinberger E, Shaw DWW, White KS, et al: Nontraumatic pediatric musculoskeletal MR imaging: comparison of conventional and fast-spin echo short inversion time inversion-recovery technique. Radiology 1995;194:721-726

Desmoid and Other Fibrous Tumors

Casillas J, Sais GJ, Greve JL, et al: Imaging of intra- and extraabdominal desmoid tumors. Radiographics 1991; 11:959-968

Coffin CM, Hornick JL, Zhou H: Gardner Fibroma: a clinicopathologic and immunohistochemical analysis of US patients with 57 Fibromas. Am J Surg Pathol 2007;31:410-416

Eich GF, Hoeffel J-C, Tschäppeler H, et al: Fibrous tumours in children: imaging features of a heterogeneous group of disorders. Pediatr Radiol 1998;28:500-509

Humar A, Chou S, Carperter B: Fibromatosis in infancy and childhood: the spectrum. J Pediatr Surg 1993;28:1446-1450

Kingston CA, Owens CA, Jeanes A, et al: Imaging of desmoid fibromatosis in pediatric patients. AJR Am J Reontgenol 2002;178:191-199

Koujok K, Ruiz RE, Hernandez RJ: Myofibromatosis: imaging characteristics. Pediatr Radiol 2005;35:374-380

Kransdorf MJ, Jelinek JS, Moser RP, et al: Magnetic resonance appearance of fibromatosis: a report of 14 cases and review of the literature. Skeletal Radiol 1990;19:495-499

Patrick LE, O'Shea P, Simoneaux SF, et al: Fibromatosis of childhood: the spectrum of radiographic findings. AJR Am J Roentgenol 1996;166:163-169

Rao BN, Horowitz ME, Parham DM, et al: Challenges in the treatment of childhood fibromatosis. Arch Surg 1987; 122:1296-1298

Robbin MR, Murphey MD, Temple HT, et al: Imaging of musculoskeletal fibromatosis. Radiographics 2001;21:585-600

Romero JA, Kim EE, Kim C-G, et al: Different biologic features of desmoid tumors in adult and juvenile patients: MR demonstration. J Comput Assist Tomogr 1995;19:782-787

Soper JR, DeSilva M: Infantile myofibromatosis. Pediatr Radiol 1993;23:189-194

Spiegel DA, Dormans JP, Meyer JS, et al: Aggressive fibromatosis from infancy to adolescence. J Pediatr Orthop 1999;19:776-784

Peripheral Nerve Sheath Tumors

Bhargava R, Parham DM, Lasater OE, et al: MR imaging differentiation of benign and malignant peripheral nerve sheath tumors: use of the target sign. Pediatr Radiol 1997;27:124-129

Burk DL Jr, Brunberg JA, Kanal E, et al: Spinal and paraspinal neurofibromatosis: surface coil MR imaging at 1.5 T. Radiology 1987;162:797-801

Dewit L, Albus-Lutter CE, De Jong ASH, et al: Malignant schwannoma with a rhabdomyoblastic component, a so-called triton tumor. Cancer 1986;58:1350-1356

Ducatman BS, Scheithauer BW, Piepgras DG, et al: Malignant peripheral nerve sheath tumors. Cancer 1986;57:2006-2021

Ferrari A, Bisogno G, Maagluso A, et al: soft-tissue sarcomas in children and adolescents with neurofibromatosis type 1. Cancer 2007;109:1406-1412

Huang G-S, Huang C-W, Lee H-S, et al: Diffuse neurofibroma of the arm: MR characteristics. AJR Am J Roentgenol 2005;184:1711-1712

Knapp TR, Struk DW, Munk PL, et al: Tumour of a peripheral nerve sheath with invasion of the lumbar spine. Can Assoc Radiol J 1994;45:469-472

Kuman AJ, Kuhajda FP, Martinez CR, et al: Computed tomography of extracranial nerve sheath tumors with pathological correlation. J Comput Assist Tomogr 1983;7:857-865

Levine E, Huntrakoon M, Wetzel LH: Malignant nerve-sheath neoplasms in neurofibromatosis: distinction from benign tumors by using imaging techniques. AJR Am J Roentgenol 1987;149:1059-1064

Lin F, Martel W: Cross-sectional imaging of peripheral nerve sheath tumors: characteristic signs on CT, MR imaging, and sonography. AJR Am J Roentgenol 2001;176:75-82

Mandell GA, Herrick WC, Harcke HT, et al: Neurofibromas: location by scanning with Tc-99m DTPA. Work in progress. Radiology 1985;157:803-806

Murphey MD, Smith WS, Smith SE, et al: Imaging of musculoskeletal neurogenic tumors: radiologic-pathologic correlation. Radiographics 1999;19:1253-1280

Ros PR, Eshaghi N: Plexiform neurofibroma of the pelvis: CT and MRI findings. Magn Reson Imaging 1991;9:463-465

Stull MA, Moser RP, Kransdorf MJ, et al: Magnetic resonance appearance of peripheral nerve sheath tumors. Skeletal Radiol 1991;20:9-14

Suh J-S, Abenoza P, Galloway HR, et al: Peripheral (extracranial) nerve tumors: correlation of MR imaging and histologic findings. Radiology 1992;183:341-346

Varma DGK, Moulopoulos A, Sara AS, et al: MR imaging of extracranial nerve sheath tumors. J Comput Assist Tomogr 1992;16:448-453

Lipoblastoma and Liposarcoma

Arkun R, Memis A, Akalin T, et al: Liposarcoma of soft tissue: MRI findings with pathologic correlation. Skeletal Radiol 1997;26:167-172

Chung EB, Enzinger FM: Benign lipoblastomatosis: an analysis of 35 cases. Cancer 1973;32:482-492

Collins MH, Chatten J: Lipoblastoma/lipoblastomatosis: a clinicopathologic study of 25 tumors. Am J Surg Pathol 1997;21:1131-1137

Cowling MG, Holmes SJK, Adam EJ: Benign chest wall lipoblastoma of infancy producing underlying bone enlargement. Pediatr Radiol 1995;25:54-55

Fisher MF, Fletcher BD, Dahms BB, et al: Abdominal lipoblastomatosis: radiographic, echographic, and computed tomographic findings. Radiology 1981;138:593-596

Katz DS, Merchant N, Beaulieu CF, et al: Lipoblastoma of the thigh: MR appearance. J Comput Assist Tomogr 1996;20:1002-1003

Miller GG, Yanchar NL, Magee JF: Tumor karyotype differentiates lipoblastoma from liposarcoma. J Pediatr Surg 1997;32:1771-1772

Moholkar S, Sebire NJ, Roebuck DJ: Radiological-pathological correlation in lipoblastoma and lipoblastomatosis. Pediatr Radiol 2006;36:851-856

Murphey MD, Arcara LK, Fanberg-Smith J: Imaging of musculoskeletal liposarcoma with radiologic-pathologic correlation. Radiographics 2005;25:1371-1395

Murphey MD, Carroll JF, Flemming DJ, et al: Benign musculoskeletal lipomatous lesions. Radiographics 2004;24:1433-1466

Shmookler BM, Enzinger FM: Liposarcoma occurring in children: an analysis of 17 cases and review of the literature. Cancer 1983;52:567-574

Rhabdomyosarcoma

Arndt CAS, Crist WM: Common musculoskeletal tumors of childhood and adolescence. N Engl J Med 1999;341:342-352

Breitfeld PP, Meyer WH: Rhabdomyosarcoma: new windows of opportunity. Oncologist 2005;10:518-527

Cogswell A, Howman-Giles R, Bergin M: Bone and gallium scintigraphy in children with rhabdomyosarcoma: a 10-year review. Med Pediatr Oncol 1994;22:15-21

Gehan EA, Glover FN, Maurer HM: Prognostic factors in children with rhabdomyosarcoma. Natl Cancer Inst Monogr 1981;56:83-92

Maurer HM: The intergroup rhabdomyosarcoma study: update, November 1978. Natl Cancer Inst Monogr 1981;56:61–68

McCarville MB, Spunt SL, Pappo AS: Rhabdomyosarcoma in pediatric patients. Am J Roentgenol 2001;176:1563-1569

Shapeero LG, Couanet D, Vanel D, et al: Bone metastases as the presenting manifestation of rhabdomyosarcoma in childhood. Skeletal Radiol 1993;22:433-438

Primitive Peripheral Neuroectodermal Tumor

Askin FB, Rosai J, Sibley RK, et al: Malignant small cell tumor of the thoracopulmonary region in childhood: a distinctive clinicopathologic entity of uncertain histogenesis. Cancer 1979;43:2438-2451

Dehner LP: Primitive neuroectodermal tumor and Ewing's sarcoma. Am J Surg Pathol 1993;17:1-13

Ibarburen C, Haberman JJ, Zerhouni EA: Peripheral primitive neuroectodermal tumors: CT and MRI evaluation. Eur J Radiol 1996;21:225-232

Kushner BH, Hajdu SI, Gulati SC, et al: Extracranial primitive neuroectodermal tumors: the Memorial Sloan-Kettering Cancer Center experience. Cancer 1991;67:1825-1829

Schmidt D, Herrmann C, Jürgens H, et al: Malignant peripheral neuroectodermal tumor and its necessary distinction from Ewing's sarcoma. Cancer 1991;68:2251-2259

Synovial Sarcoma

Blacksin MF, Siegel JR, Benevenia J, et al: Synovial sarcoma: frequency of non-aggressive MR characteristics. J Comput Assist Tomogr 1997;21:785-789

Cadman NL, Soule EH, Kelly PJ: Synovial sarcoma: an analysis of 134 tumors. Cancer 1965;18:613-627

Jones BC, Sundaram S, Kransdorf MJ: Synovial sarcoma: MR imaging findings in 34 patients. AJR Am J Roentgenol 1993;161:827-830

Mahajan H, Lorigan JG, Shirkhoda A: Synovial sarcoma: MR imaging. Magn Rason Imaging N Am 1989;7:211-216

Morton MJ, Berquist TH, McLeod RA, et al: MR imaging of synovial sarcoma. AJR Am J Roentgenol 1991;156:337-340

Tateishi U, Hasegawa T, Beppu Y, et al: Prognostic significance of MRI findings in patients with myxoid-round cell liposarcoma. Am J Roentgenol 2004;182:725-731

Infantile Fibrosarcoma

Boon LM, Fishman SJ, Lund DP, et al: Congenital fibrosarcoma masquerading as congenital hemangioma: report of two cases. J Pediatr Surg 1995;30:1378-1381

Dahlin DC: Case report 189: infantile fibrosarcoma (congenital fibrosarcoma-like fibromatosis). Skeletal Radiol 1982;8:77-78

Exelby PR, Knapper WH, Huvos AG, et al: Soft-tissue fibrosarcoma in children. J Pediatr Surg 1973;8:415-420

Fisher C: Myofibroblastic malignancies. Adv Anat Pathol 2004; 11:190-201

Lee MJ, Cairns RA, Munk PL, et al: Musculoskeletal radiology: congenital-infantile fibrosarcoma: magnetic resonance imaging findings. Can Assoc Radiol J 1996;47:121-125

Lilleng PK, Monge OR, Walløe A, et al: Fibrosarcoma in children. Acta Oncol 1997;36:438-440

Ninane J, Gosseye S, Panteon E, et al: Congenital fibrosarcoma: preoperative chemotherapy and conservative surgery. Cancer 1986;58:1400-1406

Soule EH, Pritchard DJ: Fibrosarcoma in infants and children: a review of 110 cases. Cancer 1977;40:1711-1721

Dermatofibrosarcoma Protuberans

Chung S, Frush DP, Prose NS, et al: Subcutaneous granuloma annulare: MR imaging features in six children and literature review. Radiology 1999;210:845-849

Mendenhall WM, Zlotecki RA, Scarborough MT: Dermatofibrosarcoma protuberans. Cancer 2004;101:2503-2508

Thornton SL, Reid J, Papay FA, et al: Childhood dermatofibrosarcoma protuberans: role of preoperative imaging. J Am Acad Dermatol 2005;53:76-83

Weinstein JM, Drolet BA, Esterly NB, et al: Congenital dermatofibrosarcoma protuberans. Arch Dermatol 2003;139:207-211

Alveolar Soft Part Sarcoma

Aluigi P, Sangiorgi L, Picci P: Alveolar soft part sarcoma. Skeletal Radiol 1996;25:400-402

Foschini MP, Eusebi V: Alveolar soft-part sarcoma: a new type of rhabdomyosarcoma? Semin Diagn Pathol 1994;11:58-68

Iwamoto Y, Morimoto N, Chuman H, et al: The role of MR imaging in the diagnosis of alveolar soft part sarcoma: a report of 10 cases. Skeletal Radiol 1995;24:266-270

Lorigan JG, O'Keeffe FN, Evans HL, et al: The radiologic manifestations of alveolar soft-part sarcoma. AJR Am J Roentgenol 1989;153:335-339

Pang LM, Roebuck DJ, Griffith JF, et al: Alveolar soft-part sarcoma: a rare soft-tissue malignancy with distinctive clinical and radiological features. Pediatr Radiol 2001;31:196-199

Sciot R, Cin PD, De Vos R, et al: Alveolar soft-part sarcoma: evidence for its myogenic origin and for the involvement of 17q25. Histopathology 1993;23:439-444

Temple HT, Scully SP, O'Keefe RJ, et al: Clinical presentation of alveolar soft-part sarcoma. Clin Orthop 1994;300:213-218

Zarrin-Khamen N, Kaye KS: Alveolar soft part sarcoma. Arch Pathol Lab Med 2007;131:488-491

Malignant Fibrous Histiocytoma

Munk PL, Sallomi DF, Janzen DL, et al: Malignant fibrous histiocytoma of soft tissue imaging with emphasis on MRI. J Comput Assist Tomogr 1998;22:819-826

Raney RB Jr, Allen A, O'Neill J, et al: Malignant fibrous histiocytoma of soft tissue in childhood. Cancer 1986;57:2198-2201

Ros PR, Viamonte M Jr, Rywlin AM: Malignant fibrous histiocytoma: mesenchymal tumor of ubiquitous origin. AJR Am J Roentgenol 1984;142:753-759

Epithelioid Sarcoma

Gross E, Rao BN, Pappo A, et al: Epithelioid sarcoma in children. J Pediatr Surg 1996;31:1663-1665

Hanley SD, Alexander N, Henderson DW, et al: Epithelioid sarcoma of the forearm. Australas Radiol 1996;40:254-256

Hanna SL, Kaste S, Jenkins JJ, et al: Epithelioid sarcoma: clinical, MR imaging and pathologic findings. Skeletal Radiol 2002;31:400-412

Romero JA, Kim EE, Moral IS: MR characteristics of epithelioid sarcoma. J Comput Assist Tomogr 1994;18:929-931

von Hochstetter AR, Cserhati MD: Epithelioid sarcoma presenting as chronic synovitis and mistaken for osteosarcoma. Skeletal Radiol 1995;23:636-638

Yamato M, Nishimura G, Yamaguchi T, et al: Epithelioid sarcoma with unusual radiological findings. Skeletal Radiol 1997;26:606-610

Disseminated Disease of Soft Tissue

Eustace S, Winalski CS, McGowen A, et al: Skeletal muscle lymphoma: observations at MR imaging. Skeletal Radiol 1996;23:425-430

Gomez N, Ocon E, Friera A, et al: Magnetic resonance imaging features of chloroma of the shoulder. Skeletal Radiol 1997;26:70-72

Guermazi A, Feger C, Rousselot P, et al: Granulocytic sarcoma (chloroma) imaging findings in adults and children. AJR Am J Roentgenol 2002;178:319-325

Lee VS, Martinez S, Coleman RE: Primary muscle lymphoma: clinical and imaging findings. Radiology 1997;203:237-244

Malloy PC, Fishman EK, Magid D: Lymphoma of bone, muscle, and skin: CT findings. AJR Am J Roentgenol 1992;159:805-809

Metzler JP, Fleckenstein JL, Vuitch F, et al: Skeletal muscle lymphoma: MRI evaluation. Magn Reson Imaging 1992;10:491-494

Pui MH, Fletcher BD, Langston JW: Granulocytic sarcoma in childhood leukemia: imaging features. Radiology 1992;190:698-702.

Schultz SR, Bree RL, Schwab RE, et al: CT detection of skeletal muscle metastasis. J Comput Assist Tomogr 1986;10:81-83

Willemze R, Jaffe ES, Burg G, et al: WHO-EORTC classification for cutaneous lymphomas. Blood 2005;105:3768-3785

Williams JB, Youngberg RA, Bui-Mansfield LT, et al: MR imaging of skeletal muscle metastases. AJR Am J Roentgenol 1997;168:555-557

161 Vascular Anomalies of the Soft Tissues

KARIN L. HOEG and DENISE ADAMS

OVERVIEW

The terminology used to describe vascular anomalies has been restructured over the past few decades. Previously, a wide variety of biologically diverse vascular lesions have been called *hemangiomas*, or other terms have been used to reflect their physical appearance, regardless of underlying histology or clinical course. Currently, vascular anomalies are categorized by histology, biologic behavior, and clinical course. The current classification system was first proposed by Mulliken and Glowacki in 1982 and was modified by the International Society for the Study of Vascular Anomalies (ISSVA) in 1996. This reclassification, based on the underlying biology of the lesion, is more clinically helpful in that the name of the lesion corresponds to its natural history and determines treatment options. Radiologists, pathologists, and clinicians are strongly encouraged to avoid using the confusing old terminology and to adhere to the new classification system. The diagnosis and successful treatment of vascular anomalies frequently require a multidisciplinary effort that depends on a common language (Table 161-1).

> Use of the terminology for vascular anomalies introduced by Mulliken and Glowacki and modified by the ISSVA is strongly encouraged because the diagnosis and successful treatment of vascular anomalies frequently require a multidisciplinary effort that depends on a common language.

Most vascular anomalies follow a typical clinical course, have characteristic physical examination findings, and can be diagnosed without imaging. However, when lesions are atypical, deep, near vital structures, or associated with other abnormalities or complications, imaging is extremely helpful for categorizing the type and extent of the lesion. Most vascular anomalies can be diagnosed by characteristic imaging features, especially by magnetic resonance imaging (MRI). Sonography is a useful adjunct in some circumstances, and in other instances, it is used as the primary imaging modality. Lesions occasionally require biopsy because imaging and the clinical appearance of some sarcomas may overlap with those of benign vascular anomalies.

This chapter describes the imaging and clinical features of vascular anomalies that allow radiologists to consistently and accurately classify them.

CLASSIFICATION OF VASCULAR ANOMALIES

Vascular anomalies are classified into two distinct biologic groups: vascular tumors and vascular malformations (Table 161-2). Vascular tumors are characterized by endothelial proliferation. The most common vascular tumor is the infantile hemangioma. In contrast, vascular malformations consist of dysplastic vessels that in general do not proliferate or regress (Table 161-3). Vascular malformations that result from errors in morphogenesis are named by the type of vessel that is malformed (e.g., capillary, venous, lymphatic, arteriovenous). Vascular anomalies may occur in isolation or in association with complex-combined lesions, or they may be part of a syndrome.

> Vascular anomalies are classified into two distinct biologic groups: vascular tumors and vascular malformations.

IMAGING OF VASCULAR ANOMALIES

MRI is the primary modality for characterizing vascular anomalies in the United States. The general MRI protocol (Table 161-4) for evaluating vascular anomalies includes gradient recalled echo sequence to differentiate between "fast- or high-flow" (i.e., arterial flow) and "slow-

TABLE 161-1

Accepted Terminology for Vascular Anomalies

Old Terminology	New Terminology
Capillary hemangioma	Hemangioma
Strawberry hemangioma	Hemangioma
Hepatic hemangioendothelioma	Infantile hepatic hemangioma
Cavernous hemangioma	Venous malformation
Lymphangioma	Lymphatic malformation
Cystic hygroma	Lymphatic malformation
Hemangiolymphangioma	Venolymphatic malformation
Synovial hemangioma	Synovial venous malformation
Port-wine stain	Capillary malformation

TABLE 161-2

Classification of Vascular Anomalies

VASCULAR TUMORS
Hemangioma
Infantile hemangioma
Congenital hemangioma
Rapidly involuting congenital hemangioma (RICH)
Noninvoluting congenital hemangioma (NICH)
Kaposiform hemangioendothelioma
Other
Tufted angioma
Pyogenic granuloma
Infantile (a.k.a. congenital) hemangiopericytoma

VASCULAR MALFORMATIONS
Simple
Slow-Flow
Venous malformation (VM)
Lymphatic malformation (LM)
Capillary malformation (CM)
Fast-Flow
Arteriovenous malformation (AVM)
Arteriovenous fistula (AVF)
Complex-Combined
Slow-Flow
Klippel-Trénaunay syndrome: capillary venous lymphatic
malformation (CVLM) with overgrowth
Fast-Flow
Parkes Weber syndrome: capillary arterial venous
malformation (CAVM) with overgrowth; lymphatic
malformation may also occur

VASCULAR ANOMALIES WITH SYNDROMIC ASSOCIATIONS
Bannayan-Riley-Ruvalcaba syndrome: *PTEN* suppressor
gene mutation, vascular malformations, and early
malignancies
Proteus syndrome: sporadic, congenital, progressive,
hamartomatous syndrome with overgrowth and vascular
anomalies
Maffucci syndrome: soft tissue venous malformation–like
lesions associated with multiple enchondromas

TABLE 161-3

Hemangioma Versus Vascular Malformation

Hemangioma	Vascular Malformation
Small or absent at birth	Present at birth
Exhibit endothelial proliferation (i.e., tumor)	Dysplastic vessels lined by normal endothelium (i.e., malformation)
Spontaneously regress during childhood	Grow in proportion to child and do not regress

TABLE 161-4

Magnetic Resonance Imaging Protocol for Vascular Anomalies

GENERAL PROTOCOL
Gradient recall echo (axial plane)
T1-weighted without fat suppression (longitudinal plane,
sagittal or coronal)
T2-weighted with fat suppression (axial plane)
Inversion recovery or T2-weighted with fat suppression
(longitudinal plane, sagittal or coronal)
T1-weighted with fat suppression (axial and longitudinal
plane) after intravenous contrast administration

OTHER IMAGING CONSIDERATIONS
T1-weighted with fat suppression prior to intravenous
contrast administration (for lesions with possible
lymphatic components or hemorrhage)
Contrast-enhanced magnetic resonance angiography
(performed prior to conventional T1-weighted imaging
with intravenous contrast)

VASCULAR TUMORS

Hemangioma

INFANTILE HEMANGIOMA

The most common vascular tumor of infancy is the hemangioma, also known as *infantile hemangioma* and *hemangioma of infancy*. It usually is first recognized when the infant is several weeks of age. There is a 3:1 female-to-male predominance. This benign neoplasm typically shows a rapid proliferative stage followed by a slower involutional stage. Most lesions regress by adolescence.

> **Infantile hemangiomas are benign vascular tumors that eventually involute.**

Hemangiomas that involve the superficial skin are red (Fig. 161-2). Multiple cutaneous hemangiomas are associated with concomitant visceral lesions. Large draining veins of a deep hemangioma may produce a deep, bluish hue and may develop small superficial telangiectasias.

Doppler sonography and MRI document the high-flow component of a hemangioma. The soft tissue component and the extent of the lesion are clearly seen on MRI. The mass is usually focal, well marginated, and of intermediate T1-weighted and high T2-weighted signal

or low-flow" (i.e., venous flow or only vascular flow in the wall or septations of the malformation) anomalies (Fig. 161-1).

> **Vascular anomalies are divided into two distinct imaging groups: "fast-flow" and "slow-flow."**

T2-weighted imaging with fat suppression technique delineates the extent of the lesion because most vascular anomalies are T2-weighted hyperintense. T1-weighted imaging is used to evaluate overall anatomy. T1-weighted imaging after intravenous contrast administration further characterizes the lesion, especially when fat saturation is applied to make the enhancement more conspicuous. Use of magnetic resonance (MR) angiography is becoming more widespread and frequently obviates the need for diagnostic conventional angiography.

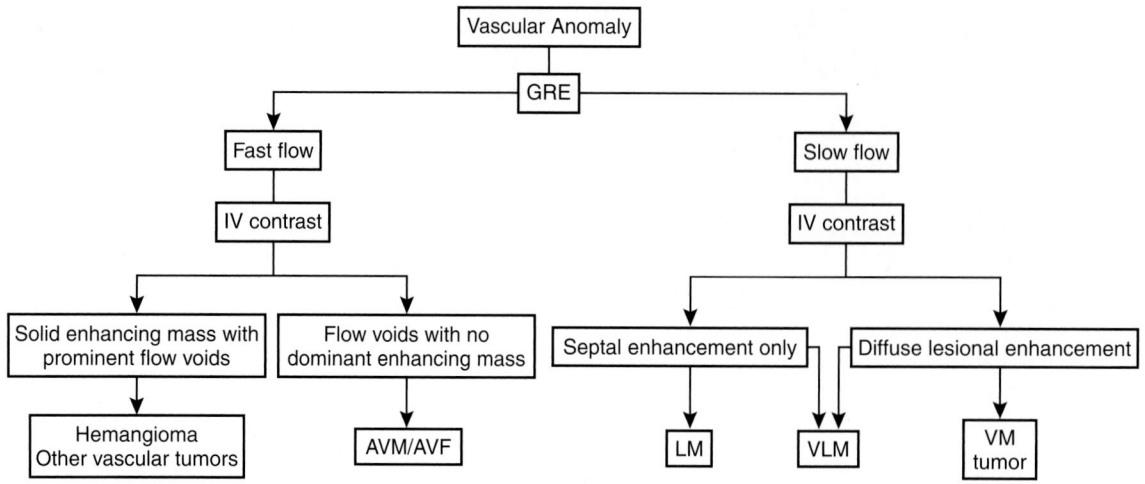

FIGURE 161-1. Vascular anomaly imaging algorithm. VLM, venolymphatic malformation.

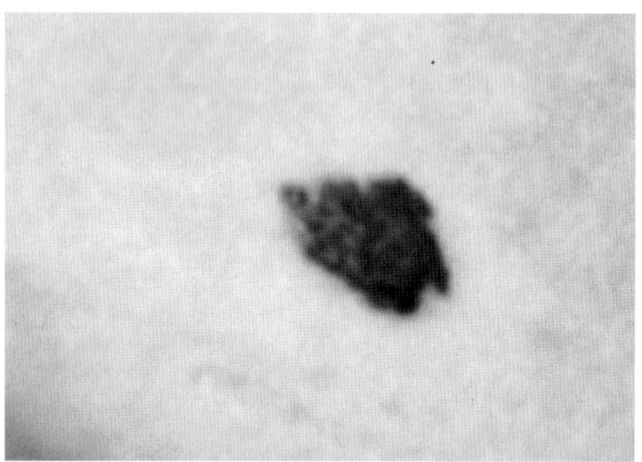

FIGURE 161-2. Superficial hemangioma in the thigh of a baby with classic red color. (*See color plate.*)

intensity (Fig. 161-3). After administration of intravenous contrast, diffuse enhancement may occur (see Fig. 161-3). Dilated feeding arteries and draining veins are seen as bright signal intensity on gradient recalled echo images and as flow voids on spin echo images (see Fig. 161-3). With involution, progressive replacement with fibrofatty tissue occurs.

Occasionally, hemangiomas are imaged by computed tomography (CT), although MRI is better. Imaging by CT reveals a lobulated mass with discrete margins and attenuation similar to muscle (Fig. 161-4). After intravenous contrast is administered, proliferating hemangiomas exhibit diffuse intense enhancement with associated prominent enhancing draining veins/feeding arteries (see Fig. 161-4).

Gray scale sonography with color Doppler spectral analysis can be used to distinguish a hemangioma from a vascular malformation. Sonograms of hemangiomas typically reveal a solid mass of variable echotexture that contains arterial and venous waveforms (Fig. 161-5). Through the presence of solid tissue, hemangiomas can be distinguished from arteriovenous malformations (AVMs), which also contain vessels that have arterial and venous waveforms. Venous malformations and lymphatic

malformations do not contain prominent vessels with arterial flow.

> **Hemangiomas can be distinguished sonographically from other vascular anomalies by their characteristic features of solid mass with arterial waveforms as seen on Doppler.**

Infantile hepatic hemangiomas are a rare manifestation of infantile hemangiomas that are typically found in the setting of multiple cutaneous hemangiomas (>5). They may be asymptomatic; if extensive, they may result in congestive heart failure. The term *infantile hepatic hemangioma* is preferred over *hemangioendothelioma* because the behavior of these lesions is similar to that of hemangiomas in other parts of the body. MRI is the imaging modality of choice for evaluating hepatic hemangiomas, although screening with abdominal ultrasonography is often performed and is sufficient in patients with multiple cutaneous hemangiomas. Imaging of infantile hepatic hemangioma is covered in greater detail in Chapters 16 and 17.

PHACES is an acronym that stands for an association of large facial hemangiomas with **P**osterior fossa abnormalities, **H**emangioma (large facial), **A**rterial anomalies, **C**oarctation of the aorta or **C**ardiac anomalies, **E**ye anomalies, and a **S**ternal cleft or **S**upraumbilical raphe. When a child has a large facial hemangioma, further imaging of the brain for eye and posterior fossa abnormalities such as a Dandy-Walker variant or other intracranial and extracranial arterial anomalies and cardiac anomalies should be considered. Hemangiomas in the beard distribution also have a very high association with airway hemangiomas.

The differential diagnosis of a hemangioma includes infantile fibrosarcoma and rhabdomyosarcoma. Infantile fibrosarcoma usually enhances more heterogeneously after intravenous contrast administration than does a hemangioma. Rhabdomyosarcoma may simulate hemangioma clinically and upon imaging. It is very rare, and if the lesion does not respond to treatment or follow the usual clinical course, biopsy is indicated.

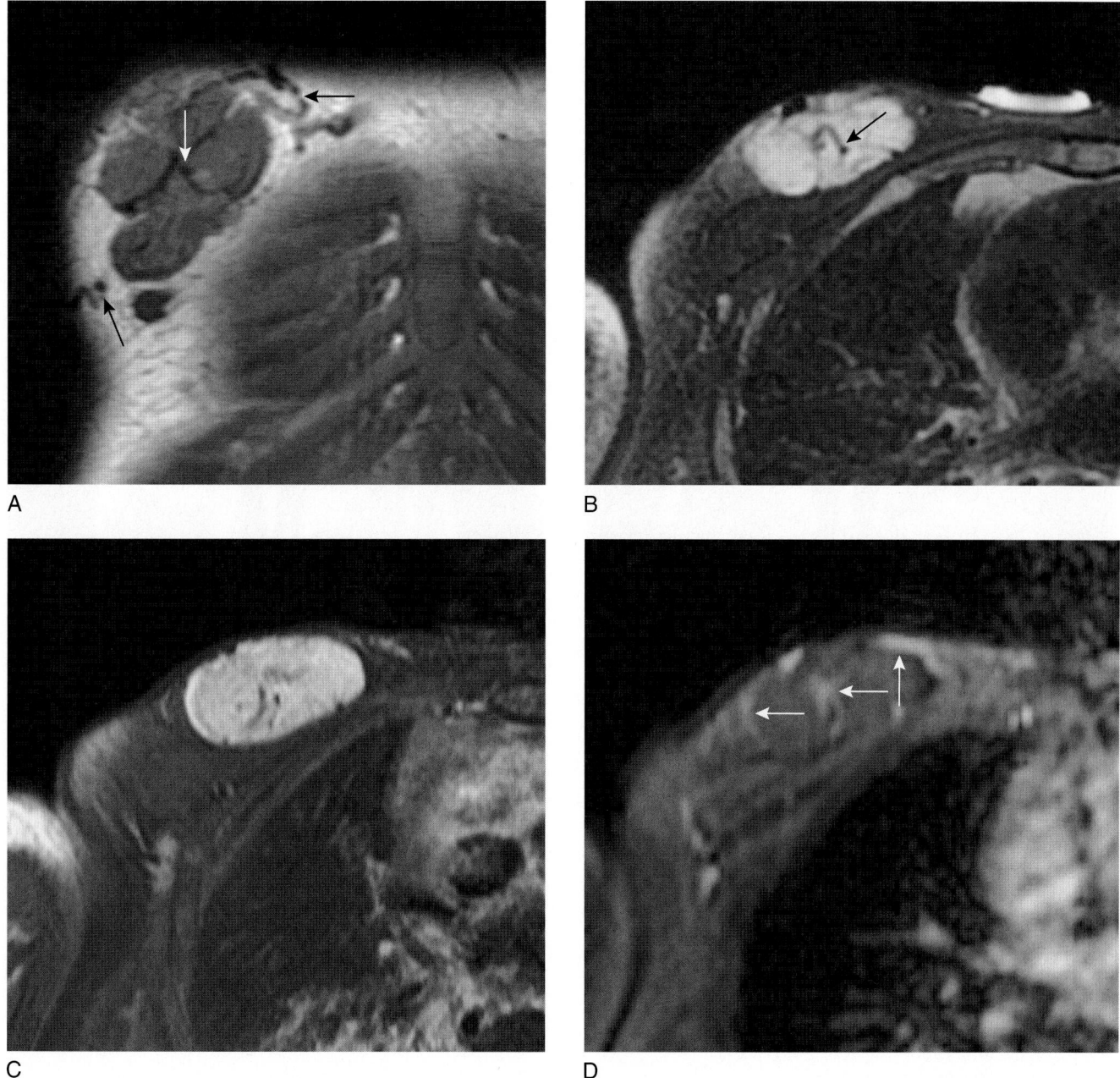

FIGURE 161-3. Classic magnetic resonance imaging features of a hemangioma in the anterior chest subcutaneous tissues. **A,** T1-weighted sequence reveals a discrete lobulated mass with signal isointense to muscle and prominent flow voids *(arrows)* near and within the mass. **B,** T2-weighted sequence shows nearly uniform high signal, with internal flow voids *(arrow)*. **C,** Postcontrast T1-weighted sequence with fat suppression reveals uniform marked enhancement of the hemangioma. **D,** Spoiled gradient recalled echo sequence shows high signal in the areas of suspected flow voids, confirming the presence of "fast flow" within and around the mass *(arrows)*.

> **Solid masses with an atypical clinical appearance or behavior for hemangioma should be biopsied to exclude malignant tumor.**

Complicated hemangiomas are treated with corticosteroids as the first line of therapy. These may be administered topically, orally, or intralesionally. Chemotherapy such as vincristine is sometimes used when corticosteroids fail, and interferon may be used only as a last resort because of its associated neurotoxicity. Surgical excision is occasionally performed for complicated hemangiomas.

Congenital Hemangioma

DESCRIPTION. Congenital hemangioma is a variant of infantile hemangioma or a related but separate vascular tumor. Congenital hemangiomas are sometimes discovered on prenatal ultrasonography. Different from infantile hemangiomas, congenital hemangiomas are fully grown at birth, are Glut-1 receptor (glucose transporter protein found in the blood of children with infantile hemangio-

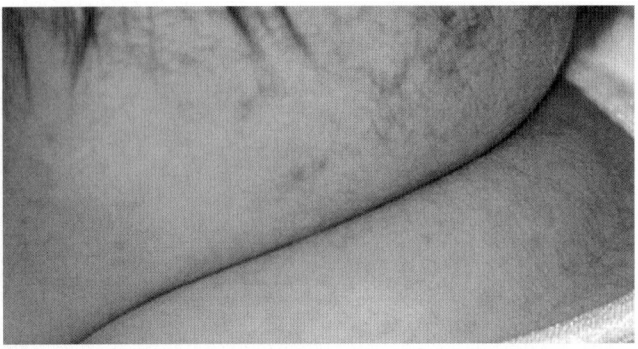

A

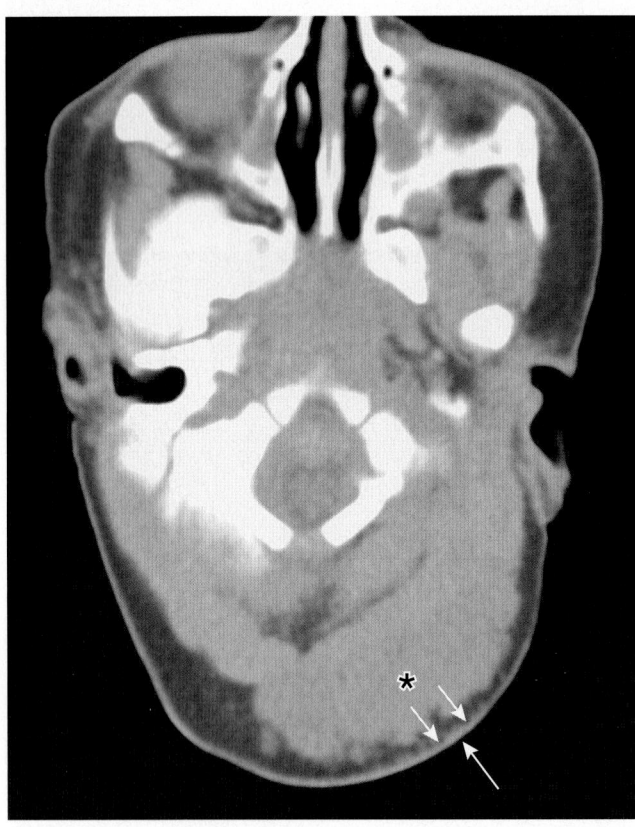

B

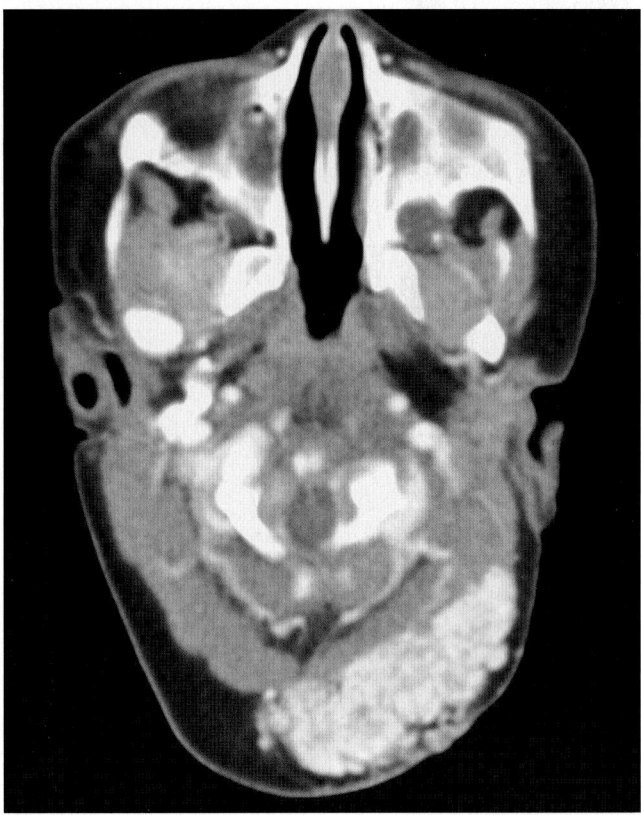

C

FIGURE 161-4. Infant with predominantly deep hemangioma of the posterior neck with a small superficial component. **A,** Deep hemangiomas with superficial telangiectasias, as shown on this photograph of the neck, can be difficult to definitively diagnose with physical examination. (**A,** *see color plate.*) **B,** Precontrast computed tomography (CT) scan shows a large subcutaneous mass *(asterisk)* with attenuation similar to muscle and subtle skin thickening *(arrows)*, corresponding to a small superficial component. **C,** Postcontrast CT image reveals uniform intense enhancement of the hemangioma.

mas) negative, and have no sex predominance. Two main subtypes of congenital hemangioma have been identified: rapidly involuting congenital hemangioma (RICH) and noninvoluting congenital hemangioma (NICH). RICH is much more common than NICH, but both lesions are extremely rare.

> **Congenital hemangioma, in contrast to infantile hemangioma, is fully grown at birth.**

RICH, which typically occurs as a single, large tumor, involutes over the first 2 to 14 months of life. Some infants develop high-output heart failure from arteriovenous shunting and require embolization.

In contrast to infantile hemangioma and RICH lesions, NICH lesions do not involute. The imaging appearance of NICH is similar to that of infantile hemangioma. NICH is typically treated with surgical excision.

IMAGING. RICH, NICH, and infantile hemangioma have similar imaging features. The literature describes angiographic differences between RICH and infantile hemangioma, including heterogeneous parenchymal staining, irregular and large feeding arteries, arterial aneurysms, direct arteriovenous shunts, and intravascular thrombi. Practically speaking, however, angiography is rarely used to evaluate these lesions. Sometimes, a biopsy is required to distinguish RICH from congenital infantile fibrosarcoma and AVM. Distinction is usually made clinically on the basis of growth and involution patterns. Clinical follow-up over the first year of life is very helpful. RICH will involute, NICH will not change, and infantile hemangioma will rapidly enlarge.

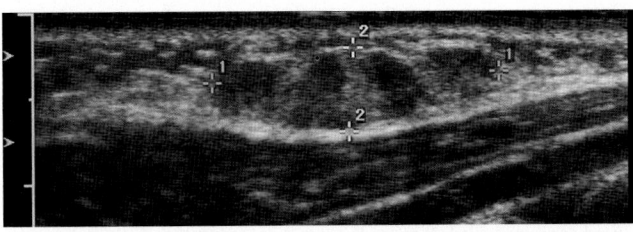

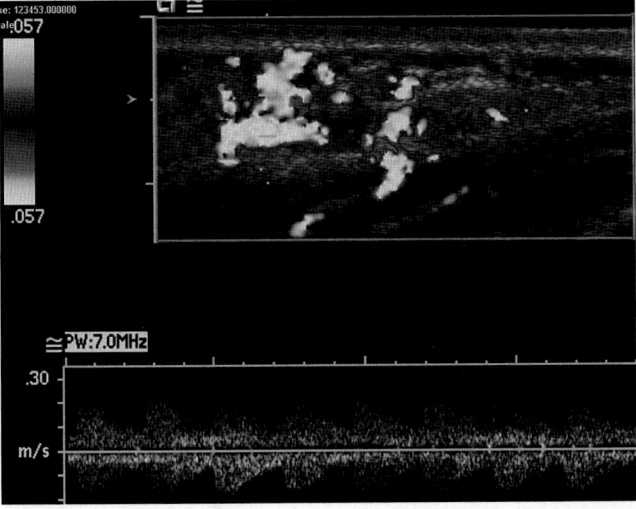

FIGURE 161-5. Soft tissue hemangioma, which presented as a nonspecific, soft, slightly blue subcutaneous mass in an infant. **A,** Gray scale sonogram reveals a fairly well-defined lobulated mass *(cursors)* with heterogeneous echotexture. **B,** Doppler imaging shows prominent vascular flow with arterial waveforms. The presence of arterial waveforms distinguishes it from a venous malformation.

> Imaging features of RICH, NICH, and hemangioma are very similar: The clinical timing of growth and involution is very helpful in distinguishing between them.

KAPOSIFORM HEMANGIOENDOTHELIOMA

DESCRIPTION. Kaposiform hemangioendothelioma (KHE) is an aggressive vascular tumor that may be present at birth or may develop during the first few months of life. It is associated with the Kasabach-Merritt phenomenon, a consumptive coagulopathy. It typically presents as an ill-defined purpuric mass with rapid enlargement and coagulopathy. A high mortality rate is associated with this.

IMAGING. In comparison with infantile hemangioma, KHE is ill defined, involves many tissue planes, and is associated more frequently with edema (Fig. 161-6). It is typically solitary. Flow-voids related to feeding and draining vessels are smaller and less common than with infantile hemangioma. Lesions are typically T2 hyperintense and enhance with intravenous contrast. KHE is more commonly associated with destructive osseous changes.

Other

TUFTED ANGIOMA

DESCRIPTION. Tufted angioma is a benign vascular tumor that is characterized by angiomatous proliferation. It may be a less aggressive version of KHE and may be associated with Kasabach-Merritt phenomenon. It is most commonly found in the skin of the neck and in the upper trunk.

> **KHE and tufted angiomas (NOT hemangiomas) are associated with the Kasabach-Merritt phenomenon.**

CONGENITAL HEMANGIOPERICYTOMA

DESCRIPTION. Congenital hemangiopericytoma is a rare benign vascular tumor with prominent vascularity that may appear clinically similar to congenital hemangioma. Debate is put forth in the literature about whether congenital hemangiopericytoma and infantile myofibromatosis are part of a spectrum of the same neoplasm rather than distinct vascular tumors. The tumor is usually found in an extremity of a young infant or child. This tumor may rarely spontaneously involute without intervention, or it may be surgically removed.

IMAGING. Most descriptions of the imaging features of hemangiopericytoma are based on tumors in adult patients. These tumors are well circumscribed, may contain calcifications, and may cause partial destruction of adjacent bone. They have no specific imaging features, but they are extremely vascular, exhibit avid enhancement with intravenous contrast, and frequently develop central necrosis. On MRI, these tumors tend to be isointense to muscle on T1-weighted images and high signal on T2-weighted and STIR images, and they enhance with intravenous gadolinium (Fig. 161-7).

VASCULAR MALFORMATIONS

Slow-Flow

VENOUS MALFORMATION

DESCRIPTION. Venous malformations are the most common vascular malformations of childhood. The confusing term, *cavernous hemangioma,* historically has been applied to these lesions. Venous malformations may be localized unifocal or multifocal masses, or they may represent diffuse dilation and varicosity of major draining veins. Venous malformations enlarge when a limb is dependent and often decompress with elevation or compression. These lesions grow at a level commensurate with growth of the child.

Venous malformations of the synovium deserve special mention. They have been mistakenly referred to in the literature as *synovial hemangiomas.* Although usually isolated, they may be associated with diffuse venous malformations. On MRI, features typical of venous malformation are seen within the knee joint, most frequently within the suprapatellar pouch. The affected child may

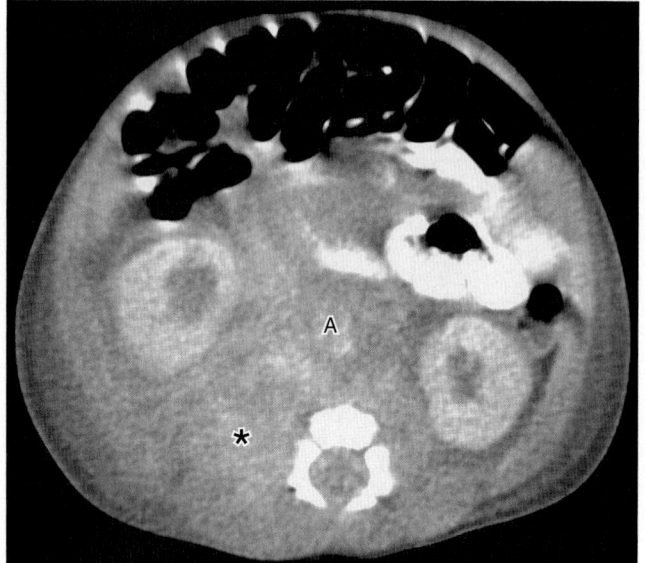

A

FIGURE 161-6. Kaposiform hemangioendothelioma presenting in a neonate as a purpuric mass and consumptive coagulopathy (Kasabach-Merritt phenomenon). **A,** Initial computed tomography scan reveals a large, ill-defined high attenuation retroperitoneal mass *(asterisk)* that displaces the right kidney anteriorly, surrounds the abdominal aorta (A), and extends posteriorly into the paraspinal muscles, crossing several tissue planes. **B,** Axial T2-weighted sequence with fat suppression shows the same mass, which has intermediate T2-weighted signal intensity (atypical, in that it is usually hyperintense). Anasarca and ascites are present. **C,** Postcontrast T1-weighted sequence with fat suppression shows mild enhancement of the mass *(asterisk)* (enhancement frequently more intense). Right hydronephrosis is noted.

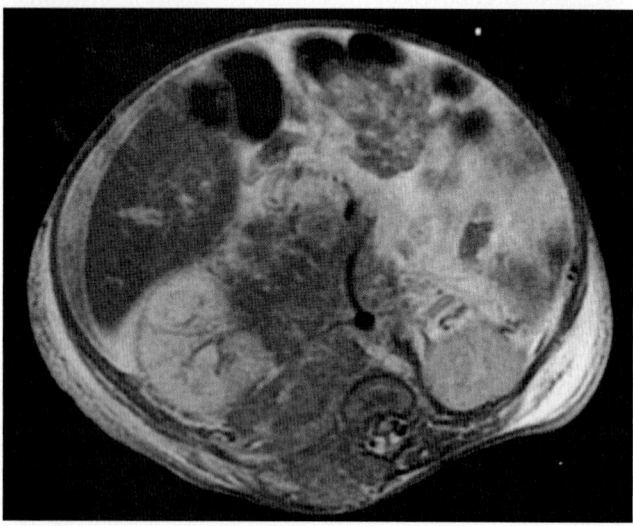

B

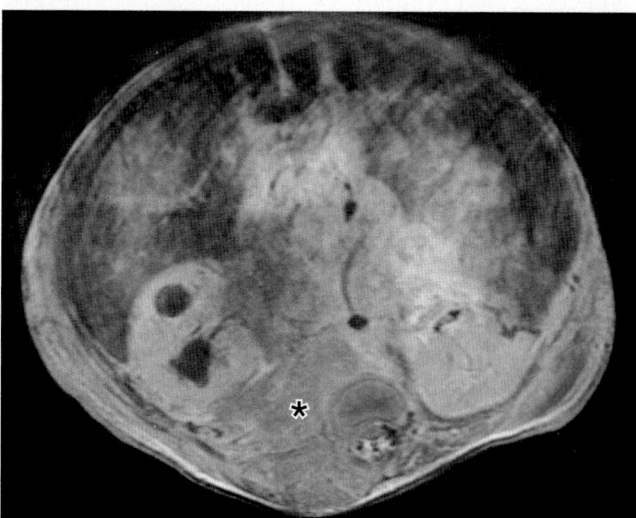

C

report recurrent, painful knee swelling. A high incidence of hemosiderin arthropathy is associated with repeated episodes of bleeding into the joint. This results in significant loss of articular cartilage and formation of subchondral cysts (Fig. 161-8). Early synovectomy is recommended to minimize articular damage.

> Synovial venous malformations often lead to hemosiderin arthropathy similar to that seen with hemophilia; thus, early synovectomy is recommended.

Extensive pure venous malformations that involve an entire upper or lower limb and adjacent trunk are rare. These malformations worsen over time, causing painful deformity and loss of function of the limb. Diffuse pure venous malformations are associated with a local coagulopathy that must be recognized prior to surgical intervention so that unexpected hemorrhage can be avoided.

IMAGING. Radiography may reveal phleboliths or a soft tissue mass. Sonography shows a lesion of mixed echogenicity with occasional phleboliths. Doppler tracings range from no flow to monophasic, low-flow patterns. A biphasic Doppler sample is due to mixed composition of vessels in the lesion (such as capillaries and lymphatics). Venous malformations are compressible, which helps in distinguishing them from soft tissue neoplasms. Angiography is not needed for diagnosis of a venous malformation. It may be normal or may show only venous stasis.

> Phleboliths are found in venous malformations (NOT hemangiomas).

MRI is useful for the diagnosis and management of venous malformations. These usually are multilocular, multiseptated masses that may be superficial or deep (Figs. 161-9 through 161-11). They are bright on T2-weighted images and enhance diffusely after intravenous

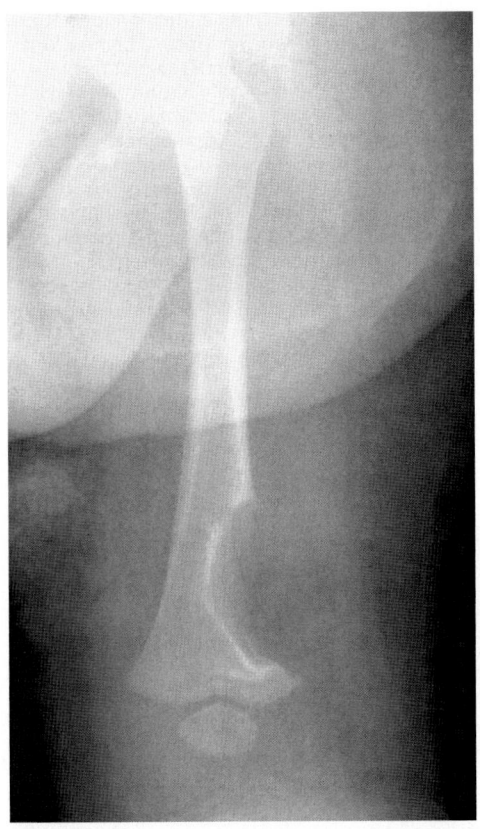
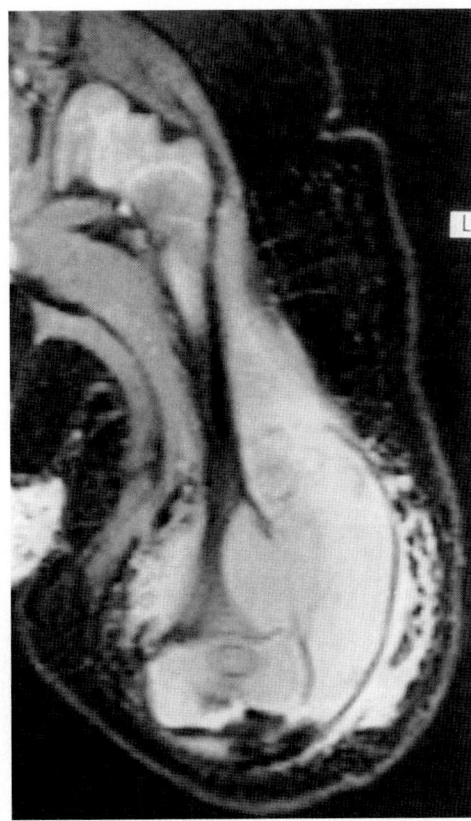

A

B

FIGURE 161-7.
Hemangiopericytoma in a
2-month-old infant. **A,** An
anteroposterior radiograph of
the femur shows a well-defined
erosion in the distal femur.
B, Coronal short tau inversion
recovery image shows a
hyperintense soft tissue mass
eroding the bony cortex and
extending into the medullary
space.

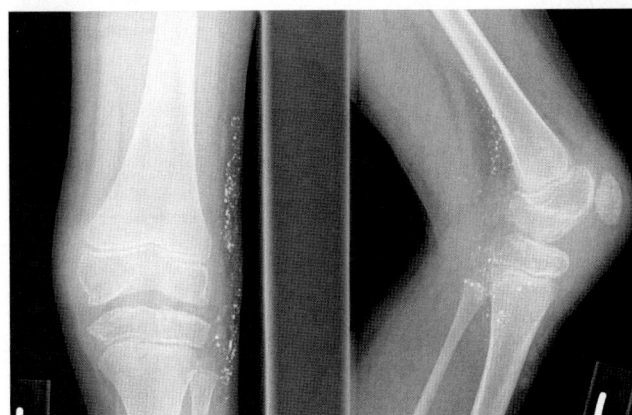

A

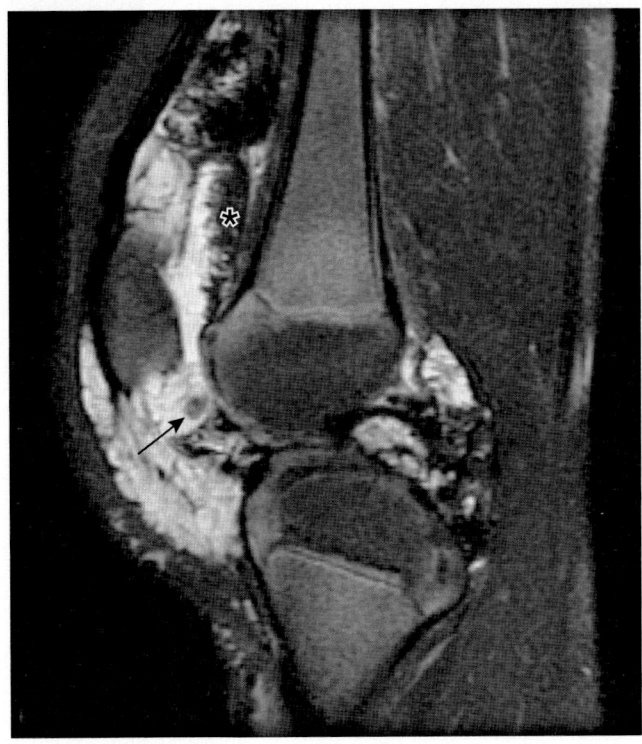

B

FIGURE 161-8. Synovial venous malformation of the knee
and surrounding soft tissues resulting in hemarthropathy.
A, Anterior-posterior and lateral left knee radiographs reveal
degenerative changes of the epiphyses caused by intra-articular
bleeding and hemosiderin deposition. (The high attenuation
material along the lateral aspect of the knee is a sclerosant from
a prior therapy.) **B,** Sagittal T2-weighted sequence with fat
suppression shows the large, high T2 signal mass distending the
knee joint, which is a venous malformation. Areas of low signal
(asterisk) represent hemosiderin deposition caused by prior
intra-articular bleeds. *Arrow* points to thrombus.

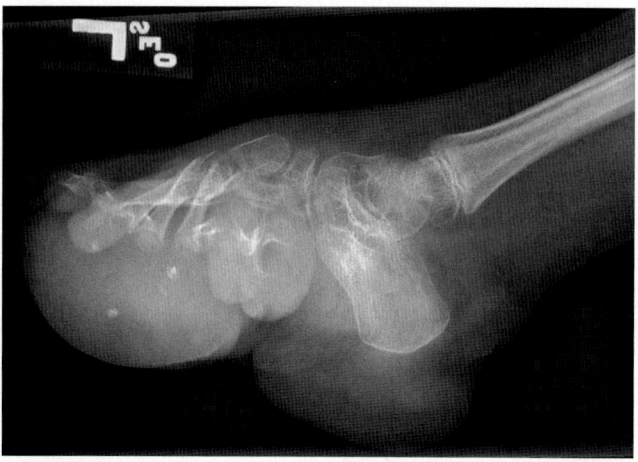

A

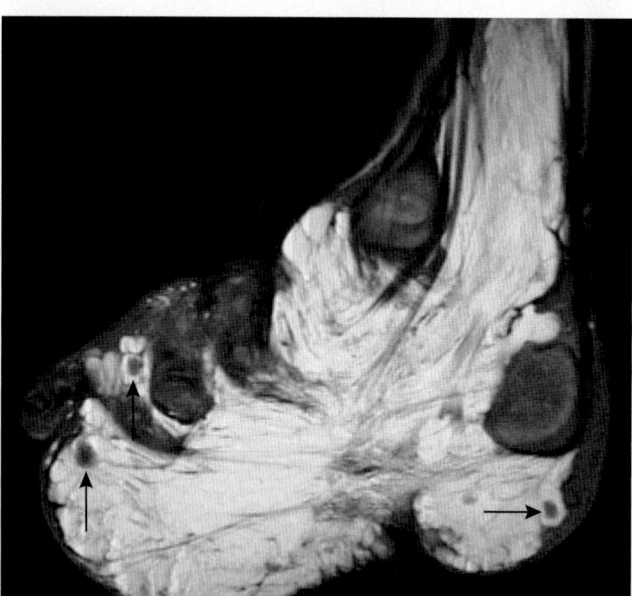

B

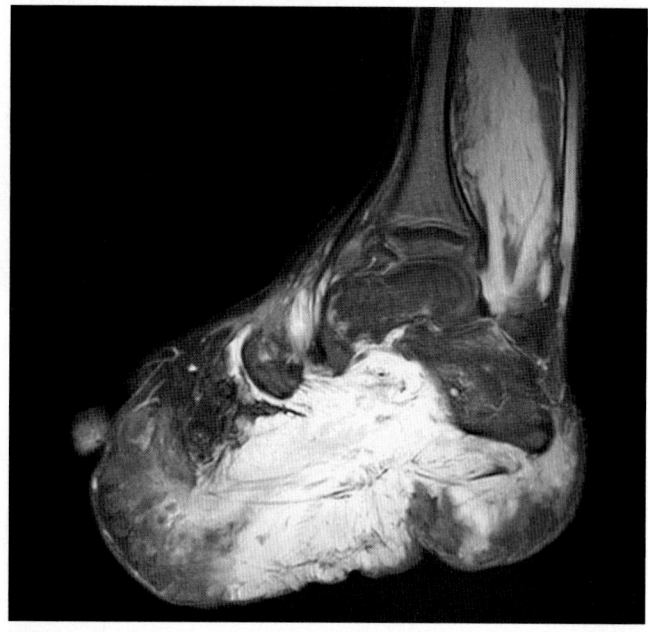

C

FIGURE 161-9. Extremely extensive foot venous malformation in a child with multifocal venous malformations. **A,** Lateral foot radiograph shows several phleboliths in the large soft tissue mass that is associated with morphologically abnormal bones. **B,** Sagittal T2-weighted sequence with fat suppression of the left foot reveals a large, nearly uniform high T2 signal mass that crosses tissue planes. Scattered low signal foci *(arrows)* represent phleboliths or thrombi within the venous malformation. **C,** Postcontrast sagittal T1-weighted sequence with fat suppression reveals intralesional enhancement of most of the mass. Areas that do not enhance may represent relatively stagnant flow or associated lymphatic malformation, which is common.

contrast administration. Small hypointense foci on T1- and T2-weighted sequences represent thrombi or phleboliths (see Figs. 161-9 and 161-10). Conventional radiography may help to confirm the presence of underlying bone abnormalities or phleboliths, which are almost pathognomonic for venous malformations (see Figs. 161-9 and 161-10). Gradient recalled echo images may show dilation and anomalies of the venous system. No enlarged arteries are seen. MR venography is usually normal in pure venous lesions.

> **Venous malformations are slow-flow vascular malformations with diffuse intralesional enhancement.**

LYMPHATIC MALFORMATION

DESCRIPTION. Misleading terms such as "cystic hygroma" and "lymphangioma" are found throughout the medical literature; the preferred term used to describe the underlying pathology is *lymphatic malformation*. Lymphatic malformations are slow-flow lesions that present as a localized mass or diffuse malformation. They may be macrocystic or microcystic. Deep lymphatic malformations may extend to the skin, resulting in superficial vesicles. Similar to venous malformations, lymphatic malformations grow at a level commensurate with growth of the child, but they may enlarge acutely as the result of hemorrhage, infection, or obstruction. Lymphatic malformations are produced by sequestered primitive lymphatic tissue that fails to communicate with peripheral drainage pathways.

> **Lymphatic malformations are produced by sequestered primitive lymphatic tissue that fails to communicate with peripheral drainage pathways.**

Gorham syndrome is a lymphatic malformation within bone that is associated with bone degeneration. It has

FIGURE 161-10. Focal venous malformation (or venolymphatic malformation) in a child with a proximal forearm mass. **A,** Anterior-posterior forearm radiograph shows a phlebolith in the proximal forearm soft tissues, nearly pathognomonic for a venous malformation. **B,** Axial postcontrast T1-weighted sequence with fat suppression reveals a mass with a fluid-fluid level and a central low signal phlebolith. The fluid-fluid level may represent stagnant blood in a venous malformation or a venolymphatic malformation with hemorrhage. **C,** Coronal postcontrast T1-weighted sequence shows the discrete soft tissue lesion that contains the phlebolith.

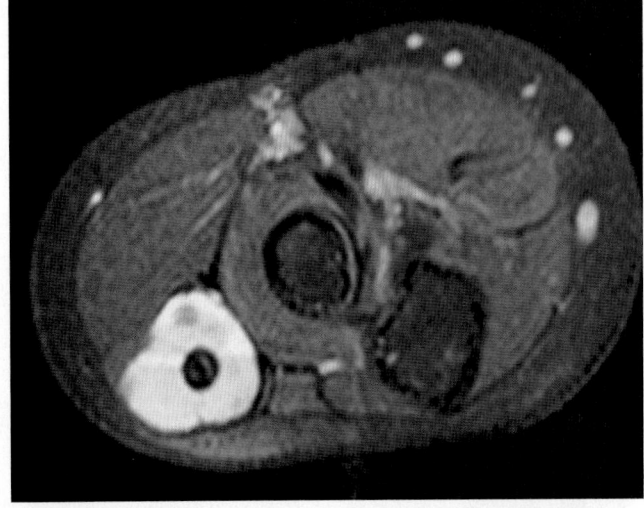

B

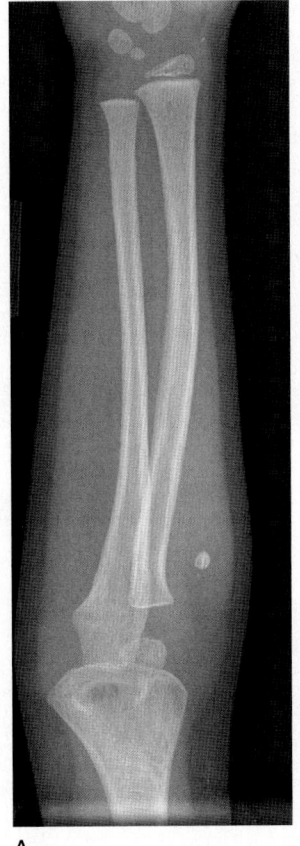

A

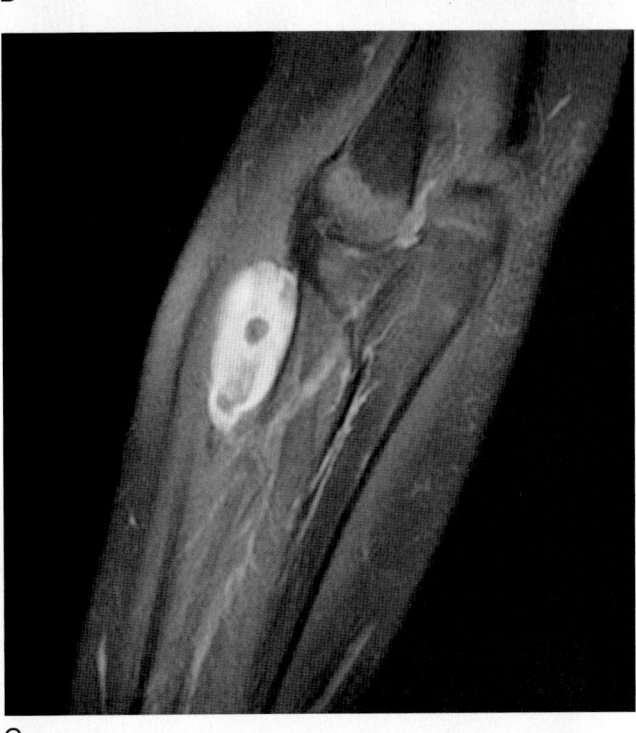

C

many synonyms, including "vanishing bone disease." Chest wall involvement is associated with a chylous effusion.

IMAGING. Lymphatic malformations can be divided into macrocystic, microcystic, and mixed malformations. Sonography of lymphatic malformations shows multilocular architecture and vascular flow that is present only in the septa (Fig. 161-12). Microcystic lesions are hyperechoic as a result of numerous interfaces. Lymphatic malformations do not show flow with Doppler interrogation.

On MRI, macrocystic lymphatic malformations are typically septated masses of low T1- and high T2-weighted signal intensity (Fig. 161-13). Variable signal intensity and fluid-fluid levels are due to hemorrhage or

infection (see Fig. 161-12). Only the septa enhance after intravenous contrast administration. No flow-voids are seen on spin echo sequences, and gradient recalled echo images show no signal from high flow. Occasionally, adjacent veins may be enlarged or anomalous. MR lymphangiography may be useful for distinguishing varicose lymphatic channels from interstitial leakage caused by lymphatic hypoplasia.

> On MRI, macrocystic lymphatic malformations are typically seen as septated masses of low T1- and high T2-weighted signal intensity, with only septal enhancement.

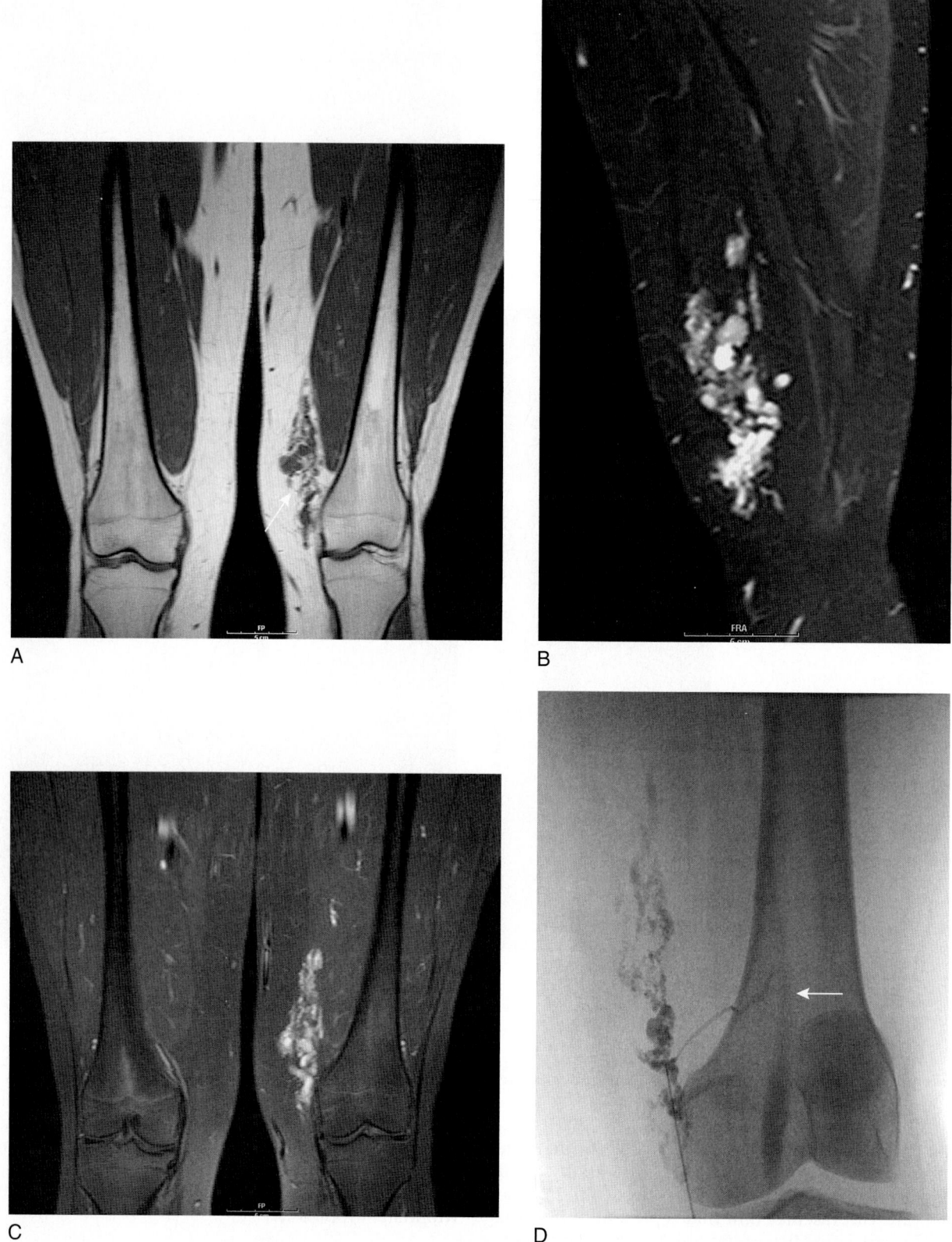

A

B

C

D

FIGURE 161-11. Venous malformation deep in the subcutaneous fat. **A,** Coronal T1-weighted sequence through the distal thighs reveals a focal serpentine mass within the medial left thigh subcutaneous fat with signal isointense to muscle *(arrow).* **B,** Sagittal short tau inversion recovery (STIR) sequence through the same lesion shows high signal. **C,** Coronal postcontrast T1-weighted sequence with fat suppression reveals uniform intralesional enhancement. **D,** Anterior-posterior radiograph obtained during percutaneous sclerotherapy of this painful venous malformation shows drainage of the venous malformation into the popliteal vein *(arrow).*

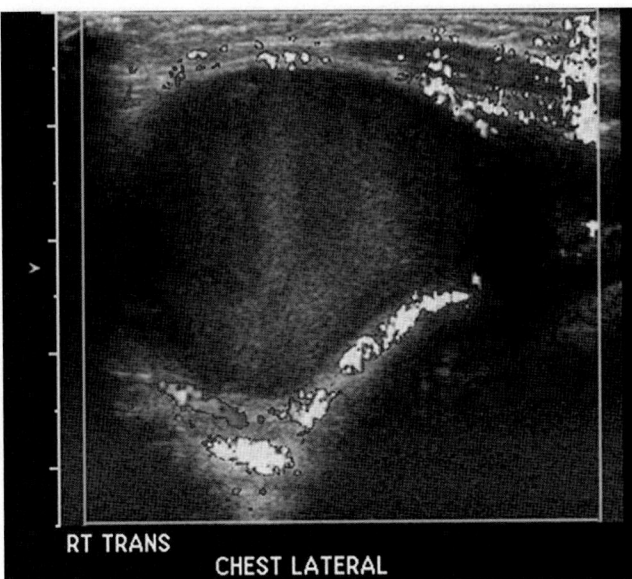

A

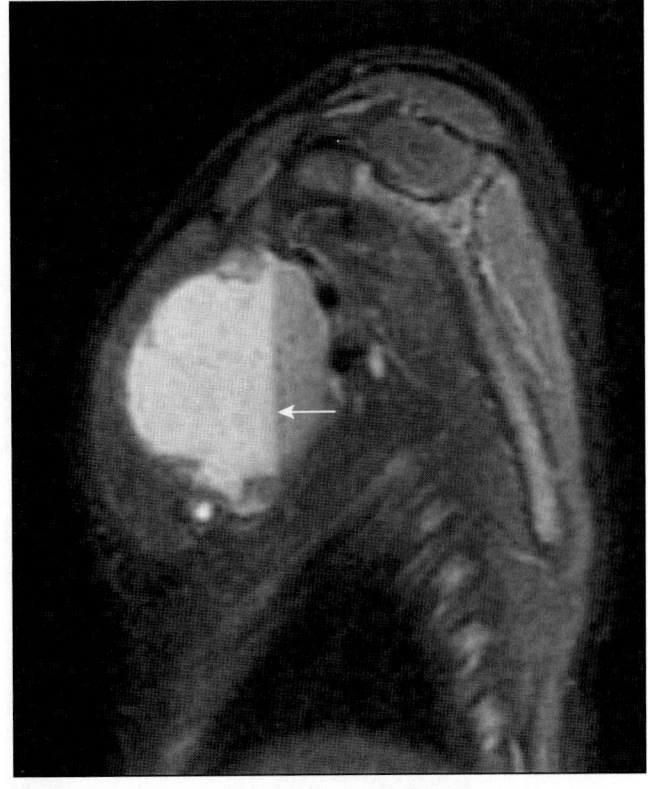

B

FIGURE 161-12. Macrocystic lymphatic malformation presented as a sudden mass with subtle blue skin discoloration in an 11-month-old infant. **A,** Transverse sonogram with color Doppler shows an ovoid hypoechoic axillary mass with increased through-transmission and peripheral flow, consistent with a lymphatic malformation with hemorrhage. Sudden development of a large mass due to internal hemorrhage of an otherwise occult lymphatic malformation is a common presentation. **B,** Sagittal magnetic resonance imaging short tau inversion recovery sequence through the right axillary mass a few days later reveals a fluid-fluid level *(arrow)* in the mass, consistent with hemorrhage.

CAPILLARY MALFORMATION

DESCRIPTION. Capillary malformations (CMs) are common birthmarks that are usually diagnosed clinically. CM may appear as a small localized lesion, or it can be extensive and may be associated with limb hypertrophy. CM may contribute to an underlying structural abnormality, such as encephalocele or spinal dysraphism, or it may be part of a syndrome such as Sturge-Weber or Klippel-Trénaunay syndrome, for which imaging studies may be required. MRI is the imaging modality of choice for these abnormalities. In Sturge-Weber syndrome, MRIs show pial vascular enhancement, enlargement and enhancement of the ipsilateral choroid plexus, and prominent cerebral sulci, suggesting regional atrophy. Gyriform calcification over the affected brain may be seen in advanced cases.

> Capillary malformations may contribute to an underlying structural abnormality such as encephalocele or spinal dysraphism, or it may be part of a syndrome for which imaging studies may be required.

IMAGING. Capillary malformations are often imperceptible on MRI, or they may result in dermal thickening. Lesions are imaged during evaluation of associated underlying abnormalities in syndromes such as Sturge-Weber, Klippel-Trénaunay, or Parkes Weber, and with some AVMs. The imaging modality of choice is MRI.

Fast-Flow

ARTERIOVENOUS MALFORMATION (AVM)

DESCRIPTION. A vascular malformation composed of channels that bypass the capillary bed with connections between feeding arteries and draining veins is termed an *arteriovenous malformation.* AVMs are high-flow lesions that can result in tissue overgrowth and limb hypertrophy. In contrast to a hemangioma, which also has high flow, an AVM exhibits no endothelial cell proliferation.

> In contrast to a hemangioma, which also has high flow, an AVM exhibits no endothelial cell proliferation.

AVMs are staged clinically as follows: stage I—pink-bluish stain and warmth; stage II—pulsations, thrill, and bruit; stage III—dystrophic skin changes, ulceration, bleeding, and pain; and stage IV—high-output cardiac failure. Staging is used to guide the timing of interventions; some clinicians wait until stage III before they treat the patient with AVM.

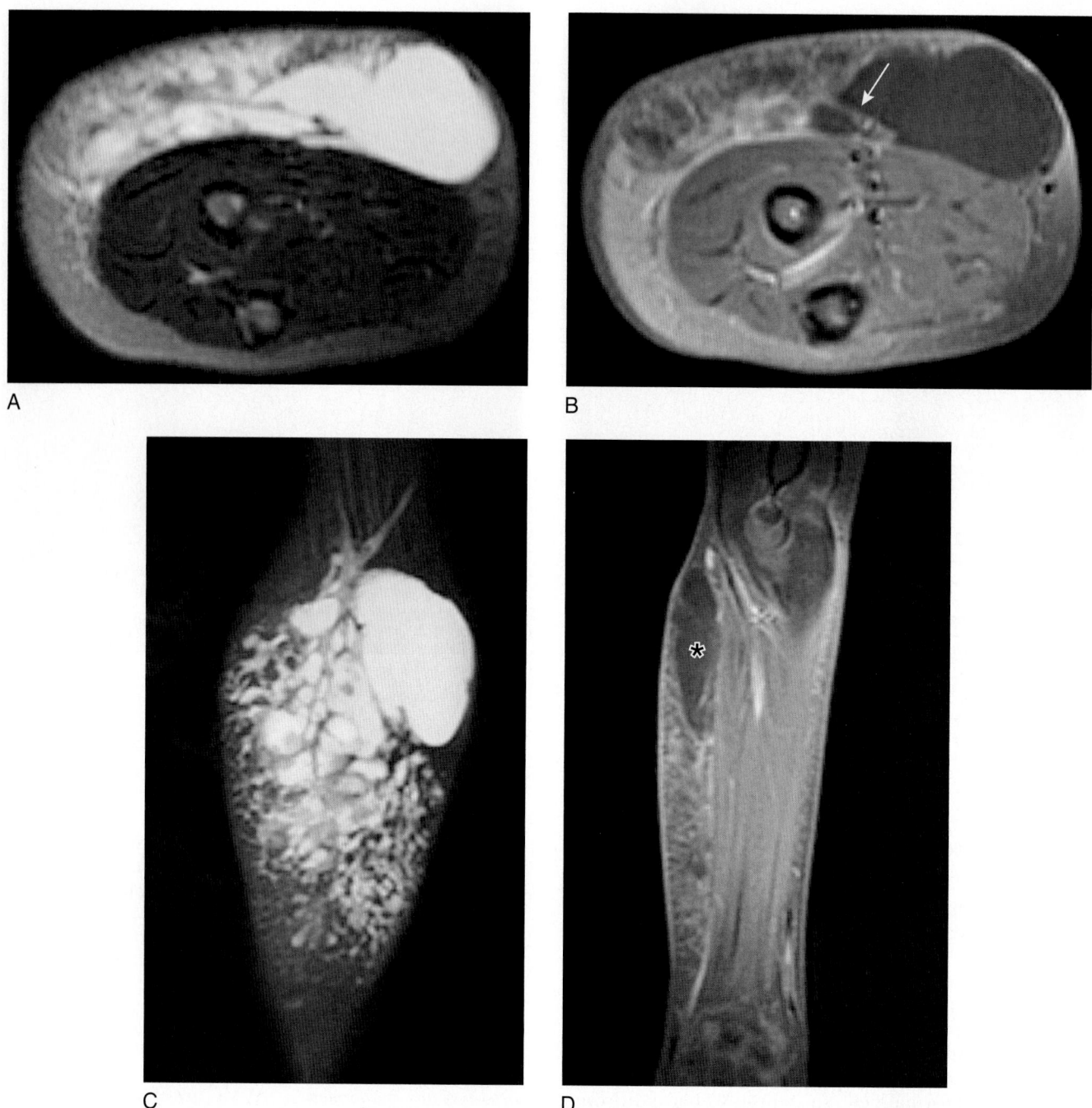

FIGURE 161-13. Multiloculated forearm lymphatic malformation with classic imaging characteristics. **A,** Axial T2-weighted image with fat suppression shows a multiloculated high T2 signal intensity mass in the subcutaneous fat. **B,** Postcontrast T1-weighted image with fat suppression at the same level reveals septal enhancement *(arrow)* around the low signal lymphatic fluid. **C,** Coronal T2-weighted sequence with fat suppression reveals high signal multiloculated cysts of varying sizes. **D,** Sagittal postcontrast T1-weighted sequence with fat suppression shows no internal enhancement *(asterisk).*

AVMs may be localized or diffuse. On physical examination, the affected area may exhibit warmth, a palpable thrill, or pulsations (Fig. 161-14). AVMs can occur anywhere. Large lesions may be complicated by congestive heart failure.

IMAGING. Sonographic evaluation of AVMs shows a heterogeneous lesion with large feeding and draining vessels. Doppler interrogation shows pulsatile tracings with high systolic flow and multiple sites of arteriovenous shunting. MRI can be used to evaluate the extent of the lesion and the extent of associated soft tissue overgrowth (Fig. 161-15; see Fig. 161-14). High-flow enlarged channels are seen as flow-voids on spin echo images, and as vessels of high signal on gradient recalled echo sequences. No surrounding mass is seen, although ill-defined surrounding high T2 signal and enhancement are common. Contrast angiography may be combined with interventional embolization and sclerotherapy.

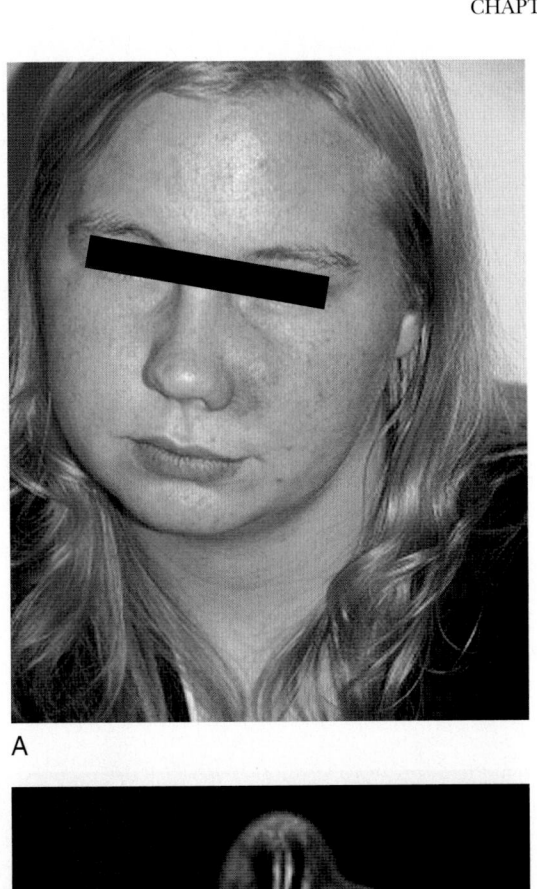

A

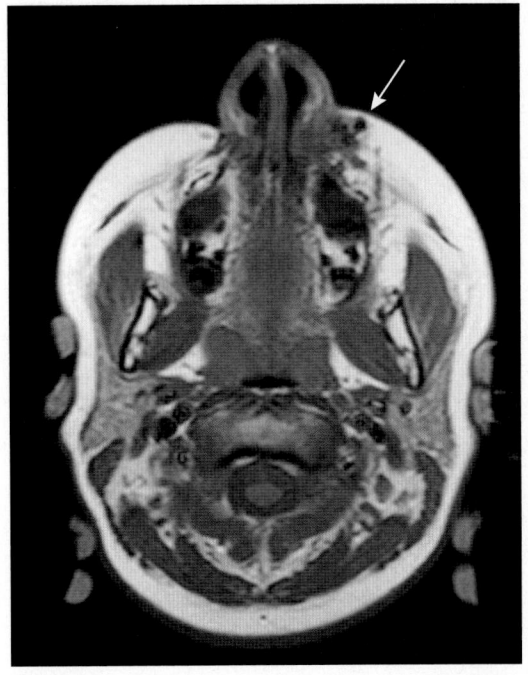

B

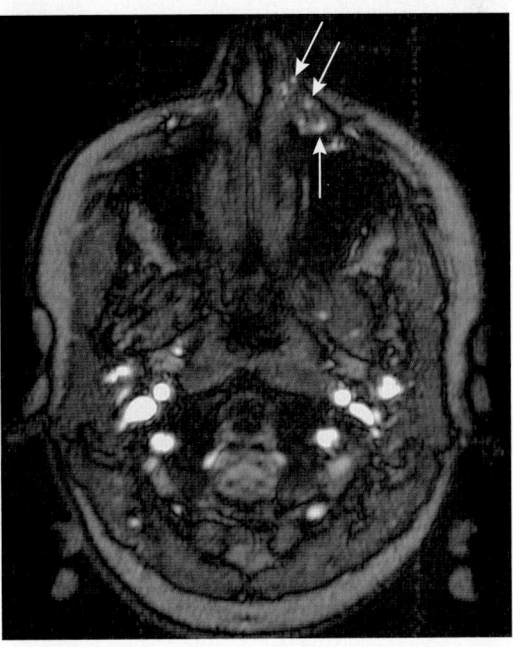

D

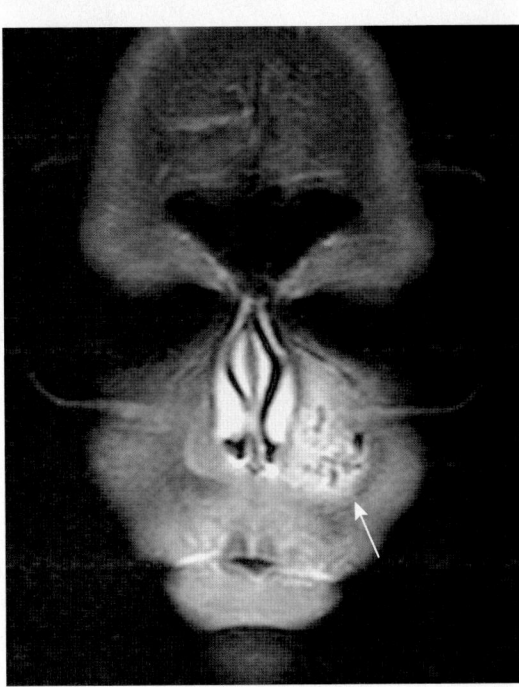

E

FIGURE 161-14. Stage II arteriovenous malformation in the soft tissues near the left nasolabial fold.
A, Photograph shows pink skin discoloration and thickening of soft tissues in the region of the underlying lesion. On physical examination, the skin was warm, and a palpable thrill was noted. (**A,** *see color plate.*) **B,** Axial T1-weighted sequence reveals a small cluster of flow voids surrounded by ill-defined intermediate signal in the subcutaneous fat lateral to the left nostril *(arrow).* **C,** Axial T2-weighted sequence with fat suppression also reveals flow voids. Ill-defined high T2 signal surrounds the flow voids, but no discrete mass is present; this differs from images seen with hemangiomas. **D,** Flow-sensitive sequence (axial two-dimensional time of flight) shows high signal *(arrows)* in the areas of low signal on T2- and T1-weighted sequences *(arrows)*, confirming fast flow. **E,** Coronal postcontrast T1-weighted sequence with fat suppression again shows ill-defined enhancement *(arrow)*.

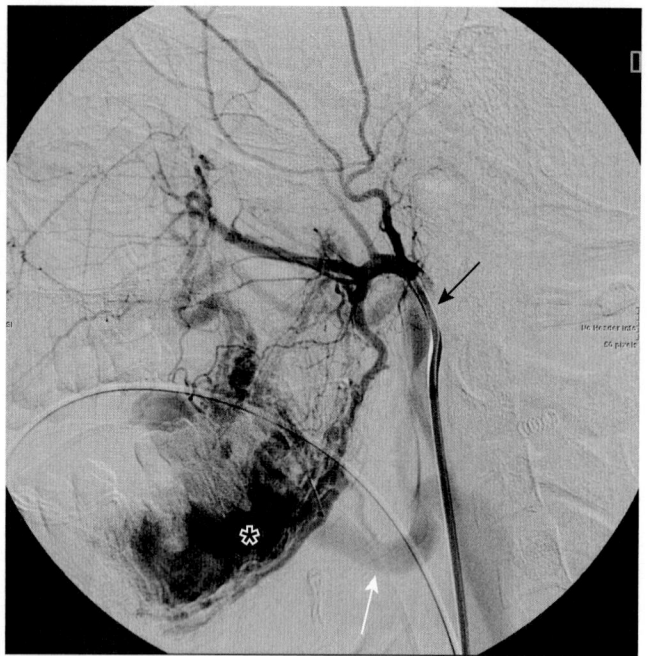

A

FIGURE 161-15. Left mandibular arteriovenous malformation that presented with uncontrolled rapid bleeding after mandibular tooth extraction. **A,** Lateral digital subtraction angiogram with catheter in the external carotid artery *(black arrow)* reveals a classic appearance of an arteriovenous malformation (AVM), including multiple abnormal enlarged feeding arteries, abnormal opacification of the mandibular bone marrow *(asterisk)*, and an early draining vein *(white arrow)*. **B,** Axial postcontrast T1-weighted sequence shows large flow voids around the left hemimandible *(arrow)*. An enhancing soft tissue mass represented by high signal within the mandible is not characteristic for an AVM but may represent granulation tissue related to the extracted tooth. **C,** Axial computed tomography with intravenous contrast reveals the enlarged draining vein *(arrow)* arising from the abnormally enhancing and expanded left hemimandible bone marrow.

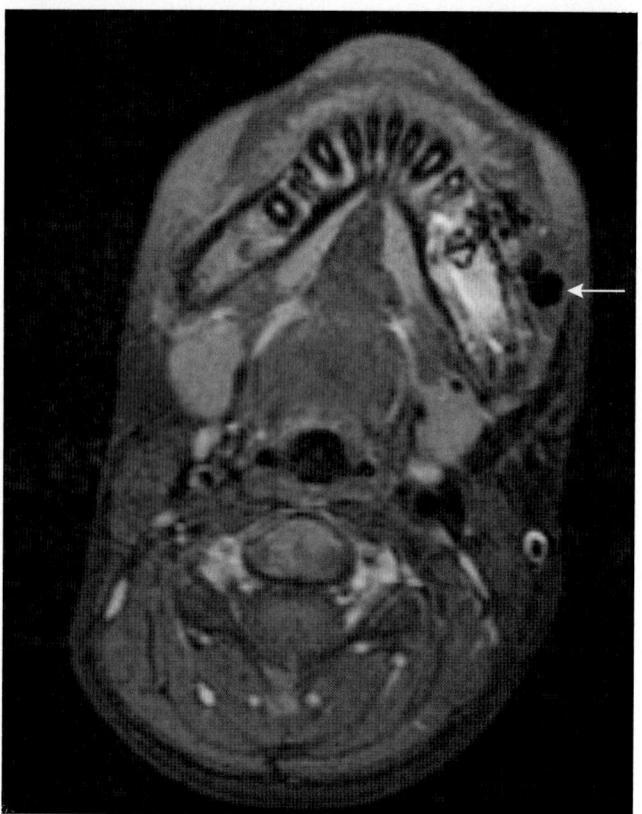

B

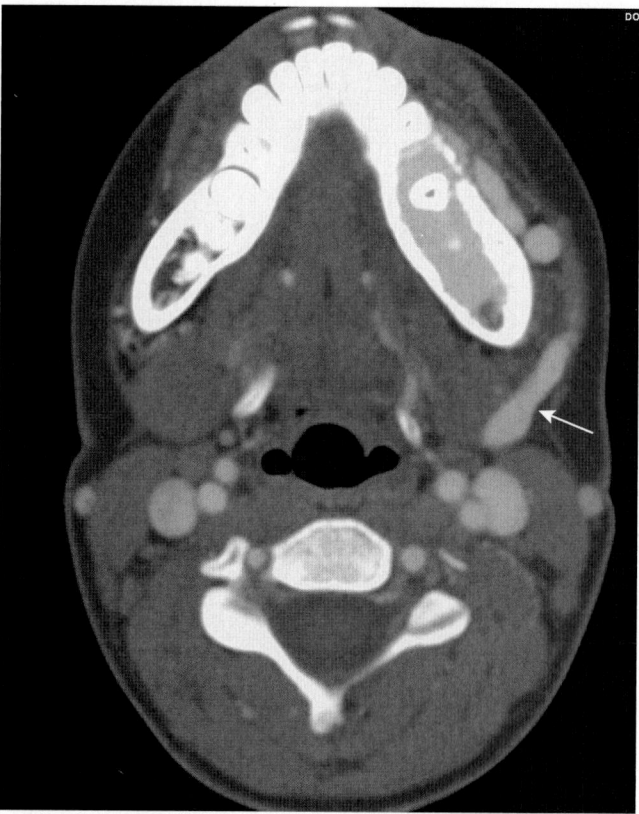

C

> High-flow enlarged channels are seen as flow-voids on spin echo images, and as vessels of high signal on gradient recalled echo sequences.

COMPLEX-COMBINED LESIONS

Klippel-Trénaunay Syndrome

Various eponyms have been assigned to vascular malformations composed of mixed channel types. *Klippel-Trénaunay (KT) syndrome* refers to a capillary-venolymphatic malformation (CVLM) with limb overgrowth. The lower limbs are more frequently involved. This syndrome includes a dermal capillary stain with lymphatic vesicles; varicosities of superficial veins and abnormal, often valveless, channels; deep venous malformations; and variable soft tissue lymphatic malformations. Affected children usually exhibit a leg length discrepancy.

> *Klippel-Trénaunay syndrome* refers to a capillary-venous-lymphatic malformation (CVLM) with overgrowth.

MRI is useful for evaluating the components and extent of the vascular malformation (Figs. 161-16 and 161-17). MR venography is particularly useful for documenting patency of the deep venous system in KT syndrome because frequently, the deep venous system may be hypoplastic or absent. In this case, intervention for abnormal superficial or collateral veins may result in a greater number of varicosities and more frequent edema. Conventional venography performed to opacify deep venous structures is difficult to complete. A

hallmark of diffuse combined vascular malformations is the persistence of embryonic channels, most often the superficial primitive lateral marginal vein of Servelle (Fig. 161-18; see Fig. 161-17). This is readily seen on MR venography. It is speculated that the Klippel-Trénaunay syndrome may be due to a somatic mutation in a factor critical to vasculogenesis and angiogenesis during embryonic development.

> MR venography is particularly useful for documenting patency of the deep venous system in KT syndrome because frequently, the deep venous system may be hypoplastic or absent.

Parkes Weber Syndrome

Parkes Weber syndrome is similar to Klippel-Trénaunay syndrome in that it is a combined vascular malformation with associated limb gigantism (Fig. 161-19). However, the vascular anomaly includes multiple small AVMs or shunts within a capillary arteriovenous lesion (Fig. 161-20). Lymphatic malformations occasionally may be present.

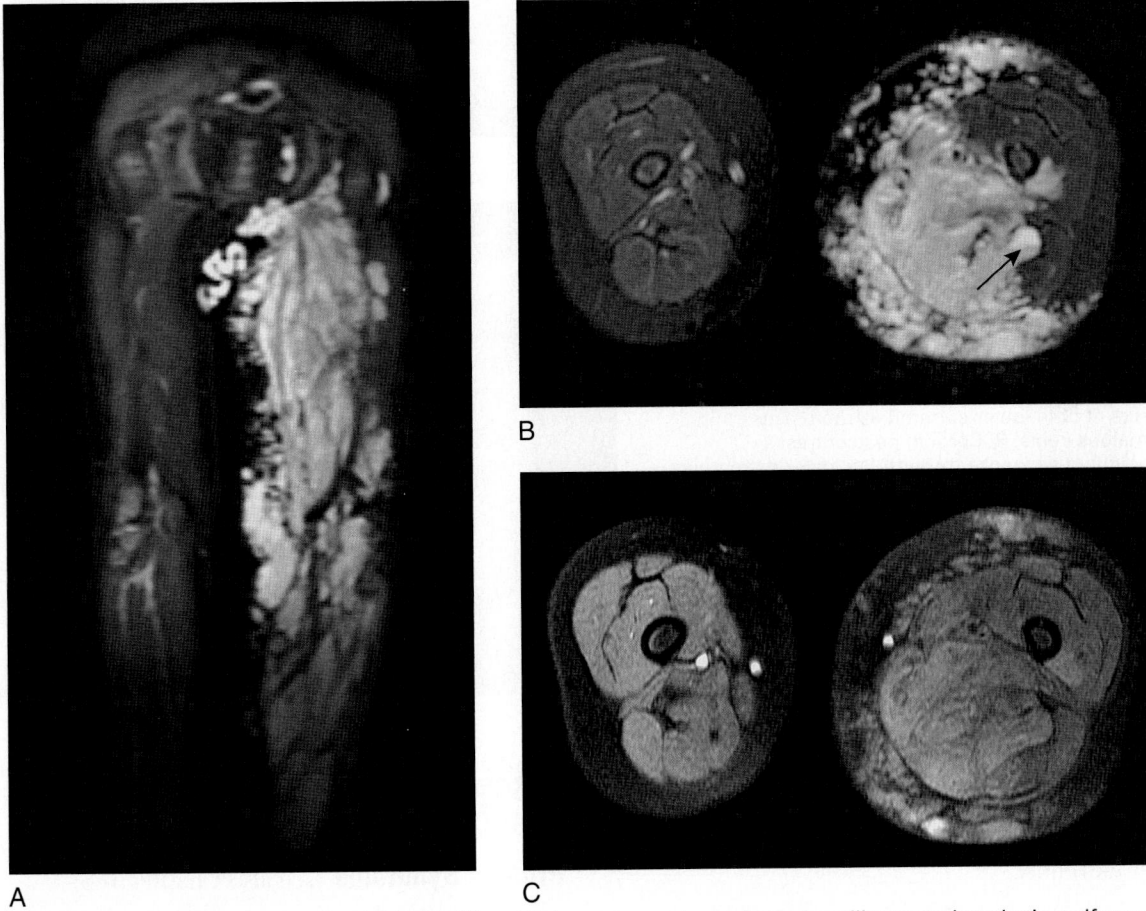

FIGURE 161-16. Left lower extremity of a child with Klippel-Trénaunay syndrome (mixed capillary venolymphatic malformation with overgrowth). **A,** Coronal fast spin echo inversion recovery (FSEIR) through the lower extremities reveals extensive abnormal infiltrative high signal throughout the enlarged left leg, which may represent venous or lymphatic malformations. **B,** Axial T2 with fat suppression shows abnormal high signal in subcutaneous fat and muscle, along with fluid-fluid levels *(arrow).* Fluid-fluid levels may be located in lymphatic malformations or venous malformations with large channels and stagnant flow. **C,** Axial postcontrast T1-weighted sequence with fat suppression shows enhancement of abnormal subcutaneous veins and abnormal high signal in portions of the thigh muscles. Some high signal may result from contrast enhancement; other high signal was present on precontrast fat-suppressed images, representing lymphatic fluid.

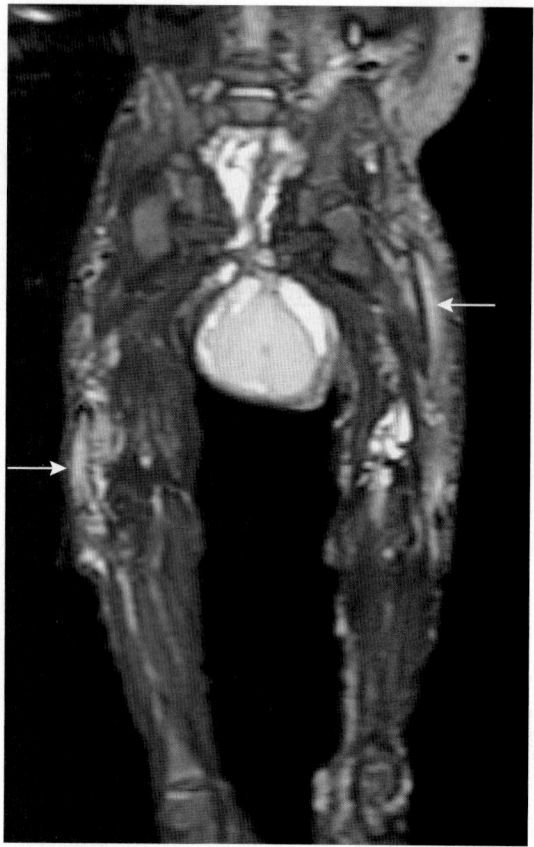

A

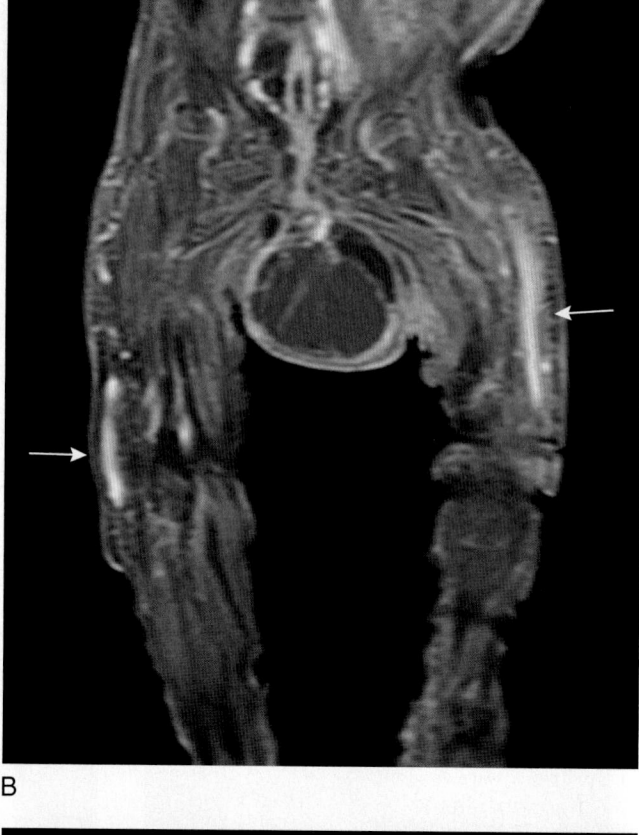

B

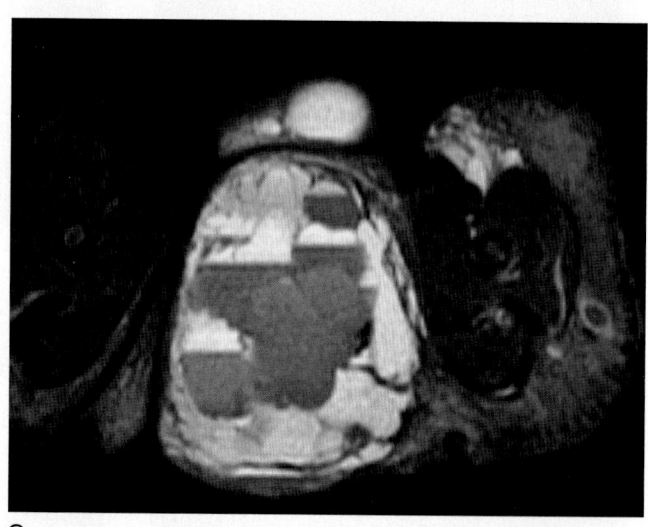

C

FIGURE 161-17. Patient with extensive bilateral lower extremity lesions associated with Klippel-Trénaunay (KT) syndrome. **A,** Coronal short tau inversion recovery (STIR) of the lower extremities shows a large mass between the legs (posterior to the scrotum) that has a mixture of high signal and intermediate signal and represents a lymphatic malformation with internal hemorrhage. Abnormal serpentine high signal *(arrows)* along the lateral aspects of both lower extremities represents anomalous veins. **B,** Coronal postcontrast T1-weighted sequence through the lower extremities reveals enhancement of the bilateral lateral marginal veins of Servelle, commonly seen with KT and sometimes associated with absence of the deep venous system. The lymphatic malformation arising from the perineum shows no internal enhancement. **C,** Axial T2-weighted sequence with fat suppression through the perineal mass reveals multiple septations with some locules containing fluid-fluid levels, consistent with blood products from hemorrhage.

Diffuse arteriovenous shunting can result in ischemic skin lesions and congestive heart failure, particularly in neonates. The lower limb is involved more often than the upper extremity.

> Parkes Weber syndrome is a combined vascular malformation that consists of capillary malformation, multiple small AVMs, and limb overgrowth.

VASCULAR ANOMALIES WITH SYNDROMIC ASSOCIATIONS

Proteus Syndrome (see also Chapter 166)

Cohen and Hayden in 1979 first described a disorder characterized by tissue overgrowth, connective tissue nevi, epidermal nevi, and hyperostosis in two patients. It was termed *Proteus syndrome* by Wiedemann and coworkers in 1983. This name refers to the variability of clinical expression seen in this congenital hamartomatous syndrome, which consists of partial gigantism of the

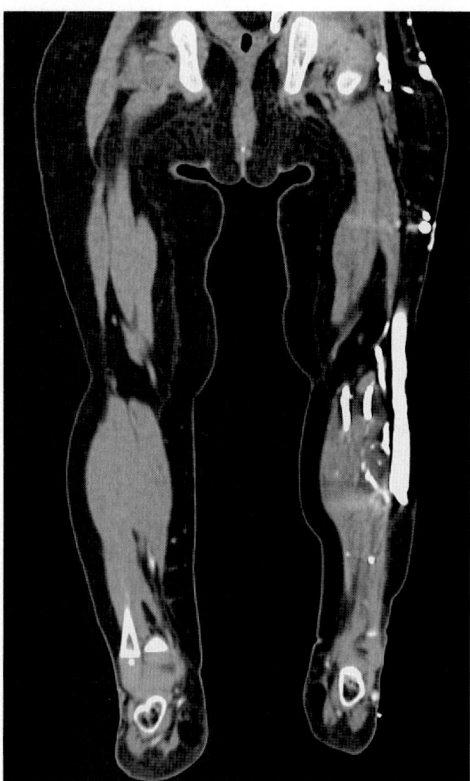

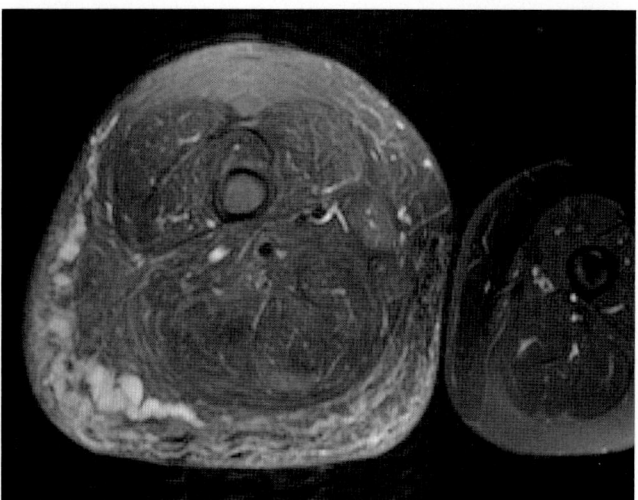

FIGURE 161-19. Child with Parkes Weber syndrome (capillary arteriovenous malformation with overgrowth) of the right lower extremity. Axial T2-weighted sequence through the thighs reveals a marked abnormally increased size of the right thigh caused by overgrowth of muscles and fat. Numerous abnormally enlarged arteries and veins in the subcutaneous fat are caused by innumerable small arteriovenous fistulas.

FIGURE 161-18. Computed tomography of the lateral marginal vein of Servelle in a child with Klippel-Trénaunay syndrome. Coronal reconstruction reveals the large left lower extremity lateral marginal vein of Servelle. The child's deep venous system within the thigh was partially absent.

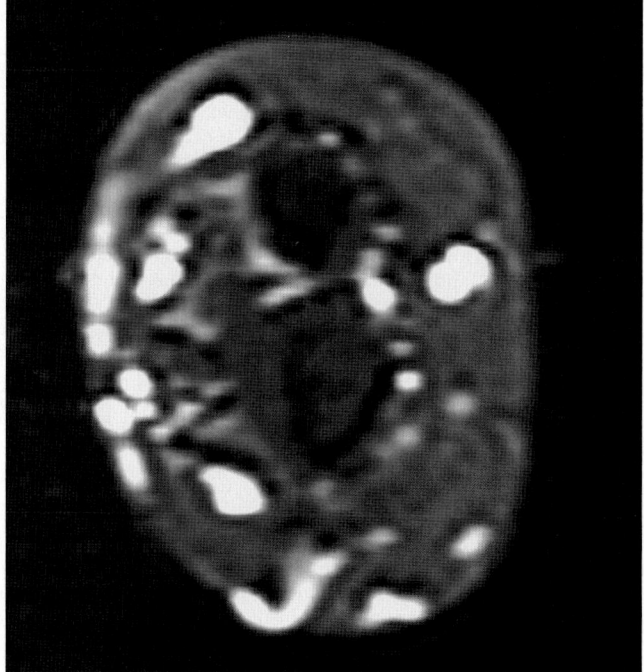

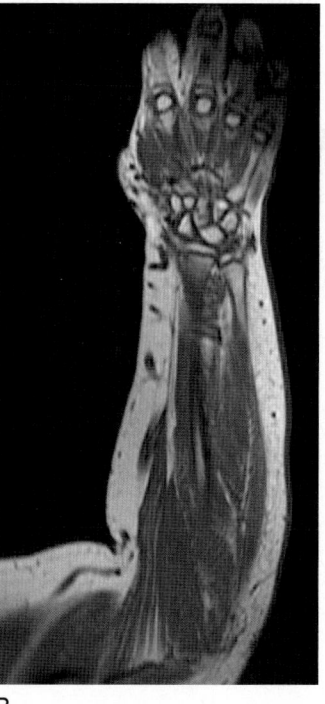

A   B

FIGURE 161-20. Child with Parkes Weber syndrome of the left upper extremity. **A,** Axial spoiled gradient recalled echo (SPGR) image through the forearm shows innumerable fast-flow vessels (high signal) in the subcutaneous tissues and muscle. **B,** Coronal T1-weighted image of the left forearm shows innumerable soft tissue flow-voids in the subcutaneous fat, which correspond to fast flow caused by multiple tiny arteriovenous fistulas.

hands and feet, pigmented nevi, hemihypertrophy, subcutaneous hamartomatous tumors, macrocephaly, and bony exostoses. The syndrome, named after the Greek god Proteus (the polymorphous), has since been expanded to include many other anomalies. A mosaic distribution of lesions, progressive course of the disorder, and infrequent occurrence are mandatory for diagnosis.

Proteus syndrome has been reported as a sporadic occurrence, whereas other hamartomatous disorders usually display a dominant inheritance pattern. Two essential features that help to reveal the diagnosis include regional gigantism and lymphangiomatous hamartoma or malformation. Other manifestations of Proteus syndrome include macrodactyly, macrocephaly or other skull abnormalities, lipoma, lymphatic and other vascular malformations (often with a diffuse cutaneous purpuric staining), subcutaneous tumors, exostoses, and scoliosis.

Gigantism results from overgrowth of the epidermis, connective tissue, endothelium, fat, and bone. Asymmetric growth of the extremities is almost always noted. Conventional radiography is used to characterize the bony abnormalities, and MRI is helpful for evaluating mesodermal malformations. MRI can be used to delineate the extensive fatty and lymphangiomatous lesions prior to surgical excision. It is particularly useful in the abdomen and pelvis, where the extent of malformation may be underestimated. Vascular abnormalities such as AVMs are frequent and should be recognized prior to resection. To avoid postoperative lymphatic leakage and recurrence, the entire lymphatic malformation must be removed.

Bannayan-Riley-Ruvalcaba Syndrome

Although it is included in the differential diagnosis of Proteus syndrome, Bannayan-Riley-Ruvalcaba syndrome (BRRS) has a different genotypic and phenotypic profile. Inheritance is autosomal dominant, and the disorder is associated with *PTEN* gene mutation on chromosome 10q. Clinical features include freckling/pigmentation of the genitalia, colorectal polyposis, lipoma, capillary malformation, macrocephaly, and thyroiditis. Some patients with *PTEN* mutations do not match the clinical spectrum of BRRS, but they do exhibit overgrowth. These patients also do not match the diagnosis of Proteus syndrome.

Maffucci Syndrome (see also Chapter 176)

Maffucci syndrome is characterized by enchondromas, bone deformities, and venous malformations. Enchondromas may appear anywhere, but they are usually found in the phalanges and the long bones of the hands. Other sites of involvement include foot, tibia, fibula, femur, humerus, ribs, and skull. The incidence of malignant degeneration of enchondroma to chondrosarcoma is relatively high (20% to 40%) in patients with Maffucci syndrome.

Glomovenous Malformation

Glomovenous malformation, also known as *glomangioma*, is an autosomal dominant condition that is characterized by multiple venous malformations in the skin. These low-flow vascular birthmarks are often tender, blue, and nodular. Lesions differ from typical venous malformations in terms of the presence of numerous glomus cells; these immature smooth muscle cells line the ectatic venous channels.

Blue Rubber Bleb Nevus Syndrome

Blue rubber bleb nevus syndrome (BRBNS) is characterized by multiple cutaneous venous malformations associated with internal venous malformations that most commonly affect the bowel. Most cases are sporadic. Bleeding from the gastrointestinal tract usually is slow, chronic, and occult and may result in iron-deficiency anemia. However, intestinal bleeding may be massive and severe.

SUGGESTED READINGS

General

Adams DM, Lucky AW: Cervicofacial vascular anomalies. I. Hemangiomas and other benign vascular tumors. Semin Pediatr Surg 2006;15:124-132

Bittles MA, Sidhu MK, Sze RW, et al: Multidetector CT angiography of pediatric vascular malformations and hemangiomas: utility of 3-D reformatting in differential diagnosis. Pediatr Radiol 2005; 35:1100-1106

Burrows PE, Laor T, Paltiel H, et al: Diagnostic imaging in the evaluation of vascular birthmarks. Dermatol Clin 1998;16:455-488

Burrows PE, Mulliken JB, Fellows KE, et al: Childhood hemangiomas and vascular malformations: angiographic differentiation. AJR Am J Roentgenol 1983;141:483-488

Chang MW: Updated classification of hemangiomas and other vascular anomalies. Lymphat Res Biol 2003;1:259-265

Cohen MM: Vascular update: morphogenesis, tumors, malformations, and molecular dimensions. Am J Med Genet 2006;140:2013-2038

Donnelly LF, Adams DM, Bisset GS 3rd: Vascular malformations and hemangiomas: a practical approach in a multidisciplinary clinic. AJR Am J Roentgenol 2000;174:597-608

Dubois J, Garel L: Imaging and therapeutic approach of hemangiomas and vascular malformations in the pediatric age group. Pediatr Radiol 1999;29:879-893

Dubois J, Garel L, Grignon A, et al: Imaging of hemangiomas and vascular malformations in children. Acad Radiol 1998;5:390-400

Enjolras O, Ciabrini D, Mazoyer E, et al: Extensive pure venous malformations in the upper or lower limb: a review of 27 cases. J Am Acad Dermatol 1997;36:219-225

Fordham LA, Chung CJ, Donnelly LF: Imaging of congenital vascular and lymphatic anomalies of the head and neck. Neuroimaging Clin N Am 2000;10:117-136

Garzon MC, Enjolras O, Frieden IJ: Vascular tumors and vascular malformations: evidence for an association. J Am Acad Dermatol 2000;42:275-279

Hand JL, Frieden IJ: Vascular birthmarks of infancy: resolving nosologic confusion. Am J Med Genet 2002;108:257-264

Herborn CU, Goyen M, Lauenstein TC, et al: Comprehensive time-resolved MRI of peripheral vascular malformations. AJR Am J Roentgenol 2003;181:729-735

Hyodoh H, Hori M, Akiba H, et al: Peripheral vascular malformations: imaging, treatment approaches, and therapeutic issues. Radiographics 2005;25(Suppl 1):S159-S171

Jackson IT, Carreno R, Potparic Z, et al: Hemangiomas, vascular malformations, and lymphovenous malformations: classification and methods of treatment. Plast Reconstr Surg 1993; 91:1216-1230

Kesava PP, Turski PA: MR angiography of vascular malformations. Neuroimaging Clin N Am 1998;8:349-370

Konez O, Burrows PE: Magnetic resonance of vascular anomalies. Magn Reson Imaging Clin N Am 2002;10:363-388

Konez O, Burrows PE: An appropriate diagnostic workup for suspected vascular birthmarks. Cleve Clin J Med 2004;71:505-510

Laor T, Burrows PE: Congenital anomalies and vascular birthmarks of the lower extremities. Magn Reson Imaging Clin N Am 1998; 6:497-519

Laor T, Burrows PE, Hoffer FA: Magnetic resonance venography of congenital vascular malformations of the extremities. Pediatr Radiol 1996;26:371-380

Marler JJ, Fishman SJ, Upton J, et al: Prenatal diagnosis of vascular anomalies. J Pediatr Surg 2002;37:318-326

Marler JJ, Mulliken JB: Current management of hemangiomas and vascular malformations. Clin Plast Surg 2005;32:99-116

Mason KP, Neufeld EJ, Karian VE, et al: Coagulation abnormalities in pediatric and adult patients after sclerotherapy or embolization of vascular anomalies. AJR Am J Roentgenol 2001;177:1359-1363

Metry DW, Hebert AA: Benign cutaneous vascular tumors of infancy: when to worry, what to do. Arch Dermatol 2000;136:905-914

Meyer JS, Hoffer FA, Barnes PD, et al: Biological classification of soft-tissue vascular anomalies: MR correlation. AJR Am J Roentgenol 1991;157:559-564

Mueller BU, Mulliken JB: The infant with a vascular tumor. Semin Perinatol 1999;23:332-340

Mulliken J, Young A: Vascular Birthmarks: Hemangiomas and Malformations. Philadelphia, WB Saunders, 1988

Mulliken JB, Fishman SJ, Burrows PE: Vascular anomalies. Curr Probl Surg 2000;37:517-584

Mulliken JB, Glowacki J: Hemangiomas and vascular malformations in infants and children: a classification based on endothelial characteristics. Plast Reconstr Surg 1982;69:412-422

Paltiel HJ, Burrows PE, Kozakewich HP, et al: Soft-tissue vascular anomalies: utility of US for diagnosis. Radiology 2000;214:747-754

Rak KM, Yakes WF, Ray RL, et al: MR imaging of symptomatic peripheral vascular malformations. AJR Am J Roentgenol 1992; 159:107-112

Robertson RL, Robson CD, Barnes PD, et al: Head and neck vascular anomalies of childhood. Neuroimaging Clin N Am 1999;9:115-132

Smith MB, Hardin WD Jr, Moynihan PC: Differentiation and treatment of hemangiomas and arteriovenous malformations. J La State Med Soc 1989;141:41-43

Teo EL, Strouse PJ, Hernandez RJ: MR imaging differentiation of soft-tissue hemangiomas from malignant soft-tissue masses. AJR Am J Roentgenol 2000;174:1623-1628

Upton J, Coombs CJ, Mulliken JB, et al: Vascular malformations of the upper limb: a review of 270 patients. J Hand Surg (Am) 1999;24:1019-1035

van Rijswijk CS, van der Linden E, van der Woude HJ, et al: Value of dynamic contrast-enhanced MR imaging in diagnosing and classifying peripheral vascular malformations. AJR Am J Roentgenol 2002;178:1181-1187

Vilanova JC, Barcelo J, Villalon M: MR and MR angiography characterization of soft tissue vascular malformations. Curr Probl Diagn Radiol 2004;33:161-170

Ziyeh S, Schumacher M, Strecker R, et al: Head and neck vascular malformations: time-resolved MR projection angiography. Neuroradiology 2003;45:681-686

Ziyeh S, Strecker R, Berlis A, et al: Dynamic 3D MR angiography of intra- and extracranial vascular malformations at 3T: a technical note. AJNR Am J Neuroradiol 2005;26:630-634

Hemangioma and Related Lesions

Barnes CM, Huang S, Kaipainen A, et al: Evidence by molecular profiling for a placental origin of infantile hemangioma. Proc Natl Acad Sci U S A 2005;102:19097-19102

Berenguer B, Mulliken JB, Enjolras O, et al: Rapidly involuting congenital hemangioma: clinical and histopathologic features. Pediatr Dev Pathol 2003;6:495-510

Boon LM, Enjolras O, Mulliken JB: Congenital hemangioma: evidence of accelerated involution. J Pediatr 1996;128:329-335

Boon LM, Fishman SJ, Lund DP, et al: Congenital fibrosarcoma masquerading as congenital hemangioma: report of two cases. J Pediatr Surg 1995;30:1378-1381

Cohen MM: Hemangiomas: Their uses and abuses. Am J Med Genet A 2007;143:235-240

Christison-Legacy FR, Burrows PE, Alomari A, et al: Hepatic menangiomas: subtype classification and development of a clinical practice algorithm and registry. J Pediatr Surg 2007;42:62-67

del Rosario ML, Saleh A: Preoperative chemotherapy for congenital hemangiopericytoma and a review of the literature. J Pediatr Hematol Oncol 1997;19:247-250

Drut RM, Drut R: Extracutaneous infantile haemangioma is also Glut1 positive. J Clin Pathol 2004;57:1197-1200

Enjolras O, Mulliken JB, Boon LM, et al: Noninvoluting congenital hemangioma: a rare cutaneous vascular anomaly. Plast Reconstr Surg 2001;107:1647-1654

Enjolras O, Wassef M, Mazoyer E, et al: Infants with Kasabach-Merritt syndrome do not have "true" hemangiomas. J Pediatr 1997; 130:631-640

Frieden IJ, Reese V, Cohen D: PHACE syndrome: the association of posterior fossa brain malformations, hemangiomas, arterial anomalies, coarctation of the aorta and cardiac defects, and eye abnormalities. Arch Dermatol 1996;132:307-311

Gampper TJ, Morgan RF: Vascular anomalies: hemangiomas. Plast Reconstr Surg 2002;110:572-585

Goldberg NS, Hebert AA, Esterly NB: Sacral hemangiomas and multiple congenital abnormalities. Arch Dermatol 1986;122:684-687

Gorincour G, Kokta V, Rypens F, et al: Imaging characteristics of two subtypes of congenital hemangiomas: rapidly involuting congenital hemangiomas and non-involuting congenital hemangiomas. Pediatr Radiol 2005;35:1178-1185

Greene AK, Rogers GF, Mulliken JB: Management of parotid hemangioma in 100 children. Plast Reconstr Surg 2004;113:53-60

Gruman A, Liang MG, Mulliken JB, et al: Kaposiform hemangioendothelioma without Kasabach-Merritt phenomenon. J Am Acad Dermatol 2005;52:616-622

Hayashi N, Masumoto T, Okubo T, et al: Hemangiomas in the face and extremities: MR-guided sclerotherapy—optimization with monitoring of signal intensity changes in vivo. Radiology 2003;226:567-572

Konez O, Burrows PE, Mulliken JB, et al: Angiographic features of rapidly involuting congenital hemangioma (RICH). Pediatr Radiol 2003;33:15-19

Maguiness S, Guenther L: Kasabach-Merritt syndrome. J Cutan Med Surg 2002;6:335-339

Marchuk DA: Pathogenesis of hemangioma. J Clin Invest 2001;107:665-666

Metry DW, Dowd CF, Barkovich AJ, et al: The many faces of PHACE syndrome. J Pediatr 2001;139:117-123

Metry DW, Hawrot A, Altman C, et al: Association of solitary, segmental hemangiomas of the skin with visceral hemangiomatosis. Arch Dermatol 2004;140:591-596

Mulliken JB, Enjolras O: Congenital hemangiomas and infantile hemangioma: missing links. J Am Acad Dermatol 2004;50:875-882

North PE, Waner M, James CA, et al: Congenital nonprogressive hemangioma: a distinct clinicopathologic entity unlike infantile hemangioma. Arch Dermatol 2001;137:1607-1620

North PE, Waner M, Mizeracki A, et al: GLUT1: a newly discovered immunohistochemical marker for juvenile hemangiomas. Hum Pathol 2000;31:11-22

Perkins P, Weiss SW: Spindle cell hemangioendothelioma: an analysis of 78 cases with reassessment of its pathogenesis and biologic behavior. Am J Surg Pathol 1996;20:1196-1204

Rogers M, Lam A, Fischer G: Sonographic findings in a series of rapidly involuting congenital hemangiomas (RICH). Pediatr Dermatol 2002;19:5-11

Sarkar M, Mulliken JB, Kozakewich HP, et al: Thrombocytopenic coagulopathy (Kasabach-Merritt phenomenon) is associated with kaposiform hemangioendothelioma and not with common infantile hemangioma. Plast Reconstr Surg 1997;100:1377-1386

Vilanova JC, Barcelo J, Smirniotopoulos JG, et al: Hemangioma from head to toe: MR imaging with pathologic correlation. Radiographics 2004;24:367-385

Wahrman JE, Honig PJ: Hemangiomas. Pediatr Rev 1994;15:266-271

Wendelin G, Kitzmuller E, Salzer-Muhar U: PHACES: a neurocutaneous syndrome with anomalies of the aorta and supraaortic vessels. Cardiol Young 2004;14:206-209

Venous Malformation

Boll DT, Merkle EM, Lewin JS: Low-flow vascular malformations: MR-guided percutaneous sclerotherapy in qualitative and quantitative assessment of therapy and outcome. Radiology 2004;233:376-384

Boon LM, Mulliken JB, Vikkula M, et al: Assignment of a locus for dominantly inherited venous malformations to chromosome 9p. Hum Mol Genet 1994;3:1583-1587

Burrows PE, Mason KP: Percutaneous treatment of low flow vascular malformations. J Vasc Interv Radiol 2004;15:431-445

Donnelly LF, Bissett GS 3rd, Adams DM: Combined sonographic and fluoroscopic guidance: a modified technique for percutaneous sclerosis of low-flow vascular malformations. AJR Am J Roentgenol 1999;173:655-657

Donnelly LF, Bisset GS 3rd, Adams DM: Marked acute tissue swelling following percutaneous sclerosis of low-flow vascular malformations: a predictor of both prolonged recovery and therapeutic effect. Pediatr Radiol 2000;30:415-419

Dubois J, Soulez G, Oliva VL, et al: Soft-tissue venous malformations in adult patients: imaging and therapeutic issues. Radiographics 2001;21:1519-1531

Goyal M, Causer PA, Armstrong D: Venous vascular malformations in pediatric patients: comparison of results of alcohol sclerotherapy with proposed MR imaging classification. Radiology 2002; 223:639-644

Puig S, Aref H, Chigot V, et al: Classification of venous malformations in children and implications for sclerotherapy. Pediatr Radiol 2003;33:99-103

Lymphatic Malformation

Hayward PG, Orgill DP, Mulliken JB, et al: Congenital fibrosarcoma masquerading as lymphatic malformation: report of two cases. J Pediatr Surg 1995;30:84-88

Konez O, Vyas PK, Goyal M: Disseminated lymphangiomatosis presenting with massive chylothorax. Pediatr Radiol 2000; 30:35-37

Laor T, Hoffer FA, Burrows PE, et al: MR lymphangiography in infants, children, and young adults. AJR Am J Roentgenol 1998;171:1111-1117

North PE, Kahn T, Cordisco MR, et al: Multifocal lymphangioendotheliomatosis with thrombocytopenia: a newly recognized clinicopathological entity. Arch Dermatol 2004; 140:599-606

Arteriovenous Malformation

Hara H, Burrows PE, Flodmark O, et al: Neonatal superficial cerebral arteriovenous malformations. Pediatr Neurosurg 1994;20:126-136

Kohout MP, Hansen M, Pribaz JJ, et al: Arteriovenous malformations of the head and neck: natural history and management. Plast Reconstr Surg 1998;102:643-654

Complex-Combined Lesions

Cha SH, Romeo MA, Neutze JA: Visceral manifestations of Klippel-Trenaunay syndrome. Radiographics 2005;25:1694-1697

Gloviczki P, Stanson AW, Stickler GB, et al: Klippel-Trenaunay syndrome: the risks and benefits of vascular interventions. Surgery 1991;110:469-479

Jacob AG, Driscoll DJ, Shaughnessy WJ, et al: Klippel-Trenaunay syndrome: spectrum and management. Mayo Clin Proc 1998; 73:28-36

Lee A, Driscoll D, Gloviczki P, et al: Evaluation and management of pain in patients with Klippel-Trenaunay syndrome: a review. Pediatrics 2005;115:744-749

Maari C, Frieden IJ: Klippel-Trenaunay syndrome: the importance of "geographic stains" in identifying lymphatic disease and risk of complications. J Am Acad Dermatol 2004;51:391-398

Noel AA, Gloviczki P, Cherry KJ Jr, et al: Surgical treatment of venous malformations in Klippel-Trenaunay syndrome. J Vasc Surg 2000;32:840-847

Samuel M, Spitz L: Klippel-Trenaunay syndrome: clinical features, complications and management in children. Br J Surg 1995; 82:757-761

Ziyeh S, Spreer J, Rossler J, et al: Parkes Weber or Klippel-Trenaunay syndrome? Non-invasive diagnosis with MR projection angiography. Eur Radiol 2004;14:2025-2029

Vascular Anomalies with Syndromic Associations

Brouillard P, Boon LM, Mulliken JB, et al: Mutations in a novel factor, glomulin, are responsible for glomuvenous malformations ("glomangiomas"). Am J Hum Genet 2002;70:866-874

Cohen MM. Proteus syndrome: an update. Am J Med Genet C Semin Med Genet 2005;15:38-52

Cohen MM, Hayden PW: A newly recognized hamartomatous syndrome. Birth Defects Orig Artic Ser 1979;15:291-296

Fernandes C, Silva A, Coelho A, et al: Blue rubber bleb naevus: case report and literature review. Eur J Gastroenterol Hepatol 1999;11:455-457

Gorlin RJ, Cohen MM Jr, Condon LM, et al: Bannayan-Riley-Ruvalcaba syndrome. Am J Med Genet 1992;44:307-314

Jamis-Dow CA, Turner J, Biesecker LG, et al: Radiologic manifestation of Proteus syndrome. Radiographics 2004;24:1051-1068

Waite KA, Eng C: Protean PTEN: form and function. Am J Hum Genet 2002;70:829-844

Wiedemann HR, Burgio GR, Aldenhoff P, et al: The proteus syndrome. Partial gigantism of the hands and/or feet, nevi, hemihypertrophy, subcutaneous tumors, macrocephaly or other skull anomalies and possible accelerated growth and visceral affections. Br J Pediatr 1983;140:5-12

CHAPTER

162

Normal Anatomy, Growth, and Development

PETER J. STROUSE and THEODORE E. KEATS

NORMAL STRUCTURE

The bones provide rigid support for the body and sites of insertion for muscles, to which they respond as levers. They are active physiologically in the infant and child, changing size and shape with growth and in response to mechanical stresses; at all ages, they serve as a reservoir of calcium for body needs.

Three types of bone are found in the limbs: (1) long and short tubular bones, (2) round bones in the wrists and ankles, and (3) sesamoids—small bones in the tendons and articular capsules. Functionally, a growing tubular bone is made up of the following segments: diaphysis, metaphysis, physis, and epiphysis (Fig. 162-1). "Long bones" have epiphyses at both ends. Short tubular bones ("short bones") have epiphyses at one end—generally, where the greater joint motion of the individual bone occurs. In the hands and feet, secondary ossification centers appear in the bases of the phalanges and in the distal ends of metacarpals and metatarsals 2 through 5. Epiphyses for the first metacarpal and first metatarsal are found in the proximal ends of the bones.

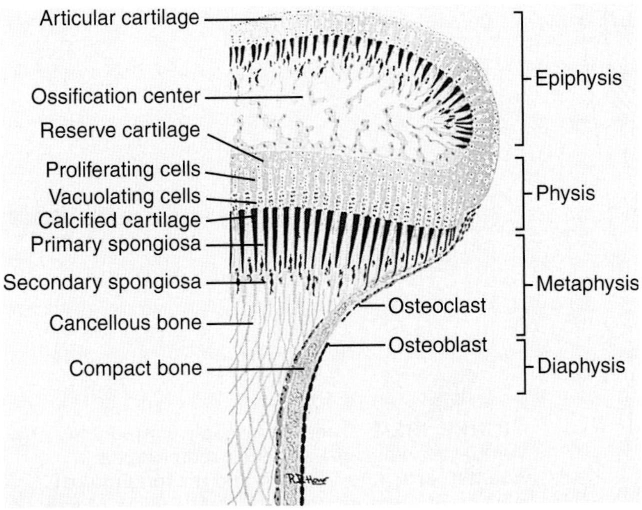

FIGURE 162-1. Functional components of the growing end of a tubular bone and their anatomic substrate.

Labels in figure:
- Articular cartilage
- Ossification center
- Reserve cartilage
- Proliferating cells
- Vacuolating cells
- Calcified cartilage
- Primary spongiosa
- Secondary spongiosa
- Cancellous bone
- Compact bone
- Osteoclast
- Osteoblast
- Epiphysis
- Physis
- Metaphysis
- Diaphysis

The location of the secondary centers appears to be related to the sites of maximal joint motion of individual bones. Apparent epiphyseal ossification centers observed at the ends of short bones, where their occurrence is not expected, are termed *pseudoepiphyses* (see Chapter 163).

> "Long bones" have epiphyses at both ends. "Short bones" have epiphyses at one end.

Bones form through two mechanisms: membranous and endochondral ossification. With membranous ossification, mesenchymal cells directly ossify to bone. Craniofacial bones, clavicle, and mandible form through membranous ossification. Endochondral ossification involves an ordered process of transformation of a cartilage model into bone. Most of the axial and appendicular skeleton is formed by endochondral ossification. Endochondral ossification occurs at the growth plates. Secondary membranous bone formation occurs at the periosteum of growing or remodeling bones. Bone formation and turnover is presented in greater detail in Chapter 167.

The diaphysis (shaft) of a tubular bone consists of a central cavity and a cortical wall. The central cavity (medullary cavity) contains blood-forming marrow during growth. Cancellous bone (spongiosa) encloses the medullary cavity at the epiphyseal ends, and a thin layer of spongy bone lines the inner surface of the cortex. The diaphysis is covered externally by a cellular and fibrous envelope, the periosteum, which is composed of an inner layer of osteoblasts and an outer layer of densely packed collagenous fibers parallel to its long axis. The inner layer deposits subperiosteal bone onto the outer surface of the cortex, increasing the girth of the diaphysis. The periosteum is bound to the cortex by its perpendicular fibers (Sharpey fibers), which are less numerous and shorter in children than in adults and are thus less effective as binding agents in young bone. Resorption of the internal surface of the cortex accounts for expansion of the medullary cavity during growth. The balance between subperiosteal apposition of bone and endosteal resorption is largely responsible for the thickness of the cortex. Except during adolescence, when endosteal apposition contributes to cortical thickness and narrows the medullary cavity, the medullary cavity widens progressively during childhood.

Periosteal new bone forms through membranous ossification. Physiologic periosteal new bone is a normal finding in healthy infants and a manifestation of the normal growing process. It is most prevalent on the diaphyses, femur, humerus, and tibia and, to a lesser degree, the radius and ulna. Physiologic periosteal new bone is most common in infants 1 to 4 months of age.

The epiphyses are terminal remnants of original cartilaginous models of bone. They are bounded by articular cartilage, where a bone articulates with an adjacent bone, and by the physis, which unites the epiphysis to the metaphysis. Longitudinal growth takes place at the junction of the physis and the metaphysis by proliferation of cartilage cells in the physis, calcification of the surrounding matrix, and transformation to bone through the activity of metaphyseal vessels and accompanying osteoblasts and osteoclasts. Ossification centers develop within the epiphyses; growth ceases when these secondary centers fuse, through the physis, with the metaphysis.

Apophyses are outgrowths of a bone that develop where muscle tendons originate or insert. Similar to the epiphyses, the apophyses develop ossification centers that eventually fuse with the main body of the underlying bone. Apophyses are different from epiphyses in that they do not contribute to longitudinal growth.

> **Apophyses do not contribute to longitudinal growth.**

RADIOGRAPHIC APPEARANCE

The macroscopic components of a long tubular bone are shown in Figure 162-2. Calcified portions of growing bone cast opaque shadows of calcium density; noncalcified components cast shadows of lesser density that are comparable with those of other noncalcified tissues apart from fat. The overall density of a bone is provided almost exclusively by cortical bone; medullary spicules (spongiosa) are poorly visible, except in the ends of bones or in disorders characterized by excess trabecular bone. The visibility of trabeculae is increased with osteomalacia, in which thick trabeculae remain faintly visible and thin trabeculae become invisible, as in rickets. Channels in bone for nutrient vessels may present as focal defects in specific areas (see Chapter 163).

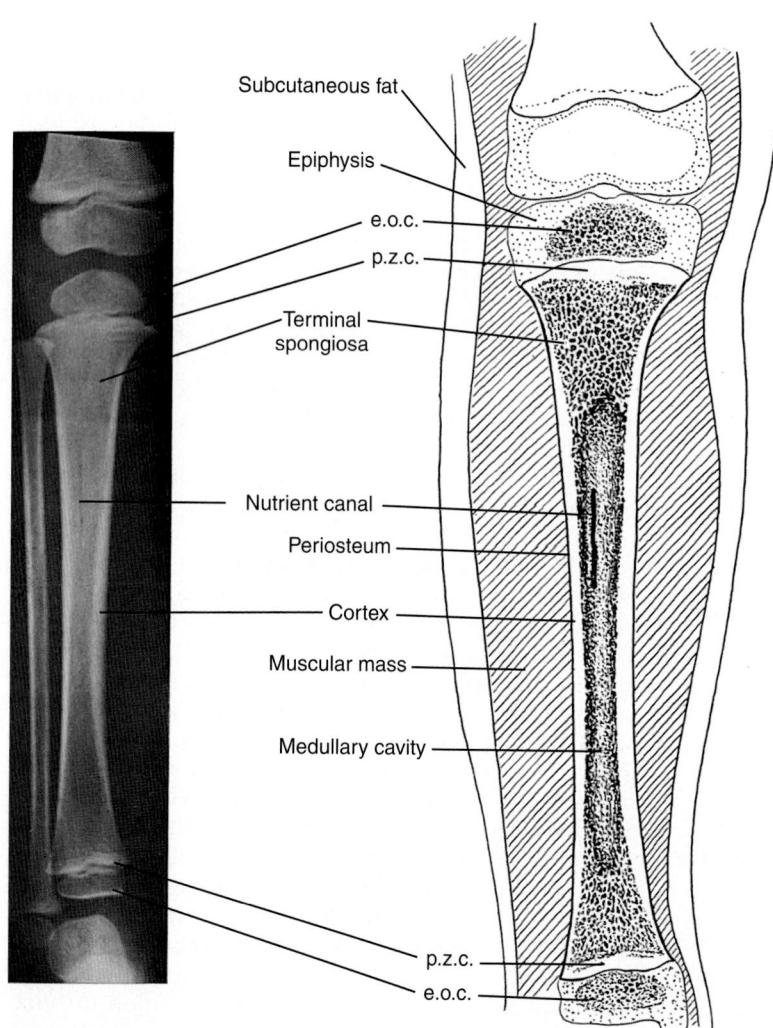

FIGURE 162-2. The macroscopic components of a normal tubular bone and their radiographic counterparts. A radiograph and the longitudinal section of the right tibia of a child 2 years of age. e.o.c., epiphyseal ossification center; p.z.c., zone of provisional calcification and cartilage plate.

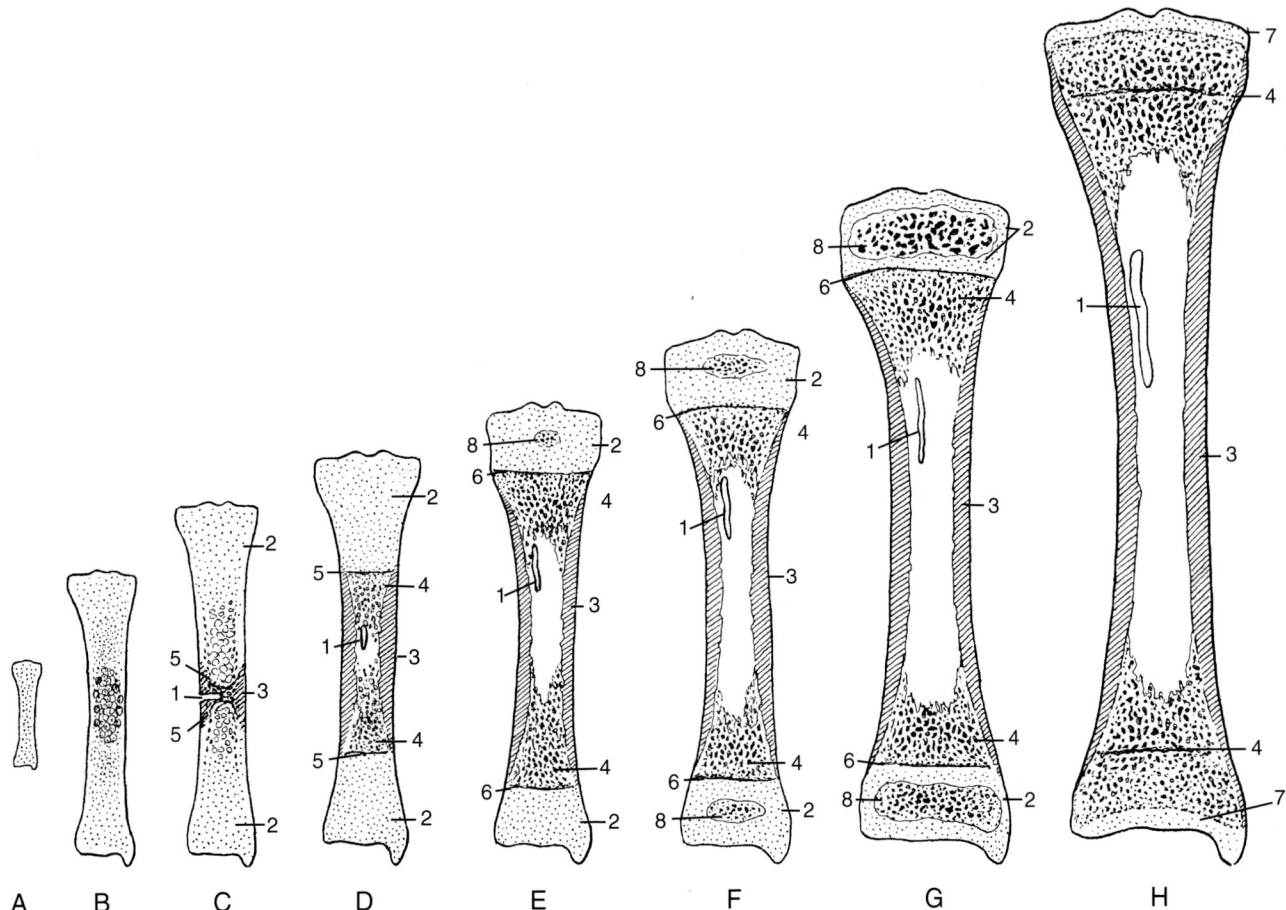

FIGURE 162-3. Schema of progressive stages in the growth and maturation of the tibia. **A,** The mass of embryonal cartilage that is the anlage of the tibia. **B,** Initial enlargement and multiplication of the central cartilage cells and an increase in cartilaginous matrix—the chondrification center that is the forerunner of the primary ossification center. **C,** The early primary ossification center shows the formation of a central belt of subperiosteal bone (early cortex) and penetration of the cartilaginous matrix by the periosteal elements; the channel of this penetration persists as the nutrient canal. **D,** Extension of ossification toward both ends of the shaft, with central resorption forming the medullary cavity. **E,** The tibia at birth, with a secondary ossification center in the proximal epiphyseal cartilage. **F,** At approximately the fourth postnatal month, ossification centers are seen in both of the epiphyseal cartilages. **G,** Juvenile tibia shows the growth of all components and enlargement of the epiphyseal secondary ossification centers. **H,** Adult tibia, with complete fusion of the shaft and both epiphyses. The narrow plates of articular cartilage that cap each end of the bone persist throughout life. 1, nutrient canal; 2, epiphyseal cartilage; 3, corticalis; 4, spongiosa; 5 and 6, provisional zones of calcification or epiphyseal plates; 7, articular cartilages; 8, secondary epiphyseal ossification centers. (Modified from an original drawing by W. M. Rogers, MD.)

GROWTH AND MATURATION

Near the end of the second month of fetal life, the embryonal cartilaginous skeleton is already subdivided into its principal segments, which are the forerunners of bones of the limbs. Primary ossification centers are formed by deposition of calcium in the cartilaginous matrix after hypertrophy and vacuolization of local cartilage cells. In tubular bones, this occurs at approximately the midpoint of the shaft and is followed by central resorption, which gives rise to the primary marrow cavity. Calcified disks proximal and distal to the primary cavity become preparatory zones of calcification after the development of advancing, proliferating shaft during growth. Cartilage proximal and distal to the zones of calcification becomes the epiphyses. A layer of cells within the epiphyses near the shaft produces new cells that are interposed between the resting cartilage of the epiphysis and the older cells and calcified cartilage

adjacent to the shaft. The matrix around the old cells calcifies and is invaded by capillaries and bone cells from the marrow. Bone is formed on the calcified cartilage, and new bone and cartilage undergo remodeling by osteoclasts and osteoblasts, so that the length of the bone is increased (Fig. 162-3). The girth of the bone and the thickness of the cortex are increased by subperiosteal accretion caused by activity of the subperiosteal osteoblasts. Peripheral resorption of bone at the advancing ends of the shaft maintains the gentle flaring that characterizes normal tubular bone, and it is the mechanism responsible for what is termed *modeling*. Disproportionate osteoclastic activity within the shaft of the bone reams out a marrow cavity. Continued, balanced activity of all these processes permits a small tubular bone to become a large tubular bone while functional shape and relations with adjacent structures are maintained.

Secondary ossification centers appear in the cartilaginous epiphyses and apophyses and enlarge by similar

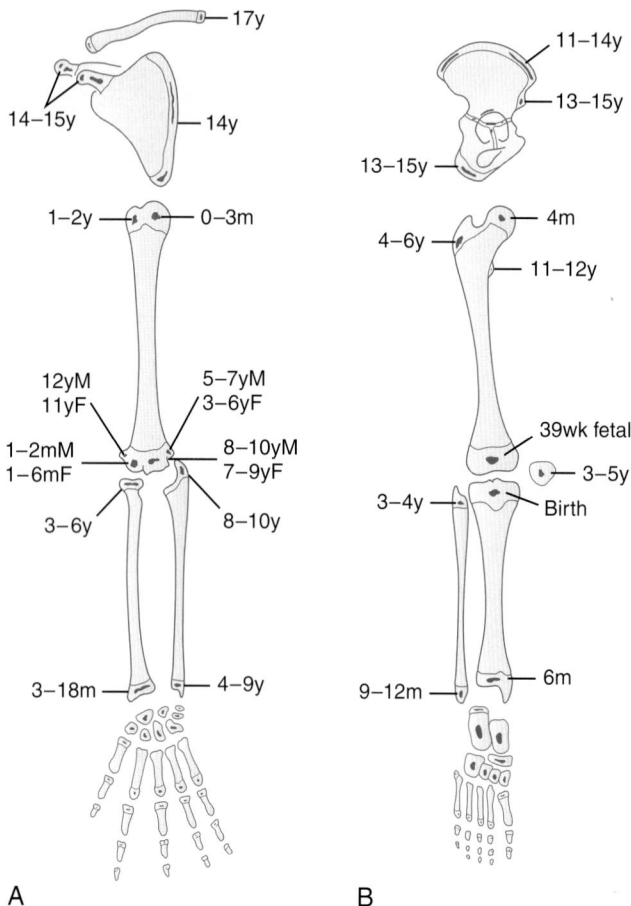

FIGURE 162-4. Ages of onset of secondary (epiphyseal and apophyseal) ossification of the major bones of the upper (**A**) and lower (**B**) extremity. (Reproduced from Ogden JA: Skeletal Injury in the Child, 3rd ed. New York, Springer, 2000:115-146.)

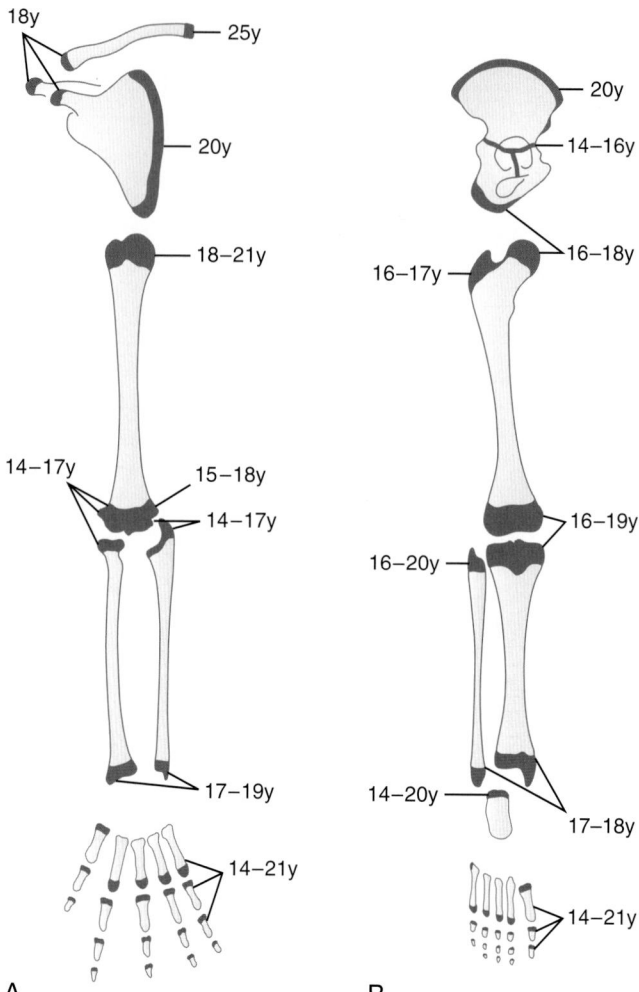

FIGURE 162-5. Ages of physeal closure of the major bones of the upper (**A**) and lower (**B**) extremities. (Reproduced from Ogden JA: Skeletal Injury in the Child, 3rd ed. New York, Springer, 2000:115-146.)

but much slower processes than those that enlarge the shaft. Irregularities in density and discontinuities in the structure of secondary ossification centers are normally frequent during mineralization of these centers and simulate the features of disease. The ages of children at first appearance and upon fusion of these ossification centers are known within limits and serve as indicators of physical maturation (Figs. 162-4 through 162-6; Table 162-1).

During the period of growth, in addition to its constant increase in length and breadth, the shaft is continuously molded or reshaped to its final form. As previously mentioned, the mechanism responsible for these changes in shape has been called *modeling* or *tubulation*. One of the most conspicuous features of modeling is progressive concentric contraction of the shaft behind the wider, advancing terminal segment (Fig. 162-7); this results in flared ends of bones. Significant disturbances in configuration of the shafts occur in many of the diseases that affect the growing skeleton. With overtubulation, a bone is abnormally narrow in caliber. Most often, this is seen in children with cerebral palsy or other neuromuscular disease, in whom normal muscular stresses are not present. With undertubulation, a bone is abnormally broad in caliber. Causes may include Gaucher disease, Pyle dysplasia, and osteochondromatosis.

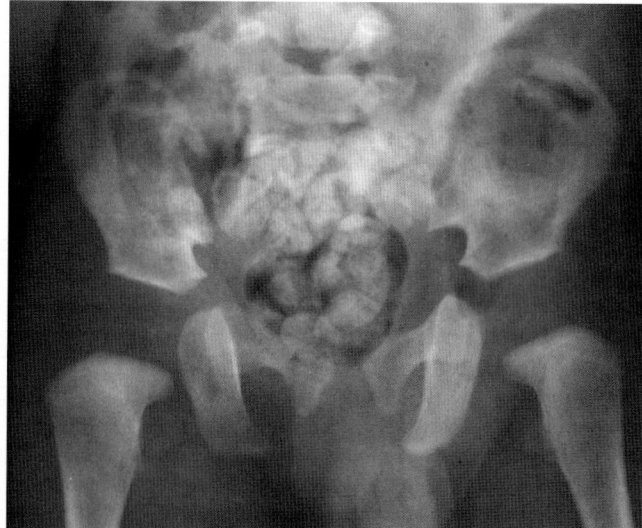

FIGURE 162-6. Hypothyroidism. Although the chronologic age of the patient was 23 months, minimal ossification of the femoral heads is present. Minimal early ossification is seen on the right. Findings indicate substantial delay in maturation.

TABLE 162-1

Epiphyseal Ossification in the Fetus and Neonate—Fifth and Ninety-Fifth Percentiles

Ossification Center	Fifth Percentile	Ninety-Fifth Percentile
Humeral head	37th week	16 post-natal weeks
Distal femur	31st week	39th week (female)
		40th week (male)
Proximal tibia	34th week	2 postnatal weeks (female)
		5 postnatal weeks (male)
Calcaneus	22nd week	25th week
Talus	25th week	31st week
Cuboid	37th week	8 postnatal weeks (female)
		16 postnatal weeks (male)

Data from Kuhns LR, Finnstrom O: New standards of ossification of the newborn. Radiology 1976;119:655-660.

VELOCITY OF GROWTH AND DEVELOPMENT

Ultrasound measurement of the fetal femur during pregnancy is usually reliable for estimation of fetal age; it can be supplemented by the revelation of ossification centers in the fetal calcaneus (24th week), talus (26th week), distal femur (32nd week), and proximal tibia (37th week), as well as by biparietal diameters. If gestational age is known, measurements may identify growth disturbances such as skeletal dysplasia. In such cases, other bones are also short when compared with the norm. Abnormal fetal dimensions or configurations of bone may reveal specific skeletal dysplasias, such as achondroplasia or osteogenesis imperfecta, or malformation syndromes. In the former, bones may be abnormally short, or initially, only mildly short with subsequent inappropriate growth. During infancy and childhood, serial examinations are necessary to ascertain the velocity of growth and development, but evaluation of images of the limbs is adequate for identifying the state of development of skeletal structures, which reflect fairly accurately the general status of the child.

The gestational age of a newborn can be estimated radiographically through several methods. The proximal humeral ossification center ossifies shortly after birth with 5% and 95% confidence intervals of 37 weeks' gestation and 16 weeks' postnatal, respectively. Because ossification before 37 weeks is not the norm, ossification in the proximal humeral ossification center is an indication that a newborn is not premature. Teeth appear at the characteristic time. The first deciduous molars form at 33 weeks, and the second deciduous molars form at 36 weeks. Finally, the height of the thoracic spine can be measured from the top of T1 to the bottom of T12. This measurement increases linearly from 21 to 41 weeks' gestation, and this method is of limited use in small-for-gestational-age infants.

> **Ossification in the proximal humeral ossification center is an indication that a newborn is not premature.**

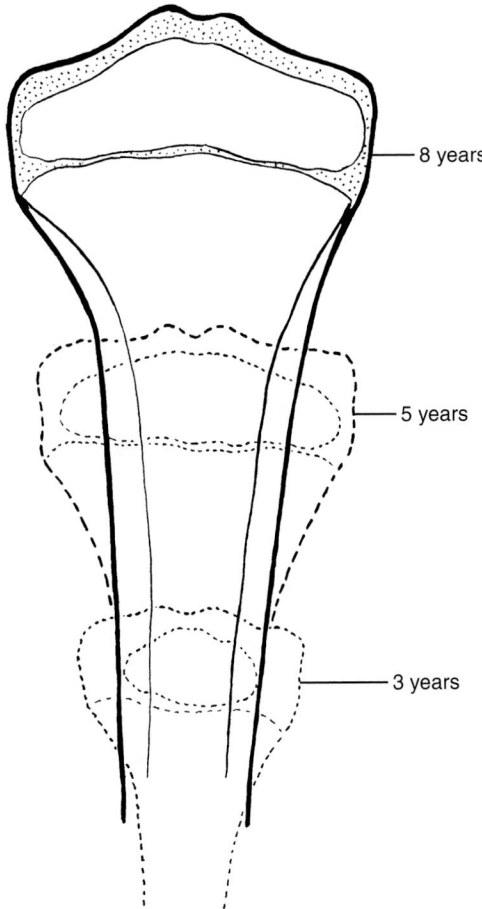

FIGURE 162-7. Growth and configuration of the tibia with advancing age. The progressive concentric constriction of the shaft away from the wider epiphyseal plate is shown schematically on superimposed tracings of radiographs.

Lengths of tubular bones, as seen on images obtained through techniques developed for these purposes, can be evaluated with the use of tables that list age standards. Values are sex dependent, and observations of bone lengths are useful for identification of growth disturbances, for planning of surgery in cases of limb length discrepancy, and in many other circumstances. Moseley converted standards from orthoroentgenograms (scanograms) to a nomogram, on which measurements from serial lower limb scanograms can be plotted. Optimal times for epiphysiodesis to correct a discrepancy are easily determined with the use of his straight-line graph. Bone age rather than chronologic age is used as a reference point for surgical procedures.

Quantities of longitudinal growth derived from the two ends of a tubular bone are unequal. In the arm, the ends of bones at the elbow grow less than their counterparts at the shoulder and wrist; in the leg, the ends of bones at the knee grow more than those at the hip and ankle (Fig. 162-8). It is not known whether rates of growth at specific sites maintain constant relations throughout childhood.

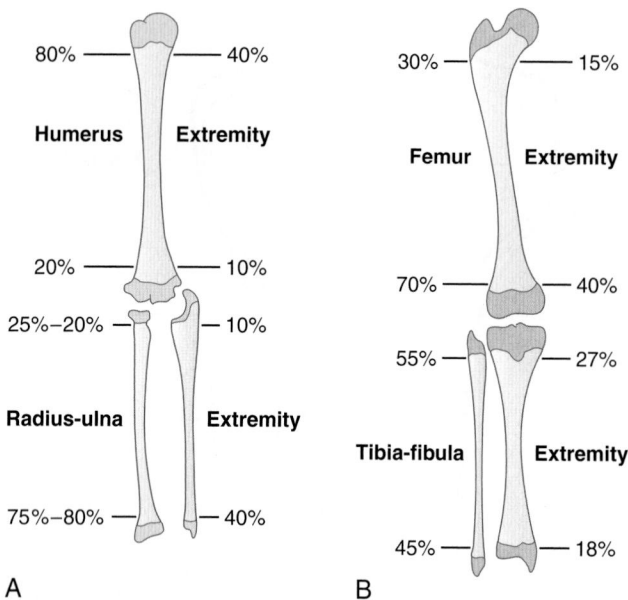

FIGURE 162-8. Relative contributions of individual growth regions to the overall length of an individual bone and the composite extremity in the arm (**A**) and leg (**B**). (Reproduced from Ogden JA: Skeletal Injury in the Child, 3rd ed. New York, Springer, 2000:115-146.)

> In the arm, the ends of bones at the elbow grow less than their counterparts at the shoulder and wrist; in the leg, the ends of bones at the knee grow more than those at the hip and ankle.

Growth in girth of tubular bones and thickness of flat bones takes place through a process that involves addition and removal of bone at external and internal surfaces, respectively. Garn and associates provided considerable data with respect to cortical bone thickness and medullary width of the second metacarpal bone as an indication of bone gain and loss in the remainder of the skeleton. Although such techniques are adequate for clinical use, much more exact information on bone density is provided today through dual-energy x-ray absorptiometry and quantitative computed tomography methods (see Chapter 169).

Measurement of metacarpal and phalangeal lengths (metacarpophalangeal pattern profile analysis), as described by Poznanski and coworkers, may be useful in the diagnosis of dysmorphic syndromes. The shape of the curve thus formed tends to be consistent in some disorders and may be diagnostic in cases equivocal on the basis of other criteria.

Evaluation of the number, size, and configuration of secondary ossification centers (bone age) is used to estimate biologic maturation relative to chronologic age. Various techniques and standards are available, and these are generally in agreement, but the procedure to be followed for each must be adhered to carefully at each examination, especially in sequential examinations. The range of values is great, even in premature infants (see Table 162-1).

The possibility of evaluating maturity through radiographic techniques was explored in the first years after the discovery of x-rays, by Lambertz and by other investigators in Europe and America. Subsequently, longitudinal growth studies were mounted in the United States and elsewhere. With increased realization in the mid-1950s that medically unnecessary radiation should be avoided, serial radiographic examinations of study populations were discontinued, and later studies of skeletal maturation used cross-sectional methods. Thus, current standards for sequential skeletal maturation in individual children are based on examinations dating from 1931 to 1942; the oldest studies were performed longer than 75 years ago. Differences in familial, racial, and socioeconomic factors limit the applicability of the standards of Greulich and Pyle to today's children. Many studies have confirmed differences from standards in children of specific ethnic groups. It is now well accepted that maturation varies between races. For instance, African American children mature faster than Caucasian children do. Overall, children of the 2000s mature more quickly than children of the 1940s.

> Differences in familial, racial, and socioeconomic factors limit the applicability of the standards of Greulich and Pyle to today's children.

Applicability of the standards of Greulich and Pyle is therefore limited; however, use of these standards is well established and is still reasonably accurate, particularly when used longitudinally to follow the growth and maturation of an individual patient. Notwithstanding limitations related to sex, race, geographic location, and socioeconomic factors, serial evaluation of bone maturation with the use of appropriate standards and in a consistent fashion can provide helpful information regarding children with medical problems that affect growth and development. None of the standards applies to patients with skeletal dysplasia in whom skeletal development, growth, and maturation deviate from norms.

The hand, with its numerous secondary centers in phalanges and metacarpals, and the wrist, with its tightly packed primary centers, are used most frequently as an index of total skeletal maturation. Genetic variability in the timing of ossification within carpal bones accounts for their elimination from some types of evaluation.

Through the method of Greulich and Pyle, the appearance, size, and differentiation (fusion) of the epiphyses and bones of the hands and wrists are assessed. The overall appearance of the hand and wrist is matched to the closest standard for the patient's sex. Occasionally, a patient will fall between two standards. Because maturation of the carpus is more variable than that of the metacarpals and phalanges, greater weight is placed on the metacarpals and phalanges in assignment of bone age; however, information provided by all bones of the hands and wrists is considered. Assessment of bone age is subjective. Standard deviations, which are based on chronologic age, are somewhat broad. A bone age within

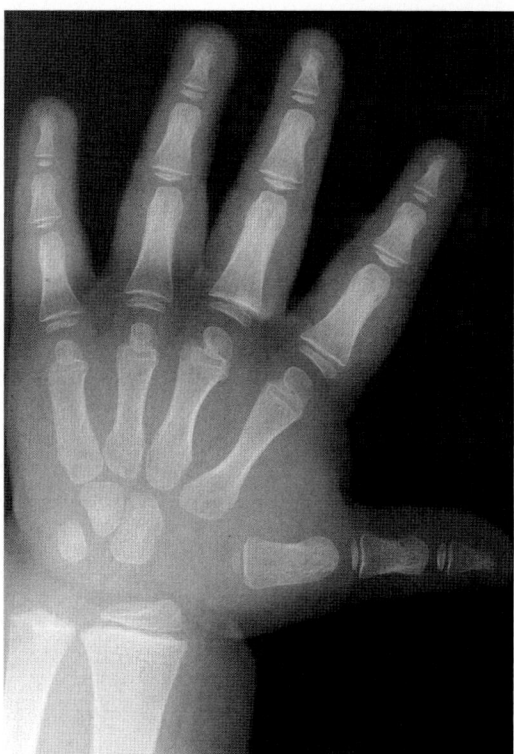

FIGURE 162-9. Hypothyroidism. Bone age of this hand was 3 years, 6 months. The patient's chronologic age was 10 years, 9 months.

the 5% to 95% confidence interval (or ±2 standard deviations) is considered normal (Fig. 162-9).

In children younger than 2 years of age, use of the standards of Greulich and Pyle is limited because relatively little change is noted in the ossification centers of the hand and wrist during this period. More rapid changes, however, may be observed in the knee or foot. Radiographs of the left knee and left foot—anteroposterior (AP) and lateral—are therefore routinely obtained in children younger than 2 years of age and are compared with published standards (for the knee, standards of Pyle and Hoerr [1969]; for the foot and ankle, standards of Hoerr, Pyle, and Francis [1962]).

The Tanner-Whitehouse method is based on a study of British children in the 1950s and 1960s. Each of 20 ossification centers in the hand and wrist is assigned a maturational stage. A fractional multiplier is applied to determine the score for each bone. A score for the radius, ulna, and phalanges is summed (radius, ulna, and short bone [RUS] score). A score for the carpus is summed (seven carpal bones, excluding the pisiform). These two scores are averaged to produce an overall score between 0 and 100. Skeletal age is obtained by plotting overall score on a chart versus skeletal age. Although it is more reproducible, the Tanner-Whitehouse method is cumbersome. Research studies that require greater precision routinely use the Tanner-Whitehouse method rather than the standards of Greulich and Pyle.

The methods of Sontag and Elgenmark assess skeletal age by counting the number of ossification centers found in half of the body (hemiskeleton). This method is most useful in very young children (<2 years old) in whom the number of ossified centers is rapidly changing. The drawback of this method is the greater radiation dose to which the patient is exposed.

The Risser classification can be used to assess skeletal maturation through evaluation of the appearance and state of fusion of the iliac crest. Ossification of the iliac crest begins laterally and proceeds medially: stage 0—no ossification; stage I—0% to 25% ossified; stage II—25% to 50% ossified; stage III—50% to 75% ossified; stage IV—75% to 100% ossified; and stage V—fully ossified and fused. Original data suggest that when the iliac crest was fully fused, vertebral growth was complete. This topic is now debated. Nevertheless, the Risser stage gives a rough assessment of maturation and is used by orthopedists for estimating further progression of scoliosis.

Ultrasonography can be used to assess bone age. One technique involves the transmission of ultrasound waves with the use of separate transmitting and receiving probes. Computerized systems have been designed to assess hand and wrist maturation on radiographs. The goal of these systems is to remove the human element of subjectivity. Computerized systems have tended toward use of the Tanner-Whitehouse scheme rather than the standards of Greulich and Pyle.

Regardless of the method selected, all studies have shown that the skeletons of girls mature faster than those of boys. Therefore, it is important that different standards be used for each sex in assessment of bone age.

> **The skeleton of girls matures faster than that of boys. It is important to use different standards for each sex in assessing bone age.**

With disharmonic maturation, different parts of the skeleton are in different stages of development. For example, disharmonic maturation may be seen in left versus right or carpus versus phalanges, or it may be noted in the advanced or delayed maturation of an individual bone or group of bones. Asymmetric maturation of the hand and wrist may be caused by Silver syndrome, idiopathic hemihypertrophy, hemiparalysis/hemiparalysis, or abnormally increased or decreased vascular supply—hemangioma, arteriovenous malformation, rheumatoid arthritis, or central surgical shunt (Fig. 162-10).

Assessment of skeletal age by radiography is useful in many clinical scenarios. Tables 162-2 and 162-3 list causes of advanced and delayed skeletal maturation, respectively. Children with overall delayed development, advanced or delayed sexual maturation, and abnormal height (both extremes) benefit from assessment of bone age because it provides information that is helpful in diagnosis, counseling, and treatment planning. Menarche typically occurs after fusion of the physes of the distal phalanges. Bone age can be used with long bone measurements to predict ultimate adult height. Assessment of bone age is valuable in the planning of orthopedic treatments, including epiphysiodesis, leg lengthening procedures, and scoliosis management.

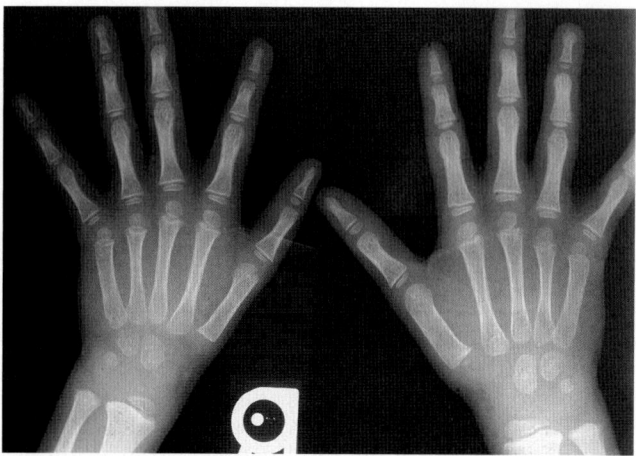

FIGURE 162-10. Disharmonious maturation in a 6-year-old with a right Blalock-Taussig shunt. The left hand is slightly larger than the right. Bones of the left hand are slightly more mature than those of the right (i.e., distal radius, first metacarpal).

TABLE 162-2

Advanced Skeletal Maturation

Acrodysostosis
Adrenogenital syndrome (adrenocortical tumor or hyperplasia)
Cerebral gigantism
Gonadal tumors (androgen or estrogen secreting)
Growth hormone excess (gigantism)
Hyperthyroidism (maternal or acquired)
Hypothalamic tumors
Idiopathic familial advanced bone age
Idiopathic isosexual precocious puberty
Lipodystrophy
Liver tumors (choriocarcinoma, hepatoma)
McCune-Albright syndrome (polyostotic fibrous dysplasia)
Medication with sex hormones
Pinealoma
Premature adrenarche
Premature thelarche
Pseudohypoparathyroidism
Various syndromes

TABLE 162-3

Delayed Skeletal Maturation

Addison disease
Chromosomal disorders (i.e., trisomy 21, trisomy 18)
Chronic illness
Chronic renal disease
Chronic severe anemia (i.e., sickle cell anemia, thalassemia)
Congenital heart disease (especially cyanotic)
Congenital malformation syndromes
Constitutional delay
Cushing syndrome
Growth hormone deficiency
Hypogonadism (i.e., Turner syndrome)
Hypothyroidism
Idiopathic causes
Inflammatory bowel disease
Intrauterine growth retardation
Juvenile diabetes mellitus
Malabsorption syndromes (i.e., celiac disease)
Malnutrition
Neurologic disorders
Panhypopituitarism
Rickets
Skeletal dysplasias (most)
Steroid therapy

GROWTH LINES

Skeletal growth and maturation are affected by a host of factors. Disease and stress inhibit skeletal growth and may slow maturation. Growth lines are a manifestation of varying health and stress. Many names have been applied to these lines. They are probably better called "growth lines" than "growth arrest lines" or "growth recovery lines" because they are a manifestation of arrest and recovery of growth. The names "lines of Park" and "Harris lines" derive from early investigators.

According to Ogden (1984), growth lines form when growth rate is slowed or temporarily halted because of a stressor. Trabeculae thicken and fuse transversely rather than propagating longitudinally. When the stressor is removed, rapid endochondral growth resumes, and a more normal longitudinal orientation of the trabeculae is produced (Fig. 162-11). With growth, lines are displaced

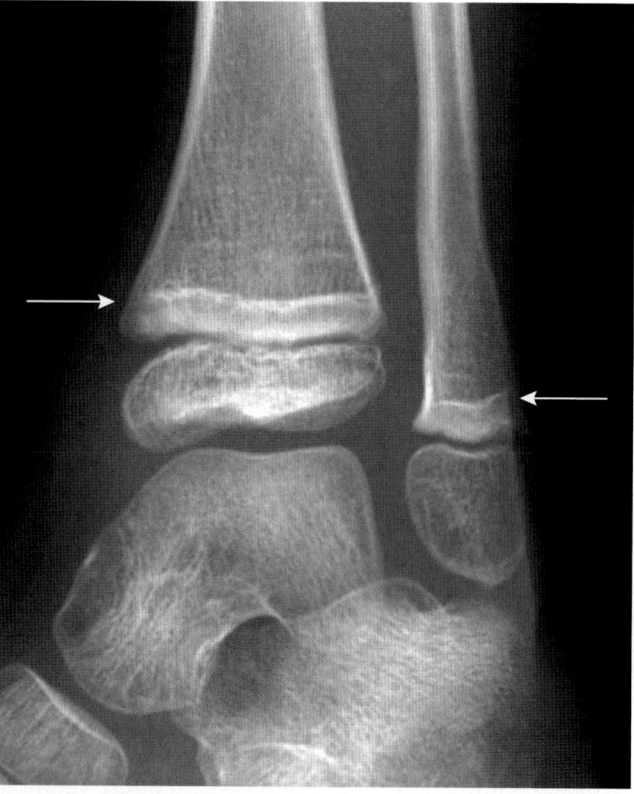

FIGURE 162-11. Growth lines *(arrows)* after healing of distal tibial epiphyseal fracture in a 6-year-old boy. Although the fracture was in the tibia, a prominent growth line is also seen in the fibula. Slight sclerosis in the distal tibial epiphysis is due to fracture healing.

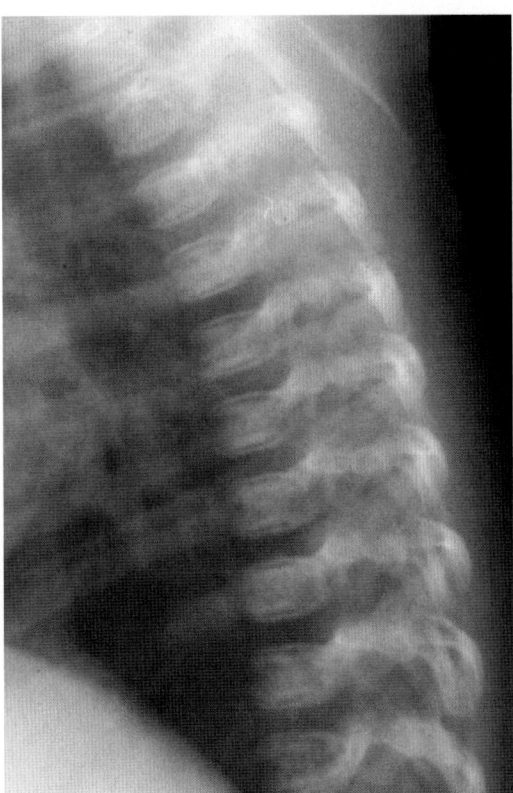

FIGURE 162-12. Bone-in-bone appearance of vertebral bodies in an infant suffering from malnutrition.

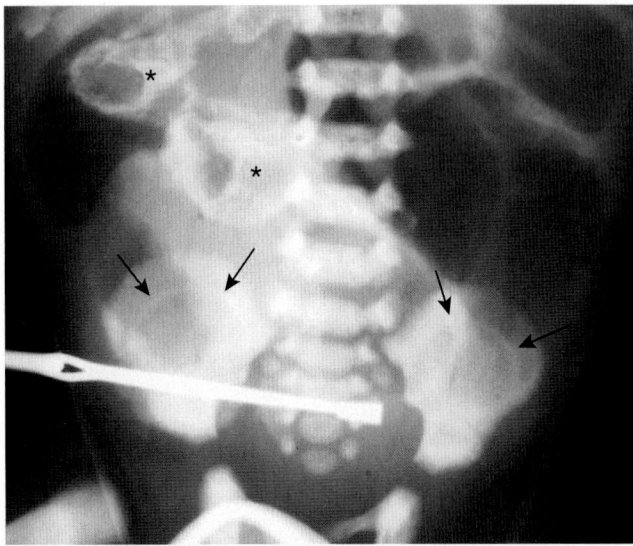

FIGURE 162-13. Growth lines *(arrows)* in the ilia ("Wolfson lines") in a child with meconium peritonitis. Note the dilated bowel and intraperitoneal calcifications *(asterisks)*.

away from the physis—actually, the physis moves away from the stationary growth line. Growth lines are gradually resorbed in the process of endosteal remodeling. Growth lines do not persist beyond skeletal maturity.

> **Growth lines reflect growth arrest and subsequent growth recovery. The physis moves away from the stationary growth line with subsequent growth.**

Growth lines are not limited to the long bones. Growth lines in the spine produce a "bone in bone" appearance (Fig. 162-12). Growth lines found in the ilia of newborn infants with bowel atresia are known as "Wolfson lines" (Fig. 162-13).

Growth lines, which are a nonspecific reflection of stress on the musculoskeletal system, may reflect systemic illness or injury of any sort, including fracture (Fig. 162-14). Growth lines also reflect varying nutritional status of patients. Important work by Hernandez and associates elucidated this point: Patients with psychosocial (deprivational) dwarfism had growth lines caused by varying periods of nutritional support and neglect; patients with hypopituitarism did not have growth lines because their pathophysiologic stress was more constant (Fig. 162-15).

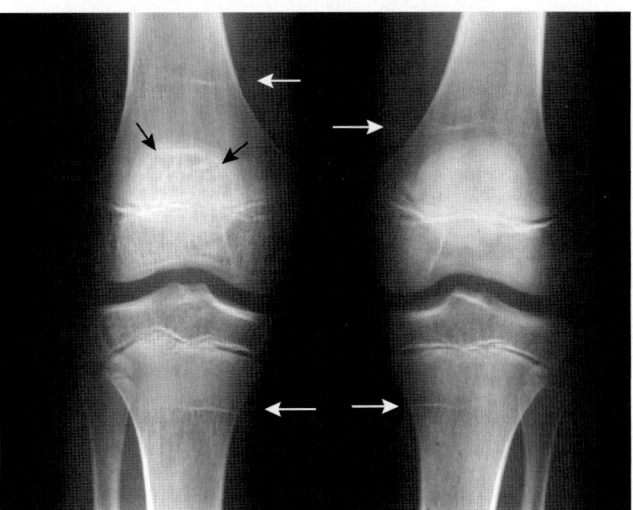

FIGURE 162-14. Growth lines after right femur fracture in a 10-year-old boy *(white arrows)*. Growth lines on the right, particularly in the femur, are farther from the physes because of accelerated growth caused by fracture healing. Concentric growth lines are seen in the patella *(black arrows)*.

A florid example of growth lines can be seen in children treated with bisphosphonate for osteogenesis imperfecta, cerebral palsy, and other disorders. Bisphosphonate causes decreased osteoclastic activity—less bone is absorbed. Because the drug is administered cyclically (i.e, every 3 months), dense metaphyseal bands form in response to the drug; these are separated by less dense bone that forms during the interval between treatments (Fig. 162-16).

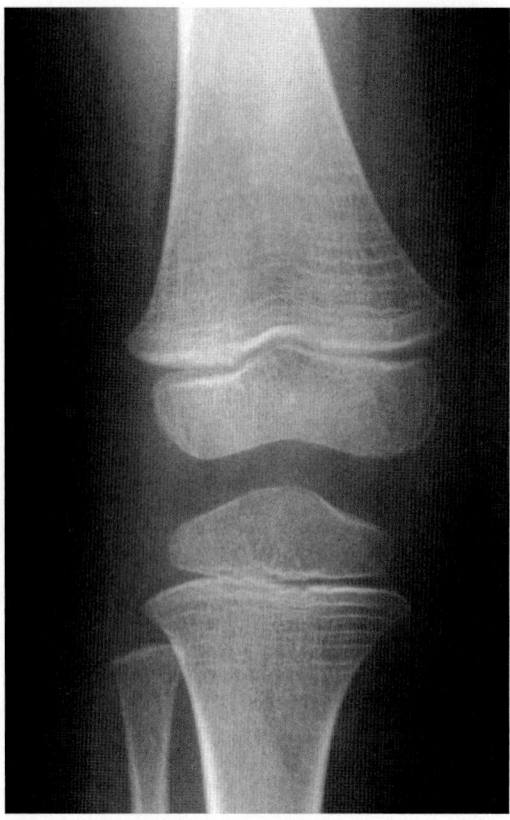

FIGURE 162-15. Growth lines in a 4-year-old girl with psychosocial (deprivational) dwarfism. Multiple growth lines are seen in the metaphyses.

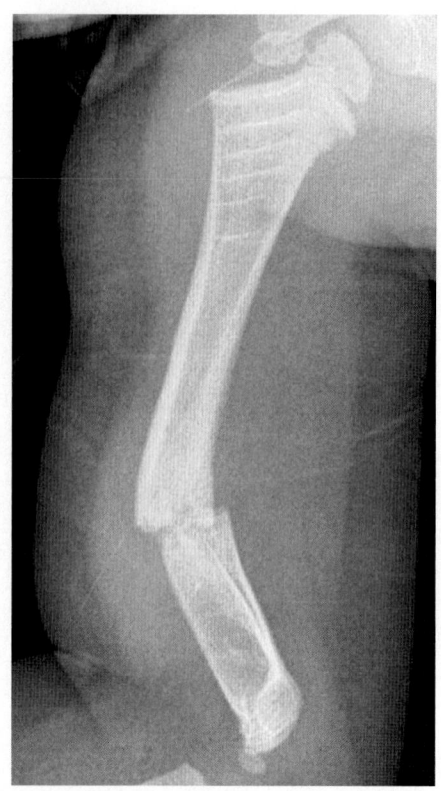

FIGURE 162-16. Growth lines in an 18-month-old patient with osteogenesis imperfecta treated with bisphosphonates on a 4-month cycle. Regularly spaced growth lines are seen in the proximal humerus. Multiple growth lines are also present in the distal humerus and are more closely spaced, indicative of slower growth of the distal humerus compared with the proximal humerus. In spite of treatment, the patient has a fracture. (Courtesy of Dr. B. H. Adler, Columbus, OH.)

SUGGESTED READINGS

Acheson RM: A method of assessing skeletal maturity from radiographs: a report from the Oxford Child Health Survey. J Anat 1954;88:498-508

Anderson M, Messner MB, Green WT: Distribution of lengths of the normal femur and tibia in children from 1 to 18 years of age. J Bone Joint Surg Am 1964;46:1197-1202

Berst MJ, Dolan L, Bogdanowicz MM: Effect of knowledge of chronologic age on the variability of pediatric bone age determined using the Greulich and Pyle standards. AJR Am J Roentgenol 2001;176:507-510

Bull RK, Edwards PD, Kemp PM, et al: Bone age assessment: a large scale comparison of the Greulich and Pyle, and Tanner and Whitehouse (TW2) methods. Arch Dis Child 1999;81:172-173

Edwards DK III: Skeletal growth lines seen on radiographs of newborn infants: prevalence and possible association with obstetric abnormalities. AJR Am J Roentgenol 1993;161:141-145

Elgenmark O: The normal development of ossific centers during infancy and childhood. Acta Paediatric Scand 1946;33(Suppl 1):1-79

Forriol F, Shapiro F: Bone development. Clin Orthop Relat Res 2005;432:14-33

Garn SM, Hertzog KP, Poznanski AK, et al: Metacarpophalangeal lengths in the evaluation of skeletal malformation. Radiology 1972;105:375-381

Garn SM, Poznanski AK, Larson K: Metacarpal lengths, cortical diameters and areas from the 10-state survey. In Jaworski ZFG (ed): Proceedings of the First Workshop on Bone Morphometry. Ottawa, University of Ottawa Press, 1976:367-391

Gilli G: The assessment of skeletal maturation. Horm Res 1996;45(Suppl 2):59-62

Girdany BR, Golden R: Centers of ossification of the skeleton. Am J Roentgenol Radium Ther Nucl Med 1952;68:922-924

Greulich WW, Pyle SI: Radiographic Atlas of Skeletal Development of the Hand and Wrist, 2nd ed. Stanford, CA, Stanford University Press, 1959

Grissom LE, Harcke HT: Radiographic features of bisphosphonate therapy in pediatric patients. Pediatr Radiol 2003;33:336-339

Hadlock FP: Computer-assisted, multiple-parameter assessment of fetal age and growth. Semin Ultrasound CT MR 1989; 10:383-385

Hadlock FP, Harrist RB, Deter RL, et al: Fetal femur length as a predictor of menstrual age: sonographically measured. AJR Am J Roentgenol 1982;138:875-878

Hansman CF: Appearance and fusion of ossification centers in the human skeleton. Am J Roentgenol Radium Ther Nucl Med 1962;88:476-482

Harris HA: The growth of long bones in childhood with special reference to certain bony striations of the metaphysis and the role of vitamins. Arch Intern Med 1926;38:785-793

Hernandez M, Sanchez E, Sobradillo B, et al: A new method for assessment of skeletal maturity in the first 2 years of life. Pediatr Radiol 1988;18:484-489

Hernandez RJ, Poznanski AK, Hopwood NJ, et al: Incidence of growth lines in psychosocial dwarfs and idiopathic hypopituitarism. AJR Am J Roentgenol 1978;131:477-479

Hoerr NL, Pyle SI, Francis CC: Radiographic Atlas of Skeletal Development of the Foot and Ankle. Springfield, IL, Charles C Thomas, 1962

Jeantry P, Kirkpatrick C, Dramaix-Wilmet M, et al: Ultrasonic evaluation of fetal limb growth. Radiology 1981;140:165-168

Johnson LC: The kinetics of skeletal remodeling: a further

consideration of theoretical biology of bone. Birth Defects Orig Artic Ser 1966;2:66-142

Kuhns LR, Finnstrom O: New standards of ossification of the newborn. Radiology 1976;119:655-660

Kuhns LR, Poznanski AK: Radiological assessment of maturity and size of the newborn. CRC Crit Rev Diagn Imaging 1980;12:245-308

Kurtz AB, Filly RA, Wagner RJ, et al: In utero analysis of heterozygous achondroplasia: variable time onset as detected by femur length measurements. J Ultrasound Med 1986;5:137-140

Kwon DS, Spevak MR, Fletcher K, et al: Physiologic subperiosteal new bone formation: prevalence, distribution, and thickness in neonates and infants. AJR Am J Roentgenol 2002;179:985-988

Lambertz: Die Entwicklung des menschlichen Knochengerüstes während des fötalen Lebens. *In* Atlas der normalen und pathologischen Anatomie in typischen Röntgenbildern. Hamburg, Lucas Gräfe & Sillem, 1900

Little DG, Suisman MD: The Risser sign: a critical analysis. J Pediatr Orthop 1994;14:569-585

Loder RT, Estle DT, Morrison K, et al: Applicability of the Greulich and Pyle skeletal age standards to black and white children of today. Am J Dis Child 1993;147:1329-1333

Maresh MM: Linear growth of the long bones of the extremities from infancy through adolescence. Am J Dis Child 1955;89:735-742

Mentzel H-J, Vilser C, Eulenstein M, et al: Assessment of skeletal age at the wrist in children with a new ultrasound device. Pediatr Radiol 2005;35:429-433

Mora S, Boechat MI, Pietka E, et al: Skeletal age determination in children of European and African descent: applicability of the Greulich and Pyle standards. Pediatr Res 2001;50:624-628

Moseley CF: A straight line graph for leg-length discrepancies. J Bone Joint Surg Am 1977;59:174-179

O'Brien GD, Queenan JT: Growth of the ultrasound fetal femur length during normal pregnancy. Part I. Am J Obstet Gynecol 1981;141:833-837

Ogden JA: Diagnostic imaging. *In* Ogden JA (ed): Skeletal Injury in the Child, 3rd ed. New York, Springer, 2000:115-146

Ogden JA: Growth slowdown and arrest lines. J Pediatr Orthop 1984;4:409-415

Ogden JA, Conlogue GJ, Rhodin AGJ: Roentgenographic indicators of skeletal maturity in marine mammals (Cetaea). Skeletal Radiol 1981;7:119-123

Ontell FK, Ivanovic M, Ablin DS, et al: Bone age in children of diverse ethnicity. AJR Am J Roentgenol 1996;167:1395-1398

Park EA: The imprinting of nutritional disturbances on the growing bone. Pediatrics 1964;33:815-862

Park EA, Richter CP: Transverse lines in bone—the mechanism of their development. Bull Johns Hopkins Hosp 1953;93:345-348

Pietka E, Gertych A, Pospiech S, et al: Computer-assisted bone age assessment: image preprocessing and epiphyseal/metaphyseal ROI extraction. IEEE Trans Med Imaging 2001;20:715-729

Poznanski AK, Garn SM, Nagy J, et al: Metacarpophalangeal pattern profiles in the evaluation of skeletal malformation. Radiology 1972;104:1-11

Pyle SI, Hoerr NL: A Radiographic Standard of Reference for the Growing Knee. Springfield, IL, Charles C Thomas, 1969

Pyle SI, Waterhouse AM, Greulich WW: A Radiographic Standard of Reference for the Growing Hand and Wrist (prepared for the National Health Examination Survey). Cleveland, OH, Case Western Reserve University Press, 1971

Risser JC: The iliac apophysis: an invaluable sign in the management of scoliosis. Clin Orthop 1958;1:111-119

Roche AF: Skeletal Maturity of Children 6-11 Years: Racial, Geographic and Socioeconomic Differentials. Bethesda, MD, U.S. National Center for Health Statistics, 1975. DHEW Publication No. (HRA) 76-1631

Russell DL, Keil MF, Bonat SH, et al: The relations between skeletal maturation and adiposity in African American and Caucasian children. J Pediatr 2001;139:844-848

Scoles PV, Salvagno R, Villalba K, et al: Relationship of iliac crest maturation to skeletal and chronologic age. J Pediatr Orthop 1988;8:639-644

Seeds JW, Cefalo RC: Relationship of fetal limb lengths to both parietal diameter and gestational age. Obstet Gynecol 1982; 60:580-585

Shuren N, Kasser JR, Emans JB, et al: Reevaluation of the use of the Risser sign in idiopathic scoliosis. Spine 1992;17:359-361

Siffert RS, Gilbert MD: Anatomy and physiology of the growth plate. *In* Rand M (ed): The Growth Plate and Its Disorders. Baltimore, MD, Williams & Wilkins, 1969

Sontag LW, Snell D, Anderson M: Rate of appearance of ossification centers from birth to the age of five years. Am J Dis Child 1939;58:949-956

Tanner JM, Whitehouse RH, Marshall WA, et al: Assessment of Skeletal Maturity and Prediction of Adult Height (TW2 Method). London, Academic Press, 1975

Wolfson JJ, Engel RR: Anticipating meconium peritonitis from metaphyseal bands. Radiology 1969;92:1055-1060

Zerin JM, Hernandez RJ: Approach to skeletal maturation. Hand Clin 1991;7:53-62

CHAPTER

163

Anatomic Variants

THEODORE E. KEATS and PETER J. STROUSE

Anatomic variants in the growing skeleton may simulate disease. Dr. Caffey was convinced that many so-called cases of osteochondrosis or osteochondritis described in the literature were normal variations in the bones rather than the result of ischemic necrosis. Conversely, Lawson later pointed out that "all that varies is not necessarily normal, and there is nothing to exempt a normal variant from harboring a pathologic process that may be symptomatic." Many so-called normal variants may predispose the patient to pathology and symptoms. In the presence of symptoms, it may be difficult to differentiate a normal variant from a true pathologic process. This is particularly true in children, in whom there is wide normal variation related to the growth and maturation of bones.

Correlation of radiographic findings with clinical symptoms is the first measure of determining the significance of the radiographic finding. Comparison views of the contralateral side may aid in confirming normalcy. Comparison views are most effective when identically positioned to the symptomatic side. In some cases, follow-up films will distinguish a normal variant from a now healing fracture. Bone scintigraphy, computed tomography (CT), magnetic resonance imaging (MRI), and even ultrasound may prove valuable in distinguishing a normal variant from pathology.

Experience and knowledge are often the best resources for successfully identifying normal variants. Compendiums of normal variants (*An Atlas of Normal Roentgen Variants That May Simulate Disease* by Keats and Anderson; *Borderlands of Normal and Early Pathological Findings in Skeletal Radiography* by Freyschmidt et al.) are invaluable resources that have a place in every reading room where pediatric bone films are interpreted.

In this chapter, significant normal variants of the pediatric musculoskeletal system are presented. The chapter thus includes normal variants that are commonly mistaken for disease and normal variants that may cause disease unto themselves. The discussion is limited to variants occurring in the pediatric skeleton. The discussion is also limited to variants in the pelvis and appendicular skeleton. Variants in the bones of the head, spine, and thorax, including the shoulder girdle, are discussed elsewhere in this text. By necessity, the presentation is by no means complete and the reader is referred to the aforementioned texts for additional examples of the presented entities and other less common variants.

GENERALIZED AND SCATTERED PROCESSES

Irregular Ossification

Many epiphyseal and apophyseal ossification centers are irregular and fragmented in their early development. Figure 163-1 illustrates common sites of irregular ossification in the developing skeleton. Specific examples of this variant are discussed within the corresponding sections on the involved anatomy. In the evaluation of the significance of irregular ossification in a single area, it is often helpful to remember that normal irregularities of ossification are usually symmetric and accompanied by similar changes in other areas of the skeleton.

> **Many epiphyseal and apophyseal ossification centers are irregular and fragmented in their early development.**

Normal Newborn Sclerosis

The long tubular bones of fetuses, premature infants, and newborn mature infants often appear sclerotic radiographically in comparison with the bones of older children because of proportionately thicker cortical bone and more abundant spongiosa during fetal and neonatal periods (Fig. 163-2). The sclerotic features disappear gradually during the first weeks of life and resolve by 2 to 3 months of age. Cortical thickening is a common finding in premature infants. Physiologic osteosclerosis of the newborn is not associated with clinical abnormality. The presence of anemia, granulocytopenia, thrombocytopenia, biochemical abnormality, hepatosplenomegaly, dysmorphism, or a positive family history suggests a possible underlying dysplasia or metabolic abnormality. The differential diagnosis includes osteopetrosis, pyknodysostosis, idiopathic hypercalcemia (Williams syndrome), erythroblastosis fetalis, and intrauterine infection (rubella, syphilis).

Physiologic Periosteal New Bone

Physiologic periosteal new bone on the long bone diaphyses of a growing infant is probably due to relatively rapid growth of the bones without adequate time for incorporation of developing bone into the underlying

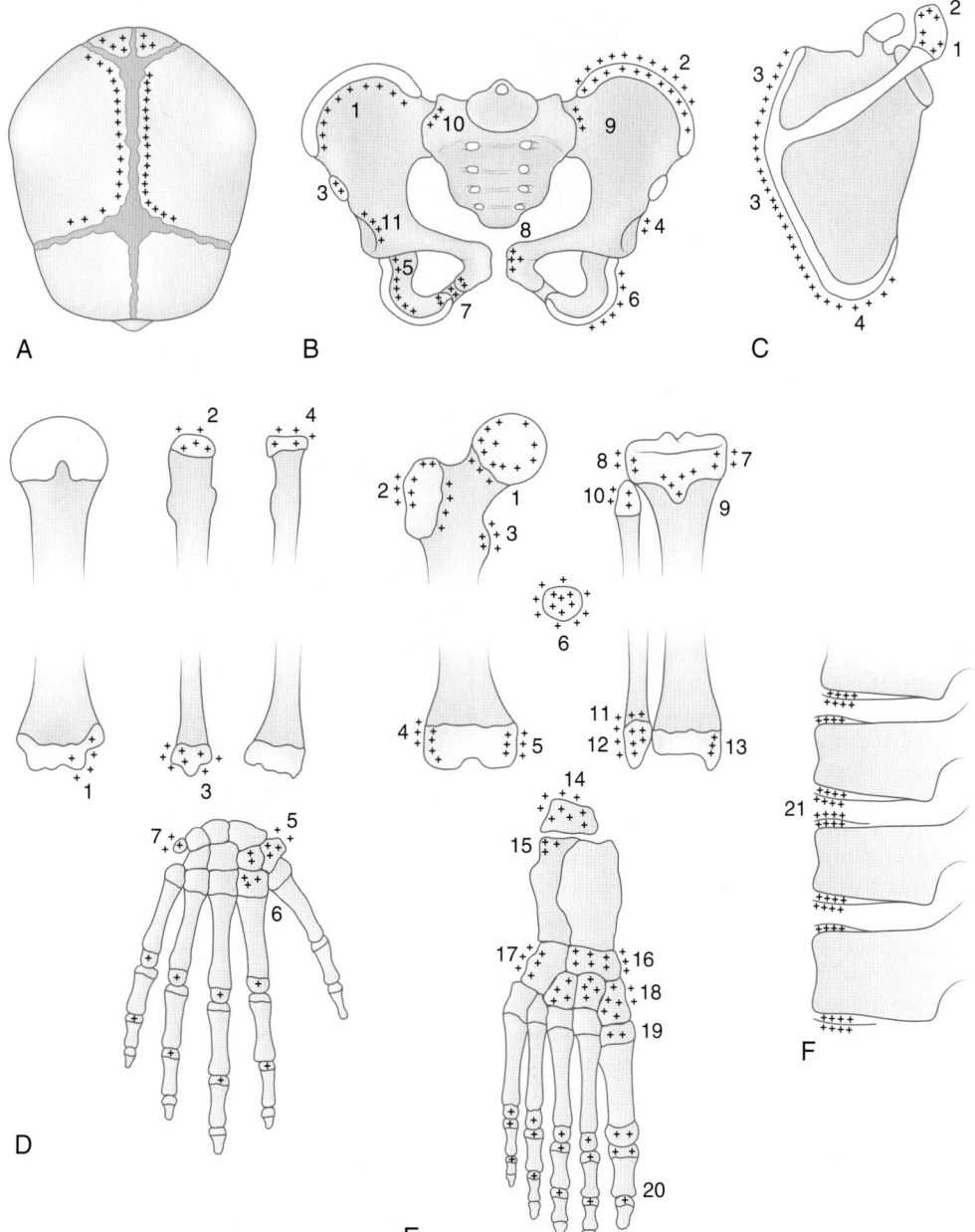

FIGURE 163-1. Common sites of normally irregular mineralization in the growing skeleton are marked by *crosses.* **A,** Cranium. During the first weeks of life and continuing for several months, edges of the bones at the great sutures are commonly irregular, and in many infants deep fissures extend from the sutures into the bodies of the bones. Irregularities are also common on the edges of the temporal suture (not shown). **B,** Pelvis: *1,* crest of ilium; *2,* secondary center in crest of ilium; *3,* secondary center of anterior superior spine; *4,* os acetabuli marginalis; *5,* body of ischium; *6,* secondary center of ischium; *7,* ischium and pubis at the ischiopubic synchondrosis; *8,* body of pubis; *9,* ilium at sacroiliac joint; *10,* sacrum at sacroiliac joint; *11,* iliac edge and roof of the acetabular cavity. **C,** Scapula: *1* and *2,* secondary centers of acromion process; *3,* secondary center of vertebral edge; *4,* secondary center of inferior angle. **D,** Upper limb: *1,* secondary center of trochlea, always irregular; *2* and *3,* proximal and distal epiphyseal centers of ulna; *4,* proximal epiphyseal center of radius; *5,* greater and lesser multangulars; *6,* inconstant center of second metacarpal (pseudoepiphysis); *7,* pisiform. **E,** Lower limb; *1,* proximal metaphysis of femur; *2* and *3,* secondary center and edges of shaft at greater and lesser trochanters, respectively; *4* and *5,* lateral and medial edges, respectively, of distal epiphyseal center of femur; *6,* patella; *7* and *8,* medial and lateral edges, respectively, of proximal epiphyseal center of tibia; *9,* secondary center in anterior tibial process; *10,* proximal epiphyseal center of fibula; *11* and *12,* distal metaphysis and distal epiphyseal center of fibula, respectively; *13,* internal malleolus of distal epiphyseal center of tibia; *14,* apophysis of calcaneus; *15,* primary center of calcaneus; *16,* navicular; *17,* cuboid; *18,* cuneiform; *19,* proximal epiphyseal center of first metatarsal; *20,* epiphyseal centers of phalanges. **F,** Spine; *21,* marginal centers (end plate apophyses).

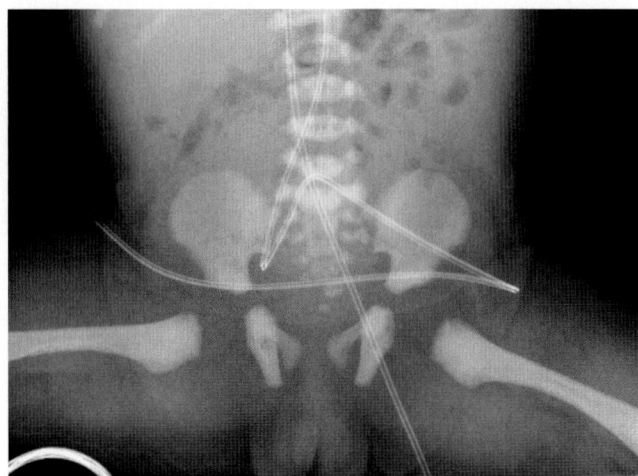

FIGURE 163-2. Normal osteosclerosis of the newborn. All of the bones appear dense. The medullary cavities of the pubic bones and proximal femurs are obscured.

cortices. Physiologic periosteal new bone is seen in infants from 1 to 5 months of age. This age range holds for both premature and full-term infants. Physiologic periosteal new bone is diaphyseal, smooth, regular, and 2 mm or less in thickness (Fig. 163-3). It is most common in the tibia, femur, and humerus and occasionally seen in the radius and ulna. In most infants, physiologic periosteal new bone is symmetric; however, it may be asymmetric in one third to one half of patients. Asymmetric positioning also may make symmetric physiologic periosteal new bone appear asymmetric. There are many pathologic causes for periosteal new bone that need be differentiated from physiologic periosteal new bone (see Chapter 175). Traumatic periosteal new bone tends to be asymmetric, metaphyseal, thicker, and irregular in comparison to physiologic periosteal new bone.

> Physiologic periosteal new bone is seen in infants from 1 to 5 months of age. Physiologic periosteal new bone is diaphyseal, smooth, regular, and 2 mm or less in thickness.

Normal Metaphyseal Irregularities

A variety of normal variants in the metaphyses of infants may simulate injury. It is important to distinguish these findings from the *classic metaphyseal lesions* of child abuse. A detailed discussion of these variants is found in Kleinman's text, *Diagnostic Imaging of Child Abuse*. A "step-off" due to apparent abrupt angulation of the metaphyseal cortex as it approaches the physis is due to the junction of subperiosteal bone collar with adjacent cortex. This is most common in the distal radius and distal femur. Tiny spurs due to extension of the subperiosteal bone collar beyond the metaphysis are most common in the distal radius and distal ulna and are occasionally evident in the proximal tibia and distal femur (Fig. 163-4). Normal beaking is seen at the medial margin of the proximal humeral metaphysis. Apparent

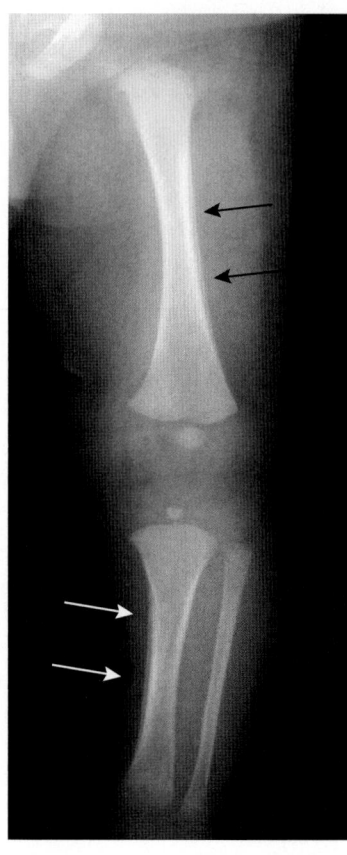

FIGURE 163-3. Physiologic periosteal new bone on the lateral aspect of the femoral diaphysis and medial aspect of the tibial diaphysis *(arrows)* in a 9-week-old boy.

cupping of the distal ulnar metaphysis is due to oblique positioning. Subtle undulation of the medial proximal tibial metaphyseal margin is a normal finding in approximately 25% of infants and is usually symmetric. For each of these variants, follow-up radiographs may help. On follow-up, the normal variant persists unchanged, whereas a subtle fracture will heal and disappear.

Bone Islands

"Bone islands" or enostoses are hamartomatous foci of cancellous structure that usually are resorbed but may occasionally enlarge. Bone islands may be round or oval, small or occasionally large, foci of opaque bone occurring in various sites in round, tubular, and flat bones (Fig. 163-5). The lesions may grow slowly over time. The larger islands are generally observed in tubular bones. The presence of thick, intersecting, marginal trabeculae in smaller lesions helps to distinguish bone islands from infarcts or tumors. Bone islands are most commonly identified in the pelvis, proximal femur, carpus (particularly the hamate), and tarsus (particularly the calcaneus). Bone islands and individual lesions of osteopoikilosis have been said to show similar histologic features. Bone scans are usually negative, but in up to a third of large lesions, bone scans may be positive.

Fibrous Cortical Defects

Benign fibrous cortical defects are the most common pediatric bone tumor (see Chapter 176). In fact, they are

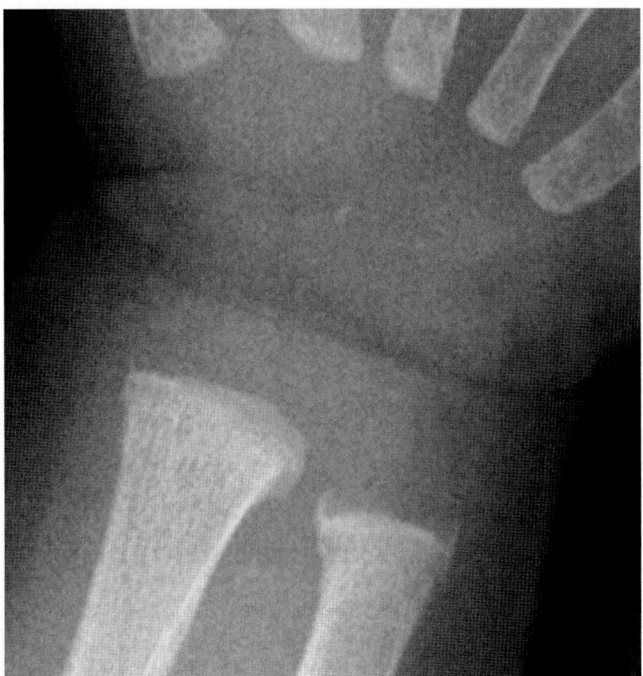

A

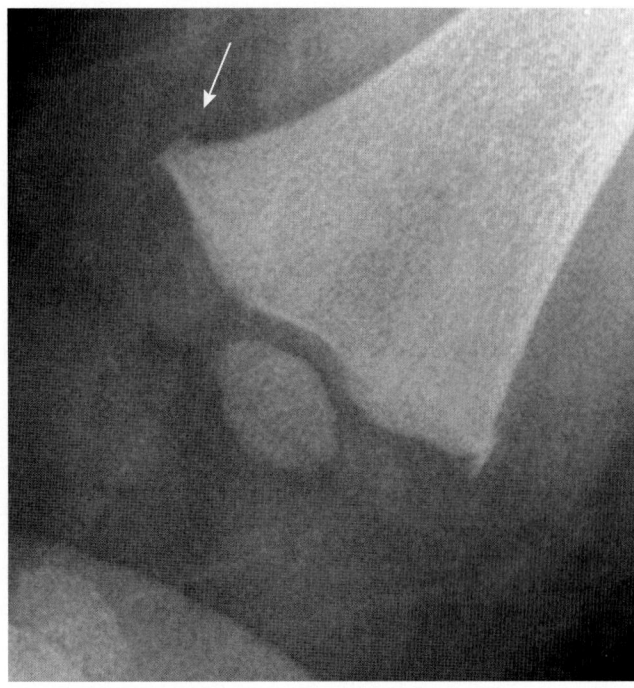

B

FIGURE 163-4. Small spurs on the distal ulnar **(A)** and distal femoral **(B)** metaphyses in a 5-month-old girl due to extension of the subperiosteal bone collar beyond the metaphysis. A normal "step-off" is also noted on the distal femur *(arrow)*.

so common as to be considered a normal variant. Up to 40% of children have fibrous cortical defects. These lesions are most common in the metaphyses of the tibia, fibula, and distal femur. Lesions are less than 2 cm, are cortically based, and have a well-defined sclerotic margin (Fig. 163-6). Sclerosis occurs with involution.

Vascular Channels and Foramina

"Nutrient" canals or grooves and foramina for vascular structures can be identified throughout the skeleton. Some canals or foramina are seen at characteristic anatomic locations such as the proximal femur, ilium, ischium, skull, proximal ulna, and proximal and mid-tibial diaphysis (Fig. 163-7). Most are symmetric. The nutrient foramen of the distal femoral epiphysis is often clearly visible in frontal projections in children older than 4 years (Fig. 163-8); bilateral symmetry may not be present. Foramina and canals are often visible in complementary projections (Fig. 163-9). Although the veins for the cancellous tissue run separately from the arteries, one or two may accompany the main nutrient artery. The others leave the bone through apertures near the ends of the bone and may contribute to some of the irregularities of cortex in these regions.

The walls of vascular canals are not as sharp as an acute fracture line and may be slightly sclerotic. The canals do not completely traverse the bone and do not create a sharp discontinuity in the cortex. If the exit point of a vascular canal is in profile, the cortex may appear slightly indistinct or irregular. Findings persist without change on follow-up imaging.

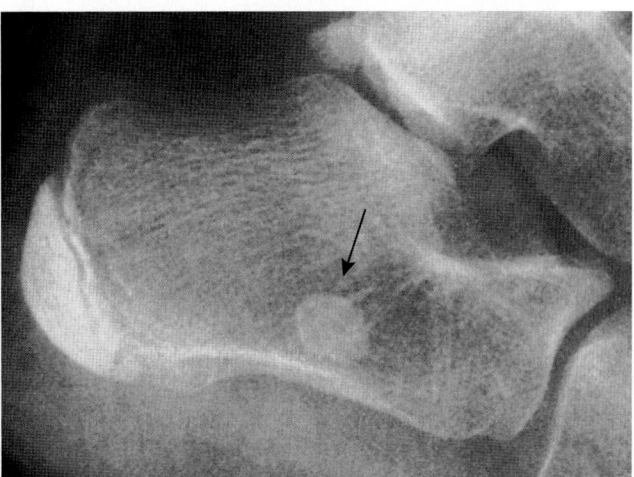

FIGURE 163-5. An oval area of bone density *(arrow)* in the medullary cavity of the body of the calcaneus of an asymptomatic 9-year-old boy. Such lesions are known as "bone islands" or enostoses and have no clinical significance. The calcaneal apophysis is normally sclerotic.

Provisional Zone of Calcification

The thickness of the zone of provisional calcification in the metaphyses of long bones and at the metaphyseal-equivalent regions of flat and round bones is extremely variable in healthy children (Fig. 163-10). In healthy children, the zone of provisional calcification may appear as a dense band, most prominent between the second and fifth years, possibly reflecting the flattening of the growth curve at that time, and simulating the dense lines of lead intoxication.

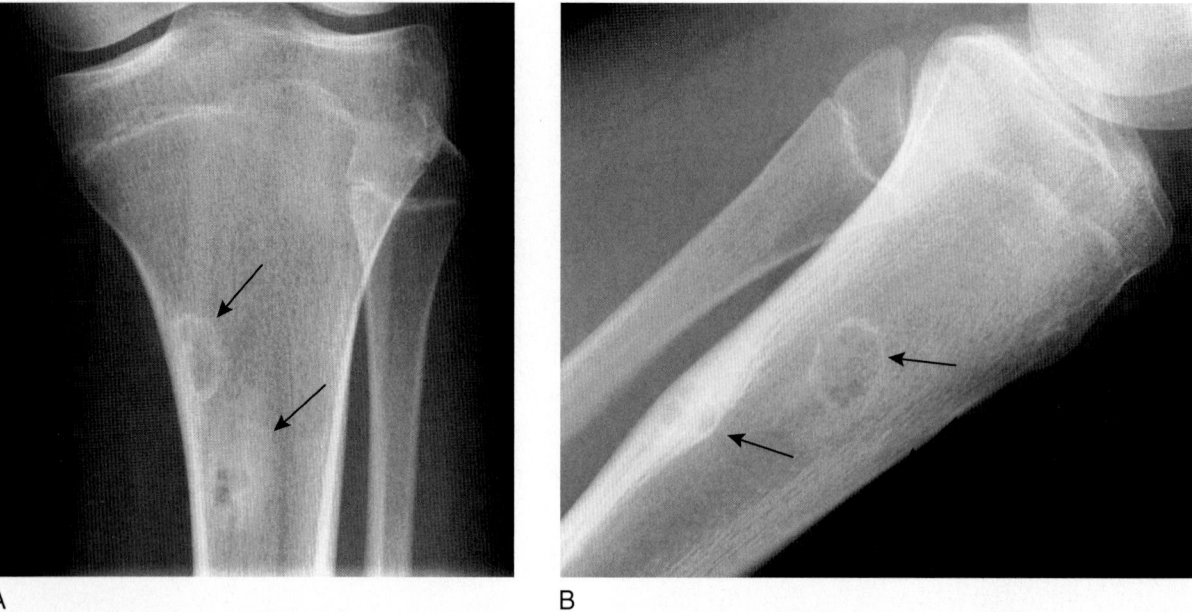

A   B

FIGURE 163-6. Fibrous cortical defects of varying age in a 14-year-old girl. The proximal lesion *(upper arrow)* is newer and appears lucent with a well-defined sclerotic margin. The distal lesion *(lower arrow)* is involuting and sclerotic. En face **(A)**, the distal lesion appears as ill-defined sclerosis with a small residual lucency. Tangentially **(B)**, the lesion appears well-defined and cortically based.

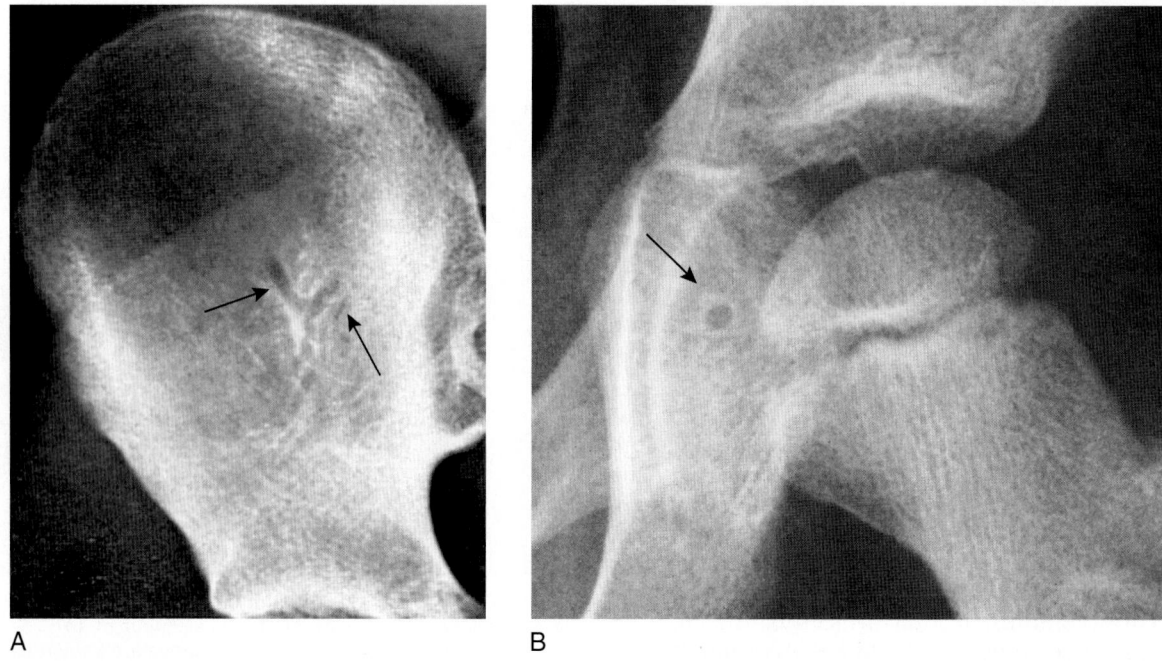

A   B

FIGURE 163-7. Normal vascular markings in the pelvic bones. **A,** Y-shaped tubular shadow *(arrows)* in the ilium of a 4-year-old boy. **B,** Circular vascular foramen *(arrow)* in the body of the ischium of another asymptomatic 4-year-old boy. Sometimes several small circular foramina are present in the same site instead of a single large foramen, as in this patient.

> In healthy children, the zone of provisional calcification may appear as a dense band, most prominent between the second and fifth years.

Vacuum Joint

Gas is commonly seen in a joint due to traction in positioning a young child for radiographs. The gas is nitrogen. The finding is most commonly seen at the shoulder and hip. The finding is normal. In fact, the presence of a vacuum joint on radiography strongly mitigates against the presence of an effusion.

HAND AND WRIST

Ivory Epiphyses

Sclerotic epiphyseal ossification centers of the phalanges are called "ivory epiphyses" when they are large enough

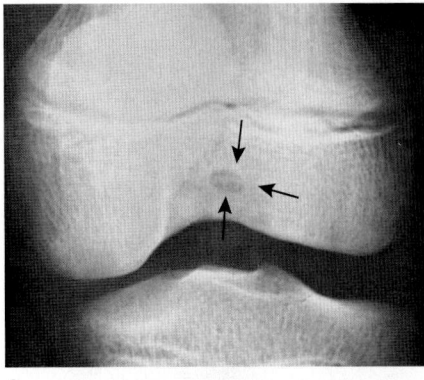

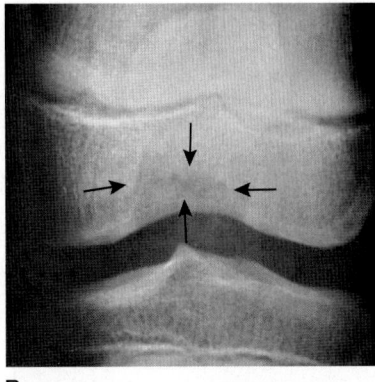

FIGURE 163-8. Normal radiolucent shadow of the nutrient foramen of the distal femoral epiphysis *(arrows)* on the posterior wall of the intercondylar fossa. **A,** Sharply defined foramen in an 11-year-old girl. **B,** Long transverse foramen in a 10½-year-old girl.

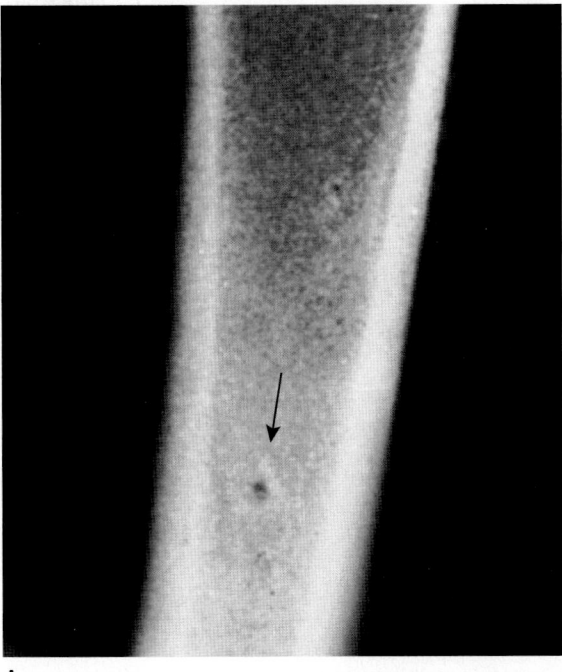

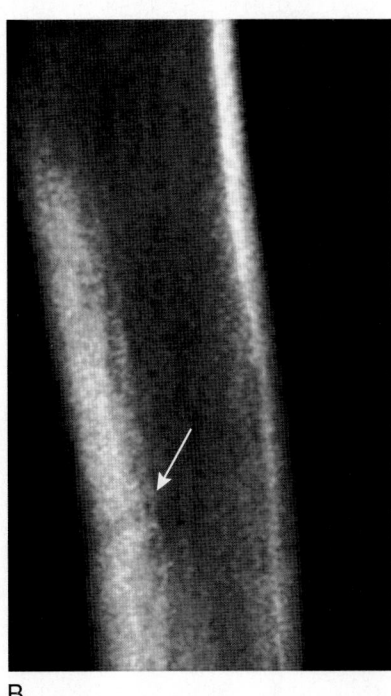

FIGURE 163-9. Superior foramina for femoral nutrient arteries in frontal **(A)** and lateral **(B)** projections. **A,** The foramen casts a small circular radiolucent image. **B,** The canal perforates the anterior cortical wall and could be interpreted as a cortical fracture line. Similar foramina and canals were present in the other femur at the same level in this asymptomatic 3½-year-old boy.

to be trabeculated but are not (Fig. 163-11). They occur in approximately 1 in every 300 patients. Ivory epiphyses are usually found in the distal phalanges and in the middle phalanx of the fifth digit. Maturation may be retarded. Ivory epiphyses may also occur in association with cone-shaped epiphyses in dysplastic syndromes.

Cone-Shaped Epiphyses

Cone-shaped epiphyses of the phalanges (Fig. 163-12) occur most frequently, singly or in combination, in the distal phalanx of the first digit or the middle phalanx of the fifth in normal children and are frequently associated with shortening of the latter, especially in girls. They are seen only in disease states in the proximal phalanges and in the middle phalanges of the third and fourth digits, but occur in the second through fifth middle phalanges and the second middle phalanx in

both normal and diseased children. Giedion described 38 types of cone-shaped epiphyses and indicated those most commonly seen in both groups. Dysplastic renal disease has been noted in association with his types 28, 37, and 38; he has designated disease entities showing the association as "conorenal syndromes."

Pseudoepiphyses

Extra and false epiphyseal ossification centers may appear in the proximal cartilaginous portion of the growing second through fifth metacarpal bones and in the distal cartilage of the first metatarsals—the "nonepiphyseal ends" (Figs. 163-13 and 163-14). They are formed from a thin rod of osteogenic tissue that invades the proximal cartilage from the shaft. The end of the rod enlarges to form a mushroom-shaped mass of bone that appears radiographically as the "pseudoepiphysis." Unlike true

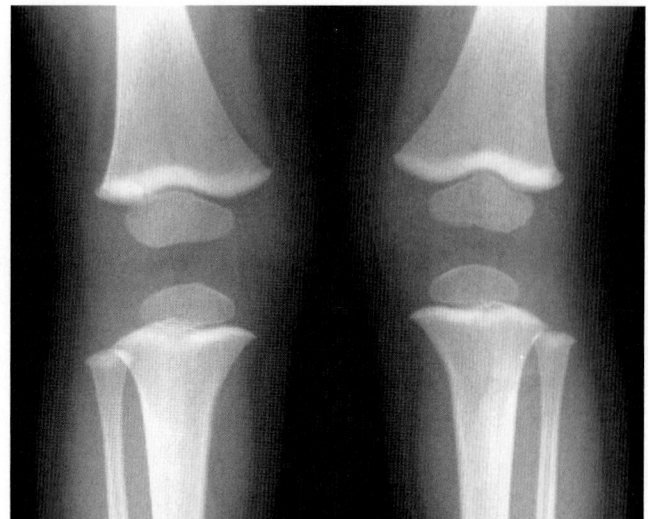

FIGURE 163-10. Dense metaphyseal bands due to relative sclerosis in the zones of provisional calcification in a healthy 2-year-old boy. (From Keats TE: An Atlas of Normal Roentgen Variants That May Simulate Disease, 7th ed. St. Louis, Mosby, 2001.)

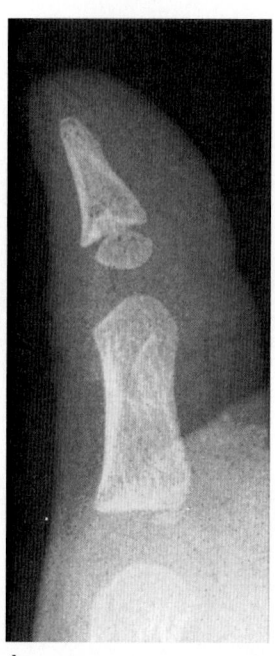
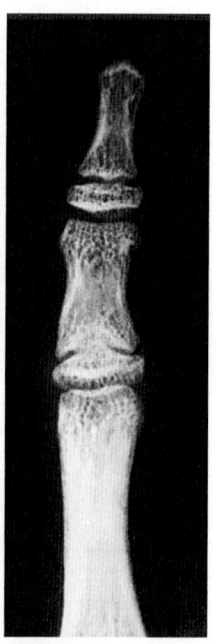

A   B

FIGURE 163-12. Cone-shaped epiphyses as incidental findings in healthy children. **A,** Distal phalanx of the thumb. **B,** Middle phalanx of the fifth digit. (From Poznanski AK: The Hand in Radiologic Diagnosis, 2nd ed. Philadelphia, Saunders, 1984.)

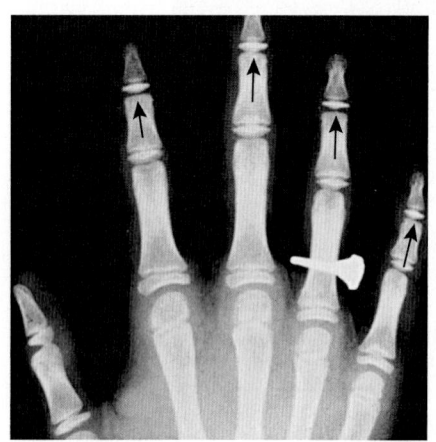
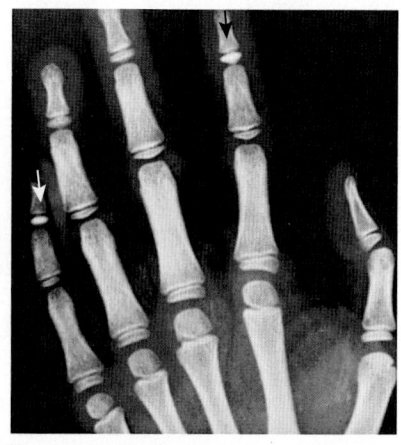

A   B

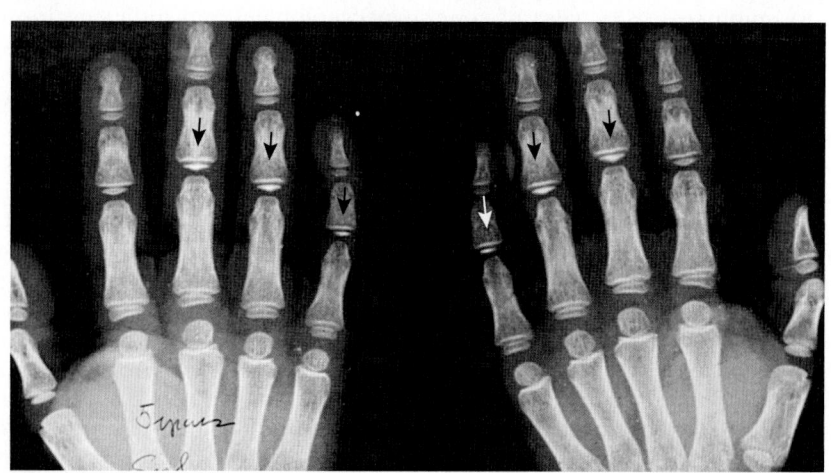

C

FIGURE 163-11. Physiologic sclerosis of the epiphyseal ossification centers *(arrows)* in the phalanges of asymptomatic children. **A,** Sclerosis in the distal phalanges of digits 2, 3, 4, and 5 of an 8-year-old girl. **B,** Sclerosis in the terminal phalanges of digits 2 and 5 of a 6-year-old boy. **C,** Symmetric sclerosis in both hands, digits 3, 4, and 5 of the middle phalanges, of a 5-year-old girl.

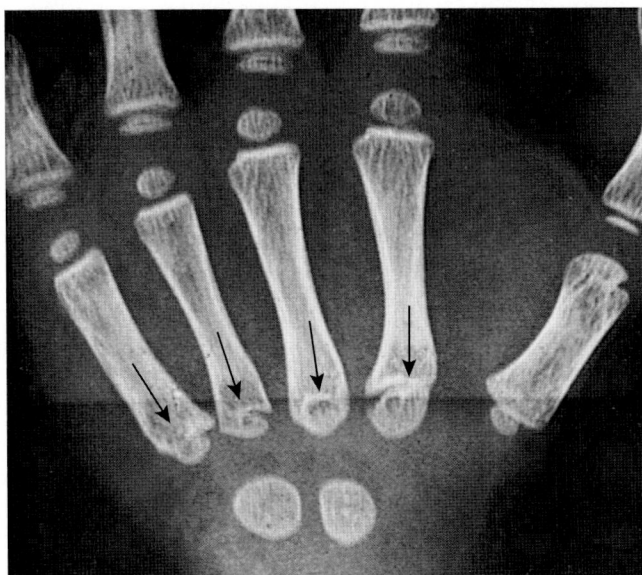

FIGURE 163-13. False centers (pseudoepiphyses) in the second, third, fourth, and fifth metacarpals of a 2-year-old child *(arrows)*; similar false centers were present in the other hand.

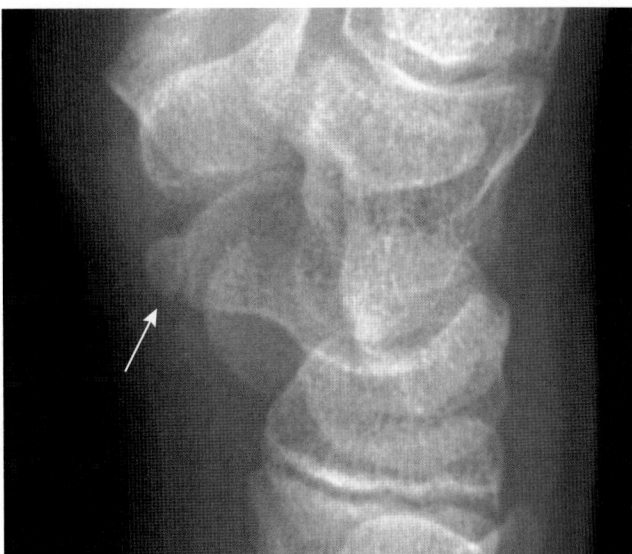

FIGURE 163-15. Accessory ossification center of the distal pole of the scaphoid *(arrow)* in an 11-year-old girl.

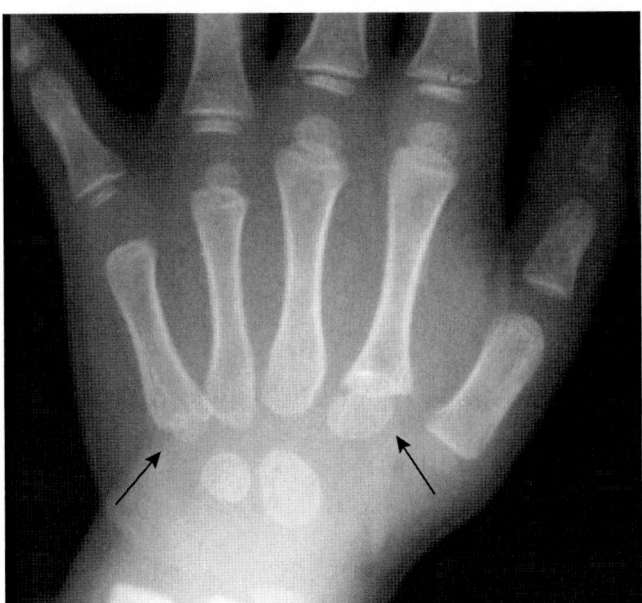

FIGURE 163-14. Pseuodepiphyses in the proximal second and fifth metacarpals of a 3-year-old boy.

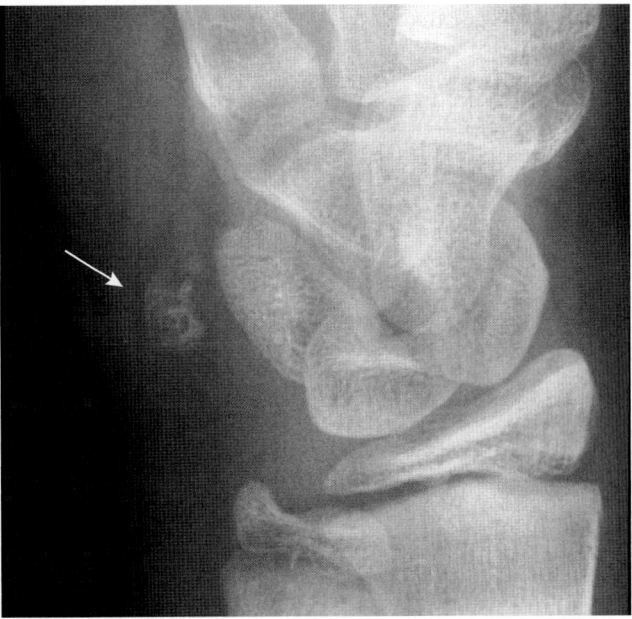

FIGURE 163-16. Irregular ossification of the pisiform *(arrow)* in a 12-year-old boy.

epiphyses, there is bony continuity with the shaft from the beginning of their development and they contribute little or nothing to longitudinal growth. The site of fusion of the bone mass with the shaft is often indicated by a notch; notches have been found in the base of the second metacarpal in up to 60% of normal children, and in the distal end of the first metacarpal in up to 85%. Pseudoepiphyses are well formed by 4 to 5 years of age and coalesce with the rest of the underlying bone at the time of skeletal maturation. Pseudoepiphyses are frequent in children with hypothyroidism and in cleidocranial dysplasia.

Irregular Carpal Ossification

Irregularity of mineralization occasionally occurs in the carpal bones during development. These result from the onset of ossification in several centers, which is generally followed by coalescence to a single center (Fig. 163-15). The pisiform is the bone most frequently affected (Fig. 163-16).

Accessory Carpal Ossification Centers

Approximately 25 separate, well-defined bones can appear as accessory carpal ossification centers in normal

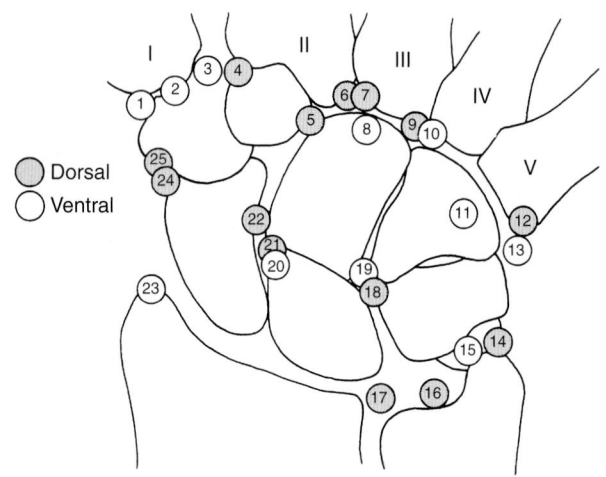

FIGURE 163-17. Schematic diagram of sites for best known accessory ossicles of the wrist: *1,* paratrapezium; *2,* praetrapezium; *3,* trapezium secundarium; *4,* trapezoideum secundarium; *5,* metastyloideum; *6,* parastyloideum; *7,* styloideum; *8,* subcapitatum; *9,* capitatum secundarium; *10,* os Gruberi; *11,* ununited hamulus; *12,* vesalianum; *13,* ulnare externum; *14,* ulnostyloideum; *15,* pisiforme secundarium; *16,* triangulare; *17,* small radioulnar ossicle; *18,* epitriquetrum; *19,* hypotriquetrum; *20,* hypolunatum; *21,* epilunatum; *22,* os centrale; *23,* radiostyloideum; *24,* radiale externum; *25,* epitrapezium.

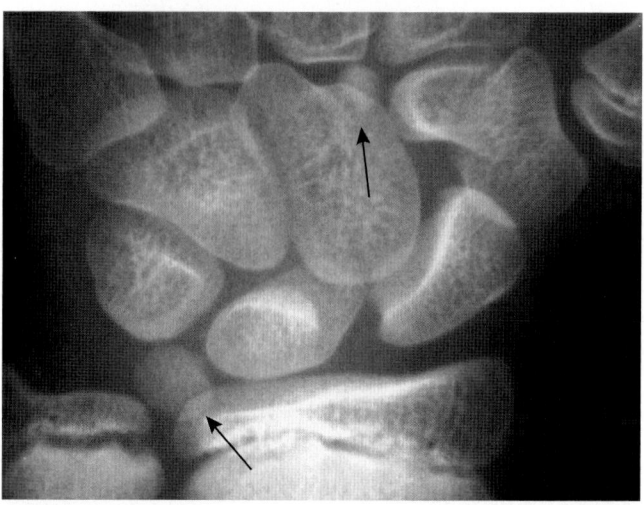

FIGURE 163-18. Accessory ossicles of the carpus *(arrows).*

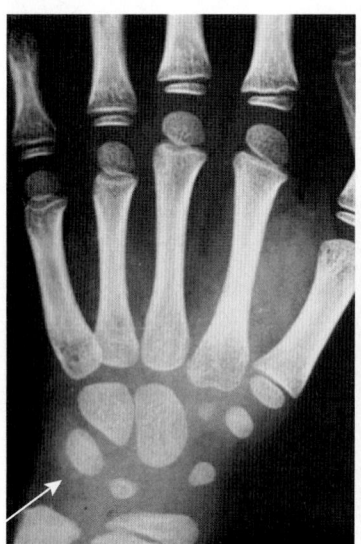
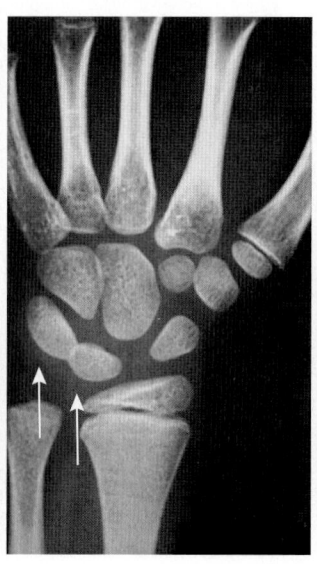
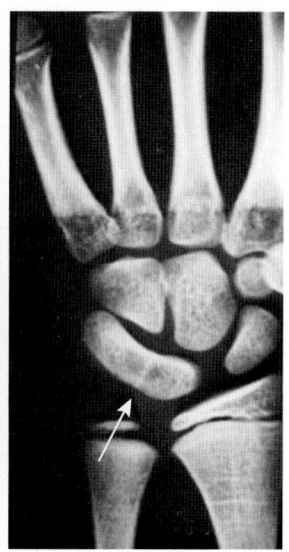

FIGURE 163-19. Lunotriquetral "fusion" *(arrows)* observed in serial films of an African American child with sickle cell anemia at (from left) ages 6, 7, and 8 years.

people (Figs. 163-17 and 163-18). Others occur in certain dysplastic disorders. In the normal person, the ossicles can simulate (and be simulated by) sequelae of injury.

Carpal Fusion

Fusions of ossification centers of adjacent carpal bones probably result from segmentation errors in early embryonic development. Carpal fusions occur in 0.1% of whites and 1.6% of people of black African descent. Triquetral-lunate fusion is the most common (Fig. 163-19). Capitate-hamate fusion is next in frequency. Fusions of any pair of adjacent carpal bones, and even of adjacent

carpal and metacarpal bones, have been observed. Most are isolated anomalies, but some are associated with other malformations or dysplastic syndromes.

Sesamoid Bones

Named for their resemblance to sesame seeds, sesamoid bones in the hands are found on the palmar surface of the distal ends of the metacarpal bones and, less frequently, in the regions of the interphalangeal joints. They lie within the insertions of tendons, articulating with the palmar surface of the adjacent bone. They appear at the first metacarpophalangeal joint at about 11 years in girls and 13 years in boys. Ossification may occur from multiple centers; failure of these centers to unite is probably responsible for partite sesamoid bones. A bipartite sesamoid may mimic a fracture; however, fractures of the sesamoids are rare in the hands. The number and distribution of the sesamoids of the hand are shown in Figure 163-20.

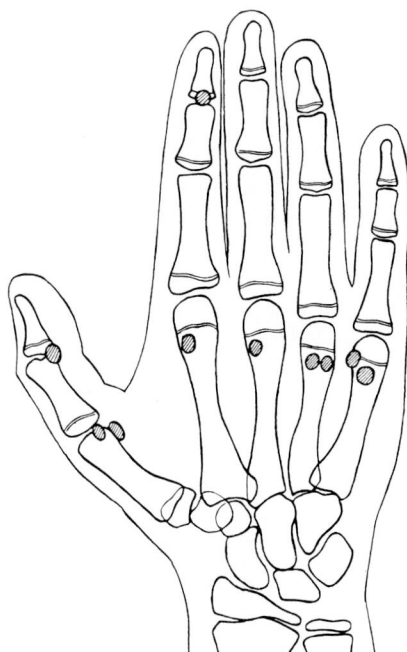

FIGURE 163-20. Location and distribution of the constant and inconstant sesamoid bones of the hands. Five sesamoids are of almost constant occurrence: the pair at the base of the thumb that appears just before adolescence, the single sesamoid more distal in the thumb, and the solitary sesamoids at the bases of the second and fifth digits. Five additional sesamoids are shown.

Os Styloideum (Carpal Boss)

The os styloideum ("the ninth carpal bone") is a mobile bony protrusion at the dorsum of the wrist between the trapezoid, capitate, and second and third metacarpals. It may be isolated or fused to an adjacent bone. The os styloideum is present in 1% to 3% of patients, but rarely causes symptoms (pain) until later adolescence or adulthood. In symptomatic cases, bone scanning will be positive. CT or MRI delineates the anatomy (Fig. 163-21).

Tendon Sheath Insertion on the Phalanges

At the insertion of tendon sheaths on the phalanges, there may be small, smooth osseous protrusions, which may simulate periosteal new bone. Symmetry, lack of symptom correlation, and characteristic location differentiate these protrusions from pathology.

FOREARM
Radial and Ulnar Styloid Processes

Separate ossification centers may appear in the regions of the ulnar (Fig. 163-22) and radial (Fig. 163-23) styloid processes before uniting with the main ossification center.

Variations of Radial and Ulnar Contour

In infants, normal indistinctness of the outer margins of the radius and ulna may simulate disease. During the latter half of childhood, the shafts of the radius and ulna may terminate in wavy, irregular surfaces (Fig. 163-24) in normal children whose other bones show normally

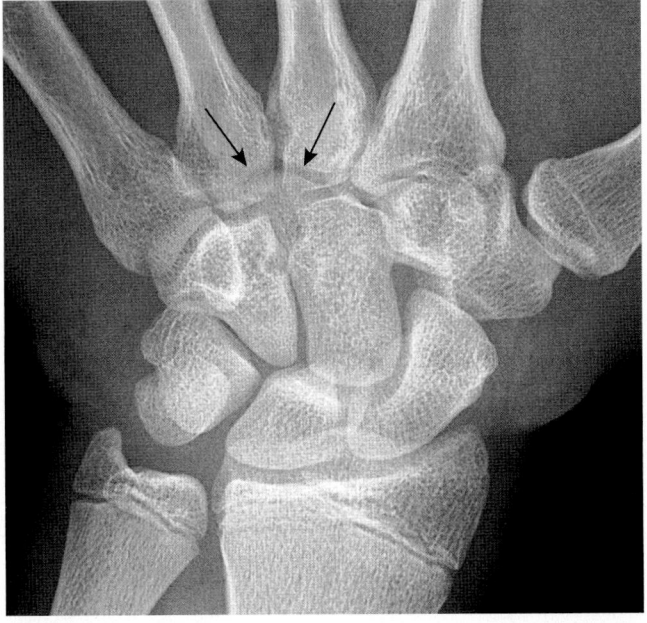

A

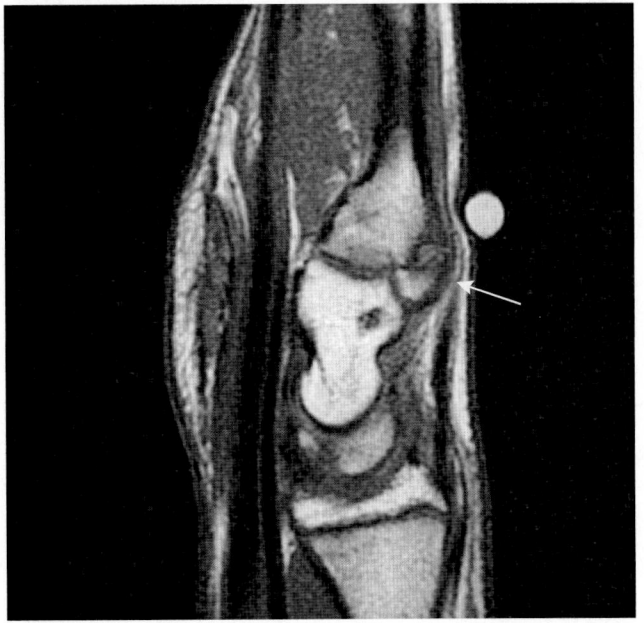

B

FIGURE 163-21. Os styloideum ("carpal boss") in a 14-year-old boy. **A,** Anteroposterior radiograph—the accessory bone is barely visible (arrow). **B,** Sagittal T1-weighted MR image shows the accessory ossicle (arrow) at the dorsum of the wrist. Note that the ossicle causes a "bump" on the dorsum of the wrist.

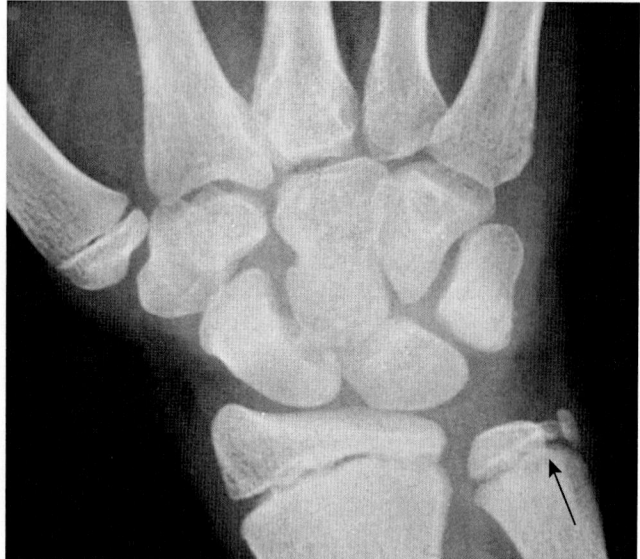

FIGURE 163-22. Separate secondary epiphyseal ossicles *(arrow)* for the styloid in the distal epiphyseal cartilage of the ulna of an asymptomatic 11-year-old boy. Ossicles of this type should not be mistaken for fracture fragments in cases of injury. Such separate ossification centers may later fuse with the main epiphyseal ossification center or may persist throughout life as separate ossicles.

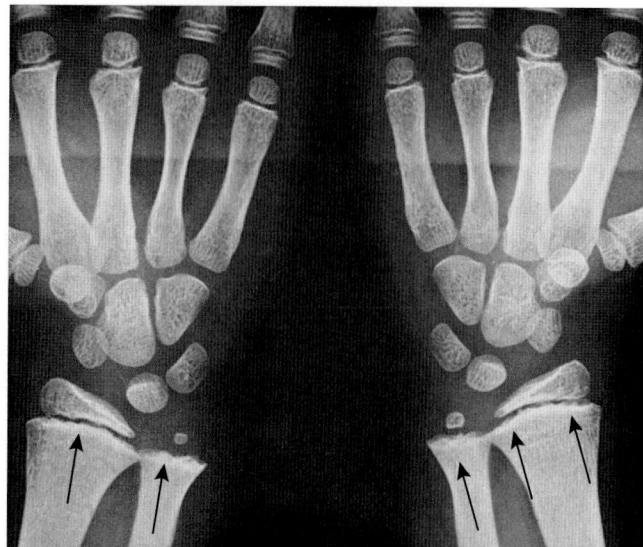

FIGURE 163-24. Physiologic wavy irregularities *(arrows)* in the distal metaphyses of the radii and ulnae in an asymptomatic 9-year-old girl; none of the other bones showed similar changes.

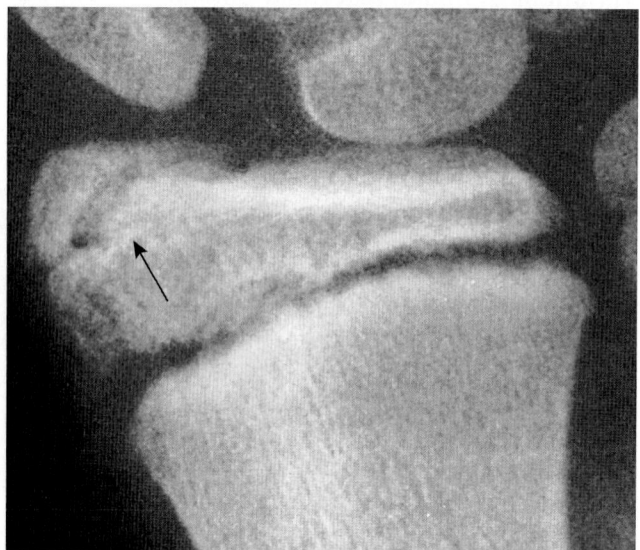

FIGURE 163-23. A large accessory ossification center *(arrow)* in the styloid process of the radial epiphyseal ossification center of a healthy 13-year-old boy simulates a fracture fragment.

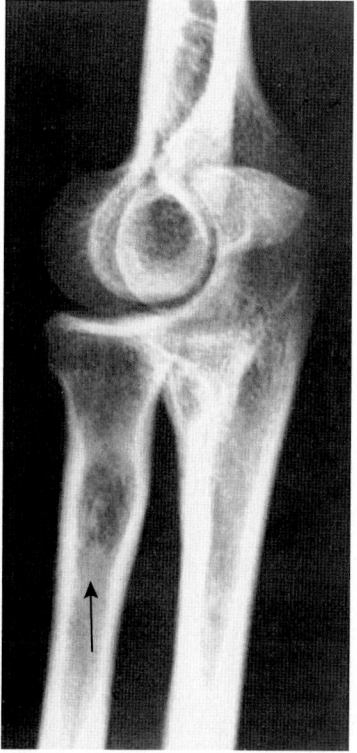

FIGURE 163-25. Slightly oblique projection of the elbow with the forearm extended in a teenage boy. The bicipital tuberosity of the radius is projected en face and simulates a destructive lesion in the proximal shaft just distal to the neck *(arrow).* The cortical bone of the tuberosity is projected parallel to the direction of the x-ray beam and provides a contrasting dense margin for the portion of the medullary cavity that extends into the tuberosity. (From Keats TE: An Atlas of Normal Roentgen Variants That May Simulate Disease, 7th ed. St. Louis, Mosby, 2001.)

smooth metaphyseal ends. In the shafts of these bones, interosseous ridges related to the interosseous membrane may produce external cortical thickening encroaching on the interosseous space, which may simulate pathologic productive bone reaction. The radial tuberosity projected en face may simulate a destructive lesion (Fig. 163-25).

ELBOW

Ossification Centers

The six major secondary epiphyseal centers in the elbow cannot be satisfactorily identified with a single projection. Their positions are indicated in Figure 163-26. In frontal projections, the ulnar centers are superimposed

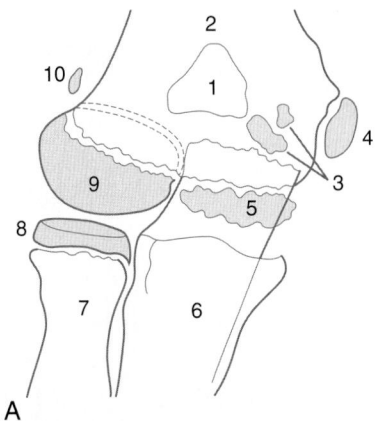
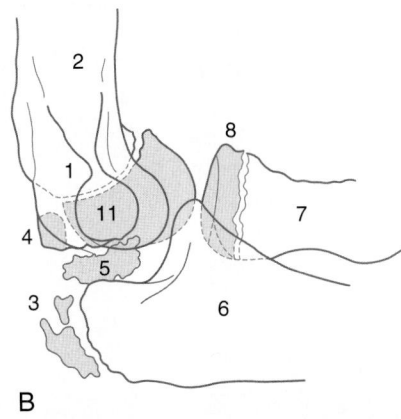

FIGURE 163-26. Normal secondary epiphyseal ossification centers at the elbow in frontal **(A)** and lateral **(B)** projections: *1,* olecranon fossa; *2,* shaft of the humerus; *3,* centers of the olecranon process; *4,* medial epicondyle; *5,* trochlea; *6,* shaft of the ulna; *7,* shaft of the radius; *8,* capitulum of the radius; *9,* capitulum of the humerus; *10,* lateral epicondyle; *11,* lateral projection of the diaphyseal end below the olecranon fossa.

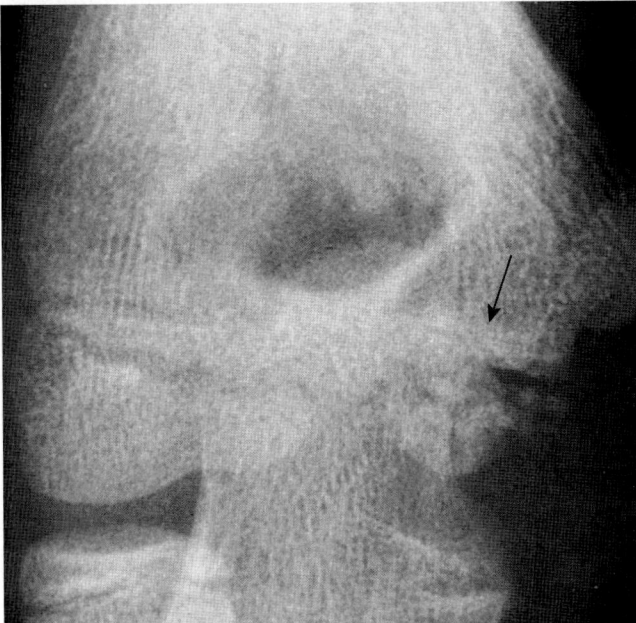

FIGURE 163-27. Normal irregular ossification center *(arrow)* of the trochlea of a healthy 13-year-old boy. This irregular ossification of the trochlea persists throughout the growth period and should always be recognized as a normal variant; actually, it is the norm. The capitulum, in contrast, ossifies uniformly as it expands during the growth period.

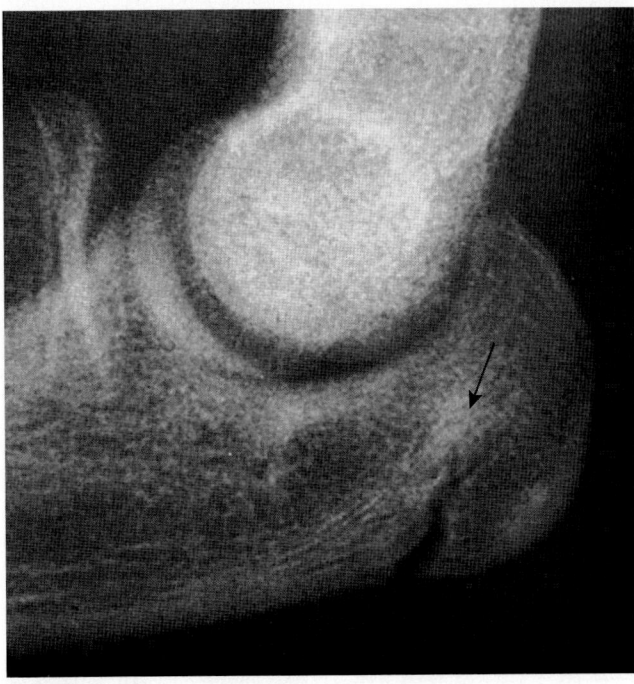

FIGURE 163-28. Synchondrosis of a partially fused single normal secondary ossification center of the olecranon that simulates an incomplete fracture line *(arrow).* The patient was a healthy 13-year-old boy.

on the supracondylar portions of the humerus. Trochlear ossification is very irregular (Fig. 163-27). Likewise, the olecranon centers tend to be grossly irregular during the early years after their appearance and may simulate fractures (Figs. 163-28 and 163-29). The olecranon ossification center varies considerably in size, and the olecranon growth plate thus varies considerably in position and orientation. Findings are usually symmetric. The lateral epicondyle does not fuse directly with the humeral shaft, as the medial epicondyle does, but fuses first with the adjacent capitellum; their fused mass then joins with the end of the humeral shaft (Fig. 163-30). With early ossification, the lateral epicondylar ossification center appears like a small, irregular flake of bone, easily mistaken for an avulsion fragment (Fig. 163-31). Avulsions of the lateral epicondylar ossification center itself are very rare. The medial epicondyle occasionally has an

irregular, fragmented appearance. This finding must be differentiated from an avulsion with widening or irregularity, or both, of the medial epicondylar growth plate. Superimposition of the capitellar growth plate on the lateral condyle may simulate a lateral condylar fracture.

Accessory Ossification Centers

Accessory ossification centers for the named centers may persist ununited even into adult life (Fig. 163-32).

Bifid Radial Head

The radial head center may occasionally originate as two moieties that subsequently unite. In all projections and positions of the normal elbow, the radial head and its

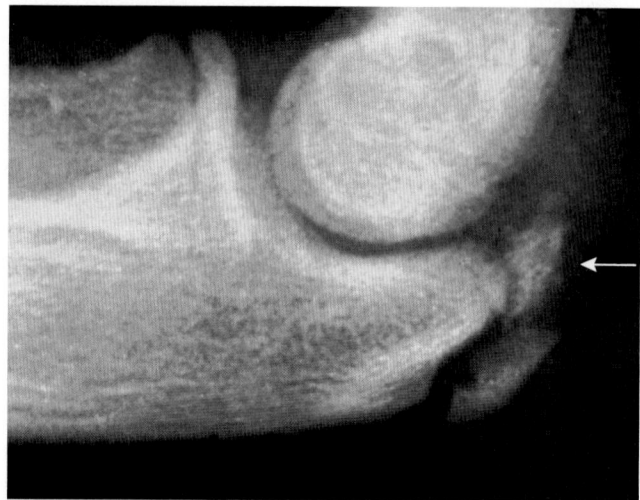

FIGURE 163-29. Multiple ossification centers in the olecranon epiphysis *(arrow)* that simulate multiple fracture fragments at the elbow. The patient was a healthy 11-year-old boy.

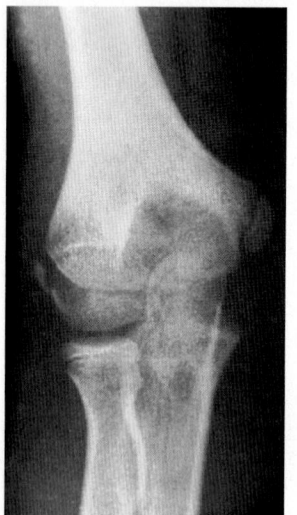 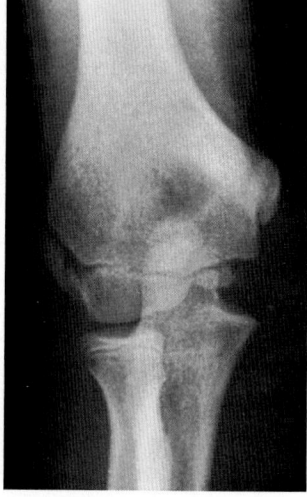

A   B

FIGURE 163-30. The lateral epicondyle center is independent of both the capitulum and the shaft at 11 years **(A)**; it has already fused with the capitulum at 12½ years **(B)**, and these combined ossification centers will later fuse with the shaft. The medial epicondyle center is fusing directly with the shaft in **A** and **B**. In **B**, the trochlea is normally irregular.

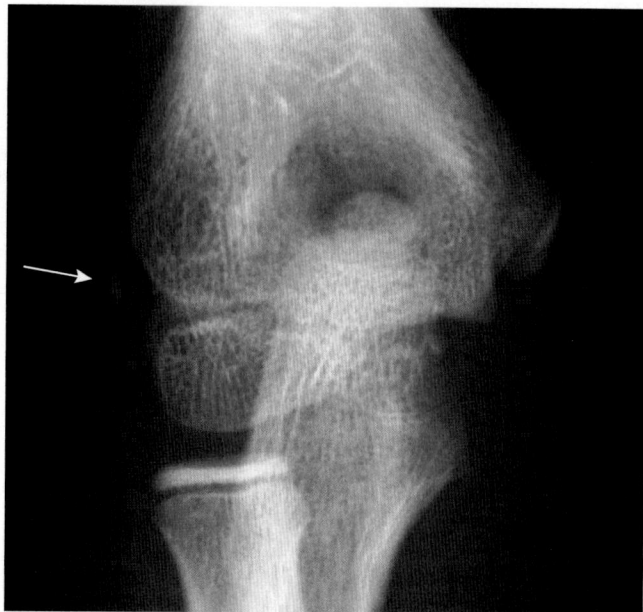

FIGURE 163-31. Early ossification of a normal lateral epicondyle in a 10-year-old girl. The ossification center falsely appears separated from the underlying bone *(arrow)*.

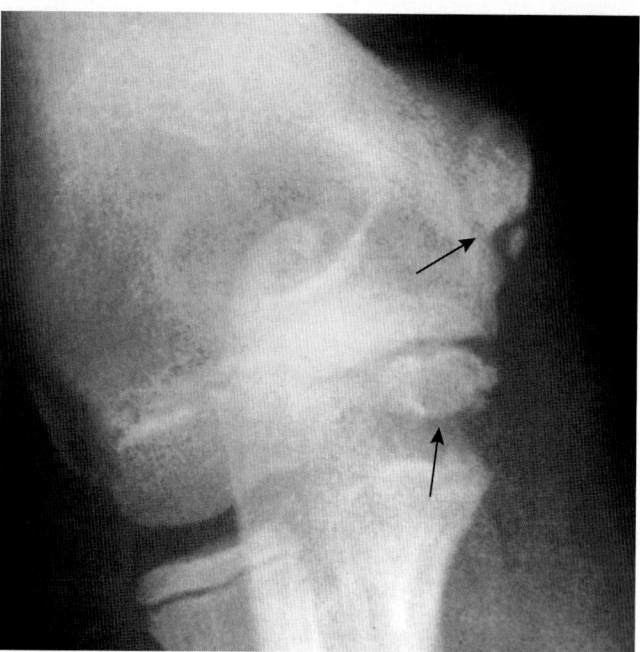

FIGURE 163-32. Accessory ossification center *(proximal arrow)* at the lower pole of the medial epicondyle of a healthy boy 12 years of age, which simulates a fracture fragment. *Distal arrow* points to the normal irregular edges of the trochlear center of the humerus.

subjacent shaft should be in line with the capitulum. As opposed to fracture, no elbow effusion will be present, unless there is other pathology to produce one.

Sequence of Ossification

The six major ossification centers at the elbow ossify in an expected sequence—*c*apitulum, *r*adial head, *i*nternal (*m*edial) epicondyle, *t*rochlea, *o*lecranon, and *e*xternal (*l*ateral) epicondyle. The sequence of ossification can be remembered with the acronym *CRITOE (CRMTOL)*. If a bony density is seen in one area when an earlier appearing center is lacking, a traumatic fragment is very likely the cause. This is most useful in identifying avulsions of the medial epicondyle. Rarely, variations in the order of ossification occur. The most common variation is the medial epicondyle appearing prior to the radial head. Fortunately, ossification of the trochlea before the medial epicondyle is very rare. The sequence of ossification is usually symmetric.

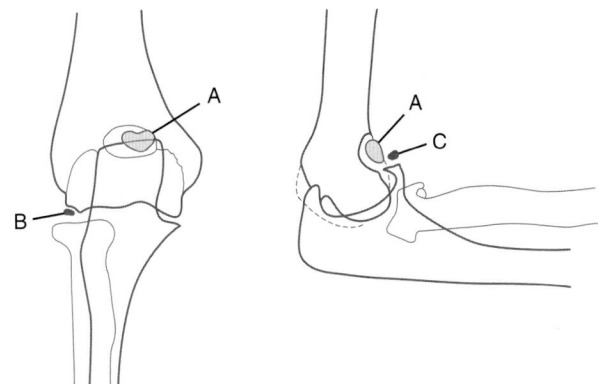

FIGURE 163-33. Rare accessory ossicles at the elbow: A, antecubital bone; B, paratrochlear bone; C, accessory coronoid. (From Schwarz GS: Bilateral antecubital ossicles [fabella cubiti] and other rare accessory bones of the elbow: with a case report. Radiology 1965;69:730-734.)

> *C*apitellum, *R*adial head, *I*nternal (*M*edial) epicondyle, *T*rochlea, *O*lecranon, and *E*xternal (*L*ateral) epicondyle—*CRITOE* (*CRMTOL*).

Accessory Ossicles

Rarely, a sesamoid bone develops in the triceps tendon *(patella cubiti)*. Other rare anomalous ossicles may be seen in the elbow: *antecubital bone* (within the antecubital fossa), *paratrochlear bone* (adjacent to the radiocapitellar joint at the lateral aspect of the trochlea), and *accessory coronoid* (at the tip of the coronoid process) (Fig. 163-33). The absence of a history of injury and of symptoms differentiates them from identically appearing osteochondral loose bodies that can follow injury.

Os Supratrochleare Dorsale

The os supratrochleare dorsale is a large ossicle within the olecranon fossa that is probably the sequela of chronic trauma and an osteochondral loose body rather than an accessory ossicle. It is most common in the dominant arm of males, 15 to 40 years of age.

Supratrochlear Foramen

At the distal humerus, the bony septum separating the olecranon fossa behind from the coronoid fossa in front varies in thickness. An area of variable lucency is seen on radiographs. Defects in the septum are called supratrochlear foramina and appear lucent.

Supracondylar Process

The supracondylar process of the humerus is a vestigial structure that projects from the medial aspect of the anterior surface of the humeral shaft 5 to 7 cm proximal to the medial epicondyle (Figs. 163-34 through 163-36). It occurs in 1% of individuals. The supracondylar process may be connected by the ligament of Struthers to the medial epicondyle. Portions of pronator teres and

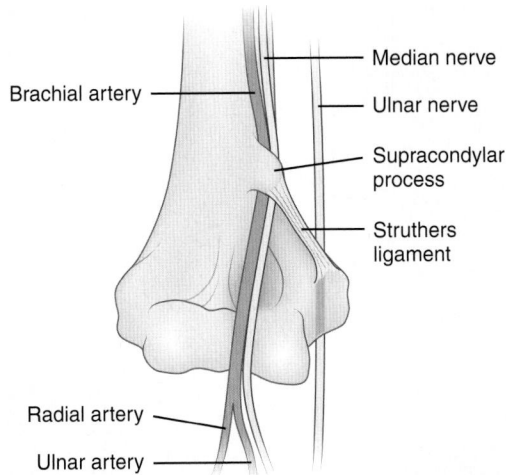

FIGURE 163-34. Drawing of the supracondylar process on the anterior surface of the humerus that shows the relationship of the process to the brachial artery and its branches and to the median nerve. (From Spinner RJ, Lins RE, Jacobson SR, et al: Fractures of the supracondylar process of the humerus. J Hand Surg [Am] 1994;19;1038-1041.)

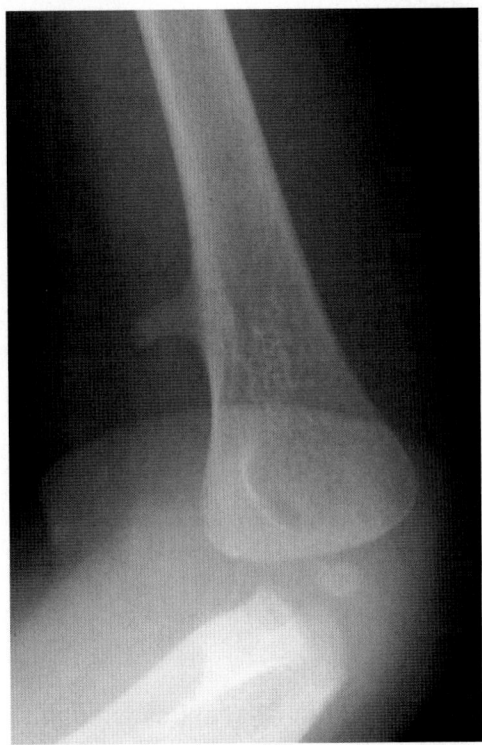

FIGURE 163-35. Supracondylar process of the distal humerus in a 21-month-old girl.

brachioradialis muscles may attach to the process, to the ligament of Struthers, or to both. The ligament may ossify. Occasionally, median nerve neuralgia occurs due to entrapment or compression of the median nerve as it passes through the tunnel created by the supracondylar process, the ligament of Struthers, and associated structures. The supracondylar process is best demonstrated by a slightly oblique, internally rotated projection of the distal humerus. The supracondylar process may fracture.

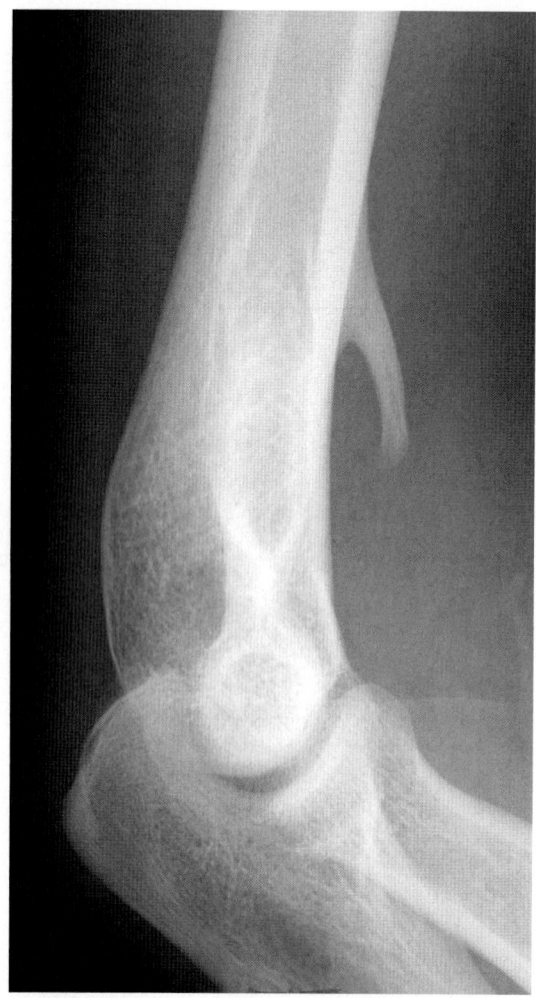

FIGURE 163-36. Large supracondylar process of the distal humerus in a skeletally mature patient. (From Keats TE: An Atlas of Normal Roentgen Variants That May Simulate Disease, 7th ed. St. Louis, Mosby, 2001.)

> The supracondylar process is usually asymptomatic. Occasionally, symptoms develop due to median nerve entrapment.

SHOULDER

Proximal Humeral Epiphyseal Ossification

At the upper end of the humerus, two and occasionally three secondary ossification centers can be observed. The first center (humeral head proper) to appear develops in the medial half of the epiphysis at about 2 weeks of age; because of its eccentric location, it shifts to a factitious lateral position when the arm is rotated (Fig. 163-37). The second center appears laterally in the greater tuberosity during the second half of the first year. A rare third center occurs in the lesser tuberosity during the third year and fuses with the humeral head during the sixth to seventh years. This center may be seen in axillary views of the shoulder and may simulate a fracture fragment.

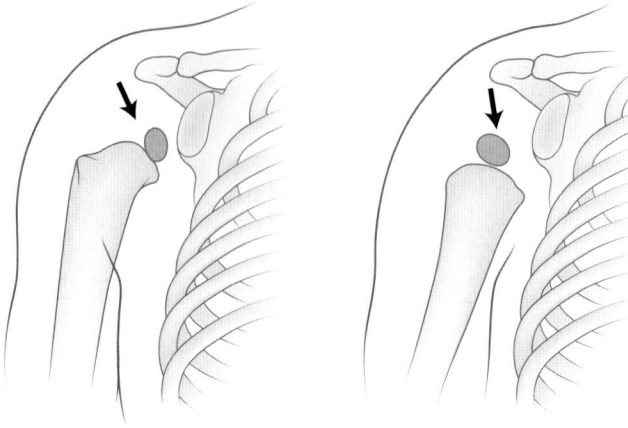

A   B

FIGURE 163-37. Factitious shift in position *(arrows)* of the normally eccentric proximal ossification center of the humerus caused by rotation of the bone. **A,** Anatomic position of the humerus with the ossification center in the medial segment of the epiphysis. **B,** With the humerus in internal rotation, the ossification center appears to be displaced laterad.

Proximal Humeral Physis

The physis at the upper end of the humerus is "tented," with the apex well above the pitched anterior and posterior segments (Fig. 163-38). In rotated positions of the humerus, these segments are projected at different levels and may simulate fracture. Offset of the epiphyseal ossification center relative to the lateral metaphyseal margin may simulate a Salter fracture.

Bicipital Groove

The bicipital groove in the anterior surface of the humerus may simulate local bone destruction or production (Fig. 163-39).

Muscular Insertions

Local cortical thickening, resembling a pathologic periosteal reaction, occurs frequently at sites of insertion of major muscles of the upper arm, possibly resulting from minor trauma of heavy muscular efforts in physically active children. This finding is most common at the site of the deltoid insertion at the lateral aspect of the humeral diaphysis (Fig. 163-40).

Notched Proximal Metaphysis of the Humerus

The medial cortical wall of the proximal humeral metaphysis may be notched in the absence of disease (Fig. 163-41). This may simulate a disease process.

Humeral Head Pseudocyst

When the humeral head is well ossified, the region of the greater tuberosity appears relatively radiolucent and devoid of trabeculation. This may be mistaken for a destructive lesion (see Fig. 163-41).

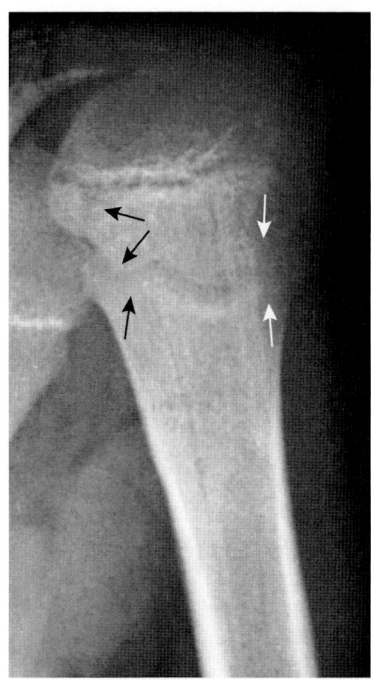

A

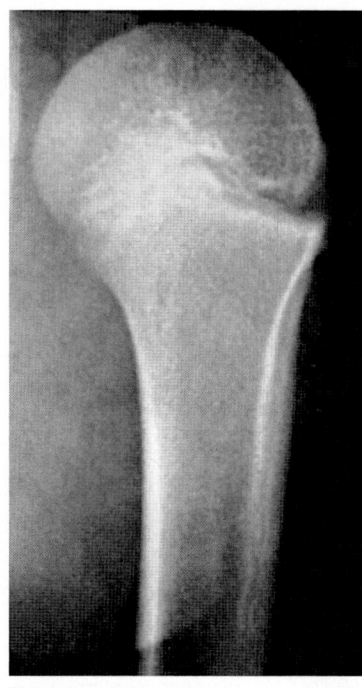

B

FIGURE 163-38. A, False fracture *(arrows)* of the humeral neck on internal rotation to 90 degrees. **B,** There is no fracture line in the anatomic position. The anterior pitch of the upper end of the humeral shaft is wider and deeper than the posterior, and it is the image of the segment below the posterior end of the shaft that casts the factitious fracture line.

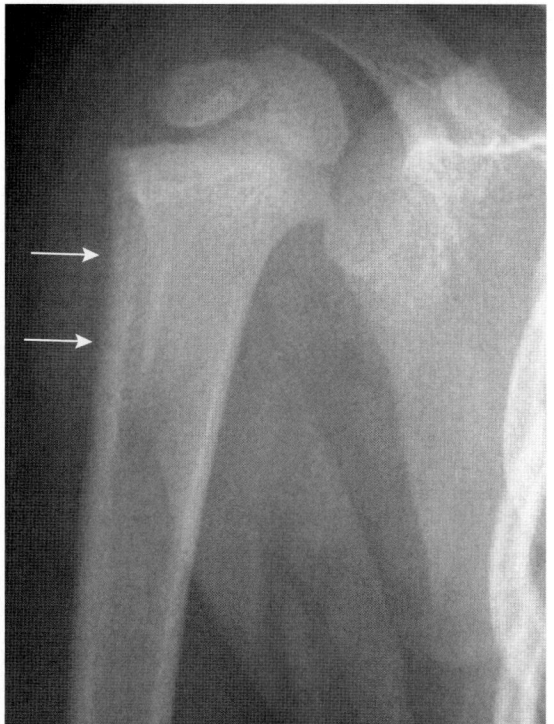

FIGURE 163-39. Pseudolesion of the proximal humeral metaphysis *(arrows)* due to bicipital groove in a 16-month-old girl.

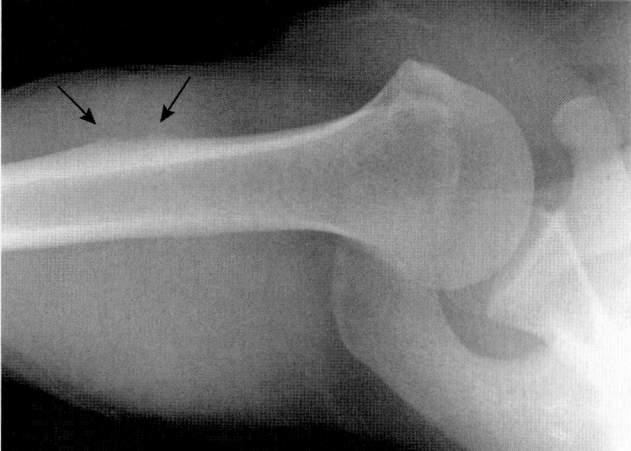

FIGURE 163-40. Irregularity of the anterior cortex of the proximal humeral diaphysis *(arrows)* due to muscle insertion in a 16-year-old boy. Similar findings were seen on the opposite side.

PELVIS

Normal Pelvic Osseous Anatomy

The pelvis of a fetus, infant, or child is conspicuously small and funnel-shaped. During the neonatal period, the vertical pelvic diameter is elongated in proportion to the transverse and sagittal diameters. At birth, the acetabular cavities are relatively larger and shallower than in older children and the obturator foramina are proportionately smaller and situated nearer together. The sacrum makes up a larger segment of the pelvic girdle during the early years and is situated higher in relation to the ilia than later in life. The infantile sacral promontory is less marked than in the adult until the infant assumes an erect posture, when the sacrum descends between the ilia and tilts forward. Pelvic growth is most rapid during the first 2 years of life, after which growth is slow until puberty.

Anatomists claim that sexual differences in pelvic morphology can be recognized as early as the fourth fetal month but, from the radiographic standpoint, the

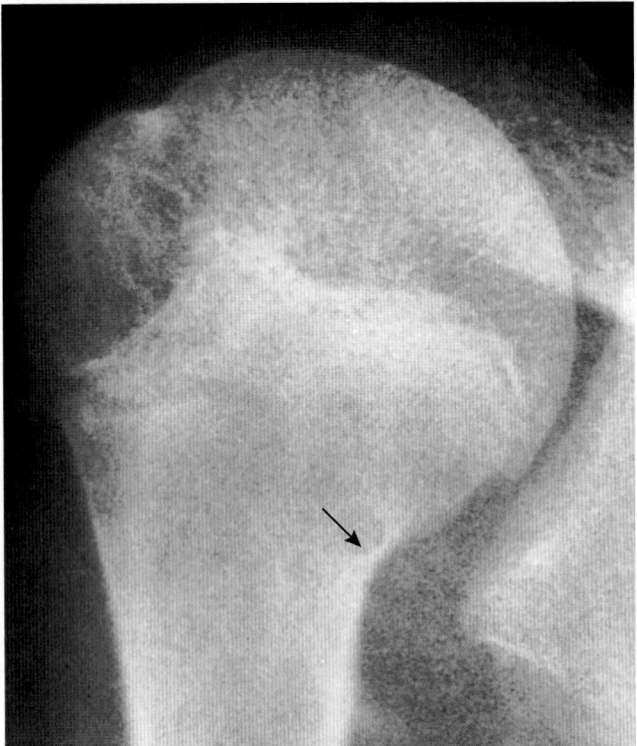

FIGURE 163-41. Normal shallow notching of the humeral cortical wall at the surgical neck *(arrow)* in a 14-year-old girl. Note the normal radiolucency of the greater tuberosity.

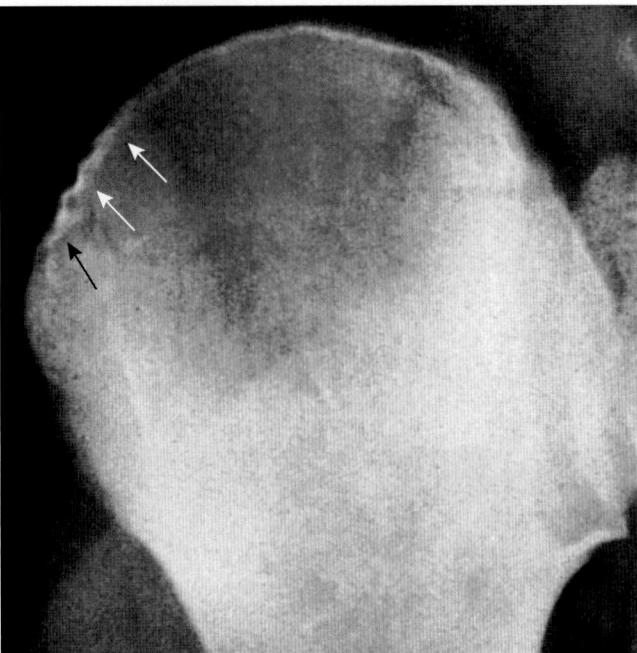

FIGURE 163-42. Normal marginal scalloping *(arrows)* in the ventral segment of the iliac crest of an asymptomatic 6-year-old girl.

bony pelves of young boys and young girls are practically indistinguishable. Later, the male pelvis tends to be larger, but the major gender differences are not obvious until after puberty. In girls, the ossification centers for the iliac crests usually appear within 6 months of menarche. It is possible that similar changes in the ilia of boys represent an analogous level of maturation.

Secondary ossification centers in the pelvis include the iliac crests, ischial tuberosities, anterior superior iliac spine, and anterior inferior iliac spine. These ossification centers may be sites of variation or disease (fracture, infection).

Iliac Crest

The iliac crest apophysis often develops from several foci that fuse with one another before fusing with the underlying iliac bone. The margin of the ilium is smooth at birth but often becomes wavy and irregular after the second or third year (Fig. 163-42). The ventral segment of the ilium is always the most affected, and in many instances the scalloping of the ilium is confined to the anterior portions. Such irregularities may persist until puberty, after which they are obliterated by fusion of the ilium with the iliac crest apophysis.

Acetabulum

Irregular ossification into the cartilaginous roof of the acetabulum is a normal phenomenon during growth (Fig. 163-43). The regular smooth configuration of the

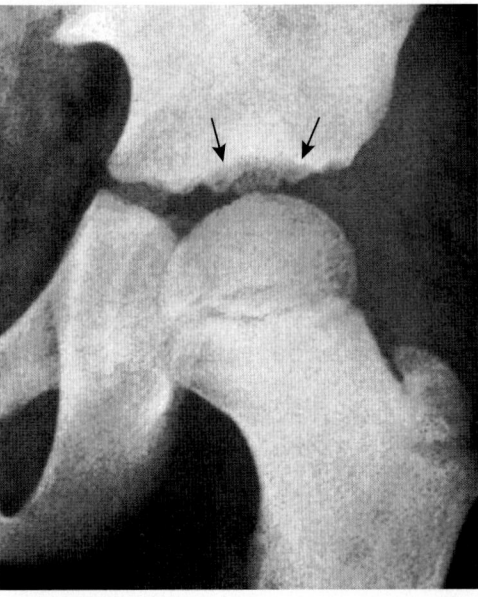

FIGURE 163-43. Normal irregular margins of the acetabulum *(arrows)* in a 6-year-old boy.

roof develops from confluence of individual bony foci near the end of the first decade.

Accessory Ossification Centers

Accessory centers of ossification may develop in cartilage in the spine of the ischium and also in the rim of the acetabulum (*"os acetabuli"* or *"os marginale superius acetabuli"*) just below the anterior inferior iliac spine. Os acetabuli may be seen in up to 20% of patients. These centers usually become visible between the 14th and

18th years (Fig. 163-44), after which they fuse with the main body of the ischium and ilium, respectively. Rarely, an os acetabuli persists as a separate ossicle. The rare *os acetabuli centrale* is a separate ossification center, or group of centers, that appears during puberty in the central portion of the triradiate in the wall of the acetabulum. Accessory ossification centers may also form at the pubic symphysis and superior pubic ramus.

Ischiopubic Synchondrosis

Ossification of the cartilage in the ischiopubic synchondrosis is extremely variable in both velocity and pattern.

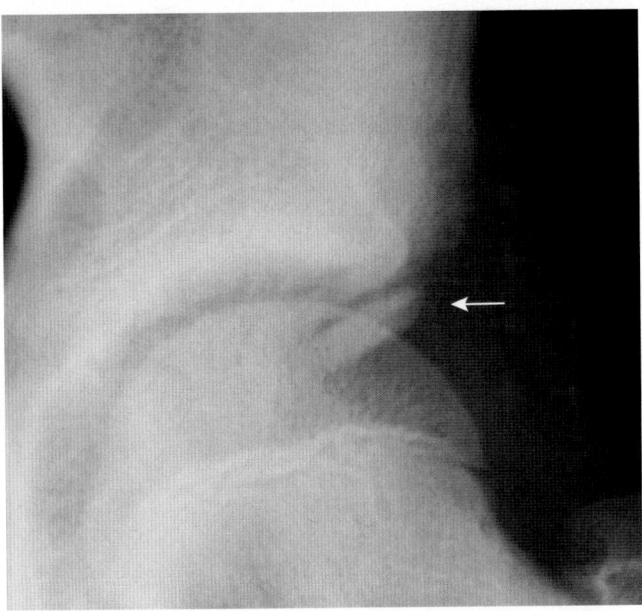

FIGURE 163-44. Os acetabuli marginalis superior *(arrow)* in the cartilaginous rim of the acetabulum of a 14-year-old girl. These normal separate marginal ossicles should not be mistaken for fracture fragments or calciferous foci in the soft tissues. (From Keats TE: An Atlas of Normal Roentgen Variants That May Simulate Disease, 7th ed. St. Louis, Mosby, 2001.)

Enlargement of the ischiopubic synchondrosis is usually an asymptomatic normal variant; however, this finding has received considerable attention in the literature. Regardless of its etiology, the prognosis of the finding of a swollen ischiopubic synchondrosis appears to be uniformly favorable.

Caffey and Ross found that bilateral fusion of the ischiopubic synchondrosis was complete in 6% of children at 4 years of age and in 83% of children at 12 years. At 6 to 8 years of age during its peak, unilateral swelling was seen at the ischiopubic synchondrosis (Fig. 163-45) in 22% of children and bilateral swelling in 45%. Caffey and Ross concluded that swelling preceded closure of the synchondrosis in most, and perhaps all, cases. The swellings lasted from 1 to 3 years. Irregular mineralization was present in about 42% of all subjects between ages 4 and 11, but was never present without swelling and tended to develop in the more pronounced examples of swelling. Occasionally, an independent supernumerary ossification center developed in the ischiopubic synchondrosis (Fig. 163-46).

Cawley and associates found accumulation of radionuclide on bone scans to vary in intensity and, frequently, to be asymmetric in the ischiopubic synchondrosis area in healthy children during the period of beginning, but incomplete, fusion (see Fig. 163-45). Uptake is less than at the adjacent triradiate cartilage. On MRI, slightly increased T2 signal and mild enhancement may be seen within an enlarged ischiopubic synchondrosis (Fig. 163-47).

Patients have been reported in whom regional pain and tenderness and impaired locomotion were associated with irregular mineralization and swelling of the ischiopubic synchondrosis. This clinical picture and the associated roentgen findings have previously been called ischiopubic osteochondrosis (van Neck disease) in the belief that it is analogous in pathogenesis to an ischemic necrosis, such as Perthes disease. Junge and Heuck noted the considerable frequency with which the radiographic changes occur in asymptomatic school-age children, beginning about the age of 5 years. These

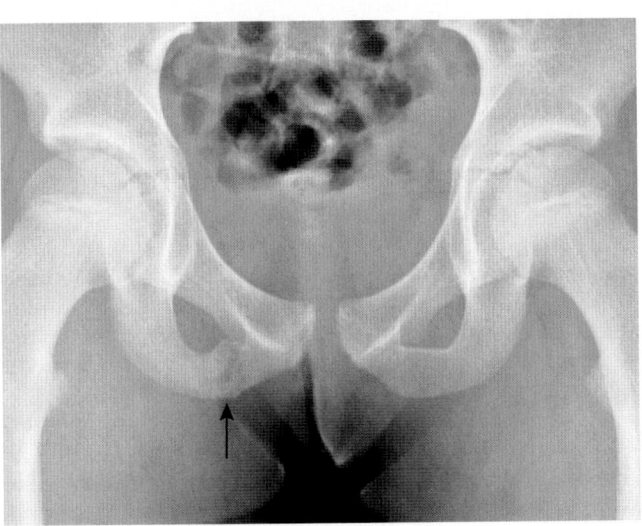

A

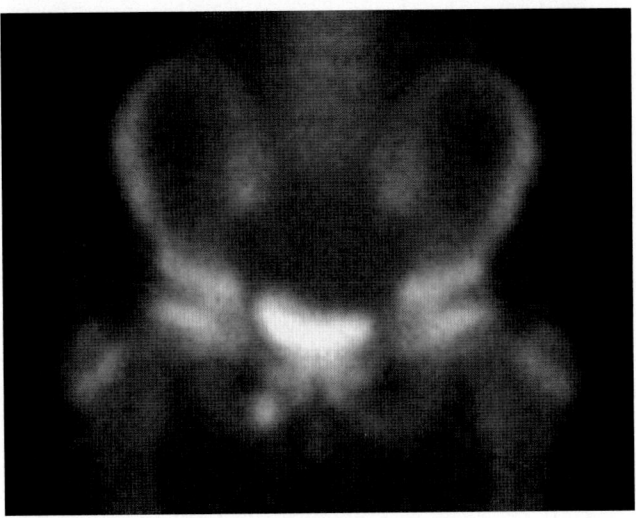

B

FIGURE 163-45. Asymmetric ischiopubic synchondrosis in an asymptomatic 12-year-old girl. **A,** The right ischiopubic synchondrosis *(arrow)* is enlarged on radiography. **B,** Corresponding increased activity is seen on bone scan.

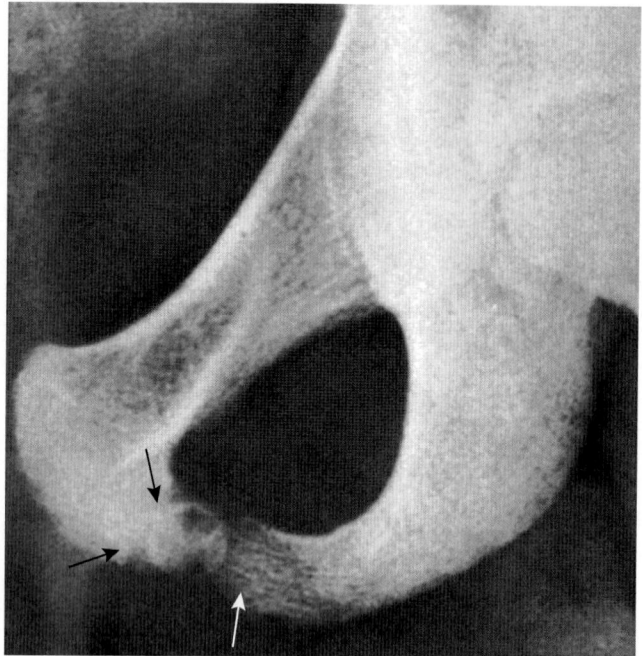

FIGURE 163-46. Independent supernumerary circular ossification center *(arrows)* in the ischiopubic synchondrosis of an asymptomatic 8-year-old boy.

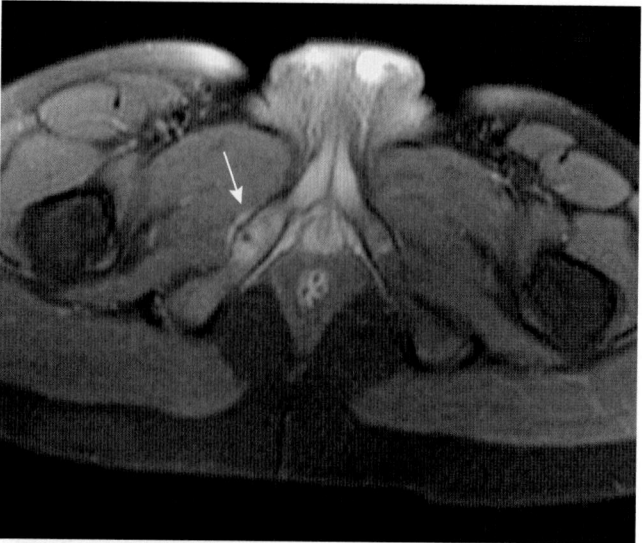

FIGURE 163-47. Asymmetric enlargement of the right ischiopubic synchondrosis in an asymptomatic 4-year-old boy. T1-weighted MR image with fat saturation and gadolinium shows mild enhancement of bone and soft tissues at the enlarged synchondrosis *(arrow)*.

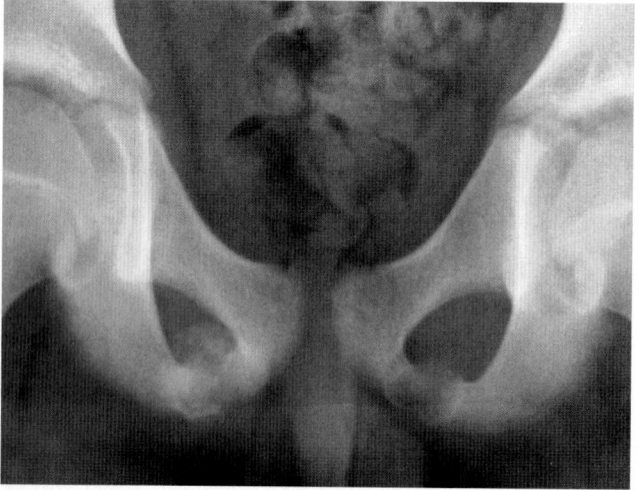

A

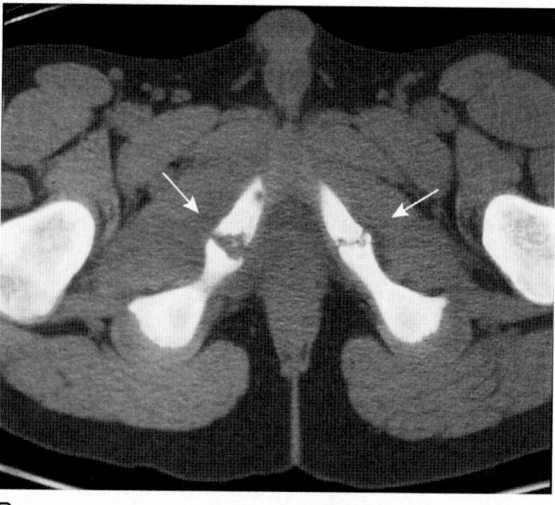

B

FIGURE 163-48. A, Radiograph showing bilaterally enlarged ischiopubic synchondroses in an 11-year-old male soccer player with right groin pain. The ischiopubic synchondrosis is larger on the symptomatic side. **B,** Irregularity of the ischiopubic synchondroses is seen on CT *(arrows)*.

authors, as well as Byers, reported no evidence of inflammation or other pathologic change in material removed from a "swollen" ischiopubic synchondrosis. Current thinking is that the swollen ischiopubic synchondrosis is not related to ischemia. The abnormality is believed to arise, near the time of fusion, from microtrauma resulting from excessive or repeated activity of the adductor muscles that insert into the region of the synchondrosis. This region is also a classic site of stress fracture in the adult, and the lesion has been considered a pediatric equivalent of this in an appropriate clinical setting of local pain and progressive radiographic signs. This

theory is supported by a recent study from Europe by Herneth and colleagues, in which unilaterality of swollen ischiopubic synchondroses was associated with the footedness (right vs. left dominant) of child soccer players (Fig. 163-48).

As the ischiopubic synchondrosis is a metaphyseal equivalent, it is a potential site for osteomyelitis. The diagnosis of osteomyelitis has also been made in some children with swelling of the ischiopubic junction, supported by patient symptoms and physical examination, positive blood cultures, elevated erythrocyte sedimentation rates, change from normal radiographs to

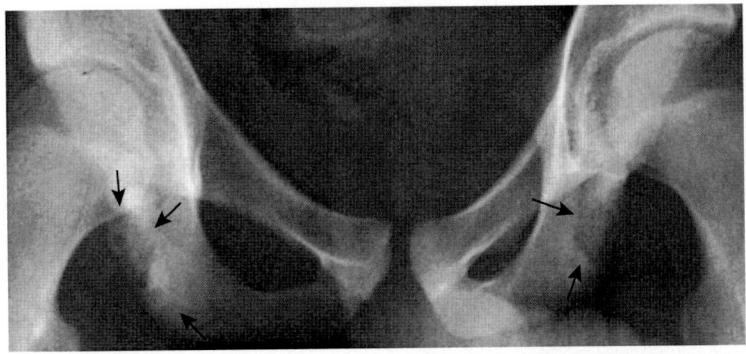 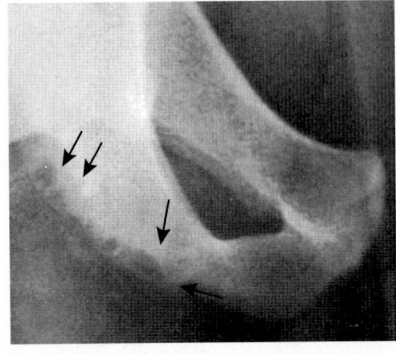

FIGURE 163-49. Irregularities in both ischia of asymptomatic 12- and 11-year-old boys. **A,** The right ischium is irregularly rarefied at the tuberosity and slightly caudad into the ramus *(arrows)*. The tuberosity of the left ischium is evenly rarefied. **B,** There is "bubbly" rarefaction in the right tuberosity and caudad into the ramus *(arrows)*.

focal irregularity before healing, and scintigraphic findings that differed from those in normal ischiopubic synchondroses (positive blood pool images and activity equal to or exceeding the triradiate cartilage on delayed images). In these cases, too, the prognosis has been favorable with appropriate antibiotic treatment.

Notwithstanding the previous comments, in most cases, however, identification of an enlarged ischiopubic synchondrosis on radiographs is an incidental finding unrelated to patient symptoms and unrelated to the reason for imaging. The lesion is usually of no clinical consequence, but may be mistaken by inexperienced readers for a traumatic, infectious, or neoplastic lesion.

> Asymmetry of the ischiopubic synchondrosis is a very common normal variant and is usually an incidental finding unrelated to patient symptoms.

Ischium

Irregularities in the posterolateral edge of the ischium may also be observed; occasionally during preadolescence, the lateral borders of the body of the ischium and its inferior ramus show marked irregularity both in the margin and in density (Fig. 163-49). The two sides may be unequally affected. During growth and before fusion of the body of the ischium, the ischial apophysis is scalelike at the inferior margin of the ischium. The adjacent ischial metaphyseal equivalent is a provisional zone of calcification analogous to the provisional zones of calcification in the metaphyses of all the long bones; it is not cortical lamellar bone.

The ischial spine, projecting posteriorly, usually is not visible in frontal radiographs of the pelvis. The lesser sciatic notch lies below it and sometimes appears as an indentation on the lateral margin of the ischium (Fig. 163-50), at the region where the ischial irregularities are most common.

Some of the "variations" in mineralization are almost certainly sequelae to the normal vigorous activity of children and the response to minor tendon avulsions from sites where cartilage has yet to change to bone.

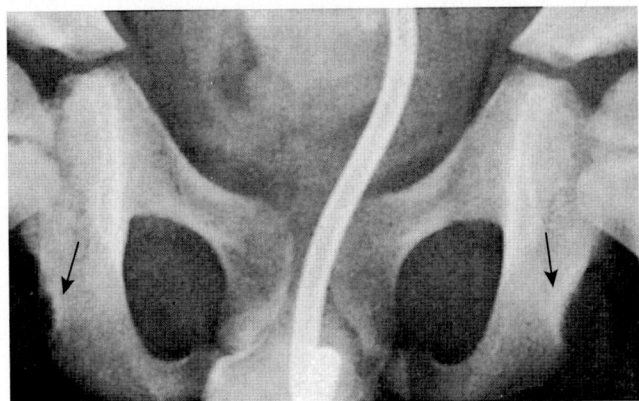

FIGURE 163-50. Conspicuously deep and large lesser sciatic notches with sclerotic edges *(arrows)* in an asymptomatic 4-year-old boy.

These findings are comparable to minor epiphyseal separations. A few weeks of clinical observation during limited activity serve to resolve the significance of the findings when local symptoms were the reason for examination.

Pubic Rami

Delayed and irregular mineralization of the pubic rami may be present at birth, with subsequent mineralization from several ossification centers (Fig. 163-51). Vertical, radiolucent clefts occasionally noted as incidental findings in pelvis radiographs (Fig. 163-52) probably represent bars of nonossified cartilage between expanding ossification centers. Caffey and Madell identified this anomaly in 1.6% of children studied. The medial edges of the bodies of the pubic bones are often irregularly mineralized during the growth period.

Pseudotumors

Radiolucent pseudotumors may be seen in areas of the pelvis that are relatively radiolucent and devoid of trabeculae— the pubis, iliac fossa, and sacral ala.

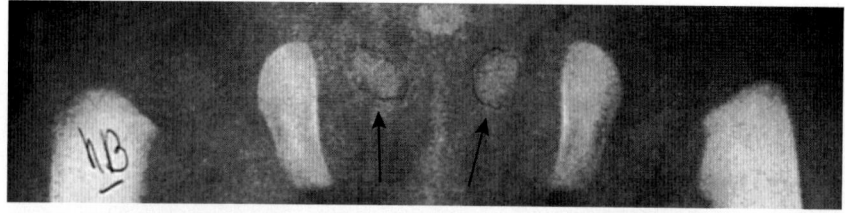

A

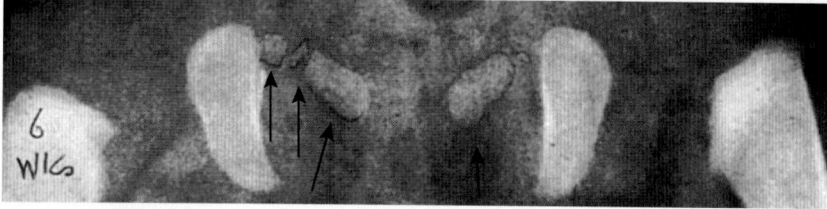

B

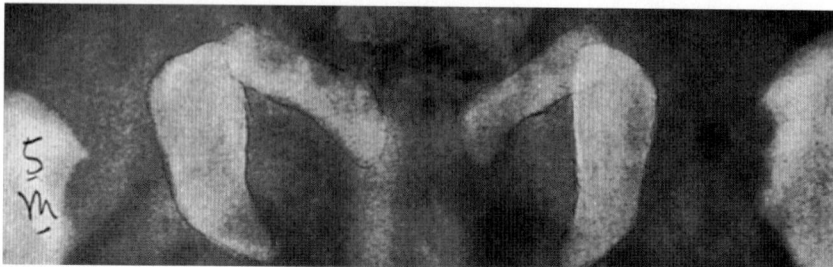

C

FIGURE 163-51. Retarded and irregular mineralization of both superior pubic rami. **A,** Neonatal. In the pubic rami, ossification is confined on each side to a round center *(arrows)*; most of the superior pubic rami are entirely radiolucent because ossification has not yet occurred. **B,** At 6 weeks. Ossification is now increased in both superior rami, but it is still incomplete and irregular *(arrows)*. On the right side there are at least three large independent ossification centers with radiolucent clefts between them. **C,** At 5 months. The superior rami are evenly and extensively ossified, but there is still cartilage between the dorsal ends of the rami and their ischial bodies. The changes in the pubic bones are chance findings in a patient who also had bilateral dysplasia and dislocation of the hips. (From Ribbing S: Zur ätlologie der osteochondrosis dissecans. Acta Radiol 1944;25:732-755.)

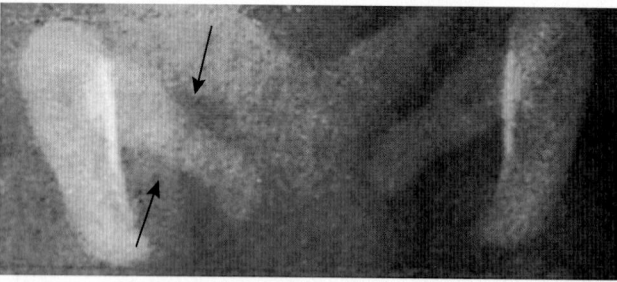

A

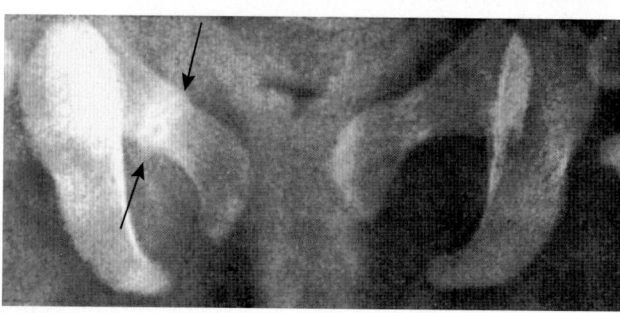

B

FIGURE 163-52. Congenital "strip" defect in the superior ramus of the pubis; these lesions may be unilateral or bilaterally symmetric. **A,** At birth, there is a vertical band of diminished density in the middle third of the pubic ramus *(arrows)*. **B,** At 6 months, at the same site there is a narrower radiolucent band, which is now bordered by strips of increased density *(arrows)*. The patient was always asymptomatic, and palpation disclosed no signs of fracture at this site.

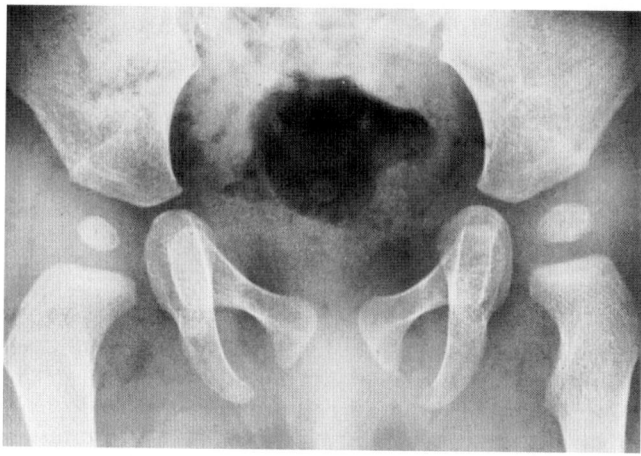

FIGURE 163-53. Slight asymmetry in development of the femoral heads in an infant. (From Keats TE: An Atlas of Normal Roentgen Variants That May Simulate Disease, 7th ed. St. Louis, Mosby, 2001.)

HIP

Asymmetric Appearance of Femoral Head Ossification

A slight disparity in the timing of ossification, the size of the femoral head ossifications centers, or both is normal (Fig. 163-53). In up to 30% of infants 3 to 6 months of age, there is a disparity of at least 2 mm between the two sides.

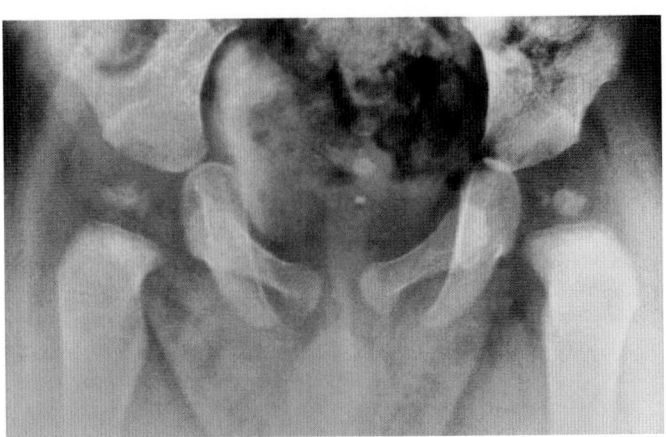 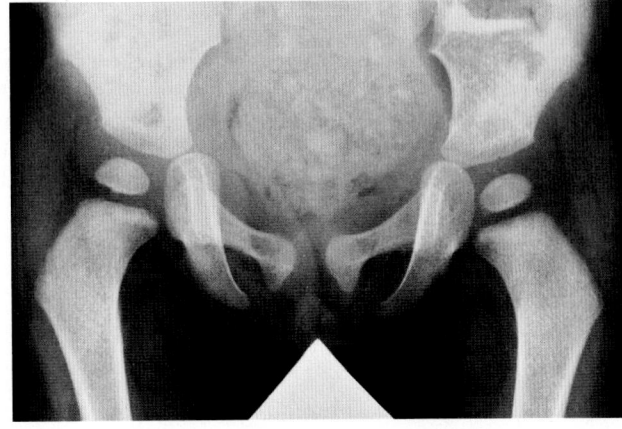

FIGURE 163-54. A, Irregular ossification of the femoral head in an 18-month old infant. **B,** By 30 months, the femoral heads had coalesced into a normal single nucleus. (From Keats TE: An Atlas of Normal Roentgen Variants That May Simulate Disease, 7th ed. St. Louis, Mosby, 2001.)

Irregularity of Femoral Head Ossification

The ossification center for the head of the femur appears at about 4 months of age and enlarges with time. As ossification fills in the hemispheric cartilage of the head, the center may exhibit irregularities of form and density in the absence of disease (Fig. 163-54). Ossification may begin with coarse stippling and progress, as the size increases, to irregularities along the margin. A bifid or split femoral head is a rare variant (Fig. 163-55). A notch (separate from the fovea capitis) at the vertex of the femoral head is not uncommon. The variations may occur unilaterally, but generally they are bilateral so that comparison with the asymptomatic side, in questions of disease, may avoid misdiagnosis. Before the ossification center has rounded out fully, some flattening of the contour may be observed where subsequently the fovea capitis can be recognized. Variations in ossification and contour of the femoral head may mimic avascular necrosis (Perthes disease) or skeletal dysplasia.

Consideration must also be given to density changes caused by superimposition of components of the bone constituting the acetabular cavity and channels for nutrient vessels in the ischium, which can simulate destructive lesions in the femoral head when superimposition occurs.

Femoral Neck-Shaft Angle

The femoral neck has an anterior deviation from the coronal plane (the angle of anteversion) greatest in early infancy and decreasing to approximately 23 degrees in late childhood. The angle of the femoral neck and the shaft in frontal projection decreases from approximately 180 degrees at birth to 120 to 140 degrees in later childhood. Ambulation plays a role in these changes, and abnormal angulation and anteversion are usually evident in older children who are nonambulatory. A child who is non–weight bearing from infancy usually retains large angles between the shaft and the neck of the femur (coxa valga). Coxa valga can be the consequence of many disease processes.

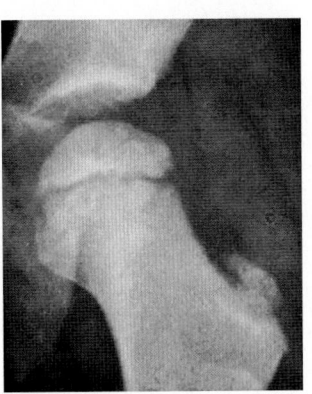 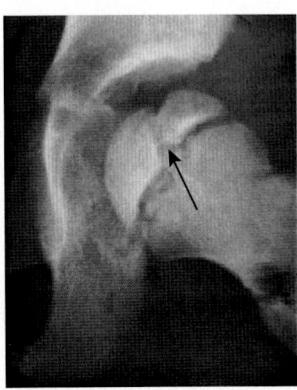

FIGURE 163-55. Factitious splitting of the femoral head in an asymptomatic 4-year-old girl. **A,** In frontal projection, the femoral head image is normal. **B,** In lateral externally rotated position, the femoral head image is divided longitudinally into two unequal segments by a strip of decreased density *(arrow)* that represents the synchondrosis between the two ossification centers that developed one behind the other ventrodorsally.

Rotation of the femur affects the neck-shaft angle, which is displayed on a radiograph. External rotation of the femur increases the femoral neck-shaft angle and may factitiously suggest coxa valga. The position of the greater trochanter may help differentiate true coxa valga from external rotation. With true coxa valga, the greater trochanter projects laterally rather than being superimposed on the underlying femur, whereas with external rotation, the greater trochanter is rotated posteriorly and projects over the underlying femur.

Radiolucent Defects in the Femoral Neck

Occasionally, radiolucent defects with sclerotic borders are observed incidentally in the femoral neck; some that have been followed radiographically have resolved much as those of benign cortical defects. Herniation pits ("Pitt's pits") may occasionally be seen in older children.

Trochanters

The centers for the greater and lesser trochanters are frequently irregularly mineralized (Fig. 163-56). The growth plate for the lesser trochanter sometimes appears wide. Avulsions of the lesser trochanter are uncommon. When they do occur, the lesser trochanteric fragment is displaced.

KNEE

Cortical Irregularity of the Distal Femoral Metaphysis

Irregularity of the cortex of the posteromedial distal femoral metaphysis is a common normal finding that can

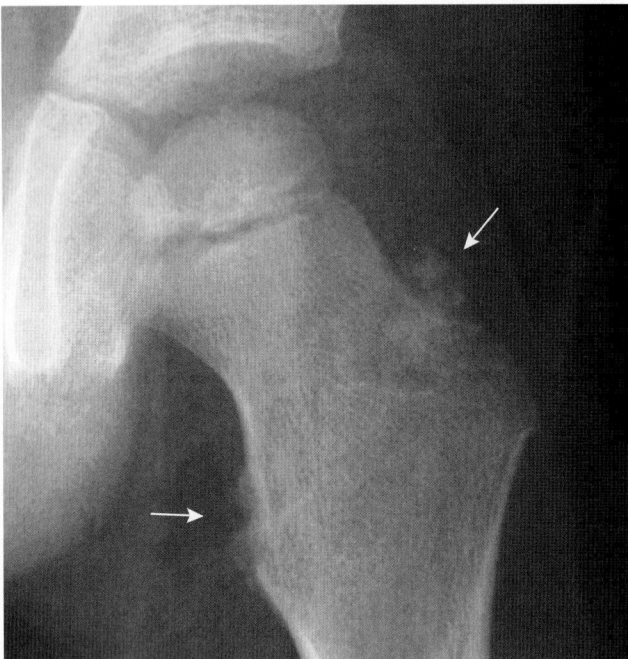

FIGURE 163-56. Normal irregularities in ossification *(arrows)* of the trochanteric ossification centers.

easily be mistaken for disease. Cystlike cortical defects are common at this location, as are proliferative tuglike lesions probably related to the adductor muscle insertions. Particularly on anteroposterior radiographs, these findings may have a misleading ominous appearance.

Cystlike cortical defects ("*cortical desmoids*") occur frequently at the posteromedial aspect of the distal metaphysis of the femur, lateral to the supracondylar ridge. Histologically, cortical desmoids are similar, if not identical, to fibrous cortical defects occurring elsewhere, with whorls of connective tissue and frequent multinuclear giant cells. These defects are most commonly identified in the latter half of the first decade and early in the second decade of life. The frequency of these defects in normal children (up to 40% or greater) indicates that they will be found in children suffering from a variety of diseases associated with destructive lesions of bone and will be a common finding on radiographs obtained for any indication. Generally, their benign nature can be recognized by the radiographic characteristics and location (Fig. 163-57). CT or MRI may provide more definitive information about their nature (Fig. 163-58). Cortical desmoids may show increased activity on bone scans.

The defects have a round or oval, radiolucent, cystlike appearance when projected en face. When projected in profile, they appear most frequently as shallow superficial defects in the cortex extending into it from the outer surface (see Fig. 163-57). Classic fibrous cortical defects appear similar and are common at this location. Fibrous cortical defects are less consistent in location, are often asymmetric, and migrate away from the growth plate with maturation. Cortical desmoids are more consistent in location, do not migrate away from the growth plate with maturation, and tend to be symmetric.

Local external thickenings with irregular margins ("*avulsive cortical irregularity*") are common findings at the posteromedial aspect of the distal femoral metaphysis along the medial supracondylar ridge in healthy adolescents (Fig. 163-59). This site corresponds to the

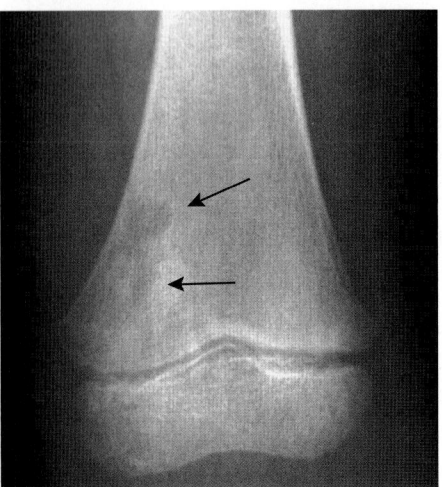 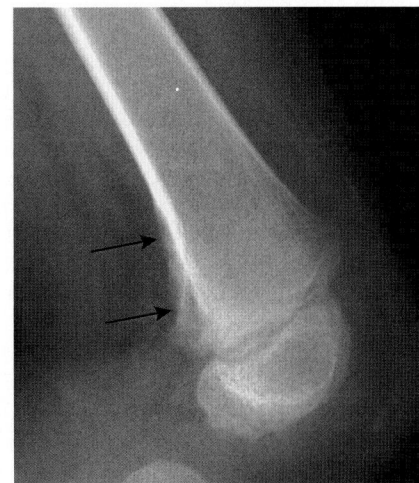 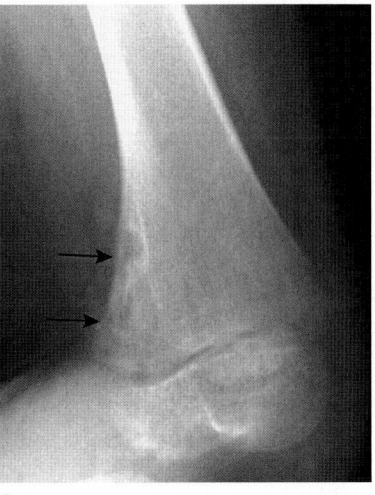

A   B   C

FIGURE 163-57. "Cortical desmoid" of the distal femoral metaphysis in a 4-year-old girl. The defect is posteromedial. **A,** The anteroposterior view shows an ill-defined lucency *(arrows)*. **B,** The lateral view shows irregularity *(arrows)* of the posterior margin of the distal humeral metaphysis. **C,** An oblique view shows the cortical lucencies *(arrows)*.

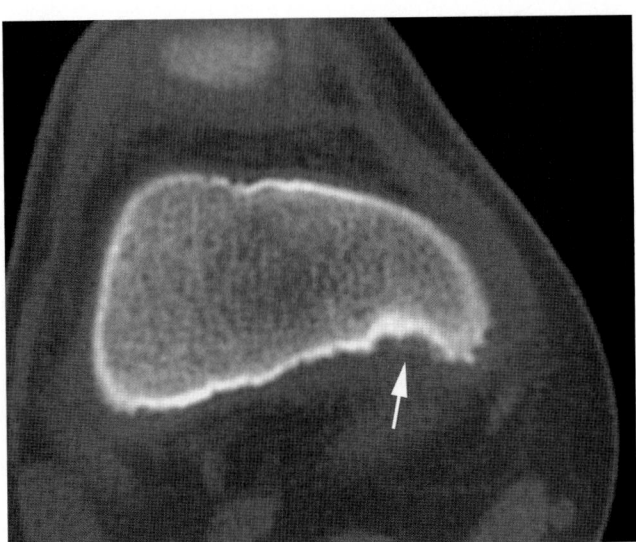

FIGURE 163-58. CT of a cortical desmoid *(arrow)* in an asymptomatic 6-year-old girl.

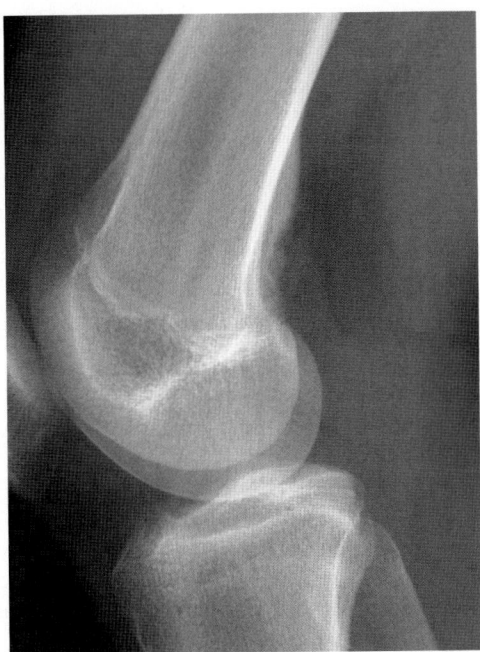

FIGURE 163-59. Avulsive cortical irregularity of the posteromedial distal femoral metaphysis in an adolescent.

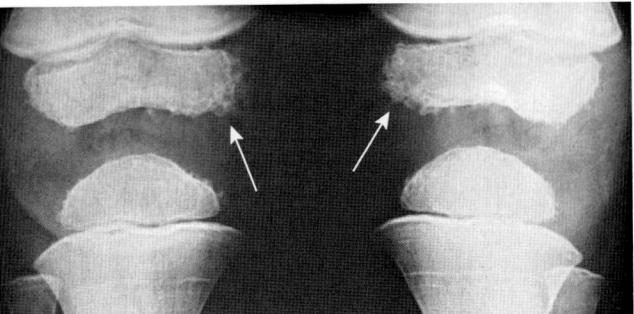

FIGURE 163-60. Normal irregular mineralization on the margins of the ossification centers *(arrows)* in the distal epiphyses of the femurs of a 3-year-old boy.

cluded that the pathogenic mechanism responsible for the lesion was repeated microavulsions of cortical fragments at the site of insertion of a portion of the tendon of the adductor magnus muscle. This opinion has been supported by others. In any case, this finding is of no clinical significance other than the potential for misidentification as a more ominous process.

> Cortical desmoids, or avulsive cortical irregularity, are common findings at the distal femoral metaphysis. Characteristic posteromedial location, characteristic appearance, and lack of correlating symptoms aid in differentiation from true pathology.

Irregular Ossification of the Distal Femoral Epiphysis

In the epiphyseal ossification center that is present at the lower end of the femur in almost all term infants at birth, extension in width occurs rapidly between the second and sixth years. As a result, the lateral and medial margins are commonly irregular and ragged (Fig. 163-60). In lateral projection, normal distal femoral ossification centers may have a rough, fringelike margin (Fig. 163-61). Accessory ossification centers may persist at the margins of cartilage-shaft junctions when ossification is almost complete (Fig. 163-62). In older children, marginal mineralization of the femoral condyles is characteristically uneven and is often associated with independent ossification centers beyond the edge of the main bony mass (Fig. 163-63). The radiographic appearance simulates that of osteochondritis dissecans. Caffey and colleagues found this variant in approximately 30% of healthy children when the knees were examined in tunnel and lateral projections. The pattern and distribution of these extra, normal, independent ossification centers in the distal femoral epiphyseal cartilage is shown schematically in Figure 163-64. This defect is much more common on the lateral than on the medial condyle, in contradistinction to the findings in osteochondritis dissecans. In addition, these irregularities are seen in children younger than the usual age for this disease.

The posterior margin of the lateral femoral condyle ossification center may be irregular and slightly flattened

insertion of the adductor magnus muscle. Findings are often present on both sides, but may not be symmetric. The abnormality is probably the result of repetitive, vigorous, muscular activity. The finding may mimic neoplasm, but usually can be differentiated by its bilaterality, characteristic appearance, absence of any adjacent soft tissue swelling, and lack of related symptoms. Bufkin pathologically found the lesion to be a localized segment of periosteal thickening embedded within the cortical wall. It was made up of proliferating fibrous tissue that merged imperceptibly with the overlying thickened periosteum. Small fragments of resorbing bone were often present in the proliferating mass of fibrous tissue near the periosteum. He con-

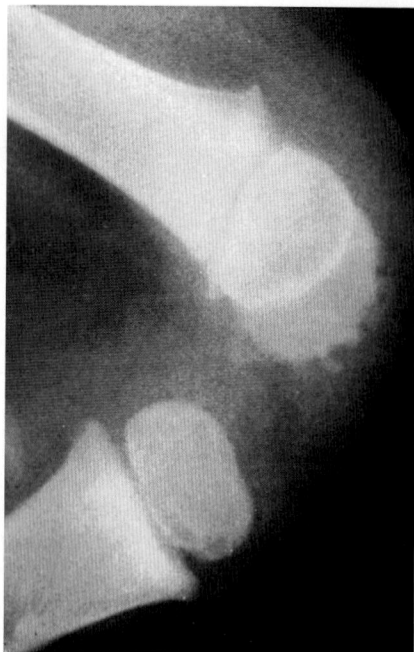

FIGURE 163-61. Lateral projection of the left knee of an asymptomatic 3½-year-old boy. The femoral condyle has a rough, fringelike edge as a result of partial fusion with several marginal accessory ossification centers in the contiguous epiphyseal cartilage. Similar marginal centers were present at both ends of the ossification center in the frontal projection.

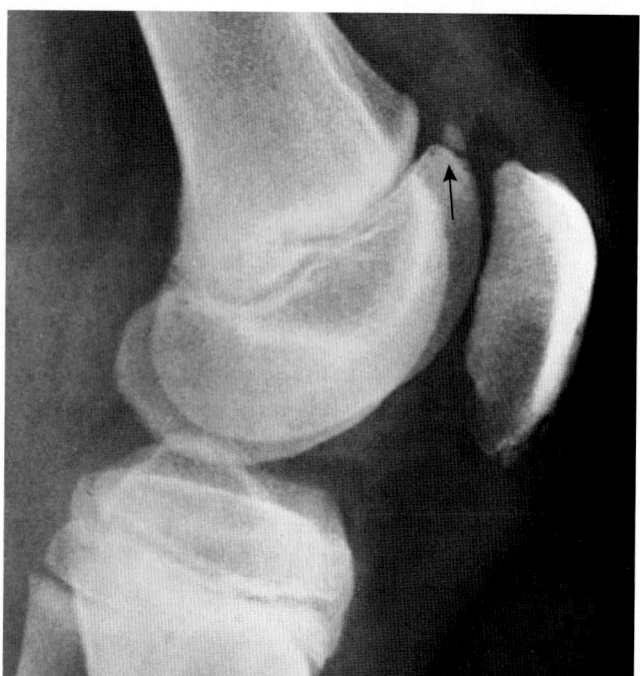

FIGURE 163-62. Small triangular independent accessory ossification center at the proximal ventral edge of the greater condyle (arrow) of an asymptomatic 13-year-old boy. Smaller scale accessory centers are also visible at the ventral edge of the lower pole of the patella.

in appearance. This finding may be evident on radiographs, CT, or MRI. The finding simulates osteochondritis dissecans. Normal developmental irregularity tends to be more posterior and symmetric and occurs in younger children. It is most common at 8 to 10 years of

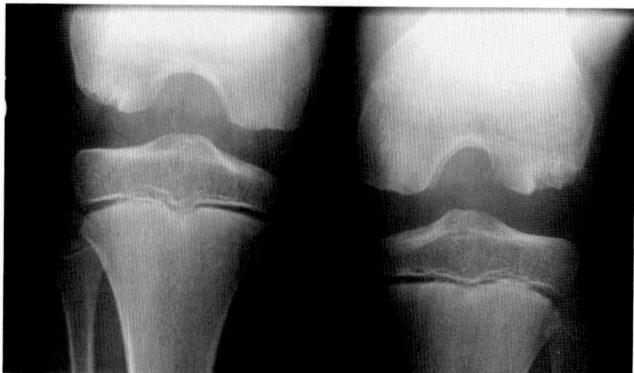

FIGURE 163-63. Normal developmental irregularity of the posterior aspect of the femoral condyles seen on a notch view in a 10-year-old boy. The defects are most prominent in the lateral condyles.

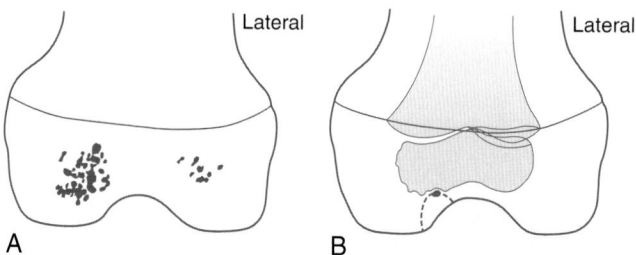

FIGURE 163-64. A, Sites of focal extra ossification centers in the left distal femoral epiphyseal cartilages of 291 children recorded on a tracing of an adult femur. **B,** Tracing of the distal ends of a child's femur, superimposed on a tracing of the distal end of an adult femur, that shows an accessory ossification center (black dot) in the cartilage of the epiphysis just beyond the caudal edge of the main ossification center. The dotted line indicates projected growth of the accessory center. (From Ribbing S: Zur ätlologie der osteochondrosis dissecans. Acta Radiol 1944;25:732-755.)

age. The normal variant is differentiated from osteochondritis dissecans on MRI by its position in the inferocentral posterior femoral condyles, intact overlying cartilage, a large residual cartilage model, accessory ossification centers and spiculation, and absence of adjacent bone marrow edema (Fig. 163-65).

> **Developmental irregularity of the femoral condyles is much more common on the lateral than on the medial condyle, in contradistinction to the findings in osteochondritis dissecans. In addition, these irregularities are seen in children younger than the usual age for osteochondritis dissecans.**

Popliteal Groove

The popliteal groove is a normal marginal defect that appears on the posterolateral aspect of the outer condyle in the prepubertal period (Fig. 163-66); at times it may be very prominent. This groove carries the tendon of the popliteal muscle and is never visible during infancy or early childhood.

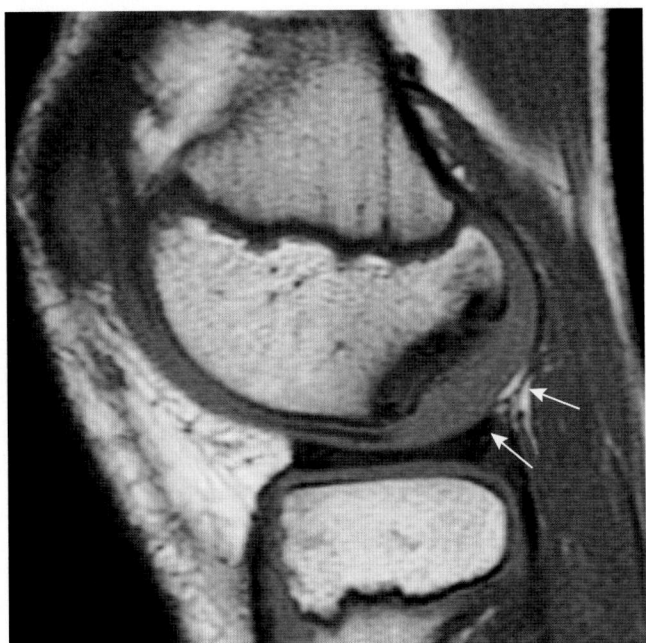

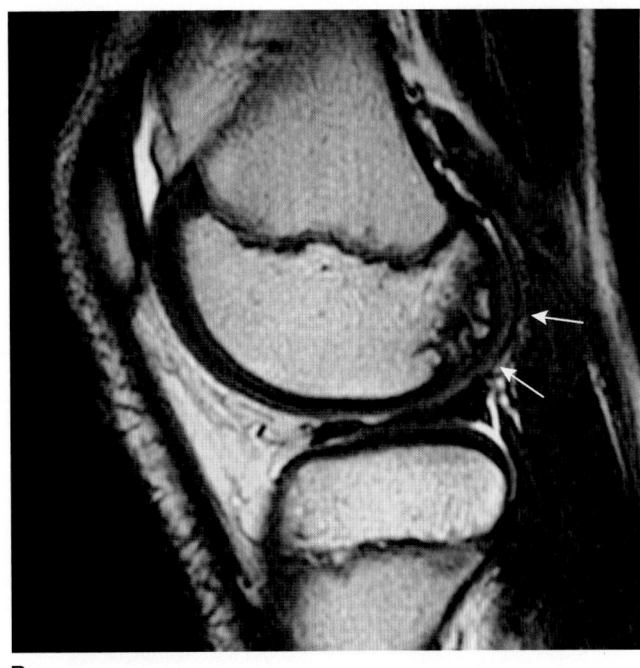

A   B

FIGURE 163-65. Irregular ossification of the posterior aspect of the femoral condyles in an 11-year-old boy. **A,** T1-weighted MR image shows large defect *(arrows)*. Cartilage fills the defect and has a normal contour over the defect. **B,** T2-weighted MR image shows a defect that is not as large; however, multiple small accessory ossification centers are present within the defect *(arrows)*.

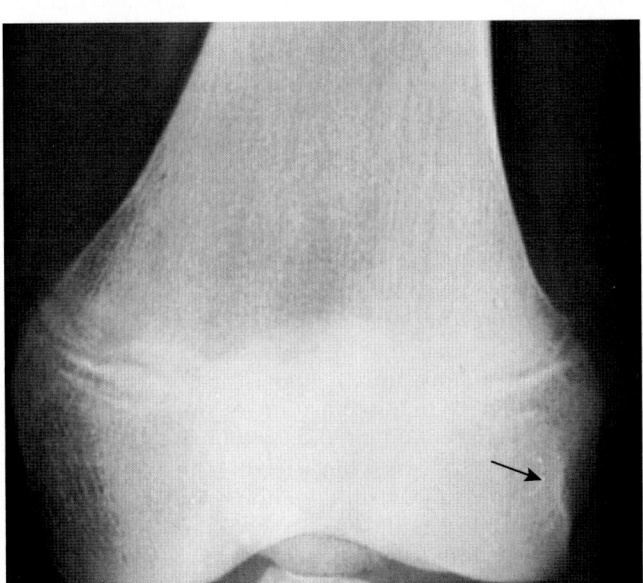

FIGURE 163-66. Normal popliteal groove *(arrow)* in the posterolateral wall of the lateral femoral condyle of an asymptomatic 11-year-old girl.

Femoral Condyles

During late childhood, when the intercondylar fossa becomes deeper, lateral projections of the distal femoral epiphysis show the anterior segment to be more radiolucent than the remainder. This reflects the fact that the posterior portion of the epiphysis is wider than the anterior, and the x-rays have to traverse four layers of cortex (the lateral and medial walls of each of the two condyles) instead of only two anteriorly. The lateral condyle can be differentiated from the medial in lateral projections of the knee because it is relatively flat in comparison with the rounded configuration of the latter.

Sesamoid Bones

The patella is the largest sesamoid bone of the body, lying within the tendon of the quadriceps muscle. Variations of the patella are discussed later. Two other sesamoids of the knee occur as normal variants, the fabella and cyamella. The fabella (more common) forms in the tendon of the lateral head of the gastrocnemius muscle. The cyamella (less common) forms in the tendon of the popliteus muscle. A fabella is best seen on a lateral view (Fig. 163-67). The cyamella is found at the edge of the lateral condyle of the femur in the popliteal groove (Fig. 163-68). Fabellar syndrome is characterized by intermittent pain at the posterolateral knee accentuated by extension and localized tenderness over the fabella accentuated by compression.

Irregular Patellar Ossification

The patellar ossification normally develops from several foci. The patella is often granular early. Its edges may be irregular during childhood (Fig. 163-69). Following fusion of the focal centers, another center may develop in the superolateral portion of the bone and may persist as a distinct ossicle (Fig. 163-70). This variant, known as *bipartite patella*, is very common, occurring in 1% to 6% of the population. Ninety percent of those affected are male, and 40% have bilateral findings. Stress injury or acute fracture may occur at the synchondrosis between the superolateral ossicle and the patellar body, pro-

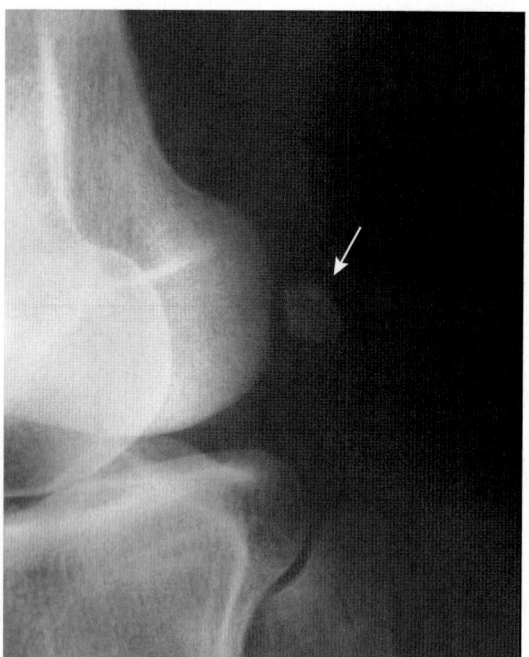

FIGURE 163-67. Fabella *(arrow)* in the lateral head of the gastrocnemius in its normal position, well separated from the femur itself.

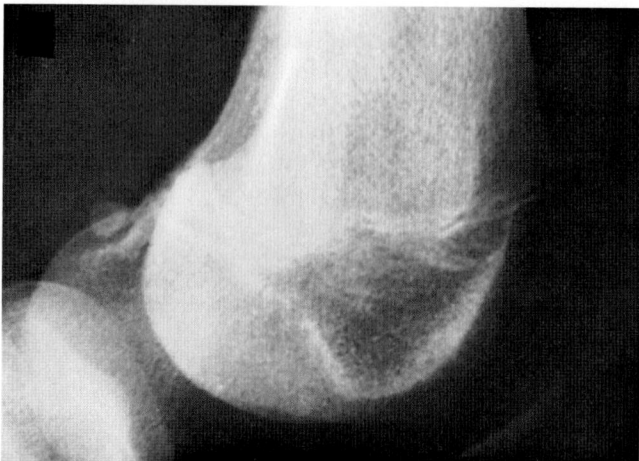

FIGURE 163-68. Sesamoid (cyamella). Small, partially embedded ossicle in the edge of the lateral femoral condyle of an asymptomatic 16-year-old boy. This ossicle appears to be in the position of the head of the popliteal muscle near its site of origin on the lateral femoral condyle. This is the normal position for this rare sesamoid of the popliteus.

ducing symptoms. Bipartite patella may be related to aberrant traction by the vastus lateralis muscle, which inserts into the patella at its upper and outer quadrant. The patella may also be tripartite.

Segmentation of the patella into anterior and posterior components has been described in multiple epiphyseal dysplasia, but has also been reported without reference to any associated skeletal abnormalities.

Irregular ossification of the lower pole of the patella is a common finding. It may be impossible to distinguish variation in ossification from old traumatic avulsion. Acute injuries will be symptomatic and accompanied by soft tissue swelling.

> **Although usually asymptomatic, bipartite patella may be complicated by stress injury or acute fracture at the synchondrosis between the superolateral ossicle and the patellar body, producing symptoms.**

Dorsal Defect of the Patella

Dorsal defect of the patella occurs in 1% of individuals. It is usually asymptomatic, but occasionally produces a dull ache. Focal defects of the patella occasionally occur in asymptomatic children, most commonly indenting the posterior aspect of the patella and seen as radiolucent defects in frontal projection (Fig. 163-71). The defects are 5 to 25 mm in diameter. On MRI, overlying cartilage is intact. As with bipartite patella, dorsal defects also occur in the superolateral portion of the bone, and also may relate to aberrant traction by the vastus lateralis muscle. Dorsal defect of the patella may be seen concomitantly with bipartite patella.

TIBIA AND FIBULA

Irregular Proximal Tibial Ossification Center

Anatomic variants are more common in the tibia than in the fibula at the knee. Irregular mineralization along the margins of the tibial ossification center is similar to that in the distal femoral epiphysis during periods of rapid transformation of cartilage to bone.

Tibial Tuberosity

A steplike notched defect appears in the upper anterior border of the tibia in lateral projection before ossification proceeds into the cartilaginous anterior tibial tubercle from the main proximal tibial ossification center. The tubercle may also be ossified from accessory centers that, before union, may simulate avulsed fragments of bone. When ossification of the anterior tibial process is nearly complete, the radiolucent cartilage still separating the process from the shaft may appear as a notch or a horizontal strip depending on the projection used (Figs. 163-72 and 163-73). Asymmetry of development on the two sides is common. External rotation tends to superimpose the thick cortex, extending to the anterior tibial crest, onto the lateral aspect of the bone. Projection of the partially fused tibial tubercle over the proximal tibial metaphysis produces a sclerotic pseudotumor.

Fibular Head Pseudotumor

The fibular head may have a lucent, expansile appearance mimicking a cystic lesion.

Variations in Tibial and Fibular Contour

Irregularity of the interosseous membrane may produce undulations of the lateral tibial or medial fibular cortex.

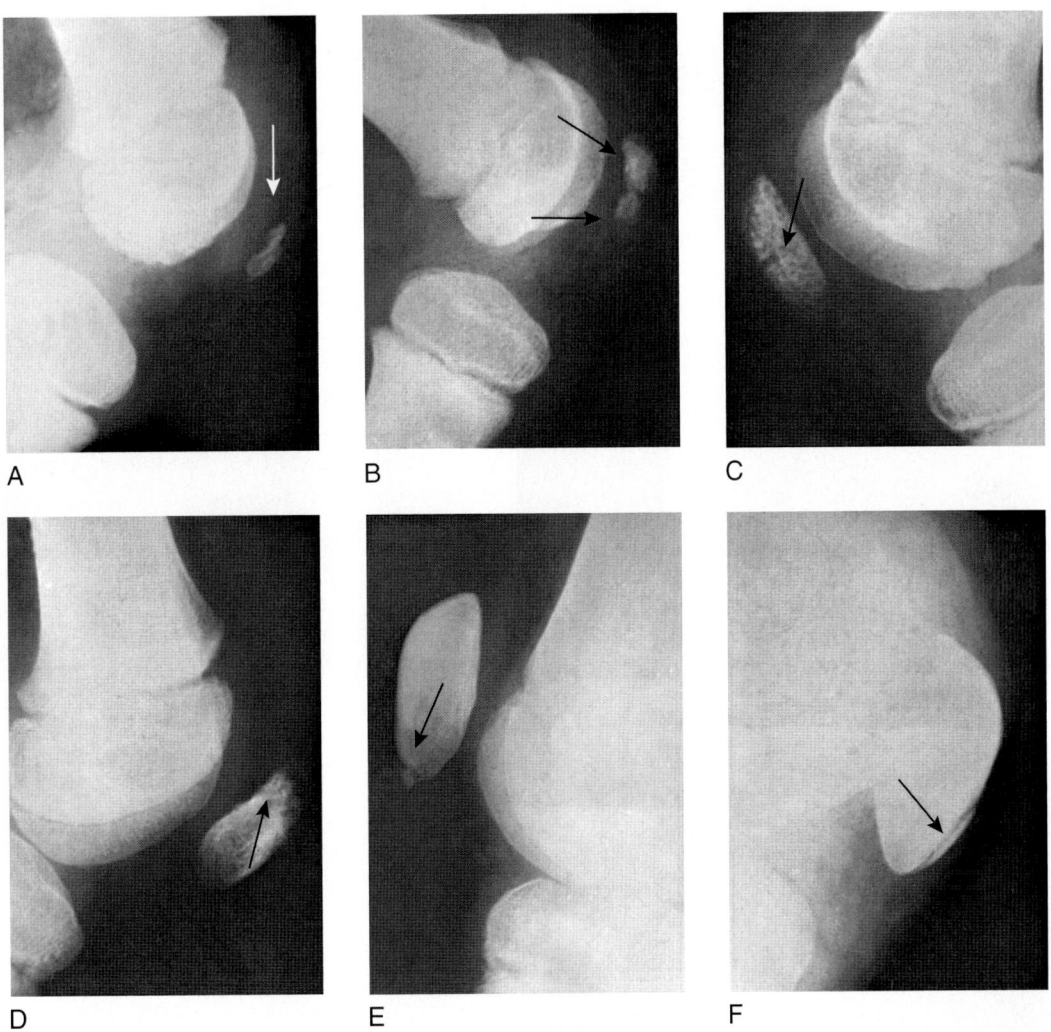

FIGURE 163-69. Normal variations in size, shape, and density of the patella *(arrows)* in healthy children at different ages. **A,** Small irregular patella of a 5-year-old boy. **B,** Multiple irregular centers in a 6-year-old girl. **C,** Generalized granular texture with partial segmentation in an 8-year-old girl. **D,** Irregularity in density of the superior third of the patella in an 8-year-old boy. **E,** Small separate ossicle at the inferior pole of the patella of an 11-year-old boy. **F,** Scalelike marginal ossicle on the anterior edge of the patella in a 9-year-old girl.

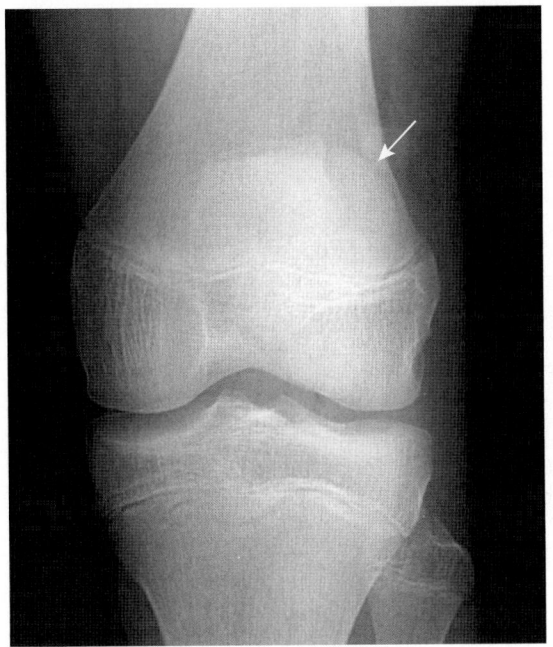

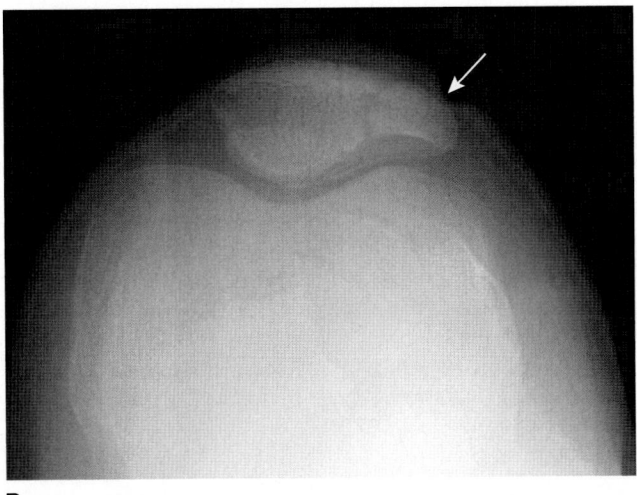

FIGURE 163-70. Anteroposterior **(A)** and sunrise **(B)** views of a bipartite patella in a 13-year-old boy. The accessory ossification center is superolateral *(arrows)*.

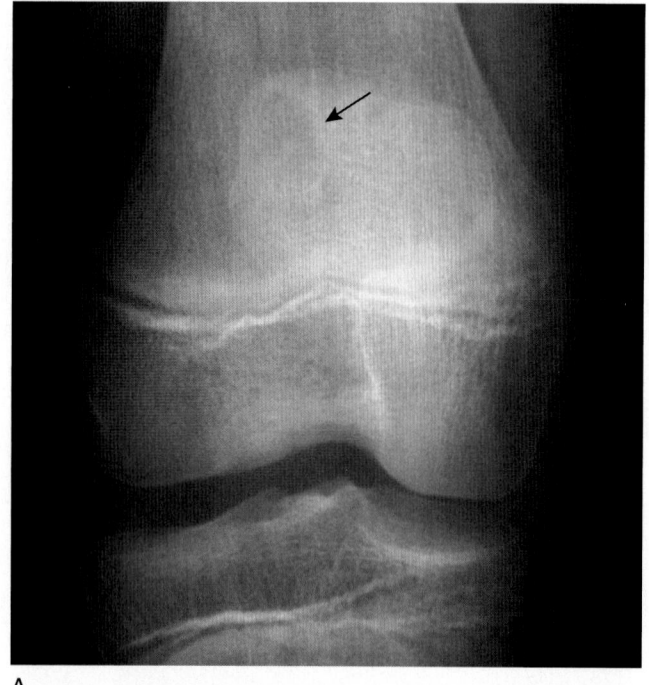

A

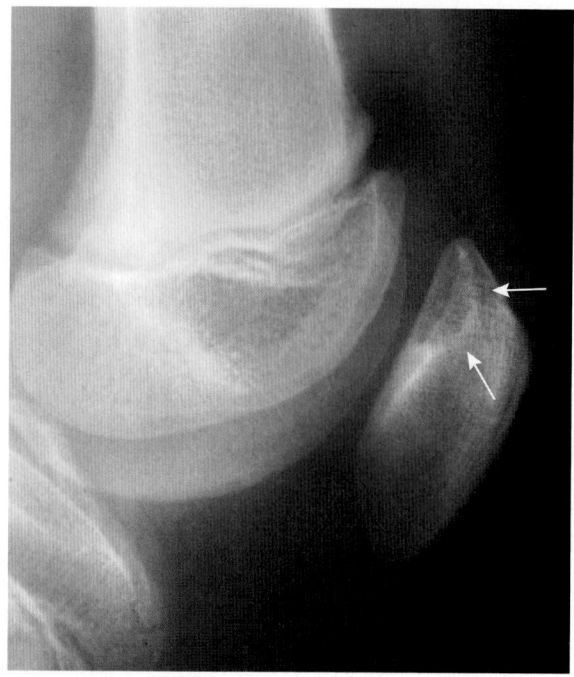

B

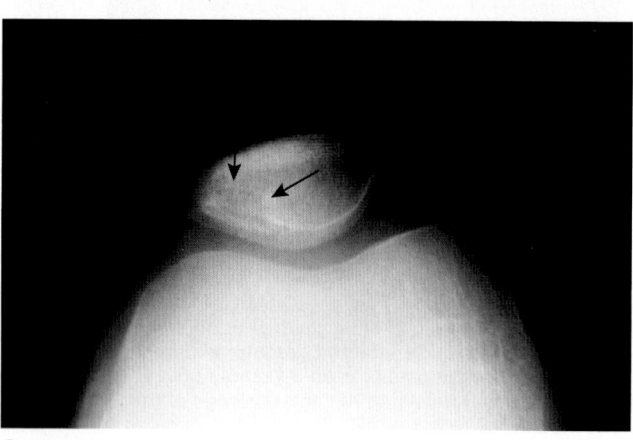

C

FIGURE 163-71. Dorsal defect of the patella. Anteroposterior **(A)**, lateral **(B)**, and sunrise **(C)** views of an 11-year-old girl with dorsal defect of the patella. The defect is at the posterior aspect of the superolateral portion of the patella *(arrows)*.

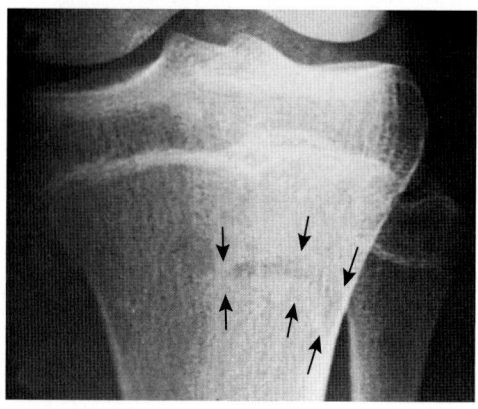

A

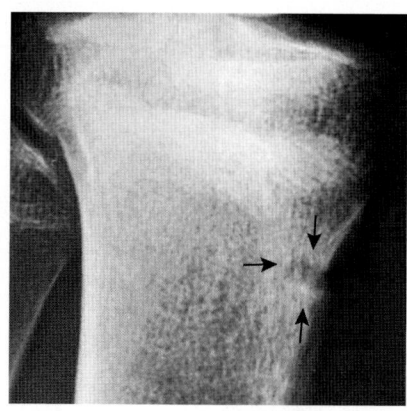

B

FIGURE 163-72. Frontal **(A)** and lateral **(B)** projections of the tibia of a 13-year-old boy showing radiolucent shadow of the notch on the anterior surface of the tibia that the anterior tibial process overlies *(arrows)*. The peripheral portions of this depression in the tibial shaft that are not covered by the opaque anterior tibial process appear as a strip of diminished density in the anteromedial segment of the tibia. This shadow is never visible in infants and younger children.

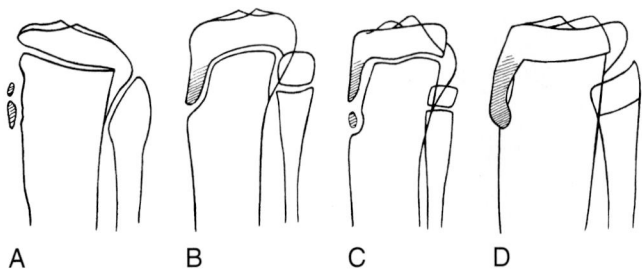

FIGURE 163-73. A-D, Normal variations in the size and configuration of the anterior tibial process. (Modified from Köhler A, Zimmer EA: Borderlands of the Normal and Early Pathologic in Skeletal Roentgenology, 4th ed. New York, Grune & Stratton, 1993.)

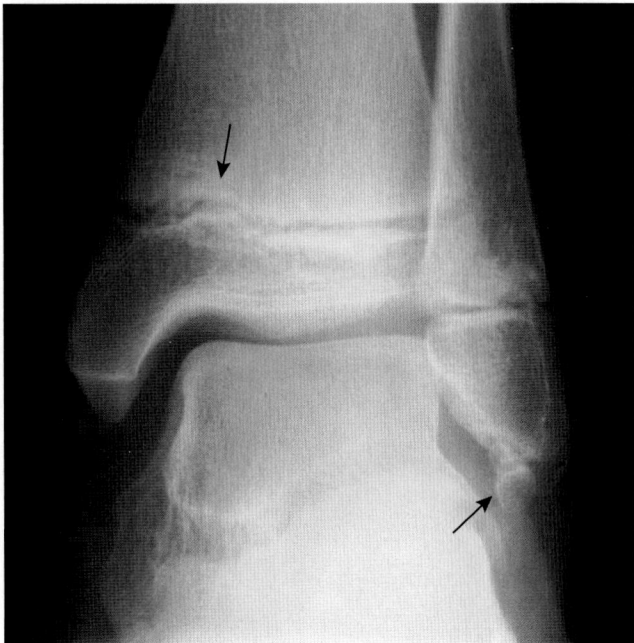

FIGURE 163-75. Accessory ossification centers (os subfibulare) of the lateral malleolus *(lower arrow)* in a 14-year-old boy. *Upper arrow*—a Kump bump.

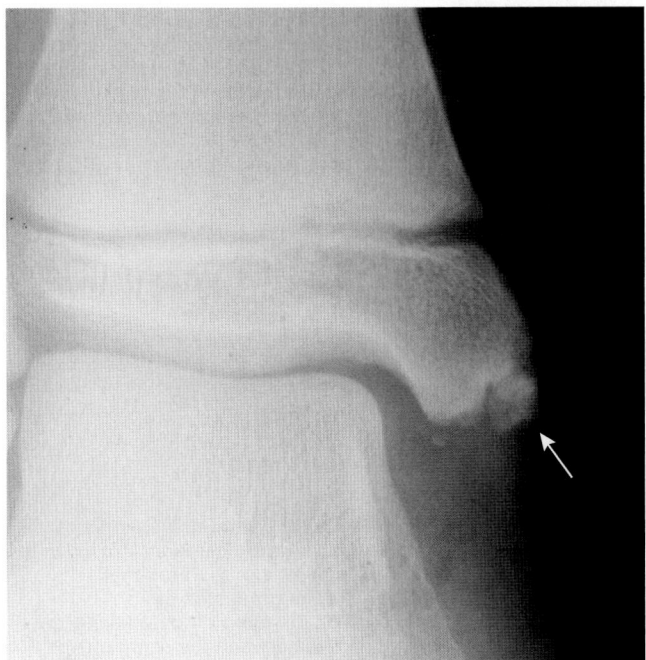

FIGURE 163-74. Accessory ossification center of the medial malleolus *(arrow)* in a 10-year-old girl.

The proximal fibular metaphysis may have a phlanged appearance, possibly due to muscular tug.

Irregular Ossification of the Medial and Lateral Malleoli

Separate accessory ossification centers are common in the cartilage of the medial malleolus *(os subtibiale)* and less common in the lateral malleolus *(os subfibulare)* (Figs. 163-74 and 163-75). At each location, the differential diagnosis is an avulsed fragment. Acute avulsed fragments will have an irregular shape and a sharp, noncorticated margin. Old avulsion fragments appear similar to ossification centers—both appear rounded and corticated. Accessory ossification centers are much more common medially than laterally. Debate persists as to whether lateral findings are accessory ossification centers or the sequelae of old avulsion fractures. When there is evidence of ligamentous laxity, it is more likely that an "os subfibulare" is the sequela of a fracture rather than a variant of ossification.

Kump Bump

The cephalad notching of the distal tibial physis in its medial aspect is a normal phenomenon (Kump bump; see Fig. 163-75).

Fibular Ossicle

The provisional zone of calcification in the distal fibular metaphysis may be notched upward, and a tiny extra ossicle may develop in the notch (Fig. 163-76). The notching is usually bilateral.

FEET

Bifid Epiphyses

Accessory ossification centers may occur in the epiphyses of phalanges and metatarsal bones. Bifid epiphysis is most common in the great toes, where examination before fusion of the centers is complete may simulate fracture (Fig. 163-77). The affected epiphysis is relatively sclerotic.

Pseudoepiphyses

Incompletely fused pseudoepiphyses of metatarsal bones are common. Analogous to the metacarpals, the pseudoepiphyses are located distally in the first metatarsal and proximally in the second through fifth metatarsals (Fig. 163-78).

Absent Epiphyses

The pedal phalanges, especially the middle group, frequently lack epiphyseal centers in healthy children;

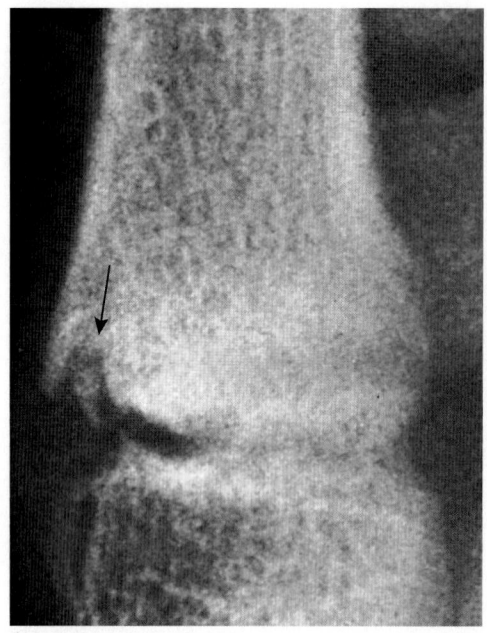
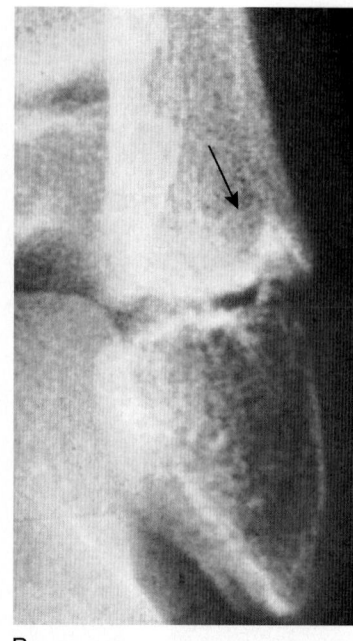

A   B

FIGURE 163-76. A, Extra ossicle in a notched marginal recess *(arrow)* in the lateral segment of the distal fibular metaphysis in an asymptomatic 9-year-old boy. Similar changes were present in the right fibula. In cases of injury, this small variant ossicle must not be mistaken for a fracture fragment or osteochondrosis dissecans. **B,** Similar ossicle with a notch *(arrow)* in an asymptomatic boy 10 years of age.

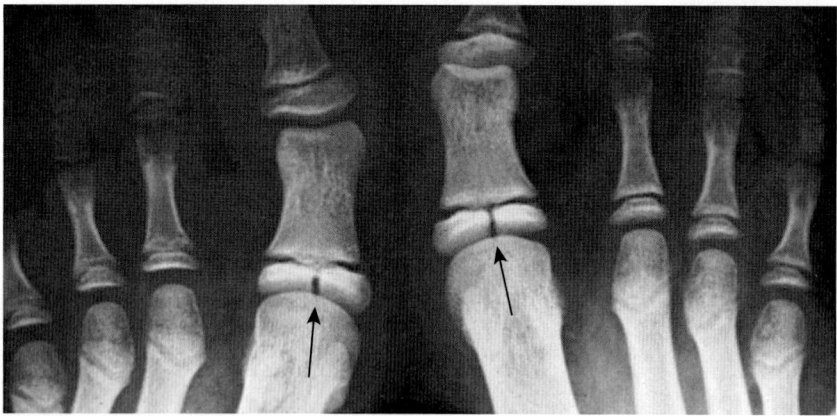

FIGURE 163-77. Symmetric fissures of the secondary ossification centers *(arrows)* in the proximal epiphyses of the proximal phalanges of the great toes of an asymptomatic 11-year-old boy. Radiolucent synchondroses between the segments of each center must not be mistaken for fracture lines.

this absence may be associated with symphalangism at the affected joints. Fifty percent of the population has a biphalangeal fifth toe.

Cone-Shaped Epiphyses

Cone-shaped epiphyses of the pedal phalanges are shown in Figure 163-79. They are more frequent than cone-shaped epiphyses of the hands but apparently do not have the association with specific disorders that occurs with similar findings in the hands. Premature fusion and shortening of the affected bones probably occurs. Cone-shaped epiphyses can affect the great toe.

Fifth Metatarsal Apophysis

During puberty, a longitudinally oriented, scalelike secondary center appears within the proximal apophyseal cartilage of the fifth metatarsal (Fig. 163-80). Irregular ossification of the apophysis is common. The normal apophyseal ossification center may appear widely spaced from the underlying fifth metatarsal, simulating fracture. Absence of associated symptoms and symmetry exclude a fracture. The fifth metatarsal apophysis may be bifid (Fig. 163-81).

Sesamoid Bones

Sesamoid bones are present in the foot as in the hand. Sesamoids of the great toe reside within the medial and lateral slips of the hallux brevis tendon overlying the head of the first metatarsal. The medial great toe sesamoid is bipartite in 4% to 33% of patients (Fig. 163-82). Sesamoids of the feet do fracture. In general, there is an absence of local complaints when the separation is a variant as opposed to the case of local injury. A bipartite sesamoid is larger than a fractured normal sesamoid. To complicate matters, bipartite sesamoids can fracture through the synchondrosis uniting the two parts.

Sesamoiditis may develop due to chronic stress. This is associated with high-heeled shoes, dancing, and some sporting activities.

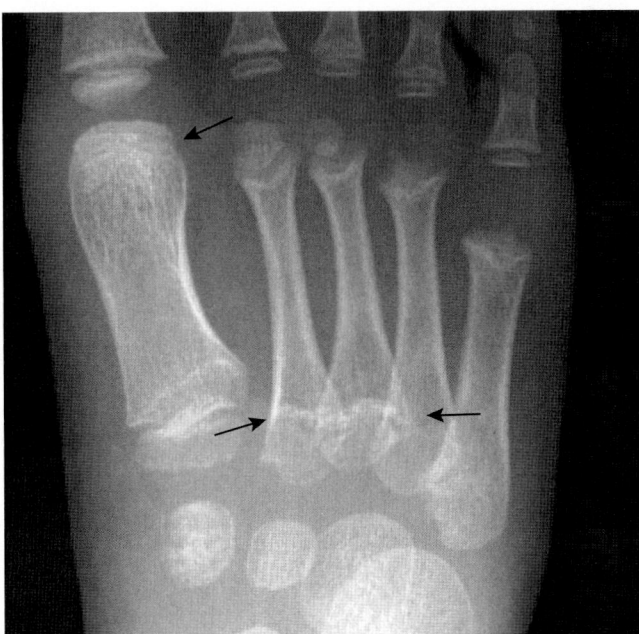

FIGURE 163-78. Pseudoepiphyses of the first metatarsal *(distal arrow)* and the second and third metatarsals *(proximal arrows)* in a 6-year-old boy.

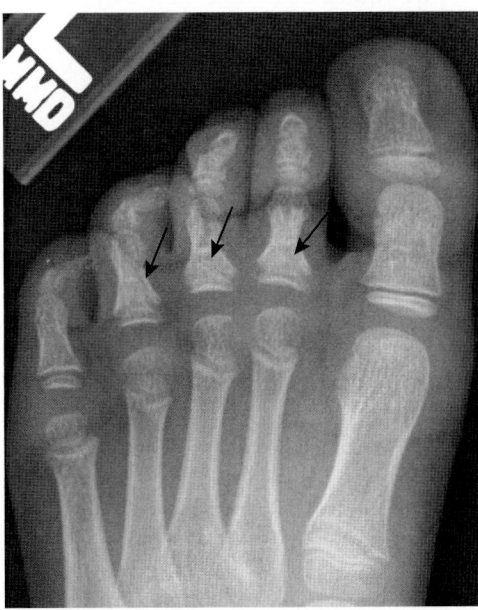

FIGURE 163-79. Symmetric bilateral conical or bell-shaped epiphyseal ossification centers *(arrows)* in the proximal phalanges of the second, third, and fourth toes of both feet of an asymptomatic 5-year-old girl. The contiguous distal end of each shaft is recessed to receive its elongated ossification center. The epiphyseal ossification centers in the proximal phalanges of the first and fifth toes are the normal, flat, shallow, transverse disks usually present in all of the phalanges.

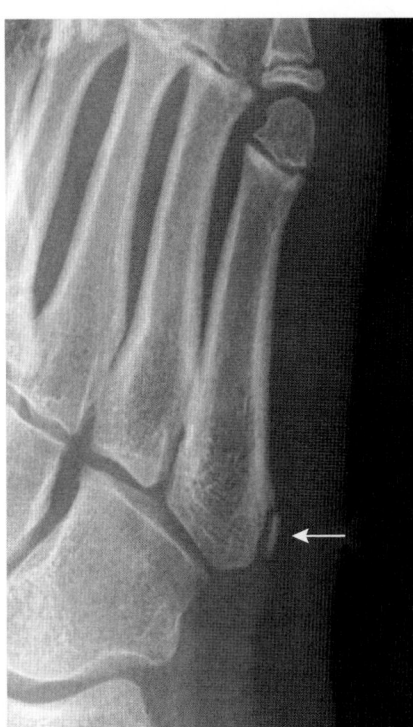

FIGURE 163-80. Normal apophysis of the fifth metatarsal in a 10-year-old girl *(arrow)*. The apophyseal growth plate is longitudinal in orientation and the apophysis appears "scalelike."

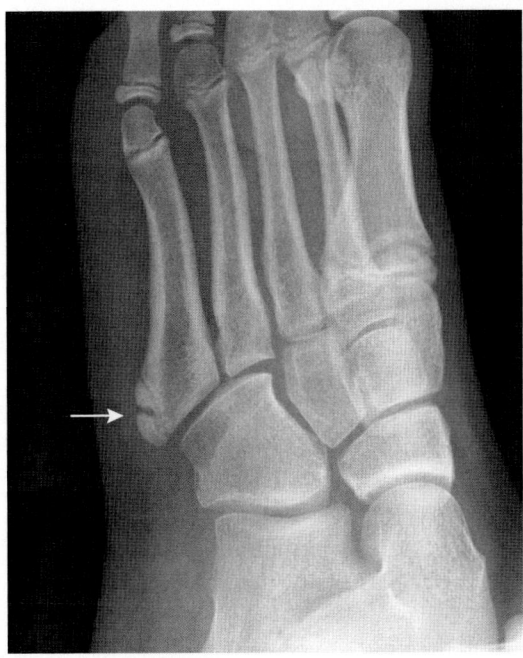

FIGURE 163-81. Bifid apophysis of the fifth metatarsal in a 13-year-old girl *(arrow)*. Findings persisted on follow-up examinations without change.

Accessory Ossicles

In addition to the sesamoids, there are numerous other supernumerary ossicles of the foot and ankle (Fig. 163-83).

Bifid Calcaneus

The ossification center for the calcaneus is present at birth. Occasionally, the body of the calcaneus may ossify from two or more independent centers (Fig. 163-84).

This finding is rare as a normal variant. More often it is associated with an underlying disorder, such as Down syndrome, mucolipidosis, or Larsen syndrome.

Calcaneal Apophysis

The ossification centers for the apophysis of the calcaneus appear in the cartilage behind its normally irregular border about the middle of the first decade and maintain their fragmented or sclerotic character well into the second decade until fusion with the body of the calcaneus is complete (Fig. 163-85). The normal calcaneal apophysis may appear remarkably sclerotic and frag-

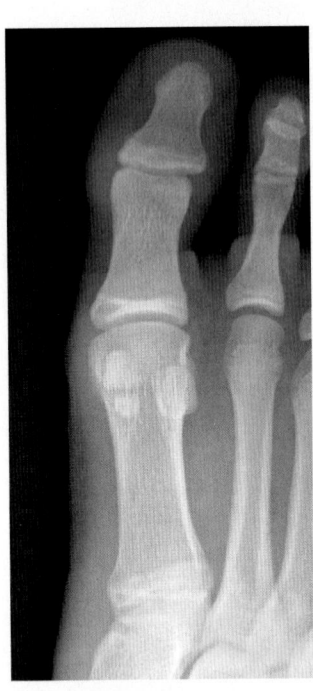

FIGURE 163-82. Bipartite sesamoid of the great toe in a 15-year-old boy.

mented. Sclerosis is diminished or lacking only in the case of nonuse or absence of weight bearing. Calcaneal apophysitis (Sever disease) is a poorly understood cause of heel pain in children. A study by Ogden et al suggests that the etiology is a chronic repetitive stress injury of the apophysis rather than an inflammatory or ischemic process. Sever disease is usually a clinical diagnosis, although increased signal from edema may be evident on MRI.

Calcaneus Secondarius

The calcaneus secondarius (Fig. 163-86) may simulate a fracture fragment. The ossicle is located in between the anteromedial calcaneus, cuboid, talar head, and navicular. It is rare and of no clinical significance other than possibly being mistaken for a fracture.

Calcaneal Pseudocyst

A pseudocystic triangular area of radiolucency is present in the anterior half of the laterally imaged calcaneus. At this location, there is a normal deficiency of spongy bone (see Fig. 163-85). The pseudocyst is of no clinical significance in itself; however, it must be differentiated from true bone cysts that can develop at this site. True cysts are more round in contour and have better defined margins than pseudocysts.

Os Trigonum

An os trigonum is located at the posterior margin of the talus in 15% to 25% of individuals. The primary ossification center for the talus is also present at birth. A secondary center appears in the dorsal process during the 5th and 6th postnatal years and fuses with the body of the talus between the 16th and 20th years. Before

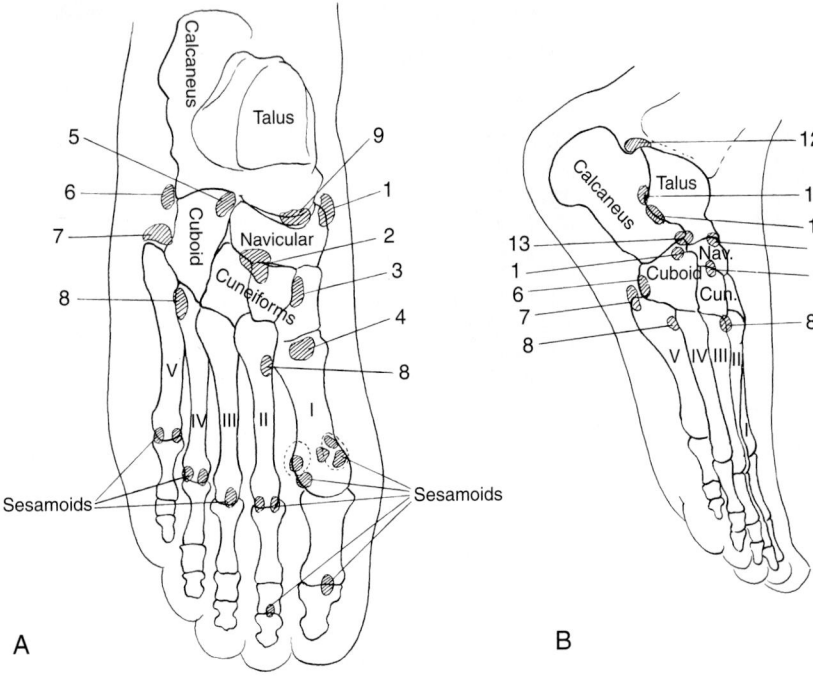

FIGURE 163-83. Normal supernumerary ossicles of the feet in ventrodorsal (**A**) and lateral (**B**) projections: *1,* os tibiale externum; *2,* processus uncinatus; *3,* os intercuneiforme; *4,* pars peronea metatarsalia; *5,* os cuboideum secundarium; *6,* os peroneum; *7,* os vesalianum pedis; *8,* os intermetatarseum; *9,* accessory navicular; *10,* talus accessorius; *11,* sustentaculum tali; *12,* os trigonum tarsi; *13,* calcaneus secundarius.

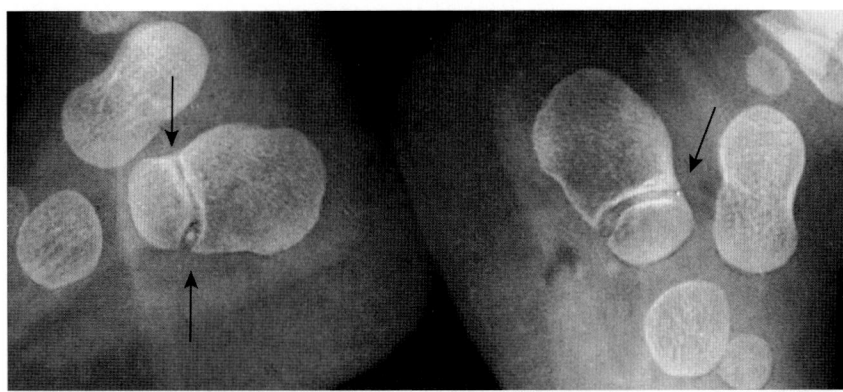

FIGURE 163-84. Double ossification centers *(arrows)* in the body of the calcaneus on each side of a 20-month-old infant. The infant was normal, and films were made only because of an injury to the left ankle a few hours before. We have seen similar double ossification centers in the body of the calcaneus in patients with Down syndrome and with mucolipidosis type I.

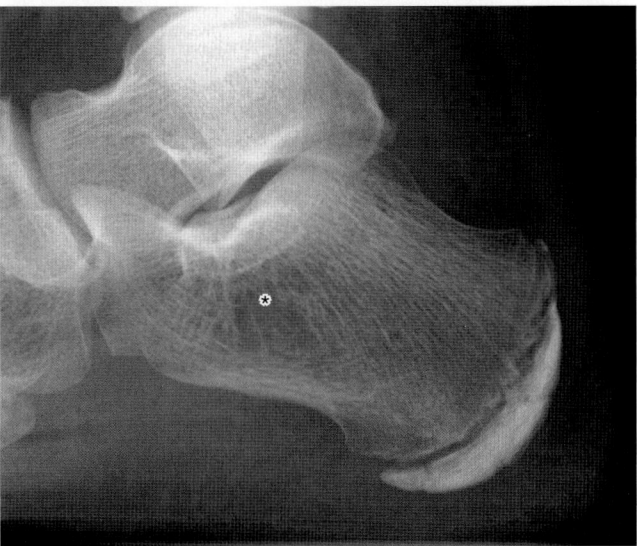

FIGURE 163-85. Normal, sclerotic, slightly fragmented appearance of the calcaneal apophysis in a 13-year-old boy. *Asterisk,* area of normal deficiency of trabecular bone, appearing radiolucent.

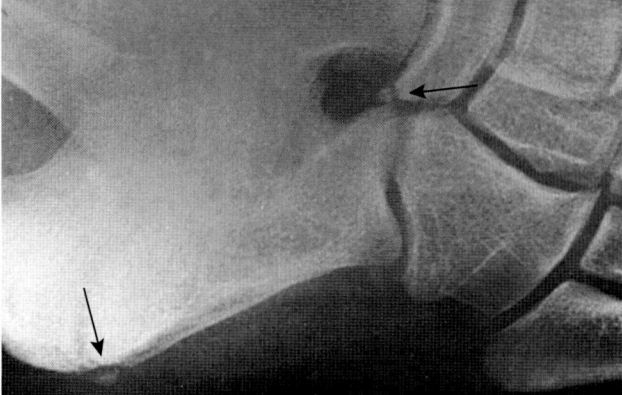

FIGURE 163-86. Small, round, smooth calcaneus secundarius *(arrow at right)* in the center of the space between the calcaneus, cuboid, navicular, and talus on lateral oblique projection. The patient was an asymptomatic 12-year-old boy. The *posterior arrow* points to a center in the apophysis. Similar ossicles were present in the other foot.

fusion, it may simulate pathologic changes (Fig. 163-87); if it fails to fuse, it is called the os trigonum. Repetitive forced flexion may cause a syndrome of posterior ankle impingement or "os trigonum syndrome." This occurs most commonly in ballet dancers, soccer players, and basketball players. Trauma may cause a fracture at the synchondrosis between the ossification center and the underlying talus or may cause a fracture after fusion occurs (Shepherd fracture). In symptomatic patients, bone scans will be positive and MRI will show edema in the os trigonum, talus, and adjacent soft tissues.

Os Supratalare

The os supratalare on the crest of the head of the talus may simulate injury or be simulated by injury (Fig. 163-88).

Os Supranaviculare

The center for the navicular bone is frequently irregular up to about 5 years of age, and occasionally later (Fig. 163-89). The os supranaviculare (Fig. 163-90) is an accessory ossicle that can be confused with an accessory

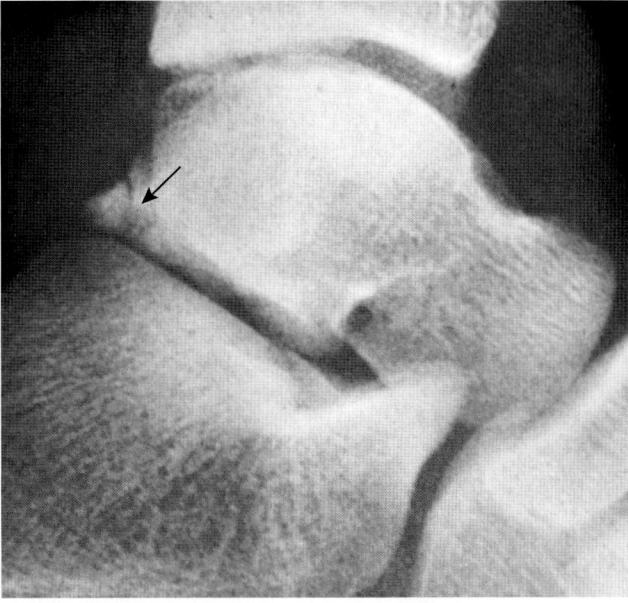

FIGURE 163-87. Normal apophyseal ossification center *(arrow)* in the dorsal process of the talus in a healthy 11-year-old boy. The radiolucent strip between the body of the talus and the ossification center is a normal synchondrosis, not a fracture line. When the synchondrosis persists after the normal age for its fusion with the body of the talus, the persistent ossification center is called the os trigonum.

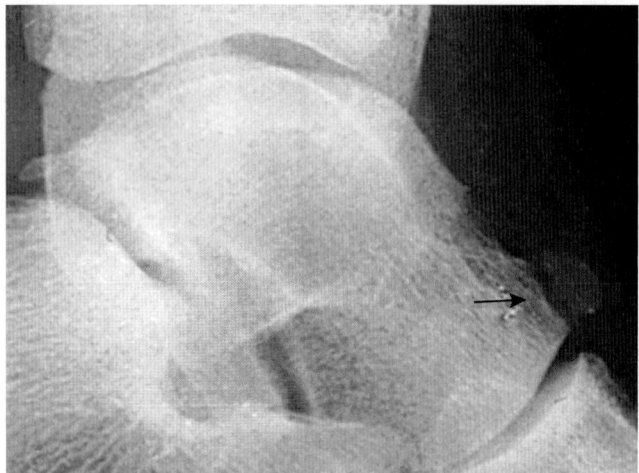

FIGURE 163-88. Os supratalare *(arrow)* on the dorsal edge of the talus just proximal to the talonavicular joint in an asymptomatic 18-year-old girl.

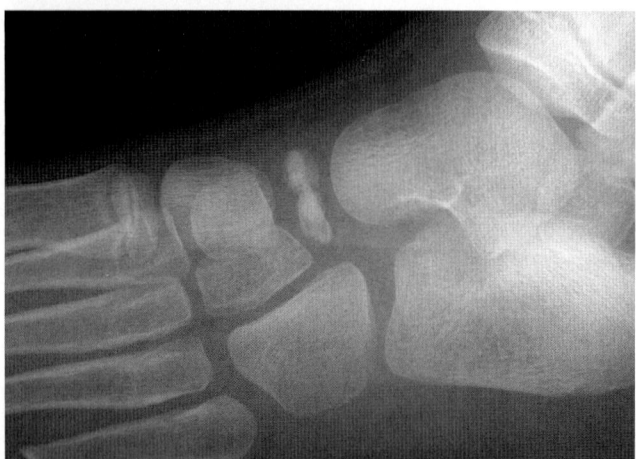

FIGURE 163-89. Irregular ossification of the navicular in a 2-year-old boy.

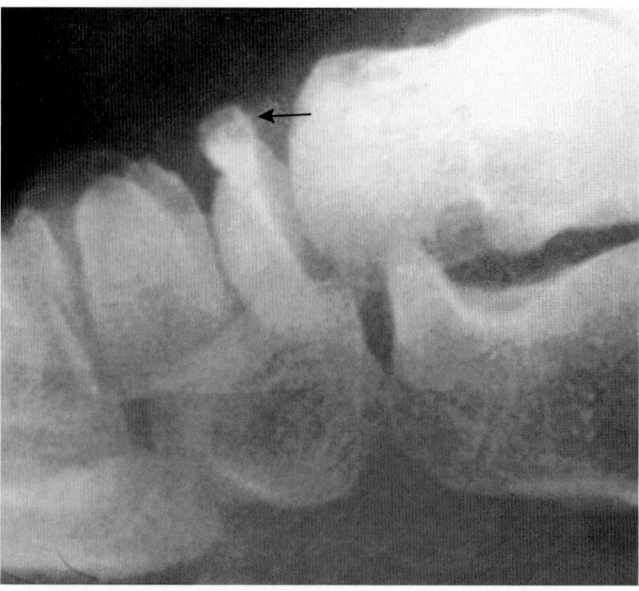

FIGURE 163-90. Large supranavicular bone *(arrow)* that seems to be partially fused with the main mass of the navicular itself. This appears to be an accessory ossification center in the periphery of the navicular cartilage; similar changes were present in the other foot. The patient was an asymptomatic 8-year-old boy.

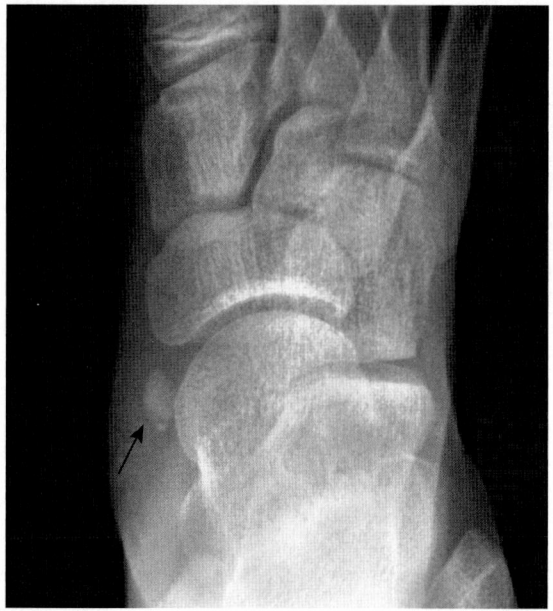

FIGURE 163-91. Type I accessory navicular *(arrow)* in a 10-year-old girl.

ossification center before the latter fuses with the parent bone, and both must be differentiated from fracture. The variant is usually bilateral.

Accessory Navicular

The accessory navicular is the best known and one of the most important variants in the foot. Accessory navicular bones are seen in approximately 15% of patients; 50% to 90% are symmetric. Two types have been described.

Type I ("os tibiale externum" or "navicular secundarium") is a true rounded sesamoid bone measuring 2 to 6 mm that lies within the tendon of the posterior tibialis muscle and approximately 3 mm separate from the navicular bone (Fig. 163-91). Type I variants are asymptomatic and do not fuse with the navicular. Type I accounts for 10% to 15% of cases in children.

Type II variants ("prehallux" or "bifurcated hallux") are united to the navicular by a cartilaginous or fibrocartilaginous bridge and represent an accessory ossification center for the tubercle of the navicular (Fig. 163-92). The ossicle is larger (9 to 12 mm), triangular or heart shaped, and congruent with and closely apposed to the adjacent navicular. It is connected to the navicular by a synchondrosis. Injury to the synchondrosis produces pain. Females are affected four times as frequently as males; symptoms generally develop in the second decade. In symptomatic patients, bone scans are positive and MRI shows increased signal. Fusion with the navicular bone occurs in the great majority of these cases, often producing a "cornuate navicular." Cornuate navicular and type II accessory navicular can also cause symptoms due to irritation of overlying soft tissues.

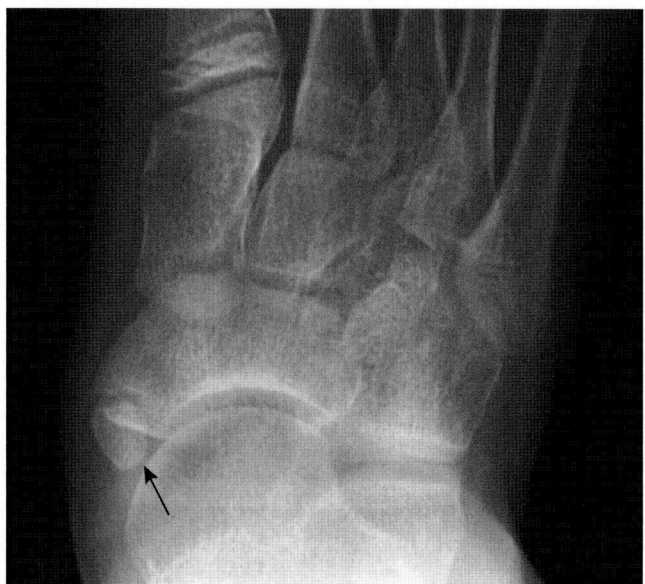

A

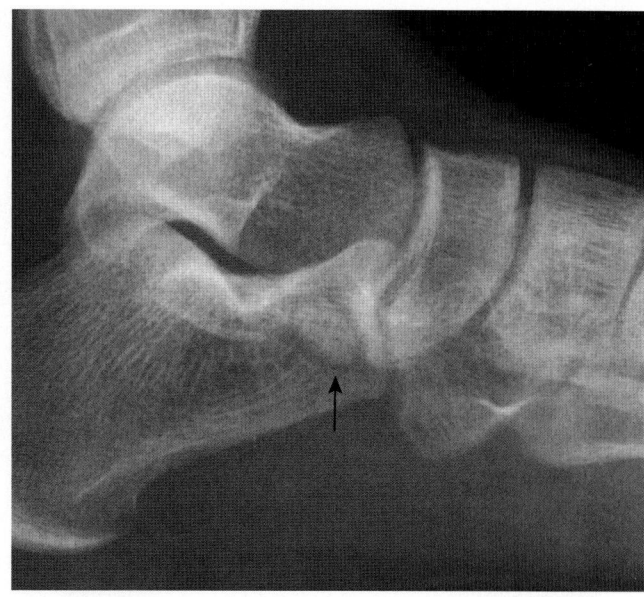

B

FIGURE 163-92. Type II accessory naviculars *(arrows)*. **A,** 11-year-old girl. **B,** 13-year-old girl.

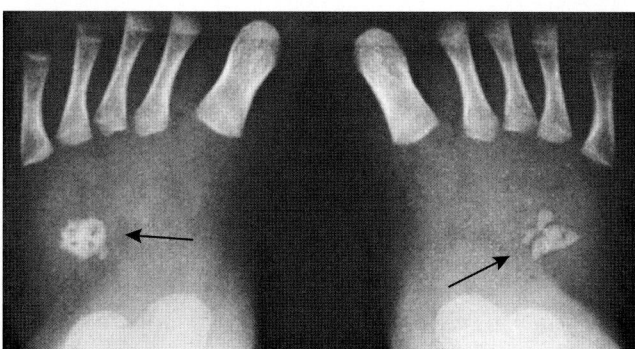

FIGURE 163-93. Normal bilateral irregular mineralization of the cuboids *(arrows)* of an asymptomatic 3-day-old infant. The left cuboid contains 9 or 10 separate small bony centers; the right cuboid is a single, relatively large bony mass of irregular density and rough edges.

> Os trigonum and accessory navicular are relatively common accessory ossicles. Although usually asymptomatic, each of these variants may produce symptoms.

Bipartite Navicular

Bipartite navicular is an uncommon cause of dorsal foot pain and stiffness. A smaller fragment is dorsally subluxed and a larger fragment is medially subluxed.

Cuboid

The early cuboid is often composed of multiple fine ossification centers (Fig. 163-93) that later slowly fuse to form a single bony mass.

Cuneiforms

The three cuneiforms may ossify irregularly in children who are healthy and have no clinical evidence of local disease in the feet. A bipartite medial cuneiform has a coronal cleft separating it into proximal and distal portions. A duplicate cuneiform may be longitudinal in form, as is shown in Figure 163-94.

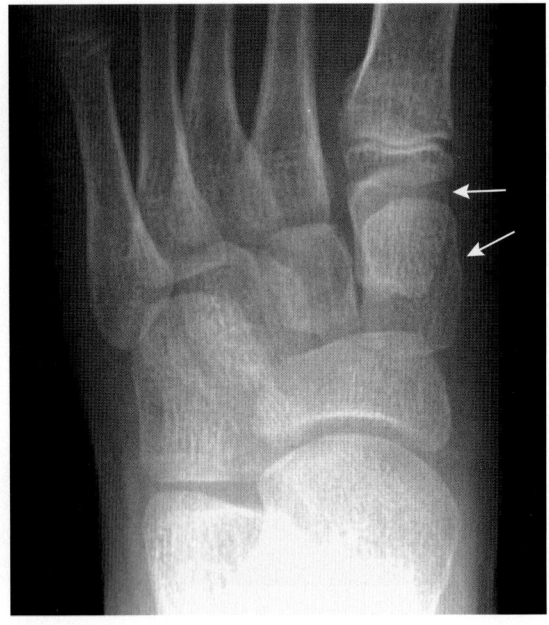

A

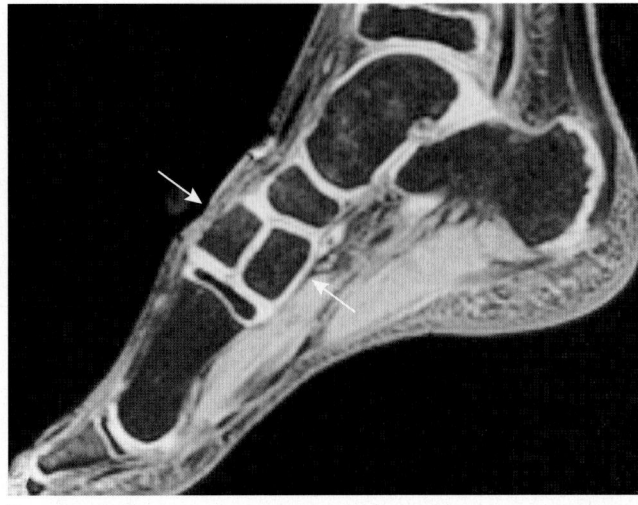

B

FIGURE 163-94. Radiography (**A**) and proton density with fat saturation MR image (**B**) show longitudinal duplication of the medial cuneiform *(arrows)*.

SUGGESTED READINGS

General References

Duncan AW: Normal variants—an approach. *In* Carty H, Brunelle F, Stringer D, Kao SCS (eds): Imaging Children, 2nd ed. Philadelphia, Elsevier, 2005:47-63

Freyschmidt J, Brossman J, Wiens J, Sternberg A: Borderlands of Normal and Early Pathological Findings in Skeletal Radiography, 5th ed. New York, Thieme, 2003

Gould CF, Ly JQ, Lattinn GE, et al: Bone tumor mimics: avoiding misdiagnosis. Curr Probl Diagn Radiol 2007;36:124-141

Keats TE, Anderson MW: An Atlas of Normal Roentgen Variants That May Simulate Disease, 7th ed. St. Louis, Mosby, 2001

Kleinman PK: Differential diagnosis IV: normal variants. *In* Kleinman PK (ed): Diagnostic Imaging of Child Abuse, 2nd ed. St. Louis, Mosby, 1998:225-236

Lawson JP: Symptomatic radiographic variants in extremities. Radiology 1985;157:625-631

Lawson JP: Not-so-normal variants. Orthop Clin North Am 1990;21:483-495

Lawson JP: Clinically significant radiologic anatomic variants of the skeleton. AJR Am J Roentgenol 1994;163:249-255

Ozonoff MB: Pediatric Orthopedic Radiology, 2nd ed. Philadelphia, Saunders, 1992

Generalized and Scattered Variants

Kim SK, Barry WF Jr: Bone islands. Radiology 1968;90:77-78

Kleinman PK, Belanger PL, Karellas A, et al: Normal metaphyseal radiologic variants not to be confused with findings of child abuse. AJR Am J Roentgenol 1991;156:781-783

Kwon DS, Spevak MR, Fletcher K, et al: Physiologic subperiosteal new bone formation: prevalence, distribution, and thickness in neonates and infants. AJR Am J Roentgenol 2002;179:985-988

Lagier R, Nussle D: Anatomy and radiology of a bone island. Rofo 1978;128:261-264

Oestreich AE, Ahmad BS: The periphysis and its effect on the metaphysis: I. Definition and normal radiographic pattern. Skeletal Radiol 1992;21:283-286

Simon K, Mulligan ME: Growing bone islands revisited. J Bone Joint Surg Am 1985;67:809-811

Hand and Wrist

Cockshott WP: Carpal fusions. Am J Roentgenol Radium Ther Nucl Med 1963;89:1260-1271

Conway WF, Destouet JM, Gilula LA, et al: The carpal boss: an overview of radiographic evaluation. Radiology 1985;156:29-31

Cope JR: Carpal coalition. Clin Radiol 1974;25:261-266

Delaney TJ, Eswar S: Carpal coalitions. J Hand Surg [Am] 1992; 17:28-31

Giedion A: Phalangeal cone-shaped epiphyses of the hands (PhCSEH) and chronic renal disease—the conorenal syndromes. Pediatr Radiol 1979;8:32-38

Hubay CA: Sesamoid bones of the hands and feet. Am J Roentgenol Radium Ther 1949;61:493-505

Karmazyn B, Siddiqui AR: Painful os styloideum in a child. Pediatr Radiol 2002;32:370-372

Kuhns LR, Poznanski AK, Harper HA, et al: Ivory epiphyses of the hands. Radiology 1973;109:643-648

Ogden JA, Ganey TM, Light TR, et al: Nonepiphyseal ossification and pseudoepiphysis formation. J Pediatr Orthop 1994;14:78-82

Ogden JA, Ganey TM, Light TR, et al: Ossification and pseudoepiphysis formation in the "nonepiphyseal" end of bones of the hands and feet. Skeletal Radiol 1994;23:3-13

O'Rahilly R: Developmental deviations in the carpus and the tarsus. Clin Orthop 1957;10:9-18

Poznanski AK: The Hand in Radiologic Diagnosis, 2nd ed. Philadelphia, Saunders, 1984

Senecail B, Perruez H, Colin D: Numerical variants and congenital fusions of carpal bones. Morphologie 2007 Jun 5 [Epub ahead of print]

Forearm, Elbow, and Shoulder

Barnard LB, McCoy SM: The supracondyloid process of the humerus. J Bone Joint Surg Am 1946;28:845-850

Bilge T, Yalaman O, Bilge S, et al: Entrapment neuropathy of the median nerve at the level of the ligament of Struthers. Neurosurgery 1990;27:787-789

Levine MA: Patella cubiti. J Bone Joint Surg Am 1950;32:686-687

Mellado JM, Calmet J, Domenech S, et al: Clinically significant skeletal variations of the shoulder and the wrist: role of MR imaging. Eur Radiol 2003;13:1735-1743

Obermann WR, Loose HW: The os supratrochleare dorsale: a normal variant that may cause symptoms. AJR Am J Roentgenol 1983;141:123-127

Ozonoff MB, Zeiter FM Jr: The upper humeral notch: a normal variant in children. Radiology 1974;113:699-701

Resnik CS, Hartenberg MA: Ossification centers of the pediatric elbow: a rare normal variant. Pediatr Radiol 1986;16:254-256

Resnick D, Cone RO III: The nature of humeral pseudocysts. Radiology 1984;150:27-28

Schwarz GS: Bilateral antecubital ossicles (fabella cubiti) and other accessory bones of the elbow. Radiology 1965;69:730-734

Silberstein MJ, Brodeur AE, Graviss ER, et al: Some vagaries of the olecranon. J Bone Joint Surg Am 1981;63:722-725

Spinner RJ, Lins RE, Jacobson SR, et al: Fractures of the supracondylar process of the humerus. J Hand Surg [Am] 1994;19:1038-1041

Pelvis and Hip

Byers PD: Ischiopubic "osteochondritis": a report of a case and a review. J Bone Joint Surg Br 1963;45:694-702

Caffey J, Madell SH: Ossification of the pubic bones at birth. Radiology 1956;67:346-350

Caffey J, Ross SE: The ischiopubic synchondrosis in healthy children: some normal roentgenologic findings. Am J Roentgenol Radium Ther Nucl Med 1956;76:488-494

Cawley KA, Dvorak AD, Wilmot MD: Normal anatomic variant: scintigraphy of the ischiopubic synchondrosis. J Nucl Med 1983;24:14-16

Freedman E: Os acetabuli. Am J Roentgenol Radium Ther 1934;32:492-495

Hergan K, Oser W, Moriggl B: Acetabular ossicles: normal variant or disease entity? Eur Radiol 2000;10:624-628

Herneth AM, Philipp MO, Pretterklieber ML, et al: Asymmetric closure of ischiopubic synchondrosis in pediatric patients: correlation with foot dominance. AJR Am J Roentgenol 2004;182:361-365

Herneth AM, Trattnig S, Bader TR, et al: MR imaging of the ischiopubic synchondrosis. Magn Reson Imaging 2000;18:519-524

Iqbal A, McKenna D, Hayes R, et al: Osteomyelitis of the ischiopubic synchondrosis: imaging findings. Skeletal Radiol 2004;33:176-180

Junge H, Heuck F: Die Osteochondropathia ischiopubica (gleichzeitig ein Beitrag zur normalen Entwicklung der Scham-Sitzbeingrenze in Wachstumsalter). Fortschr Geb Rontgenstr 1953;78:656-668

Kloiber R, Udjus K, McIntyre W, et al: The scintigraphic and radiographic appearance of the ischiopubic synchondroses in normal children and in osteomyelitis. Pediatr Radiol 1988;18:57-61

Lemperg R, Liliequist B, Mattson S: Asymmetry of the epiphyseal nucleus in the femoral head in stable and unstable hip joints. Pediatr Radiol 1973;1:191-195

Reynolds EL: The bony pelvic girdle in early infancy: a roentgenometric study. Am J Phys Anthropol 1945;3:321-354

Zander G: "Os acetabuli" and other bone nuclei: periarticular calcifications at hip-point. Acta Radiol 1943;24:317-327

Knee

Bufkin WJ: The avulsive cortical irregularity. Am J Roentgenol Radium Ther Nucl Med 1971;112:487-492

Caffey J, Madell SH, Royer C, et al: Ossification of the distal femoral epiphysis. J Bone Joint Surg Am 1958;40:647-654

Gebarski K, Hernandez RJ: Stage-I osteochondritis dissecans versus normal variants of ossification in the knee in children. Pediatr Radiol 2005;35:880-886

Jung C, Choi YY, Cho S, et al: Symptomatic cortical desmoids detected on knee SPECT. Clin Nucl Med 2002;27:437-438

Kavanagh EC, Zoga A, Omar I, et al: MRI findings in bipartite patella. Skeletal Radiol 2007;36:209-214

Mellado JM, Salvado E, Ramos A, et al: Dorsal defect on a multi-partite patella: imaging findings. Eur Radiol 2001;11:1136-1139

Nawata K, Teshima R, Morio Y, et al: Anomalies of ossification in the posterolateral femoral condyle: assessment by MRI. Pediatr Radiol 1999;29:781-784

Ogden JA, Lee J: Accessory ossification patterns and injuries of the malleoli. J Pediatr Orthop 1990;10:306-316

Ogden JA, McCarthy SM, Jokl P: The painful bipartite patella. J Pediatr Orthop 1982;2:263-269.

Oohashi Y, Noriki S, Koshino T, et al: Histopathological abnormalities in painful bipartite patellae in adolescents. Knee 2006;13:189-193

Pennes DR, Braunstein EM, Glazer GM: Computed tomography of cortical desmoid. Skeletal Radiol 1984;12:40-42

Resnick D, Greenway G: Distal femoral cortical defects, irregularities, and excavations. Radiology 1982;143:345-354

Suh JS, Cho JH, Shin KH, et al: MR appearance of distal femoral cortical irregularity (cortical desmoid). J Comput Assist Tomogr 1996;20:328-332

van Holsbeeck M, Vandamme B, Marchal G, et al: Dorsal defect of the patella: concept of its origin and relationship with bipartite and multipartite patella. Skeletal Radiol 1987;16:304-311

Weiner DS, Macnab I: The "fabella syndrome": an update. J Pediatr Orthop 1982;2:405-408

Ankle and Foot

Berg EE: The symptomatic os subfibulare: avulsion fracture of the fibula associated with recurrent instability of the ankle. J Bone Joint Surg Am 1991;73:1251-1254

Berquist TH: Anatomy, normal variants and biomechanics. In Berquist TH (ed): Radiology of the Foot and Ankle, 2nd ed. Philadelphia, Lippincott, Williams & Wilkins, 2000:1-40

Bureau NJ, Cardinal E, Hobden R, et al: Posterior ankle impingement syndrome: MR imaging findings in seven patients. Radiology 2000;215:497-503

Carty H: Accessory ossicles at the lateral malleolus: a review of the incidence. Eur J Radiol 1992;14:181-184

Frankel JP, Harrington J: Symptomatic bipartite sesamoids. J Foot Surg 1990;29:318-323

Griffiths JD, Menelaus MB: Symptomatic ossicles of the lateral malleolus in children. J Bone Joint Surg Br 1987;69:317-319

Harrison RB, Keats TE: Epiphyseal clefts. Skeletal Radiol 1980;5:23-27

Hubay CA: Sesamoid bones of the hands and feet. Am J Roentgenol Radium Ther 1949;61:493-505

Karasick D, Schweitzer ME: The os trigonum syndrome: imaging features. AJR Am J Roentgenol 1996;166:125-129

Lawson JP, Ogden JA, Sella E, et al: The painful accessory navicular. Skeletal Radiol 1984;12:250-262

Lyritis G: Developmental disorders of the proximal epiphysis of the hallux. Skeletal Radiol 1983;10:250-254

Mellado JM, Ramos A, Salvado E, et al: Accessory ossicles and sesamoid bones of the ankle and foot: imaging findings, clinical significance and differential diagnosis. Eur Radiol 2003; 13:L164-L177

Miller TT: Painful accessory bones of the foot. Semin Musculoskelet Radiol 2002;6:153-161

Miller TT, Staron RB, Feldman F, et al: The symptomatic accessory tarsal navicular bone: assessment with MR imaging. Radiology 1995;195:849-853

Ogden JA, Lee J: Accessory ossification patterns and injuries of the malleoli. J Pediatr Orthop 1990;10:306-316

Ogden JA, Ganey TM, Hill JD, et al: Sever's injury: a stress fracture of the immature calcaneal metaphysis. J Pediatr Orthop 2004; 24:488-492

O'Rahilly R: Developmental deviations in the carpus and tarsus. Clin Orthop 1957;10:9-18

Powell H: Extra centre of ossification for the medial malleolus in children: incidence and significance. J Bone Joint Surg Br 1961;43:107-113

CHAPTER

164

Congenital Malformations of Bone

TAL LAOR

The most obvious congenital malformations of the skeleton are those that involve size, shape, and number of bones. These malformations are frequently accompanied by soft tissue abnormalities. Occasionally, a soft tissue abnormality may occur as an isolated finding. Most limb malformations are classified as reduction (deficiency), excess, and fusion (malsegmentation) deformities. The last group often occurs in association with reduction deformities. Congenital malformations that result in abnormalities of limb size, configuration, and segmentation are reviewed here.

ABNORMAL SIZE: SMALL LIMBS

Congenital deficiencies are more common than acquired amputations in children. Frantz and O'Rahilly developed a system of classification that is still commonly used to evaluate congenital anomalies of the extremities. Each malformation is defined by the part that is deficient. For example, the fibula is deficient in fibular hemimelia. The abnormality is considered *terminal* if the deformity extends to the distal aspect of the extremity; it is *intercalary* if the limb distal to the deformity is normal. For example, in fibular hemimelia, if the foot is abnormal, the deficiency is terminal, and if the foot is normal, it is intercalary. Likewise, a defect may be classified as *longitudinal (paraxial)* or *transverse*. The malformation is paraxial if only the fibular side is affected. If both the tibia and the fibula are affected, the deformity is considered transverse.

Aplasia and hypoplasia of the long bones occur in the following descending order of frequency: fibula, radius, femur, ulna, and humerus. Deficiencies of the tibia are very uncommon. The cause of reduction malformations is known in only a small number of cases. A few abnormalities are inheritable, but most are sporadic. Environmental factors are infrequently implicated. A drug that is firmly associated with anomalies is thalidomide. This drug, which was introduced as an antipyretic and sedative, had potential teratogenic effects on the human embryo if ingested by the mother early in pregnancy.

Induced malformations were usually reduction deformities that ranged from severe amelias to mild muscular hypoplasia. Most malformations were on the radial or tibial side, and the upper limbs were affected more often than were the lower extremities. Infrequently, excess deformities such as polydactyly were observed. Deprivation of factors necessary for normal development may also result in reduction deformities, as shown by Warkany and Nelson in the case of maternal riboflavin deficiency. Paraxial congenital malformations of the extremities also have been attributed to early compromise of embryonic vascular structures.

Regardless of origin, abnormal limb development tends to fall into patterns that can be recognized clinically and radiographically (Fig. 164-1). Most classification systems of congenital malformations are based on osseous structures, but it is well recognized that anomalous conditions of surrounding soft tissues are certain to be present. Although one deficiency is usually dominant, dysplasia often involves the entire limb. Deficiencies may involve both lower and upper extremities.

> Each malformation is defined by the part that is deficient. For example, the fibula is deficient in fibular hemimelia.

LOWER EXTREMITY DEFICIENCIES

Congenitally Short Femur

Femoral shortening can be unilateral or bilateral, and it is often associated with reduction defects elsewhere in the same limb. Abnormality ranges from mild hypoplasia to complete absence of the femur. Most cases are sporadic, but several external factors have been implicated in more complex deformities. Known causes include drugs (such as thalidomide), trauma, irradiation, infection, and focal ischemia.

Anterolateral bowing and medial cortical thickening are seen in hypoplasia of the femur (Fig. 164-2). The

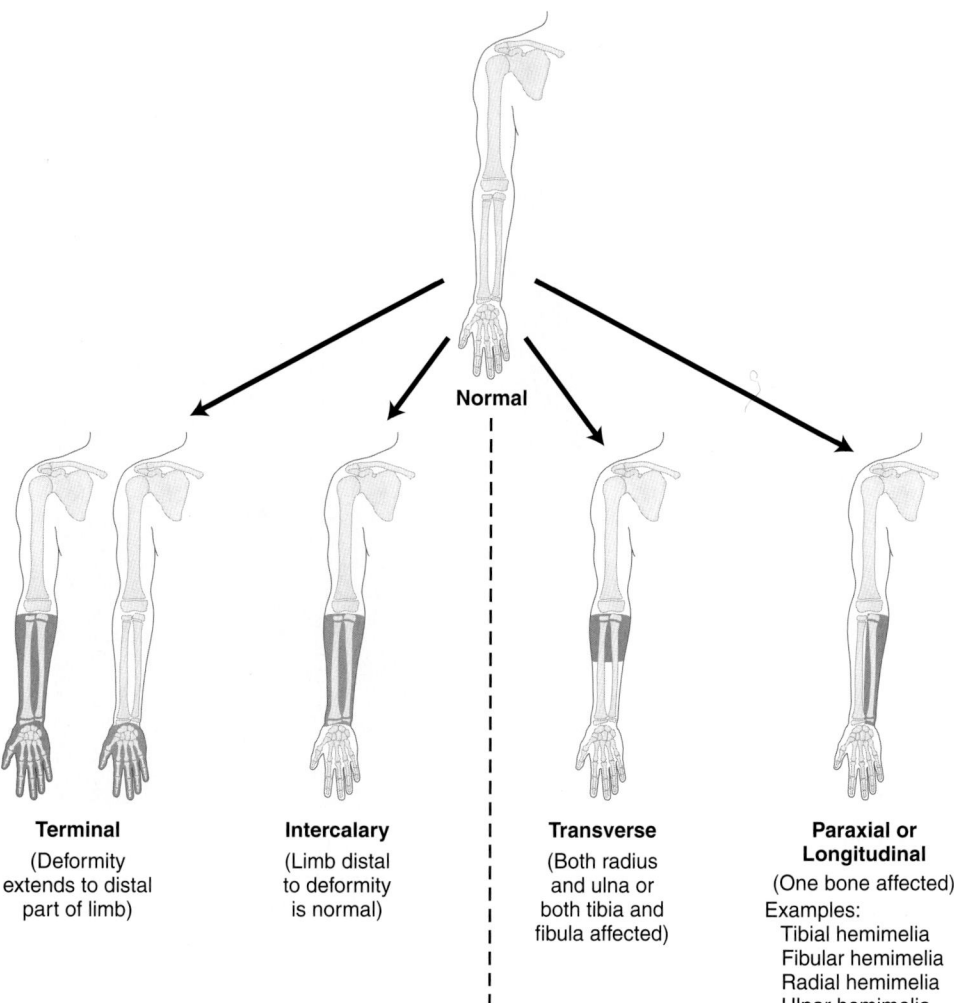

Normal

Terminal
(Deformity
extends to distal
part of limb)

Intercalary
(Limb distal
to deformity
is normal)

Transverse
(Both radius
and ulna or
both tibia and
fibula affected)

**Paraxial or
Longitudinal**
(One bone affected)
Examples:
   Tibial hemimelia
   Fibular hemimelia
   Radial hemimelia
   Ulnar hemimelia

FIGURE 164-1. Skeletal deformities of the limbs. The *shaded blackened areas* indicate deficient parts.

femoral and tibial condyles are flattened. The knee joint often is lax and may have an accentuated valgus alignment. In contrast to proximal femoral focal deficiency (PFFD) (see later), the hip is stable. A coxa vara alignment of the femoral neck may be present. The hypoplastic femur grows at the same rate as, or at a slower rate than, the contralateral normal femur, so that leg length discrepancy persists or increases. Degree of hypoplasia of the femur and instability of the knee joint guide therapy. Leg lengthening can be performed if shortening is less than 20 cm.

> **Different from proximal femoral focal deficiency, in congenitally short femur, the proximal femur and the acetabulum are not significantly affected.**

Proximal Femoral Focal Deficiency

PFFD refers to abnormalities that range from mild shortening and hypoplasia of the femur to severe deficiency of the bone and dysplasia of the acetabulum. The defect is thought to be due to altered proliferation and maturation of the chondrocytes of the proximal femoral physis in utero, which, in turn, result in underdevelopment of

the ipsilateral acetabulum. The child with PFFD usually presents in infancy with a short extremity. A well-formed acetabulum implies the presence of a femoral head, which might be cartilaginous and therefore is not apparent radiographically early in life. Most cases are sporadic; however, the combination of bilateral femoral deficiencies and abnormal facies, known as the femoral hypoplasia–unusual facies syndrome, is thought to be an autosomal dominant disorder.

Numerous attempts have been made to classify PFFD; all were based on radiographic findings. Historically, the most commonly used classification is that of Aitken (Fig. 164-3). The least severe type is class A, which refers to an adequate or only mildly dysplastic proximal femur and acetabulum. The femoral head is present but is separated from the shortened distal femoral segment. With age, a fibrous connection between the head and the distal femoral segment ossifies—usually, not completely. A subtrochanteric varus deformity is invariably present. In the most severe form, class D, most of the femur and the ipsilateral acetabulum are absent (Fig. 164-4).

PFFD is associated with other ipsilateral deformities, including fibular hemimelia (in more than 50% of affected children), shortening of the tibia, equinovalgus

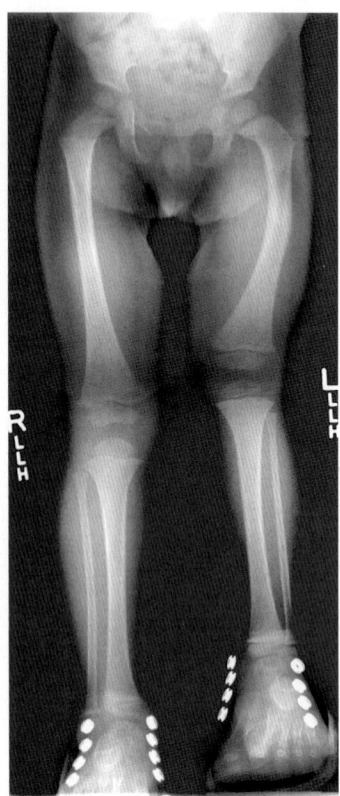

FIGURE 164-2. Two-year-old child with a short left femur. The distal femoral epiphysis is mildly hypoplastic and flattened, and the proximal femoral epiphysis and the acetabulum are relatively normally developed. Bowing of the left femur is noted, along with medial cortical thickening and a significant leg length discrepancy.

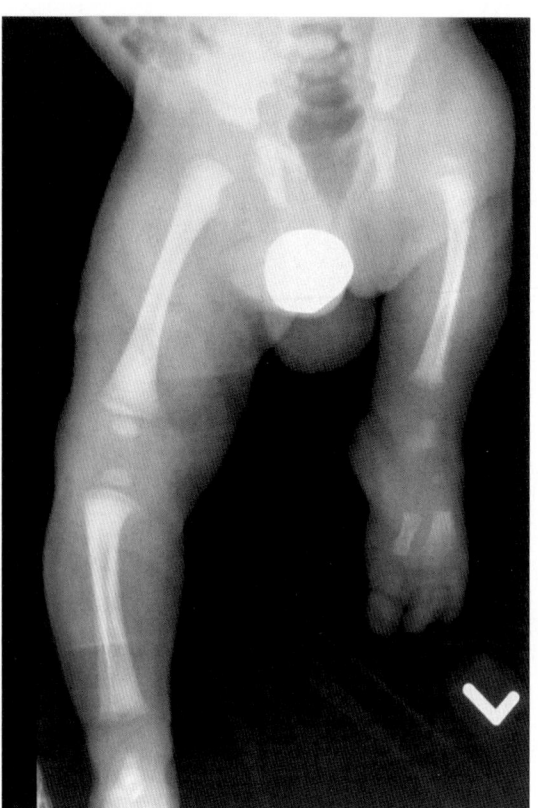

FIGURE 164-4. Two-month-old boy with severe proximal femoral focal deficiency, Aitken type D. Radiographic absence of the left femur is noted, along with associated ipsilateral acetabular hypoplasia. The left ankle joint is located at approximately the same level as the right knee joint.

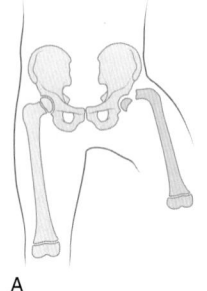
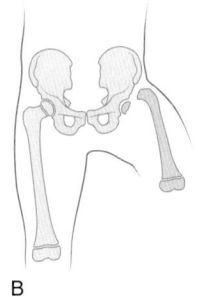
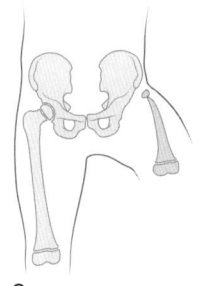
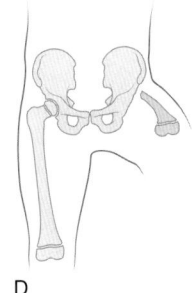

A   B   C   D

FIGURE 164-3. Aitken classification of proximal femoral focal deficiency.

deformity of the foot (more often than equinovarus deformity), and deficiency of the lateral rays of the foot. PFFD is bilateral in 15% of affected children.

Sonography can be used to delineate radiographically inapparent structures at an early age. If a cartilaginous femoral head and its connection to the femoral shaft can be shown, the stability of the hip joint is likely greater than is implied from radiographs. Similar to sonography, magnetic resonance imaging (MRI) is useful for defining the anatomy of the hip joint and associated deformities of the limb (Fig. 164-5). It also allows for appropriate early classification of deformity in a young child, in whom structures may be radiographically inapparent. Although the acetabulum might appear developed, even the least severe forms of PFFD are associated with acetabular deficiency. In contrast to the predominantly

anterior deficiency of developmental acetabular dysplasia, the acetabulum in PFFD usually has an insufficient posterior wall. Most of the muscles about the affected hip are hypoplastic when compared with the contralateral normal side, with the exception of the sartorius muscle, which is often hypertrophied. This results in the characteristic flexion deformity of the hip and knee. MRI also defines the anatomy of soft tissues that can guide surgical exposure and preparation of the limb stump for fitting of a prosthesis.

Therapy for children with PFFD is based on severity of the deficiency and projection of growth and final limb length discrepancy at maturity. Objectives for treatment are to maximize the length of the extremity; to promote stability of the hip, knee, and ankle; and to optimize anatomic alignment. Mild deformities may not require

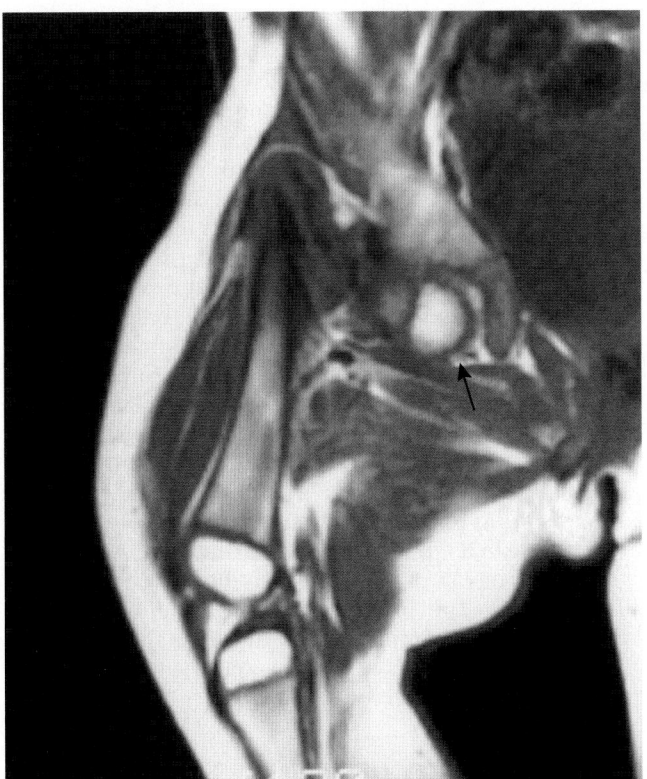

FIGURE 164-5. Coronal T1-weighted magnetic resonance image of a girl with proximal focal femoral deficiency. The femoral head *(arrow)* is ossified, and the acetabulum is well developed. Marked angulation is seen at the site of a proximal femoral fibrous pseudarthrosis. The distal femoral condyle is well developed.

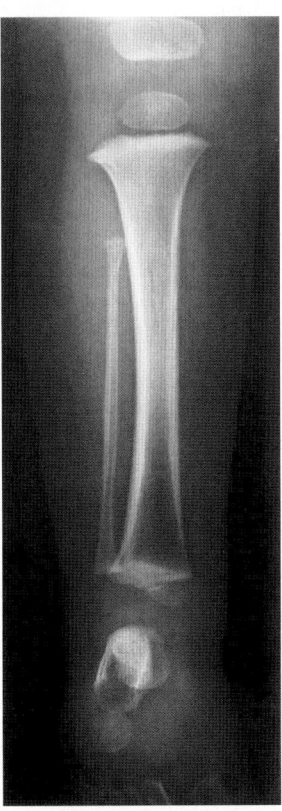

FIGURE 164-6. Three-year-old boy with fibular hemimelia. The fibula is short, predominantly at its proximal end.

surgery. Stabilization of the upper femoral defect is controversial and usually is indicated if a deformity is progressive. Children with more severe deformities benefit from amputation of the foot and fusion of the knee. Rotationplasty of the tibia, in which the foot is rotated 180 degrees (so that the toes face posteriorly and the ankle now serves as a knee joint), allows the ankle and foot to control a distal prosthesis. Intact sensory feedback from the foot provides proprioceptive control of the knee. Thus, it is imperative to assess the morphology of the proximal femur and acetabulum and the cartilaginous epiphyses of the knee, as well as supporting soft tissue structures. For example, instability of the knee can result from absence of the anterior cruciate ligament. In the rare case of bilateral PFFD, amputation is contraindicated, and therapy is based on extension prostheses that improve the child's height.

> **PFFD is associated with extensive bone and soft tissue deformities of the ipsilateral lower extremity.**

Fibular Hemimelia

Deformities of the fibula range from mild deficiency of the proximal end of the bone (Fig. 164-6) to complete absence accompanied by multiple malformations of neighboring structures.

Fibular hemimelia is the most common hemimelia and the most common congenital anomaly of the fibula. It is also referred to as congenital short tibia with absent fibula syndrome. Unilateral absence is more frequent than bilateral deformity. A band of strong connective tissue may replace all or most of the fibula. Fibular hemimelia is associated with a short, bowed tibia; absence of lateral rays of the foot; tarsal abnormalities (particularly coalitions); and femoral shortening or deficiency in 15% of patients. Caskey and Lester reported a clubfoot deformity in 16% of patients with fibular hemimelia. Other associations include small, subluxed, or dislocated patellae, hypoplastic femoral condyles, and absent cruciate ligaments. MRI can document these associated abnormalities, particularly if surgery is contemplated. One of the most frequently used classification schemes is that of Achterman and Kalamchi, which is based on the radiographic appearance of the fibula, but it does not address associated ankle joint and foot deformities. Stanitski and Stanitski have proposed a new classification method that assesses ankle and foot morphologies, in addition to fibular deformity.

The talipes equinovalgus deformity of the foot and severe shortening of the limb associated with fibular hemimelia result in poor function of the limb. Children with extensive abnormalities involving the fibula, ipsilateral tibia, femur, and foot benefit the most from early amputation of the foot and often the more proximal structures. If the deformity is less severe, lengthening of the affected side, realignment of the talotibial articulation, and epiphysiodesis of the contralateral limb are often undertaken. Attempts at lengthening a severely dysplastic limb are often unsatisfactory.

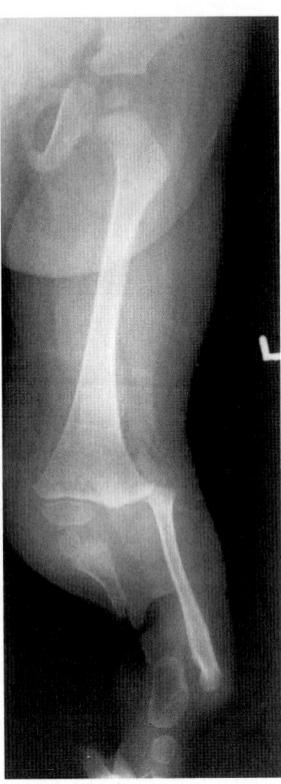

FIGURE 164-7. Two-year-old girl with tibial hemimelia. A dysplastic proximal tibial remnant is evident, as are fibular deformity and absence of multiple tarsal bones.

Vascular anomalies associated with congenital malformations of the extremities, including fibular hemimelia, can be delineated with magnetic resonance (MR) arteriography. Preoperative knowledge of the vascularity of the limb can help to prevent ischemic complications related to vascular injury during surgery.

Tibial Hemimelia

Most cases of tibial hemimelia are sporadic, although reported forms (particularly bilateral deformities) display an autosomal dominant inheritance pattern. Jones and coworkers classified the spectrum of tibial dysplasia into four groups. In type I, which is the most severe form, the tibia is not recognized radiographically at birth. Lack of ossification of the distal femoral epiphysis implies that no proximal tibia is present. The least severe form, type IV, involves congenital tibial diastasis. In these children, the tibia is short and diverges from the fibula at the ankle. The talus is displaced proximally. No normal distal tibial articulation surface is present (Fig. 164-7).

As with other deformities of the extremities, radiography is insensitive to unossified structures, and the true extent of the malformation may be overestimated. An unossified tibial remnant may not be recognized. Sonography can be used to document a tibial anlage and the integrity of the patellar tendon. MRI may identify a tibial remnant and associated osteocartilaginous abnormalities. The patella may be absent or hypoplastic. Epiphyses of the knee are often dysplastic, and tarsal bone abnormalities such as coalition may be present. Additional deformities include foot malalignment, muscular hypoplasia (especially of the quadriceps muscle), fibular displacement, and vascular anomalies.

Treatment of tibial hemimelia varies with the severity of the deformity. A knee disarticulation is recommended for complete tibial absence. Brown pioneered centralization of the fibula with a Syme amputation of the foot in children with complete tibial hemimelia. This produces adequate results in the rare cases in which the quadriceps muscles are well developed. Knee instability and flexure contracture caused by unopposed hamstring pull caused by hypoplastic quadriceps muscles are complications of knee salvage procedures. When the quadriceps mechanism is abnormal, the patella is often absent. MRI can be used to assess deficiencies preoperatively, allowing the clinician to discern who will function better with primary knee disarticulation (most patients) rather than knee reconstruction. Some cultures do not accept amputation. Hosny described the use of an external fixator to centralize the fibula and lengthen the limb, resulting in functional improvement.

If the tibial deficiency is partial (Jones type II deformity), fusion of the proximal fibula to the proximal tibial remnant can provide excellent function. In these cases, the foot is amputated to alleviate accompanying distal instability. This usually is performed after the proximal tibia has ossified.

UPPER EXTREMITY DEFICIENCIES

Radial Deficiency

Congenital radial deficiency, also referred to as *radial clubhand,* ranges from hypoplasia of the thumb to various degrees of radial hypoplasia. Complete absence is the most common longitudinal deficiency. This deformity usually is accompanied by radial and volar deviation of the hand, which results in part from unopposed pull by the flexor carpi radialis and brachioradialis muscles. In most cases of radial aplasia, the forearm is bowed to the radial side and the distal ulna is prominent (Fig. 164-8). The forearm is short (usually approximately two thirds the length of the normal contralateral side) and remains proportionately so throughout growth. Often, only the capitate, hamate, and triquetral bones and the metacarpals and phalanges of the four ulnar rays are present and normal. The trapezium, scaphoid, and first ray often are deformed or absent. If a remnant of the radius is present proximally, it usually is fused to the ulna, which is curved, shortened, and thickened. Bilateral deficiency occurs in approximately 50% of affected children. The degree of deformity of the hand is related to the severity of deficiency of the forearm. Conditions associated with radial dysplasia are listed in Table 164-1. Usually, the entire limb is involved to some degree, which often results in joint dysfunction of the shoulder, elbow, wrist, carpus, and small joints of the hand. Associated muscular deficiencies also are proportionate to the degree of skeletal abnormality. Neurovascular abnormalities include an absent radial artery and superficial radial nerve.

Whether radial dysplasia is isolated or is associated with a syndrome, the primary malformation is likely the result of a vascular abnormality in the embryo that occurred prior to differentiation of mesenchyme into muscle and bone. In humans, the critical time for radial

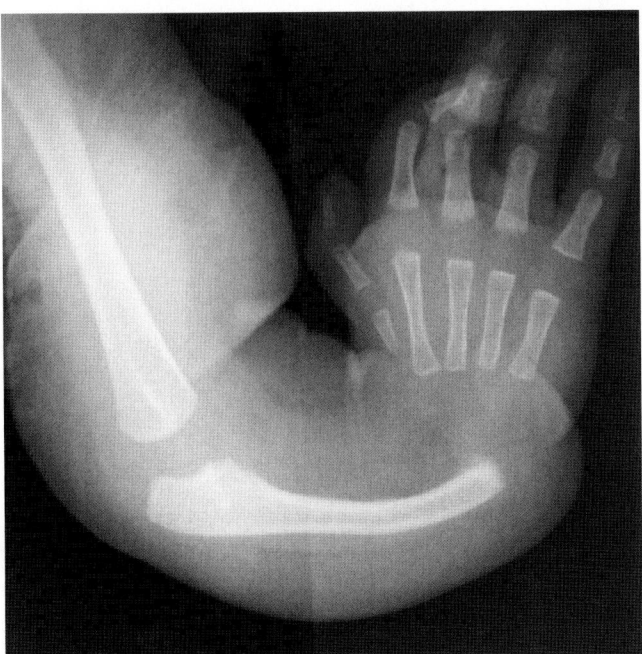

FIGURE 164-8. Radial clubhand in a 10-month-old boy with complete absence of the radius. The ulna is short and bowed. The thumb is hypoplastic and is displaced proximally.

TABLE 164-1

Conditions Associated with Radial Dysplasia

SYNDROMES ASSOCIATED WITH CONGENITAL HEART DISEASE
Holt-Oram syndrome

SYNDROMES ASSOCIATED WITH BLOOD DYSCRASIAS
Fanconi anemia (pancytopenia–dysmelia syndrome)
Thrombocytopenia—absent radius syndrome

SYNDROMES ASSOCIATED WITH MENTAL RETARDATION
Brachmann-de Lange (Cornelia de Lange) syndrome
Seckel syndrome

SYNDROMES ASSOCIATED WITH CHROMOSOMAL ABNORMALITIES
Trisomy 13
Trisomy 18

SYNDROMES ASSOCIATED WITH TERATOGENS
Thalidomide embryopathy
Varicella embryopathy

OTHER: VACTERL ASSOCIATION

Modified from Goldberg MJ, Bartoshevsky LE: Congenital hand anomaly: etiology and associated malformations. Hand Clin 1985;1:405-415.
VACTERL, vertebral, anal, cardiac, tracheal, esophageal, renal, limb.

development occurs between the fifth and sixth post-ovulatory weeks. Most cases are sporadic, but some autosomal dominant and autosomal recessive inheritance patterns are reported. Other cases are likely the result of various environmental insults from viruses, chemicals, radiation, and drugs during limb bud development.

Treatment of a longitudinal radial deficiency begins with serial casting and splinting intended to improve radial deviation by stretching the soft tissues. This often is followed by surgical centralization of the hand over the ulna to improve function and appearance. Thumb reconstruction and pollicization of the index finger are often indicated. Experimental work with vascularized epiphyseal transplantation has shown promising results and may become part of established treatment.

Radial dysplasia may be isolated or associated with a syndrome; it usually involves the entire limb to some degree.

Ulnar Deficiency

Deficiency that occurs along the ulnar or postaxial border of the upper extremity is known as *ulnar clubhand*. This is a relatively uncommon disorder that occurs much less frequently than radial clubhand. Approximately 25% of cases are bilateral. Most cases are sporadic, but associations with many other syndromes have been reported; one of the most common of these is Brachmann-de Lange syndrome.

In ulnar hypoplasia or aplasia, abnormalities are almost always present in the ulnar carpal, metacarpal, and phalangeal rays (Fig. 164-9). The pisiform is always absent, and the hamate frequently is not detected.

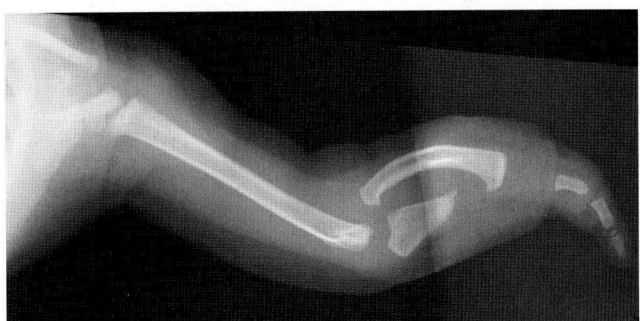

FIGURE 164-9. Ulnar deficiency. Partial formation of the proximal ulna is evident, as is aplasia of the distal portion. The radius is bowed, and only a single digit of the hand is present. The humerus is normal.

Syndactyly, carpal fusion, and radiohumeral fusion are frequently noted. The forearm is shortened and bowed, with a concavity to the ulnar side. The hand is deviated in an ulnar direction, and elbow abnormalities are common. Hypoplasia of the shoulder girdle and the upper arm can coexist with ulnar deficiencies. Anomalies of the contralateral upper limb and the lower limbs (such as proximal femoral focal deficiency) have been reported.

Treatment for ulnar deficiency includes early correction of ulnar deviation of the hand achieved with serial casting. Surgical treatment is reserved for those cases with significant limitation of function. Forearm instability and associated hand deformities must be addressed.

GENERALIZED DEFICIENCIES AND CONTRACTURES

Congenital Constriction Bands

Constricting rings around limbs present at birth are known as *Streeter bands, congenital constriction bands,* or

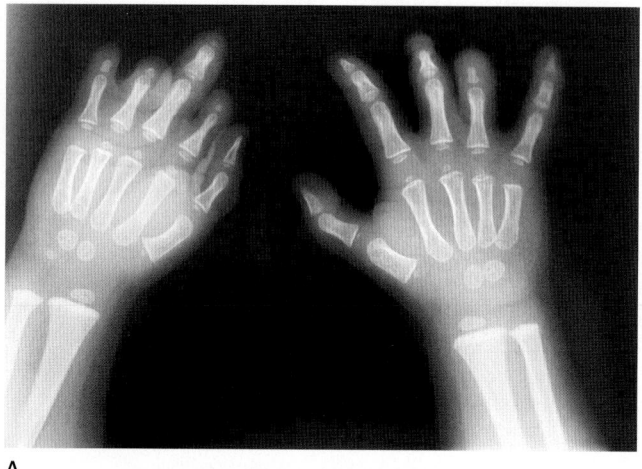

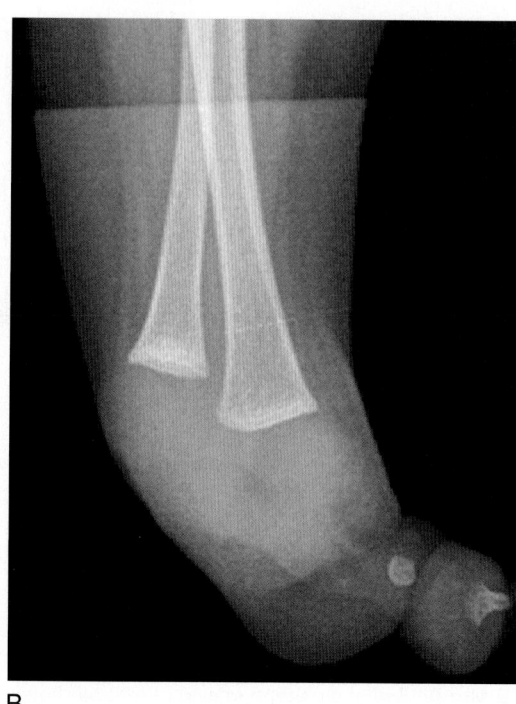

FIGURE 164-10. Amniotic band syndrome. **A,** Two-year-old girl with absence of several distal phalanges bilaterally. Several small middle phalangeal remnants are seen. The thumbs are nearly normal. **B,** Oblique view of the distal leg and foot in an infant shows near-complete absence of the bones of the foot and a constriction band of a solitary digit.

annular or *amniotic bands*. These bands occasionally are associated with loss of the limb distal to the constriction. Various theories have attempted to explain these malformations. Streeter proposed one of the most popular early theories. He believed that ring contractions of the limbs, often associated with intrauterine amputations, were the result of local dysplasias that occurred early in fetal life. This dysplasia caused the soft tissue to slough and eventually heal, resulting in the constricting ring. Ring tissue was unable to expand while the tissue on each side of the ring continued to grow.

Now, evidence strongly suggests that the bands result from intrauterine rupture of the amnion and subsequent mechanical constriction of fetal limbs. Various body parts become entangled in the amnion as it separates from the surrounding chorion. In some instances, adjacent structures are pulled together by the bands and ultimately become fused, producing a soft tissue syndactyly. Bony syndactyly is very rare. The earlier the amnion ruptures, the more severe are the malformations. Limb abnormalities range from slight soft tissue grooves to transverse intrauterine amputations (Fig. 164-10). Acrosyndactyly, craniofacial and visceral anomalies, and fetal death are part of the spectrum of congenital constriction band syndrome. Sporadic congenital constriction band syndrome is estimated to occur at an incidence of 1:1200 to 1:15,000 births.

Radiography may result in underestimation of the degree of soft tissue compromise, and associated anomalous vascular anatomy may go unrecognized. MRI can be used to evaluate the depth of the constriction band, the degree of resultant lymphedema, and the integrity of the involved musculature. Delineation of vascular anatomy with the use of MR arteriography may help to prevent injury to the vessels during surgery.

Surgical treatment is usually cosmetic, although it may be needed to relieve massive edema distal to a constriction band or to improve neurovascular function. Intervention for patients with acrosyndactyly may result in partial correction of the deformity and improved longitudinal growth. With more accurate prenatal identification of isolated extremity involvement by congenital constriction bands, attempts at fetoscopic lysis in utero suggest promise for limb salvage. Three-dimensional sonography may prove useful for prenatal diagnosis and counseling of parents.

> The earlier in utero rupture of the amnion occurs with subsequent mechanical constriction, the more severe is the limb malformation.

Arthrogryposis

Multiple congenital contractures presenting in infants was termed *arthrogryposis multiplex congenita* early in the last century. *Arthrogryposis*, derived from the Greek for "crooked or curved joint," is also referred to as *amyoplasia congenita fetalis deformans, multiple congenital articular rigidities,* and *multiple congenital contractures.* However, the term is a descriptive diagnosis and does not specify a cause. It is used loosely to refer to any condition that results in congenital contractures, such as conditions that limit intrauterine movement of joints. The earlier in gestation that movement is limited, and the longer the restriction lasts, the more severe will be the contractures at birth. Normal in utero motion is necessary for normal development of joints. Girls and boys are affected equally.

TABLE 164-2

Causes of Arthrogryposis: Causes of Limited Fetal Joint Mobility

Neurologic	Disorders of cerebrum
	Anterior horn cell deficiency
	Abnormalities of nerve function or structure (central or peripheral)
Muscular	Abnormal formation or function
	Congenital muscular dystrophy
	Mitochondrial disorders
Connective tissue or skeletal	Primary disorders
Vascular compromise	Severe bleeding
	Monozygotic twins
	Amniotic bands
Mechanical compression	Fetal crowding from multiple births
	Oligohydramnios
	Uterine fibroids/other tumors
	Amniotic bands
	Trauma
Maternal	Diabetes mellitus
	Hyperthermia
	Infection
	Drug use and abuse

Adapted from Jones K: Smith's Recognizable Patterns of Human Malformation, 5th ed. Philadelphia, WB Saunders, 1997:688.

It has been postulated that most cases of multiple congenital contractures are the result of abnormal muscles (such as myopathies), abnormal nerve function or innervation, abnormal connective tissues, or mechanical limitation of movement (such as oligohydramnios or multiple fetuses). Indirect evidence suggests that intrauterine damage to the anterior horn cells of the spinal cord may be responsible for the congenital contractures. Other possible causes include mutagenic agents, mitotic abnormalities, and toxic chemicals or drugs (Table 164-2). More than 150 different conditions have been reported in association with multiple congenital contractures. Arthrogryposis is also associated with genetic syndromes and other malformations. Incidences of clubfeet, dysplastic hips, and hyperextensibility are increased in the families of children with arthrogryposis.

Radiography is used to evaluate the skeleton for bony anomalies. Contractures that are present at birth are often symmetric and most commonly affect distal parts of limbs. The lower extremities are usually involved, but more than half of patients have upper limb abnormalities as well. Rigid joints and hypotonia contribute to frequent perinatal fractures. Soft tissue dimples may be seen over the affected joints, and muscle mass is decreased in affected limbs (Fig. 164-11). Affected muscles are partially or completely replaced by fatty or fibrous tissue.

Many children eventually develop a scoliosis. MRI can be used to assess joint integrity when surgery to maximize joint function is planned. The long-term prognosis for most children with arthrogryposis is good. However, children with associated central nervous system abnormalities usually have a limited life span. A neuromuscular workup is recommended for all children with arthrogryposis. Early therapy administered prior to 12 months of age, which includes manipulation to increase range of motion as well as surgery, is advocated for best results.

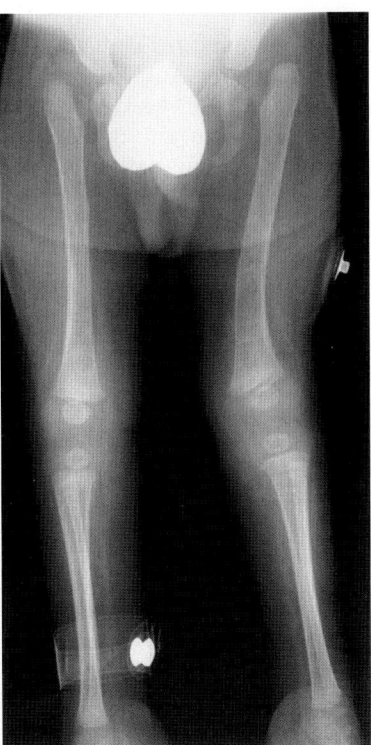

FIGURE 164-11. Lower extremities of a child with arthrogryposis. The bones are gracile and demineralized, and muscle mass is reduced. The proximal femora are dislocated, and the acetabula are dysplastic. Femoral bowing on the left is the result of previous fractures.

Arthrogryposis is a descriptive term that refers to any condition that results in congenital contractures, including abnormal nerves, muscles, and connective tissues, or mechanical limitation to fetal movement.

ABNORMAL SIZE: LARGE LIMBS

Overgrowth of the body ranges from involvement of a whole side (hemihypertrophy) to involvement of a limb (macromelia) or only a digit (macrodactyly). Abnormal growth may be confined to a single tissue or may involve all tissues of the affected body part. Children with asymmetry that results from hemihypertrophy are predisposed to develop neoplasms, most commonly within the abdomen. Congenital causes of localized or general body asymmetry include vascular disorders (vascular birthmarks and combined vascular lesions), phakomatoses, asymmetry associated with neoplasia, and bone dysplasia, or the condition may be idiopathic. Various disorders that result in abnormally large limbs are reviewed in other chapters (Chapters 161 and 166).

ABNORMAL CONFIGURATION

Unilateral Congenital Tibial Bowing and Congenital Tibial Dysplasia

Posteromedial congenital bowing is also referred to as *kyphoscoliosis tibia*. This congenital deformity affects the tibia, fibula, and soft tissues of the lower extremity. The tibia and the fibula show marked posteromedial bowing at the middle or distal one third of the shaft (Fig. 164-12). Rarely is the bowing lateral. At birth, the foot is held in a calcaneovalgus (dorsiflexed) position. The origin and pathogenesis remain uncertain and may be related to abnormal early embryologic development rather than to abnormal fetal positioning or intrauterine fracture.

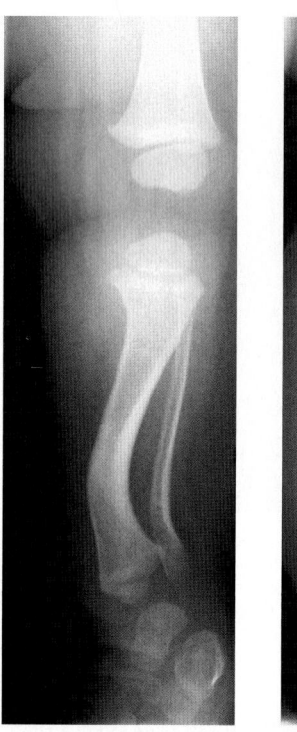 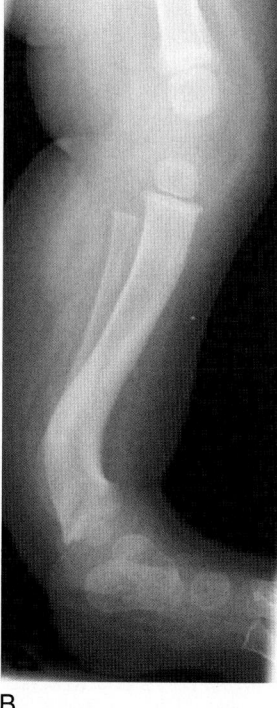

A   B

FIGURE 164-12. One-year-old girl with congenital posteromedial bowing. **A,** On the frontal radiograph, medial bowing is seen at the junction of the middle and distal one third of the tibia. The fibula is similarly bowed. **B,** The posterior component of the bowing is seen on the lateral radiograph.

Fetal vascular insufficiency may also play a role. After examination of a fetus with congenital bowing, De Maio and associates suggested that compressive events associated with amnion rupture may be responsible for the deformity. As the child grows, tibial bowing and shortening often partially resolve. Treatment is conservative, such as corrective casts or splints to hold the foot and support the leg during growth and remodeling. If severe persistent deformity continues beyond toddler age, a leg length discrepancy, usually on the order of 3 to 7 cm, may result, requiring osteotomies and lengthening procedures. Occasionally, epiphysiodesis of the contralateral side may be needed.

Anterolateral bowing of the tibia has been termed *congenital pseudarthrosis*. This is a misnomer because the pseudarthrosis or fracture is rarely congenital. The deformity is almost always unilateral. The preferred term is *congenital tibial dysplasia* (CTD). It is a rare anomaly (1 in 140,000 live births), but it occurs in 1% to 2% of children with neurofibromatosis type 1 (NF1). However, at least 70% of children with CTD have NF1. This may be an underestimation because clinical features of NF1 may appear only later in life. CTD presents as anterolateral bowing or fracture of the tibia, often before other manifestations of NF1 present. Lack of involvement of the fibula suggests that the bowing will resolve spontaneously. In anterolateral bowing associated with NF1, fracture and refracture rates are very high. Limb length inequality is frequent and results from disuse atrophy and abnormal growth at the distal tibial physis. Often, a valgus deformity is noted at the ankle. Surgical management can be frustrating because nonunion or pseudarthrosis after osteotomy is frequent.

Radiographic changes seen with CTD are variable and include anterolateral bowing of the tibia, fracture, pseudarthrosis, hourglass-like constriction of the midshaft of the tibia, cystic changes usually at the junction of the upper and middle thirds of the tibia, sclerosis that narrows the medullary canal, and, infrequently, involvement of the fibula alone (Fig. 164-13). Several classifications of CTD have been proposed, all of which include sclerotic, cystic, and dysplastic types. Pathologic studies show abnormal, highly cellular fibrovascular tissue with variable amounts of fibrocartilage and hyaline cartilage within the tibia. Bone growth and repair are abnormal. The pattern of abnormal fibrous tissue results in the dysplastic or cystic changes characteristic of the disorder.

> **Congenital bowing of the tibia and fibula is almost always posteromedial, whereas congenital tibial dysplasia (congenital pseudarthrosis) shows anterolateral bowing.**

ABNORMAL SEGMENTATION (FUSION DEFORMITIES)

Tarsal Coalition

Tarsal coalition is a congenital failure of segmentation of the primitive mesenchyme that results in the union of two or more tarsal bones. Intertarsal bridges have been

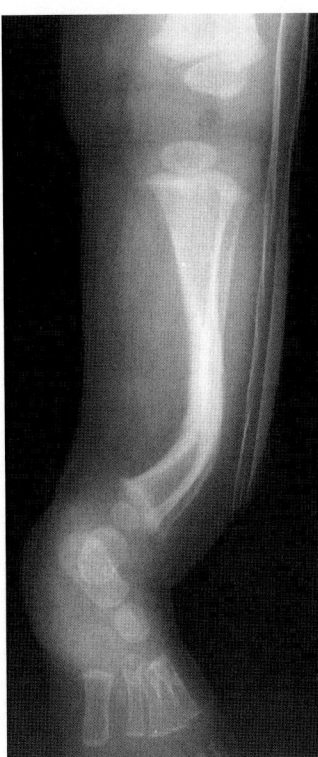 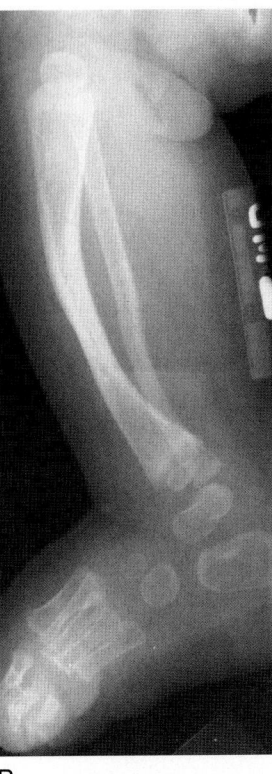

A   B

FIGURE 164-13. Anteroposterior **(A)** and lateral **(B)** radiographs of anterolateral tibial bowing in a child with congenital tibial dysplasia and neurofibromatosis type 1. The medullary canal is nearly obliterated, but no fracture is apparent.

found in fetal tissue. A preadolescent or adolescent child with pain in the midfoot and hindfoot that is associated with lack of motion in the subtalar region should be suspected of having a tarsal coalition. Prevalence in the U.S. population is approximately 1% or less. At least 50% of patients with coalitions have bilateral findings. An autosomal dominant inheritance pattern with a high level of penetrance is reported, although the coalition need not involve the same joint. Although it typically presents during the second decade of life, tarsal coalition may not manifest until adulthood.

Tarsal coalition is defined on the basis of anatomic location and completeness of ossification. A complete ossific bar forms a *synostosis*, a cartilaginous bar forms a *synchondrosis*, and a fibrous union is termed a *syndesmosis*. The most common of fusions are talocalcaneal and calcaneonavicular. The middle facet is the most common location for a talocalcaneal coalition. Talonavicular and calcaneocuboid coalitions are much less common. Synostoses can occur between other bones of the foot but frequently are associated with other limb abnormalities, such as fibular hemimelia or short femur, or disorders such as Apert syndrome.

Symptoms from a tarsal coalition present with advancing ossification. Pain with activity usually is the presenting symptom. The child may have a peroneal spastic flatfoot, which involves pain and rigid valgus deformity of the hindfoot and forefoot, along with peroneal muscle spasm. This condition is not a true spasticity

but reflects peroneal shortening to adjust for heel valgus and to maintain a less painful position for the subtalar joint. However, any abnormality of the subtalar joint that restricts motion, such as fracture, arthritis, or tumor, also can result in a peroneal spastic flatfoot. Inflammatory arthrofibrosis mimicking a talocalcaneal coalition has been described in the middle subtalar facet.

Imaging evaluation of all children suspected of having a tarsal coalition should begin with conventional radiographs. Anteroposterior (AP), lateral, and 45-degree lateral oblique views should be obtained. The oblique radiograph is used to show a calcaneonavicular bar (Fig. 164-14). Although the AP view rarely directly delineates a coalition, it can be used to exclude other causes of peroneal spastic foot. A "ball-and-socket" articulation of the distal tibia and talus is an uncommon association with tarsal coalition. This configuration at the ankle joint is nonspecific and may be associated with congenital long bone deficiencies. The lateral radiograph is useful for showing secondary signs of tarsal coalition. These include a hypoplastic talar head, a talar beak (flaring of the superior margin of the talar head), and broadening or rounding of the lateral talar process. An "anteater nose" on a lateral radiograph, which represents an anterior prolongation of the superior calcaneus, is a consistent sign of a calcaneonavicular coalition (see Fig. 164-14). A continuous "C-line" formed by the medial outline of the talar dome and the inferior aspect of the sustentaculum tali (see Fig. 164-14) is suggestive of a talocalcaneal coalition but may be found in other causes of flatfoot deformity as well.

A talar beak (see Fig. 164-14) should not be confused with the talar ridge that forms more proximally or at the mid-neck of the talus—the site of attachment of the anterior tibiotalar joint capsule. Additional radiographic signs for a talocalcaneal coalition recently have been reported, including nonvisualization of the middle facet on lateral radiograph, a dysmorphic (ovoid and enlarged) sustentaculum tali, and a short talar neck. Additional signs for a calcaneonavicular coalition include a wide navicular, which shows a proximal articular cortex wider than the adjacent cortex of the talar head, and a laterally tapering navicular bone. Secondary radiographic signs that may be seen in tarsal coalition are summarized in Table 164-3.

The axial or Harris-Beath view is used to evaluate for a talocalcaneal coalition. In this projection, the normal middle and posterior talocalcaneal facets are relatively parallel to each other. Because most subtalar coalitions involve the middle facet, most abnormalities are seen medially. A frank bony bridge may be seen. In nonosseous fusion, the facet surfaces may be irregular and angled inferomedially. Because the axial view may be difficult to angle correctly for optimal visualization of the subtalar joint, children suspected of having subtalar fusion are commonly referred for cross-sectional imaging.

Computed tomography (CT) and MRI help to define the nature and cross-sectional area of a fusion. Either modality can be used, and a high percentage of agreement has been found between imaging findings obtained through these modalities. CT is more cost-effective if the clinical suspicion for coalition is high (see Fig. 164-14).

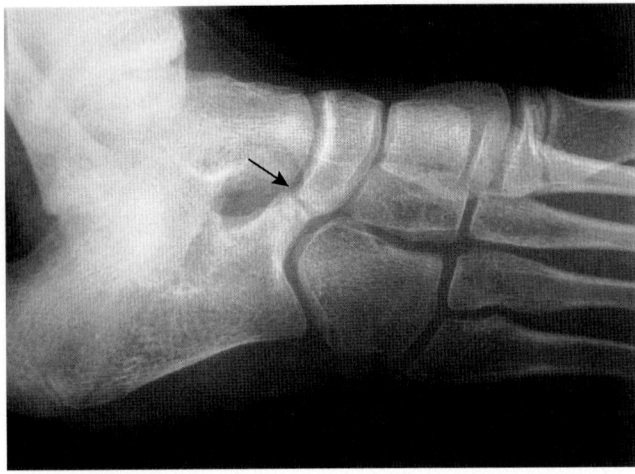

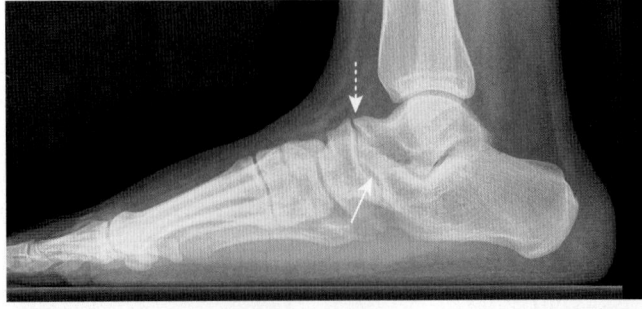

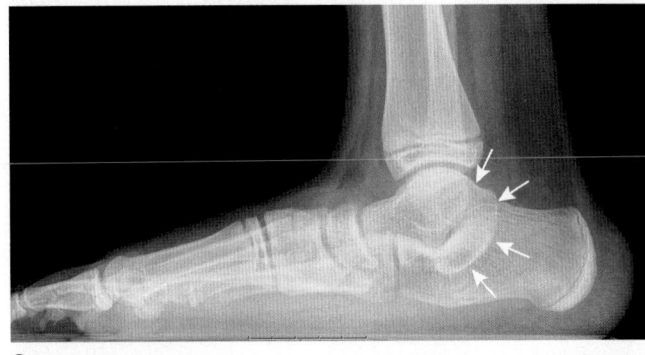

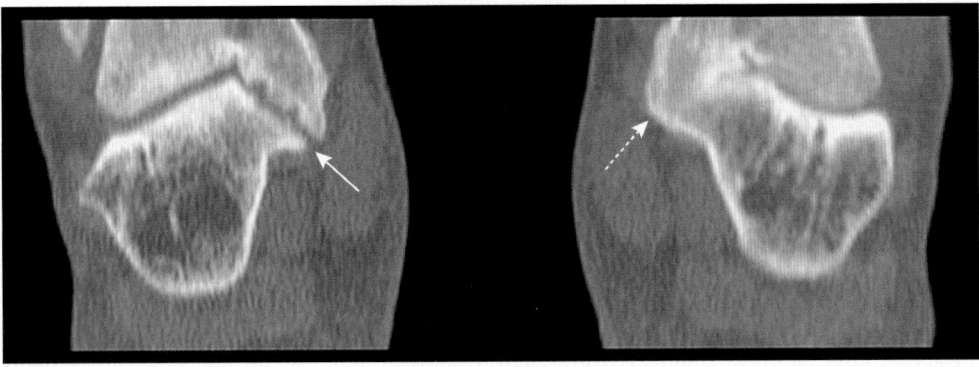

FIGURE 164-14. Tarsal coalition. **A,** Calcaneonavicular incomplete osseous coalition *(arrow)* is seen on an oblique view of the foot. **B and C,** Upright foot. **B,** Prominent talar beak *(dashed arrow)*, an elongated anterior process of the calcaneus, and "the anteater nose sign" *(arrow)* are seen in this child with a calcaneonavicular tarsal coalition. **C,** A continuous C-shaped outline of increased density is present *(arrows)* on the lateral radiograph of a child with a talocalcaneal tarsal coalition. Flatfoot alignment is noted. **D,** Direct coronal computed tomography image shows a nonosseous talocalcaneal coalition (evidenced by bony enlargement, irregularity, and sclerosis) of the middle facet of the right foot *(arrow)* and an almost complete osseous coalition of the left foot *(dashed arrow)*.

TABLE 164-3
Radiographic Secondary Signs Associated with Tarsal Coalition

Talar beaking
Posterior subtalar facet narrowing
Rounding or flattening of the lateral talar process
Hypoplasia of the talus/shortening of the talar neck
"Anteater nose" sign
Ball-and-socket ankle joint
Continuous "C-sign"
Flatfoot deformity
Altered navicular morphology (wide or laterally tapering)
Dysmorphic sustentaculum tali (enlarged and ovoid on
    lateral radiograph)

CT imaging should include coronal (perpendicular to the long axis of the foot) and axial (parallel to the long axis of the foot) images. These can be obtained directly or through reformations. Occasionally, sagittal reformations also can be useful. Both feet should be imaged simultaneously and symmetrically. However, if other causes of pain and limited hindfoot mobility are considered, then MRI may be indicated. MRI can directly show bony, cartilaginous, and fibrous unions. Bone marrow edema often is noted adjacent to the fused articulation. Bone scintigraphy is abnormal in patients with tarsal coalition but generally is not used as the primary diagnostic modality.

Casting and nonsteroidal anti-inflammatory medications are often the initial treatment for symptomatic children. Steroid injections and physical therapy also may be used. If symptoms are not relieved and no degenerative changes have occurred, then surgical resection of the abnormal tarsal bridging is often attempted. Regrowth of a calcaneonavicular coalition can be halted by interposition of the extensor digitorum brevis tendon. Fat is frequently interposed after resection of a subtalar coalition. Subtalar fusion or triple arthrodesis may be indicated in refractory cases.

Carpal Fusion

Fusion of the carpal bones is a normal variant that is seen in approximately 0.1% of the population (Fig. 164-15).

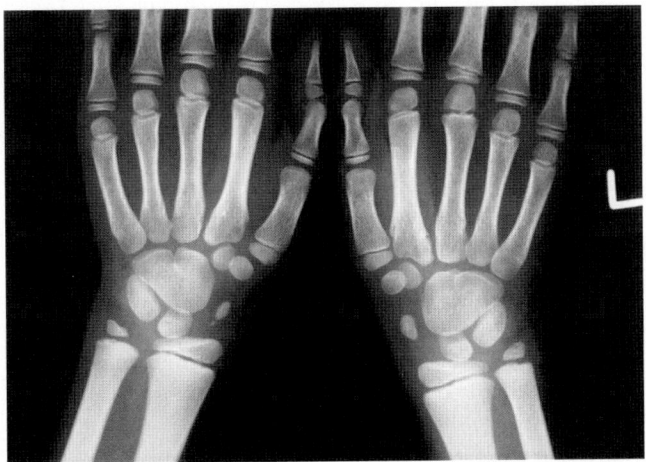

FIGURE 164-15. Fusion of the hamate and capitate bones bilaterally.

Carpal fusion is most frequently seen between the lunate and triquetrum bones. Fusion between bones of the proximal and distal carpal rows usually is associated with a syndrome. Fusions also may be acquired, as in juvenile rheumatoid arthritis.

Syndactyly

Fusion between adjacent digits resulting from intra-uterine failure to separate is termed *syndactyly* (also referred to as "webbed toes or fingers"). These fusions may involve only soft tissue (simple syndactyly), or they may also involve bone (complex syndactyly). If the entire length of the digit is involved, syndactyly is termed *complete,* and if only a partial length is bridged, it is *incomplete.* Syndactyly is easily diagnosed at birth. Fusion may be unilateral or bilateral and most often involves the second, third, and fourth digits. Syndactyly may be isolated or may be associated with congenital disorders such as Poland, Apert (Fig. 164-16), and Carpenter syndromes. Syndactyly is thought to have an autosomal dominant inheritance pattern. Surgery is performed early in life to improve function and appearance.

Symphalangism

Symphalangism is an uncommon autosomal dominant disorder of fusion of the interphalangeal joints of the hands and feet (Fig. 164-17). Although proximal interphalangeal joint fusion is more common, fusion can also be more distal. The anomaly is usually bilateral, and the little finger is affected most often. Fusion may not be recognized radiographically until later in childhood. Despite the radiographic appearance of the digits, seldom

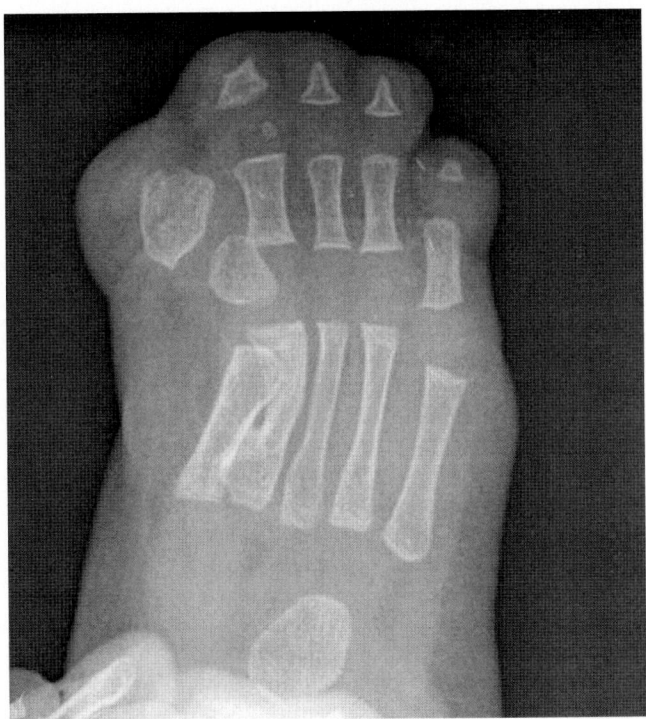

A

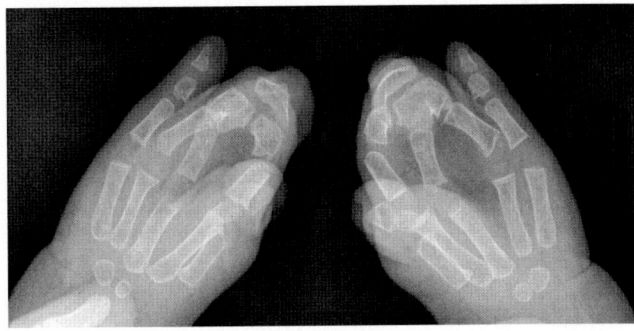

B

FIGURE 164-16. One-year-old child with Apert syndrome. **A,** Frontal view of the foot shows syndactyly of the digits. Hypoplasia of many bones of the foot is seen with absent middle phalanges. The first and second metatarsals are partially fused. **B,** Frontal radiograph of both hands of the same child shows syndactyly, synostosis, and symphalangism bilaterally.

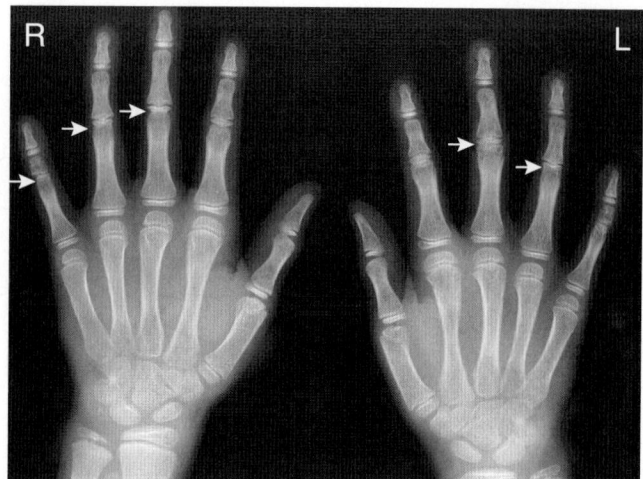

FIGURE 164-17. Symphalangism, or absence of joints, in the hands of a 9-year-old girl with stiff fingers and toes since birth. Fusion of the proximal and middle phalanges of the third, fourth, and fourth digits of the right hand, and of at least the third and fourth digits of the left hand is seen *(arrows).* (The horizontal lucencies are the patent physes of the middle phalanges.) The remaining digits are suboptimally seen. Carpal fusion is also present bilaterally. Fusion of the calcaneus and cuboid and the middle and lateral cuneiform bones was present in the feet bilaterally (not shown).

is disability or loss of function of the hand reported. Symphalangism may be associated with other skeletal abnormalities, various digit deformities (e.g., brachydactyly, clinodactyly, camptodactyly), radioulnar fusion, hip dislocation, tarsal coalition, and spinal anomalies.

> Although they are occasionally associated with syndromes, fusion deformities are often isolated findings. Fusion can occur between the tarsal bones, carpal bones, adjacent digits (syndactyly), interphalangeal joints (symphalangism) and long bones (synostosis).

Radioulnar Synostosis

Congenital radioulnar synostosis anomaly is due to failure of longitudinal segmentation between the radius and the ulna. In utero, cartilaginous anlagen of the humerus, radius, and ulna are connected. During the course of normal separation, which progresses from the distal end of the forearm to the proximal end, at some point the proximal ends of the radius and ulna are connected by a common perichondrium. An insult to segmentation during early in utero development can lead to bony or fibrous synostosis (Fig. 164-18). Boys are affected slightly more frequently than girls, and synostosis may be bilateral.

Cleary and Omer subclassified various forms of congenital radioulnar synostosis on the basis of radiographic appearance. Type I is a fibrous synostosis with a reduced, normal-appearing radial head. Type II is a visible bony synostosis with a reduced radial head. Type III is a bony synostosis with a posteriorly dislocated and hypoplastic radial head, and type IV is a short bony synostosis with an

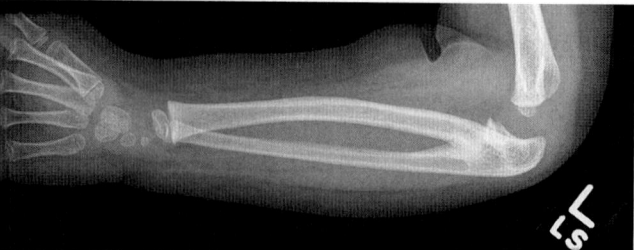

FIGURE 164-18. Radioulnar synostosis in a 4-year-old child with limited pronation. The proximal ends of the bones of the forearm are fused. A bowing deformity is noted in the radius.

anteriorly dislocated, mushroom-shaped radial head. The more common disorder of isolated congenital radial head dislocation can be confused with a proximal radioulnar synostosis. Radioulnar synostosis is associated with disorders such as Apert and Carpenter syndromes, as well as with other upper extremity abnormalities such as polydactyly, syndactyly, and carpal coalition.

On clinical examination, the child is observed to have a fixed degree of pronation and a mild degree of flexion at the elbow. Pain usually occurs during the teen years, when progressive and symptomatic radial head subluxation may be seen. Surgical treatment is usually reserved for patients with a severe pronation deformity or symptomatic radial head subluxation. A derotational osteotomy through the fusion mass must be performed with consideration of the degree of associated soft tissue contracture and neurovascular bundle compromise. Interposition of a vascularized fascio-fat graft, in addition to radial osteotomy, has shown favorable results.

MISCELLANEOUS CONGENITAL MALFORMATIONS

Digits

CLINODACTYLY

Clinodactyly is a curvature of the finger in a radial or ulnar direction (in the mediolateral plane) away from the axis of joint flexion and extension. Although it may involve any digit, clinodactyly most often refers to radial curvature of the distal interphalangeal joint of the fifth digit (Fig. 164-19). Clinodactyly is associated with a short middle phalanx and most often is bilateral. It may be seen in the normal population as a sporadic variant but also can be inherited in an autosomal dominant pattern. It has been described in numerous syndromes, in bone dysplasias, after trauma, and in many miscellaneous conditions. It frequently is seen in Down syndrome. Treatment is undertaken for cosmesis or for excessive scissoring of the digits.

CAMPTODACTYLY

Camptodactyly refers to a congenital or acquired flexion contracture of the finger. It usually is located at the proximal interphalangeal joint of the fifth finger but also can involve the second through fourth digits (Fig. 164-20). Occasionally, the distal interphalangeal joints may be affected. The cause remains unknown but may relate

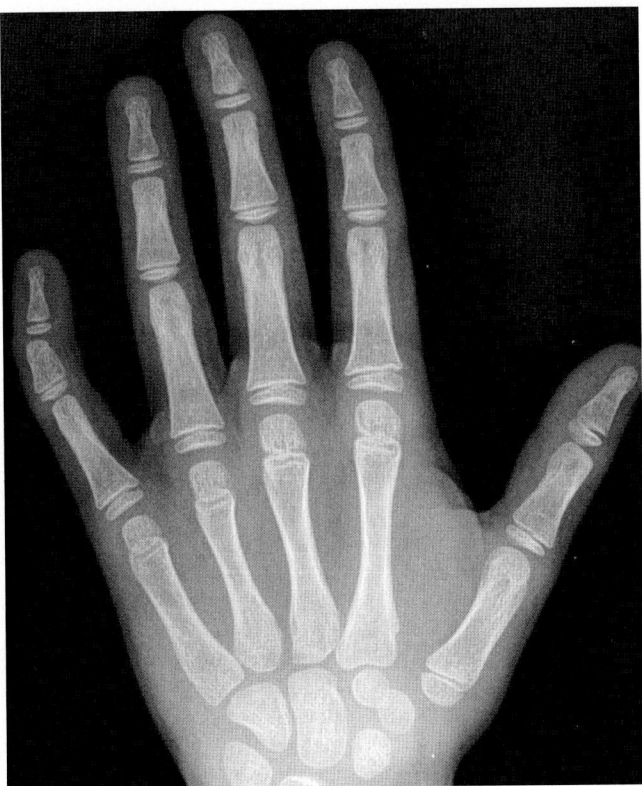

FIGURE 164-19. Seven-year-old girl with clinodactyly of the fifth digit. Medial bending of the finger and a short middle phalanx are noted.

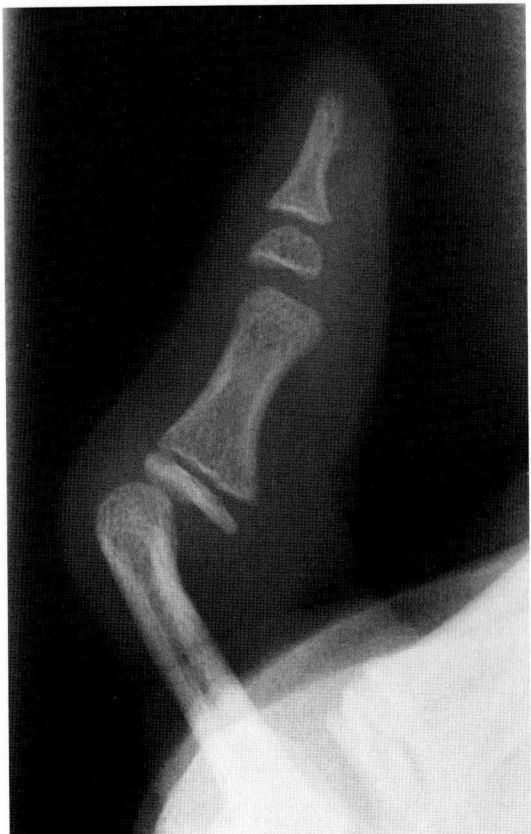

FIGURE 164-20. Flexion of the proximal interphalangeal joint of the fifth digit is seen in this child with camptodactyly. No skin crease is seen, and palmar subluxation of the middle phalanx is evident.

to abnormal insertion of the lumbrical muscles or the flexor digitorum superficialis tendon. Similar to clinodactyly, camptodactyly may be sporadic or may show an autosomal dominant inheritance pattern. It occasionally is associated with a chromosomal abnormality, a bony dysplasia, or other syndrome. Treatment includes bracing or, infrequently, surgical release.

KIRNER DEFORMITY

Palmar bending of the distal phalanx of the fifth digit is termed *Kirner deformity*. It usually is an isolated abnormality that is bilateral and symmetric. The long axis of the distal phalanx is bent toward the palm, and the epiphysis is normally oriented (Fig. 164-21). The physis is widened. With skeletal maturation, the physis fuses on an angle. The distal phalanx exhibits a permanent palmar curvature. Similar to the other digit deformities, Kirner deformity can be a sporadic or an autosomal dominant inherited anomaly.

LONGITUDINAL EPIPHYSEAL BRACKET

Abnormal longitudinal development of the diaphyseal–metaphyseal segment of a phalanx, metacarpal, or metatarsal that often results in a triangular shape has been termed a *delta phalanx*. However, because a metatarsal or a metacarpal may be involved, this term is not entirely correct. The phrase *longitudinal epiphyseal bracket* is more accurate for describing the pathologic anatomy.

This congenital deformity affects the short tubular bones that normally develop a proximal epiphyseal ossification center (e.g., phalanges, first metacarpal, first metatarsal). The involved bone is trapezoid or triangular in shape. The diaphyseal–metaphyseal osseous unit is bracketed along the longitudinal side by a physis and an epiphysis. The physis is arclike, extending from the medial proximal surface along the longitudinal margin of the bone to the distal medial surface, and is similar in configuration to a bracket (Fig. 164-22). The thumb most commonly is affected. Other anomalies of the digits are frequently associated with the longitudinal epiphyseal bracket. The deformity may be sporadic but also is found in the Rubinstein-Taybi syndrome and with fibrodysplasia ossificans progressiva. The cause is likely incomplete development of the primary ossification center of the bone during embryonic or early fetal growth. The growth disturbance relates to the longitudinally oriented cartilaginous bracket, which causes growth to follow a "C-shaped" curve. MRI can be helpful for delineating the size and location of the bracket when it has not yet ossified (see Fig. 164-22). Corrective splinting in infancy is not effective. Early surgical intervention, often a wedge osteotomy, is recommended for better remodeling.

DUPLICATION

Duplication of digits may result from an insult in utero to the apical ectodermal ridge during development. The deformity is more than likely of a "splitting" nature, with

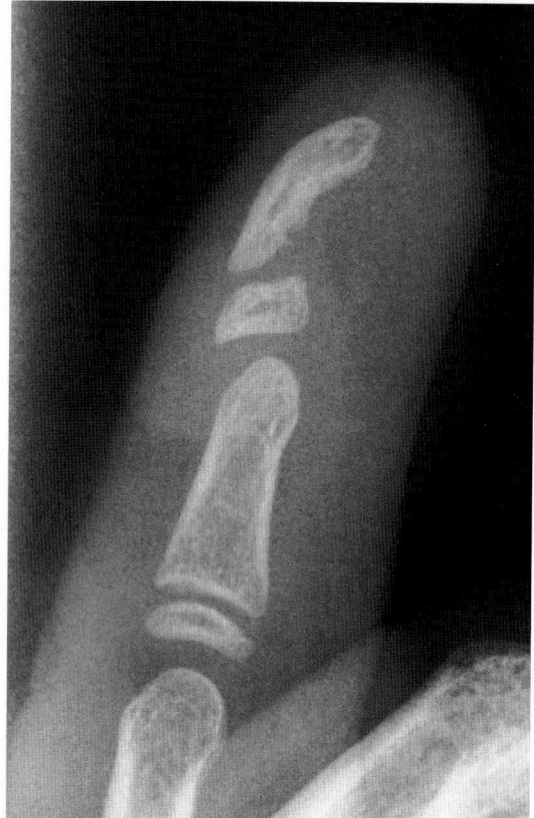

FIGURE 164-21. Palmar bending of the distal phalanx of the fifth digit is revealed in this girl with Kirner deformity. The epiphysis is in a normal position. (From Oestreich AE, Crawford AH: Atlas of Pediatric Orthopedic Radiology. New York, Thieme, 1985:166.)

resultant parts being mildly or severely hypoplastic rather than truly duplicated. Polydactyly or supernumerary digits are a common congenital anomaly most often involving the thumb or small finger. Extra digits may be bilateral and may involve both fingers and toes (Fig. 164-23). Simultaneous polydactyly of the hand and foot is present in approximately one third of cases. The incidence is similar in boys and girls. African Americans are affected more commonly than Caucasians. The malformation may be isolated or may be associated with a syndrome. Duplication can be of soft tissue alone, or of soft tissue and bone. The most accepted classification of polydactyly is based on the position of the extra digit in the hand or foot. An anomaly on the radial or thumb side, previously termed *preaxial*, is now referred to as *radial* or *tibial polydactyly*. An abnormality on the ulnar side, previously called *postaxial*, is now referred to as *ulnar* or *fibular polydactyly*. If the three central digits are affected, the term *central polydactyly* is used; this is the least common type. Additional subclassifications depend on the severity of the defect. Radial polydactyly is more frequently seen in Caucasians and is associated with various disorders, such as Holt-Oram syndrome, Fanconi anemia, and the VACTERL (vertebral, anal, cardiac, tracheal, esophageal, renal, limb) association. Extra digits frequently are fused to the neighboring digit, resulting in syndactyly, which was described previously.

> An anomaly on the radial or thumb side, previously termed *preaxial*, is now referred to as *radial* or *tibial polydactyly*. An abnormality on the ulnar side, previously called *postaxial*, is now referred to as *ulnar* or *fibular polydactyly*.

Split Hand-Foot Malformation

Split hand-foot malformation (SHFM) refers to the congenital cleft splitting of the hands or feet into two halves. It is due to hypoplasia or aplasia of the phalanges, metacarpals, or metatarsals of one or more fingers or toes. The deformity is also referred to as *ectrodactyly, cleft hand* or *cleft foot*, or *lobster* or *crab claw deformity*. The malformation likely results from abnormal cellular and molecular processes that occur between the sixth and seventh weeks of gestation.

SHFM is highly variable in presentation. It can range from mild digital changes to the most severe monodactyly with only the fifth digit remaining. Two distinctive clinical forms have been described—*typical* and *atypical* forms. The typical form has an autosomal dominant inheritance pattern and involves the lack of phalanges and metacarpals, resulting in a deep V-shaped cleft with the two halves resembling a lobster claw (Fig. 164-24). The much less frequent atypical form is sporadic and results in a much wider cleft, which forms a U-shaped central defect. The atypical form rarely involves the feet. Vascular disruption has been implicated as the cause. In most forms, the digits frequently curve in toward the cleft. Syndactyly or synostosis often is present.

SHFM may be isolated, may be associated with congenital constriction band syndrome or, most commonly, may occur as a component of the ectrodactyly–ectodermal dysplasia–cleft lip/palate syndrome (EEC). More than 75 syndromes have been associated with SHFM. EEC most commonly has an autosomal dominant inheritance pattern with incomplete penetrance and variable expression, although autosomal recessive forms have been described. SHFM has been detected on prenatal ultrasonography, which can guide counseling and reconstructive efforts.

Duplication of the Femur

Duplication of the femur is a rare anomaly that more often occurs in the distal portion of the bone. Bifurcation of the femur almost always is associated with tibial dysplasia (partial or complete hemimelia), as well as with other abnormalities such as absence of the patella, hand ectrodactyly, severe clubfoot, and tarsal anomalies. The femur is Y-shaped, and the anteromedial limb forms a protuberance in the medial thigh (Fig. 164-25). At birth, the limb can resemble an exostosis, but with growth, it may become the longer of the two limbs. The lateral limb usually forms an unstable articulation with the proximal fibula. No true knee joint is present. The patella may be absent, and complex foot deformities can be seen. An autosomal recessive form of this complex limb deformity has been reported.

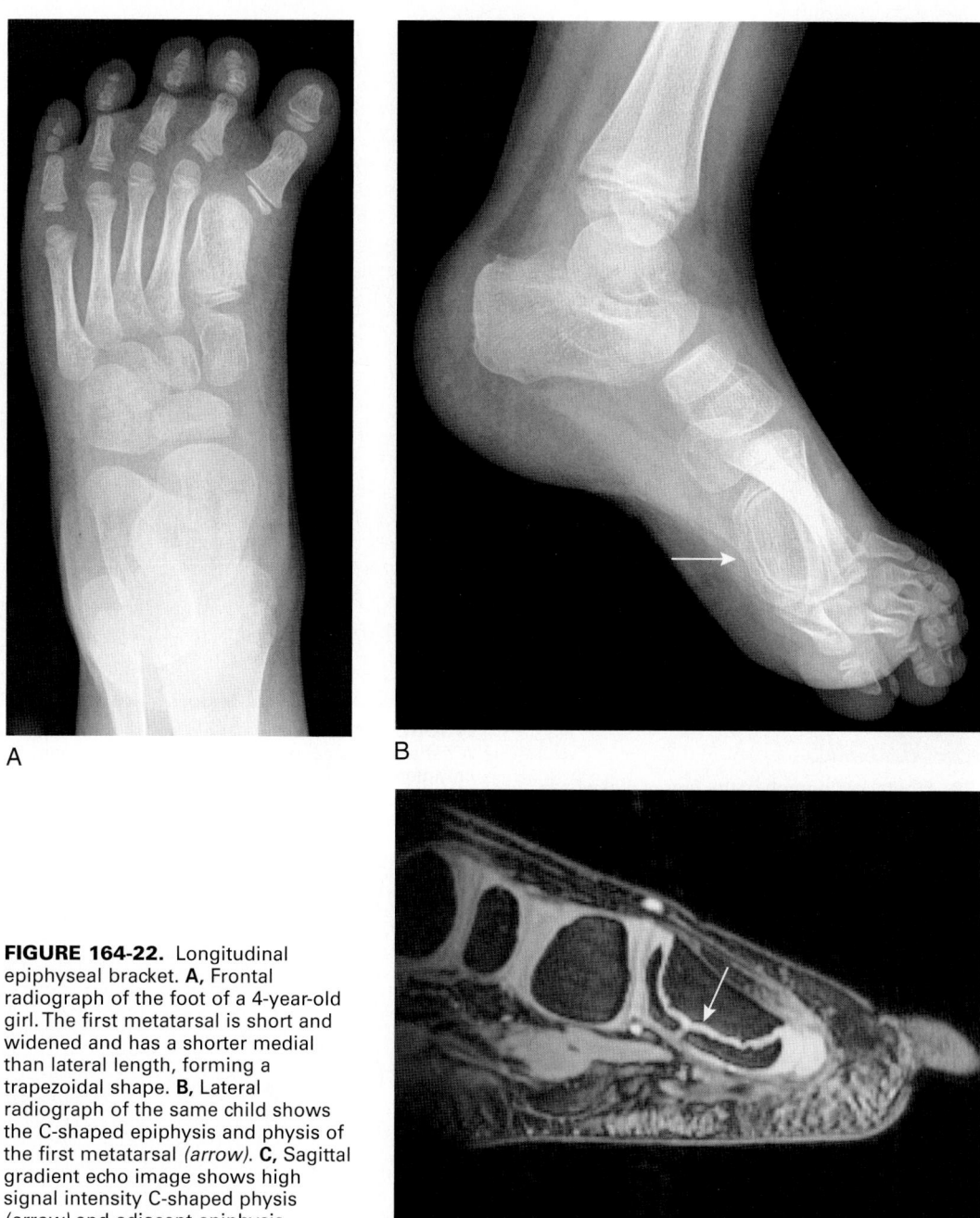

FIGURE 164-22. Longitudinal epiphyseal bracket. **A,** Frontal radiograph of the foot of a 4-year-old girl. The first metatarsal is short and widened and has a shorter medial than lateral length, forming a trapezoidal shape. **B,** Lateral radiograph of the same child shows the C-shaped epiphysis and physis of the first metatarsal *(arrow)*. **C,** Sagittal gradient echo image shows high signal intensity C-shaped physis *(arrow)* and adjacent epiphysis.

Congenital Radial Head Dislocation

Congenital radial head dislocation is the most commonly identified congenital abnormality of the elbow. More than half of cases are associated with other conditions, such as anomalies of the lower extremities, scoliosis, and various syndromes (e.g., Klippel-Feil). Whether it is an isolated abnormality or is associated with other conditions, congenital radial head dislocation is believed to have an autosomal dominant inheritance pattern. The deformity can be unilateral or bilateral.

Congenital radial head dislocation is associated with a small, underdeveloped forearm, a flattened and hypo-plastic capitellum, and a short ulna. The radial head is elongated and thinned or rounded, and most commonly is dislocated in a posterior direction (Fig. 164-26). Radiographs should be carefully evaluated for concomitant radioulnar synostosis. In the young child, the deformity is painless, but motion is usually limited.

Asymptomatic dislocations are not treated. If the child has pain, the radial head can be excised. However, excision of the radial head frequently is accompanied by pain from abnormal mechanics at the wrist. Recent work suggests that open reduction of the proximal radius at an early age may be beneficial.

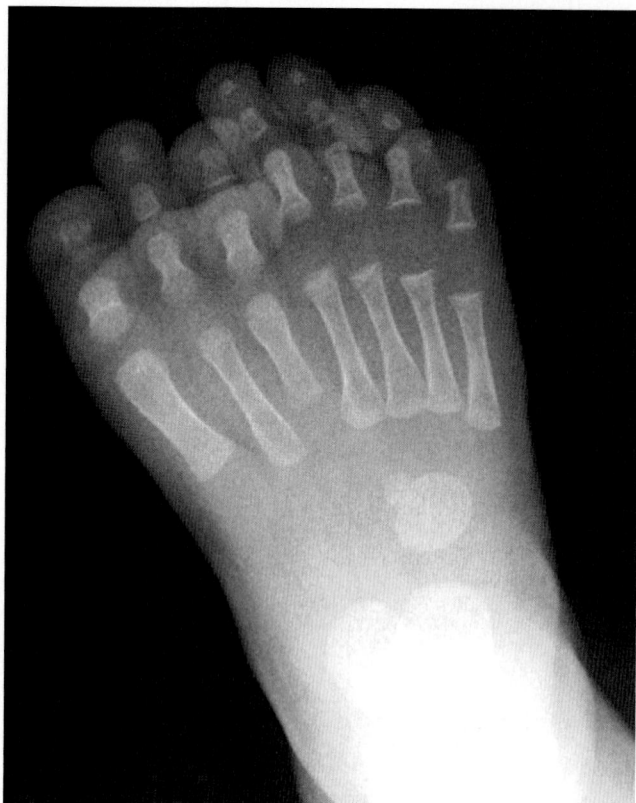

FIGURE 164-23. Frontal radiograph of the foot of a newborn girl with polydactyly. The first and third digits have smaller metatarsals, and each has two phalanges.

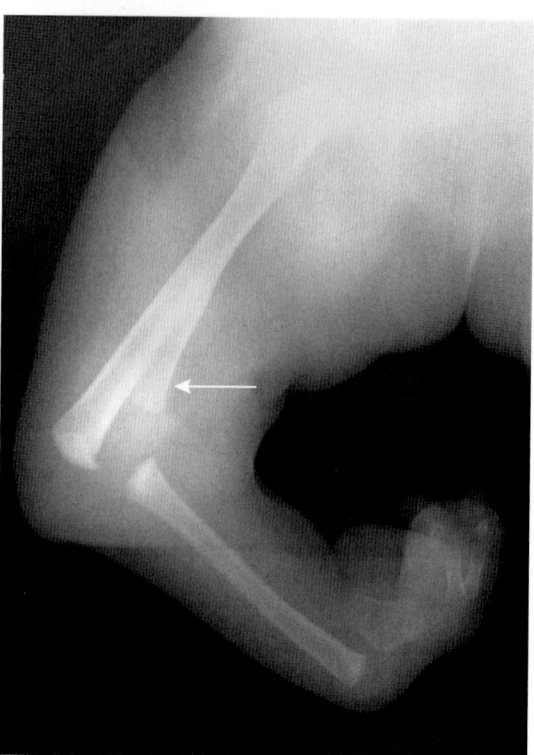

FIGURE 164-25. One-year-old girl with femoral duplication. A Y-shaped medial protuberance *(arrow)* is seen, along with complete tibial hemimelia, two rays in the foot, and absent talus. (From Laor T, Jaramillo D, Hoffer FA, et al: MR imaging in congenital lower limb deformities. Pediatr Radiol 1996;26:384.)

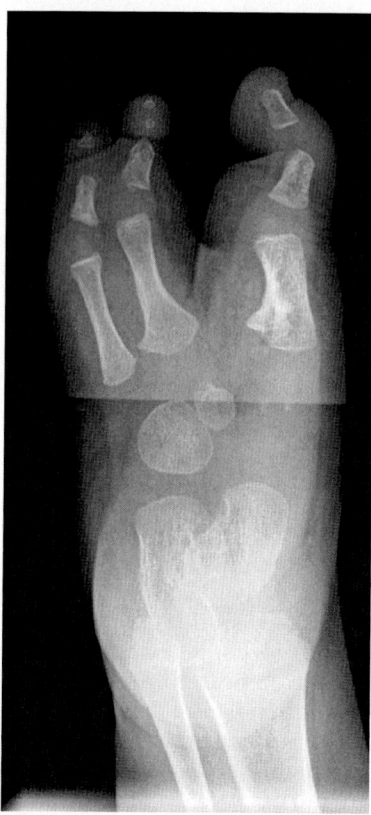

FIGURE 164-24. Frontal radiograph of the foot of a child with split hand-foot malformation. A V-shaped cleft and near-complete absence of the central two rays are evident.

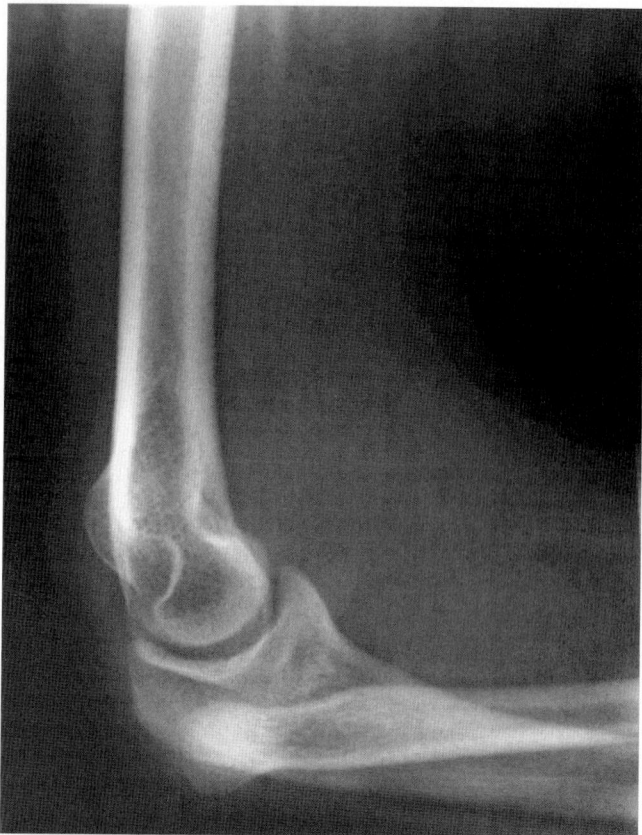

FIGURE 164-26. Congenital dislocation of the proximal radius. The radial head is rounded and dislocated in a posterior direction. Similar findings were noted in the contralateral elbow.

SUGGESTED READINGS

General

Frantz C, O'Rahilly R: Congenital limb deficiencies. J Bone Joint Surg Am 1961;43:1202-1224

Laor T, Jaramillo D, Oestreich AE: Musculoskeletal system. In Kirks D, Griscom N (eds): Practical Pediatric Imaging: Diagnostic Imaging of Infants and Children, 3rd ed. Philadelphia, Lippincott-Raven, 1998:327-510

Lenz W: Malformations caused by drugs in pregnancy. Am J Dis Child 1966;112:99-106

Lie RT, Wilcox AJ, Skjaerven R: A population-based study of the risk of recurrence of birth defects. N Engl J Med 1994;331:1-4

McCredie J: Sclerotome subtraction: a radiologic interpretation of reduction deformities of the limbs. Birth Defects Orig Artic Ser 1977;13:65-77

McGuirk CK, Westgate MN, Holmes LB: Limb deficiencies in newborn infants. Pediatrics 2001;108:E64

O'Rahilly R: Morphological patterns in limb deficiencies and duplications. Am J Anat 1951;89:135-193

Ozonoff MB: Pediatric Orthopedic Radiology, 2nd ed. Philadelphia, WB Saunders, 1992

Rypens F, Dubois J, Garel L, et al: Obstetric US: watch the fetal hands. Radiographics 2006;26:811-829

Smith JG, Weiss AP, Weiss YS: Congenital anomalies of the hand. Clin Pediatr (Phila) 1998;37:459-467

Soltan HC, Holmes LB: Familial occurrence of malformations possibly attributable to vascular abnormalities. J Pediatr 1986;108:112-114

VanHeest AE: Congenital disorders of the hand and upper extremity. Pediatr Clin North Am 1996;43:1113-1133

Warkany J, Nelson R: Skeletal abnormalities induced in rats by maternal nutritional deficiency. Arch Pathol 1942;34:375-384

Lower Extremity Deficiencies

Achterman C, Kalamchi A: Congenital deficiency of the fibula. J Bone Joint Surg Br 1979;61:133-137

Aitken G (ed): Proximal femoral focal deficiency—definition, classification, and management. In Proximal Femoral Focal Deficiency: A Congenital Anomaly. Washington, DC, National Academy of Sciences, 1969:1-22

Anton CG, Applegate KE, Kuivila TE, et al: Proximal femoral focal deficiency (PFFD): more than an abnormal hip. Semin Musculoskelet Radiol 1999;3:215-226

Boden SD, Fallon MD, Davidson R, et al: Proximal femoral focal deficiency: evidence for a defect in proliferation and maturation of chondrocytes. J Bone Joint Surg Am 1989;71:1119-1129

Christini D, Levy EJ, Facanha FA, et al: Fibular transfer for congenital absence of the tibia. J Pediatr Orthop 1993;13:378-381

Clark MW: Autosomal dominant inheritance of tibial meromelia: report of a kindred. J Bone Joint Surg Am 1975;57:262-264

Daentl DL, Smith DW, Scott CI, et al: Femoral hypoplasia—unusual facies syndrome. J Pediatr 1975;86:107-111

Davidson WH, Bohne WH: The Syme amputation in children. J Bone Joint Surg Am 1975;57:905-909

Dora C, Buhler M, Stover MD, et al: Morphologic characteristics of acetabular dysplasia in proximal femoral focal deficiency. J Pediatr Orthop B 2004;13:81-87

Fordham LA, Applegate KE, Wilkes DC, Chung CJ: Fibular hemimelia: more than just an absent bone. Semin Musculoskelet Radiol 1999;3:227-238

Gillespie R, Torode IP: Classification and management of congenital abnormalities of the femur. J Bone Joint Surg Br 1983;65:557-568

Grissom LE, Harcke HT: Sonography in congenital deficiency of the femur. J Pediatr Orthop 1994;14:29-33

Grissom LE, Harcke HT, Kumar SJ: Sonography in the management of tibial hemimelia. Clin Orthop Relat Res 1990;251:266-270

Hamanishi C: Congenital short femur: clinical, genetic and epidemiological comparison of the naturally occurring condition with that caused by thalidomide. J Bone Joint Surg Br 1980; 62:307-320

Herring A, Cummings DR: The limb deficient child. In Morrissy RT, Weinstein SL (eds): Lovell and Winter's Pediatric Orthopaedics, 4th ed. Philadelphia, Lippincott-Raven, 1996:1137-1176

Hillmann JS, Mesgarzadeh M, Revesz G, et al: Proximal femoral focal deficiency: radiologic analysis of 49 cases. Radiology 1987; 165:769-773

Hootnick DR, Levinsohn EM, Randall PA, Packard DS Jr: Vascular dysgenesis associated with skeletal dysplasia of the lower limb. J Bone Joint Surg Am 1980;62:1123-1129

Hosny GA: Treatment of tibial hemimelia without amputation: preliminary report. J Pediatr Orthop B 2005;14:250-255

Jayakumar SS, Eilert RE: Fibular transfer for congenital absence of the tibia. Clin Orthop 1979;139:97-101

Jones D, Barnes J, Lloyd-Roberts GC: Congenital aplasia and dysplasia of the tibia with intact fibula: classification and management. J Bone Joint Surg Br 1978;60:31-39

Kalamchi A, Cowell HR, Kim KI: Congenital deficiency of the femur. J Pediatr Orthop 1985;5:129-134

Kohn G, el Shawwa R, Grunebaum M: Aplasia of the tibia with bifurcation of the femur and ectrodactyly: evidence for an autosomal recessive type. Am J Med Genet 1989;33:172-175

Kritter AE: Tibial rotation-plasty for proximal femoral focal deficiency. J Bone Joint Surg Am 1977;59:927-934

Laor T, Burrows PE: Congenital anomalies and vascular birthmarks of the lower extremities. Magn Reson Imaging Clin N Am 1998;6:497-519

Laor T, Jaramillo D, Hoffer FA, Kasser JR: MR imaging in congenital lower limb deformities. Pediatr Radiol 1996;26:381-387

Levinson ED, Ozonoff MB, Royen PM: Proximal femoral focal deficiency (PFFD). Radiology 1977;125:197-203

Loder RT, Herring JA: Fibular transfer for congenital absence of the tibia: a reassessment. J Pediatr Orthop 1987;7:8-13

Maldjian C, Patel Ty, Klein RM, et al: Efficacy of MRI in classifying proximal focal femoral deficiency. Skeletal Radiol 2007;36:215-220

Manner HM, Radler C, Granger R, et al: Knee deformity in congenital longitudinal deficiencies of the lower extremity. Clin Orthop Relat Res 2006;448:185-192

McCarthy JJ, Glancy GL, Chang FM, Eilert RE: Fibular hemimelia: comparison of outcome measurements after amputation and lengthening. J Bone Joint Surg Am 2000;82:1732-1735

Naudie D, Hamdy RC, Fassier F, et al: Management of fibular hemimelia: amputation or limb lengthening. J Bone Joint Surg Br 1997;79:58-65

Pappas AM: Congenital abnormalities of the femur and related lower extremity malformations: classification and treatment. J Pediatr Orthop 1983;3:45-60

Patel M, Paley D, Herzenberg JE: Limb-lengthening versus amputation for fibular hemimelia. J Bone Joint Surg Am 2002;84:317-319

Pirani S, Beauchamp RD, Li D, et al: Soft tissue anatomy of proximal femoral focal deficiency. J Pediatr Orthop 1991;11:563-570

Roux MO, Carlioz H: Clinical examination and investigation of the cruciate ligaments in children with fibular hemimelia. J Pediatr Orthop 1999;19:247-251

Sanpera I Jr, Sparks LT: Proximal femoral focal deficiency: does a radiologic classification exist? J Pediatr Orthop 1994;14:34-38

Simmons ED Jr, Ginsburg GM, Hall JE: Brown's procedure for congenital absence of the tibia revisited. J Pediatr Orthop 1996;16:85-89

Stanitski DF, Stanitski CL: Fibular hemimelia: a new classification system. J Pediatr Orthop 2003;23:30-34

VanNes C: Rotation-plasty for congenital defects of the femur: making use of the ankle of the shortened limb to control the knee joint of a prosthesis. J Bone Joint Surg Br 1950;32:12-16

Westin GW, Sakai DN, Wood WL: Congenital longitudinal deficiency of the fibula: follow-up of treatment by Syme amputation. J Bone Joint Surg Am 1976;58:492-496

Wolfgang GL: Complex congenital anomalies of the lower extremities: femoral bifurcation, tibial hemimelia, and diastasis of the ankle: case report and review of the literature. J Bone Joint Surg Am 1984;66:453-458

Yetkin H, Cila E, Bilgin Guzel V, Kanatli U: Femoral bifurcation associated with tibial hemimelia. Orthopedics 2001;24:389-390

Upper Extremity Deficiencies

Bayne LG, Klug MS: Long-term review of the surgical treatment of radial deficiencies. J Hand Surg Am 1987;12:169-179

Goldberg MJ, Bartoshesky LE: Congenital hand anomaly: etiology and associated malformations. Hand Clin 1985;1:405-415

Goldfarb CA, Manske PR, Busa R, et al: Upper-extremity phocomelia reexamined: a longitudinal dysplasia. J Bone Joint Surg Am 2005;87:2639-2648

Goldfarb CA, Wall L, Manske PR: Radial longitudinal deficiency: the incidence of associated medical and musculoskeletal conditions. J Hand Surg (Am) 2006;31:1176-1182

Lourie GM, Lins RE: Radial longitudinal deficiency: a review and update. Hand Clin 1998;14:85-99

Swanson AB, Tada K, Yonenobu K: Ulnar ray deficiency: its various manifestations. J Hand Surg Am 1984;9:658-664

Van Allen MI, Hoyme HE, Jones KL: Vascular pathogenesis of limb defects. I. Radial artery anatomy in radial aplasia. J Pediatr 1982;101:832-838

Generalized Deficiencies and Contractures

Askins G, Ger E: Congenital constriction band syndrome. J Pediatr Orthop 1988;8:461-466

Davidson R, Drummond D: Arthrogryposis. In Drennan JC (ed): The Child's Foot and Ankle. New York, Raven Press, 1992:253-266

Fisher RM, Cremin BJ: Limb defects in the amniotic band syndrome. Pediatr Radiol 1976;5:24-29

Hall JG: An approach to congenital contractures (arthrogryposis). Pediatr Ann 1981;10:15-26

Hall JG: Arthrogryposis. Am Fam Physician 1989;39:113-119

Keswani SG, Johnson MP, Adzick NS, et al: In utero limb salvage: fetoscopic release of amniotic bands for threatened limb amputation. J Pediatr Surg 2003;38:848-851

Mennen U, van Heest A, Ezaki MB, et al: Arthrogryposis multiplex congenita. J Hand Surg Br 2005;30:468-474

Paladini D, Foglia S, Sglavo G, et al: Congenital constriction band of the upper arm: the role of three-dimensional ultrasound in diagnosis, counseling and multidisciplinary consultation. Ultrasound Obstet Gynecol 2004;23:520-522

Poznanski AK, La Rowe PC: Radiographic manifestations of the arthrogryposis syndrome. Radiology 1970;95:353-358

Shapiro F, Specht L: The diagnosis and orthopaedic treatment of childhood spinal muscular atrophy, peripheral neuropathy, Friedreich ataxia, and arthrogryposis. J Bone Joint Surg Am 1993;75:1699-1714

Stern WA: Arthrogryposis multiplex congenita. JAMA 1923;81:1507-1510

Streeter G: Focal deficiencies in fetal tissues and their relation to intra-uterine amputation. Contrib Embryol 1930;22:1-44

Swinyard CA, Bleck EE: The etiology of arthrogryposis (multiple congenital contractures). Clin Orthop 1985;194:15-29

Wiedrich TA: Congenital constriction band syndrome. Hand Clin 1998;14:29-38

Large Limbs

Kirks DR, Shackelford GD: Idiopathic congenital hemihypertrophy with associated ipsilateral benign nephromegaly. Radiology 1975;115:145-148

Levine C: The imaging of body asymmetry and hemihypertrophy. Crit Rev Diagn Imaging 1990;31:1-80

Pfister RC, Weber AL, Smith EH, et al: Congenital asymmetry (hemihypertrophy) and abdominal disease: radiological features in 9 cases. Radiology 1975;116:685-691

Tibial Bowing and Congenital Tibial Dysplasia

Crawford AH Jr, Bagamery N: Osseous manifestations of neurofibromatosis in childhood. J Pediatr Orthop 1986;6:72-88

Crawford AH, Schorry EK: Neurofibromatosis in children: the role of the orthopaedist. J Am Acad Orthop Surg 1999;7:217-230

Crawford AH, Schorry EK: Neurofibromatosis update. J Pediatr Orthop 2006;26:413-423

Hall BD, Spranger J: Congenital bowing of the long bones: a review and phenotype analysis of 13 undiagnosed cases. Eur J Pediatr 1980;133:131-138

Hefti F, Bollini G, Dungl P, et al: Congenital pseudarthrosis of the tibia: history, etiology, classification, and epidemiologic data. J Pediatr Orthop B 2000;9:11-15

Ippolito E, Corsi A, Grill F, et al: Pathology of bone lesions associated with congenital pseudarthrosis of the leg. J Pediatr Orthop B 2000;9:3-10

Klatte EC, Franken EA, Smith JA: The radiographic spectrum in neurofibromatosis. Semin Roentgenol 1976;11:17-33

Pappas AM: Congenital posteromedial bowing of the tibia and fibula. J Pediatr Orthop 1984;4:525-531

Tuncay IC, Johnston CE 2nd, Birch JG: Spontaneous resolution of congenital anterolateral bowing of the tibia. J Pediatr Orthop 1994;14:599-602

Abnormal Segmentation (Fusion Deformities)

Emery KH, Bisset GS 3rd, Johnson ND, et al: Tarsal coalition: a blinded comparison of MRI and CT. Pediatr Radiol 1998;28:612-616

Harris RI: Retrospect—peroneal spastic flat foot (rigid valgus foot). J Bone Joint Surg Am 1965;47:1657-1667

Hochman M, Reed MH: Features of calcaneonavicular coalition on coronal computed tomography. Skeletal Radiol 2000;29:409-412

Kulik SA Jr, Clanton TO: Tarsal coalition. Foot Ankle Int 1996;17:286-296

Lateur LM, Van Hoe LR, Van Ghillewe KV, et al: Subtalar coalition: diagnosis with the C sign on lateral radiographs of the ankle. Radiology 1994;193:847-851

Leonard MA: The inheritance of tarsal coalition and its relationship to spastic flat foot. J Bone Joint Surg Br 1974;56:520-526

Letts M, Davidson D, Beaule P: Symphalangism in children: case report and review of the literature. Clin Orthop 1999;366:178-185

Newman JS, Newberg AH: Congenital tarsal coalition: multimodality evaluation with emphasis on CT and MR imaging. Radiographics 2000;20:321-332

Oestreich AE, Mize WA, Crawford AH, et al: The "anteater nose": a direct sign of calcaneonavicular coalition on the lateral radiograph. J Pediatr Orthop 1987;7:709-711

Pachuda NM, Lasday SD, Jay RM: Tarsal coalition: etiology, diagnosis, and treatment. J Foot Surg 1990;29:474-488

Sachar K, Akelman E, Ehrlich M: Radioulnar synostosis. Hand Clin 1994;10:399-404

Sakellariou A, Claridge RJ: Tarsal coalition. Orthopedics 1999;22:1066-1073

Stormont DM, Peterson HA: The relative incidence of tarsal coalition. Clin Orthop 1983;28-36

Takakura Y, Tamai S, Masuhara K: Genesis of the ball-and-socket ankle. J Bone Joint Surg Br 1986;68:834-837

Vincent KA: Tarsal coalition and painful flatfoot. J Am Acad Orthop Surg 1998;6:274-281

Miscellaneous Congenital Malformations

Arbues J, Galindo A, Puente JM, et al: Typical isolated ectrodactyly of hands and feet: early antenatal diagnosis. J Matern Fetal Neonatal Med 2005;17:299-301

Cornah MS, Dangerfield PH: Reduplication of the femur: report of a case. J Bone Joint Surg Br 1974;56:744-745

Duijf PH, van Bokhoven H, Brunner HG: Pathogenesis of split-hand/split-foot malformation. Hum Mol Genet 2003;12:R51-R60

Elliott A, Evans J, Chudley AE: Split hand foot malformation (SHFM). Clin Genet 2005;68:501-505

Elliott AM, Evans JA: Genotype-phenotype correlations in mapped split hand foot malformation (SHFM) patients. Am J Med Genet 2006;140:1419-1427

Light TR, Ogden JA: The longitudinal epiphyseal bracket: implications for surgical correction. J Pediatr Orthop 1981;1:299-305

Mahboub, S, Davidson R: MR imaging in longitudinal epiphyseal bracket in children. Pediatr Radiol 1999;29:259-261

Oestreich AE, Crawford AH: Atlas of Pediatric Orthopedic Radiology. New York, Thieme, 1985:166

Ogden JA, Light TR, Cinlogue GJ: Correlative roentgenography and morphology of the longitudinal epiphyseal bracket. Skeletal Radiol 1981;6:109-117

Poznanski A: The Hand in Radiologic Diagnosis, 2nd ed. Philadelphia, WB Saunders, 1984:204-208

Poznanski AK, Pratt GB, Manson G, et al: Clinodactyly, camptodactyly, Kirner's deformity, and other crooked fingers. Radiology 1969;93:573-582

Sachar K, Mih AD: Congenital radial head dislocations. Hand Clin 1998;14:39-47

Talamillo A, Bastida MF, Fernandez-Teran M, et al: The developing limb and the control of the number of digits. Clin Genet 2005;67:143-153

165 Skeletal Dysplasias

RALPH S. LACHMAN

The skeletal dysplasias (bone dysplasias, osteochondro-dysplasias) are a group of more than 250 well-defined disorders, of which about 70 are often lethal in the perinatal period. Therefore, the thrust of this text is to acquaint the reader with an approach to the skeletal dysplasias and describe 49 of the most important and common of these disorders. The dysplasias covered here are those that pediatric radiologists are most likely to encounter in practice and therefore need to know about (Table 165-1).

Most of the bone dysplasias result in clinically disproportionate short stature. Therefore, the clinician cannot consider the imaging evaluation of these disorders without first considering the radiologic assessment of all instances of significant short stature. With short stature in the pediatric age group, it is crucial to clinically determine whether the condition is proportionate or disproportionate short stature.

When the clinician has determined that the patient has *proportionate short stature,* the differential diagnosis generally consists of constitutional delay, familial short stature, a small group of endocrinopathies, and some dysmorphology syndromes. The beginning clinical imaging assessment usually warrants a left hand-and-wrist radiograph for bone age determination. A complete "genetic skeletal survey" is not necessary in these cases and perhaps even contraindicated, because ionizing radiation doses in pediatric patients should be kept as low as possible. However, if the patient in question has normal proportions and is dysmorphic or manifests multiple congenital anomalies on clinical evaluation, then one of the dysmorphology syndromes is present, and a modified genetic skeletal survey may be appropriate.

TERMINOLOGY

Certain terms are very important in the assessment of the skeletal dysplasias. Aside from the truncal shortening ("spine shortening"), extremity shortening may occur in total and/or in parts. This shortening may be evident radiologically and/or clinically. *Rhizomelia* (short upper arms/humeri and thighs/femurs), *mesomelia* (short middle segments, radii and ulnas, and tibias and fibulas), and *acromelia* (short hands and feet) play a major role not only in clinical and radiologic assessment but also in nomenclature. Pediatricians are aware of the key areas in growing bone, and so abnormal development of epi-

physes, metaphyses, and diaphyses has given rise to nomenclature with those site names (Fig. 165-1). The term *micromelic* should be reserved for very severe shortening of all four limbs and their limb parts. Abnormal development of the vertebral bodies signifies a "spondylo-" abnormality.

RADIOLOGIC ASSESSMENT

In the history of the delineation and classification of many of the specific skeletal dysplasias, radiologic assessment has played, and continues to play, a major role, because most of the skeletal dysplasias have distinctive radiographic features (e.g., stippled ossification centers), are dense or osteopenic bone disorders, or entail pathophysiologic abnormalities at or near the developing growth plates. An organized evaluation of the radiographs in the skeletal dysplasia survey includes the following steps.

Step I: Assessment of Disproportion

The clinician assesses for the presence of disproportion, this time from a radiographic point of view. A quick look at the films helps the clinician decide whether significant generalized *platyspondyly* is present, contributing to shortness of the trunk. Then the clinician looks at the extremities to ascertain whether rhizomelia, mesomelia, or acromelia is present. Rhizomelia, mesomelia, and acromelia are not always confirmed by the radiographic findings, however, because the clinical visual evaluation

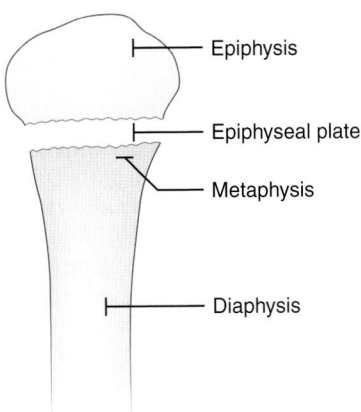

FIGURE 165-1. Drawing of key areas of the growing bone.

TABLE 165-1

Selected Skeletal Dysplasias

ACHONDROPLASIA GROUP
Thanatophoric dysplasia
Achondroplasia
Hypochondroplasia

METROPIC DYSPLASIA GROUP
Metatropic dysplasia
Schneckenbecken dysplasia

SHORT RIB–POLYDACTYLY GROUP
Short rib–polydactyly dysplasias (types I to IV)
Asphyxiating thoracic dysplasia (Jeune dysplasia)
Chondroectodermal dysplasia (Ellis–van Creveld syndrome)

DIASTROPHIC DYSPLASIA GROUP
Diastrophic dysplasia
Multiple epiphyseal dysplasia: multilayered patella/
   brachydactyly/clubfeet (AR MED)
Achondrogenesis type I [IA, IB]

TYPE II COLLAGENOPATHIES
Achondrogenesis type II/hypochondrogenesis
Spondyloepiphyseal dysplasia congenita (SEDC)
Kniest dysplasia

OTHER SPONDYLOEPI(META)PHYSEAL DYSPLASIAS
Spondyloepiphyseal dysplasia tarda (SED X-linked)
Dyggve-Melchior-Clausen dysplasia

MULTIPLE EPIPHYSEAL DYSPLASIA AND PSEUDOACHONDROPLASIA GROUP
Multiple epiphyseal dysplasia (MED)
Pseudoachondroplasia

CHONDRODYSPLASIA PUNCTATA GROUP
Rhizomelic chondrodysplasia punctata
Conradi-Hünermann syndrome/dysplasia
Brachytelephalangic chondrodysplasia punctata

METAPHYSEAL CHONDRODYSPLASIA GROUP
Jansen-type metaphyseal chondrodysplasia
Schmid-type metaphyseal chondrodysplasia
McKusick-type metaphyseal chondrodysplasia
   (cartilage-hair hypoplasia)
Shwachman-Diamond syndrome (metaphyseal
   chondrodysplasia with pancreatic insufficiency and cyclic
   neutropenia)

SPONDYLOMETAPHYSEAL DYSPLASIA GROUP
Kozlowski-type spondylometaphyseal dysplasia

MESOMELIC DYSPLASIA GROUP
Dyschondrosteosis (Leri-Weill syndrome)

ACROMELIC/ACROMESOMELIC DYSPLASIA GROUP
Trichorhinophalangeal syndrome types I and II
   (Langer-Giedion syndrome)
Acromesomelic dysplasia of Maroteaux

DYSPLASIAS WITH PROMINENT MEMBRANEOUS BONE INVOLVEMENT
Cleidocranial dysplasia

BENT-BONE DYSPLASIA GROUP
Campomelic dysplasia

DYSOSTOSIS MULTIPLEX GROUP
Hurler syndrome (mucopolysaccharidosis type IH)
Morquio syndrome (mucopolysaccharidosis types IVA
   and IVB)
Mucolipidosis type II (I-cell disease)

DYSPLASIAS WITH DECREASED BONE DENSITY
Osteogenesis imperfecta type II
Osteogenesis imperfecta, other types

DYSPLASIAS WITH DEFECTIVE MINERALIZATION
Hypophosphatasia, perinatal lethal/infantile type
Hypophosphatasia, adult type

INCREASED BONE DENSITY WITHOUT MODIFICATION OF BONE SHAPE GROUP
Osteopetrosis
Pyknodysostosis

CRANIOTUBULAR DYSPLASIAS
Craniodiaphyseal dysplasia
Craniometaphyseal dysplasia
Pyle dysplasia

DISORGANIZED DEVELOPMENT OF CARTILAGINOUS, BONY, AND FIBROUS COMPONENTS OF THE SKELETON
Multiple exostoses*
Enchondromatosis*
Metachondromatosis*
Fibrous dysplasia*
Osteopoikilosis
Osteopathia striata
Melorheostosis
Spondyloenchondromatosis
Dysspondyloenchondromatosis

OSTEOLYSIS GROUP†

PATELLA DYSPLASIA GROUP
Nail–patella syndrome

*Covered in Chapter 176.
†Covered in Chapter 166.

is guided by the skin creases and folds rather than the underlying bone length. A significantly curved long bone may appear much shorter externally than radiographically. Significant shortening of the femurs and humeri in comparison with the other segments constitutes *rhizomelia*, which is very important, for example, to confirm the specific diagnosis of the rhizomelic form of chondrodysplasia punctata. Very significant *mesomelia*, alone, suggests a group of specific disorders loosely classified as the mesomelic dysplasias. *Acromelia* is found in many disorders but is important to recognize because,

for example, if it is associated with a particular form of vertebral abnormality, then the clinician can make the rather specific diagnosis of the most common form of spondyloperipheral dysplasia. Of course, acromelia may be present by itself, and various disorders are possible, including skeletal dysplasias such as acrodysostosis and acromicric dysplasia or nonskeletal dysplasia; brachydactyly of any sort, especially brachydactyly type E; pseudohypoparathyroidism with cyclic adenosine monophosphate or cyclic guanosine monophosphate abnormalities; or even a chromosomal disorder (Turner syndrome). Acromelia is found as part of other shortening in many specific skeletal dysplasias (e.g., achondroplasia), whereas the lack of significant hand and foot shortening is a significant feature of spondyloepiphyseal dysplasia congenita (SEDC).

Step II: Assessment of Epiphyseal Ossification

Next, an overall assessment of epiphyseal ossification is made. If the *ossified epiphyses* are very small and/or irregular for age, then an epiphyseal dysplasia of some sort is present. If the *metaphyses* are widened, flared, and/or irregular, the diagnosis of a metaphyseal chondrodysplasia is entertained. Finally, the presence of *diaphyseal* abnormalities, such as widening or cortical thickening or marrow space expansion, implies a diaphyseal dysplasia of some sort. Traditionally, combinations of the aforementioned abnormalities with or without platyspondyly were ascribed not only to specific disorders but also to nonspecific types of disorders such as congenital forms of spondyloepiphyseal dysplasia and the nonspecific group of spondyloepi(meta)physeal dysplasias (SE[M]Ds). This rough estimation of type of disorder helps narrow down the diagnosis to a specific, well-described entity. Figure 165-2 is a crude depiction of these radiographic manifestations. If only the vertebral bodies are affected, with no significant changes in any of the growth plate regions, then the diagnosis is brachyolmia. Which one of the three well-described types of brachyolmia is present is ascertained from the type of vertebral involvement and other clinical findings, as described by Shohat, Lachman, and Gruber (1989). At this point, it is important to reemphasize that although the radiologic findings may play a major role in the diagnosis, other *clinical manifestations* are often very important for making a correct and complete diagnosis.

All the skeletal structures available in the skeletal dysplasia survey should then be more precisely evaluated. As a result, a specific, well-described skeletal dysplasia may be recognized, from a previous broad categorization into a nonspecific group. This is crucial for genetic counseling. Another possibility from this precise evaluation is that a single pathognomonic finding implies a precise diagnosis (e.g., the snail-shaped iliac bones of Schneckenbecken dysplasia).

Step III: Differentiation of Normal Variants from Pathologic Abnormalities

This next step is more difficult, and the examiner must have at least some quite significant radiologic experience, preferably in pediatric radiologic imaging. It is necessary to recognize the difference between normal variations and pathologic abnormalities in the growing skeleton (see also Chapter 163). *All* the skeletal structures must be assessed. I believe that this is best performed in an organized manner, each structure assessed separately. Although every portion of every structure is looked at for any possible abnormal features, the examiner should concentrate especially on certain abnormalities that are related specifically to the skeletal dysplasias. The examiner must also recognize pathognomonic and other singular findings suggestive of a specific diagnosis or a narrow group of differential diagnostic possibilities that, in turn, may lead to a specific diagnosis from other features.

DIAGNOSIS

After all the pathologic findings in every area have been established, a gamut search of some or all of these abnormalities, in conjunction with the clinical findings, may lead to the specific diagnosis. If the "group" of dysplasias has been established, then the specific disorder diagnosis can often be made by referring to a differential diagnosis table, such as that developed by Taybi and Lachman (1996, 2006).

Molecular Nomenclature

There have been remarkable breakthroughs in the study of genetics of the skeletal dysplasias. These new findings are primarily molecular in nature. These molecular abnormalities now govern a new nomenclature, by Lachman in 1998. In this text, I follow that molecular nomenclature in presenting the 49 specific bone dysplasias. The presentation is focused primarily on the radiologic rather than other clinical findings. For completeness regarding any entity described, refer to other, more complete texts (i.e., Lachman, 2007).

Fetal Diagnosis

Ultrasonography plays a critical role in the prenatal diagnosis of skeletal dysplasias. Most lethal dysplasias and many nonlethal dysplasias may be suggested by findings on ultrasonography of the fetus. In some cases ultrasound findings suggest a specific diagnosis (i.e., thanatophoric dysplasia or osteogenesis imperfecta type II). More commonly, nonspecific findings (e.g., long bone shortening) suggest that a dysplasia may be present and prompt further prenatal and postnatal evaluation. Fetal magnetic resonance imaging does not yet play a significant role in the prenatal diagnosis of bone dysplasias.

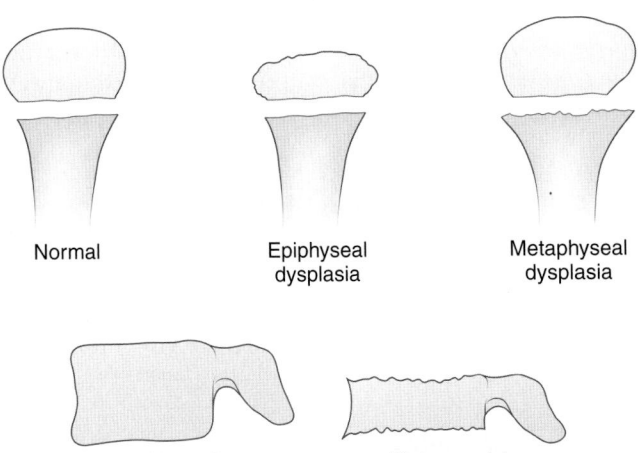

FIGURE 165-2. Drawing of radiographic manifestations of the dysplasias.

In lethal dysplasias, postmortem radiographic study is valuable in confirming or suggesting a diagnosis. This information may be extremely useful for genetic counseling.

ACHONDROPLASIA GROUP

In the achondroplasia group of disorders, three specific entities are important: thanatophoric dysplasia, achondroplasia, and hypochondroplasia. They all have the same chromosomal locus (4p16.3). The gene/protein abnormality in all of them is a different mutation or group of mutations in fibroblast growth factor receptor 3 (FGFR3).

Thanatophoric Dysplasia

Thanatophoric dysplasia, or thanatophoric dwarfism, actually represents at least two molecularly distinct disorders that have been termed *thanatophoric dysplasia types I and II.* They share common radiographic features, except that type II is characterized by straight, not quite as short femurs and a kleeblattschädel (cloverleaf skull) (Fig. 165-3). This delineation may not be that important because both types are new autosomal dominant mutations and are almost invariably lethal. This dysplasia perhaps represents the most common lethal bone dysplasia.

RADIOLOGIC FINDINGS*

1. Skull: proportionately large skull in relation to the body, narrow skull base, *kleeblattschädel*
2. Thorax: long, narrow trunk; very short ribs; handlebar clavicles
3. Spine: *flat, small vertebral bodies with round anterior ends; U-, H-, and upside-down U-shaped vertebrae in the anteroposterior projection*
4. Pelvis: *small, flared iliac bones; very narrow sacrosciatic notches; flat, dysplastic acetabula*
5. Extremities: generalized micromelia; *French telephone receiver–shaped femurs,* round proximal femoral metaphyses with medial spike

Achondroplasia

Achondroplasia is by far the most common form of nonlethal skeletal dysplasia. Most cases are manifested at birth. Patients with this disorder have the combination of rhizomelia, mesomelia, and acromelia on radiographic studies, but rhizomelia is more obvious at clinical inspection (Fig. 165-4). This is an autosomal dominant condition with a spontaneous mutation rate of about 80%.

RADIOLOGIC FINDINGS

1. Skull: enlarged, with significant midface hypoplasia; hydrocephalus rarely present; small skull base with tight foramen magnum
2. Thorax: small; shortened and anteriorly splayed ribs

---

*Throughout the text, pathognomonic radiologic findings are in italics.

3. Spine: vertebral bodies only slightly flattened, short and slightly round anteriorly, but normalizing from late childhood on; very short pedicles with *decreased interpediculate distance* most marked in lumbar spine; *posterior vertebral scalloping* that persists through life
4. Pelvis: *elephant ear–shaped iliac wings* (flared, superiorly and laterally flattened ilia), *narrow sacrosciatic notches, flat acetabular roofs*
5. Extremities: *rhizomelia, mesomelia, and acromelia*
6. Hands: brachydactyly, metacarpal metaphyseal cupping, phalangeal metaphyseal widening
7. Knees: *Chevron deformity and upside-down chevron deformity* (tibia/femur)
8. Hips: *proximal femoral fadeout* (infancy); *hemispheric capital femoral epiphyses,* short femoral necks
9. Legs: prominent tibial tubercle apophyseal region, *proximal and distal fibula overgrowth*
10. Arms: very prominent deltoid insertion area

> **Achondroplasia is the most common form of nonlethal skeletal dysplasia.**

Hypochondroplasia

Hypochondroplasia, also a very common disorder, arises from the same alleles as does achondroplasia, and the two disorders share many features. It is often difficult to distinguish severe hypochondroplasia from mild achondroplasia. Of molecularly proven cases of achondroplasia, 97% have the identical gene abnormality; however, multiple different molecular changes in fibroblast growth factor receptor 3 have been noted in hypochondroplasia. Hypochondroplasia usually manifests after 2 years of age (Fig. 165-5). The clinician should be *very wary* of making this diagnosis in a newborn. The diagnosis is often a clinical one in mild cases.

RADIOLOGIC FINDINGS

The imaging findings of hypochondroplasia are identical to those of achondroplasia but to a milder degree of abnormality. The overall experience with this disorder suggests that all cases, no matter how mild, exhibit *interpediculate narrowing in the lumbar spine.* There may be some brachydactyly, fibula overgrowth, and even short femoral necks. Other achondroplasia-like changes may or may not be present.

METATROPIC DYSPLASIA GROUP

The metatropic dysplasia group includes several disorders that appear to be linked because of their similar clinical and radiographic findings. Thus far, no molecular breakthrough discovery has occurred. The important disorder in this group is metatropic dysplasia.

Metatropic Dysplasia

Metatropic dysplasia, or metatropic dwarfism, is discoverable in the newborn with a relatively long trunk and

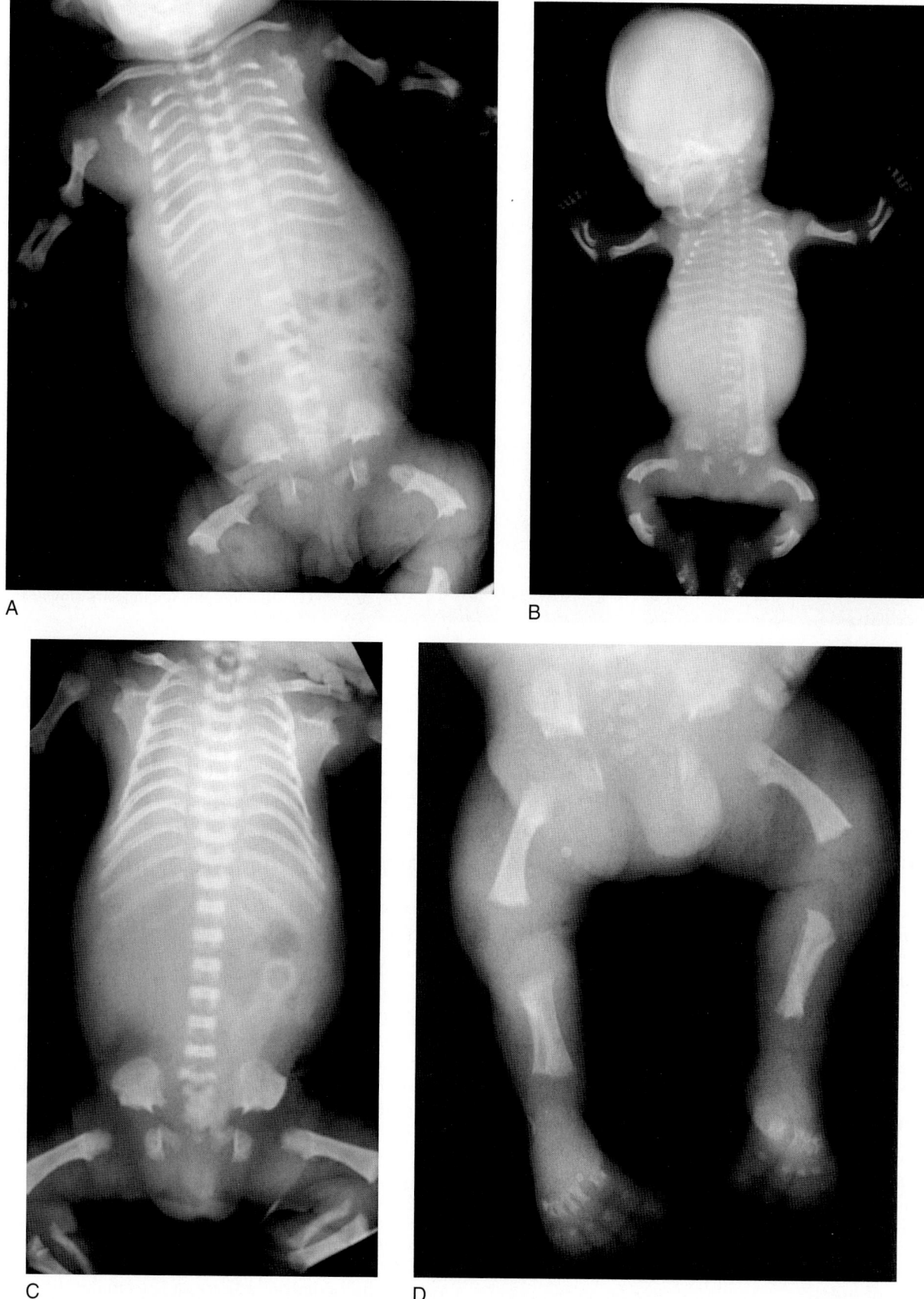

FIGURE 165-3. **A** and **B,** Radiographic findings in thanatophoric dysplasia type I. In an affected fetus of 30 weeks' gestation (**A**), there is a long, narrow trunk; very short ribs; U- and H-shaped vertebral bodies; small, flared iliac wings; narrowed sacrosciatic notches; dysplastic (trident) acetabular roofs; and French telephone receiver–shaped femurs. At 22 weeks' gestation in another affected fetus (**B**), there is a proportionally large skull, micromelia, and other findings similar to those in **A. C** to **F,** Radiologic findings in thanatophoric dysplasia type II. An affected preterm fetus (**C**) exhibits findings similar to those in type I except for higher vertebral bodies and straighter femurs. Another affected fetus (**D**) also shows the same findings as in type I but straighter femurs.

Continued

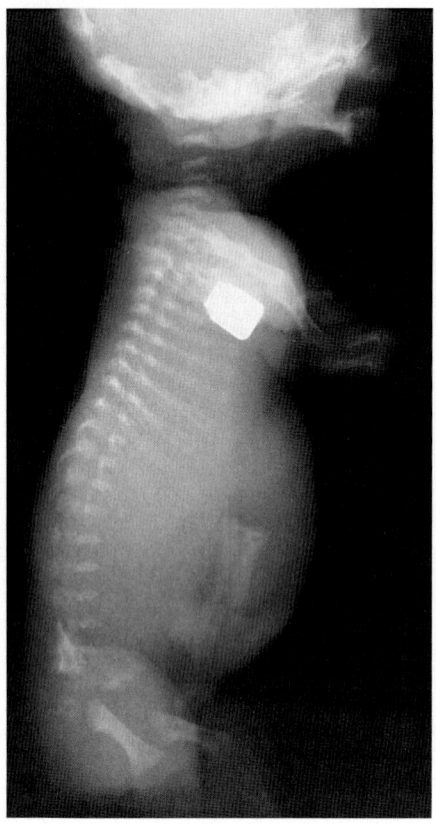

E

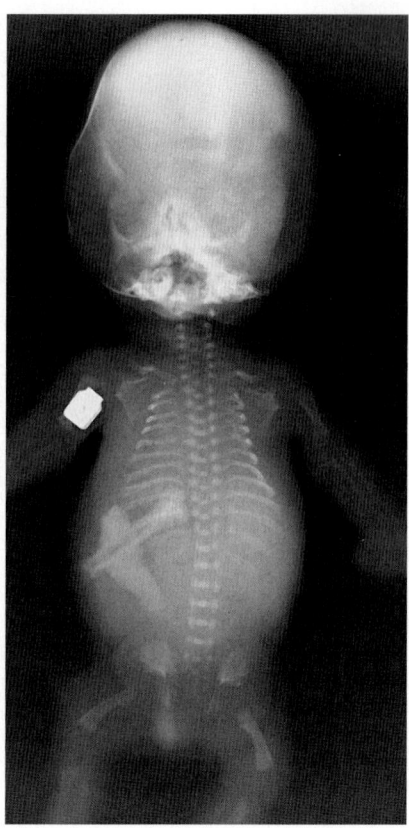

F

FIGURE 165-3, *cont'd*. E, Radiograph of affected infant with severe platyspondyly, anteriorly rounded vertebrae, straight femurs, and severely constricted skull base. **F,** Cloverleaf skull and almost straight femurs; otherwise, radiographic findings are similar to those in **C.**

markedly shortened limbs (Fig. 165-6). This "changing" dysplasia over time produces a short-trunk/short-limb form of dwarfism (severe scoliosis) with a "tail." Although heterogeneous, most cases are nonlethal and are autosomal dominant.

RADIOLOGIC FINDINGS

1. Thorax: small; short ribs
2. Spine: *dense wafer vertebral bodies* (in affected newborns), reconstituted platyspondyly (in affected children and adults), *scoliosis* (in affected adults)
3. Pelvis and hips: *short, squared iliac wings;* flat, irregular acetabular roof; narrow sacrosciatic notches; *halberd (hunting ax)–shaped proximal femurs*
4. Extremities: *trumpet-shaped metaphyses* (in affected newborns), dumbbell-shaped short tubular bones of hands and feet

Schneckenbecken (Snail Pelvis) Dysplasia

This dysplasia, although relatively uncommon, has a very interesting radiographic feature, as the name of this disorder implies (Fig. 165-7). It is a lethal skeletal dysplasia but can be diagnosed from the short limbs and with small thorax on second-trimester ultrasonography, which is especially valuable in assessing for this autosomal recessive disorder.

RADIOLOGIC FINDINGS

1. Thorax: small; short, anteriorly cupped ribs; handlebar clavicles; hypoplastic scapulas

2. Vertebrae: small, *round vertebral body ossification* (unossified posterior portion)
3. Pelvis: *snail-shaped iliac bones (Schneckenbecken)*
4. Extremities: micromelia, *dumbbell-shaped* long bones, especially *femurs*

SHORT RIB–POLYDACTYLY GROUP

The short rib dysplasia with or without polydactyly (short rib–polydactyly [SRP]) group of disorders is a rather diverse group, but they are linked at least radiologically. The chromosomal locus for at least one of this group (chondroectodermal dysplasia) has been established as 4p16. The entire group is important because it is rather common in occurrence. The group consists of all the SRP disorders (types I through IV), asphyxiating thoracic dysplasia (ATD), and chondroectodermal dysplasia. All are autosomal recessive.

Short Rib–Polydactyly Dysplasia

SRP dysplasia is a subgroup of disorders that are typed largely on radiographic grounds (Fig. 165-8). Types I and III are quite similar, as are types II and IV. The important role of the pediatric radiologist is to make the diagnosis of this subgroup as separate from ATD and chondroectodermal dysplasia. This usually can be done rather easily because the SRP dysplasias have the shortest ribs of any of the skeletal dysplasias.

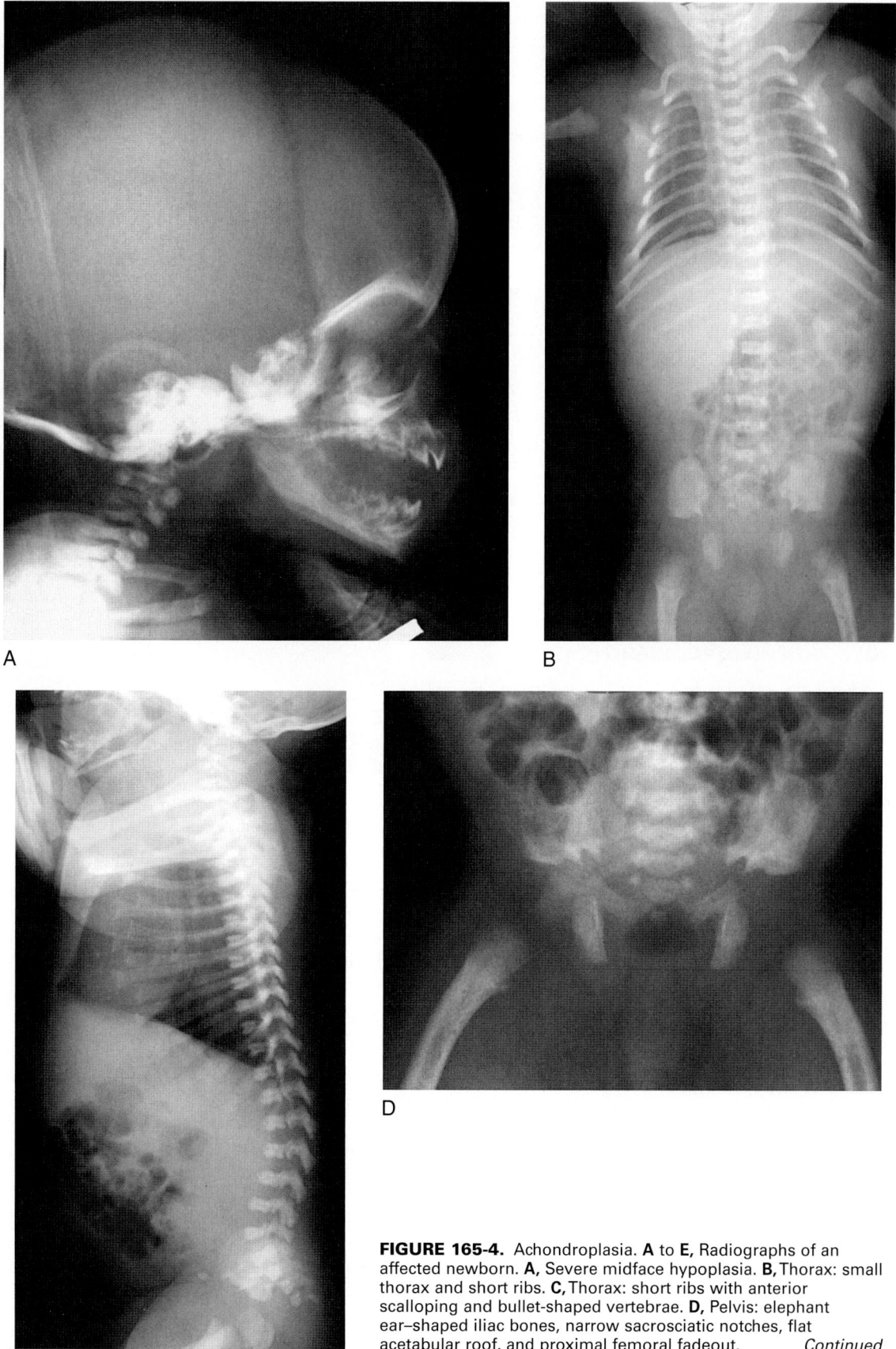

FIGURE 165-4. Achondroplasia. **A** to **E**, Radiographs of an affected newborn. **A**, Severe midface hypoplasia. **B**, Thorax: small thorax and short ribs. **C**, Thorax: short ribs with anterior scalloping and bullet-shaped vertebrae. **D**, Pelvis: elephant ear–shaped iliac bones, narrow sacrosciatic notches, flat acetabular roof, and proximal femoral fadeout. *Continued*

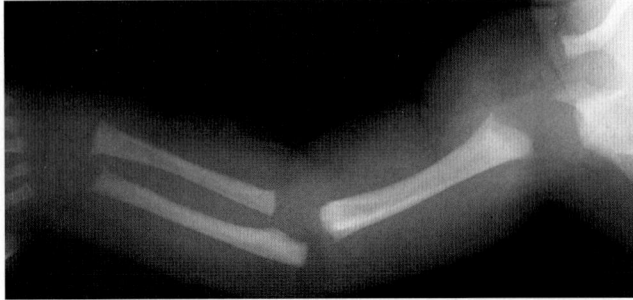

E

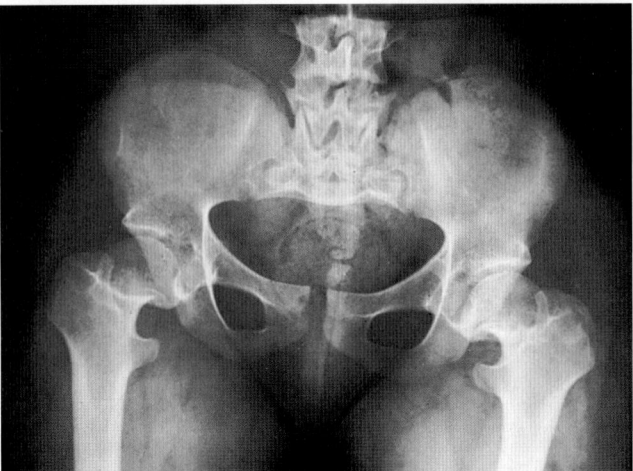

G

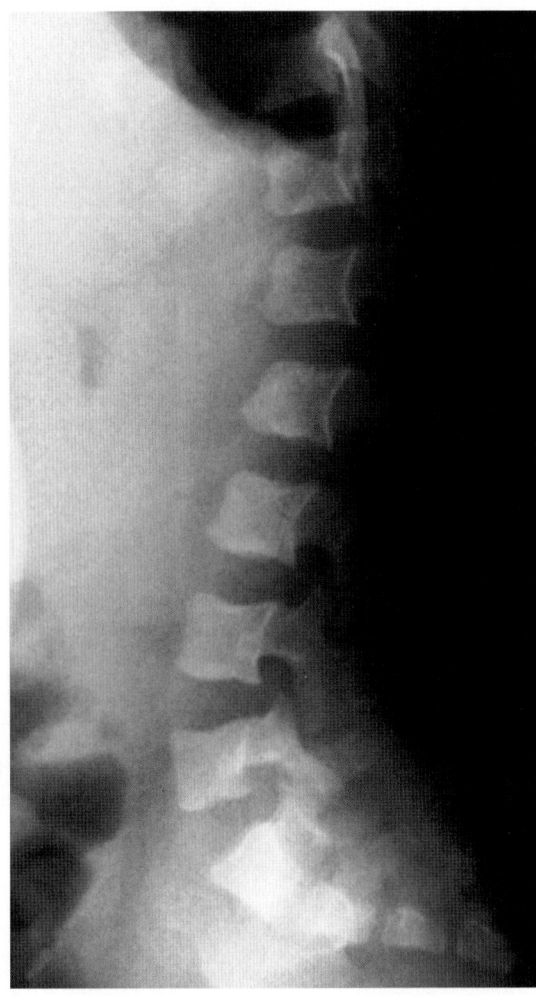

F

FIGURE 165-4, cont'd. Achondroplasia. **E,** Extremities: rhizomelia and mesomelia. **F,** Radiograph in an affected 1¹⁄₂-year-old with classic vertebrae with short pedicles, posterior scalloping, and somewhat short vertebral bodies. **G,** Radiograph in an affected woman with flat acetabular roofs, elephant ear–shaped iliac wings, and short femoral necks (compare with **D**). (**G** from Silverman FN: Achondroplasia. Prog Pediatr Radiol 1973;4:94-124.)

RADIOLOGIC FINDINGS

1. Thorax: small; *very, very short horizontal ribs*
2. Spine: relatively normally shaped
3. Pelvis: small, dysplastic ilia
4. Extremities: *micromelia; rolling pin–shaped or round-ended or metaphyseally spiked femurs; ovoid* or tiny, normal-shaped *tibias;* severe brachydactyly with hypoplastic middle and distal phalanges; *polydactyly commonly present*

> **Short rib–polydactyly dysplasia is characterized by the shortest ribs of any of the skeletal dysplasias.**

Asphyxiating Thoracic Dysplasia (Jeune Syndrome)

ATD is a disorder with a mixed prognosis. Many affected patients die in the perinatal period from respiratory complications (small chest) (Fig. 165-9). Survivors may die from renal complications (progressive nephropathy) later in life. Other internal organs may also be involved. In uncommon cases, polydactyly is present. There

are definite radiographic (but not clinical) similarities to chondroectodermal dysplasia (Ellis–van Creveld syndrome), a possible allelic disease. Some cases are so alike radiologically that they are best termed *ATD/Ellis–van Creveld syndrome complex.*

RADIOLOGIC FINDINGS

1. Thorax: long and *barrel-shaped,* handlebar clavicles, short horizontal ribs with bulbous anterior ends
2. Spine: normal
3. Pelvis: small; short, flared iliac wings; *trident acetabular roof; narrowed sacrosciatic notches*
4. Extremities: generalized shortening, *precocious proximal femoral epiphyseal ossification,* cone-shaped epiphyses in hands

Chondroectodermal Dysplasia (Ellis–van Creveld Syndrome)

Ellis–van Creveld syndrome is a nonlethal skeletal dysplasia. The nonskeletal involvement in this disorder is extremely important in defining this condition. Signs include hair, nail, and teeth abnormalities, as well as congenital heart disease. Polydactyly is almost invariably

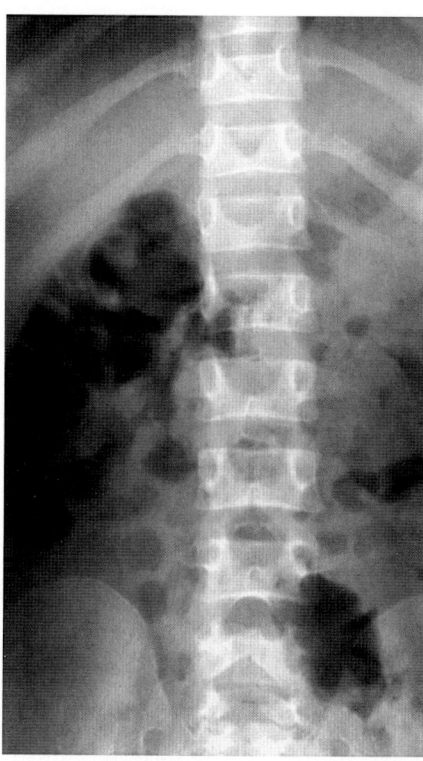 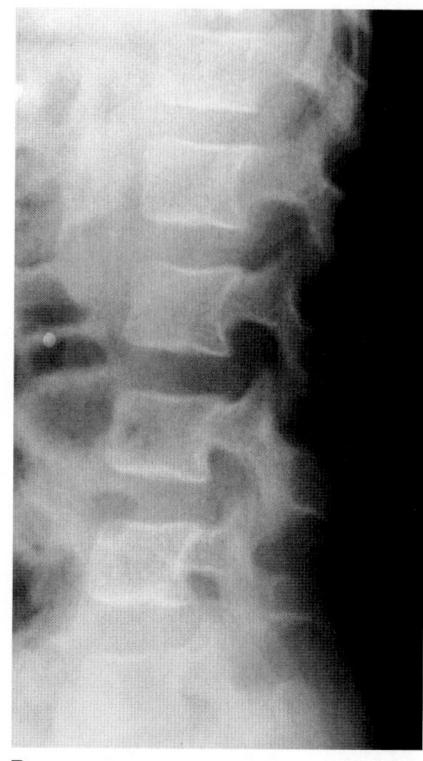 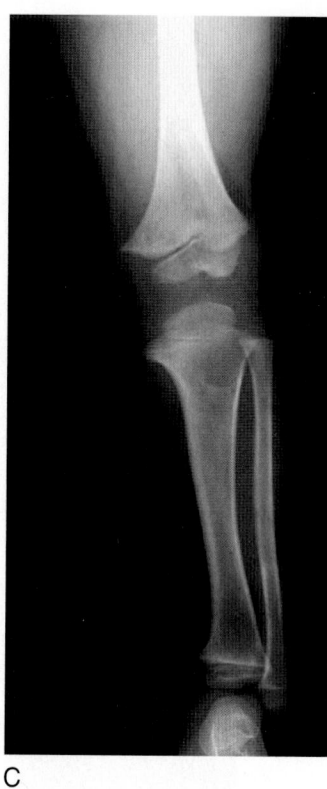

A   B   C

FIGURE 165-5. Radiographs in a 3-year-old with hypochondroplasia. **A,** Lumbosacral interpediculate narrowing. **B,** Posterior vertebral body scalloping with normal pedicles. **C,** Proximal and distal fibular overgrowth. There are mild beginning chevron deformity changes in distal femur.

present. The radiologic findings are very similar to those of ATD (Fig. 165-10). The genes involved in this autosomal recessive condition have been identified (*EvC* genes *1, 2*). The chromosome location of these genes is 4p16.

RADIOLOGIC FINDINGS

1. Thorax: small; moderately short ribs
2. Pelvis: small; short, flared iliac wings; *trident acetabula; narrowed sacrosciatic notches*
3. Spine: almost normal
4. Extremities: generalized shortening with more mesomelia and acromelia; premature ossification of capital femoral epiphyses; delayed ossification of proximal tibial epiphyses; humeral and femoral bowing; *exostosis of proximal/medial portion of tibia*
5. Hands: characteristic: *postaxial polydactyly, capitate/hamate* (and other carpal) *fusions, extra carpal bone, cone-shaped epiphyses*
6. Feet: polydactyly

DIASTROPHIC DYSPLASIA GROUP

The diastrophic dysplasia group is a molecularly defined group of disorders with a defect on chromosome 5 in *DTDST*, a sulfate transporter gene. This group comprises not only diastrophic dysplasia but also multiple epiphyseal dysplasia (MED)–multilayered patellae/brachydactyly/clubfeet, as well as achondrogenesis type IB and atelosteogenesis type II. This reveals how sometimes the radiologic findings do not point to molecular grouping, because there is no *DTDST* gene abnormality in achon-

drogenesis type IA—in which radiographic changes are almost identical to those of type IB—or in the other forms of atelosteogenesis. For radiographic clarity, I discuss both forms of achondrogenesis type I together.

Diastrophic Dysplasia

Diastrophic dysplasia is, like all the other disorders of this group, an autosomal recessive condition. It is commonly identifiable at birth and usually nonlethal. Early on it was called *achondroplasia with clubfeet*, which alluded to some of its distinctive clinical features: severe foot abnormalities (talipes equinovarus), neonatal cauliflower ear development, hitchhiker thumb, and cleft or high-arched palate. The chondro-osseous structure (resting chondrocyte death and fibro-ossification) explains some of the characteristic clinical and radiographic findings (Fig. 165-11).

RADIOLOGIC FINDINGS

1. Head: *Ear pinna calcification*
2. Thorax: moderately small
3. Spine: *progressive scoliosis, kyphosis,* upper cervical subluxation (odontoid hypoplasia), *cervical kyphosis, posterior process clefting* (cervical and sacral)
4. Extremities: often micromelia; *short, thick tubular bones;* generalized brachydactyly (*short ovoid first metacarpal, twisted metatarsals, accessory and irregular carpal bones*); problems in joint regions (epiphyseal dysplasia, especially hips; joint dislocations)

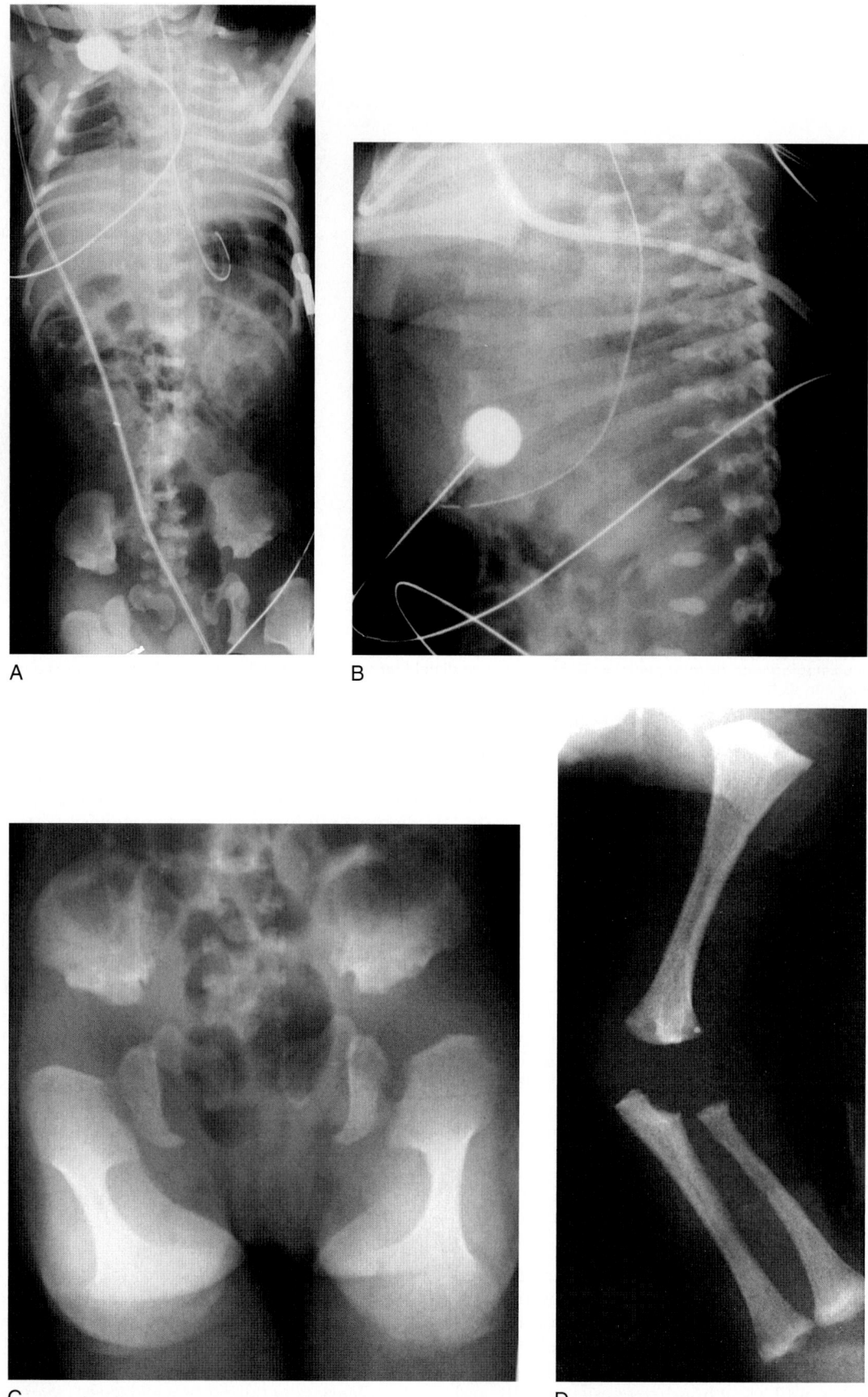

FIGURE 165-6. Radiographs in a newborn with metatropic dysplasia. **A,** Thorax: long trunk and small chest. **B,** Spine: dense wafer vertebral bodies and short ribs with anterior splaying. **C,** Pelvis: short iliac wings, narrow sciatic notches, irregular acetabular roofs, and halberd (hunting ax)–shaped femurs with trumpet-shaped metaphyses. **D,** Upper extremities: flared proximal humeral and distal radial and ulnar metaphyses; shortened long bones.

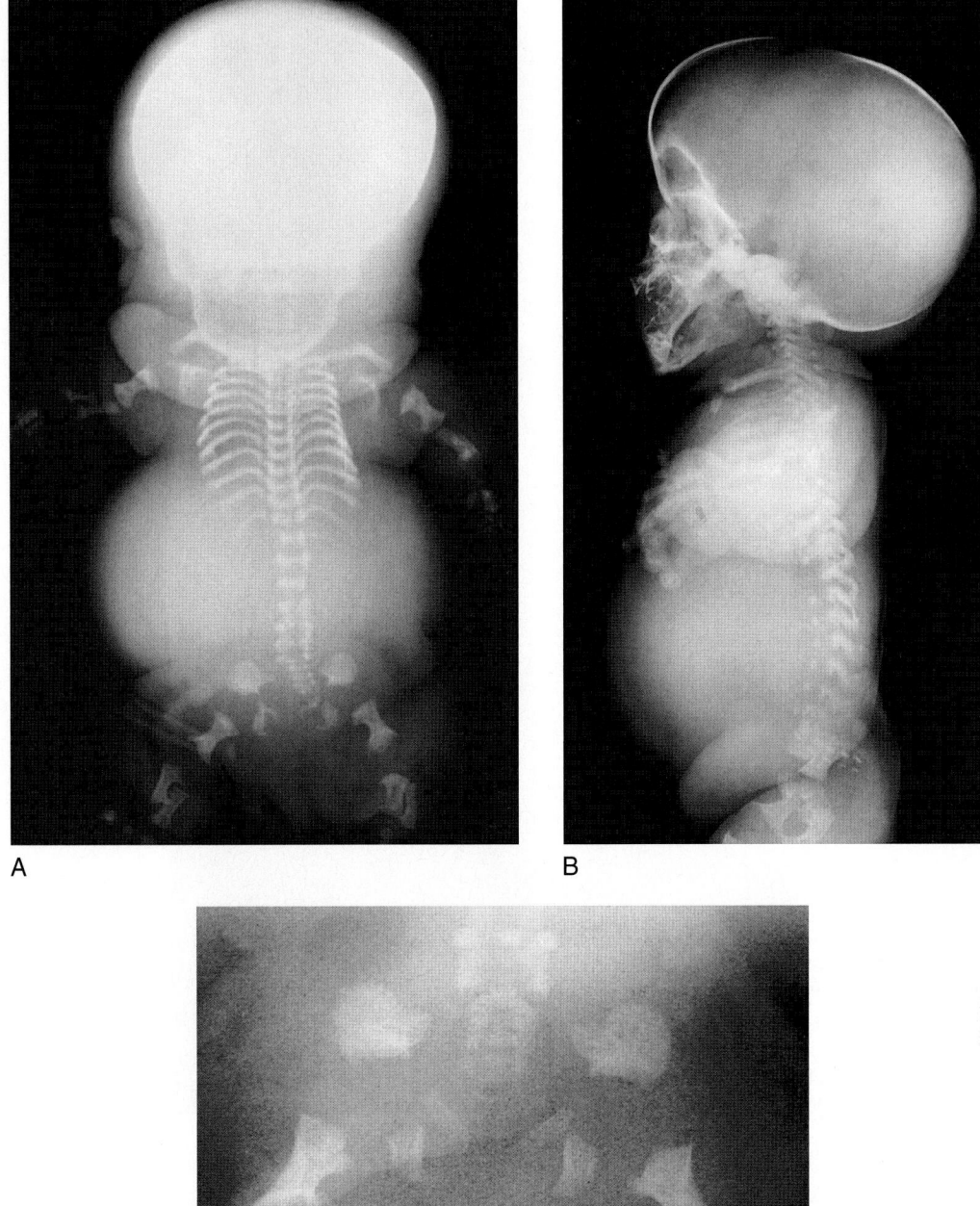

FIGURE 165-7. Schneckenbecken dysplasia. **A,** Radiograph of an affected stillborn infant with large head; short trunk; micromelia; small, barrel-shaped thorax; snail-shaped iliac bones; and dumbbell femurs and humeri. **B,** Radiograph of an affected stillborn infant with round vertebral bodies with posterior ossification failure; the hands are proportionally large. **C,** Radiograph of the "Schneckenbecken" (snail-shaped iliac bones). (**C** courtesy of A. Giedion, Zurich, Switzerland.)

5. Other sites: *precocious* costochondral and laryngeal area *cartilage calcification;* multiple sternal and patella centers

Multiple Epiphyseal Dysplasia: Multilayered Patellae/Brachydactyly/Clubfeet

In some cases of MED, there are *DTDST* gene abnormalities. Radiographs reveal MED changes, but patients also exhibit mildly short or normal stature and clubfeet

(see also multiple epiphyseal dysplasia and pseudo-achondroplasia group).

RADIOLOGIC FINDINGS

1. *Epiphyseal dysplasia, especially at hips* (half- or quarter-moon–shaped)
2. *Double/multilayered patella* (visible on lateral knee radiograph)
3. *Mild brachydactyly*
4. *Clubfeet/*twisted metatarsals

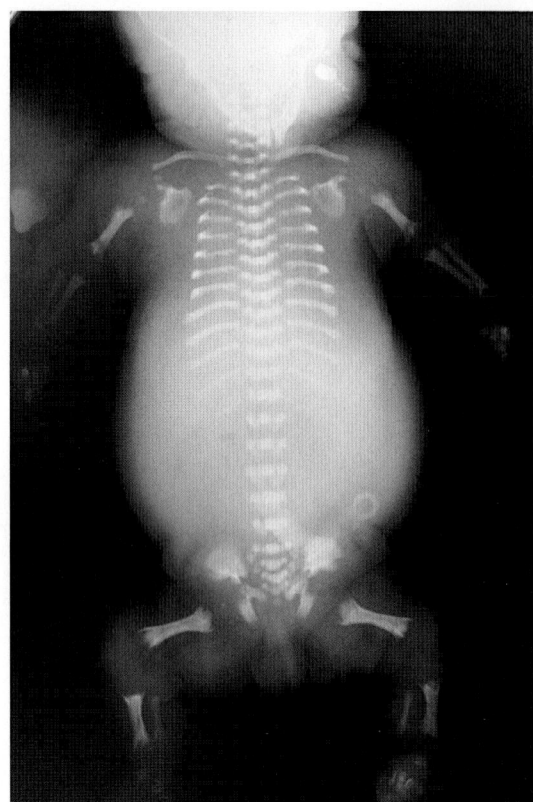

A

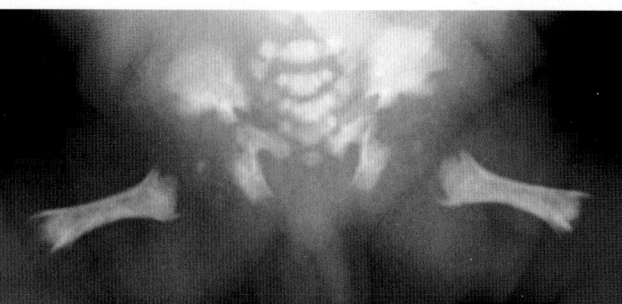

B

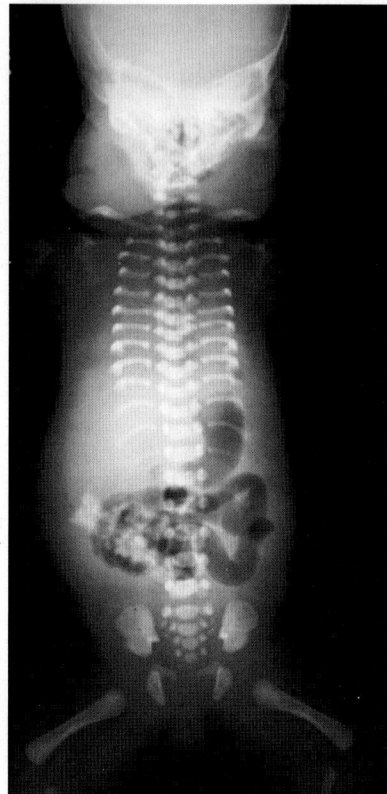

C

FIGURE 165-8. Short rib–polydactyly dysplasia. **A,** Radiograph in a stillborn infant with type I/III form, demonstrating very short ribs, handlebar clavicles, hypoplastic pelvis with notched acetabula, and metaphyseal-spiked femurs. **B,** Magnified, coned view of pelvis. **C,** Radiograph in a stillborn infant with short rib–polydactyly dysplasia type II. Findings are similar to those in type I/III but with round-ended femurs and hypoplastic acetabula.

Achondrogenesis Type I

Achondrogenesis type I is actually two separate disorders that appear almost identical radiographically (Fig. 165-12). Achondrogenesis type IB belongs to this diastrophic dysplasia (molecular) group. In achondrogenesis type IA, a molecular or gene abnormality has not yet been identified. Clinically, the two types appear identical: proportionately large skull; micromelic, hydropic, pear-shaped trunk; polyhydramnios; and lethality.

RADIOLOGIC FINDINGS

1. Skull: decreased ossification
2. Thorax: *tiny; very short ribs with anterior splaying*
3. Spine: *absent or minimal vertebral body ossification*
4. Pelvis: *short iliac bones with concave acetabular roofs, absent pubic (ischial) ossification*
5. Extremities: *severe micromelia* with broadened ends of limbs, *trapezoidal or wedge-shaped femurs*

Note: Radiographic findings in achondrogenesis type IA include *multiple fractured, beaded ribs; wedged femurs;* those in achondrogenesis type IB, *no rib fractures or beading; trapezoidal femurs.*

TYPE II COLLAGENOPATHIES

The type II collagenopathies are a heterogeneous group of disorders, all of which show some relationship to each other not only molecularly but also clinically and radiographically. Although they range from invariably lethal to mildly affected, they have in common involvement of the spine (platyspondyly/deficiency of vertebral ossification) and epiphyseal (epiphyseal equivalent) ossification delay or dysplasia. Clinically, normal type II collagen is important not only for the development of the epiphyseal plate region of developing bone but also for hyaline cartilage, nucleus pulposus, and even the vitreous of the eye (myopia). The type II collagenopathies range from

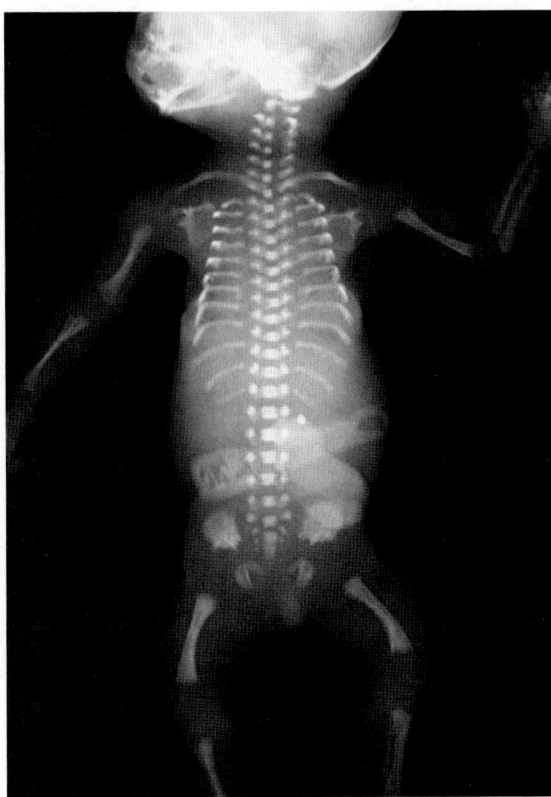
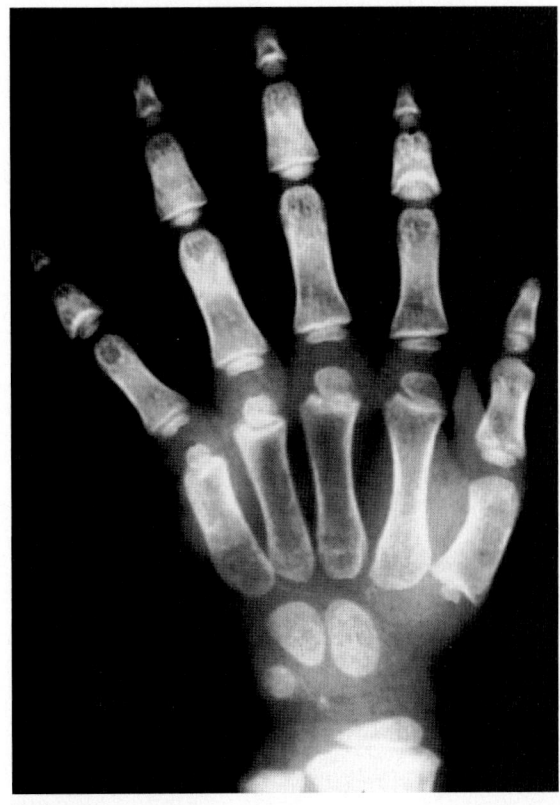

A   B

FIGURE 165-9. Asphyxiating thoracic dysplasia. **A,** Radiograph in an affected preterm stillborn infant with small thorax, short ribs, trident acetabula, narrow sacrosciatic notches, and normal spine. **B,** Radiograph in an affected infant aged 26 months with cone-shaped epiphyses in the hand, especially involving the second and fifth middle phalanges. (**B** courtesy of T. Coburn, Memphis, TN.)

lethal and severe achondrogenesis type II/hypochondrogenesis through SEDC, Kniest dysplasia, and Strudwick type SE(M)D to more mildly affected Stickler dysplasia (some Stickler cases are a type XI collagenopathy). All these disorders are autosomal dominant and, in lethal conditions, new mutations with very little likelihood of recurrence.

Achondrogenesis Type II/Hypochondrogenesis

Achondrogenesis type II is invariably lethal. Clinically, affected stillborns and fetuses appear very similar to those with achondrogenesis types IA and IB. Radiographically, however, the condition is easily diagnosed correctly (Fig. 165-13). The clinical appearance is a micromelic dwarf, somewhat hydropic, with a nuchal cystic hygroma. A cleft palate is not uncommon, as in other type II collagenopathies.

Hypochondrogenesis is just a slightly milder form of achondrogenesis type II, and, by definition, affected infants survive the immediate perinatal period but often cannot be extubated and invariably die from respiratory complications in the first month or two of life. There is obviously a spectrum of severity, but this diagnosis is important both to the family and to the physician in trying to prognosticate for the infant. Patients who survive beyond these time periods are given the diagnosis of SEDC. The pediatric radiologist can be helpful by analyzing the chest films for thoracic size, lung volume, and rib length.

RADIOLOGIC FINDINGS

In achondrogenesis type II:
1. Skull: proportionately large
2. Thorax: *very small; very short ribs*
3. Spine: *almost complete lack of mineralization of most vertebral bodies; cervical and sacral posterior elements also often unossified*
4. Pelvis: small iliac wings with concave inferior and medial margins; absence of ischia, pubic bones, and sacral elements
5. Extremities: *micromelia, mostly rhizomelia and mesomelia, with relative sparing of hands and feet;* almost normally modeled long bones with metaphyseal flare; *absence of talus and calcaneal ossification* (epiphyseal equivalents)

In hypochondrogenesis:
1. Thorax: larger, with longer ribs
2. Spine: more vertebral body ossification (*hypoplasia and platyspondyly*)

Note: Hypochondrogenesis is otherwise similar to achondrogenesis type II.

Spondyloepiphyseal Dysplasia Congenita

Most cases of spondyloepiphyseal dysplasia with a congenital onset are type II collagenopathies. SEDC is part of the previously discussed spectrum and is not lethal (cause of respiratory death). The clinical presentation in the newborn is that of a dwarf with a severely short trunk; short limbs; and normal hands, feet, and skull. There

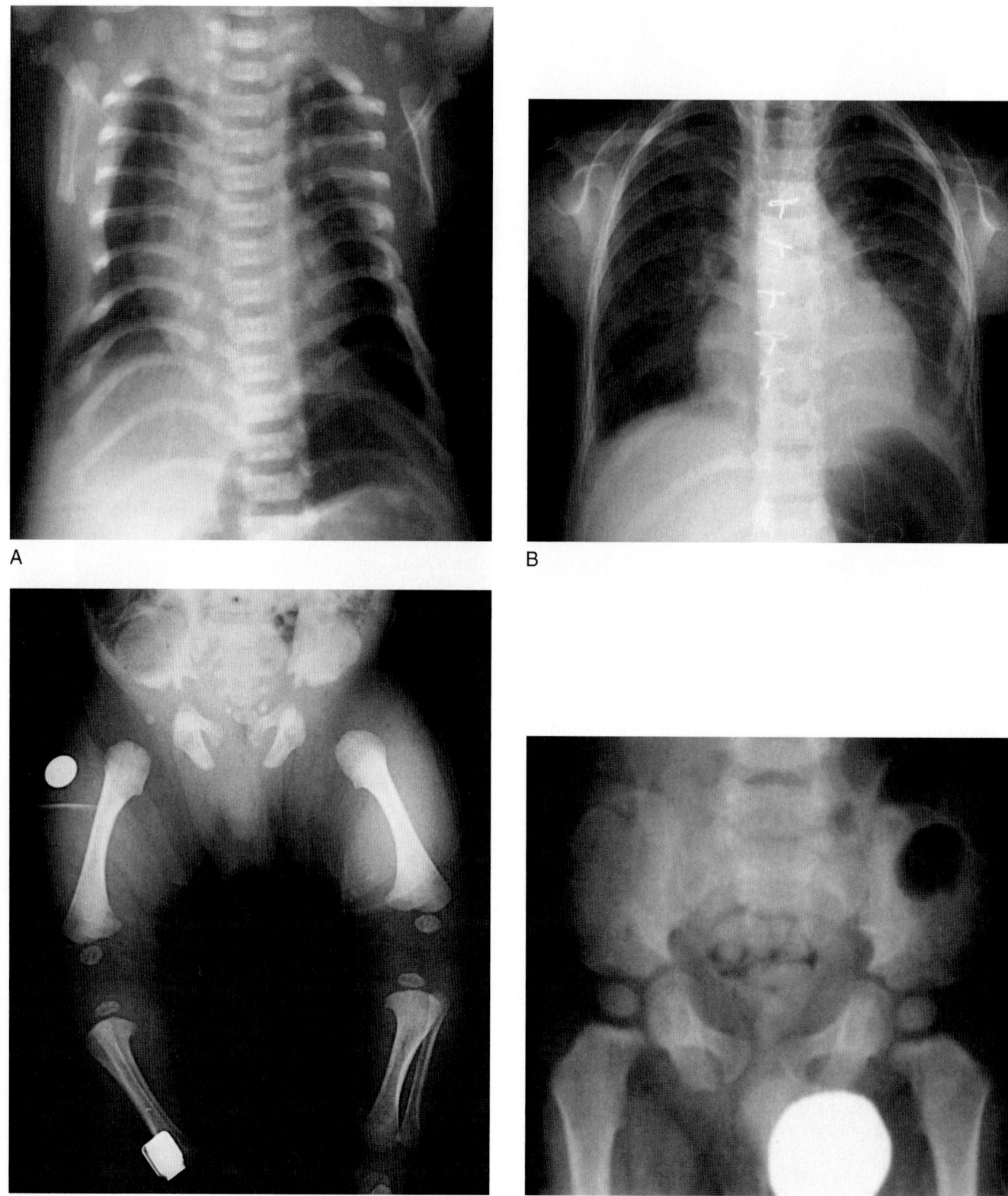

A

B

C

D

FIGURE 165-10. Chondroectodermal dysplasia (Ellis–van Creveld syndrome). **A,** Radiograph in an affected 3-month-old infant with a narrow thorax, short ribs, anterior rib flaring, and a normal spine. **B,** Radiograph in an affected 5-year-old with similar chest configuration; there is cardiomegaly with sternal sutures from a primum defect repair. **C,** Radiograph in an affected 3-month-old with short, flared iliac wings; trident acetabula; and mesomelia and rhizomelia. **D** and **E,** Radiographs of an affected child at 2½ (**D**) and 12 years of age (**E**), showing normalization of pelvis with residual "red wine glass" configuration.   *Continued*

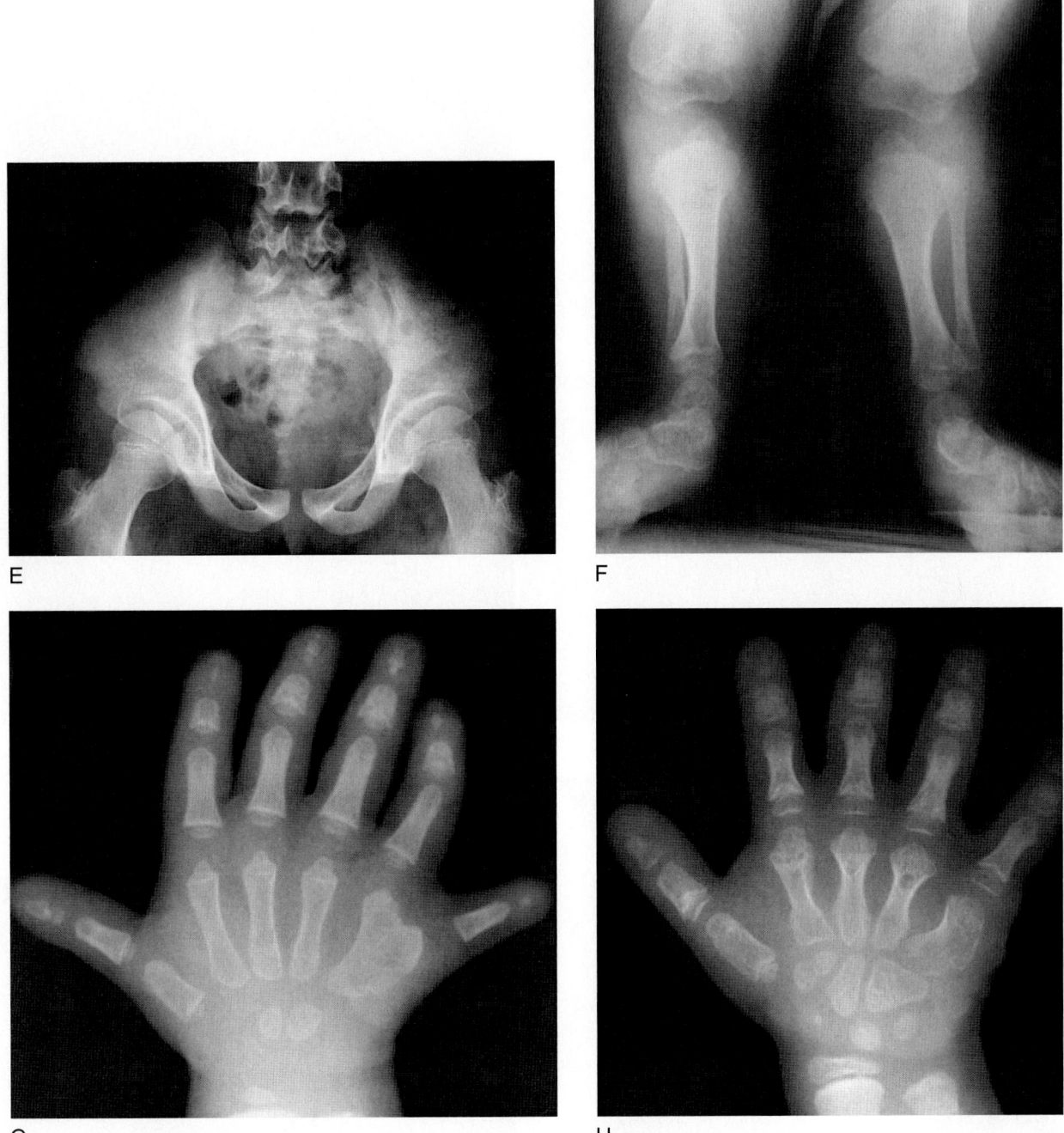

E

F

G

H

FIGURE 165-10, *cont'd*. Chondroectodermal dysplasia (Ellis–van Creveld syndrome). **F,** Radiograph in an affected 2½-year-old with remarkable mesomelia. **G,** Radiograph in an affected 2-year-old with characteristic hands: polydactyly, middle and distal phalangeal hypoplasia, cone-shaped epiphyses of middle phalanges, and beginning carpal coalition. **H,** Radiograph in the same child as in **G** at 6 years of age. After polydactyly repair, there is a residual wide fifth metacarpal; other findings are similar except that there is no carpal coalition.

may be major problems with the upper cervical spine (Fig. 165-14). Degenerative arthrosis of the hips can be a significant concern in the affected adult.

RADIOLOGIC FINDINGS

1. Thorax: small; short ribs
2. Spine: *pear-shaped or oval vertebral bodies* (at birth), anteriorly rounded *platyspondyly* (later)
3. Pelvis: *absent pubic ossification* (at birth and during infancy)
4. Extremities: normally modeled but *shortened long bones, significant generalized ossification delay* (early) and *hypoplastic-appearing/dysplastic epiphyses* (later), *unossified talus/calcaneus* in the newborn, normal hands and feet with ossification delay (epiphyses/carpal, tarsal)

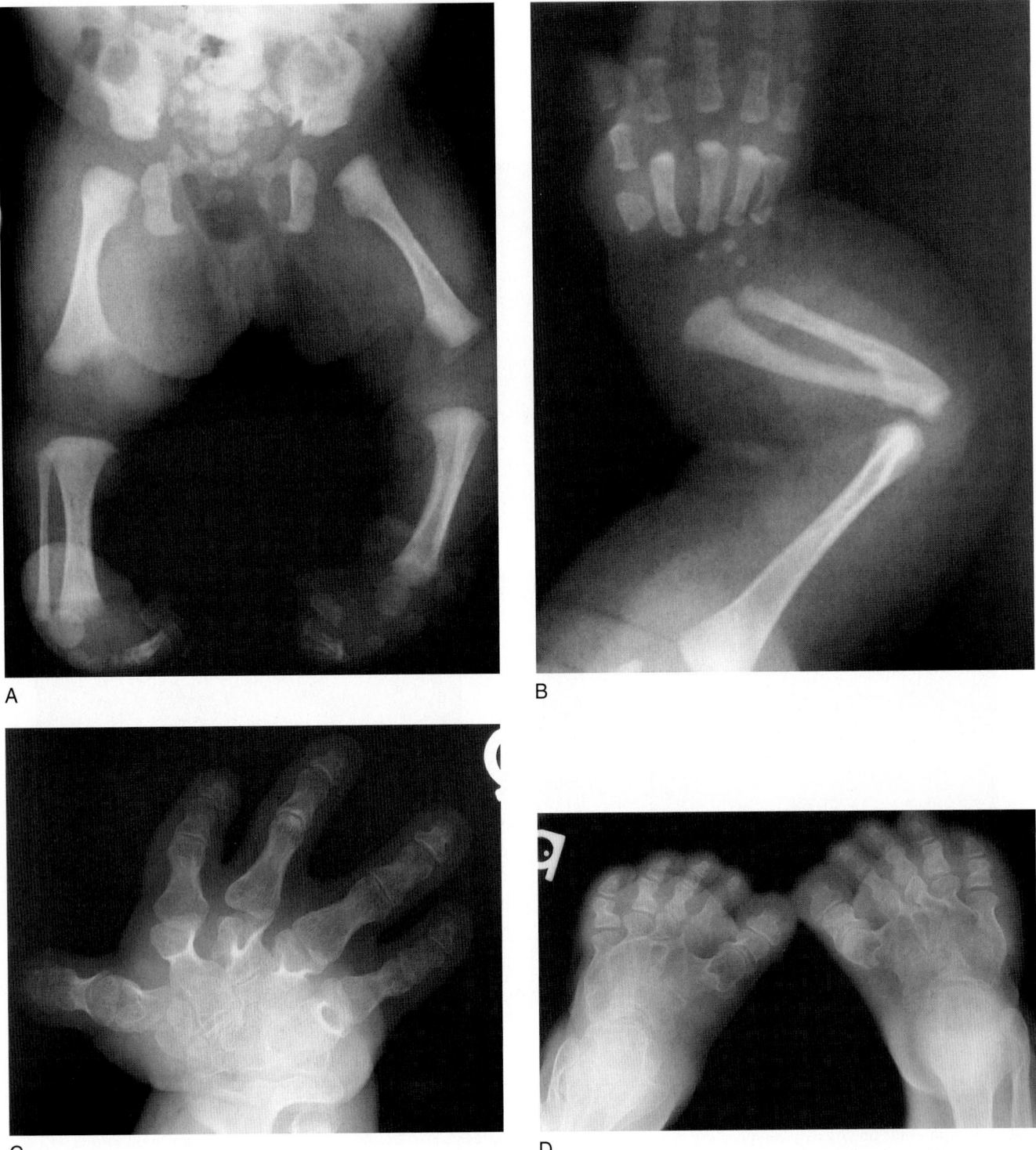

FIGURE 165-11. Diastrophic dysplasia. **A** and **B,** Radiographs in an affected newborn. **A,** Lower extremities: rhizomelia and mesomelia and severe clubfeet. **B,** Upper extremity: elbow dislocation and short, ovoid first metacarpal. **C** and **D,** Radiographs in an affected 21-year-old. **C,** Upper extremity: hitchhiker thumb, ovoid first metacarpal, brachydactyly, and irregular and extra carpal bones. **D,** Lower extremities: unusual clubfoot and twisted metatarsals.

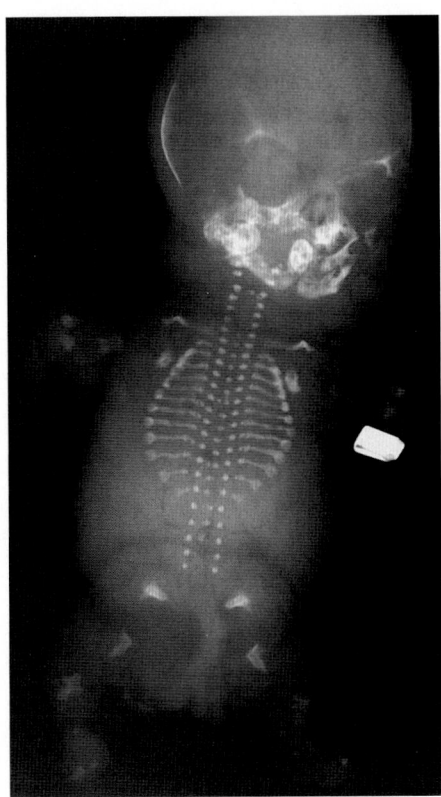

A

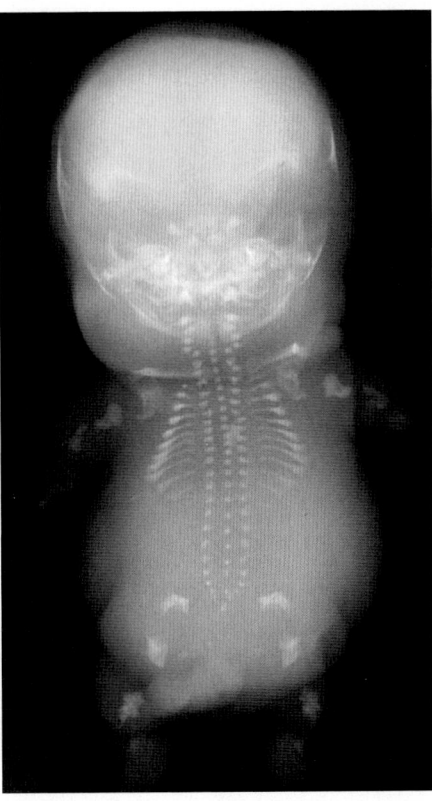

B

FIGURE 165-12. Achondrogenesis. **A,** Radiograph in a stillborn infant with type IA achondrogenesis demonstrates a tiny thorax; short, anteriorly cupped ribs with beading; micromelia; wedged femurs; and poor to absent vertebral body ossification. **B,** Radiograph in a stillborn infant with type IB achondrogenesis. Findings are similar to those in type IA but with arched iliac wings, no rib beading, and trapezoidal femurs.

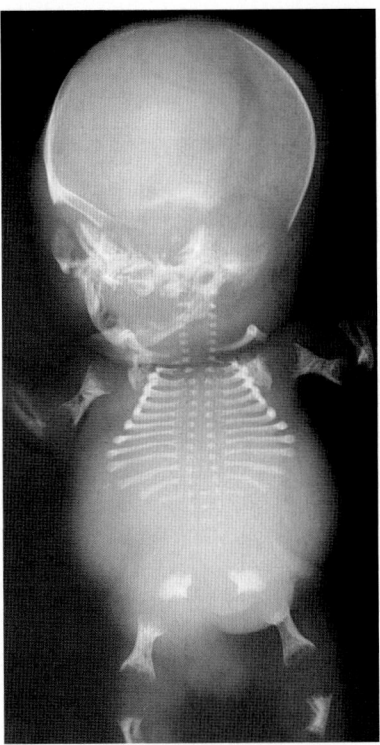

A

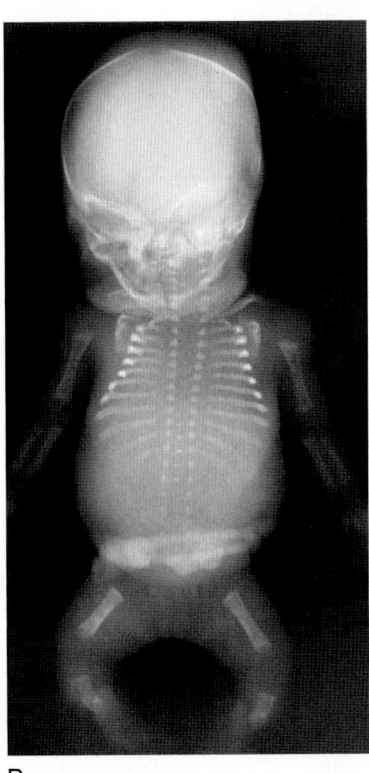

B

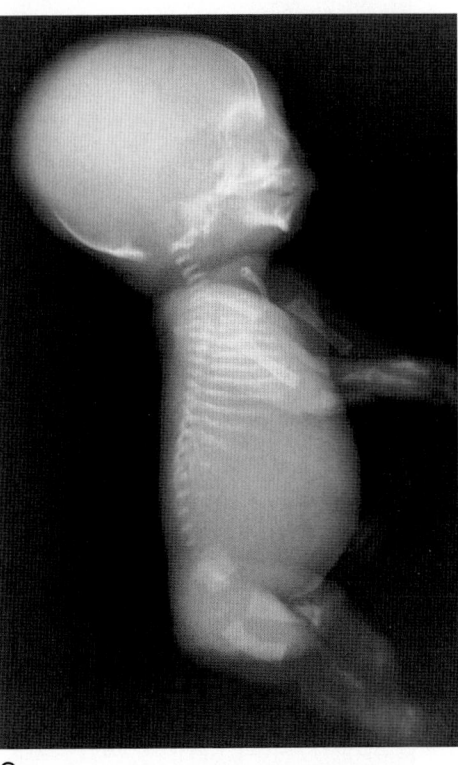

C

FIGURE 165-13. A, Radiograph in a stillborn infant with achondrogenesis type II. Findings include a proportionately enlarged skull; a tiny thorax with short ribs; almost no vertebral body ossification with lower pedicle ossification deficiency; small wide ilia, notched acetabular roofs, and absence of ischial and pubic ossification; micromelia; and normally modeled femurs with metaphyseal flaring and cupping. **B** and **C,** Radiographs in a fetus of 21 weeks' gestation with hypochondrogenesis, revealing better vertebral ossification, with more and better long bone modeling.

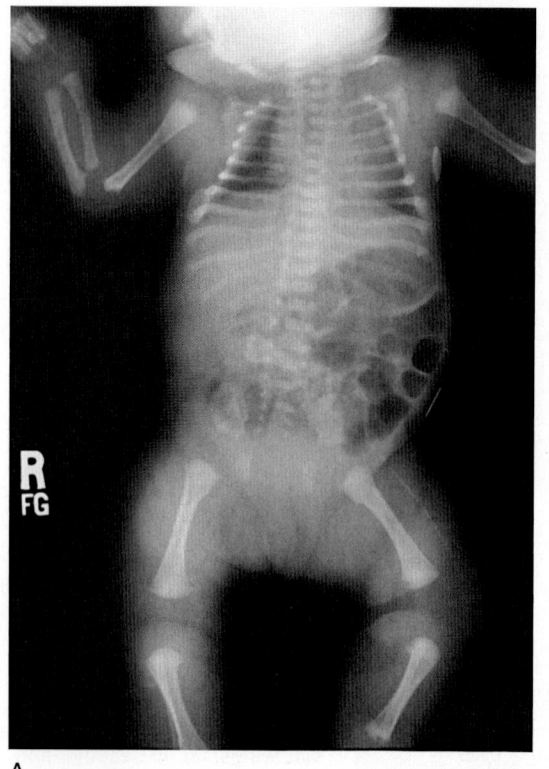

A

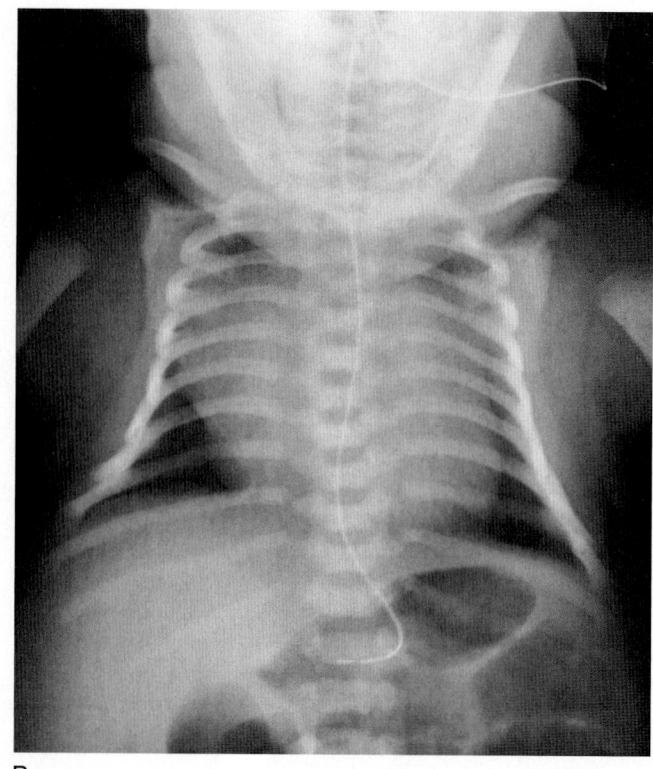

B

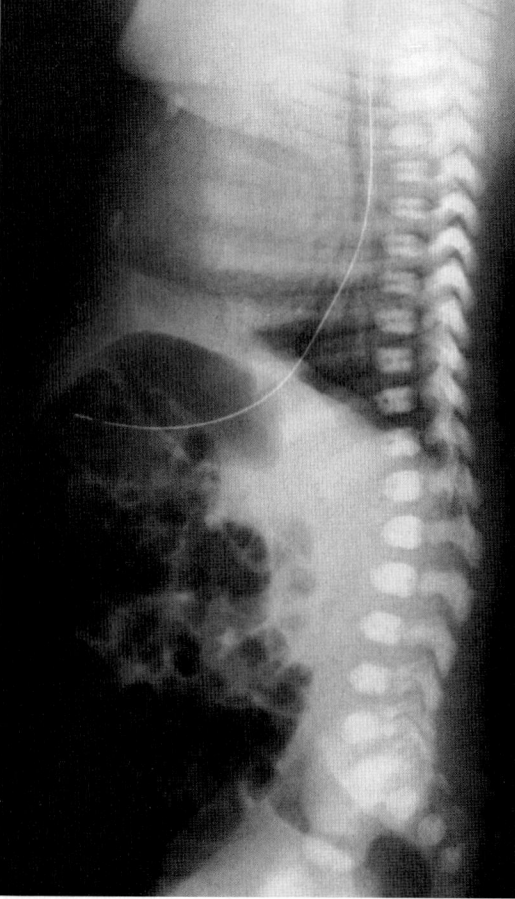

C

FIGURE 165-14. Spondyloepiphyseal dysplasia congenita.
A, Radiograph in an affected newborn with a small thorax,
rounded iliac wings, vertical ischia, absence of pubic ossification,
short femurs with metaphyseal rounding, and comparable other
long bones. **B,** Radiograph in an affected newborn with
bell-shaped chest, short ribs, and elongated clavicles.
C, Radiograph in an affected newborn with moderately short ribs
with mild anterior splaying and anteriorly rounded vertebral
bodies with minimal flattening and no coronal clefts.

> Achondrogenesis type II, hypochondrogenesis, and SEDC are related disorders along a spectrum of severity.

Kniest Dysplasia

This uncommon entity manifests in the newborn in a manner almost identical to that of SEDC, again as a nonlethal dysplasia. Over time, however, radiographic (and clinical) changes occur and help diagnose this condition (Fig. 165-15). Salient clinical findings include cleft palate, myopia (retinal detachment), deafness, limited joint motion with enlarged and painful joints, occipitoatlantal instability, and progressive kyphoscoliosis.

RADIOLOGIC FINDINGS

1. Thorax: small to normal
2. Spine: *coronal clefts* (at birth and during infancy), *platyspondyly with end plate irregularity* (later)
3. Extremities: *dumbbell femurs;* generalized ossification delay, epiphyses becoming hypoplastic/dysplastic and then later even *megaepiphyses, fluffiness/irregular calcification (cloud effect) in physeal plate regions* (in late childhood and early adulthood); hands' bulbous joints (*metaphyseal flare/epiphyseal fragmentation*) mimicking rheumatoid arthritis.

Note: In the newborn, Kniest syndrome is radiographically identical to SEDC except for *coronal clefts and dumbbell femurs.*

OTHER SPONDYLOEPI(META)PHYSEAL DYSPLASIAS

The other SE(M)Ds are an indistinctly classified group of disorders whose molecular bases have generally not been completely identified. As the name of the group implies, some of the disorders entail metaphyseal changes, and others do not. There are at least two members of this group that are important or interesting: spondyloepiphyseal dysplasia tarda and Dyggve-Melchior-Clausen syndrome.

Spondyloepiphyseal Dysplasia Tarda

This is an X-linked disorder. The *SEDL* gene is located on the short arm of the X chromosome (Xp22). Spondyloepiphyseal dysplasia tarda is often diagnosed in an adolescent or in a young adult (Fig. 165-16) with nonsevere short stature, especially a short trunk. There is early-onset degenerative arthrosis of the hips.

RADIOLOGIC FINDINGS

1. Spine: mild platyspondyly with *centrally humped end plates* with intervertebral disk space narrowing
2. Extremities: *mild to moderate "epiphyseal dysplasia" (small and irregular epiphyseal centers),* sparing of hands and feet

Dyggve-Melchior-Clausen Syndrome

This autosomal recessive disorder is uncommon but rather interesting. The alternative eponym *pseudo-Morquio syndrome* explains why. Dyggve-Melchior-Clausen syndrome is usually diagnosed in the first year of life. Affected individuals have short trunks and short limbs, and all three limb components, including hands and feet, are affected (Fig. 165-17). Although 80% have severe psychomotor retardation and the rest have normal mentation (*Smith-McCort syndrome*), it is suspected that all cases are a single entity.

RADIOLOGIC FINDINGS

1. Skull: *microcephaly*
2. Thorax: broad; anterior rib widening
3. Spine: *double-humped vertebral bodies* with end plate notching and posterior scalloping
4. Pelvis: small iliac wings with irregularly calcified apophyseal regions (lacy iliac crests)
5. Extremities: moderate shortening with epiphyseal/metaphyseal changes, generalized brachydactyly with cone-shaped epiphyses and small carpal bones (*no proximal metacarpal pointing* as in mucopolysaccharidosis [MPS]).

MULTIPLE EPIPHYSEAL DYSPLASIA AND PSEUDOACHONDROPLASIA GROUP

The MED and pseudoachondroplasia group is rather well delineated molecularly and proves that radiology does not play the definitive role in every disorder. Pseudoachondroplasia and some cases of typical MED are cartilage oligomeric protein (*COMP*) gene defects on chromosome 19 and share some commonality of radiographic findings. However, many other cases of MED (with the same apparent radiologic abnormalities) represent type IX collagen defects on chromosome 1, or matrilin 3 defects. It appears that all the described entities within this group are autosomal dominant disorders, except for MED-multilayered patellae/brachydactyly/clubfeet (see also section on the diastrophic dysplasia group).

Multiple Epiphyseal Dysplasia

MED has customarily been divided into two types: the Fairbanks and Ribbing forms (Figs. 165-18 and 165-19). Molecularly, this classification has turned out to be incorrect. Ribbing MED, the milder type, may entail only hip involvement and can be confused with bilateral Legg-Calvé-Perthes disease and Meyer dysplasia. Differentiation from these entities is possible because almost all patients with MED have clinically significant short stature. Many patients with MED later go through an asymptomatic phase of avascular necrosis of the capital femoral epiphyses. The Fairbanks form has involvement of all the long bone epiphyses to some degree. MED manifests after about 2 years of age but is most commonly diagnosed in an adolescent or young adult. Involvement is always bilateral and symmetric. The shortening is quite mild.

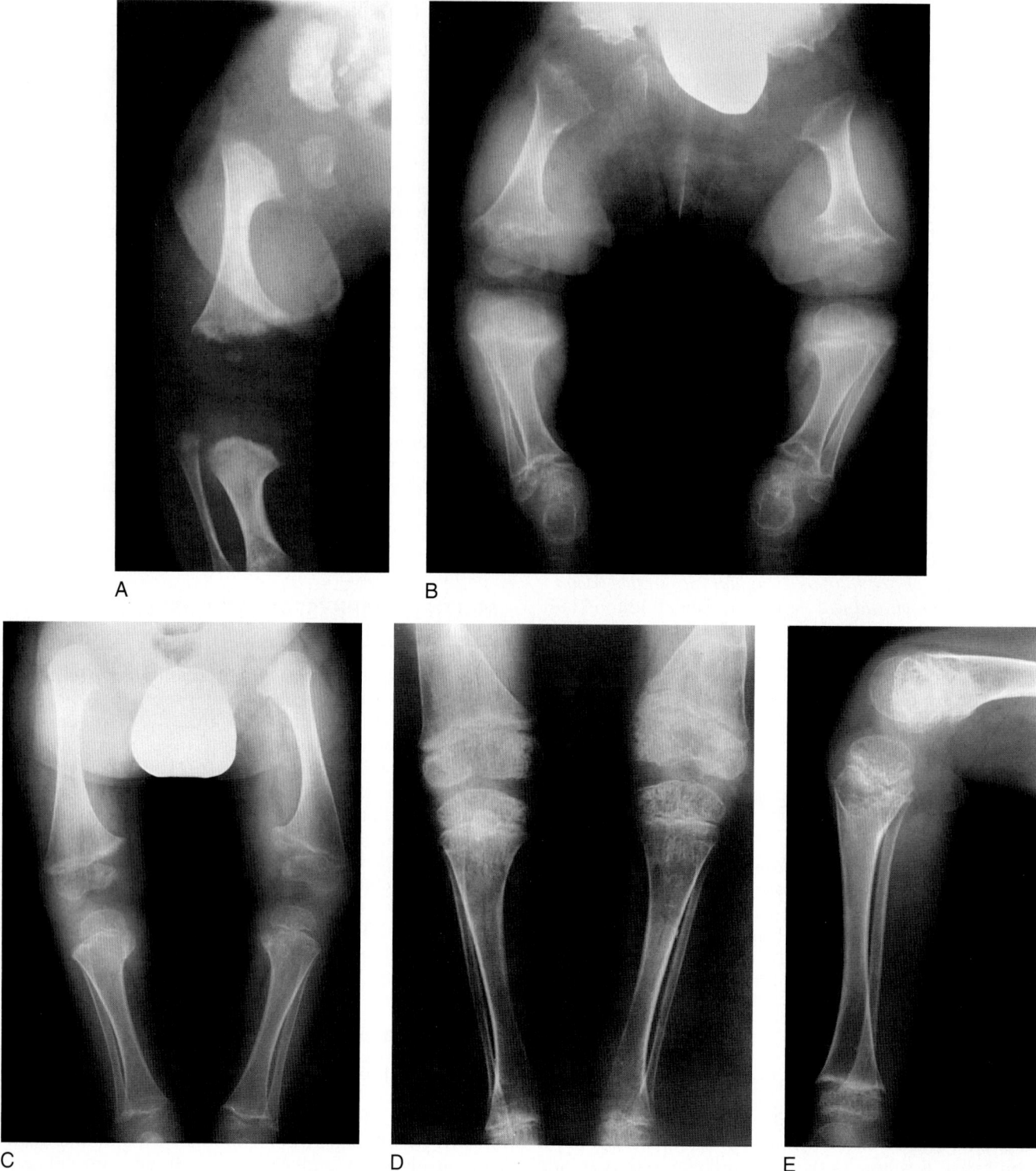

A

B

C

D

E

FIGURE 165-15. Radiographic findings in Kniest dysplasia. In two affected infants at 5 months (**A**) and 1 year of age (**B**), there are shortened femurs and tibias with metaphyseal widening, absence of femoral head ossification, knee epiphyseal ossification delay in the 5-month-old (**A**), beginning megaepiphyses in the 1-year-old (**B**), and fibular overgrowth. In three other affected children aged 1½ years (**C**), 5 years (**D**), and 4 years (**E**), there is no femoral head ossification and the beginning of woolly metaphyseal calcification with enlarging knee ossification.

Continued

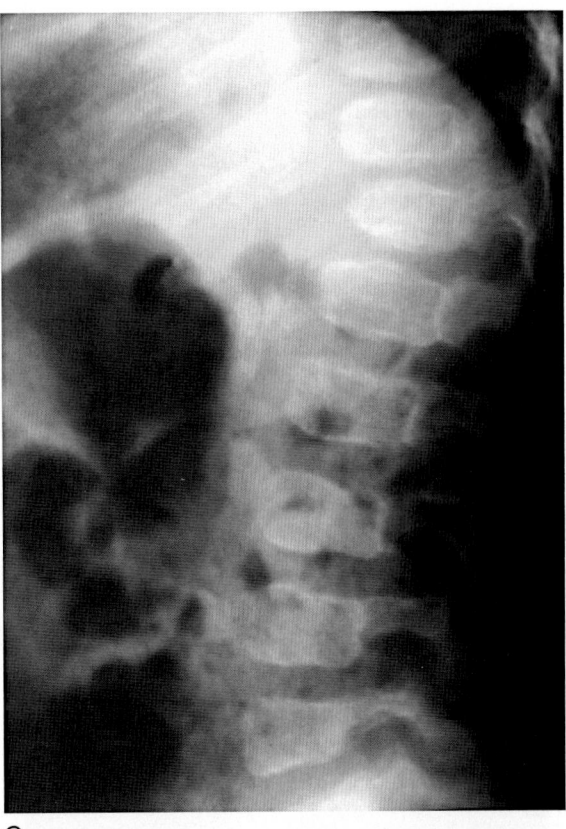

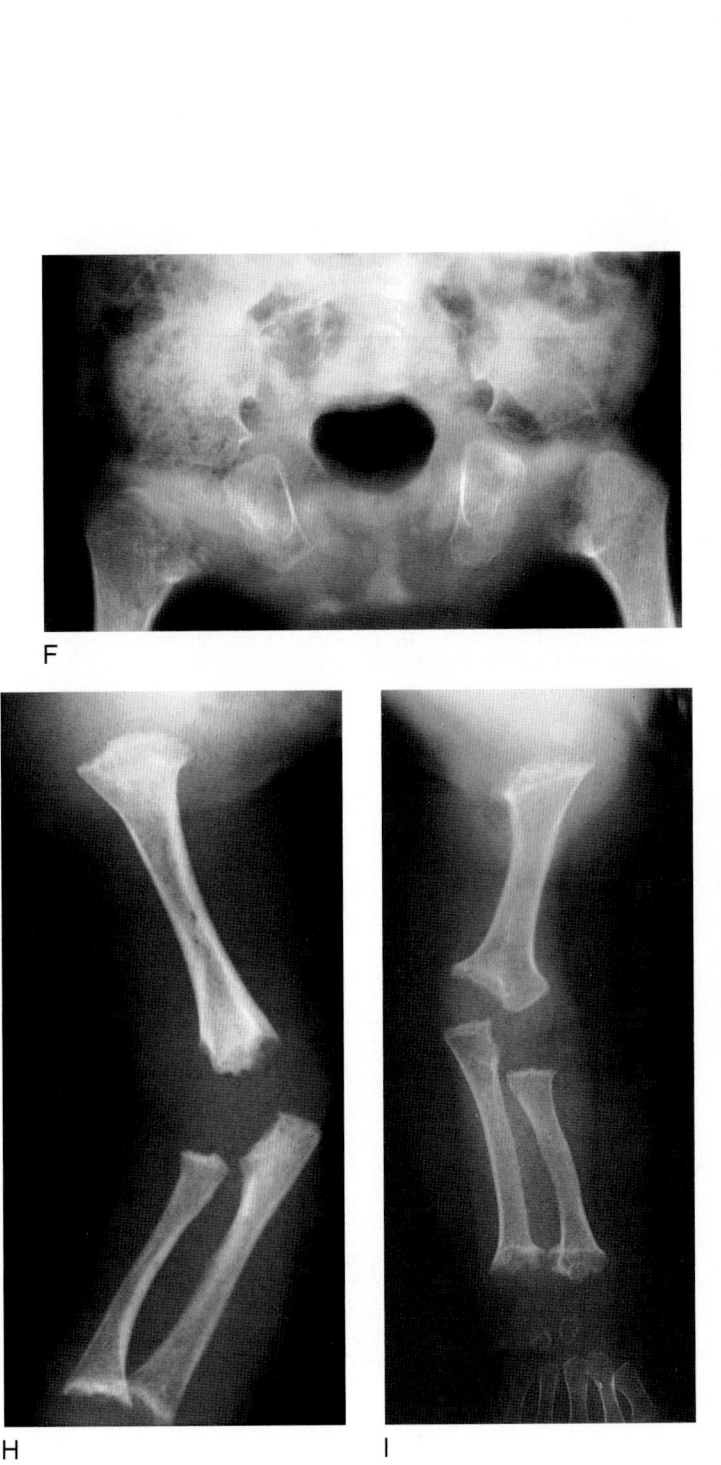

F

G

H

I

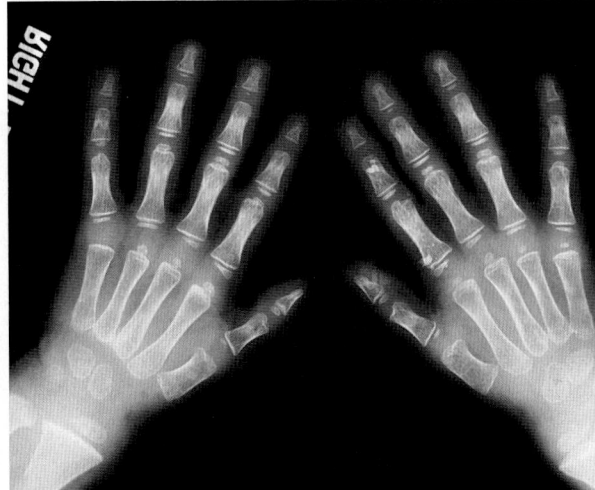

J

FIGURE 165-15, *cont'd*. Radiographic findings in Kniest dysplasia. **F** and **G,** Radiographs in an affected 1½-year-old child. **F,** Pelvis: wide iliac wings, narrowed sacrosciatic notches, downward-angled pubic bones, and small femoral heads. **G,** Spine: platyspondyly and end plate indentations (residua of coronal clefts). In another affected patient at birth (**H**) and at age 1 year (**I**), there is progression from metaphyseal rounding to metaphyseal flaring and irregularity, with proximal humeral ossification delay. **J,** Hands: in an affected 6-year-old, there are small epiphyses, widened metaphyses (bulbous joints), and no significant brachydactyly.

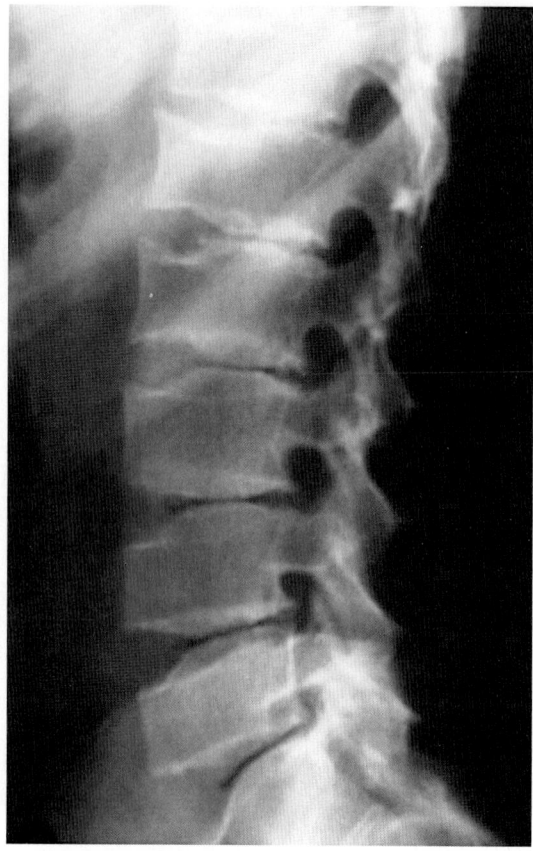

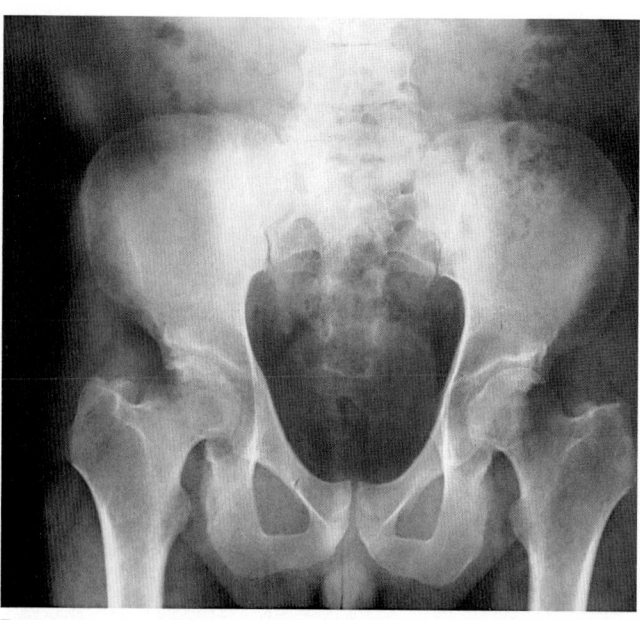

A

B

FIGURE 165-16. Radiographs in a 24-year-old with spondyloepiphyseal dysplasia tarda. **A,** Platyspondyly and centrally humped end plates. **B,** Dysplastic capital femoral epiphyses and degenerative arthrosis (joint space narrowing).

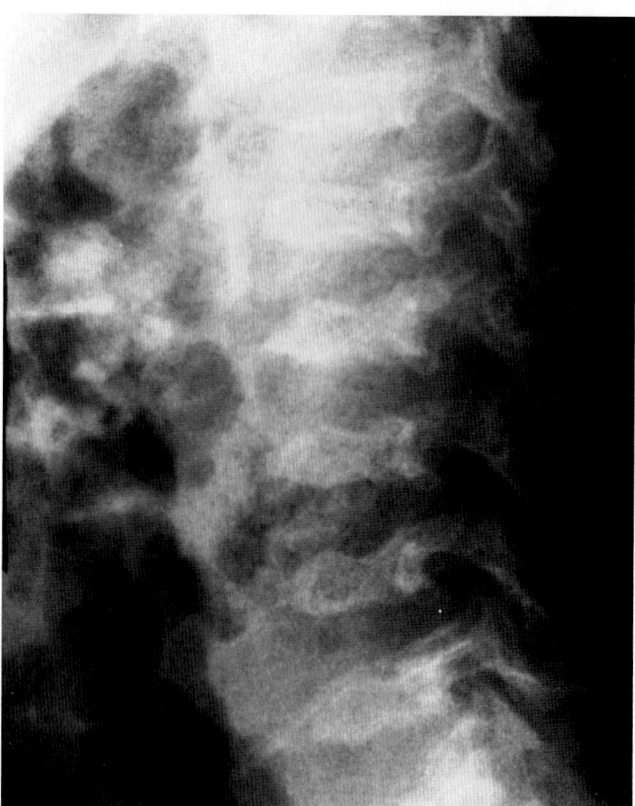

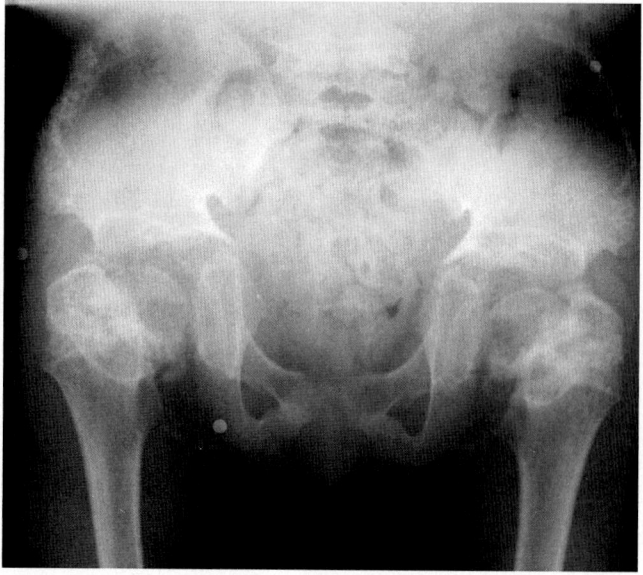

A

B

FIGURE 165-17. Dyggve-Melchior-Clausen syndrome. **A,** Radiograph in an affected 3-year-old with severe platyspondyly with residual double-humped end plates and anterior beaking. **B,** Radiograph in an affected 10-year-old with rounded iliac wings, lacy iliac crests, narrow sciatic notches, flat acetabular roofs, and epiphyseal/metaphyseal hip changes.

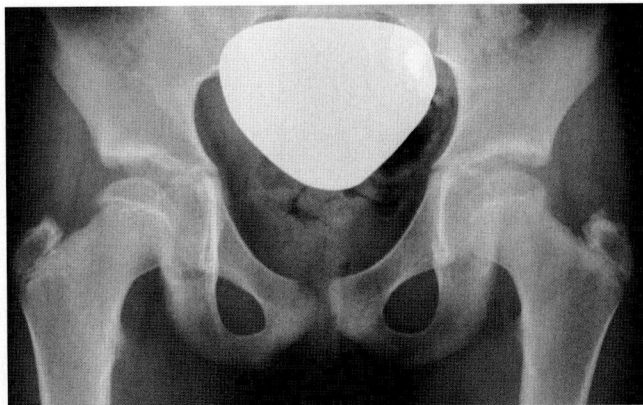

A

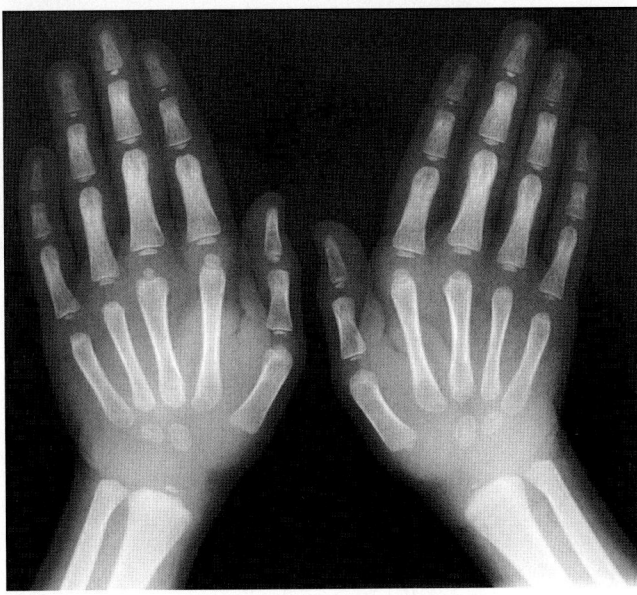

C

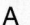

B

FIGURE 165-18. Fairbanks-type multiple epiphyseal dysplasia. **A,** Radiograph in an affected 10-year-old with small ossified proximal femoral epiphyses (ossification defect). **B** and **C,** Radiographs in an affected 6-year-old. **B,** Similar epiphyseal ossification defects in the knee. **C,** Small epiphyses of the short tubular bones of the hands and carpal ossification delay (epiphyseal equivalents), but no brachydactyly.

RADIOLOGIC FINDINGS

1. Spine: in young adults, disk herniations into vertebral end plates (*Schmorl nodes*)
2. Extremities: *small, irregular, flattened ossification centers (epiphyses);* small, irregular carpal (and tarsal) centers

Pseudoachondroplasia

This short-limb, short-trunk form of skeletal dysplasia was referred to at first as "achondroplasia with a normal face." In actuality, the facial appearance in affected individuals is usually the most beautiful or most handsome in the family. There is often mild to moderate brachydactyly (Fig. 165-20).

RADIOLOGIC FINDINGS

1. Skull: normal
2. Thorax: mild anterior rib widening
3. Spine: *superiorly and inferiorly rounded vertebral bodies, anterior central tongue (exaggerated ring epiphyses),* normalization of vertebrae (later)

4. Pelvis: *rounded iliac wings; hypoplastic, poorly formed acetabular roofs*
5. Extremities: *mini-epiphyses in the hips,* moderate to severe generalized epiphyseal "dysplasia" (small, irregular, poorly ossified), metaphyseal widening and irregularity in the knees, *proximally rounded metacarpals* with mini-epiphyses in the hands, *irregular carpal* (tarsal) *bones*

CHONDRODYSPLASIA PUNCTATA GROUP

The chondrodysplasia punctata (stippled epiphyses) group is very diverse, united by the radiographic commonality of epiphyseal stippling. Several but not all of these entities are related to each other. The rhizomelic form of chondrodysplasia punctata is a peroxisomal enzyme abnormality; the Conradi-Hünermann type is associated with a gene on the long arm of the X chromosome (*EBP* gene defect); and the brachytelephalangic type is on the short arm of the X chromosome (a defect in the ARSE gene). Because of their different genetic characteristics, it is very important to make a correct and complete diagnosis.

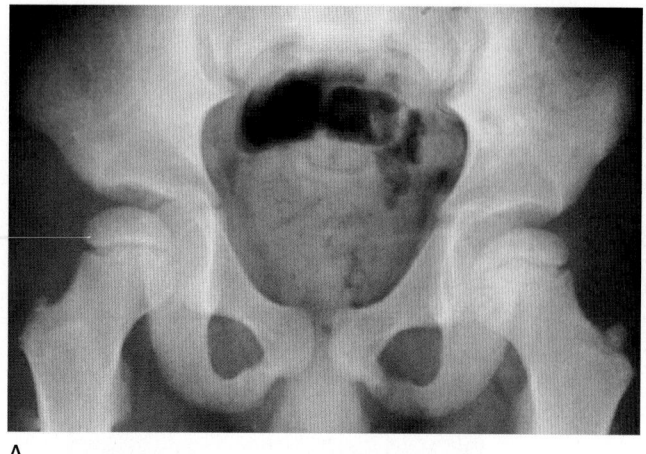

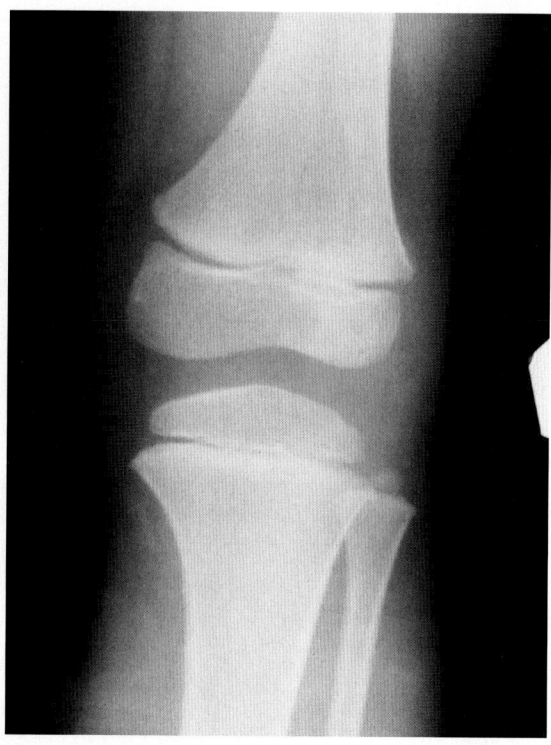

FIGURE 165-19. Radiographs in a 7-year-old with Ribbing-type multiple epiphyseal dysplasia reveal small-appearing hip epiphyses (**A**) and relatively normal-sized knee epiphyses (**B**).

Rhizomelic Chondrodysplasia Punctata

This is a distinct form of chondrodysplasia punctata and has an autosomal recessive inheritance pattern. It is a symmetric rhizomelic skeletal dysplasia manifesting in the neonatal period (Fig. 165-21). Affected infants usually die in the first year of life. Associated clinical findings include cataracts, skin lesions, alopecia, and joint contractures. Later manifestations are severe psychomotor retardation and spasticity. These infants appear to be in constant pain. Three gene abnormalities have been noted thus far (*PEX7, DHPAT, AGPS*).

RADIOLOGIC FINDINGS

1. Spine: *coronal clefting,* anteriorly rounded vertebral bodies
2. Extremities: *stippling, symmetric bilateral shortening of femurs* (and humeri) with less severe shortening of all the remaining long bones

Conradi-Hünermann Syndrome/Dysplasia

This is a *specific entity* within the group of chondro-dysplasia punctata disorders; it is incorrect for just any dysplasia with stippling to be labeled "Conradi disease." The Conradi-Hünermann type of chondrodysplasia punctata is an X-linked dominant disorder. The facies include midface hypoplasia and a high-arched palate. Cataracts and other ocular abnormalities may occur, as may skin lesions. Asymmetric shortening of limbs (one side versus the other) is an important diagnostic feature (Fig. 165-22). This dysplasia is compatible with a normal life span.

RADIOLOGIC FINDINGS

1. Spine: *diffuse stippling,* scoliosis in childhood, abnormal vertebral body formation
2. Extremities: mild symmetric or *asymmetric* shortening, diffuse generalized stippling in epiphyseal (and epiphyseal-equivalent) areas as well as periarticular and other locations; hands and feet are normal aside from stippling

Note: *Stippling resolves* during infancy to develop into *normal or malformed epiphyseal centers.*

> **Rhizomelic chondrodysplasia punctata**
> • **Autosomal recessive**
> • **Death in first year of life**
> **Conradi-Hünermann syndrome/dysplasia**
> • **X-linked dominant**
> • **Normal life span**

Brachytelephalangic Chondrodysplasia Punctata

This distinctive disorder with characteristic hand changes is also an X-linked disorder but is recessively inherited. It is far less common than the previously described disorders but quite easily diagnosed. Affected patients manifest severe midface hypoplasia with short hands and feet, as the name of the disorder suggests (Fig. 165-23).

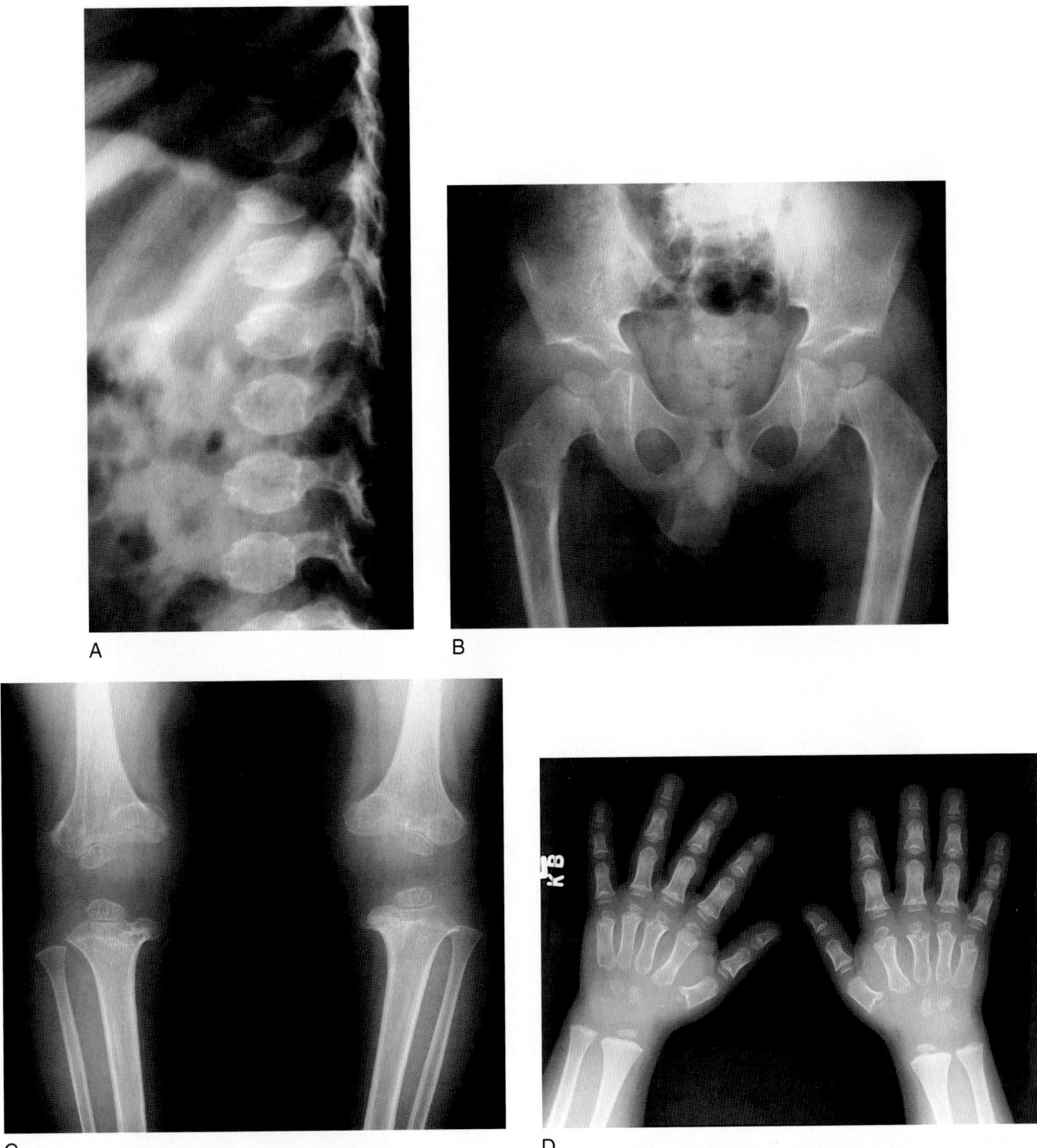

FIGURE 165-20. Pseudoachondroplasia. Radiologic findings at ages 3 years (**A** and **C**) and 4 years (**B** and **D**). **A,** Central anterior tonguing and superior and inferior rounding of vertebral bodies. **B,** Acetabular roof hypoplasia and mini-epiphyses. **C,** Small knee epiphyses and metaphyseal widening with ossification defects. **D,** Proximal metacarpal rounding, small epiphyseal centers, metaphyseal widening and irregularity, and carpal ossification delay.

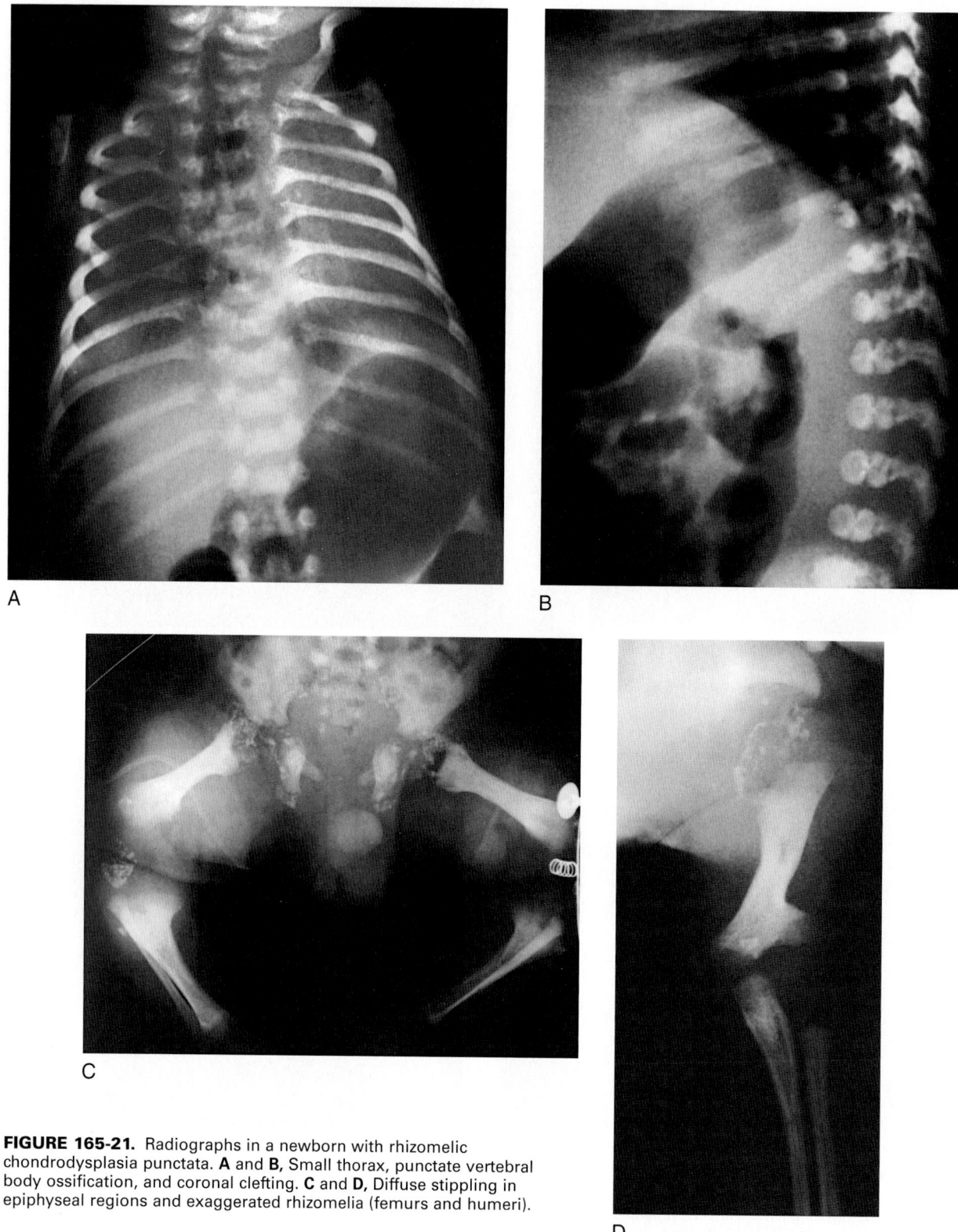

FIGURE 165-21. Radiographs in a newborn with rhizomelic chondrodysplasia punctata. **A** and **B**, Small thorax, punctate vertebral body ossification, and coronal clefting. **C** and **D**, Diffuse stippling in epiphyseal regions and exaggerated rhizomelia (femurs and humeri).

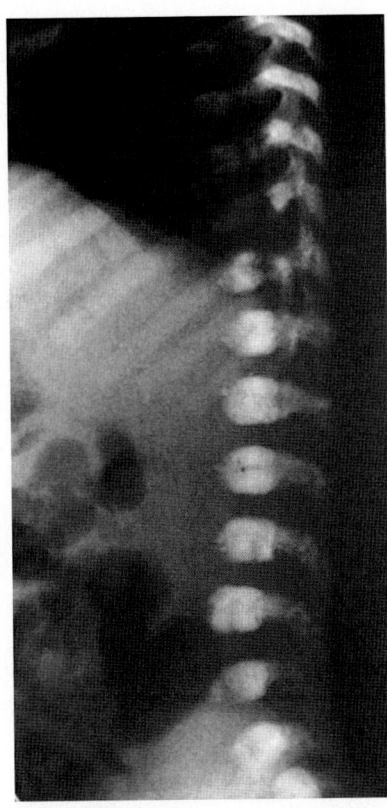 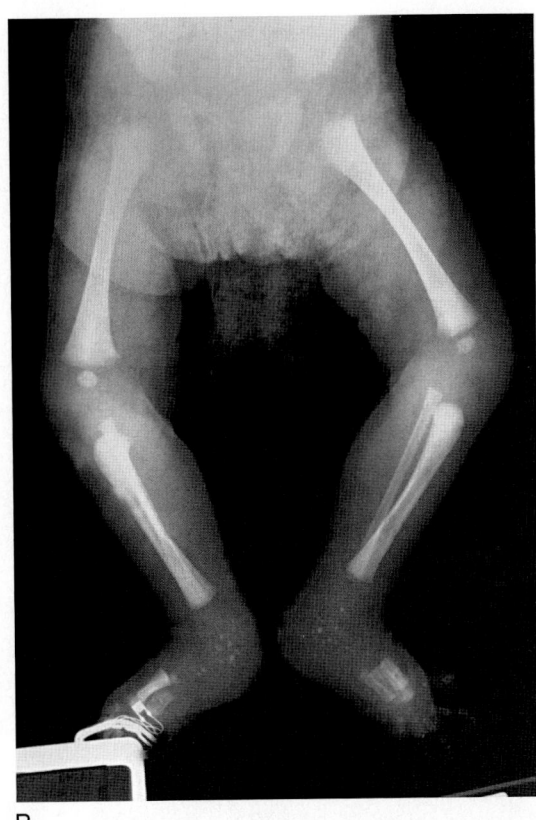

A   B

FIGURE 165-22. Radiographs in a newborn with Conradi-Hünermann syndrome/dysplasia. **A,** Mildly hypoplastic vertebral bodies and stippling (residua of coronal clefts). **B,** Stippling of ankles and hips, normal knee epiphyses, no rhizomelia.

RADIOLOGIC FINDINGS

- Spine: *hypoplastic vertebral bodies with posterior scalloping and anterior rounding; stippling, especially in the sacrococcygeal area; sagittal clefting*
- Extremities: normal length (mild shortening); *distinctive brachydactyly with hypoplastic tufts and deformed hypoplastic proximal phalanx of the second digit in the hand and the first metatarsal of the foot*

METAPHYSEAL CHONDRODYSPLASIA GROUP

The metaphyseal chondrodysplasias (MCDs) are also a heterogeneous group of disorders that have radiologic features in common. This is a rather large group, and I cover only several common and interesting entities. In two, the molecular defect has been identified. In most members of this group, spines should be normal; it has been shown that transient but significant spine changes occur in Schmid-type MCD.

Jansen-Type Metaphyseal Chondrodysplasia

This MCD was described in 1934, with a follow-up report on the same patient by Silverthorn and associates. It represents the severest form of MCD. The presentation is in the neonatal period or during late infancy, with marked short stature and a waddling gait. This is a distinct autosomal dominant disorder with an abnormality in a parathyroid receptor gene (*PTHR*), which explains the findings of hypercalcemia and its complications. The

radiographic findings in the skeleton are *not* those of typical hyperparathyroidism or hypoparathyroidism (Fig. 165-24). (See also Chapter 167.)

RADIOLOGIC FINDINGS

1. Skull: brachycephaly, platybasia, underdeveloped mandible
2. Thorax: normal size; expanded irregular anterior rib ends
3. Extremities: *extensive irregularity of markedly expanded metaphyses involving all metaphyseal regions; hands exhibit wide separation of epiphyses from metaphyses*

Note: As in other parathyroid abnormalities, pathologic fractures (in 45% of affected patients) and subperiosteal bone resorption (in 50%) are common.

Schmid-Type Metaphyseal Chondrodysplasia

This form of MCD is also a specific disorder. It is an autosomal dominant condition and represents a defect in collagen type X, the gene for which is located on chromosome 6. This disorder is the mildest of the MCDs. Presentation is usually at about 2 years of age or later with a waddling gait or bowed legs, or both (Fig. 165-25). Mild short stature is present.

RADIOLOGIC FINDINGS

1. Thorax: *widened anterior rib ends*
2. Spine: transient vertebral changes in middle childhood

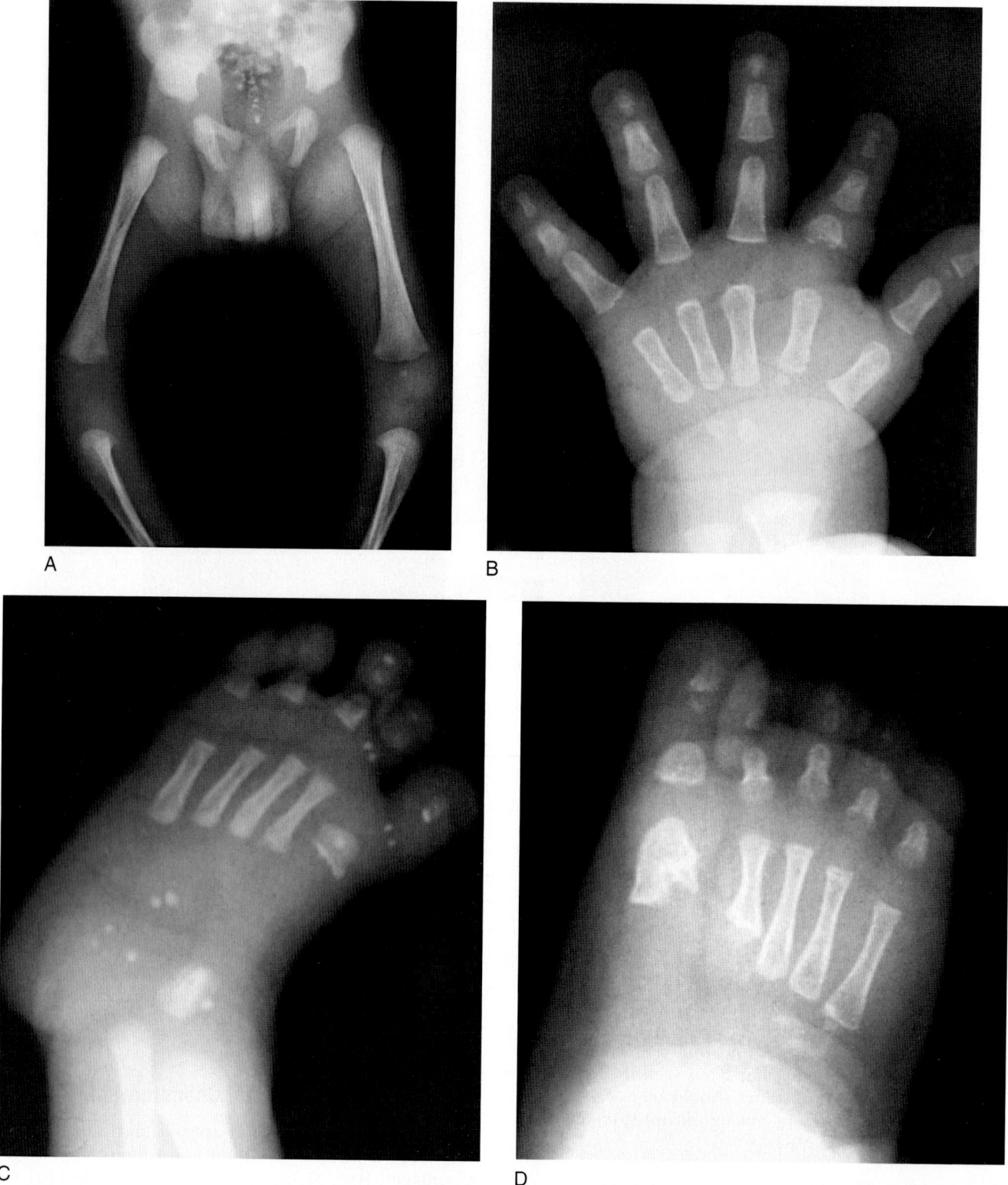

FIGURE 165-23. Brachytelephalangic chondrodysplasia punctata. **A,** Radiograph in an affected newborn with rhizomelia but intense sacral stippling. **B,** Radiograph in an affected 5-month-old with characteristic hand, demonstrating hypoplastic malformed proximal phalanx of second digit with hypoplastic tufts. **C,** Radiograph in an affected newborn with foot stippling and hypoplastic deformed metatarsals of great and other toes. **D,** Radiograph in an affected older infant with characteristically shaped first metatarsal and stippling.

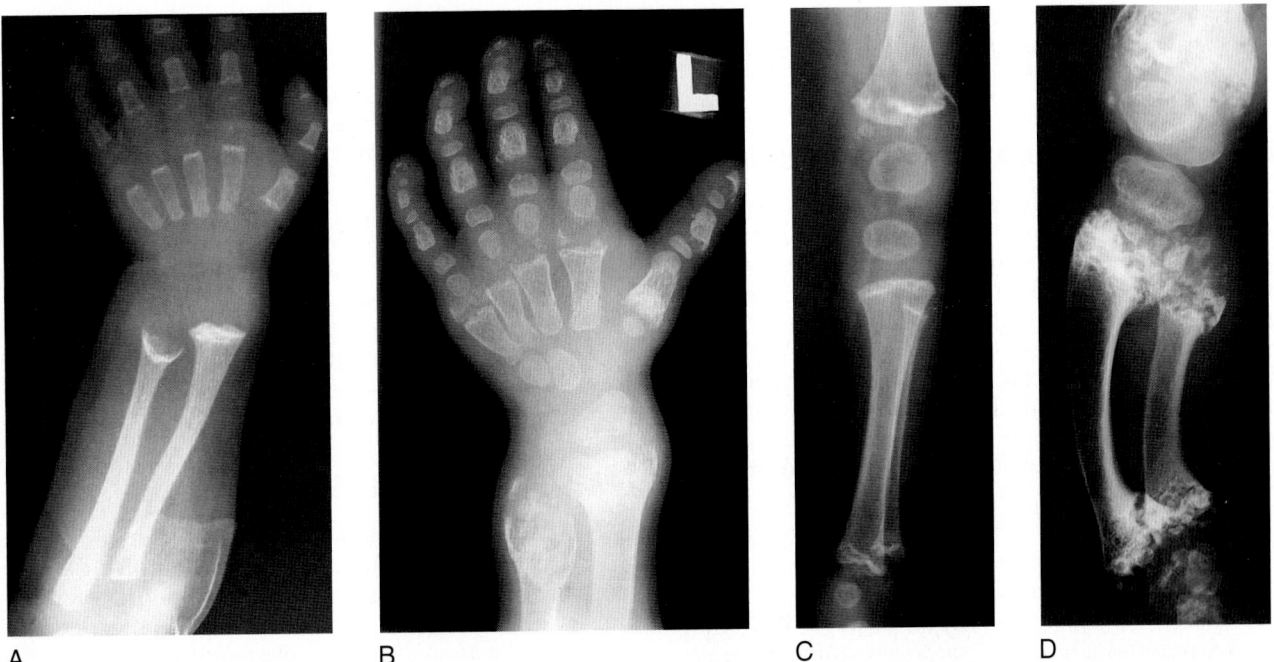

A   B   C   D

FIGURE 165-24. Radiographic findings in Jansen-type metaphyseal chondrodysplasia. **A,** At 1 year, there is severe metaphyseal cupping and splaying at the wrists and also in the hand bones. **B,** At 7 years, there is increasing metaphyseal change at the wrists with enlarged epiphysis; enlarged epiphyses with wide epiphyseal plates are also present in the hands. **C,** At 1 year, there are severe metaphyseal irregularities at knees and ankles (femur, tibia, and fibula) and enlarged, rounded epiphyses. **D,** At 7 years, there are severely fragmented, sclerotic metaphyses, wide epiphyseal plates, and enlarged epiphyses.

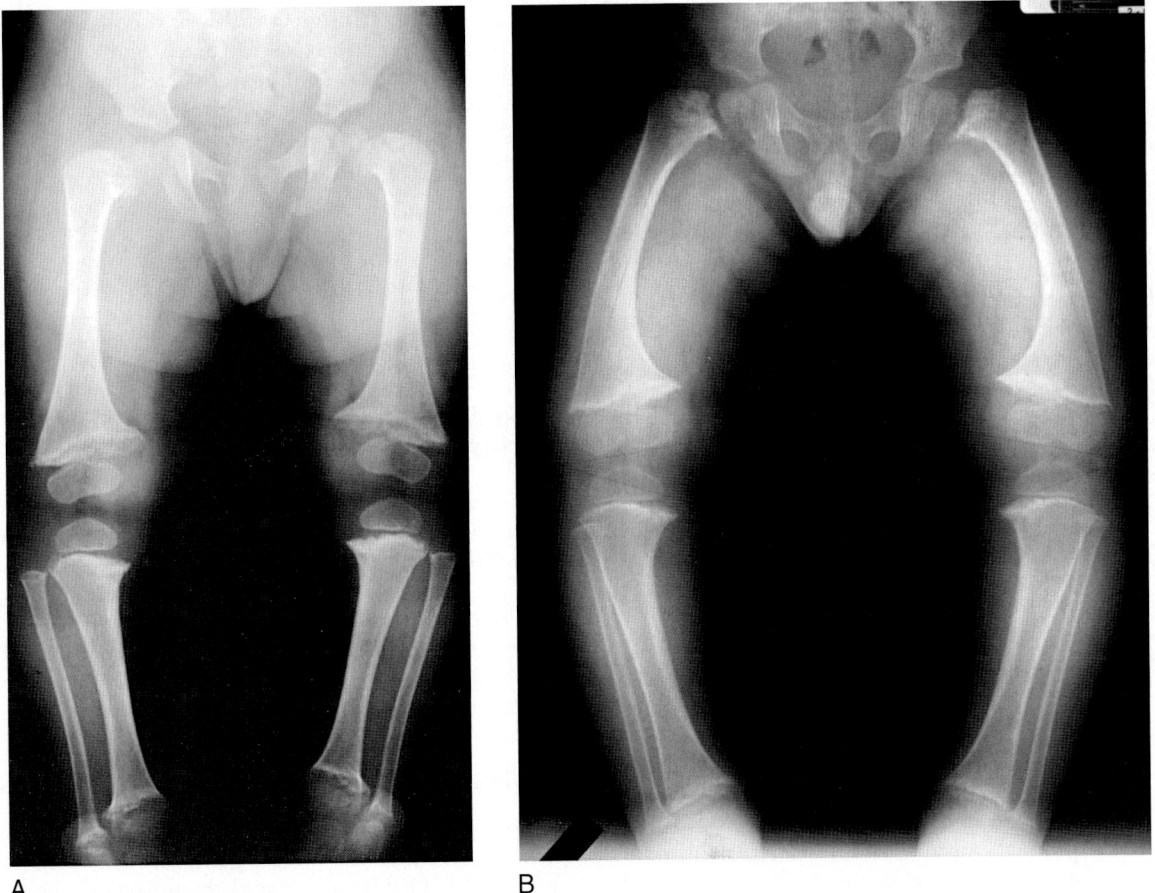

A   B

FIGURE 165-25. Schmid-type metaphyseal chondrodysplasia. **A,** Radiograph in an affected 19-month-old with severe coxa vara and moderate metaphyseal changes (cupping irregularity, widening) at the knees (and, not pictured here, ankles). **B,** Radiograph in an affected 3-year-old with coxa vara, genu varum, and moderate metaphyseal changes at hips and knees (widening, irregularity).

3. Extremities: *metaphyseal flaring, especially at the knees; rounded capital femoral epiphysis with widened growth plate; usually no hand involvement*

McKusick-Type Metaphyseal Chondrodysplasia

Cartilage-hair hypoplasia, as this entity is also known, is an autosomal recessive disorder, and, although the chromosome site has been established at the 9p region (*RMRP* gene), it has a high frequency among the Amish and Finnish populations. The presentation is of variable short-limbed dwarfism in early childhood (Fig. 165-26). There are significant clinical features that indicate the diagnosis and are important for medical management: sparse, thin, light-colored hair; Hirschsprung disease; immune mechanism problems; and increased incidence of malignancy.

RADIOLOGIC FINDINGS

1. Thorax: anterior rib widening/flaring
2. Spine: slightly small *square* vertebral bodies
3. Extremities: *flaring and cupping* fragmentation *of metaphyses (especially knees), hips usually spared;* hands exhibit *marked shortening with metacarpal and phalangeal cupping* and coning

Shwachman-Diamond Syndrome/Dysplasia

This rare autosomal recessive disorder, also known as MCD with pancreatic insufficiency and cyclic neutropenia, entails helpful diagnostic clinical clues of malabsorption and recurrent infections. It manifests in infancy, but its radiographic features are quite mild. The defect, involving the *SBDS* gene, is located on chromosome 7q11 (Fig. 165-27).

RADIOLOGIC FINDINGS

1. Thorax: *anterior rib irregularity/splaying*
2. Extremities: *metaphyseal changes (irregularity and sclerosis), especially at knees (hips)*
3. *Malabsorption pattern* evident on small bowel examination
4. *Lipomatosis of pancreas* evident on computed tomography

SPONDYLOMETAPHYSEAL DYSPLASIA GROUP

This group comprises disorders in which the specific spine and metaphyseal changes warrant that terminology. Although this is a very large and diverse group, the only important and relatively common entity is Kozlowski-type spondylometaphyseal dysplasia.

Kozlowski-Type Spondylometaphyseal Dysplasia

This bone dysplasia is an autosomal dominant disorder manifesting usually in early childhood. Clinical manifestations include moderate dwarfism, progressive kyphoscoliosis, and limited joint mobility. The mutation abnormality has not been identified (Fig. 165-28).

RADIOLOGIC FINDINGS

1. Spine: *severe platyspondyly, anteriorly rounded/wedged vertebral bodies, increased intervertebral disk spaces, overfaced (close-set) pedicles ("open staircase spine")*
2. Pelvis: short, flared iliac wings; *irregular hypoplastic acetabular roofs*
3. Extremities: widening, sclerosis, and irregularity of metaphyses; *hemispheric capital femoral epiphysis and widened proximal femoral growth plate with irregularity on both sides;* hands exhibit mild shortening with metaphyseal cupping and irregularity, disharmonious ossification (*marked carpal ossification delay*—i.e., bone age at 5 or 6 years without carpal ossification)

MESOMELIC DYSPLASIA GROUP

The mesomelic dysplasia (mesomelic dwarfism) group consists of a large number of disorders involving shortening of the middle segment bones. Milder shortening of other segments may also be noted. The most common entity by far in this group is dyschondrosteosis.

Dyschondrosteosis

This skeletal dysplasia, also known as Leri-Weill syndrome, is an apparent dominant condition. Belin and colleagues identified the molecular defect producing this genetically strange condition. It consists of a pseudo-autosomal homeobox gene (*SHOX* gene) found on the short arm of the X chromosome. Dyschondrosteosis manifests with mild to moderate short stature, usually with both forearm and shank shortening. A clinical Madelung deformity may be present (Fig. 165-29).

RADIOLOGIC FINDINGS

1. Extremities: *symmetric bowing and shortening of both radii, shortened ulnas, radiographic Madelung deformity changes, variable tibial and fibular shortening*

ACROMELIC/ACROMESOMELIC DYSPLASIA GROUP

The acromelic/acromesomelic dysplasia group consists of a large, heterogeneous collection of disorders in which those types of shortening of the limbs are present. For a number of these dysplasias, the molecular defect has been delineated, but they are too rare to discuss here. Only trichorhinophalangeal syndrome (TRP) types I and II, and the interesting acromesomelic dysplasia of Maroteaux (acromesomelic dwarfism) are detailed.

Trichorhinophalangeal Syndrome Types I and II

Both of these disorders have been located on the long arm of chromosome 8. The gene implicated in TRP type I is *TRPS1*. TRP type II is slightly more complicated. TRP type II, also known as Langer-Giedion syndrome, is the result of a contiguous gene abnormality resulting from the loss of not only *TRPS1* but also *EXT1*, an exostosis

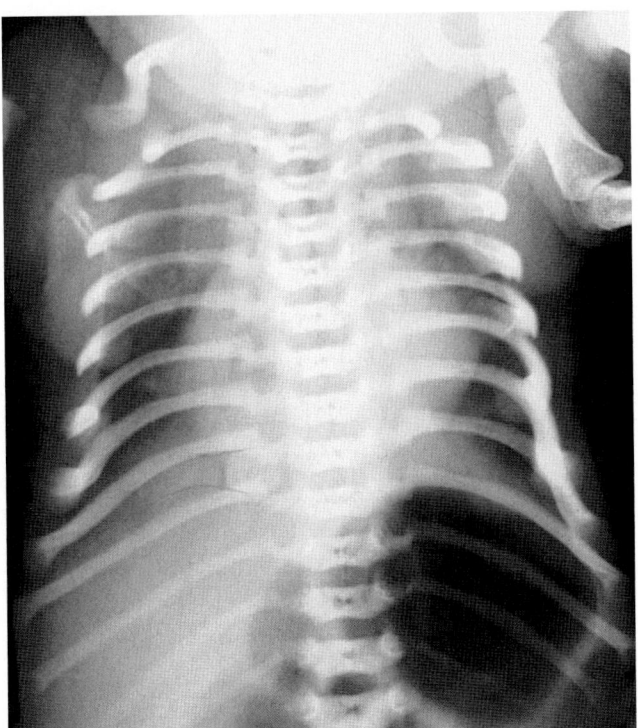

FIGURE 165-26. McKusick-type metaphyseal chondrodysplasia (cartilage-hair hypoplasia). **A** and **B**, Radiographs in an affected newborn. **A**, Thorax: anterior rib end widening and cupping. **B**, Lower extremities: mild femoral bowing with minimal distal femoral flare. **C** and **D**, Radiographic findings in late infancy. **C**, Lower extremity: metaphyseal flaring and irregularity at the knees and ankles (but the hips are spared). **D**, Upper extremity: similar metaphyseal changes at the wrists (the shoulders are spared). **E**, At 6 months of age, there is metaphyseal widening and cupping of the short tubular bones of the hand, with similar metaphyseal changes in the wrist.

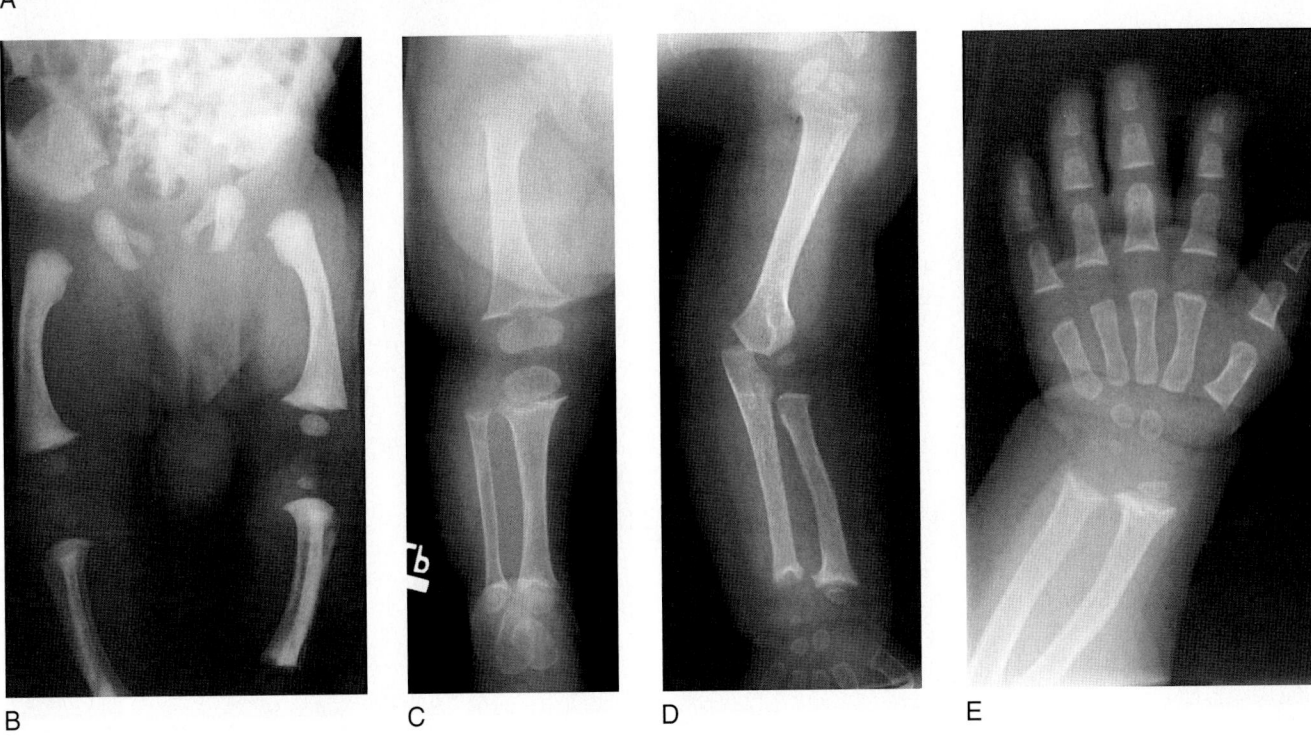

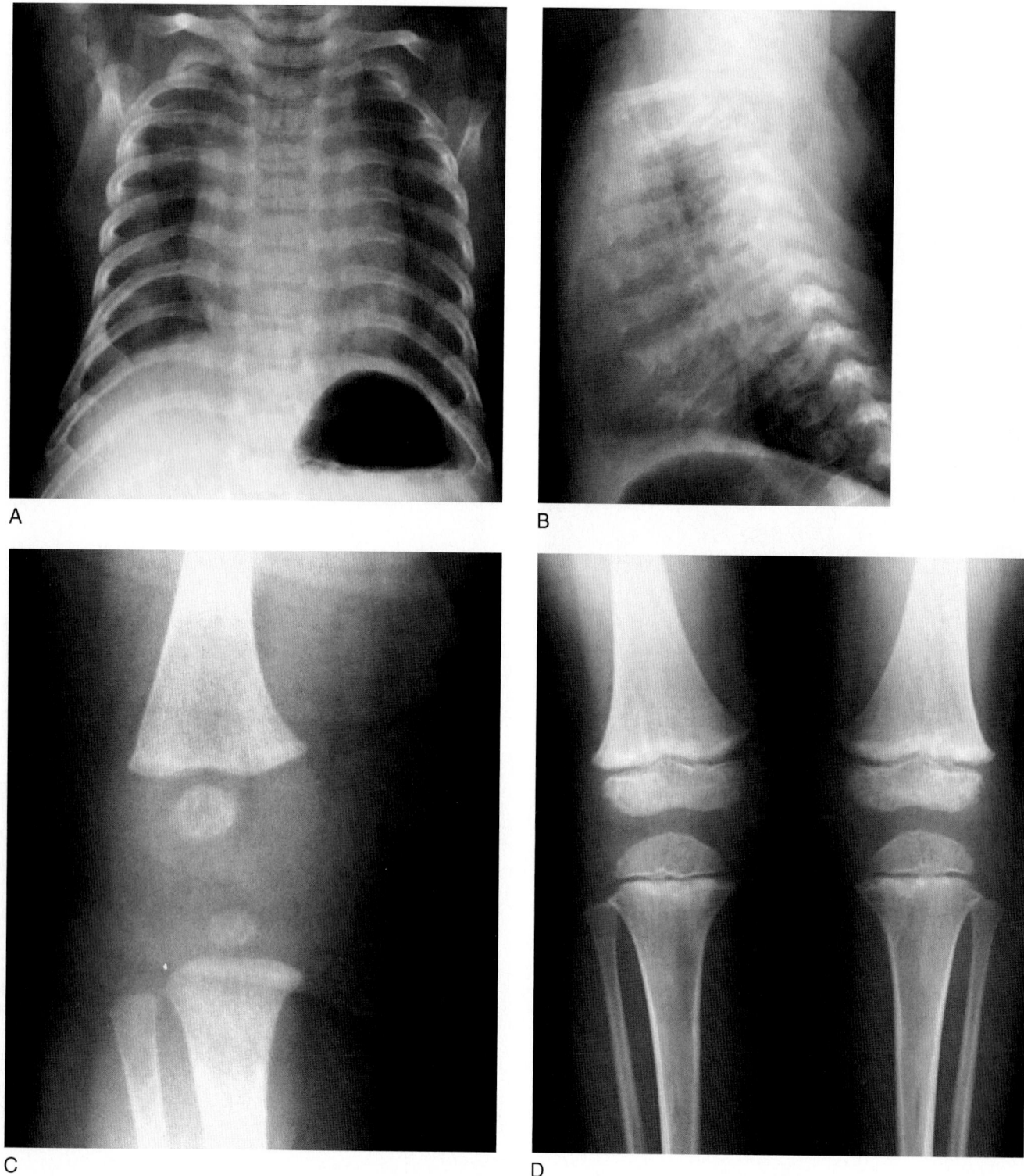

FIGURE 165-27. Radiographic findings in Shwachman-Diamond syndrome. **A** and **B,** At 2 months, there is a narrow thorax with anterior rib splaying. **C,** At 2 months, the knees are normal. **D,** At 4 years, there are sclerotic, irregular, widened metaphyses in the knees.

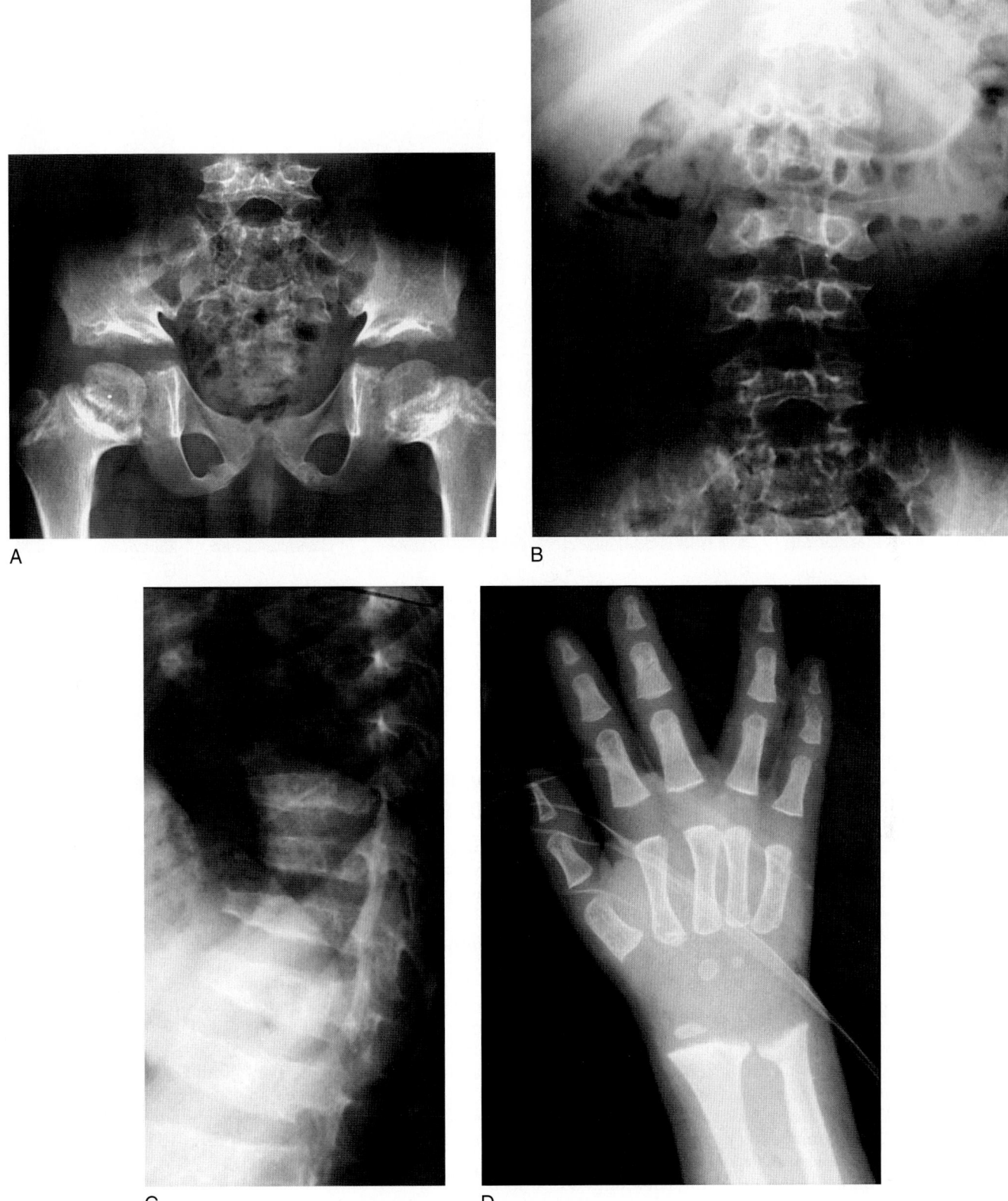

FIGURE 165-28. Kozlowski-type spondylometaphyseal dysplasia. **A** to **C,** Radiographs in an affected 8-year-old. **A,** Pelvis: narrow sacrosciatic notches, ossification defect (acetabular roofs), and widened epiphyseal plates. **B** and **C,** Spine: overfaced vertebral bodies ("open staircase," or closely set pedicles) and flattened, irregular vertebral bodies (platyspondyly). **D,** In an affected 2-year-old, there is metaphyseal widening and irregularity at the wrist and short tubular bones of the hands, with almost no carpal bone ossification.

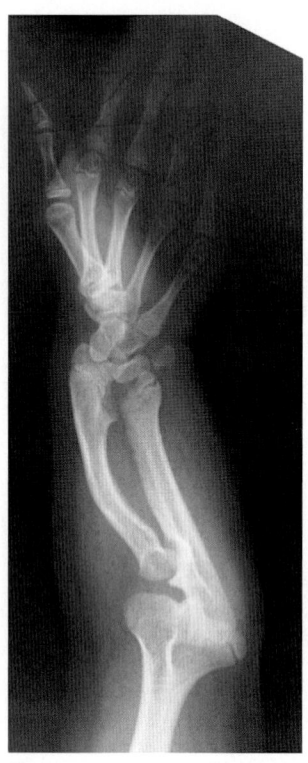
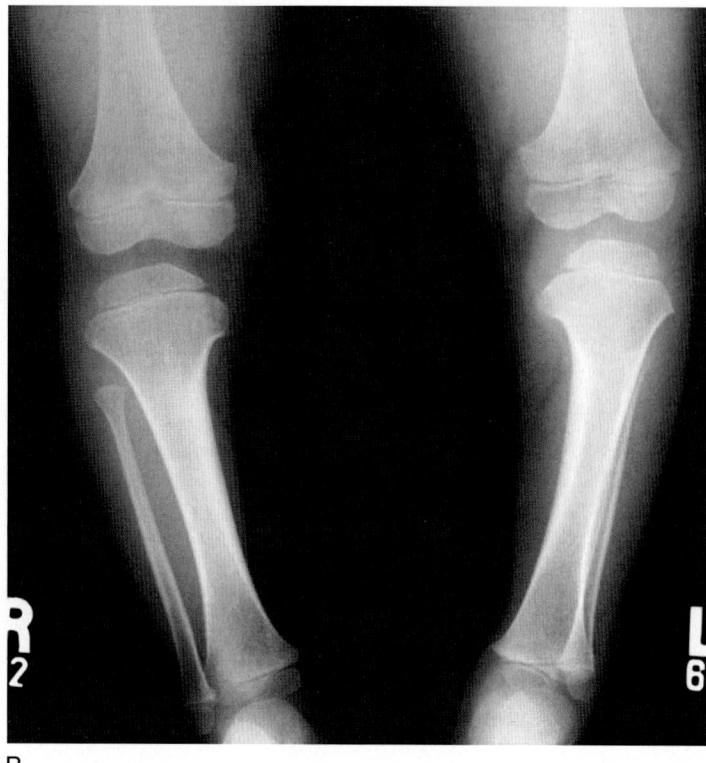

A   B   C

FIGURE 165-29. Dyschondrosteosis. **A,** Radiograph in a 12-year-old with severe mesomelia and Madelung deformity. **B** and **C,** Radiographs in two affected children aged 4 years (**B**) and 9 years (**C**) with mesomelia (short tibia and fibula).

gene distal to *TRPS1*. TRP type I is autosomal dominant, whereas most cases of TRP type II are sporadic. The clinical manifestations of both disorders include mild short stature; sparse, slow-growing hair; pear-shaped nose ("hose nose"); and short, crooked fingers (Fig. 165-30). The contiguous gene abnormality explains the added features in TRP type II, which include multiple exostoses and mental retardation.

RADIOLOGIC FINDINGS

1. Extremities: Perthes-like changes at the hips, *cone-shaped epiphyses in the phalanges of both hands*
   Note: *Multiple exostoses* in TRP type II

Acromesomelic Dysplasia of Maroteaux

This skeletal dysplasia is actually a misnomer in that the changes in this disorder are hardly just acromelic and mesomelic. There are significant spinal abnormalities (Fig. 165-31). The disorder is autosomal recessive with a defect in *NPR2*, which maps to chromosome 9p. Abnormalities are discoverable at birth but are quite significant by 1 year of age. Clinical findings include moderate short stature, short forearms, stubby hands and feet, and short shanks.

RADIOLOGIC FINDINGS

1. Spine: oval vertebral bodies (early), anterior beaking and posterior wedging (later), *gibbus and/or kyphoscoliosis* ultimately
2. Extremities: shortening of all tubular bones,

especially radius/ulna and tibia/fibula; very short tubular bones of hands and feet with cone-shaped epiphyses and large great toes

DYSPLASIAS WITH PROMINENT MEMBRANOUS BONE INVOLVEMENT

Among the dysplasias with prominent membranous bone involvement, only cleidocranial dysplasia is common enough to include.

Cleidocranial Dysplasia

In this autosomal dominant disorder, the chromosome locus is at 6p21 and a gene called *CBFA1* (core binding factor α1), also known as *RUNX2*. This dysplasia is quite common, with marked clinical variability, and is often diagnosable at birth. The clinical findings include enlarged skull with large, late-closing fontanelles; dental abnormalities; drooping, hypermobile shoulders; mild short stature; and narrow chest (Fig. 165-32).

RADIOLOGIC FINDINGS

1. Skull: large, brachycephalic; wormian bones; wide sutures; *persistently open anterior fontanelle*
2. Thorax: *absence/hypoplasia of clavicles,* mildly shortened ribs with downward slope, 11 ribs
3. Spine: *significant posterior wedging of thoracic vertebrae*
4. Pelvis: *high narrow iliac wings, absence/hypoplasia of pubic bones*

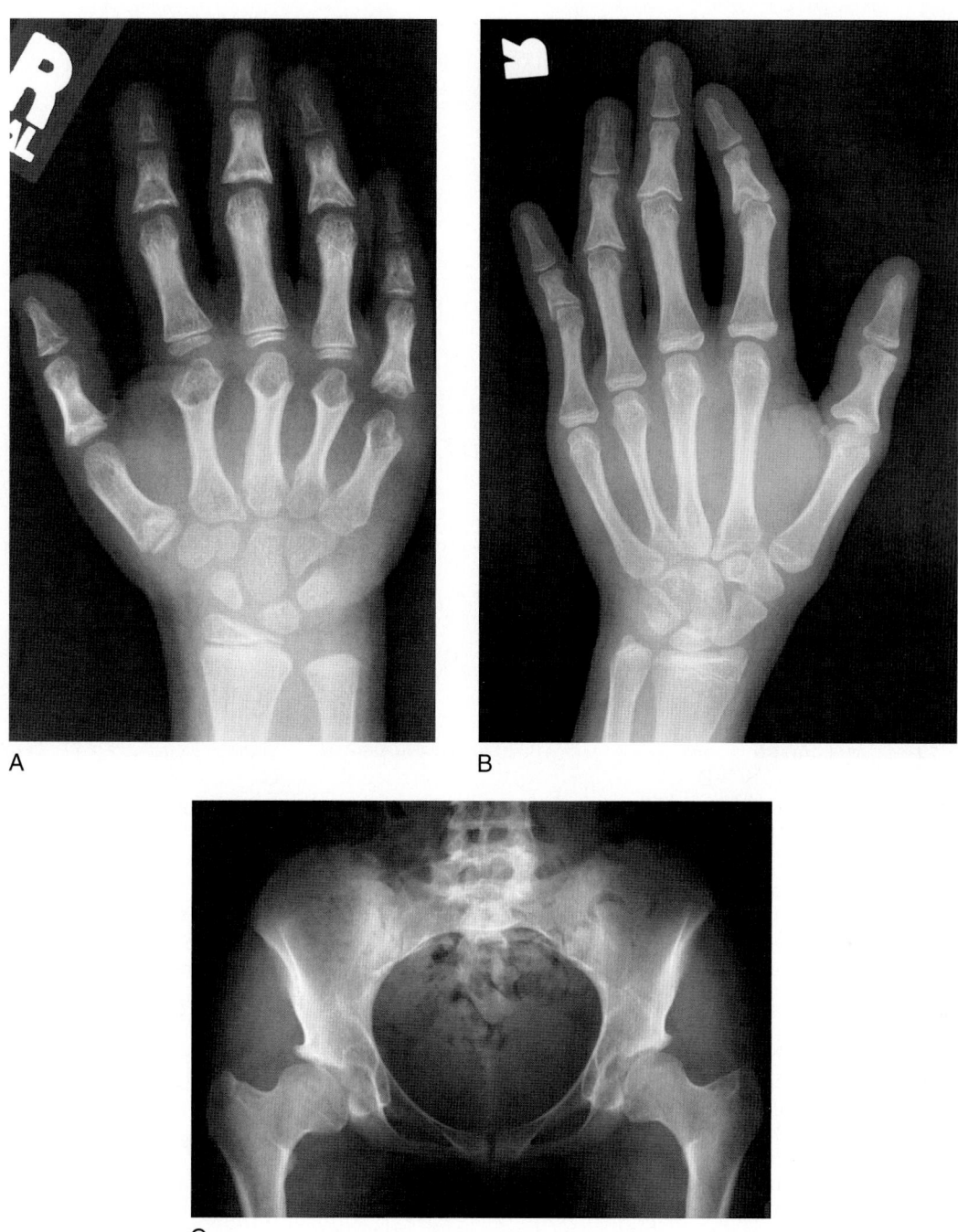

A

B

C

FIGURE 165-30. Radiographic findings in trichorhinophalangeal syndrome. **A,** In an affected 8-year-old, there are cone-shaped epiphyses involving the first metacarpal, the proximal fifth phalanx, and all middle phalanges and metacarpals in the second through fifth digits (early fusion). **B,** Radiograph in an affected 18-year-old shows result of similar changes. **C,** In an affected young adult, there are coxa vara and small capital femoral epiphyses (residua of avascular necrosis).

5. Extremities: numerous pseudoepiphyses of metacarpals and *tapered distal phalanges* in the hands

BENT-BONE DYSPLASIA GROUP

The bent-bone dysplasia group of disorders is a rather small but diverse group with an important and not uncommon entity, campomelic dysplasia (campomelic dwarfism), that has been well described molecularly.

These dysplasias have been grouped together because of their radiographic expression.

Campomelic Dysplasia

This unusual entity is an autosomal dominant disorder diagnosable at birth, manifesting with bent thighs, clubfeet, respiratory distress, and unusual small facies (Fig. 165-33). Sex reversal is often present. All the extremities are moderately short. Neonatal/perinatal

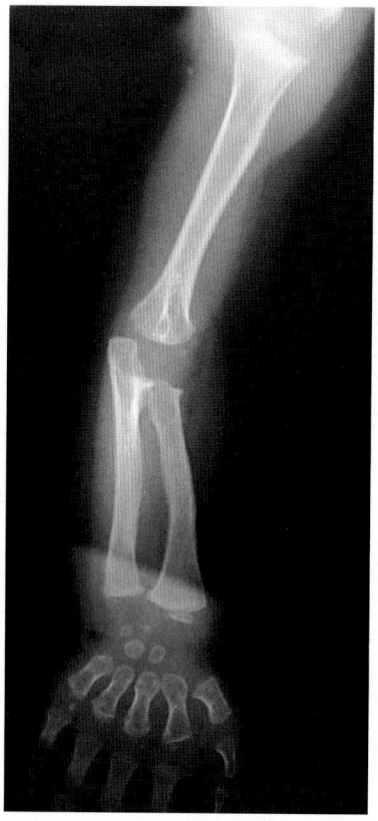 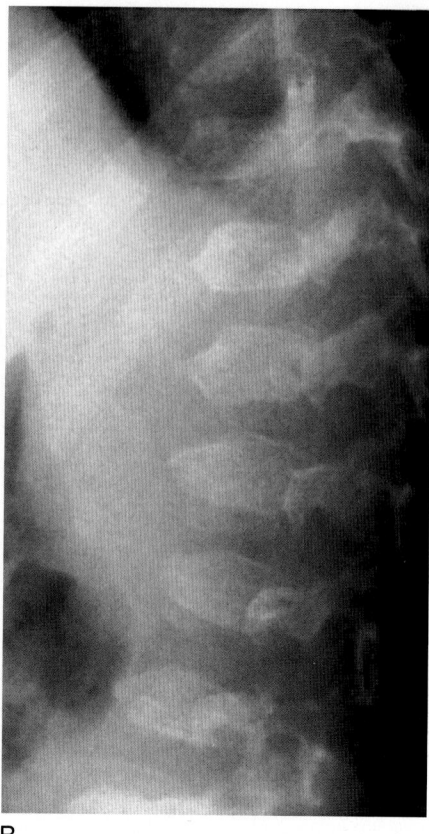 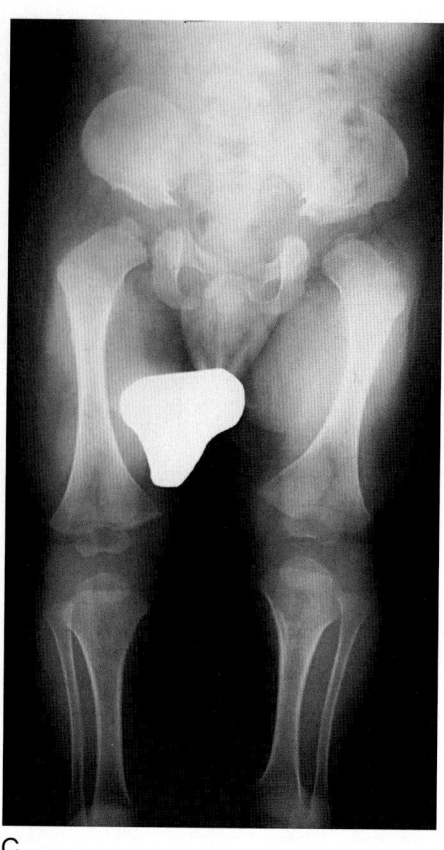

A   B   C

FIGURE 165-31. Radiographs in a 2½-year-old with acromesomelic dysplasia of Maroteaux. **A,** Upper extremities: primarily meso- and acromelia (short radius and ulna, short tubular bones of the hand). **B,** Spine: almost ovoid vertebral bodies with anterior central spike. **C,** Lower extremities: mild rhizomelia but primarily mesomelia.

death occurs in most cases. The molecular defect is a homeobox gene abnormality called *SOX9*, found on chromosome 17.

RADIOLOGIC FINDINGS

1. Skull: enlarged, narrow with a small face
2. Thorax: mildly short ribs, *numbering 11; severe hypoplasia of the bodies of the scapulae*
3. Spine: *nonossification of thoracic pedicles, cervical kyphosis,* hypoplasia of cervical vertebral bodies
4. Pelvis: *narrow, tall iliac wings*
5. Extremities: *proportionately long, bowed femurs with shortened bowed tibias;* shortened upper extremity long bones

DYSOSTOSIS MULTIPLEX GROUP

The dysostosis multiplex group contains all the muco-polysaccharidoses (MPSs), mucolipidoses, and multiple other storage diseases that produce a skeletal dysplasia. The abnormalities in this entire group consist of well-described enzymatic defects that can be rather easily diagnosed by appropriate urine, blood, or fibroblast culture analyses. These diseases act similarly on the skeleton to produce a dysostosis multiplex picture of varying severity. The term *dysostosis multiplex* was coined for the radiologic findings in this group of conditions. Therefore, the real role of the radiologist is to suggest the likelihood of one of these disorders; the geneticist

biochemically determines which exact dysplasia it is. I use Hurler syndrome (MPS type IH) as the stereotypical example of this group. Morquio syndrome (MPS types IVA and IVB) has some slightly different abnormalities and thereby can often be differentiated from the other MPS entities radiographically. Separately, I discuss the unusual findings in I-cell disease (mucolipidosis type II).

Hurler Syndrome (Mucopolysaccharidosis Type IH)

The enzyme abnormality in this specific form of MPS is in αL-iduronidase, located on chromosome 4p. As with all the other members of this group, the inheritance pattern is recessive. Most of the MPS entities manifest clinically in late infancy or early childhood (Fig. 165-34).

RADIOLOGIC FINDINGS (DYSOSTOSIS MULTIPLEX)

1. Skull: enlarged neurocranium, *abnormal J-shaped sella*
2. Thorax: *short, thick clavicles; paddle (oar)–shaped ribs;* hypoplastic glenoid
3. Spine: gibbus, *superior notched (inferior beaked)* thoracolumbar vertebral bodies, upper cervical subluxation
4. Pelvis: *flared, small iliac wings with inferior tapering; steep acetabular roofs*
5. Extremities: *diaphyseal widening of long bones ("marrow expansion");* dysplastic epiphyses; hands characteristically exhibit brachydactyly, *proximal*

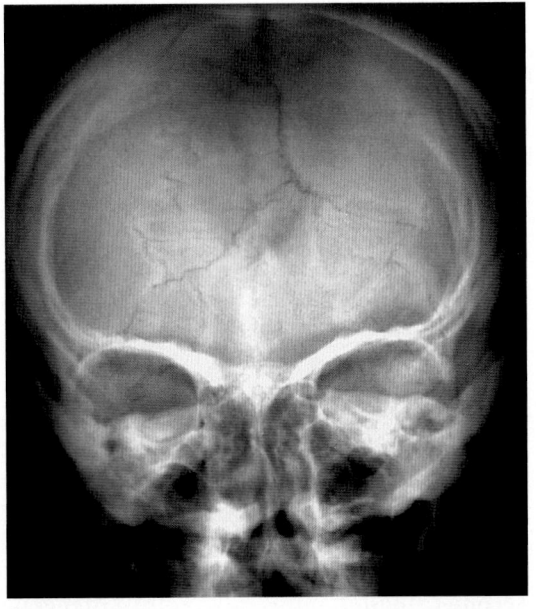

A

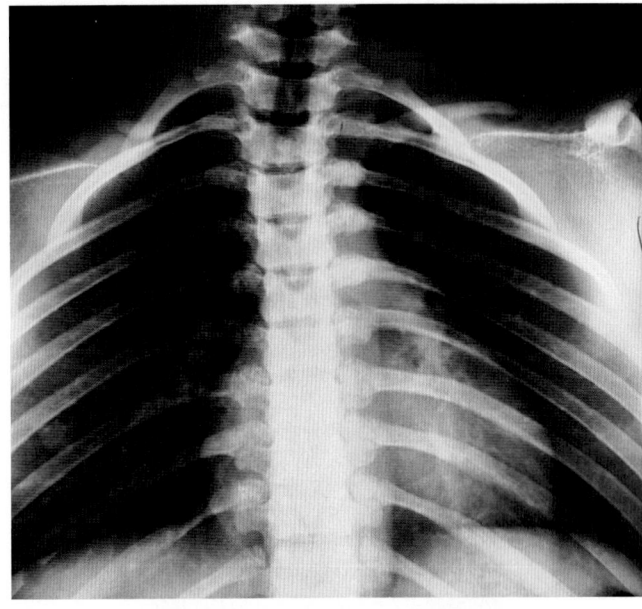

B

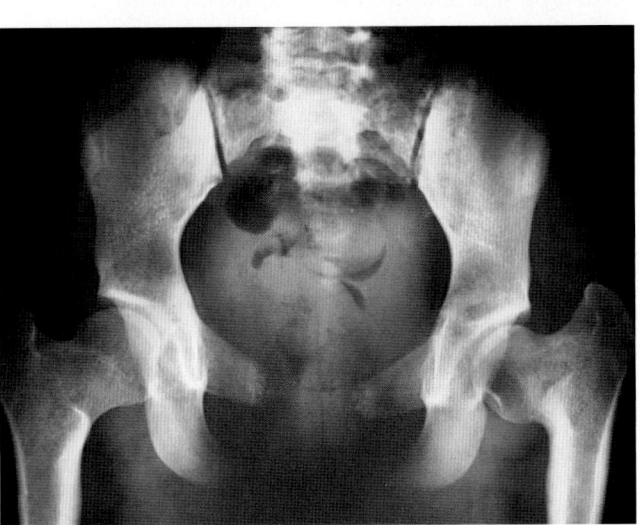

C

FIGURE 165-32. Radiographs in a 15-year-old with cleidocranial dysplasia. **A,** Skull: large open anterior fontanelle and multiple wormian bones. **B,** Thorax: asymmetric hypoplastic/absent clavicles and downward-sloping ribs. **C,** Pelvis: tall, narrow ilia and hypoplastic pubic bones. **D,** Spine: posteriorly wedged but otherwise normal vertebral bodies.

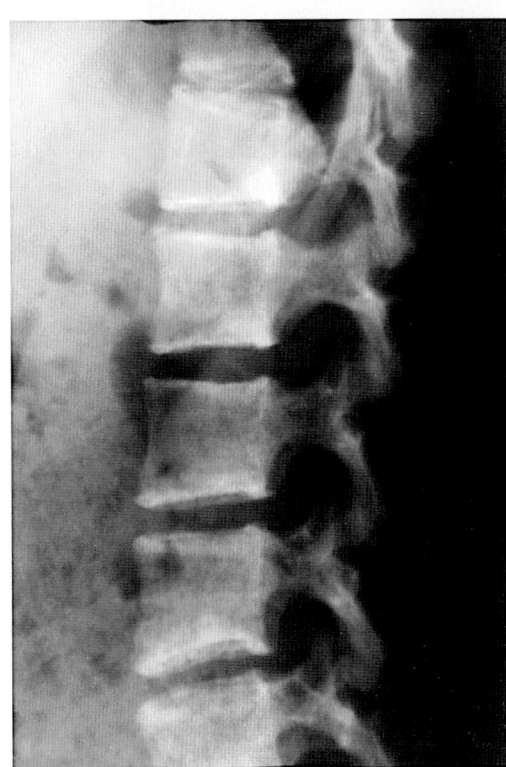

D

metacarpal "pointing," diaphyseal widening of metacarpals and proximal/middle phalanges, small irregular carpal bones

Morquio Syndrome (Mucopolysaccharidosis Types IVA and IVB)

In MPS type IVA, the enzyme abnormality is in galactose-6-sulfatase, resulting in the accumulation of excess MPS material in multiple organ systems, including the skeletal system (Fig. 165-35). This is the most common form of Morquio syndrome, and there are radiographically and clinically rare mild cases. There is some unpublished evidence that suggests that Morquio chondrocytes do not grow normally in vitro, which perhaps indicates that the cause of the skeletal abnormalities differs from those of other forms of MPS.

RADIOLOGIC FINDINGS (DIFFERENTIATING FEATURES FROM OTHER MUCOPOLYSACCHARIDOSES)

1. Skull: *no J-shaped sella*
2. Thorax: *widened,* not oar-shaped, *ribs*

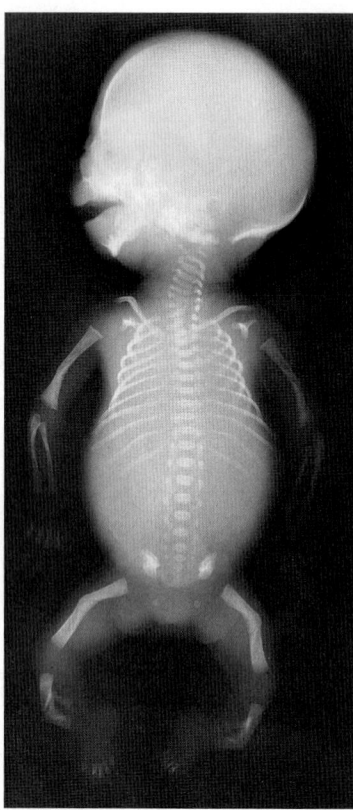

FIGURE 165-33. Radiograph in a fetus of 21 weeks' gestation with campomelic dysplasia. Findings include a large skull with a small face; hypoplastic/absent scapular bodies; 11 ribs; poorly ossified thoracic pedicles; tall, narrow iliac wings; and short extremities with proportionately long, bent femurs.

3. Spine: *middle tonguing,* not inferior beaking
4. Pelvis: no tapering of ileum
5. Extremities: *proximal metacarpal rounding,* not pointing, of hands

Mucolipidosis Type II (I-Cell Disease)

Mucolipidosis type II is another enzyme abnormality, of *N*-acetylglucosamine phosphotransferase, the gene for which is found on chromosome 4q. It clinically (and radiographically) manifests in the newborn (and prenatally). Most affected patients die in infancy. Certain radiographic features are quite unique (Fig. 165-36). (See also Chapter 168.)

RADIOLOGIC FINDINGS

1. Extremities: *severe osteopenia, poorly defined cortices, "periosteal cloaking"* (newborn)

Note: The changes of dysostosis multiplex occur later.

Dysostosis multiplex

- **Mucopolysaccharidoses, mucolipidoses, and other "storage" diseases**
- **Similar radiographic findings**
- **Biochemistry is diagnostic**

DYSPLASIAS WITH DECREASED BONE DENSITY

The dysplasias with decreased bone density are represented primarily by *osteogenesis imperfecta,* a very large group of disorders of which all entail a type I collagen abnormality. The affected genes, *COLA1* and *COLA2,* are found on chromosomes 17q and 7q, respectively. The clinical classification is not well corroborated by the molecular findings. The radiographic findings help to delineate mild and severe cases for management and prognosis. Osteogenesis imperfecta type II is almost the most common lethal skeletal dysplasia.

Osteogenesis Imperfecta Type II

This disorder is a specific autosomal dominant condition and occurs as a spontaneous new mutation, but there is a high rate of germ cell mosaicism (6% to 8%), which results in the potential for other affected fetuses in the same family. Affected fetuses can be identified on second-trimester ultrasonography. Osteogenesis imperfecta type II is specific radiographically as an invariable lethal disorder with no significant intrafamilial variability (Fig. 165-37).

RADIOLOGIC FINDINGS

1. Skull: *very poor to no ossification*
2. Thorax: small, narrow chest; *beaded ribs*
3. Spine: severe deossification, collapsed vertebral bodies
4. Extremities: generalized osteoporosis with or without fractures; shortened, widened long bones with thin cortices; *accordion-shaped femurs*

Osteogenesis Imperfecta, Other Types

It is difficult to type osteogenesis imperfecta radiographically. From the radiologic point of view, the clinician can suggest this diagnosis and ascertain whether it is mild or severe. This is the important role for the pediatric radiologist to play, letting the typing be determined on associated clinical grounds.

RADIOLOGIC FINDINGS

1. Skull: abnormal number of wormian bones (>8 to 10), variable decrease in ossification
2. Spine: wedged or collapsed vertebrae
3. Remaining skeleton: at least some osteoporosis, variable number of fractures (*especially pathologic fractures*)

Osteogenesis imperfecta

- **Type I collagen abnormality**
- **Osteogenesis imperfecta type II: prenatal diagnosis, radiographically specific, lethal**
- **Osteogenesis imperfecta, other types: varying severity, typing difficult by radiography**

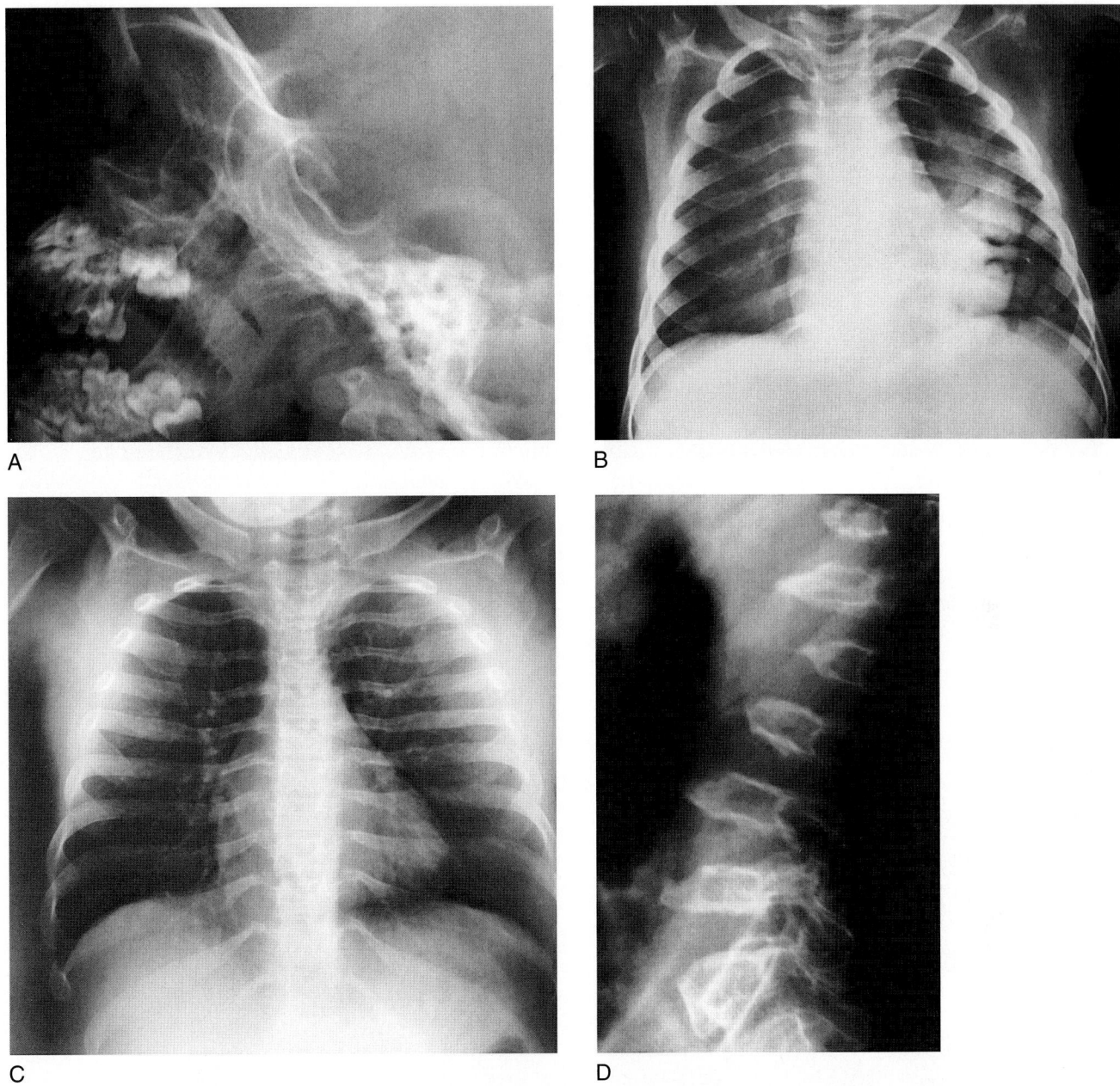

FIGURE 165-34. Radiographic findings in Hurler syndrome (mucopolysaccharidosis type IH). **A,** Skull of an affected 3-year-old with abnormal, excavated J-shaped sella turcica. **B** and **C,** Thoraces of an affected 3-year-old (**B**) and an affected 8-year-old (**C**) with thick clavicles and paddle-shaped ribs (thin posteriorly and thick anteriorly). **D,** Spine of an affected 8-year-old with superiorly notched (inferiorly beaked) vertebral bodies. *Continued*

DYSPLASIAS WITH DEFECTIVE MINERALIZATION

Among the dysplasias with defective mineralization, one important entity to recognize and discuss is hypophosphatasia. Hyperparathyroidism and rickets are well covered elsewhere in this book (see Chapters 167 and 168).

Hypophosphatasia

There are two distinct genetic forms of hypophosphatasia: the autosomal recessive perinatal lethal/infantile type and a later-onset autosomal dominant adult type (Fig. 165-38). These conditions constitute an

enzyme abnormality (alkaline phosphatase). The chromosome loci for both conditions are 1p36.1-34 and involve *TNSALP*. The perinatal/lethal form appears to represent autosomal recessive inheritance, whereas the adult form is probably autosomal dominant (see also Chapter 167).

RADIOLOGIC FINDINGS

Perinatal lethal/infantile form:
1. Skull: decreased ossification with *single island-like centers* for frontal occipital and parietal bones
2. Thorax: poorly ossified ribs; *sporadic dropout of ribs* (lack of ossification); thin, wavy, fractured ribs

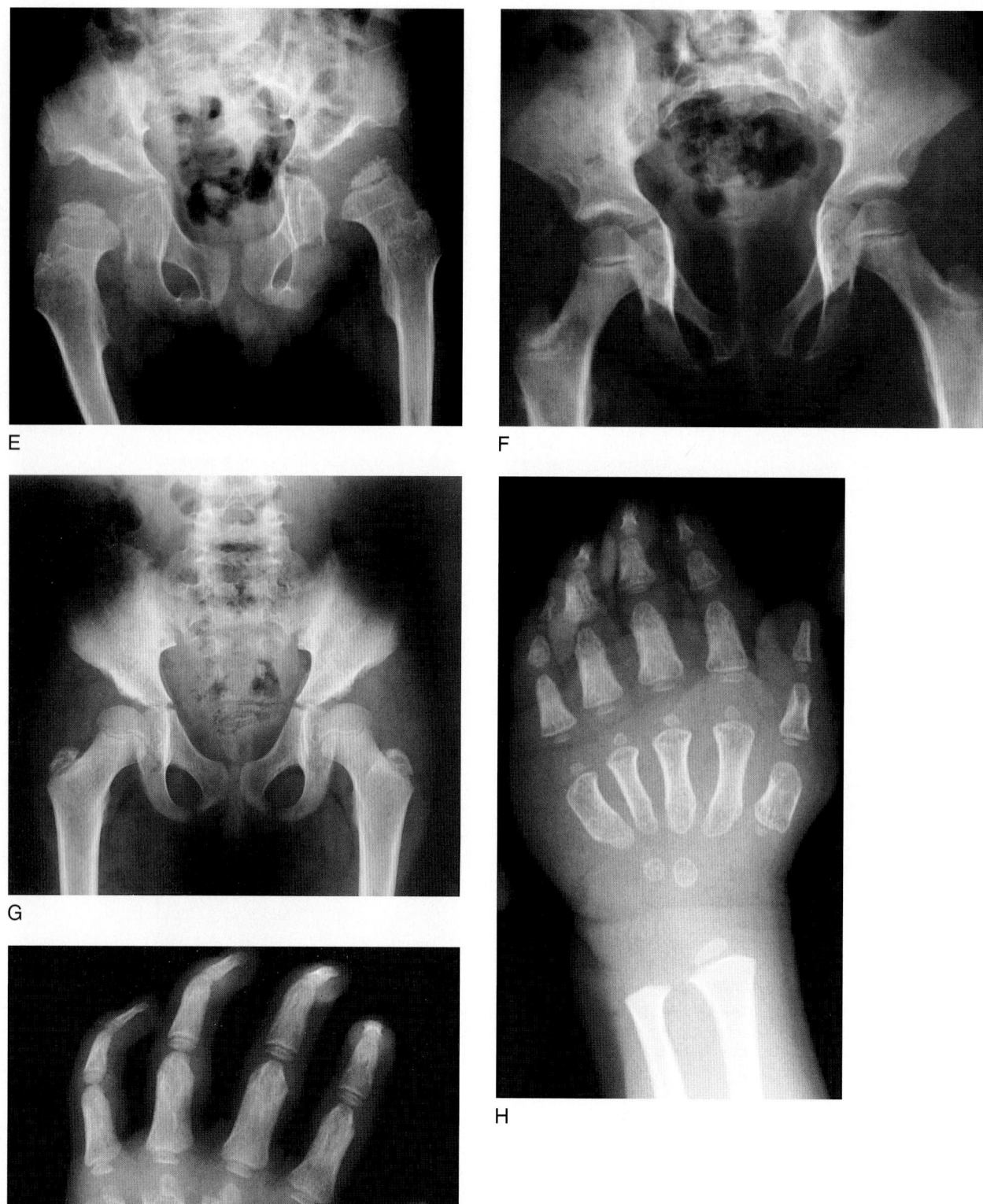

FIGURE 165-34, *cont'd.* Radiographic findings in Hurler syndrome (mucopolysaccharidosis type IH). **E** to **G,** Pelvis of an affected 8-year-old (**E**), another affected 8-year-old (**F**), and an affected 12-year-old (**G**) with small iliac wings with inferior tapering, and a slanted, irregular acetabular roof (**E** and **G**). **H** and **I,** Hands of an affected 6-year-old (**H**) and an affected 10-year-old (**I**) with proximal metacarpal pointing and epiphyseal ossification delay.

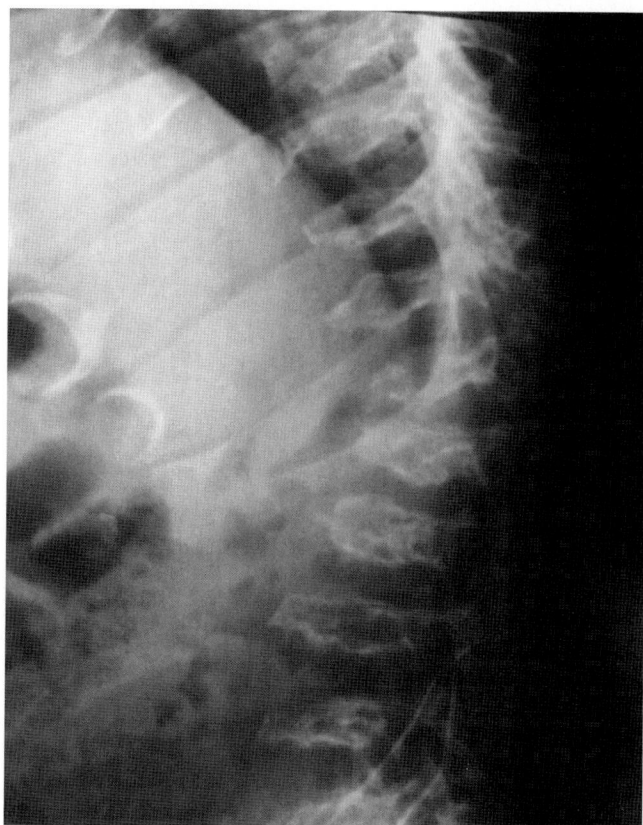

A

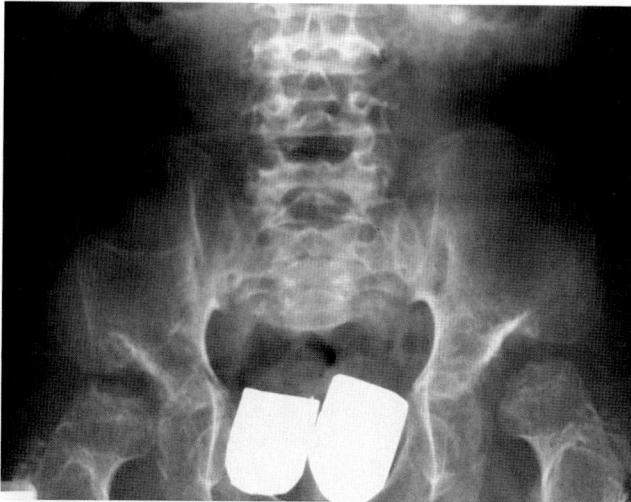

B

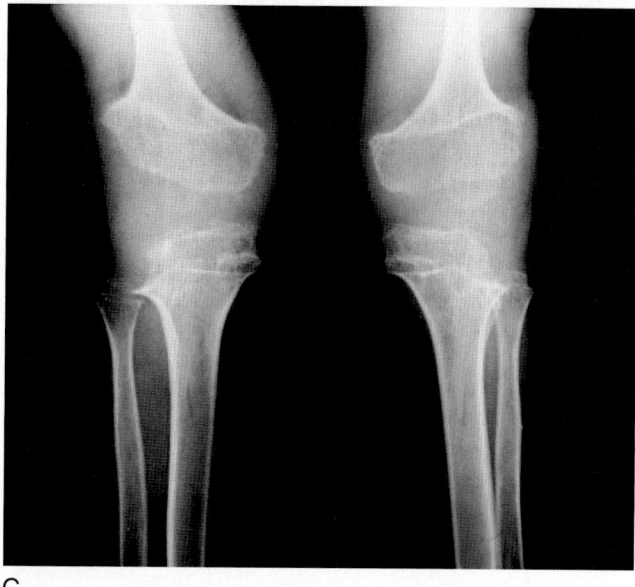

C

FIGURE 165-35. Morquio syndrome (mucopolysaccharidosis types IVA and IVB). **A,** Radiograph in an affected 7-year-old with platyspondyly with central beaking (tongue). **B,** Radiograph in an affected 18-year-old with severe capital femoral epiphyseal and acetabular dysplasia but no inferior iliac tapering. **C,** Radiograph in an affected 15-year-old with lateral distal femoral and proximal tibial epiphyseal ossification defects with genu varum.

3. Spine: *sporadic unossified vertebral bodies, dense and osteopenic vertebrae, sporadic platyspondyly, butterfly-shaped vertebral bodies, sporadic missing pedicles*
4. Extremities: generalized decreased ossification, *chromosome-shaped femurs, metaphyseal cupping* and irregularity, central lucent defect, "campomelic femurs," *sporadic "missing" short tubular bones of hands and feet*

Note: Clavicles are not affected; *infantile form is less severe.*

Adult form:
1. Generalized osteopenia
2. Extremities: *metaphyseal widening* (rickets-like changes), *punched-out metaphyseal lesions,* pathologic fractures

DISORDERS OF INCREASED BONE DENSITY WITHOUT MODIFICATION OF BONE SHAPE

The disorders of increased bone density without modification of bone shape include several entities of interest.

These disorders are still grouped by their radiographic expression. The osteopetrosis subgroup contains at least three separate entities. Pyknodysostosis is a rare but fascinating dysplasia.

Osteopetrosis

Osteopetrosis is a subgroup of disorders in which the chromosomal loci are apparently on several different chromosomes. The very severe *precocious type,* which is autosomal recessive (as is the intermediate form), is located on chromosomes 11q, 16p, and 6q. The three genes involved are *TCIRG1, CLCN,* and *GL(OSTM1).* The *delayed type (late-onset form),* which is autosomal dominant, is located at both chromosomes 11q and 16p and involves either *LRP5* or *CLCN7.* The condition known as *osteopetrosis with renal tubular acidosis (carbonic anhydrase II deficiency)* is well clarified as to chromosomal locus (8q) and gene (*CA2*—carbonic anhydrase II). Although the third dysplasia is a rare entity, certain radiographic findings suggest the correct diagnosis (Figs. 165-39 and 165-40).

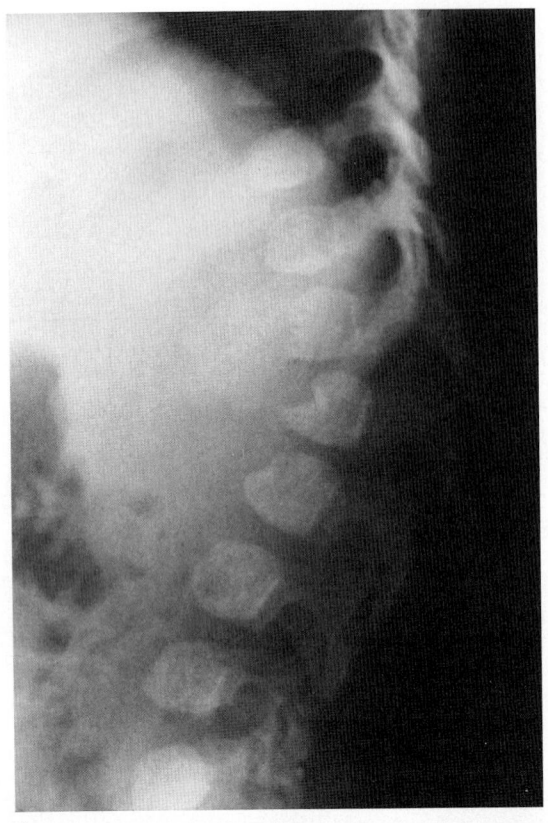

A

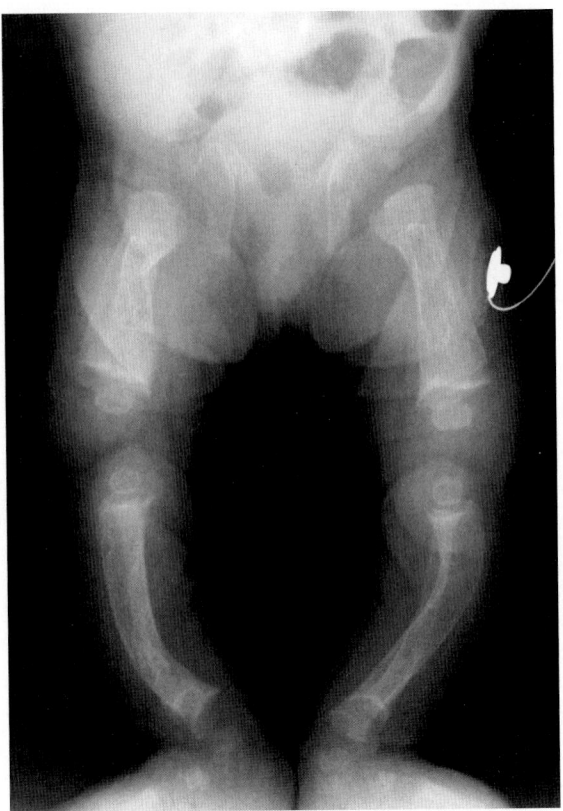

B

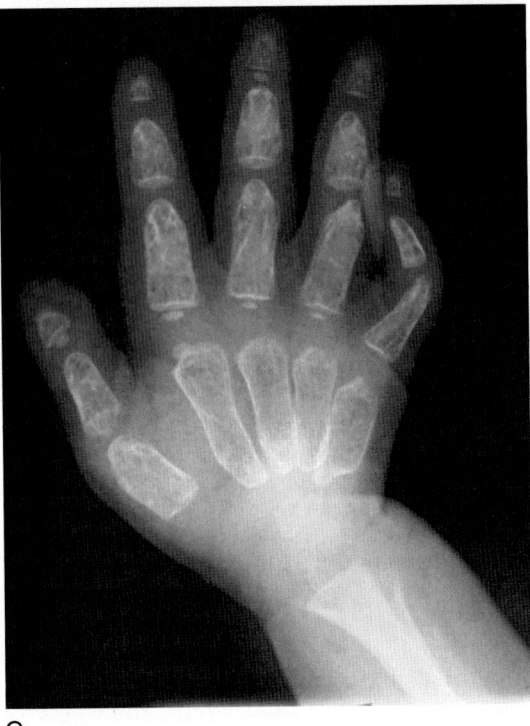

C

FIGURE 165-36. Radiographic findings in mucolipidosis type II (I-cell disease). **A,** Several hypoplastic superiorly notched vertebral bodies (mucopolysaccharidosis-like). **B,** Characteristic periosteal cloaking. **C,** Proximal metacarpal pointing and expanded short tubular bones with thin cortices.

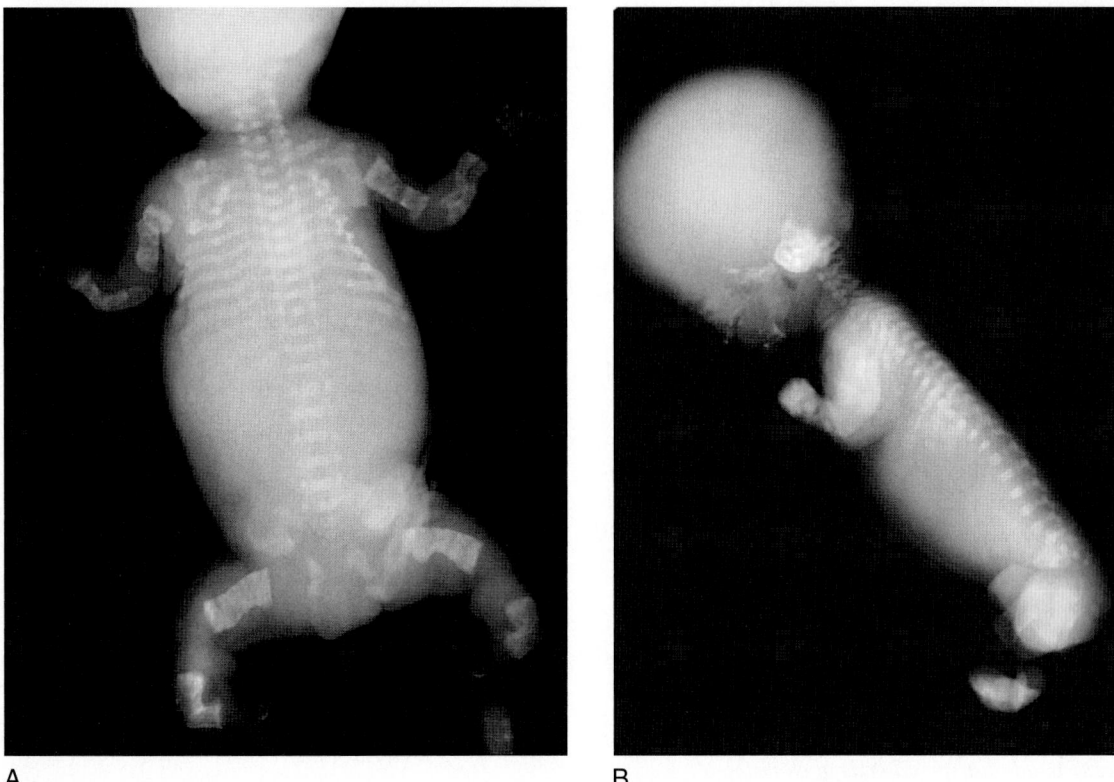

A   B

FIGURE 165-37. Radiographic findings in a stillborn full-term fetus with osteogenesis imperfecta type II. **A** and **B,** Findings include generalized osteoporosis, absence of skull ossification, beaded ribs, and crumpled long bones, including accordion-shaped femurs.

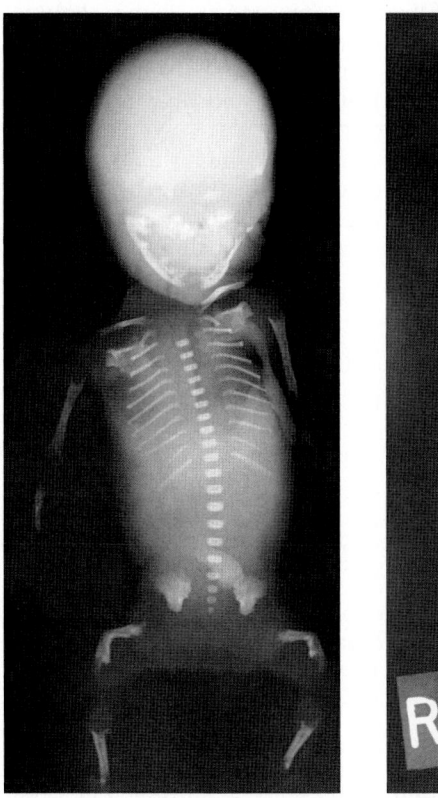

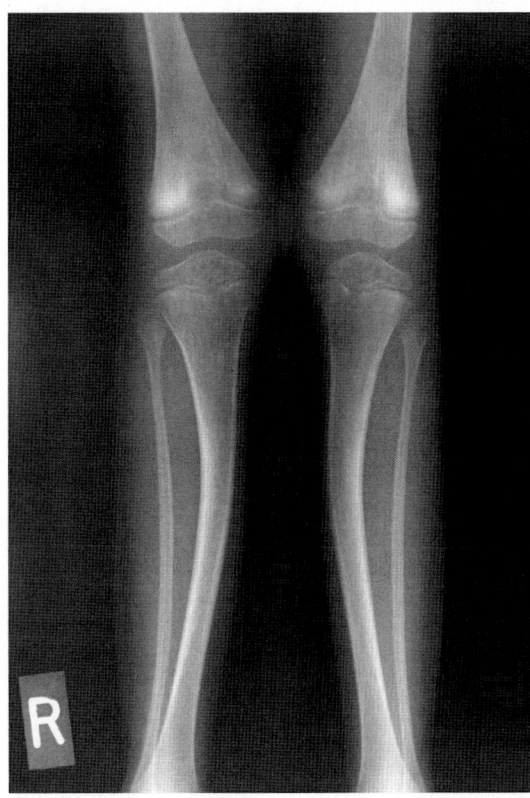

A   B

FIGURE 165-38. Hypophosphatasia. **A,** Radiograph in a fetus with perinatal lethal type demonstrates island-like skull ossification (parietal); thin, wavy ribs; platyspondyly and missing cervical vertebrae ossification; no pedicles; and bent femurs. **B,** Radiograph in a 7-year-old with adult-type hypophosphatasia demonstrates osteopenia, bent tibias, and punched-out metaphyseal lesions.

RADIOLOGIC FINDINGS

1. *Generalized increased bone density*
2. Skull: *thick and dense, especially at the base*
3. Thorax: splayed anterior ribs
4. Spine: *"sandwich" vertebral bodies, "picture frame" vertebral bodies*
5. Extremities: *splayed metaphyses,* bone-within-bone configuration, *dense metaphyseal bands*

Note: Pathologic fractures, rickets, and osteomyelitis can be present. Carbonic anhydrase II deficiency has *diffuse dense cerebral calcifications.*

Pyknodysostosis

This appears to represent the malady of the painter Toulouse-Lautrec. It is an autosomal recessive disorder that often manifests in infancy. Clinical findings include short-limbed dwarfism, micrognathia, fractures, and short fingertips (Fig. 165-41).

RADIOLOGIC FINDINGS

1. Generalized osteosclerosis
2. Skull: *marked delay in closure of fontanelles and sutures, wormian bones, obtuse or absent mandibular angle,* dense skull
3. Thorax: *resorbed acromial ends of clavicles*
4. Extremities: *resorbed phalangeal tufts*

CRANIOTUBULAR DYSPLASIAS

The *craniotubular dysplasias* are actually found in two separate nomenclature groups: increased bone density with diaphyseal involvement and increased bone density with metaphyseal involvement. Within these two groups, I only cover craniodiaphyseal dysplasia, craniometaphyseal dysplasia, and Pyle dysplasia.

Craniodiaphyseal Dysplasia

This rather rare autosomal recessive condition manifests in early infancy with progressive facial and calvarial thickening (Fig. 165-42). Sudden death, as the result of cranial foraminal narrowing, is frequent.

RADIOLOGIC FINDINGS

1. Skull: *marked thickening and sclerosis of calvaria and facial bones, obliteration of foramina* and sinuses
2. Thorax: *diffusely widened, sclerotic ribs and clavicles*
3. Extremities: *straightened, undermodeled long bone diaphyses with metaphyseal sparing; "flame" sclerosis (cortical thickening) of the short-tubular bones (hands)*

Craniometaphyseal Dysplasia

This is also an autosomal recessive craniotubular bone dysplasia. There is cranial and facial thickening, often with *nasal obstruction* (Fig. 165-43). There can be improvement with age. Cranial encroachment–induced neurologic abnormalities may develop. The chromosome site is 6q21-22.

RADIOLOGIC FINDINGS

1. Skull: diffuse *hyperostosis of cranial vault base and facial bones,* obliterated paranasal sinuses
2. Extremities: sclerosis of diaphyses (early), *undermodeled flared metaphyses* of long bones (later)

Pyle Dysplasia

This entity, also known as familial metaphyseal dysplasia, is somewhat similar to craniometaphyseal dysplasia but differs in its minimal craniofacial involvement. Patients are often asymptomatic or develop genu valgum (knock knee). This is also an autosomal recessive condition.

RADIOLOGIC FINDINGS

1. Skull: *mild skull and facial involvement,* minimal base-of-skull sclerosis, prominent supraorbital ridging
2. Thorax: mildly thickened clavicles and ribs
3. Pelvis: thickened ischium and pubis
4. Extremities: marked undertubulation of long bones, *especially distal femurs (Erlenmeyer flask deformity); distal flaring of metacarpals and proximal flaring of phalanges* (Fig. 165-44)

DISORGANIZED DEVELOPMENT OF CARTILAGINOUS, BONY, AND FIBROUS COMPONENTS OF THE SKELETON

The disorders of disorganized development of cartilaginous, bony, and fibrous components of the skeleton include many important entities that are covered elsewhere in this text, including multiple exostosis, enchondromatosis, metachondromatosis, and fibrous dysplasia. However, I cover several others in this section (osteopoikilosis, osteopathia striata, and melorheostosis) and include two other members of this group that consist of entities with significant spine involvement: spondyloenchondromatosis and dysspondyloenchondromatosis.

Osteopoikilosis

This is an autosomal dominant condition caused by mutations in *LEMD3.* It is often asymptomatic and identified on routine plain films. These lesions are often "hot" on bone scans. When skin lesions of dermatofibrosis are also present, the combination is called *Bushke-Ollendorff syndrome.*

RADIOLOGIC FINDINGS

1. Small foci of bone sclerosis (round, oval, lenticular) located primarily in cancellous bone areas (Fig. 165-45)

Osteopathia Striata

This is an asymptomatic sporadic condition, but when associated with cranial sclerosis, it is an X-linked dominant disorder. It is often identified on routine

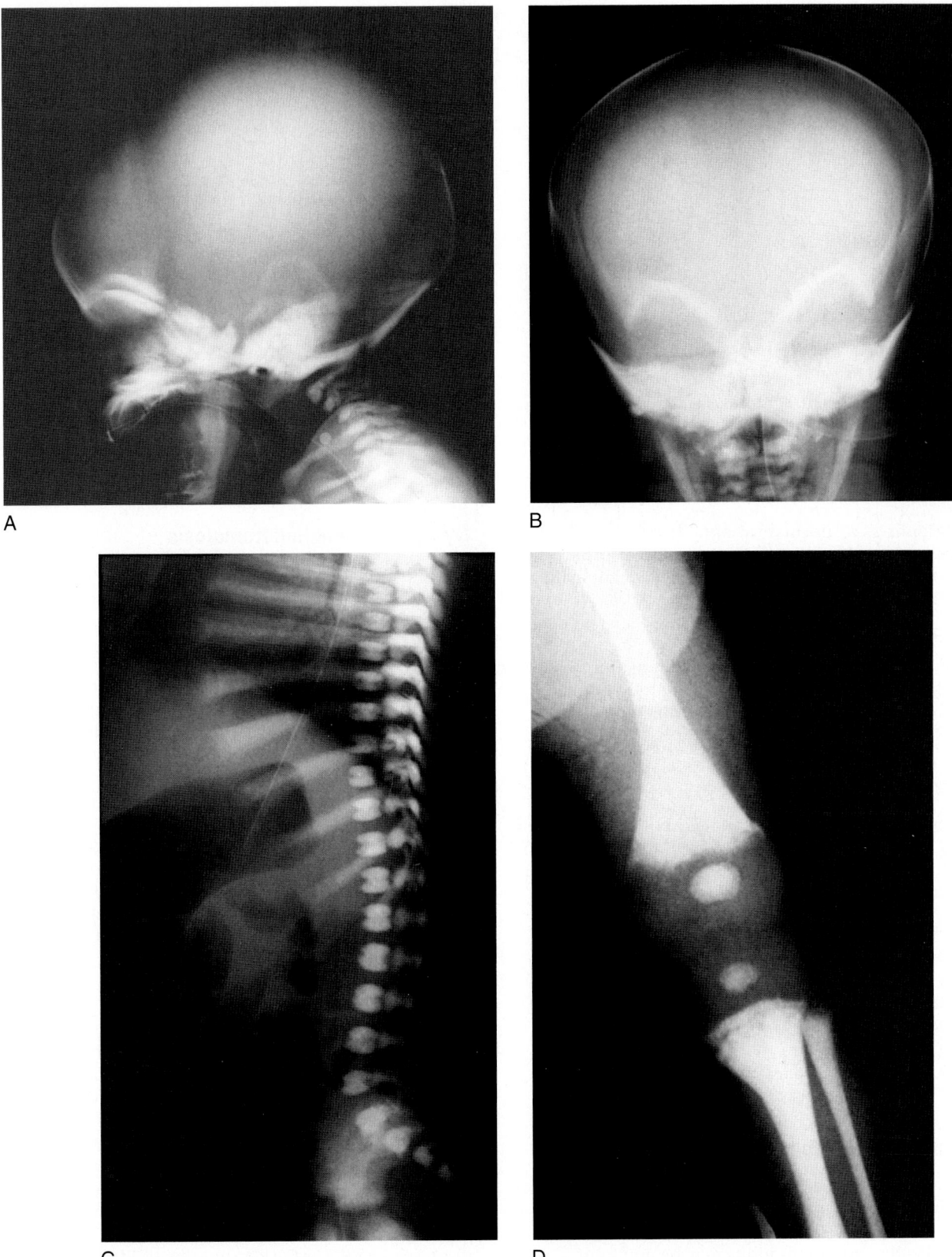

FIGURE 165-39. Precocious-type osteopetrosis (autosomal recessive). **A** to **C,** Radiographs in a newborn. **A** and **B,** Dense skull and face, especially skull base. **C,** Dense spine and ribs. **D,** At 3 months, there are very dense long bones, medullary obliteration, and frayed metaphyses (rickets).

Continued

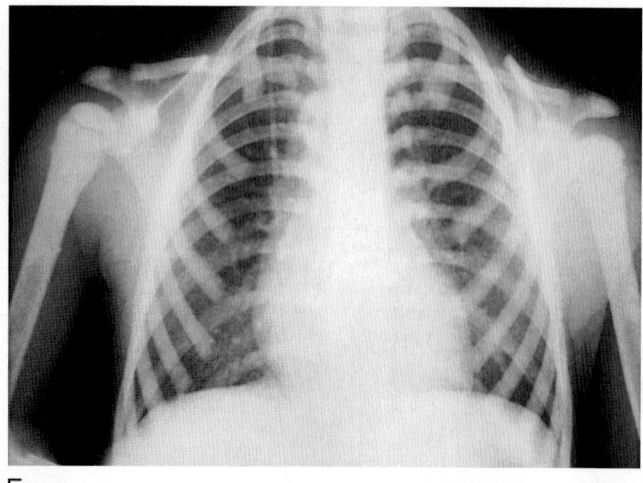
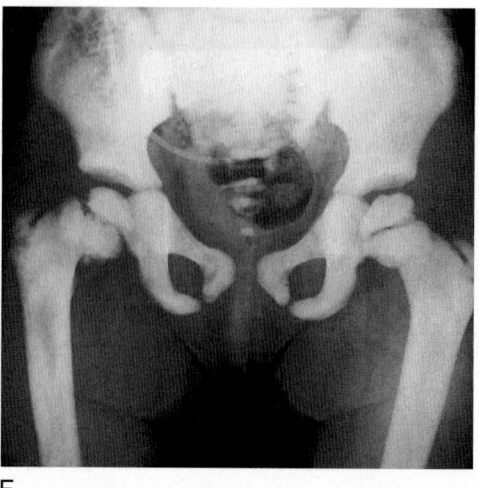

FIGURE 165-39, cont'd. Precocious-type osteopetrosis (autosomal recessive). **E** and **F**, Radiographic findings at 4 years. **E**, Dense thorax (ribs, clavicles, scapulas) and upper extremity long bones (note: less medullary obliteration). **F**, Dense pelvis and lower extremity long bones (including capital femoral epiphyses), and bilateral pathologic femoral neck fractures.

radiographs as a "normal variant." It can be seen, however, as a manifestation of other discrete disorders, such as the dysplasia of spondylar changes, nasal anomaly, and striated metaphyses (SPONASTRIME).

RADIOLOGIC FINDINGS

1. Vertical, fine, dense, linear striations (Fig. 165-46)
2. Most common at the ends of the long tubular bones, only skull and clavicles unaffected
3. Not "hot" on bone scans

Melorheostosis

This entity is often sporadic but can be seen as an autosomal dominant in families with an *LEMD3* gene mutation. Patients can experience bone pain and joint stiffening, as well as limb asymmetry.

RADIOLOGIC FINDINGS

1. Monostotic or polyostotic
2. Linear dense cortical hyperostosis following the long axis of bones
3. Resembles *melting/dripping candle wax* (Fig. 165-47)
4. Can cross joint space
5. "Hot" on bone scans

Spondyloenchondromatosis

This autosomal recessive disorder is also known as spondyloenchondrodysplasia. There is low-normal or mild short stature, with kyphosis or lordosis, or both (Fig. 165-48). Prominent joints may be apparent.

RADIOLOGIC FINDINGS

1. Spine: *severe platyspondyly with end plate irregularity*
2. Extremities: *typical enchondromata*

Note: Enchondromas may be present in all enchondral bone areas but rarely involve the hands and feet.

Dysspondyloenchondromatosis

This entity is also called dysspondylochondromatosis. The patients have short stature, kyphoscoliosis, and abnormal facies (Fig. 165-49).

RADIOLOGIC FINDINGS

1. Spine: vertebral anomalies, *hemivertebrae, anisospondyly,* and end plate irregularity
2. Extremities: *typical enchondromata,* including hand and foot involvement, with *long bone asymmetry*

OSTEOLYSIS GROUP

The osteolysis group of disorders is very large and diverse and lacks significant clarification. No molecular identification has occurred for this group, and only one chromosome site has been found in a rather rare member. See Chapter 166 for a detailed discussion of the osteolysis syndromes.

PATELLAR DYSPLASIA GROUP

The patellar dysplasia group contains only two members: the newly described scyphopatellar dysplasia and the not uncommon and important nail–patella syndrome.

Nail–Patella Syndrome

This autosomal dominant disorder is also known by a variety of synonyms, including Fong disease and onycho-osteodysplasia, among several others. The gene for this disorder (*NPS1*[*LMX1B*]) has been identified and is located on chromosome 9q. The major clinical manifestations include dysplastic nails, small or absent patellae on palpation, and a nephropathy with onset in childhood or in the young adult and characteristic electron microscopic changes. The "iliac horns" (Fig. 165-50) are sometimes palpable.

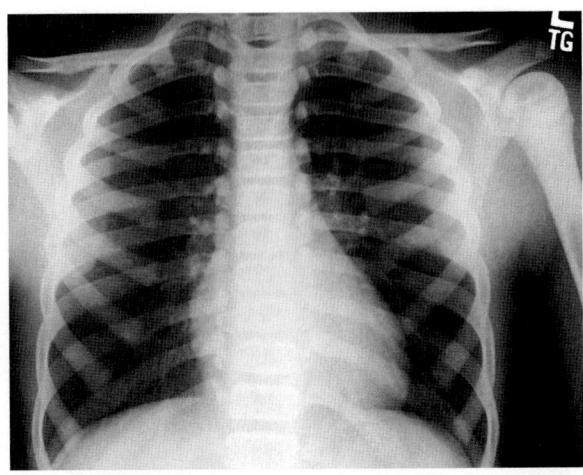

A

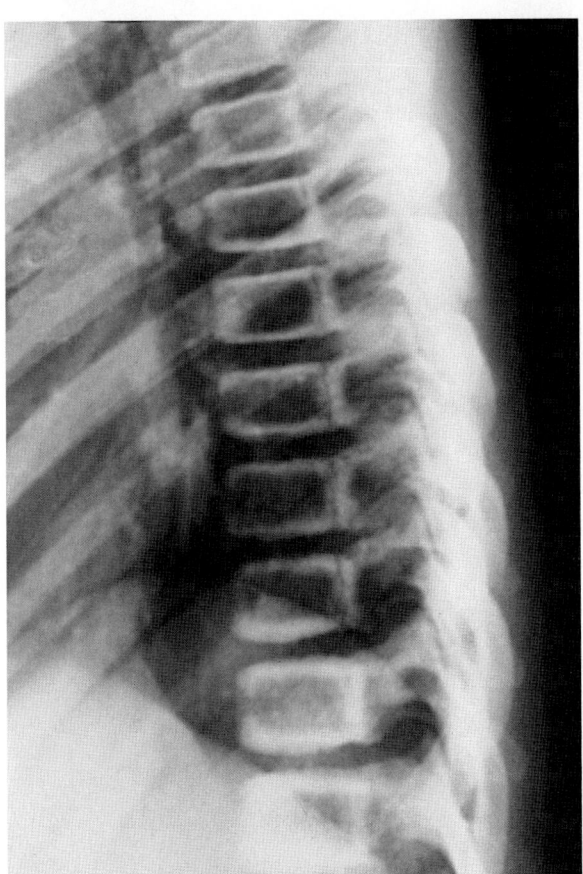

B

FIGURE 165-40. Radiographic findings in an 8-year-old with delayed-type osteopetrosis (autosomal dominant). **A,** Dense thoracic bones without medullary encroachment of left humerus. **B,** "Sandwich," almost "picture frame" vertebral bodies (dense outer borders). **C,** Increased bone density outlining ileum, including supra-acetabular regions, and pubic symphysis region, as well as dense proximal femoral epiphyses and femoral necks with sparing of lower medullary space.

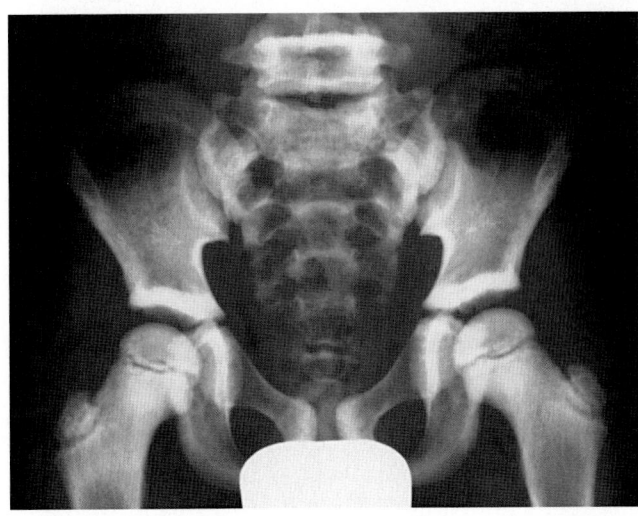

C

RADIOLOGIC FINDINGS

1. Pelvis: *iliac horn* in the center of the iliac wing extending posteriorly

2. Extremities (knees and elbows): *hypoplastic or absent patellae*, radial head and capitellum hypoplasia/elbow dislocation

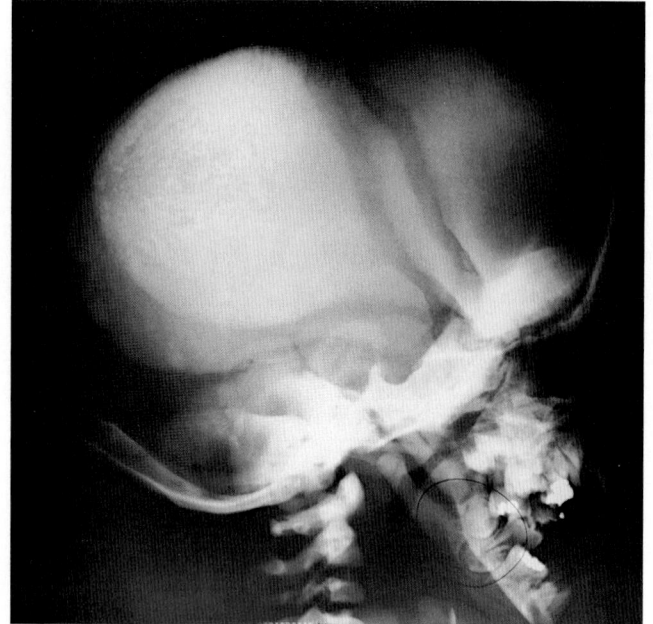

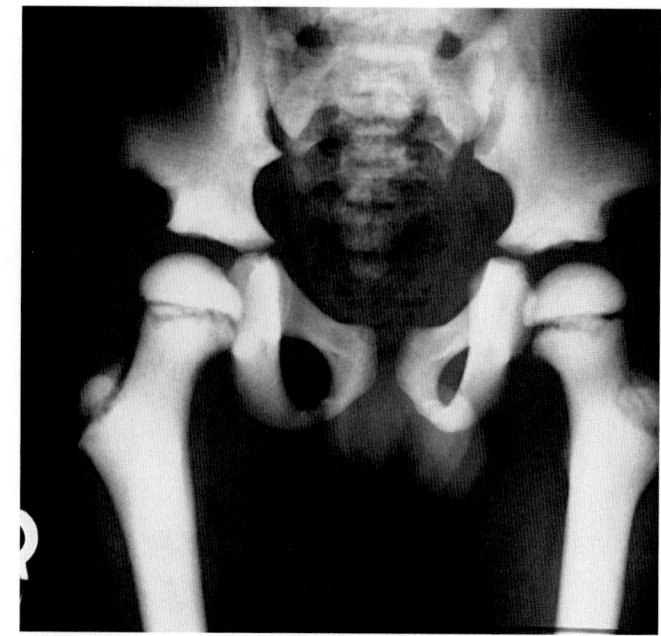

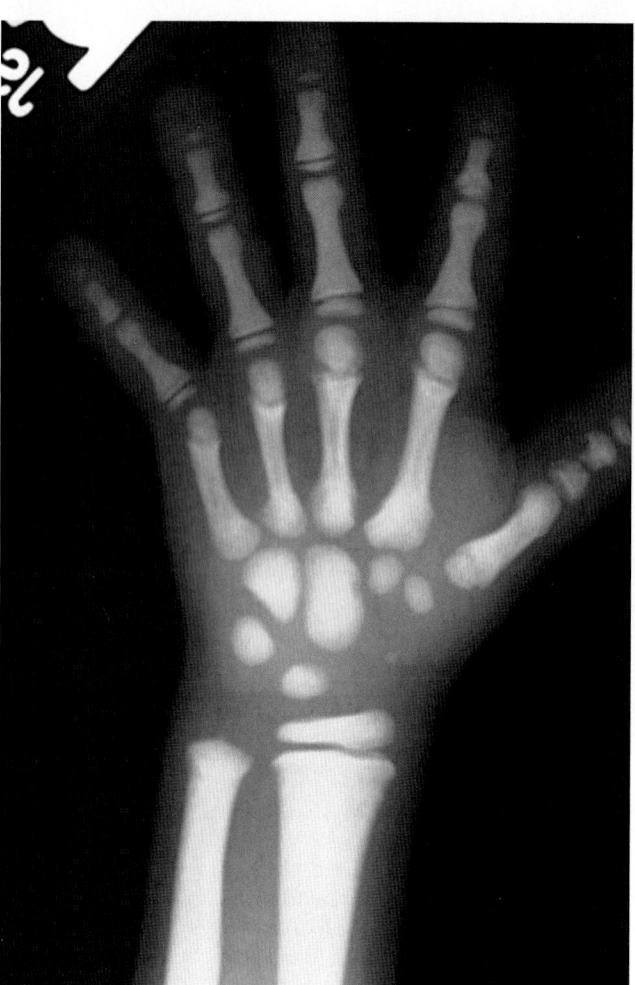

FIGURE 165-41. Radiographic findings in an 8-year-old with pyknodysostosis. **A,** Dense skull convexity and base, widely separated sutures with open fontanelle, and absence of mandibular angle. **B,** Hip and pelvis: generalized increased bone density with long, overmodeled (resorbed) femoral necks. **C,** Hands: dense bones, overmodeled metacarpals and phalanges, phalangeal tuft resorption.

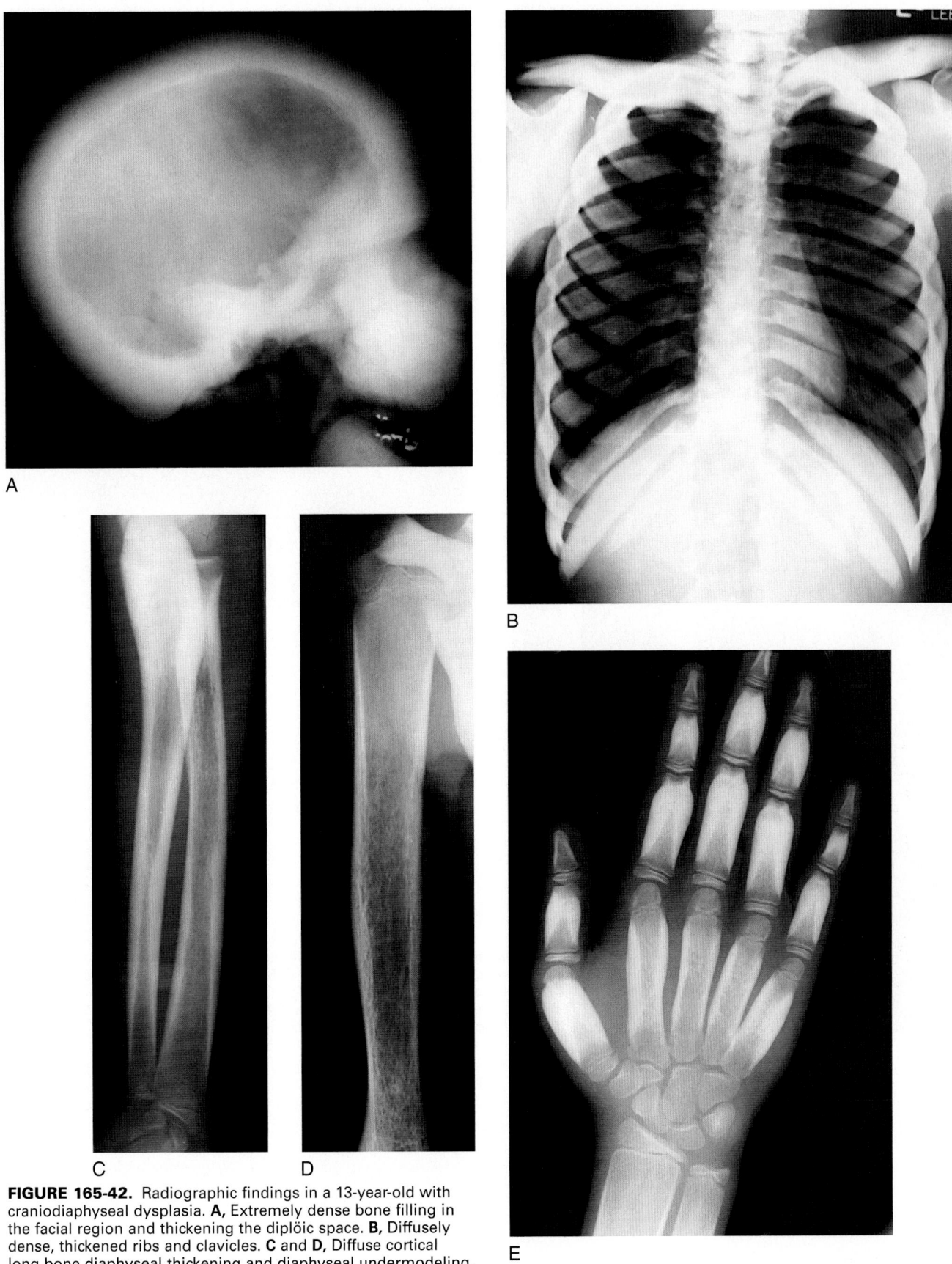

FIGURE 165-42. Radiographic findings in a 13-year-old with craniodiaphyseal dysplasia. **A,** Extremely dense bone filling in the facial region and thickening the diplöic space. **B,** Diffusely dense, thickened ribs and clavicles. **C** and **D,** Diffuse cortical long bone diaphyseal thickening and diaphyseal undermodeling. **E,** "Flame" sclerosis (cortical thickening) of the tubular bones of the hand.

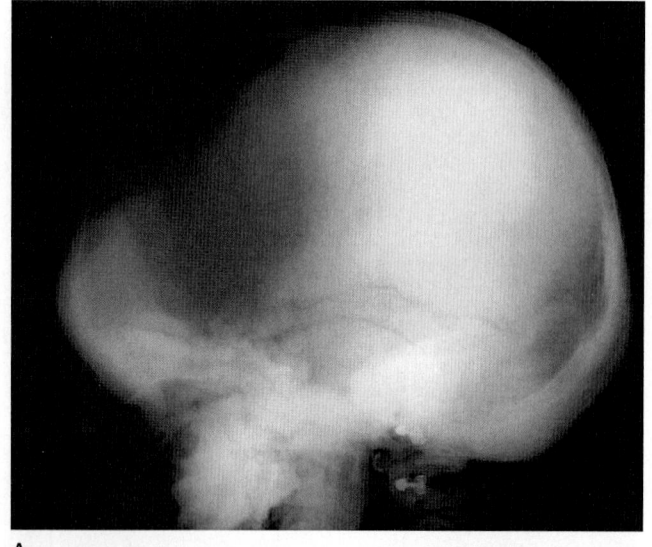

A

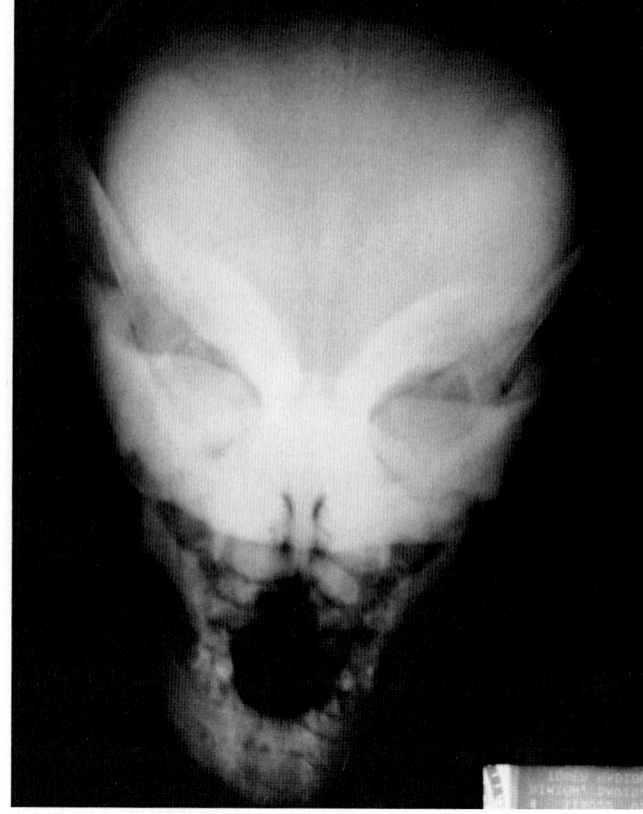

B

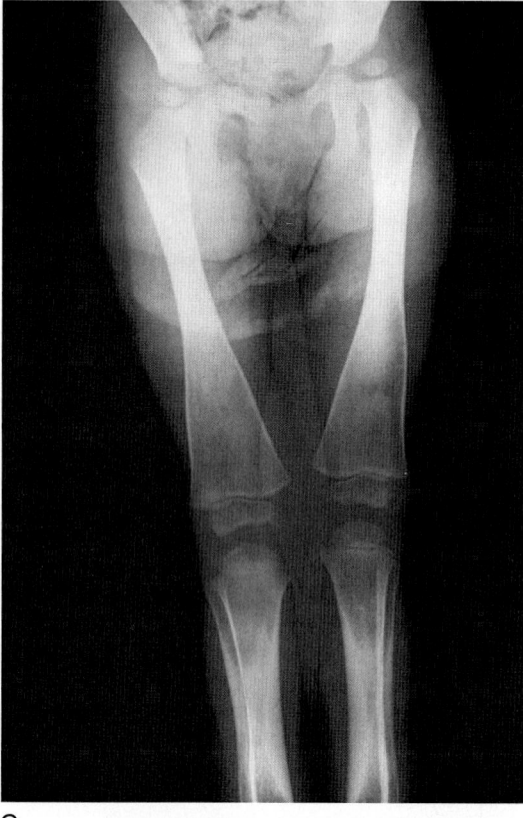

C

FIGURE 165-43. Radiographic findings in a 2-year-old with craniometaphyseal dysplasia. **A** and **B,** Marked increased bone density of cranial base and vault, and dense facial bones with obliteration of sinuses. **C,** Undermodeled flared metaphyses (Erlenmeyer flask deformity) of distal femurs, especially with sparing of diaphyses.

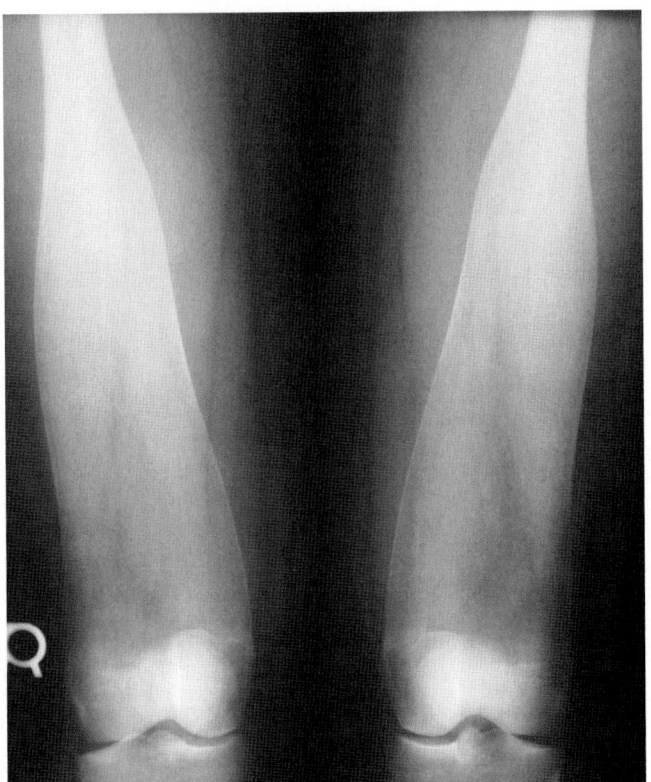

A

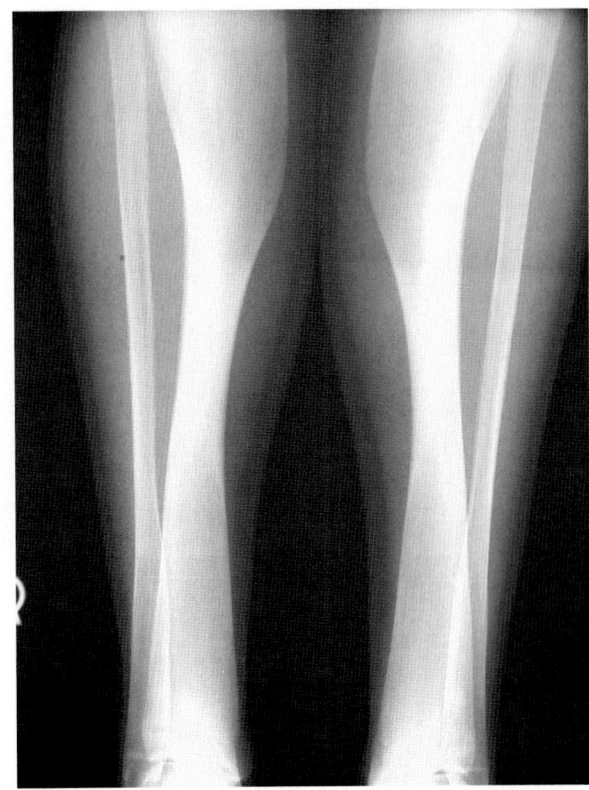

B

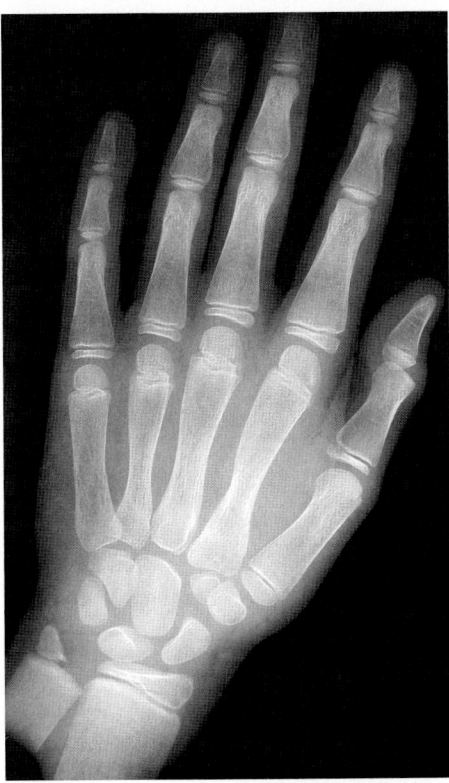

C

FIGURE 165-44. Radiographic findings in Pyle dysplasia. **A** and **B,** In an affected 17-year-old, markedly broad, undertubulated distal femurs (**A**) and markedly broad, undertubulated proximal and distal tibias with mild medial bowing proximally (**B**). **C,** In a different affected patient, distal flaring of metacarpals and proximal flaring of phalanges. The distal radial and ulnar metaphyses are broadened.

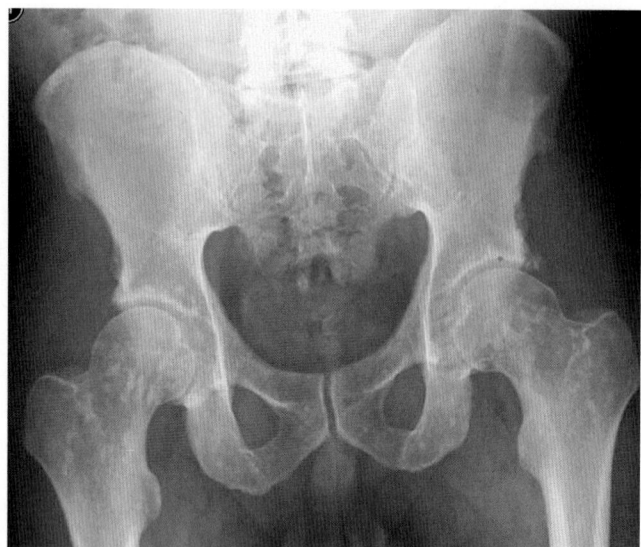

FIGURE 165-45. Radiographic findings in osteopoikilosis. Anteroposterior view of pelvis and hips reveals scattered small sclerotic lesions involving the proximal femurs, ilia, and ischia in an affected man.

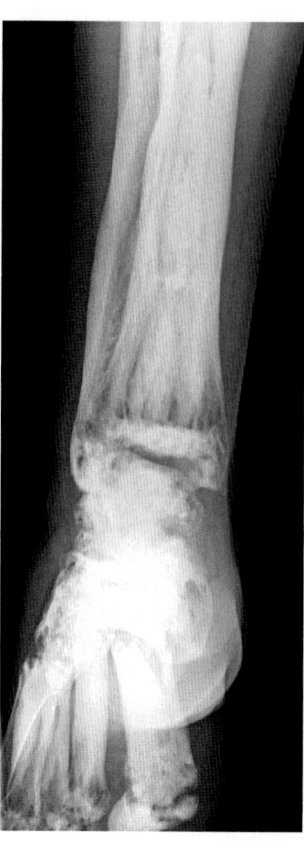

FIGURE 165-47. Radiographic findings in a 14-year-old boy with melorheostosis. Image of the tibia/fibula and ankle shows dense "candle-wax dripping" changes involving both tibia and fibula, extending into the epiphyses and across the joint into the tarsal/ metatarsal bones.

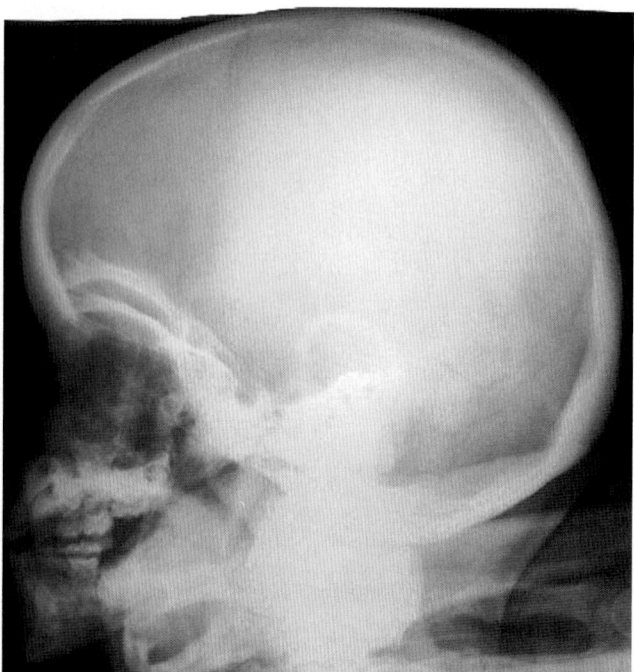

A

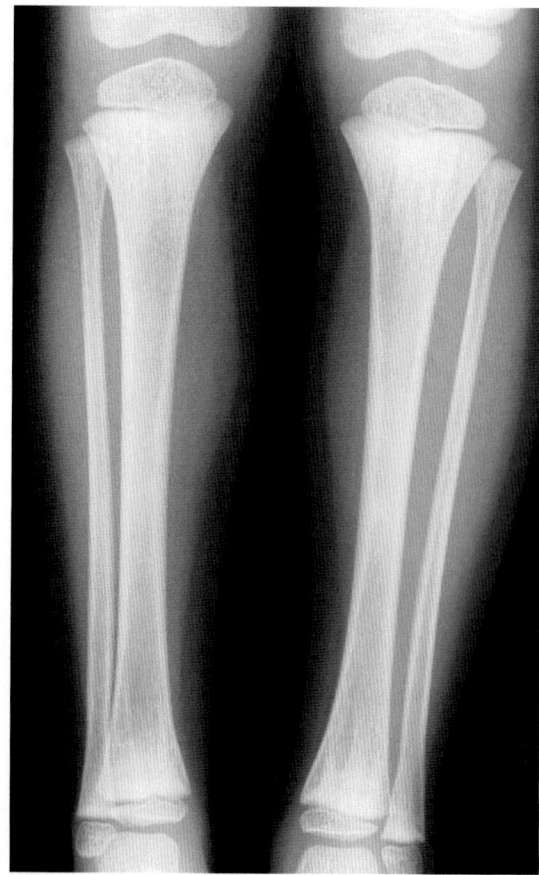

B

FIGURE 165-46. Radiographic findings in osteopathia striata with cranial sclerosis. **A,** Lateral skull film revealing dense thickening of the calvaria with increased basilar and orbital sclerosis. **B,** Anteroposterior radiograph of the lower extremity reveals linear striations of the metadiaphyseal regions of both ends of the tibias and fibulas.

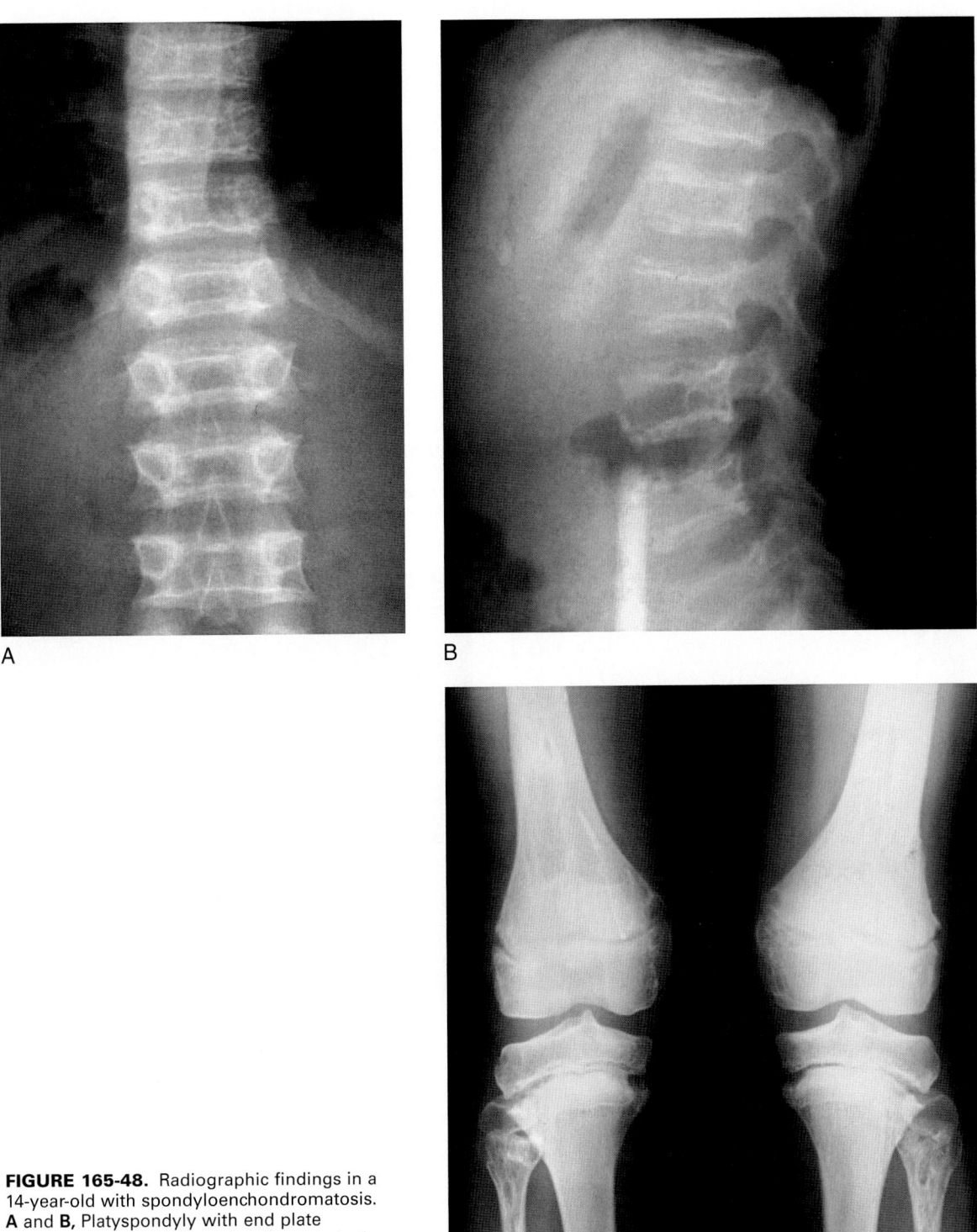

A

B

C

FIGURE 165-48. Radiographic findings in a 14-year-old with spondyloenchondromatosis. **A** and **B**, Platyspondyly with end plate irregularity. **C**, Multiple enchondromata in the long bones.

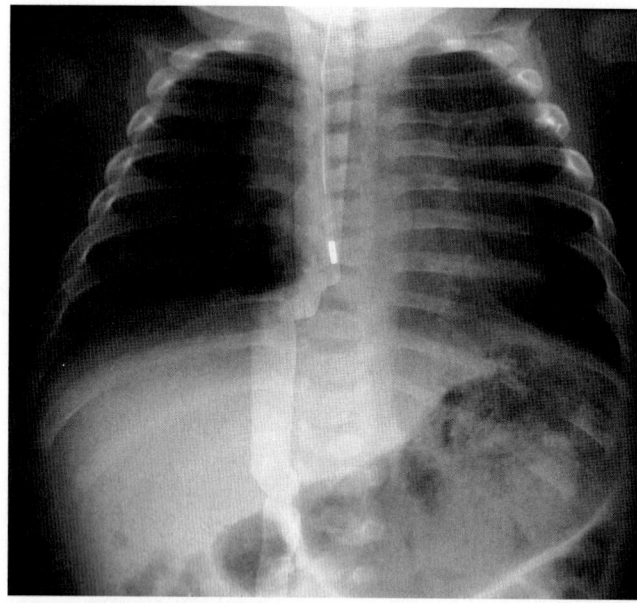

FIGURE 165-49. Radiographic findings in a 6-month-old with dysspondyloenchondromatosis include multiple hemivertebrae in thoracolumbar junctional area. (The patient also had many enchondromata in his appendicular skeleton.)

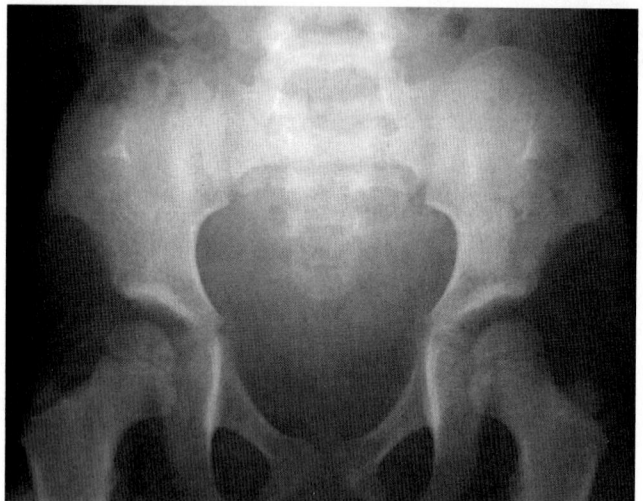

A

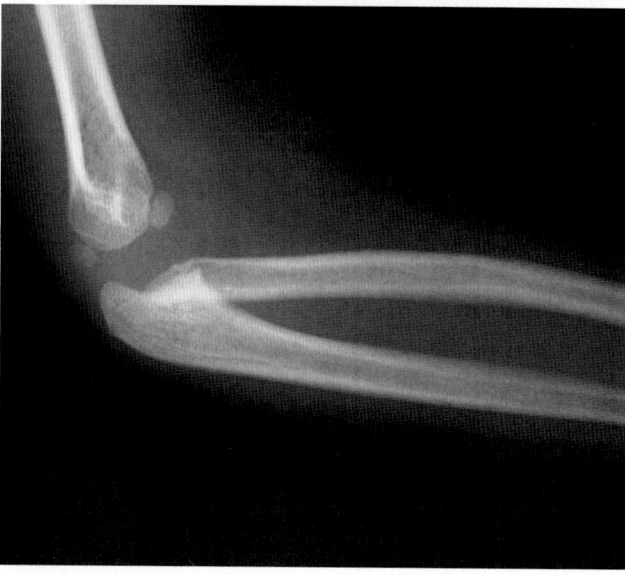

C

FIGURE 165-50. Radiographic findings in a 5-year-old with nail–patella syndrome. **A,** Iliac horn in the center of each iliac wing. **B,** Tiny (hypoplastic) patella in this sunrise view of the knee. **C,** Congenital elbow (radial head) dislocation.

SUGGESTED READINGS

General

Lachman RS: International nomenclature and classification of the osteochondrodysplasias (1997). Pediatr Radiol 1998;28:737

Shohat M, Lachman R, Gruber HE, et al: Brachyolmia: clinical, radiographic and genetic evidence of heterogeneity. Am J Med Genet 1989;33:209

Lachman RS: Taybi and Lachman's Radiology of Syndromes, Metabolic Disorders, and Skeletal Dysplasias, 5th ed. St. Louis, Mosby, 2007

Fetal Diagnosis

Avni EF, Rypens F, Zappa M, et al: Antenatal diagnosis of short-limb dwarfism: sonographic approach. Pediatr Radiol 1996;26:171

Budorick NE: The fetal musculoskeletal system. In Callen PW (ed): Ultrasonography in Obstetrics and Gynecology, 4th ed. Philadelphia, WB Saunders, 2000:331

Jeanty P, Valero G, Bircher AM, et al: Skeletal dysplasias. In Nyberg DA, McGahan JP, Pretorius DH, et al (eds): Diagnostic Imaging of Fetal Anomalies. Philadelphia, Lippincott Williams & Wilkins, 2003:661

Schumacher R, Seaver LH, Spranger J: Fetal radiology: a diagnostic atlas, New York, Springer, 2004

Teele RL: A guide to the recognition of skeletal disorders in the fetus. Pediatr Radiol 2006;36:473

Thanatophoric Dysplasia

Brodie SG, Kitoh H, Lachman RS, et al: Platyspondylic lethal skeletal dysplasia, San Diego type, is caused by FGFR3 mutations. Am J Med Genet 1999;84:476

Langer LO Jr, Spranger JW, Greinacher I, et al: Thanatophoric dwarfism: a condition confused with achondroplasia in the neonate, with brief comments on achondrogenesis and homozygous achondroplasia. Radiology 1969;92:285

Langer LO Jr, Yang SS, Hall JG, et al: Thanatophoric dysplasia and cloverleaf skull. Am J Med Genet Suppl 1987;3:167

Norman AM, Rimmer S, Landy S, et al: Thanatophoric dysplasia of the straight bone type (type 2). Clin Dysmorphol 1992;1:115

Wilcox WR, Tavormina PL, Krakow D, et al: Molecular, radiologic, and histopathologic correlations in thanatophoric dysplasia. Am J Med Genet 1998;78:274

Achondroplasia

Caffey J: Achondroplasia of pelvis and lumbosacral spine: some roentgenographic features. Am J Roentgenol Radium Ther Nucl Med 1958;80:449

Langer LO Jr, Baumann PA, Gorlin RJ: Achondroplasia. Am J Roentgenol Radium Ther Nucl Med 1967;100:12

Lemyre E, Azouz EM, Teebi AS, et al: Bone dysplasia series. Achondroplasia, hypochondroplasia and thanatophoric dysplasia: review and update. Can Assoc Radiol J 1999;50:185

Hypochondroplasia

Hall BD, Spranger J: Hypochondroplasia: clinical and radiological aspects in 39 cases. Radiology 1979;133:95

Le Merrer M, Rousseau F, Legeai-Mallet L, et al: A gene for achondroplasia-hypochondroplasia maps to chromosome 4p. Nat Genet 1994;6:318

Maroteaux P, Falzon P: Hypochondroplasia: review of 80 cases [in French]. Arch Fr Pediatr 1988;45:105

Metatropic Dysplasia

Beck M, Roubicek M, Rogers JG, et al: Heterogeneity of metatropic dysplasia. Eur J Pediatr 1983;140:231

Shohat M, Lachman R, Rimoin DL: Odontoid hypoplasia with cervical spine subluxation and ventriculomegaly in metatropic dysplasia. J Pediatr 1989;114:239

Schneckenbecken (Snail Pelvis) Dysplasia

Borochowitz Z, Jones KL, Silbey R, et al: A distinct lethal neonatal chondrodysplasia with snail-like pelvis: Schneckenbecken dysplasia. Am J Med Genet 1986;25:47

Giedion A, Biedermann K, Briner J, et al: Case report 693: Schneckenbecken dysplasia. Skeletal Radiol 1991;20:534

Short Rib–Polydactyly Dysplasia

Beemer FA, Langer LO Jr, Klep-de Pater JM, et al: A new short rib syndrome: report of two cases. Am J Med Genet 1983;14:115

Lungarotti MS, Martello C, Marinelli I, et al: Lethal short rib syndrome of the Beemer type without polydactyly. Pediatr Radiol 1993;23:325

Naumoff P, Young LW, Mazer J, et al: Short rib–polydactyly syndrome type 3. Radiology 1977;122:443

Saldino RM, Noonan CD: Severe thoracic dystrophy with striking micromelia, abnormal osseous development, including the spine, and multiple visceral anomalies. Am J Roentgenol Radium Ther Nucl Med 1972;114:257

Sillence D, Kozlowski K, Bar-Ziv J, et al: Perinatally lethal short rib–polydactyly syndromes. 1. Variability in known syndromes. Pediatr Radiol 1987;17:474

Spranger J, Grimm B, Weller M, et al: Short-rib–polydactyly (SRP) syndromes, types Majewski and Saldino-Noonan. Z Kinderheilkd 1974;116:73

Asphyxiating Thoracic Dysplasia (Jeune Syndrome)

Langer LO: Thoracic-pelvic-phalangeal dystrophy: asphyxiating thoracic dystrophy of the newborn, infantile thoracic dystrophy. Radiology 1968;91:447

Chondroectodermal Dysplasia (Ellis–van Creveld Dysplasia)

Caffey J: Chondroectodermal dysplasia (Ellis–van Creveld syndrome): report of three cases. Am J Roentgenol Radium Ther Nucl Med 1952;68:875

McKusick VA: The Amish. Endeavour 1980;4:52

McKusick VA: Ellis–van Creveld syndrome and the Amish. Nat Genet 2000;24:203

Diastrophic Dysplasia

Horton WA, Rimoin DL, Lachman RS, et al: The phenotypic variability of diastrophic dysplasia. J Pediatr 1978;93:609

Lachman R, Sillence D, Rimoin D, et al: Diastrophic dysplasia: the death of a variant. Radiology 1981;140:79

Taybi H: Diastrophic dwarfism. Radiology 1963;80:1

Multiple Epiphyseal Dysplasia: Multilayered Patellae/Brachydactyly/Clubfeet

Lachman RS, Krakow D, Cohn DH, et al: MED, COMP, multilayered, and NEIN: an overview of multiple epiphyseal dysplasia. Pediatr Radiol 2005;35:116

Achondrogenesis Type I

Borochowitz Z, Lachman R, Adomian GE, et al: Achondrogenesis type 1: delineation of further heterogeneity and identification of two distinct subgroups. J Pediatr 1988;112:23

Achondrogenesis Type II/Hypochondrogenesis

Borochowitz Z, Ornoy A, Lachman R, et al: Achondrogenesis II–hypochondrogenesis: variability versus heterogeneity. Am J Med Genet 1986;24:273

Eyre DR, Upton MP, Shapiro FD, et al: Nonexpression of cartilage type II collagen in a case of Langer-Saldino achondrogenesis. Am J Hum Genet 1986;39:52

Lachman RS, Tiller GE, Graham JM Jr, et al: Collagen, genes and the skeletal dysplasias on the edge of a new era: a review and update. Eur J Radiol 1992;14:1

Saldino RM: Lethal short-limbed dwarfism: achondrogenesis and thanatophoric dwarfism. Am J Roentgenol Radium Ther Nucl Med 1971;112:185

Spondyloepiphyseal Dysplasia Congenita

Harding CO, Green CG, Perloff WH, et al: Respiratory complications in children with spondyloepiphyseal dysplasia congenita. Pediatr Pulmon 1990;9:49

Lachman RS: Fetal imaging in the skeletal dysplasias: overview and experience. Pediatr Radiol 1994;24:413

Spranger J, Langer LO Jr: Spondyloepiphyseal dysplasia congenita. Radiology 1970;94:313

Spranger J, Wiedemann HR: Dysplasia spondyloepiphysaria congenita. Helv Paediatr Acta 1966;21:598

Tiller GE, Rimoin DL, Murray LW, et al: Tandem duplication within a type II collagen gene (COL2A1) exon in an individual with spondyloepiphyseal dysplasia. Proc Natl Acad Sci U S A 1990;87:3889

Kniest Dysplasia

Kniest W: Zur Abgrenzung der Dysostosis enchondralis von der Chondrodystrophie [Differential diagnosis between dysostosis enchondralis and chondrodystrophy]. Z Kinderheilkd 1952;70:633

Lachman RS, Rimoin DL, Hollister DW, et al: The Kniest syndrome. Am J Roentgenol Radium Ther Nucl Med 1975;123:805

Spranger J, Menger H, Mundlos S, et al: Kniest dysplasia is caused by dominant collagen II (COL2A1) mutations: parental somatic mosaicism manifesting as Stickler phenotype and mild spondyloepiphyseal dysplasia. Pediatr Radiol 1994;24:431

Wilkin DJ, Bogaert R, Lachman RS, et al: A single amino acid substitution (G103D) in the type II collagen triple helix produces Kniest dysplasia. Hum Mol Genet 1994;3:1999

Spondyloepiphyseal Dysplasia Tarda

Giedeon AK, Colley A, Jamieson R, et al: Identification of the gene (SEDL) causing X-linked spondyloepiphyseal dysplasia tarda. Nat Genet 1999;22:400

Langer LO: Spondyloepiphyseal dysplasia tarda, hereditary chondrodysplasia with characteristic vertebral configuration in the adult. Radiology 1964;82:833

Dyggve-Melchior-Clausen Syndrome

Beighton P: Dyggve-Melchior-Clausen syndrome. J Med Genet 1990;27:512

Dyggve HV, Melchior JC, Clausen J: Morquio-Ulrich's disease. Arch Dis Child 1962;37:525

Schorr S, Legum C, Ochshorn M, et al: The Dyggve-Melchior-Clausen syndrome. Am J Roentgenol 1977;128:107

Multiple Epiphyseal Dysplasia

Deere M, Sanford T, Francomano CA, et al: Identification of nine novel mutations in cartilage oligomeric matrix protein in patients with pseudoachondroplasia and multiple epiphyseal dysplasia. Am J Med Genet 1999;85:486

Hulvey JT, Keats T: Multiple epiphyseal dysplasia: a contribution to the problem of spinal involvement. Am J Roentgenol Radium Ther Nucl Med 1969;106:170

Lohiniva J, Paassilta P, Seppanen U, et al: Splicing mutations in the COL3 domain of collagen IX cause multiple epiphyseal dysplasia. Am J Med Genet 2000;90:216

Pseudoachondroplasia

Heselson NG, Cremin BJ, Beighton P: Pseudoachondroplasia: a report of 13 cases. Br J Radiol 1977;50:473

Rimoin DL, Rasmussen IM, Briggs MD: A large family with features of pseudoachondroplasia and multiple epiphyseal dysplasia: exclusion of seven candidate gene loci that encode proteins of the cartilage extracellular matrix. Hum Genet 1994;93:236

Wynne-Davies R, Hall CM, Young ID: Pseudachondroplasia: clinical diagnosis at different ages and comparison of autosomal dominant and recessive types. A review of 32 patients (26 kindreds). J Med Genet 1986;23:425

Chondrodysplasia Punctata

Brites P, Motley A, Hoganhout E, et al: Molecular basis of rhizomelic chondrodysplasia punctata type 1: high frequency of the Leu-292 stop mutation in 38 patients. J Inherit Metab Dis 1998;21:306

Gilbert EF, Opitz JM, Spranger JW, et al: Chondrodysplasia punctata—rhizomelic form: pathologic and radiologic studies of three infants. Eur J Pediatr 1976;123:89

Maroteaux P: Brachytelephalangic chondrodysplasia punctata: a possible X-linked recessive form. Hum Genet 1989;82:167

Silengo MC, Luzzati L, Silverman FN: Clinical and genetic aspects of Conradi-Hünermann disease. J Pediatr 1980;97:911

Spranger JW, Bidder U, Voelz C: Chondrodysplasia punctata (chondrodystrophia calcificans). II: the rhizomelic type [in German]. Forschr Geb Rontgenstr Nuklearmed 1971;114:327

Wells TR, Landing BH, Bostwick FH: Studies of vertebral coronal cleft in rhizomelic chondrodysplasia punctata. Pediatr Pathol 1992;12:593

Jansen-Type Metaphyseal Chondrodysplasia

de Haas WHD, de Boer W, Griffioen F: Metaphyseal dysostosis: a late follow-up of the first reported case. J Bone Joint Surg Br 1969;51:290

Kruse K, Schute C: Calcium metabolism in the Jansen type of metaphyseal dysplasia. Eur J Pediatr 1993;152:912

Nazará Z, Hernandez A, Corona-Rivera E, et al: Further clinical and radiological features in metaphyseal chondrodysplasia Jansen type. Radiology 1981;140:697

Ozonoff MB: Metaphyseal dysostosis of Jansen. Radiology 1969;93:1047

Schipani E, Langman CB, Parfitt AM, et al: Constitutively activated receptors for parathyroid hormone and parathyroid hormone-related peptide in Jansen's metaphyseal chondrodysplasia. N Engl J Med 1996;335:708

Silverthorn KG, Houston CS, Duncan BP: Murk Jansen's metaphyseal chondrodysplasia with long-term follow-up. Pediatr Radiol 1987; 17:119

Schmid-Type Metaphyseal Chondrodysplasia

Lachman RS, Rimoin DL, Spranger J: Metaphyseal chondrodysplasia, Schmid type: clinical and radiographic delineation with a review of the literature. Pediatr Radiol 1988;18:93

McIntosh I, Abbott MH, Warman ML, et al: Additional mutations of type X collagen confirm COL10A1 as the Schmid metaphyseal chondrodysplasia locus. Hum Mol Genet 1994;3:303

McKusick-Type Metaphyseal Chondrodysplasia

Mäkitie O, Kaitila I: Cartilage-hair hypoplasia—clinical manifestations in 108 Finnish patients. Eur J Pediatr 1993;152:211

Mäkitie O, Marttinen E, Kaitila I: Skeletal growth in cartilage-hair hypoplasia: a radiological study of 82 patients. Pediatr Radiol 1992;22:434

van der Burgt I, Haraldsson A, Oosterwijk JC, et al: Cartilage hair hypoplasia, metaphyseal chondrodysplasia type McKusick: description of seven patients and review of the literature. Am J Med Genet 1991;41:371

Shwachman-Diamond Syndrome

McLennan TW, Steinbach HL: Shwachman's syndrome: the broad spectrum of bony abnormalities. Radiology 1974;112:167

Robberecht E, Nachtegaele P, Van Rattinghe R, et al: Pancreatic lipomatosis in the Shwachman-Diamond syndrome: identification by sonography and CT-scan. Pediatr Radiol 1985;15:348

Shwachman H, Diamond L: The syndrome of pancreatic insufficiency and bone marrow dysfunction. J Pediatr 1964;65:645

Taybi H, Mitchell AD, Friedman GD: Metaphyseal dysostosis and associated syndrome of pancreatic insufficiency and blood disorders. Radiology 1969;93:563

Kozlowski-Type Spondylometaphyseal Dysplasia

Kozlowski K, Maroteaux P, Spranger JW: La dysostose spondylo-métaphysaire. Presse Med 1967;75:2769

Lachman R, Zonana J, Khajavi A, et al: The spondylometaphyseal dysplasias: clinical, radiologic and pathologic correlation [in French]. Ann Radiol (Paris) 1979;22:125

Dyschondrosteosis

Belin V, Cusin V, Viot G, et al: SHOX mutations in dyschondrosteosis (Leri-Weill syndrome). Nat Genet 1998;19:67

Carter AR, Currey HL: Dyschondrosteosis (mesomelic dwarfism)—a family study. Br J Radiol 1974;47:634

Young LW, Goldberg EE, Morrison J: Radiological case of the month: Dyschondrosteosis. Am J Dis Child 1978;132:1038

Trichorhinophalangeal Syndrome Types I and II

Fryns JP, Logghe N, van Eygen M, et al: Langer-Giedion syndrome and deletion of the long arm of chromosome 8. Hum Genet 1981;58:231

Giedion A: Das tricho-rhino-phalangeale syndrome. Helv Paediatr Acta 1966;21:475

Hamers A, Jongbloet P, Peeters G, et al: Severe mental retardation in a patient with tricho-rhino-phalangeal syndrome type I and 8q deletion. Eur J Pediatr 1990;149:618

Ludecke HJ, Wagner MJ, Nardmann J, et al: Molecular dissection of a contiguous gene syndrome: localization of the genes involved in Langer-Giedion syndrome. Hum Mol Genet 1995;4:31

Momeni P, Glockner G, Schmidt O, et al: Mutations in a new gene, encoding a zinc-finger protein, cause tricho-rhino-phalangeal syndrome type I. Nat Genet 2000;24:71

Parizel PM, Dumon J, Vossen P, et al: The tricho-rhino-phalangeal syndrome revisited. Eur J Radiol 1987;7:154

Zaletaev DV, Kuleshov NP, Lur'e IV, et al: Langer-Giedion syndrome and a deletion in the long arm of chromosome 8 [in Russian]. Genetika 1987;213:907

Acromesomelic Dysplasia of Maroteaux

Borrelli P, Fasanelli S, Marini R: Acromesomelic dwarfism in a child with an interesting family history. Pediatr Radiol 1983;13:165

Kant SG, Polinkovsky A, Mundlos S: Acromesomelic dysplasia Maroteaux type maps to human chromosome 9. Am J Hum Genet 1998;63:155

Langer LO, Garrett RT: Acromesomelic dysplasia. Radiology 1980;137:349

Langer LO Jr, Beals RK, Solomon IL, et al: Acromesomelic dwarfism: manifestations in childhood. Am J Med Genet 1977;1:87

Maroteaux P, Martinelli B, Campailla E: Le nanisme acromésomélique. Presse Med 1971;79:1839

Cleidocranial Dysplasia

Keats TE: Cleidocranial dysostosis: some atypical roentgen manifestations. Am J Roentgenol Radium Ther Nucl Med 1967;100:71

Mundlos S: Cleidocranial dysplasia: clinical and molecular genetics. J Med Genet 1999;36:177

Campomelic Dysplasia

Khajavi A, Lachman R, Rimoin D, et al: Heterogeneity in the campomelic syndromes: long and short bone varieties. Radiology 1976;120:641

Macpherson RI, Skinner SA, Donnenfeld AE: Acampomelic campomelic dysplasia. Pediatr Radiol 1989;20:90

Tommerup N, Schempp W, Meinecke P, et al: Assignment of an autosomal sex reversal locus (SRA1) and campomelic dysplasia (CMPD1) to 17q24.3-q25.1. Nat Genet 1993;4:170

Mucopolysaccharidoses

Nelson J, Broadhead D, Mossman J: Clinical findings in 12 patients with MPS IV A (Morquio's disease): further evidence for heterogeneity. Part I: Clinical and biochemical findings. Clin Genet 1988;33:111

Schmidt H, Ullrich K, von Lengerke HJ, et al: Radiological findings in patients with mucopolysaccharidosis I H/S (Hurler-Scheie syndrome). Pediatr Radiol 1987;17:409

Spranger J: Mini review: inborn errors of complex carbohydrate metabolism. Am J Med Genet 1987;28:489

van der Horst GTJ, Kleijer WJ, Hoogeveen AT, et al: Morquio B syndrome: a primary defect in β-galactosidase. Am J Med Genet 1983;16:261

Mucolipidosis Type II (I-Cell Disease)

Babcock DS, Bove KE, Hug G, et al: Fetal mucolipidosis II (I-cell disease): radiologic and pathologic correlation. Pediatr Radiol 1986;16:32

Lemaitre L, Remy J, Farriaux JP, et al: Radiological signs of mucolipidosis II or I-cell disease: a study of nine cases. Pediatr Radiol 1978;7:97

Osteogenesis Imperfecta

Byers PH, Wallis GA, Willing MC: Osteogenesis imperfecta: translation of mutation to phenotype. J Med Genet 1991;28:433

Lachman RS: Fetal imaging in the skeletal dysplasias: overview and experience. Pediatr Radiol 1994;24:413

Sillence DO, Barlow KK, Garber AP, et al: Osteogenesis imperfecta type II: delineation of the phenotype with reference to genetic heterogeneity. Am J Med Genet 1984;17:407

Tabor EK, Curtin HD, Hirsch BE, May M: Osteogenesis imperfecta tarda: appearance of the temporal bones at CT. Radiology 1990;175:181

Hypophosphatasia

Oestreich AE, Bofinger MK: Prominent transverse (Bowdler) bone spurs as a diagnostic clue in a case of neonatal hypophosphatasia without metaphyseal irregularity. Pediatr Radiol 1989;19:341

Shohat M, Rimoin DL, Gruber HE, et al: Perinatal lethal hypophosphatasia: clinical, radiologic and morphologic findings. Pediatr Radiol 1991;21:421

Osteopetrosis

Andersen PE Jr, Bollerslev J: Heterogeneity of autosomal dominant osteopetrosis. Radiology 1987;164:223

el-Tawil T, Stoker DJ: Benign osteopetrosis: a review of 42 cases showing two different patterns. Skeletal Radiol 1993;22:587

Horton WA, Schimke RN, Iyama T: Osteopetrosis: further heterogeneity. J Pediatr 1980;97:580

Kaibara N, Katsuki I, Hotokebuchi T, et al: Intermediate form of osteopetrosis with recessive inheritance. Skeletal Radiol 1982;9:47

Kaplan FS, August CS, Fallon MD, et al: Osteopetrorickets: the paradox of plenty. Pathophysiology and treatment. Clin Orthop Relat Res 1993;294:64

Otsuka N, Fukunaga M, Ono S, et al: Bone marrow scintigraphy and MRI in a patient with osteopetrosis. Clin Nucl Med 1991;16:443

Rao VM, Dalinka MK, Mitchell DG, et al: Osteopetrosis: MR characteristics at 1.5 T. Radiology 1986;161:217

Schroeder RE, et al: Longitudinal follow-up of malignant osteopetrosis by skeletal radiographs and RLFP analysis after bone marrow transplantation. Pediatr 1992;88:986

Pyknodysostosis

Currarino G: Primary spondylolysis of the axis vertebra (C2) in three children, including one with pyknodysostosis. Pediatr Radiol 1989;19:535

Maroteaux P, Lamy M: La pycnodysostose. Presse Med 1962;70:999

Yousefzadeh DK, Agha AS, Reinertson J: Radiographic studies of upper airway obstruction with cor pulmonale in a patient with pycnodysostosis. Pediatr Radiol 1979;8:45

Craniodiaphyseal Dysplasia

Brueton LA, Winter RM: Craniodiaphyseal dysplasia. J Med Genet 1990;27:701

Tucker AS, Klein L, Antony GJ: Craniodiaphyseal dysplasia: evolution over a five-year period. Skeletal Radiol 1976;1:47

Craniometaphyseal Dysplasia

Carnevale A, Grether P, del Castillo V, et al: Autosomal dominant craniometaphyseal dysplasia: clinical variability. Clin Genet 1983;23:17

Holt JF: The evolution of cranio-metaphyseal dysplasia. Ann Radiol 1966;9:209

Penchaszadeh VB, Gutierrez ER, Figueroa E: Autosomal recessive craniometaphyseal dysplasia. Am J Med Genet 1980;5:43

Pyle Dysplasia

Heselson NG, Raad MS, Hamersma H: The radiological manifestations of metaphyseal dysplasia (Pyle disease). Br J Radiol 1979;52:431

Shibuya H, Suzuki S, Okuyama T, et al: The radiological appearances of familial metaphyseal dysplasia. Clin Radiol 1982;33:439

Osteopoikilosis

Günal I, Kiter E: Disorders associated with osteopoikilosis: 5 different lesions in a family. Acta Orthop Scand 2003;74:497

Lagier R, Mbakop A, Bigler A: Osteopoikilosis: a radiological and pathological study. Skeletal Radiol 1984;11:161

Osteopathia Striata

Lee RD: Clinical images of osteopathia striata. Pediatr Radiol 2004;34:753

Ward LM, Rauch F, Travers R, et al: Osteopathia striata with cranial sclerosis: clinical, radiological, and bone histological findings in an adolescent girl. Am J Med Genet A 2004;129:8

Melorheostosis

Freyschmidt J: Melorheostosis: a review of 23 cases. Eur Radiol 2001;11:474

Hellemans J, Preobrazhenska O, Willaert A, et al: Loss-of-function mutations in LEMD3 result in osteopoikilosis, Buschke-Ollendorff syndrome and melorheostosis. Nat Genet 2004;36:1213

Spondyloenchondromatosis

Frydman M, Bar-Ziv J, Preminger-Shapiro R, et al: Possible heterogeneity in spondyloenchondrodysplasia: quadriparesis, basal ganglia calcifications, and chondrocyte inclusions. Am J Med Genet 1990;36:279

Menger H, Kruse K, Spranger J: Spondyloenchondrodysplasia. J Med Genet 1989;26:93

Schorr S, Legum C, Ochshorn M: Spondyloenchondrodysplasia: enchondromatosis with severe platyspondyly in two brothers. Radiology 1976;118:133

Dysspondyloenchondromatosis

Azouz EM: Case report 418: multiple enchondromatosis (Ollier disease) with severe vertebral changes. Skeletal Radiol 1987;16:236

Freisinger P, Finidori G, Maroteaux P: Dysspondylochondromatosis. Am J Med Genet 1993;45:460

Kozlowski K, Brostrom K, Kennedy J, et al: Dysspondyloenchondromatosis in the newborn: report of four cases. Pediatr Radiol 1994;24:311

Osteolysis Group

Macpherson RI, Walker RD, Kowall MH: Essential osteolysis with nephropathy. J Can Assoc Radiol 1973;24:98

Tuncbilek E, Besim A, Bakkaloglu A, et al: Carpal-tarsal osteolysis. Pediatr Radiol 1985;15:255

Nail–Patella Syndrome

Dreyer SD, Morello R, German MS, et al: LMX1B transactivation and expression in nail-patella syndrome. Hum Mol Genet 2000;9:1067

Guidera KJ, Satterwhite Y, Ogden JA, et al: Nail patella syndrome: a review of 44 orthopaedic patients. J Pediatr Orthop 1991;11:737

Reed D, Nichols DM: Computed tomography of "iliac horns" in hereditary osteo-onychodysplasia (nail-patella syndrome). Pediatr Radiol 1987;17:168

166 Selected Syndromes and Chromosomal Disorders

WILLIAM H. MCALISTER, THOMAS E. HERMAN, and
KEITH A. KRONEMER

Our knowledge base in the realm of developmental biology and pathobiology of inherited and acquired conditions continues to expand at a remarkable pace. In this chapter, we have chosen to present the syndromes and chromosomal disorders (Table 166-1) that we believe would be of greatest interest and usefulness to radiologists. Although this chapter focuses on the musculoskeletal findings in these syndromes and chromosomal disorders, major findings in other organ systems are also presented and occasionally illustrated.

BARDET-BIEDL SYNDROME

Bardet-Biedl syndrome (BBS) is an autosomal recessive condition now separated from the Lawrence-Moon syndrome, a very rare condition with some features of BBS but characterized additionally by progressive spastic paralysis and ataxia. However, BBS remains genetically heterogeneous, with linkage to eight loci (*BBS1* through *BBS8*). These genes have been shown to have gene products involved in normal cilia formation. As a consequence of this association, a high frequency of anosmia is now noted among patients with BBS, because the olfactory system is one of the most cilia-rich parts of the body. Previously, anosmia was not frequently mentioned by patients or recognized as a problem since it was present from birth or shortly after birth. Characteristic features of BBS are obesity (92%), retinitis pigmentosa (92%), mental retardation (82%), polydactyly (72%), hypogenitalism (67%), and renal disease (approximately 100%). Other occasional features include heart disease (7%), diabetes mellitus (32% of patients by age 55 years), hearing loss, speech impairment, hepatic fibrosis, situs inversus, and Hirschsprung disease. In infancy, before obesity (at a mean age of 2 years) and retinitis pigmentosa (at a mean age of 8 years) develop, BBS may be confused with McKusick-Kaufman syndrome, which is an allelic disorder due to *BBS6* mutations.

Complications of BBS are often severe. Almost all patients are blind by age 30 years. Approximately 25% of patients die before 44 years of age, with renal failure frequently being the cause of death.

Calyceal clubbing and blunting in the absence of reflux, persistent fetal lobulation, small kidneys with parenchymal thinning, multiple renal calyceal diverticula (multidiverticular renal dysplasia) (Fig. 166-1), and histologic findings of glomerulopathy and tubulointerstitial nephropathy are the most frequent renal findings. Urinary tract infection and stone formation are common complications of the multidiverticular renal dysplasia. An early clinical manifestation of renal disease is polydipsia and polyuria due to a concentrating deficiency resulting from decreased responsiveness to vasopressin. In some cases, this may progress to nephrogenic diabetes insipidus.

Multidiverticular renal dysplasia is characteristically a stable, congenital anomaly not related to reflux. Cavities seen in renal tuberculosis, isolated calyceal diverticula, and renal papillary necrosis may appear radiographically similar. The congenital nature and multiplicity of the diverticula excludes these diagnoses relative to BBS.

Hypogonadism is more obvious in male patients with BBS than in female patients. Hydrocolpos and vaginal atresia are common in females with this syndrome.

BECKWITH-WIEDEMANN SYNDROME

Beckwith-Wiedemann syndrome (BWS) is a genetically complex condition characterized by exomphalos (anterior abdominal wall defects), macroglossia, hemihypertrophy, nephromegaly, islet cell hyperplasia, nephroblastomatosis, adrenal cytomegaly, neonatal adrenal macrocysts, linearly grooved earlobes, intestinal malrotation, and an increased incidence of benign and malignant tumors.

BWS is a complex disorder genetically. It is associated with alterations in imprinted genes at chromosome 11p15. Imprinted genes are genes that are expressed exclusively or at least predominantly from either the maternal or paternal allele. Abnormalities of chromosome 11p15 are present in 85% of patients with BWS. These abnormalities are usually in regulation of imprinting and not chromosomal alterations. There are two large imprinted domains at chromosome locus 11p15. Two imprinted genes occur in domain 1: the paternally expressed, maternally imprinted insulin-like growth factor II (*IGF2*), and *H19*, a maternally expressed, paternally imprinted tumor suppressor gene. Multiple genes are associated with BWS in the imprinted domain 2. BWS can be associated with abnormalities in either domain, but tumor risk is highest with paternal uniparental disomy (both alleles of some imprinted gene derived from the father) or hypermethylation of *H19*. Eighty-five percent of BWS

TABLE 166-1

Selected Syndromes and Chromosomal Disorders

SYNDROMES

Bardet-Biedl
Beckwith-Wiedemann
Brachmann-de Lange (Cornelia de Lange)
Cerebrocostomandibular (rib-gap)
Cerebrohepatorenal (Zellweger)
Cockayne
Congenital contractural arachnodactyly
Congenital insensitivity to pain
Currarino triad
Diamond-Blackfan
Ehlers-Danlos
Epidermolysis bullosa
Fanconi anemia
Fetal alcohol
Freeman-Sheldon ("whistling face")
Gaucher
Hadju-Cheney
Hallermann-Streiff
Holt-Oram
Homocystinuria
Hypertrophic osteoarthropathy
Idiopathic (isolated) hemihypertrophy
Larsen
Marfan
Marshall-Smith
McKusick-Kaufman
Meckel
Neurofibromatosis
Nevoid basal cell carcinoma

Niemann-Pick
Noonan
Occipital horn
Opitz (G/BBB)
Oral-facial-digital
Osteolysis
Otopalatodigital
Pachydermoperiostosis
Pena-Shokeir, types I & II
Poland
Progeria
Proteus
Rubinstein-Taybi
Russell-Silver
Smith-Lemli-Opitz
Sotos
Thrombocytopenia–absent radius
Tuberous sclerosis
VACTERL association
Warfarin embryopathy
Weill-Marchesani
Werner

CHROMOSOMAL DISORDERS

Cri du chat
Klinefelter
Trisomy 13
Trisomy 18
Trisomy 21
Turner
Wolf-Hirschhorn

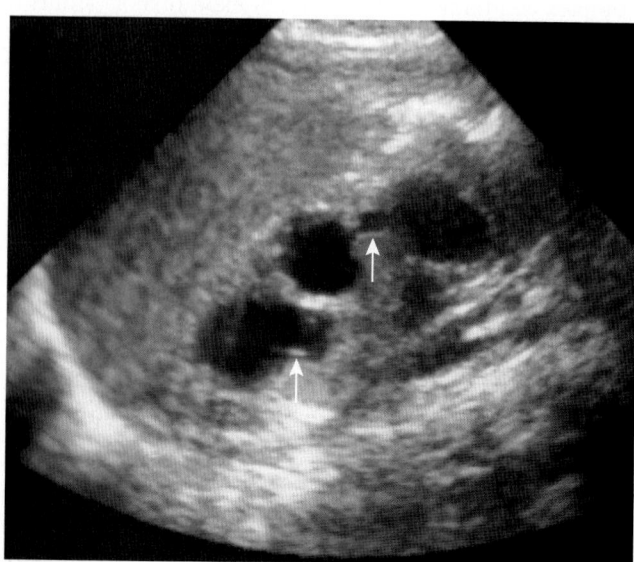

FIGURE 166-1. Bardet-Biedl syndrome. Longitudinal right renal sonogram shows caliectasis with cortical thinning and a small calyceal diverticulum from a lower pole calyx and a larger one from an upper pole calyx consistent with multidiverticular renal dysplasia seen in this syndrome. *Arrows* indicate diverticula.

cases are sporadic. Another 10% to 15% have a pedigree of autosomal dominant inheritance with preferential maternal transmission. However, the inheritance of the syndrome may be complex because imprinting is common. Imprinting is the functional difference between maternally and paternally derived chromosomes. The paternal mutation is associated with an excess of growth promoter and the maternal mutation with a deficiency of growth suppression.

Originally, BWS was described as a triad of exomphalos, macroglossia, and gigantism. The most characteristic of these abnormalities is macroglossia, which occurs in 99% of patients and often requires surgical reduction due to feeding and respiratory difficulties (Fig. 166-2). Gigantism, defined as postnatal size over the 90th percentile, is present in 87% of patients. Anterior abdominal wall defects occur in 50% to 70% of patients. Hemihypertrophy is found in 25% and is the only clinical feature highly associated with the development of malignancy (see later section on idiopathic [isolated] hemihypertrophy). Neonatal nephromegaly may be associated with an increased risk of Wilms tumor. Neonatal hypoglycemia is usually transient but in severe cases may be prolonged and associated with neurologic damage if not appropriately treated.

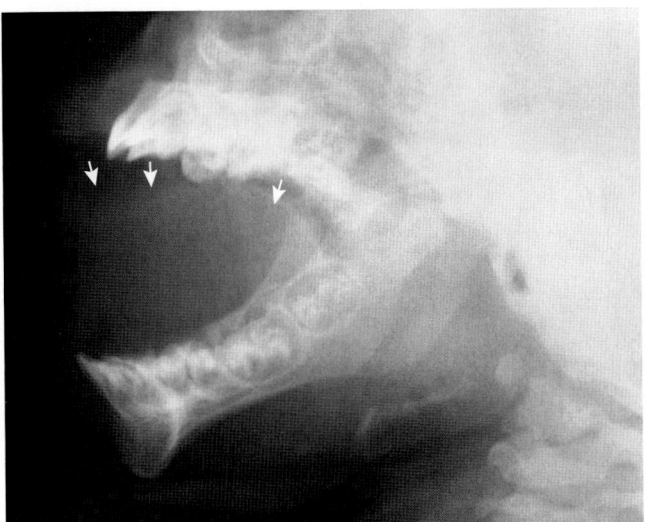

FIGURE 166-2. Beckwith-Wiedemann syndrome. Lateral facial radiograph shows a massively enlarged tongue *(arrows)* is present in the oral cavity holding the mouth open. In addition, the child had an omphalocele and a birth weight of over 4 kg.

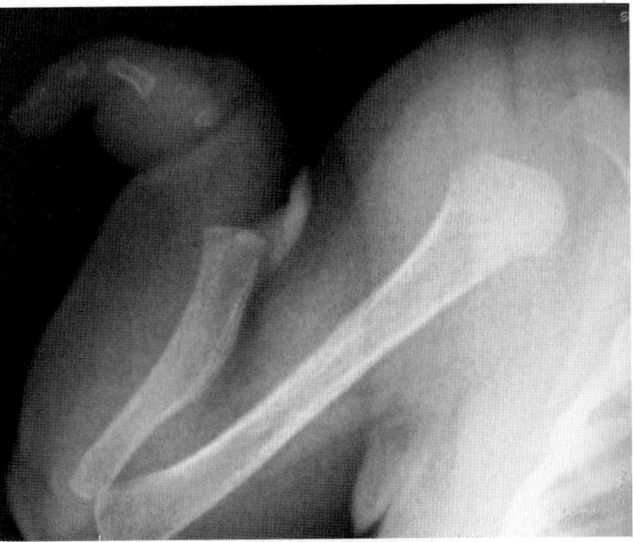

FIGURE 166-3. Brachmann-de Lange (Cornelia de Lange) syndrome. Radiograph of right upper extremity showing absent ulna, shortened radius, and a single digit, the thumb.

The risk of malignant tumor in patients with BWS is approximately 7%. The most common malignant tumors are Wilms tumor, adrenal carcinoma, hepatoblastoma, and neuroblastoma. Other reported tumors that may occur include rhabdomyosarcoma, pancreatoblastoma, breast fibroadenoma, gastric teratoma, hepatic hemangioendothelioma, and splenic hemangioma. Most BWS patients with tumors have been found to have a relatively favorable outcome. Although controversial, tumor surveillance screening in BWS is widely practiced, with current recommendations for abdominal sonography to evaluate for renal, adrenal, pancreatic, and hepatic masses every 3 to 6 months to at least the age of 6 years and possibly to 12 years of age.

BRACHMANN-DE LANGE (CORNELIA DE LANGE) SYNDROME

The Brachmann-de Lange syndrome is characterized by mental retardation, a low birth weight, postnatal growth retardation, characteristic facies (synophrys, low anterior hairline, long eyelashes, microbrachycephaly, short upturned nose, and "carp mouth"), and upper limb anomalies. Clinical findings vary considerably. Mutations in *NIPBL*, the human analog of the *Drosophila Nipped B* gene, have been identified as a cause of this syndrome. More severe phenotypes are related to truncating mutations.

The radiographic changes in the upper limbs may be severe but variable, and include micromelia, phocomelia, dislocation, deformity of the radial heads, and ulnar dysgenesis. Severe cases have reduction deformities of the ulna and ulnar portion of the hand (Fig. 166-3). Most other syndromes have a radial rather than an ulnar deficiency. Digital findings are most common and are variable but often symmetric. Findings include proximally placed thumbs, short and broad first metacarpals, syndactyly, clinodactyly, oligodactyly, ectrodactyly, abnormal metacarpophalangeal pattern profile, small

digits, and delayed skeletal maturation. Findings in the thorax are increased anteroposterior diameter, short sternum with reduced number of ossification centers and premature fusion, slender and sloping ribs, fusion of first two ribs, laterally hooked clavicles, and tracheomegaly. Gastrointestinal problems are common, can be severe, and include reflux esophagitis, aspiration pneumonia, esophageal stenosis, Barrett esophagus, cecal volvulus, and Sandifer complex. Miscellaneous findings include clubfoot, flattened acetabuli, Legg-Perthes disease, supracondylar spurs, large anterior fontanelle, and small brachycephalic skull. First-trimester nuchal translucency has been described with Brachmann-de Lange syndrome, as has congenital dysgenesis in the brain. Structural abnormalities involving the kidneys are common.

Based on the clinical variability of Brachmann-de Lange syndrome, the following classification has been proposed:

Type I (classic form)—characteristic and skeletal changes, growth deficiency, and severe psychomotor retardation

Type II—milder clinical manifestations.

Type III (phenocopy type)—causally related to chromosomal aneuploidies or teratogenic exposures.

There are no biochemical/genetic tests that can make the diagnosis; therefore, the diagnosis of Brachmann-de Lange syndrome is based on characteristic facial features, prenatal and postnatal growth retardation, mental retardation, and the deficiency defects of the upper limbs.

CEREBROCOSTOMANDIBULAR (RIB-GAP) SYNDROME

Cerebrocostomandibular syndrome, also called rib-gap syndrome, is characterized by features of the Pierre Robin syndrome (small mandible, cleft palate, glossoptosis), and posterior rib gaps. Rib gaps usually occur in

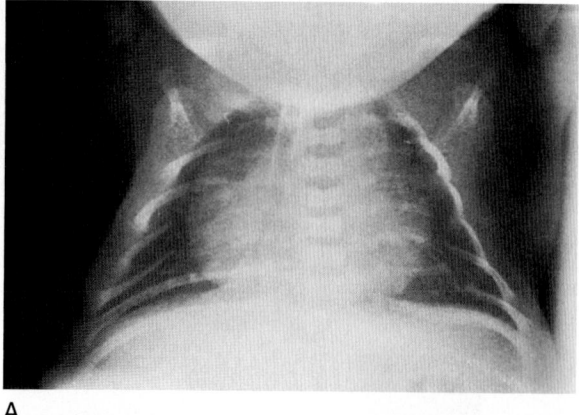

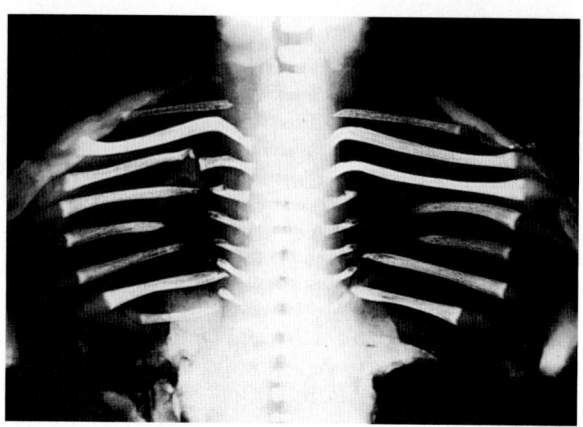

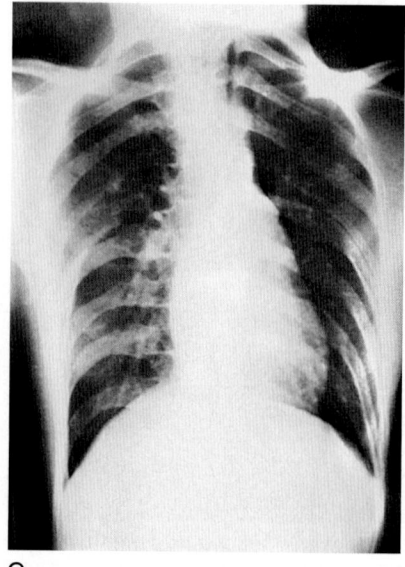

FIGURE 166-4. Cerebrocostomandibular syndrome. **A,** Posterior rib defects are seen in infancy on chest radiograph. **B,** An outfolded chest wall at necropsy shows multiple rib gaps after removal of the thoracic contents. **C,** In the survivors, the chest radiograph shows that some of the defects may fill in, resulting in a deformed but intact thoracic cage. (From Silverman FN, Strefling AM, Stevenson DK, et al: Cerebro-costo-mandibular syndrome. J Pediatr 1980;97:408-416.)

the third through the seventh ribs, although all levels have been reported (Fig. 166-4). Neonatal respiratory distress is the usual presenting sign. Eventually the rib gaps, which can be symmetric, will partially heal and may give rise to pseudoarthrosis (see Fig. 166-4). The rib gaps are filled with fibrovascular tissue. Mental retardation is seen in one half of the patients and microcephaly in 20%. Miscellaneous findings include stippled epiphyses, clubfoot, elbow dysplasia, scoliosis, progressive kyphosis, multiple ossification centers of the calcaneus, vesicoureteral reflux, and renal cysts. The diagnosis has been made prenatally. The syndrome is likely autosomal recessive, but evidence of autosomal dominant inheritance has also been reported.

CEREBROHEPATORENAL (ZELLWEGER) SYNDROME

Cerebrohepatorenal (Zellweger) syndrome is the result of mutation of genes involved in peroxisome biogenesis. Knowledge of the exact *PEX1* gene mutation helps predict the course of the disease, which is more severe than adrenoleukodystrophy or infantile Refsum disease. Findings include characteristic flat facies with a high forehead, severe hypotonia, seizures, mental retardation, liver enlargement and dysfunction, stippled epiphyses, and renal cysts. Infants, because of the facies, have been confused with those with Down syndrome. The most helpful radiographic findings are stripped calcifications,

typically affecting the patellae and the Y cartilages of the pelvis. The calcifications may involve many areas and may be periarticular (Fig. 166-5). The renal cysts tend to be small and in the periphery of the kidneys (see Fig. 166-5). Prenatal sonography may show the cysts and renal hyperechogenicity. Hyperoxaluria may occur and give rise to urolithiasis and nephrocalcinosis.

Within the central nervous system, findings include dysmyelination and neuronal migration derangements resulting in microgyria, pachygyria, heterotopic dysplasia, cortical malformations (greatest in the prerolandic and presylvian cortices), ventricular dilation, periventricular and caudothalamic groove cysts, and leukoencephalopathy. Skull findings include widened cranial sutures and dolichocephaly. Proton magnetic resonance spectroscopy has shown findings suspicious for this syndrome. Gastrointestinal abnormalities include anorectal malformations, intestinal lymphangiectasia, and hepatomegaly with abnormal liver function studies. Extremity abnormalities include contractures, clubfoot, and delayed skeletal maturation. Fetal hypokinesia and increased nuchal translucency have been noted in utero. Patients with cerebrohepatorenal syndrome typically die in infancy; however, some patients have lived into the teenage years.

COCKAYNE SYNDROME

Manifestations of Cockayne syndrome usually begin at birth with progressive growth failure. Findings include

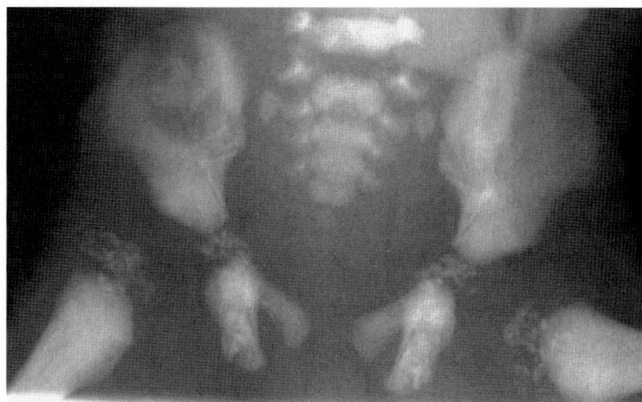

A

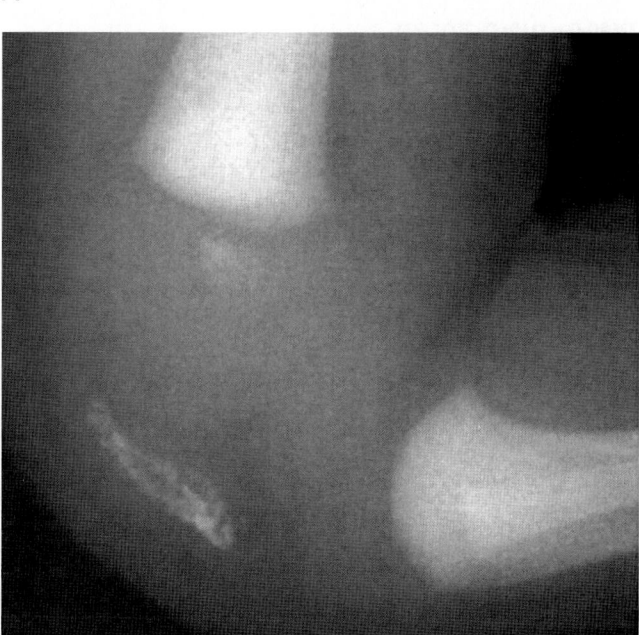

B

FIGURE 166-5. Cerebrohepatorenal (Zellweger) syndrome. **A,** Pelvic radiograph of a newborn shows stippled calcifications in the femoral heads and the Y cartilage of the pelvis. **B,** Lateral knee radiograph of a different patient shows small calcifications within the patella. **C,** Transverse sonogram of left kidney shows cysts, the largest of which is indicated by an *arrow*.

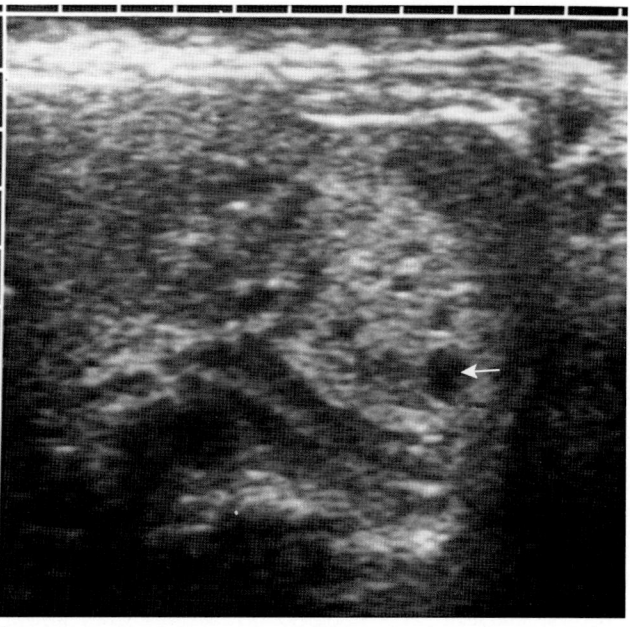

C

microcephaly, mental retardation, sun sensitivity, premature aging (Fig. 166-6), sensorineural hearing loss, abnormal nerve conduction, dwarfing with a short trunk and relatively large hands and feet, flexion contractures, and eye abnormalities (enophthalmos, retinal pigmentation and degeneration, optic atrophy, and cataracts). Exposure of cells to ultraviolet light results in chromosomal breakage. Cockayne syndrome is autosomal recessive. Radiographic findings include microcephaly, thin long bones with narrow medullary cavities and flared metaphyses, large-appearing ossification centers, large carpal and tarsal bones, hypoplasia of the iliac wings and acetabular roofs, slender clavicles, brachydactyly, ivory epiphyses in the distal phalanges, short and broad metacarpals and metatarsals, thin ribs (Fig. 166-7), coxa valga, fibular bowing, and abnormal vertebral bodies with anterior notching with resultant kyphosis or posterior scalloping. Progressive osteolysis may occur.

In addition to microcephaly, the sella is small and the calvaria is thick. Calcification in the cerebral cortex and basal ganglia, ventricular dilation, demyelination, leukodystrophy, and atrophy are common. The classic

form of Cockayne syndrome is called type I, an early-onset, more severe form associated with early death is called type II, and a mild form of the disease is called type III. The diagnosis can be confirmed by a biochemical transcription assay.

CONGENITAL CONTRACTURAL ARACHNODACTYLY

Congenital contractural arachnodactyly, also called Beals syndrome, is an autosomal dominant disorder of connective tissue that is characterized by arachnodactyly, multiple congenital flexion contractures, external ear malformations (crumpled ears), and progressive kyphoscoliosis. It is phenotypically related to Marfan syndrome. Mutations in the fibrillin-2 (*FBN2*) gene cause this syndrome. This gene has been mapped to the 5q23-31 region of chromosome 5, making prenatal diagnosis possible.

The imaging findings consist of arachnodactyly (Fig. 166-8), camptodactyly, and flexion contractures. The flexion contractures are usually symmetric and

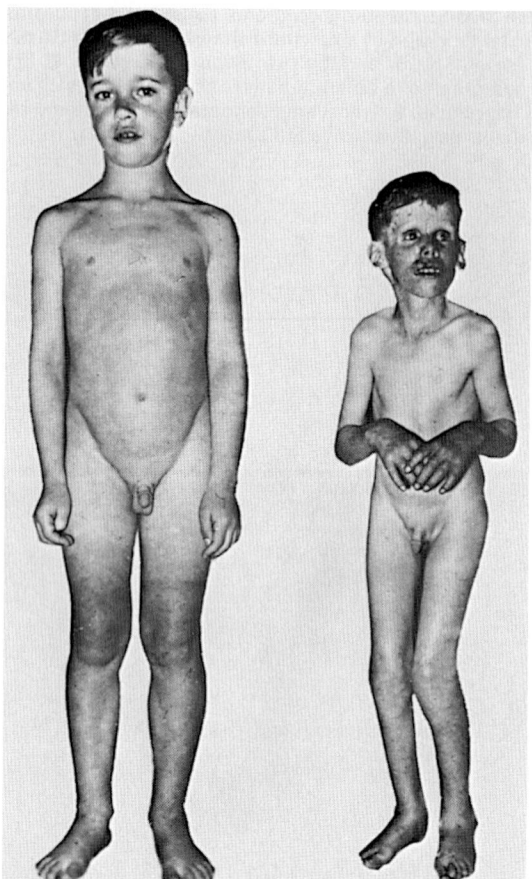

FIGURE 166-6. Cockayne syndrome. Normal boy **(left)** and affected boy **(right)**, both age 10 years. The patient with Cockayne syndrome has short stature, shriveled facies, microcephaly, large ears and large lower jaw, and disproportionately large hands and feet. (From MacDonald WB, Fitch KD, Lewis IC: Cockayne's syndrome: an heredofamilial disorder of growth and development. Pediatrics 1960;25:997-1007.)

affect the knees most severely. Elbow and proximal interphalangeal joints are also prone to have flexion contractures. As the contractures improve during childhood, scoliosis or kyphoscoliosis appears, although it may be present in infancy. Kyphoscoliosis is progressive, usually starts before age 5 years, and may be associated with restrictive lung disease. The long bones are long and narrow, and, along with normal-width epiphyses, make the joints appear prominent. Slight long bone bowing and protrusio acetabuli may be present. Skeletal adaptive changes are seen in the joints secondary to contractures. The muscles are hypoplastic. Congenital limb deficiencies may be seen, as may heart abnormalities, particularly mitral valve prolapse and aortic root dilation. The gastrointestinal abnormalities include duodenal atresia, esophageal atresia, and intestinal malrotation.

CONGENITAL INSENSITIVITY TO PAIN

Congenital insensitivity to pain is an autosomal recessive syndrome characterized by decreased sensitivity to pain without affecting touch or proprioception. Congenital insensitivity is due to a mutation on chromosome 1 that leads to a defect in nerve growth factor-β (*NGFB*). The typical clinical presentation is an insidious progressive joint swelling. The foot and ankle tend to be the most common areas of involvement. Subperiosteal hemorrhages may occur in neonates, with later development of fractures, epiphyseal separations, periosteal new bone formation, and dislocations of weight-bearing joints (Fig. 166-9). Avascular necrosis, Charcot arthropathy, and heterotopic ossification can occur (see Fig. 166-9). Skin ulcerations or surgical interventions may lead to osteomyelitis. Child abuse has been misdiagnosed in patients with congenital insensitivity to pain. Spinal Charcot arthropathy and spondylolisthesis may also occur.

CURRARINO TRIAD

Currarino triad (hereditary sacral agenesis syndrome) consists of congenital anal stenosis or low imperforate anus, sickle or scimitar hemisacrum (Fig. 166-10), and a presacral mass. The presacral mass may be a teratoma (two thirds of cases), a lipoma, a dermoid cyst, an enteric cyst, or an anterior meningocele (see Fig. 166-10). An intact first sacral segment and a sickle-shaped sacrum is a distinctive anomaly in this syndrome. Myelodysplasia with tethered cord and intradural lipoma also occur frequently. The syndrome is linked to the mutations in the *HLXB9* homeobox gene at 7q36. Currarino triad is autosomal dominant syndrome. Approximately 50% of the cases are familial. Approximately one third of patients with anal stenosis have Currarino triad. In these patients, spinal magnetic resonance imaging (MRI) is helpful to exclude associated lesions such as tethered cord or meningomyelocele. Although constipation is the most frequent symptom, life-threatening meningitis and sepsis may occur, particularly with presacral anterior meningoceles. In fact, anoplasty should be preceded by neurosurgical repair and colostomy in patients with anterior meningoceles to reduce the risk of meningitis. Moreover, approximately 50% of presacral tumors communicate with the spinal canal in Currarino triad, making surgical repair difficult without neurologic complications. Although most presacral masses in Currarino syndrome are benign, malignant presacral masses may occur. Such tumors are primarily malignant presacral teratomas, but leiomyosarcoma and malignant neuroendocrine tumors have been reported. The risk of presacral malignancy is particularly high in patients presenting after the first decade of life. However, malignant teratoma has occurred in children as young as 2 years of age.

> **Currarino Triad:**
> - **Congenital anal stenosis or low imperforate anus**
> - **Sickle or scimitar hemisacrum**
> - **Presacral mass (teratoma, lipoma, dermoid cyst, enteric cyst, or anterior meningocele)**

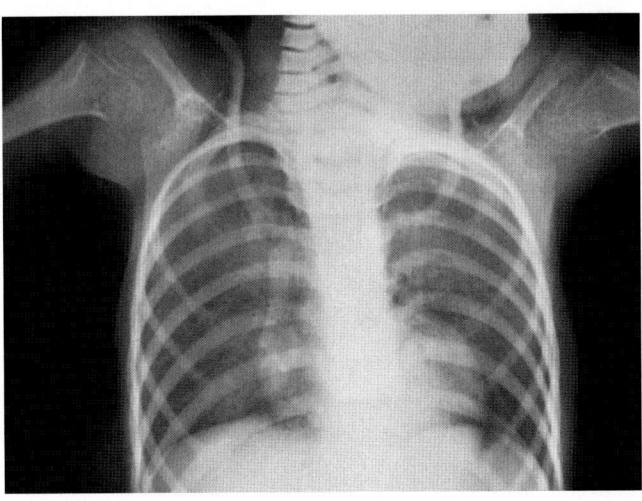

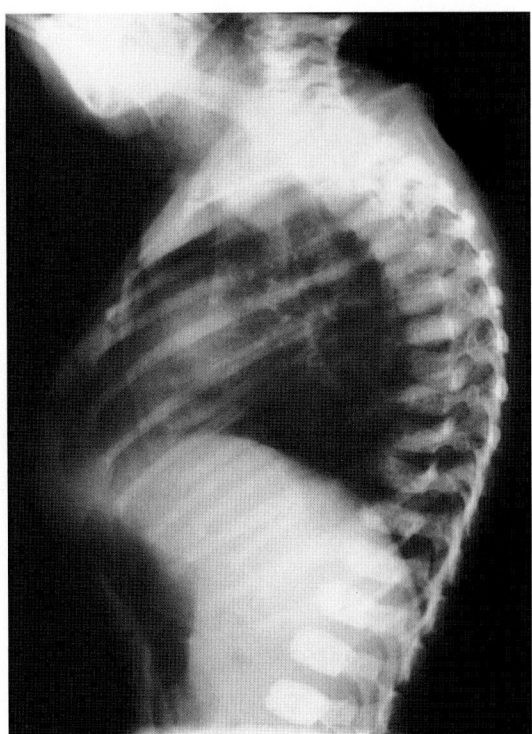

FIGURE 166-7. Cockayne syndrome. Frontal **(A)** and lateral **(B)** radiographs of the chest on an extremely small 5-year-old showing thin, sclerotic ribs and clavicles and proximal humeri, osteopenia, and an increased anteroposterior diameter of the chest.

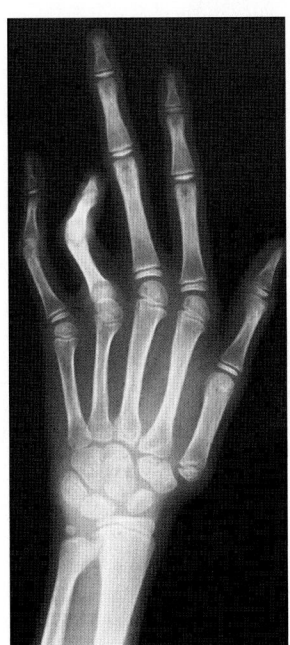

FIGURE 166-8. Contractural arachnodactyly. Posteroanterior radiograph of the right hand of a 9-year-old girl demonstrating the arachnodactyly and flexion deformities of the fourth and fifth digits and mild osteopenia.

DIAMOND-BLACKFAN SYNDROME

Diamond-Blackfan anemia is a constitutional erythroblastopenia characterized by absent or decreased erythroid precursors, usually presenting in the first year of life. Most cases are sporadic, but autosomal dominant and recessive inheritance have also been reported. Often, there is an association with mutations encoding ribosomal protein S19 and with a variety of malformations. Physical abnormalities are seen in one third of patients and are more prevalent in boys (50%) than girls

(25%). Thumb abnormalities, especially a triphalangeal thumb, are the most characteristic radiographic feature but are found in only 18% of the patients (Fig. 166-11). Other findings in the thumb include hypoplasia, duplication, subluxation, absence, and flat thenar eminence. Radial ray anomalies, Klippel-Feil syndrome, Sprengel deformity, and growth retardation may be seen. Renal findings include horseshoe kidney, renal dysplasia, and hypoplasia. Abnormal facial features include snub nose, thick upper lips, widely separated eyes, and cleft palate. Patients with Diamond-Blackfan syndrome have a predisposition to cancer. Successful stem cell transplantation has occurred.

EHLERS-DANLOS SYNDROME

Ehlers-Danlos syndrome (EDS) is a heterogeneous group of inherited anomalies of connective tissue characterized by varying degrees of skin hyperextensibility, joint hypermobility, and connective tissue fragility. Mutations in genes affecting collagen seem to be the cause of EDS. Variable expression of the features, different modes of inheritance and distinctive associated manifestations distinguish 11 types of the syndrome. Joint laxity, hypermobility, and dislocation are most often seen with types I, III, VI, VII, and XI, while scoliosis is associated with types I, VI, and XI, being most severe with type VI. Aneurysms and spontaneous arterial rupture are typically associated with type IV. Vessel rupture (both arterial and venous) is a hazard when performing angiography in patients with EDS, especially type IV. Supporting structures of the colon, bladder, and uterus may be weakened by defective collagen and may spontaneously rupture, especially in EDS types I and IV. Recurrent inguinal

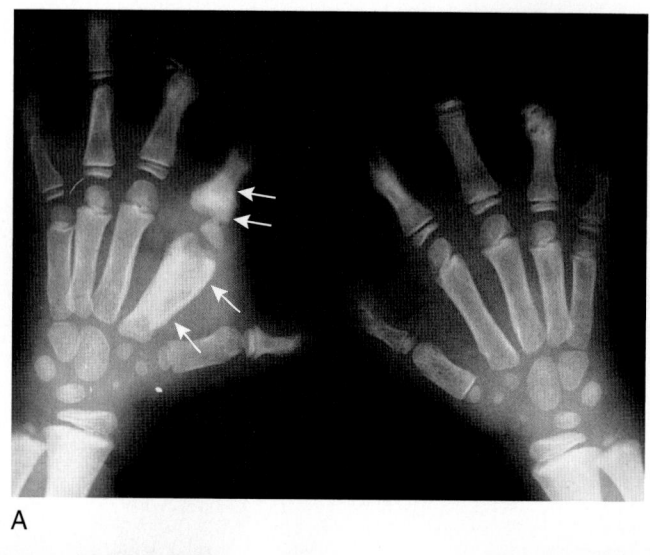

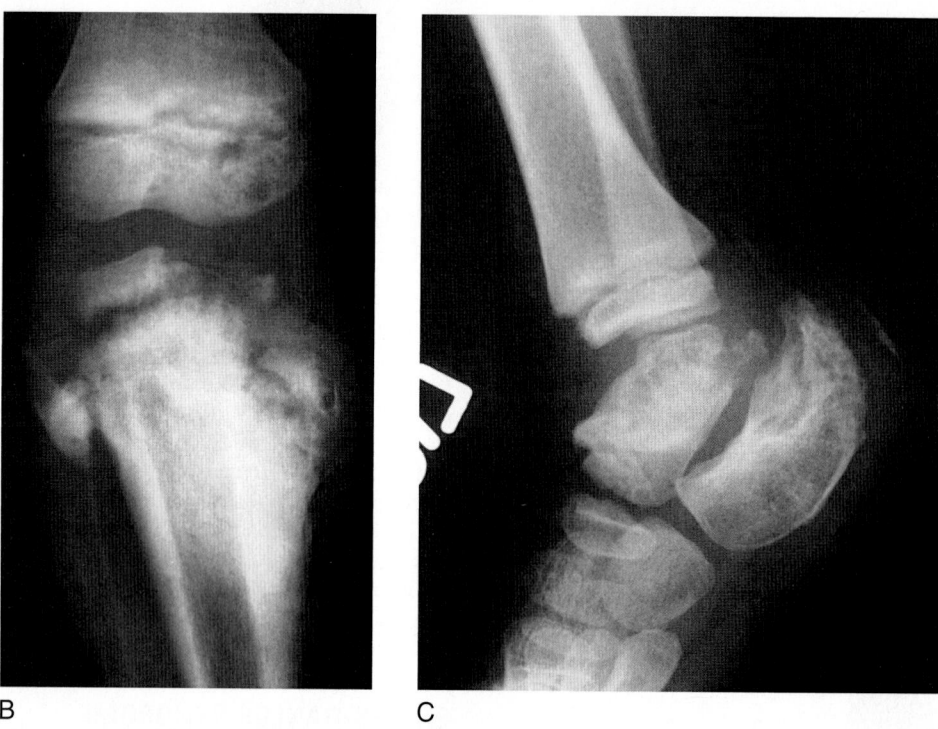

FIGURE 166-9. Congenital insensitivity to pain. **A,** Posteroanterior radiograph of the hands demonstrates extensive digital bone loss, with marked periostitis involving the right second metacarpal and the remaining portion of the second proximal phalanx *(arrows).* Posteroanterior knee radiograph **(B)** and lateral ankle radiograph **(C)** demonstrate fragmentation and irregularity typical of neuropathic joints.

hernias should raise suspicion for EDS, as should un-explained bladder or bowel diverticula in children.

Joint dislocation or subluxation may involve any joint and be acute, chronic, or repetitive (Fig. 166-12). The hip may be dislocated at birth, particularly in EDS type VII. Premature polyarticular arthritis is the result of dislocations. Affected joints may be large (e.g., hip, knee, shoulder) or small (e.g., in the thumb). Flatfoot, club-foot, and hallux valgus are common. Round subcutane-ous soft tissue calcifications are characteristic of EDS. Especially in children, joint laxity may be associated with pain, suggesting arthritis. In addition to scoliosis or kyphoscoliosis (EDS types I, VI, and XI), patients may have spondylolisthesis and a widened spinal canal. A lateral upper spine radiograph may show the cervical and upper thoracic vertebrae due to the downward-sloping shoulders.

Other clinical manifestations of EDS include re-current pneumothorax, cystic lung disease (Fig. 166-13), mitral valve prolapse, and aortic and mitral valvular in-sufficiency. Periventricular heterotopia and polymicro-gyria may be seen in the brain.

EPIDERMOLYSIS BULLOSA

Epidermolysis bullosa (EB) is the name applied to several conditions in which there is extreme fragility of the skin because of breakdown of tissues at the junction

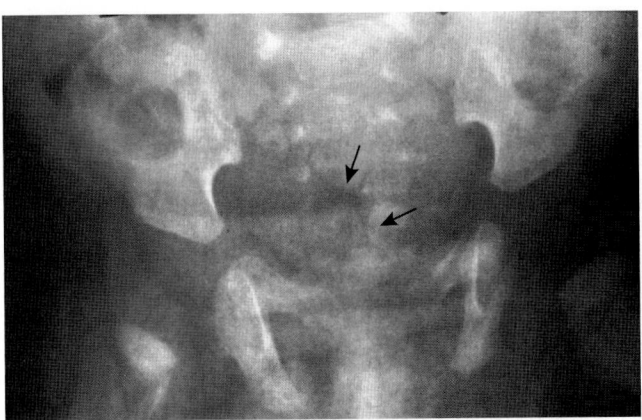

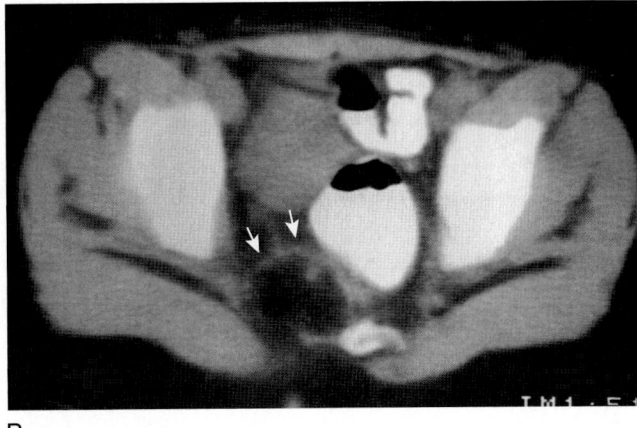

A   B

FIGURE 166-10. Currarino triad. **A,** Anteroposterior radiograph of the pelvis. A crescentic defect is present in the right inferior sacrum *(arrows)*, producing a so-called scimitar sacrum. **B,** CT scan of the pelvis at the level of the sacral defect in a patient with anal stenosis demonstrates a small fat-containing mass *(arrows)* at the level of the sacral defect. This was surgically removed and proved to be a teratoma.

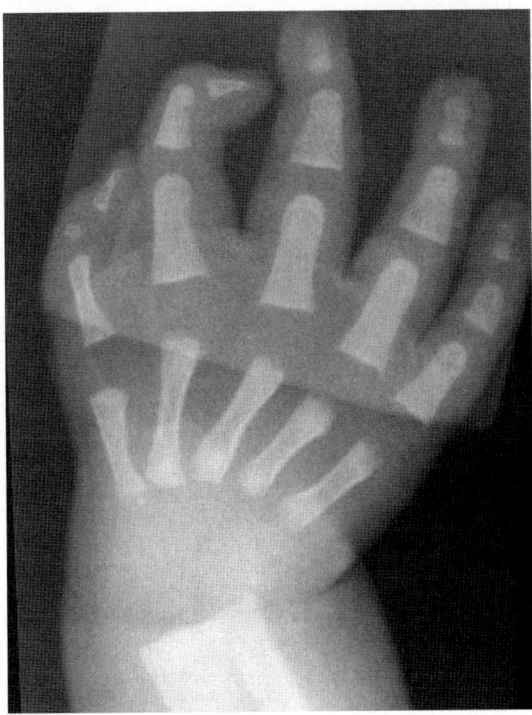

FIGURE 166-11. Diamond-Blackfan syndrome. Posteroanterior hand radiograph in a 1-week-old shows a triphalangeal thumb.

between the epidermis and dermis. EB is traditionally divided into three disorders on the basis of the tissue level of separation, or blistering, within the basement membrane:

1. Epidermolysis bullosa simplex: Autosomal dominant EB simplex is usually a fairly benign disease associated with mutations in the keratin 5 and 14 genes. Autosomal recessive EB simplex is a lethal variant often complicated by muscular dystrophy.
2. Junctional epidermolysis bullosa: A severe disease, junctional EB is usually autosomal recessive and is associated with mutations in genes for the

anchoring filament proteins laminin 5 and integrin α6 and β4.
3. Dystrophic epidermolysis bullosa: Both dominant and recessive varieties exist and are due to mutations in the gene for type VII collagen.

Congenital pyloric atresia is associated with EB. It occurs most frequently in patients with junctional EB with α6 and β4 integrin mutations, but also occurs occasionally in patients with recessive EB simplex. The pathogenesis of the pyloric atresia in these cases remains unclear. Recessive dystrophic EB is associated with severe cutaneous and gastrointestinal involvement, including pseudosyndactyly of hands ("mitten hands") and feet (Fig. 166-14), oral ulcers, microstomia, esophageal strictures, squamous cell carcinoma, and constipation and bladder outlet obstruction due to perianal and periurethral scarring. Esophageal strictures may cause high-grade obstruction and malnutrition. These strictures can occur in patients as young as 4 years old with recessive dystrophic EB, and frequently occur in the upper esophagus.

FANCONI ANEMIA

Fanconi anemia is a rare autosomal recessive disease characterized by multiple congenital abnormalities, pancytopenia, and cancer susceptibility, especially for leukemia, although an increased incidence of malignancy occurs in many organs. It is a genetically heterogeneous chromosome instability syndrome. The mean age of onset is 8 years. Mean survival is 16 years. Skeletal abnormalities are seen in 70% of patients, with 50% having radial ray abnormalities ranging from bilateral absent thumbs and radii to a unilateral hypoplastic thumb or bifid thumb (Fig. 166-15). Renal abnormalities occur in about one third of the patients and include unilateral renal agenesis, horseshoe kidney, hypoplasia, double ureters, and hydronephrosis. Microcephaly, microphthalmia, mental retardation, mild hearing loss, ear malformations, café au lait spots, brown pigmenta-

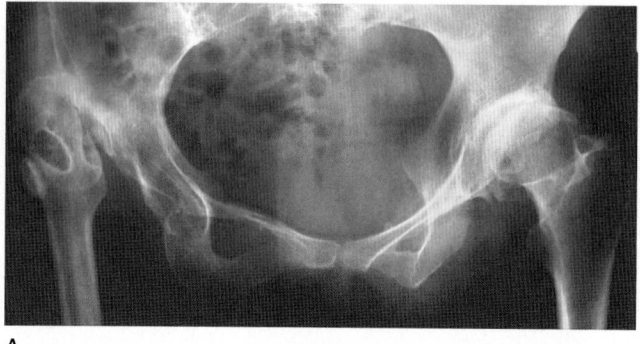

A

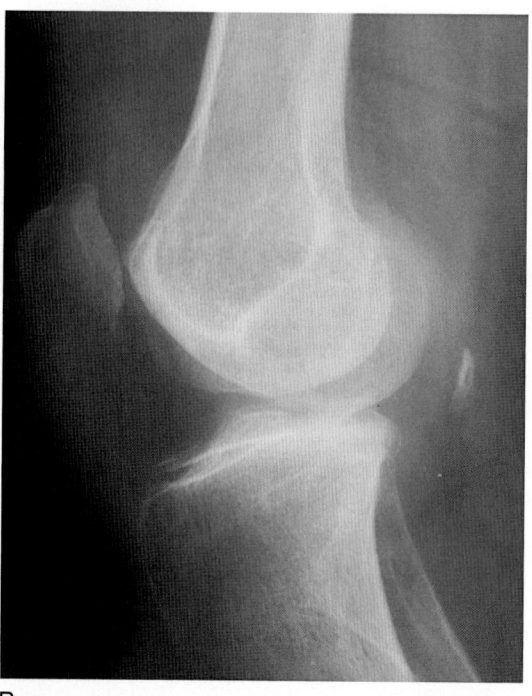

B

FIGURE 166-12. Ehlers-Danlos syndrome. **A,** Radiograph of the pelvis shows late findings of a developmental dislocation of the right hip with absorption of much of the femoral head and neck, soft tissue calcification, and secondary acetabular dysplasia. Lateral subluxation of the femoral head with joint space narrowing is noted on the left. **B,** Lateral knee radiograph demonstrates anterior subluxation of the tibia relative to the femur.

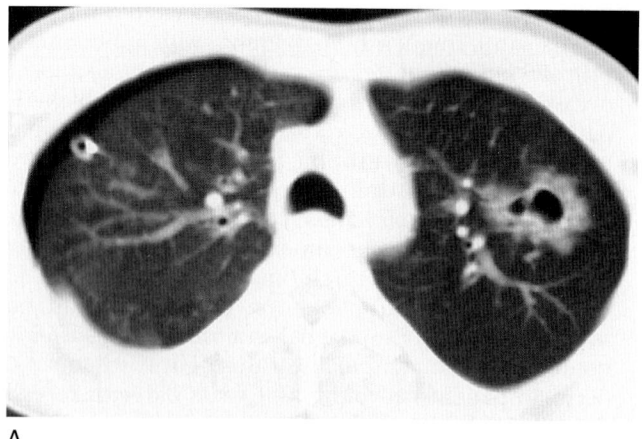

A

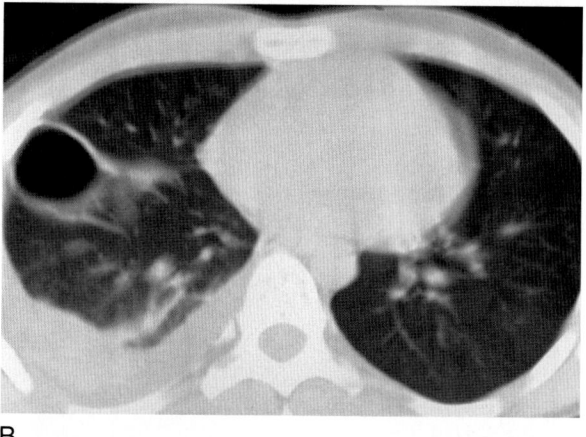

B

FIGURE 166-13. Ehlers-Danlos syndrome. Chest CT in a teenager who presented with a spontaneous right pneumothorax. Axial CT images (**A** and **B**) show multiple cystic areas in the lung, in addition to a right pleural effusion. A right pneumothorax is also present.

tion of the skin, and short stature are features of this condition.

Other imaging findings of Fanconi anemia include syndactyly, brachydactyly, pseudoepiphysis of the first metacarpal, delayed bone age, hooked clavicles, Sprengel deformity, Klippel-Feil deformity, clubfoot, hip dislocation, scoliosis, kyphosis, sacral agenesis, and nonossifying fibroma with osteomalacia. Gastrointestinal findings occasionally seen include tracheoesophageal fistula, duodenal atresia and stenosis, malrotation, and anorectal malformations. Central nervous system abnormalities include brain tumors, Arnold-Chiari malformation, hydrocephalus, microcephaly, and moyamoya disease.

FETAL ALCOHOL SYNDROME

Fetal alcohol syndrome (FAS) has a wide range of expression. The characteristic facies includes short palpebral fissures, flat upper lip, and flattened philtrum and midface.

Central nervous system developmental abnormalities include microcephaly, partial or complete agenesis of the corpus callosum, cerebellar hypoplasia, brain shape abnormalities, morphologic abnormalities in cortical and subcortical regions, and reduction in size of basal ganglia. Functional abnormalities include impaired fine motor skills, neurosensory hearing loss, and poor hand-eye coordination.

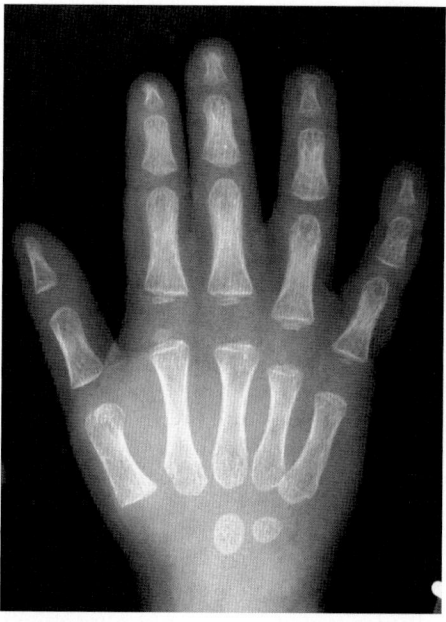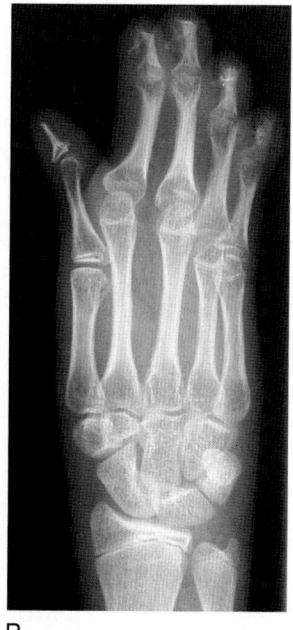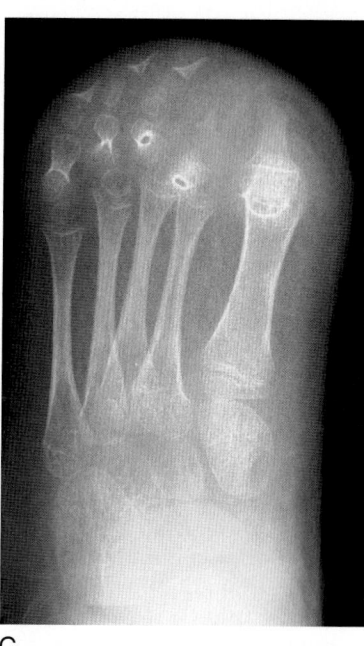

A   B   C

FIGURE 166-14. Epidermolysis bullosa. **A,** Radiograph at 2 years of age shows mild soft tissue pseudosyndactyly between the index and middle and between the middle and ring fingers. Slight resorption is noted at the tuft of the distal phalanx of the index finger. **B,** Radiograph of the same patient at 20 years of age shows more diffuse pseudosyndactyly, contractures, and "pencilling" of the distal phalanges. **C,** Foot radiograph in a different patient (8 years old) shows complete fusion of the digits with phalangeal contractures and distal bone resorption (acro-osteolysis).

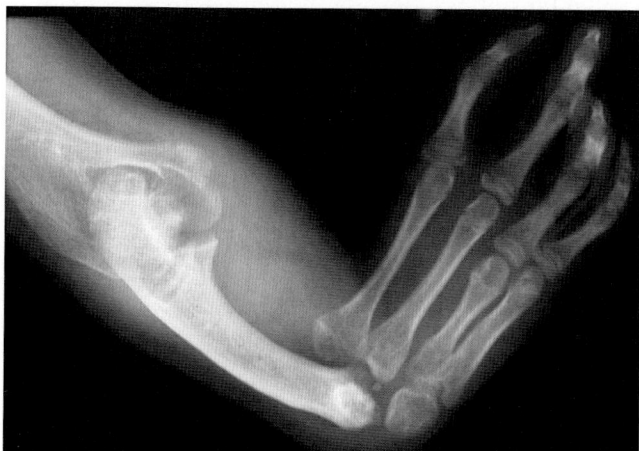

FIGURE 166-15. Fanconi anemia. Posteroanterior radiograph of the hand and forearm shows an absence of the first ray, the radius, and some of the carpal bones. The ulna is short and bowed. The patient also had only one kidney.

Skeletal abnormalities are found in 20% of FAS patients and include clinodactyly, camptodactyly, ectrodactyly, carpal fusions, flexion contractures, shortening of metacarpals and phalanges, radioulnar synostosis, epiphyseal calcifications, tibial exostoses, scoliosis, hemivertebra, Klippel-Feil deformity, hip dislocation, pectus excavatum and carinatum, rib defects, delayed bone age, and growth retardation. Cardiac defects include ventricular and atrial septal defects, tetralogy of Fallot, aberrant great vessels, hypoplastic pulmonary arteries, and aortic arch interruption.

Urogenital anomalies associated with FAS include horseshoe kidneys, hydronephrosis, ureteral duplications, calyceal diverticulum, fused kidneys, bladder diverticula, and renal aplasia, dysplasia, and hypoplasia. Gastrointestinal tract abnormalities include esophageal atresia with tracheoesophageal fistula, anal and small bowel atresias, diaphragmatic hernia, and intestinal pseudo-obstruction. Hepatobiliary abnormalities include hepatic dysfunction, biliary atresia, and hepatic fibrosis. Cystic adenomatous malformation of the lung and eye abnormalities may be seen.

FAS is weakly associated with a wide variety of tumors, including hepatoblastoma, neuroblastoma, Wilms tumor, adrenal cortical carcinoma, rhabdomyosarcoma, sacrococcygeal teratoma, leukemia, and lymphoma.

FREEMAN-SHELDON ("WHISTLING FACE") SYNDROME

Freeman-Sheldon syndrome is a congenital contracture syndrome with characteristic facies. Lip protrusion with the lips held as if whistling is due to facial muscle involvement. Brain anomalies and hearing loss have also been reported. Radiologic findings include craniofacial disproportion with brachycephaly, ulnar deviation of the hands, equinovarus feet, digital contractures, and delayed skeletal maturity. The syndrome can be inherited with genetic heterogeneity, and has been diagnosed on prenatal sonography in an affected family. Patients may also have scoliosis that may be severe, strabismus, and hearing loss. The patients are cognitively normal.

GAUCHER DISEASE

Gaucher disease is an autosomal recessive glycogen storage disease caused by one of over 200 mutations of a gene locus on chromosome 1 that leads to a defect in the acid β-glucocerebrosidase enzyme and to an accumulation of glucosylceramide in tissue throughout the body. There are three distinct phenotypic subtypes. Patients with type 1 (non-neuropathic), most common in Ashkenazi Jews, typically survive to adulthood. Patients with type 2 (infantile) and type 3 (juvenile) present with neurotoxicity due to deposition of the metabolite glucosphingosine in the brain and typically die in early infancy or childhood.

Type 1 Gaucher disease typically presents in childhood or early adolescence with hepatosplenomegaly and bone pain. Serial MR images to access liver and spleen volumes are used as a marker of response to enzyme replacement therapy (Fig. 166-16). Enzyme replacement therapy has been a useful treatment, especially in patients with type 1 disease. MRI of the spleen demonstrates infarcts, scars, and nodules, which are low signal on T1- and T2-weighted images and represent nodal clusters of glucosylceramide-laden macrophages. Bone changes include marked osteopenia (often with pathologic fractures and vertebral compression fractures), undertubulation of the long bones with Erlenmeyer flask deformity of the distal femur (see Fig. 166-16), focal "moth-eaten" areas of destruction or sclerosis, subperiosteal new bone formation, widened medullary cavities, thin ribs, degenerative joint disease, and osteomyelitis. Avascular necrosis is common (see Fig. 166-16). Bone densitometry studies are used to document osteopenia, and MRI may be useful in documenting marrow infiltration (see Fig. 166-16) and characterizing avascular necrosis. Pulmonary changes, though more common in types 2 and 3, are sometimes seen in type 1 Gaucher disease. Chest radiographs may demonstrate recurrent infiltrates or reticulonodular changes. High-resolution computed tomography (CT) may show a range of abnormal patterns, including widespread ground-glass opacification, consolidation, interstitial involvement, alveolar opacities, and bronchial wall thickening. Despite profound clinical neuropathology in types 2 and 3 Gaucher disease, cranial MRI demonstrates relatively mild findings. Mild cerebral atrophy is most commonly reported, with no parenchymal signal abnormality seen in the absence of anoxic brain injury. Dural thickening with enhancement has been reported. Hydrops fetalis may be seen in patients with type 2 disease.

Gaucher Disease:

- **Etiology: Defect in the acid β-glucocerebrosidase enzyme leads to an accumulation of glucosylceramide in tissues throughout the body.**
- **Three types:**
  - **Type 1 (non-neuropathic): responds to enzyme replacement therapy; survival to adulthood**
  - **Type 2 (infantile): neuropathic; survival to infancy**
  - **Type 3 (Juvenile): neuropathic; survival to childhood**

HADJU-CHENEY SYNDROME

Hadju-Cheney syndrome is an autosomal dominant disorder with characteristic facial features, osteolysis of the distal phalanges of the hands and feet, and multiple wormian bones. Many similar features are found in serpentine fibula polycystic syndrome. The face is broad with low-set ears, bushy eyebrows, coarse hair, enlarged outer supraorbital ridges, long philtrum, hypoplastic midface, receding chin, early tooth loss, and prominent occiput. Craniofacial findings include multiple wormian bones, bathrocephaly, cranial suture persistence, hypoplastic sinuses, an elongated sella, progressive basilar impression, absorption of the anterior nasal spine, and anteriorly positioned mandibular condyles (Fig. 166-17). In over 90% of the patients, the hands and feet show bandlike osteolysis in the midportion of the distal phalanges, especially the hands. This finding may be seen as early as age 3 to 4 years, but typically occurs in later childhood (Fig. 166-18). Occasionally the middle phalanges are involved. Osteolysis may also be seen in the radial heads. The disease may respond to bisphosphonates.

Other skeletal findings include high-bone-turnover osteoporosis with atraumatic fracture, scoliosis, kyphosis, vertebral body variation in height (including biconcave vertebral flattening), coxa valga, dislocated hips and elbows, joint laxity, bowing of the bones, elongated curved fibulas, and short stature. Cystic kidney disease resembling adult polycystic disease can be seen in up to 10% of the patients, as can glomerulonephritis, which can lead to chronic renal failure.

Central nervous system findings include Arnold-Chiari malformation, hydrocephalus, changes associated with the progressive basilar impression, and syringomyelia, which can regress. Cardiovascular abnormalities include valvular disease and heart block.

HALLERMANN-STREIFF SYNDROME

Hallermann-Streiff syndrome is a sporadic condition associated with a birdlike face, microphthalmia, beaked nose, hypotrichosis, and proportionally small stature. Radiographic findings include thinning of the calvaria with widened sutures, delayed fontanelle closure, and brachycephaly (Fig. 166-19). Long bones are gracile with thinning of the cortex. The spine is affected by scoliosis and platyspondyly. Respiratory obstruction, particularly of the upper airway, may lead to respiratory compromise, pulmonary hypertension, and death, especially in infancy. MRI may be useful in evaluating ocular changes, including microphthalmia and congenital cataracts. Agenesis of the corpus callosum may be seen.

HOLT-ORAM SYNDROME

Holt-Oram syndrome is a high-penetrant autosomal dominant condition in which anomalies of the upper extremities and shoulders are associated with congenital heart disease. Holt-Oram syndrome is linked to the *TBX5* gene, a member of the T-box gene family, which is encoded at chromosome locus 12q2. The disease is

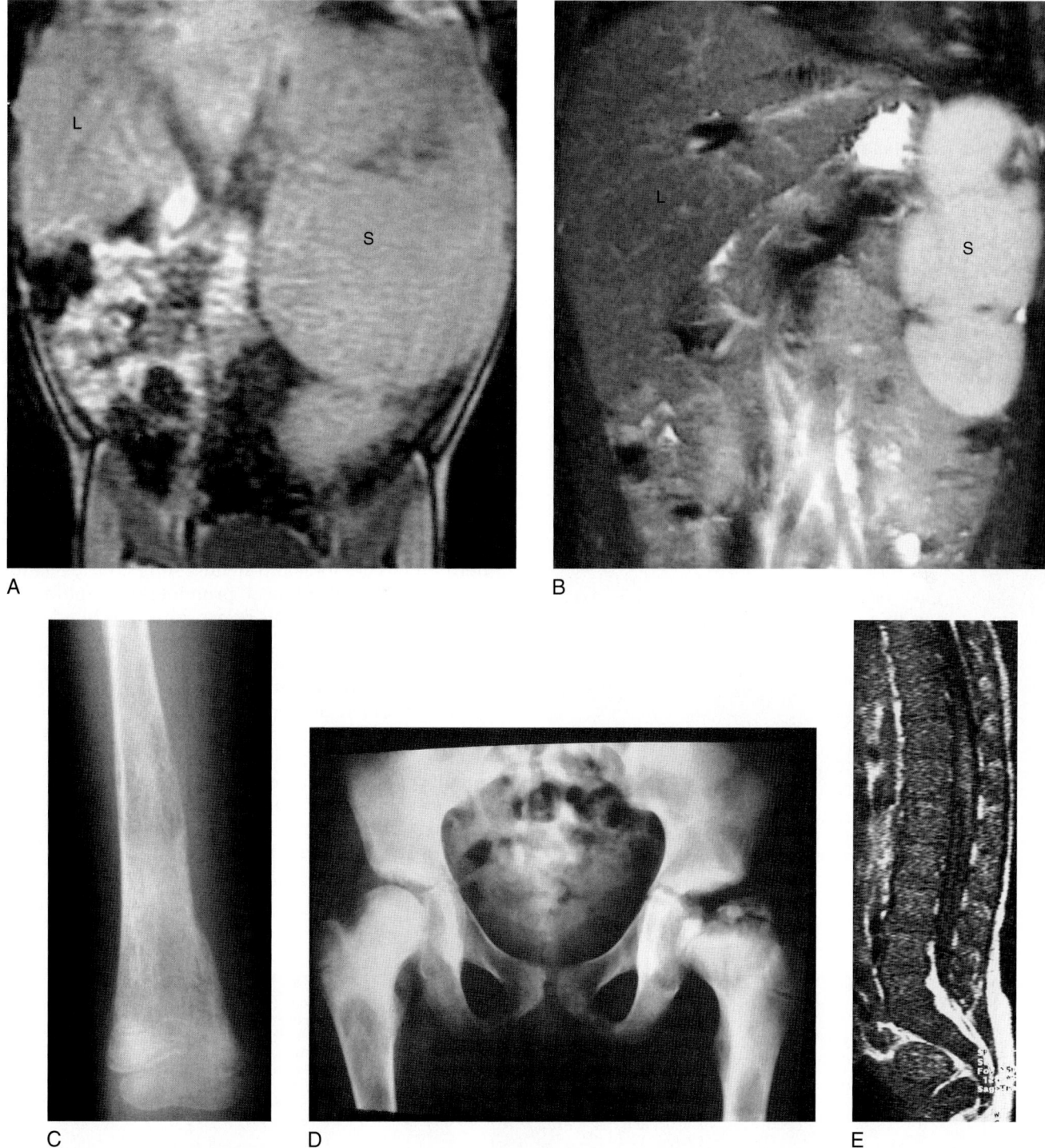

FIGURE 166-16. Gaucher disease. **A,** Coronal MR abdominal image of a 7-year-old child demonstrates moderate hepatomegaly (L) with massive splenomegaly (S). The spleen also has a nodular contour with peripheral scarring. **B,** Coronal MR abdominal image of the same child at age 19 after enzyme replacement therapy demonstrates significant interval resolution of the hepatosplenomegaly. L, liver; S, spleen. **C,** Distal femur radiograph of a different patient shows osteopenia, undertubulation (Erlenmeyer flask deformity), and focal areas of destruction in the cortex and medulla. **D,** Pelvic radiograph demonstrates patchy areas of osteopenia and sclerosis with advanced avascular necrosis of the left femoral head. **E,** Sagittal short tau inversion recovery (STIR) MR image of the spine of an 8-year-old child demonstrates near-complete marrow replacement.

familial in 60% to 70% of cases; new mutations account for the remainder. Limb anomalies range from phocomelia with absent or hypoplastic humerus (10% of patients in some series) to triphalangeal thumbs. The most common limb anomalies are radial ray anomalies (Fig. 166-20), including triphalangeal thumb, hypoplastic thumb, abnormal scaphoid (bipartite or hypoplastic), extra carpal bones, absent or hypoplastic radii, and laterally hooked clavicles. The limb anomalies tend to be bilateral and asymmetric, and are more severe on the left. Cardiac anomalies occur in 76% to 95% of patients.

The most common anomalies are atrial septal defects (58%), ventricular septal defects (28%), and conduction defects (18%). However, more severe anomalies such as tetralogy of Fallot, atrioventricular defect, hypoplastic left heart, truncus arteriosus, and total anomalous pulmonary venous return may occur.

HOMOCYSTINURIA

Homocystinuria is a metabolic disorder caused by cystathionine-β-synthetase deficiency and inherited as an autosomal recessive trait. Clinical manifestations are related to the central nervous system, eyes, and skeletal and vascular systems. Affected individuals are tall and thin. The most common central nervous system manifestation is mental retardation, which may result from vascular occlusions in the brain or in the carotid arteries, infarctions, white matter abnormalities, and atrophy. Magnetic resonance spectroscopy has been used to show biochemical abnormalities in the brain. The most common skeletal manifestation of homocystinuria is osteoporosis, which may become severe and can result in biconcave vertebral bodies, compression fractures of the spine, scoliosis, and thoracic kyphosis (Fig. 166-21). Other findings are long and slender long bones, relative epiphyseal and metaphyseal prominence resulting in part from the slender long bones, mild arachnodactyly (not as severe as in Marfan syndrome), genu valgum, humerus varus, bony spicules in the distal radial and ulnar physes, cupped metaphyses, short fourth metacarpals, malformed and enlarged carpal bones, advanced skeletal maturation, and pes cavus. The skull is small but has large paranasal sinuses. Chest deformities are common, usually pectus excavatum or carinatum. The typical eye finding is ectopia lentis, but myopia and glaucoma can be seen. Thrombosis and embolism are the life-threatening complications, and can involve any vessel in the body and both arteries and veins. Coronary

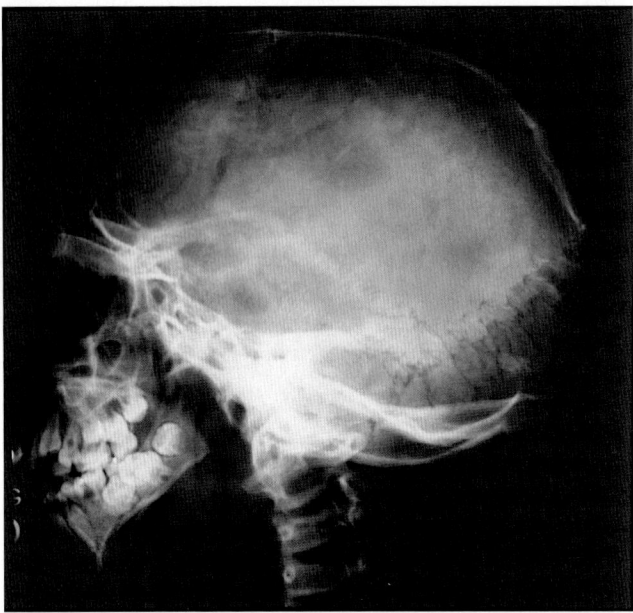

FIGURE 166-17. Hajdu-Cheney syndrome. The skull is large with prominence and bowing of the occipital bone. The lambdoid suture contains multiple wormian bones and there is basilar impression.

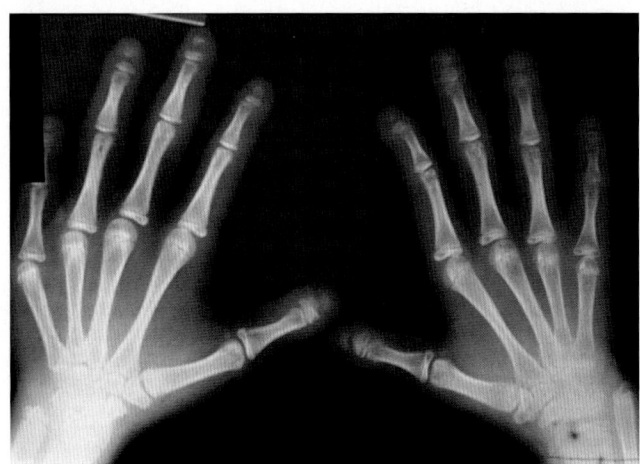
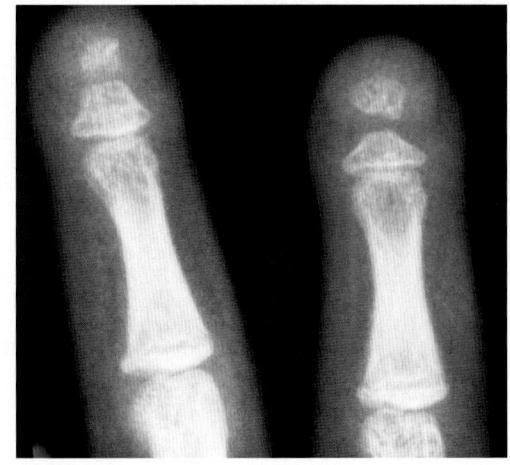

A   B

FIGURE 166-18. Hajdu-Cheney syndrome. **A,** Posteroanterior radiograph of the hands demonstrates osteolysis of the midportion of the distal phalanges. There is irregularity and decreased size of the carpal bones with elongation and displacement of the right distal ulna. **B,** Radiograph of the distal phalanges of the third and fourth digits showing the bandlike osteolysis through the midportion of the distal phalanges.

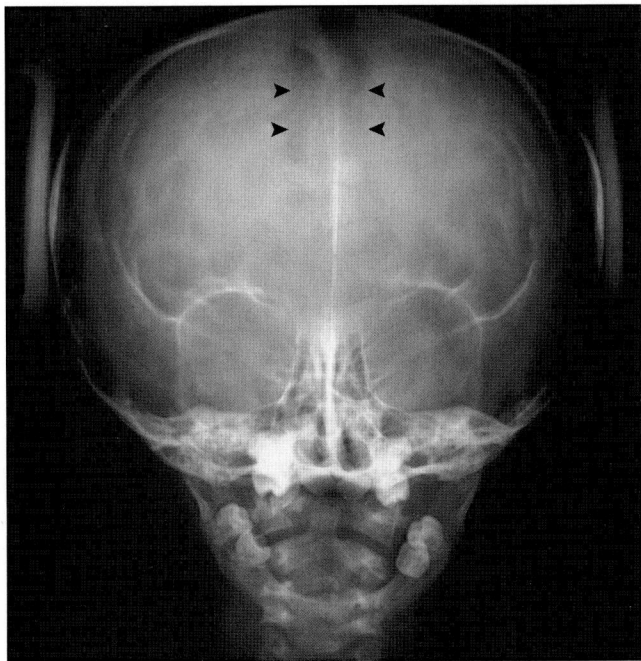

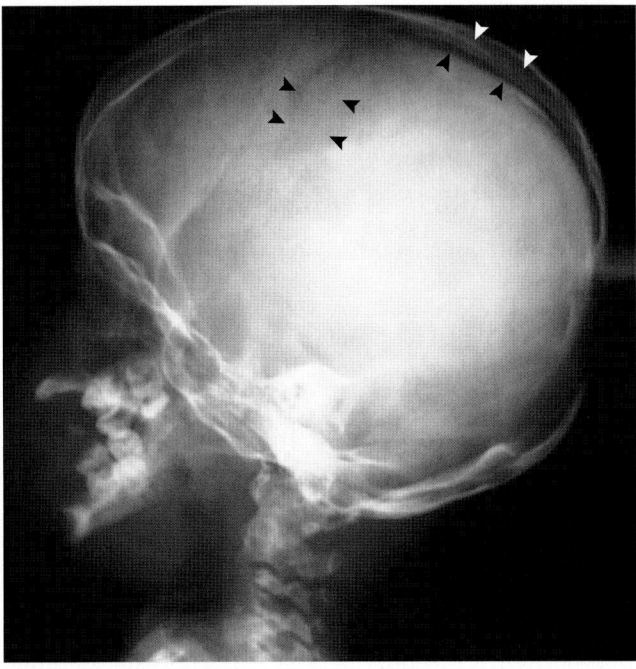

A   B

FIGURE 166-19. Hallermann-Streiff syndrome. Frontal **(A)** and lateral **(B)** skull radiographs demonstrate brachycephaly with sutural widening *(arrowheads)*, hypotelorism, micrognathia, and calvarial thinning.

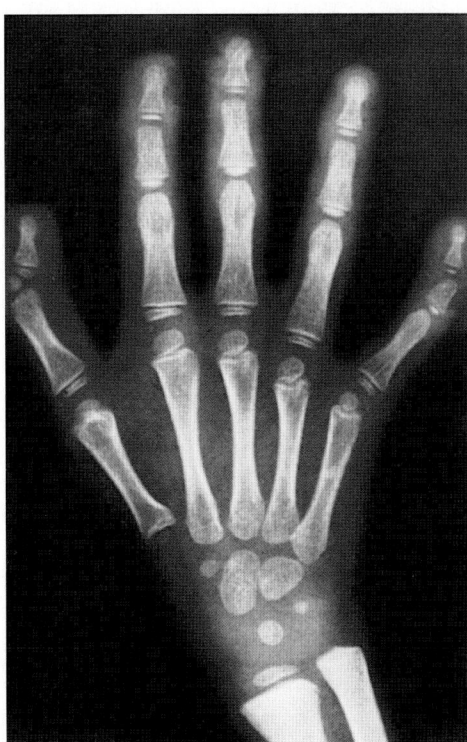

FIGURE 166-20. Holt-Oram syndrome. Radiograph of right hand of a patient with a known family history of Holt-Oram syndrome and a ventricular septal defect. Hypoplasia of first ray and adjacent carpal bones are shown along with a triphalangeal thumb. The middle thumb phalanx is very small. Clinodactyly of the fifth digit is also shown.

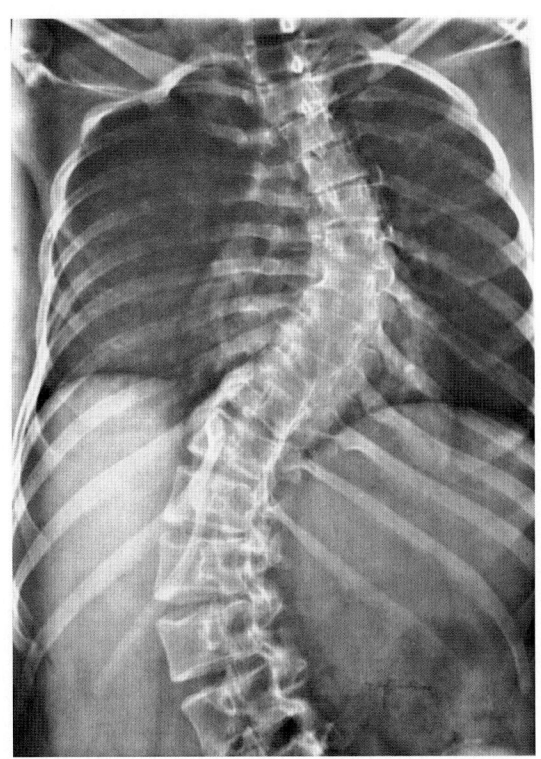

FIGURE 166-21. Homocystinuria. Anteroposterior radiograph of the spine of a teenager shows osteopenia and scoliosis.

artery occlusions, renal artery stenoses with resultant hypertension, and other arterial thromboses are of potentially great clinical importance. In addition to occlusion, corrugated arterial walls may be seen on vascular imaging.

HYPERTROPHIC OSTEOARTHROPATHY

Secondary hypertrophic osteoarthropathy (HOA) is characterized by clubbing of the fingers and toes, periostitis, and painful and swollen joints. The periostitis is both diaphyseal and metaphyseal, and can be seen as elevated and smooth, laminated, irregular, or merging with underlying cortex (Fig. 166-22). There may be periarticular osteopenia. The periostitis is best seen in the tibia, fibula, radius, ulna, femur, humerus, metacarpals, metatarsals, and phalanges. The epiphyses are usually spared. In addition to clubbing and soft tissue swelling of the fingers and toes, the tufts may hypertrophy or be absorbed. HOA can occur without clubbing. There may be peripheral hypervascularization associated with the clubbing seen by MRI. MRI has demonstrated generalized periosteal reaction, paraosseous soft tissue swelling, and muscular and septal edema.

The associations with HOA are many. Pulmonary problems associated with chronic infection are the most common—cystic fibrosis, abscess, bronchiectasis, tuberculosis, and *Pneumocystis jiroveci* (*P. carinii*) and lymphocytic pneumonitis. Other pulmonary causes are primary and metastatic tumors, inflammatory pseudotumor, sarcoidosis and histiocytosis, cyanotic congenital heart, and Eisenmenger syndrome. Abdominal associations include cirrhosis, biliary atresia, ulcerative colitis, polyposis coli, colon neoplasms, Crohn disease, cholestatic liver disease, cholangitis, pseudomembranous colitis, sprue, dysentery, achalasia, liver rhabdomyosarcoma,

and esophageal stricture. Miscellaneous causes include infected vascular grafts, nasopharyngeal carcinoma, and deep infections.

The cause of the clubbing and periostitis is unknown but maybe related to vascular endothelial growth factor-A and platelet-derived growth factor. Treatment of an associated condition, such as a lung abscess or neoplasm, can cure the HOA. Pamidronate therapy may help alleviate symptoms.

IDIOPATHIC (ISOLATED) HEMIHYPERTROPHY

Hemihypertrophy refers to asymmetric overgrowth of one side of the body. This may be total, segmental, or crossed, depending on whether an entire half of the body is involved, only a segment such as a single extremity or side of the face is involved, or opposite extremities such as the right upper extremity and the left lower extremity are involved. The asymmetric overgrowth involves osseous, muscular, and neurovascular elements of the body part involved. These elements, however, are structurally and functionally normal. Hemihypertrophy can be noted at birth or become evident during periods of somatic growth. It can occur as a manifestation of several well-defined syndromes such as BWS, Sotos syndrome, Russell-Silver syndrome, Proteus syndrome, macrocephaly–cutis marmorata–telangiectasia syndrome, Simpson-Golabi-Behmel syndrome, Perlman syndrome, neurofibromatosis type 1 (NF1), McCune-Albright syndrome, epidermal nevus syndrome, Netherton syndrome, and Klippel-Trénaunay syndrome.

Idiopathic or isolated hemihypertrophy (IH) is a condition in which hemihypertrophy occurs in the absence of manifestations of these other syndromes, such as omphalocele, hypoglycemia, and lipomatosis. There is evidence that IH is related genetically to BWS in that uniparental paternal disomy for 11p15 has been described in patients with IH. However, the epigenetic regulation is different in IH than in BWS, resulting in a distinctly different phenotype. IH has an incidence of approximately 1 in 86,000.

IH more frequently affects the right side of the body and more frequently affects boys (Fig. 166-23). IH may be associated with genitourinary anomalies, including renal hypertrophy, medullary sponge kidney, cryptorchidism, hypospadias, and clitoral or penile enlargement. IH patients are usually mentally and developmentally normal. Orthopedic surgery may be required because of limb length discrepancy and scoliosis.

IH is associated with an increased risk of malignancy. This is also true of several of the syndromes in which hemihypertrophy is a manifestation. The associated malignancies that can develop are primarily embryonal tumors: Wilms tumor, hepatoblastoma, and adrenocortical carcinoma occur in childhood. Leiomyosarcoma and renal cell carcinoma may occur later. The lifetime risk of malignancy in IH is approximately 6%. The risk of malignancy in patients with BWS and hemihypertrophy is 24% to 27%. Surveillance sonography similar to that performed in BWS should be performed in patients with IH, with scans of the abdomen performed every 3 months until at least 6 years of age and possibly longer.

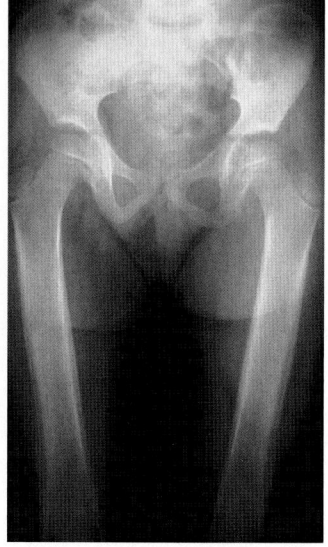

A   B

FIGURE 166-22. Hypertrophic pulmonary osteoarthropathy. There is extensive periosteal reaction on the left forearm bones (**A**) and femurs (**B**).

Idiopathic Hemihypertrophy:

- **Isolated: not associated with NF1 or another syndrome**
- **Related to BWS: uniparental disomy for 11p15 is frequent**
- **Malignancy risks: embryonal tumors (Wilms tumor, hepatoblastoma, adrenal cortical carcinoma)**
- **Surveillance sonography for tumor**

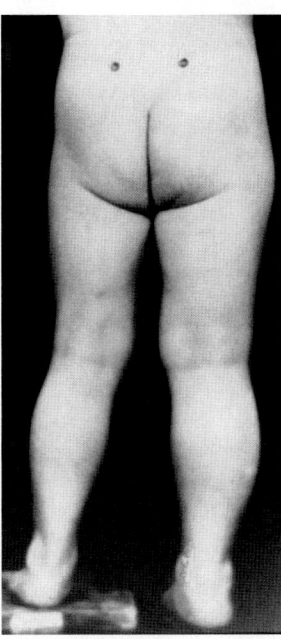

FIGURE 166-23. Idiopathic hemihypertrophy. Erect posterior legs showing right hemihypertrophy.

LARSEN SYNDROME

Larsen syndrome is characterized by multiple joint dislocations, especially of the knees, hips, and elbows; clubfoot; and a typical facies with a prominent forehead, flat nasal bridge, and hypertelorism. In knee dislocations, which are the most frequent, the tibia is displaced anteriorly. Considerable epiphyseal deformity can occur secondary to the dislocations (Fig. 166-24). Other osseous abnormalities include accessory carpal bones (Fig. 166-25), bifid calcaneus (see Fig. 166-24), short terminal phalanges of the hands, irregular shortening of some metacarpals, abnormal pattern profile analysis, kyphoscoliosis, delayed epiphyseal ossifications, coronal vertebral clefts, and delayed bone age.

Cervical kyphosis can be seen as a result of dysplastic cervical vertebrae, usually at C4 and C5, and anteroposterior subluxation in the cervical spine. Although uncommon, kyphosis may be life-threatening due to cord compression. Other findings include cleft palate, tracheomalacia, genital anomalies, cystic kidneys, aortic dilation, and valvular insufficiency and mitral valve prolapse.

Larsen syndrome is caused by mutations in the gene encoding filamin B. It is usually autosomal recessive, but dominant inheritance is also seen. Atelosteogenesis, type 3 maps to the same site and has many radiographic features in common with Larsen syndrome.

MARFAN SYNDROME

Marfan syndrome, inherited as an autosomal trait, is a connective tissue disorder caused by mutations in the extracellular matrix protein fibrillin 1, a component of elastin. The typical patient is tall with disproportionate long, slender limbs and digits. The cardiovascular, ocular, and skeletal systems are commonly involved. Common defects include pectus deformities (excavatum

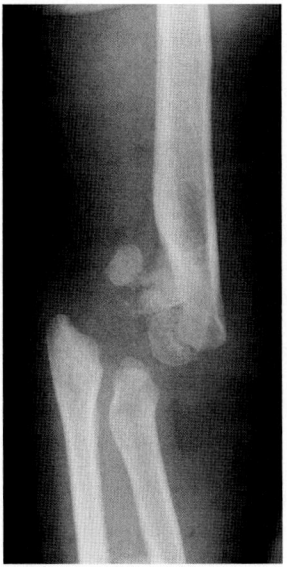
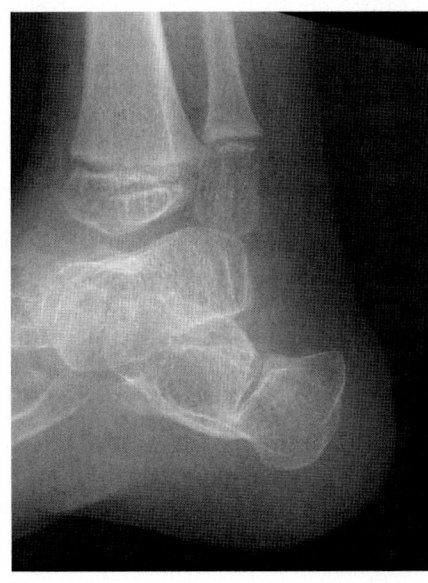

A   B

FIGURE 166-24. Larsen syndrome. **A,** Anteroposterior elbow radiograph of a 5-year-old girl shows chronic dislocation with secondary deformity of the bones. **B,** Lateral radiograph of an ankle in a 5-year-old boy shows a bifid calcaneus and some deformity of the distal tibial epiphysis and talus.

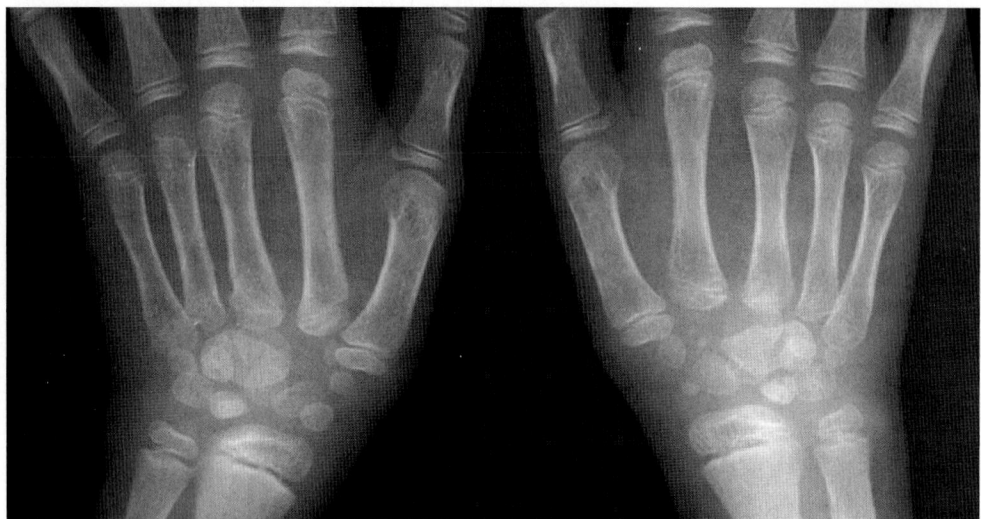

FIGURE 166-25. Larsen syndrome. Posteroanterior radiograph of the hands of an 8-year-old girl shows multiple extra carpal bones with slight deformity of the distal head of the second metacarpals. An accessory ossification center is seen at the base of the second metacarpal.

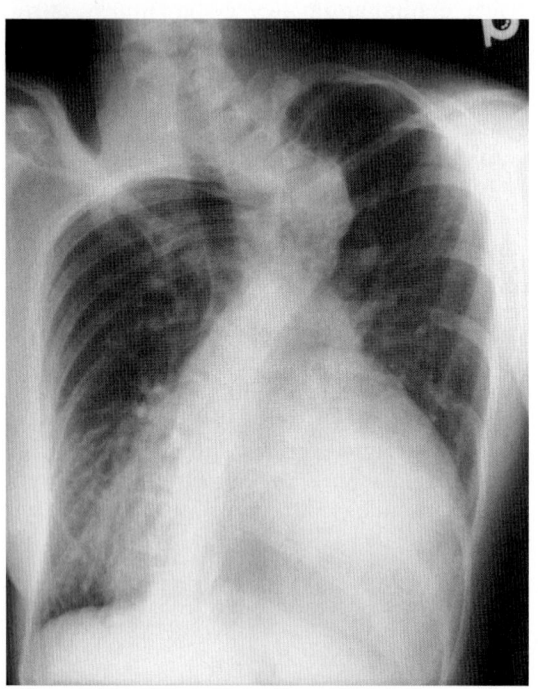

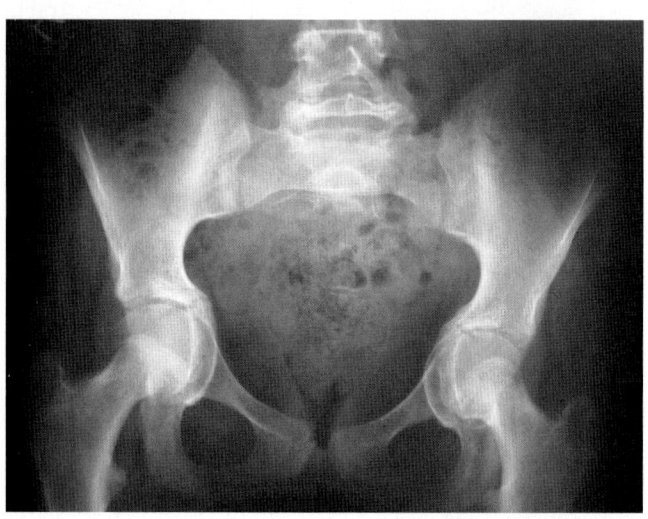

A

B

FIGURE 166-26. Marfan syndrome. **A,** Chest radiograph (14 years old) shows an acute upper thoracic scoliosis and cardiomegaly. **B,** Pelvic radiograph of the same patient (12 years old) shows bilateral protrusio acetabuli.

or carinatum), joint laxity, ocular problems (usually ectopia lentis from lax suspensory ligaments and myopia), and spinal deformity (scoliosis, which may be severe and progressive; kyphosis; flat back; and spondylolisthesis) (Fig. 166-26).

Cardiovascular manifestations, which are common, result from loss of tensile strength of the supporting tissue of the aortic and cardiac valves. These are the most devastating aspect of Marfan syndrome, leading to aortic dilation, regurgitation, and dissection and mitral valve prolapse. A measurement of aortic root growth may have prognostic value for aortic complications. Serious cardiovascular abnormalities may be present at birth.

Gastrointestinal tract complications are few but include diaphragmatic and intestinal hernias, diverticulosis coli, and Zenker diverticulum. Pulmonary complications are blebs and recurrent pneumothoraces. Liver and renal cysts occur more frequently in Marfan syndrome.

Other findings include high-arched palate, crowding of teeth, dural ectasia occurring in a majority of the patients (Fig. 166-27), spinal arachnoid cysts or diverticula, protrusio acetabuli (see Fig. 166-26), joint laxity, reduced arm span–to-height ratio, and arachnodactyly. Joint laxity can result in joint dislocations. Arachnodactyly (Fig. 166-28) may be determined by an abnormal (>9) metacarpal index (sum of the lengths of metacarpals 2 through 5 divided by the sum of the widths of the same bones), middle phalanges 50% longer than the corresponding metacarpals, and an abnormal metacarpophalangeal pattern profile, with a long first metacarpal and short first distal phalanx.

MARSHALL-SMITH SYNDROME

Marshall-Smith syndrome is characterized by accelerated skeletal maturity associated with failure to thrive. In addition to prenatal development of ossification centers, radiologic findings include "bullet-shaped" proximal and middle phalanges with narrow distal phalanges (Fig. 166-29), narrow vertebral bodies with anterior wedging, and hypoplasia of the dens with prominence of the supraoccipital bone above the foramen magnum and the posterior arch of C1 (see Fig. 166-29). Patients may have blue sclera and are prone to atraumatic fractures. Clinically, patients often do poorly, with death in infancy due to respiratory compromise; however, long-term survival has been reported.

MCKUSICK-KAUFMAN SYNDROME

McKusick-Kaufman syndrome is an autosomal recessive condition described originally in an Old Order Amish population. The syndrome consists of hydrometrocolpos usually due to vaginal atresia, anorectal malformation, mesoaxial or postaxial polydactyly, and congenital heart disease. The disease is frequently found in Old Order

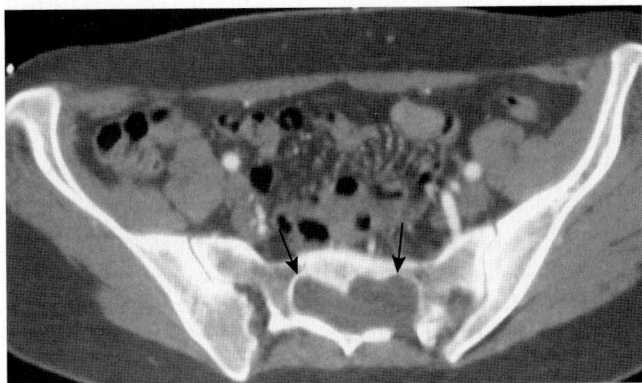

FIGURE 166-27. Marfan syndrome. CT shows dural ectasia in the sacral canal *(arrows)*.

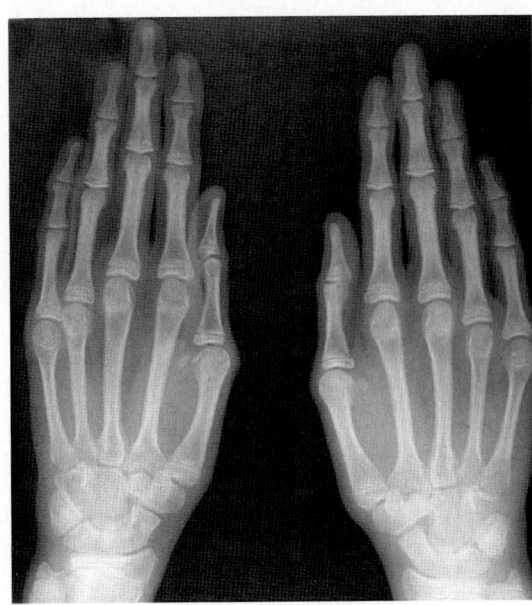

FIGURE 166-28. Marfan syndrome. Posteroanterior radiograph of the hand shows arachnodactyly.

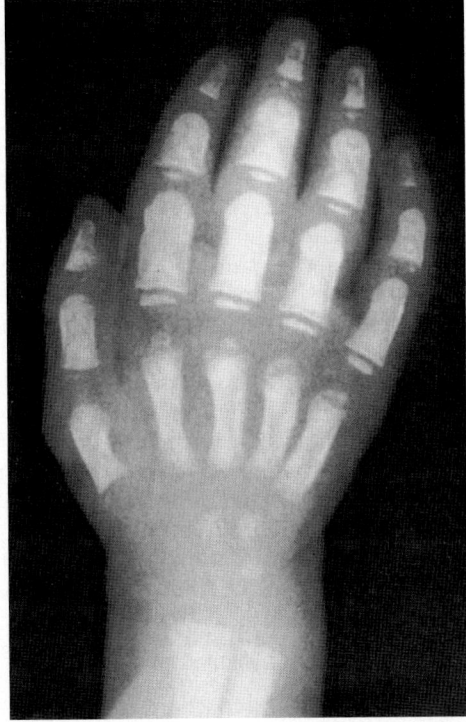

A

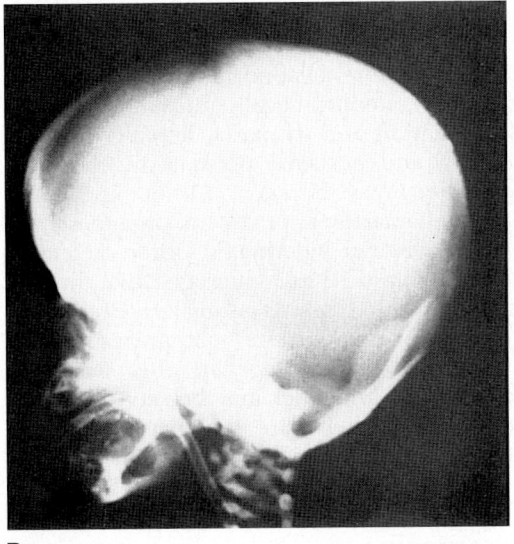

B

FIGURE 166-29. Marshall-Smith syndrome. **A,** Hand radiograph shows bullet-shaped proximal and middle phalanges. Skeletal maturation was accelerated. **B,** Lateral skull radiograph shows a hypoplastic mandible, prominent supraoccipital bone, and shallow orbits. (Courtesy of Dr. A. H. Felman, Jacksonville, FL.)

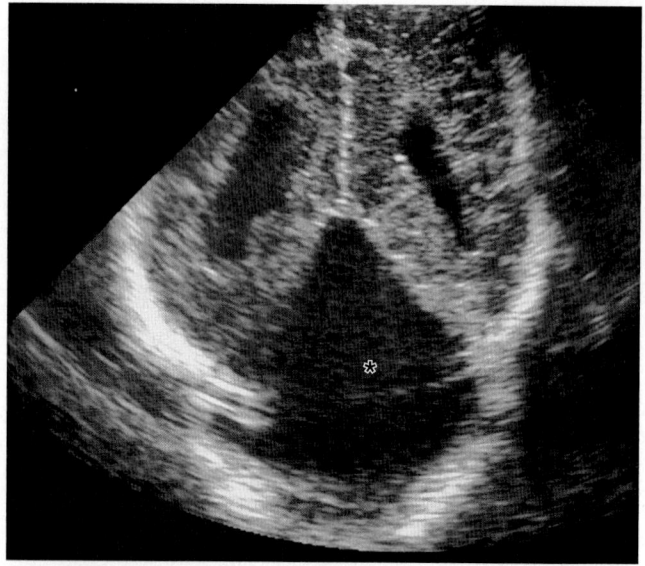

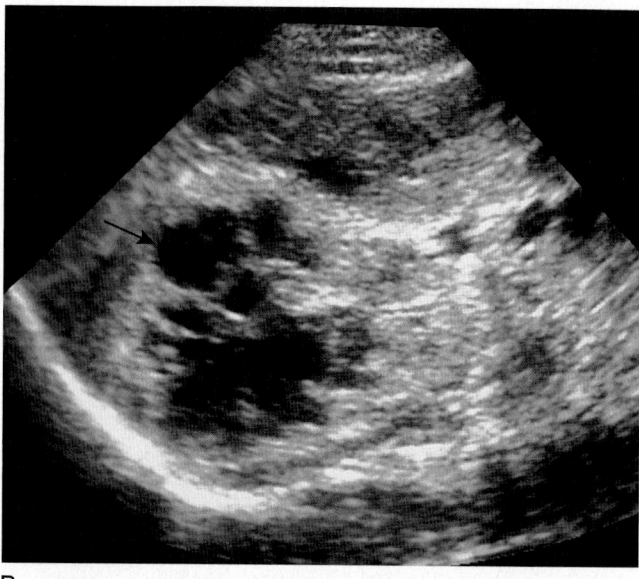

A   B

FIGURE 166-30. Meckel syndrome. **A,** Cranial sonogram of the head demonstrates a large occipital encephalocele *(asterisk)*. **B,** Transverse renal sonogram demonstrates a cyst *(arrow)* in the right kidney. Renal parenchymal echogenicity is increased and there is mild hydronephrosis.

Amish families in the United States. Males with the syndrome are diagnosed if there are affected female siblings, although postaxial polydactyly and hypospadias occur. Imperforate anus occurs in approximately 50% of patients, often with a rectovaginal fistula. Congenital heart disease includes ventricular septal defects, atrial septal defects, and single atria. There appears to be an increased incidence of long-segment Hirschsprung disease in patients with this syndrome. This syndrome is allelic to BBS. The *BB6* locus encodes for the McKusick-Kaufman syndrome gene.

MECKEL SYNDROME

Meckel syndrome, also known as Meckel-Gruber syndrome, is an autosomal recessive malformation syndrome characterized by developmental defects in the central nervous system (most commonly occipital encephalocele (Fig. 166-30), renal abnormalities including cysts (see Fig. 166-30), nephromegaly, unusual corticomedullary differentiation and dysplasia, hepatic ductal dysplasia and cysts, and postaxial polydactyly. Dandy-Walker malformation may be seen. Other findings include fibrosis and hamartomas of visceral organs, cleft lip and palate, and visceral heterotaxy. Other skeletal changes include dysplastic hips, micrognathia, limb bowing, short limbs, and vertebral anomalies. Prenatal sonographic evaluation demonstrates oligohydramnios and typical morphologic findings in the second trimester. The renal abnormalities may be seen late in the first trimester. The patients are stillborn or die in infancy. The transmembrane protein meckelin (MKS3) is mutated in patients with Meckel syndrome.

NEUROFIBROMATOSIS

Neurofibromatosis is divided into two separate and genetically distinct diseases: NF1 or von Recklinghausen

disease and neurofibromatosis type 2 (NF2). Other so-called types of neurofibromatosis and overlap syndromes have been described and are discussed in the differential diagnosis of NF1 and NF2.

Neurofibromatosis 1

NF1 (von Recklinghausen disease) is the most common of the phakomatoses or neurocutaneous syndromes. It is an autosomal dominant condition with an occurrence of 1 in 4000 individuals, with approximately 100% penetrance. Approximately 50% to 60% of patients inherit the disease. The remainder of patients have new mutations. The mutation accounting for NF1 occurs in the gene encoding for neurofibromin, a tumor suppressor gene mapped to 17q11.2. The inactivation of neurofibromin, a negative regulator of the *RAS* proto-oncogene, results in inadequate suppression of the Ras oncoprotein. Unsuppressed Ras stimulation results in excess cell proliferation and tumor formation.

The criteria for diagnosis of NF1 were established by the National Institutes of Health (NIH) Consensus Development Conference of 1987 and are listed in Table 166-2. The patient must have two of the seven characteristics to establish the diagnosis of NF1.

The manifestations of NF1 are due to the presence of tumors and neuroectodermal, mesodermal, and endodermal dysplasia. These manifestations can be broken down into groups: cutaneous–soft tissue, musculoskeletal, thoracic, abdominal, vascular, hematologic, and central nervous system.

CUTANEOUS–SOFT TISSUE MANIFESTATIONS

The soft tissue and skin changes of NF1 include those listed in Table 166-1. Café au lait macules numbering more than six can be found in 97% of children with NF1. However, café au lait macules also occur frequently in NF2, McCune-Albright syndrome, Jaffe-Campanacci

TABLE 166-2

Diagnostic Criteria for NF1

1. Six or more café au lait spots or macules
2. Two or more neurofibromas of any type, or one or more plexiform neurofibromas
3. Axillary or groin freckling
4. Optic glioma
5. Lisch nodules (benign iris hamartomas)
6. Distinctive bone lesions such as sphenoid wing dysplasia or long bone cortical thinning with or without pseudarthrosis
7. First-degree relative with NF1

syndrome, Fanconi anemia, ataxia-telangiectasia, Russell-Silver syndrome, and Watson syndrome. Many of these conditions have findings that might be confused with those in NF1. Axillary and inguinal freckling are essentially pathognomic for NF1 and are found in 81% of patients younger than 6 years of age with NF1. Lisch nodules, which are pigmented iris hamartomas, are also pathognomonic for NF1 and are found in 90% of NF1 patients. Soft tissue neurofibromas, neurolemmomas, and malignant peripheral nerve sheath tumors occur in NF1. Neurofibromas and neurolemmomas are more common as isolated lesions not associated with NF1 or NF2; however, when they are multiple and involve deep nerves, they are more often associated with NF1. Malignant peripheral nerve sheath tumors are equally divided between patients with NF1 and sporadically occurring cases in patients without NF1.

Neurofibromas are benign nerve sheath tumors and are classified as localized, diffuse, or plexiform. Only the plexiform neurofibroma is characteristic of NF1. Approximately 90% of diffuse and isolated neurofibromas occur sporadically in patients without NF1. The most common tumor in NF1, however, is the isolated neurofibroma, which tends to be large and involves deeper nerves such as the sciatic and brachial plexuses as opposed to the isolated neurofibroma (Figs. 166-31 and 166-32). Neurofibromas are concentrically located around and inseparable from the nerve of origin, making their resection impossible without loss of nerve function. A "split fat sign" is frequently seen on CT or MRI. This sign is due to a well-defined rim of fat around neurogenic tumors, unlike other soft tissue tumors. Muscles involved by the tumor may show atrophy with increased fat, also a finding unusual with other soft tissue tumors. Neurofibromas characteristically have a target appearance on MRI imaging, with a low signal center and bright periphery on T2-weighted imaging (see Fig. 166-32). The target sign is seen in 58% of neurofibromas, but also in 15% of neurolemmomas and in some malignant peripheral nerve sheath tumors. Central enhancement on T1-weighted images is also common in neurofibroma, occurring in 75% of lesions but only 8% of neurolemmomas. Neurofibromas are usually hypodense on unenhanced CT (20 to 25 Hounsfield units) and enhance (by 3 to 35 Hounsfield units). Plexiform neurofibromas are characteristic of NF1, but are rare in children less than 10 years of age. Plexiform neurofibromas resemble finger-like fronds of tissue along the involved nerve. They are also low in attenuation due to the adipose tissue and cystic and myxoid degeneration of the lesions. Plexiform neurofibromas occur in 27% of NF1 patients. It is estimated that 1% to 29% of these undergo malignant degeneration. Plexiform neurofibromas may be associated with massive enlargement or focal gigantism of the associated extremity, producing so-called elephantiasis neuromatosa. The presence of a plexiform neurofibroma allows differentiation of elephantiasis neuromatosa from the focal gigantism of macrodystrophia lipomatosa, which is associated with a neural fibrolipoma, a benign tumor unrelated to neurofibromatosis.

A neurolemmoma is a nerve sheath tumor that usually occurs as an isolated lesion not associated with either NF1 or NF2. Neurolemmomas arise eccentrically from the involved nerve. Their differentiation from neurofibroma is very helpful in surgical planning because neurolemmomas can be resected without loss of nerve function, unlike neurofibromas, and very infrequently recur. Neurolemmomas are often multiple in NF1; 18% of patients with multiple neurolemmomas have NF1. The neurolemmoma often produces the "fascicle sign" on T2-weighted imaging, appearing as multiple small ringlike structures with a peripheral high signal. This fascicular appearance is seen in 63% of neurolemmomas. A thin hyperintense rim is seen around neurolemmomas on T1-weighted imaging in 58% of cases, and diffuse enhancement with contrast occurs in 67% of lesions.

Malignant peripheral nerve sheath tumor (MPNST) occurs both in NF1 patients and sporadically. The lifetime risk of MPNST in NF1 is 8% to 13%. MPNST is found at an earlier age in NF1 patients (average age of 26 years) than in patients with sporadic tumors (average age of 62 years). Moreover, the 5-year survival in NF1 patients with MPNST is only 21%, whereas the 5-year survival is 42% in patients with sporadic lesions. MPNST frequently occurs in pre-existing plexiform neurofibromas; however, the tumor may also arise de novo. Radiation of the involved region increases the risk of MPNST. Radiotherapy is therefore avoided in NF1 patients unless absolutely necessary. The latent period after radiation therapy before the appearance of MPNST has varied from 5 to 17 years. Differentiation of a plexiform neurofibroma from a MPNST may be difficult by imaging. Imaging findings suggestive of malignancy in a patient with NF1 are lesion size larger than 5 cm, ill-defined borders, and lack of target sign on T2-weighted images.

Embryonal rhabdomyosarcoma also has an increased incidence in NF1 patients. All reported patients with rhabdomyosarcoma and NF1 have been less than 18 years of age. The malignant triton tumor is a rare variant of MPNST originally thought to be a rhabdomyosarcoma because of its rhabdomyoblastic differentiation. Approximately one third of malignant triton tumors occur in patients with NF1. These lesions often occur in the third decade of life and have a very poor prognosis. There may be a slightly increased incidence of neuroblastoma and Wilms tumor in neurofibromatosis, but this has not been satisfactorily confirmed statistically.

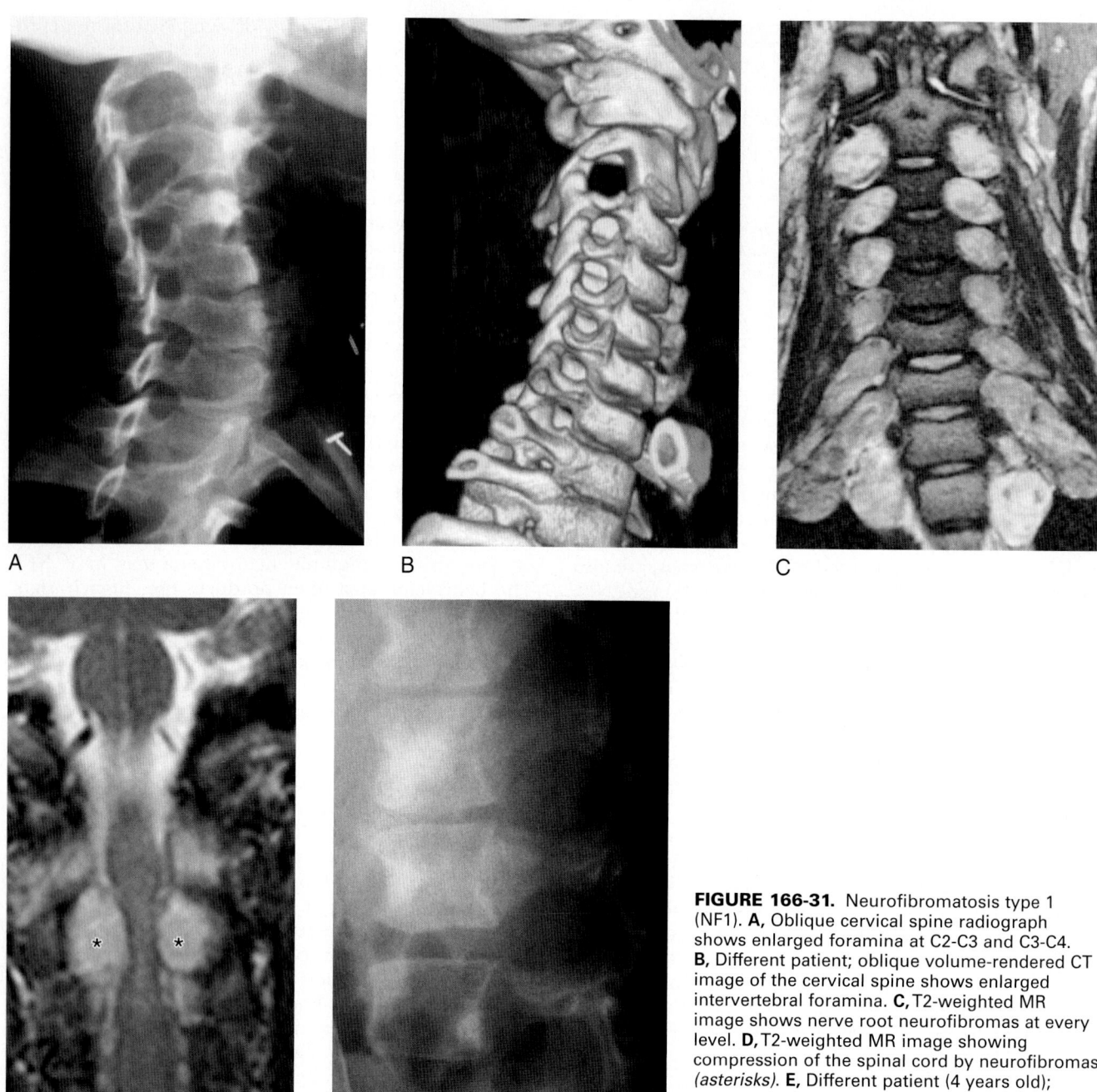

FIGURE 166-31. Neurofibromatosis type 1 (NF1). **A,** Oblique cervical spine radiograph shows enlarged foramina at C2-C3 and C3-C4. **B,** Different patient; oblique volume-rendered CT image of the cervical spine shows enlarged intervertebral foramina. **C,** T2-weighted MR image shows nerve root neurofibromas at every level. **D,** T2-weighted MR image showing compression of the spinal cord by neurofibromas *(asterisks).* **E,** Different patient (4 years old); posterior vertebral body scalloping in the lumbar spine due to dural ectasia.

MUSCULOSKELETAL MANIFESTATIONS

Musculoskeletal manifestations of NF1 are very frequent, occurring in approximately 50% to 70% of patients with NF1. Most musculoskeletal findings are the result of mesodermal dysplasia or direct erosive changes on bone by adjacent soft tissue tumors. Mesodermal dysplasia manifests in the spine as pedicle hypoplasia, usually involving three or more contiguous vertebrae; as congenital pseudarthrosis of long bones; and as sphenoid wing dysplasia. Erosive bone changes include vertebral posterior scalloping, rib deformity (although some instances of rib deformity may be mesodermal dysplasia without adjacent masses), transverse process spindling, vertebral wedging, enlarged neural foramina, thinned pedicles, and widened interpediculate distances. Because the number of neurofibromas increases throughout life, osseous deformities due to these masses also increase.

The most common skeletal abnormality in NF1 is scoliosis (Fig. 166-33), occurring in 26% to 71% of patients. Scoliosis in neurofibromatosis is usually divided into nondystrophic and dystrophic forms. The nondystrophic form is a curve resembling idiopathic scoliosis with normal-appearing vertebra in the scoliotic segment. Dystrophic scoliosis is that associated with significant dysplastic vertebral bodies. The typical dysplastic curve is

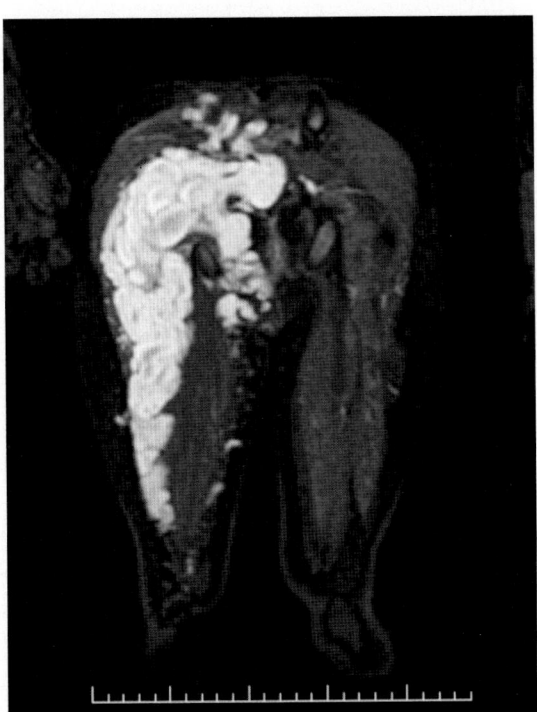

FIGURE 166-32. Neurofibromatosis type 1 (NF1). Coronal T2-weighted MR image with fat saturation shows a large plexiform neurofibroma along the course of the right sciatic nerve. Note the lobular appearance of the mass with central low signal in the lobules.

TABLE 166-3

Tibial Bowing and Pseudarthrosis in NF1

Type 1: anterolateral bowing with dense medullary canal
Type 2: anterolateral bowing with increased medullary canal
Type 3: anterolateral bowing with cystic lesion at apex (possibly a healing fracture)
Type 4: anterolateral bowing with fracture, cysts, and frank pseudarthrosis, often producing a characteristic hourglass deformity with pointed ends of bone meeting at the pseudarthrosis

a severe, angular, short-segment scoliosis with often with an acute "hairpin" appearance. The scoliosis is usually a right dextroconvex scoliosis. Nondystrophic scoliosis responds better to treatment than dystrophic scoliosis. Kyphosis is often severe in patients with dystrophic curves and may lead to paraplegia.

In NF1, congenital pseudarthrosis most commonly occurs in the distal third of the tibia and fibula (Fig. 166-34). Approximately 5% of patients with NF1 have tibial pseudarthrosis. Approximately 70% of patients with tibial pseudarthrosis have NF1. Pseudarthroses may also occur in the ulna, femur, radius, and humerus (see Fig. 166-34). Pseudarthrosis of the tibia is associated with anterolateral bowing of the tibial shaft ("tibial kyphosis"). In fact, some believe that pseudarthrosis of the tibia is the result of tibial bowing. Tibial pseudarthrosis and anterolateral tibial bowing are believed to be due to mesodermal dysplasias and, except for a single case report, no neurofibromatous tissues have been found at the site of pseudarthrosis. Patients become symptomatic between 1.5 and 8 years of age. Fractures of the bowed tibia are believed to lead to the pseudarthrosis and usually occur within the first 2 years of life. Congenital tibial bowing and pseudarthrosis has been classified into four radiologic subtypes (Table 166-3). Treatment of tibial pseudarthrosis is a challenging orthopedic surgical problem. Treatment of type 1 has the best prognosis and type 4 has the worst prognosis.

Fibular bowing and pseudarthrosis is frequently also present in patients with tibial pseudarthrosis. Approximately half of patients with tibial pseudarthrosis have fibular dysplasia. Fibular pseudarthrosis without tibial involvement is much less common.

Sphenoid wing dysplasia with absence of the greater wing of the sphenoid (see Chapter 48) is an uncommon but characteristic manifestation of NF1. It occurs in less than 1% of patients with NF1. Sphenoid wing dysplasia allows the temporal lobe and cerebrospinal fluid to prolapse into the orbit, producing a pulsating exophthalmos. Other cranial findings include macrocrania, choroid plexus calcifications, and holes in the left lambdoid suture.

Erosive bone changes due to adjacent neurofibromas and dural ectasia are very common manifestations of NF1 and are considered by many to be the most characteristic lesions in NF1 (Fig. 166-35). The posterior scalloping of vertebral bodies may be due to either intraspinal neurofibromas or to dural ectasia.

Intraosseous benign bone lesions found in patients with NF1 are usually multiple and histologically are nonossifying fibromas (NOFs). Multiple NOFs occur in less than 5% of patients with NF1. Jaffe-Campanacci syndrome is a consideration in a patient with multiple NOFs and café au lait macules. The NOFs of Jaffe-Campanacci syndrome are large, bilateral, and symmetric and involve both the upper and lower extremities, whereas those of NF1 are not usually as large, are less frequently symmetric, and less frequently involve the arms. Neurofibromas do not occur in Jaffe-Campanacci syndrome.

Polydactyly (both pre- and postaxial), clinodactyly, and vertebral segmentation anomalies occur statistically more frequently in patients with NF1 than in the general population; however, these are uncommon manifestations of NF1. Polydactyly occurs in 2.2% of NF1 patients, while it only occurs in 0.5% of the general population.

THORACIC MANIFESTATIONS

Posterior mediastinal intrathoracic lateral and anterior meningoceles are rare lesions occurring primarily in NF1. These meningoceles arise due to dural ectasia and enlarged neural foramina and are almost always associated with scoliosis. Recognition that the lesions are cystic continuations with the spinal canal can be accomplished by CT or MRI.

Mediastinal and chest wall neurofibromas may be isolated or plexiform. Isolated paraspinal, elliptical neurofibromas are often correctly diagnosed by CT or MRI due to their posterior mediastinal location. However, thoracic neurofibromas may also occur along the vagus,

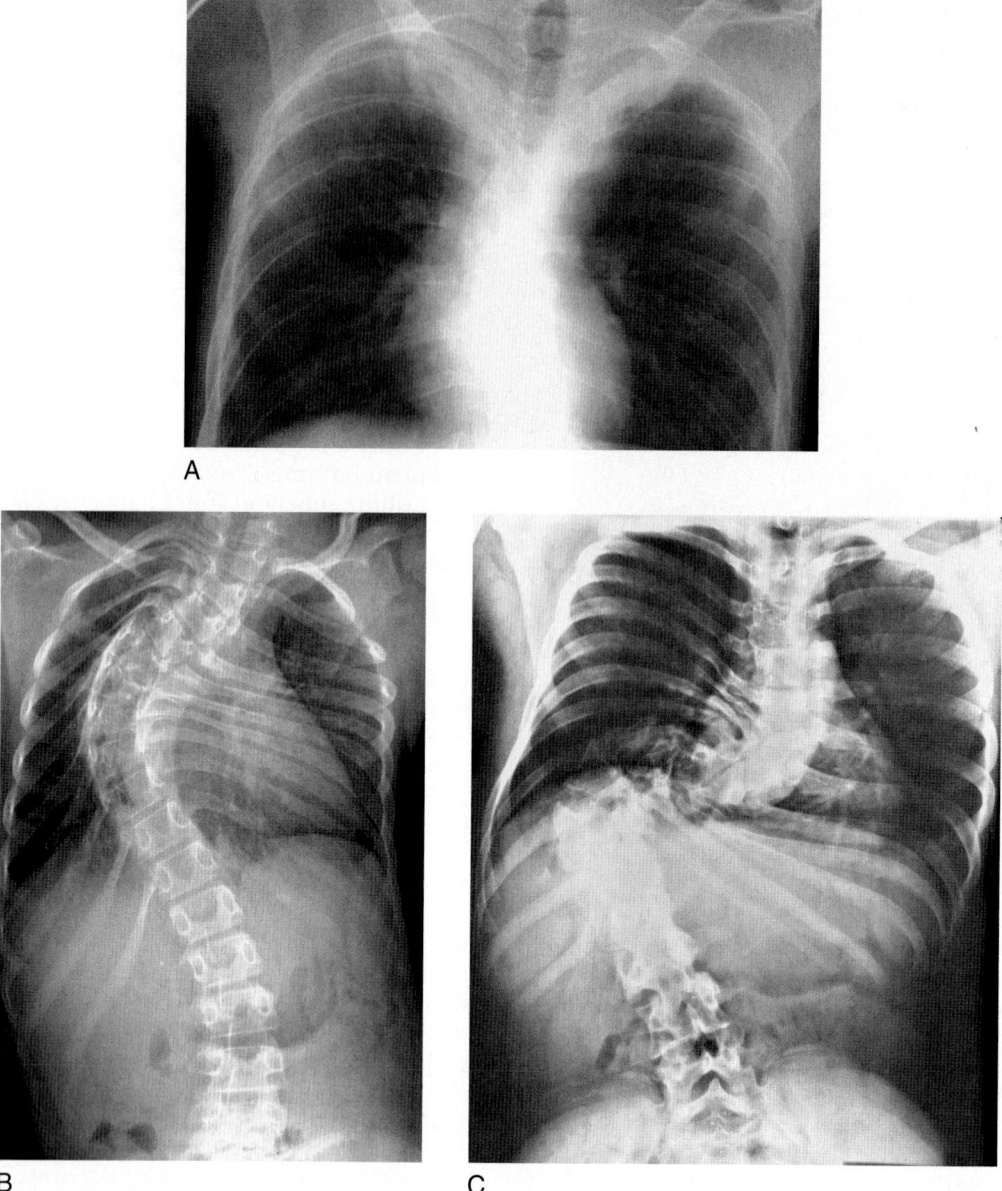

FIGURE 166-33. Neurofibromatosis type 1 (NF1). **A,** Anteroposterior chest radiograph showing thinned ribs with wavy inferior caudal surfaces, soft tissue masses at the apices (neurofibromas), and scoliosis. **B,** Nondystrophic scoliosis. No dysplastic vertebra are seen. **C,** Dystrophic scoliosis. Dysplastic vertebra contribute to an acute curvature.

phrenic, recurrent laryngeal, or intercostals nerves, locations where non-neurogenic tumors are much more common (see Fig. 166-33A). In addition, neurofibromas in the chest are hypodense by CT (usually 10 to 25 Hounsfield units), hypointense on T1-weighted MRI images, and heterogeneous high signal on T2-weighted images. Therefore, they may mimic adenopathy in the mediastinum, Ewing sarcoma in the chest wall, or metastatic lesions of the ribs. Plexiform mediastinal neurofibromas often mimic lymphoma.

There is no increased incidence of pulmonary fibrosis and bullous disease in NF1 patients. The interstitial disease originally described in older patients with neurofibromatosis subsequently has been shown to be related to manifestations of smoking.

Heart disease occurs with slightly increased frequency in NF1. Heart disease occurs with greater frequency in related syndromes (neurofibromatosis–Noonan syndrome, familial neurofibromatosis microdeletion syndrome, Watson syndrome). Patients with neurofibromatosis–Noonan syndrome manifest features of both syndromes. Familial neurofibromatosis microdeletion syndrome (FNMS) is due to deletion of the entire NF1 gene, with breakpoints at flanking repetitive sequences on either side of the gene. Microdeletions occur in 5% to 10% of NF1 patients. FNMS patients have a more severe phenotype with coarse, dysmorphic facies and heart disease. The facies of FNMS patients resembles Noonan syndrome facies. Patients with FNMS may have hypertrophic cardiomyopathy, ventricular septal defect, and mitral insufficiency, but usually not pulmonic stenosis, which is common in Noonan syndrome. FNMS patients also have a very high frequency of severe mental retardation (39%), whereas mental retardation in classic NF1 is un-

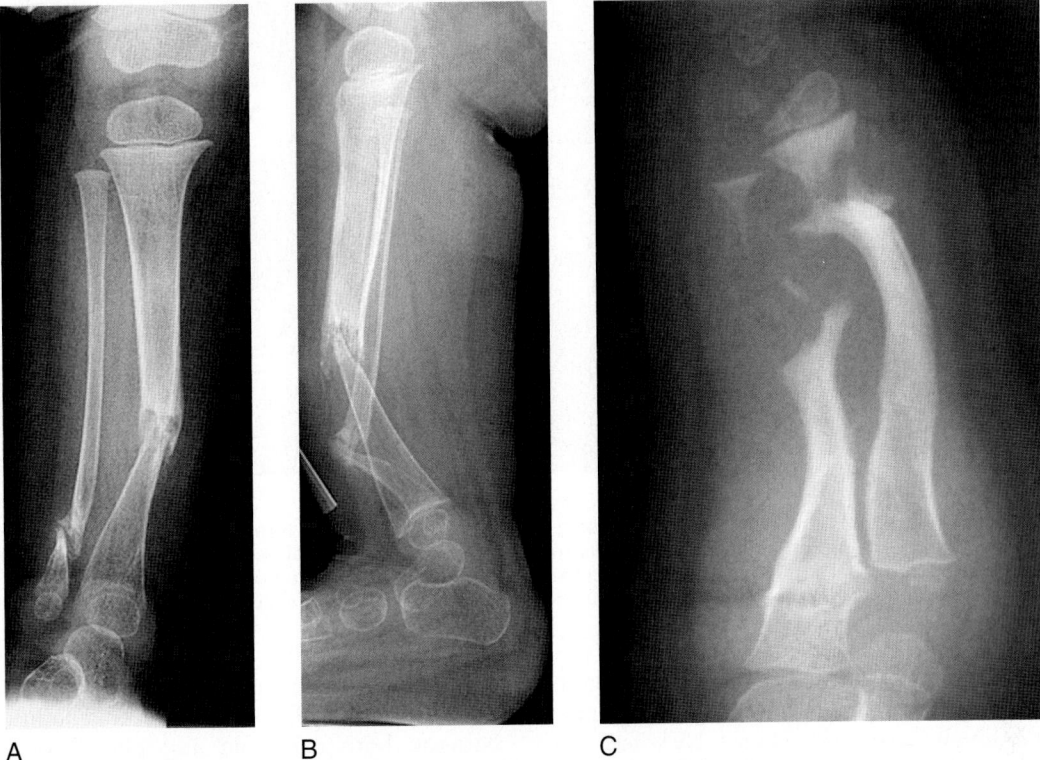

FIGURE 166-34. Neurofibromatosis type 1 (NF1). Anteroposterior **(A)** and lateral **(B)** radiographs of the tibia and fibula show congenital pseudarthroses of the tibial and fibular diaphyses. **C,** Different patient; congenital pseudarthroses of the radius and ulna in a 5-year-old boy.

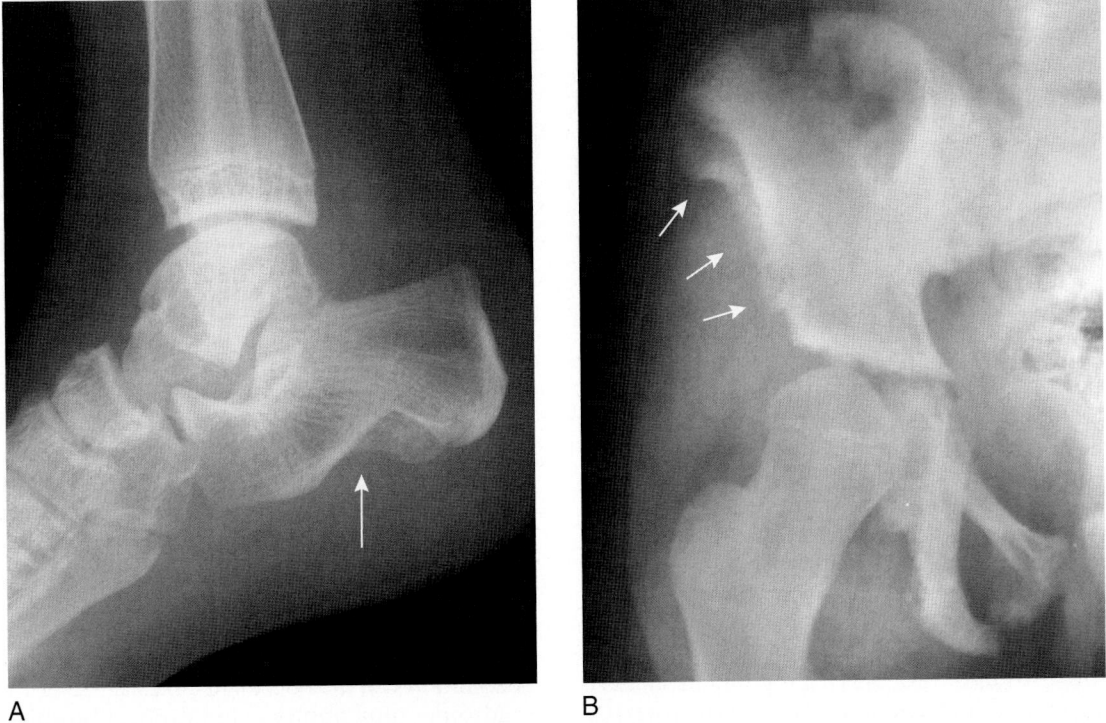

FIGURE 166-35. Neurofibromatosis type 1 (NF1). **A,** Lateral radiograph shows deformity of the undersurface of the calcaneus *(arrow)* with suggestion of an adjacent soft tissue tumor. **B,** Anteroposterior radiograph of the pelvis of a 10-year-old with deformity of the right iliac bone *(arrows)*, ischium, and pubic bone.

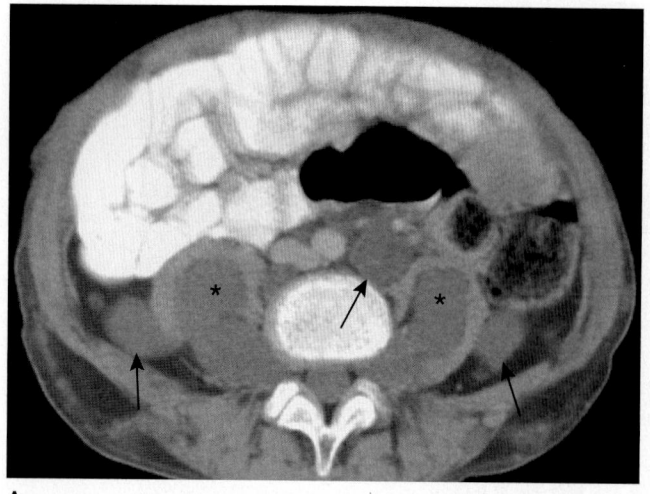
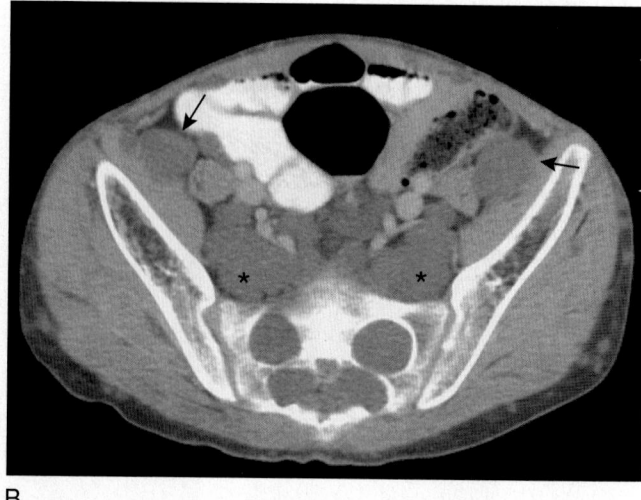

FIGURE 166-36. Neurofibromatosis type 1 (NF1) in a 16-year-old boy. **A,** Axial CT image through the lower lumbar spine shows large neurofibromas *(asterisks)* undermining each psoas muscle. Additional retroperitoneal neurofibromas are seen *(arrows)*. **B,** Axial CT image through the pelvis shows large presacral neurofibromas *(asterisks)* and expansion of the sacral spinal canal and neural foramina due to neurofibromas. Additional neurofibromas are seen adjacent to the external iliac vessels bilaterally *(arrows)*.

common in the absence of structural brain abnormalities. FNMS patients have a much higher risk of malignancy occurring at younger age than classic NF1 patients. Malignancies reported in FNMS patients have included rhabdomyosarcoma, juvenile chronic myeloid leukemia, and MPNST. The association of congenital heart disease with FNMS suggests that neurofibromin may have some role in heart development.

Watson syndrome is an autosomal dominant condition associated with valvar pulmonic stenosis, café au lait macules, short stature, mental retardation, and macrocephaly. Neurofibromas and Lisch nodules have been described in many Watson syndrome patients. Watson syndrome is closely linked to chromosome 17 and is either allelic or a contiguous gene syndrome with NF1.

ABDOMINAL MANIFESTATIONS

Neurofibromas, both isolated and plexiform, occur in the abdomen, retroperitoneum, and pelvis. Mesenteric lesions may be very large. Retroperitoneal neurofibromas and lateral meningoceles are often bilateral and symmetric within or undermining the psoas muscles. Neurofibromas are lower in attenuation than the muscle (Fig. 166-36). Pelvic presacral plexiform neurofibromas tend to be infiltrative (see Fig. 166-36).

In addition to nerve sheath tumors, there is an increased incidence in NF1 of other abdominal tumors: ganglioneuroma, intestinal carcinoid, pheochromocytoma, gastrointestinal stromal tumors (GISTs), adenocarcinoma, and embryonal sarcoma. In ganglioneuromatosis, there are multifocal or diffuse colonic polypoid ganglioneuromas. In addition to NF1, ganglioneuromatosis also occurs in multiple endocrine neoplasia type IIB. Clinically, patients have constipation and a Hirschsprung disease–like picture.

Carcinoids in NF1 occur most commonly in African Americans and are located at the ampulla of Vater. The incidence of adenocarcinoma of the pancreas, gallbladder, and stomach has been said to be higher in

NF1 patients than in the general population; however, this is unproven. There is, however, a definite association between both carcinoid and pheochromocytoma and NF1. Both tumors frequently occur in the same patient. Pheochromocytoma is found in 20% to 50% of hypertensive patients with NF1. The pheochromocytoma is usually unilateral (84%) and adrenal in origin (96%).

GISTs are tumors with immunoreactivity with CD117 (KIT) and CD34. They resemble leiomyomas, arising in the bowel wall and extending into the mesentery. The most characteristic features of GISTs in NF1 are their small bowel location and multiplicity.

Genitourinary neurofibromatosis is rare in infancy and adolescence. Neurofibromas can arise from the bladder trigone, ureters, and urethra. Hematuria and urinary tract obstruction are common presentations. Involvement of the vagina, cervix, seminal vesicles, spermatic cord, prostate, testes, and external genital has also been described.

VASCULAR MANIFESTATIONS

The vasculopathy of neurofibromatosis is associated with intimal hypertrophy with fragmentation of the media and elastic laminas and small nodules of smooth muscle. This results in arterial aneurysms and stenoses most frequently involving the thoracoabdominal aorta and mesenteric and renal arteries. Vasculopathy is found in approximately 2% of NF1 patients. Aortic and renal lesions frequently cause systemic hypertension, often producing the middle aortic syndrome or abdominal aortic coarctation (Fig. 166-37). Similar abdominal coarctation can also occur in Takayasu arteritis, Williams syndrome, mucopolysaccharidosis, fibromuscular dysplasia, and tuberous sclerosis.

HEMATOLOGIC MANIFESTATIONS

Patients with NF1 are predisposed to leukemia, primarily juvenile chronic myelogenous leukemia (JCML). JCML is a rare malignancy accounting for less than 5% of

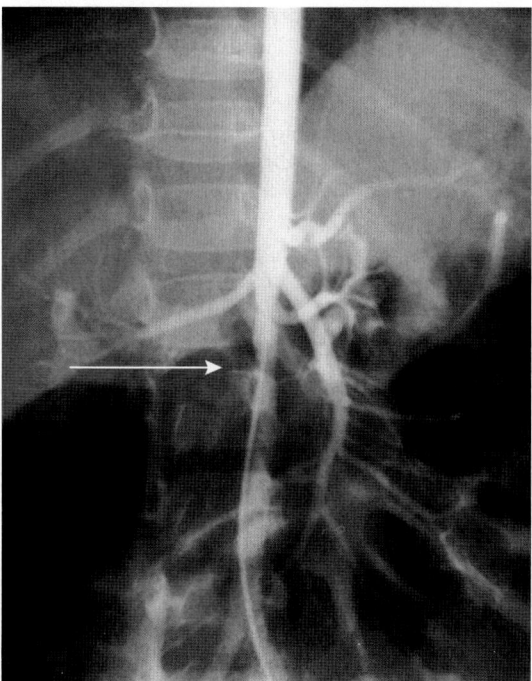

FIGURE 166-37. Neurofibromatosis type 1 (NF1). Abdominal aortogram shows an abdominal aortic coarctation in a hypertensive patient. The aorta is narrow at the level of the renal arteries and caudally *(arrow)*.

childhood leukemia. It occurs in children less than 3 years old and is characterized by marked hepatosplenomegaly, severe thrombocytopenia, extreme leukocytosis, absence of the Philadelphia chromosome, and a very poor prognosis. Approximately 15% of all patients with JCML have neurofibromatosis.

CENTRAL NERVOUS SYSTEM MANIFESTATIONS

Central nervous system manifestations of neurofibromatosis are very frequent (see Section III). The most common intracranial tumors of NF1 are optic glioma, cerebellar and cerebral astrocytomas, brainstem gliomas, ependymomas, and third ventricular glioma. Other findings include macrocrania, extracranial neurofibromas, internal auditory canal ectasia, sphenoid wing dysplasia, aqueductal stenosis, and high signal lesions on T2-weighted MRI images in the basal ganglia, brainstem, and cerebellum. These high signal lesions are believed to be the most common central nervous system manifestations of NF1, occurring in 66% of patients. The lesions may regress and are believed to be due to intermittent intramyelinic edema. Precocious puberty occurs in NF1, but only in the presence of optic glioma.

Neurofibromatosis Type 1 (NF1):

- **Soft tissue tumors: neurofibroma, neurolemmomas, malignant peripheral nerve sheath tumor, rhabdomyosarcoma, malignant triton tumor**
- **Skeletal manifestations: erosive changes due to neurofibromas, scoliosis, congenital tibial**

---

pseudarthrosis, sphenoid wing dysplasia, multiple nonossifying fibromas
- **Abdominal tumors: ganglioneuromatosis, intestinal carcinoid, pheochromocytoma, GISTs**
- **Vascular/hematologic: abdominal aortic coarctation, leukemia (juvenile chronic myelogenous leukemia)**

Neurofibromatosis 2

Neurofibromatosis type 2 is an autosomal dominant condition, first described by Wishart in 1820 in a patient with bilateral acoustic neuromas, and then confused with von Recklinghausen disease after that was described in 1865. NF2 was only definitively differentiated from NF1 in 1987 when the gene loci for NF2 was identified. NF2 is also called bilateral acoustic neuroma syndrome, central neurofibromatosis, and MISME syndrome (multiple inherited schwannomas, meningiomas, and ependymomas). The gene locus for NF2 is located on the long arm of chromosome 22 at 22q12.2 and encodes for the tumor suppressor protein merlin or schwannomin. Approximately 50% of patients have a new mutation and 50% have familial NF2.

Bilateral eighth nerve tumors are the essential feature of NF2. Originally, these tumors were called acoustic neuromas. The 1991 NIH Consensus Conference on Acoustic Neuroma preferred the name vestibular schwannoma because the lesion involves more often the vestibular than the acoustic branch of the eighth nerve and because it is pathologically a schwannoma.

The 1988 NIH Consensus Conference on Neurofibromatosis developed criteria for the diagnosis of NF2 (Table 166-4), revised by Gutmann into criteria for definitive and presumptive NF2. The reasoning behind these criteria is the difficulty in making a definitive diagnosis of NF2 in a patient who does not have bilateral vestibular schwannomas at initial presentation.

The incidence of NF2 is between 1 in 33,000 and 1 in 87,000. Approximately 100 new cases occur in the United

---

TABLE 166-4

Diagnostic Criteria for NF2

DEFINITIVE DIAGNOSIS
- Bilateral VIIIth nerve schwannomas on MRI or CT
- First-degree relative with NF2 and early-onset vestibular schwannoma (younger than 30 years) or any two of the following: meningioma, glioma, schwannoma, juvenile posterior cortical cataract

PRESUMPTIVE DIAGNOSIS
- Early-onset unilateral VIIIth nerve schwannoma on MRI or CT (younger than 30 years) and one of the following: meningioma, glioma, schwannoma, juvenile cortical cataract
- Multiple meningiomas (>2) and vestibular schwannoma and one of the following: glioma, schwannoma, juvenile cortical cataract

States each year. Nonpenetrance is rare. Symptoms may occur as early as 5 years of age; almost all patients have symptoms by age 60. NF2 can be divided into a severe variety (sometimes called Wishart type) that is symptomatic before 20 years of age with bilateral vestibular schwannomas and multiple other tumors, and a mild variety (sometimes called Gardner type) with only late-developing bilateral vestibular schwannomas.

Other tumors occurring in NF2 include intramedullary low-grade ependymomas, schwannomas of other cranial nerves (especially the fifth), meningiomas, and neurofibromas. The risk of malignancy in NF2 is much less than that in NF1, but is increased by radiation. Therefore, CT scanning should be limited in these patients. MRI is thus the preferred method to follow NF2 patients. Meningiomas are frequently supratentorial but may be spinal; 63% to 67% of patients with NF2 have spinal tumors. Approximately half are intramedullary and half are extramedullary. Approximately 45% of NF2 patients have at least one intramedullary and one extramedullary tumor. Ependymoma, astrocytoma, and schwannoma are the most common intramedullary tumors. Schwannoma and meningioma are the most common extramedullary.

Schwannomatosis is a condition believed to be separate from NF2 in which there are multiple peripheral and cranial nerve schwannomas, but not vestibular schwannomas. This disease is probably due to a mutation in the long arm of chromosome 22 and may be allelic to NF2.

Meningioangiomatosis is a hamartomatous condition often associated with intractable seizures. Cortical meningovascular fibroblastic proliferation with leptomeningeal calcification is present. Meningioangiomatosis may be a forme fruste of NF2, occurring both in patients with NF2 and patients without other manifestations of NF2. Meningioangiomatosis is differentiated from Sturge-Weber syndrome by the presence of cortical calcification in the latter condition.

Non–central nervous system manifestations of NF2 are not common. They include café au lait macules in 41% of patients, skin tumors in 68% of patients (although areolar neurofibroma, plexiform neurofibroma, and Lisch nodules do not occur), and juvenile cortical cataracts in 38% of patients. Posterior subcapsular lenticular opacities, or juvenile cortical cataracts, may antedate any of the other findings and are the presenting abnormality in more than 10% of patients. Children at risk for NF2 by family history should be followed with MRI, audiologic, and ophthalmologic examinations beginning by at least 10 years of age.

NEVOID BASAL CELL CARCINOMA SYNDROME

Nevoid basal cell carcinoma syndrome (NBCCS) or Gorlin syndrome is an autosomal dominant condition characterized by basal cell skin carcinomas, odontogenic keratocysts of the jaw (Fig. 166-38), palmar and plantar pits, and lamellar calcifications in the falx cerebri (Fig. 166-39), the diaphragma sellae and the tentorium cerebelli. In addition to basal cell carcinoma, there is an increased incidence of multiple neoplastic conditions, including medulloblastoma, Hodgkin disease, fibrosarcoma, bilateral calcified ovarian fibromas, intra-abdominal lymphangioma, and cardiac fibroma. Associated skeletal malformations include bifid anterior ribs, cervical spine segmentation anomalies, Sprengel deformity, spotty sclerotic skeletal lesions, and phalangeal cysts.

The genetic locus for NBCCS is the *PTCH* tumor suppressor gene mapped to 9q22. Patients may develop basal cell carcinomas in great numbers. The tumors are found in over 90% of patients over 40 years of age, but are rare before 20 years of age. The basal cell carcinomas in this syndrome are related to ultraviolet radiation and

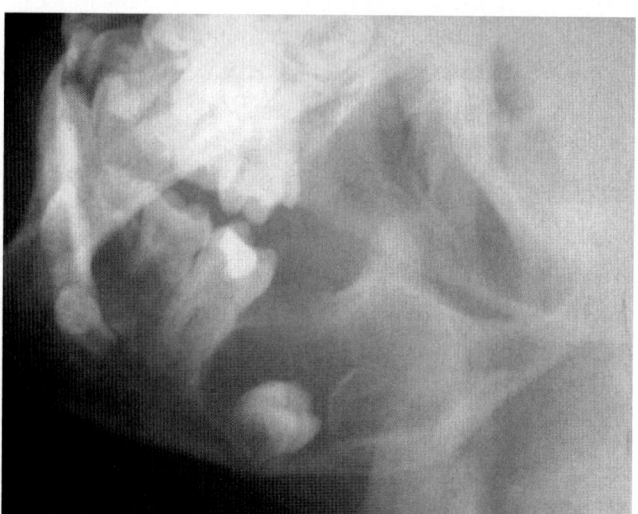

FIGURE 166-38. Nevoid basal cell carcinoma syndrome. Oblique mandible radiograph shows a lucent lesion of a keratocyst with distortion of surrounding teeth.

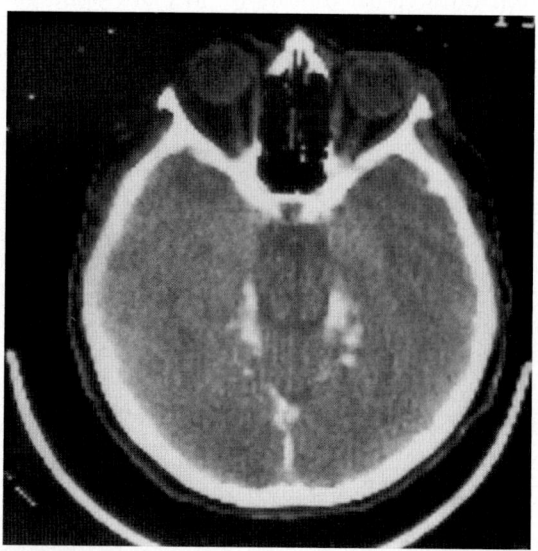

FIGURE 166-39. Nevoid basal cell carcinoma syndrome. Axial noncontrast CT scan of the brain shows extensive dural calcifications along the falx cerebri and the edges of the tentorium cerebelli.

are significantly less common in dark-skinned individuals affected by the syndrome. Patients with NBCCS who have had spinal radiation for medulloblastoma may develop hundreds of scalp basal cell carcinomas and also meningiomas. The meningiomas occur only after therapeutic radiation and are not otherwise associated with NBCCS. It has been suggested that patients with NBCCS with medulloblastoma receive chemotherapy in lieu of radiation therapy. Odontogenic keratocysts are much more common in the mandible than the maxilla, are infrequently symptomatic, and begin to appear between the ages of 7 and 40 years.

NIEMANN-PICK DISEASE

Niemann-Pick disease is a group of autosomal recessive congenital lipidoses in which sphingolipids accumulate in cells, especially reticuloendothelial cells, throughout the body—in the liver, spleen, bone marrow, lungs, and, to varying degrees, central nervous system. Several subtypes have been described. Types A and B (most common in people of Ashkenazi Jewish descent) result from the deficient activity of sphingomyelinase, a lysosomal enzyme encoded by a gene located on chromosome 11. Patients with type A have neurodegenerative disease, are typically normal at birth, but may present with hydrops fetalis and have prolonged neonatal hyperbilirubinemia. They typically develop hepatosplenomegaly, lymphadenopathy, and psychomotor retardation by age 6 months, followed by developmental regression, and, in later stages, spasticity and rigidity. Most type A patients die by 3 years of age due to respiratory failure. Patients with type B do not have nervous system involvement. They typically present with hepatosplenomegaly, pulmonary reticulonodular interstitial changes and alveolar infiltrates, and pancytopenia, and typically survive to adulthood. Type C is a phenotypically milder form of the neuropathic type with hepatosplenomegaly and longer survival (to approximately 7 years of age). Diffusion tensor imaging has been used to follow the progression of type C disease. Other forms of Niemann-Pick disease have been described.

The skeletal findings of Niemann-Pick disease consist of widening of the medullary cavities, thin cortices, undertubulation of long bones, osteopenia, delayed bone age, mild gibbus at the thoracolumbar junction, and coxa valga. Abdominal imaging will demonstrate hepatosplenomegaly, and may show adrenal calcifications. High-resolution CT of the lungs shows ground-glass opacities in the upper lungs with smooth thickening of the interlobular septae in the lower lungs. Lipid abnormalities in types A and B disease may lead to premature atherosclerosis with elevated coronary artery calcium scores.

NOONAN SYNDROME

Noonan syndrome is an autosomal dominant condition associated with proportionate short stature, dysmorphic facial features, and specific congenital heart defects. The diagnostic features of Noonan syndrome are distinctive heart disease (either pulmonic stenosis or hypertrophic cardiomyopathy), hypertelorism, down-slanting palpebral fissures, ptosis, neck pterygia, short stature, psychomotor retardation, bleeding diathesis, thoracic deformity (especially pectus carinatum), cubitus valgus, low-set ears, low posterior hairline, perinatal lymphedema, and a family history of Noonan syndrome. Approximately 20% of Noonan syndrome patients have lymphatic abnormalities such as pulmonary lymphangiectasia, intestinal lymphangiectasia, and/or lymphedema. Bleeding diathesis occurs in 50% of Noonan syndrome patients and has been associated with complex platelet defects, partial factor XI deficiency, and von Willebrand disease. Other, less typical cardiac lesions may occur in Noonan syndrome, including atrial septal defect, atrioventricular canal, and tetralogy of Fallot.

Noonan syndrome is genetically heterogeneous. Approximately 50% of patients have point mutations in the gene *PTPN11* which is involved in the *RAS* protooncogene transduction pathway. Mutations in another Ras pathway gene, the *KRAS* gene, have also been found to occur in some Noonan syndrome patients. The phenotype of Noonan syndrome patients with *PTPN11* mutations is strongly associated with pulmonic stenosis and very infrequently with hypertrophic cardiomyopathy. *PTPN11* mutation patients more frequently have short stature, characteristic Noonan facies, easy bruisability, and sternal abnormalities than Noonan patients without *PTPN11* mutations. Interestingly, *PTPN11* mutations are also known to occur in some hematologic malignancies, including juvenile myelomonocytic leukemia. An increased incidence of leukemia, particularly juvenile myelomonocytic leukemia, does occur in patients with Noonan syndrome. There is also an increased incidence of rhabdomyosarcoma and neuroblastoma.

In addition to classical Noonan syndrome, there are several conditions that are genetically and phenotypically similar to Noonan syndrome. Neurofibromatosis–Noonan syndrome occurs with a phenotype overlapping NF1 and Noonan syndrome. A few patients have been shown to have both the *PTPN11* mutation and the neurofibromin mutation of NF1. Other so-called neurofibromatosis–Noonan syndrome patients have only NF1 with some features of Noonan syndrome, probably explained by the fact that both neurofibromin and *PTPN11* are involved in the Ras activation pathway. LEOPARD syndrome (*l*entigenes, *e*lectrocardiographic conduction defects, *o*cular hypertelorism, *p*ulmonic stenosis, *a*bnormal genitalia, *r*etardation of growth, and sensorineural *d*eafness) is an autosomal recessive condition, and a majority of studied patients had mutations in the *PTPN11* gene. Interestingly, approximately one third of LEOPARD syndrome patients with *PTPN11* mutations have had hypertrophic cardiomyopathy. Patients who have features of both syndromes—Noonan syndrome plus lentigenes and deafness—are believed to have mutations in the *PTPN11* gene specific for both syndromes. A small number of patients with Noonan syndrome have features characteristic of Turner syndrome, including coarctation of the aorta and horseshoe kidney. It is thought that these Noonan syndrome patients might have mutations in a putative *Xp-Yp* lymphogenic gene.

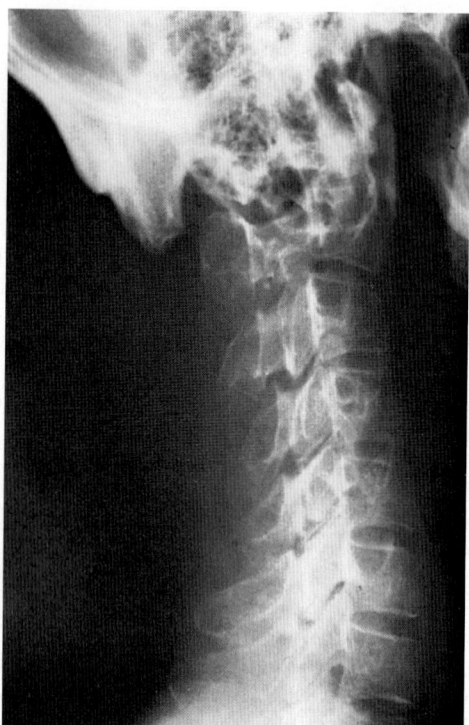

FIGURE 166-40. Occipital horn syndrome. Lateral radiograph of the skull base shows an occipital horn. (Courtesy of Dr. D. Sartoris, Stanford, CA.)

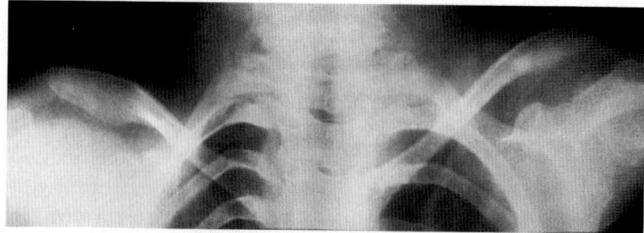

A

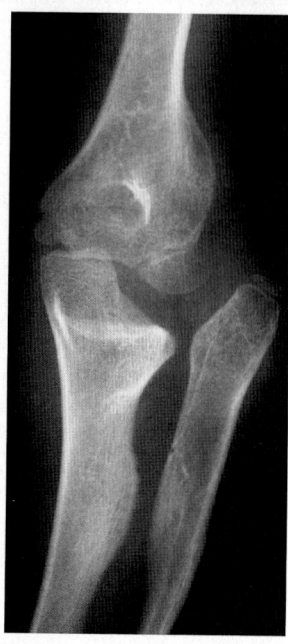

B

FIGURE 166-41. Occipital horn syndrome. **A,** Anteroposterior (AP) radiograph shows the abnormally shaped outer ends of the clavicles. **B,** AP elbow radiograph shows lateral radial head dislocation and bulbous distal humerus, proximal ulna, and proximal radius.

OCCIPITAL HORN SYNDROME

The occipital horn syndrome, previously called X-linked cutis laxa or type IX EDS, is an X-linked recessive condition associated with a pathognomonic skeletal dysplasia, chronic diarrhea, obstructive uropathy, bladder diverticula, hypermobile fingers and joints, characteristic facies, and soft, velvety, easily bruised skin. Occipital horn syndrome is an allelic disorder to Menkes disease, with both associated with mutations in *ATP7A*, an X-linked cellular copper transport gene. Patients with both diseases have elevated levels of copper in fibroblasts, decreased serum copper, and decreased serum ceruloplasmin levels. It is believed that the milder phenotype of occipital horn syndrome occurs with mutations that allow expression of 2% to 5% or more of *ATP7A* function. The major manifestations of occipital horn syndrome may be due to the copper-dependent enzyme lysyl oxidase, which is required to produce cross links in collagen. The pathognomonic radiographic features of this condition include occipital horns (Fig. 166-40) and short broad clavicles with hammer-shaped ends (Fig. 166-41). Occipital horns are bilateral parasagittal ectopic bone within the trapezium and sternocleidomastoid insertions that extend caudally from the occiput and probably increase in size with age. Other radiographic manifestations include abnormal elbows (see Fig. 166-41), capitate-hamate fusion, mild platyspondyly, undulating thickness of long bone cortices, flat acetabular roofs osteopenia, and wormian bones. The facies are also said to be characteristic, with a narrow face, high forehead, and long neck. The etiology of the chronic diarrhea is not known. Obstructive uropathy and bladder

diverticula may lead to recurrent infections and require surgical reconstruction of the urinary tract. Vascular tortuosity, kinking and dilation of cranial and extracranial vessels, vascular occlusions, and cystic medial degeneration occur in occipital horn syndrome, similar to the vascular abnormalities in Menkes disease.

OPITZ (G/BBB) SYNDROME

Opitz (G/BBB) syndrome is a heterogeneous malformation characterized by the triad of hypertelorism, cleft lip and palate, and hypospadias. Additional manifestations include characteristic facies, swallowing dysfunction, and stridor due to laryngeal abnormalities, including hypoplastic epiglottis, hypoplastic larynx, and congenital laryngo-tracheoesophageal cleft (Fig. 166-42). The syndrome has two identified forms: X-linked recessive (type I) and autosomal dominant (type II). The laryngeal abnormalities are limited to type I, only occur in males, and are associated with a high morbidity due to aspiration pneumonia and airway obstruction. Hypospadias of variable severity is present in 100% of males. Genitourinary anomalies are not present in females. Imperfo-

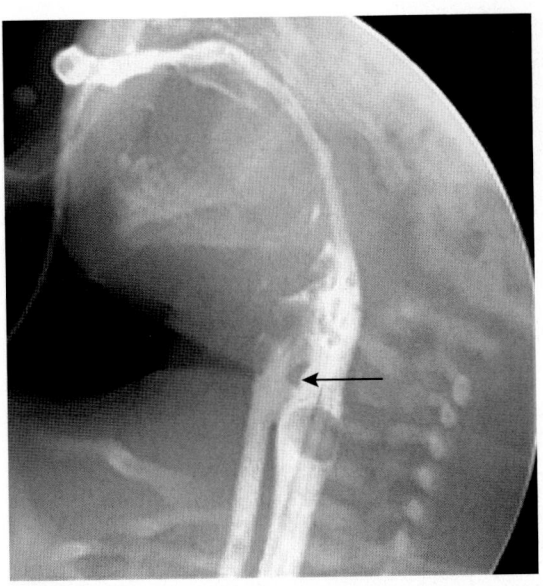

A

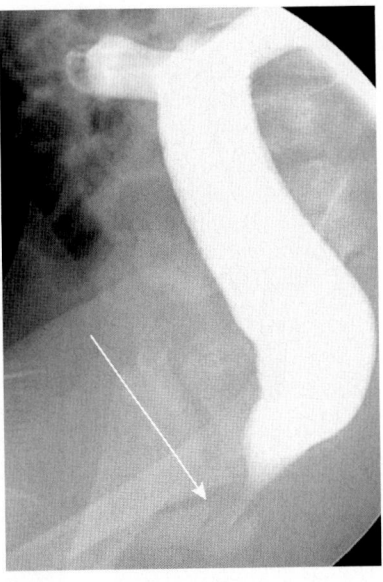

B

FIGURE 166-42. Opitz (G/BBB) syndrome. **A,** Esophagram shows laryngotracheoesophageal cleft *(arrow)* with contrast in both the trachea and esophagus. **B,** A mucus fistulogram shows an imperforate anus with a rectobulbar urethral fistula *(arrow).* The patient also had hypospadias.

rate anus has been occasionally reported both in affected males and female carriers (see Fig. 166-42). Cardiac lesions occur in approximately 20% of patients, but are not characteristic. Reported lesions include atrioseptal defect, partial anomalous pulmonary venous return, and patent ductus arteriosus. The most characteristic abnormality in Opitz (G/BBB) syndrome is hypertelorism, measured by the bony interorbital distance between the dacryons (medial orbit at the lacrimomaxillary suture). This finding is present in 100% of patients and may occur in female carriers of X-linked Opitz (G/BBB) syndrome. Other craniofacial abnormalities include cleft lip, palate, or uvula in 40%; broad, high nasal bridge; and short, posteriorly angled ears, and neonatal teeth. Midline central nervous system anomalies include agenesis/hypoplasia of the corpus callosum, large cisterna magna, and cerebellar vermian atrophy. The gene locus for the autosomal dominant type II disease is 22q11.2. The gene locus for the X-linked variety (Xp22.3) encodes for MID1, which is expressed in microtubular stabilization of the embryonic ventral midline.

ORAL-FACIAL-DIGITAL SYNDROMES

The oral-facial-digital (OFD) syndromes are a heterogeneous group. Multiple types are described. All have facial anomalies, oral findings (cleft or lobulated tongue, oral frenula, and/or cleft palate) (Fig. 166-43), and digital anomalies (brachy-, syn-, clino-, and polydactyly). Types I and II are discussed here.

OFD syndrome type I has dominant X-linked inheritance, multiple mutations, and a distinctive facies. Malformations of the fingers are seen in 50% to 70% and also include some slightly malformed, wide, short tubular bones; Y-shaped metatarsals; and cone-shaped epiphyses (see Fig. 166-43). Irregular mineralization is seen in the metacarpals, metatarsals, and proximal and middle phalanges, and spiculated areas on the middle parts of some phalanges. Toe malformations (25%) also include preaxial polydactyly.

Central nervous system findings include neuronal migration defects, intracerebral cysts and porencephaly or arachnoid cysts, abnormal gyration, heterotopic gray matter, brainstem abnormalities, hydrocephalus, vermian hypoplasia, Dandy-Walker malformation, and agenesis of the corpus callosum (40%). The nasion-sella-basion angle is increased from a normal 133 degrees (1 SD = 4.5) to 144 degrees. Renal abnormalities include polycystic kidneys (50%). The kidneys look like those of adult polycystic disease except that the cysts form from both the tubules and glomeruli, whereas, in adult polycystic kidney disease, the cysts are only from the tubules.

OFD syndrome type II (Mohr syndrome) is distinguished from type I in that it is autosomal recessive, is seen in females, and has median cleft lip, polylobed tongue, and medial cleft tongue more frequently. The medial incisors may be absent, and patients may have a conductive hearing loss and a bifid nasal tip. Polydactyly is more common, being present in more than 80% of patients. The polydactyly is postaxial in the hands and preaxial in the feet. Bilateral bifid great toes are common in OFD type II (Fig. 166-44).

OSTEOLYSIS SYNDROMES

The osteolysis syndromes are difficult to classify but can be roughly divided into five forms based on the areas of bone absorption and associated malformations.

1. Multicentric, affecting predominantly the carpal and tarsal bones with and without nephropathy
2. Multicentric, predominantly carpal, tarsal, and interphalangeal forms: Francois, Winchester, Torg, Whyte-Hemingway, NAO (*n*odulosis-*a*rthropathy-*o*steolysis), Singh syndromes
3. Forms affecting primarily the distal phalanges: Hajdu-Cheney, mandibular-acral form
4. Forms involving the diaphyses and metaphyses: familial expansile osteolysis, juvenile hyaline fibromatosis
5. Massive osteolysis of Gorham

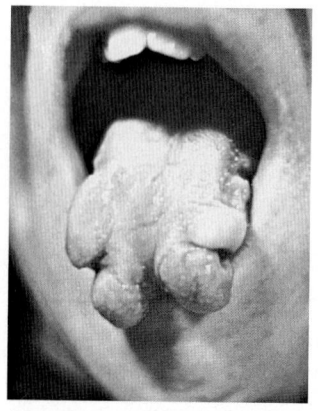

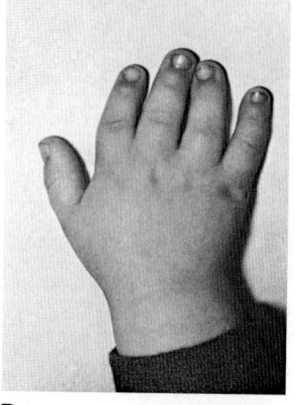

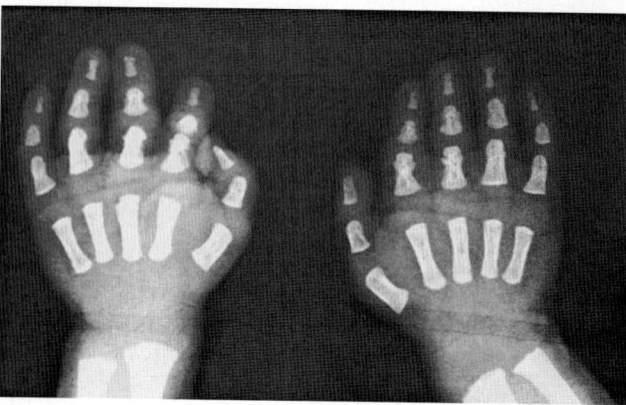

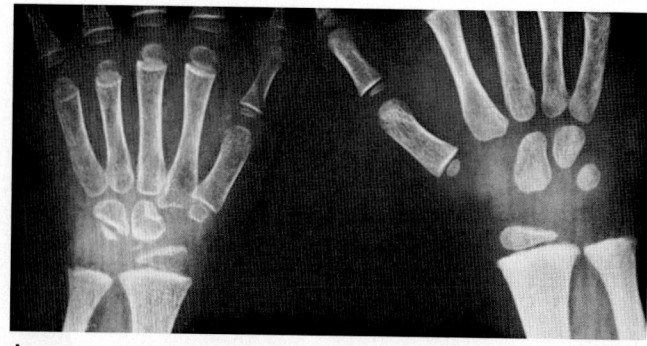

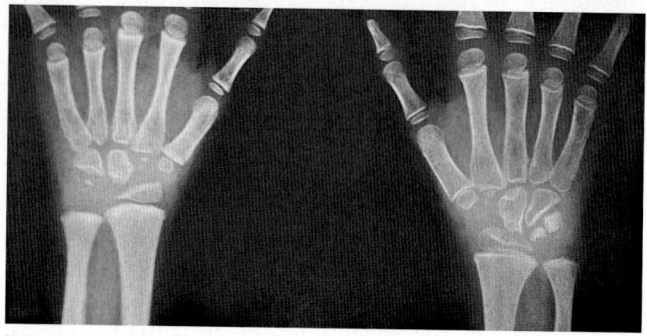

FIGURE 166-43. Oral-facial-digital syndrome, type I.
A, Longitudinal and lateral clefts and fibrous swellings are seen in the tongue of a 14-year-old girl. **B,** The fingers in the hand are broad and short, and some of the fingers are bent. The fourth and fifth fingers are relatively long in this girl of age 10. **C,** Posteroanterior radiograph of the hands shows shortening and bending of the proximal and middle phalanges of the second and third digits and relative elongation of the fourth and fifth fingers despite some deformity of these proximal phalanges. (**A** and **B** from Gorlin RJ, Psaume J; Orodigitofacial dysotosis—a new syndrome: a study of 22 cases. J Pediatr 1962;61:520-530. **C** from Schwarz E, Fish A: Roentgenographic features of a new congenital dysplasia. Am J Roentgenol Radium Ther Nucl Med 1960;84:511-517.)

FIGURE 166-45. Multicentric osteolysis syndrome (tarsocarpal osteolysis). **A,** The patient's left hand had been caught in a washing machine wringer, and the deformity of the carpal bones noted 10 months after injury had been attributed to the accident. **B,** The development of similar changes in the right hand 18 months later indicates the intrinsic nature of the changes.

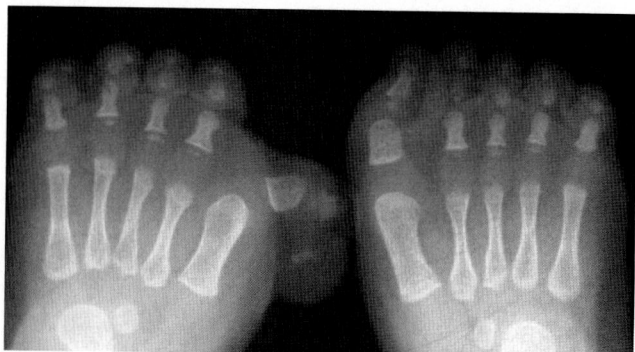

FIGURE 166-44. Oral-facial-digital syndrome, type II. Anteroposterior foot radiograph at 11 months old demonstrates preaxial polydactyly of the first digit on the right.

Hereditary multicentric osteolysis involving the carpal and tarsal bones starts in early childhood, usually by age 3 or 4 years, with arthritis-like symptoms of the wrists and feet. There develops a progressive absorption of the carpal and tarsal bones, which become crenated and eventually disappear, with marked narrowing of the carpal and tarsal areas (Fig. 166-45). The adjacent metacarpals and metatarsals are often involved, showing erosions and pencilling. Unlike rheumatoid arthritis, the mineral content of the bones remain good. Despite severe wrist and foot deformities, there may be few symptoms related to these areas.

Lesions are bilateral but not necessarily symmetric. The ankles (Fig. 166-46), elbows (Fig. 166-47), and knees may be involved, but the phalanges are generally spared. The metatarsophalangeal and the metacarpophalangeal joints can be involved. The disease becomes quiescent in adulthood. Both autosomal dominant and autosomal recessive forms can be seen. When associated with nephropathy, the disease can be fatal in the third decade. The pathogenesis is unknown, and on biopsy the tissues have fibrous elements and increased vascularity with little inflammation.

Imaging and clinical features help separate the group of osteolysis syndromes involving the carpal, tarsal, and interphalangeal areas: Francois, Torg, Winchester, Whyte-Hemingway, NAO, and Singh. Torg, Winchester, and NAO are autosomal recessive and are mutations in the MMP2 gene.

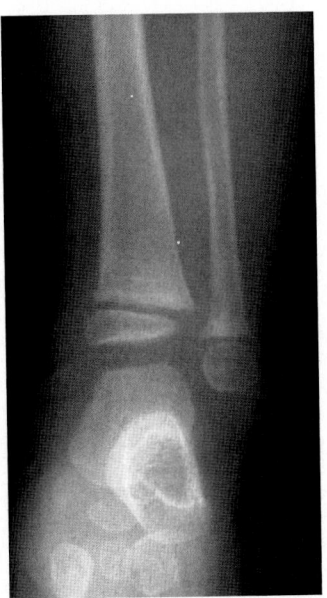 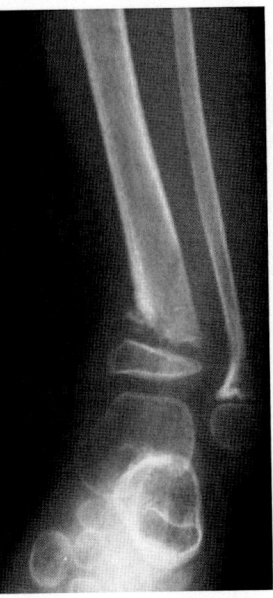

FIGURE 166-46. Osteolysis syndrome. Left ankle radiographs at age 15 months **(A)** and age 18 months **(B)**. There has been significant progressive absorption of the metaphyseal area on the distal tibia with bowing of the distal fibula.

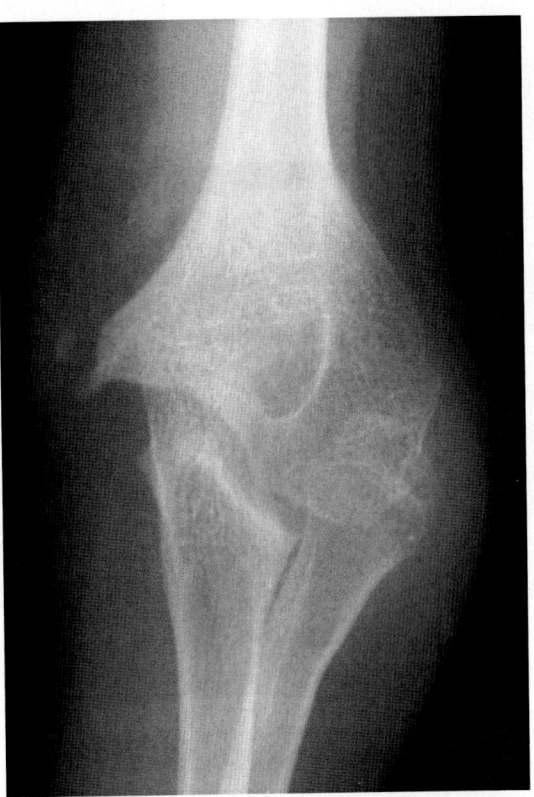

FIGURE 166-47. Osteolysis syndrome (hereditary multicentric osteolysis). Elbow radiograph of a 7-year-old boy with destructive changes about the elbow, most notable in the distal medial aspect of the humerus.

The forms principally involving the distal phalanges are also progressive and can be called acro-osteolysis. The lesions may stabilize in adult life. The more proximal phalanges can also exhibit absorption. Hadju-Cheney syndrome is discussed elsewhere in this chapter. Some osteolysis syndromes are difficult to classify.

Gorham, or Gorham-Stout, syndrome or "vanishing bone disease" is a condition usually starting gradually or abruptly before the age of 40 years that has striking radiographic findings of massive osteolysis and with proliferation of vascular and lymphatic vessels that involves soft tissues and bones. In the first stage of this disease, there is patchy osteoporosis with intramedullary and subcortical radiolucent foci. These foci enlarge with the development of new foci in the second stage. The third stage is cortical erosion and invasion of an angiomatous mass into surrounding tissues (Fig. 166-48). Finally, the bone disappears with lack of new bone formation (see Fig. 166-48). The remaining osseous tissue is tapered, and the destructive process may involve a whole region (i.e., shoulder or hip) with the adjacent bones being severely affected. The shoulder region is the most commonly affected.

OTOPALATODIGITAL SYNDROME

Two types of otopalatodigital (OPD) syndrome are described, and there are many similarities in facial features and radiologic findings. Type II is more severe. The syndrome's main features are abnormal facies, thumb and great toe deformity, cleft palate, and conductive hearing loss. There is some support for mapping the *OPD* gene to Xq28.

In type I, the typical face has prominent supraorbital ridges, a broad nasal root, poorly formed ears, and small nose and mouth, all giving the impression of a prize

fighter. The skull radiographs show thickening of the frontal and occipital regions, sclerotic skull base, large anterior fontanelle, unpneumatized sinuses and mastoids, and a small mandible. The deformities of the fingers and toes include shortening of the thumb and great toe and wide spacing between the first and second toes, giving the foot a resemblance to that of a tree frog. Broad, short first toes and thumbs associated with fusions of accessory ossification centers of the second metacarpals and metatarsals with adjacent carpal and tarsal bones are characteristic (Fig. 166-49). Other radiographic findings in the hands and feet include relatively long second and fifth metacarpals, clinodactyly, duplication of the terminal phalanges of the index finger and second toe, cone-shaped epiphyses of the terminal phalanges of the thumbs, carpal fusions, comma-shaped trapezoid, transverse capitate, tarsal fusions, and extra carpal and tarsal bones. Other radiographic findings include dislocation of radial heads, pectus excavatum, thin undulating posterior ribs, and hip subluxation.

Type II OPD is X-linked recessive and has more severe changes in the face, hands, and feet. The latter two show hypoplastic metacarpals and metatarsals, hypoplasia of the phalanges (especially the first), and camptodactyly. The ribs showed more marked waviness and angulation, sloping clavicles, and fused sternal segments. The long bones are dense, undermodeled, and bowed and may have irregular surfaces, and there may be hypoplastic fibulas. The ilia are flared, the acetabula flat, and the fibulas may be hypoplastic. Coronal cleft vertebra, dislo-

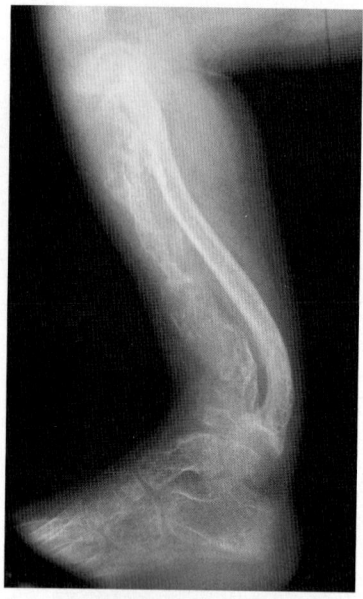

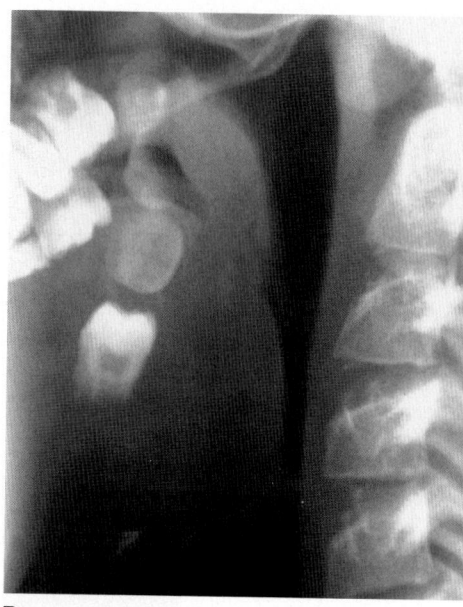

FIGURE 166-48. Gorham syndrome. **A,** Radiograph of a 7-year-old with diffuse osteolysis of the tibia. (Courtesy of Dr. Richard M. Shore, Chicago, IL.) **B,** Radiograph of a 9-year-old with complete osteolysis of the mandible, producing "floating teeth."

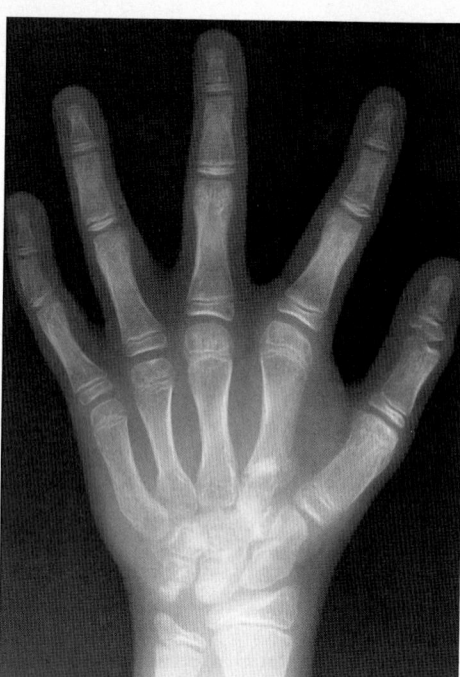

FIGURE 166-49. Otopalatodigital syndrome. Right hand radiograph shows typical findings of fusion of the accessory ossification centers of the second metacarpal with the adjacent deformed carpal bones. There is widening or abnormal tubulation of the metacarpals. The distal phalanx of the thumb is shortened with a coned-shaped epiphysis. Clinodactyly is present.

cated hips, and postaxial polydactyly can be seen. There may be an overlap of OPD type II and Melnick-Needles syndrome.

PACHYDERMOPERIOSTOSIS

Pachydermoperiostitis is a form of primary HOA having no causal associations as are found in secondary HOA.

This form is much rarer than the secondary form. It is autosomal dominant, mostly found in males. In the complete syndrome there is clubbing of the fingers and toes, large hands and feet, enlarged extremities from periarticular and osseous proliferation, and painful and swollen joints. There are coarse facial features with thickening and folding of the skin. The disease typically has an insidious onset around puberty but can occur earlier and then arrests after 10 years. Differences from the secondary form of the disease are earlier onset, family history, nonpainful bone proliferations, extension of the periostitis into the epiphyses, and more irregular bone proliferations. Osseous proliferations can occur in the pelvis and would be unusual in the secondary form. Also the diaphyses of the tubular bones, along with the ribs and clavicles, may be expanded and have coarse trabeculae, sclerotic islands, and a thick cortex. Ligamentous ossifications can occur. Osseous bridges between bones can lead to ankylosis. Hypertrophy and then osteolysis of the tufts are more common in primary HOA, but articular inflammation occurs less often. The skull may be thickened, and may have delayed suture closure and wormian bones. While increased peripheral blood flow is thought to be a factor in secondary HOA, in pachydermoperiostosis, the blood flow is decreased.

Myelofibrosis has occurred in association with pachydermoperiostosis. Primary HOA without cutaneous involvement is called Currarino's disease. Bisphosphonates may be useful in treatment.

PENA-SHOKEIR SYNDROME TYPE I (FETAL AKINESIA SEQUENCE)

Pena and Shokeir originally described a syndrome of arthrogryposis and facial anomalies that is now divided into two distinct entities. Pena-Shokeir syndrome type I or fetal akinesia sequence is a phenotype and not a nosologic entity, due to decreased fetal movement and belonging to the overall category of arthrogryposis

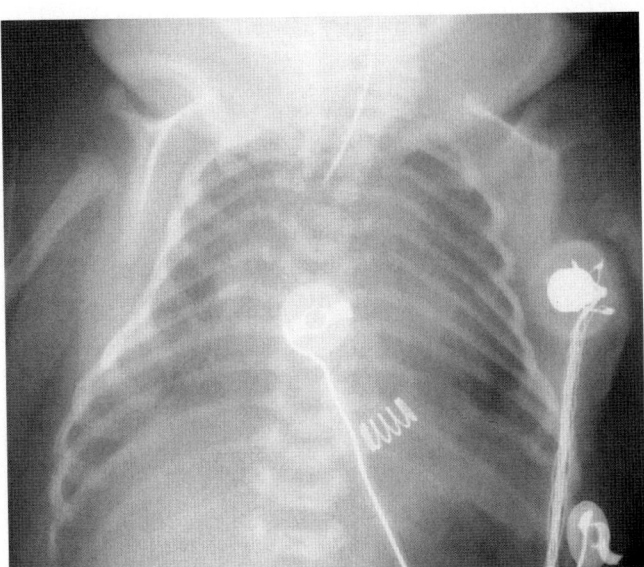

FIGURE 166-50. Pena-Shokeir syndrome type I. Chest radiograph of a newborn shows hypoplastic lungs, hypoplastic glenoid fossae, and dislocated proximal humerii.

multiplex congenita (AMC) syndromes. AMC refers to multiple joint contractures at birth with an intact skeleton. Pena-Shokeir syndrome type I is additionally characterized by camptodactyly and pulmonary hypoplasia. It is a genetically heterogeneous disease. The major findings of Pena-Shokeir syndrome type I include a history of maternal polyhydramnios, fetal growth retardation and short umbilical cord, pulmonary hypoplasia (Fig. 166-50), micrognathia, thin ribs, arthrogryposis, clubfoot, and camptodactyly. Moessinger demonstrated that the findings of the Pena-Shokeir syndrome type I can be produced by fetal akinesia in experiments with curarized fetal rats. Neuropathologic studies have demonstrated many abnormalities of the spinal motor neurons, pyramidal tracts, and muscles and of the central nervous system, including reactive gliosis, multicystic encephalopathy, polymicrogyria, persistent meningeal vascularization, agenesis of the septum pellucidum, and hydranencephaly. These cerebral lesions probably play a role in the development of the spinal muscular atrophy, which in turn leads to fetal akinesia.

PENA-SHOKEIR SYNDROME TYPE II (CEREBRO-OCULOFACIAL-SKELETAL SYNDROME)

Pena-Shokeir syndrome type II is a distinct autosomal recessive condition with a phenotype somewhat similar to that of type I, but with microphthalmia as a constant feature. Pena-Shokeir syndrome type II is also frequently called cerebro-oculofacial-skeletal (COFS) syndrome. It is characterized by microcephaly, cataracts, microphthalmia, blepharophimosis, characteristic facies, camptodactyly, kyphoscoliosis, joint contractures of the elbows and knees (arthrogryposis), vertical tali with rocker-bottom feet, failure to thrive, and progressive central nervous system demyelination. Frequently associated findings include hypoplasia or agenesis of the corpus callosum, cerebral calcifications, and hypoplasia of the

second tarsal cuneiform with a proximally positioned second metatarsal. COFS is an allelic disorder to Cockayne syndrome (severe retardation, leukodystrophy, intracranial calcifications, photosensitivity). Mutations in the excision repair cross-complementing group 6 gene (*ERCC6*) are found in 75% of patients with Cockayne syndrome and in most patients with COFS.

POLAND SYNDROME

Poland syndrome is characterized by partial or complete absence of the pectoral muscles associated with anomalies of the ipsilateral upper extremity. It is occasionally associated with development of neoplasm and may have familial inheritance. Extremity changes range from syndactyly, polydactyly, or phalangeal hypoplasia to radial ray anomalies and shoulder girdle anomalies (Fig. 166-51). Other reported anomalies include scoliosis, rib anomalies, and renal hypoplasia/agenesis. Plain radiographs demonstrate relative thoracic hyperlucency as well as skeletal extremity changes (see Fig. 166-51). CT and MRI better demonstrate the musculoskeletal anomalies and also possible breast hypoplasia (see Fig. 166-51). Poland syndrome is thought to arise from subclavian arterial compromise in fetal life.

PROGERIA

Progeria is a rare condition causing premature aging. Mutations in the lamin A/C (*LMNA*) gene are responsible for this syndrome. There is growth retardation and accelerated degenerative changes in the cutaneous, cardiovascular, and musculoskeletal systems. Affected infants are normal at birth, but the changes are evident by the first or second year of life when progressive signs of aging appear, such as alopecia, craniofacial disproportion, beaklike nose, atrophic skin, decreased subcutaneous tissue, prominent eyes, and "horse-riding" stance.

The radiographic findings include osteopenia, fish-mouth vertebrae, coxa valga, thin long bones with widened metaphyses, genu valgum, hypoplastic mandible with tooth loss, thin diploic space in the skull, craniofacial disproportion, open fontanelles, thin and sloping ribs, small thoracic cage, hip subluxation or aseptic necrosis, and cerebrovascular occlusions (Fig. 166-52). An unusual feature is that certain parts of the skeleton undergo progressive osteolysis. This occurs in the clavicles, distal phalanges, upper ribs, and proximal humeri. In the clavicle, the absorption progresses from lateral to medial and the clavicle can completely resorb. The distal phalanges of the fingers and toes can disappear, leaving only the proximal phalanges. The most commonly involved ribs are the second and third posteriorly. Most patients die by the teenage years, but the condition can be lethal at birth.

PROTEUS SYNDROME

Proteus syndrome is a congenital hamartomatous disorder that may be autosomal dominant. Most cases are sporadic and the result of new mutations. Patients have overgrowth of the hands or feet, asymmetry of the limbs,

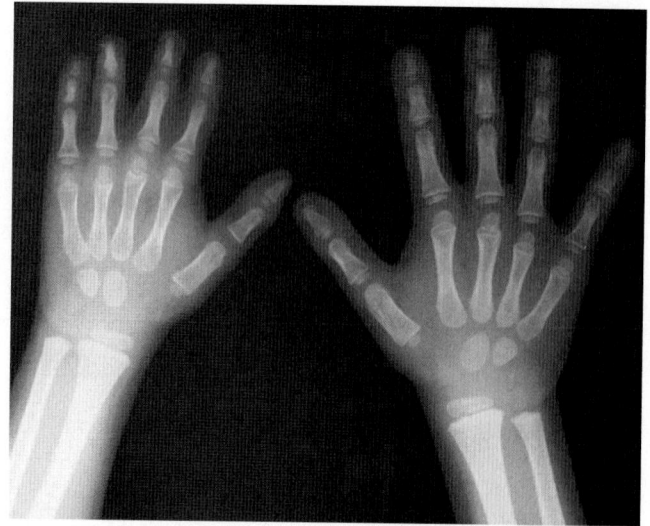

A

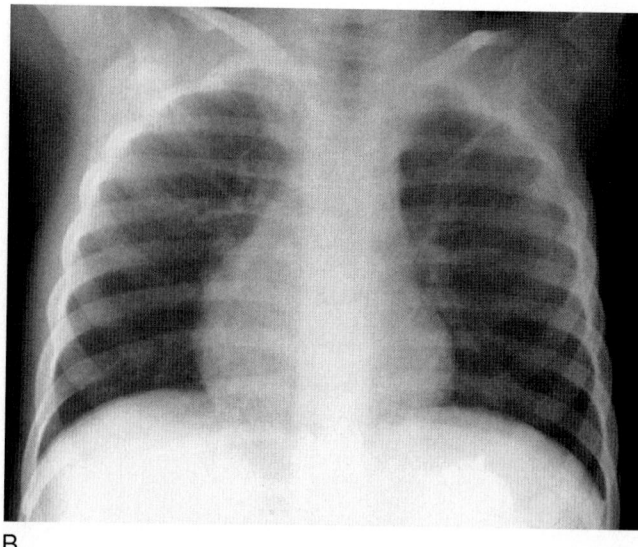

B

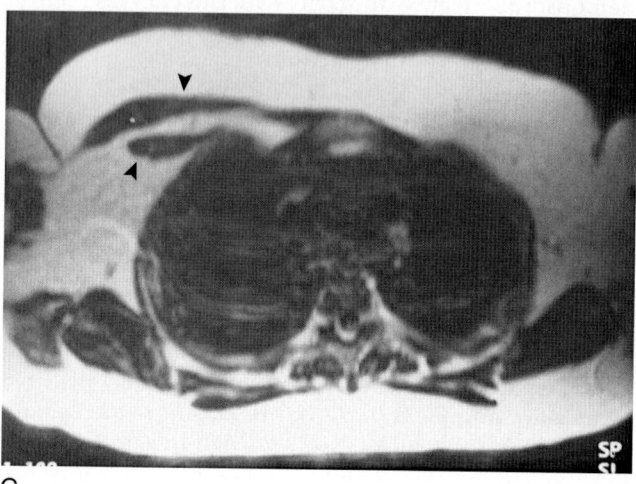

C

FIGURE 166-51. Poland syndrome. **A,** Hand radiograph shows generalized hypoplasia of the right hand with soft tissue syndactyly affecting the second through fourth digits. **B,** Anteroposterior chest radiograph on a different patient shows relative lucency of the left hemithorax with loss of the pectoral shadow. **C,** Axial T1-weighted MR image shows absence of the left anterior chest wall musculature (*arrowheads* indicate normal musculature on the right).

connective tissue nevi, epidermal nevi, vascular and lymphatic malformations, and cranial hyperostosis. The tissue overgrowth is progressive but tends to plateau after puberty.

Patients with Proteus syndrome may have marked craniofacial abnormalities with facial and ocular asymmetry. A hyperplastic plantar overgrowth called "moccasin lesion" is characteristic in the feet. The hands and feet are large and often have macrodactyly.

The radiographic findings of Proteus syndrome reflect what is seen clinically, namely overgrowth of limbs and digits from both bone and soft tissues. The hands and feet are particularly involved. There may be postaxial polydactyly, clinodactyly, cubitus valgus, radial head subluxation, hip dysplasia, coxa valga, coxa vara, coxa plana, genu recurvatum, and long bone bowing. Abnormal and asymmetric fat distribution and asymmetric muscle development may occur. The skull may be large, asymmetric, and dolichocephalic and have hyperostosis. Hydrocephalus and hemimeganencephaly can be seen. The spine may show large vertebral bodies and neural arches, asymmetric vertebral bodies, scoliosis, and kyphosis. Lung cysts (12% to 13% of cases), progressive

diffuse cystic lung disease, pectus excavatum, pulmonary embolism, and respiratory failure can occur. Several types of tumors are associated with the Proteus syndrome, including lipomas that tend to grow aggressively, ovarian cystadenoma, monomorphic parotid adenoma, testicular tumors, and central nervous system tumors (especially meningiomas).

RUBINSTEIN-TAYBI SYNDROME

Rubinstein-Taybi syndrome is a sporadic condition due to a mutation on chromosome 16, or less commonly on chromosome 22, characterized by facial dysmorphism, mental retardation, and broadening of the thumbs and great toes. Characteristic broadening of the distal phalanges of the thumb and great toe is a diagnostic marker for the syndrome (Fig. 166-53). Additional radiographic findings include delayed skeletal maturation and dislocations, flared iliac wings, large foramen magna, and cervical instability with odontoid malformation. Visceral malformations include malrotation and vesicoureteral reflux. Intracranial lesions include agenesis of the corpus callosum and Dandy-Walker malformation.

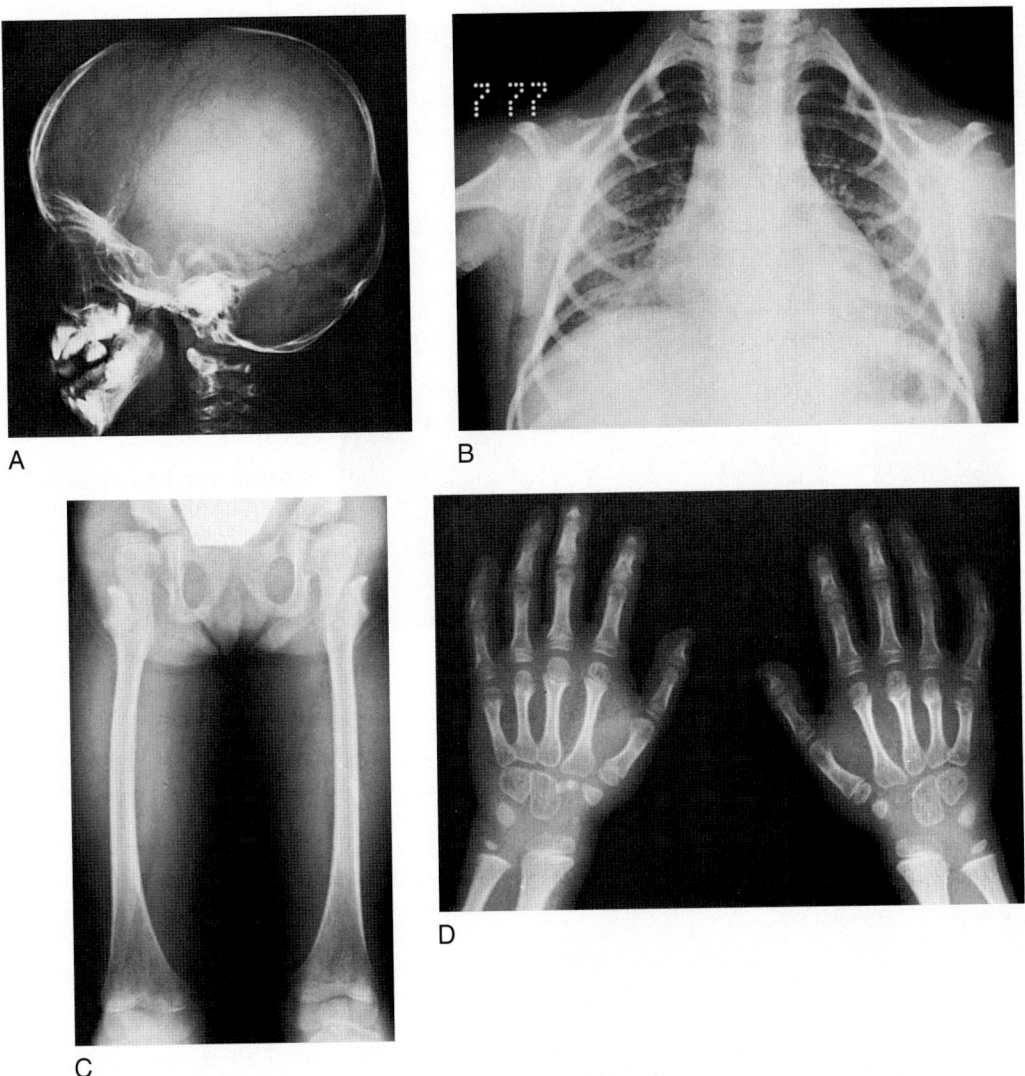

FIGURE 166-52. Progeria in a 7-year-old girl. **A,** Lateral skull radiograph shows small facial structures in relation to the neurocranium, with a persistent open anterior fontanelle. The ascending rami of the mandible are very short. **B,** The clavicles are miniscule, in part due to osteolysis of the lateral portions. The clavicles thus appear widely separated from the acromion processes. The ribs are abnormally gracile. **C,** Coxa valga deformity is marked, with the femoral necks continuous with the axes of the femoral shafts with no angulation. The femoral heads are only partially in their acetabuli. The greater trochanters are bizarre in shape and position. **D,** Acro-osteolysis is prominent in the terminal phalanges. Some carpal ossification centers are sclerotic, while others participate in the generalized osteopenia. Skeletal maturation is appropriate for the age.

RUSSELL-SILVER SYNDROME

The Russell-Silver syndrome is characterized by body asymmetry, low birth weight, and variable dysmorphic features. Both autosomal dominant and X-linked inheritance have been described. Additional features include intrauterine growth retardation, postnatal retardation of height and weight (hence the occasional reference to "Russell-Silver dwarfism"), clinodactyly, toe syndactyly, delayed bone age, scoliosis, developmental dysplasia of the hip, triangular facies, and urogenital anomalies. Body asymmetry with leg length discrepancy is found in approximately 50% of patients (Fig. 166-54). Discrepancies of up to 6 cm may occur. The bone age is delayed in childhood, averaging 69% of chronologic age, but at puberty is approximately 95% of the chronologic age. Hand anomalies include ivory epiphyses of the distal phalanges, brachymesophalangy of the fifth digit, and clinodactyly. Genitourinary anomalies include ureteropelvic junction obstruction, reflux, renal ectopia, renal fusion anomalies, hypospadias, cryptorchidism (42% of males), posterior urethral valves, hydroceles, and scrotal hypoplasia. There may be an increased incidence of Legg-Calvé-Perthes disease, which, like Russell-Silver syndrome, is associated with delayed bone age, and of malignancies, which interestingly also occur in some other syndromes of growth disturbance and asymmetric growth, such as BWS.

SMITH-LEMLI-OPITZ SYNDROME

Smith-Lemli-Opitz syndrome or RSH/Smith-Lemli-Opitz syndrome, is an autosomal recessive condition with two phenotypes. The classic, or type I, phenotype is asso-

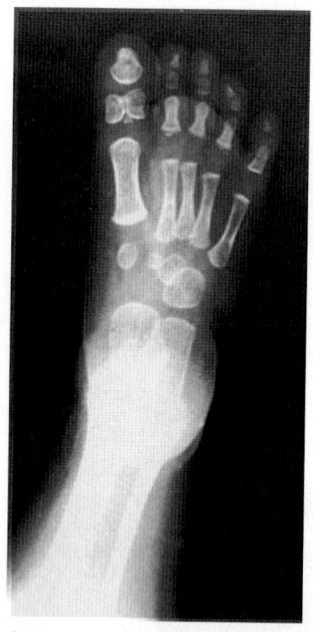
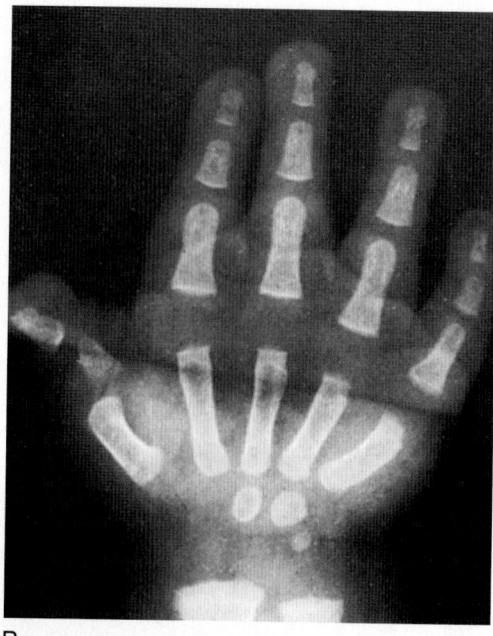

FIGURE 166-53. Rubenstein-Taybi syndrome. Radiographs of hand **(A)** and foot **(B)** in patients with Rubinstein-Taybi syndrome show the great toe and thumb to have short, wide phalanges. Partial duplication of the proximal phalanx of the great toe is noted.

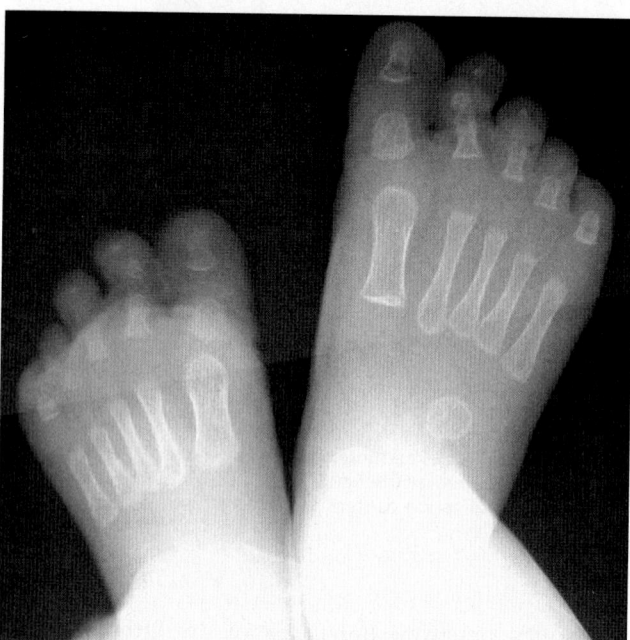

FIGURE 166-54. Russell-Silver syndrome. Radiograph of a 9-month-old boy with marked asymmetry of the feet.

Malformations of the central nervous system include agenesis of the corpus callosum, cerebellar hypoplasia, fusion of the cerebral hemispheres, arhinencephaly, and holoprosencephaly.

Cardiovascular malformations include atrioventricular canal defects and anomalous pulmonary venous return. An increased incidence of pyloric stenosis has been described. Both type I and type II are associated with markedly reduced activity of the enzyme converting 7-dehydrocholesterol to cholesterol. This deficiency is more marked in the type II patients. The higher the level of plasma cholesterol, the greater the chance of survival of the infant; the lower the level, the greater the number of malformations present. Because of the marked variability of expression, including very mild forms, it is suggested that children with mental retardation, developmental delay, any degree of cleft palate, micrognathia, and second/third toe syndactyly should have plasma cholesterol levels drawn to exclude Smith-Lemli-Opitz syndrome.

SOTOS SYNDROME

Sotos syndrome, or cerebral gigantism, is an autosomal dominant condition associated with somatic gigantism, with height, weight, and head circumference all greater than the 97th percentile for age, advanced bone age with the phalanges being more advanced that the carpals, abnormal metacarpophalangeal pattern profile, large hands and feet, craniofacial abnormalities (usually a large dolichocephalic skull with frontal bossing), and mental retardation. Patients have an increased risk of malignancy between 2% and 7%. Reported tumors include Wilms tumor, hepatocellular carcinoma, small cell carcinoma of the lung, leukemia, neuroblastoma, and lymphoma. Hydronephrosis has also been reported. Haploinsufficiency of *NSD1* is the major cause of Sotos syndrome.

ciated with microcephaly, mental retardation, growth delay, characteristic facies with anteverted nostrils, ptosis and high-arched palate, hypotonia, cryptorchidism, and syndactyly of the second and third toes. The lethal, or type II, phenotype is characterized by features of the type I phenotype but also male pseudohermaphrodism with complete sex reversal, postaxial polydactyly of the hands and/or feet, small tongue, Hirschsprung disease or total colonic aganglionosis, and high lethality. Other anomalies described in type II Smith-Lemli-Opitz syndrome include unilobar lungs, renal hypoplasia, and testicular dysgenesis with diminished number of Leydig cells.

THROMBOCYTOPENIA–ABSENT RADIUS (TAR) SYNDROME

Thrombocytopenia with absent radius is a congenital malformation syndrome characterized by bilateral absence of radii and thrombocytopenia. The thrombocytopenia is early onset, but usually transient, and may be associated with a marked leukemoid reaction. Absent radii is a constant feature. A distinguishing feature from other absent radius conditions is the presence of the thumb (Fig. 166-55). Other clinical features can also help distinguish other causes of absent radii, including Holt-Oram syndrome, Fanconi anemia, Roberts syndrome, and thalidomide embryopathy. Other upper extremity abnormalities may be present in TAR syndrome, including phocomelia, hypoplasia or absence of any of the other bones, and shoulder anomalies.

Up to 50% of patients with TAR syndrome may have very significant lower extremity abnormalities, including absent fibula, phocomelia, fusion of the femur and tibia, short long bones, clubfoot, and dislocated knees, ankles, and hips. Approximately, 30% have congenital heart disease, primarily tetralogy of Fallot and septal defects. Central nervous system abnormalities include hypoplasia of the vermis and corpus callosum and delay in myelination. Infrequent abnormalities include müllerian agenesis, horseshoe kidney, absent kidney, and esophageal atresia. A first-trimester diagnosis is possible. Early diagnosis and treatment of the thrombocytopenia is the key to preventing death from internal bleeding, which can be intracerebral. The inheritance pattern is unclear.

> **Thrombocytopenia–absent radius syndrome: A distinguishing feature from other absent radius conditions is the presence of the thumb.**

TUBEROUS SCLEROSIS

Tuberous sclerosis is a neurocutaneous syndrome characterized by hamartomatous growths involving virtually all organ systems. Diagnosis is based on radiographic, dermatologic, or histologic evidence of at least two major features or one major feature and two minor features. Major features are facial angiofibromas, nontraumatic ungual or periungual fibromas, shagreen patches, cortical tubers in the brain, subependymal nodules or giant cell astrocytoma, multiple renal hamartomas or angiomyolipomas, cardiac rhabdomyoma, and lymphangiomyomatosis. Minor features are bone cysts, renal cysts, nonrenal hamartomas, cerebral white matter "migration tracts," hamartomatous rectal polyps, gingival fibromas, "confetti" skin lesions, retinal achromic patches, and random pitting dental enamel. Tuberous sclerosis has an autosomal dominant mode of inheritance with variable expression, with up to 50% of cases believed to be sporadic. It is genotypically heterogeneous, with two distinct genes identified that are associated with the syndrome: *TSC1*, located on chromosome 9, and *TSC2*, located on chromosome 16.

> **Tuberous Sclerosis:**
>
> **For diagnosis, the patient must demonstrate two major features or one major plus two minor features:**
>
> **Major Features:**
> - Facial angiofibromas
> - Nontraumatic ungual or periungual fibroma
> - Shagreen patch
> - Cortical tuber
> - Subependymal nodule or giant cell astrocytoma
> - Multiple renal hamartomas or angiomyolipomas
> - Cardiac rhabdomyoma
> - Lymphangiomyomatosis
>
> **Minor Features:**
> - Bone cysts
> - Renal cysts
> - Nonrenal hamartoma
> - Cerebral white matter "migration tracts"
> - Hamartomatous rectal polyps
> - Gingival fibromas
> - "Confetti" skin lesions
> - Retinal achromic patch
> - Random pitting of dental enamel

Skeletal findings of tuberous sclerosis include patchy cortical thickening or sclerotic areas involving both the axial and appendicular skeleton; bone cysts, which are most commonly seen in the hands; periosteal thickenings; and rib expansion and sclerosis (Fig. 166-56). Intracranial findings of tuberous sclerosis have been diagnosed by fetal MRI. Imaging of the neonatal head with ultrasound may demonstrate subependymal nodules. CT, or preferably MRI, will show giant cell astrocytomas, cortical tubers and white matter heterotopias (Fig. 166-57). Echocardiography, multidetector cardiac CT, and MRI can be useful in characterizing rhabdomyomas. Renal hamartomas and angiomyolipomas are readily characterized by ultrasound, CT, or MRI (Fig. 166-58). Angiomyolipomas are heterogeneous vascular renal masses

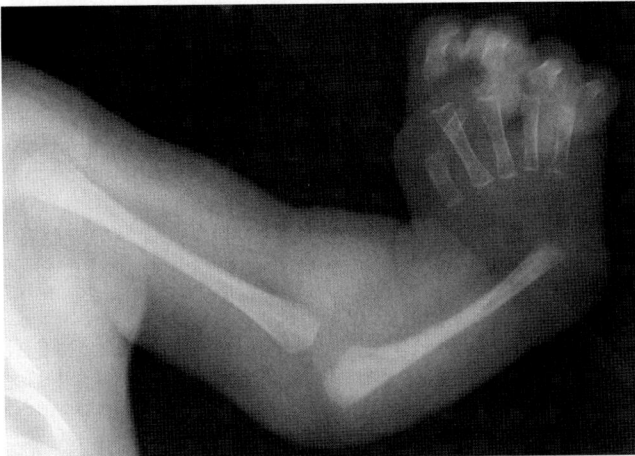

FIGURE 166-55. Thrombocytopenia–absent radius (TAR) syndrome. Radiograph of right upper extremity shows an absent radius, slightly short ulna, radial deviation of the hand, and five digits, including a thumb.

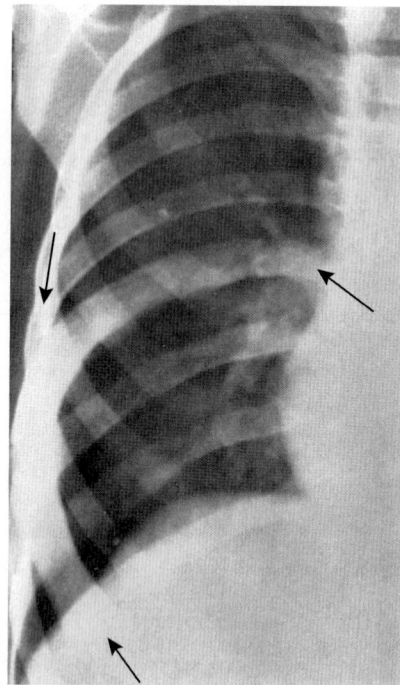

FIGURE 166-56. Tuberous sclerosis. Diffuse thickening and sclerosis of the right sixth rib *(arrows)* of a 3-year-old child who suffered from convulsions and adenoma sebaceum, characteristic of tuberous sclerosis. Intracranial lesions were also found. (Courtesy of Dr. Harold G. Jacobson, New York City, NY.)

with soft tissue and fat attenuation or signal characteristics. These tumors may bleed or rupture. They can also occasionally occur in other organs such as the liver (see Fig. 166-58). The earliest renal ultrasound finding is subcapsular echogenic foci. The kidneys may also develop cysts, and there appears to be a slight increase in the incidence of both Wilms tumor and renal cell carcinoma in patients with tuberous sclerosis. Pulmonary lymphangiomyomatosis, rare in children, produces a multicystic appearance on CT of the lungs. Miscellaneous findings may include coarctation of the aorta, pulmonary artery aneurysm, renal artery stenosis, interstitial lung disease that can progress to honeycomb lung, pulmonary cysts, and spontaneous pneumothorax.

VACTERL ASSOCIATION

The acronym VATER (later expanded to VACTERL) was first used by Quan and Smith to describe the anomalies in multiple organ systems believed to arise from mesodermal defects occurring by the fifth week of fetal life, probably from a defect in blastogenesis. VACTERL is believed to be a primary, polytopic, developmental field defect that is causally heterogeneous and rarely familial. The mnemonic acronym denotes the following: *v*ertebral anomalies, *a*norectal anomalies, *c*ardiac lesions, *t*racheo-*e*sophageal anomalies (especially esophageal atresia), *r*enal anomalies, and *l*imb anomalies (especially radial ray anomalies). The possible diagnosis of VACTERL association is often raised by the presence of either esophageal atresia or imperforate anus. VACTERL association has a low risk of recurrence in siblings or offspring of the

proband case. It is not associated with facial dysmorphism, learning disability, growth failure, or abnormal head size or shape. If any of these features is present, a genetic condition associated with either esophageal atresia, such as Feingold syndrome or CHARGE association, or with imperforate anus, such as Townes-Brocks syndrome, needs to be excluded.

The vertebral anomalies may occur in any part of the spine, although sacral anomalies are most common in patients with imperforate anus (Fig. 166-59). Thirteen rib-bearing vertebral bodies is the most common anomaly in some series of esophageal atresia patients. Hemivertebra and hypoplastic vertebra are the next most common. Limb anomalies are variable, including radial segment hypoplasia, proximal focal femoral deficiency, fibular hemimelia, and amelia. The VACTERL association is present in 4% of infants with limb reduction defects. Renal anomalies include agenesis, dysplasia, hypoplastic kidneys, horseshoe kidney, and pelvic kidney. Cardiovascular anomalies include isolated ventriculoseptal defect (most frequent), atrial septal defect, tetralogy of Fallot, and transposition of the great arteries. Central nervous system anomalies are not included in the VACTERL acronym but are not uncommon in affected patients. As many as 34% of patients with imperforate anus have spinal dysraphism, including tethered cord, intradural lipoma, and lipomeningocele. Hydrocephalus associated with the VACTERL association is known to have a high rate of recurrence in subsequent pregnancies. This is referred to as VACTERL-H association, with hydrocephalus added to the acronym. VACTERL-H is frequently an X-linked disorder, particularly when aqueductal stenosis is present and the prognosis is poor.

Defects in at least three organ systems of the VACTERL acronym should be present in order to apply the diagnosis and to avoid misdiagnosing other conditions such as Goldenhar syndrome or Holt-Oram syndrome.

> **VACTERL association:** *v*ertebral, *a*norectal, *c*ardiac, *t*racheo*e*sophageal, *r*enal, and *l*imb anomalies

WARFARIN EMBRYOPATHY

Warfarin, an anticoagulant commonly in use, can have marked teratogenic effects when taken during the first trimester of pregnancy. Common findings include nasal hypoplasia, epiphyseal calcifications, stippled calcification of the axial skeleton, and mental retardation (Fig. 166-60). Other skeletal changes include shortening of the tubular bones, especially the phalanges. Occipital prominence and frontal bossing can be seen. Other less commonly reported findings include dextrocardia and situs inversus, atrial septal defect, patent ductus arteriosus, asplenia, intracranial hemorrhage, ventriculomegaly, and diaphragmatic hernia. Fetal MRI can demonstrate some of these abnormalities, including the stippled cervical spine calcifications that can appear as hypoplasia (see Fig. 166-60). The radiographic appearance can resemble chondrodysplasia punctata.

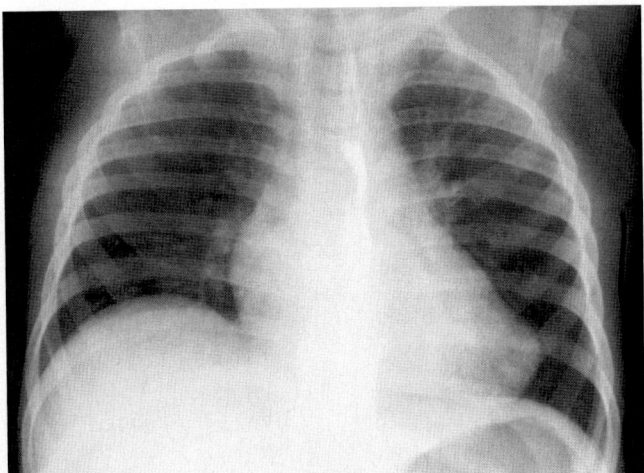

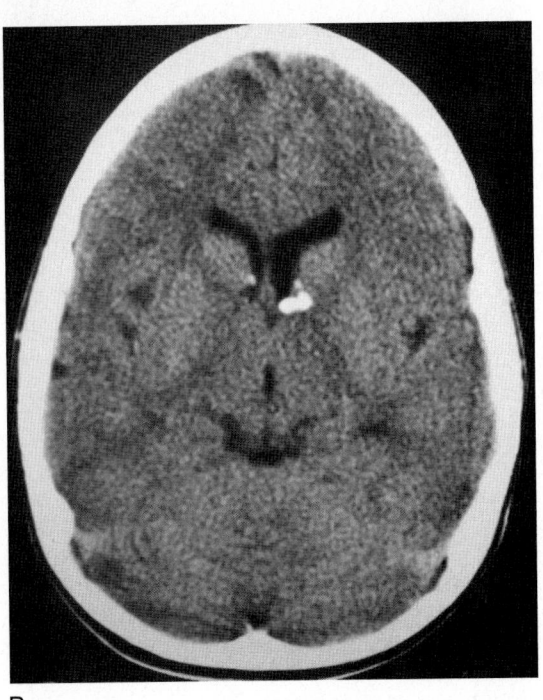

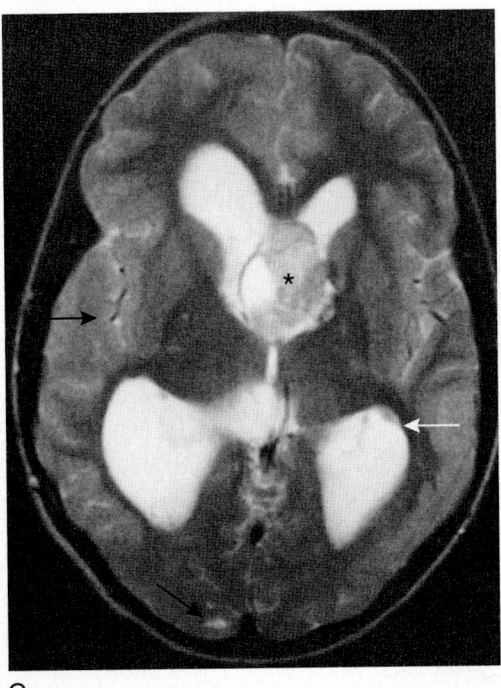

FIGURE 166-57. Tuberous sclerosis. **A,** Anteroposterior chest with a bulging lower left cardiac heart border from a rhabdomyoma. **B,** Axial CT demonstrates calcified subependymal nodules. **C,** Axial T2-weighted MR image of a different patient shows a large giant cell astrocytoma in the region of the foramen of Monro *(asterisk)*, a hypointense subependymal nodule *(white arrow)*, and subcortical tubers *(black arrows)*.

WEILL-MARCHESANI SYNDROME

Weill-Marchesani syndrome is an autosomal recessive syndrome associated with short stature, brachydactyly, misshapen small lenses, and glaucoma. Radiographs demonstrate brachycephaly with hypotelorism and shortened metacarpals, metatarsals, and phalanges with a delayed bone age. Undertubulation of bones with thinning of the cortices, widened ribs, rounding of vertebral bodies, and osteoporosis have also been reported (Fig. 166-61). The etiology appears to be a mutation on chromosome 19 related to the ADAMTS10 protease.

WERNER SYNDROME

Werner syndrome, or progeria adultorum, is a condition of premature aging and susceptibility to cancer that begins sometime after puberty. It is an autosomal recessive syndrome caused by the loss of function of a single gene product, WRN. It is most common in Japan. Typical radiographic features include generalized osteopenia with osteosclerosis of the phalanges. Soft tissue calcification may be seen. Generalized muscle atrophy and osteoarthritis are often seen, as well as markedly advanced atherosclerosis. Advanced brain atrophy is also associated.

CHROMOSOMAL DISORDERS

Cri du Chat Syndrome

Cri du chat syndrome is a chromosomal disorder caused by partial deletion of the short arm of chromosome 5 where the telomerase reverse transcriptase gene is localized. The syndrome is characterized clinically by severe growth and mental retardation associated with a

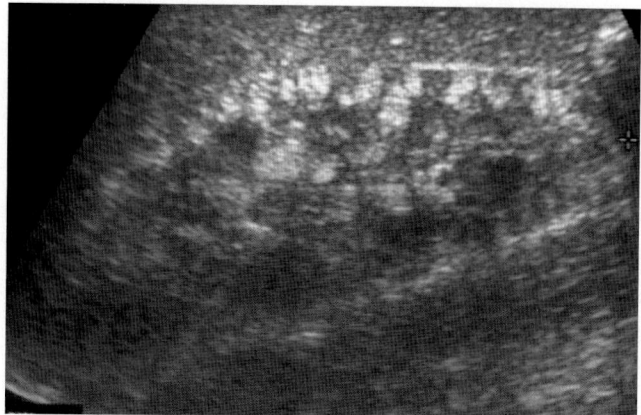

A

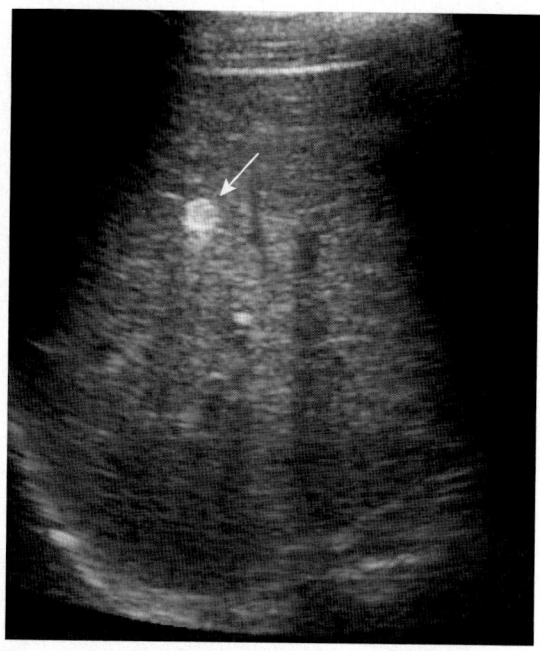

B

FIGURE 166-58. Tuberous sclerosis. **A,** Longitudinal ultrasound image of the right kidney of an 11-year-old shows multiple small echogenic lesions within the kidney consistent with angiomyolipomas. The kidney is mildly large for age. **B,** Longitudinal ultrasound image of the liver in a 10-year-old shows a focal hyperechoic lesion *(arrow)* in the liver consistent with an angiomyolipoma. The patient also had innumerable angiomyolipomas in the kidneys.

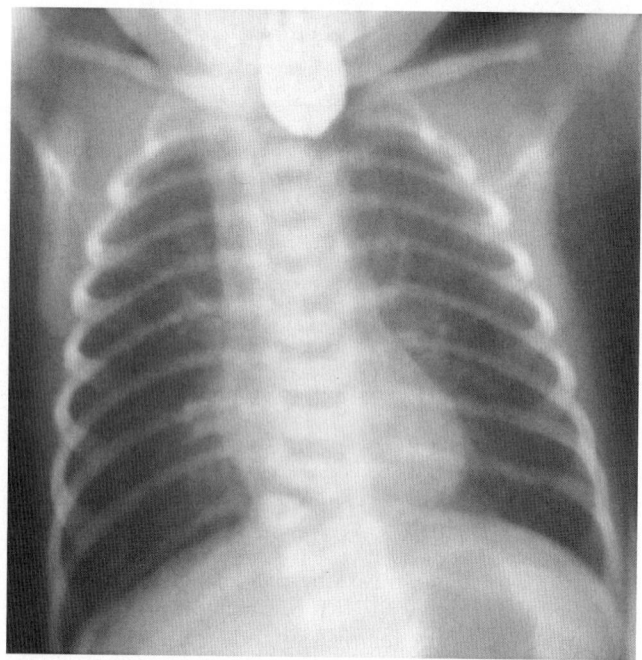

FIGURE 166-59. VACTERL association. Chest radiograph of a newborn with tracheoesophageal fistula and esophageal atresia. Contrast medium is in the proximal esophageal pouch. Air in the stomach indicates the presence of a distal tracheoesophageal fistula. A hemivertebra is noted. The patient also had a pelvic kidney.

encephalocele, Dandy-Walker syndrome, ventriculomegaly, and choroid plexus cysts. However, these findings are too nonspecific to suggest the diagnosis, and karyotyping is required. There is a higher incidence of congenital cardiac defects in cri du chat syndrome.

Klinefelter Syndrome

Klinefelter syndrome, the most common sex chromosome disorder, affects 1 in 600 males, and is characterized by additional (one or more) X chromosomes. It manifests as maldevelopment of the testes, resulting in hypogonadism and infertility. Patients have increased height with long legs and arms, gynecomastia, feminine distribution of fat, small testes, and elevated levels of follicle-stimulating hormone. There is an increased incidence of male breast cancer, mediastinal germ cell tumor, leukemia, non-Hodgkin lymphoma, and lung cancer, and a decreased risk of prostate cancer. Patients have an increased incidence of dying from circulatory and cerebrovascular diseases, and a higher incidence of diabetes mellitus, mitral valve prolapse, and autoimmune diseases, especially lupus. Osteopenia is seen after puberty. In adolescence and adulthood, sonography of the small testes shows abnormal echogenicity and increased intratesticular blood flow resistance.

Skeletal abnormalities include scoliosis, kyphosis, cubitus valgus, radioulnar synostosis or dislocation, elongated distal ulna, delayed bone age, pseudoepiphysis in the hands, positive metacarpal sign, and clinodactyly. The skeletal findings are more often seen when the number of X chromosomes exceeds two.

Radiographic abnormalities of the skull include temporal flattening, reduced width, short anterior fossa, increased pituitary size, and reduced cranial base angle. The brain shows areas of hypoperfusion, most frequently in the temporal regions.

classic "catlike" cry ("cri du chat"). Radiographic findings include microcephaly with hypertelorism, micrognathia, gracile bones, and shortened metacarpals with elongated proximal phalanges (Fig. 166-62). Hirschsprung disease, malrotation, and developmental dysplasia of the hip have been reported. Prenatal sonography may demonstrate varied central nervous system abnormalities, including

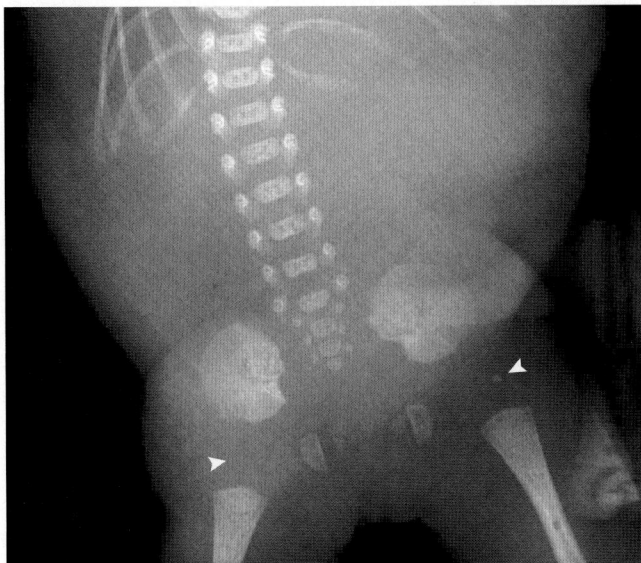

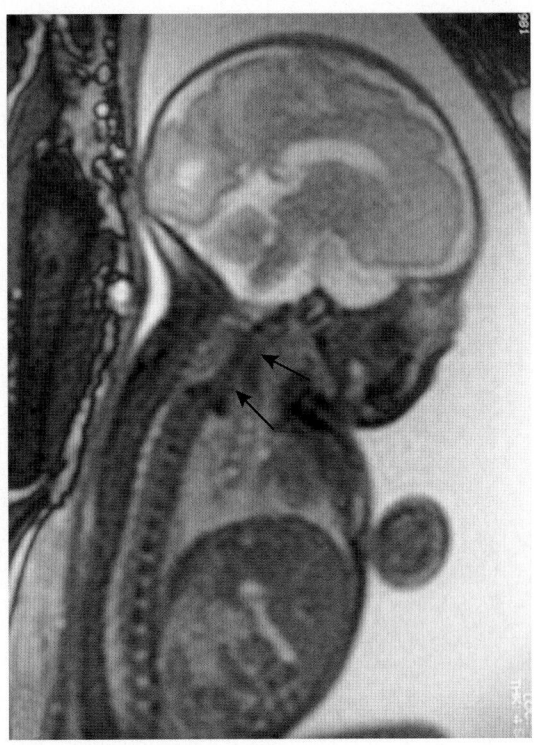

FIGURE 166-60. Warfarin embryopathy. **A,** Fetal radiograph of the pelvis demonstrates punctate early ossification in the area of the femoral head epiphyses *(arrowheads)*. **B,** Fetal MR true fast imaging with steady-state precision (FISP) image of a different fetus in utero demonstrates cervical vertebral hypoplasia *(arrows)*.

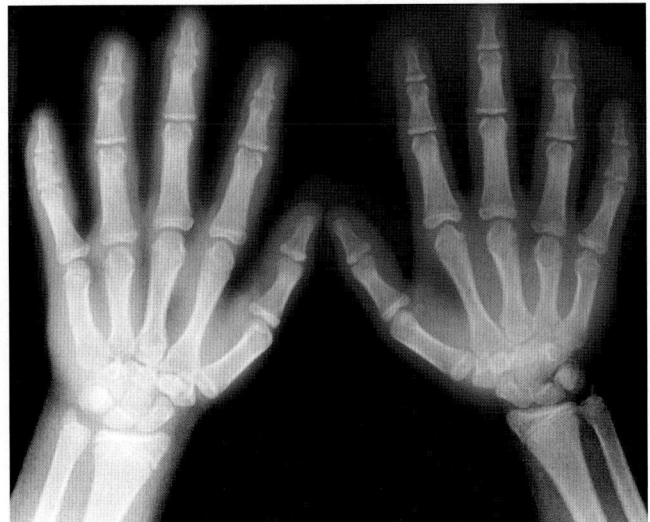

FIGURE 166-61. Weill-Marchesani syndrome. Shortened metacarpals and phalanges and delayed bone age are seen in this 18-year-old female.

Trisomy 13 (Patau Syndrome)

Trisomy 13 is characterized by low birth weight, craniofacial dysmorphism, and mental retardation. Prenatally detected sonographic abnormalities are common, including structural abnormalities of the face and of the central nervous system, most often ventriculomegaly and holoprosencephaly. Other intracranial abnormalities include agenesis of the corpus callosum and Dandy-Walker malformation. Cardiovascular anomalies are common. Other findings include diaphragmatic hernia,

microcephaly, brachycephaly, facial clefts, a variety of hand and foot anomalies (including postaxial polydactyly and rocker-bottom feet), cystic hygroma, webbed neck, thin ribs, and hypoplasia of the pelvis with shallow acetabular angles (Fig. 166-63). Prenatal sonography can detect many of the morphologic findings of trisomy 13, as well as echogenic intracardiac foci, increased nuchal translucency, and echogenic bowel, suggesting further evaluation or karyotyping. Life expectancy is usually short, with most patients dying in infancy, though long-term survival has been reported.

Trisomy 18 (Edwards Syndrome)

Trisomy 18 is characterized by low birth weight, hypotonia followed by hypertonia, craniofacial dysmorphism, and mental retardation. The three most common clinical findings are clenched hands, rocker-bottom feet, and low-set or malformed ears. Common radiographic findings include gracile ribs, congenital heart disease (ventricular septal defect, patent ductus arteriosus, atrial septal defect), and a small pelvis with narrow iliac crests with high iliac and acetabular angles (Fig. 166-64). Other radiographic findings include thinning of the calvaria, hypoplasia of the mandible and maxilla, dolichocephaly, aplasia of the medial thirds of the clavicles, rocker-bottom feet, and changes of the hand, including short thumb and index finger with ulnar deviation of the digits (see Fig. 166-64). Intracranial findings include gyral and lobar dysplasia often involving the hippocampus, cerebellum, and midbrain; cerebellar hypoplasia; choroid plexus cysts; and an enlarged cisterna magna. Neonatal hepatitis and biliary atresia have also been reported.

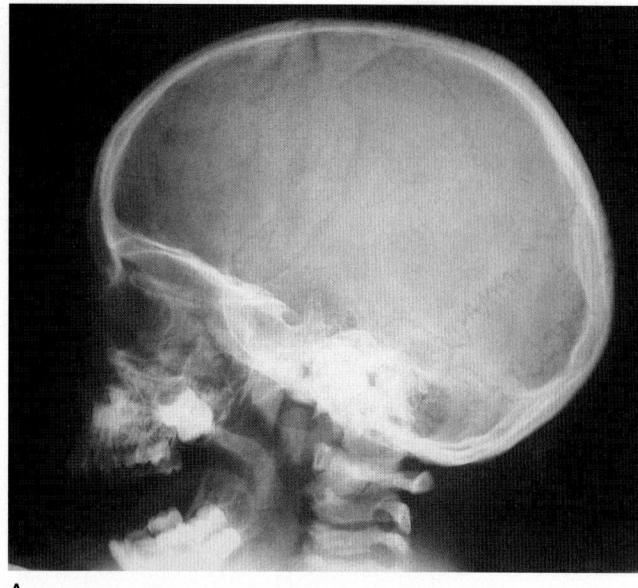

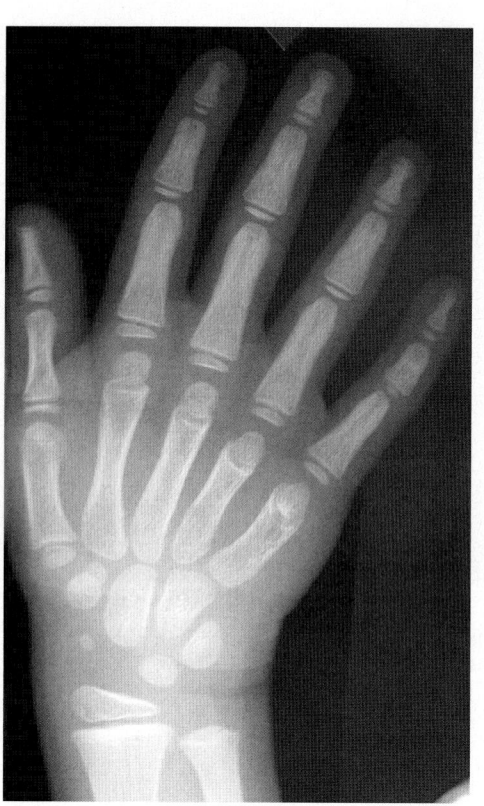

FIGURE 166-62. Cri du chat syndrome. **A,** Skull radiograph shows mild microcephaly. **B,** Hand radiograph shows shortening of the fourth and fifth metacarpals and relatively long proximal phalanges.

Trisomy 18 patients generally have poor long-term survival. Prenatal sonography can detect many of the morphologic findings of trisomy 18, as well as intrauterine growth retardation, suggesting further evaluation or karyotyping.

Trisomy 21 (Down Syndrome)

Trisomy 21 is the most common chromosomal syndrome. The syndrome is characterized by mental retardation, low birth weight, craniofacial dysmorphism, and a host of anomalies involving virtually all organ systems.

Pelvic radiographs demonstrate characteristics of trisomy 21 early in life. Flaring of the iliac wings and flattening of the acetabular roofs are seen and can be quantified by measuring the iliac index (Fig. 166-65). The iliac index is the sum of the acetabular angle (the angle between the roof of the acetabulum and a line drawn through the triradiate cartilages) and the iliac angle (the angle between the iliac wing and a line drawn through the triradiate cartilages). In trisomy 21 patients, the iliac index is less than 60 degrees.

Skeletal abnormalities include brachycephaly with micrognathia, hypoplastic atlas, cervical spondylosis in older patients, a systemic arthropathy similar to JRA, hypersegmentation of the sternum, gracile ribs, 11 ribs, bell-shaped thorax, congenital hip dislocation, absence of widening of the interpediculate distance of the lumbar spine, and slightly diminished bone mass. The occipitoatlantal and atlantoaxial instability found in Down syndrome is controversial both for diagnosis and therapy.

Anteroposterior occipitoatlantal instability is defined as more than 2 mm of motion on extension of the occipitoatlantal joints. An MRI is recommended of the neck to evaluate for signal changes in the cord if the motion is greater than 2 mm. An atlantoaxial distance of 4.5 mm or less is considered normal. However, from 4.5–10 mm and a normal neurological exam avoidance of high risk sports (diving, football) is recommended (see Fig. 166-65). If more than 4.5 mm and a neurological deficit, activities are restricted and MRI recommended to evaluate for cord changes. At greater than 10 mm surgical fusion is recommended. However, the poor reproducibility of findings and both intraobserver and interobserver variability may make it difficult to base surgical and clinical treatment protocols for upper cervical spine instability on measurements alone.

Other radiographic findings in trisomy 21 include congenital heart disease, most often endocardial cushion defect or ventricular septal defect, duodenal atresia or stenosis, malrotation, tracheoesophageal fistula, imperforate anus, and Hirschsprung disease. Nasopharyngeal cine MRI during sleep is useful in evaluating patients with persistent sleep apnea after tonsillectomy and adenoidectomy in Down syndrome. Patients with trisomy 21 have an increased incidence of leukemia, most commonly acute lymphocytic leukemia (ALL). Prenatal sonography may be helpful in screening for characteristic sonographic markers, including a thickened nuchal fold, limb shortening, echogenic bowel, and echogenic intracardiac foci, which are nonspecific findings seen in trisomy 21 fetuses.

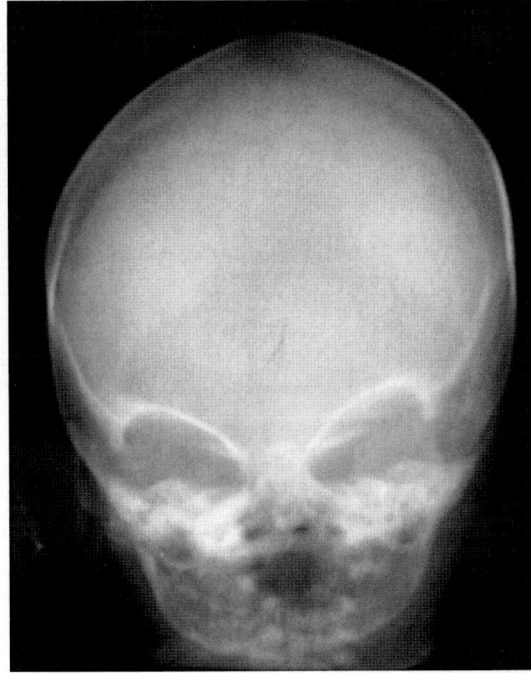

A

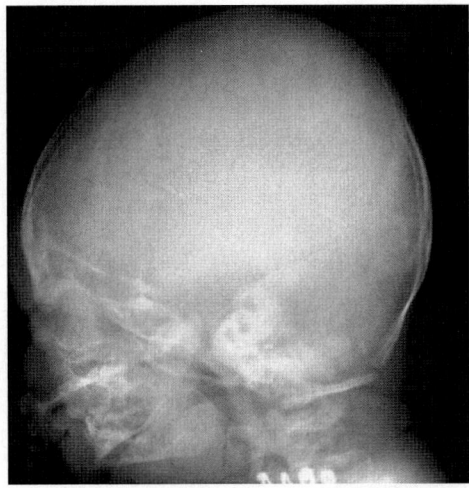

B

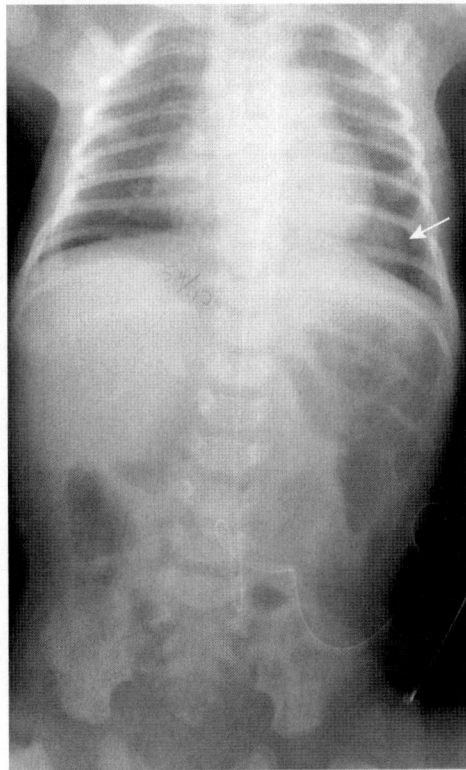

C

FIGURE 166-63. Trisomy 13. Anteroposterior **(A)** and lateral **(B)** skull radiographs demonstrate microcephaly, brachycephaly, micrognathia, and a J-shaped sella. **C,** Chest and abdominal radiograph shows 11 pairs of gracile ribs, mild cardiomegaly, a left diaphragmatic hernia *(arrow)*, and a dysplastic pelvis with high iliac angles.

Trisomy 21:

- **Skeletal findings**
  - **Flared iliac wings**
  - **Flat acetabular roofs**
  - **Iliac index <60 degrees**
  - **Brachycephaly**
  - **Atlantoaxial instability**
- **Duodenal atresia**
- **Congenital heart disease**
  - **Endocardial cushion defect**
  - **Ventricular septal defect**
- **Increased risk for leukemia (ALL)**

TURNER SYNDROME

Turner syndrome, or isochromosome X, was initially described as a triad of infertility, webbing of the neck, and cubitus valgus deformity of the elbow. Since that time, a multitude of associated findings have been described involving most organ systems. In addition to the classic valgus deformity of the elbow, skeletal findings include brachycephaly, thin lateral clavicles, hypoplasia of the sacrum, pectus carinatum, platyspondyly, over-tubulation of long bones, and flattening of the medial tibial condyle with associated patellar dislocation and proximal tibial exostosis (Fig. 166-66). Hand radiographs demonstrate typical changes with osteopenia, shortening of the fourth and fifth metacarpals, delayed

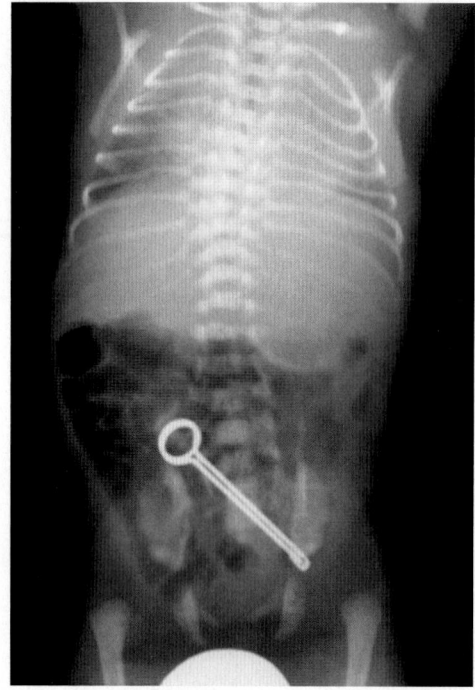

A

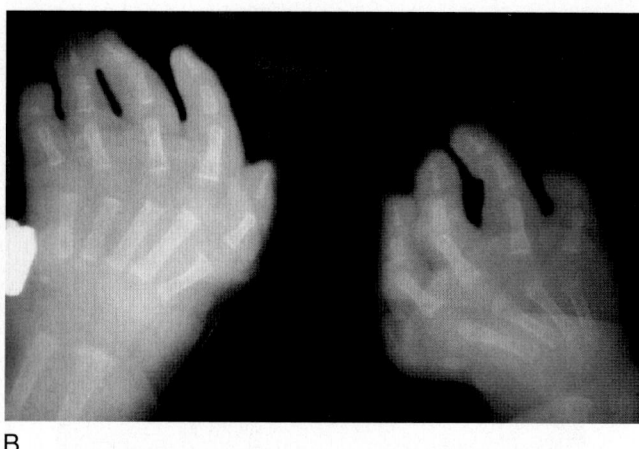

B

FIGURE 166-64. Trisomy 18. **A,** Chest and abdominal radiograph shows cardiac enlargement from complex heart disease, a transverse liver, asplenia, and a small pelvis with high acetabular and iliac angles. **B,** Posteroanterior hand radiograph shows ulnar deviation of the digits, flexion deformities, and hypoplasia of some phalanges and the right first metacarpal.

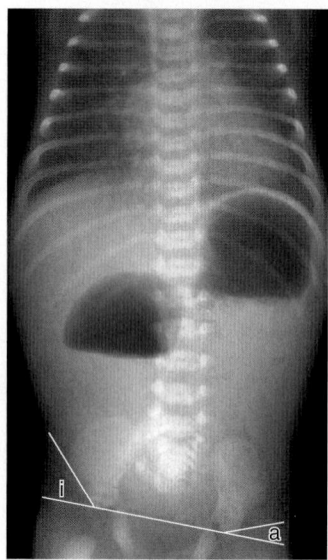

A

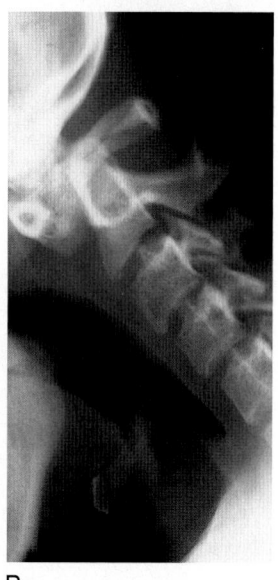

B

FIGURE 166-65. Trisomy 21. **A,** Newborn chest and abdominal radiograph shows many findings typical of trisomy 21, including pulmonary overcirculation due to the patient's atrioventricular canal defect, double bubble sign typical of duodenal atresia, lack of widening of the intrapedicular distances in the lumbar region and decreased iliac index. The iliac index is the sum of the acetabular angle (a) and the iliac angle (i). **B.** Flexion lateral radiograph of cervical spine demonstrates widening of the predental space.

maturation, phalangeal predominance, a V-shaped deformity of the distal radiocarpal joint, and drumstick-shaped distal phalanges (see Fig. 166-66). Cardiovascular findings include cardiac septal defects, aortic coarctation and dissection, and mitral valve prolapse. Renal anomalies include rotational anomalies, bifid renal pelvis,

horseshoe kidney, and multicystic dysplastic kidney. Autoimmune conditions, including hypothyroidism, diabetes, and juvenile rheumatoid arthritis, have been associated with Turner syndrome. Genital abnormalities, best evaluated with pelvic ultrasound or MRI, include ovarian and uterine absence or hypoplasia. Vascular abnormalities also include intestinal telangiectasia, lymphedema, and an increased incidence of vascular tumors (hemangioma, lymphangioma).

Wolf-Hirschhorn Syndrome

Wolf-Hirschhorn syndrome is a chromosomal syndrome caused by partial deletion of the short arm of chromosome 4 (chromosome 4p– deletion), and characterized by mental retardation, epilepsy, growth delay, and severe craniofacial anomalies. The deletion of the Wolf-Hirschhorn syndrome critical region (WHSCR) is variable, but always appears to include the *WHSC1* gene. However, *WHSC1* gene absence, in itself, is insufficient to cause the syndrome. Cranial findings include microcephaly with hypertelorism and micrognathia with proportionately small maxilla. The axial skeleton demonstrates 13 rib pairs, scoliosis, vertebral segmentation anomalies, and widely separated pubic bones (Fig. 166-67). The appendicular skeleton shows gracile long bones with a tendency toward radioulnar synostosis, hip dysplasia, and clubfoot along with multiple other malformations. Visceral abnormalities include malformations of the heart and great vessels and diaphragmatic hernia. Intracranial malformations include agenesis of the corpus callosum and other midline defects, ventriculomegaly, cerebellar disorders, and disorders in gyration, including microgyria. Prenatal diagnosis can be suggested with intrauterine growth retardation and facial dysmorphism.

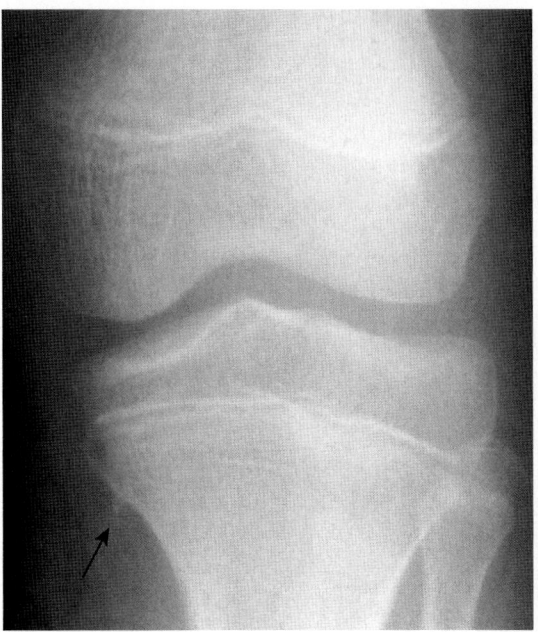
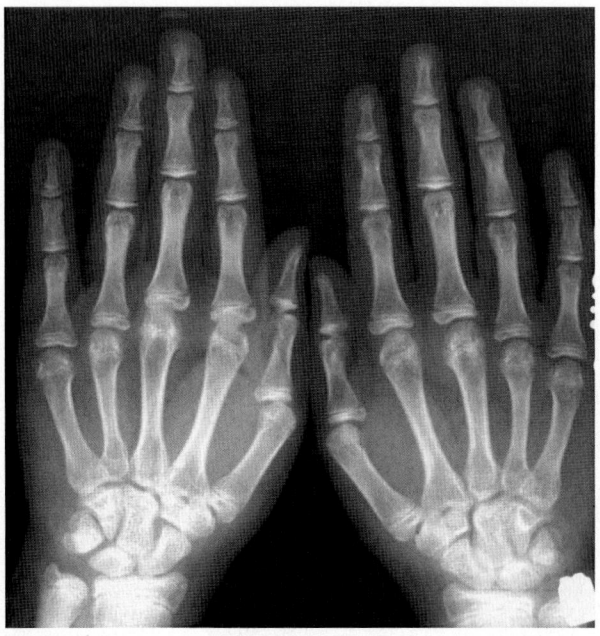

A   B

FIGURE 166-66. Turner syndrome. **A,** Knee radiograph shows flattening of the medial tibial condyle with an exostosis *(arrow)* along the medial metaphysis. **B,** Hand radiograph demonstrates shortening of the fourth and fifth metacarpals with phalangeal predominance, typical of Turner syndrome.

Syndrome	Defect
Cri du chat	5p- deletion
Klinefelter	Usually XXY
Patau	Trisomy 13
Edwards	Trisomy 18
Down	Trisomy 21
Turner	Usually XO
Wolf-Hirschhorn	4p- deletion

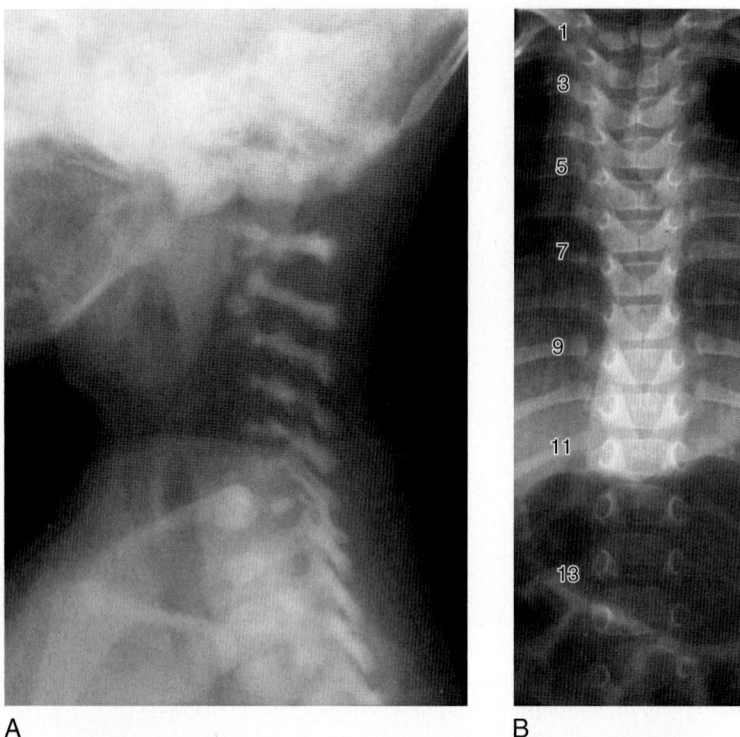

A   B

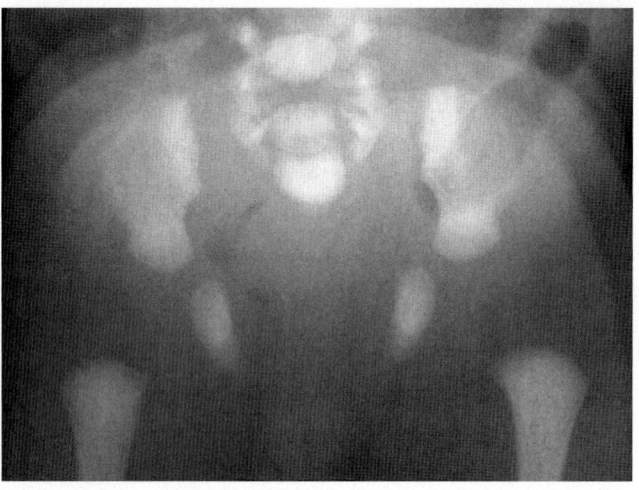

C

FIGURE 166-67. Wolf-Hirschhorn syndrome.
A, Lateral cervical spine radiograph shows hypoplastic vertebrae. **B,** The thoracic spine in an older patent has 13 rib pairs and spina bifida occulta in some of the upper thoracic vertebrae. **C,** Pelvic radiograph shows poorly ossified, widely separated pubic bones, small iliac bones, and a hypoplastic sacrum.

SUGGESTED READINGS

General Reading

Lachman RD (ed): Taybi and Lachman's Radiology of Syndromes, Metabolic Disorders and Skeletal Dysplasias, 5th ed. Philadelphia, Elsevier, 2006

McAlister WH, Herman TE: Osteochondrodysplasias, dysostoses, chromosomal aberrations, mucopolysaccharidoses, and mucolipidoses In: Bone and Joint Disorders, Resnick D (ed), 4th ed. WB Saunders, Philadelphia, Elsevier, 2002

Bardet-Biedl Syndrome

Beales PL, Elcioglu N, Woolf AS, et al: New criteria for improved diagnosis of Bardet-Biedl syndrome: results of a population survey. J Med Genet 1999;36:437-446

Bitoun DA, Lacombe D, Lambert JC, et al: Hydrometrocolpos and polydactyly: a common neonatal presentation of Bardet-Biedl and McKusick-Kaufman syndromes. J Med Genet 1999;36:599-603

Cramer B, Green J, Harnett J, et al: Sonographic and urographic correlation in Bardet-Biedl syndrome. Urol Radiol 1988; 10:176-180

Fralick RA, Leichter HE, Sheth KJ: Early diagnosis of Bardet-Biedl syndrome. Pediatr Nephrol 1990;4:264-265

Kulaga HM, Leitch CC, Eichers ER, et al: Loss of BBS proteins causes anosmia in humans and defects in olfactory cilia structure and function in the mouse. Nat Genet 2004;36:994-998

Lorda-Sanchez I, Ayuso C, Ibanez A: Situs inversus and Hirschsprung disease: two uncommon manifestations in Bardet-Biedl syndrome. Am J Med Genet 2000;90:80-81

Mehrota N, Taub S, Covert TF: Hydrometrocolpos as a neonatal manifestation of the Bardet-Biedl syndrome. Am J Med Genet 1997;69:220

Mykytyn K, Sheffield VC: Establishing a connection between cilia and Bardet-Biedl syndrome. Trends Mol Med 2004;10:106-109

Stoler JM, Herrin JT, Holmes LB: Genital abnormalities in females with Bardet-Biedl syndrome. Am J Med Genet 1995; 55:276-278

Tieder M, Levy M, Gulber MC: Renal abnormalities in the Bardet-Biedl syndrome. Int J Pediatr Nephrol 1982; 3:193-203

Tobin JL, Beales PL: Bardet Biedl syndrome – beyond the cilium. Pediatr Nephro 2007;7:926-936

Beckwith-Wiedemann Syndrome

Andrews MW, Ampar EG: Wilms tumor in a patient with Beckwith Wiedemann syndrome: onset detected with 3 months serial sonography. AJR Am J Roentgenol 1992;159:835-836

Azouz EM, Larsen EJ, Patel J, et al: Beckwith Wiedemann syndrome: development of nephroblastoma during the surveillance period. Pediatr Radiol 1990;20:550-552

Biljoen D, Ramesar R: Evidence for paternal imprinting in familial Beckwith Wiedemann syndrome. J Med Genet 1992;29:221-225

DeBaun MR, Tucker MA: Risk of cancer during the first four years of life in children from the Beckwith Wiedemann Syndrome Registry. J Pediatr 1998;132:398-400

Drut R, Celina Jones M: Congenital pancreatoblastoma in Beckwith Wiedemann syndrome: an emerging association. Pediatr Pathol 1988;8:331-339

Elliott M, Maher ER: Beckwith Wiedemann syndrome. J Med Genet 1994;31:560-564

Hedborg F, Holmgren L, Sandstedt B, et al: Cell type specific *IGF2* expression during early human development correlates to the pattern of overgrowth and neoplasia with the Beckwith Wiedemann syndrome. Am J Pathol 1994;145:802-817

McCauley RGK, Beckwith JB, Elias ER, et al: Benign hemorrhagic adrenocortical macrocysts in Beckwith Wiedemann syndrome. AJR Am J Roentgenol 1991;157:549-552

Vaughn WG, Sanders DW, Grosfeld JL, et al: Favorable outcome in children with Beckwith-Wiedemann syndrome and intraabdominal malignant tumors. J Pediatr Surg 1995;30:1042-1045

Weksberg R, Shuman C, Smith AC: Beckwith Wiedemann syndrome. Am J Med Genet 2005;137C:12-23

Worth LL, Slopis JM, Herzog CE: Congenital hepatoblastoma and schizencephaly in an infant with Beckwith Wiedemann syndrome. Med Pediatr Oncol 1999;33:591-593

Brachmann-de Lange (Cornelia de Lange) Syndrome

Allanson JE, Hennekam RCM, Ireland M: De Lange syndrome: subjective and objective comparison of the classical and mild phenotypes. J Med Genet 1997;34:645-650

Bhuiyan Z, Klein M, Hannond P, et al: Genotype-phenotype correlations of 39 patients with cornelia de Lange syndrome: the Dutch experience. J Med Genet 2006;43:568-575

Braddock SR, Lachman RS, Stoppenhagen CC, et al: Radiological features in Brachmann-de Lange syndrome. Am J Med Genet 1993;47:1006-1013

Roposch A, Bhaskar AR, Lee F, et al: Orthopaedic manifestations of Brachmann-de Lange syndrome: a report of 34 patients. J Pediatr Orthop B 2004;13:118-122

Yamaguchi K, Ishitobi F: Brain dysgenesis in Cornelia de Lange syndrome. Clin Neuropathol 1999;18:99-105

Cerebrocostomandibular (Rib-Gap) Syndrome

Flodmark P, Wattsgard C: Cerebro-costo-mandibular syndrome. Pediatr Radiol 2001;31:36-37

James PA, Aftimos S: Familial cerebro-costo-mandibular syndrome: a case with unusual prenatal findings and review. Clin Dysmorphol 2003;12:63-68

Megier P, Ayeva-Derman M, Esperandieu O, et al: Prenatal ultrasonographic diagnosis of the cerebro-costo-mandibular syndrome: case report and review of the literature. Prenat Diagn 1998;18:1294-1299

Plotz FB, van Essen AJ, Bosschaart F, et al: Cerebro-costo-mandibular syndrome. Am J Med Genet 1996;62:286-293

Cerebrohepatorenal (Zellweger) Syndrome

Barkovich AJ, Peck WW: MR of Zellweger syndrome. AJNR Am J Neuroradiol 1997;18:1163-1170

Barth PG, Majoie CB, Gootjes J, et al: Neuroimaging of peroxisome biogenesis disorders (Zellweger spectrum) with prolonged survival. Neurology 2004;62:439-444

Crane DI, Maxwell MA, Paton BC: *PEX1* mutations in the Zellweger spectrum of the peroxisome biogenesis disorders. Hum Mutat 2005;26:167-175

Luisiri A, Sotelo-Avila C, Silberstein MJ, et al: Sonography of the Zellweger syndrome. J Ultrasound Med 1988;7:169-173

Poznanski AK, Nosanchuk JS, Baublis J, et al: The cerebro-hepato-renal syndrome (CHRS): (Zellweger's syndrome). Am J Roentgenol Radium Ther Nucl Med 1970;109:313-322

Cockayne Syndrome

Dabbagh O, Swaiman KF: Cockayne syndrome: MRI correlates of hypomyelination. Pediatr Neurol 1988;4:113-116

Nance MA, Berry SA: Cockayne syndrome: review of 140 cases. Am J Med Genet 1992;42:68-84

Nishio H, Kodama S, Matsuo T, et al: Cockayne syndrome: magnetic resonance images of the brain in a severe form with early onset. J Inherit Metab Dis 1988;11:88-102

Pasquier L, Laugel V, Lazaro L, et al: Wide clinical variability among 13 new Cockayne syndrome cases confirmed by biochemical assays. Arch Dis Child 2006;91:178-182

Congenital Contractural Arachnodactyly

Currarino G, Friedman JM: A severe form of congenital contractural arachnodactyly in two newborn infants. Am J Med Genet 1986;25:763-773

Martin AG, Foguet PR, Marks DS, et al: Infantile scoliosis in Beals syndrome: the use of a non-fusion technique for surgical correction. Eur Spine J 2006;15:433-439

McClure SD, Vande Velde S, Fillman R, et al: New finding of protrusio acetabuli in two families with congenital contractural arachnodactyly. A report of seven cases. J Bone Joint Surg Am 2007;89:849-854

Ramos Arroyo MA, Weaver DD, Beals RK: Congenital contractural arachnodactyly: report of four additional families and review of literature. Clin Genet 1985;27:570-581

Congenital Insensitivity to Pain

Bar-On E, Weigl D, Parvari R, et al: Congenital insensitivity to pain: orthopaedic manifestations. J Bone Joint Surg Br 2002;84:252-257

Minde J, Swensson O, Holmberg M, et al: Orthopedic aspects of familial insensitivity to pain due to a novel nerve growth factor beta mutation. Acta Orthop 2006;77:198-202

Rosemberg S, Marie SK, Kliemann S: Congenital insensitivity to pain with anhidrosis (hereditary sensory and autonomic neuropathy type IV). Pediatr Neurol 1994;11:50-56

Spencer JA, Grieve DK: Congenital indifference to pain mistaken for non-accidental injury. Br J Radiol 1990;3:308-310

Currarino Triad

Cretolle C, Zerah M, Jaubert F, et al: New clinical and therapeutic perspectives in Currarino syndrome (study of 29 patients). J Pediatr Surg 2006;46:126-131

Currarino G, Coln D, Votteler T: Triad of anorectal, sacral and presacral anomalies. AJR Am J Roentgenol 1981;137:395-398

Gudinchet F, Maeder P, Laurent T, et al: Magnetic resonance detection of myelodysplasia in children with Currarino triad. Pediatr Radiol 1997;27:903-907

Kirks DA, Merten DF, Filston HC, et al: Currarino triad: complex of anorectal malformation, sacral bony abnormality and presacral mass. Pediatr Radiol 1984;14:220-225

Lee SC, Chun YS, Jung SE, et al: Currarino triad: anorectal malformation, sacral bony abnormality and presacral mass—a review of 11 cases. J Pediatr Surg 1997;32:58-61

Masuno M, Imaizumi K, Aida N, et al: Currarino triad with terminal deletion 7q35→qter. J Med Genet 1996;33:877-878

Ross AJ, Ruiz Perez V, Wang Y, et al: A homeobox gene *HLXB9* is the major locus for dominantly inherited sacral agenesis. Nat Genet 1998;20:358-361

Urisote M, Garcia Andrade MC, Valle L, et al: Malignant degeneration of presacral teratoma in the Currarino anomaly. Am J Med Genet 2004;128:299-304

Diamond-Blackfan Syndrome

Ball SE, McGuckin CP, Jenkins G, et al: Diamond-Blackfan anaemia in the U.K.: analysis of 80 cases from a 20-year birth cohort. Br J Haematol 1996;94:645-653

Ellis SR, Massey AT: Diamond Blackfan anemia: A paradigm for a ribosome-based disease. Med Hypotheses 2006;66:643-648

Flygare J, Karlsson S: Diamond-Blackfan anemia: erythropoiesis lost in translation. Blood 2007;109:3152-3160

Ehlers-Danlos Syndrome

Beighton P: The Ehlers-Danlos syndromes. *In* McKusick's Heritable Disorders of Connective Tissue, 5th ed. St. Louis, Mosby–Year Book, 1993:189-251

Herman TE, McAlister WH: Cavitary pulmonary lesions in type IV Ehlers-Danlos syndrome. Pediatr Radiol 1994;24:263-265

Malfaiar F, De Paepe A: Molecular genetics in classic Ehlers-Danlos syndrome. Am J Med Genet Part C Semin Med Genet 2005;139:17-23

Pepin M, Schwarze U, Superti-Furga A, et al: Clinical and genetic features of Ehlers-Danlos syndrome type IV, the vascular type. N Engl J Med 2000;342:673-380

Epidermolysis Bullosa

Azizkhan RG, Stehr W, Cohen AP, et al: Esophageal strictures in children with recessive dystrophic epidermolysis bullosa: an 11-year experience with fluoroscopically guided balloon dilatation. J Pediatr Surg 2006;41:55-60

Dolan CR, Smith LT, Sybert VP: Prenatal detection of EB lethalis with pyloric atresia. Am J Med Genet 1993;47:395-400

Lin AN, Carter DM: Epidermolysis bullosa. J Pediatr 1989;114:349-355

Nakamura H, Sawamura D, Goto M, et al: Epidermolysis bullosa simplex associated with pyloric atresia is a novel clinical subtype caused by mutation in the plectin gene (PLEC1). J Mol Diag 2005;7:28-35

Orlando RC, Bozymski EM, Birggman RA, et al: Epidermolysis bullosa: gastrointestinal manifestations. Ann Intern Med 1974;81:203-206

Smith PK, Davidson GP, Moore L, et al: Epidermolysis bullosa and severe ulcerative colitis in an infant. J Pediatr 1993;122:600-603

Wong WL, Pemberton J: The musculoskeletal manifestations of epidermolysis bullosa: an analysis of 19 cases with a review of the literature. Br J Radiol 1992;65:480-484

Fanconi Anemia

Alter BP: Fanconi's anemia, transplantation, and cancer. Pediatr Transplant 2005;7(Suppl):81-86

Nookala RK, Hussain S, Pellegrini L: Insights into Fanconi anemia from the structure of human FANCE. Nucleic Acids Res 2007;35:1638-1648

Rogers PC, Desai F, Karabus CD, et al: Presentation and outcome of 25 cases of Fanconi's anemia. Am J Pediatr Hematol Oncol 1989;11:141-145

Fetal Alcohol Syndrome

Chudley AE, Conry J, Cook JL, et al: Fetal alcohol spectrum disorder: Canadian guidelines for diagnosis. CMAJ 2005;172:S1-S21

Martinez-Frias ML, Bermejo E, Rodriguez-Pinilla E, et al: Risk for congenital anomalies associated with different sporadic and daily doses of alcohol consumption during pregnancy: a case-control study. Birth Defects Res A Clin Mol Teratol 2004;70:194-200

Freeman-Sheldon ("Whistling Face") Syndrome

Stevenson DA, Carey JC, Palumbos J,et al: Clinical characteristics and natural history of Freeman-Sheldon syndrome. Pediatrics 2006;117:754-762

Vimercati A, Scioscia M, Burattini MG, et al: Prenatal diagnosis of Freeman-Sheldon syndrome and usefulness of an ultrasound fetal lip width normogram. Prenat Diagn 2006;26:679-683

Zampino G, Conti G, Balducci F, et al: Severe form of Freeman-Sheldon syndrome associated with brain anomalies and hearing loss. Am J Med Genet 1996;62:293-296

Gaucher Disease

Beutler E, Gelbart T, Scott CR: Hematologically important mutations: Gaucher disease. Blood Cells Mol Dis 2005;35:355-364

Chang YC, Huang CC, Chen CY, Zimmerman RA: MRI in acute neuropathic Gaucher's disease. Neuroradiology 2000;42:48-50

Elsayes KM, Narra VR, Mukundan G, et al: MR imaging of the spleen: spectrum of abnormalities. Radiographics 2005;25:967-982

Goitein O, Elstein D, Abrahamov A, et al: Lung involvement and enzyme replacement therapy in Gaucher's disease. QJM 2001;94:407-415

Grabowski GA: Recent clinical progress in Gaucher disease. Curr Opin Pediatr 2005;17:519-524

Hermann G, Pastores GM, Abdelwahab IF, et al: Gaucher disease: assessment of skeletal involvement and therapeutic responses to enzyme replacement. Skeletal Radiol 1997;26:687-696

Hill SC, Damaska BM, Tsokos M, et al: Radiographic findings in type 3 b Gaucher disease, Pediatr Radiol 1996;26:852-860

McHugh K, Olsen E OE, Vellodi A: Gaucher disease in children: radiology of non-central nervous system manifestations. Clin Radiol 2004;59:117-123

Mignot C, Doummar D, Maire I, et al; French Type 2 Gaucher Disease Study Group: Type 2 Gaucher disease: 15 new cases and review of the literature. Brain Dev 2006;28:39-48

Hadju-Cheney Syndrome

Albano LMJ, Bertola DR, Barba MF, et al: Phenotypic overlap in Melnick-Needles, serpentine fibula-polycystic kidney and Hajdu-Cheney syndromes: a clinical and molecular study in three patients. Clin Dysmorph 2007;16:27-33

Drake WM, Hiorns MP, Kendler DL: Hadju-Cheney syndrome: response to therapy with bisphosphonates in two patients. J Bone Miner Res 2003;18:131-133

Kaplan P, Ramos F, Zackai EH, et al: Cystic kidney disease in Hajdu-Cheney syndrome. Am J Med Genet 1995;56:25-30

Kawamura J, Miki Y, Yamazaki S, et al: Hajdu-Cheney syndrome: MR imaging. Neuroradiology 1991;33:441-442

Hallermann-Streiff Syndrome

Christian CL, Lachman RS, Aylsworth AS, et al: Radiological findings in Hallermann-Streiff syndrome: report of five cases and a review of the literature. Am J Med Genet 1991;41:508-514

Cohen MM Jr: Hallermann-Streiff syndrome: a review. Am J Med Genet 1991;41:488-499

Robinow, M: Respiratory obstruction and cor pulmonale in the Hallermann-Streiff syndrome. Am J Med Genet 1991:41:515-516

Sigirci A, Alkan A, Bicak U, et al: Hallermann-Streiff syndrome associated with complete agenesis of the corpus callosum. J Child Neurol 2005;20:691-693

Holt-Oram Syndrome

Basson CT, Huant T, Lin RC, et al: Different TBX235 interactions in heart and limb defined by Holt-Oram syndrome mutations. Proc Natl Acad Sci U S A 1999;96:2919-2924

Hurst JA, Hall CM, Baraister M: The Holt-Oram syndrome. J Med Genet 1991;28:406-410

Newbury-Ecob RA, Leanage R, Raeburn JA, et al: Holt-Oram syndrome: a clinical genetic study. J Med Genet 1996;33:300-307

Poznanski AK, Gall JC, Stern AM: Skeletal anomalies of the Holt-Oram syndrome. Radiology 1970;94:45-53

Sletten LJ, Pierpont MEM: Variation in severity of cardiac disease in Holt-Oram syndrome. Am J Med Genet 1996;65:128-132

Spranger S, Ulmer H, Troger J, et al: Muscular involvement in Holt-Oram syndrome. J Med Genet 1997;34:978-981

Homocystinuria

Longo D, Fariello G, Gionisi-Vici C, et al: MRI and 1H-MRS findings in early-onset cobalamin C/D defect. Neuropediatrics 2005;36:366-372

Mudd SH, Skovby F, Levy HL, et al: The natural history of homocystinuria due to cystathionine beta-synthase deficiency. Am J Hum Genet 1985;37:1-31

Van Guldener C, Stehouwer CD: Homocysteine and large arteries. Adv Cardiol 2007;44:278-301

Hypertrophic Osteoarthropathy

Atkinson S, Fox SB: Vascular endothelial growth factor (VEGF)-A and platelet-derived growth factor (PDGF) play a central role in the pathogenesis of digital clubbing. J Pathol 2004;203:721-728

Augarten A, Goldman R, Laufer J, et al: Reversal of digital clubbing after lung transplantation in cystic fibrosis patients: a clue to the pathogenesis of clubbing. Pediatr Pulmonol 2002;34:378-380

Pineda CJ, Martinez-Lavin M, Goobar JE, et al: Periostitis in hypertrophic osteoarthropathy: relationship to disease duration. AJR Am J Roentgenol 1987;148:773-778

Sainani NI, Lawande MA, Parikh VP, et al: MRI diagnosis of hypertrophic osteoarthropathy from a remote childhood malignancy. Skeletal Radiol 2007;36:S63-S66

Idiopathic (Isolated) Hemihypertrophy

Abraham P: What is the risk of cancer in a child with hemihypertrophy? Arch Dis Child 2005;90:1312-1313

Eisenberg RL, Pfister RC: Medullary sponge kidney associated with congenital hemihypertrophy (asymmetry). Am J Roentgenol Radium Ther Nucl Med 1972;116:773-777

Memon MA, Mohanty S, Das K, et al: Hemihypertrophy, renal dysplasia, and benign nephromegaly. Pediatr Nephrol 2005;20:821-823

Niemitz EL, Feinberg AP, Brandenburg SA, et al: Children with idiopathic hemihypertrophy and Beckwith Wiedemann syndrome have different constitutional epigenotypes associated with Wilms tumor. Am J Hum Genet 2005;77:887-891.

Larsen Syndrome

Forese LL, Berdon WE, Harcke HT, et al: Severe mid-cervical kyphosis with cord compression in Larsen's syndrome and diastrophic dysplasia: unrelated syndromes with similar radiologic findings and neurosurgical implications. Pediatr Radiol 1995;25:136-139

Houston CS, Reed MH, Desansch JEL: Separating Larsen's syndrome from the 'arthrogryposis basket.' J Can Assoc Radiol 1981; 32:206-214

Katz DA, Hall JE, Emans JB: Cervical kyphosis associated with anteroposterior dissociation and quadriparesis in Larsen's syndrome. J Pediatr Orthop 2005;25:429-433

Laville JM, Lakermance P, Limouzy E: Larsen's syndrome: review of the literature and analysis of thirty-eight cases. J Pediatr Orthop 1994;14:63-73

Marfan Syndrome

Baumgartner C, Matyas G, Steinmann B, et al: Marfan syndrome: a diagnostic challenge caused by phenotypic and genetic heterogeneity. Methods Inf Med 2005;44:487-497

Chow K, Pyeritz RE, Litt HI: Abdominal visceral findings in patients with Marfan syndrome. Genetics in Med 2007;9:208-212

Ha HI, Seo JB, Lee SH, et al: Imaging of Marfan syndrome: multisystemic manifestations. Radiographics 2007;27:989-1004

Judge DP, Dietz HC: Marfan's syndrome. Lancet 2005;366:1965-1976

Knirsch W, Kurtz C, Haffner N, et al: Dural ectasia in children with Marfan syndrome: a prospective, multicenter, patient-control study. Am J Med Genet Part A 2006;140:775-781

Moura B, Tubach F, Sulpice M, et al: Bone mineral density in Marfan syndrome. A large case-control study. Joint Bone Spine 2006; 73:733-735

Sponseller PD, Hobbs W, Riley LH III, et al: The thoracolumbar spine in Marfan syndrome. J Bone Joint Surg Am 1995;7:867-876

Marshall-Smith Syndrome

Adam M, Hennekam R, Keppen L, et al: Marshall-Smith syndrome: natural history and evidence of an osteochondrodysplasia with connective tissue abnormalities. Am J Med Genet Part A 2005;137:117-124

Eich GF, Silver MM, Weksberg R, et al: Costa T. Marshall-Smith syndrome: new radiographic, clinical, and pathologic observations. Radiology 1991;181:183-188

Williams DK, Carlton DR, Green SH, et al: Marshall-Smith syndrome: the expanding phenotype. J Med Genet 1997;34:842-845

McKusick-Kaufman Syndrome

Davenport M, Taitz LS, Dickson JAS: The Kaufman-McKusick syndrome: another association. J Pediatr Surg 1989;24:1192-1194

David A, Bitou P, Lacombe D, et al: Hydrometrocolpos and polydactyly: a common neonatal presentation of Bardet-Biedl and McKusick-Kaufman syndromes. J Med Genet 1999;36:599-603

Kaufman RL, Hartmann HF, McAlister WH: Family studies in congenital heart disease II: a syndrome of hydrometrocolpos, post axial polydactyly and congenital heart disease. Birth Defects Orig Artic Ser 1972;8:85-87

Nakane T, Biesecker LG: No evidence for triallelic inheritance of MKKS/BBS loci in Amish McKusick Kaufman syndrome. Am J Med Genet Part A 2005;13:32-34

Robinow M, Shaw A: The McKusick-Kaufman syndrome. J Pediatr 1979;94:776-778

Stone DL, Agarwala R, Schaffer AA, et al: Genetic and physical mapping of the McKusick-Kaufman syndrome. Hum Mol Genet 1998;7:475-481

Meckel Syndrome

Ickowicz V, Eurin D, Maugey-Laulom B,et al: Meckel-Gruber syndrome: sonography and pathology. Ultrasound Obstet Gynecol 2006;27:296-300

Kjaer KW, Fischer HB, Keeling JW, et al: Skeletal malformations in fetuses with Meckel syndrome. Am J Med Genet 1999;84:469-475

Rapola J, Salonen R: Visceral anomalies in the Meckel syndrome. Teratology 1985;31:193-201

Salonen R, Paavola P: Meckel syndrome. J Med Genet 1998; 35:497-501

Smith UM, Consugar M, Tee LJ, et al: The transmembrane protein mecklein (MKS3) is mutated in Meckel-Gruber syndrome and the wpk rat. Nat Genet 2006;38:191-196

Neurofibromatosis

Bass JC, Korobkin M, Francis IR, et al: Retroperitoneal plexiform neurofibroma: CT findings. AJR Am J Roentgenol 1994; 163:617-620

Buckley PG, Mantripragada KK, Diazde Stahl T, et al: Identification of genetic aberrations on chromosome 22 outside the NF2 locus in schwannomatosis and neurofibromatosis type 2. Hum Mutat 2005;26:540-549

Cordeiro NJ, Gardener KR, Huson SM, et al: Recent vascular disease in neurofibromatosis 2: association or coincidence? Dev Med Child Neurol 2006;48:58-59

Evans DGR, Baser ME, McGaughran J, et al: Malignant peripheral nerve tumors in NF1. J Med Genet 2002;39:311-314

Evans DGR, Huson SM, Donnai D, et al: A genetic study of type 2 neurofibromatosis in the United Kingdom: prevalence, mutation, rate, fitness and confirmation of maternal transmission effect on severity. J Med Genet 1992;29:841-846

Ferner RE: Neurofibromatosis 1 and neurofibromatosis 2: a 21st century perspective. Lancet Neurol 2007;4:340-351

Fortman BJ, Kuszyk BS, Urban BA, et al: Neurofibromatosis type 1: a diagnostic mimicker at CT. Radiographics 2001;21:601-612

Holt JF: 1977 Edward B.D. Neuhauser lecture: neurofibromatosis in children. AJR Am J Roentgenol 1978;130:615-639

Jee WH, Oh SN, McCauley T, et al: Extraaxial neurofibromatosis versus neurolemmomas: discrimination with MRI. AJR Am J Roentgenol 2004;183:629-633

Lampe AK, Seymour G, Thompson PW, et al: Familial neurofibromatosis microdeletion syndrome complicated by rhabdomyosarcoma. Arch Dis Child 2002;87:444-445

Levy AD, Patel N, Dow N, et al: Abdominal neoplasms in patients with neurofibromatosis type 1: radiologic-pathologic correlation. Radiographics 2005;25:455-480

Listernick R, Charrow J, Greenwald M, et al: Natural history of optic pathway tumors in children with neurofibromatosis type 1: a longitudinal study. J Pediatr 1994;125:63-66

Mautner VF, Tatagiba M, Lindenau M, et al: Spinal tumors in patients with neurofibromatosis type 2: MR imaging study of frequency, multiplicity and variety. AJR Am J Roentgenol 1995;165:951-955

Pinna A, Demontis S, Maltese G, et al: Absence of the greater sphenoid wing in neurofibromatosis 1. Arch Ophthalmol 2005; 123:1454

Restropo CS, Riascos RF, Hatta AA, et al: Neurofibromatosis type 1: spinal manifestations of a systemic disease. J Comput Assist Tomgr 2005;29:532-540

Rossi SE, Erasmus JJ, McAdams HP, et al: Thoracic manifestations of neurofibromatosis 1. AJR Am J Roentgenol 1999;173:1631-1638

Ruggieri M, Pavone V, DeLuca D, et al: Congenital bone malformations in patients with neurofibromatosis type 1 (NF1). J Pediatr Orthop 1999;19:301-305

Ryan A, Hurley M, Brennan P, et al: Vascular dysplasia in neurofibromatosis type 2. Neurology 2005;65:163-164

Ryu JH, Parambil JG, McGrann PS, et al: Lack of evidence of an association between neurofibromatosis and pulmonary fibrosis. Chest 2005;128:2381-2386

Nevoid Basal Cell Carcinoma Syndrome

Evans DGR, Ladusans EJ, Rimmer S, et al: Complications of nevoid basal cell carcinoma syndrome. J Med Genet 1993;30:460-464

Fukushima Y, Oka H, Utsuki S, et al: Nevoid basal cell carcinoma with medulloblastoma and meningioma. Neurol Med Chir 2004; 44:665-668

Gorlin RJ: Nevoid basal-cell carcinoma syndrome. Medicine 1987;66:98-113

Gorlin RJ: Nevoid basal cell carcinoma (Gorlin) syndrome: unanswered issues. J Lab Clin Med 1999;134:551-552

Kimonis VE, Goldstein AM, Pastakia B, et al: Clinical manifestations in 105 persons with nevoid basal cell carcinoma syndrome. Med Genet 1997;369:299-308

Korczak JF, Brahim JS, DiGiovanna JJ, et al: Nevoid basal cell carcinoma syndrome with medulloblastoma: a rare case illustrating gene-environment interaction. Am J Med Genet 1997;69:309-314

Kulkarni P, Brashear R, Chuang TY: Nevoid basal cell carcinoma syndrome in a person with dark skin. J Am Acad Dermatol 2003;49:332-335

Niemann-Pick Disease

Chang MJ, Lee KS, Franquet T, et al: Metabolic lung disease: imaging and histopathologic findings. Eur J Radiol 2005;54:233-245

Elleder M: Niemann-Pick disease. Pathol Res Pract 1989;185:293-328

Kolodny EH: Niemann-Pick disease. Curr Opin Hematol 2000; 7:48-52

McGovern MM, Pohl-Worgall T, Deckelbaum RJ, et al: Lipid abnormalities in children with types A and B Niemann Pick disease. J Pediatr 2004;145:77-81

Mendelson DS, Wasserstein MP, Desnick RJ, et al: Type B Niemann-Pick disease: findings at chest radiography, thin-section CT, and pulmonary function testing. Radiology 2006;238:339-345

Trouard TP, Heidenreich RA, Seeger JF, et al: Diffusion tensor imaging in Niemann-Pick type C disease. Pediatr Neurol 2005;33:325-330

Wraith JE: Lysosomal disorders. Semin Neonatol 2002;7:75-83

Noonan Syndrome

Digilio MC, Barino B, Giannotti A, et al: Noonan syndrome with cardiac left-sided obstructive lesions. Hum Genet 1997;99:289

Hagekawa T, Ogata T, Hasegawa Y, et al: Coarctation of the aorta and renal hypoplasia in a boy with Turner/Noonan surface anomalies and a 46 XY karyotype: a clinical model for the possible impairment of a putative lymphogenic gene for Turner somatic stigmata. Hum Genet 1996;97:564-567

Moschovi M, Touliatou V, Papadopoulu A, et al: Rhabdomyosarcoma in a patient with Noonan syndrome phenotype and review of literature. J Pediatr Hematol Oncol 2007;5:341-344

Noonan JA: Noonan syndrome: an update and review for the primary pediatrician. Clin Pediatr 1994;33:548-555

Schorry EK, Lovell AM, Milatovich A, et al: Ullrich-Turner syndrome and neurofibromatosis. Am J Med Genet 1996;66:423-425

Schubbert S, Zenker M, Rowe SL, et al: Germline KRAS mutations cause Noonan syndrome. Nat Genet 2006;38:331-336

Tanaka Y, Masuno M, Kwamoto H, et al: Noonan syndrome and cavernous hemangioma of the brain. Am J Med Genet 1999; 82:212-214

Vander Burgt I, Thoonen G, Roosenboom N, et al: Patterns of cognitive functioning in school-aged children with Noonan syndrome associated with variability in phenotypic expression. J Pediatr 1999;135:707-713

Zenker M, Buheitel G, Rauch R, et al: Genotype-phenotype correlations in Noonan syndrome. J Pediatr 2004;144:368-374

Occipital Horn Syndrome

Dagenais SL, Adam AN, Innis JW, et al: A novel frameshift mutation in exon 23 of ATP7A (MNK) results in occipital horn syndrome and not in Menkes disease. Am J Hum Genet 2001;69:420-427

Herman TE, McAlister WH, Boniface A: Occipital horn syndrome: additional radiographic findings in two new cases. Pediatr Radiol 1992;22:363-365

Mentzel HJ, Seidel J, Vogt S, et al: Vascular complications (splenic and hepatic artery aneurysms) in the occipital horn syndrome: report of a patient and review of the literature. Pediatr Radiol 1999;29:19-22

Palmer CA, Percy AK: Neuropathology of occipital horn syndrome. J Child Neurol 2001;16:764-766

Tsukahara M, Kmaizumi K, Kawai S, et al: Occipital horn syndrome: report of a patient and review of the literature. Clin Genet 1994;45:32-35

Opitz (G/BBB) Syndrome

Berti C, Fontanella B, Ferrentino R, et al: Mig12, a novel Opitz syndrome gene product partner, is expressed in the embryonic ventral midline and cooperates with Mid1 to bundle and stabilize microtubules. BMC Cell Biol 2004;5:9

de Silva EO: The hypertelorism-hypospadias syndrome. Clin Genet 1983;23:30-34

Funderburk SJ, Stewart R: The G and BBB syndromes: case

presentations, genetics and nosology. Am J Med Genet 1978; 2:131-144

MacDonald MR, Olney AH, Kolodziej P: Opitz syndrome (G/BBB). Ear Nose Throat J 1998;77:528-529

McDonald MR, Schaefer GB, Olney A, et al: Brain magnetic resonance imaging findings in the Opitz G/BBB syndrome: extension of the spectrum of midline brain anomalies. Am J Med Genet 1993;46:706-711

Parashar SYU, Anderson PJ, Cox TC, et al: Multidisciplinary management of Opitz G BBB syndrome. Ann Plast Surg 2005;55:402-408

Shaw A, Longman C, Irving M, et al: Neonatal teeth in X-linked Opitz (G/BBB) syndrome. Clin Dysmorphol 2006;3:185-186

Oral-Facial-Digital Syndromes

Anneren G, Arvidson B, Gustavson KH, et al: Oro-facio-digital syndromes I and II: radiological methods of diagnosis and the clinical variations. Clin Genet 1984;26:178-186

Holub M, Potocki L, Bodamer OA: Central nervous system malformations in oral-facial-digital syndrome, type 1. Am J Med Genet Part A 2005;136:218

Sakai N, Nakakita N, Yamazaki Y, et al: Oral-facial-digital syndrome type II (Mohr syndrome): clinical and genetic manifestations. J Craniofac Surg 2002;13:321-326

Thauvin-Robinet C, Cossee M, Cormier-Daire V, et al: Clinical, molecular, and genotype-phenotype correlation studies from 25 cases of oral-facial-digital syndrome type 1: a French and Belgian collaborative study. J Med Genet 2006;43:54-61

Osteolysis Syndromes

Al-Otaibi L, Al-Mayouf SM, Majeed M, et al: Radiological findings in NAO syndrome. Pediatr Radiol 2002;32:523-528

Collucci S, Taraboletti G, Primo L, et al: Gorham-stout syndrome: a monocyte-mediated cytokine propelled disease. J Bone Miner Res 2006;21:207-218

Singh JA, Williams CB, McAlister WH: Talo-patello-scaphoid osteolysis, synovitis, and short fourth metacarpals in sisters: a new syndrome? Am J Med Genet Part A 2003;121:118-125

Zankl A, Pachman L, Poznanski A, et al: Torg syndrome is caused by inactivating mutations in MMP2 and is allelic to NAO and Winchester syndrome. J Bone Mineral Res 2007;22:329-333

Otopalatodigital Syndrome

Brewster TG, Lachman RS, Kushner DE, et al: Oto-palato-digital syndrome, type II—an X-linked skeletal dysplasia. Am J Med Genet 1985;20:249-254

Hidalgo-Bravo A, Pompa-Mera EN, Kofman-Alfaro S, et al: A novel filamin A D203Y mutation in a female patient with otopalatodigital type 1 syndrome and extremely skewed X chromosome inactivation. Am J Med Genet Part A 2005;136:190-193

Kondoh T, Okamoto N, Norimatsu N, et al: A Japanese case of oto-palato-digital syndrome type II: an apparent lack of phenotype-genotype correlation. J Hum Genet 2007;52:370-373

Langer LO Jr: The roentgenographic features of the oto-palato-digital (OPD) syndrome. Am J Roentgenol Radium Ther Nucl Med 1967;100:63-70

Pachydermoperiostosis

Bachmeyer C, Blum L, Cadranel JF, et al: Myelofibrosis in a patient with pachydermoperiostosis. Clin Exp Dermatol 2005;30:646-648

Diren HB, Kutluk MT, Karabent A, et al: Primary hypertrophic osteoarthropathy. Pediatr Radiol 1986;16:231-234

Latos-Bielenska A, Marik I, Kuklik M, et al: Pachydermoperiostosis—critical analysis with report of five unusual cases. Eur J Pediatr 2007;Feb 7: Epub [ahead of print]

Pena-Shokeir Syndrome Type I (Fetal Akinesia Sequence)

Agapitos M, Theodoropoulou M, Kouselinis A, et al: Athrogryposis multiplex congenita, Pena Shokeir phenotype with gastroschisis and agenesis of the leg. Pediatr Pathol 1988;8:409-413

Choi BH, Ruess WR, Kim RC: Disturbances in neuronal migration and laminar cortical formation with multicystic encephalopathy in Pena Shokeir syndrome. Acta Neuropathol 1986;69:177-183

Eguiluz I, Barber MA, Martin A, et al: Fetal akinesia deformation sequence: Pena Shokeir type I syndrome: new features of uncommon condition. J Obstet Gynaecol 2006;8:818-820

Hageman G, Willemse J, van Ketel BA, et al: The heterogeneity of the Pena Shokeir syndrome. Neuropediatrics 1987;18:45-50

Pena SDJ, Shokeir MHK: Autosomal recessive cerebro-oculo-facial-skeletal (COFS) syndrome. Clin Genet 1974;5:285-293

Porter HJ: Lethal arthryogryposis multiplex congenita. Pediatr Pathol Lab Med 1995;15:617-637

Pena-Shokeir Syndrome Type II (Cerebro-Oculofacial-Skeletal Syndrome)

Gorlin RJ, Cohen MM, Hennekam RCM (eds): Syndromes of the Head and Neck. 4th Edition, New York, Oxford University Press, 2001

Linna SL, Finni K, Simila A, et al: Intracranial calcifications in cerebro-oculo-facial-skeletal (COFS) syndrome. Pediatr Radiol 1982;79:282-284

Meira LB, Graham JM, Greenberg CR, et al: Manitoba aboriginal kindred with original COFS has a mutation in the Cockayne group B (*CSB*) gene. Am J Hum Genet 2000;66:1221-1228

Sakai T, Kikuchi F, Takashima S, et al: Neuropathological findings in the COFS (Pena Shokeir II) syndrome. Brain Dev 1997;19:58-62

Poland Syndrome

Azouz EM, Oudjhane K: Disorders of the upper extremity in children. Magn Reson Imaging Clin N Am 1998;63:6776-6795

Bavinck JN, Weaver DD: Subclavian artery supply disruption sequence: hypothesis of a vascular etiology for Poland, Klippel-Feil, and Mobius anomalies. Am J Med Genet 1986;234:903-918

Fokin A, Robicsek F: Poland's syndrome revisited. Ann Thorac Surg 2002;74:2218-2225

Wright AR, Milner RH, Bainbridge LC, et al: MR and CT in the assessment of Poland syndrome. J Comput Assist Tomogr 1992;163:442-447

Progeria

Ackerman J, Gilbert-Barness E: Hutchinson-Gilford progeria syndrome: a pathologic study. Pediatr Pathol Mol Med 2002;21:1-13

McClintock D, Gordon LB, Djabali K: Hutchinson-Gilford progeria mutant lamin A primarily targets human vascular cells as detected by an anti-Lamin A G608G antibody. Proc Natl Acad Sci U S A 2006;103:2154-2155

Ramirez CL, Cadinanos J, Varela I, et al: Human progeroid syndromes, aging and cancer: new genetic and epigenetic insights into old questions. Cell Mol Life Sci 2007;64:155-170

Proteus Syndrome

Jamis-Dow CA, Turner J, Biesecker LG, et al: Radiologic manifestations of Proteus syndrome. Radiographics 2004;24:1051-1068

Pazzaglia UE, Beluffi G, Bonaspetti G, et al: Bone malformations in Proteus syndrome: and analysis of bone structural changes and their evolution during growth. Pediatr Radiol 2007;37:829-835

Turner JT, Cohen MM Jr, Biesecker LG: Reassessment of the Proteus syndrome literature: application of diagnostic criteria to published cases. Am J Med Genet Part A 2004;130:111-122

Rubinstein-Taybi Syndrome

Mazzone D, Milana A, Pratico G, et al: Rubinstein-Taybi syndrome associated with Dandy-Walker cyst: case report in a newborn. J Perinat Med 1989;175:381-384

Roelfsema JH, White SJ, Ariyurek Y, et al: Genetic heterogeneity in Rubinstein-Taybi syndrome: mutations in both the *CBP* and *EP300* genes cause disease. Am J Hum Genet 2005;76:572-580

Rubinstein JH: Broad thumb-hallux Rubinstein-Taybi syndrome 1957–1988. Am J Med Genet Suppl 1990;6:3-16

Stevens CA: Patellar dislocation in Rubinstein-Taybi syndrome. Am J Med Genet 1997;722:188-190

Yamamoto T, Kurosawa K, Masuno M, et al: Congenital anomaly of cervical vertebrae is a major complication of Rubinstein-Taybi syndrome. Am J Med Genet Part A 2005;135:130-133

Russell-Silver Syndrome

Abraham E, Altiok H, Lubicky JP: Musculoskeletal manifestations of Russell-Silver syndrome. J Pediatr Orthop 2004;24:552-564

Al Fifi S, Teebi AS, Shevell M: Autosomal dominant Russell-Silver syndrome. Am J Med Genet 1996;61:96-97

Bruckheimer E, Abrahamov A: Russell-Silver syndrome and Wilms tumor. J Pediatr 993;122:165-166

Herman TE, Crawford JD, Cleveland RJ, et al: Hand radiographs in Russell-Silver syndrome. Pediatrics 1987;79:743-744

Hotokebuchi T, Miyahara H, Sugioka Y: Legg Calve Perthes' disease in Russell-Silver syndrome. Int Orthop 1994;18:32-37

Nakabayashi K, Fernandez BA, Teshima I, et al: Molecular genetic studies of human chromosome 7 in Russell-Silver syndrome. Genomics 2002;79:186-196

Ortiz C, Cleveland RH, Jaramillo D: Urethral valves in Russell-Silver syndrome. J Pediatr 1991;119:776-778

Patton MA: Russell-Silver syndrome. J Med Genet 1988;25:557-560

Saal HM, Pagon RA, Pepin MG: Reevaluation of the Russell-Silver syndrome. J Pediatr 1985;107:733-778

Tanner JM, LeJarraga H, Cameron N: Natural history of the Silver-Russell syndrome: a longitudinal study of 39 cases. Pediatr Res 1975;9:611-623

Smith-Lemli-Opitz Syndrome

Craig WY, Haddow JE, Palomaki GE, et al: Major fetal abnormalities associated with positive screening test for Smith-Lemli-Opitz syndrome (SLOS). Prenat Diag 2007;27:409-414

Curry CJR, Carey JC, Holland JS, et al: Smith-Lemli-Opitz syndrome type II. Am J Med Genet 1987;26:45-57

Herman TE, Siegel MJ, Lee BCP, et al: Smith-Lemli-Opitz syndrome type II: report of a case with additional radiographic findings. Pediatr Radiol 1993;23:37-40

Lin AE, Ardinger HH, Ardinger RH, et al: Cardiovascular malformations in Smith-Lemli-Opitz syndrome. Am J Med Genet 1997;68:270-278

Nowaczyk MJM, Whelan DT, Hill RE: Smith-Lemli-Opitz syndrome. Am J Med Genet 1998;78:419-423

Yu H, Patel SB: Recent insights into the Smith-Lemli-Opitz syndrome. Clin Genet 2005;68:383-391

Sotos Syndrome

Bhalala US, Parekh PR, Tullu MS: Soto's [sic] syndrome with bilateral hydronephrosis and hydroureters. Indian J Pediatr 2002;69:913-915

Cole TRP, Hughes HE: Sotos syndrome. J Med Genet 1994;31:20-22

Cole TRP, Hughes HE, Jeffreys MJ, et al: Small cell lung carcinoma in a patient with Sotos syndrome. J Med Genet 1992;29:338-341

Hersh HM, Cole TRP, Bloom AS, et al: Risk of malignancy in Sotos syndrome. J Pediatr 1992;120:572-574

Kurotaki N, Imaizumi K, Harada N, et al: Haploinsufficency of *NSD1* causes Sotos syndrome. Nat Genet 2002;30:365-366

Thrombocytopenia–Absent Radius (TAR) Syndrome

Greenhalgh KL, Howell RT, Bottani A, et al: Thrombocytopenia-absent radius syndrome: a clinical genetic study. J Med Genet 2002;39:876-881

Hall JG: Thrombocytopenia and absent radius (TAR) syndrome. J Med Genet 1987;24:79-83

Klopocki E, Schulze H, Straub G, et al: Complex inheritance pattern resembling autosomal recessive inheritance involving a microdeletion in thrombocytopenia-absent radius syndrome. Am J Hum Gene 2007;80:232-240

Tuberous Sclerosis

Carette MF, Antoine M, Bazelly B, et al: Primary pulmonary artery aneurysm in tuberous sclerosis: CT, angiography and pathological study. Eur Radiol 2006;16:2369-2370

Elsayes KM, Narra VR, Lewis JS Jr, et al: Magnetic resonance imaging of adrenal angiomyolipoma. J Comput Assist Tomogr 2005;29:80-82

Evans JC, Curtis J: The radiological appearances of tuberous sclerosis. Br J Radiol 2000;73:91-98

Lendvay TS, Marshall FF: The tuberous sclerosis complex and its highly variable manifestations. J Urol 2003;169:1635-1642

Muhler MR, Rake A, Schwabe M, et al: Value of fetal cerebral MRI in sonographically proven cardiac rhabdomyoma. Pediatr Radiol 2007;37:467-474

O'Callaghan FJ, Osborne JP: Advances in the understanding of tuberous sclerosis. Arch Dis Child 2000;83:140-142

Pallisa E, Sanz P, Roman A, et al: Lymphangioleiomyomatosis: pulmonary and abdominal findings with pathologic correlation. Radiographics 2002;22:S185-S198

Roach ES, Sparagana SP: Diagnosis of tuberous sclerosis complex. J Child Neurol 2004;19:643-649

VACTERL Association

Appignani BA, Jaramillo D, Barnes PD, et al: Dysraphic myelodysplasia associated with urogenital and anorectal anomalies: prevalence and types seen with MRI imaging. AJR Am J Roentgenol 1994;163:1199-1203

Day DL: Aortic arch in neonates with esophageal atresia. Radiology 1985;155:99-10

Kuo MF, Tsai Y, Hsu WM, et al: Tethered spinal cord and VACTERL Association. J Neurosurg 2007;3:201-204

Lomas FE, Dahlstrom JE, Ford JH: VACTERL with hydrocephalus: family with X-linked VACTERL-H. Am J Med Genet 1998;76:74-78

Martinez-Frias ML, Frias JL: VACTERL as primary, polytopic developmental field defects. Am J Med Genet 1999;83:13-16

Nezarati MM, McLeod DR: VACTERL manifestation in two generations of a family. Am J Med Genet 1999;82:40-42

Onyeije CI, Sherer DM, Handwerker S, et al: Prenatal diagnosis of sirenomelia with bilateral hydrocephalus: report of a previously undocumented form of VACTERL-H association. Am J Perinatol 1998;15:193-197

Quan L, Smith DW: The VATER association: vertebral defects, anal atresia, T-E fistula with esophageal atresia, radial and renal dysplasia: a spectrum of associated defects. J Pediatr 1973;28:104-107

Shaw-Smith C: Oesophageal atresia, tracheo-esophageal fistula, and the VACTERL association: review of genetics and epidemiology. J Med Genet 2006;43:545-554

Warfarin Embryopathy

Barker DP, Konje JC, Richardson JA: Warfarin embryopathy with dextrocardia and situs inversus. Acta Paediatr 1994;83:411

Chan KY, Gilbert-Barness E, Tiller G: Warfarin embryopathy. Pediatr Pathol Mol Med 2003;22:277-283

Tongsong T, Wanapirak C, Piyamongkol W: Prenatal ultrasonographic findings consistent with fetal warfarin syndrome. J Ultrasound Med 1999;18:577-580

Zakzouz MS: The congenital warfarin syndrome. J Laryngol Otol 1986;100:215-219

Weill-Marchesani Syndrome

Dagoneau N, Benoist-Lasselin C, Huber C, et al: *ADAMTS10* mutations in autosomal recessive Weill-Marchesani syndrome. Am J Hum Genet 2004;75:801-806

Faivre L, Dollfus H, Lyonnet S, et al: Clinical homogeneity and genetic heterogeneity in Weill-Marchesani syndrome. Am J Med Genet Part A 2003;123:204-207

Giordano N, Senesi M, Battisti E, et al: Weill-Marchesani syndrome: report of an unusual case. Calcif Tissue Int 1997;60:358-360

Harasymowycz P, Wilson R: Surgical treatment of advanced chronic angle glaucoma in Weill-Marchesani syndrome. J Pediatr Opthalmol Strabismus 2004;41:295-299

Werner Syndrome

Goto M, Kindynis P, Resnick D, et al: Osteosclerosis of the phalanges in Werner syndrome. Radiology 1989;172:841-843

Kakigi R, Endo C, Neshige R, et al: Accelerated aging of the brain in Werner's syndrome. Neurology 1992;42:922-924

Laroche M, Ricq G, Cantagrel A, et al: Bone and joint involvement in adults with Werner's syndrome. Rev Rhum Engl Ed 1997; 64:843-846

Machwe A, Xiao L, Orren DK: Length-dependent degradation of single-stranded 3' ends by the Werner syndrome protein (WRN): implications for spatial orientation and coordinated 3' to 5' movement of its ATPase/helicase and exonuclease domains. BMC Mol Biol 2006;7:6

Cri du Chat Syndrome

Fenger K, Niebuhr E: Measurements on hand radiographs from 32 cri-du-chat probands. Radiology 1978;129:137-141

Hills C, Moller JH, Finkelstein M, et al: Cri du chat syndrome and congenital heart disease: a review of previously reported cases and presentation of an additional 21 cases from the Pediatric Cardiac Care Consortium. Pediatrics 2006;117:924-927

James AE Jr, Atkins L, Feingold M, et al: The cri du chat syndrome. Radiology 1969;92:50-52

Niebuhr E: The cri du chat syndrome: epidemiology, cytogenetics, and clinical features. Hum Genet 1978;44:227-275

Stefanou EG, Hanna G, Foakes A, et al: Prenatal diagnosis of cri du chat (5p-) syndrome in association with isolated moderate bilateral ventriculomegaly. Prenat Diagn 2002;22:64-66

Zhang A, Zheng C, Hou M, et al: Deletion of the telomerase reverse transcriptase gene and haploinsufficiency of telomere maintenance in cri du chat syndrome. Am J Hum Genet 2003;72:940-948

Klinefelter Syndrome

Bojesen A, Gravholt CH: Klinefelter syndrome in clinical practice. Nat Clin Pract Urol 2007;4:192-204

Junik R, Kosowicz J: Reduced brain perfusion and neurocranial shape abnormalities of the temporal regions in patients with Klinefelter syndrome. Neurol Endocrinol Lett 2005;26:593-598

Swerdlow AJ, Schoemaker MJ, Higgins CD, et al: Cancer incidence and mortality in men with Klinefelter syndrome: a cohort study. J Natl Cancer Inst 2005;97:1204-1210

Trisomy 13 (Patau Syndrome)

Iliopoulos D, Sekerli E, Vassiliou G, et al: Patau syndrome with a long survival (146 months): a clinical report and review of literature. Am J Med Genet Part A 2006;140:92-93

James AE Jr, Merz T, Janower ML, et al: Radiological features of the most common autosomal disorders: trisomy 21-22 (mongolism or Down's syndrome), trisomy 18, trisomy 13-15, and the cri du chat syndrome. Clin Radiol 1971;22:417-433

Kumar AJ, Naidich TP, Stetten G, et al: Chromosomal disorders: background and neuroradiology. AJNR Am J Neuroradiol 1992;13:577-593

Nyberg DA, Souter VL: Sonographic markers of fetal trisomies: second trimester. J Ultrasound Med 2001;20:655-674

Papp C, Beke A, Ban Z, et al: Prenatal diagnosis of trisomy 13: analysis of 28 cases. J Ultrasound Med 2006;25:429-435

Trisomy 18 (Edwards Syndrome)

James AE Jr, Merz T, Janower ML, et al: Radiological features of the most common autosomal disorders: trisomy 21-22 (mongolism or Down's syndrome), trisomy 18, trisomy 13-15, and the cri du chat syndrome. Clin Radiol 1971;22:417-433

Kumar AJ, Naidich TP, Stetten G, et al: Chromosomal disorders: background and neuroradiology. AJNR Am J Neuroradiol 1992;13:577-593

Lin HY, Lin SP, Chen YJ, et al: Clinical characteristics and survival of trisomy 18 in a medical center in Taipei, 1988–2004. Am J Med Genet Part A 2006;140:945-951

Niedrist D, Riegel M, Achermann J, et al: Survival with trisomy 18—data from Switzerland. Am J Med Genet Part A 2006; 140:952-959

Singleton EB, Rosenberg HS, Yang SJ: The radiographic manifestations of chromosomal abnormalities. Radiol Clin North Am 1964;2:281-295

Viora E, Zamboni C, Mortara G, et al: Trisomy 18: Fetal ultrasound findings at different gestational ages. Am J Med Genet A 2007;143:553-557

Trisomy 21 (Down Syndrome)

Ali FE, Al-Bustan MA, Al-Busairi WA, et al: Cervical spine abnormalities associated with Down syndrome. Int Orthop 2006;30:284-289

Hayes A, Batshaw ML: Down syndrome. Pediatr Clin North Am 1993;40:523-535

James AE Jr, Merz T, Janower ML, et al: Radiological features of the most common autosomal disorders: trisomy 21-22 (mongolism or Down's syndrome), trisomy 18, trisomy 13-15, and the cri du chat syndrome. Clin Radiol 1971;22:417-433

Kriss VM: Down syndrome: imaging of multiorgan involvement. Clin Pediatr 1999;38:441-449

Nybert DA, Hyett J, Johnson JA, et al: First Trimester screening. Radiol Clin North Am 2006;44:837-861

Pizzutillo PD, Herman MJ: Cervical spine issues in Down syndrome. J Pediatr Orthop 2005;25:253-259

Ross JA, Spector LG, Robison LL, et al: Epidemiology of leukemia in children with Down syndrome. Pediatr Blood Cancer 2005; 44:8-12

Wellborn CC, Sturm PF, Hatch RS, et al: Intraobserver reproducibility and interobserver reliability of cervical spine measurements. J Pediatr Orthop 2000;20:66-70

Turner Syndrome

Bondy CA: New issues in the diagnosis and management of Turner syndrome. Rev Endocr Metab Disord 2005;6:269-280

Haber HP, Ranke MB: Pelvic ultrasonography in Turner syndrome: standards for uterine and ovarian volume. J Ultrasound Med 1999;18:271-276

Hall JG, Gilchrist DM: Turner syndrome and its variants. Pediatr Clin North Am 1990;37:1421-1440

Ho VB, Bakalov VK, Cooley M, et al: Major vascular anomalies in Turner syndrome: prevalence and magnetic resonance angiographic features. Circulation 2004;110:1694-1700

Subramaniam PN: Turner's syndrome and cardiovascular anomalies: a case report and review of the literature. Am J Med Sci 1989;297:260-262

Wihlborg CE, Babyn PS, Schneider R: The association between Turner's syndrome and juvenile rheumatoid arthritis. Pediatr Radiol 1999;29:676-681

Wolf-Hirschhorn Syndrome

Bergemann AD, Cole F, Hirschhorn K: The etiology of Wolf-Hirschhorn syndrome. Trends Genet 2005;21:188-195

Kumar AJ, Naidich TP, Stetten G, et al: Chromosomal disorders: background and neuroradiology. AJNR Am J Neuroradiol 1992;132:577-593

Magill HL, Shackelford GD, McAlister WH, et al: 4p– Wolf-Hirschhorn syndrome. AJR Am J Roentgenol 1980; 1352:283-288

Sase M, Hasegawa K, Honda R, et al: Ultrasonographic findings of facial dysmorphism in Wolf-Hirschhorn syndrome. Am J Perinatol 2005;22:99-102

Sergi C, Schulze BR, Hager HD, et al: Otto HF. Wolf-Hirschhorn syndrome: case report and review of the chromosomal aberrations associated with diaphragmatic defects. Pathologica 1998; 903:285-293

CHAPTER

167

Metabolic Bone Disease

RICHARD M. SHORE

An overlap exists between the metabolic bone diseases, endocrine bone diseases, and many skeletal dysplasias, necessitating arbitrary decisions regarding which disorders to cover in these categories. In some instances, it is convenient to categorize these disorders by mechanism, such as abnormalities of mineralization, whereas in other cases they are categorized by etiology, such as toxic disorders. Table 167-1 outlines the organization of this chapter and Chapter 168 and indicates where related conditions are included in other chapters. To keep the major aspects of parathyroid disorders in one chapter, renal osteodystrophy is included with parathyroid disorders in Chapter 168.

OVERVIEW OF BONE BIOLOGY AND DEVELOPMENT

The major functions of the skeleton are structural support and the interaction of the skeleton with muscle for motion. The skeleton also contains most of the total body calcium and phosphorus, and serves as a reserve for these minerals, which can be mobilized when needed.

Bone is a specialized connective tissue containing cells, bone matrix, minerals, and water. The cellular component includes osteoblasts, osteoclasts, and osteocytes. Osteoblasts secrete bone matrix known as osteoid. Osteoclasts are multinucleated giant cells involved in bone resorption. Osteocytes, formed from osteoblasts, are embedded in small lacunae in bone. These lacunae are connected by an extensive network of canaliculi providing a large surface area between bone and extracellular fluid for mineral exchange.

Bone matrix (osteoid) is composed of type I collagen (90% to 95%) and ground substance. Ground substance contains glycoproteins and proteoglycans, which are involved in mineralization and fixation of hydroxyapatite to the collagen framework. Grossly, bone is divided into compact bone, which form the cortices, and cancellous or trabecular bone, which fills the medullary space, and their proportions vary by site. Long bone diaphyses are more than 95% cortical bone, whereas the lumbar spine is more than 66% trabecular bone. Trabecular bone has a greater surface area, making it more active metabolically as a site for mineral mobilization when needed.

Histologically, bone is divided into lamellar and woven bone. Lamellar bone, formed during bone modeling and remodeling, is highly organized with alternating layers of parallel cross-linked collagen fibers, a structure allowing for the highest concentration of collagen and greatest strength. These lamellae are parallel at bone surfaces and concentric surrounding vessels in haversian systems. Conversely, in woven bone the collagen fibers are randomly and more loosely organized, resulting in a lower collagen density. Although woven bone is not as structurally strong as lamellar bone, its looser collagen meshwork permits more mineral to be deposited, so that it is more opaque radiographically. Woven bone is produced during initial ossification and with rapid bone formation, as with callus and tumor bone.

Bone is initially formed by two mechanisms: intramembranous ossification, with bone produced directly by a surrounding membrane, and endochondral ossification, in which a cartilage model (anlage) is initially produced and subsequently replaced by bone. Some flat bones are formed entirely by intramembranous ossification, whereas all long bones, and many other bones, including the spine, pelvis, and skull base, are formed by endochondral ossification. In endochondral bone formation, the cartilaginous anlage is formed by chondroblasts, which secrete cartilaginous matrix. The primary ossification center usually forms at the center of the cartilage anlage and expands toward both ends of the bone. The secondary ossification centers arise in the epiphyses at the bone ends. The growth plate, or physis, is located between the epiphysis and shaft, and it is the site of most rapid growth. Physeal cartilage is highly organized into several zones. The layer of cartilage closest to the epiphysis is the reserve zone. On the metaphyseal side of the reserve zone, the chondroblasts proliferate in columns, each of which arises from a single cell,

TABLE 167-1

Metabolic and Endocrine Bone Disorders

METABOLIC DISORDERS (CHAPTER 167)
Overview of Bone Formation and Mineralization
Insufficient Mineralization of Organic Matrix
- Rickets/osteomalacia (insufficient Ca × P product)
  - Vitamin D abnormalities
    - Nutritional deficiency or malabsorption
    - Vitamin D metabolic disorders
      - Hepatic and renal disease
      - Vitamin D–dependent rickets type I
    - Abnormal response to vitamin D
      - Vitamin D–dependent rickets type II
  - Mineral deficiency
    - Metabolic bone disease of prematurity
  - Hypophosphatemic rickets
    - X-linked hypophosphatemia (vitamin D resistant rickets)
    - Renal tubular disease
    - Oncogenic rickets
    - Miscellaneous causes of rickets
- Hypophosphatasia
Insufficient Organic Matrix Production
- Osteogenesis imperfecta
- Scurvy
- Copper disorders
Disorders of Bone Resorption
- Increased resorption
  - Hyperparathyroidism (discussed in Chapter 168)
  - Hyperphosphatasia
- Decreased resorption
  - Osteopetrosis (discussed in Chapter 165)
  - Toxic/pharmacologic (discussed in next section)
Miscellaneous Disorders
- Nutritional
  - Vitamin deficiency

- C (discussed with scurvy)
- D (discussed with rickets)
- Vitamin toxicity
  - A, D
- Toxic, pharmacologic, and other disorders
  - Heavy metal
  - Bisphosphonates
  - Prostaglandins (discussed in Chapters 28 and 175)
  - Oxalosis

ENDOCRINE DISORDERS (CHAPTER 168)
Hyperparathyroidism/Renal Osteodystrophy
- Primary hyperparathyroidism
- Renal osteodystrophy
- Neonatal hyperparathyroidism and related conditions
  - Williams syndrome
  - Idiopathic infantile hypercalcemia
  - Familial hypocalciuric hypercalcemia
  - Jansen metaphyseal chondrodysplasia
  - I-cell disease (mucolipidosis II)
Other Parathyroid Disorders
- Hypoparathyroidism
- Pseudohypoparathyroidism and pseudopseudohypoparathyroidism
Other Endocrine Disorders
- Thyroid disorders: hypothyroidism and hyperthyroidism
- Growth hormone disorders: growth hormone deficiency and excess
- Adrenal disorders
  - Glucocorticoid excess
  - Adrenogenital syndrome
  - Pheochromocytoma
- Gonadal disorders

forming the proliferative zone. These cells then hypertrophy, forming the hypertrophic zone, and finally they undergo terminal differentiation, resulting in mineralization of the cartilage and apoptosis of the chondroblasts. The calcified cartilage formed at the metaphyseal side of the physis is the zone of provisional calcification, seen radiographically as the opaque line separating the metaphysis from the lucent cartilaginous physis. Deficient mineralization of this zone is the most important initial finding in rickets. The calcified cartilage is then resorbed by osteoclasts (or possibly specific chondroclasts), blood vessels enter from the metaphysis, and osteoblasts secrete osteoid. In the presence of an adequate *calcium × phosphate* product and tissue-nonspecific alkaline phosphatase, osteoid becomes calcified with hydroxyapatite crystals deposited along the collagen fibers. Bone initially formed by this process is woven bone, with a random arrangement of collagen fibers. This woven bone, along with the framework of calcified cartilage that it is formed on, comprises the primary spongiosa. Of interest for the radiologist, the primary spongiosa is the region through which the characteristic metaphyseal fractures of nonaccidental trauma occur. The primary spongiosa is then resorbed by osteoclasts and replaced by lamellar bone. In the

medullary space, this more mature bone is the secondary spongiosa. In intramembranous ossification, osteoblasts arise from the surrounding periosteum and secrete osteoid, which then becomes mineralized.

Following initial bone formation, the skeleton is continuously renewed throughout life by bone remodeling, a process that repairs damaged bone and adapts the skeleton to changes in physical load. With remodeling, old bone is removed by osteoclastic resorption and new osteoid is then secreted, which must then become mineralized. Deficient mineralization during this process is the hallmark of osteomalacia. The relative rates of bone resorption and formation are important determinants of bone size and shape. Periosteal appositional bone formation contributes to growth of bone width, and bone may be resorbed along the endosteal surface. If these processes proceed at the same rate, cortical thickness remains constant and there is a gradual increase in width of the bone and its medullary canal. Imbalance of these processes leads to increased or decreased cortical thickness. Bone may also be resorbed by osteoclasts along the outer subperiosteal surface. This is responsible for "metaphyseal cutback," which narrows the bone from the relatively wide metaphysis to the narrower diaphysis. Osteopetrosis, a sclerotic bone dysplasia, is caused by defective osteoclast resorption, and deficient subperiosteal osteoclastic resorption accounts for the lack of metaphyseal cutback and decreased tubulation in that disorder.

ABNORMALITIES OF MINERALIZATION: RICKETS AND RELATED DISORDERS

Physiology of Mineralization

To form structurally competent bone, osteoid must be mineralized. In endochondral bone formation, cartilage also becomes calcified prior to being replaced by bone. Normal calcification requires the presence of an adequate circulating calcium × phosphate product. Conditions resulting in an inadequate calcium × phosphate product produce rickets and/or osteomalacia, terms that are distinguished by the location of the mineralization abnormality. In rickets, this defect occurs at the growth plate and involves deficient mineralization of cartilage and osteoid. Osteomalacia refers to deficient mineralization of osteoid produced during the process of bone turnover and remodeling. Since the growth plate exists only during childhood, rickets is unique to children; osteomalacia occurs in both children and adults. Forms of rickets due to low circulating calcium (calcipenic rickets) are mostly due to abnormalities of vitamin D.

> **Rickets is due to an insufficient calcium × phosphate product. Calcipenic rickets are mostly due to abnormalities of vitamin D, which acts to maintain a normal circulating calcium concentration.**

Other causes of rickets are inadequate mineral intake, most frequently seen in metabolic bone disease of prematurity, and phosphopenic disorders, mostly due to with renal tubular phosphate wasting. In addition to an adequate calcium × phosphate product, mineralization also requires the presence of tissue-nonspecific alkaline phosphatase; a defect in this enzyme produces the related disorder hypophosphatasia.

The major function of vitamin D is to maintain an adequate calcium × phosphate product. Effective vitamin D insufficiency may be due to insufficient vitamin D production and intake, malabsorption, abnormal transformation of vitamin D to its active form, or failure of the end organs to respond to vitamin D. Vitamin D is synthesized in the skin from 7-dehydrocholesterol upon exposure to sunlight containing ultraviolet B radiation (290 to 315 nm). In the absence of sufficient sunlight exposure, vitamin D can also be provided in the diet. Natural dietary sources of vitamin D are quite limited, with significant vitamin D supplied only by oily fish and fish liver oil. Most dietary vitamin D is derived from fortification of certain foods. Once produced in the skin or absorbed from the gut, vitamin D undergoes hepatic hydroxylation in the 25 position, producing $25(OH)D$, a step that is not tightly regulated. The next step, which occurs in the kidney and is highly regulated, is 1-α-hydroxylation producing $1,25(OH)_2D$, the active form

of vitamin D. $1,25(OH)_2D$ has been named calcitriol (both its trivial chemical name and pharmaceutical name), which will used in this chapter. Calcitriol has many biologic functions, the most important of which is promoting gastrointestinal absorption of calcium by inducing transcription of the gene for calcium-binding protein. Additionally, it increases renal tubular reabsorption of phosphate in the presence of parathyroid hormone (PTH), and it decreases PTH synthesis and secretion. The major effect of calcitriol for bone is promotion of mineralization by maintaining adequate calcium and phosphate levels. It also has seemingly paradoxical direct effects on bone, both promoting calcium mobilization from bone (which requires PTH) and directly promoting mineralization, with partial healing of rickets even before normalization of serum mineral levels. Hypocalcemia is a major stimulus to calcitriol production (an indirect effect). Calcitriol then acts to increase the circulating calcium concentration, achieving homoeostasis.

Vitamin D–Deficiency Rickets

ETIOLOGY AND EPIDEMIOLOGY

Vitamin D deficiency requires both inadequate sunlight exposure and dietary intake. The first and most severe epidemic of rickets occurred during the industrial revolution, with urbanization and darkened skies limiting sunlight exposure. This epidemic ended with food fortification following the discovery by Harry Steenbock in 1923 that vitamin D can be produced by ultraviolet irradiation of certain foods. However, this did not entirely eliminate rickets. Risk factors included migration of dark-skinned populations to northern latitudes with decreased sunlight intensity, decreased exposure to sunlight related to specific cultural practices, and diets low in vitamin D, particularly dairy-free vegetarian diets. Breast milk contains relatively little vitamin D, and a smaller but not insignificant epidemic of rickets developed in the United States in the mid-1990s with increased breastfeeding in the African American and Hispanic populations. Although the vast majority of dietary rickets is due to vitamin D deficiency, dietary calcium deficiency is occasionally responsible for rickets. This was initially recognized in parts of Africa where sunlight exposure is plentiful but dietary calcium is very limited, and children with rickets responded to calcium supplementation but not to vitamin D supplementation. It has more recently been recognized that some rickets in the United States may also be due to calcium deficiency in infants weaned to a dairy-free diet, although this is quite uncommon.

CLINICAL FEATURES

Because $25(OH)D$ readily crosses the placenta, infants born to vitamin D–replete mothers have sufficient stores so that vitamin D–deficiency rickets is usually not manifest before 3 to 6 months. However, if the mother is vitamin D deficient, nutritional rickets may be seen in early infancy. Clinical features of rickets include prominence of anterior rib ends causing a "rachitic rosary,"

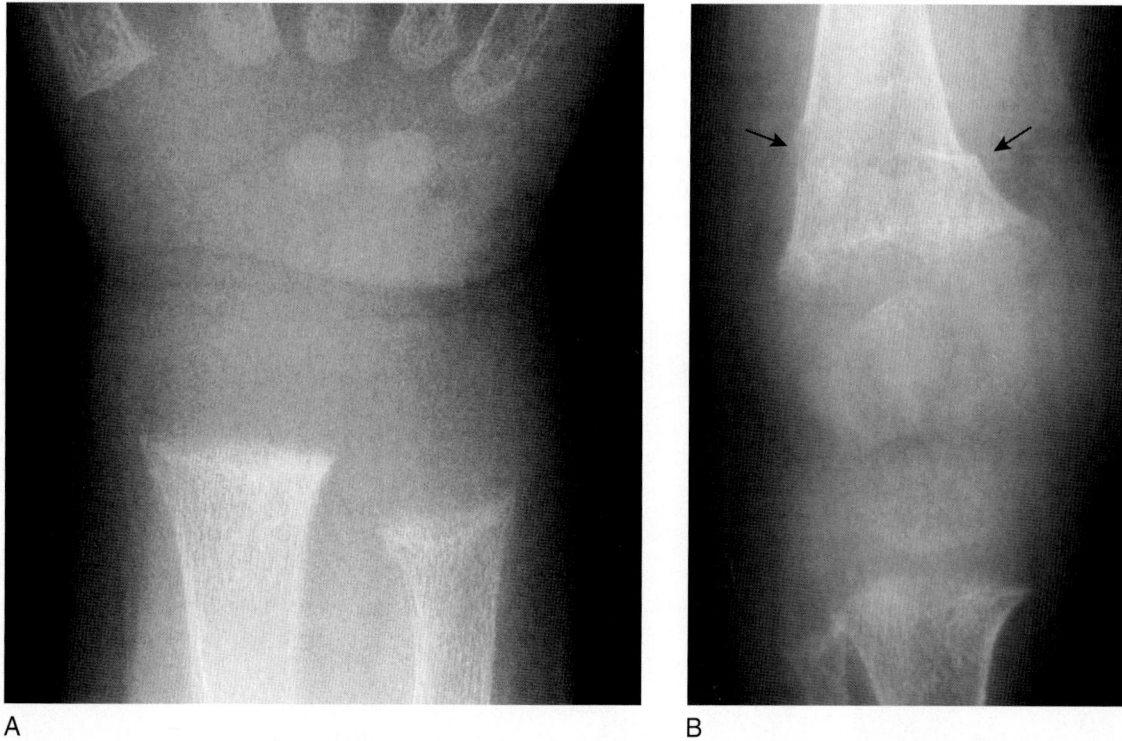

A   B

FIGURE 167-1. Severe vitamin D–deficiency rickets in a 17-month-old child. **A,** The wrist shows loss of definition of the zone of provisional calcification for the distal radius and ulna, with metaphyseal bone fading into the lucent growth plate. The cortical margins of the distal forearm bones are poorly delineated, suggesting subperiosteal resorption from hyperparathyroidism secondary to rickets. **B,** Severe findings are noted in the knee. In addition to loss of the zone of provisional calcification for the distal femoral and proximal tibial metaphyses, there is also loss of definition of the white line usually surrounding the epiphyses. A pathologic distal femoral fracture is also present *(arrows).*

prominent metaphyseal regions in the wrists and knees, craniotabes (ping-pong ball deformity of the skull), and frontal bossing. Deformities (which are largely due to the osteomalacia accompanying rickets) include lower extremity bowing (especially the tibias), chest wall (Harrison) grooves related to diaphragmatic insertions, scoliosis, and kyphosis.

Pathologic and Radiographic Findings

The pathologic and radiographic features of rickets are most pronounced in regions of greatest bone growth, particularly the distal radius and ulna at the wrist, the distal femur and proximal tibia at the knee, and the proximal humerus and anterior rib ends, which may be noted on chest radiographs. Conversely, the findings of rickets are masked by poor linear growth, even in the presence of significant biochemical abnormality.

An insufficient calcium × phosphate product leads to decreased mineralization of the zone of provisional calcification and lack of normal chondrocytic terminal differentiation. The initial radiographic finding is rarefaction of the normally sharply defined zone of provisional calcification on the metaphyseal side of the growth plate so that metaphyseal bone fades gradually into the lucent physeal and epiphyseal cartilage (Fig. 167-1). There is also loss of definition of the Laval-Jeantet collar of new bone formed by periosteal intramembranous ossification at the margin of the metaphysis in young infants. With failure of chondrocytic terminal differentiation and apoptosis, which occurs in a patchy

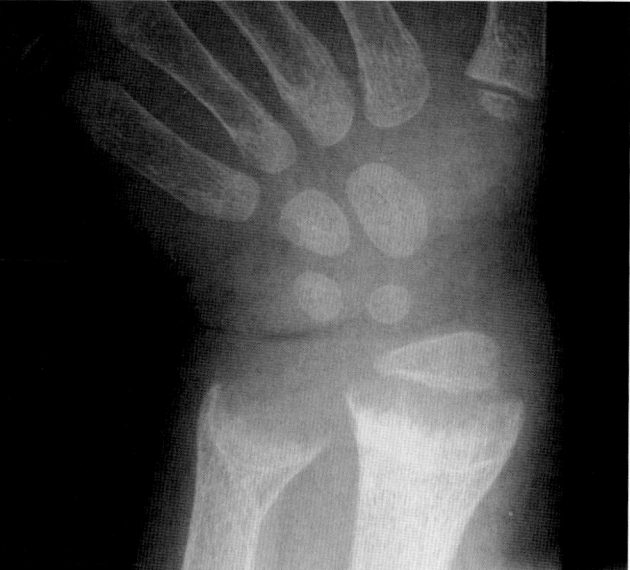

FIGURE 167-2. Metaphyseal cupping in a 23-month-old child with vitamin D–deficiency rickets from prolonged breastfeeding. In addition to the cupping, note the loss of visualization of the zone of provisional calcification and the irregular calcification at the base of the cup related to disorganized, irregularly calcified cartilage.

distribution, there is lack of normal vascular ingrowth and accumulation of disorganized cartilage lacking the normal columnar pattern of the hypertrophic zone. The affected metaphysis then becomes widened and cupped (although cupping of the distal ulnar metaphysis is often a normal finding in young infants, and this finding alone is not indicative of rickets). With further accumulation of disorganized cartilage and osteoid, the metaphysis becomes markedly frayed and irregular and there is widening of the distance between mineralized bone in the metaphysis and epiphysis, producing an appearance pathognomonic of rickets. Metaphyseal concavity

(cupping) varies by site, being most pronounced in the distal forearm bones (Fig. 167-2). Cupping may also be absent in an atrophic variety of rickets in which muscular weakness decreases limb activity and weight bearing, decreasing mechanical forces on the metaphyses. The classic metaphyseal findings of rickets are often best illustrated by comparison of active and healed or healing phases (Fig. 167-3).

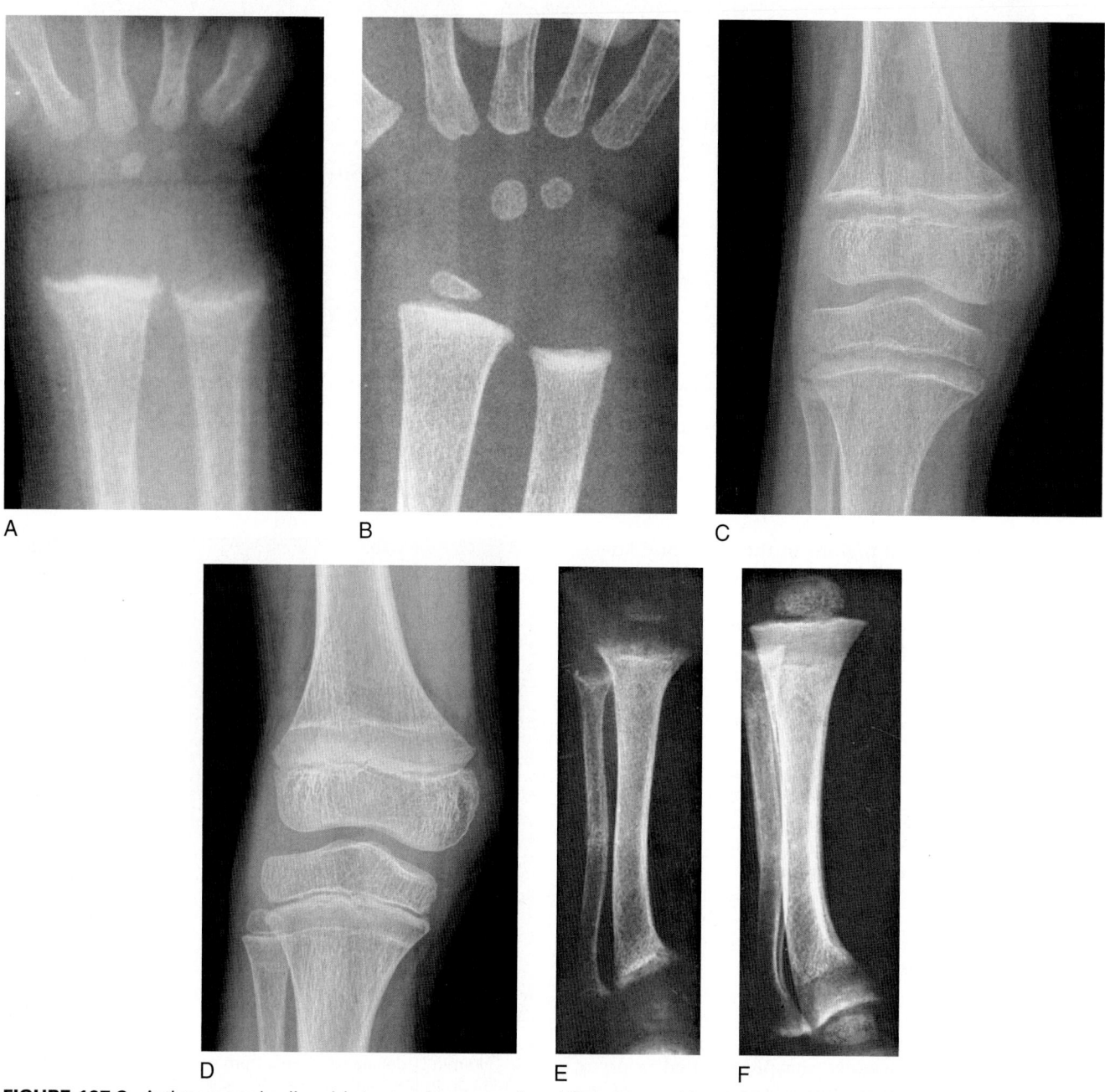

FIGURE 167-3. Active versus healing rickets at various ages. **A** and **B,** Active nutritional rickets in the wrist at 4 months **(A)** versus healed at 7 months **(B)**. In addition to the classic findings at the physis, **A** also shows periosteal new bone along the radial and ulnar diaphyses and the metacarpal shafts. Although periosteal new bone is more typically seen with healing rickets, it may also be seen in untreated rickets as an anabolic effect of associated hyperparathyroidism. The flaring of the metaphyses (more pronounced for the ulna than the radius) in **A** has resolved in **B. C** and **D,** Active **(C)** versus healing **(D)** rickets in the knee at 9.5 and 10 years. With treatment, there is visualization of the zone of provisional calcification in the metaphyses. The growth plate widening in **C** has resolved in **D. E** and **F,** An infant with nutritional rickets at presentation **(E)** and following 3 months of treatment **(F)**. Note that, with healing, a large amount of previously nonmineralized metaphyseal osteoid has become calcified and visible, giving the false impression of rapid bone growth.

The ossification centers of the carpal and tarsal bones and long bone epiphyses (see Fig. 167-1) may show findings similar to those in the metaphyses, although they are not seen as early since these areas are not as rapid growing. The margins of these small bones are analogous to the zones of provisional calcification and may become indistinct and disappear. In most cases, the trabecular regions are relatively preserved. These findings are opposite to those of scurvy, which shows loss of internal trabeculae but maintenance of the peripheral white line. In severe cases with progressive osteopenia of the trabecular regions from osteomalacia, these small bones may become invisible. This appearance simulates delayed skeletal maturation, and acceleration of maturation may be erroneously suggested when this bone becomes mineralized with healing of rickets.

In the calcipenic forms of rickets (primarily those due to vitamin D abnormality), PTH rises in an attempt to restore a normal serum calcium concentration, producing a secondary hyperparathyroidism (2° HPTH). This term is also used in renal osteodystrophy, in which PTH rises to correct hypocalcemia caused by phosphate retention in chronic renal failure. When 2° HPTH develops with rickets, typical radiographic findings of HPTH are seen, including subperiosteal bone resorption, intracortical tunneling, and overall demineralization (Fig. 167-4).

The radiographic findings of rickets in the shaft lag behind those in the metaphysis, and are largely those of associated osteomalacia and 2° HPTH (see Fig. 167-4). The entire shaft shows diffuse rarefaction from loss of bone mineral. The cortex becomes thin and its texture coarsens with intracortical lucent striations from 2° HPTH, which also produces subperiosteal bone resorption. Paradoxically, periosteal new bone formation may also be seen in rickets even prior to healing, which is likely due to an anabolic effect of PTH (see Fig. 167-3). With ongoing bone remodeling, as nonmineralized osteoid replaces mineralized bone (osteomalacia), the smaller trabeculae are no longer seen, producing a coarse trabecular pattern from the remaining larger trabeculae. Associated cortical thinning allows this coarse trabecular pattern to be even more prominent. Insufficiency fractures may develop in rachitic bones. Bowing of long bones, most pronounced in the tibias, is a major manifestation of rickets (Fig. 167-5). Bowing in rickets is related to loss of normal bone rigidity and may involve both the metaphyses and shafts. At the ends of bones, the rachitic metaphysis contains a large zone of nonmineralized cartilage and osteoid that is particularly deformable and subject to bending. Bowing may also develop in the shaft due to osteomalacia or as a consequence of fracture. Additional deformities that are the result of osteomalacia include Harrison grooves, kyphoscoliosis, platybasia, and pelvic deformity. Looser zones (also called pseudofractures) may be seen, but are more common with more chronic forms of rickets, such as X-linked hypophosphatemia (vitamin D–resistant rickets), and are discussed in that section. Craniosynostosis may also occur in rickets and hypophosphatasia, although this may be difficult to recognize during the acute phase because of the associated demineralization. Findings that

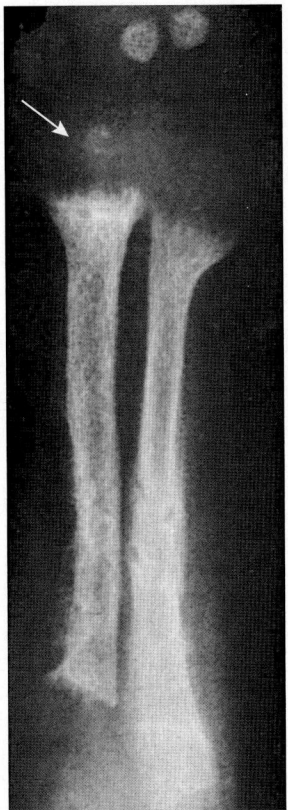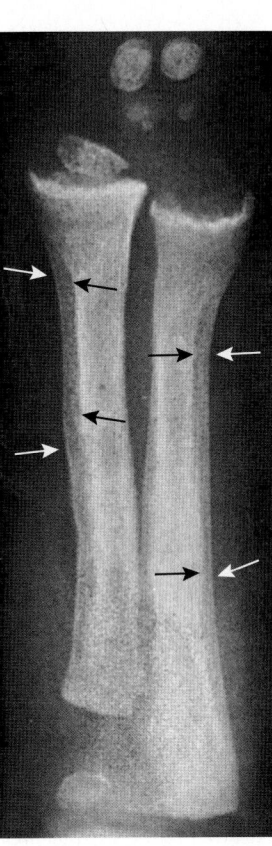

A   B

FIGURE 167-4. Diaphyseal findings in rickets. Same patient as in Figure 3E and 3F. **A,** During the active phase, there is coarse demineralization and subperiosteal bone resorption indicative of hyperparathyroidism secondary to rickets. The distal radial epiphyseal ossification center is small and barely visible *(arrow).* **B,** With healing 3 months later, there is visible extensive subperiosteal new bone formation *(arrows).* Previously, nonmineralized osteoid was present that was not radiographically identifiable.

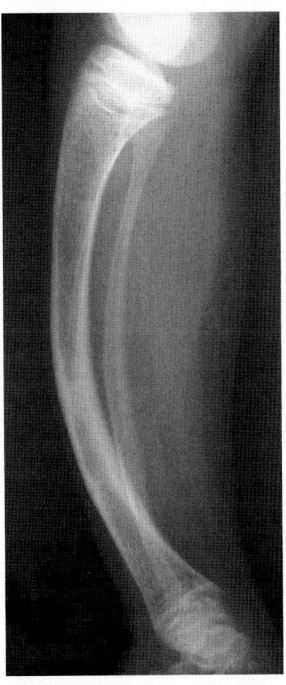

FIGURE 167-5. Radiograph of a 9-year-old with vitamin D–resistant rickets. The tibia is markedly bowed anteriorly.

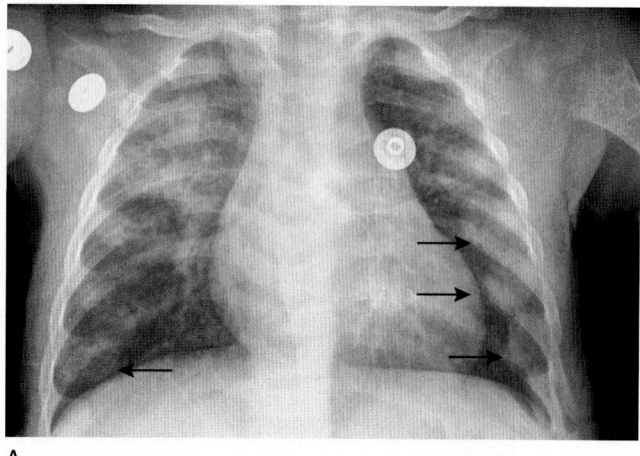
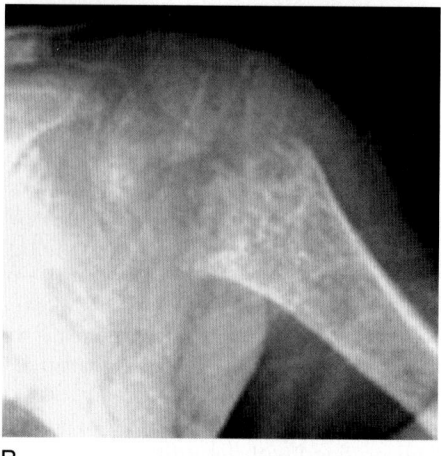

A   B

FIGURE 167-6. Chest radiograph findings in a 17-month-old child with vitamin D–deficiency rickets. **A,** Widening of the rib ends *(arrows)* produces the "rachitic rosary," which is often more apparent on physical examination. **B,** Severe rickets is also noted in the close-up view of the proximal humerus.

may be recognized on chest radiographs include involvement of the proximal humeral metaphyses and the anterior rib ends, producing the rachitic rosary (Fig. 167-6).

With healing (see Fig. 167-3), there is mineral deposition in the zone of provisional calcification, restoration of normal chondrocytic terminal differentiation, and ingrowth of metaphyseal vessels. The initial radiographic finding of healing is reidentification of the zone of provisional calcification as a thin opaque line that is separated from the identifiable shaft by the intervening lucent nonmineralized cartilage and osteoid in the rachitic metaphysis. With further healing, the zone of provisional calcification thickens and metaphyseal trabecular bone recalcifies, filling in the previously lucent region (see Fig. 167-3). This recalcification of the terminal segment of the shaft may give the false impression rapid bone growth. Healing of cortical bone is usually slower and less conspicuous. In the process of appositional bone growth, osteoid is produced by the periosteum, which does not become properly calcified in the active phase of rickets. With healing, this osteoid becomes calcified, producing either a uniform or lamellated layer surrounding the previous cortical boundary (see Fig. 167-4). Although not as often seen in the epiphysis as in the metaphysis, mineralization of the zone of provisional calcification surrounding the epiphyses may also be seen with healing rickets, producing a ring separated from bone in the center of the epiphysis by nonmineralized osteoid (Fig. 167-7).

Although rickets usually heals with restoration of normal anatomy, in some cases there is residual distortion and sclerosis in the previously affected metaphyseal regions related to the previous disorganized cartilage (Fig. 167-8). This may persist for years in the shaft as the physis continues to grow away from it. Central rarefaction of the epiphyses may persist, although not to the degree noted in scurvy. There may also be residual bowing deformity of the lower extremities with convex anterior bowing of the tibias and genu valgum. The radiographic findings of rickets are summarized in Table 167-2.

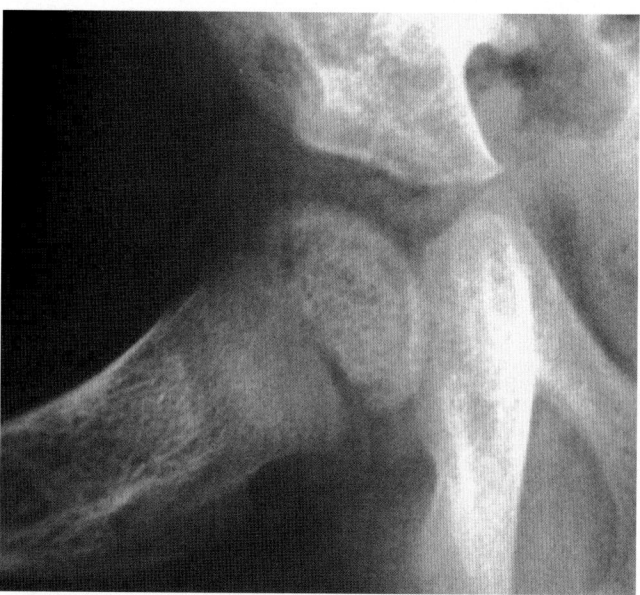

FIGURE 167-7. Remineralization of the zone of provisional calcification surrounding the epiphysis in a 4-year-old child with treated rickets.

Other Forms of Rickets

There are many conditions in addition to vitamin D deficiency that result in an insufficient calcium × phosphate product causing rickets. These are divided into calcipenic and phosphopenic disorders. The major radiographic manifestations of rickets described previously are nonspecific for the cause of rickets; similar findings are also present in the other forms of rickets, unless otherwise indicated.

OTHER FORMS OF CALCIPENIC RICKETS

MALABSORPTION AND HEPATOBILIARY DISEASE. Vitamin D insufficiency may be present for reasons other than insufficient dietary intake. In malabsorption states such as celiac disease and cystic fibrosis, there is malabsorption of vitamin D, leading to rickets. Rickets in hepato-

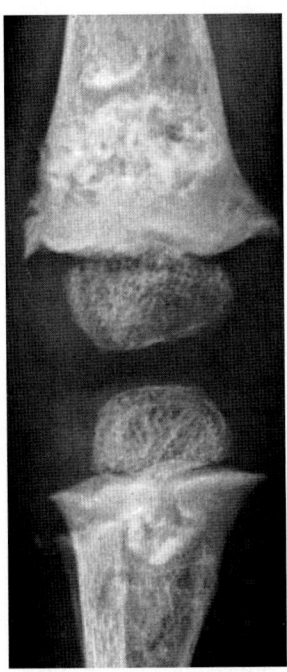

FIGURE 167-8. Residual chondroid calcifications in metaphyses from previous disorganized cartilage in rickets ("chambering").

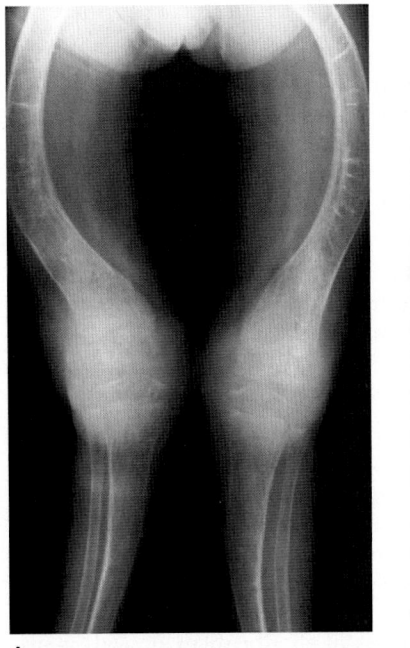

A

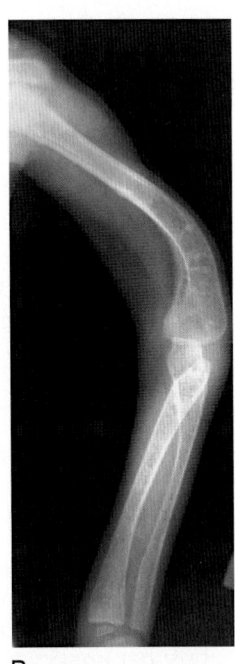

B

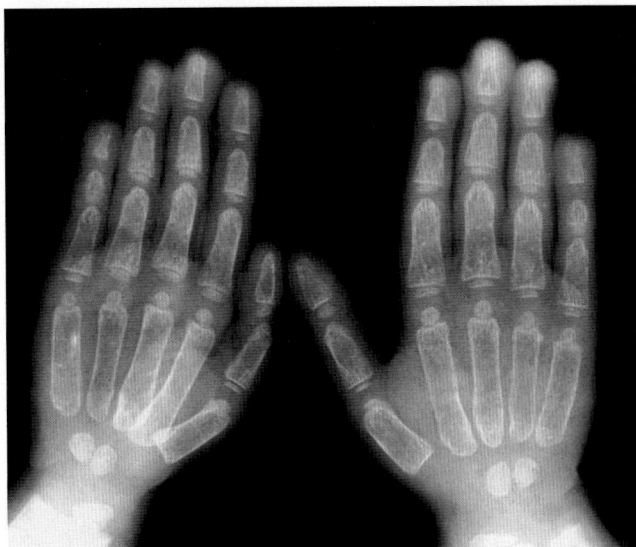

C

FIGURE 167-9. Hepatic rickets and osteomalacia in a 15-year-old boy who had a Kasai operation for extrahepatic biliary atresia during the perinatal period. Severe generalized osteopenia, bowing of the long tubular bones, slight irregularities of the metaphyses, and swelling of both knees secondary to hemarthroses (**A** and **B**), caused by associated vitamin K deficiency, and clubbing of the digits (**C**) are characteristic of hepatic osteodystrophy. In infants and children with poor muscular power and decreased activity, cupping and flaring of the metaphyses may be less evident or absent.

TABLE 167-2
Rickets: Major Radiographic Features (Excluding Rickets of Prematurity)
Demineralization of zone of provisional calcification
Metaphyseal cupping, fraying, flaring
Diffuse coarse demineralization
Deformity from osteomalacia
Bowing, platybasia, kyphoscoliosis
Associated hyperparathyroidism (calcipenic rickets)
Subperiosteal resorption
Intracortical tunneling

biliary disease is related primarily to decreased intake and intestinal absorption of fat-soluble vitamins (A, D, E, and K). Although decreased hepatic hydroxylation of vitamin D to 25(OH)D may also occur, this is usually not the cause of rickets. Associated vitamin K deficiency in hepatobiliary disease leads to recurrent hemarthrosis, most frequently involving the knee. The unusual combination of clubbing of the digits, evidence of hemarthrosis, rickets, and osteomalacia is characteristic of hepatic osteodystrophy (Fig. 167-9).

VITAMIN D–DEPENDENT RICKETS, TYPES I AND II. Vitamin D–dependent rickets (VDDR) type I is an autosomal recessive defect in the renal enzyme 1-α-hydroxylase, which converts 25(OH)D to calcitriol. Serum levels of calcitriol are undetectable or very low. The rickets in VDDR I are severe and often present in the first few months of life, which is earlier than most dietary rickets. Findings of 2° HPTH may be particularly prominent in this form of rickets. VDDR I responds to physiologic doses of calcitriol.

Rickets can also be due to end organ nonresponsiveness to vitamin D, a rare autosomal disorder. Although this condition has been named VDDR type II, this designation is inappropriate since the rickets are resistant to vitamin D, including calcitriol. Hence the preferred name for this disorder is calcitriol-resistant rickets. In addition to severe rickets beginning in early infancy, approximately half of the patients have alopecia. Other manifestations of ectodermal dysplasia, including dental abnormalities, may be present.

PHOSPHOPENIC RICKETS

Phosphopenic rickets results from disorders of renal tubular phosphate wasting, including: (1) X-linked hypophosphatemia, (2) renal tubular diseases, and (3) tumor-induced (oncogenic) rickets. Additionally, a major component of rickets of prematurity (metabolic bone disease of prematurity) is likely phosphate deficiency.

> **Phosphopenic rickets includes X-linked hypophosphatemia, renal tubular disease, oncogenic rickets, and phosphate depletion conditions.**

X-LINKED HYPOPHOSPHATEMIA. X-linked hypophosphatemia (XLH), also know as familial vitamin D–resistant rickets, is an inherited defect in renal tubular phosphate reabsorption due to a mutation of the gene *PHEX* (phosphate-regulating endopeptidase on the X chromosome). Phosphate wasting in XLH, and some other forms of phosphopenic rickets, is caused by a circulating "phosphatonin," which is likely fibroblast growth factor 23 (FGF23). This factor inhibits resorption of phosphate in the proximal tubule, and also downregulates 1-α-hydroxylase, leading to calcitriol levels that are inappropriately low for the degree of hypophosphatemia. In XLH, the *PHEX* mutation results in an abnormal endopeptidase that is unable to degrade normal FGF23, whereas in the rare autosomal dominant variety of hypophosphatemic rickets, a mutation of FGF23 prevents its degradation by a normal endopeptidase. In tumor-induced rickets, phosphate wasting is caused by production of FGF23 by certain mesenchymal tumors.

XLH is often less severe in female heterozygotes than male hemizygotes and is clinically characterized by short stature and prominent bowing deformities of the lower extremities. Radiographs show bowing and rachitic changes in the most rapidly growing bones (Fig. 167-10). The rachitic findings in XLH are often (but not always) relatively mild compared to other causes of rickets. Since XLH involves hypophosphatemia rather than hypocalcemia, findings of 2° HTPH are usually absent. The prominent bowing in XLH is often associated with cortical thickening or "buttressing" on the concave side of the bowing. Looser zones (a feature of osteomalacia) are present more often in XLH than in vitamin D–deficiency rickets, likely because of the chronicity of XLH. Looser zones, or pseudofractures, are radiolucent lines oriented perpendicular to the cortex that occur at sites of stress with or without an actual stress fracture. Stress leads to increased bone turnover with bone resorption followed by new bone production. In osteomalacia, osteoid in the newly formed bone is not mineralized properly, causing the radiolucent Looser zone. Characteristic sites for Looser zones, which are often bilaterally symmetric, include the medial aspect of the femoral neck (Fig. 167-11), the extensor surface of the ulna, the axillary border of the scapula, and the pubic rami. Osteopenia is not as prominent in XLH as in many other forms of rickets. Bone mineral studies in XLH have shown that the appendicular skeleton is often demineralized, whereas bone mineral density in the axial skeleton may be increased. In older patients, XLH may be associated with enthesopathy, causing calcification and ossification at joint capsules and sites of muscular, tendinous, or ligamentous insertion into bone. Older patients may also have paravertebral ossification, which is similar to diffuse idiopathic skeletal hyperostosis.

Treatment of XLH includes oral phosphate replacement and vitamin D, with calcitriol yielding the best results. This therapy leads to healing of rickets and also

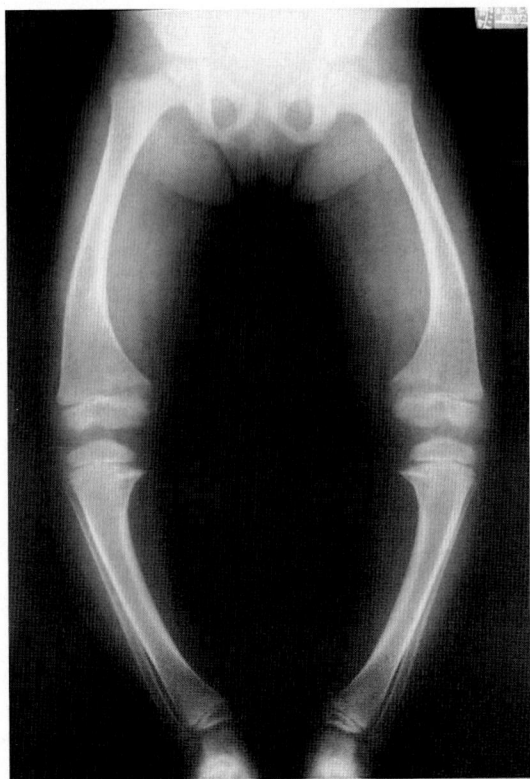

FIGURE 167-10. X-linked hypophosphatemia in a 3.5-year-old girl. There is prominent convex lateral bowing of the femurs and tibias as well as rachitic findings in the metaphyses.

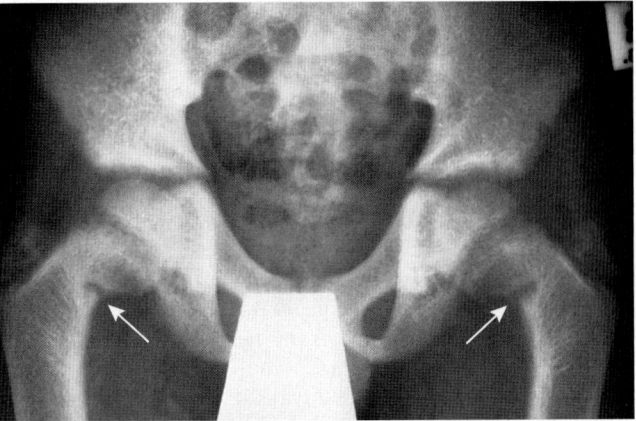

FIGURE 167-11. Looser zones in a child with X-linked hypophosphatemia. Symmetric transverse lucent areas in medial aspect of the femoral necks *(arrows)* are a manifestation of osteomalacia. Also note the patchy increased density, coarse trabeculations, and rachitic irregularity of the metaphyses.

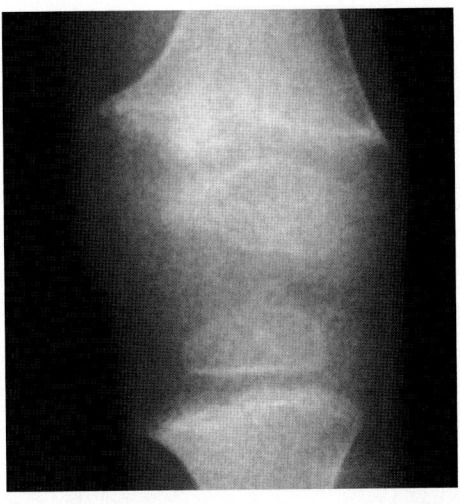 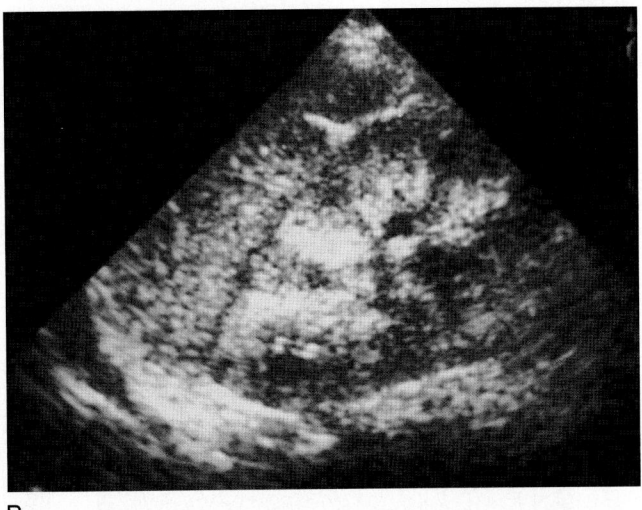

A   B

FIGURE 167-12. Hypophosphatemic rickets in renal tubular disease. **A,** Rachitic findings in the knees are nonspecific in this 3.7-year-old boy with renal tubular acidosis. **B,** Renal ultrasound shows extensive medullary hyperechogenicity, indicative of medullary calcinosis.

improved growth. It carries a risk of nephrocalcinosis, and renal ultrasonography is often used to screen for this complication. Even combined therapy with phosphate and calcitriol is not sufficient to normalize height, and growth hormone has also been used in these patients with resulting improved growth, including improved final adult height.

RENAL TUBULAR DISEASE. Renal tubular diseases may cause wasting of phosphate as well as other substances. Fanconi syndrome is a physiologic condition (not an anatomic syndrome) characterized by hyperphosphaturia, amino-aciduria, renal tubular acidosis, and renal glycosuria. It is not a specific diagnosis, but rather may be caused by several diseases, including cystinosis, tyrosinemia, galactosemia, Lowe syndrome, Wilson disease, and toxins, including heavy metals. It may also be seen as an isolated condition with autosomal dominant, autosomal recessive, and X-linked recessive forms. Rickets in renal tubular disease due to hypophosphatemia is not distinguishable from other causes of rickets (Fig. 167-12). However, depending on the severity of renal disease, there may be associated findings of renal osteodystrophy.

ONCOGENIC RICKETS AND OSTEOMALACIA. Rickets and osteomalacia with hypophosphatemia may occasionally be due to neoplasms, although this is relatively rare in children. Healing of rickets in response to removal of the tumor suggests that the mineralization defect is due to a substance produced by the tumor. The "phosphatonin" produced by these tumors is likely FGF23 (see previous discussion of XLH). Oncogenic rickets and osteomalacia have been associated with a variety of benign and malignant soft tissue and bone neoplasms, most of which are mesenchymal, although some are epithelial. These are often quite vascular, and there is a particularly high association with hemangiopericytoma. Other tumors include giant cell tumor, osteoid osteoma, osteosarcoma, chondrosarcoma, angiosarcoma, and a variety of fibrous lesions, including ossifying fibroma, nonossifying fibroma,

and fibrous dysplasia. Neurofibromatosis, epidermal nevus syndrome, and McCune-Albright syndrome have also been implicated. Figure 167-13 illustrates a rare case of oncogenic rickets caused by Gorham syndrome (massive osteolysis).

Patients with oncogenic rickets and osteomalacia may present with chronic vague symptoms, including generalized pain and muscle weakness. With recognition of hypophosphatemic rickets or osteomalacia and no specific etiology, a search should be made for a causative tumor, although these are often small and slowly growing. Evaluation should begin with a through physical examination followed by a skeletal survey. Skeletal scintigraphy may be a useful screening examination, with magnetic resonance imaging (MRI) and computed tomography (CT) used to further evaluate any regions that are either clinically suspicious or abnormal on scintigraphy.

MISCELLANEOUS FORMS OF RICKETS

CONGENITAL RICKETS. Congenital rickets is very uncommon, but has been described in infants of mothers with severe malnutrition or other causes of vitamin D deficiency, such as malabsorption. These mothers have osteomalacia, low levels of 25(OH)D, and a low circulating calcium × phosphate product that is reflected in the fetus. Maternal untreated chronic renal insufficiency, preeclampsia, and hypoparathyroidism have also been associated with congenital rickets.

RICKETS OF PREMATURITY. Rickets of prematurity, also known as metabolic bone disease of prematurity, is most common in infants with birth weight below 1 kg or gestational age less than 28 weeks. During normal gestational development, 80% of bone mineral accretion occurs during the third trimester. Hence prematurely born infants would have to accumulate bone mineral at a high rate to prevent falling behind. Metabolic bone disease of prematurity is primarily due to inadequate nutrition. Although mineral deficiency is rare in term

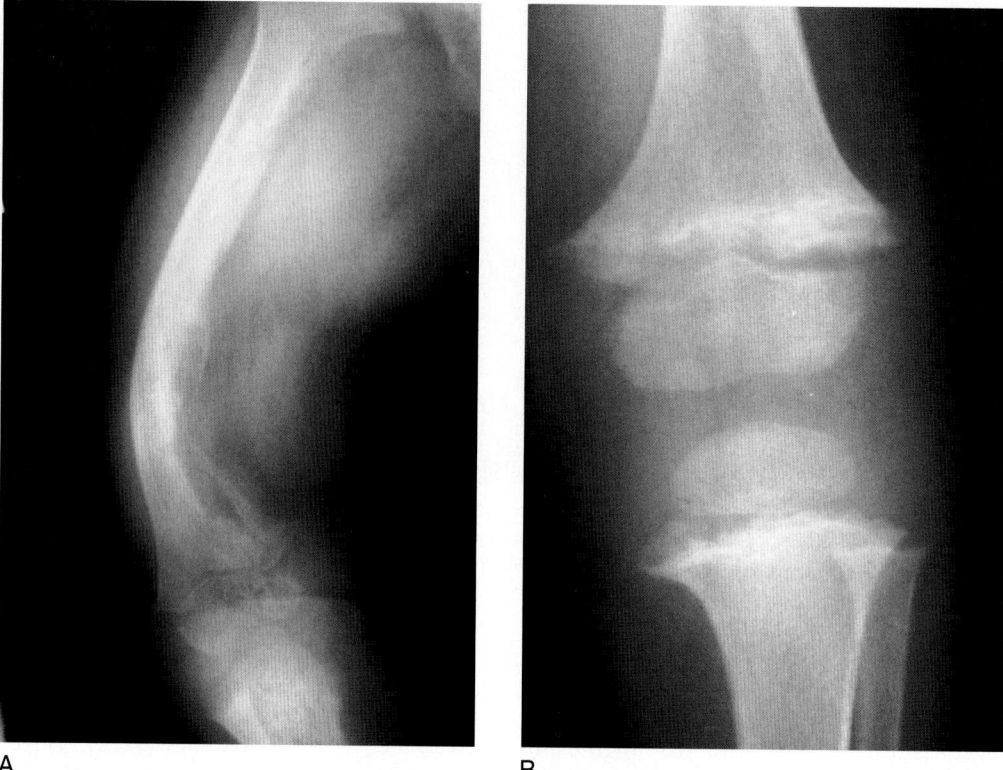

A
B

FIGURE 167-13. "Oncogenic" hypophosphatemic rickets in a 2.4-year-old girl with Gorham syndrome (massive osteolysis). **A,** The right femur shows osteolysis. **B,** The left knee reveals typical findings of rickets.

infants and older children, inadequate intake of calcium and especially phosphorus is the major cause of metabolic bone disease of prematurity. Breast milk and infant formulas do not supply sufficient calcium and phosphorus for premature infants, and this deficiency becomes most pronounced during the period of "catch-up" growth, often near the time of hospital discharge. Radiographic features include generalized osteopenia, fractures, and rachitic changes in the metaphyses (Fig. 167-14). However, the rachitic metaphyses will be seen only during periods of growth and will be masked when the infant is not growing. The fractures are often not recognized acutely and, if first discovered after discharge, may be confused with nonaccidental trauma. Rib fractures may exacerbate respiratory distress from neonatal lung disease. Extremity fractures are common and usually do not lead to long-term morbidity since there is ample opportunity for remodeling.

Metabolic bone disease of total parenteral nutrition (TPN) is an overlapping condition, with pediatric cases described predominantly in preterm infants. Pathogenesis includes calcium and phosphate deficiency, aluminum toxicity, the nonphysiologic manner in which TPN is administered, the underlying condition requiring TPN, and medications. Excessive vitamin D supplementation may paradoxically impair mineralization in these patients.

DRUG-INDUCED RICKETS. Anticonvulsants, particularly phenytoin and phenobarbital, are the most common cause of drug-induced rickets. Although the pathophysiology of anticonvulsant rickets is not clear, it may involve induction of hepatic microsomes with production of multihydroxylated inactive forms of vitamin D. Phenytoin also inhibits calcium absorption in the gut by decreasing production of calcium-binding protein, the protein normally induced by calcitriol. Patients on anticonvulsants are also often neurologically impaired and may have associated dietary deficiency and lack of sunlight exposure. The radiographic findings of rickets are nonspecific, but these patients may also show other skeletal manifestations of neuromuscular disease, including severe osteopenia and overtubulation of bones. Nephrotoxicity from the cancer chemotherapeutic agent ifosfamide may cause rickets from renal tubular phosphate wasting. Rickets has also been described in infants treated for gastroesophageal reflux and colic with aluminum hydroxide gel antacids, which bind phosphate in the gut, leading to phosphate depletion.

RICKETS IN OSTEOPETROSIS. Rickets is a common and paradoxical feature of infantile osteopetrosis. Osteopetrosis (discussed further in Chapter 165) is a condition characterized by markedly increased mineral deposition in bone caused by decreased osteoclastic bone resorption. As a result, the serum levels of calcium and phosphate are decreased, leading to rickets, and this may be exacerbated by attempts to decrease the excessive bone mineralization by restricting dietary calcium.

Hypophosphatasia

Hypophosphatasia, like rickets, is a disorder characterized by deficient mineralization of cartilage and osteoid.

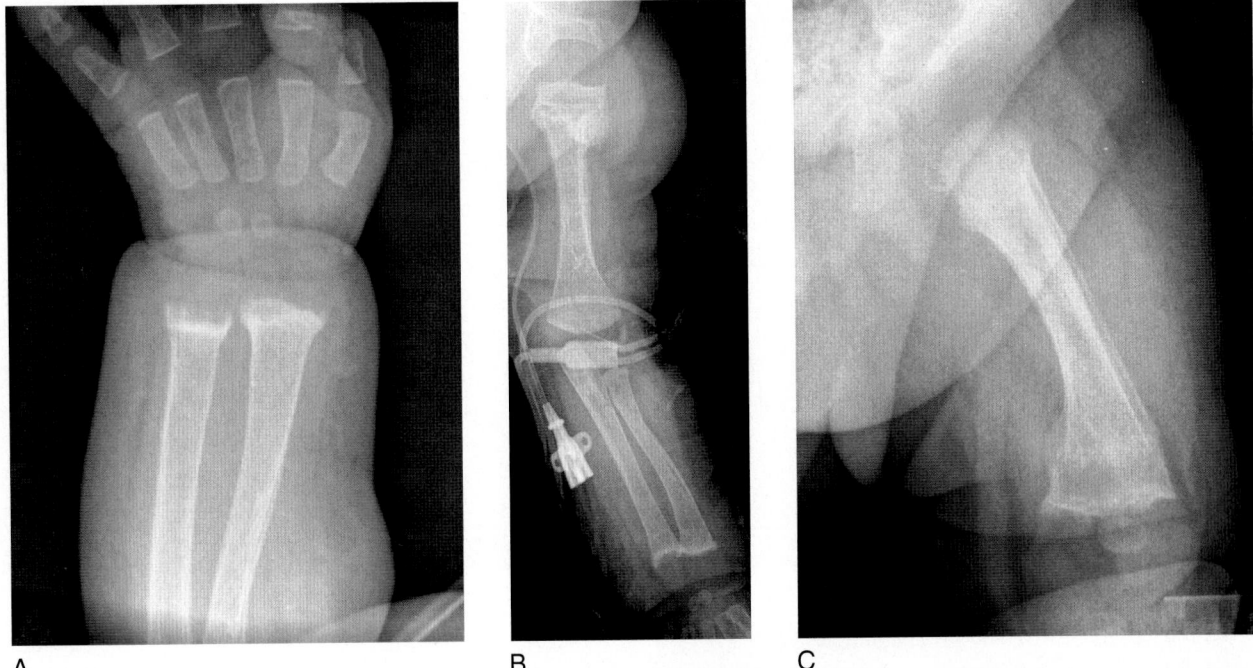

A   B   C

FIGURE 167-14. Metabolic bone disease of prematurity. Former 26 weeks' gestational age infant. **A,** At 6 months of age, the wrist shows prominent demineralization and rachitic changes in the distal radius and ulna. **B** and **C,** Radiographs from a skeletal survey 1 month later demonstrate these findings plus multiple fractures including both proximal humeri (left shown in **B**) and both proximal and distal femurs (left shown in **C**).

However, in hypophosphatasia, the calcium × phosphate product is normal and the mineralization defect is due to deficiency of tissue-nonspecific alkaline phosphatase (TNSALP; "tissue-nonspecific" distinguishing it from placental-, germ cell–, and intestinal-specific forms of alkaline phosphatase). TNSALP is an enzyme that functions at cell surfaces to break down several phosphate compounds, including inorganic pyrophosphate (PP_i), which accumulates in hypophosphatasia. Although PP_i enhances precipitation of amorphous calcium phosphate, it interferes with conversion of calcium phosphate to hydroxyapatite crystals, and adherence of PP_i to hydroxyapatite prevents further growth of these crystals.

> In hypophosphatasia, alkaline phosphatase deficiency causes pyrophosphate accumulation, which inhibits mineralization by preventing deposition of hydroxyapatite crystals.

Laboratory tests used to establish this diagnosis include low serum levels of alkaline phosphatase and elevated urinary excretion of phosphoethanolamine, a compound that accumulates in hypophosphatasia due to deficient breakdown by TNSALP.

CLINICAL FEATURES

Hypophosphatasia is divided clinically into perinatal, infantile, childhood, and adult forms, with decreasing severity as the age of presentation increases. The severe perinatal and infantile forms are due to autosomal recessive mutations in the gene for TNSALP. The perinatal form has severe lack of mineralization of the skeleton with short and deformed limbs. Absence of structural support for the thorax leads to respiratory insufficiency and early death. Accumulation of nonmineralized osteoid in the medullary canal causes myelophthisic anemia. Dimpling may be present overlying short bone spurs. The perinatal form is invariably fatal. The infantile form has a less severe mineralization defect. Patients present before 6 months of age with clinical features that are similar to rickets, with lethargy leading to poor feeding and failure to thrive. Rachitic-appearing ribs and multiple rib fractures may lead to pneumonia. Craniosynostosis is often present and may be associated with increased intracranial pressure despite a wide appearance of the sutures radiographically. Prognosis for the infantile form is variable. Approximately half die from pneumonia and respiratory distress and others improve spontaneously. Progression of skeletal findings suggests a poor and likely fatal outcome.

The childhood and adult forms are milder, and both autosomal dominant and recessive inheritance has been described for these. Extremity pain, stiffness, and gait disturbance are often present, and weakness may simulate myopathy. Premature loss of deciduous teeth is frequent and due to absence or underdevelopment of the dental cementum that attaches the tooth to the periodontal ligament. The entire tooth falls out of its socket without root resorption. Craniosynostosis is also present in this form. The skeletal manifestations of childhood hypophosphatasia improve during adolescence, but symptoms of the "adult" form recur later in life. The adult form often presents in middle age with features simulating osteomalacia, including recurrent metatarsal stress fractures, femoral pseudofractures, and

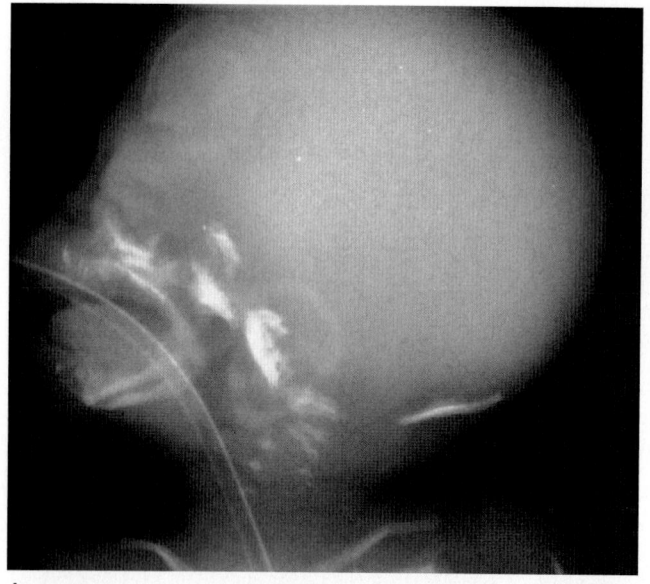

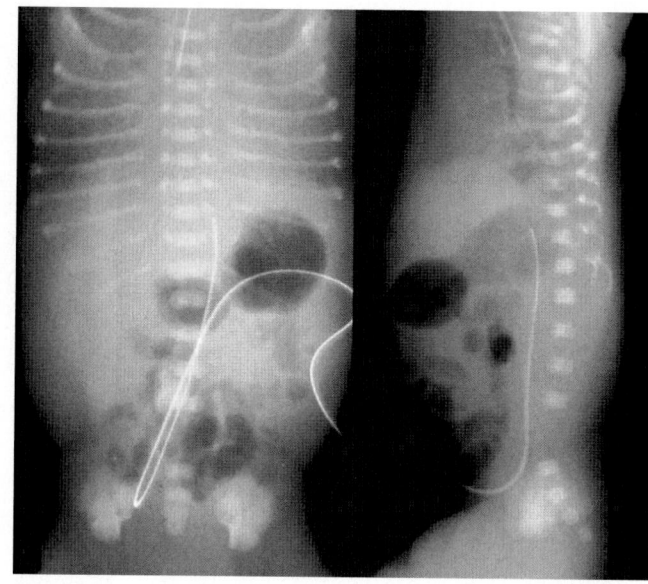

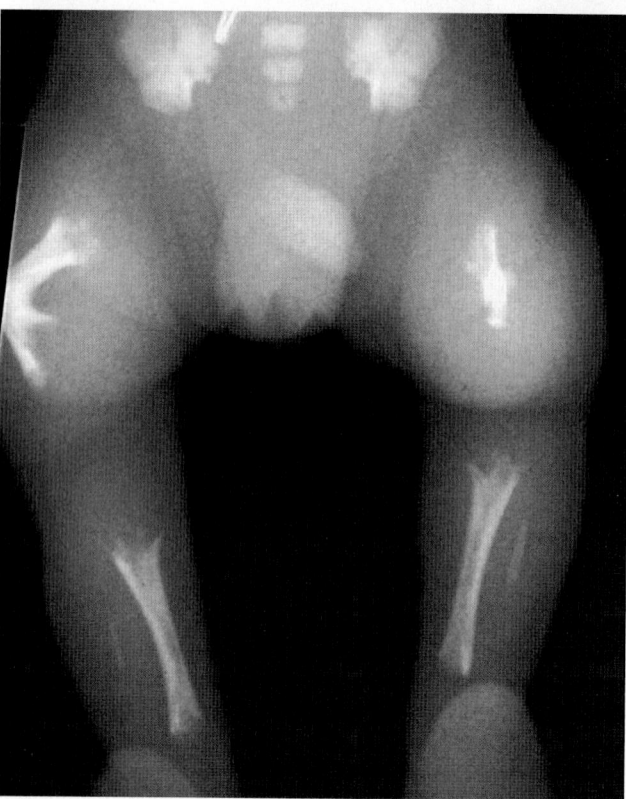

FIGURE 167-15. Perinatal hypophosphatasia. **A,** The skull is nonmineralized except for part of the base, a portion of the occipital bone, and very minimal mineralization of the frontal bone. **B,** In the trunk, the posterior elements of the entire spine and the lower lumbar vertebral bodies are nonmineralized. In the pelvis, the iliac bones are seen but the pubic and ischial bone are not. **C,** The lower extremities demonstrate marked deficiency of the femurs and fibulas, with less severe involvement of the tibias. (Case courtesy of Ellen Benya, MD, Chicago, IL.)

other recurrent orthopedic symptoms. Accumulation of PP_i may lead to calcium pyrophosphate crystal deposition arthropathy. These patients may have a history of "rickets" during childhood or premature loss of deciduous teeth, indicating overlap with the childhood form.

Attempted treatment of hypophosphatasia with alkaline phosphatase is ineffective, supporting the concept that the enzyme functions at the cell surface rather than in the circulation. Bone marrow transplantation has been used successfully in the treatment of infantile hypophosphatasia, although the variable prognosis of that form complicates assessment of this experimental therapy. The milder forms are treated symptomatically, and slow healing of orthopedic manifestations should be expected.

RADIOGRAPHIC FINDINGS

The perinatal form is characterized by severe failure of mineralization of much of the skeleton (Fig. 167-15). Although the skull base is usually mineralized, the calvarium may be completely or nearly completely non-mineralized. The rest of the axial skeleton has varying regions of present or absent mineralization. The extremities are short and incompletely mineralized, and have small bone spurs from the ulnar and fibular diaphyses. The mineralization defect in perinatal hypophosphatasia is significantly more pronounced than in osteogenesis imperfecta. Infantile hypophosphatasia not as severe as the perinatal form. The diaphyses appear normal and the metaphyses are poorly mineralized, suggesting a process similar to rickets. The "rachitic" changes of hypophosphatasia in the infantile and childhood forms differ from true rickets in that the process is not uniform across the growth plate. Rather, it involves a more localized portion of the growth plate with deficient mineralization extending into the metaphysis, creating a more localized "chewed out" appearance (Fig. 167-16). Because of poor mineralization of the calvarium, the sutures may appear widened despite actual premature sutural closure. The resultant increased intracranial pressure of sutural synostosis may produce a "beaten-metal" appearance of the calvarium with increased convolutional markings, although these may be difficult to distinguish from the variable normal appearance of the skull. The adult form simulates osteomalacia with a coarse trabecular pattern, Looser zones, and metatarsal fractures. The Looser zones in adult hypophosphatasia have more of a tendency to involve the lateral aspects of the bones, whereas those of osteomalacia are usually located medially.

ABNORMALITIES OF BONE MATRIX FORMATION

Bone matrix (osteoid) is the organic framework upon which mineral, in the form of hydroxyapatite, is deposited. The most common disorder that causes decreased bone mineral due to insufficient matrix formation is osteogenesis imperfecta, the various types of which are due to either qualitative or quantitative defects in the synthesis of type I collagen. Osteogenesis imperfecta is discussed in Chapter 165. Normal collagen synthesis depends on ascorbic acid (vitamin C) and ascorbic acid oxidase, a copper-dependent enzyme, and hence matrix synthesis is impaired in vitamin C deficiency (scurvy), copper deficiency, and some abnormalities of copper metabolism.

> Collagen synthesis requires ascorbic acid and copper-dependent ascorbic acid oxidase, accounting for osteoid deficiency in scurvy and copper deficiency or metabolic disorders.

Scurvy

Scurvy, caused by deficiency of vitamin C, is now quite rare, although occasional reports suggest that it may be underdiagnosed. Historically, infantile scurvy occurred almost exclusively in babies fed pasteurized or boiled milk, with heat destruction of vitamin C. Scurvy nearly always presents after 6 months of age; when similar findings are seen earlier, alternative diagnoses such as congenital syphilis should be considered.

The skeletal findings of scurvy are due to diminished collagen synthesis needed for osteoid. Mineral deposition in the zone of provisional calcification is not disturbed. There is also deficiency of intercellular cement substance in the endothelial layer of the capillaries, causing a hemorrhagic tendency leading to subperiosteal hematomas. Decreased osteoid formation causes an imbalance between bone production and resorption, leading to generalized atrophy of the cortex and spongiosa. At the growth plate, chondrocyte proliferation is decreased but terminal differentiation and cartilage calcification are normal, forming a well-mineralized zone of provisional calcification. On the diaphyseal side of the physis, resorption of calcified cartilage is diminished or stops, leading to thickened zone of provisional

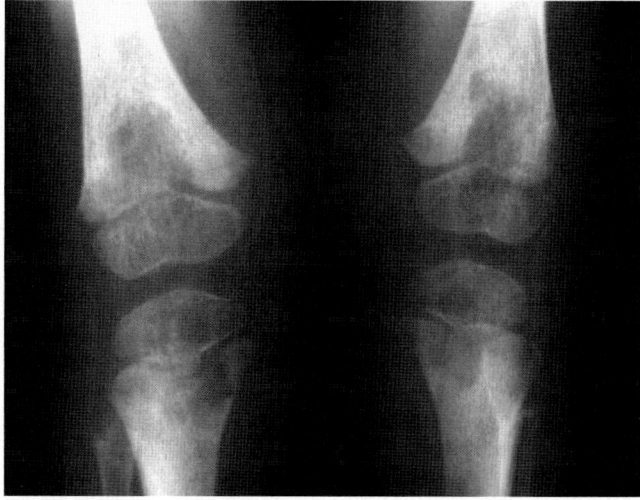
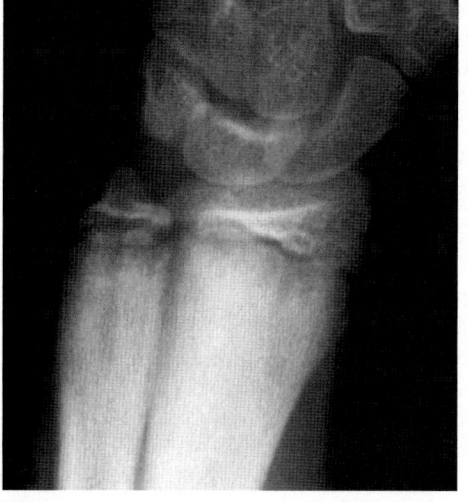

A   B

FIGURE 167-16. Childhood hypophosphatasia. **A,** Prominent lucent defects extend into the metaphyses from the growth plates with a more focal and "chewed out" appearance than the uniform mineralization defect of rickets. **B,** A much milder example with a few streaklike lucencies extending into the distal radial and ulnar metaphyses.

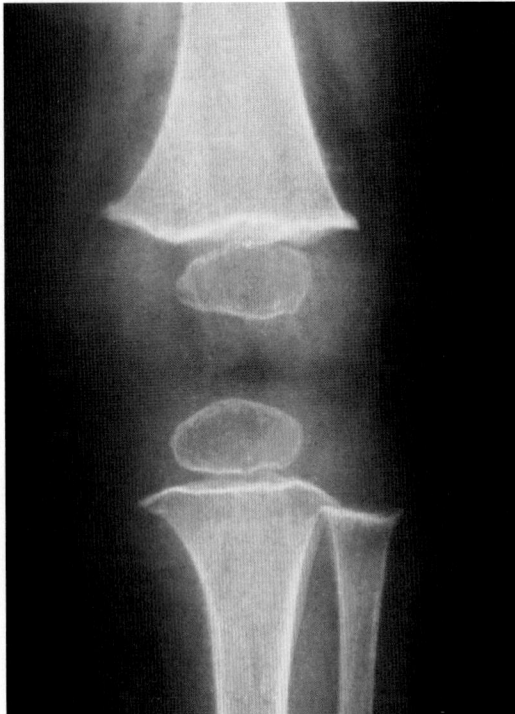

FIGURE 167-17. Scurvy. The zones of provisional calcification are prominent and form the white line of scurvy. These stand out in high contrast compared to the subjacent demineralized scurvy zone. Similar findings are also present at the margins of the epiphyses where the epiphyseal zone of provisional calcification forms the Wimberger ring surrounding the centrally lucent epiphysis. A small spur is present at the lateral aspect of the distal femoral metaphysis, and a proximal tibial spur is partially obscured by the fibula.

TABLE 167-3
Radiolucent Metaphyseal Bands: Major Causes

Severe stress (below age 2 yr)
   Transplacental infection
   Congenital heart disease
   Respiratory distress syndrome
Other systemic illness
Leukemia
Metastatic neuroblastoma
Scurvy

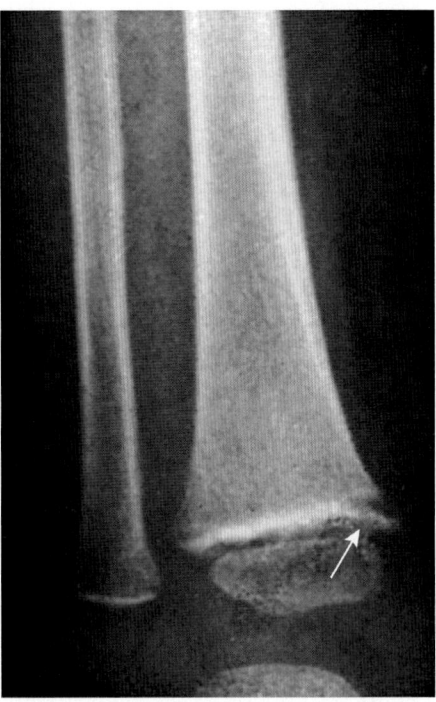

FIGURE 167-18. Peripheral metaphyseal cleft in a 14-month-old child with scurvy. An eccentric lucent cortical and trabecular defect produces a cleft *(arrow)* just beneath the zone of provisional calcification, with the peripheral aspect of the zone of provisional calcification separated from the shaft and tilted off the shaft toward the epiphysis.

calcification. Radiographically, this thickened zone is seen as a prominent opaque line (Fig. 167-17), designated as the white line of scurvy (white line of Fränkel). Despite its thickness, this zone is brittle rather than strong and may develop fissures and fractures. The trabeculae just beneath the thickened provisional zone are sparse, brittle, and irregularly disposed in a random network, having lost much of their normally longitudinal parallel pattern. This region of demineralized bone causes a prominent lucent zone adjacent to the zone of provisional calcification (see Fig. 167-17) known as the scurvy zone (Trümmerfeld zone). The heightened contrast between the prominent opaque zone of provisional calcification and lucent adjacent metaphysis alone is nonspecific as it may be difficult to distinguish from diffuse osteopenia and other causes of lucent metaphyseal bands (Table 167-3). Later, transverse fractures may develop through the brittle zone of provisional calcification and the demineralized metaphyseal scurvy zone. If such a fracture is limited to a peripheral portion of the scurvy zone, a subepiphyseal marginal lucent cleft will be seen between the zone of provisional calcification and the shaft, forming the "corner" or "angle" sign of scurvy (Fig. 167-18). With transverse displacement of the epiphysis and zone of provisional calcification from the rest of the shaft, the heavily mineralized zone of provisional calcification projects peripherally beyond the usual limits of the shaft, forming a metaphyseal spur (Pelkan

spur), another characteristic radiographic feature of scurvy (Fig. 167-19). Fractures through the thickened provisional zone are nearly diagnostic of scurvy (Figs. 167-20 and 167-21) when syphilis can be excluded.

Rarely the combination of diffuse bone atrophy and multiple spurs at the cartilage-shaft junction may also be seen in patients treated with methotrexate. Compression fractures of the brittle zone of provisional calcification may also occur by axial loading (Fig. 167-22). All of these metaphyseal changes appear earliest and are most marked at the sites of most rapid growth and most active endochondral bone formation, especially at the distal femur, proximal humerus, proximal and distal tibia and fibula, and distal radius and ulna.

In the ossification centers, the changes are analogous to those in the metaphyses. The thickened zone of provisional calcification produces a thickened peripheral shell of calcified cartilage surrounding the ossification

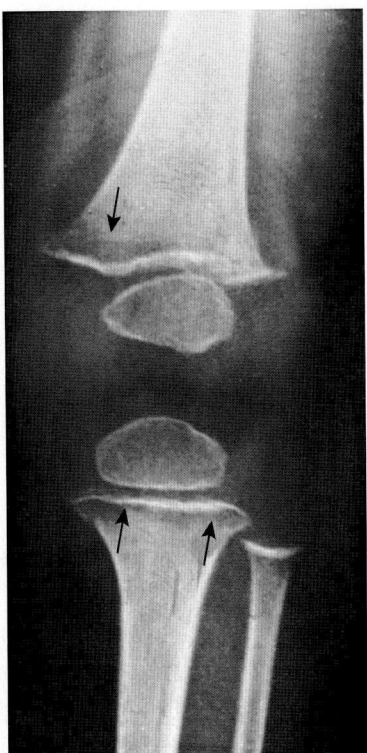

FIGURE 167-19. Metaphyseal spur in a 7-month-old child with scurvy. The distal femoral metaphyseal spur is more prominent than that in Figure 167-17. Note the opaque white lines of scurvy and lucent scurvy zones *(arrows)*.

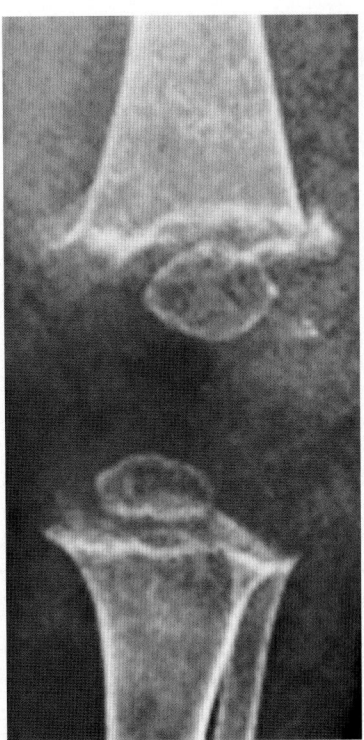

FIGURE 167-20. Advanced scurvy with fractures of thickened, brittle provisional zones of calcification. There are multiple infractions in the provisional zone, with peripheral spurring. The epiphysis and a portion of the zone of provisional calcification are displaced laterally.

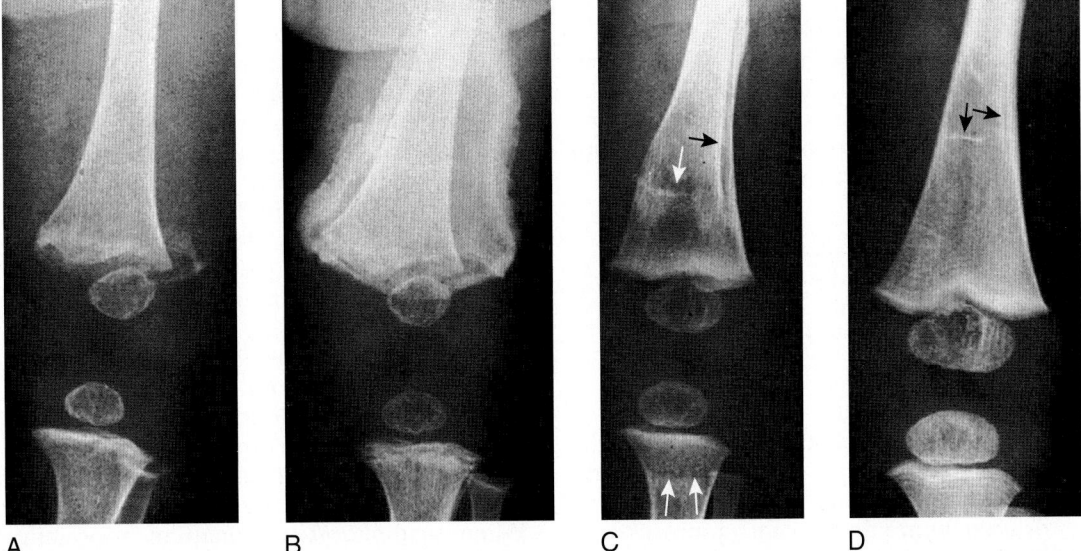

A   B   C   D

FIGURE 167-21. Healing scurvy in an infant 6 months of age with formation of a new cortex and realignment with the displaced epiphyses of the left femur. **A,** Active stage: There is a fracture through the distal femoral zone of provisional calcification with lateral displacement of the epiphysis. **B,** Fourteen days after the administration of ascorbic acid, a heavy shell of subperiosteal bone has formed around the subperiosteal hematoma. **C,** Four months after **A,** the shell of bone around the subperiosteal hematoma has shrunk and now forms the new cortex. The old cortex and provisional zone are gradually being resorbed *(arrows)*. The new shaft is now aligned with the displaced epiphyses. **D,** One year after **A.** The old cortex *(horizontal arrow)* is barely visible, and the old provisional zone is buried deeply in the shaft as a "transverse line" *(vertical arrow)*. Alignment of the shaft and epiphysis is normal.

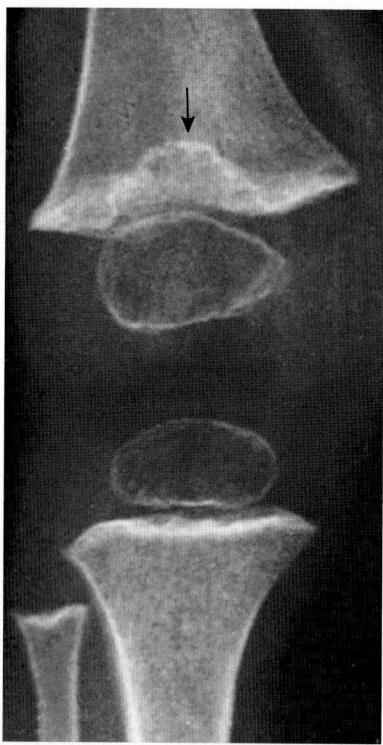

FIGURE 167-22. Scurvy with a "crumpling fracture" *(arrow)* of the brittle zone of provisional calcification.

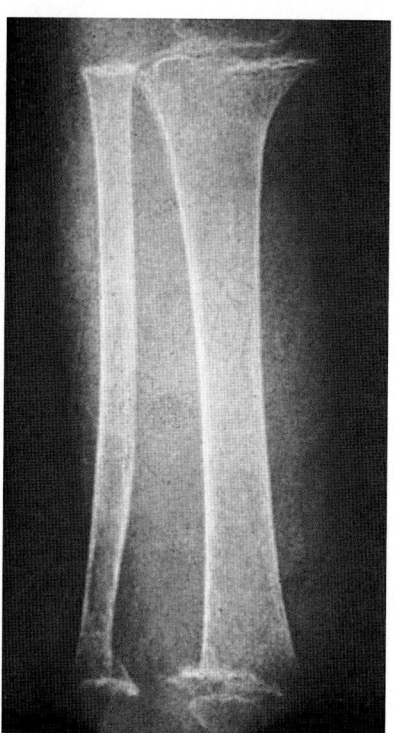

FIGURE 167-23. Fresh subperiosteal hematoma surrounding the distal half of the tibia and spreading apart the distal ends of the tibia and fibula. Transverse fractures are present in the distal tibia and fibula.

center. Atrophy of the spongiosa is responsible for central rarefaction and heightens the contrast between the two components. The prominent white line surrounding the internally rarefied epiphysis produces the Wimberger ring (see Figs. 167-17 and 167-22), one of the most characteristic findings of scurvy (this should not be confused with the Wimberger sign of congenital syphilis, which is erosion of the medial aspect of the proximal tibial metaphyses). This appearance is opposite that of rickets, in which the peripheral ring is lost with relative sparing of the central trabecular bone.

> **In scurvy, a peripheral mineralized ring is maintained around the centrally demineralized epiphysis, whereas in rickets the peripheral ring is lost with relative sparing of central trabecular bone.**

Although the carpal and tarsal bones are anatomically similar to the epiphyses, the contrast between central rarefaction and the surrounding opaque line is less pronounced for these bones than for the epiphyses.

In the shaft, the findings are those of generalized osteopenia. The spongiosa becomes atrophic, which may produce a ground-glass texture radiographically, and there is generalized cortical thinning. Despite severe cortical atrophy in scurvy, diaphyseal cortical fractures are uncommon, particularly compared to fractures through the zone of provisional calcification and subjacent demineralized scurvy zone in the metaphysis.

Subperiosteal hemorrhage is a frequent manifestation of scurvy and is most common in the larger tubular

bones such as the femur, tibia, and humerus. Occasionally, subperiosteal hematomas form on the flat bones of the calvarium, orbit, and shoulder girdle. Intraorbital hematoma may be a cause of proptosis. The hemorrhages vary greatly in size; they may extend the entire length of the shaft from one epiphyseal plate to the other. Hemorrhage does not occur around the epiphyses in scurvy, and hemarthrosis is also exceedingly rare during infancy and childhood. Large subperiosteal hemorrhages present as areas of increased opacity in the soft tissues surrounding the bone and may spread adjacent bones (Fig. 167-23). Acutely, surrounding edema exaggerates the soft tissue findings, and the true extent of the subperiosteal hematoma is delineated later by periosteal new bone.

With the onset of healing, the cortex becomes thicker and the spongiosa more clearly defined. The transverse band of diminished density in the metaphysis regains its normal density and disappears. As growth proceeds, the thickened provisional zone of calcification is buried within the shaft as a "transverse line" (see Fig. 167-21). When a subperiosteal hematoma is present, the raised periosteum produces a layer of subperiosteal bone along the periphery of the hematoma (see Fig. 167-21). Concurrent with resorption of a hematoma, this new layer of bone thickens and shrinks down onto the shaft to become the new cortex (see Fig. 167-21). Residues of this cortical thickening may persist for years. In the event of epiphyseal displacement, longitudinal growth after healing proceeds from the displaced proliferating cartilage with shift of newly formed bone to this new position, leading to remodeling of the deformity.

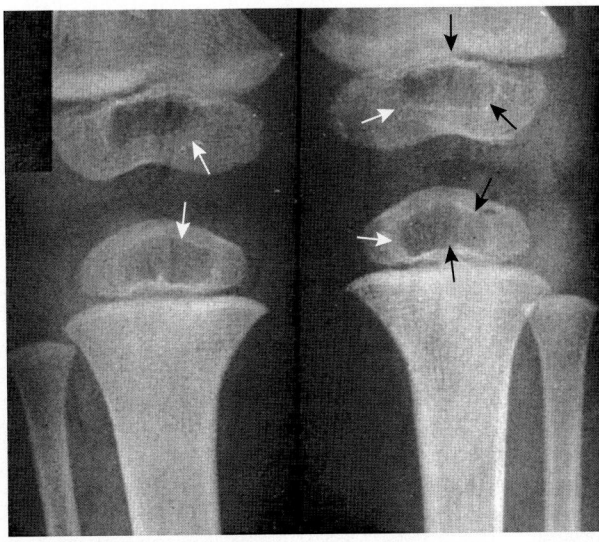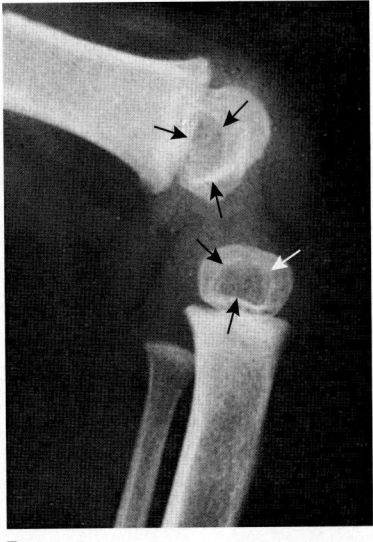

A   B

FIGURE 167-24. Frontal **(A)** and lateral **(B)** projections of healed scurvy, showing the epiphyseal insets of central rarefaction *(arrows)*, 20 months after the active stage of the disease, in distal ossification centers of the femora and proximal centers of the tibias.

The healed epiphyseal ossification center may exhibit a central region of rarefaction that persists for years after the beginning of healing (Fig. 167-24). These rarefied regions correspond to the size and contour of the rarefied epiphyseal centers during the active stage of the disease. The major radiographic findings of scurvy are given in Table 167-4.

Although nutritional deficiencies are usually described individually, multiple deficiencies are often present. When scurvy and rickets are both present, the scurvy features usually predominate because of the diminished osteoblastic activity with low rather than elevated serum alkaline phosphatase levels.

Copper Deficiency and Menkes Disease

Ascorbic acid oxidase is a copper-dependent enzyme and hence copper deficiency results in deficient matrix formation and osteopenia. These findings are nonspecific, and copper deficiency has been confused with metabolic bone disease of prematurity, although neutropenia and anemia serve as other markers of copper deficiency.

Menkes disease is an X-linked condition that is characterized by kinky hair, osteopenia and bone fragility, mental retardation, seizures, and intracranial hemorrhage due to widespread arterial abnormalities. It is due to deficiency of a cation-transporting enzyme needed for transport of copper from the gut and its intracellular delivery to copper-dependent enzymes, including lysyl oxidase, which is needed for proper cross-linking of collagen and elastin. This results in abnormal collagen and elastin, leading to osteopenia and increased bone fragility. Fractures in Menkes disease may follow minor trauma, and metaphyseal fractures with spurring may also occur that appear very similar to those seen in nonaccidental trauma and have erroneously led to that diagnosis (Fig. 167-25).

TABLE 167-4
Scurvy: Major Radiographic Features
Diffuse demineralization
Washed-out trabecular pattern
Prominent zone of provisional calcification
White line of scurvy in metaphyses
Wimberger ring around epiphyses
Demineralized metaphyseal scurvy zone
Metaphyseal fractures with spur formation
Subperiosteal hematoma

ABNORMALITIES OF BONE RESORPTION

Physiology of Bone Resorption

Bone resorption is mediated by osteoclasts. Osteoclasts are likely derived from monocyte-macrophage lineage, with differentiation and fusion leading to multinucleated giant cells. Many factors regulate osteoclast differentiation and activation. Many of these act through a membrane-bound receptor named RANK, which binds and is activated by osteoclast differentiation factor (also called RANK-ligand or RANKL), which is produced by osteoblasts. PTH has a major role in stimulating osteoclastic bone resorption, probably acting through stimulation of RANKL, although PTH may also stimulate osteoclasts directly.

> Osteoclastic bone resorption is regulated by PTH and other factors, many of which cause osteoblasts to secrete an osteoclast differentiation factor called RANKL.

Calcitriol also stimulates osteoclastic differentiation and function through RANKL, whereas calcitonin

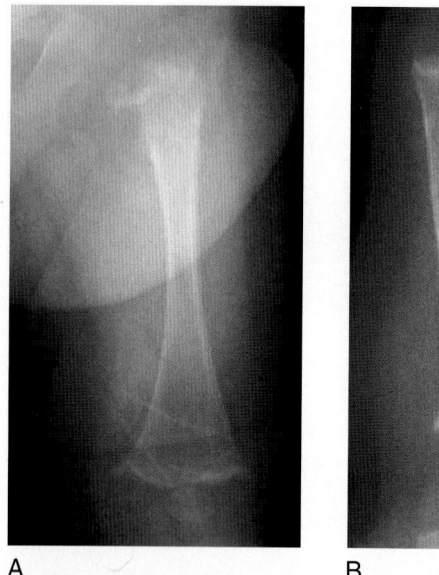

A

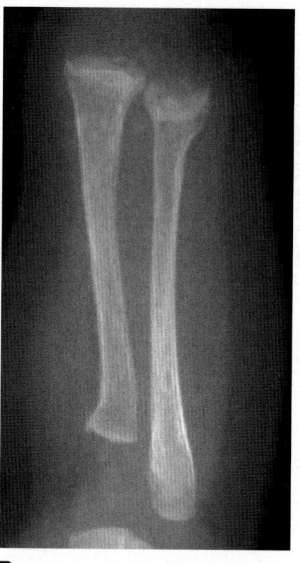

B

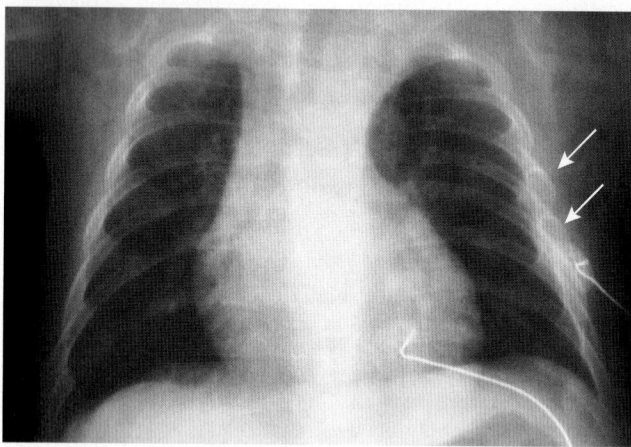

C

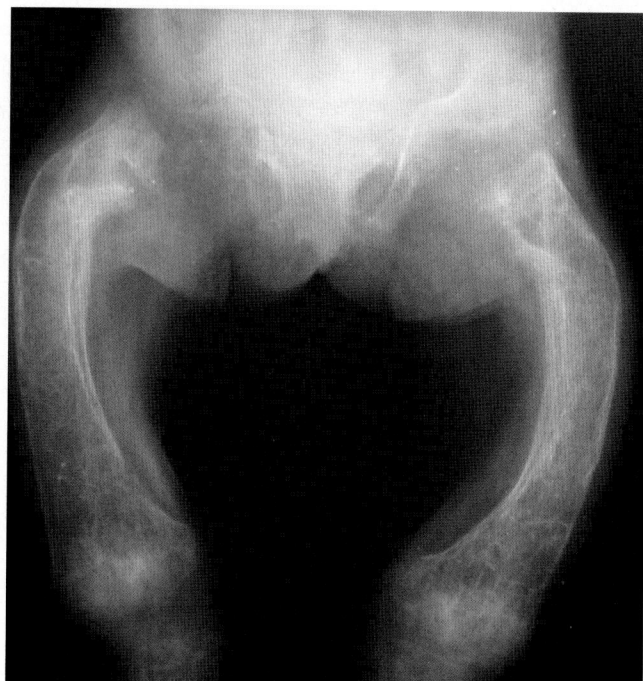

FIGURE 167-26. Hyperphosphatasia. The diaphyses are expanded and bowed. There is marked demineralization with a very heterogeneous pattern. The findings are symmetric, unlike the more focal appearance of adult Paget disease.

FIGURE 167-25. Menkes syndrome. **A,** Fracture of the proximal femur. The distal femoral metaphysis is irregular with prominent spurs at its margins. **B,** The distal radial and ulnar metaphyses have rickets-like changes. A small spur is seen on the proximal radius. **C,** Chest radiograph in which the bones are osteopenic. Two healing left rib fractures are seen *(arrows).* The infant presented with subdural hygromas related to the associated central nervous system disease and was initially suspected to be the victim of child abuse.

transiently inhibits osteoclastic resorption. Activated osteoclasts, which are recognized histologically by a ruffled border, form a sealed-off compartment along the resorption surface. Within this localized compartment, bone is dissolved by highly concentrated enzymes in acidified extracellular fluid.

Increased Resorption

The major cause of increased bone resorption is hyperparathyroidism, which is covered in Chapter 168.

HYPERPHOSPHATASIA

Hyperphosphatasia, also known as juvenile Paget disease, is a rare autosomal recessive condition with increased bone turnover, elevated serum alkaline phosphatase,

increased urinary hydroxyproline, and normal levels of calcium and phosphate. It appears to be due to deficiency of osteoprotegerin, which normally suppresses bone turnover by acting as a "decoy receptor" for the osteoclast differentiation factor RANKL. In the absence of this decoy receptor, osteoclast differentiation factor excessively stimulates osteoclast differentiation and activity, causing accelerated bone resorption and hence bone turnover.

Clinically, hyperphosphatasia often presents at 2 to 3 years of age and is characterized by short stature, bone fragility, and deformity, including long bone bowing, kyphoscoliosis, and pectus carinatum. Unlike adult Paget disease, which involves limited portions of the skeleton, hyperphosphatasia is more generalized. The radiographic features may be striking, with overall demineralization, coarse trabecular pattern, cortical thickening, widened cylindrical long bones with decreased tubulation, and markedly variable bone texture with osteosclerosis intermixed with regions of cystic-appearing lucency (Fig. 167-26). Bowing and pathologic fractures are common. The skull shows thickening and regions of lucency combined with "cotton-wool" sclerosis, similar to adult Paget disease. Like adult Paget disease, hyperphosphatasia has been treated with calcitonin, with variable results.

Expansile skeletal hyperphosphatasia and familial expansile osteolysis are related conditions characterized by deafness, loss of teeth, episodic hypercalcemia, expansion of bones, painful phalanges, and episodic hypercalcemia. These disorders have been associated with a duplication of the gene encoding RANK, the osteoclast membrane-bound receptor that is activated by RANKL.

Decreased Resorption

OSTEOPETROSIS

Osteopetrosis is a sclerosing disorder that is covered in Chapter 165 and is mentioned here because of its pathogenesis. It has several forms, all of which are caused by an abnormality of osteoclastic resorption, usually due to heritable mutations. Although osteoclasts are present, and often abundant, they lack ruffled borders and are ineffective in bone and calcified cartilage resorption. Histologically, residual calcified cartilage is found within mature bone.

OTHER CAUSES OF DECREASED RESORPTION

Decreased resorption of bone and calcified cartilage are also present in heavy metal toxicity and bisphosphonate therapy, discussed later in the section on toxic, pharmacologic, and other disorders.

ADDITIONAL METABOLIC DISORDERS

Hypervitaminoses

Vitamins are essential nutrients without which specific diseases or metabolic disorders become manifest. While vitamins are thus defined by their deficiency states, some vitamins may also have toxic effects in higher doses. With very rare exceptions (most notably extremely high levels of vitamin A in polar bear liver), the amounts of vitamins in naturally foods are far below levels that would cause toxicity. Vitamin toxicity has been best described primarily for the fat-soluble vitamins A and D.

HYPERVITAMINOSIS A

Vitamin A (retinol and related compounds) is a fat-soluble vitamin needed for vision and epithelial differen-tiation. It also has many other effects on the immune system and cancer suppression. For vision, it is essential for the function of the light-sensitive opsins. Also essential for vision is its role in epithelial differentiation of mucus membranes, with deficiency leading to xerophthalmia (dry ulcerating eye) which is the leading cause of blindness worldwide. For prevention and treatment of this disorder, fish liver oil had been used. Vitamin A toxicity historically had been due to over-dosage of vitamin A formulations given to prevent deficiency. More recently, toxicity has been from the use of high-potency vitamin A analogs used for dermatologic disorders, when given for their pharmacologic rather than physiologic effects.

Chronic vitamin A toxicity usually presents at least 6 months following the beginning of excessive vitamin A intake. Initial symptoms are nonspecific, with anorexia and irritability. Dry, pruritic skin with desquamation is common. Hair loss, lip fissuring, hepatomegaly, and other manifestation of hepatic disease may be present. The extremities demonstrate focal painful, hard regions of swelling that overlie the skeletal changes (Fig. 167-27). The clinical manifestations of chronic vitamin A toxicity often resolve within 3 days of stopping excessive vitamin A ingestion, even though a longer time is needed for blood vitamin A levels to fall to normal.

Radiographic recognition of the skeletal manifesta-tion of hypervitaminosis A may be extremely helpful in establishing this diagnosis in a child with a confusing clinical picture. Hyperostosis of the long bones is the most frequent and most well-recognized finding. It is characterized by periosteal new bone formation leading to undulating diaphyseal cortical thickening most frequently involving the ulnae (Fig. 167-28) and metatarsals.

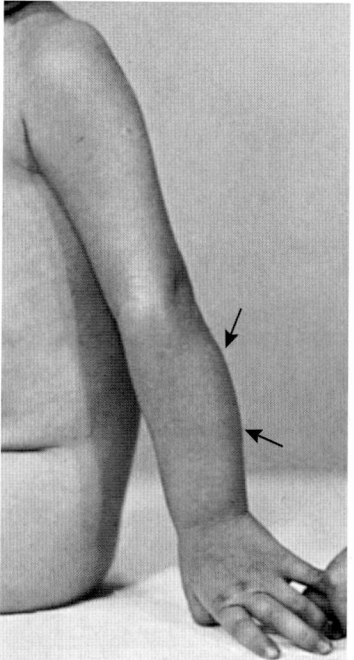
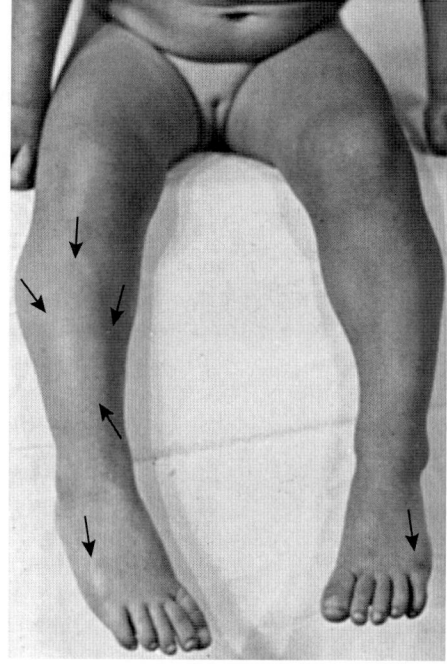

FIGURE 167-27. Soft tissue swellings in a 21-month-old girl with hypervitaminosis A, 5 weeks after onset. **A,** Swelling of the left forearm *(arrows)*; there was a similar swelling in the right forearm. **B,** Pretibial swelling on the right shank and symmetric swelling over the fifth metatarsals in both feet *(arrows)*.

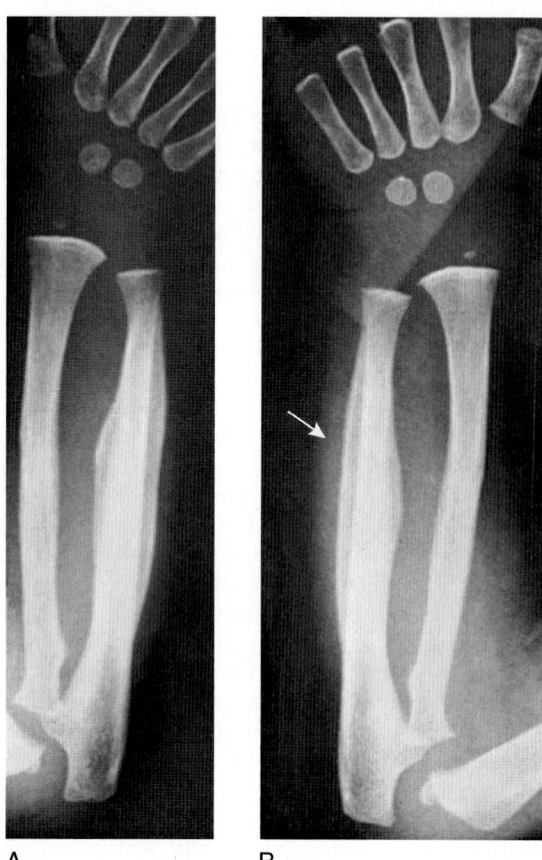

A   B

FIGURE 167-28. Symmetric cortical hyperostosis *(arrow)* of the right **(A)** and left **(B)** ulnas in poisoning due to vitamin A, 5 weeks after onset of clinical signs.

> **The major radiographic feature of vitamin A toxicity is hyperostosis, most characteristically involving the ulnae and metatarsals.**

Radiographically, this has been confused with infantile cortical hyperostosis (Caffey disease), although distinct differences were initially delineated by Caffey. Age alone distinguished these conditions, with infantile cortical hyperostosis presenting before 5 months of age and vitamin A toxicity presenting over 11 months. Mandibular involvement was present in all patients with infantile cortical hyperostosis and none with vitamin A toxicity, whereas metatarsal involvement was seen in all patients with vitamin A toxicity and infrequently with infantile cortical hyperostosis. The soft tissue swelling and tenderness were also more prominent with infantile cortical hyperostosis. While symptoms of vitamin A toxicity abated relatively quickly after stopping vitamin A administration, infantile cortical hyperostosis is characterized by recurrent exacerbations over several months. The imaging diagnosis of hypervitaminosis A is usually made from radiographs, although corresponding diaphyseal findings on skeletal scintigraphy may also be suggestive.

Growth plate damage is also a manifestation of hypervitaminosis A. Premature central growth plate closure

leading to cone-shaped epiphyses invaginated into the metaphysis may mimic the appearance of prior meningococcemia (Fig. 167-29). Similar findings have also been shown in cows given high doses of vitamin A. Early work suggested that vitamin A caused release of proteolytic enzymes in the growth plate, leading to cartilage degradation and subsequent physeal closure. More recent studies have shown that retinoic acid also promotes chondrocyte terminal differentiation, leading to cartilage calcification, chondrocyte apoptosis, and endochondral ossification, all steps leading to replacement of growth plate cartilage by bone.

Acute vitamin A poisoning is rare and presents primarily with central nervous system signs and symptoms of increased intracranial pressure, including vomiting, mental status changes, a bulging fontanelle, and widened cranial sutures.

High-potency synthetic analogs of vitamin A (e.g., isotretinoin), used in prolonged treatment of keratinizing disorders such as ichthyosis and keratoderma, have caused hyperostosis and premature physeal closure. The hyperostoses caused by these drugs differ from those usually seen in vitamin A toxicity and resemble those of diffuse idiopathic skeletal hyperostosis. The common sites of involvement include the cervical, thoracic, and lumbar spine. The anterior longitudinal ligament, other spinal ligaments, and iliolumbar ligaments may be ossified. Beaklike ossifications occur at margins of the vertebral bodies, at the calcaneus, and near the ends of the long bones. This differs from vitamin A toxicity, in which the periosteal new bone formation affects the diaphyses but spares the ends of bones. The costal cartilages may be diffusely calcified. These agents are highly teratogenic, having caused the "isotretinoin dysmorphic syndrome," characterized by anomalies of the ears, face, central nervous system, and heart.

HYPERVITAMINOSIS D

Although vitamin D toxicity exists, some protection against it is afforded by the fact that vitamin D, dietary or produced in the skin, is a precursor rather than an active substance. It requires hydroxylation in the liver and kidney for conversion to the active hormone calcitriol, with the final step, renal 1-α-hydroxylation, being highly regulated to achieve normal mineral homeostasis. Hepatic 25-hydroxylation is not as regulated, and 25(OH)D levels are indicative of vitamin D sufficiency, insufficiency, or excess. Although not nearly as potent as calcitriol, 25(OH)D does have some physiologic effect. Hence, vitamin D toxicity results either from sufficient overdosage that 25(OH)D levels are high enough to have an excessive physiologic effect or from ingestion of calcitriol. In addition to that produced pharmaceutically, calcitriol is also present in four known "calcinogenic" plants that may produce vitamin D poisoning if ingested. Iatrogenic vitamin D poisoning has occurred in patients with physiologic bowlegs who were mistakenly thought to have XLH (vitamin D–resistant rickets) and were given escalating doses of vitamin D (Fig. 167-30). Metaphyseal chondrodysplasia type Schmid can also mimic XLH, and large vitamin D doses will not "cure" the bowing or metaphyseal irregularity.

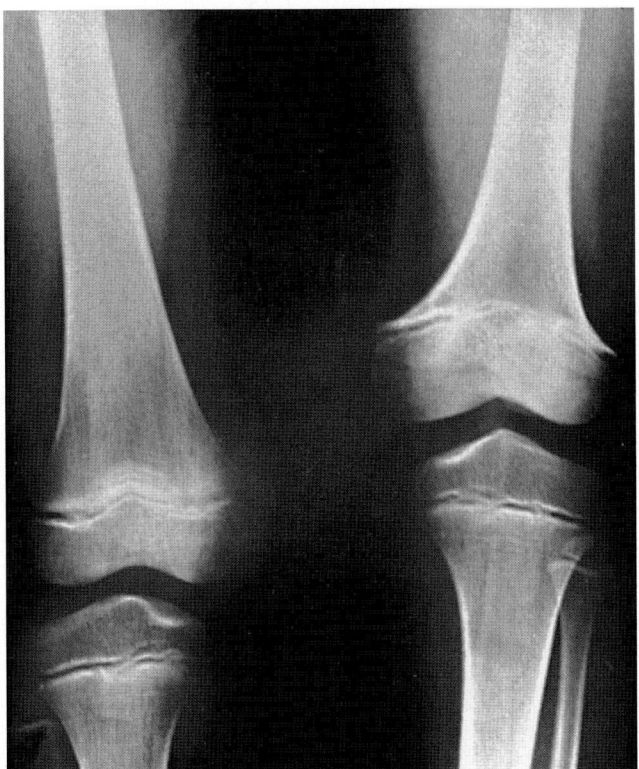
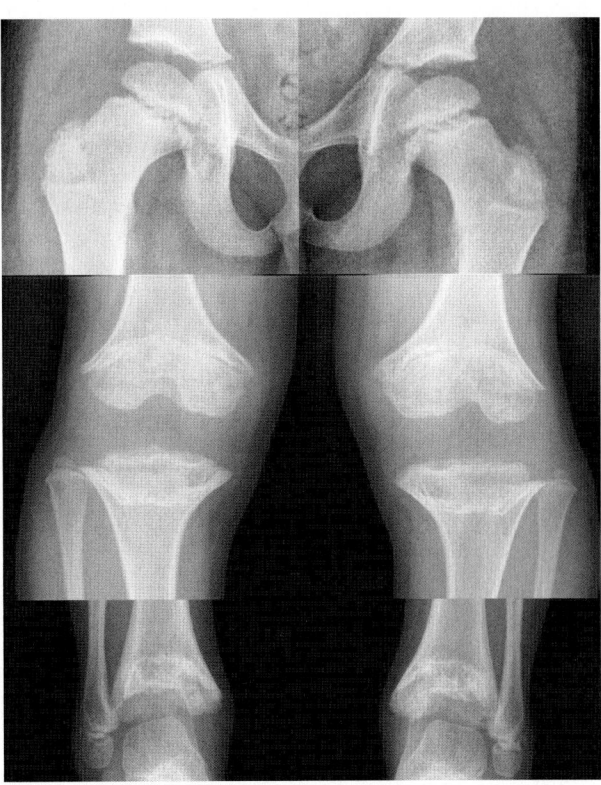

A   B

FIGURE 167-29. Growth plate symmetric damage in vitamin A toxicity. **A,** Isolated left distal femoral growth plate injury. **B,** More extensive damage in a 5-year-old boy with symmetric involvement of both distal femurs proximal tibias, and distal tibias. The proximal femurs and fibulas are normal. The upper extremities were also normal. (Case in **A** provided by Dr. Charles N. Pease, Chicago, IL, who initially described this finding.)

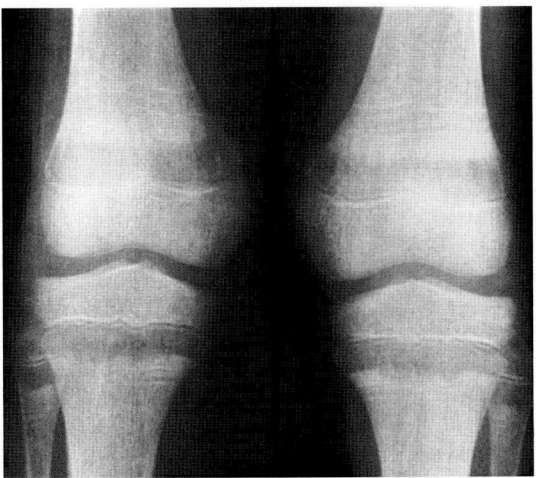
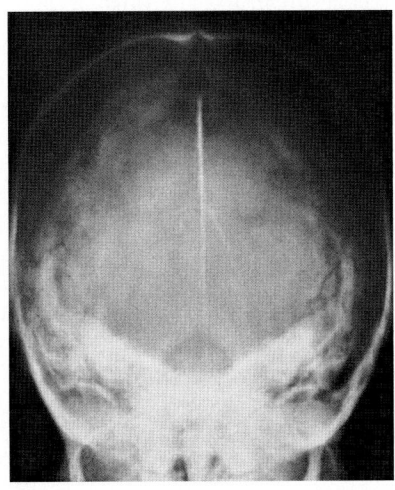
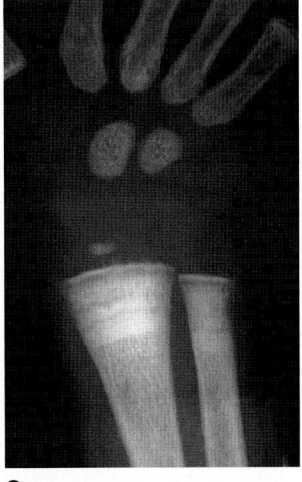

A   B   C

FIGURE 167-30. **A** and **B,** Fatal vitamin D poisoning in a 9-year-old boy who had diabetes mellitus and had been on a high-vitamin diet as part of his general treatment. **A,** The metaphyses at the knees have a series of radiolucent and radiopaque transverse bands. The epiphyseal ossification centers are not affected. **B,** The Towne projection of the skull demonstrates calcification of the falx cerebri and tentorium cerebelli. **C,** Iatrogenic vitamin D poisoning in another child with physiologic bowleg mistakenly though to have X-linked hypophosphatemia (vitamin D–resistant rickets). Multiple opaque metaphyseal bands are present in the distal radial metaphysis.

Vitamin D poisoning may be acute or chronic. Most symptoms and signs are associated with manifestations of hypercalcemia. Massive overdosage (4 to 18 million U/day) may cause severe illness or even death within 3 to 9 days. Vomiting followed by dehydration and high fever is common in the severely ill patient. Other manifestations in some patients include coma, convulsions, abdominal cramps, and "bone pain." In chronic poisoning, the common early symptoms are lethargy, thirst, anorexia, and urinary urgency, with or without polyuria. Later symptoms are vomiting, diarrhea, and abdominal discomfort. Renal damage with renal calcification is due to increased urinary excretion of calcium. Serum levels of calcium and phosphate are increased, and the urine contains albumin, casts, blood, and an excess of calcium. Radiographic changes include metastatic calcifications in the media of blood vessels, kidneys (especially the tubules), heart, gastric wall, alveoli of the lungs, bronchi, adrenals, and even the falx cerebri. Renal ultrasound may demonstrate medullary nephrocalcinosis. In the long bones, the initial change is an increase in width of the zone of provisional calcification. Subsequently, there is cortical thickening and, later, osteoporosis with deep zones of diminished density in the ends of the shafts and, often, alternating bands of increased and diminished density (see Fig. 167-30).

Toxic, Pharmacologic, and Other Disorders

HEAVY METAL POISONING

Lead poisoning is the most common form of heavy metal poisoning. Other heavy metals may produce similar findings. In children, lead poisoning is most often from ingesting lead contained in paint chips. Inhalation of fumes from burning storage batteries may result in severe acute toxicity. Lead bullets result in toxicity only if within a serous space such as a synovium-lined joint, where the presence of lead will cause both systemic toxicity and synovitis causing lead arthropathy. Clinically, lead poisoning is characterized by abdominal pain, encephalopathy (including varying degrees of altered mental status and seizures), peripheral neuropathy, and anemia with basophilic stippling. Chronic lead toxicity causes bands of increased opacity (lead lines) in the metaphyses (Fig. 167-31). Although these bands are caused by lead in the metaphyses, the opacity seen radiographically is not due to the lead, which is present in quantities far below that required to be seen. Rather, the opacity represents increased calcium caused by defective resorption of calcified cartilage in the primary spongiosa.

> The opacity of lead lines is due to excessive calcified cartilage, with lead toxicity causing defective resorption.

When first formed, these bands are located along the zone of provisional calcification of long bone metaphyses and other metaphyseal equivalent regions, such as the iliac crests. The major differential diagnostic considera-

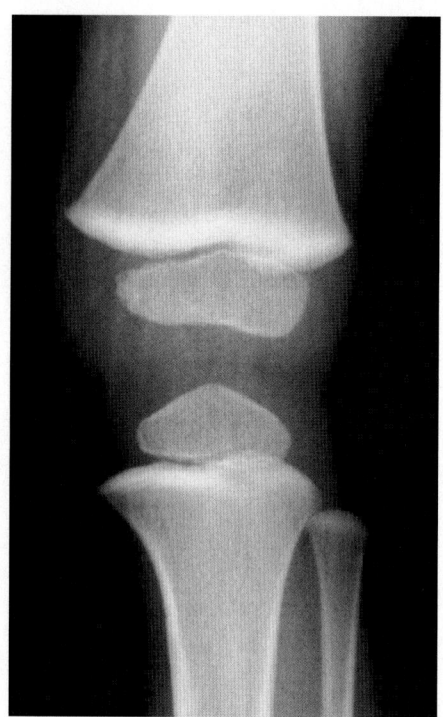

FIGURE 167-31. Lead lines. Typical band of increased opacity, most pronounced in the distal femur. Although lead is present in this region, its amount is not sufficient to account for the opacity, which instead is due to deficient resorption of calcified cartilage.

tion is normal-variant opaque metaphyseal bands. Distinguishing true lead lines from normal opaque metaphyseal bands is not easy radiographically, and this distinction is best made by measurement of the blood lead level. In general, the more opaque the metaphyseal band, the more likely it is to be pathologic. Although it has been suggested that involvement of the fibula is key to making this distinction, this may not be reliable. However, lead lines can be clearly distinguished from normal opaque metaphyseal bands once interval bone growth separates the abnormally sclerotic bone from the zone of provisional calcification. Normal opaque metaphyseal bands are always contiguous with the zone of provisional calcification, and the sclerotic bone is resorbed by the time that it "migrates away" from the physis (Fig. 167-32). The major causes of opaque metaphyseal bands are given in Table 167-5.

> Migration of the opaque band away from the physis with growth distinguishes pathologic from normal-variant opaque metaphyseal bands.

BISPHOSPHONATES

Bisphosphonates, which include drugs such as pamidronate, are agents used to treat osteopenia. In children they have been used mainly to treat osteogenesis imperfecta and lead to not only increased bone density, but also decreased fracture incidence. These drugs are chemically similar to pyrophosphate, but have an added

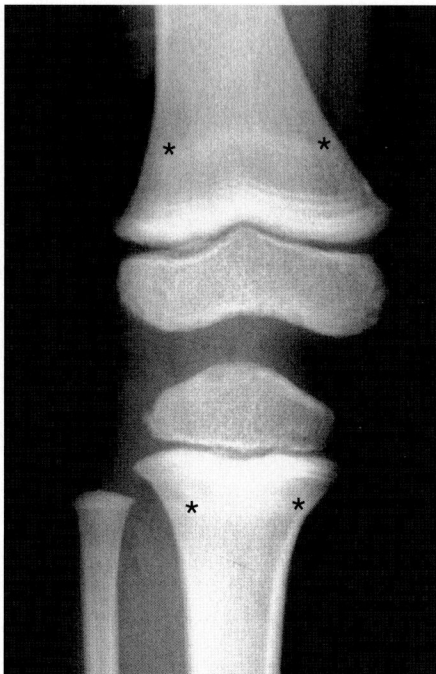

FIGURE 167-32. Lead toxicity. In addition to the opaque bands at the zones of provisional calcification, there are also faint opaque bands (between *asterisks*) that have "migrated away," clearly establishing that they are abnormal rather than normal-variant opaque metaphyseal bands, which are always in continuity with the zone of provisional calcification.

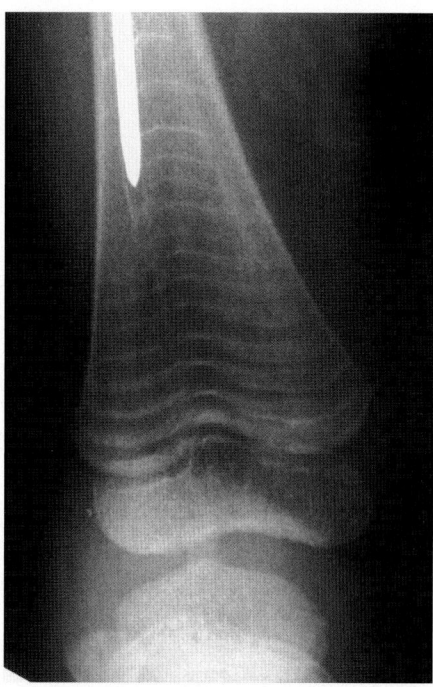

FIGURE 167-33. Multiple opaque lines due to cyclic bisphosphonate therapy in a 3-year-old girl with osteogenesis imperfecta. In addition to the opaque lines, there is also less than the normal amount of osteoclast-mediated "metaphyseal cutback," leading to abnormal modeling with undertubulation.

TABLE 167-5
Opaque Metaphyseal Bands: Major Causes

Normal variant
Toxicity
   Lead and other heavy metals
   Vitamin D
   Bisphosphonates
Healed rickets
Healed leukemia/neuroblastoma

amino side chain that prevents their breakdown and leads to prolonged action at bone surfaces. Their major effect is inhibition of osteoclast-mediated resorption. Additionally, through transient lowering of serum ionized calcium, they may also cause increased PTH secretion. Although the major effect of PTH on bone is to stimulate resorption, PTH also has a positive effect on bone osteoblastic formation, and this may become particularly important when its influence on bone resorption is blocked by bisphosphonates. An expected effect of bisphosphonate therapy is the production of sclerotic metaphyseal lines at the time of administration. Similar to lead lines, these are due to failure of resorption of calcified cartilage, and they "migrate away" from the growth plate with subsequent bone growth. As bisphosphonates are typically administered cyclically, this results in a series of multiple sclerotic "bisphosphonate lines" (Fig. 167-33) that are usually of no clinical significance other than serving as a record of prior treatment.

Of greater concern, bisphosphonate therapy has also caused an induced form of osteopetrosis with typical radiographic and histologic features. Radiographic features include multiple sclerotic metaphyseal bands, decreased tubulation, sclerotic vertebral end plates, and increased bone fragility. Histologic features include abnormal osteoclast morphology and failure of resorption of calcified cartilage in the primary spongiosa. Although this form resulted from a greater dosage of bisphosphonate than usually given, therapy in other patients has also been associated with decreased metaphyseal modeling leading to a convex rather than concave metaphyseal contour, suggesting a similar defect in osteoclast mediated modeling (see Fig. 167-33).

PROSTAGLANDINS

Prostaglandins have many effects on bone, including stimulation of both bone resorption and periosteal new bone formation. These are briefly discussed in Chapters 28 and 175.

OXALOSIS

In primary oxalosis, there is abnormal deposition of calcium oxalate due to oxalate overproduction. In primary oxalosis type 1, this results from increased production of glycolic acid in the liver due to deficiency of alanine glyoxylate aminotransferase. In type 2 primary oxalosis, there is increased production of glyceric acid. Both of these are subsequently metabolized to oxalate. Deposition of calcium oxalate crystals causes nephrocalcinosis, nephrolithiasis, and progressive renal failure

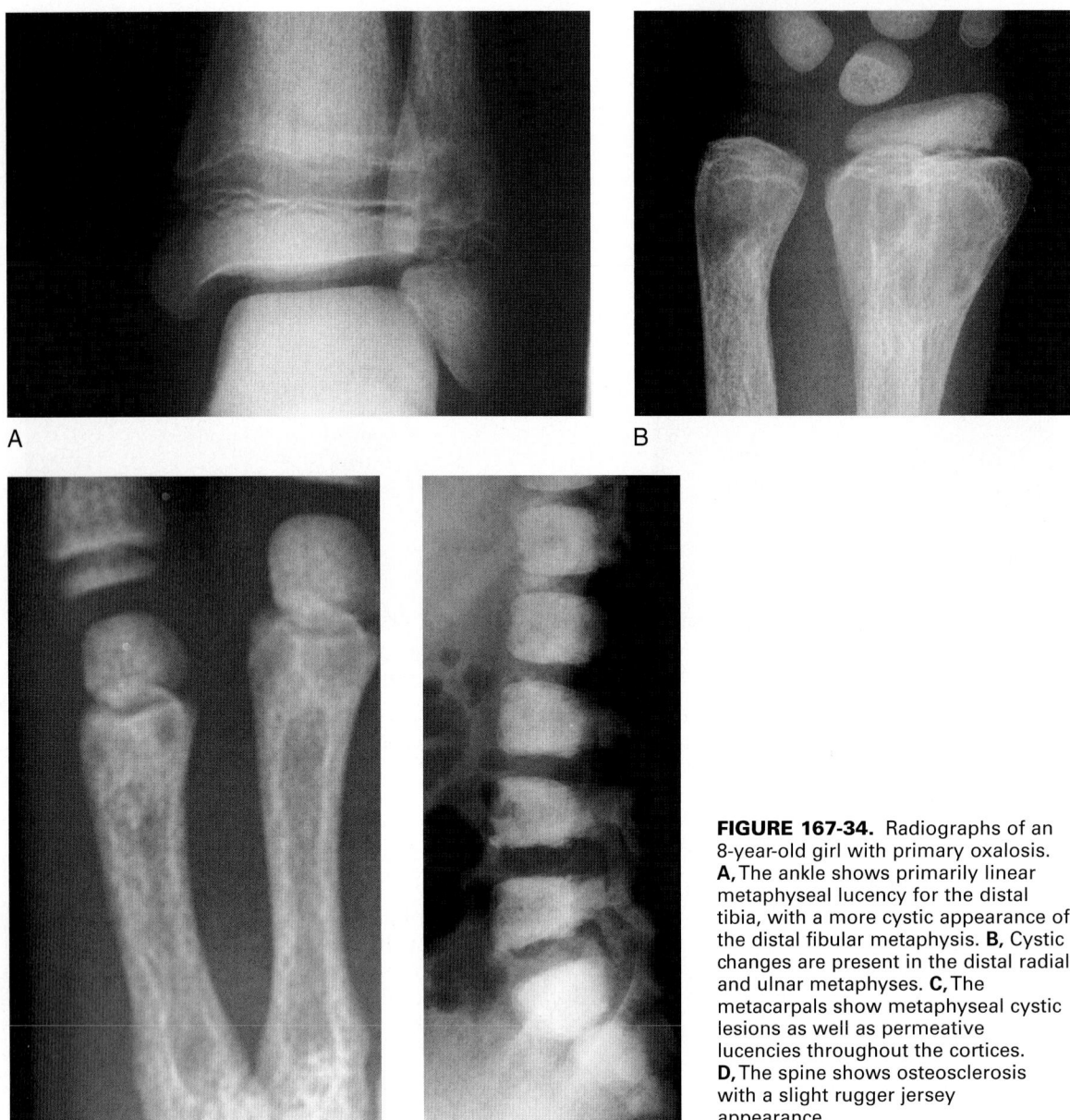

FIGURE 167-34. Radiographs of an 8-year-old girl with primary oxalosis. **A,** The ankle shows primarily linear metaphyseal lucency for the distal tibia, with a more cystic appearance of the distal fibular metaphysis. **B,** Cystic changes are present in the distal radial and ulnar metaphyses. **C,** The metacarpals show metaphyseal cystic lesions as well as permeative lucencies throughout the cortices. **D,** The spine shows osteosclerosis with a slight rugger jersey appearance.

with small calcified kidneys. Crystal deposition also occurs in many other organs and bone. Crystal deposition in bone leads to a giant cell granulomatous inflammatory response, which may lead to both sclerosis and bone resorption. These findings are usually symmetric and most pronounced in the metaphyses of both long and short tubular bones. Initially this causes transverse lucent metaphyseal bands (Fig. 167-34). With greater resorption, more cystic lesions develop (see Fig. 167-34). With further enlargement, pathologic fractures that heal poorly develop through these lesions. The spine may demonstrate diffuse osteosclerosis (see Fig. 167-34) or a rugger jersey appearance. As chronic renal failure is also present in these patients, subperiosteal resorption and other findings of renal osteodystrophy may also be seen.

SUGGESTED READINGS

Bone Biology

Baron R: General principles of bone biology. *In* Favis MJ (ed): Primer on the Metabolic Bone Diseases and Disorders of Mineral Metabolism, 5th ed. Washington, DC, American Society for Bone and Mineral Research, 2003:1-8

Mundy GR, Chen D, Oyajobi BO: Bone remodeling. *In* Favis MJ (ed): Primer on the Metabolic Bone Diseases and Disorders of Mineral Metabolism, 5th ed. Washington, DC, American Society for Bone and Mineral Research, 2003:46-58

Resnick D, Manolagas SC, Niwayama G, et al: Histogenesis, anatomy, and physiology of bone. *In* Resnick D (ed): Diagnosis of Bone and Joint Disorders, 4th ed. Philadelphia, Saunders, 2002:647-687

Rickets

General, Pathophysiology, Vitamin D Deficiency

Chesney RW: Rickets: an old form for a new century. Pediatr Int 2003;45:509-511

Holick MF: Vitamin D: photobiology, metabolism, mechanism of action, and clinical applications. *In* Favis MJ (ed): Primer on the Metabolic Bone Diseases and Disorders of Mineral Metabolism, 5th ed. Washington, DC, American Society for Bone and Mineral Research, 2003:129-137

Le May M, Blunt JW Jr: A factor determining the location of pseudofractures in osteomalacia. J Clin Invest 1949;28:521-525

Pettifor JM: Rickets and vitamin D deficiency in children and adolescents. Endocrinol Metab Clin North Am 2005;34:537-553

Pitt MJ: Rickets and osteomalacia. *In* Resnick D (ed): Diagnosis of Bone and Joint Disorders, 4th ed. Philadelphia, Saunders, 2002:1901-1946

Steinbach HL, Kolb FO, Gilfillon A: A mechanism of the production of pseudofractures in osteomalacia (milkman's syndrome). Radiology 1954;62:388-395

Other Calcipenic Forms (Low Circulatory Calcium) of Rickets

Donnelly LF, Johnson JF 3rd, Benzing G: Infantile osteopetrosis complicated by rickets. AJR Am J Roentgenol 1995;164:968-970

Gradus D, LeRoith D, Karplus M, et al: Congenital hyperparathyroidism and rickets: secondary to maternal hypoparathyroidism and vitamin D deficiency. Isr J Med Sci 1981;17:705-708

Kaplan FS, August CS, Fallon MD, et al: Osteopetrorickets: the paradox of plenty. Pathophysiology and treatment. Clin Orthop 1993;294:64-78

Milhaud G, Labat ML, Litwin I, et al: Osteopetro-rickets: a new congenital bone disorder. Metab Bone Dis Relat Res 1981;3:91-97

Oliveira G, Boechat MI, Amaral SM, Young LW: Osteopetrosis and rickets: an intriguing association. Am J Dis Child 1986;140:377-378

Rosen JF, Fleishman AR, Feinberg L, et al: Rickets with alopecia: an inborn error of vitamin D metabolism. J Pediatr 1979;94:729-735

Tsuchiya Y, Matsuo N, Cho H, et al: An unusual form of vitamin D-dependent rickets in a child: alopecia and marked end-organ hyposensitivity to biologically active vitamin D. J Clin Endocrinol Metab 1980;51:685-690

Young LW, Forbes GB, Borgstedt AD, et al: "Antiepileptic therapy" rickets: roentgenologic implications. Ann Radiol 1974;17:375-383

Metabolic Bone Disease of Prematurity

Greer FR: Osteopenia of prematurity. Annu Rev Nutr 1994;4:169-185

James JR, Congdon PJ, Truscott J, et al: Osteopenia of prematurity. Arch Dis Child 1986;61:871-876

Klein GL: Metabolic bone disease of total parenteral nutrition. Nutrition 1998;14:149-152

Laing IA, Glass EJ, Hendry GMA, et al: Rickets of prematurity: calcium and phosphorus supplementation. J Pediatr 1985; 106:265-268

Ryan S: Nutritional aspects of metabolic bone disease in the newborn. Arch Dis Child 1996;74:F145-F148

Hypophosphatemic Rickets

Asnes RS, Berdon WE, Bassett CA: Hypophosphatemic rickets in an adolescent cured by excision of a nonossifying fibroma. Clin Pediatr 1981;20:646-648

Avila NA, Skarulis M, Rubino DM, et al: Oncogenic osteomalacia— lesion detection by MR skeletal survey. AJR Am J Roentgenol 1996;167:343-345

Baroncelli GI, Bertelloni S, Ceccarelli C, et al: Effect of growth hormone treatment on final height, phosphate metabolism, and bone mineral density in children with X-linked hypophosphatemic rickets. J Pediatr 2001;138:236-243

Berndt TJ, Schiavi S, Kumar R: "Phosphatonins" and the regulation of phosphorus homeostasis. Am J Physiol Renal Physiol 2005;289:F1170-F1182

Evans A, Caffey J: Metaphyseal dysostosis resembling vitamin D-refractory rickets. Am J Dis Child 1958;95:640-648

Glorieux FH: Hypophosphatemic vitamin-D resistant rickets. *In* Favis MJ (ed): Primer on the Metabolic Bone Diseases and Disorders of Mineral Metabolism, 5th ed. Washington, DC, American Society for Bone and Mineral Research, 2003:414-417

Haffner D, Nissel R, Wuhl E, Mehls O: Effects of growth hormone treatment on body proportions and final height among small children with X-linked hypophosphatemic rickets. Pediatrics 2004;113:e593-e596

Jan de Beur SM: Tumor-induced osteomalacia. *In* Favis MJ (ed): Primer on the Metabolic Bone Diseases and Disorders of Mineral Metabolism, 5th ed. Washington, DC, American Society for Bone and Mineral Research, 2003:418-422

Lee HK, Sung WW, Solodnik P, et al: Bone scan in tumor-induced osteomalacia. J Nucl Med 1995;36:247-249

Pivnick EK, Kerr NC, Kaufman RA, et al: Rickets secondary to phosphate depletion: a sequela of antacid use in infancy. Clin Pediatr (Phila) 1995;34:73-78

Renton P, Shaw DG: Hypophosphatemic osteomalacia secondary to vascular tumors of bone and soft tissue. Skeletal Radiol 1976; 1:21-24

Hypophosphatasia

Currarino G: Hypophosphatasia. Prog Pediatr Radiol 1973;4:469-494

Oestreich AE, Bofinger MS: Prominent transverse (Bowdler) bone spurs as a diagnostic clue in a case of neonatal hypophosphatasia without metaphyseal irregularity. Pediatr Radiol 1989;19:341-342

Scriver C, Cameron P: Pseudohypophosphatasia. N Engl J Med 1969;281:604-606

Shohat M, Rimoin DL, Gruber HE, et al: Perinatal lethal hypophosphatasia; clinical, radiologic and morphologic findings. Pediatr Radiol 1991;21:421-427

Whyte MP: Hypophosphatasia: nature's window on alkaline phosphatase function in man. *In* Bilezikian JP, Raisz LG, Rodan GA (eds): Principles of Bone Biology, 2nd ed. San Diego, Academic Press, 2002:1229-1248

Whyte MP: Hypophosphatasia. *In* Favis MJ (ed): Primer on the Metabolic Bone Diseases and Disorders of Mineral Metabolism, 5th ed. Washington, DC, American Society for Bone and Mineral Research, 2003:423-425

Whyte MP, Kurtzberg J, McAlister WH, et al: Marrow cell transplantation for infantile hypophosphatasia. J Bone Miner Res 2003;18:624-636

Scurvy and Copper Abnormalities

Grewar O: Infantile scurvy. Clin Pediatr 1965;4:82-89

Hess AF: Scurvy, Past and Present. Philadelphia, Lippincott, 1920

Kanumakala S, Boneh A, Zacharin M: Pamidronate treatment improves bone mineral density in children with Menkes disease. J Inherit Metab Dis 2002;25:391-398

Park EA, Guild HG, Jackson D: Recognition of scurvy with especial reference to early x-ray changes. Arch Dis Child 1935;10:265-294

Schwartz AM, Leonidas JC: Methotrexate osteopathy. Skeletal Radiol 1984;11:13-16

Hyperphospatasia

Whyte MP, Mills BG, Reinus WR, et al: Expansile skeletal hyperphosphatasia: a new familial metabolic bone disease. J Bone Miner Res 2000;15:2330-2344

Whyte MP, Obrecht SE, Finnegan PM, et al: Osteoprotegerin deficiency and juvenile Paget's disease. N Engl J Med 2002;347:175-184

Congenital Hyperphosphatasia (Juvenile Paget's Disease)

Eroglu M, Taneli NN: Congenital hyperphosphatasia (juvenile Paget's disease): eleven years follow-up of three sisters. Ann Radiol (Paris) 1977;20:145-150

Nutritional/Toxic/Pharmacologic Disorders

Caffey J: Chronic poisoning due to excess of vitamin A. Am J Roentgenol Radium Ther 1951;65:12-26

De Luca F, Uyeda JA, Mericq V, et al: Retinoic acid is a potent regulator of growth plate chondrogenesis. Endocrinology 2000;141:346-353

Knudson AG Jr, Rothman PE: Hypervitaminosis A: a review with discussion of vitamin A. Am J Dis Child 1953;85:316-334

Langman CB: Improvement of bone in patients with osteogenesis imperfecta treated with pamidronate—lessons from biochemistry. J Clin Endocrinol Metab 2003;88:984-985

MacKay RJ, Woodard JC, Donovan GA: Focal premature physeal closure (hyena disease) in calves. J Am Vet Med Assoc 1992;201:902-905

Miller JH, Hayon II: Bone scintigraphy in hypervitaminosis A. AJR Am J Roentgenol 1985;144:767-768

Morrice G Jr, Havener WH, Kapetansky F: Vitamin A intoxication as a cause of pseudotumor cerebri. JAMA 1960;173:1802-1805

Pease CN: Focal retardation and arrestment of growth of bones due to vitamin A intoxication. JAMA 1962;182:980-985

Resnick D: Disorders due to medications and other chemical agents. *In* Resnick D (ed): Diagnosis of Bone and Joint Disorders, 4th ed. Philadelphia, Saunders, 2002:3423-3455

Resnick D: Heavy metal poisoning and deficiency. *In* Resnick D (ed): Diagnosis of Bone and Joint Disorders, 4th ed. Philadelphia, Saunders, 2002:3464-3478

Resnick D: Hypervitaminosis and hypovitaminosis. *In* Resnick D (ed): Diagnosis of Bone and Joint Disorders, 4th ed. Philadelphia, Saunders, 2002:3456-3464

Wang W, Xu J, Kirsch T: Annexin-mediated Ca^{2+} influx regulates growth plate chondrocyte maturation and apoptosis. J Biol Chem 2003;278:3762-3769

Woodard JC, Donovan GA, Fisher LW: Pathogenesis of vitamin (A and D)-induced premature growth-plate closure in calves. Bone 1997;21:171-182

Whyte MP, Wenkert D, Clements KL, et al: Bisphosphonate-induced osteopetrosis. N Engl J Med 2003;349:457-463

Oxalosis

Danpure CJ: Primary hyperoxaluria. *In* Scriver CR, Beaudet AL, Sly WS, et al (eds): The Molecular and Metabolic Basis of Inherited Disease, New York, McGraw-Hill, 2001:3323-3367

Fisher D, Hilleer N, Drukker A: Oxalosis of bone: report of four cases and a new radiological staging. Pediatr Radiol 1995;25:293-295

Resnick D: Other crystal-induced diseases. *In* Resnick D (ed): Diagnosis of Bone and Joint Disorders, 4th ed. Philadelphia, Saunders, 2002:1692-1703

Several endocrine glands have significant effects on normal and abnormal skeletal growth, maturation, modeling, and remodeling. Additionally, the parathyroid glands are directly involved in mineral homeostasis and have major effects on bone mineralization and resorption.

HYPERPARATHYROIDISM, RENAL OSTEODYSTROPHY, AND RELATED CONDITIONS

Hyperparathyroidism (HPTH) in children is most often caused by chronic renal failure. Renal osteodystrophy (ROD) refers to the many skeletal abnormalities caused by chronic renal insufficiency, which are predominantly those of HPTH caused by renal insufficiency (2° HPTH). Hence, ROD is discussed in this section on HPTH. Other neonatal hypercalcemic and hyperparathyroid conditions are also included in this section.

Causes of Hyperparathyroidism

Primary HPTH (1° HPTH) may be caused by diffuse parathyroid hyperplasia or parathyroid adenoma. Parathyroid adenomas are infrequent in children and are usually associated with multiple endocrine neoplasia (MEN) I. Parathyroid hyperplasia may be seen with MEN II and MEN III.

In 2° HPTH, PTH secretion is increased in response to hypocalcemia. In children, 2° HPTH is much more common than 1° HPTH, and the most frequent cause is chronic renal failure. Rickets and some other disorders of calcium metabolism may also cause 2° HPTH.

> **Hyperparathyroidism in children is most often caused by chronic renal failure.**

Pathophysiology

Maintenance of normal serum calcium concentration by parathyroid hormone (PTH) secretion is controlled by calcium sensing receptors (CASRs) of parathyroid chief cells. Binding of calcium to this receptor triggers a series of events that involve the G-protein system of signal transduction and lead to inhibition of PTH secretion. As calcium concentration falls, this inhibition is released, leading to PTH secretion. The CASR controls serum calcium concentration by establishing the "set point" for inhibition of PTH secretion by calcium. Although it is less important than calcium concentration in regulating PTH secretion, decreased calcitriol (1,25[OH]$_2$D) also stimulates PTH. PTH has effects on bone, kidney, and intestine that help to regulate calcium and phosphate levels. For bone, PTH stimulates calcium and phosphate mobilization through osteoclastic bone resorption. In the kidney, PTH stimulates the synthesis of calcitriol, decreases urinary calcium excretion, and increases phosphate excretion. PTH enhances the gut absorption of minerals directly and through calcitriol.

In chronic renal failure, as the glomerular filtration rates falls low enough, phosphate excretion also falls, leading to mild hyperphosphatemia with associated hypocalcemia. Slightly decreased calcium triggers increased PTH secretion, which acts to reverse hyperphosphatemia and hypocalcemia. Although this restores the calcium concentration to normal, it does so at the expense of producing PTH elevations and causing associated mobilization of calcium and phosphate from bone. With advancing renal failure, decreased renal mass also reduces calcitriol synthesis, leading to rickets and osteomalacia. However, this effect on the skeleton is less pronounced than is hyperparathyroidism, and many of the manifestations of "renal rickets" are actually those of hyperparathyroidism.

> **Many of the manifestations of "renal rickets" are actually those of hyperparathyroidism.**

Pathologic and Radiographic Findings

BONE RESORPTION

PTH stimulates bone resorption by osteoclasts. The most specific radiographic manifestation of HPTH is subperiosteal resorption, which is initially seen along the radial aspects of the index and the middle finger middle phalanges (Fig. 168-1). The distal phalangeal terminal tufts are also involved relatively early. With progression, subperiosteal resorption is noted along the ulnar aspects of the phalanges and other bones. Additional "target sites" for subperiosteal resorption include the medial aspects of the humeral (Fig. 168-2) and femoral necks and the medial aspects of the proximal tibial metaphyses.

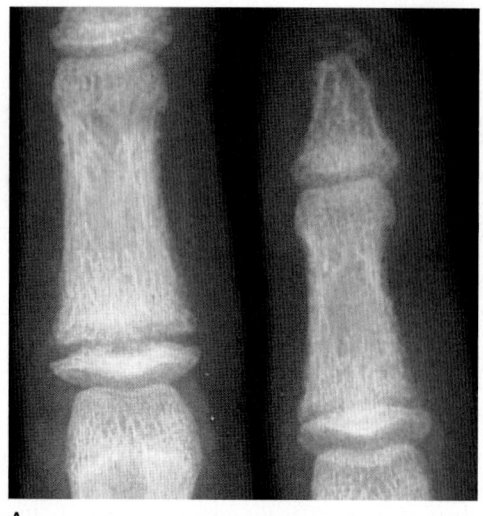
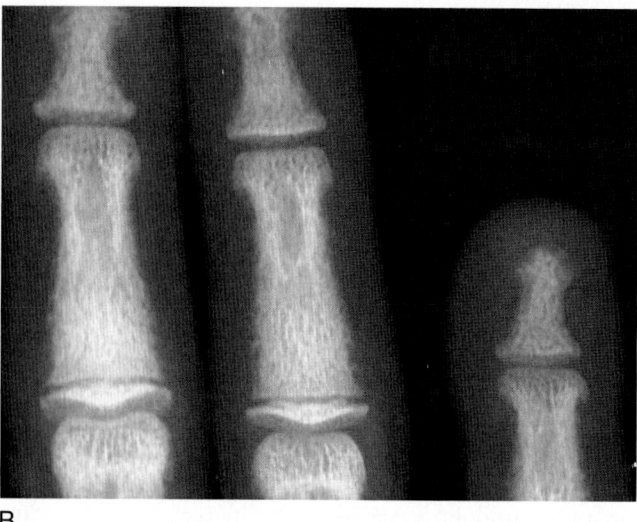

A   B

FIGURE 168-1. Subperiosteal bone resorption of secondary hyperparathyroidism in renal osteodystrophy. **A,** A 15-year-old in whom resorption is primarily seen along the radial aspects of the middle phalanges with mild involvement of the ulnar aspects. **B,** A 13-year-old with more extensive involvement of both sides.

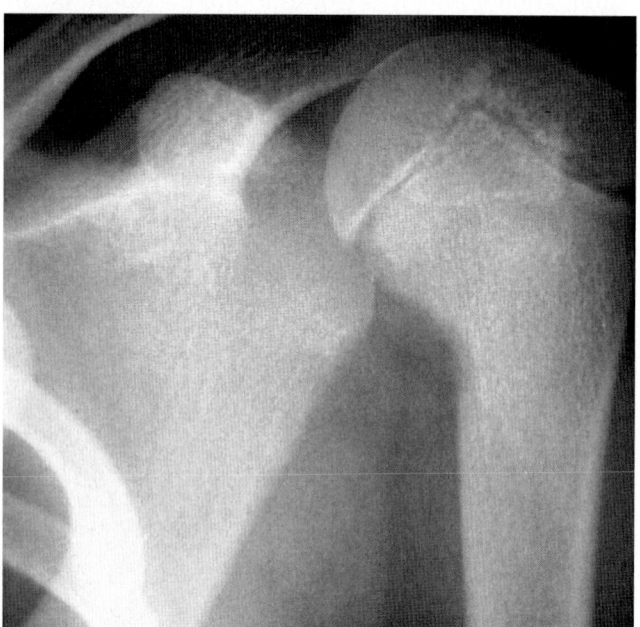

FIGURE 168-2. Proximal humeral subperiosteal resorption in a 15-year-old. Same patient as Figure 168-1, **A.**

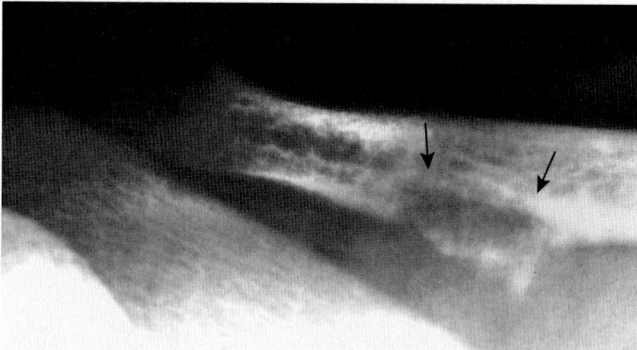

FIGURE 168-3. Subligamentous resorption at coracoclavicular ligament *(arrows)* in secondary hyperparathyroidism of renal osteodystrophy.

Although less specific than subperiosteal resorption, HPTH may lead to intracortical resorption or "tunneling," causing a striated appearance of the cortex, endosteal resorption, and subchondral, subligamentous (Fig. 168-3), and subtendinous resorption. In infancy, bone resorption from HPTH may lead to loss of anatomic detail and poorly defined bone ends, which have been likened to the "rotten stump" appearance of a wooden log (Fig. 168-4). Subphyseal resorption (a form of subchondral resorption) leads to resorption of the zone of provisional calcification and metaphyseal bone beneath the physis, simulating the appearance of rickets. An important distinction from true rickets is that the radiolucent material beneath the growth plate does not represent nonmineralized cartilage and osteoid, but rather fibrous tissue related to osteitis fibrosa cystica. Additional findings of HPTH include resorption of the lamina dura, which forms the thin opaque line surrounding tooth roots (Fig. 168-5), cystic-appearing "brown tumors" (osteoclastomas) (Fig. 168-6), and bone sclerosis. Although brown tumors are more characteristic of 1° HPTH, overall they are seen more often in 2° HPTH because it is much more common than 1° HPTH in children. Osteosclerosis is more frequent with 2° HPTH than with 1° HPTH and may be due to a stimulatory effect of PTH on osteoblasts. Osteosclerosis in ROD may be generalized or may be most pronounced subjacent to the vertebral end plates, resulting in a "rugger jersey" appearance (Fig. 168-7). Because overall bone mineral is decreased rather than increased in ROD, osteosclerosis may be due to redistribution of cortical bone to trabecular bone.

SLIPPED EPIPHYSES

Slipped epiphyses are an important manifestation of ROD in children. The incidence of slipped epiphyses in

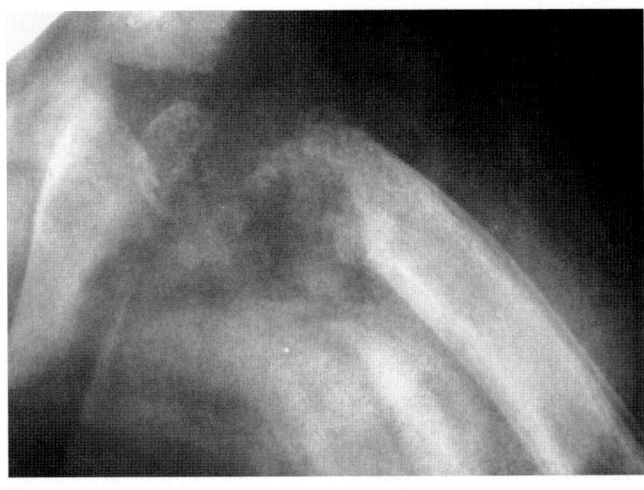

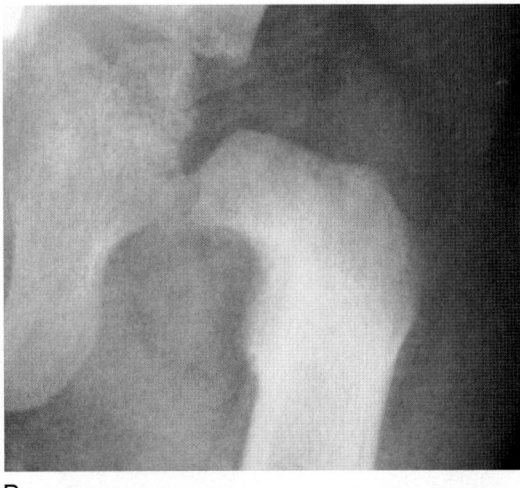

A   B

FIGURE 168-4. "Rotten stump" appearance of secondary hyperparathyroidism in renal osteodystrophy. **A,** At 2 years 2 months, severe resorption of the proximal femur separates the shaft from the femoral head, which remains seated in the acetabulum. **B,** At 3 years 10 months, much of this region has healed with residual widening of the physis. On long-term follow-up, the hips are normal.

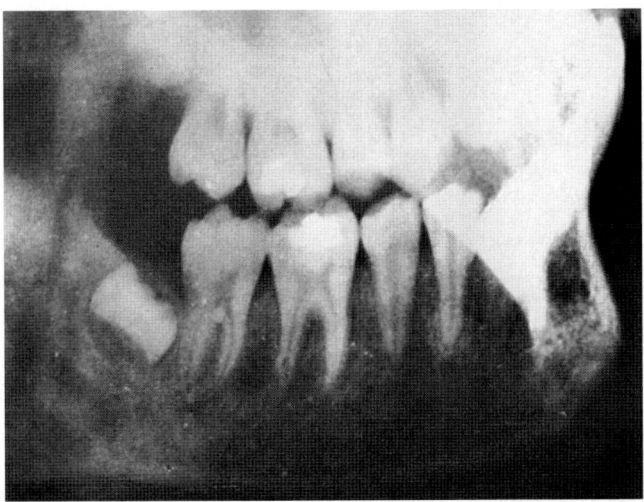

FIGURE 168-5. Loss of lamina dura surrounding tooth roots in secondary hyperparathyroidism.

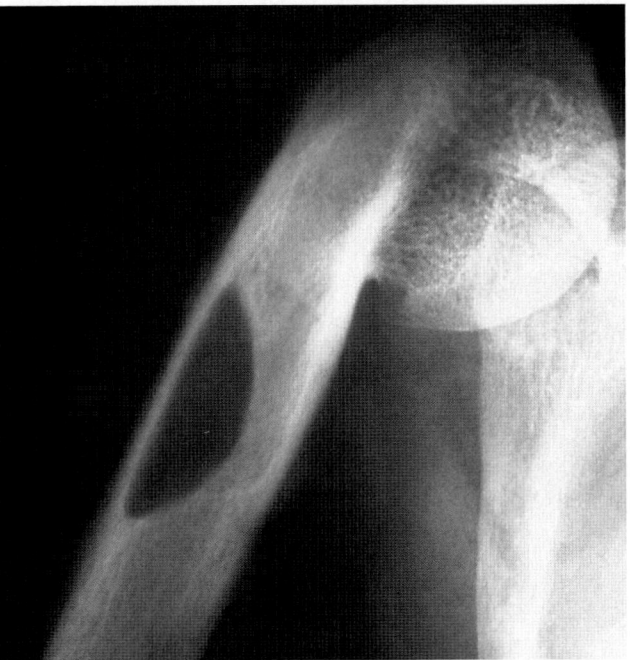

FIGURE 168-6. Proximal humeral diaphyseal brown tumor in secondary hyperparathyroidism. Also note deformity of proximal humeral metaphysis from prior slipped humeral head epiphysis.

ROD is greater than in other predisposing conditions, including hypothyroidism, hypogonadism, and growth hormone deficiency. This predisposition to slipped epiphyses in ROD is due to weakness of the fibrous tissue (osteitis fibrosa cystica) subjacent to the growth plate. Slipped epiphyses are not usually seen in true rickets, where the lucent material is mechanically stronger cartilage and osteoid, thus supporting the concept that the radiographic appearance of "renal rickets" is mostly related to HPTH.

> **Slipped epiphyses are common in renal osteodystrophy but are not usually seen in true rickets.**

In ROD, slippage occurs through the fibrous tissue and disorganized woven bone of the metaphysis affected by osteitis fibrosa cystica, whereas in idiopathic slipped capital femoral epiphysis, the fracture occurs through the hypertrophic zone of the cartilaginous growth plate. Radiographic findings indicating a particularly high risk of slippage include coxa vara with reorientation of the physis from horizontal toward vertical, increased width of the growth plate, and subperiosteal resorption of the adjacent metaphysis. The risk of epiphyseal slippage is particularly high when growth hormone is used to treat short stature, a major clinical problem in children with chronic renal failure. Although slipped epiphyses are seen most frequently in the proximal femur (Fig. 168-8), other sites may be involved; these include the proximal humerus (see Fig. 168-6), distal femur, distal tibia and

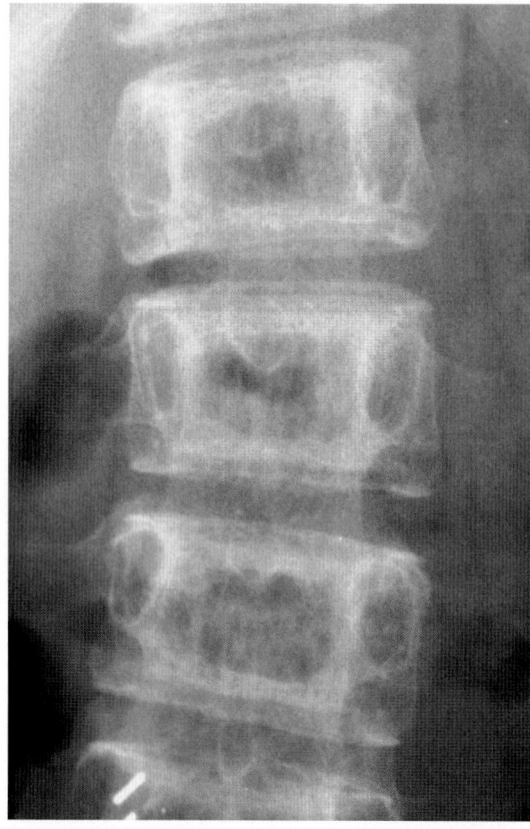

A

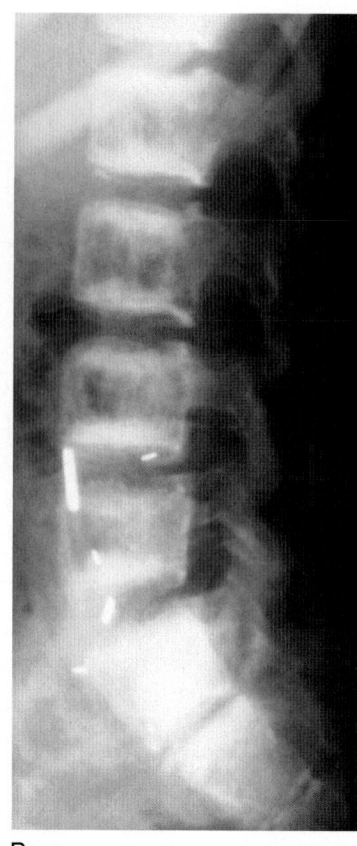

B

FIGURE 168-7. Rugger jersey spine. Anteroposterior (**A**) and lateral views (**B**) of the lumbar spine show vertebral end plate sclerosis producing rugger jersey appearance. Same patient as in Figure 168-6.

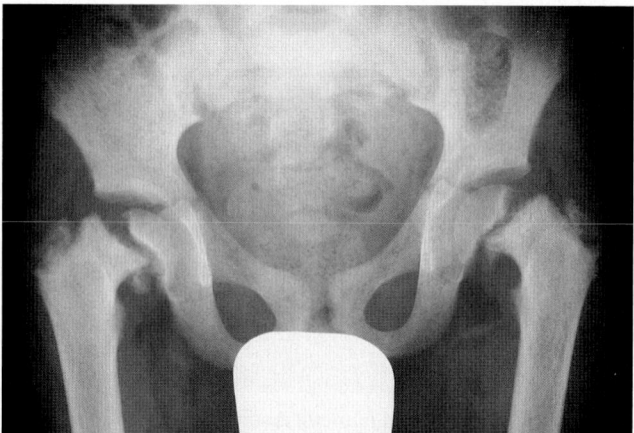

FIGURE 168-8. Bilateral slipped capital femoral epiphyses due to secondary hyperparathyroidism and renal osteodystrophy in an 11-year-old boy. This finding was made at the time of presentation with previously undiagnosed end-stage renal failure.

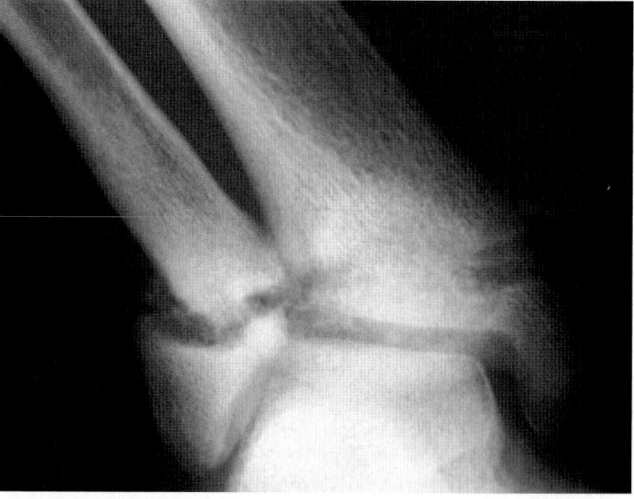

FIGURE 168-9. Slipped distal fibular epiphysis with tibial physeal abnormality and valgus deformity in a 13-year-old with severe secondary hyperparathyroidism of renal osteodystrophy. Same patient as in Figure 168-1, **B**.

fibula (Fig. 168-9), distal forearm bones, and, occasionally, the small tubular bones of the hands and feet.

Renal Osteodystrophy: Additional Manifestations

Renal osteodystrophy describes the constellation of skeletal abnormalities caused by chronic renal insufficiency. Although the major manifestations of ROD are those of 2° HPTH, other manifestations of this disorder include the following: (1) true rickets and osteomalacia, (2) aluminum toxicity and other causes of adynamic bone disease, (3) osteopenia and fractures, and (4) soft tissue calcifications. The features of ROD are summarized in Table 168-1.

Rickets and osteomalacia are due to decreased production of calcitriol caused by decreased renal mass. It is usually difficult or not possible to distinguish true rickets from the rachitic appearance of osteitis fibrosa cystica. Looser zones, if present, indicate osteomalacia.

TABLE 168-1

Findings in Renal Osteodystrophy

Secondary hyperparathyroidism
  Subperiosteal bone resorption
  Bone resorption at other sites (e.g., subligamentous, endosteal)
  Intracortical tunneling
  "Rachitic-appearing" metaphyseal changes of osteitis fibrosa
  Brown tumors
  Slipped epiphyses
Osteosclerosis
True rickets and osteomalacia
Adynamic bone disease
  Aluminum toxicity
  Parathyroid hormone suppression
  Malnutrition, debility
Fractures
  Metaphyseal, others
Soft tissue calcification
  Vascular
  Periarticular
  Visceral

Metabolic bone disease may be divided into "high turnover" and "low turnover" states. High turnover is generally associated with HPTH and is present in most patients with ROD. However, an adynamic form of metabolic bone disease may also be present in ROD. In the past, aluminum toxicity was a major cause of adynamic bone disease in patients with chronic renal failure. This resulted from aluminum contamination of dialysis solutions or aluminum-containing agents used to bind phosphate in the intestinal tract. Aluminum has many effects on bone metabolism, all of which are detrimental. It inhibits osteoblast differentiation, proliferation, and function, leading to decreased collagen synthesis. It also directly inhibits mineralization, leading to rickets and osteomalacia, and it suppresses PTH secretion, which leads to a low turnover rather than high turnover state. Aluminum toxicity is now less common. However, the use of calcium as an intestinal phosphate–binding agent and vitamin D metabolites, particularly calcitriol, may lead to adynamic bone disease caused by the suppression of PTH. Other factors implicated in adynamic bone disease include malnutrition, immobilization, corticosteroid therapy, and prior parathyroidectomy.

Fractures may occur in ROD as a complication of HPTH, rickets/osteomalacia, and other causes of osteopenia such as aluminum bone disease. In children, HPTH is associated with a predisposition to metaphyseal fracture (Fig. 168-10). Soft tissue calcifications seen in ROD include vascular calcifications, periarticular calcifications, which may be similar to those of tumoral calcinosis, and metastatic calcifications involving the lung and other organs.

NEONATAL HYPERCALCEMIC AND HYPERPARATHYROID CONDITIONS

Several conditions are associated with hypercalcemia during the neonatal period—a potentially life-threatening condition. Primary HPTH in neonates is rare; fewer than 100 cases have been reported. It causes severe hypercalcemia for which emergent parathyroidectomy is required, and it is usually due to hyperplasia rather

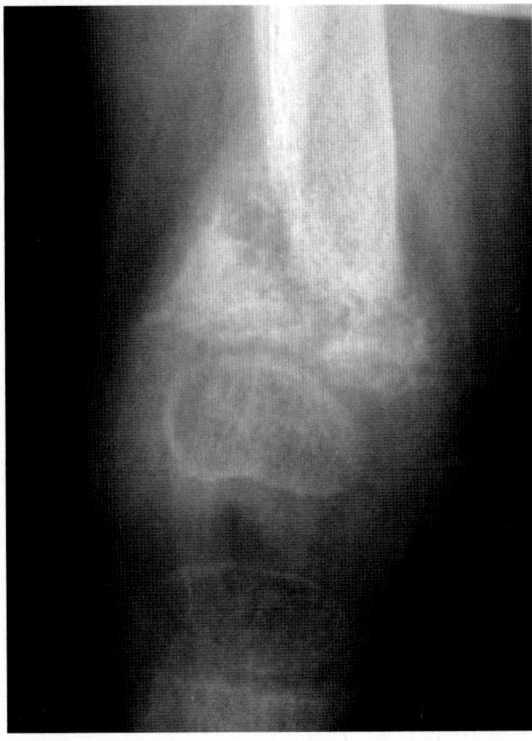

A

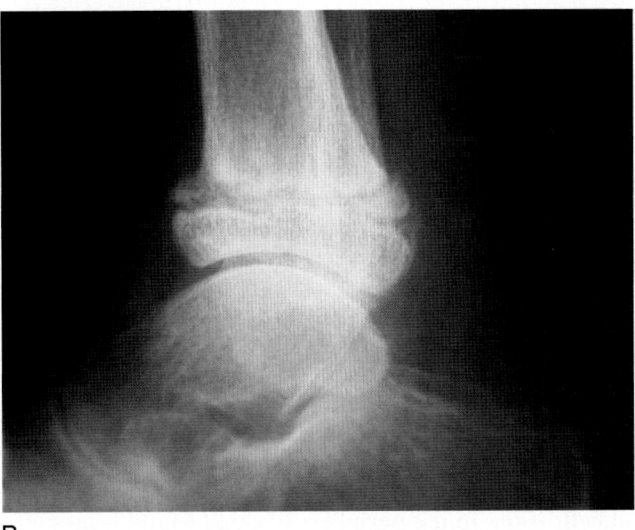

B

FIGURE 168-10. Metaphyseal fractures in renal osteodystrophy. **A,** Distal femur in a 2.6-year-old child (same patient as in Fig. 168-4). **B,** Distal tibial fracture in an 18-year-old (same patient as in Figs. 168-6 and 168-7).

than to a parathyroid adenoma. Neonatal HPTH may be related to the more benign condition, familial hypocalciuric hypocalcemia (FHH), for which an autosomal dominant inactivating mutation of the calcium-sensing receptor gene produces an elevation of the "set point," at which circulating ionized calcium inhibits PTH secretion. Although FHH usually causes asymptomatic hypercalcemia in adults, cases of severe neonatal hypercalcemia have occurred in families with FHH, most of which are believed to be due to inheritance of two mutant alleles. This may be the same condition as neonatal 1° HPTH. Maternal hypocalcemia resulting from hypoparathyroidism may also cause neonatal HPTH.

Williams Syndrome and Idiopathic Infantile Hypercalcemia

Williams syndrome and idiopathic infantile hypercalcemia are related conditions that are associated with hypercalcemia during the neonatal period. Williams syndrome has many morphologic features involving the cardiovascular system and distinct facial features. Hypercalcemia in Williams syndrome is not constant, and when present, it is usually limited to the first year of life. The cause of hypercalcemia is uncertain, but the condition may be related to altered vitamin D metabolism; high levels of calcitriol have been noted during episodes of hypercalcemia but not at other times. In utero vitamin D poisoning in rabbits has produced findings similar to those of Williams syndrome, but such poisoning is not believed to be the cause of this syndrome in children.

In England in the early 1950s, idiopathic infantile hypercalcemia (IIH) was described in a series of several infants with severe hypercalcemia. Most of these cases were associated with excessive maternal vitamin D intake from heavily fortified foods; the incidence of this disorder has decreased substantially since the amounts of vitamin D added to food have decreased. Some afflicted infants also had morphologic features of Williams syndrome; thus, it was unclear whether these are the same or different conditions. Several children with idiopathic infantile hypercalcemia have been shown to have elevated levels of parathyroid hormone–related peptide (PTHrP), which has the same actions as PTH and is the substance secreted by several malignant tumors (most often, squamous carcinomas in adults) that causes hypercalcemia of malignancy. Elevation of PTHrP has not been found in Williams syndrome. Hypercalcemia in IIH may persist later into childhood than does Williams syndrome.

Skeletal findings of IIH and Williams syndrome include generalized bone sclerosis, bands of increased or decreased opacity in the metaphyses, and peripheral radiolucent zones in the periphery of small round bones and epiphyses, which represent metaphyseal equivalent regions (Fig. 168-11). These findings are similar to those reported in vitamin D poisoning. Nephrocalcinosis may be identified by detection of increased renal medullary echogenicity in 20% of patients with IIH or Williams syndrome; calcifications also may be seen in blood vessels, intramuscular septa, and other soft tissues. Premature craniosynostosis may occur.

Jansen Metaphyseal Chondrodysplasia

Jansen metaphyseal chondrodysplasia is an autosomal dominant condition that is characterized by hypercalcemia and other findings suggestive of severe HPTH during the neonatal period and of short-limbed dwarfism later in life. It is due to a mutation of the receptor for PTH and PTHrP that causes the receptor to be always activated. Hence, even though no PTH or PTHrP is detectable, kidney and bone respond as though PTH were elevated, producing hypercalcemia and bone resorption suggestive of HPTH (Fig. 168-12). The "hyperparathyroid phase" usually occurs only during early infancy; the reason for its resolution is not known. The PTH/PTHrP receptor is also active in growth plate chondrocytes, where it inhibits endochondral ossification. This leads to the characteristic features of Jansen metaphyseal chondrodysplasia, which are first seen later in infancy. With impaired endochondral ossification, a large distance develops between the epiphysis and the ossified portion of the shaft. This gap is composed of cartilage that has not yet entered terminal differentiation, resulting in endochondral ossification. This defect also impairs bone growth, causing dwarfism. Subsequently, bizarre chondroid calcifications develop within these regions, which become widened and dysplastic. Eventually, the skeleton becomes fully ossified with residual shortening and deformity.

Mucolipidosis II

Mucolipidosis II (I-cell disease) is an autosomal recessive storage disorder caused by inability to localize lysosomal enzymes in lysosomes, resulting in high enzyme levels in serum but low levels in cells. It produces clinical features similar to those of Hurler syndrome and dysostosis multiplex, which describes the characteristic bone findings of mucopolysaccharidoses and mucolipidoses (see Chapter 165). In addition, some infants with mucolipidosis II have skeletal features of HPTH, including generalized demineralization and subperiosteal bone resorption (Fig. 168-13). Periosteal new bone formation and rachitic changes may also be seen, and serum PTH is elevated. Unlike many of the other causes of neonatal HPTH, serum calcium is not elevated, indicating that this is a form of 2° HPTH. It is speculated that the HPTH in mucolipidosis II is due to involvement of the placenta with the storage disorder, resulting in impaired transplacental calcium transport. This leads to fetal and neonatal calcium deficiency, causing 2° HPTH; PTH is secreted to maintain extracellular calcium concentration by mobilizing it from the skeleton. The findings of 2° HPTH in mucolipidosis II resolve with administration of calcium or vitamin D therapy. However, the overall prognosis in terms of the other manifestations of mucolipidosis II is very poor.

HYPOPARATHYROIDISM AND PSEUDOHYPOPARATHYROIDISM

Hypoparathyroidism

"Idiopathic hypoparathyroidism" in children is most commonly part of polyglandular autoimmune disease

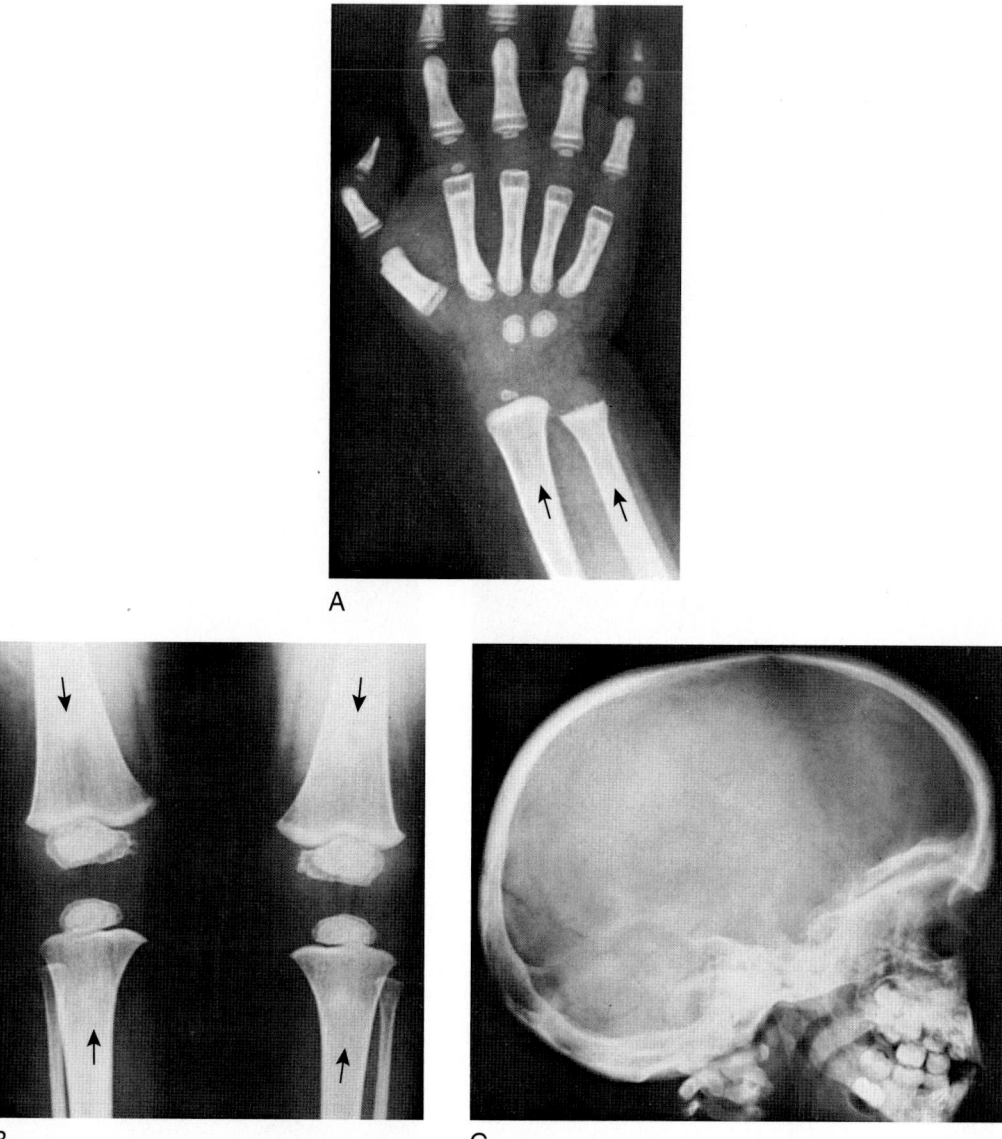

FIGURE 168-11. Chronic idiopathic hypercalcemia with generalized sclerosis of the skeleton and transverse bands in the metaphyses of a 4-year-old who had failed to grow and gain weight and had retardation of motor development; serum calcium value was 13.8 mg/100 ml when these images were made. **A,** Deep transverse radiolucent bands are seen in the metaphyses of tubular bones *(arrows)* and in peripheral radiolucent zones in the round bones of the wrists. **B,** Similar changes are evident in the bones at the knees, although the terminal radiolucent bands are much deeper in these larger and more rapidly growing metaphyses *(arrows).* **C,** All parts of the skull (i.e., calvarium, base, and facial segment) are sclerotic. Both renal regions were stippled with fine foci of calcium density.

type I, also known as candida endocrinopathy. This autosomal recessive autoimmune disorder targets multiple endocrine glands and is associated with chronic mucocutaneous candidiasis. Hypoparathyroidism and adrenal cortical insufficiency (Addison disease) are the most frequent endocrine manifestations, and hypoparathyroidism often precedes adrenal insufficiency and candidiasis. Less frequent manifestations include gonadal insufficiency, autoimmune thyroiditis, Graves disease, diabetes mellitus, malabsorption, and chronic active hepatitis. Other causes of hypoparathyroidism in children include congenital absence of the parathyroids, which may accompany thymic absence in DiGeorge syndrome, surgical removal during thyroidectomy, and transient

suppression of fetal parathyroids by maternal hyperparathyroidism.

Skeletal manifestations of hypoparathyroidism include osteosclerosis, dense metaphyseal bands, cranial vault thickening, intracranial calcifications such as basal ganglia and choroid plexus, and dental abnormalities. Vertebral findings, including marginal sclerosis, "bone within bone" appearance (Fig. 168-14), and paravertebral ossification, are similar to those of diffuse idiopathic skeletal hyperostosis. When hypoparathyroidism is due to congenital absence in DiGeorge syndrome, additional findings of the disorder include thymic aplasia causing retrosternal hyperlucency on lateral chest radiograph or absence of the thymus on cross-sectional imaging,

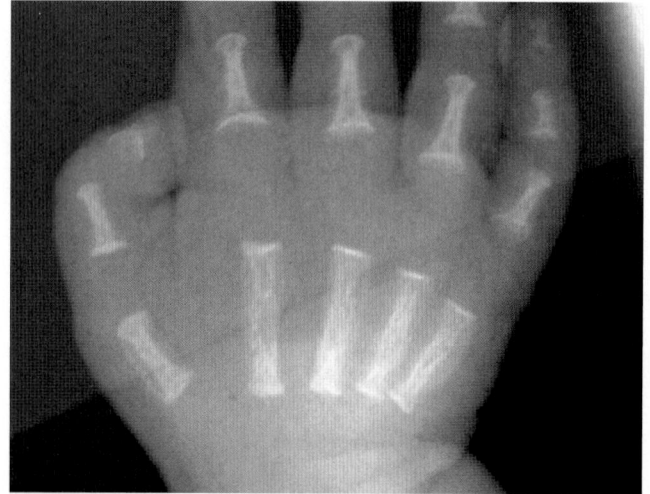

A

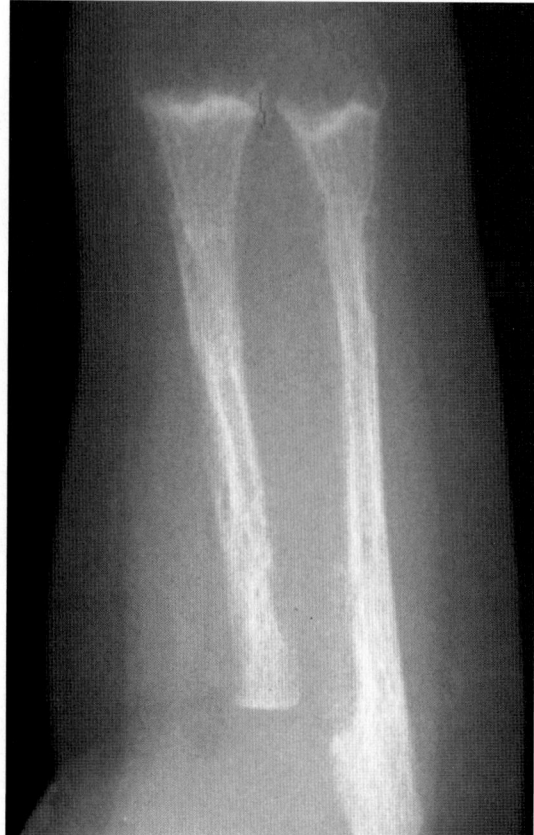

B

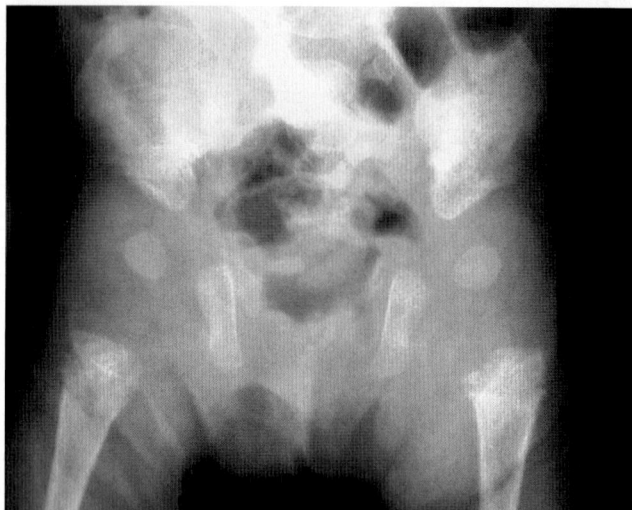

C

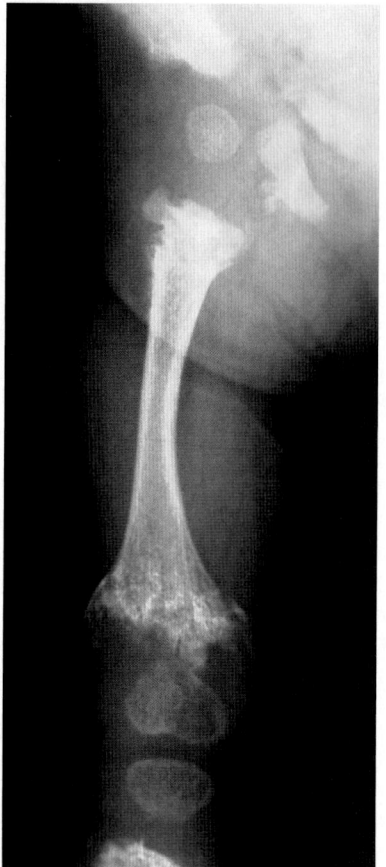

D

FIGURE 168-12. Jansen metaphyseal chondrodysplasia. At
5 days of age, the hand (**A**) and the forearm (**B**) show severe
demineralization and subperiosteal resorption indicative of a
hyperparathyroid state due to a constitutively activated
parathyroid hormone/parathyroid hormone related peptide
(PTH/ PTHrP)receptor. Also prominent are rachitic findings in the
metaphyses. At 7 months, large lucent gaps are apparent
between the femoral heads and the femoral shafts (**C**); these are
due to nonossified cartilage. At 15 months, the right femur (**D**)
shows persistent gaps between the shaft and the epiphyses,
although these have begun to fill in with chondroid
calcifications, which are most apparent distally.   *Continued*

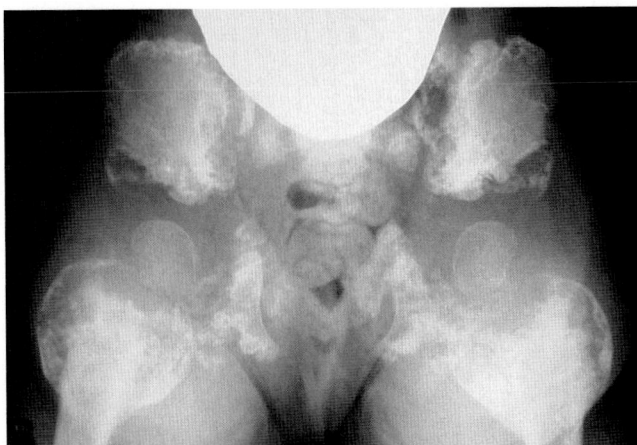

E

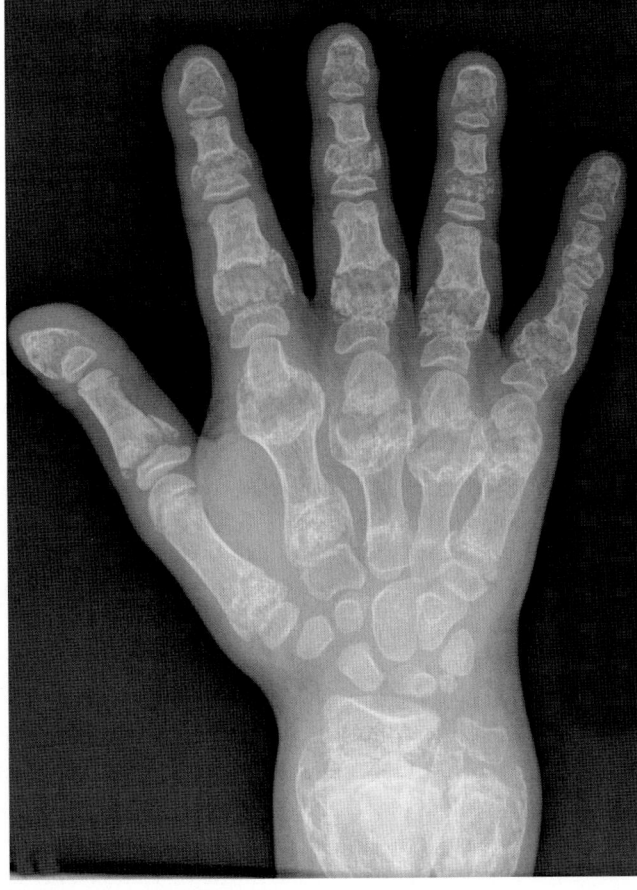

G

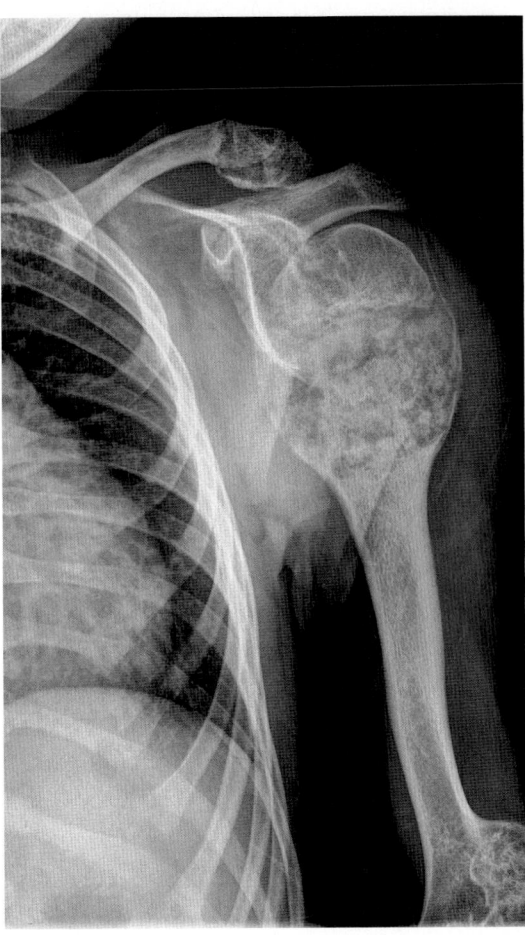

F

FIGURE 168-12, *cont'd*. Jansen metaphyseal chondrodysplasia. At 4.5 years, the pelvis (**E**) shows marked expansion and deformity of the proximal femora with extensive bizarre chondroid calcifications, also present in the pelvic bones. Another patient, who is 11 years of age, shows expansion of the proximal humeral metaphysis (**F**) and of multiple metaphyses in the hand (**G**) that contain chondroid calcifications

nonvisualization of the hyoid bone early in life, and associated aortic arch abnormalities.

Pseudohypoparathyroidism

Pseudohypoparathyroidism (PHP) includes several related conditions that involve varying degrees of resistance to PTH and in some cases other hormones. The most common form, designated as PHP 1a, consists of hormone resistance and characteristic somatic features known as Albright hereditary osteodystrophy (AHO). PHP 1a

mimics true hypoparathyroidism with hypocalcemia, hyperphosphatemia, and soft tissue and basal ganglia calcifications. However, PTH levels are elevated rather than low or absent, and mineral abnormalities are due to end organ resistance to PTH. Hormone resistance is caused by an autosomal dominant, inactivating mutation of the *GNAS1* gene, which codes for the Gsα subunit of a G protein involved in transmitting the signal from the cell surface hormone receptor to adenylyl cyclase. Despite high levels of PTH and adequate binding of PTH to its receptor, adenylyl cyclase is not activated, cyclic

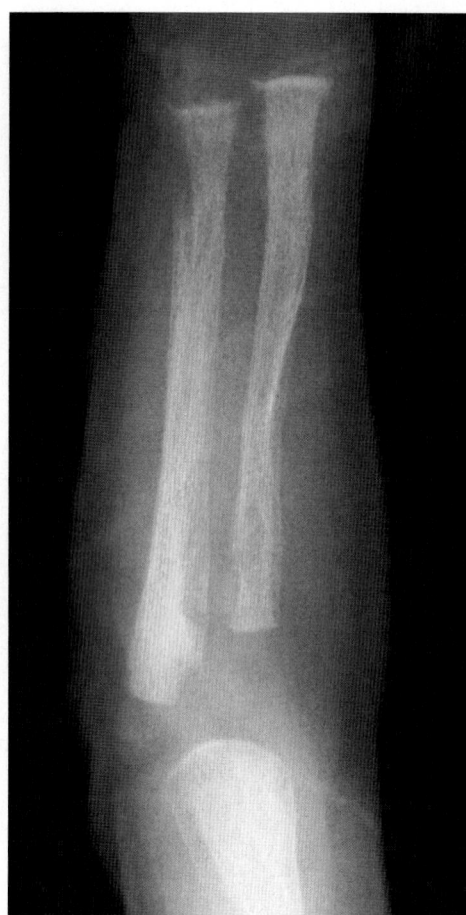

FIGURE 168-13. Mucolipidosis II (I-cell disease). Forearm in newborn shows demineralization and subperiosteal resorption indicative of hyperparathyroidism. (Case courtesy of Ron Glass, MD, New York, NY.)

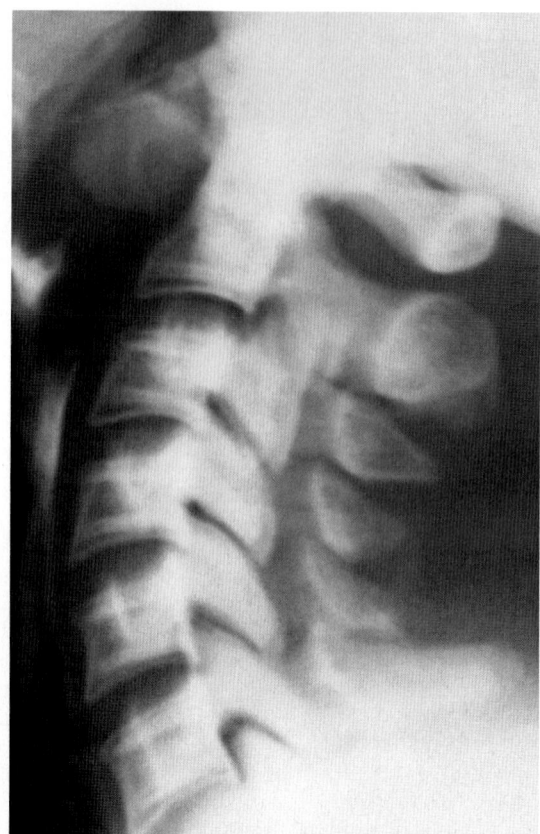

FIGURE 168-14. Idiopathic hypoparathyroidism. Bone-within-bone appearance and patchy osteosclerosis of cervical vertebrae are observed in a patient with idiopathic hypoparathyroidism.

adenosine monophosphate (cAMP) is not generated, the kidney does not respond with increased phosphate excretion, and hypocalcemia occurs. In PHP 1a, varying degrees of skeletal responsiveness to PTH may lead to skeletal manifestations of HPTH, such as subperiosteal bone resorption or slipped capital femoral epiphyses, despite hypocalcemia from renal nonresponsiveness to PTH (Fig. 168-15).

Somatic features of AHO include short stature, obesity, a round face, variable degrees of subnormal intelligence, subcutaneous calcification and ossification (Fig. 168-16), lower extremity bowing, small exostoses, and brachydactyly of the hands and feet (Fig. 168-17). In the hands, the most frequently affected bones are the thumb distal phalanx and the fourth and fifth metacarpals. The first metacarpal and other bones also may be involved. Brachydactyly is often associated with cone epiphyses and premature growth plate closure. Brachydactyly E, Turner syndrome, and acrodysostosis are differential considerations.

Pseudopseudohypoparathyroidism (PPHP), also within the spectrum of PHP 1a, is characterized by somatic features of AHO with absence of resistance to PTH and hence absence of hypocalcemia. PHP and PPHP may coexist in the same family; in some cases, this is determined by genetic imprinting with differences noted between maternal and paternal transmission of the same gene. Maternal inheritance of the *GNAS1* gene leads to resistance to PTH and the somatic features of AHO (PHP), whereas paternal transmission of the same gene leads to characteristic somatic features with absence of hormone resistance (PPHP).

> **PHP includes somatic features of AHO and hypocalcemia from PTH resistance. PPHP consists of AHO without PTH resistance. For the same gene, maternal transmission causes PHP and paternal transmission causes PPHP.**

Other combinations of hormone resistance and somatic features are also possible. PHP 1b exhibits resistance to PTH with hypocalcemia but lacks the somatic features of AHO. Patients are even more likely than those with PHP 1a to have skeletal responsiveness to PTH and manifestations of HPTH. PHP 1b is due to a tissue-specific imprinting abnormality that occurs in renal proximal tubular cells and results in effective Gsα deficiency in those cells. PHP 1c has manifestations similar to PHP 1a, but it does not have a known G-protein abnormality. In PHP 2, adenylyl cyclase is stimulated normally by the G-protein system, but inability of cyclic AMP to increase renal phosphate excretion leads to effective PTH resistance with hypocalcemia. PHP 2 lacks the somatic features of AHO.

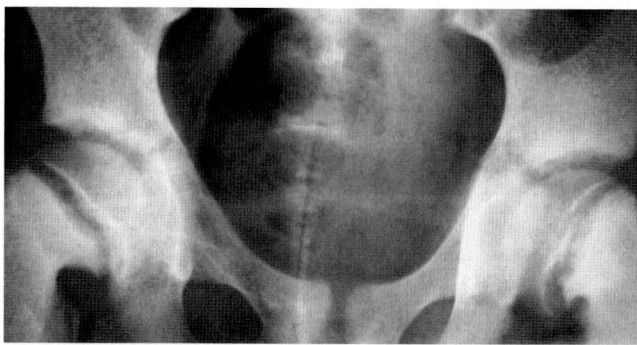

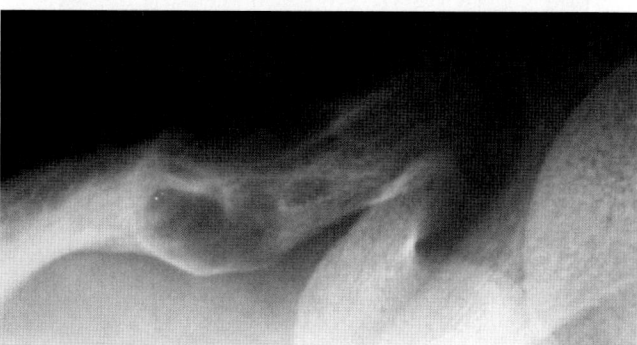

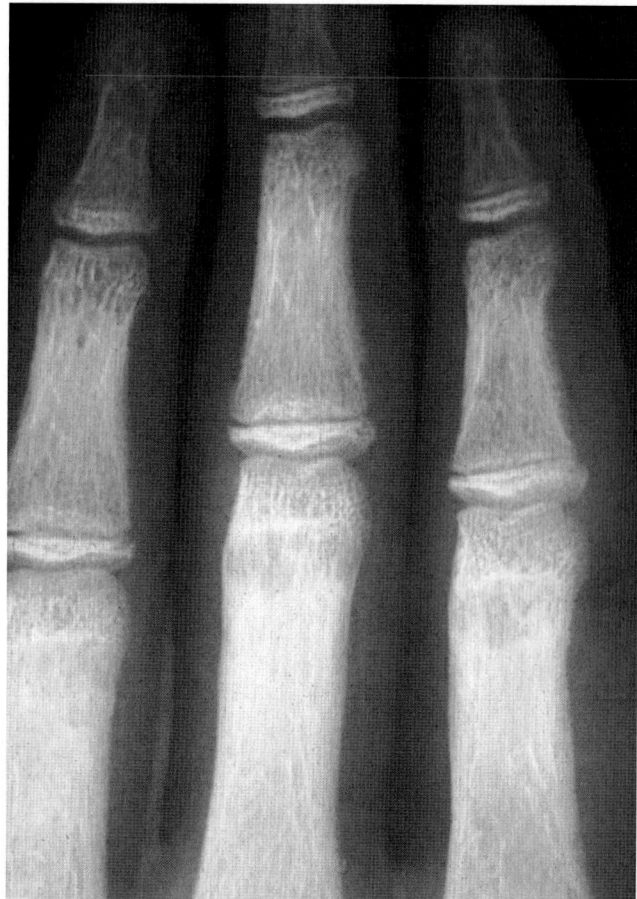

FIGURE 168-15. Pseudohypoparathyroidism with skeletal responsiveness leads to findings of hyperparathyroidism. The hips (**A**) reveal findings of hyperparathyroidism, including bilateral slipped femoral capital epiphyses combined with subphyseal lucency, representing osteitis fibrosa cystica. Phalangeal subperiosteal resorption (**B**) and a distal clavicular brown tumor (**C**) are also noted. (Case courtesy of Andrew K. Poznanski, MD, Chicago, IL.)

Although paternal transmission of a *GNAS1* mutation causes PPHP in most families, in other families, paternal transmission of the same mutation leads to progressive osseous heteroplasia (Fig. 168-18). This relatively rare disorder is characterized by heterotopic soft tissue ossification that usually begins in the subcutaneous tissues during infancy and may progress to involve deeper tissues. It is distinguished from fibrodysplasia ossificans by intramembranous rather than endochondral ossification, absence of edema and inflammation, and lack of central-to-peripheral and dorsal-to-ventral progression.

NONPARATHYROID ENDOCRINE DISORDERS

Several other endocrine disorders have important effects on skeletal development. Although these effects on bone mineralization are generally not as great as those on PTH, several disorders may have serious consequences in terms of skeletal maturation and development.

Thyroid Disorders

HYPOTHYROIDISM

Thyroid hormone is essential for normal brain development during the first 2 to 3 years of life and for normal skeletal growth and maturation until skeletal maturity is attained. Of the many endocrine disorders and other conditions that may cause retarded skeletal growth and maturation, hypothyroidism is the most severe, and maturation is even more retarded than is linear growth.

> Hypothyroidism causes a more severe delay in skeletal maturation than is caused by other endocrine disorders.

Maturation in hypothyroidism is more delayed than is linear growth as assessed by measurement of either height or second metacarpal length; in other endocrine disorders, such as growth hormone deficiency, retardation of maturation is more concordant with delayed linear growth. The development of secondary ossification centers is grossly retarded in hypothyroidism, and growth plates may remain open into adulthood. Dependence on thyroid hormone for skeletal development is less pronounced in utero; size at birth is normal, although delayed maturation is manifest at birth and becomes increasingly severe in the absence of treatment. Dental development is also delayed, although not as severely as skeletal maturation. Ossification of the epiphyses in hypothyroidism is delayed and also is often irregular, yielding a fragmented and stippled appearance referred to as *epiphyseal dysgenesis*. Instead of developing

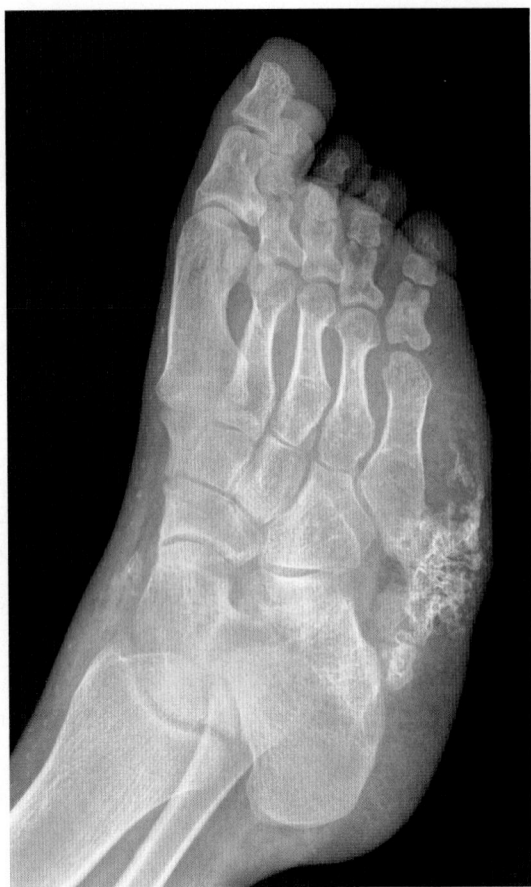

FIGURE 168-16. Pseudohypoparathyroidism in a 14-year-old with extensive heterotopic ossification along the lateral aspect of foot. Also note brachydactyly involving some of the metatarsals.

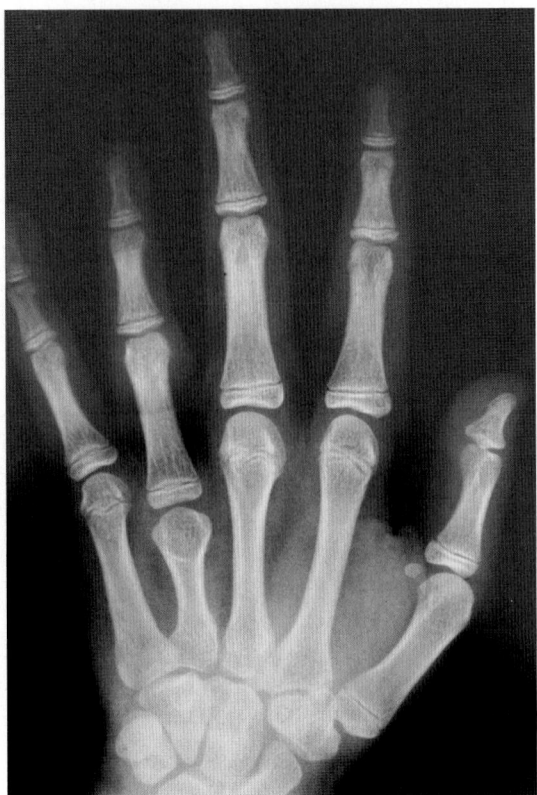

FIGURE 168-17. Brachydactyly in pseudohypoparathyroidism. Note the short thumb distal phalanx and fourth metacarpal with premature growth plate closure.

from a single focus of ossification that is followed by uniform marginal extension, as in the normal infant, ossification centers in children with hypothyroidism may begin in numerous small foci within the cartilage. Later, these grow larger and coalesce to form a single center of uneven density with irregular margins (Fig. 168-19). Other conditions also associated with fragmented-appearing epiphyses are listed in Table 168-2. Although the term "stippled" is often used for these epiphyses, the appearance is distinct from the epiphyseal puncta seen in chondrodysplasia punctata (congenital stippled epiphyses), which are associated with a different set of differential diagnoses.

Epiphyseal dysgenesis is more common in the hips than in the hands and feet. In older untreated hypothyroid patients, the metaphyses are sometimes irregularly mineralized. In hypothyroid children, the proximal femoral epiphyses may be flattened and irregularly mineralized, the neck of the femur may be broadened, and coxa vara deformity may be observed; delay in ossification of cartilage may result in features resembling those of congenital hip dislocation (Fig. 168-20). With treatment, the findings of epiphyseal dysgenesis resolve. Slipped capital femoral epiphysis (SCFE) may be a presenting manifestation of hypothyroidism; it often occurs prior to puberty (hence, younger than idiopathic SCFE) and frequently is bilateral. SCFE may occur after initiation of thyroid replacement therapy; this may be due to a transient increase in pituitary growth hormone secretion. In the skull, hypothyroidism may cause multiple Wormian bones, enlargement of the sella from pituitary hyperplasia, and brachycephaly from decreased growth at the spheno-occipital synchondrosis. Vertebrae may be short, and kyphotic deformity may be associated. Hand radiographs may show small projections of bone extending from the distal phalangeal metaphyses into the growth plates (Fig. 168-21). Additional findings of hypothyroidism include generalized osteoporosis and erosive arthritis, the latter usually seen in adults.

HYPERTHYROIDISM

Hyperthyroidism in the pediatric age range is most frequent in adolescent girls. It is extremely uncommon in infancy. Hyperthyroidism may also occur as a manifestation of McCune-Albright syndrome (polyostotic fibrous dysplasia and endocrinopathies), although precocious puberty is most frequent. Iatrogenic hyperthyroidism may result from excessive thyroid hormone therapy.

Skeletal maturation in hyperthyroidism may be normal or advanced. The degree of advancement in maturation in hyperthyroidism is usually less pronounced than that caused by excessive sex hormones. Accelerated maturation may be seen in infants born to mothers with uncontrolled hyperthyroidism during the last trimester of pregnancy. Although hyperthyroidism is uncommon in infancy, acceleration of skeletal maturation is greatest in this group and may include premature craniosynostosis.

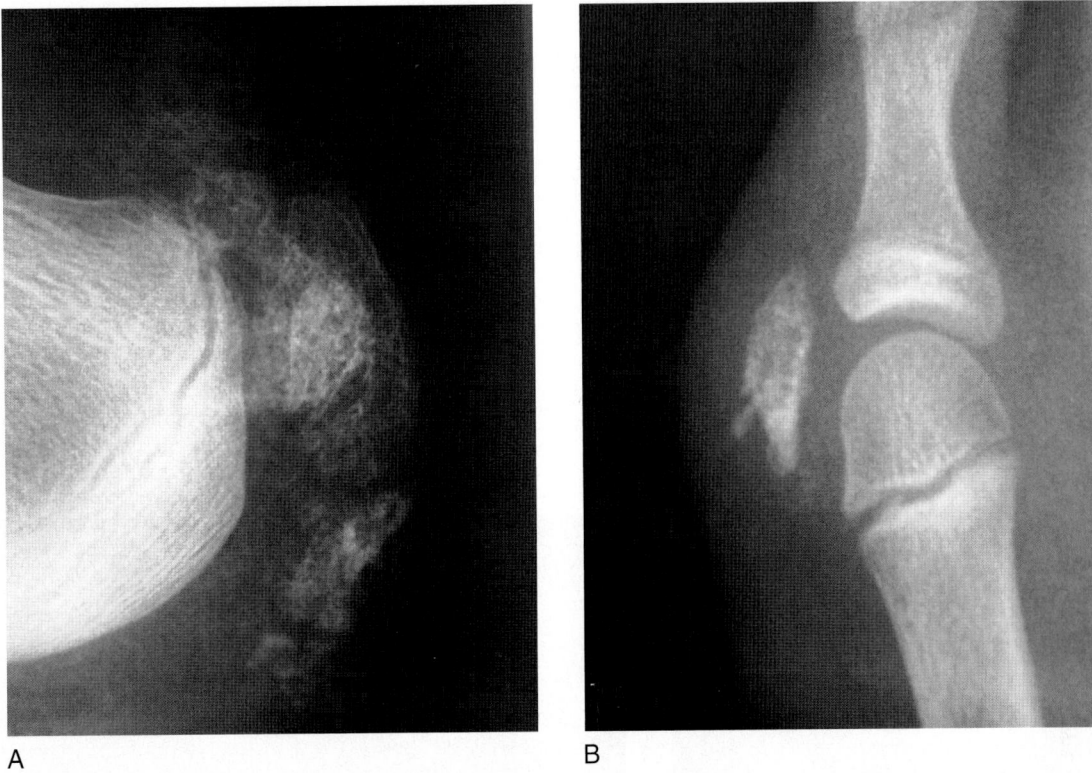

FIGURE 168-18. Progressive osseous hyperplasia in a 12-year-old with heterotopic ossification posterior to the calcaneus (**A**) and lateral to the little toe metatarsophalangeal joint (**B**) that had been present since 1 year of age.

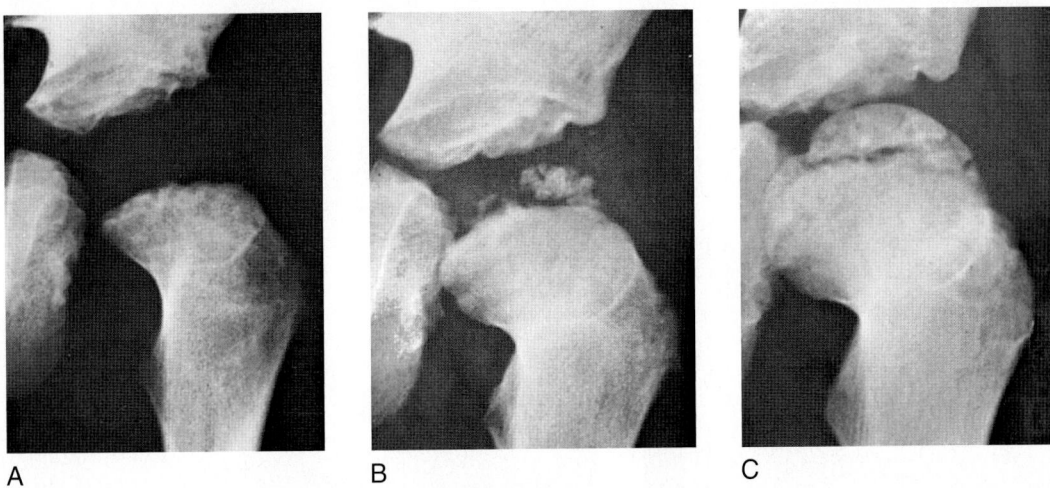

FIGURE 168-19. Epiphyseal dysgenesis in a hypothyroid girl 8 years of age. **A,** Before treatment, the proximal femoral epiphyseal center is not visible radiographically. **B,** After 1 year of treatment, at 9 years of age, an irregularly mineralized, fragmented, small femoral head has appeared. **C,** After 3 years of treatment, at 11 years of age, the femoral epiphyseal center is flattened, and the femoral neck is broadened into a coxa plana deformity. A narrow irregular strip of ossification is evident in the medial segment of the epiphyseal center. Similar changes are present in the other femur. On serial examinations, similar dysgenesis was revealed in the proximal and distal epiphyses of the humeri, the distal epiphyses of the femora, and both ends of the tibias.

Brachydactyly may result from early physeal closure. Other skeletal manifestations of hyperthyroidism include calcification of costal cartilage and tracheal rings, diffuse osteopenia, and cortical striations, which are indicative of increased bone turnover. Hyperthyroidism may mimic osteomalacia including the presence of Looser zones, although excessive nonmineralized osteoid is due to overproduction rather than impaired mineralization. Although it is predominantly an adult disorder, thyroid acropachy may be seen in adolescents. This condition manifests clinically as exophthalmos, pretibial myxedema, clubbing, and soft tissue swelling of the distal extremities. Radiographically, periosteal new bone most often is seen to involve the metacarpals, metatarsals, and proximal and middle phalanges. This periosteal new bone often has a spiculated or feathery appearance, which contrasts with the more linear appearance of most other conditions.

TABLE 168-2

Irregular Fragmented Epiphyseal Ossification Centers

Normal variant
Hypothyroidism
Multiple epiphyseal dysplasia
Spondyloepiphyseal dysplasia
Avascular necrosis
Trisomy 21
Mucopolysaccharidoses
Stickler syndrome (hereditary arthro-ophthalmopathy)
Osteopoikilosis
Osteopathia striata
Dysplasia epiphysialis hemimelica (Trevor disease)

Growth Hormone Disorders

Growth hormone is an important positive regulator of postnatal longitudinal growth; it acts directly and indirectly, through insulin-like growth factor (IGF)-I, to stimulate proliferation of physeal chondrocytes. Prenatally, growth is more dependent on IGF-II, a fact that accounts for the relative preservation of prenatal growth in growth hormone deficiency. Growth hormone also stimulates endosteal and periosteal bone formation; this accounts for acromegaly that occurs after skeletal maturity is attained.

GROWTH HORMONE DEFICIENCY

Growth hormone deficiency causes decreased skeletal linear growth and maturation. In isolated growth

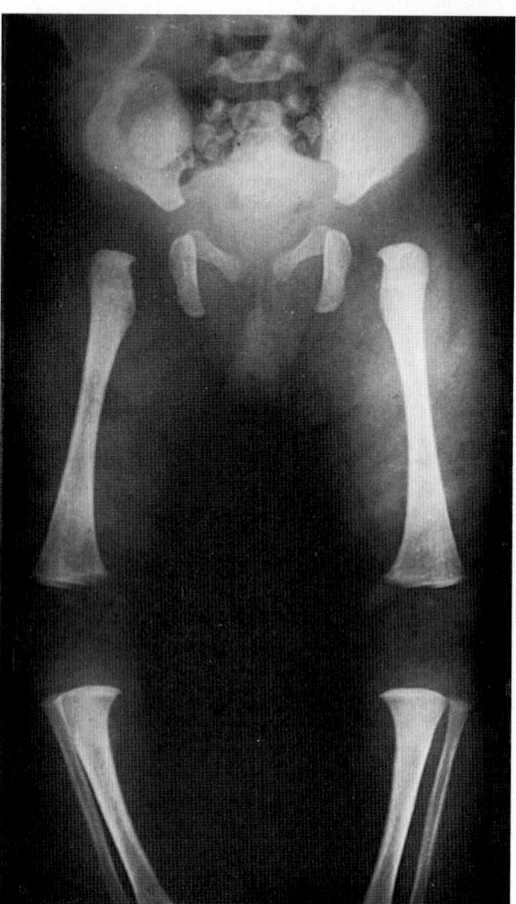

A

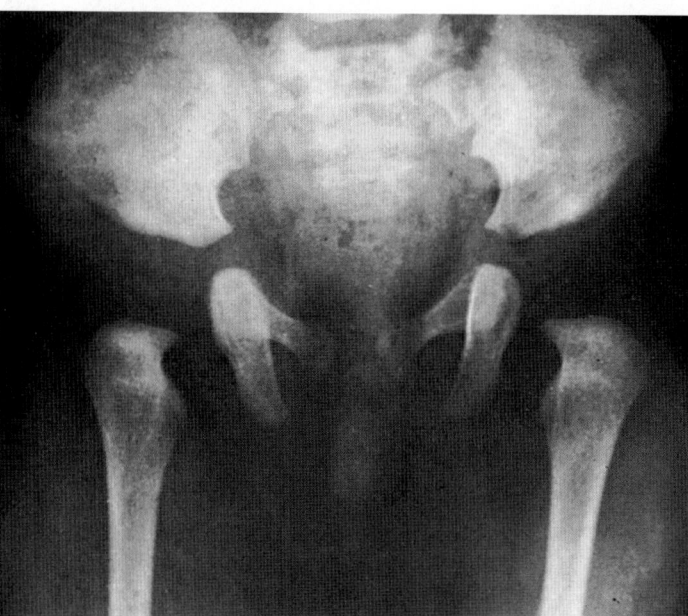

B

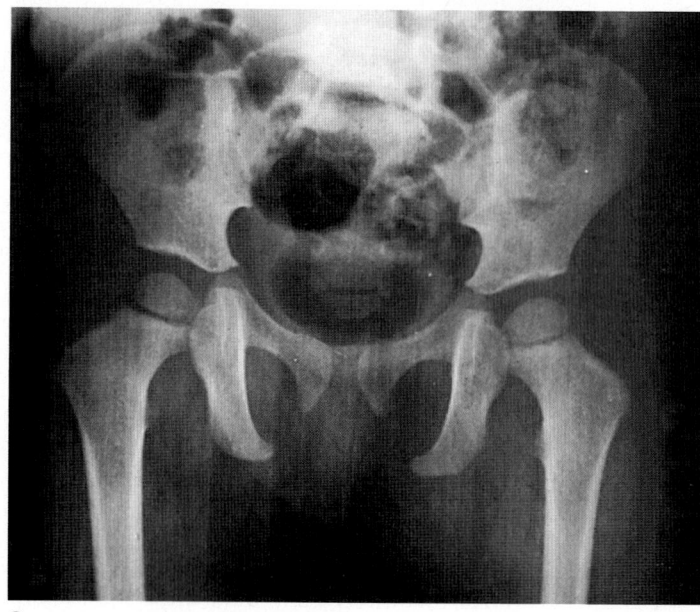

C

FIGURE 168-20. Hypothyroidism simulating congenital dislocation of the hips on radiographs. **A,** Apparent dislocation at the time of diagnosis at 4 months. Delayed ossification of the acetabular roofs accounts for the resemblance to acetabular dysplasia. **B** and **C,** "Spontaneous recovery" with thyroid medication alone at 9 and 30 months, respectively. (From Silverman FN, Currarino G: Roentgen manifestations of hereditary metabolic diseases in childhood. Metabolism 1960;9:248-283.)

hormone deficiency, the degree of retarded maturation is less pronounced than in hypothyroidism. Carpal maturation is often more delayed than maturation of the phalanges. SCFE may be seen with growth hormone deficiency prior to or after completion of growth hormone therapy. Similar to hypothyroidism, this

condition is often bilateral and is more frequently seen in younger patients than is idiopathic SCFE. The retarded growth and maturation of growth hormone deficiency may be mimicked by deprivational dwarfism ("psychosocial dwarfism"). The presence of multiple growth restart lines favors a diagnosis of deprivational dwarfism; this likely reflects the intermittent growth that occurs with alternating periods of nutritional sufficiency and insufficiency (Fig. 168-22).

> Deprivational dwarfism, which may simulate growth hormone deficiency, should be suspected by the presence of multiple growth restart lines.

GROWTH HORMONE EXCESS

Prior to skeletal maturity, growth hormone excess causes gigantism with increased linear growth. After physeal closure has occurred, increased appositional growth leads to acromegaly.

Gigantism due to growth hormone excess prior to skeletal maturity is relatively rare. Most cases are due to an isolated pituitary adenoma. Approximately 20% of cases of gigantism are associated with McCune-Albright syndrome (polyostotic fibrous dysplasia and endocrin-

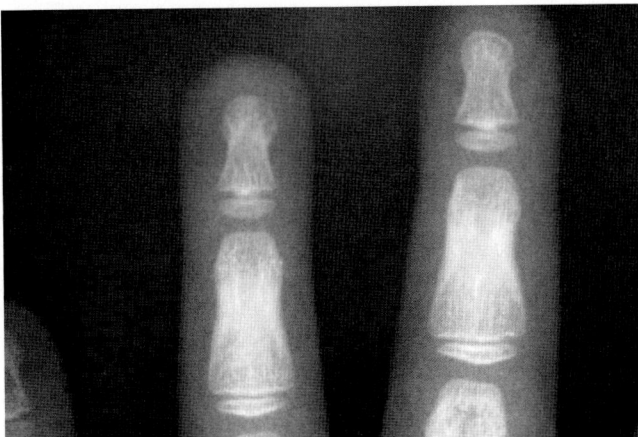

FIGURE 168-21. Hypothyroidism in an 11-year-old boy. Small spikelike projections of bone extend into the growth plates from the distal phalangeal metaphyses.

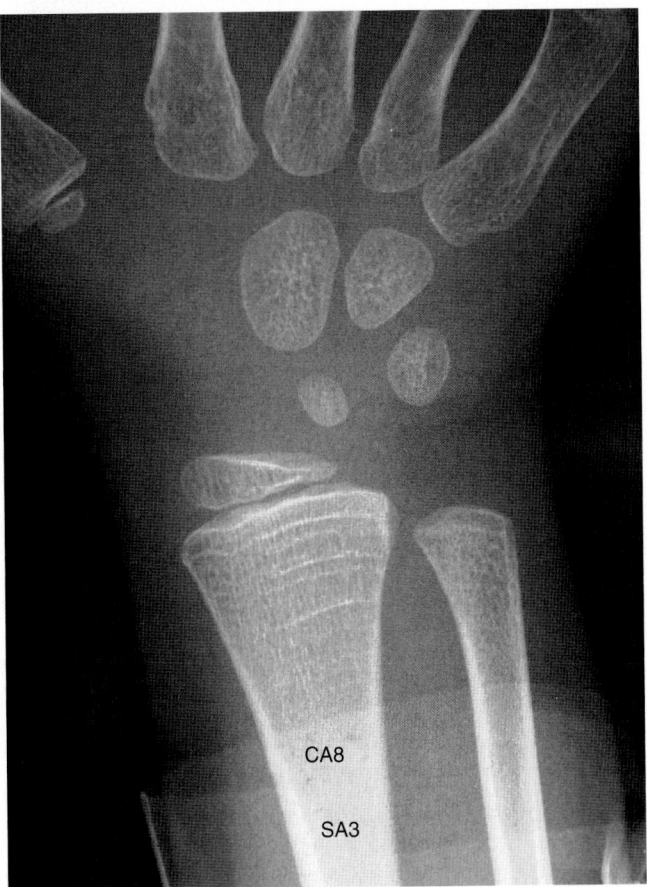
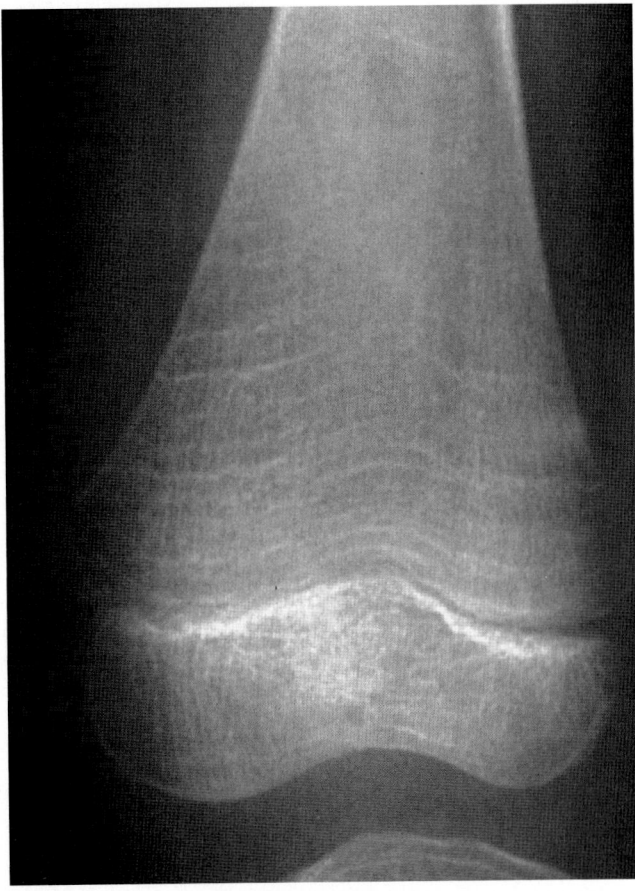

FIGURE 168-22. Deprivational dwarfism. The hand (**A**) reveals severely delayed skeletal maturation with a skeletal age of 3 years (SA3). Chronologic age was 8 years (CA8). **B,** Multiple growth restart lines in the distal radius and the distal femur. (Case courtesy of Andrew K. Poznanski, MD, Chicago, IL.)

opathy), with growth hormone excess due to either adenoma or hyperplasia. Linear growth is increased and body proportions are normal. In most cases, skeletal maturation is normal. With increased linear growth and advanced skeletal maturation, other endocrinopathies should be considered, such as excessive gonadal or adrenal androgens.

After skeletal maturity has been attained, increased growth hormone and IGF-I lead to increased periosteal bone formation, reactivation of endochondral bone formation at chondro-osseous junctions, and cartilage and soft tissue hypertrophy. These processes lead to acromegaly, which is predominantly an adult disorder but may rarely be seen in children. Enlargement of bone and soft tissue is particularly prominent in the hands and feet, as suggested by the designation of acromegaly. The face is also involved with enlargement of the jaw, prominence of the forehead, large paranasal sinuses, and coarse facial features. Tubular bones are thickened by subperiosteal bone formation, and excrescences arise from the trochanters and tuberosities through subtendinous and subligamentous bone formation. Enlargement of the terminal tufts is characteristic. Reactivation of endochondral bone formation at the costochondral junctions may produce an "acromegalic rosary." Proliferation of hyaline cartilage and fibrocartilage may lead to arthropathy in acromegaly. Spinal findings include enlargement of transverse and anteroposterior (AP) diameters of the vertebrae and osteophytosis. A more complete description of the radiographic findings in acromegaly can be found in textbooks on adult skeletal radiology.

Adrenal Disorders

Adrenal cortical disorders with radiographic abnormalities that occur in children include Cushing syndrome (glucocorticoid excess) and adrenogenital syndrome. Pheochromocytoma, arising in the adrenal medulla, may also exhibit skeletal findings.

CUSHING SYNDROME

The term *Cushing syndrome* has come to be used to describe the many manifestations of glucocorticoid excess, whereas *Cushing disease* refers specifically to adrenal cortical hyperfunction caused by an adrenocorticotropic hormone (ACTH)-secreting pituitary adenoma. Most cases of Cushing syndrome in children are iatrogenic and result from pharmacologic dosages of glucocorticoids used for treatment of chronic inflammatory or autoimmune disorders. Endogenous Cushing syndrome may result from a primary adrenal cortical lesion such as carcinoma, adenoma, or hyperplasia, or it may be caused by increased ACTH, usually resulting from a pituitary adenoma. In infancy, most cases are due to primary adrenal lesions, whereas beyond 5 years of age, pituitary lesions predominate.

Glucocorticoids have many effects on the skeleton. In children, they decrease linear growth and maturation, acting at multiple levels to negatively regulate physeal chondrogenesis by decreasing growth hormone secretion and downregulating growth hormone and IGF-I

receptors in growth plate chondrocytes. Glucocorticoids also impair skeletal mineralization in children and adults through systemic effects and by direct action on bone. Systemically, glucocorticoids decrease sex hormone secretion and hence negate the positive influence of sex steroids on mineralization. They also decrease absorption of calcium in the gut, an effect that is partially independent of vitamin D, resulting in negative calcium balance and subsequent 2° HPTH. Direct actions of glucocorticoids on bone include decreasing bone formation and increasing resorption. Decreased bone formation is the result of reduced osteoblast replication, increased osteoblast apoptosis, and decreased synthesis of organic bone matrix. Increased bone resorption results from increased expression of RANKL (receptor activator of NF-κB ligand) and decreased expression of osteoprotegerin.

Osteonecrosis is an additional complication of endogenous or exogenous glucocorticoid excess. The pathogenesis of glucocorticoid-induced osteonecrosis is not well understood; potential mechanisms include compromise of intraosseous perfusion caused by increased intraosseous pressure from fat deposition in marrow, fat embolization resulting from fatty liver, and increased blood viscosity. Trabecular microfractures related to osteopenia may also be contributory.

Skeletal radiographic findings are similar in endogenous and exogenous corticosteroid excess. Major findings are nonspecific and are related to generalized osteopenia with cortical thinning, trabecular rarefaction, and vertebral compression fracture. In addition, more specific findings include sclerosis of the vertebral end plates (Fig. 168-23), abundant formation of callus at fracture sites, and osteonecrosis. Excessive callous formation associated with compression fractures of vertebral bodies probably accounts for sclerosis along their end plates and is an important clue in the diagnosis of Cushing's syndrome in a patient with osteopenia. Osteonecrosis caused by endogenous or exogenous steroids most frequently involves the femoral head, with the humeral head and the femoral condyles being next in frequency. Radiographic findings include subcortical fracture, bone collapse, fragmentation, and patchy osteosclerosis. It has been suggested that "steroid osteopathy" is different from other forms of avascular necrosis such as Perthes disease, in that it often does not go through a phase during which the femoral head is morphologically normal yet avascular, as would be demonstrated by "coldness" on scintigraphy or lack of enhancement with gadolinium on magnetic resonance imaging (MRI). However, this may be related to a more patchy distribution of the process rather than to a fundamental difference in pathology.

ADRENOGENITAL SYNDROME AND OTHER CAUSES OF ADRENAL ANDROGEN EXCESS

Adrenogenital syndrome is caused by a biosynthetic defect in the production of cortisol that leads to a compensatory increase in ACTH secretion and increased production of adrenal androgens. Although they are weaker than testosterone, adrenal androgens cause virilization prenatally and postnatally, which is more apparent in females than in males. The presence of these

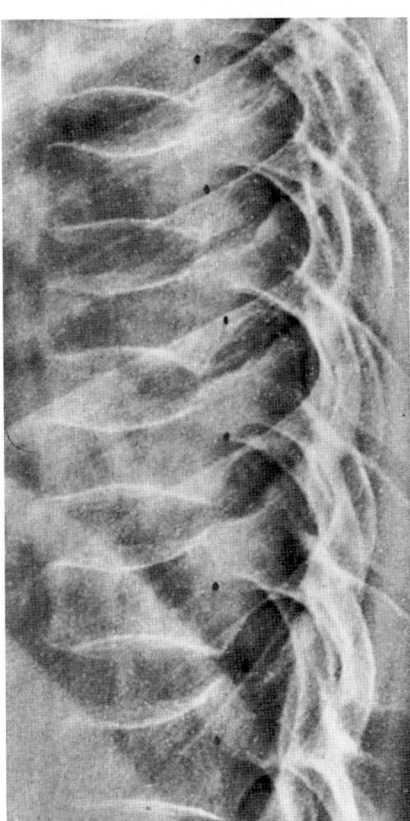

FIGURE 168-23. Diffuse osteopenia and multiple biconcave vertebral compression fractures in a 13-year-old given long-term glucocorticoid therapy for juvenile rheumatoid arthritis. Mild end plate sclerosis is noted.

androgens also leads to accelerated skeletal maturation—the only skeletal finding in this disorder. Although growth is initially accelerated, this effect is less pronounced than is advancement of maturation; therefore, physeal closure occurs prematurely, and final height is decreased rather than increased. Excessive amounts of adrenal androgens may also be secreted by adrenal cortical neoplasms. Advancement of skeletal maturation due to excessive androgens is more pronounced than that due to hyperthyroidism.

Pheochromocytoma

Pheochromocytoma, a tumor of neuroendocrine origin, most frequently arises in the adrenal medulla, although it may also occur in the sympathetic chain, the organ of Zuckerkandl or, occasionally, in neuroendocrine tissue in the bladder. These tumors have been associated with multiple sclerotic metaphyseal lesions that resolved after the pheochromocytoma was removed. Skeletal findings are believed to represent infarcts caused by hemoconcentration and microthrombi caused by excessive catecholamine production.

Gonadal Disorders

Gonadal tumors that cause increased production of androgens and estrogens may lead to acceleration of skeletal maturation, whereas gonadal insufficiency may delay maturation. It was previously thought that skeletal maturation is normally mediated by estrogens in females and androgens in males. However, recent data suggest that estrogens are responsible for adequate bone mineral development and physeal fusion and for completion of skeletal maturation, and that these processes are mediated in males by estrogens formed from peripheral conversion of androgens. This has been supported by the case of a male patient with an estrogen receptor–inactivating mutation who had severe osteopenia and delayed physeal closure, along with continued linear growth, well into adulthood.

SUGGESTED READINGS

Hyperparathyroidism and Renal Osteodystrophy

Andreoli SP, Smith JA, Bergstein JM: Aluminum bone disease in children: radiographic features from diagnosis to resolution. Radiology 1985;156:663-667

Goodman WG, Coburn JW, Slatopolsky E, et al: Renal osteodystrophy in children and adults. *In* Favis MJ (ed): Primer on the Metabolic Bone Diseases and Disorders of Mineral Metabolism, 5th ed. Washington, DC, American Society for Bone and Mineral Research, 2003:430-447

Pugh DG: Subperiosteal resorption of bone: roentgenologic manifestation of primary hyperparathyroidism and renal osteodystrophy. Am J Roentgenol Radium Ther Nucl Med 1951;66:577-586

Resnick D, Niwayama G: Parathyroid disorders and renal osteodystrophy. *In* Resnick D (ed): Diagnosis of Bone and Joint Disorders, 4th ed. Philadelphia, WB Saunders, 2002:2043-2111

Sedman A: Aluminum toxicity in childhood. Pediatr Nephrol 1992;6:383-393

Teplick JG, Eftekhari F, Haskin ME: Erosion of the sternal ends of the clavicles: a new sign of primary and secondary hyperparathyroidism. Radiology 1974;113:323-326

Neonatal Hypercalcemic, Hyperparathyroid, and Related Conditions

Aarskog D, Akanes L, Markistad T: Vitamin D metabolism in idiopathic infantile hypercalcemia. Am J Dis Child 1981;135:1021-1024

Aceto T Jr, Ball RE, Bruck ER, et al: Intra-uterine fetal hyperparathyroidism: a complication of untreated maternal hypoparathyroidism. J Clin Endocrinol 1966;26:487-492

Black JA, Bonham-Carter RE: Association between aortic stenosis and facies of severe infantile hypercalcemia. Lancet 1963;2:745-749

Eftekhari F, Yousefzadeh DK: Primary infantile hyperparathyroidism: clinical, laboratory and radiographic features in 21 cases. Skeletal Radiol 1982;8:201-208

Langman CB: Hypercalcemic syndromes in infants and children. *In* Favis MJ (ed): Primer on the Metabolic Bone Diseases and Disorders of Mineral Metabolism, 5th ed. Washington, DC, American Society for Bone and Mineral Research, 2003:267-270

Marx SJ: Familial hypocalciuric hypercalcemia. *In* Favis MJ (ed): Primer on the Metabolic Bone Diseases and Disorders of Mineral Metabolism, 5th ed. Washington, DC, American Society for Bone and Mineral Research, 2003:239-242

Unger S, Paul DA, Nino MC, et al: Mucolipidosis II presenting as severe neonatal hyperparathyroidism. Eur J Pediatr 2005;164:236-243

Hypoparathyroidism and Pseudohypoparathyroidism

Burnstein MI, Kottamasu SR, Peffifor JM, et al: Metabolic bone disease in pseudohypoparathyroidism: radiologic features. Radiology 1985;155:351-356

DiGeorge AM: Congenital absence of the thymus and its immunologic consequences: concurrence with congenital hypoparathyroidism. Birth Defects 1968;4:116-123

Frame B, Hanson CA, Frost HM, et al: Renal resistance to parathyroid hormone with osteitis fibrosa: pseudohypohyperparathyroidism. Am J Med 1972;52:311-321

Levine MA: Parathyroid hormone resistance syndromes. *In* Favis MJ (ed): Primer on the Metabolic Bone Diseases and Disorders of

Mineral Metabolism, 5th ed. Washington, DC, American Society for Bone and Mineral Research, 2003:278-285

Schipani E, Langman CB, Parfitt AM, et al: Constitutively activated receptors for parathyroid hormone and parathyroid hormone–related peptide in Jansen's metaphyseal chondrodysplasia. N Engl J Med 1996;335:708-714

Spiegel AM, Weinstein LS: Inherited diseases involving G proteins and G protein–coupled receptors. Annu Rev Med 2004;55:27-39

Steinbach HL, Rudhe U, Jonsson M, et al: Evolution of skeletal lesions in pseudohypoparathyroidism. Radiology 1965;85:670-676

Weinstein LS, Liu J, Sakamoto A, et al: Minireview: GNAS: normal and abnormal functions. Endocrinology 2004;145:5459-5464

Weinstein LS, Yu S, Warner DR, et al: Endocrine manifestations of stimulatory G protein alpha-subunit mutations and the role of genomic imprinting. Endocr Rev 2001;22:675-705

Wells TR, Gilsanz V, Senac MO Jr, et al: Ossification centre of the hyoid bone in DiGeorge syndrome and tetralogy of Fallot. Br J Radiol 1986;59:1065-1068

Other Endocrine Disorders

Becker MH, Redisch W, Messina EJ: Bone and microcirculatory changes in a child with benign pheochromocytoma. Radiology 1967;88:487-490

Bonakdarpour A, Kirkpatrick JA, Renzi A, et al: Skeletal changes in neonatal thyrotoxicosis. Radiology 1972;102:149-150

Hernandez R, Poznanski AK, Kelch RP, et al: Hand radiographic measurements in growth hormone deficiency before and after treatment. AJR Am J Roentgenol 1977;129:487-492

Hernandez RJ, Poznanski AK: Distinctive appearance of the distal phalanges in children with primary hypothyroidism. Radiology 1979;132:83-84

Hernandez RJ, Poznanski AW, Hopwood NJ: Size and skeletal maturation of the hand in children with hypothyroidism and hypopituitarism. AJR Am J Roentgenol 1979;133:405-408

Heyerman W, Weiner D: Slipped epiphysis associated with hypothyroidism. J Pediatr Orthop 1984;4:569-573

Lang EK, Bessler WT: The roentgenologic features of acromegaly. Am J Roentgenol Radium Ther Nucl Med 1961;86:321-361

Murray RO: Steroids and the skeleton. Radiology 1961;77:729

Resnick D: Pituitary disorders. In Resnick D (ed): Diagnosis of Bone and Joint Disorders, 4th ed. Philadelphia, WB Saunders, 2002:2003-2025

Resnick D: Thyroid disorders. In Resnick D (ed): Diagnosis of Bone and Joint Disorders, 4th ed. Philadelphia, WB Saunders, 2002:2026-2042

Riggs W Jr, Wilroy RS Jr, Etteldorf JN: Neonatal hyperthyroidism with accelerated skeletal maturation, craniostenosis and brachydactyly. Radiology 1972;105:621-625

Schlesinger B, Fisher OD: Accelerated skeletal development from thyrotoxicosis and thyroid overdosage in childhood. Lancet 1951;2:289-290

Silverman FN, Currarino G: Roentgen manifestations of hereditary metabolic diseases in childhood. Metabolism 1960;9:248-283

van der Eerden BCJ, Marperien M, Wit JM: Systemic and local regulation of the growth plate. Endocr Rev 2003;24:782-801

CHAPTER 169

Bone Mineral Density Assessment

SUE C. KASTE

OVERVIEW

Skeletal health in adulthood is dependent on skeletal health during childhood and adolescence. Thus, the rapidly growing "epidemic" of osteoporosis in adults is likely initiated in childhood. If maximal peak bone mass, an important determinant of osteoporosis and fracture associated with aging, is not achieved, then the risk of adult-onset bone mineral density (BMD) deficits rises. In normal individuals, bone mass rises rapidly during puberty in concert with skeletal growth. BMD usually reaches its peak at the end of sexual development. Therefore, children with chronic diseases, those who undergo cancer treatment, and those with physical handicaps that limit weight bearing during the normal period of maximal bone mass accrual are at risk for future deficits in BMD and associated sequelae.

ANATOMY AND PHYSIOLOGY

The development of skeletal integrity is a dynamic process that occurs throughout life and depends upon a delicate balance between bone resorption by osteoclasts and bone deposition by osteoblasts. This process is also balanced between modeling and remodeling; the former predominates during growth and development, and the latter occurs throughout life. Modeling forms new bone at sites distant from bone resorption and results in increased bone mass, a changing configuration of the bone, and increased size. In contrast, remodeling does not affect the configuration or size of the bone but rather serves to repair microdamage and maintain skeletal integrity.

Although 70% to 80% of BMD is genetically determined, the 20% associated with environmental and lifestyle factors can be significant; these determinants include smoking, weight-bearing exercise or lack thereof, nutritional status, body habitus, long-term medications, and chronic diseases.

At birth, skeletal calcium on average weighs about 25 g; its weight increases to 900 g in adult women and 1200 g in adult men. Approximately 80% of skeletal bone mass is composed of cortical bone, whose primary functions include support and protection of subjacent structures. The remaining 20% of bone mass comprises the more metabolically active trabecular bone, which serves as a repository of available calcium. The density

of cortical bone in the appendicular skeleton remains relatively constant throughout life in the normal individual, regardless of age, gender, and race, but its thickness increases significantly. Lumbar spine trabecular density increases during puberty. To support skeletal growth during childhood and adolescence, a positive calcium balance must be maintained. Interference with a positive balance caused by inactivity, medications, chronic diseases, endocrine dysfunction, and other factors can lead to diminished accretion of bone mass and potentially places these young adults at earlier and greater risk for BMD deficits, osteoporosis, and insufficiency fractures in adulthood.

The distribution of trabecular and cortical bone varies anatomically. In the spine and proximal femur, trabecular bone accounts for about 70% and 50% of total bone, respectively. The midshaft of the long bones consists of cortical bone, almost exclusively. Thus, accurate assessment of BMD must take into account the anatomic location evaluated, as well as the changing morphology of the skeleton during growth and maturation.

> Accurate BMD assessment must take into account the anatomic location and the changing morphology of the growing skeleton.

Peak BMD occurs during early adulthood, and maximum BMD accretion occurs during adolescence and peaks during the late 20s. Thus, children and adolescents with chronic diseases, genetic defects, physical handicaps, compromised nutritional status, and other processes that can compromise bone mineral accretion should be monitored for BMD deficits (Table 169-1). Amelioration of such deficits requires identification and timely intervention.

CRITERION FOR BONE MINERAL DENSITY CHARACTERIZATION

The established criterion for a diagnosis of osteopenia or osteoporosis, which reflects the risk of fracture for a given BMD in postmenopausal women, was established by the World Health Organization (WHO) [56 National Osteoporosis Foundation 1998]. In this categorization, a T-score (i.e., BMD comparison between an individual

TABLE 169-1

Pediatric Patient Cohorts for Whom Monitoring of Bone Mineral Density Is Valuable

Survivors of childhood cancer and those with the following:
- Cerebral palsy
- Long-term steroid use
  - Asthma
  - Crohn disease
- Endocrinopathy
  - Growth hormone deficiency
  - Hypogonadism
  - Hypothyroidism and hyperthyroidism
- Chronic renal failure
- Rickets
- Osteoporosis
- Defects in bone formation
  - Osteogenesis imperfecta
  - Homocystinuria
  - Galactosemia
  - Some chondrodyplasias
  - Menkes syndrome

and maximum adult BMD) from −1 to −2.5 is considered to indicate osteopenia; a T-score that is more than 2.5 standard deviations (SDs) below the mean reveals osteoporosis. Therefore, terminology and classification bear little semblance to skeletal health in children. For these reasons, Z-scores (BMD comparisons between an individual and age- and gender-matched healthy peers) are the appropriate variable to be used in pediatrics. In contrast to the established fracture risk in adults, no association has been identified in children and adolescents for a given BMD.

> **Z-scores (not T-scores) are used for BMD comparison in children and adolescents.**

Previously, no consensus had been reached on the Z-score threshold that best reflects low bone mineral density in pediatric patients. Recently, the International Society for Clinical Densitometry (ISCD) suggested that the term "low bone density for chronological age" should be applied to children whose Z-scores are less than −2 SD. As alluded to here, skeletal strength is dependent on more than just bone mass. It also depends on bone "quality," configuration, and size. These aspects are difficult to define and are more difficult to measure, but they likely account for the ability of a young child to fall from the same height as a postmenopausal woman without fracture. Such a fall would likely result in a hip or wrist fracture in the adult woman; however, the child would be less likely to fracture.

> **No correlation between BMD and fracture risk has yet been identified in pediatric patients; this suggests the importance of "bone quality" and "bone quantity."**

IMAGING METHODS

Bone mass can be determined only by direct measurement. Numerous methods have evolved over decades and through technological advancements. Most methods are based on absorptiometric techniques of beam attenuation that reflect the characteristics of the tissues interrogated. Thus, the accuracy of most BMD techniques varies with the tissues examined and the surrounding milieu.

The leading methods of assessing bone mineral density consist of quantitative computed tomography (QCT) and dual x-ray absorptiometry (DXA); DXA is more widely used. With both of these methods, clinical treatment decisions for pediatric patients are typically based on standard deviation or Z-scores, which, despite their limitations, allow comparison of individual BMD values versus age- and gender-matched normative values. Values for peak BMD and BMD throughout life appear to be higher in African Americans than in Caucasians; the Z-scores of non-Caucasian patients are likely to be higher on QCT than on DXA because Z-scores determined by QCT are derived with the use of BMD normative data for Caucasians. Clinicians who make treatment decisions must remember the distinction between these two modalities. Clinicians should not assume that Z-scores obtained by QCT and DXA are equivalent in pediatric populations. It is important that clinicians consider the complexity of BMD assessment, particularly in growing children, so they can use the information gained for the maximal benefit of individual patients.

> **Accurate BMD assessment must include consideration of the modality used and the impact of patient race on assessment.**

A low areal (two-dimensional) BMD has a well-documented association with risk of fracture in postmenopausal women, but such a relationship has not been definitively established in healthy children. Most but not all studies suggest that BMD as measured by DXA is lower in children who have low-energy fractures than in others. In contrast, DXA measurements (including absolute BMD, Z-score, and calculated bone mineral apparent density [BMAD]) are suggested to be a weak predictor of fracture in children with acute lymphoblastic leukemia (ALL).

Dual X-ray Absorptiometry

DXA, which is available worldwide, is the most common means of assessing bone mass. It may be used to assess the bone mass of the whole body or of individual anatomic compartments and can provide values for variables of body composition. Because DXA assessment depends partially on bone size, its use in growing children is especially challenging.

This two-dimensional method provides values for "areal" BMD; changes in the third dimension are not accounted for. It has been suggested that calculation of apparent volumetric BMD of the lumbar spine (BMAD) more accurately reflects the BMD of growing children and adolescents. This disadvantage is an important consideration in growing children. When only two dimensions are measured on DXA, the volumetric BMD (BMAD) is calculated with the following formula: BMAD = Bone mineral content (BMC) ÷ (Area of lumbar vertebral bodies in cm^2). Other formulas have been suggested for reconstructing DXA-derived volumetric BMAD, which is less dependent on bone size than on areal BMD. The dependence of DXA-derived areal BMD on body size is a well-known limitation of this method that might become especially important in children who are at risk for abnormal linear growth. Normative values in the manufacturer's reference database are used to calculate the Z-score, which is generated by the DXA software program. A patient's bone mineral status is defined by its deviation from the mean age- and sex-matched reference value (i.e., the Z-score). DXA also defines bone mineral status by comparing values with race-matched references.

In addition to the fact that DXA is a two-dimensional measurement, disadvantages of its use include lack of differentiation between cortical and trabecular bone, attenuating effects of overlying soft tissues and fat on BMD measurement, and sensitivity to artifacts and scoliosis. Cross-calibration of DXA units is needed to accurately compare values obtained on different machines. One longitudinal study reported a reduction in BMC during the first 6 months of chemotherapy in patients with ALL; this variable had a 64% positive predictive value for fracture, whereas increased BMC had a negative predictive value of 82% for subsequent fracture.

Quantitative Computed Tomography

BMD values determined by QCT are true volumetric measures that are independent of bone size. Because these readings are not influenced by bone size, this is a particularly valuable method in growing children. QCT can differentiate trabecular from cortical bone, while providing additional information regarding bone health. Although standard software includes reference values for the lumbar spine, assessment of the appendicular skeleton also may be performed. Affordable QCT software can be installed on most computed tomography (CT) scanners. QCT of the lumbar spine is typically performed by obtaining direct axial images of the centers of the first and second lumbar vertebrae (L1 and L2, respectively) as localized from a sagittal scout image, as was previously described. BMD (mg/cm^3) is recorded for individual vertebral bodies, and the mean value is calculated by vendor software. Normative values in the manufacturer's reference database provide calculated Z-scores, which are generated by the QCT software program.

Software has been developed to determine hip BMD, but this method is seldom used in pediatrics. The most important advantage of QCT use in children is that measures of BMD are volumetric and are independent of bone size. QCT can also differentiate the metabolically more active trabecular bone from cortical bone, providing additional useful information regarding bone

health status. Affordable QCT software can be installed on most CT scanners, but the initial costs of CT scanners and of support staff limit its availability. Radiation dose is low for both modalities and falls considerably below background exposure.

The relationship between DXA and QCT methods used to assess BMD in young patients has not been extensively studied. In clinical practice, both methods are used, sometimes in the same patient, making it difficult for clinicians to interpret longitudinal changes in BMD and to assess the effectiveness of treatment.

Peripheral QCT

Peripheral QCT (pQCT) is growing in popularity and acceptance as an independent imaging modality for assessing BMD. This method is considerably less costly to install than QCT, and because it images the extremities (usually the radius or tibia), added radiation exposure to the trunk is avoided. This high-resolution technique allows calculation of trabecular and cortical compartments through measurement at two different sites. The distalmost radius and tibia are made up predominantly of cortical bone, whereas the midshafts consist primarily of trabecular bone. Density is estimated through attenuation of the x-ray beam by body tissues. Cortical and trabecular components are calculated from cross-sectional area and scan thickness. Bone strength can also be calculated from QCT parameters. Normative values of 371 German youths and young adults have been published. Despite the lack of normative pediatric values, BMD assessment with the use of pQCT can be valuable for comparison of patient cohorts.

Quantitative Ultrasonography

Similar to routine clinical ultrasonography, broadband quantitative ultrasonography (QUS) is particularly attractive in pediatrics because of its portability and lack of ionizing radiation. Ultrasound determination of bone density is based on soft tissue attenuation of interrogated tissue, which typically consists of the calcaneus, proximal tibia, or phalanges. In contrast to more standard ultrasound technology, QUS uses frequencies in the range of 0.1 to 1 MHz. Current QUS units typically target specific anatomic sites; therefore, information obtained from one system is not translatable to other systems. QUS has been shown prospectively to discriminate between normal and osteoporotic adults. Toward that end, QUS incorporates information attributable to bone quality with information related to bone quantity. Results may vary significantly depending on the main orientation of interrogated trabeculae. Technological development and validation of QUS variables are ongoing.

Magnetic Resonance Imaging

Similar to ultrasonography (US), magnetic resonance imaging (MRI) is an enticing modality for pediatric imaging because of its lack of ionizing radiation. However, such examinations are expensive, and sedation of the patient may be necessary for completion of the study.

Experience with MRI-determined BMD assessment, particularly in pediatrics, is thus far limited, as are available normative reference values. However, numerous publications on adult cohorts over the past decade have shown the usefulness of MRI-determined BMD assessment. Further, these reports reveal the ability of MRI to provide quantitative BMD values—as do QCT and DXA—as well as a physiologic assessment that includes fat content of vertebral marrow and vertebral perfusion. Both of these variables have been correlated with age- and gender-associated BMD changes.

Thus far, MRI sequences that seem to provide the most useful and consistent information include T2′-weighted, T2*-weighted, perfusion, and spectroscopy.

Radiographic Absorptiometry

Typically, about 40% of BMD must be lost if a deficit is to become apparent through radiographic techniques. In spite of this limitation, radiographic absorptiometry (RA) of the phalanges provides a good assessment of BMD and an accurate correlation with phalangeal ash weight (r = 0.983; accuracy, 4.8%). An aluminum alloy reference wedge is placed parallel to the middle phalanx of the left index finger. Two images are obtained of the left hand, each with a slightly different exposure, as instructed by the manufacturer. BMD is estimated by means of electronic image capture, and the estimated average density of the middle phalanges of the left second through fourth digits is reported.

SUGGESTED READINGS

Arikoski P, Komulainen J, Riikonen P, et al: Reduced bone density at completion of chemotherapy for a malignancy. Arch Dis Child 1999;80:143-148

Atkinson SA, Halton JM, Bradley C, et al: Bone and mineral abnormalities in childhood acute lymphoblastic leukemia: influence of disease, drugs and nutrition. Int J Cancer Suppl 1998;11:35-39

Bachrach LK: Bare-bones fact—children are not small adults. N Engl J Med 2004;351:924-926

Binkovitz LA, Henwood MJ: Pediatric DXA: technique and interpretation. Pediatr Radiol 2007;37:21-31

Binkovitz LA, Sparke P, Henwood MJ: Pediatric DXA: clinical applications. Pediatr Radiol 2007;37:625-635

Burnham JM, Zemel BS, Leonard MB: Sensitivity of dual x-ray absorptiometry to stature and reference data source in pediatric patients: comment on the article by Stewart et al. Arthritis Rheum 2004;50:2378-2379

Cann CE: Quantitative CT for determination of bone mineral density: a review. Radiology 1988;166:509-522

Cann CE, Genant HK: Precise measurement of vertebral mineral content using computed tomography. J Comput Assist Tomogr 1980;4:493-500

Cann CE, Genant HK, Kolb FO, et al: Quantitative computed tomography for prediction of vertebral fracture risk. Bone 1985;6:1-7

Carter DR, Bouxsein ML, Marcus R: New approaches for interpreting projected bone densitometry data. J Bone Miner Res 1992;7:137-145

Cooper C, Dennison EM, Leufkens HGM, et al: J Bone Miner Res 2004;19:1976-1981

Ellis KJ, Shypailo RJ, Hardin DS, et al: Z score prediction model for assessment of bone mineral content in pediatric diseases. J Bone Miner Res 2001;16:1658-1664

Fielding KT, Nix DA, Bachrach LK: Comparison of calcaneus ultrasound and dual x-ray absorptiometry in children at risk of osteopenia. J Clin Densitom 2003;6:7-15

Furstenberg AL, Mezey MD: Differences in outcome between black and white elderly hip fracture patients. J Chronic Dis 1987;40:931-938

Gilsanz V: Bone density in children: a review of the available techniques and indications. Eur J Radiol 1998;26:177-182

Gilsanz V, Gibbens DT, Roe TF, et al: Vertebral bone density in children: effect of puberty. Radiology 1988;166:847-850

Gilsanz V, Roe TF, Mora S, et al: Changes in vertebral bone density in black girls and white girls during childhood and puberty. N Engl J Med 1991;325:1597-1600

Goulding A, Cannan R, Williams SM, et al: Bone mineral density in girls with forearm fractures. J Bone Miner Res 1998;13:143-148

Harke HT: Pediatric bone densitometry: technical issues. Semin Musculoskelet Radiol 1999;3:371-378

Hesseling PB, Hough SF, Nel ED, et al: Bone mineral density in long-term survivors of childhood cancer. Int J Cancer Suppl 1998;11:44-47

Kaste SC: Bone-mineral density deficits from childhood cancer and its therapy. Pediatr Radiol 2004;34:373-378

Kaste SC, Chesney RW, Hudson MM, et al: Bone mineral status during and after therapy of childhood cancer: an increasing population with multiple risk factors for impaired bone health. J Bone Miner Res 1999;14:2010-2014

Kotzan JA, Martin BC, Reeves JH, et al: The impact of race and fractures on mortality in a postmenopausal Medicaid population. Clin Ther 1992;21:1988-2000

Kroger H, Kotaniemi A, Kroger L, et al: Development of bone mass and bone density of the spine and femoral neck—a prospective study of 65 children and adolescents. Bone Miner 1993;23:171-182

Landin LA: Fracture patterns in children: analysis of 8,682 fractures with special reference to incidence, etiology and secular changes in a Swedish urban population 1950-1979. Acta Orthop Scand Suppl 1983;202:1-109

Landis JR, Koch GG: The measurement of observer agreement for categorical data. Biometrics 1977;33:159-174

Lentz H, Samuelson G, Bratteby LE, et al: Differences in whole body measurements by DXA scanning using two Lunar DPX-L machines. Int J Obes Relat Metab Disord 1999;23:764-770

Leonard MB: Dual energy x-ray absorptiometry: shortcomings in the assessment of bone health in children. Calcif Tissue Int 2002;70:355-383

Leonard MB: Assessment of bone health in children and adolescents with cancer: promises and pitfalls of current techniques. Med Pediatr Oncol 2003;41:198-207

Leonard MB, Bachrach LK: Assessment of bone mineralization following renal transplantation in children: limitations of DXA and the confounding effects of delayed growth and development. Am J Transplant 2001;1:193-196

Leonard MB, Shults J, Elliott DM, et al: Interpretation of whole body dual energy x-ray absorptiometry measures in children: comparison with peripheral quantitative computed tomography. Bone 2004;34:1044-1052

Leonard MB, Shults J, Wilson BA, et al: Obesity during childhood and adolescence augments bone mass and bone dimensions. Am J Clin Nutr 2004;80:514-523

Lequin MH, van der Sluis M, van Rijn RR, et al: Bone mineral assessment with tibial ultrasonometry and dual-energy x-ray absorptiometry in long-term survivors of acute lymphoblastic leukemia in childhood. J Clin Densitom 2002;5:167-173

Liao X-P, Zhang W-L, He J, et al: Bone measurements of infants in the first 3 months of life by quantitative ultrasound: the influence of gestational age, season, and postnatal age. Pediatr Radiol 2005;35:847-853

Loro ML, Sayre J, Roe TF, et al: Early identification of children predisposed to low peak bone mass and osteoporosis later in life. J Clin Endocrinol Metab 2000;85:3908-3918

Ma DQ, Jones G: Clinical risk factors but not bone density are associated with prevalent fractures in prepubertal children. J Paediatr Child Health 2002;38:497-500

Melton LJ 3rd, Atkinson EJ, O'Fallon WM, et al: Long-term fracture prediction by bone mineral assessed at different skeletal sites. J Bone Miner Res 1993;8:1227-1233

Nevill AM, Holder RL, Maffulli N, et al: Adjusting bone mass for differences in projected bone area and other confounding variables: an allometric perspective. J Bone Miner Res 2002;17:703-708

Skaggs DL, Loro ML, Pitukcheewanont P, et al: Increased body weight and decreased radial cross-sectional dimensions in girls with forearm fractures. J Bone Miner Res 2001;16:1337-1342

van der Sluis IM, Heuvel-Eibrink MM, Hahlen K, et al: Bone mineral density, body composition, and height in long-term survivors of acute lymphoblastic leukemia in childhood. Med Pediatr Oncol 2000;35:415-420

van der Sluis IM, van den Heuvel-Eibrink MM, Hahlen K, et al:

Altered bone mineral density and body composition, and increased fracture risk in childhood acute lymphoblastic leukemia. J Pediatr 2002;141:204-210

van Rijn RR, van der Sluis IM, Link TM, et al: Bone densitometry in children: a critical appraisal. Eur Radiol 2003;13:700-710

Wren TA, Gilsanz V: Assessing bone mass in children and adolescents. Curr Osteoporos Rep 2006;4:153-158

CHAPTER

170

Skeletal Trauma

PETER J. STROUSE

In this chapter, traumatic injuries to the pediatric appendicular skeleton and pelvis are presented. Injuries to the axial skeleton, including the skull, spine, and bony thorax, are covered in separate chapters dedicated to those portions of the body. This presentation will concentrate on fractures in the child; however, other forms of trauma to the pediatric skeleton are briefly covered.

No where else does the dictum "children are not small adults" hold more weight than in regard to skeletal trauma. Fracture patterns and fracture healing are different processes within children than adults. The composition of a child's bones and the presence of the growth process both predispose the child to different types of fractures and complications of fractures than are seen in the adult. Unfortunately, a fracture may interfere with subsequent normal growth of a bone. Fortunately, such injuries are relatively uncommon. In healthy children, the process of fracture healing and remodeling is rapid. Most post-traumatic deformities readily correct with healing and remodeling.

> The composition of a child's bones and the presence of the growth process both predispose the child to different types of fractures and complications of fractures than are seen in the adult.

IMAGING MODALITIES

Plain radiographs are the mainstay of the imaging of traumatic injuries to the pediatric skeleton. As a general rule, two orthogonal views are obtained to assess for fracture. At some locations, normal anatomy limits the value of orthogonal projections (i.e., the pelvis). At other locations, unique projections are helpful for delineation of anatomy (i.e., an axillary view of the shoulder). When imaging a long bone, both the proximal and distal joints must be included so that the entirety of the bone is imaged.

Contralateral comparison views are not routinely obtained, but frequently aid in differentiating normal developmental variation from pathology. Comparison

views are most helpful in areas of complex anatomy, such as the elbow. Normal variants are common and may mimic fracture (see Chapter 163).

At certain sites and with complex patterns of injury, computed tomography (CT) is very helpful in diagnosing fractures and delineating the anatomy of fracture planes and resultant deformity. Occasionally, magnetic resonance imaging (MRI) or sonography can be used to diagnose fractures in children; however, these modalities excel in delineating associated soft tissue injury rather than osseous injury. Ultrasound, however, may be particularly helpful in the infant whose epiphyses are not yet ossified. The cartilaginous epiphysis is well seen with ultrasound, and its relationship and continuity with an adjacent metaphysis can be readily assessed.

With the increasing capabilities of cross-sectional imaging, nuclear scintigraphy is less utilized than in the past. Nonetheless, scintigraphy can be a valuable tool to identify an occult fracture. Bone scans typically become positive 24 to 48 hours after a fracture.

FRACTURE MECHANISMS

Many mechanisms may play a role in pediatric trauma. Falls, injuries at play, and motor vehicle accidents account for a majority of childhood fractures. Unfortunately, younger children may suffer fractures as a consequence of nonaccidental trauma (child abuse). These injuries are often characteristic and are covered in Chapter 171, which is devoted to this subject. Children of all ages are increasingly involved in and dedicated to athletics and competitive sports. Certain types of fractures, including stress fractures, are often associated with sporting injury. These fractures are addressed Chapter 172. Pathologic fractures may be seen with bone tumors (Chapter 176). Insufficiency fractures may be seen with metabolic bone disease (Chapter 167).

PLASTIC (INCOMPLETE) FRACTURES

The composition of the bones of a child is different than that of the bones of an adult. The plasticity of a child's bones allows for substantial deformity prior to fracture

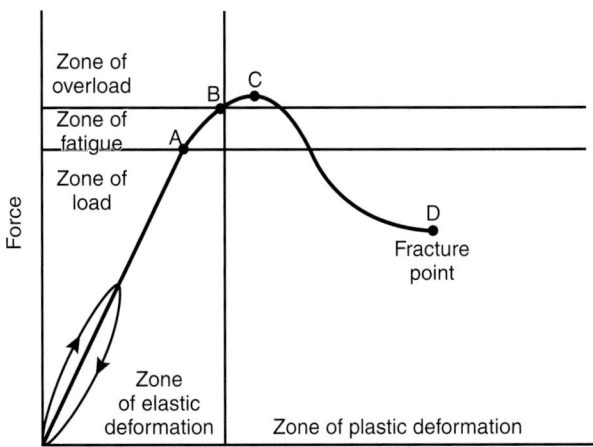

FIGURE 170-1. Graphic relation of bony deformation (bowing) and force (longitudinal compression) showing that the limit of an elastic response is not a fracture but plastic deformation. If the force continues, a fracture results. A, reversible bowing with stress; B, microfractures occur; C, point of maximal strength; between C and D, bowing fractures; D, linear fracture occurs. (Modified from Borden S IV: Roentgen recognition of acute plastic bowing of the forearm in children. Am J Roentgenol Radium Ther Nucl Med 1975;125:524-530.)

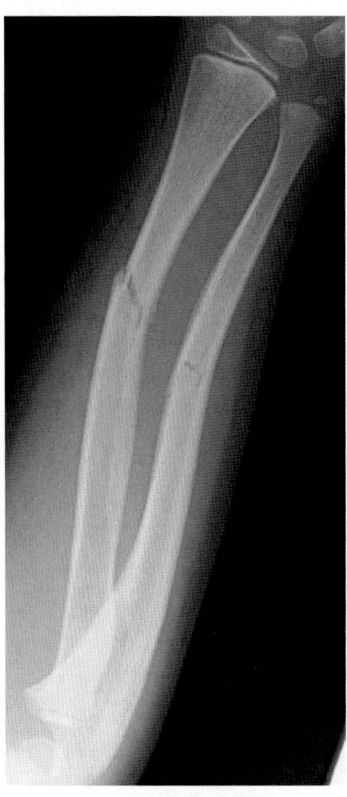

FIGURE 170-3. Greenstick fractures of the radial and ulnar diaphyses in an 8-year-old boy. The fracture lines only extend through part of the cortex.

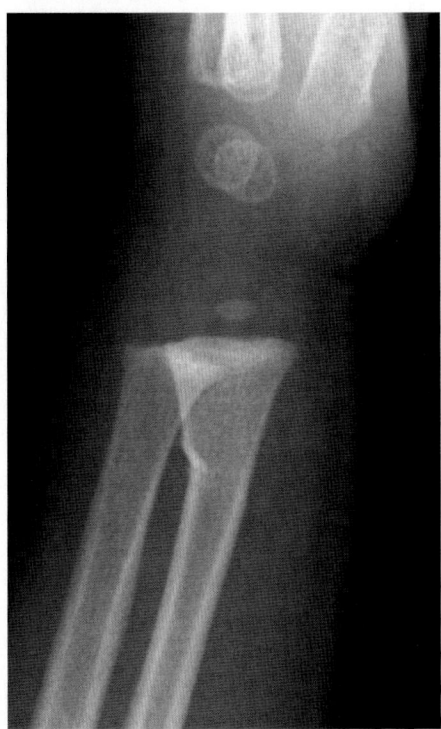

FIGURE 170-2. Buckle fracture of the distal radius in a 19-month-old boy. The distal radius is slightly angulated posteriorly.

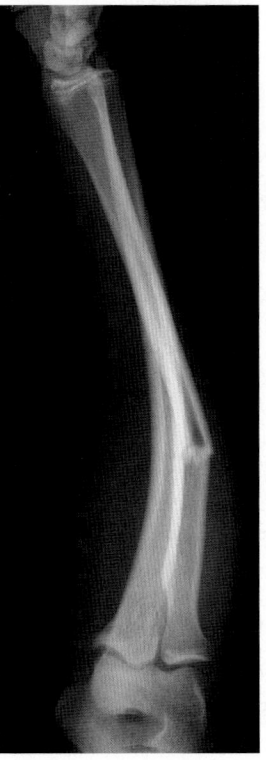

FIGURE 170-4. Bowing fracture of the ulna in a 14-year-old boy. The ulna is bowed with no fracture line or cortical buckle. A transverse fracture is seen in the radius.

(Fig. 170-1). The bone may give way and permanently deform prior to a complete break. The result is an "incomplete fracture" or a "plastic fracture." Subtypes of incomplete fractures are buckle or torus fractures (Fig. 170-2), lead pipe fractures (part transverse fracture/part buckle fracture), greenstick fractures (Fig. 170-3) and bowing fractures (Fig. 170-4). With incomplete fractures, the periosteum is also partially intact.

Plastic fractures often occur at characteristic sites. Buckle fractures are most common within the distal radius and ulna, within the tibia, and within the proximal aspect of the first metatarsal. Bowing and greenstick fractures most commonly occur in long bones, particularly the radius and ulna. Plastic fractures are most

Type I

Type II

Type III

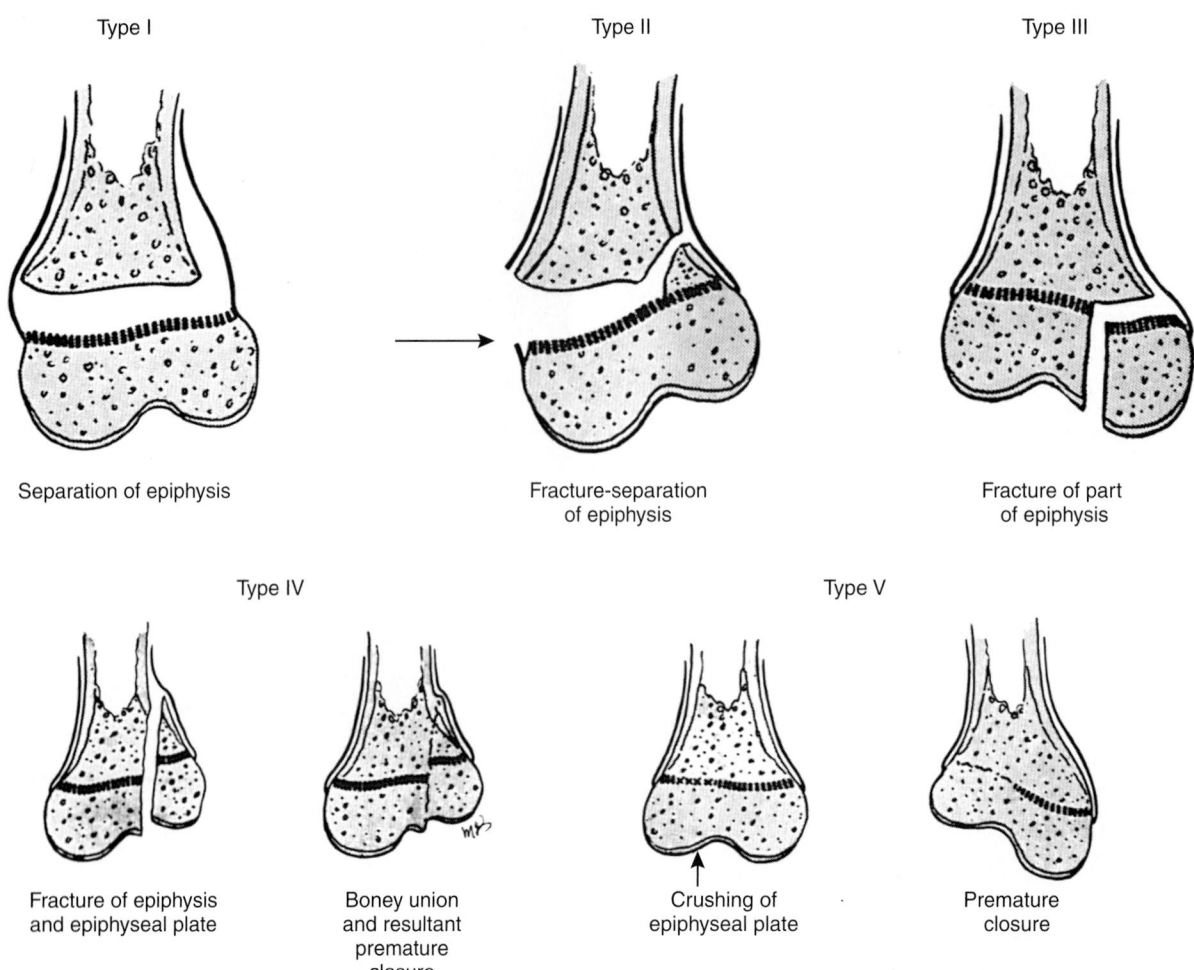

Separation of epiphysis

Fracture-separation
of epiphysis

Fracture of part
of epiphysis

Type IV

Type V

Fracture of epiphysis
and epiphyseal plate

Boney union
and resultant
premature
closure

Crushing of
epiphyseal plate

Premature
closure

FIGURE 170-5. Injuries to the cartilage plate classified according to Salter and Harris. **Type I,** Complete transverse laceration of the cartilage plate with longitudinal distraction and some transverse displacement of the epiphysis. The bone itself is not broken. **Type II,** Incomplete transverse laceration of the cartilage through a variable distance is associated with an oblique fracture of the contiguous shaft with a triangular tag of shaft attached to the displaced epiphysis. The prognosis is good. **Type III,** Short incomplete transverse laceration of the cartilage plate with longitudinal fracture extending through the epiphyseal ossification center toward the joint. This usually occurs in the cartilage plates of the tibia. The prognosis is bad if the epiphyseal fracture is not reduced with smooth joint surfaces. **Type IV,** Oblique longitudinal fracture extending from the articular cartilage through the epiphyseal ossification center, across the cartilage plate, and through a short segment of the metaphysis through the cortical wall. This type is most frequently seen at the lateral condyle of the humerus. Perfect reduction is essential for a good prognosis. **Type V,** Segmental crushing of the cartilage plate, often followed by closure of the plate prematurely and stoppage of growth. (From Salter RE, Harris WR: Injuries involving the epiphyseal plate. J Bone Joint Surg Am 1963;45:587-622.)

common in the first decade of life, are uncommon in the second decade of life, and are not seen in normally developed and mineralized bones of an adult.

Plastic fractures usually heal completely and with a good prognosis. Rarely, it may be necessary to operatively "complete" the fracture in order for reduction of deformity.

PHYSEAL FRACTURES (SALTER-HARRIS FRACTURES)

Another difference between the bones of children and adults is the presence of the growth plates or physes. Until fused, the physes represent a site of relative weakness and are thus prone to fracture. This is true for epiphyses and apophyses. Approximately 20% of pediatric fractures involve the physes. Physeal fractures are classified by the system of Salter and Harris (Fig. 170-5).

Fractures through the growth plates may pass solely and directly through the whole growth plate (Salter-Harris I; Fig. 170-6), involve the growth plate and a portion of the metaphysis (Salter-Harris II; Fig. 170-7), involve the growth plate and a portion of the epiphysis (Salter-Harris III; Fig. 170-8), or cross the growth plate in single plane involving both epiphysis and metaphysis (Salter-Harris IV; Fig. 170-9). Crushing of the growth plate (Salter-Harris V) is rare as an isolated injury to the bone and is rarely, if ever, diagnosed prospectively. Many lesser grade Salter-Harris fractures that proceed to premature growth plate fusion probably have a component of growth plate crush injury. The Salter-Harris classification serves to assign prognosis. Higher grade Salter-Harris fractures have a higher incidence of premature growth plate fusion. Most physeal fractures, however, are either Salter-Harris I (approximately 10%) or Salter-Harris II (approximately 75%). Thus, although premature growth

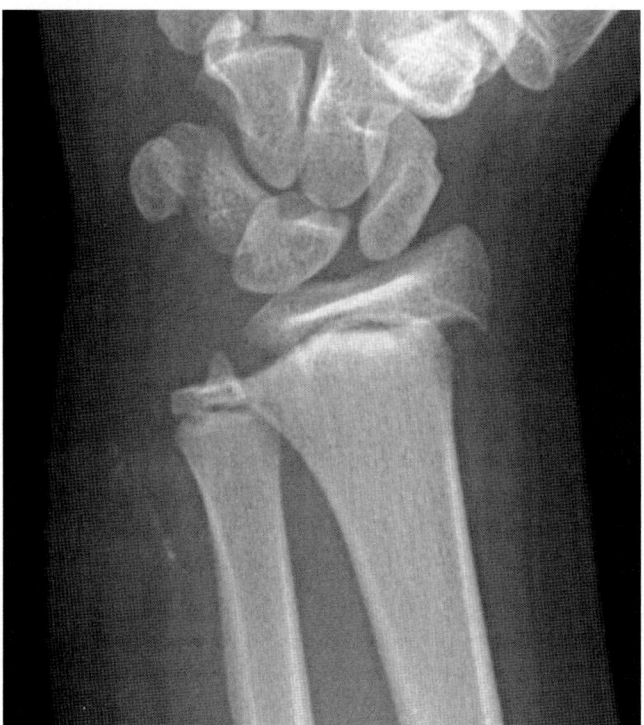

FIGURE 170-6. Salter-Harris I fracture of the distal radius in an 11-year-old girl. The distal radial epiphysis is displaced lateral.

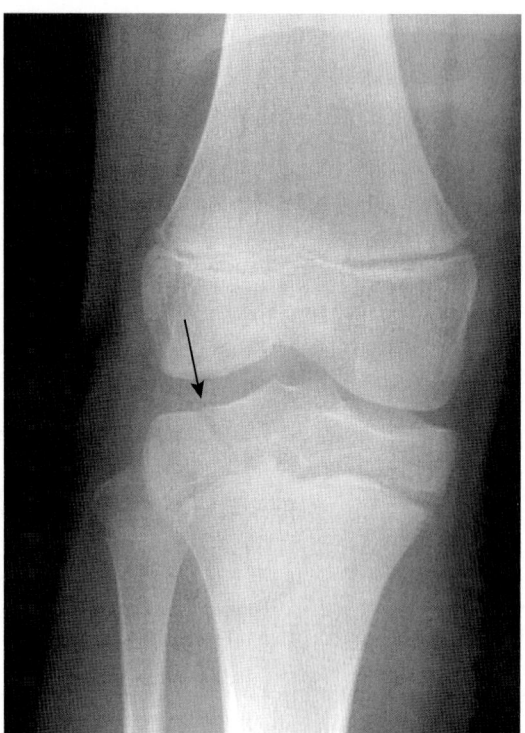

FIGURE 170-8. Salter-Harris III fracture of the proximal tibia in a 10-year-old girl. The proximal tibial growth plate is wide. The *arrow* shows the epiphyseal fracture line.

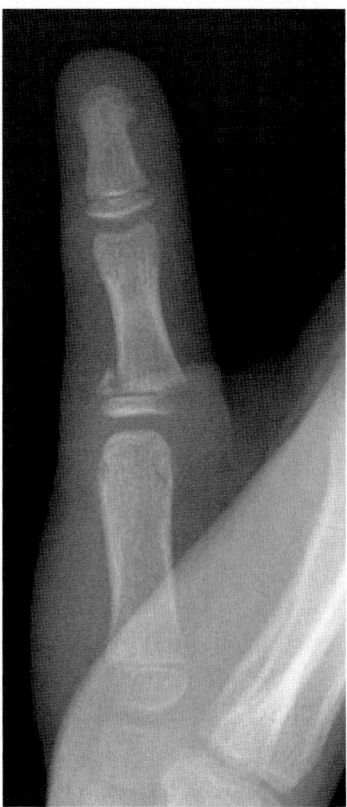

FIGURE 170-7. Salter-Harris II fracture of the proximal phalanx of the thumb in a 10-year-old boy. The distal fragment is slightly displaced medially.

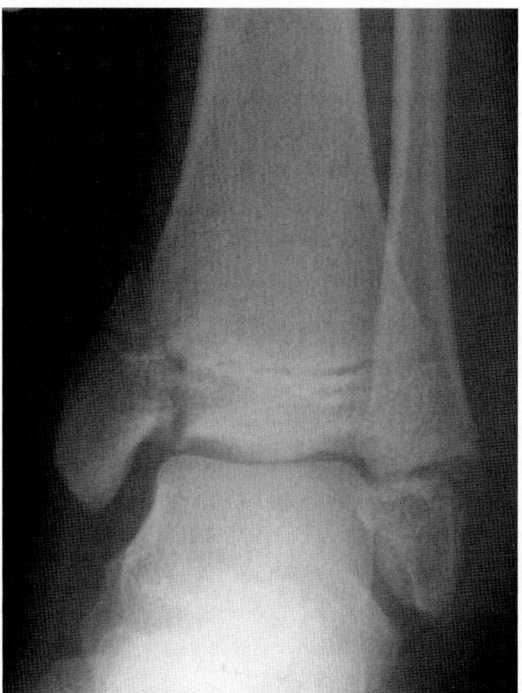

FIGURE 170-9. Salter-Harris IV fracture of the distal tibia in a 13-year-old boy who fell from a tree. There is also a Salter-Harris I fracture of the distal fibula with overlying soft tissue swelling.

plate fusion is more likely to occur with a higher grade Salter-Harris fracture, this complication is probably more commonly the result of a lower grade Salter-Harris fracture. The Salter-Harris classification is also an aid to communication.

> **Higher grade Salter-Harris fractures have a higher incidence of premature growth plate fusion.**

Fracture planes within the growth plate pass through the zone of calcified cartilage and adjacent newly formed bone, which represent the point of least resistance to fracture forces. Fracture lines that extend into the epiphysis (Salter-Harris III and IV) cross the zone of proliferating cartilage, which is more susceptible to damage leading to premature growth plate fusion. The zone of proliferating cartilage is thought to be damaged by Salter-Harris V fractures. Malalignment of Salter-Harris IV fracture fragments may promote formation of a bridge across the healing fracture from metaphysis to epiphysis.

Although not in common use, there are additional fractures within an expanded Salter-Harris classification. A Salter-Harris VI fracture occurs at the perichondral ring at the edge of the growth plate. A Salter-Harris VII fracture is confined to the epiphyses.

Apophyseal avulsions are Salter-Harris I fractures through the apophyseal growth plate. At some locations, Salter-Harris II, III, or IV fractures may occur in an apophysis. More so than with epiphyses, apophyseal injuries tend to occur within a relatively narrow range of age when the apophysis is prone to injury.

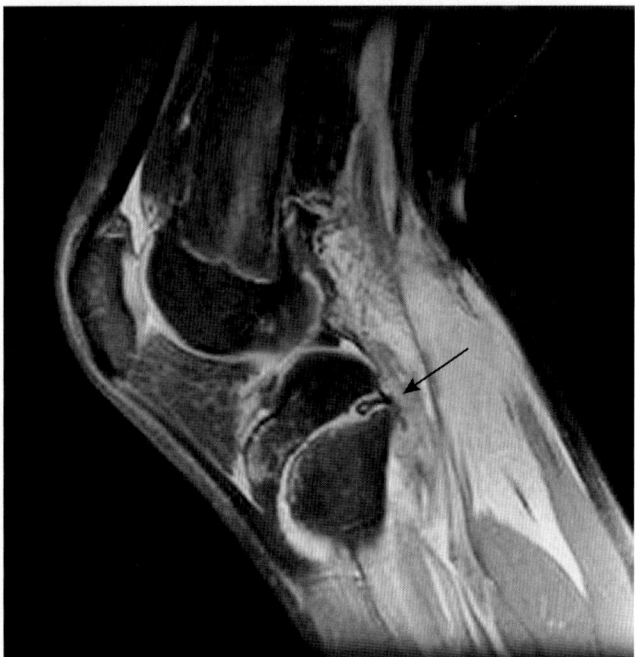

FIGURE 170-10. Proton density MR image with fat saturation of an adolescent with a Salter-Harris I fracture of the proximal tibia. Disrupted periosteum is trapped with the physeal fracture *(arrow)*. Abundant soft tissue edema is seen posteriorly. (Courtesy of Dr. D. Grattan-Smith, Atlanta, GA.)

Most physeal fractures are adequately delineated by radiography. At certain locations, CT or MRI may be used to confirm or delineate fracture. On MRI, physeal fractures are diagnosed by widening and increased T2 signal within the fractured portion of the growth plate, adjacent bone marrow edema, associated metaphyseal (Salter-Harris II) or epiphyseal (Salter-Harris III) fracture lines, and periosteal disruption. A rare complication of physeal fracture diagnosed by MRI is entrapment of periosteum within the fracture (Fig. 170-10). The entrapped periosteum will prevent complete reduction of the fracture.

Once the growth plates have fused, fracture patterns in older children are similar to fracture patterns seen in adults. This chapter does not cover such fractures in detail; rather, it concentrates on fractures and patterns of fracture that are characteristic of and unique to the pediatric age group.

FRACTURE HEALING

Fracture healing in children has been described in three phases—inflammatory, reparative, and remodeling (Fig. 170-11). At the time of fracture, bone and periosteum are disrupted. A hematoma is formed at the site of fracture enveloping the ends of the fracture bone. The hematoma may also contain necrotic fragments of bone, bone marrow, and adjacent tissues. An inflammatory response is initiated (inflammatory phase). The hematoma then begins to organize. Osteoclasts and osteoblasts arise from precursor cells of the involved tissues. Capillary beds grow into the hematoma. Initial callus is formed during the reparative phase. Osteoid and chondroid material (callus) forming within the hematoma envelops the fracture fragments, joining them and stabilizing them. Callus is immature woven bone. Endosteal callus also forms within the fracture fragments and is seen as sclerosis on radiographs. Devitalized portions of bone at the margin of the fracture fragments may undergo resorption and appear demineralized on radiographs. With time, the woven bone of callus is replaced by organized lamellar bone as the form of the bone returns to normal (remodeling phase). With remodeling, excess thickness from callus is resorbed and the medullary canal is re-established. Remodeling lasts months and, occasionally, years.

The healing process is more rapid and more complete in children than adults. Most childhood fractures heal completely and without residual deformity.

COMPLICATIONS OF FRACTURE

Complications may occur at the time of fracture, during treatment, or as a failure of normal, complete fracture healing. Table 170-1 lists potential complications of pediatric fractures. The incidence of a particular complication varies depending on many factors, including the site and severity of the fracture, complicating factors (i.e., open fracture), the age and overall health of the patient, associated injuries, and the adequacy of therapy.

In nonunion, healing stops before osseous continuity of the fracture fragments occurs. The united fragments

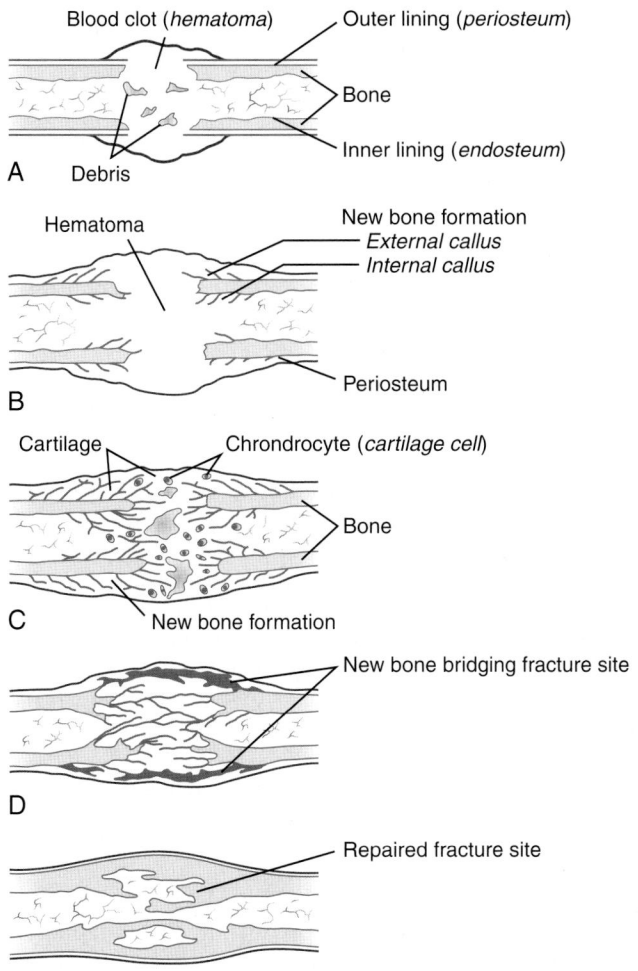

FIGURE 170-11. Stages in healing of a fracture. **A,** Hematoma under the periosteum surrounding the fracture, communicating through the fracture with blood clot within the medullary cavity. **B,** Subperiosteal and endosteal cellular proliferation encroaching on the hematoma. Islands of cartilage may be present. Bone at the margins of the fracture has been devitalized. **C,** Callus formation from osteoblastic cells in the proliferating cellular masses. The intracellular substance becomes calcified to form woven bone. The dead bone at the margins of the fracture undergoes resorption. **D,** Replacement of woven bone by lamellar bone with bone continuity across the fractured area. **E,** Remodeling. Cortical bone is organized to conform to the cortex. Resorption of excess bone results in recanalization of the medullary cavity. (From Bleck EE, Nagel DA: *Physically Handicapped Children.* New York, Grune & Stratton, 1982.)

TABLE 170-1
Complications of Fracture

ACUTE
Neurovascular injury
Hemorrhage
Fat embolism
Compartment syndrome

SUBACUTE/CHRONIC
Premature growth plate fusion
Delayed union
Nonunion/pseudarthrosis
Malunion/deformity
Synostosis (cross union)
Heterotopic ossification/myositis ossificans
Osteomyelitis/septic arthritis
Post-traumatic osteolysis
Avascular necrosis
Post-traumatic cyst
Osteochondroma
Fibrous cortical defect
Aneurysmal bone cyst
Iatrogenic
    Soft tissue infection
    Hardware misplacement/migration/infection
    Casting complications
    Hypocalcemia of immobilization
    Superior mesenteric artery syndrome
Deep venous thrombosis/pulmonary embolism
Overgrowth
Refracture
Reflex sympathetic dystrophy syndrome
Premature degenerative joint disease (osteoarthritis)

may form a pseudarthrosis. Pseudarthrosis is most common in the clavicle, humerus, and tibia. Nonunion and pseudarthroses are uncommon in normal children, but may be seen with underlying abnormalities such as neurofibromatosis or congenital insensitivity to pain. The incidence of nonunion is increased with greater injury, comminution, and distraction, and with open fractures complicated by substantial soft tissue injury, infection, or both. Delayed union is defined as failure of bone union to occur in the expected time. Malunion indicates fusion in a nonanatomic orientation. As noted, mild degrees of malalignment are well tolerated and usually result in no permanent deformity due to the

aggressive remodeling that occurs in a child. Surgical interruption of the healing process with realignment is occasionally necessary. Post-traumatic synostoses are most common in the paired bones of the forearm and distal leg. Infection may occur due to an open fracture or as a complication of surgery or percutaneous pinning.

Certain sites of fracture may be predisposed to neurovascular injury; however, such injuries are rare and usually only seen with substantial displacement and deformity. Approximately 1% to 3% of supracondylar fractures of the distal humerus result in injury to the nerves or vasculature. Compartment syndrome is an uncommon complication of extremity fractures, most commonly in the lower leg or with supracondylar fractures, which may lead to Volkmann contracture due to ischemia.

Reflex sympathetic dystrophy syndrome (RSDS; aka "Sudeck atrophy") is a poorly understood dysfunction of the autonomic nervous system. The etiologic relationship to preceding fracture is unknown. RSDS most commonly affects the lower extremities in children. Patients present with pain, swelling, joint stiffness, and exquisite sensitivity to touch. Onset of symptoms is approximately 1 month after injury. Radiographs show osteopenia that is difficult to distinguish from disuse osteoporosis. MRI shows patchy bone marrow edema. Bone scintigraphy is usually abnormal but inconsistent. Early, increased activity is seen on both flow and delayed phases. Later, decreased activity may be seen on both phases.

TABLE 170-2

Causes of Physeal Arrest

Trauma
Fracture (Salter-Harris I–IV)
Crush/compression (Salter-Harris V)
Stress fracture
Neuropathic (i.e., myelodysplasia)
Infection
Osteomyelitis
Meningococcemia
Ischemia
Thalassemia
Sickle cell anemia
Radiation therapy
Electrical injury
Burn
Frostbite
Iatrogenic (epiphysiodesis)
Disuse
Tumor
Developmental
Blount disease
Madelung deformity
Metabolic
Chronic vitamin A intoxication
Scurvy

Premature Growth Plate Fusion

Premature fusion occurs in approximately 15% of physeal fractures. A bony "bridge" or "bar" forms across the growth plate from metaphysis to epiphysis. Prognosis depends on the involved bone, the extent of fusion, the site of fusion within the growth plate, and the amount of remaining growth. Morbidity is greater when remaining growth potential is higher. Premature fusion is most common in the phalanges and distal radius; however, premature fusion in the distal femur and tibia is of greater clinical importance due to possible resultant leg length discrepancy or deformity. Other forms of trauma (i.e., burns, frostbite, and electrical injury—discussed later in this chapter) and other processes, such as ischemic damage and infection (particularly meningococcemia), can also cause premature growth plate fusion (Table 170-2).

Larger areas of fusion and central fusions cause loss of growth potential. Central fusions result in a cupped appearance of the growth plate with the epiphysis and physis invaginating into the center of the metaphysis. Peripheral fusions result in angular deformity.

Premature growth plate fusion is usually manifest 3 to 6 months after injury. Radiographs may show loss of patency of the growth plate. Comparison views are often helpful, particularly when evaluating an older child in whom the time of normal growth plate closure is near. A secondary sign of premature growth plate fusion is tethering of growth lines. Growth lines normally form during the healing process. Growth lines normally parallel the growth plate, whereas with premature fusion, growth lines are angled toward a bony bar where they are tethered.

Both CT and MRI have been used to diagnose and map areas of premature fusion. With CT, a limited scan with narrow collimation is obtained through the growth plate. A standard protocol obtains 1.25-mm images overlapping at 0.625-mm intervals. Sagittal and coronal reformats will show the area of fusion. Small bars may be seen as a sclerotic band across the growth plate, whereas with larger areas of fusion, continuity of the marrow space is seen across the fusion. Cartilage-sensitive sequences (proton density with fat saturation, three-dimensional spoiled gradient recalled [SPGR] with fat saturation) can be employed on MRI to delineate the physis (Fig. 170-12). Areas of fusion will be seen as defects with the bright signal of the cartilaginous growth plate. With either CT or MRI, maps can be created showing the degree and site of fusion.

Smaller bars may be resected. Usually a plug of fatty tissue is placed in the void. Premature fusion may recur. If greater than 50% of the growth plate is fused, resection of the bar may be impractical. Depending on the deformity and growth potential of the patient, other orthopedic techniques may be utilized to minimize morbidity from the premature fusion, including osteotomy and contralateral epiphysiodesis (surgical growth plate fusion).

TRAUMATIC INJURIES OF THE HAND AND WRIST

Phalangeal Avulsion Fracture

Avulsion injuries from epiphyses of the fingers are common. These injuries usually occur due to hyperextension, hyperflexion, or "jamming" of the finger into an object. "*Baseball finger*" or "*mallet finger*" is the result of forced flexion of a distal interphalangeal joint. Pull of the long extensor tendon avulses a small fragment at the dorsal aspect of the base of the distal phalanx, a Salter-Harris III fracture (Fig. 170-13). Other Salter-Harris fractures act as "mallet-equivalent" fractures (Fig. 170-14). Unopposed flexor tendons thus flex the finger. Additional imaging is rarely needed. Treatment is usually a brace or buddy taping of the involved digit to its neighbor.

Phalangeal/Metacarpal Salter-Harris Fracture

Salter-Harris II fractures involving the growth plates of the phalanges are very common. Injury to the metacarpal growth plates is less common. These lesions vary in displacement. The fractures may be very subtle with minimal growth plate widening or a tiny metaphyseal fragment (Fig. 170-15). Salter-Harris I and III fractures occur occasionally.

Boxer's Fracture

Boxer's fractures are common in adolescents, particularly boys who sustain the fractures by hitting an object, a wall, or another individual. The fracture plane is transverse or oblique through the metaphysis at the distal aspect of the fifth metacarpal. The distal fragment is angulated toward the palm (Fig. 170-16).

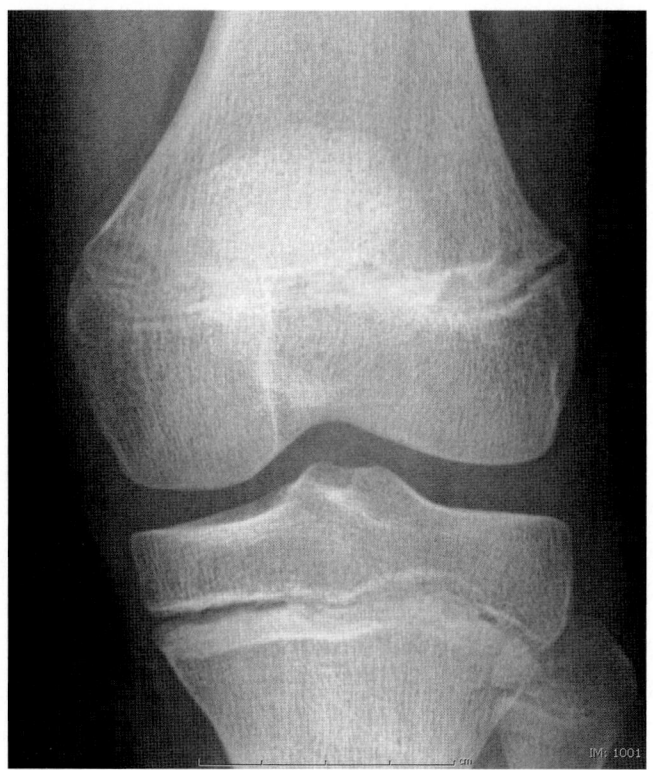

A

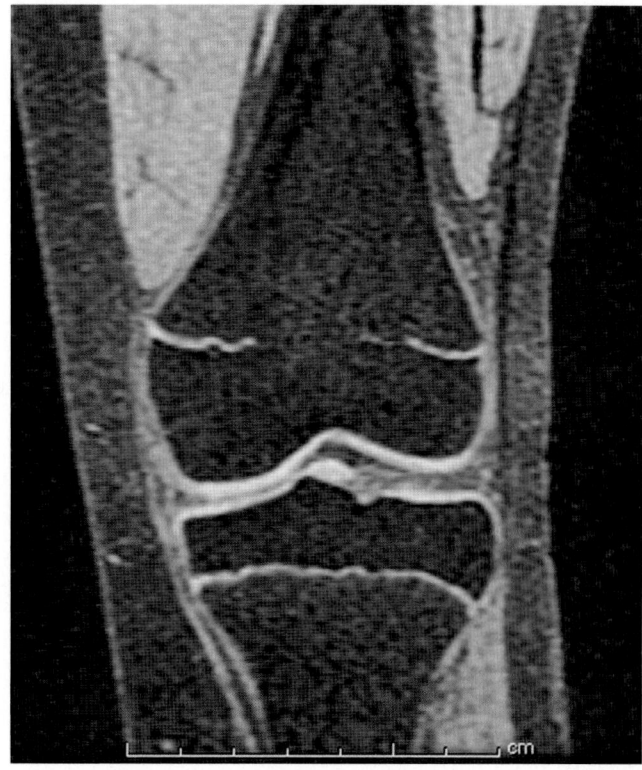

B

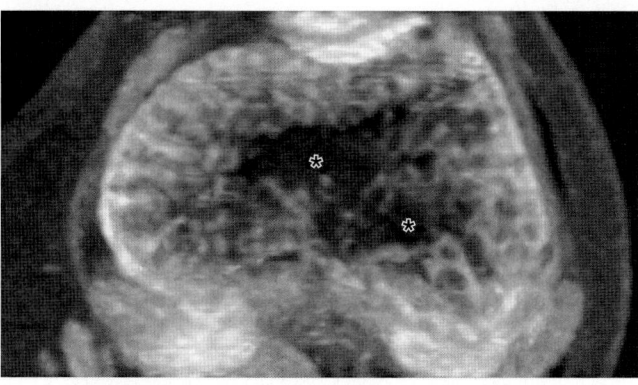

C

FIGURE 170-12. Premature growth plate fusion. **A,** On radiography, the central portion of the distal femoral growth plate is poorly defined; however, the extent of fusion is poorly delineated. **B,** Coronal SPGR MR image with fat saturation. The central growth plate is fused. **C,** Axial maximum intensity projection image constructed from the stack of coronal SPGR with fat saturation images. The area of growth plate fusion is mapped *(asterisks).* (Courtesy of Dr. K. Ecklund, Boston, MA.)

Thumb Fracture

Salter-Harris II and III fractures of the metacarpal of the thumb are common. Salter-Harris III fractures are analogous to Bennett fracture occurring after skeletal maturity (Fig. 170-17). With Bennett fracture, an intra-articular fracture is seen at the base of the thumb metacarpal with subluxation at the first metacarpal–carpal (trapezium) joint. This injury is rare in children. Salter-Harris fractures of the thumb phalanges are common. It may be difficult to distinguish between a Salter-Harris II fracture of the proximal phalanx and a bifid epiphysis, an uncommon normal variant.

Gamekeeper's thumb is a traumatic avulsion of the ulnar collateral ligament of the thumb metacarpal-phalangeal joint. Historically described in Scottish gamekeepers, this injury most commonly occurs in children due to ski pole injury or breakdancing. An avul-

sion may be seen at the ulnar volar base of the proximal phalanx of the thumb, or a Salter-Harris III fracture if the growth plate is not yet fused. Radial subluxation of the proximal phalanx may be evident, but stress views may be required to show instability in the absence of fracture. Ulnar collateral ligament avulsion may also cause a Stenor lesion with the adductor tendon interposed between the torn ulnar collateral ligament and its insertion, preventing approximation. Pseudo-gamekeeper's thumb results from a Salter-Harris I or II fracture of the proximal phalanx (see Fig. 170-7).

Buckle Fracture

Buckle fractures of the diaphyses and metaphyses of the fingers are common. Fractures of the phalangeal metaphyses may be very subtle. A loss of the smooth metaphyseal curve is seen in comparison to phalanges of

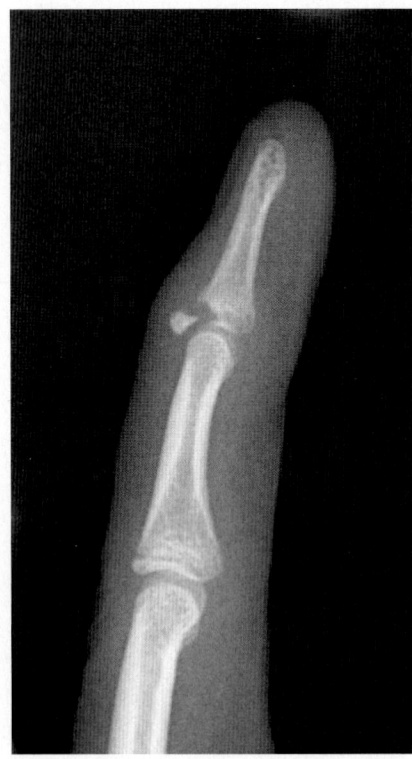

FIGURE 170-13. Mallet finger in a 13-year-old boy.

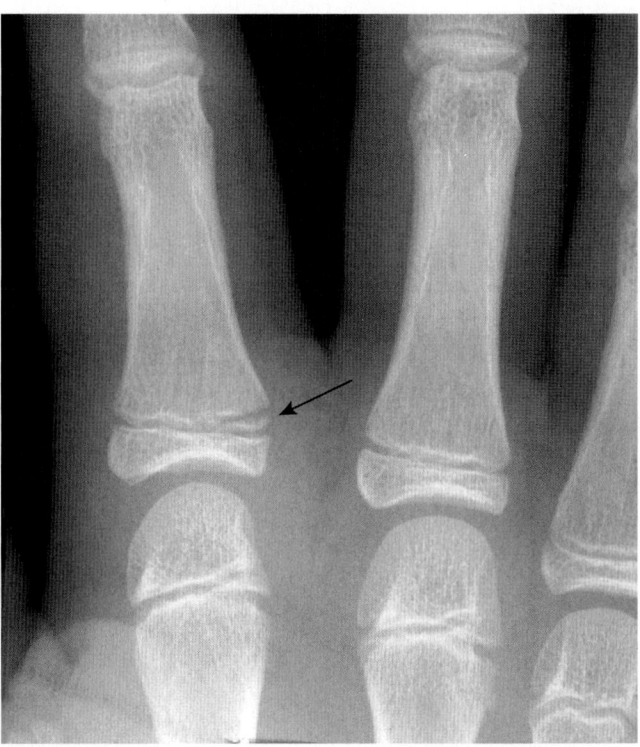

FIGURE 170-15. Salter-Harris II fracture of the proximal phalanx of the index finger *(arrow)* of a 9-year-old girl. The child was hit with a ball with the finger extended.

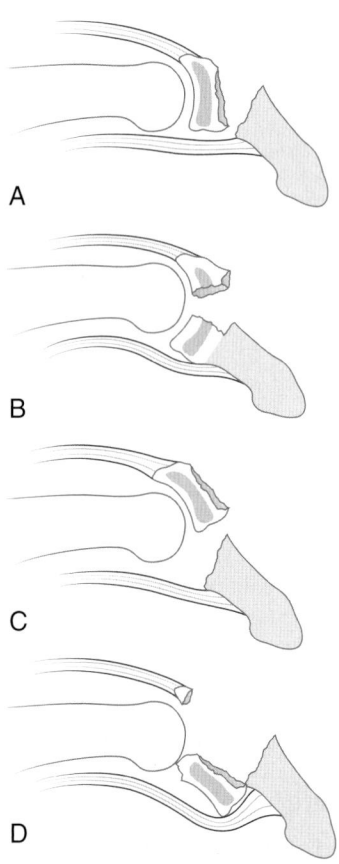

FIGURE 170-14. Mallet-equivalent fractures. (Modified from Beaty JH, Kasser JR: Rockwood and Wilkins' Fractures in Children, 6th ed. Philadelphia, Lippincott Williams & Wilkins, 2006.)

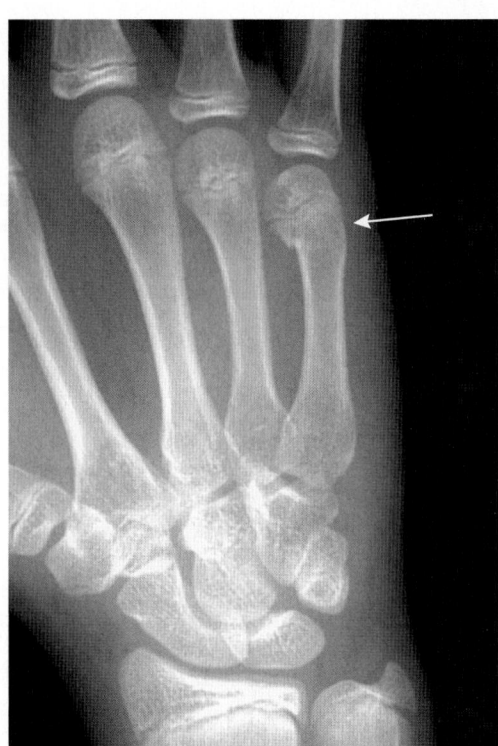

FIGURE 170-16. Boxer's fracture of the fifth metacarpal *(arrow)* in a 17-year-old boy who punched a wall. Slight palmar angulation is seen distally.

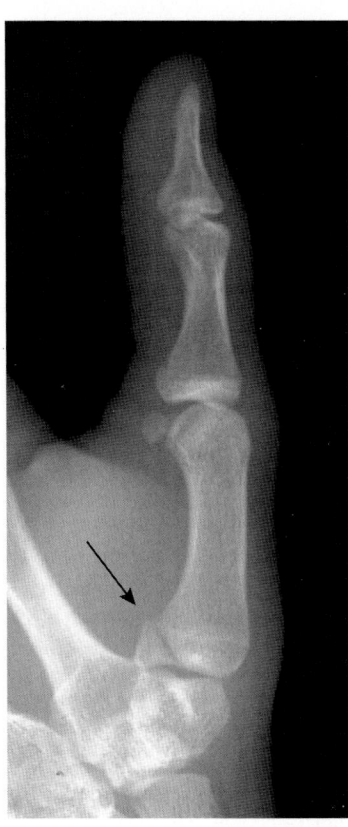

FIGURE 170-17. Salter-Harris III fracture of the base of the thumb metacarpal *(arrow)* in a 16-year-old boy, suffered when the boy's thumb caught on another player's equipment while playing football.

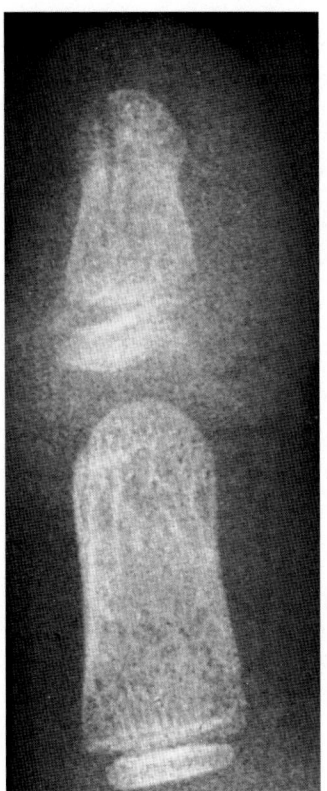

FIGURE 170-18.
Comminuted crush injury to the distal phalanx of the thumb. The shaft has two long longitudinal fracture lines. The cartilage plate is lacerated transversely, and the epiphyseal ossification center is impacted on one side of the shaft. An automobile door was slammed on the thumb of this 6-year-old boy.

adjacent digits. Some metaphyseal buckle fractures may actually be nondisplaced Salter-Harris II fractures with minimal growth plate widening.

Crush Fracture

Crush fractures may result in transverse, longitudinal, or complex comminuted fracture patterns, particularly at the tufts of the fingers (Fig. 170-18). Younger children may suffer these injuries due to fingers being slammed or caught in a door.

Scaphoid Fracture

The scaphoid is the most commonly fractured carpal bone in childhood. Scaphoid injuries typically do not occur until the bone is well ossified. This is probably due the protective cushioning effect of the unossified carpal cartilage. The incidence of scaphoid fracture increases in later childhood and adolescence. In younger children, a buckle fracture may occur. Scaphoid buckle fractures are very subtle, difficult to differentiate from normal scaphoid contour, and not associated with subsequent development of avascular necrosis. Complete fractures are more prevalent in older children (Fig. 170-19). As in adults, scaphoid fractures may be very subtle. Scaphoid views with ulnar deviation will better profile the scaphoid. CT or MRI can be used to confirm the diagnosis. Alternatively, if clinical suspicion persists due to mechanism or physical examination findings (snuff-box tenderness), then the patient can be splinted, with follow-up films to reassess for fracture usually obtained in 10 to 14 days.

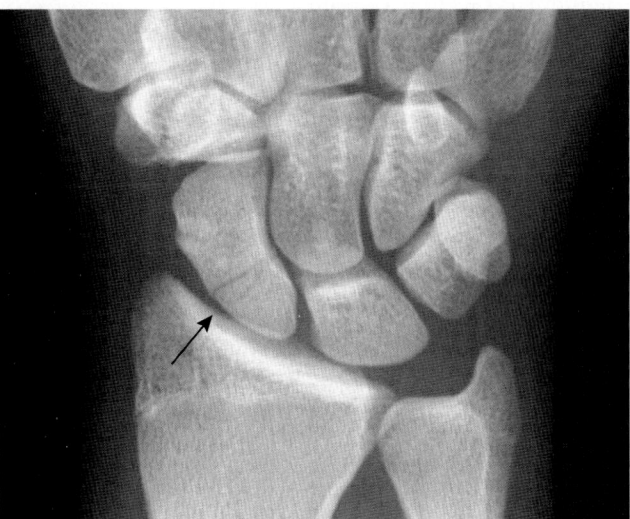

FIGURE 170-19. Transverse fracture of the scaphoid *(arrow)* in a 16-year-old boy.

Because of its recurrent blood supply, the scaphoid is prone to the development of avascular necrosis of its proximal pole after fracture (Fig. 170-20). The likelihood of avascular necrosis depends on the site of fracture, the degree of displacement, and the adequacy of immobilization. The affected proximal pole of the scaphoid will appear dense relative to the other bones of the wrist. Nonunion of the scaphoid can occur with or without avascular necrosis. The incidence of nonunion is increased with delay in diagnosis.

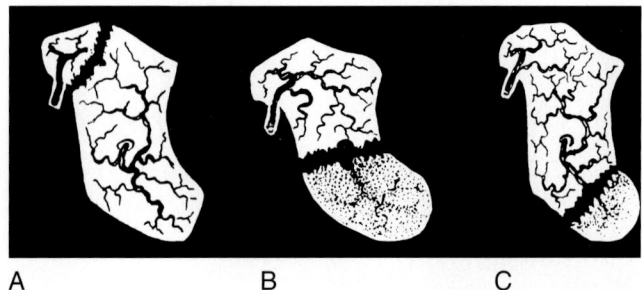

FIGURE 170-20. Schematic drawing of the different types of breaks in relation to arterial circulation in scaphoid fractures. **A,** Fracture between the two sources of arterial blood, with good prognosis because each fragment has satisfactory blood supply. **B** and **C,** Fractures at the central (**B**) and proximal (**C**) levels, in which the blood supply of the proximal fragment is impaired or lost. (From Cave FF: Fractures and Other Injuries. St. Louis, Mosby, 1958.)

> Scaphoid fractures may be very subtle. Aids to diagnosing scaphoid fractures include scaphoid views with ulnar deviation, CT or MRI, and follow-up films to reassess for fracture.

Other Carpal Fractures

Fractures of other carpal bones besides the scaphoid are rare. Fractures of the triquetrum are seen as a small fragment projecting dorsally. Fractures of the hook of the hamate may occur in athletes. Carpal dislocations are rare in children. As in adults, these dislocations may involve a fracture of the scaphoid. Carpal instability rarely manifests in childhood.

TRAUMATIC INJURIES OF THE FOREARM

Distal Radius and Ulna

Fractures of the distal radius and ulna are extremely common. The distal radius is the most common site of buckle fractures in children. These fractures usually occur due to a fall on an outstretched arm. The cortex tends to buckle dorsally. A fracture line may be present volarly. Distal radial buckle fracture may be extremely subtle and are commonly missed by inexperienced readers. It is important to look at all views for a subtle disruption of the normal smooth flared curve of the metaphyseal margin. Any extra angulation or "bump" is likely a fracture. A distal ulnar fracture may or may not be present. Even with a subtle distal radial fracture, the accompanying distal ulnar buckle fracture may be even more occult, often not identified until there are signs of healing on follow-up. Distal radial buckle fractures may also be associated with avulsions of the ulnar styloid process.

Salter-Harris fractures of the distal radius and transverse fractures of the distal radial metaphysis are also very common. As with buckle fractures, these fractures often occur due to falls on an outstretched arm. The distal fragment is usually displaced or angulated dorsally, or both. Some form of distal ulnar fracture is usually

present, usually an avulsion of the ulnar styloid process by the triangular cartilage. Growth plate fractures of the distal radius are usually Salter-Harris II. Stress injury to the distal radial growth plate occurs in gymnasts (see Chapter 172).

Radial/Ulnar Shaft Fracture

Fractures of the radial and ulnar shafts usually occur together. Plastic fractures are common. Often the fracture in one bone is complete, whereas the other bone has an incomplete fracture. As with other long bones, with complete fractures, displacement is dependent on the location of the fracture relative to muscular insertions and origins.

GALEAZZI INJURY

The Galeazzi injury is a fracture of the distal radial shaft with a dislocation of the distal radioulnar joint (DRUJ) (Fig. 170-21). These injuries seem to be rarely diagnosed in children, as DRUJ disruption is uncommon perhaps due to under-recognition. The distal ulna is most commonly subluxed or dislocated in the direction opposite of distal radial displacement. CT has been utilized to assess for DRUJ subluxation. Axial images of both wrists are obtained in neutral position, maximal supination, and maximal pronation. Various measurement criteria have been described; however, comparison to the opposite wrist is often most valuable.

MONTEGGIA INJURY

Monteggia injury is defined as fracture of the proximal third of the ulna with dislocation of the radial head (Fig. 170-22; see also Fig. 170-21). In Monteggia injury, the proximal radioulnar joint and associated ligaments are disrupted. The ulnar fracture may be complete or incomplete. Monteggia injuries are relatively common and are diagnosed much more frequently in children than Galeazzi injuries. There are several subtypes or variations of Monteggia fractures, most dependent on the anatomy of the ulnar fracture and the direction of radial head dislocation.

> Galeazzi injury = fractured radius with dislocation of distal ulna.
>
> Monteggia injury = fractured ulna with dislocation of the proximal radius.

TRAUMATIC INJURIES OF THE ELBOW

Effusion

Intra-articular fractures of the pediatric elbow produce an elbow joint effusion. The effusion causes displacement of the anterior and posterior fat pads of the elbow (Fig. 170-23). Although the anterior fat pad is seen normally, it may appear elevated by an effusion ("sail sign"). The posterior fat pad normally resides within the olecranon fossa and is not seen on radiographs of a normal elbow. Visualization of the posterior fat pad is indicative of the presence of an elbow joint effusion.

Normal

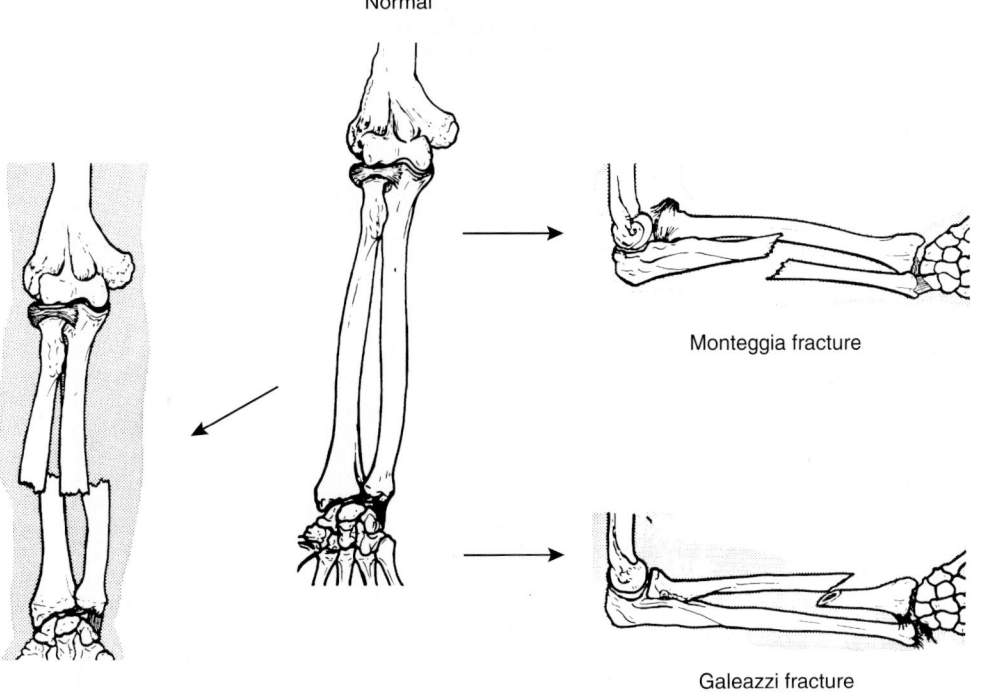

Monteggia fracture

Galeazzi fracture

Fracture

FIGURE 170-21. Effect of midshaft fracture of the radius or ulna on the elbow and wrist joints. In Monteggia's fracture of the ulna, the radial head is dislocated at the elbow. In Galeazzi's fracture of the radius, the ulna is dislocated at the wrist. When the radius and ulna are fractured simultaneously, these dislocation do not occur. (From Reckling FW, Cordell ID: Unstable fracture-dislocations of the forearm: the Monteggia and Galeazzi lesions. Arch Surg 1968;96:999-1007. © 1968 American Medical Association.)

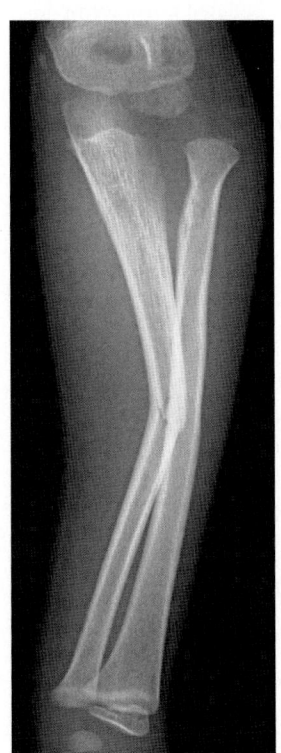

FIGURE 170-22. Monteggia lesion in a 6-year-old boy. A greenstick fracture of the ulna is present with medial angulation of the distal ulna. The radial head is dislocated.

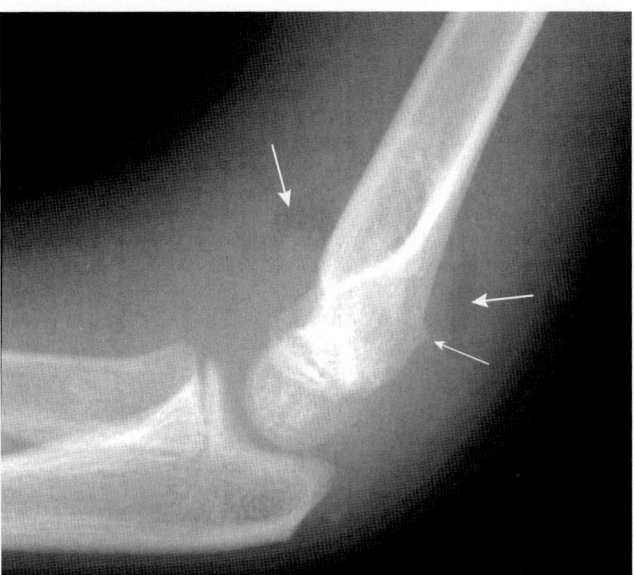

FIGURE 170-23. Buckle-type supracondylar fracture *(small arrow)* in a 6-year-old boy. The anterior and posterior fat pads *(large arrows)* are displaced by an elbow joint effusion. Note that the anterior humeral cortical line passes along the anterior margin of the capitellum, indicating posterior angulation of the distal fragment.

The presence of an elbow joint effusion is strong evidence for the presence of a fracture. Usually, the fracture is obvious. In younger children, there may be a subtle buckle or greenstick fracture of the supracondylar distal humerus. In older children, there may be a subtle fracture of the radial head or radial neck. The presence of an effusion is not unequivocal evidence for a fracture. In about 15% to 20% of cases, no fracture is identified on follow-up. However, as fractures are often subtle or occult, the presence of an effusion without an identifiable fracture usually prompts splinting of the arm with follow-up radiographs to assess for healing of an occult fracture. Alternatively, MRI has been used by some centers to evaluate for fracture; however, MRI may identify some subtle fractures that are likely of little clinical importance.

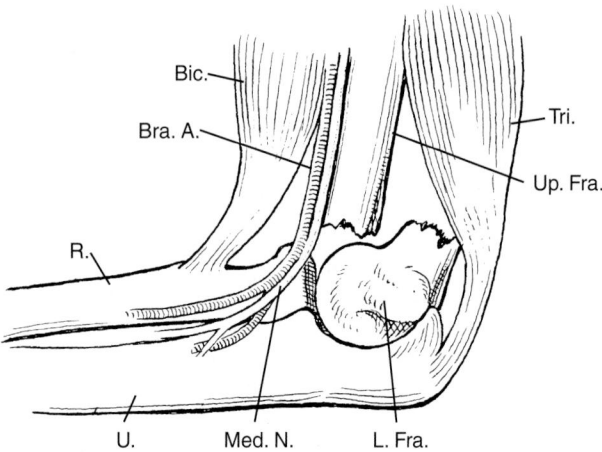

FIGURE 170-24. Morbid anatomy of supracondylar fracture of the humerus; schematic drawing. Forward displacement of the proximal fragment may puncture the brachial vessels or injure the median nerve. Bic., biceps; Bra. A., brachial artery; L. Fra., lower fragment; Med. N., median nerve; R., radius; Tri., triceps; U., ulna; Up. Fra., upper fragment.

> The presence of an elbow joint effusion is not unequivocal evidence for a fracture. In about 15% to 20% of cases, no fracture is identified on follow-up.

Supracondylar Fracture

Supracondylar fractures of the distal humerus are the most common type of fracture seen at the pediatric elbow, accounting for 60% of pediatric elbow fractures. These fractures usually occur by the mechanism of hyperextension with impingement of the olecranon on the posterior distal humerus. Fractures vary widely in severity from a faintly perceptible buckle fracture to a complete fracture with marked displacement. Approximately 1% to 3% of supracondylar fractures may be complicated by neurovascular injury, with the likelihood increased with greater severity of fracture fragment displacement (Fig. 170-24). Compartment syndrome (Volkmann contracture) is a rare complication.

The distal fragment of a supracondylar fracture is almost uniformly displaced or angulated posteriorly. As a result, the anterior humeral cortical line will not bisect the capitellum. In a normal elbow, anterior angulation of the distal humerus causes the anterior humeral cortical line to pass through the center of the capitellar ossification center. If this line passes through the anterior third of the capitellar ossification center or anterior to it, then a supracondylar fracture is likely present. It is important to assess for this finding on a properly positioned lateral view of the distal humerus. Obliquity of the distal humerus may cause the capitellar ossification center to appear falsely posterior relative to the anterior humeral cortical line.

Type I supracondylar fractures are nondisplaced (see Fig. 170-23). Type II fractures are displaced with angulation, but with an intact posterior cortex. Type III fractures are displaced with no cortical continuity (Fig. 170-25).

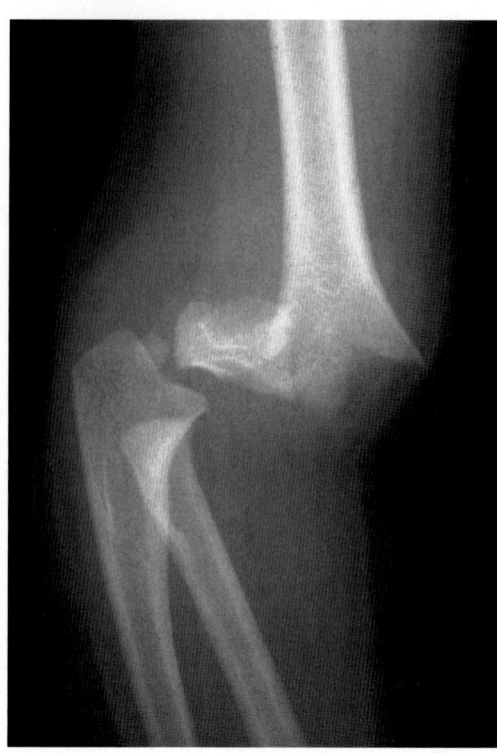

FIGURE 170-25. Supracondylar fracture in a 2-year-old boy. The distal fragment is displaced and angulated posteriorly.

Type III fractures are subdivided into posteromedial and posterolateral based on displacement.

After reduction, supracondylar fractures often demonstrate a mild degree of posterior displacement or angulation. This will not adversely affect functional outcome; however, fusion with loss of normal cubitus valgus will potentially inhibit the range of motion of the elbow. Normally, there is slight lateral angulation of the radius relative to the humerus (cubitus valgus), greater in females. The Baumann angle is created by the intersection of the humeral axis with a line tangent to the growth plate of the lateral condyle. Normal is approximately 75 degrees. With post-traumatic cubitus varus, the Baumann angle is greater than 83 degrees. Unfortunately, the Baumann angle is somewhat dependent on positioning. Severe deformity of the distal humerus with cubitus varus has been called "gun stock deformity."

Lateral Condylar Fracture

Lateral condylar fractures are the second most common type of fracture of the pediatric elbow after supracondylar fractures, accounting for 15% to 20% of pediatric elbow fractures. The mechanism is hyperextension with varus.

The severity of lateral condylar fractures varies considerably. The fracture may or may not extend through the unossified portion of the distal humeral epiphysis (Fig. 170-26). "Stable" lateral condylar fractures (type I) do not traverse the cartilaginous epiphysis and are incomplete, and thus not displaced or minimally displaced (Fig. 170-27). Type II lateral condylar fractures are complete and thus "unstable," but with little or no dis-

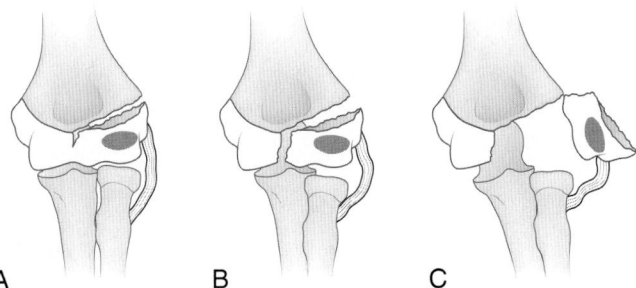

FIGURE 170-26. Classification of lateral condylar fractures according to the amount of displacement. **A,** Type I fracture. Note that the fracture line enters the cartilaginous surface of the distal end of the humerus between the capitellum and trochlea but that the fracture is not complete and to the articular surface and is therefore nondisplaced. **B,** Complete fracture (type II). The fracture is complete through the articular surface but is not displaced out of the elbow joint. **C,** Complete fracture with complete displacement of the lateral condyle (type III). (From Green NE, Swinotowski MF: Skeletal Trauma in Children, 3rd ed. Philadelphia, Saunders, 2003.)

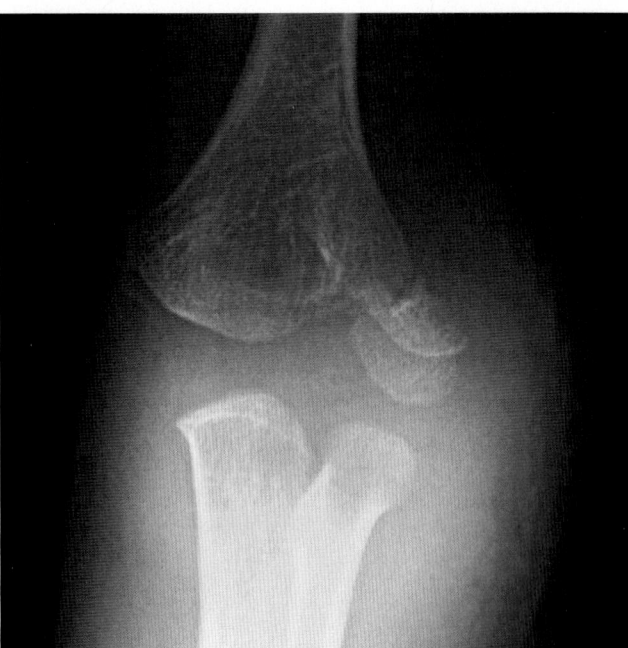

FIGURE 170-28. Displaced lateral condylar fracture in a 6-year-old boy. Marked soft tissue swelling is present.

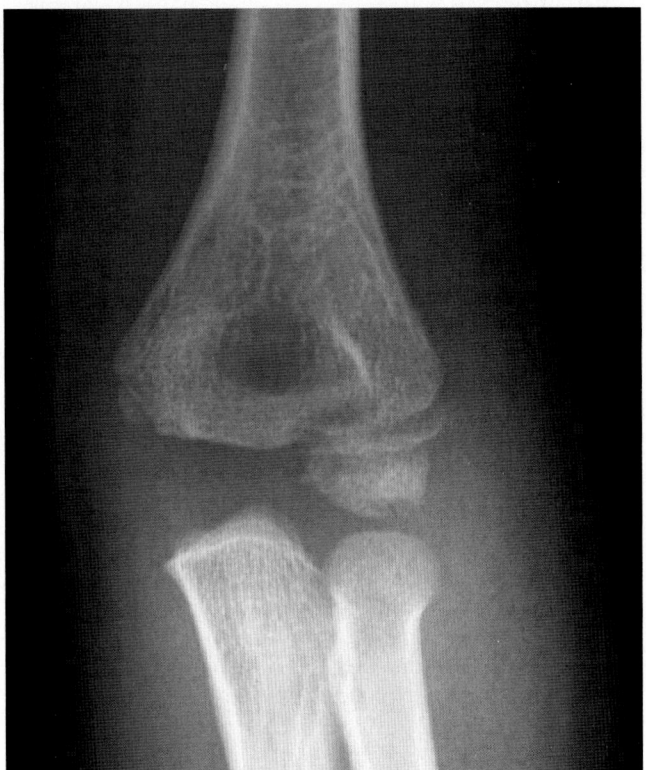

FIGURE 170-27. Nondisplaced lateral condylar fracture in a 6-year-old boy.

placement. The lateral condylar fracture line may be quite subtle, often paralleling the adjacent metaphyseal margin. With "stable" lateral condylar fractures, the limb is casted. Short-term follow-up films are obtained to assess for stability and exclude a type II fracture. In the past, arthrography (with or without CT) was occasionally used to assess for the epiphyseal fracture line. Recently, both MRI and sonography have proven capable of demonstrating the fracture through epiphyseal cartilage. With complete or "unstable" fractures, the lateral

condylar fragment is displaced and rotated (type III; Fig. 170-28). These fractures are operatively reduced and pinned.

Medial condylar fracture, not to be confused with medial epicondylar avulsion (see below), has an appearance similar to the more common lateral condylar fracture. Medial condylar fractures are uncommon and account for 1% to 2% of pediatric elbow fractures.

> In most cases, the stability of a lateral condylar fracture is evident by radiography. Ultrasound or MRI can be used to further delineate extension of the fracture through the cartilaginous distal humeral epiphysis.

Elbow Ossification Centers

There is a normal, orderly progression of the ossification of the six major ossifications centers of the elbow (Fig. 170-29): *c*apitellum (~ 1 to 2 years), *r*adial head (~ 2 to 4 years), *m*edial (*i*nternal) epicondyle (~4 to 6 years), *t*rochlea (~9 to 10 years), *o*lecranon (~9 to 11 years), and *l*ateral (*e*xternal) epicondyle (~9.5 to 11.5 years). This can be remembered by the acronyms CRMTOL or CRITOE. With very rare exceptions, the medial epicondyle ossifies prior to the trochlea. If the trochlea is ossified, so should be the medial epicondyle. Fusion of the elbow ossification centers is less orderly, occurring after puberty.

Medial Epicondyle Avulsion

The medial epicondyle ossifies by 7 years and fuses by 16 years. Avulsions thus occur within this age range, although rare avulsions of the unossified medial epicon-

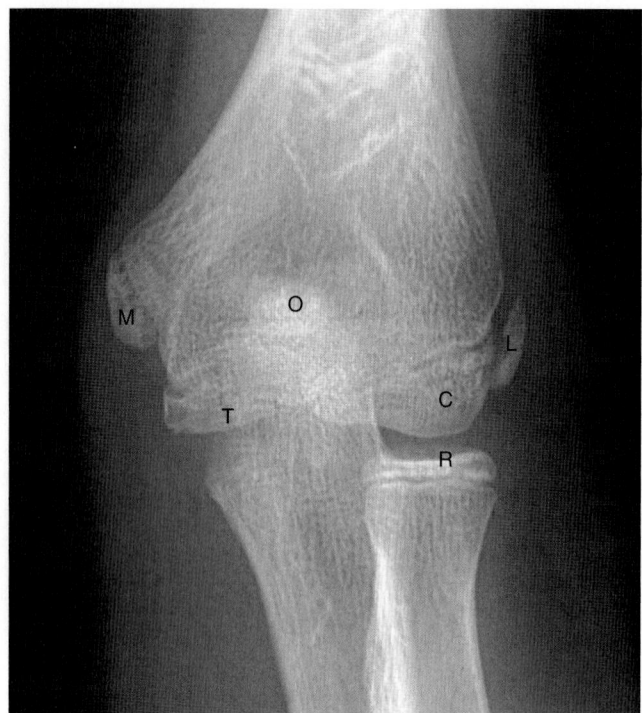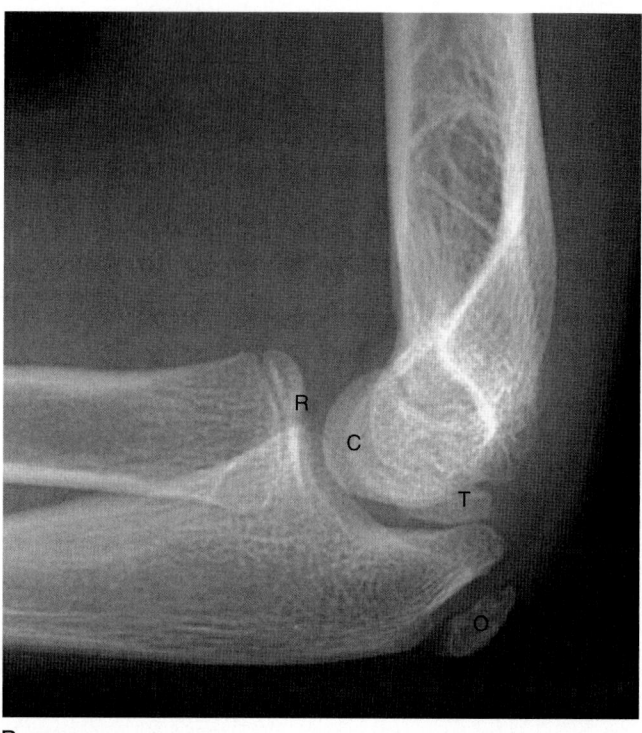

A   B

FIGURE 170-29. Radiographs of a normal elbow in a 14-year-old boy: anteroposterior **(A)** and lateral **(B)** views. C, capitellum; L, lateral epicondyle; M, medial epicondyle; O, olecranon; R, radial head; T, trochlea.

dyle have been reported. There are two chief mechanisms of acute avulsion fracture of the medial epicondyle: throwing injury and elbow dislocation.

Acute avulsion of the medial epicondyle is but one of several injuries that can occur in the elbow of a skeletally immature throwing athlete. The avulsion occurs due to hyperextension with valgus stress producing traction on the apophysis by the flexor tendons and pronators. In the setting of an acute avulsion, the child will experience sudden-onset medial elbow pain while throwing and have point tenderness over the medial epicondyle. Rarely, the medial epicondyle may displace into the joint. This occurs because the valgus stress of throwing temporarily widens the joint.

With elbow dislocation in the skeletally immature patient, the medial epicondyle is often avulsed from its normal location. When assessing the images of a dislocated elbow, the status of the medial epicondyle should be specifically addressed (Fig. 170-30): Is it in the normal location or avulsed? Some cases of medial epicondyle avulsion occur with a transient, unrecognized dislocation. When an elbow dislocation is reduced, the medial epicondyle may be trapped in the elbow joint (Fig. 170-31).

With a nondisplaced medial epicondyle avulsion, the medial epicondyle will appear abnormally separated from the distal humerus. With milder separation, comparison views may be helpful in confirming abnormality; however, they are usually not necessary. The avulsed medial epicondyle is usually pinned surgically. Displacement of 3 mm or greater is considered an indication for pinning (Fig. 170-32).

When the medial epicondyle is displaced into the joint, it may be confused with other, normal ossification centers; however, absence of the medial epicondyle at its normal location should prompt a search for it within the joint. If the trochlea is ossified, the medial epicondyle should be as well. Visualization of the trochlea without the medial epicondyle may be due to displacement of the medial epicondyle or due to a displaced medial epicondyle mistaken for trochlea.

Avulsion of the medial epicondyle prior to its ossification is distinctly rare, but reported. Sonography can be used to diagnose the avulsion.

> The medial epicondyle ossifies prior to the trochlea. In an injured elbow, visualization of an ossified trochlea without an ossified medial epicondyle in its normal location should raise suspicion for an avulsed medial epicondyle.

Distal Humeral Salter-Harris I Fracture

Distal humeral Salter-Harris I fracture is an uncommon fracture that occurs from birth to approximately 7 years of age, peaking at 2.5 years of age. Radiographically, the fracture may be mistaken for a dislocation of the elbow as the bones do not appear to align. The radial axis, however, will be normally aligned with the capitellum, and the capitellum itself will be abnormally related to the distal humeral metaphysis (Figs. 170-33 through 170-35).

Olecranon Fracture

Olecranon fractures are commonly seen in association with proximal radial fractures or dislocations. Less

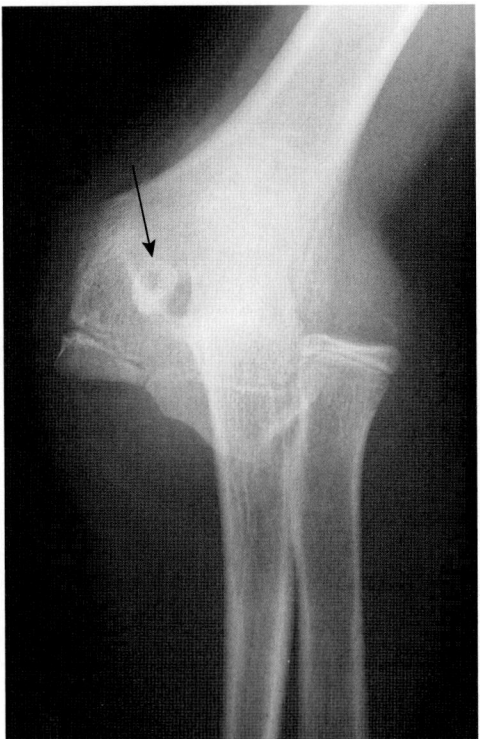

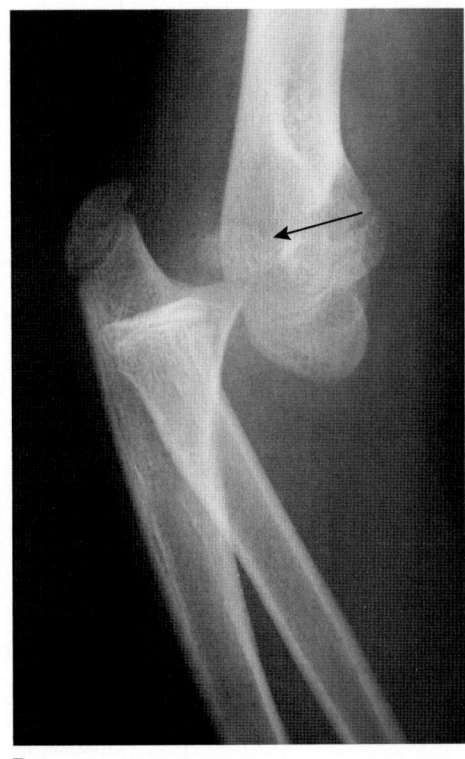

FIGURE 170-30. Anteroposterior **(A)** and lateral **(B)** radiographs of a dislocated elbow in a 12-year-old boy. The medial epicondyle *(arrows)* is avulsed.

A

B

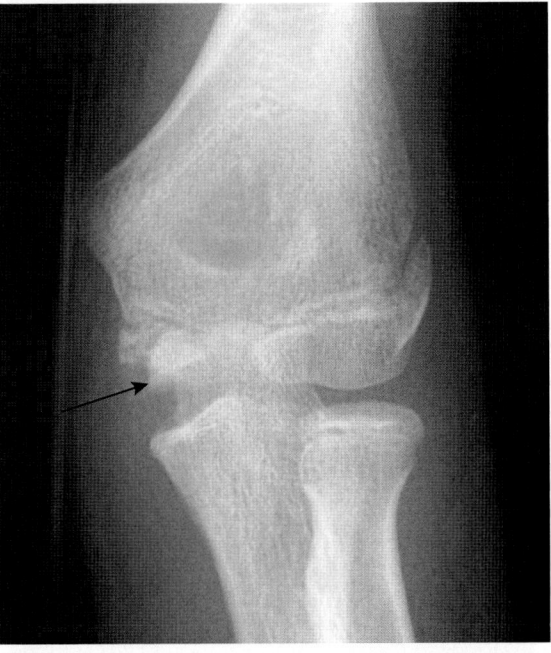

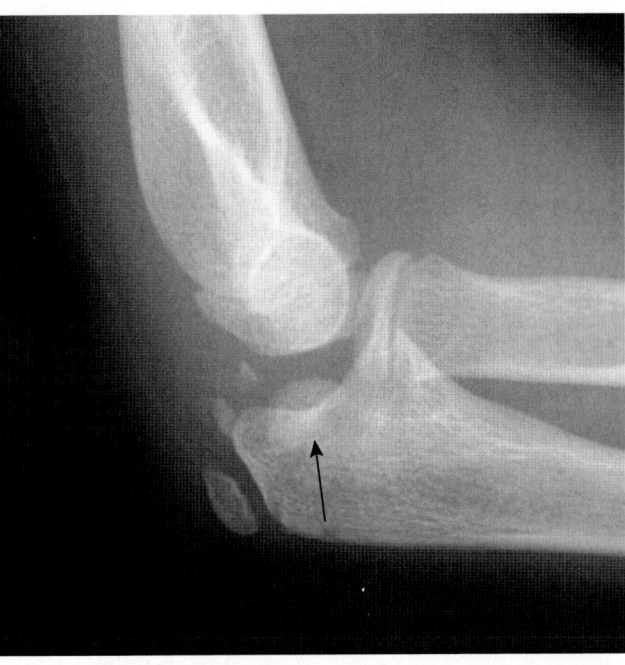

A

B

FIGURE 170-31. Anteroposterior **(A)** and lateral **(B)** radiographs after reduction of a dislocated elbow in a 10-year-old girl. The avulsed medial epicondyle *(arrows)* is trapped in the elbow joint.

commonly, there are associated fractures of the lateral or medial humeral condyle, a supracondylar fracture, or a distal radius/ulna fracture. Olecranon fractures may be transverse, oblique, or longitudinal. Buckle, bowing, or greenstick fractures are common in younger patients. Fractures may pass through the olecranon growth plate.

The olecranon growth plate varies considerably in location, and the olecranon ossification center varies considerably in size. The growth plate may be mistaken for fracture and vice versa. Comparison views are helpful. Stress fractures of the olecranon growth plate occur in adolescent baseball pitchers.

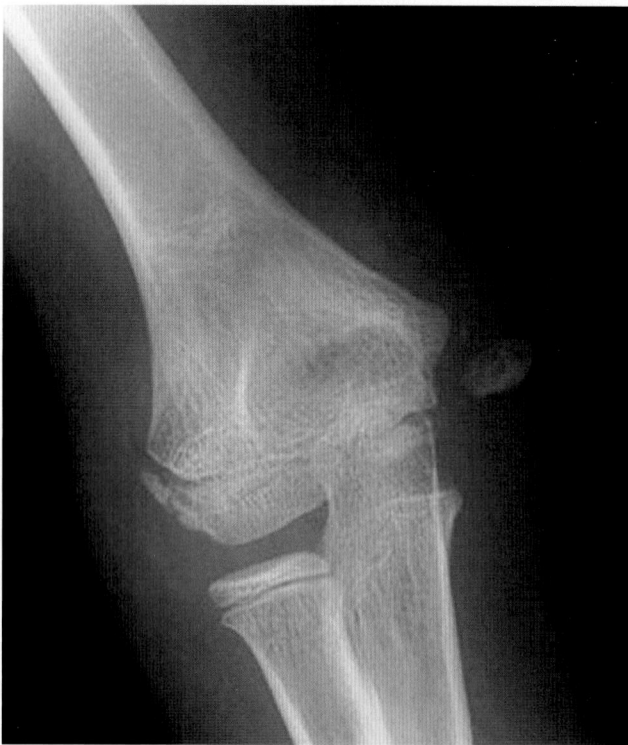

FIGURE 170-32. Avulsed medial epicondyle in an adolescent boy.

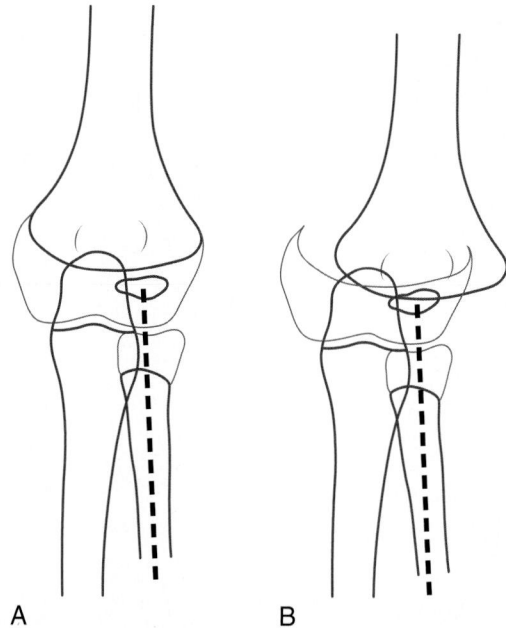

FIGURE 170-34. Separation of the entire distal humeral epiphysis. **A,** Normal elbow of a 2-year-old child. *Heavy lines* represent bony cortex, and *fine lines* the margin of the cartilaginous epiphysis of the humerus and radius. The radial capitellar line *(broken line)* defines the normal relationship of the radius and the capitellum. **B,** Salter-Harris type I separation of the entire distal humeral epiphysis. Note the medial displacement of the radius, ulna, and humeral epiphysis. The normal relationship of the radius and capitellum is maintained. (From Rogers LF: Radiology of Skeletal Trauma, 3rd ed. New York, Churchill Livingstone, 2002.)

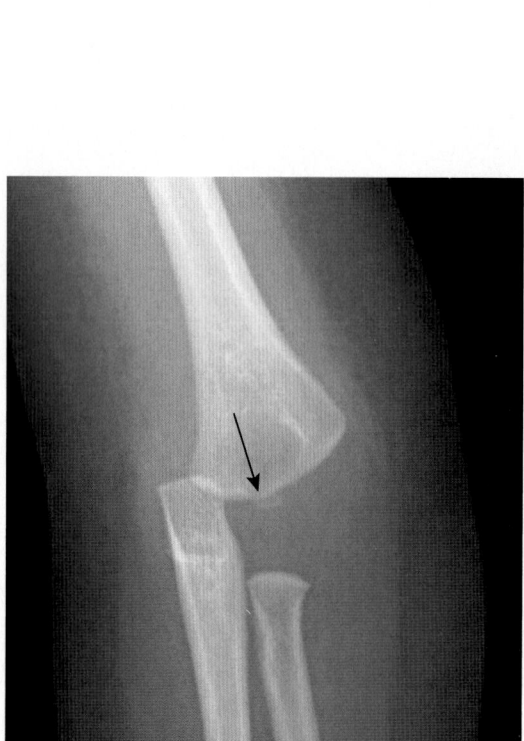

FIGURE 170-33. Salter-Harris I fracture of the distal humerus in a 16-month-old boy. The capitellum *(arrow)* is not properly aligned with the distal humeral metaphysis, and the whole forearm is shifted medially relative to the humerus. Soft tissue swelling is present.

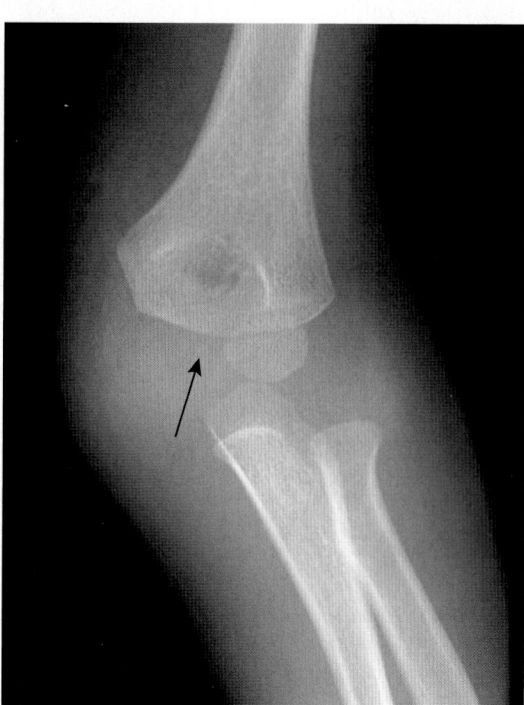

FIGURE 170-35. Dislocation of the elbow in a 5-year-old boy. Compare relationships to Figures 170-33 and 170-34. In this patient, the capitellum is normally aligned with the distal humerus; however, the radius is not properly aligned with the capitellum. Marked soft tissue swelling is seen medially. The medial epicondyle is undoubtedly avulsed and may be represented by a small ossific density *(arrow)*.

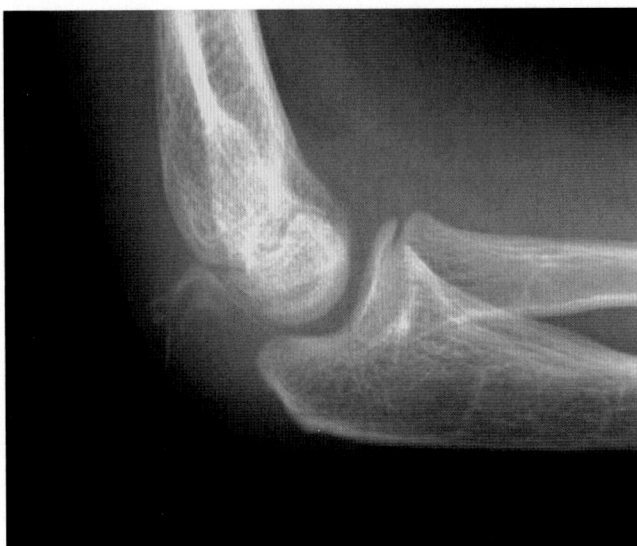

FIGURE 170-36. Olecranon sleeve fracture in an 11-year-old boy. A shell of bone is avulsed from the olecranon process and displaced proximally. Overlying soft tissues are swollen.

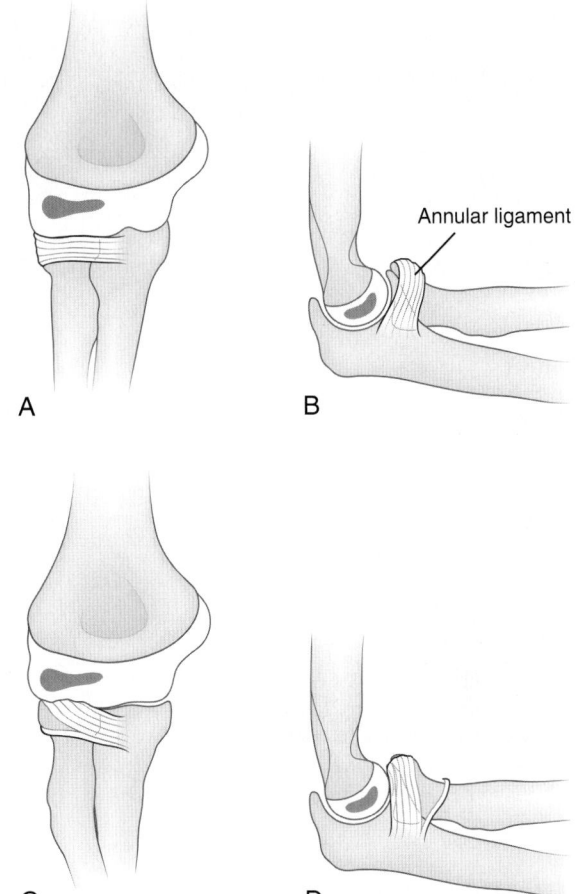

FIGURE 170-37. Pathology of pulled elbow. **A** and **B,** The normal position of the annular ligament is demonstrated in the anteroposterior **(A)** and lateral **(B)** projections. **C** and **D,** In the presence of a pulled elbow, the forearm is held in pronation **(C)** and a portion of the annular ligament is retracted proximally in to the radiocapitellar joint **(C** and **D).** (From Rogers LF: Radiology of Skeletal Trauma, 3rd ed. New York, Churchill Livingstone, 2002.)

An olecranon sleeve fracture is an avulsion of the triceps tendon from the olecranon process. A sleeve of cartilage and bone is avulsed from the margin of the olecranon ossification center (Fig. 170-36).

Radial Neck Fracture

Fractures of the radial head and neck account for 5% of pediatric elbow fractures. Fractures of the radial neck and proximal radial growth plate are commonly associated with fractures of the proximal ulna. The likely mechanism is hyperextension with valgus stress. Salter-Harris I fractures of the proximal radius are much less common than Salter-Harris II fractures. These fractures vary from subtle fractures, barely perceptible, to markedly displaced fractures. Angulated or displaced proximal radial fractures are difficult to properly reduce. The proximal radial fragment may rotate and become trapped, with the radial metaphysis preventing relocation of a displaced and rotated radial head fragment.

Isolated fractures of the radial head are more common with skeletally maturity. Salter-Harris III fractures of the radial head are uncommon.

Pulled Elbow (Nursemaid's Elbow)

Pulled elbow occurs due to an upward pull on an extended elbow in pronation. The annular ligament of the proximal radius is disrupted or displaced, allowing the radial head to subluxate or dislocate anteriorly relative to the capitellum (Figs. 170-37 and 170-38). This injury most commonly occurs in the toddler years, up to 5 years of age. An astute pediatrician will make the diagnosis clinically and reduce the radius without imaging. Oftentimes when imaging is requested, the dislocation is reduced in the course of properly positioning the patient for the anteroposterior (AP) view of the elbow.

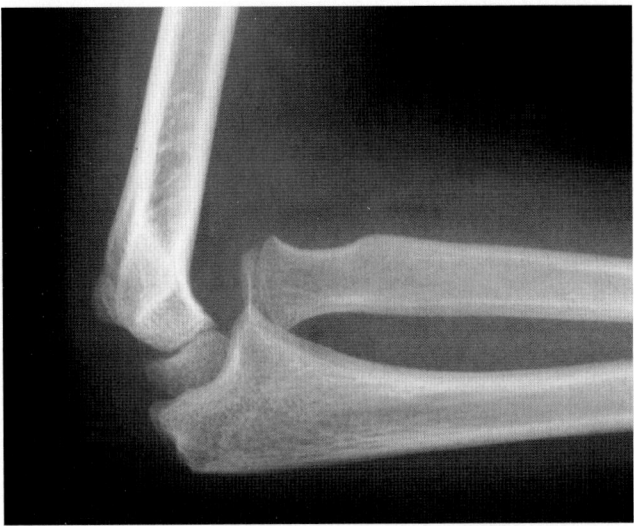

FIGURE 170-38. Dislocated radial head in a 9-year-old girl.

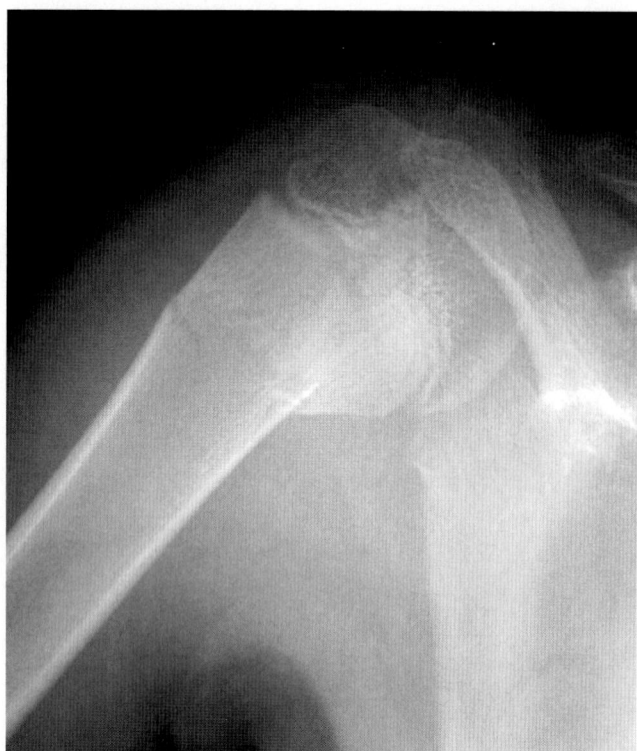

FIGURE 170-39. Incomplete fracture of the proximal humeral metaphysis in a 9-year-old girl.

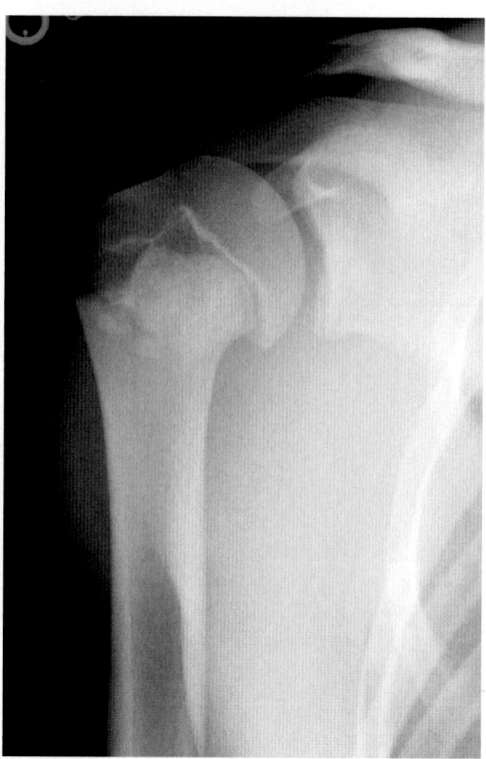

FIGURE 170-40. Salter-Harris II fracture of the proximal humerus in an adolescent. The metaphyseal fragment is small and projects through the larger distal metaphyseal fragment. There is slight medial rotation of the humeral head due to pull of the rotator cuff tendons on the greater tuberosity.

TRAUMATIC INJURIES OF THE HUMERUS

Injuries to the shoulder girdle, including the sternum, scapula, and clavicle, are covered in Chapter 80. Glenohumeral dislocation and instability is uncommon in younger children. These injuries are not uncommon in older teens, in whom patterns of injury are similar to those in young adults.

Proximal Humeral Epiphysis and Metaphyses

Injury to the proximal humerus varies with the age of the child. Infants and toddlers are likely to have a Salter-Harris I fracture of the proximal humeral physis. From 5 to 10 years of age, buckle fractures of the proximal humeral metaphysis are most prevalent (Fig. 170-39). These fractures may have considerable angulation. In older children, Salter-Harris II fractures predominate (Fig. 170-40).

The proximal humeral physis is may be a site of birth trauma. These injuries can also be seen with child abuse. Radiographically, since the humeral head is usually not ossified or only slightly ossified at birth, fracture through the growth plate mimics dislocation of the shoulder (Fig. 170-41). The humeral metaphysis may appear to align inferior to the glenoid. In the newborn, however, Salter-Harris I fracture of the proximal humerus is much more common than glenohumeral dislocation. Ultrasound may be used to diagnose the fracture by showing malalignment of the cartilaginous femoral head with the proximal femoral metaphysis and showing motion at the physis (Fig. 170-42).

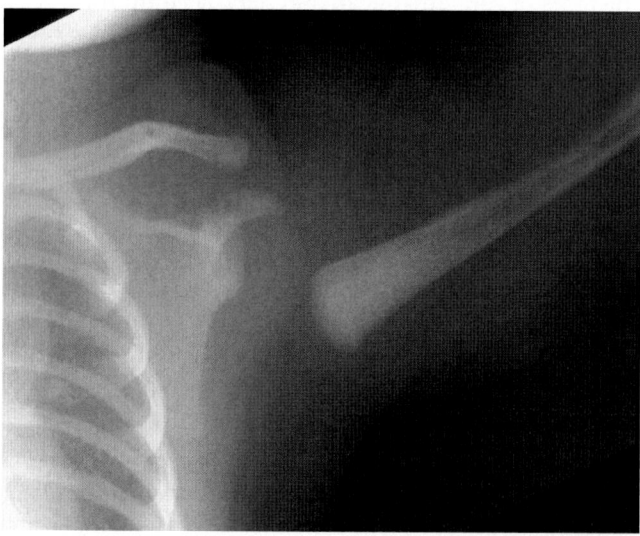

FIGURE 170-41. Proximal humeral Salter-Harris I fracture in a newborn due to birth trauma. The proximal humeral metaphysis appears malaligned with the glenoid. The humeral head is not ossified. In an infant, this finding is more likely due to fracture than dislocation.

Salter-Harris fractures of the proximal humerus are common in older children. Usually these fractures are Salter-Harris II fractures, although the metaphyseal fragment is often very small. Occasionally, there is no metaphyseal fragment. Such Salter-Harris I fractures are sometimes called "slipped capital humeral epiphysis."

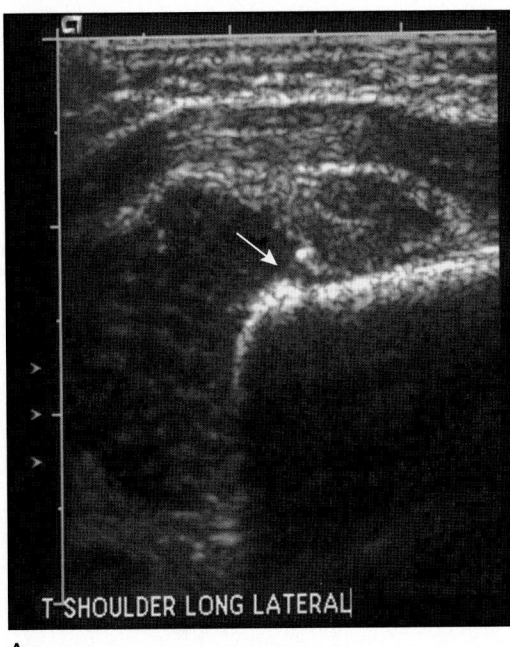
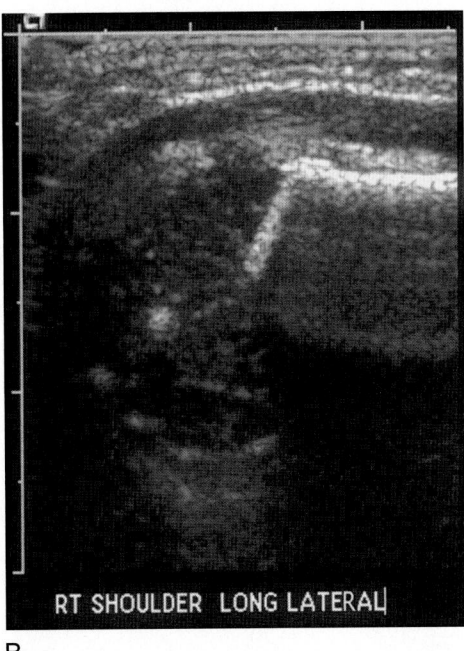

FIGURE 170-42. Proximal left humeral fracture in a 16-day-old girl with decreased arm movement and normal radiograph. Sonographic images of the shoulders were made in the coronal plane with lateral transducer positioning. **A,** In the left shoulder, the cartilaginous epiphysis is displaced laterally from the metaphysis *(arrow).* There is soft tissue swelling at the fracture site. **B,** Normal right shoulder for comparison.

Typically with a Salter-Harris I or II fracture of the proximal humerus, the epiphyseal fragment rotates medially due to unopposed pull by the rotator cuff. Salter-Harris III and IV fractures of the proximal humerus are rare. Avulsion of the greater tuberosity is a Salter-Harris III fracture. Avulsions of the lesser tuberosity are rare, due to hyperextension with avulsion of the subscapularis tendon, often delayed in diagnosis, and best delineated by an axillary view.

Humeral Diaphysis

Fractures of the humeral diaphysis are common. In very young children, these may be incomplete fractures; however, beyond the toddler years, most fractures of the humeral diaphysis are complete. Fractures may be transverse or oblique. The humerus is one of the more common sites for a pathologic fracture due to its propensity to develop bone cysts.

The positioning and alignment of the fragments of a humeral fracture are dependent upon the site of fracture and its relationship to the deltoid and pectoral muscular insertions (Fig. 170-43).

TRAUMATIC INJURIES OF THE PELVIS

Pelvic Ring Fractures

Fractures of the pelvic ring are most commonly seen with severe trauma, such as falls or motor vehicle accidents. The immature pelvis has greater elasticity and resilience to fracture, especially the sacroiliac joints and pubic symphysis. Associated injury to pelvic soft tissue structures, notably the bladder and urethra, should be suspected with severe fractures of the pubic bones with dis-

placement. Severe pelvic injuries may be accompanied by life-threatening hemorrhage; however, the incidence of such hemorrhage is considerably less than in adults with similar fractures.

In skeletally mature patients, fracture patterns may be classified as in adults. Several classifications schemes have been applied to pediatric pelvic fractures. In the classification scheme of Torode and Zieg, type I fractures are avulsions, type II are iliac wing fractures, type III are simple ring fractures with no clinical instability, and type IV are pelvic ring disruptions with instability (Fig. 170-44). Type IV fractures include straddle injuries with bilateral pubic rami fractures and Malgaigne fractures with anterior and posterior disruption on the same side. Disruption of the sacroiliac joints or pubic symphysis may accompany pelvic fractures. Plastic or incomplete fractures may be seen in children. Usually if there is one break in the obturator ring or pelvic ring, another break is also present. Younger children, however, may not follow this rule as the composition and plasticity of their bones may allow for only a single break.

CT is the preferred modality for delineation of unstable pelvic fractures. Although most fractures are seen on radiography, CT better delineates the full extent of fracture. The utility of plain radiographs for screening for pelvic fractures has been questioned. Inlet and outlet views and oblique (Judet) views do assist in delineating anatomy; however, they do not provide any information not obtainable from CT. Lesser degrees of trauma are unlikely to cause fracture, and most patients with trauma severe enough to result in a pelvic fracture will have undergone an abdominal/pelvic CT. With modern multidetector CT, there is no need for repeat imaging of the osseous pelvis. Rather, the same CT data set can be reconstructed to images with narrower slice thickness

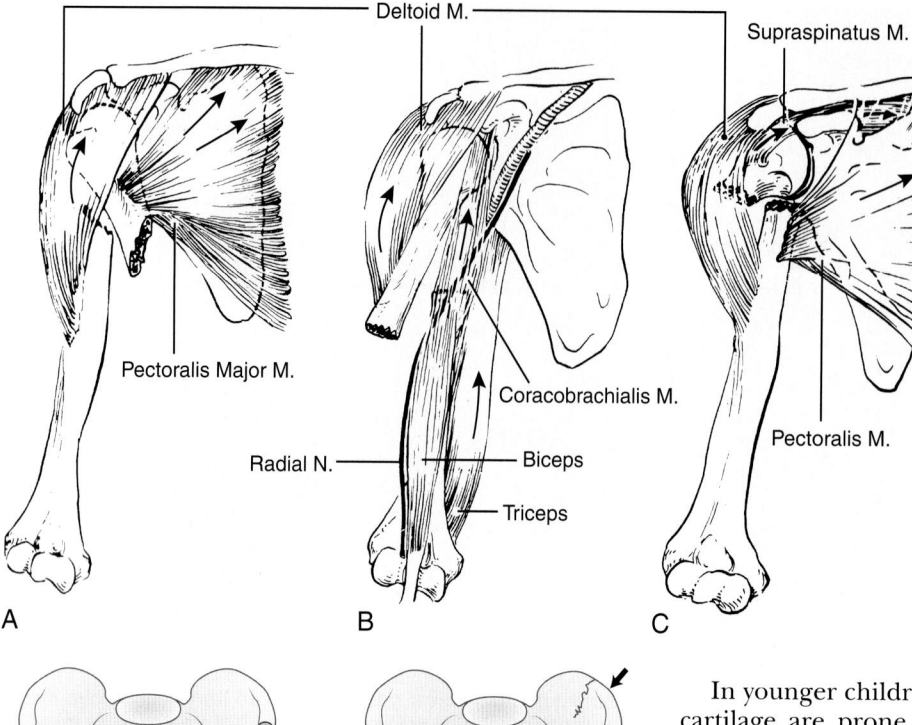

FIGURE 170-43. Fractures at the proximal end of the humerus, with characteristic deformities. **A,** Adduction of the proximal fragment as a result of pull of the pectoralis major and deltoid muscles. **B,** Abduction of the proximal fragment when the fracture is distal to the insertion of the deltoid muscle. **C,** Abduction and rotation of the proximal fragment when the fracture is proximal to the insertion of the pectoralis major and the rotator cuff. (From Cave EF: Fractures and Other Injuries. St. Louis, Mosby, 1958.)

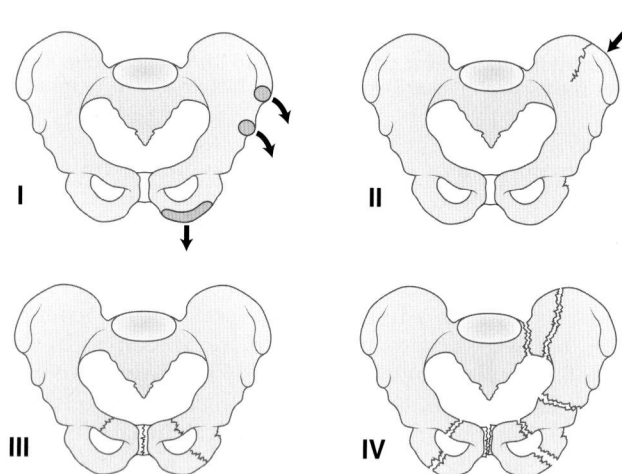

FIGURE 170-44. Pelvic fractures in children—Torode and Zieg classification. Type I, avulsion fracture; type II, iliac wing fracture; type III, simple ring fracture; type IV, ring disruption fracture. (Modified from Beaty JH, Kasser JR: Rockwood and Wilkins' Fractures in Children, 6th ed. Philadelphia, Lippincott Williams & Wilkins, 2006.)

and use of a bone algorithm to evaluate the bones. Sagittal and coronal reformats are invaluable.

> **Pelvic fractures in children may be incomplete. Single disruptions in the obturator ring may occur due to the composition of a child's bones.**

Acetabular Fracture

Fractures involving the acetabulum of young children are fortunately rare. Asymmetric widening of the triradiate cartilage may be noted (Fig. 170-45). Acetabular fractures become more common in the later teen years due to motor vehicle accidents. Fractures of the acetabulum in older children follow patterns similar to those in adults. CT is used for delineation of fracture anatomy.

In younger children, fractures involving the triradiate cartilage are prone to complications, particularly with associated dislocation or displacement of fragments. The Salter-Harris classification can be applied to acetabular fractures (Fig. 170-46). Premature fusion of the triradiate cartilage may lead to a shallow acetabulum and progressive hip disease. This complication is more common in children less than 10 years of age at the time of fracture.

> **Fractures involving the triradiate cartilage may interfere with subsequent acetabular growth.**

Apophyseal Avulsions

The apophyses of the pelvis begin to ossify early in the second decade and fuse at the time of puberty (Fig. 170-47). During this interval, the apophyseal growth plate represents a point of relative weakness and thus a potential site of fracture. The apophyses are sites of muscular origin or insertion; therefore, characteristic mechanisms of injury may lead to avulsion of a particular apophysis.

Avulsions of the anterior superior iliac spine (sartorius muscle origin) occur in sprinters. This is the most common site of pelvic apophyseal avulsion (Fig. 170-48). Patients will be point tender over the anterior superior iliac spine. Due to the similar symptoms and age, slipped capital femoral epiphysis (SCFE) may be suspected clinically. Avulsions of the ischial apophysis (hamstring muscle origin) occur in teenage hurdlers, cheerleaders, and gymnasts (Fig. 170-49). Avulsions of the iliac crest (abdominal wall muscle insertion) occur with abrupt changes in direction while running and in adolescent wrestlers. Avulsions of the iliac crest are rare and may be partial or total. Avulsions of the greater trochanter (hip rotators insertion) also occur with sudden change in direction. Avulsions also occur at the anterior inferior

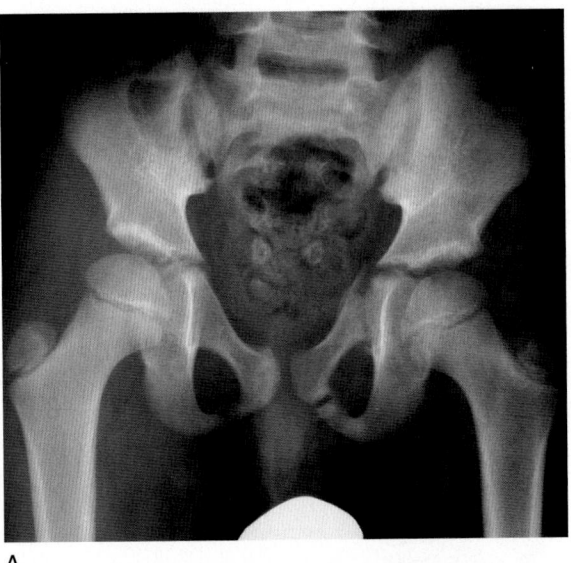
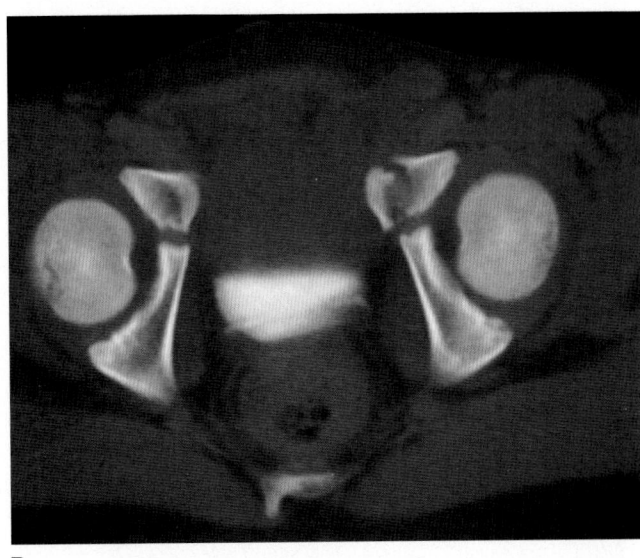

A   B

FIGURE 170-45. Acetabular fracture in an 8-year-old boy struck by an automobile. **A,** AP radiograph of the pelvis shows left pubic fractures and widening of the left triradiate cartilage. **B,** Axial CT shows the superior pubic ramus fracture to extend to involve the triradiate cartilage.

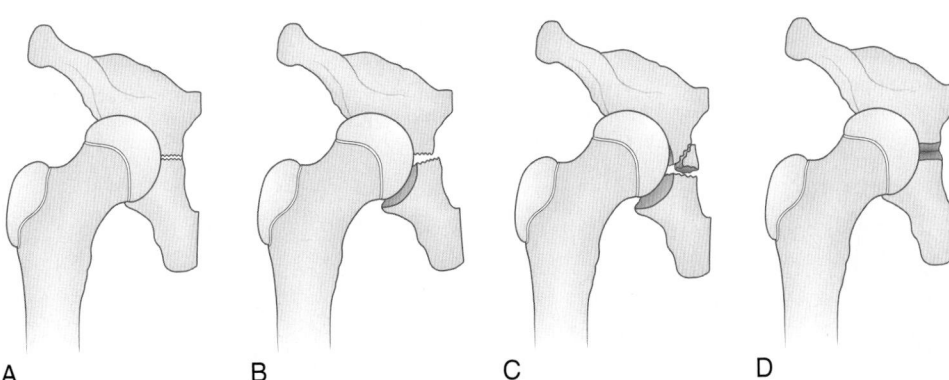

A   B   C   D

FIGURE 170-46. Types of triradiate cartilage fractures. **A,** Normal triradiate cartilage. **B,** Salter-Harris I fracture. **C,** Salter-Harris II fracture. **D,** Salter-Harris V (compression) fracture. (From Scuderi G, Bronson MJ: Triradiate cartilage injury: report of two cases and review of the literature. Clin Orthop Relat Res 1987;217:179-189.)

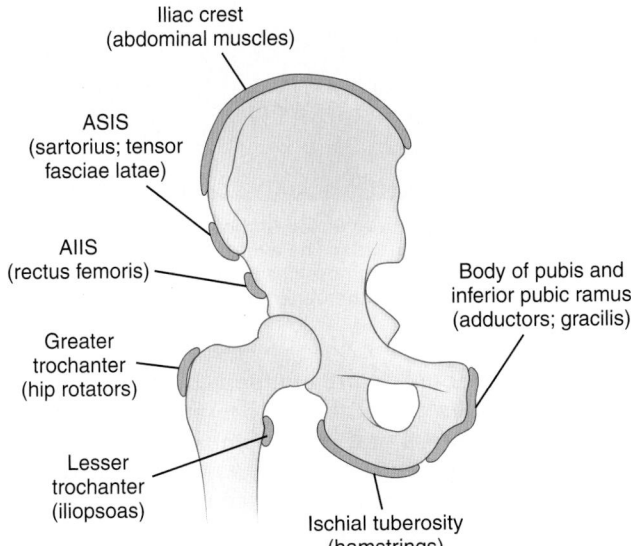

Iliac crest
(abdominal muscles)

ASIS
(sartorius; tensor
fasciae latae)

AIIS
(rectus femoris)

Greater
trochanter
(hip rotators)

Lesser
trochanter
(iliopsoas)

Body of pubis and
inferior pubic ramus
(adductors; gracilis)

Ischial tuberosity
(hamstrings)

FIGURE 170-47. Diagram showing the apophyses of the pelvis, sites of avulsion injury in adolescents. AIIS, anterior inferior iliac spine; ASIS, anterior superior iliac spine. (Modified from El-Khoury GY, Daniel WW, Kathol MH: Acute and chronic avulsive injuries. Radiol Clin North Am 1997;35:747-766.)

iliac spine (rectus femoris muscle origin; Fig. 170-50) and lesser tuberosity (iliopsoas tendon insertion). As opposed to adults, avulsions of the lesser trochanter in a skeletally immature child do not indicate an underlying pathologic lesion.

With an acute avulsion, symptoms are sudden in onset and directly related to the inciting activity. Avulsions can also be chronic. Chronic avulsions and healing, displaced acute avulsions may lead to exuberant reparative bone formation that may be mistaken for an osseous tumor (Fig. 170-51).

> Apophyseal avulsions occur at specific locations in the pelvis with characteristic injury mechanisms. These injuries characteristically occur in adolescents.

TRAUMATIC INJURIES OF THE HIP

Hip Dislocation

Traumatic hip dislocations are most common in older teenagers. Dislocations are almost always posterior.

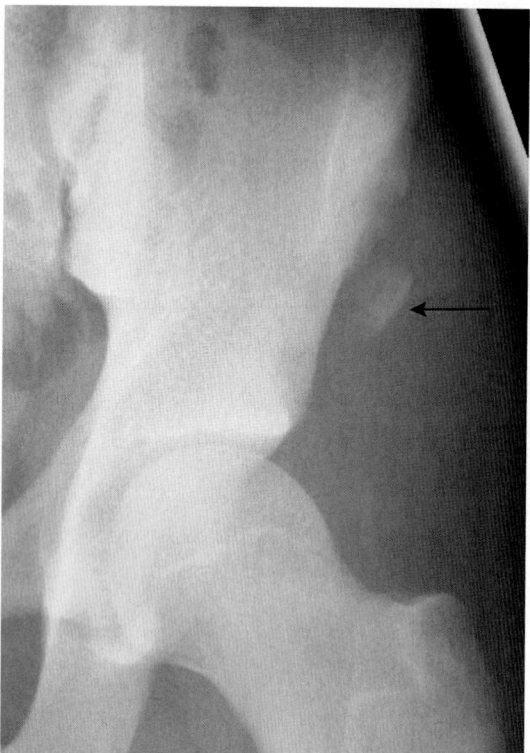

FIGURE 170-48. Avulsion of the anterior superior iliac spine *(arrow)* in a 16-year-old boy. The injury occurred with kicking.

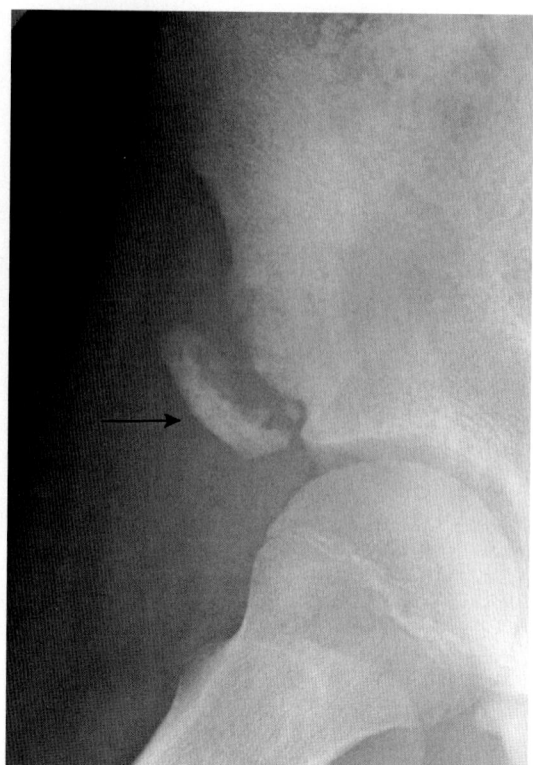

FIGURE 170-50. Avulsion of the anterior inferior iliac spine *(arrow)* in a 14-year-old boy. The injury occurred while playing soccer.

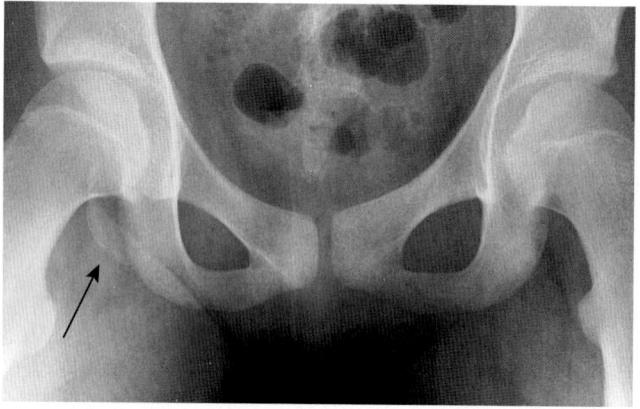

FIGURE 170-49. Avulsion of the ischial tuberosity *(arrow)* in a 14-year-old girl. The injury occurred when doing the "splits" in cheerleading.

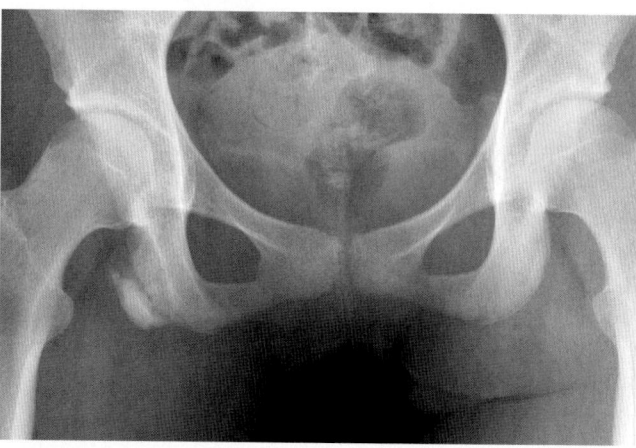

FIGURE 170-51. Chronic avulsion of the ischial tuberosity in a 17-year-old female cheerleader. The avulsed fragment is enlarged and sclerotic. Some ossification is seen within the gap between the fragment and the underlying ischium.

There may be an associated fracture of the posterior rim of the acetabulum.

Slipped Capital Femoral Epiphysis (SCFE)

SCFE is almost unique to the adolescent population; it is rare in the first decade of life. The patient may note an episode of minor trauma leading to presentation; however, in most patients a history of trauma is absent. Nonetheless, SCFE is essentially a Salter-Harris I fracture of the proximal femoral growth plate. Hence, SCFE is included within this chapter.

Twenty percent to 30% of patients will have bilateral SCFEs. In half of such patients, the SCFEs are simultan-

eous and diagnosed at presentation. In the other half, they are sequential. Risk for contralateral SCFE is greatest in the first 2 years after a unilateral SCFE.

SCFE typically occurs in boys ages 10 to 17 years and girls ages 8 to 15 years. It is more common in boys than girls. SCFE tends to occur earlier in girls due to their faster maturation than boys. SCFE is more common in African Americans than in whites. Patients are often overweight or delayed in development of secondary sexual maturation, or both. SCFE is of increased incidence in certain metabolic disorders such as hypothyroidism,

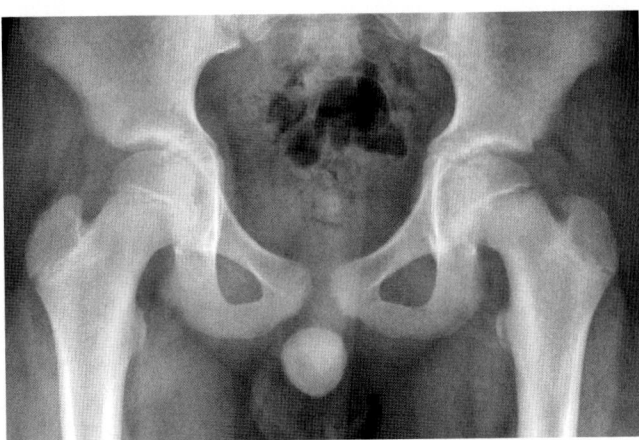

A

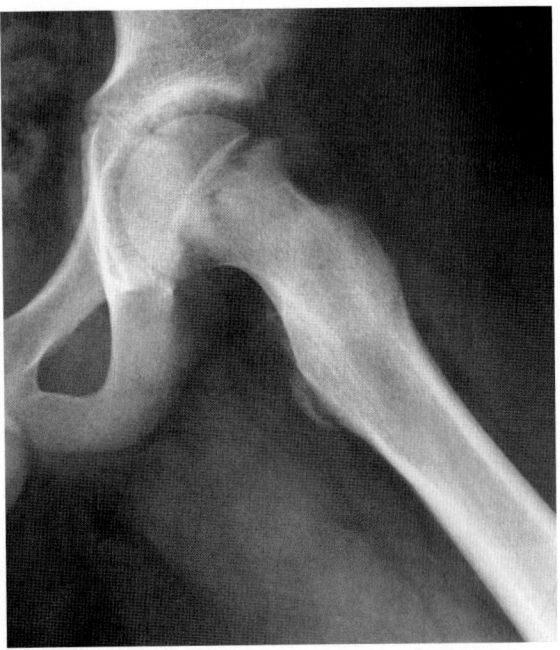

B

FIGURE 170-52. Slipped capital femoral epiphysis in an 11-year-old boy with left hip pain. **A,** On the AP view, the growth plate of the left proximal femur is wide and indistinct. No portion of the left femoral head projects lateral to Klein's line. The right proximal femur is normal. **B,** On the lateral view, malalignment of the femoral head and neck at the growth plate is better seen. The femoral head is displaced posteromedially relative to the femoral neck, but is still in continuity.

pituitary dysfunction, hypogonadism, and renal osteo-dystrophy. Hips within a radiation treatment field are at increased risk. SCFE occurs at a younger age and with greater bilaterality in patients with underlying disorders. When a child presents with bilateral symmetric SCFE or outside of the typical age range, an underlying disorder should thus be suspected.

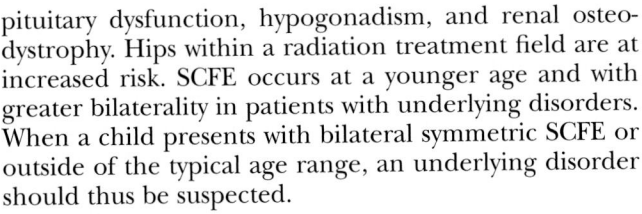

When a child presents with bilateral symmetric SCFE or outside of the typical age range, an underlying disorder should be suspected.

Children with SCFE usually present with hip, groin, or thigh pain. Pain may be referred to the knee. Up to a quarter of patients present with knee pain. Hip films are therefore recommended in the adolescent with unexplained knee pain.

By definition, children with "acute" SCFE have had symptoms for less than 3 weeks and children with "chronic" SCFE have had symptoms for greater than 3 weeks. Acute or subacute persistent hip pain in an adolescent should immediately raise suspicion for SCFE. Radiographs to evaluate for SCFE are best obtained to include both hips, one with the legs in the AP projection and the other in the lateral projection. The asymptomatic side serves as an internal control; however, it may not be normal.

SCFE can be also classified as "stable" or "unstable." With stable SCFE, there is osseous continuity across the proximal femoral growth plate. Essentially, the patient has a stress fracture of the growth plate. This has also been termed a "chronic SCFE." This is the most common type of SCFE. With unstable SCFE, there is loss of direct osseous continuity across the proximal femoral growth plate. Unstable SCFE may represent an acute Salter-

Harris I fracture of the proximal femoral growth plate without prior abnormality (an "acute SCFE") or an acute Salter-Harris I fracture of the proximal femoral growth plate superimposed on a chronic SCFE (an "acute-on-chronic SCFE"). Regardless of the type or chronicity of the slip, the femoral head tends to displace medially and posteriorly relative to the femoral neck.

On the AP view, the findings of SCFE may vary from frankly obvious to very subtle. An acute unstable SCFE will show obvious deformity of malalignment of the femoral head with the femoral neck. More indolent cases of SCFE may show widening and irregularity of the physis, demineralization, diminution of the femoral head, and increased metaphyseal density due to a healing response. Medial displacement of the femoral head on the AP view is often subtle. Klein's line is drawn parallel to the lateral margin of the femoral neck on the AP view. Normally, a small portion of the femoral head extends lateral to Klein's line. When the femoral head does not extend lateral to Klein's line, medial displacement may be suspected (Fig. 170-52). With chronic slips, sclerosis may be seen in the medial femoral neck with bone remodeling ("buttressing") in response to altered mechanics (Fig. 170-53).

Findings on the AP view may be very subtle; however, malalignment of the femoral head and neck is usually more manifest on a lateral view (see Fig. 170-52). It is thus critical to obtain a lateral view of the hips when evaluating an adolescent with hip pain, and specifically when SCFE is suspected. Either a frog-leg lateral or a true lateral view may be obtained. Patient discomfort may prohibit or limit the lateral view. Frog-leg laterals should only be obtained as tolerated by the patient; forceful positioning should be avoided. Some authors recommend avoiding the frog-leg lateral view with an acute SCFE as positioning of the patient may accentuate the degree of displacement.

CT and MRI may also be used to make the diagnosis of SCFE; however, usually plain radiographs suffice and these modalities are not called upon.

"Stable" SCFE is treated with screw fixation in situ; no reduction is attempted. Some chronic deformity therefore persists. Milder deformity is well tolerated. More severe deformity may be more debilitating in the long term, potentially leading to early-onset degenerative diseases. "Unstable" SCFE, by its nature, requires some reduction of malalignment of the femoral head and neck prior to fixation.

Due to complete loss of osseous continuity, "unstable" SCFE is associated with a higher incidence of avascular necrosis as a complication (Fig. 170-54). Chondrolysis (loss of hip joint cartilage) is a rare complication that seems to be more frequent in African American girls. While chondrolysis is said to complicate 5% to 10% of

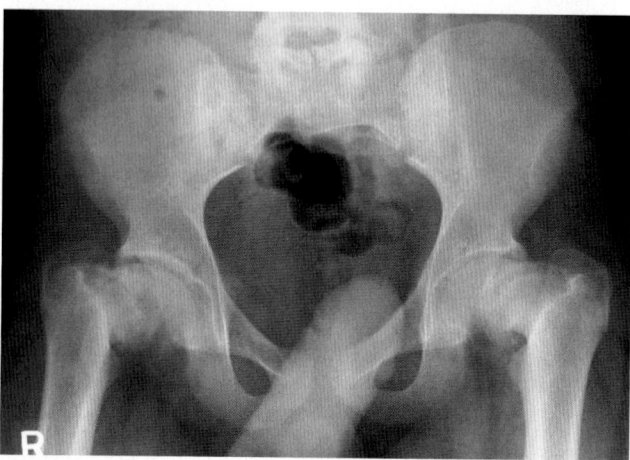

FIGURE 170-53. Advanced, chronic bilateral slipped capital femoral epiphyses at presentation in a 16-year-old boy. The femoral heads are rotated medially with varus deformity. The femoral necks are sclerotic with buttressing medially.

SCFE patients, the incidence of this complication has substantially lessened with newer fixation techniques. Complications due to malpositioning of a screw within the joint are now uncommon with modern orthopedic techniques for screw placement.

TRAUMATIC INJURIES OF THE FEMUR

Femoral Neck Fractures

Femoral neck fractures are relatively uncommon in children, particularly in comparison to the older adult. Nevertheless, femoral neck fractures may be seen at any age. The prognosis of femoral neck fractures in children is relatively good; however, avascular necrosis may occur as a complication. The risk for avascular necrosis is greater with greater displacement, greater time interval between injury and reduction, and instability of reduction/fixation.

The Delbert classification describes femoral neck fractures: type I, transphyseal; type II, transcervical; type III, basicervical; type IV, intertrochanteric; and type V, subtrochanteric (Figs. 170-55 and 170-56). Fractures are subgrouped as displaced or nondisplaced.

Femoral Diaphyseal Fractures

Femoral shaft fractures are common throughout childhood. Femoral fractures due to falls become relatively common at the time that children learn how to walk, have sufficient maneuverability to put themselves at risk, and can generate sufficient force for the fractures to occur. When a femoral shaft fracture is identified in a child who is not yet ambulatory, child abuse must be considered; it may be the etiology of fracture in as many as half of such cases.

In younger children, femoral diaphyseal fractures are occasionally incomplete. In older patients, fractures may

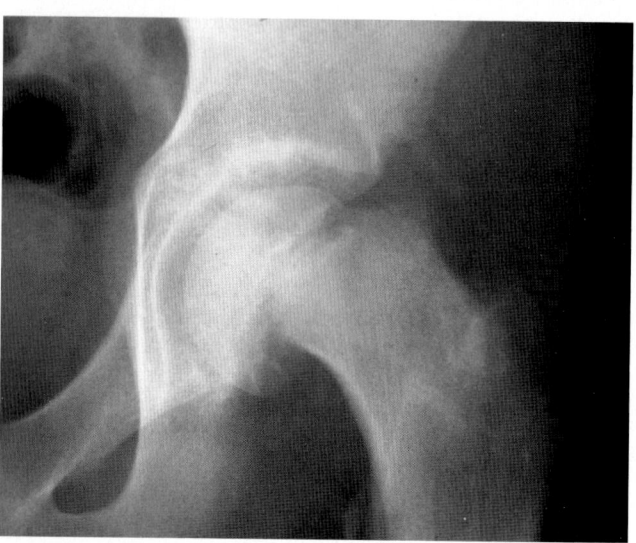

A

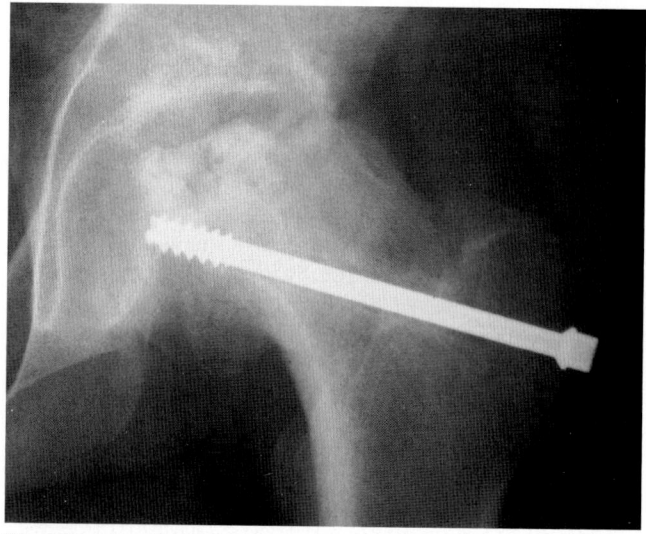

B

FIGURE 170-54. A, Unstable slipped capital femoral epiphysis in a 15-year-old boy. The femoral head is completely dissociated from the femoral neck and displaced and rotated medially. **B,** On follow-up, several months after pinning, the femoral head is deformed and sclerotic due to avascular necrosis.

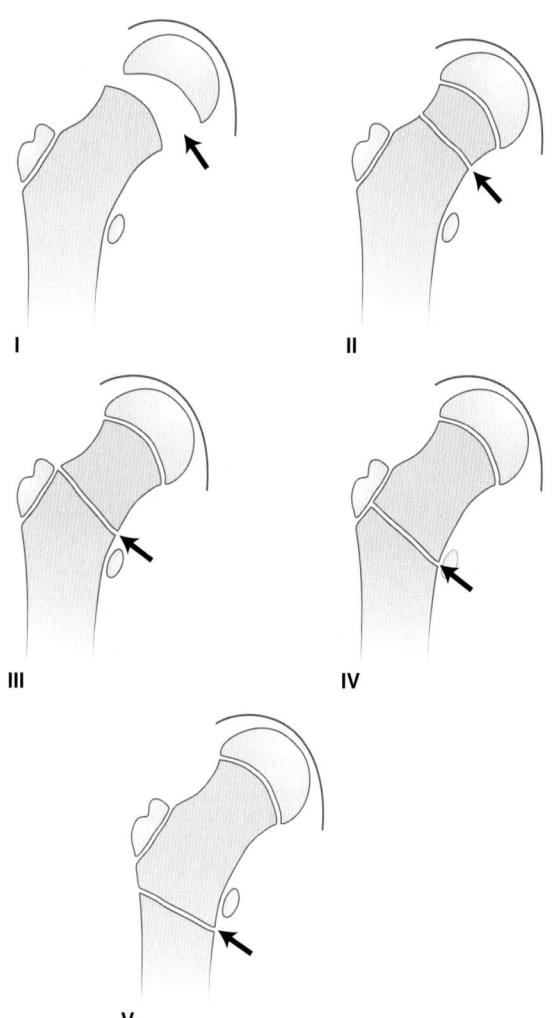

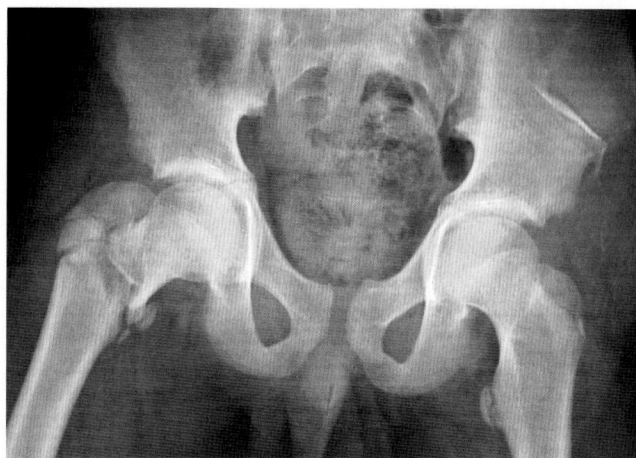

FIGURE 170-56. Type IV fracture of the proximal right femur in a 14-year-old boy due to a motorcycle accident. The facture is intertrochanteric and comminuted, with separate fragments from the lesser and greater trochanters. A fracture of the left ilium is also noted.

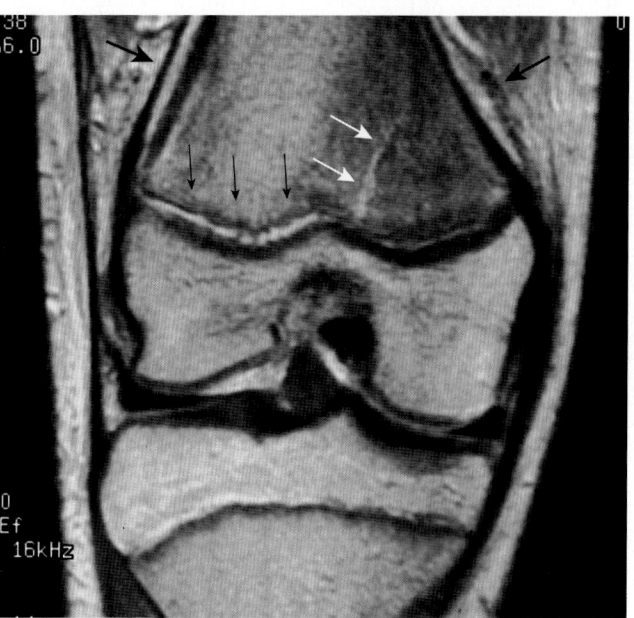

FIGURE 170-57. Salter-Harris II fracture of the distal femur in a 12-year-old girl. Proton density MR image shows widening of the distal femoral growth plate (*small black arrows*) and bone marrow edema. A small metaphyseal fracture line is seen (*white arrows*). Periosteum is elevated (*large black arrows*).

FIGURE 170-55. Classification of femoral neck fractures in children. I, transepiphyseal; II, transcervical; III, basal; IV, intertrochanteric; V, subtrochanteric. (From Azouz EM, Karamitsos C, Reed MH, et al: Types and complications of femoral neck fractures in children. Pediatr Radiol 1993;23:415-420.)

be transverse or oblique and are occasionally comminuted. Displacement of fracture fragments is dependent on positioning of the fracture relative to major sites of muscular insertion or origin.

TRAUMATIC INJURIES OF THE KNEE

Distal Femoral Metaphysis and Epiphysis

Until the growth plates of the knee fuse at puberty, they represent the weakest link within the knee and thus are the usual site of traumatic injury in the skeletally immature patient. Once the growth plates fuse, cruciate ligament injuries become much more common.

Most Salter-Harris fractures of the distal femoral metaphysis are frankly obviously on clinical examination and on radiographs; however, distal femoral Salter-Harris injuries may be deceptively subtle or occult on radiography and not diagnosed until MRI is performed (Fig. 170-57). The review of an MR image of the knee in a child with unfused growth plates must include specific attention to the physes as part of the search pattern.

> Some physeal fractures at the knee may be very subtle. The review of an MR image of the knee in a child with unfused growth plates must include specific attention to the physes to exclude a fracture.

Salter-Harris I fractures of the distal femur (distal femoral epiphyseal separation) are relatively uncommon. Usually, there is at least a small attached metaphyseal fragment. Salter-Harris II fractures are most prevalent, Salter-Harris III fractures are occasionally seen, and Salter-Harris IV fractures are rare.

Osteochondral injury ("osteochondritis dissecans") is likely a post-traumatic process. This is covered in Chapter 172.

Knee Effusion

Hemarthrosis of the knee joint is common and may be the consequence of soft tissue injury or fracture. Lipohemarthrosis is indicative of intra-articular fracture. Lipohemarthrosis may be seen on positional radiographs (cross-table lateral), MRI, or CT.

Fractures of the Patella

Fractures of the patella in children may be transverse, longitudinal, or comminuted. Transverse fractures are most common. The two poles of the transected patella are pulled apart by the quadriceps tendon. Like the scaphoid, the patella has a recurrent blood supply. Avascular necrosis of the proximal fragment is a rare complication of transverse patellar fracture. Patellar sleeve fracture represents an acute avulsion of the inferior pole of the patella. A "sleeve" of unossified cartilage is avulsed with a small fragment of bone. It may be difficult to differentiate patellar sleeve fracture from normal variation in ossification of the patella. Patellar sleeve fracture is covered in Chapter 172. Lastly, a bipartite patella may fracture at the synchondrosis between the patellar body and the smaller superolateral ossification center.

Proximal Tibial Epiphysis and Metaphysis

Salter-Harris fractures of the proximal tibia are less common than of the distal femur. Salter-Harris II fractures are most common; however, the metaphyseal fragment is often very small. Tibial spine fractures are most commonly due to athletic injury and are covered in Chapter 172.

Tibial Tuberosity Avulsion Fracture

The tibial tuberosity begins to ossify at 8 to 12 years in girls and 9 to 14 years in boys, and fuses to the underlying tibia at approximately 15 years in girls and 17 years in boys. The pattern of ossification varies considerably. Often the tuberosity has a fragmented appearance that should not be mistaken for a fracture. Acute fractures are also to be differentiated from Osgood-Schlatter disease, which is a chronic avulsion. Up to 20% of acute tibial tuberosity avulsions may be preceded by symptoms or findings of Osgood-Schlatter disease. Avulsions of the tuberosity occur due to acute pull on the tuberosity by the patellar tendon. The fracture occurs most frequently in boys 15 to 17 years old due to jumping injury.

As the tibial tuberosity is part of the same cartilaginous anlagen as the proximal tibial epiphysis, avulsions of the tuberosity are thus best defined as a Salter-Harris III fracture. Fractures of the proximal tibial growth plate may extend through the apophysis or through the apophyseal growth plate, the latter separating the proximal tibial epiphysis and tibial tuberosity from the

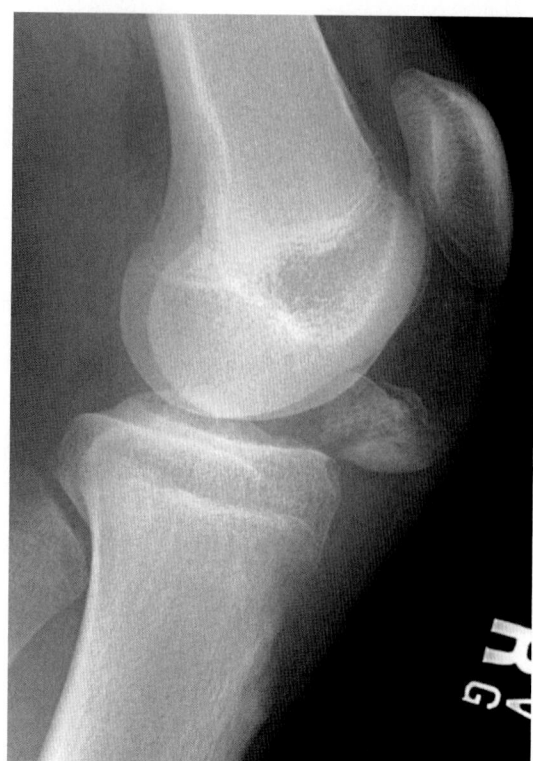

FIGURE 170-58. Tibial tuberosity avulsion in a 16-year-old after a bicycle accident. The avulsed fragment is distracted proximally and rotated.

tibial metaphysis as one single fragment (Fig. 170-58). A classification scheme for tibial tuberosity avulsion was originally developed by Watson and Jones and subsequently modified by others (Fig. 170-59). Type I injury is an avulsion of a small fragment of the apophysis. Type II avulsions occur at the junction between the tibial tubercle and the proximal tibial epiphysis. Type III avulsions course through the proximal tibial epiphysis and into the joint. Type IV fractures extend through the proximal tibial physis (Salter-Harris I). Type V fractures represent a combination of types III and IV. Types I, II, and III fractures can be further divided into subtypes A, without comminution, and B, with comminution.

TRAUMATIC INJURIES OF THE TIBIA AND FIBULA

Proximal Tibial Hyperextension Fracture

Incomplete fractures of the proximal tibia may occur in toddlers due a hyperextension force from jumping. These fractures are often subtle with a slight buckling or "scooping" of cortex anteriorly (Fig. 170-60). An incomplete fracture line may be seen posteriorly. The proximal tibial physis may be tilted anteriorly. It may be difficult to distinguish the normal contour of the anterior margin of the proximal tibia (underlying the cartilaginous tibial tuberosity) from a buckle fracture. Usually, the normal tibia has a smooth, uninterrupted curve, whereas the fracture creates a focal buckle of cortex. Comparison images may be helpful.

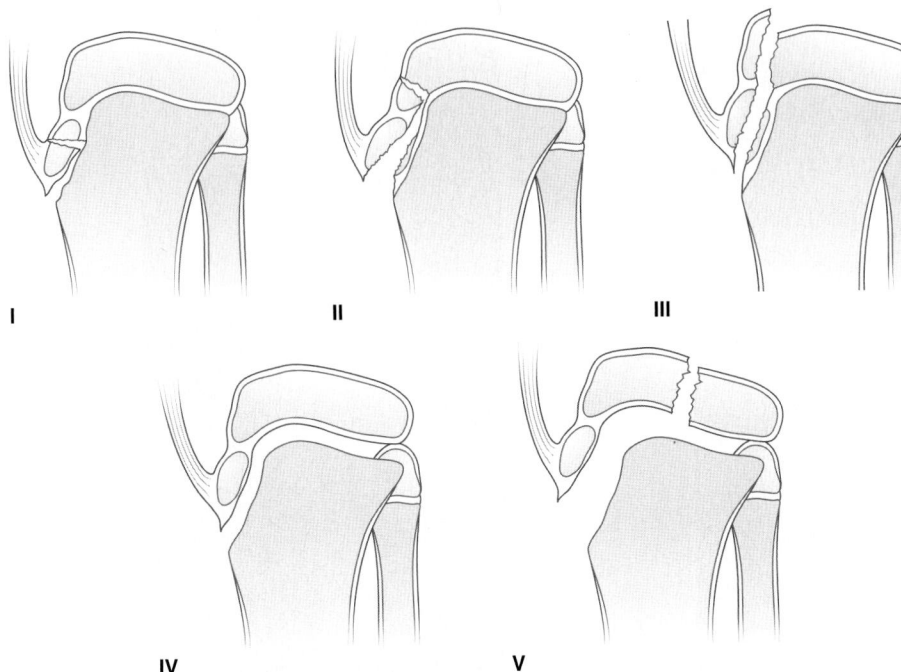

FIGURE 170-59. Tibial tuberosity fracture classification. I, avulsion of a small fragment of the apophysis; II, avulsion at junction between tibial tubercle and proximal tibial epiphysis; III, fracture extends through proximal tibial epiphysis and into joint; IV, fracture extends through proximal tibial physis (Salter-Harris I); V, combination of types III and IV. (From McKoy BE, Stanitski CL: Acute tibial tubercle avulsion fractures. Orthop Clin North Am 2003;34:397-403.)

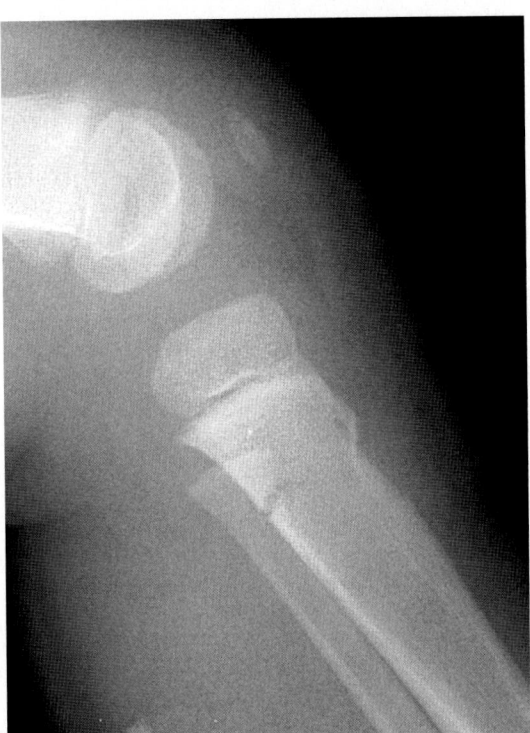

FIGURE 170-60. Proximal tibial hyperextension fracture in a 2-year-old girl. An incomplete fracture is seen with cortical buckling anteriorly and cortical break posteriorly. Compare the appearance of the surface of the anterior tibial metaphysis to that in Figure 170-61.

Toddler Fracture of the Tibia

Toddler fracture is typically seen between 9 months and 3 years of age. In this age range, the child is relatively imbalanced and prone to falling and twisting injury. In a classic toddler fracture, the child catches his or her leg on an object and twists and falls. Often a specific incident is witnessed. Some children present with pain and refusal to bear weight without a specific precipitating incident. Symptoms may be acute in onset or indolent. On physical examination, the child will be point tender over the fracture.

Toddler fractures may occur anywhere within the proximal metaphysis, diaphysis, or distal metaphysis of the tibia. The fracture line is oblique or spiral with no distraction or displacement (Fig. 170-61). Acutely, the fracture line may be very subtle. In some patients, follow-up radiographs are necessary to confirm the fracture. The healing process, with sclerosis at the margins of the fracture line and development of periosteal new bone, may increase the conspicuity of the fracture.

Because the fracture line is oblique or spiral and because there may not be a particular event leading to fracture, toddler fractures may erroneously be ascribed to child abuse. In the absence of other injury, however, the typical radiographic appearance of a toddler fracture in a child of the typical age range should not in itself raise suspicion for child abuse, even without a witnessed event. Toddler fractures are very common once children begin to cruise and walk. The presence of a similar fracture prior to the cruising or ambulatory stage should raise greater concern for abuse.

> Classic toddler fracture of the tibia is one cause of pain and refusal to bear weight. Toddlers may also incur fractures of the fibula and tarsal bones (talus and cuboid) and present similarly.

Fibular Toddler Fracture

Although tibial toddler fractures are classic and much more common, isolated fractures of the fibula can occur

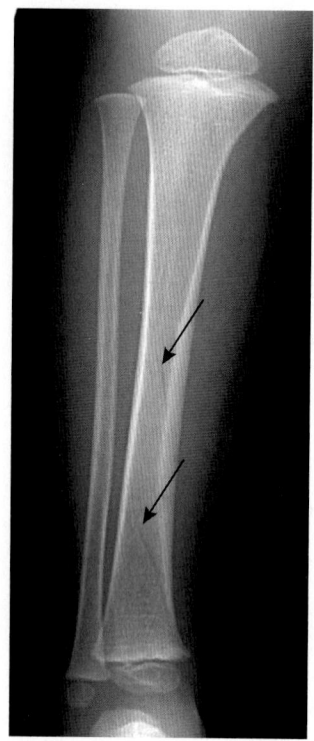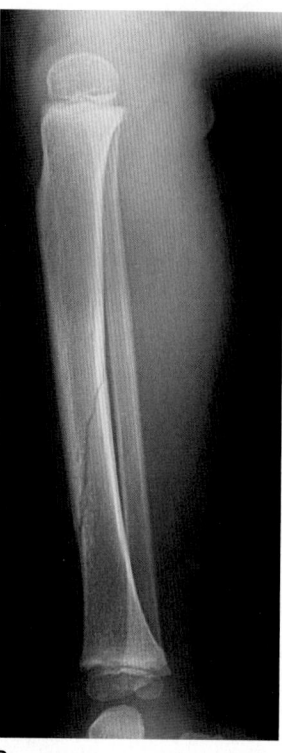

A   B

FIGURE 170-61. Anteroposterior **(A)** and lateral **(B)** views of a toddler fracture of the tibia in a 2-year-old girl. The fracture line has a spiral course as shown by two apparent fracture lines on the AP view *(arrows)* and the intervening single fracture line on the lateral view. Slight soft tissue swelling is seen anterior to the fracture on the lateral view.

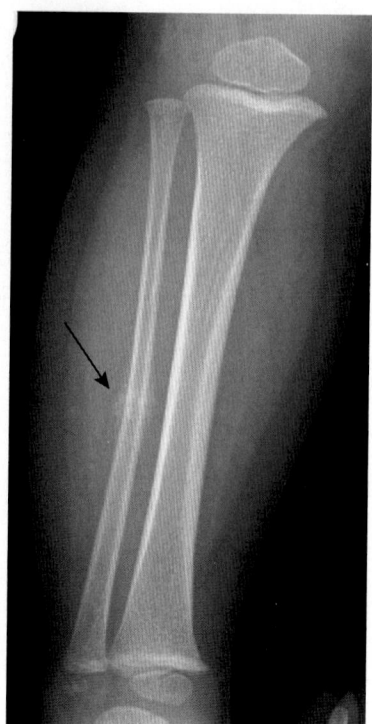

FIGURE 170-62. Fibular toddler fracture in a 19-month-old boy. Callus is present *(arrow)* with a faint transverse fracture line.

with a similar mechanism. These fractures are usually subtle buckle or bowing fractures. As with tibial toddler fractures, the fracture may become more conspicuous with healing (Fig. 170-62).

Tibial and Fibular Diaphyseal Fractures

In older children, fractures of the tibial shaft are usually complete with a transverse or oblique fracture plane. The fibula is almost uniformly fractured when there is a complete fracture of the tibial diaphysis.

Maisonneuve fracture of the proximal fibula may occur with medial ligamentous injury or medial malleolar fracture at the ankle. The fracture may also occur with juvenile Tillaux or triplane fracture of the distal tibia. With a disruption of medial support at the ankle, the injury may traverse the interosseous membrane up the leg and pass obliquely through the proximal fibular diaphysis. The presence of a Maisonneuve fracture thus indicates disruption of the interosseous membrane and potential instability without fixation. An image of the proximal fibula should always be obtained when there is injury medially at the ankle.

Distal Tibial Metaphyseal Fracture

The distal tibial metaphysis is a common site for buckle fractures in young children. As with buckle fractures at other sites, subtle disruption of the smooth normal

contour of the distal tibial metaphysis should be sought as evidence for fracture.

Salter-Harris fractures are also very common at the distal tibia. In younger children, Salter-Harris II fractures predominate. Salter-Harris III fractures may be seen medially (medial malleolar fragment; Fig. 170-63) or laterally (juvenile Tillaux fracture; see later). The distal tibial metaphysis is one of the more common locations of Salter-Harris IV fractures (Fig. 170-64; see also Fig. 170-9). Unfortunately, premature fusion at this site bears considerable potential morbidity due to deformity and leg length discrepancy.

Juvenile Tillaux Fracture

The juvenile Tillaux fracture is a Salter-Harris III fracture of the distal tibial physis and epiphysis. This "transitional" fracture occurs in the early teen years when the distal tibial growth plate is nearing the time of fusion or is already partially fused. The distal tibial growth plate begins to fuse at "Kump's bump" in the medial central physis. Fusion then proceeds medially and posteriorly (Fig. 170-65). The anterolateral portion of the growth plate is the last portion of the physis to close and thus is the plane of least resistance to fracture. Juvenile Tillaux fractures probably represent an anterolateral avulsion of the distal tibial epiphysis pulled by the anterior tibiofibular ligament due to forced external rotation. The epiphyseal component of the fracture is usually sagittal or sagittal oblique, with the physeal portion of the fracture coursing through the anterolateral aspect of the distal tibial physis (Fig. 170-66).

The epiphyseal fragment is usually not considerably displaced. The concern with a juvenile Tillaux fracture

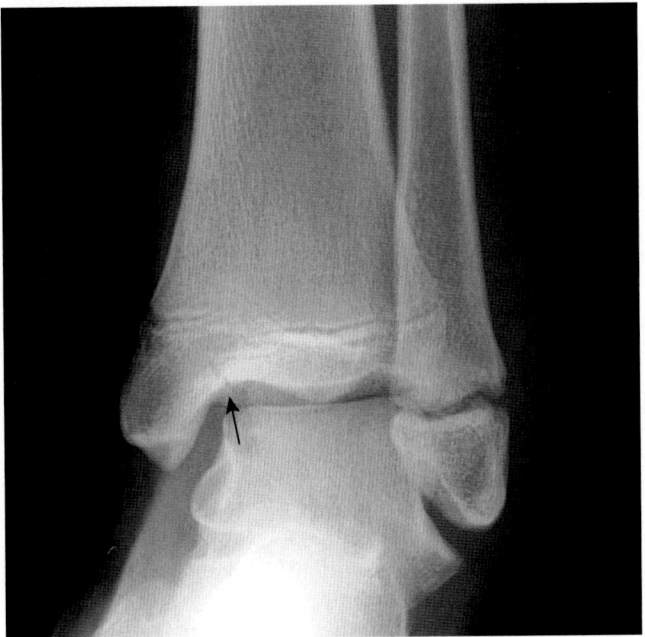

FIGURE 170-63. Radiograph of a 14-year-old boy with a skateboarding injury showing a Salter-Harris III fracture of the medial tibia *(arrow)* and a Salter-Harris I fracture of the distal fibula. Marked soft tissue swelling overlies the fibula.

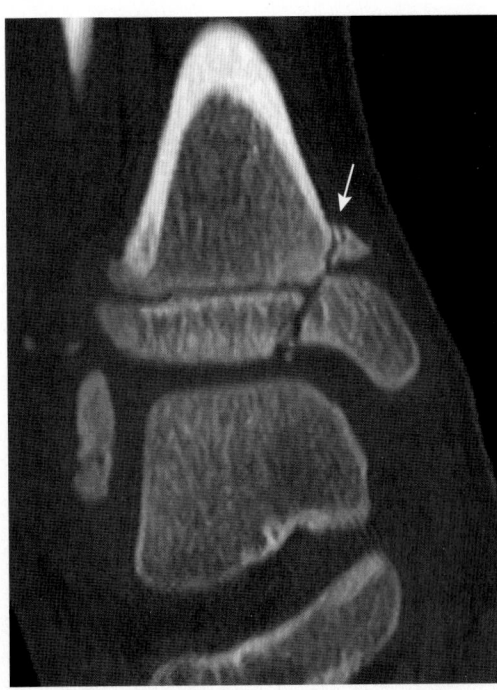

FIGURE 170-64. Salter-Harris IV fracture of the distal tibia in an 8-year-old boy. Coronal CT reconstruction shows the course of the fracture *(arrow)*. Note the apposition of metaphysis and epiphysis across the fracture.

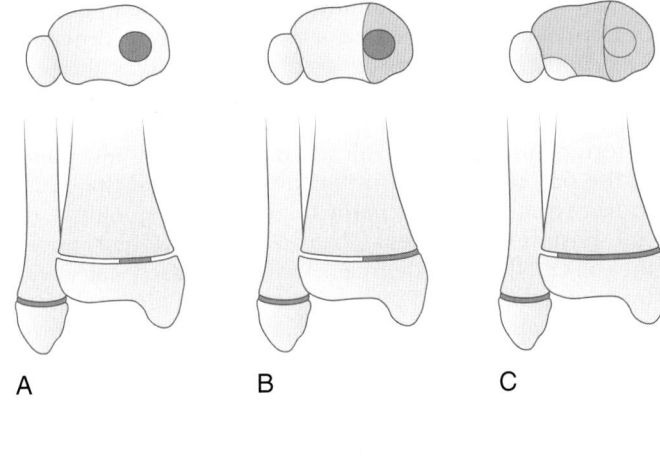

A   B   C   D

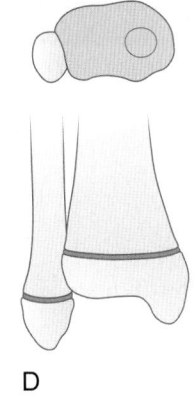

FIGURE 170-65. Diagram of the path of closure of the distal tibial physis. Closure begins centrally **(A)** and proceeds medially **(B)** and then laterally **(C)** before fusion is complete **(D)**. (Modified from Beaty JH, Kasser JR: Rockwood and Wilkins' Fractures in Children, 6th ed. Philadelphia, Lippincott Williams & Wilkins, 2006.)

of the distal tibia is not possible premature fusion of the growth plate, as the growth plate is already starting to fuse, but rather involvement of the articular surface. A significant gap or incongruity of the fracture fragments at the articular surface may portend an early progression to degenerative disease in the ankle. As a rule, if the fracture line is wider than 2 mm, a juvenile Tillaux fracture will undergo operative fixation. Practically speaking, most of these fractures are surgically fixated. CT is used in preoperative planning to measure displacement at the articular surface and to map the anatomy of the fracture planes (Fig. 170-67).

Triplane Fracture

Triplane fracture is closely related to juvenile Tillaux fracture; however, there is an additional plane of fracture of the distal tibial metaphysis, usually coronal in orientation (Fig. 170-68). The three planes of a triplane fracture are thus a sagittal fracture through the epiphysis, a transverse fracture through the physis, and a coronal fracture through the metaphysis (Fig. 170-69). The epiphyseal and metaphyseal fracture planes may vary somewhat from true orthogonal orientation. A classic triplane fracture has two parts; however, three-part and four-part variants occasionally occur. Although the triplane fracture involves both the epiphysis and the metaphysis, it is not a true Salter-Harris IV fracture as the epiphyseal and metaphyseal fracture lines are not in continuity within the same plane. More correctly, the triplane fracture is a combination of a Salter-Harris II fracture and a Salter-Harris III fracture. Prognosis and treatment of triplane fracture are analogous to that in the previous discussion for juvenile Tillaux fracture.

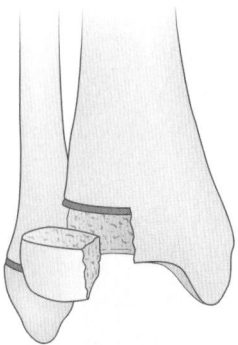

FIGURE 170-66. Juvenile Tillaux fracture. A fragment of the anterolateral epiphysis is avulsed by the anteroinferior tibiofibular ligament. (Modified from Beaty JH, Kasser JR: Rockwood and Wilkins' Fractures in Children, 6th ed. Philadelphia, Lippincott Williams & Wilkins, 2006.)

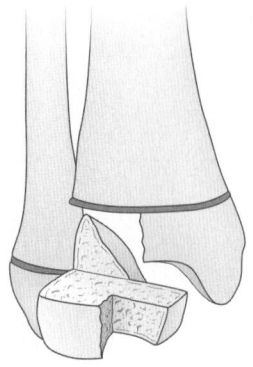

FIGURE 170-68. Triplane fracture. In a two-part triplane fracture, there are typically sagittal epiphyseal, transverse physeal, and coronal metaphyseal fracture lines. (Modified from Beaty JH, Kasser JR: Rockwood and Wilkins' Fractures in Children, 6th ed. Philadelphia, Lippincott Williams & Wilkins, 2006.)

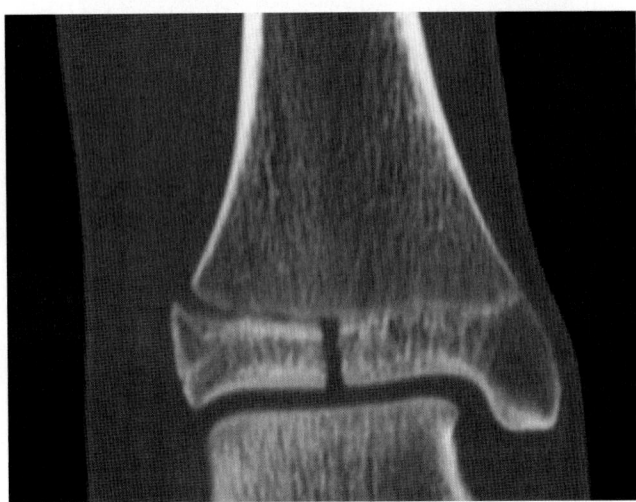

FIGURE 170-67. Juvenile Tillaux fracture in a 14-year-old boy. Coronal CT reconstruction shows the Salter-Harris III fracture of the anterolateral distal tibial epiphysis.

> Juvenile Tillaux and triplane fractures are "transitional" fractures, occurring in older children in whom the distal tibial growth plate is partially fused.

TRAUMATIC INJURIES OF THE ANKLE AND FOOT

Talus Injuries

Fractures of the talus in children are uncommon. Fractures most commonly occur in the talar neck. Complete fractures across the neck are rarely seen in older children. Younger children may have buckle fractures of the talar neck. The buckle is evident along the dorsal surface of the bone and may be very subtle. The talus is one location of so-called tarsal toddler fracture. These fractures occur due to compression of the talus neck against the anterior margin of the tibia with forced dorsiflexion. The child will refuse to bear weight. The fracture may be difficult to diagnose acutely. With healing, a band of sclerosis will be seen within the talus.

Dislocations at the tibiotalar joint are very rare compared to the incidence of fracture of the distal tibia. Subtalar dislocations or complete talar dislocations are also rare injuries. These dislocations are usually only seen in the setting of a severe traumatic injury.

Due to the talar body's recurrent blood supply, fractures may be complicated by avascular necrosis of the proximal pole. The dislocated talus is also at risk for subsequent development of avascular necrosis due to disruption of vascular supply.

A common injury of the talus is an osteochondral fracture of the talar dome. This injury is covered in Chapter 172.

Calcaneal Fractures

Calcaneal fractures most commonly occur with jumps or falls from a large height. Such fractures can cause a variable degree of comminution and variable degree of depression of the superior margin of the calcaneus. The Böhler angle can be used to assess for calcaneal depression due to fracture. This angle is the posterior angle between two lines, one drawn tangent to the anterior process of the calcaneus and the highest point of the posterior subtalar articular surface, and the other drawn from the latter point to the superior margin of the posterior calcaneus. Normally, the Böhler angle measures 30 to 35 degrees. With depressed calcaneal fractures, the Böhler angle is decreased. Calcaneal fractures are also characterized as articular verses nonarticular with reference to involvement of the subtalar joint. CT is utilized for full delineation of calcaneal fracture anatomy.

Prior to apophyseal fusion, the posterior calcaneus may experience fractures involving the apophyseal growth plate and apophysis that can be classified by the Salter-Harris system.

Subtle compression fractures of the calcaneal body are not infrequent in younger children. These injuries may be virtually impossible to diagnose acutely from radiographs unless there is a buckle of the margin of the bone. Follow-up radiographs will show an oblique band of sclerosis within the midcalcaneal body (Fig. 170-70).

Cuboid Fractures

The cuboid is the most common site of so-called tarsal toddler fractures. These fractures occur due to compression of the cuboid between the calcaneus and metatarsal bones with forced dorsiflexion as might occur with jumping from a height. Acute cuboid fractures are often

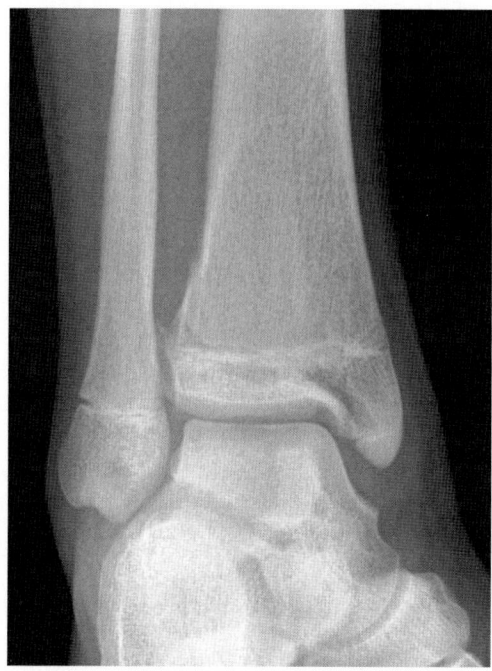
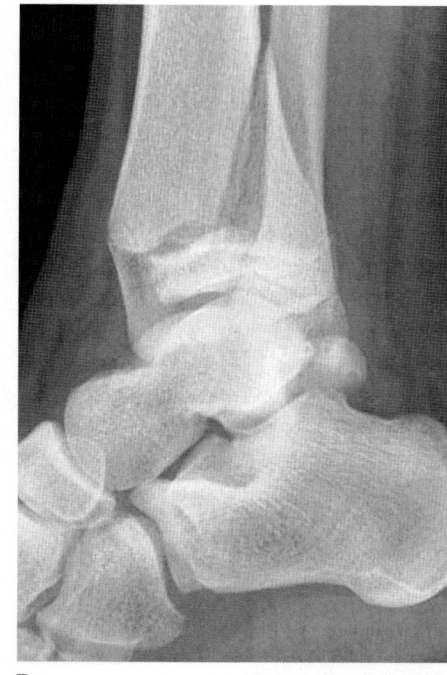

A   B

FIGURE 170-69.
Anteroposterior **(A)** and lateral **(B)** views of a triplane fracture in an adolescent. (Courtesy of Dr. B. H. Adler, Columbus, OH.)

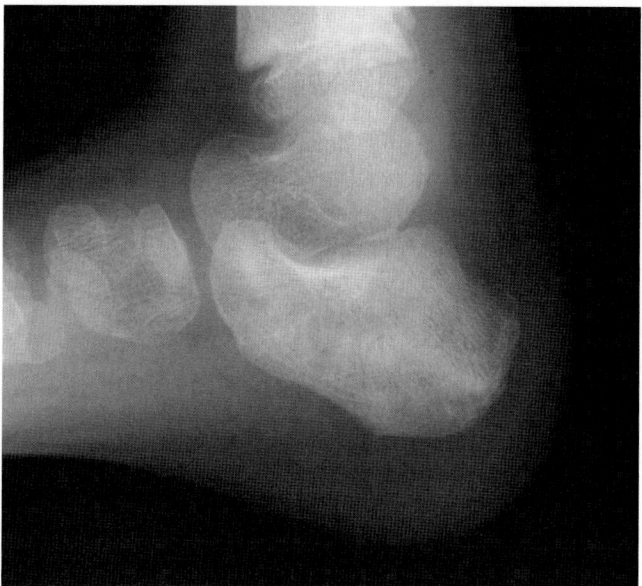

FIGURE 170-70. Healing calcaneal fracture in a 6-year-old boy. A horizontal band of sclerosis is seen within the body of the calcaneus.

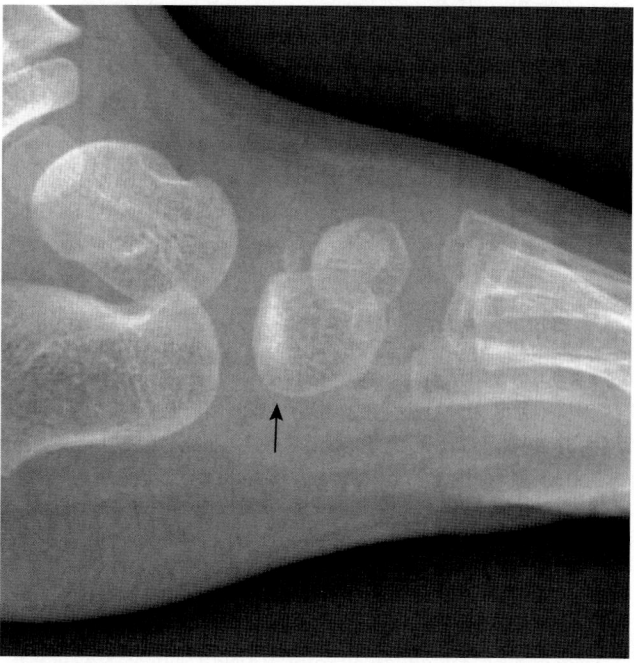

FIGURE 170-71. Healing toddler fracture of the cuboid in a 19-month-old boy. A band of sclerosis is seen within the proximal aspect of the cuboid *(arrow).*

occult at initial evaluation. With healing, a band of sclerosis is seen (Fig. 170-71).

Cuneiform Fractures

Isolated fractures of the cuneiform bones are rare. Lisfranc injuries may occur throughout childhood, but become more common in older children. The mechanism may be direct, from a falling object, or indirect, due to forced plantar flexion or abduction or both. The Lisfranc joint, which courses between the distal tarsals and the metatarsals, is disrupted. Fractures may be seen within the bases of the metatarsals or within the cuneiforms. Fracture at the base of the second metatarsal is a consistent finding. Lisfranc injuries can be classified as homolateral, with the first metatarsal displaced in the same direction as the other four metatarsals, or divergent, with the first metatarsal displaced medially and the other metatarsals displaced laterally (Figs. 170-72 and 170-73). Radiographic abnormality may be subtle. CT is used for confirmation of diagnosis and delineation of morbid anatomy.

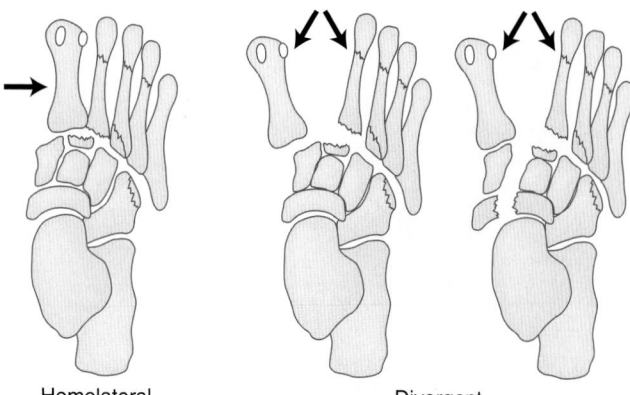

Homolateral   Divergent

FIGURE 170-72. Lisfranc tarsometatarsal fracture-dislocations. There are two basic types: homolateral and divergent. A fracture is consistently seen at the base of the second metatarsal. *Jagged lines* represent additional potential sites of fracture. (From Rogers LF: Radiology of Skeletal Trauma, 3rd ed. New York, Churchill Livingstone, 2002.)

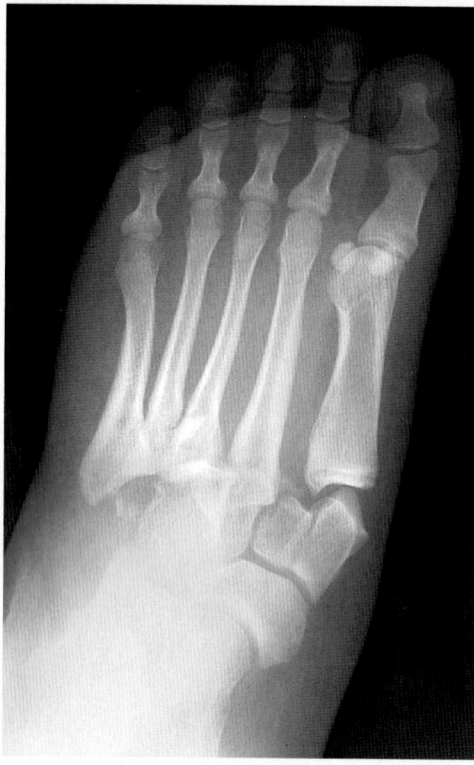

FIGURE 170-73. Lisfranc fracture-dislocation in a 15-year-old morbidly obese boy due to a motor vehicle accident. The injury is homolateral. The space between the first and second metatarsals is widened. The tarsal-metatarsal joint is completely disrupted. A fracture is present at the base of the second metatarsal as well as other metatarsals.

> **CT may be necessary to diagnose or exclude a Lisfranc injury.**

Tarsal Avulsion Fractures

Small avulsion fractures may occur at sites of tendon or ligament attachment. The most common sites are at the medial aspect of the talus and calcaneus.

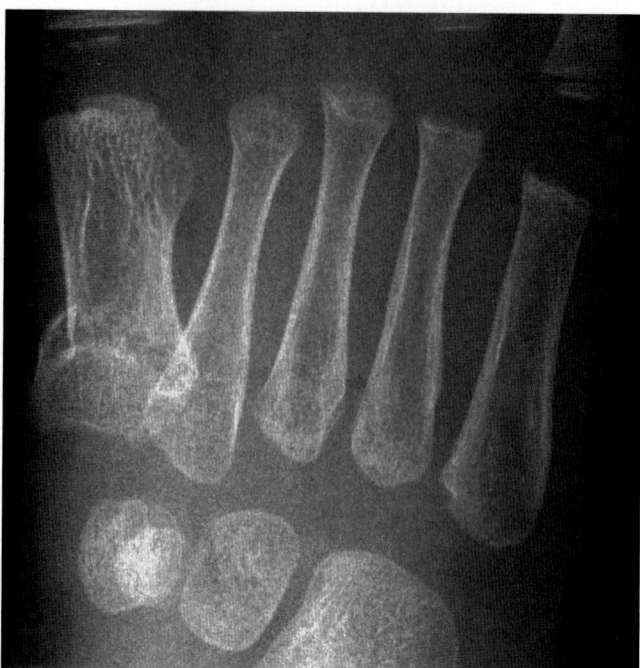

FIGURE 170-74. Bunk bed fracture of the first metatarsal in a 3-year-old boy. The cortex is buckled proximally.

Metatarsal and Phalangeal Fractures

Acute fractures of the metatarsals and phalanges of the feet are common. Salter-Harris fractures may affect the growth plates of these bones. Salter-Harris III fractures at the base of the proximal phalanx of the great toe may be mistaken for a bifid epiphysis and vice versa.

Buckle fractures of the phalanges and metatarsals are common in younger children. Often adjacent bones are fractured together. Oblique or transverse fractures of the metatarsal shafts may occur due to dropped objects, falls, or twisting injuries. In severe twisting injuries in which the foot is caught, multiple adjacent metatarsals may be fractured.

Dropped or falling objects may commonly cause distal phalangeal fractures, particularly within the great toe. Fracture lines may be transverse, longitudinal, or comminuted ("crush injury").

Bunk Bed Fracture

A bunk bed fracture is a buckle fracture within the metaphysis of the great toe, most commonly seen in children 3 to 6 years of age (Fig. 170-74). These fractures occur with a fall or a jump from a height onto a hard surface, with the prototypical injury occurring with a jump from the top bunk of a bunk bed onto a hardwood floor, landing in a tiptoe position. The child's entire weight is placed upon the first metatarsal, leading to fracture. Occasionally, the normal undulation of the growth plate of the first metatarsal may mimic a bunk bed fracture. This should not cause interruption or buckling of the metaphyseal cortex, however, as is seen with a fracture.

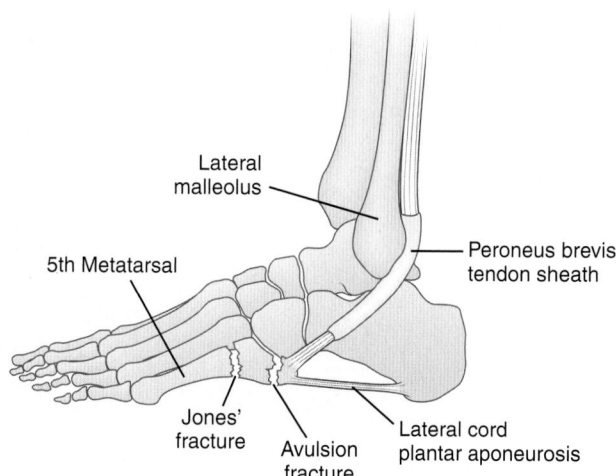

FIGURE 170-75. Fractures at the base of the fifth metatarsal. These fractures result from inversion of the foot, which places tension on the peroneus brevis tendon and the lateral cord of the plantar aponeurosis. An avulsion fracture of the proximal bulbous tip of the metatarsal is to be distinguished from the classic Jones fracture, a transverse fracture at the base of the metatarsal located 1.5 to 2 cm distal to the tip of the metatarsal. (From Rogers LF: Radiology of Skeletal Trauma, 3rd ed. New York, Churchill Livingstone, 2002.)

Fractures at the Base of the Fifth Metatarsal

Fractures at the base of the fifth metatarsal are common. Fractures at this site are usually transverse as opposed to the normal apophyseal growth plate at the lateral aspect of the fifth metatarsal, which is longitudinally oriented. A "true" Jones fracture is a transverse fracture at the base of the fifth metatarsal at the junction of the diaphysis and metaphysis approximately 2 cm distal to the tip of the tuberosity of the fifth metatarsal (Fig. 170-75). Instability occurs as the fracture is distal to attachments to the adjacent second metatarsal. Instability predisposes to delayed union or nonunion, therefore true Jones fractures are usually operatively managed.

The true Jones fracture occurs with inversion of the foot. The original description by Sir Robert Jones was of his own injury, sustained while dancing. A "dancer's fracture" is usually considered to be an avulsion fracture at the base of the fifth metatarsal; however, more distal shaft fractures have also confusingly been called dancer's fractures, as have true Jones fractures. Fractures of the tuberosity at the base of the fifth metatarsal (Fig. 170-76) are not true Jones fractures, although often erroneously labeled as "Jones fractures." Since the use of "Jones fracture" and "dancer's facture" is imprecise and often incorrect, these terms are best avoided in favor of accurately describing the site of fracture. In children, avulsions of the tuberosity are more common than true Jones fractures. Tuberosity avulsions also occur with forced flexion and inversion, often due to an unexpected step or falling when on stairs. The transverse fracture line of a tuberosity avulsion may extend through the apophysis and its growth plate.

The apophysis of the fifth metatarsal may occasionally avulse (Fig. 170-77). The growth plate of the avulsed apophysis will appear widened. A comparison view of the opposite side obtained in the same position will be confirmatory.

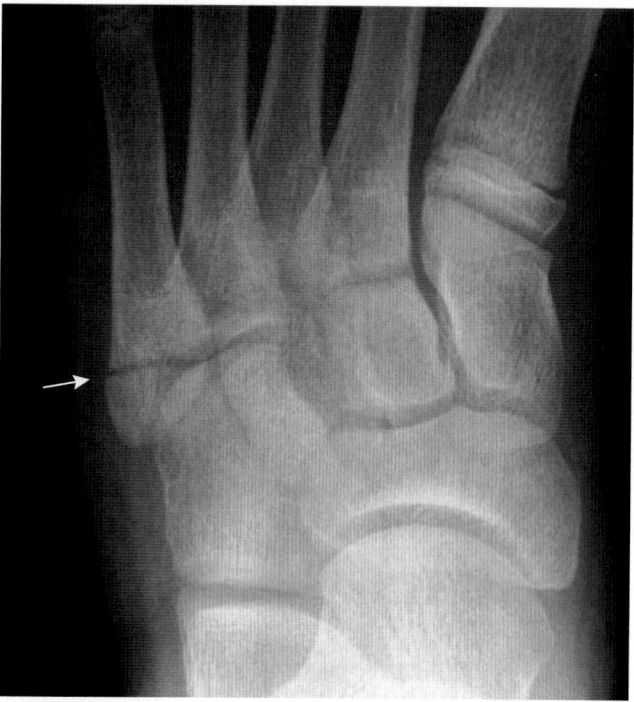

FIGURE 170-76. Transverse fracture of the tuberosity of the fifth metatarsal *(arrow)* in a 12-year-old boy.

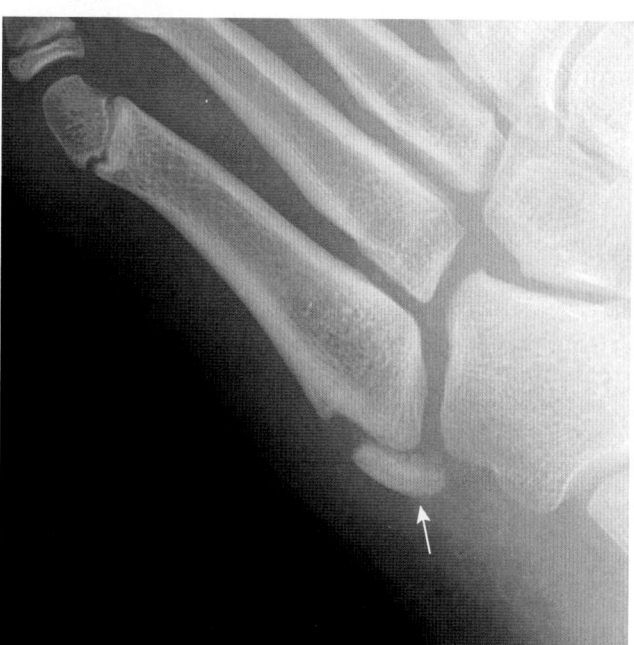

FIGURE 170-77. Avulsion of the fifth metatarsal apophysis *(arrow)* in a 13-year-old boy. The apophysis is displaced from the underlying bone.

A "true" Jones fracture is a transverse fracture at the base of the fifth metatarsal at the junction of the diaphysis and metaphysis, approximately 2 cm distal to the tip of the tuberosity of the fifth metatarsal. In children, avulsions of the tuberosity are more common than true Jones fractures.

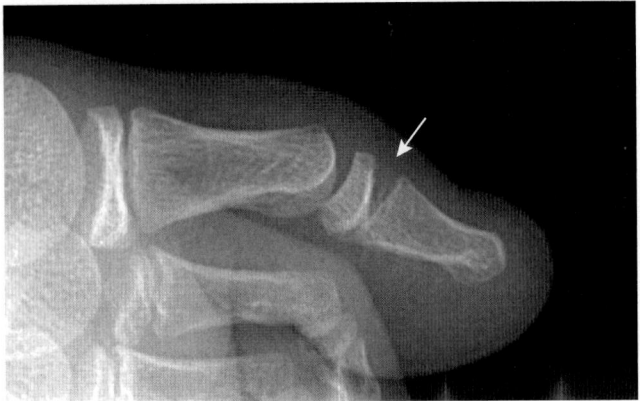

FIGURE 170-78. Stubbed great toe fracture in a 12-year-old boy *(arrow).* There is a tiny metaphyseal fragment. The patient was prophylactically placed on antibiotics.

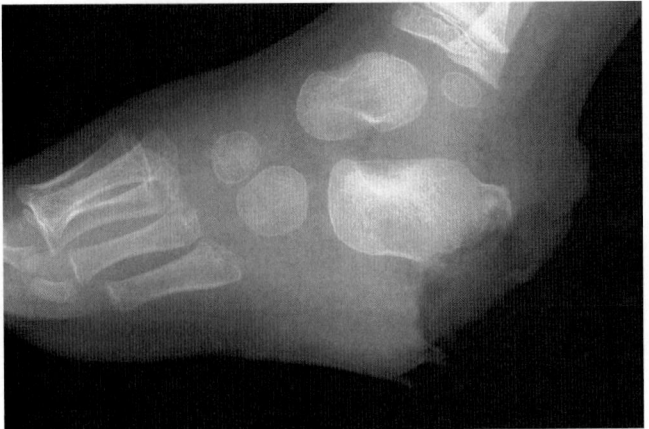

FIGURE 170-79. Lawn mower injury in a 4-year-old boy. Soft tissue and osseous defects are seen at the posterior aspect of the calcaneus.

Stubbed Great Toe Fracture

The nail bed of the great toe is closely apposed to the growth plate of the distal phalanx of the digit. In fact, the skin is directly attached to periosteum. This proximity is thought to allow seeding of a fracture with bacteria from the nail bed. Although not frankly an open fracture, physeal fractures of the distal phalanx of the great toe are therefore considered open fractures (Fig. 170-78). It is usually recommended that these patients be treated with prophylactic antibiotic therapy to prevent the development of osteomyelitis. Nonorthopedic care providers may be unaware of this relationship, warranting direct communication of the findings and their significance.

> Due to proximity to the nail bed, Salter-Harris fractures of the distal phalanx of the great toe are considered to be open fractures. Children should receive prophylactic antibiotics to prevent osteomyelitis.

SPECIFIC MECHANISMS OF INJURY

Birth Trauma

Birth fractures are usually seen with difficult deliveries of larger babies. Other risk factors include twins, breech position, prematurity, and underlying disease. Often there is a history of dystocia. Although fractures at numerous sites have been described with birth trauma, certain sites predominate and others are less frequent.

The clavicle is the bone most commonly fractured from birth trauma, with this fracture occurring in 1 in 200 births. Most clavicle fractures are suspected based on history and physical examination; however, sometimes these fractures are not diagnosed until callus develops and is palpated, or they are found incidentally on a chest radiograph performed for other reasons. Callus is usually present by 7 days after delivery and uniformly present by 11 days after delivery.

Fractures of the humerus and femur are next most common, but are rare relative to the incidence of clavicle fractures. The occurrence of humerus or femur fracture is usually recognized by the obstetrician at the time of fracture. Long bone fractures from birth trauma may be transverse or oblique shaft fractures, physeal fractures, or, very rarely, even "bucket-handle" type fractures, similar to those occurring with child abuse. In such cases, there is uniformly a history of a torsional force applied to the affected extremity during delivery.

Fractures of ribs are extremely rare, but reported. Skull fractures are not uncommon and are associated with forceps delivery and vacuum-assisted delivery. Spine injuries are very rare, but may be catastrophic.

Lawn Mower Injury

Unfortunately, children are the most common victims of traumatic injury due to lawn mowers, usually on account of neglect or poor decision making by caregivers. Lawn mowers cause devastating soft tissue and bone injury that may be life threatening due to blood loss and will be permanently deforming. Osseous injuries are complex, open, and comminuted. CT may be used to delineate anatomy. Cuts across a growth plate with loss of bone usually also result in premature fusion due to crush injury or devascularization. Injury is most common in the feet (Fig. 170-79). Infection is a common complication.

Neuropathic Injury

Neuropathic fractures and joints ("Charcot joints") are much less common in pediatric patients than in adults. Neuropathic injury is characterized by the four Ds: dislocation, debris, disorganization (deformity), and density (sclerosis). Injuries fail to heal. Causes of neuropathic injury in children include myelomeningocele, syrinx, congenital insensitivity to pain, and familial dysautonomia (Riley-Day syndrome). Neuropathic fractures are most common in the lower extremities in the diaphysis or metaphysis (Fig. 170-80). Physeal fractures may occur and are often associated with subperiosteal

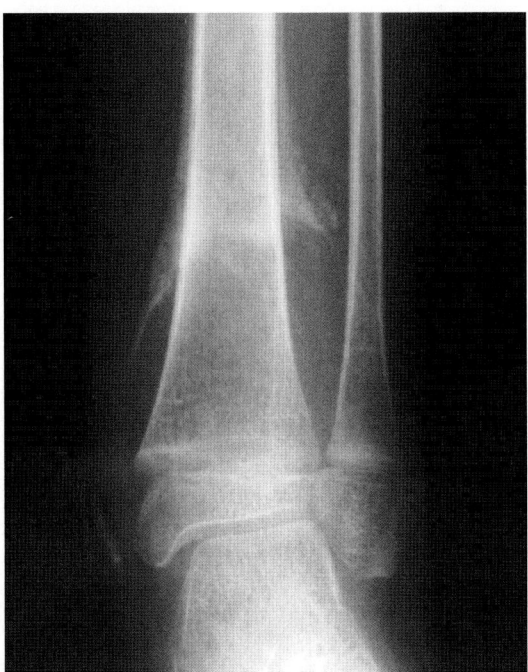

FIGURE 170-80. Neuropathic fracture of the distal tibial growth plate in an 11-year-old girl with myelomeningocele. The patient presented with swelling. The distal tibial growth plate is widened. Periosteal new bone is elevated and interrupted due to subperiosteal hemorrhage, which occurred due to delayed diagnosis and lack of immobilization.

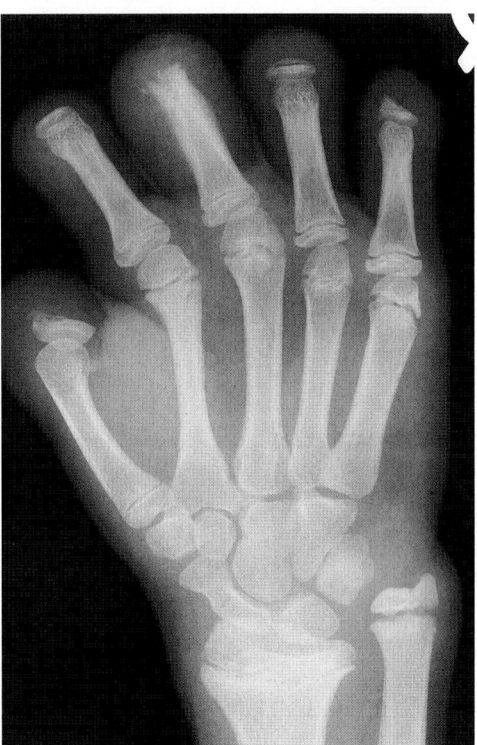

FIGURE 170-81. Sequelae of congenital insensitivity to pain in a 16-year-old boy. All of the fingers are amputated due to chronic injury. Premature fusion of the distal radial growth plate is noted with resultant shortening of the radius.

hematoma and exuberant periosteal new bone. Findings may mimic tumor or infection.

A variety of chronic abnormalities may be seen in children with insensitivity to pain (see Chapter 166). Injury to the fingertips occurs due to crush, thermal damage, and chewing (Fig. 170-81). Superimposed infection is common. Repetitive trauma may lead to chronic physeal injury that may lead to premature fusion. Other sequelae include acro-osteolysis, joint deformity, joint dislocation, and avascular necrosis.

Physical Agents

FROSTBITE

The pathophysiologic mechanism of frostbite is not well defined. There is probably a direct injury to chondrocytes within the physis. The sequela in children is premature fusion of growth plates and shortening of the involved digits. Bone fragmentation may also be due to ischemic damage. Secondary degenerative changes develop due to direct articular injury and malapposition of joint surfaces in affected digits.

Radiographic findings are manifest 6 to 12 months after injury. Frostbite injury is most common in children 5 to 10 years of age. Characteristically, the thumb is spared as at the time of exposure it is clenched and covered by the other digits. Findings are most pronounced in distal phalanges, occasionally affect middle phalanges, and rarely involve the proximal phalanges or metacarpals (Fig. 170-82).

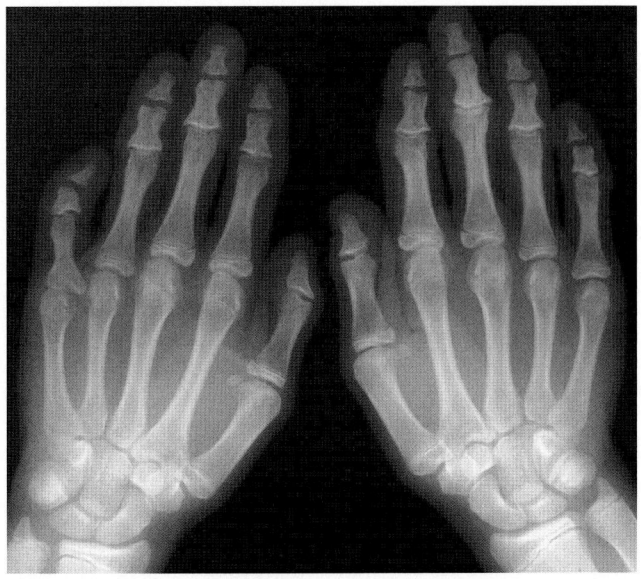

FIGURE 170-82. Sequelae of frostbite in a 15-year-old girl. The distal and middle phalanges are shortened due to premature growth plate closure. In this patient, the thumbs were not spared. The proximal phalanx of the right fifth finger is also shortened.

> Frostbite causes damage to physes and premature fusion, usually affecting the distal phalanges of the fingers. Characteristically, the thumb is spared.

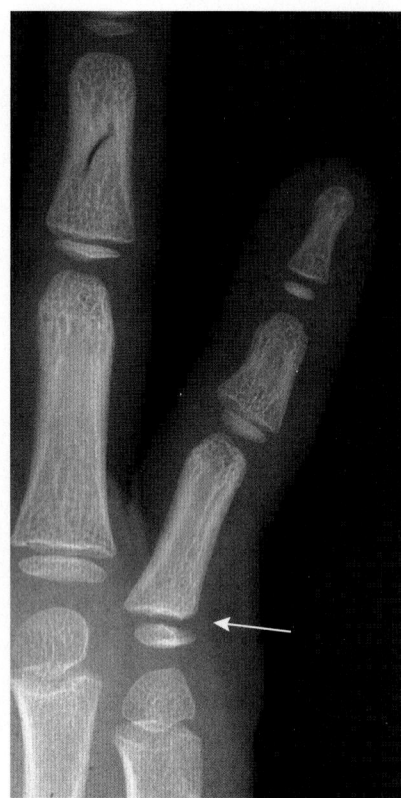

FIGURE 170-83. Sequelae of thermal injury. The child suffered a burn 7 years prior. Although the growth plate of the proximal phalanx appears patent *(arrow)*, growth disturbance has resulted in medial deviation of the phalanx.

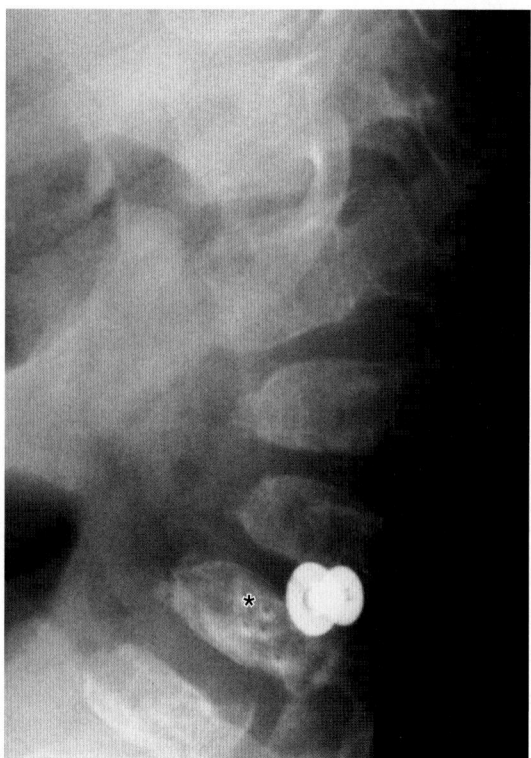

FIGURE 170-84. Stunted bone growth due to radiation therapy in an 11-year-old girl. The patient had radiation therapy 9 years previously for a primary primitive neuroectodermal tumor originating in the L4 vertebra. The L2 through L5 vertebral bodies are hypoplastic. Slight sclerosis in L4 *(asterisk)* is due to the original tumor.

BURNS

Injury from burns is usually to the soft tissues, leading to contractures and ankylosis. Heterotopic bone contributes to ankylosis, as does direct thermal injury of a joint. Direct thermal injury to the growth plate may lead to premature fusion or growth disturbance (Fig. 170-83).

ELECTRICAL INJURY

Electrical injury may lead to premature fusion and ankylosis due to tissue heating. Associated soft tissue injury and heterotopic bone formation may also proceed to ankylosis. Osteolysis may occur.

RADIATION

Therapeutic radiation doses may be sufficient to cause permanent injury to bone. Consequences include growth retardation with hypoplasia (Fig. 170-84), premature growth plate fusion, SCFE, bone marrow infarcts/avascular necrosis, osteochondroma formation, and radiation-induced sarcoma. Regarding growth retardation, microscopic changes are seen with a little as 300 cGy and growth retardation with as low as 400 cGy. Histologic recovery occurs with doses up to 1200 cGy; however, beyond this level there is almost uniformly permanent cell damage and premature growth plate fusion. Radiation-induced sarcomas are uncommon and occur with an average latent period of 10 years after therapy.

SUGGESTED READINGS

General

Beaty JH, Kasser JR: Rockwood and Wilkins' Fractures in Children, 6th ed. Philadelphia, Lippincott Williams & Wilkins, 2006
Lee P, Hunter TB, Taljanovic M: Musculoskeletal colloquialisms: how did we come up with these names? Radiographics 2004;24:1009-1027
Ogden JA: Skeletal Injury in the Child, 3rd ed. New York, Springer, 2000
Ozonoff MB: Pediatric Orthopedic Radiology, 2nd ed. Philadelphia, Saunders, 1992
Renner RR, Mauler GG, Ambrose JL: The radiologist, the orthopedist, the lawyer, and the fracture. Semin Roentgenol 1978;13:7-18
Rogers LF: Radiology of Skeletal Trauma, 3rd ed. New York, Churchill Livingstone, 2002

Plastic (Incomplete) Fractures

Borden S: Roentgen recognition of acute plastic bowing of the forearm in children. Am J Roentgenol Radium Ther Nucl Med 1975;125:524-530
Hernandez JA, Swischuk LE, Yngve DA, et al: The angled buckle fracture in pediatrics: a frequently missed fracture. Emerg Radiol 2003;10:71-75

Physeal Fractures (Salter-Harris Fractures)

Jaramillo D, Hoffer FA, Shapiro F, et al: MR imaging of fractures of the growth plate. AJR Am J Roentgenol 1990;155:1261-1265
Mizuta T, Benson WM, Foster BK, et al: Statistical analysis of the incidence of physeal injuries. J Pediatr Orthop 1987;7:518-523
Peterson H: Physeal and apophyseal injuries. *In* Rockwood CA, Wilkins KE (eds): Fractures in Children, 4th ed. Philadelphia, Lippincott–Raven, 1996:103-148

Rogers LF, Poznanski AK: Imaging of epiphyseal injuries. Radiology 1994;191:297-308

Salter RB, Harris WR: Injuries involving the epiphyseal plate. J Bone Joint Surg Am 1963;45:587-632

Fracture Healing

Islam O, Soboleski D, Symons S, et al: Development and duration of radiographic signs of bone healing in children. AJR Am J Roentgenol 2000;175:75-78

Wilkins KE: Principles of fracture remodeling in children. Injury 2005;36:S-A3-S-A11

Complications of Fractures

Boles CA, Hendrix RW: Complications of fracture. *In* Rogers LF (ed): Radiology of Skeletal Trauma, 3rd ed. Philadelphia, Churchill Livingstone, 2002:231-271

Ecklund K, Jaramillo D: Imaging of growth disturbance in children. Radiol Clin North Am 2001;39:823-841

Ecklund K, Jaramillo D: Patterns of premature physeal arrest: MR imaging of 111 children. AJR Am J Roentgenol 2002;178:967-972

Hensinger RN: Complications of fractures in children. *In* Ogden JA (ed): Skeletal Injury in the Child, 3rd ed. New York, Springer, 2000:124-151

Loder RT, Swinford AE, Kuhns LR: The use of helical computed tomographic scan to assess bony physeal bridges. J Pediatr Orthop 1997;17:356-359

Peterson HA: Partial growth plate arrest and its treatment. J Pediatr Orthop 1984;4:246-258

Roach RT, Cassar-Pullicino V, Summers BN: Paediatric post-traumatic cortical defects of the distal radius. Pediatr Radiol 2002;32:333-339

Sailhan F, Chotel F, Guibal AL, et al: Three-dimensional MR imaging in the assessment of physeal growth arrest. Eur Radiol 2004;14:1600-1608

Whan A, Breidahl W, Janes G: MRI of trapped periosteum in a proximal tibial physeal injury of a pediatric patient. AJR Am J Roentgenol 2003;181:1397-1399

Wilder RT, Berde CB, Wolohan M, et al: Reflex sympathetic dystrophy in children: clinical characteristics and follow-up of seventy patients. J Bone Joint Surg Am 1992;74:910-919

Traumatic Injuries of the Hand and Wrist

Goddard N: Carpal fractures in children. Clin Orthop Relat Res 2005;432:73-76

Hernandez JA, Swischuk LE, Bathurst GJ, et al: Scaphoid (navicular) fractures of the wrist in children: attention to the impacted buckle fracture. Emerg Radiol 2002;9:305-308

Johnson KJ, Haigh SF, Symonds KE: MRI in the management of scaphoid fractures in skeletally immature patients. Pediatr Radiol 2000;30:685-688

Nakamura R, Horii E, Imaeda T, et al: Criteria for diagnosing distal radioulnar joint subluxation by computed tomography. Skeletal Radiol 1996;25:649-653

Nofsinger CC, Wolfe SW: Common pediatric hand fractures. Curr Opin Pediatr 2002;14:42-45

Valencia J, Leyva F, Gomez-Bajo GJ: Pediatric hand trauma. Clin Orthop Relat Res 2005;432:77-86

Traumatic Injuries of the Forearm

Reckling FW, Cordell LD: Unstable fracture-dislocations of the forearm: the Monteggia and Galeazzi lesions. Arch Surg 1968;96:999-1007

Rodríguez-Merchán EC: Pediatric fractures of the forearm. Clin Orthop Relat Res 2005;432:65-72

Traumatic Injuries of the Elbow

Anderson SE, Otsuka NY, Steinbach LS: MR imaging of pediatric elbow trauma. Semin Musculoskelet Radiol 1998;2:185-198

Beltran J, Rosenberg ZS, Kawelblum M, et al: Pediatric elbow fractures: MRI evaluation. Skeletal Radiol 1994;23:277-281

Bledsoe RC, Izenstark JL: Displacement of fat pads in diseases and injury of the elbow: a new radiographic sign. Radiology 1959;73:717-724

Bretland PM: Pulled elbow in childhood. Br J Radiol 1994;67:1176-1185

Brogdon BG, Crow NE: Little leaguer's elbow. Am J Roentgenol Radium Ther Nucl Med 1960;83:671-675

Chapman V, Grottkau B, Albright M, et al: MDCT of the elbow in pediatric patients with posttraumatic elbow effusion. AJR Am J Roentgenol 2006;187:812-817

Donnelly LF, Klostermeier TT, Klosterman LA: Traumatic elbow effusions in pediatric patients: are occult fractures the rule? AJR Am J Roentgenol 1998;171:243-245

Evans MC, Graham HK: Olecranon fractures in children: Part 1: a clinical review; Part 2: a new classification and management algorithm. J Pediatr Orthop 1999;19:559-569

Griffith JF, Roebuck DJ, Cheng JCY, et al: Acute elbow trauma in children: spectrum of injury revealed by MR imaging not apparent on radiographs. AJR Am J Roentgenol 2001;176:53-60

John SD, Wherry K, Swischuk LE, et al: Improving detection of pediatric elbow fractures by understanding their mechanics. Radiographics 1996;16:1443-1460

Kamegaya M, Shinohara Y, Kurokawa M, et al: Assessment of stability in children's minimally displaced lateral humeral condyle fracture by magnetic resonance imaging. J Pediatr Orthop 1999;19:570-572

Kay RM, Skaggs DL: The pediatric Monteggia fracture. Am J Orthop 1998;27:606-609

Keenan WN, Clegg J: Variation of Baumann's angle with age, sex, and side: implications for its use in radiological monitoring of supracondylar fracture of the humerus in children. J Pediatr Orthop 1996;16:97-98

Kissoon N, Galpin R, Gayle M, et al: Evaluation of the role of comparison radiographs in the diagnosis of traumatic elbow injuries. J Pediatr Orthop 1995;15:449-453

Labelle H, Bunnell WP, Duhaime M, et al: Cubitus varus deformity following supracondylar fractures of the humerus in children. J Pediatr Orthop 1982;2:539-546

Landin LA, Danielsson LG: Elbow fractures in children: an epidemiological analysis of 589 cases. Acta Orthop Scand 1986;57:309-312

Lins RE, Simovitch RW, Waters PM: Pediatric elbow trauma. Orthop Clin North Am 1999;30:119-132

May DA, Disler DG, Jones EA, et al: Using sonography to diagnose an unossified medial epicondyle avulsion in a child. AJR Am J Roentgenol 2000;174:1115-1117

Rasool MN: Dislocations of the elbow in children. J Bone Joint Surg Br 2004;86:1050-1058

Rettig AC, Wurth TR, Mieling P: Nonunion of olecranon stress fractures in adolescent baseball pitchers: a case series of 5 athletes. Am J Sports Med 2006;34:653-656

Ring D, Jupiter JB, Waters PM: Monteggia fractures in children and adults. J Am Acad Orthop Surg 1998;6:215-224

Rogers LF, Rockwood CA Jr: Separation of the entire distal humeral epiphysis. Radiology 1973;106:393-400

Salter RB, Zaltz C: Anatomic investigations of the mechanism of injury and pathologic anatomy of "pulled elbow" in young children. Clin Orthop Relat Res 1971;77:134-143

Skaggs DL: Elbow fractures in children: diagnosis and management. J Am Acad Orthop Surg 1997;5:303-312

Traumatic Injuries of the Humerus

Bishop JY, Flatow EL: Pediatric shoulder trauma. Clin Orthop Relat Res 2005;432:41-48

Caviglia H, Garrido CP, Palazzi FF, et al: Pediatric fractures of the humerus. Clin Orthop Relat Res 2005;432:49-56

Grissom LE, Harcke HT: Infant shoulder sonography: technique, anatomy, and pathology. Pediatr Radiol 2001;31:863-868

Levine B, Pereira D, Rosen J: Avulsion fractures of the lesser tuberosity of the humerus in adolescents: review of the literature and case report. J Orthop Trauma 2005;19:349-352

Shibuya S, Ogawa K: Isolated avulsion fracture of the lesser tuberosity of the humerus: a case report. Clin Orthop Relat Res 1986;211:215-218

Traumatic Injuries of the Pelvis and Hip

Azouz EM, Karamitsos C, Reed MH, et al: Types and complications of femoral neck fractures in children. Pediatr Radiol 1993;23:415-420

Canale ST: Fractures of the hip in children and adolescents. Orthop Clin North Am 1990;21:341-352

Fernbach SK, Wilkinson RH: Avulsion injuries of the pelvis and proximal femur. AJR Am J Roentgenol 1981;137:581-584

Moeller JL: Pelvic and hip apophyseal avulsion injuries in young athletes. Curr Sports Med Rep 2003;2:110-115

Momiy JP, Clayton JL, Villalba H, et al: Pelvic fractures in children. Am Surg 2006;72:962-965

Pisacano RM, Miller TT: Comparing sonography with MR imaging of apophyseal injuries of the pelvis in four boys. AJR Am J Roentgenol 2003;181:223-230

Quick TJ, Eastwood DM: Pediatric fractures and dislocations of the hip and pelvis. Clin Orthop Relat Res 2005;432:87-96

Rees MJ, Aickin R, Kolbe A, et al: The screening pelvic radiograph in pediatric trauma. Pediatr Radiol 2001;31:497-500

Salisbury RD, Eastwood DM: Traumatic dislocation of the hip in children. Clin Orthop Relat Res 2000;377:106-111

Schlickewi W, Keck T: Pelvic and acetabular fractures in childhood. Injury 2005;36:A57-A63

Scuderi G, Bronson MJ: Triradiate cartilage injury: report of two cases and review of the literature. Clin Orthop Relat Res 1987;217:179-189

Silber JS, Flynn JM: Changing patterns of pediatric pelvic fractures with skeletal maturation: implications for classification and management. J Pediatr Orthop 2002;22:22-26

Silber JS, Flynn JM, Katz MA, et al: Role of computed tomography in the classification and management of pediatric pelvic fractures. J Pediatr Orthop 2001;21:148-151

Silber JS, Flynn JM, Koffler KM, et al: Analysis of the cause, classification, and associated injuries of 166 consecutive pediatric pelvic fractures. J Pediatr Orthop 2001;21:446-450

Stevens MA, El-Khoury GY, Kathol MH, et al: Imaging features of avulsion injuries. Radiographics 1999;19:655-672

Sundar M, Carty H: Avulsion fractures of the pelvis in children: a report of 32 fractures and their outcome. Skeletal Radiol 1994;23:85-90

Torode I, Zieg D: Pelvic fractures in children. J Pediatr Orthop 1985;5:76-84

Watts HG: Fractures of the pelvis in children. Orthop Clin North Am 1976;7:615-624

Yamamoto T, Akisue T, Nakatani T, et al: Apophysitis of the ischial tuberosity mimicking a neoplasm on magnetic resonance imaging. Skeletal Radiol 2004;33:737-740

Slipped Capital Femoral Epiphysis

Boles CA, el-Khoury GY: Slipped capital femoral epiphysis. Radiographics 1997;17:809-823

Brenkel IJ, Dias JJ, Davies TG, et al: Hormone status in patients with slipped capital femoral epiphysis. J Bone Joint Surg Br 1989; 71:33-38

Hägglund G, Hansson LI, Ordeberg G, et al: Bilaterality in slipped upper femoral epiphysis. J Bone Joint Surg Br 1988;70:179-181

Kallio PE, Mah ET, Foster BK, et al: Slipped capital femoral epiphysis: incidence and clinical assessment of physeal instability. J Bone Joint Surg Br 1995;77:752-755

Klein A, Joplin RJ, Reidy JA, et al: Roentgenographic features of slipped capital femoral epiphysis. Am J Roentgenol Radium Ther 1951;66:361-374

Loder RT: Slipped capital femoral epiphysis in children. Curr Opin Pediatr 1995;7:95-97

Loder RT: Unstable slipped capital femoral epiphysis. J Pediatr Orthop 2001;21:694-699

Loder RT, Aronson DD, Greenfield ML: The epidemiology of bilateral slipped capital femoral epiphysis: a study of children in Michigan. J Bone Joint Surg Am 1993;75:1141-1147

Loder RT, Richards BS, Shapiro PS, et al: Acute slipped capital femoral epiphysis: the importance of physeal stability. J Bone Joint Surg Am 1993;75:1134-1140

McAfee PC, Cady RB: Endocrinologic and metabolic factors in atypical presentations of slipped capital femoral epiphysis: report of four cases and review of the literature. Clin Orthop Relat Res 1983;180:188-197

Vrettos BC, Hoffman EB: Chondrolysis in slipped upper femoral epiphysis: long-term study of the aetiology and natural history. J Bone Joint Surg Br 1993;75:956-961

Traumatic Injuries of the Femur, Tibia, and Fibula

Donnelly LF: Toddler's fracture of the fibula. AJR Am J Roentgenol 2000;175:922

Dunbar JS, Owen HF, Nogrady MB, et al: Obscure tibial fracture of infants—the toddler's fracture. J Can Assoc Radiol 1964;15:136-144

Englaro EE, Gelfand MJ, Paltiel HJ: Bone scintigraphy in preschool children with lower extremity pain of unknown origin. J Nucl Med 1992;33:351-354

Hunter JB: Femoral shaft fractures in children. Injury 2005; 36:S-A86-S-A93

John SD, Moorthy CS, Swischuk LE: Expanding the concept of the toddler's fracture. Radiographics 1997;17:367-376

Loder RT, O'Donnell PW, Feinberg JR: Epidemiology and mechanisms of femur fractures in children. J Pediatr Orthop 2006;26:561-566

Poolman RW, Kocher MS, Bhandari M: Pediatric femoral fractures: a systematic review of 2422 cases. J Orthop Trauma 2006;20:648-654

Shrader MW, Jacofsky DJ, Stans AA, et al: Femoral neck fractures in pediatric patients: 30 years experience at a level 1 trauma center. Clin Orthop Relat Res 2007;454:169-173

Starshak RJ, Simons GW, Sty JR: Occult fracture of the calcaneus— another toddler's fracture. Pediatr Radiol 1984;14:37-40

Swischuk LE, John SD, Tschoepe EJ: Upper tibial hyperextension fractures in infants: another occult toddler's fracture. Pediatr Radiol 1999;29:6-9

Traumatic Injuries of the Knee

Bates DG, Hresko MT, Jaramillo D: Patellar sleeve fracture: demonstration with MR imaging. Radiology 1994;193:825-827

Davidson D, Letts M: Partial sleeve fractures of the tibia in children: an unusual fracture pattern. J Pediatr Orthop 2002;22:36-40

Edwards PH Jr, Grana WA: Physeal fractures about the knee. J Am Acad Orthop Surg 1995;3:63-69

Hunt DM, Somashekar N: A review of sleeve fractures of the patella in children. Knee 2005;12:3-7

Jones MH, Simon JE, Winell JJ: Pediatric knee fractures. Curr Opin Pediatr 2005;17:43-47

Lee J-H, Weissman BN, Nikpoor N, et al: Lipohemarthrosis of the knee: a review of recent experiences. Radiology 1989;173:189-191

McKoy BE, Stanitski CL: Acute tibial tubercle avulsion fractures. Orthop Clin North Am 2003;34:397-403

Mosier SM, Stanitski CL: Acute tibial tubercle avulsion fractures. J Pediatr Orthop 2004;24:181-184

Rogers LF, Jones S, Davis AR, et al: "Clipping injury" fracture of the epiphysis in the adolescent football player: an occult lesion of the knee. Am J Roentgenol Radium Ther Nucl Med 1974;121:69-78

Ryu RK, Debenham JO: An unusual avulsion fracture of the proximal tibial epiphysis: case report and proposed addition to the Watson-Jones classification. Clin Orthop Relat Res 1985;194:181-184

Traumatic Injuries of the Ankle and Foot

Blumberg K, Patterson RJ: The toddler's cuboid fracture. Radiology 1991;179:93-94

Brown SD, Kasser JR, Zurakowski D, et al: Analysis of 51 tibial triplane fractures using CT with multiplanar reconstruction. AJR Am J Roentgenol 2004;183:1489-1495

Cutler L, Molloy A, Dhukuram V, et al: Do CT scans aid assessment of distal tibial physeal fractures? J Bone Joint Surg Br 2004;86:239-243

Johnson GF: Pediatric Lisfranc injury: "bunk bed" fracture. AJR Am J Roentgenol 1981;137:1041-1044

Kay RM, Matthys GA: Pediatric ankle fractures: evaluation and treatment. J Am Acad Orthop Surg 2001;9:268-278

Kay RM, Tang CW: Pediatric foot fractures: evaluation and treatment. J Am Acad Orthop Surg 2001;9:308-319

Kensinger DR, Guille JT, Horn BD, et al: The stubbed great toe: importance of early recognition and treatment of open fractures of the distal phalanx. J Pediatr Orthop 2001;21:31-34

Laliotis N, Pennie BH, Carty H, et al: Toddler's fracture of the calcaneum. Injury 1993;24:169-170

Lawrence SJ, Botte MJ: Jones' fractures and related fractures of the proximal fifth metatarsal. Foot Ankle 1993;14:358-365

Munro TG: Fractures of the base of the fifth metatarsal. Can Assoc Radiol J 1989;40:260-261

Pinckney LE, Currarino G, Kennedy LA: The stubbed great toe: a cause of occult compound fracture and infection. Radiology 1981;138:375-377

Ribbans WJ, Natarajan R, Alavala S: Pediatric foot fractures. Clin Orthop Relat Res 2005;432:107-115

Senaran H, Mason D, De Pellegrin M: Cuboid fractures in preschool children. J Pediatr Orthop 2006;26:741-744

Spiegel PG, Mast JW, Cooperman DR, et al: Triplane fractures of the distal tibial epiphysis. Clin Orthop Relat Res 1984;188:74-89

Starshak RJ, Simons GW, Sty JR: Occult fracture of the calcaneus—another toddler's fracture. Pediatr Radiol 1984;4:37-40

Stefanich RJ, Lozman J: The juvenile Tillaux fracture. Clin Orthop Relat Res 1986;210:219-227

Strayer SM, Reece SG, Petrizzi MJ: Fractures of the proximal fifth metatarsal. Am Fam Physician 1999;59:2516-2522

Theodorou DJ, Theodorou SJ, Kakitsubata Y, et al: Fractures of proximal portion of fifth metatarsal bone: anatomic and imaging evidence of a pathogenesis of avulsion of the plantar aponeurosis and the short peroneal muscle tendon. Radiology 2003;226:857-865

Walling AK, Grogan DP, Carty CT, et al: Fractures of the calcaneal apophysis. J Orthop Trauma 1990;4:349-355

Wiley JJ: Tarso-metatarsal joint injuries in children. J Pediatr Orthop 1981;1:255-260

Specific Mechanisms of Injury

Balen PF, Helms CA: Bony ankylosis following thermal and electrical injury. Skeletal Radiol 2001;30:393-397

Bingham H: Electrical burns. Clin Plast Surg 1986;13:75-85

Brinn LB, Moseley JE: Bone changes following electrical injury: case report and review of literature. Am J Roentgenol Radium Ther Nucl Med 1966;97:682-686

Brown HC: Current concepts of burn pathology and mechanisms of deformity in the burned hand. Orthop Clin North Am 1973;4:987-999

Carrera GF, Kozin F, Flaherty L, et al: Radiographic changes in the hands following childhood frostbite injury. Skeletal Radiol 1981;6:33-37

Crouch C, Smith WL: Long term sequelae of frostbite. Pediatr Radiol 1990;20:365-366

DeSmet AA, Kuhns LR, Hold JF: Effects of radiation therapy on growing long bones. Am J Roentgenol 1976;127:935-939

Fletcher BD: Effects of pediatric cancer therapy on the musculoskeletal system. Pediatr Radiol 1997;27:623-636

Jaffe N, Reid HL, Cohen M, et al: Radiation induced osteochondroma in long-term survivors of childhood cancer. Int J Radiat Oncol Biol Phys 1983;9:665-670

Kumar D, Papini R, Tillman RM: Partial growth plate fusion caused by burn. Burns 2001;27:664-667

Laplaza FJ, Turajane T, Axelrod FB, et al: Nonspinal orthopaedic problems in familial dysautonomia (Riley-Day syndrome). J Pediatr Orthop 2001;21:229-232

Lee RC, Kolodney MS: Electrical injury mechanisms: dynamics of the thermal response. Plast Reconstr Surg 1987;80:663-671

Libshitz HI, Edeiken BS: Radiotherapy changes of the pediatric hip. AJR Am J Roentgenol 1981;137:585-588

Marcovici PA, Berdon WE, Liebling MS: Osteochrondromas and growth retardation in secondary to externally or internally administered radiation in childhood. Pediatr Radiol 2007;37:301-304

Oeconomopoulos CT: Electrical burns in infancy and early childhood: a review of the current literature. Am J Dis Child 1962;103:35-38

Ogden JA, Southwick WO: Electrical injury involving the immature skeleton. Skeletal Radiol 1981;6:187-192

Oppenheim WL, Davis A, Growdon WA, et al: Clavicle fractures in the newborn. Clin Orthop Relat Res 1990;250:176-180

Reed MH: Growth disturbances in the hands following thermal injuries in children. 2. Frostbite. Can Assoc Radiol J 1988;39:95-99

Riseborough EJ, Grabias SL, Burton RI, et al: Skeletal alterations following irradiation for Wilms' tumor: with particular reference to scoliosis and kyphosis. J Bone Joint Surg Am 1976;58:526-536

Roebuck DJ: Skeletal complications in pediatric oncology patients. Radiographics 1999;19:873-885

Rutan RL, Herndon DN: Growth delay in postburn pediatric patients. Arch Surg 1990;125:392-395

Schulman H, Tsodikow V, Einhorn M, et al: Congenital insensitivity to pain with anhidrosis (CIPA): the spectrum of radiological findings. Pediatr Radiol 2001;31:701-705

Vollman D, Khosla K, Shields BJ, et al: Lawn mower-related injuries to children. J Trauma 2005;59:724-728

Wenzl JE, Burke EC, Bianco AJ Jr: Epiphyseal destruction from frostbite of the hands. Am J Dis Child 1967;114:668-670

Williams HJ, Davies AM: The effect of x-rays on bone: a pictorial review. Eur Radiol 2006;11:619-633

Child Abuse

DANIELLE K. B. BOAL

OVERVIEW

In the decades since landmark articles were written by Caffey (1946) and Kempe and Silverman (1962), the medical community, law enforcement, and Child Protective Services (CPS) have developed a much greater awareness and sensitivity to the diagnosis of child abuse; these groups have also promoted a more aggressive approach to the identification and prosecution of offending individuals. Although reports of different agencies vary somewhat, according to the most recent survey from the U.S. Department of Health and Human Services (in 2004), a total of 3,503,000 children were the subject of investigations undertaken by CPS agencies as alleged victims of child abuse, and approximately 872,000 were found to be victims of abuse. Thus, in 2004, 42.6 of every 1000 children in the United States were reported as abused or neglected, and 11.9 of every 1000 children were confirmed as abused or neglected. Neglect accounts for 62.4% of confirmed cases, physical abuse 17.5%, sexual abuse 9.7%, psychological maltreatment 7%, and other forms of maltreatment 3.4%. Young children are at greatest risk for fatality; 81% are younger than 4 years of age at the time of death, and 45% are younger than 1 year of age at death. An estimated 1490 children died from abuse or neglect in 2004. Female perpetrators predominate in neglect and physical abuse; more than 90% of all confirmed perpetrators have a parental relationship to the victim (mother, father, stepparent, paramour of parent). Neglect and abuse remains a difficult and emotionally charged topic. Because it typically occurs behind closed doors, the behavior is unobserved, and confessions are rare. Presentations are varied, and abuse and neglect may mimic other disease processes.

> **In the United States, 11.9 of every 1000 children were confirmed as abused or neglected in 2004.**

Although significant morbidity and mortality are associated, the diagnosis of child abuse and the treatment of abused children are intertwined with legal issues of parental rights and family preservation. Lack of research support further impairs progress in finding practical solutions that will protect children at risk, while at the same time avoiding erroneous accusations. The current CPS system is overwhelmed, underfunded, and understaffed. Approximately 15% of children who die as a result of abuse are known to CPS agencies as current or prior clients at the time of death. Abuse and neglect is truly a societal issue. These dismal statistics will not improve until risk factors such as poverty, drugs, ignorance, and isolation have been identified and addressed.

THE ROLE OF IMAGING

Radiologic imaging has evolved to play a major role in the diagnosis of physical abuse; with the advent of nuclear medicine, ultrasonography, computed tomography (CT), and magnetic resonance imaging (MRI), its usefulness is no longer limited to identification of bony trauma. CT and MRI are the primary diagnostic modalities used in the diagnosis of abusive head trauma, including shaken baby syndrome with or without impact. The role of diagnostic imaging is threefold:

1. Recognition of physical abuse, supporting the diagnosis in suspected cases, and recognizing characteristic lesions when the possibility of child abuse has not been suspected
2. As evidence in the prosecution or defense of offenders by providing an understanding of the mechanism, pattern of healing (dating), and likelihood of such injuries with a reasonable degree of medical certainty
3. Exclusion of the diagnosis of child abuse in cases of true accidental trauma or with variants of normal and disease processes that may mimic abuse

IMAGING FINDINGS

Abused infants and children are rarely brought to medical attention with an accurate history. Often, the radiologist is the first to suggest the possibility of child abuse when characteristic lesions are identified on imaging studies. With the possible exception of the classic metaphyseal lesion and multiple rib fractures in infancy, it is risky to state unequivocally that certain patterns or types of fractures are pathognomonic of abuse. Each case must be considered individually with respect to the history provided and the possibility of underlying abnormalities that would predispose to fracture, such as history of prematurity, metabolic disease, or dysplasia. With this proviso, it can be stated that certain patterns and types of skeletal injury occur more or less commonly as a result of abuse (Table 171-1). When a child presents with an injury, it is necessary for the clinician to consider whether the explanation offered for that injury is plausible, and whether the developmental level of the child is consistent with that history.

> **Abused infants and children are rarely brought to medical attention with an accurate history.**

TABLE 171-1

Skeletal Injuries From Abuse

COMMON
Multiple fractures (unsuspected and/or varying in age)
*Classic metaphyseal lesions**
Multiple rib fractures*
Diaphyseal fractures (non-ambulatory infant/child)
Skull fractures
Subperiosteal new bone formation

LESS COMMON
Spine
Small bones of hands and feet
Clavicular fractures
Dislocations and epiphyseal separations

UNCOMMON
Scapular fractures*
Pelvic fractures
Sternal fractures
Facial and mandibular fractures

*High specificity for abuse in infants.

Multiple fractures at variable locations in different stages of healing are well described and continue to be highly specific for child abuse, unless an underlying bone dysplasia or metabolic abnormality is diagnosed (Figs. 171-1 and 171-2). Patterns of injury, including distribution, and characteristic traumatic lesions unique to abuse have been studied and reported on by various authors. It is now recognized that fractures to the rib cage, metaphyseal fractures, and skull fractures predominate in infants younger than 1 year of age, whereas diaphyseal fractures are more common in older infants and children. The appropriateness of the history in relation to the mechanism of injury(s) is usually the first and most important clue to the diagnosis of nonaccidental or abuse injuries. Any delay in seeking treatment and the amount of detail that the caretaker is able to provide are also important considerations. Infants who are not ambulatory do not normally incur fractures from unintentional injury events. A fall from 3 to 4 feet to a hard surface may result in a linear parietal skull fracture, but rarely do long bone fractures or central nervous system (CNS) injuries occur in this circumstance. Mid-shaft transverse, spiral, and oblique diaphyseal fractures of the femur and humerus are almost always inflicted in a young infant, as are rib fractures and *classic metaphyseal lesions*. Injury plausibility studies that use biomechanics and computer simulation may increase our ability to distinguish abusive from true accidental injuries in the future.

> **The appropriateness of the history in relation to the mechanism of injury is usually the first and most important clue to the diagnosis of nonaccidental or abuse injuries.**

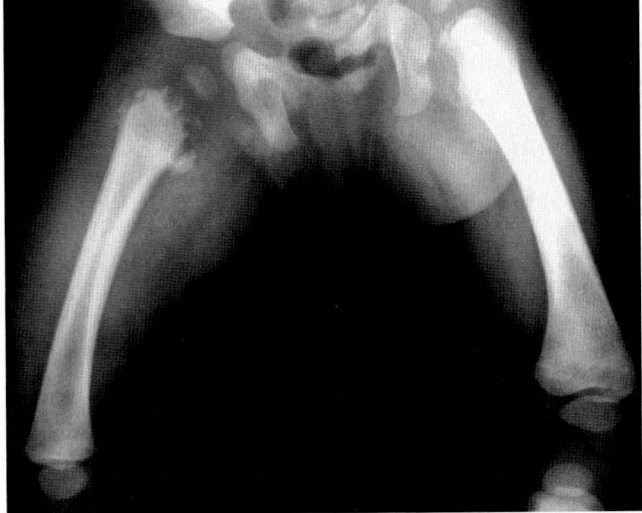 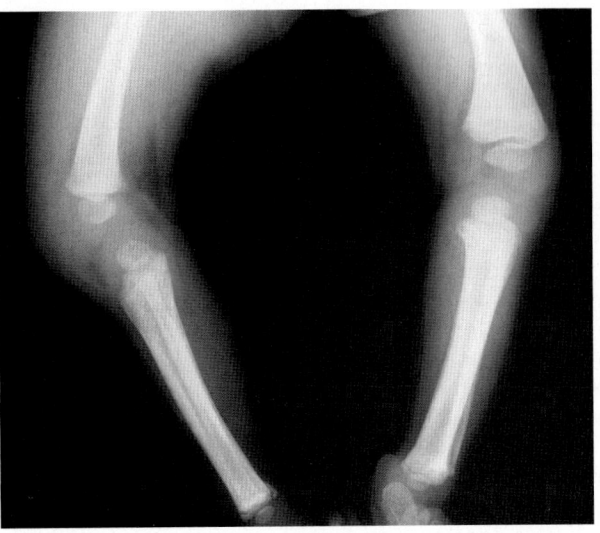

A   B

FIGURE 171-1. A 7-month-old female brought to the emergency room for swelling of the thigh. Skeletal survey revealed 54 fractures, including 35 rib fractures and 19 fractures of long bones. **A,** An anteroposterior film of the pelvis and lower extremities reveals chronic traumatic epiphysiolysis at the proximal right femur. Well-organized periosteal healing bone is seen on the shafts of both femora. **B,** Abnormal modeling of the proximal right tibia is due to healed injury. *Classic metaphyseal lesions* (**A** and **B**) are seen at the proximal left femur, both distal femora, the proximal left tibia, and both distal tibias, and the infant has a swollen right thigh.

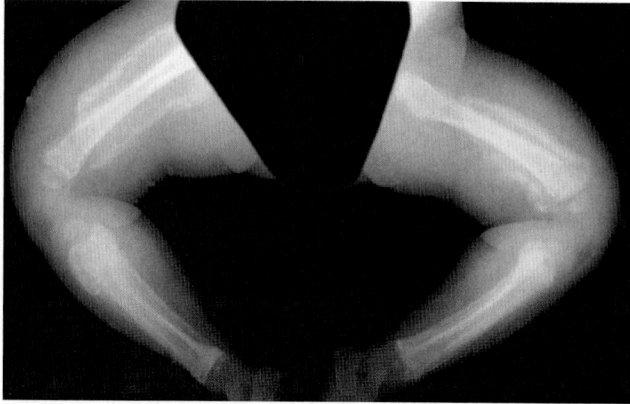

A

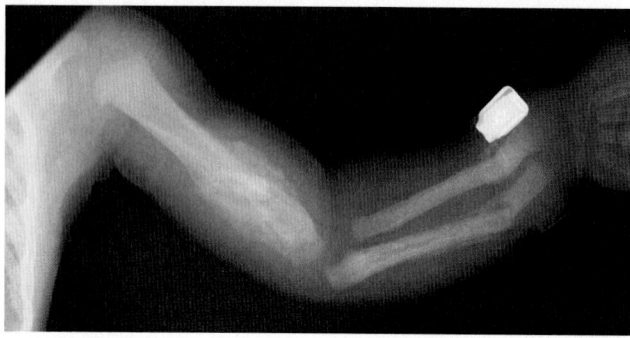

B

FIGURE 171-2. A 3-month old female with 30 fractures of long bones and ribs. **A,** Frog lateral projection of lower extremities shows extensive proliferation of callus and subperiosteal new bone with metaphyseal fractures. Callus extends into the physeal regions. Traumatic epiphysiolysis was found at the proximal right hip (not included on radiograph). Subsequent growth arrest at multiple sites required surgical intervention. **B,** Anteroposterior film of the left upper extremity shows healing transverse fractures of the distal diaphysis of the radius and ulna, a *classic metaphyseal lesion* of the proximal humerus, and a midhumeral diaphyseal healing oblique fracture.

DIAPHYSEAL FRACTURES

Solitary long bone fractures may occur after nonintentional trauma in the older infant and child; however, factors that increase the likelihood of an abuse injury include association with another fracture and other clinical features that produce a high level of suspicion for abuse, inappropriate clinical history, failure to seek medical attention, and discovery of the fracture in a healing state. Diaphyseal fractures may be transverse, oblique, or spiral. It is risky to assign significance to the type of fracture because all occur with unintentional or true accidental trauma, as well as with abuse.

Particular note is made of the spiral diaphyseal fracture because this fracture has erroneously become synonymous with abuse. The spiral nature of the fracture indicates that torque was a component of the stress applied, which resulted in fracture. The fracture is thought to occur when an infant is grabbed or shaken, with the extremity used as a handle. However, spiral fractures also occur in a child who is ambulatory, and we now know that they may occur accidentally in younger

infants. One mechanism was graphically illustrated and reported by Hymel when a 5-month-old infant was videotaped while lying prone; the extended upper extremity was unable to adduct as the baby was rolled from the prone to the supine position. What is most important to consider, when one is presented with a spiral fracture, is the explanation offered and the developmental level of the child, in addition to the age of the fracture at presentation and whether or not other injuries are apparent.

Nonaccidental fractures of the hands and feet occur in abused infants and toddlers. These fractures are often subtle, are frequently torus fractures, and may be better appreciated on oblique views.

METAPHYSEAL FRACTURES

The classic metaphyseal fracture first described by Caffey and commonly referred to as "corner" or "bucket-handle" fracture was re-examined by Kleinman in 1986 with the use of detailed histopathologic and radiographic studies. He determined that this traumatic lesion seen in infancy as a result of shaking abuse indeed represents a complete shearing or planar fracture that extends through the primary spongiosa of the metaphysis, and that it is not an avulsion injury, as described by Caffey. Depending on the amount of metaphyseal bone that is included in the fracture fragment and the radiographic projection, this highly specific metaphyseal lesion for abuse may present as a corner or bucket-handle fracture (Fig. 171-3).

The *classic metaphyseal lesion*, as coined by Kleinman, occurs with violent shaking as the infant is held by the trunk or extremities (Figs. 171-4 through 171-8). Typically, no bruising or outward sign of injury is observed. The same can be said for rib fracture, which is the most common fracture caused by abuse in infants younger than 1 year of age.

> **Typically, no bruising or outward sign of injury is evident with a classic metaphyseal lesion.**

RIB FRACTURES

Kleinman, Marks, Nimkin, and colleagues found that 51% of all fractures in 31 infants who died from abuse involved the rib cage. Rib fractures from abuse are occult; the astute clinician may palpate callus with healing, but otherwise, typically, no physical sign of injury is present. Moreover, acute rib fractures are easily overlooked on x-ray and frequently are not appreciated until evidence of healing is found (Fig. 171-9). Rib fracture may occur at any point along the arc of the rib (costovertebral, posterior, lateral, anterior, or costochondral), but frequently it involves the posterior rib. Excellent scientific evidence suggests that posterior rib fractures at the costovertebral junction have a high specificity for abuse. Boal, in a roundtable discussion, noted that when individual sites along the rib arc were compared, costovertebral junction fractures outnumbered all other individual sites in a large population of 141 abused patients with 1463 rib

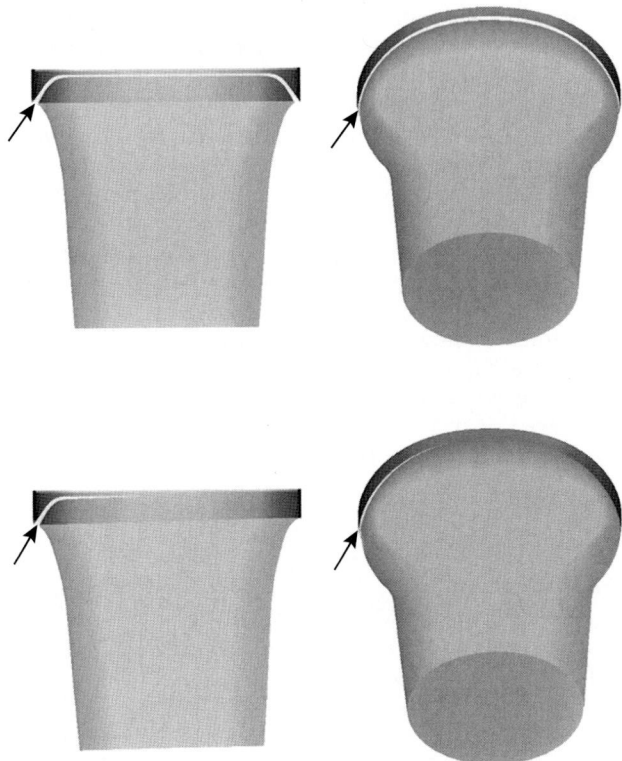

FIGURE 171-3. Diagram of corner and bucket-handle fracture patterns of the *classic metaphyseal lesion* (CML). Fractures *(arrows)* extend adjacent to the chondro-osseous junction and then veer toward the diaphysis to undercut the larger peripheral segment that encompasses the subperiosteal bone collar. When the physis is viewed tangentially, the CML appears as a corner fracture *(left images).* When a view is obtained through beam angulation, a bucket-handle pattern results *(right images). Top images,* Diffuse injury; *bottom images,* localized injury. (From Kleinman PK: Diagnostic Imaging of Child Abuse, 2nd ed. St. Louis, Mosby, 1998:18. Originally modified from Kleinman PK, Marks SC Jr: Relationship of the subperiosteal bone collar to metaphyseal lesions in abused infants. J Bone Joint Surg Am 1995;77:1471-1476.)

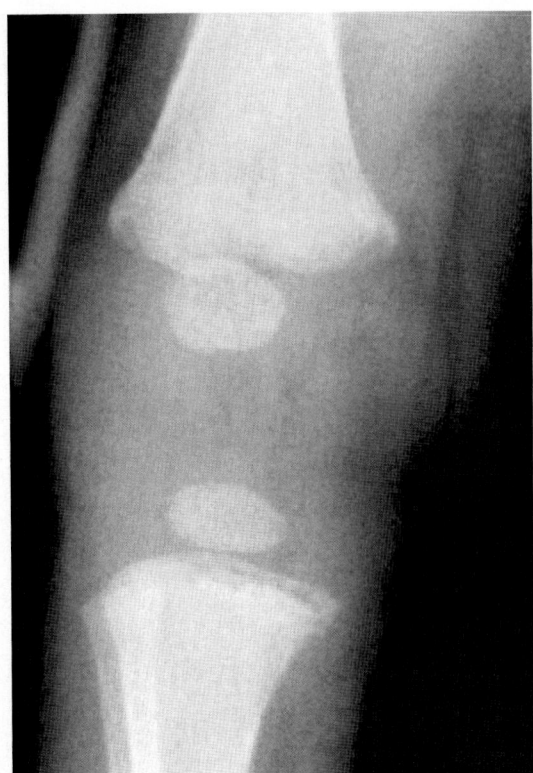

FIGURE 171-4. A 2 1/2-month-old male infant with acute and chronic subdural and 18 fractures. Anteroposterior radiograph of the right knee shows *classic metaphyseal lesions* at the distal femur and the proximal tibia.

fractures. However, if one looks at the costovertebral junction site as compared with all other fracture sites collectively, the costovertebral junction represents only 33% of the total number of rib fractures in this abuse population.

> Rib fractures from abuse are clinically occult; they may occur at any point along the arc of the rib but frequently involve the posterior rib.

A squeezing, shaking injury with compression of the sternum posteriorly results in leveraging of the posterior rib arc over the transverse process and abnormal impaction and distraction forces to the lateral and anterior rib arc and the metaphyseal equivalent at the costovertebral junction of the posterior rib (Figs. 171-10 and 171-11). Multiple fractures may involve a single rib (Fig. 171-12). Nuclear scintigraphy aids in the detection of rib fracture and plays a complementary role to that of radiography (Fig. 171-13). Oblique views of the chest and CT provide increased sensitivity. In contrast to the adult rib, fractures

do not occur in the infant rib after cardiopulmonary resuscitation (CPR); numerous reports in the literature support this finding. Although several case reports have described rib fractures that occurred as a result of birth trauma, as confirmed by personal experience, rib fractures in infants younger than 12 months of age without a predisposing condition such as prematurity or bronchopulmonary dysplasia, similar to the classic metaphyseal lesion, are highly specific for the diagnosis of abuse.

> Oblique views of the ribs increase screening sensitivity for rib fractures. Follow-up radiographs or nuclear scintigraphy may be used to detect occult rib fractures.

FRACTURE OF THE SCAPULA

Any part of the skeleton may be traumatized from abuse. Although it is uncommon, fracture of the scapula, in particular the acromion, is highly specific for abuse (Fig. 171-14).

This fracture results from abnormal indirect forces applied during shaking, and it is usually accompanied by other bony thoracic trauma. A normal anatomic variant in the ossification of the acromion may present a diagnostic dilemma. Follow-up films taken to assess whether or not healing has occurred allow discrimination between fracture and ossification variant.

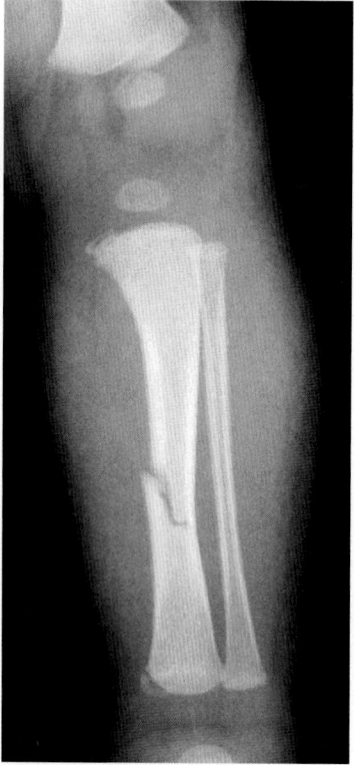
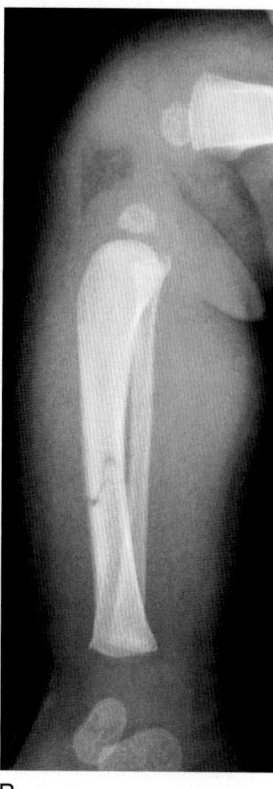

A   B

FIGURE 171-5. A 1-month-old female infant brought to the emergency department for swelling of the leg without history of trauma. **A,** Anteroposterior view of the left lower leg. **B,** Lateral view of the left lower leg shows *classic metaphyseal lesions* at the proximal and distal tibia, as well as a short oblique mid-diaphyseal fracture. Multiple rib fractures and *classic metaphyseal lesions* of the right tibia were also discovered.

SPINAL FRACTURES

Also rare, spinal fractures in infants and young children are highly associated with abuse (Fig. 171-15). The mechanism is thought to be hyperextension, hyperflexion and/or axial loading. Radiographically, these injuries manifest as compression deformities of the vertebral body, often with associated end plate defects and avulsive injuries of the spinous processes. Commonly involving multiple vertebral bodies, the injury is often located near the thoracolumbar junction. More severe fracture-dislocations have been described, including classic hangman's fracture of the C2 vertebra (Fig. 171-16). Although spinal cord injury is uncommon, severe spinal cord injury without radiographic abnormality (SCIWORA) has been described in the shaken infant.

SKULL FRACTURES

Skull fractures are frequent in abuse and are always indicative of an impact injury to the head, but poor correlation has been shown between the presence of fracture and associated intracranial injury. Skull fractures also commonly result from accidental injury. Several authors have tried to characterize specific patterns of injury that occur in abuse, thereby distinguishing abuse skull fractures from true accidental skull

fractures. Some agreement has been expressed that multiple fractures, bilateral fractures, diastasis of fractures and sutures, and fractures that cross suture lines are significantly associated with abuse (Fig. 171-17). However, no particular pattern of skull fracture is diagnostic of abuse. Bilateral complex fractures that cross the sagittal suture may result from a single high-impact blow to the midline, and simple linear fractures are seen in abuse and in accidental trauma. One must consider the appropriateness of the history with respect to the type of injury in trying to make the distinction of abuse versus accidental trauma. Anteroposterior (AP) and lateral skull films should always be part of the radiographic skeletal survey in suspected abuse; additional views may be necessary. CT alone is inadequate because skull fractures in the axial plane may be overlooked.

> Poor correlation has been shown between the presence of skull fracture and associated intracranial injury in infants and young children.
> Skull films should always be part of the radiographic skeletal survey. CT alone is inadequate because skull fractures in the axial plane may be overlooked.

DATING OF FRACTURES

Dating of fractures is dependent on many variables, including the age of the child, the state of nutrition, immobilization of the fracture or the possibility of repetitive injury, and fracture location. Fractures of the skull and spine cannot be satisfactorily dated, and the classic metaphyseal lesion is difficult to date with any degree of precision. In general, a young infant develops subperiosteal new bone much earlier and forms callus more quickly. The range for the appearance of subperiosteal new bone is 4 days to several weeks. Soft tissue swelling resolves during this same period with subsequent loss of fracture line definition and the appearance of soft callus followed by hard callus. Remodeling of fractures occurs over a span of months to years. Precise dating of fractures is not possible, but some general guidelines are provided in Table 171-2.

> A young infant develops subperiosteal new bone much earlier and forms callus more quickly

RADIOGRAPHIC EVALUATION

In all cases of suspected physical abuse in children younger than 2 years of age, a skeletal survey is mandatory (Table 171-3). A "babygram" of single or several images of the entire infant is unsatisfactory. If radiographic film is used, high-detail film without a grid is recommended; the American College of Radiology recommends imaging systems with a spatial resolution of 10 line pairs per millimeter and film speeds no greater than 200. In spite of widespread acceptance and use of a picture archiving and communication system (PACS) and filmless imaging, data at present comparing the

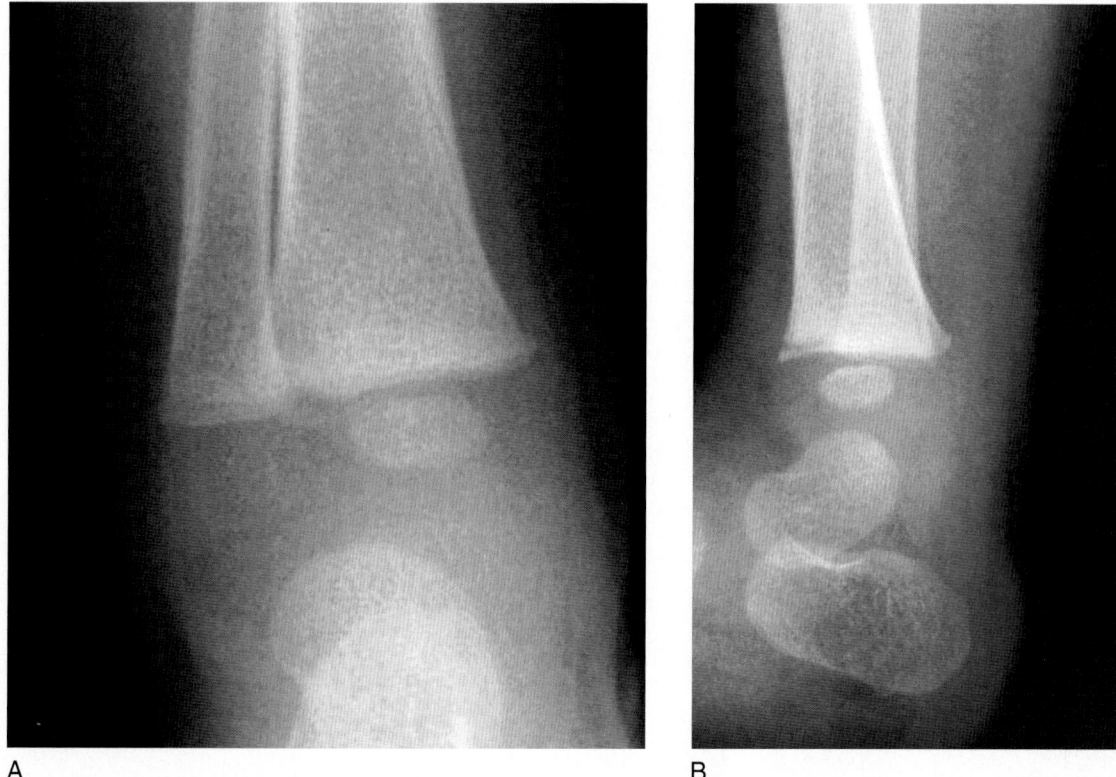

A   B

FIGURE 171-6. Anteroposterior **(A)** and lateral **(B)** radiographs of an 11-month-old infant who sustained severe closed head injury with retinal hemorrhages from shaken baby syndrome while in the care of a babysitter. The only other injury is a *classic metaphyseal lesion* of the distal right tibia, best seen on the lateral view (**B**).

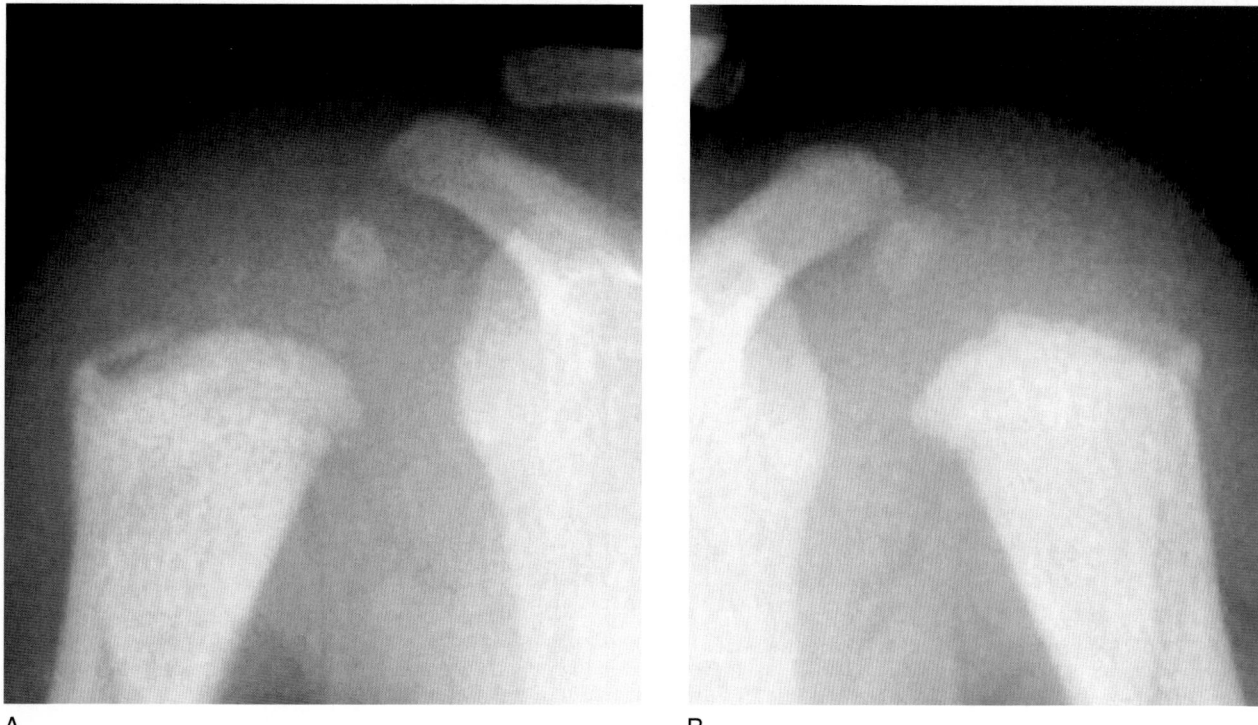

A   B

FIGURE 171-7. Anteroposterior right **(A)** and left **(B)** shoulders of a 5-month-old female infant, deceased, cause of death unknown. Eight fractures were identified at postmortem skeletal survey, including bilateral proximal humeral *classic metaphyseal lesions*.

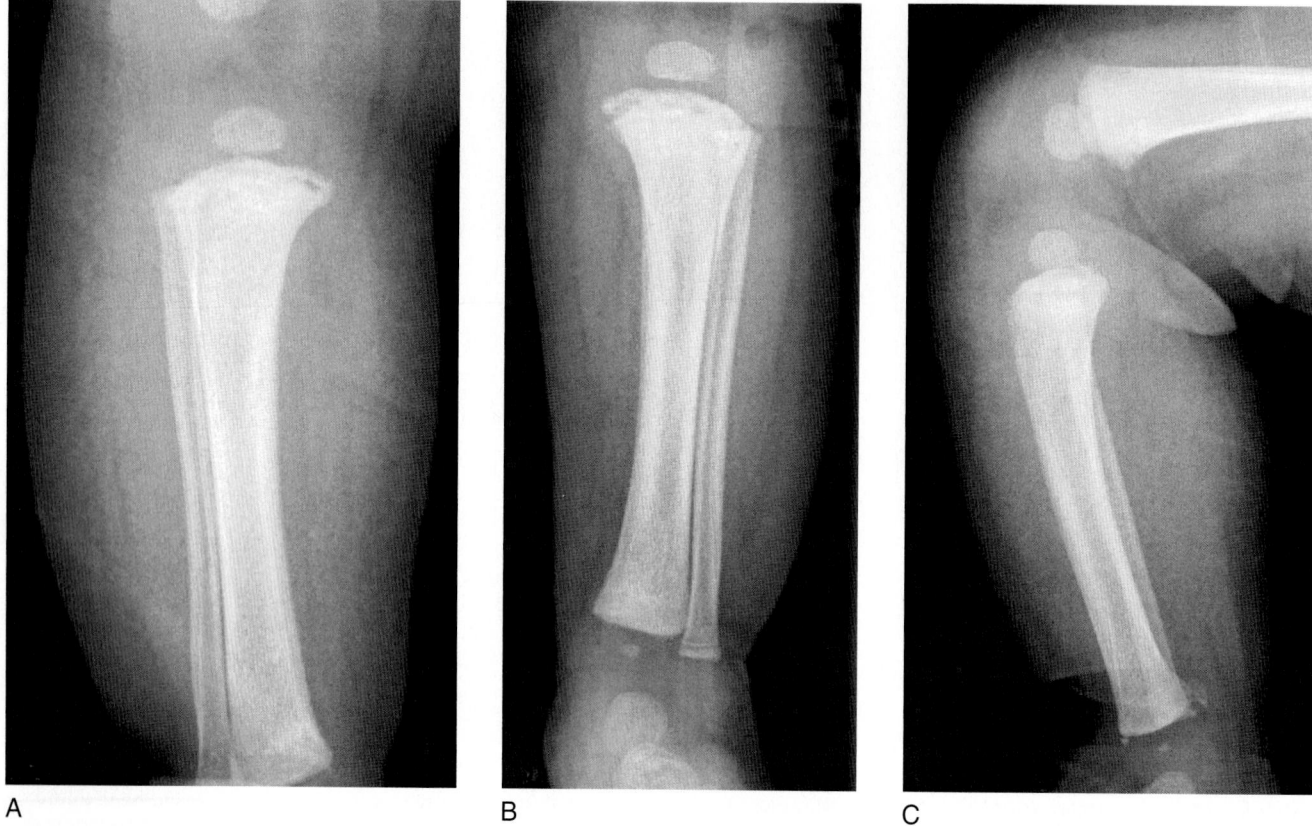

A   B   C

FIGURE 171-8. Anteroposterior right **(A)** and left **(B)** lower leg and lateral right **(C)** lower leg of 3-month-old male infant transferred with acute occipital skull fracture, *classic metaphyseal lesions* of the distal femora and proximal and distal tibias, and 23 rib fractures.

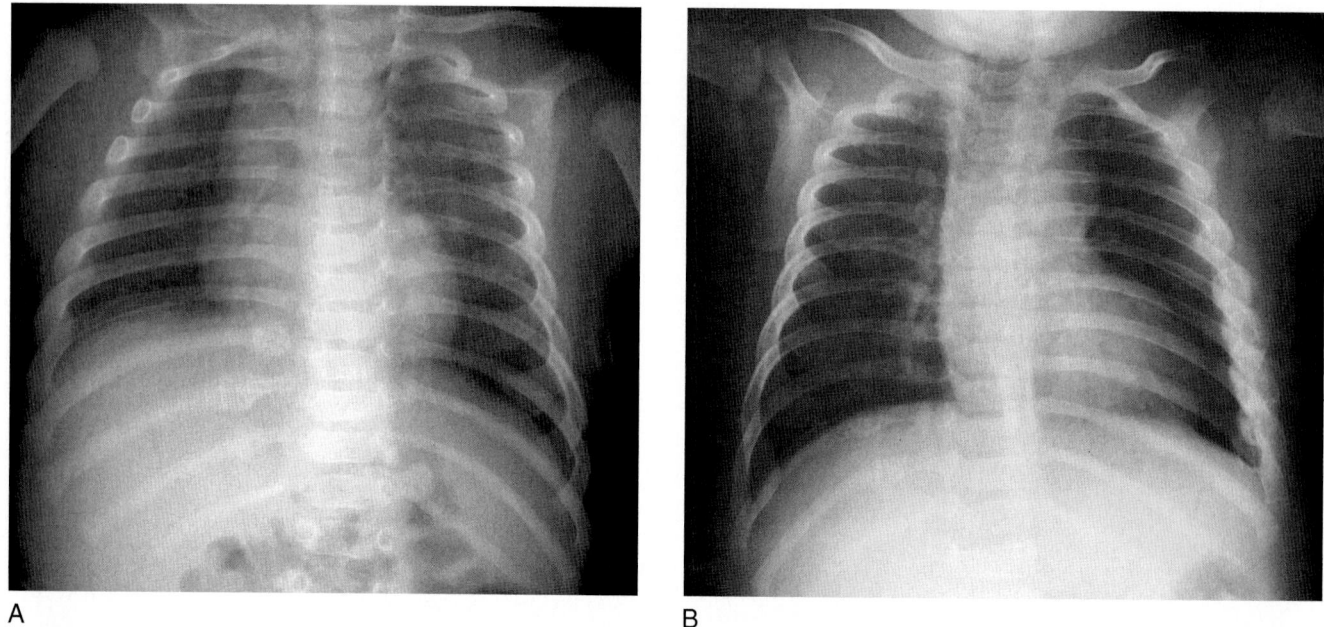

A   B

FIGURE 171-9. A 6-week-old male infant sent for an upper gastrointestinal series for evaluation of colicky pain was found to have healing rib fractures. **A,** Initial chest x-ray identifies healing fractures at the right 9th, 10th, and 11th ribs. **B,** Follow-up chest film 2 weeks later shows additional fractures, now healing, at the lateral aspect of the left third through ninth ribs. The father admitted to shaking.

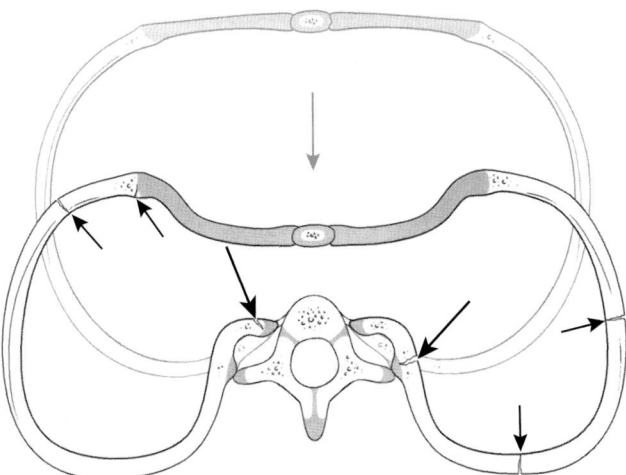

FIGURE 171-10. Diagram of mechanism of injury to ribs. With anteroposterior compression *(grey arrow)* of the chest, excessive leverage of the posterior ribs occurs over the fulcrum of the transverse processes. This places tension along the inner aspects of the rib head and neck regions, resulting in fractures at these sites *(long black arrows)*. This mechanism is consistent with morphologic patterns of injury occurring at other sites along the rib arcs and at the costochondral junctions *(short black arrows)*. (From Kleinman PK: Diagnostic Imaging of Child Abuse, 2nd ed. St. Louis, Mosby, 1998:116.)

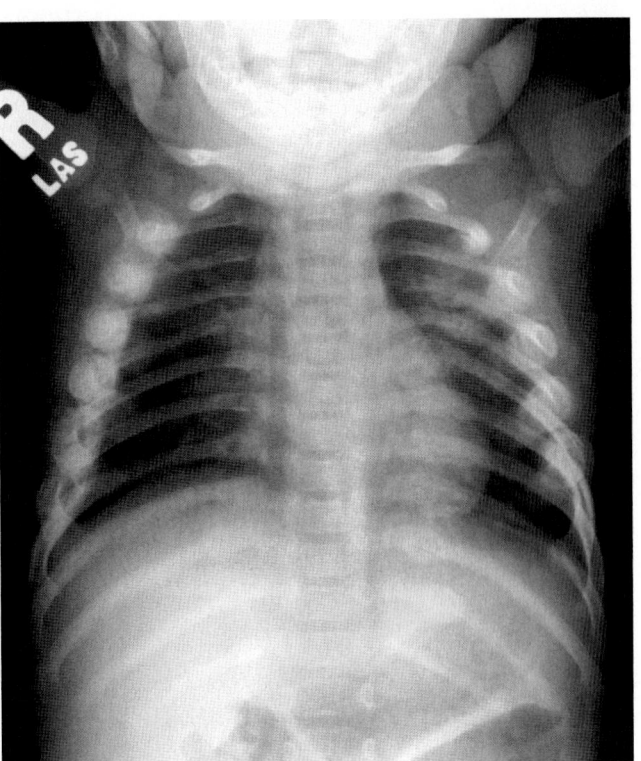

FIGURE 171-12. A 3-month-old infant returned from foster care to mother and boyfriend was found 6 weeks later to have 26 rib fractures and a linear skull fracture. Anteroposterior chest view shows multiple lateral and posterior costovertebral junction rib fractures bilaterally.

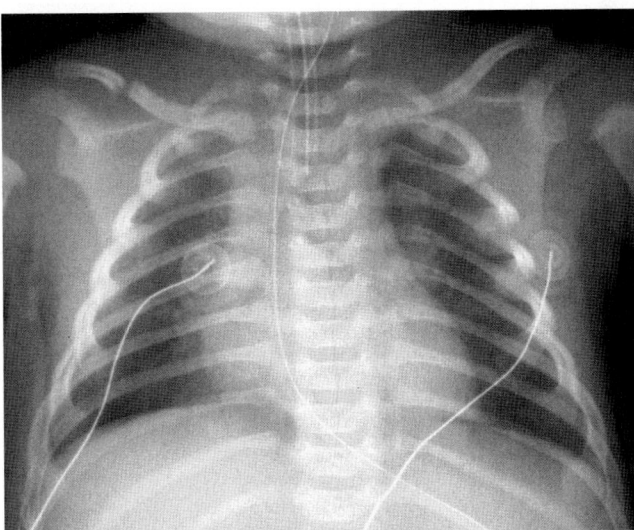

A

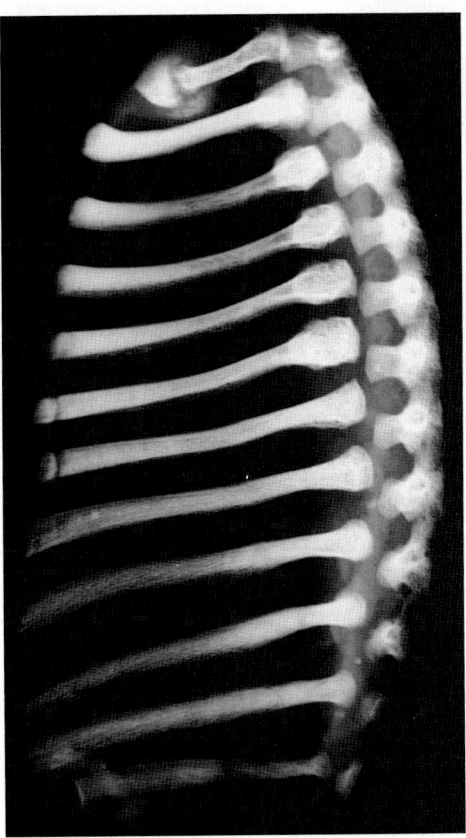

B

FIGURE 171-11. A 2-month-old infant died within 24 hours of presentation from severe closed head injury due to shaken baby syndrome. A total of 33 fractures of ribs and long bones were identified. **A,** Anteroposterior chest radiograph taken prior to death reveals multiple bilateral costovertebral junction rib fractures and fractures of both first ribs, as well as midshaft fracture of the right clavicle. **B,** Faxitron image of postmortem right ribs better shows clubbing and callus at the costovertebral junction of the first through sixth ribs and posterolateral fracture of the right first rib.

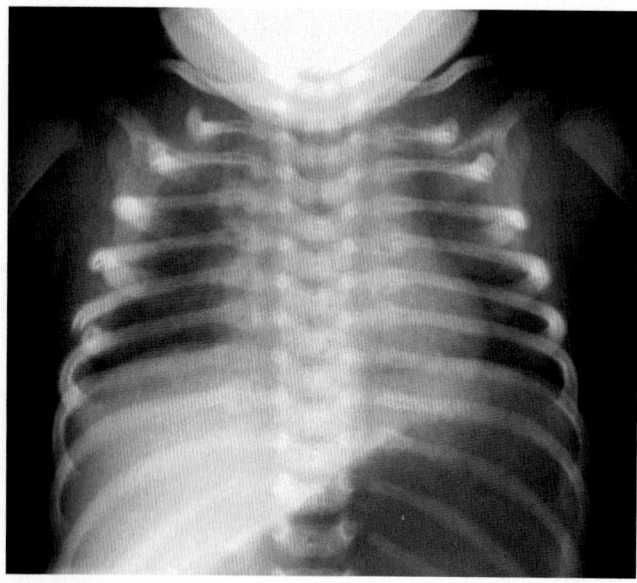

A

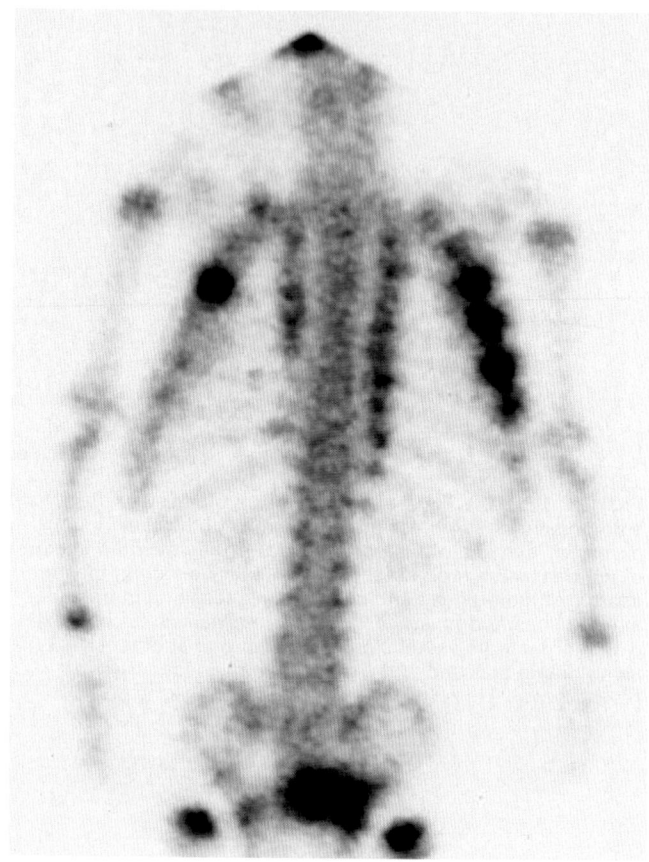

B

FIGURE 171-13. A 17-day-old infant presented with hemothorax and flail chest. The mother's paramour admitted throwing the child against a wall after shaking. **A,** Anteroposterior chest radiographs taken 6 days after injury reveal multiple healing fractures at the costovertebral junction and lateral ribs bilaterally. **B,** Posterior image from bone scintigraphy performed the same day shows multiple bilateral posterior and lateral rib fractures.

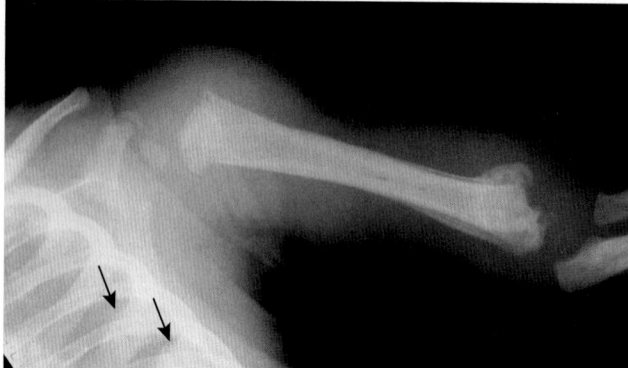

FIGURE 171-14. Anteroposterior radiograph of the left humerus in a 4-month-old male who was not using his arm reveals healing fracture of the acromion, a proximal humeral *classic metaphyseal lesion*, and a healing distal humeral fracture. Multiple other osseous injuries, including rib fractures *(arrows)*, classic metaphyseal lesions, and fracture of the right acromion, were noted.

efficacy of filmless or digital radiography versus that of conventional radiography are limited. Digital radiography will replace film screen skeletal surveys; further evaluation of the technical elements necessary to produce high-detail images is needed.

> A "babygram," a single image or limited images of the entire infant, is unsatisfactory.

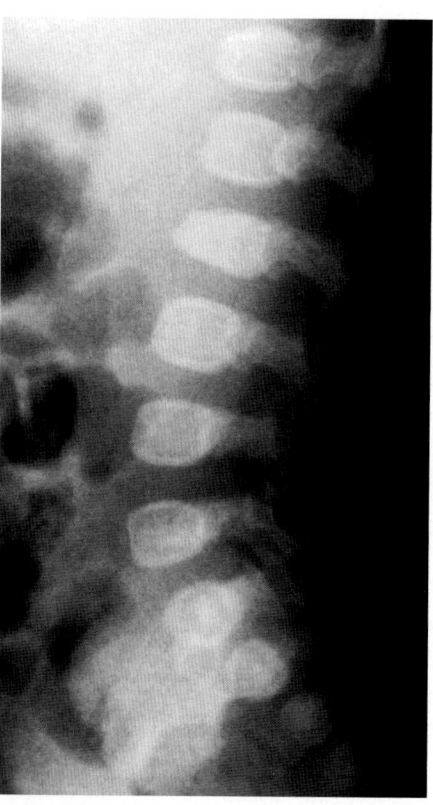

FIGURE 171-15. Lateral radiograph of the spine in a 2-month-old female infant (same patient as Fig. 171-8) shows a compression fracture L2 vertebral body.

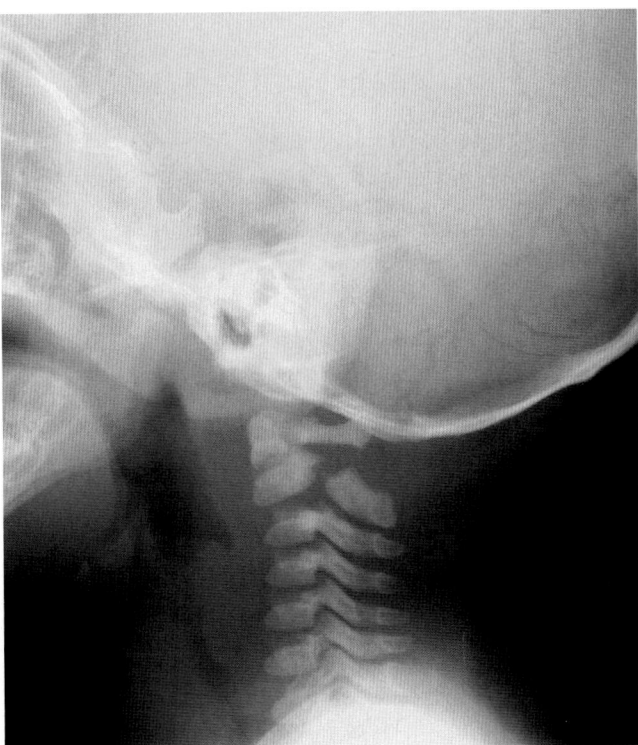

FIGURE 171-16. Lateral cervical spine radiograph of a 6-month-old infant who presented with bruising over the left neck. Although the infant is neurologically intact, 14 fractures, including hangman's fracture of C2, were identified.

TABLE 171-2
Timetable of Radiologic Changes in Children's Fractures*

Category	Early	Peak	Late
1: Resolution of soft tissue swelling	2-5 days	4-10 days	10-21 days
2: SPNBF	4-10 days	10-14 days	14-21 days
3: Loss of fracture line definition		10-14 days	14-21 days
4: Soft callus		10-14 days	14-21 days
5: Hard callus	14-21 days	21-24 days	42-90 days
6: Remodeling	3 mo	1 yr	2 yr to physeal closure

From Kleinman PK: Diagnostic Imaging of Child Abuse, 2nd ed. St. Louis, Mosby, 1998:176.
SPNBF, subperiosteal new bone formation.
*Repetitive injuries may prolong categories 1, 2, 5, and 6.

The initial survey should include AP and lateral views of the skull and spine, along with AP and lateral views of the extremities, to include hands and feet (Fig. 171-18). Additional views of any suspected abnormality must be obtained (Fig. 171-19). In addition to an AP view of the chest, it is now recognized that oblique views increase screening sensitivity for rib fractures (Fig. 171-20). A

TABLE 171-3
Skeletal Survey*

Anteroposterior (AP) and lateral of skull
AP and lateral spine
AP and both obliques (right posterior, left posterior) of chest
AP pelvis and hips
AP and frog lateral of lower extremities
AP upper extremities (shoulder through wrist)
Posteroanterior of hands
AP feet
Lateral of sternum

*Additional collimated projections are recommended for all questioned abnormalities. Follow-up films in 10 to 14 days often confirm or refute questionable findings.

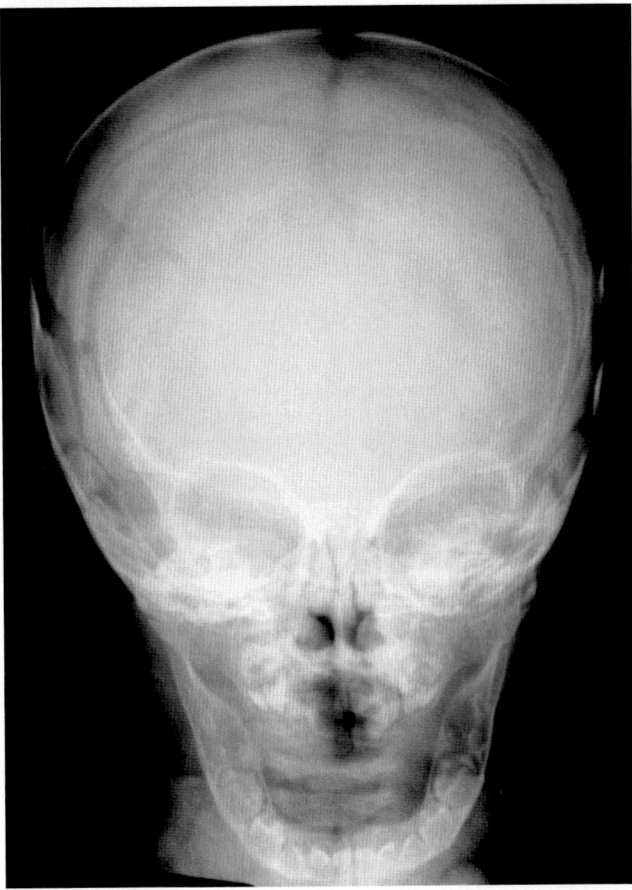

FIGURE 171-17. In a 5-month-old female infant, an anteroposterior skull radiograph shows a diastatic stellate right parietal fracture with diastasis of sutures and extension of the fracture across the sagittal suture into the left parietal bone. Associated right frontal and posterior interhemispheric subdural hematomas are evident. The mother's paramour pleaded guilty to reckless endangerment.

follow-up skeletal survey performed 2 weeks after the initial examination provides additional information (see Figs. 171-9 and 171-20). As noted by Kleinman, the follow-up survey can also do the following: (1) detect additional fractures; (2) differentiate fractures from normal developmental variants; and, (3) assist in dating injuries. In the child older than 5 years, skeletal scinti-

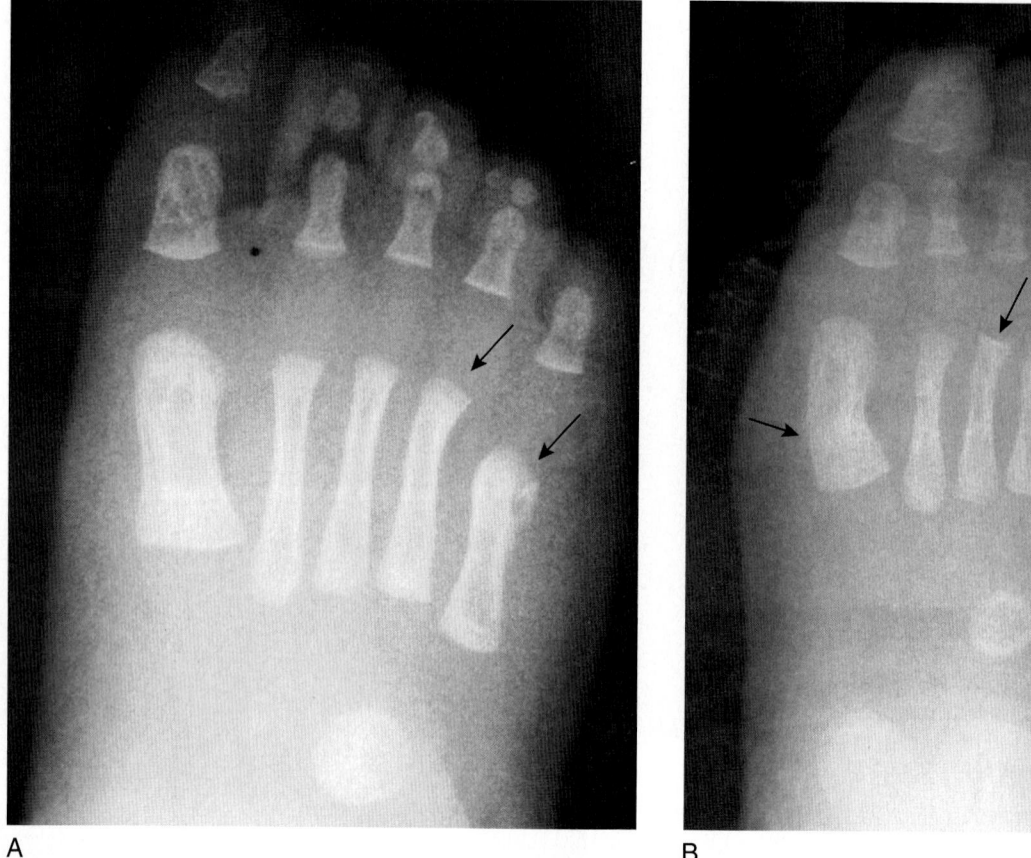

A

B

FIGURE 171-18. Three-month-old twin sisters with metatarsal fractures. **A,** One twin has healing fractures of the fourth and fifth metatarsals *(arrows)*. **B,** The other twin has healing fractures of the first, third, and fourth metatarsals *(arrows)*. Both twins also had rib fractures, classic metaphyseal lesions, and skull fractures.

graphy may be substituted, but neither radiographic nor scintigraphic screening has proved to be useful in the older child. For infants and children younger than 2 years, nuclear scintigraphy should be viewed as a complimentary modality to x-ray evaluation. The imaging of children between 2 and 5 years of age must be assessed individually.

> A follow-up skeletal survey performed 2 weeks after the initial examination is performed can detect additional fractures, can differentiate fractures from normal developmental variants, and can assist in dating injuries.

DIFFERENTIAL DIAGNOSIS

True accidental injury is not the only consideration in the differential for child abuse. Unrecognized obstetric trauma, normal metaphyseal variants, physiologic new bone formation, variation in acromion ossification, accessory skull sutures, and many other conditions may, on first inspection, initially suggest an abuse lesion. Rickets of prematurity may result in multiple rib fractures. Other disease processes, including inherited bone dysplasia, copper deficiency, congenital syphilis, neurologic disorders, and osteogenesis imperfecta, in

particular, may have radiographic features that overlap with those of abuse (Table 171-4). Most of these disorders are discussed individually in this text. Kleinman's text presents an excellent overview of the differential diagnosis and review of diseases that simulate abuse. Fortunately, it is almost always possible to make an accurate determination as to the presence or absence of genetic disease on the basis of clinical and radiographic examination, along with a review of family and social history.

A well-publicized controversy with respect to accidental versus nonaccidental fracture in infancy is that of temporary brittle bone disease (TBBD). This was proposed as a variant of osteogenesis imperfecta by Paterson and colleagues, who identified a group of young infants who were thought to have diminished bone strength, possibly due to temporary deficiency of a metalloenzyme such as copper. Evidence provided to support the existence of TBBD included denial by caregivers of wrongdoing, absence of episodes of trauma that may explain fractures, lack of bruising, absence of systemic injury, radiographs revealing normal bones, and normal laboratory studies. This particular diagnosis has been refuted by others, including the authors of a recent critical review of TBBD prepared by the Committee on Child Abuse of the Society for Pediatric Radiology. To date, no scientific proof definitively supports the existence of TBBD.

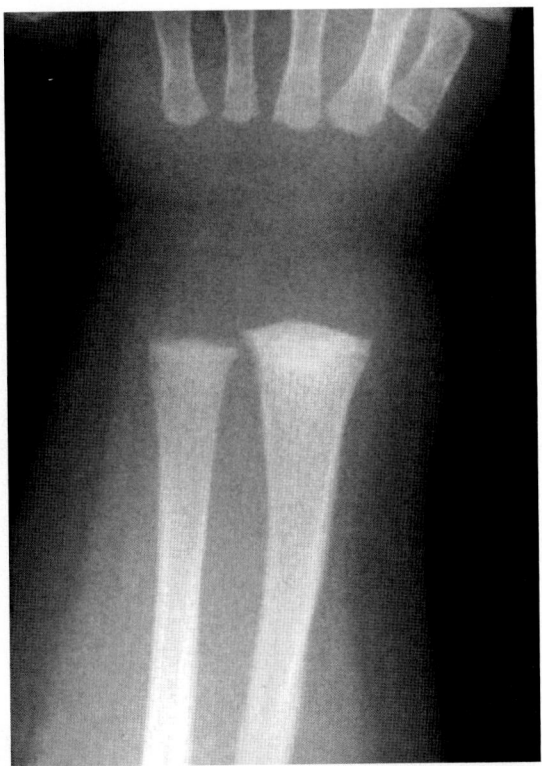 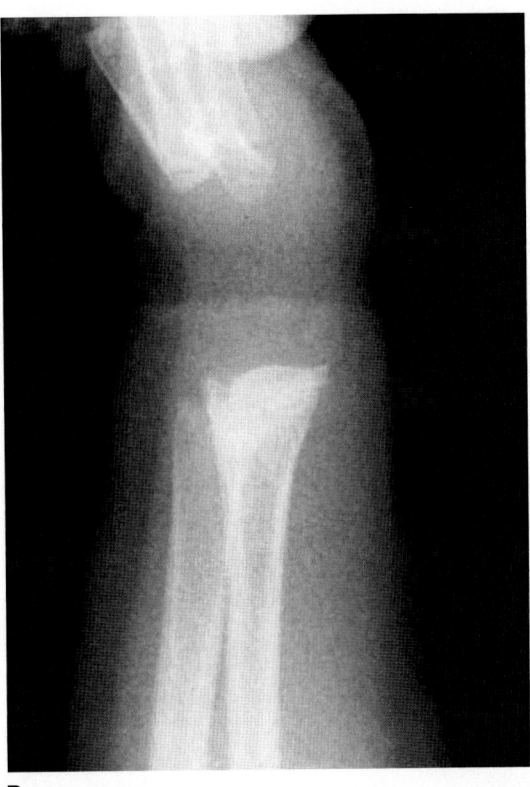

A   B

FIGURE 171-19. Images showing the value of additional views in a 2-month-old female infant. **A,** Anteroposterior view of the right wrist shows subtle irregularity of the radial metaphysis. **B,** Lateral view confirms healing *classic metaphyseal lesion.*

TABLE 171-4
Differential Diagnostic Considerations

TRAUMA True accidental Birth Trauma	**DYSPLASIA** Osteogenesis imperfecta Metaphyseal and spondylometaphyseal dysplasia
VARIANTS OF OSSIFICATION AND MATURATION Acromion Metaphyseal Accessory skull sutures Physiologic periosteal new bone	**DRUG INDUCED** Prostaglandin E_1 therapy **NEUROGENIC** Spina bifida Congenital insensitivity to pain
METABOLIC Bone disease of prematurity Copper deficiency (Menkes syndrome) Rickets Vitamin A toxicity	**MISCELLANEOUS** Caffey disease Congenital syphilis Neoplastic-metastatic round cell tumors

MORBIDITY AND MORTALITY

Morbidity and mortality associated with nonaccidental or abusive head injury have been recognized for some time. Dr. Caffey coined the term *whiplash shaken baby* longer than 30 years ago. In contrast to true accidental head injury, the neurologic deficits that occur in *shaken baby syndrome* are out of proportion to the degree of physical trauma and to changes evident on CT and MRI. Retinal hemorrhages are present in 80% to 85% of shaken babies, in addition to intracranial injury and

often skeletal trauma. Debate is ongoing about whether or not shaking alone is sufficient to result in brain injury, or whether an impact injury must accompany the shaking event. Using models equipped with accelerometers, Duhaime and associates provided experimental evidence that shaking with impact to the head increases the magnitude of angular deceleration forces by 50 times. Whether shaking is done alone or is accompanied by impact, it is the abnormal movement of the infant brain within the skull that results in diffuse axonal injury and subdural and subarachnoid hemorrhages, as

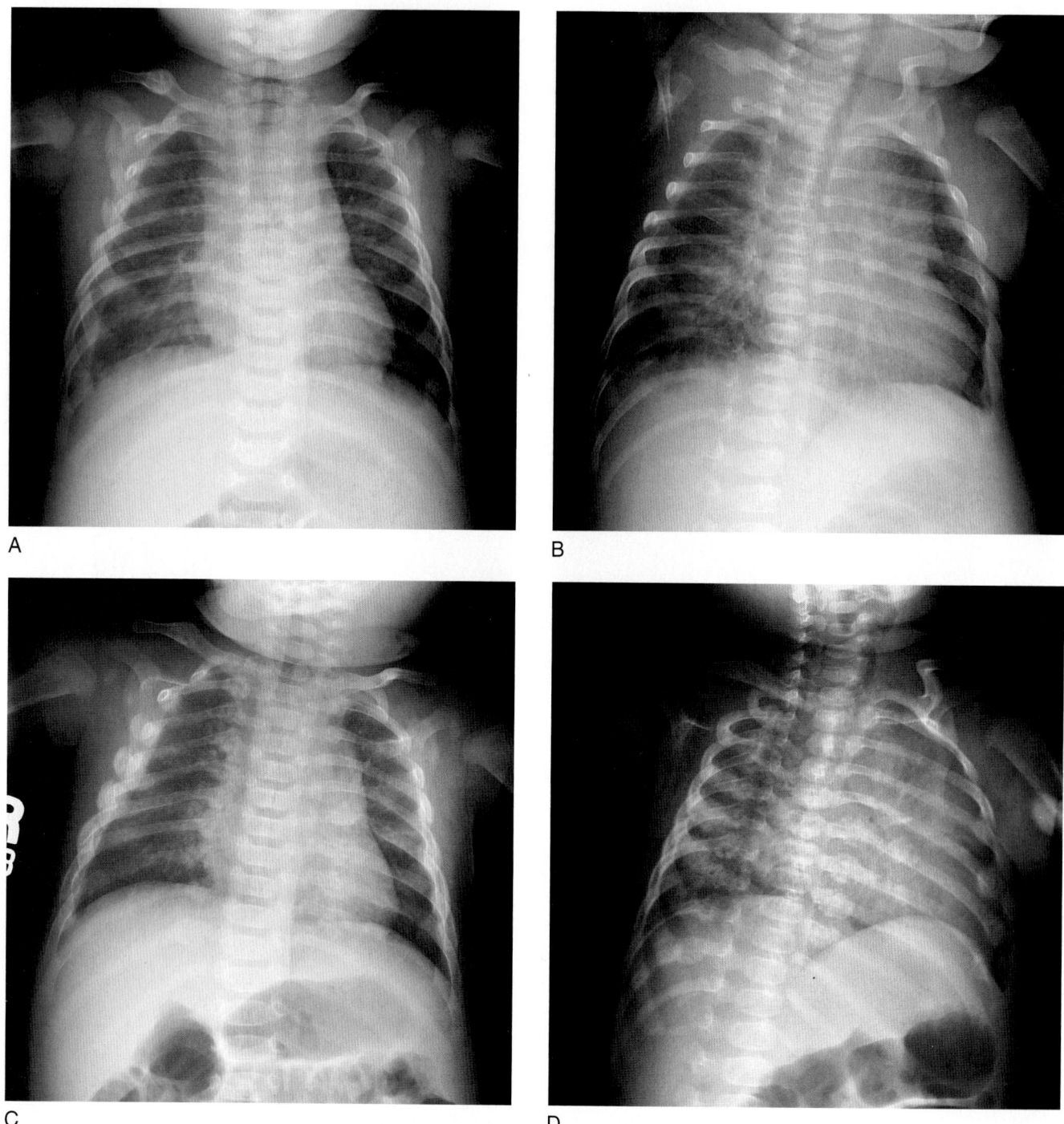

FIGURE 171-20. A, Anteroposterior radiograph of a 2-month-old male infant with right pleural effusion and healing right clavicular fracture shows nine fractures of the right ribs and four fractures of the left ribs on initial survey. Some fractures are better depicted on the left posterior oblique **(B)** view. Two weeks later, anteroposterior **(C)** and left posterior oblique **(D)** radiographs of the chest clearly show 18 right rib fractures and 11 left rib fractures, illustrating the value of a follow-up skeletal survey.

well as apnea that leads to cerebral hypoxia. Shaking an infant is a violent act, and blows to the head with or without skull fractures are frequent. The critical question is whether the head injury is inflicted or accidental. The baby may be shaken alone; shaken and impacted; or shaken, choked, and impacted. Regardless, the outcome for each event is often fatal. Neuroimaging is necessary in all infants with suspected

shaken or shaken impact injury; CT is used emergently, and MRI is used for more detailed evaluation of the brain. CT is adequate for the emergent workup of possible intracranial injury; however, MRI may reveal injuries not appreciated on CT, and it provides greater detail and understanding of the pathophysiology of abusive head injury. Intracranial injury is discussed in Chapter 50.

> Retinal hemorrhages are present in 80% to 85% of shaken babies, in addition to intracranial injury and frequent skeletal trauma.
>
> CT or MRI of the brain is necessary for any infant with suspected intracranial injury due to abuse.
>
> The critical question is whether the head injury is inflicted or accidental. The baby may be shaken alone; shaken and impacted; or shaken, choked, and impacted.

The other major cause of morbidity and mortality in child abuse is visceral injury from thoracoabdominal trauma. In contrast to CNS injury from abuse, which occurs more commonly in infants younger than 12 months, abdominal/pelvic and thoracic injury is more common in the toddler and young child. Blunt trauma from physical assault results in contusion and laceration of the solid viscera and mesentery and perforation or hematoma of the bowel. The fatality rate may be as high as 50%, usually because of shock resulting from hemorrhage or peritonitis, compounded by delay in seeking medical treatment. CT with intravenous (IV) contrast is the most readily available and efficacious way to evaluate suspected abusive trauma of the abdomen/pelvis and chest. CT is indicated in any child with suspected blunt traumatic injury to the abdominal viscera. Abdominal/pelvic trauma is discussed in Chapter 157.

> After CNS trauma, the other major cause of morbidity and mortality in child abuse is visceral injury resulting from thoracoabdominal trauma.

SUGGESTED READINGS

General

American Academy of Pediatrics: Newsletter of the section of child abuse and neglect. SCAN. 1999;2:6

American Academy of Pediatrics, Section on Radiology: Diagnostic imaging of child abuse. Pediatrics 2000;105:1345-1348

American College of Radiology: ACR standards for skeletal surveys in children: resolution 22. Reston, VA, American College of Radiology, 1997:23

Boal DKB: Child abuse roundtable discussion: controversial aspects of child abuse: 43rd Annual Meeting of the Society of Pediatric Radiology. Pediatr Radiol 2001;31:760-774

Caffey J: The whiplash-shaken-infant syndrome: manual shaking by the extremities with whiplash-induced intracranial and intraocular bleedings, linked with residual permanent brain damage and mental retardation. Pediatrics 1974;54:396-403

Carty H, Pierce A: Non-accidental injury: a retrospective analysis of a large cohort. Eur Radiol 2002;12:2919-2925

Carty HML: Fractures caused by child abuse. J Bone Joint Surg Br 1993;75:849-857

Chapman S: Non-accidental injury. Imaging 2004;16:161-173

Kellog ND, American Academy of Pediatrics Committee on Child Abuse and Neglect: Evaluation of suspected child physical abuse. Pediatrics 2007;119:1232-1241

Kempe CH, Silverman FN, Steele BF, et al: The battered child syndrome. JAMA 1962;181:17-24

Kleinman PK: Diagnostic Imaging of Child Abuse, 2nd ed. St. Louis, Mosby, 1998

Leventhal JM, Thomas SA, Rosenfield NS: Fractures in young children: distinguishing child abuse from unintentional injuries. Am J Dis Child 1993;147:87-92

Lonergan GJ, Baker AM, Morey MK, et al: Child abuse: radiologic-pathologic correlation. Radiographics 2003;23:811-845

Merten DF, Radkowski MA, Leonidas JC: The abused child: a radiological reappraisal. Radiology 1983;46:377-381

Offiah AC, Moon L, Hall CM, et al: Diagnostic accuracy of fracture detection in suspected non-accidental injury: the effect of edge enhancement and digital display on observer performance. Clin Radiol 2006;61:163-173

Silverman FN: Unrecognized trauma in infants, the battered child syndrome, and the syndrome of Amboise Tardieu: Rigler lecture. Radiology 1972;104:337-353

U.S. Department of Health and Human Services, Administration on Children, Youth and Families: Child Maltreatment 2004. Washington, DC, US Government Printing Office, 2006

Extremity Trauma

Caffey J: Multiple fractures in the long bones of infants suffering from chronic subdural hematoma. Am J Roentgenol Radium Ther 1946;56:163-173

Hymel KP: Abusive spiral fractures of the humerus: a videotaped exception. Arch Dis Child 1996;150:226-227

Kleinman PK: The metaphyseal lesion in abused infants: a radiologic-histopathologic study. AJR Am J Roentgenol 1986;146:895-905

Loder RT, O'Donnell PW, Feinberg JR. Epidemiology and mechanisms of femur fractures in children. J Pediatr Orthop 2006;26:561-566

Thoracic Trauma

Feldman KW, Brewer KD: Child abuse, cardiopulmonary resuscitation, and rib fractures. Pediatrics 1984;73:339-342

Kleinman PK, Marks SC, Nimkin K, et al: Rib fractures in 31 abused infants: postmortem radiologic-histopathologic study. Radiology 1996;200:807-810

Kleinman PK, O'Connor B, Nimkin K, et al: Detection of rib fractures in an abused infant using digital radiography: a laboratory study. Pediatr Radiol 2002;32:896-901

Spevak MR, Kleinman PK, Belanger PL, et al: Cardiopulmonary resuscitation and rib fractures in infants: a postmortem radiologic-pathologic study. JAMA 1994;272:617-618

Dating of Fractures

Prosser I, Maguire S, Harrison SK, et al: How old is this fracture? Radiologic dating of fractures in children: a systematic review. Am J Radiol 2005;184:1282-1286

Central Nervous System Trauma

American Academy of Pediatrics Committee on Child Abuse and Neglect: Shaken baby syndrome: inflicted cerebral trauma. Pediatrics 1993;92:872-875

Brown JK, Minns RA: Non-accidental head injury, with particular reference to whiplash shaking injury and medico-legal aspects. Dev Med Child Neurol 1993;35:849-869

Chen CY, Zimmerman RA, Rorke LB: Neuroimaging in child abuse: a mechanism-based approach. Neuroradiology 1999;41:711-722

Conway EE: Non-accidental head injury in infants: the shaken-baby syndrome revisited. Pediatric Ann 1998;27:677-690

Duhaime AC, Christian CW, Rorke LB, et al: Non-accidental head injury in the infants—the "shaken-baby syndrome." N Engl J Med 1998;338:1822-1829

Duhaime AC, Gennarelli TA, Thibault LE: The shaken baby syndrome. J Neurosurg 1987;66:409-415

Feldman KW, Brewer DK, Shaw DW: Evolution of the cranial computed tomography scan in child abuse. Child Abuse Negl 1995;19:307-314

Hobbs CJ: Skull fracture and the diagnosis of abuse. Arch Dis Child 1984;59:246-252

Hymel KP, Bandak FA, Partington MD, et al: Abusive head trauma? A biomechanics-based approach. Child Maltreatment 1998;3:116-128

Johnson DL, Boal D, Baule R: Role of apnea in nonaccidental head injury. Pediatr Neurosurg 1995;23:305-310

Keenan HT, Runyan DK, Marshall SW, et al: A population-based comparison of clinical and outcome characteristics of young children with serious inflicted and noninflicted traumatic brain injury. Pediatrics 2004;114:633-639

Meservy CJ, Towbin R, McLaurin RL, et al: Radiographic characteristics of skull fractures resulting from child abuse. AJNR Am J Neuroradiol 1987;8:455-457

Mogbo KI, Slovis TL, Canady AI, et al: Appropriate imaging in children with skull fractures and suspicion of abuse. Radiology 1998;208:521-524

Sato Y, Yuh WTC, Smith WL, et al: Head injury in child abuse: evaluation with MR imaging. Radiology 1989;173:653-657

Abdominal/Pelvic Trauma

Johnson K, Chapman S, Hall CM: Skeletal injuries associated with sexual abuse. Pediatr Radiol 2004;34:620-623

Differential Diagnosis

Ablin DS, Greenspan A, Reinhart M, et al: Differentiation of child abuse from osteogenesis imperfecta. AJR Am J Roentgenol 1990;154:1035-1046

Ablin DS, Sane SM: Non-accidental injury: Confusion with temporary brittle bone disease and mild osteogenesis imperfecta. Pediatr Radiol 1997;27:111-113

Bertocci GE, Pierce MC, Deemer E, et al: Computer simulation of stair falls to investigate scenarios in child abuse. Arch Pediatr Adolesc Med 2001;155:1008-1014

Carroll DM, Doria AS, Babyn SP: J Perinat Med 2007;35:[Epub ahead of print]

Chadwick DL, Chin S, Salerno C, et al: Deaths from falls in children: how far is fatal? J Trauma 1991;31:1353-1355

Helfer RE, Slovis TL, Black M: Injuries resulting when small children fall out of bed. Pediatrics 1977;60:533-535

Jenny C, American Academy of Pediatrics Committe on Child Abuse and Neglect: Evaluating infants and young children with multiple fractures. Pediatrics 2006;118:1299-1303

Kleinman PK, Belanger PL, Karellas A, et al: Normal metaphyseal radiologic variants not to be confused with findings of infant abuse. AJR Am J Roentgenol 1991;156:781-783

Lyons TJ, Oates RK: Falling out of bed: a relatively benign occurrence. Pediatrics 1993;92:125-127

Maguire S, Mann M, John N, et al: Does cardiopulmonary resuscitation cause rib fractures in children? A systematic review. Child Abuse Negl 2006;30:739-751

Mendelson KL: Critical review of temporary brittle bone disease. Pediatr Radiol 2005;35:1036-1040

Patterson CR, Burns J, McAllison SJ: Osteogenesis imperfecta: the distinction from child abuse and the recognition of a variant form. Am J Med Genet 1993;45:187-192

Pierce MC, Bertocci GE, Janosky JE, et al: Femur fractures resulting from stair falls among children: an injury plausibility model. Pediatrics 2005;115:1712-1722

Worlock P, Stower M, Barbor P: Patterns of fractures in accidental and non-accidental injury in children: a comparative study. Br Med J 1986;293:100-102

172 Sports-Related Injury in Children

KIRSTEN ECKLUND

More than 40 million children ages 5 through 18 participate in organized school and community athletic programs. This number has been increasing annually as first forays into organized sports begin at younger and younger ages. An unfortunate consequence of this unprecedented increase in athletic activity is the associated increased risk of injury from acute trauma as well as repetitive overuse mechanisms. According to the National Safe Kids Campaign, more than 3.5 million children under 15 years of age receive medical treatment for sports injuries each year. Musculoskeletal injury can lead to lifelong disability, especially when the growth mechanism is involved. Since developing bones are partially composed of radiolucent structures and supporting soft tissue structures are not well evaluated with radiographs, magnetic resonance imaging (MRI) plays an increasingly critical role in the diagnosis and management of pediatric musculoskeletal trauma. Though standard radiography, scintigraphy, computed tomography (CT), and ultrasound continue to be important, the unique ability of MRI to visualize the path of osteocartilaginous injury as well as the associated soft tissue abnormalities makes it ideally suited for evaluation of these children. This section reviews the role of imaging in common, as well as unique, pediatric musculoskeletal injuries. Most acute fractures, however, regardless of mechanism of injury, are discussed in detail in Chapter 170.

EPIPHYSEAL/OSTEOCHONDRAL INJURIES

Osteochondritis Dissecans

Juvenile osteochondritis dissecans (OCD), especially common in athletic children, involves subchondral bone as well as epiphyseal and articular cartilage. This lesion, likely secondary to chronic microtrauma, is most frequently encountered in the femoral condyles, the talar dome, and the capitellum. Radiographs may show an oval radiolucency of the articular surface, which may contain a central bony fragment (Fig. 172-1). MRI, especially T2-weighted sequences, can determine the stability of the lesion and help direct therapy. Stable lesions are treated conservatively while unstable lesions generally require surgical management. The four MRI signs of unstable OCD are linear high signal intensity between the fragment and the parent bone, linear high signal intensity through the articular cartilage, a focal high

signal articular cartilage defect, and a ≥5-mm cystic area beneath the fragment. If any one of these features is present, the lesion is considered to be unstable (Fig. 172-2). In distal femoral OCD, poor prognostic factors indicating the need for surgical interventions include large lesion size, an adjacent closed growth plate, and MRI features of instability, especially visualization of an articular cartilage defect or fracture. Large osteochondral defects in young patients, especially competitive athletes, are currently being treated with a variety of cell-based surgical therapies, including autologous chondrocyte implantation and osteochondral autograft or allograft transplantation. MRI is utilized in the follow-up of these patients to assess graft healing.

MRI Features of Unstable OCD

- Fluid signal intensity between the fragment and the parent bone
- Linear high signal through the articular cartilaginous surface
- Focal cartilage defect
- ≥5-mm cyst beneath the fragment

When imaging young children with presumed OCD of the distal femoral condyle, it is important to differentiate this lesion from the normal developmental epiphyseal irregularity, which can be indistinguishable radiographically. MRI features of developmental variants include defects in the posterior aspect of the condyle as opposed to the intercondylar notch, accessory ossification centers, spiculated osseous margins, a large amount of residual epiphyseal cartilage, and lack of bone marrow edema (Fig. 172-3). Additionally, in children less than 6 years of age, physiologic T2 hyperintensity will be seen in the posterior epiphyseal cartilage of both medial and lateral femoral condyles, likely related to advancing ossification within the cartilaginous epiphysis (see Fig. 172-3). In these young children, low signal intensity is normally seen in the inferior aspect of the cartilaginous epiphysis, presumably due to weight bearing. This normal maturation process should not be confused with osteochondral injury. Misinterpretation of developmental variants as OCD may, in part, account for the higher rate of spontaneous resolution of juvenile OCD compared to the adult form.

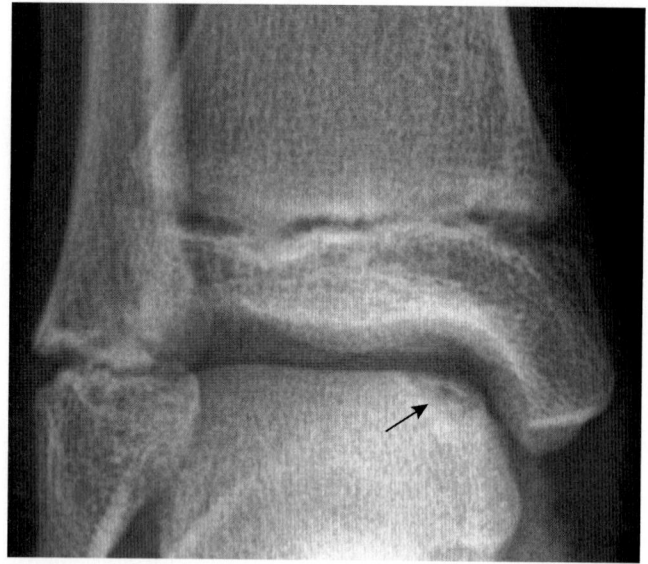

A

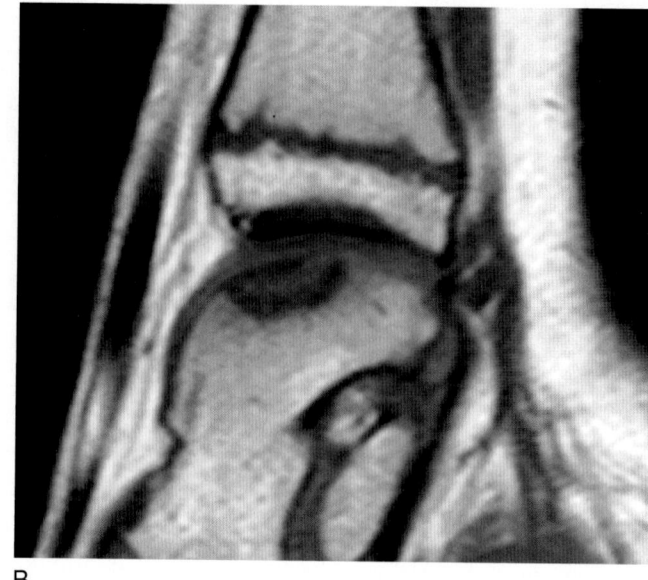

B

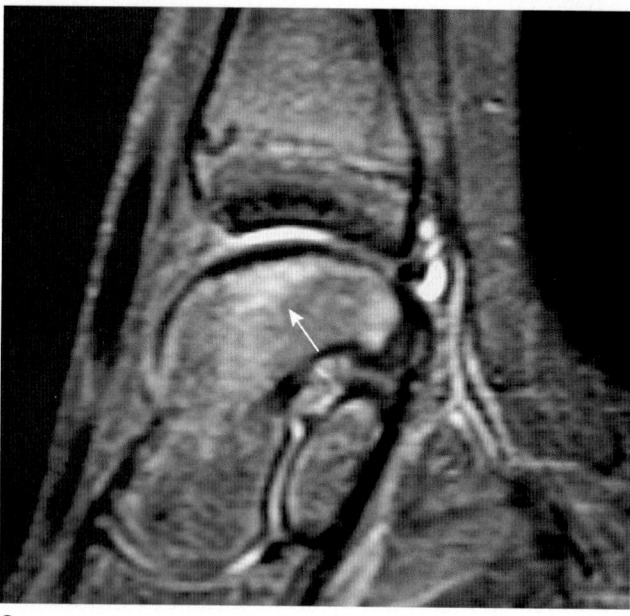

C

FIGURE 172-1. Osteochondritis dissecans of the talar dome in a 9-year-old soccer player with 6 months of pain in her right ankle. **A,** Frontal radiograph shows the medial talar lesion *(arrow)* but cannot determine stability. **B** and **C,** Sagittal T1-weighted **(B)** and inversion recovery **(C)** MR images show the sclerotic margins and intact overlying articular cartilage, confirming stability. The mild associated marrow edema *(arrow)* suggests that the lesion is active. This was treated with activity restriction, and radiographs obtained 6 months later (not shown) showed resolution.

> **MRI Features Suggesting Normal Variant Rather Than OCD**
> - Posterior location (not intercondylar)
> - No bone marrow edema
> - Accessory ossification centers and spiculated cortical margins
> - Young age; large amount of epiphyseal cartilage

OCD of the capitellum occurs in active adolescents, especially those involved in throwing sports and gymnastics. It should not be confused with Panner disease, which is an osteochondrosis of the capitellum that occurs almost exclusively in boys ages 5 to 10 years, prior to complete ossification of the capitellum (Fig. 172-4). The etiology of Panner disease is uncertain and is likely related to excessive valgus stress applied at a particularly vulnerable developmental stage.

Acute Osteochondral Injury

Acute osteochondral injury is a less commonly discussed lesion in children. With the advent of specialized, high-resolution fast spin-echo proton density–weighted MRI sequences with longer time to echo, articular cartilage is much better visualized and these lesions are more frequently recognized. A recent report found that chondral injuries are the most common lesions in children undergoing MRI evaluation for internal derangement of the knee. Subchondral bone marrow edema, best

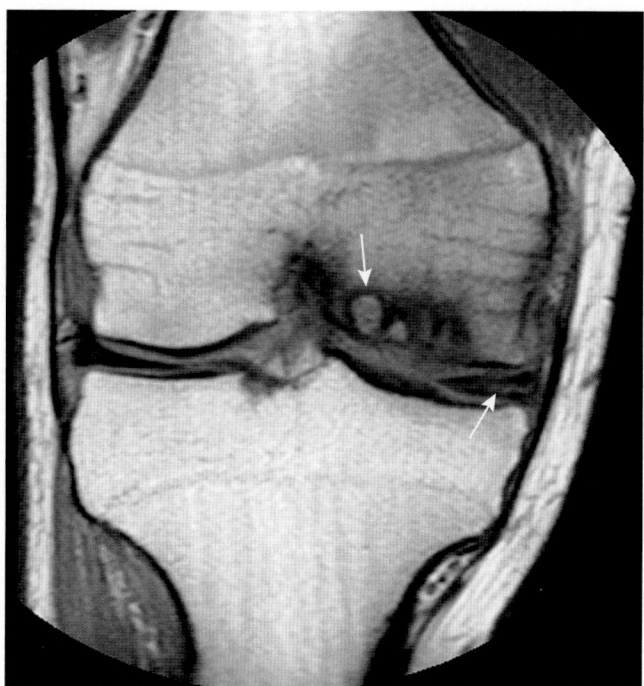
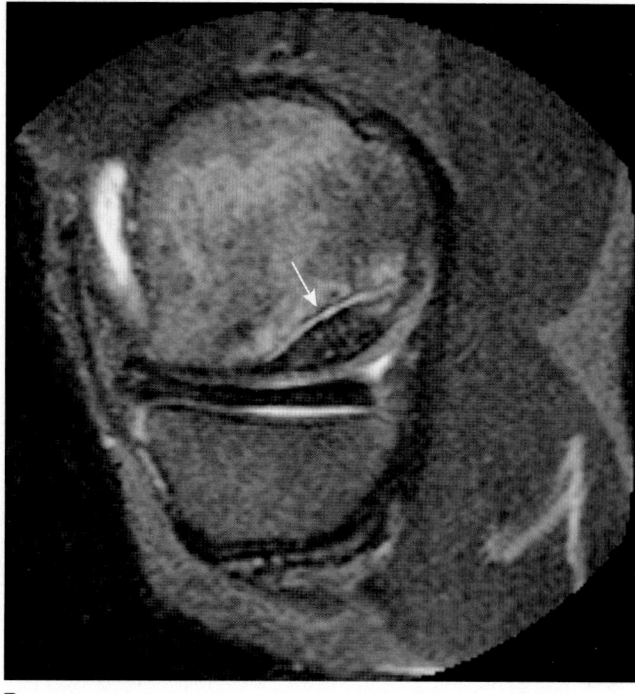

A   B

FIGURE 172-2. Osteochondritis dissecans of the right medial femoral condyle in a 16-year-old basketball player with recurrent hyperextension of the knee. Coronal T1-weighted (**A**) and sagittal inversion recovery (**B**) MR images show features of instability, including high signal intensity fluid between the osteochondral fragment and the parent bone (*white arrow* in **B**) and cysts beneath the fragment (*upper arrow* in **A**). This lesion required surgical repair, including drilling and internal fixation. A discoid medial meniscus with extensive high signal degeneration is also present (*lower arrow* in **A**).

seen on fat-suppressed T2-weighted or inversion recovery images, frequently accompanies chondral injuries. Identification of these subchondral "bone bruises" should alert the radiologist to scrutinize the overlying articular cartilage for associated injury (Fig. 172-5). Acute injury to the articular cartilage and adjacent subchondral bone occurs most frequently in the knee and ankle, but can also be seen in the capitellum and femoral head. It is important to be aware of age-related signal changes within epiphyses, especially when assessing MR images for chondral injury in young children who still have a large component of epiphyseal cartilage. Increased signal intensity on T2-weighted images is often present within the epiphysis just prior to ossification and should not be confused with pathology (Fig. 172-6).

Magnetic resonance arthrography with direct intra-articular contrast injection has increased sensitivity for the detection of articular cartilage injury and is frequently employed in the evaluation of acute hip and shoulder trauma or dislocation. MR arthrography has the added advantage of improved visualization of the acetabular and glenoid labra (Fig. 172-7). Recent reports, however, suggest that 3-Tesla MRI, with its inherent increased resolution and improved signal-to-noise ratio, has improved sensitivity for articular cartilage and labral pathology and may decrease the need for MR arthrography.

OVERUSE INJURIES

Stress Reactions and Fractures

Stress fractures and stress reactions in children, once considered rare, are seen with increasing frequency presumably due to increased participation in athletics. Stress is the force applied to a bone that arises from weight bearing or from muscular contractions. The term *stress fracture* encompasses both *insufficiency* fractures, which result from normal stresses applied to abnormal bone, and *fatigue* fractures, which occur in normal bones exposed to repetitive stresses. Often, however, the term "stress fracture" is used to describe only the fatigue variant, and it will be so used for the purposes of this discussion.

The common sites of stress fractures in children are the tibia, fibula, metatarsals, cuboid, calcaneus, and femur. Unfortunately, the sensitivity of early radiographs is as low as 15%, and delayed radiographs only reveal findings in 50% of patients. Bone scintigraphy, MRI, or CT may be necessary to help differentiate between stress reaction and other pathology. On MRI, short tau inversion recovery (STIR) sequences and T2-weighted sequences with frequency-selective fat saturation are exquisitely sensitive to the high signal intensity marrow edema that is associated with stress reactions. These long repetition

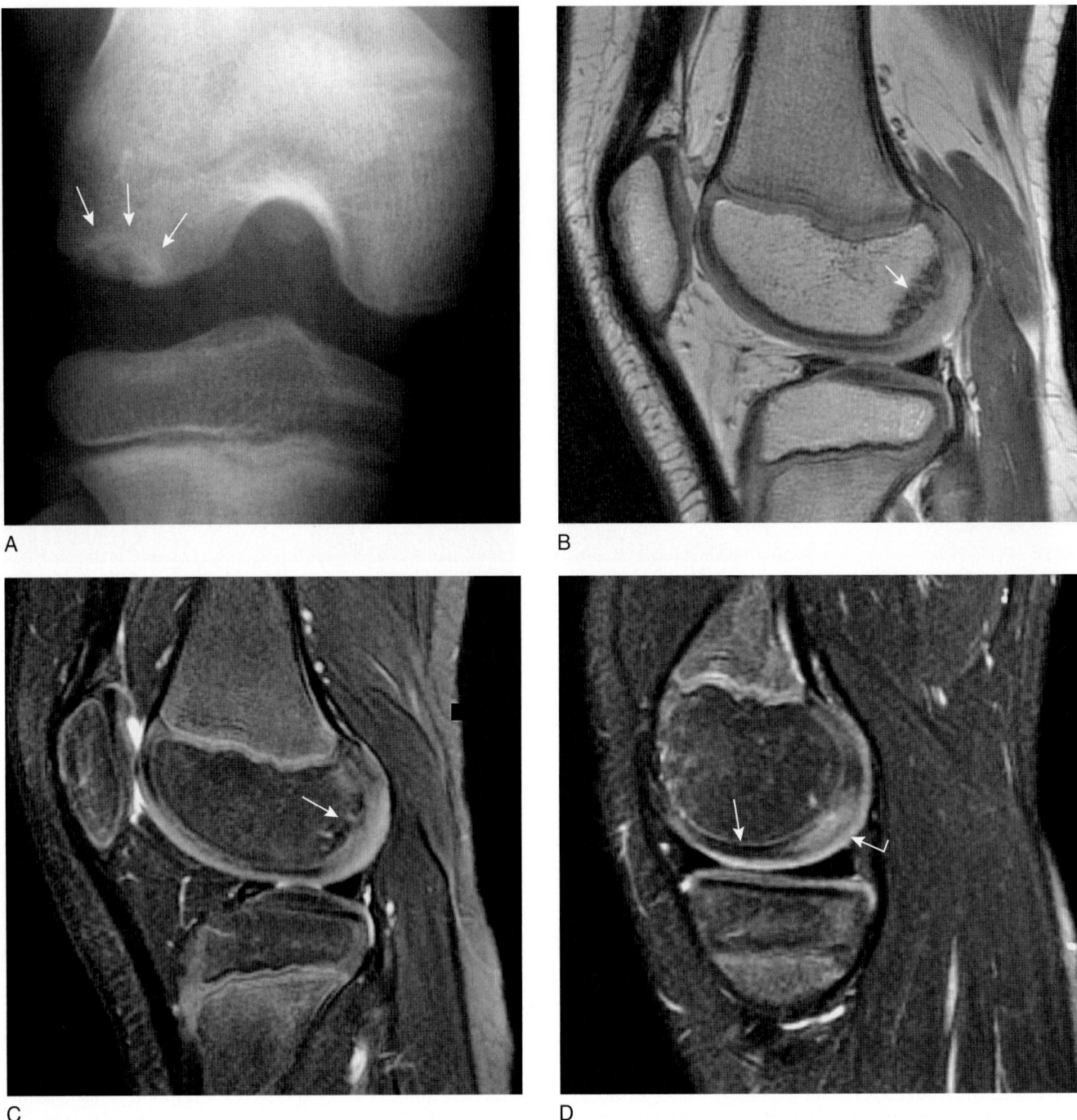

FIGURE 172-3. Normal developmental ossification variant in a 6-year-old boy with intermittent right knee pain. **A,** Frontal tunnel projection radiograph shows irregularity and fragmentation of the lateral femoral condyle *(arrows)*. **B** and **C,** Sagittal proton density–weighted **(B)** and fat-suppressed T2-weighted **(C)** MR images show the findings *(arrows)* in the posterior condyle with normal overlying epiphyseal and articular cartilage and no associated marrow edema. **D,** A sagittal fat-suppressed T2-weighted MR image through the medial femoral condyle shows normal high signal in the posterior condylar epiphyseal cartilage *(bent arrow)* and low signal in the weight-bearing epiphyseal cartilage *(straight arrow)*. This should not be confused with cartilaginous pathology.

time fat-suppressed images should be scrutinized for the presence of a low signal intensity line within the high signal marrow edema (Fig. 172-8). This line allows the lesion to be confidently identified as a stress fracture. Multidector CT with long axis reformations can also be very helpful in delineating the occult fracture lucency.

Common Sites of Stress Injury in Children
- **Tibia**
- **Femur**
- **Tarsal and metatarsal bones**

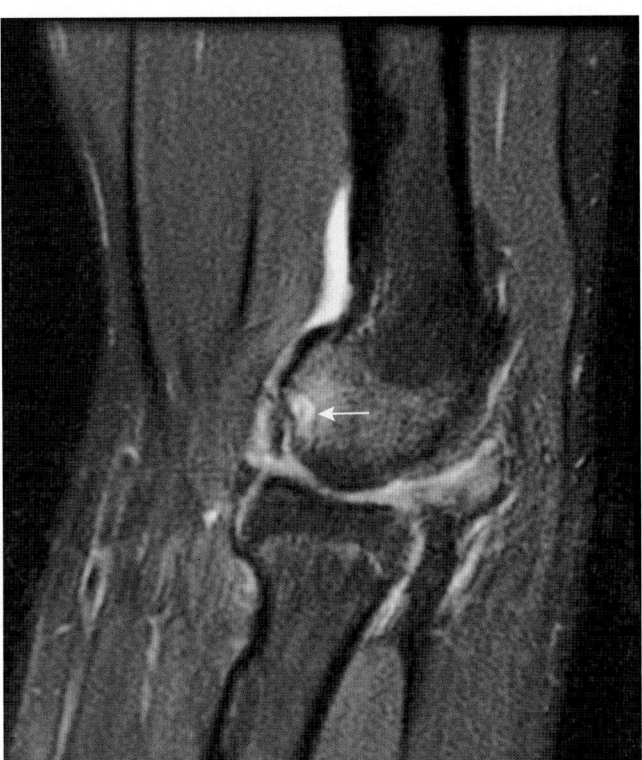
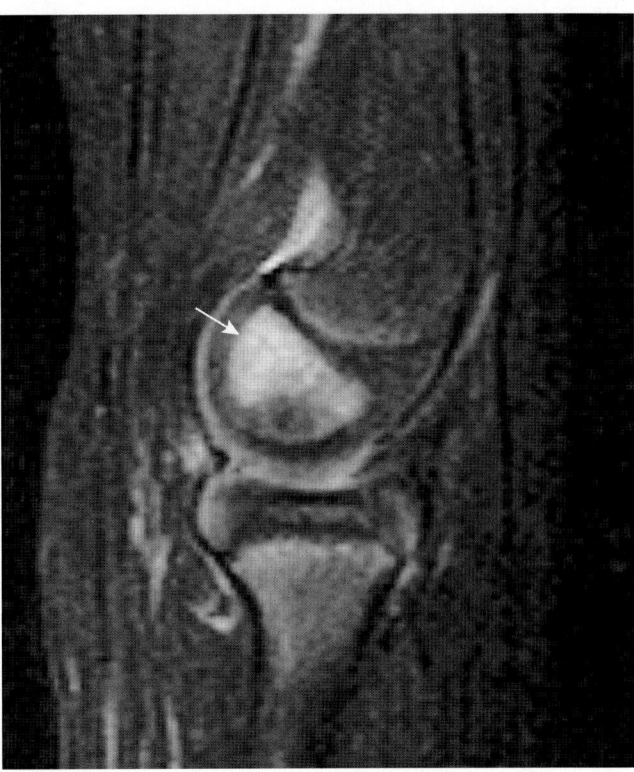

A
B

FIGURE 172-4. Osteochondritis dissecans and Panner disease of the capitellum. **A,** Sagittal fat-suppressed T2-weighted MR image of the elbow in a 16-year-old baseball catcher shows an osteochondral defect in the anterior articular surface of the capitellum associated with a focal fluid collection beneath the fragment *(arrow)*, confirming unstable OCD. **B,** In contrast, the sagittal fat-suppressed T2-weighted MR image in a 6-year-old boy with elbow pain shows high signal within the capitellar ossification center *(arrow)* and intact overlying articular and epiphyseal cartilage consistent with osteochondrosis, or Panner disease.

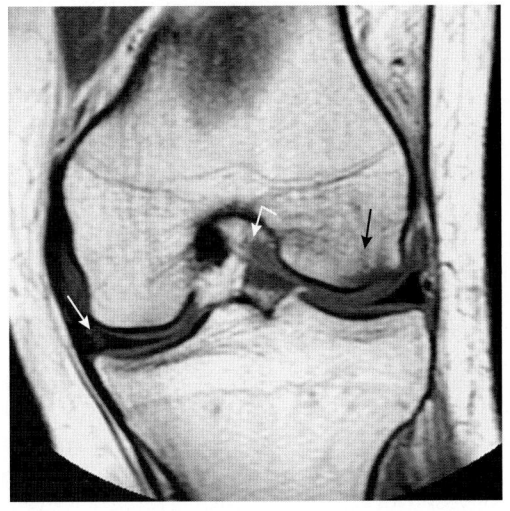
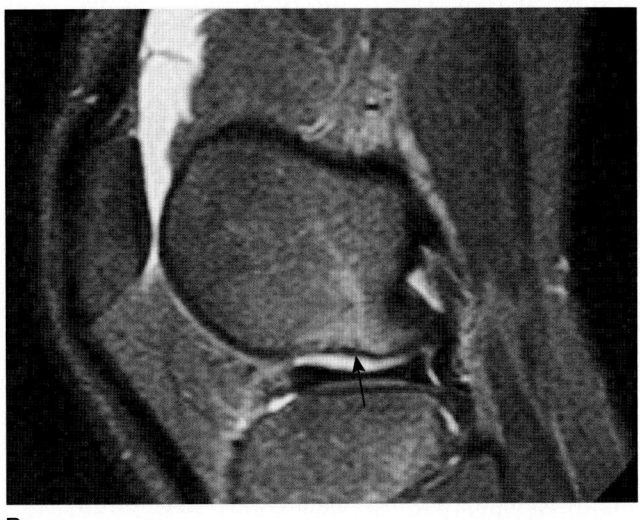

A
B

FIGURE 172-5. Acute osteochondral fracture, medial meniscal tear, and anterior cruciate ligament tear in a 17-year-old girl who sustained an injury to her left knee while skiing. Coronal T1-weighted **(A)** and sagittal inversion recovery **(B)** MR images show a focal bone contusion *(black arrow in* **A***)* in the lateral femoral condyle, with flattening and compression of the overlying articular surface *(arrow in* **B***)* related to an osteochondral fracture. High signal is also seen within the torn anterior cruciate ligament in the intercondylar notch *(bent arrow in* **A***)* and in the vertical tear at the periphery of the medial meniscus *(white arrow in* **A***)*.

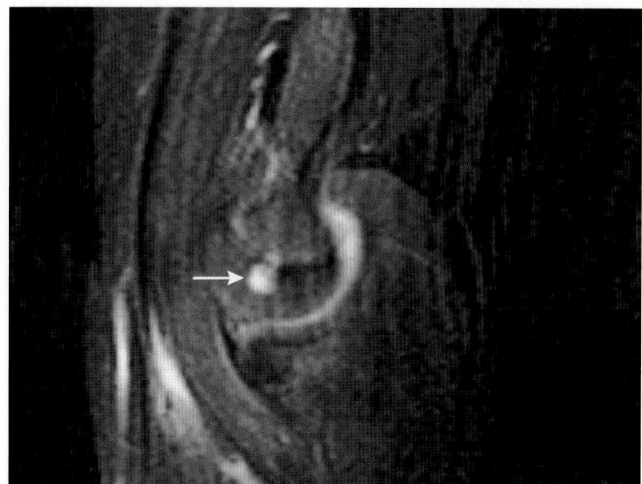

FIGURE 172-6. Normal trochlear ossification center of the distal humerus in a 6-year-old boy. Sagittal fat-suppressed T2-weighted MR image shows focal high signal within the trochlear epiphysis *(arrow)* related to impending ossification.

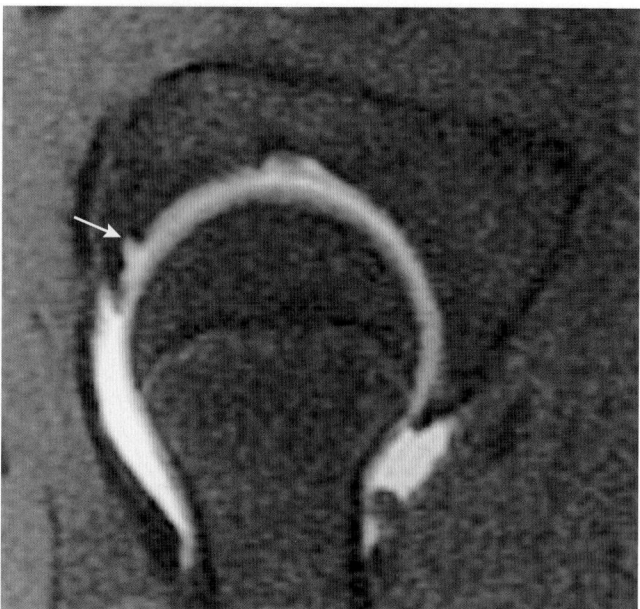

FIGURE 172-7. Acetabular labral tear in a 12-year-old ballet dancer with left hip pain. Sagittal fat-suppressed T1-weighted MR image obtained after the intra-articular injection of gadolinium demonstrates focal high signal intensity in the anterior superior labrum. A discrete labral tear as well as frayed degeneration was confirmed arthroscopically.

Stress-related changes without cortical fracture are commonly seen in young athletes, especially in the tibia ("shin splints"), femur, and bones of the feet. The exact pathogenesis of stress injury is not clear, but likely relates to the development of microfractures. Abnormal stress leads to increased osteoclastic activity. If the increased level of stress persists, the delicate balance between bone resorption and bone production is disrupted, leading to osteopenia, resorption cavities, microfracture, and edema. Periosteal and endosteal proliferation, commonly seen radiographically, may lay down bone in an attempt to buttress the weakened bone. MRI is the most sensitive technique for the early detection of these "prefracture" injuries. The MRI findings include bone marrow and periosteal edema reflected as increased signal intensity on T2-weighted and inversion recovery sequences, as well as subtler cortical hyperintensity (Fig. 172-9). Though CT is insensitive to the marrow edema associated with stress, it better demonstrates the associated cortical changes, including round or oval hypoattenuating cortical resorption cavities and low-attenuation intracortical striations. Scintigraphy is overall less sensitive than MRI but more sensitive than CT, and may demonstrate diffuse or focal increased activity at the site of stress. It is important to note that asymptomatic uptake in the lower extremities of young athletes is generally considered a normal response to stress and not of clinical significance.

A recently recognized sports-related injury in children is femoral diaphyseal periostitis due to adductor muscle strain-avulsion. The radiographic appearance of medial femoral shaft periosteal reaction may mimic more sinister diagnoses, especially Ewing sarcoma and other primary osseous neoplasms. The MR images, however, show characteristic posteromedial or anteromedial diaphyseal periosteal elevation, edema at the muscle-bone interface centered at the junction of the vastus medialis and the vastus intermedius, associated marrow edema, and absence of a soft tissue mass (Fig. 172-10).

Physeal Overuse Injuries

Physeal injuries, either acute or chronic, can substantially affect the growth mechanism and may result in lifelong disability due to subsequent malalignment or limb length discrepancy. Physeal insult may result from overuse or repetitive trauma in young athletes. Physeal dysfunction without premature transphyseal bone bridge formation occurs secondary to recurrent microtrauma leading to vascular compromise and disruption of enchondral ossification. Unossified bands or tongues of hypertrophic physeal cartilage extend into the metaphysis. Radiographically, this appears as physeal widening and irregularity. MR images in these patients show focal or bandlike physeal widening and T2 hyperintensity related to the excess unossified cartilage as well as edema. The most well-described locations of these injuries are the distal radius and olecranon in gymnasts (Fig. 172-11) and the proximal humerus in pitchers (Fig. 172-12). Recently, however, similar physeal widening has been reported in the physes of the knee in high-level child athletes involved in football, basketball, soccer, gymnastics, and tennis. Similarly, MR images in these children with knee pain show focal bands of physeal cartilage signal extending into the distal femoral, proximal tibial, and proximal fibular metaphyses (Fig. 172-13). The abnormalities are medial or lateral depending upon the sport. The clinical symptoms and imaging findings of these chronic physeal stress injuries tend to resolve in 1 to 2 months with strict rest, immobilization, or both. Continuation of athletic activity leads to persistent pain and growth disturbance with malalignment.

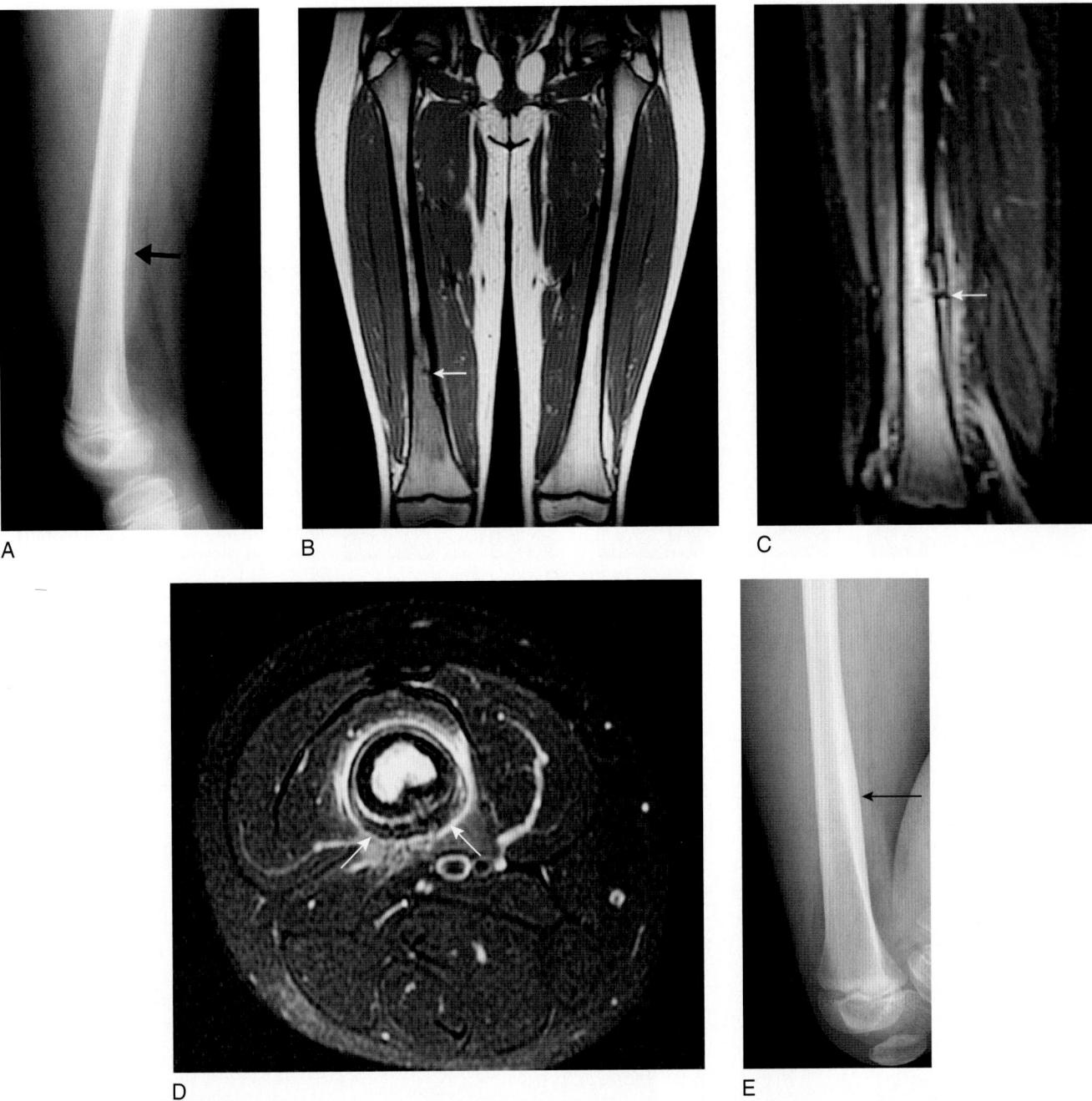

FIGURE 172-8. Stress fracture of the right femur in an 8-year-old girl who plays on a travel soccer team. **A,** Lateral radiograph of the femur shows fine, benign-appearing periosteal reaction *(arrow)* along the posterior femoral diaphysis. **B-D,** Coronal T1-weighted **(B)**, sagittal inversion recovery **(C)**, and axial fat-suppressed T2-weighted **(D)** MR images demonstrate marrow edema in the distal femoral diaphysis, posterior periosteal reaction *(arrows in D)*, and focal thickening and irregularity in the posteromedial cortex *(arrows in B and C)* corresponding to the fracture site. Note the absence of soft tissue mass or extensive surrounding soft tissue edema. **E,** Lateral radiograph of the femur obtained 2 months later shows incorporation of the periosteal reaction, now appearing as cortical thickening *(arrow)*.

AVULSION INJURIES

Avulsion injuries in children are most frequent during puberty and adolescence, when the physis is the weakest part of the musculoskeleton. In this age group, acute apophyseal avulsion fractures are more common than ligament and tendon injury. Avulsion fractures may be acute, related to sudden, forceful muscle contraction, or chronic, due to overuse and repeated insults. Most acute avulsion fractures, including the common pelvic avulsions, are discussed in greater detail in Chapter 170. Acute avulsion injuries are also common about the knee and elbow in young athletes. MRI is useful in evaluating these largely cartilaginous injuries.

Lower Extremity Avulsion Injuries

Acute patellar sleeve fracture is an avulsion of the lower pole of the patella at the patellar tendon insertion site that is being reported with increasing frequency in

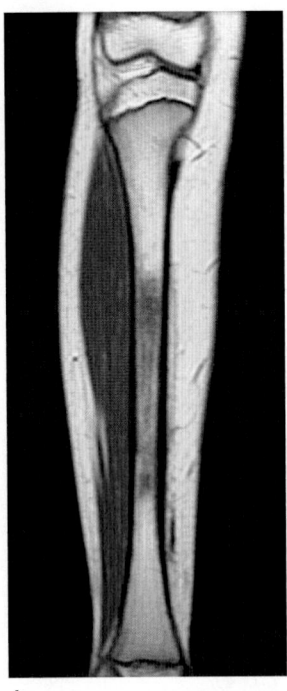

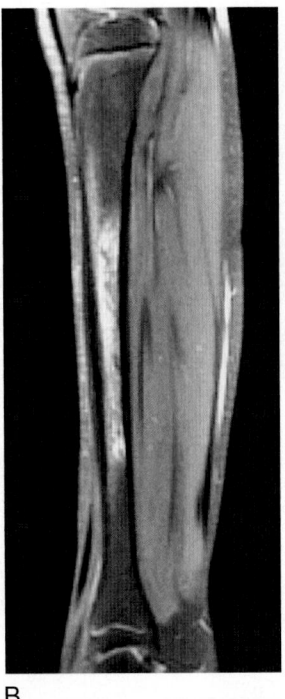

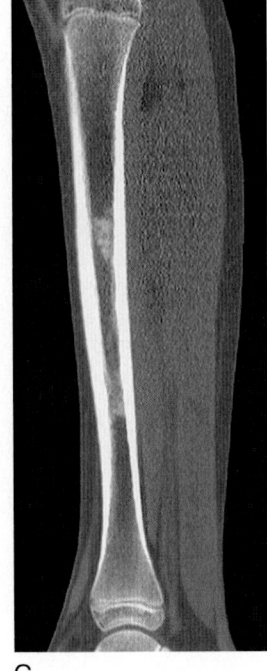

FIGURE 172-9. Stress reaction in an active 11-year-old girl with right tibial pain with activity. Radiographs (not shown) were normal. **A** and **B**, Sagittal T1-weighted **(A)** and proton density–weighted **(B)** MR images show nonspecific marrow edema within the shaft of the tibia. **C,** The corresponding sagittal CT reformation shows medullary sclerosis and anterior cortical thickening. These features are consistent with stress reaction without clear fracture. A follow-up MRI examination 3 months later (not shown) was normal.

A   B   C

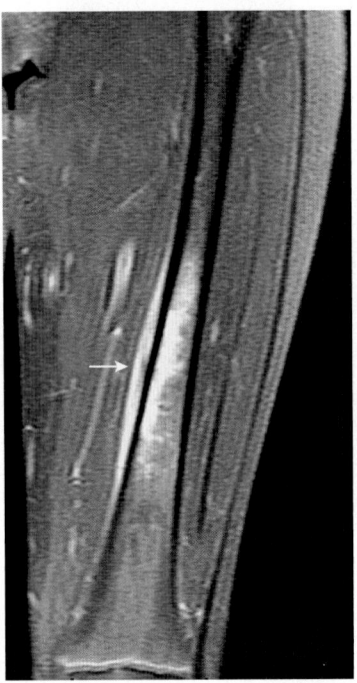

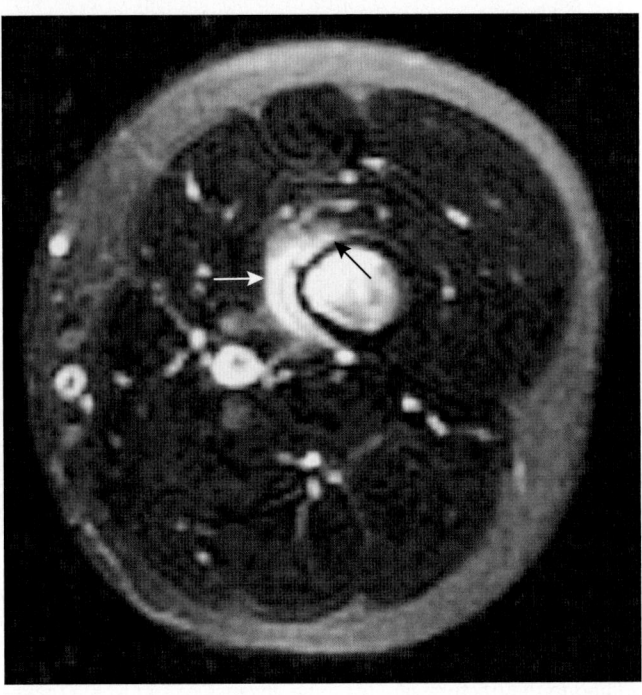

A   B

FIGURE 172-10. Adductor muscle strain secondary to overuse in a 7-year-old gymnast with left thigh pain and periostitis. Radiographs (not shown) revealed smooth periosteal reaction along the medial femur. Coronal fat-suppressed T1-weighted MR image with contrast **(A)** and axial fat-suppressed T2-weighted MR image **(B)** show medial periosteal reaction in the midfemoral diaphysis and high signal intensity edema at the interface between the bone and the inserting adductor muscles *(arrows)*. Associated marrow edema is also present asymmetrically in the medial diaphysis. There is no associated fracture line or soft tissue mass.

young athletes. With forceful quadriceps contraction against resistance, a small fragment of the patella is torn off. Lateral radiographs of the knee typically show a joint effusion, a high-riding patella, and a small avulsed lower pole fragment. The magnitude of the injury is underestimated because of the large cartilaginous component

of the patellar fracture. MR images exquisitely show the larger cartilaginous lower pole patellar fragment, the degree of distraction, and the integrity of the patellar tendon (Fig. 172-14). The displacement as seen on MR images determines the need for open surgical reduction and fixation.

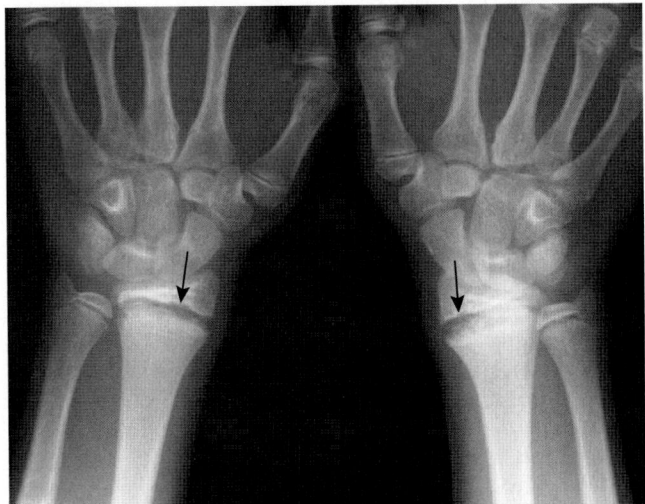

A

FIGURE 172-11. Distal radial physeal injury due to repetitive injury in an 11-year-old highly competitive gymnast who participates 15 hours per week. **A,** Frontal radiograph of the wrists demonstrates bilateral distal radial physeal widening *(arrows)*. MR imaging of the right wrist was performed because of persistent pain despite 2 months of rest. **B** and **C,** Coronal T1-weighted **(B)** and gradient recalled echo **(C)** images show distal radial physeal widening *(arrows in B)* and increased signal intensity at the physeal-metaphyseal junction *(arrows in C)* related to unossified physeal cartilage. Radiographs obtained after 2 additional months of activity restriction (not shown) showed normal distal radial physes.

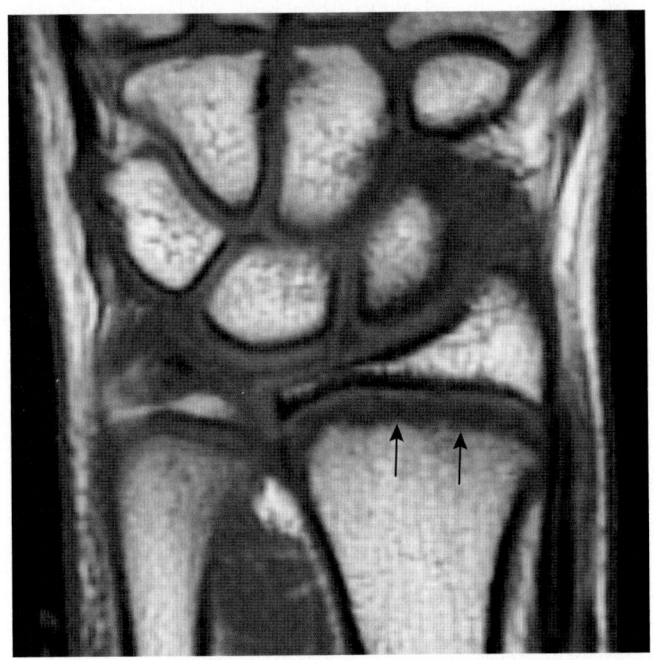

B

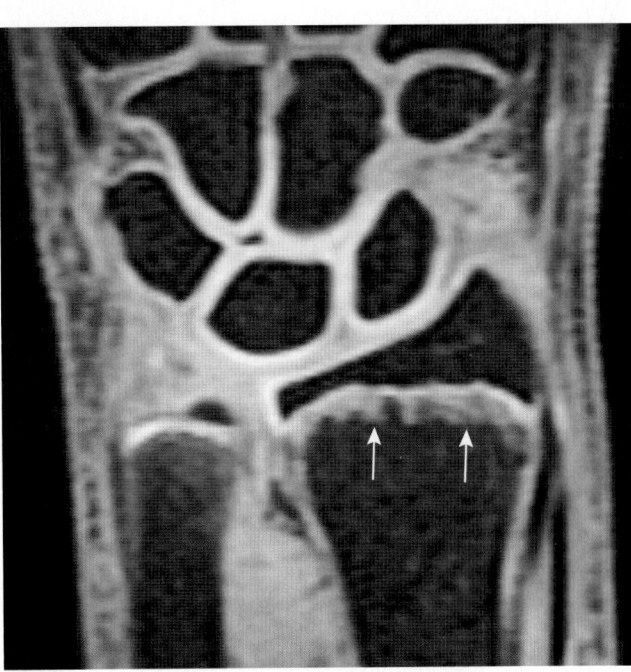

C

Acute tibial tubercle avulsion fractures typically occur in late adolescence when the proximal tibial physis is primarily fused but the anterior and inferior extent of the physis at the tubercle remains open. The fractures generally are the result of sudden hyperextension of the knee. Lateral radiographs show fragmentation and anterosuperior displacement of the tibial tubercle (Fig. 172-15). MRI may show associated distal patellar tendon injury. Chronic tibial tubercle avulsion injury, known as Osgood-Schlatter disease, is discussed later in this chapter in the section on patellar tendon injury.

Osteochondral fracture of the tibial spines due to acute anterior cruciate ligament (ACL) avulsion is also discussed later in this chapter in the section on ligament injury of the knee.

Upper Extremity Avulsion Injury

The medial epicondyle of the distal humerus is the origin of the ulnar collateral ligament. In children, excessive valgus stress on the elbow results in medial epicondylar avulsion rather than ligament tear as seen in adults. The anterior band of the ulnar collateral ligament is the prime medial stabilizer of the elbow. It arises from the inferior surface of the medial epicondyle and inserts into the medial portion of the ulnar coronoid process. Prior to complete apophyseal ossification and fusion, the ulnar collateral ligament arises from the inferior cartilaginous portion of the apophysis. On T2-weighted MR images, there is normally an area of high signal intensity at the junction of the ligament and the cartilaginous apophysis that disappears with skeletal maturity. This high signal focus should not be misinterpreted as a tear.

Avulsion injury of the medial epicondyle may be acute or chronic. Acute medial epicondylar avulsion fracture is presented in Chapter 170 in the context of other elbow fractures. Chronic medial epicondylar avulsive injury, or medial epicondylitis, in children is most frequently encountered in baseball pitchers. *Little leaguer's elbow* is a term used to describe medial elbow pathology in preadolescent and adolescent pitchers who place the elbow in extreme valgus position during the acceleration phase of throwing, placing excessive traction on the medial elbow structures. Similar pathology occurs in fielders and catchers in intensely competitive leagues as well. Several studies have shown catchers to have an even higher incidence than pitchers, perhaps due to the increased stress on the medial elbow when throwing from a squatting position. Ulnar collateral ligament injuries are most commonly diagnosed in teenage baseball pitchers and other throwing athletes (Fig. 172-16). Radiographs and MR images show irregularity, fragmentation, and hypertrophy of the medial epicondyle and occasionally complete apophyseal separation (Fig. 172-17).

Chronic avulsive stress injuries of the distal clavicle can be seen in older children and adolescents usually related to weight lifting. The coracoacromial ligaments remain intact, but there can be significant instability of the acromioclavicular joint. Radiographs show heterotopic bone formation and periosteal reaction at the distal end of the clavicle (Fig. 172-18). The findings are often bilateral. Acromioclavicular joint dislocations are rare in children.

SOFT TISSUE INJURY

Muscle Contusion and Myotendinous Strain

Injuries to muscles and the myotendinous unit deserve attention because of their increasing incidence in children, particularly adolescent athletes, and because

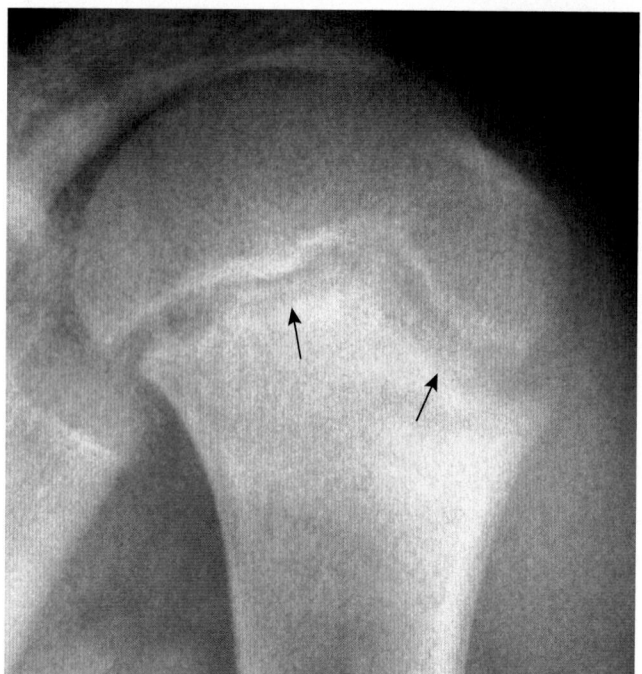

FIGURE 172-12. Left shoulder physeal stress injury in a 12-year-old left-handed pitcher who developed pain with throwing. Frontal radiograph of the shoulder obtained after approximately 4 months of symptoms shows proximal humeral physeal widening and irregularity *(arrows)*, so-called little leaguers' shoulder.

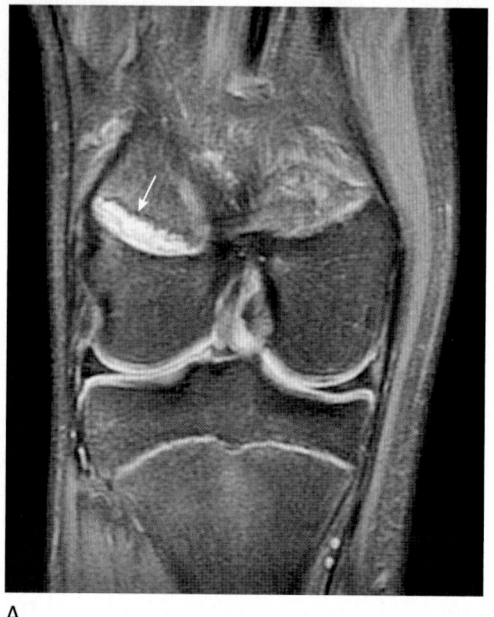
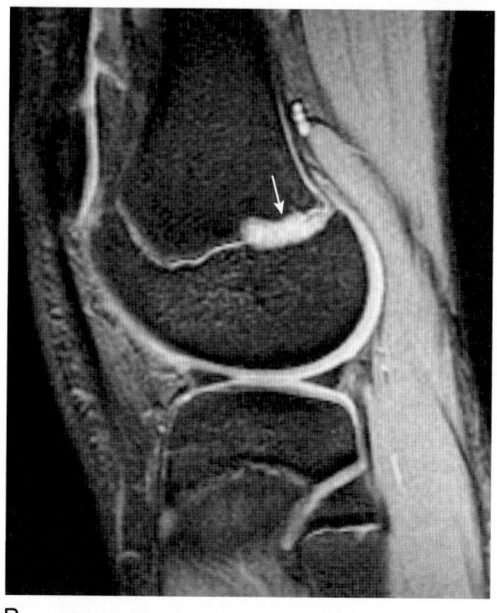

A   B

FIGURE 172-13. Distal femoral physeal overuse injury in a 14½-year-old high-level soccer player with knee pain. Coronal fat-suppressed proton density–weighted **(A)** and sagittal gradient recalled echo **(B)** MR images of the knee demonstrate bandlike high signal intensity widening *(arrows)* of the medial distal femoral physis due to extension of unossified hypertrophic physeal chondrocytes into the metaphysis.

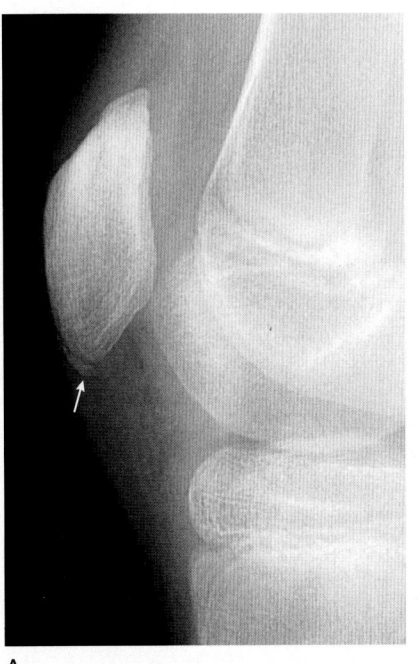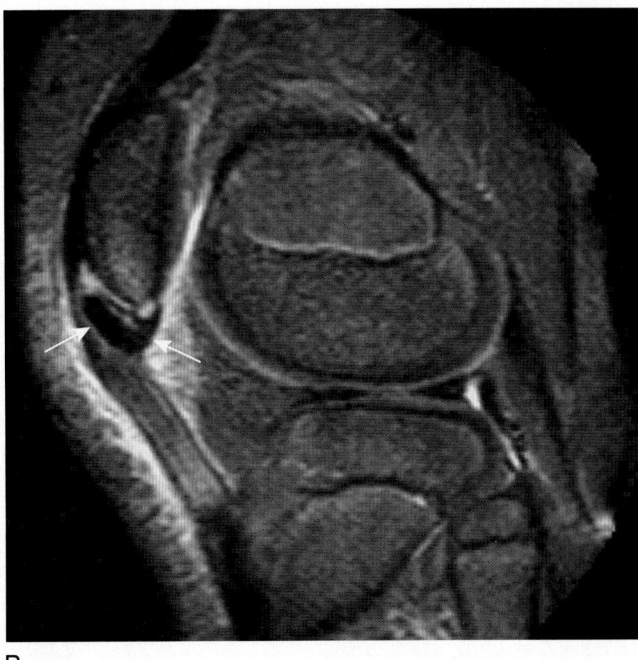

A   B

FIGURE 172-14. Patellar sleeve fracture. **A,** Lateral radiograph of the knee in an 11-year-old boy who sustained an acute hyperextension injury while playing basketball shows soft tissue swelling inferior to the patella and in the Hoffa fat pad as well as a small avulsed bony fragment minimally displaced from the inferior pole of the patella *(arrow)*. **B,** Sagittal inversion recovery MR image in another patient—a 10-year-old soccer player—shows the largely cartilaginous fracture fragment *(arrows)*, surrounding soft tissue edema, and high signal intensity edema within the proximal patellar tendon. The minimal displacement of the fracture fragments allowed both patients to be treated successfully with immobilization and no surgical fixation.

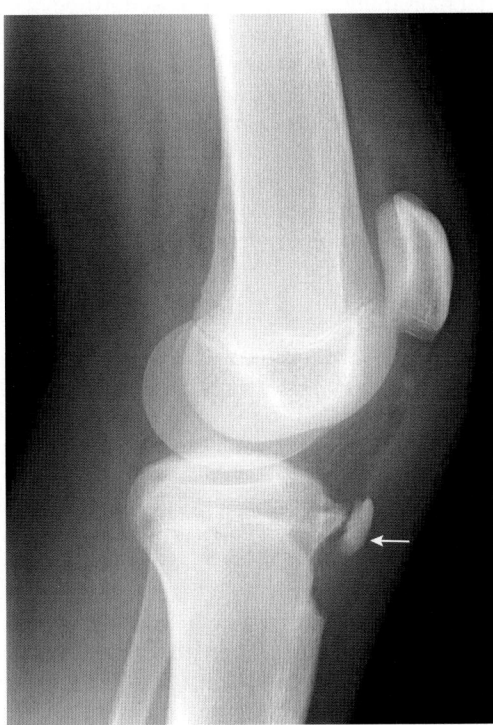

FIGURE 172-15. Tibial tubercle avulsion fracture in a 16-year-old high jumper who experienced sudden pain upon planting his left foot while hyperextending for a jump. Lateral radiograph of the left knee shows superior and anterior displacement of the avulsed tibial tubercle fracture fragment *(arrow)*, elevation of the patella, and fused proximal tibial physis. As in this case, these fractures generally require internal fixation to restore patellar tendon function.

their appearances can be misinterpreted if the radiologist is unaware of the typical imaging characteristics. The three categories of acute musculotendinous injury are muscle contusion, myotendinous strain, and tendon avulsion.

Contusions typically occur deep in the muscle belly and are the result of direct blunt trauma. MRI demonstrates intramuscular edema, seen as feathery high signal on STIR and T2-weighted images, and hemorrhage, best seen on T1-weighted images (Fig. 172-19).

Myotendinous strains occur more superficially at the myotendinous junction and are caused by a single traumatic event associated with excessive muscle stretch. These injuries are further subdivided into minor fiber disruption (first degree), partial tear (second degree), and complete tendon rupture (third degree) (Fig. 172-20). MR images in first-degree strain reveal hemorrhage and feathery high signal edema at the myotendinous junction. Second-degree partial tears demonstrate hemorrhage at the myotendinous junction and increased signal within the substance of the tendon without retraction. Complete myotendinous rupture can have a masslike quality on physical examination. MRI demonstrates the edema, hemorrhage, and retracted tendon.

Finally, the most severe of the myotendinous injuries is acute avulsion of the tendon due to forceful, eccentric muscle contraction. MR images show periosteal stripping and hematoma at the tendon insertion site. Muscles that are particularly prone to strain injuries are those that are superficial, cross two joints, have a predominance of type II fibers, and/or exhibit eccentric contraction. Examples

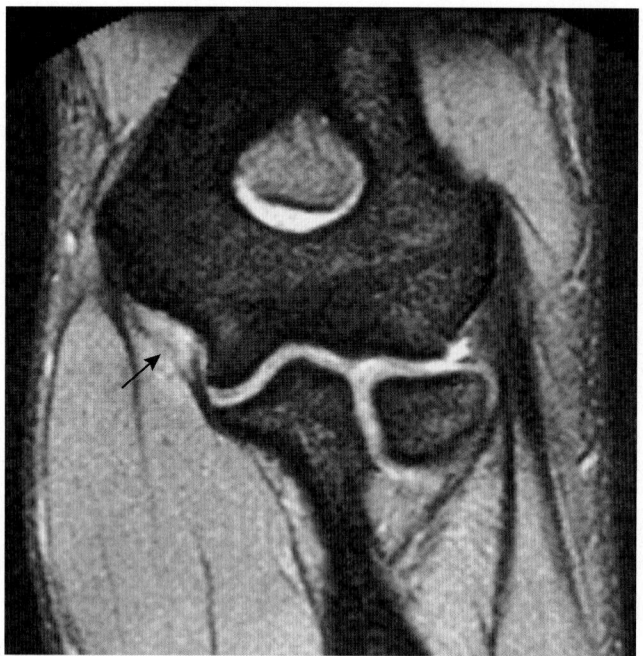 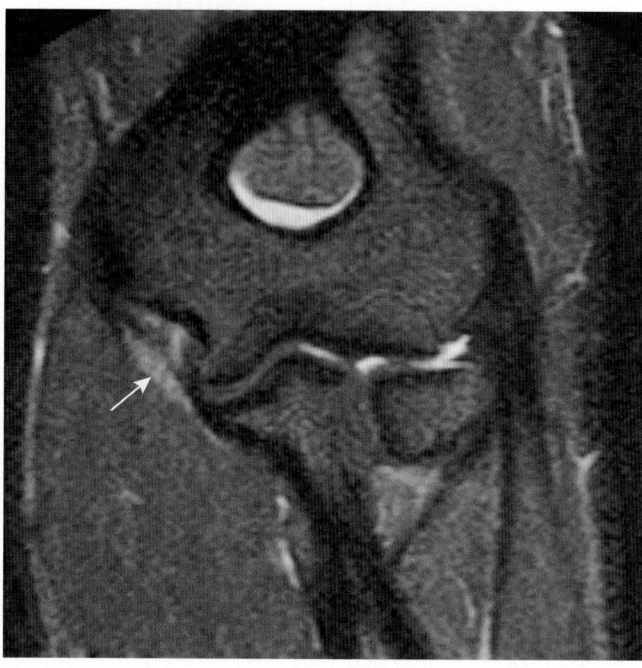

A

B

FIGURE 172-16. Chronic ulnar collateral ligament tear. This 18-year-old left-handed high school baseball pitcher complained of 2 months of left elbow pain and popping during college recruiting season. Coronal gradient recalled echo **(A)** and inversion recovery **(B)** MR images reveal complete disruption of the ulnar collateral ligament *(arrows)*, with mild associated high signal intensity soft tissue edema seen on the inversion recovery image.

of such muscles include the biceps brachii, rectus femoris, sartorius, semimembranosus, and gastrocnemius.

Myotendinous Injury—MRI Appearance

- **Contusion—hemorrhage, edema in muscle belly**
- **Strain**
  - **First degree—hemorrhage, edema at myotendinous junction**
  - **Second degree—hemorrhage at myotendinous junction, high signal within tendon**
  - **Third degree—hemorrhage, edema, and tendon retraction**
- **Tendon avulsion—hematoma and stripped periosteum at tendon insertion site**

Myositis Ossificans

Myositis ossificans is a non-neoplastic condition of heterotopic bone formation within a single muscle or muscle group. The condition is known by several other names, including myositis ossificans traumatica, myositis ossificans circumscripta, and ossifying hematoma. Most cases are post-traumatic due to a single direct insult or repeated minor trauma, although no history of trauma is present in about one third of cases. Myositis ossificans is most common in adolescents and young adults. Athletes involved in contact sports such as football, hockey, and soccer are most vulnerable. The anterior compartments of the thigh and arm are commonly involved, specifically

the quadriceps and brachialis muscles. Patients complain of pain, a palpable mass, and decreased range of motion. Myositis ossificans has a variable appearance on imaging related to a predictable evolution of the lesion from the time of injury, and unlike myotendinous strains, myositis ossificans can be confused with other lesions, including neoplasm. Unfortunately, in the event of percutaneous biopsy, the lesion can be misinterpreted histologically as well. Careful attention to the specific imaging characteristics of myositis ossificans can generally avoid misinterpretation of this benign condition as a more ominous lesion.

In the early phase, 7 to 14 days after injury, radiographs show a nonspecific soft tissue mass that may be associated with faint periosteal reaction in the adjacent bone (Fig. 172-21). MRI may be performed at this point for evaluation of the soft tissue mass if myositis ossificans is not suspected. The MR images will show extensive intramuscular edema surrounding a more focal heterogeneous mass with central T2 hyperintensity and perhaps a subtle low signal intensity rim. The appearance can be deceptively aggressive (Fig. 172-22). CT in the first 2 weeks may only show a nonspecific low-attenuation mass without calcification. Histologically, the center of the lesion corresponds to proliferating fibroblasts with hemorrhage, while osteoblasts beginning to form mature bone are present at the periphery. The differential diagnosis for the imaging features of the lesion at this early stage include hematoma, abscess, myonecrosis, and (less likely) soft tissue sarcoma because of the extensive surrounding inflammatory change.

In the subacute phase of the lesion, 3 to 4 weeks post-injury, radiographs show flocculent calcification in the

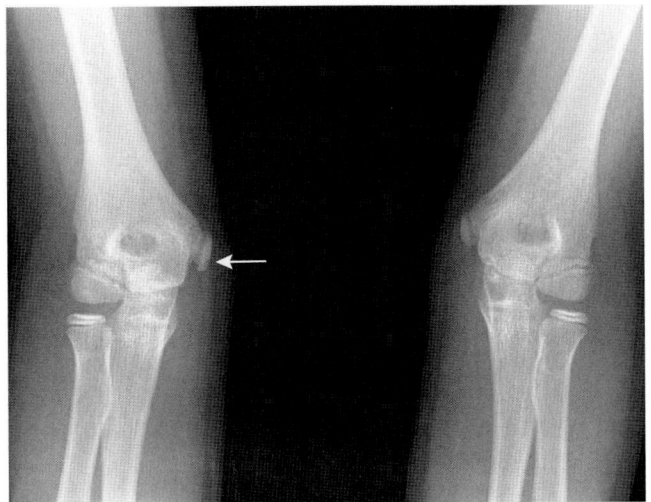

A

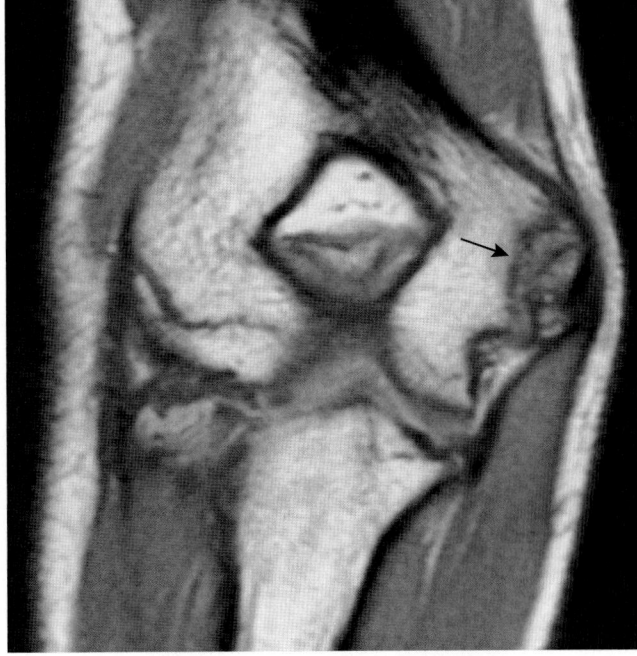

B

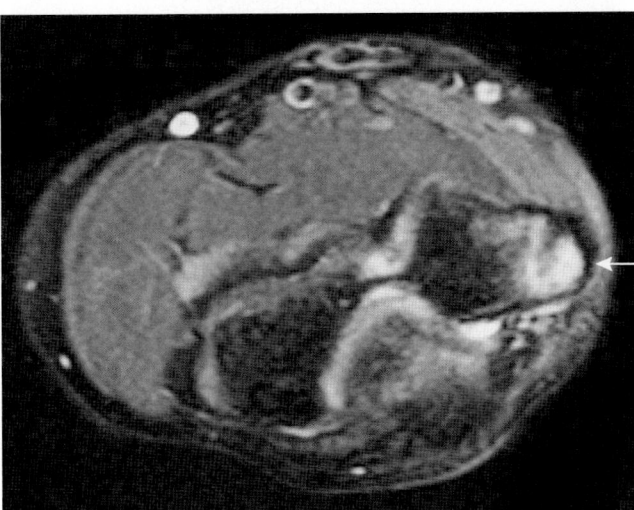

C

FIGURE 172-17. Medial epicondylitis (little leaguer's elbow) in a 14-year-old baseball pitcher with medial right elbow pain. **A,** Frontal radiographs of both elbows show an enlarged, fragmented right medial epicondyle *(arrow)* of the right elbow with overlying soft tissue swelling. The left elbow, for comparison, is normal. **B** and **C,** Coronal proton density–weighted **(B)** and axial fat-suppressed T2-weighted **(C)** MR images show widening of the medial epicondylar physis *(arrow* in **B)** and high signal intensity medial epicondylar apophyseal marrow edema *(arrow* in **C)** and overlying soft tissue edema.

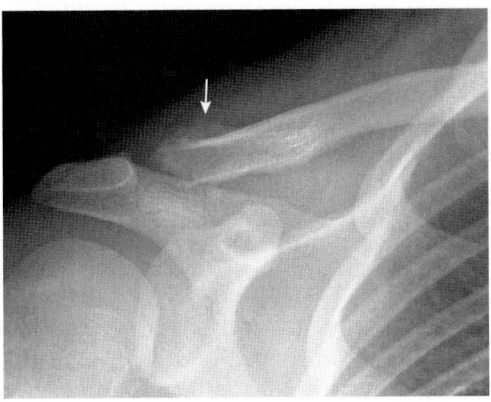

A

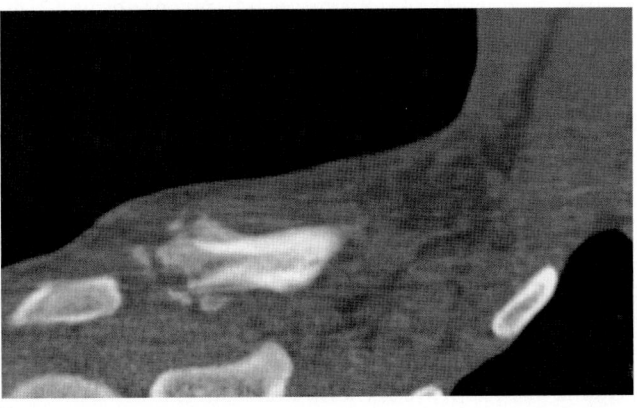

B

FIGURE 172-18. Chronic distal clavicular avulsion injury in a 14-year-old hockey player. Frontal radiograph **(A)** and coronal reformatted CT **(B)** of the right clavicle reveal fragmentation and osteolysis of the distal right clavicle with heterotopic callus formation *(arrow* in **A).** This is a chronic overuse injury related to stress at the deltoid muscle origin.

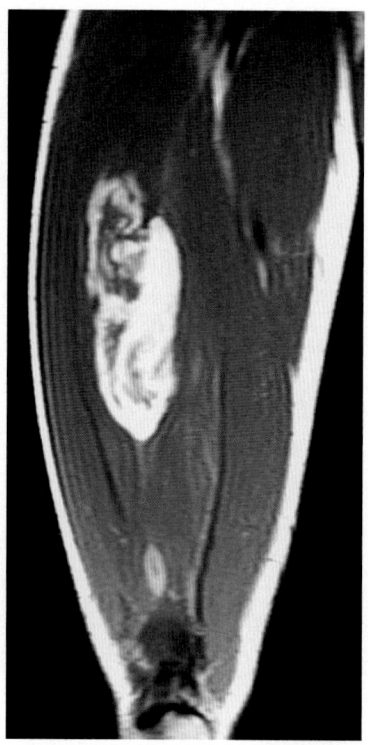

FIGURE 172-19. Vastus intermedius muscle contusion. This 16-year-old boy experienced blunt trauma to the right thigh during a football game. Coronal T1-weighted MR image obtained 1 week after the injury shows a large hematoma within the belly of the vastus intermedius muscle, distant from the myotendinous junction. The hematoma is predominately bright on T1-weighted images but does contain areas of low signal intensity likely related to a combination of hemosiderin and edema.

mass with maximum opacity at the periphery and relative radiolucency centrally. At this point, CT shows the lucent center and the rim of calcification with a cleavage plain separating it from the adjacent cortical bone. These features are diagnostic of myositis ossificans and differentiate the lesion from surface osteosarcoma. MRI at this point is often confusing, demonstrating a heterogeneous soft tissue mass with peripheral low signal and residual surrounding soft tissue edema, as well as periosteal high signal and even edema within the adjacent bone marrow.

Finally, in the late phase of the lesion, radiographs and CT will show a lacy pattern of new bone with a well-defined peripheral cortex separate from the adjacent bone. By 6 months, the lesion has reached maturity as a densely ossified mass and usually begins to shrink in size.

Myositis Ossificans—Imaging Features
- **Early (1–2 weeks): faint periosteal reaction, soft tissue mass, extensive intramuscular edema**
- **Subacute (3–4 weeks): mass with flocculent calcification densest at periphery, lucent centrally; cleavage plain between mass and adjacent bone**
- **Late (up to 6 months): lacy new bone with well-defined peripheral cortex, diminishing size**

Treatment of myositis ossificans involves rest and analgesia with nonsteroidal anti-inflammatory agents. Partial or total involution of the lesion over time is common. Excision may rarely be necessary for large lesions that limit function. Surgical excision should be delayed until the lesion has completely matured (at least 6 months) to limit the resection of healthy muscle tissue.

INJURY TO THE KNEE

Special attention is given to the knee, as it is the most frequently injured joint in athletic children seeking medical attention. Unique features of the pediatric knee predispose to certain injury patterns and associated imaging features that are different from those seen in adults.

Meniscal Injury

The menisci develop their characteristic shape prenatally. The menisci grow in size commensurate with growth of the child but should always have a semilunar configuration. Throughout postnatal life, the major change in the meniscus is progressive decrease in vascularity extending from the center to the periphery. In early childhood, the menisci are highly vascular. Coronal and sagittal MR images of the knee show high signal intensity horizontal bands throughout the menisci (Fig. 172-23). By adolescence, this normal vascular band is seen in only the peripheral one third of the meniscus. This signal related to nutrient vessels does not extend to the articular surface of the meniscus and should not be confused with a tear.

Discoid menisci, much more commonly lateral than medial, are the most common cause of knee pain in young children regardless of athletic activity or trauma. A discoid meniscus is abnormally thick with lack of the normal central tapering. As in adults, MR images of discoid meniscus in children show a diffusely thick meniscus with a slab configuration. Coronal images show the meniscus to encompass more than one half of the surface area of the tibiofemoral joint on all sections. Sagittal images reveal absence of the normal "bow tie" morphology with persistence of the body of the meniscus on greater than two consecutive 3- or 4-mm contiguous sections. A band of increased intrasubstance high signal is generally seen due to chronic trauma and degeneration (Fig. 172-24; also see Fig. 172-2). Discoid menisci are also prone to discrete linear tears.

Meniscal tears in older children are frequently sports related, commonly associated with basketball, soccer, and football. The medial meniscus is more frequently torn than the lateral meniscus, though not with as great a predominance as in adults. Meniscal tears in children are usually vertical (Fig. 172-25) and easily differentiated from the normal horizontal band of increased signal related to nutrient vessels. The complex horizontal tears seen in adults are much less common in children. Vertically oriented bucket-handle tears are frequently encountered in competitive athletes.

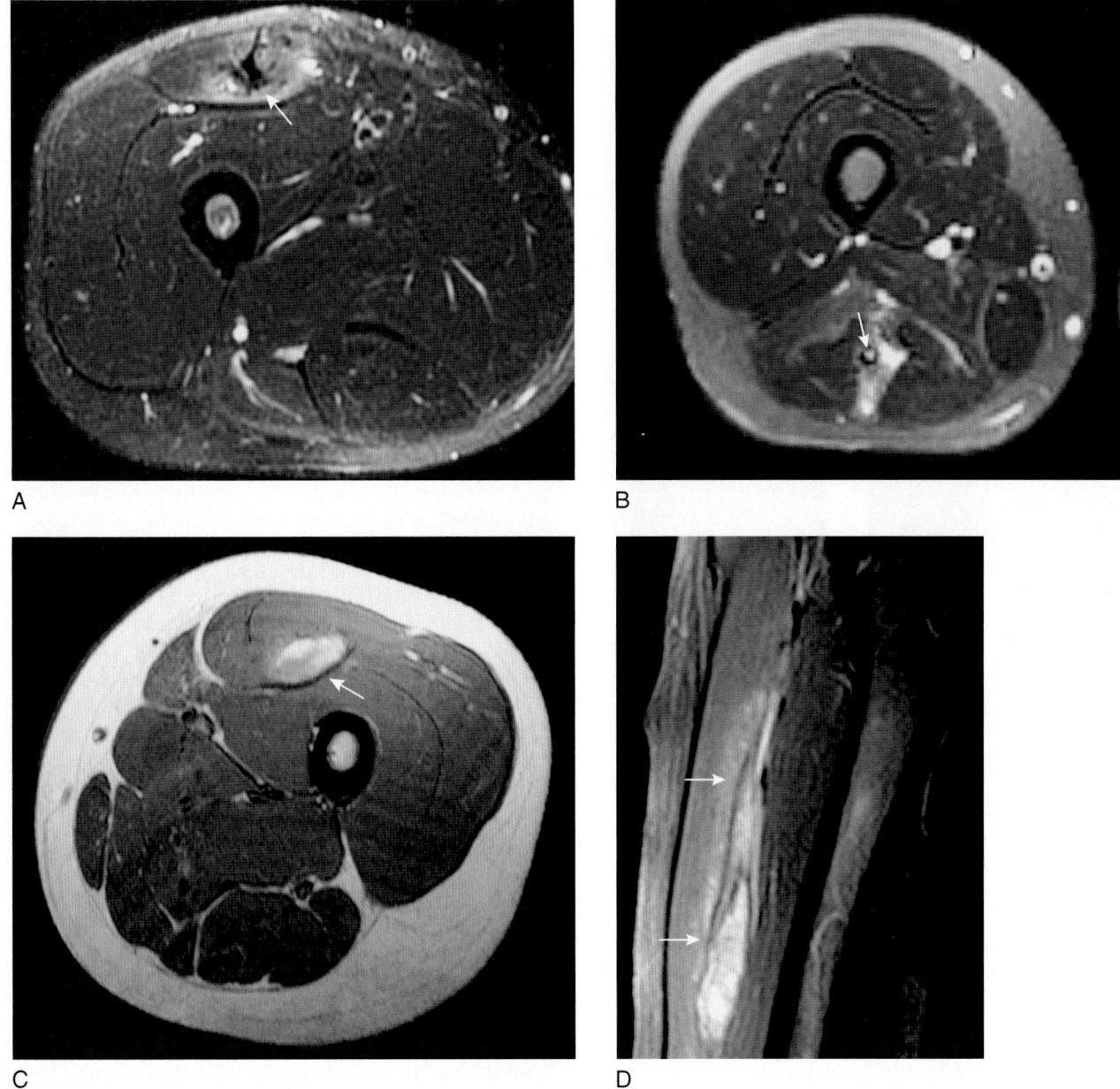

FIGURE 172-20. Myotendinous strain. **A,** Axial fat-suppressed T2-weighted MR image in a 16-year-old basketball player with right thigh pain shows feathery high signal intensity at the rectus femoris–myotendinous junction *(arrow)* but normal signal within the tendon itself, consistent with a first-degree strain. **B,** Axial fat-suppressed T2-weighted MR image in a different 14-year-old basketball player with 3 months of right posterior thigh pain and swelling shows abnormal high signal intensity edema and low signal intensity hemosiderin in the semitendinosus-myotendinous junction with intrasubstance high signal in the tendon itself *(arrow).* These findings confirm a second-degree strain with partial tendon tear. **C** and **D,** A more extensive second-degree strain with partial tendon tear is seen in a third child who is a high-level soccer player with anterior thigh pain. Axial T1-weighted **(C)** and sagittal inversion recovery **(D)** MR images show hemorrhage within the myotendinous junction of the rectus femoris *(arrow* in **C)** as well as edema and enlargement throughout the length of the tendon *(arrows* in **D).**

Ligament Injury

Generally, injury to the ligaments of the knee in preadolescent children is uncommon. The overall ligamentous strength in contrast to the relatively weak physis and bone predisposes to physeal and epiphyseal avulsion fractures as opposed to ligament tears. Generalized ligamentous laxity in young children is also protective. Osteochondral fracture of the tibial spines due to ACL avulsion occurs with forces that would result in ACL tear in the adolescent or adult. The incompletely ossified

tibial spine is weaker than the ACL and its attachments, and therefore failure occurs in the subchondral bone. Radiographically, a small bony fragment is usually seen within the intercondylar notch. MR images show the fracture path as well as the integrity of the ACL (Fig. 172-26). As with ACL tears in adults, MR images of children with tibial spine avulsion injuries may show associated collateral ligament injuries.

Recent reports, however, have shown an increase in ACL injuries in children. Young athletes participating in high-level, cutting sports such as football, basketball, and

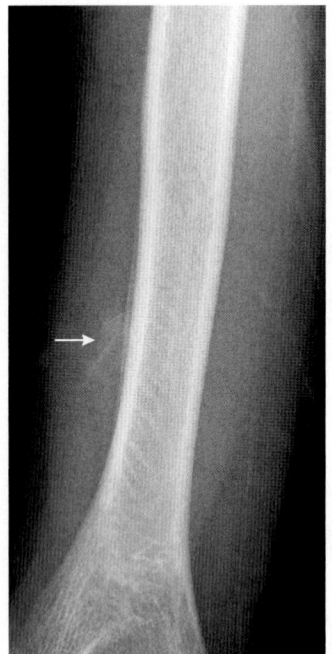
A

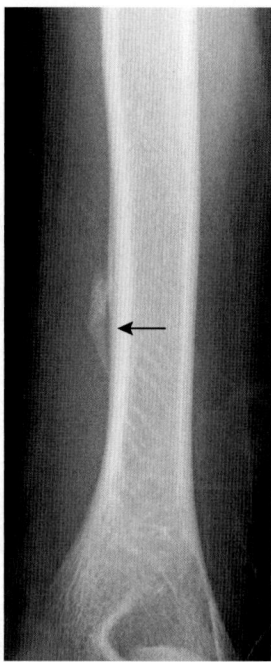
B

FIGURE 172-21. Myositis ossificans in a 12-year-old football player and weight lifter with right upper arm pain and swelling. **A,** Frontal radiograph shows smooth periosteal reaction along the lateral surface of the distal humeral shaft as well as faint, feathery calcification in the adjacent soft tissues *(arrow)*. **B,** Follow-up frontal radiograph obtained 2 months later reveals progressive ossification in the soft tissues that corresponds to the brachialis muscle. The density is highest at the periphery of the lesion. There is a clear cleavage plane *(arrow)* between the calcified soft tissue mass and the underlying humeral cortex.

soccer are at particularly high risk. Partial ACL tears and ACL avulsion with tibial spine fracture are more commonly encountered in skeletally immature boys. With skeletal maturity, complete ACL tears predominate and are more common in girls, as is seen in the adult population. Also as in adults, ACL injuries in skeletally mature children are often associated with collateral ligament tears, meniscal tears, and bone contusions. The predisposition to ACL injury in adolescent girls and women is probably multifactorial and thought to relate to a relative valgus alignment of the knee, the intercondylar notch morphology, hormonal influences, and joint laxity, as well as training techniques (Fig. 172-27). ACL tears, previously treated conservatively in children, are now more often surgically repaired, especially in female athletes. Surgical repair of the ACL in children is analogous to that in adults, except in younger children in whom special surgical techniques may be employed to avoid transgression of the distal femoral growth plate.

Collateral ligament injuries are less common in children than in adults. The deep medial and lateral collateral ligament attachments are to the distal femoral and proximal tibial epiphyses. Valgus or varus stress that would result in medial or lateral collateral ligament tear in the adult much more commonly leads to physeal fracture in skeletally immature children.

Patellar Tendon Injury

The patella is a large sesamoid bone that lies within the tendon of the quadriceps femoris muscle. It is completely cartilaginous at birth, with ossification becoming radiographically apparent at about 3 to 4 years of age in girls and 5 to 6 years of age in boys. The developing patellar ossification center often appears irregular and fragmented. Multiple ossification centers may develop normally, especially superolaterally, and should not be confused with fracture or osteochondritis.

The patellar tendon, its osseous attachments, and the adjacent soft tissues are affected by a number of different traumatic conditions that have confusing terminology and overlap. "Jumper's knee" is a term used to describe patellar tendon pathology, also called patellar tendonitis, tendinosis, and tendonopathy, that occurs in skeletally mature athletes participating in sports that require repetitive quadriceps contraction such as running, jumping, and kicking. Pathologically, involved tendons reveal microtears with chronic inflammatory changes and regeneration. The patellar tendon, with its large size and superficial location, is ideally suited for sonographic evaluation. Longitudinal and transverse images obtained with a high-frequency linear array transducer show thickening of the proximal patellar tendon, a hypoechoic area at the posterior aspect of the proximal patellar insertion, and dystrophic calcification within the tendon and inferior pole of the patella. Similarly, MRI shows high T2-weighted signal intensity edema and enlargement of the proximal tendon (Fig. 172-28). The posterior tendon fibers are predominately involved because they attach directly to the patella as opposed to the anterior fibers, which are extensions of the quadriceps tendon.

OSGOOD-SCHLATTER DISEASE

The Osgood-Schlatter lesion is a common disorder characterized by pain and swelling at the tibial tuberosity. It is most often seen in athletic boys between 11 and 15 years of age and is bilateral in 25% to 50% of cases. The condition is an overuse injury related to chronic trauma to the distal patellar tendon at its insertion into the tibial tuberosity. This causes patellar tendon microtears, hemorrhage, and small cartilaginous avulsions from the tuberosity. Osgood-Schlatter disease is a clinical diagnosis, and imaging is not necessary for the diagnosis. Radiographs, however, are often performed to exclude other diagnoses. The radiographic features of this entity are almost exclusively soft tissue related, including attenuation or loss of the infrapatellar fat pad, obliteration of the subcutaneous fat and swelling anterior to the tibial tuberosity, and thickening of the distal aspect of the patellar tendon (Fig. 172-29). Radiographic bony changes in Osgood-Schlatter disease are infrequent and should not be confused with normal multiplicity and irregularity of the tibial tubercle ossification center. Ultrasound and MRI, also unnecessary for the diagnosis, nicely demonstrate the soft tissue findings. Sagittal T2-weighted MR images can show fluid within the deep and superficial infrapatellar bursae, as well as thickening and high signal within the distal patellar tendon at the

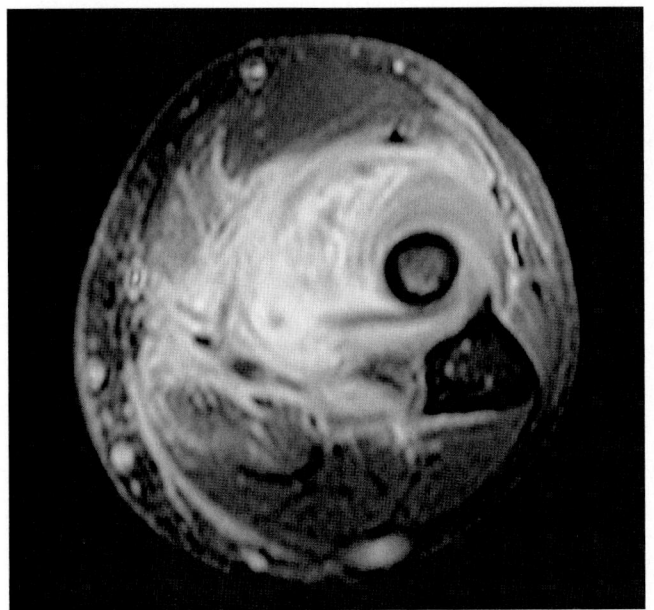

A

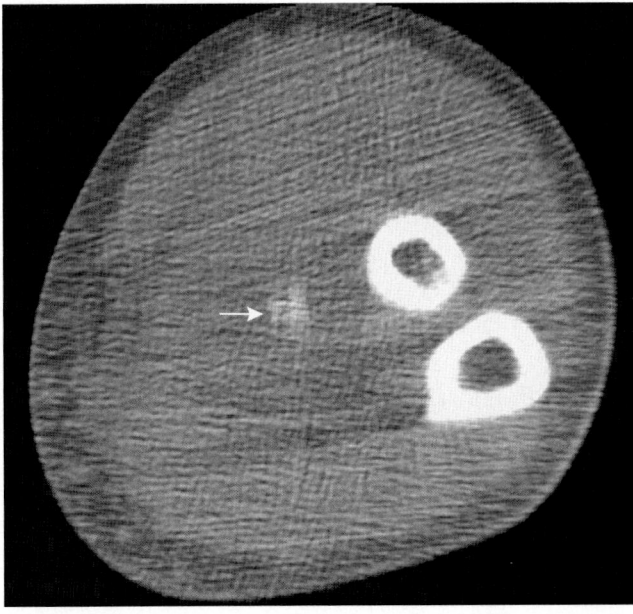

B

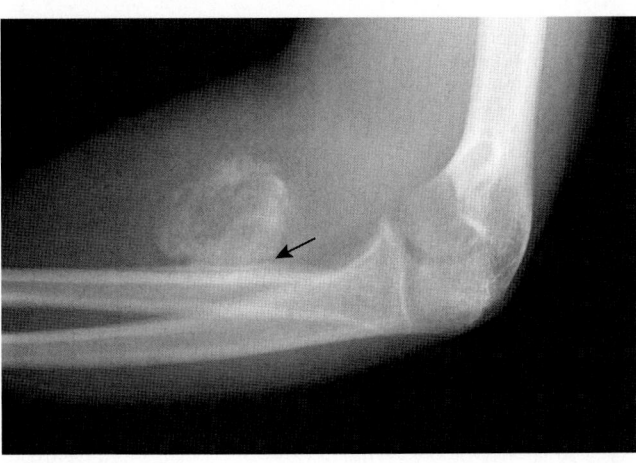

C

FIGURE 172-22. Myositis ossificans. This 12-year-old girl who plays on two travel basketball teams developed a painful swelling of her left forearm just below the elbow. **A,** An axial fat-suppressed T2-weighted MR image obtained after 4 weeks of symptoms demonstrates extensive, feathery high signal intensity edema within the pronator muscles and surrounding soft tissues. There is very little bone marrow edema in the adjacent radius. **B,** An axial CT image reveals faint soft tissue calcification anteriorly *(arrow)* and associated periosteal reaction in the radius. **C,** A lateral radiograph of the forearm obtained 3 weeks later shows evolution of the calcification into an ossifying mass that is most dense at the periphery, is lucent centrally, and has a cleavage plain with the underlying bone *(arrow).*

tibial tubercle (Fig. 172-30). Marrow edema may be seen within the tubercle itself and within the anterior tibial metaphysis. Rarely, cartilaginous ossicles surrounded by soft tissue edema are identified.

SINDING-LARSEN-JOHANSSON DISEASE

Sinding-Larsen-Johansson disease consists of pain and soft tissue swelling at the inferior pole of the patella. It can be thought of as the inferior patellar equivalent of Osgood-Schlatter disease and is related to recurrent traction forces at the superior insertion of the patellar tendon on the lower pole of the patella. Sinding-Larsen-Johansson disease is also more common in athletic boys and occurs in a similar age group, adolescents 10 to 14 years old. Radiographs reveal enlargement of the proximal patellar tendon as well as irregularity and fragmentation of the inferior pole of the patella. Ultrasound and MRI more clearly demonstrate the soft tissue findings (Fig. 172-31). Similar changes can occur, though much less frequently, at the superior pole of the patella and the quadriceps tendon insertion. Sinding-Larsen-Johansson disease is indolent and chronic, in

contrast to acute trauma at the inferior pole of the patella, which may result in a patellar sleeve fracture as discussed previously.

Chronic Patellar Tendon Injuries—Imaging Features

- **Jumper's knee: skeletally mature athletes; thickened proximal tendon at patellar insertion with increased echogenicity (ultrasound) and signal intensity (MRI).**

- **Osgood-Schlatter disease: boys ages 11 to 15 years; edema involving the distal patellar tendon, Hoffa fat pad, and tibial tubercle. Late findings include tibial tubercle fragmentation and heterotopic bone production.**

- **Sinding-Larsen-Johansson disease: adolescents ages 10 to 14 years; edema and enlargement of the proximal patellar tendon. Late findings include fragmentation of the inferior pole of the patella.**

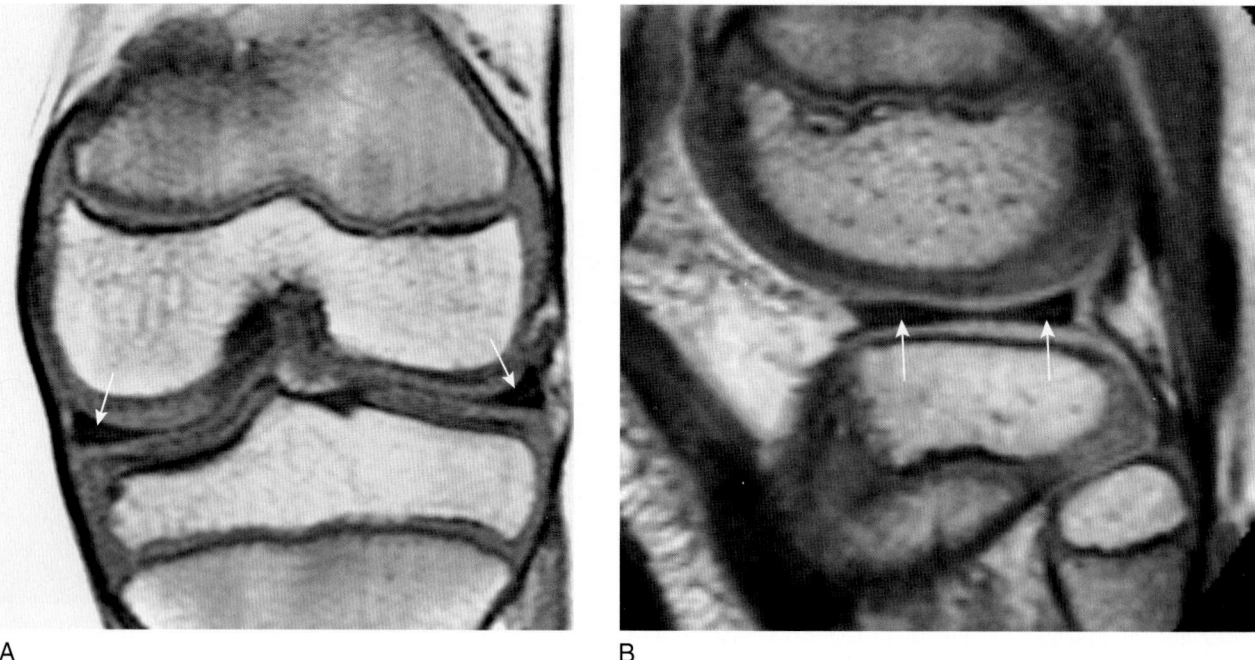

FIGURE 172-23. Normal meniscal vascularity. Coronal T1-weighted **(A)** and sagittal proton density–weighted **(B)** MR images of the knee in a 9-year-old boy show horizontal linear high signal intensity within the medial and lateral menisci *(arrows)* related to normal nutrient vessels. With increasing age, the vascularity diminishes, and this high signal is seen only in the peripheral one third of the meniscus in adolescents and young adults.

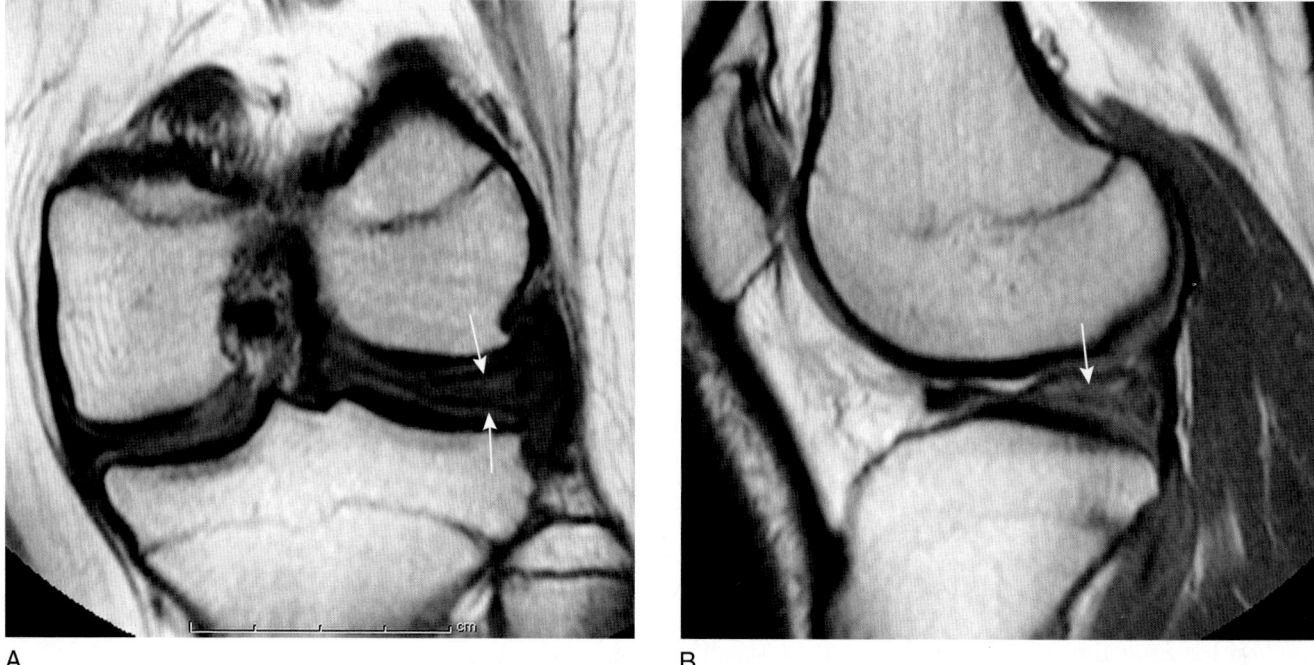

FIGURE 172-24. Discoid lateral meniscus in a 12-year-old female soccer player with more than a 1-year history of left knee pain. Coronal T1-weighted **(A)** and sagittal proton density–weighted **(B)** MR images reveal a thick, slab-shaped lateral meniscus with diffuse central high signal *(arrows)* due to chronic trauma and degeneration.

Patellar Dislocation

Acute and chronic patellar dislocations and subluxations are common in young athletes. The patellar displacement is almost always lateral, caused by a direct blow to the medial side of the patella (in contact sports) or by twisting muscular contractions when the knee is placed in valgus stress (pivoting sports). Chronic patellar subluxation is common in adolescent girls and usually associated with congenital or developmental deficiency of the extensor mechanism. These include weakness of the vastus medialis obliquus muscle, shallow trochlear

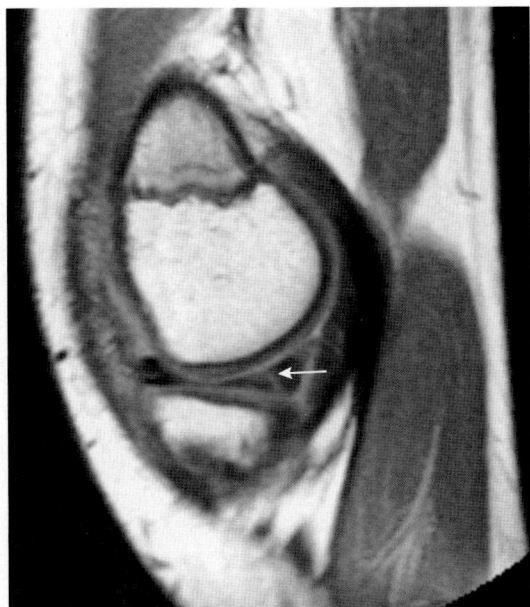

FIGURE 172-25. Medial meniscal tear in a 12-year-old boy with Down syndrome who developed left knee pain while training for the Special Olympics. Sagittal proton density–weighted MR image reveals linear vertical hyperintensity in the posterior horn of the medial meniscus *(arrow)* that extends to the superior and inferior articular surfaces. The child underwent arthroscopic débridement of the tear with resolution of his symptoms.

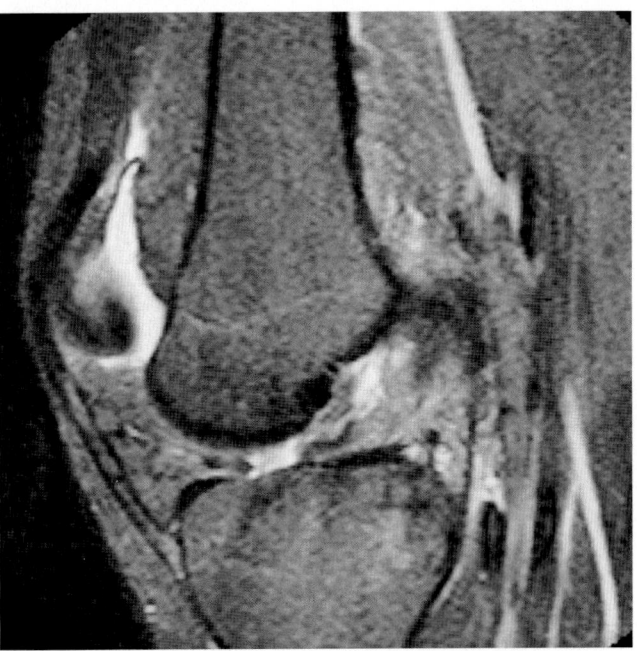

FIGURE 172-27. Anterior cruciate ligament tear in a 17-year-old female competitive skier. Sagittal inversion recovery MR image shows high signal intensity edema within the intercondylar notch and complete disruption of the anterior cruciate ligament. Associated medial meniscal tear and osteochondral fracture of the lateral femoral condyle were seen on other images (not shown).

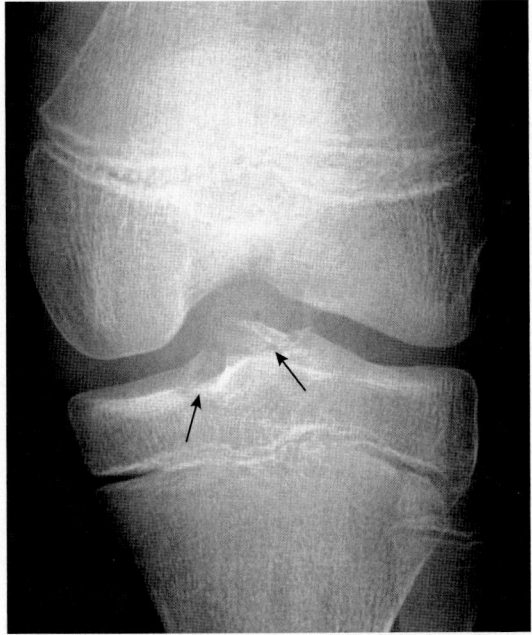

A

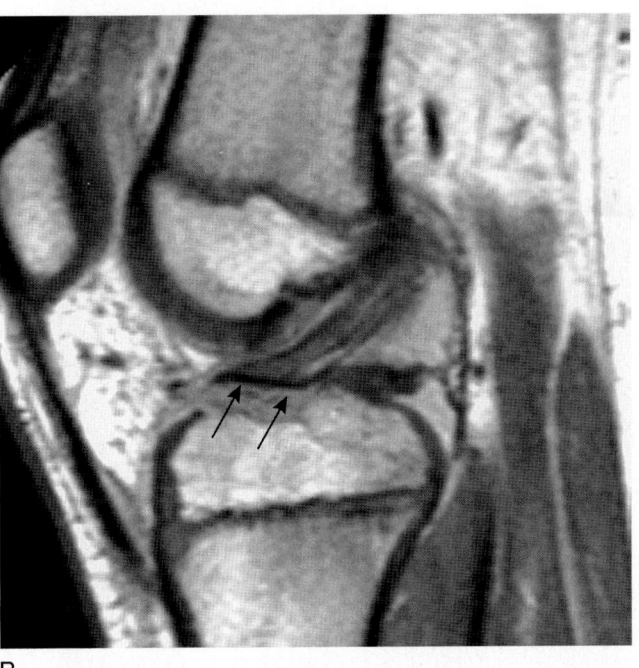

B

FIGURE 172-26. Tibial spine avulsion fracture. **A,** Frontal radiograph of the left knee in a 13-year-old boy who was injured while skiing shows a fracture of the lateral tibial spine extending into the tibial plateau *(arrows).* **B,** Sagittal proton density–weighted MR image in a 10-year-old boy who sustained a snowboarding injury shows the fracture path *(arrows),* superior displacement of the tibial spine fracture fragment, and an intact anterior cruciate ligament. The displacement of the fracture fragments in both patients necessitated surgical fixation.

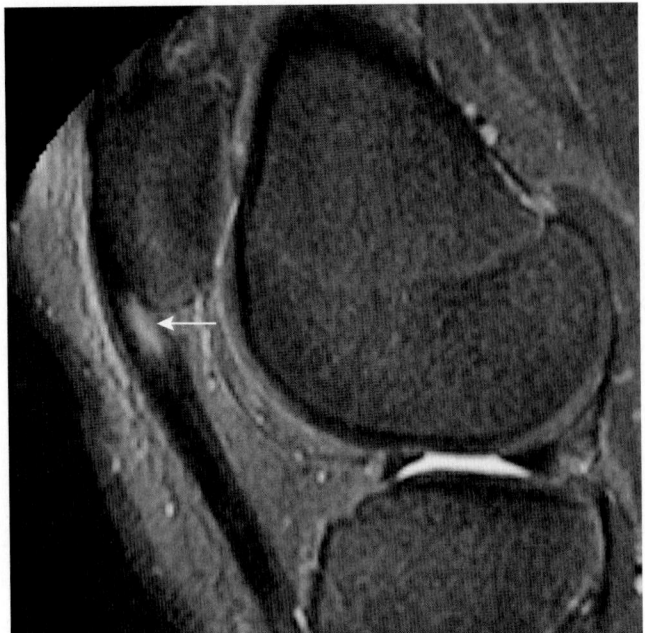

FIGURE 172-28. Jumper's knee/patellar tendonitis in a 16-year-old basketball player with persistent anterior knee pain. Sagittal inversion recovery MR image shows focal high signal intensity within the posterior fibers of the proximal patellar tendon at its insertion on the lower pole of the patella *(arrow)*. A mild amount of associated soft tissue edema is also seen anteriorly.

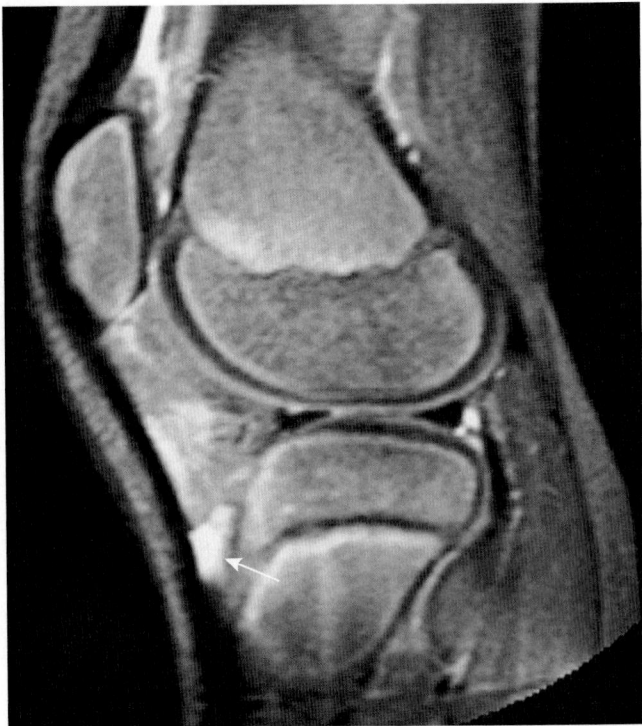

FIGURE 172-30. Osgood-Schlatter disease. Sagittal inversion recovery MR image in this 13-year-old boy shows fluid within the deep infrapatellar bursa *(arrow)* and edema in the infrapatellar fat pad.

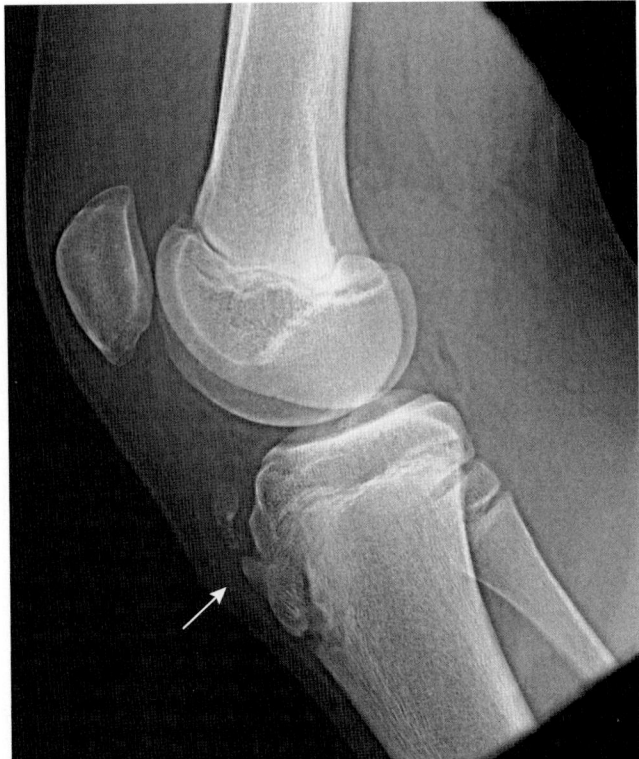

FIGURE 172-29. Osgood-Schlatter disease in an 11-year-old female soccer player. Lateral radiograph of the knee shows fragmentation of the tibial tubercle, adjacent soft tissue swelling *(arrow)*, and attenuation of the infrapatellar fat pad due to chronic microtrauma to the patellar tendon at its insertion on the tibial tubercle.

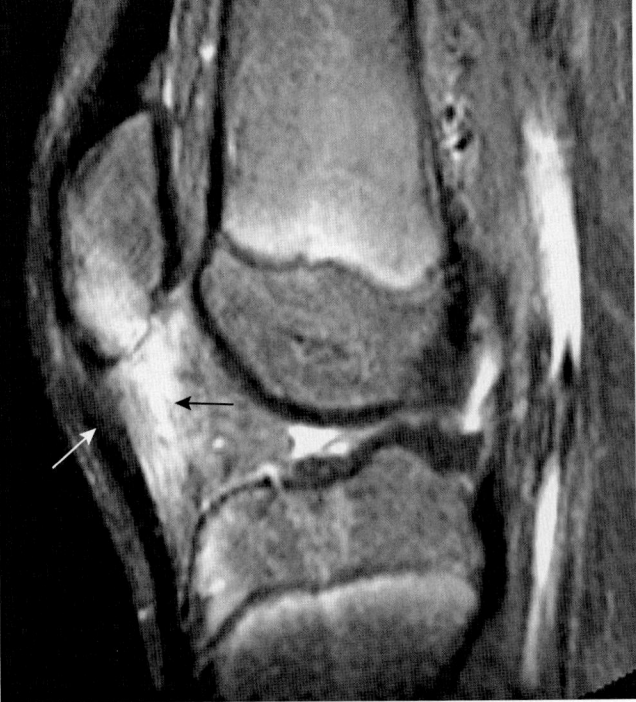

FIGURE 172-31. Sinding-Larsen-Johansson disease in an 11-year-old male tennis player. Sagittal inversion recovery MR image shows extensive marrow edema within the lower pole of the patella, intrasubstance signal abnormality within the proximal patellar tendon *(white arrow)*, and edema in the Hoffa infrapatellar fat pad *(black arrow)*.

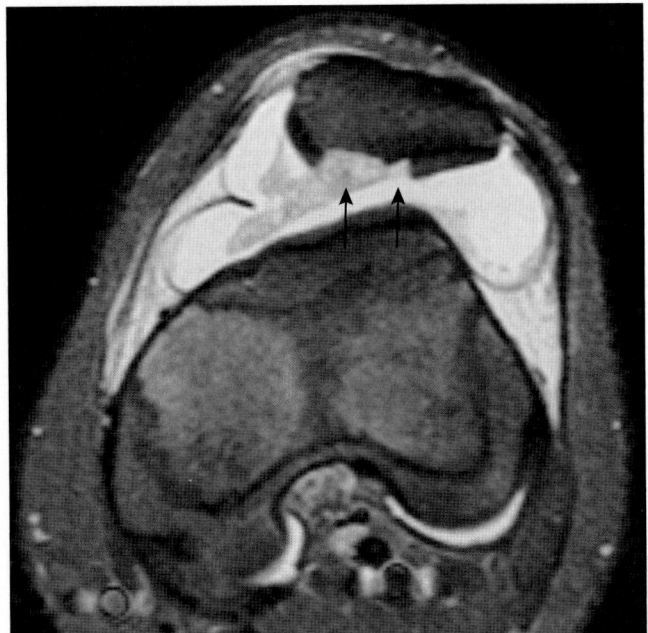
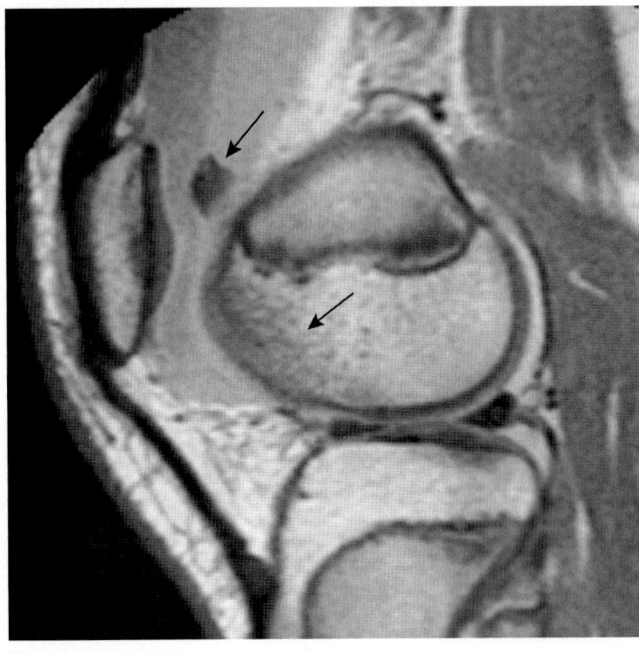

A   B

FIGURE 172-32. Acute patellar dislocation in a 15-year-old high-level ballet dancer who felt her knee collapse upon landing from a jump. Axial inversion recovery (**A**) and sagittal proton density–weighted (**B**) MR images show a large hemarthrosis with medial and lateral plicae surrounded by fluid. A large osteochondral defect is seen on the articular surface of the patella (*arrows* in **A**) associated with an intra-articular loose fragment (*upper arrow* in **B**). The sagittal image also shows abnormal signal intensity (*lower arrow* in **B**) within the anterior aspect of the lateral femoral condyle that represents a contusion from impact with the dislocated patella. The patella is relocated at the time of the MR, as is usually the case.

groove, and relative hyperextension or genu recurvatum. MRI after acute dislocation reveals a large hemarthrosis, lateral femoral condylar and medial patellar facet bone contusions, extensive medial and anterior soft tissue edema, and usually a tear of the medial patellar retinaculum. In younger patients, avulsion fracture of the medial patellar facet at the retinacular insertion is more common than complete retinacular tear. Osteochondral injuries to the articular surfaces of the medial patellar facet and lateral trochlea are also common and can lead to intra-articular loose bodies (Fig. 172-32).

SUMMARY

Evaluation of pediatric musculoskeletal trauma has always depended heavily on imaging techniques. With the increased participation of children in athletics, radiologists are more frequently asked to assist in the diagnosis and management of acute and chronic injury to the growing skeleton. Initial imaging assessment is almost always radiographic and is often sufficient. However, we are increasingly expected to accurately evaluate soft tissue, ligamentous, tendinous, and cartilaginous injuries in competitive child athletes. Advanced imaging techniques, including high-frequency ultrasound, multidetector CT with multiplanar reformations, and MRI, with its unique ability to visualize cartilage, bone marrow, and adjacent soft tissues, have become extremely valuable and relied-upon tools in the care of children with musculoskeletal injury.

SUGGESTED READINGS

Epiphyseal/Osteochondral Injuries

Brittberg M, Lindahl A, Nilsson A, et al: Treatment of deep cartilage defects in the knee with autologous chondrocyte transplantation. N Engl J Med 1994;331:889-895

De Smet AA, Fisher DR, Graf BK, et al: Osteochondritis dissecans of the knee: value of MR imaging in determining lesion stability and the presence of articular cartilage defects. AJR Am J Roentgenol 1990;155:549-553

De Smet AA, Ilahi OA, Graf BK: Untreated osteochondritis dissecans of the femoral condyles: prediction of patient outcome using radiographic and MR findings. Skeletal Radiol 1997;26:463-467

Gebarski K, Hernandez RJ: Stage-I osteochondritis dissecans versus normal variants of ossification in the knee in children. Pediatr Radiol 2005;35:880-886

Jaramillo D, Waters PM: MR imaging of the normal developmental anatomy of the elbow. Magn Reson Imaging Clin N Am 1997; 5:501-513

Klingele KE, Kocher MS: Little league elbow: valgus overload injury in the paediatric athlete. Sports Med 2002;32:1005-1015

Oeppen RS, Connolly SA, Bencardino JT, et al: Acute injury of the articular cartilage and subchondral bone: a common but unrecognized lesion in the immature knee. AJR Am J Roentgenol 2004;182:111-117

Potter HG, Deland JT, Gusmer PB, et al: Magnetic resonance imaging of the Lisfranc ligament of the foot. Foot Ankle Int 1998;19:438-446

Stoane JM, Poplausky MR, Haller JO, et al: Panner's disease: x-ray, MR imaging findings and review of the literature. Comput Med Imaging Graph 1995;19:473-476

Sundberg TP, Toomayan GA, Major NM: Evaluation of the acetabular labrum at 3.0-T MR imaging compared with 1.5-T MR arthrography: preliminary experience. Radiology 2006;238:706-711

Takahara M, Mura N, Sasaki J, et al: Classification, treatment and outcome of osteochondritis dissecans of the humeral capitellum. J Bone Joint Surg Am 2007;89:1205-1214

Yoshida S, Ikata T, Takai H, et al: Osteochondritis dissecans of the femoral condyle in the growth stage. Clin Orthop Relat Res 1998;346:162-170

Overuse Injuries

Anderson MW, Greenspan A: Stress fractures. Radiology 1996;199:1-12

Anderson MW, Ugalde V, Batt M, et al: Shin splints: MR appearance in a preliminary study. Radiology 1997;204:177-180

Anderson SE, Johnston JO, O'Donnell R, et al: MR imaging of sports-related pseudotumor in children: mid femoral diaphyseal periostitis at insertion site of adductor musculature. AJR Am J Roentgenol 2001;176:1227-1231

Barnett LS: Little League shoulder syndrome: proximal humeral epiphyseolysis in adolescent baseball pitchers. A case report. J Bone Joint Surg Am 1985;67:495-496

Caine D, De Fiori J, Maffulli N: Physeal injuries in children's and youth sports: reasons for concern? Br J Sports Med 2006;40:749-760

Chilvers M, Donahue M, Nassar L, et al: Foot and ankle injuries in elite female gymnasts. Foot Ankle Int 2007;28:214-218

Coady CM, Micheli LJ: Stress fractures in the pediatric athlete. Clin Sports Med 1997;16:225-238

Drubach LA, Connolly LP, D'Hemecourt PA, et al: Assessment of the clinical significance of asymptomatic lower extremity uptake abnormality in young athletes. J Nucl Med 2001;42:209-212

Gaeta M, Minutoli F, Scribano E, et al: CT and MR imaging findings in athletes with early tibial stress injuries: comparison with bone scintigraphy findings and emphasis on cortical abnormalities. Radiology 2005;235:553-561

Ishibashi Y, Okamura Y, Otsuka H, et al: Comparison of scintigraphy and magnetic resonance imaging for stress injuries of bone. Clin J Sport Med 2002;12:79-84

Laor T, Hartman AL, Jaramillo D: Local physeal widening on MR imaging: an incidental finding suggesting prior metaphyseal insult. Pediatr Radiol 1997;27:654-662

Laor T, Wall EJ, Vu LP: Physeal widening in the knee due to stress injury in child athletes. AJR Am J Roentgenol 2006;186:1260-1264

Niemeyer P, Weinberg A, Schmitt M, et al: Stress factures in adolescent competitive athletes with open physis. Knee Surg Sports Traumatol Arthrosc 2006;14:771-777

Obembe OO, Gaskin CM, Taffoni MJ, et al: Little leaguer's shoulder (proximal humeral epiphysiolysis): MRI findings in four boys: Pediatr Radiol 2007; In Press

Ogden JA: Injury to the growth mechanisms of the immature skeleton. Skeletal Radiol 1981;6:237-253

Ogden J: Fractures associated with pediatric disease. In Ogden J (ed): Skeletal Injury in the Child. Philadelphia, Saunders, 1990:299-303

Shih C, Chang CY, Penn IW, et al: Chronically stressed wrists in adolescent gymnasts: MR imaging appearance. Radiology 1995;195:855-859

Avulsion Injuries

Bates DG, Hresko MT, Jaramillo D: Patellar sleeve fracture: demonstration with MR imaging. Radiology 1994;193:825-827

Donnelly LF, Bisset GS, Helms CA, et al: Chronic avulsive injuries of childhood. Skeletal Radiol 1999;28:138-144

Hang DW, Chao CM, Hang YS: A clinical and roentgenographic study of Little League elbow. Am J Sports Med 2004;32:79-84

Havranek P: Injuries of distal clavicular physis in children. J Pediatr Orthop 1989;9:213-215

Sofka CM, Potter HG: Imaging of elbow injuries in the child and adult athlete. Radiol Clin North Am 2002;40:251-265

Stevens MA, El-Khoury GY, Kathol MH, et al: Imaging features of avulsion injuries. Radiographics 1999;19:655-672

Sugimoto H, Ohsawa T: Ulnar collateral ligament in the growing elbow: MR imaging of normal development and throwing injuries. Radiology 1994;192:417-422

Soft Tissue Injury

Bencardino J, Rosenberg Z, Brown R, et al: Traumatic musculotendinous injuries of the knee: diagnosis with MR imaging. Radiographics 2000;20:S103-S120

Lovell WW, Winter RB, Morrissy RT, et al (eds): Lovell and Winter's Pediatric Orthopedics, 5th ed. Philadelphia, Lippincott Williams & Wilkins, 2001

Ogden J (ed): Skeletal Injury in the Child. Philadelphia, Saunders, 1990

Palmer W, Kuong S, Elmadbouh H: MR imaging of myotendinous strain. Am J Roentgenol 1999;173:703-709

Parikh J, Hyare H, Saifuddin A: The imaging features of post-traumatic myositis ossificans, with emphasis on MRI. Clin Radiol 2002;57:1058-1066

Injury to the Knee

Baker MM: Anterior cruciate ligament injuries in the female athlete. J Womens Health 1998;7:343-349

Carr JC, Hanly S, Griffin J, et al: Sonography of the patellar tendon and adjacent structures in pediatric and adult patients. AJR Am J Roentgenol 2001;176:1535-1539

Gholve PA, Scher DM, Khakharia S, et al: Osgood-Schlatter syndrome. Curr Opin Pediatr 2007;19:44-50

McLoughlin RF, Raber EL, Vellet AD, et al: Patellar tendinitis: MR imaging features, with suggested pathogenesis and proposed classification. Radiology 1995;197:843-848

Micheli LJ, Metzl JD, Di Canzio J, et al: Anterior cruciate ligament reconstructive surgery in adolescent soccer and basketball players. Clin J Sport Med 1999;9:138-141

Prince JS, Laor T, Bean JA: MRI of anterior cruciate ligament injuries and associated findings in the pediatric knee: changes with skeletal maturation. AJR Am J Roentgenol 2005;185:756-762

Rosenberg ZS, Kawelblum M, Cheung YY, et al: Osgood-Schlatter lesion: fracture or tendinitis? Scintigraphic, CT, and MR imaging features. Radiology 1992;185:853-858

Schachter AK, Rokito AS: ACL injuries in the skeletally immature patient. Orthopedics 2007;30:365-370

Stark JE, Siegel MJ, Weinberger E, et al: Discoid menisci in children: MR features. J Comput Assist Tomogr 1995;19:608-611

Utukuri MM, Somayaji MS, Khanduja V, et al: Update on pediatric ACL injuries. Knee 2006;13:345-352

Varich LJ, Laor T, Jaramillo D: Normal maturation of the distal femoral epiphyseal cartilage: changes on MR imaging with age and weight bearing. Radiology 2000;214:705-709

Zaidi A, Babyn P, Astori I, et al: MRI of traumatic patellar dislocation in children. Pediatr Radiol 2006;36:1163-1170

Zobel MS, Borrello JA, Siegel MJ, et al: Pediatric knee MR imaging: pattern of injuries in the immature skeleton. Radiology 1994;190:397-401

Osteochondroses

JENNIFER D. SMITH and DIEGO JARAMILLO

INTRODUCTION

Osteochondroses are acquired focal disorders of endochondral ossification involving the epiphyses, apophyses, or other epiphyseal equivalents, such as the round bones of the carpal and tarsal regions. During the first half of the 20th century, osteochondroses were reported in more than 75 locations in the pediatric skeleton (Fig. 173-1), and most of these were labeled with eponyms. Over time, these entities have proved to be developmental variants (such as Van Neck disease, a normally occurring irregularity in ischiopubic synchondrosis), chronic traumatic lesions (such as Osgood-Schlatter disease involving the tibial tubercle), idiopathic avascular necrosis (such as Köhler disease), or entities that probably represent unique occurrences, such as scaphoid osteochondrosis (Preiser disease). Legg-Calvé-Perthes disease, or idiopathic avascular necrosis of the proximal femoral epiphyseal ossification center, represents the most frequent and clinically significant osteochondrosis, but similar abnormalities occur in other bones, particularly the lunate, tarsal navicular, capitellum, ring apophyses of vertebral bodies, and metatarsals. Regardless of the cause, when bones are truly abnormal, they typically show decreased perfusion that leads to radiographic sclerosis and osseous fragmentation and collapse.

LEGG-CALVÉ-PERTHES DISEASE

In children, the vascular supply of the proximal femur is fragile, and ischemic injury to the proximal epiphysis occurs frequently. Ischemia precipitates a sequence of events, including avascular necrosis, collapse of the femoral head, deformity, decreased range of motion, and early osteoarthritis. Avascular necrosis of the femoral head occurs primarily as a result of Legg-Calvé-Perthes disease (LCP), but it can also result from systemic disease or medications, abduction therapy for developmental dysplasia of the hip, and acute distention of the joint space in septic arthritis.

Epidemiology and Clinical Features

LCP is the idiopathic necrosis of the immature proximal femur in children, involving primarily the epiphysis. Incidence has been reported to be 1 in 20,000, and a recent study revealed a 4:1 male predominance. LCP occurs usually in boys between 5 and 10 years of age, but usually, the condition is diagnosed in girls at a slightly earlier age. Genetic predisposition is weak or absent; a greater incidence, however, is seen with a history of lower birth weight, delayed skeletal maturity, passive smoking, attention deficit hyperactivity disorder, and lower income. It is more common among Caucasians. A hypercoagulable state may be a contributing factor; a past history of toxic synovitis is rare (occurring in less than 1% of cases) but may be a causal factor. Bilateral involvement is seen in about 10% of cases, although it is almost always asynchronous. Symmetric involvement is atypical for LCP and should suggest the possibility of another diagnosis, such as epiphyseal dysplasia or sickle cell disease.

> LCP usually occurs in boys from 5 to 10 years of age. Girls are less commonly affected, and the condition is usually diagnosed in girls at an earlier age.
> Symmetric involvement is atypical for LCP and should suggest the possibility of another diagnosis, such as epiphyseal dysplasia or sickle cell disease.

Deformity of the femoral head, neck, and acetabulum that results from LCP is one of the main causes of degenerative disease of the hip in men. Patients with a history of LCP often develop radiographic signs of osteoarthritis by the third and fourth decades, and most have severe degenerative disease by age 70. Poor prognostic predictors include increased age at onset, female gender, and bilaterality. Children who present before 6 years of age generally have a benign course, whereas those who

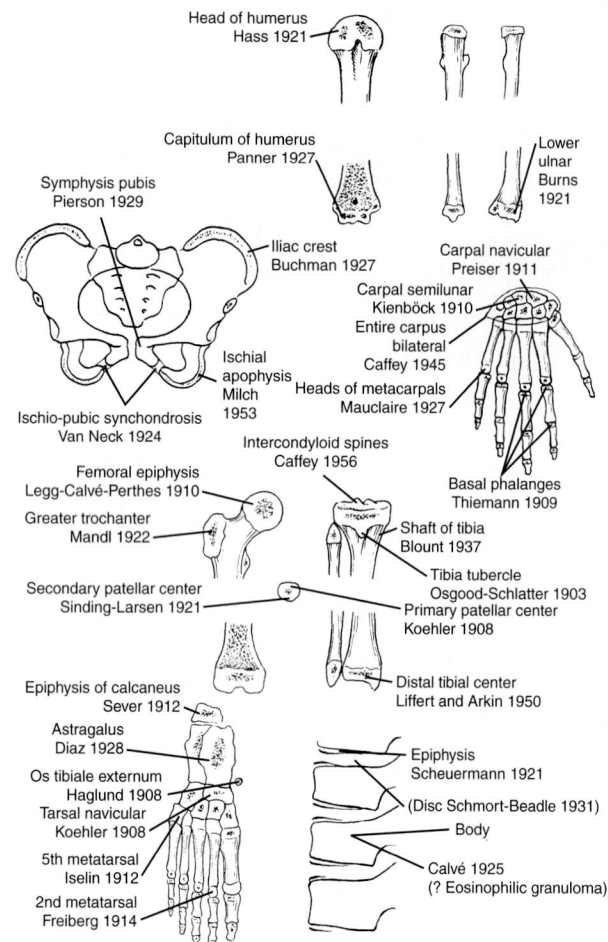

FIGURE 173-1. Schematic drawing of the growing skeleton with the supposed sites of the juvenile osteochondroses (focal ischemic necroses, names of the discovers of the various lesions, and the year that each lesion was first reported). These sites are also regions where irregularity of mineralization occurs as a normal anatomic variant in growing children.

present after 8 years of age fare less well and usually require surgery.

Children with LCP typically present after having had several weeks or months of limping, often without pain. Physical findings include spasm, limitation of abduction and internal rotation, and atrophy of the thigh and buttock in a child who is otherwise normal.

Stages

LCP lasts up to 8 years, and it progresses through four main stages: avascularity, revascularization, healing, and residual deformity (Fig. 173-2). During the months of the quiescent stage of avascularity, the child is usually asymptomatic. The ossific nucleus of the proximal femur fails to grow and gradually becomes smaller than the normal side because of absent blood flow for endochondral ossification. The articular cartilage continues to be nourished by synovial fluid and therefore grows and thickens. The ossific nucleus becomes increasingly dense—a finding that is accentuated by concomitant osteopenia of the metaphysis and periarticular structures due to increasing periepiphyseal vascularity. Magnetic

resonance imaging (MRI) during the quiescent stage reveals absence of enhancement of the epiphyseal ossification center with moderate edema of the marrow.

During the revascularization stage, which lasts from 1 to 4 years, surrounding tissues react to the dead bone. In this stage, the child experiences pain, and the most dramatic radiographic changes occur. The ossific nucleus appears even denser because of new bone formation occurring within the dead trabeculae; it is easily flattened and deformed. A pathologic subchondral fracture in the anterosuperior ossific nucleus creates the radiographic "crescent sign." The epiphyseal ossification center undergoes varying degrees of fragmentation, primarily in its central portion. The adjacent metaphysis sometimes develops cystic changes and broadening (Fig. 173-3). Disturbed endochondral ossification from ischemia probably results in residual cartilage in the metaphysis. On MRI and scintigraphy, evidence of revascularization of the femoral head may be noted through the physis or around it, along the lateral aspect of the epiphysis. The metaphyseal lucencies are avidly enhancing. This stage is characterized by highly significant synovial proliferation, usually accompanied by a small effusion; both of these events are detectable on gadolinium-enhanced MRI and result in lateral displacement of the femoral head.

During the healing phase, new bone slowly replaces granulation tissue in the ossific nucleus, and the epiphysis regains its height. The better the femoral head is contained by the acetabulum, the more spherically the femoral head will remodel. On MRI performed during the healing phase, the physeal cartilage may exhibit irregularity or bridging. Epiphyseal deformity is more pronounced anteriorly; hence, sagittal images are more useful for evaluation.

Residual deformity persists after healing, although the articular cartilage is reasonably preserved despite the changes in avascularity that have occurred in the epiphysis. As a result, joint function may be satisfactory for several years. Abnormal shape of the healed epiphysis is characterized by coxa magna, a residual enlargement of the femoral head and neck, and coxa breva, a short femoral neck due to premature physeal arrest. Subsequent varus or valgus hip deformity may occur depending on the location of the physeal fusion. Joint incongruity leads to degenerative joint disease later in life.

Imaging Diagnosis and Assessment of Prognosis

Radiographic imaging plays a key role in the diagnostic and prognostic evaluation of patients with LCP. Early radiographic diagnosis is based on the detection of periarticular osteoporosis, medial joint space widening and lateral displacement of the femoral head, and eventually, a relatively smaller and denser appearance of the femoral head. Once the disease is apparent, several radiographic features may help to reveal the severity of the disease and its prognosis. A frog-leg lateral view is important for showing the anterior "crescent sign" that is associated with a worse outcome. One key feature is the preservation of the lateral third of the femoral head, the so-called "lateral pillar." Because the lateral pillar is an

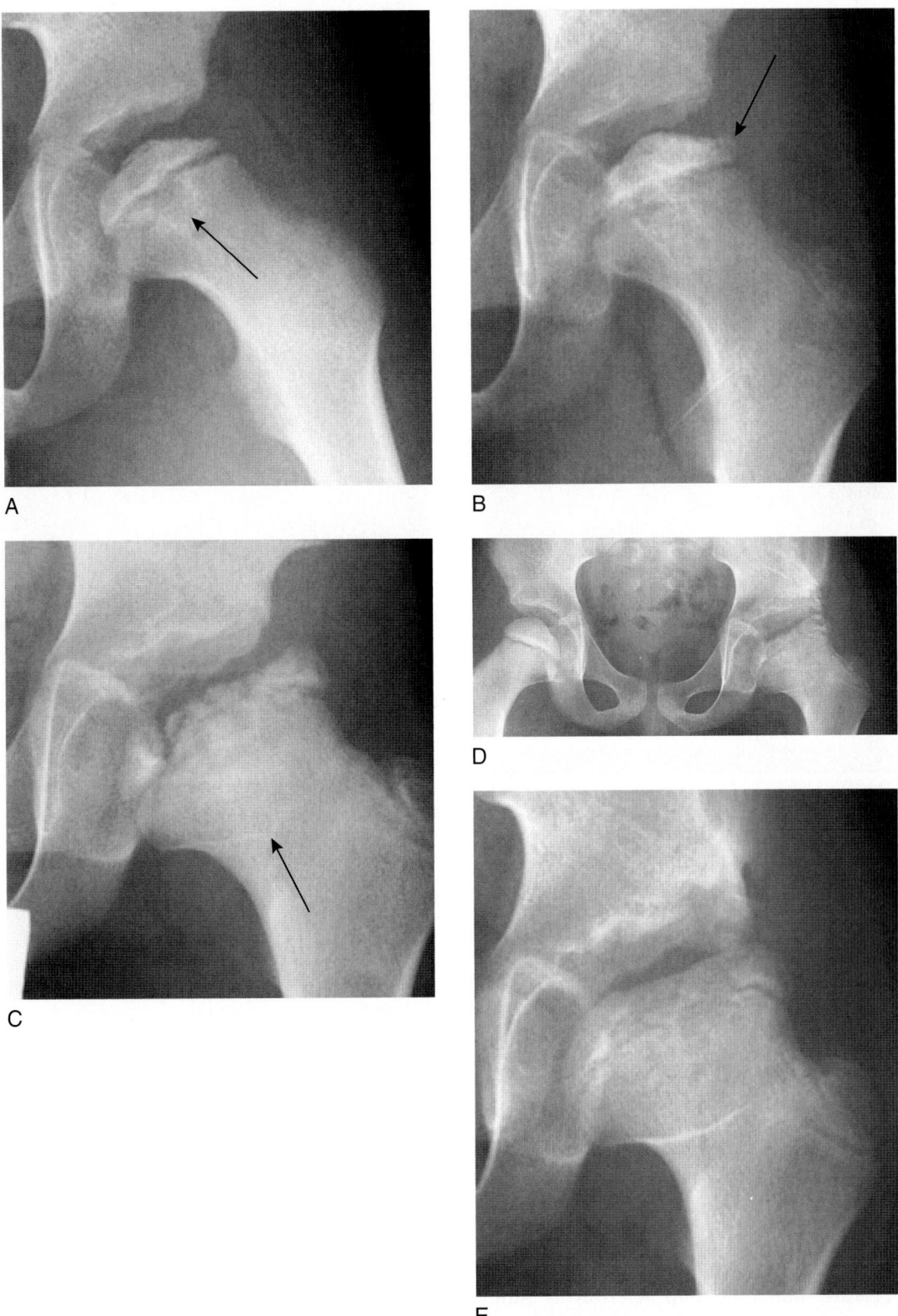

FIGURE 173-2. A 7-year-old boy with a limp and osteonecrosis of the left proximal femoral epiphysis. **A,** Radiograph of the left hip reveals a small, sclerotic proximal femoral epiphysis with an irregular joint surface. The metaphysis of the proximal femur also shows cystic changes *(arrow)*, which indicate a poor prognosis. **B,** Radiograph performed 2 months later shows continued sclerosis and flattening, particularly laterally. Very early fragmentation of the epiphysis is noted in the lateral pillar *(arrow)*. **C,** At 18 months after presentation, a radiograph of the left hip reveals further fragmentation with continued lateral extrusion of the epiphysis. The acetabulum is beginning to impinge on the portion of the lateral column that is uncovered, and incongruence of the hip joint is apparent. The "sagging rope" sign *(arrow)*, which is produced by the outline of an abnormally oriented physis, indicates growth arrest. Widening of the femoral neck is seen ("coxa magna"). **D,** At 25 months after diagnosis, there is evidence of a left iliac osteotomy attempting to cover the widened, flattened left capital femoral epiphysis that is starting to coalesce. Early sclerosis of the right proximal femoral epiphysis is seen, indicating early avascular necrosis in the contralateral hip. **E,** At 3 years after presentation, the left hip radiograph shows healed Legg-Calvé-Perthes disease with residual flattening, coxa magna, and irregular acetabulum.

FIGURE 173-3. A 10-year-old boy with left Legg-Calvé-Perthes disease. **A,** Coronal T1-weighted hip magnetic resonance image reveals crescentic low signal in the left proximal femoral epiphysis with irregularity of the joint surface. Epiphyseal height is also decreased. Some normal high signal is present, indicating preserved fat in the epiphysis. The lateral left femoral metaphysis reveals a rounded area of lower signal, indicating cystic changes. Additionally, cartilaginous hypertrophy is evident within the left hip joint that often accounts for apparent radiographic widening. **B,** Sagittal T2-weighted magnetic resonance image shows hyperintense crescentic fracture *(white arrow)*, predominantly in the anterior portion of the left femoral epiphysis. There is an associated joint effusion.

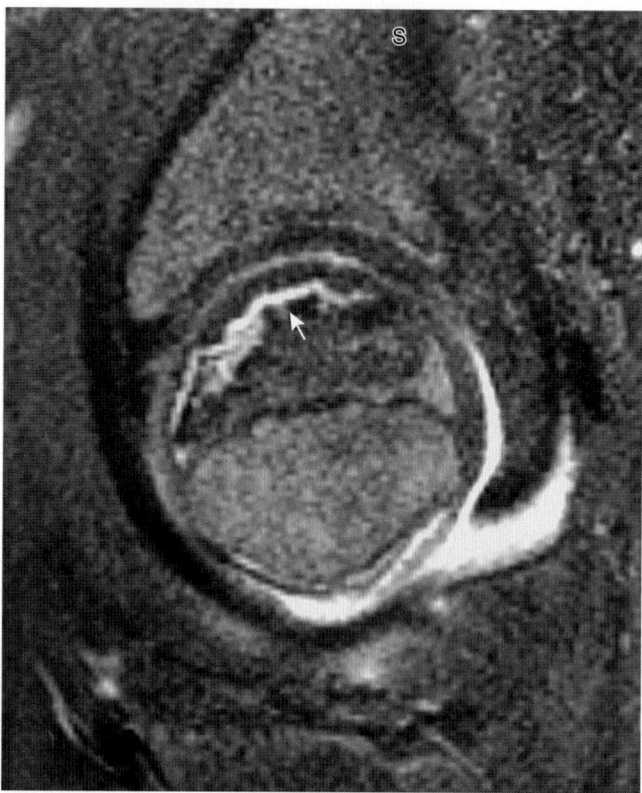

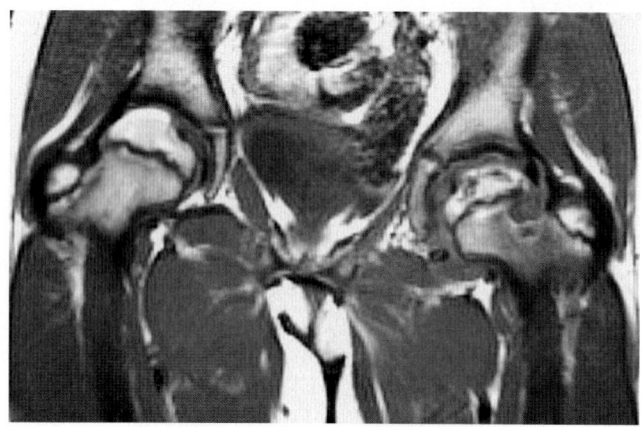

A

B

TABLE 173-1

Modified Herring Classification of Legg-Calvé-Perthes Disease

Type A: no involvement of the lateral pillar, which maintains its full height. Possible lucency and collapse of central and medial pillars
Type B: some lucency of the lateral pillar with preservation of bone density at a height between 50% and 100% of the original height of the lateral head
Type C: less than 50% of lateral pillar height is maintained, and the lateral pillar is more radiolucent than in type B; any preserved bone is at a height of <50% of the original height of the lateral pillar

After Herring et al.

TABLE 173-2

Modified Stulberg Classification of Legg-Calvé-Perthes Disease

Class I: femoral head indistinguishable from normal
Class II: a slightly deformed femoral head (less than 2 mm deviation from a circular shape)
Class III: ovoid femoral head, coxa magna, shortened femoral neck, abnormally steep acetabulum
Class IV: flattened femoral head and acetabulum, with abnormalities of the neck
Class V: flattened femoral head, usually with central collapse, with normal neck and acetabulum
Class I and II hips have spherical congruency and tend not to develop arthritis, whereas Class III and IV hips have aspherical congruency and develop mild to moderate arthritis in late adulthood. Class V hips have aspherical incongruency and develop severe arthritis before the age of 50.

important area of weight bearing and the zone where revascularization begins, collapse of the lateral pillar is perhaps the most important predictor of a poor outcome. The degree of integrity of the lateral pillar provides the basis for lateral pillar (Herring) classification (Table 173-1). Progressive flattening and sclerosis resulting from necrosis are seen. Other radiographic indicators of poor prognosis include changes in the metaphysis of the proximal femur, such as the development of well-defined radiolucent structures ("cysts") adjacent to the anterior physis. These metaphyseal changes are associated with subsequent growth arrest. The pattern of deformity of the femoral head and acetabulum is also important in the prediction of subsequent events; it forms the basis of the Stulberg classification (Table 173-2).

Other imaging modalities are seldom used, with the exception of MRI. Skeletal scintigraphy shows lack of epiphyseal perfusion early in the course. The revascularization pattern can also be evaluated later in the disease. Ultrasonography may aid in the detection of small joint effusion or synovial thickening early in the disease. Contrast-enhanced power Doppler can reveal femoral head and cartilage revascularization. Angiographic evaluation of the hip in LCP disease is usually not clinically useful.

MRI can be useful at different stages of LCP. At presentation, although it is uncommon for a symptomatic child with LCP to have normal radiographs; MRI may reveal unsuspected avascular necrosis and marrow edema that manifest as an abnormal signal intensity of the epiphyseal fatty marrow (see Fig. 173-3). Imaging during the early vascular phase approximately 2 minutes after contrast injection allows for optimal detection of the decreased enhancement indicative of the perfusion abnormality. Some children may present solely with transient abnormal signal in the femoral head that may be a self-limited mild form of LCP. In LCP, early diagnosis of osteonecrosis may not substantially alter management; however, in conditions such as sickle cell disease, steroid therapy, bone marrow transplant, malignancy, or rheumatologic disease, diagnosis of osteonecrosis may dictate a more aggressive investigation or modification of therapy.

> **MRI in LCP:** Early findings consist of epiphyseal edema and decreased or absent perfusion. Late findings include femoral head deformity and lack of full containment. MRI assesses for degree of epiphyseal involvement, femoral containment (presence of synovial hypertrophy, epiphyseal cartilage thickening), physeal interruption and bridging, and evidence of reperfusion and healing.

MRI is widely used at a more advanced stage of LCP for assessment of the degree of marrow involvement of the capital femoral epiphysis, particularly when it is performed 3 to 8 months after onset of symptoms. MRI can also detect synovial hypertrophy (Fig. 173-4) and thickening of the epiphyseal cartilage at this stage, both of which result in decreased femoral head containment. Physeal interruption as shown on MRI may occur in more than 60% of children with LCP disease and leads to growth arrest. Sagittal images best reveal the high signal intensity areas in the anterior juxtaphyseal metaphysis that also are associated with growth arrest. Reperfusion across the physis reflects neovascularization through the physis, and this pattern is associated with a worse outcome because of early physeal closure. In advanced cases of LCP, MRI or arthrography can assess the containment of the femoral head by the acetabulum and varying femoro-acetabular relationships in different positions. It is important to show whether with abduction, the lateral aspect of the femoral head hinges against the acetabular rim (Fig. 173-5). This incongruency, which may prevent a successful osteotomy, is more likely to lead to acetabular impingement and early degeneration.

Several classification schemes based on radiographs have been developed for the evaluation of LCP disease. Currently, no agreement has been reached regarding the classification scheme that will best aid in treatment and

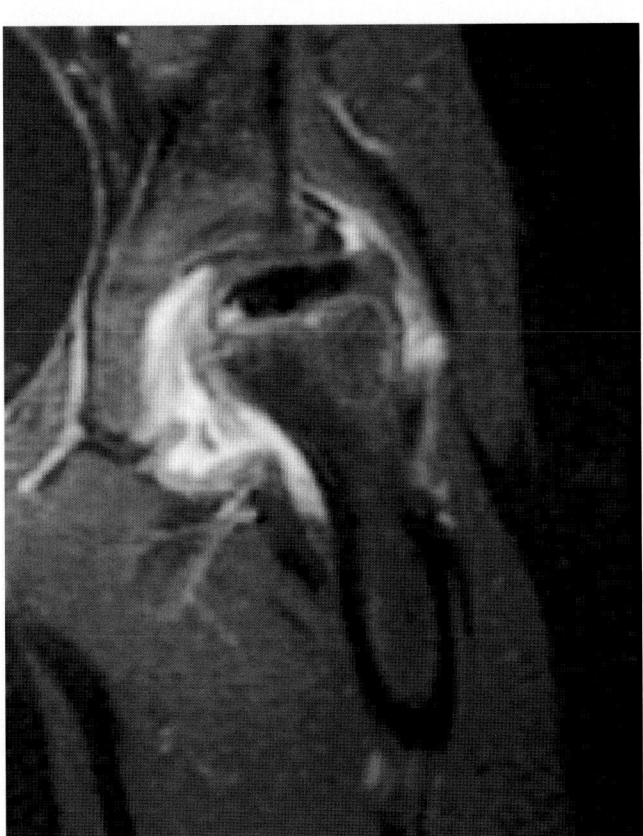

FIGURE 173-4. A 6-year-old boy with a history of left Legg-Calvé-Perthes disease. Coronal gadolinium-enhanced T1-weighted image shows lack of enhancement of the flattened femoral head and increased synovial enhancement. The head is subluxed.

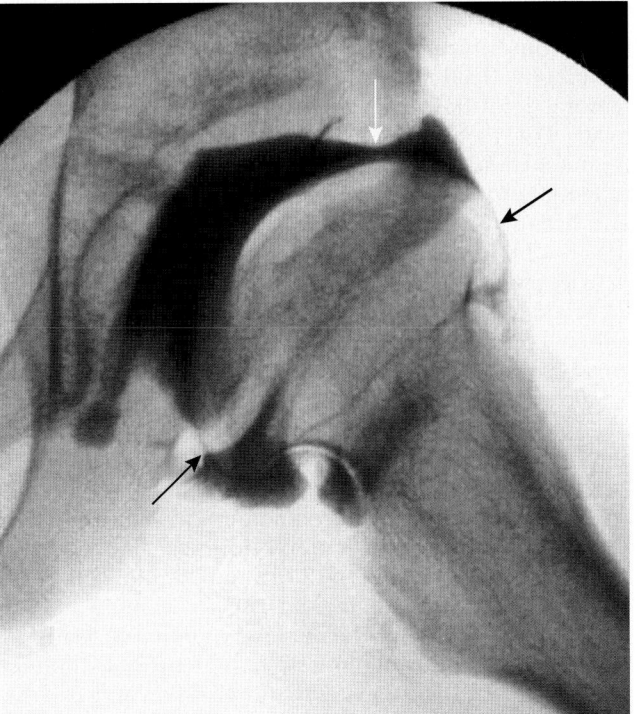

FIGURE 173-5. A 12-year-old boy with healed Legg-Calvé-Perthes disease status post iliac osteotomy with persistent pain and limited range of motion. This is the same patient as was shown in Figure 173-2, at 4 years and 8 months after initial presentation. Conventional direct arthrography of the abducted left hip performed intraoperatively reveals hinged abduction between the peripheral superior acetabulum *(white arrow)* and the deformed lateral portion of the femoral head. Note the unossified cartilaginous portion of the proximal femoral head *(black arrows).*

prognosis. One recent long-term multicenter study used two different schemes, according to the stage of disease and the age of the patient. Herring and colleagues modified the lateral pillar classification to characterize the integrity of the lateral pillar of the capital epiphysis during the fragmentation phase of LCP disease (see Table 173-1). The same study clarified the Stulberg classification and applied it to describe the residual deformity of the femoral epiphysis after skeletal maturation (see Table 173-2).

The most important predictors of patient outcome aside from age of onset are femoral head congruency within the acetabulum and range of motion of the hip joint. The acetabulum continues to have significant growth potential until age 8 or 9. Its configuration is dependent on the shape of the femoral head within the acetabulum during its growth period. If a femoral head deformity develops prior to completion of acetabular growth before the age of 6, the immature acetabulum conforms to the abnormal shape. Between the ages of 6 and 8, the acetabulum cannot conform to the shape of a deformed femoral head, and the chance that an incongruous relationship will develop is greater, leading to early degenerative joint disease. A deformed femoral head, especially with a large anterolateral segment that is uncovered, can impinge on the lateral acetabular lip, causing clinical symptoms of decreased range of motion, pain, and a clunking sensation.

Treatment of LCP disease is individualized on the basis of clinical and radiographic findings, including age of onset, range of motion in the hip joint, extent of femoral head involvement, presence or absence of femoral deformity, and lateral subluxation of the femoral head. For many patients, a combination of traction treatment with an abduction cast, nonsteroidal anti-inflammatory agents, and gentle range-of-motion exercises are used to enhance molding of the femoral head by the acetabulum. Surgery is indicated in children younger than 8 years who have femoral head deformity and in those older than 8 years even in the absence of deformity. Other indications for surgery include pain and decreased range of motion once healing has concluded. Surgical treatment consists of femoral (varus derotational) or pelvic (innominate) osteotomy. The main goals of surgical therapy are to preserve joint congruity during the active phase of the disease and to contain the femoral head within the acetabulum, preventing extrusion and subluxation. A femoral head that is contained by the acetabulum tends to heal more spherically than one that is partially subluxed. In severe cases, a vicious circle ensues in which decreased containment leads to increased deformity that in turn leads to further subluxation. Surgery can prevent this progression and can be used to maintain a full range of motion at the hip joint.

Differential Diagnosis

Differential considerations for a painful limp and stiffness in a child include osteonecrosis due to other causes such as sickle cell disease, Gaucher disease, renal disease, steroid or antineoplastic therapy; infection or inflammation around the hip; trauma including apophyseal avulsions from the pelvis; tumor (particularly osteoid osteoma); and slipped capital femoral epiphysis (in older children). Imaging findings of osteonecrosis related to other causes are indistinguishable from those of LCP. Patients with sickle cell disease show radiographic evidence of bone infarcts and osteonecrosis of other epiphyses; those with Gaucher disease show deformity related to marrow expansion. In both instances, MRI shows diffuse abnormality of the marrow. LCP should also be differentiated from Meyer dysplasia of the femoral head, an epiphyseal dysplasia limited to the femoral epiphyses that is reviewed below. This condition may be misdiagnosed as LCP disease because the ossification center is fragmented and irregular, but the radiographic appearance becomes normal, usually without significant sequelae. Epiphyseal irregularity can also occur in the absence of osteonecrosis in normal patients and in those with systemic or multifocal disorders such as hypothyroidism and epiphyseal dysplasia.

> The differential diagnosis for LCP includes avascular necrosis related to an underlying cause (e.g., sickle cell disease, steroid therapy), Meyer dysplasia, epiphyseal dysplasia, fracture/trauma, tumor (particularly osteoid osteoma), inflammation/infection of the hip or other adjacent structure, hypothyroidism, and normal developmental variation in ossification.

MEYER DYSPLASIA (FEMORAL EPIPHYSEAL DYSPLASIA)

Meyer dysplasia is a rare but benign developmental disorder of the hip that causes asymptomatic irregularity of ossification of the proximal femoral epiphysis. It usually occurs in boys younger than 4 years, and in 70% of cases, it is discovered incidentally. The abnormality occurs bilaterally approximately 50% to 60% of the time, and it is often present in those with hip disease in the immediate family. The cause of this disease is unclear. Avascular necrosis or synovitis may complicate this dysplasia, creating symptomatic pain and limited range of motion. The prognosis of Meyer dysplasia, in contrast to that of LCP, is good, and no abnormality is clinically detected during the remainder of hip growth. Risk of early degenerative disease may be increased if the proximal femoral epiphysis on the affected side is smaller. Differential diagnosis primarily includes LCP, but if the disease is bilateral, hypothyroidism, multiple epiphyseal dysplasia, and spondyloepiphyseal dysplasia should be considered.

Radiographs of children with Meyer dysplasia show a small and irregular ossific nucleus, often with multiple ossification centers that coalesce over time (Fig. 173-6). Two to four years later, the affected proximal femoral epiphysis will have a normal or nearly normal appearance with minimal residual epiphyseal height loss or mild coxa magna deformity. In contrast to LCP, the proximal femur does not develop subchondral fracture, collapse of the head, and subluxation. The absence of symptoms and progressive healing without residual

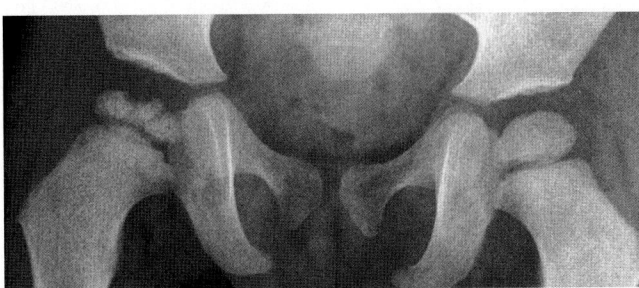

FIGURE 173-6. Meyer dysplasia. A 3-year-old boy with hypoplastic left heart after Fontan procedure. During an abdominal radiograph performed to evaluate distention, a fragmented, somewhat diminutive, right capital femoral epiphysis was found. The patient reported no symptoms referable to the hip.

deformity also suggest the diagnosis of Meyer dysplasia. Three-phase bone scans are normal. If MRI is performed, normal signal is noted in the fragments of the proximal femoral epiphysis. No treatment is required for Meyer dysplasia.

> Absence of symptoms and progressive healing without residual deformity suggest the diagnosis of Meyer dysplasia. Meyer dysplasia is usually bilateral and is discovered incidentally.

KÖHLER DISEASE

Köhler disease is a rare, idiopathic, self-limited osteochondrosis that affects the tarsal navicular bone of children approximately 5 to 6 years of age; it is more common in boys than in girls by a factor of 3. It is typically unilateral and presents with a limp, as well as pain and swelling localized to the dorsal midfoot. Although the cause is unclear, it has been speculated that the location of the navicular at a focal stress point in the arch of the foot renders it more susceptible to vascular compromise with normal activity. Usually, no history of prior foot-related complaints is documented, but one study found that approximately 25% of patients had prior injuries or other problems, including LCP. Laboratory values are normal.

Radiographs of the foot exhibit varied severity with sclerosis, fragmentation, and flattening in the longitudinal axis of the navicular, consistent with necrosis (Fig. 173-7). Scintigraphy shows decreased to absent flow in all three phases with localization to the navicular. MRI reveals findings of necrosis with abnormal bone marrow signal and no enhancement after gadolinium administration. The disease resolves with normal radiographic configuration of the navicular bone in several months to 4 years. Treatment is symptomatic and ranges from arch support to casting for patients with more severe pain. Köhler disease has an excellent prognosis with no predisposition to degenerative changes in adulthood; if pain recurs, it is usually the result of other abnormalities such as coalition.

Köhler disease should be differentiated from the asymptomatic delayed, irregular ossification of the tarsal

navicular that can occur during normal development. The normal ossific nucleus develops at between 18 and 24 months in girls and between 30 to 36 months in boys. Different from Köhler disease, developmental ossification irregularity is seen in younger children, is often bilateral and symmetric, and is not associated with symptoms.

> The differential diagnosis of Köhler disease includes irregular ossification, a normal developmental variant.

PANNER DISEASE

Panner disease consists of avascular necrosis of the capitellum of the humerus that usually follows trauma from repeated valgus stress to the elbow. It occurs in athletic patients younger than 10 years, more commonly in young baseball players and gymnasts. It presents with lateral epicondylar pain and decreased range of motion. Radiographically, the capitellum reveals irregular mineralization, sclerosis, and fragmentation; less severe changes may be seen in the radial head (Fig. 173-8). MRI exhibits findings associated with avascular necrosis, and coexistent effusion may be noted. Differential diagnosis of lateral elbow pain in this patient population includes osteochondritis dissecans and traumatic osteochondral fracture. Although the prognosis is usually favorable, Panner disease is important to recognize because it may result in joint incongruity and secondary degenerative changes in the elbow. Treatment includes restricted activity and rest; surgery is needed if loose osteochondral fragments are present.

FREIBERG DISEASE

Avascular necrosis of the second metatarsal head is called Freiberg disease. It occurs predominantly in girls aged 8 to 17 years and is likely related to chronic repetitive trauma that causes ischemia and avascular necrosis, perhaps as the result of wearing high-heeled shoes. Similar lesions can occur in other metatarsals, and associated stress fractures may be seen in either foot. Radiographs show a superficial lucency in the epiphysis of the second metatarsal head that progresses to sclerosis and fragmentation. Pinhole scintigraphy and MRI reveal avascular necrosis (Fig. 173-9). The metatarsal head may heal with a flattened configuration. In some cases, associated loose fragments require removal for relief of symptomatic pain. Osteotomy can be performed to create a new area of articulation between the metatarsal and the proximal phalanx.

KIENBÖCK DISEASE

Osteonecrosis of the lunate, or Kienböck disease, is commonly seen in adult patients from 20 to 40 years of age; it rarely occurs in children younger than 15 years. It may be caused by repetitive trauma and is commonly seen in the wrists of gymnasts and tennis players, as well as in adults who perform repetitive jobs. The blood supply to the lunate is fragile and can be affected by

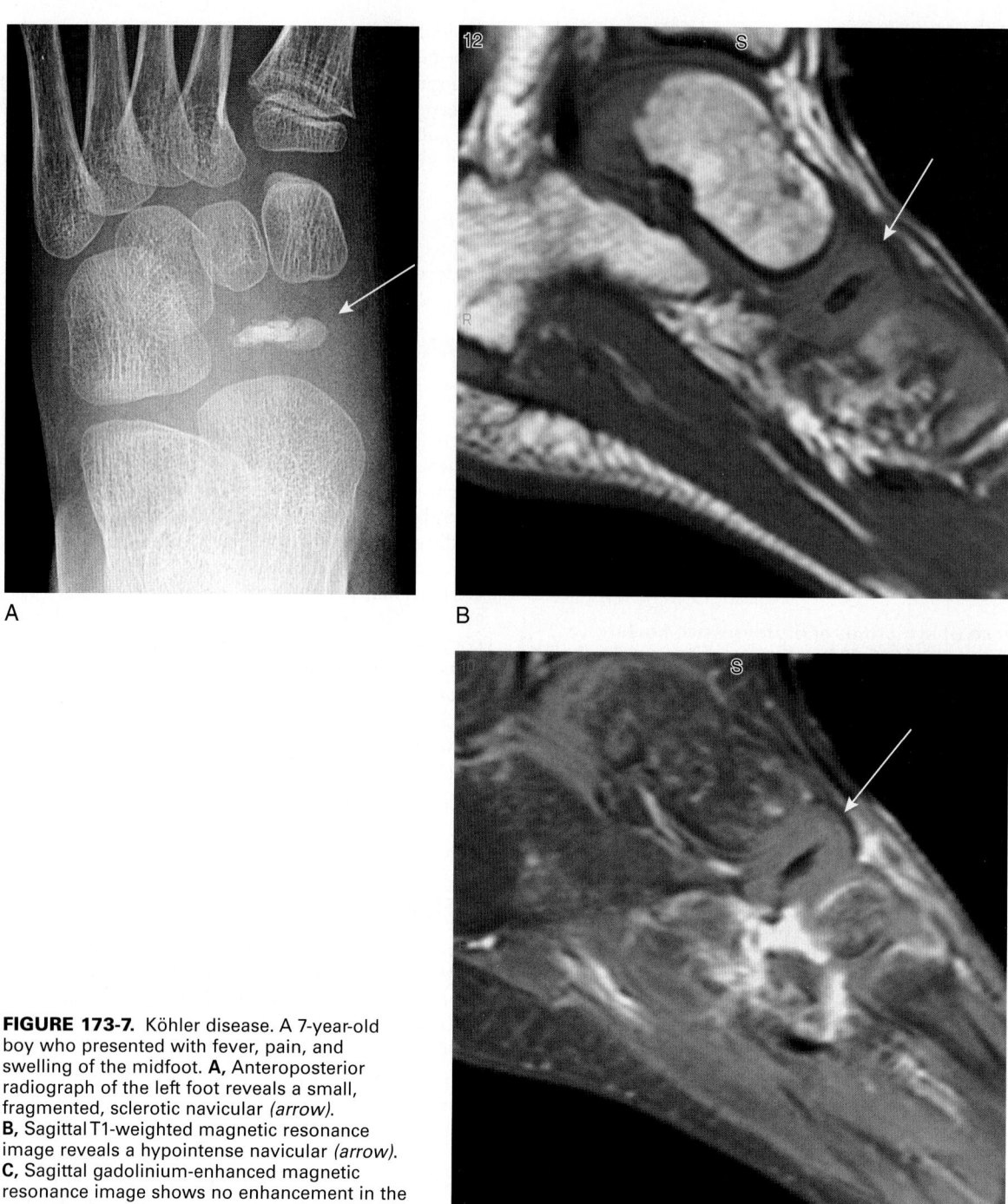

FIGURE 173-7. Köhler disease. A 7-year-old boy who presented with fever, pain, and swelling of the midfoot. **A,** Anteroposterior radiograph of the left foot reveals a small, fragmented, sclerotic navicular *(arrow).* **B,** Sagittal T1-weighted magnetic resonance image reveals a hypointense navicular *(arrow).* **C,** Sagittal gadolinium-enhanced magnetic resonance image shows no enhancement in the navicular *(arrow).*

injury or systemic disease with an associated vasculitis such as systemic lupus erythematosus or long-term corticosteroid use. The role of negative ulnar variance has been debated; it probably does not contribute to the development of lunate avascular necrosis in children. Patients present with pain and decreased range of motion.

Radiographically, the lunate progressively flattens, fragments, and becomes more sclerotic (Fig. 173-10).

Scintigraphy and MRI exhibit avascular necrosis (Fig. 173-11). In older adolescents and adults, the lunate then progresses to collapse, and proximal migration of the capitate results in eventual scapholunate dissociation. In children, healing may readily occur if the extraosseous vascular supply remains intact. Prognosis is dependent on age at presentation, and long-term casting and splinting may be especially beneficial in skeletally immature patients. Advanced deformity may require surgery.

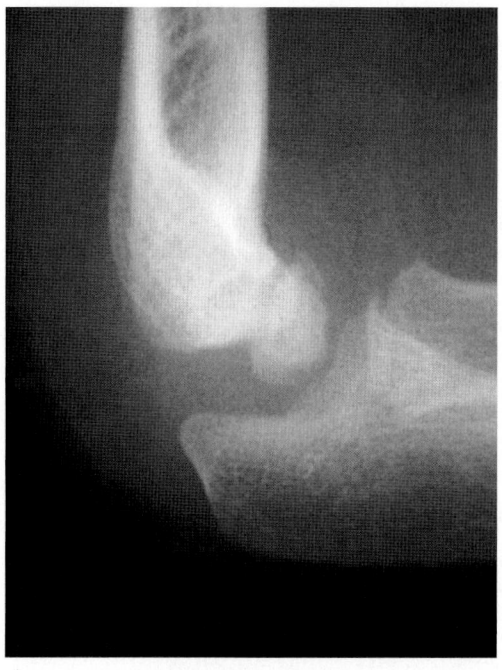

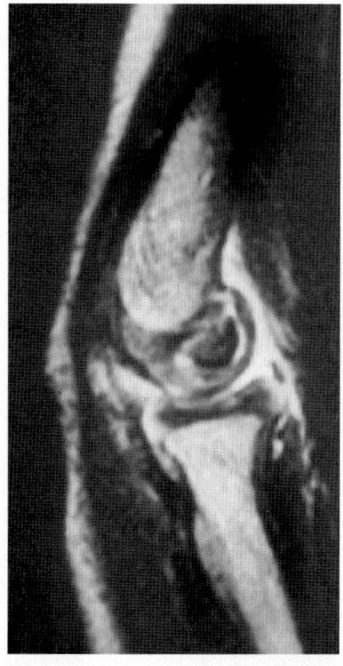

A

B

FIGURE 173-8. Panner disease. A 6-year-old boy with elbow pain. **A,** Lateral radiograph of the elbow shows mild irregularity and sclerosis of the capitellum. The adjacent radial head appears normal. **B,** Sagittal T2-weighted magnetic resonance image of the elbow in extension in the same patient with T2 weighting shows loss of normal fatty marrow signal with hypointensity in the capitellum. There is an associated joint effusion. (Reprinted from Azouz EM, Oudjhane K: Disorders of the upper extremity in children. Magn Reson Imaging Clin N Am 1998:6;677-695.)

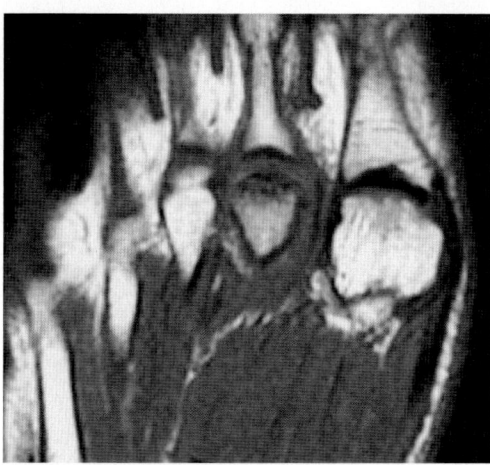

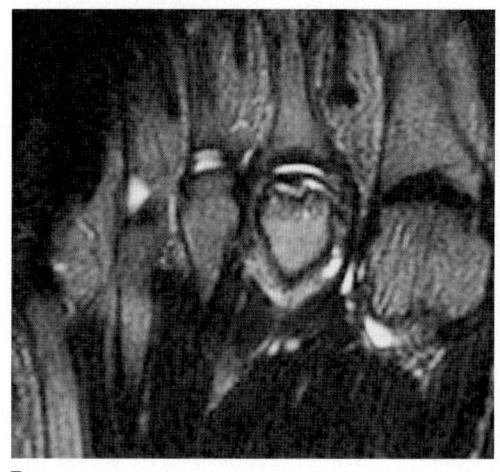

A

B

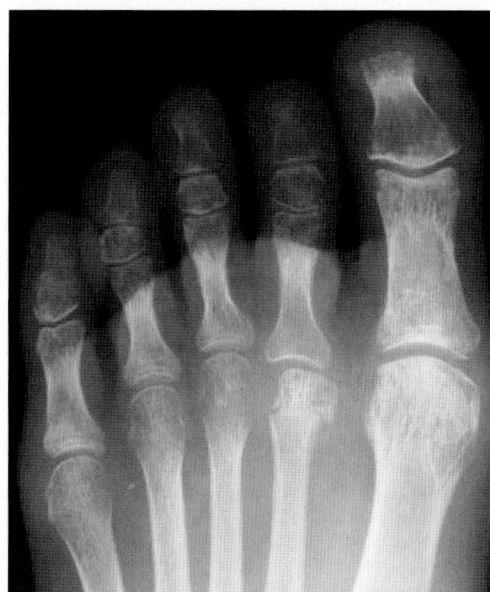

C

FIGURE 173-9. Freiberg disease. A 19-year-old woman who presented with foot pain. **A,** Coronal T1-weighted magnetic resonance image reveals hypointensity in the second metatarsal head with collapse. **B,** Coronal T2-weighted magnetic resonance image shows crescentic hyperintense subchondral fracture of the second metatarsal head. **C,** Frontal radiograph obtained 2 months after magnetic resonance imaging reveals a sclerotic, fractured second metatarsal head. Flattening of the head is noted as well with progression of disease.

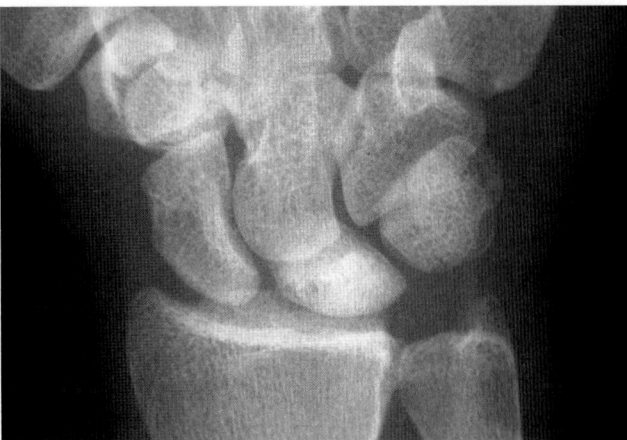

FIGURE 173-10. Kienböck disease. A 16-year-old boy with bilateral wrist pain and a family history of Kienböck disease. Sclerosis is seen in the lunate. Similar findings were present on the contralateral side.

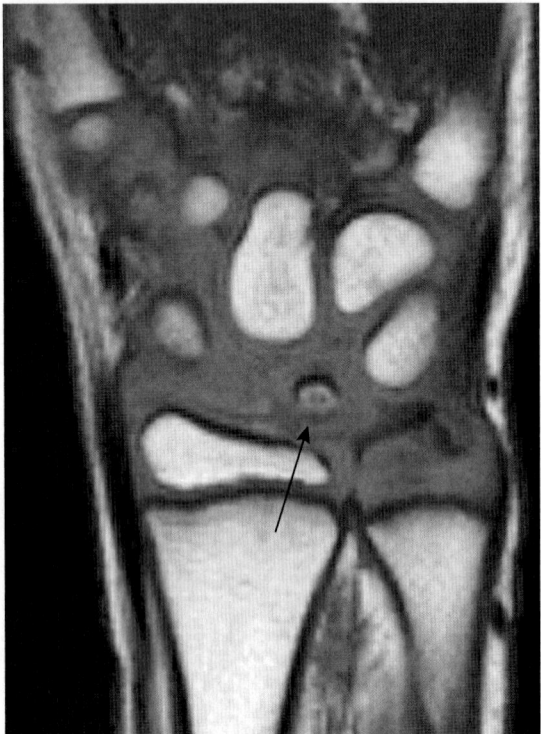

FIGURE 173-11. Kienböck disease. An 8-year-old boy who presented with wrist pain. Coronal T1-weighted magnetic resonance imaging of the left wrist reveals a small lunate *(arrow)* with an area of hypointensity. Some hyperintense bone marrow signal is preserved in the lunate.

SUGGESTED READINGS

General

Brower AC: The osteochondroses. Orthop Clin North Am 1983; 14:99-117

Siffert RS: Classification of the osteochondroses. Clin Orthop Relat Res 1981;158:10-18

Legg-Calvé-Perthes Disease

Barker DJ, Hall AJ: The epidemiology of Perthes' disease. Clin Orthop Relat Res 1986;209:89-94

Bensahel H, Bok B, Cavailloles F, et al: Bone scintigraphy in Perthes disease. J Pediatr Orthop 1983;3:302-305

Caffey J: The early roentgenographic changes in essential coxa plana: their significance in pathogenesis. Am J Roentgenol Radium Ther Nucl Med 1968;103:620-634

Catterall A: Legg-Calve-Perthes syndrome. Clin Orthop Relat Res 1981;41:152-158

Conway JJ: A scintigraphic classification of Legg-Calve-Perthes disease. Semin Nucl Med 1993;23:274-295

De Billy B, Viel JF, Monnet E, et al: Interobserver reliability in the interpretation of radiologic signs in Legg-Calve-Perthes disease. J Pediatr Orthop B 2002;11:10-14

de Sanctis N, Rega AN, Rondinella F: Prognostic evaluation of Legg-Calve-Perthes disease by MRI. Part I: The role of physeal involvement. J Pediatr Orthop 2000;20:455-462

de Sanctis N, Rondinella F: Prognostic evaluation of Legg-Calve-Perthes disease by MRI. Part II: Pathomorphogenesis and new classification. J Pediatr Orthop 2000;20:463-470

Ducou le Pointe H, Haddad S, Silberman B, et al: Legg-Perthes-Calvé disease: staging by MRI using gadolinium. Pediatr Radiol 1994;24:88-91

Eggl H, Drekonja T, Kaiser B, Dorn U: Ultrasonography in the diagnosis of transient synovitis of the hip and Legg-Calve-Perthes disease. J Pediatr Orthop B 1999;8:177-180

Eyring EJ, Bjornson DR, Peterson CA: Early diagnostic and prognostic signs in Legg-Calve-Perthes disease. Am J Roentgenol Radium Ther Nucl Med 1965;93:382-387

Forster MC, Kumar S, Rajan RA et al: Head-at-risk signs in Legg-Calve-Perthes disease: poor inter- and intra-observer reliability. Acta Orthop 2006;77:413-417

Frick SL: Evaluation of the child who has hip pain. Orthop Clin North Am 2006;37:133-140.

Herring JA, Kim HT, Browne R: Legg-Calve-Perthes disease. Part I: Classification of radiographs with use of the modified lateral pillar and Stulberg classifications. J Bone Joint Surg Am 2004; 86:2103-2120

Herring JA, Kim HT, Browne R: Legg-Calve-Perthes disease. Part II: Prospective multicenter study of the effect of treatment on outcome. J Bone Joint Surg Am 2004;86:2121-2134

Herring JA, Neustadt JB, Williams JJ, et al: The lateral pillar classification of Legg-Calve-Perthes disease. J Pediatr Orthop 1992;12:143-150

Hesse B, Kohler G: Does it always have to be Perthes' disease? What is epiphyseal dysplasia? Clin Orthop Relat Res 2003;414:219-227

Jaramillo D, Galen TA, Winalski CS, et al: Legg-Calve-Perthes disease: MR imaging evaluation during manual positioning of the hip-comparison with conventional arthrography. Radiology 1999;212:519-525

Jaramillo D, Kasser JR, Villegas-Medina OL et al: Cartilaginous abnormalities and growth disturbances in Legg-Calve-Perthes disease: evaluation with MR imaging. Radiology 1995;197:767-773

Joseph B, Varghese G, Mulpuri K, et al: Natural evolution of Perthes disease: a study of 610 children under 12 years of age at disease onset. J Pediatr Orthop 2003;23:590-600

Kaniklides C: Diagnostic radiology in Legg-Calve-Perthes disease. Acta Radiol Suppl 1996;406:1-28

Kaniklides C, Lonnerholm T, Moberg A, et al: Legg-Calve-Perthes disease: comparison of conventional radiography, MR imaging, bone scintigraphy and arthrography. Acta Radiol 1995; 36:434-439

Lamer S, Dorgeret S, Khairouni A, et al: Femoral head vascularization in Legg-Calve-Perthes disease: comparison of dynamic gadolinium-enhanced subtraction MRI with bone scintigraphy. Pediatr Radiol 2002;32:580-585

Lappin K, Kealey D, Cosgrove A: Herring classification: how useful is the initial radiograph? J Pediatr Orthop 2002;22:479-482

Loder RT, Farley FA, Herring JA, et al: Bone age determination in children with Legg-Calve-Perthes disease: a comparison of two methods. J Pediatr Orthop 1995;15:90-94

Mahnken AH, Staatz G, Ihme N, et al: MR signal intensity characteristics in Legg-Calve-Perthes disease: value of fat-suppressed (STIR) images and contrast-enhanced T1-weighted images. Acta Radiol 2002;43:329-335

Mandell GA, MacKenzie WG, Scott CI Jr, et al: Identification of avascular necrosis in the dysplastic proximal femoral epiphysis. Skeletal Radiol 1989;18:273-281

Moens P, Fabry G: Legg-Calve-Perthes disease: one century later. Acta Orthop Belg 2003;69:97-103

Nathan Sambandam S, Gul A, Shankar R, et al: Reliability of radiological classifications used in Legg-Calve-Perthes disease. J Pediatr Orthop B 2006;15:267-270

Neyt JG, Weinstein SL, Spratt KF, et al: Stulberg classification system for evaluation of Legg-Calve-Perthes disease: intra-rater and inter-rater reliability. J Bone Joint Surg Am 1999;81:1209-1216

Ponseti IV: Legg-Perthes disease: observations on pathological changes in two cases. J Bone Joint Surg Am 1956;38:739-750

Rush BH, Bramson RT, Ogden JA: Legg-Calve-Perthes disease: detection of cartilaginous and synovial change with MR imaging. Radiology 1988;167:473-476

Scoles PV, Yoon YS, Makley JT, et al: Nuclear magnetic resonance imaging in Legg-Calve-Perthes disease. J Bone Joint Surg Am 1984;66:1357-1363

Sebag G, Ducou Le Pointe H, Klein I, et al: Dynamic gadolinium-enhanced subtraction MR imaging—a simple technique for the early diagnosis of Legg-Calve-Perthes disease: preliminary results. Pediatr Radiol 1997;27:216-220

Stulberg SD, Cooperman DR, Wallensten R: The natural history of Legg-Calve-Perthes disease. J Bone Joint Surg Am 1981;63:1095-1108

Sugimoto Y, Akazawa H, Miyake Y, et al: A new scoring system for Perthes' disease based on combined lateral and posterior pillar classifications. J Bone Joint Surg Br 2004;86:887-891

Thompson GH, Price CT, Roy D, et al: Legg-Calve-Perthes disease: current concepts. Instr Course Lect 2002;51:367-384

Uno A, Hattori T, Noritake K, et al: Legg-Calve-Perthes disease in the evolutionary period: comparison of magnetic resonance imaging with bone scintigraphy. J Pediatr Orthop 1995;15:362-367

Van Campenhout A, Moens P, Fabry G: Serial bone scintigraphy in Legg-Calve-Perthes disease: correlation with the Catterall and Herring classification. J Pediatr Orthop B 2006;15:6-10

Wall EJ: Legg-Calve-Perthes' disease. Curr Opin Pediatr 1999;11:76-79

Weinstein SL: Natural history and treatment outcomes of childhood hip disorders. Clin Orthop Relat Res 1997;344:227-242

Weinstein SL: Legg-Calve-Perthes syndrome. In Morriss RT, Weinstein SL (eds): Lowell and Winter's Pediatric Orthopedics, 5th ed. Philadelphia, PA, Lippincott, Williams and Wilkins, 2001:957-998

Weishaupt D, Exner GU, Hilfiker PR, et al: Dynamic MR imaging of the hip in Legg-Calve-Perthes disease: comparison with arthrography. AJR Am J Roentgenol 2000;174:1635-1637

Wiig O, Terjesen T, Svenningsen S, et al: The epidemiology and aetiology of Perthes' disease in Norway. A nationwide study of 425 patients. J Bone Joint Surg Br 2006;88:1217-1223

Williams GA, Cowell HR: Kohler's disease of the tarsal navicular. Clin Orthop Relat Res 1981;158:53-58

Yrjonen T: Long-term prognosis of Legg-Calve-Perthes disease: a meta-analysis. J Pediatr Orthop B 1999;8:169-172

Meyer Dysplasia

Emmery L, Timmermans J, Leroy JG: Dysplasia epiphysealis capitis femoris? A longitudinal observation. Eur J Pediatr 1983;140:345-347

Harel L, Kornreich L, Ashkenazi S, et al: Meyer dysplasia in the differential diagnosis of hip disease in young children. Arch Pediatr Adolesc Med 1999;153:942-945

Khermosh O, Wientroub S: Dysplasia epiphysealis capitis femoris: Meyer's dysplasia. J Bone Joint Surg Br 1991;73:621-625

Meyer J: Dysplasia epiphysealis capitis femoris: a clinical-radiological syndrome and its relationship to Legg-Calve-Perthes disease. Acta Orthop Scand 1964;34:183-197

Rowe SM, Chung JY, Moon ES, et al: Dysplasia epiphysealis capitis femoris: Meyer dysplasia. J Pediatr Orthop 2005;25:18-21

Specchiulli F, Scialpi L, Mastrorillo G: Meyer's dysplasia epiphysealis. Chir Organi Mov 1996;81:401-405

Köhler Disease

Borges JL, Guille JT, Bowen JR: Köhler's bone disease of the tarsal navicular. J Pediatr Orthop 1995;15:596-598

McCauley RG, Kahn PC: Osteochondritis of the tarsal navicular: radioisotopic appearances. Radiology 1977;123:705-706

Stanton BK, Karlin JM, Scurran BL: Kohler's disease. J Am Podiatr Med Assoc 1992;82:625-629

Panner Disease

Adams JE: Injury to the throwing arm: a study of traumatic changes in the elbow joints of baseball players. Calif Med 1965;102:127-132

Daniel WW: Panner's disease. Arthritis Rheum 1989;32:341-342

Kobayashi K, Burton KJ, Rodner C, et al: Lateral compression injuries in the pediatric elbow: Panner's disease and osteochondritis dissecans of the capitellum. J Am Acad Orthop Surg 2004;12:246-254

Stoane JM, Poplausky MR, Haller JO, et al: Panner's disease: x-ray, MR imaging findings and review of the literature. Comput Med Imaging Graph 1995;19:473-476

Freiberg Disease

Ary KR Jr, Turnbo M: Freiberg's infraction: an osteochondritis of the metatarsal head. J Am Podiatry Assoc 1979;69:131-132

Hoskinson J: Freiberg's disease: a review of the long-term results: Proc R Soc Med 1974;67:106-107

Mandell GA, Harcke HT: Scintigraphic manifestations of infraction of the second metatarsal (Freiberg's disease). J Nucl Med 1987;28:249-251

Kienböck Disease

Allan CH, Joshi A, Lichtman DM: Kienbock's disease: diagnosis and treatment. J Am Acad Orthop Surg 2001;9:128-136

Irisarri C: Aetiology of Kienbock's disease. J Hand Surg 2004;29:281-287

Thienpont E, Mulier T, Rega F, et al: Radiographic analysis of anatomical risk factors for Kienbock's disease. Acta Orthop Belg 2004;70:406-409

Tsuge S, Nakamura R: Anatomical risk factors for Kienbock's disease. J Hand Surg (Br) 1993;18:70-75

Wagner JP, Chung KC: A historical report on Robert Kienbock (1871-1953) and Kienbock's disease. J Hand Surg 2005;30:1117-1121

CHAPTER

174 Alignment Disorders

PETER J. STROUSE and H. THEODORE HARCKE

The bones of the extremities are aligned to best serve the functions required of them by evolutionary change. Malalignment of bony components of limbs may be congenital or acquired. The defect that creates malalignment can be primary to bone or to soft tissue or secondary to neuromuscular disorders. Disorders of alignment may be congenital or acquired. Malalignment is often seen with congenital deformities characterized by embryologic failure of development. These disorders are discussed in Chapter 164. One of the most common alignment disorders is developmental dysplasia of the hip. This entity is discussed separately in Chapter 180.

The reader is referred to Dr. Ozonoff's excellent treatise, *Pediatric Orthopedic Radiology*, for a more detailed discussion than can be presented here regarding many of these alignment disorders.

UPPER EXTREMITIES

Erb Palsy

Erb palsy (or Erb-Duchenne Palsy) is due to birth trauma to the C5 and C6 nerve roots. Infants present soon after birth with decreased motion of the involved extremity. Radiographs serve to exclude fractures. Ultrasonography and magnetic resonance imaging (MRI) have been used to directly evaluate the brachial plexus. Infants may recover from mild injury. Children with a persistent defect will hold their arm in internal rotation with pronation of the forearm and flexion of the wrist. Progressive deformity may be seen at the glenohumeral joint with a small, flattened humeral head that may subluxate relative to a small, shallow, abnormally angulated glenoid (Fig. 174-1). In normal patients, the glenoid is angled approximately 5 degrees posterior relative to a line perpendicular to the axis of the scapular body. With Erb palsy, posterior glenoid version averages 25 degrees. The scapula is hypoplastic and elevated, and the acromion is tapered and inferiorly directed, as is the coracoid. The clavicle is shortened. Many of these findings are seen on radiography; however, computed tomography (CT) or MRI can be used to assess glenoid deformity

and humeral head, that is, glenoid congruence. MRI is preferred in young children (<5 years old) in whom the glenoid is not well ossified. MRI may also show blunting of the labrum. CT shows osseous deformity well in older children (see Fig. 174-1).

Klumpke palsy is due to C7-C8-T1 nerve injury and affects the lower arm. Duchenne-Erb-Klumpke palsy is rarer and is due to C5-T1 nerve root injury. The whole arm is affected and flaccid.

Madelung Deformity

In Madelung deformity, the distal articular surface of the radius is tilted in an ulnar and volar direction. The radius is short and bowed dorsal and lateral ("bayonet deformity"). The distal radial growth plate may fuse prematurely, particularly at its ulnar aspect. Secondary distortion of the carpus is observed. The distal ulna is subluxed. The cause of Madelung deformity is unknown. The process is considered congenital but often does not manifest until late childhood or adolescence. Madelung deformity occurs more often in girls than in boys. Patients may have pain; however, treatment is more often sought because of deformity or limited range of motion. In some patients, the deformity is due to prior trauma or infection that interferes with normal radial growth. A Madelung-like deformity may also be seen in patients with hereditary osteochondromatosis or enchondromatosis, also suggesting a defect in normal distal radial maturation. Other patients have an underlying syndrome in which the deformity is more likely to be bilateral. Madelung deformity is occasionally seen with Turner syndrome and is a characteristic finding in dyschondrosteosis (Léri-Weill disease) (Fig. 174-2). In all, 10% to 15% of cases are familial.

Ulnar Variance

At skeletal maturity, the distal radial and ulnar articular surfaces are nearly at the same level, and the radial styloid projects 9 to 12 mm distal to the ulnar articular surface. With negative ulnar variance, the ulna ends

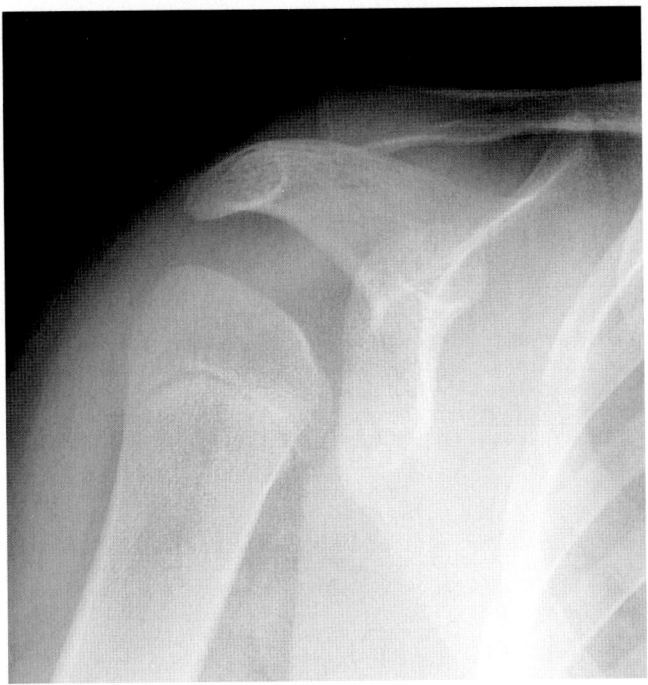

A

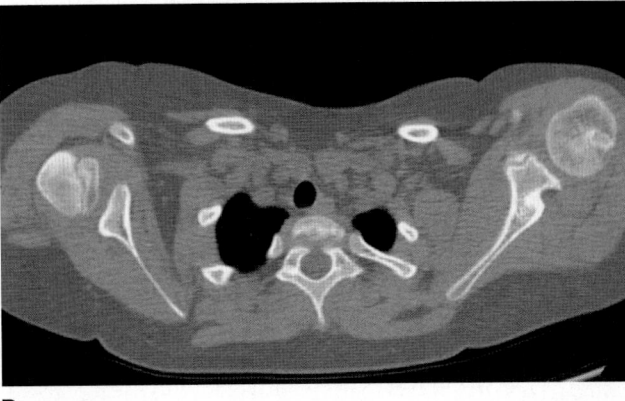

B

FIGURE 174-1. Erb palsy in a 9-year-old girl. **A,** On radiography, the humeral head appears small and abnormally contoured, the glenoid margins are indistinct, and the acromion is curved. **B,** Axial computed tomography shows the right glenoid to be small and retroverted. The right humeral head is small and squared in contour but appears normally located relative to the glenoid.

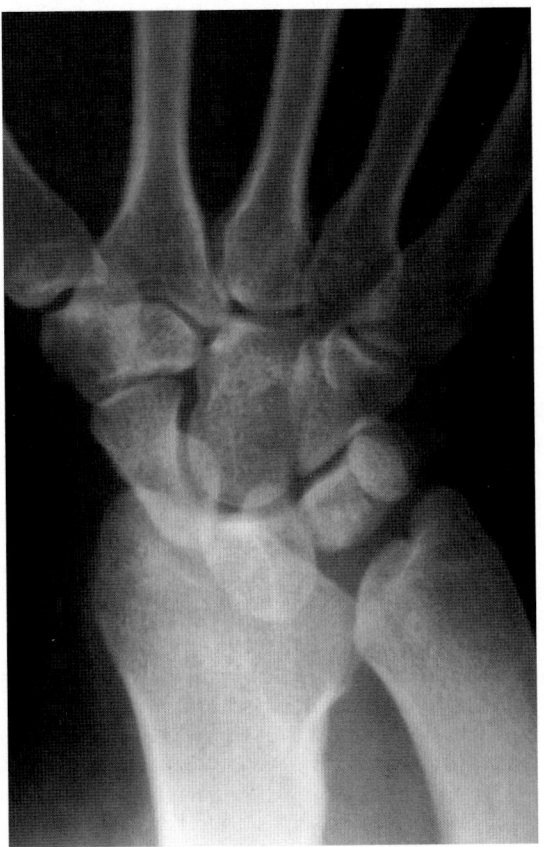

FIGURE 174-2. Madelung deformity in a 22-year-old woman with dyschondrosteosis. The distal radius is shortened medially with tilt of the distal radial articular surface toward the ulna.

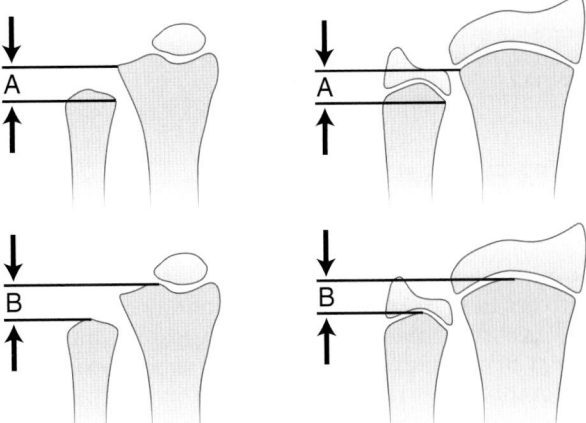

FIGURE 174-3. Method of measuring ulnar variance. A, Distance from the most proximal point of the ulnar metaphysis to the most proximal point of the radial metaphyses; B, distance from the most distal point of the ulnar metaphysis to the most distal point of the radial metaphysis. (Modified from Hafner F, Poznanski AK, Donavan JM. Ulnar variance in children—standard measurements for evaluation of ulnar shortening in juvenile rheumatoid arthritis, hereditary multiple exostosis and other bone and joint disorders of childhood. Skeletal Radiol 1989;18:513-516.)

more proximally, and with positive ulnar variance, the ulna ends more distally (Fig. 174-3). Alignment varies somewhat with age, forearm rotation, wrist deviation, and radiographic angle. Minor malalignment of the distal radial and ulnar articular surfaces is of doubtful significance. Negative ulnar variance is associated with the development of avascular necrosis of the lunate (Kienböck disease). Positive ulnar variance is associated with ulnar impaction syndrome and triangular fibrocartilage complex disruption (Fig. 174-4).

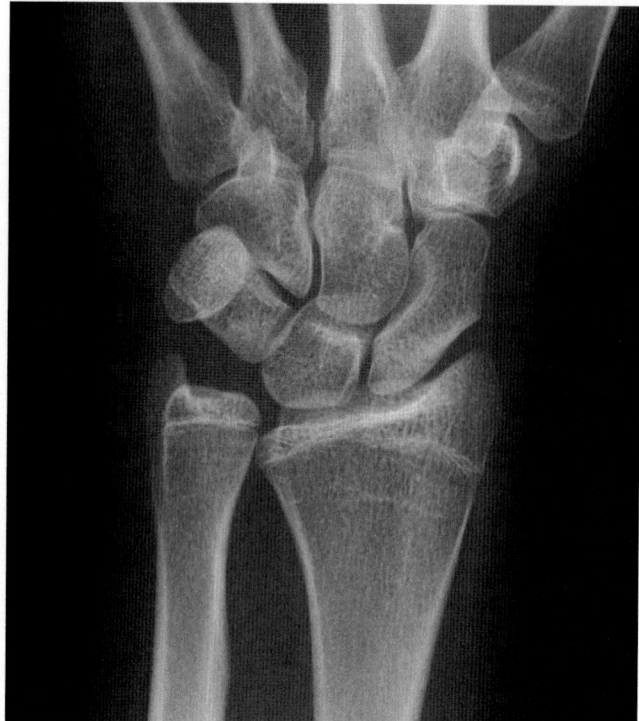

FIGURE 174-4. Positive ulnar variance in a 14-year-old with a history of prior osteomyelitis of the ulna. Presumably, resultant overgrowth of the ulna occurred. The patient required ulnar shortening because of clinical evidence of ulnar impaction syndrome.

LOWER EXTREMITIES

Hip

The normal neck-shaft angle of the proximal femur is approximately 150 degrees at birth and decreases to 120 to 130 degrees in adulthood. The "apparent" neck-shaft angle can be measured on an anteroposterior (AP) radiograph. External/internal rotation of the hip or femoral anteversion may affect this measurement. Anteversion is the anterior angulation of the femoral neck within the transverse plane (Fig. 174-5). This can be measured relative to the femoral condyles distally. Normal femoral anteversion is 35 to 50 degrees at birth, decreasing steadily to 10 to 15 degrees in adulthood (Fig. 174-6).

> **Normal femoral anteversion is 35 to 50 degrees at birth, decreasing to 10 to 15 degrees in adulthood.**

Coxa Vara

In coxa vara, the femoral neck-shaft angle is decreased from normal. A measurement below 110 degrees is considered coxa vara. Functional coxa vara occurs with disorders that result in femoral neck shortening, such as trauma, infection, or avascular necrosis. True coxa vara occurs as a congenital anomaly that is due to bone softening (e.g., rickets, osteogenesis imperfecta, fibrous dysplasia) or to abnormal growth (e.g., spondylo-

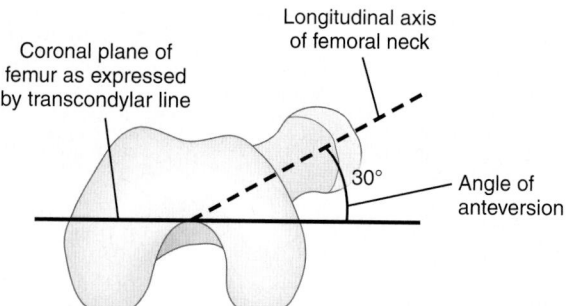

FIGURE 174-5. Schematic diagram of the right femur as viewed from below. The femoral neck is angulated anterior (anteversion) relative to the transcondylar axis of the distal femur. (Modified from: Greenspan A: Orthopedic Imaging: A Practical Approach, 4th ed, Philadelphia, Lippincott Williams & Wilkins, 2004.)

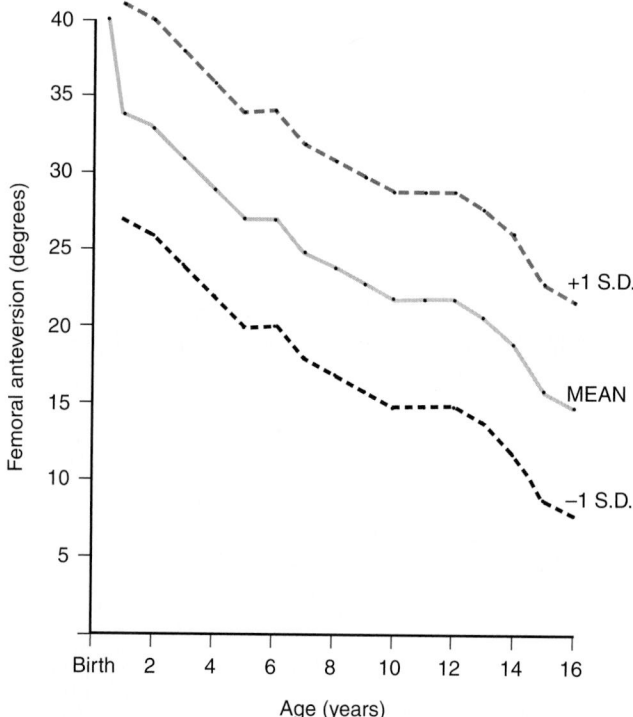

FIGURE 174-6. Normal femoral anteversion. The mean value is an average of those reported by Shands and Steele (1958), Crane (1959), and Fabry and associates (1973). Standard deviations are only an approximation based on the range of those determined by Fabry and associates. (Reprinted from Ozonoff MB: Pediatric Orthopedic Radiology, 2nd ed., Philadelphia, WB Saunders, 1992.)

epiphyseal dysplasia congenita, spondyloepimetaphyseal dysplasia, cleidocranial dysplasia). Children with developmental coxa vara present with a limp (unilateral deformity) or a waddling gate (bilateral deformities). Coxa vara may occur as the result of abnormal growth at the proximal femoral physis that results in abnormal angulation of the physis. Fragmentation and sclerosis may be seen at the medial margin of the proximal femoral metaphysis (Fig. 174-7).

Coxa vara may be subclassified as congenital, infantile, or acquired. The congenital form occurs with a congenital short femur (i.e., proximal focal femoral deficiency)

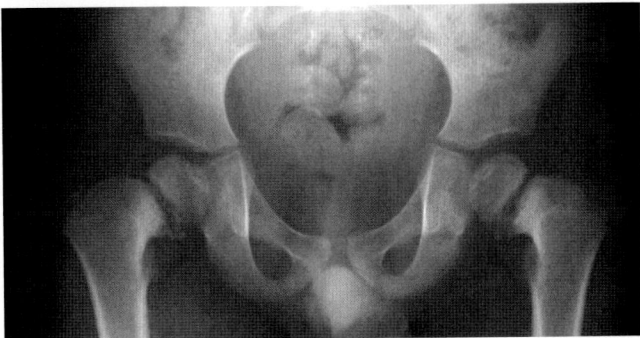

FIGURE 174-7. Bilateral congenital coxa vara in a 4-year-old boy. Proximal femoral growth plates are tilted, medial side down. Slight fragmentation is noted at the medial aspect of each proximal femoral growth plate.

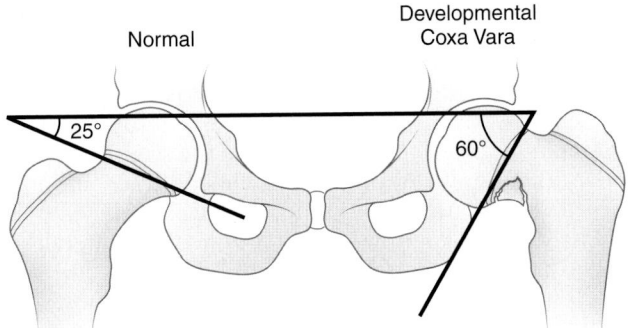

FIGURE 174-8. The Hilgenreiner epiphyseal angle is created by a single line through the triradiated cartilage and its intersection with another line through the physes. The normal angle is about 25 degrees. (Reprinted from Beals RK: Coxa vara in childhood: evaluation and management. J Am Acad Orthop Surg 1998;6:93-99.)

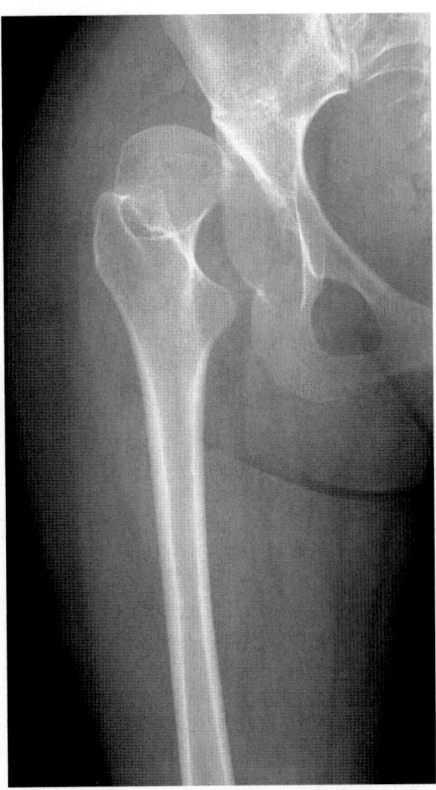

FIGURE 174-9. A 15-year-old girl with cerebral palsy. The acetabulum is markedly dysplastic. The femoral head is subluxed. Coxa valga is noted, and the lesser trochanter is hypertrophied.

and does not spontaneously resolve. With infantile or developmental coxa vara, the hip is normal at birth, and deformity is noted when the child begins to walk. Infantile coxa vara may be self-limited. Acquired coxa vara is related to another process such as trauma.

The Hilgenreiner epiphyseal angle is the angle between the Hilgenreiner line and a line drawn through the physis (Fig. 174-8). If less than 45 degrees, progression is unlikely. If over 60 degrees, progression is likely. If 45 to 60 degrees, prognosis is less predictable.

COXA VALGA

With coxa valga, the neck-shaft angle of the proximal femur is abnormally high. Because development of the proximal femur is reliant on normal weight bearing, coxa valga is most often seen in patients who are non-ambulatory and nonerect, such as those with cerebral palsy and other neuromuscular disorders (Fig. 174-9). External rotation may mimic coxa valga and can be differentiated through the positioning of the greater trochanter. With external rotation, the greater trochanter projects through the femur, whereas with true coxa valga, it is located laterally.

> **External rotation may mimic coxa valga.**

FEMORAL ANTEVERSION

Increased femoral anteversion may hinder proper localization of the femoral head relative to the acetabulum. Increased femoral anteversion is seen in hip deformity due to developmental dysplasia of the hip, Legg-Calvé-Perthes disease, and cerebral palsy. With increased anteversion, in-toeing of the feet is noted. Femoral anteversion can be estimated by physical examination techniques, or more precisely, by CT. On CT, femoral anteversion is the angle between the axis of the femoral neck and the transcondylar axis at the distal femur (Fig. 174-10). Limited low-dose axial images are needed. Femoral anteversion can also be measured with ultrasonography or MRI.

Leg

TIBIAL TORSION

Tibial torsion is the degree of rotation of the distal end of the tibia relative to the upper end of the tibia. Newborns have internal tibial torsion relative to older children and adults. Internal tibial torsion is thus the most common cause of in-toeing in the preschool age group. Normal values are 4 degrees of external rotation as a newborn, which progresses to 15 to 20 degrees of external rotation as an adult. Lack of normal progression results in in-toeing. Surgery is rarely needed because more than 95% of cases resolve spontaneously, usually by 8 years of age. Tibial torsion can be assessed by physical examination. It also can be assessed through limited low-dose axial images on CT. Tibial torsion is best measured as the angle between the posterior surface of the proximal tibia and a bimalleolar line distally. Tibial torsion can also be measured with ultrasonography or MRI.

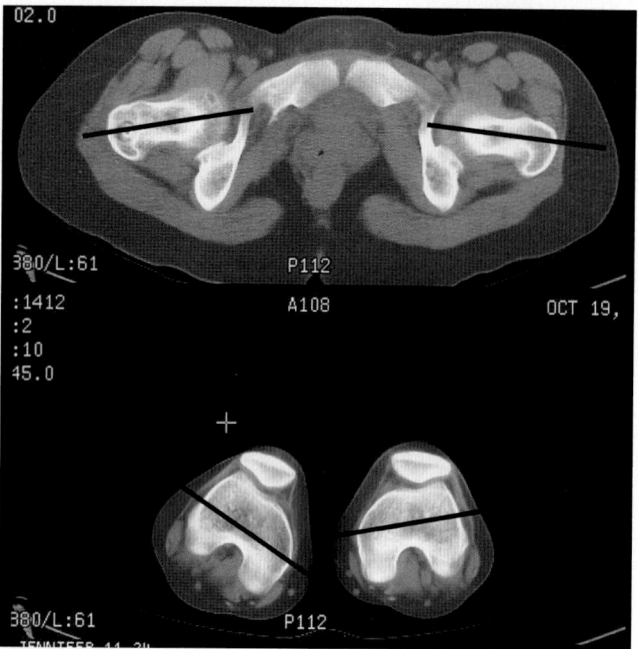

FIGURE 174-10. Computed tomography method for assessing femoral anteversion in a 17-year-old girl with a history of right femoral fracture. Lines denote the axes of the femoral necks and the transcondylar axes of the distal femora. An angle of 49 degrees of anteversion was measured on the right and an angle of 14 degrees on the left.

BOWLEG

Bowleg deformity (genu varum) is manifest by separation of the knees when the legs are placed in anatomic position. A variety of pathologic causes may be identified, including rickets, osteogenesis imperfecta, neurofibromatosis, skeletal dysplasias (i.e., camptomelic dysplasia, achondroplasia), congenital bowing, Blount disease, and, occasionally, growth plate trauma. However, most lateral bowing in otherwise normal infants and children younger than 2 years of age is normal and developmental ("physiologic") and resolves without treatment. It is important to recognize physiologic bowing as a normal process. Ozonoff details the following findings as characteristic of physiologic lower extremity bowing:

• The tibia is abducted relative to the femur, and both bones are intrinsically bowed laterally. Relative tibial torsion produces external rotation of the upper tibia relative to the distal tibia.
• Margins of the distal femoral and proximal tibial metaphyses are mildly accentuated with small beaks.
• Medial cortices of the tibia and femur are thickened.
• Distal femoral and proximal tibial epiphyses are not well ossified medially and are wedge shaped.
• The distal tibial growth plate may be tilted lateral.

Radiographically, the femur and the tibia are also mildly bowed anteriorly, and beaking is posterior (Fig. 174-11). Physiologic bowing is usually more marked in the tibias, but occasionally, bowing may almost exclusively result from lateral bowing of the distal femur (Fig. 174-12). The varus deformity is common in normal infants and converts to valgus between 18 and 36 months of age (Fig. 174-13). Degree of valgus reduces spontan-

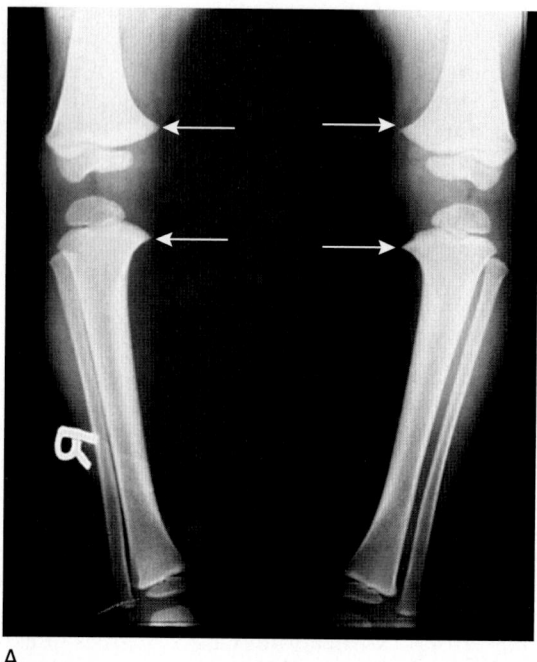

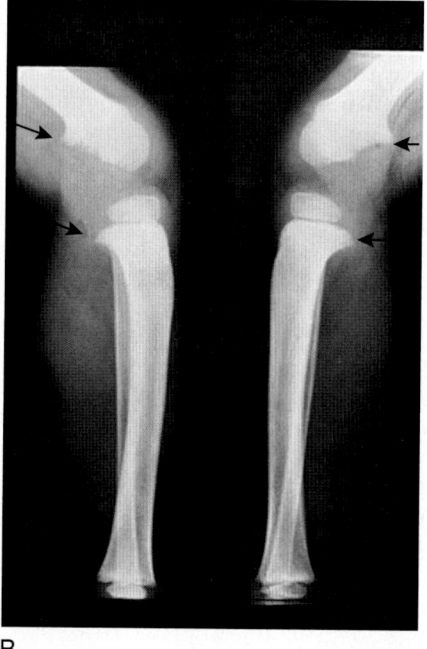

A   B

FIGURE 174-11. A, Bilateral idiopathic bowed legs (frontal projection) in a boy 22 months of age. *Arrows* point to the medial beaking of the femoral and tibial metaphyses at the knees. The increased stress of weight bearing has thickened the medial and dorsal cortical walls of the tibias inward. The femoral epiphyseal ossification centers are much too small, especially in their medial halves, which are under greater stress of weight bearing when the legs are bowed. **B,** Lateral projection. *Arrows* point to dorsal beaking of the femoral and tibial metaphyses. After correction of bowed legs, these "stress" phenomena disappear after several months.

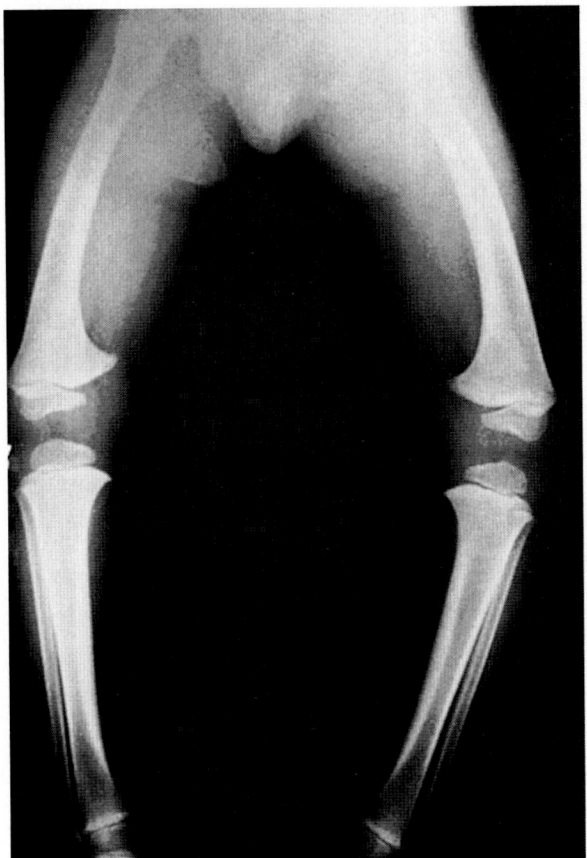
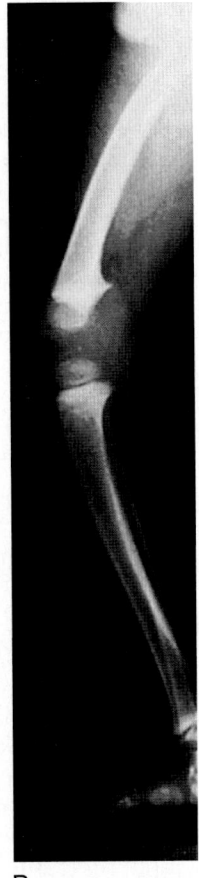

A

B

FIGURE 174-12. Femoral bowed legs (femora vara): endogenous stress trauma at the knees without weight bearing. **A,** Frontal projection shows marked bowlegs, in which the tibias are straight and both femora are bowed abruptly laterad near their distal ends (femora vara). Femoral epiphyseal ossification centers are small and flattened on their medial halves. **B,** On lateral projection, the right tibia is straight, but the femur is bowed ventrad near its distal end, and a spur projects dorsad from the same level of the femoral shaft. When possible, a frontal projection of the leg should be obtained with the patient standing and the ankles in apposition.

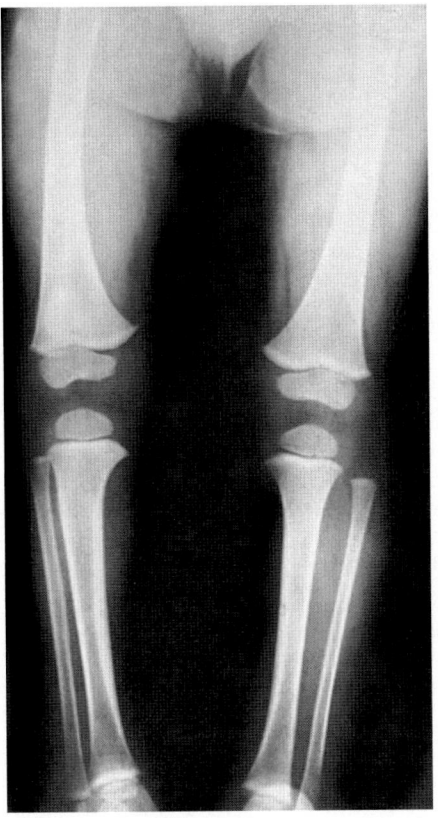
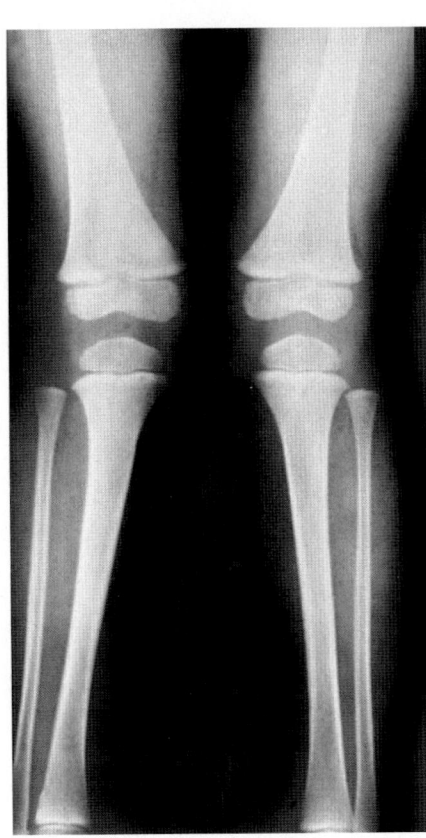

A

B

FIGURE 174-13. Spontaneous conversion of bowed legs to knock-knees. **A,** At 21 months, both femora and both tibias are bowed laterad. **B,** The same patient at 42 months exhibits symmetric knock-knees with wide spreading at the ankles.

eously by 6 to 7 years of age to a mild degree that remains throughout life. Approximate normal angles are 17 degrees varus in a newborn, 9 degrees varus at 1 year, 2 degrees valgus at 2 years, 11 degrees valgus at 3 years, and 5 to 6 degrees valgus at 13 years (Fig. 174-14). Persistent varus with delayed conversion to valgus may indicate a higher likelihood of Blount disease (tibia vara). In the second year, it may be difficult to distinguish normal physiologic bowing from Blount disease. Any varus at the knee after 2 years of age should raise

concern. Exaggerated varus during the second year is likely developmental or physiologic and does not require treatment. Such patients must be followed to exclude progression to Blount disease. Similar to Blount disease, exaggerated physiologic bowing is seen in early walkers, African Americans, and heavier children.

Radiographs should be obtained with the patient bearing weight as soon as he or she is able to stand (Fig. 174-15). The clues to pathologic causes are found principally in the distal ends of the long bones, where changes of rickets are manifest in the growth plate, and changes of dysplasia are reflected by abnormal metaphyseal or epiphyseal development. Serial radiographs are frequently necessary to reveal a pathologic condition, particularly if progressive deformity is due to Blount disease.

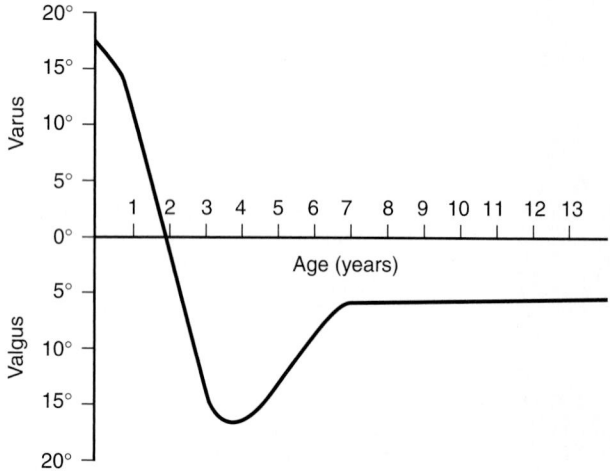

FIGURE 174-14. Development of the tibiofemoral angle during growth. This graph shows the normal physiologic progression of bowlegs to knock-knees and then to normal during the early years of growth. (Reprinted from Bruce RW Jr: Torsional and angular deformities. Pediatr Clin North Am 1996;43:867-881.)

> The most common cause of bowing of the legs in children is physiologic bowing.

BLOUNT DISEASE (TIBIA VARA)

Blount disease (tibia vara; osteochondrosis deformans tibiae) is a progressive deformity that results from changes in the proximal tibia (Fig. 174-16). It is theorized that stress on the posteromedial proximal tibial physis causes growth suppression. Blount disease is diagnosed in only a very small fraction of children assessed for bowing of the legs. Blount disease was initially considered an osteochondrosis or a result of ischemic necrosis of the medial aspect of the proximal tibial epiphysis. Later

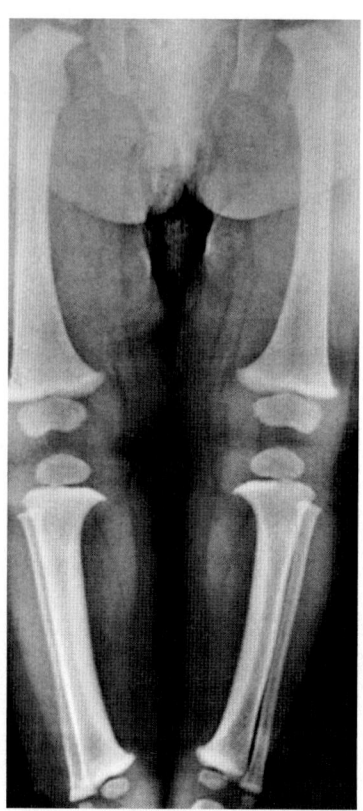

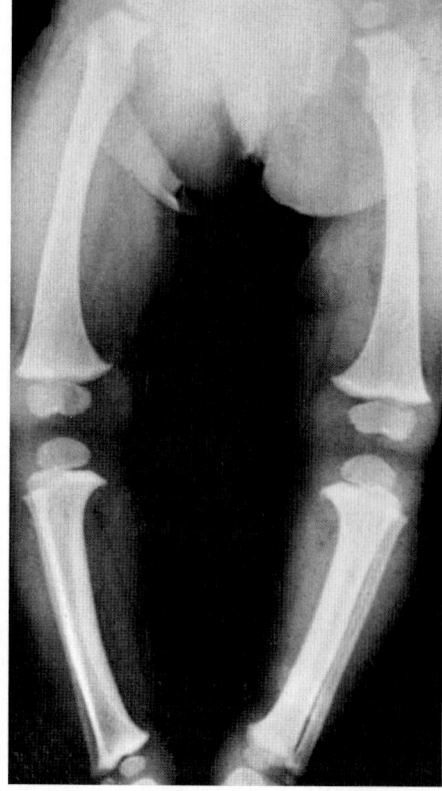

FIGURE 174-15. Bowed legs of a girl 12 months of age who started to walk at 8 months. **A,** In recumbent position, the tibias and femora are bowed, but the legs are not bowed because the knees and ankles are in apposition. **B,** In erect position during weight bearing and with ankles in apposition, the legs are bowed, with a gap of 12 cm at the knees. The real clinical deformity of bowed legs is shown most accurately radiographically when the patient is erect and is bearing weight.

A   B

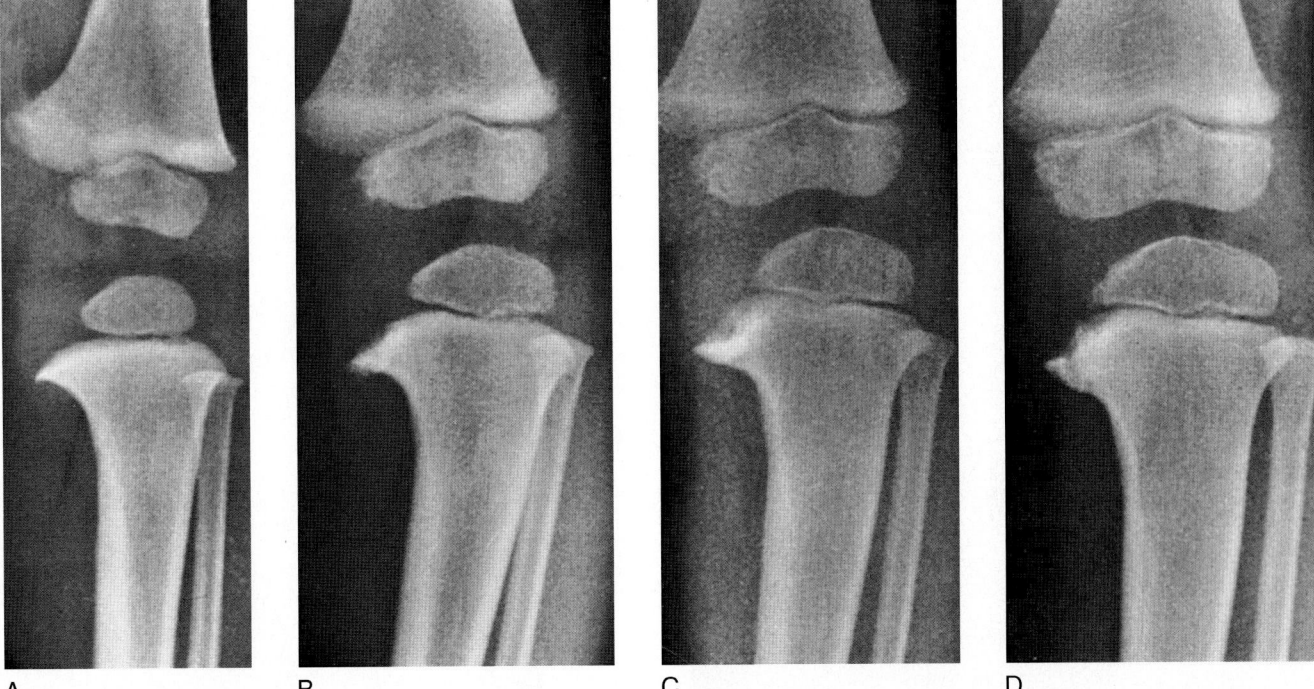

A   B   C   D

FIGURE 174-16. Progressive changes in Blount tibia vara. **A,** At 17 months, the medial segment of the tibial metaphysis is widened and sharpened into a short beak or spur that is bent slightly caudad. **B,** At 26 months, the spur is longer, sharper, and more bent; a radiolucent strip on its upper edge represents noncalcified cartilage. **C,** At 32 months, the amount of cartilage is increased and the spur thickened. **D,** At 38 months, the beak of the spur is displaced caudad, possibly owing to trauma; the medial edge of the ossification center is flattened, and the femur has shifted mediad in relation to the tibia.

evidence, however, indicates that excessive compressive stress at the proximal medial tibial physis alters endochondral bone formation. Pathologic changes are not limited to the growth plate but include abnormalities of growth in the metaphysis, epiphyseal cartilage, and osseous epiphysis. Occasionally, changes can be observed in the opposing femur at the knee (Fig. 174-17). Patients with Blount disease may be divided into those with an infantile form and those with adolescent tibia vara.

The infantile form, which develops in children between 1 and 3 years of age, must be differentiated from developmental bowing. Infantile Blount disease may represent normal developmental bowing that fails to correct and progresses. The diagnosis is made when progressive clinical bowing is seen in the presence of characteristic radiographic changes in the proximal tibia. The disease is typically bilateral (60% to 80%) but is often asymmetric and occasionally unilateral (Fig. 174-18). A family history is often reported. The disorder is more common in early walkers, African Americans, and obese children.

> Infantile Blount disease may represent normal developmental bowing that fails to correct and progresses. The diagnosis is made when progressive clinical bowing is seen in the presence of characteristic radiographic changes in the proximal tibia.

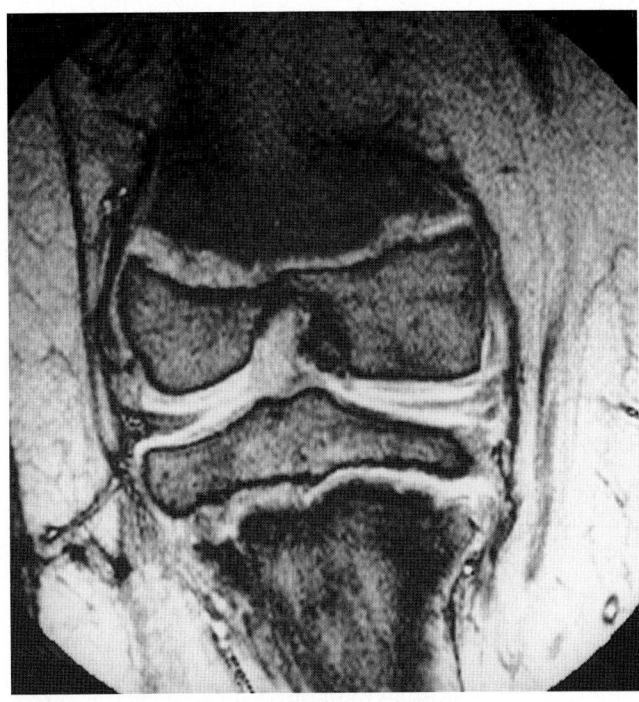

FIGURE 174-17. Growth plate changes in adolescent Blount disease. Gradient-echo coronal magnetic resonance image shows widening and irregularity of the proximal tibial growth plate medially and laterally. Note that the distal femoral growth plate shows changes of a similar nature.

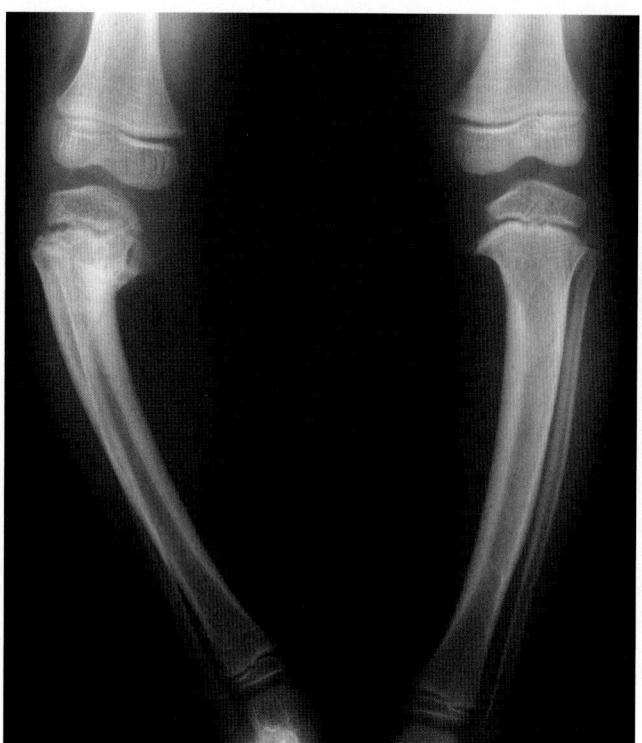

FIGURE 174-18. Bilateral Blount disease in a 3-year-old girl. Abnormality is greater on the right, where more sclerosis and irregularity of the proximal tibial metaphysis are evident.

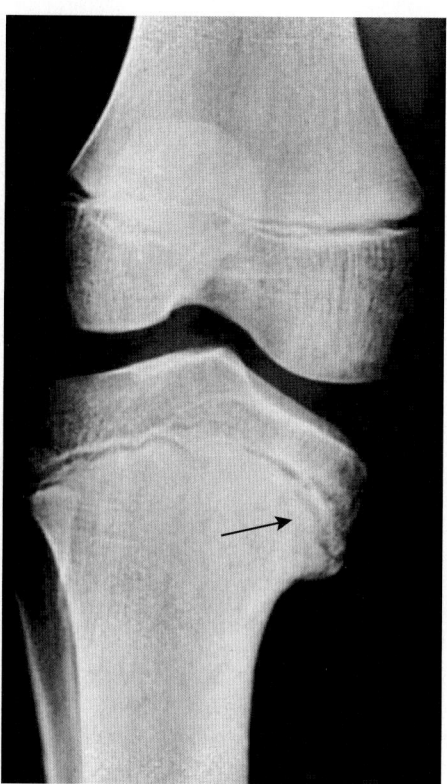

FIGURE 174-19. Blount disease in a 10-year-old girl with right bowleg. Sharp bending of the medial segment of the tibial metaphysis caudad and mediad in tibia vara *(arrow)*. The medial segment of the tibial ossification center has followed the metaphysis caudad. Irregular ossification of the medial metaphysis and early closure of the medial segment of the bent cartilaginous plate are noted. The medial femoral condyle is hypertrophied in compensation for the tibial deformity.

Adolescent or late-onset tibia vara is a separate entity from the infantile form. It occurs in children 8 to 14 years of age; obese African American males of normal height are at particular risk (Fig. 174-19). Adolescent tibia vara is commonly unilateral but may be bilateral. The degree of varus is typically less than that seen with infantile Blount disease. Adolescent Blount disease is slowly progressive and probably results from the repetitive trauma of weight bearing on the medial physis of the proximal tibia. Patients often present with knee pain. It is possible that adolescent Blount disease is due to segmental arrest of the proximal tibial growth plate. The differential diagnosis of unilateral tibial vara includes growth plate injury caused by trauma, focal fibrocartilaginous dysplasia of the proximal tibia, osteochondroma, or enchondroma of the proximal tibia or distal femur.

The characteristic radiographic feature of Blount disease is deformity of the medial metaphysis of the proximal tibia (Fig. 174-20). Irregularity with a more vertically oriented growth plate creates a beaked appearance. The severity of radiographic changes has been described by the six-stage Langenskiöld classification (Fig. 174-21). Higher stage denotes greater abnormality; bone bridging between diaphysis and metaphysis is seen with stage IV and higher. The medial portion of the epiphyseal ossification center is often smaller than the lateral portion. The tibia may subluxate laterally. Prior to the occurrence of tibial metaphyseal changes, it is often impossible to distinguish Blount disease from physiologic bowing. Metaphyseal–diaphyseal angle measurement has been proposed by Levine and Drennan as one method of differentiation. The metaphyseal–diaphyseal angle is measured by drawing a single line through the widest portion of the proximal tibial metaphysis (between the medial and lateral beaks) and another line perpendicular to the long axis of the tibia. With physiologic bowing, this angle measures approximately 5 degrees, whereas with Blount disease, average angle measurement is 16 degrees (Fig. 174-22). A metaphyseal–diaphyseal angle greater than 11 degrees is considered suggestive Blount disease. However, several studies have questioned the validity of the metaphyseal–diaphyseal angle, and measurement may be affected by tibial rotation.

Although spontaneous resolution of infantile Blount disease is reported in some instances, treatment with bracing is begun usually between ages 18 and 24 months and is continued during waking hours for an average of 2 years. If conservative management fails, the patient may undergo a realignment osteotomy, which is most effective when performed before 5 years of age. For adolescent Blount disease, the customary surgical procedure is a proximal tibial valgus osteotomy to produce normal alignment.

Cross-sectional modalities and scintigraphy are occasionally employed in the evaluation of bowleg. CT or MRI can assess the degree of proximal tibial growth plate fusion. Cartilage-sensitive MRI sequences display the cartilage model of the proximal tibial epiphysis. Focal

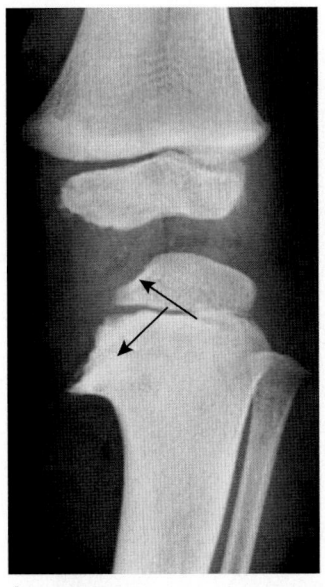
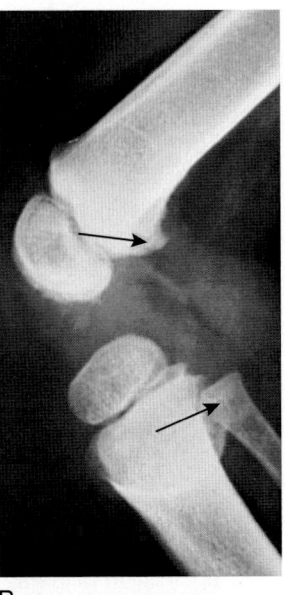

A   B

FIGURE 174-20. Blount tibia vara in a girl, 2½ years of age, who had pronounced lateral bowing of the left leg. **A,** In frontal projection, the medial end of the tibial ossification center *(upper arrow)* is flattened into a slope in place of the normal convex curve at this site. This is a hypoplasia of the medial segment of the bony nucleus rather than destruction by ischemic necrosis. The metaphysis is widened mediad by a broad horizontal spur that is roughened on its medial edge *(lower arrow),* where the previously bony terminal segment of the spur has been replaced by a radiolucent cartilage. The lateral cortical wall is not bent at the level of the medial wall. **B,** In lateral projection, spurs *(arrows)* project dorsad from the dorsal walls of the femoral and tibial shafts.

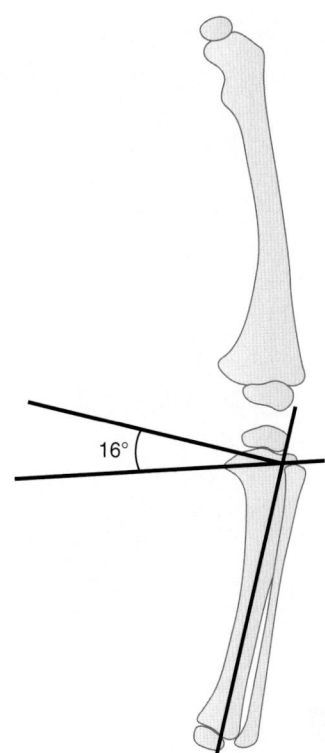

FIGURE 174-22. The metaphyseal–diaphyseal angle is defined as the angle between a line perpendicular to the axis of the tibia and a line through the most distal ossified beak of the medial and lateral beak of the tibial metaphysis. (Reprinted from Eggert P, Viemann M: Physiological bowlegs or infantile Blount's disease: some new aspects to an old problem. Pediatr Radiol 1996; 26:349-352.)

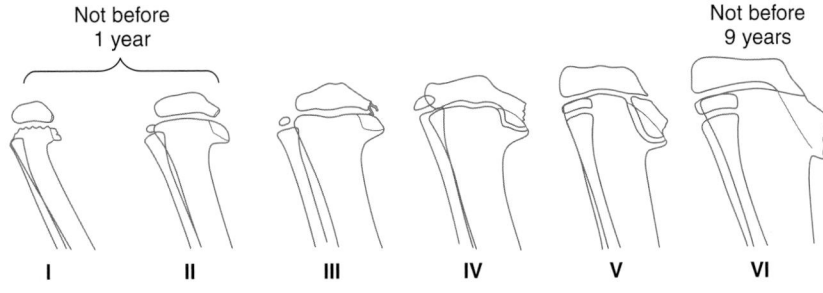

Not before 1 year

Not before 9 years

I   II   III   IV   V   VI

FIGURE 174-21. Diagram of radiographic changes seen in infantile tibia vara and their development with increasing age. (Reprinted from Langenskiöld A, Riska E: Tibia vara [osteochondrosis deformans tibiae]. J Bone Joint Surg Am 1964;46:1405-1420.)

increased activity on bone scans may help distinguish Blount disease from physiologic change.

FOCAL FIBROCARTILAGINOUS DYSPLASIA

Focal fibrocartilaginous dysplasia (FFD) is due to a rest of fibrocartilaginous tissue in the cortex of the metaphysis or metadiaphysis. On radiography, a scalloped defect with associated cortical thickening is seen with mild angulation of the bone (Fig. 174-23). On MRI, the defect appears as low signal on T1 and T2 images. FFD is most common in the proximal medial tibia near the pes anserinus insertion. Resultant varus angulation may be confused with Blount disease; however, the deformity from FFD is centered farther distal. The epiphysis and the metaphysis appear normal. Less common sites include the distal femur, proximal humerus, and distal

ulna. In 45% of tibial cases, spontaneous resolution of deformity occurs. Spontaneous resolution may be less notable with femoral and humeral lesions; however, outcomes data are limited for these sites.

KNOCK-KNEE

In knock-knee (genu valgum), the lower legs deviate laterally when the knees are placed in anatomic position. Wide separation is noted at the ankles (Fig. 174-24). As was noted in the preceding discussion of bowleg deformity, genu valgum is a normal developmental phase that lasts from 2 to 12 years age and is most apparent at 3 to 4 years of age in normal children. Persistent knock-knee can be related to pathologic causes such as trauma, skeletal dysplasia, obesity, metabolic disease, or laxity of muscles and ligaments. Renal osteodystrophy is said to

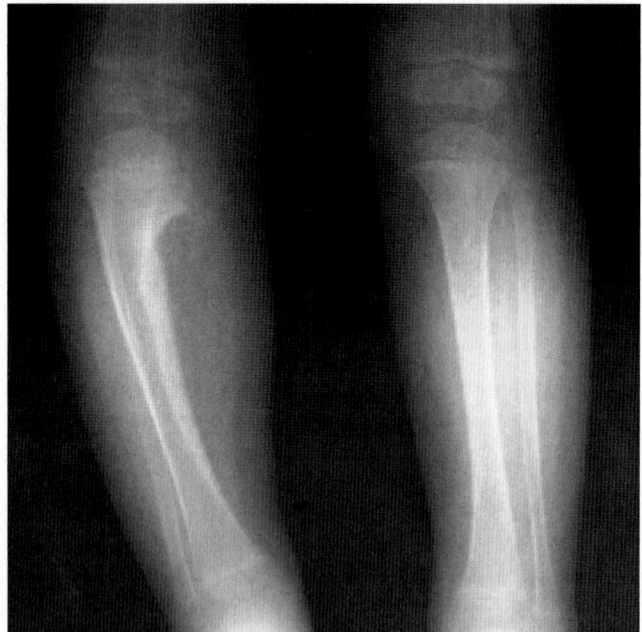

FIGURE 174-23. Focal fibrocartilaginous dysplasia in a 2-year-old boy. The proximal right tibia appears scalloped medially with adjacent cortical thickening and slight angular deformity compared with the left tibia.

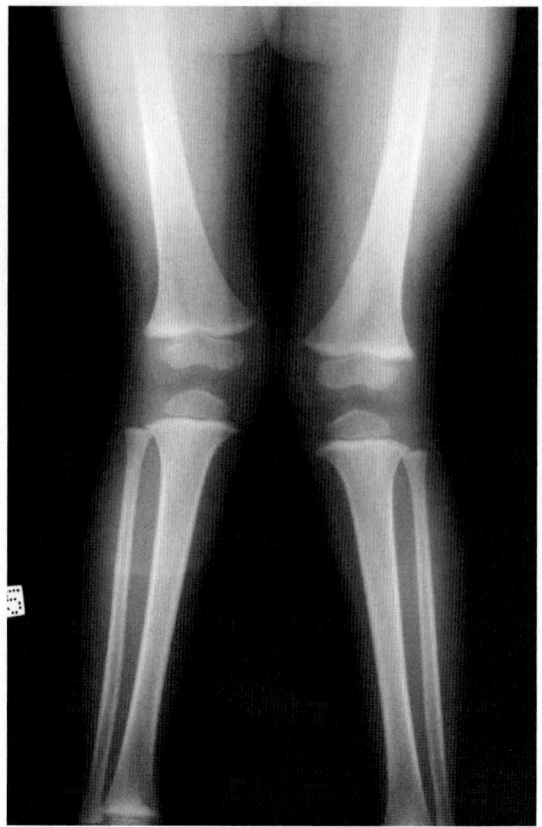

FIGURE 174-24. Physiologic knock-knee in a 3-year-old girl. In follow-up, the child's legs straightened normally, without treatment.

be the most common cause of pathologic bilateral genu valgum. Knock-knee may also be related to a foot or ankle deformity. External tibial torsion may be associated with genu valgum, so that when the patella is placed straight ahead, the feet are externally rotated.

Unilateral tibia valga may be noted after tibial metaphyseal fracture. Even when fracture does not involve the growth plate, progressive valgus deformity develops despite adequate postreduction alignment. Many mechanisms have been postulated regarding growth plate effects and soft tissue changes.

> Genu valgum (knock-knee) is a normal developmental phase that lasts from 2 to 12 years of age and is most apparent at 3 to 4 years of age in normal children.

CONGENITAL DISLOCATION OF THE KNEE

Congenital dislocation of the knee is 80 times less common than congenital hip dislocation. Congenital malalignment of the knee is actually a continuum of hyperextension, subluxation, and dislocation. Associated events are arthrogryposis, Larsen syndrome, myelodysplasia, developmental dysplasia of the hip, clubfoot, and breech birth. The cause may be a congenital postural deformity or a malformation due to an intrinsic problem within the developing knee. Many cases are characterized by atrophy, fibrosis, and shortening of the quadriceps muscle and tendon. Deformity of the knee is frankly obvious clinically. Ultrasonography or MRI may be helpful in assessing the cartilaginous structures of the knee and the quadriceps tendon.

ABNORMAL PATELLAR TRACKING

The spectrum of patellar tracking abnormalities ranges from congenital dislocation of the patella at birth to milder tracking abnormalities that occur during adolescence and in young adults.

Congenital dislocation of the patella may be irreducible. Ultrasonography is diagnostic. In developmental patellar dislocation, the dislocation is reducible. The patella drifts laterally with flexion. Findings are evident when the infant begins to walk. Milder forms of patellar instability present during adolescence with recurrent subluxation or dislocation and are much more common in girls than in boys. Patellar tracking abnormalities are associated with syndromes that produce ligamentous laxity and with excess genu valgum (Fig. 174-25).

With normal valgus of the knee, the patella normally tends toward lateral displacement. This force is counterbalanced by the retaining force of the vastus medialis. Predisposing factors toward lateral patellar subluxation include increased genu valgus, increased femoral anteversion, increased tibial torsion, an abnormally lateral location of the tibial tuberosity, a shallow patellar sulcus on the distal femur, and increased laxity (e.g., Down syndrome, Marfan syndrome). Vigorous athletic activity may accentuate symptoms. Girls approaching the age of puberty are most affected. Radiographic findings consist of lateral subluxation of the patella, a longer than normal patellar tendon (patella alta), a shallow patellar

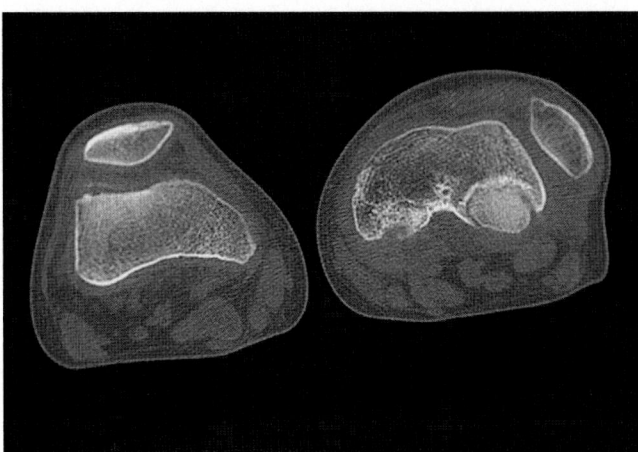

FIGURE 174-25. Chronic patellar dislocation in an 11-year-old boy with Down syndrome. Axial computed tomography image shows that the left patella is dislocated laterally. Both patellar sulci appear shallow.

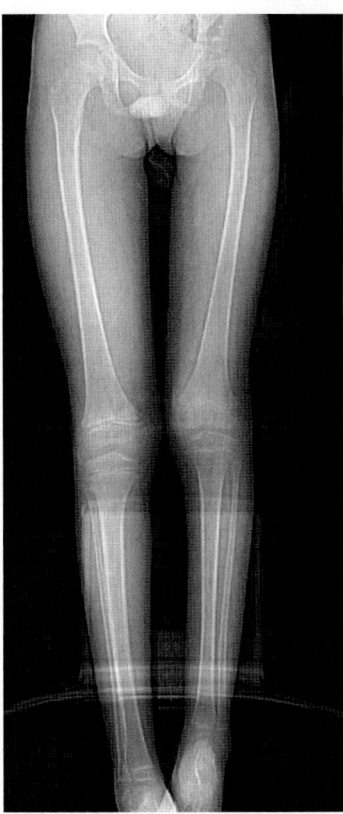

FIGURE 174-26. Leg length determination by computed tomography scout image in a 7-year-old boy with hemiplegia and leg length discrepancy. The left leg is shorter.

groove, and an abnormally faceted patella. A variety of axial views have been used; however, the usefulness of a single axial view in assessing a dynamic process is limited. Insufficiency of the patellar groove and abnormality of the patellar facets may be better appreciated with CT or MRI. Cross-sectional imaging can be used to track patellar motion and to assess for subluxation.

Abnormal patellar tracking often presents as knee pain. Traumatic transient patellar dislocation is another manifestation of abnormal patellofemoral congruence. This injury is discussed in Chapter 172.

LEG LENGTH DISCREPANCY

A leg length discrepancy of less than 1 cm is considered within normal limits; however, in most normal individuals, the legs are within 1 mm of each other in length. The presence of a leg length discrepancy may reflect overgrowth of the long limb or decreased size or growth of the short limb. Leg length discrepancy is often of clinical significance because of associated alteration of gait and resultant pelvic tilt. With significant pelvic tilt, secondary compensatory scoliosis may develop.

The differential diagnoses for overgrowth and undergrowth are too numerous to list here. Overgrowth is associated with a number of syndromes and vascular abnormalities. Mild overgrowth may occur as the result of fracture healing. In many cases, the cause is unknown. Undergrowth may be due to hypoplasia or aplasia of a segment of the limb. Acquired shortening most often occurs as a consequence of premature growth plate fusion due to trauma, infection, or vascular insufficiency.

Radiographic techniques seek to determine bone lengths in a manner that minimizes magnification and other technical factors. A standard method should be used to assess leg length inequality. The technique of orthoroentgenography uses three separate exposures collimated to the hip, knee, and ankle and made on a single image that contains a radiopaque ruler. CT digital scout images have been used to measure bone length (Fig. 174-26). These are limited by field size and are subject to errors in cursor placement on a small image.

In the literature, tables and graphs project future growth on the basis of current size and maturation. Maturation is best assessed as bone age through the standards of Greulich and Pyle or others; however, variability in the assignment of bone age limits accuracy.

Mild leg length discrepancy does not warrant treatment. More severe discrepancies are treated. The type of treatment varies with the age of the child, the amount of projected growth remaining, the site of abnormality, and the degree of leg length discrepancy. With the Ilizarov procedure, bone on either side of a diaphyseal corticotomy is distracted slowly. New bone forms within the gap to add length.

> A leg length discrepancy of less than 1 cm is considered within normal limits; however, in most normal individuals, the legs are within 1 mm of each other in length.

Feet

Alignment disorders of the foot occur on an idiopathic basis or are due to a large number of underlying disorders. The standard method of radiologic evaluation of the foot involves weight-bearing or simulated weight-bearing anteroposterior (dorsoventral) and lateral views. The talus, which is more proximal, is considered fixed at the ankle because it has no musculotendinous attachments of its own. The calcaneus, which is more distal,

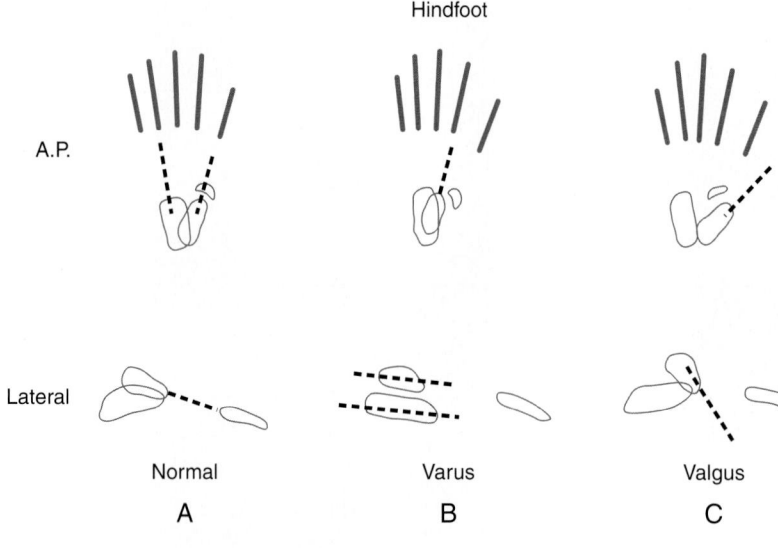

Hindfoot

A.P.

Lateral

Normal   Varus   Valgus
  A   B   C

FIGURE 174-27. Diagrammatic representation of hindfoot and forefoot relationships in the anteroposterior (A.P.) and lateral projections. **A,** Normal hindfoot. The talar axial line intersects or points slightly medial to the first metatarsal base. The navicular is situated directly opposite the head of the talus. The calcaneus points toward the fourth metatarsal base, forming a definable angle with the talus. On the lateral projection, the anterior portion of the talus is slightly plantarflexed, and the calcaneus is slightly dorsiflexed. The talar axial line points down the shaft of the first metatarsal. **B,** Hindfoot varus. The talocalcaneal angle is decreased, with these two bones more parallel to each other and actually superimposed. The navicular is medially displaced, and the axial talar line points lateral to the first metatarsal base. On lateral projection, the calcaneus and the talus are more horizontal and parallel to each other. **C,** Hindfoot valgus. The talocalcaneal angle is increased, with the navicular and other midfoot bones displaced lateral to the talus. The talar axial line passes medial to the first metatarsal base. On lateral projection, the talus is more vertical than normal. (Reprinted from Ozonoff MB: Pediatric Orthopedic Radiology, 2nd ed. Philadelphia, WB Saunders, 1992.)

is linked to the midfoot and forefoot and moves as a unit with these structures relative to the talus. In a normal foot, on the anteroposterior view, the axis of the talus extends through the base of the first metatarsal (Fig. 174-27). With hindfoot varus, the more distal calcaneus is angulated inward, and the axis of the talus passes lateral to the base of the first metatarsal. With hindfoot valgus, the more distal calcaneus is angulated outward, and the axis of the talus passes medial to the base of the first metatarsal. The normal lateral talocalcaneal angle is approximately 45 degrees, decreasing to 30 degrees in older children and adults. With hindfoot varus, the lateral talocalcaneal angle is decreased, whereas with hindfoot valgus, the angle is increased. Normal elevation of the middle metatarsals relative to the fifth metatarsal reflects the transverse arch of the foot. The anterior calcaneus is slightly inclined upward. Accentuation of this upward inclination is called "calcaneus" position of the hindfoot. Equinus is downward inclination of the distal calcaneus. Normal calcaneal tilt and normal slight downward tilt of the distal metatarsals create slight longitudinal concavity in the osseous contour of the bottom of the foot.

When foot deformity is assessed, the talus is proximal, and the calcaneus and the rest of the foot are distal. In varus, the calcaneus is angulated medial relative to the talus. In valgus, the calcaneus is angulated lateral relative to the talus.

CLUBFOOT

Talipes ("talus" = ankle; "pes" = foot) equinovarus, or clubfoot, is a common congenital anomaly that is clinically obvious at birth. It is also commonly identified on prenatal sonography and MRI. The principal components of clubfoot deformity include plantar flexion of the ankle (equinus), inversion of the heel (varus), and adduction of the forefoot (varus) (Fig. 174-28). Abnormal intrauterine pressures contribute to the development of clubfoot. Genetics also appears to play a role, with a

higher than normal incidence of the deformity reported in first-degree relatives. Most congenital clubfeet are supple, and the condition is managed conservatively with serial casting. For very stiff, inflexible clubfeet and those that fail to respond to conservative treatment, operative reduction is required.

Anteroposterior and lateral views permit determination of talocalcaneal angulation, which is a commonly used method for grading the extent of deformity and monitoring treatment. An AP radiograph shows superimposition and parallelism of the talus on the calcaneus with the talar axis directed lateral to the first metatarsal (hindfoot varus). Parallelism of the talus and calcaneus is also seen on a lateral view. The lateral view shows plantarflexion of the calcaneus (equinus) and a step-ladder arrangement of the metatarsals, with the first metatarsal highest and the fifth metatarsal at the weight-bearing surface of the foot. Ultrasonography has been used in select centers to assess the flexibility of clubfoot and to guide therapeutic decision making (Fig. 174-29).

Anatomic deformities persist after treatment of clubfoot and should be recognized as children grow. Many clubfeet have small, squared tali with flattened heads, decreased talocalcaneal angles, subtalar joint changes, and medial displacement of the navicular. Valgus deformity may result from overcorrection.

CONGENITAL VERTICAL TALUS

Congenital vertical talus (congenital rigid flatfoot) may be an isolated condition or may be seen in association with various syndromes (e.g., trisomies) or other systemic abnormalities (i.e., central nervous system defects, arthrogryposis, and neurofibromatosis). The talus is almost completely vertical in this condition (parallel with the longitudinal axis of the tibia), and the calcaneus is fixed in plantarflexion (equinus) (Fig. 174-30). In the AP projection, the talar axis is medial to the base of the first metatarsal (valgus). The navicular dislocates dorsally, and clinically, a pronated rocker-bottom foot is present.

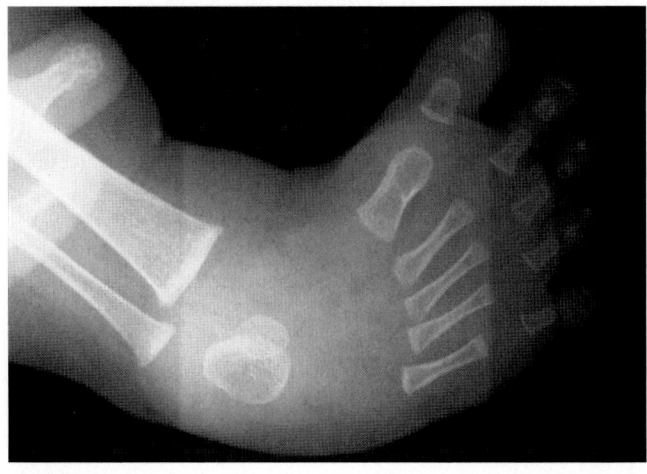
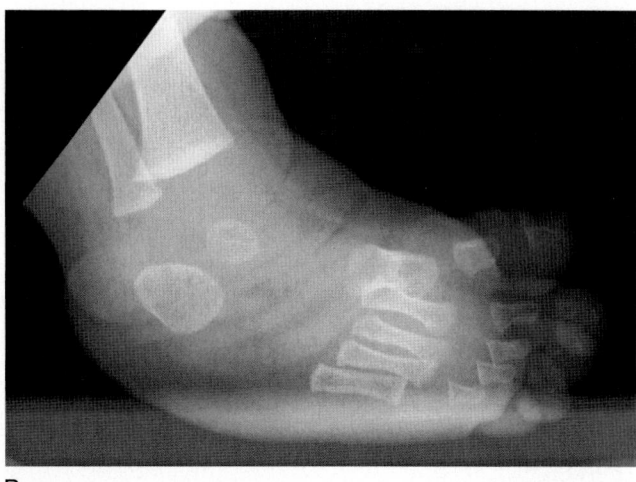

FIGURE 174-28. Radiographs of congenital clubfoot obtained with simulated weight bearing. **A,** Note inversion and forefoot adduction in the anteroposterior view. **B,** Inversion on the lateral view shows "laddering" of the metatarsals. Equinus of the hindfoot and parallelism of the talus and calcaneus are evident.

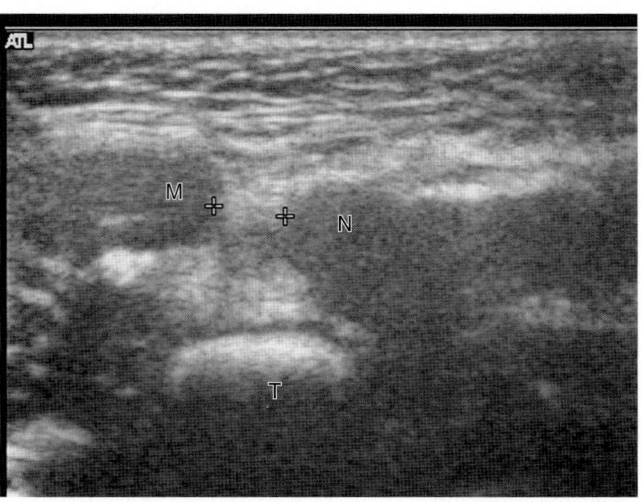
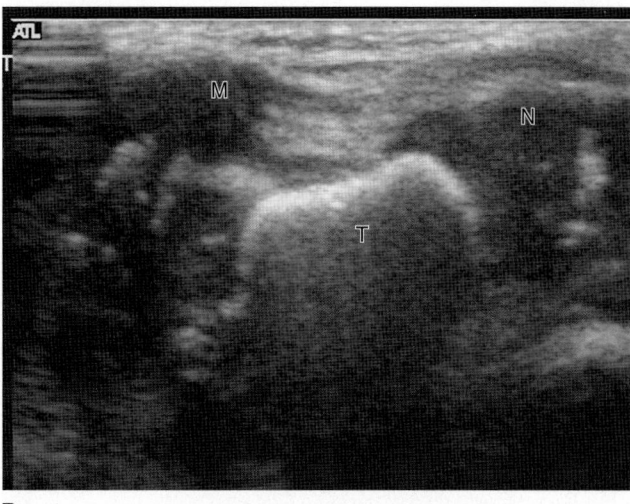

FIGURE 174-29. Ultrasonography of clubfoot in a 6-month-old girl: longitudinal scans at the medial aspect of the feet. **A,** In the clubfoot, the cartilaginous navicular (N) and the medial malleolus (M) are closely spaced *(cursors).* These structures overlie the talus (T), which is ossified. **B,** In the normal foot, the navicular and the medial malleolus are widely spaced, and the talus is not covered. The distance between the navicular and the medial malleolus is an indicator of the severity of deformity and can be followed over time. Dynamic assessment reveals the flexibility of the deformed clubfoot. (Courtesy of Dr. M. A. DiPietro, Ann Arbor, MI.)

After the navicular ossifies, its abnormal position helps to distinguish congenital vertical talus from severe planovalgus or flatfoot deformity. Prior to ossification, the position of the navicular can be determined by ultrasonography.

METATARSUS VARUS (ADDUCTUS)

Metatarsus adductus is another cause of in-toeing that is usually seen in children younger than 5 years of age. Forefoot adduction differs from clubfoot in that midfoot and hindfoot relationships are normally maintained. This condition commonly disappears with normal maturation and no treatment. The affected foot has a C-shaped contour on examination. Forefoot adduction also can occur as a result of excessive internal tibial torsion or increased femoral neck anteversion. On AP (simulated) weight-bearing radiographs, the metatarsals are adducted and hindfoot alignment is normal.

SKEWFOOT

In skewfoot (Z-foot; serpentine metatarsus adductus), the forefoot is adducted and the hindfoot is in valgus, resulting in a "Z"-like distortion of the bones of the foot (Fig. 174-31). Skewfoot is considered a severe form of metatarsus adductus. It is not congenital but develops in the young child. Skewfoot is common in otherwise normal children and also occurs in children with cerebral palsy.

FLATFOOT (PES PLANUS)

Flatfoot (pes planus) is a descriptive term. The differential diagnosis of pes planus includes flexible planovalgus

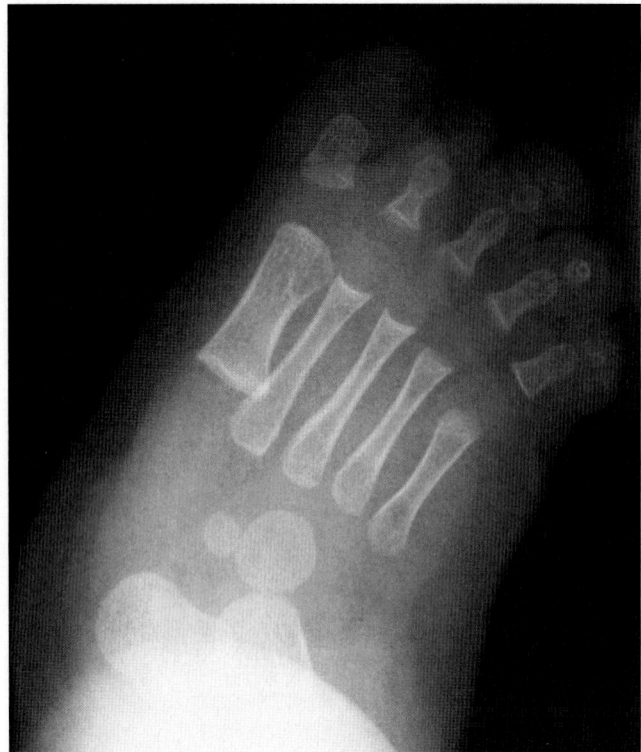

A

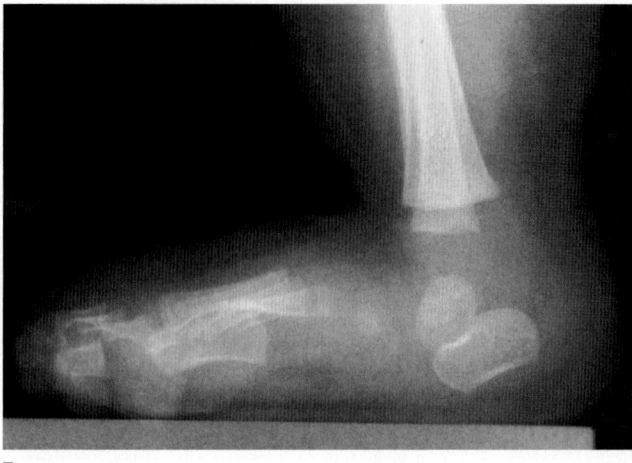

B

FIGURE 174-30. Congenital vertical talus in 7-month-old boy. **A,** In the anteroposterior view, the axis of the talus projects well medial to the base of the first metatarsal, consistent with hindfoot valgus. **B,** In the lateral view, the talus is nearly vertical in orientation, and the calcaneus is plantarflexed.

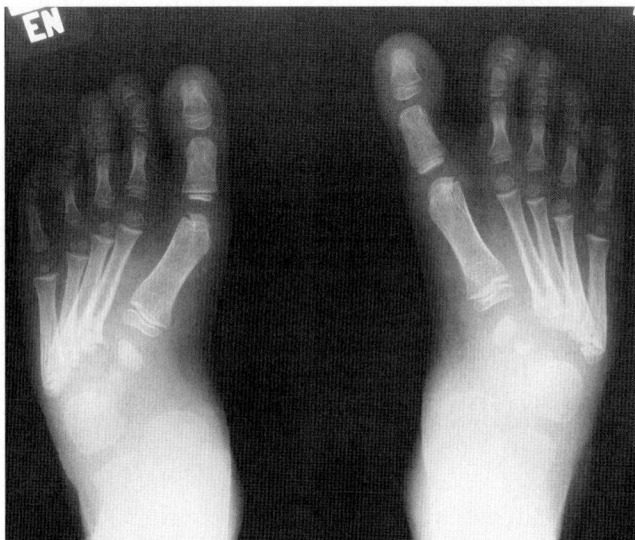

FIGURE 174-31. Bilateral skewfoot in a 4-year-old boy. The forefeet are abducted and the hindfeet are in valgus, resulting in a "Z"-like appearance of the feet.

foot, peroneal spastic (rigid) flatfoot related to tarsal coalition, congenital vertical talus (congenital rigid flatfoot), and congenital calcaneovalgus (congenital flexible flatfoot).

The common flatfoot is a painless, flexible planovalgus foot. Variable degrees of hindfoot valgus, plantar arch flattening, and forefoot pronation occur. Pathology is thought to involve excess ligamentous laxity, which allows the calcaneus to shift into a valgus position under the talus. Abduction and eversion result from loss of

calcaneal support. The AP projection shows the talocalcaneal angle to be increased as the result of abduction of the calcaneus. The midtalar line passes medial to the first metatarsal. On the lateral projection, hindfoot valgus causes the talus to be more vertical than normal. The navicular is normally located relative to the calcaneus. The calcaneus and metatarsals are horizontal longitudinally, and loss of the plantar arch is noted. Similar deformity may occur in some children with cerebral palsy (Fig. 174-32).

With rigid or painful flatfoot (peroneal spastic flatfoot), CT may be performed to detect subtalar coalition. Patients may develop peroneal muscle spasm and pain caused by irritation. Tarsal coalition is discussed in Chapter 164.

CALCANEOVALGUS

Calcaneovalgus feet are reflective of intrauterine positioning. A total of 30% to 50% of newborns have mild calcaneovalgus deformity. In severe congenital calcaneovalgus, the foot is dorsiflexed against the talus. Radiographs show the hindfoot in severe valgus position with a plantarflexed talus. The navicular is not dislocated. The defect is flexible and correctable.

ROCKER-BOTTOM FOOT

In rocker-bottom foot, the calcaneus is in equinus position and the metatarsals are dorsiflexed, producing a convex surface on the bottom of the foot. Rocker-bottom foot is seen with congenital vertical talus and severe cerebral palsy with hindfoot valgus, and it occurs as a complication of incorrectly treated clubfoot with persistent equinus.

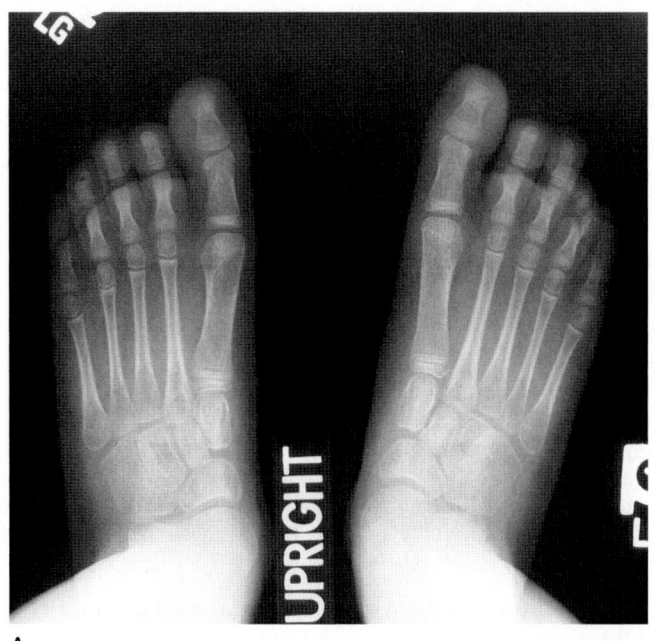

A

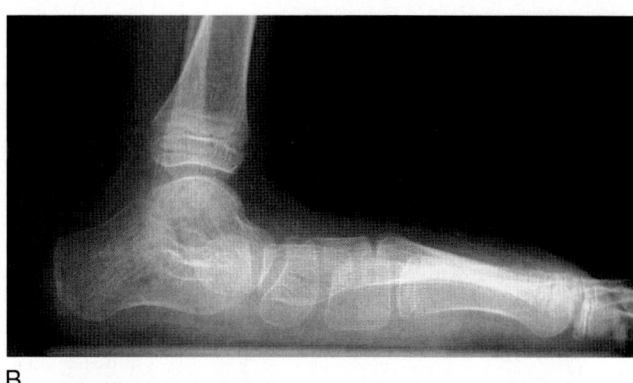

B

FIGURE 174-32. Bilateral planovalgus feet in a 9-year-old with cerebral palsy. **A,** In the anteroposterior view, hindfoot valgus is symmetric. **B,** Lateral view of the right foot shows pes planus with a mild increase in the lateral talocalcaneal angle, also consistent with hindfoot valgus. The calcaneus is horizontal in orientation.

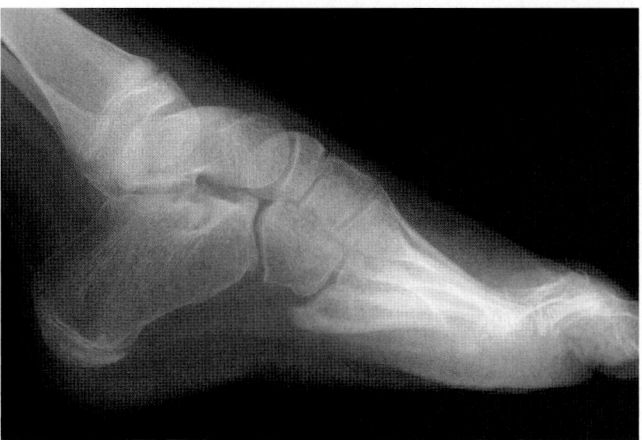

FIGURE 174-33. Marked pes cavus in an 11-year-old girl with Charcot-Marie-Tooth peroneal muscular atrophy. The talocalcaneal angle is increased, and the longitudinal arch is elevated. The metatarsophalangeal joints are extended, and the interphalangeal joints are flexed (hammertoe deformity).

CAVUS FOOT

In pes cavus, the longitudinal plantar arch is deepened. The anterior calcaneus is abnormally dorsiflexed and the metatarsals are plantarflexed (Fig. 174-33). Although an idiopathic congenital form of cavus foot exists, more commonly the finding is related to neuromuscular abnormalities. MRI of the spinal cord or central nervous system may be indicated. Differential diagnoses include peroneal muscular atrophy (Charcot-Marie-Tooth disease), Friedreich ataxia, myelomeningocele, poliomyelitis, and other paralytic conditions.

HALLUX VALGUS

Hallux valgus usually manifests during adulthood, but the deformity begins to develop and may occasionally present in childhood. Hallux valgus affects females 10 times as frequently as males. Patients present with pain and deformity that may interfere with proper shoe fitting. The upper normal limit of medial angulation of the proximal phalanx of the great toe to the first metatarsal is 14 to 16 degrees. Higher angles are considered hallux valgus (Fig. 174-34). With increasing angulation, the medial margin of the first metatarsal head may become more uncovered and protuberant.

GENERALIZED DISORDERS

Cerebral Palsy

Cerebral palsy is the consequence of injury to areas of the immature brain that control neuromuscular function. Although cerebral palsy is a static encephalopathy, resultant musculoskeletal disease may be progressive. Variable manifestations of cerebral palsy are due to variation in severity and location of the original insult. In most cases, cerebral palsy is the consequence of fetal or perinatal insult to the brain, usually hypoxic-ischemic or hemorrhagic in nature. Cerebral palsy also occurs as the result of injury to the brain matter that occurs during early childhood. A wide variety of skeletal deformities, malalignments, and dysfunction may occur. Most of these disorders are the result of imbalanced muscular forces.

Among patients with cerebral palsy, 25% have scoliosis. Scoliosis is more prevalent and severe with greater neurologic deficit. With spastic quadriplegia, 60% to 75% have scoliosis. Scoliosis occurs as the result of imbalanced forces on the two sides of the spinal column. As opposed to the S-shaped curves of idiopathic scoliosis, curves in cerebral palsy often have a long C-shaped contour. As opposed to idiopathic forms, scoliosis related to cerebral palsy may continue to progress after skeletal maturation. Associated findings may include accentuated thoracic kyphosis or lumbar lordosis,

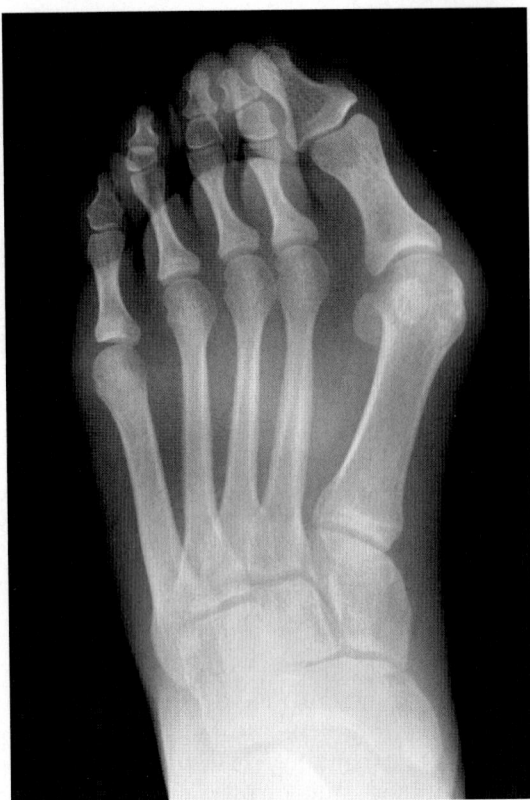

FIGURE 174-34. Hallux valgus in a 14-year-old girl. Slight sclerosis is present in the medial aspect of the first metatarsal head.

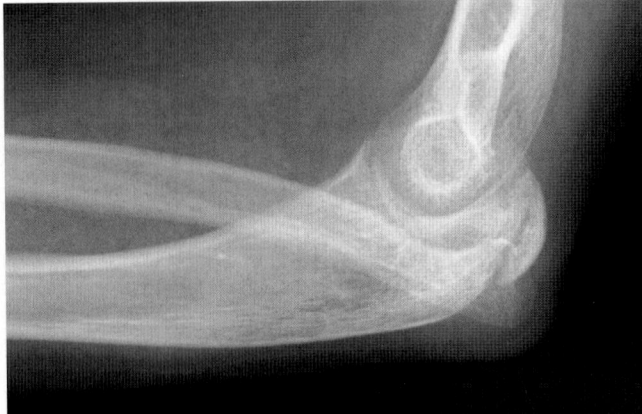

FIGURE 174-35. Chronic radial head dislocation in a 14-year-old boy with cerebral palsy. The radial head is displaced posteriorly and has a rounded contour. The radius is bowed anteriorly. Similar findings were present on the opposite side.

spondylolysis/spondylolisthesis, and pelvic obliquity. Nonambulatory patients also show caninization of the vertebral bodies (narrow anteroposterior diameter) due to lack of weight-bearing forces during development.

Upper extremity defects include radial head dislocation and contracture at the elbow (Fig. 174-35), wrist and fingers. Kienböck disease and negative ulnar variance are of increased incidence in cerebral palsy, but a link between the two findings has not been shown in these patients. Accelerated degenerative changes in the elbow and wrist are common in older patients with cerebral palsy.

Abnormalities at the hip include coxa valga due to lack of weight bearing, increased femoral anteversion, prominence of the lesser trochanter due to external rotation forces by the iliopsoas tendon, femoral head subluxation/dislocation, acetabular hypoplasia and dysplasia, and flattening of the femoral head (see Fig. 174-9). Medial femoral head flattening is more common and probably is due to pressure against the superolateral acetabulum. Lateral femoral head flattening may also occur, probably caused by pressure exerted by the hip adductors. Acetabular deficiency is posterior and superior. Hip displacement is progressive without corrective measures. Patients may experience pain with progressive hip subluxation that progresses to dislocation. The "windblown" or "windswept" pelvis is seen when one hip has an adductor contracture and the other hip has an abductor contracture. This defect reflects asymmetric neuromuscular defects and is most often

seen in nonambulatory patients with severe spasticity. Older patients with cerebral palsy show evidence of superimposed degenerative disease at the hips.

At the knee, flexion contractures may be present. The patella is often high (patella alta) and elongated. Tug lesions are common at the lower pole of the patella, producing a fragmented appearance. The tibial tuberosity may appear elevated and irregular. Genu recurvatum may be seen with rectus femoris contracture. Equinus and hindfoot valgus are common in the foot (see Fig. 174-32).

> **Deformities in patients with cerebral palsy are the result of imbalanced muscular forces. Deformity may continue to progress after skeletal maturity.**

Myelomeningocele

Patients with myelomeningocele have a defect in innervation to the lower body and lower extremities that is variable in level and severity.

Scoliosis in patients with myelomeningocele may be congenital or developmental and progressive. A total of 20% of patients have congenital scoliosis that is often due to vertebral segmentation errors. Congenital kyphosis is most common at L1-L2. Kyphosis may also be acquired. Lumbar lordosis is commonly accentuated.

One third to one half of patients with myelomeningocele have hip dysplasia. The hips are occasionally dislocated at birth; however, more often, dysplasia develops over time as the result of paralysis of the hip extensors and abductors with unopposed hip flexors and adductors (Fig. 174-36). Coxa valga and increased femoral anteversion are common. Excessive external tibial torsion with out-toeing or internal tibial torsion with in-toeing may be seen. In all, 80% to 95% of patients have foot deformities. Equinovarus (clubfoot), congenital vertical talus, and other foot deformities may be seen.

Infants with myelomeningocele have an increased incidence of fracture of a lower extremity during birth. A higher incidence of fracture is seen with contractures

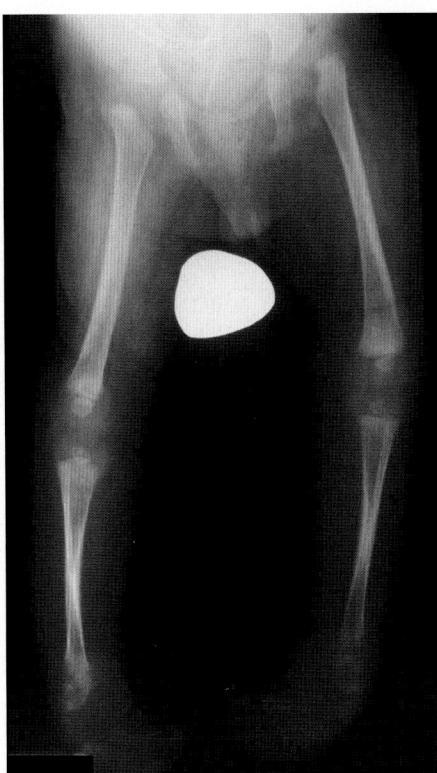

FIGURE 174-36. A 7-month-boy with myelomeningocele. Both hips are dislocated, and both feet are clubfeet. The musculature is atrophic. A ventriculoperitoneal shunt is present.

and higher levels of spinal defect. Patients with myelomeningocele may develop neuropathic injuries as the result of osteoporosis and lack of sensation. Fractures are most commonly metaphyseal or diaphyseal, but they may occur through a physis. Physeal fractures may be complicated by delayed union or growth arrest. Periosteal new bone may be exuberant because of delayed diagnosis without immobilization and abundant subperiosteal hemorrhage. Such injuries may be mistaken for tumor or infection.

SUGGESTED READINGS

General

Ozonoff MB: Pediatric Orthopedic Radiology, 2nd ed. Philadelphia, WB Saunders, 1992

Erb Palsy

Gudinchet F, Maeder P, Oberson JC, et al: Magnetic resonance imaging of the shoulder in children with brachial plexus birth palsy. Pediatr Radiol 1995;25:S125-128
Hernandez RJ, Dias L: CT evaluation of the shoulder in children with Erb's palsy. Pediatr Radiol 1988;18:333-336
Mintzer CM, Waters PM, Brown DJ: Glenoid version in children. J Pediatr Orthop 1996;16:563-566
Pollock AN, Reed MH: Shoulder deformities from obstetrical brachial plexus paralysis. Skeletal Radiol 1989;18:295-297
Waters PM, Smith GR, Jaramillo D: Glenohumeral deformity secondary to brachial plexus birth palsy. J Bone Joint Surg Am 1998;80:668-677

Wrist

Arora AS, Chung KC. Otto W. Madelung and the recognition of Madelung's deformity. J Hand Surg Am 2006:31:177-182
Hafner R, Poznanski AK, Donovan JM: Ulnar variance in children—

standard measurements for evaluation of ulnar shortening in juvenile rheumatoid arthritis, hereditary multiple exostosis and other bone or joint disorders in childhood. Skeletal Radiol 1989;18:513-516
Palmer AK, Glisson RR, Werner FW: Ulnar variance determination. J Hand Surg Am 1982;7:376-379
Schmidt-Rohlfing B, Schwobel B, Pauschert R, et al: Madelung deformity: clinical features, therapy and results. J Pediatr Orthop B 2001;10:344-348
Schuurman AH, Maas M, Dijkstra PF: Assessment of ulnar variance: a radiological investigation in a Dutch population. Skeletal Radiol 2001;30:633-638

Coxa Vara

Aarabi M, Rauch F, Hamdy RC, et al: High prevalence of coxa vara in patients with severe osteogenesis imperfecta. J Pediatr Orthop 2006;26:24-28
Beals RK: Coxa vara in childhood: evaluation and management. J Am Acad Orthop Surg 1998;6:93-99
Oh C-W, Thacker MM, Mackenzie WG, et al: Coxa vara: a novel measurement technique in skeletal dysplasias. Clin Orthop Relat Res 2006;447:125-131
Pavlov H, Goldman AB, Freiberger RH: Infantile coxa vara. Radiology 1980;135:631-640
Weinstein JN, Kuo KN, Millar EA: Congenital coxa vara: a retrospective review. J Pediatr Orthop 1984;4:70-77

Femoral Anteversion/Tibial Torsion

Bobroff ED, Chambers HG, Sartoris DJ, et al: Femoral anteversion and neck-shaft angle in children with cerebral palsy. Clin Orthop Relat Res 1999;364:194-204
Bruce RW Jr: Torsional and angular deformities. Pediatr Clin North Am 1996;43:867-881
Cibulka MT: Determination and significance of femoral neck anteversion. Phys Ther 2004;84:550-558
Davids JR, Marshall AD, Blocker ER, et al: Femoral anteversion in children with cerebral palsy: assessment with two and three-dimensional computed tomography scans. J Bone Joint Surg Am 2003;85:481-488
Dietz FR: Intoeing—fact, fiction and opinion. Am Fam Physician 1994;50:1249-1259, 1262-1264
Guenther KP, Tomczak R, Kessler S, et al: Measurement of femoral anteversion by magnetic resonance imaging—evaluation of a new technique in children and adolescents. Eur J Radiol 1995;21:47-52
Hernandez RJ, Tachdjian MO, Poznanski AK, et al: CT determination of femoral torsion. AJR Am J Roentgenol 1981;137:97-101
Joseph B, Carver RA, Bell MJ, et al: Measurement of tibial torsion by ultrasound. J Pediatr Orthop 1987;7:317-323
Karol LA: Rotational deformities in the lower extremities. Curr Opin Pediatr 1997;9:77-80
Lincoln TL, Suen PW: Common rotational variations in children. J Am Acad Orthop Surg 2003;11:312-320
Staheli LT, Corbett M, Wyss C, et al: Lower-extremity rotational problems in children: normal values to guide management. J Bone Joint Surg Am 1985;67:39-47

Bowleg, Knock-Knee, Tibia Vara

Blount WP: Tibia vara. J Bone Surg 1937;19:1-29
Blount WP: Tibia vara, osteochondrosis deformans tibiae. Curr Pract Orthop Surg 1966;3:141-156
Cheema JI, Grissom LE, Harcke HT: Radiographic characteristics of lower-extremity bowing in children. Radiographics 2003;23:871-880
Craig JG, van Holsbeeck M, Zaltz I: The utility of MR in assessing Blount disease. Skeletal Radiol 2002;31:208-213
Davids JR, Blackhurst DW, Allen BL Jr: Radiographic evaluation of bowed legs in children. J Pediatr Orthop 2001;21:257-263
Do TT: Clinical and radiographic evaluation of bowlegs. Curr Opin Pediatr 2001;13:42-46
Ducou le Pointe H, Mousselard H, Rudelli A, et al: Blount's disease: magnetic resonance imaging. Pediatr Radiol 1995;25:12-14
Eggert P, Viemann M: Physiological bowlegs or infantile Blount's disease: some new aspects on an old problem. Pediatr Radiol 1996;26:349-352
Heath CH, Staheli LT: Normal limits of knee angle in white children—genu varum and genu valgum. J Pediatr Orthop 1993;13:259-262

Holt JF, Latourette HB, Watson EH: Physiological bowing of the legs in young children. J Am Med Assoc 1954;154:390-394

Iwasawa T, Inaba Y, Nishimura G, et al: MR findings of bowlegs in toddlers. Pediatr Radiol 1999;29:826-834

Kling TF Jr: Angular deformities of the lower limbs in children. Orthop Clin North Am 1987;18:513-527

Langenskiold A: Tibia vara: a critical review. Clin Orthop Relat Res 1989;195-207

Levine AM, Drennan JC: Physiological bowing and tibia vara: the metaphyseal-diaphyseal angle in the measurement of bowleg deformities. J Bone Joint Surg Am 1982;64:1158-1163

Lin CJ, Lin SC, Huang W, et al: Physiological knock-knee in preschool children: prevalence, correlating factors, gait analysis, and clinical significance. J Pediatr Orthop 1999;19:650-654

Loder RT, Johnston CE 2nd: Infantile tibia vara. J Pediatr Orthop 1987;7:639-646

McCarthy JJ, Betz RR, Kim A, et al: Early radiographic differentiation of infantile tibia vara from physiologic bowing using the femoral-tibial ratio. J Pediatr Orthop 2001;21:545-548

Salenius P, Vankka E: The development of the tibiofemoral angle in children. J Bone Joint Surg Am 1975;57:259-261

Shopfner CE, Coin CG: Genu varus and valgus in children. Radiology 1969;92:723-732

Stricker SJ, Faustgen JP: Radiographic measurement of bowleg deformity: variability due to method and limb rotation. J Pediatr Orthop 1994;14:147-151

Focal Fibrocartilaginous Dysplasia

Bell SN, Campbell PE, Cole WG, et al: Tibia vara caused by focal fibrocartilaginous dysplasia: three case reports. J Bone Joint Surg Br 1985;67:780-784

Choi IH, Kim CJ, Cho TJ, et al: Focal fibrocartilaginous dysplasia of long bones: report of eight additional cases and literature review. J Pediatr Orthop 2000;20:421-427

Jouve JL, Kohler R, Mubarak SJ, et al: Focal fibrocartilaginous dysplasia ("fibrous periosteal inclusion"): an additional series of eleven cases and literature review. J Pediatr Orthop 2007;27:75-84

Meyer JS, Davidson RS, Hubbard AM, et al: MRI of focal fibrocartilaginous dysplasia. J Pediatr Orthop 1995;15:304-306

Smith NC, Carter PR, Ezaki M: Focal fibrocartilaginous dysplasia in the upper limb: seven additional cases. J Pediatr Orthop 2004;24:700-705

Knee

Eilert RE: Congenital dislocation of the patella. Clin Orthop Relat Res 2001;389:22-29

Elias DA, White LM: Imaging of patellofemoral disorders. Clin Radiol 2004;59:543-557

Ghelman B, Hodge JC: Imaging of the patellofemoral joint. Orthop Clin North Am 1992;23:523-543

Kamata N, Takahashi T, Nakatani K, et al: Ultrasonographic evaluation of congenital dislocation of the knee. Skeletal Radiol 2002;31:539-542

Koplewitz BZ, Babyn PS, Cole WG: Congenital dislocation of the patella. AJR Am J Roentgenol 2005;184:1640-1646

Muhle C, Brossmann J, Heller M: Kinematic CT and MR imaging of the patellofemoral joint. Eur Radiol 1999;9:508-518

Ooishi T, Sugioka Y, Matsumoto S, et al: Congenital dislocation of the knee: its pathologic features and treatment. Clin Orthop Relat Res 1993;287:187-192

Shabshin N, Schweitzer ME, Morrison WB, et al: MRI criteria for patella alta and baja. Skeletal Radiol 2004;33:445-450

Leg Length Discrepancy

Aaron A, Weinstein D, Thickman D, et al: Comparison of orthoroentgenography and computed tomography in the measurement of limb-length discrepancy. J Bone Joint Surg Am 1992;74:897-902

Aitken AG, Flodmark O, Newman DE, et al: Leg length determination by CT digital radiography. AJR Am J Roentgenol 1985;144:613-615

Green WT, Wyatt GM, Anderson M: Orthoroentgenography as a method of measuring the bones of the lower extremity. J Bone Joint Surg Am 1946;28:60-65

Kasser JR, Jenkins R: Accuracy of leg length prediction in children younger than 10 years of age. Clin Orthop Relat Res 1997;338:9-13

Terry MA, Winell JJ, Green DW, et al: Measurement variance in limb length discrepancy: clinical and radiographic assessment of interobserver and intraobserver variability. J Pediatr Orthop 2005;25:197-201

Foot

Aurell Y, Johansson A, Hansson G, et al: Ultrasound anatomy in the neonatal clubfoot. Eur Radiol 2002;12:2509-2517

Aurell Y, Johansson A, Hansson G, et al: Ultrasound anatomy in the normal neonatal and infant foot: an anatomic introduction to ultrasound assessment of foot deformities. Eur Radiol 2002; 12:2306-2312

Chami M, Daoud A, Maestro M, et al: Ultrasound contribution in the analysis of the newborn and infant normal and clubfoot: a preliminary study. Pediatr Radiol 1996;26:298-302

Coley BD, Shields WE, Kean J, et al: Age-dependent dynamic sonographic measurement of pediatric clubfoot. Pediatr Radiol 2007; In press

Cummings RJ, Davidson RS, Armstrong PF, et al: Congenital clubfoot. J Bone Joint Surg Am 2002; 84:290-308

Gore AI, Spencer JP: The newborn foot. Am Fam Physician 2004;69:865-872

Harty MP: Imaging of pediatric foot disorders. Radiol Clin North Am 2001;39:733-748

Napiontek M: Skewfoot. J Pediatr Orthop 2002;22:130-133

Oestreich AE: How to Measure Angles From Foot Radiographs: A Primer. New York, Springer-Verlag, 1990.

Schwend RM, Drennan JC: Cavus foot deformity in children. J Am Acad Orthop Surg 2003;11:201-211

Shields WE, Coley BD, Kean J, et al: Focused dynamic sonographic examination of the congenital clubfoot. Pediatr Radiol 2007; In press

Sullivan JA: Pediatric flatfoot: evaluation and management. J Am Acad Orthop Surg 1999;7:44-53

Vanderwilde R, Staheli LT, Chew DE, et al: Measurements on radiographs of the foot in normal infants and children. J Bone Joint Surg Am 1988;70:407-415

Cerebral Palsy

Flynn JM, Miller F: Management of hip disorders in patients with cerebral palsy. J Am Acad Orthop Surg 2002;10:198-209

Gordon GS, Simkiss DE: A systematic review of the evidence for hip surveillance in children with cerebral palsy. J Bone Joint Surg [Br] 2006;88:1492-1496

Kaye JJ, Freiberger RH: Fragmentation of the lower pole of the patella in spastic lower extremities. Radiology 1971;101:97-100

Kerr Graham H, Selber P: Musculoskeletal aspects of cerebral palsy. J Bone Joint Surg Br 2003;85:157-166

Leet AI, Mesfin A, Pichard C, et al: Fractures in children with cerebral palsy. J Pediatr Orthop 2006;26:624-627

Morrell DS, Pearson JM, Sauser DD: Progressive bone and joint abnormalities of the spine and lower extremities in cerebral palsy. Radiographics 2002;22:257-268

Nishioka E, Yoshida K, Yamanaka K, et al: Radiographic studies of the wrist and elbow in cerebral palsy. J Orthop Sci 2000;5:268-274

Presedo A, Dabney KW, Miller F: Fractures in patients with cerebral palsy. J Pediatr Orthop 2007;27:147-153

Sauser DD, Hewes RC, Root L: Hip changes in spastic cerebral palsy. AJR Am J Roentgenol 1986;146:1219-1222

Soo B, Howard JJ, Boyd RN, et al: Hip displacement in cerebral palsy. J Bone Joint Surg Am 2006;88:121-129

Topoleski TA, Kurtz CA, Grogan DP: Radiographic abnormalities and clinical symptoms associated with patella alta in ambulatory children with cerebral palsy. J Pediatr Orthop 2000;20:636-639

Myelomeningocele

Boytim MJ, Davidson RS, Charney E, et al: Neonatal fractures in myelomeningocele patients. J Pediatr Orthop 1991;11:28-30

Kumar SJ, Cowell HR, Townsend P: Physeal, metaphyseal, and diaphyseal injuries of the lower extremities in children with myelomeningocele. J Pediatr Orthop 1984;4:25-27

Lock TR, Aronson DD: Fractures in patients who have myelomeningocele. J Bone Joint Surg Am 1989;71:1153-1157

Westcott MA, Dynes MC, Remer EM, et al: Congenital and acquired orthopedic abnormalities in patients with myelomeningocele. Radiographics 1992;12:1155-1173

CHAPTER

175

Infections in Bone

E. MICHEL AZOUZ

OSTEOMYELITIS

Over the past decade, there seems to have been a gradual increase in bacterial virulence with diminished susceptibility to antibiotics, and infections in bone remain a diagnostic and therapeutic medical challenge. There have been great medical advances in molecular microbiology and other sophisticated diagnostic laboratory techniques, in imaging methods including magnetic resonance imaging and positron emission tomography combined with computed tomography, and in the manufacture of a broad armamentarium of powerful antibiotics. With early diagnosis, rapid initiation of medical treatment with the appropriate antibiotic for the appropriate length of time should be curative. Hematogenous osteomyelitis is preponderantly a disease of children; however, infantile and even neonatal cases are not uncommon.

Bacteria are the most common inflammatory agents, but growing bones may also be invaded by other pathogens, including viruses, spirochetes, and fungi. Rarely, osteomyelitis in children is post-traumatic, including after surgery or after accidental penetrating trauma, wounds, or foreign bodies. Adjacent joint or soft tissue infection may spread to bone and vice versa. Radiographic changes are similar regardless of the infecting agent.

The diagnosis of acute bone and joint infection is clinical, and is established by identifying the causative organism in blood and tissue culture. In the appropriate clinica setting, infection may be suggested by radiographs when early soft tissue changes, such as soft tissue swelling and deep soft tissue edema, develop.

Sources of bone infection:
- Hematogenous
- Adjacent joint or soft tissue infection
- Direct implantation
  - Trauma
  - Surgery
  - Foreign body

Radionuclide imaging is more sensitive than plain radiographs in the early detection of acute bone infection. It can also identify additional foci of disease not clinically apparent at the time of examination. Vascular phase images of the bone scan done within the first 5 minutes following injection, delayed images with pinhole collimators, and special attention to the affected area have proven of great value. Osteomyelitis appears as an area of increased tracer activity reflecting the hyperemia and bone turnover induced by the infectious process. Park found that the sensitivity and specificity of three-phase bone scans for acute osteomyelitis were 84% and 97%, respectively, in 100 children with acute limb pain. Errors arise from simulation of infection by fracture or sickle cell disease and obscuration of osteomyelitis by septic arthritis, prior antibiotic treatment, and "cold" defects resulting from ischemia. It is difficult to detect infection close to the growth plate because both the region of the physis in the growing child and the nearby area of bone infection show increased activity on the bone scan. Newer cameras, magnification, digital imaging, and better positioning of the patient allow better differentiation between the metaphysis and the growth plate.

Compared with magnetic resonance imaging (MRI), computed tomography (CT) is less sensitive with respect to identification of marrow changes. The specificity of CT is good in the appropriate clinical circumstances; however, CT is of limited clinical value in acute osteomyelitis. It is more useful in advanced or chronic disease to detect cortical destruction and delineate bone cavities and sequestra.

MRI is as sensitive as scintigraphy in the early detection of bone and bone marrow changes and delineates the anatomy and extent of marrow involvement to better advantage. Its ability to detect and define the adjacent soft tissue changes and its multiplanar capabilities further enhance its value. MRI has thus become an important tool for imaging of suspected osseous infections. However, MRI does carry additional cost and, depending on the availability of scanner time and the need for sedation or anesthesia, possible delays in definitive diagnosis and treatment. MRI does not need be used routinely in every case of suspected osteomyelitis. Imaging should aim at guiding or modifying treatment, if necessary. Some

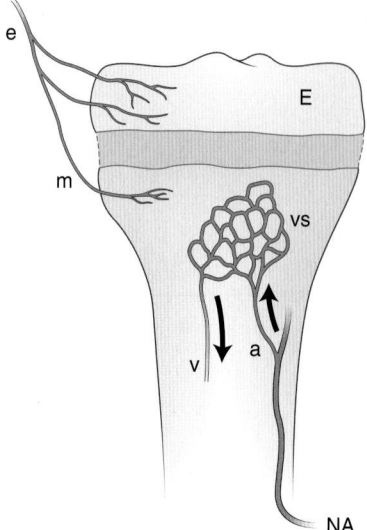

FIGURE 175-1. The blood supply to the metaphysis and epiphysis of a child and the arterial channels through which invading organisms enter the growing bone. a, arteriole; NA, nutrient artery; v. venule; vs, venous sinuses in the metaphysis. An epiphyseal artery (e) supplies the epiphysis (E) and may branch to give (minor) metaphyseal vessels (m). The major blood supply of the metaphysis comes from the nutrient artery.

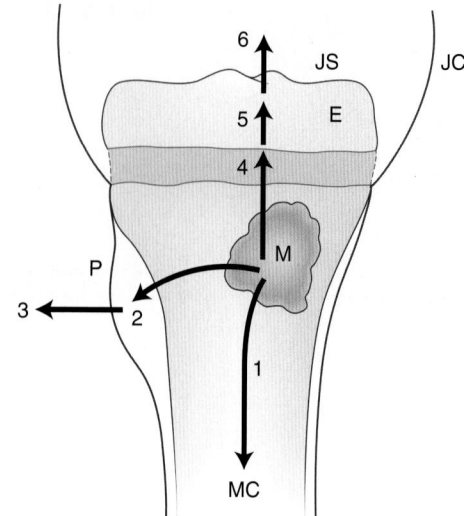

FIGURE 175-2. The pathways of infection after hematogenous implantation in the metaphysis and formation of a metaphyseal focus (M) of bone infection (bone abscess). 1, spread to the medullary canal (MC); 2, formation of a subperiosteal abscess; 3, penetration of the periosteum (P) and spread to the adjacent soft tissues; 4, 5, and 6. spread across the growth plate to the epiphysis (E), and eventually to the joint space (JS). JC, joint capsule.

specific indications for MRI include suspected osteomyelitis of the spine or pelvis, suspected osteomyelitis affecting the growth plate, and osteomyelitis that fails to respond to therapy.

Diagnosis of bone infection:
- History and clinical findings
- Blood/tissue culture
- Imaging
  - Plain radiography
  - Radionuclide scanning
  - ± Sonography
  - ± CT
  - MRI

Pyogenic Hematogenous Osteomyelitis

Bone can be infected with a variety of organisms by extension from contiguous soft tissue infection or joint infection, or through the bloodstream from a remote source. The latter is most frequent in the pediatric age group, and it results in what is known as hematogenous osteomyelitis, a true infection of the bone marrow with early extension to other bony components and potentially severe, systemic symptoms. Hematogenous osteomyelitis usually involves the highly vascularized metaphysis of the fastest growing bones, such as the distal femur, proximal tibia, proximal humerus, and distal radius. Organisms lodge most frequently in the terminal capillary loops of the metaphyses. Rarely, they may locate initially in the epiphyses or in the cortex (Fig. 175-1). In the usual case, a small abscess forms in the marrow of the metaphysis, followed by local decalcification and destruction of the adjacent bone. When focal abscesses are generated, multiple small foci of bone destruction develop and later coalesce. Inflammatory swelling increases the intraosseous pressure because of the rigid bony walls of the

marrow cavity, and can force extension of the infected exudate into several sites, as indicated in Figure 175-2. The most common route is via the haversian canals of the cortex to the subperiosteal space, where a subperiosteal abscess is formed. Simultaneously, spread also occurs further within the medullary cavity. Rupture of the periosteal abscess is responsible for extension of infection into the adjacent soft tissues. Inflammation and rapidly increased intraosseous pressure may cause thrombosis of the vascular channels. Therefore, very early bone scans may demonstrate a cold metaphyseal lesion as a result of compression or occlusion of the metaphyseal vessels. In these cases, increased activity is observed toward the diaphysis, beyond the "cold" metaphyseal area, which subsequently becomes "hot" and merges with the adjacent increased activity. The multiphase bone scan is very sensitive and is usually positive after 24 to 48 hours from the onset of symptoms. It can detect extension of metaphyseal osteomyelitis into the epiphysis through the growth plate (Fig. 175-3).

The earliest plain radiographic changes do not involve the bone. The deep soft tissues are swollen and edematous, obliterating the deep intermuscular fat septa. This occurs within the first 48 to 72 hours after infection and before the subcutaneous fat becomes edematous. Recognizable changes in bone are seldom present radiographically until the second week of the disease, but scintigraphy is very helpful in the early stages. MRI can demonstrate the marrow alterations and extent of disease in bone, soft tissues, or adjacent joint at the same time (Fig. 175-4). Subperiosteal abscess formation is an early sonographic finding in osteomyelitis, preceding radiographic bony changes (Fig. 175-5). Needle puncture of the abscess can be carried out under sonographic control and the fluid sent for microscopic and bacteriologic analysis. Subperiosteal abscess may also

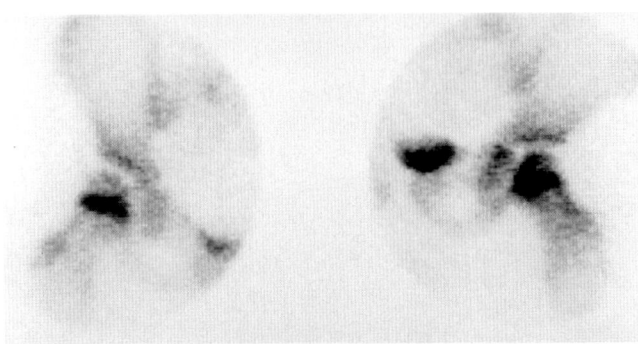

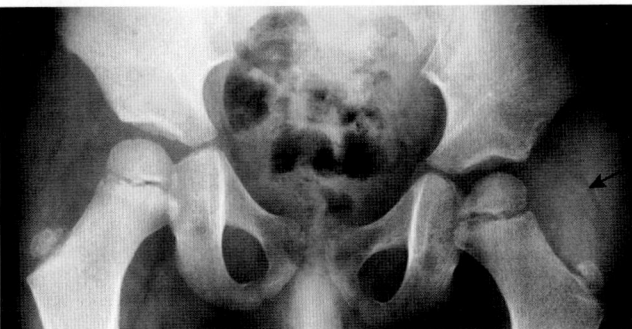

FIGURE 175-3. A 4-year-old boy with fever and "inability" to walk or move the left lower extremity for 6 days. **A,** Bone scan shows increased uptake in the femoral neck and head on the left side, likely resulting from extension of an initial metaphyseal focus of infection into the epiphysis. The right hip shows normal increased uptake in the region of the growth plate. **B,** Plain radiograph of the hips 2 weeks after the beginning of symptoms shows osteopenia on the left side, ill-defined medial metaphyseal and epiphyseal bone lucencies on each side of the growth plate, and indirect evidence of left hip joint effusion. *Arrow,* fat line displaced laterally by the joint fluid. Adjacent deep soft tissues also appear swollen and edematous compared with the normal right side.

be visualized with CT or MRI (Figs. 175-6 and 175-7), even before visible plain radiographic changes. The earliest bone changes seen on conventional images are one or more small radiolucencies, usually in the metaphyseal region, where necrosis and destruction of bone has occurred (Fig. 175-8). On serial examinations, these areas of bone destruction enlarge and become confluent.

> **The earliest change on plain radiographs with acute osteomyelitis is soft tissue swelling. Osseous changes are seldom present until the second week of disease.**

With continuing appropriate antibiotic therapy, the periosteum begins to produce new bone on its undersurface after the second or third week. The resumption of osteogenic function by the periosteum suggests that

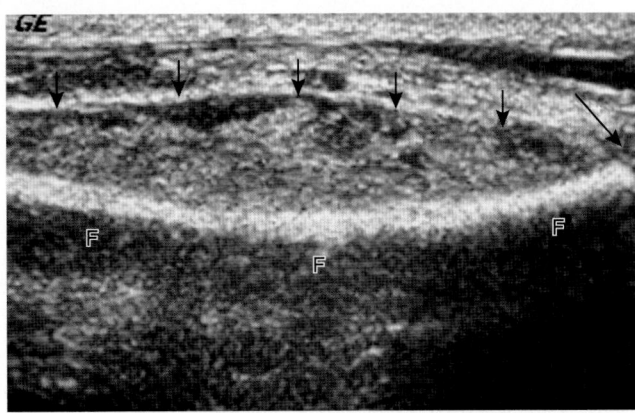

FIGURE 175-5. A 12-year-old boy with acute osteomyelitis of the distal fibula. Ultrasound shows a large subperiosteal abscess *(small arrows).* F, fibula. *Large arrow,* distal fibular growth plate.

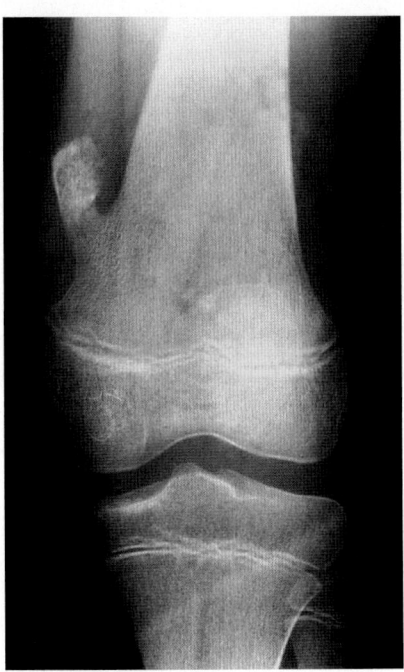

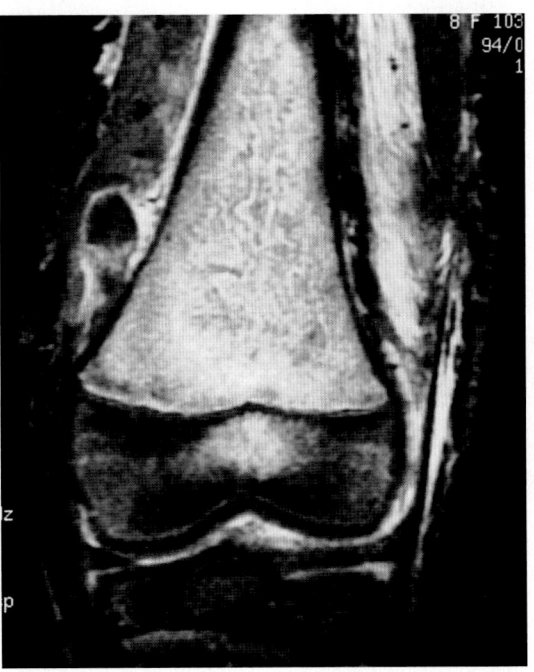

FIGURE 175-4. An 8-year-old girl with hematogenous osteomyelitis of the left distal femur. **A,** Anteroposterior plain radiograph shows generalized osteopenia of the left distal femur and proximal tibia. Note an incidental osteochondroma of the distal femoral metaphysis. **B,** Coronal short tau inversion–recovery (STIR) magnetic resonance image shows abnormal (high) bone marrow signal in the diaphysis, the metaphysis, and the central part of the epiphysis of the distal femur. There are also extensive changes in the soft tissues, especially laterally, again showing as high-signal-intensity areas on this inversion–recovery sequence.

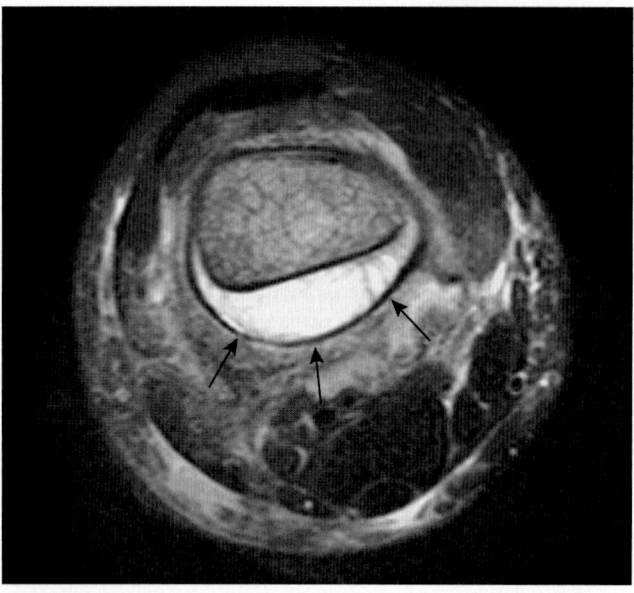

A

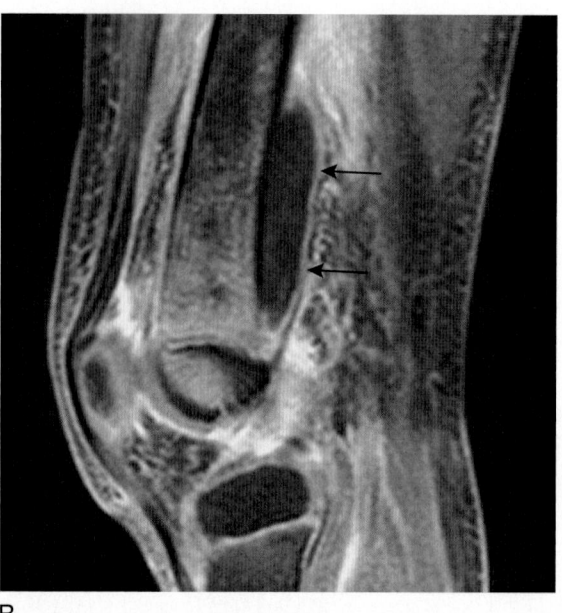

B

FIGURE 175-6. A 5-year-old boy with acute osteomyelitis of the distal femur. **A,** Axial T2-weighted magnetic resonance image with fat saturation shows a large subperiosteal abscess *(arrows)* at the posterior aspect of the femur. Mildly increased signal is seen within the bone, and there is adjacent soft tissue edema. **B,** Sagittal postgadolinium T1-weighted image with fat saturation shows the longitudinal extent of the subperiosteal abscess *(arrows)*. An enhancing rim is seen around the abscess with mild enhancement within the femur and adjacent soft tissues.

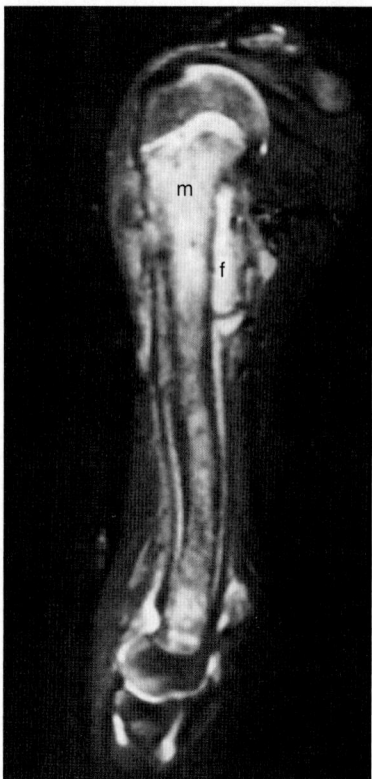

FIGURE 175-7. A 13-month-old boy with osteomyelitis of the proximal humerus. Magnetic resonance image shows no bone destruction. There is, however, abnormal increase of the bone marrow signal (m) on this STIR image, extensive linear periosteal reaction along the whole humeral diaphysis, and a fluid collection (subperiosteal abscess) at the medial aspect of the proximal humerus (f). The proximal and distal humeral epiphyses are normal.

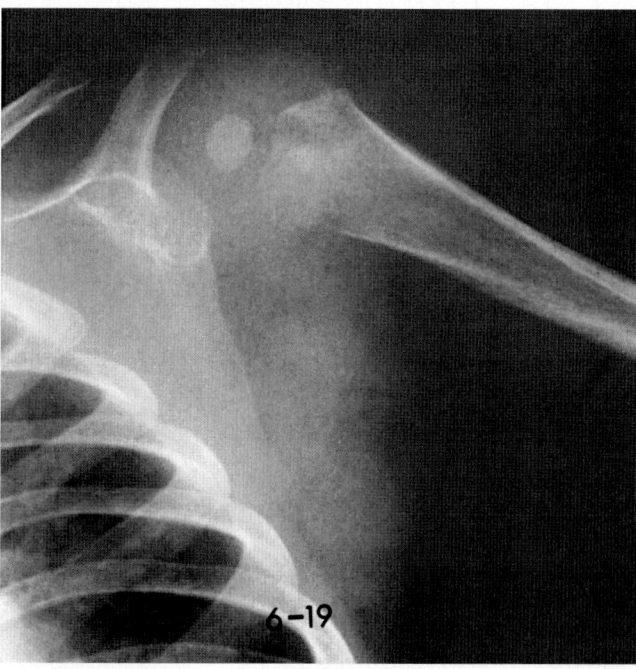

FIGURE 175-8. Early plain radiographic changes of osteomyelitis in the proximal metaphysis of the left humerus in a 9-month-old boy with fever and local signs and symptoms for 12 days. Metaphyseal areas of bone destruction are visualized as irregular, ill-defined lucencies. There is adjacent deep soft tissue swelling and edema, but there is no visible periosteal reaction.

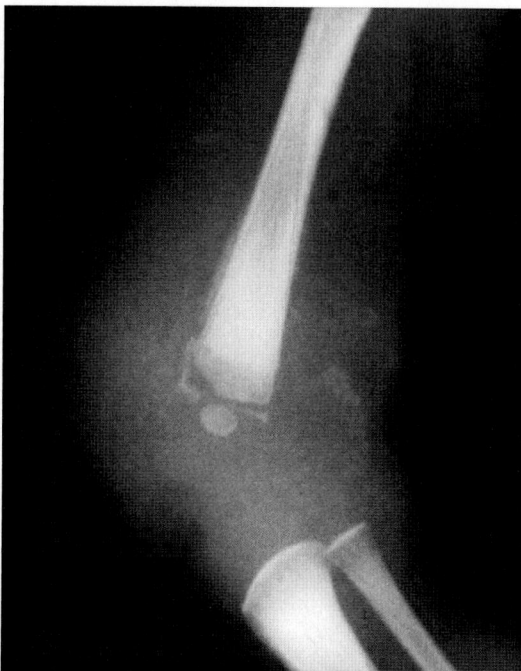

FIGURE 175-9. Osteomyelitis of the distal femur in a newborn showing distal femoral metaphyseal destructive bone changes and periosteal reaction, as well as extensive adjacent soft tissue swelling due to cellulitis and infectious arthritis of the knee joint.

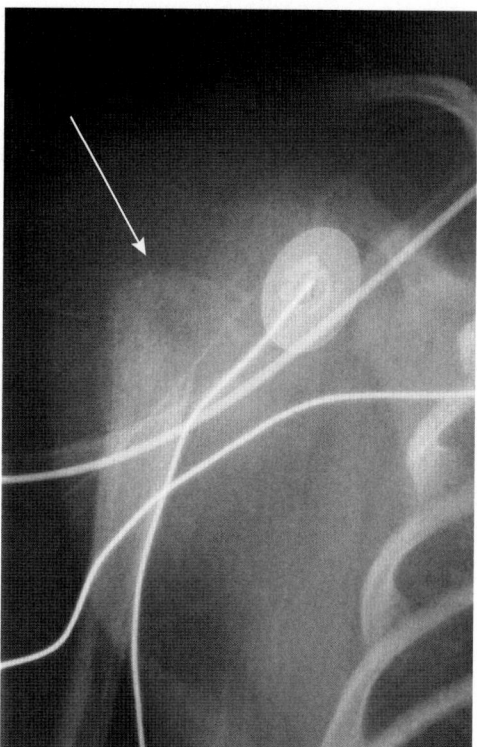

FIGURE 175-10. Neonatal osteomyelitis in a 25-day-old infant. Findings of an advanced infection with destruction of the proximal humeral metaphysis *(arrow)* were incidentally made on this chest radiograph.

the infectious process has been at least partly controlled at that site. Subsequent healing may involve remodeling of the cortical new bone and reconstitution of the underlying bone or, if damage has been extensive, increase in the amount of periosteal reaction to form an involucrum, a living bone sheath around the fragments of the old devitalized diaphyseal bone.

Although the mortality and morbidity of bone infection have decreased significantly, permanent sequelae do occur, largely as a result of delay in diagnosis or inadequate treatment. Complications of bone infection include pathologic fracture through regions of bone destruction, adjacent infectious arthritis and destruction of joints (Fig. 175-9), and premature union of an epiphysis with the metaphysis across the growth plate, with resulting growth disturbance, deformity and discrepancy of limb length.

> **Complications of bone infection:**
> - **Premature and asymmetric epiphyseal plate closure**
> - **Growth disturbance/limb deformities**
> - **Limb length discrepancy (shortening or lengthening)**
> - **Joint infection/destruction**
> - **Pathologic fracture**

NEONATAL OSTEOMYELITIS. In the neonatal period and in infants, the bone disease is generally milder and the recovery with antibiotic treatment is faster, because extension to form a subperiosteal abscess is more rapid and spontaneous rupture into the soft tissues more common.

A higher incidence of epiphyseal and joint involvement and a higher incidence of multifocal disease may portend a worse prognosis in a neonate. Also, osteomyelitis in infants is often indolent in onset or masked by other medical conditions. Particularly in a sick neonate, delayed diagnosis of osteomyelitis is not infrequent (Fig. 175-10). The high incidence of staphylococcal disease seen in older children is not seen in infant osteomyelitis, in which is found a large variety of organisms, many of which do not carry the tissue-disruptive enzymes that the staphylococci do. Group B streptococcus is a frequent pathogen in neonates.

Staphylococcus aureus remains the most common organism causing acute osteomyelitis and septic arthritis in children. Unfortunately, community-acquired methicillin-resistant strains are increasing in prevalence. *Haemophilus influenzae* osteomyelitis and septic arthritis are now less common since the availability of effective vaccination (*H. influenzae* type B vaccine).

Various organisms of low pathogenicity may be responsible for low-grade, chronic sclerosing osteomyelitis in immunosuppressed children. Bone production is usually greater than bone destruction in such cases. Osteomyelitis in the acquired immunodeficiency syndrome (AIDS) population is most often caused by common organisms such as *Staphyloccus aureus*, *Salmonella* and *Escherichia coli*.

In sickle cell disease, bone infarcts are frequent, but osteomyelitis is also a common and well-documented complication in infants and children, with involvement of a single or multiple long bones. The proposed mechanism of osteomyelitis in sickle cell disease is hematogenous with bacteria gaining entrance to blood vessels through ischemic bowel and finding suitable culture material in foci of infarcted bone marrow.

In chronic granulomatous disease of childhood, an X-linked recessive disorder of leukocyte function, repeated infections occur in lymph nodes, skin, and lungs. Osteomyelitis is seen in approximately one third of patients.

Likely causative organisms in hematogenous osteomyelitis:

1. **Neonatal period**
   - Group B streptococcus
   - *E. coli*
2. **Infancy**
   - *S. aureus*
   - *H. influenzae*
3. **Childhood**
   - *S. aureus*
4. **In acquired immunodeficiency and sickle cell disease**
   - *S. aureus*
   - *Salmonella*
   - *E. coli*

Calcaneal Osteomyelitis

Neonatal calcaneal osteomyelitis may develop after heel pad puncture for blood drawing. Although this iatrogenic complication is very rare considering the thousands of punctures performed, it is potentially preventable with strict aseptic technique for neonatal heel puncture. Bone scanning is very helpful for early diagnosis. The bone scan will be positive several days before plain radiographic findings become manifest. The disease course is usually benign if the condition is treated immediately with an adequate course of antibiotic therapy. Rarely, destruction of the calcaneus and its posterior apophysis lead to serious deformities of the hind-foot in later life.

At any age, plantar puncture wounds secondary to walking on broken glass, metal (i.e., nail) or vegetable matter (i.e., thorn, toothpick) may also result in infectious cellulitis, plantar fasciitis, and calcaneal osteomyelitis, whether the foreign body is removed or retained.

Brodie Abscess (Subacute Osteomyelitis)

Occasionally, in nonimmunologically compromised children, a focus of subacute or chronic osteomyelitis is sharply localized and minimally active, presumably because of low virulence of the infecting organism and a partial host response containing the infection. The initial purulent exudate is replaced by granulation tissue and the clinical manifestations are mild, consisting mainly of local pain. The lesion is generally in a metaphysis, commonly in the tibia (Fig. 175-11). It is characterized radiographically by a variable zone of sclerosis with a central or eccentric round, oval, or serpiginous radiolucency that tracks toward the adjacent growth plate and may occasionally cross the growth plate into the epi-

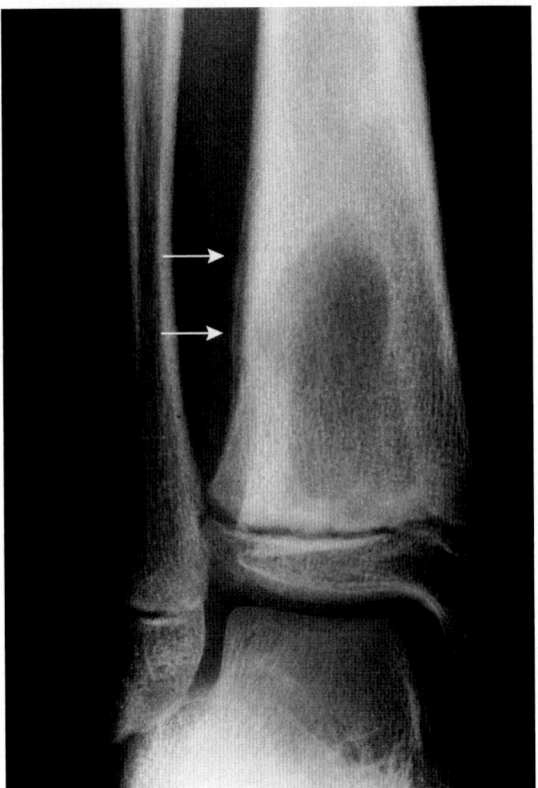

FIGURE 175-11. An 11-year-old boy with a 6-week history of pain and swelling of the right ankle. The patient was afebrile and had no leukocytosis. The erythrocyte sedimentation rate was 63 mm/hr. A large "active" Brodie abscess cavity is seen in the distal tibial metaphysis. There is no sequestrum and no visible extension into the epiphysis; however, the process abuts the metaphyseal side of the growth plate. Linear periosteal reaction *(arrows)* is seen along the lateral cortex of the distal tibia. Surgical incision and drainage were performed. *Staphylococcus aureus* was cultured. In most cases, cultures of the contents of Brodie abscesses are sterile.

physis. The growth plate is only a partial barrier against the spread of infection. The cavity may contain a small, dense sequestrum visible on plain radiographs or CT. On MRI, lesions have a characteristic layered appearance with a high-signal periphery due to edema, a low-signal rim due to sclerosis, and a high signal centrally due to granulation tissue (Fig. 175-12). Adjacent soft tissue swelling and edema as well as periosteal new bone formation may be present. Material removed from the abscess may disclose an organism of low virulence or none at all. In spite of occasional growth plate involvement, the incidence of premature growth plate fusion after subacute osteomyelitis (Brodie abscess) is low.

Subacute osteomyelitis (Brodie abscess) is likely the result of an organism of low virulence contained by a partial host response.

Chronic Osteomyelitis

If untreated or only partially treated, acute and subacute osteomyelitis may become chronic. Cortical and trabecular bone sclerosis, cavities, and sequestra are characteris-

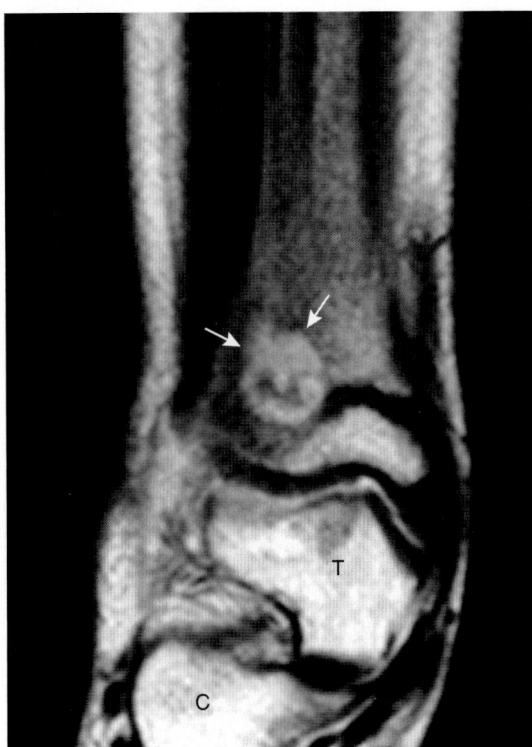

FIGURE 175-12. A 5-year-old girl with subacute osteomyelitis (Brodie abscess). Coronal T2-weighted magnetic resonance image shows a high-signal lesion *(arrows)* abutting the growth plate. A slightly decreased signal is seen at the lesion's margins. A focus of decreased signal within the center of the lesion may represent a sequestrum. C, calcaneus; T, talus.

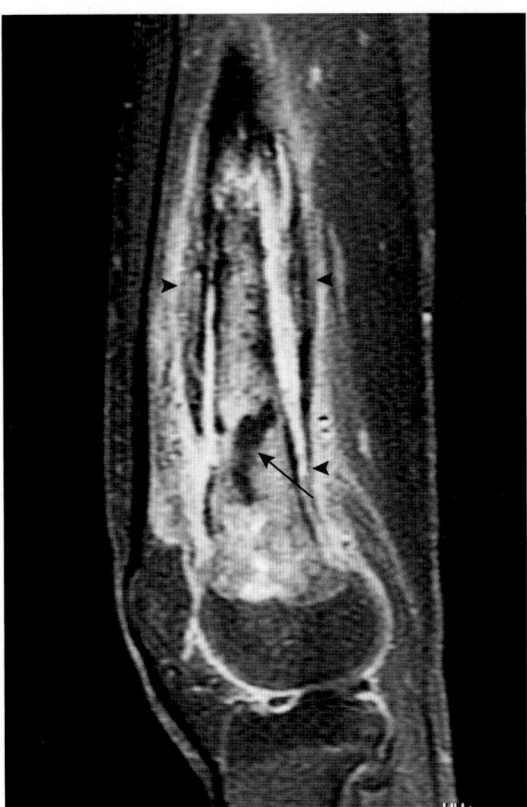

FIGURE 175-13. Postgadolinium fat-saturated T1-weighted magnetic resonance image in a 16-year-old boy with chronic osteomyelitis of the left femur shows a newly formed periosteal thick sheath or envelope called the involucrum *(arrowheads)*. A separate large, nonenhancing devitalized piece of bone *(arrow)* represents a sequestrum. Extensive areas of high signal intensity are seen in soft tissues and bone marrow.

tic of chronic osteomyelitis. The affected bone is thickened, and its outline may be wavy, with or without periosteal new bone. An involucrum of new bone may cloak an area of infection (Fig. 175-13). The involucrum may be perforated by sinus tracts (cloacae) through which infection exits toward the surrounding soft tissues and eventually to the outside through the skin. The necrotic, devitalized bone of a sequestrum is surrounded by inflammatory granulation tissue and may be located within a bone abscess cavity. The dead bone of a sequestrum is relatively sclerotic. Sequestra may be demonstrated on plain radiography, CT, or MRI. The best demonstration is usually achieved with CT (Fig. 175-14). Sequestra are foci for continued infection, and their detection and localization are crucial in view of surgical excision. Sequestration is now relatively rare owing to earlier diagnosis (largely due to imaging) and more effective modern antibiotic therapies.

Plain radiographs will suggest the diagnosis of chronic osteomyelitis and may be used to follow for gross changes. Although CT is of limited clinical value in acute osteomyelitis, it is very useful in imaging chronic disease to detect cortical metaphyseal tracts and channels, sequestra and bone destruction as well as to delineate bone abscesses and cavities. MRI will detect any reactivation or persistence of infection by showing focal active disease in the bone marrow and juxtacortical soft tissue hyperemia and edema (see Fig. 175-13). MRI is the preferred modality for showing soft tissue changes, such as fluid collections, associated with chronic osteomyelitis.

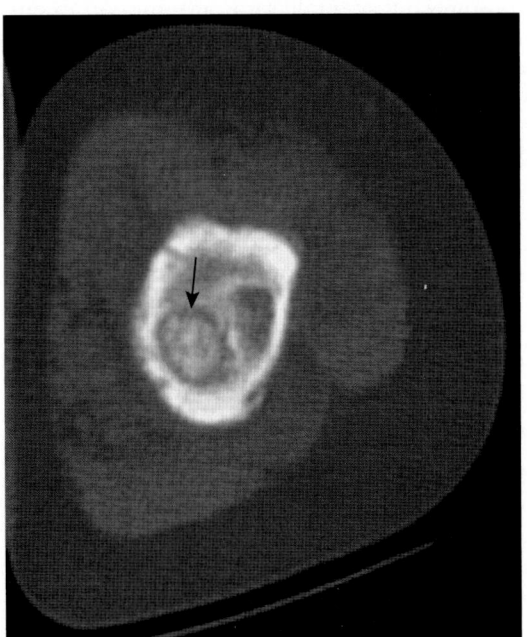

FIGURE 175-14. A 5-year-old child with chronic osteomyelitis of the proximal humeral diaphysis. The humerus is sclerotic and irregularly marginated. A sequestrum is noted *(arrow)*.

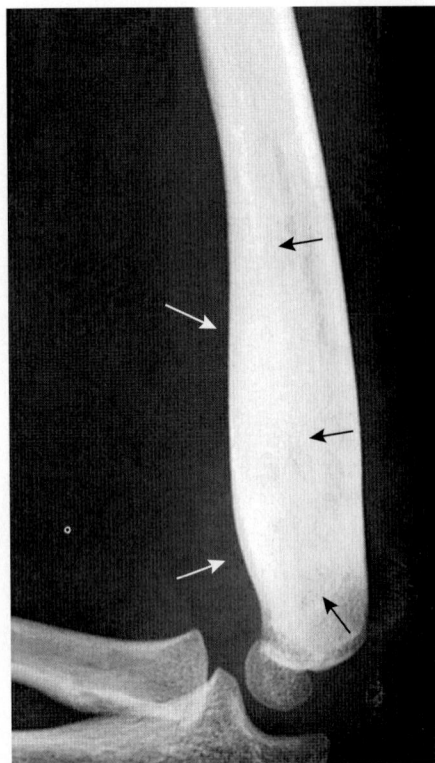

FIGURE 175-15. Chronic sclerosing osteomyelitis of Garré in the distal humerus of a 4-year-old boy. The anterior cortex is thickened internally and externally *(arrows).* Changes of this nature should also raise the question of an osteoid osteoma, in which the lucent nidus is concealed in the surrounding dense bone.

SCLEROSING OSTEOMYELITIS OF GARRÉ

Sclerosing osteomyelitis of Garré is a chronic non-suppurative osteomyelitis affecting children and young adults. The onset is insidious. Limb pain is the present-ing symptom, but systemic signs are mild or absent. The diagnosis is made by the radiographic picture of diffuse bone production with little or no bone destruction or sequestrum formation (Fig. 175-15) in the absence of other causes for these findings. Mild bowing may be present (Fig. 175-16). The diaphysis of tubular bones is the most common location. Osteoid osteoma is clinically and radiographically similar. CT aids in the search of the small lucent nidus in osteoid osteoma. Biopsy is often necessary for differentiation. In the mandible, this form of chronic osteomyelitis is often termed "*periostitis ossifi-cans,*" and onion-skin type of periosteal calcification may be seen. The cause of sclerosing osteomyelitis of Garré is believed to be a low-grade infection.

EPIPHYSEAL OSTEOMYELITIS

In tubular bones, the early changes of pyogenic hemato-genous osteomyelitis are usually localized to the meta-physis, where capillary vascularization is very rich and blood flow is slow on the venous side of the loops. As described earlier, and illustrated in Figure 175-2, infection may spread from the metaphysis, through the growth plate to the epiphysis. In children, a purely epiphyseal focus of infection is possible but very rare. Epiphyseal osteomyelitis and septic arthritis occur more

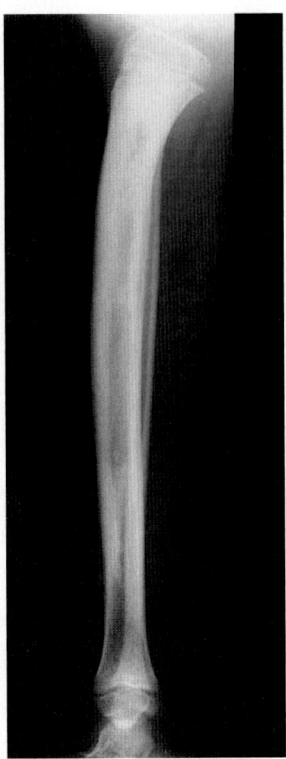

FIGURE 175-16. An 8-year-old boy with chronic sclerosing osteomyelitis of Garré. Note the increased bone density, the diffuse cortical thickening, and the mild anterior bowing of the proximal tibia.

freely in infants younger than 15 months of age because metaphyseal vessels penetrate the growth plate and enter the epiphysis.

Plain radiography usually demonstrates a focus of bone destruction localized to the epiphysis. In subacute and chronic cases, a small round or oval epiphyseal abscess cavity with well-defined borders is seen. CT is useful for imaging of the bone cavity, detecting the presence of a sequestrum or an associated joint effusion. Suspected spread of infection to the adjacent soft tissues is best imaged by MRI. This will reveal the epiphyseal focus of infection as low signal on T1-weighted images and high signal on T2-weighted images. Imaging after gadolinium injection shows rim enhancement outlining the abscess cavity (Fig. 175-17). The differential diagnosis of an epiphyseal (or apophyseal) lucent lesion mainly in-cludes infection and chondroblastoma. Epiphyseal infec-tion may also be tuberculous, fungal, or post-traumatic.

Sequelae of Infantile Meningococcemia

Late epiphysial and metaphyseal changes are sometimes seen in children years after surviving severe meningo-coccal sepsis. These changes are likely the result of occlu-sion of small blood vessels by microthrombi or septic emboli during the acute phase of the meningococcemia. Metaphyseal cupping, early and asymmetric growth plate fusion, with ball-and-socket deformities or triangle-shaped epiphyses are seen at the ends of long bones (Fig. 175-18). There is often secondary shortening and bowing of the affected tubular bones with limb length discrepancy.

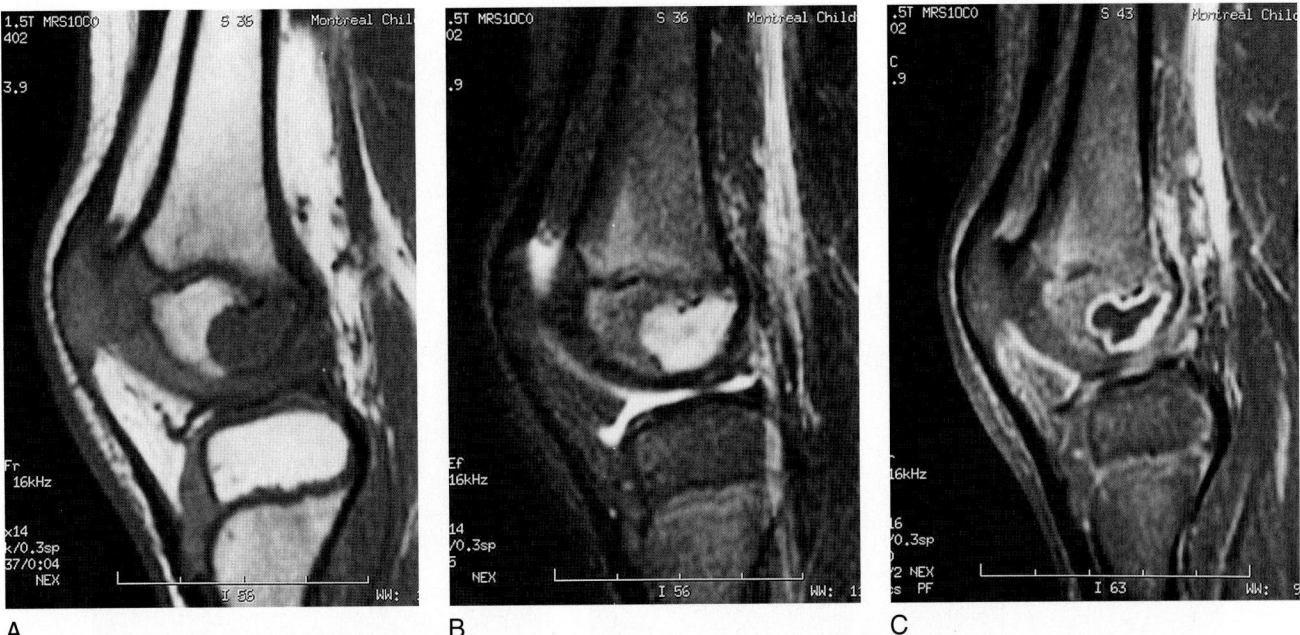

FIGURE 175-17. Magnetic resonance image of a 5-year-old boy with a primary epiphyseal focus of osteomyelitis. **A,** T1-weighted image shows low-signal-intensity area in the distal femoral epiphysis. **B,** That same area shows high signal on the fat-suppressed T2-weighted image. **C,** T1-weighted fat-suppressed image after intravenous injection of gadolinium chelate clearly outlines the enhancing wall of the abscess cavity.

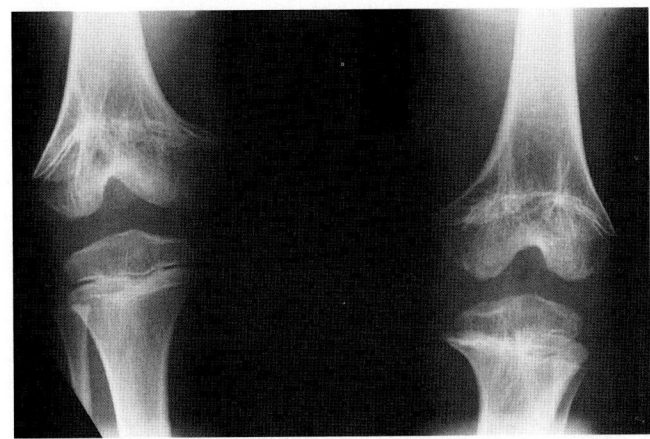

FIGURE 175-18. Late sequelae of infantile meningococcemia in an 8-year-old boy with severe changes seen in both knees. Early central fusion of the growth plates is seen in the distal femurs and left tibia, with metaphyseal cupping and secondary abnormal shape of the related epiphyses.

Osteomyelitis Resulting from Unusual Organisms

Fungal infections of bone are becoming more common as the immunosuppressed population increases. The radiographic changes are similar to those of chronic pyogenic osteomyelitis or tuberculosis (TB)—destruction of bone and periosteal reaction, with areas of cortical thickening and trabecular sclerosis. *Candida, Histoplasma, Blastomyces,* and others have been implicated.

In musculoskeletal *Candida* infections, predisposing factors include multiple broad-spectrum antibiotic administration, hyperalimentation with indwelling vascular lines, immunosuppressive therapy, prematurity, and in the newborn, maternal vaginal candidiasis. Sepsis may be present for several weeks before the skeletal complica-

tions arise. Arthritis usually precedes adjacent osteitis, in contradistinction to staphylococcal infections, in which septic arthritis generally extends from contiguous bone infection. The knee is most frequently affected, but multiple joint involvement is common. Clinical findings are primarily soft tissue swelling and effusions with pain and tenderness but little or no increase in local heat.

Bone involvement is infrequent in classic histoplasmosis, although patchy rarefaction of the skull, metaphyseal bone destruction, and periosteal reaction have been reported. It is commonplace and prominent in African histoplasmosis caused by *Histoplasma duboisii,* in which bone and joint involvement is associated with large soft tissue abscesses. Bone lesions are frequent in actinomycosis, coccidioidomycosis, and moreso in blastomycosis. Actinomycosis is a very rare cause of osteomyelitis in long bones. Coccidioidomycosis is frequently multicentric but may also involve one bone, and the lesions are usually well demarcated (Fig. 175-19). In Latin America, children infected by *Paracoccidioides braziliensis* may have bone involvement, usually in the clavicles, ribs, and forearm bones. Blastomycosis may be focal or diffuse. The focal lesions tend to have a sclerotic margin, whereas the bone lesions of diffuse blastomycosis tend to show rapid destruction with penetration into adjacent joints. Long bones and ribs are frequently involved, followed by carpal and tarsal bones. Chest wall aspergillosis is usually secondary to contiguous spread of pulmonary aspergillosis (Fig. 175-20). Multifocal hematogenous peripheral *Aspergillus* osteomyelitis is extremely rare.

Viruses, such as those of rubella (Fig. 175-21), cytomegalic inclusion disease, chickenpox (varicella), and smallpox (variola) (Fig. 175-22), have been associated with bone lesions. In variola, bizarre shortening of metacarpal bones has been observed (Fig. 175-23) mimicking

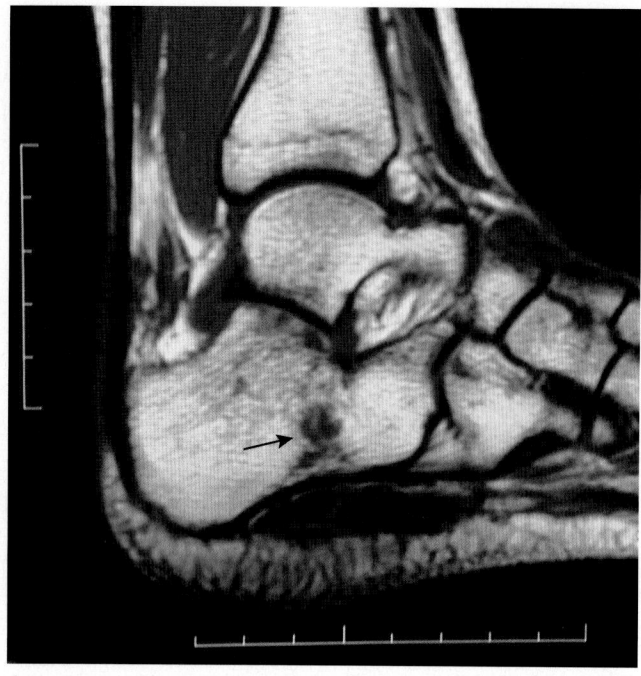
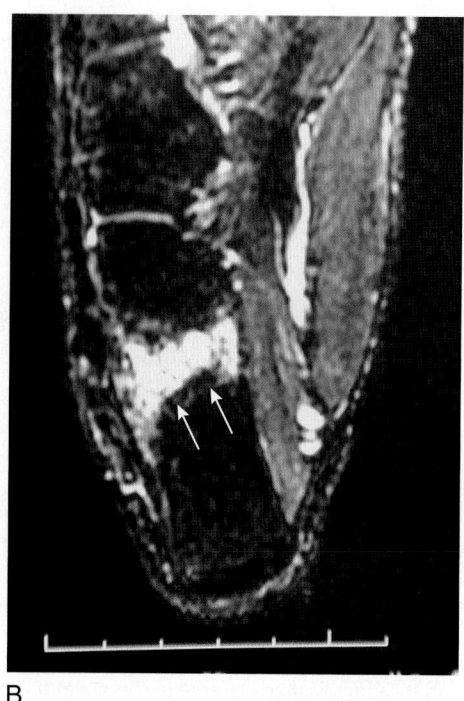

A   B

FIGURE 175-19. A 16-year-old girl with culture-proven coccidiooidomycosis of the mid-part of the calcaneus, of six months duration. **A,** Sagittal T1-weighted magnetic resonance image of the hindfoot. **B,** Coronal T2-weighted MR image of the calcaneus, with fat suppression. The lesions are intraosseous and relatively well-demarcated *(arrows),* showing as low signal on T1-weighted images and high signal on T2-weighted images. No soft tissue mass or periosteal reaction is seen. No other bone was involved.

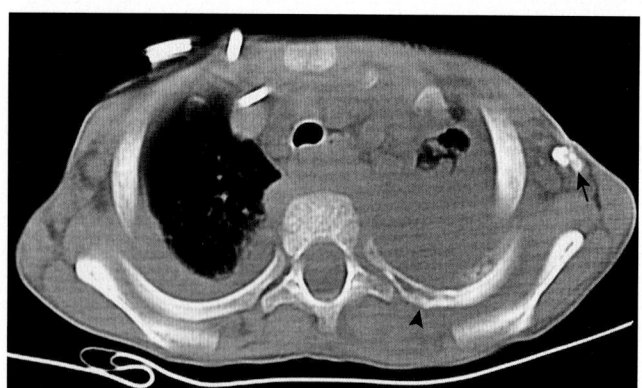

FIGURE 175-20. Axial computed tomographic image of the upper chest of a 4-year-old boy with left rib destructive changes *(arrowhead)* and periosteal reaction, the result of contiguous spread from invasive pulmonary and pleural aspergillosis. Pleural disease with significant pleural thickening is seen on the right. Note the calcified left anterior axillary lymph nodes *(arrow).*

brachydactylies of the types seen in skeletal dysplasias, sickle cell disease, and endocrinopathies. Varicella can produce cutaneous and bone lesions in fetuses of mothers infected during the first trimester. Acute osteomyelitis may rarely occur as a complication of varicella. Rubella (German measles) and cytomegalic inclusion disease may show very similar metaphyseal and metadiaphyseal changes in infected newborns with longitudinal linear sclerosis and lucencies.

Parasitic bone diseases are uncommon in Western countries and are seldom considered in the differential diagnosis of bone lesions; consequently, they may be easily overlooked. Hydatid disease can cause bone lesions, although this location is rare in comparison with other sites (e.g., liver and lung). The affected bone develops irregular cystic expansions. Lesions in the ilium, vertebral column, femur, and other tubular bones have been observed in children. No cases of bone hydatidosis have been reported in children younger than 2.5 years of age, suggesting that a lengthy period of infestation is necessary for disease of bone to declare itself.

> The differential diagnostic considerations for an osseous infection vary with geographic location.

Chronic Recurrent Multifocal Osteomyelitis

Chronic recurrent multifocal osteomyelitis (CRMO) is seen mostly in children and adolescents. It is a bone-destructive and bone-productive inflammatory disorder of, as yet, unknown cause. Recurrent episodes of local swelling and pain, low-grade fever, leukocytosis, and elevated sedimentation rate are associated with focal lytic lesions usually seen in the metaphyses of tubular bones (Fig. 175-24). Pustular lesions of the palms and soles (pustulosis palmoplantaris), often associated with exacerbations of the disease, have been noted in several instances. The tibia has been affected most frequently, followed by the clavicle, fibula, spine, and femur. The upper limb bones and the flat bones are less frequently affected. Lesions may be bilateral and symmetric. Children may rarely present with isolated spinal lesions. Vertebral involvement with findings resembling those of diskitis has been observed. Not all lesions are symptomatic. Mild to moderate progressive sclerosis may surround the initial lytic foci. Cavities and sequestra are not seen in chronic recurrent multifocal osteomyelitis.

Biopsies demonstrate only a nonspecific chronic inflammatory reaction, often with numerous plasma cells, hence the name *plasma cell osteomyelitis*. Cultures are negative. The course of the disease may extend over several years with exacerbations and remissions. Complete resolution may occur, but some patients are left with residual bone changes such as sclerosis and expansion. Epiphyseal extension across the growth plate may occasionally cause premature physeal fusion and secondary degenerative arthritis.

The differential diagnosis of CRMO includes subacute osteomyelitis, Langerhans cell histiocytosis, and neoplasm (i.e., osteosarcoma, Ewing's sarcoma, leukemia,

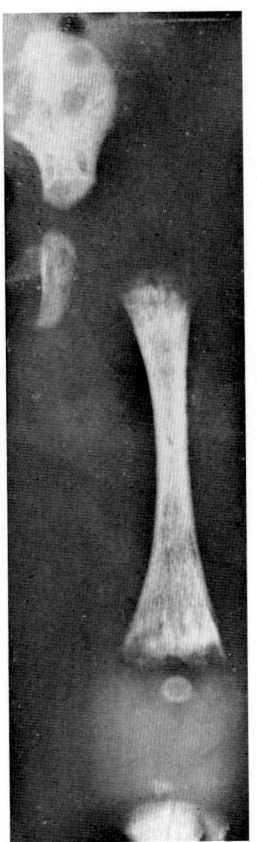 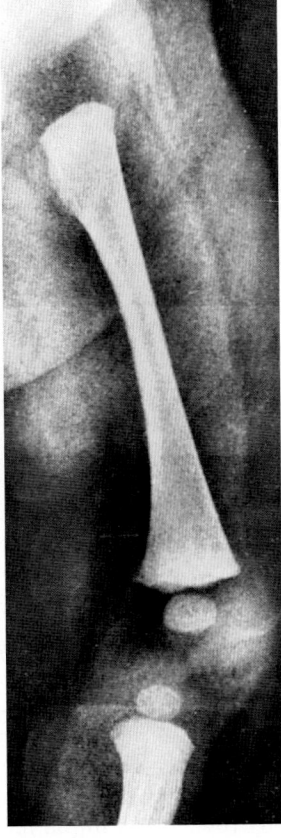

A   B

FIGURE 175-21. Radiographic changes in the bones of a newborn caused by transplacental rubella infection. **A,** On the third postnatal day, the ilium, ischium, femur, tibia, and fibula are irregularly mineralized, with large and small scattered patches of rarefaction. Deep transverse terminal bands of rarefaction, longitudinally streaked, occupy the metaphyseal zones. The absence of cortical thickening is noteworthy. The mother had typical clinical rubella during the first trimester of the pregnancy. The infant, born after gestation of 40 weeks, had thrombocytopenic purpura. Rubella virus was isolated from throat swabs. Serologic tests for syphilis were negative for infant and mother. **B,** On the 62nd postnatal day, the bones are normal radiographically. (Courtesy of Dr. Aaron R. Rausen, Elmhurst, NY.)

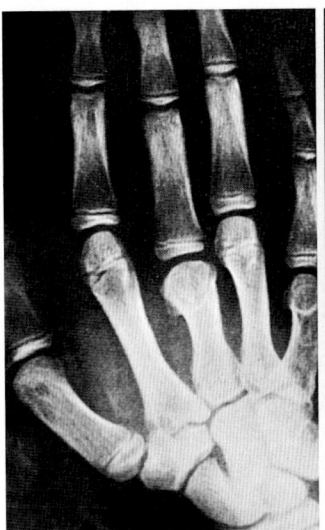 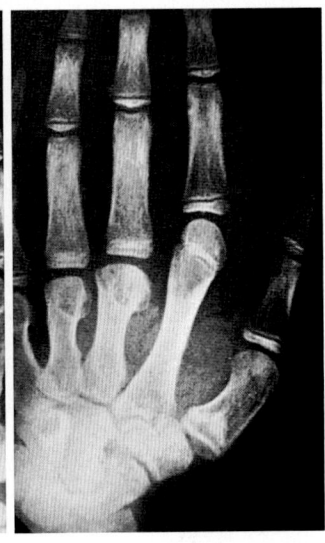

FIGURE 175-23. Late bizarre brachymetacarpia secondary to premature epiphyseal union as a complication of variola osteomyelitis (smallpox) affecting the hands. (From Cockshott WP: Osteomyelitis variolosa. Z Tropenmed Parasitol 1965; 16:199-206, with permission.)

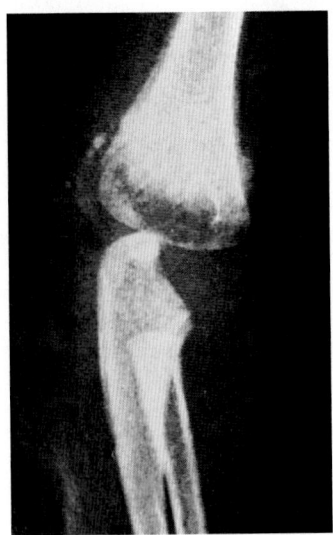 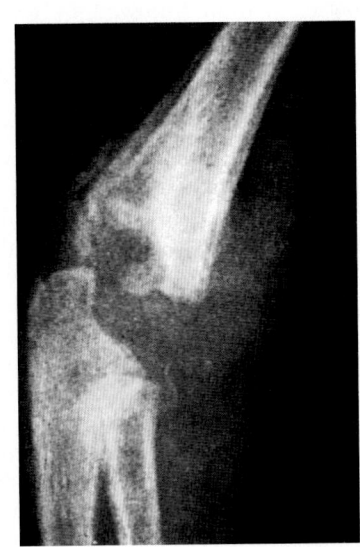 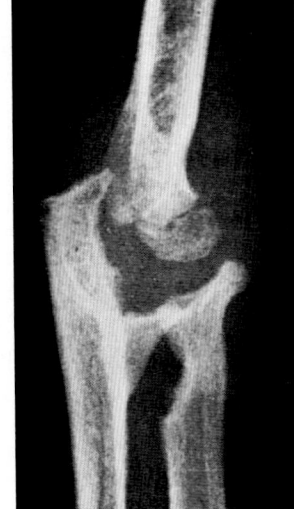

A   B   C

FIGURE 175-22. Serial changes in the elbow in variola osteomyelitis. **A,** Acute phase. **B,** Further disorganization of the joint 3 weeks later. **C,** Flail joint 2 years later. (From Cockshott WP: Osteomyellitis variolosa. Z Tropenmed Parasitol 1965;16:199-206, with permission.)

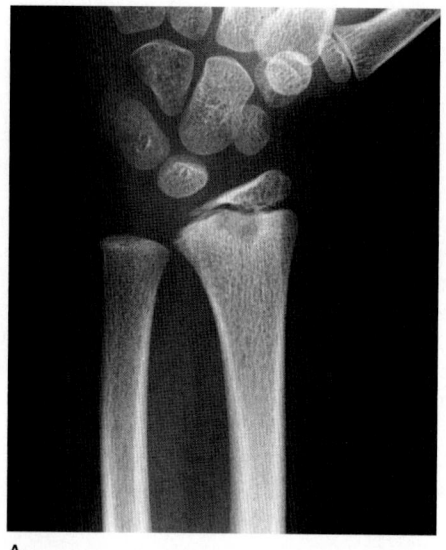 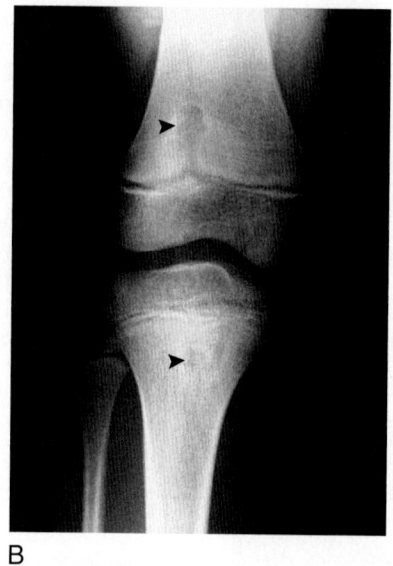 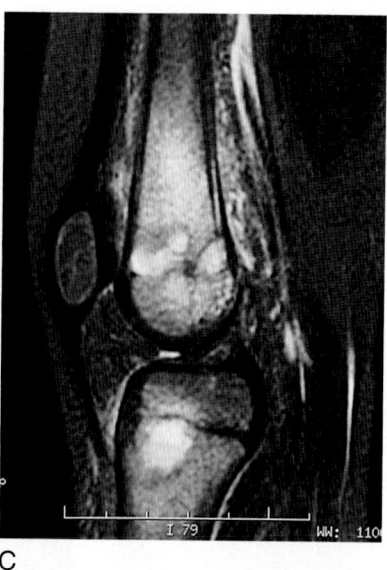

A   B   C

FIGURE 175-24. An 8-year-old girl with recurrent knee pain and swelling and biopsy-proven chronic recurrent multifocal osteomyelitis. There was simultaneous bone involvement in the left wrist and right knee. **A,** Plain radiograph of the wrist shows a metaphyseal lucent focus in the distal radius, abutting the central part of the growth plate. **B,** Anteroposterior radiograph of the right knee shows irregular lucencies in the distal femoral and in the proximal tibial metaphyses *(arrowheads).* **C,** Sagittal T2-weighted, fat-suppressed magnetic resonance image reveals relatively well-defined areas of increased signal intensity in the distal femur and proximal tibia. These are areas of active inflammation. The wrist lesion was clinically silent and was discovered after a total-body bone scan revealed an area of increased uptake in that specific region.

lymphoma, and metastases). A very similar condition, termed *sternocostoclavicular hyperostosis,* occurs more commonly in adults, is limited to the chest wall, and has a frequent association with pustulosis palmoplantaris. Some affected individuals have the human leukocyte antigen allele B27 tissue type and may also have features of a seronegative spondyloarthropathy (psoriatic arthritis). SAPHO (*s*ynovitis, *a*cne, *p*ustulosis, *h*yperostosis, and *o*steitis) is now a frequently used acronym that unifies these idiopathic inflammatory or infectious disorders of bone and skin.

Diagnosis is based on plain radiographic appearance. Scintigraphy with ^{99m}Tc-methylene diphosphonate demonstrates intense focal increased activity at affected sites and may also detect clinically silent lesions. MRI, as expected with inflammatory processes, will show low signal intensity on T1-weighted images and high signal on T2-weighted images. With chronicity and intense sclerosis, there is decreased signal on the T2-weighted images also.

> The etiology of chronic recurrent multifocal osteomyelitis is unknown. Cultures are negative.

TUBERCULOSIS

With the AIDS epidemic, there has been a significant increase in cases of TB worldwide. Although osseous TB is a relatively rare condition today, cases are still encountered that are not diagnosed until an extensive and expensive workup has been completed. Hematogenous metastases of tubercle bacilli to the skeleton may take place early during the active phase of the primary

complex in the thorax or later from postprimary tuberculous foci. After implantation in the bone, an immediate active inflammatory reaction may develop, or the bacilli may be dormant for years until activated by local factors such as trauma to the bone or joint. The synovial surface may be infected before the bones are involved; the infection may then spread from the joint into the contiguous epiphysis and metaphysis. In Cremin's experience in South Africa, the distribution of childhood skeletal TB is 60% to 70% vertebral, 20% to 25% large joints, and 10% to 15% tubular and flat bones.

TB produces a chronic inflammatory reaction in the bones that is similar in its macroscopic aspects to chronic pyogenic osteomyelitis. Local necrosis of the intraosseous tissues develops at the site of implantation and is then followed by regional decalcification and bone destruction. Spread of infection from the focus in the bone takes place through the same pathways as those described in the pathogenesis of pyogenic osteomyelitis. During infancy and early childhood, when the epiphyseal cartilages are relatively thick, direct transfer of the infection from the joint to the bone, or infection across joints, is not common. The articular cartilages are preserved longer in tuberculous osteitis and arthritis than in pyogenic arthritis because of the lack of a destructive proteolytic enzyme in tuberculous exudates. Sinus formation and cold abscesses are common in tuberculous osteitis; involucrum formation and sequestration are very rare. With the antituberculous agents available today, direct needle aspiration from a lesion for diagnosis may be done without danger of chronic sinus formation.

The radiographic findings also are similar to those of chronic pyogenic osteomyelitis in all of the principal features, so that TB should be added regularly to the differential diagnosis of focal bone disease just as are

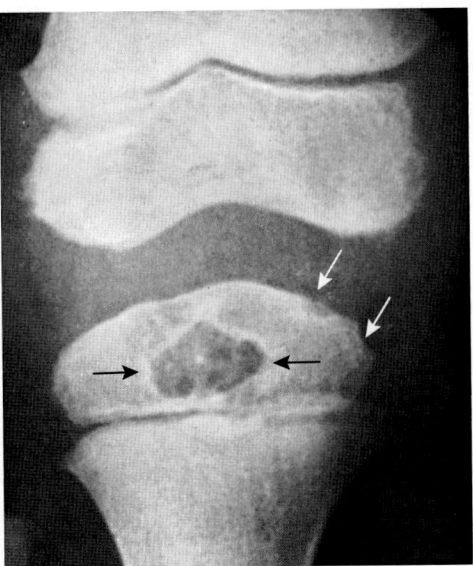 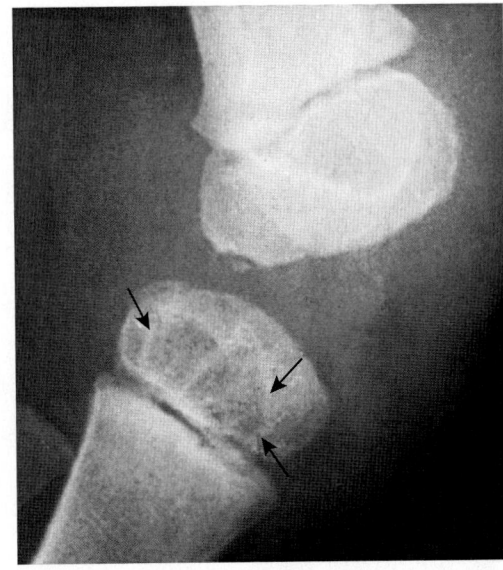

A   B

FIGURE 175-25. Destructive tuberculous epiphysitis of the tibia and arthritis of the knee in a 3-year-old boy. Frontal **(A)** and lateral **(B)** projections. Note that both central *(black arrows)* and marginal *(white arrows)* destructive changes are visible in the ossification center. Tuberculous tissue was found at biopsy.

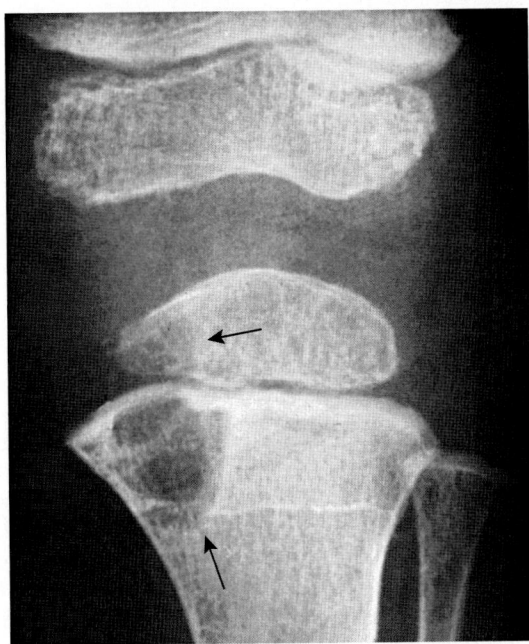

FIGURE 175-26. Tuberculous metaphysitis and epiphysitis of the tibia and arthritis of the knee in a 3-year-old boy. Large areas of destruction are present in the medial aspects of the metaphysis and the epiphyseal ossification center *(arrows).* The large metaphyseal lesion suggests that the bone was infected independently of the joint and possibly before synovial involvement.

neoplasms, neurofibromatosis, Langerhans cell histiocytosis, and osteomyelitis. Certain features do occur that can suggest the diagnosis of TB. In the metaphyses and epiphyses, destruction of bone is more prominent than production of bone (Figs. 175-25 and 175-26). The epiphysis is a site of predilection in primary skeletal TB. Nevertheless, Gardner and Azouz found 40% of solitary radiolucent epiphyseal lesions in a series of 15 children

to represent nontuberculous osteomyelitis. The joint space is characteristically preserved in the early phases of tuberculous arthritis. In the diaphyses of tubular bones, long segments may exhibit destructive and productive changes, whereas metaphyseal regions are unaffected (Fig. 175-27). Sometimes, sharply defined rarefactions are present that gave rise to the term *cystic tuberculosis of bone.* In the short bones of the hands and feet, tuberculous lesions may cause bone expansion and are called *spina ventosa* (Figs. 175-28 and 175-29). Skeletal TB may affect multiple sites, and a bone scan is recommended to detect the presence of quiescent lesions. MRI is useful in certain cases and clearly demonstrates the full extent of the bone marrow, subperiosteal, and soft tissue involvement, as well as any extension into the adjacent joint (Fig. 175-30).

Imaging signs of musculoskeletal tuberculosis

Common
- **Synovitis**
- **Osteopenia**
- **Bone destruction**
- **Sinus formation**
- **Cold abscesses**

Uncommon or rare
- **Bone sclerosis**
- **Bone expansion**
- **Dactylitis (spina ventosa)**
- **Cyst/cavity formation**
- **Sequestration (very rare)**
- **Involucrum formation (very rare)**

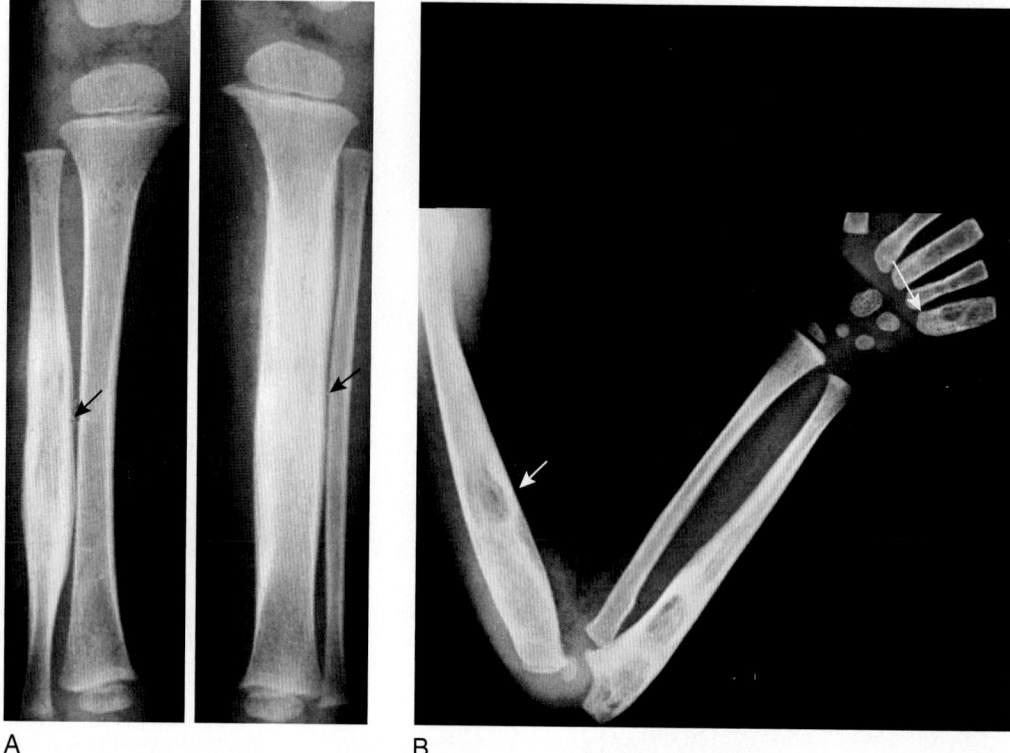

A   B

FIGURE 175-27. Multiple sites of tuberculous diaphysitis in an 18-month-old boy with cold abscesses on the dorsal surfaces of the hands. **A,** Lower extremities. The left tibia and right fibula are enlarged; the medullary canals are expanded, and the overlying cortex is thickened *(arrows).* **B,** Left upper extremity. The distal half of the humerus is enlarged into a sausage-shaped contour and the cortex is thickened; the medullary canal is expanded and exhibits cystic rarefaction *(short arrow).* The proximal half of the ulna is enlarged and irregularly cystic; its cortex is thickened. The fifth left metacarpal is expanded and irregularly lytic and osteoporotic *(long arrow).* All of these lesions healed slowly but completely. On images made 2 years later, the skeleton appeared to be normal.

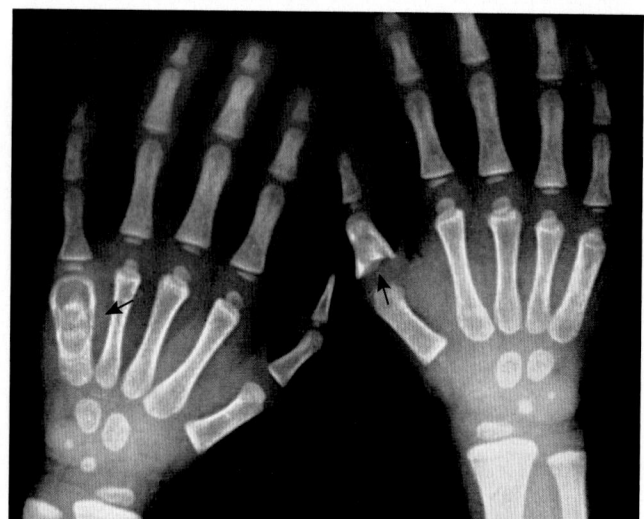

FIGURE 175-28. Tuberculous dactylitis (spina ventosa) in a 2-year-old child. Cystic swelling of the fifth metacarpal and destructive changes in the proximal phalanx of the first digit are evident *(arrows).* Spina ventosa is of historical interest because it was the first lesion described roentgenographically in a child.

Growth disturbances of bones infected with TB are common and may result from partial destruction and premature fusion of growth plates. Disuse osteopenia is a constant feature of the bones when movement has been limited for more than a few weeks. Limitation of movement may contribute to the occasional premature fusion of the growth plates on both sides of a joint with subsequent limb shortening.

Atypical Mycobacterial Infection

Atypical mycobacterial infection in humans is caused by organisms that are not *Mycobacterium tuberculosis* but are closely related to it. The best known is *Mycobacterium bovis,* causing TB in cattle and transmitted to humans through unpasteurized milk. Several other nontuberculous acid-fast organisms have been found to cause focal and disseminated infections in children and are called *atypical tubercle bacilli;* they are identified and categorized by microbiologic techniques. Bone lesions produced by these organisms are indistinguishable from those of TB, but although they are characterized clinically by chronicity and recurrent breakdown of tissue, healing usually occurs with little relation to therapy. Frequent association with skin and lymph node lesions is a helpful clue in recognizing this form of infection.

Focal, TB-like bone lesions have occurred in a few infants and young children inoculated with bacille Calmette-Guérin (BCG) vaccine (Fig. 175-31), and the attenuated organism has been recovered from some lesions. These children were not seriously ill, unlike immunodeficient children, who may develop a generalized disease with widespread, predominantly metaphyseal osteopenic lesions following BCG inoculation.

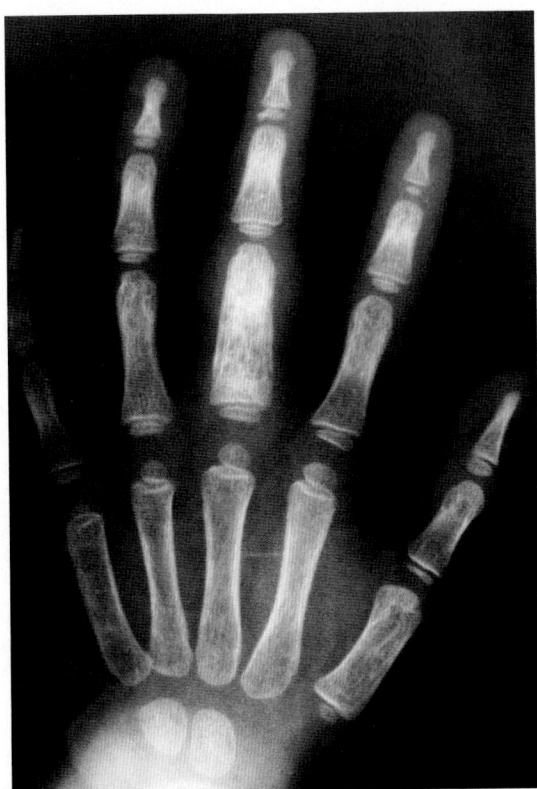

FIGURE 175-29. Tuberculous dactylitis (spina ventosa) in the proximal phalanx of the third finger of a 2-year-old girl. The whole diaphysis is involved. The epiphysis is spared. There is expansion of the rest of the phalanx, which shows mixed areas of bone destruction and sclerosis.

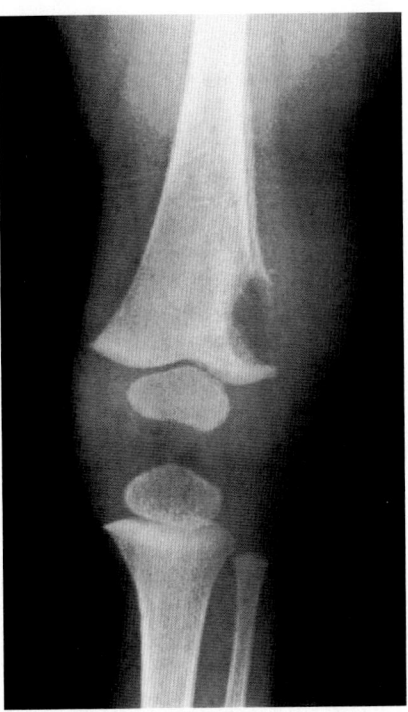

FIGURE 175-31. Bacille Calmette-Guérin osteomyelitis in a 7-month-old boy who had been immunized in the first week of life. Swelling and tenderness began 16 days before taking this film. Only focal demineralization was visible radiographically. (From Mortensson W, Eklof O, Jorulf H: Radiologic aspects of BCG osteomyelitis in infants and children. Acta Radiol 1976;17:845-855, with permission.)

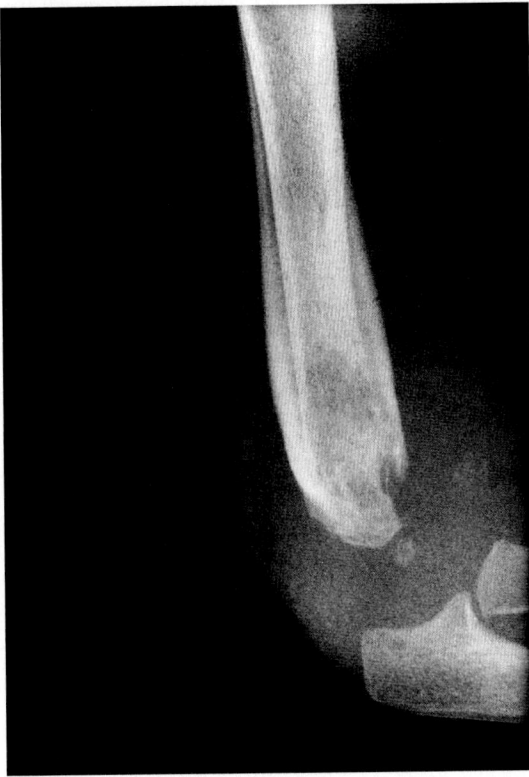

A

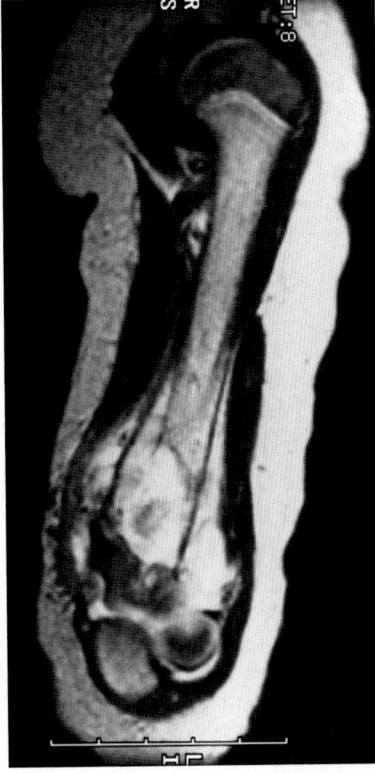

B

FIGURE 175-30. A 7-month-old Inuit boy presented with left elbow swelling. **A,** Lateral plain radiograph of the distal humerus and elbow shows an ill-defined lytic lesion in the distal humerus and thick periosteal reaction parallel to the cortex. There is also soft tissue swelling and edema. **B,** Sagittal T2-weighted magnetic resonance image shows with exquisite detail the abnormal high-signal bone marrow involvement of the distal humerus, the large subperiosteal inflammatory masses, and the extension into the elbow joint. Needle aspiration material from the distal humeral lesion grew *Mycobacterium tuberculosis.*

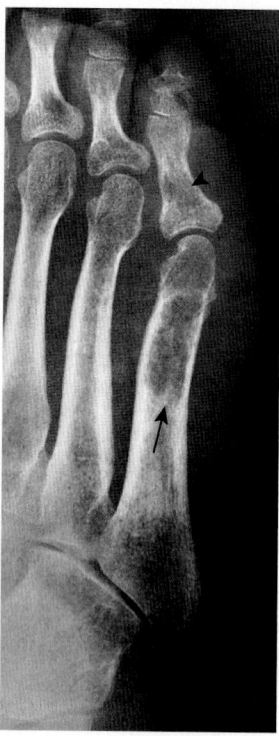

FIGURE 175-32. Lytic bone lesions of sarcoidosis in the foot of a 17-year-old girl. There is a definitely lytic destructive lesion in the distal half of the fifth metatarsal *(arrow)*, and foamy rarefaction of the base of its proximal phalanx *(arrowhead)*.

BRUCELLOSIS

Brucellosis is a zoonosis, seen all over the world. It is caused by gram-negative bacilli of the genus *Brucella*. *Brucella melitensis* is the most common cause of brucellosis. In a series of 96 Saudi patients, Madkour and colleagues found the spine to be most frequently involved (101 spinal sites showed increased uptake on the bone scan), followed by the joints (53 joints); only three long bones were involved. *Brucella* osteomyelitis of tubular bones was osteolytic, with only minimal periosteal reaction. Ruyssen and colleagues reported the case of a French child (from Yvelines), with *B. melitensis* osteomyelitis of the second metatarsal.

SARCOIDOSIS

Sarcoidosis is a chronic granulomatous disease that very rarely involves the bones of children. Skin, lungs, and lymphatic structures are often affected. In the skeleton, small, destructive cystic areas or a coarse lace-like reticulated pattern occur in the tubular bones of the hands and feet (Fig. 175-32). There is no periosteal reaction. There may be acro-osteolysis, but there is usually no osteopenia. Well-defined lytic lesions may occur in long bones or vertebral bodies, reminiscent of TB or metastatic disease. Redman and associates reported a case of sarcoidosis of the femur in a child who presented with a pathologic fracture. Occasionally, joint manifestations are present and simulate rheumatoid arthritis clinically, but there is no radiologic evidence of joint involvement in sarcoidosis. Concomitant involvement of salivary glands and eyes may suggest the diagnosis. Biopsy of skin lesions may establish the diagnosis. A causal agent has not been established.

CONGENITAL SYPHILIS

There is now an increased incidence of this transplacental infection caused by *Treponema pallidum*. Congenital syphilis causes hepatosplenomegaly, lymphadenopathy, skin rash, and anemia. Bones are often involved but may not become clinically or radiologically manifest in the first weeks of life. Bone pain in one or more extremities may be severe and may result in lack of movement of those extremities, a condition termed *Parrot pseudoparalysis*. Syphilis of bone can be suggested on the basis of radiologic signs when it has not been considered on clinical grounds. The diagnosis, however, still rests on appropriate serologic tests. Two main forms are observed, infantile and juvenile, and their radiographic features are different.

The outstanding characteristic of infantile syphilis is multiple bone involvement with almost selective localization in the metaphyses. Broad bands of metaphyseal radiolucency were considered evidence of "metaphysitis" but are now known to be nonspecific responses to the stress of disseminated infection. Syphilitic granulation tissue can occur in these regions (Fig. 175-33). Radiographically, the two causes cannot be distinguished, but when there is associated metaphyseal serration (the so-called sawtooth metaphysis) (Fig. 175-34), the diagnosis of congenital syphilis is practically assured. Similar diagnostic "specificity" is provided by the Wimberger sign after the newborn period, when focal destructive foci are found in the metaphyseal regions of tubular bones, particularly the medial tibial metaphyses at the knee (Fig. 175-35). These destructive metaphyseal lesions are not pathognomonic of congenital syphilis. They may be seen with ordinary osteomyelitis, hyperparathyroidism, skeletal infantile myofibromatosis and metastases. The epiphyses are generally spared. Diaphyseal involvement, especially with periosteal new bone formation, also tends to occur after the first month and may be associated with some destructive foci (Fig. 175-36) and even scattered focal cortical destruction and expansion of the medullary cavity (Fig. 175-37). Healing of the bone lesions in the infantile form of the disease occurs with or without therapy, usually without deformity. Metaphyseal destructive lytic lesions may lead to pathologic fractures, and child abuse is in the differential diagnosis.

Imaging signs of bone involvement in syphilis (*Treponema pallidum*)

Congenital—infantile
- **Multiple bone involvement**
- **Metaphyseal lucent bands**
- **Metaphyseal serration (sawteeth)**
- **Metaphyseal bone destruction: the Wimberger sign**
- **Diaphyseal involvement**
- **Periosteal reaction**

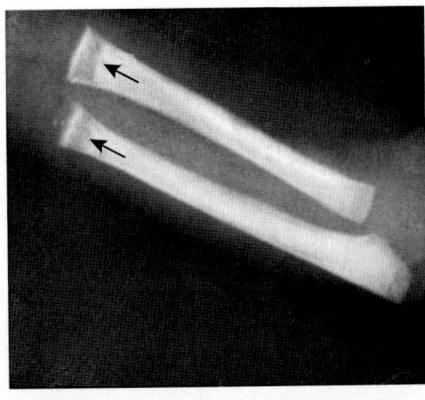

A

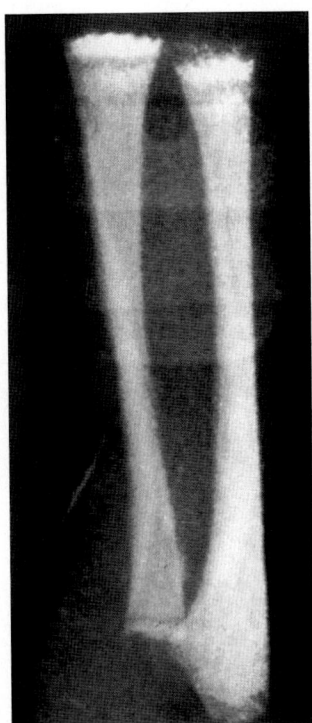

FIGURE 175-34. Sawtooth metaphysis in a newborn infant with congenital syphilis. This patient had a rash and mucocutaneous lesions characteristic of the disease.

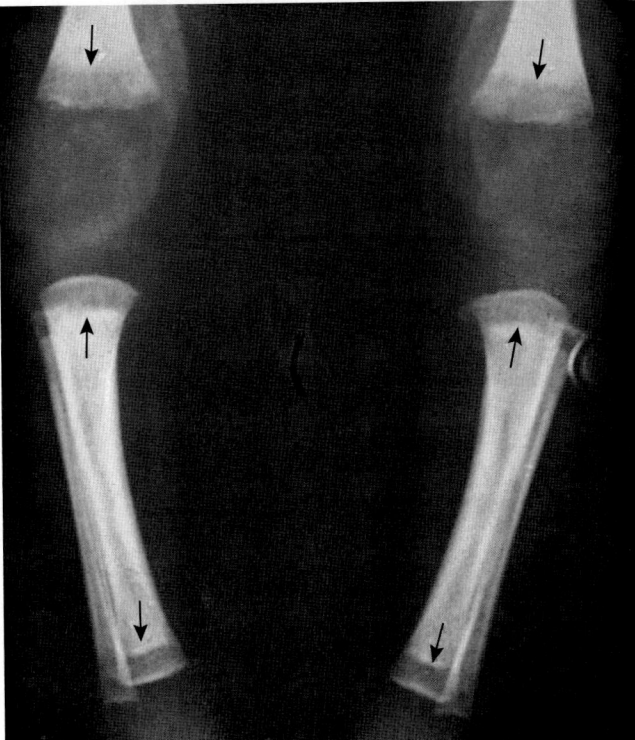

B

FIGURE 175-33. Radiographs of syphilitic metaphysitis in a premature 1-month-old infant, showing deep segments of diminished density *(arrows)*. The spongiosa in these segments has been replaced by radiolucent syphilitic granulation tissue. **A**, Upper limb. **B**, Lower limbs.

Congenital—juvenile
- Periosteal and cortical thickening: saber shin
- Focal destructive lesions

Acquired
- Gumma (an infectious granuloma)

Juvenile syphilis is observed radiographically in childhood and is manifested by diffuse or localized subperiosteal thickening of the cortex (Fig. 175-38). Associated focal destructive lesions, resembling cystic TB, occasionally are present. Thickening of the anterior cortex of the tibia is responsible for the "saber shin" deformity of congenital syphilis that appears in late childhood.

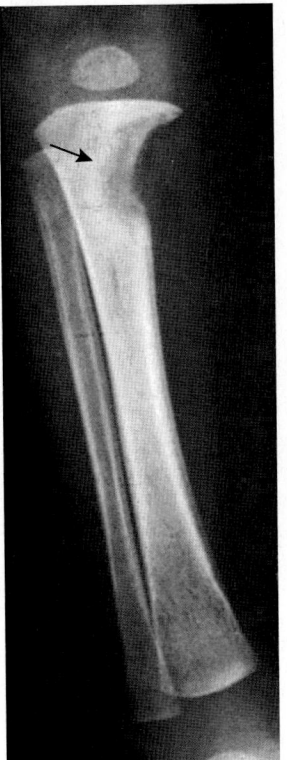
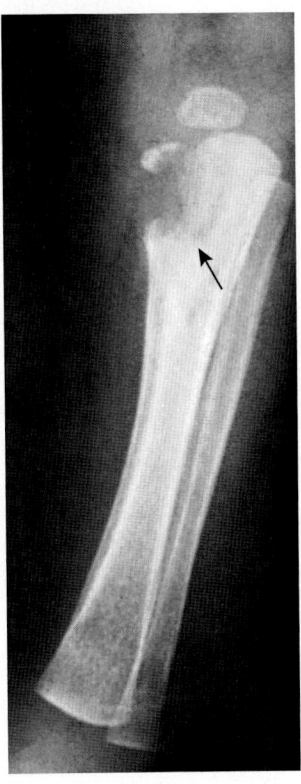

A   B

FIGURE 175-35. Bilateral symmetric destructive syphilitic metaphysitis of the proximal ends of the tibias (Wimberger sign) in a 2-month-old infant. Large areas of destruction of the spongiosa and overlying cortex are seen at the medial aspects of the tibias *(arrows)*. In the left tibia, the medial segment of the epiphyseal plate is partially destroyed. Note also diffuse periosteal thickening of the diaphyses.

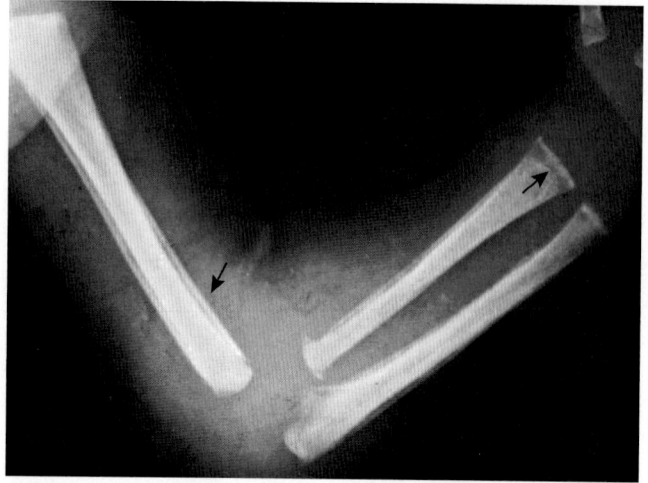

A

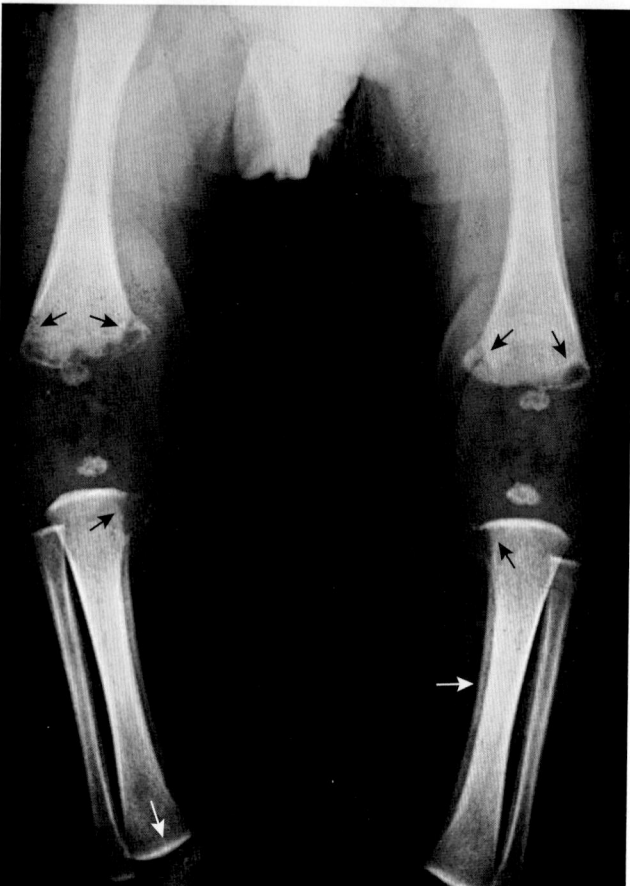

B

FIGURE 175-36. Syphilitic panosteitis in an infant 5 weeks of age. **A,** Upper limb. **B,** Lower limbs. Focal destructive changes are visible in the metaphyses, and the diaphyses show diffuse periosteal thickening. The main radiographic differential diagnosis here is non-accidental trauma (child abuse).

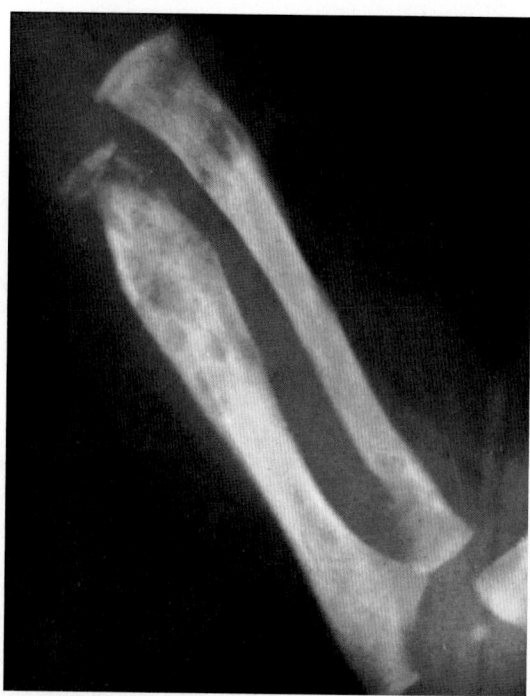

FIGURE 175-37. Expansion and destructive metaphyseal and diaphyseal changes in a syphilitic 3-month-old infant.

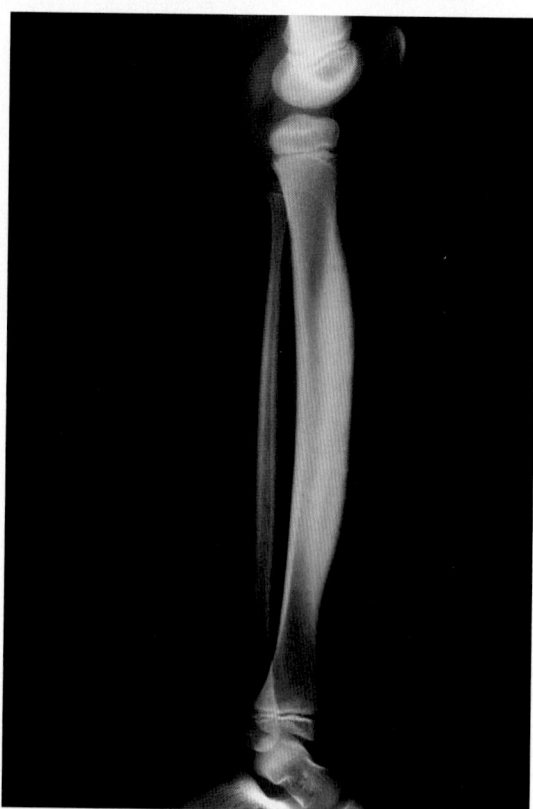

FIGURE 175-38. Lateral view of the lower leg in an 8-year-old boy with saber shin due to congenital syphilis. There is extensive anterior cortical and periosteal thickening of the tibial diaphysis.

The preceding discussion relates to congenital syphilis. However, acquired syphilis does occur in children, albeit very rarely, and its clinical manifestations are comparable to those in adults.

Yaws is a nonvenereal spirochetal disease caused by *Treponema pertenue*. Bone pain and active osteoperiostitis are common. Thick, irregular bony outlines may be clinically palpable. New bone formation may be massive, simulating a tumor. In later stages, bone destruction with sequestration and fistula formation may occur.

INFANTILE CORTICAL HYPEROSTOSIS (CAFFEY DISEASE)

Infantile cortical hyperostosis (ICH) is a disorder affecting the skeleton and some of its contiguous fasciae and muscles. For the last two decades, the incidence of ICH has been declining, and it is now a rare disease. It carries the eponymic designation Caffey disease as a result of Caffey's in-depth report of the condition in 1945, when he coined the descriptive term, as well as of his subsequent publications. Descriptions of individual cases, unknown to Caffey, preceded his initial report and were subsequently acknowledged. These include those of Roske and DeToni (hence DeToni-Caffey disease).

Since ICH was first clearly recognized and named in 1945, it has been widely reported, especially in the United States, where several cases have been observed in almost every large hospital and clinic. It has occurred in all manner of circumstances—in cities and rural communities, in all kinds of climates, in all seasons of the year, in all races, in all culture levels and in poverty and luxury.

The incidence in boys and girls is approximately equal, but there is a striking age limitation. Caffey believed that there were no valid cases in which the onset occurred later than the fifth to seventh month of life. Occasional reports now indicate initial onsets up to the middle of the first decade in patients in whom the diagnosis is acceptable by all other standards. Although several cases have been recognized in utero, most patients have been well for several weeks after birth. In some of these patients who had radiographs, the skeleton was normal before the disease appeared clinically. The average age at onset is about 9 weeks.

The occurrence of ICH in siblings, in twins, and in cousins raises the question of familial and possibly genetic transmission. Veller and Laur reported the disease in an infant 9 weeks of age whose father had productive periostitis of unknown origin when he was 4 weeks of age in 1929. The father was the patient described by Roske in 1930. Several large family studies have been reported, supporting an autosomal dominant transmission with incomplete penetrance. Saul and coworkers have illustrated 26 pedigrees with more than 100 persons affected to support this conclusion. Additional familial cases have been reported. There can be no question now that hereditary factors are involved, but the pathogenesis remains obscure. Some authors suggest that there are two major types of ICH: an autosomal dominant form and a sporadic form. Sporadic cases of ICH are on the decline. Gensure and associates have

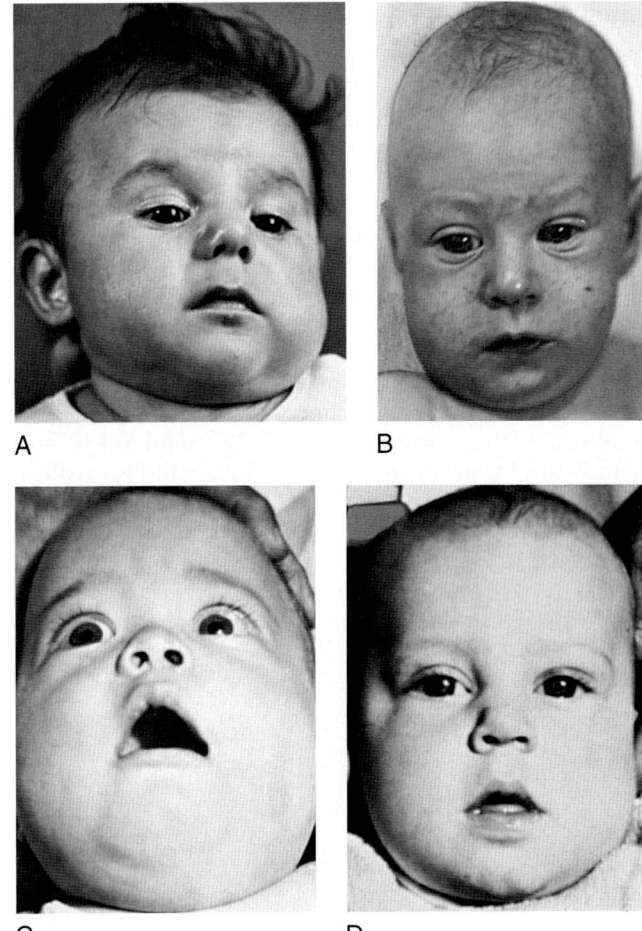

A   B

C   D

FIGURE 175-39. Facies in infantile cortical hyperostosis. In almost all cases, the changes have appeared before the fifth month of life. **A,** Unilateral swelling of the left cheek and left side of the jaw in a 12-week-old infant, five weeks after its first appearance. **B,** Unilateral swelling of the right cheek and right side of the jaw in a 15-week-old infant, eight weeks after its first appearance. **C,** Bilateral swelling of the cheeks and jaw in a 6-month-old infant, five weeks after their first appearance. **D,** Bilateral swelling of the cheeks and jaw in a 12-week-old infant, 4 days after their first appearance; hyperostosis of the mandible was not visible in films made at this time but became visible in later films. The cervical lymph nodes were not enlarged.

recently proved that autosomal dominant Caffey disease is associated with a mutation in *COL1A1* and thus belongs to the family of type I collagen-related conditions. It remains uncertain why the mutation results in a self-limited hyperostosis affecting one or a few specific bones of the infant's body.

Among the causes that have been postulated as possible precipitating factors are viral infections causing the initial fever, painful swellings, and elevated erythrocyte sedimentation rate.

> Infantile cortical hyperostosis (Caffey disease) may, in part, have a genetic basis.

Clinical Findings

There are but three manifestations common to all patients: irritability, swellings of the soft tissues, and cortical thickenings of the underlying bones. The soft tissue swellings appear suddenly at the onset. The babies present with a painful wooden, deeply situated hardness during the active phases of the disease. Early on, the swellings may be exquisitely tender but are not overly warm or discolored (Figs. 175-39 and 175-40). In rare cases, local redness has been described. Massive deep swelling in the muscular masses probably represents apparent extension of the primary periosteal reaction into the adjacent tissues. The swellings appear clinically before the hyperostoses become visible roentgenographically; they subside and lose their tenderness long before the hyperostoses resolve. The swellings involute slowly without suppuration; sometimes they recur suddenly in their original sites or in new sites either

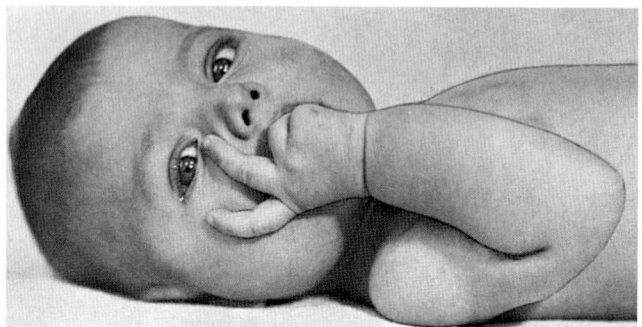

FIGURE 175-40. Swelling of the forearm and recurrent swelling of the right side of the face in a 5-month-old infant. The facial swelling first appeared at age 2 months; the forearm became swollen at age 3 months. The mandible and both bones in the forearm showed massive hyperostoses at the time this photograph was made (see Fig. 175-46*B*). All cervical, axillary, and epitrochlear lymph nodes were normal.

during or after the subsidence of the swellings that appeared at the onset of the disease. Edema and swellings around the orbits and even unilateral proptosis have been described. Other features, present in some patients but lacking in others, have been fever in the initial clinical phases of the disease, pallor, painful pseudoparalysis, and pleurisy. The condition has been found in asymptomatic persons in the course of family surveys or radiographic examination for other causes.

The uneven, protracted clinical course of the disease, with unpredictable remissions and relapses, is one of the most characteristic features and one that makes the evaluation of therapeutic agents difficult or impossible.

Caffey disease is usually self-limited, with severe symptoms lasting from 2 to 3 weeks to 2 or 3 months. Swellings may persist even longer, but generally disability is limited to the early acute phase. Occasionally, active disease in the mandible or tubular bones may persist and recur intermittently for years, with crippling deformities in the limbs and markedly delayed muscular and motor development. Hyperostoses are usually gone within 12 months (Fig. 175-41), but several cases have indicated persistence of cortical thickening and bowing even into adult life. The few deaths that have been recorded appear to result from intercurrent infection rather than from the primary disease.

Complications include pseudoparalyses, particularly of the upper limb with scapular involvement, and pleural effusion with costal involvement. Ipsilateral diaphragmatic elevation has been observed in several instances of scapular involvement. Torticollis has been associated with clavicular hyperostosis. Dysphagia has occurred in the presence of mandibular reaction. Sequelae are rare but include mandibular asymmetry, bowing deformities of the lower limbs, limb overgrowth, and bony fusions between adjacent bones such as ribs or bones of the forearm or lower leg (Figs. 175-42 and 175-43).

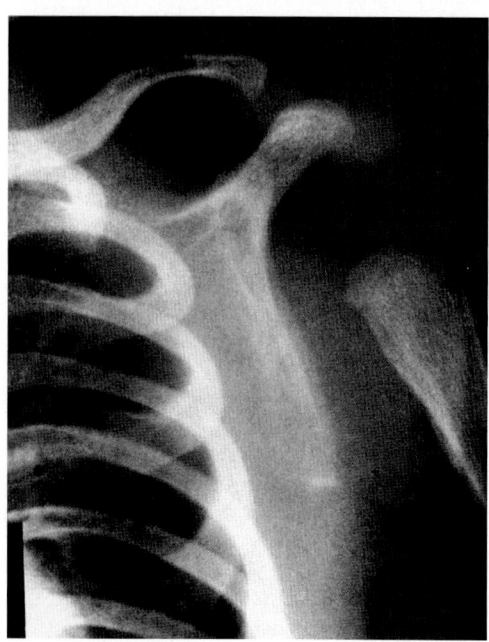

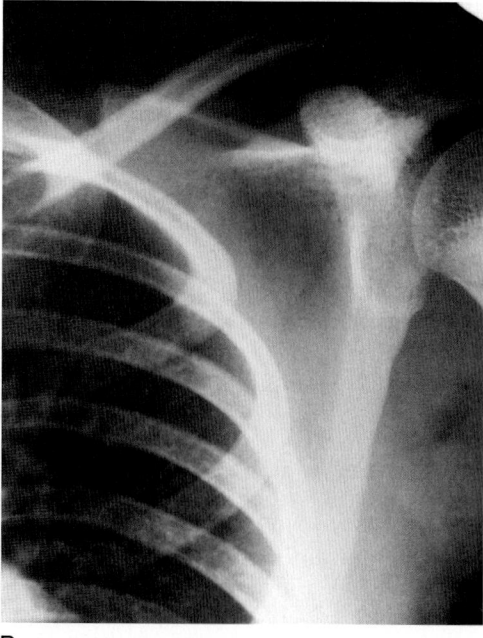

A

B

FIGURE 175-41. Infantile cortical hyperostosis (ICH) of the scapula. **A,** Periosteal thickening is seen along the lateral cortex of the left scapula. **B,** Film taken 13 years later shows a completely normal left scapula. In ICH, periosteal thickening is usually completely gone within 12 months.

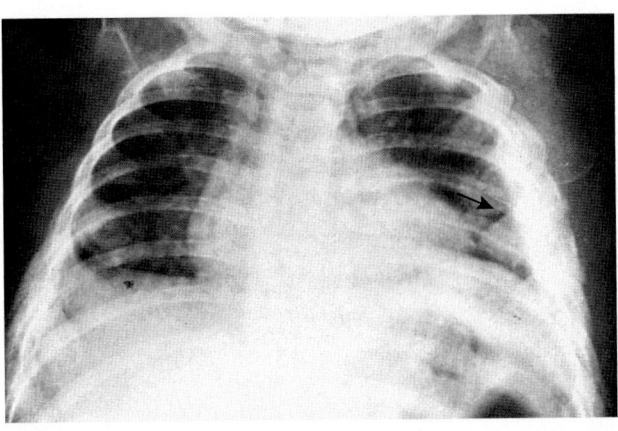 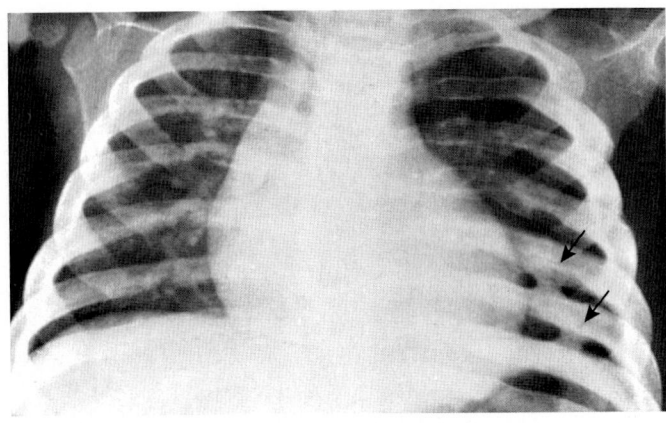

FIGURE 175-42. Multiple costal cortical hyperostoses with residual bony bridges between the fifth and sixth and the sixth and seventh left ribs. **A,** At 4½ months, 4 weeks after onset, during the active phase, there are multiple bilateral hyperostoses in the ribs and a longitudinal strip of water density *(arrow)* along the inner edges of the ribs that suggests pleural reaction. **B,** At 9 months, after subsidence of all general and local manifestations, there is still some expansion of the ribs, and bridges of bone have formed *(arrows).*

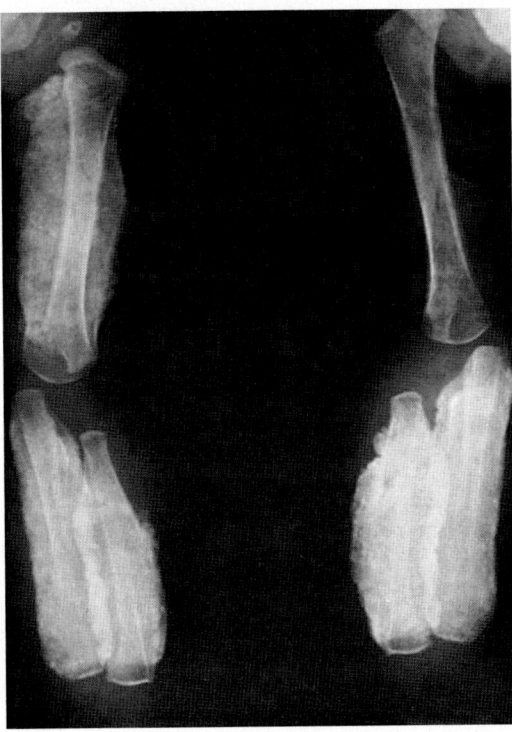 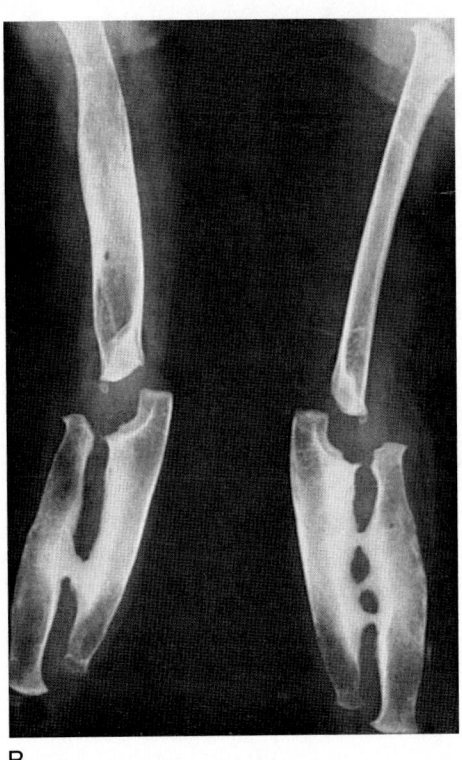

FIGURE 175-43. Residual bony bridges between each radius and ulna in infantile cortical hyperostosis. **A,** Massive cortical thickenings of the radii and ulnas at 4½ months of age. Pressure from the external thickenings has forced the radial heads laterad out of the elbows. **B,** At 12½ months, 9 months after onset, all affected bones are still enlarged, owing largely to expansion of the medullary cavities, although there are still residues of the earlier cortical thickening. The radial heads are still dislocated, and the radial diaphyses are now anchored in this ectopic position by solid bony bridges between them and the ulnar diaphyses—a single bridge on the right and three on the left. At 32 months, these bridges were still intact, although they had diminished slightly in caliber. It is possible that these bony bridges represent ossification of parts of the interosseous membrane.

Laboratory Findings

The most constant positive laboratory findings in ICH are elevated erythrocyte sedimentation rate and increased serum alkaline phosphatase activity. During active phases of the swellings and fever, these two laboratory findings are usually present. Hemoglobin level and the number of red blood cells are frequently reduced. Thrombo-cytosis has occurred in several instances and has been associated with thromboses in some infants. An increase in immunoglobulins has also been noted in some cases.

The results of serologic tests for both bacterial and viral infections have been consistently negative. All attempts to culture bacteria from the tissues and fluids of these patients have failed. In several infants, the disease has been associated with the Wiskott-Aldrich syndrome,

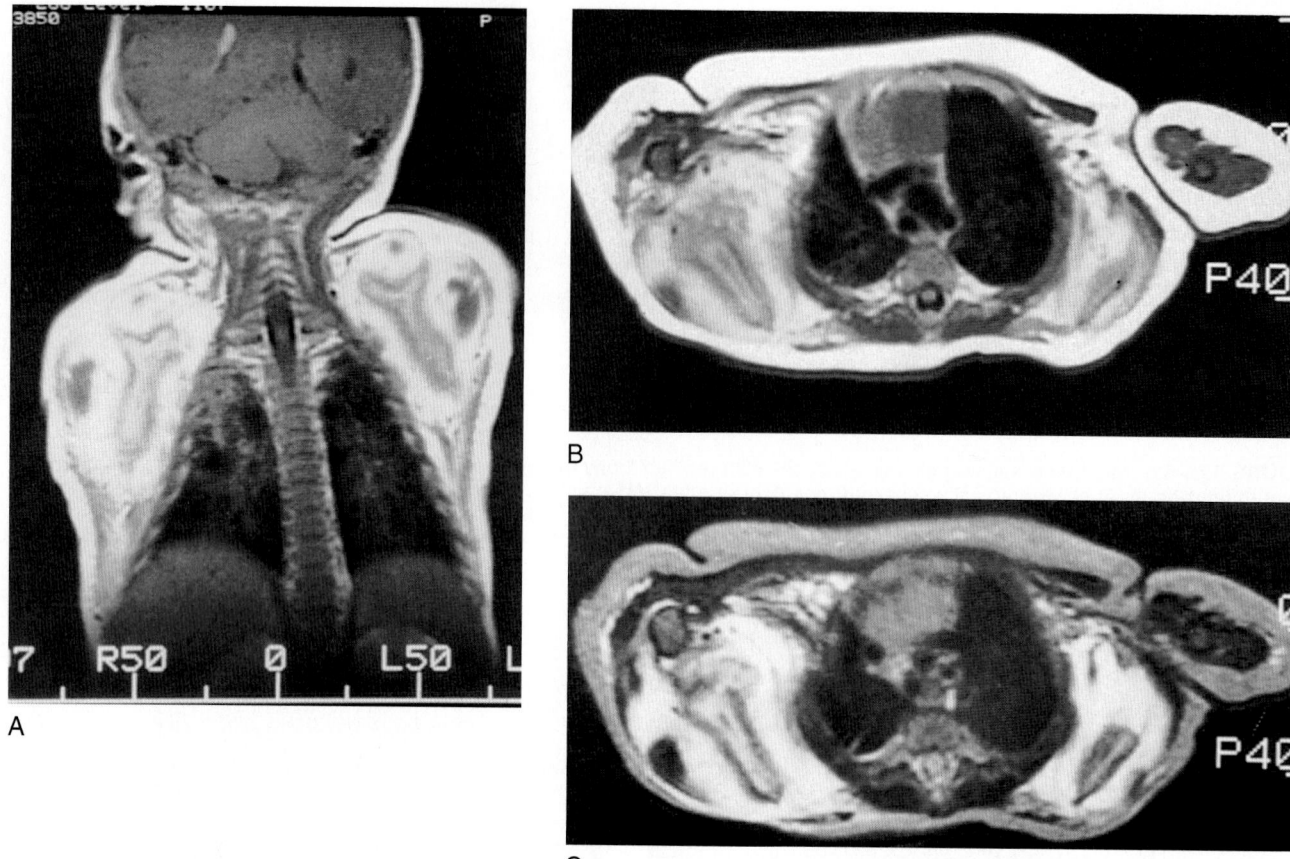

FIGURE 175-44. Magnetic resonance images of scapular involvement in infantile cortical hyperostosis. This 7-week-old boy with firm masses overlying the scapulae, bilateral Erb palsy, irritability, and generalized hypotonia was sent to the neurologist because of paralysis, and magnetic resonance imaging was requested. Skull and cervical spine were normal. Shoulders show increased marrow signal and cortical thickening of scapulas bilaterally; an extensive area of high signal completely surrounds both scapulas. **A,** Coronal contrast-enhanced T1-weighted image. **B,** Axial contrast-enhanced T1-weighted image. **C,** Axial T2-weighted image. The severity of the edema surrounding the affected bones is clearly shown, especially on the T2-weighted image, and although the brachial plexus was not clearly identified, it seemed reasonable that compression by the large swellings was responsible for the Erb palsy. (Courtesy of Dr. Drew Sullivan, San Jose, CA.)

a rare X-linked recessive immunodeficiency characterized by a triad of eczema, infections, and bleeding caused by thrombocytopenia.

Imaging Findings

The radiographic features of Caffey disease are a sine qua non for diagnosis and consist of stages in the appearance, development, and regression of hyperostotic lesions throughout the skeleton. Hyperostoses develop in contact with the external cortical surface, expand, and then remodel by resorption externally or expansion from the internal aspect of the bone. In the latter case, the affected bone may show an expanded medullary cavity and thin cortex for months or even longer.

Bone and gallium scans may be positive before the development of radiographic signs. A bone scan is usually performed to look for other lesions, even if only one bone has radiographic abnormalities suggesting the diagnosis. MRI has demonstrated the marked soft tissue reaction surrounding the affected bones with increased signal on T2-weighted images (Fig. 175-44). Diffuse enhancement after gadolinium administration has been described.

Cortical hyperostoses have been demonstrated in all of the tubular bones of the skeleton except the phalanges (Fig. 175-45). Vertebral bodies have also been spared. Of all the bones, the mandibles, clavicles, and ulnas have been involved the most frequently, the first in approximately 75% of cases. In the tubular bones, the lesions of ICH are confined to the diaphyses and metaphyses. Epiphyseal ossification centers are normal roentgenographically. In the lower limbs, distribution of lesions is asymmetric; the larger hyperostoses of the limb bones often present conspicuous marginal irregularities (Fig. 175-46). Involvement may be very marked in one of a pair of adjacent bones, whereas the other remains conspicuously normal.

Of the flat bones, the mandibles, scapulas, ilia, parietals, and frontals have all shown alterations (Figs. 175-47 and 175-48). Scapular lesions have usually been unilateral and have almost always appeared during the first 6 months of life. The scapular hypertrophy and sclerosis of ICH may be mistaken for malignant neoplasm. Cortical hyperostoses are usually most prominent in the lateral arcs of the ribs, possibly as a result of projection factors, since both vertebral and costochondral portions of the ribs may be affected (Fig. 175-49).

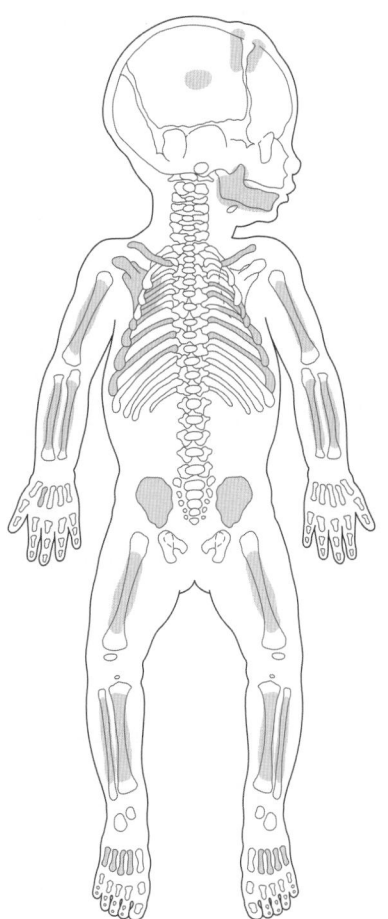

FIGURE 175-45. Distribution of the skeletal lesions in infantile cortical hyperostosis. The sites of hyperostosis are shaded. The mandible, clavicles, and ulnas are affected most frequently. Hyperostoses in the vertebrae, round bones of the wrists and ankles, and phalanges have not been observed.

Fauré and colleagues reported four cases with exclusively orbital and facial involvement. Thickenings in the calvaria have been identified in several patients, and it seems likely that many inconspicuous lesions in the calvaria have been overlooked. Focal radiolucent lesions of the flat bones of the skull also have been observed.

The distribution of the bone lesions is one of the most diagnostic features of ICH. If the disease was ever confined to one bone, other than the mandible, it would be impossible to identify it with certainty.

It is possible that most of the mild cases of ICH are overlooked clinically and are never examined radiographically. After a short course of mild fever, these patients recover without a satisfactory diagnosis. Slight swellings of the mandible are exceedingly difficult to palpate in the deep subcutaneous fat of the infantile jaw, as are deep, mild swellings of the ribs and long bones in the limbs. Many of the unexplained cortical hyperostoses encountered radiographically in healthy infants and young children may be residuals of earlier and mild unrecognized ICH. Their presence has been instrumental in case finding in several of the studies on the familial distribution of Caffey disease.

> Infantile cortical hyperostosis has been demonstrated in all tubular bones of the skeleton except the phalanges. The mandible, clavicles and ulnas are most frequently affected.

Differential Diagnosis

From the standpoint of differential diagnosis, the clinical course, laboratory findings, and radiographic features differentiate ICH from the most common diseases of infants with skeletal manifestations. Moreover, the clinical features and the serial changes in the formation of the hyperostoses are quite different from those of trauma, osteomyelitis, or scurvy. In the last-named lesions, a thin shell of bone forms first over the soft tissue swelling, separated from the bone diaphysis by a deep strip of relative radiolucency. In ICH, new bone formation begins in the soft tissue swelling, directly contiguous to the original cortex, that is, in the subperiosteal space. It then becomes progressively denser; and capped by a dense shell of limiting bone. Eversole and coworkers confirmed this feature in microscopic sections of biopsy specimens.

The periosteal reaction of congenital syphilis develops later than that of ICH, and the serologic test for syphilis is positive. The hyperostosis of vitamin A intoxication appears only after many months of excessive ingestion of large amounts of vitamin A; the mandible is not involved, and the degree of hyperostosis is relatively mild.

As mentioned earlier, neoplasm has been considered in instances of isolated scapular involvement; the infrequency of primary bone neoplasms in infants is an important diagnostic consideration.

Treatment

Heyman and associates treated patients with typical ICH and increased prostaglandin serum levels with indomethacin, a prostaglandin synthetase inhibitor, and reported clinical improvement within 48 hours and progressive decrease of soft tissue swelling subsequently. Investigation of levels of endogenous prostaglandin may be of value in typical cases of ICH. If prostaglandin is involved in the disorder, the role of treatment of undiagnosed illnesses with aspirin in the ascertainment of cases may merit study.

Because the disease is generally self-limited, no therapy has been necessary in the great majority of cases. Caffey advocated the use of steroids for severe cases, and generally a prompt clinical response was observed, although recurrence was frequent following withdrawal of the drug. Steroids are contraindicated when thrombocytosis is present because of their tendency to induce thrombosis.

OTHER CONDITIONS ASSOCIATED WITH HYPEROSTOTIC LESIONS

Other conditions associated with hyperostotic lesions have been described in children older than those usually affected with ICH (Table 175-1). Goldbloom and

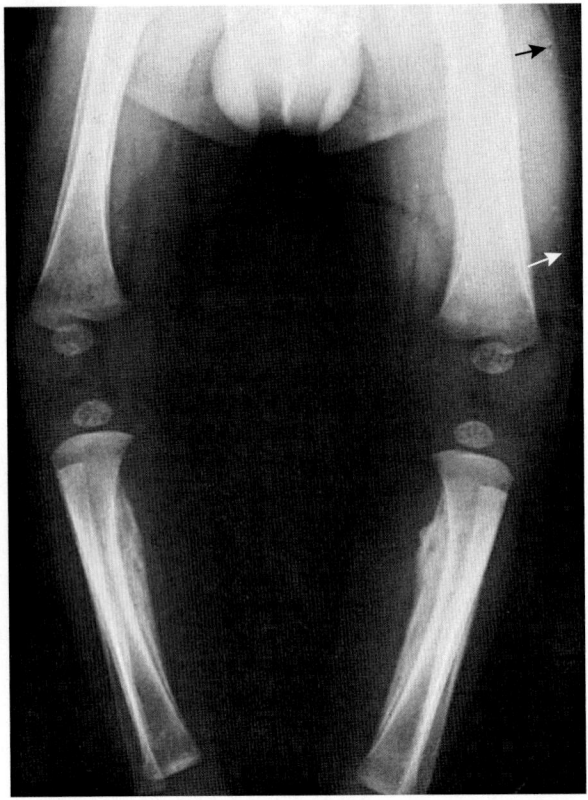
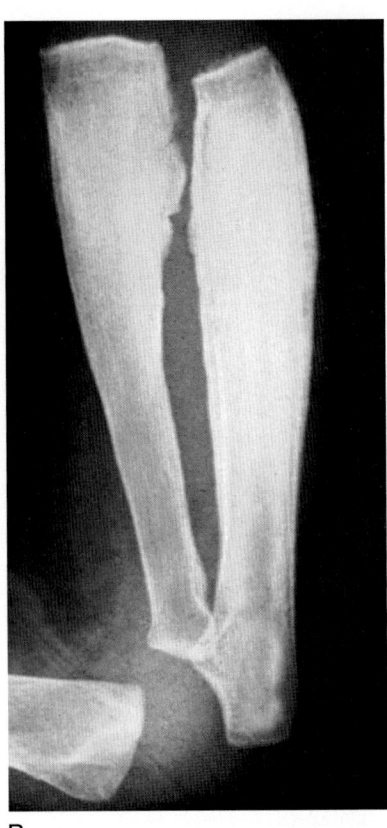

A   B

FIGURE 175-46. Massive cortical hyperostoses in tubular bones of the limbs. **A,** In the lower extremities of a 14-week-old infant, the *arrows* point to thick swellings in the soft tissues of the thigh. **B,** In the forearm of a 5-month-old infant, note the coarse and deep marginal irregularities in the distal radius.

colleagues observed cortical hyperostoses in long tubular bones and the mandible associated with dysproteinemia in two unrelated children, 10 and 14 years of age, who had fever, pain, and tenderness in bones and who were unable to walk. The serum gamma globulin content in one patient was increased, with an increase in the immunoglobulin G fraction. Plasma cells were overabundant in the bone marrow. These radiographic changes faded gradually over several months after the fever subsided.

Melhem and associates reported more prominent cortical hyperostoses in association with hyperphosphatemia in a 5½-year-old boy with migrating swellings of the limbs and face of several months' duration. A less severely affected 13-year-old girl had similar clinical and laboratory findings. Grégoire and coworkers reported older patients with a prolonged clinical course who demonstrated hyperphosphatemia and also increased immunoglobulin G and M. These older children, with protracted disease and biochemical alterations do not represent cases of ICH.

Prostaglandin administration in neonates with cyanotic congenital heart disease commonly used to maintain patency of the ductus arteriosus, has been associated with periostitis. This type of cortical/periosteal hyperostosis has been experimentally duplicated in dogs in response to long-term prostaglandin infusions. Bone changes have been observed as early as the ninth day of treatment (Fig. 175-50) and may increase and persist for weeks to months; they ultimately resolve without sequelae. In contrast with the features in ICH, the productive reactions tend to be symmetric (Fig. 175-51) and usually fail to affect the mandible. Ribs, clavicles, and scapulas may be affected.

Hypertrophic osteoarthropathy is rarely encountered in children. Most cases are associated with chronic lung suppuration with or without cystic fibrosis, congenital cyanotic heart disease, biliary atresia and cirrhosis, as well as chronic inflammatory bowel disease.

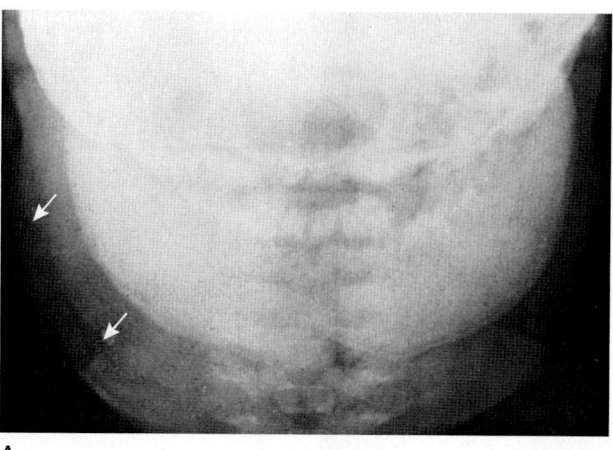

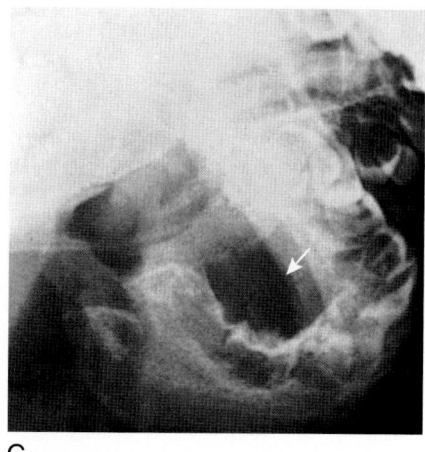

FIGURE 175-47. **A** and **B,** Massive cortical thickenings of the mandible in a 6-month-old infant whose facial swellings (*arrows* in **A**) first appeared during the fourth week of life. **A,** Mouth closed. **B,** Mouth open. **C,** Massive mandibular hyperostosis in a 7-week-old infant whose facial swelling *(arrow)* first appeared during the fourth week of life.

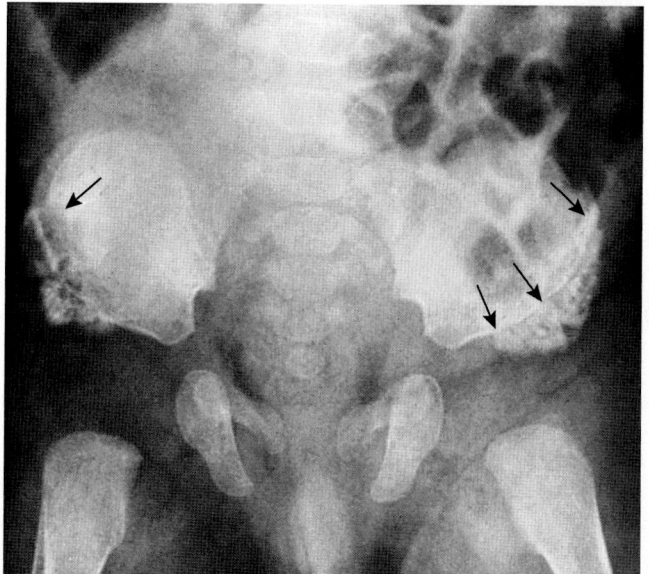

FIGURE 175-48. Massive marginal hyperostoses on the lateral edges of the iliac wings *(arrows).* The lesions stop short of the faces of the acetabular cavities and crests of the ilia. The patient, who was 6 weeks old, had classic signs of infantile cortical hyperostosis, with thick hyperostoses in the mandible and several long bones. (Courtesy of Dr. W. P. Yarbrough, Greene, MI.)

TABLE 175-1
Differential Diagnosis of Cortical Hyperostosis and Periosteal Reaction
Physiologic in the newborn
Trauma
Osteomyelitis
Vitamin A intoxication
Scurvy
Congenital syphilis
Primary bone tumor
Infantile cortical hyperostosis (Caffey disease)
Goldbloom disease
Hypertrophic osteoarthropathy
Prostaglandin administration
Hyperphosphatemia

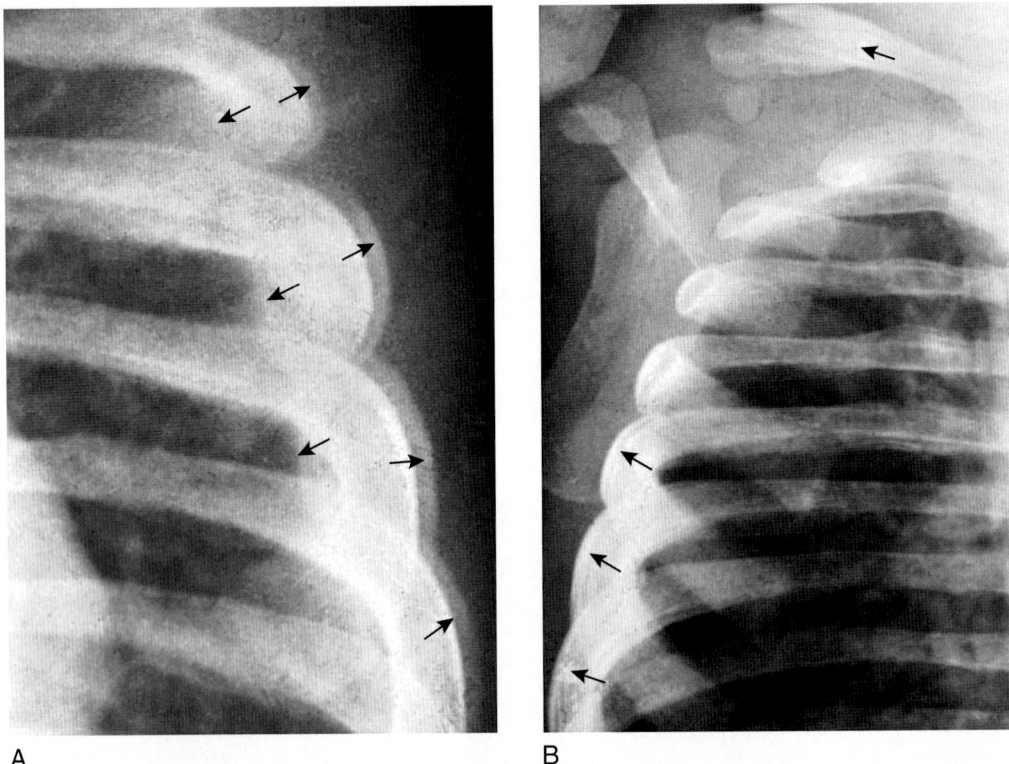

FIGURE 175-49. Costal hyperostoses. **A,** Early bilateral multiple thickenings of the ribs with underlying pleural thickening in a 14-week-old infant. **B,** Older multiple costal hyperostoses in a 5-month-old infant. The lamellations are a sign that the hyperostoses are old and beginning to involute.

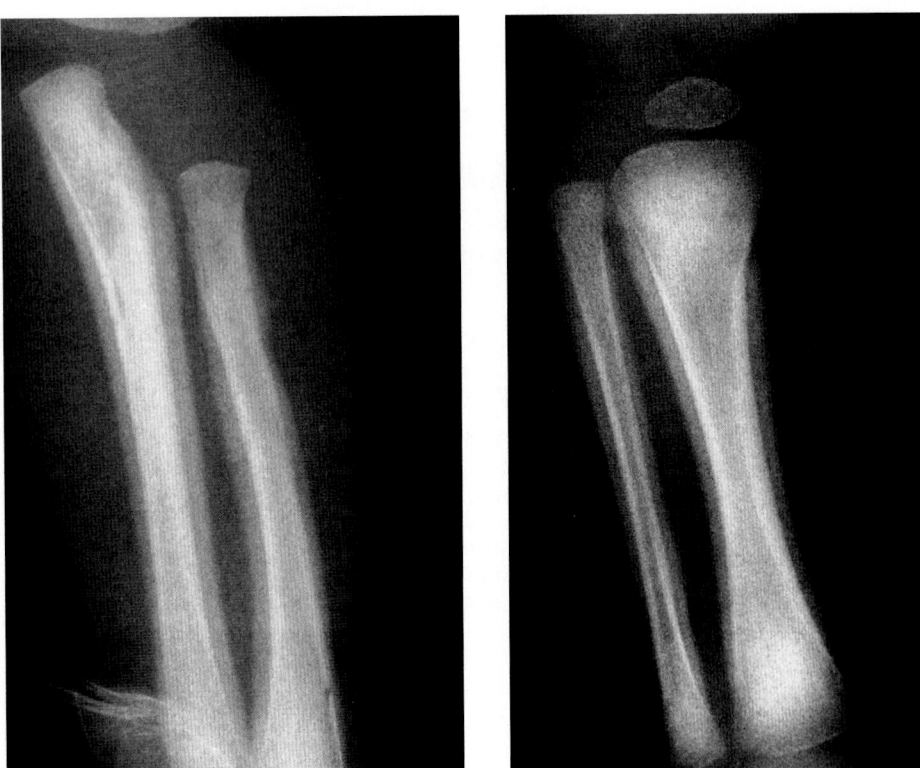

FIGURE 175-50. A 1-month-old boy with cyanotic congenital heart disease on prostaglandin E therapy. Forearm **(A)** and lower leg **(B)** radiographs show periosteal reaction along the entire length of the diaphyses of the radius, ulna, tibia, and fibula. Both sides were similarly affected.

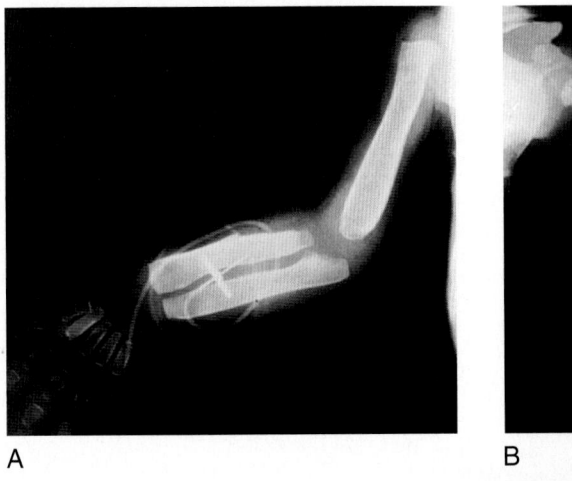
A

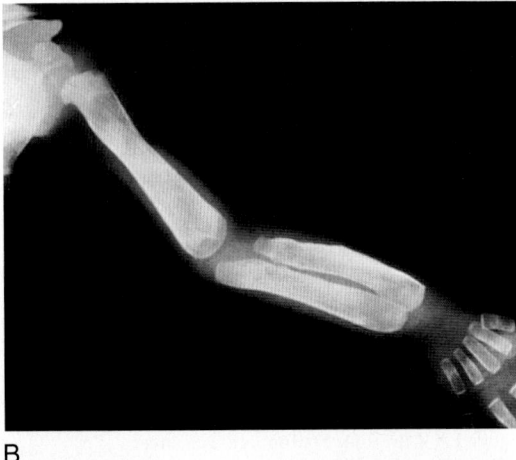
B

FIGURE 175-51. Expansion and hyperostoses of tubular bones of the upper (**A** and **B**) and lower (**C**) extremities following long-term administration of prostaglandin in an infant with congenital heart disease. (Courtesy of Dr. Y. Sato, Department of Radiology, University of Iowa, Iowa City, IA).

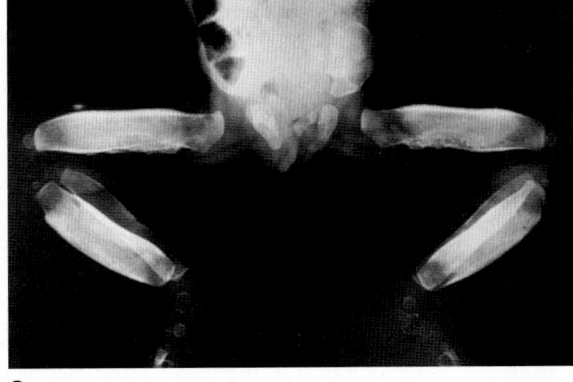
C

SUGGESTED READINGS

General

Blickman JG, van Die CE, de Rooy JW: Current imaging concepts in pediatric osteomyelitis. Eur Radiol 2004;14(Suppl 4):55-64

Bureau NJ, Chhem RK, Cardinal E: Musculoskeletal infections: US manifestations. Radiographics 1999;19:1585-1592

Connolly LP, Connolly SA: Skeletal scintigraphy in the multimodality assessment of young children with acute skeletal symptoms. Clin Nucl Med 2003;28:746-754

DeBoeck H: Osteomyelitis and septic arthritis in children. Acta Orthop Belg 2005;71:505-515

Gutierrez K: Bone and joint infections in children. Pediatr Clin North Am 2005;52:779-794

Gylys-Morin V: MR imaging of pediatric musculoskeletal inflammatory and infectious disorders. Magn Reson Imaging Clin N Am 1998;6:537-559

Keller MS: Musculoskeletal sonography in the neonate and infant. Pediatr Radiol 2005;35:1167-1173

Kocher MS, Lee B, Dolan M, et al: Pediatric orthopedic infections: early detection and treatment. Pediatr Ann 2006;35:112-122

Martinez-Aguilar G, Avalos-Mishaan A, Hulten K, et al: Community-acquired, methicillin-resistant and methicillin-susceptible *Staphylococcus aureus* musculoskeletal infections in children. Pediatr Infect Dis J 2004;23:701-706

McCarthy JJ, Dormans JP, Kozin SH, et al: Musculoskeletal infections in children: basic treatment principles and recent advancements. Instr Course Lect 2005;54:515-528

Steinbach LS, Tehranzadeh J, Fleckenstein JL, et al: Human immunodeficiency virus infection: musculoskeletal manifestations. Radiology 1993;186:833-838

Tang JS, Gold RH, Bassett LW, et al: Musculoskeletal infection of the extremities: evaluation with MR imaging. Radiology 1988;166:205-209

Waagner DC: Musculoskeletal infections in adolescents. Adolesc Med 2000;11:375-400

Acute Osteomyelitis

Bray H, Stringer DA, Poskitt K, et al: Maple tree knee: a unique foreign body—value of ultrasound and CT examination. Pediatr Radiol 1991;21:457-458

Buhne K-H, Bohndorf K: Imaging of posttraumatic osteomyelitis. Semin Musculoskel Radiol 2004;8:199-204

Canale ST, Manugian AH: Neonatal osteomyelitis of the os calcis: a complication of repeated heel punctures. Clin Orthop Relat Res 1981;156:178-182

Capitano MA, Kirkpatrick JA: Early roentgen observations in acute osteomyelitis. Am J Roentgenol Radium Ther Nucl Med 1970;108:488-496

Connolly LP, Connolly SA, Drubach LA, et al: Acute hematogenous osteomyelitis of children: assessment of skeletal scintigraphy—diagnosis in the era of MRI. J Nucl Med 2002;43:1310-1316

Dangman BC, Hoffer FA, Rand FF, et al: Osteomyelitis in children: gadolinium-enhanced MR imaging. Radiology 1992;182:743-747

Davidson D, Letts M, Khoshhal K: Pelvic osteomyelitis in children: a comparison of decades from 1980-1989 to 1990-2001. J Pediatr Orthop 2003;23:514-521

Gill PJ, Goddard E, Beatty DW, et al: Chronic granulomatous disease presenting with osteomyelitis: favorable response to treatment with interferon-γ. J Pediatr Orthop 1992;12:398-400

Gonzalez BE, Teruya J, Mahoney DH Jr, et al: Venous thrombosis associated with staphylococcal osteomyelitis in children. Pediatrics 2006;117:1673-1679

Hoffer FA, Emans J: Percutaneous drainage of subperiosteal abscess: a potential treatment for osteomyelitis. Pediatr Radiol 1996;26:879-881

Ibia EO, Imoisili M, Pikis A: Group A beta-hemolytic streptococcal osteomyelitis in children. Pediatrics 2003;112:e22-e26

Jaramillo D, Treves ST, Kasser JR, et al: Osteomyelitis and septic arthritis in children: appropriate use of imaging to guide treatment. AJR Am J Roentgenol 1995;165:399-403

Kaiser S, Rosenberg M: Early detection of subperiosteal abscess by ultrasonography: a means for further successful treatment in pediatric osteomyelitis. Pediatr Radiol 1994;24:336-339

Kaplan SL: Osteomyelitis in children. Infect Dis Clin North Am 2005;19:787-797

Karmazyn B, Loder RT, Kleiman MB, et al: The role of pelvic magnetic resonance in evaluating nonhip sources of infection in children with acute nontraumatic hip pain. J Pediatr Orthop 2007;27:158-164

Kleinman PK: A regional approach to osteomyelitis of the lower extremities in children. Radiol Clin N Am 2002;40:1033-1059

Lagard D, Dupont S, Boutry N, et al: Ostéite corticale septique. J Radiol 2000;81:54-58

Mah ET, LeQuesne GW, Gent RJ, et al: Ultrasonic features of acute osteomyelitis in children. J Bone Joint Surg Br 1994;76:969-974

Martin JCA, Rodriguez LA, Cilveti JA: Flatfoot and calcaneal deformity secondary to osteomyelitis after neonatal heel puncture. J Pediatr Orthop B 1999;8:122-124

Offah AC: Acute osteomyelitis, septic arthritis and discitis: differences between neonates and older children. Eur J Radiol 2006;60:221-232

Oudjhane K, Azouz EM: Imaging of osteomyelitis in children. Radiol Clin N Am 2001;39:251-266

Perron AD, Brady WJ, Miller MD: Orthopedic pitfalls in the ED: osteomyelitis. Am J Emerg Med 2003;21:61-67

Rasool MN: Hematogenous osteomyelitis of the calcaneus in children. J Pediatr Orthop 2001;21:738-743

Riebel TW, Nasir R, Nazarenko O: The value of sonography in the detection of osteomyelitis. Pediatr Radiol 1996;26:291-297

Rosenbaum DN, Blumhagen JD: Acute epiphyseal osteomyelitis in children. Radiology 1985;156:89-92

Saigal G, Azouz EM, Abdenour G: Imaging of osteomyelitis with special reference to children. Sem Musculoskel Radiol 2004;8:255-265

Schmit P, Glorion C: Osteomyelitis in infants and children. Eur Radiol 2004;14 Suppl 4:44-54

Solomon M, Stening M, Macdessi S et al: Occult epiphyseal bone abscess: lessons for the unwary. Australas Radiol 2003;47:181-183

Song KM, Sloboda JF: Acute hematogeneous osteomyelitis in children. J Am Acad Orthop Surg 2001;9:166-175

Weber-Chrysochoou C, Corti N, Goetshel P, et al: Pelvic osteomyelitis: a diagnostic challenge in children. J Pediatr Surg 2007;42:553-557

Wu JS, Gorbachova T, Morrison WB, et al: Image guided bone biopsy for osteomyelitis. Are there factors associated with positive or negative cultures? AJR Am J Roentgenol 2007;188:1529-1534

Yagupsky P: Kingella kinga infections of the skeletal system in children: diagnosis and therapy. Expert Rev Anti Infect Ther 2004;2:787-794

Subacute Osteomyelitis (Brodie Abscess) and Chronic Osteomyelitis

Beslikas TA, Panagopoulos PK, Gigis I, et al: Chronic osteomyelitis of the pelvis in children and adolescents. Acta Orthop Belg 2005;71:405-409

Gonzalez-Lopez JL, Soleto-Martin FJ, Cubillo-Martin A, et al: Subacute osteomyelitis in children. J Pediatr Orthop B 2001;10:101-104

Hernandez RJ: Visualization of small sequestra by computerized tomography: report of six cases. Pediatr Radiol 1985;15:238-241

Kozlowski K: Brodie's abscess in the first decade of life. Pediatr Radiol 1980;10:33-37

Marti-Bonmati L, Aparisi F, Poyatos C, et al: Brodie abscess: MR imaging appearance in 10 patients. J Magn Reson Imaging 1993;3:543-546

Pöyhiä T, Azouz EM: MR imaging evaluation of subacute and chronic bone abscesses in children. Pediatr Radiol 2000;30:763-768

Rasool MN: Primary subacute haematogenous osteomyelitis in children. JBJS 2001;83B:93-98

Segev E, Hayek S, Lokiec F, et al: Primary chronic sclerosing (Garre's) osteomyelitis in children. J Pediatr Orthop 2001;10:360-364

Unusual Infections

André C, Badoual J, Kalifa G, et al: Histoplasmose africaine. Arch Fr Pediatr 1984;41:429-431

Arkun R: Parasitic and fungal diseases of bones and joints. Sem Musculoskel Radiol 2004;8:231-242

Barter SJ, Hennessy O: Actinomycetes as the causative organism of osteomyelitis in sickle cell disease. Skeletal Radiol 1984;11:271-273

Borgen L, Kaakonsen MO, Gudmundsen TE, et al: Acute osteomyelitis as a complication of varicella. Acta Radiol 2005;46:652-656

Borzyskowski M, Harris RF, Jones RWA: The congenital varicella syndrome. Eur J Pediatr 1981;137:335-338

Cockshott P, MacGregor M: Natural history of osteomyelitis variolosa. J Fac Radiol 1969;10:57-63

Damry N, Schurmans T, Perlmutter N: MRI evaluation and follow-up of bone necrosis after meningococcal infection and disseminated intravascular coagulation. Pediatr Radiol 1993;23:429-431

Doria AS, Taylor GA: Bony involvement in paracoccidioidomycosis. Pediatr Radiol 1997;27:67-69

Gaisie G, Bowen A, Quattromani FL, et al: Chest wall invasion by aspergillus in chronic granulomatous disease of childhood. Pediatr Radiol 1981;11:203-206

Gehweiler JA, Capp MP, Chick EW: Observations on the roentgen patterns in blastomycosis of bone. Am J Roentgenol Radium Ther Nucl Med 1970;108:497-510

Gharbi HA, Ben Cheikh M, Hamza R, et al: Les localisations rares de l'hydatidose chez l'enfant. Ann Radiol (Paris) 1977;20:151-157

Grier D, Feinstein KA: Osteomyelitis in hospitalized children with chickenpox: imaging findings in four cases. AJR Am J Roentgenol 1993;161:643-646

Lachman RS, Yamauchi T, Klein J: Neonatal systemic candidiasis and arthritis. Radiology 1972;105:631-632

Patriquin HB, Trias A, Jéquier S, et al: Late sequelae of infantile meningococcemia in growing bones of children. Radiology 1981;141:77-82

Robinson JL, Vaudry WL, Dobrovolsky W. Actinomycosis presenting as osteomyelitis in the pediatric population. Pediatr Infect Dis J 2005;24:365-369

Silverman FN: Virus diseases of bone: do they exist? AJR Am J Roentgenol 1976;126:677-703

Thomas KE, Owens CM, Veys PA, et al: The radiological spectrum of invasive aspergillosis in children: a 10-year review. Pediatr Radiol 2003;33:453-460

Torricelli P, Martinelli C, Biagini R, et al: Radiographic and computed tomographic findings in hydatid disease of bone. Skeletal Radiol 1990;19:435-439

Yousefzadeh DK, Jackson JH: Neonatal and infantile candidal arthritis with or without osteomyelitis: a clinical and radiographical review of 21 cases. Skeletal Radiol 1980;5:77-90

Zeppa MA, Laorr A, Greenspan A, et al: Skeletal coccidioidomycosis: imaging findings in 19 patients. Skeletal Radiol 1996;25:337-343

Chronic Recurrent Multifocal Osteomyelitis

Azouz EM, Jurik AG, Bernard C: Sternocostoclavicular hyperostosis in children: a report of eight cases. AJR Am J Roentgenol 1998;171:461-466

Boutin RD, Resnick D: The SAPHO syndrome: an evolving concept for unifying several idiopathic disorders of bone and skin. AJR Am J Roentgenol 1998;170:585-591

Cotten A, Flipo RM, Mentre A, et al: SAPHO syndrome. Radiographics 1995;15:1147-1154

Demharter J, Bohndorf K, Michl W, et al: Chronic recurrent multifocal osteomyelitis: a radiological and clinical investigation. Skeletal Radiol 1997;26:579-588

Job-Deslandre C, Krebs S, Kahan A: Chronic recurrent multifocal osteomyelitis: five year outcomes in 14 pediatric cases. Joint Bone Spine 2001;68:245-251

Jurik AG: Chronic recurrent multifocal osteomyelitis. Semin Musculoskel Radiol 2004;8:243-253

Jurik AG, Egund N: MRI in chronic recurrent multifocal osteomyelitis. Skeletal Radiol 1997;26:230-238

Jurriaans E, Singh NP, Finlay K, et al: Imaging of chronic recurrent multifocal osteomyelitis. Radiol Clin N Am 2001;39:305-327

Laasonen LS, Karvonen SL, Reunala TL: Bone disease in adolescents with acne fulminans and severe cystic acne: radiologic and scintigraphic findings. AJR Am J Roentgenol 1994;162:1161-1165

Manson D, Wilmot DM, King S, et al: Physeal involvement in chronic recurrent multifocal osteomyelitis. Pediatr Radiol 1989;20:76-79

Mortensson W, Edeburn G, Fries M, et al: Chronic recurrent multifocal osteomyelitis in children: a roentgenologic and scintigraphic investigation. Acta Radiol 1988;29:565-570

Piddo C, Reed MH, Black GB: Premature epiphyseal fusion and degenerative arthritis in chronic recurrent multifocal osteomyelitis. Skeletal Radiol 2000;29:94-96

Tuberculosis, Brucellosis, Sarcoidosis, and Syphilis

Adler DD, Blane CE, Holt JF: Case report 220: Osseous sarcoidosis of left 5th digit in a young child with systemic sarcoidosis. Skeletal Radiol 1983;9:205-207

Centers of Disease Control and Prevention (CDC): Congenital syphilis—United States, 2002. MMWR Morb Mortal Wkly Rep 2004;53:716-719

Cockshott WP, Davies AGM: Tumoural gummatous yaws. J Bone Joint Surg Br 1960;42:785-787

Cremin BJ: Tuberculosis: the resurgence of our most lethal infectious disease—a review. Pediatr Radiol 1995;25:620-626

Engeset A, Eek S, Giljie O: On the significance of growth in the roentgenological skeletal changes of early congenital syphilis. Am J Roentgenol Radium Ther Nucl Med 1953;69:542-556

Grossman H, Merten DF, Spock A, et al: Radiographic features of sarcoidosis in pediatric patients. Semin Roentgenol 1985;20:393-399

Hugosson C, Harfi H: Disseminated BCG-osteomyelitis in congenital immunodeficiency. Pediatr Radiol 1991;21:384–385

Madkour MM, Sharif HS, Abed MY, et al: Osteoarticular brucellosis: results of bone scintigraphy in 140 patients. AJR Am J Roentgenol 1988;150:1101-1105

McClean S: Osseous lesions of congenital syphilis: summary and conclusions in one hundred and two cases. Am J Dis Child 1931;41:1411-1418

Pace JL: Treponematoses in Arabia. Saudi Med J 1983;4:211-220

Pourbagher A, Pourbagher MA, Savas L, et al: Epidemiologic, clinical and imaging findings in brucellosis patients with osteoarticular involvement. AJR Am J Roentgenol 2006;187:873-880

Rasool MN: Osseous manifestations of tuberculosis in children. J Pediatr Orthop 2001;21:749-755

Rasool MN, Govender S, Naidoo KS: Cystic tuberculosis of bone in children. J Bone Joint Surg Br 1994;76:113-117

Redman DS, McCarthy RE, Jimenez JF: Sarcoidosis in the long bones of a child: a case report and review of the literature. J Bone Joint Surg Am 1983;65:1010-1014

Shannon FB, Moore M, Houkom JA, et al: Multifocal cystic tuberculosis of bone. J Bone Joint Surg Am 1990;72:1089-1092

Solomon A, Rosen E: Focal osseous lesions in congenital lues. Pediatr Radiol 1978;7:36-39

Teo HE, Peh WC: Skeletal tuberculosis in children. Pediatr Radiol 2004;34:853-856

Vanthournout I, Quinet B, Neuenschwander S: Pediatric yaws osteoperiostitis. Pediatr Radiol 1991;21:303

Wang M, Chen W-M, Lee K-S, et al: Tuberculous osteomyelitis in young children. J Pediatr Orthop 1999;19:151-155

Wessels G, Hesseling PB, Beyers N: Skeletal tuberculosis: dactylitis and involvement of the skull. Pediatr Radiol 1998;28:234-236

Infantile Cortical Hyperostosis and Other Causes of Cortical Hyperostosis

Abinum M, Mikuska M, Filipovic B: Infantile cortical hyperostosis associated with the Wiskott-Aldrich syndrome. Eur J Pediatr 1988;147:518-519

Boyd RDH, Shaw DG, Thomas BM: Infantile cortical hyperostosis with lytic lesions in the skull. Arch Dis Child 1972;47:471-472

Caffey J: Infantile cortical hyperostoses. J Pediatr 1946;29:541-559

Caffey J: Infantile cortical hyperostosis: a review of the clinical and radiographic features. Proc R Soc Med 1957;50:347-354

Caffey J, Silverman WA: Infantile cortical hyperostoses: preliminary report on a new syndrome. Am J Roentgenol Radium Ther 1945;54:1-16

Clemett R, Williams JH: The familial occurrence of infantile cortical hyperostosis. Radiology 1963;80:409-416

DeToni G: Una nuova malattia dell'apparato ossea: la poliosteopatia deformante connatale regressive. Policlin Infant 1943; 11:1-32

Eversole SL Jr, Holman GH, Robinson RA: Hitherto undescribed characteristics of the pathology of infantile cortical hyperostosis (Caffey's disease). Bull Johns Hopkins Hosp 1957;101:80-89

Fauré C, Beyssac J-M, Montagne J-P: Predominant or exclusive orbital and facial involvement in infantile cortical hyperostosis (DeToni-Caffey's disease). Pediatr Radiol 1977;6:103-106

Gensure RC, Makitie O, Barclay C et al: A novel COL1A1 mutation in infantile cortical hyperostosis (Caffey's disease) expands the spectrum of collagen-related disorders. J Clin Invest 2005; 115:1250-1257

Gerscovich EO, Greenspan A, Lehman WB: Idiopathic periosteal hyperostosis with dysproteinemia—Goldbloom's syndrome. Pediatr Radiol 1990;20:208-211

Goldbloom RB, Stein PB, Eisen A, et al: Idiopathic periosteal hyperostosis with dysproteinemia: a new clinical entity. N Engl J Med 1966;274:873-878

Grégoire A, Combes JC, Hornung H, et al: Périostose multifocale récurrente de l'enfant: problèmes nosologiques. Pediatrie 1978;33:491-496

Heyman E, Laver J, Beer S: Prostaglandin synthetase inhibitor in Caffey disease [Letter]. J Pediatr 1982;101:314

Jorgensen HR, Svanholm H, Host A: Bone formation induced in an infant by systemic prostaglandin-E2 administration. Acta Orthop Scand 1988;59:464-466

Katz D, Eller DJ, Bergman G, et al: Caffey's disease of the scapula: CT and MR findings. AJR Am J Roentgenol 1997;168:286-287

Keeton BR: Vitamin E deficiency and thrombocytosis in Caffey's disease. Arch Dis Child 1976;51:393-395

Maclachlan AK, Gerrard JW, Houston CS, et al: Familial infantile cortical hyperostosis in a large Canadian family. Can Med Assoc J 1984;130:1172-1174

Matzinger MA, Briggs VA, Dunlap HJ, et al: Plain film and CT observations in prostaglandin-induced bone changes. Pediatr Radiol 1992;22:264-266

Melhem RE, Najjar SS, Khachadurian AK: Cortical hyperostosis with hyperphosphatemia: new syndrome? J Pediatr 1970;77: 986-990

Neuhauser EBD: Infantile cortical hyperostosis and skull defects. Postgrad Med 1970;48:57-59

Pazzaglia UE, Byers PD, Beluffi G, et al: Pathology of infantile cortical hyperostosis (Caffey's disease): report of a case. J Bone Joint Surg Am 1985;67:1417-1426

Roske G: Eine eigenartige Knochenerkrankung im Säugling-salter. Montasschr Kinderheilkd 1930;25:385-400

Saatci I, Brown JJ, McAlister WH: MR findings in a patient with Caffey's disease. Pediatr Radiol 1996;26:68-70

Saul RA, Lee WH, Stevenson RE: Caffey's disease revisited: further evidence for autosomal dominant inheritance with incomplete penetrance. Am J Dis Child 1982;136:56-60

Schweiger S, Chaoui R, Tennstedt C, et al: Antenatal onset of cortical hyperostosis (Caffey disease): case report and review. Am J Med Genet A 2003;120:547-552

Sheppard JJ, Pressman H: Dysphagia in infantile cortical hyperostosis (Caffey's disease): a case study. Dev Med Child Neurol 1988; 30:111-114

Ueda K, Saito A, Nakano H, et al: Cortical hyperostosis following long-term administration of prostaglandin E1 in infants with cyanotic congenital heart disease. J Pediatr 1980;97:834-836

Veller K, Laur A: Zur Ätiologie der infantilen kortikalen hyperostose (Caffey-Syndrom). Fortschr Geb Roentgenstr 1953;79:446-452

Wright JR Jr, Van den Hof MC, Macken MB: Prenatal infantile cortical hyperostosis (Caffey's disease): a 'hepatic myeloid hyperplasia-pulmonary hypoplasia sequence' can explain the lethality of early onset cases. Prenat Diagn 2005:25:939-944

PART 10 BONE TUMORS

CHAPTER 176

Benign and Malignant Bone Tumors

SUE C. KASTE, PETER J. STROUSE, BARRY D. FLETCHER, and MICHAEL D. NEEL

THE RADIOGRAPHIC EVALUATION OF BONE TUMORS

In this chapter, the radiologic evaluation of bone tumors is presented. The chapter begins with benign, non-aggressive lesions and finishes with malignant, aggressive lesions. In between, some lesions with variable aggressivity and variable malignant potential are presented. All common pediatric bone lesions are presented, as are some that are less common. A few extraordinarily rare or almost uniformly adult-onset lesions are better left elsewhere. Other chapters in this text cover osseous lesions that might mimic a bone tumor, such as some traumatic lesions and some infectious processes. Imaging of diffuse disorders of the bone marrow, including leukemia and metastases, is covered in the chapter on bone marrow imaging.

Regardless of the site and aggressivity of a bone lesion, the initial mode of imaging of bone tumors is radiography. Radiographs serve to confirm the presence and site of a tumor, formulate differential diagnoses, characterize the tumor, and guide in the selection of further imaging. The initial decision to obtain radiographs, however, is a clinical one, based on presentation, history, physical examination, and occasionally, laboratory tests. When put together with the clinical information, the radiographic findings determine what further imaging is necessary, if any.

It has often been said that one can narrow down the differential diagnosis of a pediatric bone tumor by asking a few simple questions:

How Old Is the Child?

Most bone tumors have a proclivity to occur within a certain age range. The differential diagnosis of a bone tumor in a 1-year-old infant is much different than that of a 16-year-old teenager, or even a 5-year-old child. Table 176-1 lists common pediatric bone tumors in accordance with the peak age at which they most commonly occur.

What Is the Location of the Lesion? What Bone? What Part of the Bone?

Many bone tumors have a proclivity to affect certain bones within the skeleton or to occur at certain locations within a bone. Some tumors tend to occur in certain bones, certain types of bones or certain regions of the

TABLE 176-1
Pediatric Bone Tumors—Peak Age of Occurrence

Infant and toddler ≤5 years old	Infantile myofibromatosis Leukemia Langerhans cell histiocytosis (multifocal) Metastatic neuroblastoma Osteofibrous dysplasia
Child 5–10 years old	Ewing sarcoma of long bone Langerhans cell histiocytosis (unifocal)
Adolescent 10–20 years old	Aneurysmal bone cyst Chondroblastoma Chondromyxoid fibroma Ewing sarcoma of axial skeleton Fibrous dysplasia Osteochondroma Leukemia (second peak) Nonossifying fibroma/fibrous cortical defect Osteoblastoma Osteoid osteoma Osteosarcoma Periosteal chondroma Primary lymphoma of bone Simple bone cyst
Adult ≥20 years old	Adamantinoma Enchondroma Giant cell tumor (rare until physes fuse) Parosteal osteosarcoma Periosteal osteosarcoma

TABLE 176-2	
Pediatric Bone Tumors—Location in Long Bones	
Epiphysis	Chondroblastoma
	Giant cell tumor (after physeal fusion)
	Langerhans cell histiocytosis
Metaphysis	Aneurysmal bone cyst
	Chondromyxoid fibroma
	Enchondroma
	Leukemia
	Metastases
	Nonossifying fibroma/fibrous cortical defect*
	Osteochondroma*
	Osteoid osteoma
	Osteosarcoma
	Parosteal osteosarcoma
	Simple bone cyst*
Diaphysis	Adamantinoma
	Ewing sarcoma/primitive neuroectodermal tumor
	Fibrous dysplasia
	Nonossifying fibroma/fibrous cortical defect (in older patients)*
	Osteochondroma (in older patients)*
	Osteofibrous dysplasia
	Osteoid osteoma
	Periosteal osteosarcoma
	Simple bone cyst (in older patients)*

*Osteochondromas, nonossifying fibromas/fibrous cortical defects and simple bone cysts begin in the metaphyses. With maturation, these lesions may "migrate" into metadiaphysis and diaphysis.

TABLE 176-3
Pediatric Bone Tumors—Multifocal Lesions
Brown tumors (hyperparathyroidism)
Cystic angiomatosis/lymphangiomatosis
Enchondroma (Ollier disease, Maffucci syndrome)
Fibrous dysplasia (McCune-Albright syndrome)
Infantile myofibromatosis
Langerhans cell histiocytosis
Leukemia
Metastases (i.e., from neuroblastoma)
Multifocal osteosarcoma
Nonossifying fibromas/fibrous cortical defects
Osteochondroma (oteochondromatosis)

TABLE 176-4	
Pediatric Bone Tumors—Aggressive vs. Nonaggressive Radiographic Appearance*	
Nonaggressive	Aneurysmal bone cyst
	Chondroblastoma
	Chondromyxoid fibroma
	Enchondroma
	Fibrous dysplasia
	Nonossifying fibroma/fibrous cortical deficit
	Osteoblastoma
	Osteoid osteoma
	Osteochondroma
	Simple bone cyst
Indeterminate	Adamantinoma
	Desmoplastic fibroma
	Giant cell tumor
	Langerhans cell histiocytosis
	Osteofibrous dysplasia
Aggressive	Ewing sarcoma/primitive neuroectodermal tumor
	Leukemia
	Lymphoma
	Metastases
	Osteoblastoma (aggressive form)
	Osteosarcoma

*Lesions are listed based on their most common radiographic presentations. With some lesions, variation from the norm is common.

skeleton. Some tumors favor the metaphysis. Others favor the diaphysis. A few even favor the epiphysis. Table 176-2 lists common pediatric bone tumors according to their preferred location in growing long bones.

Lesions also vary in their centricity relative to the involved bone. Some tumors (i.e., simple bone cyst) are central, whereas others are eccentric within bone (i.e., nonossifying fibroma [NOF]) or juxtacortical (i.e., osteochondroma, periosteal osteosarcoma).

Is the Lesion Unifocal or Multifocal?

Some lesions are always solitary. Others are usually multifocal. Some may be solitary or multifocal. Multifocal disease often implies a systemic disease or an underlying syndrome predisposing the patient to the development of a particular type of bone tumor. Table 176-3 lists common pediatric bone tumors that are multifocal.

Is the Lesion Aggressive or Nonaggressive in Appearance?

In general, benign lesions have a nonaggressive radiographic appearance. In general, malignant lesions have an aggressive radiographic appearance. Exceptions are common, and some lesions may have both aggressive and nonaggressive features. Table 176-4 lists lesions covered in this chapter by their characteristic radiographic appearance—aggressive, nonaggressive, or indeterminate.

Radiographic features of a nonaggressive, and usually benign, bone tumor are well-defined margins with a narrow zone of transition, particularly with sclerosis, expansion of bone contour from slow growth, smooth, single layered periosteal new bone and absence of an associated soft tissue mass. Radiographic features of an aggressive, and usually malignant, bone tumor are poorly defined margins with a wide zone of transition, permeative or moth-eaten bone destruction, frank destruction of bone without remodeling, aggressive forms of periosteal new bone, interrupted periosteal new bone and the presence of an associated soft tissue mass. Nonaggressive lesions tend to be geographic in appearance, and aggressive lesions tend to be ill-defined, "moth-eaten," or permeative. Aggressive forms of periosteal new bone include layering, or "onion skin," and "hair on end" periosteal new bone. Interrupted periosteal new bone may take the form of a Codman triangle, a sign of an aggressive process.

By answering the aforementioned four questions, the radiologist can often arrive at a single diagnosis or at least narrow the differential to a few lesions. Most important, the distinction of aggressive verses nonaggressive lesions is of major importance in guiding further imaging and initial therapy.

Some benign bone tumors are adequately defined by radiography and do not require any further imaging for diagnosis or treatment. Most bone tumors, however, do require additional imaging for diagnosis or to guide diagnostic procedures or therapeutic decisions. Additional imaging may take the form of computed tomography (CT), magnetic resonance imaging (MRI), bone scintigraphy, positron emission tomography (PET) scanning, and rarely, even ultrasound. The choice of imaging for a given tumor depends on the differential diagnostic considerations, possible treatment options, and whether the lesion is aggressive or nonaggressive in nature. MRI is usually the preferred modality in the delineation of aggressive and suspected malignant lesions. Radiographs followed by MRI adequately define most bone lesions. As opposed to radiography, on MRI, an aggressive lesion may have a well-defined margin, particularly with T1 weighting. Although MR is also very good at delineating nonaggressive and likely benign lesions, CT is better able to delineate ossified bone and, thus, occasionally may better define the characteristics and anatomy of many benign lesions.

Image-guided biopsy has become a viable option to determine or confirm the diagnosis of many bone lesions. CT, ultrasound, fluoroscopy, and even MRI may be used for guidance. Techniques for image guided biopsy of osseous lesions are covered in detail in Chapter 194.

> Radiographic features of a nonaggressive bone tumor are well-defined margins with a narrow zone of transition, expansion of bone contour from slow growth, smooth, single-layered periosteal new bone, and absence of an associated soft tissue mass. Radiographic features of an aggressive bone tumor are poorly defined margins with a wide zone of transition, permeative or moth-eaten bone destruction, frank destruction of bone without remodeling, aggressive forms of periosteal new bone, interrupted periosteal new bone, and the presence of an associated soft tissue mass.

BENIGN BONE TUMORS

More than 50% of all childhood bone neoplasms are benign. It is important that radiologists recognize the typical benign tumors so that appropriate therapy can be initiated and so that the patient can avoid unnecessary diagnostic procedures. The differentiation of a nonaggres-

sive lesion from an aggressive lesion will significantly affect the course of subsequent imaging evaluations, the approach to biopsy, and the preliminary choice of definitive treatment.

Cartilaginous Tumors

OSTEOCHONDROMA (EXOSTOSIS)

In pathologic series, osteochondroma is the most common pediatric bone tumor. Rather than a true tumor, osteochondromas are thought to be a developmental defect of growing bone in which an injury to the perichondrium causes bone growth in an aberrant direction. It is theorized that islets of cartilage from the physis are displaced along the metaphyseal surface and then grow. Osteochondromas occur in approximately 1% of the general population. Solitary osteochondroma is slightly more common in boys than girls. Growth ceases at skeletal maturity.

Lesions usually present in the second decade of life as they grow. Most osteochondromas are asymptomatic and discovered incidentally. However, a host of complications can occur (Table 176-5). When one of a pair of adjacent bones is affected, the osteochondroma can cause pressure deformity of the other bone. Symptomatic presentations of osteochondroma are usually due to irritation of adjacent muscles, tendons, nerves or, rarely, blood vessels. Pseudoaneurysm is a rare complication. A bursa may develop over an osteochondroma due to inflammation. A pedunculated osteochondroma may fracture. Presentation with pain due to malignant transformation of a solitary osteochondroma in a child is extraordinarily rare.

On radiography, osteochondromas are most often found on the long bone metaphyses. Thirty-five percent occur at the knee. Lesions in younger patients tend to be closer to the growth plates. Osteochondromas may also form on the pelvis, ribs, and scapula. Spinal lesions are rare. Underlying metaphyses are broadened due to disturbance of normal modeling. The shape of osteochondromas varies from sessile, plaque-like lesions (Fig. 176-1) to pedunculated lesions (Fig. 176-2) with a long stalk. The stalk of a pedunculated lesion is directed away from the adjacent joint. En face, osteochondromas may be mistaken for a sclerotic intramedullary lesion. On radiography, CT, and MRI, a hallmark of osteochondroma is continuity of cortex and medullary space from the underlying bone into the lesion.

CT nicely demonstrates the morphology of the lesions and usually confirms the diagnosis; however, MRI much better demonstrates the cartilaginous cap characteristic of the lesion (Fig. 176-3). On T2-weighting and with other cartilage sensitive sequences, the cartilaginous cap is well seen as a well-defined, thin, high signal crescent capping the osteochondroma. The cap usually measures less than 5 mm in thickness with 10 mm usually considered the upper limit of normal. The outer margin is smooth. Increased signal and enhancement may be seen in adjacent soft tissues with irritation.

Malignant transformation of solitary osteochondromas, even those that are radiation induced, is exceed-

TABLE 176-5

Complications of Osteochondroma

Cosmetic and functional deformity
    Pseudo-Madelung deformity
    Radial head subluxation/dislocation
    Coxa valga
    Genu valga
    Tibiotalar tilt
    Leg length discrepancy
    Decreased range of motion
Impingement syndrome
Muscle/tendon irritation
    Tenosynovitis
    Snapping tendon
    Tendon dislocation
Bursa formation
    Synovial (osteo)chondromatosis
Synostosis
Pseudarthrosis
Short stature

Fracture
Vascular
    Displacement
    Stenosis/occlusion
    Claudication
    Pseudoaneurysm
    Venous compression/deep venous thrombosis/pulmonary embolism
Neurologic
    Peripheral nerve compression/entrapment
    Cranial neuropathy
    Spinal stenosis
Thoracic
    Hemothorax
    Pneumothorax
    Ruptured pericardium
    Thoracic outlet syndrome
    Dysphagia
Malignant transformation

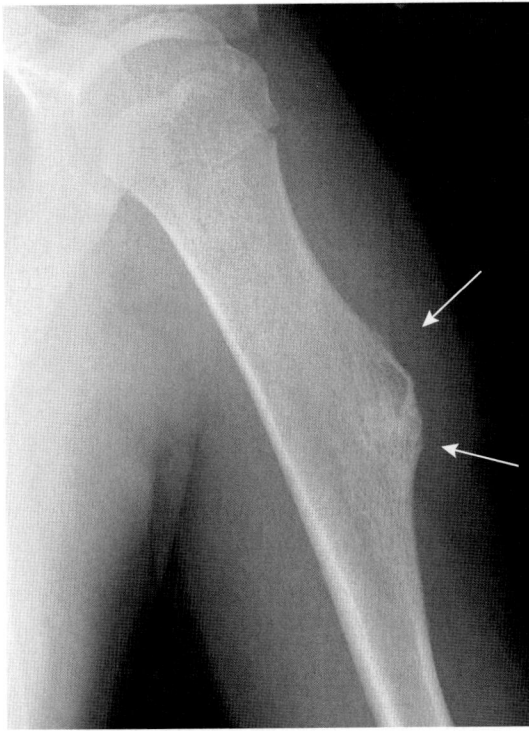

FIGURE 176-1. Sessile osteochondroma *(arrows)* of the proximal humeral diaphysis in a 16-year-old girl.

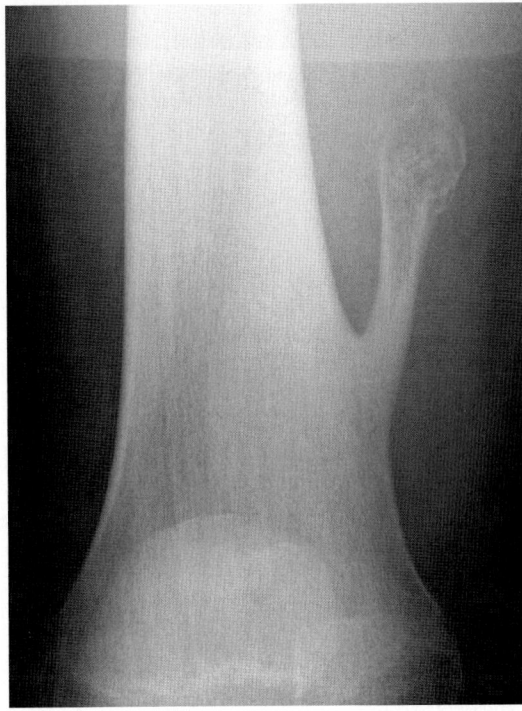

FIGURE 176-2. Pedunculated osteochondroma of the distal femoral metaphysis in a 14-year-old boy.

ingly rare, probably occurring in much less than 1% of patients. However, the reported incidence transformation to chondrosarcoma in patients with hereditary osteochondromatosis is 0.5% to 25%. Wide variation reflects patient selection biases and the actual incidence is probably less than 5%. Malignant transformation does not occur until skeletal maturity. Clinical and imaging findings suggestive of malignant transformation include an osteochondroma that grows or begins to produce symptoms after epiphyseal closure, cartilaginous cap is greater than 1.5 to 2 cm thick, indistinct lesion margins, new lucency within in an osteochondroma, and an associated soft tissue mass. Chondrosarcomas tend to arise at the periphery of an osteochondroma. The chondrosarcomas are usually of low histologic grade. A rare case of osteosarcoma arising in a long-standing osteochondroma has been described in a 17-year-old boy.

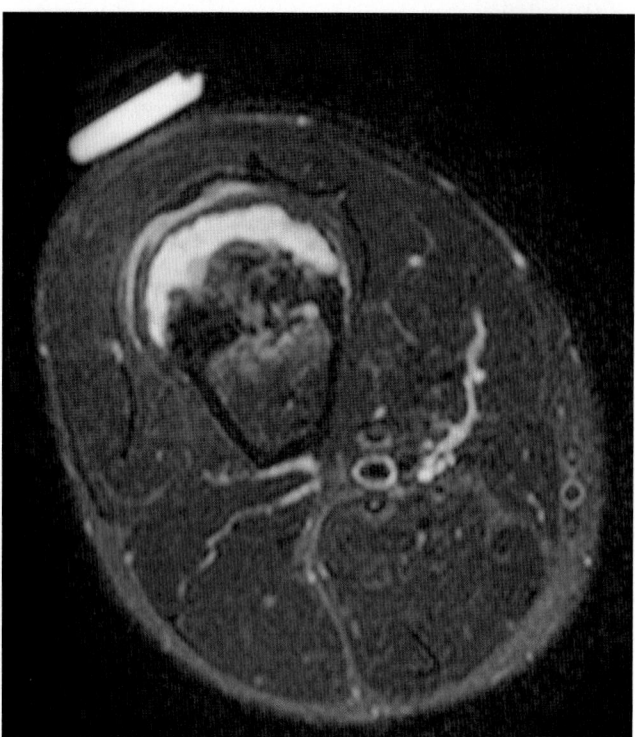

FIGURE 176-3. Sessile osteochondroma in a 14-year-old boy—T2-weighted magnetic resonance image with fat saturation. A broad, high signal cartilaginous cap covers the osteochondroma. The anterior cortex under the cartilaginous cap is thickened. An external vitamin E marker was placed anteriorly over the palpable abnormality for localization.

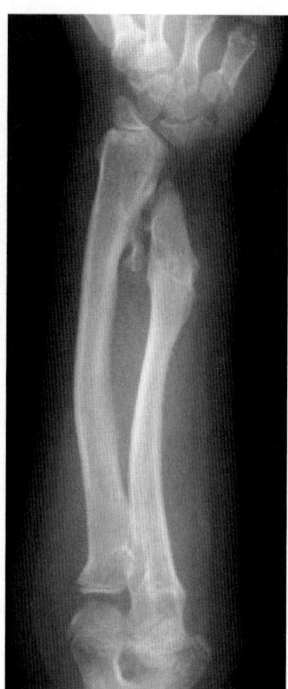

FIGURE 176-4. Osteochondromatosis in a 13-year-old girl. Multiple osseous excrescences are seen on the metaphyses of the radius and ulna. The ulna is shortened. A Madelung deformity of the distal radius is noted. Both bones are slightly bowed laterally.

> Malignant transformation of solitary osteochondromas, even those that are radiation induced, is exceedingly rare, probably occurring in much less than 1% of patients. Clinical and imaging findings suggestive of malignant transformation include an osteochondroma that grows or begins to produce symptoms after physeal closure, cartilaginous cap is greater than 1.5 to 2 cm thick, indistinct lesion margins, new lucency within in an osteochondroma and an associated soft tissue mass.

Osteochondromas develop in 6% to 12% of patients who received radiation at a young age. Latent periods vary from 3 to 16 years. Osteochondromas can occur even after low doses of radiation therapy and often occur in bones that were in the periphery of the radiation field. Multiple osteochondromas have been found in patients who received total-body irradiation as preparation for bone marrow transplantation at a young age. Sarcomatous degeneration of radiation-induced osteochondroma is very rare and of no greater incidence than with other osteochondromas.

Patients with *hereditary osteochondromatosis* (multiple exostoses; diaphyseal aclasis) develop multiple osteochondromas throughout their skeleton. The disorder is autosomal dominant, with 10% of cases arising spontaneously. Patients have a mutation of the *EXT* gene family

resulting in an error in regulation of normal chondrocyte proliferation and maturation. In most patients, the disorder becomes manifest by 10 years of age. The multiplicity of lesions in these patients may lead to substantial deformity. Axial osteochondromas are frequently seen and may cause complications. Small lesions are common on tubular the bones of the hand. Most notable is a pseudo-Madelung deformity of the wrist due to forearm exostoses causing ulnar shortening and angular deformity of the distal radius (Fig. 176-4). Multiple metaphyseal lesions may interfere with normal modelling of the metaphyses (Fig. 176-5).

Dysplasia epiphysealis hemimelica (Trevor's disease) may be a manifestation of epiphyseal osteochondroma. Patients present before 15 years of age. Seventy-five percent of patients are boys. Patients present with deformity, swelling, and pain. These patients form osteochondroma-like protuberances from the epiphyses. The lesions are usually confined to one side of the joint (medial > lateral) and may occasionally involve contiguous joints in one extremity. The lower extremity (femur, tibia, talus) is usually affected. Radiographs show deformity with irregular enlargement of one side of the epiphysis (Figs. 176-6 and 176-7). MRI is necessary to define the abnormality in younger children because the lesions may be predominantly cartilaginous. With further ossification in older children, CT is preferred (Fig. 176-8).

Subungual exostosis is a broad-based irregular osteochondroma of the tuft of the finger under the nail bed. The lesion is most common in males in the second decade of life and most commonly affects the great toe (Fig. 176-9). Unlike conventional osteochondroma,

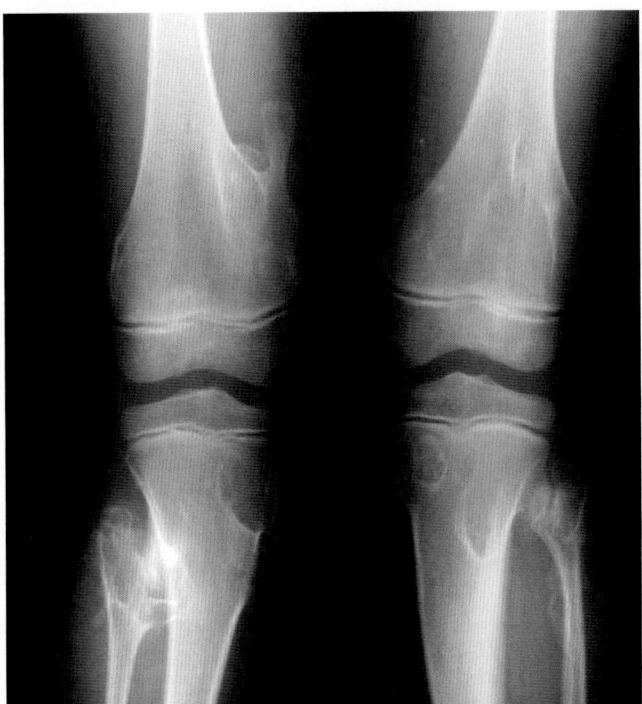

FIGURE 176-5. Osteochondromatosis in an 8-year-old girl. Multiple sessile and pedunculated osteochondromas arise from the metaphyses with mild resultant modeling deformity. The proximal right tibia is slightly bowed medial.

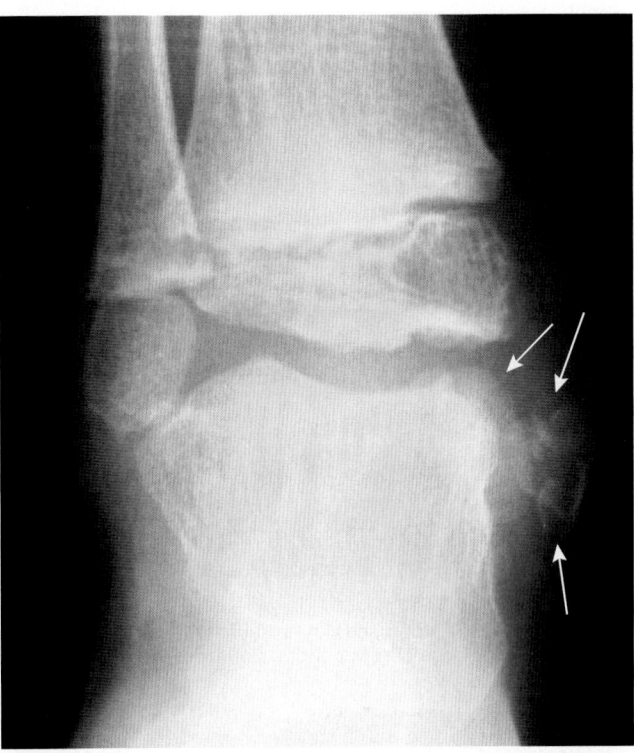

FIGURE 176-7. Trevor disease in a 4-year-old boy. The distal tibial epiphysis and talus are deformed. Osseous protrusions are noted at the lateral aspect of the talus, under the fibula, and at the medial aspect of the talus *(arrows).*

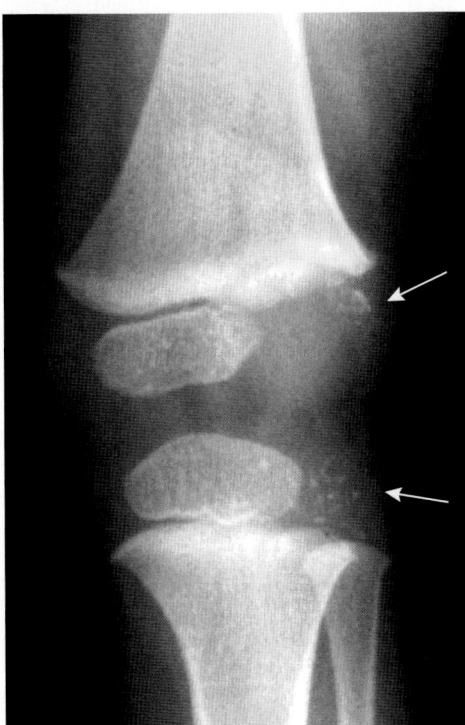

FIGURE 176-6. Trevor disease in a 20-month-old girl. Both the distal femoral and proximal tibial epiphyseal ossification centers appear medial positioned relative to their metaphyses. Speckles of cartilaginous calcification *(arrows)* are seen at the lateral aspect of each epiphysis due to epiphyseal osteochondroma-like deformity.

there is no medullary continuity of the exostosis with the underlying bone.

Nora's lesion of bone (bizarre parosteal osteochondromatous proliferation) is an irregular, predominantly ossified lesion typically occurring in the tubular bones of the hands and feet over intact underlying cortex. The lesion occurs at the proximal phalanges, metacarpals, and metatarsals. Histologically, the lesion contains "histologically aggressive and cytologically bizarre cartilage that undergoes irregular ossification" (per Nora and associates). Peak incidence is in the third and forth decades, with occasional lesions presenting in the teens. The appearance of Nora lesion varies from a globular ossification in adjacent soft tissue to an aggressive appearing cloak of osteoid enveloping the underlying bone (Fig. 176-10). The lesion has a pronounced tendency to recur but is otherwise acts like a benign tumor.

ENCHONDROMA

Enchondromas form owing to a failure of normal endochondral ossification adjacent to a physis. The tumors are composed of cartilage cells derived from the neighboring physis. Enchondromas are most frequently located in the small tubular bones of the hands and feet, and in the metaphyses and metadiaphyses of the long bones. Enchondromas represent 80% of primary hand tumors in children and can form in any bone that forms in cartilage. Rib and vertebral lesions are uncommon. In children, enchondromas become more common with age. The peak age for diagnosis is in the third decade.

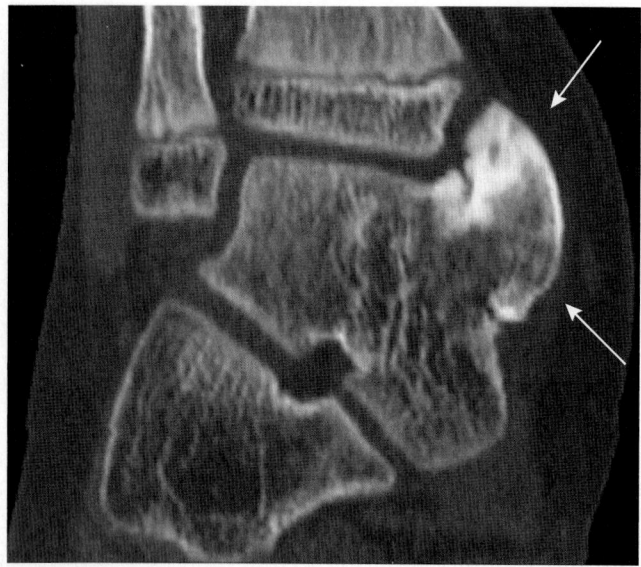

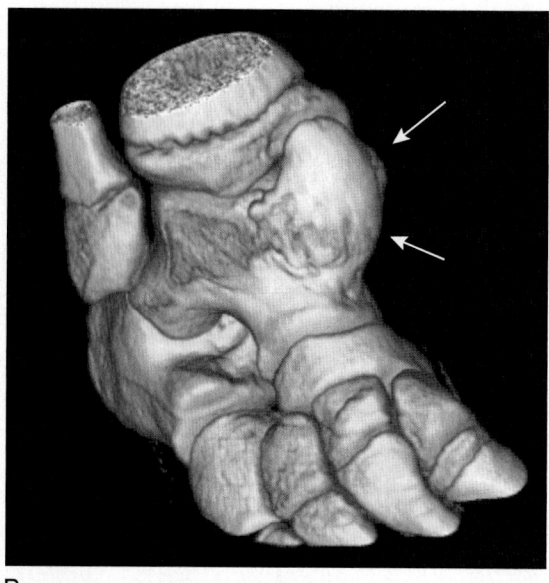

A

B

FIGURE 176-8. Trevor disease in a 10-year-old boy. Coronal reconstruction **(A)** and volume rendered **(B)** computed tomography images shows a large osseous protrusion from the medial talus *(arrows).*

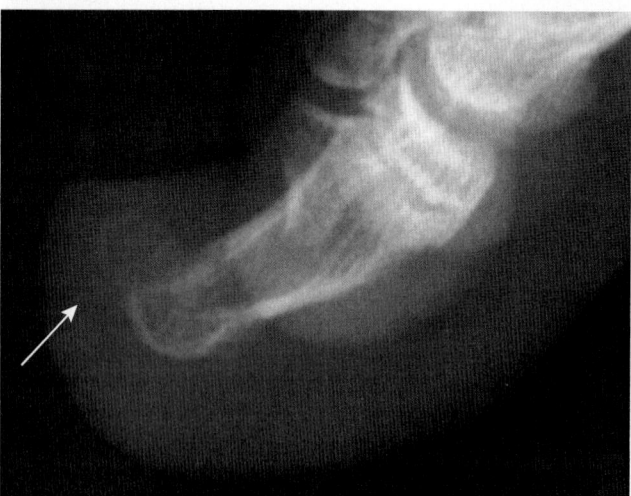

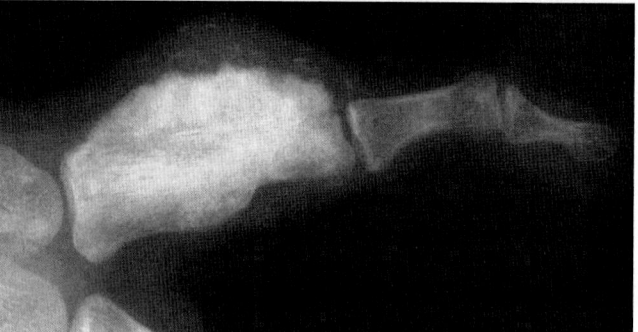

FIGURE 176-10. Nora lesion of the proximal phalanx of the index finger in a 17-year-old girl. A cloak of dense bone envelops the phalanx. The bone appears sclerotic. The appearance is indistinguishable from osteosarcoma.

FIGURE 176-9. Subungual osteochondroma in a 15-year-old boy *(arrow).*

> **Enchondromas are most frequently located in the small tubular bones of the hands and feet and in the metaphyses and metadiaphyses of the long bones.**

On radiography, as with other cartilaginous tumors, enchondromas exhibit a lobulated growth pattern that results in asymmetric expansion of the medullary cavity and endosteal scalloping. Lesions are oval, well-circumscribed, and lucent (Fig. 176-11). Focal, punctate calcifications may be evident on radiographs but are better appreciated with CT. The cartilaginous "ring and arc" pattern may be seen on CT. Margins of the lesion are sclerotic. The lesion may scallop the endosteum, erode cortex and expand or distort the bone (Fig. 176-12). Periosteal reaction is absent. On MRI, the tumor is isointense with muscle on T1-weighted MRI and exhibits

a heterogeneous, predominantly high T2-weighted signal. Signal intensity of the lesion parallels cartilage on all sequences. Enhancement with gadolinium varies, with some lesions enhancing peripherally and others more homogeneously. Adjacent bone marrow edema and enhancement is typically absent. Bone scans typically show increased activity.

Enchondroma protuberans is an enchondroma variant that can resemble either a periosteal chondroma or a sessile osteochondroma (Fig. 176-12). It has been described as an exophytic, exaggerated, eccentric from of enchondroma. This tumor arises in the medulla and expands eccentrically through the cortex so that the tumor eventually protrudes beyond it. Rather than a cartilaginous cap, the tumor is covered by a thin layer of cortex and periosteum. This variant of enchondroma most commonly occurs in the proximal humerus and in the hand.

Ollier disease (enchondromatosis) is a nonheritable disorder of cartilage proliferation in which enchondromas involve multiple bones (Figs. 176-13 and 176-14). In fact, Ollier disease is a mesodermal dysplasia and not just enchondromatosis but a broader dyschondrogenesis affecting any part of endochondrally formed bones. Ollier disease is more common in boys. The hands are most affected, but enchondromas form in any bone with a physis. The hands may be disparately affected and may be grotesquely deformed. Enchondromas are bilateral but usually asymmetric in severity. Onset during infancy or early childhood may result in severe skeletal deformity. Enchondromas may interfere with growth plate func-

tion, leading to limb shortening. The lesions of Ollier disease are expansile and lucent or trabeculated, usually with a shell of thin cortex. In the long bones, longitudinal lucent columns or streaks are characteristic.

Enchondromatosis accompanied by vascular malformations is known as *Maffucci syndrome*. Maffucci syndrome

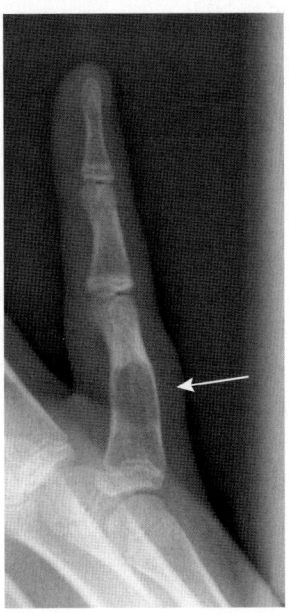

FIGURE 176-11. Solitary enchondroma in a 13-year-old girl. The lesion is well defined with thinning of the overlying cortex and slight expansion of the bone.

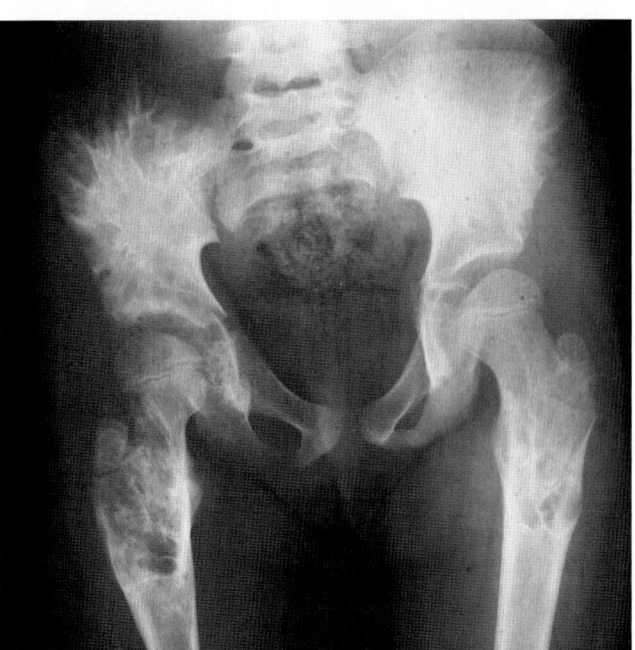

FIGURE 176-13. Enchondromatosis in a 8-year-old girl. Multiple lesions are present within the proximal femurs and the iliac bones. The iliac lesions on the right are confluent, producing a radial pattern. The proximal femoral diaphyses are mildly expanded. Some speckled cartilaginous calcification is present in some of the lesions.

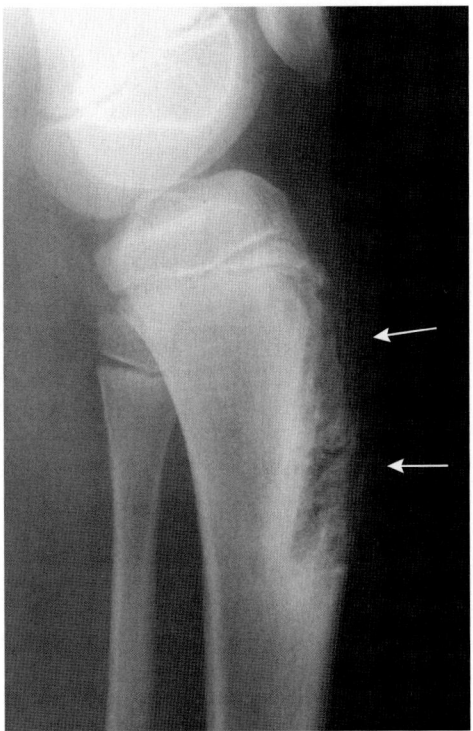

A

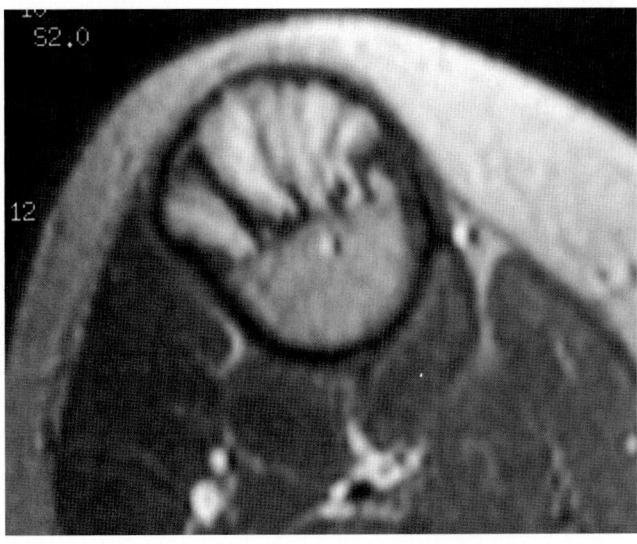

B

FIGURE 176-12. Enchondroma protuberans in an 11-year-old boy. **A,** Radiograph shows an ill-defined lucent lesion in the anterior cortex of the proximal tibia. **B,** Axial T2-weighted magnetic resonance image shows a well-defined, high-signal lesion in the anterior tibia.

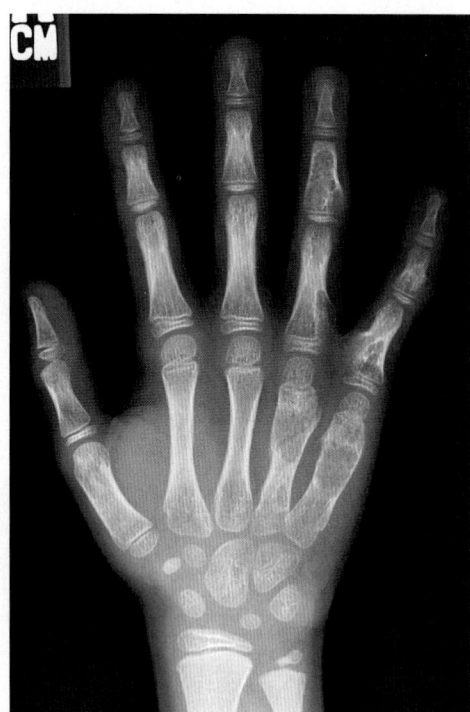

FIGURE 176-14. Enchondromatosis in a 13-year-old girl. Multiple well-defined, lucent, expansile lesions are present in the metacarpals and phalanges of the ring and little fingers. A pathologic fracture is seen through an enchondroma in the distal fourth metacarpal.

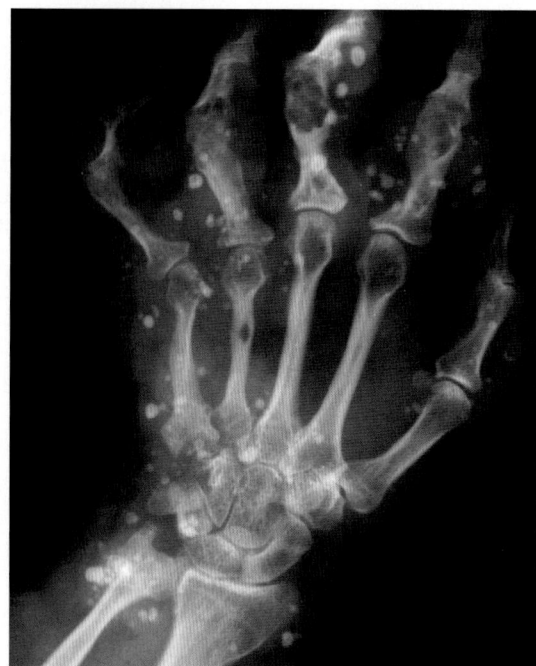

FIGURE 176-15. Maffucci syndrome in a 35-year-old woman. Innumerable phleboliths are present. Enchondromas are seen in the proximal and middle phalanges of the index, middle, and ring fingers.

is also nonhereditary and also a form of mesodermal dysplasia. The vascular malformations are predominantly venous, but also capillary and, occasionally, lymphatic. Calcified phleboliths may be demonstrated radiographically in the vascular soft tissue masses of patients with Maffucci syndrome (Fig. 176-15).

Malignant transformation is extremely rare with a solitary enchondroma, particularly in childhood. Unlike in adults, chondrosarcoma is very rare in children. Lesions associated with both Ollier disease and Maffucci syndrome carry a significant risk of malignant degeneration to chondrosarcoma. Ten to twenty percent of patients may experience a malignant transformation. Malignant transformation is extremely rare in childhood. Approximately 5% of patients with chondrosarcoma have Ollier disease. Patients with Maffucci syndrome also have an increased risk of central nervous system and intra-abdominal malignancy. Findings suggesting malignant degeneration of an enchondroma include increasing pain, bone destruction and soft tissue mass.

Metachondromatosis is a very rare disorder that is a combination of enchondromatosis and osteochondromatosis.

> **Lesions associated with both Ollier disease and Maffucci syndrome carry a significant risk of malignant degeneration to chondrosarcoma (10% to 20% of patients). Malignant transformation is extremely rare in childhood.**

PERIOSTEAL (JUXTACORTICAL) CHONDROMA

This rare tumor is a surface variant of an enchondroma that arises from the periosteal surface of the cortex of the large and small tubular bones. One theory holds that the tumor is post-traumatic in origin. The tumor is located under the periosteum and external to the cortex. Some tumors, such as within the femoral neck, are not covered with periosteum and are better labeled as "juxtacortical." Periosteal chondroma most commonly occurs in the proximal humerus metaphysis, phalanges of the hands and feet, femur, and proximal tibia. Patients are usually 10 to 30 years of age, with the peak incidence in the second decade of life. The lesion is more frequent in boys.

Patients usually present with mild pain and swelling. Radiographically, although periosteal chondroma may bear superficial similarity to a sessile osteochondroma, it is associated with sclerosis and scalloped erosion of the adjacent cortex, forming a periosteal shelf (Fig. 176-16). Focal calcifications of matrix within the lesion may be seen. Cross-sectional imaging delineates the underlying cortex and clearly distinguishes the lesion from a sessile osteochondroma. CT may show chondroid calcification (Fig. 176-17). MRI shows chondroid composition of the lesion. Peripheral enhancement is usually seen with gadolinium. The tumor is usually 1 to 3 cm in size. A shell of reactive bone may be seen around the lesion. Adjacent cortex is eroded or saucerized. Reactive bone sclerosis and buttressing is seen.

Periosteal chondroma does not have malignant potential, but biopsy may be advisable to distinguish periosteal chondroma from juxtacortical chondrosarcoma and periosteal osteosarcoma, particularly in adults. Periosteal chondromas may be seen in patients with Ollier disease.

CHONDROBLASTOMA

Chondroblastoma, an uncommon tumor composed of primitive cartilage cells, usually occurs in the second decade of life. Roughly half of chondroblastomas occur before the physes close. The most specific feature is its location in the epiphysis of a long bone, most often the proximal humerus, distal femur, or proximal tibia. Chondroblastoma may also occur in epiphyseal equivalent such as apophyses, the patella, and carpal and tarsal bones. Larger lesions may extend into an adjacent

metaphysis, particularly in skeletally mature persons. Up to 15% of chondroblastomas have a component of aneurysmal bone cyst (ABC).

> **Chondroblastoma occurs in the epiphyses of long bones, most often the proximal humerus, distal femur, or proximal tibia, and in epiphyseal equivalents such as apophyses, the patella, and carpal and tarsal bones. Larger lesions may extend into an adjacent metaphysis, particularly in skeletally mature persons.**

Patients with chondroblastoma present with pain. The tumor evokes a striking inflammatory response, which may help to distinguish it from other lesions.

Radiographically, a chondroblastoma presents as an eccentric, lucent, well-defined, smooth or lobulated lesion with sclerotic borders within an epiphysis or epiphyseal equivalent (Fig. 176-18). The lesion may expand the bone; however, the cortex is usually intact. Periosteal reaction distant from the lesion is another common feature suggesting an accompanying inflammatory process. Periosteal reaction on an adjacent metaphysis is seen in 30% to 50% of cases.

Approximately one third of chondroblastomas have a calcified chondroid matrix. This is better demonstrated by CT, which may also show cortical destruction (see Fig. 176-18). On MRI, chondroblastoma typically parallels cartilage signal intensity on all sequences. Signal intensity varies with the degree of calcification in the lesion. The rim of the tumor may have a lower intensity and some foci give no signal because of calcification. Adjacent inflammatory changes consisting of bone marrow edema, soft tissue edema and joint effusion are

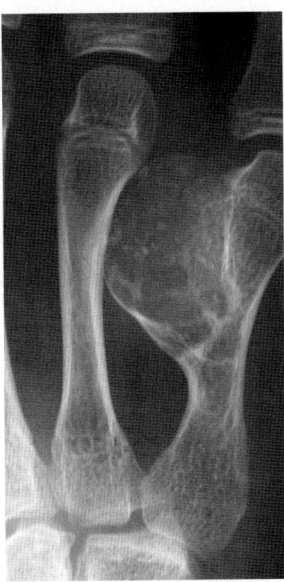

FIGURE 176-16. Periosteal chondroma in a 13-year-old girl. An expansile lesion originates at the surface of the metacarpal. Chondroid matrix is seen within the lesion. The underlying cortex is externally scalloped.

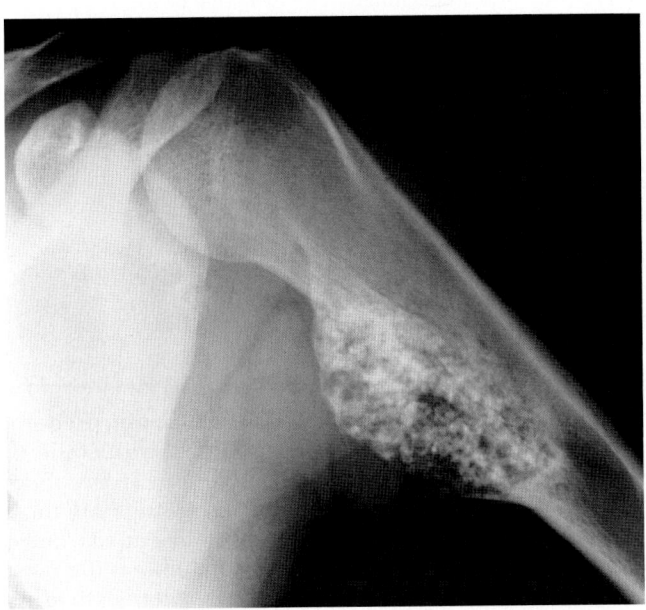

A

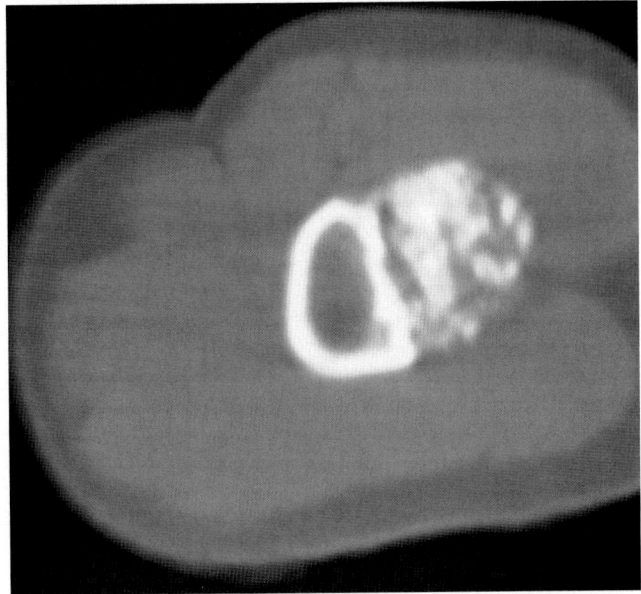

B

FIGURE 176-17. Periosteal chondroma in a 19-year-old young girl. **A,** Anteroposterior view of the humerus shows a broad-based tumor with a lobular mineralized matrix. **B,** Computed tomography shows the superficial nature of the lesion, which is separated from the medulla by cortical bone.

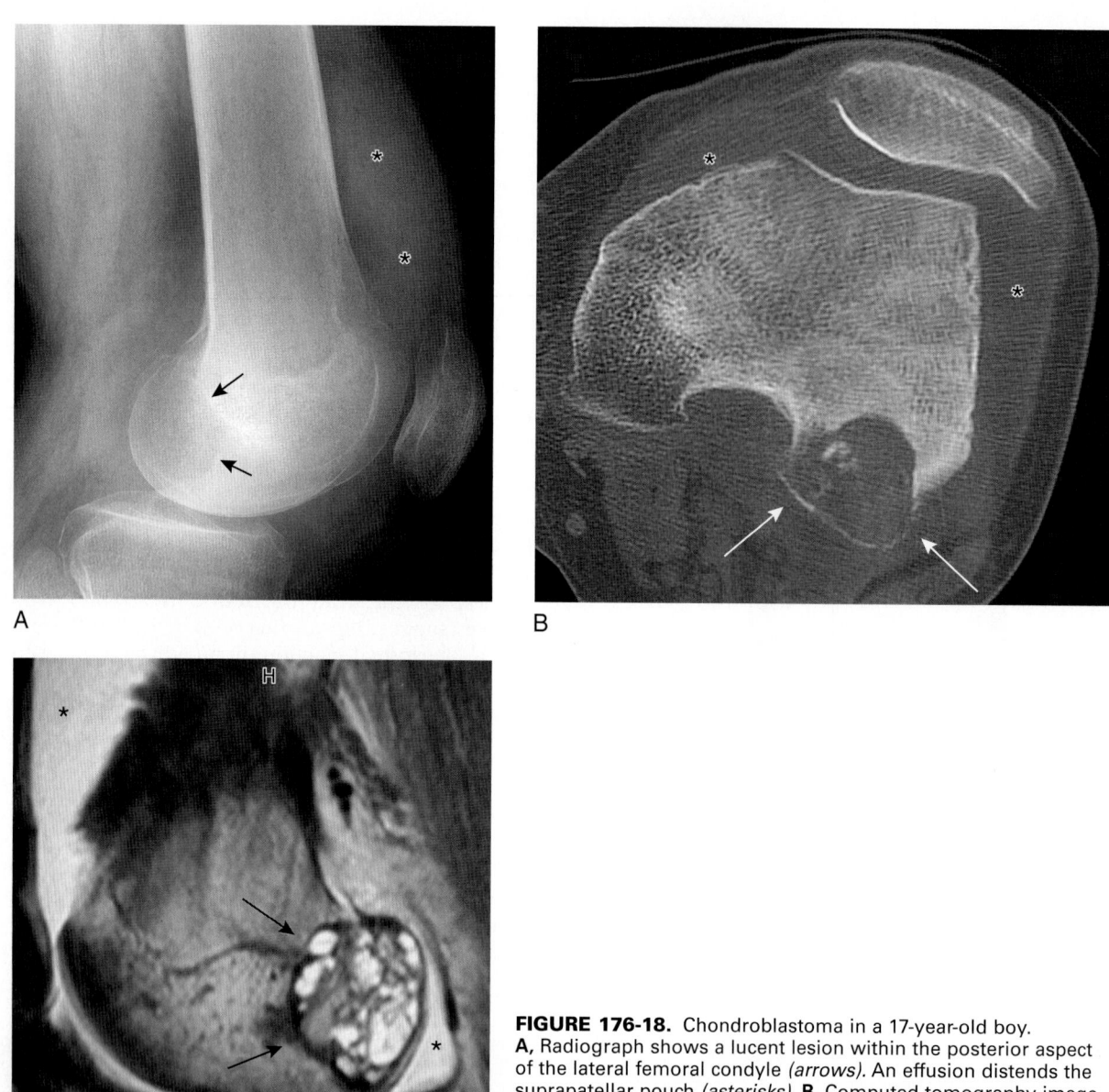

FIGURE 176-18. Chondroblastoma in a 17-year-old boy. **A,** Radiograph shows a lucent lesion within the posterior aspect of the lateral femoral condyle *(arrows)*. An effusion distends the suprapatellar pouch *(asterisks)*. **B,** Computed tomography image shows a well-defined lesion *(arrows)* with some calcified cartilaginous matrix. Asterisks, effusion. **C,** Sagittal T2-weighted magnetic resonance image with fat saturation shows the lesion to be of mixed high-signal intensity. Bone marrow edema is seen in the femur (compare with the tibia [T]). Knee joint effusion *(asterisks)* and adjacent soft tissue edema are noted.

usually prominent and seen on MR (see Fig. 176-18). On bone scans, intense activity on the blood pool phase of skeletal scintigrams is consistent with hyperemia. Delayed phase images show uptake at the lesion.

The differential diagnosis for a lucent epiphyseal lesion in a child includes chondroblastoma, osteomyelitis, giant cell tumor (GCT, after physeal closure), Langerhans cell histiocytosis (LCH), and osteoblastoma.

Chondroblastomas are treated with curettage and bone grafting. Approximately 20% of lesions recur. Otherwise, the prognosis is good. There are rare reports of metastatic chondroblastoma.

CHONDROMYXOID FIBROMA

Chondromyxoid fibroma (CMF) is a rare tumor, predominantly affecting males in the second or third decade of life. Patients present with pain. The lesion is a rubbery mix of fibrous, myxoid, and chondroid tissue. CMF most frequently arises within ilium, long bones at the knee, and tubular bones of the foot. Proximal tibia is the most common site. The tumor is metaphyseal, often extending into metadiaphysis, but very rarely extending past a physis.

On radiography, CMF has a characteristic but nonspecific appearance of a solitary, eccentric, lucent, well-defined lesion with sclerotic margins. There may

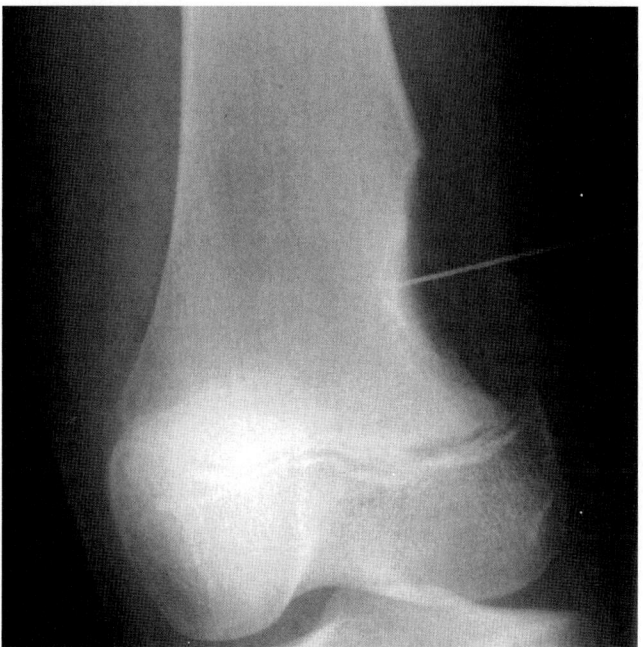

FIGURE 176-19. Chondromyxoid fibroma in a 14-year-old boy. The lesion has produced a well-defined scalloped defect in the distal tibial metaphysis. Biopsy needle is present.

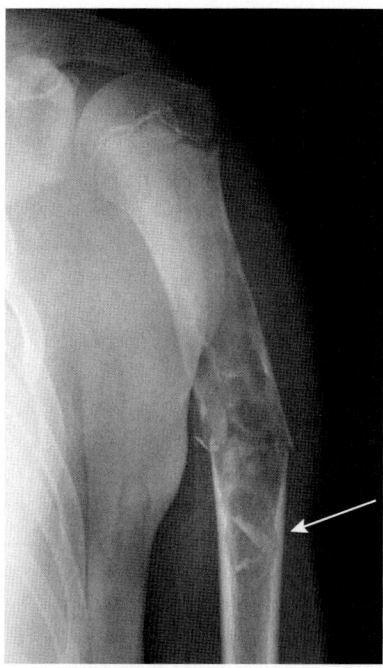

FIGURE 176-20. Simple bone cyst with pathologic fracture in a 12-year-old boy. The cyst has thinned and scalloped the overlying cortex. A fallen fragment is noted *(arrow).*

be septations within the lesion. In the short bones of the hands and feet, the lesion appears more central. The underlying cortex may be expanded, thinned, and occasionally, absent. The lesion may appear bubbly, similar to an ABC. Most lesions are elongated and oriented parallel to the long axis of the involved bone (Fig. 176-19). Matrix calcification and periosteal new bone formation usually do not occur. On MR, CMF produces variable and often heterogeneous signal intensity depending on the composition of the lesion. In general, the lesion is of low signal on T1 and intermediate to high signal on T2.

Treatment of CMF is excision. 25% of lesions recur. Multiple recurrences are common.

Cysts

SIMPLE BONE CYST

Although pathologists do not consider simple bone cysts to be true neoplasms, radiologists include them in the differential diagnosis of bone-replacing tumors. A simple bone cyst is also referred to as a solitary or "unicameral bone cyst," although the latter term is a misnomer because these cysts may be septated. One theory holds that bone cysts arise due to a defect in endochondral bone formation or altered hemodynamics with venous occlusion elevating intraosseous pressure and leading to cyst formation. Bone cysts have a membrane of loose vascular connective tissue and contain osteoclast-like giant cells and accumulations of fibrinoid material. The cyst space is usually filled with yellow, sometimes bloody fluid.

Cysts are more common in boys than girls by three-fold. Seventy-five percent of cysts are seen in patients younger than 25 years of age, and 25% are found incidentally.

Bone cysts occur centrally in the metaphyses of the long bones, most commonly involving the proximal humerus (50%) and proximal femur (20%). Cysts have an "active phase," during which they increase in size and remain in close proximity to the physis. "Latent phase" cysts are found further from the physis and usually do not continue to grow. Cysts may "migrate" into the diaphysis; actually, the growth plate migrates away from the cyst. Septations are more commonly seen in such mature cysts. Bone cysts may occur at other sites, including the axial skeleton. In older patients, pelvic and calcaneal bone cysts become more common.

Bone cysts are asymptomatic unless complicated by fracture. Seventy-five percent of patients present with a pathologic fracture. Bone cysts are the most common cause of pathologic fracture in children.

> **Bone cysts are the most common cause of pathologic fracture in children.**

On radiography, bone cysts have a central, medullary location within the metaphysis. Most cysts are less than 3 cm in diameter but may be much larger in long axis. The cyst wall is well defined and sclerotic. The overlying cortex is thinned and the lesion may be mildly expansile. With fracture, a fragment of bone may be seen dependently within the cyst. This "fallen fragment" sign is considered pathognomonic for a simple bone cyst (Fig. 176-20). CT delineates the cyst and confirms a fallen fragment, but the study is rarely necessary. In atypical cases, MRI is performed and confirms the cystic

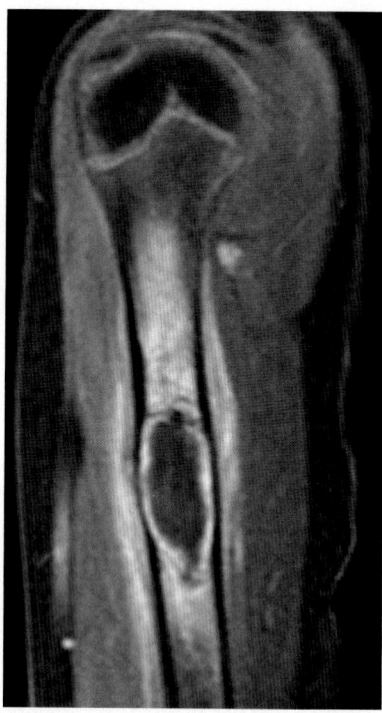

FIGURE 176-21. Simple bone cyst in an 8-year-old boy. Sagittal T1-weighted magnetic resonance image with fat saturation post gadolinium shows a lesion containing fluid with an enhancing rim. Enhancement is also seen in the adjacent marrow and soft tissues. The degree of enhancement is increased in this patient owing to a healing pathologic fracture through the lesion.

nature of the lesion. The fluid contents are low signal on T1 and high signal on T2. With contrast, the cyst contents do not enhance; however, the lining of the cyst does enhance (Fig. 176-21). Occasionally, with preceding intralesional hemorrhage from fracture, fluid-fluid levels may be seen representing settled, degraded blood products. On bone scans, bone cysts produce a cold defect, with occasional mild peripheral uptake.

Fractured cysts tend to heal spontaneously; however, larger cysts with or without fracture are usually treated with curettage and bone grafting. The prognosis is excellent. However, 35% to 50% of bone cysts recur, in some cases multiple times. Treated cysts often have a complex appearance with mixed sclerosis and lucency, septations, and mild expansion and deformity of the involved bone. Premature growth plate closure may occur as a complication of treatment but not due to the cyst itself. Cyst aspiration with corticosteroid injection has also been used for treatment.

Solitary unicameral bone cysts are occasionally found in the calcanei of pediatric patients. Often, these cysts are painless and are first detected by radiography of acute injuries to the feet. Calcaneal bone cysts are nearly always located near the base of the neck of the calcaneus. The thin, overlying lateral cortical wall of the calcaneus forms a well-defined bony border that allows differentiation from the "physiologic" pseudocystic radiolucent areas observed in the same region of normal bones (Chapter 163). Van Linthoudt and Lagier consider calcaneal cysts to be the result of organizing hemorrhages.

TABLE 176-6
Precursors of Secondary Aneurysmal Bone Cyst*
Chondroblastoma
Chondromyxoid fibroma
Eosinophilic granuloma
Fibrous dysplasia
Fibrous histiocytoma
Giant cell tumor
Giant cell reparative granuloma
Hemangioma
Malignant fibrous histiocytoma
Myositis ossificans
Nonossifying fibroma
Osteoblastoma
Osteosarcoma
Solitary bone cyst

*Modified from Dorfman HD, Czerniak B: Bone Tumors. St. Louis, Mosby, 1998:879.

ANEURYSMAL BONE CYST

ABC is a pseudolesion that occurs due to intraosseous or subperiosteal hemorrhage or as a transitional lesion secondary to an underlying primary bone tumor. Histologically, ABC is composed of anastomosing channels containing blood and variably lined with fibrous walls containing red blood cells, hemosiderin granules, foreign body giant cells, and spicules of reactive bone. The etiology of ABC is poorly understood. ABC may be primary or secondary. Most ABCs are thought to be reactive or secondary. A wide variety of lesions may act as the nidus for ABC development (Table 176-6). Underlying lesions are pathologically identified in one third of cases. A large ABC may obscure the underlying lesion. Conversely, ABC may represent only a small component of a larger tumor. In lesions without an underlying tumor, the role of antecedent trauma acting as a nidus has been proposed.

ABC is slightly more common in girls. Whether primary or secondary, the lesion is most common in the first three decades of life. It is rare in patients less than 5 years of age. Patients usually present with nonspecific pain and swelling; 10% of patients present with pathologic fracture. ABC is most common in the metaphyses of long bones, the craniofacial bones and the spine. Spinal lesions occur in the posterior elements. Long bone lesions can be subclassified as intramedullary and juxtacortical (cortical or subperiosteal). Subperiosteal ABC is rare and mimics other subperiosteal tumors and pathologies.

On radiography, ABC appears as a lucent, expansile, "blowout" or "soap-bubble" lesion with thin, smooth bony walls (Figs. 176-22 and 176-23). Lesions are multiloculated. The cortex is usually intact but may be markedly thinned to the point of not being visible. Periosteal new bone may be present.

Both CT and MRI demonstrate fluid-fluid levels, which are characteristic of the lesion. This finding is due to sedimentation of degraded blood products, especially methemoglobin, which has a much shorter T1 relaxation time than that of hemoglobin. Fluid-fluid levels may be

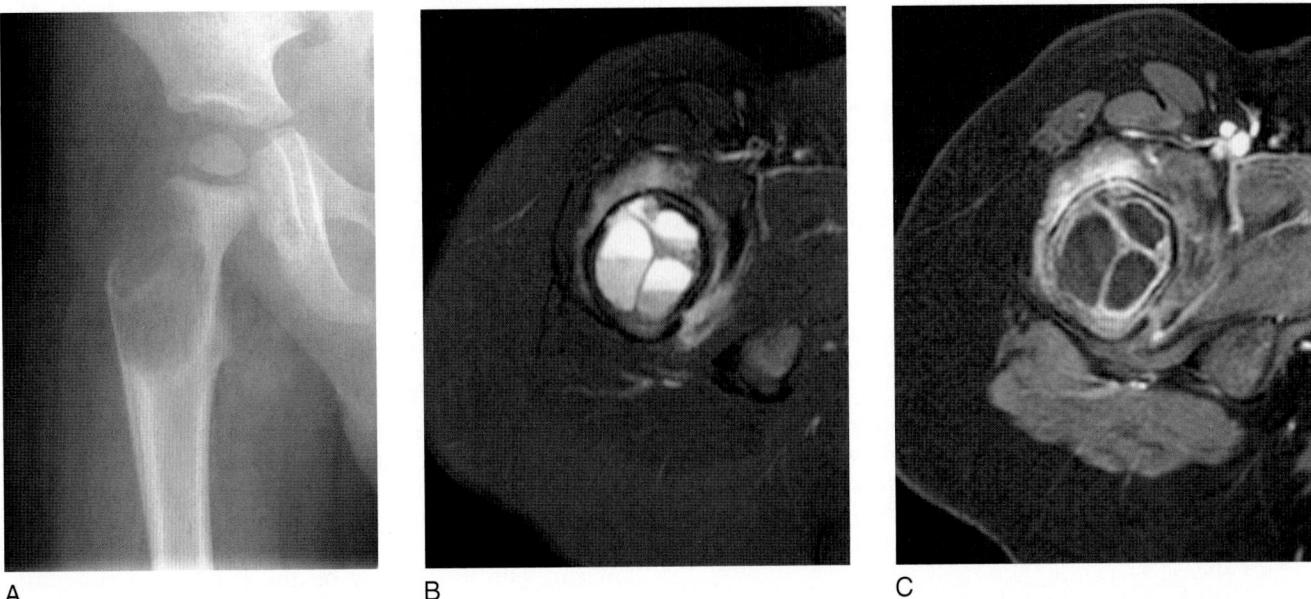

FIGURE 176-22. Aneurysmal bone cyst in a 22-month-old boy. **A,** Anteroposterior radiograph of the hip shows a large, relatively well-defined, mildly expansile lucent lesion of the proximal femur. The cortex of the lateral femoral neck is thinned and absent. Smooth periosteal new bone is present on the lateral aspect of the proximal femoral diaphysis. **B,** Axial T2-weighted magnetic image shows fluid-fluid levels within the lesion. The cortex is thinned but intact. Some edema is seen in adjacent soft tissues. **C,** Axial T1-weighted magnetic resonance image with fat saturation post gadolinium—enhancement is seen within cyst walls and septations. Slight enhancement is seen with soft tissues anteriorly.

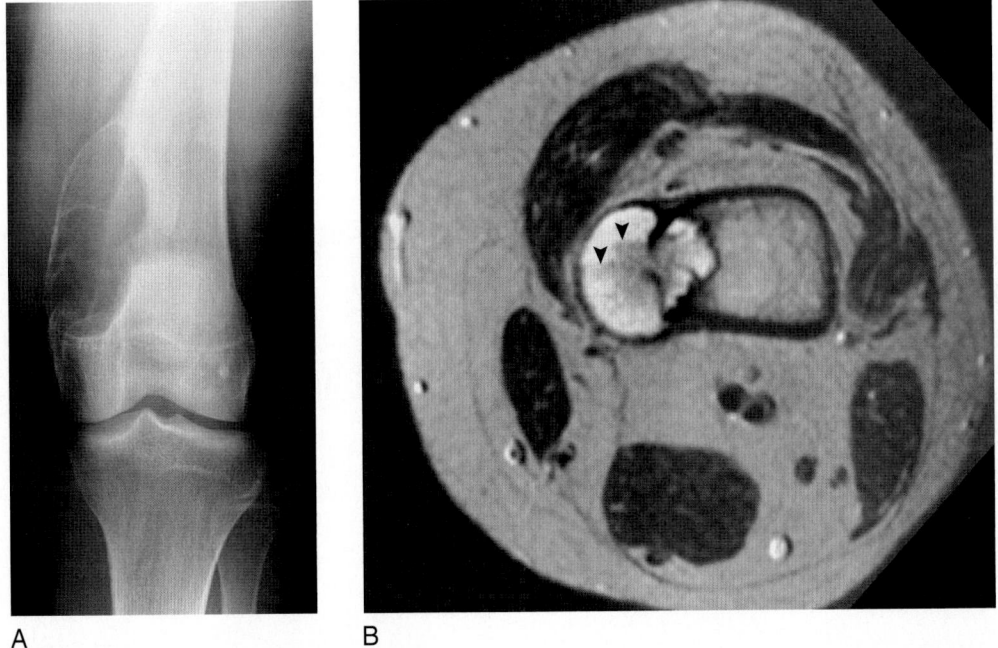

FIGURE 176-23. Aneurysmal bone cyst in a 13-year-old. **A,** Radiograph of the knee shows an eccentric, expansile lucent lesion with a thin, bony shell involving the medial aspect of the distal femur. **B,** On a transverse T2-weighted magnetic resonance image, the lesion is seen to penetrate the cortex of the femur and extend into the adjacent soft tissues. Several fluid-fluid levels are demonstrated *(arrowheads)*.

single or multiple and may be seen as varying horizontal levels within separate loculations (see Figs. 176-22 and 176-23). If the loculations are very small, fluid-fluid levels may be less apparent. The signal characteristics of the cyst contents are variable and are probably dependent on the relative age and concentration of the blood components. Abundant hemosiderin may produce foci of low signal, which may be diffuse throughout the lesion. Cyst contents do not enhance; however, the septations do enhance.

Fluid-fluid levels are characteristic of ABC; however, this finding is not pathognomonic for ABC. Fluid-fluid levels have been identified in numerous benign and malignant bone lesions, including fibrous dysplasia, chondroblastoma, GCT, NOF, simple bone cyst and osteosarcoma, particularly the telangiectatic variant. Any solid component suggests an underlying tumor. Lesions composed of a greater percentage composition of fluid-fluid levels are more likely benign in origin. Differentiation of ABC from telangiectatic osteosarcoma is particularly difficult and, at times, cannot be achieved by imaging methods. Greater bone destruction may be evident with telangiectatic osteosarcoma. It should be noted that ABC may also develop within a conventional osteosarcoma.

> **Fluid-fluid levels are characteristic of, but not pathognomonic for ABC. Fluid-fluid levels have been identified in numerous benign and malignant bone lesions, including fibrous dysplasia, chondroblastoma, GCT, NOF, simple bone cyst and osteosarcoma, particularly the telangiectatic variant.**

ABC is treated with curettage and bone grafting. Twenty percent of ABCs recur after grafting. Vascular embolization and percutaneous sclerotherapy have also been used.

An unusual *solid variant of ABC* has radiographic features similar to those of the typical ABC. The solid variant lacks cavernous, blood-containing spaces but is characterized histologically by the solid elements (proliferating fibrous tissue, benign giant cells, and newly formed osteoid matrix) found in the typical ABCs. A third of these tumors are not "aneurysmal." The solid variant of ABCs is histologically indistinguishable from extragnathic giant cell (reparative) granuloma. It is most common in the second and third decade. The lesion favors the axial skeleton over appendicular locations. Most common locations are craniofacial bones, small tubular bones of the hands and feet, and the femur. On MRI, the lesion is predominantly solid with little or no cystic component (Fig. 176-24). Signal is low on both T1 and T2 due to fibrosis. The lesion enhances with gadolinium. The solid variant of ABC may occasionally produce osteoid which may be evident on radiographs or CT.

LYMPHANGIOMA/LYMPHANGIOMATOSIS OF BONE

Osseous involvement of lymphangioma is much less common than soft tissue involvement. Osseous involvement is usually part of a multifocal process (lymphangiomatosis) and is usually associated with an adjacent soft tissue component. The etiology of lymphangioma is unclear. The lesion may be the result of a congenital obstruction of lymphatic drainage. The tumor is composed of fluid-filled spaces lined with lymphatic epithelium. Lymphangioma of bone is usually asymptomatic in itself. Patients present in early childhood. Osseous lesions usually remain stable or progress slowly. On radiography, focal lesions are rounded, well-defined and cystic in appearance. Larger, more complex lesions may appear multiseptated, "soap bubble" like or moth eaten with more variable margination (Fig. 176-25). The involved bone may be deformed or occasionally, hypoplastic. Sclerosis is minimal. CT or MRI shows a relatively nonaggressive-appearing lesion with septated fluid

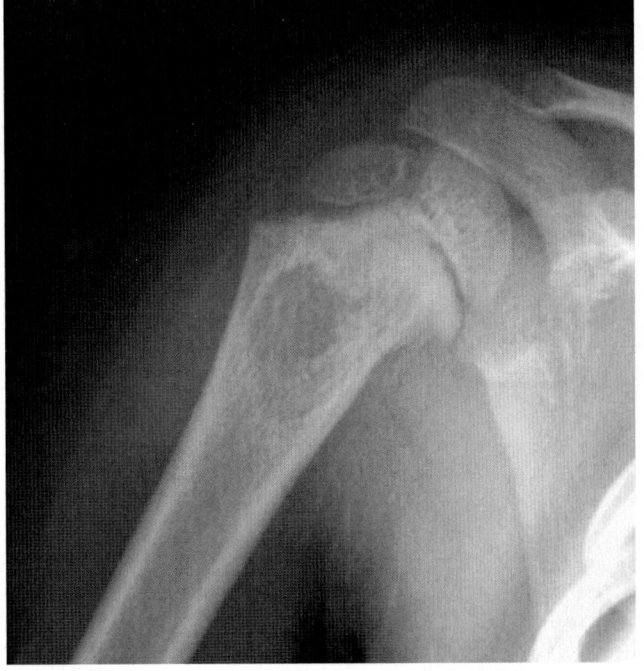

A

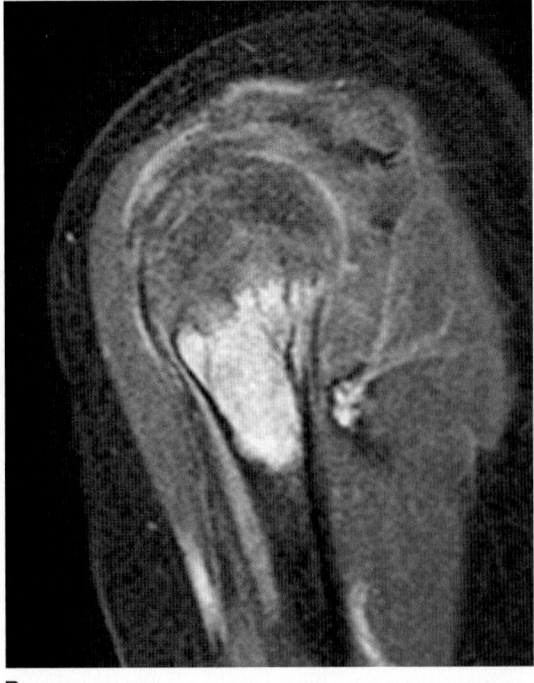

B

FIGURE 176-24. Solid variant of aneurysmal bone cyst in a 4-year-old boy. **A,** Radiograph shows an ill-defined lucent lesion in the proximal humeral metaphysis. The medial cortex is poorly defined. **B,** Sagittal T1-weighted magnetic resonance image with fat saturation post gadolinium – homogeneously enhancing soft tissue is seen with the lesion.

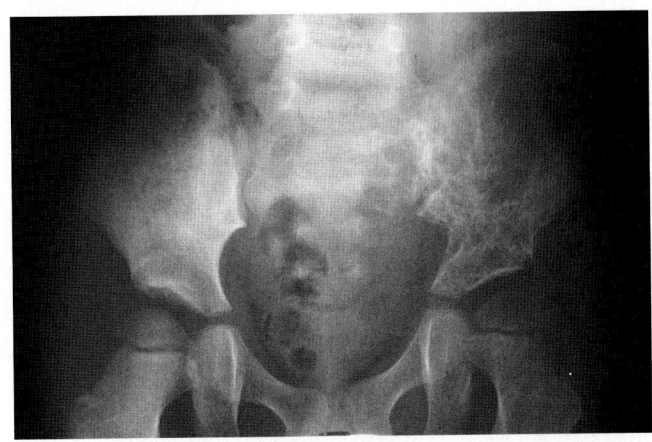
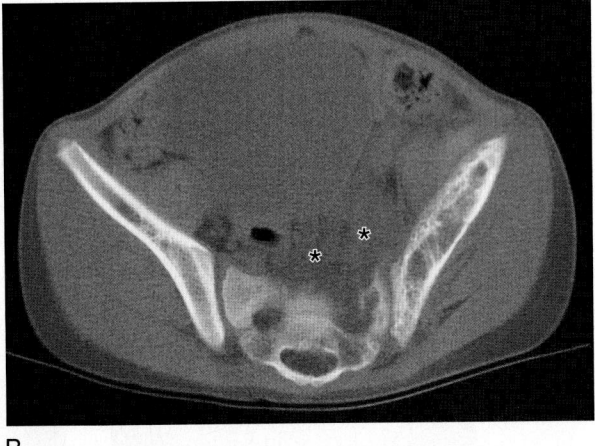

A   B

FIGURE 176-25. Lymphangioma of bone in a 4-year-old boy presenting with a limp on the left. **A,** Radiograph shows coarsened trabeculae throughout the left ilium with a "bubbly" or cystic appearance. Abnormality extends into the left sacral ala. The left hip is osteopenic. **B,** Axial computed tomographic image shows cystic expansion of the left iliac wing and left sacrum corresponding to the radiographic abnormality. Increased soft tissue anterior to the left sacroiliac joint *(asterisks)* is due to the extraosseous portion of the lesion.

spaces. There is minimal enhancement of septae and walls on MRI.

Giant Cell Tumor

GCT (osteoclastoma) is an uncommon neoplasm that rarely occurs before skeletal maturity. Approximately 5% of cases are reported before skeletal maturity, most in the second decade and rarely in the first decade of life. The lesion is most common in the long bones, particularly the distal femur and proximal tibia, is less common in the short bones of the hands and feet, and rarely occurs elsewhere in children. In skeletally mature individuals, the lesion is uniformly within the epiphysis with variable extension into the adjacent metaphysis. Epiphyseal lesions abut the articular surface. In skeletally immature patients, the lesion is almost uniformly metaphyseal, usually abutting the physis. Epiphyseal involvement is very rare before physeal closure. Multifocal GCT is very rare in children.

> In skeletally mature individuals, GCTs are uniformly found within the epiphysis, abutting the articular surface and with variable extension into the adjacent metaphysis. GCT is much less common in skeletally immature patients, in whom the lesion is almost uniformly metaphyseal, usually abutting the physis.

Patients with GCT present with pain and tenderness, swelling, and limited range of motion of the adjacent joint.

On radiographs, GCT appears as a geographic, lytic lesion (Fig. 176-26). Margins vary from sclerotic to ill defined. Frequently, there is relatively sharp but non-sclerotic margin. Periosteal new bone, expansion of bone, and pathologic fracture are common. The metaphyseal end of the lesion tends to be less well defined. CT

delineates the lesion and its margins (see Fig. 176-26). No calcified or ossified matrix is seen. MRI findings vary. In Kransdorf's large series, 56% of tumors were solid or solid with cystic change and 44% were cystic. Solid areas tend to be of intermediate signal on T1 and T2. Hemosiderin from intratumoral hemorrhage may produce foci of low signal. Occasionally, a GCT may have a more aggressive appearance with cortical penetration and soft tissue extension. Approximately 15% of GCTs have an associated component of ABC. Such lesions appear more expansile.

The prognosis of GCT is excellent; however, up to 25% of tumors recur locally. Malignant GCT and metastasizing GCT have rarely been reported in children. The pulmonary "implants" from GCT are usually of self-limited growth potential, but recurrence and disease progression is possible.

Fibrous Tumors

FIBROUS CORTICAL DEFECT / NON-OSSIFYING FIBROMA (FIBROXANTHOMA)

Fibrous cortical defect (FCD) and NOF are extremely common tumors occurring in the metaphyses of the long bones of children. FCDs are essentially a normal variant, occurring in up to 40% of children during development. FCD and NOF are histologically identical and composed of highly cellular stroma with spindle-shaped fibroblasts, osteoclast-like multinucleated giant cells and foam or xanthoma cells. Arbitrarily, lesions smaller than 2 cm are called FCD and those larger than 2 cm are called NOF. The lesions probably represent a developmental defect in the periosteum of cortical bone. Lesions are seen in the latter part of the first decade until shortly after skeletal maturation. The average time from diagnosis to spontaneous regression is 29 to 52 months. Lesions are inactive after skeletal maturity. Rarely, a NOF may persist into adulthood.

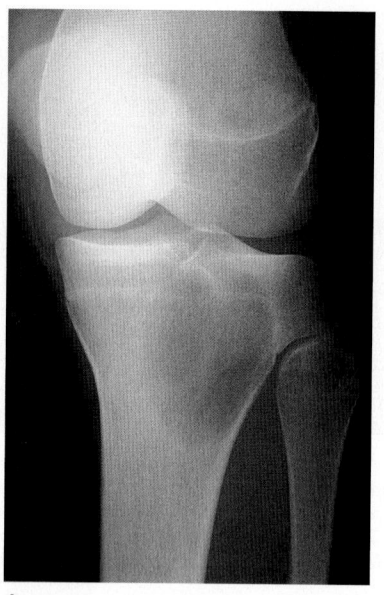
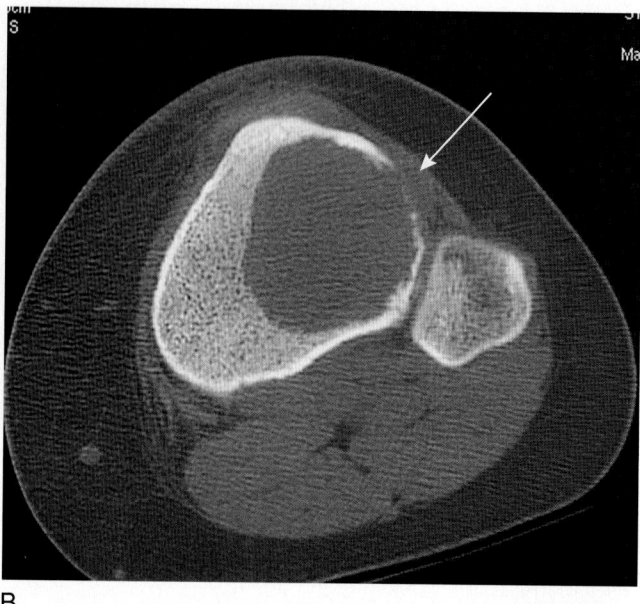

A   B

FIGURE 176-26. Giant cell tumor in a 14-year-old girl. **A,** Radiograph shows a relatively well-defined lucent lesion in the proximal tibial metaphysis and epiphysis. The lesion does not have sclerotic margins. The lesion is near the articular surface but does not abut it. **B,** Axial computed tomography shows a large lucent lesion of the tibia. The lesion margins are well-defined but not sclerotic. The anterolateral cortex is destroyed *(arrow)*.

> Arbitrarily, lesions smaller than 2 cm are called FCD and those larger than 2 cm are called NOF. The lesions are histologically identical. The radiographic appearance of FCD and NOF is sufficiently specific that neither additional imaging nor biopsy is indicated.

FCD and NOF are usually detected incidentally. The lesions are asymptomatic, with the exception of very large lesions, which may cause dull pain. Uncommonly, an NOF may be large enough to cause a pathologic fracture or lead to a stress fracture. FCD and NOF are most common in the metaphyses of the long bones of the lower extremity, especially at the knee. Lesions are more commonly posterior. FCD and cortical desmoids of the posteromedial distal femoral metaphysis are histologically similar.

On radiography, FCDs are seen as small, well-defined, ovoid, cortically based lesions. NOFs appear to be similar but are larger (Fig. 176-27), and more lobular and multi-locular. Usually, the lesions extend inward; however, the outer cortex may be thinned and bulged. In thinner bones, such as the fibula, the lesion may occupy the entire width of the bone. FCDs and NOFs originate in metaphysis near the growth plate and migrate into metadiaphysis and diaphysis with maturation. The natural history of the lesions is for involution to occur with progressive sclerosis of the lesion. Sclerosis and involution begin on the diaphyseal end of the lesion (Fig. 176-28). The radiographic appearance of FCD and NOF is sufficiently specific that neither additional imaging nor biopsy is indicated. Because the lesions are so common, they will often be incidental findings on other imaging studies. The radiographic features of FCD

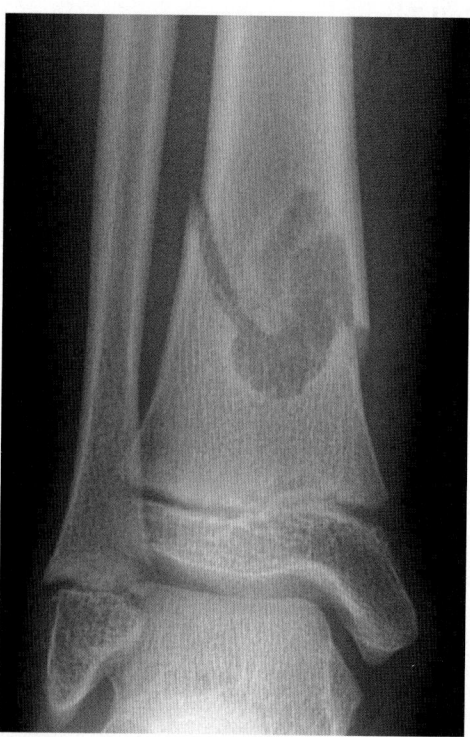

FIGURE 176-27. Pathologic fracture through a nonossifying fibroma in a 10-year-old boy. The lesion has well-defined, minimally sclerotic margins.

and NOF are also manifest on CT. On MRI, the lesions are well defined, lobular and cortically based. Low signal is seen on T1. T2 signal and enhancement with gadolinium varies with the stage of lesion development. Active, early lesions are high signal on T2 and enhance. Involuting lesions are low signal on T2 and do not enhance. No

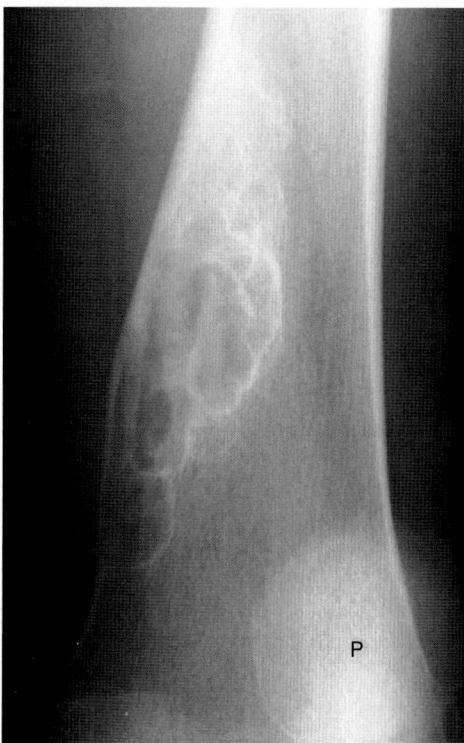

FIGURE 176-28. Large, lobulated nonossifying fibroma in a 16-year-old boy—anteroposterior view of the distal femur. The proximal portion of the lesion is sclerotic, consistent with early involution. P, patella.

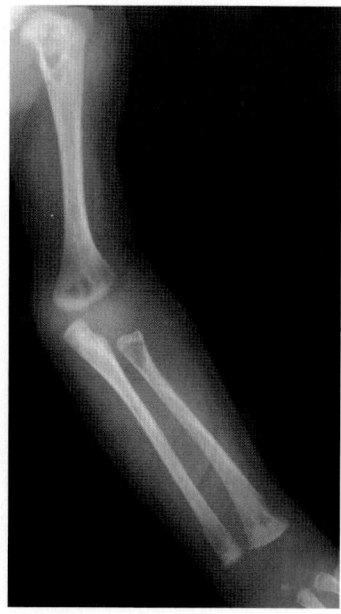

FIGURE 176-29. Infantile myofibromatosis—focal lucent lesions are seen in the proximal and distal humeral and radial metaphyses and in the distal ulnar metaphysis.

peritumoral edema is seen. Active, early lesions may also show uptake on bone scans and PET scans.

Multiple NOFs may be seen with neurofibromatosis. In *Jaffe-Campanacci syndrome*, disseminated NOFs are associated with cystic lesions of the jaw, café-au-lait skin lesions, mental retardation, ocular anomalies, hypogonadism, and cardiovascular anomalies in the absence of other signs of neurofibromatosis. There is debate that Jaffe-Campanacci syndrome is a forme fruste of neurofibromatosis.

INFANTILE MYOFIBROMATOSIS

The fibromatoses are predominantly soft tissue processes and are discussed in greater detail in Chapter 160. Patients with infantile myofibromatosis may have extensive osseous involvement with tumor. Such patients present in infancy and rarely beyond the age of 2 years. Multifocal, eccentric, geographic lesions are most common in the metaphyses of long bones (Fig. 176-29). Usually, the osseous lesions are accompanied by soft tissue lesions. The tumors regress spontaneously with complete healing of osseous abnormality.

DESMOPLASTIC FIBROMA

Desmoplastic fibroma is a rare, benign, locally aggressive neoplasm seen in the second and third decade. It is an osseous analog of soft tissue desmoid tumor. Patients present with nonspecific pain and swelling. The mandible, long bone metaphyses, and pelvis are most frequently affected. Usually, the lesion has a nonaggressive radiographic appearance but some cases show a soft tissue

mass and more aggressive-appearing bone destruction. Low signal on T2 in the absence of calcified or ossified matrix may be a differentiating feature because this is not usually seen in other soft tissue lesions in bone.

FIBROUS DYSPLASIA

Although it is not a true neoplasm, fibrous dysplasia involving a long bone may mimic a bone tumor or cyst, especially when it causes localized expansion of the bone and is monostotic. Pathologically, fibro-osseous tissue replaces the normal medullary space. Fibrous dysplasia can be monostotic or polyostotic, and monomelic or polymelic. Seventy to eighty percent of cases are monostotic. Polyostotic disease predominates on one side. Fibrous dysplasia is more common in girls than in boys. Most patients with focal disease are adolescents or young adults, with occasional patients seen in the first decade of life. Polyostotic disease tends to present in the first decade. Any bone may be affected. The most common presentation of fibrous dysplasia is monostotic and affecting craniofacial bones (especially skull base), a rib, or a long bone (most commonly the femur). Lesions may involve metaphysis and diaphysis, sparing the epiphysis before physeal fusion.

Patients with solitary lesions present with pain, edema, deformity, pathologic fracture, or fatigue fracture. Patients with polyostotic disease present similarly but often at a younger age (i.e., first decade). Polyostotic disease is often syndrome related and may be suspected based on other clinical findings.

Fibrous dysplasia in the long bones causes expansion of the medullary cavity, endosteal scalloping, coarse trabeculation, and sclerotic margins forming a "rind." Bowing of the affected bone may occur. In the femur, the resulting deformity is called a "shepherd's crook" (Fig. 176-30) Lesions may be central or eccentric. The

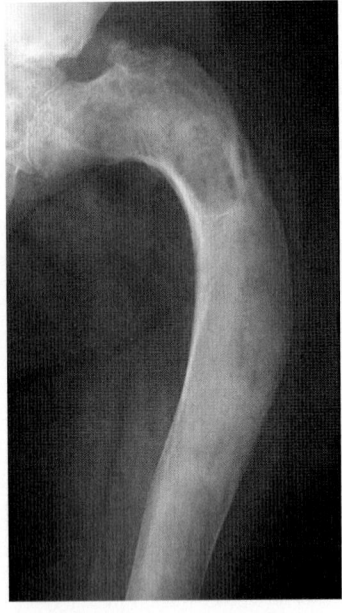
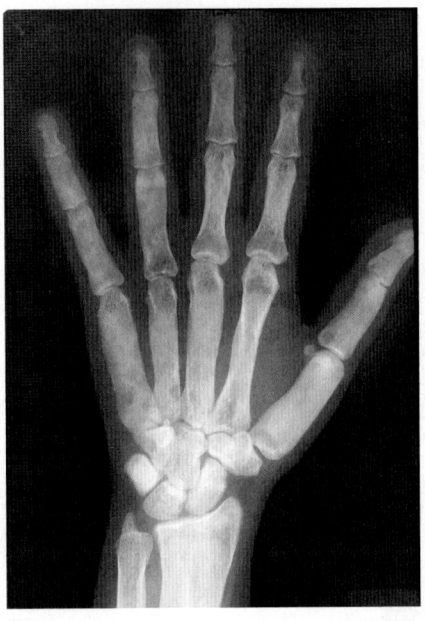

FIGURE 176-30. Polyostotic fibrous dysplasia in a 22-year-old woman. **A,** The femur is expanded and bowed with a "shepherd's crook" deformity. The femoral trabeculae are replaced by ground glass matrix. **B,** Diffuse sclerosis is seen in the hand and wrist with mild expansion and indistinct transition from cortex to medullary space.

radiographic opacity of a fibrous dysplasia lesion depends on the relative amount of dysplastic bone and fibrous material within the lesion. Therefore, lesions vary in appearance from "ground glass" to radiolucent. The ground-glass appearance is due to matrix containing a fine mesh-like pattern of delicate bone spicules (see Figs. 176-30 and 176-31). It is relatively specific for fibrous dysplasia but may be simulated by other lesions replacing the medullary trabeculae. Lucent lesions usually have a sclerotic margin. Small cartilaginous foci within the lesion may develop chondroid calcification (osteocartilaginous fibrous dysplasia). A single lesion or involved bone may demonstrate varying appearances within different areas. Active, early lesions tend to be radiolucent whereas older lesions may be more sclerotic. No periosteal reaction is present unless there is a fracture.

Lesions are well characterized on CT. On MRI, lesions are similar in signal intensity to muscle on T1. On T2, lesion signal intensity varies depending on the composition of the lesion. Pure fibrous tissue is hypointense on T2; however, lesions of fibrous dysplasia are often hyperintense. This seeming inconsistency is probably due to the inhomogeneous nature of the lesion, which consists of spindle cells, trabeculae of immature woven bone with osteoid seams, and small cysts. Fluid-fluid levels have been reported. Soft tissue extension is rare. With gadolinium, central or, less frequently, peripheral enhancement of fibrous dysplasia may occur. Lesion uptake on bone scans is variable. Bone scans may be normal.

Fibrous dysplasia lesions in the face and/or skull may be quite debilitating and clinically challenging. These manifestations are briefly discussed in Chapter 40.

Sarcomatous degeneration is rare in fibrous dysplasia, occurring in 0.5% of patients; osteosarcoma is most common followed by fibrosarcoma. Malignancy may be simulated by intralesional hemorrhage or ABC. Risk is

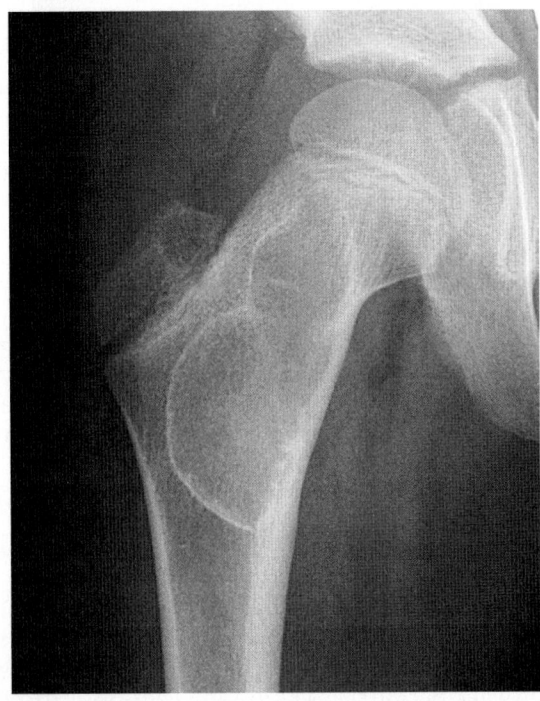

FIGURE 176-31. Focal fibrous dysplasia in an 11-year-old boy. The lesion has well-defined, sclerotic margins and a "ground-glass" matrix.

greater with polyostotic disease and prior radiation therapy.

In 2% to 3% of patients, fibrous dysplasia is associated with endocrine disorders, mostly of hypothalamic dysfunction. In *McCune-Albright syndrome*, female patients present with precocious puberty, cutaneous café-au-lait spots, and unilateral polyostotic fibrous dysplasia. *Mazabraud syndrome*, characterized by polyostotic fibrous dysplasia and intramuscular myxoma, is rare in children.

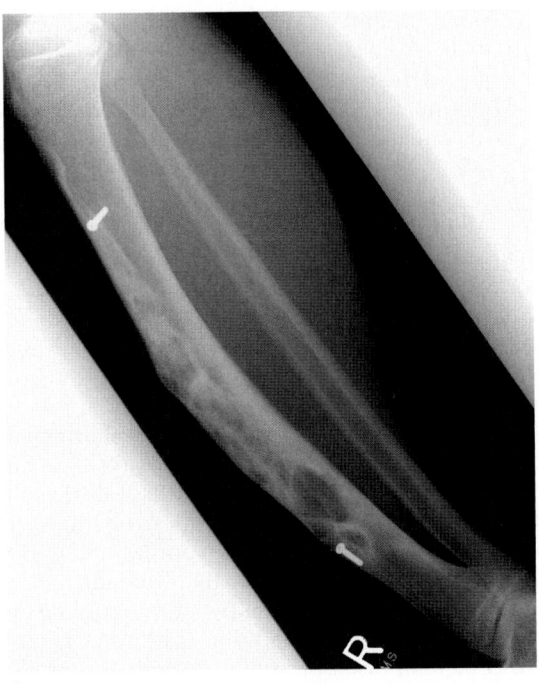

A

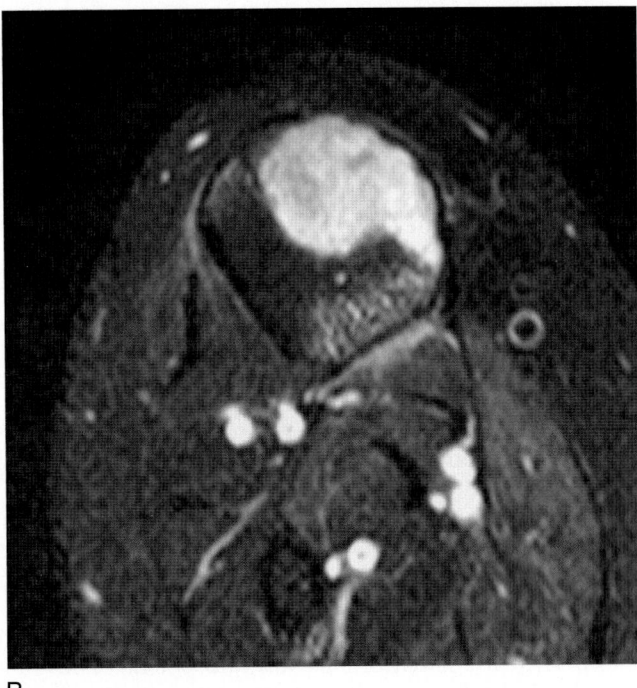

B

FIGURE 176-32. Osteofibrous dysplasia in a 15-year-old boy. Biopsies several years prior had made the diagnosis of adamantinoma, for which surgical excision with grafting had been performed. Screws are related to the prior graft. Symptoms recurred. **A,** Lateral radiograph shows anterior tibial bowing with mixed sclerosis and cystic lucencies centered anteriorly within the tibia. **B,** Axial T2-weighted magnetic resonance image with fat saturation shows homogeneous, high-signal soft tissue within the lesion. Percutaneous and excisional biopsies both showed osteofibrous dysplasia.

> McCune-Albright syndrome—female patients present with precocious puberty, cutaneous café-au-lait spots and unilateral polyostotic fibrous dysplasia.

OSTEOFIBROUS DYSPLASIA

Osteofibrous dysplasia (OFD; extragnathic ossifying fibroma; intracortical fibrous dysplasia) is a proliferation of fibro-osseous tissue. OFD is usually sporadic, although Karol and colleagues reported a kindred with six affected members by autosomal dominant inheritance. Most cases occur during the first decade of life, and some tumors have been found in newborn infants. OFD is a rare lesion that is usually confined to the diaphysis and metadiaphysis of the tibia but can also involve the fibula, sometimes synchronously in the same patient. Rarely, lesions may be multiple and bilateral.

OFD is usually painless and is characterized by deformity that can progress until the time of physeal fusion occurs. Patients may present with anterior bowing. Fracture or pseudoarthrosis may complicate its course.

By radiography, OFD is an eccentric, lucent, solitary or multiloculated lesion involving the anterior cortex of the tibia (Fig. 176-32). Involvement of the tibia is more commonly proximal, but distal lesions occur and may be complicated by pseudarthrosis. The cortex is expanded. Larger lesions will expand posteriorly, replacing the medullary cavity. Lesions appear lucent or like ground

glass. The lesion is associated with cortical thickening and anterior bowing of the bone. Cross-sectional imaging is very helpful in determining its intracortical location, an important feature in distinguishing OFD from fibrous dysplasia, which is intramedullary (see Fig. 176-32).

OFD is histologically similar to fibrous dysplasia in that it contains well-differentiated fibroblasts, collagen, and bony trabeculae. The main differentiating feature is the presence of active osteoblasts in OFD. Especially in the second decade, radiologic and even pathologic differentiation between OFD and adamantinoma is difficult. This subject is further discussed later. OFD tends to occur at a younger age than adamantinoma.

OFD exhibits tendencies both toward local recurrence and spontaneous regression. Therefore, aggressive surgical management is usually avoided.

LONG BONE ADAMANTINOMA

As opposed to OFD, adamantinoma is potentially progressive and malignant acting. Up to 15% of affected patients die of metastatic disease. On the basis of clinical, radiologic, histologic, and histochemical characteristics, long bone adamantinomas, which are unrelated to the jaw lesion of the same name, have recently been divided into two groups: classic and differentiated (OFD–like). Both types involve the tibia, the fibula, or both, but the classic form, which occurs almost exclusively in adults, is located in either the cortex or the medulla, and can expand through the cortex and periosteum. The differentiated form is seen in children and young adults up to 20 years of age and has been reported in newborn infants. The tumor is limited to the bony cortex and has a radiographic appearance identical to that of OFD (see Fig. 176-32). OFD and adamantinoma are pathologically distinct: epithelial and mesenchymal cells, which express immunoreactive cytokeratin and vimentin, are present in adamantinomas. Epithelial elements are absent in classic OFD and are minimal in differentiated adamantinoma.

> **Clinical, radiologic, and pathologic distinction of adamantinoma from OFD is challenging.**
> **Epithelial elements are absent in classic OFD and are minimal in differentiated adamantinoma.**

Long bone adamantinomas are rare tumors in children. The tumors may occur in adolescents but are more common in patients 20 to 50 years old. Patients present with pain and anterior tibial bowing. Radiographic findings are analogous to OFD. Variable features that might raise suspicion for adamantinoma are periosteal reaction, moth-eaten destruction, and soft tissue extension. MRI of adamantinoma was nonspecific. The T1- and T2-weighted signal characteristics are similar to those of other tumors. Soft tissue extension may be evident. Treatment of adamantinoma is usually en bloc resection.

Clinical, radiologic, and pathologic distinction of adamantinoma from OFD is challenging. The concept of a differentiated form implies a continuum between OFD and adamantinoma and suggests that OFD may be a regressive phase of adamantinoma. Some well-documented cases in the literature support this contention. Czerniak and associates suggested that patients with the differentiated type have a more favorable prognosis than those with classic adamantinoma—no differentiated tumors have been known to metastasize—and that long bone adamantinoma could be included among the few neoplasms that are capable of spontaneous regression.

Table 176-7 summarizes the distinguishing features of fibrous dysplasia, OFD and adamantinoma.

Langerhans Cell Histiocytosis

The unifying pathologic feature of LCH is in an inappropriate proliferation of Langerhans cells. Like the cells of monocyte-macrophage lineage, the Langerhans cell originates from CD34+ stem cells of the bone marrow. Knowledge of the derivation of these cells has made the term *histiocytosis X* obsolete. The cause of LCH is unknown. An infectious etiology was postulated in the past. Recent evidence of clonal proliferation of Langerhans cells suggests a neoplastic etiology. Histologically, the tumors are composed of Langerhans histiocytes containing characteristic cleaved nuclei and, on electron microscopy, racquet-shaped Birbeck granules in the cytoplasm adjacent to the cell membrane. The lesions also contain ordinary histocytes and eosinophils. Immunohistochemical staining for S100 protein and CD1a antigen are used in making the diagnosis.

Overall, focal LCH is a relatively common pediatric bone tumor. LCH is a continuum of disease ranging from a single, indolent, self-limited osseous lesion to a fulminant disseminated disorder involving multiple organs systems, not just bone. Approximately 80% of patients with LCH have osseous involvement.

In the past, patients with LCH pathology were divided into three diagnoses. Eosinophilic granuloma referred to localized skeletal disease, usually a single lesion. Seventy percent of patients fall into this category. Children with Hand-Schüller-Christian disease had the triad of geographic bone lesions, proptosis, and diabetes insipidus. The triad is rarely seen in an individual patient. Letterer-Siwe disease referred to the fulminant, disseminated, multisystem form, which was often fatal. Fewer than 10% of patients fall into this category. It is now recognized that LCH is a spectrum of disease rather than these three distinguishable entities.

> **LCH is a spectrum of disease rather than three distinguishable entities, as previously categorized.**

LCH is more common in Caucasians. It is twice as common in boys than in girls. LCH is seen from the neonatal period into adulthood. Most patients are younger than 15 years old at presentation. Overall, the peak incidence is at 1 to 5 years of age. Focal lesions tend to present slightly older with an average age of 10 to 12 years. Multifocal and systemic disease is most common in infants and younger children. Fulminant, life-threatening LCH is usually seen in the first two decades of life and is

TABLE 176-7

Features of Fibrous Dysplasia—Osteofibrous Dysplasia and Adamantinoma

Lesion	Location*	Histologic Features
Fibrous dysplasia	*Medulla*, long bones, face, ribs	Proliferation of fibro-osseous tissue; immature bone, fibroblasts
Osteofibrous dysplasia	*Cortex*, anterior tibia	Similar to fibrous dysplasia, but also contains active osteoblasts
Classic adamantinoma	*Cortex*, anterior tibia, fibula	Abundant epithelial elements
Differentiated adamantinoma	*Cortex*, anterior tibia, fibula	Like those of osteofibrous dysplasia; minimal scattered epithelial elements

*Italics indicate the bone region that is the primary site of each tumor.

rare beyond 3 years of age. Disseminated disease may cause lymphadenopathy, hepatosplenomegaly, skin lesions (purpuric rash), diabetes insipidus, exophthalmos, thrombocytopenia, and anemia. Pulmonary involvement of LCH in children is seen almost always in the setting of disseminated disease. Most children with osseous lesions do not have pulmonary disease. With disseminated disease, osseous lesions vary from relatively few to diffuse, confluent involvement.

Solitary LCH lesions usually present with local pain, tenderness, and occasionally, a palpable mass. Symptoms also relate to the involved bone. Mastoid lesions may present as ear disease. Spinal lesions may present with painful scoliosis or kyphosis. Patients may have a low-grade fever. Erythrocyte sedimentation rate and C-reactive protein may be elevated.

The skull is the most frequent site of LCH, followed by the femur, mandible, pelvis, ribs, and spine. Seventy percent of lesions occur in flat bones and 30% in tubular bones (long bones, clavicle, hands and feet). Lesions are usually located in the medulla. Primary lesions of the cortex are rare; however, the cortex is often secondarily affected by expansion of an intramedullary lesion. Long bone lesions occur in the diaphysis or metaphysis, with rare involvement of the epiphysis (Fig. 176-33). Rarely, lesions may cross an open growth plate. Multiple bone lesions occur in approximately 25% of patients.

In the extremities, most LCH lesions are purely osteolytic, with well-defined, minimally sclerotic borders. Many lesions are mildly expansile. Endosteal scalloping may be prominent, progressing to cortical disruption. Some lesions are permeative, and periosteal new bone formation may occur, giving them an aggressive

appearance. Periosteal new bone may be a single layer or layered. Although it is often said that LCH can have any radiographic appearance, lesions often have both aggressive and non-aggressive features. When such an indeterminate lesion is identified, LCH is high on the list of differential diagnoses.

> LCH can have any radiographic appearance; however, lesions often have both aggressive and non-aggressive radiographic features. When such an indeterminate lesion is identified, LCH is high on the list of differential diagnoses.

Radiographically, LCH of the calvaria typically appears as a lytic bone lesion with well-defined ("punched out") appearance. Skull lesions appear geographic with beveled borders due to differential destruction of the inner and outer tables (Fig. 176-34). A "button sequestrum" may be seen. Lesions of the maxilla and mandible produce "floating teeth" (Fig. 176-35) Vertebral lesions produce compression deformities, most common in the thoracic spine followed by lumbar and cervical. LCH often produces vertebra plana with marked loss of height of a single vertebral body (Fig. 176-36). With vertebral involvement, there may be soft tissue extension into the spinal canal, best assessed by MRI. The height of affected vertebral segments tends to reconstitute following therapy. Involvement of the posterior element may occur but is less common than vertebral body involvement.

The appearance of LCH lesions on imaging depends on the stage and activity of the lesions. The natural history of LCH is for spontaneous involution of some lesions. Even at the time of diagnosis, some lesions may be present which are already in a state of involution or quiescence. Involuting lesions will be less well defined and show sclerosis.

Both CT and MRI can be used for further delineation of osseous lesions. On CT, active lesions usually have a

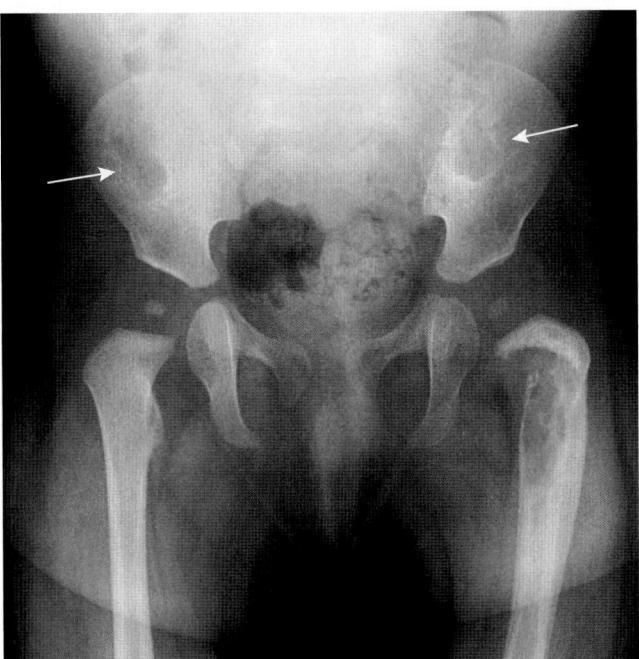

FIGURE 176-33. Langerhans cell histiocytosis in an 8-month-old girl. A large lesion in the proximal left femur has destroyed the medial cortex. Abundant smooth periosteal new bone is present laterally. Additional lesions are present in each ilium *(arrows).*

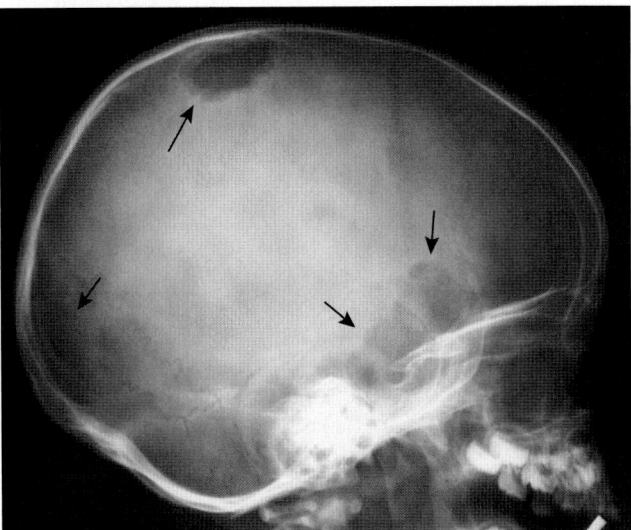

FIGURE 176-34. Langerhans cell histiocytosis in a 2-year-old girl. Lateral skull radiograph shows three lytic lesions in the skull. The lesion at the vertex has beveled edges.

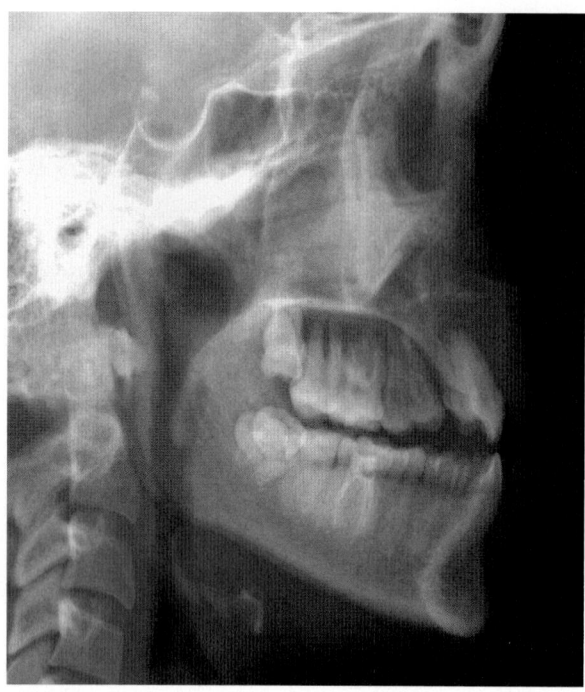

A

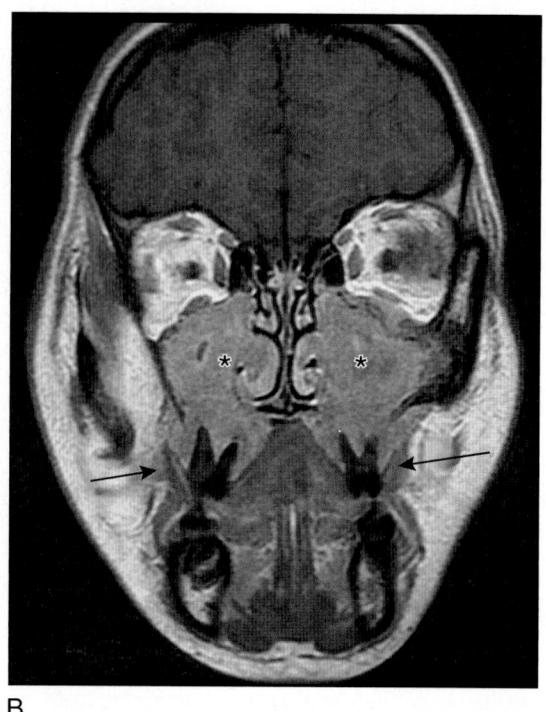

B

FIGURE 176-35. Langerhans cell histiocytosis in a 16-year-old girl. Lateral radiograph **(A)** and coronal T1-weighted magnetic resonance with gadolinium show "floating" maxillary teeth (*arrows* in **B**). Enhancing soft tissue (*asterisks* in **B**) fills the maxillary sinuses and replaces the maxilla.

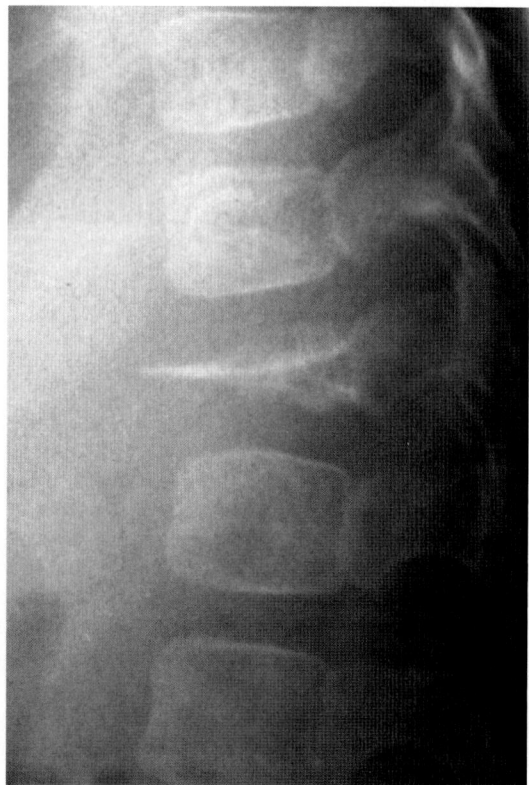

FIGURE 176-36. Vertebra plana due to Langerhans cell histiocytosis in a 20-month-old girl.

well-defined, nonsclerotic margin. Cortical break and soft tissue mass may be seen (Fig. 176-37). MRI is preferred to CT owing to the lack of ionizing radiation and superior tissue contrast. On MRI, active lesions are composed of soft tissue, which is low signal on T1 and high signal on T2, and enhances relatively homogenously (see Fig. 176-35). About half of lesions will be hyperintense to muscle on T1 images. Enhancement of the tumor with gadolinium is usually marked. Extensive bone marrow and soft tissue edema produces high signal on T2-weighted images and enhances. This prominent inflammatory reaction produces an aggressive appearance, suggesting a malignant process. LCH lesions that disrupt the cortex may also produce a sizable soft tissue mass, simulating malignancy. Thirty percent of lesions have associated soft tissue mass on MR. Older, involuted, or involuting lesions appear as low signal on T1 and T2 images.

A multiplicity of lesions is very suggestive of LCH, as opposed to many other lesions, which are usually unifocal (see Fig. 176-33). If LCH is a consideration, a radiographic skeletal survey may be beneficial in identifying other lesions. Often, the presenting lesion is not the best site for biopsy and other unsuspected sites may prove more suitable for tissue diagnosis. Because multiple skeletal lesions may coexist, skeletal imaging is necessary at the time of diagnosis and for purposes of follow-up. Some controversy exists about the relative accuracy of radiographic skeletal surveys and radionuclide bone scintigraphy. Up to 35% of lesions may be missed by bone scans. New technology has probably improved the accuracy of bone scans for LCH. Because

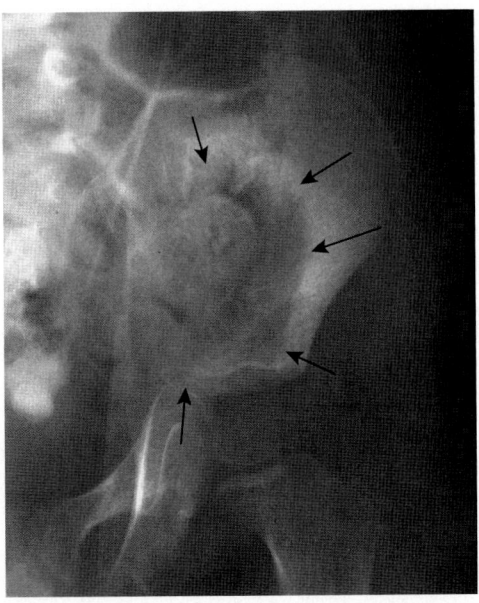 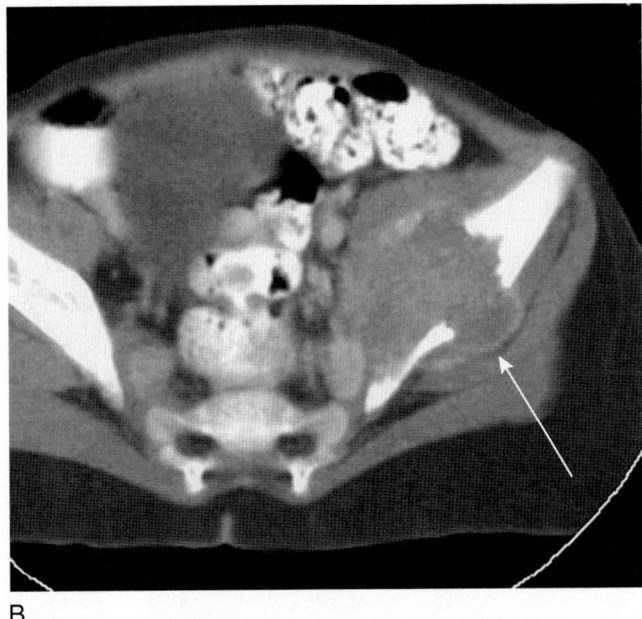

A   B

FIGURE 176-37. Langerhans cell histiocytosis in a 2-year-old boy. **A,** Radiograph shows a large lucent lesion in the right ilium. Margins of the lesion are indistinct. **B,** Axial computed tomography with contrast shows a corresponding destructive lesion. The soft tissue mass *(arrow)* extends beyond the bone both internally and externally.

bone scans may detect lesions not seen on radiography and because some eosinophilic granulomas may not be detected on bone scintigrams, both examinations are often performed at the time of diagnosis. Usually, one modality suffices for follow-up, with most centers choosing the radiographic skeletal survey. Whole-body MRI may become an alternative method for identifying and following multifocal disease. PET scans have also shown utility in identifying sites of active disease and following response to therapy.

LCH localized to the skeleton carries a favorable prognosis. Recurrences are not uncommon. Solitary lesions are watched and usually involute spontaneously. More aggressive therapy may be occasionally warranted depending on symptoms and lesion characteristics. Curettage and ablative techniques have been used. Children with multiple lesions and/or associated systemic disease are treated more aggressively with steroids and chemotherapy. The disease is thus treated similar to a malignant process. The morbidity in children with systemic disease varies depending on the organs involved and the histologic pattern of disease. Children in whom organ function is unaffected and who respond well to initial therapy show a better long-term prognosis. Mortality of disseminated disease is approximately 10%.

Osseous Tumors

Osteoid Osteoma

Osteoid osteoma is a common, benign tumor of bone that has a characteristic presentation and radiologic appearance. These tumors occur predominantly in boys, usually those in the second decade of life; however, it is not uncommon in both sexes from the first decade until the mid-fourth decade. There is a strong Caucasian prevalence.

Pathologically, osteoid osteoma consists of a nidus that is usually surrounded by dense sclerotic bone. The nidus contains interlacing trabeculae at various stages of ossification within a stroma of loose, vascular connective tissue. Three types of osteoid osteoma are recognized: cortical (most common), cancellous or medullary, and subperiosteal (least common). The latter two types produce less sclerotic bone than cortical lesions, making radiologic diagnosis difficult. Kayser proposed that osteomas originate subperiosteally and gradually become incorporated in the cortex by continual remodeling, periosteal new bone formation, and endosteal resorption ("cortical drift"). Osteoid osteomas can also be subdivided into extra-articular and intra-articular types. There is a higher incidence of medullary and subperiosteal types at juxta- and intra-articular locations.

Osteoid osteomas may develop in any bone. The single most common location of osteoid osteoma is the femur, and specifically, the femoral neck. The tibia is the next most frequent site. Osteoid osteomas occur less frequently in the upper extremities than in the lower extremities, but frequently affect the tubular bones of the hands and feet. Osteoid osteomas most commonly affect the metaphysis or metadiaphysis, less commonly the diaphysis, and rarely the epiphysis. They are less common in flat bones and the spine, where they tend to affect the posterior arches of the vertebrae. In such cases, patients usually present with painful scoliosis.

> **The most common location of osteoid osteoma is the femoral neck.**

The classic presentation of osteoid osteoma, which actually does occur in many patients, is well-localized pain that is especially severe at night and relieved by

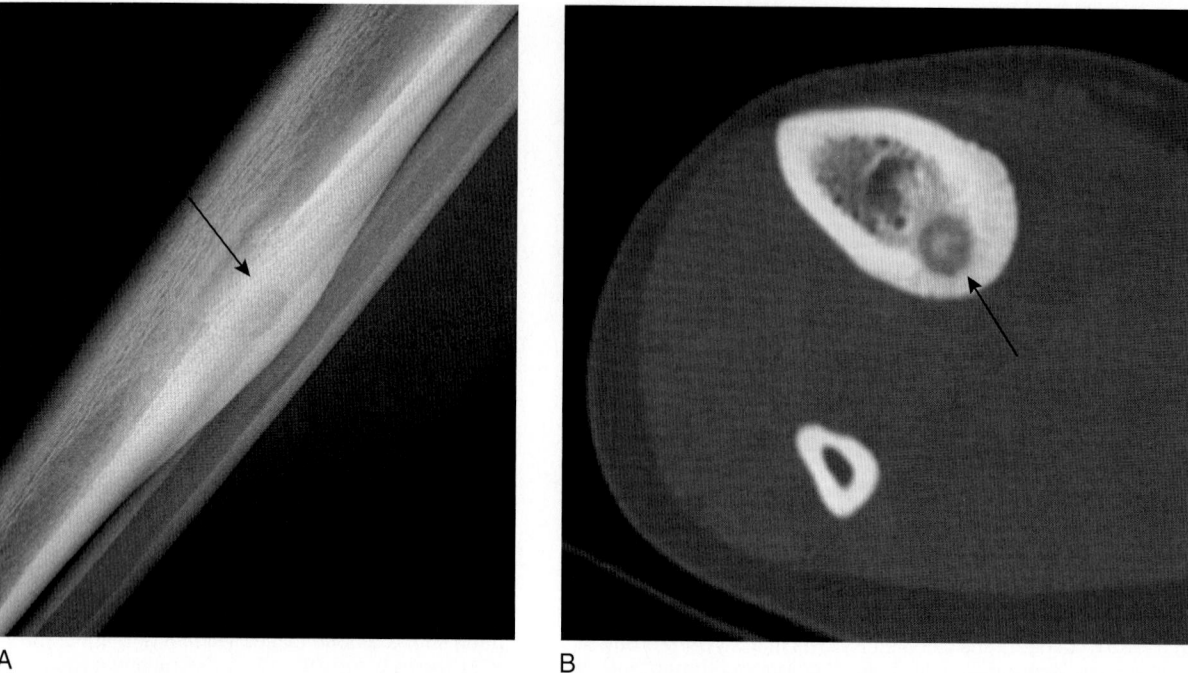

A   B

FIGURE 176-38. Osteoid osteoma of the tibia in a 15-year-old girl. **A,** Radiograph shows cortical thickening posteriorly. The lucent nidus is faintly seen *(arrow)*. **B,** Computed tomography better shows the nidus *(arrow).* A small radio-opacity (sequestrum) is present within the nidus.

aspirin or another nonsteroidal anti-inflammatory agent. Aspirin relieves the pain in 75% of patients. Lesions near a joint may mimic arthritis.

Radiographically, the nidus may be purely radiolucent or contain a dense center. The lucent nidus ranges from a few millimeters to 15 mm in diameter. With cortical osteoid osteomas, which are most common, the nidus is encased by a broad zone of dense bone (Fig. 176-38). Intra-articular osteoid osteomas tend to have little reactive bone or periosteal new bone formation. This type of osteoid osteoma most frequently affects the hip, where it causes osteopenia and joint effusion. Regardless of location, the nidus of an osteoma may be difficult to see on radiography.

CT is valuable in showing the lesion, confirming the diagnosis and determining the anatomic location of the lesion before percutaneous therapy or surgical excision. The CT appearance of a lucent nidus with central sequestrum opacity and surrounding sclerosis is usually diagnostic of osteoid osteoma, particularly if the clinical presentation is classic (see Fig. 176-38). Intramedullary and subperiosteal lesions show less sclerosis. Subperiosteal osteoid osteomas lie on top of the cortex and may erode it. Lesions may or may not have ossification within the nidus. Without the ossification, findings are less specific. CT shows the nidus of an osteoid osteoma better than MRI. On MRI, low intensity may be seen on both T1 and T2 images, depending on the relative amount of ossification and fibrovascular tissue. Although there is no signal from the sclerotic bone, the inherent contrast resolution of MRI provides precise definition of potentially extensive reactive changes in the bone marrow and adjacent soft tissues. Osteoid osteoma may produce an intense inflammatory response within adjacent bone,

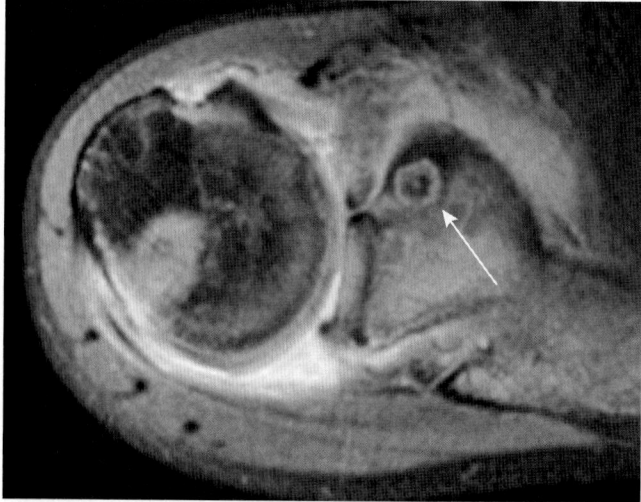

FIGURE 176-39. Osteoid osteoma at the base of the coracoid in a 12-year-old boy. Axial proton density magnetic resonance image with fat saturation shows a large nidus *(arrow).* Low signal within the nidus is consistent with a sequestrum. Bone marrow edema is present in the coracoid and adjacent scapula. Adjacent soft tissues are edematous. Synovitis affects the shoulder joint.

joint, and soft tissues (Fig. 176-39). Particularly if the nidus is not identified, a more aggressive process is suggested by these findings. Both the nidus and the adjacent inflamed tissues enhance with gadolinium. Intra-articular osteoid osteomas produce joint effusions and synovial proliferation that also appear of high intensity on T2-weighted images and enhance after gadolinium.

> CT shows the nidus of an osteoid osteoma better than MRI. Osteoid osteoma may produce an intense inflammatory response within adjacent bone, joint, and soft tissues simulating a more aggressive process.

On bone scans, increased flow activity is seen in the involved region and a "double-density" pattern represents localization of the radiotracer in the nidus surrounded by less intense activity in the reactive bone. This pattern is considered to be characteristic of osteoid osteoma. The sensitivity of bone scans for osteoid osteoma approaches 100%. In the past, angiography was also used diagnose and locate osteoid osteomas. Angiography shows increased vascularity in the region of the lesion and contrast enhancement of the nidus. A feeding vessel may also be identified.

The chief imaging differential diagnoses for osteoid osteoma are stress fracture and osteomyelitis. Usually, clinical presentation and laboratory results point towards the correct diagnosis. Imaging findings of osteoid osteoma tend to be specific.

The traditional treatment for osteoid osteoma has been surgical excision. Localization of the lesion and confirmation of excision may be challenging in the operating room. Recently, percutaneous methods of treatment have been developed. Percutaneous radiofrequency ablation is now the preferred method of treatment at many centers. Other percutaneous methods include excision with a large bore needle and cryoablation. Percutaneous treatment of osteoid osteoma is discussed in further detail in the interventional radiology section (Chapter 194). Complex lesions or lesions located where percutaneous methods are contraindicated may still require surgical excision. Surgical or percutaneous methods are successful in approximately 90% of patients on the initial attempt.

> Percutaneous radiofrequency ablation is now the preferred method of treatment of osteoid osteoma.

OSTEOBLASTOMA

Osteoblastomas are closely related to osteoid osteomas and have, in the past, been considered a larger version of that tumor (giant osteoid osteoma). The two lesions are nearly identical histologically. Osteoblastoma consists of numerous osteoblast-lined trabeculae containing osteoid. However, these trabeculae are less organized than those in osteoid osteoma. Size is an important consideration in distinguishing between the two types of tumors: tumors less than 1.5 cm in diameter are considered to be osteoid osteomas, whereas tumors larger than 1.5 cm are usually osteoblastomas (Fig. 176-40). The two types of tumors can also be distinguished by differences in clinical presentation, anatomic location, and imaging features.

Osteoblastoma most commonly occurs in patients in the second and third decades of life. It is more common

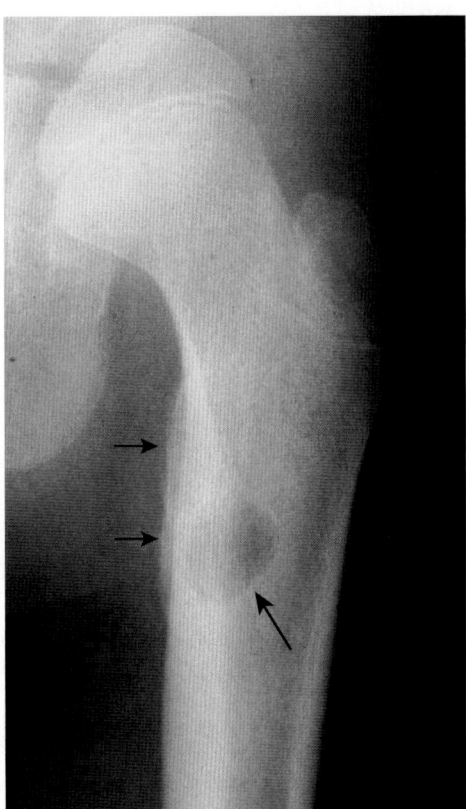

FIGURE 176-40. Osteoblastoma of the proximal femoral diaphysis in a 12-year-old boy. The lesion is lucent *(large arrow).* Smooth periosteal new bone is present medially.

in boys. Unlike osteoid osteomas, osteoblastomas are not associated with a typical pattern of pain, and if painful, do not typically respond to nonsteroidal anti-inflammatory agents. Many osteoblastomas are found in the posterior elements of the vertebrae, where they can cause scoliosis and neurologic deficits. Nearly half of these tumors occur in the appendicular skeleton, primarily in the proximal femoral diaphysis and metaphysis. Tibial lesions are next most common. Long bone lesions may be cortical or medullary in location. Another characteristic location for osteoblastoma is the neck of the talus, usually at its dorsal margin.

There are three distinct radiologic variants in the appearance of osteoblastoma: (1) an osteoid osteoma–like appearance, but larger; (2) and ABC-like appearance, most common in the spine; and, (3) an aggressive, malignant-like appearance. Aggressive-appearing osteoblastomas are uncommon.

Osteoblastomas vary from 1 to 10 cm in size. Most osteoblastomas are lytic with a well-defined sclerotic margin, but the tumor usually lacks the wide, dense rim of sclerosis that is typical of osteoid osteoma. Lesions in the spine are often expansile (Fig. 176-41). Adjacent sclerosis with spinal lesions may be minimal or absent. In the long bones, osteoblastomas appear radiologically as round or oval lucent tumors eccentric within the medulla or within cortex (see Fig. 176-40). Some sclerosis is seen adjacent to the lesion. Mineralization of the matrix is frequently present. Periosteal reaction is common and is solid or layered. Talar lesions may expand into the soft

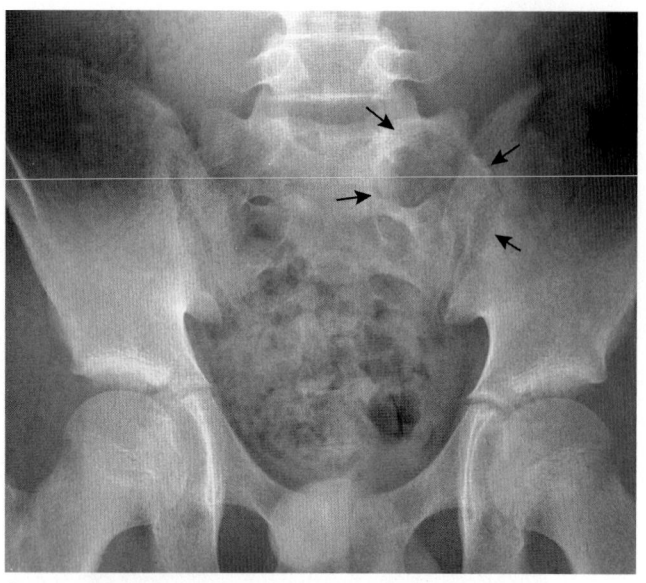
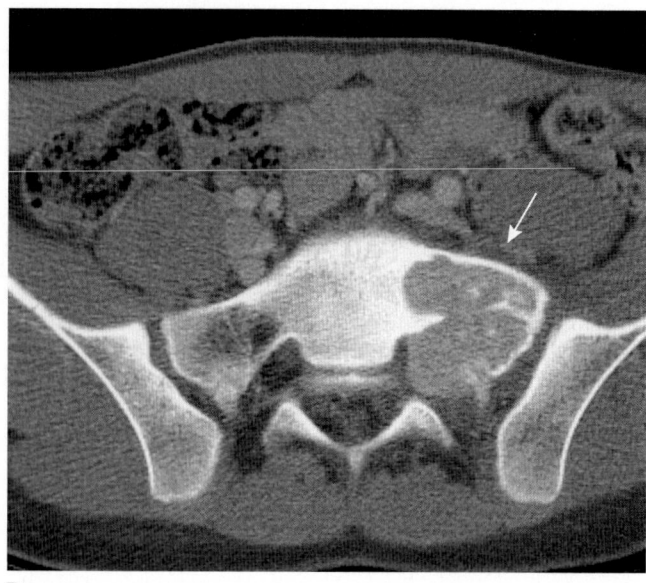

A   B

FIGURE 176-41. Osteoblastoma of the sacrum in a 12-year-old boy. A well-defined, lucent, expansile lesion *(arrows)* is seen within the left sacrum on radiography **(A)** and computed tomography **(B)**.

TABLE 176-8		
Differentiating Features of Osteosarcoma and Ewing Sarcoma		
Feature	**Osteosarcoma**	**Ewing Sarcoma**
Age range	15–25 years	0–25 years
Incidence	More common	Less common
		Rare in nonwhites
Location	Metaphyses of long bones	Metadiaphysis of long bones
		Axial, flat bone involvement more common than osteosarcoma
Matrix	Usually "cloud-like" mineralization	Not mineralized or sclerotic
Periosteal reaction	"Sunburst"	"Onion-skin"
	Codman triangles	
Metastases	Lung (80%)	Lung, rarely bone, marrow, lymph nodes
	Bone (20%)	
Other	Occasional multifocal disease	11:22 translocation
	Association with retinoblastoma	Radiation sensitive

tissues, and osteoporosis of the talus and other bones of the foot may be an associated finding.

The calcified or ossified matrix of an osteoblastoma and the tumor's thin, bony outer shell are especially well seen on CT images. Edema in the soft tissues or marrow may give high signal on T2 MR, but the signal characteristics of the lesion are not specific. Osteoid within the lesion may cause areas of decreased signal within the lesion. Bone scans may help in determining the location of a lesion. Osteoblastomas are relatively vascular, hence angiography may reveal a dense capillary blush.

Treatment of osteoblastoma is by surgical excision or curettage, but there is a moderate recurrence rate after those procedures.

MALIGNANT BONE TUMORS

Approximately 50% of all bone tumors in the pediatric age group are malignant; nearly two thirds of these are osteosarcomas. Ewing sarcomas of bone comprise most of the remainder, with 2.9 cases/million diagnosed in patients less than 20 years of age. Other types of osseous malignancies, such as chondrosarcoma, are extremely rare in children, although non-Hodgkin's lymphoma occasionally presents as a primary bone neoplasm.

Osteosarcoma and Ewing sarcoma differ sufficiently both in their clinical and imaging presentation such that they can usually be distinguished from one another. Their characteristic features, to be discussed in this chapter, are summarized in Table 176-8.

> **Osteosarcoma is the most common pediatric malignant bone tumor followed by Ewing sarcoma.**

Osteosarcoma

Osteosarcoma is the most common malignant primary bone tumor in pediatrics. The peak incidence of osteosarcoma is in patients 15 to 25 years of age, but the youngest patient described to date with osteosarcoma was a 19-month-old girl. The tumors are slightly more common in males.

Most osteosarcomas are single, primary neoplasms that arise from the medullary cavity of the metaphyses of the long bones. The diaphyses alone are less commonly involved, occurring in 2% to 11% of cases, and epiphyseal origin of osteosarcoma is extremely rare. Often referred to as conventional osteosarcomas, most are considered to be high grade because of their degree of cellular atypia and anaplasia. Other much less common categories of this tumor include well-differentiated medullary osteosarcoma, telangiectatic osteosarcoma, and surface osteosarcomas, including intracortical osteosarcoma and parosteal, periosteal, and high-grade surface osteosarcomas. Secondary osteosarcomas, which are rare in children, are usually associated with previous radiation therapy. Osteosarcoma can also arise in patients with inherited (usually bilateral) retinoblastoma who have a defect in the RB gene or in patients in whom there has been a spontaneous mutation of the gene. Although radiation therapy increases the incidence of osteosarcoma in these patients, secondary osteosarcoma may develop in sites remote from radiation fields. Osteosarcoma unassociated with other malignancies is occasionally familial and has been identified in siblings.

The long bones are affected in approximately 70% of cases; more than half of osteosarcomas are distributed about the bones of the knee. The face, mandible, cranium, and axial skeleton are among the less commonly affected sites (Fig. 176-42). Osteosarcomas can involve multiple skeletal sites synchronously; this condition is known as osteosarcomatosis. Extremely rare in children, extraskeletal osteosarcomas are found in various organs or the soft tissues of the extremities of adults. Osteosarcomas are not radiosensitive. Thus, treatment consists of preoperative chemotherapy, extirpation of resectable lesions usually by limb-sparing surgery, and postoperative chemotherapy. Prognosis is influenced by response to initial chemotherapy, which is evaluated postoperatively by histologic estimation of necrosis within the treated tumor. Little change in tumor size is expected even in tumors that respond well to chemotherapy. Imaging methods of assessing the effects of therapy include thallium-201 scintigraphy and dynamic contrast-enhanced MRI. Although PET/PET-CT appears to be useful in both staging and monitoring response, experience is currently limited in its use for osteosarcoma and other bone tumors.

Long-term follow-up of osteosarcoma and other malignant bone tumors in children is essential and extends over many months. A sample imaging protocol for osteosarcoma is shown in Table 176-9.

Intramedullary Osteosarcoma

CONVENTIONAL OSTEOSARCOMA

Approximately 75% of osteosarcomas are the high-grade variant, with 75% of cases occurring in patients between the ages of 15 and 25 years. The histologic hallmark of osteosarcoma is the presence of an osteoid matrix produced by sarcoma cells. In most cases, there is extensive immature bone formation. However, other tissues may predominate in the tumor matrix. The three main types of osteosarcoma, based on matrix type, are osteoblastic, chondroblastic, and fibroblastic. These tumors have differing mineral content.

Radiography remains the primary method of diagnosis. Other imaging methods are used mainly for staging purposes and to help the surgeon plan an en bloc resection of the tumor. Osteosarcoma typically presents as a large, mixed sclerotic–lytic mass with a "cloud-like" matrix involving the long-bone metaphyses. The tumors

TABLE 176-9			
Timeline for Imaging Evaluation of Patients with Osteosarcoma at St. Jude Children's Research Hospital			
Time	**Treatment**	**Evaluations**	**Imaging Methods***
Week 1	Begin preoperative chemotherapy	Diagnosis and pretreatment	Primary tumor: XR, MRI, BS Metastases: CXR, Chest CT, BS
Week 9	Continue chemotherapy	Interim response	Primary tumor: XR, MRI, BS Metastases: Chest CT
Week 12	Surgical resection	Preoperative response	Primary tumor: XR, MRI, BS Metastases: Chest CT, BS
Week 14	Begin postoperative chemotherapy	Postoperative monitoring	CXR: every 2 mo Chest CT at weeks 23 and 32
Week 38	End chemotherapy	Off therapy	XR primary site, CXR, Chest CT, BS
Week 38–month 86	Off therapy	Long-term follow-up	XR primary site every 2 mo for 12 mo then every 6 mo for 36 mo then once per year CXR every 4 mo for 12 mo then every 3 mo for 12 mo then every 4 mo for 12 mo then every 6 mo for 12 mo Chest CT every 4 mo for 12 mo, BS every 6 mo for 12 mo

BS, Technetium-99m MDP scintigram; CT, computed tomography; CXR, chest radiograph; MRI, magnetic resonance imaging; XR, radiograph.
*Notes: MRI includes dynamic contrast-enhanced study (DEMRI). Bone scintigraphy is single phase (skeletal equilibrium).

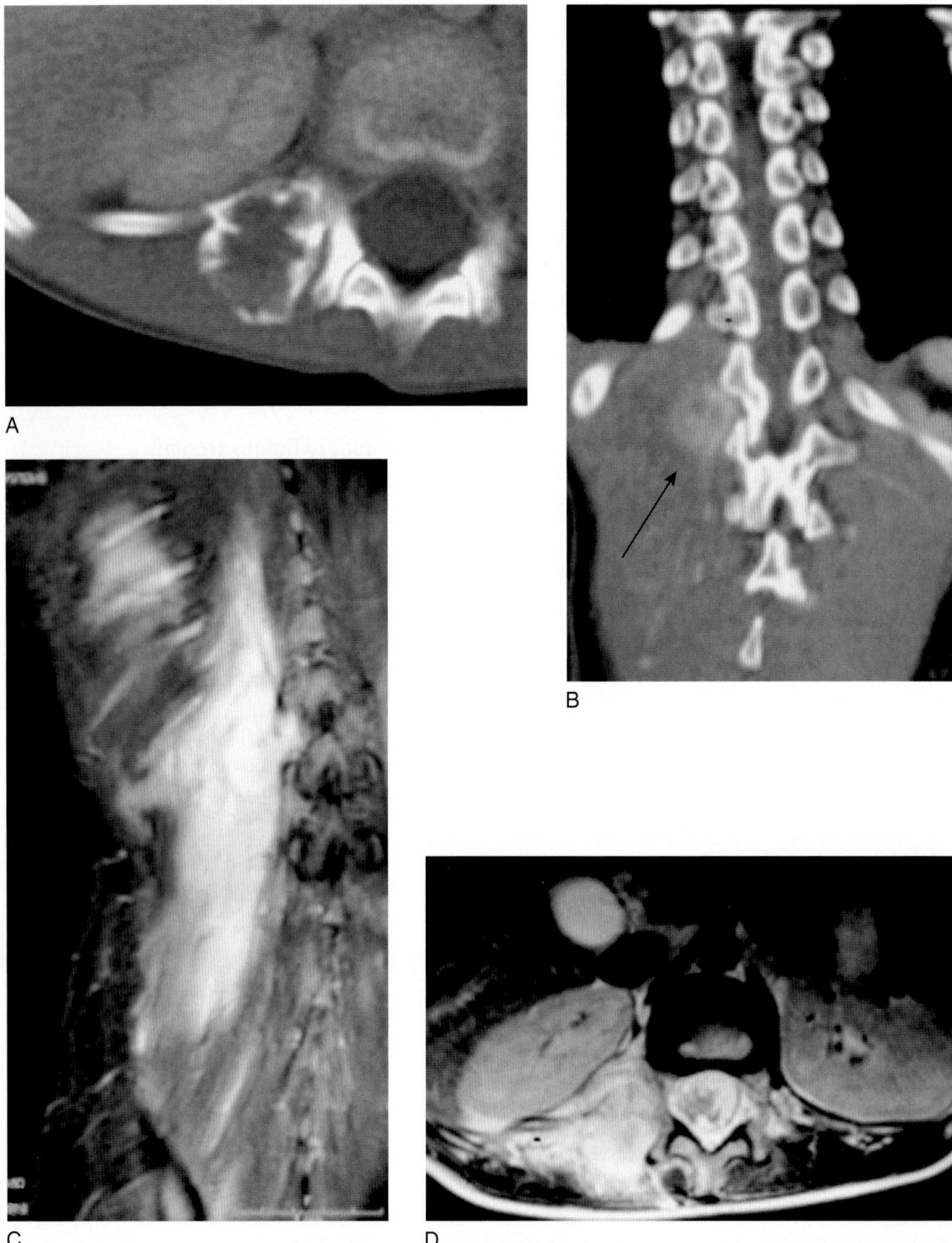

A

B

C

D

FIGURE 176-42. Osteosarcoma of the spine in an 8-year-old girl. **A,** Axial contrast-enhanced computer tomography image through T12 after 10 weeks of chemotherapy shows a peripherally sclerotic expansile mass arising from the right costovertebral junction. Note disruption of the cortex posteriorly. **B,** Coronal reconstruction shows the relationship of the mass *(arrow)* to the apex of the scoliosis. **C,** A coronal short tau inversion recovery image demonstrates the massive edema in the paraspinal muscles in response to the osteosarcoma. **D,** Axial contrast-enhanced T1-weighted magnetic resonance image with fat saturation demonstrated intense tumor enhancement and moderate enhancement of the surrounding paraspinous musculature.

cause cortical erosion and destruction rather than expansion. Resultant periosteal new bone formation, often of the spiculated "sunburst" variety, and periosteal elevation are often observed, frequently with Codman triangles (Fig. 176-43). However, occasionally conventional osteosarcomas are purely lytic and exhibit no periosteal reaction.

CT images illustrate the same features in a cross-sectional plane. Although CT is the most sensitive method for detecting subtle mineralization of the osteoid matrix; its use has been largely replaced by MR for staging, surgical planning and assessment of therapeutic response. In contrast to the normal low attenuation fatty marrow, abnormally high marrow attenuation caused by the tumor is observed on CT images (see Fig. 176-43).

MRI is used extensively to evaluate osteosarcoma. The longitudinal extent of marrow involvement, an important determinant of surgical therapy, is accurately shown as well-defined hypointense signals on T1-weighted images obtained in either coronal or sagittal planes. Normal yellow marrow is hyperintense. It is important to obtain a longitudinal T1-weighted image of the entire bone to measure intramedullary tumor length (see Fig. 176-43) to assess possible epiphyseal involvement, which can occur in as many as 80% of metaphyseal tumors, and to detect skip metastases that occur in a small percentage of cases (see Fig. 176-45 below).

On T2-weighted images, the tumor-containing marrow can be either hyperintense or, if there is sufficient bone formation, hypointense to normal fat. The soft tissue component is usually of heterogeneous, mainly high-intensity signals that contrast greatly with those of the surrounding muscles (see Fig. 176-43). Short tau inversion recovery images are very sensitive to the water content of tumors, thus markedly increasing the conspicuity of most osteosarcomas. The intramedullary length of tumor extension may be overestimated on short tau inversion recovery sequences. Contrast-enhanced T1-weighted images, preferably obtained with fat saturation, provide similar contrast and better signal-to-noise ratios than T2-weighted images. Furthermore, contrast-enhanced T1-weighted images are especially useful in determining the relationship between the tumor and the major blood vessels, in detecting joint involvement in the presence of effusion, and in estimating the amount of necrosis within the tumor (see Fig. 176-43). Osteosarcoma is frequently accompanied by edema of the adjacent soft tissues that is hyperintense to muscle on T2-weighted, short tau inversion recovery images, and contrast-enhanced T1-weighted images. This edema can be localized to the tumor periphery (paratumoral or peritumoral) or can involve whole muscle groups, as in the case of larger tumors (see Fig. 176-43). The latter finding has been associated with a poor prognosis as reported by Hanna and colleagues.

Between 10% and 20% of patients with osteosarcoma have metastases at the time of diagnosis, mainly to the lungs. Therefore, chest CT is essential in the search for pulmonary lesions at presentation. Like the primary tumor, these metastases can be calcified and, therefore, difficult to distinguish from calcified granulomas (Fig. 176-44). Pleural-based lung metastases can also produce a pneumothorax, hemothorax, or malignant pleural effusion. Such a finding may be the first sign of pulmonary metastases at the time of diagnosis or at follow-up. Bone metastases are much less frequent, but radionuclide bone scans are justified to detect these lesions and to assess the extent of the primary tumor (see Fig. 176-53). Preliminary experience, although limited, suggests that PET/PET-CT will be useful for staging. Skip metastases, which can occur in the same bone as the primary tumor or can be transarticular in location, may also be detected (Fig. 176-45). Bone scintigraphy and chest CT should also be performed periodically after treatment with chemotherapy and surgery, especially within the two years following therapy. Eighty percent of relapses occur in the lung only, and 20% in the skeleton. Local or distant lymph node involvement is extremely rare.

> **Between 10% and 20% of patients with osteosarcoma will have metastases at the time of diagnosis, mainly to the lungs. CT of the chest is therefore necessary in staging of osteosarcoma.**

TELANGIECTATIC OSTEOSARCOMA

Telangiectatic osteosarcoma is now considered to be a specific type of osteosarcoma, comprising about 2% of all osteosarcomas. Like conventional osteosarcomas, telangiectatic osteosarcoma tends to occur in the long bones adjacent to the knee and is seen more frequently in boys than in girls. These tumors contain little osteoid and do not form bone but are composed of single or multiple cavities containing blood or necrotic tumor with septa of anaplastic cells. Radiographically, they appear as lytic rather than sclerotic lesions, often having a nonaggressive appearance in that they tend to expand, rather than destroy, the cortex (Fig. 176-46). There is often little or no periosteal new bone formation. They may be associated with a soft tissue mass.

Except for the presence of malignant cells that are often at the periphery of the cavity, the pathologic appearance of telangiectatic osteosarcoma mimics that of an ABC. Indeed, on MRIs, the appearance of telangiectatic osteosarcoma and ABC may be identical; both may have single or multiple fluid-fluid levels produced by blood products of differing ages that are best demonstrated on T2-weighted images (Figs. 176-47 and 176-48). According to Murphey and associates, telangiectatic osteosarcomas are characterized by enhancing soft tissue in the periphery and septations of the tumor, a feature that is absent in ABCs. The prognosis of patients with telangiectatic osteosarcoma is similar to that of patients with conventional osteosarcoma.

> **Biopsy is necessary to differentiate telangiectatic osteosarcoma from an ABC.**

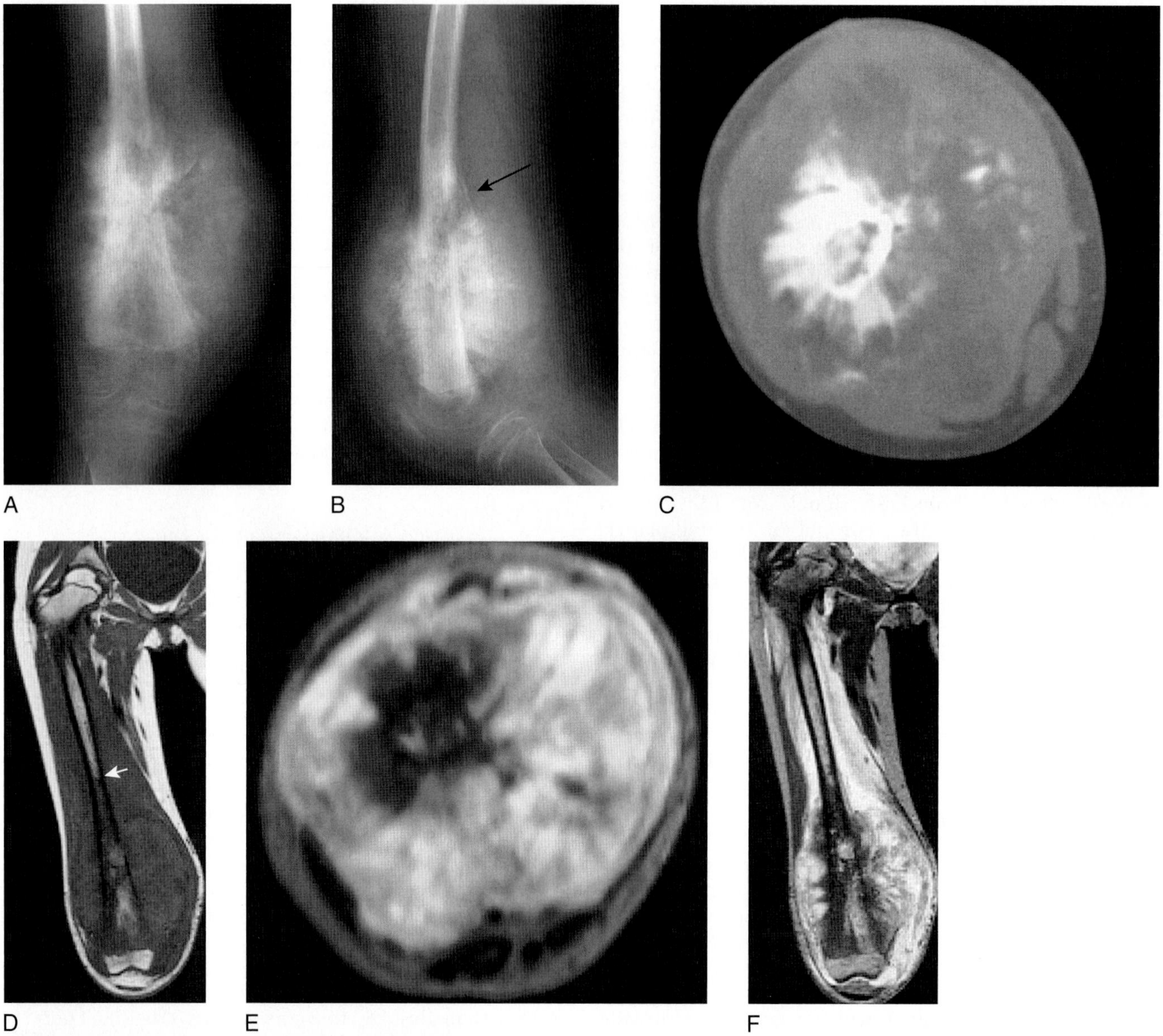

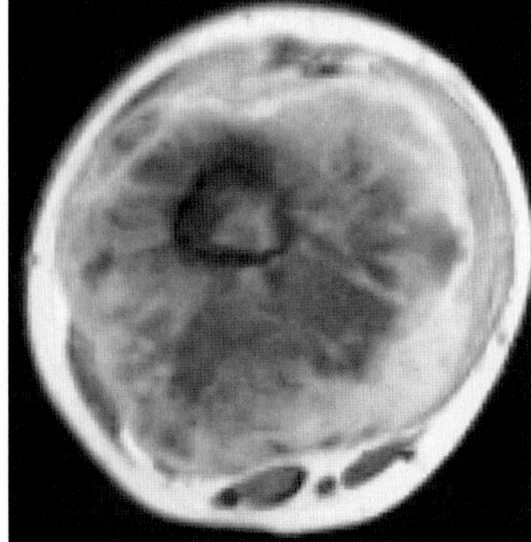

FIGURE 176-43. **A** and **B,** Radiographs of the thigh of an 11-year-old girl with osteosarcoma show a large osteoblastic tumor arising from the distal femoral diametaphysis. The epiphysis appears to be spared. "Sunburst" periosteal new bone formation and cloud-like tumor mineralization are seen in the soft tissue mass. Codman triangles are present superiorly (*arrow* in **B**). **C,** Radiating periosteal new bone and amorphous mineralization of the medulla and the soft tissue mass are demonstrated on a contrast-enhanced computed tomography. **D,** Coronal T1-weighted magnetic resonance image shows medullary involvement extending proximally to the midshaft of the femur *(arrow).* **E,** Transverse T2-weighted magnetic resonance image demonstrates a heterogeneously hyperintense soft tissue mass. Relatively little signal is seen from the medulla and radiating periosteal new bone. **F,** Coronal T2-weighted magnetic resonance image shows extensive hyperintensity of the edematous thigh muscles adjacent and proximal to the tumor. **G,** Transverse contrast-enhanced T1-weighted image shows extensive hypointensity consistent with necrosis.

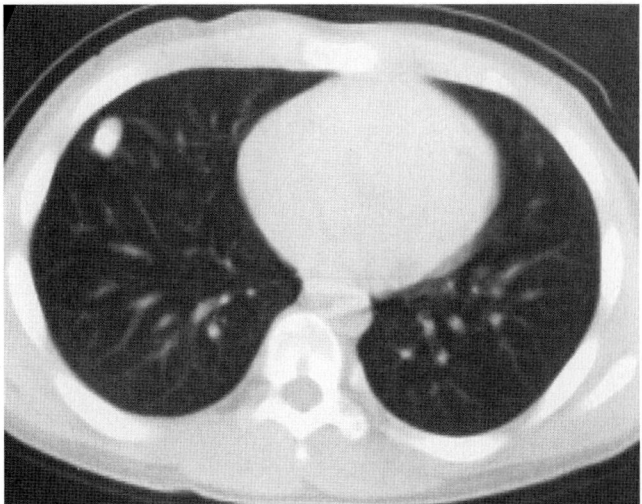

FIGURE 176-44. A computerized tomography section of the chest of a 13-year-old boy with femoral osteosarcoma shows a partially calcified metastasis in the right lung. On other computed tomography sections, several other calcified and noncalcified metastases were demonstrated in both lungs.

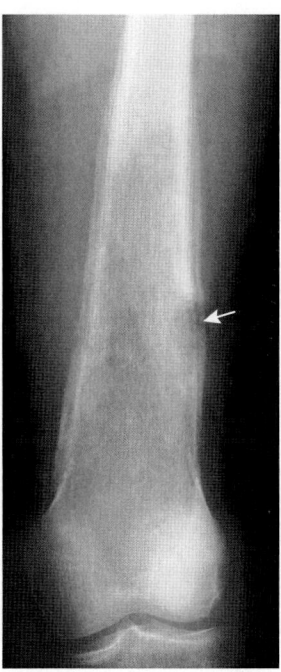

FIGURE 176-46. Radiograph of the femur of a 16-year-old boy with telangiectatic osteosarcoma shows a large lesion in the distal metadiaphysis extending into the epiphysis. The tumor is lytic rather than bone forming. There is mild periosteal reaction. There has been a recent incisional biopsy *(arrow)*.

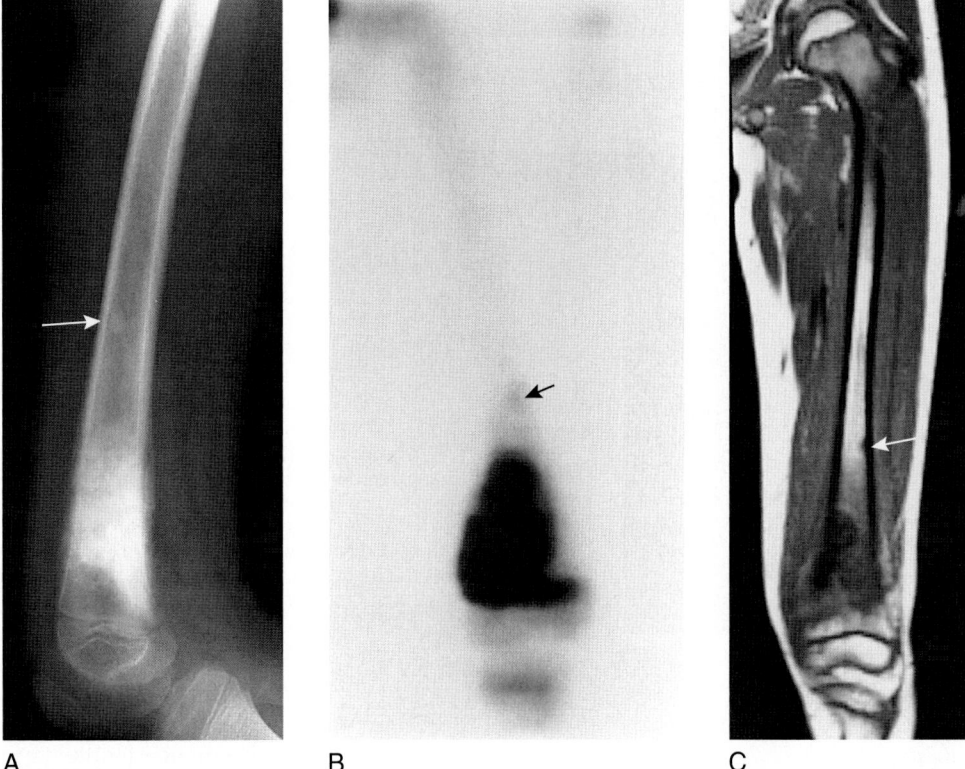

A   B   C

FIGURE 176-45. A, Lateral radiograph of the femur of a 9-year-old boy with osteosarcoma shows a sclerotic intramedullary distal femoral tumor with slight periosteal new bone formation. A small, dense skip metastasis *(arrow)* is seen proximal to the primary tumor of the main tumor mass. The skip metastasis *(arrow)* is also seen on a technetium-99m methylene diphosphonate bone scan **(B)** and is shown as a cortical-based intramedullary lesion *(arrow)* on a coronal T1-weighted magnetic resonance image **(C)**.

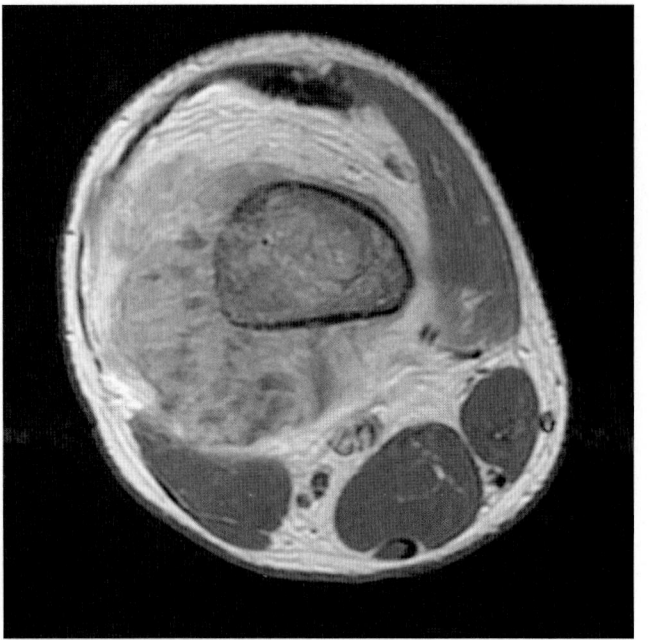

A

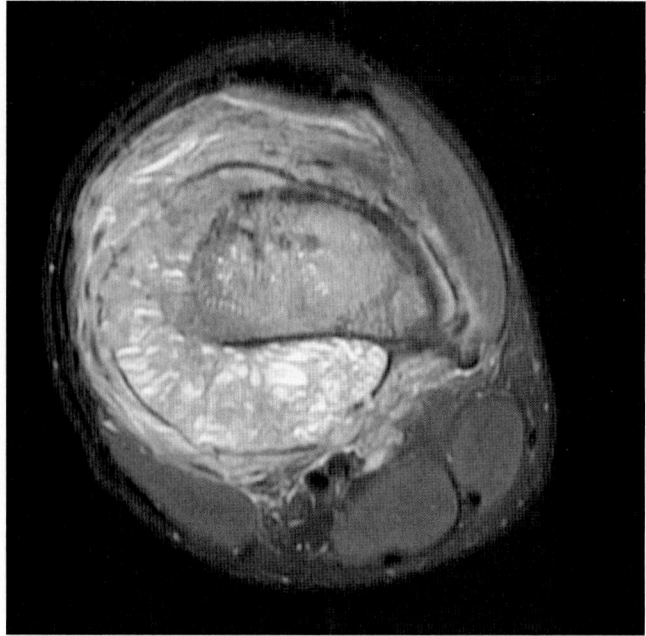

B

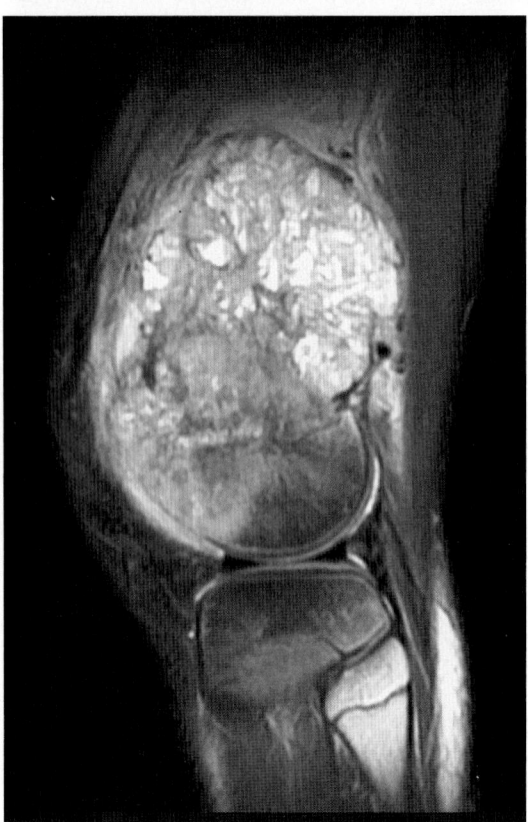

C

FIGURE 176-47. Axial noncontrast T1-weighted **(A)** and short tau inversion recovery **(B)** images through the distal femur of an adolescent boy with knee pain demonstrate a tumor containing numerous horizontally oriented fluid-fluid levels involving both the intramedullary bone and extracortical soft tissues. Note areas of discontinuous cortex from tumor breakthrough. **C,** On the sagittal short tau inversion recovery image, the fluid levels are oriented vertically. Biopsy must be performed in order to distinguish an aneurysmal bone cyst from a telangiectatic osteosarcoma.

WELL-DIFFERENTIATED MEDULLARY OSTEOSARCOMA

Unlike most medullary osteosarcomas, which display histologic features of a high-grade malignancy, this unusual variant of osteosarcoma (fewer than 2% of osteosarcoma patients in the Mayo Clinic files) is a low-grade and usually clinically indolent entity. The peak incidence is during the third decade of life, but well-differentiated medullary osteosarcoma has been found in several teenaged patients. Unlike conventional osteosarcoma, the well-differentiated variety occurs more often in females than in males. The skeletal distribution of the tumor is similar to that of conventional osteosarcoma: the most common location is the diametaphyseal region of the long bones about the knee, especially the distal femur.

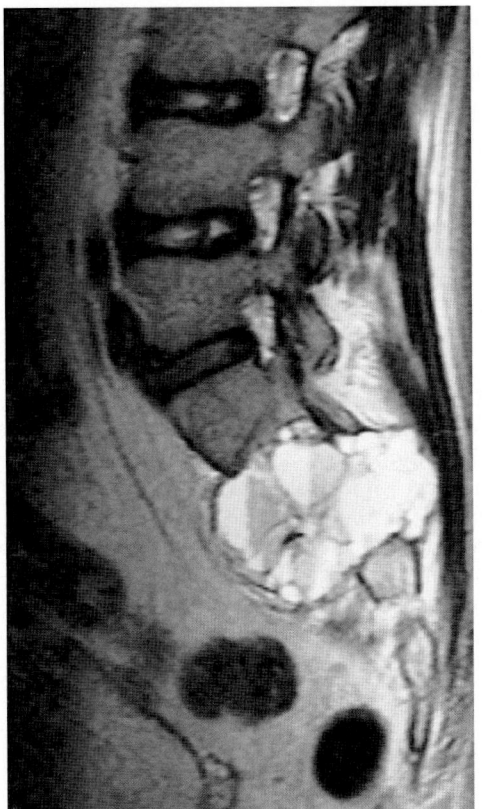

FIGURE 176-48. Sagittal T2-weighted magnetic resonance image of the sacrum of a 14-year-old girl with telangiectatic osteosarcoma shows a large, well-defined cystic lesion with fluid-fluid levels simulating an aneurysmal bone cyst.

Histologically, this tumor contains well-differentiated fibroblastic and osteoblastic components similar to those seen in parosteal osteosarcoma (see surface osteosarcomas, below). Well-differentiated medullary osteosarcoma can be mistaken for fibrous dysplasia on both pathologic and radiologic examinations. Its radiographic appearance is quite variable and ranges from that of a well-defined lesion with sclerotic margins (Fig. 176-49) to that of an expansile, poorly defined tumor with periosteal reaction and soft tissue invasion. The tumor matrix varies from dense trabecular bone to homogeneous "cloud-like" mineralization. Less often, the tumor is osteolytic. Patients with this variant of osteosarcoma have a favorable prognosis, although dedifferentiation and metastasis can occur.

INTRACORTICAL OSTEOSARCOMA

Intracortical osteosarcoma is the rarest of all osteosarcomas; only 13 cases have been reported since 1960, when the lesion was first defined histologically. It is a high-grade tumor that occurs in the diaphysis of the tibia or femur and typically may be as large as 4 cm in diameter. Radiographs show a deep or superficial cortical lucency with cortical thickening. The radiographic differential diagnosis includes osteoblastoma, osteoid osteoma, and osteomyelitis. Cross-sectional CT and MRIs reveal an expanded sclerotic cortex and no medullary involvement. However, edema of the marrow and adjacent soft tissues may be seen as high signal on T2-weighted MRI. One reported case was associated with oncogenic rickets.

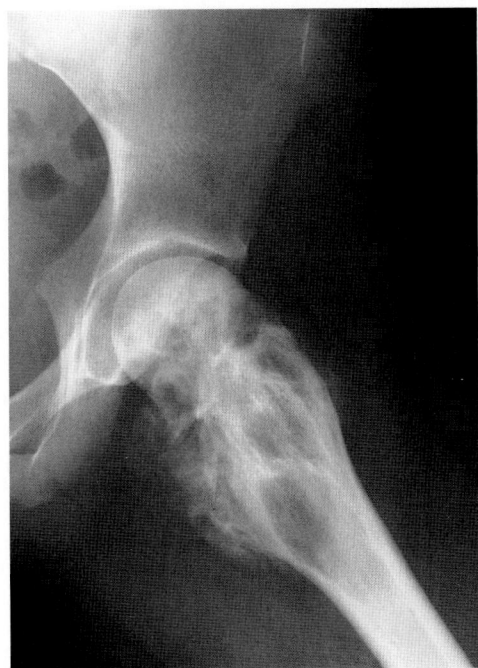
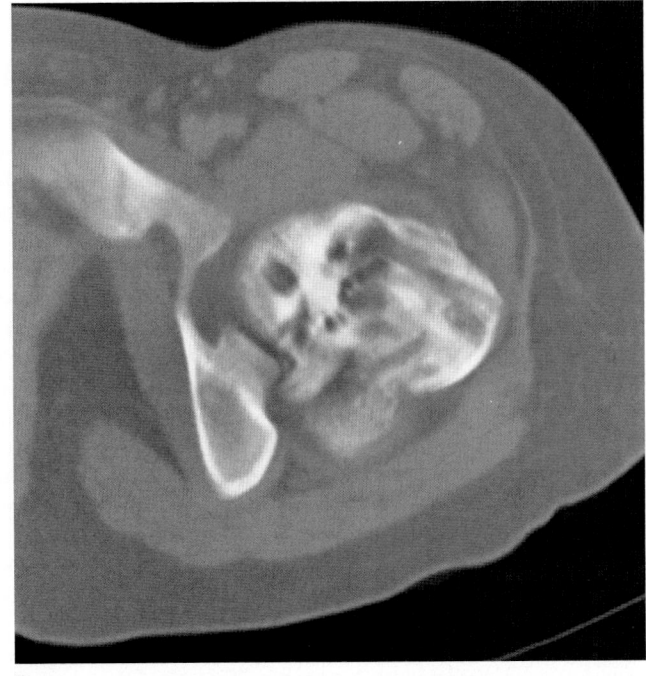

A   B

FIGURE 176-49. Radiographic **(A)** and computed tomography **(B)** images of the left hip of a 17-year-old girl show an expansile lesion of the proximal femur with osseous sclerosis. This patient had a three year history of hip pain. The resected specimen contained a mixture of low- and high-grade medullary osteosarcoma.

SURFACE OSTEOSARCOMAS

Surface osteosarcomas are classified by histologic grade as low-, intermediate-, and high-grade lesions, as reviewed by Klein and Siegal. *Parosteal osteosarcoma* is considered to be of low histologic grade and is thought to arise from the outer layer of periosteum. *Periosteal osteosarcoma* probably arises from the deep layers of periosteum or the outer cortex and is classified as an intermediate-grade osteosarcoma. The more superficial origin of parosteal osteosarcoma permits exophytic growth from the surface of the bone, usually the posterior aspect of the distal femoral metaphysis. Periosteal elevation and new bone formation are lacking. Parosteal osteosarcoma is more common in boys than in girls and tends to occur after skeletal maturity has been achieved. *High-grade surface osteosarcomas* comprise dedifferentiated parosteal osteosarcoma and high-grade surface osteosarcoma. Patients with parosteal osteosarcoma generally have an excellent prognosis, but ingrowth into the medullary cavity may adversely affect the prognosis.

Parosteal osteosarcomas are composed of extensive osteoid tissue with a fibrous stroma and form a lobulated, ossified juxtacortical mass. Early lesions may have a radiologic cleavage plane between the cortex and the tumor. As growth progresses, the mass envelops the cortex. CT and axial MR images demonstrate the superficial nature of the mass: dense ossification is seen on CT images, and diminished signal as the result of bone formation is observed on T1- and T2-weighted MRIs (Fig. 176-50). The tumor may also grow through the cortex into the medullary cavity.

The differential diagnosis includes myositis ossificans, which has a more heavily mineralized periphery than that of parosteal osteosarcoma (Chapter 172). Because parosteal osteosarcoma can also have a cartilaginous cap, it must be differentiated from osteochondroma.

The deeper origin of periosteal osteosarcoma within the cortex results in a fusiform mass with periosteal elevation and perpendicular spiculated periosteal new bone formation with Codman triangles and a scalloped cortex (Fig. 176-51). Cartilaginous differentiation causes areas of low attenuation on CT images, low signal on T1-weighted MR images, and very high signal on T2-weighted images. Hypointense rays of periosteal new bone may be seen within the mass. Medullary invasion is rare, but signal abnormalities caused by reactive changes of the marrow are common. These tumors tend to occur in the diaphysis of the tibia and femur. Patients with these tumors have a less favorable prognosis than do those with parosteal osteosarcoma. The differential features of parosteal osteosarcoma, periosteal osteosarcoma, and the benign soft tissue lesion myositis ossificans are summarized in Table 176-10.

The least common surface osteosarcoma, high-grade surface osteosarcoma, is similar in appearance to periosteal osteosarcoma, but histologically it resembles conventional intramedullary osteosarcoma (Fig. 176-52). Metastases are more common, and prognosis is consequently poorer than that associated with periosteal osteosarcoma.

MULTIFOCAL OSTEOSARCOMA

There is considerable debate as to whether simultaneously occurring osteosarcomas represent true multifocal disease or are manifestations of early metastatic spread. Some authors consider that synchronous occurrence of osteosarcomas in skeletally immature patients with symmetric skeletal involvement in the absence of a dominant mass and of early pulmonary metastases as characteristic of multifocal disease. In a review from the Armed Forces Institute of Pathology of patients with multifocal skeletal involvement, a dominant lesion was present in all patients younger than 18 years of age (Amstutz type I osteosarcomatosis); this dominant lesion almost always involved the metaphysis of the distal femur or proximal tibia. Histologic characteristics of the dominant tumors were similar to those of conventional solitary osteosarcomas. The secondary lesions were smaller, better defined, and more sclerotic, and they mainly involved the metaphyses of the long bones. Nearly 75% of the patients in this age range had pulmonary metastases that were detected by chest radiography. These investigators believed that the presence of a radiographically dominant tumor, the high incidence of pulmonary metastases, and the similar distributions of skeletal tumors and metastases indicate that this unusual presentation is due to widespread metastatic disease rather than multifocality (Fig. 176-53). In contrast to the preceding hypothesis, the association of multifocal osteosarcoma with hereditary cancer syndromes such as Rothmund-Thomson syndrome suggests that an impaired DNA repair in fibroblasts may contribute to malignant degeneration of benign cutaneous and bone lesions, as described by El-Khoury and colleagues. In any event, survival rates of pediatric patients with multiple osteosarcomas are very poor.

Ewing Sarcoma

In 1921, James Ewing described a radium-sensitive bone tumor consisting of sheets of small polyhedral cells of probable endothelial origin that he called an endothelioma. Although the origin of this undifferentiated tumor has been debated since its initial description, Ewing sarcoma has proved to be a distinct entity with characteristic histologic, radiologic, and cytogenetic features. The Ewing family of tumors includes Ewing sarcoma of bone, extraosseous Ewing sarcoma, and primitive neuroectodermal tumor (PNET), which is also known as peripheral neuroepithelioma. PNET exhibits neural differentiation and may arise from either bone or soft tissues. The Ewing family of tumors shares a distinctive cytogenetic feature: reciprocal translocation of chromosome bands q24 and q12 of chromosomes 11 and 22. This same translocation is also found in Askin tumor of the thorax (Chapter 80).

> The Ewing family of tumors includes Ewing sarcoma of bone, extraosseous Ewing sarcoma, and PNET.

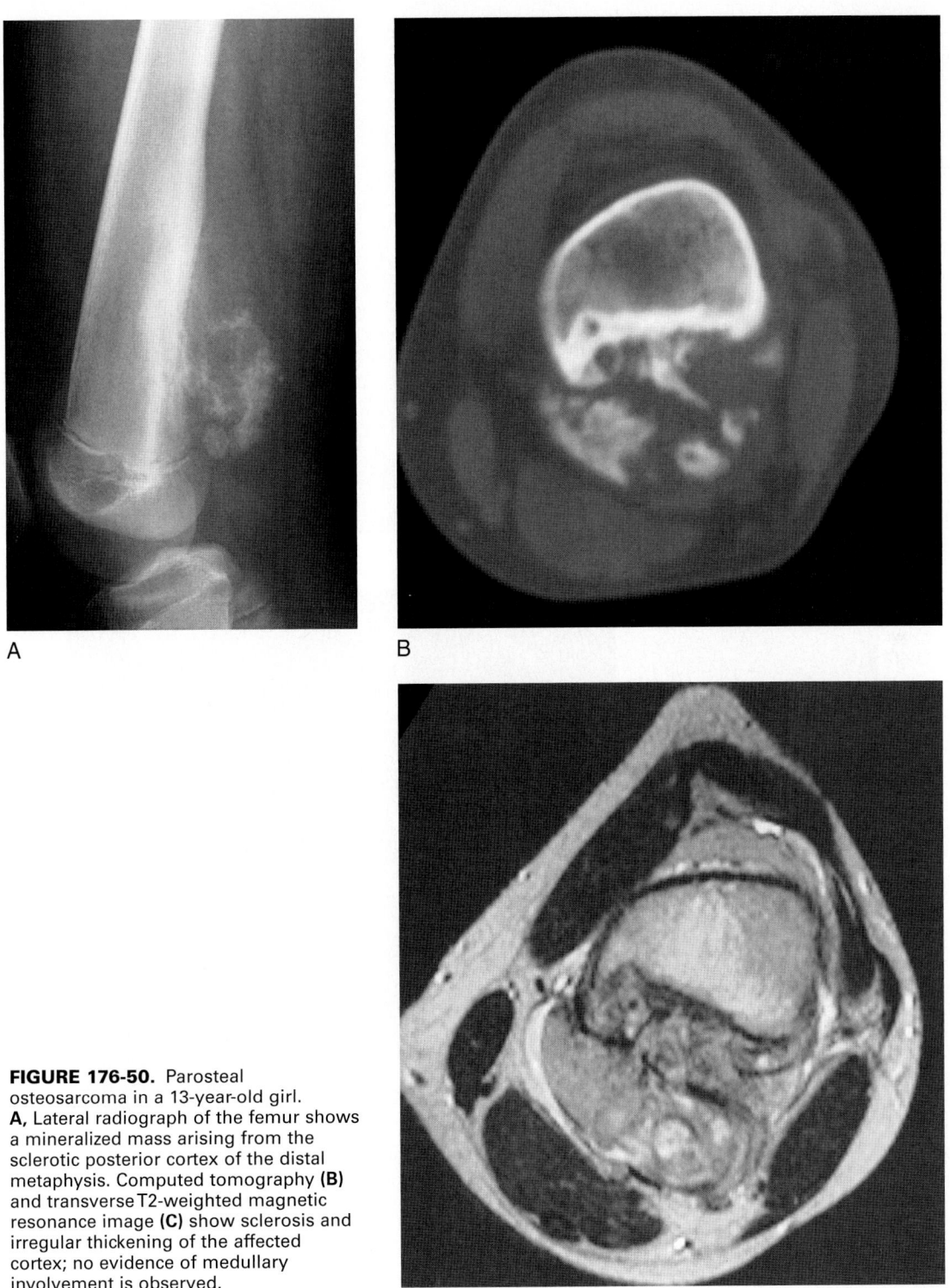

FIGURE 176-50. Parosteal osteosarcoma in a 13-year-old girl. **A,** Lateral radiograph of the femur shows a mineralized mass arising from the sclerotic posterior cortex of the distal metaphysis. Computed tomography **(B)** and transverse T2-weighted magnetic resonance image **(C)** show sclerosis and irregular thickening of the affected cortex; no evidence of medullary involvement is observed.

In younger patients, Ewing sarcoma of bone occurs less frequently than osteosarcoma; most cases are detected in patients between 10 and 25 years of age (median age, 15 years). Like osteosarcoma, Ewing sarcoma occurs more commonly in boys (55 boys: 45 girls). However, Ewing sarcoma and PNET are rarely found in black patients (six Caucasian:one African American). Fever, leukocytosis, and elevation of the erythrocyte sedimentation rate may accompany these neoplasms.

More than 50% of Ewing sarcomas involve a single long bone (Figs. 176-54 and 176-55); Ewing sarcoma involving the bones of the hands and feet, which is often initially diagnosed as an infection, is rare (Fig. 176-56). Within the long bones, the metaphysis and diaphysis are the usual locations for these types of malignancies.

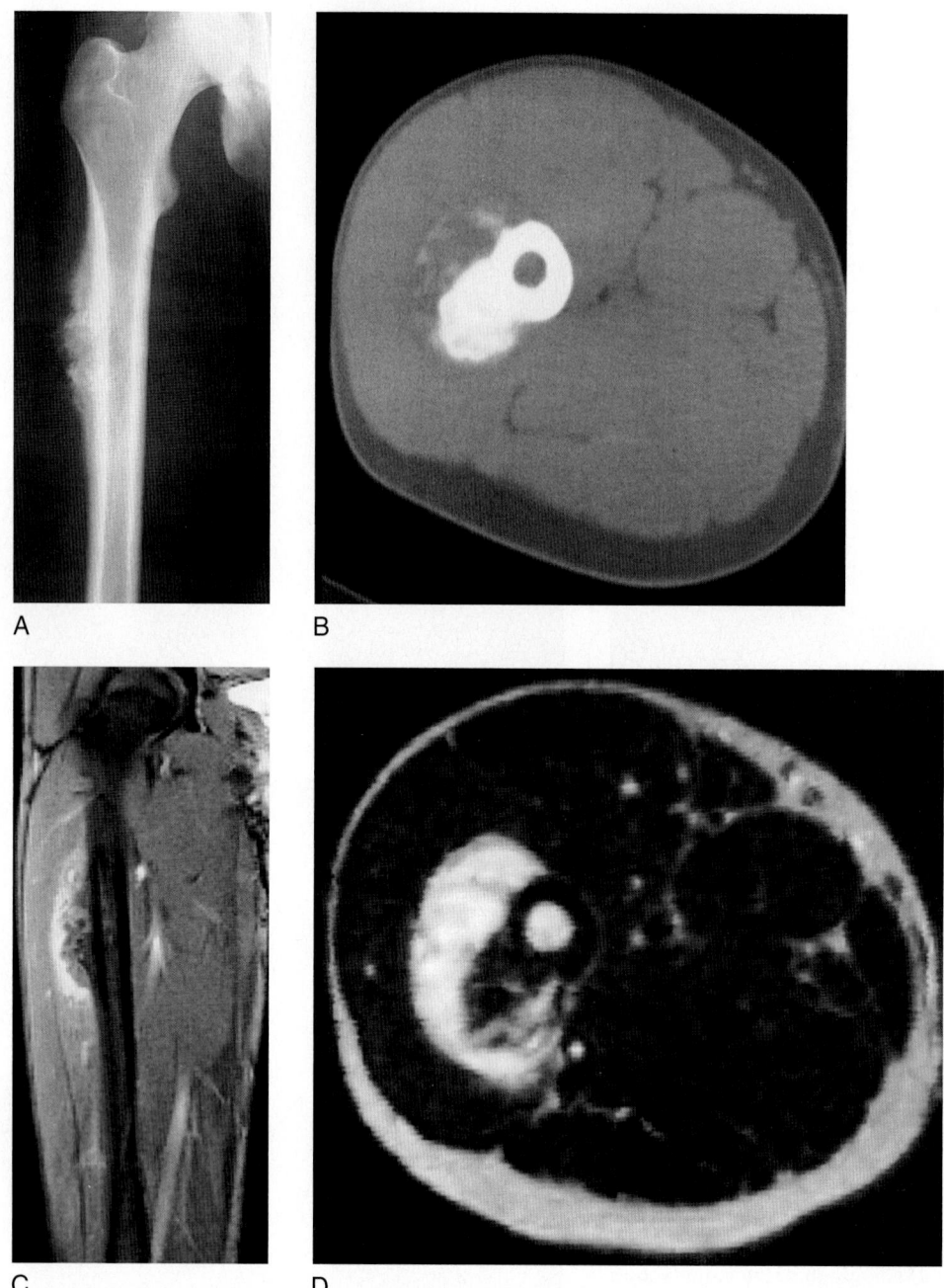

FIGURE 176-51. Periosteal osteosarcoma in a 15-year-old boy. **A,** Radiograph of the femur shows a fusiform ossified mass arising from the cortical surface of the diaphysis. Computed tomography **(B)** and contrast-enhanced coronal T1-weighted gradient-echo **(C)** and axial T2-weighted **(D)** magnetic resonance images show the close proximity of the mass to the periosteal surface of the cortex.

The flat bones, especially the ribs and pelvis, are also commonly involved. Most Ewing sarcomas appear to arise from the medullary cavity. Multifocal osseous involvement at the time of diagnosis is rare.

The typical radiographic appearance of Ewing sarcoma in the long bones is that of a permeative lesion with a lamellar "onion-skin" periosteal reaction (see Fig. 176-54). However, nearly 40% of these tumors display diffuse sclerosis, sometimes with a mixed lytic–sclerotic pattern (Fig. 176-56). The sclerosis correlates histologically with the presence of dead bone.

> The typical radiographic appearance of Ewing sarcoma in the long bones is that of a permeative lesion with a lamellar "onion-skin" periosteal reaction.

Because Ewing sarcomas do not ossify, soft tissue extension is often poorly detected by plain radiographs but is almost always apparent on contrast-enhanced CT images or on T2-weighted or contrast-enhanced T1-

TABLE 176-10

Differential Features of Myositis Ossificans, Parosteal Osteosarcoma, and Periosteal Osteosarcoma

Feature	Myositis Ossificans	Parosteal Osteosarcoma	Periosteal Osteosarcoma
Origin	Soft tissue	Outer periosteum	Deep periosteum—cortex
Common location	Thigh or arm	Metaphysis of distal femur	Diaphysis of tibia or femur
Shape	Circular	Exophytic	Fusiform
Cleavage plane	Occurs late	Occurs early	Does not occur
Periosteal reaction	Occurs frequently	Does not occur	Occurs sometimes
Cortex	Intact	Intact	Scalloped
Site of mineralization	Peripheral rim	Center of tumor	Center of tumor
Prognosis	Benign	Good	Poor

Data from Fletcher BD: Imaging pediatric bone sarcomas: diagnosis and treatment related issues. Radiol Clin N Am 1997;35:1478.

weighted MR images (see Fig. 176-54). Indeed, the soft tissue masses tend to be disproportionately large in comparison to the amount of bone destruction, and they are especially extensive in Ewing sarcoma of the pelvis (Fig. 176-56). Cortical permeation and destruction may be visible on CT or MRI. However, these tumors can permeate haversian canals and grow into the soft tissues without causing large areas of cortical loss. Extensive marrow involvement is particularly well shown as non-specific low signal, isointense to muscle on T1-weighted images. We have observed that most Ewing sarcomas found in the medullary cavity display intermediate signal that is isointense to that of fat on T2-weighted images (Fig. 176-57 and 176-58).

Rarely, Ewing sarcoma can arise from the surface of the bone rather than from the medullary cavity. In this periosteal or subperiosteal location, Ewing sarcoma resembles other surface malignancies, such as periosteal osteosarcoma with periosteal elevation and Codman triangles. The affected cortex is typically excavated or saucerized (Fig. 176-59). Cross-sectional imaging is required to exclude medullary involvement. Patients with this form of Ewing sarcoma are thought to have a relatively favorable prognosis.

With appropriate multimodality therapy, the long-term survival rate of patients with nonmetastatic medullary Ewing sarcoma approaches that of patients with osteosarcoma (about 65%). In some series, tumor volume has been shown to influence prognosis. Survival of patients with pelvic tumors may be somewhat shortened and is much reduced in patients with metastatic disease. As many as 25% of patients with Ewing sarcoma have detectable metastases at the time of diagnosis; most of these are found in the lung. Thus, chest CT is necessary for disease staging. Metastases in bone or bone marrow are less frequent. Local and regional lymph node involvement may rarely occur. Skip metastases have been reported. In addition to MRI of the primary tumor, technetium-99m methylene diphosphonate (MDP) scintigraphy, thoracic CT scanning, and bone marrow examination should be performed to detect possible disseminated disease. Early experience indicates that PET/PET-CT is useful for detection of metastatic sites of disease and monitoring therapeutic response (Fig. 176-60).

Most Ewing sarcomas respond well to initial chemotherapy: Increased bony sclerosis develops, and the soft tissue mass disappears (see Figs. 176-60 and 176-61). Percentage change in size of the soft tissue mass appears to be an important prognostic indicator. T2-weighted MRIs show an increase in intensity of the treated medullary component because of serous atrophy, with increased interstitial fluid of the yellow marrow and replacement of cytoplasmic lipid with serous material. High T2-weighted signal intensity caused by radiation-induced inflammatory reactions may also be observed in those patients treated with radiation therapy.

Chondrosarcoma

Chondrosarcomas are rare in children, but their clinical, pathologic, and radiologic features have been described in two modern series comprising a total of 126 young patients. These neoplasms may be primary or, less commonly, may be caused by previous irradiation or by malignant transformation of benign cartilaginous lesions, namely solitary or multiple osteochondromas and enchondromas (see cartilaginous tumors earlier). Several histologic types of chondrosarcoma have been described: conventional, myxoid, mesenchymal, and spindle cell. Although most chondrosarcomas have only low-grade malignant potential, up to 11% may undergo focal histologic change to a high-grade non-cartilaginous sarcoma within a low-grade chondrosarcoma. High-grade chondrosarcomas are extremely rare in children comprising two cases in a cohort of 174 cases of high-grade lesions reported by Littrell and colleagues.

Primary chondrosarcoma most frequently involves the appendicular skeleton, especially the diaphysis or metaphysis (or both) of the humerus or femur. Nearly 15% of chondrosarcomas arise in the craniofacial bones. Radiographically, these tumors are similar to chondrosarcomas of adults in that they are central lesions that grow from cancellous bone into the medulla. They are usually elongated, poorly delineated lytic lesions with variable matrix mineralization, endosteal scalloping, periosteal reaction, and soft tissue reaction (Fig. 176-62). Chondrosarcomas are capable of growing into draining veins. MRI is helpful in determining tumor extent before en bloc resection. Cartilaginous and myxoid tumor tissue is isointense to muscle on T1-weighted images and markedly hyperintense on T2-weighted images.

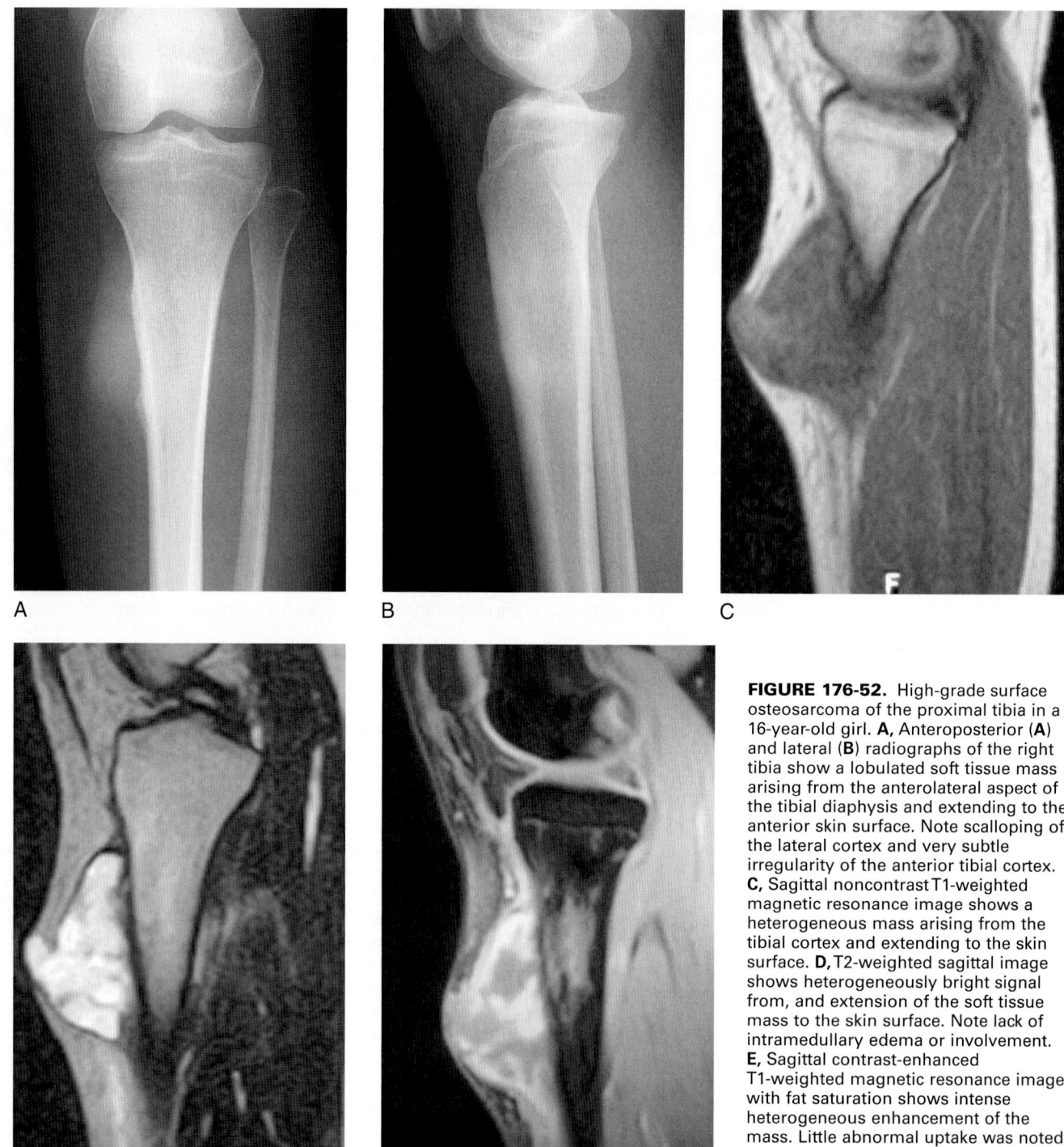

A

B

C

D

E

FIGURE 176-52. High-grade surface osteosarcoma of the proximal tibia in a 16-year-old girl. **A,** Anteroposterior (**A**) and lateral (**B**) radiographs of the right tibia show a lobulated soft tissue mass arising from the anterolateral aspect of the tibial diaphysis and extending to the anterior skin surface. Note scalloping of the lateral cortex and very subtle irregularity of the anterior tibial cortex. **C,** Sagittal noncontrast T1-weighted magnetic resonance image shows a heterogeneous mass arising from the tibial cortex and extending to the skin surface. **D,** T2-weighted sagittal image shows heterogeneously bright signal from, and extension of the soft tissue mass to the skin surface. Note lack of intramedullary edema or involvement. **E,** Sagittal contrast-enhanced T1-weighted magnetic resonance image with fat saturation shows intense heterogeneous enhancement of the mass. Little abnormal uptake was noted within this tumor site on technetium-99m methylene diphosphonate bone scan *(not shown).* Imaging cannot predict the histologic grade of surface osteosarcomas.

Secondary chondrosarcomas occur more frequently in the vertebrae than do primary tumors. In the long bones, they are most often on the periphery and may be identified by thickening of the cartilaginous cap of an osteochondroma or by the loss of the organized appearance of pre-existing benign exostotic lesions. Extraskeletal mesenchymal chondrosarcomas have also been identified in children.

Primary Osseous Lymphoma

Although secondary bone involvement in patients with non-Hodgkin lymphoma is common, primary skeletal lymphoma (formerly called reticulum cell sarcoma) is rare. In adults, non-Hodgkin lymphoma comprises 5% or fewer of all malignant bone tumors. Lymphoma can be primary in any part of the skeleton but occurs most

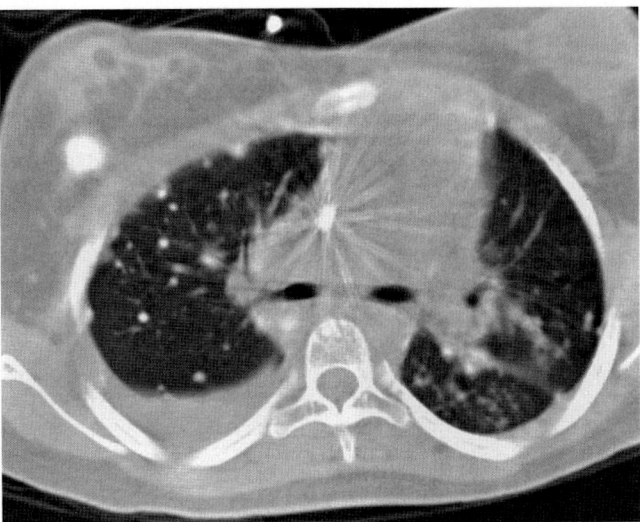

A

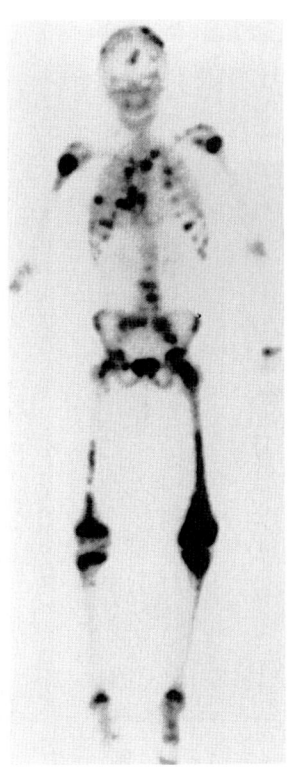

B

FIGURE 176-53. **A,** Computed tomography scan of a 9-year-old girl with osteosarcoma shows multiple calcified pulmonary metastases, a right pleural effusion, and a calcified metastasis in the right anterior chest wall. **B,** Anterior technetium-99m methylene diphosphonate bone scan shows multiple foci of abnormally increased radiotracer uptake in the soft tissues and bones. The primary tumor arose from the distal metaphysis of the left femur. This patient also had rare involvement of lymph nodes.

commonly in the lower extremities. Cases of multifocal bone lymphoma have been reported.

Both technetium-99m MDP bone scintigrams and gallium-67 scans are capable of detecting skeletal involvement. Nodal and extranodal spread from the primary lesion can occur. The image of the primary bone tumor is often subtle on radiographs: It can be either sclerotic or lytic or can display a mixture of these two features (Fig. 176-63). Periosteal reaction may be minimal or absent. Findings may mimic a primary bone malignancy.

MRI, an important method of evaluating osseous non-Hodgkin lymphoma, often unexpectedly reveals extensive bone marrow involvement. Frequently, soft tissue extension is disproportionately extensive as compared with the relatively small amount of cortical destruction. The MRI signal of lymphoma is nonspecific, heterogeneous, and somewhat variable. T1-weighted signal intensity ranges from isointense to hypointense to muscle, and T2-weighted intensities can be hypointense, isointense, or hyperintense to fat. Intermixed bone marrow fibrosis may contribute to the heterogeneity of MR signal characteristics.

Disseminated Skeletal Malignancy

The skeleton is a frequent site of leukemia, non-Hodgkin lymphoma, and Hodgkin disease in pediatric patients.

Radiographic manifestations of leukemia are discussed in Chapter 178. MR imaging manifestations of leukemia are discussed in Chapter 177. Occasionally, leukemia may produce a focal, destructive bone lesion mimicking a primary bone malignancy. Granulocytic sarcoma, also known as chloroma, is a localized collection of granulocyte precursors that affects many tissues of patients with myelogenous leukemia. Less than 10% of chloromas involve bone (Fig. 176-64). Found most frequently in the skull, spine, ribs, and sternum, chloromas cause localized expansion of bone with irregular margins. They are isointense to muscle and marrow on T1- and T2-weighted MR images and enhance homogeneously.

Many solid tumors that metastasize to bone or bone marrow are detected radiographically. Neuroblastoma is the most common source of metastatic bone disease and is the most common cause of an aggressive-appearing metaphyseal lesion in a young child (Fig. 176-65). Neuroblastoma metastases are usually osteolytic and may produce a submetaphyseal lucency resembling leukemia or a more permeative pattern (Fig. 176-66). Vertebral collapse from neuroblastoma metastases is common, and calvarial metastases appear as numerous small punctate areas of lucency. Osseous metastases from other primary lesions besides neuroblastoma in children are relatively rare. Metastases from medulloblastoma, osteosarcoma, and retinoblastoma are often blastic.

Technetium-99m MDP bone scintigraphy is an effective way of detecting skeletal metastases, but for patients with neuroblastoma, the results may be either false positive or false negative. Thus, radiographic skeletal surveys may also be performed. Iodine-131 or Iodine-123 metaiodobenzylguanidine (MIBG) scintigraphy is a useful adjunct to bone scintigrams and skeletal surveys because it further characterizes the extent of skeletal involvement resulting from neuroblastoma (see Figs. 176-65 and 176-67). Although there has thus far been little experience with ^{18}F-FDG PET/PET-CT staging

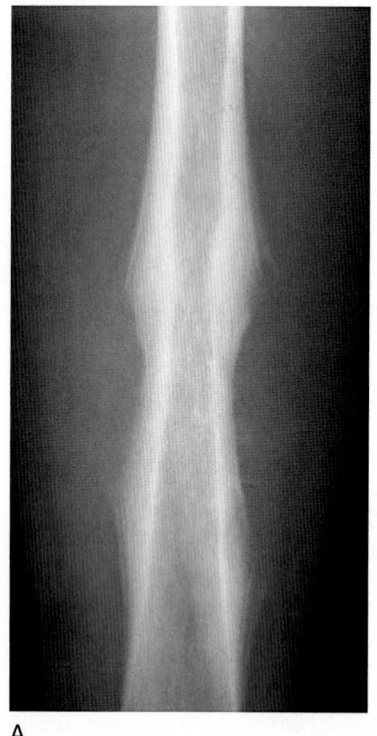

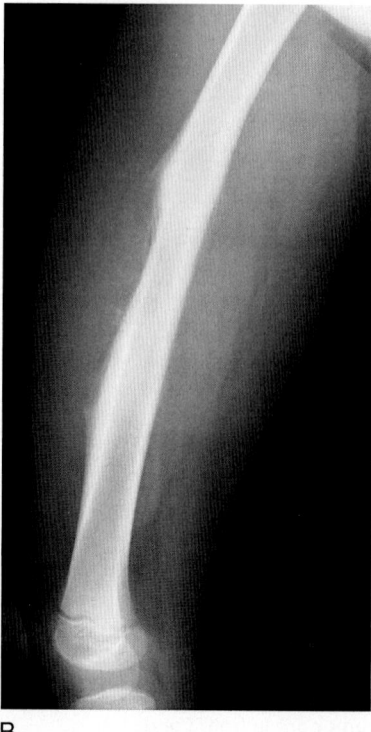

FIGURE 176-54. Anteroposterior **(A)** and lateral **(B)** radiographs of the femur of a 6-year-old girl show a Ewing sarcoma arising from the mid-diaphysis. There is lamellar periosteal reaction and new bone formation, with Codman triangles at the proximal and distal ends of the tumor. Faint periosteal new bone extends perpendicularly into the soft tissue component of the tumor. The medulla is not expanded. Contrast-enhanced computed tomography **(C)** and T2-weighted magnetic resonance image **(D)** show a large soft tissue mass.

A

B

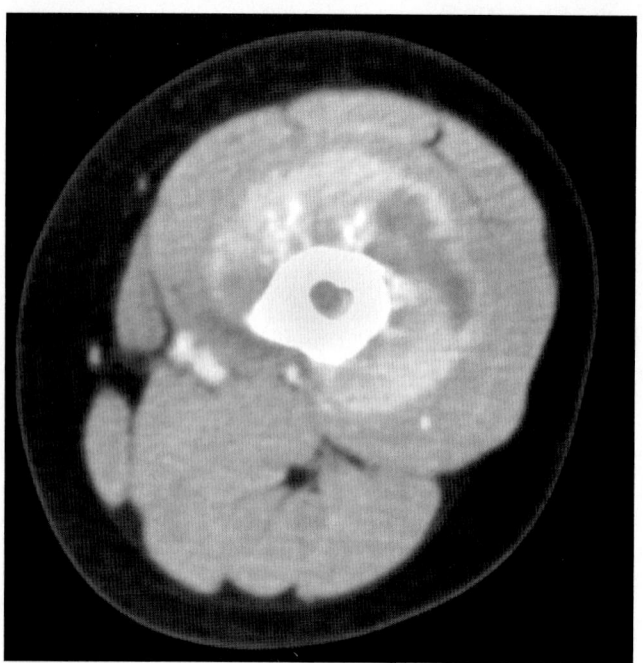

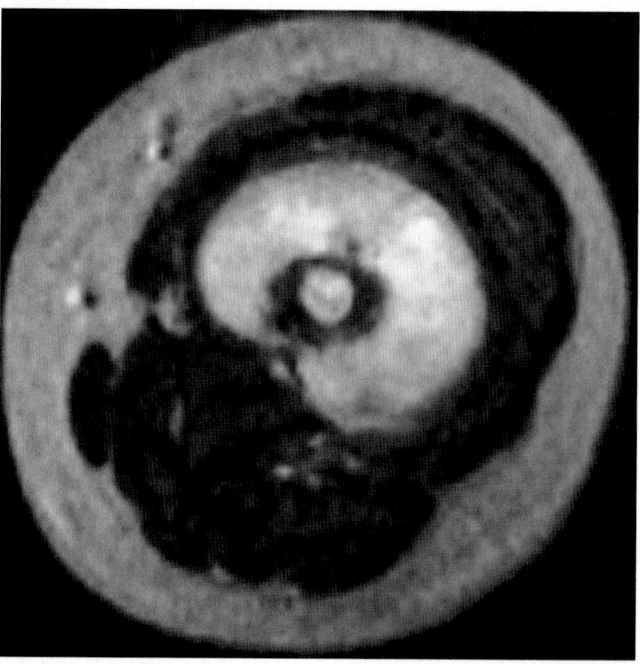

C

D

of disseminated solid tumors, preliminary experience suggests that this method may prove to be useful for staging of neuroblastoma. Recent development of faster MRI techniques has led to investigations of the use of whole-body MRI to detect bone marrow metastases that may be applicable to pediatric patients. In studies of neuroblastoma, MRIs have shown diffuse or multifocal nodular bone marrow signal abnormalities in the spine, pelvis, and proximal long bones (see Fig. 176-66). Cortical bone metastases are almost always accompanied

by marrow disease. In some cases, reactive changes with high T2-weighted signal intensities are demonstrated in adjacent soft tissues (Fig. 176-68).

> **Imaging modalities for detecting diffuse skeletal involvement by tumor include skeletal surveys, bone scan, ^{123}I MIBG, whole-body MRI, and ^{18}F-FDG PET/PET-CT.**

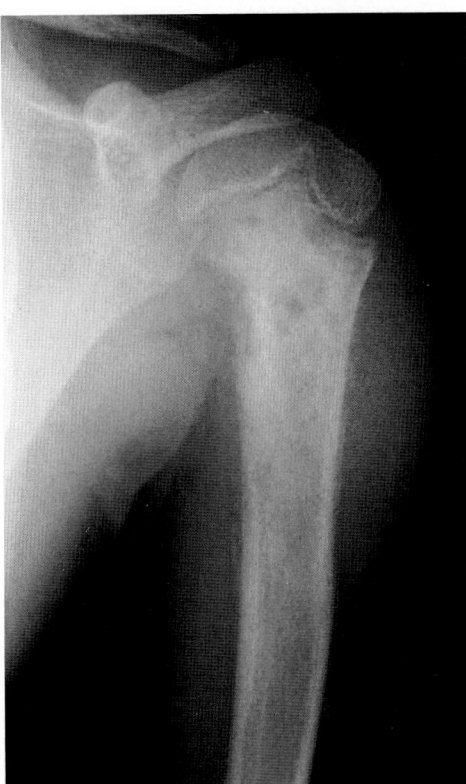

FIGURE 176-55. Ewing sarcoma of the proximal humerus of a 5-year-old boy. The tumor is predominantly sclerotic with "moth-eaten" permeation. Little periosteal reaction is apparent.

SURGICAL MANAGEMENT OF BONE TUMORS

Benign bone tumors can be classified as either latent, active, or aggressive. Frequently benign, latent tumors can simply be observed without the need for surgical intervention. Active lesions are those that are symptomatic and but have caused only minimal bone destruction. Aggressive tumors have, by definition, violated the cortex and have extended into the surrounding soft tissues; they often have a soft tissue component as well. Active and aggressive lesions require extensive surgery. Active lesions and some aggressive ones are managed surgically with curettage and bone grafting alone. A high-speed burr can be used to remove gross and microscopic tumor from within the cavity of the tumor itself, resulting in an intralesional margin. This procedure is usually sufficient for local control of either active or aggressive benign lesions. More aggressive lesions, especially those with a higher risk of local recurrence are treated with an extended curettage. An adjuvant agent such as phenol, liquid nitrogen, or polymethylmethacrylate (bone cement) may be used to "extend" the curettage along with the high speed burr, and reduce local recurrence. Bone cement or bone graft may then be used to fill the defect.

Malignant bone tumors spread by direct local extension into the surrounding bone and soft tissue and thus, require an even more aggressive approach. The local extent of micrometastatic spread is impossible to determine with imaging or intraoperatively. Therefore, a

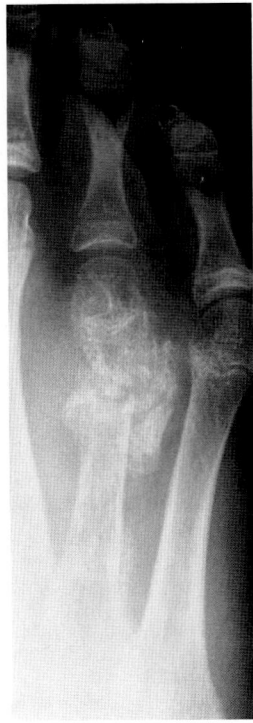

A

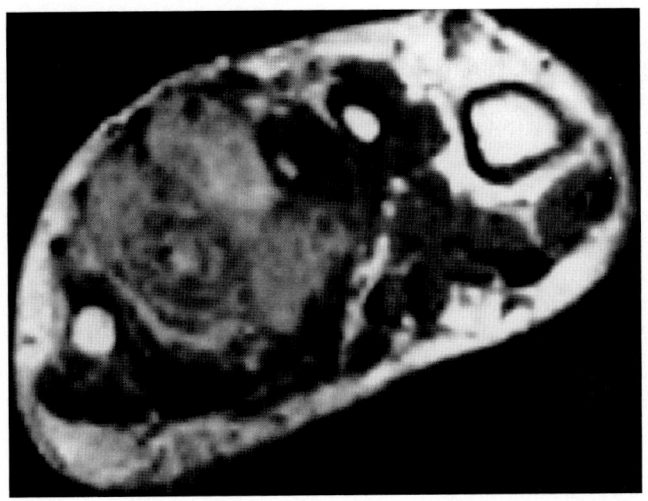

B

FIGURE 176-56. A 13-year-old boy with Ewing sarcoma of the foot. **A,** Anteroposterior radiograph shows a destructive lesion of the fourth metatarsal with a pathologic fracture. **B,** Transverse T2-weighted magnetic resonance image shows a large soft tissue mass.

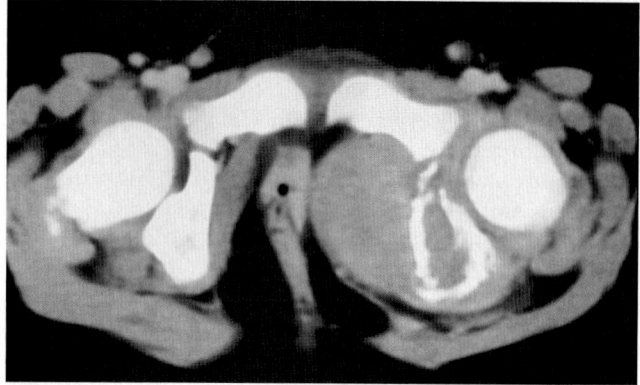

A

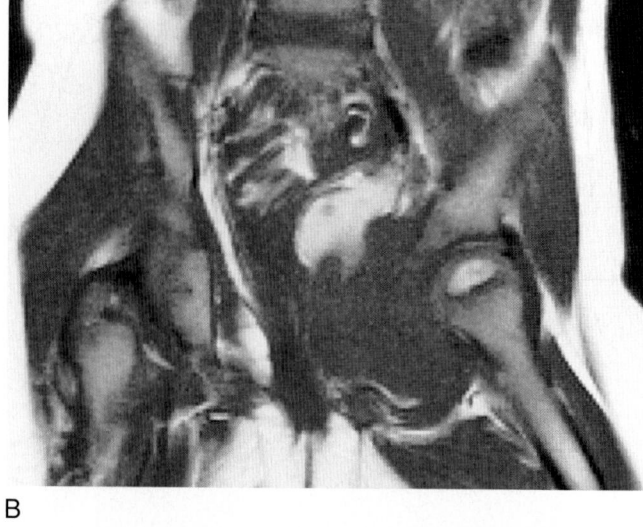

B

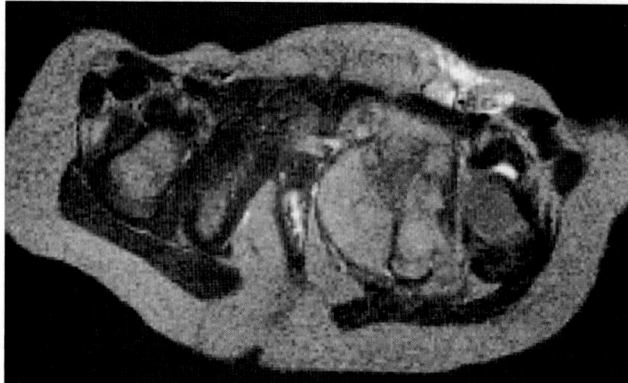

C

FIGURE 176-57. Computed tomography **(A)** and coronal T1-weighted **(B)** and transverse T2-weighted **(C)** Magnetic resonance images of the pelvis of a 3-year-old girl with Ewing sarcoma show an expansile tumor involving the medulla and cortex of the left ischium and a large soft tissue mass. In **C,** signal intensity of the tumor is similar to that of the subcutaneous fat. The high signal in the left groin is due to a recent biopsy. (**C** from Hanna SL, Fletcher BD, Kaste SC, et al: Increased confidence of diagnosis of Ewing sarcoma using T2-weighted magnetic resonance images. Magn Reson Imaging 1994;12:560, with permission.)

wide margin is required to insure that the tumor and its micrometastases are completely resected. By definition, a wide margin removes the tumor with a cuff of normal bone and surrounding soft tissue of at least 1 to 3 cm. This helps to ensure that the resection is beyond all local microscopic disease. Following resection, the defect can be reconstructed using a large modular oncology endoprosthesis, allograft, or a combination of these. Function can be good with these reconstructions despite extensive loss of bone and soft tissue.

Radiographs represent the mainstay for postoperative monitoring of the surgical resection sites for both benign and malignant bone tumors. The metal implanted in patients in which reconstructive techniques have been used (including placement of a prosthesis and intercalary reconstructions) may create significant artifact when imaging the operative site with CT or MRI (Fig. 176-69). When needed, MRI using metal suppression techniques can be performed on patients with prostheses. Particularly when coupled with contrast subtraction studies, MR examinations can provide clinically useful information regarding infection and tumor recurrence.

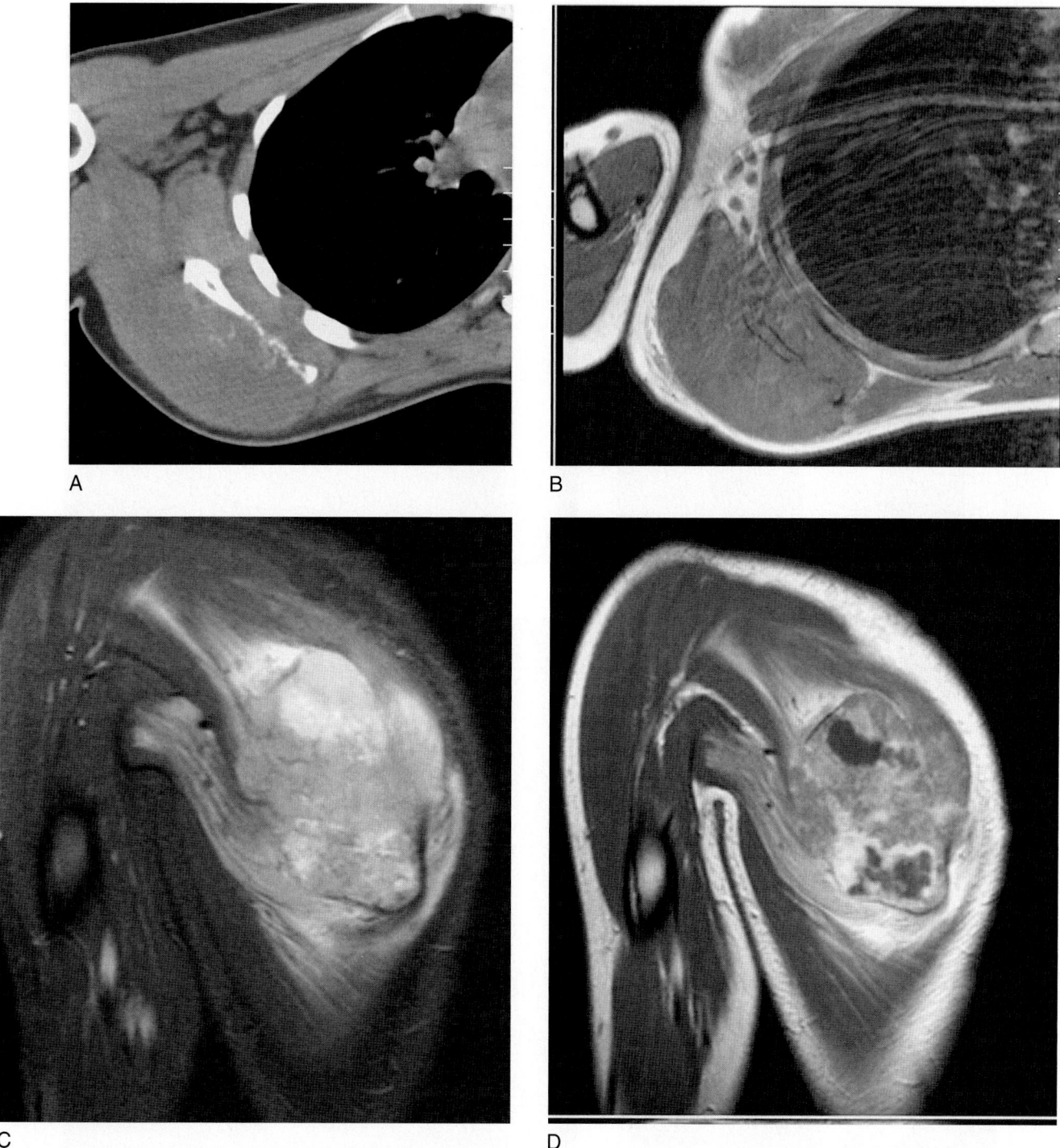

FIGURE 176-58. Ewing sarcoma of the right scapula in a 16 year-old girl. **A,** Axial computed tomography image shows a permeative pattern to the scapula with subtle calcifications within the soft tissue mass. The mass is isodense with muscle on this noncontrast study. **B,** Noncontrast axial T1-weighted magnetic image shows abnormal signal within the scapula and poor definition of the extraosseous component of Ewing sarcoma. **C,** Parasagittal short tau inversion recovery image shows encasement of the scapula by tumor that exhibits intensely increased signal. Note surrounding soft tissue edema. **D,** With intravenous administration of contrast material, this T1-weighted parasagittal image shows heterogeneous enhancement of the mass and defines areas of tumor necrosis (low-signal areas).

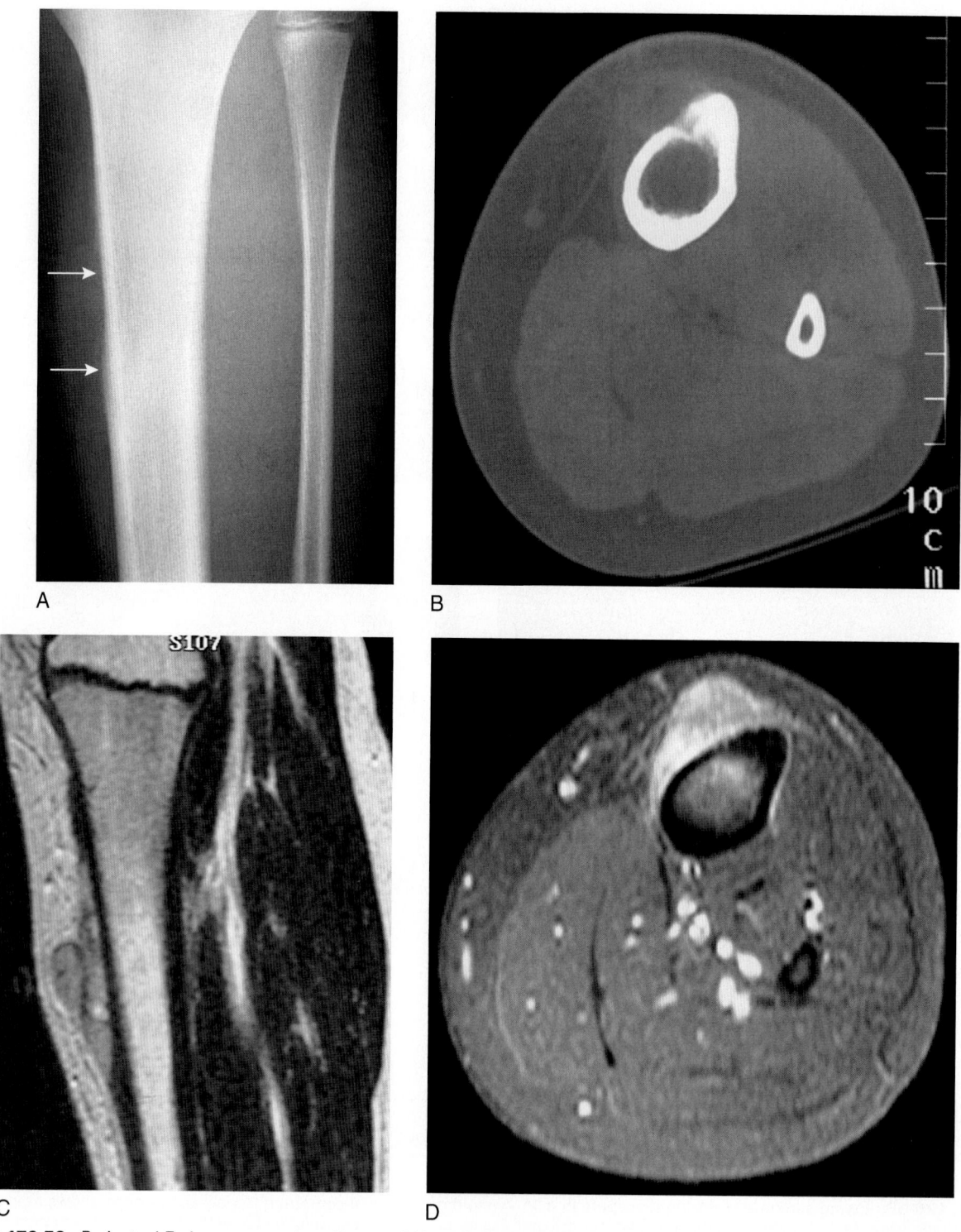

FIGURE 176-59. Periosteal Ewing sarcoma in a 12-year-old-boy. **A,** Radiograph shows very subtle excavation of the cortex, Codman triangles *(arrows),* and a soft tissue mass. **B,** Computed tomography scan obtained without the administration of contrast shows a small cortical defect. A sagittal T2-weighted magnetic resonance image **(C)** demonstrates a superficial soft tissue mass adjacent to the slightly thinned cortex that is also seen on a transverse contrast-enhanced, fat-saturated T1-weighted magnetic resonance image **(D).** The slight hyperintensity in the contiguous marrow suggests tumor extension into the medulla.

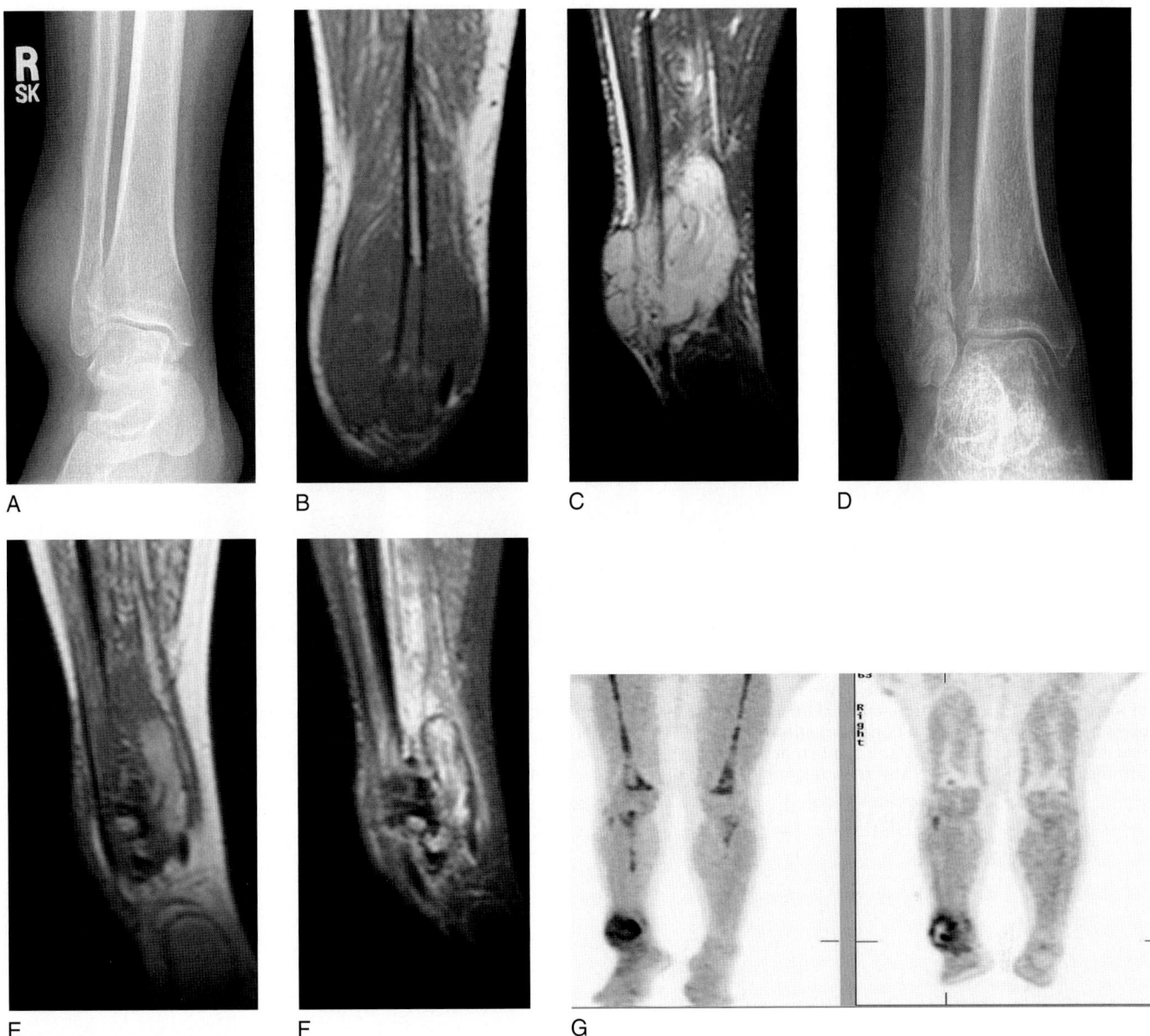

FIGURE 176-60. Ewing sarcoma of distal fibula in a 19-year-old girl undergoing chemotherapy. **A,** Anteroposterior radiograph of the right ankle demonstrates a large soft tissue mass along the lateral aspect of the distal right fibula. Note periosteal reaction along the fibula and poorly defined permeative pattern. **B,** Coronal T1-weighted magnetic resonance image shows a large soft tissue mass arising from the intramedullary canal and surrounding the distal fibula. Note line of demarcation between the normal fatty marrow of the fibula and the dark intramedullary component replaced by tumor. **C,** Coronal short tau inversion recovery image exquisitely shows the large mass but less readily demonstrates the intramedullary tumor margins. Note massive edema in the adjacent soft tissues. **D,** After 8 weeks of chemotherapy, there has been significant reduction in the soft tissue mass but development of increased conspicuity of the permeative involvement of the fibula. Also now evident is some ossification within the remaining soft tissue mass. **E,** Coronal T1-weighted image shows decrease in soft tissue mass and some areas of bright hemorrhage. **F,** corresponding short tau inversion recovery image shows decrease in the mass but with persistent soft tissue edema. **G,** Coronal ^{18}F-FDG PET image shows metabolically active areas of the mass to lie in the periphery of the tumor.

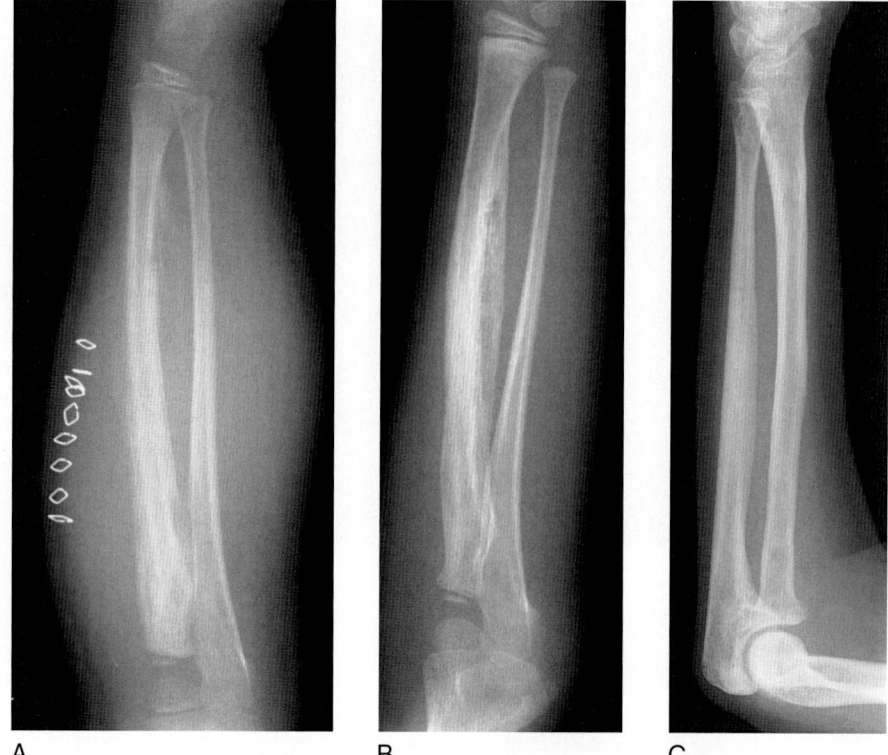

A   B   C

FIGURE 176-61. Ewing sarcoma of the radius of a 7-year-old girl who received chemotherapy and radiation therapy. **A,** Radiograph of the forearm obtained after incisional biopsy and before the initiation of therapy shows a long, permeative lesion of the radius, periosteal reaction, and new bone formation. There is a large, ill-defined soft tissue mass. **B,** There is solidification of the periosteal reaction and reduction in the soft tissue mass after completion of initial chemotherapy. **C,** One year after diagnosis, and the completion of all chemotherapy and radiation therapy, the appearance of the radius is nearly normal.

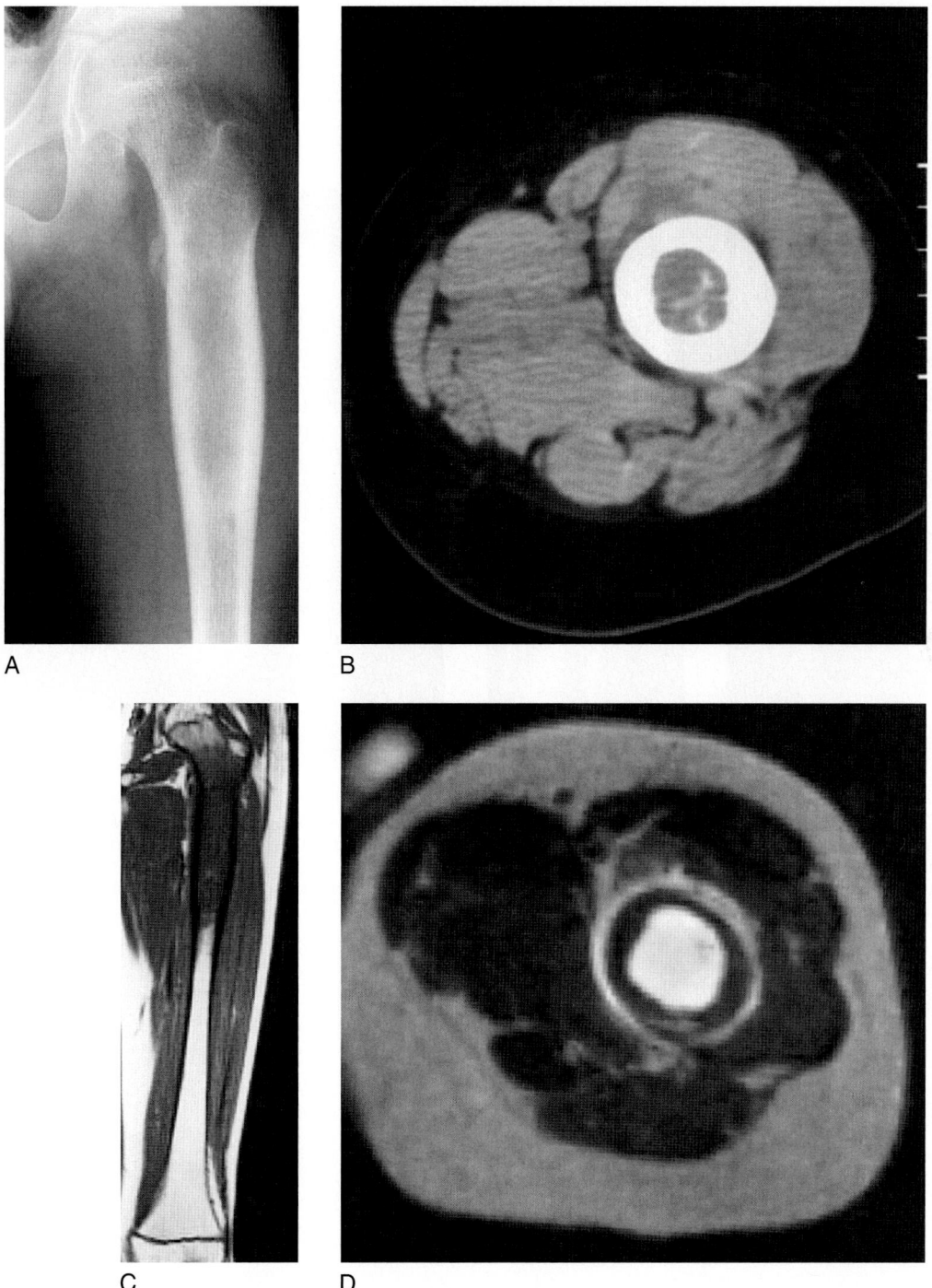

A

B

C

D

FIGURE 176-62. **A,** Radiograph of the femur of a 12-year-old boy with chondrosarcoma. The tumor has caused mild diaphyseal expansion and slight cortical thickening. **B,** Unenhanced computed tomography demonstrates slight calcification of the medullary tumor matrix. **C,** Coronal T1-weighted magnetic resonance image shows the distal and proximal limits of the low-intensity tumor. **D,** Transverse T2-weighted magnetic resonance image shows uniform high signal of the mixed cartilaginous-myxoid tumor matrix. The peritumoral high signal was due to periosteal elevation and soft tissue edema. (**A, C** and **D** from Hanna SL, Magill HL, Parham DM, et al: Childhood sarcoma: magnetic resonance imaging with Gadolinium-DTPA. Magn Reson Imaging 1990;8:670, with permission.)

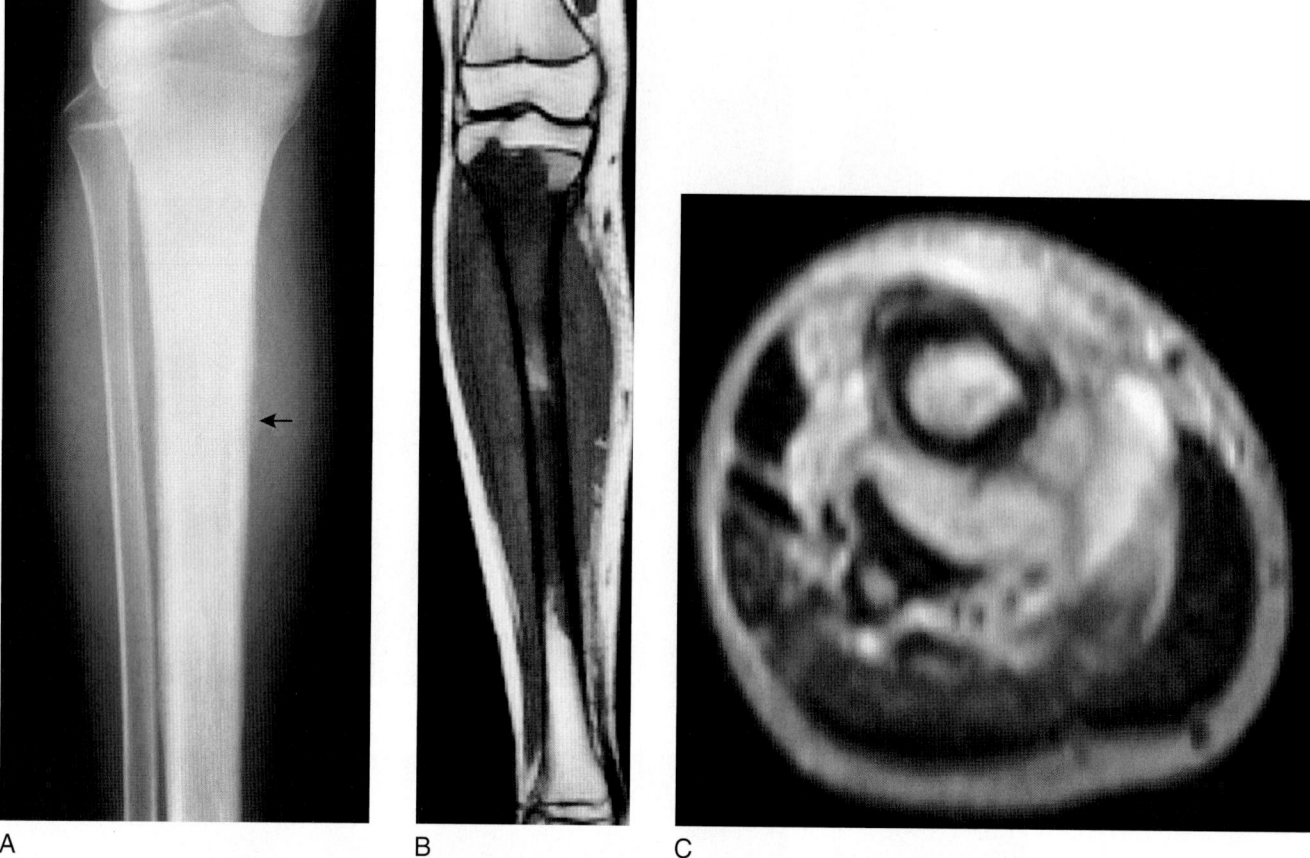

A   B   C

FIGURE 176-63. **A,** Radiograph of the tibia of a 15-year-old girl with a primary large cell lymphoma shows subtle sclerosis, medial periosteal new bone formation *(arrow),* and soft tissue swelling. **B,** Coronal T1-weighted magnetic resonance image shows extensive marrow involvement of the tibial diametaphysis with extension into the epiphysis. **C,** Transverse T2-weighted magnetic resonance image demonstrates abnormally high signal in the tibial medullary space and a large, hyperintense soft tissue mass.

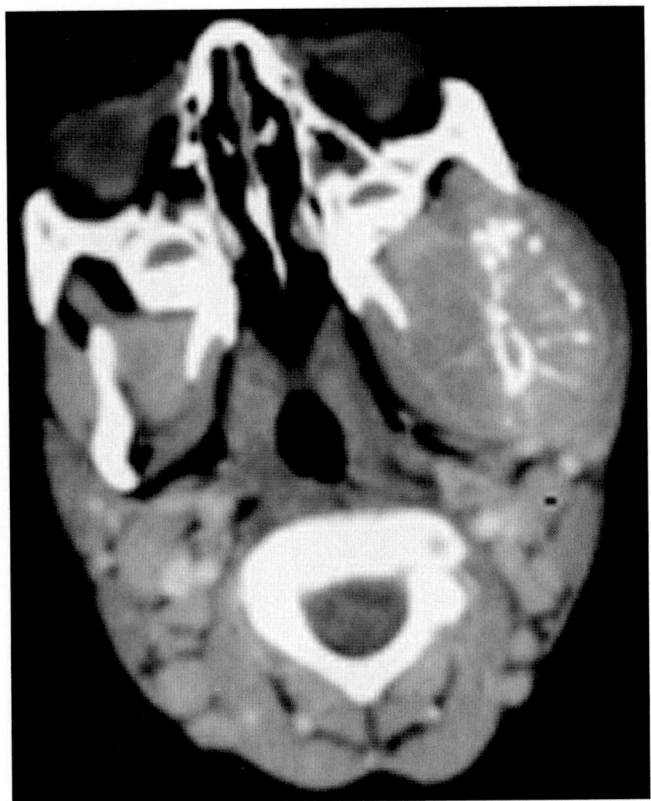

A

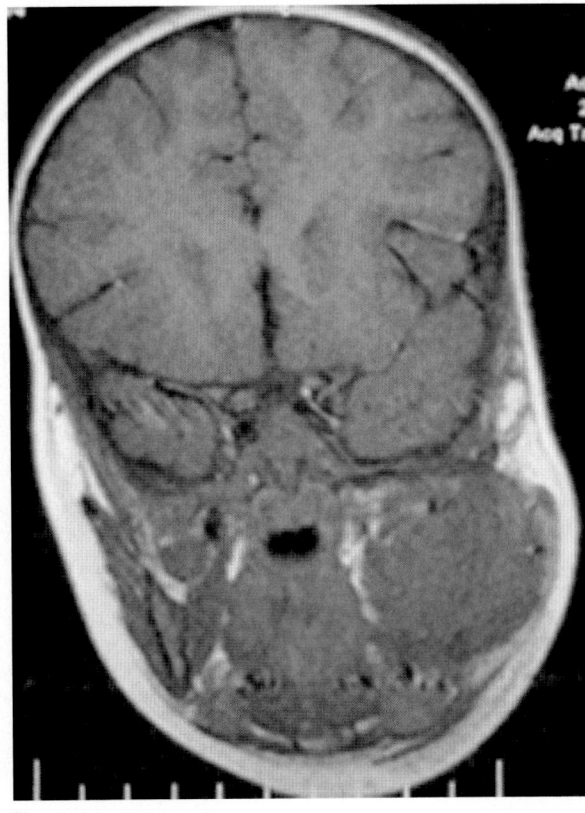

B

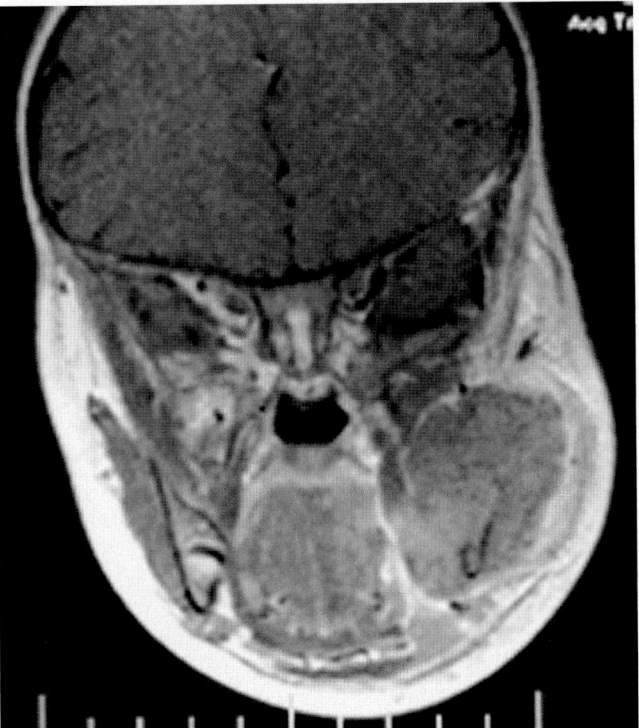

C

FIGURE 176-64. Chloroma of left mandible in a 20-month-old girl with acute M7 myelogenous leukemia at diagnosis. **A,** Axial contrast-enhanced computed tomography image of the face shows a large destructive soft tissue mass arising from the left mandible and associated with sunburst periosteal reaction. **B,** Coronal non-contrast T1- **C,** and contrast-enhanced T1-weighted magnetic resonace images through the midface show a large left face mass arising from the left mandible, having grown through the mandibular cortex and showing heterogeneous enhancement.

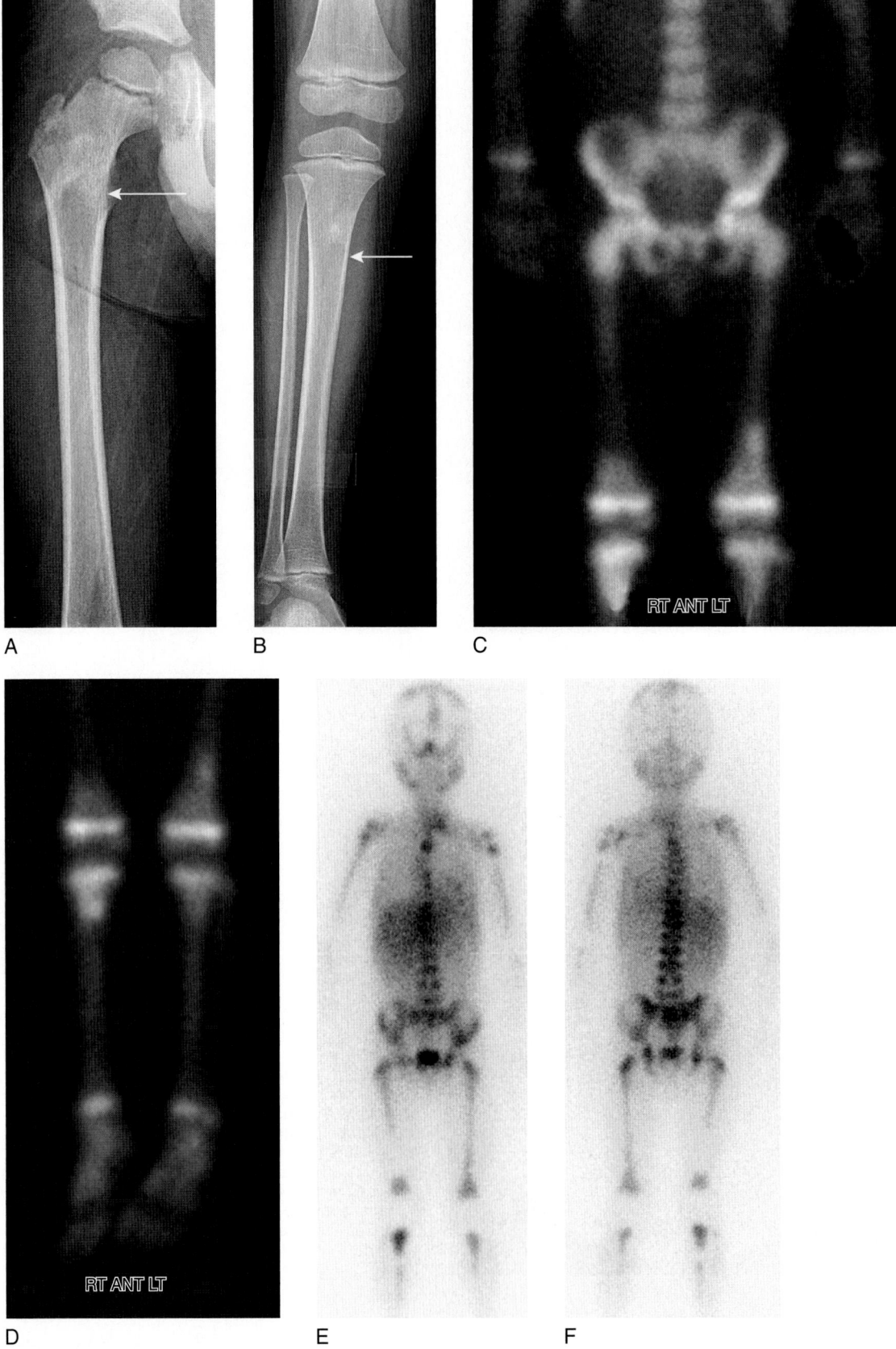

FIGURE 176-65. Anteroposterior radiograph of the right femur (**A**) and lower leg (**B**) of a 5-year-old boy with metastatic neuroblastoma. Poorly defined sclerotic metastases are present in the subtrochanteric femur *(arrow)* and proximal tibial diametaphysis *(arrow)*. Anteroposterior technetium-99m methylene diphosphonate bone scintigram of the femurs (**C**) and lower legs (**D**) show increased uptake within the spine, pelvic bones, proximal and distal femora and tibia bilaterally. Anteroposterior (**E**) and posteroanterior (**F**) whole-body ^{123}I MIBG scintigrams demonstrate diffuse abnormal skeletal uptake indicative of widespread bony metastases.

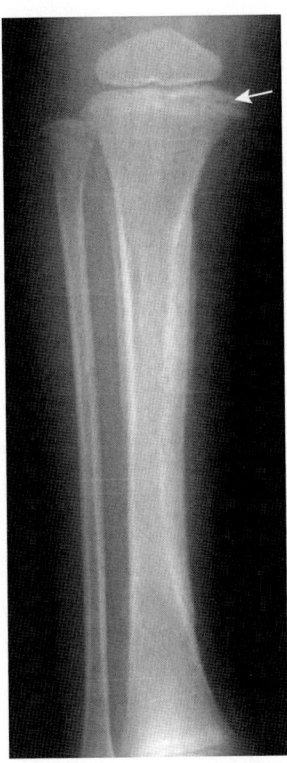

A

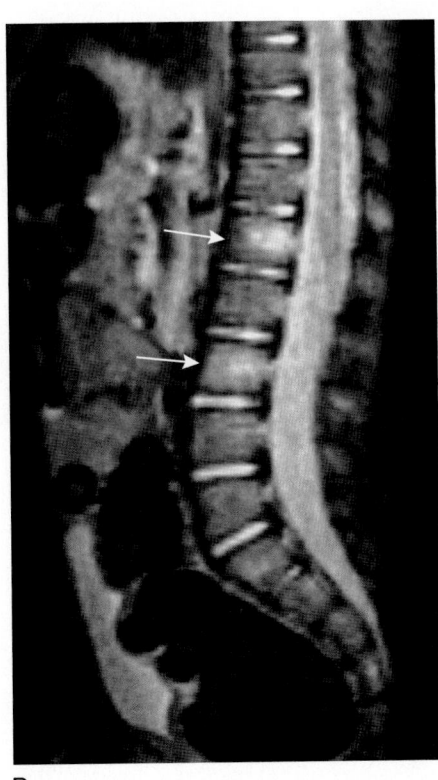

B

FIGURE 176-66. **A,** Radiograph of the lower leg of a 4-year-old boy with neuroblastoma shows an irregular proximal tibial submetaphyseal lucency (arrow) and extensive diaphyseal periosteal reaction. **B,** Sagittal short tau inversion–recovery image of the lower thoracic and lumbosacral spine shows abnormally high signal intensity in the bodies of L1 and L3, a finding consistent with metastases (*arrows*).

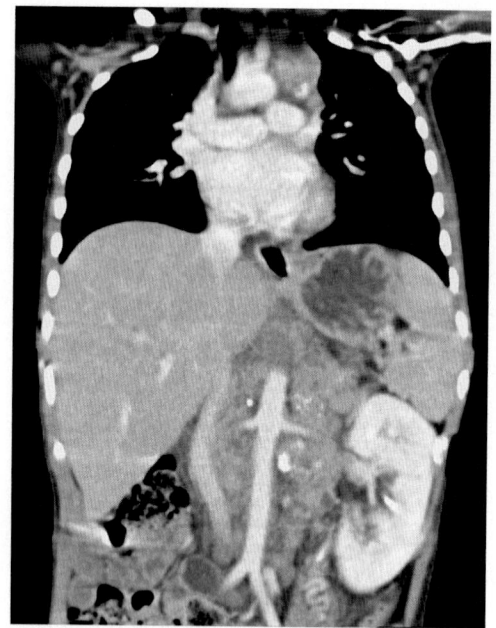

A

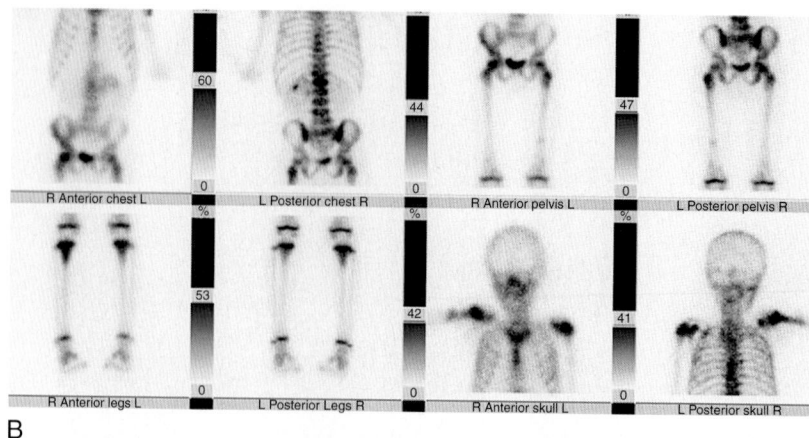

B

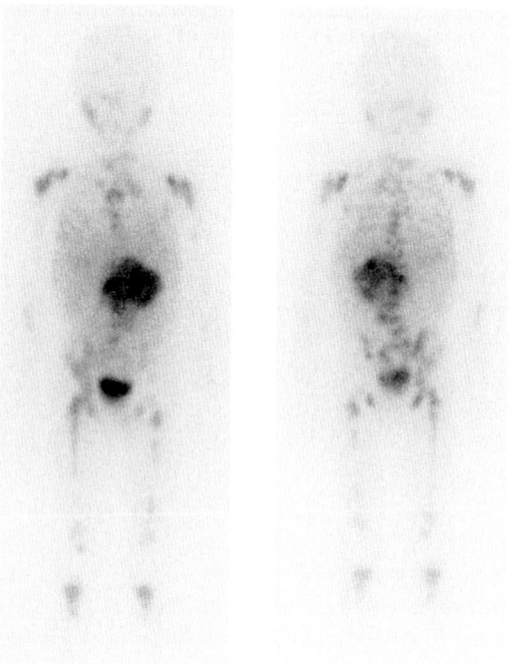

C   D

FIGURE 176-67. **A,** Coronal reconstruction of a contrast-enhanced computed tomography image of a 5-year-old boy with neuroblastoma extending from retroperitoneum into the chest. **B,** Anterior technetium-99m methylene diphosphonate bone scintigram of the entire skeletal showing diffuse bony disease. **C,** Anterior, and posterior **(D)** coronal ^{123}I MIBG image demonstrates intense tracer uptake in the primary abdominal mass, moderate uptake in the left superior mediastinal disease, and widespread bony metastases.

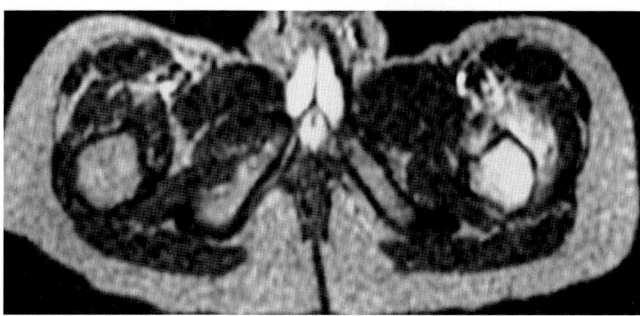

A

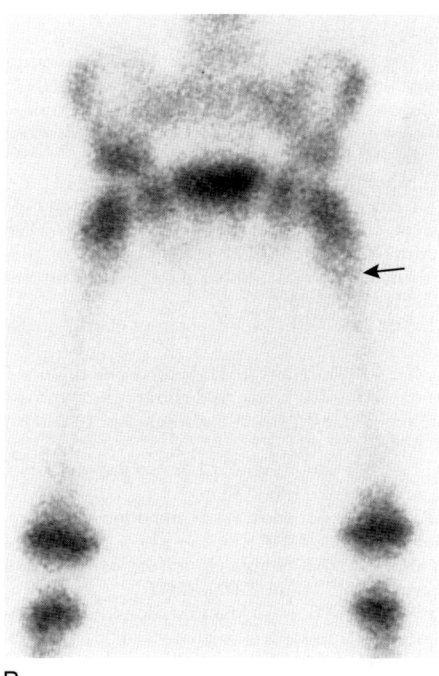

B

FIGURE 176-68. A, Transverse T2-weighted magnetic resonance image of a 2-year-old boy with neuroblastoma demonstrates abnormally high signal in the proximal left femur and adjacent musculature. B, Anterior technetium-99m methylene diphosphonate bone scintigram of the pelvis shows a subtle increase in activity in the trochanteric region of the left femur (arrow). No abnormalities were demonstrated on radiographs.

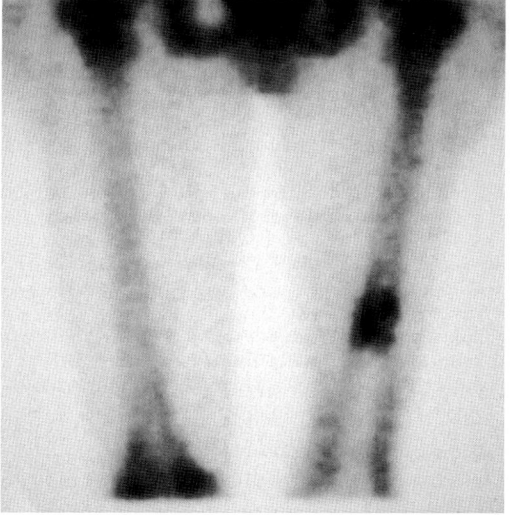

A

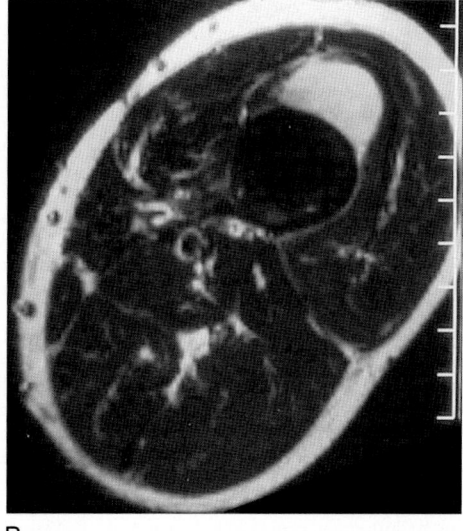

B

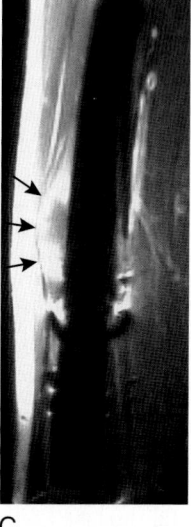

C

FIGURE 176-69. A, Anterior technetium-99m methylene diphosphonate bone scintigram showing increased uptake at the upper limit of the femoral stem in a 19-year-old patient with recurrent osteosarcoma. B, Axial and, C, sagittal non-contrast T1-weighted magnetic resonance images show a focal soft tissue mass arising from the anterior cortex of native femur at the osteotomy site (arrows). Tumor recurrence with limb-sparing procedures is similar to that of recurrence after amputation (5%). (B and C from Kaste SC, Neel MN, Rao BN, et al: Complications of limb-sparing replacements about the knee for pediatric skeletal sarcomas. Pediatr Radiol 2001:31:62-71, with permission)

SUGGESTED READINGS

General

Aoki J, Watanabe H, Shinozaki T, et al: FDG PET of primary benign and malignant bone tumors: standardized uptake value in 52 lesions. Radiology 2001;219:774-777

Daldrup-Link HE, Franzius C, Link TM, et al: Whole-body MR imaging for detection of bone metastases in children with skeletal scintigraphy and FDG PET. AJR Am J Roentgenol 2001; 177:229-236

Dorfman HD, Czerniak B: Bone Tumors. St. Louis, Mosby, 1998

Franzius C, Schober O: Assessment of therapy response by FDG PET in pediatric patients. Q J Nucl Med 2003;47:41-45

Gyorke TA, Zajic TB, Lange AB, et al: Impact of FDG PET for staging of Ewing sarcomas and primitive neuroectodermal tumours. Nucl Med Commun 2006;27:17-24

Hawkins DS, Rajendran JG, Conrad EU III, , et al: Evaluation of chemotherapy response in pediatric bone sarcomas by [F-18]-fluorodeoxy-d-glucose positron emission tomography. Cancer 2002;94:3277-3284

Hayes CW, Conway WF, Sundaram M: Misleading aggressive MR imaging appearance of some benign musculoskeletal lesions. Radiographics 1992;12:1119-1134

Levine SM, Lambiase RE, Petchprapa CN: Cortical lesions of the tibia: characteristic appearances at conventional radiography. Radiographics 2003;23:157-177

Lodwick GS: A probabilistic approach to the diagnosis of bone tumors. Radiol Clin North Am 1965;3:487-497

Mirra JM, Picci P, Gold RH: Bone Tumors: Clinical, Radiologic, and Pathologic Correlations. Philadelphia, Lea & Febiger, 1989

Ortiz EJ, Isler MH, Navia JE, et al: Pathologic fractures in children. Clin Orthop Relat Res 2005;432:116-126

Pizzo PA, Poplack DG: Principles and Practice of Pediatric Oncology, 5th ed. Philadelphia, Lippincott Williams & Wilkins, 2006

Schulte RM, Brecht-Krass D, Werner M, et al: Evaluation of neoadjuvant therapy response of osteogenic sarcoma using FDG PET. J Nucl Med 1999;40:1637-1643.

Seeger LL, Yao L, Eckardt JJ: Surface lesions of bone. Radiology 1998;206:17-33

Senac MO, Jr., Isaacs H, Gwinn JL: Primary lesions of bone in the 1st decade of life: retrospective survey of biopsy results. Radiology 1986;160:491-495

Shulkin BL, Mitchell DS, Ungar DR, et al: Neoplasms in a pediatric population: 2-[F-18]-fluoro-2-deoxy-D-glucose PET studies. Radiology 1995;194:495-500

Van Dyck P, Vanhoenacker FM, Vogel J, et al: Prevalence, extension and characteristics of fluid-fluid levels in bone and soft tissue tumors. Eur Radiol 2006;16:2644-2651

Benign Cartilaginous Tumors

Abramovici L, Steiner GC: Bizarre parosteal osteochondromatous proliferation (Nora's lesion): a retrospective study of 12 cases, 2 arising in long bones. Hum Pathol 2002;33:1205-1210

Bloem JL, Mulder JD: Chondroblastoma: a clinical and radiological study of 104 cases. Skeletal Radiol 1985;14:1-9

Brien EW, Mirra JM, Kerr R: Benign and malignant cartilage tumors of bone and joint: their anatomic and theoretical basis with an emphasis on radiology, pathology and clinical biology. I. The intramedullary cartilage tumors. Skeletal Radiol 1997;26:325-353

Brien EW, Mirra JM, Luck JV Jr: Benign and malignant cartilage tumors of bone and joint: their anatomic and theoretical basis with an emphasis on radiology, pathology and clinical biology. II. Juxtacortical cartilage tumors. Skeletal Radiol 1999;28:1-20

Brower AC, Moser RP, Kransdorf MJ: The frequency and diagnostic significance of periostitis in chondroblastoma. AJR Am J Roentgenol 1990;154:309-314

Caballes RL: Enchondroma protuberans masquerading as osteochondroma. Hum Pathol 1982;13:734-739

Crim JR, Mirra JM: Enchondroma protuberans: report of a case and its distinction from chondrosarcoma and osteochondroma adjacent to an enchondroma. Skeletal Radiol 1990;19:431-434

Fletcher BD, Crom DB, Krance RA, et al: Radiation-induced bone abnormalities after bone marrow transplantation for childhood leukemia. Radiology 1994;191:231-235

Hunter AG, Kozlowski K, Hochberger O: Metachondromatosis. Can Assoc Radiol J 1995;46:202-208

Jaffe N, Ried HL, Cohen M, et al: Radiation induced osteochondroma in long-term survivors of childhood cancer. Int J Radiat Oncol Biol Phys 1983;9:665-670

Karasick D, Schweitzer ME, Eschelman DJ: Symptomatic osteochondromas: imaging features. AJR Am J Roentgenol 1997;168:1507-1512

Keating RB, Wright PW, Staple TW: Enchondroma protuberans of the rib. Skeletal Radiol 1985;13:55-58

Lewis MM, Kenan S, Yabut SM, et al: Periosteal chondroma: a report of ten cases and review of the literature. Clin Orthop 1990;256:185–192

Libshitz HI, Cohen MA: Radiation-induced osteochondromas. Radiology 1982;142:643-647

Mahboubi S, Dormans JP, D'Angio G: Malignant degeneration of radiation-induced osteochondroma. Skeletal Radiol 1997; 26:195-198

Marcovici PA, Berdon WE, Liebling MS: Osteochondromas and growth retardation secondary to externally or internally administered radiation in childhood. Pediatr Radiol 2007;37:301-304

Marin C, Gallego C, Manjón P, et al: Juxtacortical chondromyxoid fibroma: imaging findings in three cases and a review of the literature. Skeletal Radiol 1997;26:642-649

Murphey MD, Choi JJ, Kransdorf MJ, et al: Imaging of osteochondroma: variants and complications with radiologic-pathologic correlation. Radiographics 2000;20:1407-1434

Nora FE, Dahlin DC, Beabout JW: Bizarre parosteal osteochondromatous proliferations of the hands and feet. Am J Surg Pathol 1983;7:245-250

Oxtoby JW, Davies AM: MRI characteristics of chondroblastoma. Clin Radiol 1996;51:22-26

Pierz KA, Womer RB, Dormans JP: Pediatric bone tumors: osteosarcoma, Ewing's sarcoma, and chondrosarcoma associated with multiple hereditary osteochondromatosis. J Pediatr Orthop 2001;21:412-418

Ramappa AJ, Lee FYI, Tang P, et al: Chondroblastoma of bone. J Bone Joint Surg Am 2000;82:1140-1145

Richardson RR: Variants of exostosis of the bone in children. Semin Roentgenol 2005;40:380-390

Robbin MR, Murphey MD: Benign chondroid neoplasms of bone. Semin Musculoskelet Radiol 2000;4:45-58

Saglik Y, Altay M, Unal VS, et al: Manifestations and management of osteochondromas: a retrospective analysis of 382 patients. Acta Orthop Belg 2006;72:748-755

Stieber JR, Dormans JP: Manifestations of hereditary multiple exostoses. J Am Acad Orthop Surg 2005;13:110-120

Unni KK: Cartilaginous lesions of bone. J Orthop Sci 2001;6:457-472

Vanhoenacker FM, Van Hul W, Wuyts W, et al: Hereditary multiple exostoses: from genetics to clinical syndrome and complications. Eur J Radiol 2001;40:208-217

Vasseur M-A, Fabre O: Vascular complications of osteochondromas. J Vasc Surg 2000;31:532-538

Vázquez-Flores H, Domínguez-Cherit J, Vega-Memije ME, et al: Subungual osteochondroma: clinical and radiologic features and treatment. Dermatol Surg 2004;30:1031-1034

Weatherall PT, Maale GE, Mendelsohn DB, et al: Chondroblastoma: classic and confusing appearance at MR imaging. Radiology 1994;190:467-474

Wilson AJ, Kyriakos M, Ackerman LV: Chondromyxoid fibroma: radiographic appearance in 38 cases and in a review of the literature. Radiology 1991;179:513-518

Woertler K, Blasius S, Brinkschmidt C, et al: Periosteal chondroma: MR characteristics. J Comput Assist Tomogr 2001;25:425-430

Woertler K, Lindner N, Gosheger G, et al: Osteochondroma: MR imaging of tumor-related complications. Eur Radiol 2000; 10:832-840

Wu CT, Inwards CY, O'Laughlin S, et al: Chondromyxoid fibroma of bone: a clinicopathologic review of 278 cases. Hum Pathol 1998;29:438-446

Yamamura S, Sato K, Sugiura H, et al: Inflammatory reaction in chondroblastoma. Skeletal Radiol 1996;25:371–376

Cystic Lesions

Baker DM: Benign unicameral bone cyst: a study of forty-five cases with long-term follow up. Clin Orthop Relat Res 1970;71:140-151

Bertoni F, Bacchini P, Capanna R, et al: Solid variant of aneurysmal bone cyst. Cancer 1993;71:729-734

Bonakdarpour A, Levy WM, Aegerter E: Primary and secondary aneurysmal bone cyst: a radiological study of 75 cases. Radiology 1978;126:75-83

Campanacci M, Capanna R, Picci P: Unicameral and aneurysmal bone cysts. Clin Orthop Relat Res 1986;204:25-26

Capanna R, Campanacci DA, Manfrini M: Unicameral and aneurysmal bone cysts. Orthop Clin North Am 1996;27:605-614

Hudson TM: Fluid levels in aneurysmal bone cysts: a CT feature. AJR Am J Roentgenol 1984;142:1001-1004

Ilaslan H, Sundaram M, Unni KK: Solid variant of aneurysmal bone cysts in long tubular bones: giant cell reparative granuloma. AJR Am J Roentgenol 2003;180:1681-1687

Jaffe HL, Lichtenstein L: Solitary unicameral bone cyst: with emphasis on the roentgen picture, the pathologic appearance and the pathogenesis. Arch Surg 1942;44:1004–1025

Kransdorf MJ, Sweet DE: Aneurysmal bone cyst: concept, controversy, clinical presentation, and imaging. AJR Am J Roentgenol 1995; 164:573-580

Maki DD, Nesbit ME, Griffiths HJ: Diffuse lymphangiomatosis of bone. Australas Radiol 1999;43:535-538

Mankin HJ, Hornicek FJ, Ortiz-Cruz E, et al: Aneurysmal bone cyst: a review of 150 patients. J Clin Oncol 2005;23:6756-6762

Margau R, Babyn P, Cole W, et al: MR imaging of simple bone cysts in children: not so simple. Pediatr Radiol 2000;30:551-557

Martinat P, Cotton A, Singer B, et al: Solitary cystic lymphangioma. Skeletal Radiol 1995;24:556-558

Munk PL, Helms CA, Holt RG, et al: MR imaging of aneurysmal bone cysts. AJR Am J Roentgenol 1989;153:99-101

O'Donnell P, Saifuddin A: The prevalence and diagnostic significance of fluid-fluid levels in focal lesions of bone. Skeletal Radiol 2004;33:330-336

Parman LM, Murphey MD: Alphabet soup: cystic lesions of bone. Semin Musculoskelet Radiol 2000;4:89-101

Steiner GM, Farman J, Lawson JP: Lymphangiomatois of bone. Radiology 1969;93:1093-1098

Tsai JC, Dalinka MK, Fallon MD, et al: Fluid-fluid level: a nonspecific finding in tumors of bone and soft tissue. Radiology 1990; 175:779-782

Van Linthoudt D, Lagier R: Calcaneal cysts: a radiological and anatomico-pathological study. Acta Orthop Scand 1978; 49:310-316

Winterberger AR: Radiographic diagnosis of lymphangiomatosis of bone. Radiology 1972;102:321-324

Woertler K, Brinkschmidt C: Imaging features of subperiosteal aneurysmal bone cyst. Acta Radiol 2002;43:336-339

Giant Cell Tumor

Krajca-Radcliffe JB, Thomas JR, Nicholas RW: Giant-cell tumor of bone: a rare entity in the hands of children. J Pediatr Orthop 1994;14:776-780

Kransdorf MJ, Sweet DE, Buetow PC, et al: Giant cell tumor in skeletally immature patients. Radiology 1992;184:233-237

Murphey MD, Nomikos GC, Flemming DJ, et al: Imaging of giant cell tumor and giant cell reparative granuloma of bone: radiologic-pathologic correlation. Radiographics 2001;21:1283-1309

Schajowicz F, Granato DB, McDonald DJ, et al: Clinical and radiological features of atypical giant cell tumours of bone. Br J Radiol 1991;64:877-889

Schütte HE, Taconis WK: Giant cell tumor in children and adolescents. Skeletal Radiol 1993;22:173-176

Stratil PG, Stacy GS: Multifocal metachronous giant cell tumor in a 15-year-old boy. Pediatr Radiol 2005;35:444-448

Benign Fibrous Tumors

Betsy M, Kupersmith LM, Springfield DS: Metaphyseal fibrous defects. J Am Acad Orthop Surg 2004;12:89-95

Bloem JL, van der Heul RO, Schuttevaer HM, et al: Fibrous dysplasia vs adamantinoma of the tibia: differentiation based on discriminant analysis of clinical and plain film findings. AJR Am J Roentgenol 1991;156:1017-1023

Cabral CEL, Guedes P, Fonseca T, et al: Polyostotic fibrous dysplasia associated with intramuscular myxomas: Mazabraud's syndrome. Skeletal Radiol 1998;27:278–282

Caffey J: On fibrous defects in cortical walls of growing tubular bones: their radiologic appearance, structure, prevalence, natural course, and diagnostic significance. Adv Pediatr 1955;7:13-51

Campanacci M, Laus M: Osteofibrous dysplasia of the tibia and fibula. J Bone Joint Surg Am 1981;63:367-375

Colby RS, Saul RA: Is Jaffe-Campanacci syndrome just a manifestation of neurofibromatosis type 1? Am J Med Genet A 2003;123:60-63

Czerniak B, Rojas-Corona RR, Dorfman HD: Morphologic diversity of long bone adamantinoma. The concept of differentiated (regressing) adamantinoma and its relationship to osteofibrous dysplasia. Cancer 1989;64:2319-2334

DiCaprio MR, Enneking WF: Fibrous dysplasia. Pathophysiology, evaluation, and treatment. J Bone Joint Surg Am 2005;87:1848-1864

Faivre L, Nivelon-Chevallier A, Kottler ML, et al: Mazabraud syndrome in two patients: clinical overlap with McCune-Albright syndrome. Am J Med Genet 2001; 99:132-136

Fisher AJ, Totty WG, Kyriakos M: MR appearance of cystic fibrous dysplasia. J Comput Assist Tomogr 1994;18:315–318

Fitzpatrick KA, Taljanovic MS, Speer DP, et al: Imaging findings of fibrous dysplasia with histopathologic and intraoperative correlation. AJR Am J Roentgenol 2004;182:1389-1398

Frick MA, Sundaram M, Unni KK, et al: Imaging findings in desmoplastic fibroma of bone: distinctive T2 characteristics. AJR Am J Roentgenol 2005;184:1762-1767

Goodin GS, Shulkin BS, Kaufman RA, et al: PET/CT characterization of fibroosseous defects in children: 18F-FDG uptake can mimic metastatic disease. AJR Am J Roentgenol 2006;187:1124-1128

Hazelbag HM, Taminiau AH, Fleuren GJ, et al: Adamantinoma of the long bones. A clinicopathological study of thirty-two patients with emphasis on histological subtype, precursor lesion, and biological behavior. J Bone Joint Surg Am 1994;76:1482-1499

Hindman BW, Bell S, Russo T, et al: Neonatal osteofibrous dysplasia: report of two cases. Pediatr Radiol 1996;26:303-306

Ishida T, Iijima T, Kikuchi F, et al: A clinicopathological and immunohistochemical study of osteofibrous dysplasia, differentiated adamantinoma, and adamantinoma of long bones. Skeletal Radiol 1992;21:493-502

Jee WH, Choe BY, Kang HS, et al: Nonossifying fibroma: characteristics at MR imaging with pathologic correlation. Radiology 1998;209:197-202

Kahn LB: Adamantinoma, osteofibrous dysplasia and differentiated adamantinoma. Skeletal Radiol 2003;32:245-258

Karol LA, Brown DS, Wise CA, et al: Familial osteofibrous dysplasia: a case series. J Bone Joint Surg Am 2005;87:2297-2307

Komiya S, Inoue A: Aggressive bone tumorous lesion in infancy: osteofibrous dysplasia of the tibia and fibula. J Pediatr Orthop 1993;13:577-581

Mirra JM, Gold RH, Rand F: Disseminated nonossifying fibromas in association with cafe-au-lait spots (Jaffe-Campanacci syndrome). Clin Orthop Relat Res 1982:192-205

Moser RP, Jr., Sweet DE, Haseman DB, et al: Multiple skeletal fibroxanthomas: radiologic-pathologic correlation of 72 cases. Skeletal Radiol 1987;16:353-359

Parekh SG, Donthineni-Rao R, Ricchetti E, et al: Fibrous dysplasia. J Am Acad Orthop Surg 2004;12:305-313

Robbin MR, Murphey MD, Temple T, et al: Imaging of musculoskeletal fibromatosis. Radiographics 2001;21:585-600

Ruggieri P, Sim FH, Bond JR, et al: Malignancies in fibrous dysplasia. Cancer 1994;73:1411-1424

Smith SE, Kransdorf MJ: Primary musculoskeletal tumors of fibrous origin. Semin Musculoskelet Radiol 2000;4:73-88

Taconis WK, Schütte HE, van der Heul RO: Desmoplastic fibroma of bone: a report of 18 cases. Skeletal Radiol 1994;23:283-288

Utz JA, Kransdorf MJ, Jelinek JS, et al: MR appearance of fibrous dysplasia. J Comput Assist Tomogr 1989;13:845-851

Van der Woude HJ, Hazelbag HM, Bloem JL, et al: MRI of adamantinoma of long bones in correlation with histopathology. AJR Am J Roentgenol 2004;183:1737-1744

Van Rijn R, Bras J, Schaap G, et al: Adamantinoma in childhood: report of six cases and review of the literature. Pediatr Radiol 2006;36:1068-1074

Yao L, Eckardt JJ, Seeger LL: Fibrous dysplasia associated with cortical bony destruction: CT and MR findings. J Comput Assist Tomogr 1994;18:91–94

Langerhans Cell Histiocytosis of Bone

Azouz EM, Saigal G, Rodriguez MM, et al: Langerhans' cell histiocytosis: pathology, imaging and treatment of skeletal involvement. Pediatr Radiol 2005;35:103-115

Beltran J, Aparisi F, Bonmati LM, et al: Eosinophilic granuloma: MRI manifestations. Skeletal Radiol 1993;22:157-161

David R, Oria RA, Kumar R, et al: Radiologic features of eosinophilic granuloma of bone. AJR Am J Roentgenol 1989;153:1021-1026

Egeler RM, D'Angio GJ: Langerhans cell histiocytosis. J Pediatr 1995;127:1-11

Goo HW, Yang DH, Ra YS, et al: Whole-body MRI of Langerhans cell histiocytosis: comparison with radiography and bone scintigraphy. Pediatr Radiol 2006;36:1019-1031

Hindman BW, Thomas RD, Young LW, et al: Langerhans cell histiocytosis: unusual skeletal manifestations observed in thirty-four cases. Skeletal Radiol 1998;27:177-181

Kaste SC, Rodriguez-Galindo C, McCarville ME, et al: PET-CT in Langerhans cell histiocytosis. Pediatr Radiol 2007;37:615-622

Kilborn TN, Teh J, Goodman TR: Paediatric manifestations of Langerhans cell histiocytosis: a review of the clinical and radiological findings. Clin Radiol 2003;58:269-278

Kilpatrick SE, Wenger DE, Gilchrist GS, et al: Langerhans' cell histiocytosis (histiocytosis X) of bone: a clinicopathologic analysis of 263 pediatric and adult cases. Cancer 1995;76:2471-2484

Kransdorf MJ, Smith SE: Lesions of unknown histiogenesis: Langerhans cell histiocytosis and Ewing sarcoma. Semin Musculoskel Radiol 2000;4:113-125

Meyer JS, Harty MP, Mahboubi S, et al: Langerhans cell histiocytosis: presentation and evolution of radiologic findings with clinical correlation. Radiographics 1995;15:1135-1146

Schmidt S, Eich G, Hanquinet S, et al: Extra-osseous involvement of Langerhans' cell histiocytosis in children. Pediatr Radiol 2004;34:313-321

Siegelman SS: Taking the X out of histiocytosis X. Radiology 1997;204:322–324

Stull MA, Kransdorf MJ, Devaney KO: Langerhans cell histiocytosis of bone. Radiographics 1992;12:801-823

Van Nieuwenhuyse JP, Clapuyt P, Malghem J, et al: Radiographic skeletal survey and radionuclide bone scan in Langerhans cell histiocytosis of bone. Pediatr Radiol 1996;26:734-738

Benign Osteoid-Producing Tumors

Allen SD, Saifuddin A: Imaging of intra-articular osteoid osteoma. Clin Radiol 2003;58:845-852

Assoun J, Richardi G, Railhac J-J, et al: Osteoid osteoma: MR imaging versus CT. Radiology 1994;191:217-223

Azouz EM, Kozlowski K, Marton D, et al: Osteoid osteoma and osteoblastoma of the spine in children: report of 22 cases with brief literature review. Pediatr Radiol 1986;16:25-31

Ghanem I: The management of osteoid osteoma: updates and controversies. Curr Opin Pediatr 2006;18:36-41

Greenspan A: Benign bone-forming lesions: osteoma, osteoid osteoma, and osteoblastoma: clinical, imaging, pathologic, and differential considerations. Skeletal Radiol 1993;22:485-500

Jambhekar NA, Desai S, Khapake D: Osteoblastoma: a study of 12 cases. Indian J Pathol Microbiol 2006;49:487-490

Kayser F, Resnick D, Haghighi P, et al: Evidence of the subperiosteal origin of osteoid osteomas in tubular bones: analysis by CT and MR imaging. AJR Am J Roentgenol 1998;170:609-614

Kransdorf MJ, Stull MA, Gilkey FW, et al: Osteoid osteoma. Radiographics 1991;11:671-696

Kroon HM, Schurmans J: Osteoblastoma: clinical and radiologic findings in 98 new cases. Radiology 1990;175:783-790

Lucas DR, Unni KK, McLeod RA, et al: Osteoblastoma: clinicopathologic study of 306 cases. Hum Pathol 1994;25:117-134

McLeod RA, Dahlin DC, Beabout JW: The spectrum of osteoblastoma. AJR Am J Roentgenol 1976;126:321-325.

Roach PJ, Connolly LP, Zurakowski D, et al: Osteoid osteoma: comparative utility of high-resolution planar and pinhole magnification scintigraphy. Pediatr Radiol 1996;26:222–225

Shankman S, Desai P, Beltran J: Subperiosteal osteoid osteoma: radiographic and pathologic manifestations. Skeletal Radiol 1997;26:457-462

Torriani M, Rosenthal DI: Percutaneous radiofrequency treatment of osteoid osteoma. Pediatr Radiol 2002;32:615-618

White LM, Kandel R: Osteoid-producing tumors of bone. Semin Musculoskel Radiol 2000:4;25-43

Yamamura S, Sato K, Sugiura H, et al: Magnetic resonance imaging of inflammatory reaction in osteoid osteoma. Arch Orthop Trauma Surg 1994;114:8-13.

Osteosarcoma

Bloem JL, Taminiau AHM, Eulderink F, et al: Radiologic staging of primary bone sarcoma: MR imaging, scintigraphy, angiography, and CT correlated with pathologic examination. Radiology 1988;169:805-810

Brown ML: The role of radionuclides in the patient with osteogenic sarcoma. Semin Roentgenol 1989;24:185-192

Doud TM, Moser RP Jr, Giudici MAI, et al: Case report 704: extraskeletal osteosarcoma of the thigh with several suspected skeletal metastases and extensive metastases to the chest. Skeletal Radiol 1991;20:628-632

Ellis JH, Siegel CL, Martel W, et al: Radiologic features of well-differentiated osteosarcoma. AJR Am J Roentgenol 1988; 151:739-742

Fletcher BD: Imaging pediatric bone sarcomas: diagnosis and treatment-related issues. Radiol Clin North Am 1997;35:1477-1494

Gomes H, Menanteau B, Gaillard D, et al: Telangiectatic osteosarcoma. Pediatr Radiol 1986;16:140-143

Goorin AM, Abelson HT, Frei E III: Osteosarcoma: fifteen years later. N Engl J Med 1985;313:1637-1643

Graham NJ, Cairns RA, Anderson RA: Osteosarcoma in a 19-month-old-girl. Can Assoc Radiol J 1996;47:33-35

Griffith JF, Kumta SM, Chow LTC, et al: Intracortical osteosarcoma. Skeletal Radiol 1998;27:228-232

Hanna SL, Fletcher BD, Parham DM, et al: Muscle edema in musculoskeletal tumors: MR imaging characteristics and clinical significance. J Magn Reson Imaging 1991;1:441-449

Hasegawa T, Shimoda T, Yokoyama R, et al: Intracortical osteoblastic osteosarcoma with oncogenic rickets. Skeletal Radiol 1999;28:41-45

Hopper KD, Moser RP, Haseman DB, et al: Osteosarcomatosis. Radiology 1990;175:233-239

Hudson TM, Schiebler M, Springfield DS, et al: Radiologic imaging of osteosarcoma: role in planning surgical treatment. Skeletal Radiol 1983;10:137-146

Iemoto Y, Ushigome S, Fukunaga M, et al: Case report 679: central low-grade osteosarcoma with foci of dedifferentiation. Skeletal Radiol 1991;20:379-382

Kaste SC, Fuller CE, Saharia A, et al: Pediatric surface osteosarcoma: clinical, pathologic, and radiologic features. Pediatr Blood Cancer 2006;47:152-162

Kaufman RA, Towbin RB: Telangiectatic osteosarcoma simulating the appearance of an aneurysmal bone cyst. Pediatr Radiol 1981; 11:102-104

Murphey MD, Robbin MR, McRae GA, et al: The many faces of osteosarcoma. Radiographics 1997;17:1205-1231

Olson PN, Prewitt L, Griffiths HJ, et al: Case report 703: multifocal osteosarcoma. Skeletal Radiol 1991;20:624-627

Onikul E, Fletcher BD, Parham DM, et al: Accuracy of MR imaging for estimating intraosseous extent of osteosarcoma. AJR Am J Roentgenol 1996;167:1211-1215

Panicek DM, Gatsonis C, Rosenthal DI, et al: CT and MR imaging in the local staging of primary malignant musculoskeletal neoplasms: report of the Radiology Diagnostic Oncology Group. Radiology 1997;202:237-246

Panuel M, Gentet JC, Scheiner C, et al: Physeal and epiphyseal extent of primary malignant bone tumors in childhood: correlation of preoperative MRI and the pathologic examination. Pediatr Radiol 1993;23:421-424

Schima W, Amann G, Stiglbauer R, et al: Preoperative staging of osteosarcoma: efficacy of MR imaging in detecting joint involvement. AJR Am J Roentgenol 1994;163:1171-1175

Sim FH, Kurt A-M, McLeod RA, et al: Case report 628: low-grade central osteosarcoma. Skeletal Radiol 1990;19:457-460

Sundaram M, McGuire MH, Herbold DR: Magnetic resonance imaging of osteosarcoma. Skeletal Radiol 1987;16:23-29

Sundaram M, Totty WG, Kyriakos M, et al: Imaging findings in pseudocystic osteosarcoma. AJR Am J Roentgenol 2001; 176:783-788

Tsuneyoshi M, Dorfman HD: Epiphyseal osteosarcoma: distinguishing features from clear cell chondrosarcoma, chondroblastoma and epiphyseal enchondroma. Am J Surg Pathol 1986;10:754-764

van Zanten TEG, Golding RP, Taets ven Amerongen AHM: Osteosarcoma with calcific mediastinal lymphadenopathy. Pediatr Radiol 1987;17:258-259

Vanel D, Picci P, De Paolis M, et al: Osteosarcoma arising in an exostosis: CT and MRI imaging [Letter to the Editor]. AJR Am J Roentgenol 2001;176:259-260

Weiss A, Khoury JD, Hoffer FA, et al: Telangiectatic osteosarcoma: the St. Jude Children's Research Hospital's experience. Cancer 2007;109:1627-1637

Wetzel LH, Schweiger GD, Lévine E: MR imaging of transarticular skip metastases from distal femoral osteosarcoma. J Comput Assist Tomogr 1990;14:315-317

Ewing Sarcoma

Coombs RJ, Zeiss J, McCann K, et al: Case report 360: multifocal Ewing tumor of the skeletal system. Skeletal Radiol 1986; 15:254-257

Coombs RJ, Zeiss J, Paley KJ, et al: Case report 802: Ewing's tumor of the proximal phalanx of third finger with radiographic progression documented over a 6-year-period. Skeletal Radiol 1993;22:460-463

Daugaard S, Sunda LM, Kamby C, et al: Ewing's sarcoma: a retrospective study of prognostic factors and treatment results. Acta Oncol 1987;26:281-287

Davies AM, Makwana NK, Grimer RJ, et al: Skip metastases in Ewing's sarcoma: a report of three cases. Skeletal Radiol 1997;26:379-384

Ewing J: Diffuse endothelioma of bone. Proc N Y Pathol Soc 1921;21:17; reprinted in Clin Orthop 1984;185:2-5

Hameed M: Small round cell tumors of bone. Arch Pathol Lab Med 2007;13:192-204

Hanna SL, Fletcher BD, Kaste SC, et al: Increased confidence of diagnosis of Ewing sarcoma using T_2-weighted MR images. Magn Reson Imaging 1994;12:559-568

Jaffe R, Santamaria M, Yunis EJ, et al: The neuroectodermal tumor of bone. Am J Surg Pathol 1984;8:885-898

Jürgens H, Exner U, Gadner H, et al: Multidisciplinary treatment of primary Ewing's sarcoma of bone: a 6-year experience of a European cooperative trial. Cancer 1988;61:23-32

Lemmi MA, Fletcher BD, Marina NM, et al: Use of MR imaging to assess results of chemotherapy for Ewing sarcoma. AJR Am J Roentgenol 1990;155:343-346

Kretschmar CS: Ewing's sarcoma and the "peanut" tumors. N Engl J Med 1994;331:325-327

Mueller DL, Grant RM, Riding MD, et al: Cortical saucerization: an unusual imaging finding of Ewing sarcoma. AJR Am J Roentgenol 1994;163:401-403

Reinus WR, Gilula LA, Donaldson S, et al: Prognostic features of Ewing sarcoma on plain radiograph and computed tomography scan after initial treatment: a Pediatric Oncology Group Study (8346). Cancer 1993;72:2503-2510

Shapeero LG, Vanel D, Sundaram M, et al: Periosteal Ewing sarcoma. Radiology 1994;191:825-831

Shirley SK, Gilula LA, Siegal GP, et al: Roentgenographic-pathologic correlation of diffuse sclerosis in Ewing sarcoma of bone. Skeletal Radiol 1984;12:69-78

Taber DS, Libshitz HI, Cohen MA: Treated Ewing sarcoma: radiographic appearance in response, recurrence, and new primaries. AJR Am J Roentgenol 1983;140:753-758

Vanel D, Lacombe M-J, Couanet D, et al: Musculoskeletal tumors: follow-up with MR imaging after treatment with surgery and radiation therapy. Radiology 1987;164:243-245

Wuisman P, Roessner A, Blasius S, et al: (Sub)periosteal Ewing's sarcoma of bone. J Cancer Res Clin Oncol 1992;118:72-74

Chondrosarcoma

Giuliano C, Kauffman WM, Haller JO, et al: Inferior vena cava–right atrial tumor thrombus in malignant pelvic bone tumors in children. Pediatr Radiol 1992;22:206-208

Hanna SL, Magill HL, Parham DM, et al: Childhood chondrosarcoma: MR imaging with gadolinium-DTPA. Magn Reson Imaging 1990;8:669-672

Huvos AG, Marcove RC: Chondrosarcoma in the young: a clinicopathologic analysis of 79 patients younger than 21 years of age. Am J Surg Pathol 1987;11:930-942

Shapeero LG, Vanel D, Couanet D, et al: Extraskeletal mesenchymal chondrosarcoma. Radiology 1993;186:819-826

Young CL, Sim FH, Unni KK, et al: Chondrosarcoma of bone in children. Cancer 1990;66:1641-1648

Primary Osseous Lymphoma

Häussler MD, Fenstermacher MJ, Johnston DA, et al: MRI of primary lymphoma of bone: cortical disorder as a criterion for differential diagnosis. J Magn Reson Imaging 1999;9:93-100

Hicks DG, Gokan T, O'Keefe RJ, et al: Primary lymphoma of bone: correlation of magnetic resonance imaging features with cytokine production by tumor cells. Cancer 1995;75:973-980

Melamed JW, Martinez S, Hoffman CJ: Imaging of primary multifocal osseous lymphoma. Skeletal Radiol 1997;26:35-41

Mouratidis B, Gilday DL, Ash JM: Comparison of bone and ^{67}Ga scintigraphy in the initial diagnosis of bone involvement in children with malignant lymphoma. Nucl Med Commun 1994;15:144-147

Schmidt A-G, Kohn D, Bernhards J, et al: Solitary skeletal lesions as primary manifestations of non-Hodgkin's lymphoma: report of two cases and review of the literature. Arch Orthop Trauma Surg 1994;113:121-128

Stiglbauer S, Augustin I, Kramer J, et al: MRI in the diagnosis of primary lymphoma of bone: correlation with histopathology. J Comput Assist Tomogr 1992;16:248-253

White LM, Schweitzer ME, Khalili K, et al: MR imaging of primary lymphoma of bone: variability of T_2-weighted signal intensity. AJR Am J Roentgenol 1998;170:1243-1247

Disseminated Skeletal Malignancy

Andrich MP, Shalaby-Rana E, Movassaghi N, et al: The role of 131 iodine-metaiodobenzylguanidine scanning in the correlative imaging of patients with neuroblastoma. Pediatrics 1996;97:246-250

Bohndorf K, Benz-Bohm G, Gross-Fengels W, et al: MRI of the knee region in leukemic children: Part I. Initial pattern in patients with untreated disease. Pediatr Radiol 1990;20:179-183

Cohen MD: Imaging of Children with Cancer. St. Louis, Mosby–Year Book, 1992:254

Fisher D, Ruchlemer R, Hiller N, et al: Aggressive bone destruction in acute megakaryocytic leukemia: a rare presentation. Pediatr Radiol 1997;27:20-22

Fletcher BD, Miraldi FD, Cheung N-KV: Comparison of radiolabeled monoclonal antibody and magnetic resonance imaging in the detection of metastatic neuroblastoma in bone marrow: preliminary results. Pediatr Radiol 1989;20:72-75

Kaufman RA, Thrall JH, Keyes JW, et al: False negative bone scans in neuroblastoma metastatic to the ends of long bones. AJR Am J Roentgenol 1978;130:131-135

McKinstry SC, Steiner RE, Young AT, et al: Bone marrow in leukemia and aplastic anemia: MR imaging before, during and after treatment. Radiology 1987;162:701-707

Moody A, Simpson E, Shaw D: Florid radiological appearance of megakaryoblastic leukaemia—an aid to earlier diagnosis. Pediatr Radiol 1989;19:486-488

Moore SG, Gooding CA, Brasch RC, et al: Bone marrow in children with acute lymphocytic leukemia: MR relaxation times. Radiology 1986;160:237-240

Newman AJ, Melhorn DK: Vertebral compression in childhood leukemia. Am J Dis Child 1973;125:863-865

Parker BR, Marglin S, Castellino RA: Skeletal manifestations of leukemia, Hodgkin disease, and non-Hodgkin lymphoma. Semin Roentgenol 1980;15:302-315

Pui MH, Fletcher BD, Langston JW: Granulocytic sarcoma in childhood leukemia: imaging features. Radiology 1994;190:698-702

Shulkin BL, Shapiro B, Hutchinson RJ: Iodine-131-metaiodobenzylguanidine and bone scintigraphy for the detection of neuroblastoma. J Nucl Med 1992;33:1735-1740

Steinbron MM, Heuck AF, Tiling R, et al: Whole-body bone marrow MRI in patients with metastatic disease to the skeletal system. J Comput Assist Tomogr 1999;23:123-129

Tanabe M, Ohnuma N, Iwai J, et al: Bone marrow metastasis of neuroblastoma analyzed by MRI and its influence on prognosis. Med Pediatr Oncol 1995;24:292-299

177 Imaging of Normal and Abnormal Bone Marrow

R. PAUL GUILLERMAN

NORMAL MARROW FUNCTION AND COMPOSITION

Bone marrow is one of the largest and most dynamic tissues in the body. Its functions include the production of red and white blood cells and platelets for tissue oxygenation, cellular immunity, and blood coagulation. Bone marrow occupies approximately 85% of the medullary cavity and is supported by a network of trabecular bone. In addition to hematopoietic elements, it contains stromal cells, collagen, nerves, and a variable amount of fat. On gross examination, bone marrow may be red (because of hemoglobin in the erythrocytes and their precursors), indicating active hematopoietic

marrow, or it may be yellow because of the presence of carotenoid derivatives dissolved in fat droplets in adipocytes. Red marrow is rich in vascular sinusoids, and yellow marrow is considerably less vascular. During periods of decreased hematopoiesis, fat cells increase in size and number, and during periods of increased hematopoiesis, fat cells atrophy. Hematopoietically active red marrow in the neonate contains minimal fat and few adipocytes. The cellularity of bone marrow diminishes most rapidly in the first two decades of life. The cellularity of red marrow is near 100% at birth and decreases to 50% to 75% by 15 years of age. By adulthood, red marrow is composed of approximately 40% fat, 40% water, and 20% protein, and 60% of cells are hemato-

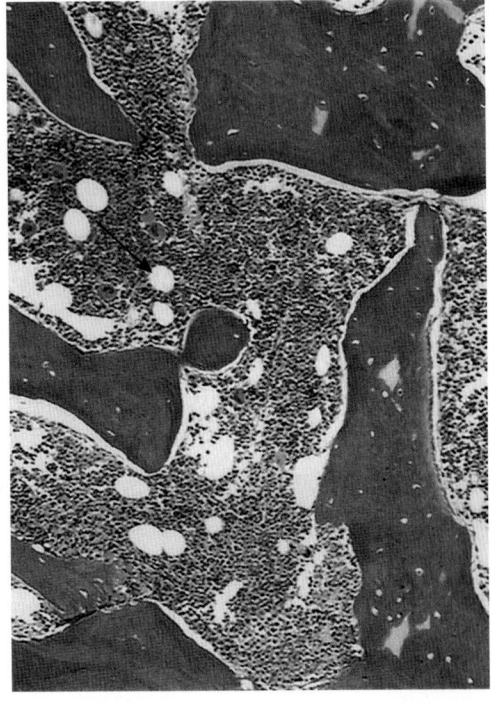
A

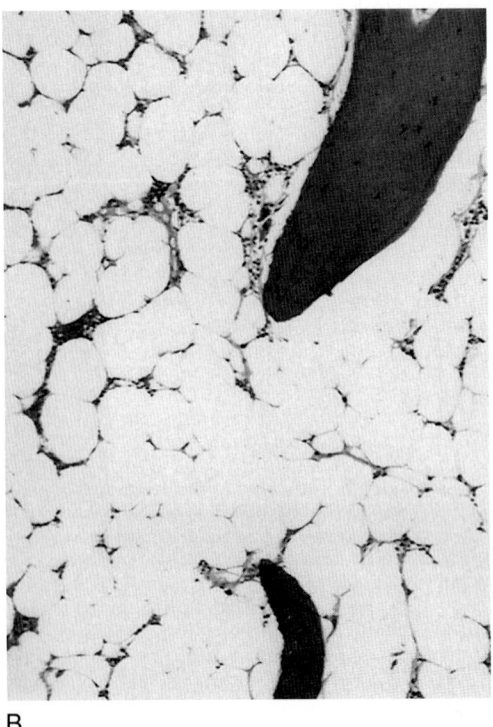
B

FIGURE 177-1. Histologic sections of normal bone marrow (hematoxylin-eosin, ×75). **A,** Hematopoietic elements and bony trabeculae of red marrow with few adipocytes *(arrow).* **B,** Yellow marrow containing numerous adipocytes. (From Babyn PS, Ranson M, McCarville ME: Normal bone marrow: signal characteristics and fatty conversion. Magn Reson Imaging Clin N Am 1998;6:473-495.)

poietic while 40% are adipocytes. In contrast, by adulthood, yellow marrow is composed of 80% fat, 15% water, and 5% protein, and 95% of cells are adipocytes (Fig. 177-1).

> **Red marrow:**
> - **Active in hematopoiesis**
> - **Highly vascularized**
> - **Cellularity diminishes with age.**
>
> **Yellow marrow:**
> - **Hematopoietically quiescent**
> - **Paucity of vasculature**
> - **Predominantly composed of adipocytes and fat**

MARROW IMAGING TECHNIQUE

Magnetic resonance imaging (MRI) is the primary imaging modality used to evaluate bone marrow. It provides a noninvasive method for visualizing the gross anatomic structure of a large sample of bone marrow and for inferring alterations in its chemical and cellular composition related to a variety of physiologic and pathologic processes. MRI can provide valuable information about regions of the bone marrow that are inaccessible or difficult to biopsy.

Constituents of bone marrow that contribute to bone marrow signal characteristics on MRI are fat, water, and, to a lesser extent, mineralized matrix. The proportion of each constituent dictates the signal characteristic of red and yellow marrow. Fat is the predominant contributor to red and yellow marrow signal intensity patterns. Most fat protons are in hydrophobic methylene ($-CH_2-$) groups of relatively heavy molecular complexes responsible for very efficient spin-lattice relaxation, resulting in a short T1 relaxation time and high signal intensity on T1-weighted sequences. The T1 relaxation time of fat varies less with magnetic field strength than do T1 relaxation times of other tissues, resulting in fewer differences in the signal intensity of marrow than are observed in other tissues when MRI scanners of different field strengths are used. The T2 relaxation time of fat is relatively long compared with that of other tissues, but it is much shorter than that of free water protons, and water contributes much more to the signal intensity of red marrow than yellow marrow. The mineralized matrix of bone has a low density of hydrogen protons that lack mobility within the crystalline structure of bone, accounting for very long T1 and short T2 relaxation times and low signal intensity of mineralized matrix on T1- and T2-weighted sequences. In addition, local field gradients at the trabecular surface are generated by the fixed dipole from immobile protons and cause magnetic field inhomogeneity. This magnetic susceptibility effect, as well as that resulting from iron deposition, can play a large role in the signal characteristics of red and yellow marrow on gradient-echo images.

Normal marrow exhibits signal intensity on MRI that varies primarily according to the proportions of fat and water protons. Normal intervertebral disks, skeletal muscle, and subcutaneous fat exhibit little interindividual and intraindividual variation in signal intensity on T1-weighted sequences during childhood; consequently, they serve as convenient internal reference standards for comparison with the signal intensity of marrow. Yellow marrow has a relatively short T1 relaxation time because it is composed predominantly of fat and appears as high signal intensity on conventional spin echo (CSE) T1-weighted sequences. The T1 relaxation time of red marrow is much more variable and depends on relative amounts of fat, water, and protein included. These substances contribute in a complex fashion to production of a longer T1 relaxation time in red marrow, with signal intensity ranging from intermediate to low (less than that of muscle or intervertebral disks) in predominantly hematopoietic marrow to intermediate to high (greater than that of muscle or intervertebral disks but less than that of subcutaneous fat) in hematopoietic marrow with larger proportions of fat. In neonates, red marrow contains minimal fat and has low signal intensity on CSE T1-weighted sequences. With aging, red marrow signal intensity progressively increases on T1-weighted sequences, reflecting a progressive increase in fat content. After the neonatal period, red marrow has signal intensity equal to or slightly greater than that of muscle and the intervertebral disks, but much less than that of subcutaneous fat on CSE T1-weighted sequences. Yellow marrow approaches the signal intensity of subcutaneous fat on CSE T1-weighted sequences. Because of the similar proton densities of red and yellow marrow, proton density sequences are less useful than T1-weighted sequences for evaluating marrow.

On T2-weighted spin echo sequences without fat suppression, the contrast between red and yellow marrow is much less apparent than on T1-weighted sequences, and red marrow shows intermediate signal intensity, similar to that of yellow marrow. Fast spin echo (FSE) or turbo spin echo (TSE) sequences are now routinely acquired in pediatric imaging to shorten imaging times. On FSE T2-weighted sequences without fat suppression, the signal intensity of fatty marrow and subcutaneous fat is higher than on CSE T2-weighted sequences because of J-coupling and magnetization transfer effects. Fat saturation techniques are often used to reduce motion and chemical shift misregistration artifacts, and to nullify the signal from fat to accentuate tissue contrast and enhance the conspicuity of lesions. However, field homogeneity is problematic on fat-suppressed FSE T2-weighted sequences, particularly with large fields-of-view. Short tau inversion recovery (STIR) sequences provide better field homogeneity and are highly sensitive for the detection of lesions associated with marrow edema, but the signal-to-noise ratio is lower and the image acquisition per unit of time is more limited than with FSE T2-weighted sequences. On fat-suppressed FSE T2-weighted and STIR sequences, normal red marrow shows higher signal intensity than yellow marrow and slightly higher signal intensity than muscle.

The signal characteristics of marrow are highly variable on gradient-echo sequences. With gradient-echo sequences, images that exploit chemical shift can be obtained by choosing an echo time when the phases of relaxing water and fat protons are opposed by 180 degrees (opposed-phase sequences) or coincide (in-phase sequences) according to differences in their resonance frequencies. When red marrow contains approximately equivalent amounts of water and fat, as in normal adults, the signal intensity is markedly diminished on opposed-phase T1-weighted sequences compared with in-phase T1-weighted sequences because of intravoxel chemical shift effect. When amounts of fat and water are no longer balanced, for example, in yellow marrow or in edematous or hypercellular red marrow, marrow signal intensity does not show such a profound difference between opposed-phase and in-phase T1-weighted images. Magnetic susceptibility effects from trabecular bone and iron lead to a lower signal intensity of the marrow on gradient echo T2*-weighted sequences than on spin echo sequences.

The degree of enhancement of the signal intensity of normal marrow after intravenous administration of a gadolinium chelate varies with the timing of image acquisition following contrast administration, the age of the patient, and the composition of the marrow. Marrow enhancement peaks within a minute of contrast administration and then slowly declines. Enhancement is greater in children than in adults, greater in the metaphyses than in the epiphyses, and greater in red marrow than in yellow marrow. Enhancement may be imperceptible by visual inspection in the marrow of adults and in the marrow of the epiphyses in those older than 2 years of age. Interindividual variation in degree of enhancement is substantial. If gadolinium-enhanced T1-weighted sequences are acquired without fat suppression, contrast between red and fatty marrow is decreased, potentially obscuring marrow lesions or age-related marrow conversion changes.

Marrow signal intensity on MRI:

- **Largely determined by the proportion of fat in the marrow.**
- **Yellow marrow signal intensity is similar to that of subcutaneous fat on CSE T1-weighted sequences.**
- **Red marrow contains minimal fat in neonates, resulting in low signal intensity on CSE T1-weighted sequences.**
- **Red marrow fat content progressively increases through childhood, with signal intensity on CSE T1-weighted sequences equal to or slightly greater than that of muscle and intervertebral disks, but much less than that of subcutaneous fat.**
- **Red marrow exhibits higher signal intensity than yellow marrow and slightly higher signal intensity than muscle on fat-suppressed FSE T2-weighted and STIR sequences.**
- **Gadolinium enhancement is greater in red marrow than in yellow marrow.**

For a basic MRI protocol for evaluation of bone marrow, the combination of T1-weighted and fat suppressed FSE T2-weighted or STIR sequences is sufficient for the detection and characterization of most marrow lesions. Contrast-enhanced T1-weighted sequences increase the cost and duration of the MRI examination while providing only modest incremental added sensitivity for marrow lesions; these should be reserved for cases with unclear findings on precontrast sequences. Image subtraction and fat suppression techniques facilitate the detection of abnormal marrow enhancement on postcontrast T1-weighted sequences. Gradient echo sequences are valuable for the assessment of the iron content of marrow, and chemical shift techniques are useful for detecting subtle changes in the fat and water fractions of marrow. Because they facilitate evaluation of symmetry and the longitudinal pattern of marrow signal intensity, coronal and sagittal imaging planes are generally preferable to the axial imaging plane.

Practical time constraints previously limited MRI scanning of the marrow to sections of the skeleton. This disadvantage has been mitigated by the development of fast whole-body MRI scanning techniques, including fast spin echo and single shot sequences, parallel imaging, and rolling table platforms with a large field of view. Obscuration of lesions by motion artifact may be overcome to some extent by the use of respiratory triggering or other motion suppression techniques and with higher field strength MRI systems that can ameliorate the lower signal-to-noise ratios in smaller children on whole-body MRI examinations. Fast whole-body MRI has great promise as a technique for global assessment of bone marrow for hematologic disorders or tumor metastases.

NORMAL MARROW DISTRIBUTION AND CONVERSION

Hematopoiesis occurs in the yolk sac during early stages of fetal development; later in gestation, it shifts to the liver and, to a lesser extent, the spleen. Bone marrow begins hematopoiesis in the fourth intrauterine month, overtakes the liver in this function by the sixth month, and is entirely responsible for red cell production by birth. Shortly before birth, conversion from red to yellow marrow begins in the distal phalanges of the hands and feet and proceeds in a centripetal fashion from the distal to the more proximal portions of the appendicular skeleton. Within the long bones, conversion from red to yellow marrow proceeds from the mid-diaphyses to the distal metaphyses and then to the proximal metaphyses. Conversion also progresses from the central medullary canal to the endosteum. Fatty transformation in the epiphyses and apophyses begins almost as soon as they begin to ossify. In infants, the skull and limbs contain about half of the total amount of red marrow. By early adulthood, red marrow is confined to the vertebrae, sternum, ribs, pelvis, skull, proximal humeri, and proximal femora, and approximately one half of bone marrow volume is yellow marrow, which is located primarily in the appendicular skeleton. The involution of red marrow gradually continues throughout adult life, although at a slower pace than during childhood. Different from the case with skeletal maturation, gender differences in rate of marrow conversion are generally not observed during childhood. Knowledge of normal age-related changes in the distribution of red and yellow marrow in the axial and appendicular skeleton is necessary for the recognition of abnormal conversion and reconversion patterns, as well as for the detection of infiltration of the marrow by tumors and other pathologic processes.

> **Marrow conversion from hematopoietic to fatty occurs in a predictable pattern:**
> - **Centripetal in the appendicular skeleton, from distal to proximal**
> - **Diaphyseal to metaphyseal in the long bones**
> - **Soon after onset of ossification in the epiphyses and apophyses**
> - **Faster pace in the appendicular skeleton than in the axial skeleton**

MRI of Marrow Conversion

MRI readily detects conversion from red to yellow marrow because of the high sensitivity of T1-weighted spin echo sequences to fat (Table 177-1). In fact, marrow conversion is observed earlier by MRI than by gross pathologic inspection because of the ability of MRI to detect microscopic fat that is present in marrow. For example, marrow composed of only 20% fat and appearing macroscopically as hematopoietic marrow may show high signal intensity on MRI. Numerous publications detail the temporal and spatial sequences of conversion from red to yellow marrow revealed by MRI. Although discrepancies are apparent among these publi-

cations in terms of the precise ages of transformation, the sequence of conversion is consistent along the long axes of individual bones and in the skeleton as a whole, and it occurs at a faster pace in the appendicular skeleton (i.e., extremities, shoulder, and pelvic girdle) than in the axial skeleton (i.e., skull, spine, ribs, and sternum).

APPENDICULAR SKELETON

Marrow conversion follows a similar pattern in the upper and lower limbs. Within the long bones, conversion initially begins within the diaphysis before it spreads to the metaphysis. In general, low signal intensity marrow on T1-weighted images within the diaphyses of long bones is unusual after 10 years of age. The metaphyseal marrow of the long bones shows high signal intensity on T1-weighted images by 15 to 25 years of age, except for low signal intensity red marrow that may persist through adulthood in the proximal femoral metaphyses, the metaphyses around the knee, and the humeral head, particularly in those with increased hematopoiesis, such as smokers, endurance athletes, and obese women.

Under normal circumstances, epiphyseal ossification centers do not participate in hematopoiesis to any appreciable degree. In early infancy, they are cartilaginous and produce a signal of intermediate intensity on T1-weighted sequences that should not be misinterpreted as abnormal marrow signal intensity. To avoid confusion, the MRI appearance of the epiphyseal ossification centers should be interpreted in conjunction with plain radiographs, when available. Soon after the onset of epiphyseal ossification, low signal intensity bony trabeculae and red marrow begin to be replaced by high signal intensity fatty marrow, with near-complete conversion

---

TABLE 177-1

T1-Weighted Signal Intensities Associated with Bone Marrow Conversion

Marrow Site*	SIGNAL INTENSITY†				
	0-1 yr	1-5 yr	6-10 yr	11-15 yr	15+ yr
Femur					
Diaphysis	L-H	M-H	H	H	H
Proximal metaphysis	L	L	M	M	M
Distal metaphysis	L	M	M	H	H
Epiphyses	L-H	H	H	H	H
Sternum	L	L	M	M	M
Clavicle	L	L	M	M	M
Humerus					
Proximal epiphysis	L-H	H	H	H	H
Proximal metaphysis	L	M	M	M	M
Diaphysis	M	H	H	H	H
Distal metaphysis	L	M	M	H	H
Pelvis	L	M	M	M	M
Vertebrae*	L-I	I-H	H	H	H
Skull					
Clivus	L	L-M	M-H	H	H
Calvarium	L	L-M	M-H	H	H

*Intensity of vertebral bodies compared with intervertebral disks. All other marrow sites compared with muscle (hypointense) and fat (hyperintense).

†H, hyperintense; I, isointense; L, hypointense; M, intermediate or heterogeneous signal intensity. "L-H" and similar indicate a transition signal intensity during the time interval.

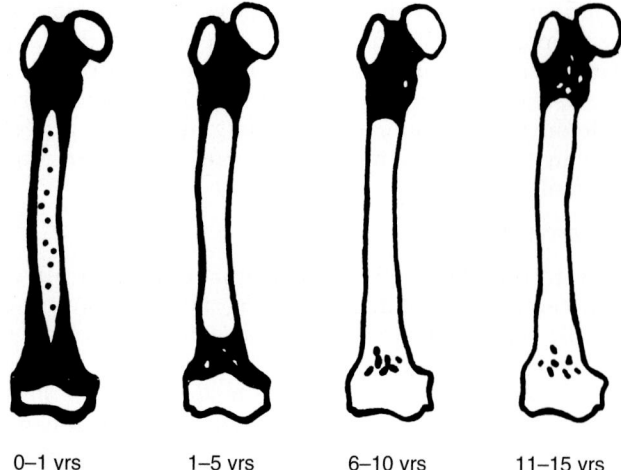

0–1 yrs   1–5 yrs   6–10 yrs   11–15 yrs

FIGURE 177-2. Diagrammatic representation of changes in magnetic resonance imaging appearance of the femoral marrow with increasing age. *Black areas* represent red marrow, *white areas* signify yellow marrow or cartilage, and *stippled areas* indicate heterogeneous red and yellow marrow. (From Waitches G, Zawin JK, Poznanski AK: Sequence and rate of bone marrow conversion in the femora of children as seen on MR imaging: are accepted standards accurate? AJR Am J Roentgenol 1994; 162:1399-1406.)

occurring within 6 to 8 months from onset of ossification of the epiphysis. Hence, fatty marrow appears earlier in the proximal humeral epiphysis than in the femur because of the earlier onset of ossification of the proximal humeral epiphysis. Apophyses and sesamoid bones follow a similar pattern to the epiphyses, with high signal intensity fatty marrow appearing soon after ossification begins.

Conversion in the skeleton first occurs within the phalanges and is complete in the fingers and toes by 1 year of age. Conversion in the femur begins during infancy. High signal intensity fatty marrow is seen in the femoral diaphyses as early as 3 months of age and is commonly observed in this location by 12 months of age. At 1 to 5 years of age, the diaphyseal fat signal becomes homogeneous and the red marrow in the distal femoral metaphyses is replaced by high signal intensity yellow marrow at 6 to 15 years of age (Fig. 177-2). However, a mottled pattern of relatively low signal intensity in the proximal femoral metaphyses may remain present, which is related to persistent red marrow and major stress-bearing bony trabeculae extending from the inferolateral aspect of the femoral neck to the superomedial aspect of the femoral head.

Bone marrow conversion in the humerus follows a similar, predictable pattern. Conversion to fatty marrow with high signal intensity on T1-weighted sequences is complete in the proximal humeral epiphyses by 1 year of age, nearly complete in the diaphyses by 5 years of age, and nearly complete in the distal metaphyses by 10 years of age. Conversion occurs less rapidly in the proximal humeral metaphyses and is nearly complete by 15 years of age. However, low signal intensity red marrow is retained in the proximal humeral metaphyses and subchondral medial aspects of the humeral heads into adulthood, particularly in women. The acromion is formed from a secondary ossification center, which

behaves similarly to an epiphysis in regard to marrow distribution and conversion rate. In the clavicle, marrow is of uniformly low signal intensity on T1-weighted sequences for the first 5 years after birth and then becomes heterogeneously higher in signal intensity, with red marrow persisting into adulthood.

Conversion of marrow in the forearm and foreleg bones lags slightly behind that in the more proximal bones of the arms and thighs. Conversion to yellow marrow begins in the diaphyses between 1 and 5 years of age and is complete in all portions of the forearm and foreleg bones by 10 to 15 years of age. Patellar marrow conversion begins around 4 years of age and is completed by 5 to 10 years of age. Marrow conversion ensues in the tarsal and carpal bones at 2 to 6 months of age and is complete by 6 years of age, with the possible exception of small foci of residual red marrow that persist in the tarsal bones up to 15 years of age.

During the first year after birth, low signal intensity red marrow is seen on T1-weighted images in the pelvis, except for the triradiate cartilage, pubic symphysis, and cartilaginous apophyses, which show intermediate signal intensity. Conversion to fatty marrow in the pelvis initially occurs in the anterior ilium and acetabulum, beginning as early as 2 years of age (Fig. 177-3). In the second decade of life, the remainder of the pelvic marrow increases to intermediate signal intensity. Heterogeneous signal intensity of the pelvic marrow is a normal finding, except in infants, and is most prominent in adolescents and adults in the acetabulum and anterior ilium because of macroscopic foci of hematopoietic and fatty marrow.

AXIAL SKELETON

During the first month after birth, vertebral marrow lacks fat and exhibits uniformly lower signal than do adjacent cartilaginous disks on T1-weighted sequences. Later in infancy, as the vertebral ossification center size increases and the cartilaginous end plates decrease in prominence, vertebral body marrow increases in signal intensity, particularly adjacent to the cartilaginous end plates. Hypointensity of the vertebral body marrow compared with the intervertebral disks and the cartilaginous end plates is seen only up to the age of 1 year. Isointensity or hyperintensity of the vertebral body marrow compared with the intervertebral disks is commonly seen at 1 to 5 years of age. After the age of 5 years, vertebral body marrow signal intensity on T1-weighted sequences is typically greater than that in the intervertebral disks, and a conspicuous band of fatty marrow may appear in the vertebral body centrally or along the basivertebral venous plexus (Fig. 177-4). The spine continues as a site of hematopoietic marrow throughout life, although the proportion of fatty marrow gradually rises by approximately 7% per decade of life.

The skull is the site where the bone marrow is most frequently imaged by MRI during childhood, typically incidentally in studies obtained to evaluate the brain. The skull contains 25% of the active hematopoietic marrow at birth, and conversion from red marrow to yellow marrow begins by 2 years of age within the facial bones and skull base before it proceeds to the calvarium.

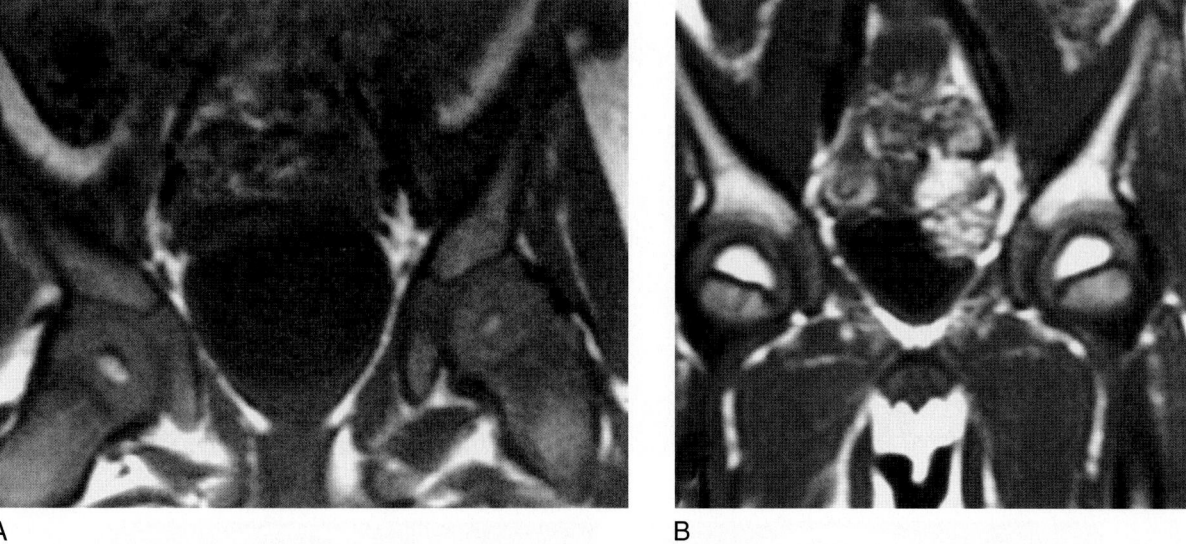

FIGURE 177-3. Coronal T1-weighted MR images of the pelvis. **A,** A 7-month-old girl. **B,** A 3-year-old boy. Note conversion from low signal intensity red marrow to high signal intensity yellow marrow in the acetabulae, anterior ilia, and proximal femoral epiphyses. (From Babyn PS, Ranson M, McCarville ME: Normal bone marrow: signal characteristics and fatty conversion. Magn Reson Imaging Clin N Am 1998;6:473-495.)

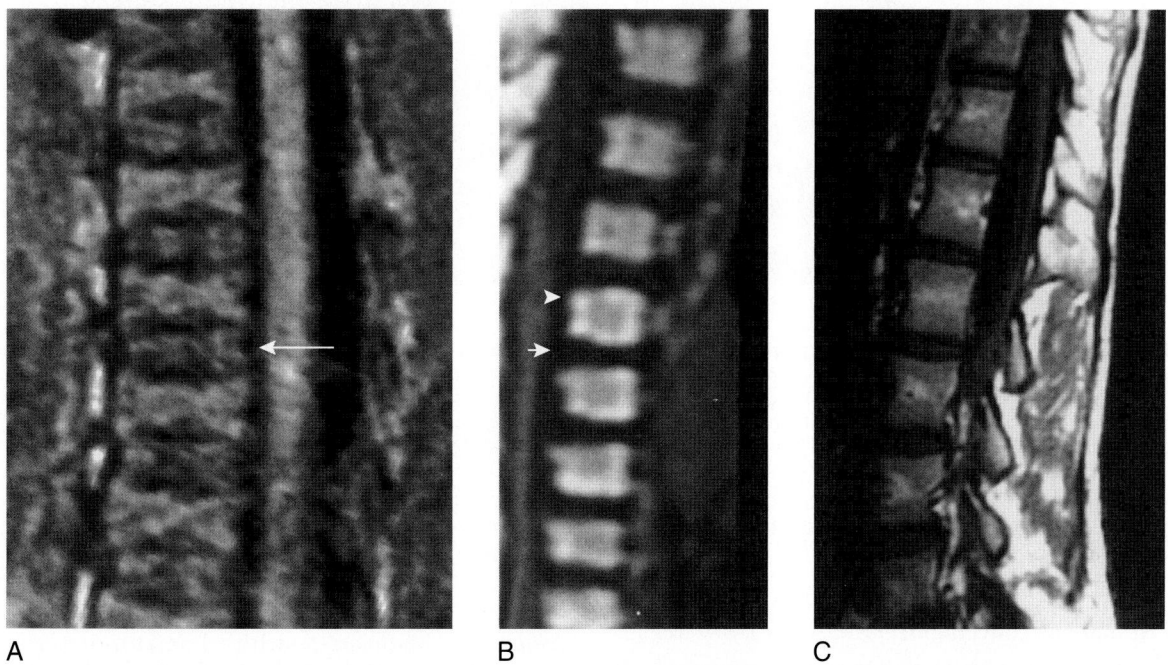

FIGURE 177-4. Sagittal T1-weighted magnetic resonance images of the lumbar spine show increase in signal intensity of vertebral body marrow with age. **A,** A 2-week-old infant. *Arrow* indicates vertebral body. The paucity of marrow fat accounts for the low signal intensity of the marrow of the vertebral bodies relative to the intervertebral disks. **B,** A 3-year-old boy. Vertebral body marrow is hyperintense compared with the intervertebral disks *(arrow)*, particularly the superior *(arrowhead)* and inferior aspects of the vertebral body medullary cavity subadjacent to the cartilaginous end plates. **C,** A 7-year-old boy. Marrow signal intensity is greater than signal intensity of the intervertebral disks; a central band of more fatty, higher signal intensity marrow is seen in the vertebral bodies. (From Babyn PS, Ranson M, McCarville ME: Normal bone marrow: signal characteristics and fatty conversion. Magn Reson Imaging Clin N Am 1998;6:473-495.)

Marrow at the site of the future paranasal sinuses becomes fatty before pneumatization. By 3 to 4 years of age, foci of high signal intensity on T1-weighted sequences are seen in the clivus, and complete conversion is typical by 15 years of age. In the calvarium, conversion begins earlier in the frontal and occipital bones than in parietal bone. Conversion in the calvarium should be obvious by 7 years of age and is complete in the great

majority by 15 years of age (Fig. 177-5). Conversion to fatty marrow in the calvarium may occur more slowly in females, which represents an exception to the rule of no gender differences in rate of marrow conversion.

Marrow conversion in the sternum precedes that in the ribs. Acquisition of intermediate to high signal intensity on T1-weighted sequences occurs in the sternum after 5 years of age and in the ribs by 10 years of

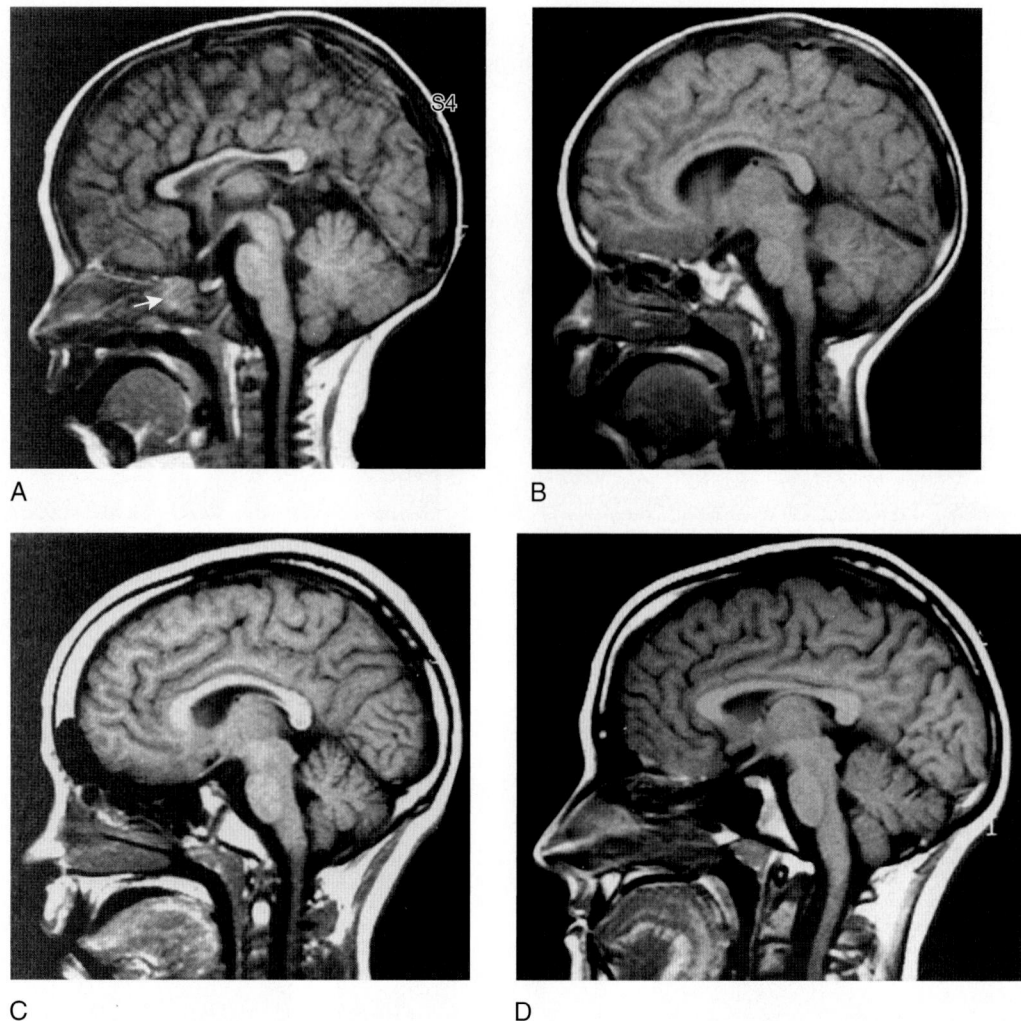

FIGURE 177-5. Sagittal T1-weighted magnetic resonance images of the head in children of ages 1 year (**A**), 3 years (**B**), 11 years (**C**), and 15 years (**D**). Note the minimal high signal intensity within the presphenoid marrow in **A** *(arrow)*. In older children (**B to D**), the marrow of the clivus is predominantly high in signal intensity, indicating conversion to yellow marrow. The calvarial marrow is hypointense at 1 year of age (**A**) and gradually increases in intensity with advancing age. (From Babyn PS, Ranson M, McCarville ME: Normal bone marrow: signal characteristics and fatty conversion. Magn Reson Imaging Clin N Am 1998;6:473-495.)

age. The sternum and the ribs, to a lesser extent, remain hematopoietic into adulthood.

> **MRI of marrow conversion:**
> - **Clearly depicted by T1-weighted spin echo sequences because of their high sensitivity for fat**
> - **Observed earlier by MRI than by gross pathologic inspection**

MARROW DISORDERS

On the basis of signal intensity changes, MRI can detect alterations in the chemical and cellular composition of bone marrow that accompany a variety of physiologic and pathologic processes. Detection of bone marrow lesions is usually easier in fatty marrow than in hematopoietic marrow. Because of the dominant effect of fat on bone marrow signal intensity on T1-weighted sequences,

the processes in which the proportion of fat is decreased relative to other components of the bone marrow appear as a focal or diffuse decrease in bone marrow signal intensity on T1-weighted sequences. These include processes associated with hematopoietic lineage hypercellularity (e.g., hemolytic anemia, hematopoietic growth factor treatment, leukemoid reaction, glycogen storage disease type 1b, myelodysplastic syndrome, leukemia), marrow infiltration (e.g., metastatic tumor cells, inflammatory cells, Gaucher cells), iron overload, and myelofibrosis. Some of these processes are also associated with an increase in free water in the marrow and manifest as abnormal signal intensity higher than that of red or yellow marrow on fat-suppressed FSE T2-weighted or STIR sequences. Signs that favor low marrow signal intensity on T1-weighted sequences as representing physiologic hematopoietic marrow rather than a pathologic process include similar signal intensity to other areas of red marrow on other sequences, signal intensity that is only slightly higher rather than much higher than that of muscle on fat-suppressed FSE

T2-weighted or STIR sequences, normal degree of enhancement on gadolinium-enhanced T1-weighted sequences, symmetry with the contralateral side, and no associated abnormalities of the cortical bone or extraosseous soft tissues. However, a low-grade infiltrative or edematous process of the marrow can be difficult or impossible to distinguish from hematopoietic marrow on MRI, particularly in settings where the hematopoietic marrow is extensive and hypercellular, such as in very young children and in states of marrow reconversion. This difficulty is further compounded by the propensity of some marrow disorders to preferentially involve red marrow because they originate from red marrow, or because the rich vascularity of red marrow favors its involvement over sparsely vascularized yellow marrow.

Processes in which the proportion of fat is increased relative to other components of bone marrow appear as a focal or diffuse increase in bone marrow signal intensity on T1-weighted sequences. This occurs physiologically during aging with conversion from hematopoietically active red marrow to hematopoietically quiescent yellow marrow. A pathologic example is the hematopoietic cell depletion associated with aplastic anemia. Some processes are associated with varying degrees of marrow cellularity and fat content, and their MRI appearances vary correspondingly. These include the myelodysplastic syndromes and the responses of marrow to chemotherapy, radiation therapy, and hematopoietic cell transplantation.

Potential sources of erroneous interpretation of a bone marrow disorder on pediatric MRI examinations are numerous and include ignorance of the normal pattern of marrow conversion, lack of awareness of the higher degree of normal contrast enhancement of marrow in children than adults, confusion of unossified growth cartilage for marrow, and spurious alterations in marrow signal intensity from volume averaging of the marrow with the bony cortex or cartilage, particularly on images of a small structure, such as an epiphysis or a narrow diaphysis in a young child. Patchy foci of marrow edema, commonly seen in the lower extremities in asymptomatic children, are possibly attributable to minor contusions or to physiologic stress response to alterations in weight bearing during growth and development. Those who interpret MRI examinations performed on children should become familiar with normal age-related changes in the distribution of red and yellow marrow and should be capable of recognizing abnormal conversion, reconversion, infiltration, or depletion of marrow.

Alterations in bone marrow composition:
- **Easier to detect in fatty marrow than in hematopoietic marrow**
- **Abnormal low signal intensity on T1-weighted sequences and high signal intensity on T2-weighted or STIR sequences**
  - **Hematopoietic marrow hyperplasia**
  - **Leukemia, lymphoma, and myeloproliferative syndromes**
- **Infiltration by solid tumor metastases or inflammatory cells**
- **Abnormal low signal intensity on T1- and T2-weighted sequences**
  - **Myelofibrosis**
  - **Osteopetrosis**
  - **Iron overload**
- **Abnormal high signal intensity on T1-weighted sequences**
  - **Aplastic anemia**
- **Variable alterations in signal intensity**
  - **Medullary infarction**
  - **Gaucher disease**
  - **Myelodysplastic syndromes**
  - **Response to chemotherapy, radiation therapy, or marrow transplant**

Marrow Hyperplasia and Reconversion

Reconversion is the process by which established yellow marrow is replaced by hyperplastic red marrow in response to conditions that create a demand for increased hematopoiesis. In children, reconversion is commonly encountered in patients with chronic anemia such as from sickle cell disease, thalassemia, and spherocytosis, and in those administered hematopoietic growth factors such as granulocyte colony-stimulating factor (G-CSF), granulocyte-macrophage colony-stimulating factor (GM-CSF), and erythropoietin. The stimulus for enhanced oxygen-carrying capacity of the blood in cyanotic patients with congenital heart disease, endurance athletes, heavy smokers, and high-altitude dwellers also induces red marrow hyperplasia and reconversion. Because marrow conversion is a process that occurs throughout childhood, some of what is construed as reconversion in children actually represents an arrest or delay in conversion from red to yellow marrow that is attributable to increased hematopoietic demands (Fig. 177-6).

Reconversion occurs in the reverse order of normal marrow conversion, beginning in the axial skeleton and limb girdles and proceeding sequentially to the proximal metaphyses, distal metaphyses, and diaphyses of the femora and humeri. The more distal long bones are the last to undergo this process. The epiphyses are usually spared but can undergo reconversion in response to very high hematopoietic demands.

Positron emission tomography with 18-fluorodeoxyglucose (FDG-PET) may reveal increased FDG uptake in areas of marrow hyperplasia, due to the metabolic demands of increased hematopoiesis. The marrow reconversion revealed by MRI is far more extensive than that suggested by technetium-99m phosphonate bone scintigraphy, which shows marrow expansion, predominantly in the metaphyses of long bones. On MRI, reconverted marrow follows the signal intensity of hematopoietic red marrow and tends to involve the appendicular skeleton in a symmetric fashion. The newly formed red marrow may be distributed in a homogeneous or patchy pattern and may have an appearance that overlaps that of patho-

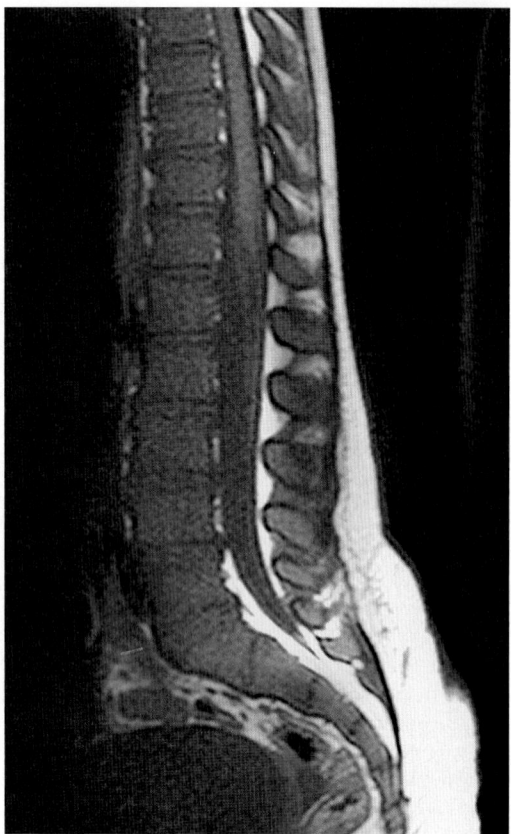

FIGURE 177-6. Sagittal conventional spin echo T1-weighted magnetic resonance image of the lumbar spine in a 7-year-old girl with homozygous sickle cell disease. The marrow signal intensity is lower than is typical for this age, because of the hematopoietic marrow hyperplasia associated with chronic hemolytic anemia.

logic processes with widespread marrow involvement, such as leukemia, disseminated lymphoma, myelodysplastic syndromes, metastases, myelofibrosis, Gaucher disease, and myeloid hyperplasia associated with leukemoid reactions or glycogen storage disease type 1b. Although MRI is very sensitive to changes in marrow fat content, disease specificity is low, and the distinction between reconverted and diseased marrow often requires clinical correlation. Also, some of the conditions that exhibit marrow reconversion consist of additional superimposed marrow processes that complicate MRI interpretation, such as marrow infarction and fibrosis in sickle cell disease and transfusional hemosiderosis in thalassemia.

Marrow reconversion:
- **Replacement of yellow marrow by hyperplastic red marrow**
- **Response to conditions that stimulate increased hematopoiesis**
  - **Chronic hemolytic anemia**
  - **Treatment with hematopoietic growth factors**
  - **Increased oxygen demands or impaired oxygen delivery**

- **Occurs in the reverse order of normal marrow conversion**
- **Can be detected by MRI or FDG-PET**
- **Appearance overlaps that of infiltrative disorders of the marrow**

Thalassemia

Thalassemia is an inherited hemoglobinopathy that is characterized by ineffective erythropoiesis, intramedullary hemolysis, and anemia. FDG-PET in patients with thalassemia shows diffuse increased uptake of FDG by the bone marrow. The appearance of bone marrow on MRI is a reflection of diffuse erythroid marrow hyperplasia, chronic transfusions, and iron chelation therapy. Transfusion therapy suppresses the marrow hyperplasia of thalassemia but at the cost of iron overload. Iron deposition in the marrow results in lowered signal intensity on T1-, T2-, and especially T2*-weighted images due to T2 relaxation time shortening and magnetic susceptibility effects. Iron deposition occurs preferentially in areas of red marrow and is reduced by chelation therapy. However, MRI can still identify excess iron deposition in some of those whose chelation is thought to be clinically adequate on the basis of serum ferritin levels.

Depending on the effectiveness of transfusion therapy, red-to-yellow marrow conversion may proceed in the extremities by puberty, although red marrow hyperplasia in the skull, spine, and pelvis may remain pronounced after puberty, and the paranasal sinuses often fail to develop because of the abrogation of normal fatty conversion of marrow that precedes sinus pneumatization. In severe cases of thalassemia, bone marrow transplantation may be pursued as a potentially curative treatment, and MRI may reveal the consequent degree of marrow conversion (Fig. 177-7).

Sickle Cell Disease

Sickle cell disease is an inherited hemoglobinopathy that is characterized by deformation of red blood cells and resultant hemolytic anemia and intravascular sludging of blood. Bone marrow imaging manifestations of sickle cell disease are primarily related to hematopoietic marrow hyperplasia, infarction, and perivascular fibrosis. Foci of low signal intensity on T1-weighted images and abnormal high intensity on fat-suppressed T2-weighted or STIR images that correlate well with pain in the acute setting commonly represent liquefactive necrosis related to acute medullary infarction (Fig. 177-8). However, acute infarction is depicted by MRI in only about one third of pain crisis episodes, suggesting that ischemia from decreased blood flow often does not lead to infarction that can be detected by conventional MRI techniques. Conversely, similar findings on MRI noted in the absence of musculoskeletal symptoms probably represent subclinical infarcts. Foci of low signal intensity on T1- and T2-weighted images correspond to fibrosis from prior infarcts. Established medullary infarcts of

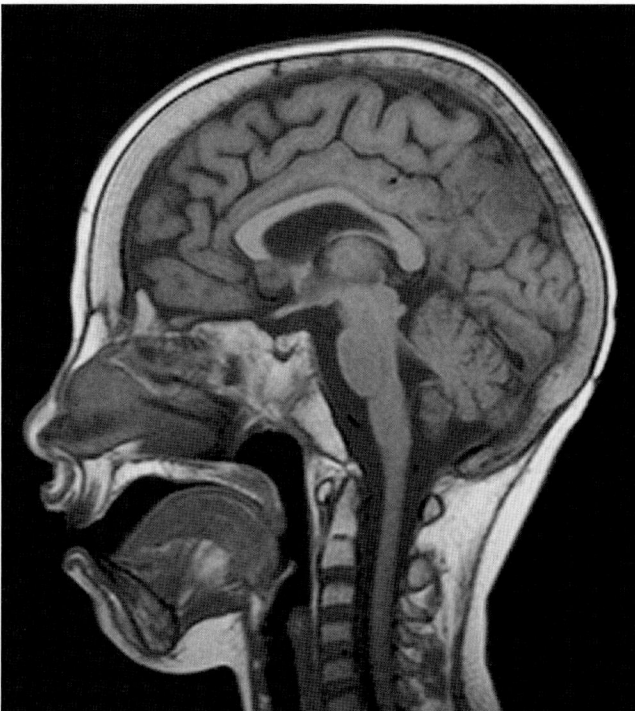

FIGURE 177-7. Sagittal conventional spin echo T1-weighted magnetic resonance image of the head in an 8-year-old girl with β-thalassemia who underwent bone marrow transplantation 6 weeks previous to the MRI examination. The diploic space of the calvarium is expanded by a mix of hematopoietic and fatty marrow, reflecting evolving fatty transformation of chronically hyperplastic marrow in response to recent bone marrow transplantation.

long bones of the extremities typically have a serpiginous margin and are commonly located in the intermediate zone between the end of the bone, which is supplied by epiphyseal arteries and perforating metaphyseal vessels, and the central portion of the shaft, which is supplied by nutrient diaphyseal arteries. Because the circulation normally passes centrifugally from the medullary cavity to the cortex, sludging of blood flow in the nutrient artery branches places increased demands on the radially arranged periosteal-cortical system of anastomosing blood vessels that supply the marrow, particularly in the peripheral subcortical region of the medullary cavity. This, coupled with increased oxygen needs from increased hematopoietic activity, accounts for the vulnerability of the bone marrow to infarction in sickle cell disease. The mottled appearance of the bone marrow on MRI with radially distributed low signal intensity areas worsens with age and represents hyperplastic hematopoietic and infarcted marrow with perivascular fibrosis. Despite chronic intravascular hemolysis in patients with sickle cell disease, iron overload in the marrow is typically seen only in those with a history of chronic transfusions, such as for cerebrovascular stroke risk reduction, and inadequate chelation therapy.

MRI cannot reliably differentiate acute osteomyelitis from the more common event of acute medullary infarction in patients with sickle cell disease. Both entities can manifest with marrow signal intensity abnormalities, periosteal reaction, and intraosseous, subperiosteal, or extraosseous soft tissue fluid collections. However, gadolinium-enhanced MRI can be useful for distinguishing vascularized inflammatory tissue from fluid collections and for guiding the aspiration of fluid collections.

> **Thalassemia and sickle cell disease:**
> - **The appearance of the marrow on MRI reflects the combined effects of red marrow hyperplasia, iron deposition, iron chelation therapy, and, in the case of sickle cell disease, medullary infarcts.**
> - **The MRI appearance of acute medullary infarction in sickle cell disease can be indistinguishable from that of acute osteomyelitis.**

Glyogen Storage Disease Type 1b

Patients with glycogen storage disease type 1b have a propensity to develop bacterial infections related to chronic neutropenia. This is a consequence of a defect in myeloid maturation that leads to bone marrow hypercellularity with hyperplasia of the myelopoietic cells and a leftward shift, although the initial stages of myeloid development are normal.

The signal intensity of bone marrow in patients with glycogen storage disease type 1b varies according to whether G-CSF has been administered for treatment. Without G-CSF treatment, patchy areas of low signal intensity on T1-weighted sequences and high signal intensity on STIR sequences are observed; these reflect patchy areas of myeloid hyperplasia. Almost complete conversion of fatty marrow to hematopoietic marrow is necessary for G-CSF to induce a small increase in circulating neutrophils in these patients; this has been corroborated by the findings of homogeneous low signal intensity on T1-weighted sequences and homogeneous high signal intensity on STIR sequences with G-CSF treatment.

With proton magnetic resonance spectroscopy (MRS), the signal from water protons correlates well with the cellularity of the bone marrow. In patients with glycogen storage disease 1b, with or without G-CSF treatment, strongly increased water signal and very low or nearly absent lipid signal from bone marrow have been observed with proton MRS. This is consistent with highly increased myelopoietic activity, even under basal conditions. Abnormal spectra in patients with glycogen storage disease type 1b are similar to those in patients with hypercellular leukemic marrow infiltration; therefore, proton MRS may not be capable of detecting myelodysplastic transformation and replacing the need for histologic assessment of bone marrow in these patients.

MARROW INFILTRATION

Gaucher Disease Type 1

Gaucher disease, the most prevalent heritable lysosomal storage disorder, results from mutations that confer a deficient level of activity of β-glucocerebrosidase,

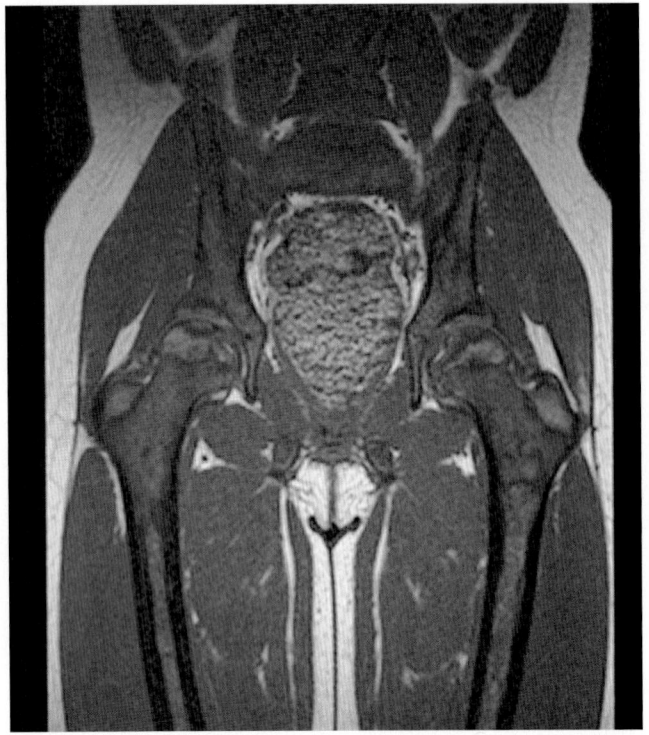

A

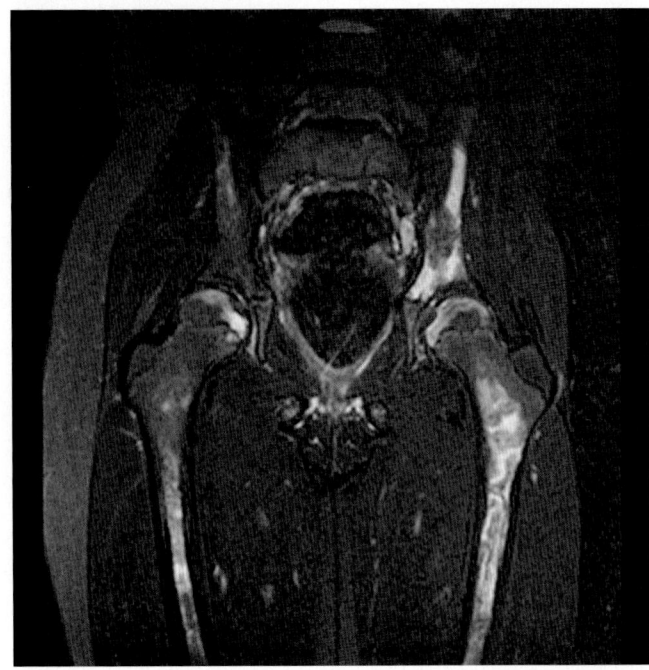

B

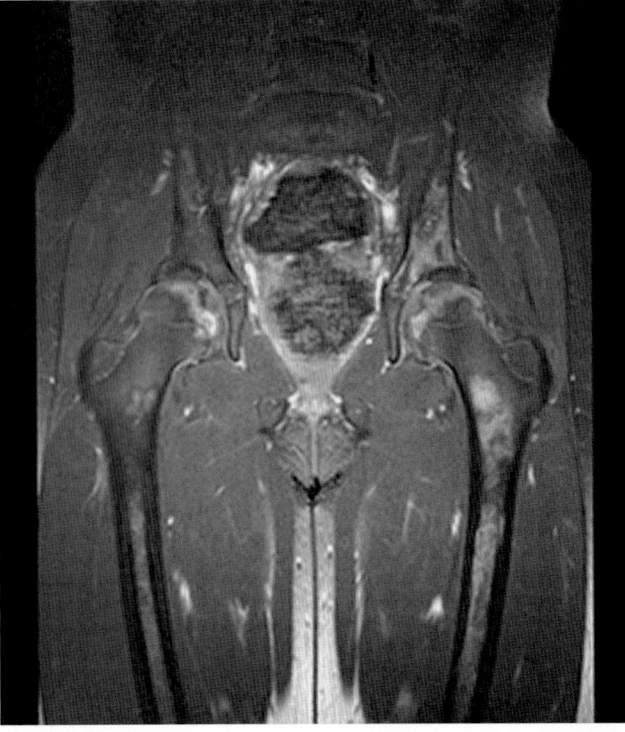

C

FIGURE 177-8. Coronal conventional spin echo T1-weighted (A), turbo spin echo T2-weighted fat-saturated (B), and postgadolinium T1-weighted fat-saturated (C) magnetic resonance imaging (MRI) of the pelvis in a 10-year-old girl with homozygous sickle cell disease who presents with left hip pain and vaso-occlusive crisis. Femoral head avascular necrosis, medullary bone infarcts, hematopoietic marrow hyperplasia, and marrow fibrosis are superimposed, resulting in heterogeneous signal intensity of the marrow that is more pronounced on the symptomatic left side. MRI findings of acute medullary infarction in the setting of vaso-occlusive crisis may be indistinguishable from those of acute osteomyelitis, and clinically occult medullary infarcts are commonly detected on MRI.

leading to accumulation of lipid glucocerebroside in the lysosomes of macrophage-like cells, called *Gaucher cells.* Symptoms and pathology of the type 1 form of Gaucher disease result from the accumulation of Gaucher cells in various organ systems, including the skeletal system.

Patients with Gaucher disease are subject to recurrent painful bone crises, similar to those with sickle cell

disease. Skeletal imaging manifestations relate to marrow infiltration by Gaucher cells, bone infarction, osteosclerosis, osteomyelitis, or fracture. Replacement of fatty marrow by Gaucher cells results in low signal intensity of the marrow on T1- and T2-weighted sequences. The presence of high signal intensity foci on gradient echo T2*-weighted, fat-suppressed FSE T2-weighted or STIR

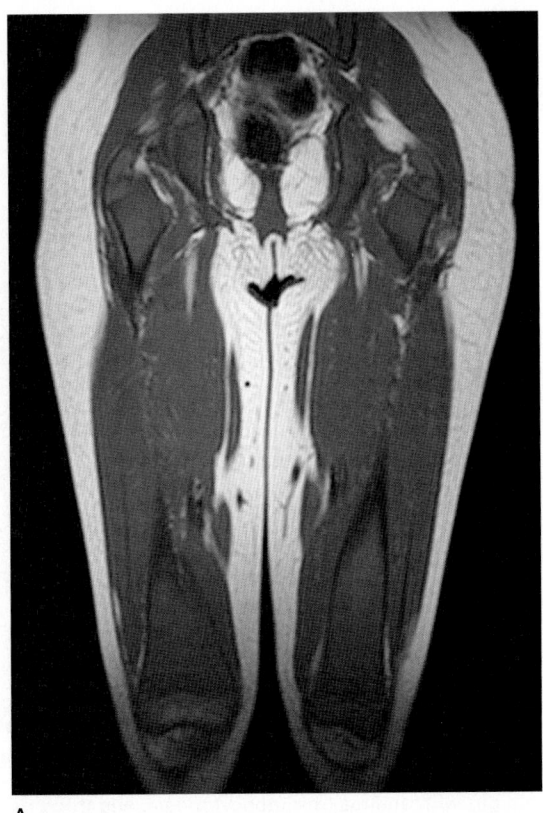

A

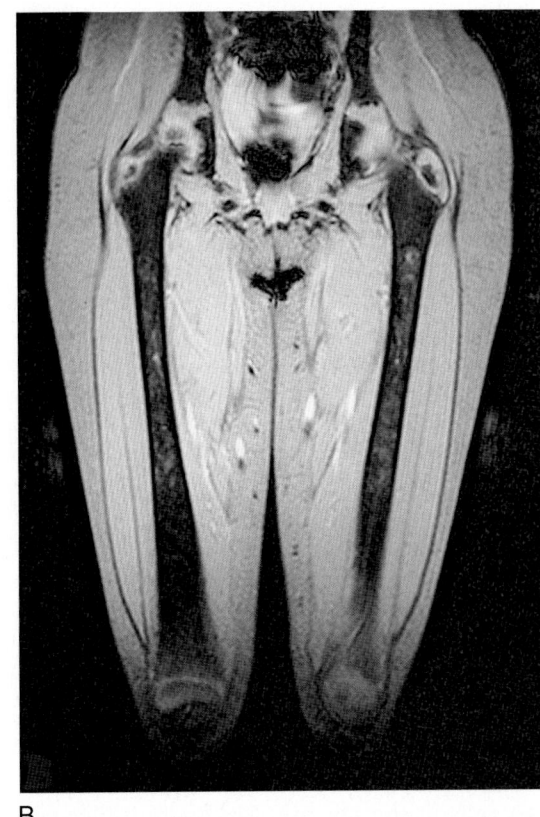

B

FIGURE 177-9. A 5-year-old girl with severe type 1 Gaucher disease, with characteristic undertubulation "Erlenymeyer flask" deformities of the distal femora and diffuse Gaucher cell infiltration and patchy marrow infarction; these account for the diffuse low signal intensity of the marrow on coronal conventional spin echo T1-weighted magnetic resonance imaging (MRI) **(A)** and patchy high signal intensity of the diaphyseal marrow on coronal fast field echo T2*-weighted MRI **(B)**.

sequences may indicate complicating bone infarction or osteomyelitis. Marrow edema induced by local production of proinflammatory cytokines in response to the presence of Gaucher cells is a possible contributing factor to abnormal marrow signal intensity on MRI (Fig. 177-9).

Gaucher disease initially involves the lumbar spine (see Fig. 16E, Chapter 166); the extremities become affected with progression of disease. The epiphyses and apophyses appear less involved than the metaphyses and diaphyses on MRI, except in severe cases. A practical approach for MRI evaluation of the skeleton in Gaucher disease is to image the lumbar spine and the lower extremities with CSE T1-weighted sequences, supplemented by fat-suppressed FSE T2-weighted or STIR sequences, for the detection of complications.

Enzyme replacement therapy results in degradation of Gaucher cell deposits and reconversion to normal fatty marrow. MRI has been advocated to monitor for an increase in the fat fraction of marrow as an indicator of response to therapy, and several MRI-based methods of quantifying bone marrow infiltration in patients with Gaucher disease are under investigation, including Dixon chemical shift imaging, T1 relaxation time calculation, and MRS. However, the normal abundance of red marrow in young children creates difficulty in detecting and quantifying the extent of Gaucher cell infiltration by MRI, and the normal developmental conversion of

red to yellow marrow can be misinterpreted as response to treatment. Also, the appearance of new low signal intensity lesions on T1-weighted sequences in more fatty marrow after enzyme replacement therapy can actually represent old infarcts that were previously obscured by diffusely infiltrated, low signal intensity marrow.

Technetium-99m sulfur colloid scintigraphy is based on uptake of radiocolloids by normal reticuloendothelial cells in the bone marrow; thus, it cannot distinguish between bone marrow infiltrated by Gaucher cells and bone marrow replaced by fibrous tissue. A promising imaging technique for the evaluation of Gaucher cell infiltration and response to enzyme replacement therapy is technetium-99m sestamibi scintigraphy. Sestamibi is a lipophilic compound that is actively accumulated in the mitochondria of glucocerebroside-laden Gaucher cells. In contrast to the pattern of marrow involvement visualized by MRI, technetium-99m sestamibi scintigraphy of the extremities reveals initial involvement of distal femoral epiphyses in the mildest cases, progressively extending to the proximal tibial epiphyses, then to the diaphyseal portion of femora and tibias, and finally, to virtually the entire femora and tibias in the most severe cases. In addition to being highly correlated with other independent parameters of disease severity, technetium-99m sestamibi scintigraphy findings correlate with response to enzyme replacement therapy.

Gaucher disease:

- **Gaucher cells initially infiltrate marrow of the lumbar spine, followed by the extremities, and produce low signal intensity of the marrow on T1-weighted MRI sequences.**

- **High signal intensity foci on fat-suppressed T2-weighted or STIR MRI sequences may represent complicating infarction or osteomyelitis.**

- **The normal abundance of red marrow in young children creates difficulty in determining the extent of Gaucher cell marrow infiltration with the use of MRI.**

Acute Leukemia

As early as 1984, publications emerged that touted the ability of MRI to reveal acute leukemia in children on the basis of alterations in marrow signal intensity. Initial studies focused on quantitative MRI methods and revealed significant prolongation of T1 relaxation time of the marrow in children with acute lymphoblastic leukemia at diagnosis compared with normal controls, as well as correlation of T1 relaxation time with the proportion of blast cells in the marrow. Malignant infiltration of the marrow by leukemia appears as decreased signal intensity on T1-weighted images and increased signal intensity on fat-suppressed T2-weighted and STIR sequences—the inverse of the appearance of normal fatty marrow. Infiltration is often diffuse and includes involvement of the epiphyses (Fig. 177-10). Findings are less conspicuous in red marrow than in yellow marrow and consequently are more difficult to appreciate in younger children, in whom marrow conversion has not yet occurred. The MRI appearance of diffuse cellular infiltration of the marrow in children is not specific for acute leukemia and can also be seen in conditions associated with hematopoietic marrow hyperplasia, in myelodysplastic and myeloproliferative syndromes, and in lymphoma and solid tumor metastases.

MRI is useful in detecting cases of so-called "aleukemic" or "subleukemic" leukemia. A substantial proportion of cases of leukemia present with a normal or low white blood cell count and no blasts on peripheral blood smear; these can masquerade clinically as aplastic anemia, osteomyelitis, or juvenile rheumatoid arthritis for several months. Many of these patients have non-specific bone or joint pain and undergo musculoskeletal MRI examinations that reveal bone marrow infiltration and prompt the correct diagnosis of leukemia.

During chemotherapy for leukemia, the bone marrow becomes hypocellular and edematous. After chemotherapy, regeneration of normal hematopoietic cells and fat is progressive (Fig. 177-11). A marked increase in the marrow fat fraction is observed by chemical shift MRI in the marrow of patients who respond to chemotherapy, and a low marrow fat fraction persists in the setting of unresponsive disease. In children with acute lymphoblastic leukemia who enter remission, marrow T1 relaxation

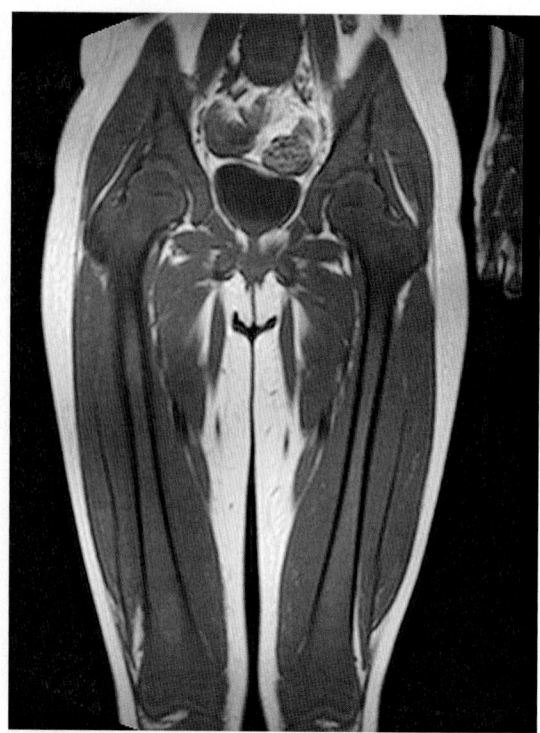

FIGURE 177-10. Coronal conventional spin echo T1-weighted magnetic resonance image of the pelvis and thighs in a 6-year-old girl with anemia, thrombocytopenia, and thigh pain shows diffuse low signal intensity of the bone marrow. Although the metaphyses and portions of the pelvis may show residual red marrow at this age, the low signal intensity of the femoral diaphyses and epiphyses is abnormal and is consistent with a diffusely infiltrative process of the marrow. Bone marrow biopsy revealed acute lymphoblastic leukemia.

time normalizes, whereas marrow T1 relaxation time remains prolonged in those who do not enter remission. These findings imply that MRI could potentially allow earlier prediction of therapeutic response, identification of residual disease, and reduced need for bone marrow biopsy. Relapsed leukemia can be detected by MRI, in some instances several weeks before it is diagnosed by iliac bone marrow aspirate or biopsy, because of iliac marrow sampling bias and earlier relapse in the vertebral marrow than in the iliac crest marrow. However, regenerating hematopoietic marrow can be indistinguishable from residual or recurrent leukemic marrow infiltration on MRI, underscoring the limited specificity of MRI in evaluation of the marrow.

Leukemia:

- **Typically manifests as widespread decreased marrow signal intensity on T1-weighted sequences and increased signal intensity on fat-suppressed T2-weighted and STIR sequences**

- **The MRI appearance can be mimicked by diffuse infiltration of the marrow by metastatic disease, myelodysplastic or myeloproliferative syndromes, or conditions associated with red marrow hyperplasia.**

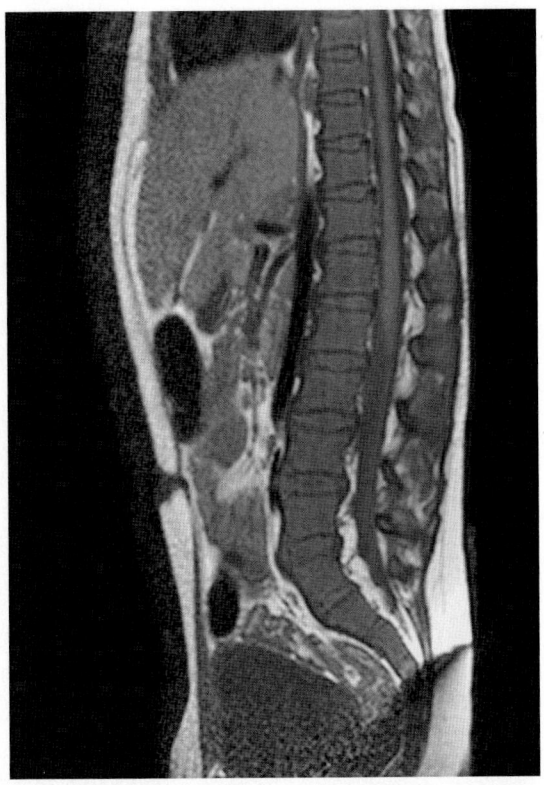
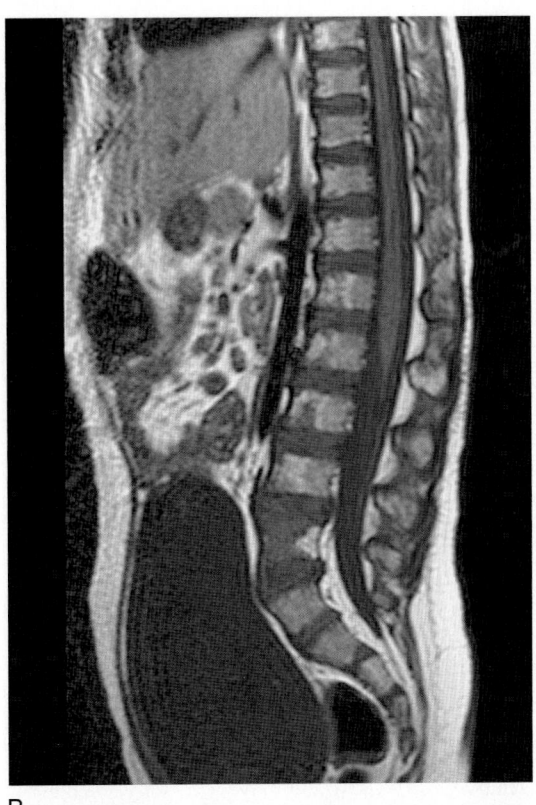

A   B

FIGURE 177-11. Sagittal conventional spin echo T1-weighted magnetic resonance images of the lower spine in a 5-year-old male with Down syndrome and acute lymphoblastic leukemia. At the time of leukemia diagnosis, the marrow is hypercellular because of diffuse infiltration of the marrow by lymphoblasts, resulting in diffuse abnormal low signal intensity of the marrow (**A**). The increase in marrow signal intensity following chemotherapy is consistent with an increase in fat content and a reduction in cellularity of the marrow (**B**).

MYELOPROLIFERATIVE SYNDROMES

The myeloproliferative syndromes (MPSs) of childhood are disorders that are characterized by excessive clonal proliferation of hematopoietic stem cells, resulting in marrow hypercellularity and elevated peripheral blood levels of one or more cell lines. Primary childhood MPS can be classified on the basis of the predominant proliferating cell lineage. Chronic myelogenous leukemia (CML) is granulocytic; juvenile myelomonocytic leukemia (JMML) is monocytic; essential thrombocythemia (ET), familial thrombocytosis, and transient myeloproliferative disorder of Down syndrome (TMD) are megakaryocytic; polycythemia vera and familial erythrocytosis are erythrocytic; idiopathic myelofibrosis (IMF) is fibroblastic; idiopathic hypereosinophilic syndrome (IHES) is eosinophilic; and mastocytosis involves mast cells. These disorders are considered neoplastic, although the transient myeloproliferative disorder that occurs in newborns with Down syndrome undergoes spontaneous remission in most cases within 3 months.

The hypercellular nature of these disorders confers low signal intensity of marrow on T1-weighted sequences. Most of these disorders are associated with high signal intensity on fat-suppressed T2-weighted and STIR sequences, although myelofibrosis can exhibit variable signal intensity, depending on the balance of the opposed effects of marrow hypercellularity and fibrosis.

Lymphoma

Marrow involvement by lymphoma in children is most strongly associated with Burkitt lymphoma, lymphoblastic lymphoma, and lymphocyte-depleted Hodgkin disease. The pattern of involvement is usually multifocal, and there is a predilection for sites of predominantly hematopoietic marrow. Involved sites typically show low signal intensity on T1-weighted sequences and high signal intensity on fat suppressed T2-weighted and STIR sequences (Fig. 177-12). When involvement is diffuse, an arbitrary threshold of neoplastic lymphoid cells constituting 25% or more of marrow cellularity differentiates the diagnosis of lymphoblastic leukemia from that of lymphoma. Although MRI is not part of the routine evaluation of bone marrow in patients with pediatric lymphoma, MRI is more sensitive than Tc-99m phosphonate bone scintigraphy for the detection of marrow involvement by lymphoma. Marrow involvement by lymphoma is often patchy, and up to one third of patients with lymphoma with negative bone marrow biopsies have marrow lymphoma involvement visible by MRI distant from the standard iliac crest biopsy sites.

Although MRI is a sensitive modality for detecting marrow infiltration, it is not routinely used for the staging of lymphoma. Positron emission tomography with 18-fluorodeoxyglucose (FDG-PET) detects lymphoma on the basis of increased glucose transporter activity and

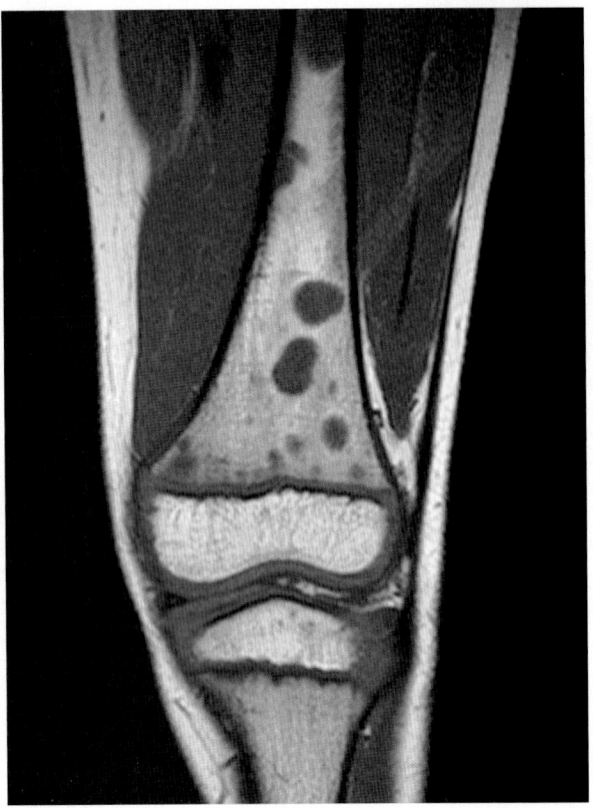
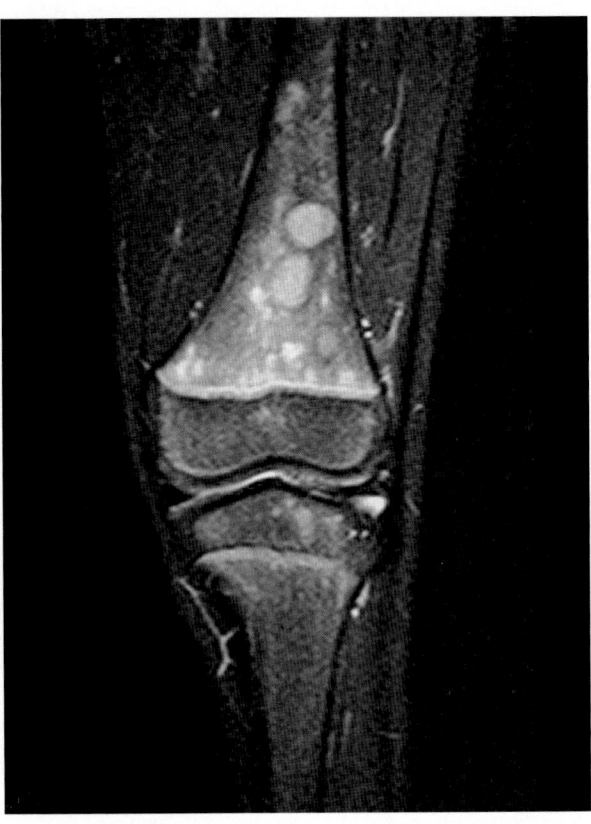

A   B

FIGURE 177-12. Coronal conventional spin echo (CSE) T1-weighted **(A)** and inversion recovery turbo spin echo (IRTSE) **(B)** magnetic resonance images of the left knee obtained on a 6-year-old male with knee pain. Multiple foci of abnormal low signal intensity on the coronal CSE T1-weighted image correspond to the multiple foci of abnormal high signal intensity on the IRTSE coronal image and represent foci of marrow involvement by Burkitt lymphoma subsequently diagnosed on bone marrow biopsy.

glycolysis in lymphoma. FDG-PET is emerging as the functional imaging study of choice for the evaluation of lymphoma and, similar to MRI, is more sensitive than technetium-99m phosphonate bone scintigraphy for the detection of bone marrow involvement by lymphoma. FDG-PET assessment of lymphoma in the marrow after therapy is hampered by reactive changes and the effect of hematopoietic growth factors on the marrow.

Solid Tumor Metastases

Infiltration of the marrow by metastases from solid tumors typically leads to decreased signal intensity of the marrow on T1-weighted images and increased signal intensity on fat-suppressed T2-weighted and STIR sequences. Metastatic infiltration is more difficult to detect by MRI in hematopoietic marrow than in fatty marrow; this is problematic because most skeletal metastases begin as intramedullary lesions in the hematopoietic marrow, and hematopoietic marrow is more extensive in younger children. Metastatic involvement of the marrow usually manifests as multiple focal lesions but can be diffusely infiltrating, most commonly from neuroblastoma (Fig. 177-13), and is also reported in rhabdomyosarcoma and Ewing sarcoma.

In children and adolescents with solid tumors, whole-body MRI has superior sensitivity compared with technetium-99m phosphonate bone scintigraphy for the detection of bone metastases, particularly in the spine, pelvis, and extremities. This is intuitive because the vast majority of bone metastases begin as intramedullary lesions, and MRI allows direct visualization of tumor deposits and tumor-related edema in the marrow before the tumor destroys bone and induces osteoblastic activity. Whole-body MRI identifies additional bone marrow lesions in Langerhans cell histiocytosis compared with radiographic skeletal survey or bone scintigraphy. Although whole-body MRI is capable of detecting tumor involvement of the bone marrow missed by conventional imaging techniques and blind marrow biopsies, the role of whole-body MRI in the routine staging of pediatric tumors remains to be defined.

MRI is more sensitive but less specific than metaiodobenzylguanidine (MIBG) scintigraphy for the detection of infiltration of the bone marrow by neuroblastoma. Although STIR sequences have been reported as the most sensitive in other studies of marrow metastases, a review of a sample of MRI examinations from the Radiology Diagnostic Oncology Group (RDOG) IV study found non–contrast-enhanced T1-weighted sequences to be the most sensitive for neuroblastoma bone marrow metastases but relatively low in specificity. Gadolinium-enhanced T1-weighted sequences were found to be the most specific but relatively low in sensitivity. The accuracy of MRI in detecting metastatic neuroblastoma in bone marrow improves in children 12 months of age

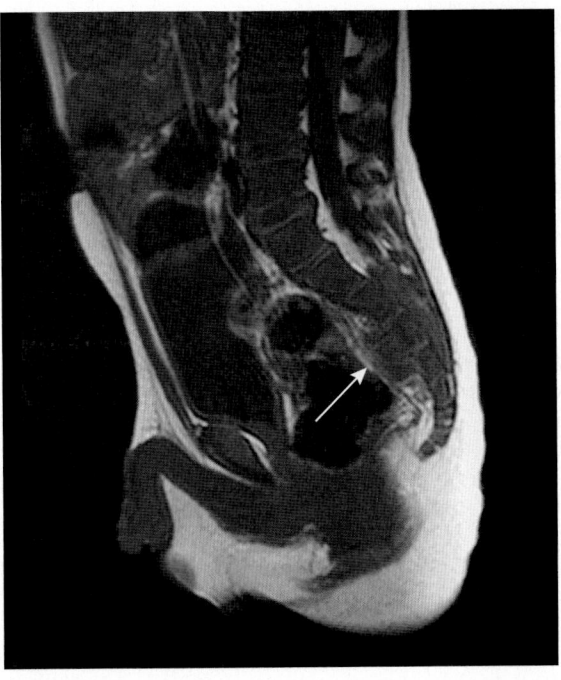

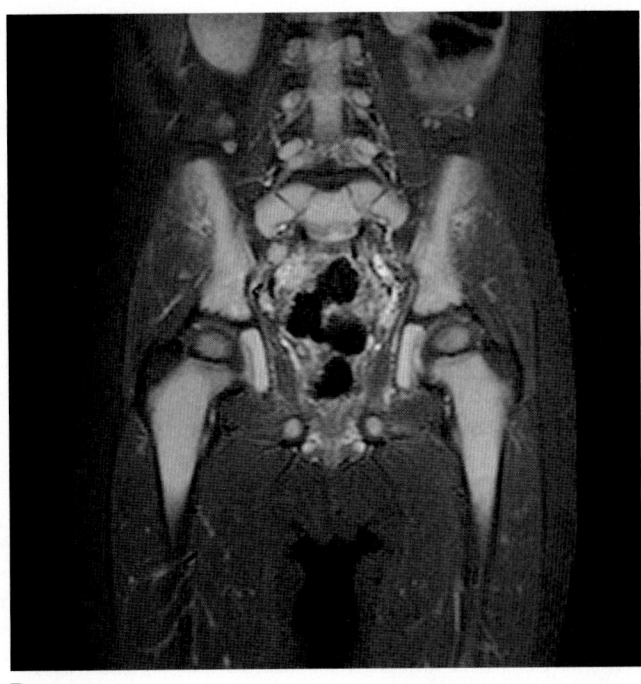

A   B

FIGURE 177-13. Pelvic magnetic resonance imaging examination performed on a 3-year-old boy with constipation reveals diffuse abnormal low signal intensity of the marrow and a perisacral extraosseous soft tissue mass *(arrow)* on a sagittal conventional spin echo T1-weighted image **(A)** and diffuse abnormal high signal intensity of the marrow on a coronal inversion recovery turbo spin echo (IRTSE) image **(B)**, corresponding to a perisacral neuroblastoma with diffuse metastatic involvement of the bone marrow.

and older, likely because of the increased proportion of yellow to red marrow and easier detection of lesions within yellow marrow than in red marrow.

FDG-PET is capable of detecting early marrow involvement by metastases because tumor generally has higher glucose utilization and FDG uptake than does normal marrow. Tumor metabolism is highly susceptible to chemotherapy, and false-negative findings for marrow metastases may occur if FDG-PET is obtained after initiation of chemotherapy. FDG-PET is less hindered by nonspecific uptake in incidental benign bone lesions compared with technetium-99m phosphonate bone scintigraphy. However, increased FDG uptake may occasionally be detected in benign lesions, especially those that contain abundant histiocytes or giant cells, and correlative radiographs should be obtained as appropriate to avoid false-positive interpretation of marrow metastases. FDG-PET has been reported to have superior sensitivity to whole-body MRI for the detection of skeletal metastases in children and adolescents with solid tumors. MRI and FDG-PET are thus complementary imaging modalities for the detection of bone metastases; most false-negative findings with FDG-PET occur in the skull and are related to obscuration by high physiologic glucose utilization of the adjacent brain. Most false-negative findings with whole-body MRI occur in the small bones, skull, and ribs and are related to signal-to-noise limitations and motion artifact.

The American College of Radiology Imaging Network (ACRIN) is sponsoring a prospective multi-institutional trial designed to compare the diagnostic performance of fast whole-body MRI versus conventional imaging (MIBG or bone scintigraphy) and FDG-PET in detecting metastases, including those in bone marrow, and in the staging of pediatric small cell solid tumors, such as neuroblastoma, rhabdomyosarcoma, and Ewing sarcoma. Whole-body MRI sequences include fast STIR and gradient-echo T1-weighted in-phase sequences (IPSs), in which the signal intensity is a summation of fat and water, and opposed out-of-phase sequences (OOPSs), in which equal fractions of fat and water are nullified, to maximize sensitivity and specificity and minimize imaging time. The MRI protocol is based on the premises that bone marrow that has only fat, such as that in the epiphyses, is bright on IPS and OOPS and dark on STIR, that bone marrow that has mixed fat and water is brighter on IPS than on OOPS and is intermediate signal intensity on STIR, and that metastases, which have water and lack fat, are as bright on OOPS as on IPS and brighter on STIR sequences than is normal marrow.

Evaluation of marrow by MRI for response to therapy and residual or recurrent metastatic disease is fraught with difficulty because of multiple potential confounding factors that may influence the signal intensity of bone marrow. Metastatic lesions may exhibit edema, hemorrhage, and necrosis in response to antitumor therapy, and myelofibrosis and alterations in the cellular and chemical composition of marrow can occur in response to antitumor therapy. In addition, marrow signal intensity changes that relate to transfusional hemosiderosis and marrow regeneration, possibly augmented by administration of hematopoietic growth factors, must be considered. Evaluation of bone marrow by FDG-PET is susceptible to similar limitations following chemotherapy and radiotherapy, and FDG uptake by regenerating red marrow is increased by hematopoietic growth factor administration, potentially masking malignant infiltration.

In patients with a history of neoplasm and a vertebral compression fracture, differentiation of a metastatic fracture versus insufficiency or traumatic fracture of the vertebra can be problematic because edema and contrast enhancement are observed in all of these conditions. Signs of metastatic fractures reported in adults include multifocal involvement of nonfractured vertebrae, infiltration of posterior elements or the entire vertebral body, sharply defined lesion borders, and a paravertebral or epidural soft tissue mass. The reliability of these signs in children is uncertain. In the case of vertebral collapse related to Langerhans cell histiocytosis, MRI or FDG-PET may be of help in differentiating active lesions from inactive healed lesions. Plain radiographs and bone scintigraphy are relatively slow in showing healing and may appear abnormal long after the lesion has become quiescent. On MRI, inactive healed lesions show mild hyperintensity of the marrow on T1-weighted sequences; active lesions show low signal intensity on T1-weighted sequences and high signal intensity on T2-weighted sequences. FDG-PET shows increased FDG uptake in active lesions and normalization of FDG in healing lesions well in advance of scintigraphic and radiographic changes.

Metastatic involvement of the marrow:

- **More difficult to detect by MRI in hematopoietic marrow than in fatty marrow.**

- **Usually multifocal but can be diffuse, most commonly from neuroblastoma.**

- **MRI is more sensitive but less specific than MIBG scintigraphy for infiltration of the marrow by neuroblastoma.**

- **Because of the effects of tumor treatment on marrow, imaging is of limited usefulness in assessing for residual metastatic disease in the marrow.**

MARROW DEPLETION AND FAILURE

A variety of disorders can reduce the amount of functioning hematopoietic tissue in the bone marrow. If hematopoietic stem cells are destroyed or altered, marrow failure or dysplasia can result, as in aplastic anemia and the myelodysplastic syndromes. In some cases, the inciting event is known and may include toxic effects of radiation, chemotherapy, or other drugs or chemicals, or extensive marrow infiltration by neoplastic or inflammatory cells and suppression or hemophagocytosis of normal hematopoietic cells. In many cases, the inciting event is unknown but is thought to be immunologically mediated. Aplastic or hypoplastic marrow exhibits high signal intensity on T1-weighted MRI sequences, related to replacement of hematopoietic marrow with fatty marrow. Fibrosis can accompany conditions associated with bone marrow depletion and appears as low signal intensity areas on all MRI sequences.

Aplastic Anemia

The incidence of idiopathic aplastic anemia peaks in adolescents and young adults. An incidence spike of aplastic anemia also occurs earlier in childhood; this is related to inherited marrow failure syndromes such as Fanconi anemia that are often accompanied by skeletal anomalies. Aplastic anemia is treated with bone marrow transplantation or immunosuppressants, and blood transfusions are used for supportive care.

Because of the paucity of hematopoietic cellular elements and the presence of abundant marrow fat, the signal intensity of bone marrow on MRI sequences in untreated aplastic anemia approaches that of subcutaneous fat (Fig. 177-14). This is easiest to appreciate in regions that normally have a relatively greater abundance of hematopoietic marrow, such as the axial skeleton and pelvis, and may be indistinguishable from normal fatty marrow in other regions of the skeleton. Because the signal intensity of bone marrow on MRI sequences reflects the relative proportion of fat and water protons and increased cellularity correlates with a higher fraction of water relative to fat, MRI can serve as a noninvasive method for determining hematopoietic cell status and therapeutic response in aplastic anemia. After treatment, islands of regenerating hematopoietic marrow in the fatty marrow appear as low signal intensity foci on T1-weighted MRI sequences.

The characteristic fatty appearance of aplastic marrow may not be observed in the presence of transfusional hemosiderosis because iron deposition causes a decrease

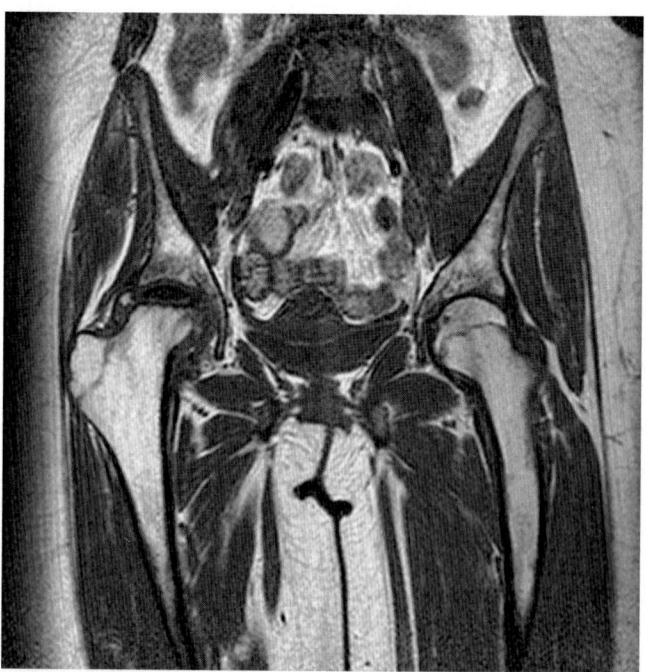

FIGURE 177-14. Coronal conventional spin echo T1-weighted image of the pelvis in a 17-year-old female with aplastic anemia and right femoral head avascular necrosis. Diffuse hypocellular fatty marrow is present that is equivalent in signal intensity to the subcutaneous fat, including the marrow of the proximal femoral metaphyses that normally contain residual red marrow at this age. Low signal and decreased height of the right femoral head are due to avascular necrosis.

in signal intensity of bone marrow on T1-weighted, T2-weighted, and particularly T2*-weighted sequences. In the absence of transfusional hemosiderosis, the presence of focal or diffuse loss of high marrow signal intensity on T1-weighted images may indicate the development of clonal disease (myelodysplastic syndrome or leukemia). Foci of hypercellular marrow due to clonal disease are difficult to differentiate from foci of regenerative hematopoietic marrow following treatment for aplastic anemia. Therefore, the patient's treatment and transfusion history must be considered for proper MRI interpretation to result. If there is clinical concern for clonal disease, MRI can help guide marrow sampling procedures to sites of relatively hypercellular marrow to enhance diagnostic yield.

> **Aplastic anemia:**
> - **MRI may reveal abnormal high marrow signal intensity on T1-weighted sequences, reflecting diminished hematopoietic marrow.**
> - **Loss of high marrow signal intensity on T1-weighted sequences suggests transfusional hemosiderosis, regenerative hematopoietic marrow, or development of clonal disease (myelodysplastic syndrome or leukemia).**

Myelodysplastic Syndromes

Myelodysplastic syndromes (MDSs) are disorders that are characterized by peripheral blood cytopenia and ineffective, dysplastic hematopoiesis. Cytogenetic abnormalities are common, and the risk of acute myelogenous leukemia (AML) is elevated. The marrow is most commonly hypercellular in MDS, but it can be hypocellular. Hypocellular marrow with scattered foci of dysplastic hematopoiesis may be misinterpreted as aplastic anemia if the bone marrow biopsy specimen is small and is not representative of the remainder of the marrow. The ability of MRI to distinguish patients with hypoplastic MDS from those with aplastic anemia rests on the finding in MDS of nodular or patchy foci of hematopoietic marrow superimposed on an otherwise diffuse background of fatty marrow.

The bone marrow blast count has a major influence on prognosis in MDS, but reduction in marrow signal intensity on T1-weighted sequences does not correlate with the percentage blast count, in contrast to the case with acute leukemia; this argues against the use of MRI for risk stratification of patients with MDS. The signal intensity of marrow shows an association with the percentage bone marrow cellularity in MDS, and the development of increased nodular or diffuse low signal intensity on T1-weighted sequences and abnormally high signal intensity on STIR suggests evolution to acute leukemia. Excess iron deposition in the marrow from frequent transfusions given for the supportive care of patients with MDS results in reduced marrow signal intensity on T1-weighted sequences that may mask or mimic the signal intensity reduction associated with marrow hypercellularity.

Myelofibrosis

Myelofibrosis is a process that is characterized by replacement of normal marrow by fibrotic tissue. In some cases, myelosclerosis (intramedullary bone formation) accompanies myelofibrosis. In children, myelofibrosis usually results from radiotherapy, chemotherapy, or neoplastic infiltration of the marrow. Idiopathic myelofibrosis is a rare clonal myeloproliferative disorder that is accompanied by elaboration of cytokines and growth factors that induce marrow fibrosis. Depending on the phase of the disorder, the marrow may be hypercellular or depleted of hematopoietic cells. Because of the range of cellularity, marrow signal intensity on MRI is variable, with fibrotic areas showing low signal intensity on all sequences.

Osteopetrosis

Osteopetrosis is a heterogeneous group of hereditary diseases characterized by abnormal osteoclast activity, defective resorption of bone, and bone sclerosis with obliteration of the marrow in the medullary cavity. The radiographic findings of osteopetrosis are presented in Chapter 165. Technetium-99m sulfur colloid scintigraphy has revealed age-dependent patterns of abnormal bone marrow distribution in the severe autosomal recessive form of the disease. In affected infants, functional marrow is found primarily in the skull base and at the ends of long bones. In patients 3 to 5 years of age, functional marrow shifts to the diaphyseal regions of long bones and to the calvarium. In older children, the calvarial diploic space is broadened with a radiographic "hair-on-end" appearance that corresponds to areas of marked hematopoietic activity on bone marrow scintigraphy. Regions of sclerotic bone show low signal intensity on T1-weighted and T2-weighted MRI sequences. Severe autosomal recessive forms of osteopetrosis can be treated by allogeneic bone marrow transplantation. Follow-up MRI after successful bone marrow transplantation shows normalization of bone marrow signal intensity.

Bone Marrow Infarction

Although it is often asymptomatic and rarely is extensive enough to impair hematopoietic function, bone marrow infarction can cause pain and disability. Epiphyseal involvement in a weight-bearing joint poses the risk of significant morbidity from articular surface collapse and degenerative joint disease. Conditions associated with an increased risk of bone marrow infarction include sickle cell disease, Gaucher disease, chronic renal failure, bone marrow transplantation, steroid therapy, pancreatitis, and highly active antiretroviral therapy for HIV infection. Putative pathophysiologic mechanisms include vascular occlusion, elevated medullary cavity pressure, coagulopathy, and altered lipid metabolism. Bone marrow infarcts most commonly occur in regions of fatty marrow and are unusual in hematopoietic marrow, except in patients with a hemoglobinopathy, possibly because of the greater vascular reserve of hematopoietic marrow compared with fatty marrow. The most commonly affected sites are the femoral, tibial, and humeral diametaphyses and epiphyses and the pelvis.

The acute phase of infarction is characterized by marrow hemorrhage, edema, and liquefactive necrosis. Marrow fibrosis and bony sclerosis later ensue. The infarction often has a geographic shape with a serpiginous margin of low signal intensity on T1-weighted sequences. T2-weighted sequences may reveal a characteristic "double line sign" that consists of an outer low signal intensity rim corresponding to sclerotic bone and an inner rim of high signal intensity corresponding to vascularized granulation tissue or chondroid metaplasia. Areas of low signal intensity on T1- and T2-weighted sequences in mature infarcts represent fibrosis or calcification. Intense contrast enhancement is commonly seen at the periphery of evolving infarcts, and dynamic contrast-enhanced MRI has been touted for early diagnosis, although the diagnosis can usually be confidently made on conventional MRI sequences without intravenous contrast (Fig. 177-15).

Bone Marrow Infarction

Associated Conditions

- **Sickle cell disease**
- **Gaucher disease**
- **Chronic renal failure**
- **Bone marrow transplantation**
- **Pancreatitis**

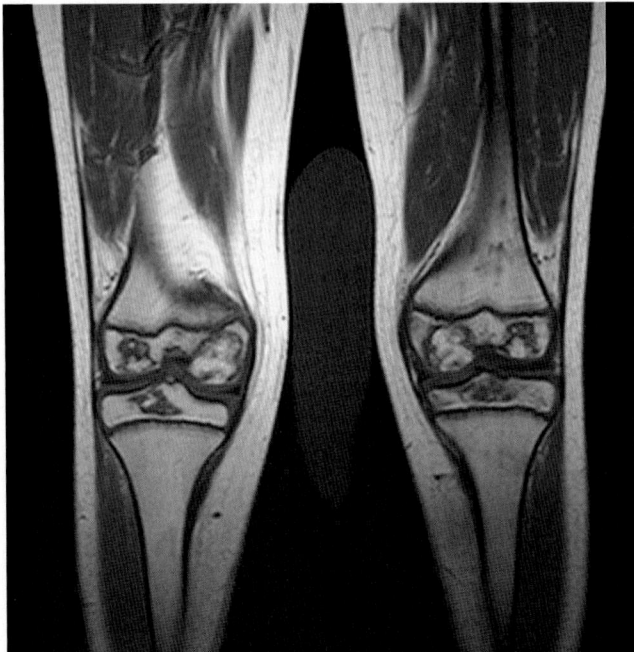

FIGURE 177-15. Coronal conventional spin echo T1-weighted magnetic resonance image of the knees in a 10-year-old girl with knee pain and a history of high-dose pulse steroid therapy for constrictive bronchiolitis. Well-marginated lesions with low signal intensity serpiginous borders characteristic of bone infarcts are present in the epiphyses of the distal femora and the proximal tibias bilaterally.

- **Steroid therapy**
- **Antiretroviral therapy for HIV infection**

Unusual in hematopoietic marrow, except in patients with hemoglobinopathy

---

EFFECTS OF THERAPY

Hematopoietic Growth Factors

Hematopoietic growth factors such as G-CSF, GM-CSF, and erythropoietin are cytokines that regulate the proliferation and differentiation of hematopoietic progenitor cells in the bone marrow. Recombinant human hematopoietic growth factors are commonly used to hasten the recovery of hematopoietic marrow from myelosuppressive chemotherapy or bone marrow failure syndromes, and to stimulate more effective myelopoiesis in glycogen storage disease type 1b.

In those treated with G-CSF or GM-CSF, MRI shows signal intensity changes associated with reconversion of fatty marrow to hypercellular hematopoietic marrow that coincide temporally with increases in absolute neutrophil count. These changes may be observed incidentally on routine imaging studies or on imaging studies prompted by bone pain accompanying G-CSF administration. As in other instances of marrow hyperplasia, imaging changes comprise diminished signal intensity on T1-weighted images and increased signal intensity on fat suppressed T2-weighted and STIR images. Increased enhancement of the marrow may be observed on gadolinium-enhanced T1-weighted sequences. Gradient echo out-of-phase sequences designed to detect altered proportions of fat and water may be most sensitive for the effects of G-CSF therapy on bone marrow. The peak of hematopoietic marrow hyperplasia observed by MRI occurs about 2 weeks after discontinuation of G-CSF administration, and bone marrow alterations normalize in most patients within 6 weeks after treatment. Marrow changes may be diffuse or patchy and can be asymmetric and simulate bone marrow involvement by leukemia, metastatic disease, or other infiltrative process. Changes can also obscure marrow lesions. Consideration of the timing of therapy and imaging is necessary to avoid misinterpretation of marrow changes (Fig. 177-16).

Similarly, FDG-PET, technetium-99m sulfur colloid scintigraphy, gallium-67 scintigraphy, and thallium-201 scintigraphy can show elevated radiopharmaceutical uptake by stimulated hematopoietic marrow (Fig. 177-17). Large interindividual variability is noted in marrow FDG uptake induced by hematopoietic growth factors. FDG uptake by the marrow returns to normal within 1 month after discontinuation of G-CSF treatment in most individuals. The effect of hematopoietic growth factors on marrow uptake of FDG also varies with the intensity of chemotherapy. In many patients treated with high-dose chemotherapy followed by bone marrow or stem cell transplantation and G-CSF or GM-CSF treatment, no significant increase is seen in marrow uptake of FDG. High-dose chemotherapy decreases the bone marrow reserve more markedly than does conventional-dose

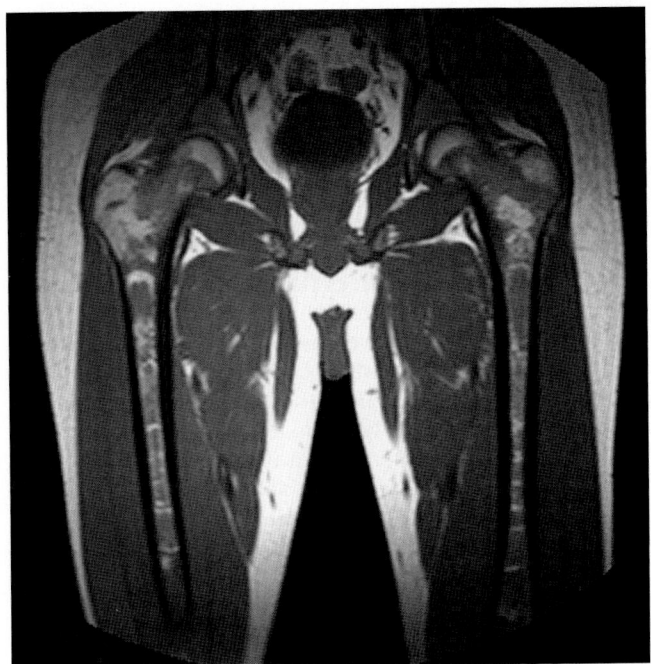
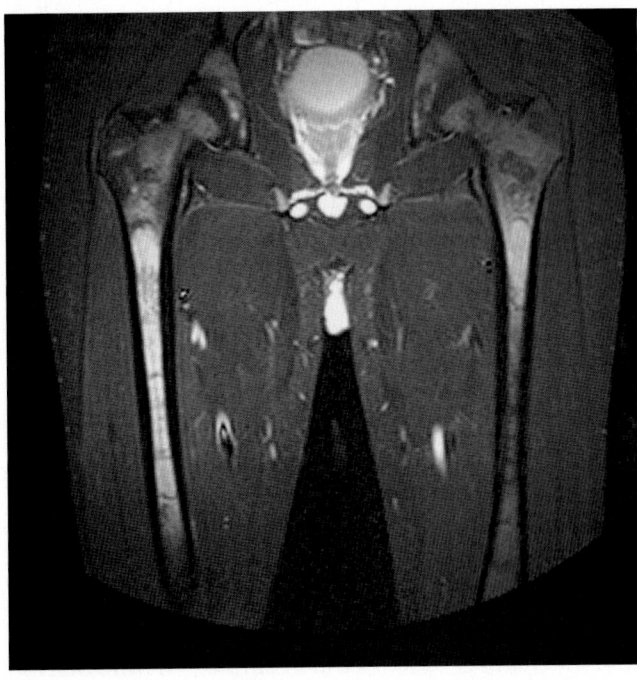

A   B

FIGURE 177-16. Coronal conventional spin echo T1-weighted **(A)** and coronal inversion recovery turbo spin echo (IRTSE) **(B)** magnetic resonance images of the thighs in a 17-year-old male on granulocyte colony-stimulating factor (G-CSF) therapy for myelosuppression related to chemotherapy for Hodgkin disease. Patchy bilateral foci of low signal intensity on the T1-weighted image and high signal intensity on the IRTSE image in the marrow represent regenerating granulopoietic marrow in response to G-CSF stimulation. Clinical correlation with the timing of therapy and imaging is necessary to distinguish these findings from neoplastic involvement of the marrow.

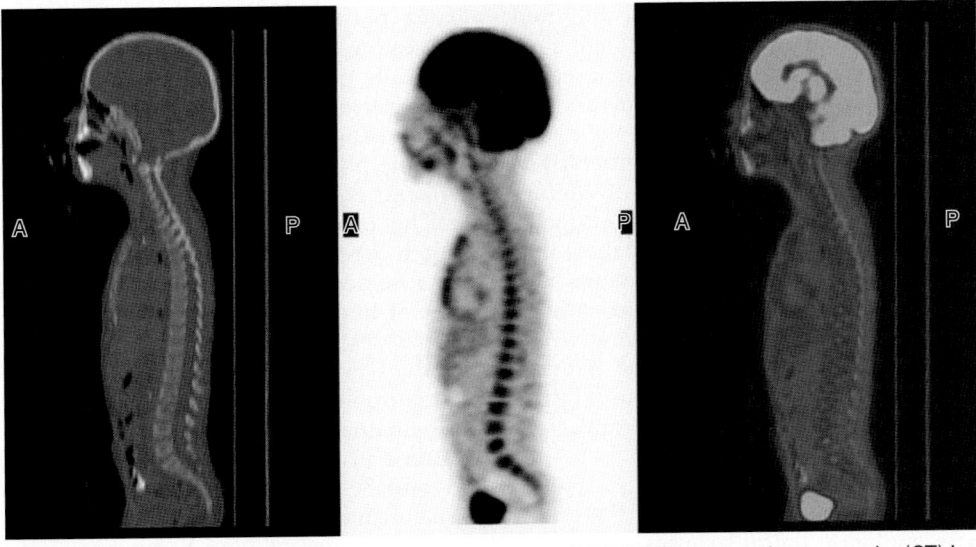

FIGURE 177-17. Positron emission tomography with fluorodeoxyglucose (FDG-PET)/computed tomography (CT) images from a 4-year-old boy on granulocyte colony-stimulating factor (G-CSF) therapy to mitigate the myelosuppressive effects of treatment for Wilms tumor. Diffuse increased uptake of FDG by the bone marrow of the spine and sternum reflects increased metabolic demand resulting from stimulation of granulopoiesis in the marrow. A, anterior; P, posterior. (Images courtesy of Dr. Barry Shulkin, St. Jude Children's Research Hospital, Memphis, TN.) (See color plate.)

chemotherapy, countering the increase in bone marrow uptake induced by G-CSF or GM-CSF. Allowing at least 1 month to elapse between discontinuation of G-CSF or GM-CSF and FDG-PET scanning in patients treated with conventional-dose chemotherapy may minimize these confounding effects on the marrow, and no wait may be necessary in patients treated with G-CSF or GM-CSF

following high-dose chemotherapy and stem cell or bone marrow transplantation.

Anemia of end-stage renal disease can be treated with recombinant human erythropoietin. Erythropoietin induces an increase in the erythropoietic marrow that manifests as decreased signal intensity on T1-weighted MRI sequences. This occurs within 2 weeks after the start of treatment and before any response is seen in the hemo-globin concentration of peripheral blood. Erythropoie-tin also increases the uptake of FDG by the bone marrow.

Effects of hematopoietic growth factor (G-CSF, GM-CSF, erythropoietin) therapy:

- **Induces hematopoietic marrow hyperplasia and reconversion that exhibits low signal intensity on T1-weighted MRI sequences and increased FDG uptake on PET**
- **Can simulate neoplastic infiltration of the marrow**
- **Usually resolves within 6 weeks after discontinuation of therapy**

Chemotherapy

Chemotherapy induces important changes in the bone marrow. During the first week of treatment with cytotoxic chemotherapy, bone marrow becomes very hypocellular and edematous, and vascular sinuses in the marrow dilate. T1-weighted MRI sequences show a decrease in signal intensity of the marrow; fat-suppressed T2-weighted and STIR sequences show an increase in marrow signal intensity, reflecting an increase in water content of the marrow. Marrow necrosis is followed by progressive regeneration of normal hematopoietic cells and adipocytes from mesenchymal progenitors, as well as variable degrees of myelofibrosis. The marrow gradually becomes higher in signal intensity on T1-weighted sequences, reflecting an increase in fat, although fatty transformation of the bone marrow may be delayed by the administration of hematopoietic growth factors (see Fig. 177-11).

Regeneration of the marrow after chemotherapy is incomplete because of chronic toxic effects of chemo-therapy on the replicative ability of marrow stem cells. This is corroborated by FDG-PET studies that show that the mean uptake of FDG by the marrow in patients with a history of chemotherapy is lower than that in patients without a history of chemotherapy. Also, several weeks after discontinuation of G-CSF or GM–CSF in patients treated with high-dose chemotherapy, FDG uptake by the bone marrow is lower than prior to chemotherapy.

Radiation Therapy

In the acute phase, radiation therapy causes depression of marrow cellularity and vascular sinusoid injury with edema and hemorrhage. During the chronic phase, vascular sinusoids are obliterated, and hematopoietic marrow is replaced by fat and fibrosis.

Before the advent of MRI, scintigraphy studies em-ploying marrow-avid radiocolloids showed suppression of bone marrow uptake immediately following 30 to 45 Gray (Gy) irradiation of the spine or pelvis, with regeneration of red marrow in most irradiated sites over a period of 1 to 2 years. The marrow of patients younger than 18 years of age has increased capacity to regenerate, although regeneration of marrow irradiated with more

than 40 Gy is infrequent. The findings of these early studies have been confirmed largely by MRI, which can depict replacement of hematopoietic marrow by fat and fibrosis.

STIR sequences represent the most sensitive conven-tional MRI technique for depicting early postradiation changes in the marrow; they can detect the effects of radiation therapy within a few days after initiation of treatment. Areas of increased signal intensity in the marrow on STIR sequences peak at 9 days post therapy and reflect edema, hemorrhage, and early influx of nonirradiated cells. T1-weighted sequences in the acute phase show a corresponding decrease in signal intensity of the bone marrow. From 2 to 6 weeks after irradiation, the signal intensity of bone marrow begins to increase on T1-weighted sequences and to decrease on STIR sequences. These changes are sharply delimited by the radiation portals and are produced by the migration of adipocytes into irradiated marrow from adjacent non-irradiated marrow (Fig. 177-18). This fatty replacement of the marrow is more conspicuous in locations prev-iously occupied by hematopoietic marrow, particularly the vertebrae and pelvis. In the vertebrae, fatty replacement of the bone marrow is first seen around the basivertebral veins. After 6 weeks, the vertebral marrow pattern becomes more homogeneous with high signal intensity on T1-weighted sequences and low signal intensity on STIR sequences, or it develops a band pattern of peripheral intermediate signal intensity surrounding central high signal intensity on T1-weighted sequences, along with reciprocal changes on STIR sequences. The band pattern is more common in young patients, suggesting that the capability of marrow for regeneration is age dependent. Within the otherwise homogeneous or band pattern, low signal intensity foci may be observed on all sequences, corresponding to sites of fibrosis. In the chronic phase, the marrow shows a marked decrease in contrast enhancement, reflecting vascular obliteration.

The process of fatty replacement of the marrow is largely irreversible for doses higher than 30 to 40 Gy because destruction of vascular sinusoids prevents migra-tion of hematopoietic cells into the irradiated marrow. For doses less than 30 to 40 Gy, fatty replacement of marrow is less complete because regeneration of hematopoietic marrow may occur. This regeneration of hematopoietic marrow manifests as a mottled or band pattern in the vertebrae of pediatric patients between 11 and 30 months after spinal irradiation at doses no greater than 40 Gy; similar findings have been observed in the marrow of long bones after irradiation. Marrow regeneration is more likely to occur with larger volumes of irradiated marrow, suggesting that partial spinal irra-diation may not provide enough stimuli for regeneration because the nonirradiated marrow is sufficient to meet hematopoietic demands.

Effects of radiation therapy on the marrow:
- **Edema and hemorrhage in the acute phase**
- **Replacement of hematopoietic marrow by fat and fibrosis in the chronic phase**

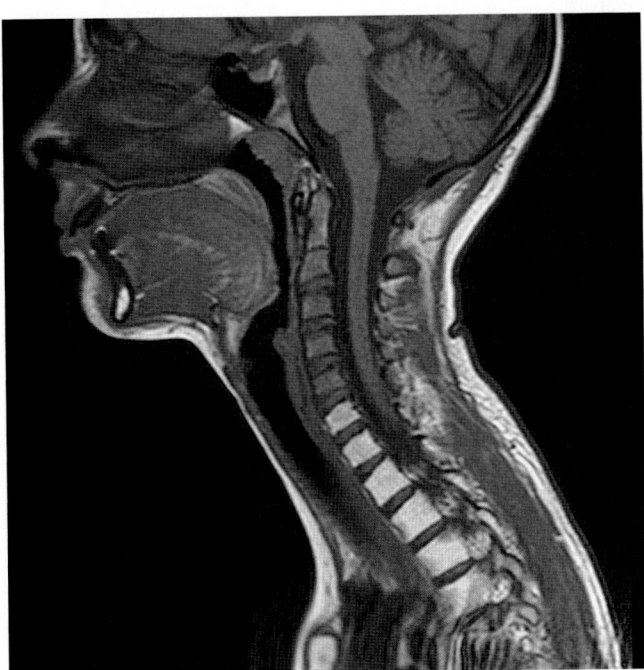

A

FIGURE 177-18. Sagittal conventional spin echo T1-weighted (A) and turbo spin echo T2-weighted (B) magnetic resonance images of the upper spine in a 15-year-old female with a history of local radiation therapy for an extraosseous Ewing sarcoma of the left supraclavicular region. Sharply demarcated homogeneous high signal intensity of the marrow of the lower cervical spine, upper thoracic spine, and upper sternum is noted, corresponding to fatty transformation of the marrow within the irradiated field.

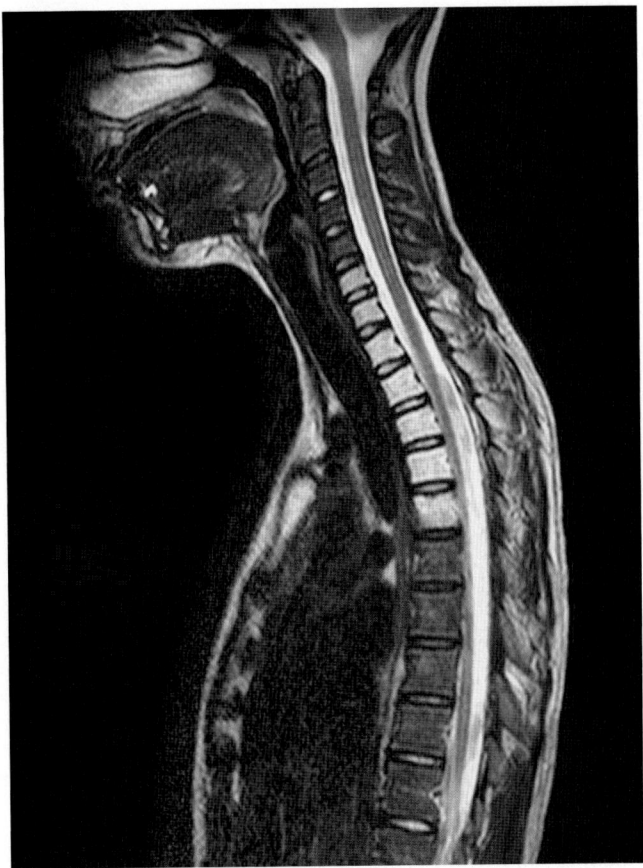

B

- **Sharply delimited by the radiation portal**
- **More conspicuous in locations previously occupied by hematopoietic marrow, particularly the vertebrae and pelvis**
- **For doses less than 30 to 40 Gy, fatty replacement of the marrow is incomplete because hematopoietic marrow regeneration may occur.**

BONE MARROW TRANSPLANTATION

Bone marrow transplantation is used in the treatment of numerous pediatric malignancies, as well as in severe aplastic anemia, hereditary hemoglobinopathies, inborn errors of metabolism, and certain immunodeficiency and autoimmune syndromes. In preparation for bone marrow transplantation, the host marrow is ablated and conditioned by chemotherapy and possibly also by fractionated total body irradiation to induce immune suppression and to eliminate residual malignant cells, if applicable. Stem cells are then infused intravenously, and they engraft in the marrow within 2 to 4 weeks. Typical fatty and hematopoietic bone marrow is usually seen within 90 days after transplantation.

Marrow necrosis from ablation therapy is seen as a slight decrease in marrow signal intensity on T1-weighted sequences and an increase in signal intensity on fat-suppressed T2-weighted and STIR sequences. In the interval following bone marrow transplantation until the recovery of hematopoiesis, hematopoietic growth factors and multiple blood transfusions may be given, and the appearance of the marrow on MRI during this time reflects the combined effects of marrow necrosis, early hematopoietic reconstitution, and possibly iron overload.

Within 90 days and as early as 40 days after transplantation, a band pattern in the vertebral bodies may develop; it consists of a peripheral zone of intermediate signal intensity and a central zone of high signal intensity on T1-weighted sequences, as well as reciprocal signal intensities on STIR sequences. This pattern corresponds to regenerating hematopoietic marrow peripherally and fatty marrow centrally. The pattern is identical to that noted in young patients after radiation therapy and is likely a consequence of the pattern of vertebral body blood flow that distributes repopulating stem cells first into the vascular sinusoids near the endosteum and then along the basivertebral venous plexus. The band pattern may gradually evolve into a homogeneous appearance of the marrow. However, hematopoietic marrow recovery after bone marrow transplantation may not achieve full reconstitution; this is corroborated by the observation that the fat fraction in vertebral and pelvic marrow determined by chemical shift MRI is higher in transplanted patients for several years after transplantation than in those without a history of bone marrow transplantation.

IRON OVERLOAD

Humans store iron as iron (III) oxyhydroxide in ferritin, a water-soluble protein complex, and hemosiderin, an insoluble complex that contains degraded ferritin. Storage occurs primarily in the reticuloendothelial system of the liver, spleen, and bone marrow. When iron levels exceed the storage capacity of the reticuloendothelial system, iron may accumulate in parenchymal cells of the liver, pancreas, heart, and endocrine glands. Unbound iron catalyzes free radical formation, resulting in cell membrane lipid peroxidation and potential hepatotoxicity, cardiotoxicity, and endocrine dysfunction. Deposition of pathologic levels of iron in the reticuloendothelial system of children occurs most often in the setting of transfusional hemosiderosis as a consequence of numerous blood transfusions administered for chronic hemolytic anemia (e.g., sickle cell disease, thalassemia, spherocytosis), aplastic anemia, myelodysplastic syndrome, bone marrow transplantation, or chemotherapy-induced marrow depletion.

Ferritin and hemosiderin are superparamagnetic and accentuate loss of transverse magnetization, resulting in shortening of T2 relaxation time and reduced signal intensity on T2-weighted sequences. At high iron concentrations, signal intensity on T1-weighted and STIR sequences is reduced (Fig. 177-19). The signal intensity reduction from the presence of iron is particularly marked on T2*-weighted gradient echo sequences because of the inherent susceptibility of gradient echo sequences to magnetic field inhomogeneity compared with spin echo sequences. Normal findings on T1-weighted spin echo sequences do not exclude iron overload, and T2*-weighted gradient echo sequences should be performed if optimal sensitivity for the detection of iron overload is desired. Evidence of iron overload may be seen on MRI within a month after transfusional

therapy begins, and MRI findings of iron deposition regress with iron chelation therapy or cessation of transfusions.

Interpretation of MRI of bone marrow can be difficult, particularly in pediatric hematology-oncology patients, because of the multiple factors that can influence the signal intensity of marrow. In addition to age-related differences in the distribution of hematopoietic and fatty marrow, considerations potentially include neoplastic infiltration of the marrow and the effects of radiation therapy, chemotherapy, hematopoietic growth factor administration, or iron overload on the marrow. Many of these processes, including iron overload, can lead to low signal intensity of the marrow on T1-weighted sequences; differentiation of these processes is facilitated by review of T2-weighted or T2*-weighted sequences. Reduction in marrow signal intensity on T1- and T2-weighted sequences generally occurs only with myelofibrosis or iron overload, and the reduction in marrow signal intensity on T2-weighted or T2*-weighted sequences is typically much more profound in iron overload than in isolated myelofibrosis.

> **Iron overload:**
> - **Most commonly a consequence of numerous blood transfusions for anemia**
> - **Reduces signal intensity of the marrow, particularly on T2*-weighted gradient echo sequences, but also on T2-weighted spin echo sequences and, at high iron concentrations, on T1-weighted spin echo sequences**
> - **May also manifest with a reduction in signal intensity in other components of the reticuloendothelial system, such as the spleen and liver**

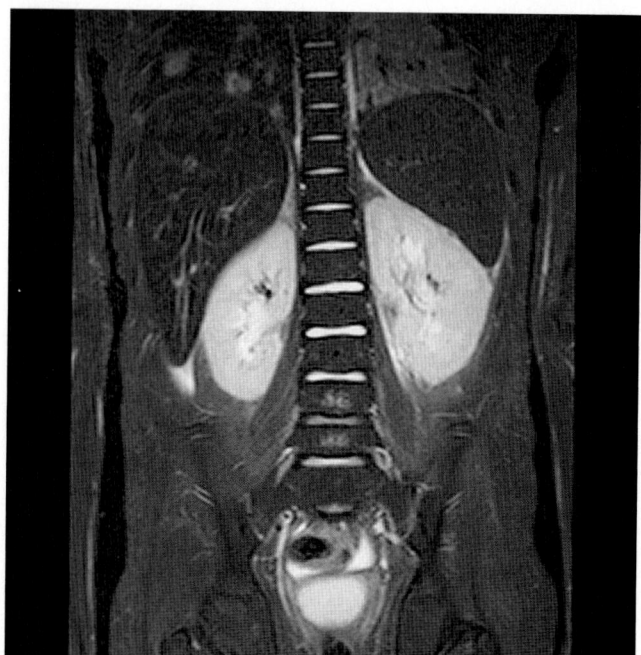

A

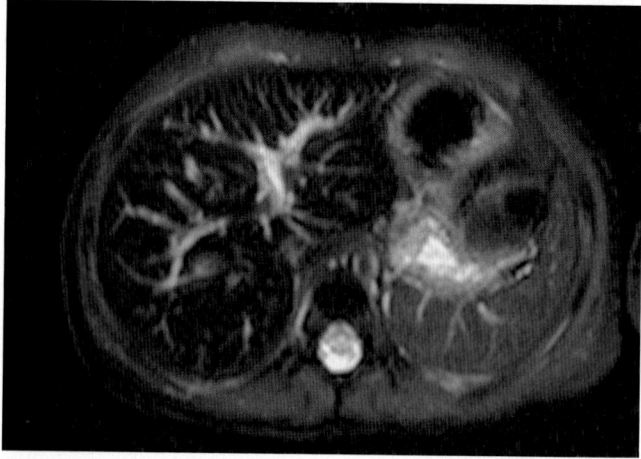

B

FIGURE 177-19. Inversion recovery turbo spin echo coronal **(A)** and turbo spin echo T2-weighted fat-saturated axial **(B)** magnetic resonance images from a 5-year-old male with a history of neuroblastoma in remission, stem cell transplantation, and markedly elevated serum ferritin levels. The reduced signal intensity of the bone marrow, liver, and spleen is consistent with iron overload.

INVESTIGATIONAL IMAGING METHODS

Magnetic Resonance Spectroscopy

Magnetic resonance spectroscopy (MRS) is a technique that allows noninvasive determination of the relative concentrations of various metabolites in vivo. MRS is based on the principle that small differences in the resonance frequencies of nuclei occur because of the chemical environment. Each metabolite is identified by the position of its peak (or chemical shift) on a frequency scale, with the area under the peak proportionate to the concentration of the metabolite within the voxel.

Proton (^{1}H) MRS can be used to measure relative peaks of water and saturated fat methylene group (-CH$_2$-) protons in vivo to assess the fat and water content of marrow. Two-point spectra represented by in-phase and out-of-phase images are added or subtracted to yield pure fat or pure water images. MRS signals from water protons correlate well with degree of cellularity of the bone marrow, as has been observed in the clinical setting of patients with glycogen storage disease type 1b and myeloid hyperplasia. This technique has been suggested as a means of increasing the volume of marrow examined compared with marrow biopsy findings, and of reducing the need for marrow biopsy.

Multiple factors have impeded the transfer of MRS from the laboratory to routine clinical use. Normal metabolite profiles of tissues vary with age, and although MRS is extremely chemical specific, the metabolic profiles of different pathologies often overlap. Proton MRS cannot distinguish between causes of marrow hypercellularity. MRS quality is highly susceptible to degradation by patient motion and magnetic field inhomogeneity, as occurs adjacent to cortical bone, and care must be taken to minimize partial volume effect and signal contamination from adjacent tissue. The higher signal-to-noise ratio and improved spectral resolution of new high field strength MRI systems promise to improve the technical quality of MRS, although more routine clinical implementation awaits the development of efficient techniques amenable to the practical time constraints of clinical practice and germane to the diagnosis and management of specific marrow disorders.

Diffusion-Weighted MRI

Molecular diffusion is a stochastic process that is characterized by brownian motion. Diffusion-weighted magnetic resonance imaging (DWI) is based on magnetic resonance signal attenuation caused by brownian motion of water molecules. In biologic tissues, diffusion of water molecules is influenced by the microstructural nature of the surrounding environment. Bone marrow is semifluid in consistency and is confined within spaces defined by the bony trabeculae and supported by reticulum cells and adipocytes. The diffusion weighting of an MRI sequence is indicated by the b-value. DWI is not pure diffusion imaging, and the apparent diffusion coefficient (ADC) reflects molecular diffusion of water and blood perfusion of the microvasculature. At b-values of 30 and 300 seconds/mm^2, the ADC values of marrow are more likely to be affected by perfusion effect than by diffusion.

A positive correlation has been noted between degree of marrow cellularity and marrow ADC. Hematopoietic marrow or marrow infiltrated by neoplastic cells has more abundant microvasculature and more intracellular and interstitial free water than does fatty marrow, and hematopoietic marrow or marrow infiltrated with neoplastic cells exhibits higher ADC values than are noted with fatty marrow.

As with MRS of the marrow, DWI of the marrow is largely investigative at present, in contrast to the routine use of these techniques in neuroimaging. The application of DWI to evaluation of the bone marrow has been impeded by technical constraints. Motion and susceptibility artifacts are especially problematic in DWI of the marrow, which is contained by bone and occurs in proximity to physiologic motions such as cerebrospinal fluid pulsations. These constraints can be ameliorated to some extent by specialized pulse sequences, but no standard sequence for DWI of the bone marrow is generally accepted; this has hampered clinical adoption of the technique.

Superparamagnetic Iron Oxide Contrast Agents

Because of similar T1 and T2 relaxation times and similar fat and water fractions, hypercellular hematopoietic marrow cannot be consistently distinguished from hypercellular neoplastic marrow by conventional MRI sequences. Phagocytic activity of the marrow serves as a marker for normal hematopoietic marrow and is typically absent or markedly reduced in the presence of neoplastic infiltration. Scintigraphy with radiocolloids tropic for the reticuloendothelial phagocytes in hematopoietic marrow can identify large lesions associated with defective marrow phagocytosis, but the limited spatial resolution of scintigraphy renders the technique insensitive for the detection of small lesions or diffuse low-grade marrow infiltration. The availability of an MRI contrast agent specific for hematopoietic marrow would be a significant advance.

Superparamagnetic iron oxide (SPIO) particles such as ferumoxide are colloid compounds with a median diameter greater than 50 nm; they are composed of a microcrystalline magnetite core and a polymer coating. Ultrasmall superparamagnetic iron oxide (USPIO) particles such as ferumoxtran also contain magnetite cores but have a median diameter less than 50 nm and confer a longer plasma half-life than is associated with SPIO particles. After intravenous injection, SPIO and USPIO particles are taken up by mononuclear phagocytes of the reticuloendothelial system, including macrophages in the hematopoietic marrow. Phagocytosed iron oxide alters the T1- and T2-relaxation times of the bone marrow, resulting in reduced signal intensity of bone marrow on T2-weighted, T2*-weighted, and STIR sequences. This negative contrast effect is observed in the bone marrow within 1 hour after injection and persists for several days. The effect increases in magnitude with greater degrees of hematopoietic marrow cellularity and is more pronounced after infusion of USPIO particles than after infusion of SPIO particles. The smaller size and greater vascular permeability of USPIO particles allow them to traverse the bone marrow sinusoids to reach interstitial macrophages in the hematopoietic marrow more readily than do SPIO particles.

Hypercellular hematopoietic marrow in patients undergoing G-CSF treatment has more numerous phagocytes and exhibits significantly greater signal intensity reduction after iron oxide particle administration compared with normocellular bone marrow in patients who are not undergoing G-CSF treatment. Replacement of the marrow by neoplastic cells reduces the number of marrow phagocytes and is associated with minimal or no signal intensity reduction of involved marrow after iron oxide particle administration. Consequently, MRI performed after iron oxide administration may be used to distinguish marrow that is infiltrated by neoplastic cells from hematopoietic marrow that is hypercellular in response to hematopoietic growth factor therapy—a distinction that is usually not possible with conventional MRI techniques. However, marrow that is infiltrated by a relatively small fraction of neoplastic cells (up to approximately 20%) may not exhibit a detectable difference in iron oxide particle uptake compared with normal hematopoietic marrow. Studies of iron oxide contrast agents for MRI have focused on adults; the efficacy and safety of iron oxide contrast agents remain to be proved in clinical trials that include children.

SUGGESTED READINGS

General and Imaging Techniques

Agool A, Schot BW, Jager PL, et al: 18F-FLT PET in hematologic disorders. A novel technique to analyze the bone marrow compartment. J Nucl Med 2006;47:1592-1598

Foster K, Chapman S, Johnson K: MRI of the marrow in the paediatric skeleton. Clin Radiol 2004;59:651-673

Kellenberger CJ, Epelman M, Miller SF, et al: Fast STIR whole-body MR imaging in children. Radiographics 2004;24:1317-1330

Mirowitz SA, Apicella P, Reinus WR, et al: MR imaging of bone marrow lesions: relative conspicuousness on T1-weighted, fat-suppressed T2-weighted, and STIR images. AJR Am J Roentgenol 1994;162:215-221

Schmidt GP, Schoenberg SO, Reiser MF, et al: Whole-body MR imaging of bone marrow. Eur J Radiol 2005;55:33-40

Zajick DC Jr, Morrison WB, Schweitzer ME, et al: Benign and malignant processes: normal values and differentiation with chemical shift MR imaging in vertebral marrow. Radiology 2005;237:590-596

Normal Marrow

Babyn PS, Ranson M, McCarville ME: Normal bone marrow: signal characteristics and fatty conversion. Magn Reson Imaging Clin N Am 1998;6:473-495

Baur A, Stabler A, Bartl R, et al: MRI gadolinium enhancement of bone marrow: age-related changes in normals and in diffuse neoplastic infiltration. Skeletal Radiol 1997;26:414-418

Dawson K, Moore S, Rowland J: Age-related marrow changes in the pelvis: MR and anatomic findings. Radiology 1992;183:47-51

Dwek JR, Shapiro F, Laor T, et al: Normal gadolinium-enhanced MR images of the developing appendicular skeleton. Part 2. Epiphyseal and metaphyseal marrow. AJR Am J Roentgenol 1997;169:191-196

Jaramillo D, Laor T, Hoffer F, et al: Epiphyseal marrow in infancy: MR imaging. Radiology 1991;180:809-812

Mirowitz SA: Hematopoietic bone marrow within the proximal humeral epiphysis in normal adults: investigation with MR imaging. Radiology 1993;188:689-693

Moore S, Dawson K: Red and yellow marrow in the femur: age-related changes in appearance at MR imaging. Radiology 1990;175:219-223

Okada Y, Aoki S, Barkovich A, et al: Cranial bone marrow in children: assessment of normal development with MR imaging. Radiology 1989;171:161-164

Richardson M, Patten R: Age-related changes in marrow distribution in the shoulder: MR imaging findings. Radiology 1994;192:209-215

Rucci C, Cova M, Kang Y, et al: Normal age-related patterns of cellular and fatty bone marrow distribution in the axial skeleton: MR imaging study. Radiology 1990;177:83-88

Sebag G, Dubois J, Tabet M, et al: Pediatric spinal bone marrow: assessment of normal age-related changes in the MRI appearance. Pediatr Radiol 1993;23:515-518

Shabshin N, Schweitzer ME, Morrison WB, et al: High-signal T2 changes of the bone marrow of the foot and ankle in children: red marrow or traumatic changes? Pediatr Radiol 2006;36:670-676

Simonson T, Kao S: Normal childhood developmental patterns in skull bone marrow by MR imaging. Pediatr Radiol 1991;22:556-559

Taccone A, Oddone M, Dell'Acqua A, et al: MRI "road-map" of normal age-related bone marrow. II. Thorax, pelvis and extremities. Pediatr Radiol 1995;25:596-606

Taccone A, Oddone M, Occhi M, et al: MRI "road-map" of normal age-related bone marrow. I. Cranial bone and spine. Pediatr Radiol 1995;25:588-595

Vande Berg BC, Malghem J, Lecouvet FE, et al: Magnetic resonance imaging of normal bone marrow. Eur Radiol 1998;8:1327-1334

Waitches G, Zawin J, Poznanski A: Sequence and rate of bone marrow conversion in the femora of children as seen on MR imaging: are accepted standards accurate? AJR Am J Reontgenol 1994;162:1399-1406

Zawin J, Jaramillo D: Conversion of bone marrow in the humerus, sternum, and clavicle: changes with age on MR images. Radiology 1993;188:159-164

Marrow Hyperplasia and Reconversion

Aflalo-Hazan V, Gutman F, Kerrou K, et al: Increased FDG uptake by bone marrow in major beta-thalassemia. Clin Nucl Med 2005;30:754-755

Allison JW, James CA, Arnold GL, et al: Reconversion of bone marrow in Gaucher disease treated with enzyme therapy documented by MR. Pediatr Radiol 1998;28:237-240

Bonnerot V, Sebag G, de Montalembert M, et al: Gadolinium-DOTA enhanced MRI of painful osseous crises in children with sickle cell anemia. Pediatr Radiol 1994;24:92-95

Levin TL, Sheth SS, Ruzal-Shapiro C, et al: MRI marrow observations in thalassemia: the effects of the primary disease, transfusional therapy, and chelation. Pediatr Radiol 1995;25:607-613

Manci EA, Culberson DE, Gardner JM, et al: Perivascular fibrosis in the bone marrow in sickle cell disease. Arch Pathol Lab Med 2004;128:634-639

Mankad VN, Williams JP, Harpen MD, et al: Magnetic resonance imaging of bone marrow in sickle cell disease: clinical, hematologic, and pathologic correlation. Blood 1990;75:274-283

Scherer A, Engelbrecht V, Neises G, et al: MR imaging of bone marrow in glycogen storage disease type IB in children and young adults. AJR Am J Roentgenol 2001;177:421-425

Scherer A, Wittsack H-J, Engelbrecht V, et al: Proton MR spectroscopy of the lumbar spine in patients with glycogen storage disease type Ib. J Magn Reson Imaging 2001;14:757-762

Marrow Infiltration

Allison JW, James CA, Arnold GL, et al: Reconversion of bone marrow in Gaucher disease treated with enzyme therapy documented by MR. Pediatr Radiol 1998;28:237-240

Baur A, Stabler A, Bartl R, et al: MRI gadolinium enhancement of bone marrow: age-related changes in normals and in diffuse neoplastic infiltration. Skeletal Radiol 1997;26:414-418

Bembi B, Ciana G, Mengel E, et al: Bone complications in children with Gaucher disease. Br J Radiol 2002;75(suppl 1):A37-A43

Binkovitz LA, Olshefski RS, Adler BH: Coincidence FDG-PET in the evaluation of Langerhans' cell histiocytosis: preliminary findings. Pediatr Radiol 2003;33:598-602

Daldrup-Link HE, Franzius C, Link TM, et al: Whole-body MR imaging for detection of bone metastases in children and young adults: comparison with skeletal scintigraphy and FDG PET. AJR Am J Roentgenol 2001;177:229-236

Even-Sapir E: Imaging of malignant bone involvement by

morphologic, scintigraphic, and hybrid modalities. J Nucl Med 2005;46:1356-1367

Gassas A, Doyle JJ, Weitzman S, et al: A basic classification and a comprehensive examination of pediatric myeloproliferative syndromes. J Pediatr Hematol Oncol 2005;27:192-196

Ghanem N, Uhl M, Brink I, et al: Diagnostic value of MRI in comparison to scintigraphy, PET, MS-CT and PET/CT for the detection of metastases of bone. Eur J Radiol 2005;55:41-55

Goo HW, Yang DH, Ra YS, et al: Whole-body MRI in Langerhans cell histiocytosis: comparison with radiography and scintigraphy. Pediatr Radiol 2006;36:1019-1031

Goo HW, Choi SH, Ghim T, et al: Whole-body MRI of paediatric malignant tumours: comparison with conventional oncological imaging methods. Pediatr Radiol 2005;35:766-773

Guillerman RP: Imaging of childhood leukemia/lymphoma. In The Society for Pediatric Radiology Postgraduate Course Syllabus. Reston, VA, Society for Pediatric Radiology, 2005:171-182

Hasle H, Niemeyer CM, Chessells JM, et al: A pediatric approach to the WHO classification of myelodysplastic and myeloproliferative diseases. Leukemia 2003;17:277-282

Hoffer FA: Magnetic resonance imaging of abdominal masses in the pediatric patient. Semin Ultrasound CT MRI 2005;26:212-223

Inoue K, Okada K, Harigae M, et al: Diffuse bone marrow uptake of F-18 FDG PET in patients with myelodysplastic syndromes. Clin Nucl Med 2006;31:721-723

Jensen KE, Thomsen C, Hernriksen O, et al: Changes in T1 relaxation processes in the bone marrow following treatment in children with acute lymphoblastic leukemia: a magnetic resonance imaging study. Pediatr Radiol 1990;20:464-468

Maas M, Poll LW, Terk MR: Imaging and quantifying skeletal involvement in Gaucher disease. Br J Radiol 2002; 75(suppl 1):A13-A24

Mariani G, Filocamo M, Giona F, et al: Severity of bone marrow involvement in patients with Gaucher's disease evaluated by scintigraphy with ^{99m}Tc-sestamibi. J Nucl Med 2003;44:1253-1262

Meyer JS, Siegel MJ, Farooqui SO, et al: Which MRI sequence of the spine best reveals bone-marrow metastases of neuroblastoma? Pediatr Radiol 2005;35:778-785

Moore SG, Gooding CA, Brasch RC, et al: Bone marrow in children with acute lymphocytic leukemia: MR relaxation times. Radiology 1986;160:237-240

Moulopoulos LA, Dimopoulos MA: Magnetic resonance imaging of the bone marrow in hematologic malignancies. Blood 1997;90:2127-2147

Nöbauer I, Uffmann M: Differential diagnosis of focal and diffuse neoplastic diseases of bone marrow in MRI. Eur J Radiol 2005; 55:2-32

Ruzal-Shapiro C, Berdon W, Cohen M, et al: MR imaging of diffuse bone marrow replacement in pediatric patients with cancer. Radiology 1991;181:587-589

Takagi S, Tanaka O, Miura Y: Magnetic resonance imaging of femoral marrow in patients with myelodysplastic syndromes or leukemia. Blood 1995;86:316-322

Tanabe M, Takahashi H, Ohnuma N, et al: Evaluation of bone marrow metastasis of neuroblastoma and changes after chemotherapy by MRI. Med Pediatr Oncol 1993;21:54-59

Vande Berg BC, Lecouvet FE, Michaux L, et al: Magnetic resonance imaging of the bone marrow in hematological malignancies. Eur Radiol 1998;8:1335-1344

Vande Berg BC, Michaux L, Scheiff J-M, et al: Sequential quantitative MR analysis of bone marrow: differences during treatment of lymphoid versus myeloid leukemia. Radiology 1996;201:519-523

Wenstrup RJ, Roca-Espiau M, Weinreb NJ, et al: Skeletal aspects of Gaucher disease: a review. Br J Radiol 2002;75(suppl 1):A2-A12

Zajick DC Jr, Morrison WB, Schweitzer ME, et al: Benign and malignant processes: normal values and differentiation with chemical shift MR imaging in vertebral marrow. Radiology 2005;237:590-596

Marrow Depletion and Failure

Bonnerot V, Sebag G, de Montalembert M, et al: Gadolinium-DOTA enhanced MRI of painful osseous crises in children with sickle cell anemia. Pediatr Radiol 1994;24:92-95

Dini G, Floris R, Garaventa A, et al: Long-term follow-up of two children with a variant of mild autosomal recessive osteopetrosis undergoing bone marrow transplantation. Bone Marrow Transplant 2000;26:219-224

Elster AD, Theros EG, Key LL, et al. Autosomal recessive osteopetrosis: bone marrow imaging. Radiology 1992;182:507-514

Kanwar VS, Wang WC, Winer-Muram HT, et al: Magnetic resonance imaging for evaluation of childhood aplastic anemia. J Pediatr Hematol Oncol 1995;17:284-289

Karimova EJ, Rai SN, Ingle D, et al. MRI of knee osteonecrosis in children with leukemia and lymphoma. Part 2: Clinical and imaging patterns. AJR Am J Roentgenol 2006;186:477-482

Kusumoto S, Jinnai I, Matsuda A, et al: Bone marrow patterns in patients with aplastic anaemia and myelodysplastic syndrome: observations with magnetic resonance imaging. Eur J Haematol 1997;59:155-161

Lewis S, Wainscoat JS, Moore NR, et al: Magnetic resonance imaging in myelodysplastic syndromes. Br J Radiol 1995;68:121-127

Negendank W, Weissman D, Bey TM, et al: Evidence for clonal disease by magnetic resonance imaging in patients with hypoplastic marrow disorders. Blood 1991;78:2872-2879

Saini A, Saifuddin A: MRI of osteonecrosis. Clin Radiol 2004; 59:1079-1093

Takagi S, Tanaka O, Miura Y: Magnetic resonance imaging of femoral marrow in patients with myelodysplastic syndromes or leukemia. Blood 1995;86:316-322

Tang YM, Jeavons S, Stuckey S, et al: MRI features of bone marrow necrosis. AJR Am J Roentgenol 2007;188:509-514

Treatment Effects

Cavenagh E, Weinberger E, Shaw D, et al: Hematopoietic marrow regeneration in pediatric patients undergoing spinal irradiation: MR depiction. AJNR Am J Neuroradiol 1995;16:461-467

Dalrup-Link HE, Henning T, Link TM: MR imaging of therapy-induced changes of bone marrow. Eur Radiol 2007; 17:743-761

Emy PY, Levin TL, Sheth SS, et al: Iron overload in reticuloendothelial systems of pediatric oncology patients who have undergone transfusions: MR observations. AJR Am J Roentgenol 1997;168:1011-1015

Fletcher BD: Effects of pediatric cancer therapy on the musculoskeletal system. Pediatr Radiol 1997;27:623-636

Fletcher BD, Wall JE, Hanna SL: Effect of hematopoietic growth factors on MR images of bone marrow in children undergoing chemotherapy. Radiology 1993;189:745-751

Jensen KE, Stenver D, Jensen M, et al: Magnetic resonance imaging of the bone marrow following treatment with recombinant human erythropoietin in patients with end-stage renal disease. Int J Artif Organs 1990;13:477-481

Jensen KE, Thomsen C, Hernriksen O, et al: Changes in T1 relaxation processes in the bone marrow following treatment in children with acute lymphoblastic leukemia: a magnetic resonance imaging study. Pediatr Radiol 1990;20:464-468

Kazama T, Swanston N, Podoloff DA, et al: Effect of colony-stimulating factor and conventional- or high-dose chemotherapy on FDG uptake in bone marrow. Eur J Nucl Med Mol Imaging 2005;32:1406-1411

Kornreich L, Horev G, Yaniv I, et al: Iron overload following bone marrow transplantation in children: MR findings. Pediatr Radiol 1997;27:869-872

Levin TL, Sheth SS, Hurlet A, et al: MR marrow signs of iron overload in transfusion-dependent patients with sickle cell disease. Pediatr Radiol 1995;25:614-619

Levin TL, Sheth SS, Ruzal-Shapiro C, et al: MRI marrow observations in thalassemia: the effects of the primary disease, transfusional therapy, and chelation. Pediatr Radiol 1995;25:607-613

Otake S, Mayr NA, Ueda T, et al: Radiation-induced changes in MR signal intensity and contrast enhancement of lumbosacral vertebrae: do changes occur only inside the radiation therapy field? Radiology 2002;180:179-183

Park JM, Jung HA, Kim DW, et al: Magnetic resonance imaging of the bone marrow after bone marrow transplantation or immunosuppressive therapy in aplastic anemia. J Korean Med Sci 2001;16:725-730

Stevens S, Moore S, Amylon M: Repopulation of marrow after transplantation: MR imaging with pathologic correlation. Radiology 1990;175:213-218

Stevens S, Moore S, Kaplan I: Early and late bone-marrow changes after irradiation: MR evaluation. AJR Am J Roentgenol 1990;154:745-750

Tanabe M, Takahashi H, Ohnuma N, et al: Evaluation of bone marrow metastasis of neuroblastoma and changes after chemotherapy by MRI. Med Pediatr Oncol 1993;21:54-59

Investigational Imaging Methods

Bao S, Guttmann CRG, Mugler JP III, et al: Spin-echo planar spectroscopic imaging for fast lipid characterization in bone marrow. Magn Reson Imaging 1999 17;1203-1210

Daldrup-Link HE, Rummeny EJ, Ihssen B, et al: Iron-oxide–enhanced MR imaging of bone marrow in patients with non-Hodgkin's lymphoma: differentiation between tumor infiltration and hypercellular bone marrow. Eur Radiol 2002;12:1557-1566

Herneth AM, Friedrich K, Weidekamm C, et al: Diffusion weighted imaging of bone marrow pathologies. Eur J Radiol 2005;55:74-83

Hundt W, Petsch R, Helmberger T, et al: Effect of superparamagnetic iron oxide on bone marrow. Eur Radiol 2000;10:1495-1500

Matuszewski L, Persigehl T, Wall A, et al: Assessment of bone marrow angiogenesis in patients with acute myeloid leukemia by using contrast-enhanced MR imaging with clinically approved iron oxides: initial experience. Radiology 2007;242:217-224

Mulkern R, Meng J, Oshio K, et al: Bone marrow characterization in the lumbar spine with inner volume spectroscopic CPMG imaging studies. J Magn Reson Imaging 1994;4:585-589

Nonomura Y, Yasumoto M, Yoshimura R, et al: Relationship between bone marrow cellularity and apparent diffusion coefficient. J Magn Reson Imaging 2001;13:757-760

Raya JG, Dietrich O, Reiser MF, et al: Techniques for diffusion-weighted imaging of bone marrow. Eur J Radiol 2005;55:64-73

Senéterre E, Weissleder R, Jaramillo D, et al: Bone marrow: ultrasmall superparamagnetic iron oxide for MR imaging. Radiology 1991;179:529-533

BONE CHANGES IN DISEASES OF BLOOD

178

Bone Changes in Hematologic Diseases

PETER J. STROUSE

Diseases of the bone marrow and blood may have a variety of effects on the appearance of bones. In this chapter, the radiographic manifestations of diseases of blood are presented. Some aspects of imaging of these disorders are covered elsewhere. Bone marrow imaging is presented in Chapter 177. Hemophilic arthropathy is discussed with other arthropathies in Chapter 179. Focal osseous lesions of lymphoma and leukemia ("chloroma") are discussed with other bone tumors in Chapter 176.

CHRONIC HEMOLYTIC ANEMIAS

Heritable hemoglobinopathies constitute a group of important clinical diseases characterized by excessive amounts of abnormal hemoglobin or fetal hemoglobin. These disorders are genetic and tend to be limited to specific racial groups. The abnormality resides in the polypeptide chains that make up the globin moiety of hemoglobin. Combinations of these hemoglobin variants give rise to different disorders.

Thalassemia

Thalassemia (Cooley's erythroblastic anemia) has strong familial and racial characteristics. It occurs with high frequency in the central and eastern Mediterranean regions and in parts of North Africa. This geographic predominance gave rise to its earlier designation as Mediterranean anemia (Greek *thalassa,* "the sea"). It is now recognized to be a common disorder of extensive distribution involving the Middle East and Southeast Asia and affecting American Indians and African Americans.

Clinically, thalassemia varies in severity. Patients with thalassemia major are homozygous for the β^o-thalassemia hemoglobin gene (β^o/β^o) and are most severely affected. Because both β-hemoglobin genes are abnormal, very little or no β-chain synthesis occurs. An excess of insoluble α-chains in red blood cells leads to intracellular precipitation that alters erythropoiesis and red blood cell life span. Patients present with a uniform clinical picture of progressive anemia and jaundice that begin during the first 2 years. Without treatment, life expectancy is only a few years. Splenomegaly is invariably present and is usually accompanied by hepatomegaly. In the most severe cases of thalassemia major, a peculiar facies occurs as a result of marrow hyperplasia involving the facial bones. Some patients also have hypogonadism. The blood is characterized by erythroblastemia and marked changes in size and shape of the red blood cells. Showers of nucleated red cells appear; this feature is aggravated by splenectomy, and these cells may persist for many months.

Patients with thalassemia minor (thalassemia trait) are heterozygous for β^o-thalassemia hemoglobin gene (β^o/β^o). In thalassemia minor, the clinical and hematologic manifestations are milder and less conspicuous, and in some cases, only the laboratory features of hemoglobinopathy are found. Thalassemia intermedia is a homozygous form of milder thalassemia (β^+/β^+); patients may have skeletal deformity but usually do not require transfusion therapy.

The radiographic findings of thalassemia major are diagnostic in severe cases. Radiographic findings are unusual before 6 months but usually manifest during the second year. The shafts of the long bones are osteopenic and undertubulated, the spongiosa is partially destroyed and deformed, and the cortex is thin (Fig. 178-1). The entire skeleton is affected, but changes are usually most conspicuous in the short and long tubular bones. Hyperplastic marrow expands the medullary cavity and interferes with normal tubulation of bones. Trabeculae are coarsened and the bones appear osteopenic. Vascular channels may appear prominent. In some cases, the spongiosa is almost completely destroyed and the bones have a widened and featureless appearance, rather than the usual coarse, trabeculated spongiosa pattern. Skeletal changes of thalassemia are indistinct in the first year of life but become more manifest as age advances. In late childhood and early adult life, the bones of some patients become sclerotic (Fig. 178-2), apparently because

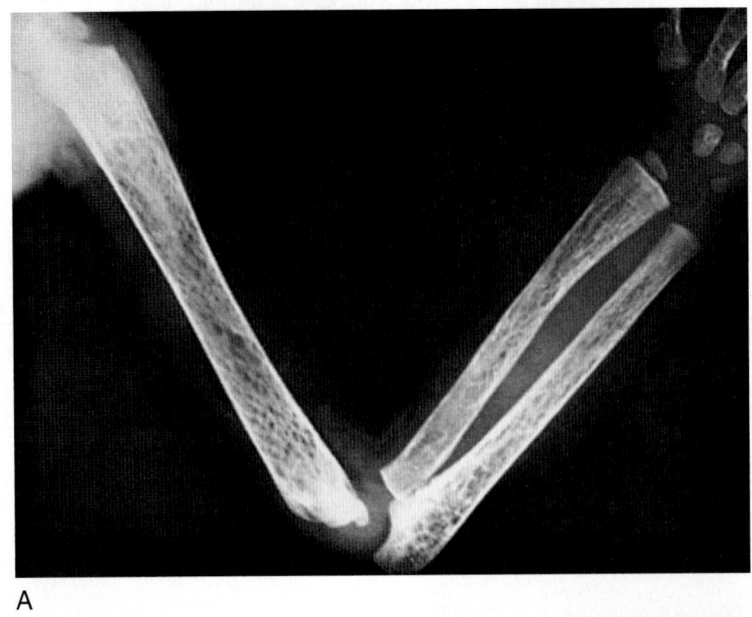

A

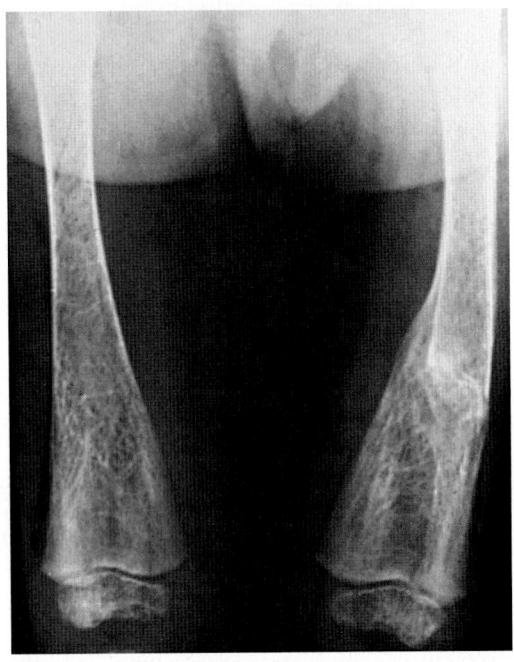

B

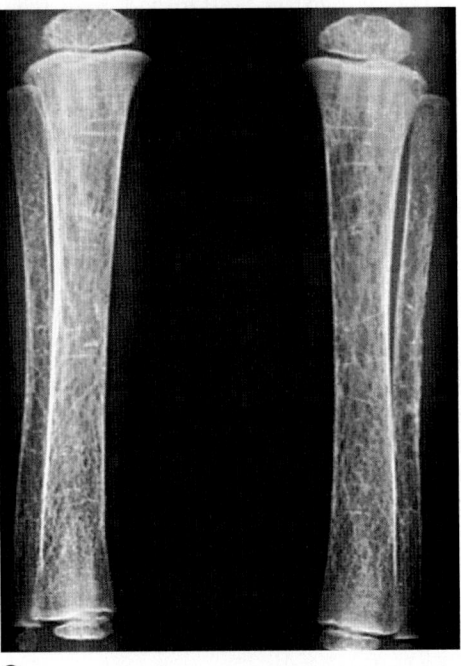

C

FIGURE 178-1. Thalassemia major in an Italian boy 3 years of age. In radiographs of the upper extremity **(A)**, femora **(B)**, and lower legs **(C)**, medullary cavities are widened, shafts are rectangular in outline, and the cortex is thin. All bones are osteoporotic and present a bizarre trabeculated appearance that results from irregular destruction of the spongiosa and irregular endosteal erosion of the cortex. Multiple transverse lines mark the tibias. Deformity of the left femur is related to an old pathologic fracture.

of increased formation of cortical bone. Caffey showed that osseous abnormalities in the limbs begin to involute during early adolescence and may then disappear, but osseous changes in the axial skeleton persist into adult life (Fig. 178-3). This probably reflects conversion of red to yellow marrow in the peripheral skeleton with advancing age and retention of red marrow in the axial skeleton throughout life.

Osseous abnormalities of thalassemia in the limbs involute and may disappear during adolescence, but osseous changes in the axial skeleton persist into adult life. This probably reflects conversion of red to yellow marrow in the peripheral skeleton with advancing age and retention of red marrow in the axial skeleton throughout life.

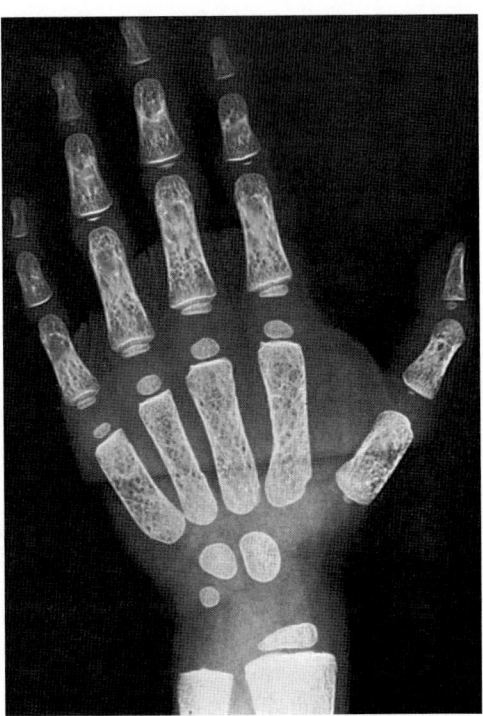 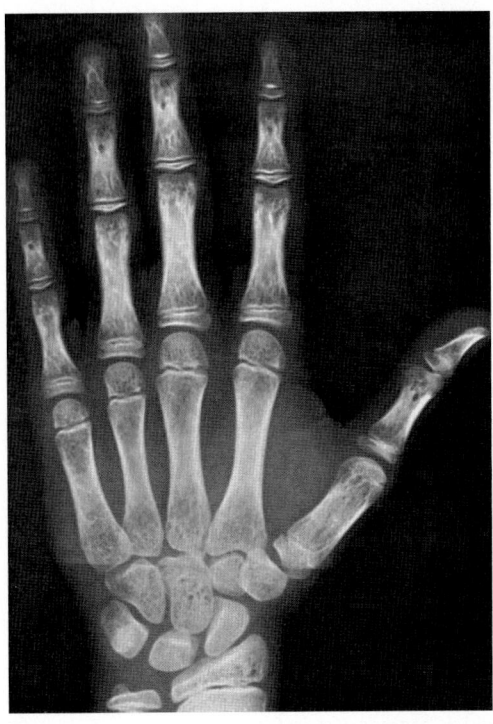

A   B

FIGURE 178-2. Radiographic changes in the hands of a Greek girl with advancing age and thalassemia major. **A,** In the third year, all characteristic changes are present, that is, cortical atrophy and widened external contours, rarefaction, and coarse reticulation. **B,** During the 12th year, all characteristic changes have disappeared despite the fact that severe hemolytic anemia persists. In our experience, characteristic infantile changes always disappear completely or partially in the long bones if the patient survives late childhood.

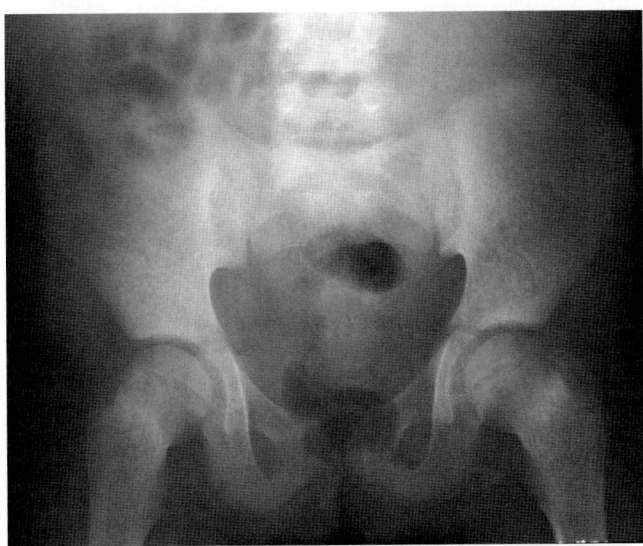

FIGURE 178-3. Thalassemia major in a 13-year-old girl. Coarsened trabeculae are seen throughout the pelvis, lower lumbar spine, and proximal femora.

In long-standing severe cases of thalassemia, skeletal maturation and growth are retarded. In a study by Currarino and Erlandson, premature fusion of epiphyseal ossification centers occurred in 23% of children older than 10 years. The proximal humerus and the distal femur were the only sites of premature fusion, except for one proximal tibia. Premature fusion is more common if treatment is not initiated early in childhood. Thus, thalassemia presents the paradox of delayed appearance of secondary centers in the epiphyseal cartilage and subsequent premature fusion of these secondary centers with the shafts. Pathologic fractures of the femur may occur in patients with extreme cortical atrophy, but they are now relatively uncommon.

Rib findings in thalassemia include widening, osteoporosis, localized lucencies, particularly subcortical, cortical erosions, and "rib in rib" appearance. Rib findings may be associated with extramedullary hematopoiesis.

Classical cranial findings in children with thalassemia major include marked widening of the diploic space, thinning of inner and outer tables, and "hair on end" appearance (Fig. 178-4). The latter finding is due to a perpendicular orientation of trabeculae within the widened diploic space that produces a radial pattern. Marrow overgrowth in the frontal, temporal, and facial bones impairs pneumatization of the sinuses. "Rodent facies" are due to marrow overgrowth in the maxillary bone that causes lateral displacement of the orbits and vertical displacement of the central incisors. This finding is considered pathognomic for thalassemia. Osteopenia and cortical thinning within vertebrae lead to compression fractures.

Thalassemia variants result from the heterozygous state of the gene. In general, skeletal abnormalities, when present, are much less marked in thalassemia variants than in thalassemia major. The thalassemia–sickle cell combination (Hb sickle-β-thal) may exhibit moderately

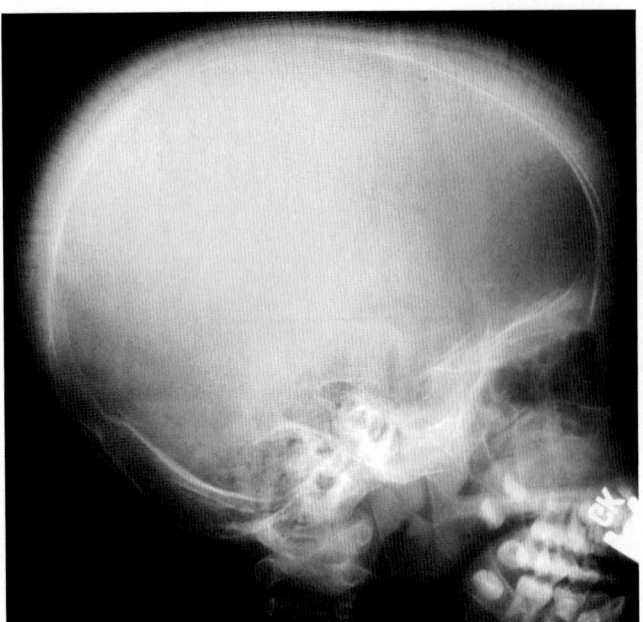

FIGURE 178-4. Thalassemia major in a 7-year-old girl. Widening of the diploic space of the skull with thinning of the inner and outer tables produces a "hair on end" appearance. The maxillary sinuses are poorly aerated.

severe bone changes that resemble those of sickle cell anemia rather than those of thalassemia. Clinical and radiographic abnormality varies substantially according to the thalassemia gene that is present. Instances of thalassemia–hemoglobin E disease have been reported with bone changes similar to those in thalassemia major, but cases involving combination with hemoglobin C and other forms of deviant hemoglobin reveal few or no skeletal abnormalities.

> **Radiographic changes in patients with thalassemia–sickle cell combination resemble those of sickle cell anemia rather than those of thalassemia.**

Bone mineral density is an important indicator of osteoporosis and gonadal function in patients with thalassemia major. Patients who require greater transfusion support tend to be more osteopenic, reflecting greater bone turnover and increased bone resorption. Decreased bone mineral density is more prevalent in patients with thalassemia who have untreated hypogonadism.

Extramedullary hematopoiesis is defined as production of blood cells outside the bone marrow. It is a common finding in patients with chronic severe anemia, such as thalassemia major. Extramedullary hematopoiesis may occur in organs such as liver and spleen and at other extraparenchymal locations; the most common site includes the lower paraspinal areas of the thorax (below T7). Lobulated or rounded masses of soft tissue density are found in the mediastinum contiguous to the spine. The vertebrae are usually not eroded by mediastinal masses. Computed tomography (CT) or magnetic

resonance imaging (MRI) can be performed to delineate the extent of abnormality. Extramedullary hematopoiesis varies in appearance on CT and MRI because of its composition. Active masses appear as soft tissue attenuation on CT and as soft tissue signal on MRI. Older, inactive masses may contain abundant iron and appear high in attenuation on CT or decreased in signal on T1- and T2-weighted MRI sequences; alternatively, they may contain abundant fat and appear low in attenuation on CT and high signal on both T1- and T2-weighted MRI sequences. Scintigraphy with technetium-99m sulfur colloid reveals intense uptake in the areas of active extramedullary hematopoiesis and confirms the diagnosis. Rare reported complications of extramedullary hematopoiesis include intraspinal extension with resultant paralysis and ileoileal intussusception due to a gastrointestinal focus.

The treatment of thalassemia major consists of three facets. Hypertransfusion is used to maintain hemoglobin levels. Iron chelation with agents such as deferoxamine prevents iron overload due to transfusion therapy. Bisphosphonates are used to treat osteoporosis. "Prophylactic" transfusions to young children with thalassemia major have tended to delay the development of skeletal signs of the disease. Nevertheless, marked accumulation of hemosiderin in lymph nodes, spleen, bone marrow, and liver is a frequent manifestation. These findings are best delineated with MRI.

Some patients with thalassemia major treated with iron-chelating drugs such as deferoxamine to reduce transfusional iron overload have been reported to develop severe osteochondrodystrophic lesions of the long bones. Chelation therapy apparently leads to damaged columnar cartilage, altered bone mineralization, and microfracture. High-dose deferoxamine chelation therapy begun early in life has been implicated in the production of radiographically evident rickets-like abnormalities of the long bones and platyspondyly.

Sickle Cell Anemia

In sickle cell anemia, affected persons are homozygous for S hemoglobin (Hb SS), which causes red blood cells to assume an elongated, curved sickle configuration under conditions of reduced oxygen tension. This disease is most common in blacks but has been found in other races as well, most notably persons of Mediterranean, Middle Eastern, and North African descent. Sickle cell anemia is characterized by acute painful crises that affect the bones and joints of the limbs, usually beginning during the second or third year of life. A total of 50% of patients have a crisis by 5 years of age. Up to that age, residual fetal hemoglobin (Hb F) apparently protects the child from the usual manifestations of the disease. Crises are associated with fever, increasing anemia, nausea, vomiting, abdominal pain, severe bone and joint pain, and prostration. Anemia frequently results in cardiomegaly and heart murmurs—findings that are frequently confused with rheumatic fever. These crises usually resolve after a time; after this, the patient may be well until another crisis supervenes.

The abnormal shape of the red cells results in a mechanical capillary stasis wherein deformed red cells

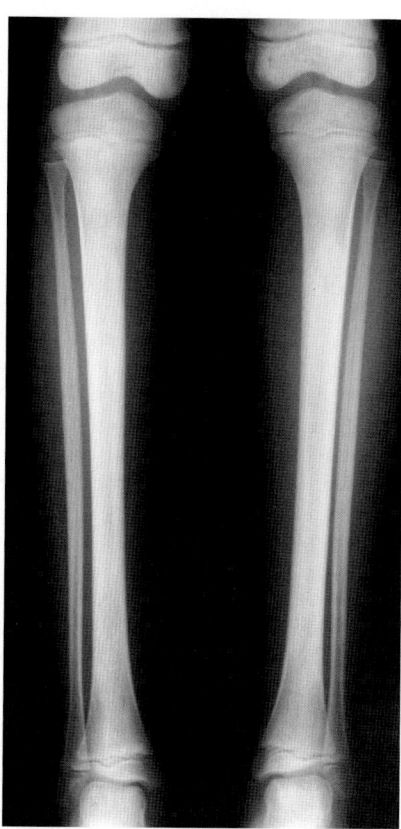

FIGURE 178-5. Sickle cell anemia in an 8-year-old boy. Patchy sclerosis is noted throughout the diaphyses and metaphyses of the tibias.

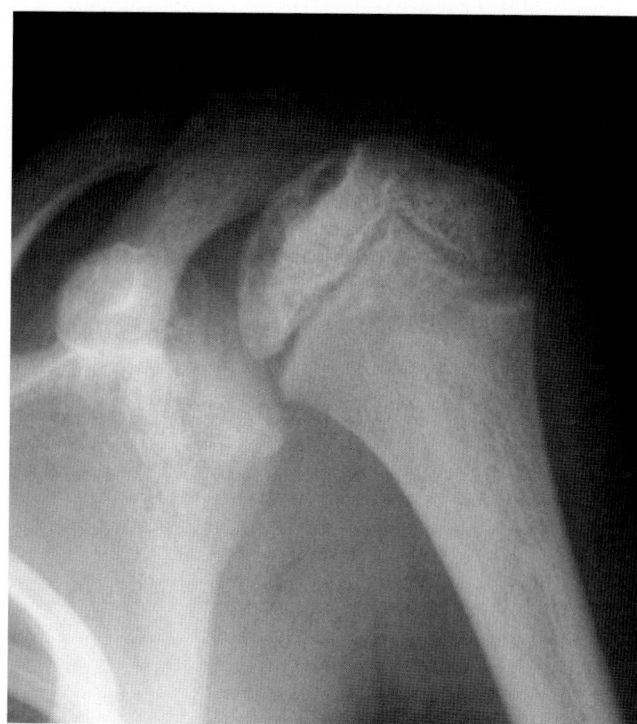

FIGURE 178-6. Sickle cell anemia in an 8-year-old boy. Avascular necrosis of the humeral head manifests as mild flattening, sclerosis, and a prominent subchondral lucency.

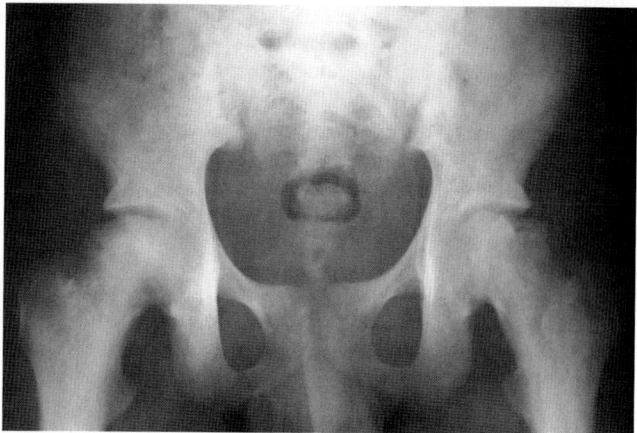

FIGURE 178-7. Sickle cell anemia in a young adult. Avascular necrosis of each femoral head is noted with sclerosis and flattening with loss of normal contour. The bones are diffusely sclerotic.

are unable to traverse the small vessels. This obstruction leads in turn to stasis and hypoxic damage of tissues distal to the obstruction, primarily bone marrow and bone, which undergo necrosis. Skeletal changes reflect infarction with focal destruction and sclerosis of medullary and cortical bone and secondary periosteal new bone formation (Fig. 178-5). Bone marrow infarction in patients with sickle cell may occur in any bone that contains marrow. Acute medullary infarctions are radiographically occult but may be seen on MRI (see Chapter 177). Older medullary infarctions produce ill-defined patches or ovals of sclerosis, most common in the metaphyses but also occurring in the diaphyses. Infarction may affect the epiphyses (avascular necrosis). The femoral heads and humeral heads are most often affected (Fig. 178-6). In the femoral heads, findings are similar to those of other causes of avascular necrosis. In all, 50% of patients develop avascular necrosis by 35 years of age. Epiphyseal abnormalities are uncommon in the age group typically affected by Legg-Perthes disease, but they become increasingly common during adolescence (Fig. 178-7).

> **Osseous abnormalities in sickle cell anemia are due largely to infarction. Any bone can be affected.**

In addition to infarction, patients with sickle cell anemia have an increased incidence of osteomyelitis.

Diminished resistance to infection probably relates to tissue injury from the infarcts and to diminished phagocytosis with lowered oxygen tension in the area of involvement, compounded by diminished splenic function. *Staphylococcus aureus* is the most common organism, but in some series of children with sickle cell anemia and osteomyelitis, *Salmonella* infection was encountered in more than 50% of cases. Radiographic findings of osteomyelitis in sickle cell disease are similar to those of osteomyelitis in children not affected by sickle cell disease, except for a higher incidence of diaphyseal infection (Fig. 178-8). Clinical and imaging differentiation of acute infarction from infection may be difficult. Neither

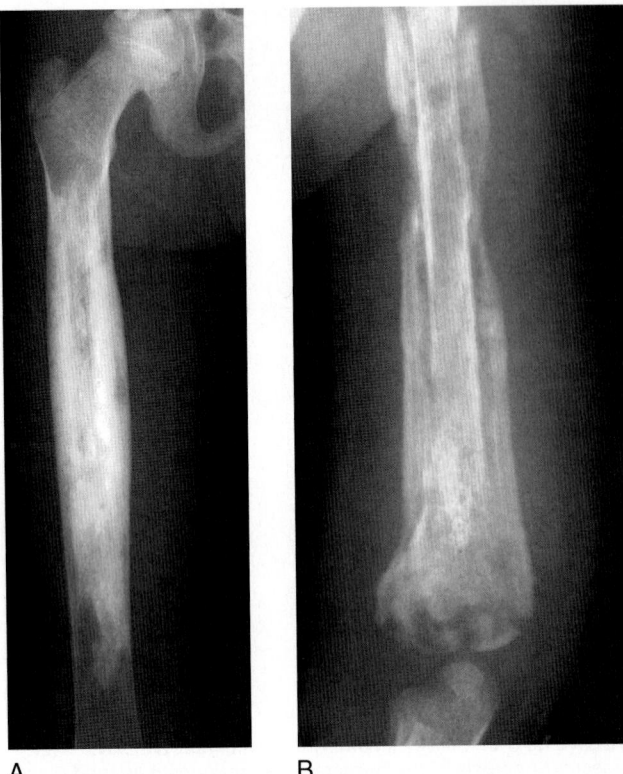

A   B

FIGURE 178-8. **A,** Osteomyelitis in the shaft of the femur of a 9-year-old girl with sickle cell anemia. The suspected causal agent was *Salmonella*; however, this was not proved bacteriologically. (Courtesy of Drs. F. J. Hodges and J. F. Holt, Ann Arbor, MI.) **B,** *Salmonella* osteomyelitis of the distal humerus in a 2-year-old boy with sickle cell anemia. A cloak of new bone ("involucrum") envelops the humerus.

MRI nor nuclear medicine techniques have proved reliable. This dilemma is discussed in Chapter 177.

> *Salmonella* accounts for more than 50% of cases of osteomyelitis in children with sickle cell anemia in some series; *Staphylococcus aureus* is the other "most common" organism.

The most common manifestation of vaso-occlusive crisis in infants and young children is hand–foot syndrome or sickle cell dactylitis, which is often the earliest manifestation of disease. It most commonly presents between 6 months and 2 years, usually by 4 years, and rarely after 7 years of age. Declining incidence with age reflects conversion of hematopoietic marrow to fatty marrow. Infarctions in the small bones of the hand and foot give rise to the term "hand-foot syndrome." In this condition, painful soft tissue swelling of the hands and feet is usually present 1 to 2 weeks prior to the development of patchy radiolucency of the shafts of short tubular bones associated with periosteal new bone formation (Fig. 178-9). Patients may have fever. Clinical and imaging differentiation from osteomyelitis is difficult, but hand–foot syndrome is more common. Reconstitution of bone generally takes place after a period of several months with no resultant deformity.

> Hand–foot syndrome, or sickle cell dactylitis, is often the earliest manifestation of disease. It most commonly presents between 6 months and 2 years, usually by 4 years, and rarely after 7 years of age.

Patients with sickle cell disease have generalized sclerosis and coarsened trabeculae due to marrow hyperplasia. Patients may have cranial changes similar to, but usually much less severe than, those observed in thalassemia. The facial bones are generally not affected because they are in thalassemia major; however, a few exceptions have been noted. Compression fractures are frequently observed in vertebrae; these are due in part to the loss of bony support that results from marrow hypertrophy and in part to infarcts that involve the vessels supplying central portions of the superior and inferior vertebral plates (Fig. 178-10). Depression of the central portion of the vertebral plate ("H vertebrae," or "Lincoln log vertebrae"), presumably as a result of central growth disturbance from vascular compromise, has been advanced as a pathognomonic sign of the disease, but similar changes have been observed occasionally in patients with other hemoglobinopathies. Vertebral changes are usually seen after 10 years of age but occasionally in children as young as 5 years. Cupping of the ends of the shafts of long bones has been observed in children who were suffering from sickle cell anemia (Fig. 178-11). Cupping of the ossification centers of the sternum may also occur (Fig. 178-12).

Sickle cell trait is found in persons who are heterozygous for hemoglobin S. Bone disease is very rare in persons with the trait, and clinical signs and symptoms are very mild if they occur at all. Combinations of sickle hemoglobin (Hb S) and other abnormal hemoglobins occur and produce disease. Patients with the combination of sickle hemoglobin and hemoglobin C (Hb SC) exhibit clinical and radiographic changes similar to, but less severe than, those reported in homozygous sickle cell disease. They usually have large spleens, in contrast to the small infarcted spleens (or functional asplenia) seen in homozygous sickle cell anemia. As was noted previously, patients with the thalassemia gene and the sickle cell gene present with clinical signs and symptoms and radiologic abnormalities more reflective of sickle cell disease than thalassemia.

Other Anemias

Other anemias may have associated skeletal changes but none as severe as those in the hemoglobinopathies already discussed. In hereditary spherocytosis (familial hemolytic anemia), an abnormality in the cell membrane of the red cell causes the cells to become spherical ("spherocyte") and, as a consequence, easily hemolyzed. The hemoglobin itself is not abnormal. Patients are anemic and have mild-to-moderate jaundice with splenomegaly. Gallstones are a frequent complication. Extramedullary hematopoiesis may be significant. Although compensatory hyperplasia of the bone marrow occurs, as in other forms of anemia, only the mildest changes are recognized in the cranial vault, with diploic widening

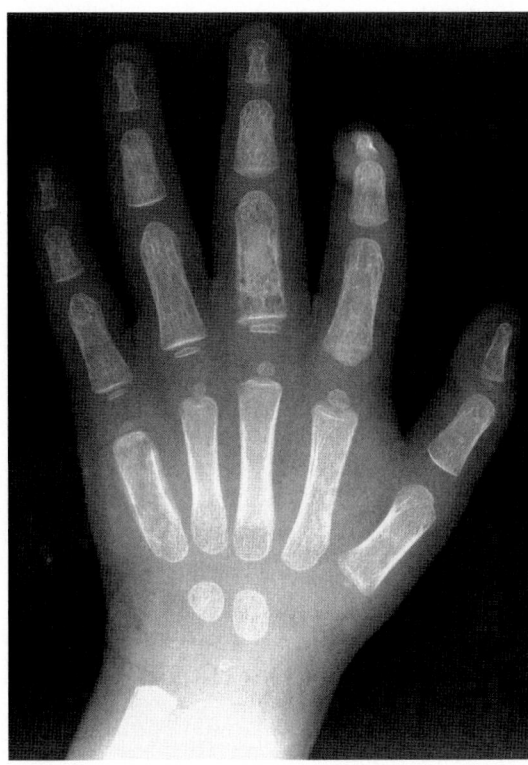
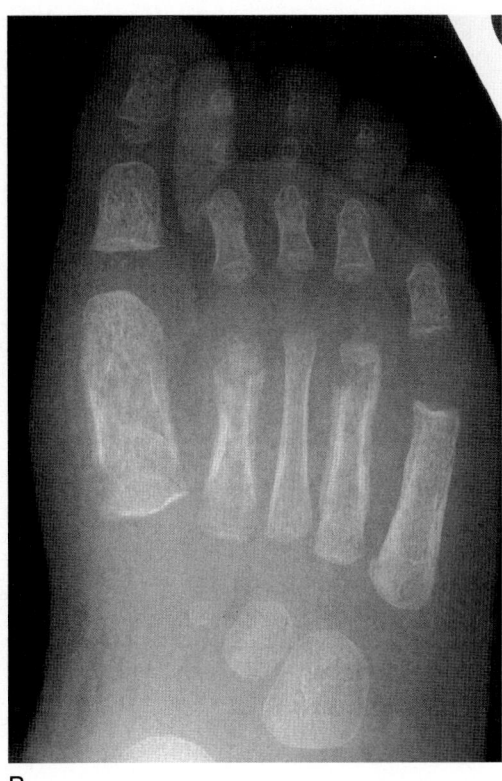

A   B

FIGURE 178-9. Hand–foot syndrome in a 20-month-old with sickle cell anemia. **A,** Digits of the hands are swollen. Osseous changes are most evident in the proximal phalanx of the index finger and the metacarpal of the little finger. Patchy radiolucency and periosteal new bone are seen. **B,** Similar abnormality is seen in the foot; it predominantly affects the metatarsals.

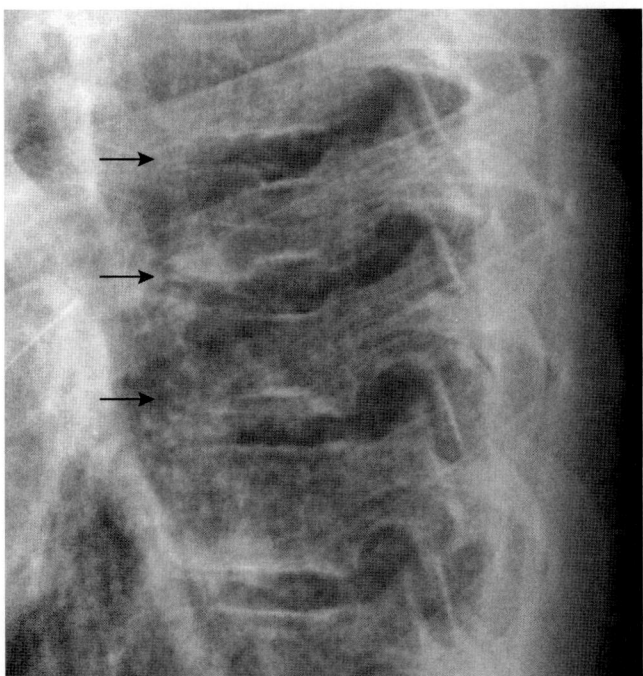

FIGURE 178-10. Radiographic spine changes in a 15-year-old boy with sickle cell anemia. Opposing central end plate depressions *(arrows)* are believed to result from local vascular occlusion and focal fracture.

and thinning of the outer table. Findings are usually not overt until later childhood or adolescence, when red marrow is disappearing from the peripheral skeleton. Radiographic changes are therefore limited to the axial skeleton. Most commonly, osteoporosis and trabecular thickening are seen in the spine and pelvis. Skeletal lesions improve after splenectomy.

Other hemolytic anemias occur without alteration in the shape of the red blood cell and are associated with enzyme deficiencies that predispose the red cell to hemolysis under certain special conditions. Pyruvate kinase–deficiency hemolytic anemia, according to Becker and associates, are associated with bone changes similar to those of thalassemia major, except that the maxillary sinuses pneumatize normally. In glucose-6-phosphate dehydrogenase deficiency, red blood cells undergo hemolysis after exposure to various drugs and foods (fava beans). In general, radiologic signs are lacking in this condition.

Erythroblastosis fetalis results from immunization of a pregnant woman of one blood type with fetal erythrocytes of another type. In the past, diffuse sclerosis of the bones were indistinguishable from physiologic osteosclerosis of the newborn, and nonspecific transverse metaphyseal bands of increased and diminished density reflecting altered endochondral ossification were reported. With almost universal monitoring of blood types and antibody levels, as well as prophylactic administration of a specific antibody to mothers following the

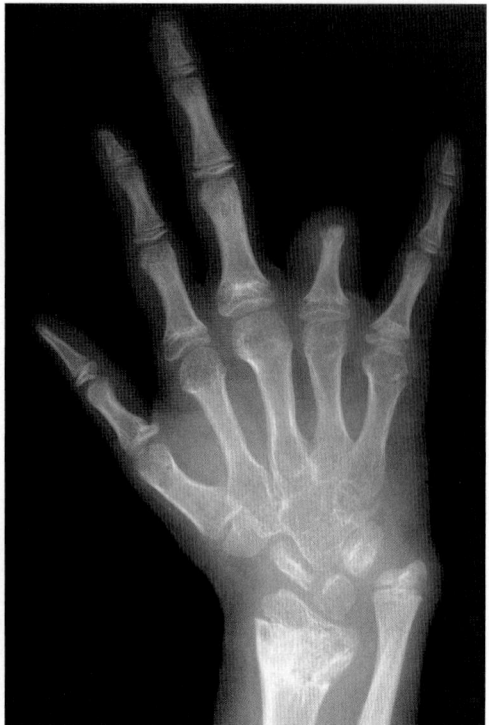
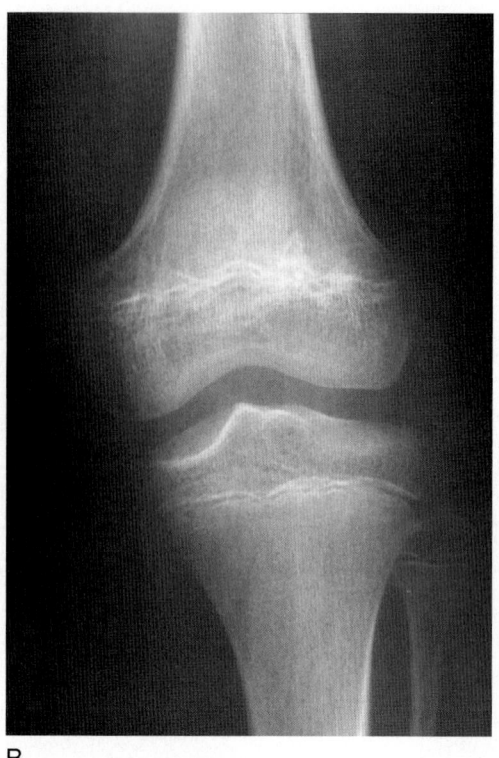

A   B

FIGURE 178-11. Premature physeal fusion in a 12-year-old girl with sickle cell anemia. **A,** Fusion is seen within the proximal phalanges and the distal radius. Digit amputations and partial carpal fusion are also the consequence of prior infarctions. **B,** Early fusion of the distal femoral growth plate.

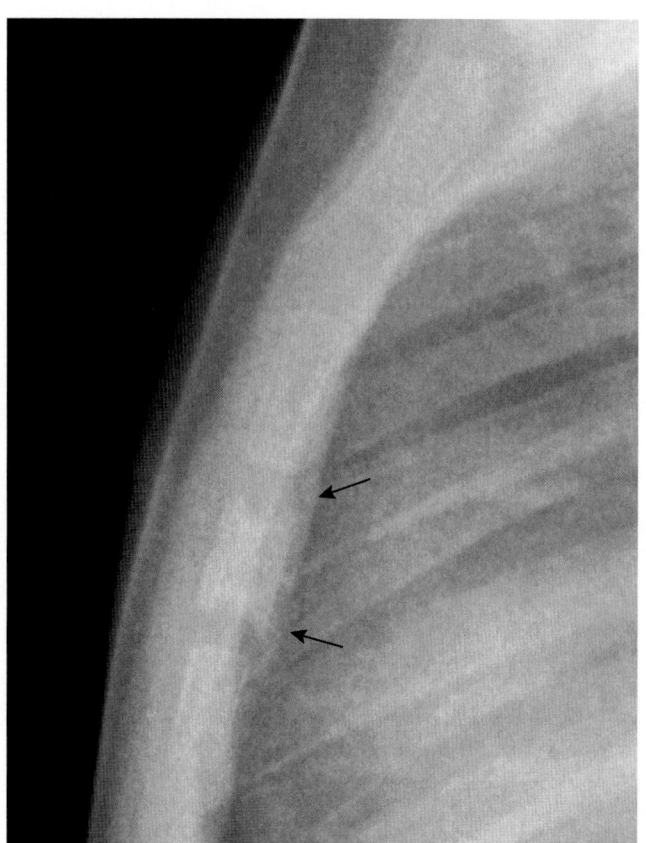

FIGURE 178-12. Cupping of sternal ossification centers *(arrows)* in an 18-month-old girl. (Courtesy of Dr. A. E. Schlesinger, Houston, TX.)

birth of an infant with the potential for causing sensitization, erythroblastosis fetalis is now rare.

Fanconi anemia is a congenital hypoplastic anemia that is associated with multiple osseous anomalies. This disorder is presented in Chapter 166.

LEUKEMIA

In the pediatric age group, acute lymphocytic leukemia (ALL) accounts for 80% of leukemia cases, acute myelogenous leukemia (AML) for 18%, and chronic myelogenous leukemia (CML) for 2%. Two peaks in presenting age have been noted: one at approximately 4 years of age and a second at 15 to 20 years of age.

The growing skeleton is an important site of proliferation of leukemic cells. In the course of the disease, multiple areas of destruction and production may appear in the bones. Recognition of bone lesions caused by leukemia is much less frequent currently than in past years because of earlier recognition of the disease and prompt effective treatment. Nevertheless, radiographic examination can be useful in suggesting the diagnosis and, occasionally, in assisting in the long-term management of the disease.

In all, 20% of patients have complaints confined to the musculoskeletal system at presentation. Up to 50% include bone or joint pain as part of their symptom complex. Osseous lesions are most common in children younger than 5 years old. In all, 75% of patients have osseous lesions at some point in the course of their disease: 45% with osseous lesions have no pain. Many

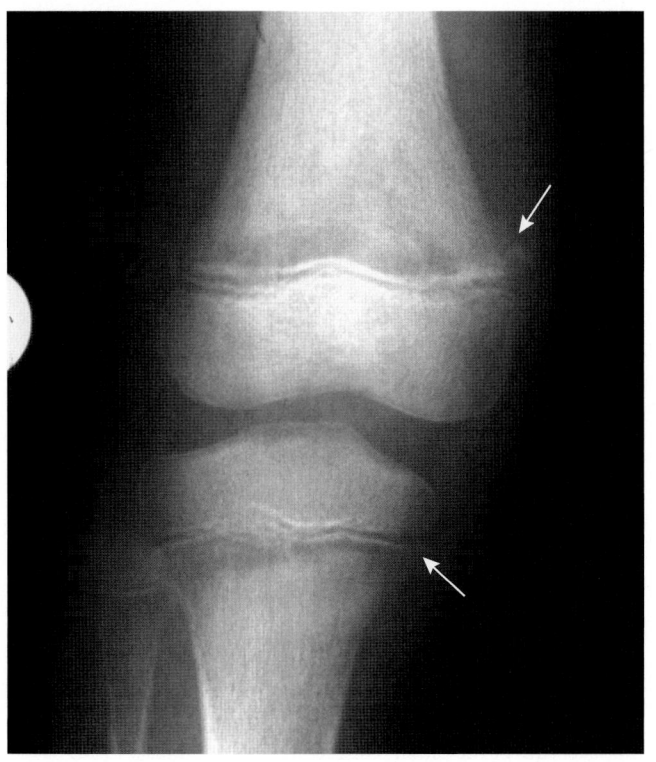
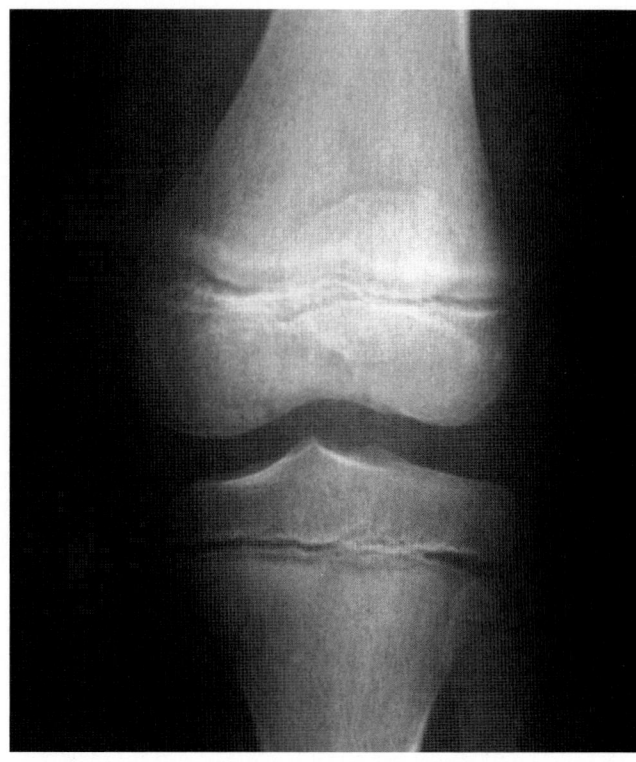

A   B

FIGURE 178-13. Lucent metaphyseal bands from acute lymphoblastic leukemia. **A,** A 4-year-old girl. **B,** An 8-year-old girl with Down syndrome. Both patients presented with knee pain. *Arrows* in **A** indicate cortical stepoff from pathologic fractures.

patients with bone pain have no radiographic abnormality. Many patients with bone pain and bone lesions have near-normal hematologic studies, potentially delaying diagnosis. The prognostic significance of osseous lesions is unclear. Various studies have shown no correlation with outcome, a poorer prognosis, or a better prognosis.

The spectrum of radiographic bony changes in patients with leukemia includes diffuse osteoporosis, focal osteolytic and osteoblastic lesions, chloroma, and arthritis. The most common abnormality is nonspecific osteoporosis. Four types of bone lesions have been traditionally described—transverse bands, periosteal new bone formations, focal destructive lesions, and diffuse osteosclerosis. These four types of lesions occur singly or in combination (Figs. 178-13 through 178-15). None is specific for leukemia. All generally resolve following successful therapy. Focal lesions may mimic neuroblastoma metastases. Pathologic fractures may occur.

> **Osseous changes in leukemia include transverse bands, periosteal new bone formation, focal destructive lesions, and diffuse osteosclerosis.**

Transverse bands of diminished density at the ends of major long bones are the most frequent recognized finding. These bands are more frequent in children younger than 10 years of age. The bands may merely indicate a metabolic dysfunction and response of growing bone to the stress of a severe disease, but they also

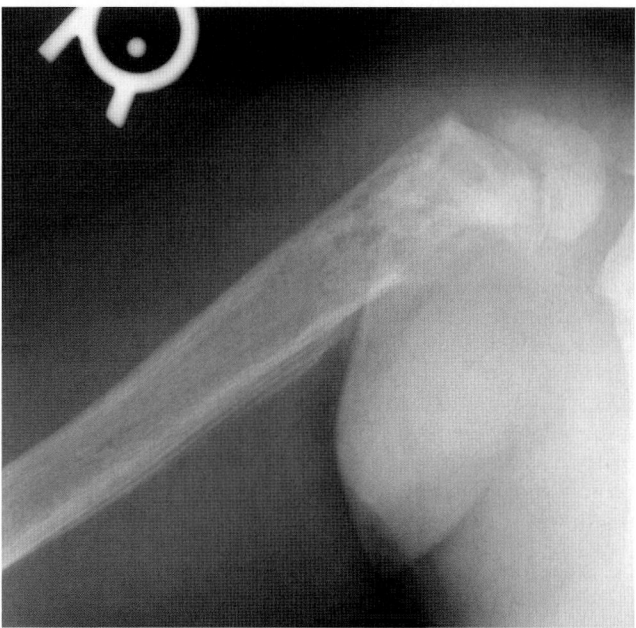

FIGURE 178-14. Acute lymphoblastic leukemia in a 17-month-old boy. An aggressive-appearing lytic lesion is seen in the proximal humeral metaphysis. Permeative changes extend into the diaphysis. Interrupted periosteal new bone is seen medially.

may indicate sites of rapidly proliferating leukemic cells within the metaphyses. Lucent bands are most common in the distal femur, proximal tibia, and distal radius—the sites of fastest growth.

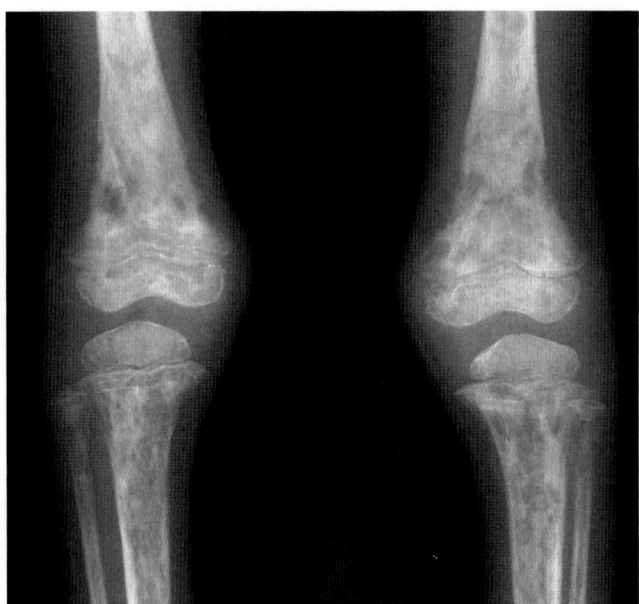

FIGURE 178-15. Diffuse, mixed lytic and sclerotic changes due to an aggressive leukemia.

> **Lucent metaphyseal bands of leukemia are most common in the distal femur, proximal tibia, and distal radius—the sites of fastest growth.**

Diffuse osteosclerosis, associated most frequently with myelogenous leukemia, may result from osteoblastic stimulation and may reflect the origin of osteoblasts from marrow cells. Patients may have mixed osteosclerosis and osteoporosis. Dense metaphyseal bands may be seen in treated patients.

Subperiosteal new bone formation along the shafts results from extension of proliferating cells from the marrow to the cortex, presumably through haversian canals, and bone production by the elevated periosteum. Subperiosteal hemorrhage may also contribute to some of these periosteal reactions. In all, 20% to 50% of patients have periosteal new bone formation.

Focal destructive lesions (chloromas) are caused by accumulations of leukemic cells and can occur in any portion of bones, but they are most common in the metaphyses (see Fig. 178-14). Chloroma (also known as myeloblastoma or granulocytic sarcoma), is a localized tumor that consists of immature myeloid cells. This uncommon tumor occurs in 2.5% to 8% patients with leukemia, most often of the myeloid type (AML). The greenish color of most of these tumors has been attributed to the presence of myeloperoxidase and the degeneration of hemoglobin. The presence of a mass together with destruction and production of bone in a patient with a known or suspected diagnosis of leukemia should suggest the possibility of chloroma. Chloromas may occur concurrently with or may present as a first manifestation of AML; they may also occur during remission or relapse. Occasionally, a chloroma presents as the first sign of a blastic crisis of chronic myeloid leukemia. The prognosis is generally poor. Chloromas also occur in other organ systems. Osseous chloromas

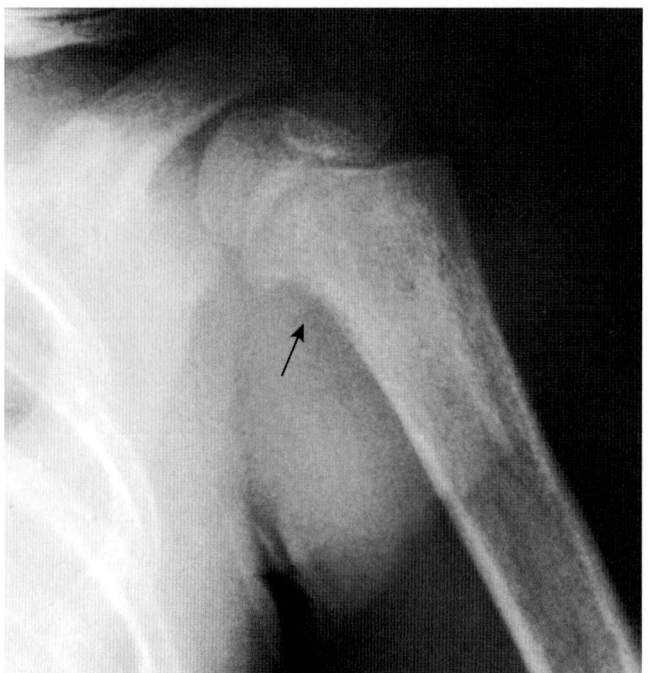

FIGURE 178-16. Erosion of the medial margin of the proximal humeral metaphysis *(arrow)* in a 2-year-old girl with acute megakaryocytic leukemia. Differential considerations include normal variant and secondary hyperparathyroidism.

may occur in any bone. Lesions usually have features of an aggressive osseous neoplasm with ill-defined margins; however, some tumors are relatively well defined. The radiologic appearance of chloroma is not specific.

Other osseous radiographic manifestations of leukemia include osteoporosis, trabecular coarsening, and permeative change. A "moth-eaten" pattern may be seen in the metaphyses and occasionally in flat bones and small bones of the hands and feet. Cortical erosions may be seen at the medial aspect of the proximal humeral or proximal tibial metaphyses, usually bilaterally (Fig. 178-16). Pathologic fractures can occur with focal chloromas or with metaphyseal infiltration. Leukemic infiltration may lead to avascular necrosis at the hip. In the spine, osteoporosis due to leukemia may lead to multiple compression fractures (Fig. 178-17). Patients may present with back pain. If no other explanation can be suggested for osteoporosis (i.e., steroid therapy), leukemia is a strong diagnostic consideration in such patients.

Osseous abnormalities and marrow infiltration may produce bone pain that is often referred to adjacent joints. Leukemia thus may be misdiagnosed as a rheumatologic condition such as juvenile rheumatoid arthritis. Up to one third of pediatric patients with ALL present with a limp, bone pain, or arthralgia. Although joint pain is usually due to metaphyseal periosteal lesions rather than direct synovial infiltration, leukemia may in itself also cause arthritis.

> **Up to one third of pediatric patients with ALL present with a limp, bone pain, or arthralgia. The presentation may thus mimic joint disease.**

Acute megakaryoblastic leukemia (AMKL; French-American British subtype M7) is a subtype of AML that accounts for 12% of AML cases in children. Patients are usually younger than 2 years of age. Patients with AMKL may have substantial radiographic findings that consist of osteoporosis, osteolytic lesions, pathologic fractures, and exuberant periosteal reaction, often symmetric (Fig. 178-18). Periosteal new bone may appear as an extensive cloak.

HEMOPHILIA

Hemophilia is a bleeding diathesis that is caused by a genetic deficiency of factor VIII (hemophilia A) or factor IX (hemophilia B). The more common hemophilia A occurs in 1 of every 10,000 live male births and hemophilia B in 1 of every 40,000 live male births. Most patients exhibit a family history that points to a bleeding disorder, although spontaneous mutations are responsible for about 30% of cases. Hemarthrosis, arthropathy, intramuscular bleeding, and pseudotumors are common manifestations of hemophilia.

Hemophilic arthropathy is an incapacitating complication of severe hemophilia that may result from recurrent bleeding within the same joint. Hemophilic arthropathy is now the most common radiographic manifestation of hemophilia. It is covered in greater detail in Chapter 179.

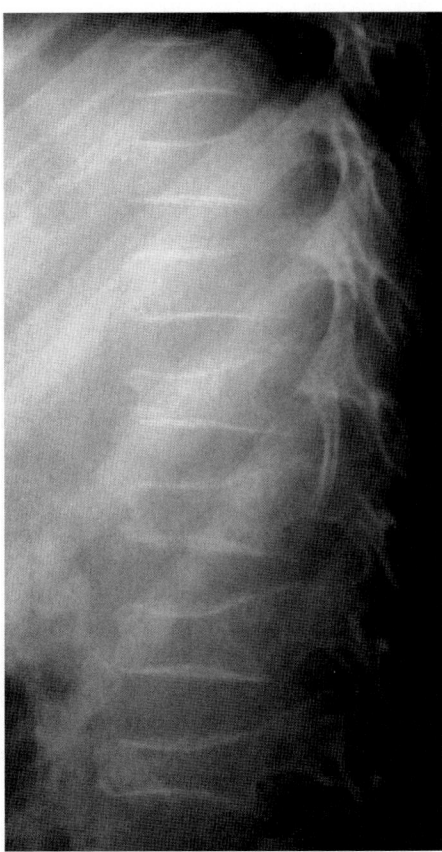

FIGURE 178-17. A 5-year-old boy with osteopenia and multiple vertebral body compression deformities at the time of presentation with acute lymphoblastic leukemia.

> **Hemophilic arthropathy is the most common radiographic manifestation of hemophilia.**

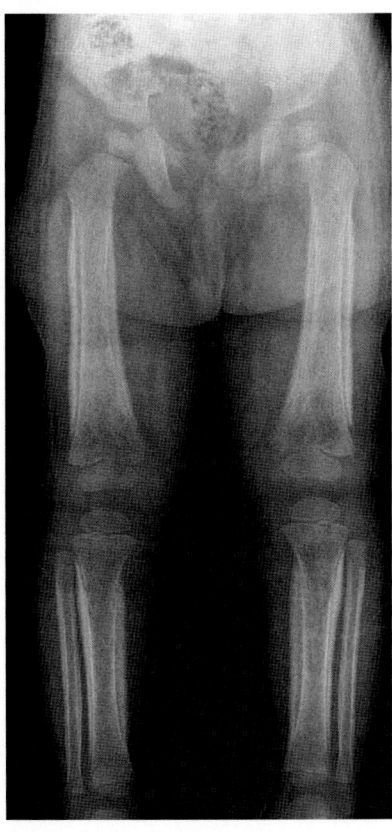

A

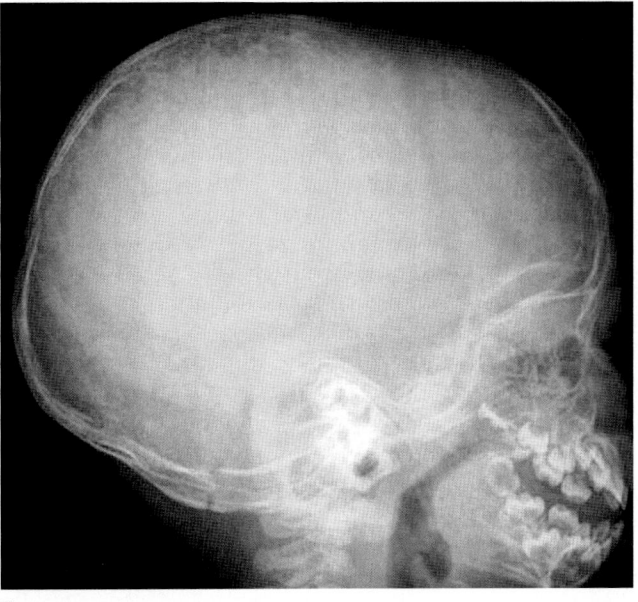

B

FIGURE 178-18. An 11-month-old boy with acute megakaryoblastic leukemia. **A,** Extensive periosteal new bone is seen on the femora and tibias and, to a lesser extent, the fibulas. Increased lucency and subtle permeative abnormality are seen at the metaphyses. **B,** Extensive lytic abnormality and permeation are seen in the skull. (Courtesy of Dr. B. B. Specter, Winston-Salem, NC.)

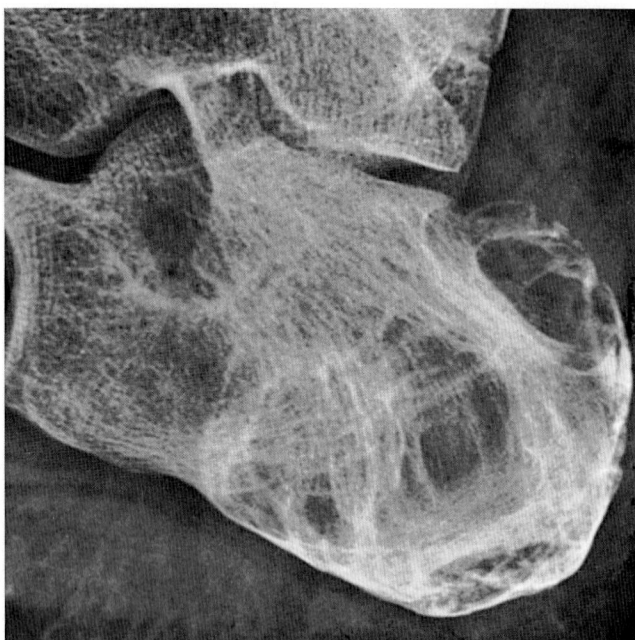

FIGURE 178-19. Hemophilia with intraosseous hemorrhages into the medullary cavity of the calcaneus of a young adult. Large radiolucent areas represent intramedullary hematomas in different stages of organization. (Courtesy of Dr. B. Ward, Grand Junction, CO.)

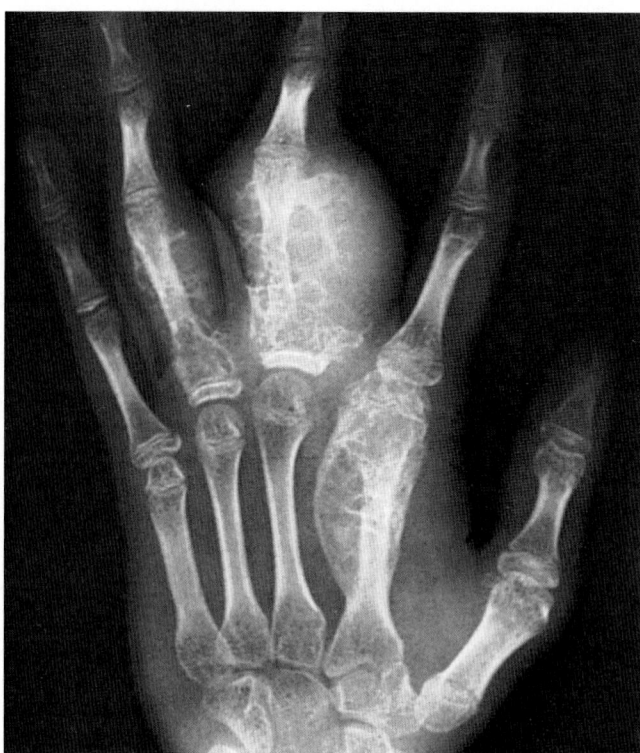

FIGURE 178-20. Hemophilia in a 14-year-old boy. Old and recent subperiosteal hemorrhages have swollen the soft tissues and destroyed the cortex of the proximal phalanx of the third and fourth digits. The old cortical walls are still visible and are surrounded by partially ossified subperiosteal hematomas. The epiphyseal ossification center at the proximal end of the proximal phalanx of the third digit is slightly displaced.

Skeletal lesions in patients with hemophilia may also occur as the result of bleeding directly into the bones (Fig. 178-19), or they may be produced by secondary changes in the bones that result from recurrent hemorrhages into adjacent joints. Hemophilic pseudotumors are well-defined masses that contain blood and blood clots in various stages of organization surrounded by a fibrous capsule in subcutaneous fat or in intramuscular, interfascial, subperiosteal, or intraosseous locations. Of these, intraosseous lesions are least common. Subperiosteal hemorrhages in hemophilia are rare and occur as the result of hemorrhage that strips the periosteum. Subperiosteal pseudotumors can result in new bone formation and pressure erosion of the underlying cortex (Figs. 178-20 and 178-21). Intramuscular pseudotumors frequently have mural nodules. Intramuscular pseudotumors are most common in the thighs, the gluteal muscles, and the iliopsoas muscles. Extramuscular pseudotumors may also occur in fascial planes and subcutaneous tissues.

> **Pseudotumors from hemophilia may develop in subcutaneous fat, or in intramuscular, interfascial, subperiosteal, or intraosseous locations.**

Intraosseous pseudotumors most commonly occur, in decreasing order of frequency, in the femur, pelvis, tibia, and small bones of the hands. A history of previous trauma is found in approximately half of patients. On radiography, intraosseous lesions are well-defined, unilocular or multilocular, expansile, lytic lesions of variable size. Lesions may mimic a variety of lucent bone tumors.

Intraosseous pseudotumors may heal spontaneously with sclerosis.

MRI allows determination of the number, size, and extent of lesions and provides evidence of neurovascular involvement and accompanying musculoskeletal alterations. MRI is not only a sensitive and accurate method for diagnosing hemophiliac pseudotumor and gaining useful information for therapeutic decision making, it can also be used to assess results of treatment of lesions in regions difficult to access by physical examination and to check for recurrent bleeding within a chronic lesion. CT is useful in evaluation of subtle bony erosions and intraosseous and extraosseous pseudotumors (Fig. 178-22), and sonography is valuable for following the progression and regression of soft tissue hematomas. On MRI, hemophilic pseudotumors have varying signal because of hemorrhage of varying age. Soft tissue pseudotumors have a peripheral low signal rim that is due to a fibrous capsule that contains hemosiderin. This low signal rim is typically absent in intraosseous lesions.

MASTOCYTOSIS

Mastocytosis (mast cell disease) is characterized by abnormal proliferation of tissue mast cells that produce histamine. Mastocytosis occurs in two main forms. The *cutaneous* form is primarily a childhood disease associated with pigmented skin lesions called *urticaria pigmentosa* that spontaneously resolve by adolescence in

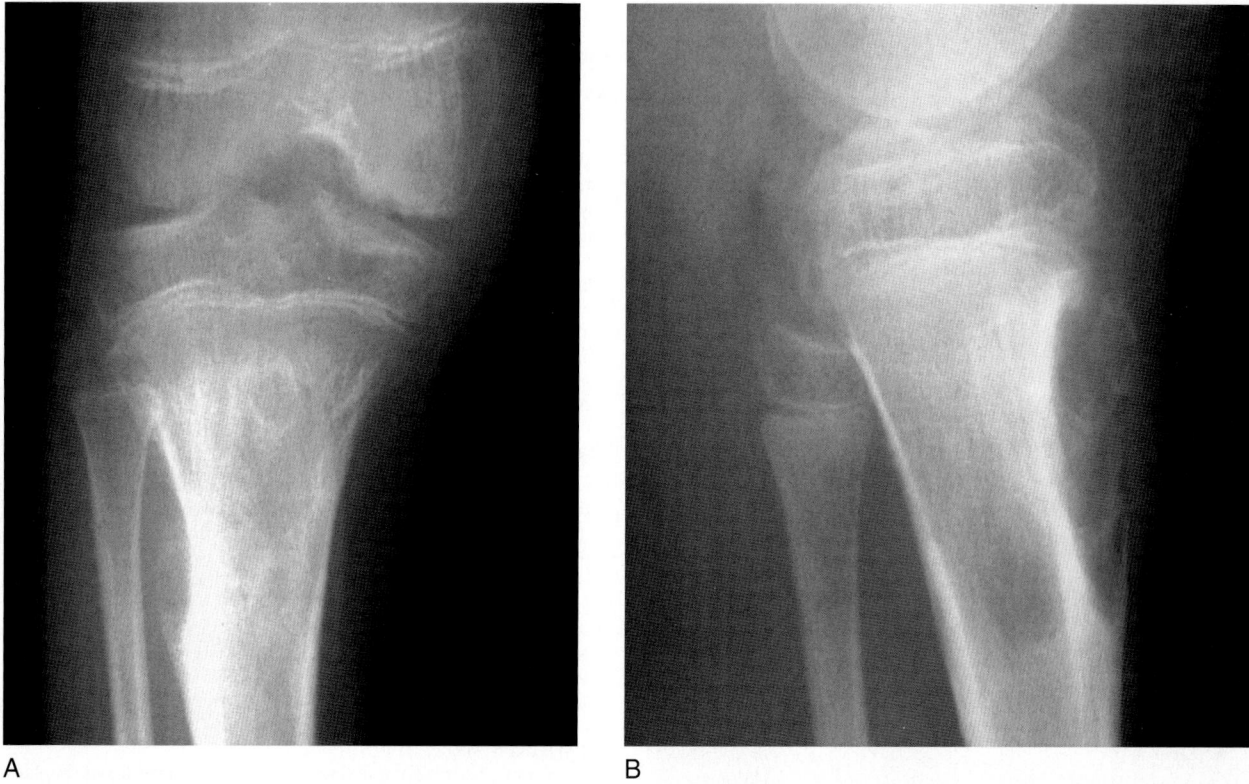

FIGURE 178-21. Proximal tibial pseudotumor in a 12-year-old boy with hemophilia. Anteroposterior **(A)** and lateral **(B)** views show an oblong subperiosteal lucent lesion at the anterior tibia. Margins of the lesion are sclerotic. Erosions due to hemophilic arthropathy are seen in the femoral condylar articular surfaces.

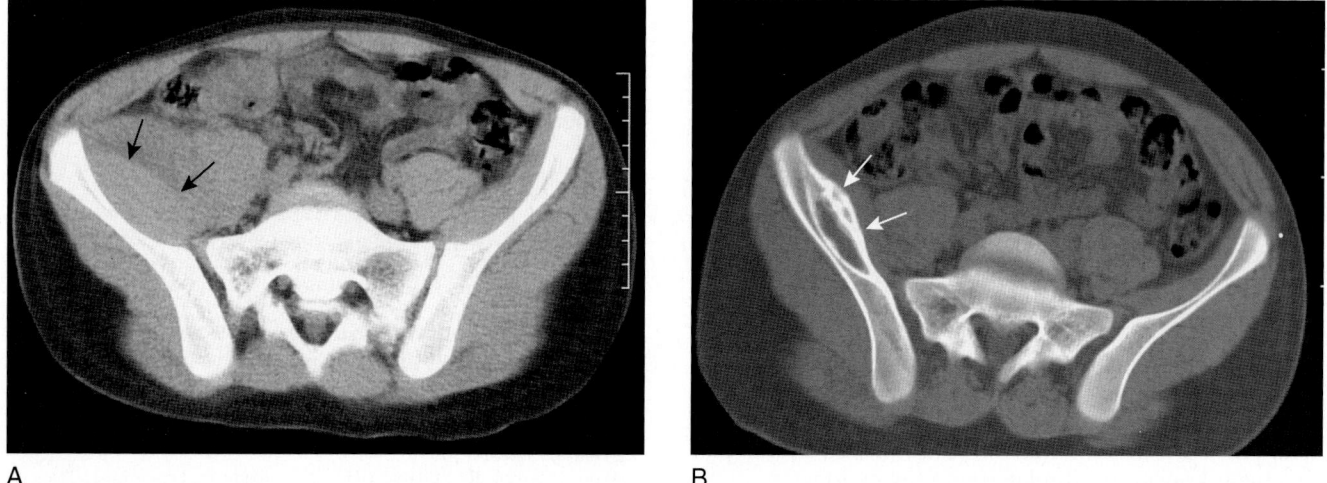

FIGURE 178-22. A 14-year-old boy with hemophilia. **A,** An acute subperiosteal hemorrhage *(arrows)* undermines the right iliacus muscle. **B,** Eight months later, new bone *(arrows)* covers the residua of the hemorrhage.

90% of instances but in about 10% of patients progress to a systemic form. The adult form with skin involvement has an onset around puberty and manifests systemic progression in about 50% of patients. *Systemic* mastocytosis accounts for about 10% of all cases of mast cell disease. In about 90% of patients with systemic mastocytosis, the bone marrow is infiltrated by mast cells. Skeletal lesions include widespread osteosclerosis mixed with osteolytic lesions, focal or generalized osteoporosis, and poorly

defined focal lytic and sclerotic lesions involving the axial and appendicular skeleton (Fig. 178-23). MRI is a sensitive method of detecting bone marrow involvement in these patients.

The pathogenesis of osteosclerosis in mastocytosis is not well understood. Ischemic injury that results from occlusion of vascular channels by mast cells may cause reactive fibrous tissue formation and osteogenesis. Various biogenic amines secreted by mast cells, such as

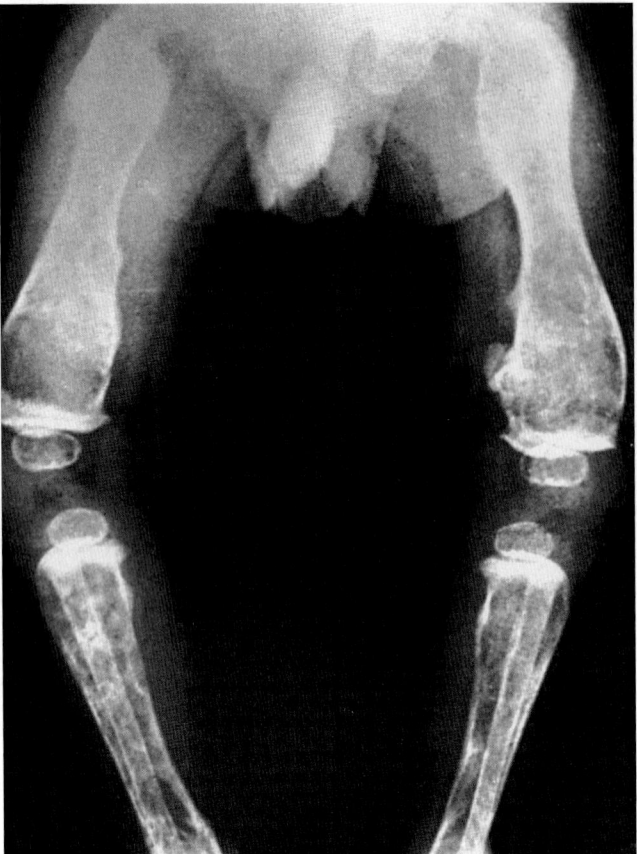

FIGURE 178-23. Radiographic evidence of mastocytosis (urticaria pigmentosa) in a 6-month-old boy who had been irritable since birth with "constant crying, vomiting, and diarrhea." Scattered urticarial pruritic skin lesions were relieved by antihistaminic medication. In several tests, histamine levels in the blood had been increased. The liver and spleen were enlarged, and the left leg and foot were paralyzed. The diagnosis was based on a biopsy study of a single femur. All long bones in the legs are widened as a result of failure of normal constriction of the shafts and hypertrophy of the marrow caused by hyperplasia of mast cells. The cortical walls are thin, and the bones demonstrate patchy lytic and sclerotic areas. Irregular bony projections on the medial aspects of the femora are not satisfactorily explained. (Courtesy of Dr. E. B. Singleton, Houston, TX.)

histamine, heparin, serotonin, and prostaglandins, have been shown to have a bone-resorbing effect and are considered to play a pathogenic role in the manifestation of osteoporosis. Prostaglandins in low concentrations have also been known to stimulate bone formation.

Proliferation of mast cells may occur in other organs such as liver, spleen, gastrointestinal tract, and lymph nodes. Clinical signs of vomiting, diarrhea, hepatosplenomegaly, and urticarial skin lesions may provide a clue to diagnosis when these bizarre skeletal features are noted on radiographs. Diagnosis is based on biopsy findings and histochemical evaluation for histamine.

Abdominal findings on CT and ultrasonography are common in patients with systemic mastocytosis. These findings include hepatosplenomegaly, retroperitoneal adenopathy, periportal adenopathy, mesenteric adenopathy, thickening of the omentum and the mesentery, and ascites.

SUGGESTED READINGS

Erythroblastosis and Fanconi Anemia

Bishop PA: The roentgenologic diagnosis of fetal hydrops. Am J Roentgenal Radium Ther Nucl Med 1961;86:415-424

Brenner G, Allen RP: Skeletal changes in erythroblastosis foetalis. Radiology 1963;80:427-429

Follis RH Jr, Jackson D, Carnes WH: Skeletal changes associated with erythroblastosis fetalis. J Pediatr 1942;21:80-92

Glanz A, Fraser FC: Spectrum of anomalies in Fanconi anemia. J Med Genet 1982;18:412-416

Juhl JH, Wesenberg RL, Gwinn JL: Roentgenographic findings in Fanconi's anemia. Radiology 1967;89:646-653

Minagi H, Steinbach HL: Roentgen appearance of anomalies associated with hypoplastic anemias of childhood: Fanconi's anemia and congenital hypoplastic anemia (erythrogenesis imperfecta). Am J Roentgenol Radium Ther Nucl Med 1966;97:100-109

Thalassemia

Alam R, Padmanabhan K, Rao H: Paravertebral mass in a patient with thalassemia intermedia. Chest 1997;112:265-267

Aliberti B, Patrikiou A, Terentiou A, et al: Spinal cord compression due to extramedullary haematopoiesis in two patients with thalassaemia: complete regression with blood transfusion therapy. J Neurol 2001;248:18-22

Bruneteau G, Fenelon G, Khalil A, et al: Spinal cord compression secondary to extramedullary hematopoiesis in a patient with thalassemia. Rev Neurol (Paris) 2000;156:510-513

Caffey J: Cooley's anemia: a review of the roentgenographic findings in the skeleton. Am J Roentgenol Radium Ther Nucl Med 1957;78:381-391

Chan Y, Li C, Chu WC, et al: Deferoxamine-induced bone dysplasia in the distal femur and patella of pediatric patients and young adults: MR imaging appearance. AJR Am J Roentgenol 2000; 175:1561-1566

Currarino G, Erlandson ME: Premature fusion of epiphyses in Cooley's anemia. Radiology 1964;83:656-664

de Sanctis V, Stea S, Savarino L, et al: Osteochondrodystrophic lesions in chelated thalassemic patients: an histological analysis. Calcif Tissue Int 2000;67:134-140

Dines DM, Canale VC, Arnold WD: Fractures in thalassemia. J Bone Joint Surg Am 1976;58:662-666

Emery JL, Follett GF: Regression of bone-marrow haemopoiesis from terminal digits in the foetus and infant. Br J Haematol 1964; 10:485-489

Images in clinical medicine: a hair-on-end skull. N Engl J Med 2001;345:e1

Kangarloo H, Dietrich RB, Taira RT, et al: MR imaging of bone marrow in children. J Comput Assist Tomogr 1986;10:205-209

Karimi M, Ghiam AF, Hashemi A, et al: Bone mineral density in beta-thalassemia major and intermedia. Indian Pediatr 2007; 44:29-32

Korsten J, Grossman H, Winchester PH, et al: Extramedullary hematopoiesis in patients with thalassemia anemia. Radiology 1970;95:257-263

Lala R, Chiabotto P, Di Stefano M, et al: Bone density and metabolism in thalassaemia. J Pediatr Endocrinol Metab 1998; 11(suppl 3):785-790

Lawson JP, Ablow RC, Pearson HA: The ribs in thalassemia. 1. The relationship to therapy. Radiology 1981;140:663-672

Levin TL, Sheth S, Berdon WE, et al: Deferoxamine-induced platyspondyly in hypertransfused thalassemic patients. Pediatr Radiol 1995;25(suppl 1):S122-S124

Long JA Jr, Doppman JL, Nienhuis AW: Computed tomographic studies of thoracic extramedullary hematopoiesis. J Comput Assist Tomogr 1980;4:67-70

Molyvda-Athanasopoulou E, Sioundas A, Karatzas N, et al: Bone mineral density of patients with thalassemia major: four-year follow-up. Calcif Tissue Int 1999;64:481-484

Moseley JR: Skeletal changes in the anemias. Semin Roentgenol 1974;9:169-184

Ozdemir A, Gungor F, Tuncdemir F, et al: Scintigraphic diagnosis of intrathoracic extramedullary hematopoiesis in a patient with beta-thalassemia. Ann Nucl Med 1998;12:149-155

Reynolds J, Pritchard JA, Ludders D, et al: Roentgenographic and clinical appraisal of sickle cell beta-thalassemia disease. Am J Roentgenol Radium Ther Nucl Med 1973;118:378-400

Ross P, Logan W: Roentgen findings in extramedullary hematopoiesis. Am J Roentgenol Radium Ther Nucl Med 1969;106:604-613

Sfikakis P, Stamatoyannopoulos G: Bone changes in thalassemia trait. Acta Haematol 1963;29:193-201

Tchang S, Tyrrell MJ, Bharadwaj B: Skeletal changes in cyanotic heart diseases simulating Cooley's anemia: report of a case with regression of the bone changes following palliative cardiac surgery. J Can Assoc Radiol 1973;24:274-279

Tsitouridis J, Stamos S, Hassapopoulou E, et al: Extramedullary paraspinal hematopoiesis in thalassemia: CT and MRI evaluation. Eur J Radiol 1999;30:33-38

Tunaci M, Tunaci A, Engin G, et al: Imaging features of thalassemia. Eur Radiol 1999;9:1804-1809

Valdez VA, Jacobstein JG: Decreased bone uptake of technetium-99m polyphosphate in thalassemia major. J Nucl Med 1980;21:47-49

Voskaridou E, Kyrtsonis MC, Terpos E, et al: Bone resorption is increased in young adults with thalassaemia major. Br J Haematol 2001;112:36-41

Winchester PH, Cerwin R, Dische R, et al: Hemosiderin laden lymph nodes: an unusual roentgenographic manifestation of homozygous thalassemia. Am J Roentgenol Radium Ther Nucl Med 1973;118:222-226

Wongwaisayawan S, Pornkul R, Teeraratkul S, et al: Extramedullary haematopoietic tumor producing small intestinal intussusception in a beta-thalassemia/hemoglobin E Thai boy: a case report. J Med Assoc Thai 2000;83(suppl 1):S17-S22

Sickle Cell Disease and Other Anemias

Becker MH, Genieser NB, Piomelli S, et al: Roentgenographic manifestations of pyruvate-kinase-deficiency hemolytic anemia. Am J Roentgenol Radium Ther Nucl Med 1971;113:491-498

Ben Dridi MF, Oumaya A, Gastli H, et al: Radiological abnormalities in the skeleton in patients with sickle-cell anemia: a study of 222 cases in Tunisia. Pediatr Radiol 1987;17:296-302

Bennett OM, Namnyak SS: Bone and joint manifestations of sickle cell anemia. J Bone Joint Surg Br 1990;72:494-499

Burke TS, Tatum JL, Fratkin MJ, Baker K: Radionuclide bone imaging findings in recurrent calvarial infarction in sickle cell disease. J Nucl Med 1988;29:411-413

Burko H, Watson J, Robinson M: Unusual bone changes in sickle cell disease in childhood. Radiology 1963;80:957-962

Cassady JR, Berdon WE, Baker DH: The "typical" spine changes of sickle cell anemia in a patient with thalassemia major (Cooley's anemia). Radiology 1967;89:1065-1068

de Gheldere A, Ndjoko R, Docquier PL, et al: Orthopaedic complications associated with sickle-cell disease. Acta Orthop Belg 2006;72:741-747

Dennis GJ, Keating RM: Muscle infarction in sickle cell anemia. Ann Intern Med 1991;115:831-832

Dhekne RD: Splenic concentration of bone imaging agents in functional asplenia. Clin Nucl Med 1981;6:313-317

Ebong WW, Kolawole TM: Aseptic necrosis of the femoral head in sickle-cell disease. Br J Rheumatol 1986;25:34-39

Ejindu VC, Hine AL, Mashayekhi M, et al: Musculoskeletal manifestations of sickle cell disease. Radiographics 2007; 27:1005-1021

Erenberg G, Rinsier SS, Fish BG: Lead neuropathy in sickle cell disease. Pediatrics 1974;54:438-441

Fernandez M, Slovis TL, Whitten-Shurney W: Maxillary sinus marrow hyperplasia in sickle cell anemia. Pediatr Radiol 1995; 25(suppl 1):S209-S211

Gellett LR, Williams MP, Vivian GC: Focal intrasplenic extramedullary hematopoiesis mimicking lymphoma: diagnosis made using liver-spleen scintigraphy. Clin Nucl Med 2001;26:145-146

Heck LL, Brittin GM: Splenic uptake of both technetium-99m diphosphonate and technetium-99m sulfur colloid in sickle cell beta (0) thalassemia. Clin Nucl Med 1989;14:557-563

Honasoge M, Kottamasu SR, Frame B: Vascular insufficiency: osteonecrosis. In Frame B, Honasoge M, Kottamasu SR (eds): Osteosclerosis, Hyperostosis and Related Disorders. New York, Elsevier Science, 1987:214-239

Hung GL, Stewart CA, Yeo E, et al: Incidental demonstration of cerebral infarction on bone scintigraphy in sickle cell disease. Clin Nucl Med 1990;15:671-672

Kahn CE Jr, Ryan JW, Hatfield MK, Martin WB: Combined bone marrow and gallium imaging: differentiation of osteomyelitis and infarction in sickle hemoglobinopathy. Clin Nucl Med 1988; 13:443-449

Kangarloo H, Dietrich RB, Taira RT, et al: MR imaging of bone marrow in children. J Comput Assist Tomogr 1986;10:205-209

Levin TL, Berdon WE, Haller JO, et al. Intrasplenic masses of "preserved" functioning splenic tissue in sickle cell disease: correlation of imaging findings (CT, ultasound, MRI, and nuclear scintigraphy). Pediatr Radiol 1996;26:646-649

Mallouh A: Acute splenic sequestration in sickle cell disease. J Pediatr 1986;108:1035-1036

Milner PF: Bone marrow infarction in sickle cell anemia. Blood 1984;63:490

Moore SG: Pediatric bone marrow and musculoskeletal imaging. In Stark DD, Bradley WG (eds): Magnetic Resonance Imaging. St Louis, Mosby–Year Book, 1991:145-157

Murphy KJ: Skull abnormalities on MR of children with sickle cell disease. AJNR Am J Neuroradiol 1997;18:596

Paknikar S, Singh A: Nonvisualization of spleen on sulfur colloid images: a sequel of massive infarction. Semin Nucl Med 1998;28:188-191

Pardoll DM, Rodeheffer RJ, Smith RR, Charache S: Aplastic crisis due to extensive bone marrow necrosis in sickle cell disease. Arch Intern Med 1982;142:2223-2225

Rao S, Solomon N, Miller S, et al: Scintigraphic differentiation of bone infarction from osteomyelitis in children with sickle cell disease. J Pediatr 1985;107:685-688

Rao VM, Fishman M, Mitchell DG, et al: Painful sickle cell crisis: bone marrow patterns observed with MR imaging. Radiology 1986;161:211-215

Reynolds J: A re-evaluation of the "fish vertebrae" sign in sickle cell hemoglobinopathy. Am J Roentgenol Radium Ther Nucl Med 1966;97:693-707

Rosner F: Hand-foot syndrome in sickle cell disease. J Clin Oncol 1998;16:808-809

Sarton CJ, Cockshott WP: Bone changes in hemoglobin SC disease. Am J Roentgenol Radium Ther Nucl Med 1962;88:523-532

Saywell WR: Bone marrow MRI in sickle cell disease. Clin Radiol 1990;41:364

Sebes JI, Massie JD, White TJ 3rd, et al: Pelvic extramedullary hematopoiesis. J Nucl Med 1984;25:209-210

Silberstein EB, DeLong S, Cline J: Tc-99m diphosphonate and sulfur colloid uptake by the spleen in sickle disease: interrelationship and clinical correlates: concise communication. J Nucl Med 1984;25:1300-1303

Snelling CE, Brown A: A case of hemolytic jaundice with bone changes. J Pediatr 1936;8:330-337

Spencer RP, Sziklas JJ, Zubi SM: Disassociation of splenic accumulation of Tc-99m MDP and radiocolloid. Clin Nucl Med 1991;16:747-749

van Zanten TE, Statius van Eps LW, Golding RP, et al: Imaging the bone marrow with magnetic resonance during a crisis and in chronic forms of sickle cell disease. Clin Radiol 1989;40:486-489

Watson RJ, Burko H, Megas H, et al: The hand–foot syndrome in sickle cell disease in young children. Pediatrics 1963;31:975-982

Wolff MH, Sty JR: Orbital infarction in sickle cell disease. Pediatr Radiol 1985;15:50-52

Worrall VT, Butera V: Sickle cell dactylitis. J Bone Joint Surg Am 1976;58:1161-1163

Leukemia

Athale UH, Kaste SC, Razzouk BI, et al: Skeletal manifestations of pediatric acute megakaryoblastic leukemia. J Pediatr Hematol Oncol 2002;24:561-565

Bassichis B, McClay J, Wiatrak B: Chloroma of the masseteric muscle. Int J Pediatr Otorhinolaryngol 2000;53:57-61

Benz G, Brandeis WE, Willich E: Radiological aspects of leukemia in childhood: an analysis of 89 children. Pediatr Radiol 1976;4:201-213

Capdeville R, Bertrand Y, Manel AM, et al: Granulocytic sarcoma (chloroma): rare extramedullary tumors associated with acute non-lymphoblastic leukemia. Pediatrie 1990;45:245-250

Crain SM, Choudhury AM, Molnar Z, et al: Destructive osteolytic bone lesions in chronic granulocytic leukemia. Ill Med J 1982;162:213-217

Hermann G, Feldman F, Abdelwahab IF, Klein MJ: Skeletal

manifestations of granulocytic sarcoma (chloroma). Skeletal Radiol 1991;20:509-512

Karimova EJ, Rai SN, Howard SC, et al: Femoral head osteonecrosis in pediatric and young adult patients with leukemia or lymphoma. J Clin Oncol 2007;25:1525-1531

Kozlowski K, Campbell JB, Leonidas JC, et al: Unusual radiographic bone abnormalities in leukaemia: report of three cases. J Belge Radiol 1987;70:229-233

Libson E, Bloom RA, Galun E, et al: Granulocytic sarcoma (chloroma) of bone: the CT appearance. Comput Radiol 1986;10:175-178

Moody A, Simpson E, Shaw D: Florid radiological appearance of megakaryoblastic leukaemia–an aid to earlier diagnosis. Pediatr Radiol 1989;19:486-488

Nijland E, Wuisman P, van Royen B, et al: Vertebral chloroma in a 1½-year-old boy with no evidence of leukemia. Med Pediatr Oncol 2001;36;341-342

Novick SL, Nicol TL, Fishman EK: Granulocytic sarcoma (chloroma) of the sacrum: initial manifestation of leukemia. Skeletal Radiol 1998;27:112-114

Pomeranz SJ, Hawkins HH, Towbin R, et al: Granulocytic sarcoma (chloroma): CT manifestations. Radiology 1985;155:167-170

Pui MH, Fletcher BD, Langston JW: Granulocytic sarcoma in childhood leukemia: imaging features. Radiology 1994;190:698-702

Rosenfield NS, McIntosh S: Prospective analysis of bone changes in treated childhood leukemia. Radiology 1977;123:413-415

Schabel SI, Tyminski L, Holland RD, et al: The skeletal manifestations of chronic myelogenous leukemia. Skeletal Radiol 1980;5:145-149

Hemophilia

Brant EE, Jordan HH: Radiologic aspects of hemophilic pseudotumors of bone. Am J Roentgenol Radium Ther Nucl Med 1972;115:525-539

Hennes H, Losek JD, Sty JR, et al: Computerized tomography in hemophiliacs with head trauma. Pediatr Emerg Care 1987;3:147-149

Hermann G, Gilbert MS, Abdelwahab IF: Hemophilia: evaluation of musculoskeletal involvement with CT, sonography, and MR imaging. AJR Am J Roentgenol 1992;158:119-123

Horton DD, Pollay M, Wilson DA, et al: Cranial hemophilic pseudotumor: case report. J Neurosurg 1993;79:936-938

Jaovisidha S, Ryu KN, Hodler J, et al: Hemophilic pseudotumor: spectrum of MR findings. Skeletal Radiol 1997;26:468-474

Kulkarni MV, Drolshagen LF, Kaye JJ, et al: MR imaging of hemophilic arthropathy. J Comput Assist Tomogr 1985;10:445-449

Lan HH, Eustace SJ, Dorfman D: Hemophilic arthropathy. Radiol Clin North Am 1996;34:446-450

Llauger J, Palmer J, Roson N, et al: Nonseptic monoarthritis: imaging features with clinical and histopathologic correlation. Radiographics 2000;20(suppl):263-278

Mathew P, Talbut DC, Frogameni A, et al: Isotopic synovectomy with P-32 in paediatric patients with haemophilia. Haemophilia 2000;6:547-555

Nuss R, Kilcoyne RF, Geraghty S, et al: Utility of magnetic resonance imaging for management of hemophilic arthropathy in children. J Pediatr 1993;123:388-392

Nuss R, Kilcoyne RF, Geraghty S, et al: MRI findings in haemophilic joints treated with radiosynoviorthesis with development of an MRI scale of joint damage. Haemophilia 2000;6:162-169

Pettersson H, Ahlberg A, Nillson IM: A radiologic classification of hemophilic arthropathy. Clin Orthop 1980;149:153-159

Pettersson H, Gillespy T, Kitchens C, et al: Magnetic resonance imaging in hemophilic arthropathy of the knee. Acta Radiol 1987;28:621-625

Plazanet F, du Boullay C, Defaux F, et al: Open synovectomy for the prevention of recurrent hemarthrosis of the ankle in patients with hemophilia: a report of five cases with magnetic resonance imaging documentation. Rev Rhum Engl Ed 1997;64:166-171

Rand T, Trattnig S, Male C, et al: Magnetic resonance imaging in hemophilic children: value of gradient echo and contrast-enhanced imaging. Magn Reson Imaging 1999;17:199-205

Reeves A, Edwards-Brown M: Intraosseous hematoma in a newborn with factor VIII deficiency. AJNR Am J Neuroradiol 2000;21:308-309

Mastocytosis

Avila NA, Ling A, Metcalfe DD, Worobec AS: Mastocytosis: magnetic resonance imaging patterns of marrow disease. Skeletal Radiol 1998;27:119-126

Avila NA, Ling A, Worobec AS, et al: Systemic mastocytosis: CT and US features of abdominal manifestations. Radiology 1997;202:367-372

Gagnon JH, Kalz F, Kadri AM, et al: Mastocytosis: unusual manifestations, clinical and radiologic changes. Can Med Assoc Journal 1975;112:1328-1332

Kiszewski AE, Alvarez-Mendoza A, Ríos-Barrera VA, et al: Mastocytosis in children: clinicopathological study based on 35 cases. Histol Histopathol 2007;22:535-539

Korenblat PE, Wedner J, Whyte MP, et al: Systemic mastocytosis. Arch Intern Med 1984;144:2249-2253

Lucaya J, Perez-Candela V, Aso C, et al: Mastocytosis with skeletal and gastrointestinal involvement in infancy: two case reports and review of the literature. Radiology 1979;131:363-366

CHAPTER

179

The Joints

MARILYN D. E. RANSON and PAUL S. BABYN

NORMAL ANATOMY

Joints comprise the tissues that allow normal motion between articulating bones. Depending on the type of interposed tissue, joints may be classified into fibrous, cartilaginous, or synovial articulations. Fibrous joints include the cranial sutures and syndesmoses, where the articulating bones are bound together either by a fibrous interosseous ligament or fibrous membrane. Cartilaginous joints have interposed cartilage connecting adjacent bones. These joints may be temporary, as in the synchondroses or growth plates between the primary and secondary ossification centers of the tubular bones, or permanent, as in the symphysis pubis. Most common are synovial joints, where the joint cavity contains synovial fluid and articular cartilage covers the opposing ends of the articulating bones (Fig. 179-1).

Synovial joints are contained within a joint capsule that arises from the periosteum near the ends of the opposing bones. The joint capsule usually originates near the epiphyseal plate to encompass the epiphysis; however, for some joints, it also contains a portion of the metaphysis (as in the hip joint), making these joints more susceptible to infection arising from the metaphysis. The outer layer of the joint capsule is fibrous tissue that develops variable thickness as surrounding capsular ligaments thicken and reinforce the capsule. The synovial membrane lies along the inner aspect of the capsule and lines the nonarticular portion of the joint. Composed of two layers, a thin cellular intima and a vascular subintima containing blood vessels and lymphatics, the synovial membrane secretes synovial fluid to both lubricate and nourish articular cartilage. Normally, the articular cartilage surfaces are in close apposition; however, in some synovial joints, an intervening disk of fibrocartilage is present (e.g., the menisci of the knee) that separates the apposing articular cartilage. The normal amount of synovial fluid is usually slight but varies with each individual joint.

Articular cartilage is derived from the immature articular epiphyseal cartilage complex. During infancy and childhood, epiphyseal and articular cartilage are directly continuous with each other. With maturation, the underlying epiphyseal cartilage is progressively ossified until only the covering articular cartilage remains when growth is completed.

Fat pads may also be present within the joint capsule. Bursae are fluid-filled spaces in the periarticular connective space. They are lined with a cellular membrane similar to the synovial covering of the articular spaces and are located at sites of maximal frictional impact

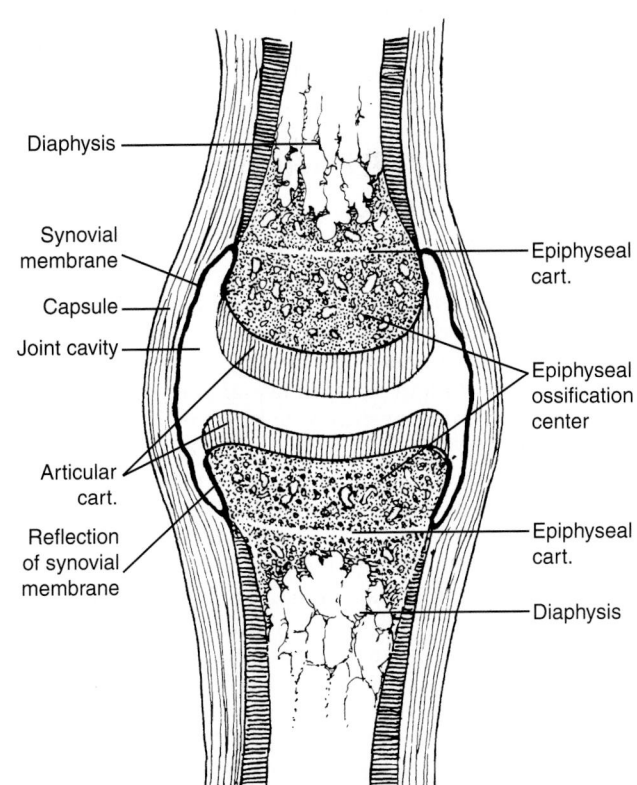

FIGURE 179-1. Schematic representation of the principal structures in a typical joint. The synovial membrane is the inner aspect of the articular capsule; it does not extend onto the articular cartilages. The joint cavity is artificially dilated to many times its normal depth.

Diaphysis

Synovial membrane

Capsule

Joint cavity

Articular cart.

Reflection of synovial membrane

Epiphyseal cart.

Epiphyseal ossification center

Epiphyseal cart.

Diaphysis

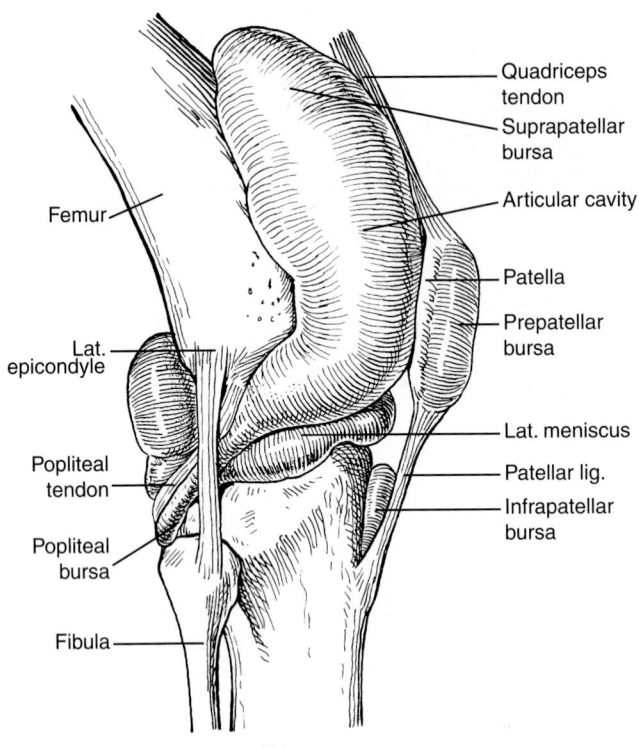

FIGURE 179-2. Normal bursae around the knee joint.

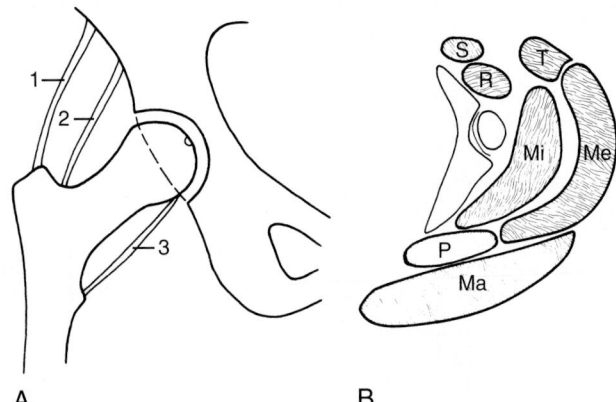

FIGURE 179-3. Diagrams of fat planes adjacent to the hip. **A,** Frontal plane. *1,* More superficial of the two lateral fat planes. *2,* More medial lateral fat plane. *3,* Fat plane medial to the hip. Plane 1 is cast by fat between the gluteus medius and minimus muscles and 2, by the fat anteriorly between the rectus femoris muscle and the tensor fasciae latae muscle and is continuous with the more narrow fat plane that overlies the capsule; plane 3 derives from fat along the medial border of the iliopsoas muscle. **B,** Horizontal section. *Ma,* gluteus maximus; *Me,* gluteus medius; *Mi,* gluteus minimus; *P,* piriformis *S,* sartorius; *R,* rectus femoris; *T,* tensor fasciae latae. (Modified from Reichmann S: Roentgenologic soft tissue appearances in hip joint disease. Acta Radiol 1967;6:167-176.)

between neighboring movable structures. Variable in number, bursae may be multilocular and often communicate with one another and the adjacent joint space. For example, the multiple bursae around the knee are shown in Figure 179-2.

NORMAL IMAGING APPEARANCE

Composed almost entirely of tissues of water density, normal articular components are all of a similar radiographic density. Thus the individual components of the normal joint cannot be clearly differentiated from each other or from neighboring muscles, fascia, tendons, ligaments, nerves, or vessels by conventional radiography. Displacement of fat deposits in fascial and intermuscular planes readily demonstrates abnormal intra-articular content, including joint effusions in the elbow and ankle. However, around the hip, the shape of these radiolucent stripes and their relationship to the underlying joint is complex (Fig. 179-3), making accurate determination of hip joint effusions difficult because they are modified by slight changes of femoral rotation and abduction.

In the newborn, radiography demonstrates wide areas between the bony structures on the two sides of the joints (Fig. 179-4). These are filled with the unossified epiphyseal cartilage that, as it ossifies, ultimately narrows the separation to the thickness of the opposing layers of articular cartilage. A vacuum phenomenon caused by the presence of gas within a joint can occur normally and appear radiographically as a crescentic lucency. This may follow a sudden lowering of intra-articular pressure by endogenous muscle pulls or from external traction. The gases move from contiguous structures to the lowered

pressure in the suddenly expanded joint space. Vacuum phenomena are most frequently evident in the shoulders and hips of infants when the extremities are suddenly abducted during positioning for a radiographic study (Fig. 179-5). The gas is rapidly absorbed or replaced by fluid even if the distraction force is maintained. In the presence of a significant joint effusion, the vacuum phenomenon cannot normally be produced, and its presence has been relied on to exclude a significant effusion. However, a recent case report has demonstrated a significant effusion sonographically following a positive traction sign. Vacuum phenomena can be seen on sonography and magnetic resonance imaging (MRI). On MRI, intra-articular gas may simulate meniscal tears, intra-articular loose bodies, or chondrocalcinosis.

Although plain images should almost always be used initially to evaluate joints, the introduction of cross-sectional imaging techniques has provided a significant improvement in anatomic delineation and diagnosis. Sonography is ideal for assessing the pediatric musculoskeletal system largely because of its ability to visualize cartilage, which is abundant in the immature skeleton. Hyaline cartilage is hypoechoic and allows through-transmission of the sound beam because of its homogeneous structure. Tiny specular echoes, which represent vascular cartilage canals, help differentiate cartilage from fluid. Cartilage canals are prominent in infancy and early childhood, and diminish with advancing age. Fibrocartilage is echogenic, especially within the acetabular labrum and menisci. Sonography is sensitive in detecting joint effusion, particularly in the hip and shoulder, where plain images are insensitive. It can demonstrate synovial thickening, which may be hypervascular with color Doppler examination. Intra-articular masses may also be detected with sonography, although the appear-

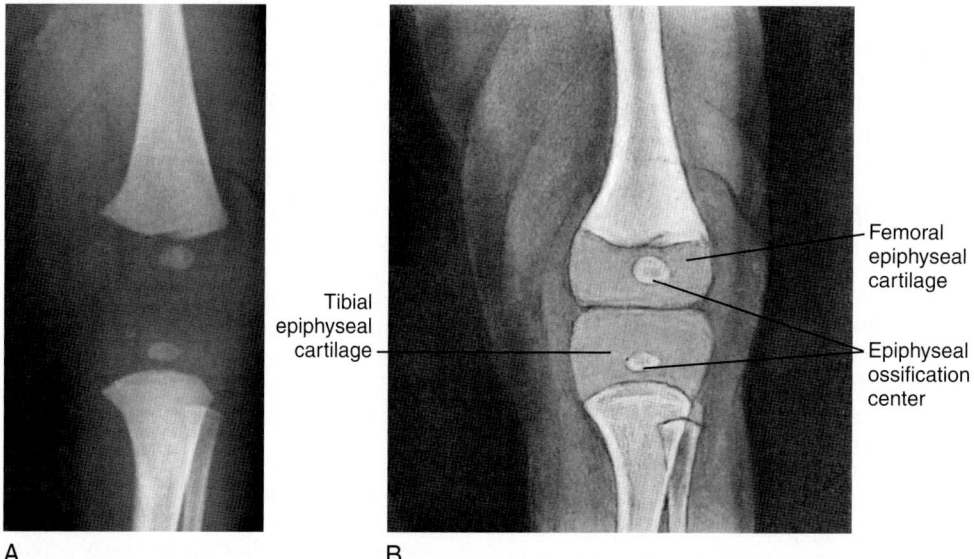

FIGURE 179-4. Cartilage space between the ends of the opposing bones at the knee joint of a newborn infant. **A,** Radiograph. **B,** Schematic drawing of **A.** The space between the ends of the opposing bones is occupied by a shadow of water density in the radiograph. In the drawing, this space is filled completely by the epiphyseal cartilages and their overlaying articular cartilages. In the normal living joint, the joint cleft is exceedingly narrow and casts an insignificant shadow in the radiograph.

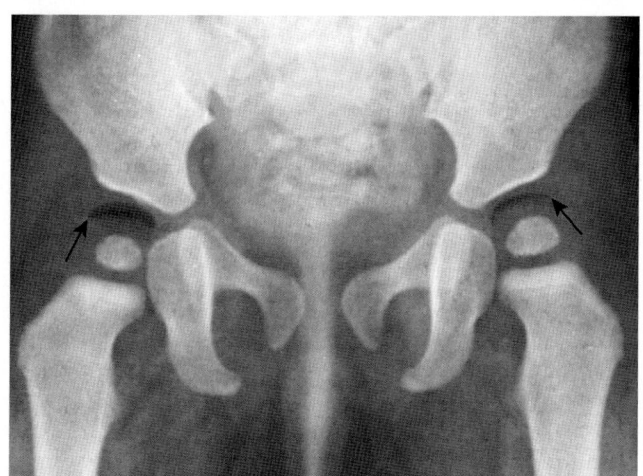

FIGURE 179-5. Bilateral natural pneumograms of the hips of a normal infant 12 months of age. The radiolucent strips *(arrows)* represent intra-articular gas between the cartilaginous edge of the acetabulum and the epiphyseal cartilage of the femoral head.

ance is often nonspecific. Ultrasound can also be used to assess tendons and ligaments with higher frequency transducers. Tendons normally have an echogenic fibrillar appearance on ultrasound. Fluid or synovial thickening within the tendon sheath appears as an anechoic or hypoechoic halo surrounding the tendon.

Computed tomography (CT) can be used to evaluate the joint space and detect adjacent bone abnormalities, including coalitions, erosions, and subchondral cysts. CT is primarily used to assess osseous structures because MRI now provides better tissue contrast with multiplanar imaging capability.

MRI has had a dramatic impact on the evaluation of joint disease. It can provide multiplanar images without radiation, achieve superb tissue contrast, and define vascular anatomy with or without contrast. However high cost, limited availability, and frequent need for sedation limit its more widespread use. It is the best modality to examine all the components of the joints, including bone marrow, cortical bone, hyaline and fibrocartilage, ligaments, menisci, synovium and joint capsule, joint fluid, and the unossified cartilaginous skeleton.

MRI technique should include multiplanar evaluation with a combination of T1- and T2-weighted sequences, fast spin-echo, and post-contrast studies tailored to the specific clinical problem. Appropriate field of view depends on the age and size of the child and the joint and structures needing to be visualized. Cartilaginous structures, including the physis, are well seen with gradient-recalled echo techniques or fat-suppressed fast-proton density sequences. Gadolinium-enhanced MRI can differentiate physeal from epiphyseal cartilage and can visualize normal vessels present within the chondro-epiphysis. MRI is useful in detecting synovial abnormalities within the joint and associated changes affecting the articular cartilage and osseous structures. The normal synovium is virtually imperceptible on MRI and enhances only minimally. Slight enhancement may be seen in richly vascularized areas such as the tissues adjacent to the posterior attachment of the temporomandibular joint. A small amount of joint fluid may normally be seen with MRI.

Multiphase bone scintigraphy can help differentiate osseous causes of pain from other causes of joint pain, including synovial, neuromuscular, or periarticular soft tissue disorders. Bone scintigraphy is helpful to establish whether an osseous lesion is solitary or multifocal and can reveal increased activity across the joint in arthritis or infection. Specialized adjuncts to routine scintigraphic imaging include magnification scintigraphy and single-photon emission CT, whereas dual-energy x-ray absorptiometry is often used in assessment of bone density.

Currently, arthrography is rarely indicated. However, intra-articular contrast injection may be combined with CT, or now more frequently with MRI, to better delineate joint detail, including the evaluation of labral tears within the shoulder or hip joint.

DISEASES OF THE JOINTS

Joint abnormalities may be caused by a wide variety of disorders, including congenital abnormalities, trauma, infection, juvenile rheumatoid arthritis (JRA) and other inflammatory arthritides, synovial disease, malignancy, and numerous noninflammatory mechanical joint lesions. A number of significant joint disorders are discussed in detail elsewhere and are not addressed here, including Legg-Calvé-Perthes disease (see Chapter 173), slipped capital femoral epiphysis (see Chapter 170), developmental hip dysplasia (see Chapter 180) and joint disease related to metabolic disorders (see Chapter 167).

CONGENITAL MALFORMATIONS

Many congenital anomalies of the joints can be encountered, including congenital dislocations, subluxation, ankylosis, and other deformities. Usually plain images suffice, but MRI may be of benefit if surgery is planned and better definition of cartilaginous structures or ligaments is needed. These anomalies are not discussed further here because they are discussed elsewhere (see Chapter 164). Contractures of one or more joints may be present at birth in a wide variety of syndromes, including arthrogryposis multiplex, fetal alcohol syndrome, chromosomal abnormalities, and nail–patella syndrome (see Chapters 165 and 166). In congenital lateral dislocation of the patella, there is typically a persistent flexion contracture with limited extension (see Chapter 174). Malposition of the patellar cartilaginous shadow may be overlooked on lateral radiographs unless specifically considered. Larsen syndrome is commonly associated with multiple congenital dislocations, particularly of the knees, hips, elbows, and feet (see Chapter 166).

ARTHRITIS

Arthritis is commonly encountered in childhood and may be defined as joint swelling or joint pain associated with limitation of joint motion in at least one joint. Arthritis may arise from a wide variety of inflammatory and noninflammatory joint disorders. The synovium is often involved, with diffuse synovitis, focal synovial proliferation, synovial infiltration, and synovial masses. Arthritis may be subdivided into acute or chronic forms. Acute arthritis is a potential medical emergency that must be investigated and treated promptly. Imaging often plays a key role in establishing the presence of disease, determining its extent, and defining the specific diagnosis. In this section, we review common and important causes of acute and chronic arthritis.

Juvenile Rheumatoid Arthritis

Clinically diagnosed, JRA is an idiopathic arthritis that begins before age 16 years and that persists for more than than 6 weeks. All other diseases that can cause arthritis need to be considered and excluded (both common and unusual) before the diagnosis of JRA is made. An approach to the significant differential diagnostic considerations of JRA is presented shown in Table 179-1. Chronic inflammatory arthritis is the most important rheumatic disease affecting children and one of the most common chronic diseases of childhood. Although JRA may be self-limited, with a majority of patients having no active synovitis in adulthood, many children have significant joint complications.

> JRA is an idiopathic arthritis that begins before age 16 years and that persists for more than 6 weeks. Many other dieases may cause arthritis and must be considered in the differential diagnosis.

Several terms are in common use to describe chronic idiopathic synovitis in children, including JRA, juvenile chronic polyarthritis, juvenile chronic arthritis (especially in Europe), chronic childhood arthritis, and Still disease. However, they are not completely synonymous in their classification, with different inclusion and exclusion criteria. This multiplicity of terms makes review of the current and historical literature difficult. In an attempt to unify diagnostic criteria, the International League of Associations for Rheumatology (ILAR) has recently proposed a new classification scheme. Because the ILAR classification has not yet received broad currency, we shall continue to use the term JRA and the recognized subgroups previously established by the American College of Rheumatology while introducing the ILAR terminology. The subgroups of JRA include systemic-onset disease, pauciarticular disease (four or fewer joints involved), and polyarticular disease (greater than four joints) as determined by their clinical features, disease onset, and response to therapy. Disease onset is characterized by the pattern of disease during the first 6 months, including number of involved joints and the nature and prominence of extra-articular manifestations. An overview of the current classification schemes is provided in Table 179-2.

> Subgroups of JRA include systemic-onset disease, pauciarticular disease (four or fewer joints involved), and polyarticular disease (greater than four joints).

Management of JRA includes use of nonsteroidal anti-inflammatory drugs for relief of pain and inflammation and to allow continued joint function; however, these drugs do not prevent radiographic progression. Joint injections with corticosteroids can be used for patients with pauciarticular joint involvement. Patients with polyarticular disease often need methotrexate, sulfasalazine, or other second-line therapy.

TABLE 179-1		
Differential Diagnosis of Juvenile Rheumatoid Arthritis		

SYNOVIAL DISORDERS
Pauciarticular
Acute   Infectious arthritis
       Septic arthritis
       Reactive arthritis
       Tuberculous arthritis
       Postinfectious arthritis
    Early rheumatic disease
       Arthritis associated with chromosomal
          abnormalities—Down, Turner
          syndromes
       Seronegative spondyloarthropathy
       Acute transient arthritis
    Other
       Foreign body arthritis
       Hemophilic arthropathy
Chronic   Rheumatic diseases
       Arthritis associated with chromosomal
          abnormalities—Down, Turner
          syndromes
    Synovial masses
       Nodular synovitis
       Pigmented villonodular synovitis
       Synovial hemangioma
       Lipoma arborescens
       Synovial osteochondromatosis
    Other
       Hemophilic arthropathy
       Sarcoidosis
       Intra-articular osteoid osteoma
Polyarticular   Seronegative spondyloarthropathies
    Infectious arthritis
       Lyme disease

    Reactive arthritis
    Arthritis associated with chromosomal
       abnormalities—Down, Turner syndromes
    Connective tissue disorders
       Systemic lupus erythematosus
       Sarcoidosis
    Inherited disorders
       Familial hypertrophic synovitis
       Hemophilic arthropathy
       Immunodeficiency

NONSYNOVIAL DISORDERS
Pauciarticular
Acute   Malignancy
       Leukemia
       Neuroblastoma
Chronic   Noninflammatory disorders
       Avascular necrosis
       Slipped epiphyses and dysplasias
    Other
       Juvenile osteoporosis
       Multifocal osteolysis
Polyarticular   Metabolic or inherited disorders
       Diabetic cheiroarthropathy
       Turner syndrome
       Lysosomal storage disease
    Others
       Kniest syndrome, Winchester syndrome,
          chondrodysplasias
       Frostbite
       Goldbloom disease

SUBTYPES

SYSTEMIC-ONSET ARTHRITIS. Systemic-onset JRA accounts for 10% to 20% of all JRA cases, affecting boys and girls almost equally. It is most frequently seen under the age of 5 years, although it may occur at any age. Systemic-onset JRA is characterized by its prominent extra-articular manifestations, including daily spiking fever (an essential diagnostic criterion), an evanescent rash, serositis, and other features, including lymphadenopathy and reticuloendothelial involvement. Although systemic-onset JRA accounts for a minority of JRA cases, there is disproportionate morbidity and mortality associated with this subtype. In systemic-onset JRA, the fever is almost always present at disease onset but infrequently may appear only after onset of arthritis. Serositis, most often pericarditis, is a classic feature, but pleuritis and peritonitis with sizable fluid collections can occur. In systemic-onset JRA, there may be hepatosplenomegaly and reticuloendothelial involvement with generalized lymphadenopathy, including para-aortic mesenteric and more peripheral nodes. Macrophage activation syndrome is a potentially fatal complication resulting from uncontrolled macrophage activation and cytokine effects on various organs.

Arthritis in systemic-onset JRA usually develops within the first few months of disease onset; however, it may be delayed for years. Chronic destructive arthritis eventually develops in 33 to 50% of cases, and the course is typically polyarticular, although the onset is usually pauciarticular. The most commonly involved joints are the knees, wrists, and ankles, but cervical spine disease and hip involvement are also common.

PAUCIARTICULAR DISEASE. Pauciarticular disease is the most common form of JRA, with a peak age of incidence in young childhood. Two main groups of pauciarticular disease are encountered; both have four joints or fewer involved within the first 6 months but may later develop more joint involvement. Joints involved include knee, ankle, elbow, and wrist. The first type is rheumatoid factor (RF) negative in 30% to 40% of cases; the hips and sacroiliac joints are spared. This type is predominantly seen in girls, with late childhood onset. Typically these patients have mild arthritis. Iridocyclitis or anterior uveitis will be present in 20% to 30% of patients.

The second type is seen in boys with late childhood onset. The hips and sacroiliac joints are often afflicted, and these patients likely have early undifferentiated spondyloarthropathy.

POLYARTICULAR DISEASE. Patients with polyarticular disease are commonly divided into two groups: those

TABLE 179-2

Classification Schemes: American College Of Rheumatology (ACR), European League against Rheumatism (EULAR), And International League of Association for Rheumatology (ILAR)

ACR	EULAR	ILAR
Juvenile Rheumatoid Arthritis Subtypes:	**Juvenile Chronic Arthritis Subtypes:**	**Juvenile Idiopathic Arthritis Subtypes:**
Systemic arthritis	*Systemic arthritis*	*Systemic arthritis*—associated with fever of 2 weeks' duration and one or more of rash, generalized lymphadenopathy, hepatosplenomegaly or serositis
Pauciarticular arthritis	*Pauciarticular disease*	
Polyarticular arthritis	*Polyarticular arthritis*	*Polyarthritis (RF positive)*—polyarticular disease, RF positive
Excludes spondyloarthritis Arthritis must be present for at least 6 weeks	*Juvenile rheumatoid arthritis (RF positive only)*	*Polyarthritis (RF negative)*—polyarticular disease, RF negative
	Spondyloarthritis	*Oligoarthritis*—less than five joints involved
	Arthritis must be present for 3 months	*Extended oligoarthritis*—initially oligoarthritis but develops polyarticular disease
		Psoriatic arthritis—arthritis and psoriasis or arthritis with two of the following: dactylitis, nail abnormalities, positive family history
		Enthesitis-related arthritis—arthritis and enthesitis or arthritis or enthesitis with two of the following: sacroiliac joint tenderness and/or inflammatory spinal pain, presence of HLA-B27, family history of HLA-B27–associated disease, anterior uveitis, onset of arthritis in a boy after the age of 8 years
		Other arthritis—idiopathic arthritis that does not fulfill other criteria or fulfills more than one set of criteria
		Arthritis must be present for at least 6 weeks

RF, rheumatoid factor.
From Petty RE: Classification of childhood arthritis: a work in progress. Baillieres Clin Rheumatol 1998;12:181-190, with permission.

who are RF positive and those who are RF negative. RF-negative disease is the most common form of polyarticular disease. There is often symmetric polyarthritis of small joints and large joints, and female preponderance with early or late childhood onset. Severe arthritis is present in 10% to 15% of patients.

RF-positive disease shows features and extra-articular manifestations similar to adult rheumatoid arthritis, with rheumatoid nodules and early erosive and symmetric polyarthritis. Arthritis involves the small joints of the hand and feet, including proximal interphalangeal joints, metacarpophalangeal joints, tarsus, and large joints, including the knees and ankles. There is female preponderance, with typically late childhood onset and severe arthritis in more than 50%.

Imaging

Imaging can be used to determine whether arthritis is indeed present, establish a specific diagnosis, and determine extent of disease. It may also be used to determine disease activity, detect disease complications, evaluate disease progression, and judge efficacy of drug treatment.

In JRA, the synovium is the target tissue for inflammation. Early in the disease course, the affected joints are clinically swollen, stiff, painful, and warm, and show limited motion. There is synovial proliferation and infiltration by inflammatory cells, including polymorpho-nuclear leukocytes, lymphocytes, and plasma cells, and increased secretion of synovial fluid. With larger areas of infiltration, lymphoid follicles and granulation tissue form, leading to synovial thickening and pannus formation. Inflammation of synovial coverings of tendons and bursae, which can also be affected, can lead to periostitis. With prolonged inflammation, destruction of cartilage, adjacent bone erosions and even joint ankylosis may be seen (Fig. 179-6).

RADIOGRAPHY

Plain images of symptomatic areas are usually obtained at initial presentation. The purpose is as much to exclude other differential diagnoses as it is to make a diagnosis of arthritis. Plain radiography in evaluation of early arthritis is of limited utility because the inflamed synovium, soft tissue changes, and cartilage erosion that precede bone erosions are not well seen. Initial radiographs are often nonspecific, reflecting early response of the soft tissues and bones to inflammation, with soft tissue swelling, osteopenia, joint effusions, and periosteal reaction (Table 179-3). Many of these findings are nonspecific (Table 179-4). The osteopenia is initially peri-articular, becoming more diffuse with time. Rarely one sees the band-like pattern observed in leukemia. Periosteal reaction is commonly seen in the phalanges, metacarpals (Fig. 179-7), and metatarsals but can occur in the long bones (Fig. 179-8).

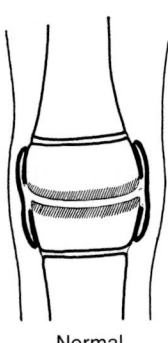 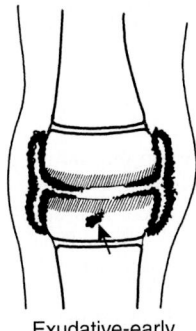 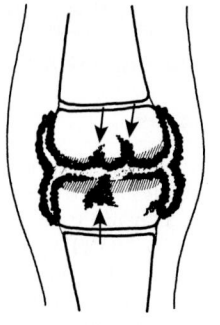 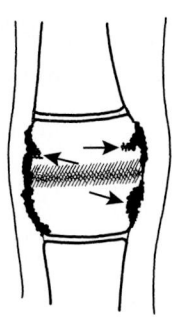

Normal	Exudative-early proliferative	Destructive	Obliterative

FIGURE 179-6. Gross progressive structural changes responsible for the radiographic findings in rheumatoid arthritis. The synovial layer is drawn in *heavy black.* In the *normal joint,* the synovium stops at the edges of the articular cartilages, which are uncovered and exposed directly to the synovial fluid and to the opposing articular cartilage. In the *early exudative and proliferative stage,* the synovial layer is thickened and the articular space laterally and medially, beyond the articular cartilages, is dilated, but the space between the cartilages themselves is not deepened. The synovium is beginning to grow over the articular cartilages from their edges and to abrade the cartilage edge on which they grow. Deep in the tibial ossification center and unrelated to the overgrowth of synovium, a patch of necrosis *(arrow)* has appeared that represents the overgrowth of mesenchymal elements in the marrow. At this time, radiographic findings include regional swelling of soft parts and beginning rarefaction of bones with destruction in the tibial epiphyseal center. In the *destructive phase,* the edges of the articular cartilages *(arrows)* are deeply abraded, with beginning destruction of subchondral bone and extension of the marrow overgrowth in the tibial center through the bone and cartilage into the joint space *(arrow).* In the *obliterative phase,* most of the articular cartilages have disappeared, and there is junction by bony union. Hypertrophic synovium is present on the sides *(arrows)* of the condyles and is growing into them and destroying them.

TABLE 179-03

Radiographic Features of Juvenile Rheumatoid Arthritis

EARLY FINDINGS
Joint effusion
Soft tissue swelling
Osteoporosis—may be juxta-articular or diffuse, may lead to insufficiency fractures, rarely metaphyseal lucent bands
Periostitis—typically in periarticular regions of phalanges, metacarpals, metatarsals; rarely metaphyses or diaphyses of long bones
Tendinitis

LATE FINDINGS
Joint space loss—reflects underlying cartilage loss
Joint malalignment—subluxation, dislocations, protrusio acetabuli; common in the wrist, hip
Bony erosions—typically late manifestation if not seropositive or systemic-onset arthritis at the margins or along the articular surface
Growth disturbances—includes epiphyseal overgrowth, premature physeal closure, short broad phalanges/ metacarpals/metatarsals, temporomandibular hypoplasia, leg length discrepancy

Ankylosis—intra-articular bone ankylosis; small joints of hand and wrist, cervical spine
Hypertrophic bursopathy
Synovial cysts—popliteal, subchondral, bicipital
Compression fractures—especially of weight-bearing epiphyses

SYSTEMIC FINDINGS
Serositis
Generalized lymphadenopathy
Macrophage activation syndrome
Hepatosplenomegaly
Interstitial lung disease
Growth retardation
Amyloidosis
Rheumatoid vasculitis
Lymphedema

> **The early radiographic changes of JRA are soft tissue swelling, osteopenia, joint effusions, and periosteal reaction. These findings are non-specific.**

Soft tissue nodules can be noted, as may periarticular calcification, although this usually is a consequence of prior intra-articular therapy. Joint space narrowing and erosions are usually seen radiographically only two years or so after disease onset (Fig. 179-9). However in polyarticular RF-positive disease and in up to one third of patients with systemic-onset JRA, early erosive disease can occur. Abnormalities in growth and maturation may be present, including accelerated osseous growth and altered maturation, leading to enlarged epiphyses (Fig. 179-10).

Late sequela of JRA are not uncommon and include deformity of epiphyses, abnormal angular carpal bones, and premature fusion of the growth plate with brachydactyly (Fig. 179-11). Other changes include large, cyst-like, well-corticated erosions (Figs. 179-12 and 179-13) that may be lobulated. At the hip, protrusio acetabuli, premature degenerative changes, coxa magna, and coxa

TABLE 179-4

Imaging Mimics of Juvenile Rheumatoid Arthritis

Imaging Findings	Differential Diagnosis
Joint effusion	Traumatic synovitis, infectious/septic arthritis, hemophilic arthropathy, acute transient synovitis, acute rheumatic fever, intra-articular tumors, connective tissue disorders, spondyloarthropathies
Soft tissue swelling	Infectious/septic arthritis, synovial hemangioma, hemophilic arthropathy, diabetic cheiroarthropathy, NOMID, sarcoidosis, PVNS, CAP syndrome
Osteoporosis	Juvenile osteoporosis, multifocal osteolysis, leukemia, collagen–vascular disease, hemophilic arthropathy, infectious arthritis
Joint space loss	Traumatic joint dislocation, septic arthritis, hemophilic arthropathy, avascular necrosis, Kniest syndrome, idiopathic chondrolysis, progressive pseudorheumatoid chondrodysplasia, slipped capital femoral epiphyses, osteoid osteoma
Ankylosis	Spondyloarthropathies, traumatic arthritis, infectious arthritis, iatrogenic
Bony erosions	Hemophilic arthropathy, septic arthritis, spondyloarthropathies, carpal osteolysis, CAP syndrome, PVNS, synovial osteochondromatosis
Periostitis	Trauma including abuse, osteomyelitis, spondyloarthropathies, osteoid osteoma, Goldbloom disease, hypertrophic osteoarthropathy, leukemia, sickle cell dactylitis
Growth disturbances	
Epiphyseal overgrowth	Hemophilic arthropathy, NOMID, trauma, tuberculous/fungal disease, spondyloarthropathies, Legg-Calvé-Perthes disease, skeletal dysplasias, Turner syndrome
Growth arrest	Turner syndrome, frostbite damage, infection
Dysplastic changes	CAP syndrome, mucopolysaccaridosis, mucolipidosis, Kniest syndrome

CAP, camptodactyly–arthropathy–pericarditis; NOMID, neonatal-onset multisystem inflammatory disease; PVNS, pigmented villonodular synovitis.

valga can be seen (Fig. 179-14). Joint space loss can progress to ankylosis, particularly in the apophyseal joints of the cervical spine (Fig. 179-15) and wrist. Subluxation of the joints, especially at the wrist, may also be evident, and atlantoaxial subluxation may also occur. Growth disturbance of the temporomandibular joint may lead to micrognathia and abnormalities of the temporomandibular disk.

BONE DENSITOMETRY

Osteopenia is often present in JRA, even in those patients not taking systemic steroids. Global effects on mineralization have been suspected because of overall poor linear and skeletal growth and an increased incidence of fractures. Bone densitometry may be used to help manage children with significantly decreased bone density.

> Osteopenia is seen with JRA, even in the absence of steroid therapy.

SONOGRAPHY

Sonography is gaining increasing utility in joint evaluation, especially with high-frequency transducers. Although total joint assessment is often hindered by acoustic barriers, sonography can be used to assess articular cartilage thickness and to detect synovial thickening, joint effusions, and associated synovial cysts. Sonography can also be used to assess tendon sheath synovial proliferation and bursal hypertrophy and to guide joint aspiration or injection. Power Doppler shows promise in evaluating the amount and activity of pannus. Sonography may also be used to identify extra-articular complications such as hepatosplenomegaly or serositis.

MAGNETIC RESONANCE IMAGING

With MRI, one can directly image synovial proliferation, joint fluid, pannus formation, and erosion of cartilage and bone (Fig. 179-16). MRI is suitable to assess disease severity or progression and is playing an increasing role in diagnosis and outcome assessment. Uncomplicated joint fluid is usually of low signal on T1- and hyperintense on T2-weighted images. Other findings in JRA include popliteal cysts and meniscal hypoplasia or atrophy (Fig. 179-17). MRI is more sensitive for detection of bone erosions than plain images.

MRI enhancement of the synovium can be used to detect early synovial proliferation, which precedes destructive changes. Normal synovium is thin and shows slight enhancement. Proliferating synovium on MRI without contrast appears as intermediate soft tissue density on T1- and T2-weighted sequences. It may have slightly higher signal than adjacent fluid on unenhanced T1-weighted images. Pannus appears as thickened synovium intermediate to low signal intensity on T2-weighted images, best seen when outlined by high signal joint fluid. Its variable signal intensity reflects its different amounts of fibrous tissue and hemosiderin.

Synovial thickening and effusion may be difficult to distinguish unless intravenous gadolinium is used to demonstrate enhancement of hypervascular synovium (Fig. 179-18). Images should be obtained immediately after contrast injection because diffusion of contrast from the synovium into the joint fluid occurs over time. Contrast enhancement improves visualization of the thickened synovium dramatically, especially with use of fat suppression, allowing the proliferating synovium to be seen in regions normally devoid of synovium as enhancing linear, villous, or nodular tissue. Hypervascular inflamed pannus enhances significantly, whereas

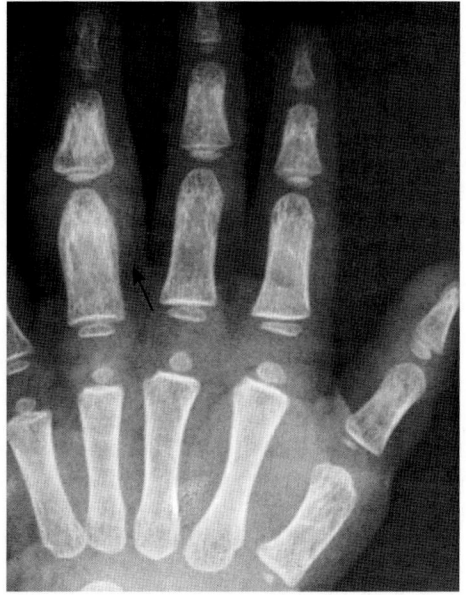

A

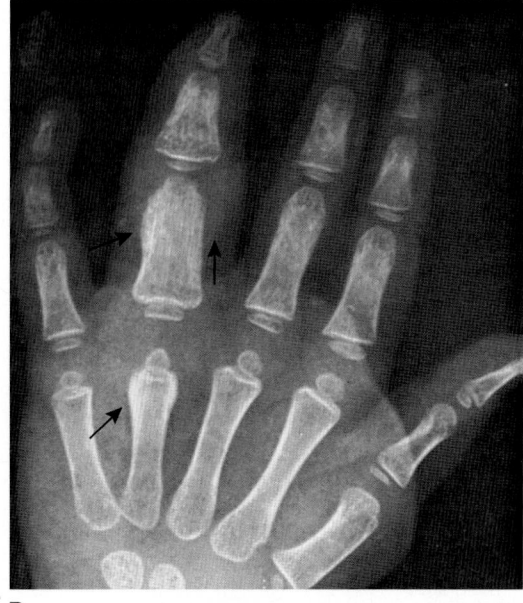

B

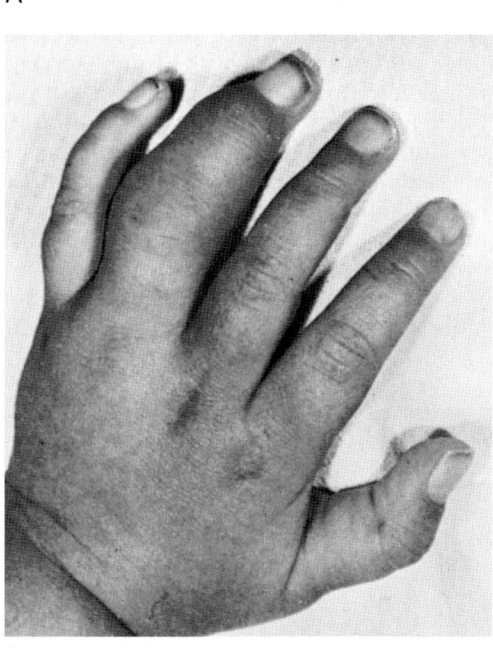

C

FIGURE 179-7. Early rheumatoid arthritis in the fourth finger that began clinically during the 14th month of life. **A,** At 20 months, the soft tissues overlying the basal and middle phalanges are swollen and have a fusiform external contour, and these two phalanges are swollen by periosteal thickening and cortical thickening. **B,** At 30 months, the soft tissues are more swollen, as are the phalanges; external cortical thickening has now begun in the distal end of the fourth metacarpal. **C,** Swelling of the fourth finger and in the hand at the distal end of the fourth metacarpal at **30 months.** (Courtesy of Dr. Sigurd Eek, Oslo, Norway.)

fibrous inactive pannus shows much less enhancement. Quantitative techniques may be used to determine synovial volume.

> **Post-gadolinium MR images are helpful to distinguish synovial proliferation from effusion.**

Hemosiderin deposition can occur in JRA, but it is more frequently is seen in disorders that are accompanied by hemarthrosis, including pigmented villonodular synovitis (PVNS), hemophilic arthropathy, synovial hemangioma, and post-traumatic synovitis. Gradient-echo sequences are most sensitive in detecting hemosiderin deposition within the synovium as signal loss resulting from increased magnetic susceptibility.

With prolonged synovial inflammation, as in JRA and tuberculosis, well-defined intra-articular nodules termed *rice bodies* (because of their characteristic macroscopic appearance) can be noted. Rice bodies likely arise from detached fragments of hypertrophied synovial villi and may lead to painless swelling of the joint. On MRI, rice bodies are of low signal on T2-weighted images. They are associated with joint effusion and synovial hypertrophy and do not usually demonstrate synovial enhancement after gadolinium administration (Fig. 179-19). Removal leads to symptomatic relief.

RESPONSE TO THERAPY

Assessment of disease activity is important for monitoring treatment efficacy and predicting outcome. Histopathologic evidence of persistent synovitis and radiologic

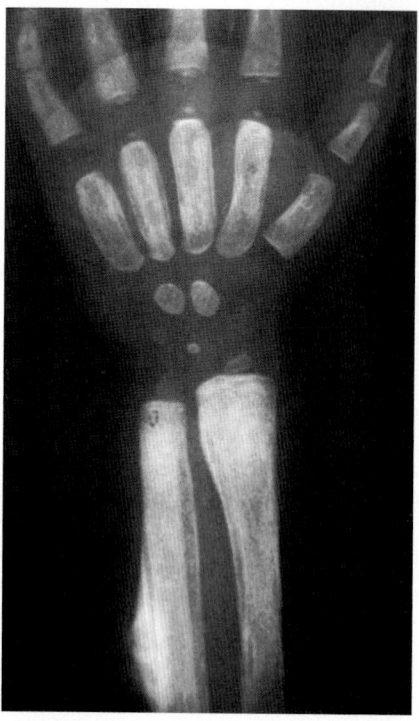

FIGURE 179-8. Radiograph showing external cortical thickenings of the tubular bones in the hands, radius, and ulna of an infant of 21 months who was reported to have had swelling periarticular soft tissues since the seventh month. Clinical and laboratory findings indicated rheumatoid arthritis. The patient did not have sickle cell anemia or familial hyperphosphatasemia. The preponderance of the evidence suggested that these changes represent the periosteal thickening of early rheumatoid arthritis. (Courtesy of La Rabida Children's Hospital and Research Center, Chicago, IL.)

deterioration has been observed in patients assumed clinically and biochemically to have inactive disease.

Radiography can be used to quantify joint destruction and assess disease treatment, with absence of change and lack of progression implying treatment success. In children who received methotrexate, Harel and associates found no interval intercarpal joint narrowing as measured by carpal length in responders versus the progressive worsening seen in nonresponders. Although joint space narrowing and erosion scores did not improve, some patients did show improvement in carpal length.

Intra-articular corticosteroids can be used to temporarily suppress local joint inflammation. Following injection of intra-articular corticosteroids, periarticular calcification can be noted. Other changes related to intra-articular therapy seem uncommon even with repeated joint injections.

Sonography may also be a useful means to noninvasively follow changes in synovitis with therapy. It may play a role in supporting clinical suspicion of disease activity in clinically mild or silent joints and in deciding on discontinuation of therapy. Increases in synovial thickening and synovial fluid accompany clinical worsening; however, the significance of residual synovial thickening and effusion seen on ultrasound in asymptomatic patients remains unclear. It may represent active silent disease or inactive fibrous pannus in a quiescent phase. Following intra-articular therapy for JRA in the hips and knees, decrease in synovial effusion, synovial proliferation, and adenopathy is noted on ultrasound.

Contrast-enhanced MRI can be used to quantitatively monitor synovial membrane volumes, effusion volumes,

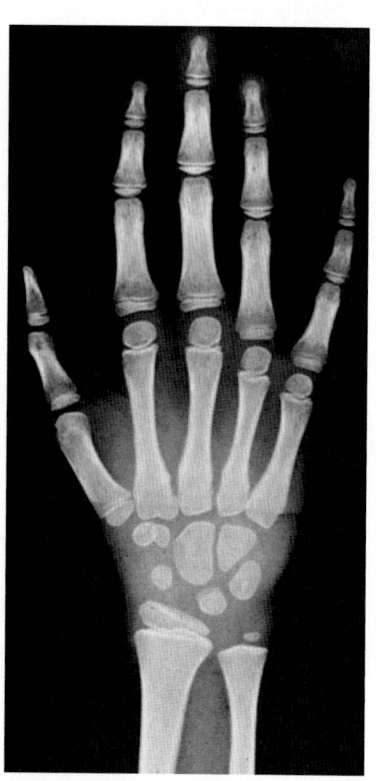

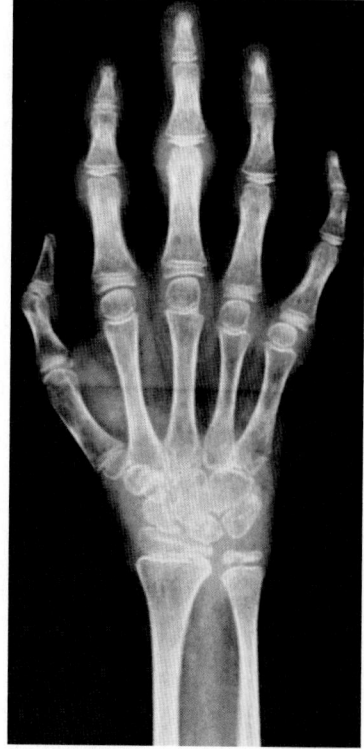

A   B

FIGURE 179-9. Rheumatoid arthritis in a 6-year-old girl. **A,** Four weeks after onset of vague pains, the radiographic findings are normal. **B,** Fifteen months later, all of the bony tissues are rarefied and the tubular bones overconstricted. The latter is best seen in the flares at the ends of the radius and ulna, with marked constriction just proximal to the flares. All of the fingers show fusiform swelling owing to the swelling of soft parts at the interphalangeal joints. The most striking change is the loss of spaces between the carpal bones owing to destruction of the articular cartilages of the intercarpal joints and the radiocarpal joint as well. Loss of cartilage is also evident at the carpometacarpal joints.

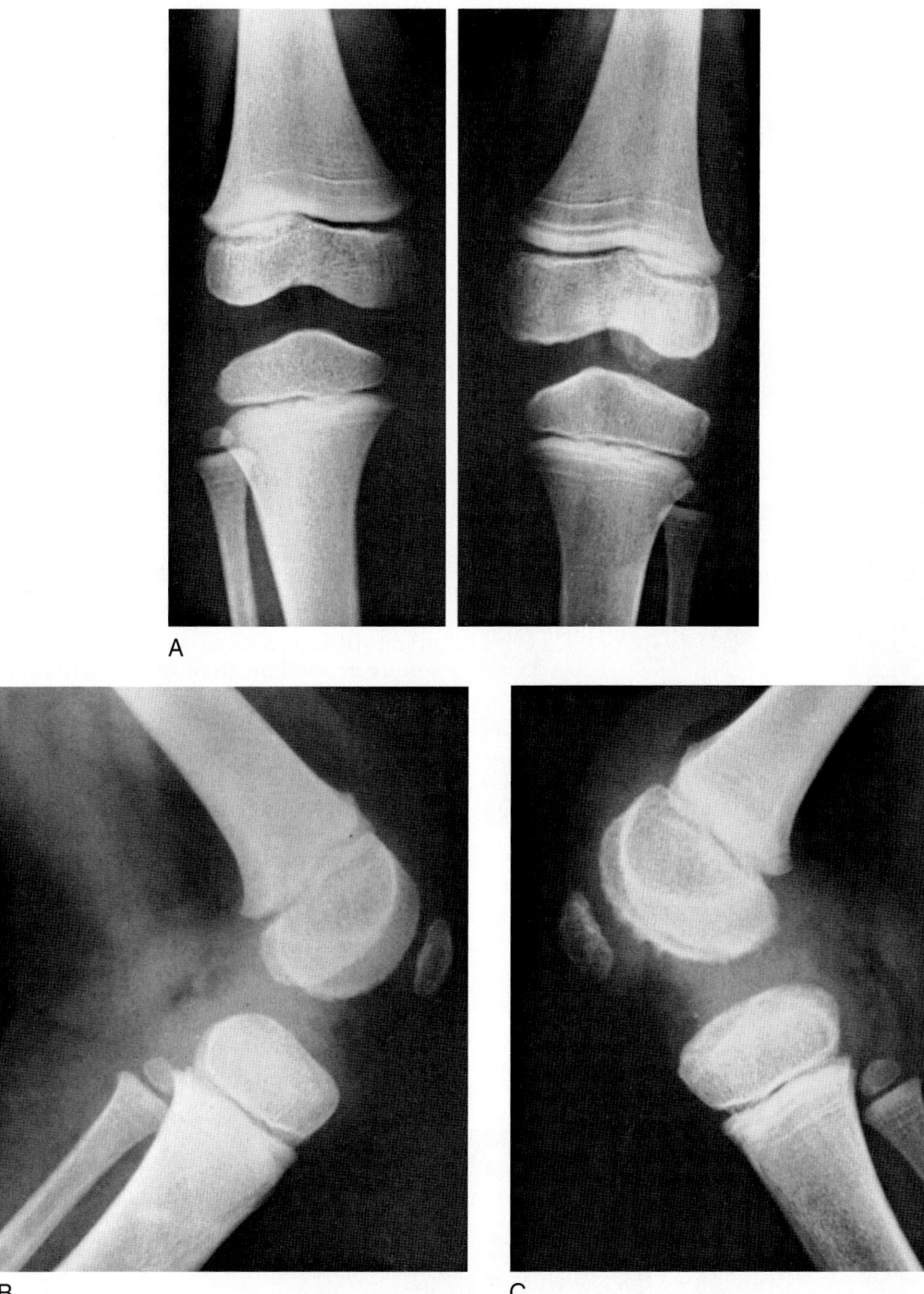

FIGURE 179-10. Radiographs showing rheumatoid arthritis in the left knee of a 3-year-old girl; the knees are in frontal (**A**) and lateral (**B** and **C**) projections. The swelling of the soft tissues at the left knee and atrophy of the muscles in the left thigh and shank are not visible in these images. The bones at the left knee are all diffusely rarefied, but there is no evidence of loss of articular cartilage or destruction of subchrondral bone. The femoral and tibial epiphyseal ossification centers and the patella on the left side are enlarged, owing presumably to the longstanding regional hyperemia induced by the chronic arthritis. Series of transverse growth lines have formed in the femoral and tibial metaphyses on both sides; the spaces between the transverse lines are deeper on the affected side, which indicates accelerated growth on that side as a result of chronic hyperemia.

and cartilage and bone erosion scores. Synovial membrane volume may reflect degree of edema, dilated vessels, and cellular infiltration in the synovial membrane and may be a measure of synovial inflammatory activity. Synovial volume, however, may also reflect the cumulative synovial proliferative disease activity and appears to correlate with duration of clinical remission. Several studies have indi-

cated a close relationship between the rate of contrast enhancement and inflammatory activity, with the enhancement rate apparently decreasing after intra-articular steroid administration, remaining low during clinical remissions, and increasing before the return of symptoms, indicating subclinical increase in synovial inflammatory activity. There may be regions of marked heterogeneity in rate of enhancement, so use of small regions of interest may be a limitation, with cases of clinical relapse showing increased enhancement back to pretreatment levels.

Autoimmune Connective Tissue Diseases

Joint findings are generally limited in connective tissue disorders. In scleroderma, which can be localized or systemic, joint changes are generally mild, with osteo-

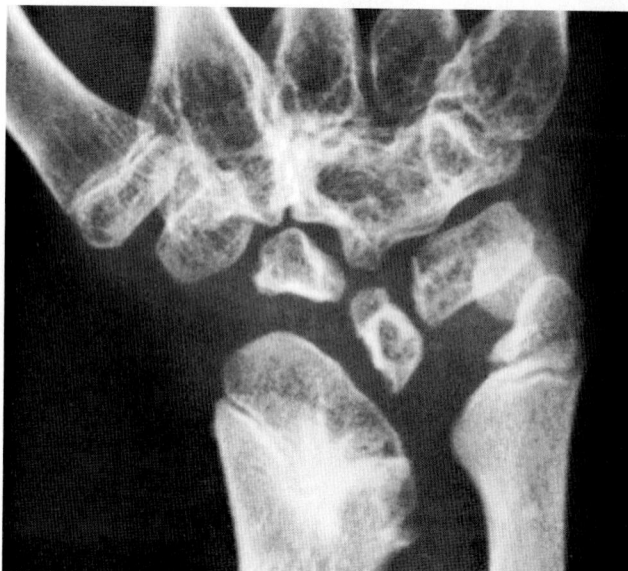

FIGURE 179-11. Radiograph showing severe rheumatoid arthritis of the left wrist of a 15-year-old girl with extensive destruction and ankylosis of second throught fifth carpometacarpal joints. The distal carpus appears fused and the proximal carpal bones are deformed. Premature union of the central portion of the distal radial epiphysis with its shaft has occurred. The ends of the radius and ulna are tipped toward each other owing to slowed longitudinal growth in the medial and lateral segments of their respective cartilage plates. (Courtesy of Dr. Fred A. Lee, Pasadena, CA.)

penia and joint contractures seen. Similarly, in juvenile dermatomyositis, a multisystem disorder primarily affecting blood vessels, there may be joint effusions, but erosions are not typically found.

Systemic lupus erythematosus is an uncommon multisystem autoimmune disease with wide variability in disease presentation and disease course. It more commonly affects women than men with median age of onset around 12 years of age. Common presentations include fever, malaise, and other systemic manifestations including lymphadenopathy and hepatosplenomegaly. The most common involved organs include skin, musculoskeletal and renal systems with skin rash, arthritis, and nephritis noted clinically. Typically lupus arthritis is a painful, symmetric polyarthritis affecting both large and small joints. Radiographic findings include joint effusion and synovitis, and subluxation may occur. Systemic lupus erythematosus arthritis is not usually associated with erosions.

Other Rheumatic or Inflammatory Diseases

Conditions with prolonged synovial inflammation may mimic JRA, and often show signs of demineralization, soft tissue swelling, joint space narrowing, and erosions.

Chromosomal Disorders

Arthritis may be associated with chromosomal disorders. There is an increased incidence of arthritis associated with both Down and Turner syndromes. Because patients with Down syndrome have various immunologic abnormalities, arthritis in these children is classified as a separate disease from JRA. It is important to be aware of the association of arthropathy with these syndromes because there is often a delay in making the diagnosis. Patients with Down syndrome usually present with polyarticular disease involving both large and small joints in a symmetric distribution, most commonly the

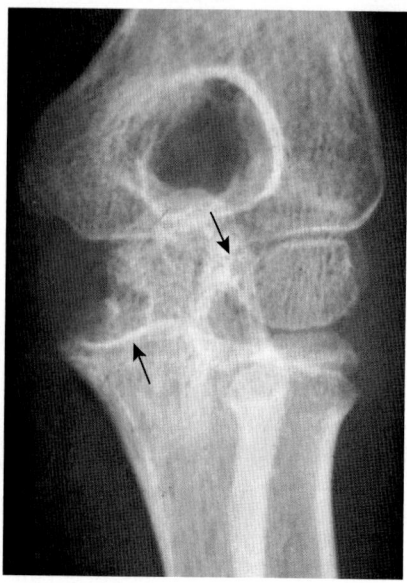

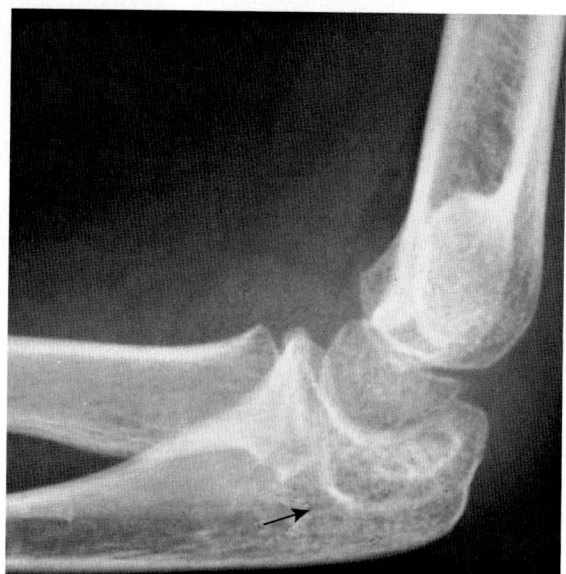

FIGURE 179-12. Anteroposterior **(A)** and lateral **(B)** radiographs showing large subchondral defects in the juxta-articular edges of the olecranon processes *(arrows)* in a girl with chronic rheumatoid arthritis of the elbow.

A

B

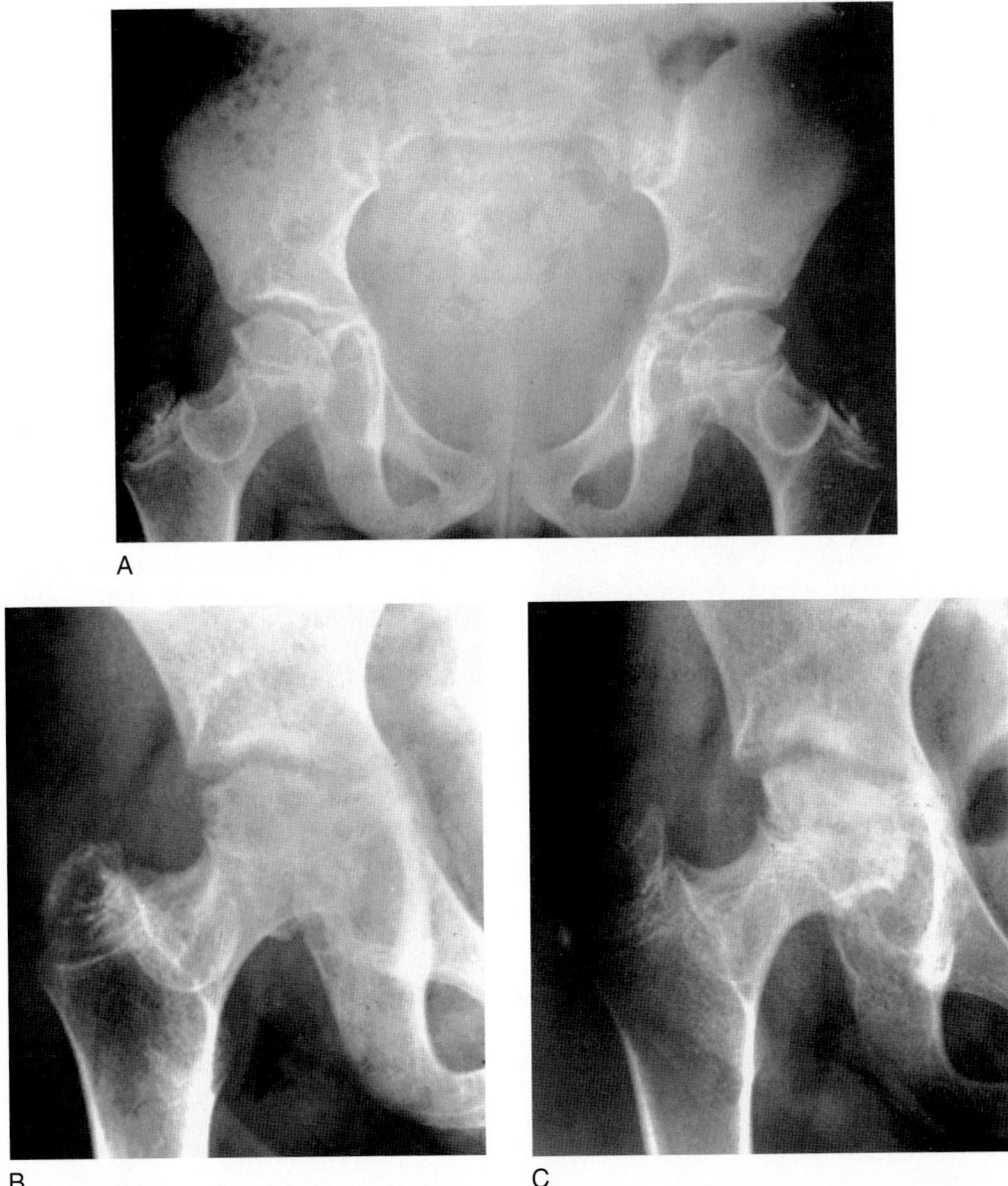

FIGURE 179-13. Rapid progression of erosive changes seen radiographically in the hips of a girl with systemic-onset juvenile arthritis beginning at 3½ years of age. **A,** Pelvis at 6 years and 8 months. Cystic erosions appear to straddle both femoral necks. Mild to moderate irregularities of ossification centers for the femoral heads and in the acetabular roofs are apparent. **B,** At 7 years and 10 months of age, there is progression of the erosions of the femoral necks from above and in front or in back. The femoral head and acetabular roof show more evidence of subchondral erosions that almost reach the medial cortex of the neck. **C,** At 8 years and 9 months, the neck has become more attenuated at the site of the enlarging erosion, and there is further progression of disease in the head and acetabulum. The patient had had multiple exacerbations and recurrences of symptoms, but her hips had been less severely affected clinically than were the small joints.

proximal interphalangeal and metacarpophalangeal joints of the hands, wrists, and knees. Joint hypermobility and subluxations occur and are most common in the cervical spine. In Turner syndrome, patients may have both radiographic bony changes of chronic inflammatory joint disease and the bony changes of Turner syndrome, including short fourth metacarpals, Madelung deformity, delayed maturation with flattening of the medial tibial plateau, and enlargement of the femoral condyle. These conditions often have overlapping features with JRA, including osteoporosis, premature fusion of bones, and metacarpal shortening. Patients with the chromosome 22q11.2 deletion syndrome (formerly known as DiGeorge syndrome or conotruncal-facial anomaly) and other immunodeficiencies also have a higher than chance probability of developing chronic polyarthritis.

> There is an increased incidence of arthritis in both Down and Turner syndromes.

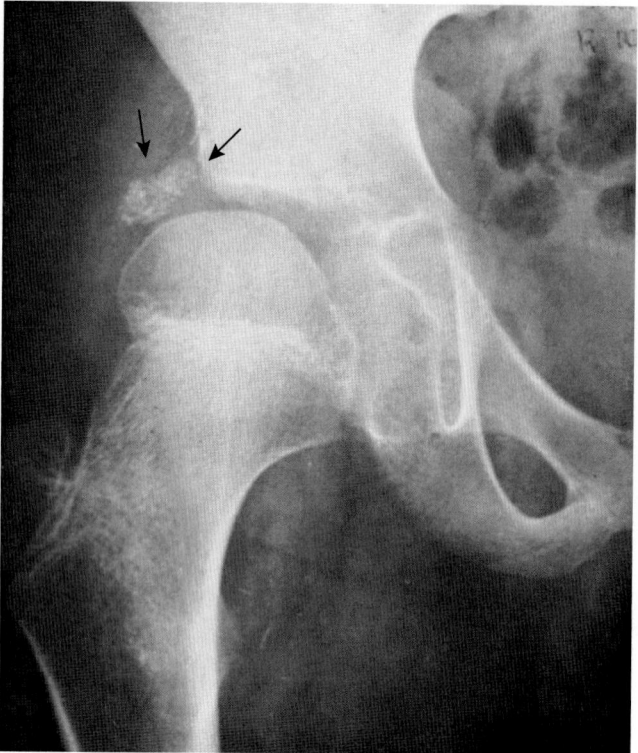

FIGURE 179-14. Radiograph showing rheumatoid arthritis with juxta-articular calcification in the soft tissues of the right hip *(arrows)* of a 9½-year-old boy. The coxa valga is noteworthy; this deformity is common in rheumatoid arthritis of the pelvis and legs and is probably due to reduced use.

Juvenile Spondyloarthropathies

The juvenile spondyloarthropathies represent a group of disorders that affect the axial and extra-axial joints. They include juvenile ankylosing spondylitis (JAS), reactive arthritis or Reiter syndrome, juvenile psoriatic arthritis (JPsA), and arthritis associated with inflammatory bowel disease, all occurring before the age of 16 years. The spondyloarthropathies share many common clinical and genetic characteristics, including positive family history, absence of subcutaneous nodules, presence of enthesitis and later sacroiliitis, and absence of RF and antinuclear antibody. Synovitis and enthesitis (inflammation at the site of attachment of ligaments or tendons to bone) are recognized as major target areas of inflammation. Enthesitis is commonly present, especially at the insertions of the Achilles tendon, plantar fascia, and patellar and quadriceps tendons (Fig. 179-20). The clinical spectrum of juvenile spondyloarthropathies is broad and includes patients with undifferentiated manifestations that do not allow specific categorization, including peripheral arthritis, enthesitis, tendinitis, dactylitis, and uveitis and patients with more characteristic features such as sacroiliitis, spinal involvement, or extra-articular manifestations, including psoriasis or gut involvement. Often specific diagnostic criteria are not initially present in children, and most will be diagnosed as having undifferentiated spondyloarthropathy. Although the juvenile spondyloarthropathies are considered separately from JRA, they can be difficult to clinically distinguish, especially

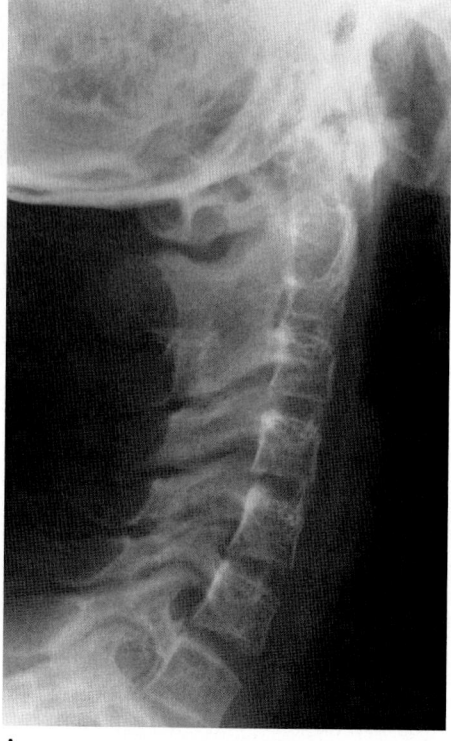

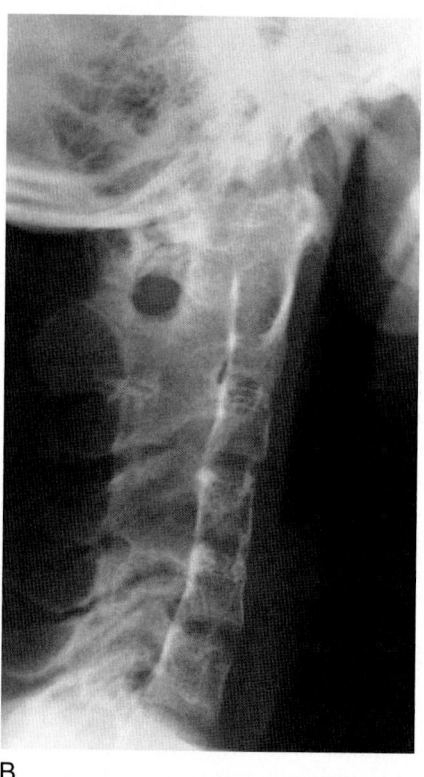

A   B

FIGURE 179-15. A, Lateral radiograph of the cervical spine of a 10-year-old girl with juvenile rheumatoid arthritis for several years shows ankylosis of C2–C3 facet joints. **B,** Subsequent radiograph 2 years later reveals progressive ankylosis at C4–C5.

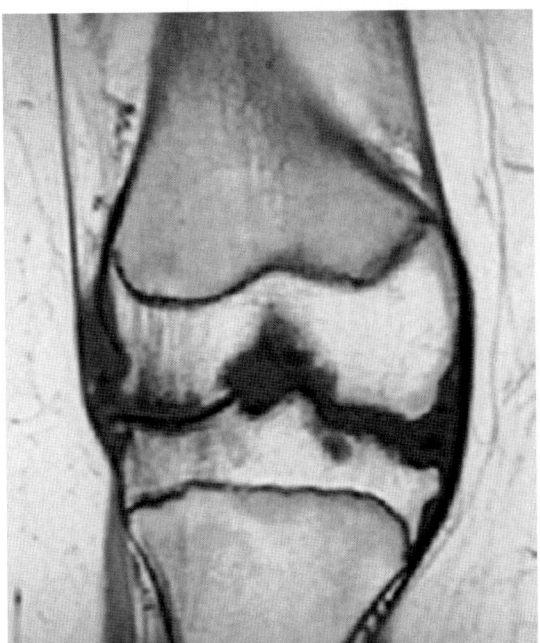

FIGURE 179-16. Magnetic resonance imaging examination of the knee in a child with JRA. Coronal T1-weighted MR image shows low signal edema and erosions along the articular surface of the knee joint.

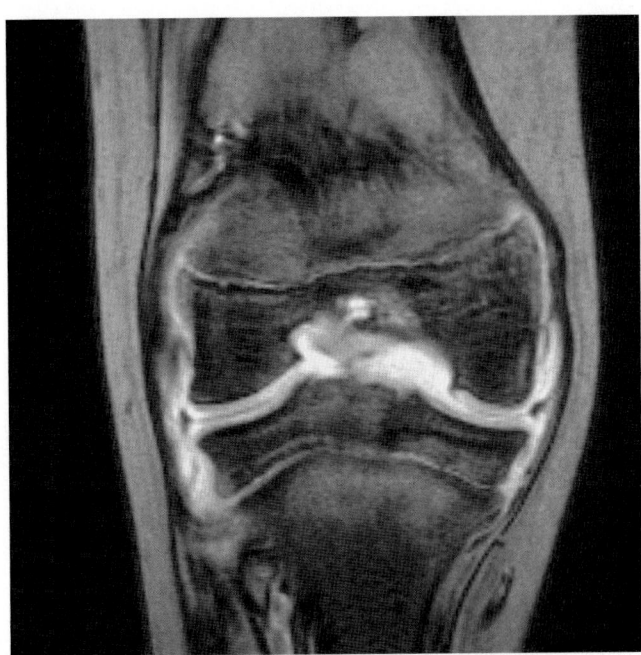

FIGURE 179-17. Magnetic resonance imaging (MRI) examination of the knee in a child with juvenile rheumatoid arthritis. Coronal gradient echo (MPGR) MRI shows high signal joint effusion, meniscal hypoplasia, and widening of the intercondylar notch.

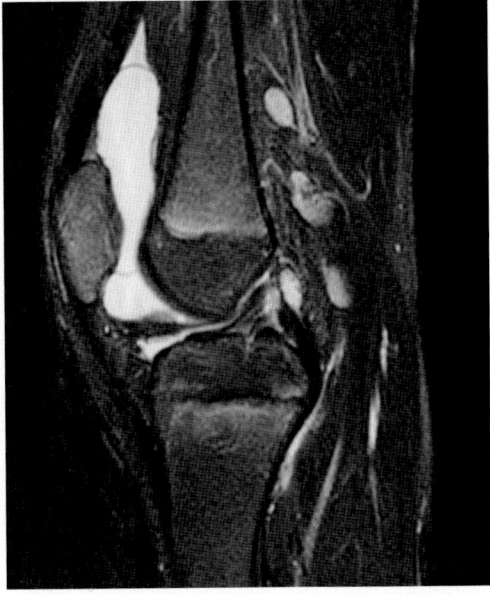
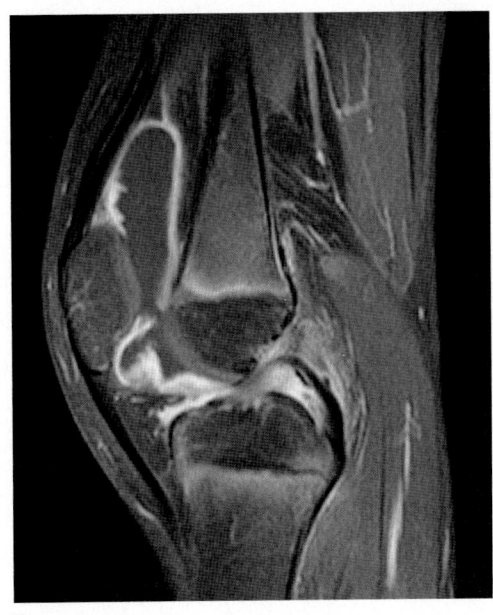

A   B

FIGURE 179-18. An 11-year-old boy with juvenile rheumatoid arthritis. **A,** Sagittal T2-weighted magnetic resonance image (MRI) of the right knee shows a few high signal popliteal lymph nodes and a large hyperintense joint effusion. **B,** Sagittal T1-weighted MRI with gadolinium shows high signal peripheral enhancement of the synovium, which is easily distinguished from the low signal knee joint effusion.

early on. The term *seronegative enthesopathy arthropathy* syndrome has been proposed to separate children, typically boys, in their early teens who present with enthesitis and peripheral asymmetric, often lower limb arthritis from those with JRA. Other entities related to the seronegative spondyloarthropathies include the arthritis associated with hyperostosis, acne or palmar pustulosis, Whipple disease, and Behçet disease.

> The juvenile spondyloarthropathies include juvenile ankylosing spondylitis, reactive arthritis or Reiter syndrome, juvenile psoriatic arthritis, arthritis associated with inflammatory bowel disease, arthritis associated with hyperostosis, acne and/or palmar pustulosis, Whipple disease, and Behçet disease.

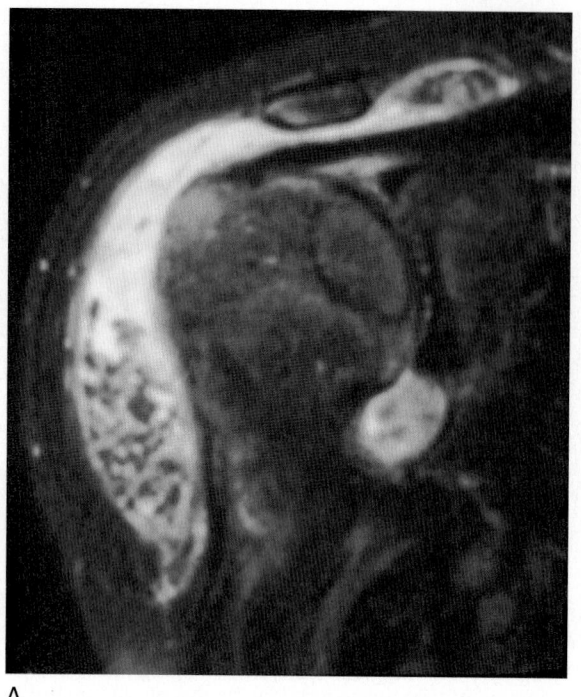

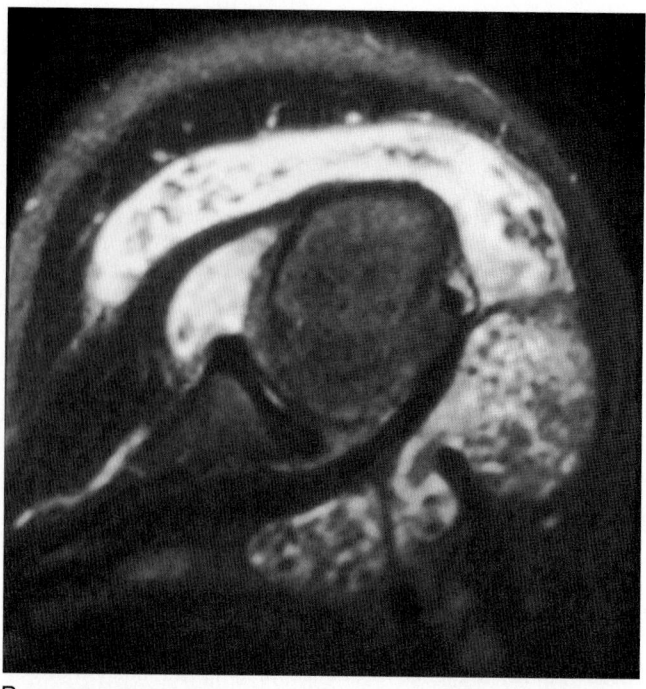

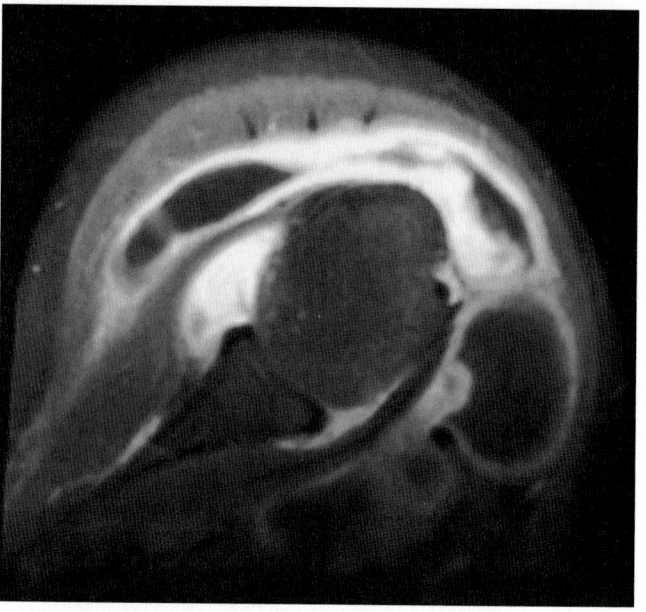

FIGURE 179-19. Magnetic resonance image (MRI) of the shoulder in a child with long-standing juvenile rheumatoid arthritis. **A,** Coronal fast inversion recovery (FIR) image, and **B,** axial fast T2-weighted MRI show large high signal shoulder joint effusion distending the subacromial and subdeltoid bursa. There are multiple small low signal foci layered dependantly in the joint fluid compatible with rice bodies. **C,** Axial T1-weighted fat-suppressed MRI following gadolinium administration shows diffuse enhancement of the synovium but no significant enhancement of the rice bodies or joint effusion.

JUVENILE ANKYLOSING SPONDYLITIS

Despite the fact that children with JAS rarely have the classic adult presentation of bilateral sacroiliitis and spondylitis, radiologic evidence of inflammation of these joints is required for definitive diagnosis. Asymmetric extra-axial arthritis is common in JAS, usually affecting the large joints of the lower extremity, including the hips, knees, and ankles. Dactylitis with finger or toe involvement may manifest as swollen red digits with painful small joints, and enthesitis is commonly found. Sacroiliitis is usually bilateral but asymmetric when present (Fig. 179-21).

REACTIVE ARTHRITIS AND REITER SYNDROME

Reactive arthritis is distinguished from the other spondyloarthropathies by its clear relationship to a precipitating infection, which may be asymptomatic. Susceptibility to reactive arthritis is closely linked to the presence of human leukocyte antigen allele B27. Infections of the gastrointestinal, genitourinary, and respiratory tract can provoke reactive arthritis, and a wide range of pathogens has been implicated. Both antigens and DNA of several microorganisms have been detected in joint material from patients with reactive arthritis. The role of these disseminated microbial elements in the provocation or

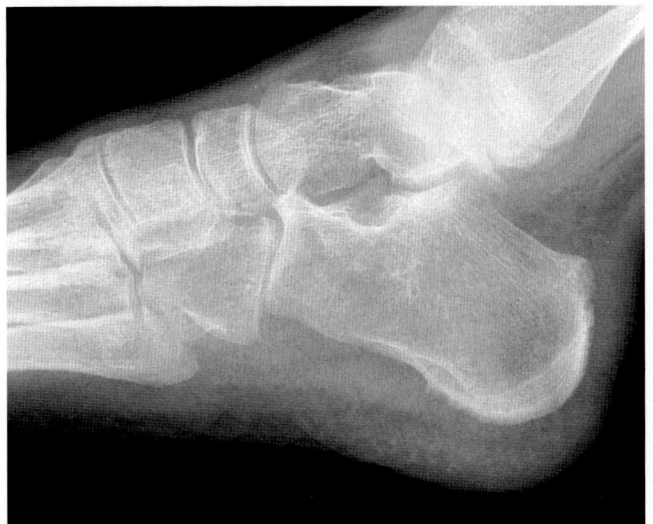

A

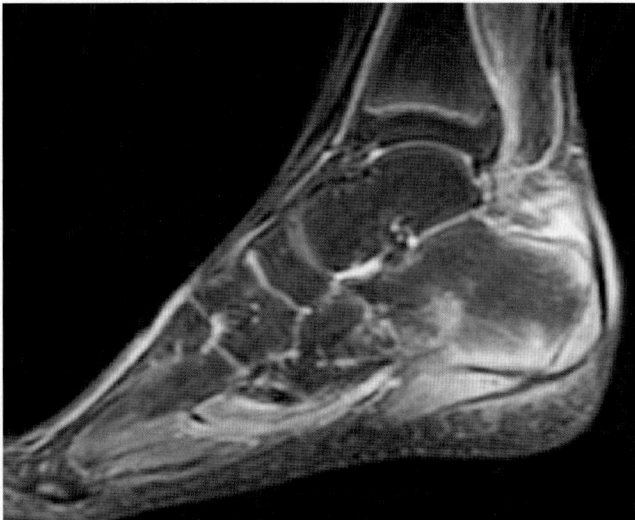

B

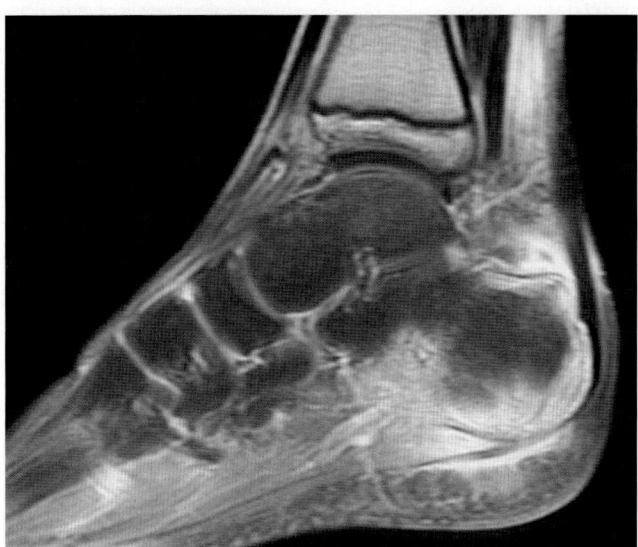

C

FIGURE 179-20. A, Radiograph of a 12-year-old boy with enthesitis related arthritis shows erosion at the insertion of the achilles tendon and new bone formation at the insertion of the plantar fascia into the calcaneus. **B,** Sagittal fast inversion recovery (FIR) magnetic resonance image (MRI) and **C,** Sagittal T1-weighted fat saturation MRI with gadolinium show retrocaneal bursitis and high signal and enhancement at the insertion of the Achilles tendon and plantar fascia.

maintenance of arthritis and the need for antibiotic therapy in the treatment of reactive arthritis remains unclear. Reiter syndrome is the association of reactive arthritis with conjunctivitis and urethritis. Although several forms of joint disease could be considered as reactive, particularly acute rheumatic fever, post–meningococcal septicemia arthritis, and Lyme disease, reactive arthritis is often restricted to an acute spondyloarthropathy, usually but not exclusively linked to an acute genitourinary or gastrointestinal infection. Reactive arthritis is usually self-limited and self-resolving. The arthritis is typically peripheral, monoarticular, or pauciarticular, but axial involvement with unilateral or bilateral sacroiliitis, enthesitis, and dactylitis can be seen.

> **Reiter syndrome is the association of reactive arthritis with conjunctivitis and urethritis.**

ARTHRITIS ASSOCIATED WITH INFLAMMATORY BOWEL DISEASE

Approximately 15% of children with inflammatory bowel disease will develop a noninfectious arthritis, which typically is pauciarticular, involving the peripheral, large joints of the lower extremity.

JUVENILE PSORIATIC DISEASE

As opposed to the other spondyloarthropathies, JPsA is more common in girls than boys, especially in childhood. It can be definitively diagnosed when patients with psoriasis have arthritis or when arthritis and three of the following—dactylitis, nail pitting, or onycholysis or family history of psoriasis—are present. The arthritis not uncommonly may precede the development of psoriasis. The arthritis most commonly is asymmetric, is pauciarticular initially, and can involve the large and small joints, including the proximal and distal interphalangeal joints. Tendon sheath involvement is common, while enthesitis seems less common than in JAS.

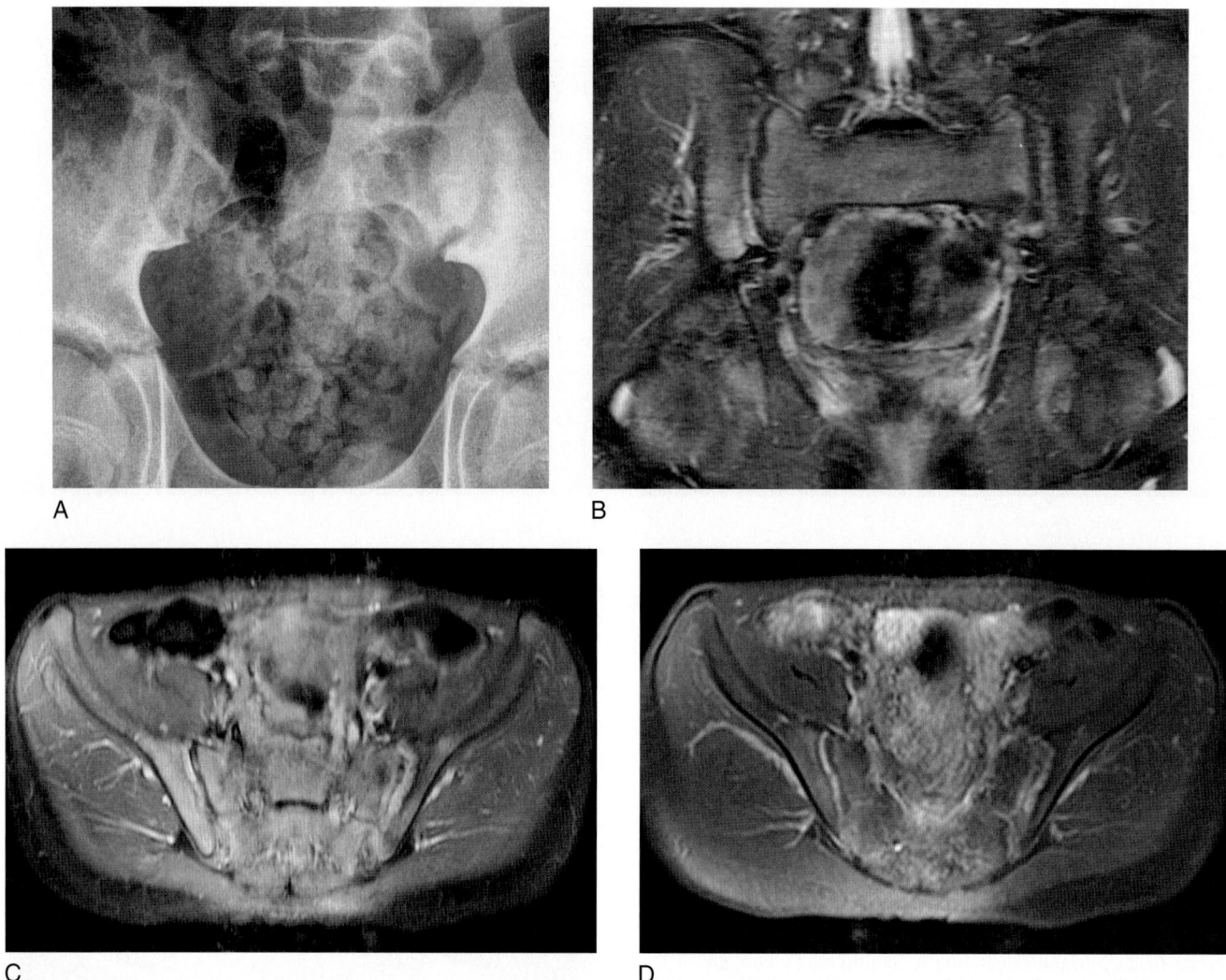

A

B

C

D

FIGURE 179-21. **A,** and **B,** 12-year-old boy with juvenile ankylosing spondyloarthritis. **A,** Frontal radiograph shows sclerosis, widening and irregularity of the left sacroiliac joint. **B,** and **C,** Coronal fast inversion recovery and axial T2-weighted magnetic resonance images (MRIs) show high signal edema along both sacroiliac joints and low signal sclerosis and irregularity on the left. **D,** Axial T1-weighted MRI post gadolinium show high signal enhancement of both sacroiliac joints.

IMAGING IN JUVENILE SPONDYLOARTHROPATHIES

Radiographic findings are common among all the spondyloarthropathies and similar to those of JRA with the exception of sacroiliitis and enthesitis, which are more specific for spondyloarthropathy (see Figs. 179-20 through 179-22). Plain images are usually normal initially but later on may demonstrate soft tissue swelling, effusion, osteopenia, joint space narrowing, or erosion and rarely fusion. Erosions are typically associated with irregular bone apposition at joint margins, referred to as "whiskering" spondyloarthropathy (see Fig. 179-22). Rapid joint destruction can be noted. With hip involvement, these proliferative changes are noted at the junction of the femoral head and neck. Dactylitis may be seen with soft tissue swelling and periosteal reaction along the shaft of metacarpals, metatarsals, or phalanges (Table 179-5). In JAS, extra-axial arthritis usually involves one or more large joints of the lower extremities (e.g., hips,

knees, and ankles). In JPsA, severe erosions can be seen, particularly in the digits (see Fig. 179-22).

Enthesitis may be revealed by soft tissue swelling, localized osteopenia, or bone erosion and spur formation, at the site of insertion of the Achilles tendon into the calcaneus, plantar aponeurosis, or patella (see Fig. 179-20). With MRI, one may see bone marrow edema, granulation tissue, or cortical erosion.

Plain images may demonstrate unilateral or bilateral sacroiliitis with indistinct articular margins, pseudo-widening, erosions, and reactive sclerosis, particularly on the iliac side of the joint (see Figs. 179-21). CT or MRI can be used if necessary to diagnose sacroiliitis earlier than radiographically present. On CT, angled scans through the sacroiliac joint should be used to lower radiation dose. On MRI, periarticular low signal may be seen on T1-weighted images with high signal on T2-weighted images from inflammatory changes in bone marrow, whereas low signal will be seen with bone

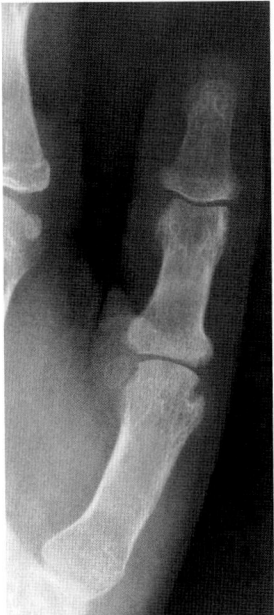 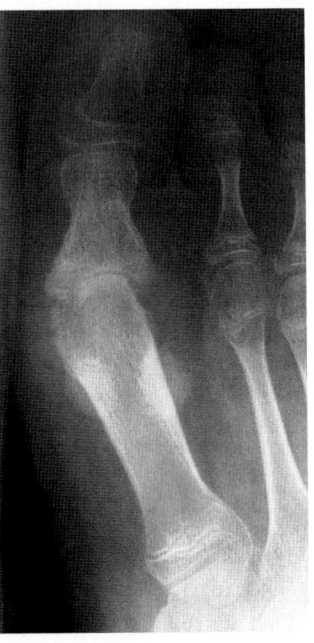

A   B

FIGURE 179-22. Radiographs of the hand and foot of a 14-year-old boy with psoriatic arthritis. **A,** Soft tissue swelling of the first digit with narrowing of the first metacarpal-phalangeal joint with marginal erosions and proliferative periostitis. **B,** Similar changes are seen at the first metatarsal-phalangeal joint.

TABLE 179-5
Radiographic Features of the Juvenile Spondyloarthropathies

AXIAL SKELETON
Sacroiliac joint
   Sacroiliitis—unilateral or bilateral
      Indistinct articular margins
      Erosions
      Reactive sclerosis
      Joint space narrowing
      Joint fusion
   Adjacent bone marrow edema and enhancement on
      magnetic resonance imaging
Vertebrae
   Apophysitis (shining corners)
   Anterior vertebral squaring
   Anterior ligament calcification

APPENDICULAR SKELETON
Enthesitis
   Soft tissue swelling
   Erosions at insertions
   Spur formation
   Bone edema
   Localized bone overgrowth
Periostitis
Tenosynovitis
Arthritis
   Synovitis
   Joint fluid
   Soft tissue swelling
   Accelerated ossification and epiphyseal overgrowth
   Joint space narrowing
   Erosions
   Demineralization
   Joint fusion
   Protrusio acetabuli

sclerosis (see Fig. 179-21). MRI may also demonstrate changes in articular cartilage with erosions. MRI evaluation, particularly with gadolinium enhancement, may allow earlier diagnosis of back pain caused by acute sacroiliitis than will conventional radiography.

In juvenile spondyloarthropathy, vertebral involvement is not usually present because it develops late. Occasionally, there may be localized osteitis, erosions, and sclerosis, particularly at vertebral margins. Syndesmophytes are rarely seen in children. Rarely, atlantoaxial subluxation can be present.

JOINT DISORDERS IN CYSTIC FIBROSIS

Joint disease is recognized as a major cause of pain and disability in 10% of children with cystic fibrosis. Two distinct types of joint disease are found in patients with cystic fibrosis, hypertrophic pulmonary osteoarthropathy and cystic fibrosis arthropathy. Hypertrophic pulmonary osteoarthropathy is the most common arthropathy of cystic fibrosis occurring in approximately 5% of patients. However, it is usually seen in adults, with only a small number of cases occurring in children. Clinical and radiologic findings include clubbing, periostitis of the long bones, and joint pain or swelling due to effusions. It often presents as a symmetric polyarthritis and most commonly involves the knees. It flares during episodes of respiratory infection and is associated with more severe pulmonary disease.

Cystic fibrosis arthropathy is a transient and recurrent arthritis occurring predominantly during childhood. Onset is usually during the second decade and it affects approximately 2% to 8% of patients with CF. Patients usually have sudden onset of severe joint pain and

swelling associated with flu-like symptoms or erythema. It presents as a monoarthritis or symmetric polyarthritis, and the knees, ankles and wrists are most commonly involved. Occasionally, the hips, shoulders and elbows may be affected and radiographs are often normal. It usually lasts 5 to 7 days and rarely results in a chronic erosive arthritis. There is no relationship between the episodes of arthritis and pulmonary disease.

> Cystic fibrosis arthropathy is a transient and recurrent arthritis occuring predominantly during childhood and affecting 2% to 8% of patients with CF.

Infectious Arthritis

Arthritis caused by infectious agents can be due to direct invasion by viable microorganisms (septic arthritis) or due to a variety of immune mechanisms (postinfectious arthritis) (Table 179-6). Infectious synovitis can be caused by various pathogens, including bacteria, viruses, and fungi. The term *septic arthritis* is reserved for bacterial infections in which bacteria are recovered from

TABLE 179-6

Infection-Related Arthritis

INFECTIOUS ARTHRITIS
Viral
  Parvovirus
  Rubella
  Epstein-Barr
  Hepatitis B
  Varicella-zoster
  Coxsackie
Bacterial
  Staphylococcus aureus
  Group B hemolytic streptococcus
  Haemophilus influenzae
  Streptococcus pneumoniae
  Streptococcus pyogenes
  Pneumococcal pneumonia
  Klebsiella pneumoniae
  Pseudomonas aeruginosa
  Neisseria meningitidis
  Neisseria gonorrhoea
Fungal
  Candida albicans
  Coccidiomycosis
Myocobacterium tuberculosis

REACTIVE ARTHRITIS (POSTINFECTIOUS)
Tuberculosis (Poncet disease)
Acute rheumatic fever (poststreptococcal)
Yersinia
Brucellosis
Rat-bite fever *(Streptobacillus moniliformis)*
Lyme borreliosis
Mycoplasma pneumonia

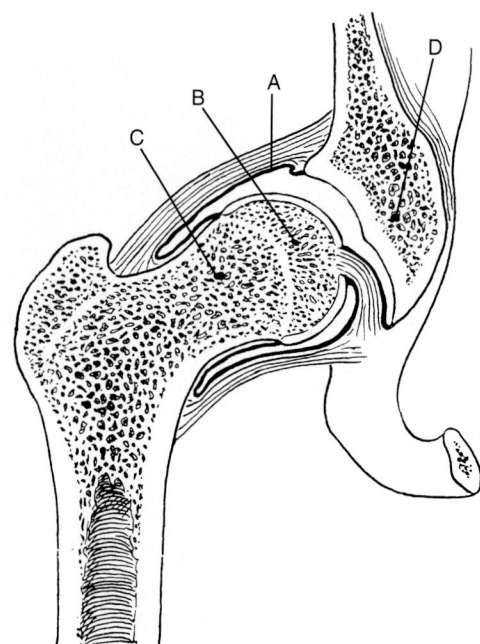

FIGURE 179-23. Primary sites of origin from which infection may extend secondarily into the hip joint. The initial focus may be in the synovium itself *(A)*, in the femoral epiphysis *(B)*, in the femoral metaphysis *(C)*, or in the innominate bone *(D)*. In some cases, the hip joint may be infected by extension from more than one of these neighboring primary foci.

the synovial fluid with the use of standard microbiologic techniques. If the synovial fluid is "sterile," the condition is termed *postinfectious arthritis* even though the triggering infection can precede (acute rheumatic fever, post-*Yersinia* arthritis) or coexist with (brucellosis, rat-bite fever) the articular symptoms. Reactive arthritides are generally defined as sterile arthritides following remote infections of the urogenital or intestinal tracts.

SEPTIC ARTHRITIS

Identification of the obvious septic joint is not much of a diagnostic challenge, although time to diagnosis is critical to avoid a poor outcome such as destruction of the femoral head, degenerative arthritis, or permanent deformity. Much more of a challenge is the diagnosis of musculoskeletal infections caused by unusual organisms or in unusual locations. Infection in the bones and joints of the back and pelvis is often difficult to diagnose because the physical examination may suggest a knee, hip, or abdominal problem, and tuberculous infections may simulate juvenile arthritis with subacute symptoms.

Acute purulent infection of the joints is more common in infancy and early childhood because of the greater blood flow to the joints during the active stages of growth. The usual cause is hematogenous dissemination related to an upper respiratory infection or pyoderma. Infection may also spread from adjacent osteomyelitis,

cellulitis, abscess, or traumatic joint invasion (Fig. 179-23). In children, septic arthritis develops commonly from osteomyelitis in metaphyses that are intra-articular, such as the hip. During infancy, septic arthritis frequently is associated with osteomyelitis because capillaries from the metaphysis traverse the physis into the epiphysis. Infants with immune dysfunction, with indwelling vascular lines, or undergoing invasive procedures are at increased risk. Neonatal septic arthritis represents a different spectrum of disease than septic arthritis of childhood. A high clinical index of suspicion is necessary because signs and symptoms may be subtle. Early signs include failure to move a limb spontaneously, while swelling, erythema, and warmth are late findings.

> **Particularly at the hip, where the metaphysis is intra-articular, septic arthritis may be due to spread of adjacent osteomyelitis.**

Staphylococcus aureus is the most common cause of bacterial arthritis, with group B streptococcus commonly seen in the neonate and *Haemophilus influenzae* in the 1- to 4-year-old age range. Children with varicella infection (chicken pox) are at increased risk of developing septic arthritis and other musculoskeletal infections secondary to group A streptococcus. Pneumococcal joint infection may be seen in children with splenic dysfunction from hemoglobinopathy or immune deficiency.

The vast majority of septic arthritides are mono-articular, with the most commonly affected joints being the knee, hip, and ankle. In septic arthritis, bacterial contamination causes hypertrophy and edema of the

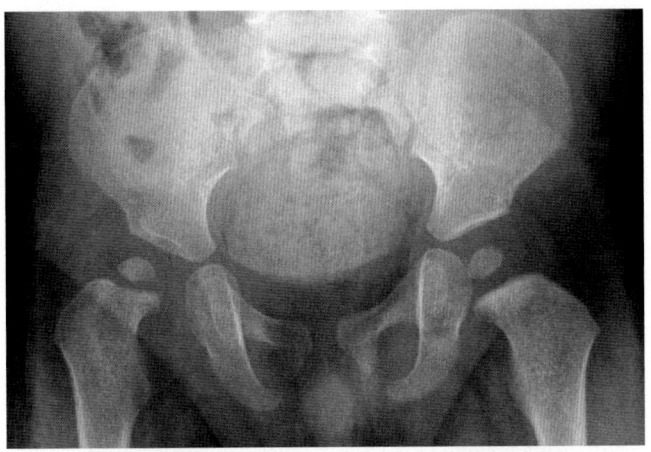

A

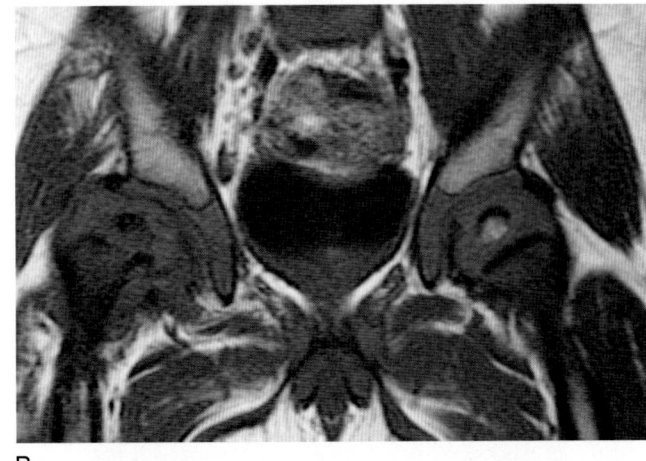

B

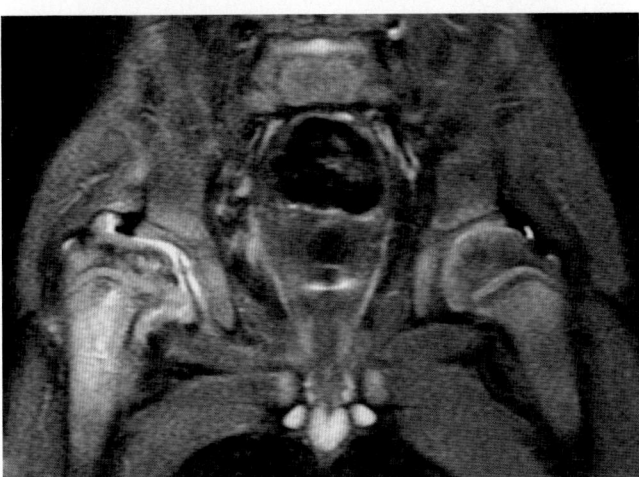

C

FIGURE 179-24. Septic arthritis in an 8-month-old infant. **A,** Frontal radiograph demonstrates subluxation of the right hip and ill-defined lucency of the proximal right femur. **B,** On follow-up magnetic resonance imaging (MRI) scan, coronal T1-weighted image of the pelvis shows low signal ossification center of the right capital femoral epiphysis and persistent subluxation of the right hip. **C,** Corresponding coronal fast inversion recovery (FIR) MRI shows high signal and flattening of the right capital femoral epiphysis related to complications of avascular necrosis. There is a residual small right hip effusion and high signal in the proximal femora related to associated osteomyelitis.

synovium. In infants with septic arthritis, distention of the joint capsule may result in pathologic dislocation, particularly in the hip or shoulder (Fig. 179-24). Joint space narrowing results from cartilage destruction by proteolytic enzymes. There may be associated bone erosion and destruction or periosteal reaction. Pus in the joint increases intra-articular pressure and may result in osteonecrosis of the epiphysis (Fig. 179-24). Other sequelae include angular deformities, leg length discrepancy, and ankylosis. Prompt diagnosis of septic arthritis is essential in infants and children to prevent complications.

The classic radiographic findings of acute septic arthritis are rapid joint space loss and erosions with relative preservation of mineralization (Fig. 179-25). These findings indicate advanced irreversible destruction of the joint but are not specific for infection. Early findings of joint effusion may be detected in the knee, ankle, or elbow, but radiographs are insensitive for detecting effusion in the shoulder, hip, or sacroiliac joints. Ultrasound, CT, and MRI are sensitive in demonstrating joint effusion but cannot distinguish infected from noninfected joint effusion, and aspiration is still necessary for diagnosis. CT is useful for guiding diagnostic aspiration or drainage of the joint and may be the best modality for evaluating certain joints such as the sternoclavicular joint. MRI may be used to demonstrate early bone erosions and cartilage destruction. In addition to joint effusions, associated findings include synovial thickening and enhancement, septations, and debris within the joint. Uncomplicated septic arthritis may cause abnormal signal within the marrow on both sides of the joint secondary to reactive edema, which may be difficult to differentiate from osteomyelitis. A secondary complication of septic arthritis is soft tissue abscess, which demonstrates localized fluid collection with peripheral enhancement following gadolinium enhancement. Edema within periarticular structures or fluid collections in tendon sheaths will also show increased signal on T2-weighted images.

Radionuclide imaging is more sensitive than radiographs in supporting the diagnosis of arthritis and may be used to screen the entire skeleton. A bone scan localizes the site of infection and is positive as early as 2 days after the onset of symptoms. In septic arthritis, there is increased articular activity in the blood flow and blood pool phases, and there may be uptake in the juxta-articular bones on the delayed phase as a result of hyperemia. Increased intra-articular pressure from joint effusion may result in reduced radionuclide uptake within the epiphysis as a result of ischemia.

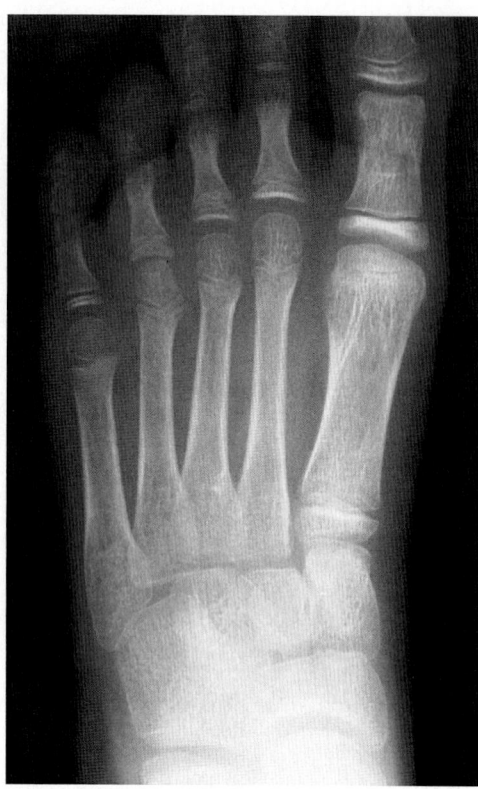

FIGURE 179-25. Frontal radiograph of right foot in a patient with septic arthritis shows joint space narrowing of the fourth metatarsal-phalangeal joint.

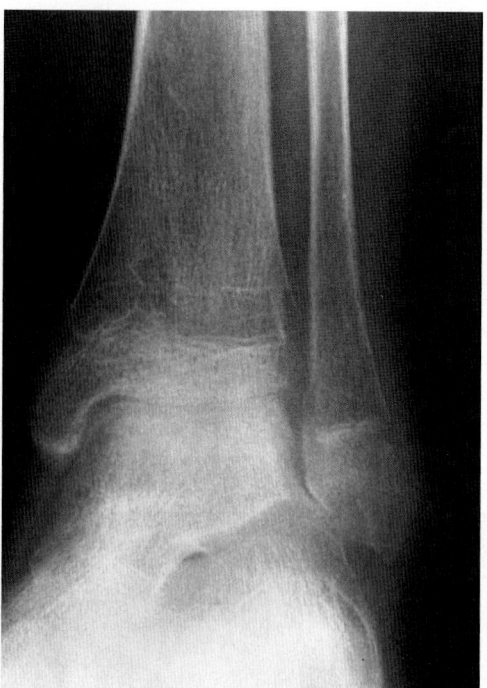

FIGURE 179-26. Tuberculosis arthritis in a 9-year-old girl with 6-month history of monoarticular arthritis of the left ankle, presumed to be juvenile rheumatoid arthritis, treated with steroid injections. Patient was lost to follow-up and returned 4 months later with marked worsening of arthritis. Radiograph of the left ankle shows soft tissue swelling, periarticular osteopenia, and severe joint space narrowing. She also had a cough, and chest radiograph showed miliary tuberculosis.

The chief differential diagnosis of septic arthritis of the hip is transient synovitis. The clinical presentation of septic arthritis of the hip ovelaps with that of transient synovitis. Fever (>38.5° during week before presentation), elevated serum white blood cell count (>12,000 cells/mm³), elevated serum erythrocyte sedimentation rate (>40 mm/hr), elevated C-reactive protein (>1 mg/dL) and non-weightbearing status are also predictors of infection. Absence of these findings mitigates strongly against infection and potentially may obviate arthrocentesis. However, there is no imaging criteria to distinguish septic arthritis from transient synovitis. If septic arthritis is suspected, arthrocentesis must be performed.

> At the hip, the chief differential diagnosis for septic arthritis is transient synovitis. Although clinical parameters may suggest the proper diagnosis, there is no imaging criteria to distinguish septic arthritis from transient synovitis.

OTHER CAUSES OF INFECTIOUS ARTHRITIS

In viral arthritis, the virus may actually invade synovial tissues, causing local inflammation and cell necrosis. Commonly encountered viruses include parvovirus, rubella, Epstein-Barr, and coxsackie. Most viral arthritides generally resolve within 6 weeks without specific therapy. Viral arthritis may also result from local host immune responses to the virus or viral products. In most cases, it is probably a systemic serum sickness type of reaction with formation of immune complexes that are demonstrable in both serum and synovial fluid. Viral arthritides may be monoarticular, pauciarticular, or polyarticular and can resemble septic arthritis or JRA.

Mycobacterium tuberculosis has made a resurgence, and in children, the frequency of bone or joint infection may be as high as 6%. Tuberculous infection usually begins as an insidious monoarticular arthritis and commonly involves the spine, hip, and knee (see Chapter 175). In children, extrapulmonary tuberculosis usually results from lymphohematogenous dissemination during a primary infection. *Mycobacterium tuberculosis* may also cause postinfectious polyarthritis or Poncet disease. Radiographs in tuberculous arthritis classically show osteopenia and periarticular erosions with relative preservation of the joint space. With chronic infection there may be joint space narrowing (Fig. 179-26), abscess formation, and draining sinuses. Tuberculous arthritis frequently causes extensive fibrous bridging and obliteration of the joint space.

Postinfectious arthritis resulting from an immune response is usually self-limited with the exception of acute rheumatic fever and Lyme disease, in which there may be significant morbidity. Rheumatic fever is secondary to group A streptococci. It usually presents as a migratory arthritis involving the large joints of the extremities, with the exception of the hip. Lyme disease is caused by *Borrelia burgdorferi*, which is a tick-transmitted spirochete. It usually presents with intermittent mono-arthritis most commonly in the knee. The radiologic findings may be similar to those of pauciarticular JRA. The diagnosis is confirmed with serology demonstrating antibodies to the infectious agent.

Other Inflammatory Arthritides

TRANSIENT SYNOVITIS OF THE HIP

Transient synovitis is a self-limited inflammatory condition specific to the hip. It affects boys more commonly than girls in all age ranges but is most common between 3 and 6 years. Its etiology is unknown, but some children have a preceding history of upper respiratory infection or trauma. Patients present with acute onset of pain and limp that generally lasts less than 2 weeks. Only 1% of patients have bilateral disease, whereas a small number of patients have a second episode, which usually occurs within the first six months after the initial symptoms. Transient synovitis is a diagnosis of exclusion, with the most common disorders in the differential including traumatic synovitis, septic arthritis, JRA, and Legg-Calvé-Perthes disease. Long-term sequelae are rare. Avascular necrosis has been described as a complication in a few patients, but it is uncertain whether these cases actually represent Legg-Calvé-Perthes disease that was initially undetectable on radiographs. Treatment consists of bed rest and nonsteroidal anti-inflammatory medications.

Radiographs are usually normal but may demonstrate evidence of a joint effusion with mild widening of the medial joint space. Scintigraphy often shows slight increase in isotope uptake in the affected hip. In approximately 25% of patients, there may be a transient decrease in uptake in the first week or two, followed by evidence of rebound hyperemia within 1 month. These findings suggest that some patients develop transient ischemia of the capital femoral epiphysis that may be secondary to the increased intracapsular pressure caused by the effusion. Sonography is a sensitive and noninvasive method of detecting joint effusion. It is performed by scanning along the anterior aspect of the femoral neck because this is where fluid tends to accumulate within the hip joint (Fig. 179-27). However, joint effusion is not specific, and aspiration is required if infection is a consideration. On MRI, there is evidence of joint effusion but no evidence of bone abnormality.

HEMOPHILIC ARTHROPATHY

Hemophilia is an X-linked recessive disorder characterized by an abnormality of the coagulation mechanism. It may be secondary to a deficiency in factor VIII, as in classic hemophilia (hemophilia A), or secondary to a deficiency of factor IX, as in Christmas disease (hemophilia B). Hemarthrosis occurs in approximately 75% to 90% of patients with hemophilia. The most commonly affected joints include the knee, elbow, and ankle. Hemorrhage may be secondary to trauma or may occur spontaneously. Recurrent hemarthrosis leads to synovial inflammation and proliferation associated with absorption of hemosiderin and red cell products. With synovial inflammation, cartilage destruction and subchondral

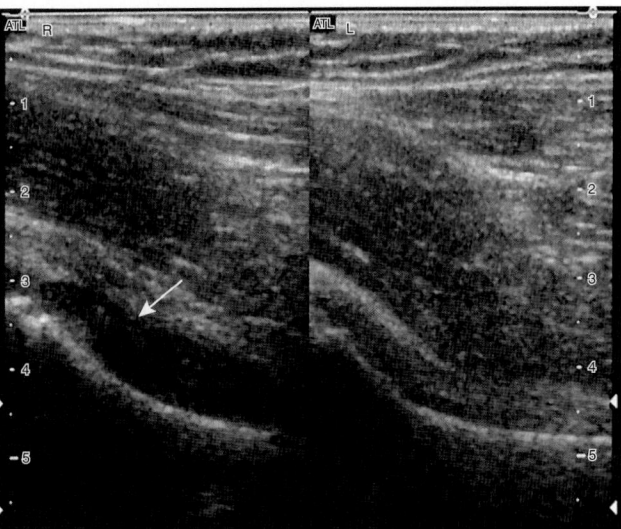

FIGURE 179-27. Sagittal sonographic images along the anterior aspect of the hips in a child with transient synovitis demonstrate a right hip joint effusion with bulging of the joint capsule *(arrow)* compared to the normal left hip.

bone damage lead to joint space narrowing. With hyperemia and prolonged inflammation, epiphyseal overgrowth, early growth plate fusion, and fibrosis of ligaments can be seen.

> **Hemophilic arthropathy is most common at the knee, elbow, and ankle.**

The radiographic changes may be identical to those of JRA, but clinical findings and typical joint involvement help distinguish these entities. Radiodense joint effusions and subchondral changes are more common in hemophilic arthropathy (Fig. 179-28). In the knee, the classic radiographic findings include squaring of the femoral condyles, a widened intercondylar notch, and squaring of the patella. In the elbow, enlargement of the radial head may result in limited movement, and there may be broadening of the distal humerus and enlargement of the olecranon fossa (Fig. 179-29).

MRI may be used to determine whether hemarthrosis has occurred, so that therapy with factor VIII can be administered to prevent chronic joint damage. Acute hemarthrosis and chronic joint effusion may be indistinguishable, with low signal on T1- and high signal on T2-weighted images. Subacute hemarthrosis is usually of high signal on both T1- and T2-weighted images related to the presence of extracellular methemoglobin (Fig. 179-30). The synovial thickening often has areas of low signal on T1- and T2-weighted images related to fibrosis or hemosiderin deposition. Gadolinium better delineates the extent of synovial thickening, which shows less enhancement compared with rheumatoid arthritis. This is likely secondary to hypovascular connective tissue and hemosiderin deposition within the synovium. MRI detects early changes within the cartilage, which may be localized or diffuse. Gradient-echo MR imaging is helpful for evaluation of hemosiderin and cartilage abnormalities. Subchondral cysts may result from intraosseous bleeding, and rarely, pseudotumours may develop secondary to hemorrhage in the periarticular soft tissues. Signal characteristics are variable depending on the age of the hematoma.

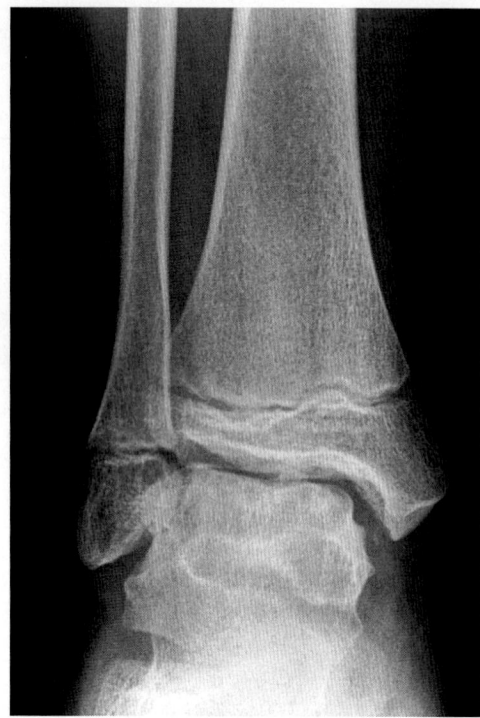

FIGURE 179-28. A 10-year-old boy with hemophilia and recurrent hemarthrosis, frontal radiograph of the right ankle demonstrates joint narrowing and slight overgrowth of the distal tibial epiphysis. There is irregularity of the talar articular surface and subchondral cyst formation.

NEUROPATHIC JOINT

Neuropathic arthritis is a destructive arthropathy secondary to long-standing repetitive trauma, frequently associated with loss of proprioception. In children, this may be related to myelomeningocele, syringomyelia, familial dysautonomia, or congenital insensitivity to pain. The most common radiographic findings include distention related to hypertrophic synovitis and effusion; degeneration of the articular surface, resulting in debris within the joint; and fracture or dislocation (Fig. 179-31). In children, there may be growth plate widening and metaphyseal fragmentation related to growth plate injury. MRI findings of neuropathic joint include fragmentation of areas of articular cartilage and subchondral bone, which are embedded in the synovium. In addition to synovial thickening and effusion, there may be associated tears of the menisci and ligaments. The periarticular bone is generally devoid of inflammation, but there may be inflammatory masses in the periarticular soft tissues that have heterogeneous signal intensity. MRI may help to distinguish infection from neuropathic destruction.

FOREIGN BODY SYNOVITIS

Foreign body synovitis usually presents with a monoarticular synovitis and may be suggested by the presence of a puncture wound. There is often a delay in diagnosis, especially if there is no history of injury and the foreign body is nonradiopaque and difficult to detect. Wood splinters, especially plant thorns such as palm or blackthorn, may dissect in from the surface and produce a chronic synovitis or tendonitis. Foreign body synovitis can simulate osteomyelitis or, rarely, primary bone

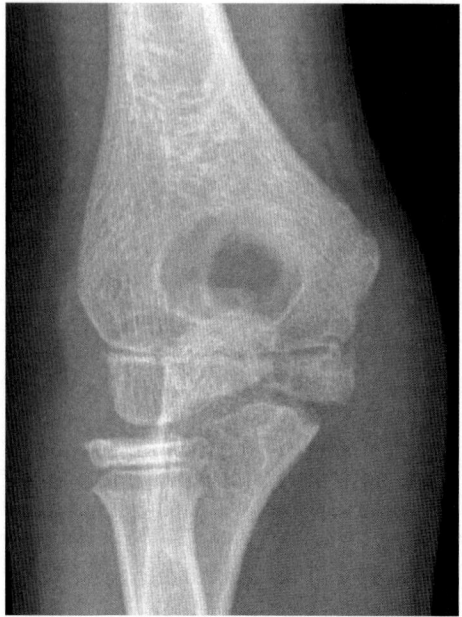
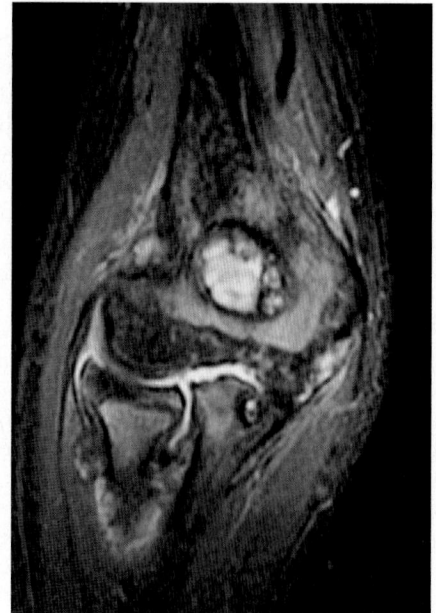
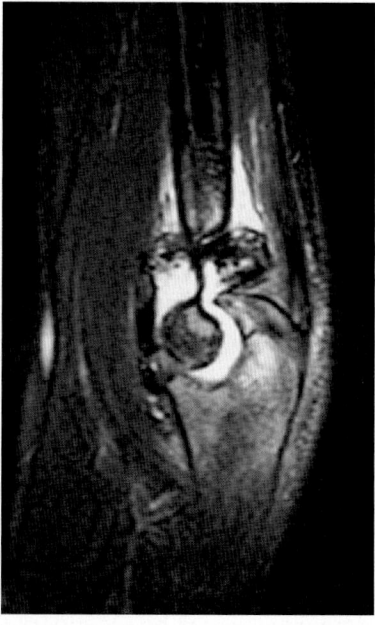

A   B   C

FIGURE 179-29. A 10-year-old boy with severe hemophilia. Frontal radiograph **(A)** of right elbow shows advanced maturation of the epiphyses, enlarged intercondylar notch and joint space narrowing. **B**, and **C**, Coronal and sagittal T2-weighted magnetic resonance images show a joint effusion with low signal foci compatible with hemosiderin due to hemarthrosis. There is associated periarticular high signal edema, subchondral irregularity, and erosions of the right elbow.

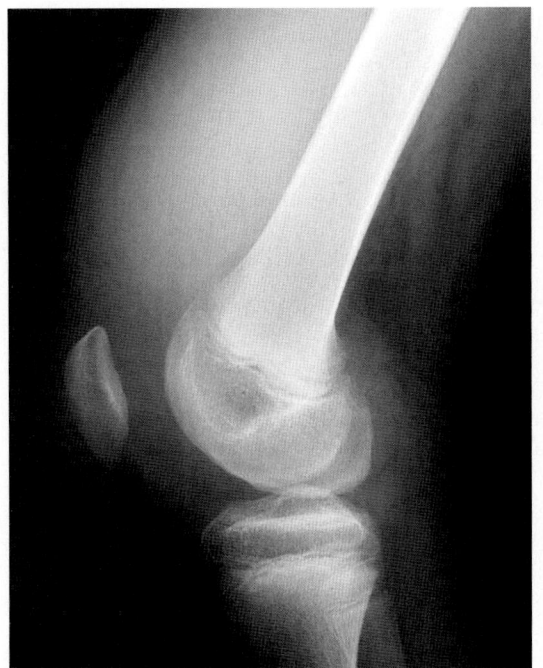

A

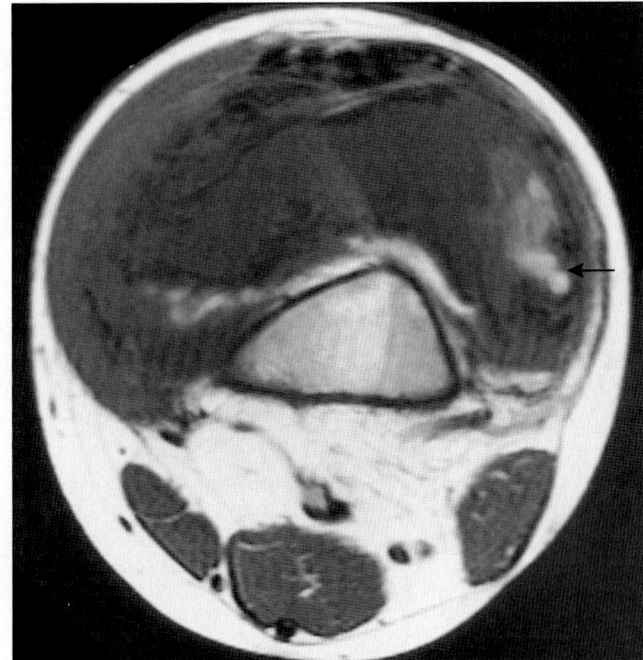

B

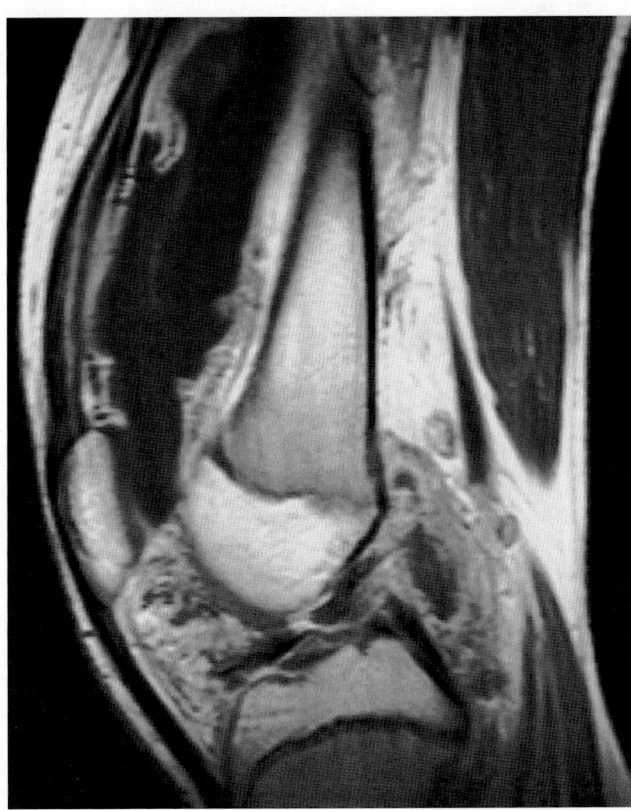

C

FIGURE 179-30. A 12-year-old boy with chronic hemophiliac arthropathy. **A,** On lateral radiograph of the left knee, there is marked soft tissue swelling in the suprapatellar bursa from extensive joint effusion. **B,** Axial T1-weighted magnetic resonance image demonstrates low-signal chronic synovial thickening and heterogeneous signal of the joint effusion, with high-signal area laterally *(arrow)* consistent with subacute hemarthrosis. **C,** Sagittal T1-weighted image following contrast enhancement shows irregular enhancing synovium in the popliteal region with several small enhancing popliteal lymph nodes.

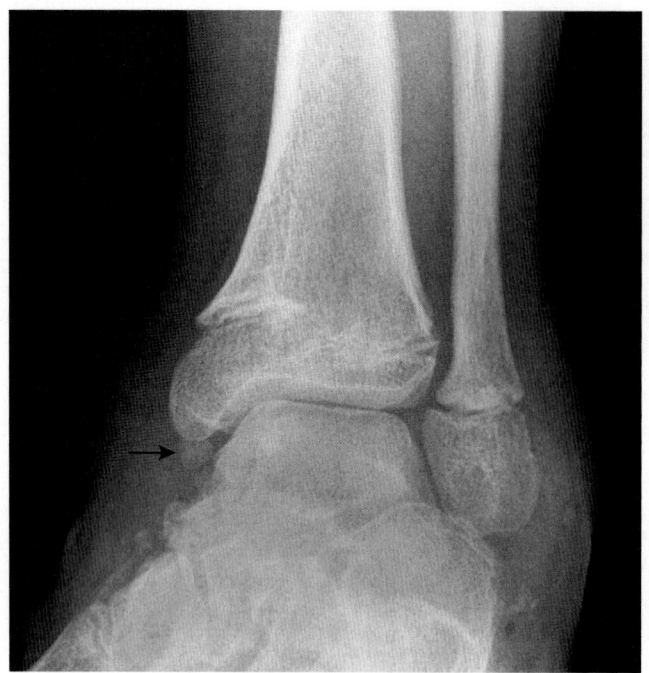

A

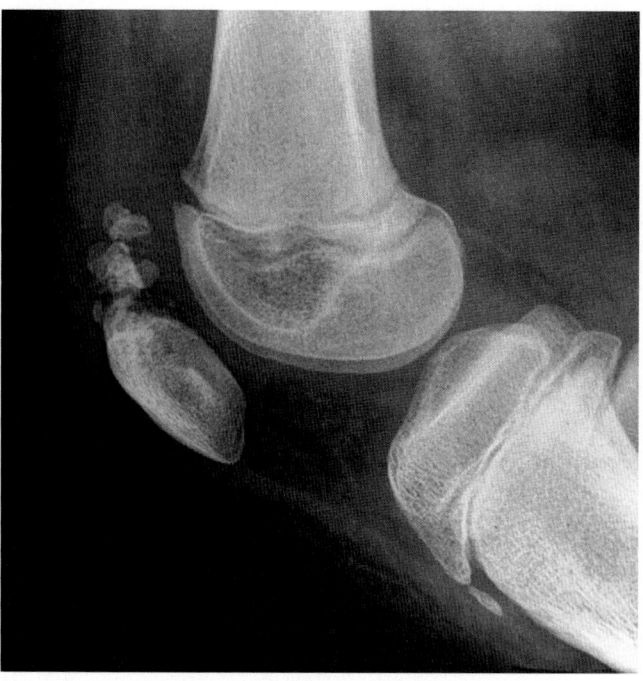

B

FIGURE 179-31. Neuropathic joints in a 10-year-old girl with congenital insensitivity to pain. **A,** Frontal oblique radiograph of the ankle demonstrates soft tissue swelling, epiphyseal overgrowth, premature growth plate fusion, and loose bodies *(arrow).* **B,** Lateral radiograph of the knee shows joint effusion with multiple ossific loose bodies in the suprapatellar region.

tumors. Extraction of the foreign body is essential for recovery, and identification of the foreign body by imaging will allow a localized synovectomy. Plant thorns have slightly higher density than soft tissue and may be detected on CT. Nonradiopaque foreign bodies may also be identified with ultrasound or MRI.

MISCELLANEOUS DISORDERS

Intra-articular Masses

A number of articular masses arise from either the synovium or capsule of a joint and lead to joint dysfunction (Table 179-7). Imaging findings may be diagnostic.

Vascular Malformations

Vascular malformations are benign lesions, usually diagnosed in childhood or young adulthood. Clinically they mimic chronic arthritis, and not uncommonly there is a delay in diagnosis. They may have associated cutaneous lesions, recurrent hemarthrosis, and arthropathy. The knee is the most commonly involved joint and the suprapatellar region is the most common location. Most commonly they are venous, and rarely arteriovenous malformations. Radiographs are normal in over half of patients; however, they may demonstrate a soft tissue mass or joint effusion. Occasionally, osteoporosis, erosions, and epiphyseal overgrowth are present, and the presence of phleboliths suggests the diagnosis. MRI findings are usually diagnostic and help in defining the extent of disease. The typical MRI appearance is of a slightly lobulated, nonencapsulated mass without significant displacement of surrounding structures. It is of low

TABLE 179-7
Intra-Articular Masses
Synovial hemangioma Pigmented villonodular synovitis Synovial osteochondromatosis Lipoma arborescens

or intermediate signal, similar to muscle, on T1-weighted images and of high signal on T2-weighted images, with low signal septa, phleboliths, or vascular channels. There may be fluid levels, low-signal hemosiderin, or bone erosions related to hemarthrosis. Vascular malformations demonstrate extensive enhancement after the administration of gadolinium (Figs. 179-32 and 179-33).

NODULAR AND PIGMENTED VILLONODULAR SYNOVITIS

Nodular synovitis and PVNS are uncommon proliferative disorders of the synovium of unknown etiology that may be post traumatic or may represent benign synovial neoplasms. Although PVNS is more common in adults, 15% of cases occur in children between 10 and 20 years of age. PVNS is usually monoarticular and only rarely polyarticular. Children may be more likely to have polyarticular involvement, and PVNS has been associated with congenital anomalies of the genitourinary, cardiac, musculoskeletal, and neurologic systems. There are two forms: a nodular type that usually involves the tendon sheath of the hand and wrist, and a less common diffuse form that involves a joint, most commonly the knee. Other joints that may be affected in the diffuse form include the hip, ankle, shoulder, and elbow in decreas-

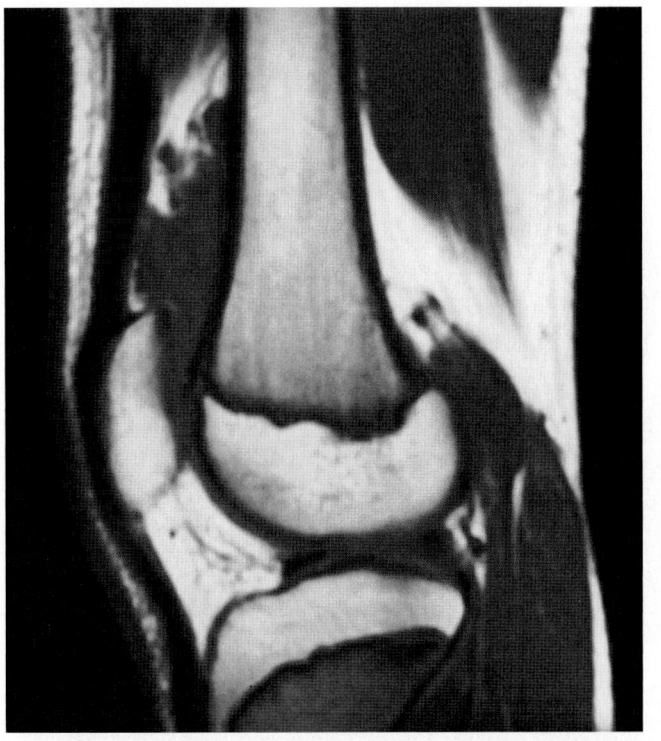

A

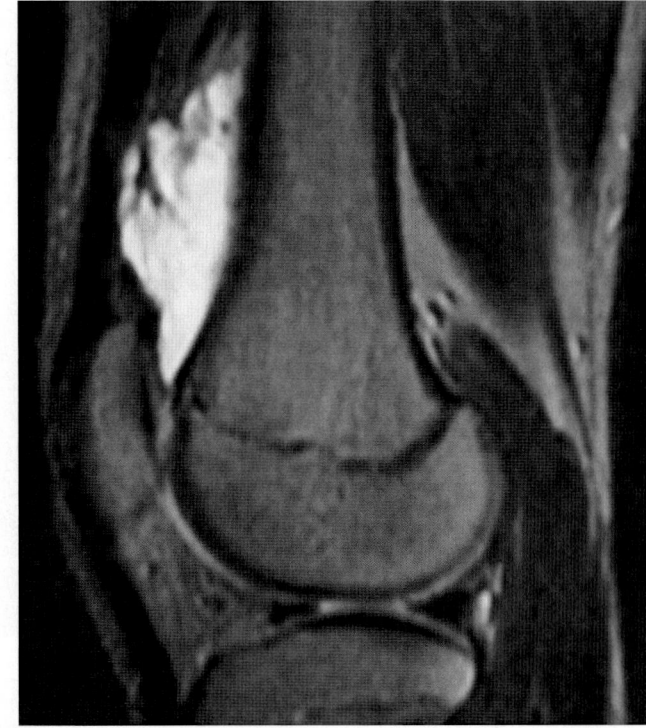

B

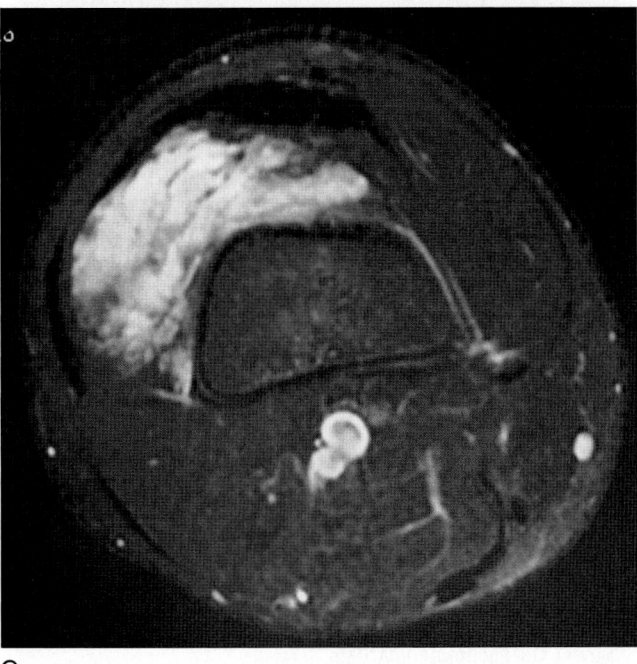

C

FIGURE 179-32. Magnetic resonance imaging of a vascular malformation in a 2-year-old girl presenting with limp and swelling in the right knee. Sagittal T1-weighted **(A)** and T2-weighted **(B)** images and fat saturation post-gadolinium axial T1-weighted image **(C)** demonstrate a lobulated suprapatellar bursal mass, which is intermediate on T1-weighted image and hyperintense on T2-weighted images, with marked heterogeneous enhancement.

ing order of frequency. The histology is identical in both types of PVNS and is characterized by synovial proliferation with an infiltrate of inflammatory cells with macrophages containing lipid and hemosiderin.

Radiographic findings are usually normal. Occasionally there are bone erosions or cysts with preservation of the joint space and bone density. There may be a joint effusion or mass of increased radiodensity on plain image or CT resulting from iron deposition, but calcification is rare. MRI demonstrates multinodular synovial masses with variable amounts of hemosiderin, which causes marked signal dropout on T2-weighted and particularly gradient-echo images. Regions of increased signal on T1-weighted images related to lipid deposition or increased signal on T2-weighted images secondary to edema may be seen. The synovial masses show prominent contrast enhancement after gadolinium administration (Fig. 179-34). If the typical features are present, the MRI appearance is diagnostic. PVNS may invade into the bone and periarticular soft tissues, and extend

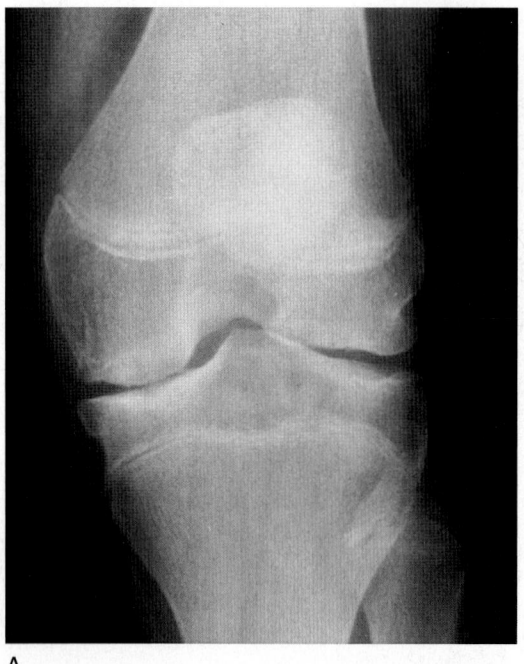

A

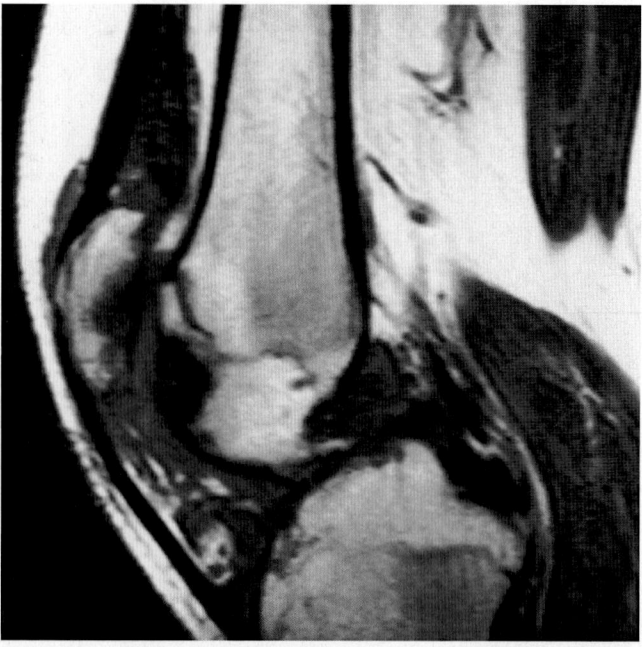

B

FIGURE 179-33. Vascular malformation with associated arthropathy related to recurrent hemarthrosis in a 16-year-old girl with right knee monoarthritis for 12 years. **A,** Frontal radiograph of right knee shows irregular joint space narrowing, erosions, and early osteophyte formation. **B,** On sagittal T1-weighted magnetic resonance (MR) image through lateral aspect of knee, there is marked joint destruction with erosions and posterior subluxation of the tibia secondary to disruption of the cruciate ligaments. **C,** Sagittal fast T2-weighted MR image with fat saturation shows large, lobulated high-signal mass involving suprapatellar bursa, Hoffa's fat pad, and the intercondylar region.

C

around neurovascular structures. MRI is useful in determining the extent of disease for surgical planning. In villonodular synovitis, a synovial mass is seen that does not have the low MRI signal associated with hemosiderin.

> **In PVNS, multinodular synovial masses are seen, with variable amounts of hemosiderin causing signal dropout on T2-weighted and gradient echo MRIs. Hemodisderin deposition can also be seen with other disease processes including hemophilic arthropathy and intra-articular vascular malformation.**

Synovial Osteochondromatosis

This is a rare benign disorder characterized by metaplastic transformation of the synovium with the formation of osteocartilaginous foci. These foci may become calcified or ossified and can detach from the synovium to become loose bodies within the joint. They are usually similar in size and may enlarge with continuing nourishment from synovial fluid. Synovial osteochondromatosis is usually monoarticular and occurs most commonly in large joints. Up to 50% of cases occur in the knee, followed in decreasing frequency by the elbow, hip, and shoulder. Less commonly, small joints such as the temporomandibular, acromioclavicular, and interphalangeal

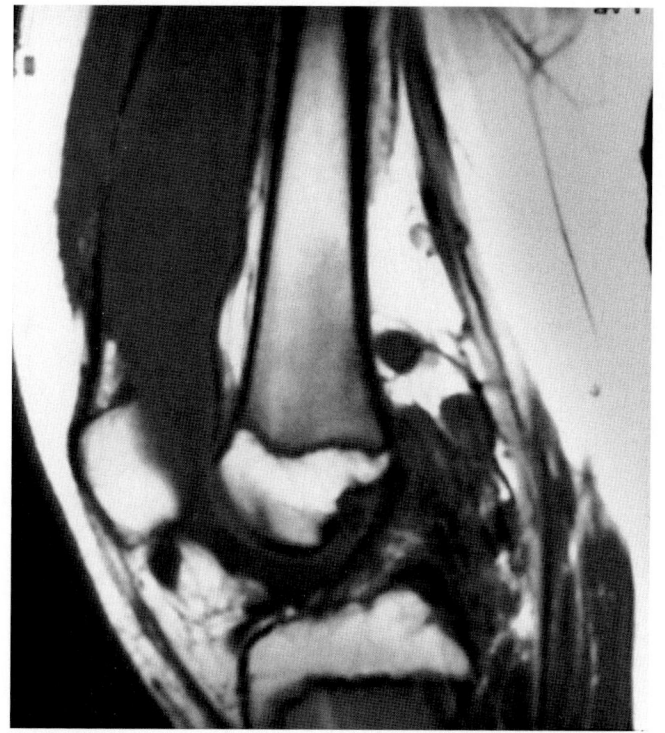

A

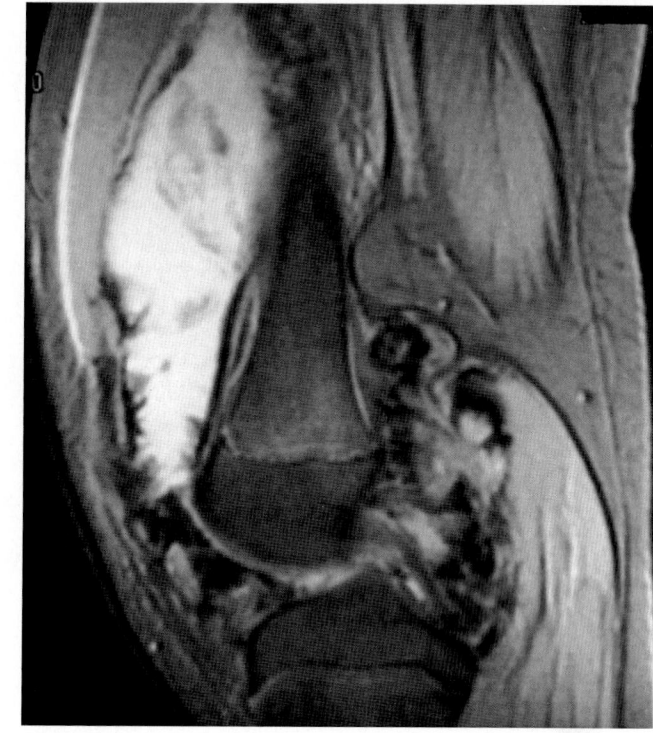

B

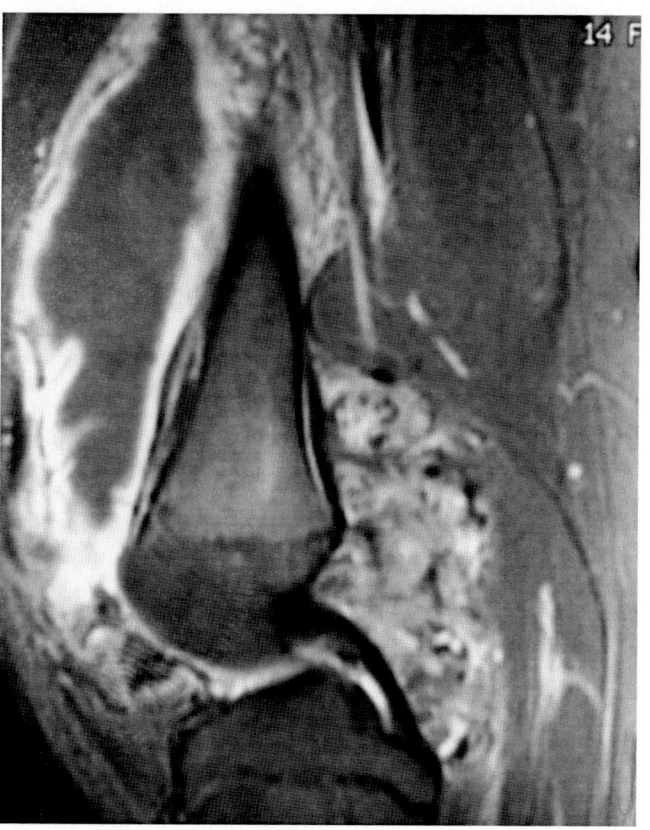

C

FIGURE 179-34. Magnetic resonance imaging findings of pigmented villonodular synovitis in a 14-year-old girl with joint swelling. On sagittal T1-weighted **(A)** and gradient echo images **(B)**, there is a large joint effusion with multiple low signal masses located predominantly in the posterior aspect of the joint related to hemosiderin deposition. **C,** Sagittal T1-weighted image post gadolinium shows heterogeneous enhancement of the masses and diffuse nodular synovial enhancement.

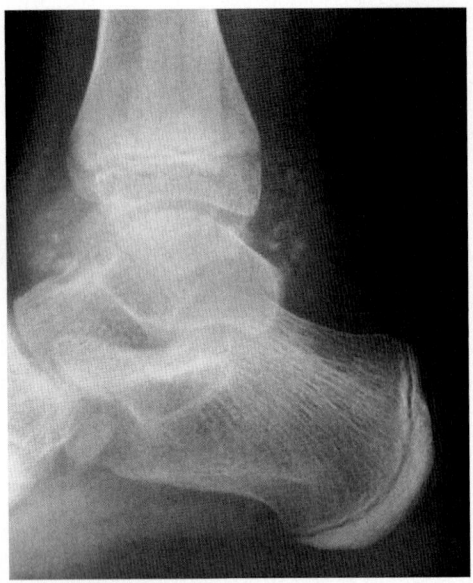
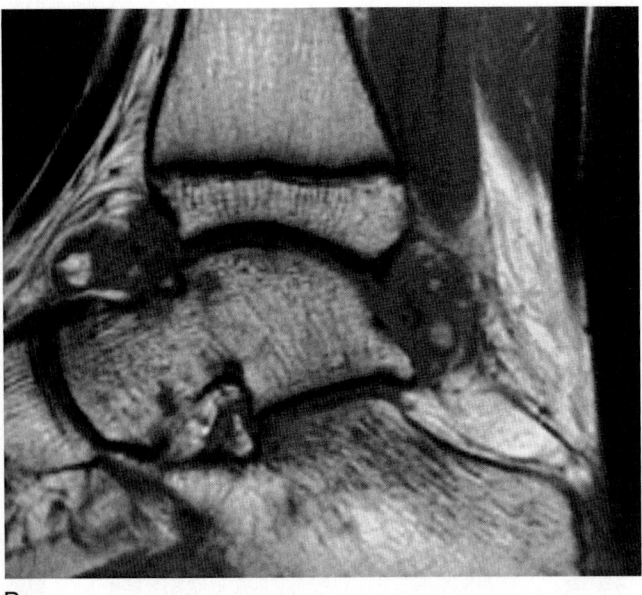

A   B

FIGURE 179-35. Synovial osteochondromatosis in an 11-year-old boy with persistent right ankle swelling. **A,** On lateral radiograph of the right ankle, there are multiple radiopaque ossific loose bodies around the ankle joint with joint space preservation. **B,** On sagittal T1-weighted magnetic resonance image of the ankle, multiple ossific foci are embedded in thickened synovium and have high signal intensity similar to adjacent marrow fat, with low signal cortical rim.

joints may be involved. Degenerative changes may occur as a late sequela, and rarely, there is transformation to chondrosarcoma. Secondary osteochondromatosis may result from underlying disorders such as osteoarthritis, osteochondrosis dissecans (OCD), avascular necrosis, neuropathic osteoarthropathy, and trauma.

The radiographic finding of multiple calcified or ossified loose bodies of uniform size in a joint free of arthritis is diagnostic. However, in up to one third of patients, no calcification is present. CT may be helpful in detecting faintly calcified loose bodies. The MRI appearance depends on the composition of the foci. MRI can better demonstrate the noncalcified cartilaginous loose bodies. Hyaline cartilaginous foci are of low to intermediate signal on T1- and high signal on T2-weighted images. With calcification, low signal on T1- and T2-weighted images is evident. Ossific foci have internal signal similar to marrow, being hyperintense on T1- and of intermediate signal on T2-weighted images, with a peripheral rim of low-signal cortical bone (Fig. 179-35). Patients usually have associated joint effusion and synovial thickening.

LIPOMA ARBORESCENS

Lipoma arborescens is a rare benign intra-articular lesion consisting of villous lipomatous proliferation of the synovium. It usually is monoarticular, but 20% of the time, the presentation is bilateral. Infrequent in children, it most commonly involves the knee joint but can be seen elsewhere, including in the glenohumeral joint, subdeltoid bursa, hip, elbow, ankle, and wrist joints. Most cases arise in an otherwise normal joint, but they may be associated with osteoarthritis, rheumatoid arthritis, Turner syndrome, or internal derangement. Of unknown etiology, it may be a nonspecific reactive

change of the synovium in response to a variety of insults, such as trauma or inflammation. Pathologically, there is marked villous proliferation of the synovial membrane with hyperplasia of the subsynovial fat.

Radiographs may demonstrate a joint effusion and mass that is of fat density, but the fat content is more easily detected with cross-sectional imaging with CT or MRI. The MRI findings are pathognomonic, with frond-like synovial masses with signal characteristics paralleling fat on all pulse sequences, with high signal on T1- and intermediate signal on T2-weighted images (Fig. 179-36) and suppression of signal with fat saturation techniques.

ARTHRITIS RELATED TO CHILDHOOD MALIGNANCIES

Any of the childhood malignancies can cause musculoskeletal complaints that mimic rheumatic disease, including the leukemias, neuroblastoma, lymphoma including Hodgkin disease, malignant histiocytosis, rhabdomyosarcoma, and the primary bone tumors, including osteosarcoma and Ewing sarcoma.

Systemic Disorders

SARCOIDOSIS

Sarcoidosis is a chronic granulomatous disease that is rare in children; the early symptoms may simulate JRA. Common manifestations include rash, ocular disease, and chronic arthritis. Pulmonary findings are uncommon in children, and other organs that may be involved include the liver, spleen, lymph nodes, and parotid gland. The arthritis in childhood appears to be divided into two phases: an insidious pauciarticular arthritis in children younger than 4 to 5 years and a second phase that develops into polyarticular arthritis in older children.

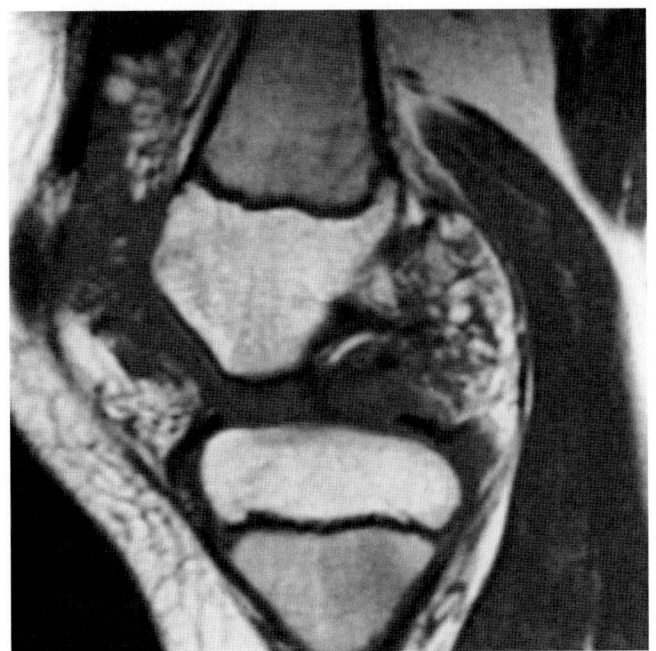

A

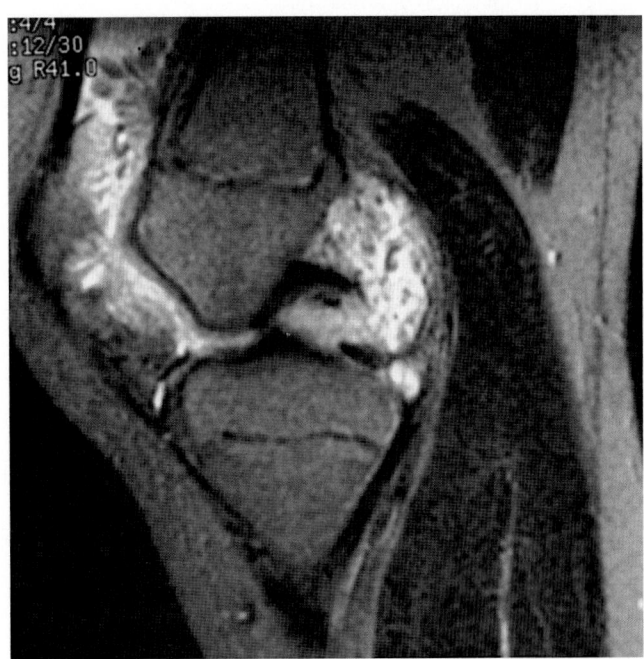

B

FIGURE 179-36. Magnetic resonance imaging findings of lipoma arborescens in an 11-year-old boy with chronic right knee swelling for 4 years. Sagittal T1-weighted **(A)** and sagittal T2-weighted **(B)** images demonstrate a lobulated soft tissue mass within the suprapatellar bursae and posterior joint space. It has high signal foci on T1-weighted and intermediate signal on T2-weighting, identical to subcutaneous fat with associated joint effusion.

Radiographs may show bone changes that include acro-osteolysis, honeycombing, or small lytic areas in the phalanges, metacarpals, and metatarsals (Fig. 179-37). In young children, sarcoidosis may result in synovial thickening that predominantly affects the large joints and tendon sheaths. Other than soft tissue swelling, radiographic findings related to the joint, including erosions, are rare (see Chapter 175).

Storage Disorders, Skeletal Dysplasias, and Syndromes

Mucopolysaccharidosis I-S (Schei disease) is a lysosomal storage disease related to a deficiency of α-L-iduronidase with excessive urinary excretion of dermatan sulfate and heparan sulfate. The biochemical abnormality is identical to Hurler syndrome (mucopolysaccharidosis I), but manifestations are less severe. Abnormalities usually appear in childhood, including corneal clouding and cardiovascular disease such as aortic valve stenosis (see Chapter 165). Joint abnormalities include stiffness with claw hand deformity and cystic changes in the carpals, metacarpals, tarsals, metatarsals, and femoral heads (Fig. 179-38). Other bone abnormalities include widening of the clavicles and ribs, which is characteristically seen in storage disorders. Inheritance is autosomal recessive, and patients have normal intelligence or mild mental retardation. Other storage disorders associated with joint abnormalities include mucolipidosis III and hyaluronidase deficiency. Abnormal low signal around affected joints can be in patients with mucolipidosis III on MRI.

Progressive pseudorheumatoid arthritis of childhood (PPAC) is an autosomal recessive noninflammatory chondrodysplasia. Initial symptoms of difficulty walking and

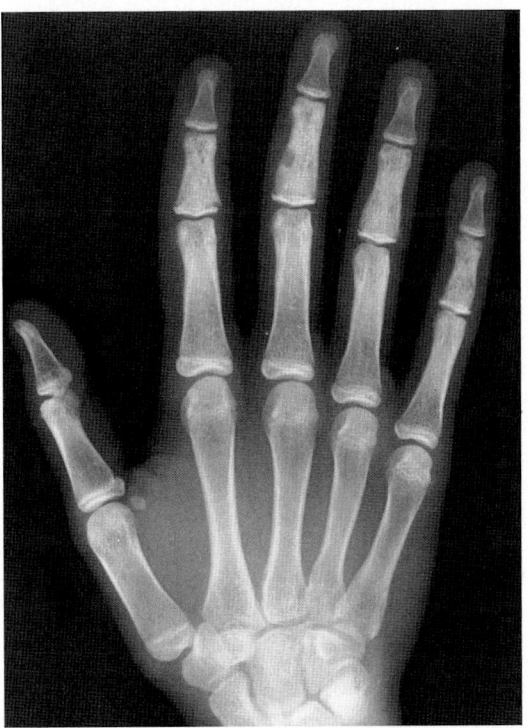

FIGURE 179-37. Sarcoidosis in a 15-year-old girl with weight loss, hypothalamic dysfunction, joint pain, and swelling in fingers for 2 years. Radiograph of left hand demonstrates soft tissue swelling of several digits and multiple small lytic lesions predominantly in the middle phalanges, which were bilateral.

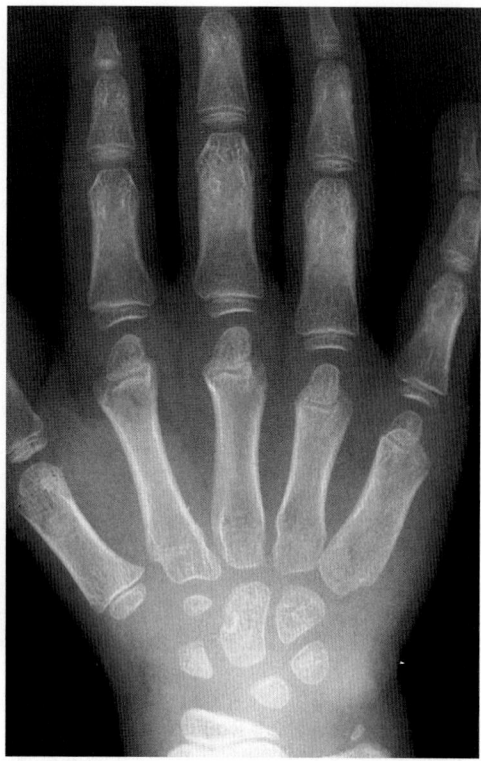

FIGURE 179-38. Mucopolysaccharidosis I-S (Scheie syndrome) in an 11-year-old male with history of chronic arthritis with multiple joint contractures treated initially as juvenile rheumatoid arthritis. Patient was noted to have corneal clouding, glaucoma, and more recently aortic insufficiency. Chest radiograph demonstrated short, broad clavicles. Hand radiograph shows short metacarpals and small carpal bones with an intraosseous cyst in the capitate, as well as soft tissue swelling and joint space narrowing.

muscular weakness develop between 3 and 8 years of age. The main clinical features are generalized, progressive joint stiffness and swelling related to osseous enlargement, which is most marked in the hands. There are characteristic dysplastic skeletal abnormalities, particularly in the spine with platyspondyly, that distinguish this disorder from JRA. Other skeletal dysplasias associated with joint symptoms include Kniest syndrome, multiple epiphyseal dysplasia, and spondyloepiphyseal dysplasia tarda with progressive arthropathy, which may represent the same disorder as PPAC.

Camptodactyly-arthropathy syndrome is a rare autosomal recessive disorder consisting of congenital camptodactyly, arthropathy, and pericarditis. The lack of inflammation and absence of joint narrowing with chronic disease help differentiate this disorder from JRA. Flexion deformities are symmetric, involving the proximal interphalangeal joint of the hands. Arthropathy predominantly affects large joints, and radiographic findings are most marked in the hips, where there is coxa vara, short broad femoral necks, and intraosseous cysts (Fig. 179-39).

Neonatal-onset multisystem inflammatory disease is a rare systemic disease characterized by arthropathy with rash, fever, hepatosplenomegaly, central nervous system and eye involvement, and deforming arthropathy of mainly large joints distinct from JRA. The typical radiographic appearance includes periarticular soft tissue swelling; enlarged, irregularly ossified epiphyses, especially around the knee; and metaphyseal splaying, osteoporosis, and metadiaphyseal periosteal new bone formation.

Goldbloom disease is a rare disorder consisting of idiopathic periosteal hyperostosis and dysproteinemia. It usually presents after infancy with an upper respiratory infection, limb pain, and joint swelling. Radiographs show lamellar periosteal reaction predominantly involving long bones but also the mandible, facial bones, metacarpals, and metatarsals. One of the distinguishing features is an abnormality of serum proteins with hypergammaglobulinemia and hypoalbuminemia. Other disorders associated with periostitis and joint swelling, such as hypertrophic osteoarthropathy, must be excluded. Treatment is symptomatic with salicylates, and recovery is complete after weeks or months.

Chondrolysis

Chondrolysis represents progressive cartilage degradation of uncertain etiology, associated with loss of joint motion and joint space narrowing. The hip is most commonly affected joint with sporadic reports of knee shoulder and ankle involvement. Most commonly seen in adolescent girls, chondrolysis is most often associated with slipped capital femoral epiphysis, but has also been observed following infection, trauma and pregnancy.

Clinically, patients present with joint pain and reduced motion. Radiographs typically show concentric joint space narrowing and juxta-articular osteopenia. Bone scintigraphy can show increased uptake on both sides of the joint. MRI findings include cartilage loss, marrow edema and muscle wasting.

In slipped capital femoral epiphysis, chondrolysis can rarely be encountered before surgical treatment but is much more common after joint pinning, particularly if there is penetration of the stabilizing pins through the articular cartilage into the joint space.

Treatment typically includes nonsteroidal anti-inflammatory medication, bed rest, and protected weight bearing.

Baker Cyst

Synovial cysts are fluid collections resulting from herniation of synovium through the joint capsule. The most common is the popliteal or Baker cyst, located within the gastrocnemius–semimembranosus bursa. Popliteal cysts may develop at any age, but up to 33% occur in children 15 years or younger and they are slightly more common in boys than in girls. They may be associated with previous injury or arthritis, but in children, the majority (95%) of popliteal cysts are isolated. In contrast to adults, popliteal cysts in children usually resolve spontaneously, and surgery is indicated only when there is associated pain or restriction of movement. Synovial cysts may simulate hematoma or tumor clinically, and, with rupture into the soft tissues of the calf, they can be confused with thrombophlebitis. Other intra-articular cysts that are not synovial in origin include ganglia and meniscal cysts. Ganglia result from myxomatous degen-

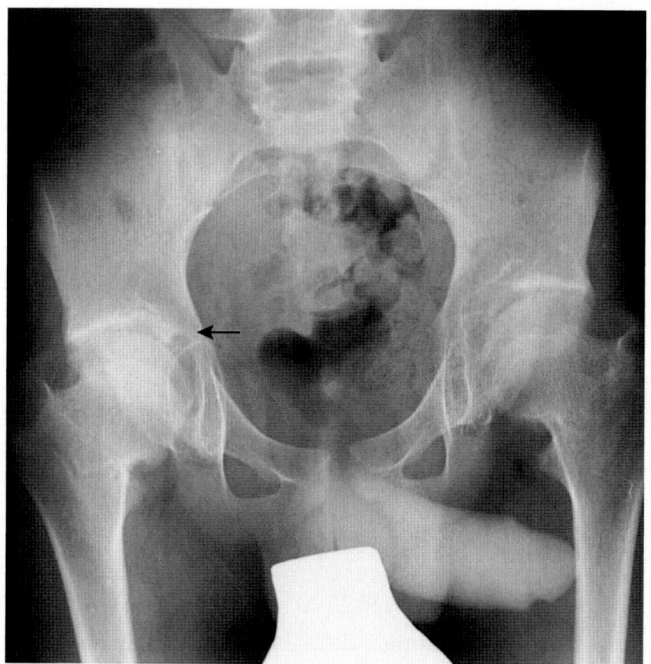

A

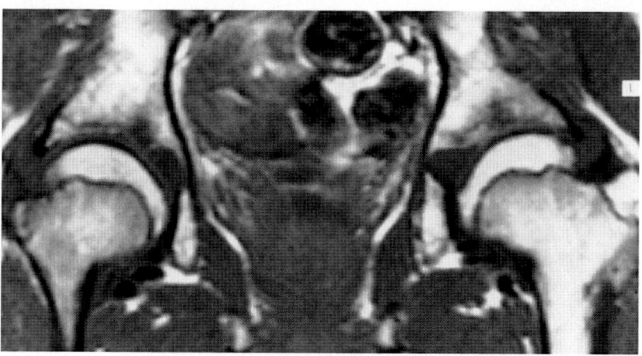

B

C

FIGURE 179-39. Camptodactyly-arthropathy syndrome in a 15-year-old boy with pericardial rub and chronic arthritis involving hips, knees, and ankles and history of flexion deformities of fingers since birth. Chest radiograph showed enlargement of pericardial silhouette secondary to pericardial effusion. **A,** Radiograph of the pelvis shows short broad femoral necks, coxa magna, and varus deformity with symmetric narrowing of hip joints, and intraosseous cysts within the acetabulum *(arrow)* better seen on magnetic resonance images (MRIs). Coronal T1-weighted **(B)** and axial T2-weighted **(C)** MR images demonstrate bilateral joint effusions with intraosseous cysts that are of intermediate signal on T1-weighted sequences and high signal on T2-weighted sequences.

eration of connective tissue and are usually associated with tendons or ligaments. Meniscal cysts are associated with horizontal tears of the menisci.

> **In children, the majority (95%) of popliteal cysts are isolated and with no association with prior injury or arthritis.**

On lateral radiographs of the knee, Baker cysts may be seen as a well-defined soft tissue mass in the popliteal

fossa. They are located along the posteromedial aspect of the knee joint, and they can be seen extending between the head of the medial gastrocnemius and the semi-membranous muscles on cross-sectional imaging. On sonography, popliteal cysts are seen as well-encapsulated, anechoic fluid collections. On MRI, they are usually homogeneous, with signal intensity identical to joint fluid, low on T1- and high on T2-weighted images (Fig. 179-40). Occasionally, they can be infected, demonstrate wall thickening or septations, or contain debris.

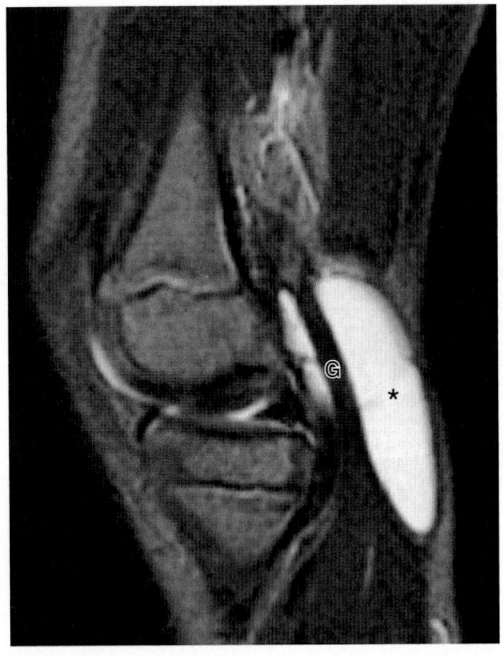
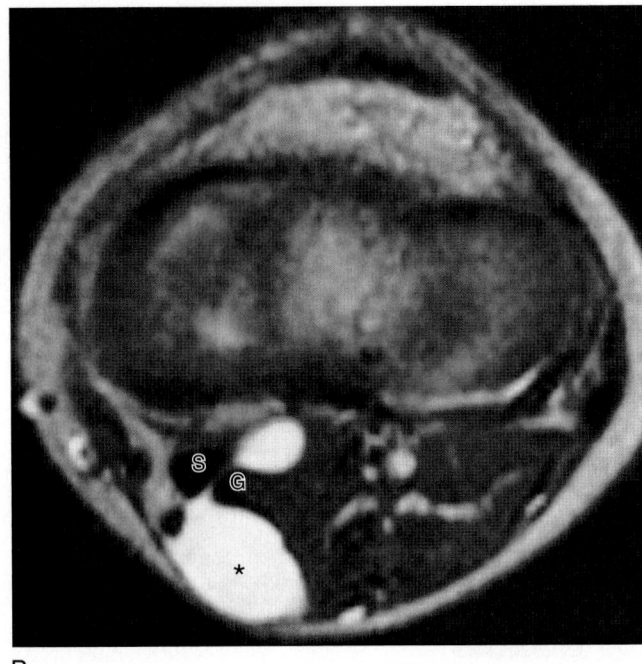

A   B

FIGURE 179-40. Magnetic resonance imaging findings with Baker cyst. Sagittal **(A)** and axial **(B)** T2-weighted images with well-defined encapsulated fluid collection (asterisks) with homogeneous high signal intensity. The neck of the Baker cyst passes between the semimembranosus tendon (S) and the medial gastrocnemius tendon (G).

SUGGESTED READINGS

Normal Anatomy and Imaging Appearance

Al-Otaibi L, Siegel MJ: The pediatric knee. Magn Reson Imaging Clin N Am 1998;6:643-660

Azouz EM, Babyn P, Chhem RK: MRI of the pediatric knee. In Munk PL, Helms CA (eds): MRI of the Knee. Philadelphia, Lippincott–Raven, 1995:281-314

Balkissoon AR: Radiologic interpretation of vacuum phenomena. Crit Rev Diagn Imaging 1996;37:435-460

Gylys-Morin VM: MR imaging of pediatric musculoskeletal inflammatory and infectious disorders. Magn Reson Imaging Clin N Am 1998;6:537-559

Smith HJ: Contrast-enhanced MRI of rheumatic joint disease. Br J Rheumatol 1996;3:45-47

Arthritis

Juvenile Rheumatoid Arthritis, Autoimmune Connective Tissue Disease, and Chromosomal Disorders

Balestrazzi P, Ferraccioli GF, Ambanelli U, et al: Juvenile rheumatoid arthritis in Turner's syndrome. Clin Exp Rheumatol 1986;4:61-62

Benseler SM, Silverman ED: Systemic Lupus Erythematosus. Pediatric Clinics of North America 2005; 443-467.

Cellerini M, Salti S, Trapani S, et al: Correlation between clinical and ultrasound assessment of the knee in children with mono-articular or pauci-articular juvenile rheumatoid arthritis. Pediatr Radiol 1999;29:117-123

Chung C, Coley BD, Martin LC: Rice bodies in juvenile rheumatoid arthritis. AJR Am J Roentgenol 1998;170:698-700

Doria AS, Babyn PS, Feldman B: A critical appraisal of radiographic scoring systems for assessment of juvenile idiopathic arthritis. Pediatr Radiol 2006;36:759-772

Dressler F: Juvenile rheumatoid arthritis and spondyloarthropathies. Curr Opin Rheumatol 1998;10:468-474

Eich GF, Halle F, Hodler J, et al: Juvenile chronic arthritis: imaging of the knees and hips before and after intraarticular steroid injection. Pediatr Radiol 1994;24:558-563

Gylys-Morin VM: MR imaging of pediatric musculoskeletal inflammatory and infectious disorders. Magn Reson Imaging Clin N Am 1998;6:537-559

Harel L, Wagner-Weiner L, Poznanski AK, et al: Effects of methotrexate on radiologic progression in juvenile rheumatoid arthritis. Arthritis Rheum 1993;36:1370-1374

Johnson K: Imaging of juvenile idiopathic arthritis. Pediatr Radiol 2006;36:743-758

Jordan A, McDonagh JE: Juvenile idiopathic arthritis: the paediatric perspective. Pediatr Radiol 2006;36:734-742

Kaye J: Arthritis: Roles of radiography and other imaging techniques in evaluation. Radiology 1990;177:601-608

Lamer S, Sebag GH: MRI and ultrasound in children with juvenile chronic arthritis. Eur J Radiol 2000;33:85-93

Lang BA, Schneider R, Reilly BJ, et al: Radiologic features of systemic onset juvenile rheumatoid arthritis. J Rheumatol 1995;22:168-173

Laxer RM, Clarke HM: Rheumatic disorders of the hand and wrist in childhood and adolescence. Hand Clin 2000;16:659-671

Olson JC, Bender JC, Levinson JE, et al: Arthropathy of Down syndrome. Pediatrics 1990;86:931-936

Ostergaard M, Stoltenberg M, Gideon P, et al: Changes in synovial membrane and joint effusion volumes after intraarticular methylprednisolone: quantitative assessment of inflammatory and destructive changes in arthritis by MRI. J Rheumatol 1996; 23:1151-1156

Patriquin HB, Camerlain M, Trias A: Late sequelae of juvenile rheumatoid arthritis of the hip: a follow-up study into adulthood. Pediatr Radiol 1984;14:151-157

Pettersson H, Rydholm U: Radiologic classification of knee joint destruction in juvenile chronic arthritis. Pediatr Radiol 1984; 14:419-421

Poznanski AK: Radiological approaches to pediatric joint disease. J Rheumatol 1992;19:78–93

Ravelli A, Martini A: Juvenile idiopathic arthritis. Lancet 2007;369:767-778

Reed MH, Wilmot DM: The radiology of juvenile rheumatoid arthritis: a review of the English language literature. J Rheumatol Suppl 1991;31:2-22

Rothschild BM: Recognition and treatment of arthritis in children. Compr Ther 1999;25:347-359

Ruhoy MK, Tucker L, McCauley RG: Hypertrophic bursopathy of the subacromial-subdeltoid bursa in juvenile rheumatoid arthritis: sonographic appearance. Pediatr Radiol 1996;26:353-355

Schanberg LE, Sandstrom MJ: Causes of pain in children with arthritis. Rheum Dis Clin North Am 1998;25:31-53, vi

Schneider R, Laxer RM: Systemic onset juvenile rheumatoid arthritis. Baillieres Clin Rheumatol 1998;12:245-271

Smith HJ: Contrast-enhanced MRI of rheumatic joint disease. Br J Rheumatol 1996;3:45-47

Sparling M, Malleson P, Wood B, et al: Radiographic follow-up of joints injected with triamcinolone hexacetonide for the management of childhood arthritis. Arthritis Rheum 1990; 33:821-826

Sureda D, Quiroga S, Arnal C, et al: Juvenile rheumatoid arthritis of the knee: evaluation with US. Radiology 1994;190:403-406

White EM: Magnetic resonance imaging in synovial disorders and arthropathy of the knee. Magn Reson Imaging Clin N Am 1994;2:451-461

Wihlborg CE, Babyn PS, Schneider R: The association between Turner's syndrome and juvenile rheumatoid arthritis. Pediatr Radiol 1999;29:676-681

Yancey CL, Zmijewski C, Athreya BH, et al: Arthropathy of Down's syndrome. Arthritis Rheum 1984;27:929-934

Juvenile Spondyloarthropathies

Azouz EM, Duffy CM: Juvenile spondyloarthropathies: clinical manifestations and medical imaging. Skeletal Radiol 1995; 24:399-408

Cabral DA, Malleson PN, Petty RE: Spondyloarthropathies of childhood. Pediatr Clin North Am 1995;42:1051-1070

Foster HE, Cairns RA, Burnell RH, et al: Atlantoaxial subluxation in children with seronegative enthesopathy and arthropathy syndrome: 2 case reports and a review of the literature. J Rheumatol 1995;22:548-551

Gensler L, Davis JC: Recognition and treatment of juvenile-onset spondyloarthritis. Curr Opin Rheumatol 2006;18:507-511

Jacobs JC: Juvenile arthritis. Am J Dis Child 1982;136:81-82

Keat A: Reactive arthritis. Adv Exp Med Biol 1999;455:201-206

Prieur AM: Spondyloarthropathies in childhood. Baillieres Clin Rheumatol 1998;12:287-307

Infectious Arthritis

Bettencourtt HL: A preterm infant with knee swelling. Clin Pediatr (Phila) 1999;38:45-47

Bradley JS, Kaplan SL, Tan TQ, et al: Pediatric pneumococcal bone and joint infections. The Pediatric Multicenter Pneumococcal Surveillance Study Group (PMPSSG). Pediatrics 1998; 102:1376-1382

Brower AC: Septic arthritis. Radiol Clin North Am 1996;34:293-309, x

Forrester DM, Feske WI: Imaging of infectious arthritis. Semin Roentgenol 1996;31:239-249

Goldenberg DL, Reed JI: Bacterial arthritis. N Engl J Med 1985;312:764-771

Gylys-Morin VM: MR imaging of pediatric musculoskeletal inflammatory and infectious disorders. Magn Reson Imaging Clin N Am 1998;6:537-559

Jacobs JC, Li SC, Ruzal-Shapiro C, et al: Tuberculous arthritis in children: diagnosis by needle biopsy of the synovium. Clin Pediatr (Phila) 1994;33:344-348

Jaramillo D, Treves S, Kasser J, et al: Osteomyelitis and septic arthritis in children: appropriate use of imaging to guide treatment. AJR Am J Roentgenol 1995;165:399-403

Jung ST, Rowe SM, Moon ES, et al: Significance of laboratory and radiologic findings for differentiating between septic arthritis and transient synovitis of the hip. J Pediatr Orthop 2003;23:368-372

Kocher MS, Zurakowski D, Kasser JR: Differentiating between septic arthritis and transient synovitis of the hip in children: an evidence-based clinical prediction algorithm. J Bone Joint Surg Am 1999;81:1662-1670

Kocher MS, Mandiga R, Zurakowski D, et al: Validation of a clinical prediction rule for the differentiation between septic arthritis and transient synovitis of the hip in children J Bone Joint Surg Am 2004;86:1629-1635

Lawson J, Rahn D: Lyme disease and radiologic findings in Lyme arthritis. AJR Am J Roentgenol 1992;158:1065-1069

Lee SK, Suh KJ, Kim YW, et al: Septic arthritis versus transient synovitis at MR imaging: preliminary assessment with signal intensity alterations in bone marrow. Radiology 1999; 211:459-465

Mitchell CS, Parisi MT: Pediatric acetabuloplasty procedures: radiologic evaluation. AJR Am J Roentgenol 1998;170:49-54

Poon AH, Terk MR, Colletti PM: The association of primary varicella infection and streptococcal infection of the cutaneous and musculoskeletal system: a case report. Magn Reson Imaging 1997;15: 131-133

Rose C, Eppes S: Infection-related arthritis. Pediatr Rheumatol 1997;23:677-695

Rutten MJ, van den Berg JC, van den Hoogen FH, et al: Nontuberculous mycobacterial bursitis and arthritis of the shoulder. Skeletal Radiol 1998;27:33-35

Spencer CH: Bone and joint infections in children. Curr Opin Rheumatol 1998;10:494-497

Strouse PJ, DiPietro MA, Adler RS: Pediatric hip effusions: evaluation with power Doppler sonography. Radiology 1998;201:731-735

White EM: Magnetic resonance imaging in synovial disorders and arthropathy of the knee. Magn Reson Imaging Clin N Am 1994;2:451-461

Yuan HC, Wu KG, Chen CJ: Characteristics and outcomes of septic arthritis in children. 2006;39:342-347

Zahraa J, Johnson D, Lim-Dunham JE, et al: Unusual features of osteoarticular tuberculosis in children. J Pediatr 1996;129:597-602

Other Inflammatory Arthritides

Baunin C, Railhac JJ, Younes I, et al: MR imaging in hemophilic arthropathy. Eur J Pediatr Surg 1991;1:358-363

Doria AS, Babyn PS, Lundin B, et al: Reliability and construct variability of the compatible MRI scoring system for evaluation of haemophilic knees and ankles of haemophilic children. Expert MRI working group of the international prophylaxis study group. Haemophilia 2006;12:503-513

Hermann G, Gilbert MS, Abdelwahab IF: Hemophilia: evaluation of musculoskeletal involvement with CT, sonography, and MR imaging. AJR Am J Roentgenol 1992;158:119-123

Koop S, Quanbeck D: Three common causes of childhood hip pain. Pediatr Clin North Am 1996;43:1053-1066

Lee SK, Suh KJ, Kim YW, et al: Septic arthritis versus transient synovitis at MR imaging: preliminary assessment with signal intensity alterations in bone marrow. Radiology 1999;211:459-465

Maillot F, Goupille P, Valat JP: Plant thorn synovitis diagnosed by magnetic resonance imaging. Scand J Rheumatol 1994;23:154-155

Marchal GJ, Van Holsbeeck MT, Raes M, et al: Transient synovitis of the hip in children: role of US. Radiology 1987;162:825-828

Nagele M, Bruning R, Kunze V, et al: Hemophilic arthropathy of the knee joint: static and dynamic Gd-DTPA-enhanced MRI. Eur Radiol 1995;5:547-552

Nuss R, Kilcoyne RF, Geraghty S, et al: Utility of magnetic resonance imaging for management of hemophilic arthropathy in children. J Pediatr 1993;123:388-392

Ozonoff MB: Pediatric Orthopedic Radiology. Philadelphia, WB Saunders, 1992

Rand T, Trattnig S, Male C, et al: Magnetic resonance imaging in hemophilic children: value of gradient echo and contrast-enhanced imaging. Magn Reson Imaging 1999;17:199-205

Ranner G, Ebner F, Fotter R, et al: Magnetic resonance imaging in children with acute hip pain. Pediatr Radiol 1989;20:67-71

Rawat B, Bell RS: Case report: rapidly progressive neuropathic arthropathy in syringohydromyelia—radiographic and magnetic resonance imaging findings. Clin Radiol 1994;49:504-507

Resnick D, Niwayama G: Diagnosis of Bone and Joint Disorders. Philadelphia, WB Saunders, 1995

Robben SG, Lequin MH, Diepstraten AF, et al: Anterior joint capsule of the normal hip in children with transient synovitis: US study with anatomic and histologic correlation. Radiology 1999; 210:499-507

Rodriguez-Merchan EC: Effects of hemophilia on articulations of children and adults. Clin Orthop 1996;328:7-13

Sequeira W: The neuropathic joint. Clin Exp Rheumatol 1994; 12:325–337

Yulish B, Lieberman J, Strandjord S, et al: Hemophilic arthropathy: assessment with MR imaging. Radiology 1987;164:759-762

Miscellaneous Disorders

Bessette PR, Cooley PA, Johnson RP, Czarnecki DJ: Gadolinium-enhanced MRI of pigmented villonodular synovitis of the knee. J Comput Assist Tomogr 1992;16:992-994

Botton E, Saraux A, Laselve H, et al: Musculoskeletal manifestations of cystic fibrosis. Joint Bone Spine 2003; 70:327-335

Bravo SM, Winalski CS, Weissman BN: Pigmented villonodular synovitis. Radiol Clin North Am 1996;34:311-326

Cameron BJ, Laxer RM, Wilmot DM, et al: Idiopathic periosteal hyperostosis with dysproteinemia (Goldbloom's syndrome): case report and review of the literature. Arthritis Rheum 1987; 30:1307-1312

Cardinal E, Dussault RG, Kaplan PA: Imaging and differential diagnosis of masses within a joint. Can Assoc Radiol 1994;45:363-372

Coles MJ, Tara HH Jr: Synovial chondromatosis: a case study and brief review. Am J Orthop 1997;26:37-40

Cotten A, Flipo RM, Herbaux B, et al: Synovial haemangioma of the knee: a frequently misdiagnosed lesion. Skeletal Radiol 1995;24:257-261

Coumas JM, Palmer WE: Knee arthrography: Evolution and current status. Radiol Clin North Am 1998;36:703-728

De Maeseneer M, Debaere C, Desprechins B, et al: Popliteal cysts in children: prevalence, appearance and associated findings at MR imaging. Pediatr Radiol 1999;29:605-609

Donnelly LF, Bisset GS 3rd, Passo MH: MRI findings of lipoma arborescens of the knee in a child: case report. Pediatr Radiol 1994;24:258-259

Eustace S, Harrison M, Srinivasen U, et al: Magnetic resonance imaging in pigmented villonodular synovitis. Can Assoc Radiol J 1994;45:283-286

Feller JF, Rishi M, Hughes EC: Lipoma arborescens of the knee: MR demonstration. AJR Am J Roentgenol 1994;163:162-164

Gerscovich EO, Greenspan A, Lehman WB: Idiopathic periosteal hyperostosis with dysproteinemia—Goldbloom's syndrome. Pediatr Radiol 1990;20:208-211

Goldbloom RB, Stein PB, Eisen A, et al: Idiopathic periosteal hyperostosis with dysproteinemia: a new clinical entity. N Engl J Med 1966;274:873-878

Goldman AB, DiCarlo EF: Pigmented villonodular synovitis: diagnosis and differential diagnosis. Radiol Clin North Am 1988;26:1327-1347

Greenspan A, Azouz EM, Matthews J 2nd, et al: Synovial hemangioma: imaging features in eight histologically proven cases, review of the literature, and differential diagnosis. Skeletal Radiol 1995; 24:583-590

Grieten M, Buckwalter KA, Cardinal E, et al: Case report 873: lipoma arborescens (villous lipomatous proliferation of the synovial membrane). Skeletal Radiol 1994;23:652-655

Hallel T, Lew S, Bansal M: Villous lipomatous proliferation of the synovial membrane (lipoma arborescens). J Bone Joint Surg Am 1988;70:264–270

Hossien RD: Progressive pseudorheumatoid chondrodysplasia. Skeletal Radiol 1994;23:411-419

Hughes TH, Sartoris DJ, Schweitzer ME, et al: Pigmented villonodular synovitis: MRI characteristics. Skeletal Radiol 1995; 24:7-12

Hugosson C, Bahabri S, McDonald P, et al: Radiological features in congenital camptodactyly, familial arthropathy and coxa vara syndrome. Pediatr Radiol 1994;24:523-526

Katz DS, Vaughn CJ, Goldschmidt AM, et al: A 15-year-old girl with a right leg mass. Clin Imaging 1995;19:65-68

Kramer J, Recht M, Deely DM, et al: MR appearance of idiopathic synovial osteochondromatosis. J Comput Assist Tomogr 1993;17:772-776

Lamon JM, Trojak JE, Abbott MA: Bone cysts in mucopolysaccharidosis I S (Scheie syndrome). Johns Hopkins Med J 1980;146:73-75

Lang IM, Hughes DG, Williamson JB, et al: MRI appearance of popliteal cysts in childhood. Pediatr Radiol 1997;27:130-132

Laxer RM, Cameron BJ, Chaisson D, et al: The camptodactyly-arthropathy-pericarditis syndrome: case report and literature review. Arthritis Rheum 1986;29:439-444

Lin J, Jacobson JA, Jamadar DA, Ellis JH: Pigmented villonodular synovitis and related lesions: the spectrum of imaging findings. AJR Am J Roentgenol 1999;172:191-197

Lindsley CB, Godfrey WA: Childhood sarcoidosis manifesting as juvenile rheumatoid arthritis. Pediatrics 1985;76:765-768

Llauger J, Monill JM, Palmer J, Clotet M: Synovial hemangioma of the knee: MRI findings in two cases. Skeletal Radiol 1995;24:579-581

Martin S, Hernandez L, Romero J, et al: Diagnostic imaging of lipoma arborescens. Skeletal Radiol 1998;27:325-329

Natowicz MR, Short MP, Wang Y, et al: Clinical and biochemical manifestations of hyaluronidase deficiency. N Engl J Med 1996;335:1029-1033

Norman A, Steiner GC: Bone erosion in synovial chondromatosis. Radiology 1986;161:749-752

North AF, Fink CW, Gibson WM, et al: Sarcoid arthritis in children. Am J Med 1970;48:449-455

Ozonoff MB: Pediatric Orthopedic Radiology. Philadelphia, WB Saunders, 1992

Poznanski AK: Radiological approaches to pediatric joint disease. J Rheumatol Suppl 1992;33:78-93

Resnick D, Niwayama G: Diagnosis of Bone and Joint Disorders. Philadelphia, WB Saunders, 1995

Resnick D, Oliphant M: Hemophilia-like arthropathy of the knee associated with cutaneous and synovial hemangiomas: report of 3 cases and review of the literature. Radiology 1975;114:323-326

Ryu KN, Jaovisidha S, Schweitzer M, et al: MR imaging of lipoma arborescens of the knee joint. AJR Am J Roentgenol 1996; 167:1229-1232

Sahn EE, Hampton MT, Garen PD, et al: Preschool sarcoidosis masquerading as juvenile rheumatoid arthritis: two case reports and a review of the literature. Pediatr Dermatol 1990;7:208-213

Sarigol SS, Hay MH, Wyllie R: Sarcoidosis in preschool children with hepatic involvement mimicking juvenile rheumatoid arthritis. J Pediatr Gastroenterol Nutr 1999;28:510-512

Spranger J, Albert C, Schilling F, et al: Progressive pseudorheumatoid arthritis of childhood (PPAC): a hereditary disorder simulating rheumatoid arthritis. Eur J Pediatr 1983;140:34-40

Sundaram M, Chalk D, Merenda J, et al: Case report 563: pigmented villonodular synovitis (PVNS) of knee. Skeletal Radiol 1989; 18:463-465

Tabyi H, Lachman RS: Radiology of Syndromes, Metabolic Disorders and Skeletal Dysplasias. St. Louis, Mosby–Year Book, 1996

Torbiak RP, Dent PB, Cockshott WP: NOMID—a neonatal syndrome of multisystem inflammation. Skeletal Radiol 1989;18:359-364

Vedantam R, Strecker W, Schoenecker P, Salinas-Madrigal L: Polyarticular pigmented villonodular synovitis in a child. Clin Orthop 1998;348:208-211

Wagner S, Bennek J, Grafe G, et al: Chondromatosis of the ankle joint (Reichel syndrome). Pediatr Surg Int 1999;15:437-439

Walls J, Nogi J: Multifocal pigmented villonodular synovitis in a child. J Pediatr Orthop 1985;5:229-231

Wihlborg CE, Babyn PS, Schneider R: The association between Turner's syndrome and juvenile rheumatoid arthritis. Pediatr Radiol 1999;29:676-681

Wong K, Sallomi D, Janzen DL, et al: Monoarticular synovial lesions: radiologic pictorial essay with pathologic illustration. Clin Radiol 1999;54:273-284

Yarbrough R, Gross R. Chondrolysis: An Update. J Pediatri Orthop 2005;25: 702-704

180

Developmental Dysplasia of the Hip

MICHAEL A. DIPIETRO and H. THEODORE HARCKE

OVERVIEW

Developmental dysplasia of the hip (DDH) is a spectrum of instability, displacement, and deformity that involves the femoral head and its acetabulum. It can occur before or after birth and can change (progress or improve) during and beyond the neonatal period. DDH thus includes but is not limited to congenital dislocation of the hip (CDH). The term *CDH* has been replaced with the more inclusive and appropriate term *DDH*.

> DDH occurs before or after birth and can change (progress or improve) during and beyond the neonatal period. DDH thus includes but is not limited to congenital dislocation of the hip.

The spectrum of DDH extends from slight hip laxity to irreducible frank hip dislocation. The description of DDH relates to the appearance of the acetabulum and the position of the femoral head relative to the acetabulum during dynamic manipulation of the leg. Thus, the spectrum of findings in DDH includes shallow immature acetabulum, subluxatable hip, subluxated relocatable hip, subluxated irreducible hip, dislocatable hip, dislocated reducible hip, and dislocated irreducible hip. These situations can exist with various degrees of acetabular immaturity or acetabular dysplasia. In general, dislocatable or dislocated hips exhibit the most severe acetabular dysplasia. However, acetabular dysplasia can exist with an unstable hip or with a stable hip. Because the severity of DDH varies, when comparing studies in the medical literature, one should be mindful of the inclusion criteria. Variable inclusion criteria limit comparison of studies in terms of frequency, detection, natural history, treatment, and outcomes of DDH.

At the mildest end of the DDH spectrum is newborn hip laxity, which resolves spontaneously by 6 to 8 weeks of age with normal hip development and with no need for intervention. Such transient laxity can be considered a normal developmental physiologic event. Nevertheless, cases of transient neonatal hip laxity are sometimes included in statistics on the frequency of DDH.

> Transient laxity of the hip in a newborn is a normal developmental physiologic event.

CAUSES, RISK FACTORS, AND ASSOCIATIONS

In utero conditions, such as fetal position and posture, maternal hormonal milieu, and genetic factors can predispose to hip laxity, acetabular underdevelopment, and hip subluxation or dislocation. Most dislocations actually occur after birth. Cultural practices influence the incidence of DDH. Swaddling of infants with the hips extended and adducted likely contributes to the greater incidence of DDH among Native Americans. Swaddling probably aggravates and accentuates the manifestation of DDH in cases where a genetic predisposition for hip laxity already exists.

Joint laxity, femoral head position, and acetabular development are interrelated, and all are affected by DDH. A normal femoral head position stimulates normal acetabular development. A normal acetabulum contains the femoral head and allows it to develop normally. If the acetabulum is shallow and cannot adequately contain the femoral head, the femoral head will be allowed to roam; this then stretches ligaments. If the acetabulum starts out as adequate but the ligaments are lax, excess motion leads to acetabular deterioration and dysplasia.

The onset of DDH occurs in late gestation (36+ weeks) or during the immediate postnatal period in 98% of cases. The structural support of the femoral head is weakest during this time because the cartilaginous femoral head has grown faster than the acetabulum. The femoral head is therefore incompletely covered. The hip is potentially unstable. However, frank dislocation at birth is unusual.

Acetabular and femoral head anatomy may be very abnormal in severe cases of DDH. Autopsies in babies at between 27 and 44 weeks' gestation with dislocatable hips reveal acetabular cartilage that is very different from that in normal hips. The labrum is everted and is stretched posteriorly and superiorly by the dislocated femoral head. Partial dislocation and subluxation correlate with restraint of the femur by the joint capsule and the ligamentum teres, both of which are stretched in hips with greater instability or dislocation. In the most severe cases, the labrum is inverted (folded down and in) between the femoral head and the acetabulum, preventing reduction, the acetabulum is shallow, and the femoral head is flattened and small.

In clinical studies, left DDH exceeds right DDH (55% left, 20% right, 25% bilateral). The left predilection may be the result of the more common vertex left posterior

TABLE 180-1
Risk Factors for Developmental Dysplasia of the Hip (DDH)
Breech delivery
Family history of DDH
First born
Female
Oligohydramnios
Foot deformities (clubfoot, metatarsus adductus)
Torticollis from fibromatosis colli
Skull-molding deformities

fetal lie. In this position, the fetal left hip is against the maternal spine, thereby restricting abduction.

> **DDH is more common on the left.**

DDH is a perinatal phenomenon in which physiologic and mechanical factors lead to deformity of otherwise normal anatomy. Dunn theorized that persistent gentle mechanical forces in utero can lead to deformations that include DDH. These deformations usually occur late in gestation because of the enlarging fetus and the relatively decreasing amniotic fluid volume. Mechanical stresses are further accentuated by breech presentation and oligohydramnios. Fetal constraint and compression from oligohydramnios, a tight uterus and taut maternal abdomen associated with primigravida, and breech presentation can restrict leg movement, predisposing to DDH. A total of 30% to 50% of DDH cases are associated with breech presentation.

In utero fetal constraint can also produce other congenital musculoskeletal deformities, including clubfoot, metatarsus adductus, torticollis from fibromatosis colli, and molding deformity of the skull, any of which might indicate a higher likelihood of DDH. Maternal hormones and genetics contribute to hip joint laxity. DDH is four to six times more common in girls than in boys. DDH is also more common when a parent or a sibling has had DDH. Table 180-1 summarizes the risk factors for DDH.

PRESENTATION AND PHYSICAL EXAMINATION

Physical signs that suggest DDH and indicate a need for diagnostic imaging include limited or asymmetric range of hip motion (usually limited abduction), asymmetric thigh or inguinal skin folds, and discrepancy of leg lengths. Missed cases can manifest later in childhood or adolescence with limp, abnormal gait, "short" leg, pain, ischemic necrosis of the femoral head, or osteoarthritis.

The newborn and infant screening physical examination for DDH includes the Ortolani and Barlow maneuvers. The Ortolani maneuver (1937) is positive in the dislocatable or dislocated but reducible hip and has been reported as being positive in 1.3 to 2.8 of 1000 births. The positive Ortolani "clunk" occurs when the dislocated hip reduces with abduction (Fig. 180-1). Therefore, this test will be falsely negative when the hip is dislocated but muscle contraction or acetabular soft tissues prevent

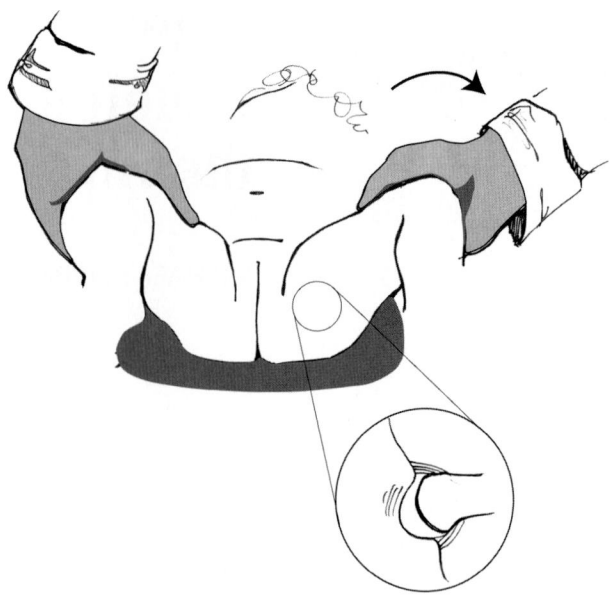

FIGURE 180-1. The Ortolani maneuver consists of pushing the femur, which is followed by abduction. The *inset* shows the femoral head reducing with abduction. Reduction of the dislocated femoral head produces the positive "clunk." Sonography can be performed during this maneuver as part of the dynamic examination.

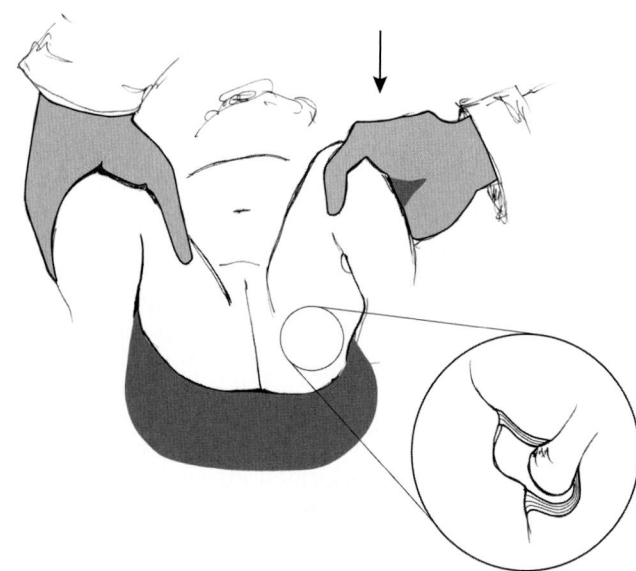

FIGURE 180-2. The Barlow maneuver consists of pulling and pushing the flexed femur, as with a piston. The *inset* shows posterolateral displacement with pushing *(arrow)* and corresponds to the transverse sonographic view. Sonography can be performed during this maneuver as part of the dynamic examination.

reduction. The Barlow maneuver (1962) for hip instability (laxity, subluxatablity, dislocatability) has been reported as positive in 7 to 25 of 1000 live births. It is performed by pulling and then pushing posteriorly (similar to a piston) on the flexed and adducted hip (Fig. 180-2). When posterior movement of the hip is excessive, the Barlow test is positive for hip laxity. Older infants and children (or newborns with teratologic hip dislocations) may have developed hip contractures that limit hip movement; therefore, they may exhibit false-negative Barlow and Ortolani maneuvers.

Many babies are referred for DDH evaluation because of high-pitched, palpable "hip clicks" that are distinct from positive Ortolani clunks. These clicks may result from stretching of the joint capsule or tendons, but they are also encountered in normal hips.

The incidence of overt infant hip dislocation is 1.5 to 1.7 per 1000 in Caucasians. If newborn hip subluxation and instability are included, the incidence of DDH may be as high as 10 infants per 1000 live births. The tendency for improvement and resolution over the first year reduces the prevalence of DDH from 1.5% to approximately 0.15%. In all, 58% of clinically unstable hips spontaneously resolved by 1 month of age and 80% by 2 months. Overall, 80% to 90% of clinically unstable hips spontaneously improve without treatment. Up to 10% of dysplastic hips are still dysplastic at 1 year of age. Spontaneous resolution on physical examination is unlikely if it has not occurred by age 2 months.

Hips with persistent instability can advance to frank subluxation or dislocation. The goal of physical examination and imaging is to identify those cases. Treatment aims to restore femoral-acetabular contact and foster capsular tightening, thereby preventing further subluxation and dislocation with subsequent irreversible sequelae.

PATHOGENESIS

Maternal estrogens remain at high levels in the newborn and may promote joint laxity with a relatively loose and elastic hip joint capsule. This laxity can lead to migration or displacement of the femoral head, usually superiorly, laterally, and posteriorly. The acetabulum, without its femoral head, does not form normally; it becomes dysplastic and remains shallow, further preventing reduction of the femoral head. If this process is not corrected, muscles eventually tighten and form contractures that limit movement of the hip. Fibrofatty tissue ("pulvinar") in the medial aspect of the acetabulum will thicken. The cartilaginous acetabular roof thickens and may invert medial to the femoral head ("labral inversion"). The ligamentum teres lengthens and thickens. All of these adaptive processes further impede or prevent reduction of the displaced femoral head. In addition, a contracted iliopsoas tendon that extends across the stretched joint capsule may constrict the capsule's midportion, creating an "hourglass" deformity that further prevents femoral head reduction.

TERATOLOGIC HIP DYSPLASIA

In most cases of newborn DDH, the hips are not actually dislocated, and osseous acetabular adaptive changes have not yet developed. In contrast, newborns with an underlying neuromuscular disorder, myelomeningocele, arthrogryposis, or caudal regression syndrome can have dislocated hips with advanced pelvic and femoral head changes at birth. These infants with teratologic hip dysplasia have a worse prognosis than those with DDH. Because this process occurs early in gestation, these "teratologic" dislocations are *not* considered part of the DDH spectrum. Teratologic hips are typically fixed dislocations. Acetabular dysplasia and pseudoacetabulum formation may already be apparent at birth, similar to unrecognized or inadequately treated DDH in the older infant.

> Teratologic DDH is not considered part of the DDH spectrum. Infants with teratologic hip dislocation may have advanced changes at birth.

LATE DDH

The term "late DDH" is confusing. It is often used to indicate DDH that is missed or ignored in early infancy and is diagnosed later, anywhere from 3 to 6 months of age until the time the child is walking. The term is not applied to children with neuromuscular disorders, including cerebral palsy, in whom the hips become progressively abnormal over time with displacement (subluxation or dislocation) and with or without acetabular dysplasia.

Also reported are rare cases in which the hips were normal on early physical examination or sonography and yet were abnormal at 6 months of age or later. Affected children seem to have acetabular deficiency, not instability. Such cases may also be referred to as "late DDH." Late-onset DDH may have a genetic basis.

RADIOGRAPHY

Since the advent of hip sonography, radiographs are no longer routinely obtained to detect DDH in neonates and very young infants. However, DDH should be recognized when present, including when incidental on abdominal, pelvic, or spinal radiographs. An anteroposterior (AP) radiograph of the hips in neutral position is preferred in the search for DDH. A view with the hips abducted in the frog lateral position can also be obtained to determine whether a subluxated or dislocated hip reduces. Unless reducibility is the specific question, the frog lateral view should function only as an adjunct to the neutral view. A subluxatable or dislocatable hip may reduce with abduction and may be missed if only a frog lateral view is obtained. A special stress view (Andren–von Rosen view) with internal rotation and 45 degree abduction of the femora was formerly used to detect DDH and laxity, but it is now seldom performed.

> A subluxatable or dislocatable hip may reduce with abduction and may be missed if only an abduction view is obtained.

The ossific nucleus of the femoral head is seen on radiographs at between 2 and 8 months of age. Ossification occurs earlier in girls than in boys. The ossific nucleus is visible on sonography several weeks before it is visible radiographically. The degree of ossification of the femoral head varies slightly with respect to age. Some slight variation from side to side may be seen in normal

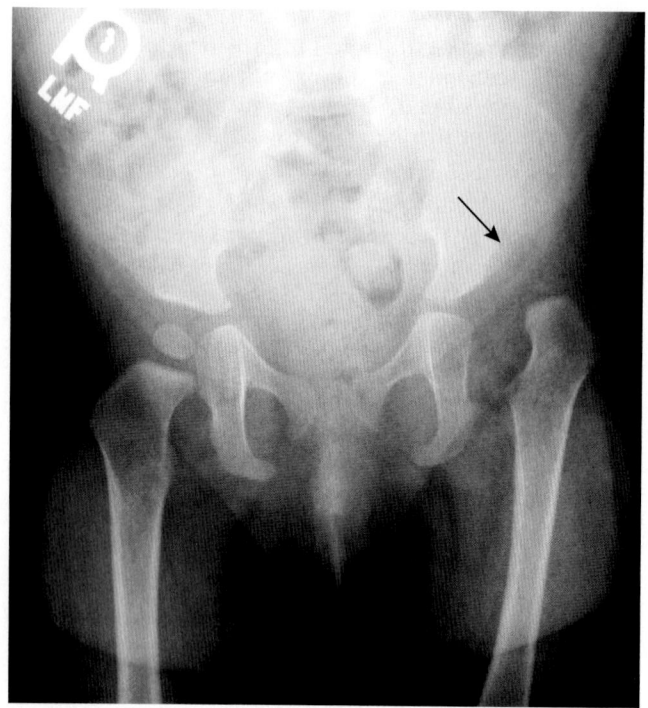

A

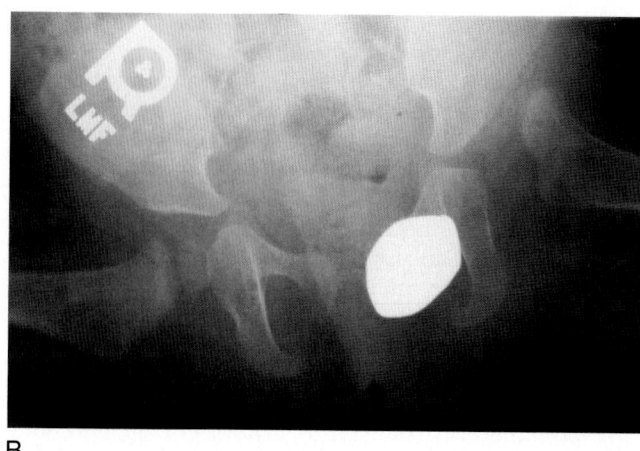

B

FIGURE 180-3. In a 10-month-old girl, the anteroposterior (AP) view **(A)** shows a dislocated left hip, left acetabular dysplasia, and pseudoacetabulum *(arrow)*. The right hip is normal. **B,** Abduction does not reduce the dislocated left hip.

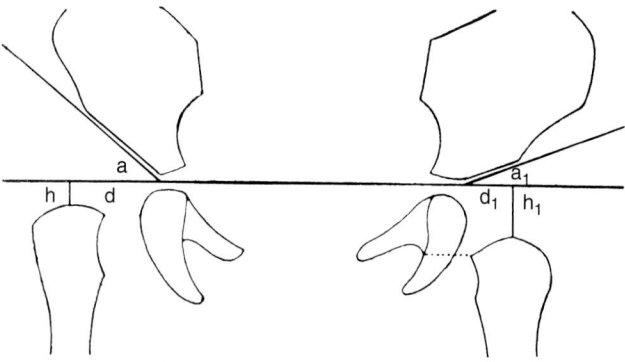

FIGURE 180-4. Schematic of an anteroposterior (AP) pelvis radiograph in a neonate or a young infant shows normal left hip and right developmental dysplasia of the hip (DDH). The increased right acetabular angle is formed by the intersection of the Hilgenreiner line (horizontal line across both triradiate cartilages) and the oblique line along the steep right acetabular roof. The right femur is also shown to be more lateral and more superior than its normal left counterpart. a, acetabular angle; h, vertical distance from the Hilgenreiner line to the femoral metaphysis; d, distance between intersection of acetabular roof lines and h-lines measuring lateral displacement of the femur. a_1, h_1, and d_1,: corresponding measurements in normal left hip.

infants. With DDH, femoral head ossification is usually delayed in the affected hip as compared with the normal side (Fig. 180-3). With maturation, the size of the femoral head ossific nucleus obscures medial acetabular sonographic landmarks, limiting the usefulness of sonography for DDH in older infants. Sonography of the hips is thus of limited value in the latter half of the first year of life. By 6 months of age, ossification of the femoral head allows better radiographic assessment of DDH.

The contour of the acetabulum can be assessed on radiographs. The normal acetabulum has a round, cup-like configuration, whereas the abnormal acetabulum is shallow with a steep roof. The acetabular angle is a measure of the steepness of the osseous acetabular roof relative to the horizontal line drawn through the right and left triradiate cartilages (the Hilgenreiner line) (Fig. 180-4). The normal acetabular angle is less than 30 degrees in newborns and is approximately 22 degrees at 1 year of age. Improper positioning of the infant for the pelvic radiograph (obliquity or tilt) can falsely make an acetabular roof appear steep and the acetabulum appear shallow.

In addition to the acetabular steep roof in DDH, the lateral edge of the ossified dysplastic acetabular roof is blunt or rounded. Acetabular dysplasia and pseudoacetabulum formation (Fig. 180-5) may occur after the neonatal period.

The lines of Hilgenreiner, Perkins, and Shenton serve as guides to recognizing the subluxated or dislocated hip, especially when the femoral head is unossified. The Hilgenreiner line was introduced previously. The Perkins line is drawn vertically, perpendicular to the Hilgenreiner line, from the ossified lateral rim of the acetabular roof. The femoral head should lie in the inferior medial quadrant produced by the intersection of these two lines. The Shenton line is a lateral continuation of the curvature of the obturator foramen that should continue smoothly along the medial aspect of the femoral neck to the lesser trochanter. With subluxation, the Shenton line is not smoothly continuous. With experience, the position of the unossified femoral head relative to the femoral neck can be inferred, and it is possible to assess whether the femoral head is centered within or displaced from the acetabulum (Fig. 180-6).

An AP radiograph with the hips in neutral position performed at about 6 months of age can be useful for

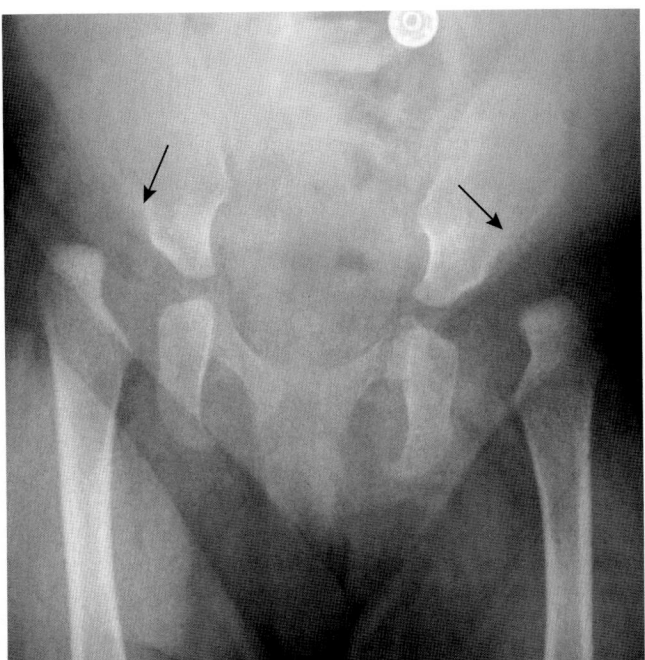

FIGURE 180-5. Neutral anteroposterior (AP) view of a 3-month-old girl shows bilateral shallow acetabula, dislocated hips, and early pseudoacetabulum formation *(arrows).*

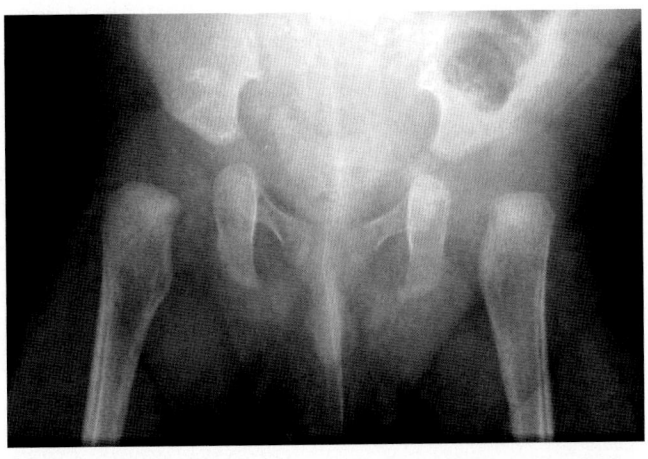

A

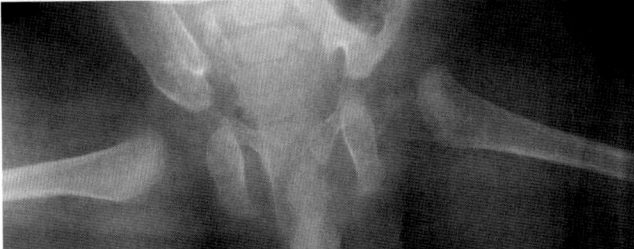

B

FIGURE 180-6. A 4-month-old girl with clubfeet. **A,** Neutral anteroposterior (AP) view shows dislocation on the left with a dysplastic left acetabulum. The right hip is slightly abnormal. **B,** The left hip does not relocate with abduction.

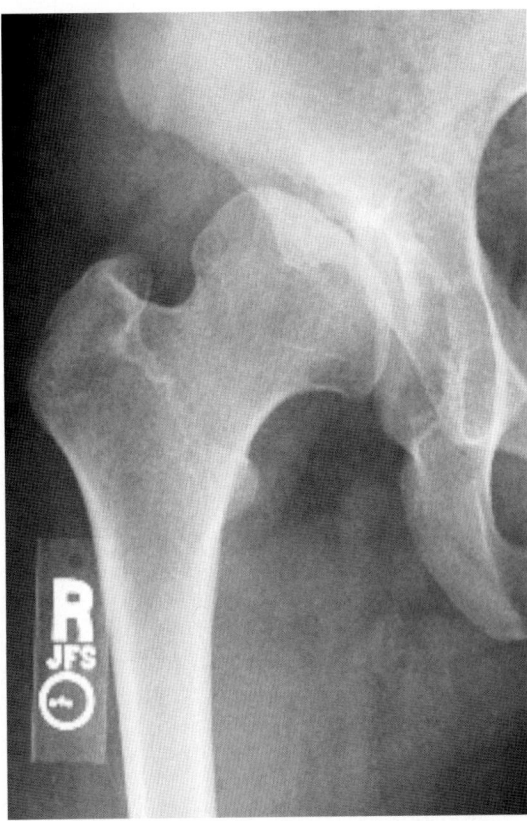

FIGURE 180-7. Anteroposterior (AP) radiograph with hips extended in a 15-year-old-girl refugee with untreated developmental dysplasia of the hip (DDH) shows dysplastic acetabulum, subluxation, and femoral head deformity.

verifying normal hip development in any infant previously evaluated for DDH or about whom the question of DDH has been raised.

> **An AP view of the hip can be obtained at 6 months of age to confirm normalcy in infants previously evaluated for DDH.**

Poor osseous coverage of the femoral head may be due to a shallow dysplastic acetabulum, lateral subluxation of the femur, or both (Fig. 180-7). In the older child, the amount of hip subluxation (displacement from the acetabulum) can be quantified in two ways: as the percentage of the femoral head with osseous acetabular roof coverage, or by the center–edge (CE) angle. A vertical straight line from the lateral edge of the ossified acetabular roof (the Perkins line) indicates what percentage of the femoral head is covered by the osseous acetabular roof (Fig. 180-8). The CE angle is formed at the center of the femoral head between a vertical line through the center and another line from the center to the lateral margin of the osseous acetabular roof (see Fig. 180-8). The normal angle is greater than 20 degrees, and it decreases with lateral subluxation of the femoral head. In the teenager, the CE angle should be greater than 26 to 30 degrees.

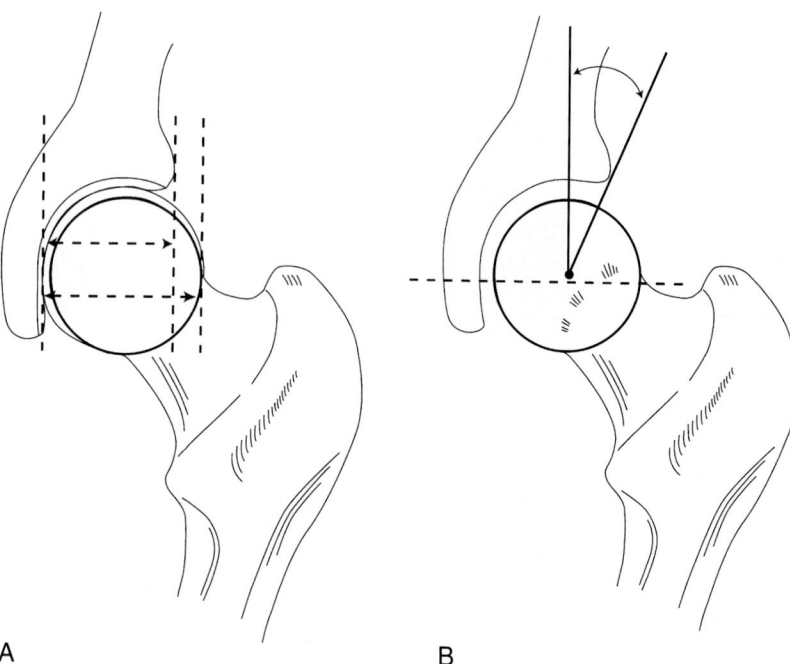

A   B

FIGURE 180-8. Osseous coverage of the femoral head can be described as the percentage of the femoral head that is covered by its osseous acetabular roof (**A**) or by the center-edge angle (**B**).

SONOGRAPHY

Sonography of the infant hip has evolved to a combination of the static method of Graf, which emphasizes acetabular morphology, and the dynamic method of Harcke, which focuses on position and stability of the femoral head within the acetabulum. Although many pediatric radiologists had combined the two methods and were already performing a combined static and dynamic study for DDH, Drs. Harcke and Graf formally proposed a minimum standard examination that incorporates morphologic and dynamic elements. The American College of Radiology (ACR) published a Hip Sonography Standard in 1998 that was modeled on this proposal. The American Institute of Ultrasound in Medicine (AIUM) and the ACR now have a joint standard that reflects this technique. The standard examination assesses the position of the femoral head relative to its acetabulum at rest and with stress and assesses the development of the acetabulum.

> A minimum standard ultrasound examination for DDH incorporates morphologic and dynamic elements of assessment.

Sonography assesses three essential features of the infant hip with respect to DDH: position, stability, and morphology. When the hip joint is regarded as a "ball in socket" this can be formulated as three questions: (1) "Is the ball in the socket?" (i.e., What is the position of the femoral head relative to the acetabulum?); (2) "Does the ball stay in the socket?" (i.e., What is the stability of the femoral head with stress maneuvers?); and (3) "Is the socket well formed?" (i.e., Is the morphology of the acetabulum adequate to cover and contain the femoral head?). The coronal view is used to assess acetabular

development and maturity, as well as acetabular coverage of the femoral head. The transverse view is used to assess laxity with stress maneuvers. Optional stress views can also be obtained in the coronal plane.

Sonography for DDH is performed through a lateral approach. A linear array transducer with the highest frequency that allows adequate penetration—usually between 7 MHz and 10 MHz—is used. In selected cases, a transducer frequency as low as 5 MHz or as high as 15MHz may be selected.

> For teaching purposes, coronal sonographic planes may be thought of as analogous to a frontal radiograph, and the transverse sonographic plane as analogous to an axial computed tomography (CT) image.

Graf Method

To ensure consistency, a standard for the coronal plane has been defined by Graf that specifies three critical sonographic landmarks: (1) the iliac line—the reflection of echoes from the ilium superior to the acetabulum (on equipment formatted with the transducer at the top of the image, the iliac line should appear horizontal on the screen); (2) the junction of the osseous acetabular roof of the ilium and the triradiate cartilage in the deepest medial aspect of the acetabulum; and, (3) the echogenic lateral tip of the cartilaginous acetabular roof—the labrum (Fig. 180-9). Graf uses these anatomic landmarks as the basis for measuring alpha and beta angles. The Graf alpha angle is formed by the intersection of a line along the lateral margin of the ilium with a line from the lower medial iliac margin in the acetabular fossa to the lateral edge of the osseous acetabular roof, all in the standard coronal plane.

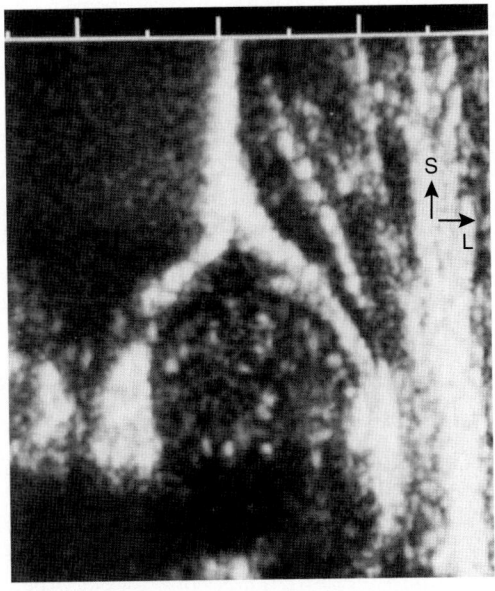 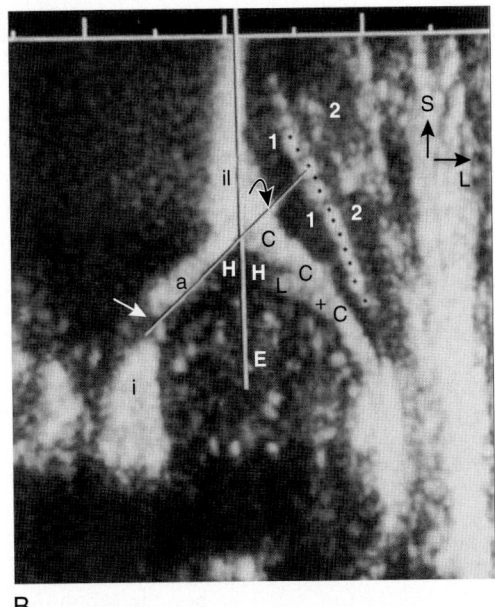

A   B

FIGURE 180-9. Coronal views of the left hip displayed vertically without **(A)** and with **(B)** labels. Black straight arrows denote superior (S) and lateral (L) directions. The unossified femoral head epiphysis (E) is well seated within the acetabulum beneath its ossified roof (a). The iliac line when extended from the lateral iliac margin (il) shows the degree of femoral head coverage by its osseous acetabular roof. More laterally, the femoral head is covered by the unossified roof, composed of hyaline cartilage (H), which will later ossify. Echogenic fibrocartilage at the lateral tip of the acetabular roof is the labrum (L), although the entire cartilaginous roof (H and L) is often referred to as "labrum." Ischium (i), triradiate cartilage *(white straight arrow)*, and joint capsule (C) are shown. The gluteus minimus (1) and the gluteus medius (2) are separated by the intermuscular septum *(dots)*. The Graf alpha angle *(black curved arrow)*, a measure of the steepness of the acetabular roof, is formed by the intersection of the iliac line (il) and a line along the osseous acetabular roof (a). The Graf beta angle (not shown), a measure of the superior deviation of the cartilaginous roof, would be drawn between the lateral aspect of the labrum (+) and the intersection of the iliac and osseous acetabular roof lines. (Reproduced from DiPietro MA, Harcke T: Pediatric musculoskeletal and spinal sonography. *In* van Holsbeeck MT, Introcaso JH (eds): Musculoskeletal Ultrasound, 2nd ed. Philadelphia, Pennsylvania, Mosby, 2001:277-323.)

The acetabular angle can be measured by radiograph or by sonography. As the steepness of the acetabular roof increases, the radiographic acetabular angle increases, and the sonographic Graf alpha angle decreases. Measured angles are roughly (but not precisely) complementary, with the radiographic acetabular angle less than 30 degrees considered normal and the sonographic acetabular angle (Graf alpha angle) greater than 60 degrees considered normal.

Graf also described a beta angle, which is a measurement of the elevation of the cartilaginous acetabular labrum within the standard coronal plane. The labrum is elevated (and the beta angle is increased) by the femoral head when it is displaced laterally and superiorly from a shallow acetabulum. When hips are categorized by the Graf classification, alpha and beta angles are measured and reported (Table 180-2). Alternatively, acetabular development can be judged by the amount of coverage of the femoral head provided by the bony acetabulum. This is determined on sonography as the percentage of the femoral head diameter that is covered by the osseous acetabular roof. Percentage coverage reflects acetabular depth. Coverage is not good if the acetabulum is too shallow to adequately contain the femoral head. At least 50% of the femoral head should be covered by the osseous acetabular roof on the coronal view. Femoral head coverage on sonography has been compared with radiographic acetabular angles. Hips with greater than 58% osseous coverage had normal radiographic aceta-

bular angles, and hips with less than 33% osseous coverage had dysplastic acetabula. Hips with osseous acetabular roof coverage of between 33% and 58% had variable acetabular angles with poor correlation of radiographic and sonographic measurements.

The alpha and beta angle measurements of Graf allow categorization into four basic hip types; additional subtypes and subdivisions are based on small angle changes

Type I morphology is normal with a deep acetabulum and with the femoral head completely covered (Fig. 180-10). The alpha angle is greater than 60 degrees. No treatment is indicated.

Type II morphology has a slightly decreased alpha angle (i.e., steeper osseous acetabular roof) and is considered immature if younger than 3 months of age and slightly dysplastic when older (Fig. 180-11). Subtypes IIa, IIb, IIc, and D are described, but clinical follow-up is recommended for all. Most will become normal (type I) by 3 months of age. In all, 1% to 2% of type II hips will not mature to normal and will require treatment.

Type III morphology involves dislocation with a shallow acetabulum (Graf alpha angle less than 43 degrees). Treatment is required.

Type IV morphology involves dislocation with a very shallow acetabulum and an interposed labrum. Treatment is required.

With mild, clinically undetectable DDH, a Graf type IIa hip has been described by Harcke and Grissom as

TABLE 180-2

Simplified Synopsis of Graf Sonographic Hip Types

Type	Description	Alpha Angle (degrees)	Beta Angle (degrees)	Comment
I	Normal	>60		Should not dislocate in the absence of a neuromuscular imbalance with altered biomechanics
IIa	Physiologic immature *(<3 mo)*	50-59		
IIb	Delayed ossification *(>3 mo)*	50-59		
IIc	Very deficient bony acetabulum but femoral head still concentric	43-49	<77	At this stage, the beta angle becomes important.
D	Femoral head *subluxed*	43-49	>77	Increased beta angle signifies an evaluated, everted labrum and subluxation.
III	*Dislocated*	<43	>77	
IV	*Severe* dysplasia/dislocation	*Not measurable*; flat, shallow, bony acetabulum		*Labrum inverted; interposed* between femoral head and ilium

Adapted from Donaldson JS: Pediatric musculoskeletal US. *In* Poznanski AK, Kirkpatrick JA Jr (eds): Diagnostic Categorical Course in Pediatric Radiology. Oak Brook, IL, Radiological Society of North America Publications, 1989:77-88; and Graf R: Guide to Sonography of the Infant Hip. New York, Thieme Medical Publishers, 1987.
Distinguishing feature of each type is in italics.

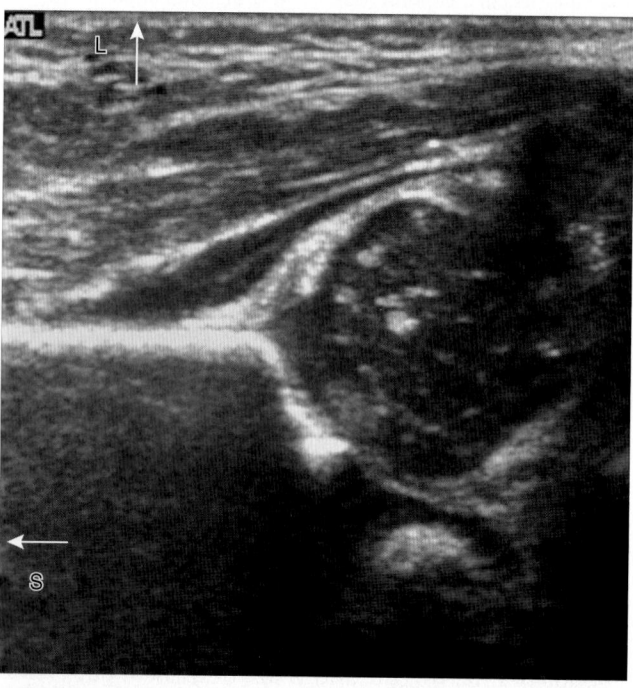

FIGURE 180-10. Normal sonogram in the standard coronal plane in a 1-week-old girl following breech delivery. *Arrows* denote lateral (L) and superior (S) directions.

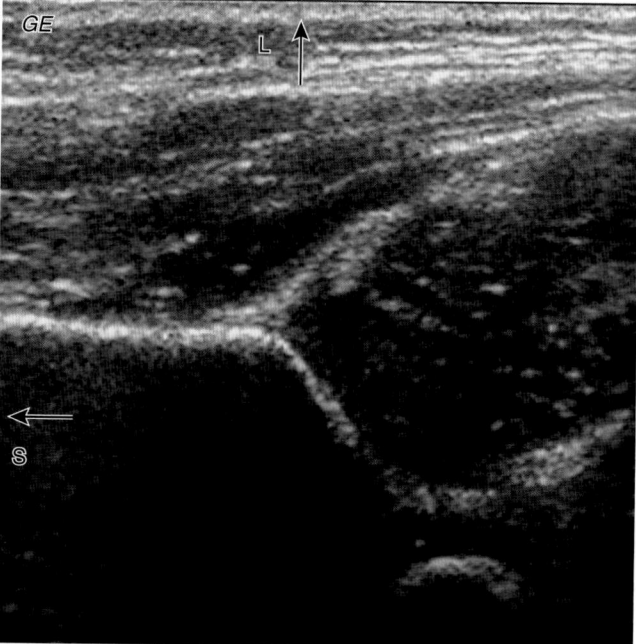

FIGURE 180-11. Sonogram of a 2-week-old girl in standard coronal plane shows a slightly steep immature acetabular roof. *Arrows* denote lateral (L) and superior (S) directions.

mild laxity, which can be regarded as physiologic (i.e., normal) with stress maneuvers in babies younger than 4 weeks of age. This milder end of the DDH spectrum with the potential to resolve spontaneously has implications for DDH diagnosis and management. Capsule laxity or mild acetabular immaturity or both, which may be seen on sonography at younger than 4 weeks of age, need not be treated but can be merely observed. A repeat sono-

gram is performed at 6 to 8 weeks of age to determine whether the hip has matured. If so, treatment is avoided.

Harcke Method

A two-view sonographic examination meets the ACR standard; however, a full four-view examination allows for a more confident diagnosis by less experienced sonographers and in difficult cases. The goals of a study are to determine the position and stability of the femoral head and to assess acetabular development. All views are obtained from the lateral aspect of the hip and are defined by transducer position relative to the position of the pelvis (coronal or transverse) and hip (neutral or flexion). "Neutral" refers to approximately 20 degrees of hip flexion (physiologic in the infant), and "flexion" refers to 90 degrees of hip flexion.

> **Standard components of the four-view examination:**
> - **Coronal neutral at rest**
> - **Coronal flexion at rest**
> - **Coronal flexion with adduction and stress (Barlow maneuver)**
> - **Transverse flexion at rest**
> - **Transverse flexion with passive abduction and adduction**
> - **Transverse flexion with adduction and stress (Barlow maneuver)**
> - **Transverse neutral at rest**

The coronal neutral view in the standard coronal plane is also the basis of the Graf technique. It allows assessment of acetabular morphology and maturity, the position of the femoral head within the acetabulum, and the degree of coverage provided by the osseous acetabular roof. The coronal flexion view is also attained in the standard coronal plane but with the hip flexed. In conjunction with the transverse flexion view, it provides a test of stability through gentle pulling and pushing of the leg, specifically pushing during adduction (Barlow maneuver), while any superior, lateral, and posterior displacement of the femoral head is observed (subluxation or dislocation).

REPORTING FOR THE HARCKE METHOD

If no acetabular coverage is noted, the hip is "dislocated." Femoral head coverage can change with position (flexion, extension, abduction, and adduction) and with stress maneuvers. Displacement of the femoral head with any acetabular coverage is "subluxation." Descriptive terminology of stability/instability as defined by the dynamic (Harcke) method includes the following:

Normal—normally seated femoral head within the acetabulum at rest, with motion, and with stress

Lax hip—normal position at rest; abnormal movement is noted with stress but femoral head remains intra-acetabular with stress

Subluxated hip—displaced laterally in the acetabulum at rest; instability present, but hip is not dislocatable with stress

Dislocatable hip—subluxated at rest, dislocates with stress

Dislocated hip—outside the acetabulum at rest; may or may not be reducible with traction and abduction

Acetabulum—normal, immature, or dysplastic

Pulvinar—noted if thickened

Acetabular roof cartilage—noted if echogenic

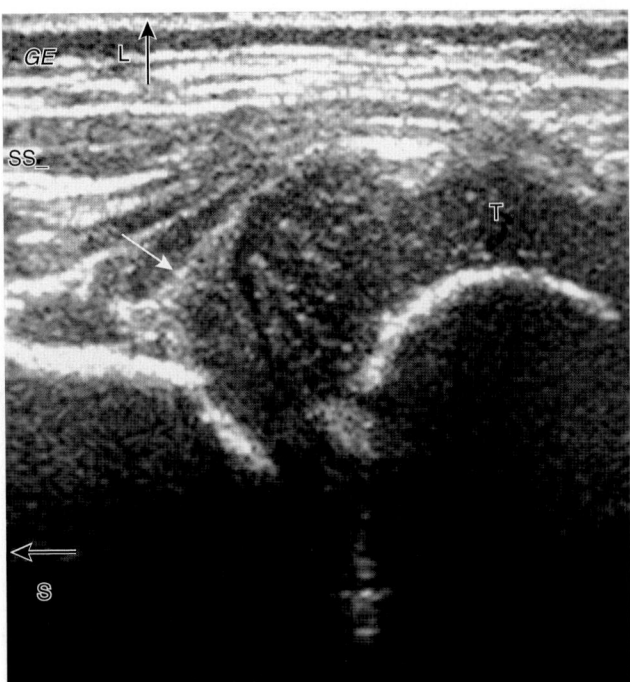

FIGURE 180-12. Coronal sonogram of a 3-month-old girl shows a steep osseous acetabular roof and marked subluxation. The displaced femoral head elevates the cartilaginous acetabular roof. The thick acetabular cartilage *(white arrow)* is slightly more echogenic than normal. *Black arrows* denote lateral (L) and superior (S) directions. T, greater trochanter.

In the standard coronal view, the acetabular roof should be concave, and its osseous portion should cover 50% or more of the femoral head if it is to be considered normal (see Fig. 180-10). The dysplastic acetabulum is shallow, and its acetabular roof is irregular and steep. Its cartilaginous roof is deflected superiorly, is thicker, and is more echogenic than normal (Fig. 180-12). In the frankly dislocated hip, the cartilaginous acetabular roof is often deformed, thickened, and echogenic, and the labrum is inverted into the acetabulum, which contains thick, echogenic fibrofatty tissue (pulvinar) (Figs. 180-13 and 180-14). The steepness of the acetabular roof and the elevation of the labrum can be described and can be measured as Graf's alpha and beta angles, respectively. The depth of the acetabulum, the position and amount of acetabular coverage of the femoral head, the thickness and echogenicity of the cartilaginous acetabular roof, and the appearance of the osseous lateral edge of the acetabular roof are all noted. The normal osseous lateral edge is sharp and angular, whereas the dysplastic edge is blunt, rounded, or flattened (see Fig. 180-13). The dysplastic acetabular roof cartilage is thicker and more echogenic than normal. Barlow and Ortolani maneuvers can be observed directly during sonography. Very lax hips might be apparent during adduction and abduction.

The dysplastic acetabular roof cartilage tends to be thicker and more echogenic than normal.

The most posterior aspect of the acetabulum is recognized on the coronal view with a small cartilage mound between the ilium and ischium (Fig. 180-15). Normally, no femoral head is present in this posterior portion of

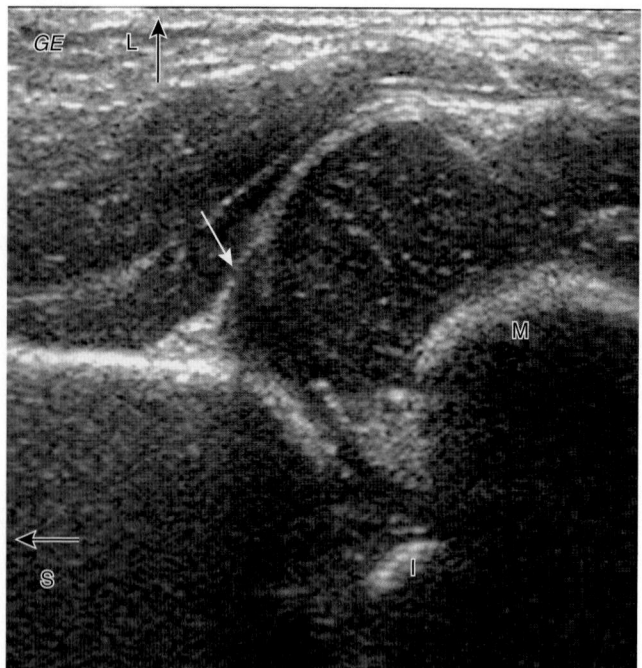

FIGURE 180-13. A 2-week-old girl with a hip "click" and marked laxity with stress maneuvers. Coronal sonogram shows marked subluxation. The acetabular cartilaginous roof is elevated by the displaced femoral head, yet the cartilaginous roof is not thick or echogenic *(white arrow)*. *Black arrows* denote lateral (L) and superior (S) directions. I, ischium; M, metaphysis.

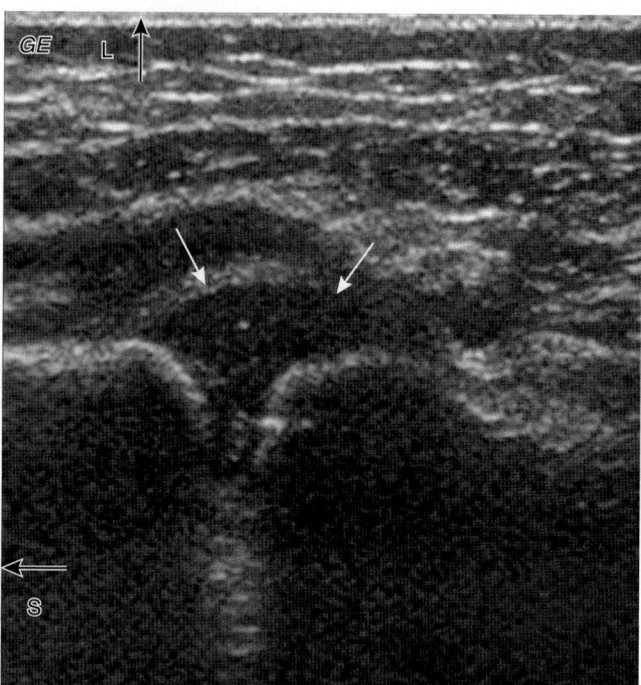

FIGURE 180-15. Normal sonographic coronal view of a breech 5-week-old girl shows the most posterior aspect of the acetabulum *(white arrows)*. No portion of the femoral head is visible this far posterior in normal hips. *Black arrows* denote lateral (L) and superior (S) directions.

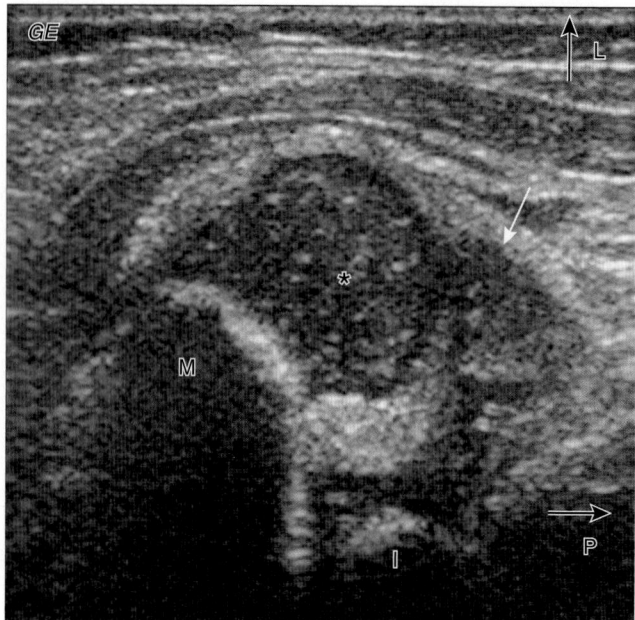

FIGURE 180-14. A 10-day-old girl. Transverse sonogram during adduction shows moderate posterolateral displacement of the femoral head *(asterisk)*. I, ischium; M, metaphysis; *white arrow*, labrum. Hyperechoic material between the femoral head and the ischium is fibrofatty pulvinar. *Black arrows* denote lateral (L) and posterior (P) directions.

the acetabulum. Visualization of the femoral head at this location indicates a subluxation or dislocation (Fig. 180-16). A markedly dislocated hip is identified by the femoral head lying along the ilium, posterior, lateral, and superior to the acetabulum (Fig. 180-17).

On the transverse view, the echogenic lines of the proximal ossified femoral metaphysis and of the ossified acetabulum form a "U" with abduction and a "V" with adduction (Fig. 180-18). Displacement from the acetabulum is seen as movement of the femoral head toward the transducer (lateral and posterior) (see Fig. 180-14). The unstable hip (subluxatable or dislocatable) is often partially intra-acetabular at rest. However, in some cases, the hip is subluxed or dislocated in its resting state, and sonography shows to what degree it can be reduced with abduction.

Sonographic Pitfalls

Pitfalls of hip sonography for DDH are often a result of the examiner's inexperience. A normal hip can be artifactually made to appear abnormal with a steep roof and a shallow acetabulum when the coronal view is obtained outside of the standard plane, or the transducer is rotated (Fig. 180-19). Less commonly, an abnormal acetabular roof can be made to appear horizontal (i.e., not steep, and therefore "normal") by scanning too far posteriorly. Errors of acetabular morphology are minimized with attention to presence in the standard coronal plane. The dynamic study may introduce some error caused by the variability of the stress applied and the degree of relaxation of the child. The transverse flexion view may be falsely abnormal if the transducer is lateral over the hip as opposed to posterolateral.

Another potential pitfall of sonography for DDH is seen in the infant with a varus deformity of the femoral neck (i.e., focal femoral deficiency) or with a hip con-

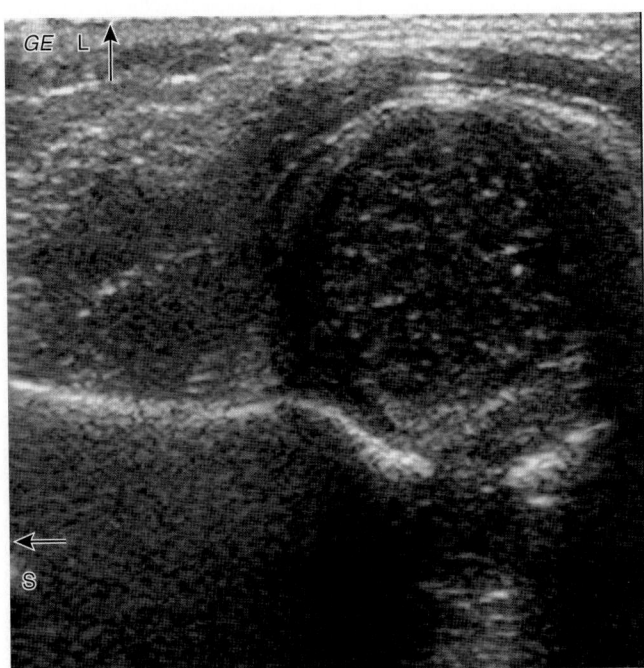

FIGURE 180-16. Same patient as Figure 180-13. The coronal sonogram in a very posterior plane (similar to the location in Fig. 180-15) shows much of the femoral head. It is markedly subluxed posteriorly because no portion of the femoral head is normally seen in this posterior plane. *Arrows* denote lateral (L) and superior (S) directions.

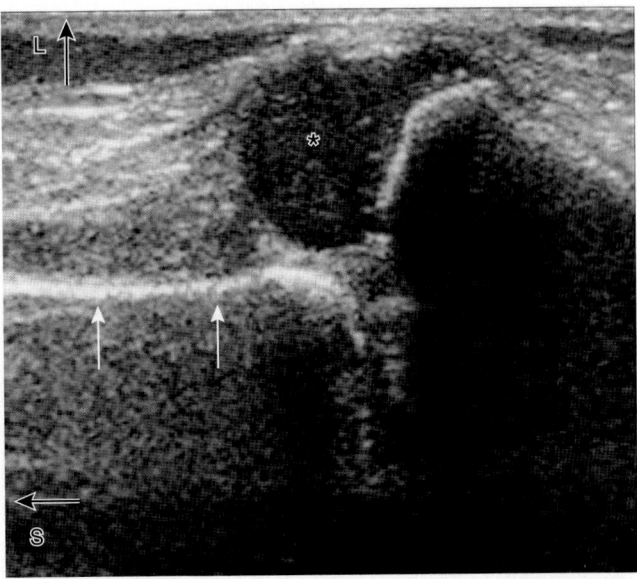

FIGURE 180-17. A 3-month-old girl with limited abduction of the hip on examination. Coronal ultrasonography shows marked dislocation of the femoral head *(asterisk)* lying along the posterolateral aspect of the ilium *(white arrows)*. *Black arrows* denote lateral (L) and superior (S) directions.

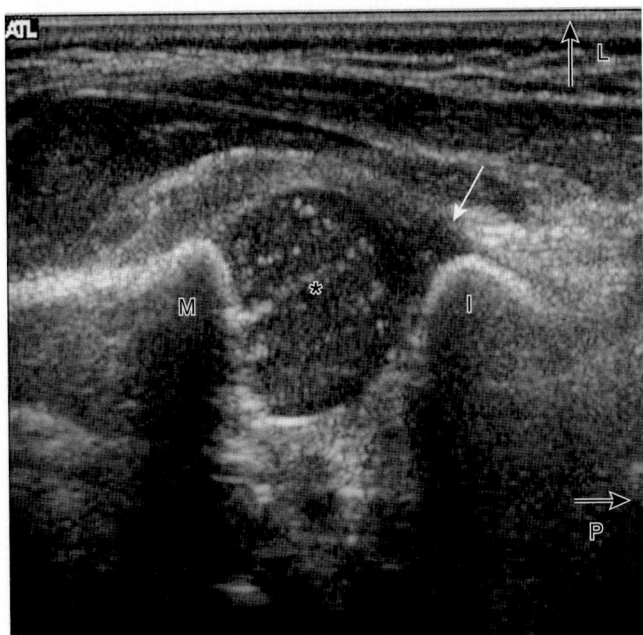

A

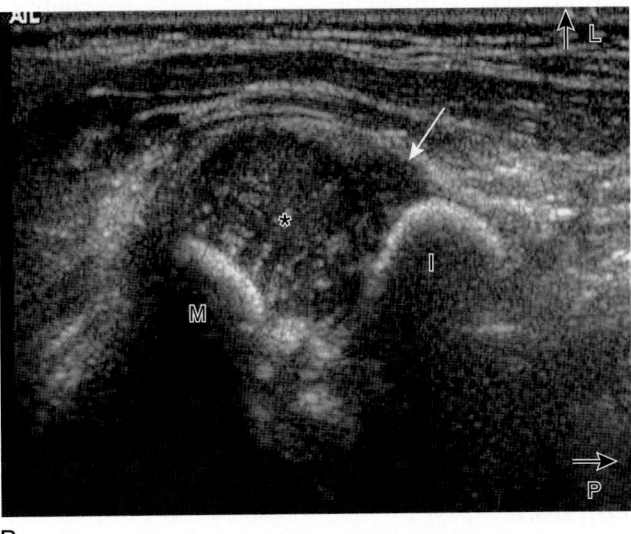

B

FIGURE 180-18. A 2-week-old girl. **A,** Normal transverse sonogram during abduction. The echogenic lines of the femoral metaphysis (M) and the ischial portion of the acetabulum (I) form a "U" configuration during abduction. **B,** Normal transverse sonogram during adduction. The echogenic lines of the femoral metaphysis and of the acetabulum form a "V" configuration during adduction. *Asterisk,* femoral head; *white arrow,* labrum. *Black arrows* denote lateral (L) and posterior (P) directions.

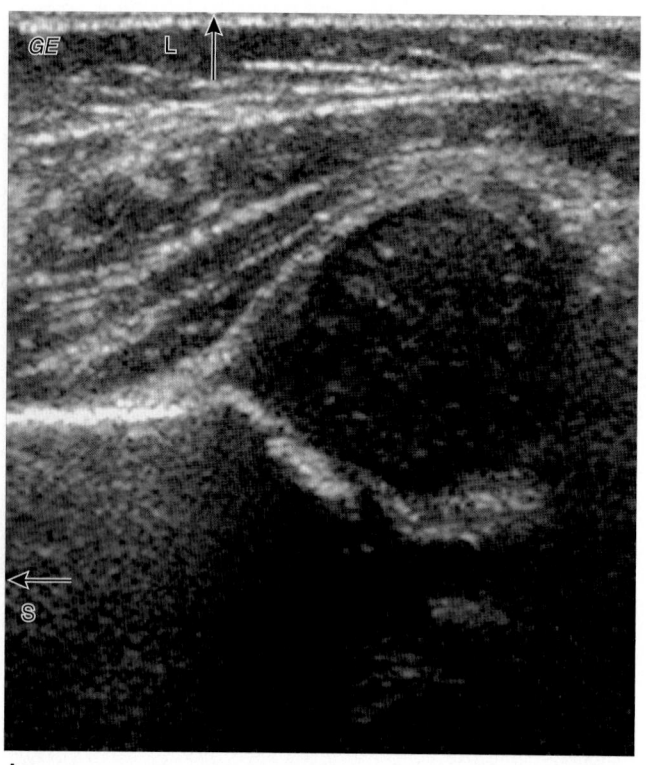
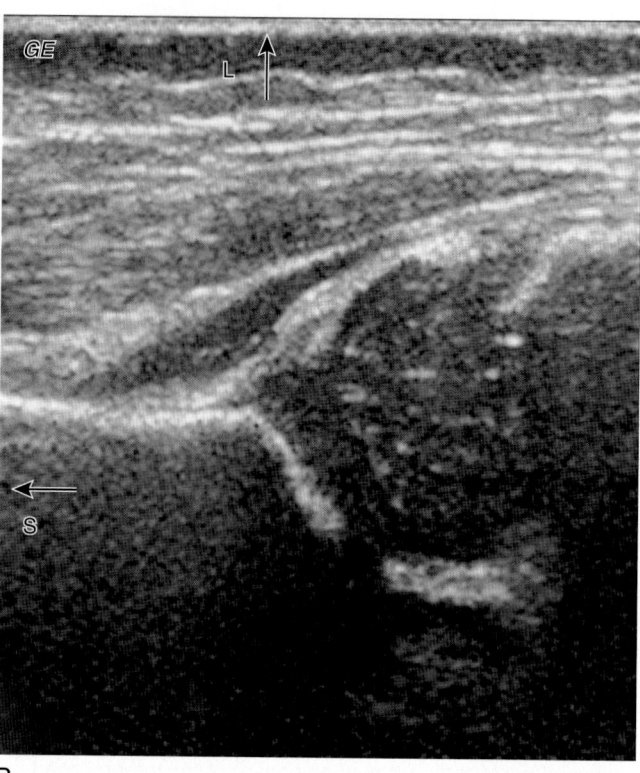

A

B

FIGURE 180-19. An 8-week-old girl. **A,** Coronal sonogram outside the standard plane appears to show a shallow acetabulum with a steep roof. **B,** Repeating the view in the standard coronal plane shows that it is normal. *Arrows* denote lateral (L) and superior (S) directions.

tracture (i.e., arthrogryposis). The varus deformity or flexion contracture causes the femur to block visualization of the acetabulum and the femoral head. In such cases, the unossified greater trochanter may be mistaken for a dislocated, small femoral head (Fig. 180-20). To avoid such a misinterpretation, the sonogram should not be interpreted without knowledge of the clinical situation and review of any plain radiographs obtained.

> Pitfalls of neonatal hip sonography: (1) assessing acetabular morphology without being present in the standard coronal plane; and (2) mistaking the greater trochanter as a displaced femoral head in children with varus deformity or contracture.

AAP CLINICAL GUIDELINES FOR SCREENING FOR DDH

In establishing guidelines, the American Academy of Pediatrics (AAP) considered that expert hip sonography may not be available to all pediatricians, and health delivery is not centrally controlled. Consequently, the algorithm incorporated clinical examination, orthopedic consultation, sonography, and plain radiography (Fig. 180-21). Although the high sensitivity of neonatal and early infant sonography for DDH has led to universal sonographic screening of all infants in some European countries, such an endeavor is impractical in the United States, where no universal health insurance is available, and where the population base is very large. Practice

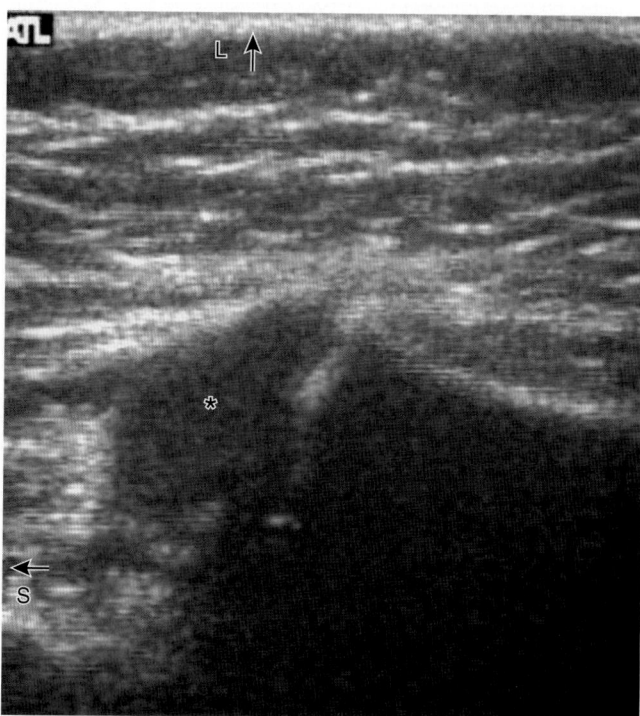

FIGURE 180-20. Coronal view of a 3-month-old girl misinterpreted as showing a dislocated small femoral head. Actually, this is the greater trochanter *(asterisk)* in a baby with a flexion contracture obscuring the acetabulum. *Arrows* denote lateral (L) and superior (S) directions.

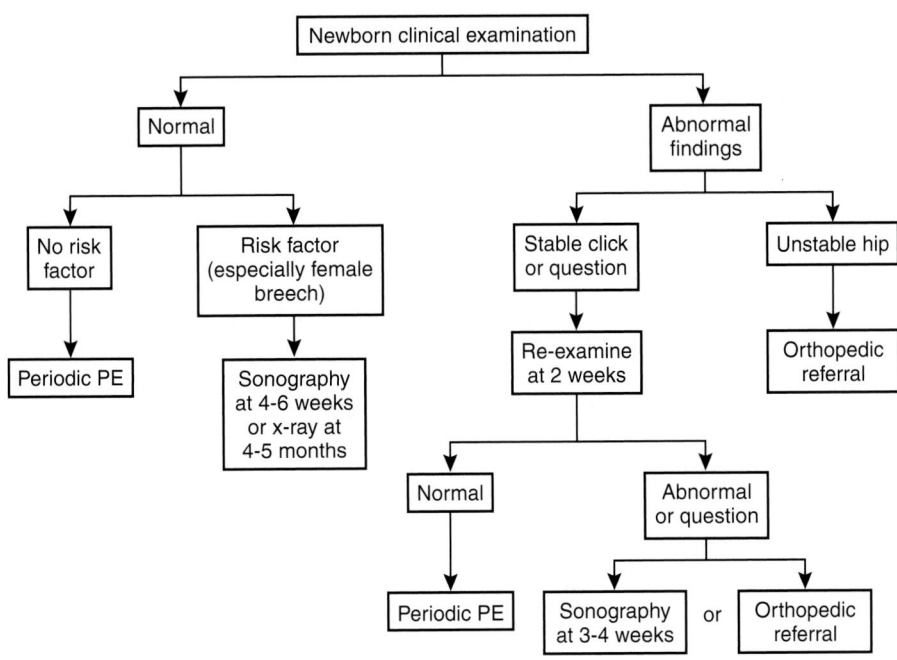

FIGURE 180-21. Guidelines for investigating developmental dysplasia of the hip (DDH). PE, physical examination.

guidelines for pediatricians in the United States, based on evidence-based literature and expert opinion, do not support the routine universal sonographic screening of newborns. Therefore, in the United States, newborn screening occurs by periodic physical examination, with ultrasonography limited to infants who are at increased risk for DDH. Increased risk includes an abnormal physical examination, a positive family history, breech delivery, clubfoot, or torticollis. These risk factors are seen in approximately 10% of all newborns.

Timing of sonography is important because DDH at birth may improve over time without treatment. When the physical examination is abnormal shortly after birth, AAP guidelines recommend orthopedic referral and delay of the sonogram until 2 to 4 weeks of age. This recommendation takes into consideration the high sensitivity of sonography and the difficulty of distinguishing "neonatal sonographic DDH" (physiologic laxity) from true DDH. The tendency for minor instability and acetabular immaturity to resolve spontaneously ("physiologic laxity and immaturity") calls in to question the need to treat such hips. Some universal newborn sonographic screening programs have led to overtreatment. With this in mind, sonography of an infant with a risk factor but with a normal physical examination should be done at 4 to 6 weeks of age, so that transient physiologic laxity or physiologic acetabular immaturity does not lead to multiple unnecessary follow-up sonograms or to unnecessary treatment.

> **Sonography of an infant with a risk factor but a normal physical examination should be done at 4 to 6 weeks of age, so that transient physiologic laxity or physiologic acetabular immaturity does not lead to multiple unnecessary follow-up sonograms or to unnecessary treatment.**

As an alternative to universal screening, sonographic screening can be performed on a limited basis in babies at risk for DDH. Such focused "screening" has been studied in the United Kingdom, where it eliminated all late cases of DDH. A Norwegian study compared physical examination screening only, selective "at risk" ultrasound screening, and universal ultrasound screening. "At risk" sonography resulted in fewer missed DDH cases than were noted with clinical screening alone, and universal sonography resulted in the fewest. However, the differences between universal and risk-based screening were not statistically significant. A study in Coventry, England reported that universal sonographic screening eliminated all late DDH cases, but a 1994 epidemiologic study of the literature based on decision analysis did not support universal sonographic screening. In summary, the case for universal sonographic screening for DDH remains controversial. Under current conditions, universal sonographic screening is impractical in the United States.

Continued clinical follow-up and a plain radiograph at 6 months of age performed to confirm continued normal maturation are helpful following sonography for DDH.

Sonography to Follow DDH and Guide Therapy

Sonography can be used to monitor DDH during observation or treatment. Soft splints, such as the commonly used Pavlik harness, allow the legs to move while keeping the hips partially flexed and partially abducted. The purpose of the harness is to maintain the femoral head within the acetabulum by limiting adduction and extension—two positions that exacerbate subluxation and dislocation of unstable hips. Serial sonograms can be performed in the harness to ascertain whether the hip is reduced properly. Sonograms can also monitor osseous maturation of the acetabulum. Sonography is easily performed without removal of the harness. Because the purposes of the harness are to prevent subluxation and dislocation and to allow loose ligaments to tighten normally, the dynamic portion of sonography during therapy in the harness is limited to gentle abduction and adduction as allowed by the harness or performed spontaneously by the infant. No Barlow or Ortolani maneuver is performed at this stage of treatment. At the conclusion of therapy, the orthopedist may request a full sonographic study out of the harness that includes stress views to confirm that stability has been achieved and the harness may be discontinued. Sonographic monitoring while in the harness is much more sensitive and specific than clinical or radiologic monitoring. The frequency of ultrasound examinations varies with DDH severity. Subluxatable hips are scanned at 2- to 3-week intervals. Sonograms in the harness are recommended weekly with frank dislocation to confirm improvement.

RISKS OF THERAPY

Ischemic necrosis may occur in treated patients with DDH. The risk of ischemic necrosis as a complication of an abduction splint is minimized by not abducting too vigorously. Extreme abduction in a soft harness or a cast can cause ischemic necrosis of the femoral head, especially when abduction is combined with internal rotation and flexion, which can press the medial circumflex artery against the intertrochanteric portion of the labrum. The risk of ischemic necrosis with splinting is approximately 2.5%. Magnetic resonance imaging (MRI) with gadolinium may be performed to detect abduction-induced vascular compromise. Theoretically, color or power Doppler sonography of the femoral head can assess femoral head vascular signals when the harness is adjusted. However, Doppler has not proved to be clinically more useful than simple avoidance of extreme abduction.

The high sensitivity of sonography relative to physical examination or radiography is associated with the risk that physiologically immature hips with slight laxity or slightly steep acetabular roofs that would mature spontaneously will be labeled as abnormal, and that the patient therefore may be subjected to needless treatment and the inconvenience, costs, and risk of ischemic necrosis that it may cause.

SUCCESS OF THERAPY

Initiation of Pavlik treatment by 3 weeks of age increases the likelihood of success, with "success" defined as attainment of stable reduction in the harness. Pavlik therapy was successful in 95% of infants with acetabular dysplasia and subluxation, but in only 80% of infants with dislocation in the European Pediatric Orthopaedic Society Multicentre study. If a frankly dislocated hip has not reduced after 3 weeks in the harness, it is unlikely that it will reduce in the harness, and a rigid splint or cast should be considered. Closed reduction or open reduction is often necessary. Prolonged use of the Pavlik harness on a frankly dislocated hip without reduction leads to erosion of the posterior acetabular wall by the dislocated femoral head, which can then lead to difficulty with subsequent attempts at closed or open reduction.

No sonographic morphologic feature of nonteratologic frankly dislocated neonatal hips reliably predicts success or failure of a harness. It has been speculated (without statistical validation) that success or failure in the harness is due to the labrum. Increased echogenicity of the labrum indicates transformation from hyaline cartilage to stiffer fibrocartilage, which does not remodel to the repositioned femoral head to allow for satisfactory reduction. Therefore, increased echogenicity of the hyaline acetabular cartilage might eventually prove to have some predictive value, but this has not yet been established.

ARTHROGRAPHY AND MRI

Arthrography with dynamic manipulation under fluoroscopy or CT arthrography can be helpful to the orthopedic surgeon, especially during treatment of older patients with adaptive acetabular and femoral head changes. The contour of the femoral head, the shape of the acetabulum, the amount of coverage throughout a range of positions, and any femoral neck anteversion or retroversion are documented. A diagnostic arthrogram with fluoroscopy is often performed in the operating room at the time of open or closed reduction (Fig. 180-22). Features of DDH that have already been discussed can be shown on arthrography, including contour and position of the femoral head, position and inversion of the

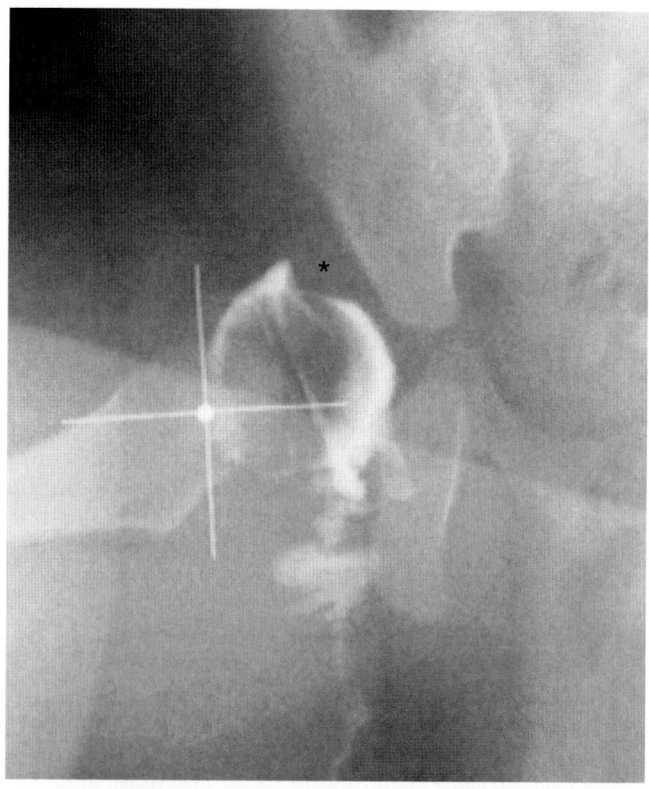

FIGURE 180-22. Intraoperative arthrogram of right developmental dysplasia of the hip (DDH) in a 6-month-old girl with a previously subluxed hip. Although the ossified acetabular roof is steep, intra-articular contrast outlines the normal contour of the cartilaginous femoral head, which is contained by the cartilaginous labrum *(asterisk)* during abduction.

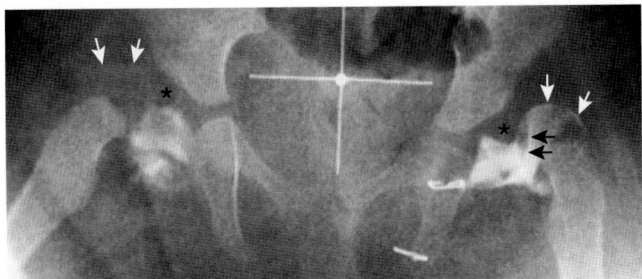

FIGURE 180-23. Bilateral hip arthrograms in a 14-month-old show bilateral developmental dysplasia of the hip (DDH) with superiorly and laterally displaced femora. Intra-articular contrast outlines the cartilaginous acetabular roofs, which are medial to the femoral heads *(white arrows)*, and the left iliopsoas tendon *(black arrows)*. *Asterisk,* labrum.

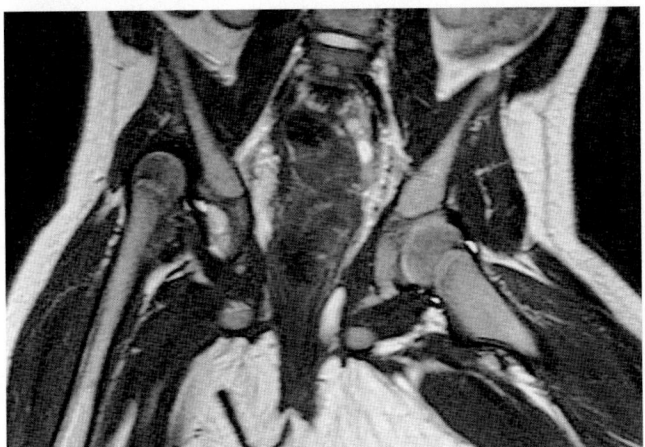

FIGURE 180-24. Coronal T2-weighted magnetic resonance image of right developmental dysplasia of the hip (DDH) with dislocation. (Courtesy of Dr. E. Stranzinger, MD, Zurich, Switzerland.)

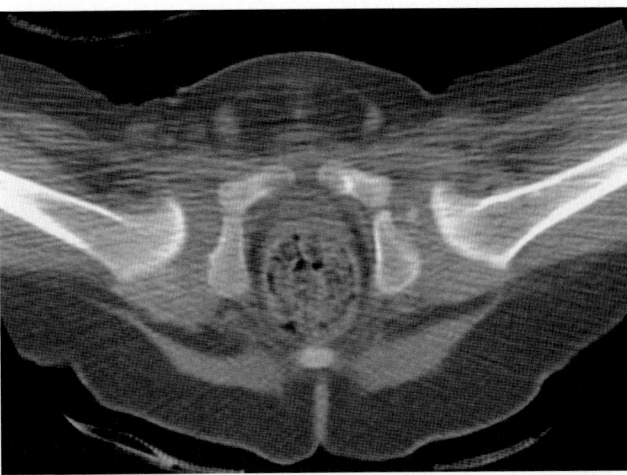

FIGURE 180-25. Low-mA axial computed tomography (CT) of a 7-month-old boy in a spica cast shows concentric reduction of both femoral heads. Although only a left femoral head ossific nucleus is present, both cartilaginous femoral heads are visible on CT. The position is also inferred by the symmetric positioning of the metaphyses relative to the triradiate cartilages.

labrum, stretching of the joint capsule with indentation by a tight iliopsoas tendon, an elongated ligamentum teres, a thick pulvinar, and reducibility of the hip with manipulation (Fig. 180-23).

Acetabular soft tissue anatomy, including interposed soft tissues that inhibit reduction, can also be detected on multiplanar MRI before reduction is attempted (Fig. 180-24). However, because dynamic evaluation is not yet possible with MRI and reduction will be attempted in the operating room anyway, often with a concurrent dynamic fluoroscopic arthrogram, the pre-reduction MRI is usually not obtained. MRI and magnetic resonance arthrography are reserved for complicated or post-operative cases or for unsuccessful reductions. MRI can also be helpful in complicated referral cases, especially when the possibility of prior ischemic necrosis exists that the orthopedist would wish to document as pre-existing prior to any intervention.

IMAGING DDH IN A CAST

Sonography can been used to assess the hips within a cast. A view via the groin or the perineum can be obtained through the opening in the cast made for urinating. Hip anatomy orientation from this perspective is not familiar to most radiologists and orthopedists, and the view is not widely used. If standard sonographic views are to be obtained, a lateral window must be made in the cast; however, this approach is not popular with orthopedists and has been largely abandoned.

Conventional radiographs are of limited value because of obstruction caused by the spica cast. However, CT provides an easy method of viewing the hips within a cast. Limited CT of the hips (a few slices at low mA) is obtained immediately after a cast is applied or changed, to confirm that the hips are reduced. If no ossification is seen within the femoral head, the configuration of the femoral neck can be used to infer the position of the femoral head and its alignment with the acetabulum and triradiate cartilage (Figs. 180-25 and 180-26). These studies can be performed quickly between scheduled CT cases. Images are read immediately, and the patient can be returned to the operating room if reduction is found to be inadequate. Because the child is in a cast, sedation is not needed. MRI can be used for the same purpose, although currently, logistical issues have prevented its widespread use. No further imaging is needed until the hips are removed from the cast, at which time sonography or radiography is obtained, depending on the age of the patient.

> Hip reduction within a cast can be quickly assessed through very limited, low-dose CT images.

SURGERY FOR DDH

The goal of early detection of DDH is to intervene before adaptive changes occur in the acetabulum and the femoral head. However, occasionally, surgery is necessary to provide adequate centering of the femoral head within its acetabulum or to improve hip biomechanics.

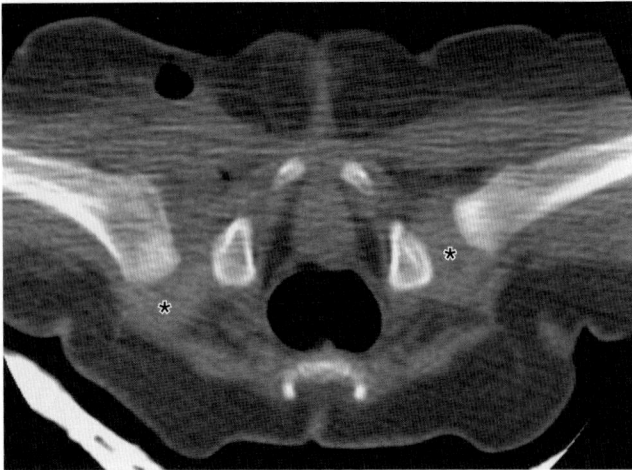

FIGURE 180-26. Low-mA axial computed tomography (CT) of a 3-month-old girl in a spica cast following right open and left closed reductions shows incomplete reduction of the left femur and nonreduction of the right femur. Both femoral necks are retroverted, right greater than left. Although both femoral heads are cartilaginous, they are visible on CT *(asterisks)*.

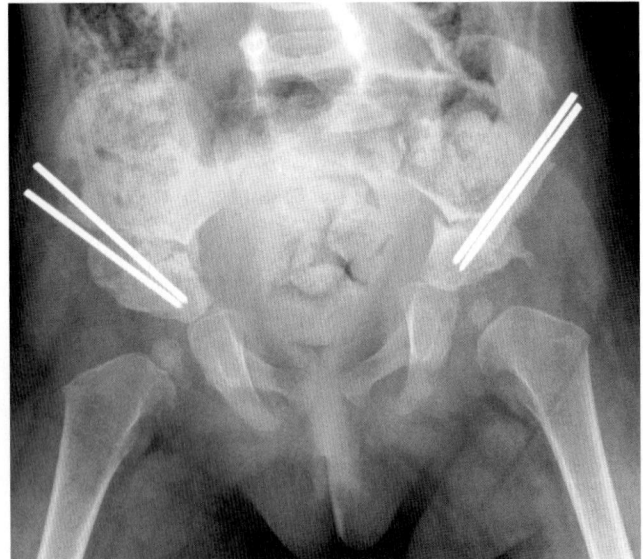

FIGURE 180-27. A 17-month-old girl with bilateral developmental dysplasia of the hip (DDH) with dislocating hips. Bilateral iliac osteotomies were preformed to realign the acetabular roofs, which now better contain the femoral heads.

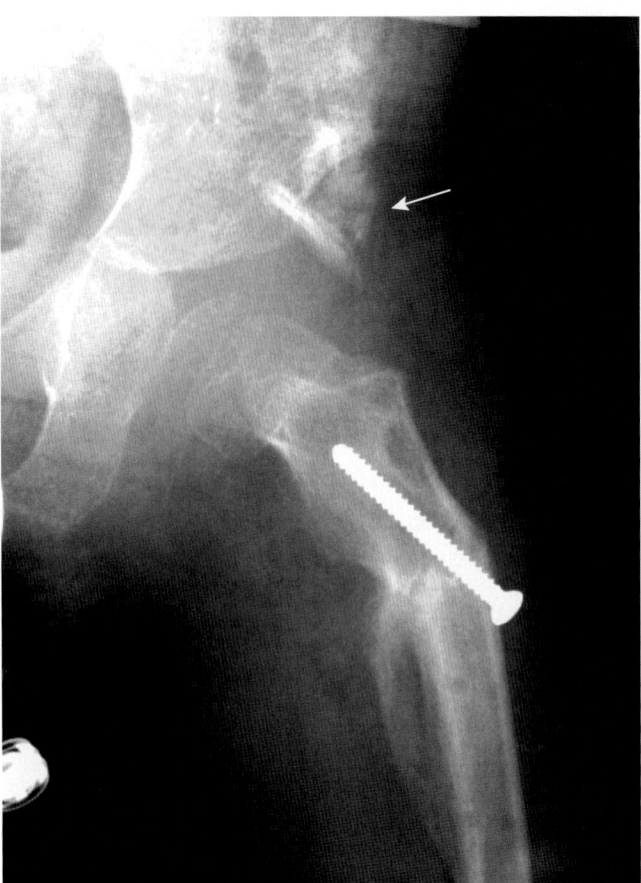

FIGURE 180-28. A 5-year-old boy with dislocatable left hip. Postoperative image shows that osseous femoral head coverage is achieved by a combination of proximal femoral varus osteotomy and lateral acetabular roof osseous augmentation *(arrow)*.

Surgical reconstruction for DDH is usually limited to chronic cases with marked soft tissue contracture and acetabular dysplasia. Operations include iliac osteotomy (Salter innominate osteotomy, Chiari median displacement pelvic osteotomy) performed to realign the acetabular roof (Fig. 180-27) and bone graft applied to the lateral aspect of the acetabular roof (acetabular augmentation) (Fig. 180-28). Both procedures improve contact of the acetabular roof with the femoral head and promote centralization of the femoral head within the acetabulum. A femoral varus osteotomy may also be performed to redirect the femoral head into the acetabulum with the same goals (see Fig. 180-28). Preoperatively, multi-

planar and volume-rendered CT reconstruction of the hip may be helpful. MRI can be used to define the configuration of the cartilage elements within the acetabulum.

SUGGESTED READINGS

Alexiev VA, Harcke HT, Kumar SJ: Residual dysplasia after successful Pavlik harness treatment: early ultrasound predictors. J Pediatr Orthop 2006;26:16-23

American Academy of Pediatrics: Clinical practice guideline: early detection of developmental dysplasia of the hip. Pediatrics 2000;105:896-905

American College of Radiology (ACR): Standards for the Performance of Ultrasound Examination for Detection of Developmental Dysplasia of the Hip. Reston, VA, American College of Radiology, 1999.

Andren L: Pelvic instability in newborns with special reference to congenital dislocation of the hip and hormonal factors: a roentgenologic study. Acta Radiol Suppl 1962;212:1-66

Andren L, Von Rosen S: The diagnosis of dislocation of the hip in newborns and the primary results of immediate treatment. Acta Radiol 1958;49:89-95

Babcock DS, Hernandez RJ, Kushner DC, et al: Developmental dysplasia of the hip: American College of Radiology ACR Appropriateness Criteria. Radiology 2000;215:819-827

Barlow TG: Early diagnosis and treatment of congenital dislocation of the hip. J Bone Joint Surg Br 1962;44:292-301

Berman L, Klenerman L: Ultrasound screening for hip abnormalities: preliminary findings in 1001 neonates. Br Med J 1986;293:719-722

Bialek V, Bialek GM, Blazer S, et al: Developmental dysplasia of the hip: a new approach to incidence. Pediatrics 1999;103:93-99

Blank E: Some effects of position on the roentgenographic diagnosis of dislocation at the infant hip. Skeletal Radiol 1981;7:59-61

Boeree NR, Clarke NMP: Ultrasound imaging and secondary screening for congenital dislocation of the hip. J Bone Joint Surg Br 1994;76:525-533

Carter CO, Wilkinson JA: Genetic and environmental factors in the etiology of congenital dislocation of the hip. Clin Orthop 1964;33:119-127

Casman JP, Round J, Taylor G, et al: The natural history of developmental dysplasia of the hip after early supervised treatment in the Pavlik harness. J Bone Joint Surg Br 2002;84:418-425

Castelein RM, Sauter AJM: Ultrasound screening for congenital dysplasia of the hip in newborns: its value. J Pediatr Orthop 1988;8:666-670

Catterall A. What is congenital dislocation of the hip [editorial]. J Bone Joint Surg Br 1984;66:469-470

Catterall A. The early diagnosis of congenital dislocation of the hip. J Bone Joint Surg Br 1994;76:515-516

Clarke NMP, Clegg J, Al-Chalabi AN: Ultrasound screening of hips at risk for CDH: failure to reduce the incidence of late cases. J Bone Joint Surg Br 1989;71:9-12

Clarke NMP, Harcke HT, McHugh P, et al: Real-time ultrasound in the diagnosis of congenital dislocation and dysplasia of the hip. J Bone Joint Surg Br 1985;67:406-412

Clegg J, Bache CE, Raut VV: Financial justification for routine ultrasound screening of the neonatal hip. J Bone Joint Surg Br 1999;81:852-857

Dahlstrom H, Oberg L, Friberg S: Sonography in congenital dislocation of the hip. Acta Orthop Scand 1986;57:402-406

Davids JR: Ultrasonography and DDH: a cost-benefit analysis of the three delivery systems. J Pediatr Orthop 1995;15:325-329

Dias JJ, Thomas IH, Lamont AC, et al: The reliability of ultrasonographic assessment of neonatal hips. J Bone Joint Surg Am 1993;75:479-482

DiPietro MA, Harcke T: Pediatric musculoskeletal and spinal sonography. In van Holsbeeck MT, Introcaso JH (eds): Musculoskeletal Ultrasound, 2nd ed. Philadelphia, Mosby, 2001:277-323

Donaldson JS, Feinstein KA: Imaging of developmental dysplasia of the hip. Pediatr Clin North Am 1997;44:591-613

Drummond DS, O'Donnell J, Breed A, et al: Arthrography in the evaluation of congenital dislocation of the hip. Clin Orthop 1989;243:148-156

Dunn PM: Perinatal observations on the etiology of congenital dislocation of the hip. Clin Orthop 1976;119:11-22

Dunn PM: The anatomy and pathology of congenital dislocation of the hip. Clin Orthop 1976;199:23-27

Eggli KD, King SH, Boal DK, et al: Low-dose CT of developmental dysplasia of the hip after reduction: diagnostic accuracy and dosimetry. AJR Am J Roentgenol 1994;163:1441-1443

Engessaeter LB, Wilson DJ, Nag D, et al: Ultrasound and congenital dislocation of the hip: the importance of dynamic assessment. J Bone Joint Surg Br 1990;72:197-201

Falliner A, Hahne HJ, Hassenpflug J: Sonographic hip screening and early management of developmental dysplasia of the hip. J Pediatr Orthop 1999;8:112-117

Fisher R, O'Brien TS, Davis KM: Magnetic resonance imaging in congenital dysplasia of the hip. J Pediatr Orthop 1991;11:617-622

Fredensborg N: The CE angle of normal hips. Acta Orthop Scand 1976;47:403-405

Gardiner HM, Duncan AW: Radiological assessment of the effects of splinting on early hip development: results from a randomized controlled trial of abduction splinting vs sonographic surveillance. Pediatr Radiol 1992;22:159-162

Garvey M, Donoghue VB, Gorman WA, et al: Radiographic screening at four months of infants at risk for congenital hip dislocation. J Bone Joint Surg Br 1992;74:704-707

Geitung JT, Rosendahl K, Sudmann E: Cost-effectiveness of ultrasonographic screening for congenital hip dysplasia in newborns. Skeletal Radiol 1996;25:251-254

Graf R: Classification of hip joint dysplasia by means of sonography. Arch Orthop Trauma Surg 1984;102:248-255

Graf R, Tschauner C, Klapsch W: Progress in prevention of late developmental dislocation of the hip by sonographic newborn hip "screening": results of a comparative follow-up study. J Pediatr Orthop 1993;2:115-121

Grill F, Bensahel H, Canadell J, et al: The Pavlik harness in the treatment of congenital dislocating hip: report on a multicenter study of the European Pediatric Orthopaedic Society. J Pediatr Orthop 1988;8:1-8

Grissom LE, Harcke HT: Pediatric musculoskeletal ultrasound. In Rumack CM, Wilson SR, Charboneau JW (eds): Diagnostic Ultrasound, 3rd ed. Philadelphia, Elsevier-Mosby, 2005:2035-2059

Grissom LE, Harcke HT, Kumar SJ, et al: Ultrasound evaluation of hip position in the Pavlik harness. J Ultrasound Med 1988;7:1-6

Hangen DH, Kasser JR, Emans JB, et al: The Pavlik harness and developmental dysplasia of the hip: has ultrasound changed treatment patterns? J Pediatr Orthop 1995;15:729-735

Hansson G, Nachemson A, Palmen K: Screening of children with congenital dislocation of the hip joint on the maternity wards in Sweden. J Pediatr Orthop 1983;3:271-279

Harcke HT: Screening newborns for developmental dysplasia of the hip: the role of sonography. AJR Am J Roentgenol 1994; 162:395-397

Harcke HT: The role of ultrasound in diagnosis and management of developmental dysplasia of the hip. Pediatr Radiol 1995;25:225-227

Harcke HT: Imaging methods used for children with hip dysplasia. Clin Orthop Relat Res 2005;434:71-77

Harcke HT, Grissom LE: Performing dynamic sonography of the infant hip. AJR Am J Roentgenol 1990;155:837-844

Harcke HT, Kumar SJ: The role of ultrasound in the diagnosis and management of congenital dislocation and dyplasia of the hip. J Bone Joint Surg Am 1991;73:622-628

Harcke HT, Lee MS, Sinning L, et al: Ossification center of the infant hip: sonographic and radiographic correlation. AJR Am J Roentgenol 1986;147:317-321

Harding MG, Harcke HT, Bowen JR, et al: Management of dislocated hips with Pavlik harness treatment and ultrasound monitoring. J Pediatr Orthop 1997;17:189-198

Hensinger RN; Congenital dislocation of the hip. Clin Symp 1979;31:1-31

Hensinger RN: Congenital dislocation of the hip: treatment in infancy to walking age. Orthop Clin North Am 1987;18:597-616

Hernandez RJ: Concentric reduction of the dislocated hip: computed-tomographic evaluation. Radiology 1984;150:266-268

Hernandez RJ, Cornell RG, Hensinger RN: Ultrasound diagnosis of neonatal congenital dislocation of the hip: a decision analysis assessment. J Bone Joint Surg Br 1994;76:539-543

Hinderaker T, Daltveit AK, Irgens LM, et al: The impact of intrauterine factors on neonatal hip instability: an analysis of 1,059,479 children in Norway. Acta Orthop Scand 1994;65:239-242

Holen KJ, Tegnander A, Bredland T, et al: Universal or selective screening of the neonatal hip using ultrasound: a prospective randomised trial of 15,529 newborn infants. J Bone Joint Surg Br 2002;84:886-890

Hubbard AM, Dormans JP: Evaluation of developmental dysplasia, Perthes disease, and neuromuscular dysplasia of the hip in children before and after surgery: an imaging update. AJR Am J Roentgenol 1995;164:1067-1073

Kilsic PJ: Congenital dislocation of the hip: a misleading term. J Bone Joint Surg Br 1984;71:136

Kocher MS: Ultrasonographic screening of developmental dysplasia of the hip: an epidemiologic analysis. Am J Orthop 2000; 29:929-933

Laor T, Roy DR, Mehlman C: Limited magnetic resonance imaging examination after surgical reduction of developmental of the hip. J Pediatr Orthop 2000;20:572-574

Lewis K, Jones DA, Powell N: Ultrasound and neonatal hip screening: the five-year results of a prospective study in high-risk babies. J Pediatr Orthop 1999;19:760-762

Lotito FM, Rabbaglietti G, Notarantonio M: The ultrasonographic image of the infant hip affected by developmental dysplasia with a positive Ortolani's sign. Pediatr Radiol 2002;32:418-422

Marks DS, Clegg J, Al-Chalabi AN: Routine ultrasound screening for neonatal hip instability. Can it abolish late-presenting congenital dislocation of the hip? J Bone Joint Surg Br 1994;76:534-538

Morin C, Harcke HT, MacEwen GD: The infant hip: real-time ultrasound assessment of acetabular development. Radiology 1985;157:673-677

Morin C, Zouaoui S, Delvalle-Fayada A, et al: Ultrasound assessment of the acetabulum in the infant hip. Acta Orthop Belg 1999; 65:261-265

Murray KA, Crim JR: Radiographic imaging for treatment and followup of developmental dysplasia of the hip. Semin Ultrasound CT MRI 2001;22:306-339

Omeroglu H, Bicimoglu A, Koparal S, et al: Assessment of variations in the measurement in developmental dysplasia of the hip. J Pediatr Orthop 2001;10:89-95

Ortolani M: The classic: congenital hip dysplasia in the light of early and very early diagnosis. Clin Orthop 1976;119:6-10

Patel H, for the Canadian Task Force on Preventive Health: Preventive healthcare, 2001 update screening and management of developmental dysplasia of the hip in newborns. Can Med Assoc J 2001;164:1669-1676

Paton RW, Srinivasan MS, Shah B, et al: Ultrasound screening for hips at risk in developmental dysplasia: is it worth it? J Bone Joint Surg Br 1999;81:255-258

Polaneur PA, Harcke HT, Bowen JR: Effective use of ultrasound in the management of congenital dislocation and/or dysplasia of the hip (DDH). Clin Orthop 1990;252:176-181

Riboni G, Bellini A, Serantoni S, et al: Ultrasound screening for developmental dysplasia of the hip. Pediatr Radiol 2003;33:475-481

Roposch A: Twenty years of hip sonography. Are we doing better today? J Pediatr Orthop 2003;23:691-692

Roposch A, Moreau NM, Ulery KE, et al: Developmental dysplasia of the hip: quality of reporting of diagnostic accuracy for US. Radiology 2006;241:854-860

Roposch A, Wright JB: Increased diagnostic information and understanding disease: uncertainty in the diagnosis of developmental hip dysplasia. Radiology 2007;242:355-359

Rosenberg N, Bialik V: The effectiveness of combined clinical-sonographic screening in the treatment of neonatal hip instability. Eur J Ultrasound 2002;15:55-60

Rosendahl K, Markestad T, Lie RT: Congenital dislocation of the hip: a prospective study comparing ultrasound and clinical examination. Acta Paediatr 1992;81:177-181

Rosendahl K, Markestad T, Lie RT: Ultrasound screening for developmental dysplasia of the hip in the neonate: the effect on treatment rate and prevalence of late cases. Pediatrics 1994;94:47-52

Rosendahl K, Markestad T, Lie RT, et al: Cost-effectiveness of alternative screening strategies for developmental dysplasia of the hip. Arch Pediatr Adolesc Med 1995;149:643-648

Rosendahl K, Toma P: Ultrasound in the diagnosis of developmental dysplasia of the hip in newborns. The European approach. A review of methods, accuracy and clinical validity. Eur Radiol 2007; 17:1960-1967

Saies AD, Foster BK, Lequesne GW: The value of a new ultrasound stress test in assessment and treatment of clinically detected hip instability. J Pediatr Orthop 1988;8:436-441

Shipman SA, Helfand M, Moyer VA, et al: Screening for developmental dysplasia of the hip: a systemic literature review for the US Preventative Services Task Force. Pediatrics 2006; 117:e557-e576

Succato DJ, John CE, Birch JG, et al: Outcome of ultrasonographic hip abnormalities in clinically stable hips. J Pediatr Orthop 1999;19:754-759

Suzuki S: Ultrasound and the Pavlik harness in CDH. J Bone Joint Surg Br 1993;75:483-487

Suzuki S, Yamamuro T: Avascular necrosis in patients treated with the Pavlik harness for congenital dislocation of the hip. J Bone Joint Surg Am 1990;72:1048-1055

Szoke N, Kuhl L, Henrichs J: Ultrasound examination in the diagnosis of congenital hip dysplasia of newborns. J Pediatr Orthop 1988;8:12-16

Taylor GR, Clarke NM: Monitoring the treatment of developmental dysplasia of the hip with the Pavlik harness: the role of ultrasound. J Bone Joint Surg Br 1997;79:719-723

Terjesen T: Ultrasonography for evaluation of hip dysplasia: methods and policy in neonates, infants and older children. Acta Orthop Scand 1998;69:653-662

Terjesen T, Holen KJ, Tegnander A: Hip abnormalities detected by ultrasound in clinically normal newborn infants. J Bone Joint Surg Br 1996;78:636-640

Toma P, Valle M, Rossi U, et al: Paediatric hip—ultrasound screening for developmental dysplasia of the hip: a review. Eur J Ultrasound 2001;14:45-55

Tonnis D, Storch K, Ulbrich H: Results of newborn screening for DDH with and without sonography and correlation of risk factors. J Pediatr Orthop 1990;10:145-152

Treadwell SJ, Bell HM: Efficacy of neonatal hip examination. J Pediatr Orthop 1981;1:61-65

Treadwell SJ, Davis LA: Prospective study of congenital dislocation of the hip. J Pediatr Orthop 1989;9:386-390

Tucci JJ, Kumar SJ, Guille JT, et al: Late acetabular dysplasia following early successful Pavlik harness treatment of congenital dislocation of the hip. J Pediatr Orthop 1991;11:502-505

Von Rosen S: Diagnosis and treatment of congenital dislocation of the hip in the newborn. J Bone Joint Surg Br 1962;44:284-291

Von Rosen S: Prevention of congenital dislocation of the hip joint in Sweden. Acta Orthop Scand 1970;130(suppl):1-64

Walker JM: Histological study of the fetal development of the human acetabulum and labrum: significance in congenital hip disease. Yale J Biol Med 1981;54:255-263

Wirth T, Stratmann L, Hinrichs F: Evolution of late presenting developmental dysplasia of the hip and associated surgical procedures after 14 years of neonatal ultrasound screening. J Bone Joint Surg Br 2004;86:585-589

Woolacott NF, Puhan Ma, Steurer J, et al: Ultrasonography in screening for developmental dysplasia of the hip in newborns: systematic review. BMJ 2005;330(7505):1413 [EPub]

Wynne-Davies R: Acetabular dysplasia and familial joint laxity: two etiologic factors in congenital dislocation of the hip. J Bone Joint Surg Br 1970;52:704-716

Wynne-Davies R: The epidemiology of congenital dislocation of the hip. Dev Med Child Neurol 1972;14:515-517

Zieger M: Ultrasound of the infant hip. II. Validity of the method. Pediatr Radiol 1986;16:488-492

Zieger M, Hilpert S, Schultz RD: Ultrasound of the infant hip. I. Basic principles. Pediatr Radiol 1986;16:483-487

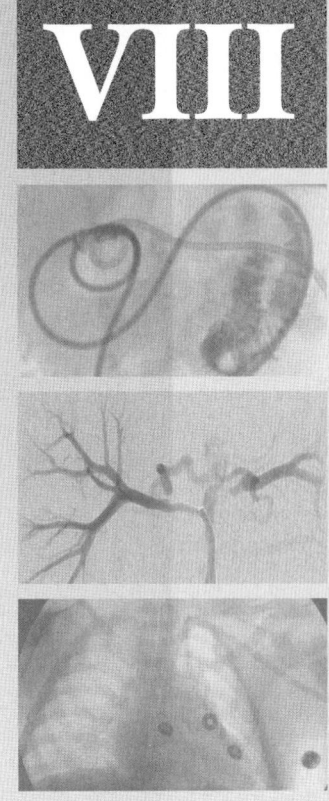

PEDIATRIC
INTERVENTIONAL
RADIOLOGY

JAMES S. DONALDSON

181 Patient Management

STANLEY T. KIM, MARTHA SAKER, and JAMES S. DONALDSON

PROCEDURE PLANNING

When a request for an interventional radiology (IR) procedure is presented to the radiologist, it should be viewed as a request for consultation on a patient. The radiologist will need to learn enough about the patient to determine the indication for the procedure, assess the risks, select the most appropriate imaging modality, make decisions about appropriate sedation or anesthesia, and coordinate scheduling. Often, physician-to-physician communication is the best way for the clinician to fully understand the clinical scenario and to judge the risks versus benefits of an invasive procedure. Existing radiographic studies must be reviewed; sometimes, additional diagnostic studies are indicated before further planning is carried out.

After it is agreed that the procedure will be performed, additional decisions must be made by the interventional radiologist. Bleeding may or may not be a significant risk, and appropriate blood clotting parameters should be ordered if they are not already available. Correction of a coagulopathy may be necessary and appropriate time may have to be allotted for administration of blood products. Preprocedure antibiotics may have to be ordered, while patient allergies are taken into account.

Consent for the procedure must be obtained from the parent or legal guardian. Requirements for consent vary from institution to institution and from state to state. The interventional radiologist must be aware of local and hospital regulations related to consent, rights of minors, including emancipated minors, and consent for administration of blood products. Families from some religious backgrounds may refuse to consent to the potential need for blood products and may refuse to sign consent for such. Local hospital policies usually include guidelines about how one should proceed in these situations.

SEDATION

Lack of patient cooperation usually mandates the use of sedation or general anesthesia. Failed sedation or lack of planning for sedation may cause the interventional radiologist to fail at the attempted procedure. Compliance in the pediatric population is such that sedation is more often needed than not for all but the most mature patients undergoing the least invasive procedures. The vast majority of our patients and those in an increasing number of other specialties are being sedated instead of undergoing general anesthesia for procedures. This led to the publication in 1992 of the Committee on Drugs of the American Academy of Pediatrics (AAP) guidelines for monitoring and management of pediatric patients during and after sedation for diagnostic and therapeutic procedures. This was followed by reaffirmation of these statements in 1995 and 1998 and an addendum in 2002.

The term *conscious sedation* has been frequently misinterpreted but is defined as "a state of sedation that permits appropriate responses by the patient to physical stimulation or verbal command." This is in comparison with the term *deep sedation*, which is defined as "a level of sedation with partial or complete loss of protective reflexes and inappropriate response to stimuli such as simple withdrawal from pain and inarticulate sounds." This state is nearly the same as general anesthesia from a monitoring and recovery perspective, as was described by the Committee on Drugs. The last level of sedation described is *mild sedation*, which is synonymous with anxiolysis. Goals of sedation stated in the original publication are as follows: (1) to guard the patient's safety and welfare; (2) to minimize discomfort and pain; (3) to minimize psychological responses to treatment by providing analgesia and to maximize the potential for amnesia; (4) to control behavior; and (5) to return the patient to a state in which safe discharge, as determined by recognized criteria, is possible.

Many pediatric practitioners would agree that conscious sedation is not adequate for procedures in children. This is true in our experience, so most of our procedures are done under deep sedation. However, the risks of deep sedation are greater than those of conscious sedation. These include airway issues such as obstruction and aspiration, breathing issues of hypoventilation and apnea, and circulatory issues of hypotension. An untreated event may lead to hypoxemia and cerebral or cardiac ischemia. Therefore, it is vital that the person who administers sedation is able to recognize when problems occur and take corrective measures.

The sedation policy of our institution closely follows the guidelines set forth by the AAP. All patients are screened prior to sedation, and information relating to acute and chronic medical problems collected. This can occur before the day of the procedure, over the telephone for outpatients or face-to-face for inpatients. Information that is important to collect includes age, allergies, perinatal history, personal or family history of problems with anesthetics, NPO (nothing by mouth) status, and current cardiac or respiratory status. If a contraindication to sedation exists, the procedure should be performed after appropriate corrective measures have been taken or under closer monitoring, as occurs when the patient is under general anesthesia. The presence of concomitant medical problems may influence the safety and efficacy of the sedation. Further consultation with the patient's primary clinical service may be needed for assessment of the ability to sedate. A medical history and physical examination with a review of the medical record should be performed prior to each episode of sedation.

> **Appropriate level of sedation after thorough screening is vital to the success of interventional procedures in children.**

Regarding NPO status, solids may be consumed until 6 hours before sedation in the 6 months of age and older group. When the patient is younger than 6 months of age, breast milk and formula are permitted until 4 hours prior to the procedure. Patients are able to take clear fluids by mouth up until 2 hours before sedation. Informed consent for the procedure and for the sedation is obtained from the parent. Dehydration is a real concern in small patients, even when the NPO period is short. Blood sugar levels also require close control in patients with poor glucose regulation.

As is recommended by the AAP, sedation should be administered by a practitioner who has been trained in pediatric advanced life support (PALS), and who is able to recognize the early signs of respiratory or cardiac complications. Additionally, an individual who is not otherwise involved in the procedure should be assigned to monitor the patient's cardiopulmonary status and to record vital signs at least as often as at 5-minute intervals. Monitoring involves continuous measurement of heart rate and pulse oximetry. Intermittent blood pressure measurement should also be performed. Although body temperature monitoring is not often performed, it should be recognized that significant hypothermia may occur, especially in small infants. Increasing the ambient room temperature or using blankets or heating devices should be considered for these patients, particularly if long procedure times or large volumes of intravenous fluids are anticipated. Emergency resuscitative equipment, including supplemental oxygen, suction apparatus, airway support, intravenous fluids, and a crash cart, should be immediately available for all sedation procedures until the patient has fully recovered from sedation and meets discharge criteria.

> **Resuscitative equipment, monitoring equipment, and life support training are required for patient safety.**

At our institution, we typically sedate patients older than 3 months of age. Before that age, patients typically respond well to an oral sucrose solution (Sweet-ease; Respironics Inc., Murrysville, PA). For those beyond that age, we use combinations of medications to provide desired levels of analgesia and sedation.

At younger ages, we often use ketamine hydrochloride for shorter procedures. It is an arycyclohexamine that has anesthetic and analgesic effects and shares properties with phencyclidine. We administer it via the intravenous or intramuscular route. Clinically, it has a rapid onset and short duration of action and causes intense analgesia, as well as amnesia, with little respiratory or cardiovascular depression. At higher doses, it can cause elevation of blood pressure and increased cardiac oxygen consumption. Because ketamine hydrochloride can cause an increase in oral secretion, we administer it with an antisialagogue such as atropine. A benzodiazepine such as midazolam hydrochloride is concomitantly given to reduce psychotropic adverse effects. Contraindications to the use of ketamine hydrochloride include uncontrolled hypertension, heart failure, increased intracranial pressure, and pre-existing psychiatric disorders.

In the presence of contraindications or longer procedure times, or when treating older patients, we use a combination of an opioid and a sedative such as fentanyl citrate and midazolam hydrochloride. Other combinations are available as well, and some alternative agents are provided in tablet form (Table 181-1). Agents used have a rapid onset of action and a short duration when given in intravenous form. This allows for frequent dosing and accurate titration of levels of sedation and analgesia. Most agents also allow for reversal if required by ventilatory or hemodynamic parameters.

For procedures of longer duration or greater difficulty, patients are placed under general anesthesia by the anesthesiology service. We also ask their assistance for critically ill patients who do not meet the criteria for sedation. Over the years, our department has fostered a relationship with the anesthesiology department to ensure that the appropriate level of sedation/anesthesia is provided according to the needs of the individual patient.

> **The sedation regimen should be chosen on the basis of patient and procedure requirements.**

RECOVERY

Recovery begins upon completion of sedation—not necessarily at the end of the interventional case. Intermittent vital sign monitoring is performed at 5-minute intervals if level of consciousness score is less than 3, and at 15-minute intervals if level of consciousness score is 3 or above (Table 181-2). Criteria for discharge at our

TABLE 181-1

Agents Commonly Used During Sedation in Pediatric Interventional Radiology

Agent	Class	Effect	Dose	Route	Onset	Comment
Ketamine hydrochloride	NA	Sedative, analgesic	2 mg/kg IV	IV	<1 min	Increased ICP, increased cardiac output, emergence phenomena
			3 mg/kg IM	IM	<5 min	Increased ICP, increased cardiac output, emergence phenomena
Midazolam hydrochloride	Benzodiazepine	Sedative, anxiolytic, amnestic	0.02-0.05 mg/kg IV, dose titrated to effect	IV (IM, PO)	1-5 min	Reduce initial dose if given with other agents.
Fentanyl citrate	Opioid	Analgesia	1 μg/kg IV with max dose of 4 μg/kg	IV	1-2 min	Can slow breathing or alter blood pressure
Morphine sulfate	Opioid	Analgesia, sedative properties	0.1-0.2 mg/kg IV with max dose of 3-4 mg	IV (IM)	3-5 min	Similar to fentanyl citrate
Meperidine	Opioid	Analgesia, sedative properties	1-2 mg/kg IV with max dose of 100 mg	IV (IM)	5-10 min	Similar to fentanyl citrate
Pentobarbital sodium	Barbiturate	Sedative	2-3 mg/kg IV titrated each 5-7 min to effect, max dose 200 mg	IV (PO, IM)	5-10 min	Can cause tolerance
Chloral hydrate	NA	Sedative	25-50 mg/kg PO	PO/PR	20-30 min	May repeat to a maximum of 100 mg/kg
Atropine sulfate	Anticholinergic	Antisialagogue	0.01 mg/kg IV 0.02 mg/kg IM	IV IM		
REVERSAL AGENT						
Naloxone	NA	Opioid antagonist	0.01-0.1 mg/kg IV	IV	1-2 min	
Flumazenil	NA	Benzodiazepine antagonist	0.01 mg/kg, max dose 0.2 mg, max total dose 1 mg	IV	1-3 min	May repeat q2-3min

ICP, intracranial pressure; NA, not applicable.

TABLE 181-2

Level of Consciousness Sedation Score

Score	Description
6	Awake/active
5	Awake/quiet, calm
4	Crying/agitated
3	Asleep, easy to arouse
2	Asleep, slow to arouse
1	Asleep, difficult to arouse

institution include the following: (1) cardiovascular function and airway patency are intact; (2) the patient is easily aroused with intact protective reflexes; (3) the patient can talk and sit up unaided (if appropriate) or has returned to presedation baseline; (4) the patient's state of hydration is adequate; and (5) the patient has attained adequate pain control. Patients who have undergone general anesthesia for procedures are recovered in the postanesthesia care unit in accordance with the standards of the anesthesiology department.

PATIENT PREPARATION

Preprocedural Laboratory Testing

The need for preprocedural laboratories is based on what procedures are being performed. In the absence of significant comorbidities, most pediatric patients do not require preprocedural laboratory testing. However, many patients who come to the interventional suite have significant pre-existing medical problems. In addition, procedures associated with a high associated risk level justify laboratory analysis. Patients who are undergoing general endotracheal anesthesia may also warrant laboratory testing prior to intubation.

> **The need for laboratory testing should be evaluated on a case-by-case basis.**

COAGULATION

All interventional procedures carry at least a small risk of bleeding. In more invasive procedures and in patients with coagulopathy, the risk is greater. Studies such as prothrombin time (PT) and partial thromboplastin time (PTT), as well as platelet counts, should be performed

and values corrected if indicated. Abnormalities in PT and PTT can be corrected by the administration of fresh frozen plasma. For procedures with risk of significant bleeding, we attempt to correct elevated PTs to an international normalized ratio (INR) of 1.5 or lower.

COMPLETE BLOOD COUNT

It is useful in cases with strong potential for bleeding complications to obtain a baseline measurement of hemoglobin/hematocrit levels, as well as platelet count. Although symptomatic anemia is often addressed prior to receipt of patients for procedures, differences in hemoglobin/hematocrit post procedure are useful as a sign of bleeding in patients undergoing solid organ biopsy or a similar procedure. Preprocedural thrombocytopenia can be corrected with platelet transfusion. Patients with platelet counts lower than $50,000/mm^3$ who are undergoing surgery have been found to have an increased risk of bleeding. We often request transfusion of platelets up to a level of $50,000/mm^3$.

Antibiotic Prophylaxis

Surgical procedures are classified into four categories that are based on level of contamination. "Clean" procedures are those in which only sterile anatomic spaces are involved. "Clean contaminated" procedures are those in which the anatomic spaces involved are colonized but are not inflamed. "Contaminated" procedures are those in which involved anatomic spaces are grossly infected. "Dirty" procedures cause spillage of infected material. Preprocedural antibiotics targeted against organisms most likely to be encountered are recommended for all but clean cases (Table 181-3). Prophylactic antibiotics are also recommended to prevent subacute bacterial endocarditis (Table 181-4). At our institution, we do not use antibiotic prophylaxis in clean procedures.

TABLE 181-3

Conditions Requiring SBE Prophylaxis

Most congenital heart malformations
Mitral valve prolapse with regurgitation
Aquired valvular disease
Prosthetic cardiac valves
Prior episodes of bacterial endocarditis
Hypertrophic cardiomyopathy

SBE, subacute bacterial endocarditis.

TABLE 181-4

Procedures for Which Antibiotic Prophylaxis Is Suggested

System	Example of Procedures	Agent (examples)
Genitourinary tract	Percutaneous nephrostomy	Cefazolin sodium
Arterial system	Bland or chemoembolization	Cefazolin sodium or cefotaxime sodium
Venous system	Transjugular intrahepatic portosystemic shunt	Cefotaxime sodium
Infected cavities	Percutaneous abscess drainage	Agent targeted against organism determined by source

TABLE 181-5

Agents Used for Anticoagulation

Medication	Route	Mode of Activity
Heparin	IV	Antithrombin III activator
Enoxaparin	Subcutaneous injection	Antithrombin III activator
Aspirin	Oral	Prevents platelet aggregation
Warfarin	Oral	Vitamin K activation inhibitor
Clopidigrel (Plavix)	Oral	Prevents platelet aggregation
Abciximab (ReoPro)	IV	Prevents platelet aggregation

TABLE 181-6

Premedication for Iodinated Contrast Allergy

Medication	Dose/Interval
Prednisone	1 mg/kg at 13 hr, 7 hr, and 1 hr prior to contrast dose
Diphenhydramine	1-2 mg/kg at 1 hr prior to contrast dose

PROCEDURAL CONSIDERATIONS

Anticoagulation

Anticoagulation with intravenous heparin should be considered for intravascular procedures, given the possibility of thrombus formation and embolism. This is especially important in smaller and younger patients with smaller vessels that are consequently more prone to vessel occlusion with catheters and wires. In procedures associated with a greater risk of thrombosis, oral and intravenous antiplatelet agents should be considered.

Oral antiplatelet medications are also commonly given to patients following arterial and venous interventions during which disruption of the vascular endothelium occurs (Table 181-5). The degree of anticoagulation can be quantified through measurement of activated clotting time (ACT), and intravenous protamine can be given to reverse the effects of heparin, if indicated.

Anticoagulation can be continued after the procedure has been performed, especially in cases where endothelial damage has occurred, or if thrombogenic material (such as a metal stent) has been placed. We often continue intravenous heparin infusion with conversion to subcutaneous enoxaparin (Lovenox; Sanofi-Aventis, Bridgewater, NJ) injections or oral medications such as warfarin (Coumadin; Bristol-Myers Squibb, Princeton, NJ) or Plavix (Bristol-Myers Squibb/Sanofi Pharmaceuticals Partnership, Bridgewater, NJ). Although warfarin doses can be titrated to desired levels of anticoagulation, enoxaparin and Plavix do not require or benefit from surveillance through coagulation studies.

Contrast Agents

Major considerations include allergic reactions and toxicity. In patients with previously documented allergic reaction, premedication with oral prednisone and diphenhydramine is used to prevent reactions (Table 181-6). If anaphylaxis or another allergic response occurs, administration of epinephrine or albuterol inhalers can be used to counter the reaction.

Contrast reactions occur more frequently at higher doses. Therefore, the dose should generally not exceed 5 mL/kg for routine cases. Higher doses can be achieved during longer procedures, but this should be accompanied by adequate levels of hydration.

SUMMARY

Infants and children present a unique set of challenges for the interventional radiologist compared with the adult patient; these include necessary level of sedation, medications and dosages, and instruments used. However, with proper preparation and familiarity with pediatric physiology, interventional radiologic procedures can be performed safely and effectively.

SUGGESTED READINGS

American Academy of Pediatrics Committee on Drugs: Guidelines for monitoring and management of pediatric patients during and after sedation for diagnostic and therapeutic procedures. Pediatrics 1992;89(6 Pt 1):1110-1115

Bravo SM, Reinhart RD, Meyerovitz MF: Percutaneous venous interventions. Vasc Med 1998;3:61-66

Connolly B, Racadio J, Towbin R: Practice of ALARA in the pediatric interventional suite. Pediatr Radiol 2006;36(Suppl 14):163-167

Mason KP, Michna E, DiNardo JA, et al: Evolution of a protocol for ketamine-induced sedation as an alternative to general anesthesia for interventional radiologic procedures in pediatric patients. Radiology 2002;225:457-465

Mehta RP, Johnson MS: Update on anticoagulant medications for the interventional radiologist. J Vasc Interv Radiol. 2006;17:597-612

Ryan JM, Ryan BM, Smith TP: Antibiotic prophylaxis in interventional radiology. J Vasc Interv Radiol 2004;15:547-556

Sanborn PA, Michna E, Zurakowski D, et al: Adverse cardiovascular and respiratory events during sedation of pediatric patients for imaging examinations. Radiology 2005;237:288-294

PART 2 — RESPIRATORY

CHAPTER 182

Empyema and Thoracic Abscess Drainage

G. PETER FEOLA

"A person with empyemata... shall die on the fourteenth day, unless something favorable supervenes."

HIPPOCRATES, 400 BCE

In all, 40% of patients who are hospitalized with bacterial pneumonia develop a parapneumonic effusion. In 5% to 10% of these patients, the effusion is complicated by extension of infection into the pleural space. The overall incidence of empyema in children appears to be increasing in the United States and the United Kingdom. Empyemas are a significant cause of morbidity but usually not mortality in children. Management remains controversial. Modern therapeutic methods and antibiotics have decreased the need for traditional surgical intervention. Although 2400 years have passed since Hippocrates observed empyema, no consensus has been reached regarding the optimal mode of therapy. Treatment goals, however, are the same:

- Sterilize the pleural cavity with antibiotics.
- Drain fluid early.
- Re-expand the lung by removing the pleural fluid.
- Return the lung to normal function.

Epidemiologically, pediatric empyema is increasing in incidence with evolving bacterial pathogens. Typical bacteria include *Streptococcus pneumoniae*, *Streptococcus pyogenes*, *Staphylococcus aureus*, and *Haemophilus influenza*. Recent years have seen the emergence of more virulent strains of resistant organisms, including methicillin-resistant *S. aureus*. Over the past decade, the incidence of empyema in our region (Utah, U.S.) has increased from approximately 1 case per 100,000 children to nearly 5 cases per 100,000 children. This dramatic increase highlights the importance of early diagnosis and aggressive treatment.

> **Early pleural drainage will prevent the progression of parapneumonic fluid to the stage III organizational phase.**

PATHOPHYSIOLOGY

Pleural infection is a continuum. It has classically been divided into three stages:

1. Exudative: Underlying inflammation in the lung from pneumonia leads to accumulation of clear fluid with a low white cell count. This is considered a simple parapneumonic effusion.
2. Fibrinopurulent: Deposition of fibrin in the pleural space leads to septations and loculations. An increase in white cells occurs with thickening of the fluid. This is considered a complicated parapneumonic effusion. As the fluid transitions to overt pus, it is considered an empyema.
3. Organizational: Fibroblasts infiltrate the pleural cavity and form a thick peel. Solid fibrous bands form and may prevent lung re-expansion, leading to a "trapped lung" and impaired function.

The pleural space normally contains approximately 0.3 ml/kg body weight of pleural fluid. Pleural fluid continually circulates as it is formed and resorbed through the visceral and parietal pleural membrane of the chest. The lymphatic system can accommodate several hundred milliliters of extra fluid. If there is an imbalance between pleural fluid formation and reabsorption, a pleural effusion will develop.

Infection alters the normal components of pleural fluid, thus activating an immune response and pleural inflammation. Pleural inflammation allows increased permeability and migration of inflammatory cells (neutrophils, lymphocytes, and eosinophils) into the pleural space, resulting in the exudative stage of pleural effusion. Progression to the fibrinopurulent stage is due to increased fluid accumulation and bacterial infection across the damaged lung. The coagulation cascade is activated, leading to procoagulant activity and decreased fibrinolysis. Deposition of fibrin leads to septations and locu-

3074

lation in the pleural space. As the inflammatory process evolves, eventual migration of fibroblasts occurs and results in formation of a pleural peel and of the fibrous bands that are apparent in the organizational stage of pleural infection.

> **Pleural infection is a continuum that can progress through three stages: (1) exudative, (2) fibrinopurulent, and (3) organizational.**

DIAGNOSIS

The child with a parapneumonic effusion/empyema usually presents with classic symptoms of pneumonia, that is, cough, fever, dyspnea, and poor appetite. These symptoms may include pleuritic chest pain or even abdominal pain. Most children who present to the hospital have already begun antibiotic therapy.

The earliest radiographic sign of pleural effusion is obliteration of the costophrenic angle on an upright frontal chest x-ray. As effusion increases, it ascends along the lateral chest wall, forming the meniscus sign. If the radiograph is performed supine, a diffuse increase in opacity may be seen over the entire hemithorax. When complete opacification of the thorax is present, it is not always possible to distinguish between consolidated lung and pleural effusion. Furthermore, chest radiographs alone cannot differentiate simple parapneumonic effusion from empyema.

Chest computed tomography (CT) and ultrasonography both detect the presence of fluid, as well as parietal pleural thickening. Ultrasonography is superior in showing the exudative nature of pleural fluid. Complex effusions with debris and thin septations are better seen with ultrasonography. Ultrasonography can also be used for therapeutic intervention. CT of the chest with contrast can delineate loculated fluid components throughout the chest and mediastinum and can better define airway or parenchymal lung abnormalities. However, the radiation dose from a CT of the chest is not trivial; therefore, routine usage should be avoided. CT should be considered in complicated cases, including those characterized by initial failure to drain pleural fluid and failure of medical management. CT is the modality of choice when intrapulmonary abscess is suspected.

TREATMENT

Conservative management of pleural infection consists of antibiotic therapy. Many small parapneumonic effusions respond to antibiotics without the need for further intervention. However, effusions that are enlarging or compromising respiratory function need drainage. Many studies over the past 10 years have shown effectiveness of chest tube drainage alone, chest tube drainage with fibrinolytics, video-assisted thoracoscopic surgery and thoracotomy (including mini-thoracotomy). Each study has its own merit; however, the length of stay in the hospital seems to be the top priority when modes of therapy are compared.

Pigtail chest tubes have become the first line of treatment in many institutions that have the personnel capable of treating children with empyema. Chest tubes should be placed under image guidance with ultrasonography and fluoroscopy to ensure proper position within the effusion and to avoid tube migration into the major fissure. Chest tubes can be placed with the use of moderate sedation and local anesthesia (see Chapter 180). To keep invasive procedures to a minimum, thoracentesis is combined with tube thoracostomy. For those children who require a general anesthetic, it is prudent to insert a pigtail drain at the onset of therapy or, alternatively, to consider early surgical drainage.

Fluid obtained should be sent for microbiologic analysis, including Gram stain and culture. Pleural fluid is often sterile because of prior antibiotics. New polymerase chain reaction techniques may be helpful for pathogen identification. Biochemical analysis is performed as well. Infection causes pleural acidosis with elevated lactate dehydrogenase (LDH) and low glucose levels. Pleural fluid pH has been used by some to assess the need for tube drainage; it has been suggested that an effusion with a pH less than 7.2 should be drained.

When a pleural drain is placed, patients should be positioned supine with the ipsilateral arm raised above the head. Ultrasonography is used to identify the most appropriate location for placement. We have found that initial needle entry should most often be 1 to 2 cm anterior to the scapular tip in the midaxillary line, with the needle trajectory posterior and cephalad. With this access, the drainage catheter will be directed into a posterior and lateral location. In our experience, this catheter location has resulted in superior drainage.

Different studies have used a variety of sizes of pigtail drains. We have standardized the tube size on the basis of patient age. Patients younger than 12 months will receive a 10F tube, and those older than 12 months a 12F tube. Small tubes require additional manipulations to achieve adequate drainage. Drains are placed at 20 to 25 cm water suction. Some centers advocate lower suction, at 5 to 10 cm water, with the thought that lower suction in the tube will lead to suctioning of less debris into the lumen, thus preventing occlusion. Fibrinolytic therapy is then initiated immediately following tube placement.

Pleural infection leads to a procoagulant effect and increased fibrin deposition in the pleural space. For this reason, a standardized protocol is recommended for fibrinolysis in all chest tubes placed in children treated for pneumonia and parapneumonic effusion. Our protocol for fibrinolysis with pigtail drainage consists of tissue plasminogen activator (tPA) at 0.1 mg/kg, maximum of 3 mg, prepared in 10 to 30 ml of normal saline. The tPA mixture is administered intrapleurally through the drain and dwells for 1 hour. The catheter is then returned to 20 to 25 cm water suction. This procedure is performed every 8 hours for 10 doses. During the duration of tPA therapy, we measure the patient's daily temperature and drainage output. Laboratory values, including complete blood count (CBC), erythrocyte sedimentation rate (ESR), and C-reactive protein (CRP), are obtained on the second day as a means of monitoring the patient's response to therapy. A chest radiograph performed on the day following chest tube placement helps the clinician to assess the stability of tube position and the quantity of residual effusion. Chest radiographs are ordered when output drops. When the chest radiograph shows a decrease in pleural fluid with a corresponding decrease in chest tube output to less than 25 ml over a 12-hour period, the drain is removed. It is important to note radiographic changes in the thorax, including parenchymal lung disease that remains after the pleural space has been evacuated, may be significant. This situation takes months to become radiographically normal. Therefore, the patient's clinical status is the most important parameter to follow. If no significant pleural fluid remains on chest radiograph, and drainage has essentially stopped, the chest tube should be removed. Other protocols have been published and all have a similar end point in mind, that is, effective evacuation of the pleural space to allow lung re-expansion (Fig. 182-1).

Analgesics and antipyretics should be given to keep the child comfortable. The chest tube can cause significant pleuritic chest pain, usually greatest during the first 48 hours. Without adequate analgesics, pleuritic pain may impede deep breathing or the willingness of the patient to cough; both of these actions are required if the lung is to be re-expanded as quickly as possible. However, a child who is completely sedated on pain medication will stay flat in bed; this leads to progressive atelectasis and delayed lung expansion. (Crying is not always a bad thing.) The smaller, softer pigtail chest tubes are generally well tolerated by most patients.

In our institution, according to the protocol as outlined, mean length of hospital stay was 9.1 days. Most patients were treated with a single catheter. Catheter duration averaged just over 6 days. We are currently between 90% and 95% effective in the primary treatment of complicated parapneumonic effusion/empyema.

It is important to identify treatment failure as early as possible. For most successful drainages, marked evacuation of fluid follows the first two doses of tPA. If less than 100 ml is evacuated and the chest radiograph or CT shows significant remaining pleural fluid, surgical intervention should be considered. This is not to say that additional tubes cannot be placed, but in keeping with the spirit of time-effective therapy, video-assisted thoracoscopy (VATS) is a worthy alternative.

Fibrinolytic (tPA) therapy in our series is associated with excellent effectiveness in breaking up loculations, improving clinical symptoms, and re-expanding the diseased lung without major complications or additional morbidity. It shows a marked improvement over the historical conventional treatment at our institution of surgical decortication, which was required to treat most patients with empyema prior to 2000. Our results are equivalent to those of VATS and thoracotomy when compared with a recently published meta-analysis of primary operative versus nonoperative therapy for pediatric empyema. Our current results and average length of hospital stay compare favorably with other reports in the literature.

Pigtail placement with intrapleural fibrinolytic administration for drainage of complicated parapneumonic effusion has become standard practice for initial therapy in our institution. The procedure is a minimally invasive and conservative approach that is used to treat children with parapneumonic effusion. It provides the benefit of avoiding both major surgery and anesthesia. We have shown it to be an effective and safe therapy that reduces morbidity and hospital stay.

> **Percutaneous drainage with intrapleural fibrinolytic therapy is an effective, safe, and minimally invasive treatment for patients with empyema.**

PNEUMATOCELES

Necrotizing pneumonia can form early pneumatoceles. These are thin walled and may be fluid filled. Rupture of a pneumatocele can lead to pneumothorax and bronchopleural fistula. This complication is almost always adequately treated with the existing chest tube. Infrequently, another chest tube must be placed to evacuate the pleural air and re-expand the lung. Physicians must not jump to surgical debridement of these cystic necrotic areas. Most resolve over the course of 3 to 4 weeks; thus, lung function is regained (Fig. 182-2).

LUNG ABSCESS

A lung abscess with coexisting empyema should be managed in the standard fashion. Antibiotics given for the empyema should also treat the lung abscess effectively. If the patient continues to spike high fevers and remains clinically ill 5 to 7 days after initiation of antibiotics, the next recommended therapy is percutaneous drainage. Pigtail drainage catheters are placed under image guidance, most often CT, directly into the abscess. The needle with catheter should traverse contiguous abnormal lung and pleura as it enters the abscess cavity. Goals are to minimize further infection and spillage into the pleural space and to decrease hemorrhagic complications and bronchopleural fistulas.

> **Most lung abscesses respond to antibiotics in 3 to 5 days. In patients who remain clinically septic beyond this point, one should consider percutaneous drainage.**

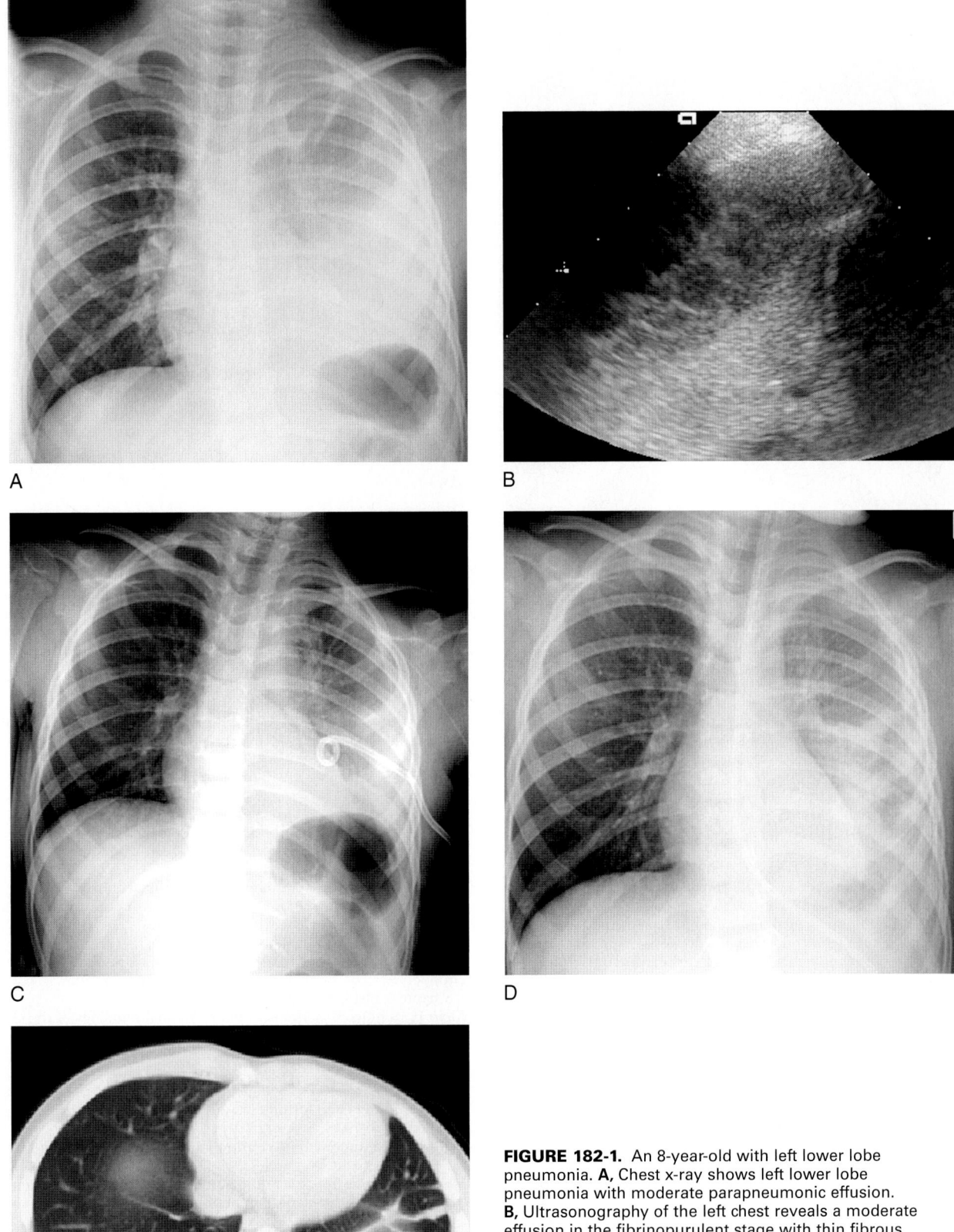

FIGURE 182-1. An 8-year-old with left lower lobe pneumonia. **A,** Chest x-ray shows left lower lobe pneumonia with moderate parapneumonic effusion. **B,** Ultrasonography of the left chest reveals a moderate effusion in the fibrinopurulent stage with thin fibrous septations and echogenic debris. **C,** Following chest tube placement, 100 ml of cloudy serous fluid with debris was immediately aspirated, resulting in improved aeration of the left lower lobe. **D,** Six days post chest tube removal; the child is clinically improved with a normalized white blood cell count. Minimal pleural fluid remains with persistent consolidation in the lower lobe. **E,** Follow-up computed tomography performed 1 month after chest tube removal shows mild fibrotic scarring.

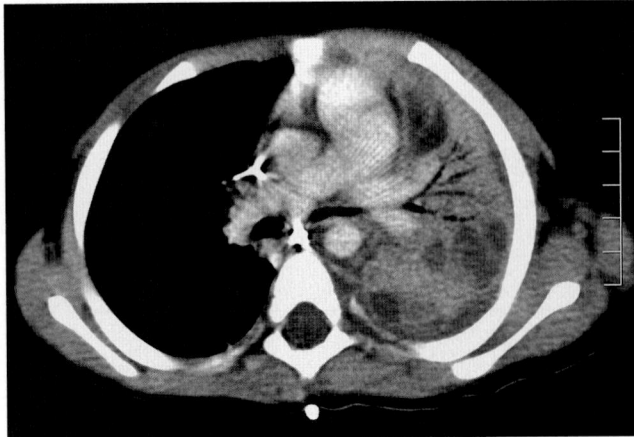

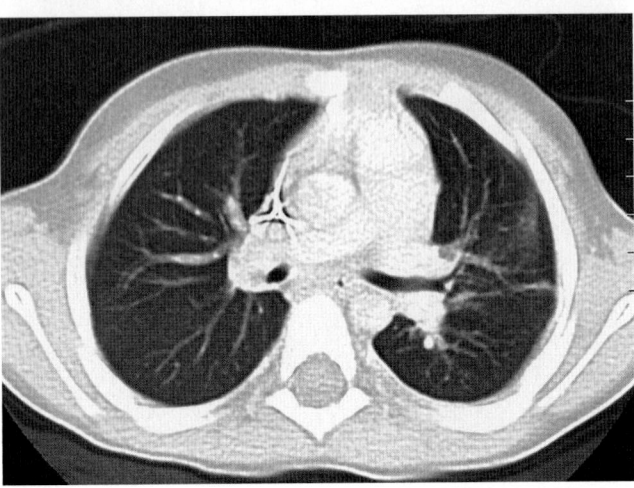

FIGURE 182-2. A 28-month-old with left upper lobe necrotizing pneumonia and complicated parapneumonic effusion. **A,** Chest tube and fibrinolytic therapy initiated 3 days prior to computed tomography (CT) evacuated more than 400 ml of pleural fluid. An area of cystic necrosis has developed in the left upper lobe. **B,** Three days following chest tube removal, residual cystic change is apparent in the left upper lobe. **C,** Follow-up CT 1 month after chest tube removal shows minimal residual inflammatory change in the left upper lobe. The pneumatoceles have resolved.

SUGGESTED READINGS

Avansino JR, Goldman G, Sawin RS, et al: Primary operative versus nonoperative therapy for pediatric empyema: a meta-analysis. Pediatrics 2005;115:1652-1659

Bailey KA, Bass J, Rubin S, et al: Empyema management: twelve years' experience since the introduction of video-assisted thoracoscopic surgery. J Laparoendosc Adv Surg Tech 2005;15:338-341

Balfour-Lynn IM, Abrahamson E, Cohen G, et al: BTS guidelines for the management of pleural infection in children. Thorax 2005;60:i1-i21

Barnes NP, Hull J, Thomson AH: Medical management of parapneumonic pleural disease. Pediatr Pulmonol 2005;39:127-134

Boland GW, Dawson SL: Interventional radiology of thoracic abscesses. *In* Baum S, Pentecost MJ (eds): Abram's Angiography, Interventional Radiology, vol III. New York, Little, Brown and Company, 1977:829-836

Byington CL, Korgenski K, Daly J, et al: Impact of the pneumococcal conjugate vaccine on pneumococcal parapneumonic empyema. Pediatr Infect Dis 2006;25:250-254

Byington CL, Samore MH, Stoddard GJ, et al: Temporal trends of invasive disease due to *Streptococcus pneumoniae* among children in the intermountain west: emergence of nonvaccine serogroups. Clin Infect Dis 2005;41:21-29

Chan P-C, Huan L-M, Wu P-S, et al: Clinical management and outcome of childhood lung abscess: a 16-year experience. J Microbiol Immunol Infect 2005;38:183-188

Colice GL, Curtis A, Deslauriers J, et al: Medical and surgical treatment of parapneumonic effusions: an evidence-based guideline. Chest 2000;118:1158-1171

de Souza A, Offner PJ, Moore EE, et al: Optimal management of complicated empyema. Am J Surg 2000;180:507-511

Feola GP, Shaw CA, Coburn LC: Management of complicated parapneumonic effusions in children. Tech Vasc Interv Radiol 2003;6:197-204

Gates RL, Hogan M, Weinstein S, et al: Drainage, fibrinolytics, or surgery: a comparison of treatment options in pediatric empyema. J Pediatr Surg 2004;39:1638-1642

Hawkins JA, Scaife ES, Hillman ND, et al: Current treatment of pediatric empyema. Semin Thorac Cardiovasc Surg 2004;16:196-200

Hippocrates: The Book of Prognostics (translated by Francis Adams), Chapters 14-18, 400 B.C.E.

Klein JS, Schultz S, Heffner JE: Interventional radiology of the chest: image-guided percutaneous drainage of pleural effusions, lung abscess, and pneumothorax. AJR Am J Roentgenol 1995; 164:581-588

Kunyoshi V, Cataneo DC, Cataneo AJM: Complicated pneumonias with empyema and/or pneumatocele in children. Pediatr Surg Int 2006;22:186-190

Light RW: Parapneumonic effusions and empyema. Proc Am Thorac Soc 2006;3:75-80

Misthos P, Sepsas E, Konstantinou M, et al: Early use of intrapleural fibrinolytics in the management of post pneumonic empyema: a prospective study. Eur J Cardiothorac Surg 2005;28:599-603

Rice TW, Ginsberg RJ, Todd TRJ: Tube drainage of lung abscesses. Ann Thorac Surg 1987;44:356-359

Tan TQ, Seilheimer DK, Kalplan SL: Pediatric lung abscess: clinical management and outcome. Pediatr Infect Dis J 1995;14:51-55

Wali SO, Shugaeri A, Samman YS, et al: Percutaneous drainage of pyogenic lung abscess. Scan J Infect Dis 2002;34:673-679

Wells RG, Havens PL: Intrapleural fibrinolysis for parapneumonic effusion and empyema in children. Radiology 2003;228:370-378

Bronchial Artery Embolization

G. PETER FEOLA

OVERVIEW

Hemoptysis in children is a relatively uncommon event, but when it occurs, it can be associated with significant morbidity and mortality. Hemoptysis has been defined as mild (<150 ml/day), large (150-400 ml/day), or massive (>400 ml/day). However, depending on the ability of the patient to maintain a patent airway, a life-threatening condition may be caused by a small amount of hemorrhage. The decision to undertake bronchial artery embolization to treat hemoptysis should be made according to a functional definition, that is, an amount sufficient to cause a life-threatening respiratory emergency.

With significant hemoptysis, asphyxiation or, less commonly, exsanguination is the usual cause of death. Severe hemoptysis most commonly presents in patients with a history of chronic inflammatory lung disease. Worldwide, this is seen more commonly with tuberculosis and aspergillus. In the West, cystic fibrosis and congenital heart disease are the most common causes of hemoptysis. Other causes include bronchiectasis, tracheobronchial vascular anomalies, respiratory tract foreign body, and tracheostomy-related bleeding. In as many as 20% of patients, no cause for hemoptysis is found.

Assessment and clinical history of the patient will lead to clues that suggest possible causes. Patients with cystic fibrosis tend to have hemoptysis as young adults. Patients with congenital heart disease have a bimodal expression of hemoptysis. One group includes patients younger than 5 years of age, and the other consists of patients 10 years old to late adolescence. Patients with hemoptysis of unknown cause who present with unexplained wheezing or paroxysmal coughing and a normal chest radiograph should be assessed for foreign body aspiration.

PATHOPHYSIOLOGY

The lungs are supplied by dual arteriovascular systems composed of the pulmonary arteries and the bronchial arteries. The pulmonary arteries account for 99% of the arterial blood supply to the lungs. The bronchial arteries provide nourishment to the supporting structures of the airways and to the pulmonary arteries themselves, as well as structures within the mediastinum, such as the esophagus. At the capillary level, connections are noted between systemic and pulmonary circulations. Communication between the bronchial and pulmonary arteries

contributes to a normal left-to-right shunt that accounts for 5% of cardiac output. Conditions that cause reduced pulmonary artery perfusion with reduction in pulmonary arterial supply lead to a gradual increase in bronchial arterial contribution. In many acute and chronic lung diseases, including cyanotic congenital heart disease, the pulmonary circulation is reduced or occluded at the level of the pulmonary arterioles because of hypoxic vasoconstriction, intravascular thrombosis, or vasculitis. As a result, bronchial arteries proliferate and enlarge to replace the pulmonary circulation. This leads to enlargement of the existing extensive anastomotic network that interconnects the bronchial circulation with mediastinal, head, neck, and spinal arteries. Enlarged bronchial vessels, which exist in an area of active or chronic inflammation, may rupture from erosion by a bacterial agent or as the result of elevated regional blood pressure. Arterial blood under systemic arterial pressure may then subsequently extravasate into the respiratory tree, causing massive hemoptysis. In most patients, hemoptysis occurs from the bronchial arteries rather than from the pulmonary arteries.

Chronic inflammation can lead to an increase in systemic arterial blood flow. Chronic inflammatory disorders such as cystic fibrosis, bronchiectasis, chronic bronchitis, and chronic necrotizing infection are associated with release of angiogenic growth factors, such as vascular endothelial growth factors and angiopoietin-1, leading to neovascularization and vascular remodeling. There is, as well, an increase in the collateral supply from nearby systemic vessels. These newly formed collateral vessels are fragile and are prone to rupture into the alveoli or bronchial airways, giving rise to hemoptysis.

IMAGING OF THE PATIENT WITH HEMOPTYSIS

Early imaging with multidetector computed tomography (CT) provides the advantage of allowing acquisition of high-quality images of the entire thorax in a rapid, safe, and noninvasive manner. The goals of multidetector CT are threefold: (1) to show underlying disease with high sensitivity, (2) to help assess the consequences of hemorrhage into the alveoli and airways, and (3) to provide a detailed road map of the thoracic vasculature by means of two-dimensional maximum intensity projection reformatted images and three-dimensional reconstructed images. These road maps are of great use to interventional radio-

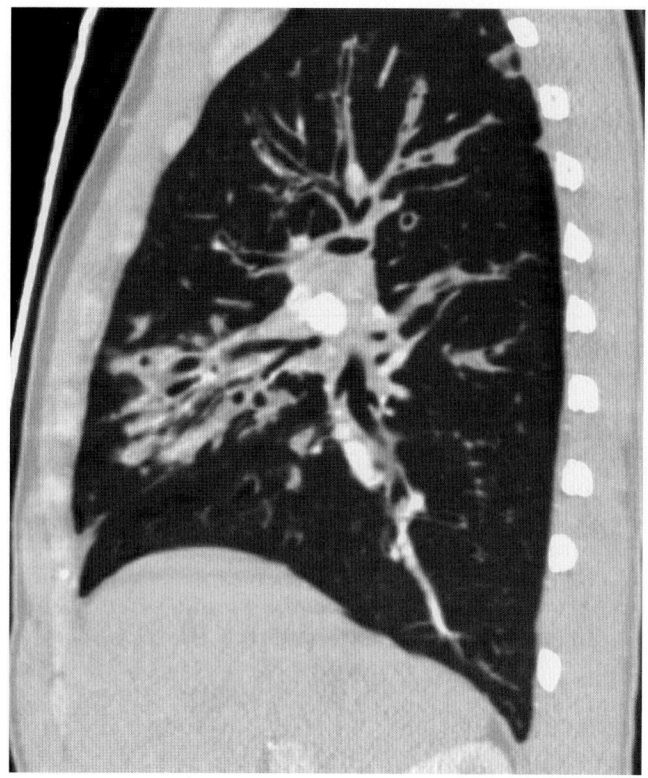

A

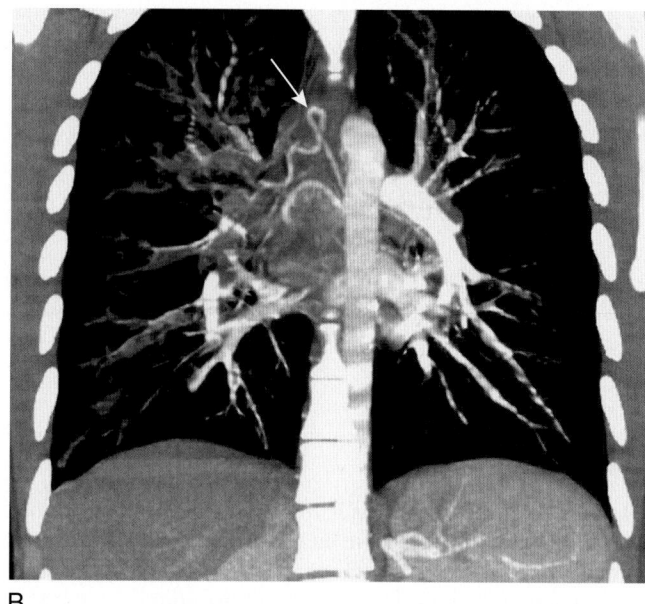

B

FIGURE 183-1. Multidetector computed tomography images in a patient with cystic fibrosis and hemoptysis. **A,** Sagittal reformation shows bronchiectasis throughout the right lung. Fluid fills the right middle lobe bronchi. **B,** Two-dimensional maximum intensity projection imaging at 12-mm slice thickness. Two enlarged right bronchial arteries are apparent. The more cephalad structure is the intercostobronchial trunk *(arrow)*.

logists who are preparing for arterial embolization and to thoracic surgeons who are contemplating lobectomy. Imaging should be carried out from the supraclavicular region to the level of the renal arteries (Fig. 183-1).

> **In 95% of cases of hemoptysis, the systemic arterial system rather than the pulmonary artery is the source of bleeding.**

Although poor correlation has been noted between bronchial artery dilation and risk of hemorrhage, a diameter greater than 2 mm is considered abnormal. A vessel of this size would warrant embolization. Although the bronchial arteries are the most common source of bleeding in hemoptysis, actual hemorrhage usually occurs from fragile, thin-walled anastomoses between distant bronchial arterial branches and pulmonary arteries that are under high systemic arterial pressure. These connections are usually too small to be directly visualized on CT. Rarely will CT reveal contrast extravasation. Bronchial artery aneurysms can be detected with contrast-enhanced CT.

Bronchial arteries of anomalous origin may be overlooked during bronchial artery embolization but are well depicted with CT angiography. Awareness of the existence, location, and anatomy of these vessels prior to the anticipated embolization can help to shorten procedure time and reduce the risk of complications.

A pulmonary arterial source of hemoptysis should be considered in addition to the more common systemic supply in settings of destructive lung disease. This is especially true with cavitary lesions that fill with blood.

A pulmonary arterial source should also be considered when bleeding continues after a technically successful bronchial artery and nonbronchial systemic artery embolization.

ANATOMY

Bronchial artery anatomy has been well described but is highly variable. In more than 70% of the population, the bronchial arteries arise from the descending thoracic aorta, most commonly between the T5 and T6 levels. Normally, one or two bronchial arteries supply each lung, arising independently or from a common trunk. On the right, an intercostobronchial trunk usually arises from the right posterior medial aspect of the aorta, coursing cranially before giving rise to one or more posterior intercostal arteries and a right bronchial artery. The bronchial component turns sharply in the caudal direction to the level of the right main stem bronchus, where it then ramifies in the lung parenchyma parallel to the bronchus and the more distal airways. The left bronchial artery usually arises from the anterior aspect of the descending thoracic aorta, either singly or as a common trunk with a second right bronchial artery.

Bronchial arteries that arise in the expected location from the descending thoracic aorta between the T5 and T6 levels are called orthotopic bronchial arteries. Anomalous bronchial arteries, defined as bronchial arteries that originate outside of the T5-6 range, can be found in 8.8% to 21% of cases of hemoptysis. These often arise from the concavity of the aortic arch. Anomalous bronchial arteries may also originate from the lower thoracic aorta, subclavian artery, internal mammary artery, thyrocervical trunk, costocervical trunk, pericardial phrenic artery, or inferior phrenic artery.

Bronchial arteries can be distinguished from nonbronchial systemic arteries in that their trajectory into the pulmonary parenchyma parallels the bronchovascular axis. In contrast, nonbronchial systemic collateral vessels do not run parallel to the airways, and they have a more unpredictable origin than do systemic branches; these collateral arteries provide systemic vessels that reach the lung via pulmonary ligaments or transpleural adhesions. Nonbronchial systemic collaterals are usually tortuous and therefore are well depicted on CT reformatted imaging. Their presence can often be predicted on the basis of pleural thickening greater than 3 mm with enhancing arteries in the extrapleural fat. These collaterals have been reported to be contributing sources of hemoptysis in 40% to 80% of cases. Failure to recognize systemic collateral arteries can lead to recurrent hemoptysis following bronchial artery embolization.

TECHNIQUE

A CT arteriogram performed prior to bronchial artery embolization will identify the number and sites of origin of abnormal bronchial arteries and of aberrant bronchial arteries. This may allow reduction in the contrast load because a preliminary descending thoracic aortogram will not be necessary. Percutaneous access is achieved at the common femoral artery with a small 4 to 5 French vascular sheath. Hook-type catheters and reverse-curve–type catheters are useful for cannulating the origins of intercostal and bronchial arteries. Coaxial microcatheters used for selective bronchial artery embolization allow a more stable catheter position beyond the origin of the spinal cord branches. Contrast is injected manually. Only nonionic contrast is used because transverse myelitis has been reported with the use of ionic contrast agents.

Two types of spinal arteries may be seen on bronchial and intercostal angiography. Dorsal and ventral radicular arteries are small vessels that arise from segmental spinal arteries and supply the dorsal and ventral aspects of the spinal cord. An average of eight anterior medullary arteries reinforce the anterior spinal artery, which is the major independent source of spinal cord perfusion. The artery of Adamkiewicz arises anywhere from T9 to T12 in 75% of cases. These anterior intramedullary arteries have a characteristic hairpin configuration. Spinal arteries will arise from the intercostal branch of the right intercostobronchial trunk in 5% to 10% of cases. However, the true prevalence is unknown.

Following injection into the bronchial arteries, one may see shunting into the pulmonary artery or vein. Bronchial artery aneurysms may be encountered; however, these are rare. The decision to embolize should be based on all available clinical information. Consideration would be given to abnormal areas of the lung seen on CT or chest radiograph, as well as areas of abnormality encountered at bronchoscopy. If these irregular areas are not visualized or abnormal bronchial arteries are not seen coursing into these areas, then one should search for systemic nonbronchial artery collaterals as a source.

The air-filled left main stem bronchus serves as a convenient fluoroscopic landmark for the general site of origin of the bronchial artery. Catheter occlusion of a bronchial artery should be avoided, especially in the right intercostobronchial trunk. This may result in spinal cord ischemia if a spinal artery branch is present.

The goal of embolization will vary depending on whether the bleeding site has been located with some degree of reliability, and whether a previous embolization procedure has been performed. If the site of hemorrhage is known, attention can be confined to embolization of the bronchial artery and collaterals supplying that area. Otherwise, bronchial artery embolization of both lungs must be attempted. In the presence of previous bronchial artery embolization, collateral pathways require special attention. When possible, any abnormal bronchial artery supplying the site of hemorrhage should be embolized. Catheter positioning distal to the site of spinal artery origin is often achievable with modern coaxial systems. Distal embolization should be performed whenever possible. When permanent proximal occlusion alone is performed, such as with coils, distal collaterals invariably develop, and future access to the main bronchial artery may be lost.

> **Distal embolization should be performed whenever possible. When permanent proximal occlusion alone is performed, such as with coils, distal collaterals will invariably develop, and future access to the main bronchial artery may be lost.**

Polyvinyl alcohol (PVA) particles are used as a nonabsorbable, permanent embolization agent. Particles 350 to 500 micrometers in diameter are most frequently used. Whatever the agent, it is essential to avoid the use of embolic material that could pass through the bronchopulmonary anastomosis. Gelatin sponge is widely used because it is inexpensive and easy to handle. However, reports have shown recanalization of the embolized artery, allowing for recurrent bleeding. An experimental study has reported a bronchopulmonary anastomosis of 325 micrometers in the human lung. For this reason, PVA particles with a diameter of 350 to 500 micrometers are recommended for bronchial artery embolization. Bronchopulmonary fistulas are often seen in patients with massive hemoptysis. However, reports describing use of the same PVA particles at 350 micrometers show no clinical problems related to pulmonary infarction or systemic embolization. Liquid embolic agents such as alcohol or cyanoacrylate are not currently used because they produce very distal embolization with occlusion of the capillary bed, leading to potential tissue infarction. Frank bronchial infarction has been reported with liquid sclerosing agents (Fig. 183-2).

RESULTS

Bronchial artery embolization is very effective in controlling acute hemoptysis. Immediate success rates

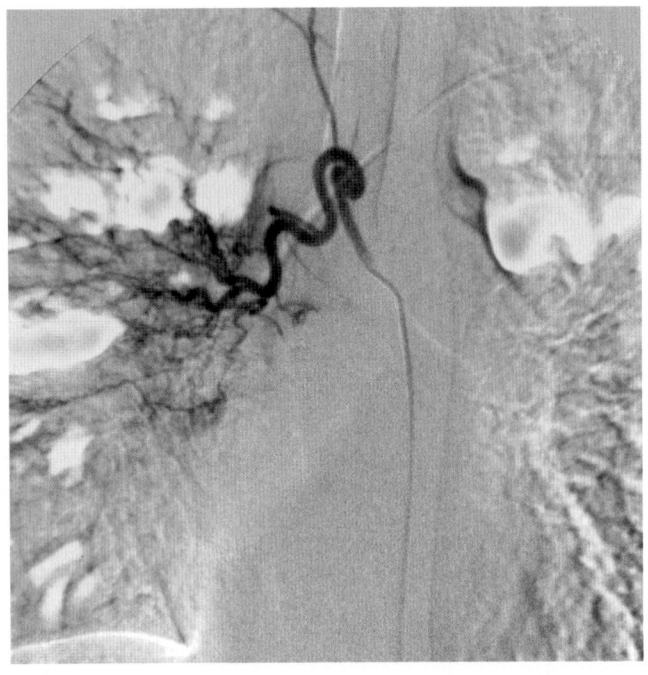

A

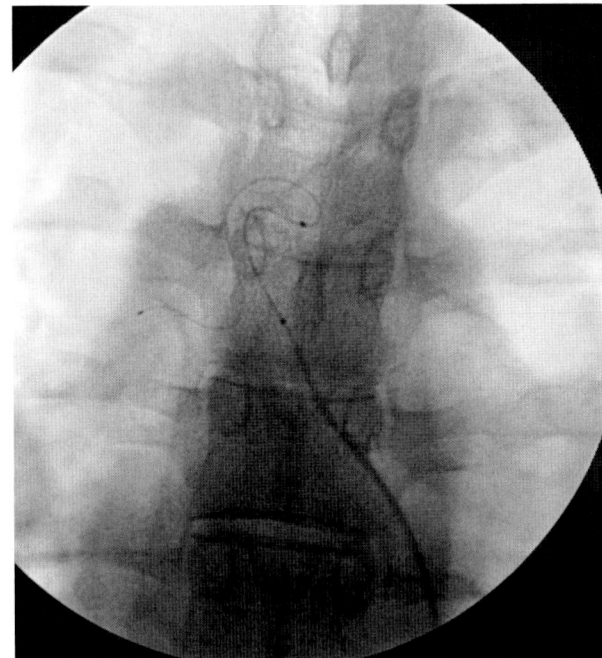

B

C

FIGURE 183-2. Selective images in the same patient with cystic fibrosis and hemoptysis. **A,** Selective catheterization of the right intercostobronchial trunk with a 4 French catheter. Hand injection of nonionic contrast. **B,** Placement of a coaxial microcatheter distally into the bronchial artery prior to embolization. **C,** Arteriogram obtained after distal embolization with 350- to 500-micrometer polyvinyl alcohol particles. Because of a shift in fluid dynamics, filling of esophageal and mediastinal artery branches is now apparent.

have been reported at 73% to 98%, with follow-up ranging from 1 day to 1 month. Long-term success rates of between 10% and 70% have been reported, with follow-up ranging from 1 to 46 months. In general, the long-term control rate of hemoptysis is largely determined by the natural progression of the underlying disease. Embolization does not address the underlying disease but rather only treats the symptoms. In this sense,

bronchial artery embolization is a palliative procedure that prepares the patient for elective surgery to address local disease, or temporizing hemoptysis to allow continued antimicrobial therapy. Recurrent bleeding may be caused by recanalization of embolized vessels, incomplete embolization, and revascularization by the collateral circulation, inadequate treatment of the underlying disease, or progression of the chronic lung disease.

COMPLICATIONS

Transverse myelitis has been reported after diagnostic bronchial arteriography performed with the use of ionic hyperosmolar contrast agents. For this reason, the use of nonionic contrast, manual injection, and avoidance of catheter occlusion of the bronchial or intercostal arteries are advised. The prevalence of spinal cord ischemia after bronchial artery embolization is reported at 1.4% to 6.5%. Visualization of radicular branches on bronchial or intercostal arteriograms is not an absolute contraindication for bronchial artery embolization. However, when the artery of Adamkiewicz is visualized, embolization should not be performed. Other complications reported in the literature include aortic and bronchial necrosis, bronchoesophageal fistula, nontarget embolization, such as ischemic colitis, and transient cortical blindness. It is hypothesized that these may occur via bronchial artery–to–pulmonary vein shunting, or through collateral vessels between the bronchial and vertebral arteries. Chest pain and dysphagia commonly occur but in general are self-limiting.

CONCLUSION

Massive hemoptysis constitutes a significant and often life-threatening respiratory emergency. Knowledge of bronchial artery anatomy, together with an understanding of the pathophysiologic features of hemoptysis, is essential for performance of safe bronchial artery embolization. CT is useful in diagnosing the disease that causes massive hemoptysis and in localizing the bleeding site. CT may also be helpful in selecting vessels for embolization and in predicting the presence of nonbronchial systemic collateral vessels, which can be a significant source of recurrent hemoptysis after successful bronchial artery embolization. Bronchial artery embolization is a palliative procedure performed to control new-onset and recurrent hemoptysis. It can be a lifesaving procedure, and when it is performed properly, good long-term results are reported with infrequent complications.

> **Bronchial and nonbronchial systemic artery embolization is a safe and effective nonsurgical treatment for patients with hemoptysis.**

SUGGESTED READINGS

Barben JU, Ditchfield M, Carlin JB, et al: Major haemoptysis in children with cystic fibrosis: a 20 year retrospective study. J Cystic Fibrosis 2003;2:105-111

Batra PS, Holinger LD: Etiology and management of pediatric hemoptysis. Arch Otolaryngol Head Neck Surg 2001;127:377-382

Bruzzi JF, Remy-Jardin M, Delhaye D, et al: Multi-detector row CT of hemoptysis. Radiographics 2006;26:3-22

Colson DJ, Mortelliti AJ: Management of pediatric hemoptysis: review and a case of isolated unilateral pulmonary artery agenesis. Int J Pediatr Otorhinolaryngol 2005;69:1161-1167

Coss-Bu JA, Sachdeva RC, Bricker JT, et al: Hemoptysis: a 10-year retrospective study. Pediatrics 1997;100:E7

Godfrey S: Pulmonary hemorrhage/hemoptysis in children. Pediatr Pulmonol 2004;37:476-484

Mauro MA, Jaques PF: Transcatheter bronchial artery embolization for inflammation (hemoptysis). *In* Baum S, Pentecost MJ (eds): Abrams' Angiography: Interventional Radiology. New York, NY, Little, Brown and Company, 1977:819-828

Yoon W, Kim JK, Kim YH, et al: Bronchial and nonbronchial systemic artery embolization for life-threatening hemoptysis: a comprehensive review. Radiographics 2002;22:1395-1409

CHAPTER

184

Neurologic Interventions

DEREK ARMSTRONG

Vascular disease involving the central nervous system (CNS) is less common in children than in adults. Although treatment pathways for individual types of neurovascular disease are the domain of the interventional neuroradiologist, their nomenclature and details should nevertheless be familiar to diagnostic radiologists. Cerebrovascular disease in those younger than 15 years is estimated at 2.5 to 3.1 per 100,000. Cerebral vasculopathy in children tends to present with clinical symptoms caused by arterial occlusion and arterial ischemic stroke (AIS) or transient ischemic attack (TIA); subarachnoid and intracerebral hemorrhage are commonly associated with intracranial vascular malformations (see Chapter 53).

Intracranial vascular lesions may be divided according to whether they are proliferative or nonproliferative. Proliferative vascular lesions include the proliferative angiopathy–Moya-moya sequence (see Chapter 54), and nonproliferative vascular malformations consist of those lesions associated with arteriovenous shunts and fistulas (see Chapter 53).

Intracranial vascular lesions, including arteriovenous shunts and fistulas, may be found in the compartments of the dura, the subarachnoid space, or the brain itself. Arteriovenous shunts in the dura are known as dural arteriovenous fistulas (DAVFs). Vascular lesions in the subarachnoid space classically consist of aneurysms and the vein of Galen malformation (VGAM). The pial or intracerebral group of intracranial vascular lesions includes vascular malformations within the brain between the pia and the ependyma. These are referred to as pial arteriovenous malformations (pial AVMs) or cerebral arteriovenous malformations (CAVMs).

The pial AVM includes a vascular nidus consisting of a large group of small arteriovenous connections or shunts, which may be focal or infiltrative within the brain substance. It may consist instead of a single or a small number of large-caliber arteriovenous connections, referred to as a fistula (pial AVF) instead of as a pial AVM. Although the pial AVM may lie adjacent to the pia or the ependyma, or may be embedded within cerebral white matter, the pial AVF typically is superficial or subpial (Table 184-1).

Venous lesions or anomalies may also occur in the compartments mentioned. Within the dura, one may find persistent primitive or anomalous venous sinuses, or communication with the extracranial venous system may involve sinus pericraniae. Subpial or intracerebral venous anomalies include cavernomas, or cavernous malformations, and developmental venous anomalies (DVAs).

DURAL ARTERIOVENOUS FISTULA

The dural arteriovenous fistula represents a large-caliber arteriovenous connection without an intervening capillary bed or the vascular nidus of an AVM; it may be single or multiple and is contained within the dura. Feeding arteries may consist of vessels of the dura, that is, the

---

TABLE 184-1

Intracranial Vascular Lesions in Children—Arterial

Proliferative
  Moya-moya—proliferative vasculopathy
Nonproliferative—Arteriovenous shunts and fistulas
  Dura
    Dural arteriovenous fistula (DAVF)
    Caroticocavernous fistula
  Subarachnoid space
    Aneurysm
      Saccular
      Mycotic
      Traumatic
    Vein of Galen malformation (VGAM)
      Choroidal
      Mural
  Pial (pial to subependymal)
    Nidus—pial AVM
    Fistula—pial AVF
  Venous (see Chapter 53)
  Sinus malformation
  Sinus pericraniae
  Developmental venous anomaly (DVA)
  Cavernoma (cavernous malformation)

meningeal arteries or branches of the internal carotid artery or the external carotid artery. Venous drainage is provided by veins within the dura, the large dural sinuses, the cavernous and petrosal sinuses, and the ophthalmic veins (Fig. 184-1). Commonly, the fistulas anastomose between the intracavernous internal carotid artery and the cavernous sinus (caroticocavernous fistula), but they may occur within the dura in any location and may have direct arterial connections to the large dural sinuses (Fig. 184-2). Uncommonly, a dural AV fistula may occur between the meningeal artery and the ophthalmic vein.

Dural arteriovenous fistulas may be high flow or low flow; dural fistulas fed by branches of the meningeal or internal maxillary artery are typically low-flow fistulas. Symptoms and signs produced by the fistula are influenced by its location, size, and pattern of venous drainage. Dural arteriovenous fistulas represent 10% to 15% of intracranial vascular malformations in adults. Involvement of the cavernous sinus is associated with proptosis, chemosis, and likely an orbital bruit; dural fistulas involving the transverse and sigmoid sinuses may produce pulsatile tinnitus. Intracranial venous hypertension may cause raised intracranial pressure and secondary glaucoma; seizures, focal CNS deficits, transient neurologic symptoms, and intracranial hemorrhage may also occur.

Dural arteriovenous fistulas are thought to be acquired lesions because of their association with dural sinus thrombosis; they may be seen initially with normal-appearing sinuses. Associated venous hypertension or hypertensive venopathy may be recognized with unusual venous exits from the intracranial space; occlusive intracranial sinus venopathy may become apparent with loss of one or both sigmoid sinuses. Compromised venous drainage and hypertensive venopathy reduce brain perfusion, causing instead signs and symptoms such as encephalopathy and dementia.

Dural arteriovenous fistulas may present in the neonate, consistent instead with a congenital origin. The arteriovenous fistula with venous hypertension and consequent compromise in cerebrospinal fluid absorption may cause hydrocephalus and macrocephaly, and arteriovenous shunting may cause cardiac failure or intracranial hemorrhage due to rupture of the abnormally pressurized venous sinus system. Fistulas involving the cavernous sinus with orbital venous drainage or direct fistulas involving the ophthalmic vein may, in addition to proptosis and chemosis, give rise to retinal hypoperfusion, thus representing an urgent to emergent situation in the developing eye with visual failure.

Anatomic classification of dural arteriovenous fistulas is dictated by arterial supply and venous drainage. Caroticocavernous fistulas are divided into the following four types, according to the origin of the arteriovenous fistula:

Type A: Direct connection between the internal carotid artery and the cavernous sinus (caroticocavernous fistula).

Type B: Meningeal branches from the internal carotid artery.

Type C: Meningeal branches from the external carotid artery.

Type D: Meningeal branches from both internal and external carotid arteries.

These may be further classified, according to direct or indirect involvement of the cavernous sinus, as follows:

Type 1: Direct drainage into the cavernous sinus.

Type 2: Indirect drainage into the cavernous sinus from a distant dural sinus.

Caroticocavernous and other dural fistulas have historically been treated with the gamut of occlusive agents, including coils, balloons, gel foam, PVA particles, and histacryl (N-butyl-2-cyanoacrylate glue). The indication for treatment and its urgency is dictated by the symptoms. Fistulas with minor symptoms may be treated conservatively; those with serious symptoms, including venous outflow obstruction with raised intracranial pressure, secondary glaucoma, seizures, focal CNS deficit, transient neurologic symptoms, and hemorrhage, are treated urgently. Treatment is provided through the endovascular transarterial or transvenous approach.

Caroticocavernous fistulas are treated with the detachable balloon technique. They may also be closed by means of transarterial or transvenous coiling or occlusion with histacryl glue. Dural arteriovenous fistulas not directly involving the cavernous sinus may be closed through the transarterial approach with PVA (polyvinyl alcohol) occlusion, but preferably with the use of cyanoacrylate occlusion or the transvenous approach. Surgical resection of the fistula and stereotactic radiation may be selected as adjunctive therapy.

ANEURYSM

Intracranial aneurysms in children are relatively uncommon in comparison with the adult population; incidence in the first two decades is approximately 2% to 5%. Intracranial aneurysms in children account for 5% of aneurysms within the general population. The occurrence of aneurysms in children may be associated with disorders associated with weakening of the blood vessel wall; in most cases, an underlying disorder is not associated (Table 184-2).

Intracranial aneurysms in childhood most often present as subarachnoid hemorrhage, which occurs in about 70% of patients. Mass effect caused by the aneurysm may be the clinical presenting symptom in approximately 20% of children; the remaining approx-

TABLE 184-2

Aneurysms and Associated Diseases

Aortic coarctation
Polycystic kidneys
Fibromuscular dysplasia
Marfan syndrome
Tuberous sclerosis
Ehlers-Danlos syndrome
Hereditary hemorrhagic telangiectasia (HHT)
Collagen deficiency
Moya-moya disease
Neurofibromatosis type 1
Pseudoxanthoma elasticum

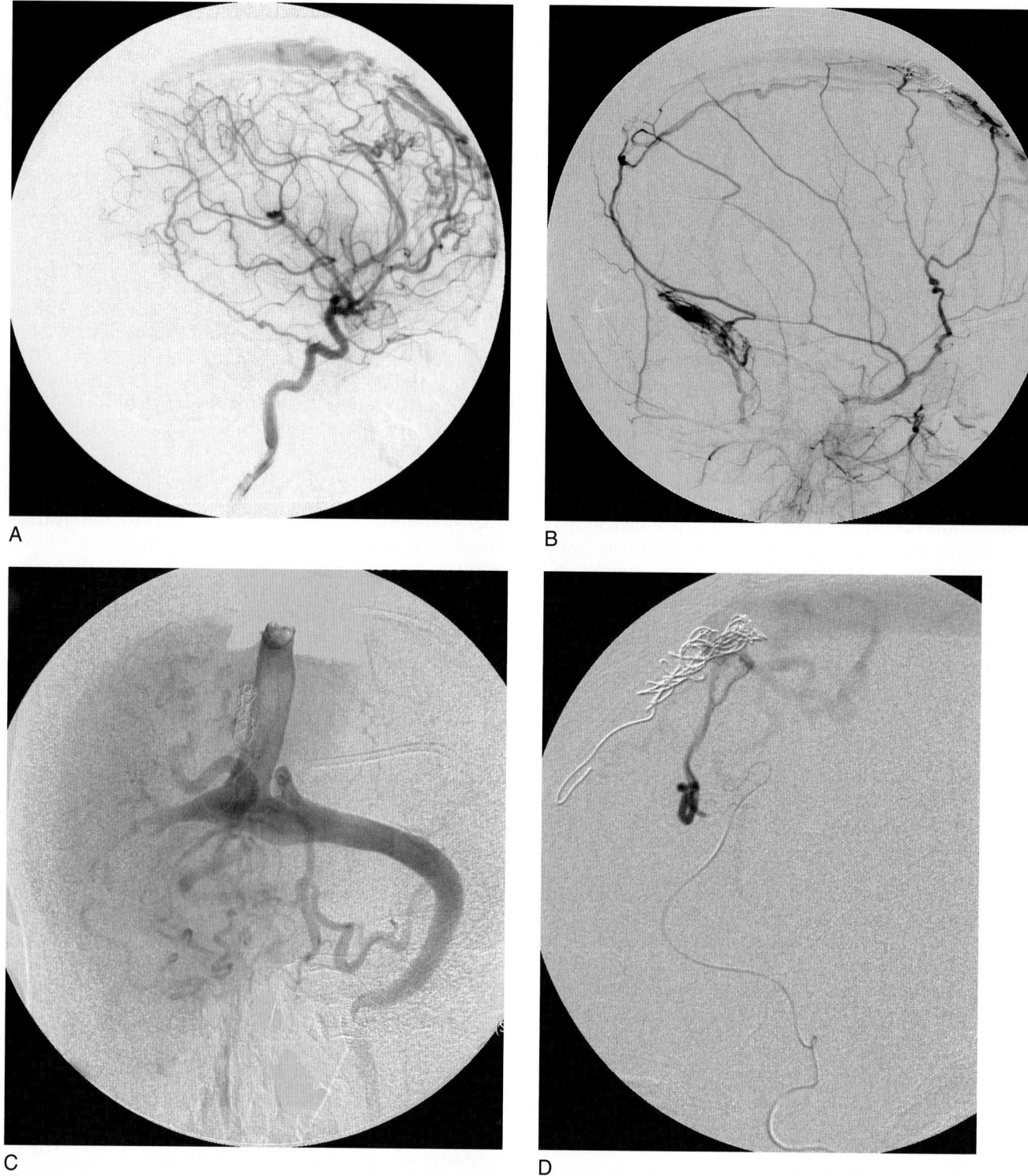

FIGURE 184-1. Dural arteriovenous fistula (DAVF). **A,** A left internal carotid artery injection reveals fistulous connections between interhemispheric branches of the anterior cerebral artery and the anterior superior sagittal sinus. The DAVF remains patent despite a prior attempt at closure made by depositing the coils visible at the site of the fistula. In addition to this pial-dural connection, the fistula is fed by a dural supply along the free edge of the tent and ascending through the falx cerebri—the artery of Bernesconi and Castinari. **B,** A left external carotid artery injection shows contribution to the fistula also by dural branches of the external carotid system. The anterior branch of the middle meningeal artery feeds the fistula, while the ascending pharyngeal artery contributes; a separate fistula in the low transverse sinus is also fed. Similar appearances were noted in the right internal and external carotid system. **C,** Intracranial hypertensive venopathy associated with fistulas is due to progressive narrowing and occlusion of the dural sinuses. The right transverse sinus is occluded, and the left has become significantly stenosed. Intracranial hypertensive venopathy causes alternative venous drainage with enlargement of basal veins and alternative exits. Venous congestion is also evident in the delayed venous drainage of the right cerebral hemisphere. Decreased perfusion caused by venous hypertension produces cerebral atrophy. **D,** Treatment by the endovascular arterial approach involves superselective catheterization of the branches from the anterior cerebral artery to the fistula. A microcatheter is positioned in a branch of the anterior cerebral artery that is dedicated entirely to the fistula, in preparation for occlusion of this branch with liquid adhesive. Ideally, the adhesive should occlude the artery as far as the arteriovenous connection but should not flow distally into the vein.

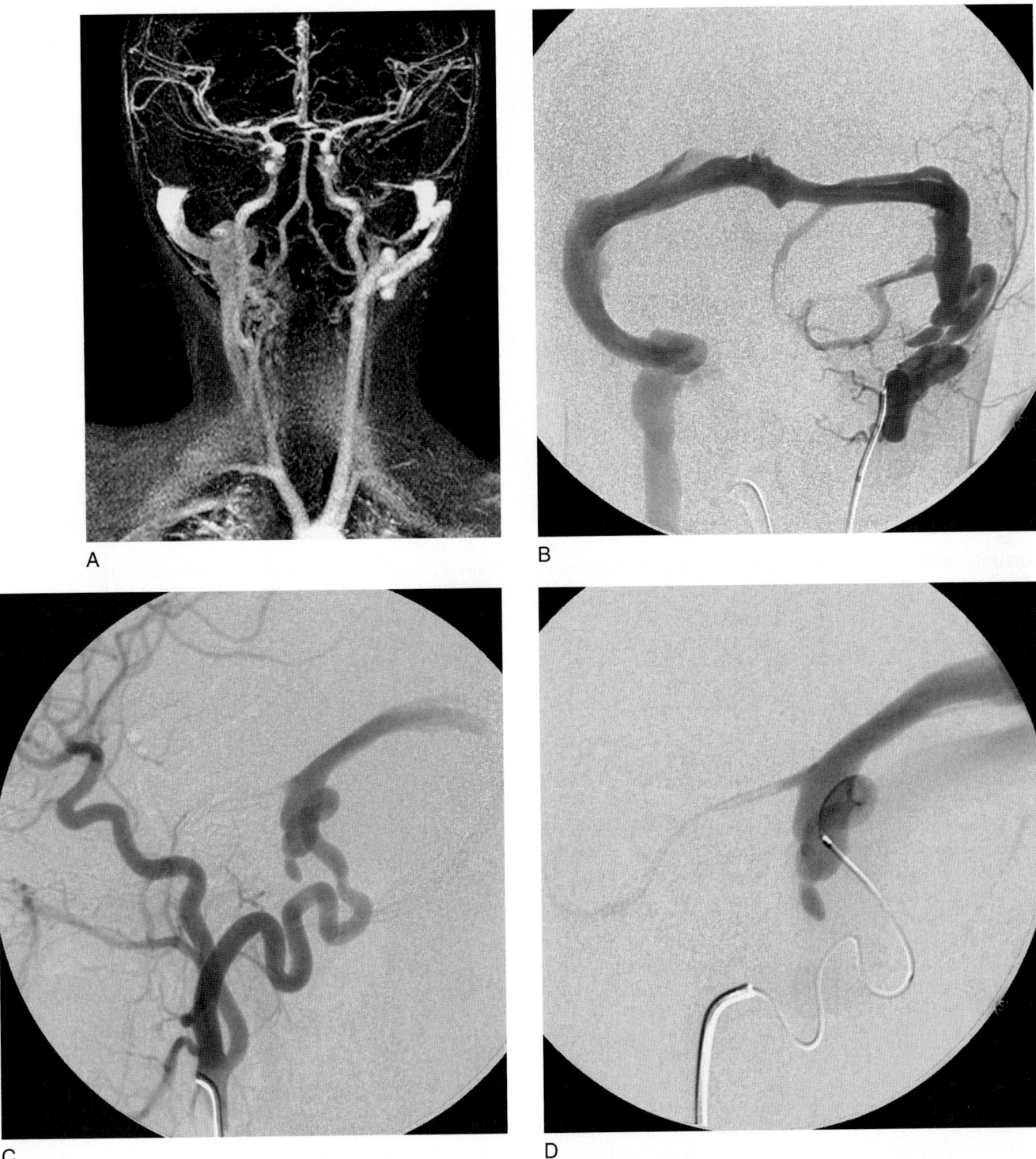

A

B

C

D

FIGURE 184-2. Large single-hole dural arteriovenous (AV) fistula. **A,** Magnetic resonance angiography reveals the dural AV fistula, along with an enlarged left occipital artery that empties into the left sigmoid sinus. The right sigmoid sinus and the internal jugular vein can be seen, while the left sigmoid sinus is occluded. **B,** Angiography with contrast injection into the left occipital artery in the anteroposterior plane shows the single-hole AV fistula between the occipital artery and the left sigmoid sinus. The left sigmoid sinus is totally occluded. A petrosal sinus fills. Drainage of the AV fistula follows the transverse sinus system to empty into the right internal jugular vein. This arterialized sinus system is the common exit pathway for venous drainage of the brain. Raised intracranial venous pressure causes cerebral venous congestion with decreased perfusion. **C,** Contrast injection into the left common carotid artery reveals a normal internal maxillary and internal carotid system with enlarged left occipital artery and fistula to the sigmoid sinus. The left sigmoid sinus is closed because of hypertensive occlusive venopathy. **D,** Superselective catheterization of the left occipital artery, with the catheter in an appropriate position for liquid adhesive occlusion of the artery immediately proximal and at the fistula.

Continued

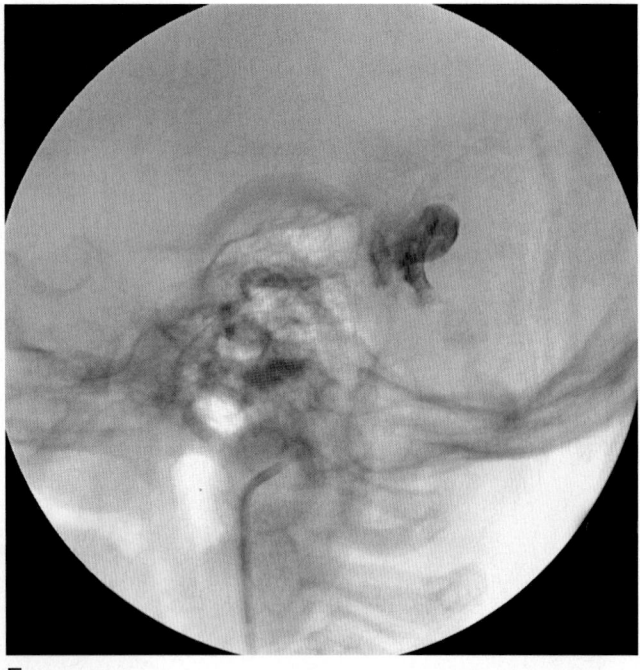
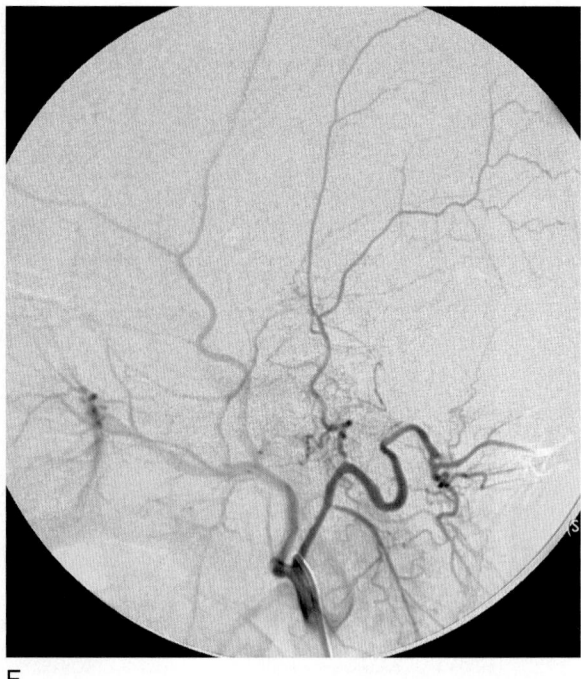

E   F

FIGURE 184-2, *cont'd*. Large single-hole dural arteriovenous (AV) fistula. **E,** Lateral view of the skull following embolization shows the glue cast. Glue opacification results from its mixture with Lipiodol and tantalum powder. The cast corresponds to the superselective position of the microcatheter and occludes the distal artery, as well as the fistula, at its window, with some entry of adhesive into the sigmoid sinus. **F,** Angiography performed 3 months later shows persistent closure of the fistula and decreased size of the occipital artery, with only muscular and scalp branches fed.

imately 10% of intracranial aneurysms present with seizures or stroke.

Aneurysms may be classified as saccular, traumatic, or mycotic. Saccular aneurysms account for 50% to 70% of aneurysms in children, and traumatic aneurysms and infectious or mycotic aneurysms represent 5% to 15% each; traumatic and mycotic aneurysms have a greater incidence in childhood than in adulthood. Traumatic aneurysms have also been reported as representing 39% of pediatric intracranial aneurysms.

Saccular aneurysms typically occur at the bifurcations of the large intracranial arteries, commonly in the anterior circulation at the carotid bifurcation. They are more common in males, in contrast to female predominance in adults, and are more commonly "giant," with a diameter of 2.5 cm or greater. The giant aneurysm typically presents with abnormal neurologic findings due to local compression by the aneurysmal sac (Fig. 184-3).

Traumatic aneurysms may follow penetrating injury with direct injury to the vessel, or blunt injury with closed head trauma. The clinical history may, however, include only mild or insignificant trauma, or the absence of any specific traumatic event. The traumatic aneurysm is typically small and irregular in shape, and it involves peripheral branches, including the distal anterior and posterior cerebral arteries in their association with the free edge of the falx cerebri or tentorium, or larger vessels with injury and fracture at the skull base (Fig. 184-4). Clinical presentation with hemorrhage from the aneurysm typically is delayed following the traumatic event. The traumatic aneurysm is considered to be a false aneurysm, or pseudoaneurysm, and the "aneurysmal sac"

represents nonclotted blood within an extravascular hematoma. Rarely, traumatic aneurysms may be related to birth.

Mycotic or infectious aneurysms arise from septic involvement of the arterial wall, with focal arteritis and weakening of the vessel wall observed with subsequent aneurysmal dilation. Local arteritis may be due to bacterial, fungal, or protozoan sepsis; bacterial endocarditis is the most common cause. Mycotic aneurysms are also typically small and irregular; they may be fusiform and may be peripherally located.

Treatment of intracranial aneurysms in children has historically been provided through a surgical approach for clipping of the aneurysmal neck. Reduced morbidity and mortality are noted with the endovascular approach in comparison with the open surgical approach with clipping. For endovascular management, a microcatheter system is navigated to a position within the aneurysm, and the aneurysm is packed with electrolytically detachable coils. The intention is to occlude the lumen of the aneurysm by filling it with coils as far as its neck and preserving the parent vessel. Aneurysms less suitable for intra-aneurysmal coiling because of a wide neck, or fusiform aneurysms, lend themselves better to stenting techniques designed to preserve the parent vessel.

Traumatic and mycotic aneurysms historically have been surgically treated, but currently, they are managed by the endovascular approach. Because of their irregular shape, ill-defined neck, and possible fusiform configuration, with a false aneurysm wall, endovascular treatment commonly involves coil occlusion of the parent vessel adjacent and immediately proximal to the aneurysm.

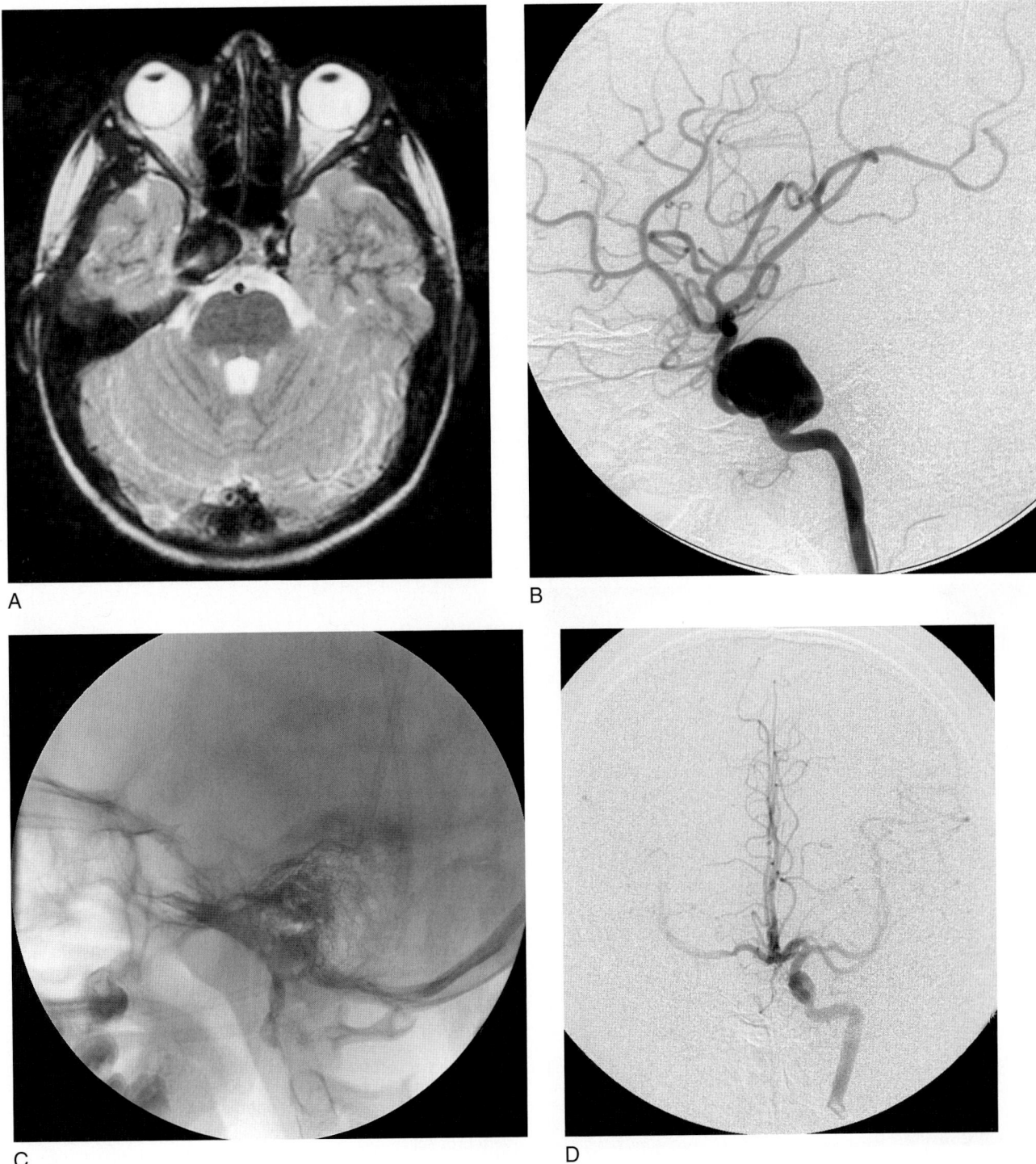

FIGURE 184-3. Aneurysm. **A,** Axial T2-weighted imaging in a 10-year-old girl reveals a large saccular cavernous-suprasellar right internal carotid artery aneurysm, with clinical cranial nerve compression. **B,** Angiography with right internal carotid artery contrast injection shows the large saccular aneurysm and normal filling of the suprasellar internal carotid artery and its branches. **C,** Treatment by sacrifice of the internal carotid artery was performed. A lateral view of a right common carotid artery injection reveals an inflatable balloon in position within the cervical internal carotid artery. With this inflated for balloon test occlusion, the cerebral circulation and perfusion were examined. **D,** Anteroposterior projection with contrast injection into the left internal carotid artery and the right internal carotid artery balloon inflated reveals crossover to the right middle cerebral artery.   *Continued*

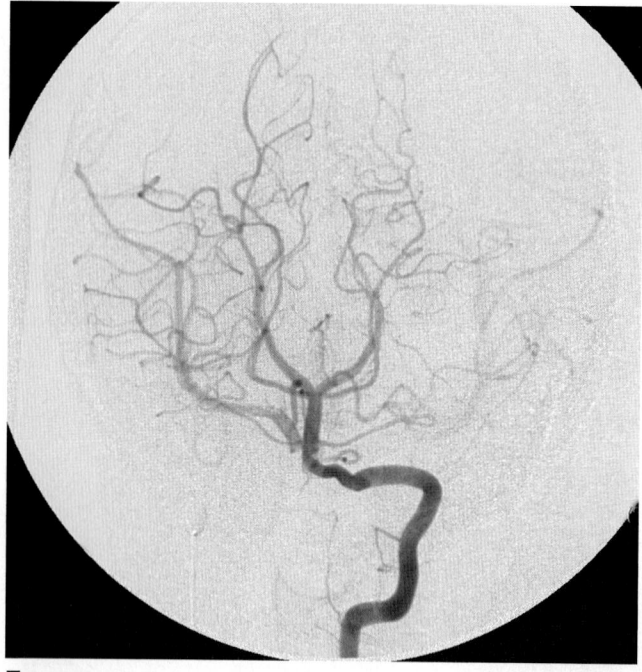

E

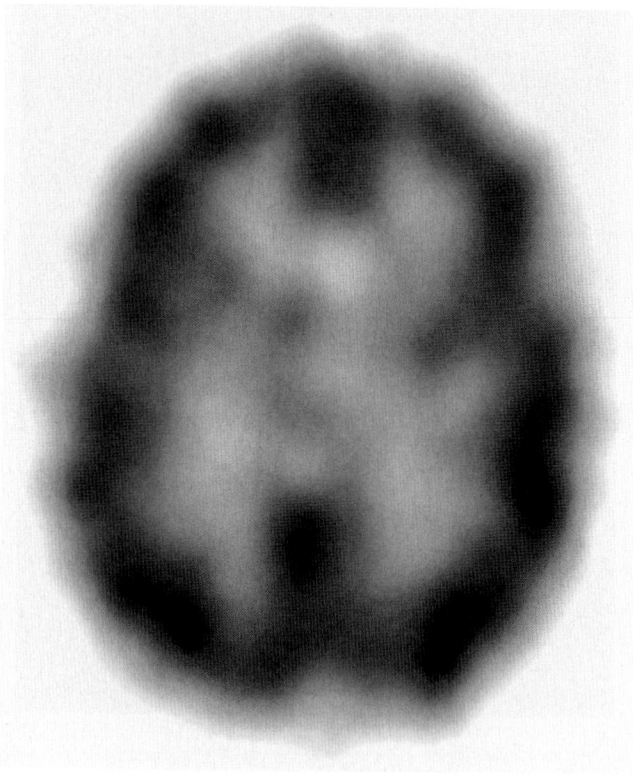

F

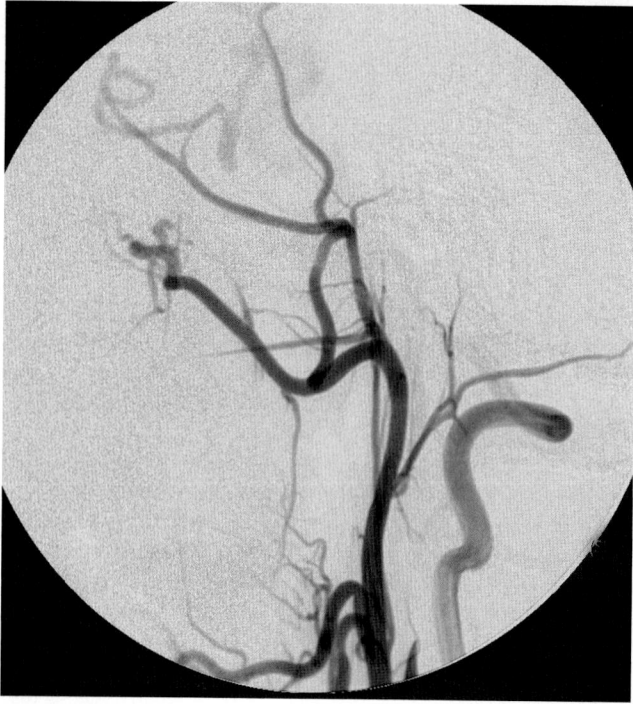

G

FIGURE 184-3, *cont'd.* Aneurysm. **E,** Left vertebral artery contrast injection with the balloon inflated shows flow by the right posterior communicating artery into the right middle cerebral artery. **F,** With the right internal carotid artery balloon inflated, radiopharmaceutical injection for cerebral perfusion assessment shows normal perfusion. **G,** The right internal carotid artery was then permanently occluded with an inflated detachable balloon. Contrast injection into the right common carotid artery system shows occlusion of the right internal carotid artery and closure of the aneurysm. The right internal carotid artery above the aneurysm fills via the congenital meningeal–to–ophthalmic artery anastomosis and via the posterior communicating artery from the vertebrobasilar system.

Patients with a mycotic aneurysm and endovascular occlusion should be investigated and treated for the likely systemic cause and site of septic emboli to the intracranial vessels.

VEIN OF GALEN MALFORMATION

The vein of Galen malformation (VGAM), which is located in the subarachnoid space, represents an uncommon intracranial vascular lesion. It consists mostly of large-caliber arteriovenous fistulas with the vein of Galen. Contributing arteries include choroidal and perforator vessels from the basilar circulation; enlarged anterior cerebral arteries are also present (Fig. 184-5). VGAM is associated with anomalous venous drainage, which may occur via the straight sinus to the torcula via a large anomalous interhemispheric vein that drains into the superior sagittal sinus; apparent absence of the straight sinus has been noted. This may be due to prior thrombosis of the straight sinus with drainage instead

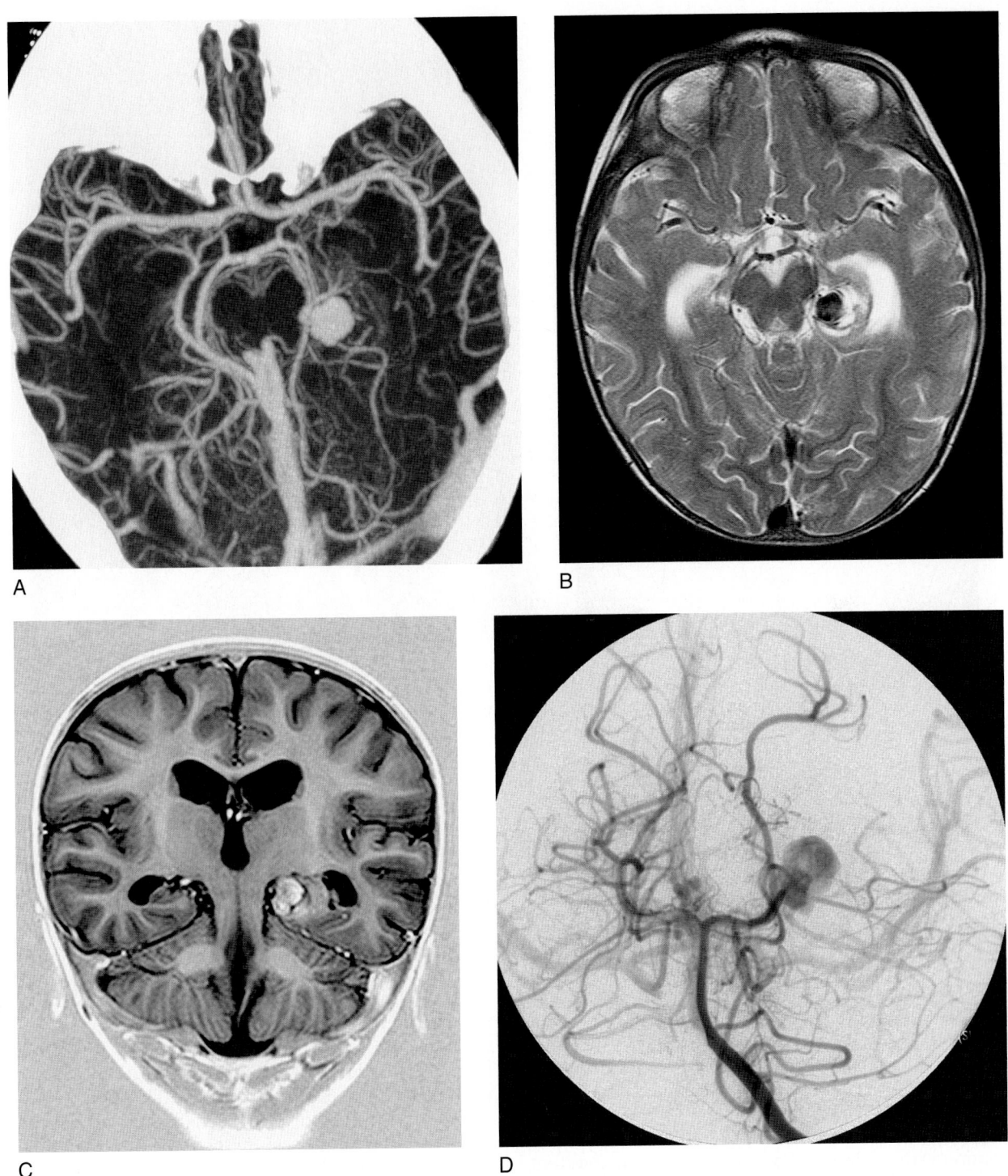

FIGURE 184-4. Traumatic aneurysm. **A,** Computed tomography angiography shows an aneurysm adjacent to the left posterior cerebral artery in its course over the free edge of the tent. **B,** Axial T2-weighted magnetic resonance imaging (MRI) shows the flow void of the aneurysm with adjacent hippocampal edema. The opposite posterior cerebral artery can be seen. **C,** Coronal short tau inversion recovery imaging reveals the aneurysm within the ambient cistern in the course of the left posterior cerebral artery over the edge of the tent. A traumatic aneurysm may develop at this site as the result of injury to the artery caused by the free edge of the tent. **D,** Angiography with left vertebral artery injection shows the aneurysm arising from a branch of the left posterior cerebral artery, while the main branch extends posteriorly.

Continued

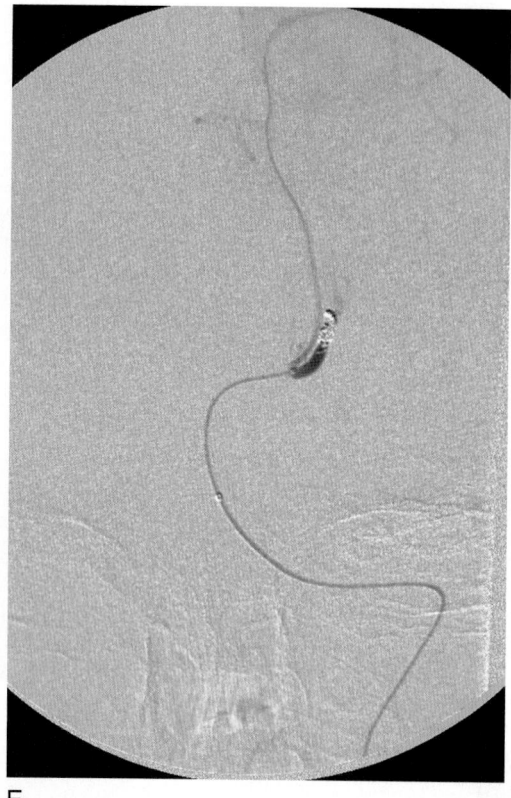
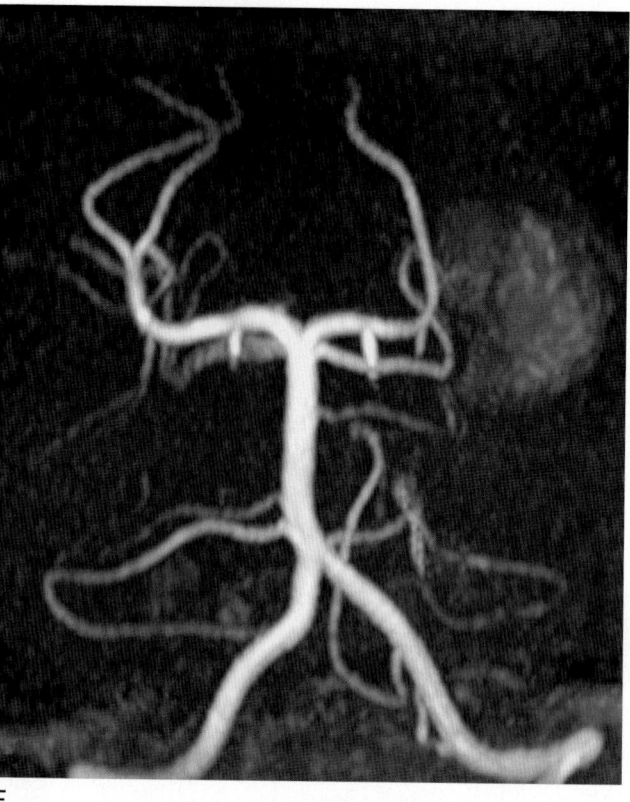

E   F

FIGURE 184-4, *cont'd*. Traumatic aneurysm. **E,** Superselective microcatheter cannulation of the branch feeding the aneurysm shows the coil positioned for occlusion of the aneurysm neck. The main posterior cerebral artery is seen flash-filling with contrast. **F,** MRI with magnetic resonance angiography a week after coil occlusion reveals persistent occlusion of the aneurysm with residual signal caused by clot within it.

to the higher vein—the interhemispheric median prosencephalic vein of Markowski.

The choroidal type of VGAM is much more common than the mural type. In the choroidal type, multiple enlarged choroidal and perforator arteries empty into the dilated vein, and significant arteriovenous shunting predisposes to neonatal or infantile high-output cardiac failure. In the mural type of malformation, a small number of large arteriovenous connections are typically present and neonatal cardiac failure is not associated; instead, the clinical presentation includes developmental delay and macrocrania with hydrocephalus. Rarely, spontaneous thrombosis of the VGAM may occur, in association with venous outflow obstruction due to retention of the fetal venous system or caused by acquired occlusion of the dural sinuses.

VGAM may present in the neonate, during infancy, or later in childhood. The neonate may present on the day of birth or within the following days with high-output cardiac failure. Cardiac failure may be medically managed but may worsen, leading to a fatal outcome within days of birth. Evidence of encephalomalacia and brain volume loss may be apparent at birth as the result of in utero arteriovenous shunting with decreased brain perfusion. Intervention through endovascular therapy is indicated if medical management fails to control cardiac failure.

Historically, management has been surgical and has included ligation of the arterial feeders intracranially, or of the internal carotid arteries in the neck; results have been poor. Currently, endovascular management for transarterial embolization has been provided through the femoral artery approach. Occlusive agents include, historically, PVA particle embolization and coil or detachable balloon occlusion; occlusion by liquid adhesive is the preferred technique. A femoral artery sheath, typically of 4 French size despite the neonate's size, is positioned in the femoral artery. Through a guiding catheter, a microcatheter system is advanced intracranially and the larger arterial feeders are addressed. The intention is to reduce flow through the fistula without necessarily intending to completely close it. Additional endovascular techniques and embolization are best performed at about 6 months of age; the opportunity for the best possible embolization is balanced against the risk of delay in cerebral maturation.

Follow-up includes magnetic resonance imaging (MRI) at approximately 3-month intervals to assess maturation and myelination, along with measurement of head circumference. Head circumference indicates whether head growth has been excessive or decreased. The latter condition indicates encephalomalacia with brain damage due to abnormal flow dynamics of the fistula with raised venous pressure and decreased brain

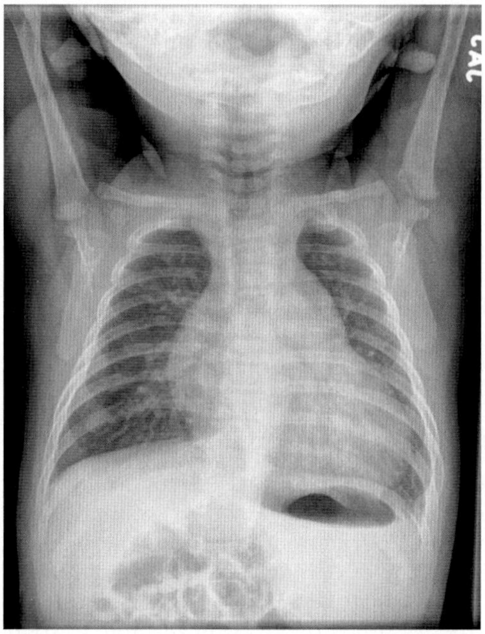

A

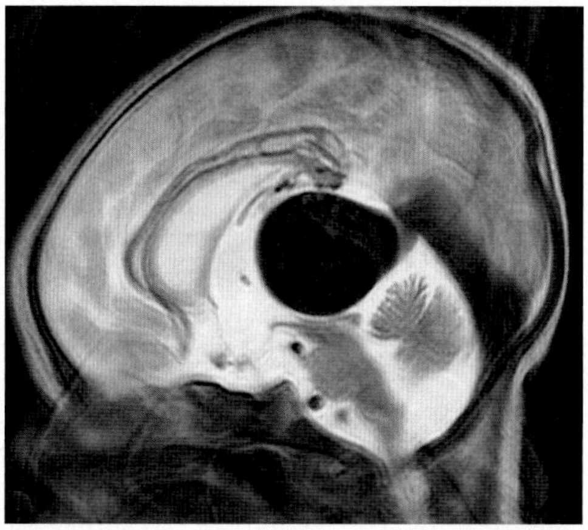

B

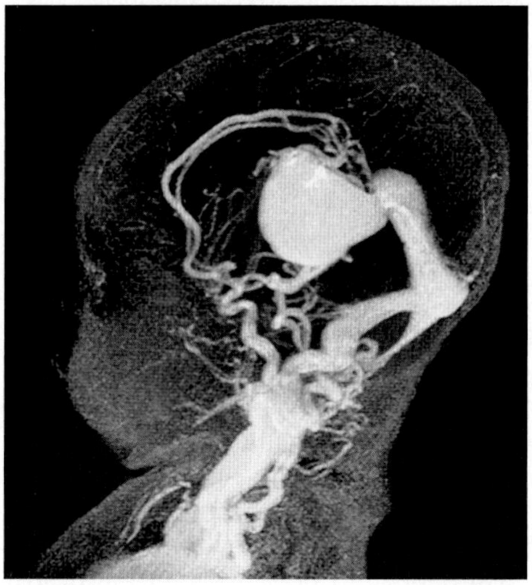

C

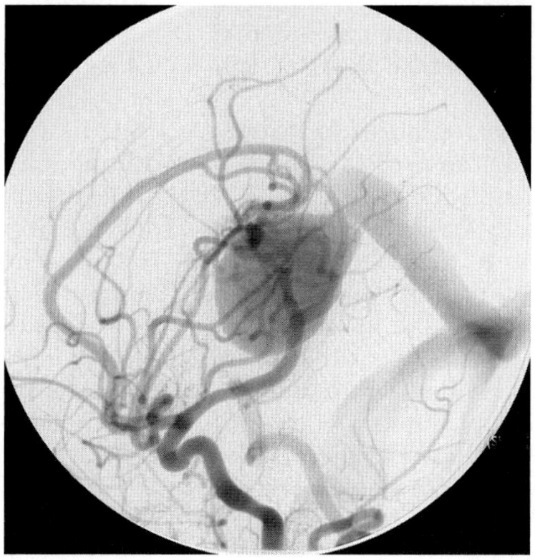

D

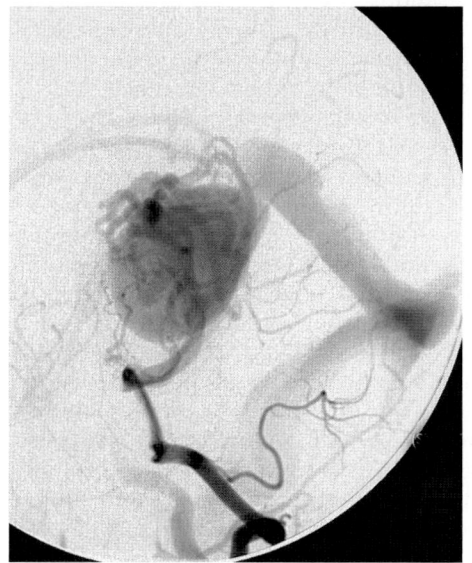

E

FIGURE 184-5. Vein of Galen malformation. **A,** Chest x-ray shows cardiomegaly in a 4-month-old with a vein of Galen malformation. Hyperdynamic high-output failure may occur with this malformation because of lack of capillary resistance in the malformation circuit. Venous return under arterial pressure increases right side loading and pulmonary hypertension, producing increased pulmonary vasculature. **B,** Sagittal T2-weighted magnetic resonance imaging shows the enlarged vein of Galen malformation. Feeders from the anterior cerebral system can be seen emptying into the dome of the malformation. Intraventricular obstructive hydrocephalus is due to compression of the aqueduct by the distended malformation, and extraventricular obstructive hydrocephalus is due to arterialization of the venous sinuses and elevation of their pressure to or above the level of cerebrospinal fluid pressure. **C,** Lateral magnetic resonance angiography image provides an overall view of the arterial supply and venous drainage of the malformation. Arterial and venous structures are seen in the same image. **D,** Internal carotid artery contrast injection shows the supply via enlarged anterior and posterior cerebral arteries with entry into the dome of the malformation and rapid entry into the draining sinuses. **E,** Following embolization by superselective microcatheter occlusion of some of the posterior cerebral artery branches, postembolization contrast injection reveals a decreased number of branches and decreased opacification in the malformation. Staged occlusion may be performed and is further indicated by a state of hydrocephalus or onset of encephalomalacia.

perfusion. Macrocrania is due to hydrocephalus. This occurs because of raised intracranial venous pressure caused by the fistula or because of progressive occlusive venopathy, which is also due to high flow in the sinovenous system; further endovascular occlusion may be required. Persistence of high pressure downstream from the fistula along with chronic venous congestion and compromised cerebrospinal fluid (CSF) flow may give rise to delayed neurologic findings in childhood, including neurodevelopmental delay and seizures, likely associated with delayed or incomplete management of the fistula.

PIAL ARTERIOVENOUS MALFORMATION

With pial AVM, the pial or subpial compartment extends from the pial covering of the cerebral cortex through the brain parenchyma to the venticular ependyma. The AVM consists of a nidus of abnormally thin-walled vessels that directly connect the arterial side of the nidus to the venous side in the absence of capillary circulation. The absence of a capillary bed and of capillary resistance causes the AVM to occur as a low-resistance circuit in parallel to adjacent normal circulation through a capillary bed with capillary resistance. Cerebral ischemia may result from shunting and preferential flow through the AVM.

The venous exit of the AVM is arterialized, or carries blood under arterial pressure, because of the absence of both capillary circulation and capillary resistance. Cerebral venous drainage locally or diffusely may be compromised as normal venous drainage with low venous pressure due to the intervening capillary bed meets and competes for drainage with the venous exit of the AVM. This impairment of normal venous drainage may cause cerebral venous congestion, which may be recognized as tortuous venous channels. As venous pressure rises, brain perfusion pressure, which is the difference between systemic arterial pressure and venous exit pressure, decreases, with consequent reduction in brain perfusion (Fig. 184-6).

As is observed with the dural AV fistula, the pial AVM may cause hyperdynamic cardiac output and associated danger of hyperdynamic cardiac failure. Local or diffuse brain ischemia with atrophic change may be seen. Preferential flow through the lower resistance circuit of the AVM and venous congestion with decreased perfusion pressure may give rise to local or diffuse cerebral atrophic change. Aneurysmal change in the feeding vessels may be seen proximally at the nidus as the result of rapid flow within the circuit (Fig. 184-7). Venous pouches or venous aneurysms distal to the nidus may result from arterialized venous exit pressure (Fig. 184-8). High flow may cause stenosis and occlusion of the draining veins, further increasing venous pressure and compromising venous exit.

The patient with a pial AVM is likely to present with seizure activity or spontaneous hemorrhage, which may be intraparenchymal, intraventricular, or subarachnoid. Surgery has historically been the treatment approach used for resection of the AVM, and resection with surgical cure remains one of the treatment approaches

used in children and in adults. Alternative approaches to the management of pial AVMs—radiation and endovascular occlusion—may be deemed suitable for the individual AVM or may be used in combination with each other and with surgical resection. Focused beam radiation therapy is especially the treatment of choice if the AVM is 3 cm or less in greatest diameter, if it consists of small vessels unsuitable for the endovascular approach, or if it lies in an eloquent area. After radiation treatment is provided to the AVM, 1 to 2 years is required for fibrosis and closure of vessels of the nidus; during this time, the risk of hemorrhage persists. Radiation management may follow as an adjunct to endovascular occlusion if embolization can reduce the AVM to 3 cm or less.

The arterial approach to the AVM and endovascular occlusion has become the primary treatment arm for pial AVMs. For smaller AVMs, a single interventional treatment may totally and permanently occlude the feeding vessels and nidus, but in larger AVMs, subsequent or staged embolizations may be necessary. If the residual component of the AVM is difficult or impossible to treat through further embolization, then surgical resection or radiation management for the residual may follow.

Catheter angiography performed under anesthesia with microcatheter superselective cannulation of the feeding vessel or vessels to the nidus is required for embolization. Biplane angiography with simultaneous subtraction is considered necessary for assessment and understanding of the flow through the nidus via individual feeding vessels and during embolization. In the interventional neuroangiographic procedure, the patient is heparinized with 50 to 100 IU of heparin per kilogram; the larger dose is typically used. Repeated doses of half the original dose are given at 2-hour intervals depending on the duration of the procedure. The embolic material of choice is liquid adhesive—N-butyl-2-cyanoacrylate (NBCA)—which causes permanent occlusion of the arterial branch. Other embolic agents, including PVA sponge and particles, are not appropriate for high-flow lesions because recannalization occurs. Liquid adhesive is preferable to coil occlusion because it occludes the malformation at its nidus; coil embolization causes occlusion only at the position of the coil, with possible distal collateralization, and the lesion may be subsequently untreatable through the endovascular approach.

The microcatheter is advanced through the single or multiple branches that feed the lesion, as closely as possible, beyond branches to normal brain parenchyma, where the liquid adhesive is injected. The intention is to occlude the nidus without passing the adhesive beyond into the draining venous system, and particularly into the large sinovenous system. Embolization of adhesive to the large sinuses may cause their occlusion and acute cerebral venous congestive ischemia. The liquid adhesive is mixed with tantalum powder or Lipiodol to opacify it. The liquid adhesive–Lipiodol mixture ratio depends on the flow characteristics of the feeding branch; a greater concentration of adhesive is appropriate for high volume and rate of flow, for proximity of the nidus, and for proximity of the draining veins. In children and even

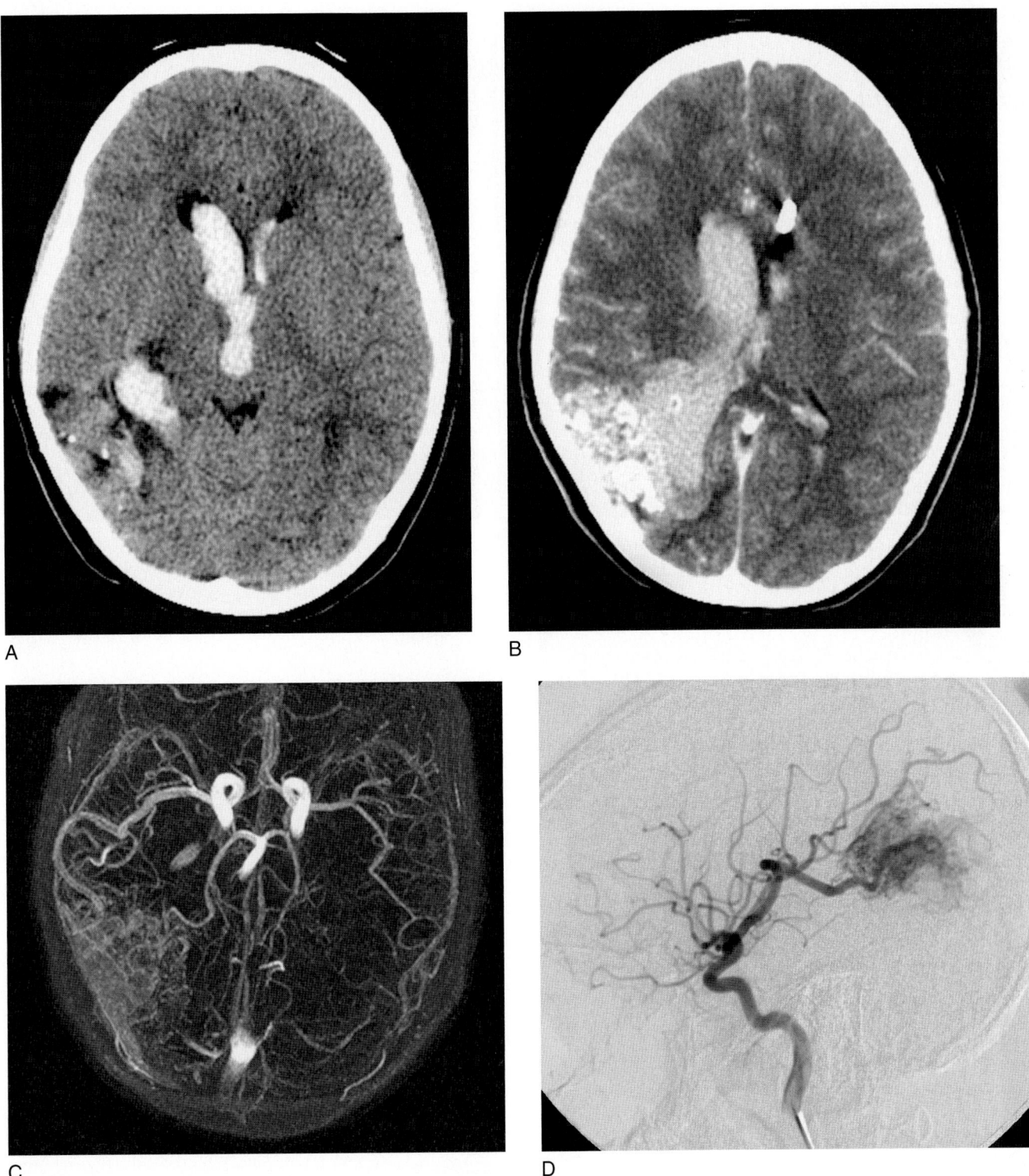

A

B

C

D

FIGURE 184-6. Cerebral arteriovenous malformation (AVM). **A,** Computed tomography scanning following a history of sudden onset of seizures reveals inventricular hemorrhage and a right parieto-occipital lesion with local encephalomalacia and calcification. **B,** Intravenous contrast enhancement shows the agent to consist of a dense rete or nidus of enhancing vessels of variable caliber, indicating the presence of a cerebral arteriovenous malformation. **C,** Magnetic resonance angiography imaging shows the nidus and the feeders rising from enlarged right middle cerebral and posterior cerebral arteries. **D,** Cerebral angiography with contrast injection into the right internal carotid reveals the enlarged sylvian branch of the middle cerebral system and dense opacification of the nidus of the AVM.

Continued

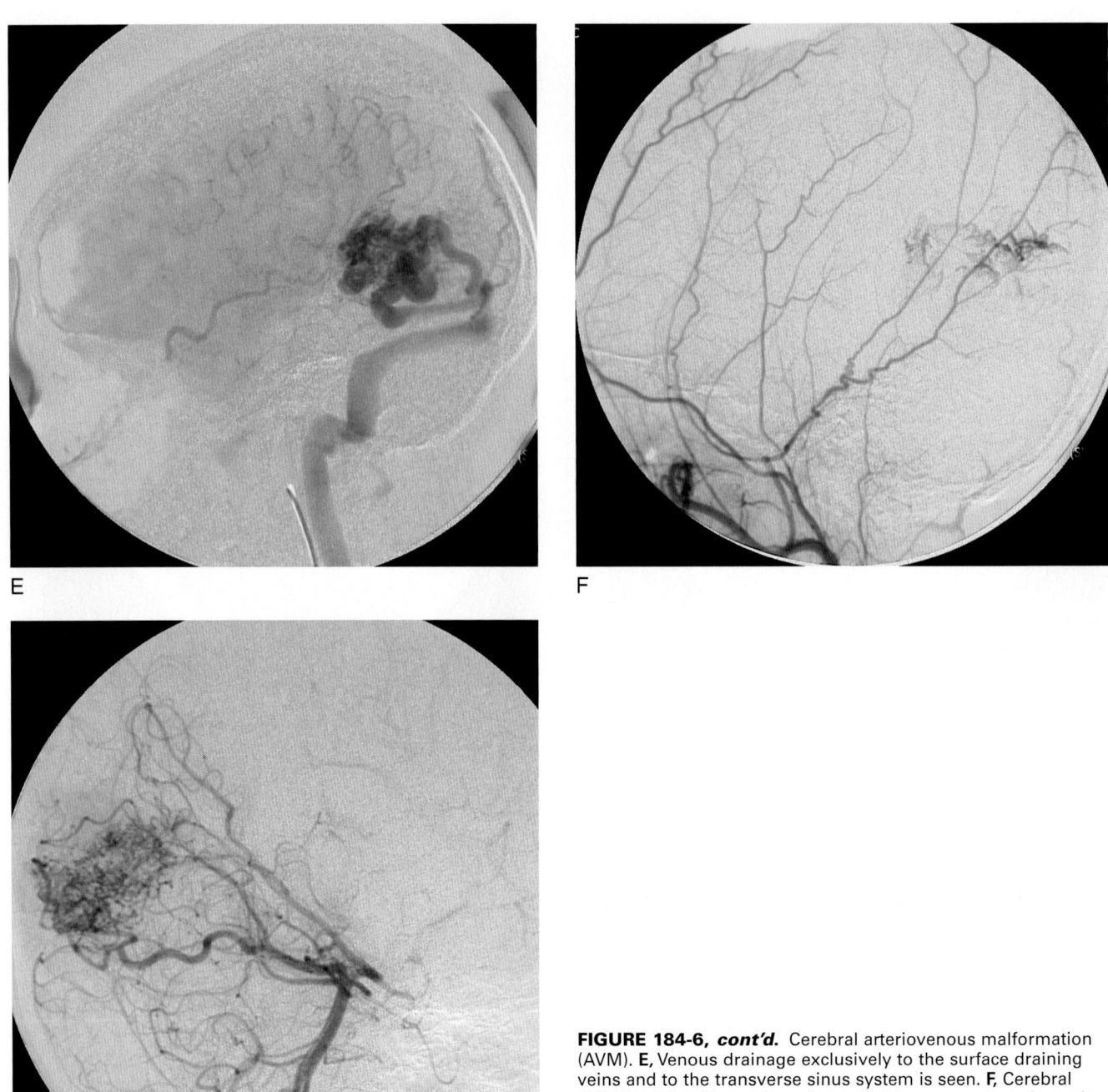

FIGURE 184-6, *cont'd*. Cerebral arteriovenous malformation (AVM). **E,** Venous drainage exclusively to the surface draining veins and to the transverse sinus system is seen. **F,** Cerebral AVM involving the surface pia may pick up a meningeal supply. Contrast injection in to the right internal maxillary system reveals acquired supply from the posterior branch of the middle meningeal artery. **G,** In correlation with the magnetic resonance imaging study, contrast injection into the left vertebral artery with oblique projection reveals the supply to the nidus via the right posterior cerebral artery.

neonates, a 4 French sheath and catheter system may be used for interventional procedures because the 4 French catheter has an internal diameter that is suitable for accepting microcatheter systems. In small infants and neonates, the femoral artery containing the sheath may be occluded for the duration of the angiogram, with

notable change in perfusion and color of the leg, but typically, return to normal circulation occurs after the sheath system has been removed. Rarely, permanent occlusion of the femoral artery occurs, with collateral vessels feeding the artery distal to the occlusion.

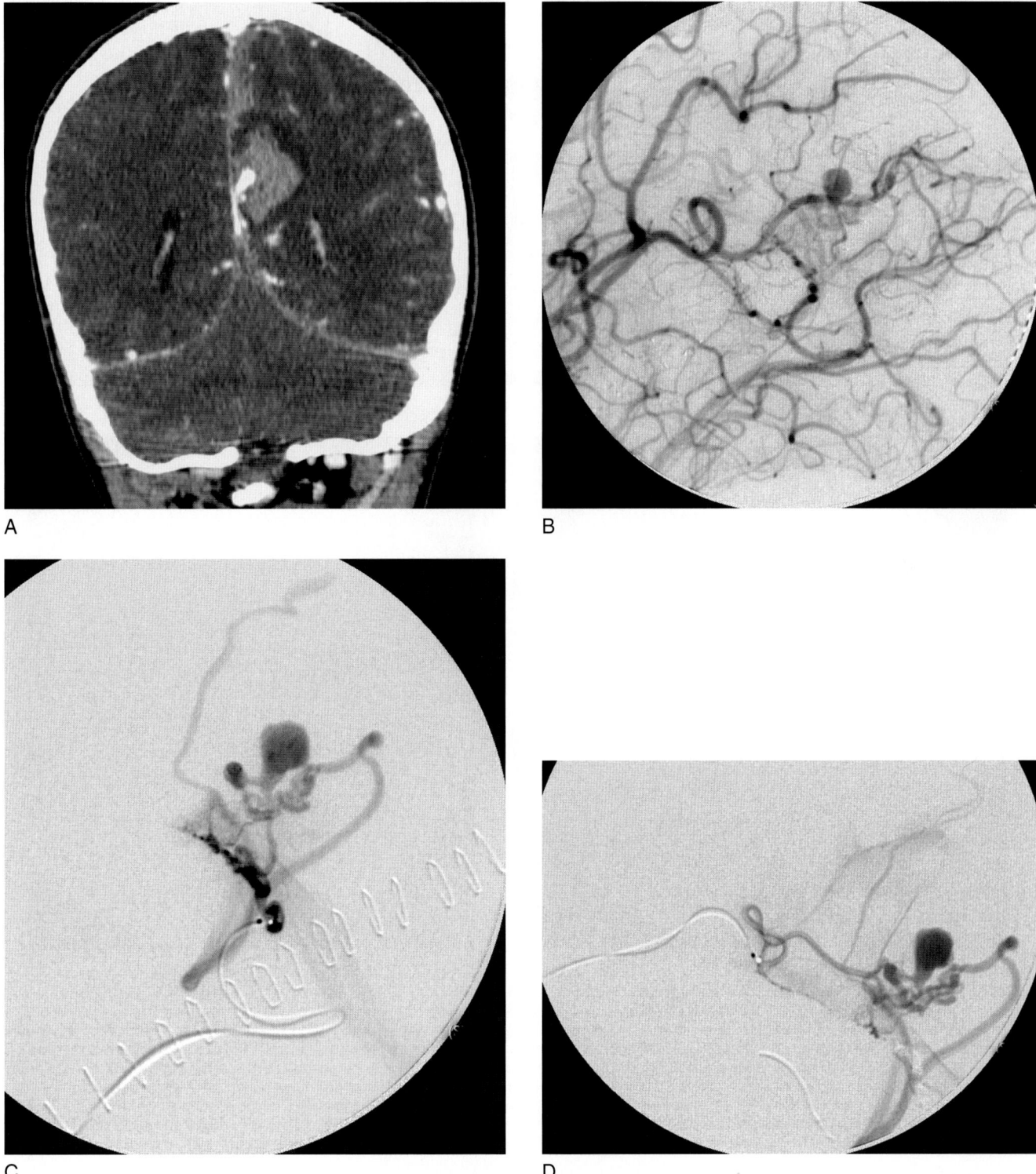

FIGURE 184-7. Cerebral arteriovenous malformation (AVM) with aneurysm pouch. **A,** Coronal contrast-enhanced computed tomography scanning reveals a left parasagittal intracerebral hematoma with a spherical vessel and associated vascular structures. **B,** Angiography with lateral projection of a left internal carotid artery contrast injection shows the vascular pouch associated with a small AVM. **C,** Superselective microcatheter investigation through the left middle cerebral supply reveals the vascular pouch within the nidus; this indicates that the pouch, which fills in the arterial phase, is associated with a small AVM, the venous drainage of which also can be seen. **D,** Superselective catheterization of the anterior cerebral artery contribution reveals the small nidus of the AVM; distal venous drainage indicates that the aneurysmal pouch is associated with the AVM.

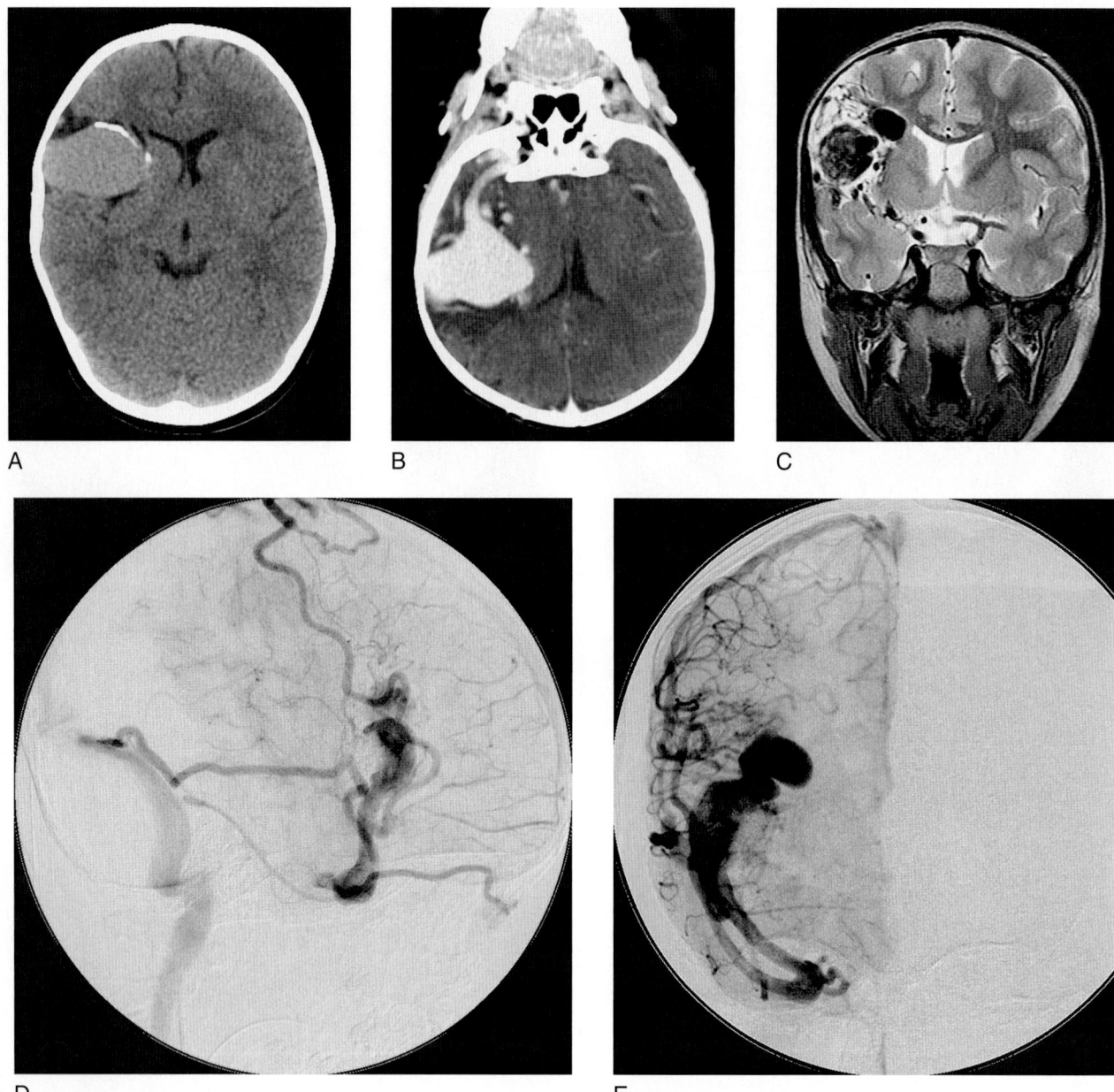

FIGURE 184-8. Cerebral arteriovenous malformation (AVM) with venous pouch. **A,** Axial computed tomography (CT) scanning reveals the hyperdense vascular pouch filled with blood, as well as calcification due to mature clot within its wall. **B,** Coronal contrast-enhanced CT scanning shows filling of the large pouch and a large sylvian draining vein descending to the cavernous sinus; this indicates that the large vascular pouch represents a venous structure associated with the AVM. **C,** Coronal T2-weighted magnetic resonance imaging (MRI) shows the large vascular structure with its flow void appearance and bilobed configuration contained within the sylvian fissure; these are associated with the abnormal vessels of the AVM. **D,** Venous drainage of the AVM shows the pouch located on the venous side of the AVM. Venous drainage via a sylvian vein to the cavernous sinus and to a vein of Labbe and a vein of Trolard can be seen. **E,** Anteroposterior projection of the venous drainage phase reveals the bilobed configuration of the large irregular venous pouch in comparison with the MRI. Cerebral AVMs may be associated with arterial aneurysms or venous varices.

SUGGESTED READINGS

Agid R, Souza M, Reitamm G, et al: The role of endovascular treatment of pediatric aneurysms. Child's Nerv Syst 2005; 21:1030-1036

Albright AL, Latchaw RE, Price RA: Posterior dural arteriovenous malformations in infancy. Neurosurgery 1983;13:129-135

Barrow DL, Spector RH, Braun IF, et al: Classification and treatment of spontaneous carotid-cavernous sinus fistulas. Neurosurgery 1985;62:248-256

Batnitsky S, Muller J: Infantile and juvenile cerebral aneurysms. Neuroradiology 1978;16:61-64

Chaudhary M, Sachdev V, Cho S, et al: Dural arteriovenous malformations of the major venous sinuses: an acquired lesion. AJNR Am J Neuroradiol 1982;3:13-19

Choux M, Lena G, Genitori L: Intracranial aneurysms in children. In Raimondi A, Choux M, Di Rocco C (eds): Cerebrovascular Disease in Children. New York, Springer-Vienna, 1992:123-131

De Marinis P, Punzo A, Colangelo M, et al: Giant aneurysm of the callosomarginal artery. Child's Nerv Syst 1991;7:353-355

Debrun G, Vinuela F, Fox A, et al: Embolization of cerebral arteriovenous malformations with bucrylate. J Neurosurg 1982;56:615-627

Debrun M, Vinuela F, Fox A, et al: Indication for treatment and classification of 132 carotid-cavernous fistulas. Neurosurgery 1988;22:285-289

Halbach VV, Higashida RT, Hieshima G, et al: Treatment of dural arteriovenous malformations involving the superior sagittal sinus. AJNR Am J Neuroradiol 1988;9:337-343

Halbach VV, Higashida RT, Hieshima GB, et al: Transvenous embolization of dural fistulas involving the transverse and sigmoid sinuses. AJNR Am J Neuroradiol 1989;10:385-392

Halbach VV, Higashida RT, Hieshima GB, et al: Transvenous embolization of dural fistulas involving the cavernous sinus. AJNR Am J Neuroradiol 1989;10:377-383

Hoffman HJ, Chuang S, Hendrick EB, et al: Aneurysms of the vein of Galen: experience at the Hospital for Sick Children, Toronto. J Neurosurg 1982;51:316-322

Holmes B, Harbaugh RE: Traumatic intracranial aneurysms: a contemporary review. J Trauma 1993;35:855-860

Humphreys RP: Intracranial arterial aneurysms. In Edwards MSB, Hoffman HJ (eds): Cerebral Vascular Disease in Children and Adolescents. Baltimore, William & Wilkins, 1989

Hurst RW, Kagetsu NJ, Berenstein A: Angiographic findings in two cases of aneurysmal malformation of vein of Galen prior to spontaneous thrombosis: therapeutic implications. AJNR Am J Neuroradiol 1992;13:1446-1450

Hurst W, Bagley L, Galetta S, et al: Dementia resulting from dural arteriovenous fistulas: the pathological findings of venous hypertensive encephalopathy. AJNR Am J Neuroradiol 1998;19:1267-1273

Johnston IH, Whittle IR, Besser M, et al: Vein of Galen malformation: diagnosis and treatment. Neurosurgery 1987;20:747-758

Kanaan I, Lasjaunias P, Coates R: The spectrum of intracranial aneurysms in pediatrics. Minim Invasive Neurosurg 1995;38:1-9

Kessava P, Turski P: Magnetic resonance angiography of vascular malformations. MRI Clin N Am 1998;6

Kiyosue H, Hori Y, Okahara M, et al: Treatment of intracranial dural arteriovenous fistulas: current strategies based on location and hemodynamics, and alternative techniques of transcatheter embolization. Radiographics 2004;24:1637-1653

Lasjaunias P: Vascular Diseases in Neonates, Infants and Children. Berlin, Heidelberg, Springer-Verlag, 1997

Lasjaunias P, Chiu M, TerBrugge K, et al: Neurological manifestations of intracranial dural arteriovenous malformations. J Neurosurg 1986;64:724-730

Lasjaunias P, Wuppalapati S, Alvarez H, et al: Intracranial aneurysms in children aged under 15 years: a review of 59 consecutive children with 75 aneurysms. Child's Nerv Syst 2005;21:437-450

Malek AM, Halbach VV, Higashida RT, et al: Treatment of dural arteriovenous malformations and fistulas. Neurosurg Clin North Am 2000;11:147-166

Martin NA, Edwards M, Wilson CB: Management of intracranial vascular malformations in children and adolescents. Concepts Pediatr Neurosurg 1983;4:264-290

Milhorat TH: Vascular disorders. In Milhorat TH (ed): Pediatric Neurosurgery. Philadelphia, Davis, 1978

Molyneux A, Kerr R, Stratton I, et al: International Subarachnoid Aneurysm Trial (ISAT) of neurosurgical clipping versus endovascular coiling in 2,143 patients with ruptured intracranial aneurysms: a randomized trial. Lancet 2002;360:1267-1274

Myer FB, Sundt TM Jr, Fode NC, et al: Cerebral aneurysms in childhood and adolescents. J Neurosurg 1989;70:420-425

Newton TH: Dural arteriovenous shunts in the region of the cavernous sinus. Neuroradiology 1970;1:71-81

Osborne AG: Intracranial vascular malformations. In Diagnostic Neuroradiology. St. Louis, Mosby-Year Book, 1994:303

Ostergaard JR: Etiology of intracranial saccular aneurysms in children. Br J Neurosurg 1991;5:575-580

Ostergaard JR, Voldby B: Intracranial arterial aneurysms in children and adolescents. J Neurosurg 1983;58:832-837

Parkinson D, Bachers G: Arteriovenous malformations: summary of 100 consecutive supratentorial cases. J Neurosurg 1980;53:285-299

Piatt J, Clunie D: Intracranial arterial aneurysm due to birth trauma. J Neurosurg 1992;77:799-803.

Pollock BE, Gorman DA, Coffey RJ: Patient outcomes after arteriovenous malformation radiosurgical management: results based on a 5-14 years follow-up study. Neurosurgery 2003;52:1291-1296; discussion:1296-1297

Raybaud CA, Strother CM, Hald JA: Aneurysms of the vein of Galen: embryonic consideration and anatomic features relating to the pathogenesis of the malformation. Neuroradiology 1989;31:109-128

Schoenberg BS, Mellinger JF, Schoenberg DG: Cerebrovascular disease in infants and children: a study of incidence, clinical features, and survival. Neurology 1978;28:763-768

Schoenberg BS, Schoenberg DG: Spectrum of pediatric cerebrovascular disease. In Rose FC (ed): Clinical Neuroepidemiology. New York, State Mutual Books, 1980:151-162

Seidenwurm D, Berenstein A, Hyman A, et al: Vein of Galen malformation: correlation of clinical presentation, arteriography and MR imaging. AJNR Am J Neuroradiol 1991;12:347-354

Tang D, Kerber C, Biglan A, et al: External carotid-cavernous fistula in infancy: case report and review of the literature. Neurosurgery 1981;8:212-218

Ventureyra EC, Higgins MJ: Traumatic intracranial aneurysms in childhood and adolescence: case reports and review of the literature. Child's Nerv Syst 1994;10:361-379

CHAPTER

185 Pediatric Vascular Procedures: Arterial and Venous

JAMES S. DONALDSON

INTRODUCTION

A substantial need continues for gaining intravascular access (venous and arterial) for appropriate delivery of medical care to children. Venous access for medication delivery and blood sampling is essential, but the use of other vascular diagnostic and therapeutic procedures in pediatric care is on the rise. These include such procedures as transvenous biopsies, portal or hepatic vein interventions, venous and arterial thrombolysis, angioplasty, and embolization. In this chapter, basic elements of diagnostic arteriography are discussed, and a brief overview of vascular access devices is presented.

VASCULAR ACCESS

Obtaining vascular access in children through the use of palpation and anatomic landmarks can be very challenging. Image-guided vascular access techniques have been shown to improve success rates and reduce complications. Ultrasound (US) guidance has proved to be a very reliable means of attaining vascular access in children. This is not to say that all standard intravenous (IV) access in uncomplicated patients has been or should be replaced by US-guided techniques, but the imaging tools available provide a reliable backup in difficult situations and should serve as standard practice in high-risk situations.

> Image-guided vascular access techniques have been shown to improve success rates and reduce complications.

Imaging Guidance for Vascular Access

Contrast venography with fluoroscopic guidance is used by some as a method for gaining venous access. Although this technique is used successfully by many, is has many disadvantages compared with US. It cannot be used for jugular, portal, or hepatic venous access, or for arterial access, because none of these vascular structures can be directly opacified with contrast material for fluoroscopy-guided access. In some children, a peripheral IV needed for the contrast venogram cannot be obtained; thus, the ability to achieve access with the use of this technique is limited. Additionally, the need for contrast and added fluoroscopy and procedure time make this technique less desirable. One advantage of venography in children with a history of prior venous lines is its usefulness in assessment of veins for patency and stenoses. Fluoroscopy-guided vein puncture is a technique that is somewhat easier to learn than US, and it may be preferred by radiologists who are not as familiar with US-guided techniques.

ULTRASONOGRAPHY-GUIDED ACCESS TECHNIQUE

The transducer can be oriented longitudinally to the vessel that is being punctured, but a transverse orientation is preferred by many operators. With the transducer orientated transversely over the vein, the needle tip can be precisely centered over the vein for the puncture (Fig. 185-1). Needle and transducer are advanced simultaneously toward the target vessel. When the needle tip approaches the target vessel (indenting the front wall of a vein but not an artery), an attempt is made to change the angle of puncture such that the needle is more parallel to the vessel. Advancing the needle almost parallel to the vessel usually ensures that the puncture will be a single-wall puncture, not a two-wall puncture. When one is puncturing deeper vessels, it is important to carefully watch the needle tip and avoid puncturing the back wall. Achieving a single-wall puncture ensures a successful catheterization.

ARTERIAL PROCEDURES

Diagnostic arteriography is gradually being replaced with noninvasive imaging. This is happening in all organ systems from neurovascular to extremity imaging. Indications for diagnostic studies alone still occur, but many times, a diagnostic study is done in conjunction with a

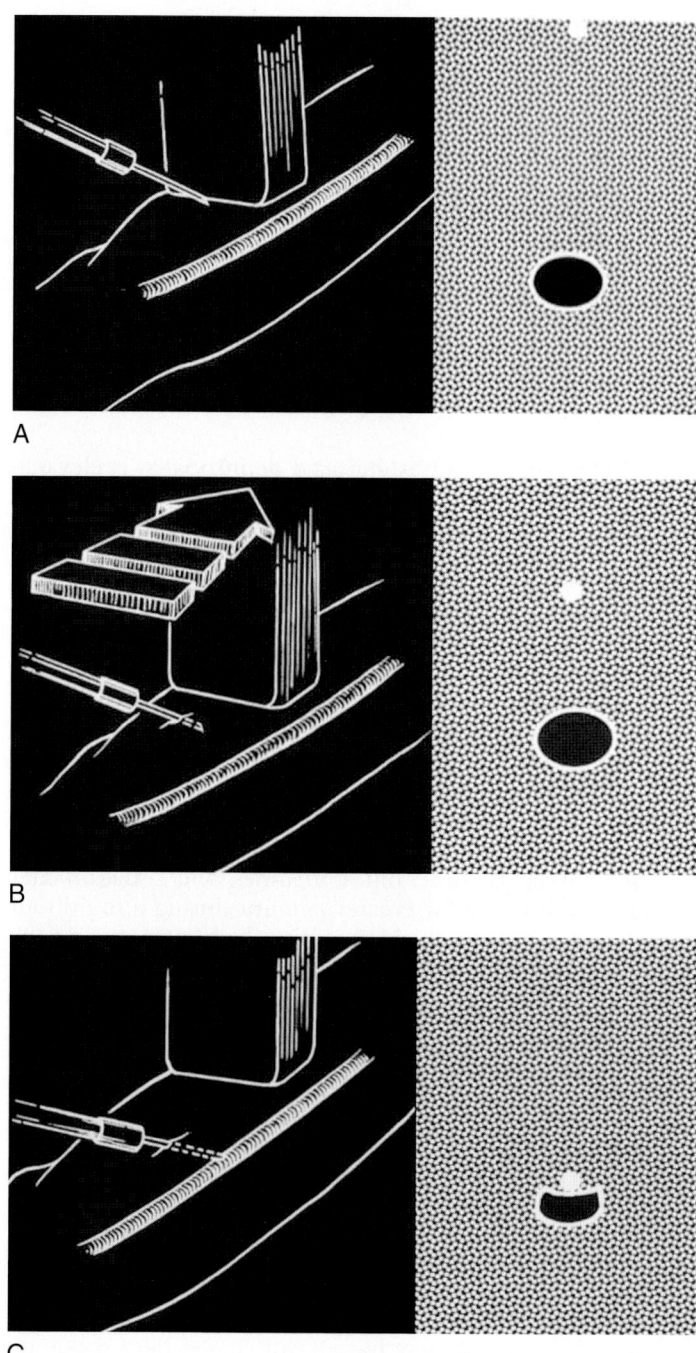

A

B

C

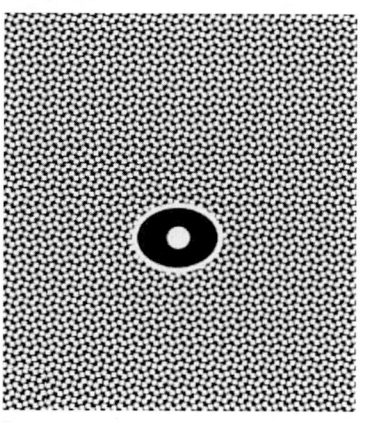

D

FIGURE 185-1. Ultrasonic placement of needle puncture. **A,** Diagram of ultrasound (US) transducer over needle puncture site centered over target vessel is seen on left. Schematic of US image on right illustrates needle tip just below skin surface and centered over circular, transversely imaged vessel below. **B,** Diagram on left of the transducer that is being advanced after needle tip as it penetrates soft tissues toward target vessel. Schematic on right shows needle tip closer to the vein. **C,** Diagram and schematic both show needle just above target vessel. Note indentation of anterior vessel wall. Needle should be advanced as parallel to the vein as possible beyond this point to avoid two-walled puncture. **D,** Needle tip has punctured vessel wall and is seen as a bulls-eye within the vessel lumen. The needle with or without an outer sheath can be advanced farther into the vein, ensuring a successful catheterization, before an attempt is made to introduce the guidewire.

therapeutic intervention (e.g., angioplasty, embolization). The added challenges associated with performing arteriography in children have made the transition to non-invasive imaging occur that much faster, even though a different set of obstacles is involved when one is performing good noninvasive imaging in children.

Technique

Arterial access is frequently attained with the use of a 22 gauge micropuncture needle; this is often done under ultrasound guidance. Arterial access in older children and adolescents may be attained through palpation alone, if a pulse is easily palpable. Ultrasound guidance facilitates the use of only a single-wall puncture. An 0.018″ guidewire is introduced, and the needle is exchanged for a coaxial introducer set that allows upsizing to a 0.035″ wire. If a single catheter will be used during the procedure, a vascular sheath is not necessary; however, if catheter exchanges are anticipated during the arteriogram, then a vascular sheath should be used. Arterial access into the brachial artery can be attained if groin access is not possible. Size of the vascular sheath depends on the size of the catheters needed. Generally, 4 or 4.5 French sheaths are used, except in the smallest infants.

If catheterization of the superficial femoral artery becomes occlusive to the artery, heparin is given immediately after vascular access is achieved. The heparin dose is between 50 and 100 µ/kg, with 75 µ/kg being a common dose. If an examination is lengthy, an activated clotting time (ACT) measurement can be obtained during the procedure and additional heparin given accordingly; a minimum time of 250 to 300 seconds is targeted. Arterial closure devices have not been widely used in pediatrics, and direct pressure to the arterial puncture site has been standard for achieving hemostasis. If the child has been anticoagulated, an ACT may be repeated until the time is less than 200 seconds before the catheter will be pulled.

> If catheter exchanges are anticipated during the arteriogram, then a vascular sheath should be used.

Contrast Agents

Currently, four classes of iodinated contrast media are available for clinical use: high osmolar ionic monomers, low osmolar nonionic monomers, low osmolar ionic dimers, and iso-osmolar nonionic dimers. All contrast media are distributed during the extracellular phase; they do not penetrate an intact blood-brain barrier, and all are excreted via glomerular filtration. Most diagnostic radiology departments have switched to exclusive use of one of several nonionic contrast agents, thus reducing the incidence of severe life-threatening reactions. The prevalence of adverse reactions with low osmolar contrast media is lower in comparison with high osmolar contrast media by a factor of 5 to 6. Lethal reactions rarely occur.

TABLE 185-1
Risk Factors for Contrast-Induced Nephropathy

Chronic kidney disease
Diabetes mellitus (type 1 or type 2)
Volume depletion
Nephrotoxic drug use (nonsteroidal anti-inflammatory drugs [NSAIDs], cyclosporine, aminoglycosides)
Preprocedural hemodynamic instability
Other comorbidities
Anemia
Congestive heart failure
Hypoalbuminemia

The risk of contrast-induced nephropathy is elevated and becomes important in patients with chronic kidney disease characterized by an estimated glomerular filtration rate <60 mL/min/1.73 m². Evidence suggests that the risk for contrast-induced nephropathy in high-risk patients is greater among patients receiving low osmolar nonionic monomeric rather than iso-osmolar nonionic dimeric contrast media. However, various studies have reported conflicting results. A list of risk factors for contrast-induced nephropathy is provided in Table 185-1.

The maximum dose of contrast media that is allowable in a pediatric patient who is undergoing arterial intervention is not an absolute number. A target limit of 4 ml/kg is ideal, but sometimes, the situation may require use of a far greater amount during a multihour complex procedure. Maintaining hydration during the procedure is important.

> It is most important to maintain hydration; a contrast media target limit of 4 ml/kg is ideal.

Catheters

Catheters and guidewires needed for pediatric arteriography are similar to those needed for general adult work. Improved catheter materials allow completion of many procedures with the use of 4 French catheters, but in larger patients, 5 French systems may be used. The use of 3 French catheters has all but ceased, and these are seldom used by most pediatric interventionalists. The reverse-curve shaped catheters are made in tiny sizes and are ideal for selecting downward directed arteries off of the aorta.

THORACIC AORTOGRAPHY

Indications for thoracic aortography still occasionally may include evaluation of trauma, aneurysm, dissection, aortitis, and congenital abnormalities. Thoracic aortography is also performed as a road map for bronchial artery catheterization and embolization (see Chapter 182). Thoracic aortography remains the definitive study for traumatic injury to the aorta from blunt or penetrating chest trauma, and it may be necessary if computed tomography (CT) angiography is equivocal (Fig. 185-2).

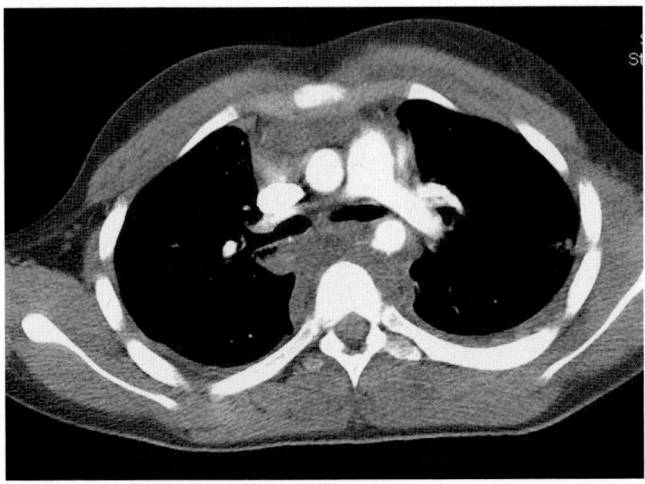

A

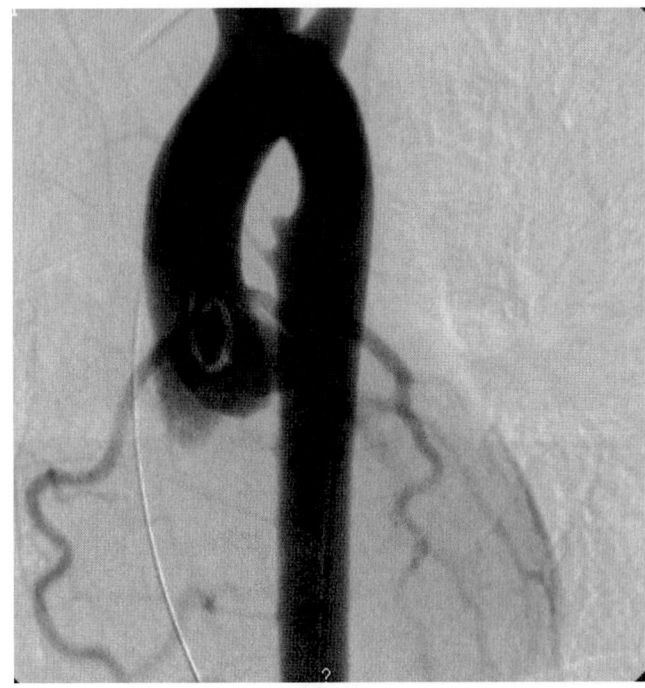

B

FIGURE 185-2. Traumatic aortic laceration. **A,** Computed tomography image through the mediastinum reveals aortic wall irregularity and mediastinal hematoma, raising suspicion for aortic laceration. **B,** A confirmatory aortogram reveals traumatic injury to the aorta on the inferior aspect of the arch distal to the subclavian artery.

Other indications include evaluation of vasculitis such as Takayasu arteritis, or Kawasaki disease (Figs. 185-3, 185-4).

A thoracic aortogram is performed with a pigtail catheter that allows sufficient flow rates to opacify the aorta. During the procedure, 4 to 7 French pigtails are placed within the ascending aorta just superior to the sinuses of Valsalva. A vigorous hand injection can confirm catheter position prior to the power injection. Injection rates depend on the size of the child; a general rule is provided in Table 185-2.

For trauma, at least two views of the aorta are necessary to ensure adequate evaluation. The most important view is a 30 degree to 45 degree left anterior oblique, which images the aortic arch en face. Other views include a straight anteroposterior (AP) view and a 30 degree right anterior oblique view. Rapid sequence filming rates are important, and a rate of at least 3 to 4 films per second is required.

> **For trauma, at least two views of the aorta are necessary.**

UPPER AND LOWER EXTREMITY ANGIOGRAPHY

Indications for extremity angiography include trauma, assessment of certain vascular malformations, vasculitis, ischemic peripheral vascular disease, and evaluation of thoracic outlet syndrome (Figs. 185-5, 185-6). The examination begins with an arch angiogram that is focused on the great vessels. A selective catheter is used to catheterize the innominate or left subclavian artery. Evaluation of the central arteries is done first, followed by evaluation of the peripheral extremity. Lower extremity examination begins with pelvis arteriography.

Long, slow injections of contrast medium are necessary for adequate opacification of the distal arteries of the hand and foot. Vasodilator injection of nitroglycerin 100 to 200 micrograms or tolazoline 10 to 25 mg can be used to enhance blood flow to the extremity.

ABDOMINAL AORTOGRAPHY

The most frequent indication for abdominal aortography is for it to be completed as part of the evaluation for renovascular hypertension. Other indications include evaluation of hepatic artery patency in liver transplantation patients, vascular anomalies, mesenteric ischemia, and gastrointestinal (GI) bleeding (Fig. 185-7). Lateral aortography is obtained in mesenteric ischemia and in evaluation of vasculitis.

RENAL ANGIOGRAPHY

Renal angiography is performed in the evaluation of hypertension. See Chapter 192 for a complete discussion of renovascular hypertension.

MESENTERIC ANGIOGRAPHY

Mesenteric angiography is the study of the celiac, superior mesenteric, and inferior mesenteric vessels. The most common indication in pediatrics is the evaluation of GI bleeding, trauma, vasculitis, and malformations (Figs. 185-8, 185-9).

A reverse-curve catheter (Sos 0) is usually preferred for selection of celiac and mesenteric arteries. Cobra or simple-angle tip catheters may also be used to easily select the visceral arteries. Long, slow injections are needed to opacify the entire mesenteric vascular bed or to visualize the splenic vascular bed.

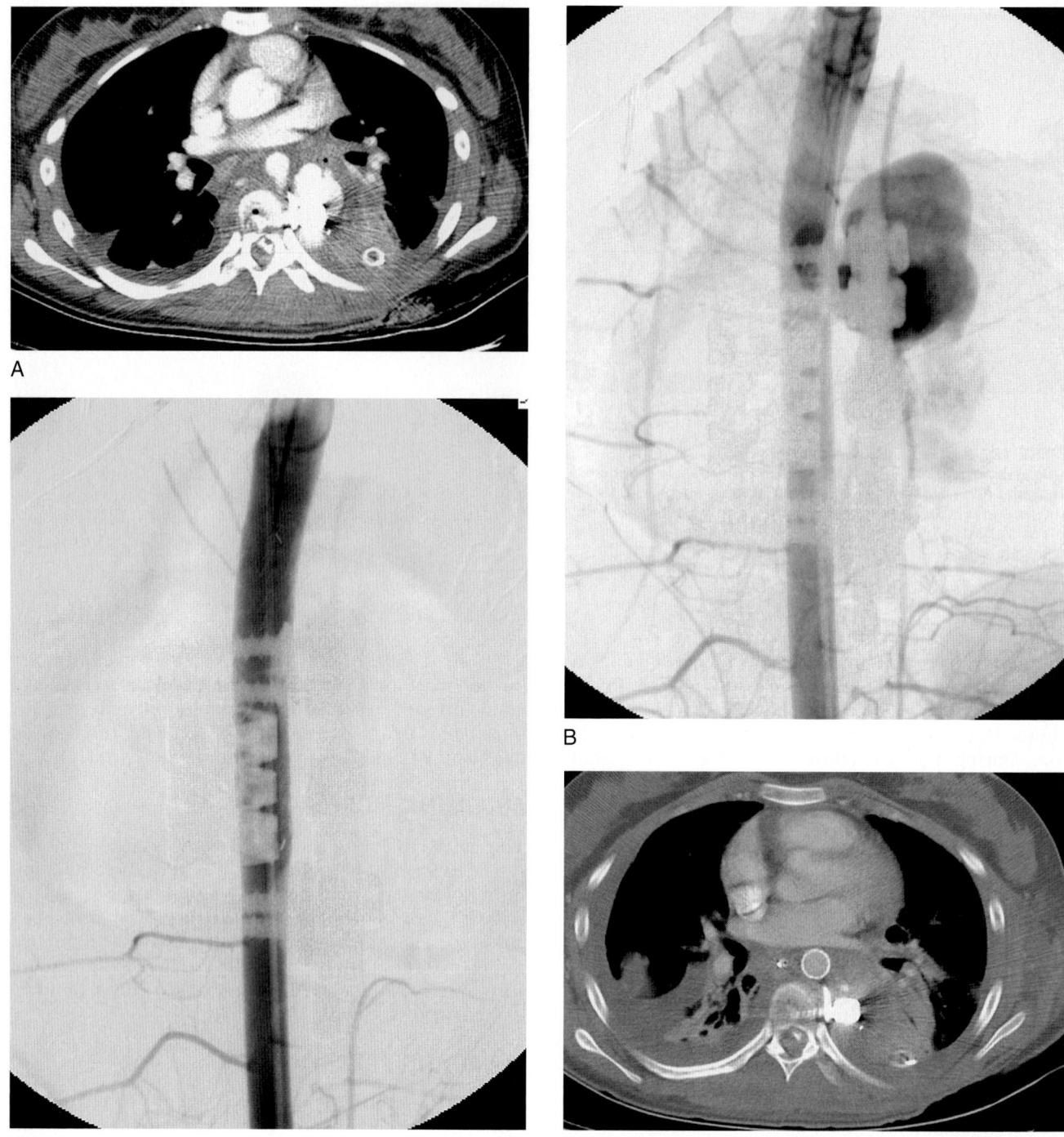

FIGURE 185-3. Aortic pseudoaneurysm. **A,** Computed tomography (CT) of the chest in this 14-year-old girl reveals aortic pseudoaneurysm caused by erosion of orthopedic hardware implanted after traumatic spine injury. **B,** The large pseudoaneurysm is contrast filled on the aortogram. Artifact is from the orthopedic hardware. **C,** Covered stent/graft was implanted in the descending aorta. A poststent aortogram shows a normal descending aortogram, except that the intercostal arteries are not visualized in the segment where the stent covers their origins. The pseudoaneurysm is not opacified. **D,** CT after stent deployment reveals the stent lining the aortic wall and hematoma surrounding the aorta but no enhancement of the pseudoaneurysm. The orthopedic hardware posterior to the aorta was removed.

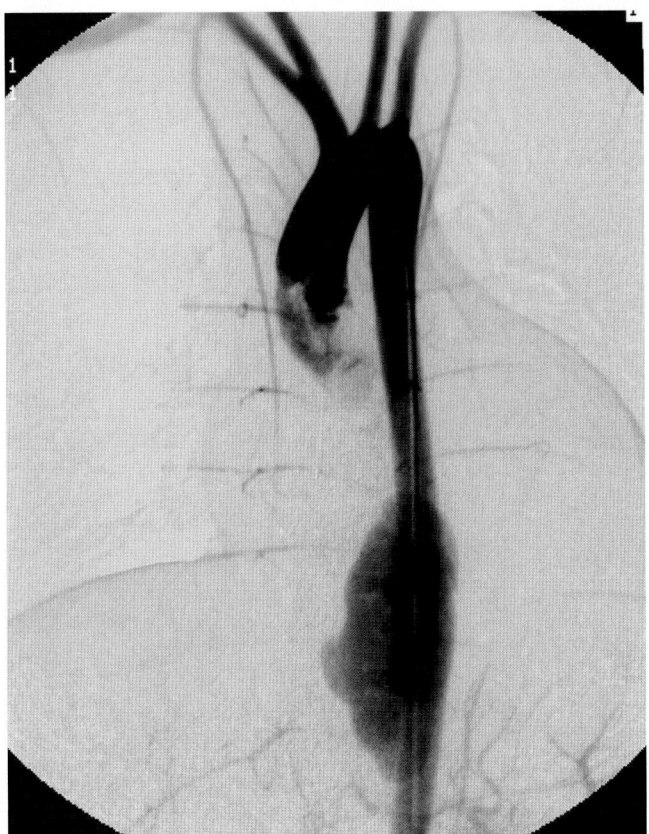

FIGURE 185-4. Mycotic pseudoaneurysm. An aortogram reveals a pseudoaneurysm of the descending aorta. The pseudoaneurysm was repaired surgically.

Detection of GI bleeding may require angiography if endoscopy and other diagnostic studies have not identified the site. The critical rate of bleeding is no different in children than in adults, and a minimum rate of bleeding for detection by angiography is 0.5 ml/min. Embolization is the treatment of choice for upper GI bleeding because of the rich collateral blood supply, which prevents ischemic complications. Embolization is also considered safe in lower GI bleeding, if it is done in a subselective location. Vasopressin therapy is less widely used because of the high rebleeding rate, and because ischemic complications may occur during vasopressin infusions.

> **Embolization is the treatment of choice for upper GI bleeding.**

VENOUS ACCESS DEVICES

Various types of access devices that may be placed include peripheral intravenous (peripheral IV) lines, peripherally inserted central (PIC) lines, tunneled central venous catheters, and subcutaneously implanted venous ports.

A PIC line is a catheter that is placed via a peripheral arm (and occasionally, leg, neck, or scalp) vein with the catheter tip positioned in a central vein (subclavian vein, innominate vein, superior or inferior vena cava). PIC lines can be used for all types of medication or blood product administration and also can be used for blood sampling. The relative ease of placing PIC lines has allowed their use for long-term therapies, often as a replacement for tunneled central lines or ports.

PIC lines are available in a large range of sizes from 2 to 7 French and in single- or dual-lumen designs (see Table 185-1). The catheters are each cut to appropriate length during insertion, so that the tip is in the desired location, usually at the superior vena cava (SVC)–right atrial junction (Fig. 185-10). An anatomic landmark for this site is usually the sixth posterior intercostal space. Resistance in small-caliber PIC lines can be very high when catheters are long, and rupture may occur when these are used with power injectors for CT or magnetic resonance imaging (MRI) contrast administration. Power injectable catheters are available from several manufacturers; most tolerate up to 25 pounds per square inch (PSI), allowing injection rates up to 3, 4, and 5 ml/sec. PIC lines can remain in place for several weeks or months, or in some cases, longer than a year.

The preferred vein for access is the basilic vein, which is the most superficial vein that runs in the groove between the brachialis and biceps muscles (Fig. 185-11). Access gained midway between the elbow and the axilla keeps the catheter well above the elbow and well tolerated by patients. The second choice for vein access varies from institution to institution; some prefer the brachial vein, and others the cephalic vein. The cephalic vein presents two challenges: (1) venospasm, and (2) difficulty maneuvering the wire and catheter across the acute angle at the junction of the cephalic and subclavian veins (Fig. 185-12).

One of the biggest concerns surrounding PIC line usage is overusage, resulting in exhaustion of upper extremity vein access in young children (Fig. 185-13). The other concern involves the patient's upper extremity vessel patency for future dialysis fistulas and grafts. Grove evaluated the incidence of extremity thrombosis in adults after PIC line placement and found an overall rate of 3.9%. He found that catheter size was a factor in predicting thrombosis after PIC line placement, and that no thromboses occurred with catheters of 3 French size or smaller. Allen reported an overall incidence of vein thrombosis after PIC line placement of 38%. Our experience would suggest that in children, the true thrombosis rate is closer to 38% than 3.9%. Central stenoses occur as result of long-standing catheter placement and can prevent future line placement. Gonsalves reported 7% central vein stenosis as a direct result of prior central venous access device in a series of adult patients. It is clear that PIC line placement has an effect on the upper extremity and on central vein patency. Authors of the Dialysis Outcomes Quality Initiative (DOQI) guidelines are concerned about patients who may need upper extremity access in the future for dialysis fistulas or grafts.

> **One of the biggest concerns surrounding PIC line usage is overusage, resulting in loss of upper extremity venous access.**

TABLE 185-2

General Injection Rates and Volumes for Arteriography (based on weight [wt] of patient in kilograms [kg])

Artery	Rate of Injection	Volume of Injection
Ascending aorta	ml/sec = wt in kg × 1.2	ml = wt in kg × 1.2
Descending aorta (thoracic and upper abdomen)	ml/sec = wt in kg	ml = wt in kg
Lower abdominal aorta	ml/sec = wt in kg × 0.8	ml = wt in kg × 0.8
Superior mesenteric artery	2-4 ml/sec	ml = wt in kg × 0.6

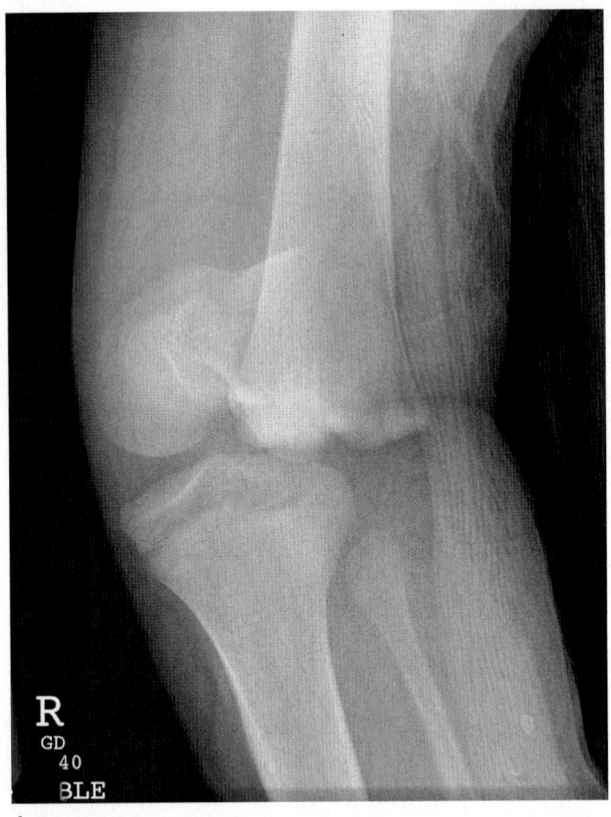
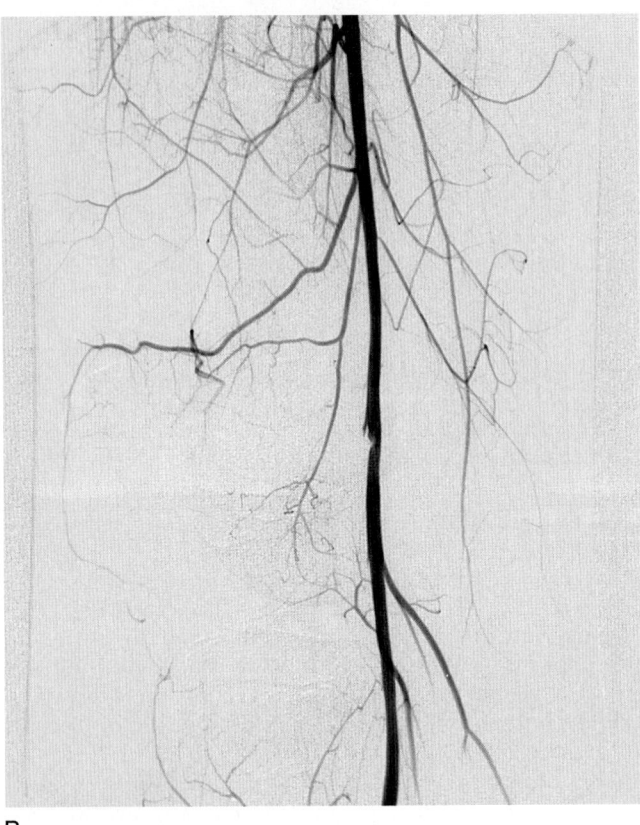

FIGURE 185-5. Intimal injury of the popliteal artery after physeal fracture. **A,** A radiograph of the knee reveals a physeal fracture of the distal femur. **B,** An arteriogram was performed because of absent pulses in the foot. An intimal injury of the popliteal artery is seen, but distal runoff of the leg was excellent. The lesion was observed and was followed with Doppler and subsequent computed tomographic angiography; no surgical repair was required.

Tunneled central lines, sometimes referred to as permanent central lines, are inserted so that the catheter exits through a subcutaneous tunnel onto the skin several centimeters from the vein puncture site (Fig. 185-14). A Dacron cuff mounted on the catheter within the subcutaneous tunnel scars into the tissues after several days or weeks and prevents inadvertent dislodgement or removal of the catheter. Insertion technique is more involved and presents higher risks than are associated with placement of a PIC line; these catheters are generally used only when the need for venous access is anticipated to last longer than 6 weeks. Catheters are available in a wide range of sizes but may be significantly larger than PIC lines because of direct puncture into a larger central vein. The largest catheters are used for pheresis or hemodialysis.

Insertion Technique

The risk of bleeding is greater with tunneled central lines because of the more central venipuncture, creation of the subcutaneous tunnel, and the usual placement of larger catheters. A risk of air embolism is also present during insertion of tunneled central lines; therefore, most are inserted with the patient under general anesthesia and with positive-pressure ventilation, thus helping to avoid this complication.

The preferred vein for access is one of the internal jugular veins, usually the right, as recommended by DOQI guidelines. These guidelines recommend that subclavian puncture should be avoided for any central line, particularly in those patients who may need hemodialysis. Subclavian vein stenosis precludes later use of

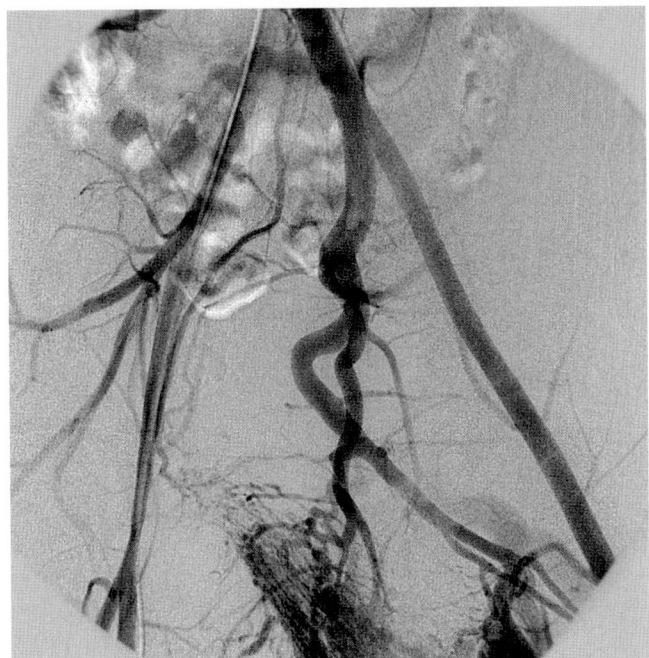

A

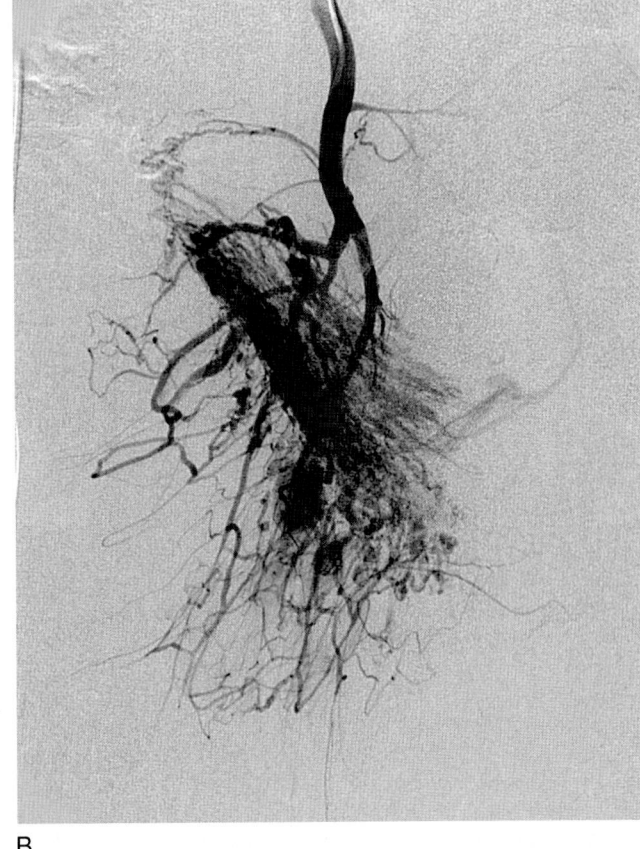

B

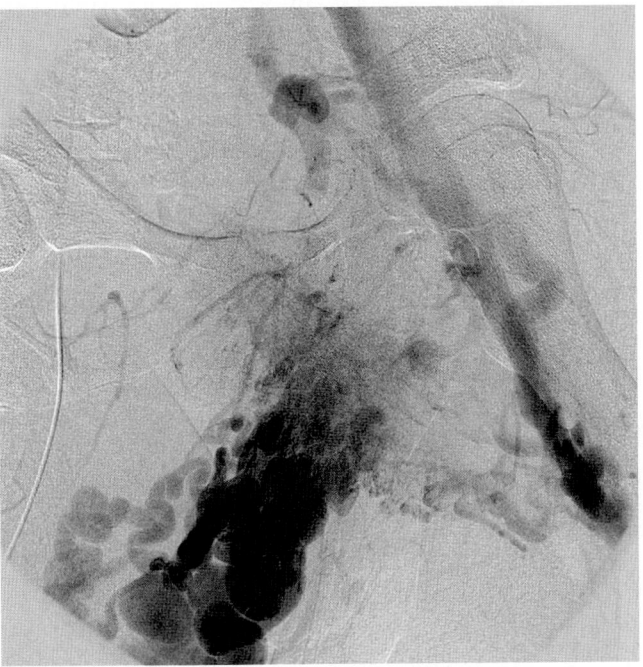

C

FIGURE 185-6. Arteriovenous malformation of the left gluteal muscles. **A,** An arteriogram of the left common iliac artery in this 16-year-old boy reveals marked enlargement of the internal iliac artery and an extensive arteriovenous malformation involving the gluteus minimus muscle. Aortogram reveals enlarged internal iliac artery. **B,** Selective injection of internal iliac artery reveals an extensive malformation within gluteal muscles. **C,** Extensive venous drainage to the iliac veins is seen in the pelvis. The lesion was embolized with ethanol.

the ipsilateral arm for creation of a dialysis fistula or graft.

A US-guided puncture is made into the internal jugular vein, a subcutaneous tunnel is created with a separate blunt needle, and the catheter is pulled through the subcutaneous tunnel (Fig. 185-15). A peel-away sheath is introduced into the venipuncture site, and while the patient is maintained in an apneic state, the dilator is removed and the catheter introduced. The risk for air embolism may be minimized by several maneuvers such as Trendelenburg positioning or clamping of the sheath, but the most certain way to avoid generation of

negative intrathoracic pressure during this exchange is to have the patient suspend respiration or to provide positive-pressure ventilation with anesthesia.

Removal of tunneled catheters requires blunt dissection to free the Dacron cuff from the subcutaneous tissues. This procedure generally requires sedation or general anesthesia in younger children.

Complications

Placement of tunneled catheters by interventional radiologists has proved safe, with complication rates

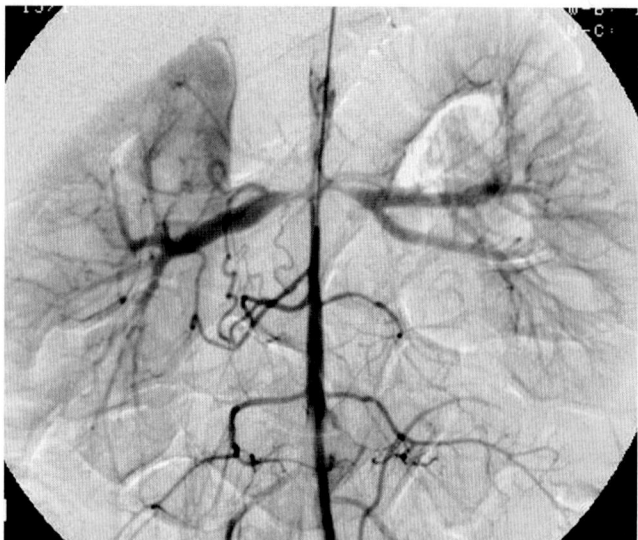

FIGURE 185-7. Midaortic syndrome. An aortogram in this 3-month-old boy performed because of severe hypertension reveals a hypoplastic abdominal aorta and bilateral renal artery stenoses. Both renal arteries were dilated with balloon angioplasty through a brachial artery approach.

lower than or equal to those associated with surgically placed lines. Image guidance adds a dimension of safety and improves success rates over those attained with non–image-guided techniques.

Air embolism is one of the most serious complications, and death can ensue if the embolism is large. Managing breathing with the use of general anesthesia and positive-pressure ventilation is the best method of preventing air embolism. Peel-away sheaths with one-way valves can prevent air embolism during the dilator/catheter exchange, but currently, these are available only

in large sizes. Central veins or the SVC can rupture, particularly when large hemodialysis catheters are inserted.

> **Air embolism is one of the most serious complications.**

DIALYSIS/PHERESIS CATHETERS

Temporary or permanent hemodialysis/pheresis catheters can be safely and efficiently placed by the interventional radiology (IR) service (Figs. 185-16, 185-17, 185-18). Temporary catheters are almost exclusively used for inpatients or for outpatients undergoing stem cell harvesting who required only one or two harvesting sessions. Permanent catheters (tunneled catheters) are used almost exclusively for patients undergoing chronic hemodialysis.

These catheters are distinct from other central lines in that they always have two equal-sized lumina, and they must provide high flow rates for their intended use as venous blood circulators. This requires that large catheters be used. Catheter caliber is selected on the basis of flow rates needed and weight of the child (see Table 185-2). Catheter length is selected on the basis of size of the child at the time of insertion.

Permanent catheters are placed through the same technique as is used for tunneled central line insertion. Temporary catheters are placed directly into the internal jugular or femoral vein. US guidance is necessary and fluoroscopy is preferred for tract dilation and over-the-wire insertion of the catheter. The right internal jugular (IJ) vein, which is preferred, provides straight access to the SVC and right atrium. The left IJ vein is to be avoided if possible because of the "S" curve created by the course

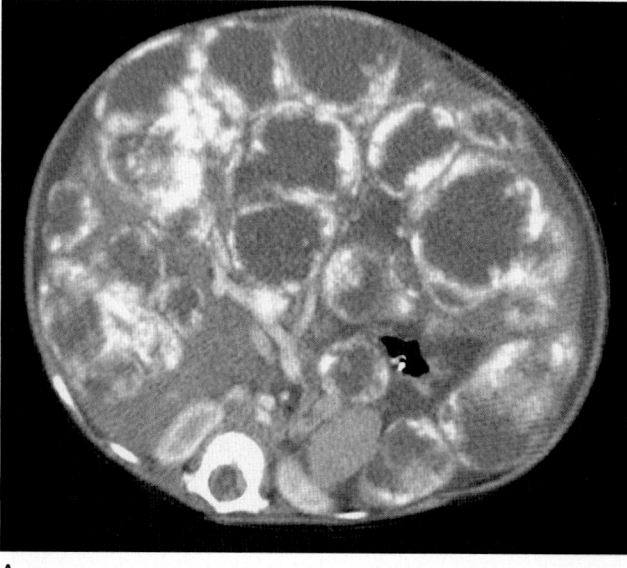
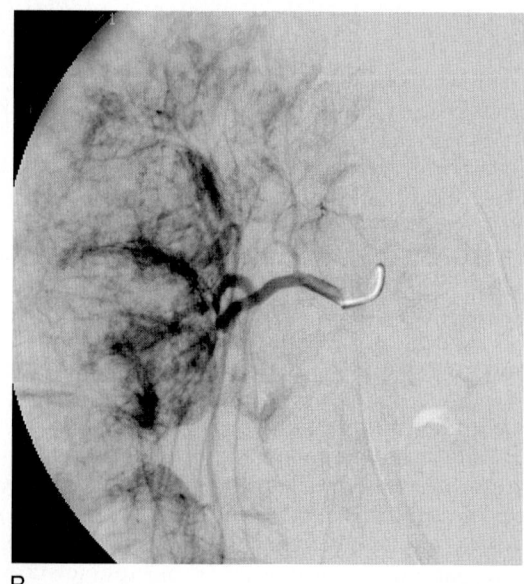

A   B

FIGURE 185-8. Hemangioendothelioma of the liver. **A,** Computed tomography during the arterial phase reveals peripheral enhancement of numerous masses replacing most of the hepatic parenchyma. **B,** A right hepatic angiogram performed because of high output failure and respiratory distress from the large abdominal mass preceded subtotal embolization of the hepatic arteries. Minimal improvement was noted after embolization, and the patient underwent liver transplantation.

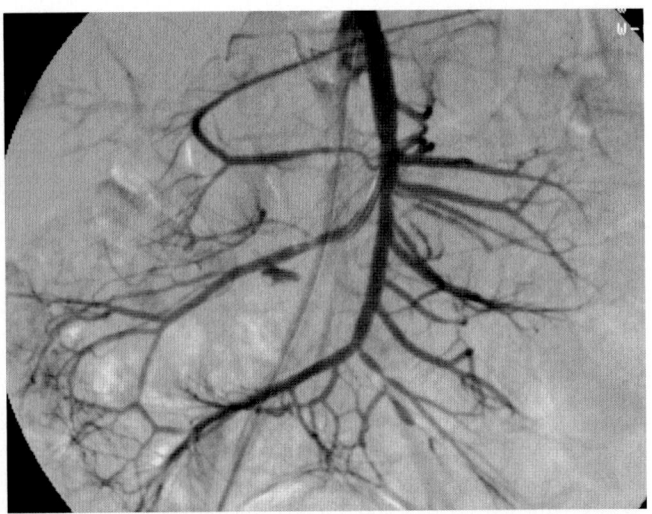
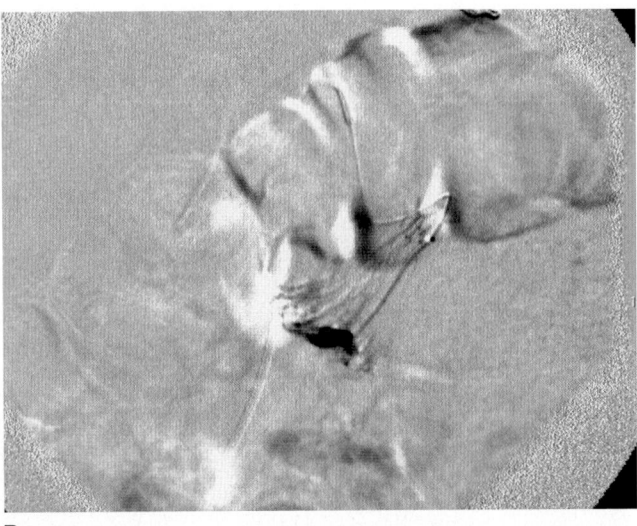

A   B

FIGURE 185-9. Gastrointestinal bleeding. **A,** Superior mesenteric angiography reveals a site of active arterial bleeding in this 24-month-old child with lymphoblastic lymphoma. **B,** Subsequent superselective catheterization with microcatheter was performed and the bleeding site isolated in a small jejunal arterial branch. The artery was embolized with a microcoil, and bleeding was successfully stopped.

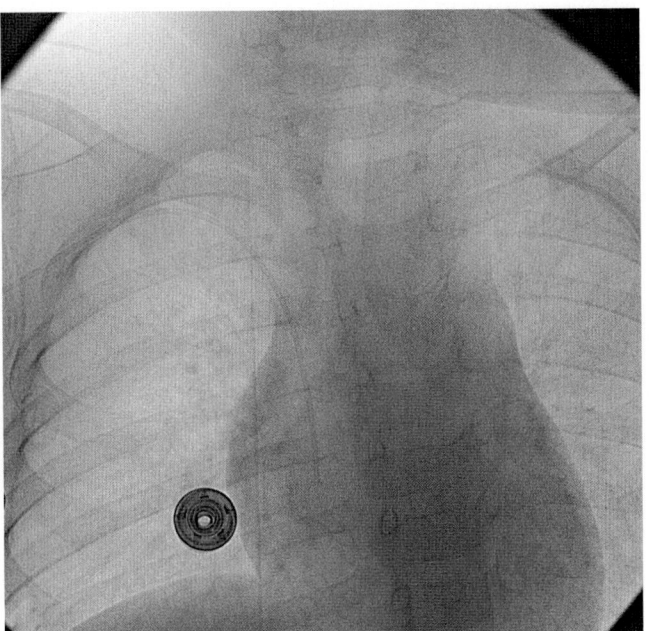
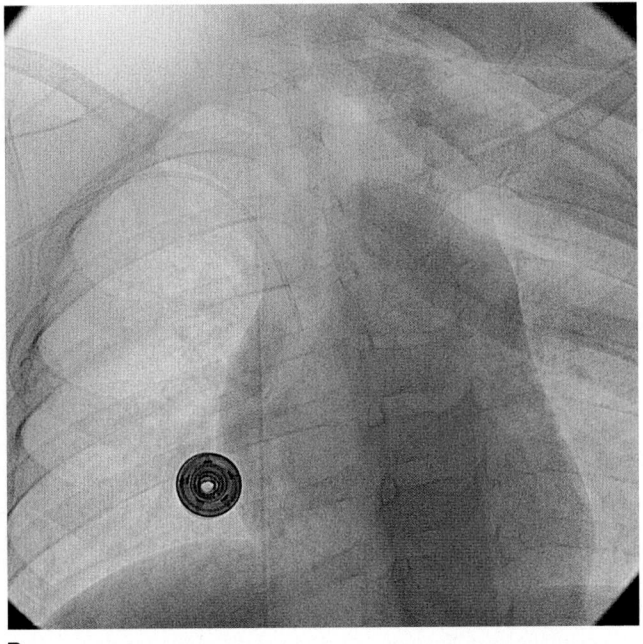

A   B

FIGURE 185-10. Peripherally inserted catheter (PIC) line. **A,** PIC line with catheter tip in the mid-right atrium. Note the catheter course along the axillary and subclavian veins. **B,** The catheter has been slightly withdrawn, and the tip is at the cavoatrial junction.

of the veins. Left IJ access often leaves the catheter tip against the SVC wall, where flow rates are suboptimal. Femoral veins may also be used in intensive care unit patients through placement at the bedside with US guidance alone; fluoroscopy is not required for catheter insertion. The subclavian veins are to be avoided as access sites per DOQI guidelines, thus preserving the upper veins for future use with dialysis shunts and fistulas.

Implantable venous ports are safely placed by pediatric interventional radiologists, and in some institutions, they are now placed exclusively by IR staff (Figs. 185-19,

185-20). Indication for venous port placement includes the need for long-term intermittent access, usually of several months' duration. Most ports are of the single-lumen type, although some large-profile dual-lumen ports are manufactured. Ports are made of plastic or metal; some titanium ports may cause minimal artifact during CT studies. Venous ports can be placed in the upper arm in older children, but fewer complications result when they are placed in the upper chest wall. Many institutions have abandoned the practice of placing ports in arms because of associated complications such

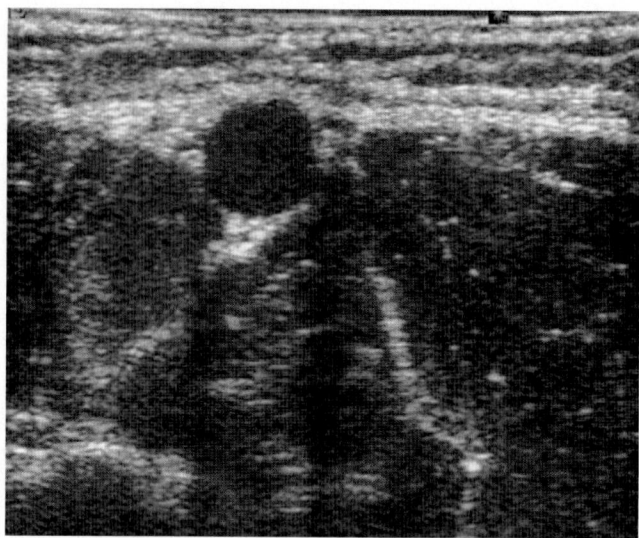

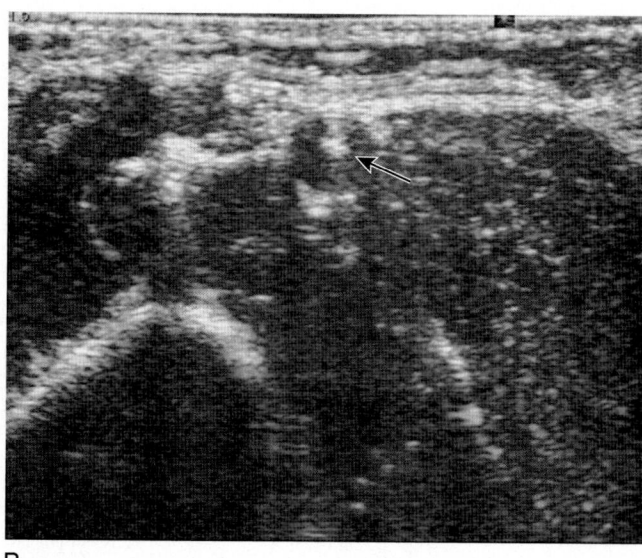

A B

FIGURE 185-11. Ultrasonography (US)-guided intravenous access. **A,** Transverse US image across upper arm reveals a large basilic vein superficial to the muscle fascia in the groove between the brachialis and biceps muscles. **B,** After puncture of the basilic vein, the echogenic needle tip is seen within the lumen of the vein *(arrow)*.

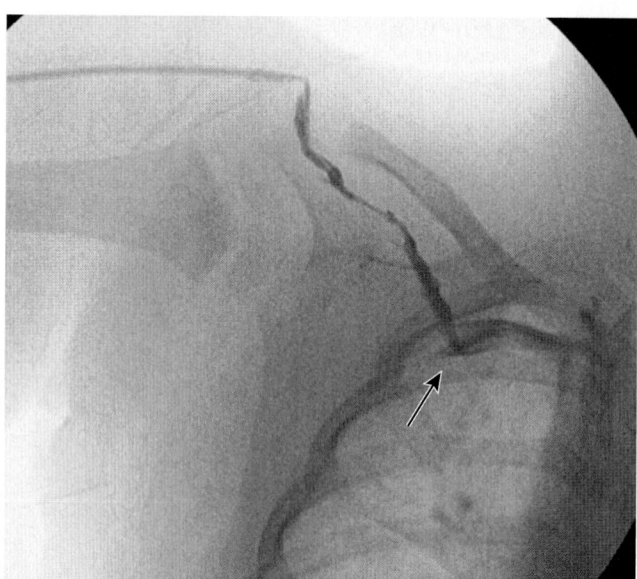

FIGURE 185-12. Cephalic vein access. A venogram performed during insertion of a peripherally inserted catheter line through the cephalic vein illustrates an acute angle at the junction with the subclavian vein *(arrow)*. Negotiating the angle with the subclavian vein often requires use of a directional guidewire.

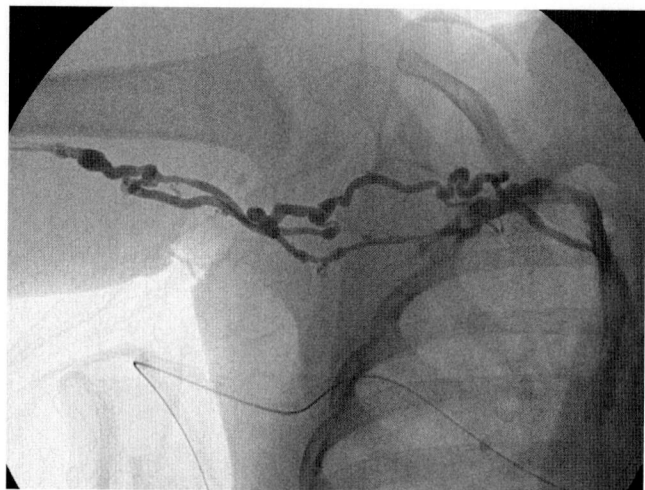

FIGURE 185-13. Stenoses of central veins. A venogram performed because a peripherally inserted catheter (PIC) line could not be advanced reveals collateral veins due to occlusion of the axillary and subclavian veins. The patient had had several PIC lines previously.

as wound dehiscence, skin erosion over the port, and difficulty accessing the port in the upper arm.

Insertion Technique

It is important to check coagulation parameters prior to port placement and to try to correct any coagulopathy. Preferred venous access for a chest port is gained via the right jugular vein, in the same manner described for a tunneled central line. The selected site for port placement is usually lateral on the flat anterior chest wall, thereby avoiding breast tissue and axillary crease. The

second anterior rib, which is marked fluoroscopically, helps provide stability for later access to the port. The incision for the pocket is created above or below the planned pocket location, depending on operator preference, and anesthesia is achieved with lidocaine with or without epinephrine. The incision is made with a No. 13 scalpel blade for smoothly cut edges. The pocket between the subcutaneous fat and the muscle fascia layer is then created with the use of blunt dissection performed with curved clamp instruments and one's own finger inserted to expand the pocket. When the port fits into the pocket easily, then the subcutaneous tunnel is created and connects the pocket to the venipuncture site at the neck. The catheter is pulled through the tunnel by a similar approach to that used for tunneled catheters.

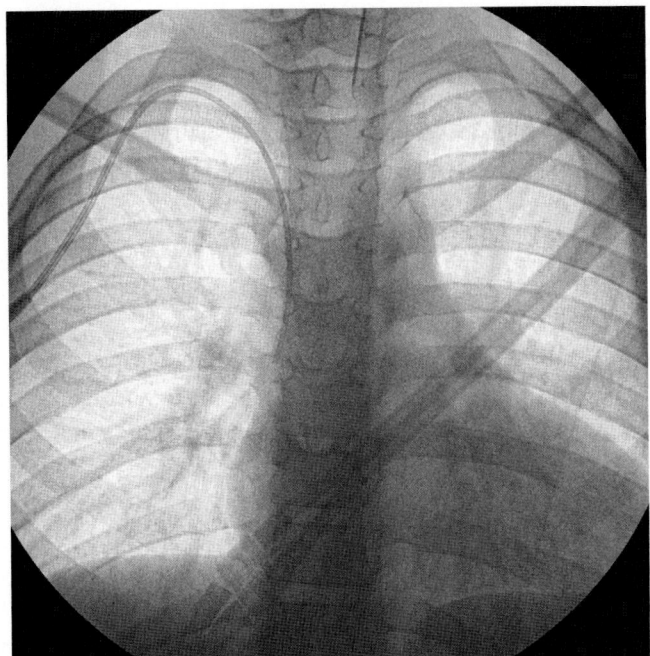

FIGURE 185-14. Tunneled central line placement. A radiograph confirms catheter tip location at the cavoatrial junction. Note the catheter course above the clavicle indicating insertion via the internal jugular vein. The catheter exits on the patient chest through a subcutaneous tunnel created during insertion.

The catheter is connected to the port, and the port is placed into the pocket. The catheter must be introduced through the peel-away sheath at the neck with adherence to the same precautions as those recommended for tunneled catheters, while measures are taken to eliminate risk for air embolism. The port should be immediately accessed and flushed with heparin 100 μ/ml.

The port pocket is then closed with two layers of suture. The first is a series of interrupted stitches, usually 3.0 absorbable, applied to close the subcutaneous tissues. The second is a running subcuticular stitch made with 4.0 absorbable suture to close the skin. Dermabond (Ethicon, Inc., Johnson & Johnson, Somerville, NJ), the equivalent of Superglue, is then used to cover the skin incision. Dermabond is allowed to wear off and is not removed. The neck incision is closed with one subcutaneous stitch, or simply with Dermabond.

ALTERNATIVE VENOUS ACCESS SITES

Additional sites are available for vascular access if stenoses should prevent standard access to the central veins. Translumbar and transhepatic inferior vena cava catheters may be placed with the use of a combination of US, fluoroscopy, and sometimes CT guidance for placement (Fig. 185-21). Catheters may be tunneled on the abdominal wall for secure placement.

CATHETER MAINTENANCE

Most external central venous catheters are flushed with heparin solution after each use, or at least once a day. In catheters that are used regularly during the day, 100 μ/ml heparin solution is used for children weighing >10 kg, 10 μ/ml heparin solution for children weighing between 3 and 10 kg, and 1 μ/ml for infants who weigh less than 3 kg. Venous ports are flushed with heparin solution of 100 μ/ml. Dialysis catheters are packed with 5000 μ/ml heparin solution at precise catheter volume.

Clotted catheters are injected with tissue plasminogen activator 1 mg slowly infused into the catheter. The thrombolytic is allowed to stay in the catheter for 1 hour before the catheter is flushed.

Fibrin sheaths may form on catheter tips, usually several weeks or months after insertion. Catheters may be stripped with the use of a snare inserted through the femoral vein, or they may be exchanged out over a

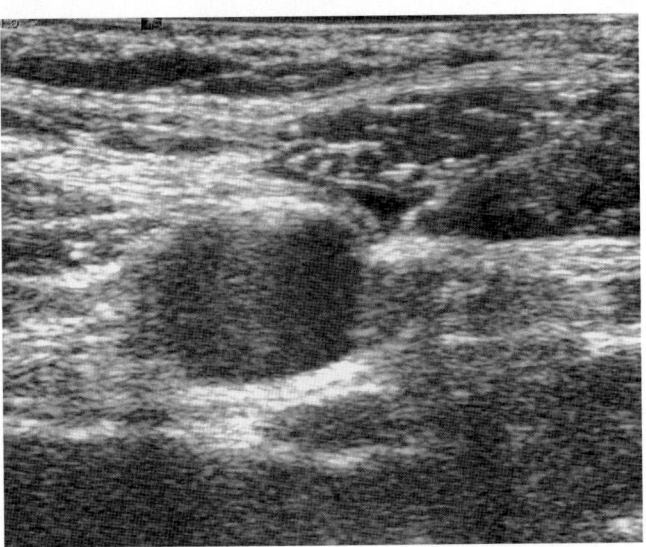

A

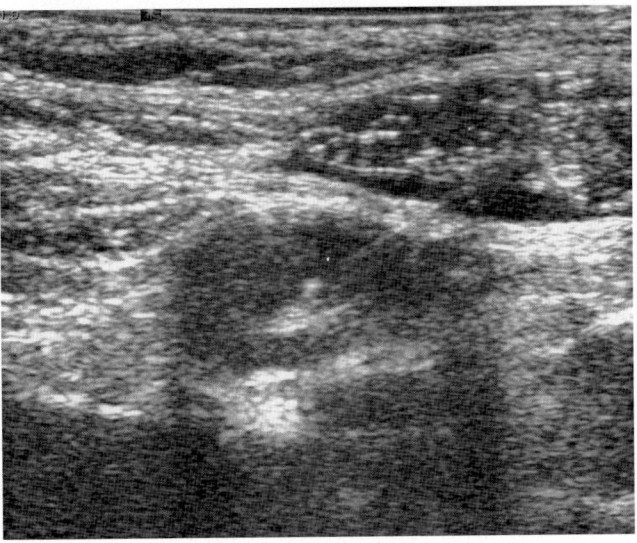

B

FIGURE 185-15. Internal jugular vein and lateral wall puncture. **A, B,** Access to internal jugular vein can be gained with ultrasound guidance by puncturing the vein in a transverse orientation similar to extremity access, or longitudinal to the transducer, thereby achieving a lateral approach to the vein. In **B,** lateral wall puncture of the vein with the needle tip is seen centrally within the vein.

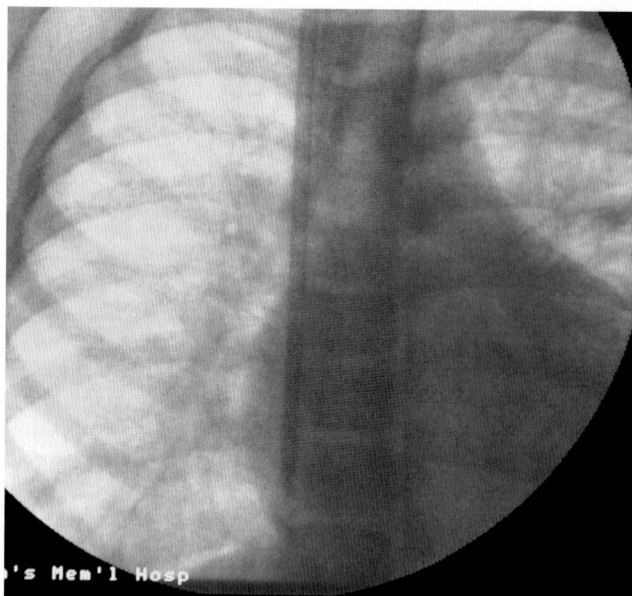

FIGURE 185-16. Perforation of the right atrium. This temporary hemodialysis catheter perforated the right atrium 1 day after insertion when the patient had a seizure. During emergent surgery to alleviate cardiac tamponade, two punctures were noted in the atrial wall. The catheter tip was left too low in the right atrium.

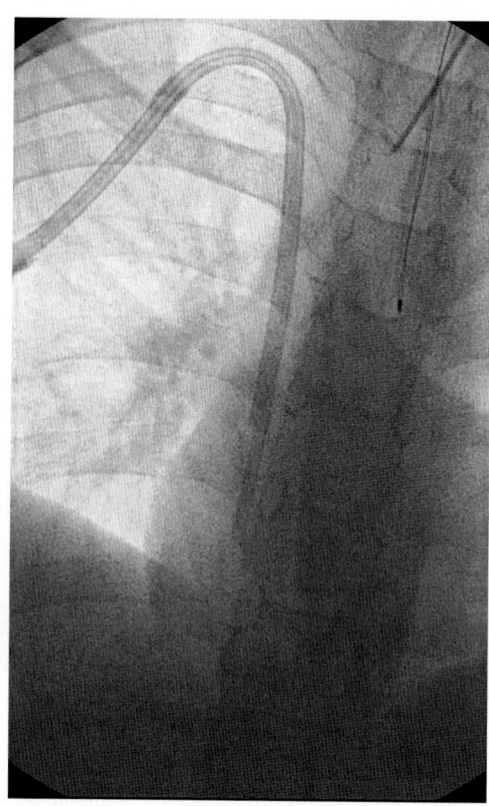

FIGURE 185-17. Permanent hemodialysis catheter. Radiograph after insertion of the permanent hemodialysis catheter illustrates ideal positioning of the catheter. Both lumina are within the right atrium, where dialysis flow rates are optimal.

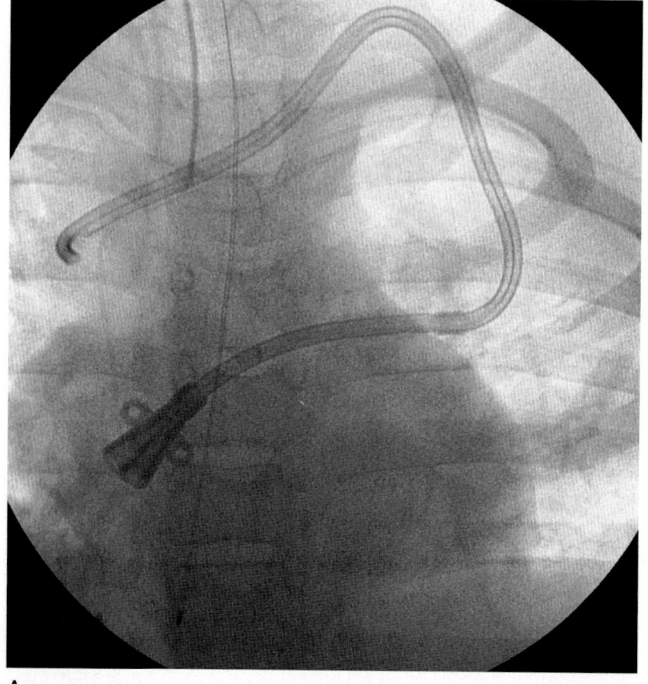

A

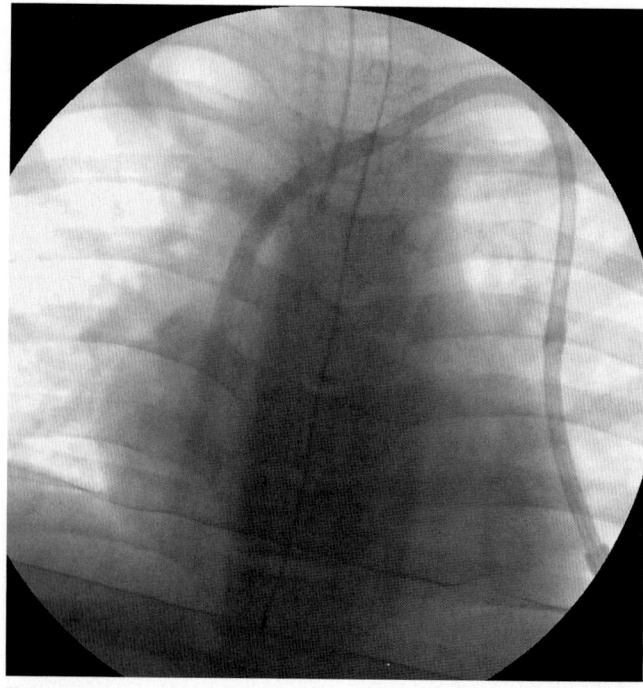

B

FIGURE 185-18. Malposition of catheter. **A,** One of many possible malpositions of hemodialysis catheters. This catheter has flipped into the azygos vein. **B,** After manipulation from the femoral vein, the catheter is correctly positioned in the superior vena cava (SVC).

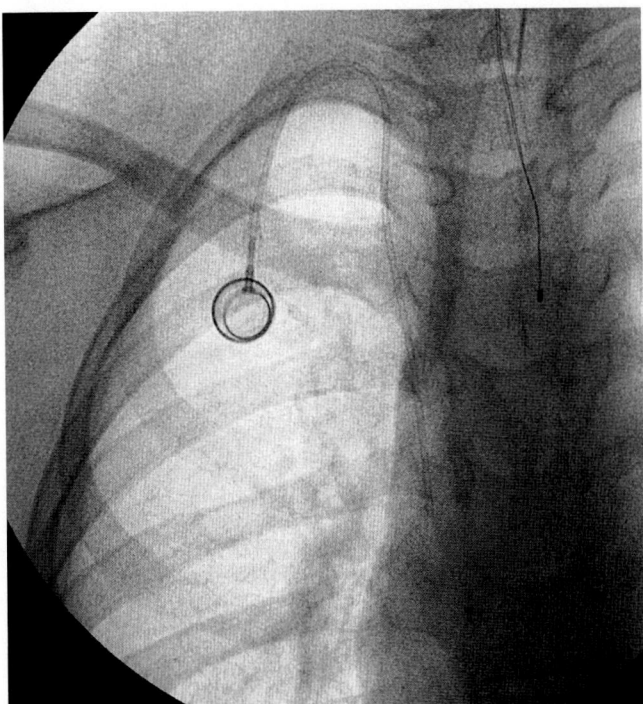

FIGURE 185-19. Venous port placement. Port is positioned over the right second anterior rib. This location is selected to provide stability to the port during needle access by nursing service.

guidewire or guidewires. Balloon inflation done over the wire before reinsertion of the new catheter may rupture the fibrin sheath and prevent malfunction of the newly replaced catheter.

VENOUS INTERVENTION PROCEDURES

Direct percutaneous access into the portal vein is necessary for a variety of procedures. Transplantation patients with portal vein anastomotic strictures requiring angioplasty, Rex shunt patients requiring intervention for the shunt, and patients with portal vein anomalies may require direct access to the portal vein for intervention. Access is attained directly into the right or left portal branches, thereby avoiding central access near the hilum. The preferred access route runs from a subcostal or subxiphoid location, thus avoiding the pleural space with inherent risks of hemothorax or pleural contamination. A puncture is usually made with a 22 gauge needle; this is followed by introduction of an 0.018″ guidewire. The wire is usually upsized to 0.035″ with a coaxial introducer system. Portal vein access can be confirmed with contrast injection or by passing the guidewire directly after performing US-guided puncture.

Similar technique and precautions are used when hepatic vein access is attained. Hepatic vein access may be used for interventions for the hepatic vein anastomosis after transplantation and for alternative central line placement in patients with no standard options

because of many prior lines; occasionally, such access may be needed for cardiac catheterization in patients with interruption of the inferior vena cava (IVC).

Parenchymal tract embolization is recommended after most portal vein interventions. Embolization can be completed with Gelfoam torpedoes or metallic coils.

Complications

Complications during catheter placement may occur during any of the procedures described in this chapter (see Figs. 185-16, 185-22). Complications from PIC line placement are few, beyond catheter infection and catheter malfunction, each of which has proved no worse than other types of central venous access. In Crowley's series of 523 pediatric PIC lines, an infection rate of 0.93 infections per 1000 catheter days was reported. Incidence of thrombophlebitis was 0.4%. In another pediatric series of PIC lines placed by pediatric radiologists, Dubois reported a catheter infection rate of 3.02/1000 catheter days. When PIC lines placed by radiologists are compared with those placed by nursing services or other staff physicians, the results are again favorable. Graham found bacteremia in 2% of PIC lines (4.6/10,000 catheter days) in lines placed by nonradiologist physicians and nurses. PIC line fracture and embolization are rare (occurred in 3 of more than 5000 central lines at Children's Memorial Hospital in Chicago) but can occur if occluded catheters are forcefully injected. If a catheter becomes fragmented, the free piece can usually be retrieved with a snare (see Fig. 185-14). Others have reported the need for thoracotomy and arteriotomy for catheter fragment removal. Other complications include inadvertent placement of catheters in arteries.

With tunneled central line placement, surgically placed catheters can be compared. In a review from the Hospital for Sick Children in Toronto, Ingram reported 2.9 infections per 1000 catheter days for surgically placed tunnel lines in children (Hickman and Broviac catheters). Nosher reported that outcomes of pediatric tunneled central lines placed by radiologists compared favorably with those placed by surgeons. He reported 1.23 infections per 1000 catheter days for lines placed by radiologists and 2.24 infections per 1000 catheter days for those placed surgically.

> **The infection rate is low for indwelling catheters placed percutaneously.**

Air embolism is a potentially fatal complication that may occur during direct central venous access, such as for tunneled lines and ports. Morello reported three cases that occurred during tunneled central line placement when sedation was used in small children. As a result of this complication, general anesthesia is recommended for children when deep sedation is required but the child is not able to breath-hold on command during final insertion of the catheter.

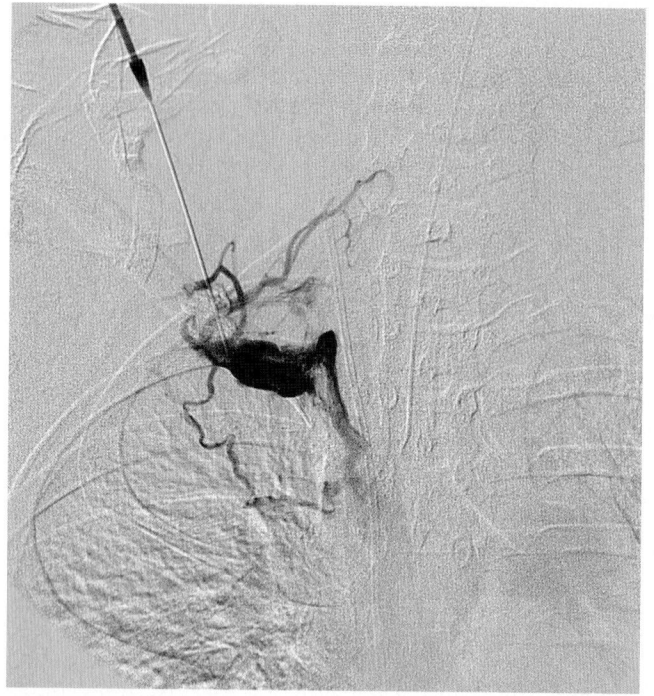

A

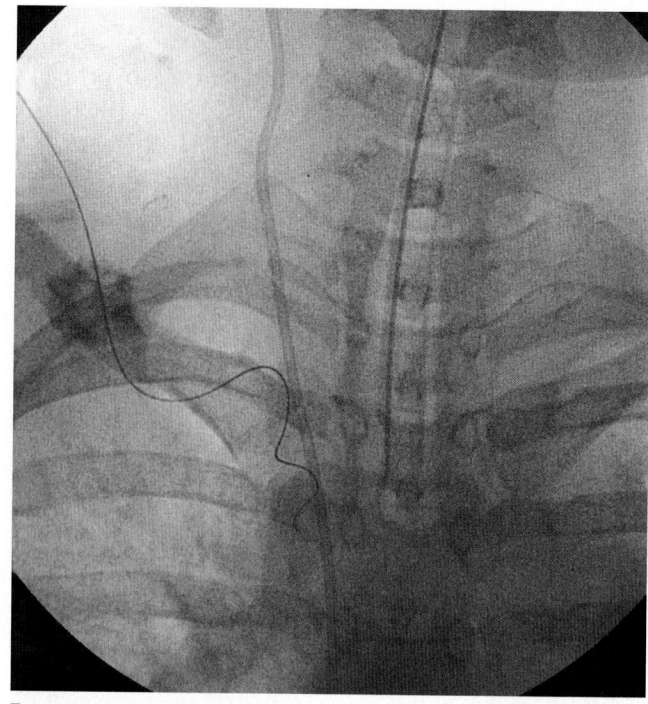

B

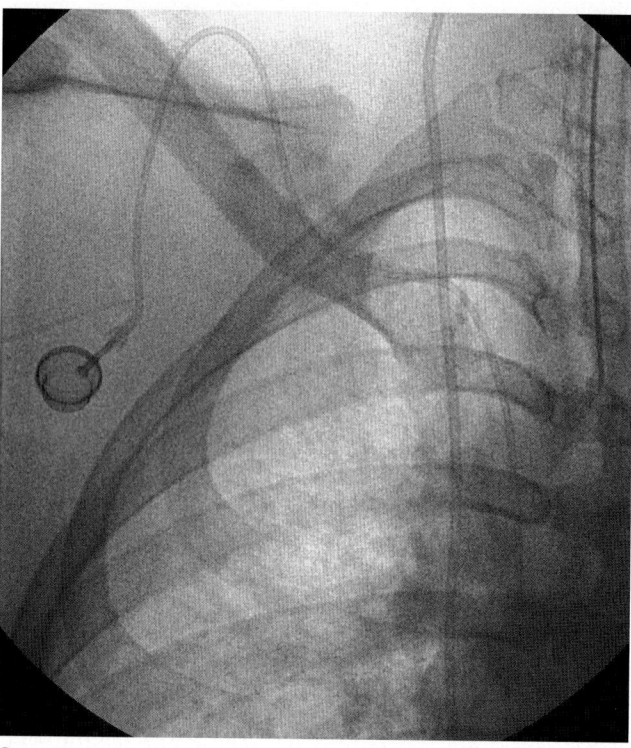

C

FIGURE 185-20. Stenoses of upper extremity veins. **A,** A venogram performed after failed surgical attempt to place central line reveals stenoses of subclavian and innominate veins. **B,** A directional guidewire was successfully manipulated through the stenoses into the superior vena cava. **C,** A venous port was successfully implanted and the catheter advanced centrally through the stenoses.

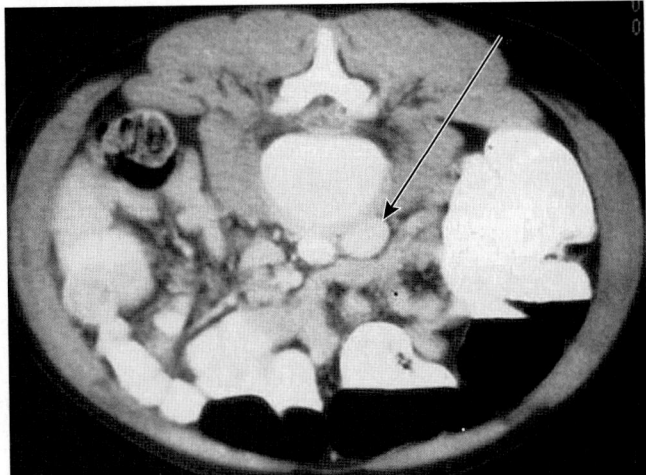

A

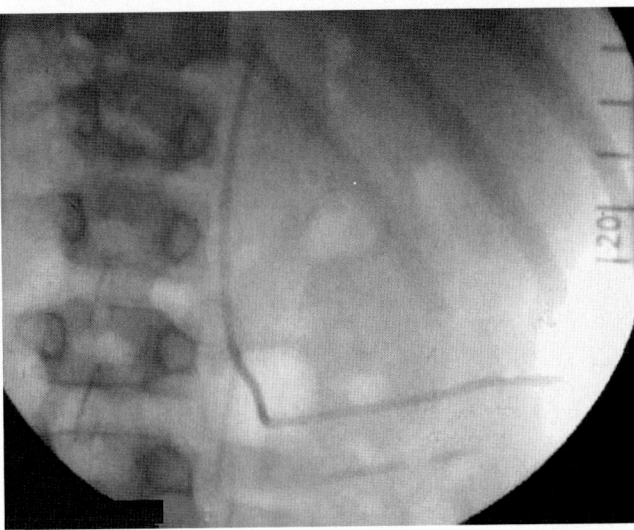

C

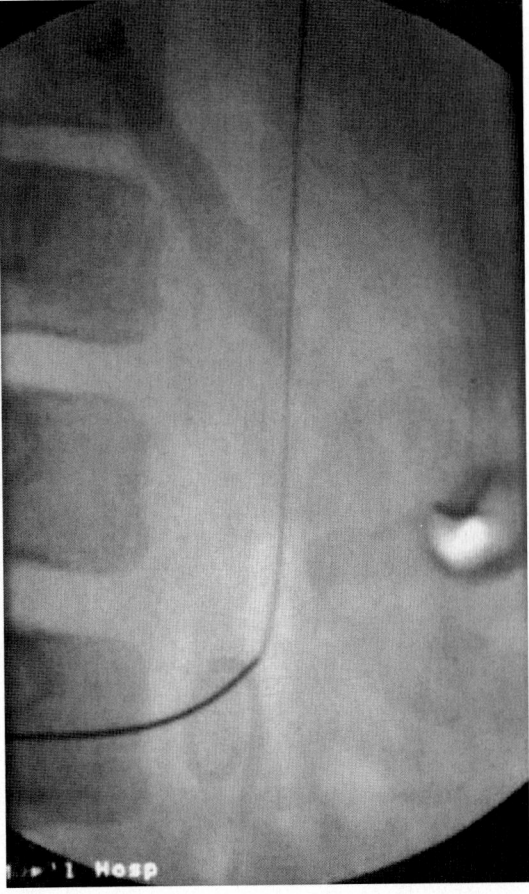

B

FIGURE 185-21. Translumbar inferior vena cava (IVC) central line placement. **A,** Computed tomography of the abdomen shown inverted illustrates the course of access for an IVC puncture for central line placement. A paraspinous approach is taken through the psoas muscle *(arrow).* (From: Donaldson JS. Pediatr Radiol 2006; 36:386-397.) **B,** Fluoroscopic image reveals dilator and guidewire directed through the pigtail catheter that was placed into the IVC as a target for fluoroscopic needle puncture. A guidewire has been advanced into the IVC. **C,** Final image of the translumbar IVC central catheter. The catheter was tunneled around the lateral aspect of the abdominal wall.

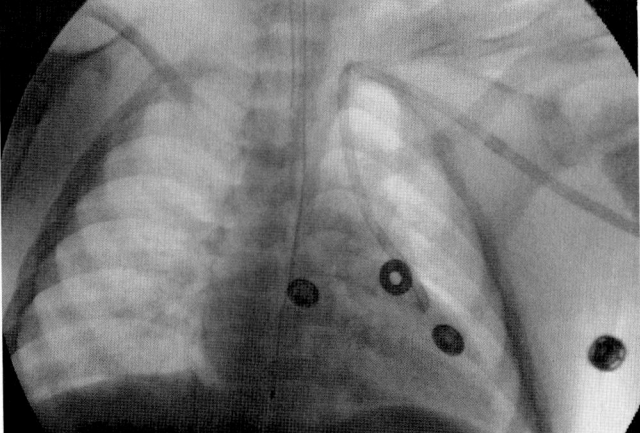

FIGURE 185-22. Laceration of stenotic left innominate vein. During insertion of a left permanent hemodialysis catheter in a child with a history of previous catheters, the left innominate vein was lacerated during dilation of the insertion site. After it was inserted through the peel-away sheath, the catheter exited the vein laceration, entering the left side of the mediastinum. The innominate vein was repaired operatively as a massive hemothorax occurred after catheter removal.

SUGGESTED READINGS

Allen AW, Megargell JL, Brown DB, et al: Venous thrombosis associated with the placement of peripherally inserted central catheters. J Vasc Interv Radiol 2000;11:1309-1414

Azizkhan RG, Taylor LA, Jaques PF, et al: Percutaneous translumbar and transhepatic inferior vena caval catheters for prolonged vascular access in children. J Pediatr Surg 1992;27:165-169

Chait PG, Ingram J, Phillips-Gordon C, et al: Peripherally inserted central catheters in children. Radiology 1995;197:775-778

Crowley JJ, Pereira JK, Harris LS, et al: Peripherally inserted central catheters: experience in 523 children. Radiology 1997;204:617-621

Donaldson JS, Morello FP, Junewick JJ, et al: Peripherally inserted central venous catheters: US-guided vascular access in pediatric patients. Radiology 1995;197:542-544

Dubois J, Garel L, Tapiero B, et al: Peripherally inserted central catheters in infants and children. Radiology 1997;204:622-626

Gonsalves CF, Eschelman DJ, Sullivan KL, et al: Incidence of central vein stenosis and occlusion following upper extremity PICC and port placement. Cardiovasc Intervent Radiol 2003;26:123-127

Grove JR, Pevec WC: Venous thrombosis related to peripherally inserted central catheters. J Vasc Interv Radiol 2000;11:837-840

Ingram J, Weitzman S, Greenberg ML, et al: Complications of indwelling venous access lines in the pediatric hematology patient: a prospective comparison of external venous catheters and subcutaneous ports. Am J Pediatr Hematol Oncol 1991;13:130-136

Jaques PF, Mauro MA, Keefe B: US guidance for vascular access: technical note. J Vasc Interv Radiol 1992;3:427-430

Johnston TA, Donnelly LF, Frush DP, et al: Transhepatic catheterization using ultrasound-guided access. Pediatr Cardiol 2003;24:393-396

Kairaitis LK, Gottlieb T: Outcome and complications of temporary haemodialysis catheters. Nephrol Dial Transplant 1999; 14:1710-1714

Lameris JS, Post PJ, Zonderland HM, et al: Percutaneous placement of Hickman catheters: comparison of sonographically guided and blind techniques. AJR Am J Roentgenol 1990;155:1097-1099

Lorenz JM, Funaki B, Van Ha T, et al: Radiologic placement of implantable chest ports in pediatric patients. AJR Am J Roentgenol 2001;176:991-994

Lund GB, Trerotola SO, Scheel PF Jr, et al: Outcome of tunneled hemodialysis catheters placed by radiologists. Radiology 1996;198:467-472

Malmgren N, Cwikiel W, Hochberg P, et al: Percutaneous translumbar central venous catheter in infants and small children. Pediatr Radiol 1995;25:28-30

Morello FP, Donaldson JS, Saker MC, et al: Air embolism during tunneled central catheter placement performed without general anesthesia in children: a potentially serious complication. J Vasc Interv Radiol 1999;10:781-784

NKF-DOQI clinical practice guidelines for vascular access: National Kidney Foundation–Dialysis Outcomes Quality Initiative. Am J Kidney Dis 1997;30(4 Suppl 3):S150-S191

Nosher JL, Bodner LJ, Ettinger LJ, et al: Radiologic placement of a low profile implantable venous access port in a pediatric population. Cardiovasc Interv Radiol 2001;24:395-399

Nosher JL, Shami MM, Siegel RL, et al: Tunneled central venous access catheter placement in the pediatric population: comparison of radiologic and surgical results. Radiology 1994;192:265-268

Thiagarajan RR, Ramamoorthy C, Gettmann T, et al: Survey of the use of peripherally inserted central venous catheters in children. Pediatrics 1997;99:E4

Trerotola SO, Johnson MS, Harris VJ, et al: Outcome of tunneled hemodialysis catheters placed via the right internal jugular vein by interventional radiologists. Radiology 1997;203:489-495

Vascular Anomalies in Children

JOSÉE DUBOIS

CLASSIFICATION

Persistent improper terminology often is used to produce inappropriate descriptions of vascular anomalies; the confusion between tumors and malformations leads to inadequate and at times dangerous therapeutic procedures. Proper identification is essential for establishing the diagnosis and guiding the management of vascular anomalies.

The author follows the classification described by Mulliken and Glowacki and adopted by the International Society for the Study of Vascular Anomalies (ISSVA). Angiogenesis and molecular biology are currently actively explored; such research should increase our knowledge of vascular tumors and vascular malformations and should contribute to the development of new, more "physiologic" treatment.

This classification differentiates vascular anomalies into vascular tumors and vascular malformations (Table 186-1). Tumors are characterized by initial cellular proliferation and hyperplasia. Vascular tumors most frequently reported in infancy are infantile hemangiomas. Other vascular tumors reported in children include congenital hemangiomas (i.e., NICH, noninvoluting congenital hemangiomas, or RICH, rapidly involuting congenital hemangiomas), hemangioendotheliomas, tufted angiomas, and sarcomas.

> This classification differentiates vascular anomalies into vascular tumors and vascular malformations.

Malformations are caused by dysplastic vessels with no cellular proliferation. These are subcategorized according to flow (high- or slow-flow malformations) and predominantly involved vessels (capillary, venous, lymphatic, and arteriovenous malformations). Complex-combined malformations are found in some syndromes such as Klippel-Trenaunay, Parkes-Weber, blue rubber bleb, Proteus, and Maffuci.

Most hemangiomas and vascular malformations are recognized on clinical grounds. Imaging is needed in cases of clinical uncertainty or when treatment is required.

IMAGING

Doppler ultrasonography is the easiest modality used to assess the hemodynamics of a vascular lesion and to clarify a doubtful diagnosis when the choice must be made between hemangiomas and malformations. Magnetic resonance imaging (MRI) is best used for evaluating the extent of lesions and their relationships to adjacent structures. Angiography and percutaneous phlebography are reserved for therapeutic purposes (Table 186-2).

HEMANGIOMAS AND OTHER VASCULAR TUMORS

The hemangiomas are infantile or congenital. Infantile hemangiomas are the most common tumors in children younger than 1 year of age. Congenital hemangiomas were first described by Boon and colleagues and are divided into noninvoluting congenital hemangiomas (NICH), which undergo proportionate growth with the child but no regression, and rapidly involuting congenital hemangiomas (RICH), which regress completely within 14 months after birth.

Infantile Hemangiomas

The incidence of infantile hemangiomas is 10% to 12% in full-term babies and over 20% in premature babies, with a definite female predominance (3:1). Hemangiomas usually appear during the first week of life and are located in the head and neck (60%), the trunk (25%), and the extremities (15%). Clinically, hemangiomas may appear as subcutaneous well-circumscribed bluish-red masses that resemble the surface of a strawberry. The spontaneous course of hemangiomas is characterized by rapid postnatal proliferation of 3 to 12 months' duration and variable stability, followed by slow involution (2 to 10 years). Histologically, during the proliferative phase, a hemangioma is made of plump, hyperplastic endothelial cells, pericytes, and dendritic cells, and it contains a large number of mast cells. During the involutive phase, cellular turnover is diminished and deposition of perivascular and interlobular fibrous tissue is progressive. Recent studies of the pathogenesis of vascular disease focus on the role of cell proliferation as a determinant of vessel cellularity. A growing body of evidence suggests that vascular structure and lesion formation are determined

TABLE 186-1		
Vascular Anomalies		
VASCULAR TUMORS	*VASCULAR MALFORMATIONS*	
Hemangiomas	**Simple Malformations**	**Combined Malformations**
Others	Capillary Lymphatic Venous Arterial	Arteriovenous fistulas Arteriovenous malformations Capillary venous malformations Capillary lymphaticovenous malformations Lymphaticovenous malformations Capillary arteriovenous malformations Capillary lymphatico-arteriovenous malformations

by a balance between cell death caused by apoptosis and cell proliferation. During the involutive phase of hemangiomas, apoptosis of endothelial cells announces the switch from uncontrolled growth to spontaneous tumor resorption.

Recent advances in the physiology of angiogenesis have shown the role of basic fibroblast growth factor (BFGF), the proliferating cell nuclear antigen, type IV collagenase, E-selectin, and the monocytic chemoattractant protein during the proliferative phase. Conversely, during the involutive phase, the tissue inhibitor of metalloproteinase is increased (thereby inhibiting new blood vessel formation). Accordingly, BFGF is elevated in the urine initially and tends to decrease as the hemangioma begins to regress. These markers monitor the activity of angiogenesis within the hemangioma. Research is active in exploring histopathology and molecular phenotypes. North and coworkers have discovered an immunohistochemical marker for infantile hemangiomas: the GLU1. The diagnostic is then established precisely when the positive marker immunophenotype GLU1 is positive.

Reports have described associated lesions, including central nervous system anomalies (Dandy-Walker, microcephaly, agenesis of the Corpus Callosum, filum terminale syndrome), ocular anomalies (microphthalmos, cataract, optic nerve hypoplasia), vascular anomalies (coarctation of aorta), and visceral malformations (biliary atresia, imperforated anus, bladder exstrophy). The PHACE association consists of posterior fossa malformations, hemangiomas, arterial and cardiac anomalies, and eye anomalies.

IMAGING FEATURES

On ultrasonography, a variable, well-defined echogenic mass can be seen during the proliferative phase. Sometimes, one or a few vessels are visible in the soft tissue mass; these most often correspond to arteries. The lesion displays enhanced color flow caused by numerous arteries and veins. High vessel density (more than 5 vessels/cm^2) with high Doppler shift (>2 kHz) and low resistance are characteristic of infantile hemangiomas. Arteriovenous shunting, which can be seen on spectral Doppler analysis, is frequently misinterpreted as indicative of an arteriovenous malformation (Figs. 186-1, 186-2).

Hemangioma is a high-flow lesion.

During the involutive phase, the lesion appears as a sonographically heterogeneous mass. This mass decreases in volume with a reduced number of vessels, but most of the time, the high Doppler shift persists in the remaining vessels.

MRI typically shows a well-defined noninfiltrating lesion with an intermediate signal intensity on T1-weighted sequences, and increased signal intensity on T2-weighted sequences (see Figs. 186-1 and 186-2). Fast-flow vessels are identified by the presence of flow voids within and around the soft tissue mass on spin echo (SE) sequences and as high signal intensity on gradient recalled echo sequences. Perilesional edema should not be seen. Vessels with fast-flowing blood are often at the periphery of the mass. After gadolinium injection, high enhancement is observed. MRI signal in involuting hemangiomas depends on the amount of fibrosis, hypointense on T1 and T2, and the quantity of fat, hyperintense on T1 and T2. Gadolinium enhancement decreases significantly (see Fig. 186-2).

Angiography shows a well-circumscribed mass with intense, persistent tissue staining, well organized in a lobular pattern, with enlargement of the branches of the normal adjacent systemic arteries.

Imaging is also useful for determining the presence of some associated lesions, such as urogenital and anorectal anomalies in cases of perineal hemangioma, or the PHACE syndrome (cystic malformation of the posterior fossa, anomalous or dysplastic cerebral arteries, aortic arch and cardiac anomalies, and defects of the eye or ear). Cerebrovascular occlusive disease can occur in infants with associated arterial abnormalities. Underlying occult spinal dysraphism similar to lipomeningocele, tethered spinal cord and diastematomyelia can be seen when the hemangioma is located in the paraspinal area.

Liver hemangiomas are the most common hepatic vascular tumors. The differential diagnosis includes hepatic angiosarcoma, hepatic epithelioid hemangioendothelioma, and metastatic disease such as neuroblastoma.

DIFFERENTIAL DIAGNOSIS

Some nonvascular tumors can mimic the appearance of infantile hemangiomas. When clinical and imaging features, particularly Doppler ultrasound and MRI criteria, are not fully present, a biopsy has to be performed to rule out infantile myofibromatosis, fibrosarcoma, rhabdomyosarcoma, metastatic neuroblastoma, and other tumors.

TABLE 186-2

Imaging Features of Congenital Vascular Anomalies

	Hemangiomas (Tumors)	Venous	AV	Lymphatic
		MALFORMATIONS		
Ultrasonography (US)	Mass of variable echogenicity	Mixed echogenicity lesion—phleboliths (16%) Compressible	Heterogeneous lesion with visible feeders at gray scale US without a well-delimited tissular mass	Macrocystic: multilocular cystic mass Microcystic: hyperechoic lesions
Doppler	High vessel density (>5 vessels/cm²) High Doppler shift (>2 kHz) Low resistance Possible arteriovenous (AV) shunting	Low monophasic venous flow No flow (16%)	High vessel density High systolic flow, low resistance AV shunts Arterialization of veins	Macrocystic: no flow except in septa Microcystic: no flow
Magnetic resonance imaging (MRI)	T1W SE: iso to intermediate possible signal, vascular flow voids T2W SE: high signal intensity (no perilesional edema) GRE: high intensity flow enhancement SE T1W post gadolinium: enhancement	T1W: heterogeneous intermediate signal, absent flow voids T2 FSE fat-sat or STIR: high signal intensity Flash 2D: venous system 3D FISP: venous system Dynamic VIBE: slow enhancement T1W SE post gadolinium: enhancement	T1W + T2W FSE/STIR serpiginous signal voids; absence of dominant mass Bright blood GRE 3D GRE gadolinium: multiple AV fistulas with mixed arterial and venous opacification	Macrocystic: T1W SE: low intermediate T2W SE: high signal Microcystic: T1W SE: intermediate T2W SE: intermediate to high SE T1W post gadolinium: no enhancement, except septa
Angiography	Well-circumscribed masses with intense persistent staining organized in lobular pattern; enlarged branches of normal adjacent arteries	Percutaneous phlebography: spongious cavities, dysplasic channels	Dilation and lengthening of afferent arteries; early opacification of enlarged efferent veins	Percutaneous approach for therapeutic purpose

2D, two-dimensional; 3D, three-dimensional; FSE, fast spin echo; FISP, fast imaging with steady precision; GRE, gradient recalled echo; SE, spin echo; STIR, short tau inversion recovery; T1W, T1 weighted; T2W, T2 weighted; VIBE, volume-interpolated breath-hold examination.

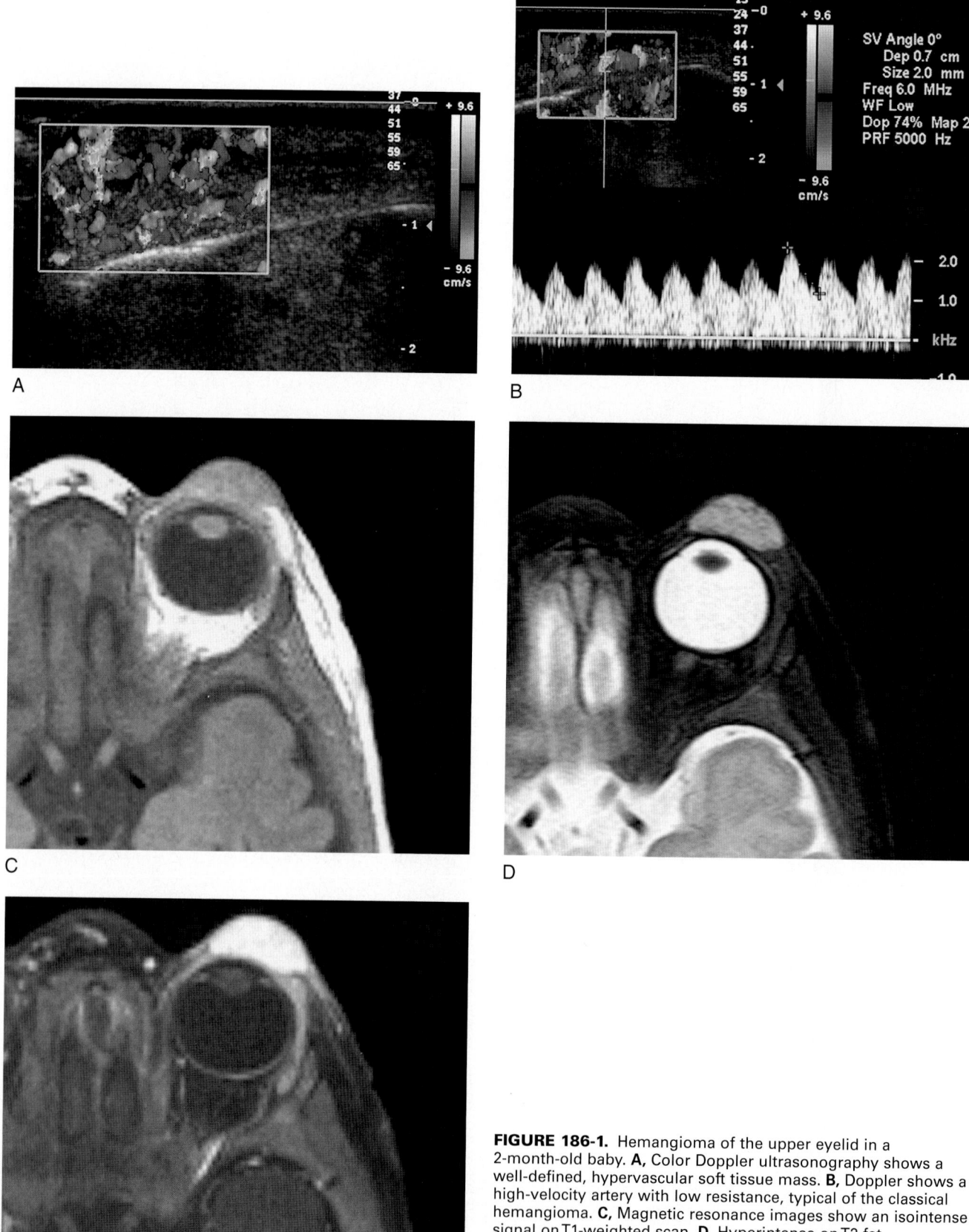

FIGURE 186-1. Hemangioma of the upper eyelid in a 2-month-old baby. **A,** Color Doppler ultrasonography shows a well-defined, hypervascular soft tissue mass. **B,** Doppler shows a high-velocity artery with low resistance, typical of the classical hemangioma. **C,** Magnetic resonance images show an isointense signal on T1-weighted scan. **D,** Hyperintense on T2 fat suppression–weighted images. **E,** An important enhancement with T1 spin echo–fat-suppressed gadolinium injection. (**A,** *see color plate.*)

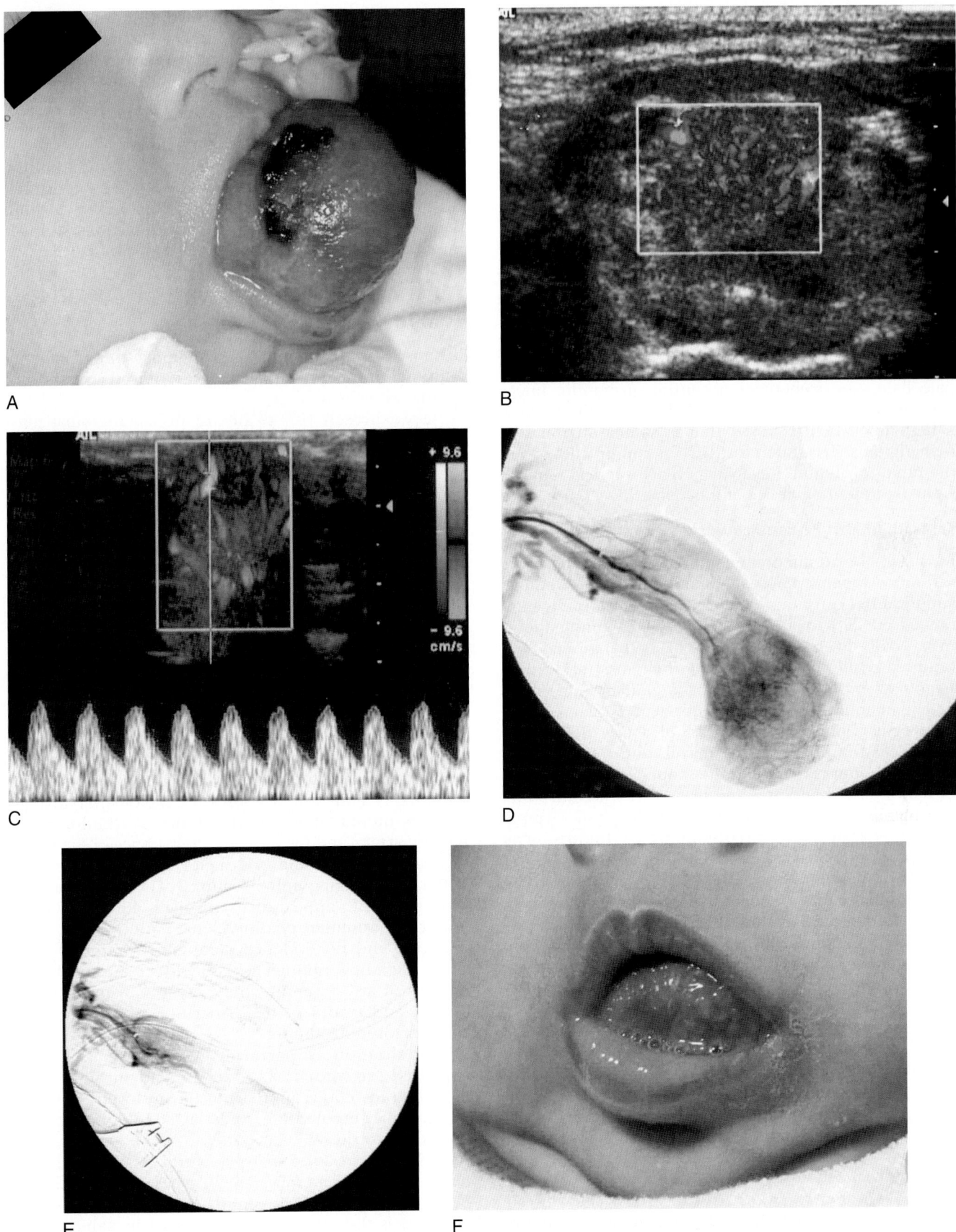

FIGURE 186-2. A 7-month-old infant with voluminous hemangioma of the tongue refractory to steroid and interferon.
A, Photograph of the tongue. **B** and **C,** Doppler ultrasonography reveals a high-flow lesion with high systolic shift and low resistance.
D, Angiogram shows a vascular tumor supplied by the lingual artery with stagnation of contrast and normal draining veins.
E, Embolization was performed with particles. Postembolization opacification of both lingual arteries shows significant devascularization of the tumor. **F,** Photograph of the tongue 1 month after embolization and medical treatment. (**A, B, F,** *see color plate.*)

> Some nonvascular tumors can mimic the appearance of infantile hemangiomas. When clinical and imaging features, particularly Doppler ultrasound and MRI criteria, are not fully present, a biopsy has to be performed.

Congenital Hemangiomas

Two types have been reported: the noninvolutive hemangioma (NICH) and the rapidly involutive hemangioma (RICH). Congenital hemangiomas are GLU1 negative. They are present at birth with an equal sex distribution, are usually solitary, and have a similar average diameter and a predilection for the same cutaneous locations (head or limbs near a joint). Color is violaceous with multiple tiny or coarse telangiectasias, often with a surrounding pale halo, and sometimes a central ulceration, linear scar, or central nodule. Imaging characteristics include a high-flow vascular lesion that is similar to infantile hemangioma. Treatment for RICH is conservative, given the rapid involution. Regarding NICH, surgical removal is the treatment of choice, if it becomes necessary.

KASABACH-MERRITT PHENOMENON AND HEMANGIOENDOTHELIOMAS

Kasabach-Merritt phenomenon (KMP) consists of severe thrombocytopenia, microangiopathic hemolytic anemia, and localized consumption coagulopathy. Mortality rates range from 20% to 30%. It is now clear that most patients with KMP do not have classical hemangiomas but rather kaposiform hemangioendotheliomas (also called *spindle cell hemangiomas*) or tufted angiomas. Kaposiform hemangioendotheliomas are more aggressive, are made of irregular lobules, and consist of a lacy network of sheet cells that infiltrate the dermis and the subcutaneous fat. Tumor cells are spindle-shaped endothelial cells with diminished pericytes and mast cells, microthrombi, and hemosiderin deposits. Dilated, hyperplastic, lymphaticoid channels are predominant in tumors. The immunohistochemical marker GLU1 is negative.

Tufted angiomas can also present with Kasabach-Merritt phenomenon, especially if associated with slitlike lymphatic vessels. Kaposiform hemangioendotheliomas and tufted angiomas may be congenital or may develop during infancy and childhood. They may spontaneously shrink and disappear, or they may persist with progressive worsening. Enjolras and colleagues reported 41 patients with residual lesions after thrombocytopenia and coagulopathy had resolved. Because of its mortality rate, KMP requires aggressive treatment.

Imaging of Hemangioendotheliomas

On ultrasonography, hemangioendotheliomas are seen as ill-defined soft tissue masses with variable echogenicity. Calcifications were present in 3 of 5 cases in our series. Color Doppler shows a high, moderate, or low vessel density, and most hemangioendotheliomas have a high Doppler shift >2 kHz.

T1-weighted MRI sequences show a heterogeneous soft tissue mass that is isointense or hypointense compared with the muscle. T2-weighted sequences show an hyperintense lesion with subcutaneous stranding. Signal voids can be seen on gradient recalled echo. Post-gadolinium imaging displays a diffuse, heterogeneous enhancement in the soft tissue mass. In contrast to infantile hemangiomas, destruction of adjacent bones can be seen with hemangioendotheliomas.

In our experience with hemangioendotheliomas, angiography shows an increased number of arterial vessels without delimitation of the lesion and without stagnation of contrast medium. Arteriovenous shunt is rarely seen within the lesion.

TREATMENT OF PATIENTS WITH VASCULAR TUMOR

In most cases of infantile hemangioma and hemangioendothelioma, no treatment is required because of spontaneous involution.

Approximately 10% to 20% of all hemangiomas must be treated. Major indications for treatment include periocular location with compromised vision, high-output cardiac failure, ulceration, compression of the airway, facial hemangiomas with rapid growth and distortion (presumed to result in important cosmetic sequelae), and symptomatic muscular hemangiomas.

Medical treatment is usually attempted first, with the use of steroids, interferon, or vincristine. Laser is used in ulceration and particularly in subglottic hemangiomas.

Embolization or surgery is required if medical alternatives are ineffective, most often in cases of liver hemangioma with cardiac failure that does not respond to pharmacologic treatment, hemangioendothelioma complicated by Kasabach-Merritt phenomenon, and uncontrolled proliferative hemangioma with functional disorder (e.g., tongue with feeding problem).

In cases of liver hemangioma, precise pre-embolization mapping is mandatory for assessing the possible involvement of intercostal or phrenic arteries, in addition to the hepatic artery, and for verifying the patency of the portal system. Kassarjian and colleagues have described five patterns of angiographic features. The first type, the most classical appearance, involves early filling of abnormal vascular channels, stagnation of contrast material, and no evidence of direct shunting. Type 2 shows high-flow nodules without direct shunts. Type 3 consists of arteriovenous shunts, type 4 of portovenous shunts, and type 5 of the association of arteriovenous with portovenous shunts.

Embolization is performed through the arterial approach for types 1, 2, 3, and 5, and through transhepatic transvenous approaches for portovenous shunts in type 4. Embolization material should be selected according to the vascular patterns of the lesions. Large particles can be used in types 1 and 2. Platinum fiber microcoils are generally safe in types 3, 4, and 5 and permit occlusion of the shunts. Glue (N-butyl-2-cyanoacrylate) is the most effective material in patients with direct arteriovenous and arterioportal shunting arising from multiple sources. Medical antiangiogenesis drugs should be continued after embolization until nearly complete regression of the lesions has occurred.

For soft tissue infantile hemangioma or hemangioendothelioma, we favor the use of gelfoam or polyvinyl alcohol (PVA) particles and complete the embolization with microcoils, if necessary. Because of the patient's weight and related limitations in the amount of contrast, the procedure can be repeated if symptoms of cardiac failure persist.

VASCULAR MALFORMATIONS

As embryonic anomalies of the vascular system, malformations are subdivided into high-flow arteriovenous malformations and low-flow capillary, venous, lymphatic, or combined malformations (see Table 186-2). Vascular malformations are present at birth but can also appear during infancy or puberty. They grow with the patient. Hormonal modulations of vascular malformations can be seen during puberty or the menstrual cycle or when the patient is under anovulant therapy. Surgery or trauma can also lead to progression of vascular malformations.

> As embryonic anomalies of the vascular system, malformations are subdivided into high-flow arteriovenous malformations and low-flow capillary, venous, lymphatic, or combined malformations.

Histologically, vascular malformation cells are stable and have a slow (normal) turnover and a flat endothelium with a normal thin basal membrane. Malformations, to the contrary of hemangiomas, do not regress spontaneously and can produce venous stasis, ischemia, localized consumptive coagulopathy, and skeletal anomalies. Boys and girls are equally affected.

VENOUS MALFORMATIONS

Venous malformations (VMs) are due to abnormal development of the vein wall. Venous malformations occur sporadically, but some cases can be inherited. A locus for autosomal dominant multiple cutaneous and mucosal VMs, VMCM1, was identified on chromosome 9p21. A mutation was found in the endothelial cell–specific receptor tyrosine kinase TIE-2. This mutation is likely to occur in VMs. VMs with glomus cells show linkage to chromosome 1p21-p22.

VMs are characterized by a soft, compressible, non-pulsatile mass that expands after Vasalva maneuver and after compression. Often asymptomatic, VMs grow in proportion with the child. They may become painful in cases of thrombophlebitis or muscular or articular involvement. VMs are sometimes associated with bony abnormalities or occur as part of a diffuse syndrome (Klippel-Trenaunay, Gorham Stout, Maffuci, blue rubber bleb nevus).

A chronic form of consumptive coagulopathy, as shown by positive D-dimer levels, and normal or low platelets and fibrinogen value can cause episodes of thrombosis that result in phleboliths or bleeding (e.g., hemarthrosis, hematomas, severe intraoperative bleeding).

Histopathology reveals multiple thin-walled vessels with flattened endothelial cells, without proliferative features, and with smooth muscle wall deficiency.

Imaging of Venous Malformations (Figs. 186-3, 186-4)

Plain radiographs show a soft tissue mass with occasional phleboliths; adjacent bone may become thinned, demineralized, hypoplastic, or eroded.

Doppler ultrasonography is the initial modality of choice for differentiating VMs from other vascular abnormalities. On gray scale images, VMs appear as compressible hypoechoic or heterogeneous lesions. Calcifications (shown in less than 20% of cases) are specific for VM; anechoic channels may be seen. Doppler examination reveals a monophasic low-velocity flow. In 20% of VMs, no flow can be exhibited. Dynamic maneuvers such as Valsalva or manual compression are sometimes necessary to induce a visible Doppler flow. In the few lesions that exhibit a biphasic component to their vascular flow, a mixed VM is likely (e.g., capillary-venous malformation, lymphatic-capillary-venous malformation).

MRI is an excellent technique for defining the extent of lesions and determining their relationship to adjacent structures. On T1-weighted images, VMs are hypointense or isointense compared with muscle. They may present with a heterogeneous or intermediate signal caused by thrombosis or hemorrhage. Absence of flow voids is mandatory for the diagnosis of venous malformation. On T2 fat-saturation–weighted sequences or short tau inversion recovery (STIR), high signal intensity is observed; sometimes, low signal intensity is due to thrombosis or phleboliths. Small fluid-fluid levels can be seen.

T2-weighted gradient echo sequences can be useful for exhibiting calcification or hemosiderin. On gradient echo sequences, the absence of intravascular signal suggests a slow-flow malformation. Three-dimensional FISP (fast imaging with steady precision) phlebographic sequence, or Flash 2D, permits evaluation of draining veins. T1-weighted sequences with fat suppression and gadolinium injection must be performed to evaluate perfusion of the malformation. Postgadolinium sequences are useful for assessing residual perfusion. Heterogeneous enhancement is seen. MRI is very helpful for delimitation and assessment of the extension, but it is not specific for VMs. MRI results must be correlated with clinical findings and Doppler examination results to reinforce the diagnosis.

Angiography is not required for diagnosis of VMs. Usually, the arteries are normal, and only evidence of venous stasis is seen. Sometimes, the angiogram is completely normal. Percutaneous direct phlebography under fluoroscopy is the best way to document the anatomy of venous malformations and their draining veins. Phlebography is often the initial therapeutic step.

Three different phlebographic patterns may be observed. The most common is a cavitary pattern with late filling of venous drainage and no evidence of abnormal veins. The second pattern consists of a spongy appearance with small honeycomb cavities, and the third appears as rapid opacification of dysmorphic veins.

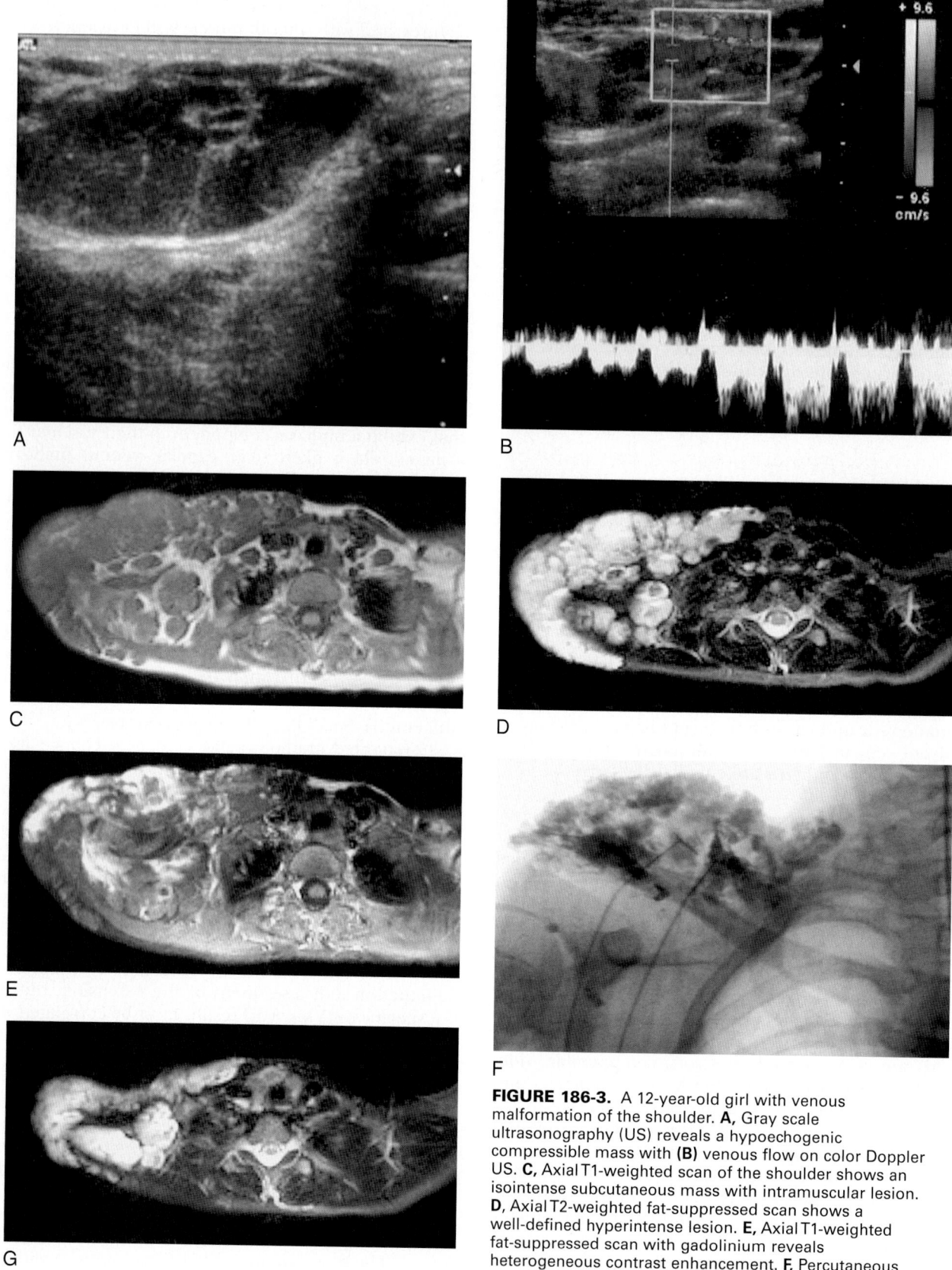

FIGURE 186-3. A 12-year-old girl with venous malformation of the shoulder. **A,** Gray scale ultrasonography (US) reveals a hypoechogenic compressible mass with **(B)** venous flow on color Doppler US. **C,** Axial T1-weighted scan of the shoulder shows an isointense subcutaneous mass with intramuscular lesion. **D,** Axial T2-weighted fat-suppressed scan shows a well-defined hyperintense lesion. **E,** Axial T1-weighted fat-suppressed scan with gadolinium reveals heterogeneous contrast enhancement. **F,** Percutaneous sclerotherapy shows multiple cavities filled with blood. **G,** Eight months post three sessions of foam injection, significant regression is noted on axial short tau inversion recovery scan.

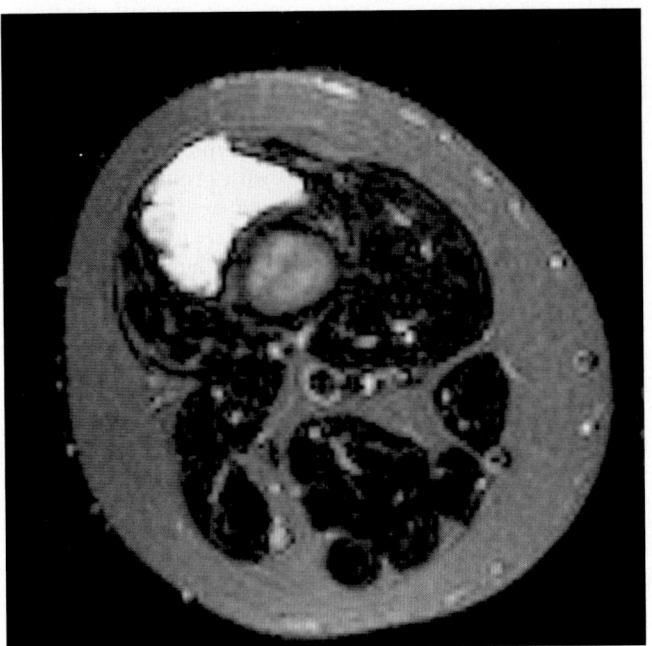
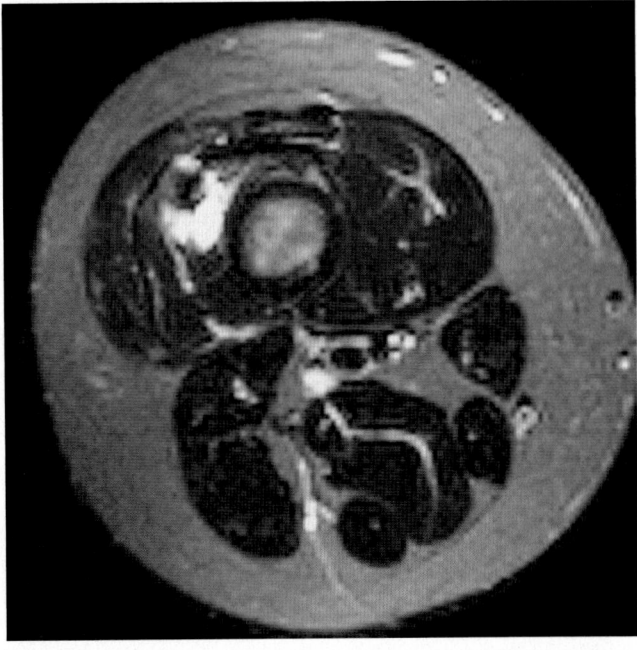

A   B

FIGURE 186-4. A 9-year-old boy with intramuscular venous malformation. **A,** Short tau inversion recovery (STIR) sequence before sclerotherapy. **B,** STIR sequence after two sessions of foam injection. Significant regression was observed.

Treatment of Venous Malformations

No medical treatment has been effective for the treatment of VMs. Prior to any intervention, the patient should be evaluated for low-grade disseminated intravascular coagulopathy (DIC) with platelet count, prothrombin time, partial thromboplastin time, fibrinogen levels, and D-dimer. Enjolras and associates have reported a high incidence of DIC in patients with VM. DIC can be exacerbated with the use of a tourniquet; this can result in postoperative hematoma, compartment syndrome, and tissue loss.

Conservative treatment with elastic stockings can provide comfort, protection of skin, and improvement of coagulopathy. Low molecular weight heparin helps to minimize the risk of hemorrhage during treatment in patients with chronic localized intravascular coagulation.

Sclerotherapy with or without surgery is the treatment of choice for symptomatic venous malformations. Sclerotherapy is performed in the angiographic suite, with the patient under sedation or general anesthesia. Direct percutaneous puncture of the lesion with or without ultrasound guidance is made with a Teflon-sheathed needle (Angiocath 21, 20 gauge; 2 inches; Becton Dickinson Vascular Access, Sandy, Utah) or a 25-gauge butterfly needle. Contrast injection documents the size of the lesion and its morphologic type, that is, varicose with dilated or dysplasic channels, lobulated with rounded vascular cavities, or spongious, infiltrating lesions and draining veins (normal or ectatic dilated veins). Tourniquet or manual compression is useful for minimizing the passage of the sclerosing agent into the systemic circulation. A progressive decompression is then paramount to avoiding pulmonary emboli. The author tends to avoid the tourniquet or manual compression.

> Sclerotherapy, with or without surgery, is the treatment of choice for symptomatic venous malformations.

Reported sclerosant agents include chemical agents (iodine or absolute alcohol), osmotic agents (salicylates or hypertonic saline), detergents (morrhuate sodium, sotradecol, polidocanol), and diatrizoate sodium. Ethibloc, histoacryl, and coils are also used for the treatment of venous malformations.

In the literature, absolute ethanol and foam (5 ml sotradecol with 2 ml of lipiodol and 10 to 20 ml of air) are the most commonly used agents. The amount of absolute alcohol used should be limited to 0.5 to 1 ml/kg. The amount of foam that should be used has not been well established.

The main complications of sclerothrerapy are cutaneous necrosis and neural toxicity. With alcohol, systemic complications, such as hemolysis with potential neurotoxicity and cardiac arrest, are rare but are reported.

For large VMs with serious danger of compromised airways, a tracheostomy is indicated for patients who require multiple sclerotherapeutic sessions. Analgesic and anti-inflammatory medications (nonsteroidal anti-inflammatories [NSAIs] or corticoids) must be given to alleviate symptoms.

We recommend 8 to 12 weeks between subsequent sclerotherapy sessions.

ARTERIOVENOUS MALFORMATIONS

Arteriovenous malformations (AVMs; high-flow malformations) are abnormal communications between arteries and veins. These present clinically as a pulsatile mass, with a thrill, a bruit, and occasionally, local hyperthermia, skeletal overgrowth, trophic changes, congestive heart failure, and functional impairment due to arterial ischemia. Some AVMs at a quiescent stage can mimic clinically port-wine capillary malformations or hemangiomas; the risk then is to trigger acute exacerbations through biopsy or partial local treatment. Most patients with AVMs experience flare-up before puberty. AVMs are isolated anomalies, or they may occur as part of a syndrome such as Parkes-Weber or Rendu-Osler-Weber.

Imaging of Arteriovenous Malformations

(Fig. 186-5)

On ultrasonography, AVMs are poorly defined, and no or little tissue mass is visible. The lesion is made up largely of vessels with multiple arteriovenous shunts on Doppler ultrasonography.

Color Doppler and spectral analysis show high vessel density of 2 to 5 vessels/cm^2 and high systolic flow, as well as characteristic multiple feeding arteries with increased diastolic flow and high-velocity venous return with systolic/diastolic flow. In contrast to hemangiomas, arterialization of all veins (i.e., pulsatile flow) is consistent in AVMs.

MRI shows low signal intensity caused by the flow-void phenomenon of rapid or turbulent blood flow on T1- and T2-weighted SE sequences or STIR. A hypersignal is observed on gradient echo and angiographic sequences. Occasionally, numerous interspersed small punctuated areas of high signal intensity are caused by hemorrhage and thrombosis.

Angiography is strongly recommended for planning therapy. Angiographic features of AVM include dilation and lengthening of afferent arteries with early opacification (shunting) of enlarged efferent veins. Selective and superselective injections are essential for determining the extent of the AVM; the precise mapping of feeding vessels is used to plan treatment.

Treatment of Arteriovenous Malformations

AVMs represent an important challenge for interventional angiographers. Some AVMs respond well to embolization, but others progress despite embolotherapy. That is the reason why we recommend conservative management in cases of quiescent AVM. However, treatment is required in cases of severe cosmetic consequences, of ulceration, of pain associated with distal steal phenomenon, or of gangrene. Less commonly, bleeding, compartment syndrome, severe overgrowth, congestive heart failure, and failure to thrive could lead to intervention.

Embolization is the first choice for the treatment of AVMs. The procedure should be performed by well-trained angiographers with the patient under general anesthesia. To destroy the AVM and reduce the risk of recurrence, a superselective catheterization is necessary; this should be combined with percutaneous direct puncture of the nidus, when feasible.

> **Embolization is the first choice for the treatment of arteriovenous malformations.**

The best agent used to destroy the nidus is dehydrated alcohol. Ethanol should be used with great caution. The amount of ethanol and the pressure of injection are evaluated on contrast material test injections. The maximum dose is 1 ml/kg. In cases of large AVM, Swan-Ganz and arterial line monitoring is recommended.

Several complications have been reported to occur after ethanol embolization (10% to 30% of cases); these include pulmonary emboli, cardiopulmonary collapse, neuropathy (motor or sensory nerve injuries), skin blisters, tissue necrosis, and vascular spasm. Also, coagulopathy disorders have been reported with ethanol that can increase the risk of bleeding, thrombosis, or hematoma. In these patients, in whom surgery followed the embolization procedure, histoacryl (N-butyl-2-cyano-acryl; not approved by the U.S. Food and Drug Administration [FDA]) is recommended.

LYMPHATIC MALFORMATIONS

Because of a defect in the connection of lymphatics with the venous system, or the abnormal development of lymphatic vessels, lymphatic malformations are most often located in the head and neck area (70% to 80%). These may be associated with Turner, Noonan, multiple pterygium syndrome, fetal alcohol syndrome, and some trisomies. Sudden enlargement indicates bleeding or inflammation. Cystic lymphatic malformations can be subdivided into macrocystic, microcystic, and mixed types.

Imaging of Lymphatic Malformations

On ultrasonography, macrocystic lymphangiomas consist of multiloculated cystic lesions with vascular channels in the septa with low arterial or venous blood flow (Fig. 186-6). Pure microcystic lymphangiomas are ill-defined and hyperechoic because of numerous interfaces of the microcystic walls.

MRI shows a septated mass with low signal intensity on T1 and high signal intensity on T2 (Fig. 186-7). Because of varying amounts of protein or hemorrhage within the lesion, lymphangiomas occasionally present with variable signal intensity on T1 and T2 sequences. No gadolinium enhancement is seen, except in the septa. Pure microcystic lymphangiomas are isointense on T1 and display a heterogeneous signal on T2, with or without slight heterogeneous enhancement on T1 postgadolinium. Stranding of adjacent subcutaneous fat may be noted. MRI with lymphangiography shows dilated or interrupted lymphatic channels, especially evident in the limbs.

Treatment of Lymphatic Malformations

Many authors have proposed primary surgical excision as the treatment of choice for lymphatic malformation (LM); however, mortality ranges from 2% to 6%, perma-

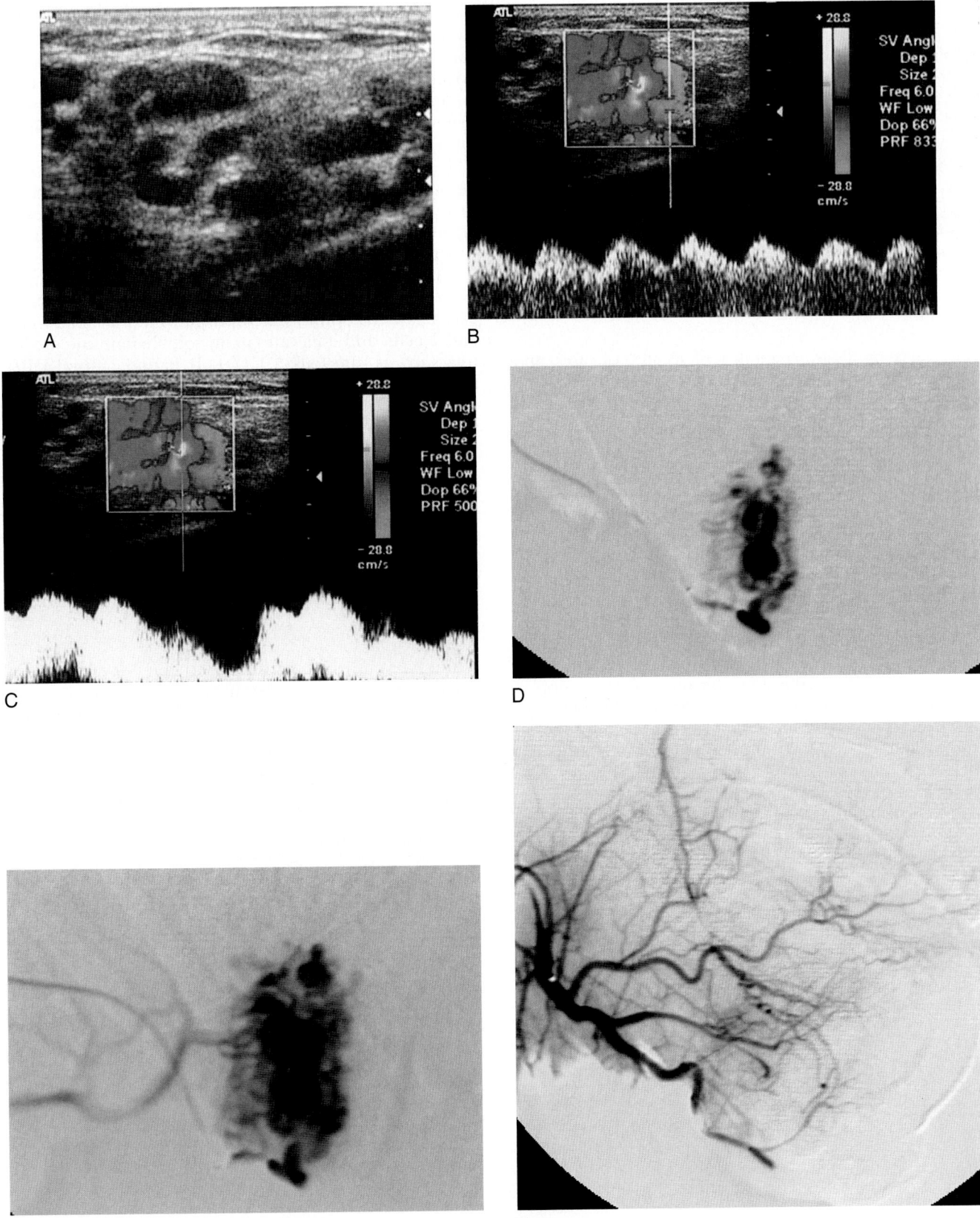

FIGURE 186-5. A 14-year-old girl with arteriovenous malformation (AVM) of the chin. **A,** Ultrasonography of the chin lesion reveals numerous vessels. **B,** Color Doppler with spectral analysis shows high-velocity arteries with a low resistance index. **C,** Pulsatile venous flow. **D,** Angiogram reveals a high-flow lesion with numerous abnormal dilated arteries from distal branches of mandibular arteries. **E,** Early draining through huge veins. **F,** Control angiogram after embolization with alcohol shows occlusion of the AVM.

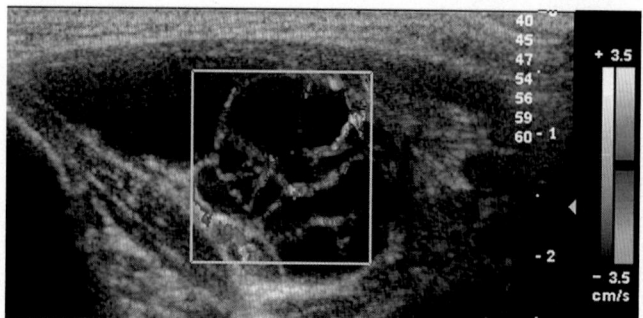

FIGURE 186-6. A 3-year-old boy with a cervical lymphatic malformation. Color Doppler ultrasound (US) shows a septated cystic mass with arteries and veins in the septa. (*See color plate.*)

nent nerve paralysis occurs in 12% to 33% of cases, and the recurrence rate is quoted at between 11.8% and 52.9%.

Several therapeutic alternatives to surgery have been described for the treatment of LM; these include simple puncture, irradiation, chemotherapy, and intracystic administration of sclerosing substances. We favor a sclerosing percutaneous approach for the macrocystic and mixed types with less recurrence and fewer complications than are reported after surgery. Sometimes, we must complete sclerosing treatment with a subsequent surgical procedure.

Sclerosing treatment is performed with the patient under sedation or general anesthesia. Under ultrasonographic guidance, we puncture the cyst with a 22 to 24 gauge sheath needle. Opacification of the lesion is essential for establishing its volume. In most lymphangiomas, intercystic communications occur. Many sclerosing agents have been reported, but the most frequently used include Ethibloc, fibrin sealant, Picibanil (OK-432), doxycycline, and bleomycin.

In our institution, we have chosen Ethibloc because of its effectiveness and safety. Ethibloc (Ethicon, Hamburg), which is not available in the United States, is a mixture of zein (corn protein), alcohol, and contrast medium. The slerosing effect is due to the gigantocellular inflammatory reaction. The product is available in a preloaded syringe (7.5 ml). External leakage of Ethibloc occurs frequently. However, no major sequelae have been reported, and patients with extruded material have favorable outcomes.

Fibrin sealant, which is FDA approved, appears also to be safe with no evidence of transmission of hepatitis or human immunodeficiency virus (HIV). This adhesive agent can effectively seal tissue surfaces and eliminate potential dead spaces.

The sclerosing ability of Picibanil (OK-432) appears to be related to its immunomodulatory activity. Picibanil activates neutrophils, macrophages, natural killer cells, and T cells, and it elevates many soluble immune mediators such as interleukin (IL)-1, IL-2, and natural killer activating factor. Additional studies are required if we are to gain a full understanding of the precise pathways used for induction of sclerosis. No significant toxicity of Picibanil was recorded in the various series. In situ Bleomycin was also reportedly used in the treatment of lymphangiomas. The dose of medication used ranges from 1 to 9 mg, and procedures can be repeated at 1- to 6-week intervals.

Whatever the agent used, failed sclerotherapy does not hinder subsequent surgical procedures.

CONCLUSION

While new drugs continue to be developed in angiogenesis research laboratories, radiologists have an important role in the treatment of hemangiomas and vascular malformations. Intervention remains crucial in cases of alarming hemangioma, VM, LM, and AVM.

A multidisciplinary team, including pediatricians, hematologists, surgeons, and radiologists, must manage problem cases in terms of diagnostic workup and therapeutic options.

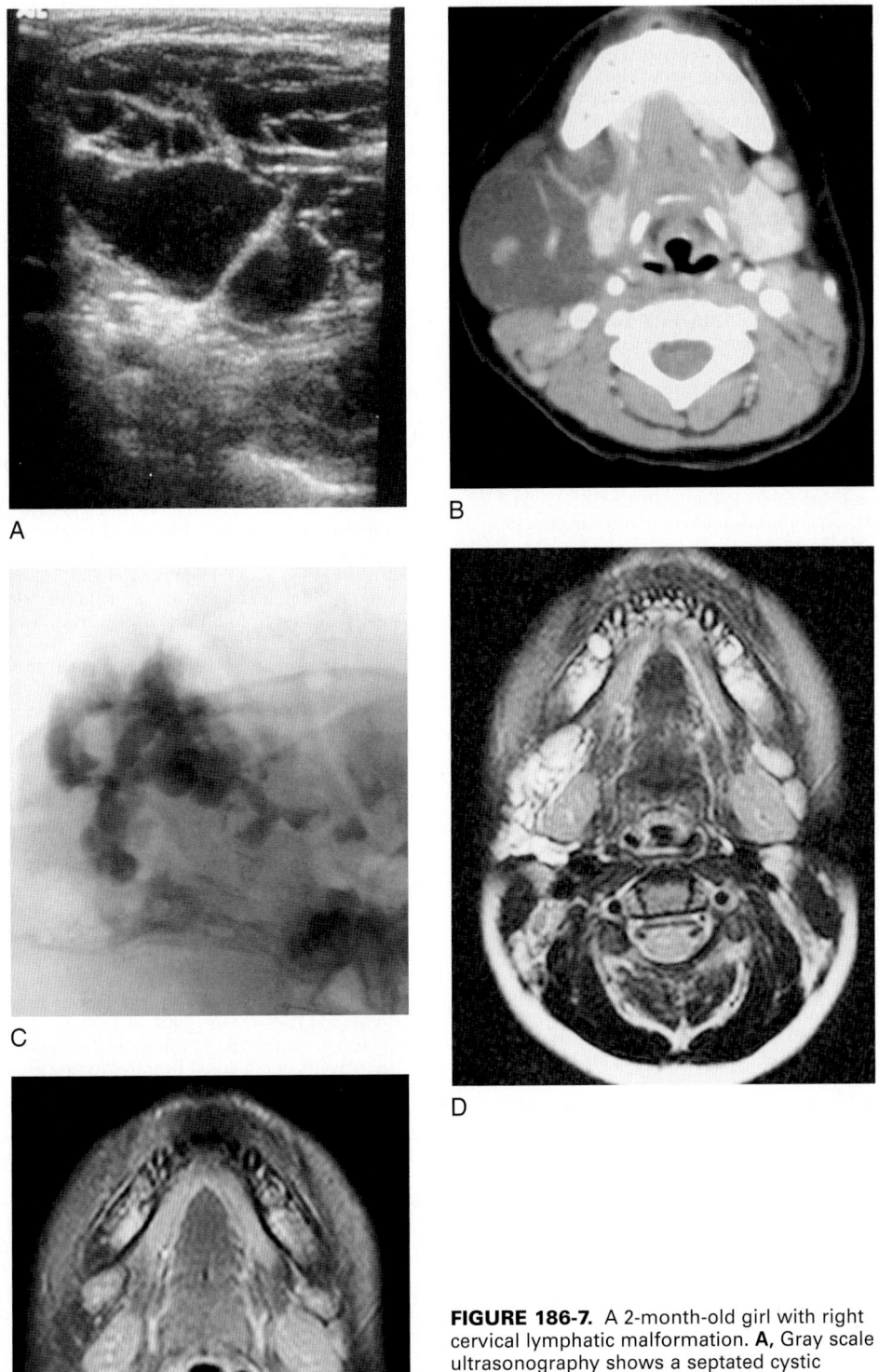

FIGURE 186-7. A 2-month-old girl with right cervical lymphatic malformation. **A,** Gray scale ultrasonography shows a septated cystic mass. **B,** Computed tomography scan of the right cervicofacial lymphangioma before sclerotherapy treatment with Ethibloc. **C,** Percutaneous puncture of the cystic mass shows communication between the cysts. Ethibloc (3 ml) was injected after the opacification. **D,** Magnetic resonance scan was performed 3 years later. T2-weighted images reveal significant regression of the lymphangioma with residual cystic lesions. **E,** T1-weighted scan with gadolinium shows no enhancement of the residual lesion.

SUGGESTED READINGS

Boon LM, Brouillard P, Irrthum A, et al: A gene for inherited cutaneous venous anomalies ("glomangiomas") localizes to chromosome 1p21-22. Am J Hum Genet 1999;65:125

Boon LM, Enjolras O, Mulliken JB: Congenital hemangioma: evidence of accelerated involution. J Pediatr 1996;128:329

Brouillard P, Boon LM, Mulliken JB, et al: Mutations in a novel factor, glomulin, are responsible for glomuvenous malformations ("glomangiomas"). Am J Hum Genet 2002;70:866

Burrows PE, Dubois J, Kassarjian A: Pediatric hepatic vascular anomalies. Pediatr Radiol 2001;31:533

Burrows PE, Mason KP: Percutaneous treatment of low flow vascular malformations. J Vasc Interv Radiol 2004;15:431

Cabrera J, Cabrera J Jr, Garcia-Olmedo MA, et al: Treatment of venous malformations with sclerosant in microfoam form. Arch Dermatol 2003;139:1409

Castanon M, Margarit J, Carrasco R, et al: Long-term follow-up of nineteen cystic lymphangiomas treated with fibrin sealant. J Pediatr Surg 1999;34:1276

Choi YH, Han MH, O-Ki K, et al: Craniofacial cavernous venous malformations: percutaneous sclerotherapy with use of ethanolamine oleate. J Vasc Interv Radiol 2002;13:475

Dickerhoff R, Bode VU: Cyclophosphamide in non-resectable cystic hygroma. Lancet 1990;335:1474

Dubois J, Garel L: Practical aspect of intervention in vascular anomalies in children. Semin Interv Radiol 2002;19:73

Dubois J, Garel L, Abela J, et al: Lymphangiomas in children: percutaneous sclerotherapy with an alcoholic solution of zein. Radiology 1997;204:651

Dubois J, Garel L, David M, et al: Vascular soft-tissue tumors in infancy: distinguishing features on Doppler sonography. AJR Am J Roentgenol 2002;178:1541

Dubois J, Patriquin HB, Garel L, et al: Soft-tissue hemangiomas in infants and children: diagnosis using Doppler sonography. AJR Am J Roentgenol 1998;171:247

Enjolras O: Vascular tumors and vascular malformations: are we at the dawn of a better knowledge? Pediatr Dermatol 1999;16:238

Enjolras O, Ciabrini D, Mazoyer E, et al: Extensive pure venous malformations in the upper or lower limb: a review of 27 cases. J Am Acad Dermatol 1997;36(2 Pt 1):219

Enjolras O, Mulliken JB, Wassef M, et al: Residual lesions after Kasabach-Merritt phenomenon in 41 patients. J Am Acad Dermatol 2000;42(2 Pt 1):225

Enjolras O, Wassef M, Mazoyer E, et al: Infants with Kasabach-Merritt syndrome do not have "true" hemangiomas. J Pediatr 1997;130:631

Ezekowitz RA, Mulliken JB, Folkman J: Interferon alfa-2a therapy for life-threatening hemangiomas of infancy. N Engl J Med 1992;326:1456

Folkman J: Seminars in Medicine of the Beth Israel Hospital, Boston. Clinical applications of research on angiogenesis. N Engl J Med 1995;333:1757

Frieden IJ, Haggstrom AN, Drolet BA, et al: Infantile hemangiomas: current knowledge, future directions. Proceedings of a research workshop on infantile hemangiomas. Pediatr Dermatol 2005;22:383

Frieden IJ, Reese V, Cohen D: PHACE syndrome: the association of posterior fossa brain malformations, hemangiomas, arterial anomalies, coarctation of the aorta and cardiac defects, and eye abnormalities. Arch Dermatol 1996;132:307

Gorincour G, Kokta V, Rypens F, et al: Imaging characteristics of two subtypes of congenital hemangiomas: rapidly involuting congenital hemangiomas and non-involuting congenital hemangiomas. Pediatr Radiol 2005;35:1178

Greinwald JH Jr, Burke DK, Sato Y, et al: Treatment of lymphangiomas in children: an update of Picibanil (OK-432) sclerotherapy. Otolaryngol Head Neck Surg 1999;121:381

Hammer FD, Boon LM, Mathurin P, et al: Ethanol sclerotherapy of venous malformations: evaluation of systemic ethanol contamination. J Vasc Interv Radiol 2001;12:595

Han MH, Seong SO, Kim HD, et al: Craniofacial arteriovenous malformation: preoperative embolization with direct puncture and injection of n-butyl cyanoacrylate. Radiology 1999;211:661

Hancock BJ, St-Vil D, Lukes FI, et al: Complications of lymphangiomas in children. J Pediatr Surg 1992;27:220

Herbreteau D, Riche MC, Enjolras O, et al: Percutaneous embolization with Ethibloc of lymphatic cystic malformations with a review of the experience in 70 patients. Int Angiol 1993;12:34

Kohout MP, Hansen M, Pribaz JJ, et al: Arteriovenous malformations of the head and neck: natural history and management. Plast Reconstr Surg 1998;102:643

Konez O, Burrows PE: Magnetic resonance of vascular anomalies. Magn Reson Imaging Clin N Am 2002;10:363

Marrocco-Trischitta MM, Guerrini P, Abeni D, et al: Reversible cardiac arrest after polidocanol sclerotherapy of peripheral venous malformation. Dermatol Surg 2002;28:153

Mason KP, Neufeld EJ, Karian VE, et al: Coagulation abnormalities in pediatric and adult patients after sclerotherapy or embolization of vascular anomalies. AJR Am J Roentgenol 2001;177:1359

Mazoyer E, Enjolras O, Laurian C, et al: Coagulation abnormalities associated with extensive venous malformations of the limbs: differentiation from Kasabach-Merritt syndrome. Clin Lab Haematol 2002;24:243

Mulliken JB, Enjolras O: Congenital hemangiomas and infantile hemangioma: missing links. J Am Acad Dermatol 2004;50:875

Mulliken JB, Fishman SJ, Burrows PE: Vascular anomalies. Curr Probl Surg 2000;37:517

Mulliken JB, Glowacki J: Hemangiomas and vascular malformations in infants and children: a classification based on endothelial characteristics. Plast Reconstr Surg 1982;69:412

North PE, Waner M, James CA, et al: Congenital nonprogressive hemangioma: a distinct clinicopathologic entity unlike infantile hemangioma. Arch Dermatol 2001;137:1607

North PE, Waner M, Mizeracki A, et al: GLUT1: a newly discovered immunohistochemical marker for juvenile hemangiomas. Hum Pathol 2000;31:11

Ogita S, Tsuto T, Nakamura K, et al: OK-432 therapy in 64 patients with lymphangioma. J Pediatr Surg 1994;29:784

Orford J, Barker A, Thonell S, et al: Bleomycin therapy for cystic hygroma. J Pediatr Surg 1995;30:1282

Pollman MJ, Naumovski L, Gibbons GH: Vascular cell apoptosis: cell type–specific modulation by transforming growth factor-β_1 in endothelial cells versus smooth muscle cells. Circulation 1999;99:2019

Razon MJ, Kraling BM, Mulliken JB, et al: Increased apoptosis coincides with onset of involution in infantile hemangioma. Microcirculation 1998;5:189

Sarkar M, Mulliken JB, Kozakewich HP, et al: Thrombocytopenic coagulopathy (Kasabach-Merritt phenomenon) is associated with kaposiform hemangioendothelioma and not with common infantile hemangioma. Plast Reconstr Surg 1997;100:1377

Tessari L, Cavezzi A, Frullini A: Preliminary experience with a new sclerosing foam in the treatment of varicose veins. Dermatol Surg 2001;27:58

Vikkula M, Boon LM, Mulliken JB: Molecular genetics of vascular malformations. Matrix Biol 2001;20:327

Yakes WF, Rossi P, Odink H: How I do it: arteriovenous malformation management. Cardiovasc Intervent Radiol 1996;19:65

187 Vasculitis in Children and Adolescents

FRANK P. MORELLO

INTRODUCTION

Vasculitis is a clinical and pathologic systemic process that is characterized by inflammation in the walls of blood vessels with reactive damage to the mural structures. This ultimately leads to vessel necrosis and occlusion with end-organ tissue ischemia. Vasculitis may occur as a primary process or may be secondary to an underlying disease. It may be the predominant manifestation or just one aspect of a multisystem disease process. Initially, it is important to sort out from a systemic vasculitis syndrome other processes such as infection, thrombosis, or neoplasia that may have similar clinical manifestations, or disease processes that have vasculitis as a component. This is important because some vasculitic disorders can be severe or life-threatening if prompt and appropriate treatment is not provided. Once it has been established that a vasculitis is present, distinguishing the type of vasculitis becomes the next goal.

> **Vasculitis may be the predominant feature or just one aspect of a multisystem disease process.**

This chapter focuses on the approach of the health care provider to the child or adolescent with vasculitis; a review of the pathophysiologic mechanisms, classification of the vasculitides, and clinical and radiographic manifestations are discussed. Specific cases in which vasculitis is the primary or predominant feature are reviewed.

Radiographic images obtained with computed tomography (CT), magnetic resonance imaging (MRI), magnetic resonance angiography (MRA), and conventional catheter angiography serve as illustrative examples. Disease processes and differential diagnoses are discussed.

CLINICAL AND RADIOLOGIC APPROACHES

The diagnosis of vasculitis should be considered in children and adolescents who present with systemic symptoms and evidence of single organ or multiorgan dysfunction. Common symptoms include fatigue, weakness, fever, arthalgias, and abdominal pain. Common signs include hypertension, neurologic dysfunction, and renal insufficiency, as well as urine sediment that contains red cells and cellular or granular casts. However, these findings are neither sensitive nor specific for

vasculitis. Because of the variability and overlap of vasculitic diseases, a single method of evaluation is difficult to incorporate.

To start, a detailed history is important for assessing whether the patient has been exposed to drugs that may produce hypersensitivity vasculitis; a history of hepatitis C, which is responsible for some cases of polyarteritis, is sought, along with information on whether a coexisting disease is present, especially a connective tissue disorder such as systemic lupus erythematosus. Some vasculitides have a propensity to occur in certain age, gender, or ethnic groups; this information can be helpful to the clinician in making a diagnosis.

A thorough physical examination helps reveal the distribution and extent of vascular involvement. The presence of particular physical findings or a particular pattern of findings may strongly indicate a specific vasculitis. As an example, palpable purpura in a child with complaints of abdominal and joint pain suggests a diagnosis of Henoch-Schönlein purpura. However, mucocutaneous inflammation with diffuse palmar and plantar erythema in an infant suggests a diagnosis of Kawasaki disease.

Laboratory tests should be used to ascertain the type of vasculitis, whether it is infectious or is associated with a rheumatic disease, which organ systems are affected, and the extent of involvement. Basic laboratory tests include serum creatinine, muscle enzyme concentrations, and liver function studies. More specific tests include antinuclear antibody and serum complement. Many of these tests, however, are not specific for any one type of vasculitis. Arteriography and other radiologic imaging approaches are helpful in identifying and characterizing vasculitis of large and medium-sized arteries, as well as distribution and extent of disease. Radiographic abnormalities are often not pathognomonic but may support a diagnosis when combined with other data. A biopsy, when possible, of the most clinically involved tissue is indispensable. Most frequently, elements derived from the history, physical examination findings, laboratory test results, and imaging evaluation reports are used to arrive at a diagnosis.

PATHOGENESIS AND PATHOPHYSIOLOGY

Most vasculitides are considered to represent an immune response to a causative antigen, although vascular damage can also be caused by an infectious agent. The presence of a causative agent alone, however, is not sufficient to produce the extensive vascular complications encountered in the vasculitides. Multiple host factors must also be involved in the spectrum of pathologic events to render an individual susceptible to acute or chronic progressive inflammation. The common denominator in all the vasculitides is the accumulation of inflammatory cells in the endothelium and the blood vessel wall. Recruitment and accumulation of the inflammatory infiltrate, including the expression of adhesion molecules and the secretion of peptides and hormones, are controlled by the endothelial cells and their specific interaction with the inflammatory cells. Some endothelial cells are able to attract inflammatory cells, whereas others are not. The accumulation of these inflammatory cells is an essential and normal immune response that results in restriction and elimination of infectious agents and antigens or damaged tissue. Inflammatory cells are equally important in the tissue repair process. The destructive inflammation of vasculitis may represent a failed attempt at maintenance of tissue integrity or, after a proper response is initiated, a failure in down-regulation that leads to tissue damage rather than triggering the proper healing process. In keeping with our current understanding of the inflammatory response, it can be postulated that cytokine-mediated changes in the expression and function of adhesion molecules coupled with inappropriate activation of leukocytes and endothelial cells are the primary factors influencing vessel damage in the vasculitis syndromes. Nonendothelial structures of the vessel wall are also involved in controlling the inflammatory process. In addition to the endothelial cells, which provide a co-stimulatory function, other cellular components serve as antigen-presenting cells and contribute proinflammatory mediators.

> **Most vasculitides are considered to represent an immune response to a causative antigen or an infectious agent.**

Inflammation within blood vessel walls may result in ischemia and necrosis of tissue and a compromised lumen. The inflammatory response may weaken the vessel wall, causing aneurysms and rupture with occult or life-threatening bleeding. The extent and site of vascular involvement vary, depending on the particular vasculitic syndrome that is occurring. The distribution of the antigen responsible for vasculitis determines the pattern of vessel involvement. Some vasculitides have a predilection for large arteries, others for small and medium-sized vessels. Symptomatic involvement of affected organs may occur in isolation or in combination with multiorgan involvement. The distribution of affected organs may suggest a particular vasculitic disorder, but significant overlap is frequently observed. The duration of disease is variable as well. Although some cases, such as those occurring as a drug reaction, may be very brief, chronic forms may persist with varying degrees of activity for longer than 20 years.

TABLE 187-1

Classification of Necrotizing Vasculitis in Children

Leukocytoclastic (hypersensitivity or allergic)
  Henoch-Schönlein purpura
  Hypersensitivity angiitis and other small-vessel disease
Polyarteritis
  Kawasaki disease (infants)
  Polyarteritis nodosa (older children)
Isolated central nervous system vasculitis
Associated with rheumatic disease
  Systemic lupus erythematosus
  Mixed connective tissue disease
  Dermatomyositis
  Juvenile rheumatoid arthritis
  Scleroderma
  Sjögren syndrome
Allergic granulomatous angiitis
Wegener granulomatosis
Lymphoid granulomatosis
Churg-Strauss syndrome
Giant cell arteritis
  Takayasu arteritis
  Temporal arteritis
Secondary to viral infection
  Hepatitis
  Essential mixed cryoglobulinemic vasculitis
  Epstein-Barr
  Cytomegalovirus

Modified from Fink CW: Vasculitis. Pediatr Clin North Am 1986;33:1203-1219

CLASSIFICATION

The Fink classification of the vasculitides (Table 187-1) has proved useful because it focuses on the pathologic presentation of the respective disorders.

Leukocytoclastic Vasculitis

HENOCH-SCHÖNLEIN PURPURA

In the pediatric age group, Henoch-Schönlein purpura (HSP) vasculitis is one of the most commonly encountered vasculitic disorders. The cause is unknown, but exposure to infectious agents, drugs, or allergens may play a role. For example, the disease is often preceded by an upper respiratory infection, and it is more common in the winter. However, clustering of cases with no obvious inciting agent has been reported. Most cases occur in children 2 to 8 years of age, and boys are affected twice as often as girls.

Characteristic skin lesions consisting of palpable purpura, which results from extravasation of red blood cells from the capillaries and venules, are present in all patients. Lesions are typically distributed on dependent and pressure-bearing areas of the lower extremities and buttocks and cannot be blanched in the way that erythema can. Biopsy of skin lesions reveals a small vessel angiocentric acute leukocytoclastic inflammatory reaction of polymorphonuclear and round cells. A unique feature of HSP is the finding of immunoglobulin (Ig)A complexes in the involved skin and glomeruli of patients.

Gastrointestinal manifestations appear in more than half of affected children. The most common symptom is colicky abdominal pain, which at times can be very severe. Gross or occult blood is found in the stools, indicating lesions in the bowel that are similar to the skin lesions. About 3% of patients develop an intussusception, with submucosal hemorrhage acting as a lead point. This complication must be considered in all children with severe or prolonged abdominal pain. Although gastrointestinal bleeding can be severe, even requiring transfusion, bowel necrosis is rare.

> **Intramural hemorrhage in the bowel may act as a lead point for intussusception.**

Renal involvement, which occurs in 20% to 25% of children, is seen as a glomerulonephritis that manifests as microscopic hematuria, usually without significant renal function impairment. Rarely, nephritic syndrome, azotemia, or hypertension may occur.

The natural history of HSP is that of a self-limiting disease; treatment is supportive with maintenance of hydration and nutrition. If significant renal disease is present in the form of progressive glomerulonephritis, steroid and immunosuppressive therapy may have a place.

HYPERSENSITIVITY ANGIITIS

The most common vasculitis after Henoch-Schönlein purpura is hypersensitivity angiitis. This usually occurs as a reaction to an antigenic stimulus such as a drug, foreign or endogenous protein, chemical, or infectious agent. Although the antigenic stimuli associated with hypersensitivity angiitis are heterogeneous, these disorders involve the small vessels, most commonly the post-capillary venules. Patients with hypersensitivity angiitis have fever, macules, papules, or palpable purpura, myalgias, and arthralgias. Predominant and almost exclusive involvement of the vessels of the skin is observed, without involvement of major organs.

The course of disease is usually short, and treatment is directed at identifying and removing the causative agent.

Polyarteritis

KAWASAKI DISEASE

Kawasaki disease, also known as mucocutaneous lymph node syndrome, is a systemic vasculitis that involves small and medium-sized arteries and is notable for its association with vasculitis of the coronary arteries. Children 5 years of age and younger are primarily affected. Although distribution is worldwide and Kawasaki disease has been described in all racial groups, a substantially higher incidence has been reported in Japan. The cause remains unknown, but epidemiologic features such as seasonal incidence, time–space clusters of cases, and age-related susceptibility, as well as clinical features resembling those of viral or bacterial exanthematous diseases, all point to an infectious origin.

Histologic examination of fatal cases during the acute or subacute phase reveals edema and intense inflammatory infiltration of the vessel wall. In vessels that are severely affected, inflammation is transmural, and destruction of the internal elastic lamina may occur. Weakening and loss of structural integrity may result, along with dilation or aneurysm formation. Thrombi may then form in the lumen of the vessel and may obstruct flow. With healing, progressive fibrosis and intimal proliferation result in stenotic occlusion of the vessel.

Diagnosis depends on the visualization of characteristic clinical signs and symptoms (Table 187-2). Other significant symptoms of Kawasaki disease are provided in Table 187-3.

Cardiac involvement is the most important manifestation and is characteristic of Kawasaki disease. Virtually all of the morbidity and mortality attributed to Kawasaki disease has been related to involvement of the cardiovascular system. Coronary arteritis, which may be asymptomatic, ranges from 20% to 30% in untreated patients and those treated with aspirin alone; it manifests in the coronary arteries as dilation or aneurysm formation. The prevalence of coronary artery aneurysms is reduced to 4% to 5% in patients treated within the first 10 days with intravenous immunoglobulin (IVIg). In addition,

---

TABLE 187-2

Diagnostic Criteria for Kawasaki Disease

- Fever lasting for at least 5 days*
- Presence of four of the five following conditions:
  1. Bilateral nonpurulent conjunctival injection
  2. Changes in the mucosa of the oropharynx, including infected pharynx, infected or fissured lips, or strawberry tongue
  3. Changes in the peripheral extremities, such as edema or erythema of the hands or feet and desquamation, which usually begins subungually
  4. Rash, primarily truncal; polymorphous but nonvesicular
  5. Illness not explained by another known disease process

*Many experts believe that, in the presence of classical features, the diagnosis of Kawasaki disease can be made (and treatment instituted) before the fifth day of fever by experienced individuals. Management of Kawasaki syndrome: a consensus statement prepared by the North American participants of the Third International Kawasaki Disease Symposium, Tokyo, Japan, December, 1998. Pediatr Infect Dis J 1989;8:663

TABLE 187-3

Kawasaki Disease Multisystem Involvement

Musculoskeletal—transient arthritis, painful large and small joint swelling, myositis
Gastrointestinal—diarrhea, vomiting, abdominal pain, hydrops of the gallbladder, hepatosplenomegaly
Neurologic—aseptic meningitis, seizures, cranial and peripheral nerve palsies
Hematologic—leukocytosis, thrombocytosis, anemia
Genitourinary—meatitis, pyuria, proteinuria
Cardiovascular—cardiomegaly, valvular disease, arrhythmias, pericarditis, pericardial effusion, coronary artery aneurysm, myocardial infarction

patients who receive IVIg rarely develop the giant aneurysms that are associated with a high risk of future ischemic heart disease. Patients who develop medium (3 to 6 mm) to large (>6 mm) coronary artery aneurysms during the acute phase of Kawasaki disease require follow-up and diagnostic tests. However, children who do not have coronary artery abnormalities during the first 6 to 8 weeks of illness are very unlikely to develop coronary artery disease in the future and are not required to undergo additional diagnostic studies.

> **The major cause of morbidity and mortality in Kawasaki disease is the occurrence of coronary artery aneurysms.**

The natural history of coronary artery aneurysms in patients with Kawasaki disease may include regression, rupture, thrombosis and recanalization, stenosis, or myocardial infarction. Fusiform and smaller aneurysms are those most likely to regress, whereas saccular and giant aneurysms (>8 mm) are less likely to regress. The mechanism of regression is characterized by proliferation of intimal smooth muscle cells. Rupture of coronary artery aneurysms is rare and usually results in sudden death.

Patients with Kawasaki disease often have an increased platelet count and enhanced platelet aggregability during the acute phase, both of which are predisposing conditions for thrombosis of coronary aneurysms. The thrombosed aneurysm may undergo recanalization, or the thrombosed artery may stimulate the formation of collateral arteries.

Coronary artery aneurysms may undergo remodeling with intimal thickening from accumulation of fibrous tissue and proliferated smooth muscle cells, resulting in localized stenosis. Stenosis is more likely to occur in large aneurysms and may be progressive.

Acute myocardial infarction is the main cause of death in Kawasaki disease. One study found that most deaths due to acute myocardial infarction (MI) occurred within 1 year of disease onset and were associated with obstruction of the main left coronary artery or disease involving the right coronary and left anterior descending coronary arteries.

The gold standard for the diagnosis of coronary artery aneurysm is angiography (Fig. 187-1), but its routine use is limited because of its invasiveness, exposure to radiation, and expense. Its use in the acute phase is not advised. Echocardiography has been shown to be highly sensitive and specific for identification of proximal coronary aneurysms (Fig. 187-2), although its sensitivity is less for distal lesions. All children with known or suspected Kawasaki disease should have an echocardiogram at the time of presentation and again after 2 to 3 weeks of illness. A possible noninvasive imaging alternative is coronary MRA. In a comparative study of 13 patients with coronary aneurysms, MRA was as accurate as conventional angiography in defining lesions.

Occasionally, arteriography of other vessels may be warranted by the clinical findings (Fig. 187-3).

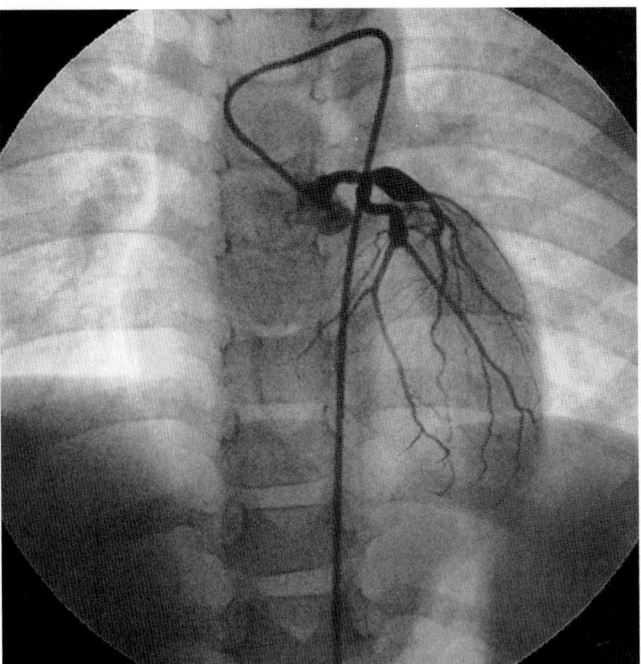

FIGURE 187-1. Kawasaki disease. Giant fusiform aneurysms of the left coronary artery and the left anterior descending artery.

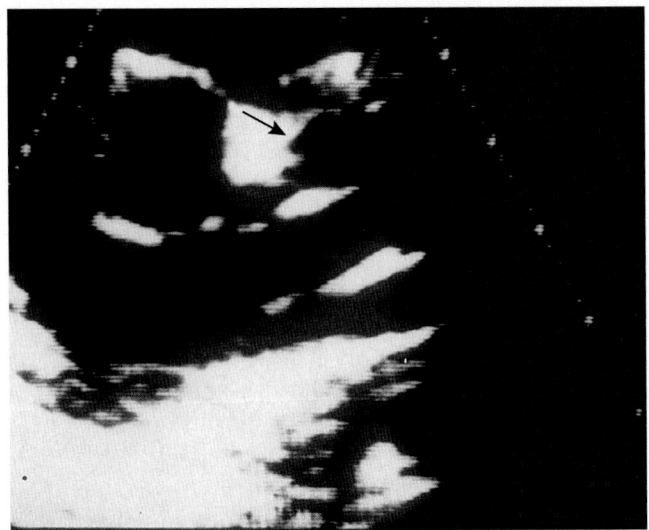

FIGURE 187-2. Echocardiogram of a patient with Kawasaki disease. A fusiform aneurysm of the proximal left coronary artery (arrow) is apparent.

> **Patients in whom Kawasaki disease is diagnosed should be screened for coronary artery aneurysms with an echocardiogram.**

Standard treatment of patients with Kawasaki disease during the acute phase includes IVIg and aspirin. Usually, a dramatic response to therapy is noted, along with abatement of fever and other systemic manifestations. This regimen has also been shown to significantly decrease the development of coronary artery dilation. In contrast to treatment for other forms of vasculitis,

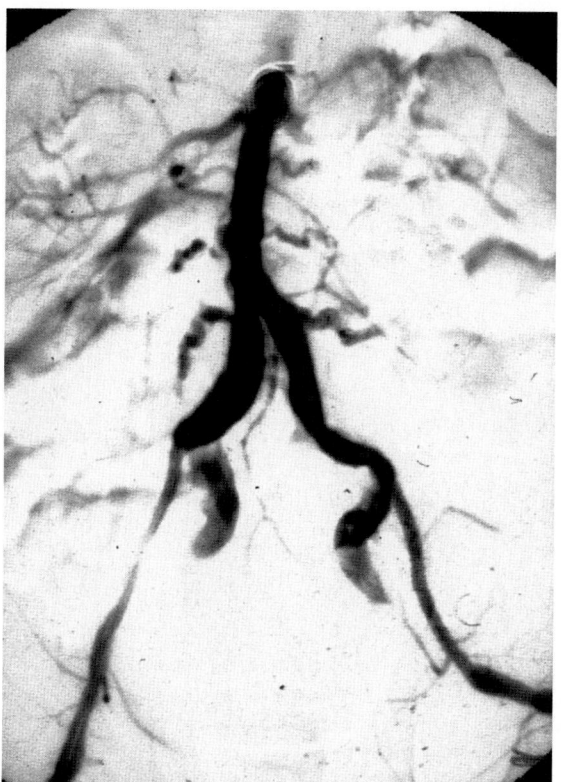

FIGURE 187-3. Abdominal aorta and iliac angiogram of a 1-year-old boy with Kawasaki disease and lower extremity ischemia. Diffuse dilation and ectasia of the abdominal aorta and iliac arteries are noted, along with diminished runoff into the external iliac arteries.

corticosteroid therapy is rarely used in Kawasaki disease, and some consider it contraindicated. Long-term treatment may be different in patients who develop coronary artery disease; aspirin continues to be sufficient in some patients, although anticoagulation and surgery must be considered in others.

POLYARTERITIS NODOSA

Vasculitides that affect small and medium-sized vessels make up a heterogeneous group with no firm consensus about a specific disease or syndrome. The classic form of polyarteritis, often referred to as polyarteritis nodosa (PAN), is an acute necrotizing vasculitis that is associated with aneurysm nodules along the walls of medium-sized and small muscular arteries. Classic polyarteritis does not involve the lung; however, some authors include glomerular (microscopic) involvement in the definition of PAN. Polyarteritis associated with hepatitis B and hepatitis C has been described but accounts for only a minority of cases. It is this association of hepatitis antigen–antibody complexes with polyarteritis that provides support for the hypothesis that the vasculitides in general are the result of immune complex deposition. PAN is one of the childhood vasculitides that differs in presentation and origin from that seen in adults, although the pathology of the lesions is similar.

The lesions of PAN have a predilection for small and medium-caliber arteries in an irregular and segmental distribution, particularly involving areas where arteries bifurcate. The inflammatory process involves the media with infiltration of polymorphonuclear leukocytes, edema, fibrinous exudates, and necrosis. Subsequently, replacement with granulation tissue and intimal proliferation occurs. These changes produce partial occlusion, thrombosis, ischemia, and aneurysm formation. The inflammatory cycle may be in multiple stages at the same time in any one patient, so that one vessel might have early inflammatory changes, while in other areas, arteries may already have undergone necrosis and thrombosis and have begun to recanalize.

> **Polyarteritis nodosa affects small and medium-caliber arteries in a segmental distribution.**

Clinical presentation varies with disease distribution and reflects the particular organ system that is involved. Early, constitutional symptoms of fever, weight loss, and malaise may be noted in classic PAN. Specific signs and symptoms are related to involvement of the affected organ system.

With musculoskeletal involvement, migratory myalgias and arthralgias are frequent. Muscle pain or weakness reflects compromised vascular supply or a peripheral neuropathy (Fig. 187-4).

Gastrointestinal involvement is common in PAN, with arterial lesions present in the blood supply to one or more abdominal organs (Fig. 187-5). Bowel ischemia can result in mucosal ulceration, infarction, or perforation. Acalculous cholecystitis, hepatic necrosis, hemorrhagic pancreatitis, and appendicitis may also result from direct involvement with PAN.

Nearly 75% of patients with PAN have renal involvement at the time of diagnosis or during the course of their disease. Renal involvement occurs in two forms, either separately or together: renal polyarteritis (macroscopic) and glomerulitis (microscopic). Renal polyarteritis (Fig. 187-6) is the most common lesion. Manifestations of renal involvement include microscopic hematuria and proteinuria. Hypertension is very common with renal involvement and may be a significant continuing problem long after other manifestations of PAN have become quiescent. With microscopic involvement and accompanying gomerulitis, progressive renal failure may result.

Central nervous system (CNS) involvement is generally a late occurrence in the course of PAN. This particular manifestation reflects the specific area of the CNS that is involved, as in focal neurologic deficits, hemiplegia, ataxia (Fig. 187-7), and vision loss. Peripheral neuropathy resulting from arteritis of the vasa nervorum is usually asymmetric, and both sensory and motor fibers are affected.

A definitive diagnosis of PAN is preferably based on typical pathologic findings observed in biopsy specimens obtained from involved areas. Renal biopsy may be helpful and is frequently undertaken when patients have evidence of renal involvement. However, it is necessary to see vasculitis in small and medium-sized arteries because changes of glomerulitis alone may not be separable from those of other diseases. Steroids, in some cases combined

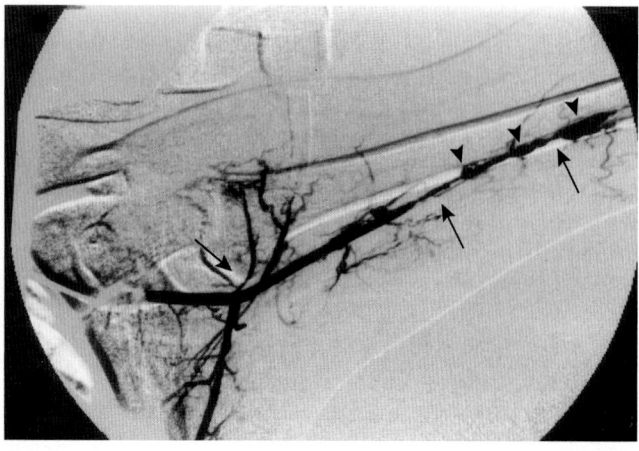
A

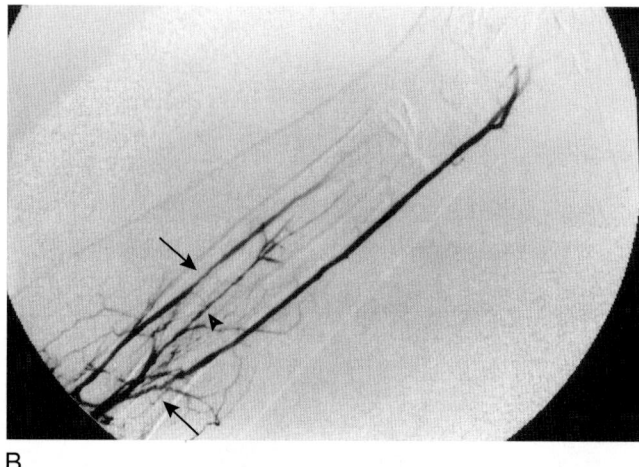
B

FIGURE 187-4. A 3-year-old boy with polyarteritis nodosa. **A,** Segmental arterial narrowing and irregularity *(arrows),* along with aneurysms *(arrowheads),* are present in the brachial artery. **B,** The process extends distally and also involves the radial, ulnar, and interosseous arteries *(arrows).*

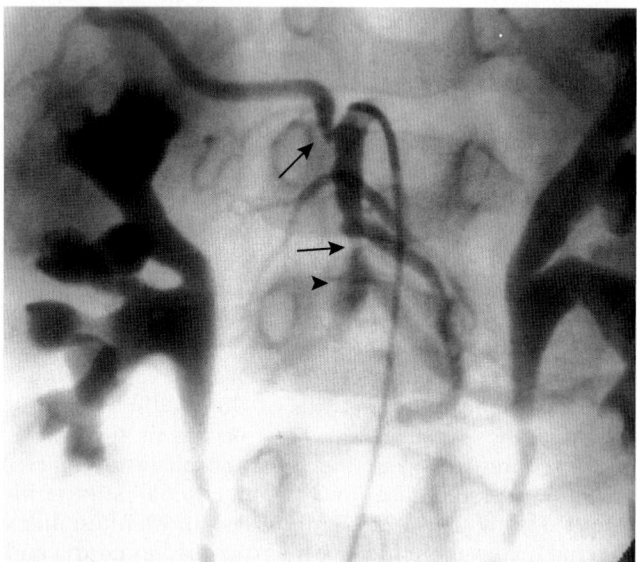

FIGURE 187-5. Polyarteritis nodosa. A 7-year-old girl presented with postprandial abdominal pain. The superior mesenteric artery and proximally replaced hepatic arteries are involved, along with segments of stenosis *(arrows)* and fusiform aneurysm formation *(arrowhead).*

with immunosuppressive and antiplatelet drugs, are the treatment of choice.

Allergic Granulomatosis Angiitis

Churg-Strauss syndrome, Wegener granulomatosis, and lymphoid granulomatosis are the three major diseases in the group that is characterized by a granulomatous vascular exudate.

Patients with Churg-Strauss syndrome may have asthma, allergic rhinitis, eosinophilic pulmonary infiltrates, peripheral eosinophilia, and a small-vessel granulomatous vasculitis. Onset of the vasculitis may be delayed by several years from the onset of asthma. Skin lesions include purpura and subcutaneous nodules of the extremities and scalp. These subcutaneous nodules

contain granulomatous necrotizing vasculitis of small arteries or veins with a predominantly eosinophilic infiltrate.

Wegener granulomatosis is typically characterized by necrotizing granulomas of the upper and lower respiratory tract and a disseminated small-vessel vasculitis in which any organ can be involved. Renal involvement is most common, occurring in up to 85% of cases in which a segmental necrotizing glomerulitis is present. Renal involvement may be asymptomatic, or it may be symptomatic with hypertension, edema, and overt nephritic syndrome. When extensive and acute, the syndrome may be rapidly fatal.

Upper respiratory manifestations include necrotizing sinusitis and nasal mucosal ulceration with epistaxis. This may be accompanied by serous otitis media. In severe nasal or sinus disease, secondary bacterial infection may predominate, especially when immunosuppressive therapy is initiated. Subglottic tracheal inflammation may lead to airway stenosis in almost 50% of children with this disease.

Other organ involvement includes that directly related to vasculitis or to granulomatous disease. Eye, neurologic, cutaneous, and musculoskeletal involvement has been described.

The treatment combination of cyclophosphamide and prednisone is effective in controlling Wegener granulomatosis, although relapses may occur.

Lymphoid granulomatosis is primarily a pulmonary vasculitis that is characterized by an angiocentric destructive inflammatory infiltrate composed of lymphoid cells. About 15% of patients develop a lymphoproliferative malignancy, usually non-Hodgkin lymphoma.

Vasculitis Associated with Rheumatic Disease

Vascular inflammation is characteristic of many of the rheumatic diseases, including systemic lupus erythematosus, juvenile rheumatoid arthritis, mixed connective tissue disease, dermatomyositis, and scleroderma. Vasculitis generally involves cutaneous vessels, producing

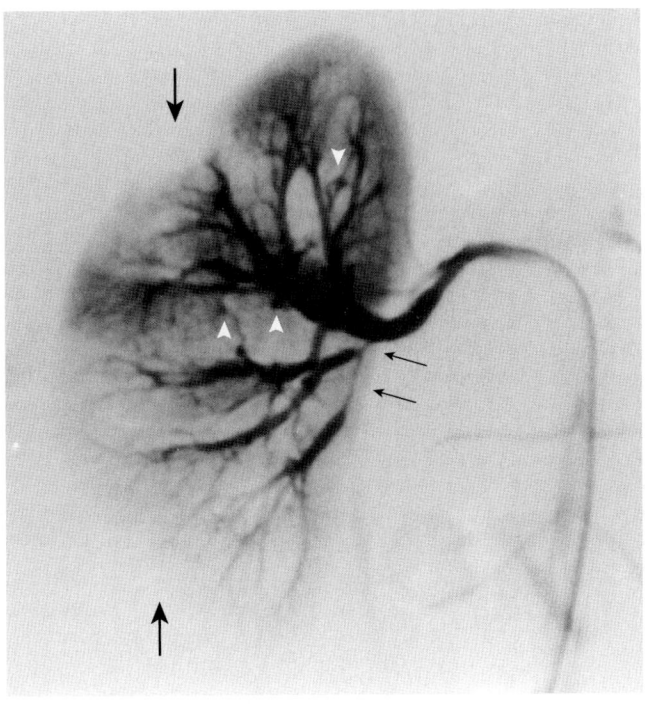
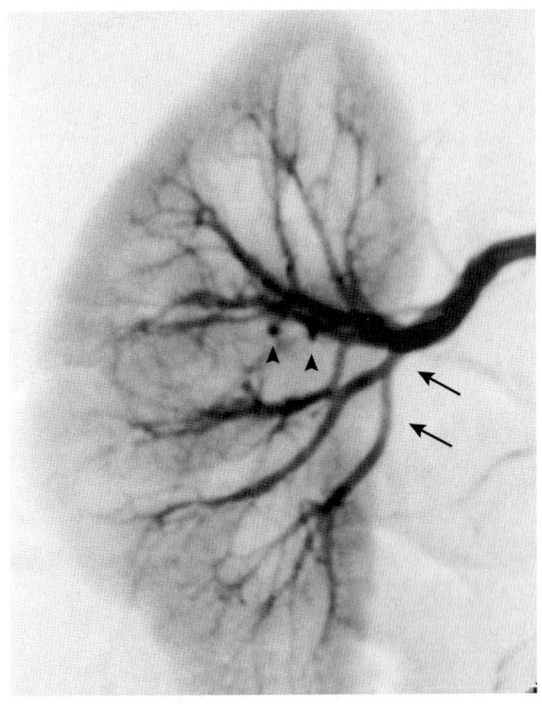

A   B

FIGURE 187-6. This patient had an established diagnosis of polyarteritis nodosa for 1 year and new onset of hypertension. **A,** Right renal angiogram shows segmental narrowing of the intrarenal branch to the lower pole *(arrows)*, small secular aneurysms at vessel branch points *(arrowheads)*, and patchy perfusion deficits in the upper and lower poles *(large arrows)*. **B,** Repeat study after 6 months of steroid therapy shows resolution of vessel stenosis *(arrows)* and perfusion abnormalities. Aneurysms at arterial bifurcations persisted *(arrowheads)*, as did the patient's hypertension.

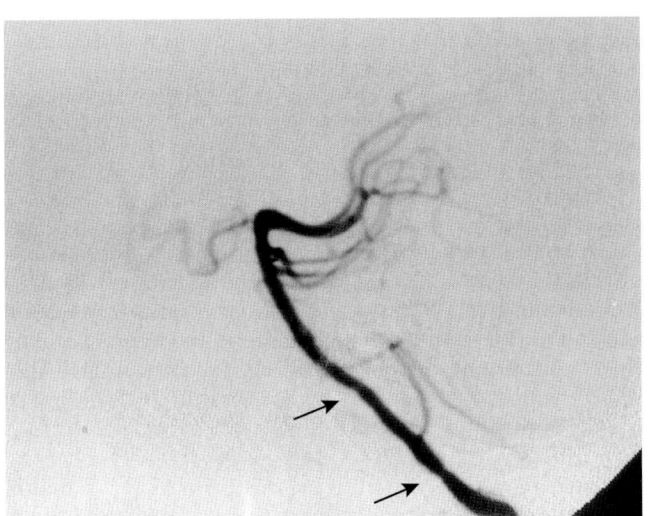

FIGURE 187-7. Polyarteritis nodosa involvement of the basilar artery *(arrows)* in a patient presenting with cerebellar ataxia.

ulcerations of the skin and subcutaneous tissues. Because vasculitis often occurs around nail beds, skin infarction and loss of fingers and toes, possibly accompanied by peripheral neuropathy, may occur (Fig. 187-8).

In children, the vasculitis of rheumatic disease is usually overshadowed by clinical and pathologic multisystem manifestations of the underlying disease process, which is nonvasculitic in nature. Therefore, the diagnosis is typically known at the time of imaging. Treatment

directed to the underlying condition may lessen or ameliorate the vasculitis.

GIANT CELL ARTERITIS

Takayasu Arteritis

The giant cell arteritis that affects children and young adults is Takayasu arteritis. Segmental inflammatory vasculitis preferentially involves the aorta and its branches. This produces stenosis and aneurysms of the large muscular arteries. Any part of the aorta may be involved. The thoracic aorta and its branches, as well as the pulmonary arteries, are generally affected (Fig. 187-9), but the abdominal aorta and the iliac arteries may be involved as well (Fig. 187-10). Takayasu arteritis has been classified into four types: (1) The aortic arch variety involves one or more of the three arch vessels, (2) the thoracoabdominal variety affects the descending thoracic or abdominal aorta and their branches, (3) the combined variety affects both the arch vessels and the thoracoabdominal aorta, and (4) the pulmonary variety involves the pulmonary arteries in combination with any of the above three types.

> **Takayasu arteries is a vasculitis that affects the aorta and its branches.**

The histopathology is that of an inflammatory reaction with lymphocytes, histiocytes, and multinucleated

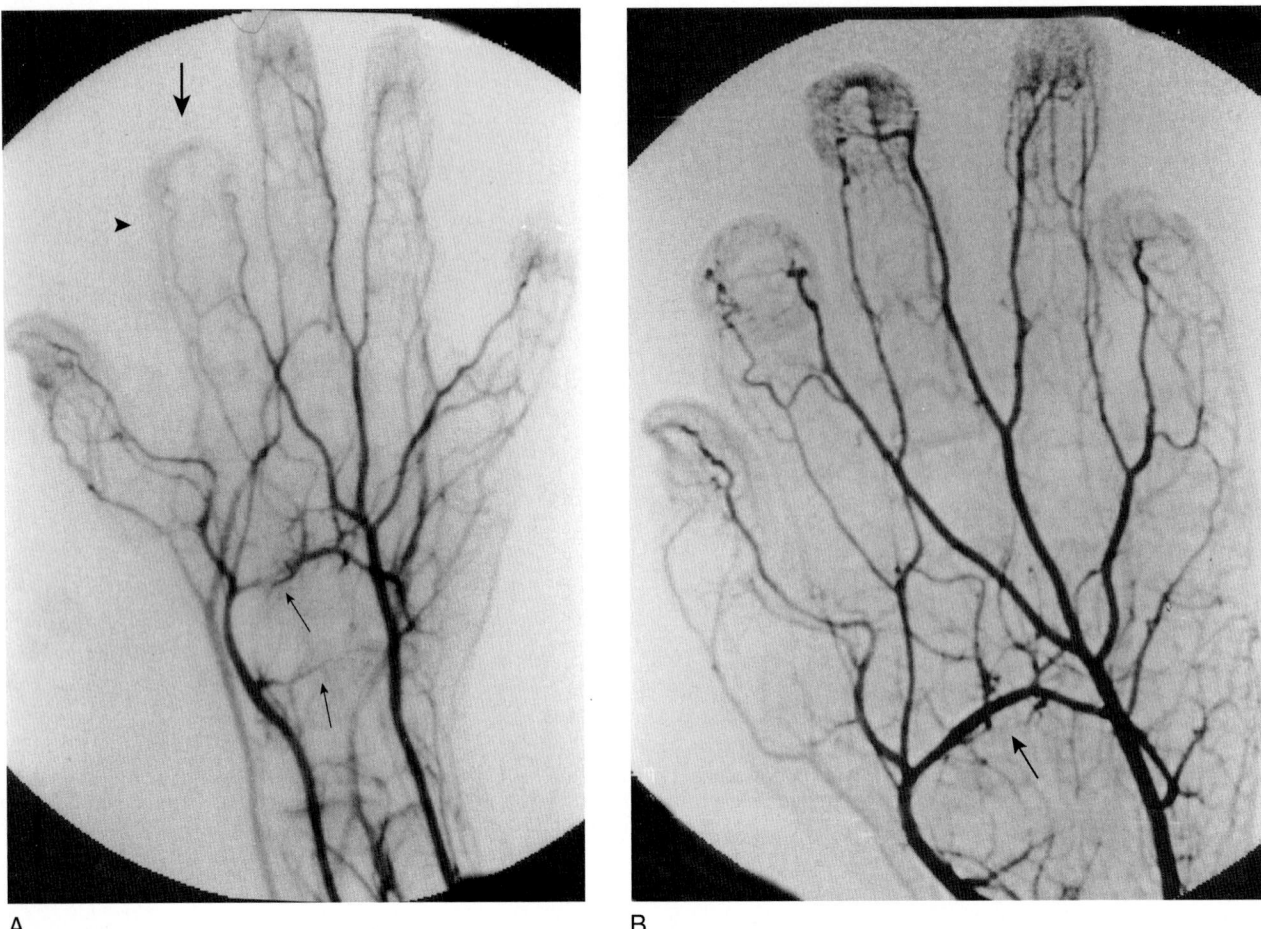

A   B

FIGURE 187-8. A 6-year-old girl with a known diagnosis of dermatomyositis and progressive ischemic changes in the fingers of the right hand. **A,** Attenuation is noted in the digital arteries, especially in the index finger *(arrowhead)*, where ischemic amputation was performed at the tip of the finger *(large arrow)*. Narrowing of the palmar arch arteries is also apparent *(arrows)*. **B,** Repeat angiogram following high-dose pulse steroids shows reversal of the changes in the palmar arch *(arrow)* and better perfusion in the digital branches.

giant cells. Focal or diffuse loss of muscular and elastic tissue is noted with extensive fibrosis of the media and destruction of the elastic lamina. The artery wall becomes irregularly thickened and the lumen narrowed as the result of intimal hyperplasia and thrombus formation. When the disease is advanced, the vessel wall consists only of acellular collagen, which leads to dilation or to aneurysm formation.

Takayasu arteritis is more prevalent in Oriental and Southeast Asian countries, although its distribution is worldwide. Young women are affected more often than men. Early manifestations of Takayasu arteritis include fever, night sweats, myalgia, and weight loss. With severe or progressive disease, hypertension, heart failure, and pulse deficits become apparent (Fig. 187-11). The origin of the disease is unknown. It is presumed to be auto-immune in nature, although genetic and infectious factors, including exposure to tuberculosis, have been proposed.

Treatment usually consists of high-dose cyclophospha-mide (Cytoxan). Transluminal angioplasty of the descending thoracic and the abdominal aorta, with or without endovascular stent placement, has been useful in the management of stenotic lesions in Takayasu arteritis.

SUMMARY

Diseases in which vasculitis is the primary or a major component may appear similar at first presentation. A number of vasculitic diseases may affect children, and overlap is noted in their presentations. Clinical features and the use of appropriate imaging modalities when biopsy is not possible usually facilitate establishment of the diagnosis and initiation of therapy to control disease activity, although associated morbidity and mortality are not inconsequential.

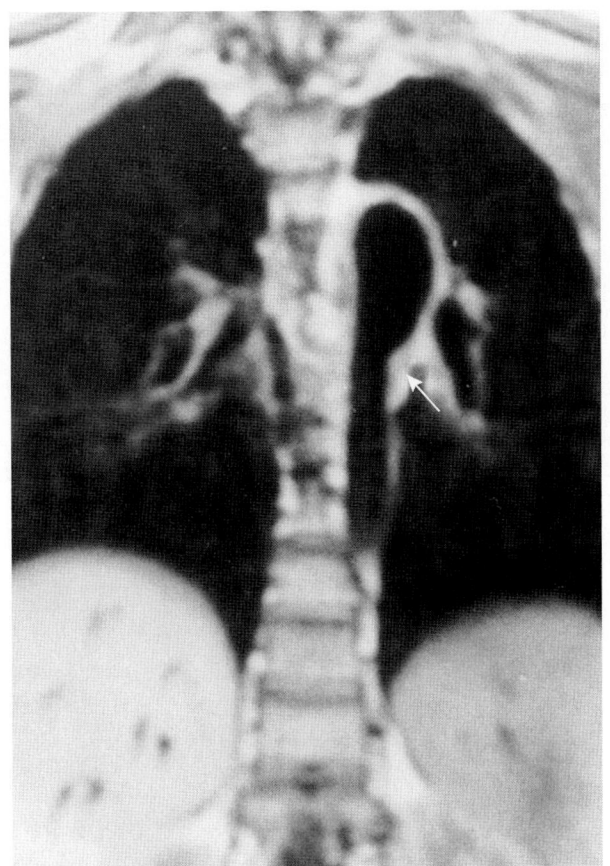

A

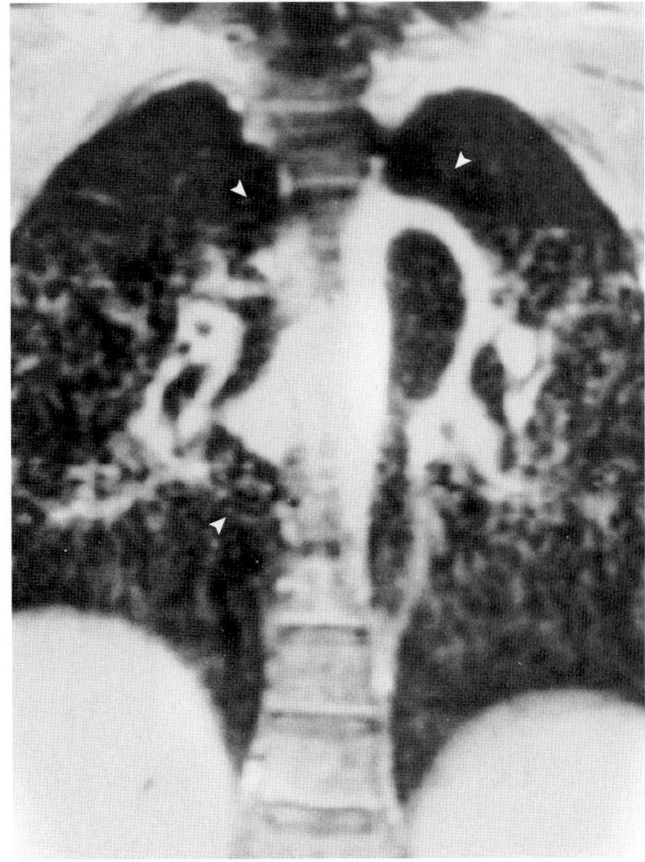

B

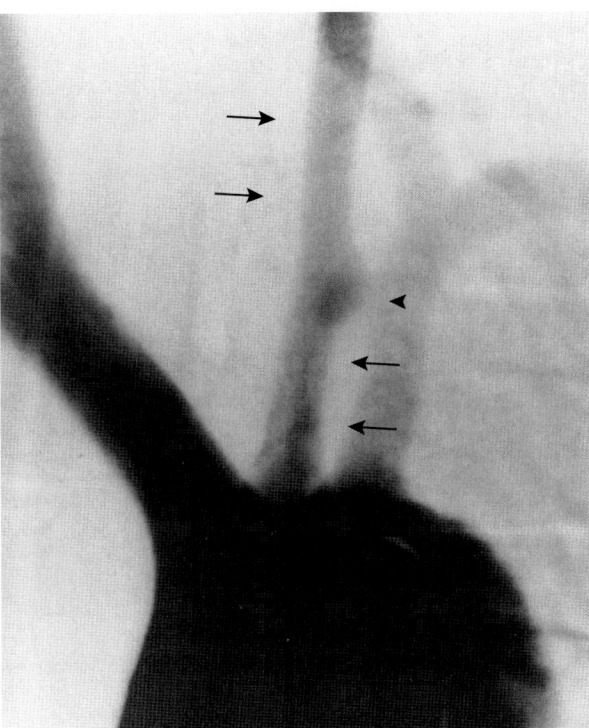

C

FIGURE 187-9. Coronal T1 pregadolinium **(A)** and postgadolinium **(B)** images show focal stenosis of the proximal descending thoracic aorta *(arrow)* with intense perivascular and mediastinal enhancement *(arrowheads)* typical of Takayasu arteritis. A corresponding arch angiogram **(C)** shows involvement of the left common carotid artery, which has an aneurysm *(arrowhead)* in the middle of a tapered segment of narrowing *(arrows)*.

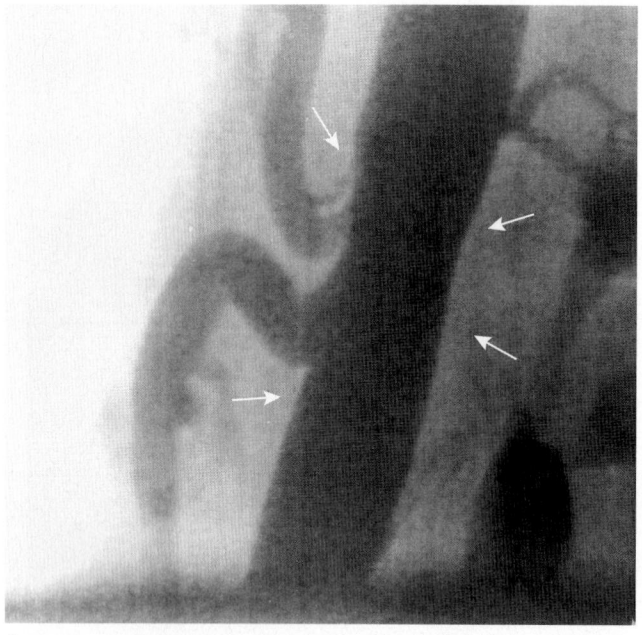

A

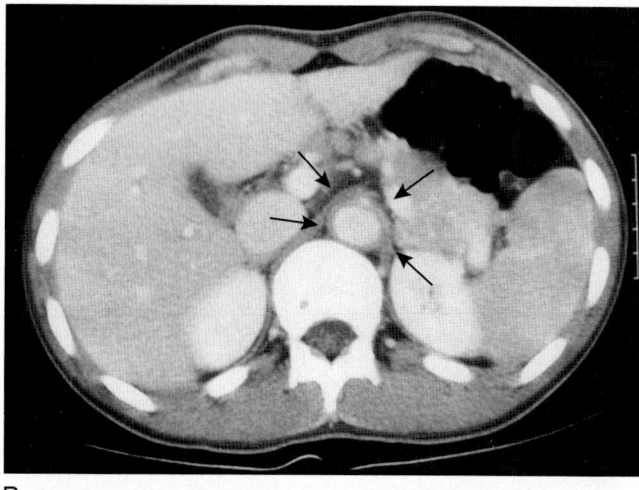

B

FIGURE 187-10. Same patient as in Figure 187-9. Disease has progressed after completion of 6 months of steroid therapy. **A,** Involvement of the abdominal aorta can be seen around the celiac and superior mesenteric arteries *(arrows)*. **B,** Computed tomography scan shows mural thickening of the aorta *(arrows)*.

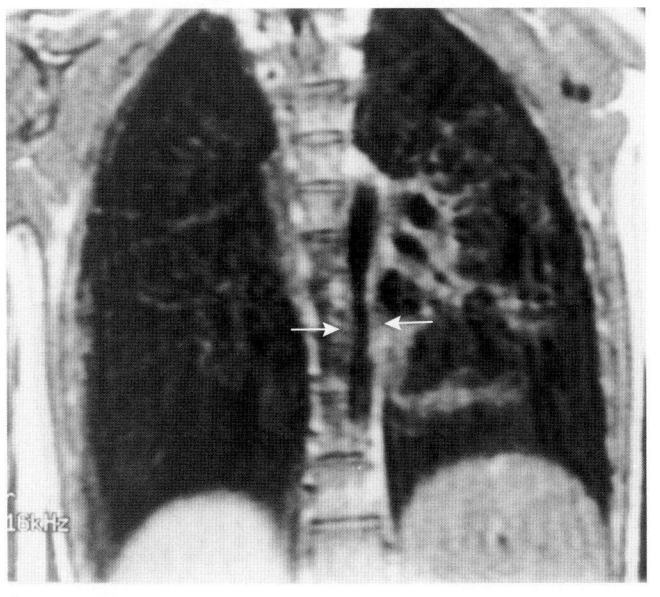

A

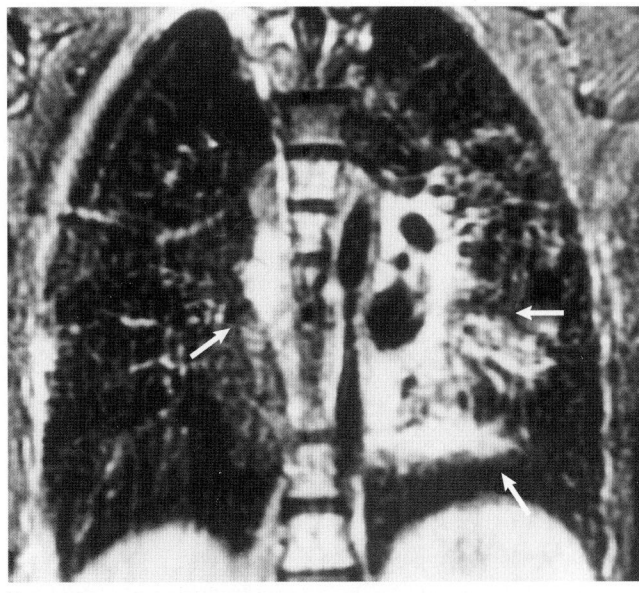

B

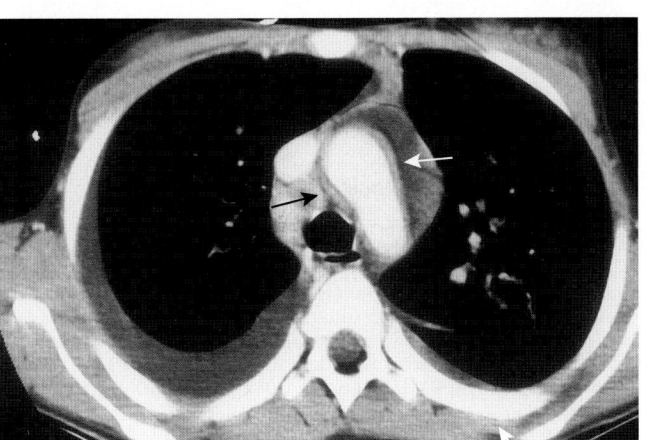

C

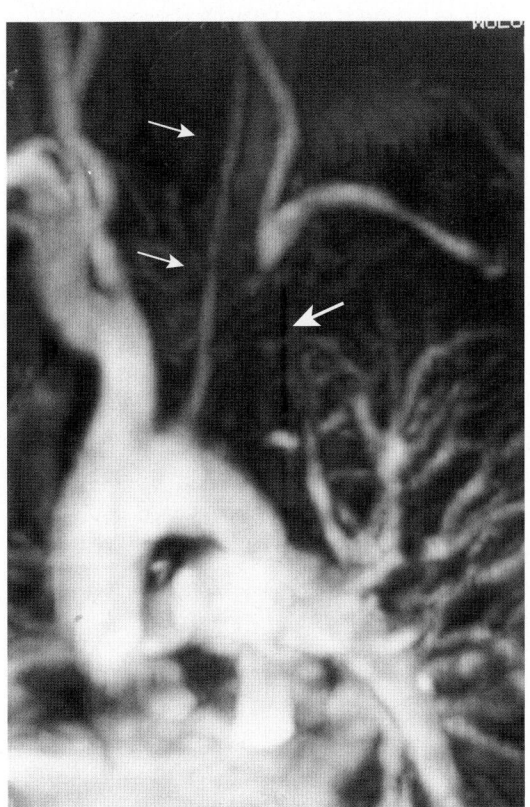

D

FIGURE 187-11. Takayasu arteritis. Pregadolinium **(A)** and postgadolinium **(B)** images of a 12-year-old girl with Takayasu arteritis who presented with heart failure and a pulseless left upper extremity. A long segment of narrowing is seen in the descending thoracic aorta *(arrows* in **A)** with characteristic perivascular and mediastinal enhancement *(arrows* in **B).** **C,** Contrast-enhanced computed tomography shows marked mural thickening of the aortic arch *(arrows).* **D,** Magnetic resonance angiography shows marked luminal narrowing of the left common carotid artery *(arrows)* and absent flow in the proximal left subclavian artery *(large arrow).* The left vertebral and subclavian arteries are filled by retrograde flow.

SUGGESTED READINGS

General

Dillon MJ, Ansell BM: Vasculitis in children and adolescents. Rheum Dis Clin North Am 1995;21:1115-1137

Fink CW: Polyarteritis and other diseases with necrotizing vasculitis in childhood. Arthritis Rheum 1977;20:378

Fink CW: Vasculitis. Pediatr Clin North Am 1986;33:1203-1219

Hunder G: Vasculitis: diagnosis and therapy. Am J Med 1996;100(suppl 24):37-45

Larsson L-G, Baum J: Treatment of the child with vasculitis syndromes. *In* Hicks RV (ed): Vasculopathies of Childhood. Littleton, MA, PSG, 1988:347

Mandell BF, Hoffman GS: Differentiating the vasculitides. Rheum Dis Clin North Am 1994;20:409-441

Schaller JG: Vasculitis syndromes. *In* Behrman RE (ed): Nelson Textbook of Pediatrics, 15th ed. Philadelphia, WB Saunders, 1996:677-678

Sneller MC, Fauci AS: Pathogenesis of vasculitis syndromes. Med Clin North Am 1997;81:222-242

Sunday JS, Haynes BF: Pathogenic mechanisms of vessel damage in vasculitis syndromes. Rheum Dis Clin North Am 1995;21:861-881

Henoch-Schönlein Purpura

Barratt TM, Drummond KN: The vasculitis syndromes: Henoch-Schönlein syndrome or anaphylactoid purpura. *In* Kelly VC (ed): Practice of Pediatrics, vol 8, Chap 63. Hagerstown, MD, Harper & Row, 1981:1-13

Kawasaki Disease

Akagi T, Rose V, Benson LN, et al: Outcome of coronary artery aneurysms after Kawasaki disease. J Pediatr 1992;121:689

Beiser AS, Takahashi M, Baker AJ, et al, for the US Multicenter Kawasaki Disease Study Group: A predictive instrument for coronary artery aneurysms in Kawasaki disease. Am J Cardiol 1998;81:1116

Consensus statement prepared by the North American participants of the Third International Kawasaki Disease Symposium, Tokyo, Japan, December 1998. Pediatr Infect Dis J 1989;8:663

Iemura M, Ishii M, Sugimura T, et al: Long-term consequences of regressed coronary aneurysms after Kawasaki disease: vascular wall morphology and function. Heart 2000;83:307

Kato H, Ichinose E, Kawasaki T: Myocardial infarction in Kawasaki disease: clinical analysis of 195 cases. J Pediatr 1986;108:923

Kato H, Ichinose E, Yoshioka F, et al: Fate of coronary aneurysms in Kawasaki disease: serial coronary angiography and long-term follow-up study. Am J Cardiol 1982;49:1758

Kato H, Sugimura T, Akagi T, et al: Long-term consequences of Kawasaki disease: a 10- to 21-year follow-up study of 594 patients. Circulation 1996;94:1379

Laupland KB, Davies HD: Epidemiology, etiology, and management of Kawasaki disease: state of the art. Pediatr Cardiol 1999; 20:177-183

Mavrogeni S, Papadopoulos G, Douskou M, et al: Magnetic resonance angiography is equivalent to x-ray coronary angiography for the evaluation of coronary arteries in Kawasaki disease. J Am Coll Cardiol 2004;43:649

Newburger JW, Takahashi M, Burns JC, et al: The treatment of Kawasaki syndrome with intravenous gamma-globulin. N Engl J Med 1986;315:341-347

Newburger JW, Takahashi M, Gerber MA, et al: Diagnosis, treatment, and long-term management of Kawasaki disease: a statement for health professionals from the Committee on Rheumatic Fever, Endocarditis, and Kawasaki Disease, Council on Cardiovascular Disease in the Young, American Heart Association. Circulation 2004;110:2747

Rowley AH, Shulman ST: Kawasaki syndrome. Clin Microbiol Rev 1998;11:405-419

Rowley AH, Shulman ST: Kawasaki disease. *In* Behrman RE (ed): Nelson Textbook of Pediatrics, 16th ed. Philadelphia, WB Saunders, 2000:726-727

Sundel RP, Newburger JW: Management of acute Kawasaki disease. Prog Pediatr Cardiol 1997;6:203-209

Yanagawa H, Nakamura Y, Sakata K, et al: Use of intravenous gamma-globulin for Kawasaki disease: effects on cardiac sequelae. Pediatr Cardiol 1997;18:10-23

Polyarteritis Nodosa

Blau EB, Morriss RF, Yunis EJ: Polyarteritis in older children. Pediatrics 1977;60:227-234

Ettlinger RE, Nelson AM, Burke EC, et al: Polyarteritis nodosa in childhood: a clinical-pathologic study. Arthritis Rheum 1979; 22:820-825

Rosenwasser LJ: Polyarteritis nodosa group. *In* Goldman L (ed): Cecil Textbook of Medicine, 21st ed. Philadelphia, WB Saunders, 2000:1527-1529

Allergic Granulomatosis Angiitis

Allen NB, Bressler PB: Diagnosis and treatment of the systemic and cutaneous necrotizing vasculitis syndromes. Med Clin North Am 1997;81:243-259

Churg J, Strauss L: Allergic granulomatosis, allergic angiitis, and periarteritis nodosa. Am J Pathol 1951;27:277-301

Hoffman GS, Kerr GS, Leavitt RY, et al: Wegener's granulomatosis: an analysis of 158 patients. Ann Intern Med 1992;116:488-498

Hoffman GS, Leavitt RY, Kerr GS, et al: The treatment of Wegener's granulomatosis with glucocorticoids and methotrexate. Arthritis Rheum 1992;35:1322-1329

Takayasu Arteritis

Gotsman MS, Beck W, Schrire V: Selective angiography in arteritis of the aorta and its major branches. Radiology 1967;88:232-248

Lupi-Herrera E, Sanchez TG, Marcushamer J, et al: Takayasu's arteritis: clinical study of 107 cases. Am Heart J 1977;93:94-103

Yamada I, Numano F, Suzuki S: Takayasu arteritis: evaluation with MR imaging. Radiology 1993;188:89-94

PART 5

ABDOMEN AND GASTROINTESTINAL TRACT

Image-Guided Biopsy in Pediatric Patients

BRIAN E. SCHIRF, STANLEY T. KIM, and JAMES S. DONALDSON

INTRODUCTION

Percutaneous biopsy is an established method of obtaining tissue diagnosis in adult and pediatric patients, but it is currently performed less in the pediatric population than is open surgical biopsy. Use of percutaneous needle biopsy for primary diagnosis and confirmation of tumor recurrence in the pediatric population varies widely across different institutions. The biggest concern may have come from pediatric pathologists, who fear making inaccurate diagnoses with limited amounts of tissue. Needle biopsies generally will have a greater rate of sampling error, and it can be more difficult to obtain sufficient tissue for the many special stains often necessary for complete diagnosis. Other concerns include needle tract seeding, insufficient tissue for banking, and concern that a child may require a second procedure if the needle biopsy is nondiagnostic.

Biopsy procedures are separated into two categories that consist of targeted lesion biopsies or nonlesion organ biopsies. Biopsies of identified lesions may be performed for primary diagnosis or for confirmation of a recurrent neoplasm (Figs. 188-1 through 188-8). Potentially infectious processes also can be biopsied if a specimen is needed for microbiologic analysis (Figs. 188-9 through 188-13). Nonlesion biopsies are performed for tissue evaluation in patients with solid organ transplantations or inflammatory processes such as hepatitis (Figs. 188-14 through 188-17).

When biopsy of a lesion is requested, the studies are reviewed by the interventional radiologist and the appropriateness of the biopsy procedure determined. The procedure may be scheduled, or further consultation with the requesting physician may be needed. Appropriate clotting parameters are evaluated and coagulopathy correction planned if necessary. A discussion with the pathologist regarding specimen handling is often valuable. It is important to anticipate how many passes may be necessary and how much tissue will be needed, as well as which media must be available for placement of the specimens.

BIOPSY PROCEDURE

The percutaneous biopsy procedure is performed under sterile technique. After the patient is optimally positioned and the appropriate level of sedation or anesthesia is reached, the access site is prepped and draped in sterile fashion. Instruments to be used during the biopsy, such as the ultrasound probe, are also draped. After the skin and subcutaneous tissues are anesthetized, the biopsy instrument is passed to the lesion and the specimen obtained. After adequate tissue has been obtained, the procedure is terminated, hemostasis is achieved, and the patient is sent for recovery. The patient should be observed for delayed complications. The length of observation should be based on the size of

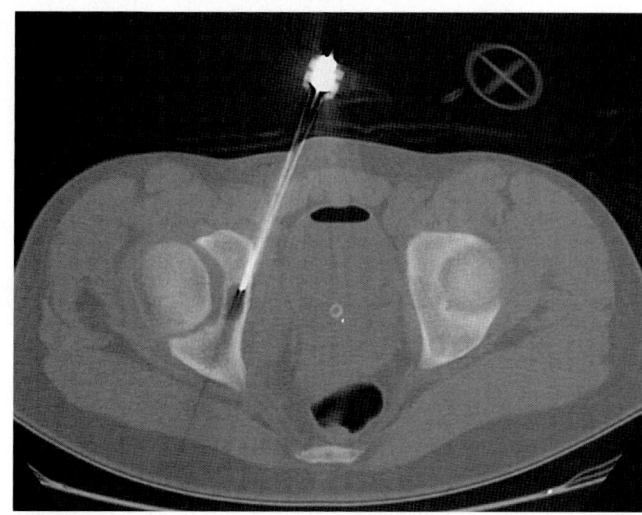

FIGURE 188-1. Langerhans cell histiocytosis (LCH). A 14-year-old male patient who presented with right hip pain was found to have a focal lytic lesion on plain film that was confirmed with computed tomography (CT) imaging. Under general anesthesia, the patient underwent CT-guided right acetabular biopsy performed with a bone biopsy needle and coaxial insertion of small-gauge (20 to 22 g) core needles. Final pathology confirmed Langerhans cell histiocytosis.

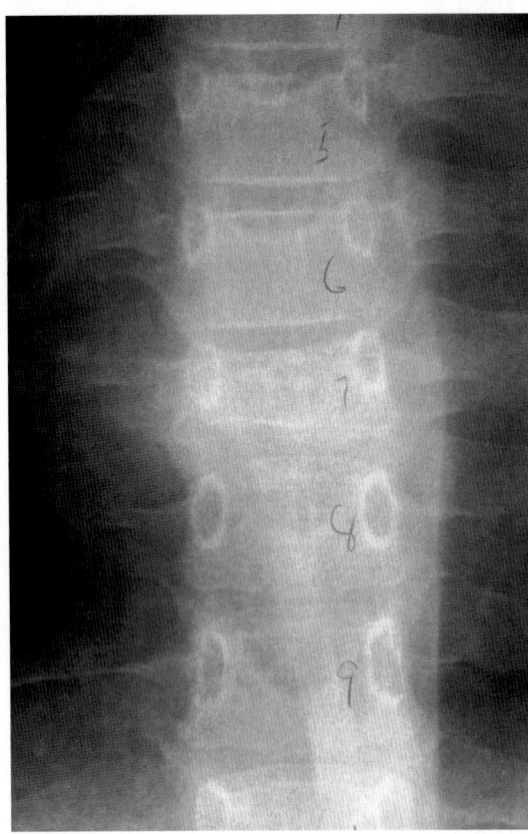

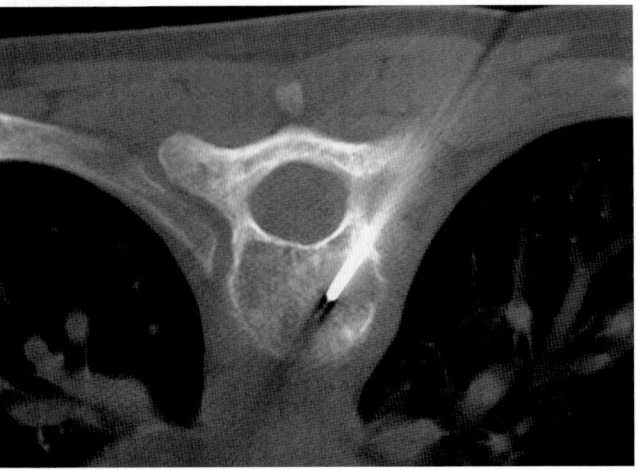

FIGURE 188-2. Langerhans cell histiocytosis (LCH).
A, A 12-year-old male patient with back pain and lesion with compression deformity of the T7 vertebral body seen on initial anteroposterior plain film imaging. **B,** Computed tomography–guided biopsy performed with a bone biopsy core needle obtained adequate material for a diagnosis of LCH.

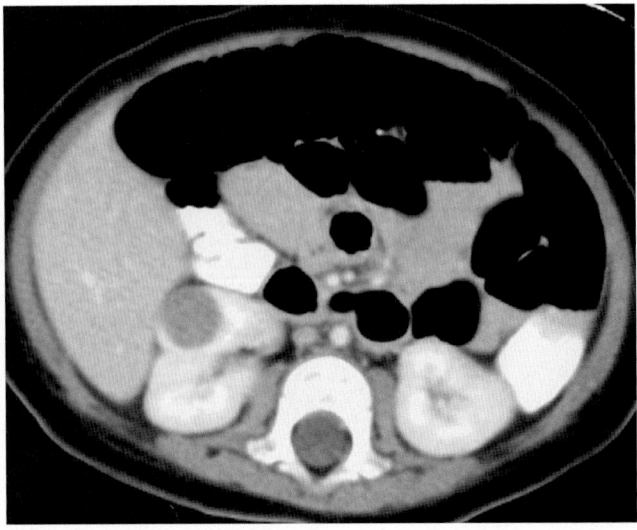

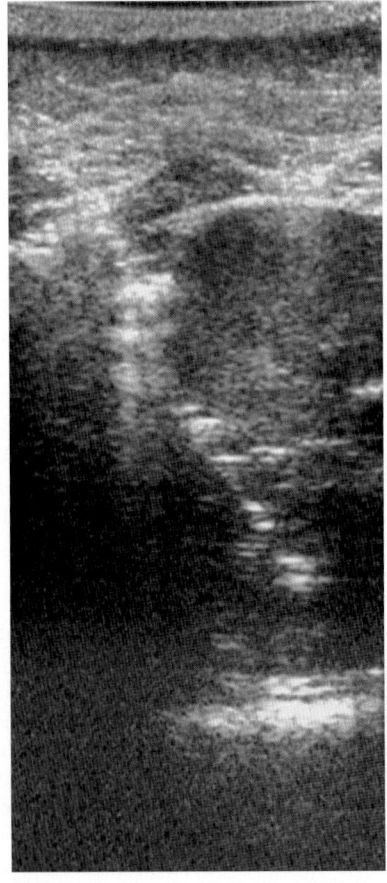

FIGURE 188-3. Primitive neuroectodermal tumor (PNET). In this 4-year-old male patient evaluated for hematuria, **(A)** contrast-enhanced computed tomography scan revealed an enhancing, right renal mass. **B,** Ultrasonography-guided biopsy of the hypoechoic solid lesion confirmed the diagnosis of a rare renal primitive neuroectodermal tumor.

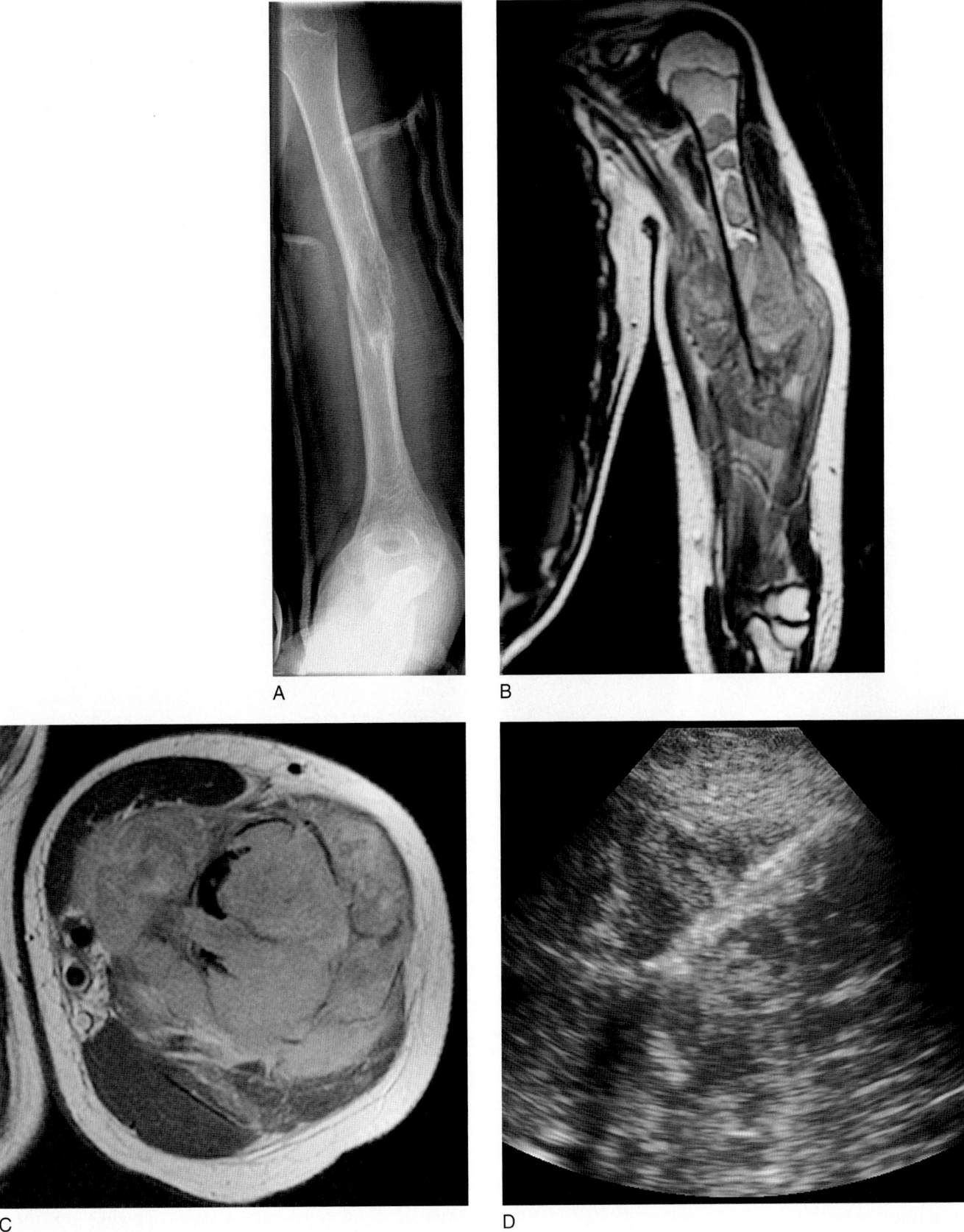

FIGURE 188-4. Ewing sarcoma. **A,** Left arm plain film image of a 13-year-old female patient with prior history of osteomyelitis diagnosed through open surgical biopsy. The patient presented again months later with pathologic fracture and soft tissue swelling. **B, C,** Coronal T1 precontrast and axial T1 fat-saturated postcontrast images reveal the fracture with enhancing soft tissue mass and extensive osseous destruction. **D,** Ultrasonography-guided core biopsy of this lesion showed small blue cells on initial staining, with a final diagnosis of Ewing sarcoma.

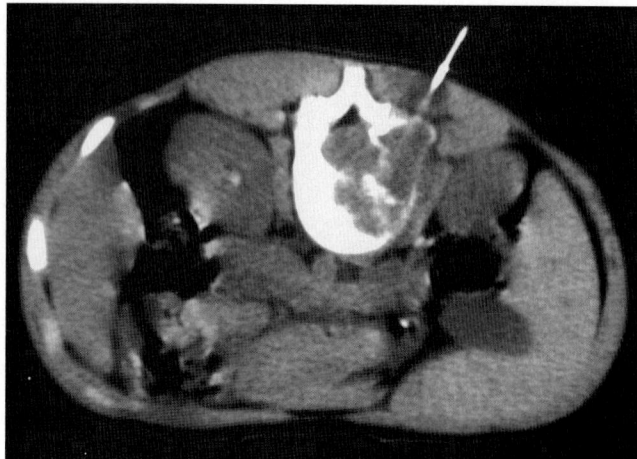

FIGURE 188-5. Ewing sarcoma spine. Axial computed tomography biopsy image reveals a destructive osseous vertebral body lesion with soft tissue component in this 4-year-old female patient. Final pathology proved that the lesion represented Ewing sarcoma.

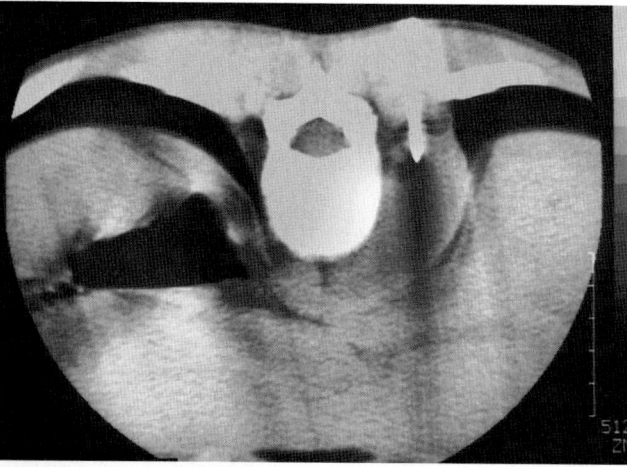

FIGURE 188-7. Neurofibroma. A 4-year-old boy presented with left back pain and was found to have a soft tissue mass in the left paraspinal region. A computed tomography–guided core needle tip is seen within the outer edge of the soft tissue mass. Coaxial needle biopsies were obtained with a pathology diagnosis of neurofibroma.

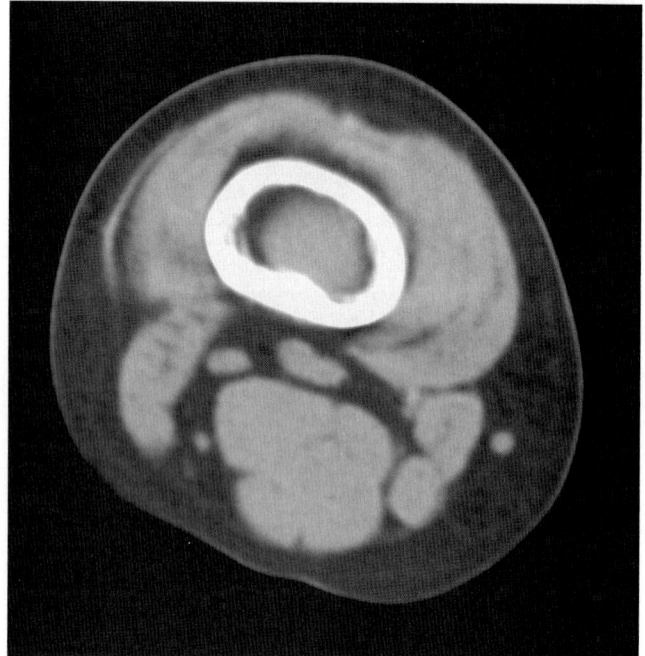

A

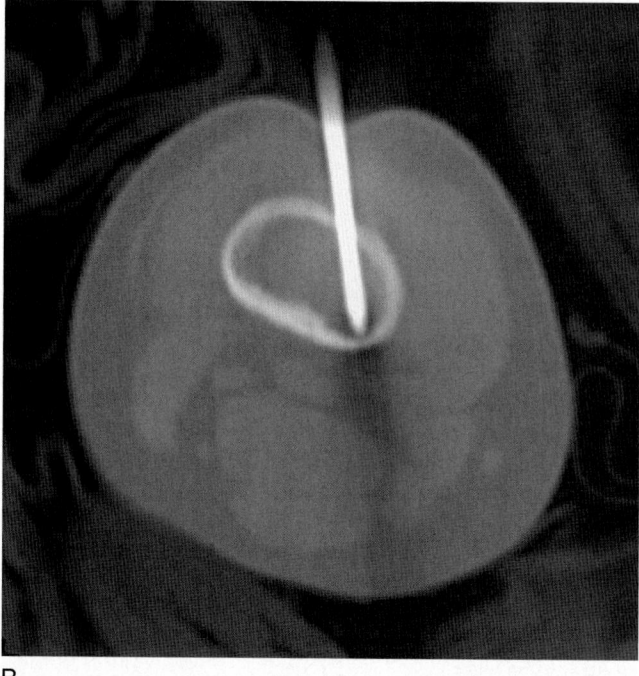

B

FIGURE 188-6. Neuroblastoma recurrence. **A,** Axial computed tomography (CT) image of the femur in this 8-year-old male patient with a prior history of neuroblastoma resection shows an intramedullary soft tissue mass with attenuation similar to that of adjacent muscle. **B,** CT-guided bone core needle access with subsequent coaxial needle sampling confirmed the diagnosis of metastatic neuroblastoma.

the biopsy specimen obtained and the location from which it was taken.

Needles

Needle sizes for core needle specimens can range from 22 gauge to 14 gauge. Fine-needle aspiration (FNA) needles typically range from 25 gauge to 20 gauge. FNA needles typically have a stylet within the needle that is

removed once the needle tip has been guided to the tissue of interest, to prevent the capture of nontarget tissue. Small fragments of tissue are then obtained by a series of short, quick passes under imaging guidance. Gentle negative pressure on a syringe attached to the FNA biopsy needle or simple capillary attraction may allow adequate sampling for cytology, although this is not always needed. The specimen can then be transferred to a slide for preparation at the time of the procedure, if a

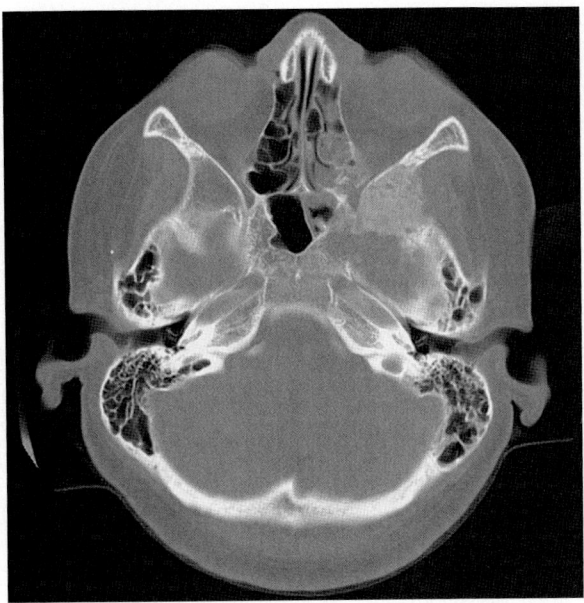
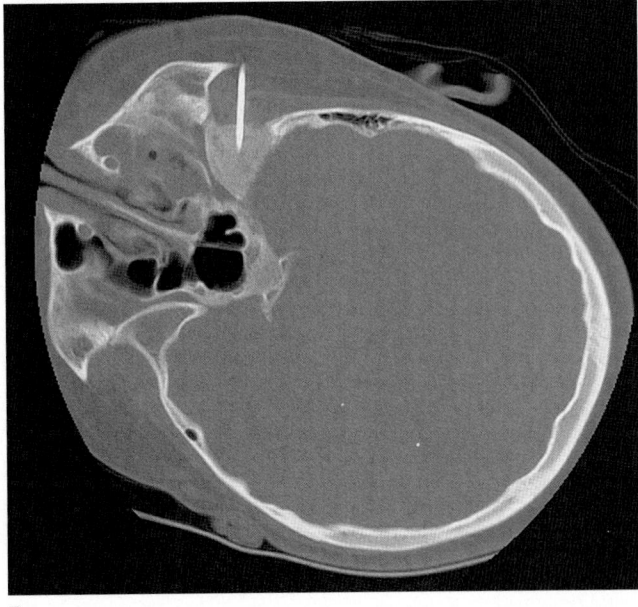

A   B

FIGURE 188-8. Sphenoid fibrous dysplasia. **A,** A 12-year-old male patient with headache was found on axial computed tomography (CT) to have an expansive lesion of the left sphenoid bone with erosion of the lateral cortical margin. **B,** CT-guided biopsy shows that the tip of the coaxial needle is well depicted within the sphenoid osseous lesion. Although the outer guided needle remained in excellent position, several small coaxial needle samples were obtained with final pathology of fibrous dysplasia.

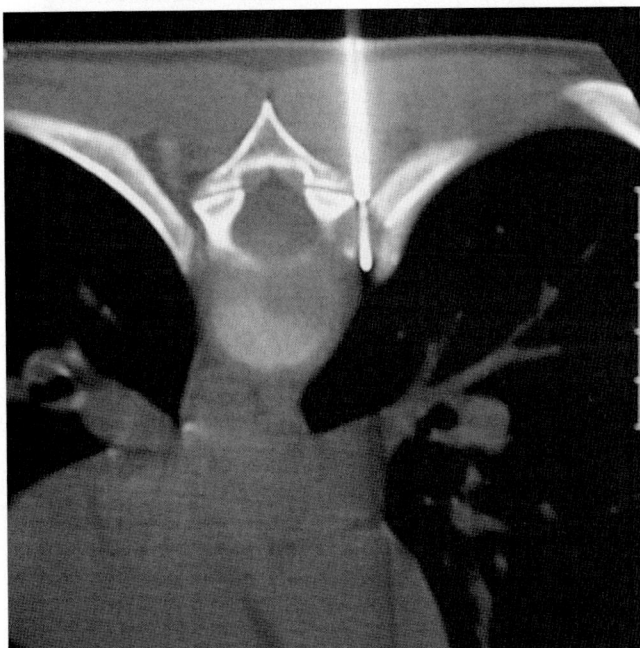

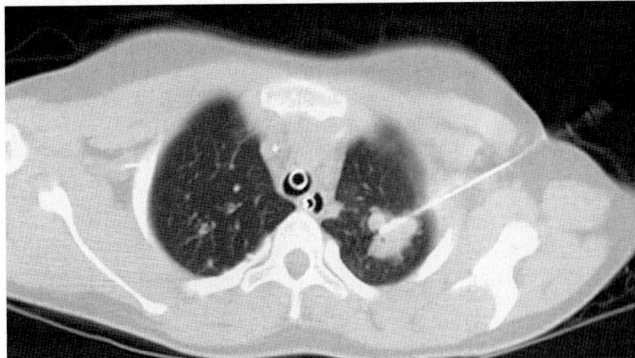

FIGURE 188-10. Aspergillosis. An 11-year-old female patient presented with fever and cough with a left upper lobe lesion on chest x-ray that did not resolve after a course of oral antibiotics was completed. Subsequent chest computed tomography (CT) revealed an irregular left apical lung lesion. Coaxial technique CT-guided biopsy of this lesion showed fungal hyphae on initial staining and culture growing *Aspergillus*.

FIGURE 188-9. Osteomyelitis. A 6-year-old female immunocompromised patient presented with left posterior back/rib pain and was found to have an irregular erosive lesion along a thoracic rib. An axial computed tomography (CT) image from a posterior approach with the patient supine shows the outer guide needle advanced to the lesion. A coaxially inserted smaller core needle is shown sampling the full width of the lesion. Final pathology and cultures showed this lesion to represent osteomyelitis.

cytopathologist is available. This allows assessment of the biopsy sample and the potential need for additional tissue for proper diagnosis. Gentle needle rinse in appropriate media such as RPMI (Roswell Park Memorial Institute) and spinning of cells may contribute to further analysis.

For many pediatric tumor types, larger tissue samples are usually required and can be obtained through single or multiple passes with readily available, spring-loaded core needle biopsy devices (20 to 14 gauge). Core biopsy specimens can be immediately evaluated with touch preparation or frozen section to confirm adequate needle localization, to assess for further tissue sampling, or to conclude a biopsy procedure when an adequate specimen has been obtained.

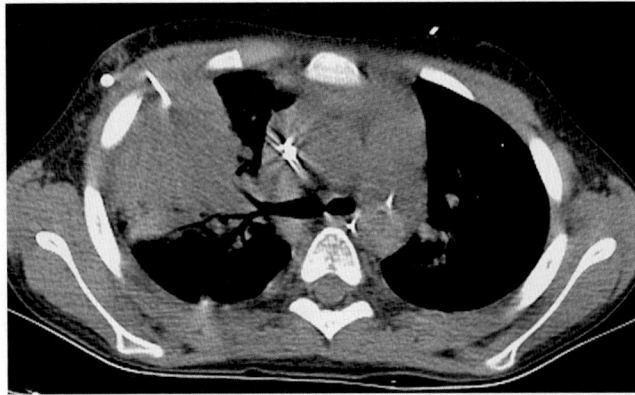

FIGURE 188-11. Lung abscess. Computed tomography–guided fine-needle aspiration of this right upper lobe–organizing process confirmed fungal hyphae; final culture results showed *Aspergillus*.

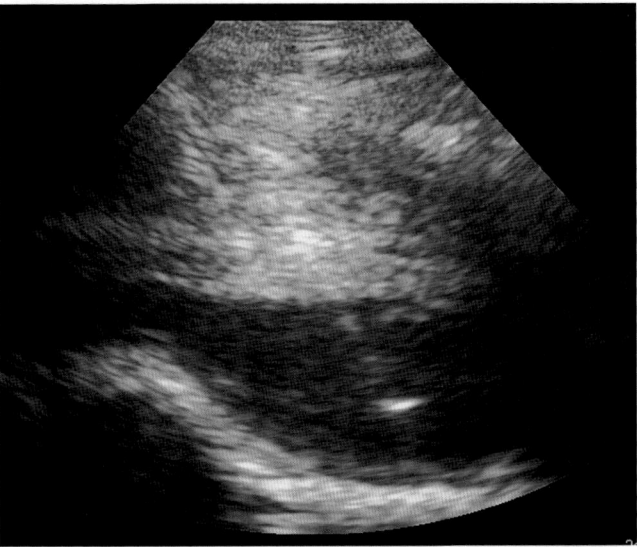

FIGURE 188-13. Hip effusion. A 14-year-old female patient with lupus presented with a painful left hip. Joint effusion was subsequently well visualized on ultrasound (US) imaging. A successful fine-needle aspiration (22 g) with real-time US guidance resulted in clinical improvement in the patient's symptoms. The effusion proved to be noninfectious.

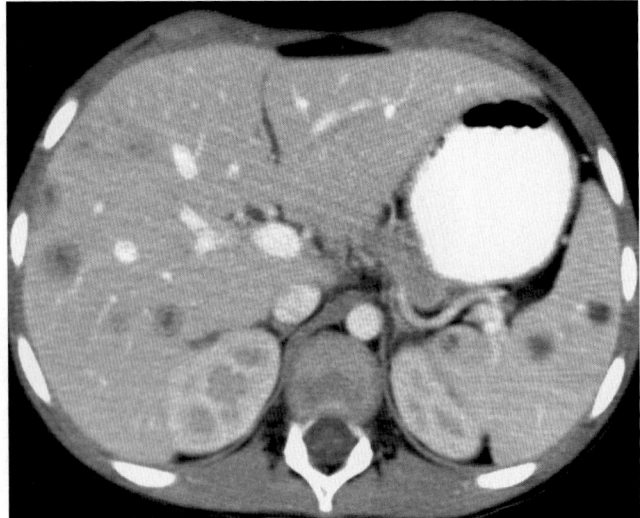

A

FIGURE 188-12. Disseminated fungal infection. **A,** A 9-year-old female patient underwent abdominal contrast-enhanced computed tomography wherein multiple hepatic and splenic lesions were identified. **B,** Ultrasonography-guided aspiration of one of the hepatic lesions was performed; histology and culture confirmed disseminated *Candida* fungal infection.

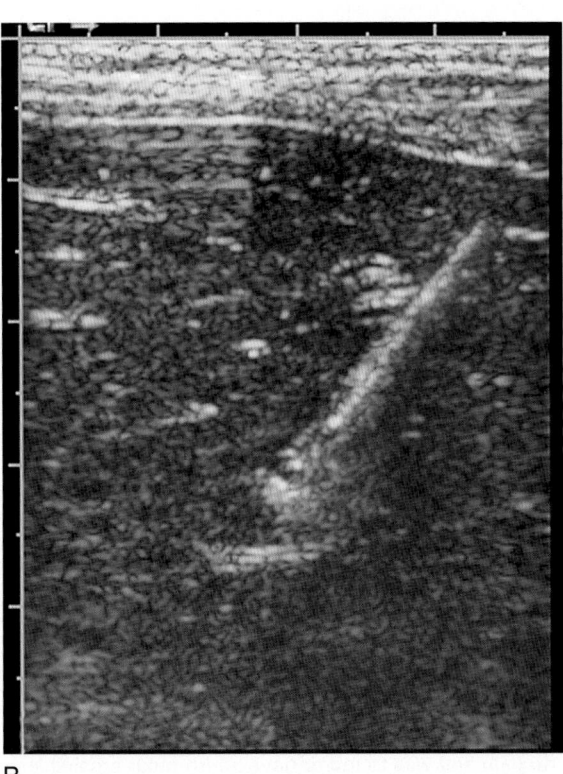

B

In cases in which multiple tissue specimens may be required, a guiding needle sheath with a smaller core biopsy needle, such as a 19 gauge guide or a 20 gauge core needle, may be used. This coaxial technique is useful for taking multiple core samples through a single access site. In lung and liver biopsies, one pass for the guiding needle is recommended across the target organ surface to reduce the risk of pneumothorax or capsular hemorrhage, respectively.

Various needle types and sizes are available for biopsy.

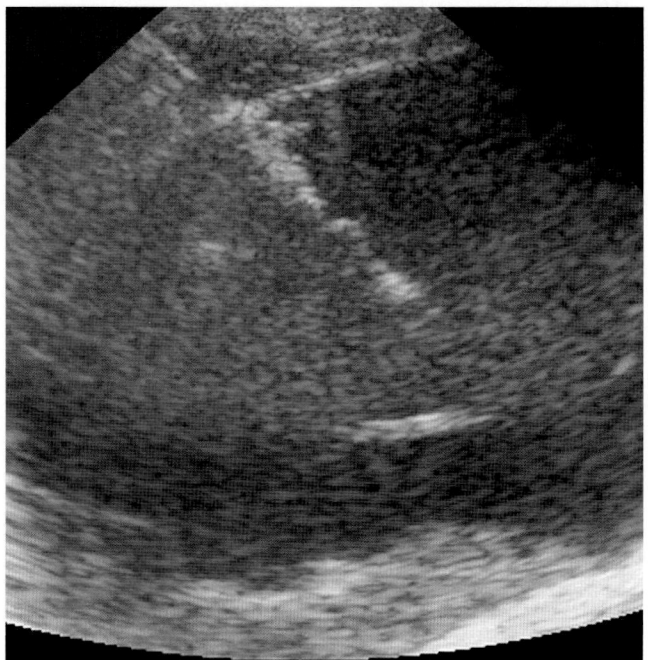

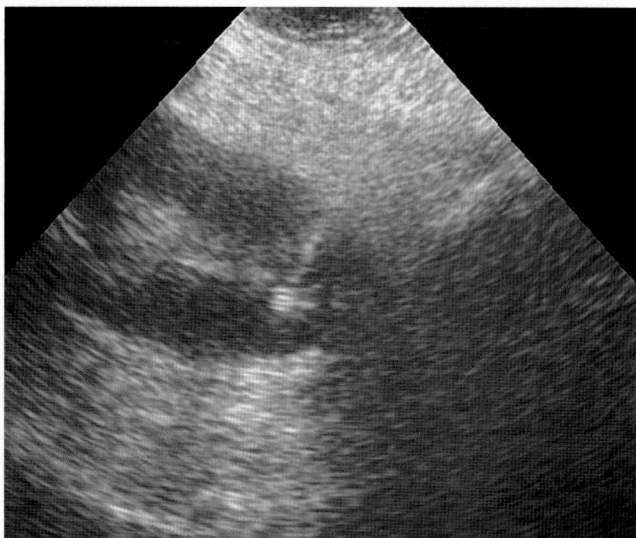

FIGURE 188-16. Kidney transplant. A 13-year-old female patient with cadaveric renal transplantation who was found to have elevated creatinine underwent real-time ultrasonography-guided renal transplant biopsy. Core needle biopsy specimens (16 or 18 gauge) are preferred to allow for a minimal number of biopsy passes while providing adequate tissue for the transplant pathologist to make a determination of rejection, drug toxicity, or other causes.

FIGURE 188-14. Liver (native). High-frequency ultrasound transducer image of a native liver undergoing percutaneous 18 gauge core biopsy in this 6-year-old male patient with elevated liver function tests.

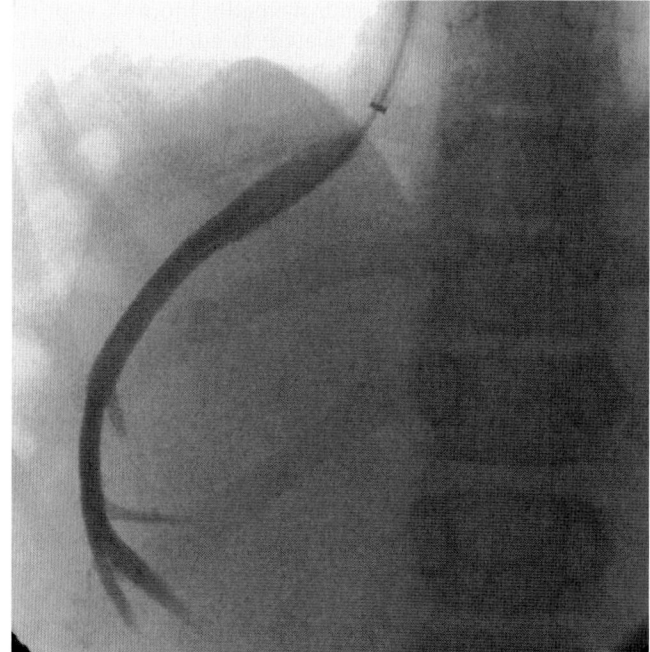

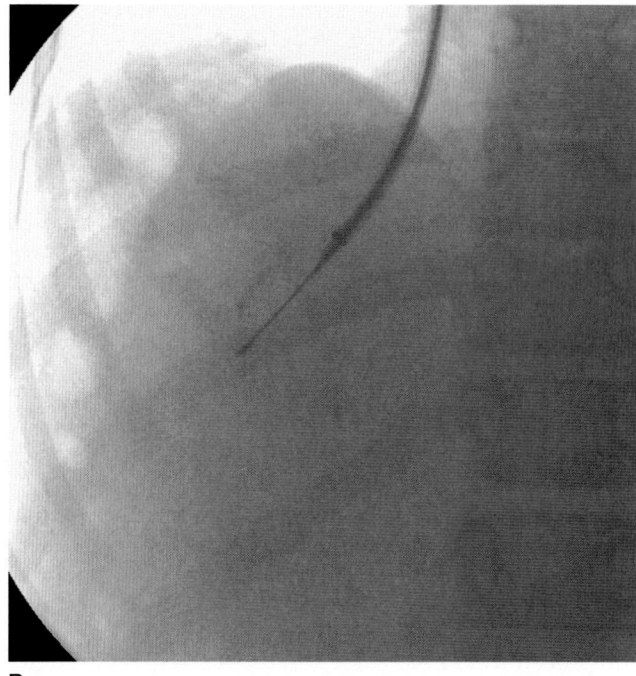

A   B

FIGURE 188-15. Liver transplantation. A 7-year-old male recipient of a left lobe split liver transplantation with elevated liver function tests was referred for transjugular liver biopsy with portosystemic pressure gradient measurements. **A,** Contrast injection confirms catheter position within the donor hepatic vein. **B,** A 19 gauge core needle advanced along the course of the hepatic vein without rotation of the base catheter allows tissue sampling far away from the capsular surface.

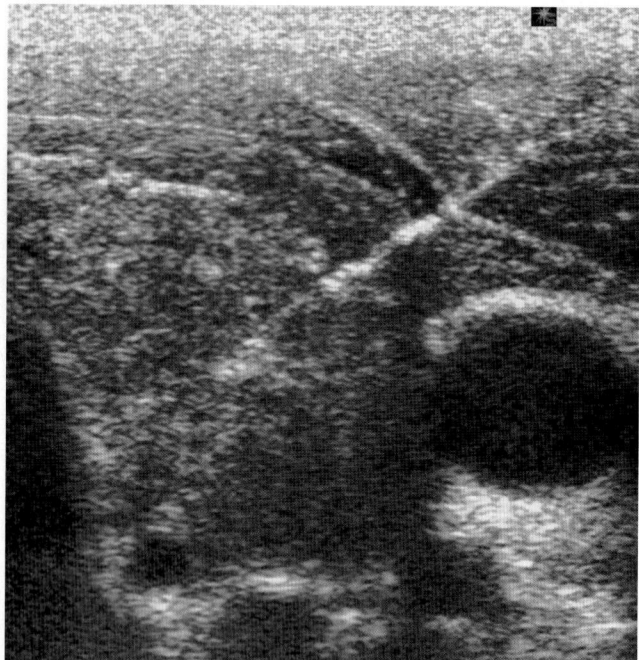

FIGURE 188-17. Thyroid. A 14-year-old female patient with diffusely swollen thyroid gland was referred for biopsy with low free thyroxine (T4), low triiodothyronine (T3), and elevated thyroid-stimulating hormone levels. Ultrasonography-guided 25 gauge fine-needle aspiration and 22 gauge core biopsies provided adequate material for diagnosis of Hashimoto thyroiditis.

TISSUE ANALYSIS

Standard light microscopy is the mainstay of pathologic analysis. Aside from standard histopathology and cytopathology, additional molecular pathology and cytogenetic analysis may be required for primary diagnosis of many pediatric malignancies. Flow cytometry can be used to investigate lymphoid tumors. Reverse transcriptase–polymerase chain reaction (RT-PCR) analysis can be used to evaluate tumor-specific fusion products. Cytogenetic analysis such as karyotyping, fluorescence in situ hybridization (FISH), and DNA index/ploidy status can be performed on core biopsy specimens.

MODALITIES

Ultrasound (US) is the ideal modality for image-guided biopsy because of real-time imaging and the lack of ionizing radiation. Attachable needle guides are available for many ultrasound probes that provide optimal alignment and visualization of the biopsy needle during the procedure. These guides can be set to specific angles relative to the transducer surface for passage of the needle to a specified depth. Alternatively, the "free-hand" technique, without limitations in three-dimensional space, may allow access to more difficult to reach lesions.

Fluoroscopy is useful for guiding biopsies of radio-dense or osseous lesions, or for performing liver biopsies via a transjugular route. Lesions are localized in orthogonal planes and the biopsy instrument advanced in stepwise fashion under real-time visualization.

Computed tomography (CT) technology has advanced in recent years (CT fluoroscopy) and provides additional soft tissue and osseous visualization in comparison with standard fluoroscopy. CT guidance can be provided in sequential stepwise fashion or under real-time imaging.

Magnetic resonance imaging (MRI)-guided biopsies may offer an additional option that avoids patient exposure to ionizing radiation. Each imaging modality has its strengths and limitations. Ultimately, the choice of guidance modality is made on the basis of the experience of the procedural physician, the imaging characteristics of the lesion, and the location of the lesion to be biopsied.

> Imaging guidance for biopsy procedures should be selected in accordance with the location of the lesion and the experience of the procedural physician.

PEDIATRIC SOLID TUMORS—PRIMARY DIAGNOSIS

Use of needle biopsy for primary diagnosis of pediatric solid tumors is not a uniform practice across institutions. If it is expected that a tumor will be resectable, it is logical that only one procedure must be done, that being surgery. However, when it is clear from imaging that complete surgical resection is not possible, consideration should be given to obtaining tissue through needle biopsy techniques. Arguments against needle biopsy for primary diagnosis are largely related to smaller specimens and sampling errors. With coaxial techniques, multiple core specimens can be safely obtained through a single outer needle puncture, which yields more tissue for analysis. This also enhances the safety of the biopsy procedure in that it permits single passage of the needle to the periphery of the lesion, and it decreases the time required for the procedure because the outer needle is poised to take the subsequent specimen without potentially lengthy retargeting. Image guidance often allows safe sampling of different sites within the same tumor. Doppler with color flow helps to differentiate necrotic portions of tumor from viable tissue more likely to yield diagnostic specimens. Other imaging modalities such as positron emission tomography (PET) help to distinguish viable from necrotic tissue. In a study with a population of 103 patients, Garrett and associates showed that core needle biopsy (when performed for primary diagnosis) had a sensitivity of 97%, a specificity of 100%, and an accuracy of 98%.

> Imaging aids in needle guidance and in determination of optimal sampling sites for ensuring high sensitivity and specificity.

In primary diagnostic core biopsies of neuroblastoma, additional prognostic information regarding N-myc Oncogene and ploidy status can be obtained. N-myc Oncogene status, 17p chromosome abnormalities, and chromosome 1p deletions affect neuroblastoma prognosis to a greater extent than histology does, and this information can readily be obtained through percutaneous biopsy. A potential disadvantage of percutaneous biopsy of neuroblastoma is that a smaller tissue sample is available for tumor banking.

Hepatic tumors such as hepatoblastoma may be diagnosed through percutaneous biopsy to help guide preoperative chemotherapy. Fibrolamellar hepatocellular carcinoma (HCC), with its fibrous/inflammatory rim, can also be diagnosed. In undifferentiated embryonal liver sarcoma, a sample from the enhancing viable rim of the tumor is recommended to avoid a necrotic/hemorrhagic center. Placing the needle through normal liver parenchyma prior to reaching the tumor mass is recommended to avoid extracapsular tumor spread.

RECURRENCE

To confirm the recurrence of a known primary pediatric malignancy, a smaller amount of tissue is usually required. Percutaneous biopsy techniques (rather than open surgical biopsy) are more often used in evaluating recurrent disease for a number of reasons, including the availability of a prior pathologic specimen for comparison, the need for smaller tissue samples, and decreased morbidity from percutaneous biopsies in a prior surgical field.

> **Percutaneous biopsy is ideal in the evaluation of recurrent malignancy.**

RELATIVE CONTRAINDICATIONS

The safety of image-guided biopsy has been well established. However, it is important to know when the percutaneous route should be avoided. In specific locations, such as the retroperitoneum, a safe path for the biopsy needle to pass through to the lesion may not exist because of the presence of vital structures. Additionally, some lesions may not be visible on imaging. A lesion seen only on contrast-enhanced CT may not be visible on ultrasonography or on noncontrast CT. Patient-specific factors such as uncorrectable coagulopathy are also contraindications.

COMPLICATIONS

Complications can be categorized according to the Society of Interventional Radiology Guidelines published by Cardella and colleagues. Complications resulting from percutaneous biopsy consist primarily of hemorrhage, organ-specific complications (such as bile leak within the liver), and pneumothorax (when lung biopsy is performed); infections such as peritonitis are less common. Needle tract seeding is a rare complication that has been reported in the literature by Nolsoe and associates; it occurs at a rate of 1 in 20,000 patients. An overall complication rate of 13.4% has been recently reported in a 202-patient study with no biopsy-related deaths or permanent adverse events. In a recent study by Garrett and coworkers, no needle tract tumors were identified.

In an effort to limit hemorrhage from solid organ/tissue biopsies and to theoretically reduce tumor needle tract seeding, solutions of microfibrillar collagen (Avitene; MedChem Products, Inc., Woburn, MA) or gelfoam slurry have been used.

> **Image-guided percutaneous biopsy is very safe and is associated with a very low risk of complications.**

CONCLUSION

Image-guided percutaneous biopsy is a safe and effective means of obtaining a diagnosis in initial disease presentations and in recurrences. Factors most responsible for successful percutaneous biopsy include the experience and skill of the interventional radiologist who is performing the procedure and the experience and skill of the pathologist who is analyzing the obtained tissue. In the future, as greater numbers of neoadjuvant and nonsurgical treatment options become available, the need will be greater to obtain tissue for primary diagnosis via less invasive percutaneous routes.

SUGGESTED READINGS

Cahill AM, Baskin KM, Kaye RD, et al: CT-guided percutaneous lung biopsy in children. J Vasc Interv Radiol 2004;15:955-960

Cardella JF, Bakal CW, Bertino RE, et al: Quality improvement guidelines for image-guided percutaneous biopsy in adults. J Vasc Interv Radiol 2003;14:S227-S230

Cohen MB, Bottles K, Ablin AR, et al: The use of fine-needle aspiration biopsy in children. West J Med 1989;150:665-667

Diament MJ, Stanley P, Taylor S: Percutaneous fine needle biopsy in pediatrics. Pediatr Radiol 1985;15:409-411

Dupuy DE, Mayo-Smith WW, Cronan JJ: Imaging-guided biopsy and radiofrequency ablation of renal masses. Semin Interv Radiol 2000;17:373-379

Fletcher JA, Kozakewich HP, Hoffer FA, et al: Diagnostic relevance of clonal cytogenetic aberrations in malignant soft tissue tumors. N Engl J Med 1991;324:436-443

Garrett KM, Hoffer FA, Behm FG, et al: Interventional radiology techniques for the diagnosis of lymphoma or leukemia. Pediatr Radiol 2002;32:653-662

Graf N, Tournade MF, de Kraker J: The role of preoperative chemotherapy in the management of Wilms' tumor: the SIOP studies. International Society of Pediatric Oncology. Urol Clin North Am 2000;27:443-454

Hardaway BW, Hoffer FA, Rao BN: Needle localization of small pediatric tumors for surgical biopsy. Pediatr Radiol 2000; 30:318-322

Hoffer FA: Liver biopsy methods for pediatric oncology patients. Pediatr Radiol 2000;30:481-488

Hoffer FA, Chung T, Diller L, et al: Percutaneous biopsy for prognostic testing of neuroblastoma. Radiology 1996; 200:213-216

Hoffer FA, Gianturco LE, Fletcher JA, et al: Percutaneous biopsy of peripheral primitive neuroectodermal tumors and Ewing's sarcomas for cytogenetic analysis. AJR Am J Roentgenol 1994;162:1141-1142

Hoffer FA, Gow K, Flynn PM, et al: Accuracy of percutaneous lung biopsy for invasive pulmonary aspergillosis. Pediatr Radiol 2001;31:144-152

Hoffer FA, Shamberger RC, Kozakewich H: Percutaneous chest biopsies in children. Cardiovasc Interv Radiol 1990;13:32-35

Hugosson CO, Nyman RS, Cappelen-Smith JM, et al: Ultrasound-guided biopsy of abdominal and pelvic lesions in children: a comparison between fine-needle aspiration and 1.2-mm needle core biopsy. Pediatr Radiol 1999;29:31-36

Jelinek JS, Murphey MD, Welker JA, et al: Diagnosis of primary bone tumors with image-guided percutaneous biopsy: experience with 110 tumors. Radiology 2002;223:731-737

Jennings PE, Donald JJ, Coral A, et al: Ultrasound-guided core biopsy. Lancet 1989;8651:1369-1371

Kaye R, Sane SS, Towbin RB: Pediatric intervention: an update. Part II. J Vasc Interv Radiol 2000;11:807-818

Kim SH, Lim HK, Lee WJ, et al: Needle-tract implantation of hepatocellular carcinoma: frequency and CT findings after biopsy with a 19.5-gauge automated biopsy gun. Abdom Imaging 2000;25:246-250

Morrissey B, Adams H, Gibbs AR, et al: Percutaneous needle biopsy of the mediastinum: review of 94 procedures. Thorax 1993;48:632-637

Nolsoe C, Nielsen L, Torp-Pederson S, Holm HH: Major complications and deaths due to interventional ultrasonography: a review of 8000 cases. J Clin Ultrasound 1990;18:179-184

Pohar-Marinsek Z, Anzic J, Jereb B: Topical topic: value of fine needle aspiration biopsy in childhood rhabdomyosarcoma: twenty-six years of experience in Slovenia. Med Pediatr Oncol 2002;38:416-420

Sabbah R, Ghandour M, Ali A, et al: Tru-cut needle biopsy of abdominal tumors in children: a safe and diagnostic procedure. Cancer 1981;47:2533-2535

Schaller RT Jr, Schaller JF, Buschmann C, et al: The usefulness of percutaneous fine-needle aspiration biopsy in infants and children. J Pediatr Surg 1983;18:398-405

Shakoor KA: Fine needle aspiration cytology in advanced pediatric tumors. Pediatr Pathol 1989;9:713-718

Shimada H: The International Neuroblastoma Pathology Classification. Pathologica 2003;95:240-241

Sklair-Levy M, Lebensart PD, Applbaum YH, et al: Percutaneous image-guided needle biopsy in children—summary of our experience with 57 children. Pediatr Radiol 2001;31:732-736

Skoldenberg EG, Jakobson A, Elvin A, et al: Diagnosing childhood tumors: a review of 147 cutting needle biopsies in 110 children. J Pediatr Surg 2002;37:50-56

Smith EH: Complications of percutaneous abdominal fine-needle biopsy. Radiology 1991;178:253-258

Somers JM, Lomas DJ, Hacking JC, et al: Radiologically-guided cutting needle biopsy for suspected malignancy in childhood. Clin Radiol 1993;48:236-240

Udayakumar AM, Sundareshan TS, Appaji L, et al: Rhabdomyosarcoma: cytogenetics of five cases using fine-needle aspiration samples and review of the literature. Ann Genet 2002;45:33-37

Van Sonnenberg E, Wittich GR, Edwards DK, et al: Percutaneous diagnostic and therapeutic interventional radiologic procedures in children: experience in 100 patients. Radiology 1987;162:601-605

Welch TJ, Sheedy PF 2nd, Stephens DH, et al: Percutaneous adrenal biopsy: review of a 10-year experience. Radiology 1994;193:341-344

Welker JA, Henshaw RM, Jelinek J, et al: The percutaneous needle biopsy is safe and recommended in the diagnosis of musculoskeletal masses. Cancer 2000;89:2677-2686

Willman JH, White K, Coffin CM: Pediatric core needle biopsy: strengths and limitations in evaluation of masses. Pediatr Dev Pathol 2001;4:46-52

Yamagami T, Iida S, Kato T, et al: Usefulness of new automated cutting needle for tissue-core biopsy of lung nodules under CT fluoroscopic guidance. Chest 2003;124:147-154

CHAPTER 189

Gastrostomies and Gastrojejunostomies in Children

BAIRBRE CONNOLLY

TERMINOLOGY

In this chapter, the following terminology is used:

Gastrostomy (G) refers to a tube that passes through the abdominal wall into the stomach.

Gastrojejunostomy (GJ) refers to a longer tube that passes through the abdominal wall, traversing the stomach, out the pylorus, and into the small bowel.

Jejunostomy (J) refers to a tube that passes through the anterior abdominal wall directly into a loop of jejunum.

PEG refers to a gastrostomy tube that is placed endoscopically, from within the stomach out through the anterior abdominal wall.

Nasogastric (NG) tube refers to a temporary straight tube that is passed from the nose to the stomach and is usually placed at the bedside.

Nasojejunal (NJ) tube refers to a long, fine tube that is passed from the nose to the jejunum, may be weighted at the inner end, and is placed at the bedside or under fluoroscopy.

INTRODUCTION

Feeding is an important component of a child's development, nutritional status, and well-being. Nutritional support should ideally be achieved through the gastrointestinal tract, if it is functional. Some children are unable to feed by mouth, either temporarily or on a long-term basis. For those unable to feed orally over the short term, alternative routes are employed (e.g., nasogastric [NG] or oral gastric [OG] tube). In those with short-term needs in whom gastroesophageal reflux is an issue, the alternative of a nasojejunal (NJ) tube may be considered. Tube feeding by these means is ideal for short-term problems only (<8 to 12 weeks) because prolonged nasal intubation may be associated with esophagitis, gastroesophageal reflux, accidental dislodgement, and poor psychosocial acceptance

For children who require longer term feeding (>8 to 12 weeks) or who are unsafe or unable to feed by mouth, other options should be considered. Traditionally, treatment use to be provided with a surgical gastrostomy (G) tube. In recent years, endoscopic placement of a G tube, known as PEG (percutaneous endoscopic gastrostomy), has been well described. This involves passing an endoscope from the mouth down the esophagus to the stomach

and antegradely placing a tube across the gastric wall to the anterior abdominal wall. A third method involves image-guided insertion of a G tube under fluoroscopy combined with ultrasonography, followed by placement of the G tube from the skin retrogradely through the anterior abdominal wall into the stomach (retrograde radiologic G tube), or an antegrade "push-pull technique." Each type of G tube has inherent advantages, disadvantages, and complications that have been outlined in a meta-analysis performed by Wollman and associates. Unfortunately, no method of enteral feeding is risk free. In those in whom gastroesophageal reflux is such a significant problem that the child cannot tolerate NG feedings, the following approaches are available: (1) the patient may undergo a trial of G feeds, and if he or she fails to tolerate G tube feeds, the radiologic G tube can readily be converted to a gastrojejunostomy (GJ) tube, (2), a GJ tube can be placed from the outset, or (3) alternatively, the child may undergo a surgical fundoplication and insertion of a G tube.

SCALE OF PROBLEM

As medical care becomes more sophisticated in the Western world, the scale of this issue is increasing, as are the numbers of technologically dependent children and adults. The past two decades have seen an increase in the number of patients of all ages who are fed through enterostomy tubes. Children with a variety of severe neurologic disorders and syndromes are surviving longer and require supportive nutrition.

The purpose of this chapter is to outline some important steps involved in placement of enterostomy feeding tubes in children, with emphasis on the imaging associated with placement, tube maintenance, and complications.

CLINICAL INDICATIONS

Placement of a G or GJ tube is indicated in those children in whom an alternative to oral nutrition is required for longer than 8 weeks. Most are children who are unsafe to feed by mouth with some or all food or liquid consistencies. Other indications include requirement for nutritional intake that is greater than that which can be achieved by mouth (e.g., high metabolic needs, congestive heart failure, chronic renal failure), specific intake needs (e.g., specific metabolic disorders, absorption difficulties, inflammatory bowel diseases), the occasional requirement for long-term unpleasant medications that are difficult to take by mouth (e.g., human immunodeficiency virus [HIV], hypoaldosteronism), and requirement for a feeding tube primarily for the maintenance of hydration. Within these broad clinical indications, a wide variety of diagnoses are included. More than 50% involve some form of central nervous system disorder (e.g., cerebral palsy, acquired brain disorders, various syndromes associated with neurologic impairment).

CONTRAINDICATIONS

Few absolute contraindications to percutaneous G/GJ tube placement have been identified. They include incorrectable coagulopathy and severe, resistant, or malignant ascites. Unfavorable anatomy may be a relative contraindication because of solid organ position. If it is due to overlying bowel, it can change with time and peristalsis, so that another attempt at another date may be successful. Alternatively, decompression of the dilated gas-filled bowel is possible.

PROCEDURE

Preprocedure Planning

The following description focuses on the radiologic technique of retrograde image-guided G or GJ tube placement. Slight variation may be observed between centers. This description outlines the current practice at the Hospital for Sick Children in Toronto, Ontario.

Initial assessment of the appropriateness of the indication is important. This frequently requires a formal or informal multidisciplinary approach involving a pediatrician, a dietitian or a nutritionist, an occupational therapist, and a radiologist. It is imperative that parental expectations are realistic, and that they are fundamentally in agreement with the decision to place a G tube. A G tube has significant psychological and emotional implications, because for many caregivers of the neurologically impaired child, feeding is perceived to represent significant pleasure for the child, despite the inordinate amount of time spent in this activity and the inherent risk of aspiration in children with oral motor disabilities.

> **The decision to place an enterostomy tube usually requires a multidisciplinary approach.**

At the assessment visit, details of the procedure are explained and risks outlined; these include failure to find a safe access route (approximately 1%), peritonitis (1.2%), injury to bowel or transfixing of small or large bowel (<1%), bleeding (rare), and death (very rare). Common tube maintenance issues (e.g., blocking, kinks, leakage, dislodgement) and site issues are outlined. Written consent may be obtained by the interventionalist at that time or on the day of the procedure. The procedure

is booked with plans for the level of analgesia deemed most appropriate (i.e., local anesthetic alone, local anesthetic and sedation, or general anesthetic).

Procedural Technique for G Tube

On the day of the procedure, the child is kept fasting. Formal written consent is obtained. It is our practice to give one dose of antibiotics immediately prior to enterostomy tube placement (e.g., cephazolin, 30 mg/kg). The patient is placed on a C-arm fluoroscopy table. A limited mapping ultrasound (linear probe, 7 to 12 MHz) is performed to outline the lower limits of the liver, the position of the spleen, and the left costal margin, which are all marked on the abdominal wall with indelible marker. A soft tube (e.g., a large Foley catheter) is placed into the rectum, and the bowel is filled with very dilute liquid barium as far as the transverse colon (Fig. 189-1). The abdomen is cleaned and draped as for a sterile procedure. A nasogastric tube is placed, with the tip in the stomach. Glucagon is administered intravenously (i.e., 0.2 mg for a neonate, 0.3 mg for a toddler, 0.4 mg for a young child, and 0.5 mg for a larger child) to achieve gastric paresis and pyloric constriction. Air is then instilled into the stomach via the NG tube to create gastric distention, which usually displaces the colon inferiorly and the liver edge superiorly, thus creating an access window (see Fig. 189-1). It is imperative that the stomach be somewhat tense with air so that it can be punctured easily. The ideal site is chosen inferior to the costal margin (≥1 cm), lateral to the rectus muscle, and above the transverse colon. Alternative sites are midline through the linea alba, and less ideally through the rectus muscle. Superior displacement of the liver can be confirmed with ultrasound in a sterile cover, to ensure that the chosen site is clear of liver. Once a site has been chosen, with the use of a combination of frontal ± caudocranial angulation, along with lateral fluoroscopy, local anesthetic is infiltrated into the skin, down to the peritoneum. A small 3-mm incision is made with a blade. An 18 gauge puncture needle loaded with a pediatric retention suture (a small piece of metal with a thread attached in the middle of it in the shape of a T) is advanced into the anterior abdominal wall, and the stomach is punctured under live fluoroscopic control, ± real-time ultrasound guidance. The intragastric position is confirmed by a contrast injection through the needle (see Fig. 189-1). A 0.035″ wire is advanced down through the puncture needle, thus deploying the metal component of the retention suture into the stomach; the wire is then coiled within the stomach. The needle is withdrawn and slight tension is placed on the thread of the retention suture, which tacks up the gastric wall to the anterior abdominal wall. Over the wire, the tract is dilated with a gentle "push-and-twist motion," while slight traction on the retention thread is maintained. The dilator is removed, and over the wire, a pigtail catheter of appropriate size (8, 10, or 12 French) is placed. The wire is then removed and the pigtail coiled within the stomach. The intragastric position is confirmed with the use of contrast, which drops freely into the air-filled stomach (see Fig. 189-1). Ancillary signs of correct intra-

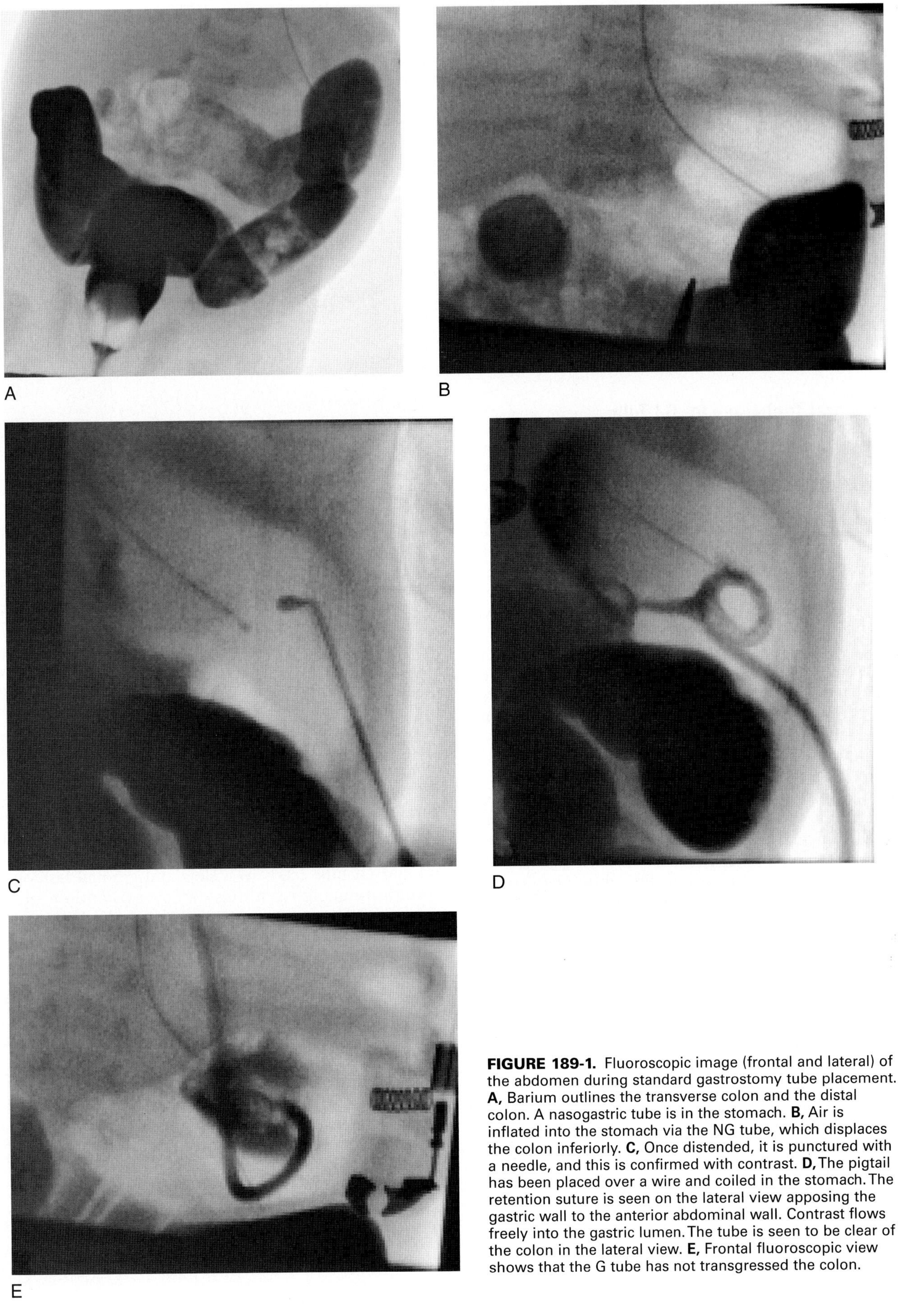

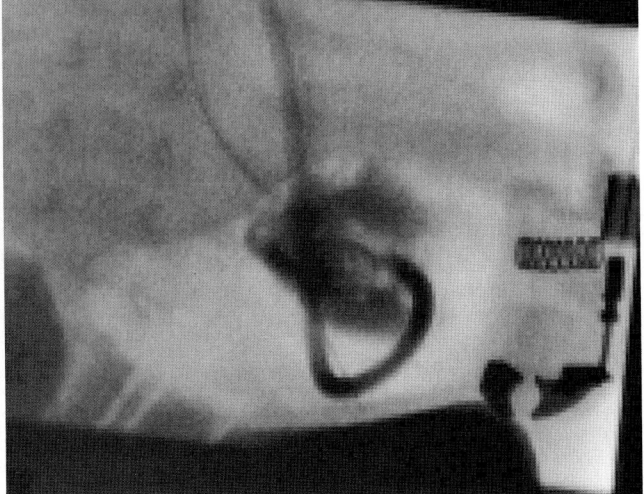

A

B

C

D

E

FIGURE 189-1. Fluoroscopic image (frontal and lateral) of the abdomen during standard gastrostomy tube placement. **A,** Barium outlines the transverse colon and the distal colon. A nasogastric tube is in the stomach. **B,** Air is inflated into the stomach via the NG tube, which displaces the colon inferiorly. **C,** Once distended, it is punctured with a needle, and this is confirmed with contrast. **D,** The pigtail has been placed over a wire and coiled in the stomach. The retention suture is seen on the lateral view apposing the gastric wall to the anterior abdominal wall. Contrast flows freely into the gastric lumen. The tube is seen to be clear of the colon in the lateral view. **E,** Frontal fluoroscopic view shows that the G tube has not transgressed the colon.

gastric position include the ability to freely rotate the pigtail, displacement or movement of the nasogastric tube by the pigtail, and ability to deflate and reinflate the stomach with air with the use of a syringe on the end of the G tube. Recorded imaging with the use of last image hold should show the intragastric position on a frontal and lateral view, which shows that the tube does not transgress the colon or the small bowel (see Fig. 189-1); absence or presence of a pneumoperitoneum and its size should also be revealed. Our practice is to then wind the retention thread taut over a small roll of gauze that is secured with steri-strips. The G tube is secured with some form of retention device or tape.

It is the interventionalist's responsibility to ensure that the tube is within the stomach at the end of the procedure. Inadvertent intraperitoneal placement can occur at any stage during this procedure and must be recognized (Fig. 189-2).

Procedural Technique for GJ Tube

Initial steps involved in placement of a GJ tube are the same as for a G tube; however, one should avoid excessive amounts of barium per rectum. Initially, one may or may not opt to use glucagon; however, it is the author's personal practice to do so to achieve adequate distention of the stomach. Once the needle has punctured the stomach, the retention suture is deployed with the use of an .035″ floppy-tipped wire (e.g., Bentson wire). Over this, a 5 French directional catheter (e.g., JB1-type catheter) is advanced, and the catheter and wire are steered toward the pylorus, into the duodenum, around to the duodenojejunal junction, and down into the proximal jejunum. The JB1 catheter is then removed. Over the wire, the gastric tract is dilated to the appropriate size for the gastrojejunostomy tube. The GJ tube is then advanced over the wire and is positioned with the tip in the jejunum; the gastric retention component (balloon, malecot, or coil—the latter requires a clockwise rotation of the gastric coil) is positioned within the stomach. Some GJ tubes require cutting to an appropriate length. The retention thread is secured in the usual manner. If it proves excessively difficult to negotiate the pylorus, a G tube can be placed instead. At a subsequent procedure, the G tube can be converted to a GJ tube without the need for sedation or local anesthetic.

Postprocedure Care

Postprocedure care and protocols may vary from institution to institution.

The patient must be seen post procedure (e.g., on the evening post enterostomy tube insertion) and daily thereafter until tube feeds are established. The patient is assessed daily for development of any complications: temperature, pulse rate, and blood pressure are reviewed; the abdomen is examined for tenderness, guarding, the presence of bowel sounds, and condition of the dressing. The patient's flowchart is reviewed for volume of gastric drainage (via NG and G) and any vomiting. The amount of analgesia required is usually small; 1 or 2 doses of morphine are required in the first

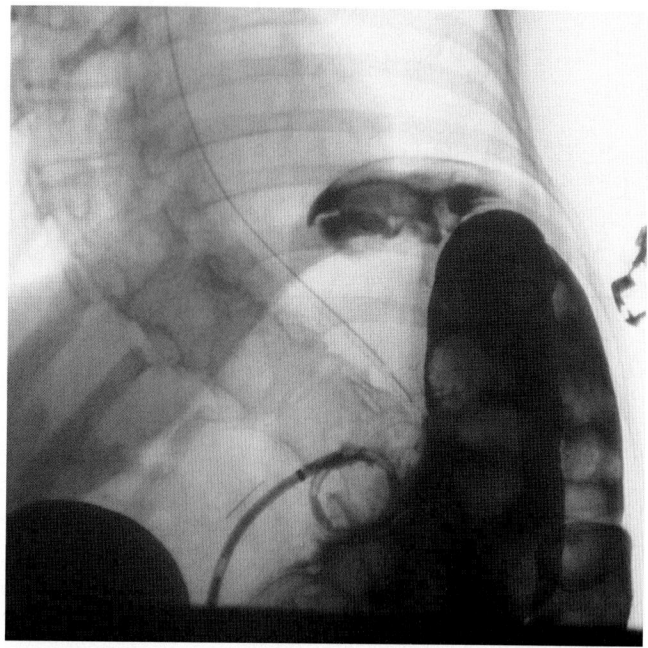

FIGURE 189-2. Fluoroscopic image (frontal) shows air in the stomach, the metal component of the retention suture in the stomach, and the coil of the gastrostomy tube in the peritoneum. This can occur at the time of placement or after a pull or displacement into the peritoneum. Contrast is seen in the peritoneum in the left subphrenic space.

24 hours. Acetaminophen is usually sufficient thereafter. It is our practice to keep the patient nil per mouth for the first 12 hours with G tube and NG tube to gravity drainage. Once active or vigorous bowel sounds are heard, clear fluids are advanced through the G tube at a slow, increasing rate (e.g., 5 ml 2 hourly initially, for 6 hours, with a switch then to small-volume feeds). Full feeds are usually achieved after about 48 to 72 hours. Once G tube feeds are being tolerated, the NG tube is removed (after 24 to 36 hours). In those in whom some oral feeding is permitted or safe, oral feeding is resumed once full feeds have been achieved per G tube, which is usually not before 48 hours. It is our practice to advance G and GJ tube feeds in a slow and gradual fashion, to avoid inducing vomiting or overdistention of the stomach. The retention thread should be kept taut, to ensure that the anterior gastric wall is held in apposition to the anterior abdominal wall and is not permitted to fall away. This helps to ensure that the healing tract is short and reduces the chance of leakage. The thread is cut after 14 days.

COMPLICATIONS

Complications may arise with any type of tube. It behooves the pediatrician to be vigilant for potential complications, and the radiologist to be alert and recognize the imaging findings of some of these possibilities. A low threshold for a tube check is required in the early postprocedure period.

> **A low threshold for a G tube or GJ tube check is required in the early postprocedure period.**

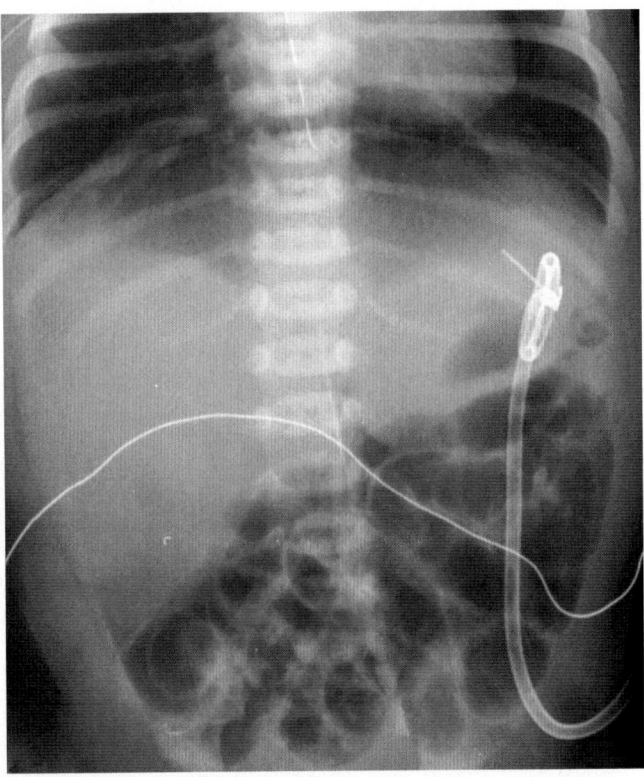
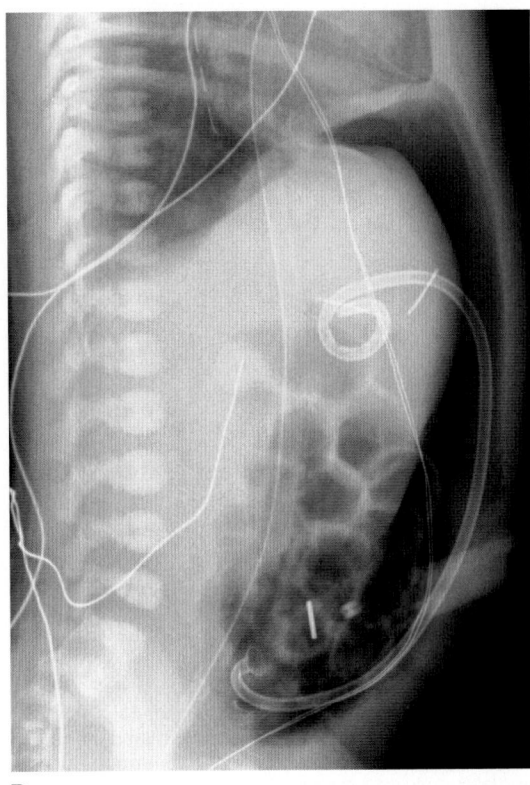

A   B

FIGURE 189-3. Abdominal x-ray shows a pneumoperitoneum in frontal (**A**) and lateral (**B**) projections. A pigtail gastrostomy tube and a retention suture are seen in the stomach. Air is observed under the diaphragm, lucency in the flanks, and a positive Rigler sign on the anteroposterior view in the right iliac fossa (**A**); clearly free air is seen on the lateral shoot-through (**B**).

Peritonitis is a very important potential complication in the first few days. This can be chemical or infectious, resulting from a small leak of gastric contents. The incidence is about 1%. Fever, abdominal distention, scant bowel sounds, tachycardia, vomiting, and pain or discomfort with feeds are signs of peritonitis. Vomiting may result from peritonitis or may itself precipitate a leak and induce peritonism. If any difficulties are noted in the first 72 hours, G or GJ tube check with contrast should be done. Any suggestion of peritonitis prompts aggressive management. Feeds should be discontinued and the NG tube and G tube put to drainage; the patient is maintained on IV fluids, and triple antibiotics are commenced. A G/GJ tube check (including postero-anterior [PA] and lateral views under fluoroscopy) is performed to ensure that no displacement of the G tube has occurred since insertion (i.e., outward into the peritoneum or inward into the duodenum), that any pneumoperitoneum is decreasing in size, and that no leak of contrast has occurred (Fig. 189-3). The child must be regularly reassessed to ensure that symptoms and signs are improving. Other sources of fever must be excluded.

> **Early post–G tube placement, peritonitis that results from a leak in the presence of a correctly placed G tube, can usually be treated with aggressive medical treatment.**
>
> **Post G tube insertion, pneumoperitoneum is common; it should be small and decreasing in size.**

A common problem post G tube insertion is constipation because of the barium used to outline the colon. Suppositories per rectum are frequently required to relieve constipation.

At the time of placement, the needle can inadvertently traverse a loop of small or large bowel. The G tube therefore traverses from the abdominal wall, through the interposed loop of bowel, and into the stomach. Subsequently, at the time of tube change, as the new tube is replaced down the tract, it enters the more superficial loop of bowel. If this is proximal jejunum, it may fortuitously be used as a primary jejunostomy. However, if this is distal jejunum, ileum, or colon, it will not function adequately for feeding (Fig. 189-4). Persistent diarrhea may result.

> **If symptoms of profuse diarrhea after a G tube change should occur, one should consider a colonic position of the tube.**

Depending on the design of the GJ tube used, a leak at the gastric coil site is a common cause of vomiting of feeds. This is readily diagnosed with the use of water-soluble contrast with careful attention to the gastric pigtail in PA and lateral positions. This requires a GJ tube exchange (Fig. 189-5).

Migration of the gastric retention component (i.e., a coil, malecot, or balloon) through the pylorus into the duodenum leads to discomfort and feeding intolerance or bilious vomiting. This event can be recognized on

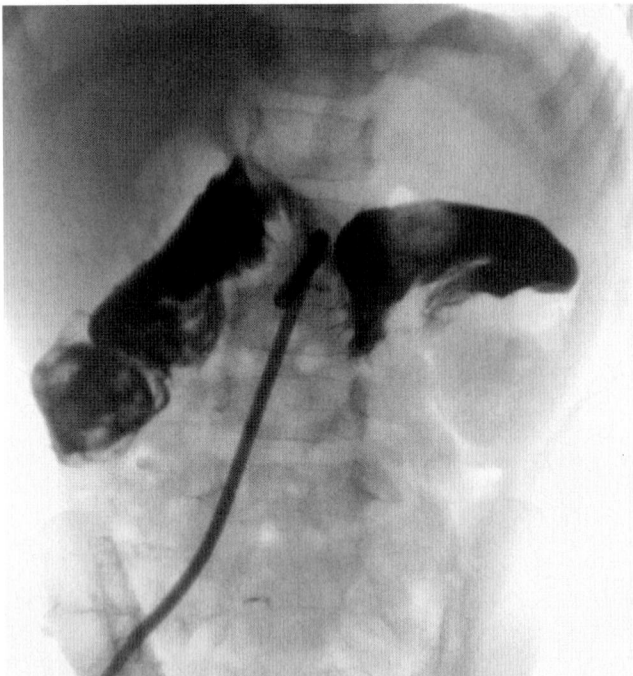

FIGURE 189-4. The gastrostomy tube is seen on a fluoroscopic image sitting in the colon, inferior to the air-filled stomach. The original tube a few months earlier had inadvertently passed through the colon, into the stomach. Colonic interposition was detected at the time of this tube change.

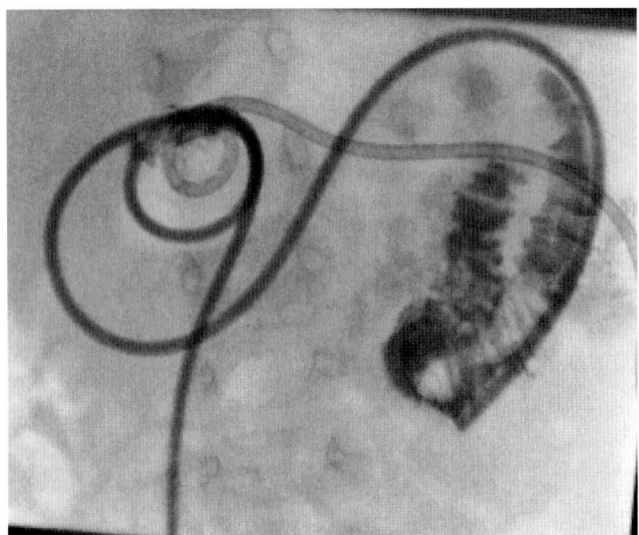

FIGURE 189-5. A frontal fluoroscopic image of a patient with both a gastrostomy tube and a gastrojejunostomy tube is shown. The GJ tube is filled with contrast and shows a leak from the coil into the stomach, as well as contrast in the jejunum. The G tube is not opacified.

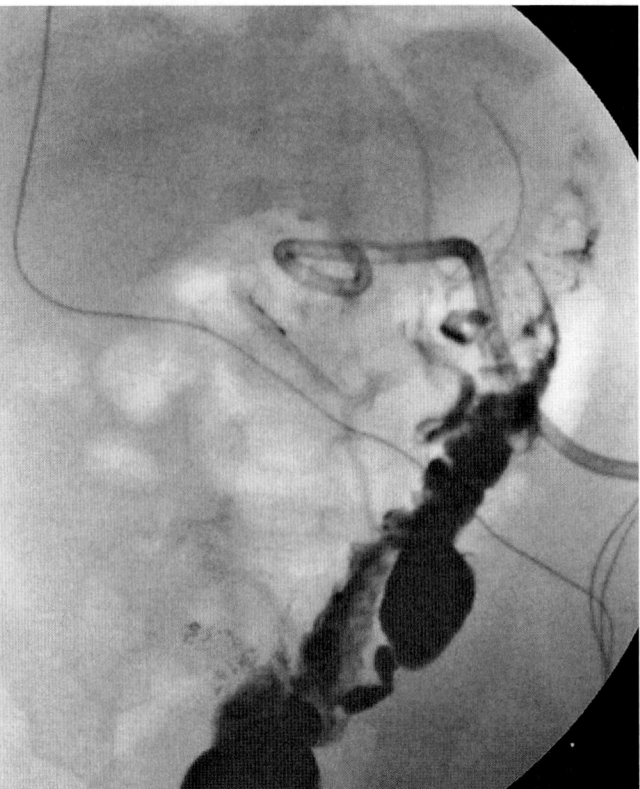

FIGURE 189-6. Frontal fluoroscopic image of a child recently postgastrostomy tube with residual barium in the colon. The pigtail of the G tube has migrated through the pylorus into the duodenum and is distant from the retention suture. This may be asymptomatic or may cause feeding intolerance, vomiting, discomfort, or even perforation of the duodenum. The tube may be positioned to the right of the spine on the frontal view, and in a posterior position on a lateral view.

> The coil of a G tube or the gastric coil of a GJ tube can migrate through the pylorus into the duodenum and cause abdominal discomfort, irritability and vomiting. When pulled back, one must ensure that the retention component passes back through the pylorus and does not intussuscept the pylorus into the stomach.

Loss of tension on the retention suture may result in falling away of the gastric anterior wall from the abdominal wall, along with a significant pneumoperitoneum (Fig. 189-7). Alternatively, the retention suture may cut through the gastric wall to lie in the peritoneum or in the abdominal wall, resulting in a similar separation. Aspiration of the pneumoperitoneum can help reappose the stomach wall to the abdominal wall; tension is then reapplied to the retention thread or the gastric coil.

Perforation of the small bowel may occur during GJ tube primary insertions or changes. A floppy-tipped wire is very important, and gentleness is imperative when one is handling the bowel, especially in a baby or a young patient. Excessive centrifugal force of the shaft of the wire causes undue stretching of the bowel and perforation of the duodenum (Fig. 189-8).

fluoroscopy in that the gastric retention component may be evident to the right of the spine and posterior on the lateral view (Fig. 189-6). It is important to ensure that when the tube is pulled back into the stomach, it truly is pulled back through the pylorus rather than retrogradely intussuscepting the pylorus in the stomach.

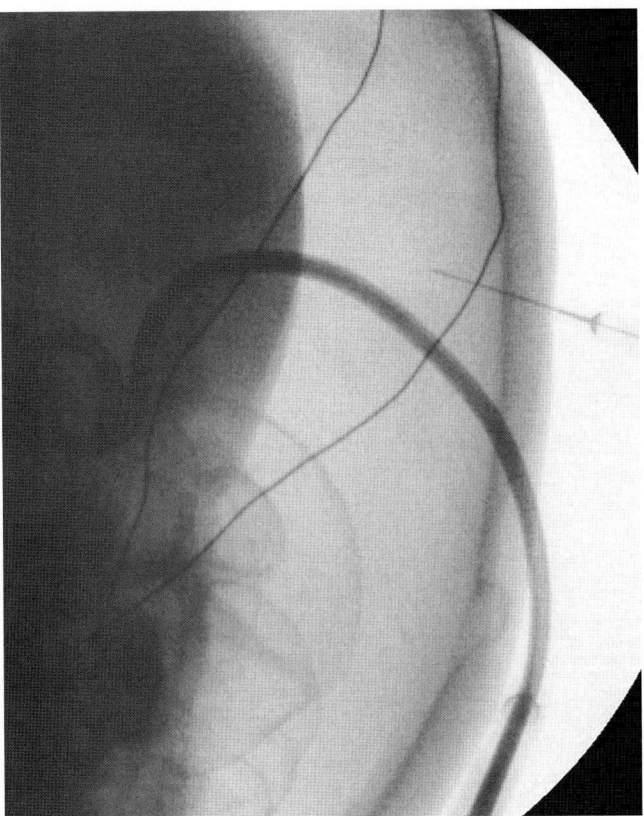

FIGURE 189-7. Lateral fluoroscopic image of the abdomen. The anterior gastric wall has fallen away from the abdominal wall, resulting in marked pneumoperitoneum. This is aspirated with the use of a small 27 gauge needle, to promote adhesion of the gastric wall to the abdominal wall and a short tract. Tension is then reapplied to the thread and the gastrostomy tube.

Occasionally, a pigtail G tube may be so blocked that it will not be possible to exchange it over a wire. Use of a glide wire, saline irrigations, or carbonated fluids may achieve patency. A peel-away sheath over the cut tube may help to uncoil a fixed pigtail and remove the blocked tube. Rarely, one must cut the tube for the child to pass per rectum. If the tube is broken, snaring from the mouth or through the stoma can also be performed.

Children with a tracheoesophageal fistula and a new, venting G tube are at risk for a massive pneumoperitoneum if the tube occludes. The stomach distends with air ventilation and air leaks around the new tube into the peritoneum. Similarly, gastric pressure may increase with excessive air when a child is ventilated or is vigorously bagged.

In our experience, whether a straight or a pigtail tube is used, intussusception is seen frequently in the small bowel around a GJ tube, either at the tip or along its length (Fig. 189-9). We currently treat this with replacement of the tube over a wire. The uncoiling force of the wire opens out the bowel, undoing the intussusception. It is then replaced with a shorter GJ tube. The vast majority of tube-related intussusceptions are transient or intermittent; rarely, they become ischemic.

> **Intussusception (diagnosed on US) around a GJ tube can cover the length of the tube or just its tip. It may present with bilious vomiting or feed intolerance or may be entirely asymptomatic.**

Issues of tube migration, blocking, kinking, and dislodgement pose a more significant problem within the first 6 weeks, because the tract is not considered healed, and any manipulation or replacement may be associated

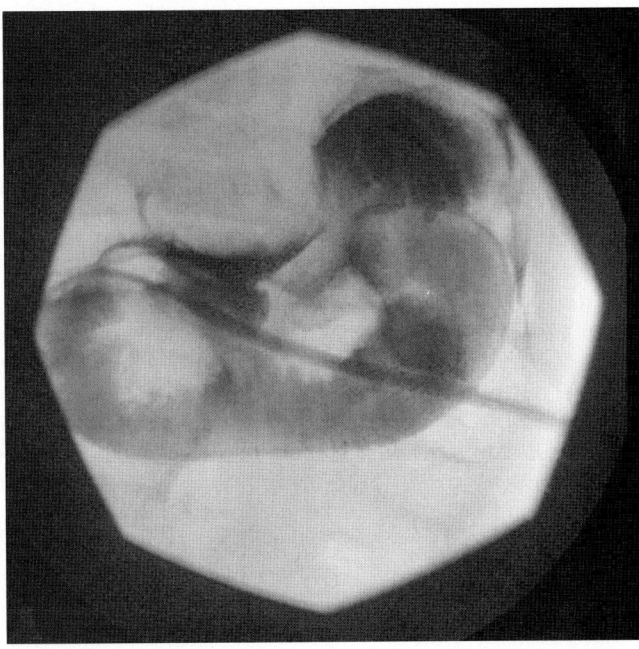
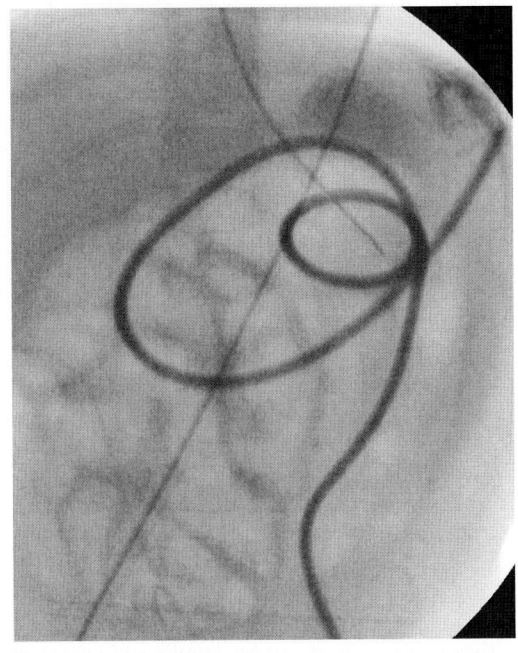

A   B

FIGURE 189-8. A, A fluoroscopic image (frontal) at the time of gastrojejunostomy tube placement. Peritoneal spill of contrast indicates acute perforation of the bowel. **B,** Imaging several days after a GJ tube change shows a small late perforation on fluoroscopy. (**A** *courtesy Dr. S. Marco.*)

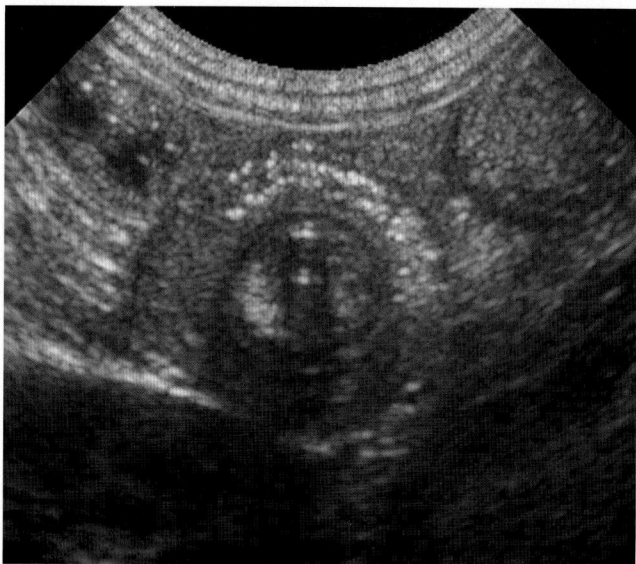

FIGURE 189-9. Intussusception around the tip of a gastrojejunostomy tube or along its length is best recognized on ultrasonography in a transverse view. The intussusceptions are usually transient but may persist and may even become necrotic. The tube is best seen as an echogenic focus that casts a shadow in the center of the doughnut sign.

with tract disruption and leakage. Some crushed medications are known to block G tubes (Fig. 189-10). It is our practice to perform a contrast tube check if any tube has been replaced during the first 6 weeks prior to resumption of feeds.

> **Replacement of a tube through a new immature tract can result in a peritoneal position. Replacement should be done gently, and the position of the tube should be confirmed with contrast before it is used for feeds.**

Late complications include site issues of irritation, infection, granulation tissue, stomal enlargement, and pain (Fig. 189-11). These are best handled through the use of a multidisciplinary enterostomy access service in consultation with the interventional radiologist. Mechanical problems with the tube (e.g., blocks, cracks, migration in or out) are considered part of normal tube maintenance. Inflammation of the tract may warrant ultrasonography to exclude abscess formation.

Migration of the metal component of the retention thread into the abdominal wall tract can lead to infection and inflammation (Fig. 189-12). This may even be hazardous if the child undergoes MRI while the metal is migrating.

Over time, the course of a GJ tube within the duodenum may be altered, and this should not be confused with malrotation (Fig. 189-13).

> **The duodenal course of a GJ tube can change over time; this should not be misdiagnosed as malrotation. Comparison with earlier imaging that shows the initial course is imperative.**

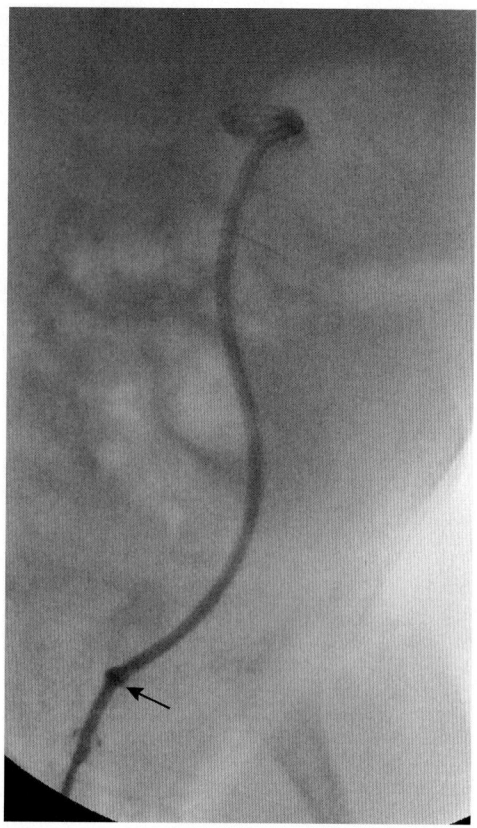

FIGURE 189-10. Tubes may block during feeds or medications. Vigorous attempts to flush these tubes against a complete block may result in breaking, cracking, or aneurysmal dilation of the tube at a point of weakness, as is shown in this fluoroscopic image.

VARIATIONS

- The vast majority of G and GJ tubes are placed in a supracolic position; however, an infracolic position can be used, if needed, although this happens very infrequently.
- Situs inversus represents an unusual but otherwise insignificant variation, in which the stomach is right-sided, rather than left-sided. Occasionally, accurate identification of pigtail catheters as G tubes or biliary, pancreatic, or abscess drains may be difficult with the use of an abdominal x-ray without contrast.
- Children with esophageal atresia without fistula may require gastrostomy tube feeds for growth, while the esophageal gap narrows. The tube can be inserted under image guidance. Inflation of the stomach with air is required; this can be achieved with the use of ultrasonography to identify the stomach, along with puncture of the stomach directly with a small-gauge needle (e.g., 27 or 25 gauge) or adoption of a transhepatic approach to the stomach (Fig. 189-14).
- In children with a mesh or graft in the anterior abdominal wall (from a repaired omphalocele or abdominal wall defects), it is imperative to avoid puncturing the graft because this may result in infection of the prosthetic material.
- Children who have a superior mesenteric artery syndrome or duodenal obstruction or web may

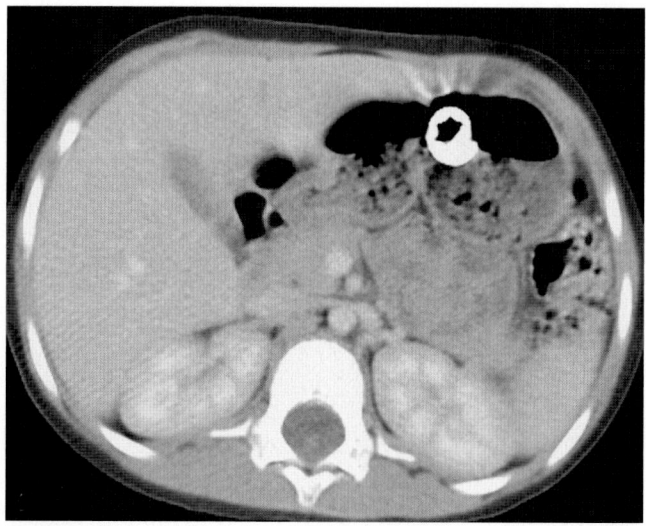

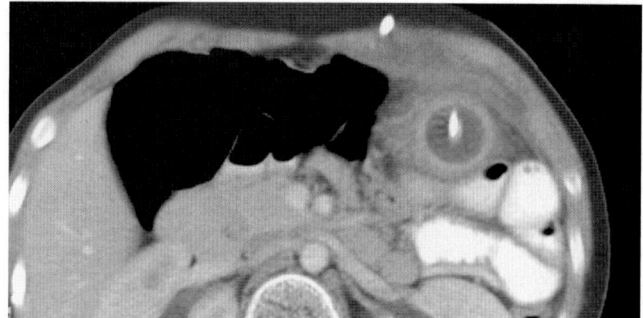

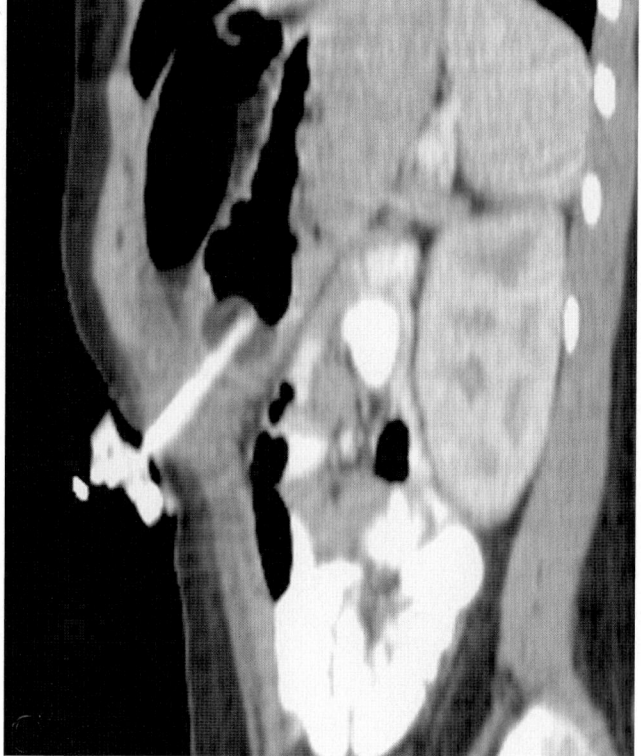

FIGURE 189-11. **A,** Axial image from a computed tomography scan of the abdomen shows a pigtail gastrostomy tube in the stomach. No thickening or inflammation is noted in the abdominal wall. **B,** Axial image from a computed tomography scan shows a balloon G tube in the stomach with inflammatory changes in the surrounding soft tissues. **C,** A sagittal reformatted image of the G tube shows thickening of the abdominal wall related to inflammation of the G tube tract.

require GJ feeding beyond the obstruction. This can be achieved by placement of a GJ tube beyond the obstruction.

- Children with ventriculoperitoneal (VP) shunts who are referred for G tube placement are at risk for ventriculitis, should they develop peritonitis. The G tube can be placed successfully and safely, with as much distance as possible between the VP shunt tubing and the G tube.

- Children with chronic renal failure who are on peritoneal dialysis (PD) may require enteral feeding for growth. Increased vigilance is required for the complication of peritonitis, related to the PD catheter or G tube.

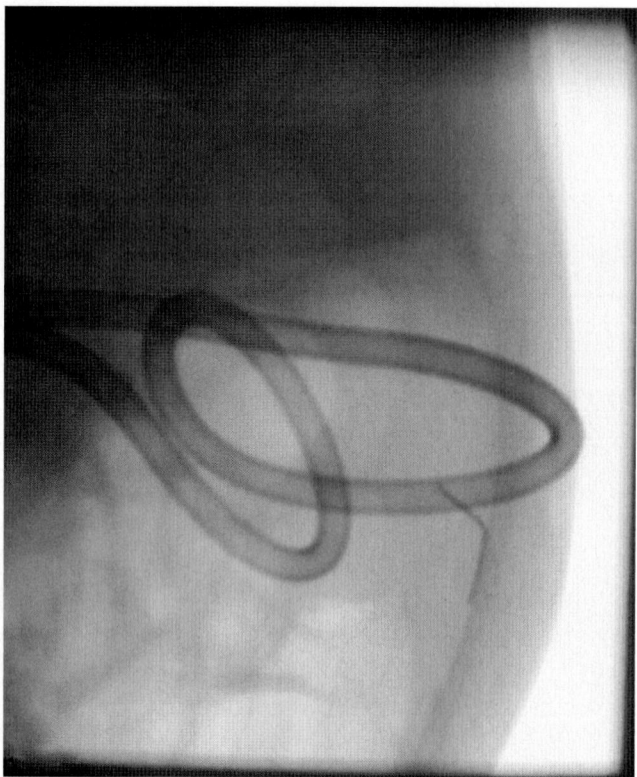

A

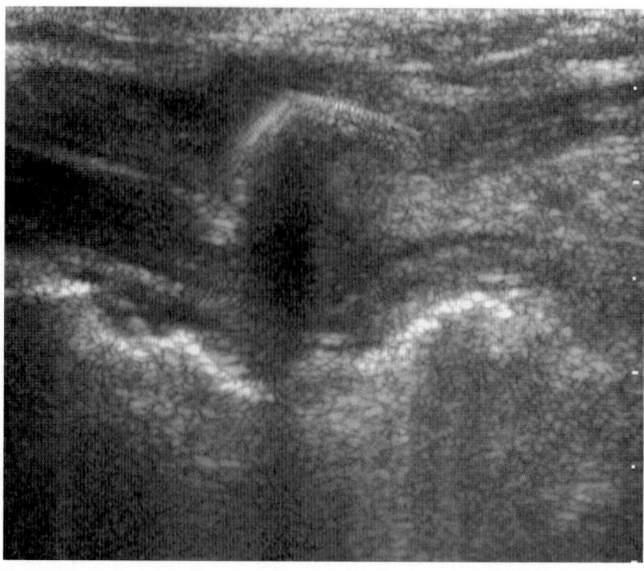

B

FIGURE 189-12. **A,** Fluoroscopic image of the metal component of a retention suture seen in the gastrostomy tube tract. The retention suture is usually passed per rectum without difficulty. It may occasionally remain in the stomach or peritoneum, or it may extrude through the abdominal wall tract and become a focus of inflammation, as shown here. **B,** Ultrasound image of the inflamed G tube tract shows the retention suture, bent within the tract. This extruded further and was subsequently removed without difficulty through the stoma.

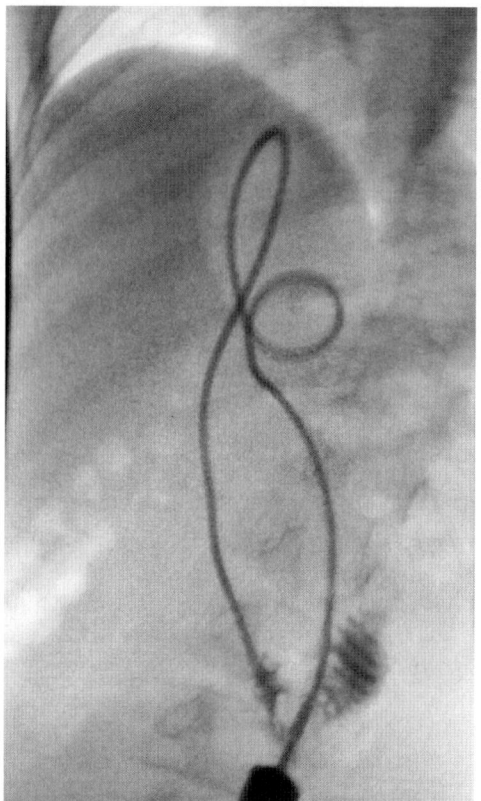

FIGURE 189-13. Over time, the course of the duodenum may be distorted by the gastrojejunostomy tube or by progression of scoliosis. This should not be misinterpreted as a malrotation.

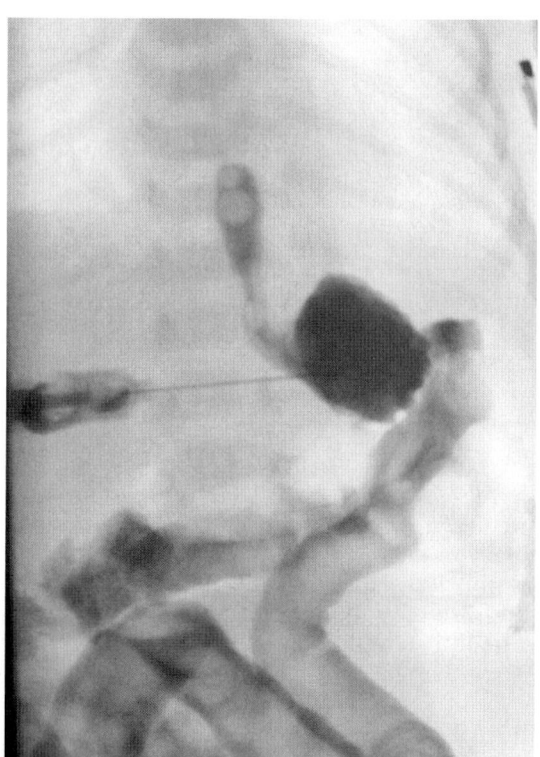

FIGURE 189-14. Fluoroscopic image of a 27 gauge needle in the stomach of a baby with esophageal atresia. The stomach was accessed transhepatically under ultrasound guidance, and position was confirmed with contrast. The stomach was subsequently distended with air to enable percutaneous placement of the gastrostomy tube.

SUGGESTED READINGS

Axelrod D, Kazmerski K, Iyer K: Pediatric enteral nutrition. J Parenter Enter Nutr 2006;30(suppl 1):S21-S26

Carey TS, Hanson L, Garrett JM, et al: Expectations and outcomes of gastric feeding tubes. Am J Med 2006;119:e11-e16

Chait PG, Weinberg J, Connolly BL, et al: Retrograde percutaneous gastrostomy and gastrojejunostomy in 505 children: a 4¹/₂ year experience. Radiology 1996;201:691-695

Chernoff R: An overiew of tube feeding: from ancient times to the future. Nutr Clin Pract 2006;21:408-410

Daveluy W, Guimber D, Mention K, et al: Home enteral nutrition in children: an 11-year experience with 416 patients. Clin Nutr 2005;24:48-54

Denzer U, Mergener K, Kanzler S, et al: Mini–laparoscopically guided percutaneous gastrostomy and jejunostomy. Gastrointest Endosc 2003;58:434-438

Ellett ML: Important facts about intestinal feeding tube placement. Gastroenterol Nurs 2006;29:112-124; quiz 124-125

Faries MB, Rombeau JL: Use of gastrostomy and combined gastrojejunostomy tubes for enteral feeding. World J Surg 1999;23:603-607

Fortunato JE, Darbari A, Mitchell SE, et al: The limitations of gastro-jejunal (G-J) feeding tubes in children; a 9-year pediatric hospital database analysis. Am J Gastroenterol 2005;100:186-189

Friedman JN, Ahmed S, Connolly B, et al: Complications associated with image-guided gastrostomy and gastrojejunostomy tubes in children. Pediatrics 2004;114:458-461

Hazel R: The psychosocial impact on parents of tube feeding their child. Paediatr Nurs 2006;18:19-22

Hughes UM, Connolly BL, Chait PG, et al: Further report of small bowel intussusceptions related to gastrojejunostomy tubes. Pediatr Radiol 2000;30:614-617

Hui GC, Gerstle JT, Weinstein M, et al: Small-bowel intussusception around a gastrojejunostomy tube resulting in ischemic necrosis of the intestine. Pediatr Radiol 2004;34:916-918

Kaye RD, Towbin RB: Imaging and intervention in the gastrointestinal tract in children. Gastroenterol Clin N Am 2002;31:897-923

Kelleher DK, Laussen P, Teixeira-Pinto A, et al: Growth and correlates of nutritional status among infants with hypoplastic left heart syndrome (HLHS) after stage 1 Norwood procedure. Nutrition 2006;22:237-244

Khattak IU, Kimber C, Kiely EM, et al: Percutaneous endoscopic gastrostomy in paediatric practice: complications and outcome. J Pediatr Surg 1998;33:67-72

Lochs H, Dejong C, Hammarqvist F, et al, for the German Society for Nutritional Medicine: ESPEN guidelines on enteral nutrition: gastroenterology. Clin Nutr 2006;25:260-274

Lopez-Herce J, Sanchez C, Carrillo A, et al: Transpyloric enteral nutrition in the critically ill child with renal failure. Intensive Care Med 2006;32:1599-1605; Jul 7, Epub ahead of print

McLoughlin RF, So B, Gray RR: Fluoroscopically guided percutaneous gastrostomy: current status. Can Assoc Radiol J 1996;47:10-15

O'Sullivan M, O'Morain C: Nutrition in inflammatory bowel disease. Best Pract Res Clin Gastroenterol 2006;20:561-573

Sanchez C, Lopez-Herce J, Carrillo A, et al: Transpyloric enteral feeding in the postoperative of cardiac surgery in children. J Pediatr Surg 2006;41:1096-1102

Sullivan PB: Gastrointestinal problems in the neurologically impaired child. Bailliere's Clin Gastroenterol 1997;11:529-546

Sullivan PB, Juszczak E, Bachlet AME, et al: Gastrostomy tube feeding in children with cerebral palsy: a prospective, longitudinal study. Dev Med Child Neurol 2005;47:77-85

Wales PW, Diamond IR, Dutta S, et al: Fundoplication and gastrostomy versus image-guided gastrojejunal tube for enteral feeding in neurologically impaired children with gastroesophageal reflux. J Pediatr Surg 2002;37:407-412

Wiebe S, Cohen J, Connolly B, et al: Percutaneous decompression of the bowel with a small-caliber needle: a method to facilitate percutaneous abdominal access. Am J Roentgenol 2005; 184:227-229

Wollman B, D'Agostino HB, Walus-Wigle JR, et al: Radiologic, endoscopic, and surgical gastrostomy: an institutional evaluation and meta-analysis of the literature. Radiology 1995;197:699-704

CHAPTER

190

Drainage of Infected Abdominal Fluid Collections

MARK J. HOGAN

OVERVIEW

Infected abdominal fluid collections are a common indication for image-guided drainage in children. Etiologies include abscesses from appendicitis, necrotizing enterocolitis (NEC), or post-surgical collections. Drainage is also often required for infected cerebrospinal fluid (CSF) pseudocysts, post-traumatic hematomas, and biliary collections including the gallbladder in acalculous cholecystitis, often seen in septic patients.

> **Causes of Infected Abdominal Fluid Collections**
> - **Appendicitis**
> - **Post-surgical**
> - **NEC**
> - **CSF pseudocysts**
> - **Biliary collections**
> - **Hematomas**

Appendicitis is the most common cause of abdominal sepsis in children, and subsequently the most common cause of intra-abdominal abscesses. Appendicitis usually occurs in school age or adolescent children, and appendicitis is more common in children than adults. Perforation occurs in 23% to 73%, which is higher than in adults, with up to 10% developing an abscess. Abscess formation can be at presentation or after surgery. Increased perforation incidence in children may be due to a different immune response, or difficulty in diagnosing appendicitis in children. The physical examination can be confusing, as the signs and symptoms can overlap with acute gastroenteritis or gynecological disease. Laboratory studies are nonspecific. In addition, there is an increased incidence of perforation in patients of lower socioeconomic status, and children disproportionately fall into this category. Although NEC is a unique cause of abscess formation in children (Fig. 190-1), other infected collections seen in children are similar to adults. Regardless of the etiology, almost all of these collections are amenable to image guided drainage, which can obviate or postpone surgery in acutely ill children.

Abscess drainage and broad spectrum antibiotics are alternatives to immediate operation which may result in prolonged drainage, an increase in postoperative

abscesses, and require a larger incision. Although smaller abscesses (2 cm or less) may respond to intravenous antibiotics alone, drainage or aspiration when possible may expedite recovery. Delayed surgery is often minimally invasive, and done as an outpatient. Some authors advocate abscess drainage and antibiotics as the definitive treatment for ruptured appendicitis, although recurrent appendicitis occurs in 3% to 21%.

IMAGING

Imaging of the patient with suspected abdominal sepsis requires multiple decisions. These are based on the suspected etiology, the size of the patient, the clinical presentation, and the ability to be transported to the radiology department. The main choices are ultrasound and computed tomography (CT). Although the presence of abdominal sepsis can usually be identified with either,

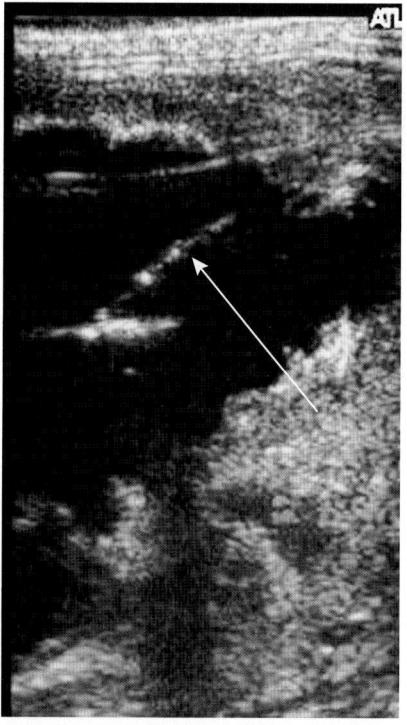

FIGURE 190-1. Ultrasound guided aspiration of an abscess from necrotizing enterocolitis with a needle *(arrow).* This was performed portably in the neonatal intensive care unit.

they may not answer specific questions needed by the interventional radiologist (IR). Image-guided drainage requires an acceptable window to the collection, without critical intervening structures such as bowel. Some abscesses are better treated surgically, especially with multiple interloop abscesses or with a concomitant small bowel obstruction. The imaging in the setting of a suspected abscess or infected collection should address all of these issues to best provide information for IR or surgical intervention.

> **Preprocedural Imaging Requirements**
> - **Identify all abscesses**
> - **Determine appropriate access to abscess**
> - **Minimize risks**

Ultrasound has several advantages in children including the lack of ionizing radiation, portability, and the ability to visualize most of the abdomen in the smaller pediatric patient. Radiation and its risks in children are real, and any technique to avoid unnecessary radiation should be pursued. Fragile neonates can be examined in the neonatal intensive care unit, and NEC abscesses are often readily visualized in these patients. Ultrasound is the preferred modality to diagnose cholecystitis in septic patients in the pediatric intensive care unit. CSF pseudocysts are usually readily identified. Ultrasound in acute appendicitis has a sensitivity of 56% to 94% and specificity of 47% to 95%, although it is difficult to evaluate the entire abdomen due to gas filled bowel loops, which may be prominent with bowel obstruction or ileus. Although an inflammatory process may be identified, this limits the ability to visualize abscesses and distinguish between aperistaltic dilated bowel loops and fluid collections.

CT scanning has been increasingly used to diagnose abdominal pain, particularly acute appendicitis. This is due to the limitations with ultrasound as well as the reported improvement in sensitivity (74% to 100%) and specificity (89% to 99%). There are multiple scanning techniques for appendicitis. Intravenous, oral, or rectal contrast may be used. The whole abdomen may be examined, or a focused study of the lower abdomen and pelvis might be performed instead. Many examinations are being performed without oral contrast in order to expedite imaging. With abscesses, the lack of bowel opacification with the limited CT technique makes therapeutic planning more difficult. Bowel loops may be interposed between the anticipated puncture site and the abscess, and it may be difficult to distinguish an abscess from an abnormally dilated fluid filled bowel loop (Fig. 190-2). If the number or position of abscesses is not clear, the CT scan may have to be repeated with oral contrast increasing radiation dose and risk. Owing to these issues, if symptoms have been present for greater than 48 hours, when a surgeon suspects an abscess, or when symptoms continue after surgery, a CT scan should be performed with both IV and oral contrast for diagnosis and therapeutic planning. The entire abdomen and pelvis are scanned as abscesses can occur anywhere

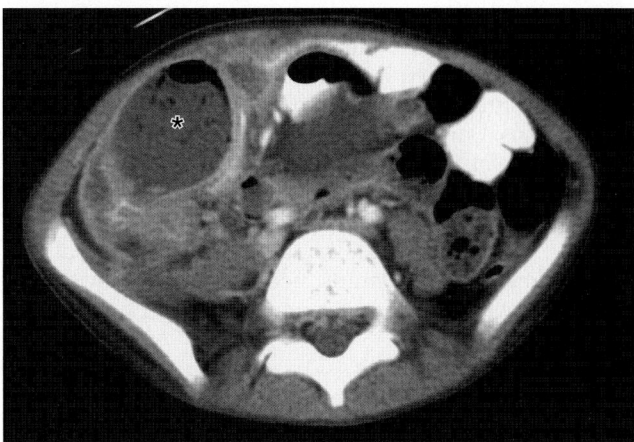

FIGURE 190-2. A computed tomographic image depicts an abscess (*) in the right lower quadrant from ruptured appendicitis. Without oral contrast, this could be mistaken for the colon.

from the diaphragms to the pelvis. The mA and kVP should be adjusted for the patient's age and size according to established protocols.

> **IV and oral contrast during CT scans aids interventional planning.**

PREPARATION

The patient's diagnosis, treatment plan, and therapeutic options are discussed with the referring physicians, surgeons, and parents. The potential benefits and risks (including sedation) are outlined, and informed written consent is obtained. No routine laboratory tests are obtained before the drainage procedure unless the patient has a history of abnormal bleeding or other medical problems. A standard sterile scrub is performed, and a hat, mask, and gown are required for blood and body fluid precaution standards.

Sedation

The sedation procedure is well known to the pediatric radiologist. However, certain pertinent issues are present during drainage procedures for abdominal collections. The patients are often in considerable discomfort already, and poor blood flow surrounding the abscess may decrease the effect of local anesthesia. Therefore, drainage procedures in these patients may require a higher level of sedation than for other procedures. Patients may benefit from general anesthesia if the procedure is expected to be particularly painful, if adequate sedation is unlikely (prior history of sedation failure or reaction to sedation medications), or if the patient is at high risk for apnea or other respiratory compromise.

IMAGE GUIDANCE

Ultrasound guidance is ideal in children owing to multiplanar capability, real-time imaging ability, portability, and avoidance of radiation. Pediatric patients tend to have a thinner body habitus, enhancing the ability of ultrasound to penetrate the tissues; however, there are limitations including the inability to view through bone or bowel gas. Correlation with a previous CT scan is often helpful to plan a successful procedure. Both freehand and biopsy guide techniques can be used depending on the preference of the radiologist. Ultrasound guidance can be transabdominal, transrectal, transgluteal, or transvaginal. Multiple transducers should be available, and endocavitary probes are necessary for transrectal or transvaginal guidance.

> **Most abscesses can be drained with ultrasound guidance. Multiple imaging windows are available.**
> * **Transabdominal**
> * **Transrectal**
> * **Transgluteal**
> * **Transvaginal**

CT has the disadvantage of radiation and limited planes. Traditional CT guidance uses intermittent imaging during the procedure. The needle is advanced incrementally, with scans performed after each advancement to confirm position and allow redirection. CT fluoroscopy can be used for continuous imaging; however, owing to the high radiation dose from this technique, it should be avoided unless absolutely necessary.

Fluoroscopy facilitates wire placement, tract dilatation, and catheter insertion, and usually requires only minimal fluoroscopy time. Updated radiation reduction techniques such as pulsed fluoroscopy should be used, if available. Ultrasound guidance can substitute for fluoroscopy if the procedure is done portably. A spot film is obtained after the procedure to document catheter position.

EQUIPMENT

Standard equipment includes an access needle, guiding wire, dilators, and catheters. Multiple vendors supply this equipment, and the interventionalist should use those with which they have the most experience.

Access needle sizes range from small (21 or 22 gauge) to large (up to 5 French). The larger needles often have a flexible outer sheath. In neonates, smaller needles or intravenous (IV) catheters can be used for aspiration. In addition, direct trocar techniques are available, and may be preferred in certain circumstances. With larger children, size is not an important limiting factor. Real-time sonographic guidance adds to control and confidence during needle placement allowing a larger initial needle to be placed, and avoiding additional dilatation steps. The small needle techniques are most useful with neonates, when the access window is small or when using CT guidance.

Wires range from 0.018″ to 0.038″. Most catheters of adequate size require larger wires. Wires with a stiff shaft and floppy atraumatic tip facilitate dilatation and catheter placement.

Pigtail catheters are typical, and locking catheters help avoid dislodgment. A hydrophilic coating can facilitate placement, and are also more easily removed. Catheter size depends on the viscosity of the fluid obtained; however, 8 to 12 Fr are typical. Although smaller catheters (5 and 6 Fr) have been designed for use in infants and smaller pediatric patients, they do not typically allow for adequate drainage except with thin collections.

PROCEDURE

The approach to the drainage is based on the site of the abscess, interposed organs, and the preference and expertise of the operator. The collection should be accessed the most direct way, while providing for the best patient comfort. Although a percutaneous abdominal transperitoneal approach is most common, abscesses are often situated deep in the pelvis, with multiple bowel loops between the abdominal wall and the abscess. In these cases, a transrectal, transgluteal, or transvaginal approach is indicated. Puncture site planning includes placing the catheter in the most dependent portion of the abscess to facilitate complete drainage.

> **Abscesses can be accessed via transabdominal, transrectal, transgluteal, and transvaginal approaches.**

If an abdominal approach is available, the patient is positioned to place the entry site towards the interventionalist. Ultrasonographic guidance is most common (Fig. 190-3), with CT guidance reserved for abscesses not visible sonographically (Fig. 190-4). With direct real-time ultrasonographic visualization, the needle is advanced into the abscess cavity. After obtaining a small sample for laboratory analysis, the wire is advanced into the cavity, serial dilatation is performed, and the catheter is

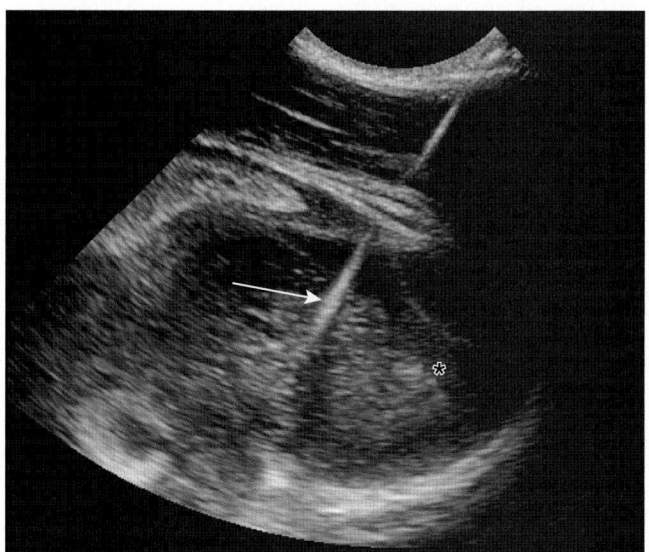

FIGURE 190-3. Ultrasound guidance allows access to a large abdominal abscess (*) with a 3.5 French sheathed needle *(arrow).*

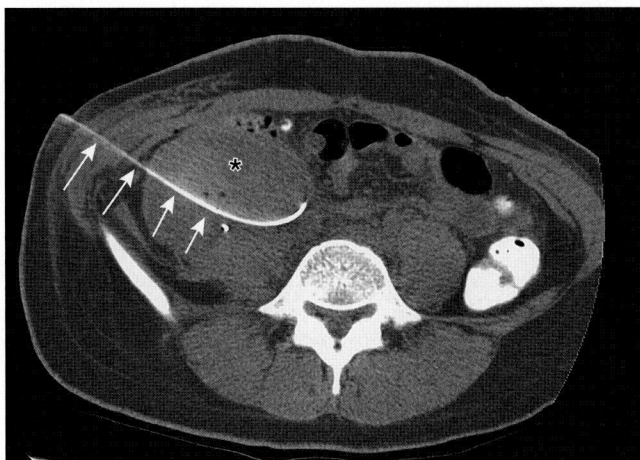

FIGURE 190-4. An infected postoperative hematoma (*) is drained with computed tomographic guidance. The wire *(arrows)* is coiled in the collection.

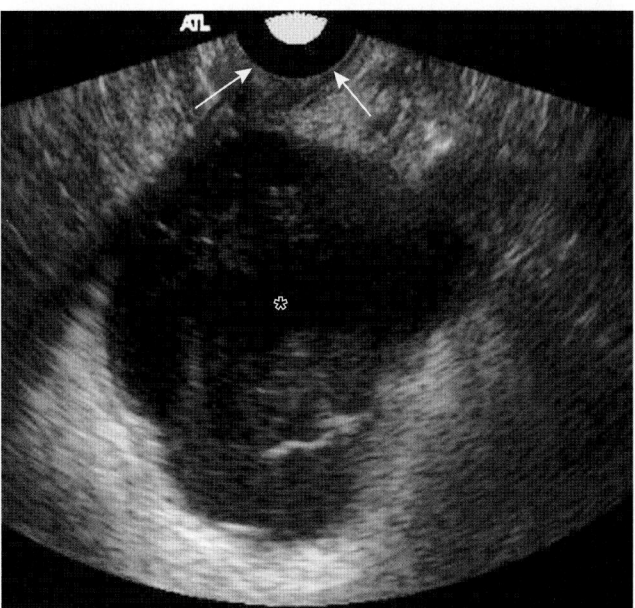

FIGURE 190-6. Transrectal drainage with transrectal ultrasound guidance. The abscess (*) is readily identified with the transducer in the rectum (arrows). This allows accurate needle placement using a needle guide.

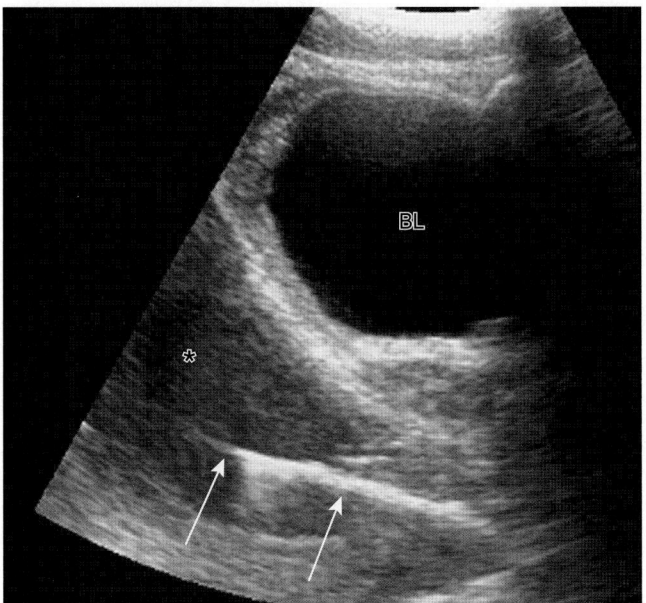

FIGURE 190-5. Transrectal drainage of a pelvic abscess (*) with transabdominal ultrasound guidance. The bladder (BL) is used as an acoustic window during advancement of a drainage catheter *(arrows)* into the abscess.

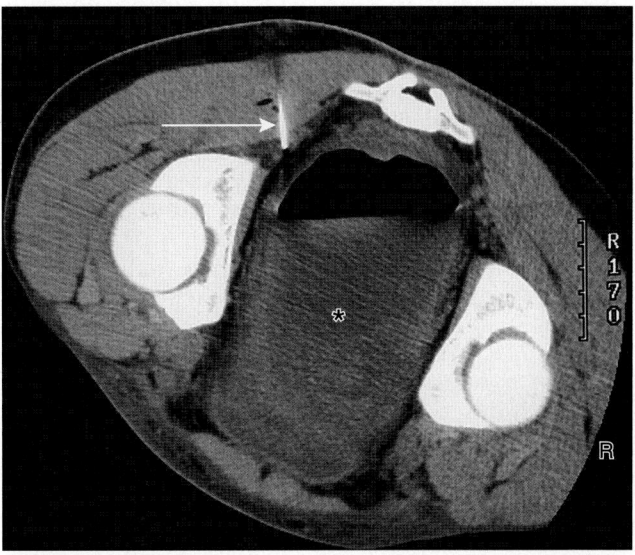

FIGURE 190-7. CT guided transgluteal drainage. A needle *(arrow)* is advanced into the pelvic abscess (*) with CT guidance.

inserted over the wire and coiled in the collection with fluoroscopic guidance.

Transrectal drainage is well tolerated because the rectum has few pain receptors. Some radiologists may hesitate to perform transrectal drainage in a child; however, this technique is well accepted by patients and parents with proper education. Many patients prefer this approach because they do not want an additional abdominal scar. Ultrasound guidance uses a sagittal midline transabdominal transducer (Fig. 190-5), or transrectal scanning with a needle guide (Fig. 190-6). The abscess is usually located anterior to the rectum a variable distance from the anus, and may be palpable, causing a mass effect. Traditionally, palpable pelvic abscesses were drained through the rectum by the surgeon in the operating room; however, image guided drainage allows access to non-palpable abscesses distal to the digital exam, direct visualization during drainage, and avoidance of general anesthesia. The patient is placed in either a left decubitis or lithotomy position for the procedure.

Transgluteal drainage is traditionally performed with CT guidance, although ultrasound guidance is possible (Fig. 190-7). The patient is placed in a prone or prone oblique position. Seldinger or trocar techniques can be used as with other approaches, and wire insertion, tract dilatation, and catheter placement is performed similarly. Care must be taken to avoid the nerves and blood vessels in the greater sciatic foramen. This procedure can be more painful than other approaches, and postoperative pain may also be more prominent. The increased risk of hemorrhage due to the position of the gluteal vessels can usually be avoided with image guidance.

Transvaginal drainage is reserved for adult women or in teenagers with known prior pregnancy or admitted sexual activity. However, with the availability of transrectal drainage, it is rarely indicated.

Percutaneous cholecystostomy with aspiration or tube placement can be performed in critically ill patients with unexplained fever, sepsis, and a distended gallbladder. This is best diagnosed with ultrasound. This procedure is well accepted in adults and is useful in selected pediatric patients. Percutaneous cholecystostomy is performed with a transabdominal approach and ultrasonographic guidance. Most commonly, these catheters are placed portably in the PICU. Typically, the catheter is placed through a portion of the liver, to avoid intra-abdominal biliary leak after catheter removal (Fig. 190-8). This procedure can resolve the sepsis, while avoiding a surgical cholecystectomy in a compromised patient.

Catheter Fixation, Dressing, and Care

Primary fixation of the catheter is with the locking loop. This is the only fixation typically performed with transrectal or transvaginal approaches. External fixation to the patient can be with sutures or with adhesive appliances, although the security of sutures is rarely necessary as dislodgment of the catheter is uncommon. Ostomy discs and other types of adhesive appliances are available from a variety of manufacturers.

The catheter entry site is covered with a transparent sterile occlusive dressing. Gauze sponges may be placed under the dressing to prevent adherence to the catheter. The dressing is changed weekly unless it becomes soiled.

The catheter is attached to either a bag for gravity drainage or to bulb suction. With gravity drainage, the bag must be kept below the level of the abscess. Bulb suction is useful in patients who are not compliant. The catheter is flushed with 10 mL of sterile normal saline each shift to keep the drain open. The flush volume must be subtracted from the overall drainage amount, a common mistake in chart recordings.

POSTPROCEDURAL EVALUATION

The patient is closely monitored on the ward. Pain can usually be controlled with IV narcotics, although when severe a patient-controlled anesthesia (PCA) pump may be necessary. The abscess cultures are noted to make sure the bacteria are sensitive to the administered antibiotics. Fever curves and tube output are evaluated at least daily. Persistent fevers without significant tube output may represent an incompletely drained abscess or additional abscesses. Follow up imaging is then indicated, and a CT scan with both oral and IV contrast is the most productive study. Conversely, if a large amount of tube output continues, a catheter injection should be performed to evaluate for an enteric fistula (Fig. 190-9).

When the patient's fever has resolved, and when the tube output is less than 20 cc/day, the tube can be removed. Post drainage imaging for documentation of abscess resolution is not usually necessary, and avoidance of this imaging can reduce the radiation exposure. A dose of narcotic analgesic is often given prior to drain removal, but the patient is not fully sedated.

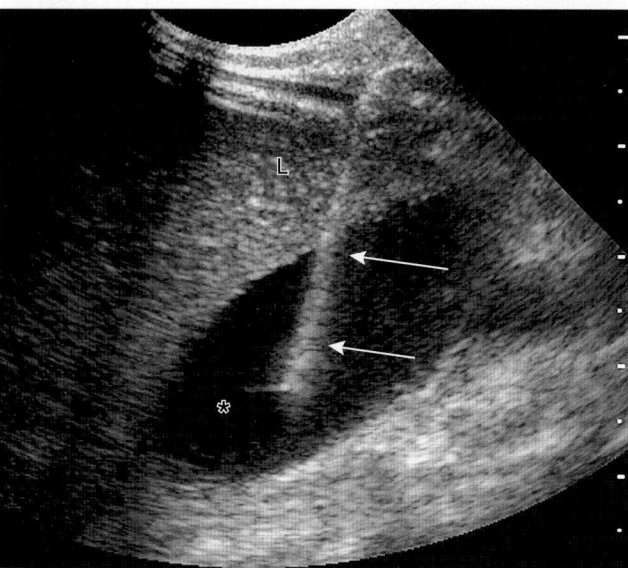

FIGURE 190-8. Percutaneous cholecystostomy. Ultrasound guidance is used to place the needle (arrows) into the gallbladder (*). A small portion of the liver (L) is traversed during placement of the needle to reduce the risk of bile leak.

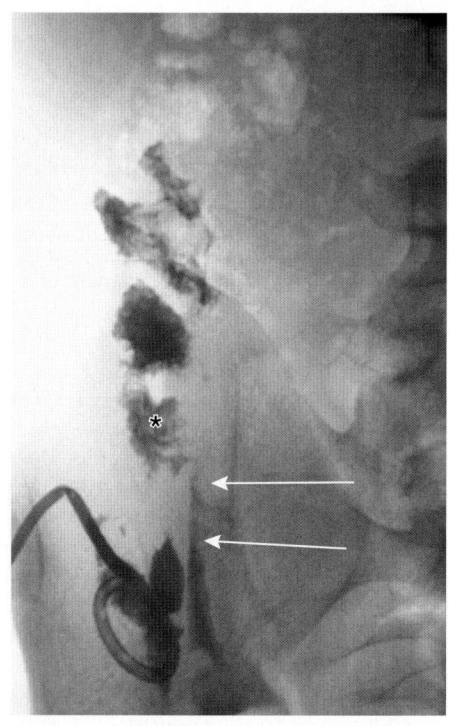

FIGURE 190-9. This patient had persistent drain output after several days. Injection of the drain demonstrates a fistula (*arrows*) to the cecum (*) after ruptured appendicitis.

> **Catheter removal should be based on clinical evaluation. Avoid unnecessary radiation from follow-up CT scans unless fever remains.**

COMPLICATIONS

Complications from abscess drainage occur in up to 11% of patients. Catheter migration is the most common problem encountered. Bloody pus is almost universal, but significant hemorrhage is rare. Vascular injury can occur from any approach but is probably more common with the transgluteal technique due to the proximity of the gluteal vessels. The inferior epigastric artery can be injured during transabdominal drainage but can usually be identified and avoided with ultrasound during guidance for the procedure. Bowel perforation is another risk, but some authors traverse bowel when necessary without significant consequences. Inadvertent injury to other organs and the female reproductive tract are possible but rare.

SUMMARY

Children have multiple causes of abdominal sepsis, with appendicitis being the most common. Image-guided drainage techniques are successful in resolving associated infected fluid collections when combined with appropriate antibiotic treatment, and complication rates are low. Imaging should be tailored for an appropriate diagnosis as well as planning for therapeutic intervention. Multiple techniques are applicable to the pediatric patient including transabdominal, transrectal, transgluteal, and rarely transvaginal approaches. Ultrasound guidance is ideal for use in children and can be used for all of these approaches.

SUGGESTED READINGS

Alexander AA, Eschelman DJ, Nazarian LN, Bonn J: Transrectal sonographically guided drainage of deep pelvic abscesses. AJR Am J Roentgenol 1994;162:1227-1230

Cahill AM, Kaye RD, Towbin RB, et al: Pelvic abscess drainage in children: The trans-gluteal approach [abstract]. Pediatr Radiol 2003;33(Suppl):S81

Curran TJ, Muenchow SK: The treatment of complicated appendicitis in children using peritoneal drainage: results from a public hospital. J Pediatr Surg 1993;28:204-208

Even-Bendahan G, Lazar I, Erez I, et al: Role of imaging in the diagnosis of acute appendicitis in children. Clin Pediatr 2003;42:23-27

Fishman SJ, Pelosi L, Klavon SL, O'Rourke EJ: Perforated appendicitis: prospective outcome analysis for 150 children. J Pediatr Surg 2000;35:923-926

Gervais DA, Hahn PF, O'Neill MJ, Mueller P: CT-guided transgluteal drainage of deep pelvic abscesses in children: selective uses as an alternative to transrectal drainage. AJR Am J Roentgenol 2000;175:1393-1396

Harisinghani MG, Gervais DA, Hahn PF, et al: CT-guided transgluteal drainage of deep pelvic abscesses: indications, technique, procedure-related complications, and clinical outcome. Radiographics 2002;22:1353-1367

Hogan MJ: Appendiceal abscess drainage. Tech Vasc Interv Radiol 2003;6:205-214

Jamieson DH, Chait PG, Filler R: Interventional drainage of appendiceal abscesses in children. AJR Am J Roentgenol 1997;169:1619-1622

Lasson A, Lundagards J, Loren I, Nilsson PE: Appendiceal abscesses: primary percutaneous drainage and selective interval appendicectomy. Eur J Surg 2002;168:264-269

Newman, K, Ponsky T, Kittle K, et al: Appendicitis 2000: variability in practice, outcomes, and resource utilization at thirty pediatric hospitals. J Pediatr Surg 2003;38:372-379

Pereira JK, Chait PG, Miller SF: Deep pelvic abscesses in children: transrectal drainage under radiologic guidance. Radiology 1996;198:393-396

Samelson SL, Reyes HM: Management of perforated appendicitis in children-revisited. Arch Surg 1987;122:691-696

Schmit PJ, Hiyama DT, Swisher SG, et al: Analysis of risk factors of postappendectomy intra-abdominal abscess. J AM Coll Surg 1994;179:721-726

Shuler FW, Newman CN, Angood PB, et al: Nonoperative management for intra abdominal abscesses. Am Surg 1996;62:218-222

Sivit CJ, Applegate KE: Imaging of acute appendicitis in children. Semin Ultrasound CT MR 2003;24:74-82

Towbin R: Interventional procedures in pediatrics. Semin Pediatr Surg 1992;1:296-307

Walser E, Rzaz S, Hernandex A, Ozkan O, Kathuria M, Akinci D: Sonographically guided transgluteal drainage of pelvic abscesses. AJR Am J Roentgenol 2003;181:498-500

Interventional Radiology of the Liver and Biliary System

JAMES S. DONALDSON and CYNTHIA K. RIGSBY

INTERVENTIONAL RADIOLOGY OF THE LIVER AND BILIARY SYSTEM

Interventional radiology (IR) plays a small role in diagnostic abnormalities of the liver but can have a significant role in therapy of various liver and biliary diseases. IR plays a major role in the patient undergoing transplant surgery and is an integral part of the care of the patient undergoing liver transplant surgery. The following section addresses some of the settings in which IR may be used.

Congenital Abnormalities

Congenital liver cysts are uncommon in children; they are benign and are usually incidental findings on imaging studies. They may be symptomatic if large, presenting as a palpable abdominal mass or with obstructive jaundice caused by mass effect on adjacent structures. Sclerotherapy can be successful in ablating simple hepatic cysts, with a variety of agents (doxycycline, ethanol, betadine) successfully used. Contrast studies should be performed to confirm that the cyst does not communicate with the biliary tree before sclerosis. Polycystic disease and hydatid disease should be considered when planning any sclerosis procedure to ensure that the procedure is appropriate for the diagnostic setting.

Infections of the Liver

Pyogenic infection with abscess formation after the neonatal period is most commonly found in immunocompromised patients, with *Staphylococcus aureus* being the most common pathogen. Patients with chronic granulomatous disease of childhood, a syndrome of leukocyte dysfunction, or those who have had bone marrow transplantation are at high risk for pyogenic abscesses.

Percutaneous abscess drainage is initial treatment of choice for most such abscesses (Fig. 191-1). Ultrasound guidance is preferred over computed tomography (CT) with placement of a large pigtail drainage catheter. When selecting catheter size, it is important to keep in mind that although the patient may be small, pus drains best through a large-bore catheter. Placement of catheters smaller than 10 Fr increases the risk of inadequate drainage and failure of the percutaneous technique. Multiple catheters may be necessary to adequately drain a multilocular abscess. Fibrinolytics (tissue plasminogen activator or urokinase) are also helpful and enhance debridement of the cavity.

Patients with chronic granulomatous disease (CGD) and liver abscesses present a significant management challenge. In past years, treatment of hepatic abscess in these children has improved with antibiotic therapy combined with percutaneous drainage. Intralesional granulocyte infiltration and also ethanol instillation have been tried with some success. Overall however, results of percutaneous management alone have been disappointing and many centers recommend surgery as the best means of treatment of liver abscesses in children with CGD.

Echinococcus (hydatid disease) has been successfully managed percutaneously with administration of hypertonic saline, ethanol and other sclerosing agents into the cysts. Pretreatment with albendazole is recommended as prophylaxis for anaphylactic reactions. The techniques for percutaneous management vary. Some authors puncture the cyst, instill the treating agent, and aspirate the cyst 20 to 30 minutes later with no drain left in place. Other authors describe leaving a drain in place and repeating the instillation two to three times over several days before removing the drain.

Amebic abscesses caused by *Entamoeba histolytica* are commonly solitary and are most frequently found in the right lobe of the liver. Percutaneous drainage is not always needed because most patients respond very quickly to metronidazole treatment. Rupture of amebic abscesses into the peritoneal cavity or into the pericardium has also occurred when lesions are near the liver surface. Percutaneous aspiration for diagnosis or in settings of large lesions with risk of perforation is recommended.

> **Management of liver abscess in CGD is probably handled best by surgical treatment.**

Diffuse Parenchymal Disease

An ultrasound-guided biopsy is one of the procedures in which IR is involved in patients with diffuse parenchymal disease. Generally, a 15-gauge biopsy core is requested for adequate sampling, but two or more 18-gauge cores can be safely obtained through a coaxial outer needle.

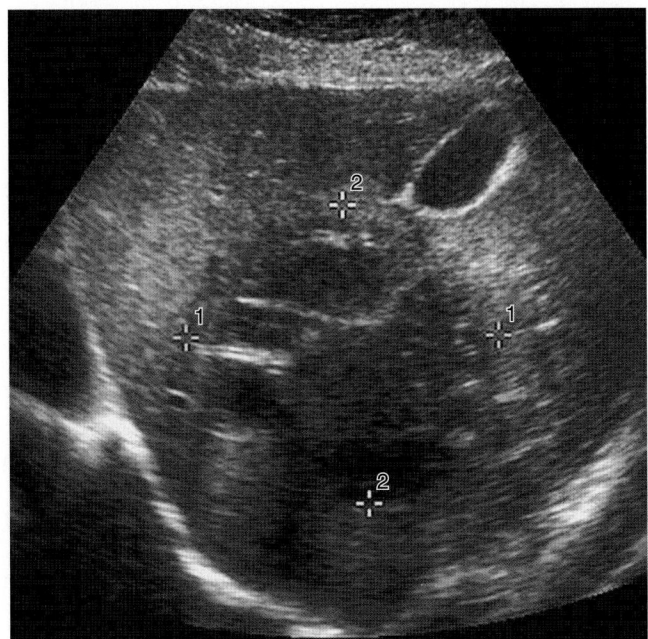

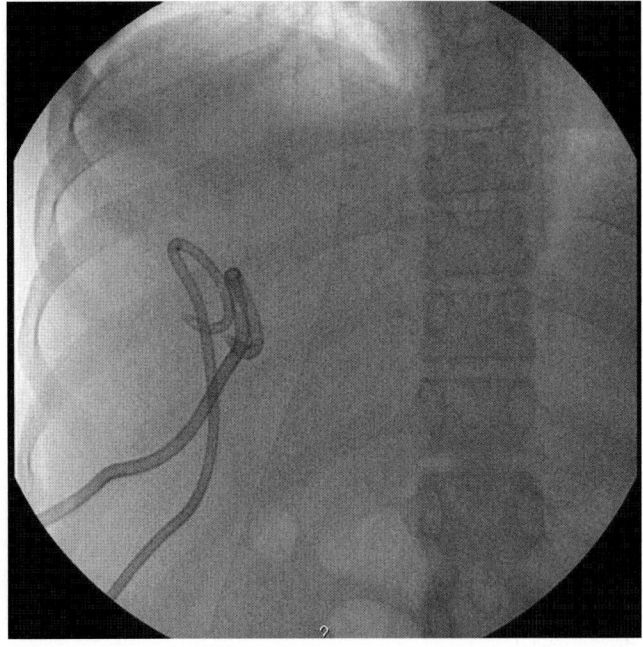

A   B

FIGURE 191-1. Multilocular liver abscess. **A,** Ultrasound of the right upper quadrant shows a complex mass containing multiple cystic areas in addition to solid surrounding inflammatory tissue. **B,** Two percutaneous drains were placed, and *Staphylococcus aureus* was cultured. The patient was successfully managed with the catheter drainage and antibiotics.

If coagulation parameters are abnormal (INR >1.5), and thrombocytopenia or ascites are present then a transjugular liver biopsy is indicated (Fig. 191-2). This procedure can be safely performed in children using smaller pediatric biopsy sets with shorter biopsy cannulas and sheaths. The biopsy spring-loaded needle in the pediatric sets is 19 gauge and is adequate for diagnosis in diffuse liver disease. We usually obtain two to three core samples during transjugular biopsy. Habdank reported 74 transjugular hepatic biopsies in children with adequate sampling in 98.6%. Overall, 8.1% of patients had procedural complications including neck hematomas, small subcapsular hematomas, subclavian artery puncture, and capsular perforation.

Wedged portal vein pressures can also be obtained in a patient being evaluated for portal hypertension. Literature review of multiple studies concludes that wedged hepatic pressure measurement correlates well with direct portal pressure measurement and the agreement is sufficiently good to use this as a surrogate measurement. A retrograde wedged hepatic venogram usually opacifies the intrahepatic portal system (Fig. 191-3). This diagnostic procedure is sometimes done in patients with extrahepatic portal vein obstruction who are being considered for Rex (superior mesenteric vein to left intrahepatic portal vein) shunts. Usually right, middle, and certainly the left hepatic veins must be catheterized and wedged venograms performed in each in order to visualize the entire portal system well. Rather than wedging a small angiographic catheter into the parenchyma, use of a flexible vascular sheath usually gives a much better portogram.

Transjugular intrahepatic portosystemic shunt (TIPS) procedure can be used in children to help manage complications of portal hypertension (see Fig. 191-3). The

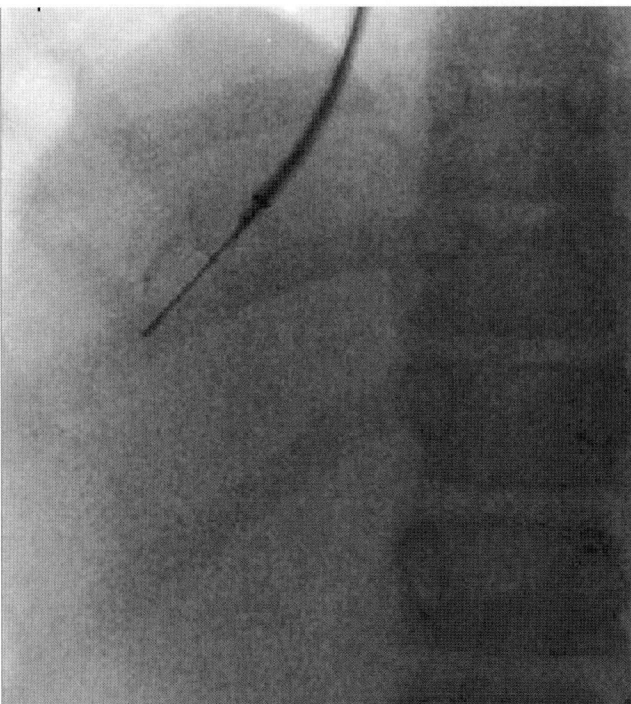

FIGURE 191-2. Transjugular liver biopsy. A radiograph confirms the needle position during performance of transjugular liver biopsy. The 18-gauge needle tip is seen protruding beyond the end of the curved guiding canula that is positioned within the right hepatic vein. Position had been confirmed with a venogram prior to the biopsy.

TIPS procedure is usually considered a bridge measure until liver transplantation can be undertaken. We have found that because most pediatric liver allografts are now obtained from a living related donor and can be

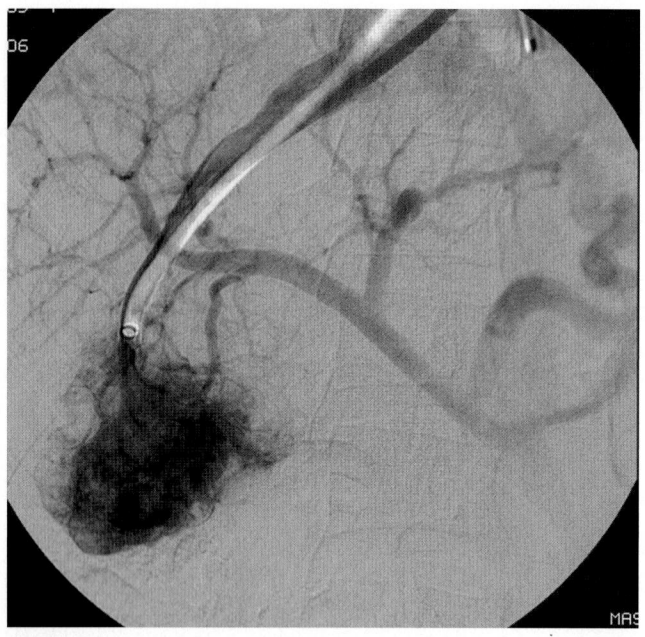

A

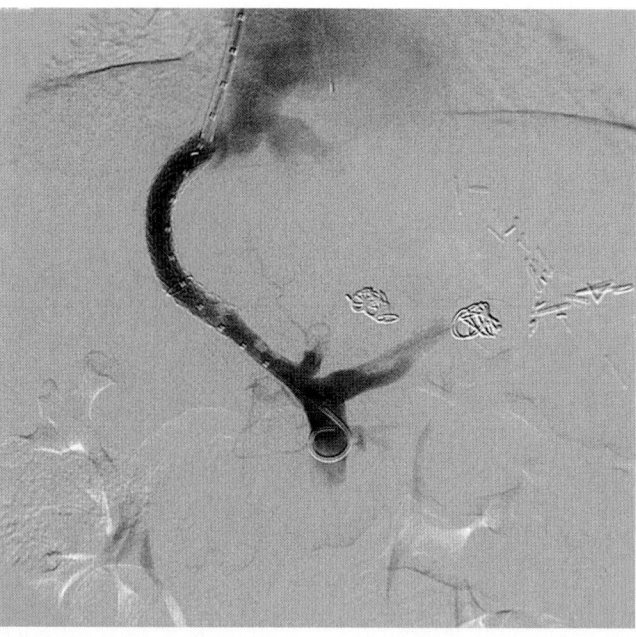

B

FIGURE 191-3. Transjugular intrahepatic portosystemic shunt (TIPS). **A,** This 17-year-old patient with autoimmune hepatitis presented with massive UGI bleeding and gastric varices that could not be banded. A wedged hepatic venogram was initially performed providing a map of the portal vein. **B,** A TIPS procedure was then performed using a Goretex-covered stent, and the large varices were embolized through the TIPS stent. A post-TIPS and postembolization portal venogram shows good flow through the shunt into the hepatic veins and IVC.

obtained relatively quickly, the need for TIPS procedures in children has diminished. Indications still include the child with good synthetic liver function and bleeding or ascites from portal hypertension not controlled by medical and endoscopic means.

Budd-Chiari syndrome is a rare disorder developing from obstruction of the hepatic veins or from obstruction of the intrahepatic or suprahepatic portions of the inferior vena cava (IVC). Obstruction secondary to congenital webs inside the hepatic veins or IVC has been reported. Although the diagnosis is usually made with noninvasive imaging, venography can still play a role when nonsurgical intervention is considered. Angioplasty of congenital webs can be curative. Usually, we have seen Budd-Chiari syndrome in the setting of liver transplantation and occasionally a stent has been needed to maintain patency.

> **TIPS procedure is usually considered a bridge measure until liver transplant can be undertaken.**

Biliary Diseases

Percutaneous transhepatic cholangiography (PTC) is occasionally useful in the evaluation of congenital abnormalities of the liver such as bile plug syndrome, Caroli disease or choledochal cyst (Fig. 191-4). PTC with biliary drainage has been used to help patients with Caroli disease and acute cholangitis. Endoscopic retrograde cholangiopancreatography (ERCP) is generally not feasible in infants and newborns because of the

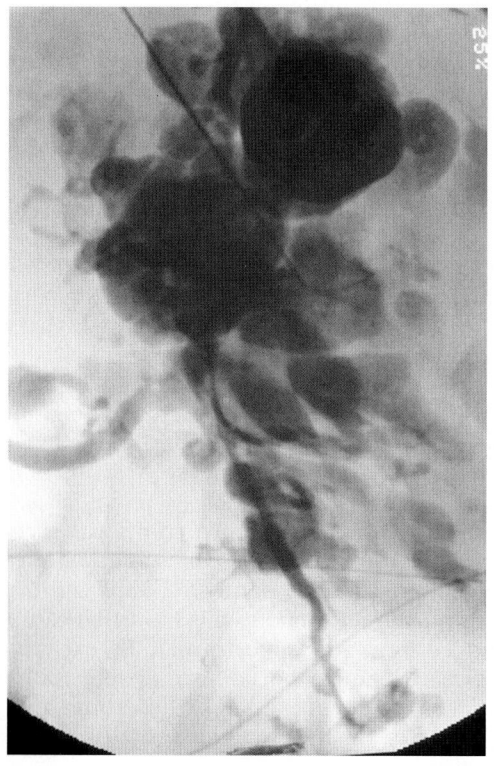

FIGURE 191-4. Caroli disease. Percutaneous transhepatic cholangiogram (PTC) in patient with Caroli disease and *Klebsiella sepsis.* The study confirmed the suspected diagnosis and was used to obtain a culture.

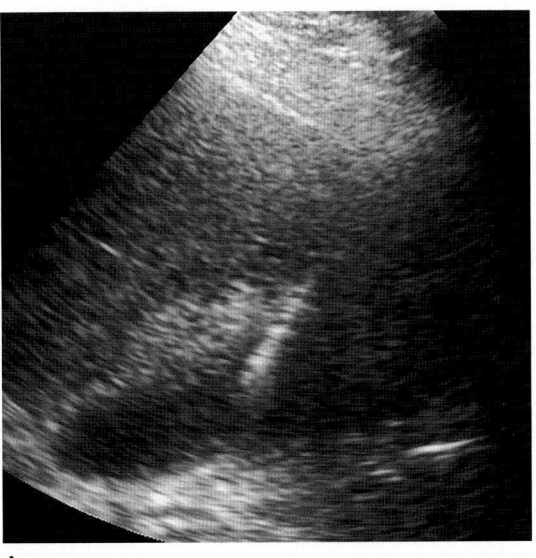
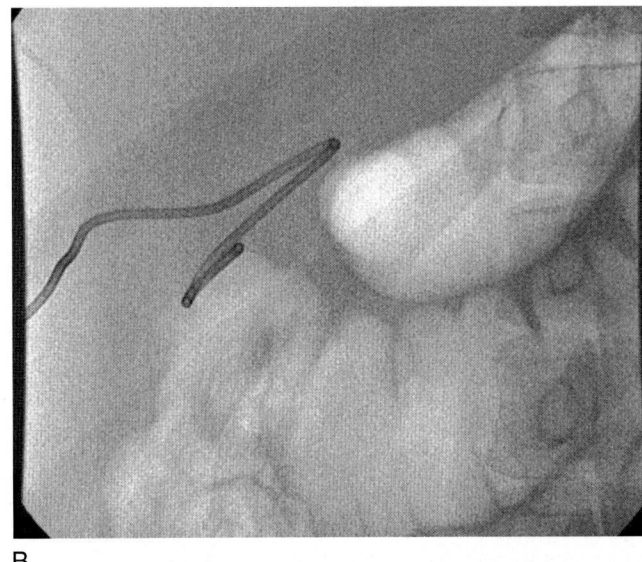

A   B

FIGURE 191-5. Percutaneous cholecystostomy. **A,** Ultrasound image during gallbladder puncture shows the transhepatic approach. The needle tip is seen within the gallbladder lumen. **B,** A radiograph obtained after placement of an 8 Fr catheter shows the catheter coiled within the gallbladder.

size of the scopes and small size of the child. ERCP is reserved for older children in whom contrast imaging of the biliary tree is necessary. PTC is reserved for select situations in which noninvasive imaging and ERCP are not feasible. Because of the fragile nature of the neonatal liver, caution should be taken when performing any percutaneous procedure on the liver of the neonate. Puncture of the gallbladder can be done using a transhepatic approach in order to opacify the biliary system in the small child with nondilated bile ducts.

Percutaneous cholecystostomy can be performed for the following indications: treatment of acute cholecystitis including empyema and perforation, drainage of common bile duct obstruction, and for performance of diagnostic cholangiography (Fig. 191-5). Percutaneous cholecystostomy is a procedure that is technically quite safe with few complications. A transhepatic approach should be taken when puncturing the gallbladder. The procedure has been done using trocar access; however, we prefer Seldinger technique with placement of an 8 Fr catheter. The catheter needs to be left in place for several weeks before removal to ensure that a fibrous tract has formed around the catheter and that bile will not leak into the peritoneal cavity on catheter removal. A tractogram can be performed over a guidewire before catheter removal to confirm an intact tract.

Trauma

Nonoperative management of blunt hepatic injury is the standard of care in the hemodynamically stable pediatric patient. Liver trauma can result in bilomas and hepatic artery pseudoaneurysms with hemobilia. Percutaneous drainage of a biloma alone may be sufficient to allow the biliary injury to heal. Percutaneous drainage or ERCP may be necessary to establish free bile drainage in select instances. Most bleeding from liver laceration will stop with conservative management, and arteriogram is

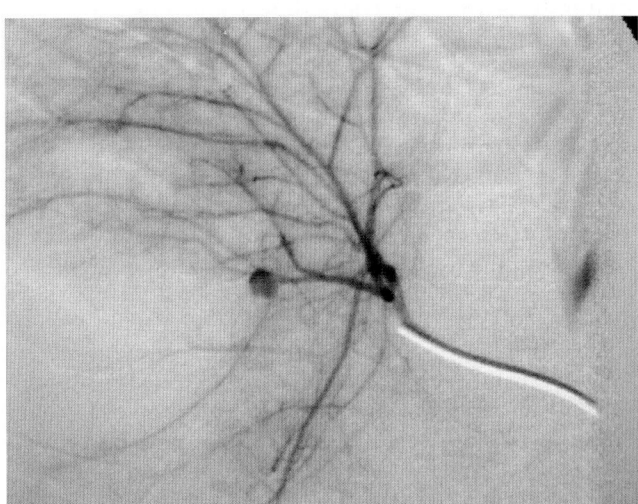

FIGURE 191-6. Traumatic pseudoaneurysm of hepatic artery. An arteriogram was obtained 2 weeks after blunt abdominal injury resulting in a liver laceration when the child presented with melena. The pseudoaneurysm causing hemobilia was successfully embolized.

seldom indicated. Hepatic artery injury from blunt trauma can result in formation of a pseudoaneurysm and may cause hemobilia (Fig. 191-6). Gastrointestinal bleeding after blunt abdominal trauma and liver laceration should raise the suspicion for a hepatic artery pseudoaneurysm. CT angiography should be the first diagnostic study for the detection of a pseudoaneurysm, with catheter angiography reserved for treatment. Hepatic artery pseudoaneurysm may be embolized successfully.

PEDIATRIC LIVER TRANSPLANT

Liver transplantation plays a major role in the treatment of end-stage liver disease in children, with reduced-size liver transplant surgical techniques allowing increasing numbers of children to undergo transplantation. As more children undergo liver transplantation, there is a growing need for radiologic diagnosis of and intervention in post-transplantation complications in these patients.

Liver transplantation is an effective and widely accepted treatment of end-stage liver disease in infants and children, with 10-year actuarial patient survival rates as high as 76%. Common indications for liver transplantation include extrahepatic biliary atresia, metabolic disease, fulminant hepatic failure, cryptogenic cirrhosis, intrahepatic cholestasis, chronic hepatitis, cystic fibroses, and tumors. Most liver transplant patients experience postoperative complications at some time. Interventional radiologists are playing an increasing role in the diagnosis and management of these complications in pediatric patients.

> Liver transplant is the accepted treatment of end-stage liver disease, with a 10-year survival rate as high as 76%.

Reduced-Size Liver Transplant Anatomy

The limited availability of appropriate size donor whole organs has led to the development of reduced-size liver transplant techniques that are now widely used to treat end-stage liver disease in infants and children. Knowledge of the unique surgical anatomy of the reduced-size liver transplant is essential to assess and treat pediatric liver transplant patients. Reduced-size liver transplants are based on the surgical segmental anatomy described by Couinaud and Bismuth (Fig. 191-7). This classification scheme divides the liver into vertical and oblique planes forming eight segments that are separated vertically by the three main hepatic veins and transversely by a plane drawn from the right to left portal veins. Reduced-size transplants include left lobe transplants (segments 2 to 4), left lateral segmental transplants (segments 2 and 3), and right lobar transplants (segments 5 to 8) (Fig. 191-8). The lateral segment of left lobe is frequently resected from a living donor for transplantation into a child.

The surgical anatomy in these reduced-size grafts differs from adult whole graft transplant anatomy in that they have a cut surface, an enteric Roux-en-Y loop for biliary drainage, and an alteration in the position and number of hepatic vessels. Five anastomoses are performed for standard liver transplantation: one portal venous, one hepatic arterial, one biliary, and two caval anastomoses. The arterial anastomosis may vary depending on the donor or recipient anatomy, but most commonly the anastomosis is end-to-end between the donor celiac axis or hepatic artery and the recipient hepatic artery. The donor and recipient portal veins are ideally attached through an end-to-end anastomosis unless the recipient portal vein is thrombosed. In this case, the recipient superior mesenteric vein can be anastomosed to the portal vein through an interposition graft. Biliary reconstruction is achieved with an end-to-end choledochojejunostomy. A biliary stent is not

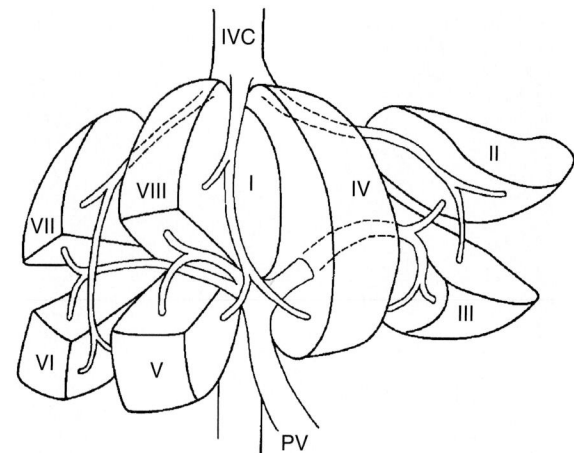

FIGURE 191-7. Liver segments described by Couinaud and Bismuth.

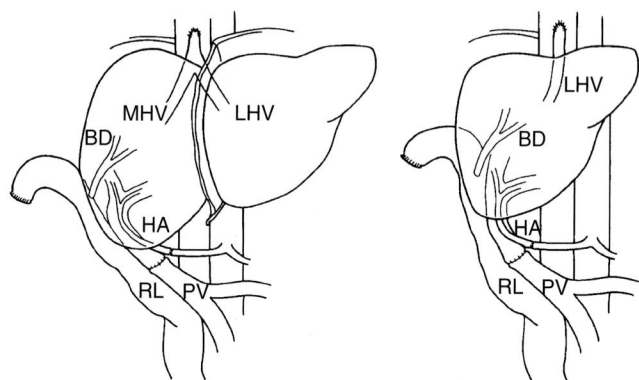

FIGURE 191-8. The whole left (segments II, III and IV) and the reduced left lobe (segments II and III) allografts. (From Rigsby CK, Superina R, Alonso EM: Interventional Radiology in the Pediatric Liver Transplant Patient. Seminars in Interventional Radiology 2002;19:59-72.)

routinely placed. A caval-sparing "piggyback" technique is used for the caval anastomosis for cadaveric organ and living donor transplantation.

Arterial Complications

Hepatic arterial thrombosis is the most common vascular complication following liver transplantation, occurring in 4% to 12% of adult liver transplantations and in as many as 50% of pediatric liver transplantations (Fig. 191-9). Thrombosis is more likely to occur in children because the small arterial size makes the anastomosis technically difficult. Arteriography remains the "gold standard" for confirmation of thrombosis but noninvasive imaging is increasingly used.

Most cases of acute thrombosis require emergent operation for revascularization and surgical revision of the anastomosis. If the arterial thrombosis is detected early, there is a high rate of graft survival with these surgical techniques. There are few reports of successful percutaneous thrombolysis or thrombolysis with angioplasty for hepatic arterial thrombosis. We have had no experience with these percutaneous techniques in children.

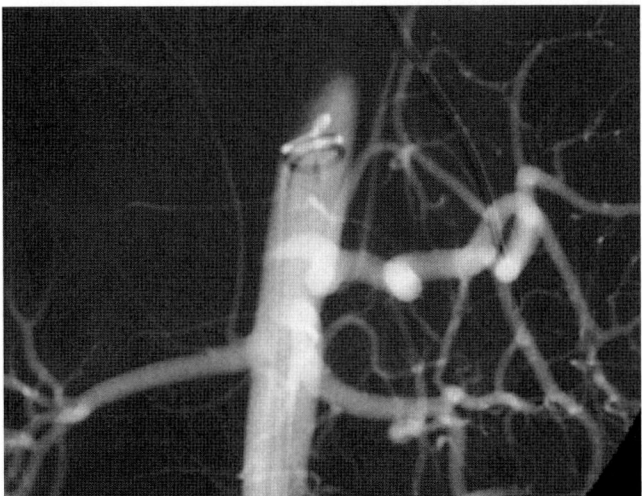

FIGURE 191-9. Hepatic artery occlusion. An abdominal angiogram shows the occluded hepatic artery in this patient one day after liver transplant surgery. The patient was re-explored surgically and the hepatic artery revascularized.

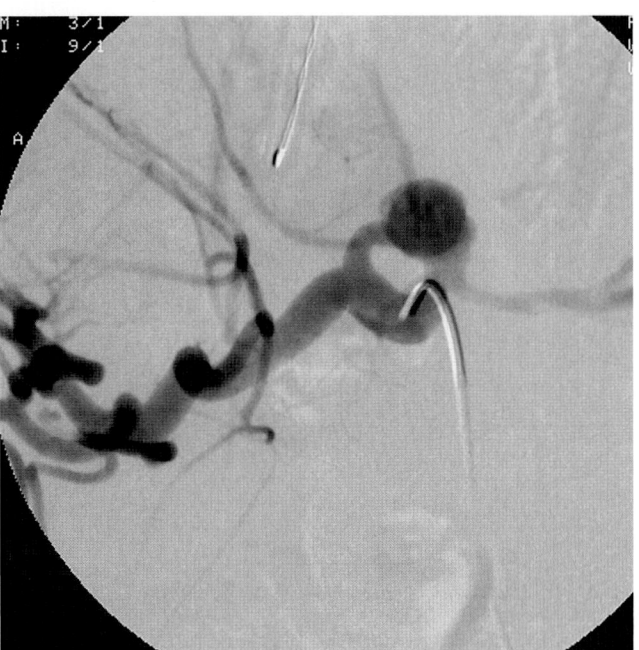

FIGURE 191-10. Hepatic artery pseudoaneurysm. This pseudoaneurysm was detected on post-transplant surveillance several months after transplantation. The pseudoaneurysm ruptured during attempts to embolize it and the artery had to be completely embolized causing the graft to fail. The patient was underwent a second transplant surgery.

Hepatic arterial stenosis can lead to arterial thrombosis. Stenoses generally occur at or within a few centimeters of the arterial anastomotic site. Percutaneous transluminal angioplasty has been reported to be successful in treating hepatic arterial stenosis in adults and in a limited number of pediatric patients. Caution should be used if performing percutaneous transluminal angioplasty in the immediate postoperative period to avoid vessel rupture.

Hepatic arterial pseudoaneurysms can occur but are rare and potentially fatal complications in liver transplant patients (Fig. 191-10). They can occur in the extrahepatic hepatic artery at the hepatic arterial anastomotic site as a result of technical factors or infection or can involve the intrahepatic hepatic artery as a result of biopsy or infection. Ruptured pseudoaneurysms can be fatal. Clinically, patients may be asymptomatic or may present with gastrointestinal bleeding or infection. These lesions may be treated surgically or embolized with percutaneous transcatheter techniques.

> **Hepatic arterial thrombosis is the most common vascular complication following liver transplantation.**

Portal Venous Complications

The incidence of portal venous thrombosis and stenosis in children following liver transplantation ranges from 0% to 33% and is higher than the 1% to 13% complication rate reported in adults. Multiple factors influence this higher complication rate in children, including the type of graft used (cadaveric versus living donor), the recipient portal vein size, the type of anastomosis used, and the position of the graft.

Portal venous thrombosis occurring in the immediate postoperative period requires emergent surgical thrombectomy or retransplantation. Late-occurring portal

venous thrombosis and stenosis were treated in the past with retransplantation, venous reconstruction, or portacaval shunting. The Rex shunt (superior mesenteric vein to left intrahepatic portal vein bypass) is now the surgical treatment of choice for late post-transplantation extrahepatic portal venous thrombosis with patent intrahepatic portal venous branches.

Percutaneous transhepatic venoplasty with or without metallic stent placement has become the treatment of choice for portal venous stenoses following reduced-size liver transplantation (Fig. 191-11). Technically, the procedure requires ultrasound-guided percutaneous access into the portal vein, manipulation across the stenosis, and confirmation of the stenosis. Angioplasty is then performed with success confirmed with venography and pressure measurements. A persistent pressure gradient of greater than 5 mm Hg is considered significant, and stent placement should be considered. The transhepatic parenchymal tract is then embolized with Gelfoam pledgets.

> **The Rex shunt (superior mesenteric vein to left intrahepatic portal vein bypass) is now the surgical treatment of choice for late post-transplantation extrahepatic portal venous thrombosis with patent intrahepatic portal venous branches.**

Hepatic Vein and Inferior Vena Cava Anastomotic Complications

IVC stenosis or thrombosis is seen in less than 1% of liver transplantations. Usual factors include anastomotic

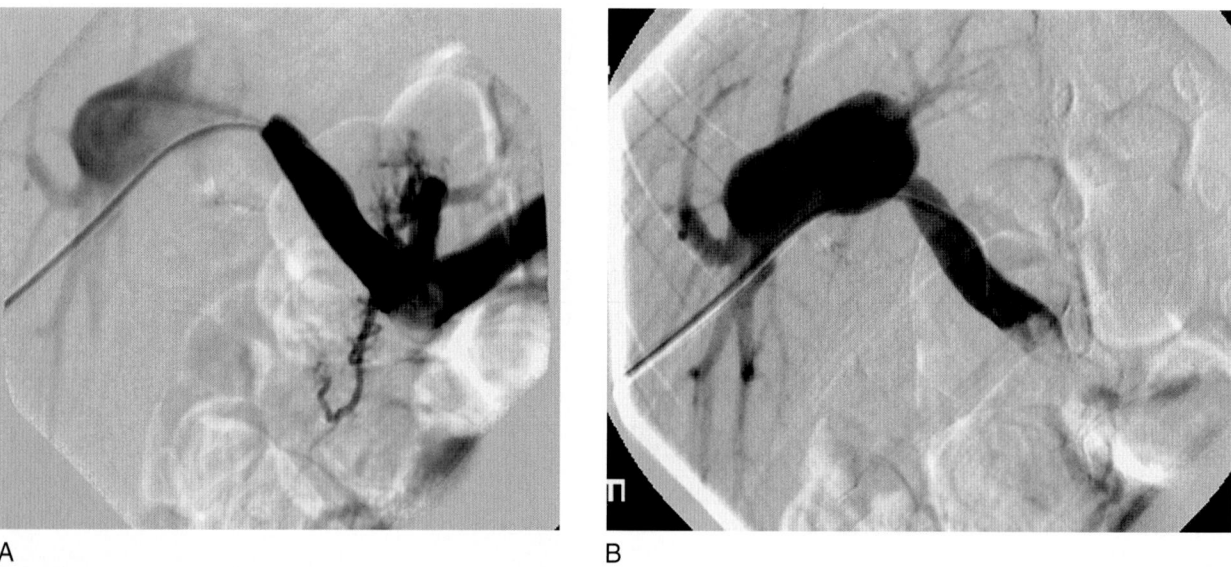

FIGURE 191-11. Liver transplant with portal vein anastomotic stenosis. **A,** A transhepatic portal venogram reveals a tight stenosis at the site of anastomosis with post-stenotic dilation of the portal vein within the liver. **B,** The stricture was successfully dilated, and the improved angiographic appearance is seen on the subsequent image.

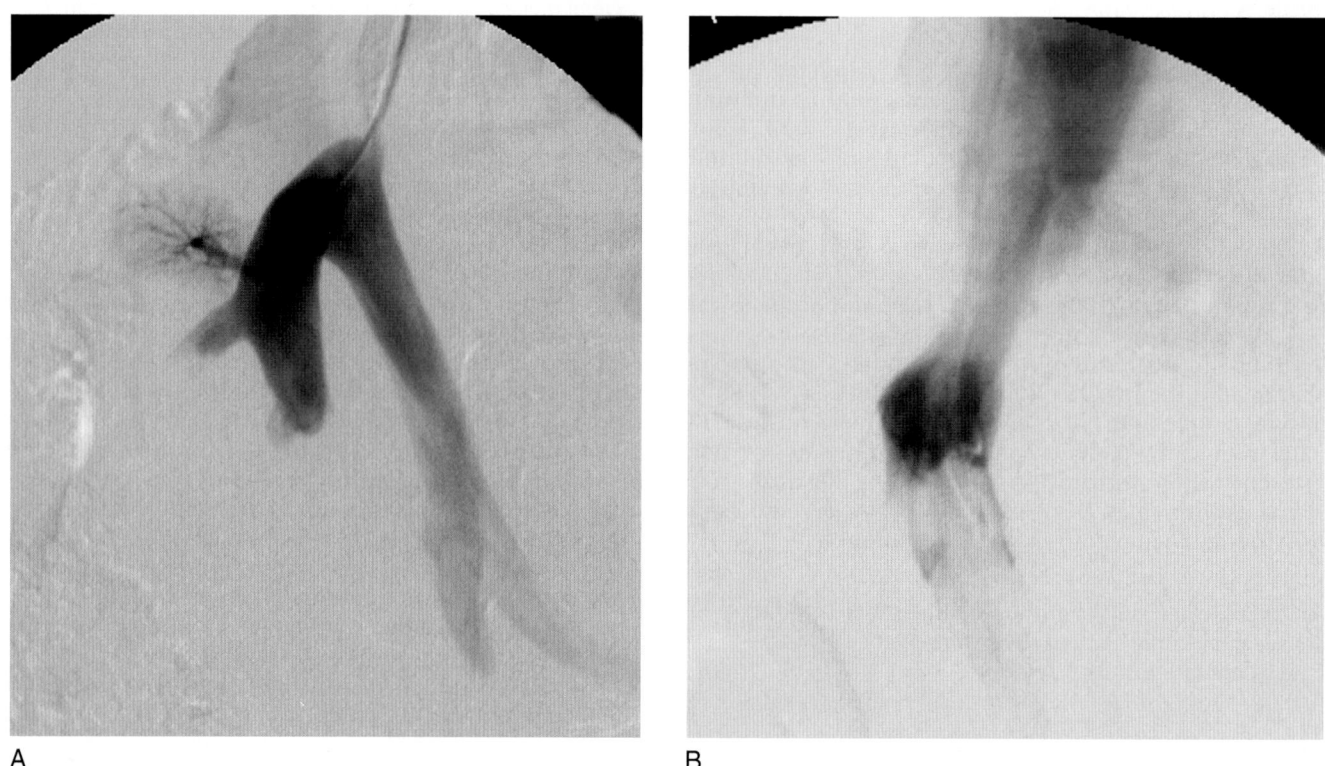

FIGURE 191-12. Liver transplant with hepatic vein–inferior vena cava stricture. **A,** A venogram performed from the femoral approach reveals a very tight stricture. **B,** After balloon dilation, the improved angiographic appearance is noted.

technical difficulties and/or extrinsic compression. Patients with stenosis or thrombosis of the IVC present clinically with symptoms resembling those of Budd-Chiari syndrome if the venous obstruction includes the hepatic venous return or may present with truncal or lower extremity edema if the obstruction is below the level of the hepatic venous confluence.

The diagnosis of occlusion of the IVC or hepatic veins can be made sonographically and confirmed with angiography, if necessary. If the occlusion is related to an underlying stenosis, treatment with percutaneous transluminal angioplasty with or without stent placement can be successful. Repeat dilatations may be necessary to achieve long-term patency (Fig. 191-12).

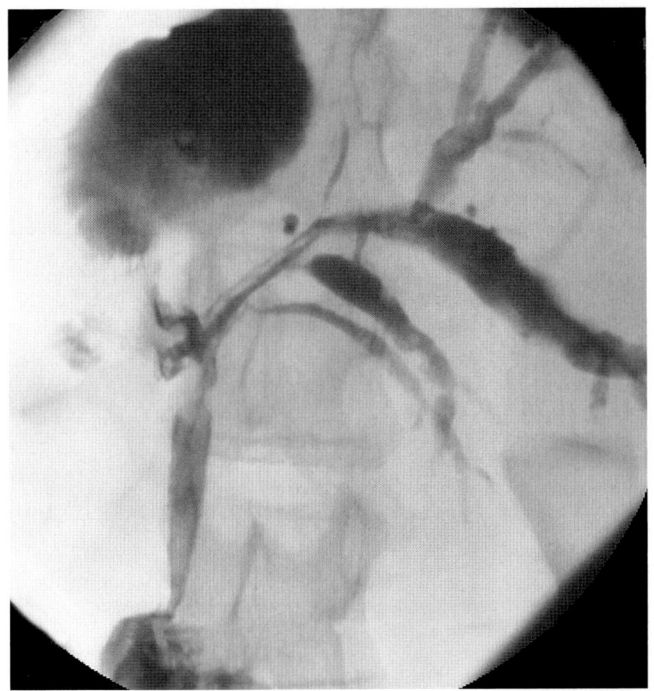
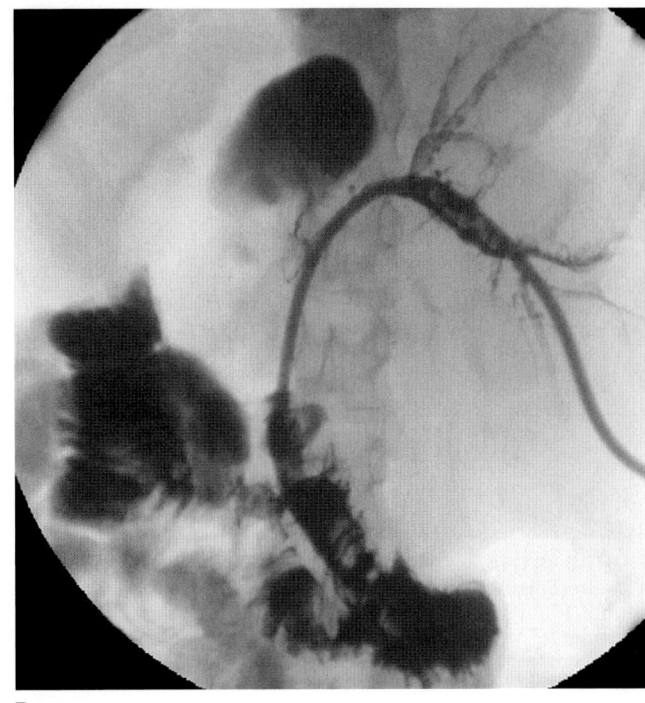

A   B

FIGURE 191-13. Biliary leak from split liver transplant. **A,** A large bile leak is seen in this patient with situs inversus (transplant in left upper quadrant) during a percutaneous transhepatic cholangiogram. The allograft was a split liver type leaving a whole left lobe and common bile duct. The leak is seen from the site of the right bile duct and right lobe resection. **B,** An internal-external biliary stent was placed across the leak into the bowel and the leak closed spontaneously after several weeks.

Biliary Complications

Biliary tract complications after liver transplantation are common and are a significant cause of morbidity after liver transplantation. The incidence of biliary complications in children after liver transplantation ranges from 11.5% to 38%. Bile leaks and biliary tract obstruction occur most commonly.

The causes of biliary complications include vascular, technical, and immunologic factors. The allograft bile duct relies solely on hepatic arterial flow and hepatic arterial thrombosis or stenosis can lead to biliary stricture or necrosis either at the anastomosis or in any portion of the donor biliary tree. With reduced-size liver grafts, the biliary enteric anastomosis is very small, leading to frequent anastomotic stricture formation. Immunologic mechanisms such as ABO incompatibility between allograft and patient may lead to an increase in the incidence of biliary strictures. Infection with cytomegalovirus and chronic rejection may also play significant roles in the development of biliary strictures.

Bile leaks are generally discovered in the immediate postoperative period and can occur at the biliary enteric anastomosis from the cut edge of the allograft or as a result of perforation of the Roux limb of the jejunum (Fig. 191-13). Early postoperative hepatic arterial thrombosis leads to allograft ischemia and leads to intrahepatic biliary ductal injury and resultant bile lakes or multiple intrahepatic and extrahepatic strictures. PTC may demonstrate anastomotic biliary leaks as contrast extravasation out of the expected location of the biliary tree or bowel. Placement of a biliary stent is indicated to decompress the biliary tree and allow closure of the leaking bile duct nonoperatively. Bile leaks associated with arterial thrombosis are more difficult to manage because of the associated bile duct necrosis, and despite biliary stent placement, these patients may require transplantation. If the extrahepatic bile collection is large, a percutaneous drainage catheter should also be placed into the biloma.

Bile leaks from the cut surface are visualized most commonly with cross-sectional imaging and may be seen with percutaneous transhepatic cholangiography if the nonoccluded bile duct leading to the leak fills adequately with contrast material. Placement of a percutaneous catheter directly into the bilomas can be performed but often surgical re-exploration and ligation of the source of the leaks is necessary.

Biliary strictures at the anastomotic site often occur relatively late in the post-transplantation course, can occur years after the initial surgery, and may not be related to hepatic arterial thrombosis (Fig. 191-14). Patients with anastomotic strictures present with a cholestatic profile on liver function tests, show evidence of biliary obstruction on biopsy, and may have frank cholangitis. Sonography may or may not show a dilated biliary tree.

> **Sonography may or may not show a dilated biliary tree when there is a biliary stricture.**

Biliary strictures are managed with percutaneous techniques. Access to the biliary tree is obtained using sonographic guidance into a primary or secondary biliary

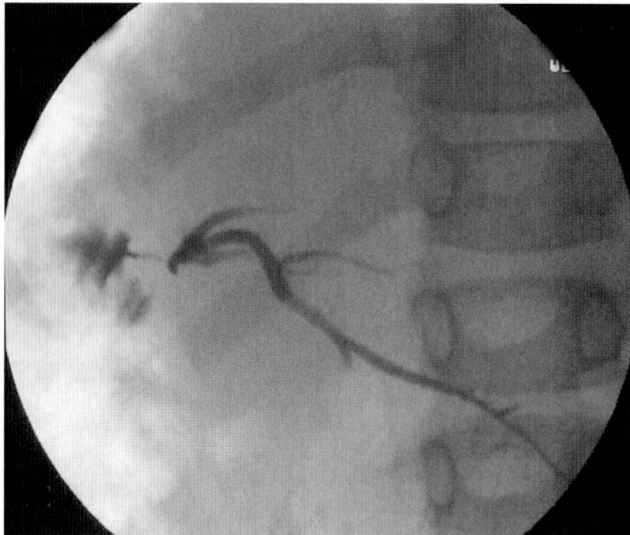

FIGURE 191-14. Liver transplant with anastomotic biliary stricture. This PTC reveals the tight anastomotic stricture in a patient 18 months after reduced left lobe living related transplant. The stricture was dilated with a balloon; a plastic internal-external biliary stent was placed for 3 months and subsequently removed.

radicle for opacification of the biliary tree. Contrast injection with appropriate angulation demonstrates the anastomotic stricture. It is important to review the type of transplant used (either whole or reduced size) to ensure opacification of all ducts because undrained obstructed ducts may not be opacified on the cholangiogram. The stricture is then crossed and dilated with a balloon usually 4 to 6 mm diameter. Usually, 8 to 14 Fr transanastomotic internal external biliary drainage catheters are placed. Follow-up cholangiograms are performed every 6 weeks with prophylactic catheter exchange. The catheters are generally left in place for 3 months.

Transhepatic cholangiography is generally highly successful, with 23/25 patients successfully accessed and drained in one series from Chicago. In some settings, the stricture may not be successfully crossed on initial attempt, but subsequent attempts are usually successful.

Biopsy Considerations

The allograft position in patients with reduced-size liver transplants is altered and may be entirely subcostal. The location of the major vessels is also altered, with the portal hepatis located on the right posterior or posterolateral aspect of the graft. If this alteration in position and anatomy is not understood, an increase in complications after liver biopsy will result. Sonographic localization or guidance for these biopsies is ideal, with a midline subxiphoid approach most often used.

SUGGESTED READINGS

Infections of the Liver

Akhan O, Ozmen MN: Percutaneous treatment of liver hydatid cysts. Eur J Radiol 1999;31:76-85

Goktay AY, Secil M, Gulcu A, et al: Percutaneous treatment of hydatid liver cysts in children as a primary treatment: long-term results. J Vasc Interv Radiol 2005;16:831-839

Pineiro-Carrero VM, Andres JM: Morbidity and mortality in children with pyogenic liver abscess. Am J Dis Child 1989;143:1424-1427

Diffuse Parenchymal Disease

Habdank K, Restrepo R, Ng V, et al: Combined sonographic and fluoroscopic guidance during transjugular hepatic biopsies performed in children: a retrospective study of 74 biopsies. AJR Am J Roentgenol 2003;180:1393-1398

Smith TP, Presson TL, Heneghan MA, Ryan JM: Transjugular biopsy of the liver in pediatric and adult patients using an 18-gauge automated core biopsy needle: a retrospective review of 410 consecutive procedures. AJR Am J Roentgenol 2003;180:167-172

Trauma

Christensen R: Invasive radiology for pediatric trauma. Semin Pediatr Surg 2001;10:7-11.

Giss SR, Dobrilovic N, Brown RL, Garcia VF: Complications of nonoperative management of pediatric blunt hepatic injury: Diagnosis, management, and outcomes. J Trauma 2006;61:334-339

Transplantation

Abad J, Hidalgo E, Cantarero J, et al: Hepatic artery anastomotic stenosis after transplantation: treatment with percutaneous transluminal angioplasty. Radiology 1989;171:661-662

Balistreri W: Transplantation for childhood liver disease: an overview. Liver Transpl Surg 1998;4:S18-S23

Bambini DA, Superina R, Almond PS, et al: Experience with Rex shunt (mesenterico-left portal bypass) in children with extrahepatic portal hypertension. J Pediatr Surg 2000;35:13-19

Ben-Ami T, Martich V, Yousefzadeh D, et al: Anatomic features of reduced-size liver transplant: postsurgical imaging characteristics. Radiology 1993;187:165-170

Bismouth H: Surgical Anatomy on Anatomical Surgery of the Liver. In: Blumgart LH, ed: Surgery of the Liver and Biliary Tract. Edinburgh: Churchill Livingstone, 1994

Couinad L: Le Foie Etudes Anatomique et Chiurgicales. Paris: Masson, 1957

Cron K, Strife J, Babcock D, et al: Left-lobed hepatic transplants: spectrum of normal imaging findings. AJR Am J Roentgenol 1992;159:497-501

De Ville de Goyet J, Gibbs P, Clapuyt P, et al: Original extrahilar approach for hepatic portal revascularization and relief of extrahepatic port hypertension related to late portal vein thrombosis after pediatric liver transplantation. Transplantation 1996;62:71-75

Edmond J, Whitington P. Thistlehwaite R, et al: Reduced-size orthotopic liver transplantation: use in the management of children with chronic liver disease. Hepatology 1989;10:867-872

Egawa H, Uemoto S, Inomata Y, et al: Biliary complications in pediatric living related liver transplantation. Surgery 1998;124:901-910

Funaki B, Rosenblum J, Leef J, et al: Angioplasty treatment of portal vein stenosis in children with segmental liver transplants: mid-term results. AJR Am J Roentgenol 1997;169:551-554

Funaki B, Rosenblum J, Leef J, et al: Percutaneous treatment of portal venous stenosis in children and adolescents with segmental hepatic transplants: long-term results. Radiology 2000;215:147-152

Heffron T, Emond J, Whitington P, et al: Biliary complications in pediatric liver transportation. Transplantation 1992;53:391-395

Hesselink EJ, Klompmaker IJ, Pruim J, et al: Hepatic artery thrombosis after orthotopic liver transplantation—a fatal complication or an asymptomatic event. Transplant Proc 1989;21:2462

Karani JB, Yu DF, Kane PA: Interventional radiology in liver transplantation. Cardiovasc Intervent Radiol 2005;28:271-283

Millis M, Seaman D, Piper J, et al: Portal vein thrombosis and stenosis in pediatric liver transplantation. Transplantation 1996;62:748-754

Orons P, Hari A, Zajko A, Marsh JW: Thrombolysis and endovascular stent placement for inferior vena caval thrombosis in a liver transplant recipient. Transplantation 1997;64:1357-1361

Orons P, Zajko A: Angiography and interventional procedures in liver transplantation. Radiol Clin North Am 1995;33:541-558

Peclet M, Rychman F. Pedersen S, et al: The spectrum of bile duct complications in pediatric liver transplantation. J Pediatr Surg 1994;29:214-220

Raby N, Karani J, Thomas S, et al: Stenoses of vascular anastomoses after hepatic transplantation: treatment with balloon angioplasty. AJR Am J Roentgenol 157;1991:167-171

Stratta R, Wood P, Langnas A, et al. Diagnosis and treatment of biliary tracts complications after orthotopic liver transplantation. Surgery 1989;106:675-684

Valera R, Cotton P, Clavien PA: Biliary reconstruction for liver transplantation and management of the biliary complications: overview and survey of current practices in the United States. Liver Transpl Surg 1995;1:143-152

Xajko A, Campbell W, Logsdon G, et al: Cholangiographic findings in hepatic artery occlusion after liver transplantation. AJR Am J Roentgenol 1987;149:485-489

Zajko A, Tobben P, Esquivel C, et al: Pseudoaneurysms following orthotopic liver transplantation: clinical and radiologic manifestations. Transplant Proc 1989;21:2457-2459

Sunku B, Salvalaggio PRO, Donaldson J, et al: Outcomes and risk factors for failure of radiologic treatment of biliary strictures in pediatric liver transplant recipients. Liver Transpl 2006;12:281-286

Shibata T, Itoh K, Kubo T, et al: Percutaneous transhepatic balloon dilation of portal venous stenosis in patients with living donor liver transplantation. Radiology 2005;235:1078-1083

CHAPTER

192

Pediatric Genitourinary Intervention

MARY BETH MOORE and CHARLES A. JAMES

Cooperative efforts of urologists and interventional radiologists are required for effective management of many genitourinary problems in children. Percutaneous techniques are necessary when retrograde approaches fail or are not attempted because likelihood of success is small or the size of the infant urethra precludes safe retrograde instrumentation. Percutaneous access to the urinary tract can be used for many procedures including stone removal, ureteral instrumentation, dilation, stenting and of course drainage. Retrograde catheterization of the urethra may be done by interventional radiology and foreign bodies including ureteral stents may be retrieved. Combined procedures involving the interventional radiologist and urologist sometimes allow completion of complicated procedures that may otherwise not be successful by either service alone.

The request for involvement by the interventional radiologists usually requires a direct consultation with the urologist and a mutually agreed-upon plan. Radiographic studies must be reviewed, patient condition taken into consideration, risk/benefit discussed, and goals of treatment clearly understood before the procedure is attempted.

PREPROCEDURE CONSIDERATIONS

Detailed information regarding management of the pediatric interventional patient can be found in Chapter 181. For routine procedures, intravenous (IV) sedation is administered by trained pediatric interventional nurses. However, for prolonged sedation or for patients with either complex anatomic issues or medical histories, general anesthesia is employed. At some pediatric hospitals, a dedicated hospital sedation service may provide sedation.

> **Detailed patient work-up before the procedure and a sedation or anesthesia plan tailored to each patient is essential for patient safety.**

Coagulation parameters and platelet count are assessed to determine the risks for bleeding. Platelet counts must be at least 50,000 and preferably more than 100,000 especially for nonvascular interventions and the International Normalized Ratio should be less than 1.5.

There are several parameters to consider in treating a patient with chronic renal disease in order to reduce procedural and periprocedural morbidity and mortality. For example, correction of severe anemia and hyperkalemia is suggested prior to the procedure. In order to combat platelet dysfunction in uremic patients, desmopressin can be administered 1 hour before the procedure.

There are special sedation concerns in infants. The infant's body temperature must be maintained in order to prevent cardiopulmonary collapse. Use of a warming device should be considered. Before the patient is placed in the prone or decubitus position, small rolls should be placed longitudinally under the chest and abdomen to facilitate respiration and to help decrease renal mobility during percutaneous nephrostomy.

> **To help prevent cardiopulmonary collapse in infants during long procedures, body temperature must be maintained.**

The use of prophylactic antibiotics is controversial. Options for urologic procedures should be based on the child's clinical condition and include no prophylaxis versus a weight- and age-appropriate IV dose of ceftriaxone, ampicillin/sulbactam, or the combination of ampicillin and gentamicin. Prophylactic antibiotics given 1 hour before the procedure are indicated or strongly suggested for patients with signs of infection or who have factors predisposing to infection such as stones, indwelling catheter, bacteriuria, ureterointestinal conduit, or pyonephrosis. Urine culture can be obtained during the procedure.

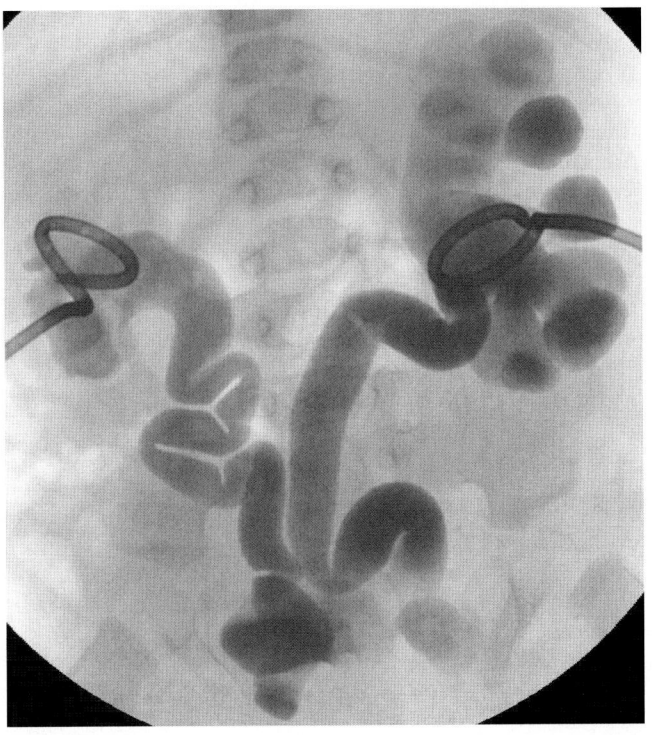
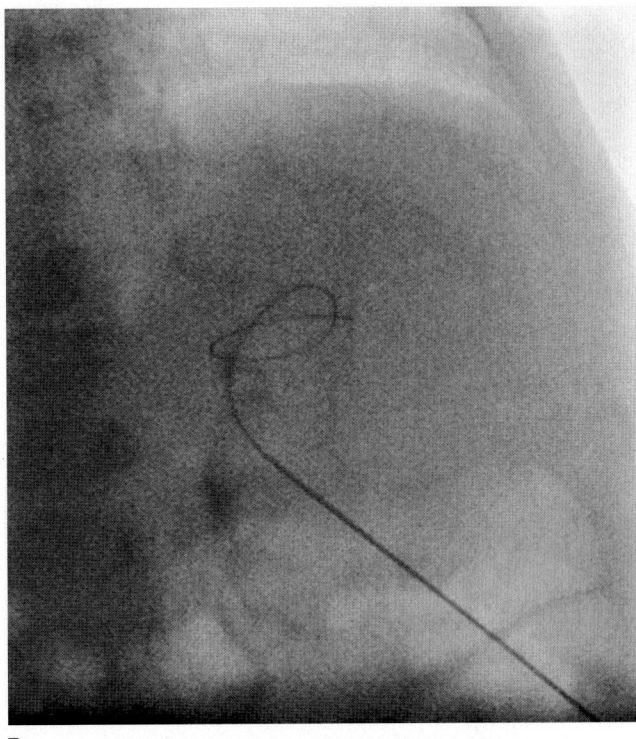

A   B

FIGURE 192-1. Bilateral nephrostomy tube placement **(A)** in a 5-month-old boy for distal obstruction showed bilateral hydroureteronephritis with debris. He had bladder repair 5 months before nephrostomy placement. Access to each kidney was through a micropuncture needle and 0.018 inch wire under ultrasound guidance **(B)**. The patient was uremic with suspected platelet dysfunction. Desmopressin and antibiotics were administered before the procedure.

PERCUTANOUS NEPHROSTOMY IN THE OLDER CHILD

The conventional technique is similar to adult nephrostomy placement. A micropuncture needle is advanced under sonographic guidance into a posterior renal calyx, preferably in the mid to lower pole. Needle placement is confirmed with aspiration of urine and a small amount of contrast is injected to opacify the collecting system. A guidewire is coiled in the renal collecting system or advanced down the ureter. Exchange for a sturdier guide wire is made. In most cases, 8 Fr nephrostomy tubes suffice.

PERCUTANEOUS NEPHROSTOMY IN THE INFANT

Nephrostomy placement in an infant can be technically difficult. Micropuncture access can be arduous because the retroperitoneal tissues and renal parenchyma have greater elasticity and the collecting system may decompress during guidewire exchange and tract dilatation. A modified technique suggests initial puncture with a 19-G needle. A small amount of urine is aspirated, and a small amount of contrast is injected. Through the needle, a stiff guidewire is passed with fluoroscopic guidance. A 6 Fr nephrostomy tube is then advanced over the wire. Alternatively, one could use the conventional micropuncture technique especially for nondilated systems, dilated systems with distal obstruction (Fig. 192-1), and patients with coagulopathy.

> Percutaneous nephrostomy in the infant can be challenging because of elastic retroperitoneal tissues and renal parenchyma, as well as collecting system decompression that occurs during the procedure.

PERCUTANEOUS NEPHROLITHOTOMY

Percutaneous nephrolithotomy is usually a multistage procedure that takes place over several days in order to remove large stones and staghorn calculi (Fig. 192-2). Less morbidity, mortality, and shorter hospital stays are expected compared with open surgery. Removal of ureteral stones can also be performed with slight modifications of the following technique. IV Mannitol may be infused before the procedure to induce diuresis and caliceal distention. The goal is to access the stone through the involved calyx with a mildly lateral approach that is inferior to the 12th rib. Rotational fluoroscopy and three-dimensional reconstruction may facilitate an interventional genitourinary procedure such as this. An access sheath needle is advanced under fluoroscopic guidance toward the stone. A hydrophilic guidewire is advanced around the stone and into the ureter. A catheter is advanced to the bladder.

In the operating room, C-arm fluoroscopy and appropriate endourologic equipment are required. Fascial tract dilatation up to 30 Fr is performed through

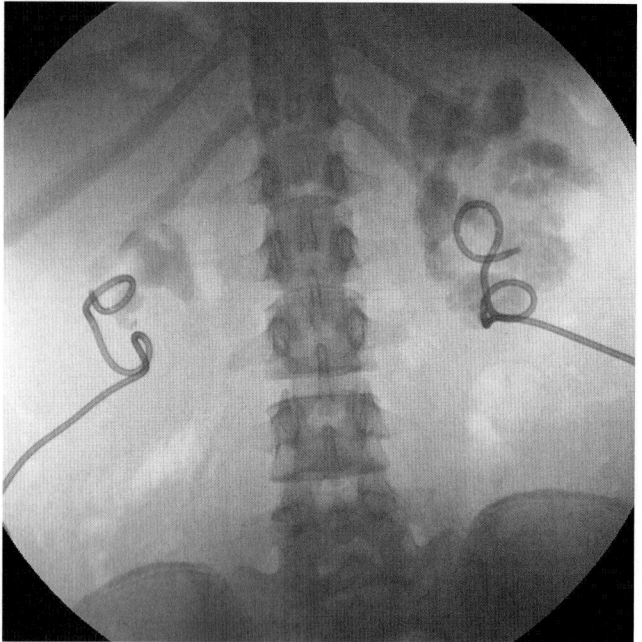

FIGURE 192-2. Bilateral nephrostomy tube placement to allow for drainage prior to nephrolithotomy in a 12-year-old girl with bilateral staghorn calculi and infundibular stenoses. She had signs of sepsis and acute renal failure. Antibiotics were administered before the procedure.

the nephrostomy access to the level of the stone. In a small child, tract dilatation with a 9 or 10 Fr peel-away sheath may suffice. A urologist then approaches the stone endoscopically through a sheath with a rigid or flexible endoscope. Endoscopic instruments are used to fragment then remove stones as well as blood clots. Laser fragmentation of stones is an option. Following completion of endoscopic treatment, a nephrostomy catheter is advanced over the working guidewire into the collecting system. A postoperative nephrostogram performed the following day assesses for contrast extravasation, residual stone burden, and ureteral patency.

ANTEGRADE URETERAL STENTING

Indications include ureteral stenosis (Fig. 192-3), ureteral calculus, and extrinsic compression by tumor. The technique includes contrast opacification of the ureter, manipulating a guidewire across the obstruction, exchange for a stiff guidewire, then placement of a ureteral stent. A back-up nephrostomy catheter can usually be removed within 24 hours.

FLUID COLLECTION DRAINAGE: URINOMA

Percutaneous drainage may be required for diagnostic sampling, drainage of infected fluid, or to relieve mass effect on nearby structures. Urinomas secondary to

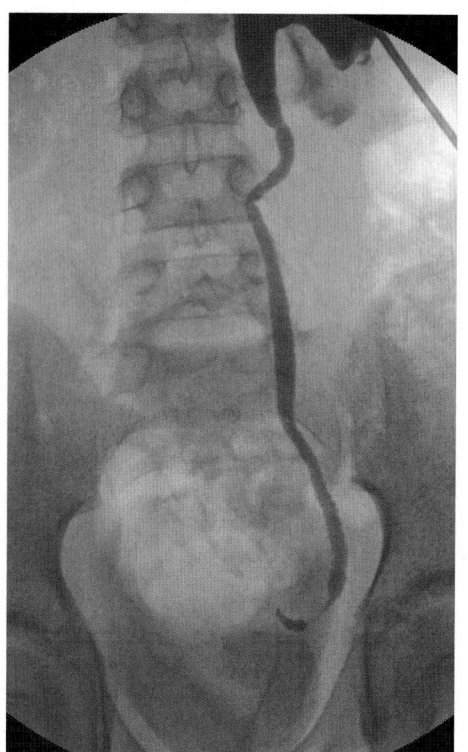

A

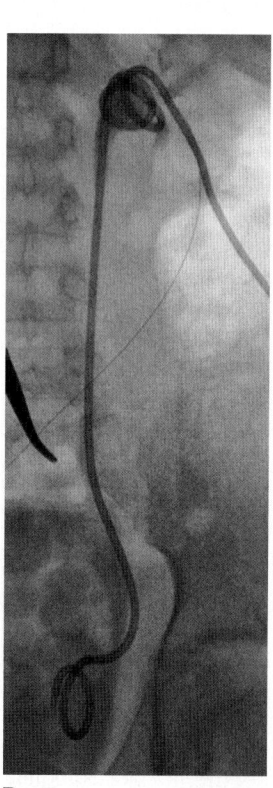

B

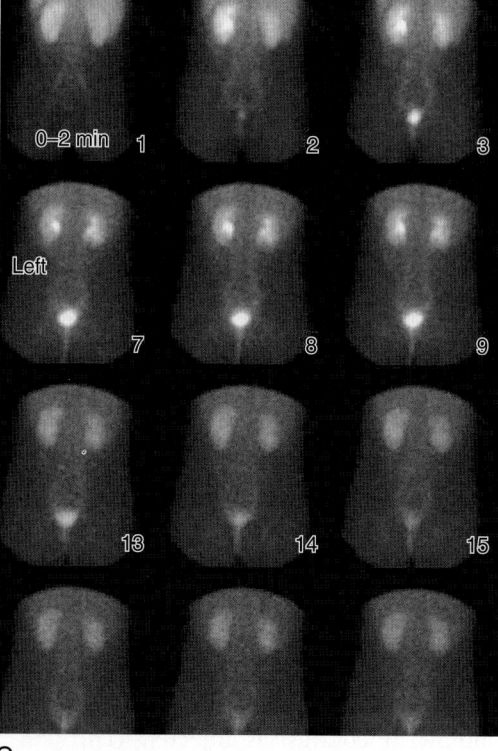

C

FIGURE 192-3. A 10-year-old girl with right obstructive nephropathy 1 week after bilateral ureteral reimplant surgery for vesicoureteral reflux. Right nephrostomy was placed to relieve the obstruction. Antibiotics were given before the procedure. Procedural nephrostogram **(A)** shows severe distal right ureteral narrowing and kinking. Follow-up nephrostogram 2 weeks later demonstrated no improvement. Therefore, a right ureteral stent was placed **(B)** as well as a nephrostomy tube. (The small caliber safety wire was removed after the nephrostomy was placed.) Ureteral stent was removed after 6 weeks. Representative images from a subsequent renogram **(C)** show no obstruction.

urinary tract obstruction in children are most commonly related to anomalies such as posterior urethral valves, ureteropelvic junction (UPJ) obstruction, or ureterovesical obstruction. Calyceal perforation results in generalized urine ascites or a localized urinoma. If hydronephrosis is significant and the urine leak is secondary, then percutaneous nephrostomy may be the initial intervention.

PERCUTANEOUS INTERVENTIONS IN NEONATES WITH *CANDIDA* INFECTION

Candida urinary tract infections are commonly seen in neonates requiring intensive care. Systemic antifungal medications are administered. Renal abscesses can be percutaneously aspirated or drained. For the rarely occurring obstructing fungal balls or bezoars, percutaneous nephrostomy can be performed to relieve the obstruction as well as provide a conduit for local irrigation with antifungal agents. There are also reports of mechanical thrombectomy devices being employed to remove the bezoars.

RENOVASCULAR INTERVENTION

Renovascular intervention includes techniques such as arterial angiography, angioplasty, stenting, embolization, ethanol ablation, and venous sampling. Techniques are similar to that used in adults but the equipment is of lower profile. Three-dimensional rotational angiography may enable visualization of small or peripheral diseased vessels. Renovascular hypertension is discussed further in Chapter 193.

EMERGING TECHNIQUES

Percutaneous biopsy is useful in the diagnosis of pediatric solid renal tumors. Additionally, radiofrequency ablation of small pediatric renal tumors can obviate surgery. In the effort to decrease the effects of ionizing radiation from interventional procedures, magnetic resonance guidance can also enable pediatric interventions. UPJ obstruction repair has classically been performed by open surgical procedure. However, an alternative treatment for UPJ combines the endoscopic skill of the urologist with the percutaneous skill of the interventional radiologist.

> Interventional radiologists and urologists can cooperate in joint procedures to reduce morbidity, mortality, and hospital stay in patients who have staghorn calculi or UPJ obstruction.

SUGGESTED READINGS

Campbell JB, Seidel FG, Gonzales ET Jr: Use of a mechanical thrombectomy catheter for percutaneous extraction of renal fungal bezoars in a premature infant. Urology 2004;64:589

Garrett KM, Fuller CE, Santana VM, Shochat SJ, Hoffer FA: Percutaneous biopsy of pediatric solid tumors. Cancer 2005;104:644-652

Hoffer FA: Interventional radiology in pediatric oncology. Eur J Radiol 2005;53;3-13

Koral K, Saker MC, Morello FP, et al: Conventional versus modified technique for percutaneous nephrostomy in newborns and young infants. J Vasc Interv Radiol 2003;14:113-116

Krishnan M: Preoperative care of patients with kidney disease. Am Fam Physician 2002;66:1471-1476

Racadio JM, Donnelly LF, Johnson ND: Non-vascular applications of 3D rotational angiography in children. Scientific presentation at the Annual Meeting of the Radiological Society of North America, Chicago, November 30-December 5, 2003

Ryan JM, Ryan BM, Smith,TP: Antibiotic prophylaxis in interventional radiology. J Vasc Interv Radiol 2004;15:547-556

Schmidt MB, James CA: Genitourinary intervention in children. Seminars in Interventional Radiology 2002;19:51-57

Schulz T, Trobs RB, Schneider JP, et al: Pediatric MR-guided interventions. Eur J Radiol 2005 Jan;53:57-66.

Towbin RB, Baskin KM, Cahill AM, Kaye RD: Interventional radiology: a modular approach. Pediatr Radiol 2006;36:378-385

William JM, Racadio JM, Johnson ND, et al: Embolization of renal angiomyolipomata in patients with tuberous sclerosis complex. Am J Kidney Dis 2006;47:95-102

CHAPTER

193

Interventional Radiology of Renovascular Hypertension

CLARE A. MCLAREN and DEREK J. ROEBUCK

BACKGROUND

The syndromes most commonly associated with renovascular hypertension (RVH) are neurofibromatosis type 1 and Williams syndrome (see Chapter 150). When no syndrome or other cause is identified, the diagnosis of fibromuscular dysplasia is usually made, although it is unusual to have biopsy proof of this. Mid-aortic (or "middle-aortic") syndrome (MAS) is a morphologic term used to describe narrowing of the abdominal aorta and one or more of its major branches.

Disease of segmental and small intrarenal arteries is a common cause of hypertension in children, and it is difficult to diagnose with noninvasive imaging techniques. Selection of children for angiography is, therefore, usually based on clinical factors, and may be appropriate even when noninvasive imaging is normal. Blood pressure should be carefully measured; matched to normal ranges for age, sex, and height; and confirmed on repeated measurements.

Indications for angiography in children with hypertension, when other causes of secondary hypertension have been excluded.

- **Syndrome known to include renovascular disease**
- **Blood pressure difficult to stabilize**
- **Need for two or more antihypertensive drugs**
- **Unacceptable adverse effects of antihypertensive drugs**
- **Strong evidence of renal artery stenosis at noninvasive imaging**

Although antihypertensive drugs are usually successful in controlling RVH, the prospect of life-long drug treatment with possible progression of disease means that some other form of intervention is usually contemplated. Endovascular treatments include angioplasty, stenting, and ethanol ablation. Surgical options include in situ revascularization, with transposition of native arteries or synthetic grafts, or autotransplantation to the pelvis. Simple lesions such as isolated unilateral renal artery stenosis usually respond well to angioplasty. Very complex abnormalities (multiple stenoses with aneurysm formation, MAS) may require surgical reconstruction.

Referral to a multidisciplinary RVH service is essential for optimal treatment.

RENAL VEIN RENIN SAMPLING (RVRS)

RVRS appears to be more useful in children than in adults, probably because bilateral and segmental disease is so common. It is usually performed through a femoral approach at the same time as diagnostic angiography. Samples are taken from the infrarenal inferior vena cava and main renal veins. Selective sampling is easier using a coaxial thin-walled microcatheter (e.g., Renegade, Boston Scientific, Natick, Massachusetts). Care must be taken to avoid nonrenal (suprarenal, capsular, and left gonadal) tributaries of the renal veins. A ratio of renin activity between the main renal veins of greater than 1.5 lateralizes the hypertensive drive. It may also be possible to identify a segmental focus (Fig. 193-1).

DIAGNOSTIC ANGIOGRAPHY

Digital subtraction angiography is still the best imaging technique for RVH, and it is the basis of endovascular treatment. Great care should be taken with technique.

Suggested angiographic technique for children with renovascular hypertension.

- **Intra-arterial heparin (50 to 100 U kg^{-1}) for children <10 kg**
- **Biplane aortography**
- **Images of common hepatic, gastroduodenal, splenic, and iliac arteries**
- **Images of all renal arteries (including oblique projections where appropriate)**
- **Optional techniques**
  renal vein renin sampling
  rotational angiography
  carbon dioxide angiography
  thoracic aortography and cerebral angiography
  intravascular ultrasound

General anesthesia is appropriate for diagnostic angiography in young children (<10 years) and for most

3184

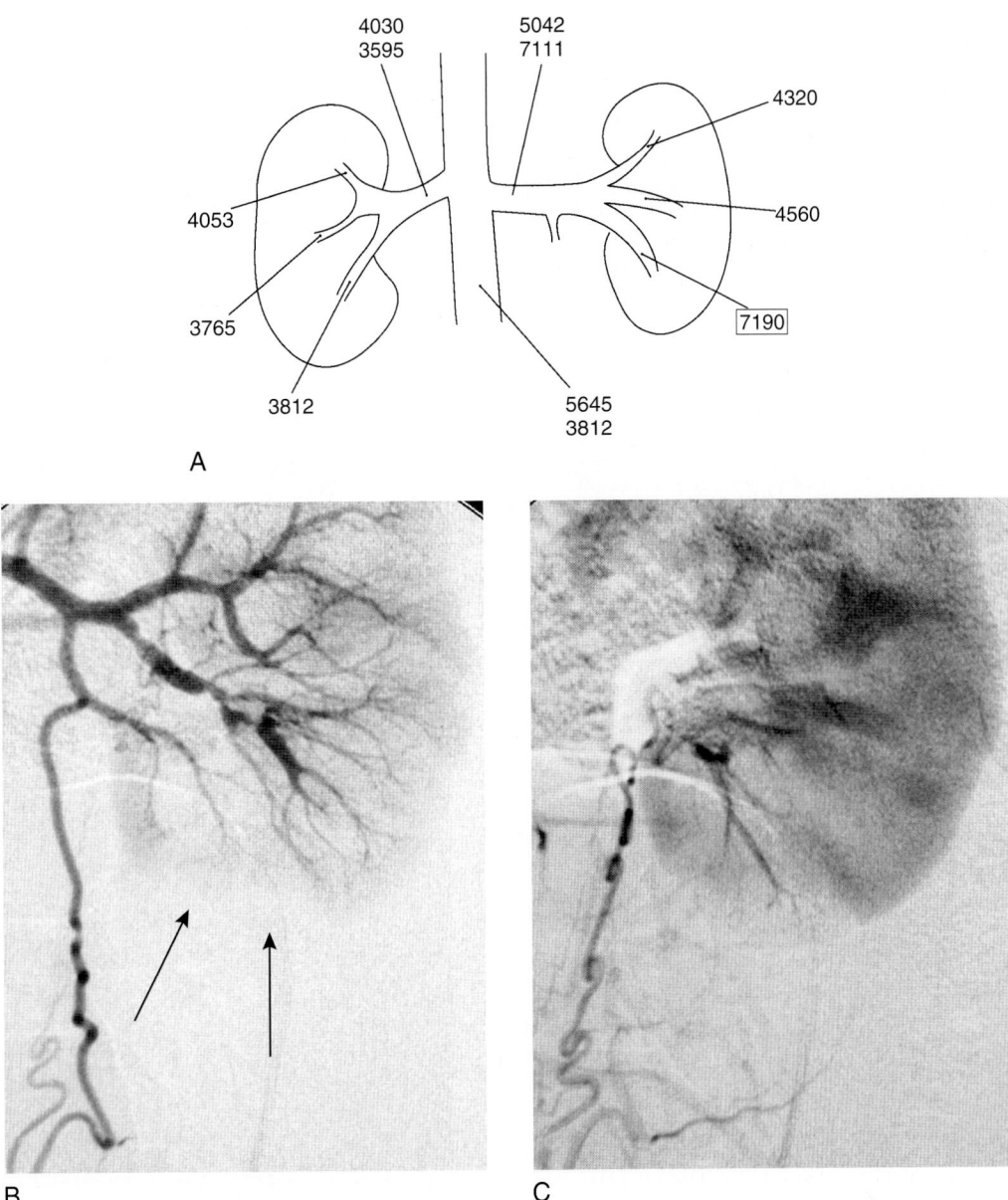

FIGURE 193-1. An 11-year-old girl with hypertension. **A,** Map of renal vein renin activity shows that the hypertension is driven by a focus in the left lower pole. **B,** Arterial phase angiography shows complex segmental stenoses, an area of delayed perfusion owing to a "missing vessel" *(arrows),* and a prominent collateral ureteric artery. **C,** Capillary phase angiography shows that the "missing vessel" is reconstituted by the ureteric artery collateral, completing the nephrogram. It is unlikely that this artery could be successfully recanalized, but segmental ethanol ablation might be possible. (From Roebuck DJ: Paediatric interventional radiology. Imaging 2001;13:302-320.)

pediatric angioplasties. The use of muscle relaxants and endotracheal intubation allows suspension of ventilation and is therefore ideal for digital subtraction angiography. A femoral approach is used in almost all cases. Diagnostic angiography and simple angioplasty can be performed through a 4-French sheath, but difficult angioplasty and stenting may require the use of a 6-Fr sheath and guiding catheter. We give heparin (50 to 100 U kg^{-1}) for small children (<10 kg) and all interventional procedures.

Aortography is primarily used to assess the caliber of the aorta and the number of renal arteries and their origins. It also provides information about the celiac trunk, superior mesenteric artery, and the iliac arteries, which may be useful for surgical planning. Selective angiography of all renal arteries is performed, with

oblique projections as appropriate. The presence of a small accessory renal artery, overlooked on the aortogram, may be identified by a defect in the nephrographic phase of a selective renal angiogram.

Various technical refinements are possible. Intravascular ultrasound may contribute useful information not evident at angiography (Fig. 193-2). Contrast nephrotoxicity is not important in children with normal (or absent) renal function, but may be a concern in those with renal impairment. In this context (e.g., failing renal transplant), or when a very prolonged procedure is anticipated, carbon dioxide angiography may be helpful. Rotational angiography can be particularly helpful in children with complex disease, such as large aneurysms or occluded vessels.

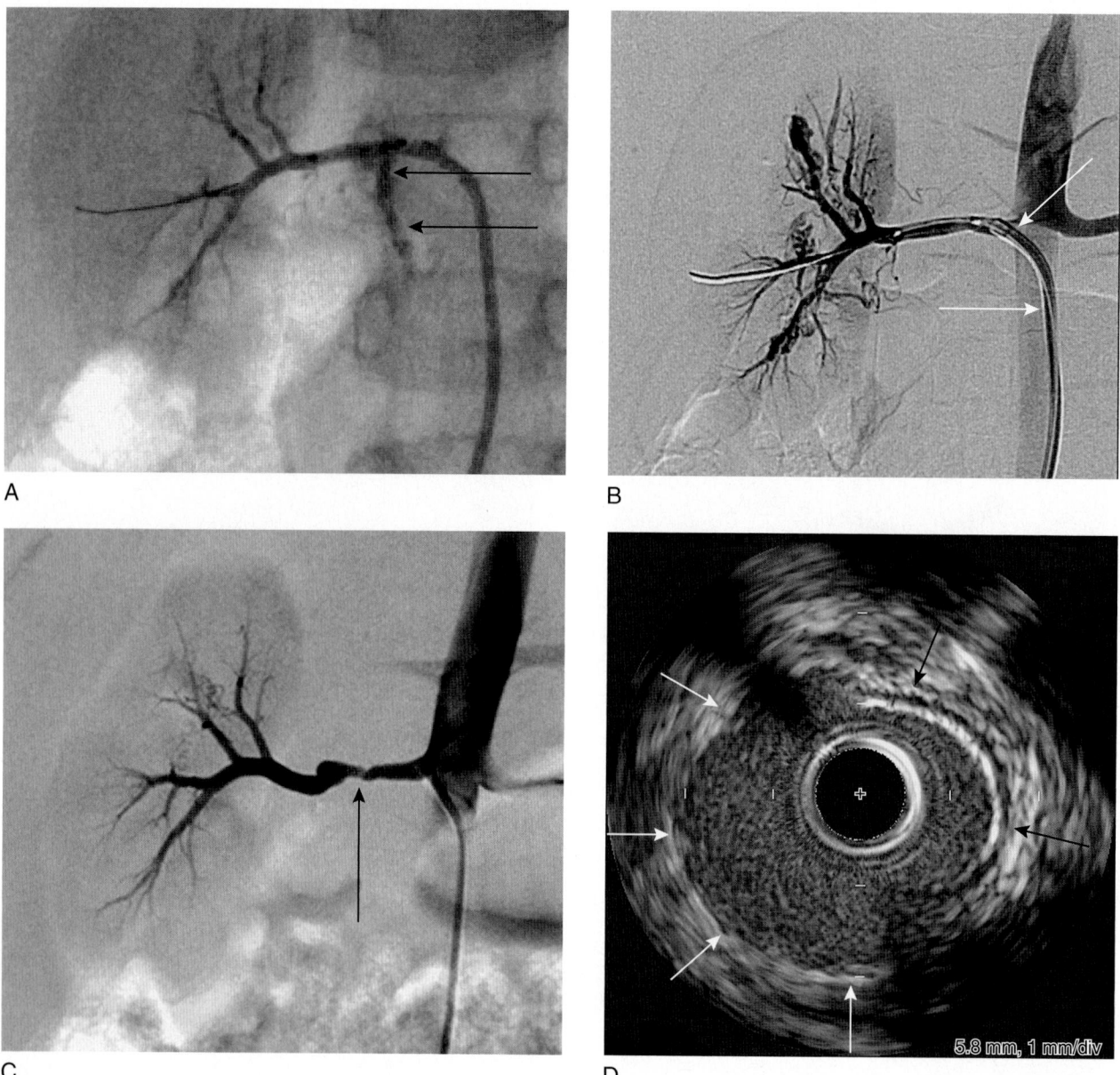

FIGURE 193-2. A 5-year-old boy with hypertension. **A,** A 2.5-mm cutting balloon has been used to dilate a resistant right renal artery stenosis. There is extravasation of contrast *(arrows)* as a consequence of arterial rupture. **B,** Following balloon tamponade, the extravasation has ceased and the right renal artery stenosis is improved. Several segmental branches are occluded, and there are prominent intrarenal collateral arteries. Note that acceptable angiographic images can be obtained by injecting contrast through the guiding catheter *(arrows).* **C,** The patient's hypertension improved at first, but then gradually worsened. Twenty-two months later, angiography shows recurrent stenosis of the right renal artery *(arrow),* with poststenotic dilation. **D,** Intravascular ultrasound image (40 MHz transducer) shows the poststenotic dilation to be a pseudoaneurysm, presumably related to the earlier angioplasty and rupture. The *black arrows* indicate intact arterial wall. The pseudoaneurysm *(white arrows)* has no normal arterial wall.

ANGIOPLASTY

The aim of renal angioplasty is to normalize blood pressure. It is important to recognize that this may be achieved without a perfect angiographic result. Angioplasty is usually performed from a common femoral artery approach, but occasionally a radial, brachial, or axillary sheath is required.

There are two main approaches for access. A long sheath can be placed with its tip at the renal artery ostium (Fig. 193-3). This provides less support for the catheters and guidewire but requires a smaller hole in the femoral artery. A guiding catheter (see Fig. 193-2) gives maximum support and allows better angiography during the procedure at the price of a larger arteriotomy. The guidewire and catheter systems used vary from 0.014 to 0.035 inch. Systems designed for use in adult coronary arteries are ideal for use in small children or segmental arteries.

The diameter of the angioplasty balloon is chosen to be equal to or slightly smaller than the artery proximal to the stenosis. The significance of the vessel diameter

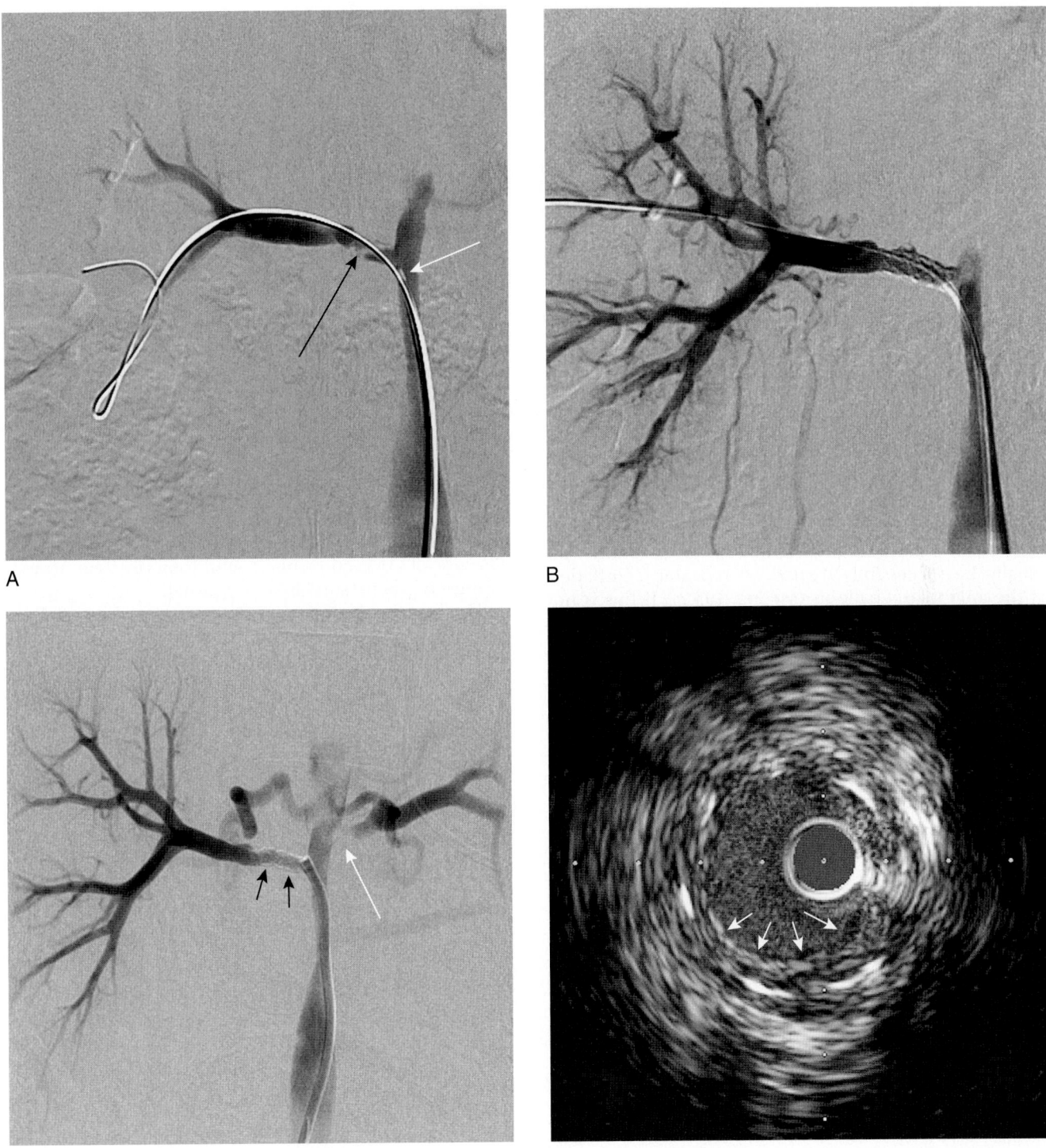

FIGURE 193-3. A 13-year-old girl with neurofibromatosis type 1 and midaortic syndrome. **A,** A tight stenosis of the right renal artery has been dilated with a 3.5-mm balloon. This has caused a significant dissection *(black arrow).* There is also stenosis of the abdominal aorta. The *white arrow* indicates the tip of a long arterial sheath. **B,** Repeat inflation of the angioplasty balloon did not improve the dissection, and a balloon-expandable stent was inserted. **C,** Angiography performed 16 months later shows tight stenosis of the left renal artery *(white arrow)* and possible in-stent restenosis *(black arrows).* **D,** Intravascular ultrasound shows the in-stent restenosis clearly *(arrows).*

distal to the stenosis is more difficult to interpret because poststenotic dilation is common. When inflation does not abolish the waist of a standard angioplasty balloon, a high-pressure balloon or a cutting balloon (see Fig. 193-2) may be used. It is not clear which of these is more likely to cause arterial rupture.

It is sometimes stated that endovascular treatment is contraindicated in MAS, and certainly the abdominal aortic stenosis tends to respond poorly to angioplasty. There are, however, many MAS patients (particularly very young children) who have significant complications of RVH and limited surgical options. In these circumstances it may be appropriate to attempt aortic and renal angioplasty. These procedures require multiple arterial access points to allow the insertion of "safety" guidewires into visceral arteries in case of ostial occlusion.

Procedural complications of angioplasty are not unusual. Arterial spasm is usually self-limiting. Dissection is almost inevitable but is usually not hemodynamically significant. Flow-limiting dissections can be treated by reinflation of the angioplasty balloon to pin back the intimal flap. If this is unsuccessful, stent insertion will be required (see Fig. 193-3). Arterial rupture with retroperitoneal extravasation of contrast is unusual and can usually be successfully treated by repeated reinflation of the angioplasty balloon (see Fig. 193-2). If this is not successful, a covered stent may be deployed across the ruptured segment. Irrecoverable renal artery occlusion or rupture are uncommon, but it is wise to have an experienced vascular surgeon available when angioplasty is performed.

Close postoperative monitoring is required after angioplasty. Heart rate and blood pressure should be recorded frequently for at least 12 hours. Fluctuations in blood pressure are not unusual, and children with cerebrovascular disease are at particular risk during the post-operative period.

It is usual to try to minimize the risk of thrombotic complications by giving low-molecular-weight heparin or, alternatively, intravenous unfractionated heparin (at 10 U kg^{-1} h^{-1} for 12 to 24 hours). Aspirin (1 mg kg^{-1} d^{-1}) is usually prescribed for 3 to 6 months.

The results of pediatric renal angioplasty depend strongly on case selection. In general, only about one in four children discontinue all antihypertensive therapy after angioplasty, but the number of drugs required is reduced in a further 60%. Restenosis occurs in about a quarter of cases, usually within 1 year, and can be treated by repeat angioplasty. Even if endovascular treatment eventually fails, angioplasty may serve to delay the need for surgery until the child is almost fully grown, and this is a worthwhile achievement.

STENTING

Renal artery stenting in children is controversial because the long-term behavior of these devices is unknown, and indications for their use are consequently limited.

Potential indications for renal artery stenting in children.
- **Failed angioplasty**
  - **immediate recoil**
  - **flow-limiting dissection (failed repeat inflation of balloon)**
- **Early recurrence of renal artery stenosis after successful angiography**
- **Kinked transplant renal artery**

As long as there is no compromise of future surgical options, renal artery stenting is an attractive option in certain situations where angioplasty is unsuccessful. Balloon-expandable stents (see Fig. 193-3) are generally preferred in children because they can be post-dilated to some extent to allow for future growth of the patient.

Stenting is technically more difficult than angioplasty in small children, because it is harder to advance the rigid stent from the aorta into a small renal artery. For this reason, a guiding catheter is used where possible. The use of covered stents in children (to treat arterial rupture or aneurysms) is very unusual.

The results of renal artery stenting in children have only been reported in small series and case reports. There is a clear tendency to develop early and sometimes severe in-stent stenosis, especially in small stents, probably because the thickness of neointimal hyperplasia is not proportional to the diameter of the stent.

Absorbable metal stents are currently being evaluated for coronary and peripheral arterial indications in adults. It may be that these devices will find appplications in children with RVH.

ETHANOL ABLATION

Although intra-arterial ethanol is sometimes used to ablate an entire kidney, laparoscopic nephrectomy is now usually preferred for this purpose. Segmental ethanol ablation may be appropriate when angioplasty fails to cure an intrarenal branch stenosis or occlusion that has been confirmed as the hypertensive focus by RVRS (see Fig. 193-1). This technique may be preferable to partial nephrectomy because it minimizes the loss of normal renal tissue. Ethanol causes severe, irreversible endothelial injury from the point of injection to the capillary bed. Embolization coils cause occlusion at the level of medium-sized arteries, and should never be used for this purpose because they will not destroy the ischemic focus, which is supplied by collaterals.

SUGGESTED READINGS

Goonasekera CD, Shah V, Wade AM, Dillon MJ: The usefulness of renal vein renin studies in hypertensive children: a 25-year experience. Pediatr Nephrol 2002;17:943-949

McLaren CA, Roebuck DJ: Interventional radiology for renovascular hypertension in children. Tech Vasc Interv Radiol 2003;6:150-157

National High Blood Pressure Education Program Working Group on High Blood Pressure in Children and Adolescents. The fourth report on the diagnosis, evaluation, and treatment of high blood pressure in children and adolescents. Pediatrics 2004;114:555-576.

Shroff R, Roebuck D, Gordon I, et al: Angioplasty for renovascular hypertension in children—20-year experience. Pediatrics 2006;118:268-275

Tyagi S, Kaul UA, Satsangi DK, Arora A: Percutaneous transluminal angioplasty for renovascular hypertension in children: initial and long-term results. Pediatrics 1997;99:44-49

CHAPTER 194

Pediatric Musculoskeletal Interventional Procedures

JOHN M. RACADIO

Musculoskeletal procedures in children have routinely been performed as open surgical procedures by orthopedic surgeons. With improved musculoskeletal imaging, some procedures have shifted to a percutaneous imaging–guided approach. The spectrum of such musculoskeletal procedures in children includes aspiration and drainage of fluid collections, biopsies of soft tissue and bone lesions, embolization of osseous tumors, vertebroplasty, ablation or drilling of benign tumors, and pain management techniques for malignant tumors.

The transition from surgery to percutaneous techniques has been slower in the musculoskeletal system than in other organ systems. This may be due to a number of unique aspects of bone work that make these procedures different from other traditional interventional radiology (IR) procedures. Most bone procedures require computed tomographic (CT) imaging, and CT time is a scarce resource. Bone procedures require a different set of tools than the traditional "needle, guidewire, catheter" trio needed for most interventional radiology techniques. There has always been a fear that the sterile environment of a radiology department is not a high enough standard to perform orthopedic work and fear of bone infections is justifiably high. The old school teaching that all pediatric osteomyelitis must be drained surgically is also slowly changing. With standards of care for other organ systems now routinely including IR techniques, IR musculoskeletal procedures are also changing.

Just as with every other field of IR, each patient and procedure must be approached with consultation with the appropriate referring physician. Initially, an orthopedic surgeon was always involved, but because some IR procedures have become the standard, sometimes consultation is with a general pediatrician or infectious disease specialist. An orthopedic surgeon is almost always consulted for the more complicated procedures.

MUSCULOSKELETAL BIOPSY

Image-guided percutaneous techniques have obviated the need for many open surgical biopsies of the musculoskeletal system. Advantages of a percutaneous approach include cost-effectiveness, minimal activity limitation following the procedure, rapid recovery time, and usually a decreased need for immobilization. However, if performed without full understanding of lesion anatomy, image guidance, and biopsy equipment, misdiagnosis and complications can occur. Therefore, careful planning and a multidisciplinary approach are critical to the success of percutaneous musculoskeletal biopsy.

> Careful planning and a multidisciplinary approach are critical to the success of percutaneous musculoskeletal biopsy.

Indications for percutaneous biopsy include histologic identification of a suspicious musculoskeletal lesion, confirmation of metastatic disease, or diagnosis of infection such as osteomyelitis or septic arthritis. Contraindications are rare but include inaccessible site adjacent to major structures such as the spinal cord or sciatic nerve, or serious noncorrectable clotting dysfunction. The patient's coagulation status is especially important during deeper biopsies for which direct pressure cannot be applied. An international normalized ratio greater than 1.5 should be treated with fresh frozen plasma, and a platelet count less than 50,000 mm^3 should be treated with platelet transfusion before deep biopsy. In addition, lesions with a classic benign appearance ("do not touch" lesions) should not be biopsied.

Musculoskeletal biopsies must be carefully planned and coordinated with the orthopedic surgeon to avoid transgressing tissue planes that will make later surgery difficult, especially in cases of bone malignancy. In this regard, the radiologist must first examine the lesion composition, and be knowledgeable about which area of the tumor would yield the most productive biopsy. For example, solid tumor components generally yield more diagnostic material than fluid or necrotic areas. Doppler ultrasound (US) is often helpful in determining the viable areas of large tumors. Second, the lesion location and surrounding anatomy should be considered. Any musculoskeletal biopsy of a malignant lesion involves the risk of seeding the needle track with malignant cells, and therefore, the track must be removed during later surgical tumor resection. The local anatomy should also be reviewed in order to define the shortest path, while avoiding neurovascular bundles and unperturbed compartments. Finally, it is imperative that appropriate tests be ordered on the biopsy specimen. This requires coordination of the radiologist with the clinicians and the orthopedic pathologist before performing the biopsy.

As a general rule, most soft tissue lesions are sampled with cutting needles and core biopsy devices. The majority of sclerotic osseous lesions are biopsied with larger needles such as the 14-gauge Bonopty (RADI Medical Systems, Uppsala, Sweden) or the 11-gauge Jamshidi (Kormed C., Minneapolis, MN). The 11-gauge and 8-gauge Gallini devices (Gallini US, Grand Rapids, MI) are also useful because they have a large and comfortable handle and the cutting tip is slightly tapered, allowing a long biopsy specimen without jamming of the specimen within the device. For access through long segments of bone, a surgical mallet or manual or electric drill may be necessary.

The radiologist must also carefully consider choice of imaging modality. US is convenient and effective for superficial soft tissue lesions. Fluoroscopy is fast and easy to use, and can be used for radiographically visible lesions for which adjacent neurovascular structures are not a concern. However, fluoroscopy has low tissue contrast and therefore is not useful for lesions with large cystic or necrotic areas. CT fluoroscopy allows excellent visualization of tissue types and local anatomy, while still providing the convenience of real-time guidance. Finally, magnetic resonance (MR) guidance is beginning to be used for lesions that are not visible with other modalities.

With careful planning, including coordination between radiologists, clinicians, surgeons, and pathologists, percutaneous musculoskeletal biopsy can be highly successful and be performed with minimal risk or discomfort.

OSTEOID OSTEOMA

Osteoid osteoma is a small, painful, benign osteogenic tumor that occurs primarily in children and young adults. Surgical excision has traditionally been the treatment of choice for these lesions; however, intraoperative localization can be difficult and large bone resection may be necessary, resulting in bone weakness and risk of fractures. Therefore, percutaneous treatments have been developed, and radiofrequency (RF) ablation has now become the first line treatment for osteoid osteomas.

> **Radiofrequency (RF) ablation has become the first line treatment for osteoid osteomas.**

RF ablation is usually performed under general anesthesia and with CT guidance (Fig. 194-1). A biopsy needle is introduced through the bone using a cannula or a drill when necessary. A biopsy can be performed in cases in which the diagnosis is in doubt. An RF electrode (5-mm noncooled tip or 1-cm cooled tip) connected to a

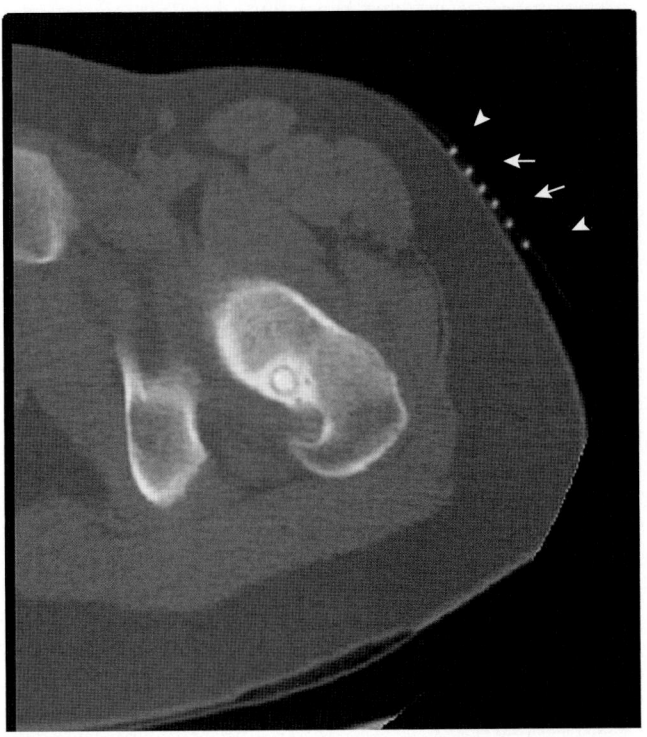
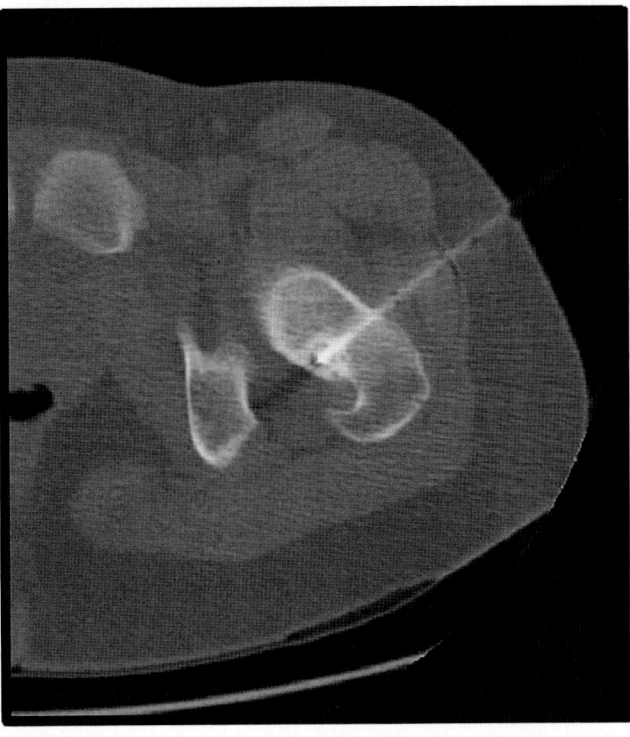

A   B

FIGURE 194-1. Osteoid osteoma. **A,** Axial CT shows the classic appearance of an osteoid osteoma in left femoral neck. Markers on the skin *(arrows)* help plan the best percutaneous approach. **B,** After drilling down to the nidus, an RF probe is positioned with the active tip in the center of the lesion and ablation is performed.

generator is introduced. The tip temperature is slowly increased, with a goal of maintaining lesion temperature at about 95°C for approximately 6 minutes. Large or elongated lesions may require treatment at two adjacent levels to ensure complete tumor ablation.

Reported primary success rates of RF ablation for osteoid osteoma range from 79% to 97%. Success rates are similar to those noted with surgical excision; however, recovery is much shorter. Patients are usually able to bear full weight and resume normal activity immediately. In cases of recurrent or persistent symptoms, RF ablation can be repeated, although the success rate decreases. Complications are rare but include local burns, cellulitis, and sympathetic dystrophy. RF ablation should be used very cautiously or not at all within 1 cm of articular cartilage or major nerves. Percutaneous CT-guided manual removal and curettage is indicated in these areas.

JOINT INJECTION

Intra-articular corticosteroids have been successfully used to treat children with juvenile idiopathic arthritis. Traditionally, injections have been reserved for children in whom non-steroidal anti-inflammatory drugs have been unsuccessful in controlling disease. However, many pediatric rheumatologists now recommend intra-articular steroid injection early in the disease to rapidly resolve synovitis, offer pain relief, facilitate physical therapy, and allow avoidance or withdrawal of regular systemic treatment. Most reports in the literature have focused on steroid injection of knee joints; they have demonstrated full remission for more than 6 months in 70% to 80% of patients. Other studies have shown a mean duration of clinical improvement of up to 74 weeks. Although knee joint injection is most commonly reported, other joints have also been shown to be effectively treated in juvenile idiopathic arthritis, including the wrist, elbow, shoulder, hip, ankle, hindfoot, interphalanges, and even temporomandibular joints and tendon sheaths.

Most joint injections can be performed using local skin anesthesia such as 1% lidocaine. Conscious sedation or even general anesthesia may be required for very young or anxious children or for multiple joint injections. Adult series have demonstrated that non–image-guided injection of even superficially palpable large joints such as the knee results in intra-articular delivery of medication in only 70% of cases. Although typically fluoroscopy with minimal contrast injection is used to confirm intra-articular needle tip position, US can also be useful, particularly with tendon sheath injections, where microbubbles can be seen flowing freely into tendon sheath fluid. In general, the smallest diameter (highest gauge) needle should be used to minimize leakage of steroid back along the needle tract into the surrounding soft tissues. A 25- to 27-G needle is usually effective for injection, although a larger needle may be necessary if aspiration of a joint effusion is anticipated.

Although relatively insoluble preparations such as triamcinolone acetonide (Kenalog) and triamcinolone hexacetonide (Aristospan) are believed to have a longer duration of action and are most commonly used, injection into periarticular soft tissues can cause local skin and fat atrophy, muscle wasting, or tendon weakening and rupture. Multiple steroid injections (10 or more including large joints) may have sufficient systemic absorption to produce a transient cushingoid appearance and transient adrenal suppression, although no long-term adverse effects have been reported. A 0.002% risk of septic arthritis with intra-articular steroid injections has been reported in the adult literature. Although this risk is very low, strict aseptic technique should always be used. Typical dosage regimen for Aristospan is 1 mg/kg for large joints (knees, hips, and shoulders), 0.5 mg/kg for smaller joints (ankles, wrists, and elbows), 1 to 2 mg/joint for MCPs/MTPs, and 0.6 to 1 mg/joint for proximal interphalangeals (PIPs). Although there is no consensus recommendation, rest and reduction in weight bearing for 24 to 48 hours is commonly advised.

Although US and fluoroscopy are the preferred imaging modalities for injection of most joints of the extremities, CT is particularly effective in guiding precise intra-articular access into vertebral facet joints and sacroiliac joints (Fig. 194-2). Percutaneous injection into these joints can help determine whether or not the accessd joint is involved in the patient's pain syndrome. Injection of steroid/anesthetic mixtures can also provide significant pain relief.

JOINT ASPIRATION

Although fluoroscopy uses bony landmarks to help identify joint spaces, US can directly visualize joint effusions and direct intra-articular needle advancement. US-guided arthrocentesis has been reported to have success rates of greater than 95% for both large and small joints. Generally 20- to 22-gauge needles are used. Sonography can be particularly helpful in guiding arthrocentesis of hip joint effusions. With the US probe parallel to the long axis of the femoral neck, an anterior parasagittal approach is chosen such that the femoral neurovascular structures lie medial to the intended needle path. With this longitudinal approach the entire needle length can be visualized as the needle tip is advanced through the distended capsule into the hip joint effusion at the junction of the femoral head and neck (Fig. 194-3).

> **Sonography can be particularly helpful in guiding arthrocentesis of hip joint effusions.**

US is also helpful in guiding most soft tissue fluid aspirations of suspected infection or abscess. If needed, percutaneous drainage catheters can be placed using standard "over-the-wire" techniques; in these cases, the addition of fluoroscopy can help guide soft tissue tract dilation to avoid kinking of the wire.

ARTHROGRAPHY

MR arthrography enhances the imaging sensitivity of MR in the evaluation of shoulder instability by providing

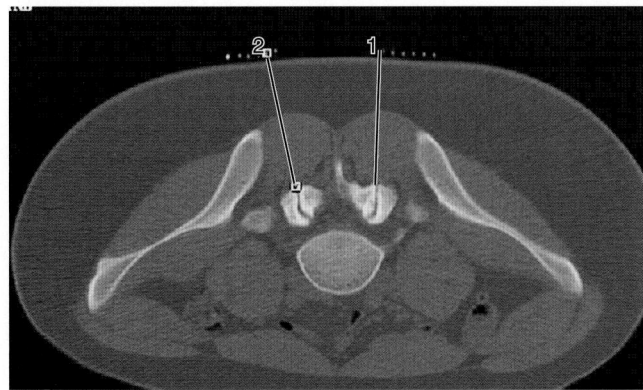

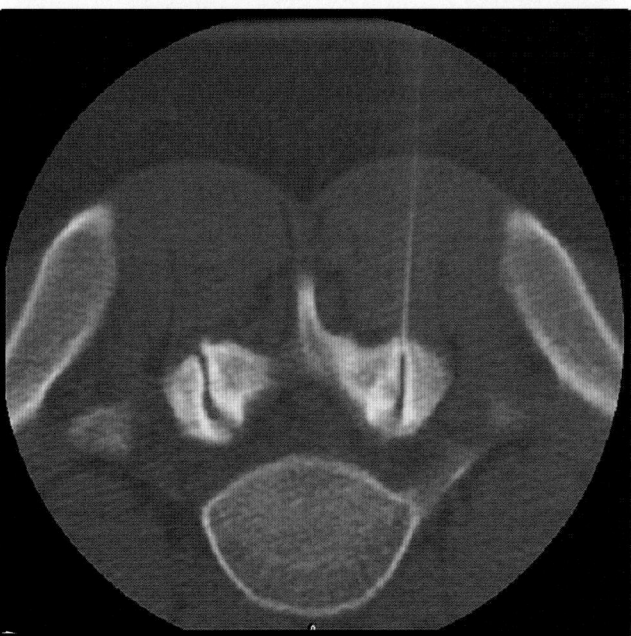

FIGURE 194-2. Joint injection. **A,** With the patient in a prone position, preprocedural computed tomographic (CT) scan with skin markers allows optimal planning of angle and depth of anticipated needle approach. **B,** CT scan confirms intra-articular needle tip position.

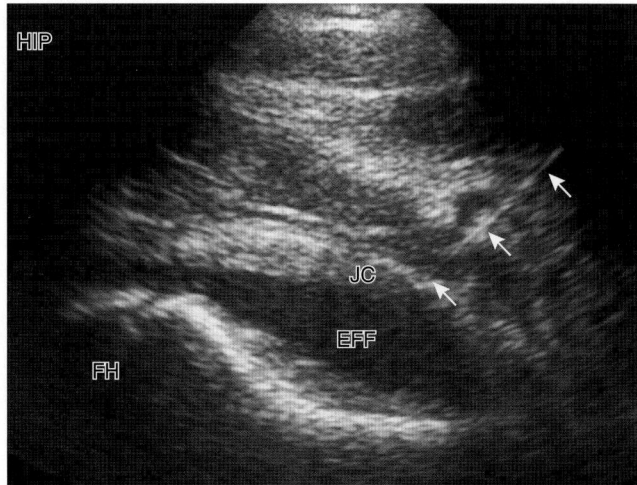

FIGURE 194-3. Joint aspiration. Longitudinal ultrasound at the femoral head and neck junction allows real-time visualization of the needle *(arrows)* as it pierces the distended joint capsule to enter the effusion. FH, femoral head; JC, joint capsule, EFF; effusion.

capsular distension and separation of intra-articular structures to better visualize the labroligamentous complex. The joint is most often accessed under fluoroscopic guidance, but US can be used as well. Although shoulder arthrography has been traditionally performed through an anterior approach, the posterior approach has recently gained popularity for several reasons. Most patients have anterior instability; if an anterior approach is performed, any contrast that is inadvertently injected into the extracapsular soft tissues may cause interpretive difficulties. With an anterior needle approach, it may be difficult to discern if some abnormalities in the anterior labroligamentous complex represent true pathology or could possibly be iatrogenic related to the procedure itself. A posterior approach (for patients with suspected anterior instability) avoids the potential for these interpretive difficulties (Fig. 194-4). In children, the posterior approach also has the added benefit of decreasing anxiety that may be provoked when a child sees a long needle advancing toward his or her shoulder. In most cases, MR arthrography can be performed with only local skin or soft tissue lidocaine anesthesia.

ANEURYSMAL BONE CYST

Traditional open surgical treatment of aneurysmal bone cysts involving extensive curettage and bone grafting or in bloc resection can still have a relatively high rate of lesion recurrence. CT and fluoroscopically guided percutaneous injections of sclerosing agents have been used successfully to treat these lesions. The most widely used agent has been Ethibloc (an emulsion of an alcoholic solution of zein, a contrast medium; oleum papaveris; and propylene glycol). One recent study reported a high rate of major local and general complications including extrusion of agent into surrounding soft tissues, aseptic abscess, and even pulmonary embolus; one death from embolization of Ethibloc into the vertebral artery has also been reported. Proponents insist that these types of complications can be prevented if meticulous technique is followed including fluoroscopic evaluation during contrast injection to verify contrast distribution, venous opacification, and leakage into soft tissues prior to the Ethibloc sclerosant injection.

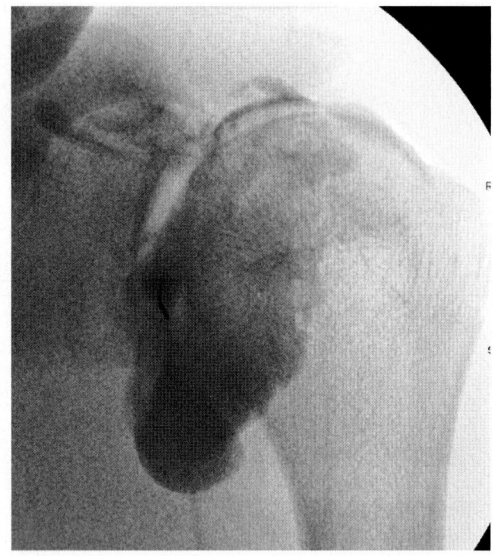
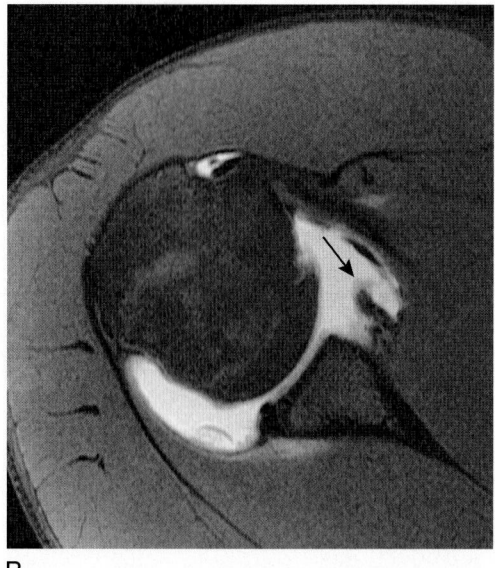

A **B**

FIGURE 194-4. Arthrography. **A,** With the patient in a prone oblique position, fluoroscopy helps guide advancement of a 20-gauge spinal needle into the shoulder joint through a posterior approach. Iodinated contrast and gadolinium injection confirms intra-articular needle tip position. **B,** Axial T1 MRI with fat saturation following intra-articular gadolinium injection demonstrates a displaced osteochondral fracture of the anterior labrum *(arrow)*.

SUGGESTED READINGS

Adamsbaum C, Kalifa G, Seringe R, et al: Direct Ethibloc injection in benign bone cysts: preliminary report on four patients. Skeletal Radiol 1993;22:317-320

Anderson MW, Temple HT, Dussault RD, et al: Compartmental anatomy: Relevance to staging and biopsy of musculoskeletal tumors. Am J Roentgenol 1999;173:1663-1671

Arabshahi B, Dewitt EM, Chill AM, et al: Utility of corticosteroid injection for temporomandibular arthritis in children with juvenile idiopathic arthritis. Arthritis Rheum 2005; 52:3563-3569

Balint PV, Kane D, Hunter J, et al: Ultrasound guided versus conventional joint and soft tissue fluid aspiration in rheumatology practice: a pilot study. J Rheumatol 2002;29:2209-2213

Breit W, Frosch M, Meyer U, et al: A subgroup-specific evaluation of the efficacy of intraarticular triamcinolone hexacetonide in juvenile chronic arthritis. J Rheumatol 2000;27:2696-2702

Cardinal E, Chhem RK, Beauregard CG: Ultrasound-guided interventional procedures in the musculoskeletal system. Radiol Clin North Am 1998;36:597-604

Centeno LM, Moore ME: Preferred intraarticular corticosteroids and associated practice: a survey of members of the American college of Rheumatology. Arthritis Care Res 1994;7:151-155

Choi JJ, Davis KW, Blankenbaker DG: Percutaneous musculoskeletal biopsy. Semin Roentgenol 2004;39:114-128

Chou MC, Yeh LR, Chen CK, et al: Comparison of plain MRI and MR arthrography in the evaluation of lateral ligamentous injury of the ankle joint. J Chin Med Assoc 2006;69:26-31

Cioni R, Armillotta N, Bargellini I, et al: CT-guided radiofrequency ablation of osteoid osteoma: long-term results. Eur Radiol 2004;14:1203-1208

Cleary AG, Murphy HD, Davidson JE: Intra-articular corticosteroid injections in juvenile idiopathic arthritis. Arch Dis Child 2003;88:192-196

Davis KW, Choi JJ, Blankenbaker DG: Radiofrequency ablation in the musculoskeletal system. Semin Roentgenol 2004;39:129-144

deGauzy JS, Abid A, Accadbled F, et al: Percutaneous Ethibloc injection in the treatment of primary aneurismal bone cysts. J Pediatr Orthop B 2005;14:367-370

Falappa P, Fassary FM, Fanelli A, et al: Aneurysmal bone cysts. Treatment with direct percutaneous Ethibloc injection: long term results. Cardiovasc Intervent Radiol 2002;25:282-290

Farmer KD, Hughes PM: MR arthrography of the shoulder: Fluoroscopically guided technique using a posterior approach. AJR 2002;178:433-434

Garg NK, Carty H, Walsh HP, et al: Percutaneous Ethibloc injection in aneurysmal bone cysts. Skeletal Radiol 2000;29:211-216

Ghanem I, Collet LM, Kharrat K, et al: Percutaneous radiofrequency coagulation of osteoid osteoma in children and adolescents. J Pediatr Orthop B 2003;12:244-252

Guibaud L, Herbreteau D, Dubois J, et al: Aneurysmal bone cysts: percutaneous embolization with an alcoholic solution of zein— series of 18 cases. Radiology 1998;208:369-373

Hoffer FA: Biopsy, needle localization, and radiofrequency ablation for pediatric patients. Tech Vasc Interv Radiol 2003;6:192-196

Huppertz HI, Tschammler A, Horwitz AE, Schwab KO: Intraarticular corticosteroids for chronic arthritis in children: efficacy and effects on cartilage and growth. J Pediatr 1995;127:317-321

Jackson DW, Evans NA, Thomas BM: Accuracy of needle placement into the intra-articular space of the knee. J Bone Joint Surg Am 2002;84:1522-1527

Johnson ND: Pediatric bone biopsy and therapeutic procedures. Seminars in Interventional Radiology 2002;19:99-109

Lanyon P, Doherty M: Intra-articular therapy. *In* Firestein GS, Panayi GS, Wollheim FA (eds): Rheumatoid Arthritis: Frontiers in Pathogenesis and Treatment. Oxford, UK, Oxford University Press, 2000:361-369

Martel J, Bueno A, Ortiz E. Percutaneous radiofrequency treatment of osteoid osteoma using cool-tip electrodes Eur J Radiol 2005;56:403-408

Padeh S, Passwell JH: Intraarticular corticosteroid injection in the management of children with chronic arthritis. Arthritis Rheum 1998;41:1210-1214

Ravelli A, Manzoni SM, Viola S, et al: Factors affecting the efficacy of intraarticular corticosteroid injection of knees in juvenile idiopathic arthritis. J Rheumatol 2001;28:2100-2102

Raza K, Lee CY, Pilling D, et al: Ultrasound guidance allows accurate needle placement and aspiration from small joints in patients with early inflammatory arthritis. Rheumatology 2003;42:976-979

Rosenthal DI, Hornicek FJ, Torriani M, et al: Osteoid osteoma: Percutaneous treatment with radiofrequency energy. Radiology 2003;229:171-175

Rosenthal DI, Hornicek FJ, Wolfe MW, et al: Percutaneous radiofrequency coagulation of osteoid osteoma compared with operative treatment. J Bone Joint Surg Am 1998;80:815-821

Schumacher HR, Chen LX: Injectable corticosteroids in treatment of arthritis of the knee. Am J Med 2005;118:1208-1214

Silbergleit R, Mehta BA, Sanders WP, Talati SJ: Imaging-guided injection techniques with fluoroscopy and CT for spinal pain management. Radiographics 2001;21:927-939

Sofka CM, Saboeiro G, Adler RS: Ultrasound-guided adult hip injections. J Vasc Interv Radiol 2005;16:1121-1123

Southwood TR: ABC of rheumatology: arthritis in children. BMJ 1995;310:728-732

Stallmeyer MJ, Ortiz AO: Facet blocks and sacroiliac joint injections. Tech Vasc Interv Radiol 2002;5:201-206

Stetson WB, Phillips T, Deutsch A: The use of magnetic resonance arthrography to detect partial-thickness rotator cuff tears. J Bone Joint Surg Am 2005;87:81-88

Thanos L, Mylona S, Kalioras V, et al: Percutaneous CT-guided interventional procedures in musculoskeletal system (our experience). Eur J Radiol 2004;50:273-277

Topouchian V, Mazda K, Hamze B, et al: Aneurysmal bone cysts in children: Complications of fibrosing agent injection. Radiology 2004;232:522-526

Weidner S, Kellner W, Kellner H: Interventional radiology and the musculoskeletal system. Best Pract Res Clin Rheumatol 2004; 18:945-956

INDEX

Note: Page numbers followed by the letter f refer to figures, and those followed by t refer to tables.

Angiogenesis
  in vascular development, 1511
  physiology of, 3118
Angiography
  airway and neck, 1057
  cardiovascular
    aortic coarctation, 369f
    iliac artery malformation, 3107f
    Kawasaki disease, 3134, 3134f, 3135f
    vascular rings, 1593
    venovenous collaterals, 1754f
    ventricular, balloon valvuloplasty for,
      1748
  cerebral, 643, 643f, 825, 827, 3088,
      3089f-3090f
    aneurysm, 829, 3088, 3089f-3090f
    arteriovenous fistula, 832f
    arteriovenous malformations, 825,
      3095f, 3097f-3098f, 3127f
    computed tomography, 624-625
    dural arteriovenous fistula, 3086f-3088f
    hemangioma, 3121f
    magnetic resonance, 636-638, 637f
    moyamoya disease, 835f-836f
    moyamoya pattern, 833, 838f, 839f
    mycotic aneurysm, 772f
    PHACES syndrome, 838f
    polyarteritis nodosa, 3137f
    primary angiitis, 833, 835, 840f
    sinus pericranii, 842f
    tumors, 790
    varicella-mediated vasculitis, 841f
    vascular malformations, 830t
    vasculitis, 834f, 839f
    vasculopathy, 831, 835f-836f
    vein of Galen malformation, 3093f
    venous angioma, 829f
    venous anomalies, 844f
  computed tomography. See Computed
      tomography angiography (CTA).
  hepatobiliary, 1860
    hemangioendothelioma, 3108f, 3122
    hemangioma, 3118
    hepatic artery pseudoaneurysm, 3175f
    hepatic artery trauma, 3173f
  magnetic resonance. See Magnetic
      resonance angiography (MRA).
  mesenteric, 3103, 3105, 3108f, 3109f
  musculoskeletal
    dermatomyositis, 3138f
    extremities, 3103, 3106f, 3107f
    osteoid osteoma, 2937
    polyarteritis nodosa, 3136f
    popliteal artery injury, 3106f
  pulmonary
    bronchial artery embolization, 3081,
      3082f
    hereditary hemorrhagic telangiectasia,
      1302f, 1303
    polysplenia, 1609f
    pulmonary embolism, 1265, 1678
  renal, 2235f
    polyarteritis nodosa, 3137f
    renovascular hypertension, 2306-2307,
      3184-3185, 3186f
    stenosis, 2308, 2308f
  spinal, 935, 966-967
  unspecified location
    arteriovenous malformations, 3126
    vascular anomalies, 3117, 3119t
    venous malformations, 3123
  vascular access for. See Vascular access.
Angioma
  cavernous, 825, 828f, 830t
  intracranial, 825, 829f, 830t
  scalp, 519

Angioma—cont'd
  tufted, 2529, 3122
  venous, 825, 829f, 830t
Angiomatosis, encephalotrigeminal.
    See Sturge-Weber syndrome.
Angiomyolipoma
  abdominal wall, 1827, 1827f
  hepatic, 1936-1937, 1937f
  in tuberous sclerosis, 680, 2255, 2709-2710
  renal, 2255, 2287-2288, 2288f
Angio-osteohypertrophy syndrome. See
    Klippel-Trénaunay syndrome.
Angiopathy. See Vasculopathy.
Angioplasty
  aortic, 1729, 1749-1750
  cerebral
    aneurysm, 3088, 3089f-3090f
    dural arteriovenous fistula, 3085
  pulmonary artery, 1749
  renal, 3186, 3187f, 3188
Angiosarcoma
  hepatic, 1943, 1944f
  littoral cell, splenomegaly in, 1979, 1981
  splenomegaly in, 1979, 1981
Angiotensin-converting enzyme
  in renovascular hypertension, 2305-2306
  in sarcoidosis, 1888
Angiotensin-converting enzyme inhibitors, in
    renography, 1801
"Angle" sign, in scurvy, 2740, 2740f
Angular artery, angiography of, 643f
Aniridia, nephroblastomatosis with, 2281
Anisospondyly, in
    dysspondyloendochondromatosis,
    2658, 2666f
Ankle
  in clubfoot, 2876, 2877f
  in congenital insensitivity to pain, 2676,
    2678f
  in hemophilia, 3035
  in Larsen syndrome, 2687, 2687f
  in McKusick-type metaphyseal
    chondroplasia, 2643f
  in metaphyseal chondrodysplasia, 2641f
  in osteochondritis dissecans, 2831, 2832f
  in osteolysis syndromes, 2702, 2703f
  in oxalosis, 2750f
  in proximal femoral focal deficiency, 2596f
  in septic arthritis, 3034f
  in synovial osteochondromatosis, 3042f
  in tarsal coalition, 2603
  neuropathic, 3038f
Ankylosing spondylitis, juvenile, 3028, 3030f
Ankylosis, in juvenile rheumatoid arthritis,
    3020
Annular bands, 2599-2600, 2600f
Annular cartilage, spinal, 872
Annular pancreas, 141, 1986-1987, 1987f,
    2106
Anomalous pulmonary connection
  partial, 1550-1551, 1551f, 1552f
  total. See Total anomalous pulmonary
    venous connection.
Anophthalmia, 536, 536f
Anorchidism, 2402, 2409, 2462
Anorectum
  anatomy of, 2158
  atresia of, 2162
  bleeding from, 216t
  congenital anomalies of, horseshoe kidney
    with, 2247
  duplications of, 2164-2165, 2168, 2168f,
    2169f
  imperforate, 142. See also Currarino
    triad/syndrome.
    in McKusick-Kaufmann syndrome, 2690

Anorectum—cont'd
  imperforate—cont'd
    in spinal dysraphism, 444f
    prostatic utricle with, 2383
  in functional constipation, 2174-2176,
    2175f
  in Hirschsprung disease, 2161, 2163f
  in VACTERL association. See VACTERL
    (vertebra, anal atresia, cardiac,
    tracheal, esophageal, renal, limb)
    association.
  malformations of, 216, 218-219, 219f-225f
  stenosis of, 2162-2164, 2167f
Anorexia, cardiovascular manifestations of,
    1686t, 1694-1695
Anovulation, 2446, 2456
"Anteater nose" appearance, in tarsal
    coalition, 2603, 2604f
Antecubital bone, 2569, 2569f
Antegonial notching, of mandible, 607
Anterior cruciate ligaments, injury of,
    2845-2846, 2849f
Anterior junction line, mediastinal, 1325,
    1325f, 1326f
Anterior urethral diverticulum, 2386-2387,
    2387f
Antibiotic(s), prophylactic
  for gastrostomy tube, 3154
  for interventional procedures, 3072, 3072t
  for urinary procedures, 3180
Antibiotic-associated diarrhea
    (pseudomembranous colitis),
    2193-2194, 2194f
Antibody(ies). See also Immunoglobulin(s).
  dysfunction of, immunodeficiency in,
    1231-1232, 1232f, 1233f
Anticoagulation, for interventional
    procedures, 3073, 3073t
Anticonvulsants, rickets due to, 2736
Antireflux surgery
  for gastroesophageal reflux, 2045-2046,
    2046f, 2047f
  for vesicoureteral reflux, 2349-2350, 2349f,
    2350f
Antronasal polyps, 555, 557f
Antropyloric web, 2065-2066, 2066f
Anulus fibrosus, 873, 873f, 876f, 884f
Anuria, in acute tubular necrosis, 2291
Aorta
  anastomosis of, for coarctation, 1729
  anatomy of, 1667, 1668f, 1669t
  aneurysms of, 1368, 1374f
    clinical manifestations of, 1668t
    formation of, 1668
    in Ehlers-Danlos syndrome, 1674-1675,
      1674f, 1675t
    in infection, 1669-1670, 1669f
    in Loeys-Dietz syndrome, 1675
    in Marfan syndrome, 1610, 1672-1674,
      1672f
    in neurocutaneous diseases, 1676-1677,
      1677f
    in Takayasu arteritis, 3137-3138, 3140f,
      3141f
    in tuberous sclerosis, 1677
    mycotic, 1485f, 1642, 1643f
  angioplasty of, 1749-1750
  circumflex
    left aortic arch with, 1597
    right aortic arch with, 1593, 1596f, 1597
  coarctation of. See Aortic coarctation.
  congenital anomalies of
    aorticopulmonary window, 1329f, 1330,
      1354, 1528-1529, 1528f, 1529f
    in Marfan syndrome, 2688
    prenatal diagnosis of, 356, 357f

Spine—cont'd
in dysspondyloendochondromatosis, 2658, 2666f
in Ehlers-Danlos syndrome, 2678
in Gaucher disease, 2683f, 2981
in Hadju-Cheney syndrome, 2682
in Hallermann-Streiff syndrome, 2682
in hematopoietic growth factor therapy, 2989f
in homocystinuria, 2684, 2685f
in Hurler syndrome, 2648, 2651f
in hyperparathyroidism, 2756f
in hypochondrogenesis, 2625
in hypoparathyroidism, 2762f
in hypophosphatasia, 2651, 2653
in hypothyroidism, 2764
in juvenile rheumatoid arthritis, 3020, 3026f
in Kniest dysplasia, 2631, 2633f
in Kozlowski-type spondylometaphyseal dysplasia, 2642, 2645f
in Langerhans cell histiocytosis, 2933, 2934f
in leukemia, 2983f, 3006, 3007f
in McKusick-type metaphyseal chondroplasia, 2642
in Marfan syndrome, 2688, 2688f
in Marshall-Smith syndrome, 2689
in metaphyseal chondrodysplasia, 2639
in metatropic dysplasia, 2618, 2622f
in Morquio syndrome, 2650
in mucolipidosis, 2654f
in mucopolysaccharidoses, 2692-2693, 2692f, 2694f
in multiple epiphyseal dysplasia, 2635
in neurofibromatosis, 2692-2693, 2692f, 2694f
in osteogenesis imperfecta, 2650
in osteopetrosis, 2656, 2657f, 2659f
in oxalosis, 2750f
in pseudoachondroplasia, 2635, 2637f
in rhizomelic chondrodysplasia punctata, 2636
in short rib–polydactyly dysplasia, 2620
in sickle cell disease, 3002, 3003f
in spondyloenchondromatosis, 2658, 2665f
in spondyloepiphyseal dysplasia congenita, 2627
in spondyloepiphyseal dysplasia tarda, 2631, 2634f
in thanatophoric dysplasia, 2616, 2617f-2618f
in trisomy 21, 2714
in VACTERL association, 2710
in vitamin A excess, 2746
in Wolf-Hirschhorn syndrome, 2716, 2718f
length of, 872
metastasis to, 2963f, 2986
neuroblastoma of, 2218-2219, 2220f, 2222f
osteosarcoma of, 2940f
physiology of, 431-432
radiotherapy effects on, 17t, 2990, 2991f
stenosis of, 695, 696f
trauma to. See Spinal trauma.
tumors of. See Spinal tumors.
"Spinnaker" sign, in pneumomediastinum, 1333
"Spinning top" urethra, 2374, 2375, 2376f, 2391
Spinous process
fractures of, 917-918, 922f
vertebral, 871, 871f
Spiral fractures, 2818
Spiral organ of Corti, anatomy of, 581

Spleen, 1970-1982
abscess of, 1976-1977, 1976f
absence of. See Asplenia syndrome.
accessory, 1971-1972
anatomy of, 1970
calcification in, 1976
congenital anomalies of, 182, 1971-1974, 1973f-1975f
cysts of, 1976, 1977, 1978f
dysfunction of, immunodeficiency in, 1238
embryology of, 1970
enlarged. See Splenomegaly.
fungal infections of, 3148f
hemorrhage of, 2470f
imaging of, 1970-1971, 1971f
in Gaucher disease, 1886, 1887f, 2682, 2683f
in situs abnormalities, 1972-1974, 1975f
in splenogonadal syndrome, 1972, 1974f
infections of, 1976-1977, 1976f
iron deposition in, 1884, 1884f
kidney relationship to, 2237f
mediastinal, 1385f
metastasis to, 1981, 1981f
multiple. See Polysplenia.
pseudocyst of, 1977, 1979f
scintigraphy of, 1773, 1775
size of, 1970
trauma to, 1979f, 2466-2467, 2466f, 2467f
tumors and tumor-like conditions of
benign, 1977, 1978f, 1979f
malignant, 1978-1979, 1980f, 1981, 1981f
wandering, 1972, 1973f
Splenectomy, immunodeficiency after, 1230t, 1238
Splenic artery
imaging of, 1971, 1971f
in wandering spleen, 1972, 1973f
Splenic flexure, 2158, 2158f
Splenic sequestration scintigraphy, 1770t, 1775
Splenic vein
imaging of, 1971, 1971f
in portal hypertension, 1908, 1914f
in portosystemic shunt, 1901f, 1902f
Splenogonadal syndrome, 1972, 1974f
Splenoma (hamartoma), 1977
Splenomegaly
definition of, 1974
differential diagnosis of, 1975-1976, 1975t
fatty liver with, 1882f
in infections, 1976-1977, 1976f
in juvenile rheumatoid arthritis, 3017
in neoplasms
benign, 1977, 1978f, 1979f
malignant, 1978-1979, 1980f, 1981, 1981f
in Niemann-Pick disease, 2699
in peliosis hepatis, 1886
in portal hypertension, 1909
in sarcoidosis, 1888, 1889f
in thalassemia, 2997
in tyrosinemia, 1891
versus hypersplenism, 1974-1975
Splenuli (accessory spleens), 1971-1972
Split cord malformation
neonatal, 443
prenatal diagnosis of, 438, 439f
"Split fat sign," in neurofibromatosis, 2691
Split hand-foot malformation, 2608, 2610f
Split notochord, 445t, 2016-2017, 2063
"Split pleura" sign, 1440
"Spoke wheel" appearance, in polycystic kidney disease, 294, 295f
SPONASTRIME acronym, for osteopathia striata, 2658

Spondylitis, mediastinal masses in, 1379
Spondyloarthropathies, juvenile, 3026-3031
clinical features of, 3026
imaging of, 3013t, 3030-3031, 3031f
in cystic fibrosis, 3031
in inflammatory bowel disease, 3029
juvenile ankylosing spondylitis, 3028, 3030f
psoriatic arthritis, 3029
reactive arthritis, 3028-3029
seronegative, 3027
spectrum of, 3026
types of, 3026-3027
whiskering, 3030
Spondylocostal dysostosis, 897
Spondyloenchondromatosis, 894, 2658, 2665f
Spondyloepiphyseal dysplasia congenita, 886, 2614t, 2625, 2627, 2630f, 2631
Spondyloepiphyseal dysplasia tarda, 2631, 2634f
Spondylolysis, 918, 920, 923f
Spondylometaphyseal dysplasia
Kozlowski-type, 2642, 2645f
vertebral malformations in, 894
Spondylometaphyseal dysplasia group, 2614t, 2642, 2645f
Spongiosa, 872, 2546, 2546f, 2547f
Sports-related injuries, 2831-2852
avulsion, 2837-2849, 2841f-2843f
epiphyseal, 2831-2833, 2832f-2836f
knee, 2844-2851
ligament injury, 2845-2846, 2849f
meniscal injury, 2844, 2848f, 2849f
patellar dislocation, 2848, 2851, 2851f
patellar tendon injury, 2846-2847, 2859f
osteochondral, 2831-2833, 2832f-2836f
osteochondritis dissecans, 2831-2832, 2832f-2835f
overuse, 2833-2836, 2837f-2840f
soft-tissue, 2840-2844, 2844f-2847f
statistics on, 2831
"Spot weld" formation, in dorsal dermal sinus, 973
Sprengel deformity, 889, 890f, 1410, 1412f
"Spring onion" appearance, in ureterocele, 2329, 2333f
Sprue, nontropical (celiac disease), 2125-2126, 2148
Squamoparietal suture, 465f
Squamosal suture, neonatal, 454f, 455f
Squamous bone, 579, 580f
Squamous cell carcinoma, abdominal wall, 1829
Squamous cells, of temporal bone, 580f, 581f
Staghorn calculi, 2275, 2275f, 2277
Stapedial artery, persistent, 589, 592f
Stapes
anatomy of, 580, 581f
congenital anomalies of, 583, 585f
Staphylococcal aortitis, 1669
Staphylococcus aureus infections
cerebritis, 760f
diskitis, 925
empyema, 3074
hepatic abscess in, 1871
in cystic fibrosis, 1155, 1163
liver abscess, 3170, 3171f
necrotizing fasciitis/cellulitis, 2493
osteomyelitis, 926, 928, 928f, 2887, 2888, 2888f, 3001
pneumonia, 1193-1194, 1199, 1202f, 1203f, 1434, 1439, 3074
pyelonephritis, 2266
pyomyositis, 2491
septic arthritis, 3032